THE
MERCK
MANUAL
OF
MEDICAL
INFORMATION

SECOND
HOME EDITION

THE
MERCK
MANUAL
OF
MEDICAL INFORMATION

SECOND
HOME EDITION

Mark H. Beers, MD, EDITOR-IN-CHIEF
Andrew J. Fletcher, MB, BChir, Thomas V. Jones, MD, MPH,
and Robert Porter, MD, SENIOR ASSISTANT EDITORS
Michael Berkwits, MD, and Justin L. Kaplan, MD, ASSISTANT EDITORS

Published by
MERCK RESEARCH LABORATORIES
Division of
MERCK & CO., INC.
Whitehouse Station, NJ
2003

FOREIGN LANGUAGE TRANSLATIONS OF

THE MERCK MANUAL—Home Edition

Chinese
Croatian
Dutch
German
Greek
Hebrew
Hungarian
Japanese
Portuguese
Russian
Slovenian
Spanish

Library of Congress Catalog Number 2002115250
ISBN 0-911910-35-2

First Edition—1997

Printed in the United States of America

PREFACE

In this, the "information age," an interested reader can easily locate information on everything from movies to medical care. When it comes to health and disease, however, the *quality* of information is vital. A reader should ask: Is the information I have found correct, reliable, and up-to-date? Is it complete, or has it left out something vital? Does the information reflect proven science or only the opinion of the writer? Is the writer an expert in the area? Does the writer have good credentials? These questions are not trivial. If information about health care is wrong, the reader who relies on it risks grave harm.

The Merck Manual of Medical Information—Home Edition (Second Edition) aims to meet the growing demand of the general public for highly detailed, complete, authoritative medical information. The book covers many difficult medical concepts, but it does so in everyday language.

This 2nd edition is more than a revision of the 1st edition. It has been completely rewritten. The authors and editors of the 2nd edition have updated every topic, added many new ones, improved explanations, added more illustrations, and expanded captions to provide more information.

The Merck Manual of Medical Information—Home Edition was not the first home medical book. Many fine books have been published during the last two decades to meet the needs of the public for more medical information. However, *The Merck Manual of Medical Information—Home Edition* covers more topics in greater detail than all other home medical books. The book explains what a disorder is, who is likely to get it, what its symptoms are, how it is diagnosed, how it might be prevented, and how it can be treated. Information about prognosis, including what can and cannot be done, is given when possible. Background information that helps readers understand disorders is provided. This information includes anatomy, function, diagnostic tests, and medical procedures, to name a few. Medical terms are defined, so that people can better understand their doctors.

The Merck Manual of Medical Information—Home Edition is based on the world's most widely used textbook of medicine, *The Merck Manual.* Millions of health care professionals worldwide rely on *The Merck Manual.* Published for more than 103 years, it is now in its 17th edition. The 2nd edition of *The Home Edition* covers almost all the topics included in the 17th edition of *The Merck Manual.* Like all of The Merck Manuals, *The Home Edition* is published on a not-for-profit basis by Merck Research Laboratories, a division of Merck & Co, Inc.

The strength of *The Merck Manual of Medical Information—Home Edition* lies in the knowledge, experience, and judgment of its more than 300 outstanding authors, consultants, and editorial board members. Their names are listed on the pages that follow the table of contents. They deserve a degree of thanks that cannot be adequately expressed here.

Readers are urged to spend a few minutes reviewing the Guide for Readers on page xxxv. The index, which is comprehensive, is usually the best way to locate specific information.

No book can replace the expertise and advice of health care professionals who have direct contact with a patient. *The Home Edition* is meant to supplement that relationship, not replace it. This book is not meant for self-diagnosis or self-treatment. Rather it is a source of accurate, reliable information that should stimulate better communication between patients and their doctors, nurses, pharmacists, therapists, and other health care professionals. We hope that you use this book in good health and welcome your comments and suggestions.

Mark H. Beers, MD
Editor-in-Chief

Special Note to Readers

The authors, reviewers, editors, and publisher have made extensive efforts to ensure that the information is accurate and conforms to the standards accepted at the time of publication. However, constant changes in information resulting from continuing research and clinical experience, reasonable differences in opinions among authorities, unique aspects of individual situations, and the possibility of human error in preparing such an extensive text require that the reader exercise judgment when making decisions and consult and compare information from other sources. In particular, the reader is advised to discuss information obtained in this book with a doctor, pharmacist, nurse, or other health care practitioner.

CONTENTS

A Guide for Readers xxxv

Understanding Medical Terms xxxvii

| Section 1 | FUNDAMENTALS | ....1 |

1   The Human Body   *Mark H. Beers, MD*   2

2   Genetics   *Andrew J. Fletcher, MB, BChir*   8

3   The Aging Body   *Richard W. Besdine, MD*   16

4   Communicating With Health Care Professionals
    Marjorie A. Bowman, MD, MPA   21

5   Prevention   *Mirza I. Rahman, MD, MPH* and
    Albert A. Rundio, Jr., PhD   25

6   Exercise and Fitness   *Steven Jonas, MD, MPH*   31

7   Rehabilitation   *Masayoshi Itoh, MD, MPH* and
    Mathew H. M. Lee, MD   36

8   Death and Dying   *Joanne Lynn, MD*   45

9   Legal and Ethical Issues   *Nancy Neveloff Dubler, LLB*   53

| Section 2 | DRUGS | ....59 |

10   Overview of Drugs   *G. Victor Rossi, PhD*   60

11   Drug Administration and Kinetics
     Thomas N. Tozer, PhD   64

12   Drug Dynamics   *G. Victor Rossi, PhD*   69

13   Factors Affecting Response to Drugs
     Daniel A. Hussar, PhD   73

14   Drugs and Aging   *Mark Monane, MD*   79

15   Adverse Drug Reactions   *G. Victor Rossi, PhD*   82

16   Compliance With Drug Treatment
     Daniel A. Hussar, PhD   86

17   Trade-Name and Generic Drugs
     Harold Silverman, PharmD   88

18   Over-the-Counter Drugs   *Daniel A. Hussar, PhD*   93

19   Medicinal Herbs and Nutraceuticals
     Ara DerMarderosian, PhD   103

Section 3   HEART AND BLOOD VESSEL DISORDERS 113

20   Biology of the Heart and Blood Vessels
     Paul H. Tanser, MD   114

21   Symptoms and Diagnosis of Heart and Blood Vessel Disorders
     Paul H. Tanser, MD   118

22   High Blood Pressure   *George L. Bakris, MD*   131

23   Low Blood Pressure   *Lewis A. Lipsitz, MD*   141

24   Shock   *Scott Manaker, MD, PhD*   148

25   Heart Failure   *Malcolm Arnold, MD*   150

26   Cardiomyopathy   *Paul H. Tanser, MD*   158

27   Abnormal Heart Rhythms   *L. Brent Mitchell, MD*   163

28   Heart Valve Disorders   *Paul H. Tanser, MD*   175

29   Infective Endocarditis   *Lawrence L. Pelletier, Jr., MD*   184

30   Pericardial Disease   *Brian D. Hoit, MD*   187

31   Heart Tumors   *M. Jay Goodkind, MD*   191

32   Atherosclerosis   *Jules Y. T. Lam, MD*   194

33   Coronary Artery Disease   *J. Wayne Warnica, MD*   199

34   Peripheral Arterial Disease   *Alan T. Hirsch, MD*   216

35   Aneurysms and Aortic Dissection
     John W. Hallett, Jr., MD   226

36   Venous Disorders   *Ronald Dee, MD*   231

37   Lymphatic Disorders   *Ronald Dee, MD*   239

Section 4   LUNG AND AIRWAY DISORDERS 243

38   Biology of the Lungs and Airways   *Joseph D. Brain, ScD*   244

39   Symptoms and Diagnosis of Lung Disorders
     Richard G. Masson, MD   248

40   Pulmonary Rehabilitation   *Bartolome R. Celli, MD*   259

41   Bronchitis   *Gordon L. Snider, MD*   262

42   Pneumonia   *John G. Bartlett, MD*   264

43   Lung Abscess   *John G. Bartlett, MD*   272

44   Asthma   *Richard J. Martin, MD*   274

45   Chronic Obstructive Pulmonary Disease
     Gordon L. Snider, MD   281

46 Pulmonary Embolism   *James K. Alexander, MD*   285

47 Bronchiectasis   *Anne L. Davis, MD*   289

48 Atelectasis   *Anne L. Davis, MD*   292

49 Occupational Lung Diseases   *David Christiani, MD*   294

50 Infiltrative Lung Diseases   *Talmadge E. King, Jr., MD*   301

51 Allergic Diseases of the Lungs   *Hal B. Richerson, MD*   308

52 Pleural Disorders   *Steven A. Sahn, MD*   312

53 Cystic Fibrosis   *Beryl J. Rosenstein, MD*   317

54 Pulmonary Hypertension   *Harrison W. Farber, MD*   322

55 Respiratory Failure   *Richard G. Masson, MD*   325

56 Acute Respiratory Distress Syndrome
    B. Taylor Thompson, MD   326

57 Lung Cancer   *Waun Ki Hong, MD*   328

Section 5   BONE, JOINT, AND MUSCLE DISORDERS 333

58 Biology of the Musculoskeletal System
    Walter H. Ettinger, MD   334

59 Symptoms and Diagnosis of Musculoskeletal Disorders
    Michael Jacewicz, MD   339

60 Osteoporosis   *Lawrence G. Raisz, MD*   343

61 Paget's Disease of Bone   *Roy D. Altman, MD*   346

62 Fractures   *Tobin N. Gerhart, MD*   348

63 Bone Tumors   *Douglas J. Pritchard, MD*   359

64 Avascular Necrosis of the Bone   *Thomas M. Zizic, MD*   362

65 Bone and Joint Infections   *Maren L. Mahowald, MD*   364

66 Osteoarthritis   *Roy D. Altman, MD*   367

67 Rheumatoid Arthritis and Other Types of Inflammatory
    Arthritis   *H. Ralph Schumacher, Jr., MD*   370

68 Autoimmune Disorders of Connective Tissue
    H. Ralph Schumacher, Jr., MD   378

69 Vasculitic Disorders of Connective Tissue
    H. Ralph Schumacher, Jr., MD   386

70 Gout and Pseudogout   *Daniel J. McCarty, MD*   391

71 Hand Disorders   *David R. Steinberg, MD*   395

72   Foot Problems   *Kendrick Alan Whitney, DPM*   403

73   Muscular Dystrophy and Related Disorders
      Michael Rubin, MD   412

74   Disorders of Muscles, Bursas, and Tendons
      Alfonse T. Masi, MD, DrPH   415

75   Sports Injuries   *Pekka Mooar, MD*   419

Section 6   **BRAIN, SPINAL CORD, AND NERVE DISORDERS 431**

76   Biology of the Nervous System
      Steven A. Goldman, MD, PhD   433

77   Diagnosis of Brain, Spinal Cord, and Nerve Disorders
      Michael Jacewicz, MD   439

78   Pain   *Russell K. Portenoy, MD*   447

79   Headaches   *Jeffrey B. Reich, MD*   456

80   Dizziness and Vertigo   *Michael Jacewicz, MD*   461

81   Sleep Disorders   *Gabriele M. Barthlen, MD*   467

82   Brain Dysfunction   *Norman R. Relkin, MD, PhD*   475

83   Delirium and Dementia
      Edward R. Marcantonio, MD   480

84   Stupor and Coma   *John J. Caronna, MD*   490

85   Seizure Disorders   *Daniel L. Menkes, MD*   495

86   Stroke   *John J. Caronna, MD*   502

87   Head Injuries   *John J. Caronna, MD*   513

88   Tumors of the Nervous System
      William R. Shapiro, MD   519

89   Infections of the Brain and Spinal Cord
      Michael Jacewicz, MD   529

90   Prion Diseases   *Pierluigi Gambetti, MD*   541

91   Movement Disorders   *David Eidelberg, MD*   544

92   Multiple Sclerosis and Related Disorders
      Brian R. Apatoff, MD, PhD   556

93   Spinal Cord Disorders   *Michael Rubin, MD*   561

94   Low Back Pain   *Jerome B. Posner, MD*   568

95   Peripheral Nerve Disorders   *Michael Rubin, MD*   575

96   Cranial Nerve Disorders   *Michael Rubin, MD*   588

97   Smell and Taste Disorders   *Michael Jacewicz, MD*   594

Section 7   MENTAL HEALTH DISORDERS **597**

98   Overview of Mental Health Care
     Glen O. Gabbard, MD   598

99   Somatoform Disorders   *Katharine A. Phillips, MD*   601

100 Anxiety Disorders   *John H. Greist, MD* and
     James W. Jefferson, MD   605

101 Depression and Mania   *Norman Sussman, MD*   613

102 Suicidal Behavior   *Robert M. A. Hirschfeld, MD*   622

103 Eating Disorders   *Albert J. Stunkard, MD*   624

104 Sexuality   *George R. Brown, MD*   627

105 Personality Disorders   *John Gunderson, MD*   631

106 Amnesia and Related Disorders   *Richard P. Kluft, MD*   636

107 Schizophrenia and Delusional Disorder
     Wayne S. Fenton, MD   640

108 Drug Use and Abuse   *Marc Galanter, MD*   646

Section 8   MOUTH AND DENTAL DISORDERS...........................**661**

109 Biology of the Mouth   *Linda P. Nelson, DMD, MScD*   661

110 Lip and Tongue Disorders   *Robert B. Cohen, DMD*   664

111 Salivary Gland Disorders   *Robert B. Cohen, DMD*   666

112 Mouth Sores   *Robert B. Cohen, DMD*   667

113 Growths in the Mouth   *Robert B. Cohen, DMD*   670

114 Tooth Disorders   *David F. Murchison, DDS*   674

115 Periodontal Diseases   *James T. Ubertalli, DMD*   681

116 Temporomandibular Disorders   *Noshir R. Mehta, DMD*   685

117 Urgent Dental Problems   *J. D. Overton, DDS*   690

Section 9   DIGESTIVE DISORDERS **693**

118 Biology of the Digestive System
     Douglas A. Drossman, MD   694

119 Symptoms and Diagnosis of Digestive Disorders
     Douglas A. Drossman, MD and
     Nicholas J. Shaheen, MD, MPH   699

120 Disorders of the Esophagus   *Joel E. Richter, MD*   706

121 Peptic Disorders   *William D. Chey, MD*   711

122   Gastroenteritis   *Thomas G. Boyce, MD*   719

123   Hiatus Hernia, Bezoars, and Foreign Bodies
      William D. Chey, MD   727

124   Pancreatitis   *Eugene P. DiMagno, MD*   729

125   Malabsorption   *Atenodoro Marciano R. Ruiz, Jr., MD*   734

126   Inflammatory Bowel Diseases   *David B. Sachar, MD* and
      Jacob S. Walfish, MD   738

127   Antibiotic-Associated Colitis   *David B. Sachar, MD* and
      Jacob S. Walfish, MD   745

128   Diverticular Disease   *Ronald G. Tompkins, MD, ScD* and
      John T. Schulz III, MD, PhD   747

129   Bowel Movement Disorders   *Sidney F. Phillips, MD*   750

130   Disorders of the Anus and Rectum   *Norman Sohn, MD*   759

131   Tumors of the Digestive System   *Elliot M. Livstone, MD*   764

132   Gastrointestinal Emergencies
      Ronald G. Tompkins, MD, ScD   776

Section 10   **LIVER AND GALLBLADDER DISORDERS** 785

133   Biology of the Liver and Gallbladder
      Jerome B. Simon, MD   786

134   Diagnostic Tests for Liver and Gallbladder Disorders
      Eldon A. Shaffer, MD   788

135   Clinical Manifestations of Liver Disease
      Jerome B. Simon, MD   791

136   Fatty Liver, Cirrhosis, and Related Disorders
      Eldon A. Shaffer, MD   797

137   Hepatitis   *Jerome B. Simon, MD*   802

138   Blood Vessel Disorders of the Liver
      Eldon A. Shaffer, MD   806

139   Liver Tumors   *Jerome B. Simon, MD*   810

140   Gallbladder Disorders   *Eldon A. Shaffer, MD*   813

Section 11   **KIDNEY AND URINARY TRACT DISORDERS**..........819

141   Biology of the Kidneys and Urinary Tract
      Ralph E. Cutler, MD   820

142   Symptoms and Diagnosis of Kidney and Urinary Tract Disorders
      Ralph E. Cutler, MD   823

143   Kidney Failure   *Ralph E. Cutler, MD*   828

144 Nephritis *Ralph E. Cutler, MD* 837

145 Blood Vessel Disorders of the Kidneys
Stewart Shankel, MD 844

146 Tubular and Cystic Kidney Disorders
Peter C. Brazy, MD 849

147 Urinary Incontinence *Joseph G. Ouslander, MD* and
H. Roger Hadley, MD 857

148 Urinary Tract Obstruction *Glenn M. Preminger, MD* 862

149 Urinary Tract Infections *Stewart Shankel, MD* 866

150 Injury to the Urinary Tract *Noel A. Armenakas, MD* 872

151 Cancers of the Kidney and Urinary Tract
David A. Swanson, MD 875

Section 12 **DISORDERS OF NUTRITION AND METABOLISM....879**

152 Overview of Nutrition *Amy Lee, MD* 880

153 Undernutrition *David R. Thomas, MD* 887

154 Vitamins *Larry E. Johnson, MD, PhD* 890

155 Minerals and Electrolytes *Larry E. Johnson, MD, PhD* and
James L. Lewis III, MD 900

156 Obesity *Albert J. Stunkard, MD* 914

157 Disorders of Cholesterol *Anne Carol Goldberg, MD* 920

158 Water Balance *James L. Lewis III, MD* 927

159 Acid-Base Balance *James L. Lewis III, MD* 930

160 Porphyrias *Karl E. Anderson, MD* 933

Section 13 **HORMONAL DISORDERS** **937**

161 Biology of the Endocrine System
John E. Morley, MB, BCh 937

162 Pituitary Gland Disorders *Ian M. Chapman, MBBS, PhD* 940

163 Thyroid Gland Disorders *Lewis E. Braverman, MD* 948

164 Adrenal Gland Disorders *Ashley B. Grossman, MD* 956

165 Diabetes Mellitus *Nir Barzilai, MD* 962

166 Hypoglycemia *Nir Barzilai, MD* 970

167 Multiple Endocrine Neoplasia Syndromes
Patricia A. Daly, MD and *Lewis Landsberg, MD* 972

168 Carcinoid Tumors *Courtney M. Townsend, Jr., MD* 974

Section 14   BLOOD DISORDERS..977

169   Biology of Blood   *Eugene P. Frenkel, MD*   978

170   Symptoms and Diagnosis of Blood Disorders
      Steven H. Kroft, MD   979

171   Blood Transfusion   *Harold S. Kaplan, MD* and
      Donna L. Skerrett, MD   982

172   Anemia   *Eugene P. Frenkel, MD*   987

173   Bleeding and Clotting Disorders   *Joel L. Moake, MD*   995

174   White Blood Cell Disorders   *Mary Territo, MD*   1001

175   Plasma Cell Disorders   *James R. Berenson, MD*   1006

176   Leukemias   *Charles A. Schiffer, MD*   1010

177   Lymphomas   *Arthur T. Skarin, MD* and
      Arnold S. Freedman, MD   1016

178   Myeloproliferative Disorders
      Steven M. Fruchtman, MD   1023

179   Spleen Disorders   *Harry S. Jacob, MD*   1027

Section 15   CANCER..1031

180   Overview of Cancer   *Eugene P. Frenkel, MD*   1031

181   Symptoms and Diagnosis of Cancer   *David G. Pfister, MD*
      and *Timothy Aliff, MD*   1035

182   Prevention and Treatment of Cancer   *Bruce A. Chabner, MD*
      and *Elizabeth Chabner Thompson, MD, MPH*   1042

Section 16   IMMUNE DISORDERS..1049

183   Biology of the Immune System
      Dhavalkumar D. Patel, MD, PhD   1049

184   Immunodeficiency Disorders   *E. Richard Stiehm, MD*   1057

185   Allergic Reactions   *Elizabeth A. Erwin, MD* and
      Thomas A. E. Platts-Mills, MD   1063

186   Autoimmune Disorders   *Philip L. Cohen, MD*   1073

187   Transplantation   *Paul S. Russell, MD*   1075

Section 17   INFECTIONS..1085

188   Biology of Infectious Disease   *Gerald L. Mandell, MD*   1086

189   Immunization   *Fred H. Rubin, MD*   1092

190   Bacterial Infections   *Paul D. Hoeprich, MD*   1095

191   Bacteremia, Sepsis, and Septic Shock
      Lowell S. Young, MD   1118

192   Antibiotics   *Matthew E. Levison, MD*   1120

193   Tuberculosis   *Edward A. Nardell, MD*   1125

194   Leprosy   *Robert H. Gelber, MD*   1130

195   Rickettsial and Ehrlichial Infections
      William A. Petri, Jr., MD, PhD   1132

196   Parasitic Infections   *Richard D. Pearson, MD*   1135

197   Fungal Infections   *John E. Edwards, Jr., MD*   1148

198   Viral Infections   *Spotswood L. Spruance, MD*   1154

199   Human Immunodeficiency Virus Infection
      J. Allen McCutchan, MD   1168

200   Sexually Transmitted Diseases
      J. Allen McCutchan, MD   1176

Section 18   **SKIN DISORDERS** 1185

201   Biology of the Skin   *Matthew J. Stiller, MD*   1186

202   Diagnosis and Treatment of Skin Disorders
      Matthew J. Stiller, MD   1188

203   Itching and Noninfectious Rashes
      Matthew J. Stiller, MD   1191

204   Acne   *Matthew J. Stiller, MD*   1204

205   Pressure Sores   *Marilyn Wright, MS, MPH*   1208

206   Sweating Disorders   *Matthew J. Stiller, MD*   1210

207   Hair Disorders   *Matthew J. Stiller, MD*   1211

208   Pigment Disorders   *Matthew J. Stiller, MD*   1214

209   Blistering Diseases   *Matthew J. Stiller, MD*   1216

210   Parasitic Skin Infections
      Barbara Braunstein Wilson, MD   1218

211   Bacterial Skin Infections   *E. Dale Everett, MD*   1220

212   Fungal Skin Infections   *Barbara Braunstein Wilson, MD*   1225

213   Viral Skin Infections   *Barbara Braunstein Wilson, MD*   1228

214   Sunlight and Skin Damage   *Matthew J. Stiller, MD*   1230

215   Noncancerous Skin Growths   *Ercem S. Atillasoy, MD*   1233

216   Skin Cancers   *Ercem S. Atillasoy, MD*   1238

Section 19   EARS, NOSE, AND THROAT DISORDERS 1243

217   Biology of the Ears, Nose, and Throat
Harold C. Pillsbury III, MD and *Austin S. Rose, MD*   1244

218   Hearing Loss and Deafness   *Robert J. Ruben, MD*   1247

219   Outer Ear Disorders   *Itzhak Brook, MD*   1253

220   Middle and Inner Ear Disorders   *Bruce J. Gantz, MD*   1255

221   Disorders of the Nose and Sinuses
Rodney J. Schlosser, MD and *David W. Kennedy, MD*   1262

222   Throat Disorders   *Robert J. Ruben, MD*   1267

223   Nose and Throat Cancers   *Richard V. Smith, MD*   1271

Section 20   EYE DISORDERS 1275

224   Biology of the Eyes   *James Garrity, MD*   1276

225   Symptoms and Diagnosis of Eye Disorders
Kathryn Colby, MD, PhD   1278

226   Refractive Disorders   *Melvin I. Roat, MD*   1286

227   Eye Injuries   *Kathryn Colby, MD, PhD*   1290

228   Eyelid and Tear Gland Disorders
Mitchell H. Friedlaender, MD   1292

229   Disorders of the Conjunctiva and Sclera
Mitchell H. Friedlaender, MD   1296

230   Corneal Disorders   *Melvin I. Roat, MD*   1299

231   Cataract   *Kathryn Colby, MD, PhD*   1303

232   Uveitis   *Melvin I. Roat, MD*   1305

233   Glaucoma   *Annette Terebuh, MD* and
Josip Terebuh, MD   1306

234   Retinal Disorders   *Scott Steidl, MD*   1309

235   Optic Nerve Disorders   *James Garrity, MD*   1315

236   Eye Socket Disorders   *James Garrity, MD*   1317

Section 21   MEN'S HEALTH ISSUES 1321

237   Male Reproductive System   *Ralph E. Cutler, MD*   1321

238   Disorders of the Penis and Testes   *Paul Lui, MD*   1324

239   Prostate Disorders   *Paul Lui, MD*   1329

240   Sexual Dysfunction   *Fran E. Kaiser, MD*   1335

Section 22   WOMEN'S HEALTH ISSUES...1341

241   Biology of the Female Reproductive System
      Pamela A. Moalli, MD, PhD   1343

242   Symptoms and Diagnosis of Gynecologic Disorders
      Paula J. Adams Hillard, MD   1349

243   Menopause   *Susan L. Hendrix, DO*   1356

244   Menstrual Disorders and Abnormal Vaginal Bleeding
      Susan L. Hendrix, DO   1361

245   Endometriosis   *Robert W. Rebar, MD*   1369

246   Fibroids   *Susan L. Hendrix, DO*   1372

247   Vaginal Infections   *Susan L. Hendrix, DO*   1374

248   Pelvic Inflammatory Disease   *Susan L. Hendrix, DO*   1377

249   Pelvic Floor Disorders   *Susan L. Hendrix, DO*   1379

250   Sexual Dysfunction   *Susan L. Hendrix, DO*   1382

251   Breast Disorders   *Victor G. Vogel, MD*   1387

252   Cancers of the Female Reproductive System
      Hervy E. Averette, MD   1401

253   Violence Against Women   *Norah C. Feeny, PhD*   1410

254   Infertility   *Robert W. Rebar, MD*   1414

255   Family Planning   *Daniel R. Mishell, Jr., MD*   1419

256   Detection of Genetic Disorders   *Sherman Elias, MD*   1429

257   Normal Pregnancy   *Michael F. Greene, MD*   1434

258   High-Risk Pregnancy   *Michael F. Greene, MD*   1444

259   Drug Use During Pregnancy   *Michael R. Foley, MD*   1458

260   Normal Labor and Delivery   *David B. Acker, MD*   1464

261   Complications of Labor and Delivery
      David B. Acker, MD   1470

262   Postdelivery Period   *David B. Acker, MD*   1476

Section 23   CHILDREN'S HEALTH ISSUES 1481

263   Normal Newborns and Infants
      Ruth A. Lawrence, MD   1483

264   Problems in Newborns   *Arthur E. Kopelman, MD*   1494

265   Birth Defects   *Gregory S. Liptak, MD, MPH*   1511

266   Chromosomal and Genetic Abnormalities
      Gregory S. Liptak, MD, MPH   1527

267 Problems in Infants and Very Young Children
     Elizabeth J. Palumbo, MD   1531

268 Normal Preschool and School-Aged Children
     *Eve R. Colson, MD, Yasmin Suzanne N. Senturias, MD, and
     Francoise Thierfelder, MD*   1538

269 Behavioral and Developmental Problems in Young Children
     Nancy Ebbesmeyer Lanphear, MD   1543

270 Normal Adolescents   *Cheryl M. Kodjo, MD, MPH*   1552

271 Problems in Adolescents   *Cheryl M. Kodjo, MD, MPH*   1555

272 Bacterial Infections   *Geoffrey A. Weinberg, MD*   1561

273 Viral Infections   *Mary T. Caserta, MD*   1568

274 Respiratory Disorders   *John T. McBride, MD*   1583

275 Digestive Disorders   *Thomas M. Rossi, MD*   1586

276 Ear, Nose, and Throat Disorders   *John D. Norante, MD*   1593

277 Eye Disorders   *J. Raymond Buncic, MD*   1600

278 Bone Disorders   *H. Ralph Schumacher, Jr., MD*   1603

279 Hereditary Connective Tissue Disorders
     H. Ralph Schumacher, Jr., MD   1607

280 Juvenile Rheumatoid Arthritis
     H. Ralph Schumacher, Jr., MD   1612

281 Diabetes Mellitus   *Nicholas Jospe, MD*   1613

282 Hereditary Disorders of Metabolism
     Nicholas Jospe, MD   1616

283 Childhood Cancers   *David N. Korones, MD*   1622

284 Cerebral Palsy   *Hart Peterson, MD*   1624

285 Mental Retardation   *Stephen Brian Sulkes, MD*   1626

286 Mental Health Disorders   *John P. Glazer, MD*   1630

287 Social Issues Affecting Children and Their Families
     Moira Szilagyi, MD   1638

288 Child Neglect and Abuse   *Ann S. Botash, MD*   1643

Section 24   ACCIDENTS AND INJURIES.....................................1647

289 Burns   *John F. Burke, MD*   1648

290 Heat Disorders   *Charles S. Houston, MD*   1652

291 Cold Injuries   *Charles S. Houston, MD*   1654

292 Radiation Injury   *Tracey Schefter, MD*   1657

293   Electrical and Lightning Injuries
      Mary Ann Cooper, MD   1661

294   Near Drowning   *Norman L. Dean, MD*   1665

295   Diving and Compressed Air Injuries
      Alfred A. Bove, MD, PhD   1666

296   Altitude Illness   *Charles S. Houston, MD*   1672

297   Poisoning   *William O. Robertson, MD*   1674

298   Bites and Stings   *Barry Steven Gold, MD*   1681

299   First Aid   *Justin L. Kaplan, MD*   1687

Section 25   SPECIAL SUBJECTS 1695

300   Medical Decision Making
      Thomas V. Jones, MD, MPH   1695

301   Surgery   *Robert G. Johnson, MD*   1698

302   Complementary and Alternative Medicine
      Brian M. Berman, MD and *John A. Astin, PhD*   1704

303   Travel and Health   *Daniel Levinson, MD*   1708

304   Amyloidosis   *Alan S. Cohen, MD*   1715

305   Familial Mediterranean Fever
      Stephen E. Goldfinger, MD   1716

306   Diseases of Unknown Cause
      Margaret-Mary G. Wilson, MD   1717

        APPENDIXES 1721

  I   **Weights and Measures**   1721

 II   **Common Medical Tests**   1724

III   **Drug Names: Generic and Trade**   1732

IV   **Resources for Help and Information**   1756

        INDEX 1769

EDITORIAL BOARD

CONSULTANTS

Robert B. Cohen, DMD
Clinical Assistant Professor, Tufts University
School of Dental Medicine

Ralph E. Cutler, MD
Professor of Medicine and Pharmacology,
Loma Linda University School of Medicine

Thomas Habif, MD
Adjunct Professor of Medicine (Dermatology),
Dartmouth Medical School

Melvin I. Roat, MD, FACS
Assistant Surgeon, Wills Eye Hospital,
Philadelphia

Robert J. Ruben, MD
Distinguished University Professor, Professor
of Otolaryngology and Professor of Pediatrics,
Albert Einstein College of Medicine; Chairman (Emeritus), Montefiore Medical Center
and Albert Einstein College of Medicine

Bruce C. Paton, MD, FRCP(E)
Clinical Professor of Surgery (Emeritus), University of Colorado Health Sciences Center

---

Reviewers for Selected Chapters

Ercem S. Atillasoy, MD
Steven Berney, MD
John J. Caronna, MD
Jules Constant, MD
Julie Abrams Faude, PhD
Christine Goertz, PhD
Mateel Graham, MD
George Grames, MD
Donald Hanson, DMD
Jerry Hershman, MD
Randall Hughes, MD
Daniel A. Hussar, PhD

Robert K. Jackler, MD
Brian D. Johnston
Peter Laibson, MD
Matthew E. Levison, MD
Paul Lui, MD
Howard Mertz, MD
John S. Oghalai, MD
Enyi Okereke, MD
Roy M. Poses, MD
Hal B. Richerson, MD
Robert A. Sinkin, MD

Acknowledgments

We thank David G. Armstrong, DPM, and Andrew JM Boulton, MD, who wrote the sidebar "The Foot in
Diabetes" in Chapter 165. We also thank Mirza I. Rahman, MD, MPH, who assisted with initial editing
of this book.

CONTRIBUTORS

David B. Acker, MD
Associate Professor of Obstetrics, Gynecology, and Reproductive Biology, Harvard University; Chief of Obstetrics, Brigham and Women's Hospital

James K. Alexander, MD
Professor of Medicine, Baylor College of Medicine

Timothy Aliff, MD
Clinical Assistant, Memorial Sloan-Kettering Cancer Center

Roy D. Altman, MD
Professor of Medicine and Chief of Rheumatology and Immunology, University of Miami; Director of Clinical Research, Geriatric Research, Education, and Clinical Center, Miami VA Medical Center

Karl E. Anderson, MD
Professor of Preventive Medicine and Community Health, Internal Medicine and Pharmacology and Toxicology, University of Texas Medical Branch at Galveston

Brian R. Apatoff, MD, PhD
Director of Multiple Sclerosis Clinical Care and Research Center, Department of Neurology and Neuroscience, New York-Presbyterian Hospital-Cornell Medical Center

Noel A. Armenakas, MD
Clinical Associate Professor, Weill Medical College of Cornell University; Attending Surgeon, Lenox Hill Hospital and New York-Presbyterian Hospital

Malcolm Arnold, MD
Professor of Medicine, University of Western Ontario; Head of Research Affairs, Division of Cardiology, London Health Sciences Center; Program Leader, Circulation Group, Lawson Health Research Institute, London, Ontario, Canada

John A. Astin, PhD
Scientist, California Pacific Medical Center

Ercem S. Atillasoy, MD, FAAD
Adjunct Clinical Faculty, Departments of Dermatology, Thomas Jefferson University and Yale University School of Medicine; Senior Director, Merck & Co., Inc.

Hervy E. Averette, MD
Professor of Clinical Oncology, University of Miami; American Cancer Society Professor and Sylvester Professor of Gynecologic Oncology

George L. Bakris, MD
Professor of Preventive Medicine and Internal Medicine, Rush Presbyterian-St. Luke's Medical Center; Director of Hypertension/Clinical Research Center, Chicago

Gabriele M. Barthlen, MD
Technische Universitaet, Muenchen, Germany

John G. Bartlett, MD
Professor of Medicine and Chief, Division of Infectious Diseases, Johns Hopkins University School of Medicine

Nir Barzilai, MD
Director of Institute for Aging Research, Albert Einstein College of Medicine

Mark H. Beers, MD
Editor-in-Chief, The Merck Manuals and Executive Director of Geriatrics and Clinical Literature, Merck & Co., Inc.; Clinical Professor of Medicine, Drexel University

James R. Berenson, MD
Professor of Medicine, University of California, Los Angeles; Director of Multiple Myeloma and Bone Metastasis Programs, Cedars-Sinai Medical Center

Brian M. Berman, MD
Professor of Family Medicine, University of Maryland School of Medicine; Director, University of Maryland Complementary Medicine Program

Richard W. Besdine, MD
Professor of Medicine and of Community Health; Interim Dean of Biology and Medical Sciences; and Director, Center for Gerontology and Health Care Research, Brown Medical School

Ann S. Botash, MD
Associate Professor of Pediatrics, SUNY Upstate Medical University; Director of Child Abuse Referral and Evaluation Program, Syracuse, NY

Alfred A. Bove, MD, PhD
Professor of Medicine (Emeritus), Temple University School of Medicine

Marjorie A. Bowman, MD, MPA
Professor and Chair of Family Practice and Community Medicine, University of Pennsylvania School of Medicine

Thomas G. Boyce, MD
Assistant Professor of Pediatrics, Mayo Medical School; Senior Associate Consultant, Mayo Clinic, Rochester, MN

Joseph D. Brain, ScD
Drinker Professor of Environmental Physiology and Chair of Environmental Health, Harvard School of Public Health

Lewis E. Braverman, MD
Professor of Medicine, Boston University School of Medicine; Chief, Section of Endrocrinology, Diabetes and Nutrition, Boston Medical Center

Peter C. Brazy, MD
Professor of Medicine, University of Wisconsin at Madison

Itzhak Brook, MD, MSc
Professor of Pediatrics, Georgetown University School of Medicine

George R. Brown, MD, FAPA
Professor and Associate Chairman of Psychiatry, East Tennessee State University; Chief of Psychiatry, Mountain Home VA Medical Center

J. Raymond Buncic, MD
Professor of Ophthalmology, University of Toronto; Ophthalmologist-in-Chief, Hospital for Sick Children, Toronto, Ontario, Canada

John F. Burke, MD
Helen Andrus Benedict Professor of Surgery (Emeritus), Harvard University; Chief of Trauma Services (Emeritus), Massachusetts General Hospital

John J. Caronna, MD
Professor of Clinical Neurology, Weill Medical College of Cornell University; Attending Neurologist, New York-Presbyterian Hospital

Mary T. Caserta, MD
Associate Professor of Pediatrics, University of Rochester School of Medicine; Attending Physician, Golisano Children's Hospital at Strong

Bartolome R. Celli, MD
Professor of Medicine, Tufts University; Chief of Pulmonary and Critical Care Medicine, St. Elizabeth's Medical Center, Boston

Bruce A. Chabner, MD
Professor of Medicine, Harvard Medical School; Clinical Director, Massachusetts General Hospital Cancer Center

Ian M. Chapman, MBBS, PhD
Senior Lecturer in Endocrinology, University of Adelaide, Department of Medicine, Royal Adelaide Hospital, Australia

William D. Chey, MD, FACG, FACP
Associate Professor of Internal Medicine and Director of Gastrointestinal Physiology Laboratory, University of Michigan Health System

David Christiani, MD
Professor of Medicine, Harvard Medical School; Professor of Occupational Medicine and Epidemiology, Harvard School of Public Health; Physician, Massachusetts General Hospital

Alan S. Cohen, MD
Distinguished Professor of Medicine in Rheumatology (Emeritus), Boston University School of Medicine; Editor-in-Chief of *Amyloid, The Journal of Protein Folding Disorders*

Philip L. Cohen, MD
Professor of Medicine, University of Pennsylvania; Staff Physician, Philadelphia VA Medical Center

Robert B. Cohen, DMD
Clinical Assistant Professor, Tufts University School of Dental Medicine

Kathryn Colby, MD, PhD
Director, Clinical Research Center, Department of Ophthalmology, Massachusetts Eye and Ear Infirmary, Harvard Medical School

Eve R. Colson, MD
Assistant Professor of Pediatrics, Yale University School of Medicine; Director of Well Newborn Nursery, Yale-New Haven Children's Hospital

Mary Ann Cooper, MD
Professor of Emergency Medicine, University of Illinois at Chicago; Director of Lightning Injury Research Program, University of Illinois at Chicago

Ralph E. Cutler, MD
Professor of Medicine and Pharmacology, Loma Linda University School of Medicine

Patricia A. Daly, MD
Clinical Endocrinologist, Warren Memorial Hospital, Front Royal, VA

Anne L. Davis, MD
Associate Professor of Clinical Medicine, New York University School of Medicine; Attending Physician, Bellevue Hospital Center

Norman L. Dean, MD
Director of Airway Clinics, North Carolina Correctional Institution for Women

Ronald Dee, MD
Associate Clinical Professor of Surgery, Albert Einstein College of Medicine; Attending Surgeon, The Stamford Hospital

Ara DerMarderosian, PhD
Professor of Pharmacognosy and Medicinal Chemistry, Roth Chair of Natural Products and Scientific Director of Complementary and Alternative Medicine Institute, University of the Sciences in Philadelphia, College of Pharmacy

Eugene P. DiMagno, MD
Professor of Medicine, Mayo Medical School; Consultant of Gastroenterology and Internal Medicine, Mayo Clinic, Rochester, MN

George E. Downs, PharmD
Professor of Clinical Pharmacy and Dean, Philadelphia College of Pharmacy, University of the Sciences in Philadelphia

Douglas A. Drossman, MD
Professor of Medicine and Psychiatry and Codirector of Center for Functional and Gastrointestinal Motility Disorders, University of North Carolina School of Medicine

Nancy Neveloff Dubler, LLB
Professor of Epidemiology and Social Medicine, Albert Einstein College of Medicine; Director, Division of Bioethics, Montefiore Medical Center

John E. Edwards, Jr., MD
Professor of Medicine, University of California, Los Angeles School of Medicine; Chief of Infectious Diseases, Harbor-UCLA Medical Center

David Eidelberg, MD
Professor of Neurology and Neurosurgery, New York University School of Medicine; Head, Center for Neurosciences, North Shore-LIJ Research Institute, Manhasset

Sherman Elias, MD
G. William Arends Chair and Phillip C. and Beverly Goldstick Professor and Head, Department of Obstetrics and Gynecology; Professor, Department of Molecular Genetics, University of Illinois at Chicago

Elizabeth A. Erwin, MD
Fellow, University of Virginia

Walter H. Ettinger, MD
Executive Vice President, Virtua Health, Inc.

E. Dale Everett, MD
Professor of Medicine, University of Missouri-Columbia

Harrison W. Farber, MD
Professor of Medicine, Boston University School of Medicine

Norah C. Feeny, PhD
Assistant Professor, Case Western Reserve University; Assistant Professor, University Hospitals of Cleveland

Wayne S. Fenton, MD
National Institute of Mental Health, Bethesda, MD

Andrew J. Fletcher, MB, BChir
Adjunct Professor of Pharmaceutical Health Care, Temple University School of Pharmacy; Senior Assistant Editor, The Merck Manuals, Merck & Co., Inc.

Michael R. Foley, MD
Clinical Professor of Obstetrics and Gynecology, University of Arizona at the Health Sciences Center; Medical Director, Phoenix Perinatal Associates/Obstetrix Medical Group

Arnold S. Freedman, MD
Associate Professor of Medicine, Harvard Medical School

Eugene P. Frenkel, MD
Professor of Internal Medicine and Radiology, Patsy R. and Raymond D. Nasher Distinguished Chair in Cancer Research, and A. Kenneth Pye Professorship in Cancer Research, The University of Texas Southwestern Medical Center at Dallas

Mitchell H. Friedlaender, MD
Adjunct Professor, The Scripps Research Institute; Head of Ophthalmology, Scripps Clinic, La Jolla

Steven M. Fruchtman, MD
Director, Myeloproliferative Disease Program and Director (Emeritus) of Stem Cell Transplant, Mount Sinai Medical Center, New York; Associate Professor of Medicine, Mount Sinai School of Medicine

Glen O. Gabbard, MD
Professor of Psychiatry, Baylor College of Medicine

Marc Galanter, MD
Professor of Psychiatry and Director of Alcoholism and Drug Abuse, New York University School of Medicine

Pierluigi Gambetti, MD
Professor and Director of Neuropathology, Case Western Reserve University; Director of National Prion Disease Pathology Surveillance Center, Cleveland

Bruce J. Gantz, MD
Professor and Head, Department of Otolaryngology-Head and Neck Surgery, and Brian F. McCabe Distinguished Chair in Otolaryngology-Head and Neck Surgery, University of Iowa Hospitals and Clinics

James Garrity, MD
Professor of Ophthalmology, Mayo Clinic, Rochester, MN

Robert H. Gelber, MD
Clinical Professor of Medicine and Dermatology, University of California at San Francisco

Tobin N. Gerhart, MD
Assistant Clinical Professor, Orthopaedic Surgery, Harvard Medical School

John P. Glazer, MD
Professor of Psychiatry and Pediatrics and Director of Child and Adolescent Psychiatry, University of Rochester Medical Center

Barry Steven Gold, MD
Assistant Professor of Medicine, Johns Hopkins University School of Medicine; Assistant Professor of Medicine, University of Maryland School of Medicine

Anne Carol Goldberg, MD
Associate Professor of Medicine, Washington University School of Medicine, St. Louis

Stephen E. Goldfinger, MD
Professor of Medicine, Harvard Medical School

Steven A. Goldman, MD, PhD
Professor of Neurology and Neuroscience, Weill Medical College of Cornell University; Attending Neurologist, New York-Presbyterian Hospital

M. Jay Goodkind, MD
Clinical Associate Professor of Medicine, University of Pennsylvania; Chief (Retired) of Cardiology, Mercer Medical Center

Michael F. Greene, MD
Associate Professor of Obstetrics, Gynecology, and Reproductive Biology, Harvard Medical School; Director of Maternal-Fetal Medicine, Massachusetts General Hospital

John H. Greist, MD
Clinical Professor of Psychiatry, University of Wisconsin Medical School; Distinguished Senior Scientist, Madison Institute of Medicine

Ashley B. Grossman, MD, FRCP, FMedSci
Professor of Neuroendocrinology, St. Bartholomew's and The Royal London School of Medicine and Dentistry, London, UK

John Gunderson, MD
Professor of Psychiatry, Harvard Medical School; Director of Personality and Psychosocial Research, McLean Hospital

H. Roger Hadley, MD
Professor of Urology, Loma Linda University School of Medicine; Chief of Urology, Loma Linda University Medical Center

John W. Hallett, Jr., MD
Clinical Professor of Surgery, Tufts Medical School; Director of Vascular Center, Eastern Maine Medical Center

Susan L. Hendrix, DO
Associate Professor of Obstetrics and Gynecology and Principal Investigator and Director of Women's Health Initiative, Wayne State University School of Medicine

Paula J. Adams Hillard, MD
Professor of Obstetrics/Gynecology and of Pediatrics, Children's Hospital Medical Center, Cincinnati; Director of Women's Health, University of Cincinnati College of Medicine

Alan T. Hirsch, MD
Associate Professor of Medicine and Radiology, Vascular Medicine Program, Minnesota Vascular Diseases Center, University of Minnesota Medical School

Robert M. A. Hirschfeld, MD
Titus H. Harris Chair, Professor and Chair of Psychiatry and Behavioral Sciences, University of Texas Medical Branch at Galveston

Paul D. Hoeprich, MD
Professor of Medicine (Emeritus), School of Medicine, University of California, Davis

Brian D. Hoit, MD
Professor of Medicine, Case Western Reserve University; Director of Echocardiography, University Hospitals of Cleveland

Waun Ki Hong, MD
American Cancer Society Professor and Head, Division of Cancer Medicine, University of Texas, M.D. Anderson Cancer Center

Charles S. Houston, MD
Professor of Medicine (Emeritus), University of Vermont College of Medicine

Daniel A. Hussar, PhD
Remington Professor of Pharmacy, Philadelphia College of Pharmacy, University of the Sciences in Philadelphia

Masayoshi Itoh, MD, MPH
Clinical Professor of Rehabilitation Medicine, New York University; Senior Management Consultant, Coler/Goldwater Specialty Hospital and Nursing Facility, New York

Michael Jacewicz, MD
Professor of Neurology, University of Tennessee College of Medicine; Assistant Chief of Neurology, VA Medical Center, Memphis

Harry S. Jacob, MD
Professor of Medicine, University of Minnesota Medical School

James W. Jefferson, MD
Clinical Professor of Psychiatry, University of Wisconsin Medical School; Distinguished Senior Scientist, Madison Institute of Medicine

Larry E. Johnson, MD, PhD
Associate Professor of Geriatric Medicine and Family and Community Medicine, University of Arkansas for Medical Sciences; Medical Director, Extended Care, Central Arkansas Veterans Healthcare System

Robert G. Johnson, MD
Chair and C. Rollins Hanlon Professor of Surgery, Saint Louis University Health Sciences Center

Steven Jonas, MD, MPH, MS
Professor of Preventive Medicine, School of Medicine, State University of New York at Stony Brook

Thomas V. Jones, MD, MPH
Clinical Associate Professor of Medicine, Temple University School of Medicine; Senior Assistant Editor, The Merck Manuals, Merck & Co., Inc.

Nicholas Jospe, MD
Associate Professor of Pediatrics, University of Rochester School of Medicine and Dentistry

Fran E. Kaiser, MD
Senior Medical Director, South Central Region, Merck & Co., Inc.; Clinical Professor of Medicine, University of Texas Southwestern Medical Center; Adjunct Professor of Medicine, Saint Louis University

Harold S. Kaplan, MD
Professor of Clinical Pathology and Director of Laboratory Medicine, Columbia University-New York-Presbyterian Hospital

Justin L. Kaplan, MD
Clinical Associate Professor of Emergency Medicine, Thomas Jefferson University; Assistant Editor, The Merck Manuals, Merck & Co., Inc.

David W. Kennedy, MD
Professor and Chairman of Otorhinolaryngology, Vice Dean for Professional Affairs, University of Pennsylvania; Senior Vice President, University of Pennsylvania Health System

Talmadge E. King, Jr., MD
Constance B. Wofsy Distinguished Professor of Medicine, University of California at San Francisco; Chief of Medical Services, San Francisco General Hospital

Richard P. Kluft, MD
Clinical Professor of Psychiatry, Temple University School of Medicine

Cheryl M. Kodjo, MD, MPH
Senior Instructor in Pediatrics and Adolescent Medicine, University of Rochester

Arthur E. Kopelman, MD
Professor of Pediatrics and Neonatology, The Brody School of Medicine at East Carolina University

David N. Korones, MD
Associate Professor of Pediatrics and Oncology, Golisano Children's Hospital at Strong, University of Rochester School of Medicine and Dentistry

Steven H. Kroft, MD
Associate Professor of Pathology, University of Texas Southwestern Medical School; Director of Hematology Laboratory, Parkland Memorial Hospital

Jules Y. T. Lam, MD, FRCP(C)
Associate Professor of Medicine, University of Montreal; Cardiologist, Montreal Heart Institute, Montreal, Quebec, Canada

Lewis Landsberg, MD
Vice President for Medical Affairs and Dean, Northwestern University, The Feinberg School of Medicine

Nancy Ebbesmeyer Lanphear, MD
Assistant Professor of Pediatrics, University of Cincinnati, Cincinnati Children's Hospital Medical Center

Ruth A. Lawrence, MD
Professor of Pediatrics, Obstetrics and Gynecology, University of Rochester School of Medicine and Dentistry; Director of Normal Newborn Nursery, Strong Memorial Hospital

Amy Lee, MD
Associate Clinical Professor, Department of Medicine, University of California, Irvine

Mathew H. M. Lee, MD
Howard A. Rusk Professor of Rehabilitation Medicine, New York University School of Medicine

Daniel Levinson, MD
Associate Professor (Emeritus) of Family and Community Medicine and Clinical Assistant Professor of Psychiatry, University of Arizona College of Medicine

Matthew E. Levison, MD
Professor of Medicine and Public Health, Division of Infectious Diseases, Drexel University School of Medicine

James L. Lewis III, MD
Nephrology Associates, PC, Birmingham

Lewis A. Lipsitz, MD
Professor and Director, Harvard Division on Aging; Usen Codirector of the Hebrew Rehabilitation Center for Aged, Research and Training Institute, Boston; Chief, Gerontology Division, Beth Israel Deaconess Medical Center

Gregory S. Liptak, MD, MPH
Associate Professor of Pediatrics, University of Rochester Medical Center; Medical Director of Andrew J. Kirch Developmental Services Center

Elliot M. Livstone, MD, FACP, FACG
Attending Physician, Sarasota Memorial Hospital

Paul Lui, MD
Associate Professor of Surgery, Division of Urology, Loma Linda University School of Medicine

Joanne Lynn, MD
Director, The Washington Home Center for Palliative Care Studies, Washington, DC; President of Americans for Better Care of the Dying

Maren L. Mahowald, MD
Professor of Medicine, University of Minnesota; Chief of Rheumatology, Minneapolis VA Medical Center

Scott Manaker, MD, PhD
Associate Professor of Medicine and Pharmacology, University of Pennsylvania

Gerald L. Mandell, MD, MACP
Owen R. Cheatham Professor of the Sciences and Professor of Medicine, University of Virginia Health Center

Edward R. Marcantonio, MD
Assistant Professor of Medicine, Harvard Medical School; Director of Quality and Outcomes Research, Hebrew Rehabilitation Center for Aged

Richard J. Martin, MD
Professor of Medicine, University of Colorado Health Sciences Center; Head of Pulmonary Division and Vice Chair of Department of Medicine, National Jewish Medical and Research Center

Alfonse T. Masi, MD, DrPH
Professor of Medicine, University of Illinois College of Medicine at Peoria; Professor of Epidemiology, University of Illinois School of Public Health

Richard G. Masson, MD
Associate Professor of Medicine, University of Massachusetts School of Medicine; Chief of Pulmonary Medicine, Framingham Union Hospital

John T. McBride, MD
Professor and Vice Chair, Department of Pediatrics, Northeastern Ohio Universities College of Medicine; Vice Chair, Department of Pediatrics, Children's Hospital Medical Center of Akron

Daniel J. McCarty, MD
Will and Cava Ross Professor of Medicine (Emeritus), Medical College of Wisconsin

J. Allen McCutchan, MD
Professor of Medicine, University of California at San Diego

Noshir R. Mehta, DMD, MDS, MS
Chairman of General Dentistry, Tufts University School of Dental Medicine; Director of Gelb Orofacial Pain Center, Boston

Daniel L. Menkes, MD
Associate Professor of Neurology and Director of Clinical Neurophysiology Services, University of Tennessee, Memphis

Daniel R. Mishell Jr., MD
Lyle G. McNeile Professor and Chairman of Department of Obstetrics and Gynecology, Keck School of Medicine, University of Southern California, Los Angeles

L. Brent Mitchell, MD
Professor of Medicine, University of Calgary; Head, Department of Cardiac Sciences, Calgary Regional Health Authority, Calgary, Alberta, Canada

Joel L. Moake, MD
Professor of Medicine, Baylor College of Medicine; Associate Director, Biomedical Engineering Laboratory, Rice University

Pamela A. Moalli, MD, PhD
Assistant Professor, University of Pittsburgh School of Medicine; Assistant Professor, Magee-Womens Hospital

Mark Monane, MD, MS
Adjunct Associate Clinical Professor, Rutgers College of Pharmacy; Principal, Biotechnology & Life Sciences, Needham and Company, Inc., New York

Pekka Mooar, MD
Associate Professor of Orthopaedic Surgery, Drexel University School of Medicine

John E. Morley, MB, BCh
Director of Geriatric Medicine, Saint Louis University Health Sciences Center; Director of Geriatric Research, Education and Clinical Center, St. Louis VA Medical Center

David F. Murchison, DDS, MMS
Colonel, USAF, DC; Commander, 35th Dental Squadron, Misawa Air Base, Japan

Edward A. Nardell, MD
Associate Professor, Harvard Medical School and Harvard School of Public Health; Director, Tuberculosis Research, Program in Infectious Disease and Social Change

Linda P. Nelson, DMD, MScD
Assistant Professor of Oral and Developmental Biology, Harvard School of Dental Medicine; Senior Attending Pediatric Dentist, Children's Hospital, Boston

John D. Norante, MD
Associate Professor of Otolaryngology, University of Rochester Medical Center

Joseph G. Ouslander, MD
Professor of Medicine and Nursing, Director, Division of Geriatric Medicine and Gerontology, and Chief Medical Officer, Wesley Woods Center of Emory University; Director, Emory Center for Health in Aging; Clinical Director, Atlanta VA Rehabilitation Research and Development Center

J. D. Overton, DDS
Private Dental Practice, Biloxi, MS

Elizabeth J. Palumbo, MD
Private Practice, The Pediatric Group, Fairfax, VA

Dhavalkumar D. Patel, MD, PhD
Associate Professor of Medicine and Chief of Allergy and Clinical Immunology, Duke University Medical Center

Richard D. Pearson, MD
Professor of Medicine and Pathology, Divisions of Geographic and International Medicine and Infectious Diseases, University of Virginia School of Medicine

Lawrence L. Pelletier, Jr., MD
Professor of Internal Medicine, University of Kansas School of Medicine; Staff Physician, Wichita VA Medical Center

Hart Peterson, MD
Clinical Professor of Neurology in Pediatrics (Retired), Cornell University; Attending Neurologist and Pediatrician (Retired), New York Hospital

William A. Petri, Jr., MD, PhD
Professor of Medicine, Microbiology and Pathology and Attending Physician and Chief, Division of Infectious Diseases, University of Virginia Health System

David G. Pfister, MD
Associate Professor, Weill Medical College of Cornell University; Associate Attending Physician/Associate Member and Co-Leader of the Head and Neck Cancer Disease Management Team, Memorial Sloan-Kettering Cancer Center

Katharine A. Phillips, MD
Associate Professor of Psychiatry, Brown University School of Medicine; Director of the Body Dysmorphic Disorder Program, Butler Hospital, Providence

Sidney F. Phillips, MD
Professor of Medicine (Emeritus), Karl F. and Marjory Hasselmann Professor of Research, Mayo Medical School; Consultant, Mayo Clinic, Rochester, MN

Harold C. Pillsbury III, MD
Thomas J. Dark Distinguished Professor and Chairman of Otolaryngology-Head and Neck Surgery, University of North Carolina School of Medicine

Thomas A. E. Platts-Mills, MD
Professor of Internal Medicine and Microbiology and Head of Asthma and Allergic Disease Center, University of Virginia

Russell K. Portenoy, MD
Professor of Neurology, Albert Einstein College of Medicine; Chairman, Department of Pain Medicine and Palliative Care, Beth Israel Medical Center

Jerome B. Posner, MD
Professor of Neurology and Neurosciences, Weill Medical College of Cornell University; Attending Neurologist, Memorial Sloan-Kettering Cancer Center

Glenn M. Preminger, MD
Professor of Urologic Surgery and Director of Duke Comprehensive Kidney Stone Center, Duke University Medical Center

Douglas J. Pritchard, MD
Consultant of Orthopedic Surgery, Mayo Clinic, Rochester, MN

Mirza I. Rahman, MD, MPH, FAAFP, FACPM
Adjunct Professor of Pharmacoepidemiology, Temple University School of Pharmacy; Director, Medical Services, Merck & Co., Inc.

Lawrence G. Raisz, MD
Professor of Medicine and Director of UConn Center for Osteoporosis, University of Connecticut Health Center

Robert W. Rebar, MD
Associate Executive Director of American Society for Reproductive Medicine, Birmingham; Volunteer Clinical Professor, Department of Obstetrics and Gynecology, University of Alabama, Birmingham

Jeffrey B. Reich, MD
Assistant Professor of Neurology, Cornell University Medical College

Norman R. Relkin, MD, PhD
Associate Professor of Clinical Neurology and Neuroscience, Weill Cornell Medical College; Director, Cornell Memory Disorders Program, New York-Presbyterian Hospital

Hal B. Richerson, MD
Professor of Internal Medicine (Emeritus), University of Iowa

Joel E. Richter, MD
Professor of Medicine, Ohio State University Health Science Center at the Cleveland Clinic; Chair of Gastroenterology, Cleveland Clinic Foundation

Melvin I. Roat, MD, FACS
Assistant Surgeon, Wills Eye Hospital, Philadelphia

William O. Robertson, MD
Professor of Pediatrics, University of Washington; Medical Director, Washington Poison Center

Austin S. Rose, MD
Fellow, Pediatric Otolaryngology, Department of Otolaryngology-Head and Neck Surgery, Johns Hopkins University School of Medicine

Beryl J. Rosenstein, MD
Professor of Pediatrics, Johns Hopkins University School of Medicine; Director of Cystic Fibrosis Center, Johns Hopkins Hospital

G. Victor Rossi, PhD
Leonard and Madlyn Abramson Professor of Pharmacology, Philadelphia College of Pharmacy and Science, University of the Sciences in Philadelphia

Thomas M. Rossi, MD
Professor of Pediatrics, Division of Gastroenterology and Nutrition, University of Rochester School of Medicine and Dentistry

Robert J. Ruben, MD
Distinguished University Professor, Professor of Otolaryngology and Professor of Pediatrics, Albert Einstein College of Medicine; Chairman (Emeritus), Montefiore Medical Center and Albert Einstein College of Medicine

Fred H. Rubin, MD
Visiting Professor of Medicine, University of Pittsburgh School of Medicine; Chairman of Medicine, University of Pittsburgh Medical Center, Shadyside Hospital

Michael Rubin, MD
Professor of Clinical Neurology, Weill Medical College of Cornell University; Attending Physician of Neurology, New York-Presbyterian Hospital

Atenodoro Marciano R. Ruiz, Jr., MD
Attending Physician, Division of Gastroenterology, Christiana Care Hospital, Newark, DE; Affiliate, Institute of Digestive Diseases, St. Luke's Medical Center, Quezon City, Philippines

Albert A. Rundio, Jr., PhD
Associate Professor of Nursing, Drexel University of the Health Sciences

Paul S. Russell, MD
John Homans Distinguished Professor of Surgery, Harvard Medical School; Senior Surgeon, Massachusetts General Hospital

David B. Sachar, MD
Clinical Professor of Medicine, Mount Sinai School of Medicine; Director (Emeritus) of Gastroenterology, The Mount Sinai Hospital

Steven A. Sahn, MD
Professor of Medicine and Director of Pulmonary and Critical Care Medicine, Medical University of South Carolina

Tracey Schefter, MD
Assistant Professor of Radiation Oncology, University of Colorado Cancer Center

Charles A. Schiffer, MD
Professor of Medicine and Oncology, Karmanos Cancer Institute, Wayne State University School of Medicine

Rodney J. Schlosser, MD
Assistant Professor, Director of Rhinology and Sinus Surgery, Department of Otolaryngology, Medical University of South Carolina

John T. Schulz III, MD, PhD
Intructor in Surgery, Harvard Medical School; Attending Physician, Burn, Trauma, and General Surgery, Massachusetts General Hospital

H. Ralph Schumacher, Jr., MD
Professor of Medicine, University of Pennsylvania School of Medicine; Director of Arthritis-Immunology Center, VA Medical Center, Philadelphia

Yasmin Suzanne N. Senturias, MD
Postdoctoral Fellow of Developmental and Behavioral Pediatrics, Yale University School of Medicine

Eldon A. Shaffer, MD, FRCP(C)
Professor of Medicine, University of Calgary, Calgary, Alberta, Canada

Nicholas J. Shaheen, MD, MPH
Assistant Professor of Medicine, University of North Carolina

Stewart Shankel, MD
Clinical Professor of Medicine, University of California at Riverside; Director of Clinical Instruction, UCR/UCLA Thomas Haider Program in Biomedical Sciences

William R. Shapiro, MD
Chief, Neuro-Oncology, Barrow Neurological Institute, Phoenix; Professor of Clinical Neurology, University of Arizona College of Medicine, Tucson

Harold Silverman, PharmD
Medical Director, Healthcare Practice, Manning, Selvage and Lee, Washington, DC

Jerome B. Simon, MD, FRCP(C), FACP
Professor of Medicine, Queen's University, Kingston, Ontario, Canada

Arthur T. Skarin, MD
Associate Professor of Medicine, Harvard Medical School; Attending Physician of Medical Oncology, Dana-Farber Cancer Institute; and Department of Medicine, Brigham and Women's Hospital

Donna L. Skerrett, MD
Assistant Professor of Pathology and Associate Director of Transfusion Medicine, Columbia Presbyterian Medical Center

Richard V. Smith, MD
Associate Professor and Vice-Chair of Otolaryngology, Albert Einstein College of Medicine; Director of Head and Neck Surgery, Montefiore Medical Center

Gordon L. Snider, MD
Maurice B. Strauss Professor of Medicine, Boston University School of Medicine

Norman Sohn, MD
Clinical Assistant Professor of Surgery, New York University School of Medicine

Spotswood L. Spruance, MD
Professor of Medicine, Adjunct Professor of Dermatology, and Adjunct Professor of Pharmaceutics and Pharmaceutical Chemistry, University of Utah

Scott Steidl, MD, DMA
Director of Vitreoretinal Disease, University of Maryland Medical Center

David R. Steinberg, MD
Associate Professor of Orthopaedic Surgery and Director of Hand and Microsurgery Fellowship Program, University of Pennsylvania

E. Richard Stiehm, MD
Professor of Pediatrics and Chief of Immunology, Allergy, and Rheumatology, Mattel Children's Hospital at UCLA

Matthew J. Stiller, MD
Associate Professor of Clinical Dermatology, College of Physicians & Surgeons, Columbia University

Albert J. Stunkard, MD
Professor of Psychiatry, University of Pennsylvania

Stephen Brian Sulkes, MD
Associate Professor of Pediatrics, Strong Center for Developmental Disabilities, Golisano Children's Hospital at Strong, University of Rochester School of Medicine and Dentistry

Norman Sussman, MD
Clinical Professor of Psychiatry, New York University School of Medicine; Director of Psychopharmacology Research and Consultation Service, Bellevue Hospital Center

David A. Swanson, MD
N.G. and Helen Hawkins Distinguished Professor for Cancer Research and Chairman of Urology, The University of Texas, M.D. Anderson Cancer Center

Moira Szilagyi, MD
Assistant Professor of Pediatrics, University of Rochester; Medical Director of Foster Care, Monroe County Health Department, Rochester, NY

Paul H. Tanser, MD, FRCP(C), FRCP (Glasgow)
Professor (Emeritus) of Medicine, McMaster University; Senior Staff Cardiologist, St. Joseph's Hospital, Hamilton, Ontario, Canada

Annette Terebuh, MD
Mary Rutan Hospital, Bellefontaine, OH

Josip Terebuh, MD
Eye Physician and Surgeon, Mary Rutan Hospital, Bellefontaine, OH

Mary Territo, MD
Professor of Medicine, University of California, Los Angeles

Francoise Thierfelder, MD
Fellow of Developmental and Behavioral Pediatrics, Yale University School of Medicine

David R. Thomas, MD, FACP, FAGS
Professor of Medicine, Saint Louis University

B. Taylor Thompson, MD
Associate Professor of Medicine, Harvard Medical School; Director of Medical Intensive Care Unit, Massachusetts General Hospital

Elizabeth Chabner Thompson, MD, MPH
21st Century Oncology, Yonkers, NY

Ronald G. Tompkins, MD, ScD
John F. Burke Professor of Surgery, Harvard University; Visiting Surgeon, Massachusetts General Hospital

Courtney M. Townsend, Jr., MD
Professor and John Woods Harris Distinguished Chairman of Surgery, The University of Texas Medical Branch at Galveston

Thomas N. Tozer, PhD
Professor (Emeritus) of Biopharmaceutical Sciences and Pharmaceutical Chemistry, University of California at San Francisco

James T. Ubertalli, DMD
Assistant Clinical Professor of Periodontology, Tufts University School of Dental Medicine; Private Practice, Hingham, MA

Victor G. Vogel, MD, MHS
Professor of Medicine and Epidemiology, University of Pittsburgh School of Medicine; Director, Magee/University of Pittsburgh Cancer Institute Breast Program, Magee-Womens Hospital

Jacob S. Walfish, MD
Assistant Clinical Professor of Medicine, Mount Sinai School of Medicine

J. Wayne Warnica, MD, FRCP(C)
Professor of Medicine, University of Calgary; Director of Cardiac Intensive Care Unit, Foothills Medical Centre, Calgary, Alberta, Canada

Geoffrey A. Weinberg, MD
Associate Professor of Pediatrics, University of Rochester School of Medicine and Dentistry; Attending Physician and Director of Pediatric HIV Program, Strong Memorial Hospital

Kendrick Alan Whitney, DPM
Assistant Professor, Department of Orthopedics, Temple University School of Podiatric Medicine

Barbara Braunstein Wilson, MD
Edward P. Cawley Associate Professor of Dermatology, University of Virginia

Margaret-Mary G. Wilson, MD
Assistant Professor of Internal and Geriatric Medicine, Saint Louis University Health Sciences Center, St. Louis VA Medical Center

Marilyn Wright, MS, MPH
Director of Community Case Management, Beth Israel Deaconess Medical Center, Boston

Lowell S. Young, MD
Clinical Professor of Medicine, University of California at San Francisco; Director, Kuzell Institute for Arthritis and Infectious Diseases, San Francisco

Thomas M. Zizic, MD
Associate Professor of Medicine, Johns Hopkins University School of Medicine; Codirector, Chesapeake Medical Research

A Guide for Readers

The Merck Manual of Medical Information—Home Edition is organized into sections and chapters. Understanding this organization will help the reader navigate through the book and find the most information. Topics of interest may be quickly located by consulting the Table of Contents or Index.

Sections

The first section—Fundamentals—covers many general topics important to health care, such as aging, communicating with health care professionals, prevention of disease and disability, exercise and fitness, rehabilitation, and death and dying. The Accidents and Injuries section includes a chapter on first aid. The last section—Special Subjects—provides an overview of medical decision making, surgery, complementary and alternative medicine, and travel and health, among other topics.

Most sections in the book cover the disorders of one organ or organ system, such as those of the eye, skin, or heart and blood vessels. A few sections cover one type of disorder, such as hormonal disorders or infectious diseases. Three separate sections cover health issues of men, women, and children.

Chapters

Some chapters describe a single disorder. Other chapters cover a group of related disorders. In either case, the discussion of a disorder usually starts with a definition of that disorder, printed in italics. The information that follows is typically organized under headings, such as causes, symptoms, diagnosis, prevention, treatment, and prognosis. Bold-faced type within the text indicates topics of major importance.

In sections about disorders of an organ or organ system, the first chapter describes the organ's normal structure and function. Reading about how the heart works or looking at illustrations of the heart, for example, may make a specific heart disorder more understandable. Many sections also include a chapter describing symptoms and the medical tests used to diagnose the disorders discussed in that section.

Cross-references

Throughout the book are cross-references that identify other important or related discussions of a subject. Cross-references are marked with a symbol within the text (▲, ■, ★, ●, ◆, ▼). Corresponding symbols, along with the page number where more information can be found, are located at the bottom of the page. Some cross-references point the reader to an illustration, sidebar, or table on a specific page.

Medical Terms

Medical terms are often provided, usually in parentheses after the common term. On page xxxvii is a list of prefixes, roots, and suffixes used in medical terminology. This list can help take the mystery out of medicine's multisyllabic vocabulary.

Illustrations, Sidebars, and Tables

The book contains many illustrations, sidebars, and tables. They help explain material in the text or give additional, related information. The reader can also refer to the 8 pages of full-color anatomical drawings to locate different parts of the body and see how they relate to each other.

Drug Information

The Drugs section provides comprehensive information about drugs, as well as medicinal herbs and nutraceuticals. Also, scattered throughout the book are many drug tables, marked by an Rx symbol. These drug tables provide additional information about a class or group of drugs.

In this book, individual drugs are almost always referred to by their generic name rather than by their brand or trade names. Appendix III contains a table of the generic drugs mentioned in the book along with some of their corresponding trade names. Appendix III also provides a separate table of trade names with their corresponding generic name.

The book does not provide drug doses because doses can vary greatly, depending on individual circumstances. For example, doses are affected by age, sex, weight, height, the presence of more than one disorder, and the use of other drugs. Therefore, health care professionals tailor the dose of a drug to the individual.

Diagnostic Tests

Diagnostic tests are mentioned throughout the book. Usually, an explanation is provided the first time a test is mentioned in a chapter. In addition, Appendix II lists many common diagnostic tests and procedures, explains what they are used for, and provides cross-references to where more detailed discussions of a test or procedure can be found.

Resources for Help and Information

Appendix IV lists contact information of many organizations that help people who have specific disorders. These organizations can provide additional information about a disorder or help locate support services.

Understanding Medical Terms

At first glance, medical terminology can seem like a foreign language. But often the key to understanding medical terms is focusing on their components (prefixes, roots, and suffixes). For example, *spondylolysis* is a combination of "spondylo," which means vertebra, and "lysis," which means dissolve, and so means dissolution of a vertebra.

The same components are used in many medical terms. "Spondylo" plus "itis," which means inflammation, forms *spondylitis,* an inflammation of the vertebrae. The same prefix plus "malacia," which means soft, forms *spondylomalacia,* a softening of the vertebrae.

Knowing the meaning of a small number of components can help with interpretation of a large number of medical terms. The following list defines many commonly used medical prefixes, roots, and suffixes.

a(n)	absence of	cut	skin
acou, acu	hear	cyan(o)	blue
aden(o)	gland	cyst(o)	bladder
aer(o)	air	cyt(o)	cell
alg	pain	dactyl(o)	finger or toe
andr(o)	man	dent	tooth
angi(o)	vessel	derm(ato)	skin
ankyl(o)	crooked, curved	dipl(o)	double
ante	before	dors	back
anter(i)	front, forward	dys	bad, faulty, abnormal
anti	against	ectomy	excision (removal by cutting)
arteri(o)	artery		
arthr(o)	joint	emia	blood
articul	joint	encephal(o)	brain
ather(o)	fatty	end(o)	inside
audi(o)	hearing	enter(o)	intestine
aur(i)	ear	epi	outer, superficial, upon
aut(o)	self	erythr(o)	red
bi, bis	double, twice, two	eu	normal
brachy	short	extra	outside
brady	slow	gastr(o)	stomach
bucc(o)	cheek	gen	become, originate
carcin(o)	cancer	gloss(o)	tongue
cardi(o)	heart	glyc(o)	sweet, or referring to glucose
cephal(o)	head		
cerebr(o)	brain	gram, graph	write, record
cervic	neck	gyn	woman
chol(e)	bile, or referring to gall-bladder	hem(ato)	blood
		hemi	half
chondr(o)	cartilage	hepat(o)	liver
circum	around, about	hist(o)	tissue
contra	against, counter	hydr(o)	water
corpor	body	hyper	excessive, high
cost(o)	rib	hypo	deficient, low
crani(o)	skull	hyster(o)	uterus
cry(o)	cold	iatr(o)	doctor

infra	beneath	phleb(o)	vein
inter	among, between	phob(ia)	fear
intra	inside	plasty	repair
itis	inflammation	pleg(ia)	paralysis
lact(o)	milk	pnea	breathing
lapar(o)	flank, abdomen	pneum(ato)	breath, air
latero	side	pneumon(o)	lung
leuk(o)	white	pod(o)	foot
lingu(o)	tongue	poie	make, produce
lip(o)	fat	poly	much, many
lys(is)	dissolve	post	after
mal	bad, abnormal	poster(i)	back, behind
malac	soft	presby	elder
mamm(o)	breast	proct(o)	anus
mast(o)	breast	pseud(o)	false
megal(o)	large	psych(o)	mind
melan(o)	black	pulmon(o)	lung
mening(o)	membranes	pyel(o)	pelvis of kidney
my(o)	muscle	pyr(o)	fever, fire
myc(o)	fungus	rachi(o)	spine
myel(o)	marrow	ren(o)	kidneys
nas(o)	nose	rhag	break, burst
necr(o)	death	rhe	flow
nephr(o)	kidney	rhin(o)	nose
neur(o)	nerve	scler(o)	hard
nutri	nourish	scope	instrument
ocul(o)	eye	scopy	examination
odyn(o)	pain	somat(o)	body
oma	tumor	spondyl(o)	vertebra
onc(o)	tumor	steat(o)	fat
oophor(o)	ovaries	sten(o)	narrow, compressed
ophthalm(o)	eye	steth(o)	chest
opia	vision	stom	mouth, opening
opsy	examination	supra	above
orchi(o)	testes	tachy	fast, quick
osis	condition	therap	treatment
osse(o)	bone	therm(o)	heat
oste(o)	bone	thorac(o)	chest
ot(o)	ear	thromb(o)	clot, lump
path(o)	disease	tomy	incision (operation by cutting)
ped(o)	child		
penia	deficient, deficiency	tox(i)	poison
peps, pept	digest	uria	urine
peri	around	vas(o)	vessel
phag(o)	eat, destroy	ven(o)	vein
pharmaco	drug	vesic(o)	bladder
pharyng(o)	throat	xer(o)	dry

FUNDAMENTALS

1 The Human Body 2

Cells ▪ Tissues and Organs ▪ Organ Systems ▪ Barriers on the Outside and the Inside ▪ Mind-Body Interactions ▪ Anatomy and Disease

2 Genetics...8

Gene Abnormalities ▪ Gene Technology ▪ Gene Therapy

3 The Aging Body 16

Disease Versus Aging ▪ Longevity ▪ Bodily Changes ▪ Implications of Illness ▪ Diseases of Accelerated Aging

4 Communicating With Health Care Professionals 21

Having a Primary Care Doctor ▪ When to Contact the Doctor ▪ Making the Most of a Doctor Visit ▪ Keeping Medical Records ▪ Researching a Personal Illness ▪ Understanding Managed Care

5 Prevention..25

Value of Prevention ▪ Components of Prevention ▪ Barriers to Prevention

6 Exercise and Fitness 31

Benefits of Exercise ▪ Starting an Exercise Program ▪ Preventing Injury ▪ Choosing the Right Exercise

7 Rehabilitation 36

Treatment of Pain and Inflammation ▪ Physical Therapy ▪ Occupational Therapy ▪ Rehabilitation for Specific Problems

8 Death and Dying 45

Time Course of Dying ▪ Making Health Care Choices ▪ Symptoms During a Fatal Illness ▪ Financial Concerns ▪ Legal and Ethical Concerns ▪ Coming to Terms ▪ When Death Is Near ▪ When Death Occurs

9 Legal and Ethical Issues..53

Competency and Capacity ▪ Informed Consent ▪ Confidentiality and Disclosure ▪ Advance Directives ▪ Surrogate Decision Making ▪ Do-Not-Resuscitate Orders ▪ Management of Property

CHAPTER 1

The Human Body

The human body is a complex, highly organized structure made up of unique cells that work together to accomplish the specific functions necessary for sustaining life. The biology of the human body includes the study of its structure (anatomy) and the study of its function (physiology). Physiology is discussed in greater detail in the first chapter of each section of this book.

Anatomy is organized by levels, from the smallest components of cells to the largest organs and their relationships to other organs. Gross anatomy is the study of the body's organs as seen with the naked eye during visual inspection and when the body is cut open for examination (dissection). Cellular anatomy is the study of cells and their components, which can be observed only with the use of special techniques and special instruments such as microscopes. Molecular anatomy (often called molecular biology) is the study of the smallest components of cells on the biochemical level.

Cells

Often thought of as the smallest unit of a living organism, a cell is made up of many even smaller parts, each with its own function. Human cells vary in size, but all are quite small. Even the largest, a fertilized egg, is too small to be seen with the naked eye.

Human cells have a membrane that holds the contents together. However, this membrane is not just a sac. It has receptors that identify the cell to other cells. The receptors also react to substances produced in the body and to drugs taken into the body, selectively allowing these substances or drugs to enter and leave the cell. Reactions that take place at the receptors often alter or control a cell's functions. An example of this is when insulin binds to receptors on the cell membrane to maintain appropriate blood sugar levels and to allow glucose to enter cells.

Within the cell membrane are two major compartments, the cytoplasm and the nucleus. The cytoplasm contains structures that consume and transform energy and perform the cell's functions. The nucleus contains the cell's genetic material and the structures that control cell division and reproduction. Inside every cell are mitochondria. Mitochondria are tiny structures that provide the cell with energy.

The body is composed of many different types of cells, each with its own structure and function. Some, such as white blood cells, move freely, unattached to other cells. Others, such as muscle cells, are firmly attached one to another. Some cells, such as skin cells, divide and reproduce quickly; others, such as nerve cells, do not divide or reproduce at all under usual circumstances. Some cells, especially glandular cells, have as their primary function the production of complex substances, such as a hormone or an enzyme. For example, some cells in the breast produce milk, some in the pancreas produce insulin, some in the lining of the lungs produce mucus, and some in the mouth produce saliva. Other cells have primary functions that are not related to the production of substances—for example, muscle cells contract, allowing movement. Nerve cells conduct electrical impulses, allowing communication between the central nervous system (brain and spinal cord) and the rest of the body.

Tissues and Organs

Related cells joined together are collectively referred to as a tissue. The cells in a tissue are not identical, but they work together to accomplish specific functions. A sample of tissue removed for examination under a microscope (biopsy) contains many types of cells, even though a doctor may be interested in only one specific type.

Connective tissue is the tough, often fibrous tissue that binds the body's structures together and provides support. It is present in almost every organ, forming a large part of skin, tendons, and muscles. The characteristics of connective tissue and the types of cells it contains vary, depending on where it is found in the body.

Inside the Torso

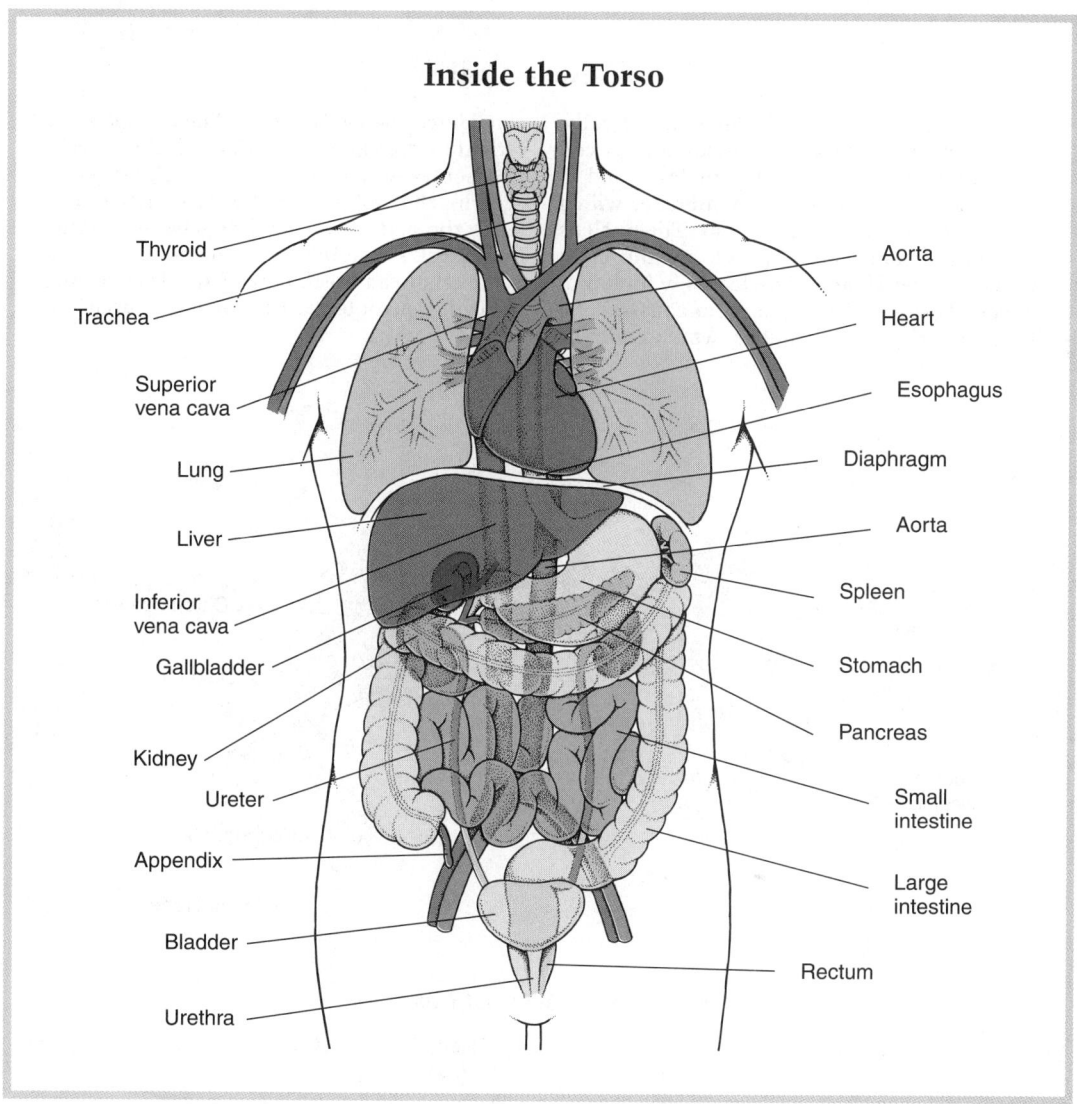

Thyroid

Trachea

Superior
vena cava

Lung

Liver

Inferior
vena cava

Gallbladder

Kidney

Ureter

Appendix

Bladder

Urethra

Aorta

Heart

Esophagus

Diaphragm

Aorta

Spleen

Stomach

Pancreas

Small
intestine

Large
intestine

Rectum

The body's functions are conducted by organs. Each organ is a recognizable structure—for example, the heart, lungs, liver, eyes, and stomach—that performs specific functions. An organ is made of several types of tissue and therefore several types of cells. For example, the heart contains muscle tissue that contracts to pump blood, fibrous tissue that makes up the heart valves, and special cells that maintain the rate and rhythm of heartbeats. The eye contains muscle cells that open and close the pupil, clear cells that make up the lens and cornea, cells that produce the fluid within the eye, cells that sense light, and

nerve cells that conduct impulses to the brain. Even an organ as apparently simple as the gallbladder contains different types of cells, such as those that form a lining resistant to the irritative effects of bile, muscle cells that contract to expel bile, and cells that form the fibrous outer wall holding the sac together.

Organ Systems

Although an organ has a specific function, organs also function as part of a group, called an organ system. The organ system is the orga-

Inside a Cell

Although there are different types of cells, most cells have the same components. A cell consists of a nucleus and cytoplasm and is contained within the cell membrane, which regulates what passes in and out. The nucleus contains chromosomes, which are the cell's genetic material, and a nucleolus, which produces ribosomes. The cytoplasm consists of a fluid material and organelles, which could be considered the cell's organs. The endoplasmic reticulum transports materials within the cell. Ribosomes produce proteins, which are packaged by the Golgi apparatus so that they can leave the cell. Mitochondria generate energy for the cell's activities. Lysosomes contain enzymes that can break down particles entering the cell. Centrioles participate in cell division.

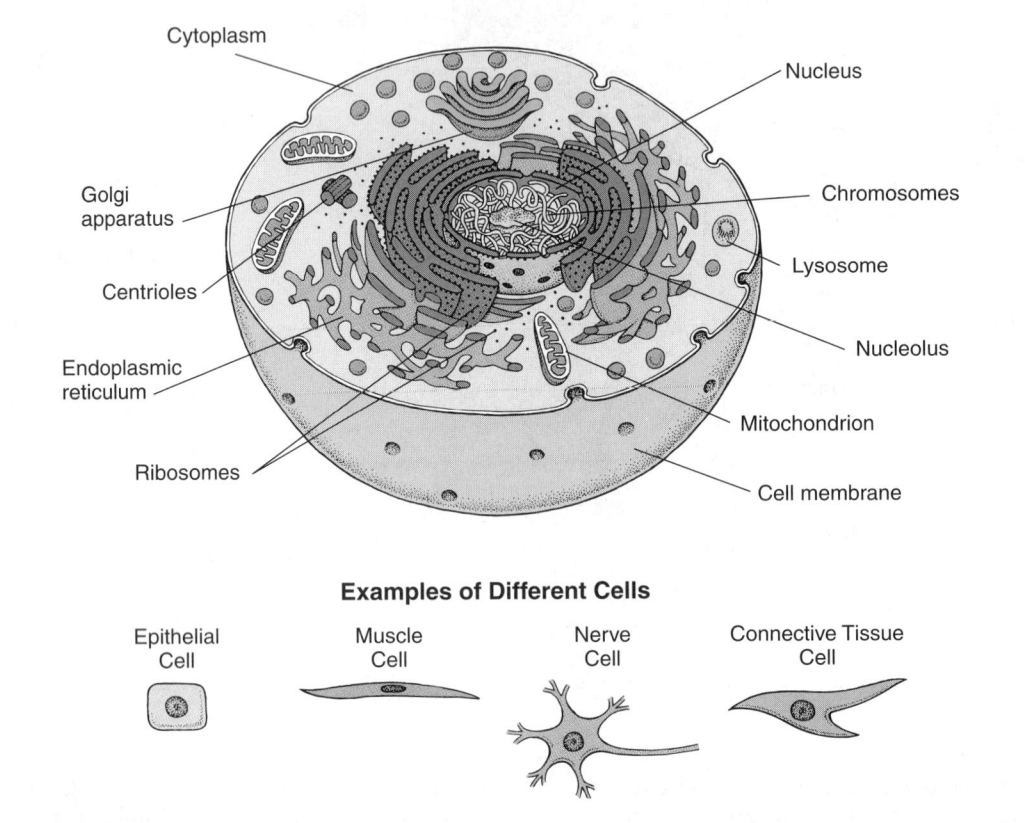

Examples of Different Cells

Epithelial Cell   Muscle Cell   Nerve Cell   Connective Tissue Cell

nizational unit by which medicine is studied, diseases are generally categorized, and treatments are planned. This book is, in large part, organized around the concept of organ systems.

An example of an organ system is the cardiovascular system, which includes the heart (cardio) and blood vessels (vascular). The cardiovascular system is responsible for pumping and circulating the blood. The digestive system, extending from the mouth to the anus, is responsible for receiving and digesting food and excreting waste. This system includes not only the stomach, small intestine, and large intestine, which move food, but also associated organs such as the pancreas, liver, and gallbladder, which produce digestive enzymes, remove toxins, and store substances necessary for digestion. The musculoskeletal system includes the bones, muscles, ligaments, tendons, and joints, which support and move the body.

Of course, organ systems do not function in isolation. For example, after a large meal is eaten, the digestive system needs more blood to perform its functions. Therefore, it enlists the aid of the cardiovascular and nervous systems. Blood vessels of the digestive system widen to transport more blood. Nerve impulses are sent to the brain, notifying it of the increased work. The digestive system even directly stimulates the heart through nerve impulses and chemicals released into the bloodstream. The heart responds by pumping more blood; the brain responds by perceiving less hunger, more fullness, and less interest in vigorous activity.

Communication between organs and organ systems is vital. Communication allows the body to adjust the function of each organ according to the needs of the whole body. The heart must know when the body is resting so that it can slow down and when organs need more blood so that it can speed up. The kidneys must know when the body has too much fluid so that they can produce more dilute urine and when the body is dehydrated so that they can conserve water.

Through communication, the body keeps itself in balance—a concept called homeostasis. Through homeostasis, organs neither underwork nor overwork, and each organ facilitates the functions of every other organ.

Communication to maintain homeostasis can occur through the nervous system or through chemical stimulation. The autonomic nervous system, in large part, controls the complex communication network that regulates bodily functions. This part of the nervous system functions without a person's thinking about it and without much noticeable indication that it is working. Chemicals used to communicate are called transmitters. Transmitters that are produced by one organ and travel to other organs through the bloodstream are called hormones. Transmitters that conduct messages between parts of the nervous system are called neurotransmitters.

One of the best known transmitters is the hormone epinephrine (adrenaline). When a person is suddenly stressed or frightened, the brain instantly sends a message to the adrenal glands, which quickly release epinephrine. Within moments, this chemical has the entire body on alert, a response sometimes called the fight-or-flight response. The heart beats more rapidly and powerfully, the eyes dilate to allow more light in, breathing quickens, and the activity of the digestive system decreases to allow more blood to go to the muscles. The effect is rapid and intense.

Other chemical communications are less dramatic but equally effective. For example, when the body becomes dehydrated and needs more water, the volume of blood circulating through the cardiovascular system decreases. This decreased blood volume is perceived by receptors in the arteries in the neck. They respond by sending impulses through nerves to the pituitary gland, at the base of the brain, which then produces antidiuretic hormone. This hormone signals the kidneys to concentrate urine and retain more water. Simultaneously, the brain senses thirst, stimulating a person to drink.

The body also has a group of organs—the endocrine system—whose primary function is to produce hormones that regulate the function of other organs. For example, the thyroid gland produces thyroid hormone, which controls the metabolic rate (the speed at which the body's chemical functions proceed); the pancreas produces insulin, which controls the use of sugar; and the adrenal glands produce epinephrine, which stimulates many organs to prepare the body for stress.

Barriers on the Outside and the Inside

As strange as it may seem, defining what is outside and what is inside the body is not always easy, because the body has many surfaces. The skin, which is actually an organ system, is obviously outside the body. It forms a barrier that prevents many harmful substances from entering the body. Although covered by a thin layer of skin, the ear canal is usually thought of as inside the body, because it penetrates deep into the head. The digestive system is a long tube that begins at the mouth, winds through the body, and exits at the anus. Is food as it passes through this tube inside or outside of the body? Nutrients and fluid are not really inside the body until they are absorbed into the bloodstream.

Air passes through the nose and throat into the windpipe (trachea), then into the exten-

MAJOR ORGAN SYSTEMS

System	Organs in the System	System	Organs in the System
Cardiovascular	Heart Blood vessels (arteries, capillaries, veins)	Digestive	Mouth Esophagus Stomach Small intestine
Respiratory	Nose Mouth Pharynx Larynx Trachea Bronchi Lungs		Large intestine Rectum Anus Liver Gallbladder Pancreas (the part that produces enzymes) Appendix
Nervous	Brain Spinal cord Nerves (both those that carry impulses to the brain and those that carry impulses from the brain to muscles and organs)	Endocrine	Thyroid gland Parathyroid gland Adrenal glands Pituitary gland Pancreas (the part that produces insulin) Stomach (the cells that produce gastrin) Pineal gland Ovaries Testes
Skin	Skin (both the surface that is generally thought of as skin and the underlying structures of connective tissue, including fat, glands, and blood vessels)	Urinary	Kidneys Ureters Bladder Urethra
Musculoskeletal	Muscles Tendons and ligaments Bones Joints	Male reproductive	Penis Prostate gland Seminal vesicles Vasa deferentia Testes
Blood	Blood cells and platelets Plasma (the liquid part of blood) Bone marrow (where blood cells are produced) Spleen Thymus	Female reproductive	Vagina Cervix Uterus Fallopian tubes Ovaries

sive, branching airways of the lungs (bronchi). At what point does this passageway stop being outside and become inside the body? Oxygen in the lungs is not useful to the body until it enters the bloodstream. To enter the bloodstream, oxygen must cross through a thin layer of cells lining the lungs. This layer acts as a barrier to viruses and bacteria, such as those that cause tuberculosis, which may be carried into the lungs with air. Unless these organisms penetrate the cells or enter the bloodstream, they generally do not cause disease. Because the lungs have many protective mechanisms, such as antibodies to fight infection and cilia to sweep debris out of the airways, most airborne infectious organisms never cause disease.

Body surfaces not only separate the outside from the inside but also keep structures and substances in their proper place so that they can function properly. For example, internal organs do not float in a pool of blood; blood is normally confined to blood vessels. If blood leaks out of the vessels into other parts of the body (hemorrhage), it not only fails to bring oxygen and nutrients to tissues but also can cause severe harm. For example, a very small amount of blood leaking into the brain destroys brain tissue because there is no room for expansion within the confines of the skull. On the other hand, a similar amount of blood leaking into the abdomen does not destroy tissue because the abdomen has room for expansion.

Saliva, so important in the mouth, can cause severe damage if inhaled into the lungs, because saliva carries bacteria that can cause an abscess to form in the lung. The hydrochloric acid produced by the stomach rarely causes harm there. However, the acid can burn and damage the esophagus if it flows backward and can damage other organs if it leaks through the stomach wall. Stool, the undigested part of food expelled through the anus, can cause life-threatening infections if it leaks through the intestinal wall into the abdominal cavity.

Mind-Body Interactions

The mind and body interact in powerful ways that affect a person's health. The digestive system is profoundly controlled by the mind (brain); anxiety, depression, and fear dramatically affect the function of this system.▲ Social and psychologic stress can trigger or ag-

gravate a wide variety of diseases, such as diabetes mellitus, high blood pressure, and possibly multiple sclerosis. However, the relative importance of psychologic factors varies widely among different people with the same disorder.

Most people, on the basis of either intuition or personal experience, believe that emotional stress can precipitate or alter the course of even major physical diseases. How these stressors do this is not clear. Emotions obviously can affect certain body functions, such as heart rate, blood pressure, sweating, sleep patterns, stomach acid secretion, and bowel movements, but other relationships are less obvious. For example, the pathways and mechanisms by which the brain and immune system interact are only beginning to be identified. It is remarkable that the mind (brain) can alter the activity of white blood cells and thus an immune response, because white blood cells travel through the body in blood or lymph vessels and are not attached to nerves. Nevertheless, research has shown that the brain does communicate with the white blood cells. For example, depression may suppress the immune system, making a depressed person more susceptible to infections, such as those by the viruses that cause the common cold.

Stress can cause physical symptoms even though no physical disease may be present, because the body responds physiologically to emotional stress. For example, stress can cause anxiety, which then triggers the autonomic nervous system and hormones such as epinephrine to speed up the heart rate and to increase the blood pressure and the amount of sweating. Stress can also cause muscle tension, leading to pain in the neck, back, head, or elsewhere.

The mind-body interaction is a two-way street. Not only can psychologic factors contribute to the onset or aggravation of a wide variety of physical disorders, but also physical diseases can affect a person's thinking or mood. People with life-threatening, recurring, or chronic physical disorders commonly become depressed. The depression may worsen the effects of the physical disease and add to a person's misery.

A possible link between the mind, body, and risk of death suggests that people who are pessimistic, that is, people who interpret bad

▲ see page 694

events as permanent and pervasive, are more likely to feel relatively helpless and depressed than those who are relatively optimistic. Feelings of helplessness and hopelessness have been associated with illness, and pessimistic people are more often in poor health and prone to depression. A pessimistic outlook on life events has been linked in one study with a 19% increased risk of death.

Anatomy and Disease

The human body is remarkably well designed. Most of its organs have a great deal of extra capacity or reserve: They can still function adequately even when damaged. For example, more than two thirds of the liver must be destroyed before serious consequences occur, and a person can survive after an entire lung is surgically removed as long as the other lung is functioning normally. Other organs can tolerate little damage before they malfunction and symptoms occur. For example, if a stroke destroys a small amount of vital brain tissue, a person may be unable to speak, move a limb, or maintain balance. A heart attack, which destroys heart tissue, may slightly impair the heart's ability to pump blood or may result in death.

Disease often affects anatomy, and changes in anatomy can cause disease. If the blood supply to a tissue is blocked or cut off, the tissue dies (infarction), as in a heart attack (myocardial infarction) or stroke (cerebral infarction). An abnormal heart valve can cause heart malfunction. Trauma to the skin may damage its ability to act as a barrier, which may lead to infection. Abnormal growths, such as cancer, can directly destroy normal tissue or produce pressure that ultimately destroys it.

Because of the relationship between disease and anatomy, methods of seeing into the body have become a mainstay of the diagnosis and treatment of disease. The first breakthrough came with x-rays, which enabled doctors to see into the body and examine internal structures without surgery. Another major advance was computed tomography (CT), in which x-rays are linked with computers. A CT scan produces detailed cross-sectional (two-dimensional) images of the body's interior.

Other methods of producing images of internal structures include ultrasound scanning, which uses sound waves; magnetic resonance imaging (MRI), which uses the movement of atoms in a magnetic field; and radionuclide imaging, which uses radioactive chemicals injected into the body.▲ These are noninvasive ways to see into the body, in contrast to surgery, which is an invasive procedure.

Anatomy in This Book

Because anatomy is so important to medicine, almost every section of this book begins with a description of the anatomy of an organ system. Illustrations throughout the book focus on the part of the anatomy being discussed. Additionally, color pictures are located in two separate areas in the book to help illustrate various important aspects of the human body.

CHAPTER 2

Genetics

The body's genetic material is contained within the nucleus of each of its cells, which in an adult person number over 5 trillion. The genetic material consists of coils of DNA (deoxyribonucleic acid) arranged in a complex way to form chromosomes. Human cells each contain 22 pairs of nonsex (autosomal) chromosomes, and one pair of sex chromosomes, for a total of 46 chromosomes.

Each **DNA** molecule is a long double helix that resembles a spiral staircase. The steps of

▲ see page 1728

the staircase, which determine a person's genetic code, consist of pairs of four types of molecules called bases (nucleotides). In each step, adenine (A) is paired with thymine (T), or guanine (G) is paired with cytosine (C). The genetic code is written in triplets, so each group of three bases codes the production of one of 20 possible amino acids, which are the building blocks of proteins. For example, "GCT" codes for the amino acid alanine, while "AAA" codes for the amino acid lysine.

A **gene** consists of the code required to construct one protein. Thus, a gene is a collection of DNA in sequence. Genes vary in size, depending on the size of the protein they code for. All inherited characteristics (traits) are encoded by genes (although many traits are governed by more than one gene). Some genetically determined characteristics, such as hair color, simply distinguish people from one another; variations in hair color are not considered abnormal. However, other genetically determined characteristics are important for the body's normal structure or function; variations in the genes controlling such characteristics may result in a hereditary disease.

A **chromosome** is a collection of genes. Genes are arranged in a precise sequence on the chromosomes; the location of a particular gene on a chromosome is called its locus.

Telomeres are like tiny caps at the ends of each chromosome and protect the chromosome from damage. Before a cell divides, it must replicate all its DNA. However, the cell has difficulty replicating the telomeres (which are also made of DNA), and each time it does so the telomeres get slightly shorter. Eventually, on any given chromosome, the telomeres disappear completely. The disappearance of the telomeres seems to lead to cell death, thus one cause of aging might be the gradual shortening of the telomeres. Curiously, some cancer cells either manage to preserve the length of the telomeres or manage to survive despite loss of the telomeres.

A person's genetic makeup is called the **genotype.** The genotype is a complete set of instructions on how the body is "supposed" to be built. The body's response to having these genes—that is, the expression of the genotype (how the body is actually built)—is called the **phenotype.**

Many genetically determined characteristics are the result of more than one gene. For example, a person's height is likely to be determined by genes affecting growth, appetite, muscle mass, and activity level along with myriad nongenetic influences. Susceptibility to disease is often the combination of multiple genetic influences as well. Thus, it is not always easy to determine which hereditary influences most affect phenotype.

Transferring Information from DNA

When a part of the DNA molecule is actively controlling some function of the cell, the DNA helix splits open along its length. One strand of the open helix is inactive; the other strand is active and acts as a template against which a complementary strand of RNA (ribonucleic acid) forms. The RNA bases are arranged in the same sequence as bases of the inactive strand of the DNA, except that RNA contains uracil (U) instead of thymine (T). The RNA copy, called messenger RNA (mRNA), separates from the DNA, leaves the nucleus, and travels into the cytoplasm of the cell. There, it attaches to a ribosome; ribosomes are the cell's factories for manufacturing proteins. The messenger RNA instructs the ribosome as to the sequence of amino acids for constructing a specific protein. Amino acids, which are floating free in the cytoplasm, are brought to the ribosome by transfer RNA (tRNA), a much smaller type of RNA. Each molecule of transfer RNA brings one amino acid to be incorporated into the growing chain of protein, which is folded into a precise shape under the influence of nearby "chaperone" molecules.

When cells divide (either for growth or for replacing cells that die), DNA replicates itself. The DNA helix unravels, and through a stepwise process, a new molecule of DNA forms. If all goes as planned, each new cell has DNA that is identical to what was in the cell from which it derived. If a mistake occurs, a mutation develops. Often, a mutation is lethal to the cell, and the cell dies. In some cases, a mutation is trivial and there is no noticeable consequence. In other cases, the mutation does not kill the cell but introduces a change that is either detrimental or advantageous to the cell.

Sex Chromosomes

The two sex chromosomes determine whether a fetus becomes male or female. Males have one X and one Y chromosome; females have two X chromosomes, only one of which is active.

There are other genes on the X and Y chromosomes besides those that control sex. How-

Structure of DNA

DNA (deoxyribonucleic acid) is the cell's genetic material, found in jumbled, loosely coiled threads called chromatin in the nucleus of each cell. Just before a cell divides, the chromatin becomes tightly coiled, forming chromosomes.

Human cells contain 23 pairs of chromosomes. Each chromosome is divided into two chromatids, held together by the centromere.

A chromatid is divided into bands, each of which contains many genes. A gene is a segment of DNA that provides the code to construct one protein.

The DNA molecule is a long, coiled double helix that resembles a spiral staircase. In it, two strands, composed of sugar (deoxyribose) and phosphate molecules, are connected by pairs of four molecules called bases, which form the steps of the staircase. In the steps, adenine is paired with thymine, and guanine with cytosine. Each pair of bases is held together by a hydrogen bond. Thus, a gene consists of a sequence of bases, each sequence of three bases coding for one amino acid (amino acids are the building blocks of proteins).

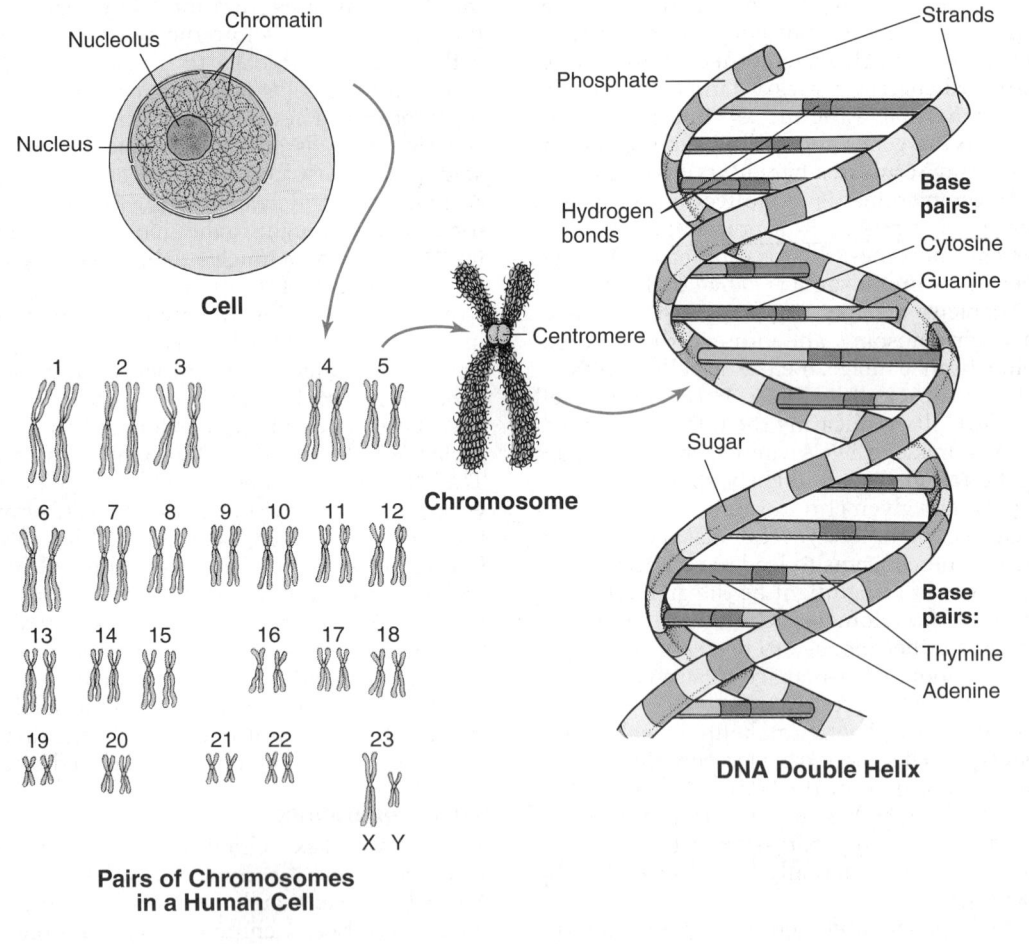

Chromatin

Nucleolus

Nucleus

Cell

Phosphate

Hydrogen bonds

Strands

Base pairs:

Cytosine

Guanine

Sugar

Base pairs:

Thymine

Adenine

Centromere

Chromosome

DNA Double Helix

1 2 3 4 5

6 7 8 9 10 11 12

13 14 15 16 17 18

19 20 21 22 23

X Y

**Pairs of Chromosomes
in a Human Cell**

ever, the Y chromosome carries relatively few genes other than the ones that determine male sex. The X chromosome contains many more genes than the Y chromosome. Genes on the X chromosome are referred to as sex-linked, or X-linked, genes. In males, virtually all of the genes on the X chromosome, whether dominant or recessive, are expressed, because there is no second X chromosome to offset the instructions of recessive genes on the one X chromosome.

Because a female has two X chromosomes, she has twice as many X-chromosome genes as does a male. This would seem to result in an overdose of some genes. However, one of the two X chromosomes in each cell of the female—except in the eggs in the ovaries—is thought to be inactivated early in the life of the fetus. The inactive X chromosome (the Barr body) is visible under a microscope as a dense lump in the nucleus of the cell.

The inactivation of the X chromosome explains certain observations. For example, extra X chromosomes cause far fewer developmental abnormalities than extra nonsex (autosomal) chromosomes, because no matter how many X chromosomes a person has, all but one seem to be inactivated. Women with three X chromosomes (triple X syndrome) are often physically and mentally normal.▲ In contrast, an additional nonsex chromosome can be fatal during early fetal development or can lead to many severe physical and mental abnormalities (for example, Down syndrome).■ Similarly, the absence of a nonsex chromosome is invariably fatal to the fetus, but the absence of one X chromosome usually results in relatively minor abnormalities (Turner syndrome).★

Gene Abnormalities

Abnormalities of one or more genes, particularly recessive genes, are fairly common. Every human being carries an average of six to eight abnormal recessive genes. However, these genes do not cause cells to function abnormally unless two copies of an abnormal recessive gene are present. In the general population, the chance of a person having two copies of an abnormal recessive gene is very small, but in children of close relatives, the chances are higher. Chances are also high among groups that intermarry, such as the Amish or Mennonites.

An abnormal gene may be inherited or may arise spontaneously as a result of a mutation (a

EXAMPLES OF GENETIC DISORDERS

GENE	DOMINANT	RECESSIVE
Non–X-linked	Marfan's syndrome Huntington's disease	Cystic fibrosis
X-linked	Familial rickets Hereditary nephritis	Red–green color blindness Hemophilia

sudden change in a gene arising as a result of any one of a number of causes or for no apparent cause at all). Depending on whether the mutation affects the reproductive cells or not, the mutation may be passed on to future generations or may simply die out with the person who has the mutation.

Whether or not a particular gene is "abnormal" can be a matter of interpretation. For example, the sickle cell gene produces disease (sickle cell anemia) but also confers protection against malaria. This so-called abnormal gene may therefore be of significant benefit in certain regions of the world.

Gene Expression

The effects of a single-gene abnormality depend on whether the gene is dominant or recessive. For a dominant gene to be expressed, only one copy of the gene is needed. For a recessive gene to be expressed, two copies are necessary. Some genes, dominant or recessive, have only partial penetrance, meaning that even if present, they do not always or do not fully cause a change. Finally, all genes residing on the X chromosome (X-linked) are expressed in males; only dominant ones are expressed in females (unless two copies of a recessive gene are present).

Because each gene directs the production of a particular protein, an abnormal gene produces an abnormal protein or an abnormal amount of protein, which may cause an abnormality in cell function and ultimately in physical appearance or bodily function.

▲ see page 1529   ■ see page 1527
★ see page 1528

Inheriting Abnormal Recessive Genes

Some diseases result from an abnormal recessive gene. To have the disease, a person must receive two genes for it, one from each parent. If both parents carry one abnormal gene and one normal gene, they do not have the disease but they can pass the abnormal gene to their children. Each child has a 25% chance of inheriting two abnormal genes (and thus of developing the disease), a 25% chance of inheriting two normal genes, and a 50% chance of inheriting one normal and one abnormal gene (thus becoming a carrier of the disease like the parents).

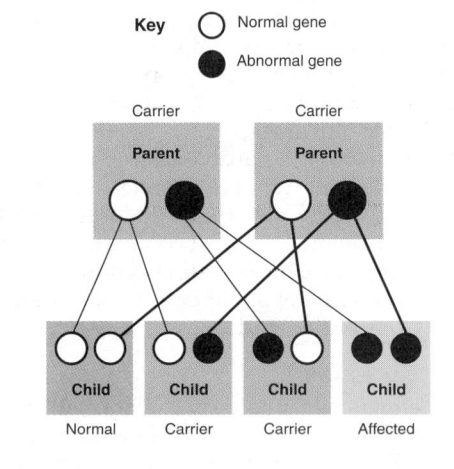

The effect (trait) produced by an abnormal dominant gene may be a deformity, a disease, or a tendency to develop certain diseases.

The following principles generally apply to traits determined by a **dominant non–X-linked gene:**

• People with the trait have at least one parent with the trait, unless it is caused by a new mutation.

• Abnormal genetic traits are often caused by new genetic mutations rather than by inheritance from the parents.

• When one parent has an abnormal trait and the other does not, each child has a 50% chance of inheriting the abnormal trait. However, if the parent with the abnormal trait has two copies of the abnormal gene—a rare occurrence—all of their children will have the abnormal trait.

• A person who does not have the abnormal trait, but whose siblings do have it, does not carry the gene and cannot pass the trait on to his offspring.

• Males and females are equally likely to be affected.

• The abnormality can, and usually does, appear in every generation.

Dominant genes that cause severe diseases are rare. They tend to disappear because the people who have them are often too ill to have children. However, there are a few exceptions, such as Huntington's disease, which causes severe deterioration in brain function that usually begins after age 35. By the time symptoms occur, the person may already have had children.

The following principles generally apply to traits determined by a **recessive non–X-linked gene:**

• Virtually everyone with the trait has parents who both have the gene, even though neither parent may have the trait (because two copies of the abnormal gene are necessary for the gene to be expressed).

• Mutations are highly unlikely to result in expression of the trait (because the mutation would have to have occurred in both parents).

• When one parent has the trait and the other has one recessive gene but does not have the trait, half of their children are likely to have the trait; the others will be carriers with one recessive gene. If the parent without the trait does not have the abnormal recessive gene, none of their children will have the trait, but all of their children will inherit an abnormal gene that they can pass on to their offspring.

• A person who does not have the abnormal trait but whose siblings do have it is likely to carry one abnormal gene.

• Males and females are equally likely to be affected.

• The abnormality can appear in every generation but usually does not unless both parents have the trait.

The following principles generally apply to traits determined by a **dominant X-linked gene:**

• Affected males transmit the abnormality to all of their daughters but to none of their sons. (The sons of the affected male receive his Y chromosome, which does not carry the abnormal gene.)

Inheriting Abnormal Recessive X-Linked Genes

If a gene is X-linked, it appears on the X chromosome and not on the Y chromosome. Diseases that result from an abnormal recessive X-linked gene usually develop only in males. This is because males have only one X chromosome. Females have two X chromosomes, so they usually receive a normal gene on the second X chromosome. The normal gene is dominant, preventing females from developing the disease.

If the father has an abnormal recessive gene on his X chromosome and the mother has two normal genes, all of their daughters receive one abnormal gene and one normal gene, making them carriers. None of their sons receive the abnormal gene.

If the mother is a carrier and the father has the normal gene, any son has a 50% chance of receiving the abnormal gene from the mother. Any daughter has a 50% chance of receiving one abnormal gene and one normal gene (becoming a carrier) or of receiving two normal genes.

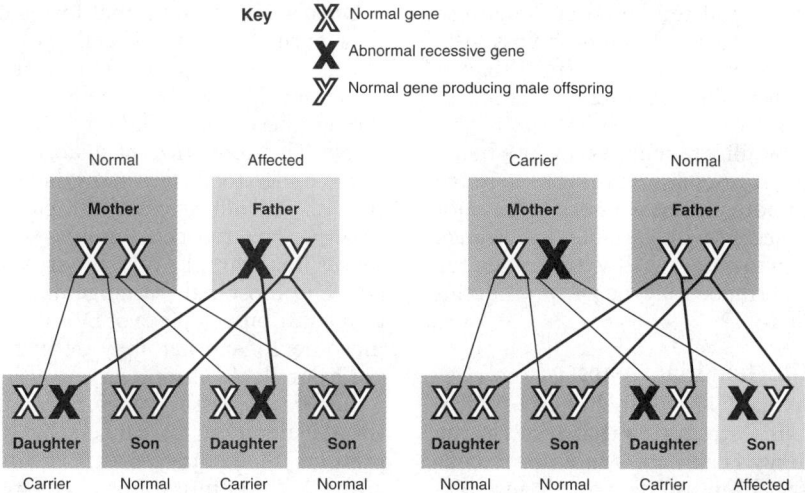

• Affected females with only one abnormal gene transmit the abnormality to, on average, half their children, regardless of sex.
• Affected females with both abnormal genes transmit the trait to all of their children.
• Twice as many females as males will have the disorder unless it is lethal in males.

As with dominant non–X-linked genes, dominant X-linked genes that cause severe diseases are rare. Examples are familial rickets (familial hypophosphatemic rickets)▲ and Alport's syndrome (hereditary nephritis).■ Females with hereditary rickets have less bone symptoms than do affected males. Females with hereditary nephritis usually have no symptoms and little abnormality of kidney function, whereas affected males develop kidney failure in early adult life.

The following principles generally apply to traits determined by a **recessive X-linked gene:**
• Nearly everyone affected is male.
• All daughters of an affected male will be carriers.
• An affected male never transmits the trait to his sons.
• Females who carry the gene do not have the trait (unless they have the abnormal gene on both X chromosomes) but transmit the gene to half their sons, who usually have the trait. None of their daughters have the trait, but half are carriers.

▲ see page 852   ■ see page 856

An example of a common X-linked recessive gene trait is red-green color blindness, which affects about 10% of males but is unusual among females. In males, the gene for color blindness comes from a mother who usually has normal vision but is a carrier of the color-blind gene. It never comes from the father, who instead supplies the Y chromosome. Daughters of color-blind fathers are rarely color-blind but are always carriers of the color-blind gene.

Codominant Genes and Penetrance

Codominant genes are both expressed. An example is sickle cell anemia: If a person has one normal gene and one abnormal gene, both normal and abnormal red blood cell pigment (hemoglobin) is produced. Nonetheless, the disease is less severe (sickle cell trait) than if the person has two abnormal genes (sickle cell disease).

To further complicate matters, even when a gene is dominant or codominant (or recessive but present on both chromosomes), it may not be expressed because of variable penetrance (the degree or frequency with which a gene is expressed). Penetrance may vary from individual to individual.

Abnormal Mitochondrial Genes

Inside every cell are mitochondria. Mitochondria are tiny structures that provide the cell with energy. Each mitochondrion contains a circular chromosome. Several rare diseases are caused by abnormal genes carried by the chromosome inside a mitochondrion. An example is Leber's hereditary optic neuropathy, which causes a variable but often devastating loss of vision in both eyes that typically occurs during the teenage years. Another example is a syndrome characterized by type 2 diabetes and deafness.

When an egg is fertilized, only mitochondria from the egg become part of the developing fetus; all mitochondria from the sperm are discarded. Therefore, diseases caused by abnormal mitochondrial genes are transmitted by the mother. A father with abnormal mitochondrial genes cannot transmit any such diseases to his children.

Unlike the DNA in the nucleus of cells, mitochondrial DNA varies from cell to cell throughout the body. It may even vary among mitochondria within a single cell. Thus an abnormal mitochondrial gene in one body cell does not necessarily mean it will cause disease in another cell. Even when two people appear to have the same mitochondrial gene abnormality, the expression of disease may be very different in the two people. This makes genetic testing and genetic counseling of limited value in making predictions for people with known or suspected mitochondrial gene abnormalities.

Genes That Cause Cancer

Certain genes are partially responsible for the development and reproduction of cancer cells. These genes may alter the quantity or behavior of the proteins encoded by genes that regulate growth and alter cell division. Two major categories of such genes are oncogenes and tumor suppressor genes.

Oncogenes are abnormal forms of the genes that normally regulate cell growth. Usually, oncogenes are inactive. However, if they become active and signal cells to divide—even though these cells should not—cancer may develop. The activation of oncogenes is not entirely understood, but many factors may contribute, including chemical carcinogens (for example, in tobacco smoke) and infectious agents (for example, certain viruses). Additionally, chromosomal rearrangements such as the translocation of a piece of DNA from one chromosome to another may activate oncogenes (for example, in chronic myelocytic leukemia).

Tumor suppressor genes normally suppress the development of cancers by encoding for proteins that suppress cancer initiation and growth. When mutations occur in tumor suppressor genes, appropriate regulation of the cell cycle (reproduction, growth, and death) may stop, allowing affected cells to divide continuously, leading to cancer.

Gene Technology

Rapidly changing technology is improving the detection of genetic diseases, both before and after birth.

One effort currently under way, called the Human Genome Project, is the identification and mapping of all the genes on human chromosomes. The project is essentially complete, and the entire human genetic code has been mapped. The hope is that this information will allow better prediction of health risk and better approaches to therapy, tailored much more to each individual. However, concerns have been raised that this information might be used improperly to deny health insurance coverage to people at high risk of particular diseases.

Other efforts involve studying individual genes to learn more about specific diseases. There are several ways to produce enough copies of a gene to study. In a laboratory, the gene to be copied is usually spliced into pieces of DNA inside a bacterium. Each time the bacterium reproduces, it makes an exact copy of all its DNA, including the spliced gene. Bacteria multiply very rapidly, so billions of copies of the original gene can be produced in a very short time.

Another technique for copying DNA uses the polymerase chain reaction (PCR). A specific segment of DNA, such as a specific gene, can be copied (amplified) in a laboratory. Starting with one DNA molecule, at the end of 30 doublings (only a few hours later) about a billion copies will be produced.

A gene probe can be used to locate a specific gene in a particular chromosome. A gene that has been cloned or copied becomes a labeled probe when a radioactive atom is added to it. The probe will seek out its mirror-image segment of DNA and bind to it. The radioactive probe can then be detected by sophisticated photographic techniques. With gene probes, a number of diseases can be diagnosed before or after birth. In the future, gene probes will probably be used to test people for many major genetic diseases. However, not everyone who

has the gene for a given disease will actually develop that disease.

A technique called the Southern blot test is widely used to identify DNA. DNA is extracted from the cells of a person being studied and is cut into precise fragments with a type of enzyme called a restriction endonuclease. The fragments are separated in a gel by a technique called electrophoresis, placed on filter paper, and covered with a labeled probe. Because the probe binds only to its mirror image, it identifies any DNA fragment matching the probe.

Gene Therapy

Gene therapy involves the insertion of normal copies of genes into the cells of a person with a specific genetic disease. The normal copies can be manufactured, using PCR, from normal DNA donated by another person. Because most diseases are recessive, in most cases an inserted copy of a normal gene is dominant and takes over the functions controlled by that particular gene.

There are two forms of gene therapy—somatic and germline. In somatic therapy, gene expression is corrected in the patient but does not affect future generations (somatic refers to

And Then There Were Two

A clone is a group of genetically identical cells or organisms derived from a single cell or individual. Cloning (the producing of clones) has been commonplace for many years in agriculture. A plant can be propagated (cloned) by simply taking a small piece of the original plant and growing a new one from it; the new plant is thus an exact genetic copy (clone) of the original one. Such propagation is also possible with simple animals such as flatworms: cut a flatworm in two, and the tail grows a new head and the head grows a new tail. However, such simple techniques do not work with higher animals, such as sheep or humans.

In the now-famous "Dolly" experiments, cells from a sheep (donor cells) were fused with unfertilized sheep eggs from another sheep (recipient cells) from which the natural genetic material had been removed by microsurgery. Thus the genetic material from the donor cells was transferred into the unfertilized eggs, which then contained a complete set of genes (as if they had been fertilized in the usual way by sperm). The eggs then started to develop into embryos. The developing embryos were transplanted into a female sheep (the surrogate mother), where they developed naturally. One of the embryos survived, the resulting lamb being called "Dolly." As ex-

pected, Dolly was an exact genetic copy (clone) of the original sheep from which the donor cells had been taken, not of the sheep that had provided the eggs.

Research on cloning continues, but no known cloning of humans has so far been attempted, due partly to technical difficulties and partly to ethical concerns and governmental attempts to make it illegal. However, cloning need not only be used to create a whole organism. It can, theoretically, also be used to create a single organ. Thus, one day a person may be able to receive "spare parts" manufactured in the laboratory, using the person's own genes.

the entire body other than the germ cells). In germline therapy, the beneficial genetic change is inserted into the cells responsible for reproduction (eggs or sperm, which are also known as germ cells). Thus, the beneficial changes are passed on to the next generation. However, germline therapy is generally considered an inappropriate way to deal with genetic diseases because of ethical issues, cost, lack of research in humans, lack of knowledge about whether changes would be maintained in the growing embryo, and the relative ease of using somatic therapy. Currently, gene therapy is most likely to be effective in the prevention or cure of single-gene defects, such as cystic fibrosis.

The transfer of the normal DNA into abnormal cells can be done in a number of ways. One way is to use a virus. The normal DNA is spliced into the virus, which then infects the abnormal cells, thereby transmitting the DNA into the nucleus of those cells. Another method uses liposomes, which are tiny sacs containing the DNA that are absorbed by the abnormal cells and thereby deliver their DNA to the cell nucleus. A third method is called naked plasmid DNA injection, in which plasmid DNA (a special circular form of DNA) is injected into a muscle.

A totally different approach to gene therapy is the use of antisense technology, in which, rather than altering abnormal genes, the abnormal genes are simply switched off (antisense drugs combine with specific sequences on the DNA that prevent the affected genes from functioning). Antisense technology is currently being tried for cancer therapy but is still very experimental.

Gene therapy is also being studied experimentally in transplantation surgery; by altering the genes of the transplanted organs, the organ recipient would not need to receive immunosuppressive drugs, which have significant side effects.

CHAPTER 3

The Aging Body

Aging is a process of gradual and spontaneous change, resulting in maturation through childhood, puberty, and young adulthood and then decline of many bodily functions through middle and late age. Aging is a continuous process that begins at birth and continues throughout all stages of life. It involves both the positive component of development and the negative component of decline.

There is no specific age at which a person becomes "elderly." Traditionally, age 65 has been so designated because it is the age at which people in industrialized societies generally leave the work force, though this is changing.

Aging can be classified into three categories: senescence, normal aging, and successful aging. **Senescence** describes the many changes that occur with age as a result of biologic, psychologic, and environmental factors as well as lifestyle choices. It is often difficult to separate the aspects of senescence that are purely biologic, and thus to be expected and difficult to avoid, from those that are nonbiologic, and thus preventable.

Normal aging refers to the common complex of diseases and impairments that affect many older people. It encompasses a wide spectrum, because people age very differently, including how they develop diseases and impairments.

Successful (healthy) aging refers to a process by which aging is not accompanied by debilitating disease and disability. People who age successfully may maintain an active healthy life until death and are said to have died of old age. In addition, people who age successfully do not experience many of the unwanted features of aging. For example, they may avoid extensive tooth loss, which used to be (and still is in some societies) common among older people. There is evidence that a greater percentage of people in the United States are aging successfully. For example, the percentage of older people residing in nursing homes has decreased, although the percentage of people over age 65 and, of those people, the proportion over age 85 have both increased. Furthermore, the percentage of people aged 75 to 84 who report disabilities has decreased, as has the percentage of people over age 65 with debilitating disease. Although there may be alternative explanations for these changes in health status, one viable explanation is an increase in the proportion of people who are aging successfully.

Disease Versus Aging

With age, many of the body's functions decline. The decline that occurs in normal aging, however, is not usually considered the same as disease, although the distinction is not always clear. As people age, blood sugar levels increase more after eating carbohydrates than they do in younger people; however, the very large increases that occur in diabetes are not considered normal aging.▲ Mental decline that includes more difficulty learning new languages and increased forgetfulness is nearly universal with advanced age and is considered normal aging; however, the serious mental decline of dementia, with its extreme loss of short-term memory, ability to learn, and understanding of the environment, although common in late life, is considered a disease.■ Alzheimer's disease is an abnormal process distinct from normal aging, a conclusion supported by analysis of brain tissue at autopsy.

Longevity

The average life expectancy of Americans has been increasing dramatically over the past century. A male child born in 1900 could expect to live only 46 years; a female child, 48 years. Today, however, a male child can expect to live more than 73 years; a female child, nearly 80 years. Although many of these gains in longevity can be attributed to the significant decrease in childhood mortality, life expectancy at every age beyond 40 has also increased dramatically. For example, a 70-year-old man can now expect to live until age 83, and a 70-year-old woman to age 85.

Despite the increase in average life expectancy, the maximum life span—the oldest age to which people can live—has changed little since records have been kept. Despite the best genetic makeup and medical care, no one seems to live much beyond 125 years, although some experts suggest that this number may be slowly increasing. Currently, a person

has a 1 in 2 billion chance of living to the age of 120.

Several factors influence longevity. One is heredity, which primarily influences whether an individual will contract a disease. For example, inheriting an increased risk of developing high cholesterol levels is likely to result in a shorter life, whereas inheriting genes that protect against heart disease and cancer can help to ensure a longer life. Another important influence on longevity is lifestyle; avoiding smoking, avoiding drug and alcohol abuse, maintaining a healthy weight and diet, and exercising appropriately help people avoid disease. Exposure to environmental toxins can shorten life expectancy even among people with the most robust genetic makeup. Medical care contributes to increased survival by preventing or treating diseases after they are contracted, especially when the diseases (for example, infectious diseases, cancer) are cured.

Bodily Changes

The human body changes in many noticeable ways with age. Often, the first signs of aging involve the musculoskeletal system. By age 35, peak performance, even among superior athletes, begins to decline. Sensory organs also begin to change early in mid-life. A common development, for example, is presbyopia, in which the eye can no longer focus easily on close objects. By age 40 or so, many people find it difficult to read without using reading glasses or changing to bifocals. Another, if later, common development is presbycusis, or age-associated hearing loss, which initially affects the ability to hear the highest pitches and, gradually, the lower pitches as well. Therefore, older people may find that violin music no longer sounds as exciting as it did when they were younger. Also, because most of the closed consonants of speech are high tones (sounds such as k, t, s, p, and ch), older people may think that others are mumbling.

In most people, the proportion of body fat increases by more than 30% by late age. The distribution of fat also changes: There is less fat under the skin and more in the abdominal area. Thus, skin becomes thinner, wrinkled (although sun exposure and smoking have a greater influence on wrinkling), and more fragile, and the shape of the torso changes.

Not surprisingly, most internal functions also decline with age. These functions gener-

---

▲ see page 962   ■ see page 484

EXAMPLES OF HOW THE BODY CHANGES WITH AGE

Organ System	Normal Age-Associated Changes	Consequences
Brain	Decreased blood flow	Fainting occurs more often
	Levels of many chemicals change	Confusion occurs more often
	Decreased central nervous system function	Mental functions decrease; ability to maintain good balance and to walk properly decrease
Eyes	Lens stiffens	Difficulty focusing on close objects
	Retina is less sensitive to light	Difficulty seeing in dim light
	Pupils react more slowly	Difficulty adjusting quickly to changes in light levels
Ears	Less able to hear high frequencies	Difficulty in understanding voices
Mouth	Fewer taste buds	Many foods taste bitter or lack taste
Smell	Less able to detect odors	Many foods taste bland
Heart	Lowered acceleration of pulse	Fainting occurs more often
	Decreased maximal output of blood	Less able to perform strenuous exercise
	Heart muscle stiffens	Heart failure is more common
	Lower response to certain stimulants	Less increase in heart rate
Lungs	Less air movement with each breath	Less able to perform strenuous exercise
	Less oxygen transferred to blood	Difficulty breathing at high altitudes
Liver	Liver shrinks; decreased blood flow	Effects of medications last longer; decreased ability to clear toxins
	Less active enzyme system	Drugs reach higher levels in body, increasing risk of side effects
Kidneys	Kidneys shrink; decreased blood flow	Effects of medications last longer; decreased ability to clear toxins
	Urine is less concentrated	Dehydration is more common
	Decreased ability to excrete salt	Abnormal salt levels occur commonly
Bladder	Muscles of wall weaken	Becomes more difficult to urinate
	Less ability to delay urination	Incontinence is more common
Large intestine (colon)	Ability to pass stool decreases	Constipation
Skin	Underlying fat begins to thin	Wrinkles are more prominent; skin tears more easily; hypothermia is more common
Immune system	Less antibody produced	Infections occur more often, are more severe, and spread more quickly
Metabolism	Blood sugar level rises after eating	Increased tendency towards diabetes
	Body fat increases	Increased risk of diabetes
	Decreased vitamin D levels; calcium absorption decreases; excretion of calcium increases	Osteoporosis
Male reproductive organs	Prostate enlarges	Urinary retention is more common
	Decreased testosterone levels	Erectile dysfunction
	Decrease blood flow to the penis	Erectile dysfunction

EXAMPLES OF HOW THE BODY CHANGES WITH AGE *(Continued)*

ORGAN SYSTEM	NORMAL AGE-ASSOCIATED CHANGES	CONSEQUENCES
Female reproductive organs	Decreased estrogen production (uterus and ovaries shrink) Breasts become more fatty and fibrous	Increased risk of coronary artery disease, osteoporosis, hot flashes, vaginal wall thinning Harder to examine breasts for breast cancer
Blood	Decreased red blood cell production	Slower response to blood loss or low oxygen

ally peak shortly before age 30 and then begin a gradual but continuous decline. Even with this decline, however, most functions remain adequate throughout life, because most organs have considerably more functional capacity than the body needs (functional reserve). For example, even if half the liver is destroyed, more than enough liver tissue remains to maintain normal function. Disease, rather than normal aging, usually accounts for loss of function in old age. Even so, the decline in function means that older people are more likely to experience side effects from drugs, changes in the environment, toxins, and illness.

Although the decline in function of many organs has little effect on how people live, the decline in some organs can greatly affect health and well-being. For example, although the amount of blood that the heart can pump at rest is not greatly reduced in old age, the heart cannot pump as much when pushed to its maximum. This means that older athletes will not be able to perform as well as younger athletes. Changes in kidney function can dramatically affect how well older people are able to eliminate certain drugs from their body.▲

Determining which changes are purely age-associated and which are the result of how a person has lived is often difficult. A sedentary lifestyle, poor diet, cigarette smoking, and alcohol and drug abuse can damage many organs over time, often more so than aging alone. People who have been exposed to toxins may experience a more significant or more rapid decline in the function of some organs, especially the kidneys, lungs, and liver. People who worked in loud environments are likely to lose more of their hearing. Some decline in function can be prevented by adopting a healthier lifestyle. For example, stopping smoking at any age, even in one's 80s, helps

improve lung function, decrease the chance of developing lung cancer, and decrease the risk of heart disease. Weight-bearing exercise helps maintain muscle and bone strength regardless of age and helps prevent falls and debilitation.

Implications of Illness

Gerontology is the study of aging. Geriatrics is the branch of medicine that specializes in the care of older people. A number of disorders occur almost exclusively in older people and are sometimes called geriatric syndromes or geriatric diseases. Other disorders that affect people of all ages may cause different symptoms or complications in older people. For example, an underactive thyroid gland usually causes younger people to gain weight and feel sluggish, whereas in older people it may initially or predominantly cause a state of confusion. An overactive thyroid usually causes younger people to become agitated and lose weight; in older people, it may cause them to become sleepy, withdrawn, depressed, and confused. Depression usually causes younger adults to become tearful, withdrawn, and noticeably unhappy. In older people, depression sometimes causes confusion, loss of memory, and apathy without a sense of sadness. The confusion that results from these conditions is often mistaken for dementia in older people.

Acute illnesses that were once likely to result in death for older people, such as heart attacks, hip fractures, and pneumonia, are now often treatable and controllable. In addition, a chronic illness no longer necessarily means disability. Many people with diabetes, kidney problems, heart disease, and other chronic illnesses now find that they can remain functional, active, and independent.

▲ see page 79

DISORDERS THAT MAINLY AFFECT OLDER PEOPLE

Disease or Condition	Explanation	Disease or Condition	Explanation
Alzheimer's disease and other dementias	Brain disorders that lead to progressive loss of memory and other intellectual functions	Hypothyroidism	Thyroid gland is underactive and produces too little thyroid hormone, which can eventually result in anemia, a low body temperature, and heart failure
Aortic aneurysm	Dilation of the wall of the aorta that can rupture and lead to death if left untreated	Monoclonal gammopathies	A group of diverse conditions in which abnormal proliferation of a single type of cell produces high levels of an immunoglobulin
Atrophic urethritis and vaginitis	Thinning of the tissue of the urethra and vagina that can lead to burning on urination and painful intercourse	Osteoarthritis	Degeneration of the cartilage that lines the joints, causing pain. Begins in middle age
Bedsores	Breakdown of skin from prolonged pressure	Osteoporosis	Loss of calcium from the bones, which makes the bones fragile and can lead to fractures
Benign prostatic hyperplasia	Enlargement of the prostate gland, which blocks the flow of urine	Parkinson's disease	Slowly progressive degenerative brain disease that leads to tremor, muscle rigidity, difficulty moving, and postural instability
Cataracts	Clouding in the lens of the eye, which impairs vision		
Chronic lymphocytic leukemia	A type of leukemia that usually has a long phase with little growth or progression (indolent phase) but that has many other characteristic features of cancer (malignancy)	Prostate cancer	A cancer of the prostate gland
		Shingles (herpes zoster)	A reawakening of the dormant chickenpox virus, which causes a skin rash and can cause prolonged pain
Diabetes, type 2 (adult onset)	A type of diabetes that may not require insulin treatment. Usually begins in middle age	Stroke	A blockage or bleeding of a blood vessel in the brain that leads to weakness, loss of sensation, difficulty talking, or other neurologic problems
Glaucoma	Elevation of the pressure in one of the chambers of the eye that can decrease vision and lead to blindness. Usually begins in middle age	Urinary incontinence	Inability to control urine flow

Social factors play a major role in the health care of older people. Older people who maintain social contact, whether it be with a spouse, with friends, or through outside interests, have been shown to have fewer medical problems. For example, older people who are married or who live with a roommate tend to be in better health than those who live alone. Older people who do not live alone also have lower rates of hospitalization and nursing home admissions than those who do live alone.

Education also plays a role in the health of older people. Higher levels of education are associated with earlier detection of disease and better health outcomes, even when disease is not detected early.

Economic factors affect the way in which older people access health care. Poverty is more common among older people than among the general population. Despite the implementation of such programs as Medicare, Medicaid, and Social Security, some older people do not have adequate health insurance and find it difficult to pay for uncovered aspects of medical care, including drugs. Consequently, otherwise treatable diseases go untreated or are treated at a later stage.

Older people often have more than one disease at a time, each of which may have an effect on the other. For example, depression may make dementia worse, and an infection may worsen diabetes. Additionally, many older people tend to conceal minor problems and do not seek medical care until the problems become major.

Psychologic factors coexist with and may complicate disease in older people. An older person may become depressed if his illness leads to temporary or permanent loss of independence or as he sees his aging friends and loved ones die. For these reasons, geriatricians often recommend multidisciplinary care. With this type of care, a team of medical personnel, which may consist of doctors, nurses, social workers, therapists, pharmacists, and psychologists, plan and implement care—including social services—under the leadership of a primary doctor.

Diseases of Accelerated Aging

Progeroid Syndromes: The progeroid syndromes are conditions that produce premature aging and a shortened life expectancy. The most striking feature of these rare disorders is extremely accelerated aging. Affected children develop all of the external signs of old age, including baldness, hunched posture, and dry, wrinkled skin. Unlike normal aging, however, progeroid syndromes also include such features as lack of ovarian or testicular activity (including sterility and absence of menstrual periods) and unusually short stature. Thus, progeria is not an exact model of accelerated aging.

Two forms of progeroid syndromes are Hutchinson-Gilford syndrome (commonly referred to as progeria), which begins in early childhood, and Werner's syndrome, which begins in adolescence or early adult life. Both syndromes are hereditary, but the exact genetic basis of Hutchinson-Gilford syndrome remains undetermined. However, recent advances have been made in understanding the genetic basis of Werner's syndrome. Hutchinson-Gilford syndrome produces scleroderma, baldness, and other conditions normally associated with aging (for example, diseases of the heart, kidneys, and lungs). Similarly, Werner's syndrome produces the skin changes of scleroderma and baldness and a high rate of atherosclerosis. The central nervous system, and therefore daily activities dependent on brain function, is largely spared in both Hutchinson-Gilford syndrome and Werner's syndrome, unless an affected person has a stroke. Other features of Werner's syndrome include premature cataracts, muscle wasting, and a high rate of cancer (including some types that are rare in unaffected people).

Down Syndrome:▲ More common than the progeroid syndromes, Down syndrome also produces in younger adults conditions typical of old age, including glucose intolerance, blood vessel disease, a high rate of cancer, hair loss, degenerative bone disease, and premature death. In contrast to Werner's syndrome, Down syndrome greatly impairs the central nervous system, usually producing retardation and, later in life, brain changes characteristic of Alzheimer's dementia.■

CHAPTER 4

Communicating With Health Care Professionals

People who communicate effectively with their doctors and other health care professionals tend to enjoy better health than people who do not. Effective communication requires active participation in one's own health care. Active participation includes learning about health care issues, visiting a doctor regularly,

obtaining appropriate preventive care,★ and remaining observant for signs of ill health or

---

▲ see page 1527

■ see page 487

★ see page 25

bodily changes, such as a change in the color of a mole or detection of a lump in the breast or testicle. Active participation also means monitoring one's health in the case of a specific disease. For example, a person with hypertension would regularly monitor blood pressure; a person with diabetes would regularly check blood sugar level.

Having a Primary Care Doctor

A primary care doctor should be the entry point into the health care system. Having a primary care doctor has many advantages and usually leads to better care. People who do not have a primary care doctor are more likely to inappropriately seek help in a hospital's emergency department or to be seen by a doctor they do not know. In such cases, medical information that could be important to the treatment of the problem is often forgotten or unknown.

Communication is often better, and medical decisions are more easily made, when an established relationship exists with a primary care doctor. People are more likely to trust doctors they know and, in turn, are likely to experience less anxiety when a medical problem arises. Additionally, doctors who are familiar with their patients are less likely to make mistakes and more likely to provide better health care at lower cost. Primary care doctors often have long-standing relationships with their patients and are familiar with their wishes, the manner in which their patients best receive information, how they cope with adversity, their ability to purchase prescribed drugs, and which family members they rely on.

When to Contact the Doctor

Generally, everyone should routinely visit their doctor, dentist, and eye care professional (for example, an optometrist or an ophthalmologist, if applicable) for preventive care.▲ The primary care doctor should provide a schedule of what type of care is required, why it is necessary, and how often visits should be scheduled. In general, preventive visits are needed most frequently in infancy and in later life, but the recommended frequency varies depending on personal risk factors (for exam-

ple, a person with genetic risk factors for a particular disease may need to have more frequent check-ups).

Between preventive visits, people may experience a variety of symptoms that require medical care. Many symptoms and problems, however, can be handled at home without visiting the primary care doctor. For example, most routine colds do not require the attention of a doctor; over-the-counter cold medicine can be used to relieve symptoms, and ibuprofen or acetaminophen can be used to reduce fever. Most small cuts and abrasions can be handled by first cleaning with a mild soap and water, and then applying an antibiotic ointment and a protective covering.■

When unsure about the need for medical attention, a person can call the primary care doctor to clarify the urgency of the problem and determine whether a doctor's visit is required. Some doctors offer e-mail access for nonemergency questions; others prefer contact by phone. In general, true emergencies should be handled by calling the local emergency service to provide ambulance service to the nearest hospital. However, deciding what qualifies as an emergency is sometimes difficult. Good judgment is often required, and under some insurance plans, a doctor's permission to visit an emergency department is required unless the situation is life threatening.

Making the Most of a Doctor Visit

Preparing for the health care visit allows a person to get the most out of time spent with a doctor. During a first visit, the person may wish to inform the doctor of any personal, religious, or ethnic considerations that might affect his health care decisions. If the person already has an advance directive such as a living will or a durable power of attorney agreement,★ a copy for the doctor's records should be made. If the person does not already have an advance directive, he may wish to discuss reasons for having one and how to proceed if planning to prepare one. Also, the person should ask questions about the doctor's practice, such as whether to expect other professionals (for example, other doctors, nurse practitioners, or physician's assistants) to participate in his care from time to time and how to handle sudden urgent health problems that occur at night or during weekends.

Information about being hospitalized, using home health services, or receiving care from any specialists or other health care profession-

▲ see page 1278
■ see page 1691
★ see page 55

als should be given to the primary care doctor. Providing the names, addresses, and phone numbers of other sources of health care can facilitate communication and obtaining copies of medical records. Any plans for upcoming diagnostic testing or new treatment should be disclosed.

Arriving at the doctor's office 10 to 15 minutes before the scheduled appointment helps the office staff ensure that insurance information is current and that any required forms are completed. Current insurance cards, any required referrals, and money for payment of any required fees should be brought along. Just as patients have a responsibility to arrive on time, doctors also have a responsibility to run on or close to schedule except when medical urgencies upset the routine.

Before any visit, the person should collect all drugs currently being taken, including herbals, vitamins, and other over-the-counter drugs, to bring to the doctor. Any forms that will need to be completed by the doctor's office should also be brought. Any significant medical symptoms or questions about medical issues should be written down; it is easy to forget a question during a busy office visit.

The person should listen carefully to the doctor and should respond as honestly and completely as possible. A common topic that requires clear and honest communication involves the taking of prescribed drugs. For example, if a person has not been taking a drug as prescribed, he needs to tell the doctor and provide an explanation (for example, "I seem to get stomach cramps from the medicine" or "I can't afford the medicine"). Other common topics requiring honest disclosure include sexual practices and drug, alcohol, and substance use.

If tests are ordered, the person should ask how and when he will be informed of both abnormal and normal results. It is particularly important that the person understand who is responsible (the doctor or the patient) for initiating follow-up of results. For example, some doctors telephone the patient promptly about abnormal results but mail normal results or discuss them at the next visit.

If treatment for a medical problem is discussed, the person should ask about different treatment options, including their effectiveness and possible side effects. Also, questions should be asked about the specific goals for the selected treatment and how the response to treatment will be followed or monitored.

The person should request an explanation of anything that is not understood and ask for an education sheet or handout on the subject if one is available. Having the doctor write out instructions and having the patient read those instructions back to the doctor at the end of the visit is one way to help clarify communication. It offers the doctor the opportunity to correct any miscommunication. If the patient cannot use written materials, other approaches may be needed to keep track of the information (for example, tape recording the instructions or having a family member or friend agree to read the instructions). The same suggestions apply to a trip to the pharmacy for medications.

A person should refer to the list of symptoms and questions made before the visit and ask the doctor about anything not covered. If many issues remain, the doctor may have to schedule another appointment or may refer the person to another health care professional, such as a nurse, pharmacist, or dietitian, for further information and education.

After the visit, the person should schedule any recommended follow-up appointments. Any prescriptions should be filled, and any material distributed by the pharmacist about the drug should be read. Finally, the person may want to consider keeping a diary of important aspects of his care (for example, a person with constant headaches may want to record when headaches occur, their timing and associations, and their response to medication).

Keeping Medical Records

Keeping a personal record that includes hospitalizations (dates, location, attending doctor's name, diagnoses), a family medical history, and significant medical problems is important, because memory alone is not always accurate, and institutional medical records from long ago may be lost.

Immunization records, which are traditionally kept for children, are important to keep on an ongoing basis throughout life. Complicated medical regimens should be written out on one sheet of paper; these can be updated as new events occur and the information changes. Copies of laboratory results are also useful to keep for future reference.

Laws vary from state to state regarding what parts of the medical record in the doctor's office are available to patients. Doctors often have ownership of the records but can be required by the courts to submit copies or summaries of the records for specific legal situations. Upon patient request, doctors' offices usually copy and release medical records or create a summary of portions or all of the record to send to other health care professionals. A patient who wants a copy of all of his medical records for personal use may or may not be entitled to these records, depending on state law. Generally, a complete record is not needed. Rather, a file should be maintained regarding the most important items, as noted above.

Researching a Personal Illness

When the diagnosis of an illness is first made, the patient is often given a handout at the doctor's office that summarizes key points of information. The person may also have some general knowledge of the condition from newspaper or magazine articles or television or radio shows.

Additional sources of information are available to the person who wants to learn more about the condition beyond what is provided by the doctor. There are many books that provide helpful, general information about illnesses. Some local libraries have helpful sources. However, judging the reliability of printed materials is not always easy.

The Internet provides a lot of information, but much of it is unreliable. Some internet sites are credible; some are not. The National Institutes of Health (NIH) and the Centers for Disease Control and Prevention (CDC) have internet sites available to the public that provide useful and accurate information. In addition, many disease-specific, patient-oriented sites (such as the National Multiple Sclerosis Society) provide information for people with a particular disease. On the other hand, sites designed to sell specific products or a specific service may provide biased or inaccurate information.

Support groups provide both psychologic support and important information. A person with a serious illness can find such groups through local newspapers, phone directories, hospitals, doctors' offices, other health care professionals' offices, and the Internet. People facing the same situation or illness have many practical and useful suggestions on how to live with a chronic illness day-to-day, such as where to find pieces of specialized equipment, what equipment works best, and how to interact with or care for someone with an illness. Additionally, chat rooms on the Internet may allow people with a specific illness to communicate with one another and to learn more about their condition and possible resources.

Understanding Managed Care

Managed care is a general term that can be confusing and is not particularly descriptive of any one specific health insurance plan. Each insurance plan is different, and these differences can lead to many problems (often in communication) for patients and their health care providers. Anyone insured through managed care should keep a copy of the description of the insurance plan readily available. The restrictions on what is covered is often an area for discussion between patients and doctors.

Many plans have requirements regarding where health care is to be received. If health care is not received at an approved location or is not provided by an enrolled doctor or other health care professional, the co-pay may be higher, or the services may not be covered at all. However, true emergencies handled through the closest hospital are usually partially or fully covered.

Referral forms approved by the primary care doctor are sometimes required before a person can see a specialist or undergo certain diagnostic tests. If this is the rule in the person's insurance plan, the specialist or testing facility will generally refuse to see the person without the referral or will require the person to pay directly for the service. Each person is responsible for having the correct referral form.

Most insurance programs limit coverage regarding some aspect of medical care. For example, certain diagnoses (such as attention deficit disorder) and certain procedures (such as cosmetic surgery) may not be covered. In addition, sometimes the total number of treatments (for example, physical therapy treatments) is limited during a year or over a lifetime. Insurance companies claim that they do not deny a person the right to a specific procedure; however, they can deny payment, which often means that, effectively, the person has been denied care.

CHAPTER 5

Prevention

The traditional practice of medicine focuses on evaluating symptoms, determining what disease is causing those symptoms, and treating the disease. In contrast, preventive medicine aims to prevent diseases from occurring in the first place or to diagnose disease at an early stage, often when there are no symptoms and when recovery is most achievable. Prevention is the area of medicine and health care that focuses on promoting health and reducing risk through specific measures taken to avoid illness, disability, and premature death.

Preventive medicine depends heavily on a person's **risk profile,** that is, the person's risk of developing a disease based on such factors as age, sex, family history, lifestyle, and physical and social environment. Once a person is made aware of his risks based on the risk profile, he can take steps to minimize them.

Everyone is subject to the good or bad fortunes of chance, and ill health sometimes is the result of injuries or other exposures that cannot be predicted. However, genetic makeup and family history are factors that can predict some risks and, although they cannot be controlled, can provide valuable clues as to a person's risk for certain diseases. For example, a person with a family history of diabetes is at higher risk than most people of developing diabetes and thus would be wise to undergo blood sugar monitoring periodically and receive additional counseling in ways to help avoid the onset of diabetes. A person with a family history of colorectal cancer or with a disease that increases the chances of developing colorectal cancer, such as ulcerative colitis, would be advised to undergo a screening sigmoidoscopy or colonoscopy▲ more often than is normally recommended for people at average risk. A woman with a family history of breast cancer would likely be advised to undergo screening mammography at an earlier age.

A person's **lifestyle choices** are also considered when determining the risk profile. For example, how well a person handles stress is important; reducing stress helps reduce blood pressure, which reduces the risk of stroke and heart attack. Smoking cigarettes and not exercising regularly can greatly increase a person's risk of many deadly diseases, and these factors are clearly controllable. A person who smokes or is sedentary, especially if there is a family history of heart disease, may be offered additional counseling about the risks of smoking or the benefits of exercise. A person who eats large amounts of fatty foods may be at increased risk of atherosclerosis■ and thus might benefit from dietary counseling and more frequent checks of blood cholesterol level.★

Social and physical environment (for example, violence in the community, lead paint in the home, a dangerous work environment) can also affect a person's health; these factors are also considered when determining a person's risk profile. For example, a person who works with asbestos is at increased risk of developing lung disease, so a health care professional may suggest periodic chest x-rays and may strongly counsel against smoking. Recommendations may also include using safety devices at work, such as a filtered respirator–style mask. Another example would be people whose jobs involve repeated movements with the wrists extended, such as performing assembly line work or using a computer keyboard; such work may increase the risk of carpal tunnel syndrome or other injuries (to nerves, tendons, and ligaments) associated with repetitive use of certain parts of the body. A health care professional may recommend reducing the amount of uninterrupted time spent doing the activity that triggers the problem and modifying workplace furniture and equipment in order to reduce physical stress on the affected parts of the body.

Value of Prevention

Preventive medicine may improve overall health and has the potential to reduce health care costs. One of the most dramatic success stories in preventive medicine is the development and widespread use of vaccines. Infectious diseases such as diphtheria, pertussis, tetanus, mumps, measles, rubella, and polio have decreased by more than 99% from their peak number of cases, thanks to the availabil-

▲ see page 770　　■ see page 194
★ see page 920

HEALTH RISK ASSESSMENT

CATEGORY	SOME RISK FACTORS
Genetic	Family predisposition to specific disease, such as heart disease, colon cancer, breast cancer, cervical cancer, diabetes, mental health disorders, substance abuse
Race and sex	White men: higher risk of heart attack; black men: higher risk of high blood pressure
Weight	Obesity (weight 20% above ideal body weight for height and build)
Diet	Eating an imbalanced, improper diet
Physical activity	Sedentary lifestyle (exercising much less than the recommended 3 times weekly for 20–30 minutes each time)
Tobacco use	Smoking cigarettes, cigars, or pipes or chewing tobacco
Stress	Stressful situations such as a new job, difficulty at work, death of a loved one, not getting sufficient sleep, getting married or divorced
Mental health	Depression, rapid or frequent mood swings, thoughts of suicide, problems sleeping, alcohol or drug abuse
Social environment	High-risk sexual behavior (multiple partners, not using a condom); difficulty getting along with others
Physical environment	Failure to maintain a safe environment, which would include keeping firearms locked; using bicycle helmets and seat belts; having working smoke detectors and fire extinguishers in the home; having heating systems and fireplaces inspected and cleaned periodically. For children: Using child safety seats, bicycle helmets, flame-retardant sleepwear, window and chair guards; assessing the home for leaded paint and removing if applicable; safely storing drugs and toxic substances. For older people: Protecting against falls, fire, and other physical harm
Vaccinations	Not being current on vaccinations appropriate to specific age group

ity of effective and safe vaccines and their widespread use. Furthermore, vaccinations save about $14 in health care costs for every $1 spent.

Preventive medicine also involves screening programs, which have greatly reduced the number of deaths associated with various diseases. For example, cervical cancer, which was once the most common cause of cancer death among American women, has decreased by 75% since 1955 after the implementation of a screening program using the Papanicolaou (Pap) smear. Although most women should have a Pap smear every few years, women at higher risk need to have them more often.▲

Efforts on the part of health care professionals to encourage people to adopt healthier lifestyles have not been as successful. The three leading causes of death in the United States—heart disease, cancer, and stroke—are associated with poor lifestyle choices, especially smoking, eating a diet high in fat and cholesterol, and not exercising regularly. Avoiding these risky behaviors could help prevent heart disease, cancer, or stroke from developing. However, the effect that doctors, nurses, and other health care professionals have in getting people to stop or never start these risky behaviors is relatively small. A doctor or other health care professional can explain a person's risk and encourage better behaviors, but only the individual person can do what it takes to change his or her lifestyle.

Although prevention can offer great benefits, it does carry risks of its own. While rare, even such a test as a sigmoidoscopy can cause serious problems, such as a perforated colon. Indirect risks stem from such things as the anxiety and financial burden of having to undergo additional tests to follow up on a test result that incorrectly indicated a person might have a particular disease. Sometimes screening reveals abnormalities that cannot or need not be treated. In such cases, this knowledge may cause anxiety without improving health. Thus, health care professionals aim for balance in providing preventive services, with the focus on selecting people most likely to benefit from intervention.

Components of Prevention

There are four major components of preventive medicine: (1) vaccinations to prevent infectious diseases (such as polio and measles);

▲ see art on page 1353

STRATEGIES FOR PREVENTING MAJOR HEALTH PROBLEMS

HEALTH PROBLEM	PREVENTIVE MEASURES
Heart disease	Maintain normal cholesterol level through diet, exercise, and drugs (if necessary); maintain normal blood pressure through diet, exercise, stress reduction, and drugs (if necessary); consume a balanced diet high in fiber and limited in fat and cholesterol; avoid smoking
Cancer	Avoid smoking (lung cancer); eat a balanced diet high in fiber and limited in fat and cholesterol (breast cancer, colorectal cancer); perform regular breast exams (women age 20 and over) or testicular exams (men age 12 to about age 40); avoid too much sun exposure and use sunscreens with a high sun-protection factor (skin cancer); observe skin for changing and bleeding skin lesions, perhaps having another person (such as a spouse) look at locations that are difficult to see, such as the back or behind the ears (skin cancer); observe for unusual bleeding or for bleeding from the rectum (colorectal cancer)*
Stroke	Avoid smoking; maintain normal blood pressure through diet, exercise, stress reduction, and drugs (if necessary); maintain normal cholesterol through diet, exercise, and drugs (if necessary); avoid stress and fatigue
Chronic obstructive pulmonary disease	Avoid smoking; avoid exposure to toxic substances (especially in industrial settings)
Injuries	Wear a seat belt in motor vehicles (children should not ride in front seat and should be in a child safety seat); wear a helmet when riding a bicycle or motorcycle; wear safety gear when skating; store firearms safely; keep drugs and toxic substances out of reach of children; make sure smoke detector is functioning; never swim alone; learn cardiopulmonary resuscitation (CPR) and other methods to relieve airway obstruction, such as the Heimlich maneuver; remove or secure throw rugs, maintain adequate lighting, and install handrails/grab bars to prevent falls; review medications to eliminate unnecessary ones and reduce others to lowest effective dose; exercise; moderate or eliminate alcohol intake
Diabetes	Exercise regularly; eat a balanced diet; avoid obesity; measure weight intermittently and attempt to maintain an ideal body weight; control blood sugar levels through monitoring and education
Pneumonia	Receive pneumonia (pneumococcal) vaccine once, repeated once after 5 years, based on risk profile
Influenza	Receive influenza vaccine every year
Tooth loss	Brush teeth and use dental floss regularly; avoid frequent sweets; visit a dentist regularly
Sexually transmitted diseases	Practice abstinence; limit the number of sex partners; use condoms and follow safe sex practices
Liver disease	Drink alcohol in moderation; receive vaccination against hepatitis B if at high risk
Stress	Observe mental health, such as for unusual irritability, anxiety, depressive symptoms, thoughts of suicide or violence, or excessive alcohol or substance abuse

*In addition to these preventive measures, screening programs are available for breast, cervical, colorectal, and prostate cancer.

(2) screening programs (such as for high blood pressure, diabetes, and cancer); (3) chemoprevention (drug therapy—for example, cholesterol-lowering drugs to prevent atherosclerosis, aspirin to prevent heart attacks or strokes, antihypertensive drugs to reduce blood pressure and prevent strokes); and (4) counseling aimed at helping people make healthy lifestyle choices (such as not smoking, wearing seat belts, and eating a healthy diet).

The components of prevention are provided to achieve one of three levels of prevention: primary, secondary, or tertiary. In **primary prevention,** disease is stopped before it starts, often by reducing or eliminating risk factors for a health problem. Vaccinations, chemoprevention, and counseling are types of primary prevention. The type of primary preventive care given usually depends on the person's age and risk profile.

In **secondary prevention,** disease is detected and treated early, often before symptoms are present, thereby minimizing adverse outcomes. Secondary prevention can involve screening programs, such as mammography to detect breast cancer and prostate-specific antigen (PSA) testing to detect prostate cancer, and tracking down the sex partners of a person diagnosed with a sexually transmitted disease (contact tracing) to treat these people, if necessary, and to minimize spread of the disease.

In **tertiary prevention,** an existing, usually chronic disease is managed to prevent further functional loss. For example, tertiary prevention for people with diabetes focuses on tight control of blood sugar, excellent skin care, and frequent exercise to prevent heart and blood vessel disease. Tertiary prevention can involve providing supportive and rehabilitative services to maximize quality of life, such as rehabilitation from injuries, heart attack, or stroke. It also includes preventing complications among people with disabilities, such as preventing bed sores among those confined to bed.

Prevention in Children and Teenagers: Most of the medical care that children receive is preventive in nature.▲ In fact, the standard "well-child" visits are geared to primary prevention. For example, most vaccinations are given during childhood. Height and weight are checked periodically to make sure a child is

growing at an appropriate pace. Other screening measures, such as blood pressure measurements and vision checks, are done at specific intervals. Health care professionals counsel parents about appropriate safety measures, such as child safety seats, bicycle helmets, smoke and carbon monoxide detectors, fire extinguishers, flame-retardant sleepwear, regular cleaning and inspection of heating systems and fireplaces, window and stair guards, locked storage of unloaded firearms, removal of leaded paint in older homes, and safe storage of drugs and toxic substances. Parents are also counseled about the dietary and exercise requirements of children, about the effects of passive smoking, and about the need for children to receive regular dental checkups.

The care given to teenagers and young adults is also mostly preventive in nature. Some vaccinations, such as tetanus/diphtheria (Td) booster, measles-mumps-rubella vaccine, and hepatitis B vaccine (HBV) (if not previously vaccinated), are given to preadolescents. Screening measures almost always include measurements of height, weight, and blood pressure. Another important screening measure is checking for depression and suicidal tendencies. Other screening measures may include recommending a Pap smear for young women, checking the immunity of young women to the rubella virus, and assessing for problem drinking and other substance abuse.

Health care professionals should counsel teenagers and young adults on seat belt usage, bicycle or motorcycle helmet usage, the importance of avoiding tobacco and illicit drugs, underage drinking, the importance of avoiding alcohol when driving or swimming, and how to prevent sexually transmitted diseases and unwanted pregnancies. The importance of a balanced diet limited in fat and cholesterol and with adequate calcium (especially for girls) and the need for regular physical activity are also the focus of doctor visits. Chemoprevention (drug therapy to prevent disease) is not a mainstay for this age group, but young women who plan on becoming pregnant are usually advised to take a multivitamin containing folic acid.

Prevention in Young to Middle-aged Adults: Preventive care measures are also needed for the population of people 25 to 64 years of age. The major areas of risk for people this age are established by periodic screenings of blood pressure, height, weight, and cholesterol levels. Some experts recommend measuring

▲ see pages 1492, 1543, and 1554

SELECTED SCREENING SCHEDULE FOR ADULTS*

TEST	AGE (YEARS)	HOW OFTEN
Blood pressure	18 and older	Every office visit or annually
Height and weight	18 and older	Height: periodically; weight: every office visit or annually
Cholesterol	35 and older (men); 45 and older (women)	Every 5 years if levels are within normal limits
Hearing	65 and older	Periodically
Mammography	40 and older (women)	Annually
Papanicolaou (Pap) smear	18 and older (women)	Every 1 to 3 years
Sigmoidoscopy	50 and older	Every 3 to 5 years
Stool occult (hidden) blood	50 and older	Annually
Dental, oral health exam	18 and older	Annually
Breast exam	40 and older	Annually
Bone density	65 and older	Periodically

*Based on recommendations by most major authorities in the United States. However, differences do exist among the recommendations of the various authorities.

blood sugar levels. A health care professional may screen for depression and stress by asking questions about mood and sleep patterns. The person may also be asked questions about the work environment to determine if there are any health hazards.

Pap smears (for cervical cancer) and mammograms (depending on the woman's age or family history of breast cancer) are recommended for women, and breast self-examination is encouraged. After the age of 50 (or younger if there is a family history suggesting increased risk), some experts recommend that men receive an annual rectal examination to screen for prostate cancer. A blood test for prostate-specific antigen (PSA) is sometimes recommended instead of or in addition to the rectal examination. Self-examination of the testicles is discussed as a means to help detect testicular cancer, especially among males from adolescence through age 40. An annual test of the stool for hidden (occult) blood and periodic sigmoidoscopy or another colon cancer screening method are recommended for men and women over the age of 50.

Depending on the person's risk profile, the health care professional may offer counseling on stopping smoking, avoiding alcohol or certain drugs (illicit drugs and drugs that cause sedation) while driving, wearing seat belts, using motorcycle or bicycle helmets, having working smoke and carbon monoxide detectors in the home, having heating systems and fireplaces cleaned and inspected periodically, and making sure all firearms are safely stored. People who spend a lot of time outdoors in areas where Lyme disease is common are advised to take precautions.▲

The health care professional will also likely emphasize the importance of a balanced diet (including whole grains, fresh fruits and vegetables, and adequate calcium) limited in fat and cholesterol and the need for regular exercise. Sexual behavior is discussed; again, depending on the person's risk profile, the focus of the discussion may be on preventing sexually transmitted diseases and unintended pregnancies. Women who are planning on becoming pregnant are advised to take a multivitamin with folic acid, to stop smoking, and to limit alcohol intake.

Vaccinations are not central to this age group, although tetanus/diphtheria (Td) boost-

▲ see page 1105

ers are recommended every 10 years, and people at high risk of complications of the flu or pneumonia would benefit from the influenza vaccine every year and pneumonia (pneumococcal) vaccine. The pneumonia vaccine should be repeated once, at least 5 years after the first immunization with the vaccine. Hepatitis B vaccine (HBV) is recommended for health care workers, people at high risk of exposure to blood and blood products, and people at increased risk of exposure due to risky sexual practices. All young adults previously not vaccinated should receive the hepatitis B vaccine.

Women who are experiencing certain symptoms of menopause are counseled about the possibility of receiving short-term hormone replacement therapy.▲ Other possibilities for chemoprevention include aspirin for people at risk of heart attacks, cholesterol-lowering drugs for people with high cholesterol levels that have not responded to diet and exercise, and drugs that improve or preserve bone density for people with or at risk of osteoporosis.■

Prevention in Older Adults: Preventive care also plays a big role in the health of people over age 65. Many screening measures (blood pressure, height, weight, blood sugar level, cholesterol level, vision and hearing tests, stool tests for hidden blood, colon cancer screening, mammograms, Pap smears, and bone density tests for women, prostate-specific antigen tests for men) may be undertaken.

Counseling measures may include smoking cessation, alcohol curtailment, injury prevention (such as removing throw rugs and installing bathtub rails and grab bars to prevent falls, installing devices such as large-numbered telephones, and setting the hot water heater at not more than 130 degrees to prevent burns), ways to prevent sexually transmitted diseases, and the need for regular dental visits.

A balanced diet limited in fat and cholesterol is emphasized, as is adequate calcium, vitamin D, and vitamin K, especially for women for prevention of osteoporosis. Regular exercise is still beneficial at this age to help prevent heart disease, diabetes, stroke, osteoporosis, and cancer, among other health problems.

Three vaccinations are recommended for people of this age group. The pneumonia (pneumococcal) vaccine is recommended for every person once after reaching 65 years of age, to prevent the most common community-acquired pneumonia, unless the person had the same vaccine before age 65 and less than 5 years previously. The influenza vaccine is recommended every year, and a tetanus/diphtheria (Td) booster is recommended every 10 years.

Possibilities for chemoprevention are cholesterol-lowering drugs to prevent atherosclerosis, antihypertensive drugs to control blood pressure and prevent stroke, and drugs that improve or preserve bone density to prevent osteoporosis or the broken bones (fractures) that may result if a person already has osteoporosis.

Barriers to Prevention

There are a number of barriers to providing preventive care. These barriers can be divided into three categories: barriers involving health care professionals, patients, or health care systems. For example, a doctor may decide against ordering a mammogram, the patient may not go for the mammogram because she is afraid or forgets, or the insurance company may not pay for the mammogram and the patient cannot pay for it because it is too expensive. To be effective, a preventive medicine program has to overcome these barriers and be workable in real-world conditions.

Barriers involving health care professionals include the training of doctors and other health care professionals, which emphasizes acute care over preventive care. Other barriers include uncertainty as a result of conflicting recommendations, a perceived lack of time, sometimes a lack of interest, forgetfulness in the context of many other problems to deal with, little gratification from providing preventive care (since there is no immediate feedback or results to evaluate how well the preventive care has worked), and low reimbursement rates from health insurance companies or Medicare for preventive services.

Barriers involving patients include lack of knowledge as to what preventive services are needed along with ignorance of the potential benefits. People may doubt that a disease that has no symptoms can be detected or that anything can or should be done about it. The mass media often fuels the overall confusion by supplying conflicting messages about what preventive care is needed and how lifestyle actually affects health (for example, Is red wine a help or hindrance to health? Is it okay to eat bacon once in a while?). Also, patients may

▲ see page 1358   ■ see page 343

have other priorities, such as getting treatment for an existing medical problem, or may worry about any potential discomfort associated with the performance of a procedure. Economic factors often present barriers as well. Patients may be unable to afford preventive screening or treatment. In addition, a diagnosis may disqualify a person from receiving health, life, or disability insurance benefits (for example, if a policy does not cover preexisting conditions).

The greatest change regarding prevention will come from patients. Since the leading causes of death are related to lifestyle choices, people will have to change their behavior (for example, stop smoking, increase exercise, wear seat belts) to increase the number of years of healthy life. It is especially difficult for an adult to make a lifestyle change; dietary, smoking, and exercise habits become deeply embedded in a person's psyche early on.

People can increase their chances of receiving preventive services by knowing which ones are appropriate for them and requesting these services from their doctors and other health care professionals. Many managed care organizations are distributing pocket-sized health guides to better inform people about which preventive services they need, based on their risk factors.

Barriers involving the health care system encompass a broad range. Within a doctor's or other health care professional's office, there may be disorganized medical records, no systematic way to provide preventive services, and an inadequate system with which to determine which patient needs what type of preventive service. Additionally, people frequently move, making it difficult to assess what preventive service they have had and what service they may need. Many people do not have a primary care doctor or other health care professional to provide them with comprehensive, coordinated preventive care. More broadly, over 45 million people in the United States lack health insurance. Even for some people who do have health insurance, preventive services may not be covered.

CHAPTER 6

Exercise and Fitness

Exercise is physical activity performed repetitively to develop or maintain fitness; fitness is the capacity to perform physical activities. Regular exercise is one of the best things that a person can do to help prevent illness and preserve health. Exercise comes in many forms and can vary in intensity. With so many ways to exercise, almost everyone can participate in some way.

Benefits of Exercise

Regular exercise makes the heart stronger and the lungs fitter, enabling the cardiovascular system to deliver more oxygen to the body with every heartbeat and increasing the maximum amount of oxygen that the body can take in and use. Exercise lowers blood pressure and reduces the levels of total and low density lipoprotein (LDL) cholesterol (the bad cholesterol), which in turn reduces the risk of heart attack, stroke, and coronary artery disease. Other conditions that are less likely to occur with regular exercise include colon cancer and some forms of diabetes.

Exercise makes muscles stronger, allowing people to perform tasks that they otherwise might not be able to do. Most everyday tasks require muscle strength and good range of motion in joints, and regular exercise can improve both.

Exercising stretches muscles and joints, which in turn can increase flexibility and help prevent injuries. Weight-bearing exercise strengthens bones and helps prevent osteoporosis. Exercise can improve function and reduce pain in people with osteoarthritis, although exercises that put undue stress on joints, such as running, may need to be avoided.

Athletic Heart Syndrome

Athletic heart syndrome refers to the normal changes that the heart undergoes in people who regularly perform strenuous aerobic exercise (for example, very well conditioned athletes).

In a person with athletic heart syndrome, the heart is larger and its walls thicker than in nonathletes. The chambers inside the heart, through which the blood passes, get somewhat larger. This increase in size and thickening of walls allow the heart to pump out substantially more blood per heartbeat without much increase in heart rate. The large volume of blood flowing through the heart results in a slower, stronger pulse (which can be felt at the wrist and elsewhere on the body) and sometimes in a heart murmur. These murmurs, which are specific sounds created as blood flows through the valves of the heart, are perfectly normal in an athlete and are not dangerous. The heartbeat of a person with athletic heart syndrome may be irregular at rest but becomes regular when exercise begins. Blood pressure is virtually the same as in any other healthy person.

The enlarged heart can be seen on a chest x-ray. A variety of changes are detectable on an electrocardiogram. These changes would be considered abnormal in a nonathlete but are perfectly normal in the athlete with athletic heart syndrome.

When an athlete stops training, the athletic heart syndrome slowly disappears—that is, heart size and heart rate tend to return gradually to that of the nonathlete.

Athletic heart syndrome is not thought to affect health in any way. The rare sudden deaths of athletes are usually due to underlying heart disease that was not previously detected rather than to any danger resulting from athletic heart syndrome.

Exercise increases the body's level of endorphins. Endorphins are chemicals in the brain that reduce pain and induce a sense of well-being. Thus, exercise appears to help improve mood and energy levels and may even help alleviate depression. Exercise also helps boost self-esteem by improving a person's overall health and appearance.

Besides the ways in which exercise benefits people of any age, regular exercise helps older people remain independent by improving functional ability and by preventing falls and fractures. It can strengthen the muscles of even the frailest older person living in a nursing home. It tends to increase appetite, reduce constipation, and promote sleep.

The benefits of exercise diminish within months after a person stops exercising. Heart strength, muscle strength, and the level of high-density lipoprotein (HDL) cholesterol (the good cholesterol) decrease, whereas blood pressure and body fat increase. Even former athletes who stop exercising do not retain measurable long-term benefits. They have no greater capacity to perform physical activities those who have never exercised, nor do they regain fitness any faster.

Starting an Exercise Program

Many people can begin an exercise program without consulting their doctor. However, people who have heart and lung disease, diabetes, or any other serious medical condition should talk with their doctor first, as should older people. People taking medication, especially for chronic illness, should consult with their doctor as well. Certain drugs may limit the ability to exercise, such as beta-blockers, which slow the heart rate▲, and sedatives, which can cause drowsiness and increase the risk of falling.

People who have done no exercise previously and who are seriously out of shape may benefit from consulting their doctor before starting an exercise program. In some cases, exercise must be supervised by a physical therapist or other health care professional or by an experienced, licensed trainer.

The safest way to start an exercise program is to perform the chosen exercise or sport at a low intensity until the legs or arms ache or feel heavy. If muscles ache after just a few minutes, the first workout should last only that long. As fitness increases, a person should be able to exercise longer without feeling muscle pain. However, some discomfort is necessary for developing stronger, larger muscles. Over time, a person can increase the intensity and duration of exercise.

▲ see table on page 138

Type of Exercise

A major distinction among different types of exercise is whether they are aerobic ("with oxygen") or anaerobic ("without oxygen"). Most forms of exercise have components of both.

Aerobic Exercise: This term refers to exercise that requires oxygen from the air to get to the muscles, thus the heart and lungs are forced to work harder than normal. Running, biking, swimming, and skating are examples of aerobic exercise. Aerobic exercise tends to burn a great deal of calories and improves cardiac function more than does anaerobic exercise. However, it is less effective at building strength and muscle mass.

Anaerobic Exercise: This term refers to exercise that requires intense straining for short periods of time. Weight lifting and isometrics (in which one part of the body is used to resist the movement of another part) are examples of anaerobic exercise. Anaerobic exercise relies on energy sources that are stored in the muscle and, unlike aerobic exercise, is not dependent on oxygen from the air. Overall, anaerobic exercise burns fewer calories than does aerobic exercise and may be somewhat less beneficial for cardiovascular fitness. However, it is better at building strength and muscle mass and still benefits the heart and lungs. In the long run, increased muscle mass helps a person become leaner and lose weight, because muscle uses large amounts of calories.

Intensity, Duration, and Frequency

Exercise is always a balance between intensity (how hard the exercise is), duration (how long a person exercises), and frequency (how often a person exercises). For most people, intensity should continue to increase as they get stronger, whereas duration and frequency remain constant once a certain level is reached.

To strengthen the heart, exercise must be performed at a reasonably high intensity. Intensity can be assessed in several ways. In one method, intensity is considered adequate (that is, enough to be beneficial) if the heart rate (measured in beats per minute) increases at least 20 beats above the resting heart rate. In another, more complex, method, intensity is considered adequate if the heart rate is between 70% and 85% of a person's estimated maximum heart rate, which is 220 minus the person's age. However, this calculation is somewhat conservative, especially for people who are physically fit. A less quantitative approach is to consider intensity to be adequate

if exercise is accompanied by reasonably heavy breathing and sweating, assuming that the environmental temperature is not inordinately hot. Very heavy breathing and profuse sweating indicate a high level of intensity. Another method by which intensity is considered adequate is to work to failure. This approach is often used by weight lifters, who continue lifting until they cannot possibly do one more repetition.

At first, most people can exercise for only a few minutes before they fatigue. For most people, exercise eventually should be performed at the most tolerable intensity for about 30 to 60 minutes at a time. This duration provides optimal benefits both for training muscles and for cardiovascular conditioning. Extending the duration much beyond this amount of time does not substantially improve muscle strength or endurance.

Most people do not benefit from exercising more than 3 to 4 times a week. Although the heart can be exercised several times a day every day, skeletal muscles start to break down when exercised intensely more often than every other day. The day after an adequate workout, bleeding and microscopic tearing can be seen in muscle fibers, which is why muscles feel sore. Exercisers should allow about 48 hours for muscles to recover after exercise. After very vigorous exercise, a muscle group may take several days to heal completely. Allowing the muscles to heal makes them stronger.

Different exercises stress different muscle groups. In aerobic exercise, for example, running stresses primarily the lower leg muscles; landing on the heels and rising on the toes exerts the greatest force on the ankle. Riding a bicycle stresses primarily the upper leg muscles; pedaling works the front thigh muscles (quadriceps) and hips. Rowing and swimming stress the upper body and back. These exercises can be alternated daily to avoid injury. In anaerobic exercise, such as weight lifting, it is usually best to alternate the muscle groups being trained. An ideal schedule, for example, alternates exercise for the upper body on one day with exercise for the lower body on the next.

Additionally, people should vary the way they train their muscles over time. The body adapts to routine, so that performing the same exercises over time becomes less effective in building strength and cardiovascular fitness. Therefore, weight lifters should alter their routines every few weeks, and aerobic exercisers should alternate among the different forms of aerobic exercise available.

Preventing Injury

More than 6 out of 10 people who start an exercise program drop out in the first 6 weeks, often because of an injury. Injuries can be prevented by scheduling workouts 48 hours apart, as described above. In addition, people should stop exercising immediately if they feel pain.

Two types of muscle discomfort may be felt after exercise. The desirable type, delayed-onset muscle soreness, does not start until several hours after exercising intensely. Usually it affects both sides of the body equally, goes away 48 hours later, and feels better after

CALORIES BURNED DURING EXERCISE

Activity	AVERAGE CALORIES EXPENDED IN 1 HOUR*	
	125-lb person	175-lb person
Aerobics	283	396
Biking	453	635
Cross-country skiing	453	635
Downhill skiing	340	476
Golf		
Riding cart	198	277
Carrying clubs	311	436
Hiking	340	476
Ice skating	396	555
In-line skating	283	396
Running		
8-minute mile	708	992
12-minute mile	453	635
Softball	283	396
Swimming	453	635
Swing dancing	226	317
Tae kwon do	283	396
Tennis (singles)	453	635
Walking	198	277
Weight lifting	170	238
Yoga	226	317

*Calories burned are calculated based on moderate intensity.

the warm-up for the next workout. The undesirable type, in which pain indicates injury, is usually felt soon after it occurs, is worse on one side of the body, does not disappear 48 hours later, and becomes much more severe if a person tries to exercise.

Injury is best prevented by warming up the muscles before exercising, followed by stretching and cooling down after exercising.

Warming Up: Starting exercise at lower intensity (for example, walking rather than running or using lighter weights) raises the temperature of muscles by increasing blood flow. Warm muscles are more pliable and less likely to tear than cold muscles, which contract sluggishly. Therefore, warming up helps prevent injuries.

Stretching: Stretching lengthens muscles and tendons, and thereby improves flexibility. Longer muscles can generate more force around joints, helping a person jump higher, lift heavier weights, run faster, and throw farther. However, stretching, unlike exercising against resistance (as in weight training), does not strengthen muscles. There is scant evidence that stretching prevents injuries or delayed-onset muscle soreness, which is caused by muscle fiber damage. A person should stretch only after warming up or exercising, when the muscles are warm and less likely to tear.

Cooling Down: Slowing down gradually (cooling down) at the end of exercise helps prevent dizziness. When the leg muscles relax, blood collects (pools) in the veins near them. To return the blood toward the heart, the leg muscles must contract. When exercise is suddenly stopped, blood pools in the legs and not enough blood goes to the brain, causing dizziness. By preventing blood from pooling, cooling down also helps the bloodstream to speed up its removal of lactic acid, a waste product that builds up in the muscles after exercise. Lactic acid does not cause delayed-onset muscle soreness, so cooling down does not prevent this soreness.

Choosing the Right Exercise

There are many forms of exercise, and each type of exercise has its advantages and disadvantages. For example, walking is relatively easy on the joints; during walking, at least one foot is on the ground at all times, so the force with which the foot strikes the ground is never much more than the person's weight. However, walking burns fewer calories than does running. Swimming rarely results in muscle tears, because the muscles are supported by the water. However, because swimming is not a weight-bearing exercise, it does not help prevent osteoporosis. Bicycles are pedaled in a smooth circular motion that does not jolt the muscles, but bicycling requires balance, and it is not always possible to enjoy this sport free of traffic and the dangers of cars.

Other choices regarding exercise exist as well. Some people prefer to exercise in a gym or at home, whereas others prefer to exercise outdoors. Some people have a very structured exercise routine, whereas others simply incorporate exercise into their lifestyle, for example, by walking rather than driving. Choosing the right exercise is a matter of finding an activity that is fun, safe, and sustainable.

Walking is a well-balanced form of exercise for most people, regardless of age. Many older people are able to keep fit through regular walking programs. However, walking slowly will not make a person very fit. To walk faster, a person can take longer steps in addition to moving the legs faster. Steps can be lengthened by swiveling the hips from side to side so that the feet can reach further forward. Swiveling the hips tends to make the toes point outward when the feet touch the ground, so the toes do not reach as far forward as they would if they were pointed straight ahead. Therefore, a walker should always try to point the toes straight ahead. Moving the arms faster helps the feet move faster. To move the arms faster, a person bends the elbows to shorten the swing and reduce the time the arms take to swing back and forth from the shoulder. People with instability or severe joint injury may find walking difficult.

Swimming exercises the whole body—the legs, arms, and back—without stressing the joints and muscles. Often, swimming is recommended for people who have muscle and joint problems. Swimmers, moving at their own pace and using any stroke, can gradually work up to 30 minutes of continuous swimming. If weight loss is one of the main goals of exercise, however, swimming is not the best choice. Exercise out of water is more effective because air insulates the body, increasing body temperature and metabolism for up to 18 hours. This process burns extra calories after exercise as well as during exercise. In contrast, water conducts heat away from the body, so that body temperature does not rise and metabolism does not remain increased after swimming.

Riding a bicycle is good exercise for cardiovascular fitness. Pedaling a bicycle strengthens the upper leg muscles. With a stationary bicycle, the tension on the bicycle wheel should be set so that the rider can pedal at a cadence of 60 rotations per minute. As they progress, riders can gradually increase the tension and the cadence up to 90 rotations per minute. A regular bicycle adds the challenges and joys of balance and coping with changes in terrain but adds the dangers of dealing with traffic. However, some people cannot maintain their balance, even on a stationary bicycle, and others will not use one because the pressure of the narrow seat against the pelvis feels uncomfortable.

A recumbent stationary bicycle is both secure and comfortable. It has a contoured chair that even a person who has had a stroke can sit in. Also, if one leg is paralyzed, toe clips can hold both feet in place, so that the person can pedal with one leg. A recumbent stationary bicycle is a particularly good choice for older people, many of whom have weak upper leg muscles. As a result of having weak upper leg muscles, many older people have difficulty rising from a squatting position, getting up from a chair without using their hands, or walking up stairs without holding on to the railing.

Aerobic dancing, a popular type of exercise offered in many communities, exercises the whole body. People can exercise at their own pace with guidance from experienced instructors. Lively music and familiar routines make the workout fun, and committing to a schedule and exercising with friends can improve motivation. Aerobic dancing also can be done at home with videotapes. Low-impact aerobic dancing eliminates the jumping and pounding of regular aerobic dancing, thus decreasing stress on the knee and hip joints. However, the benefits of aerobic dancing, especially in terms of weight loss, are proportional to the intensity.

Step aerobics stresses primarily the muscles in the front and back of the upper legs (the quadriceps and hamstrings) as a person steps up and down on a raised platform (a step) in a routine set to music at a designated pace. As soon as these muscles start to feel sore, exercisers should stop, do something else, and return to step aerobics a couple of days later.

Water aerobics is an excellent choice for older people and for those with weak muscles because it prevents falls on a hard surface and provides support for the body. It is often used for people with arthritis. Water aerobics involves doing various types of muscle movements or simply walking in waist- to shoulder-deep water.

Cross-country skiing exercises the upper body and the legs. Many people enjoy using machines that simulate cross-country skiing, but others find the motions difficult to master. Because using these machines requires more coordination than most types of exercise, a person should try out a machine before buying one. Cross-country skiing outdoors is more enjoyable to some people but adds the challenges of exercising in the cold.

Rowing strengthens the large muscles of the legs, shoulders, and back and helps protect a healthy back from injury. More people use rowing machines than row on water, although rowing outdoors adds the challenge of coordinating the oars and the joys of spending time in a boat. However, a person who has back problems should not row without a doctor's approval.

Resistance training is an anaerobic exercise meant to build strength and muscle mass. It is far more effective than other forms of exercise for achieving these goals but is less effective than aerobic exercise for burning calories (and thus losing weight) or improving cardiovascular performance at similar intensity. However, increased muscle mass may eventually help maintain a lean body weight, because muscle uses more calories than fat. The aerobic component of resistance training can be increased by increasing the repetitions performed at each station and by decreasing the time for rest between each set.

Weight lifting carries a higher risk of injury to muscles and joints if exercises are not done properly. Most people who intend to lift weights benefit from initial supervision that includes instruction on how to set the weights and seat levels and how to breathe during repetitions (out as one pushes or pulls; in during relaxation). For most people, weights should be set so 10 to 15 repetitions of each exercise can be performed. Weights that are too heavy increase the risk of injury. The part of the body trained should be varied so that a particular body part is not exercised more than every few days.

CHAPTER 7

Rehabilitation

Rehabilitation services are needed by people who have sustained severe injury, often due to trauma, a stroke, an infection, a tumor, surgery, or progressive disease. A pulmonary rehabilitation program▲ is often appropriate for people who have chronic obstructive long disease. People whose bodies become severely weak after prolonged bed rest (for example, because of a heart attack or surgery) are also in need of rehabilitation. Physical therapy, occupational therapy, and the treatment of any pain and inflammation are the focus of rehabilitation.

The need for rehabilitation crosses all age groups, although the type, level, and goals of rehabilitation often differ. People with chronic impairments, often older people, have different goals, require less intensive rehabilitation or a longer period of rehabilitation, and need different types of therapy than do younger people. For example, the goal of an older person with severe heart failure who has had a stroke may be to restore the ability to perform as many self-care activities (eating, dressing, bathing, transferring between a bed and a chair, using the toilet, controlling bladder and bowel) as possible. The goal of a younger person who has had a heart attack or been in a car accident is often to restore full, unrestricted function. Nonetheless, age alone is not a reason to alter goals or the intensity of rehabilitation; the presence of disease and limitations, however, may be.

▲ see page 259

Intensive rehabilitation that involves several components, such as physical therapy, occupational therapy, and speech therapy, usually requires continued sessions of one-on-one training for weeks to be of benefit. Sometimes, more immediate health concerns must be attended to before rehabilitation can be addressed.

To initiate a formal rehabilitation program, a doctor writes a referral (similar to a prescription) to a physiatrist (a doctor who is board-certified in rehabilitation medicine), an occupational or physical therapist, or a rehabilitation center. The referral establishes the goals of therapy, a description of the type of illness or injury, and its date of onset. The referral also specifies the type of therapy needed, such as ambulation training (help with walking) or training in activities of daily living (for example, help with eating, dressing, grooming, or toileting).

Where the rehabilitation takes place varies according to the person's needs. Care in a hospital or rehabilitation center may be necessary for people with severe disabilities. In such settings, a rehabilitation team provides care. Along with the doctor or therapist, this team may include nurses, psychologists, social workers, other health care practitioners, and family members.

The rehabilitation team or therapist establishes specific short-term goals for each of the person's problems, which may include restricted range of motion, an uncoordinated gait, and the inability to open a jar or feed himself. The person is encouraged to achieve each short-term goal, and the team closely monitors the person's progress. The goals of therapy may be changed if the person is unwilling or unable (financially or otherwise) to undergo lengthy rehabilitation. Setting a long-term overall goal at the beginning helps people understand what can be expected of rehabilitation and where they can expect to be in several months.

People who require less care, such as those who can transfer from bed to a chair or from a chair to a toilet, can often obtain rehabilitation services in an office or at home. In such cases, however, family members or friends must be willing to participate in the rehabilitative care process. Providing rehabilitation at home with the help of family members is highly desirable, but it can be physically and emotionally taxing for all involved. Sometimes, a visiting physical therapist or occupational therapist can help with home care.

Regardless of the severity of the disability or the skill of the rehabilitation team, the final outcome of the rehabilitation process depends on the person's motivation. In some cases, a person may prolong recovery in order to gain attention from family or friends.

Treatment of Pain and Inflammation

Techniques used to treat pain and inflammation include heat therapy, cold therapy, electrical stimulation, traction, massage, and acupuncture. Whether to use heat or cold therapy is often a personal choice, although cold therapy seems to be more effective for acute pain.

Heat Therapy: Heat increases blood flow and the manipulability of connective tissue. It decreases joint stiffness, pain, and muscle spasms. Heat also helps lessen inflammation and the buildup of fluid in tissues (edema). Heat therapy is used for inflammation and acute and chronic injuries, such as sprains, strains, muscle spasm, back pain, whiplash, and various forms of arthritis. The application of heat may be superficial or deep. Hot packs, infrared heat, paraffin (heated wax) baths, and hydrotherapy (agitated warm water) provide superficial heat. Diathermy (the generation of heat in tissues by electric currents) and ultrasound (the use of high-frequency sound waves) provide deep heat.

Cold Therapy (Cryotherapy): Application of cold may help relieve muscle spasms, acute low back pain, and acute inflammation. Cold may be applied using an ice bag, a cold pack, or fluids (such as ethyl chloride) that cool by evaporation. The spread of cold on the skin depends on the skin's thickness, the thickness of underlying fat and muscle, the water content of the tissue, and the rate of blood flow. The therapist takes care to avoid tissue damage and abnormally low body temperature (hypothermia).

Electrical Stimulation: Muscles that lack proper nerve function can be stimulated electrically to help prevent muscle wasting (atrophy) and spasticity. People with one-sided paralysis (such as after a stroke), those with peripheral nerve injuries, or those who have lost use of their legs (paraplegic) or of all four limbs (quadriplegic) after a traumatic injury may benefit from electrical stimulation in which electrodes are placed on the skin. For people with chronic back pain, rheumatoid arthritis, a sprained ankle, shingles, or a localized area of pain, a type of electrical stimulation that uses

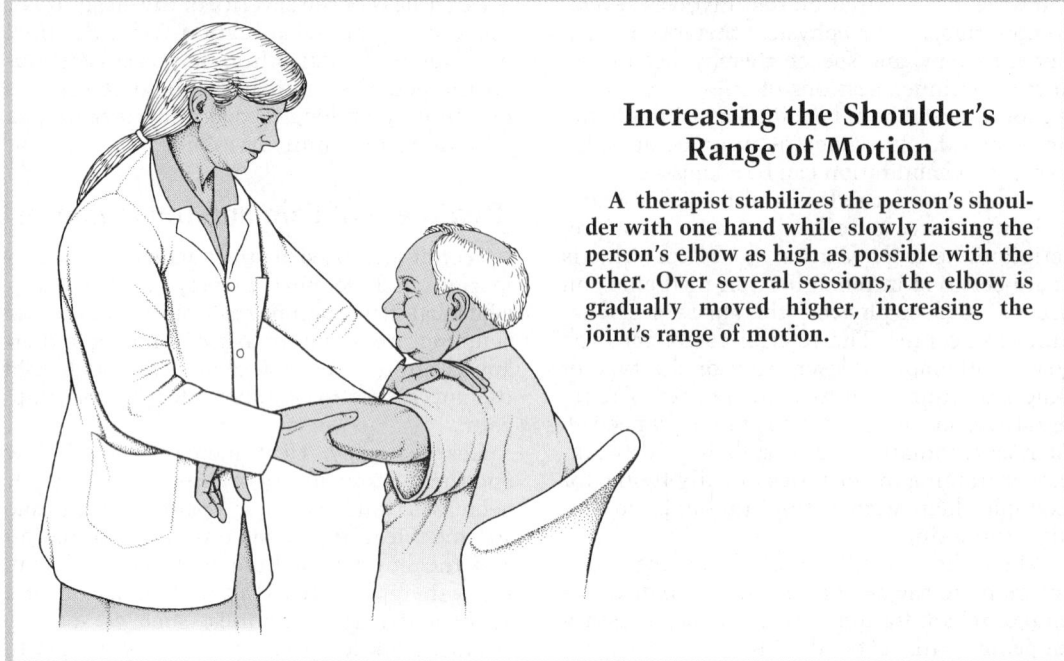

Increasing the Shoulder's Range of Motion

A therapist stabilizes the person's shoulder with one hand while slowly raising the person's elbow as high as possible with the other. Over several sessions, the elbow is gradually moved higher, increasing the joint's range of motion.

low current, called transcutaneous electrical nerve stimulation (TENS), may be helpful. TENS may be applied several times a day for 20 minutes to several hours, depending on the severity of the pain. The TENS device produces a tingling sensation without increasing muscle tension. Often, people can be taught to use the TENS device at home as needed. Most people tolerate the therapy well, but its effectiveness varies greatly.

Traction: Spinal traction is used to overcome muscle spasm and to keep bones aligned while fractures heal. A weight-and-pulley system, the patient's weight, or manual or motorized force may be used. Cervical traction is used for chronic neck pain.

Massage: Massage may relieve pain, reduce swelling, and help mobilize contracted tissues. Massage may help people with low back pain, arthritis, bursitis, neuritis, fibrositis, multiple sclerosis, cerebral palsy, or various degrees of paralysis.

Acupuncture: With acupuncture, thin needles are inserted through the skin at specific body sites, often far from the site of pain. The needles are twirled rapidly and intermittently for a few minutes, or a low electric current is applied through the needles. It is believed that acupuncture stimulates the production of endorphins (chemicals with analgesic properties that are found naturally in the brain), thus generating pain-relieving and anti-inflammatory effects.▲

Physical Therapy

Physical therapy involves exercising and manipulating the body. Techniques include range-of-motion exercises, muscle-strengthening exercises, coordination exercises, ambulation (walking) exercises, general conditioning exercises, transfer training, and use of a tilt table.

Range-of-Motion Exercises: Range of motion commonly becomes restricted after a stroke or prolonged bed rest. Restricted range of motion can cause pain, reduce a person's functional level, and predispose a person to bedsores.

Range of motion is evaluated with an instrument, called a goniometer, that measures angles of joint motion. Range of motion typically declines with age; even so, the decrease in range of motion does not usually prevent healthy older people from being able to perform self-care activities.

▲ see page 1705

Range-of-motion exercises may be active, for people who can exercise a muscle or joint without assistance; active-assistive, for people whose muscles are too weak to exercise without assistance or for people who experience pain during joint movement; or passive, for people who cannot actively participate. Active-assistive and passive range-of-motion exercises are performed very gently to avoid injury, although some discomfort may be unavoidable.

Before beginning therapy, the physical therapist determines if restricted motion is the result of tight ligaments and tendons or of tight muscles. If tight muscles are the cause, a joint may be stretched more vigorously. If tight ligaments or tendons are the cause, gentle stretching is attempted, but surgery is sometimes needed before progress can be made with range-of-motion exercises. An affected joint is moved beyond the point of pain, but the movement should not cause residual pain (pain that continues once the movement is stopped). Sustained moderate stretching is more effective than momentary forceful stretching. For sustained stretching, weights with pulleys are applied for about 20 minutes per day.

Muscle-Strengthening Exercises: Many forms of exercise increase muscle strength; all involve progressively increased resistance. When a muscle is very weak, gravity alone is sufficient. As muscle strength increases, resistance is gradually increased, either with stretchy bands or weight training. In this way, muscle mass and strength are increased, and endurance improves.

Coordination Exercises: These task-oriented exercises are for people who have problems with coordination and balance, usually as a result of a stroke or brain injury. The exercises involve repeating a meaningful movement that works more than one joint and muscle, such as picking up an object or touching a body part.

Ambulation Exercises: The purpose of these exercises is to improve a person's ability to walk independently or to walk with assistance. Before starting ambulation exercises, some people need to improve a joint's range of motion or muscle strength. Some people need an orthotic device such as a brace. Training may begin on parallel bars, especially if the person's balance is impaired, and progress to walking with mechanical aids, such as a walker, crutches, or a cane. Some people must wear an assistive belt, which the therapist uses to prevent the person from falling.

As soon as a person can walk safely on a level surface, training to step over curbs or to climb stairs may be initiated. A person being taught to climb up stairs is instructed to step up with the uninjured leg first. To climb down stairs, the person is instructed to step down with the injured leg first. These instructions can be memorized with the phrase "good is up, bad is down."

General Conditioning Exercises: A combination of range-of-motion, muscle-strengthening, and ambulation exercises is used to counter the effects of prolonged bed rest or immobilization. General conditioning exercises help restore proper blood flow and increase heart and lung function.

Transfer Training: Transfer training is often a critical goal of rehabilitation, because people who cannot transfer safely and independently from bed to chair, chair to toilet, or chair to a standing position generally require 24-hour assistance. The techniques used in transfer training depend on whether the person can bear weight on one or both legs, has sound balance, or is paralyzed on one side of the body. Assistive devices can sometimes help. For example, people who have difficulty standing from a seated position may benefit from a self-lifting chair, a chair with a raised seat, or another assistive device.

Tilt Table: For people who have low blood pressure and who get dizzy when they stand up (orthostatic hypotension▲), a tilt table may help. The person lies face up on a padded table with a footboard and is held in place with a safety belt. The table is tilted so that the angle is very slowly increased until the person is nearly upright. By slowly increasing the angle, the person's blood vessels regain the ability to constrict. How long the position is maintained depends on the person's tolerance, but it should not exceed 45 minutes. The tilt-table procedure is performed once or twice a day; its effectiveness varies depending on the person's disability.

Occupational Therapy

Occupational therapy is intended to enhance a person's ability to perform basic self-care activities, useful work, and leisure activities. Even simple tasks require the coordination of many abilities: the ability to feel

▲ see page 146

and move sufficiently (sensorimotor ability), the ability to create and execute a plan (cognitive ability), and the ability to want to do the task and to persevere until it is completed (psychologic ability).

Impairment of one of these abilities may affect task performance. Sensorimotor impairments include problems in sensation, perception, range of motion, muscle strength, muscle tone, endurance, balance, dexterity, and coordination. Cognitive impairments include inattention, distractibility, loss of concentration, impaired judgment, indecision, memory problems, and poor problem-solving skills. Psychologic impairments include apathy, depression, anxiety, perceived incompetence, frustration, a lack of persistence, and decreased coping skills. An occupational therapist may note impairments through direct observation, by specific tests, and with the aid of information provided by others.

Occupational therapists assess a person's needs by watching him perform a task in a natural environment. They also assess potential problems with the social environment (such as the effect of family members' attitudes on the person's ability to perform a task) and the physical environment (such as inadequate lighting, electrical cords obstructing walkways, and other hindrances that affect task performance).

Choice of intervention depends on the type of impairment. A person works with the occupational therapist to determine and prioritize intervention goals and select therapeutic tasks that are meaningful. For example, activities that develop fine motor skills (such as bilateral hand activities or inserting pegs on a peg board) may be used to improve coordination and the ability to use utensils when eating. A memory game may enhance recognition and recall. Adaptive techniques can help the person use his strengths to compensate for dysfunction (for example, a person with a paralyzed arm can learn new ways to dress, tie shoes, and fasten buttons). The level of difficulty increases as performance improves.

An occupational therapist is knowledgeable about devices that can help people with disabilities function more independently. For example, a person can be fitted with a splint to prevent deformity or promote function, such as the pinch needed to hold a utensil. Commonly used assistive devices are canes, grab bars on the side and back of the bathtub or toilet, shower chairs, built-up handles on eating utensils or shoehorns, and "grabbers" that help people pick items off the floor or from a shelf. Tools with built-up handles or with spring-loaded or electronic controls compensate for reduced hand mobility. Raised toilet seats and chair leg extenders compensate for diminished back or leg mobility. Sophisticated computer-assisted devices are available for people with quadriplegia and other disorders that severely limit function.

Other devices can help people with impaired vision, hearing, or memory. Larger dials can be added to telephones; a telephone ring can be replaced with a flashing light. Memory aids include automatic dialing telephones, drug organizers and reminders, and pocket devices that record and play back messages (reminders, instructions, lists) at the appropriate time.

Rehabilitation for Specific Problems

For many problems—for example, heart disease, stroke and other brain injuries, spinal injuries, hip fracture, amputation, and loss of hearing, speech, or vision—specific rehabilitation programs are available. Rehabilitation is sometimes needed for other types of fractures.▲

Heart Disease

Cardiac rehabilitation may be useful for some people who have had a recent heart attack,■ a sudden onset or worsening of heart failure, or cardiac surgery. The goal is to maintain or regain independence, at least with activities of daily living, within the constraints of abnormal heart function.

Remaining in bed for longer than 2 or 3 days can lead to deconditioning and even depression. Therefore, cardiac rehabilitation is started as soon as medical care for an event such as a heart attack has been stabilized, usually while the person is still in the hospital. Rehabilitation programs typically begin with light activity, such as transferring to and sitting in a chair. When these activities can be performed comfortably, usually by the second or third day, more moderate activities, such as dressing, grooming, and walking short distances, are begun. If fatigue or discomfort occurs as a person increases his activity (for example, walking the length of the hall), the person is instructed to stop immediately and rest until symptoms disappear. The doctor then reassess the person's readiness to continue rehabilitation.

▲ see page 353   ■ see also page 215

After discharge, the amount and intensity of activity is slowly increased, and a full range of normal activities can be resumed after about 6 weeks. However, most people benefit from an outpatient cardiac rehabilitation program, which is usually about 12 weeks long, because of the instruction and monitoring they receive. Cardiac rehabilitation programs include help with handling the psychologic effects of having had a heart attack or heart surgery. They also include instruction about why changes in lifestyle are necessary and how to make them—so that risk factors are modified. Quitting smoking, losing weight, controlling blood pressure, reducing blood cholesterol levels through diet or drugs, and performing daily aerobic exercises all help prevent or slow the progression of coronary artery disease and reduce the risk of another heart attack. Similarly, modification of risk factors may help slow the progression of heart failure.

Brain Injuries

Rehabilitation can help people who have had a stroke or other brain injury regain some or all of their functional abilities. Although rehabilitation helps people recover lost function, the extent of functional recovery depends heavily on the brain's natural repairing of the damaged area. Most of this natural healing process occurs during the first 6 months after the stroke or injury but may continue for as long as 2 years. The amount and rate of natural healing cannot be predicted with certainty. Because of this unpredictability, and to prevent other disabilities (such as muscle contractures) and depression, rehabilitation is begun as soon as the person is medically stable.

What part of the brain was injured affects what functions are lost. A detailed evaluation of the person, including psychologic testing, helps the rehabilitation team identify the type and severity of damage. The members of the rehabilitation team then assess which lost functions may benefit from rehabilitation therapy and create a program addressing the person's specific needs. The success of rehabilitation depends on the person's general condition, range of motion, muscle strength, bowel and bladder function, functional ability before the brain injury, social situation, learning ability, motivation, coping skills, and ability to participate in a rehabilitation program.

The damaged areas of the brain after stroke are limited to where the blocked or bleeding arteries are located in the brain. Thus, the area

damaged and the symptoms of stroke are relatively well defined. The extent of brain damage due to a traumatic brain injury depends on the severity and direction of force and what part of the brain was injured. The brain can also be injured during surgery performed to remove a brain tumor. The extent and location of the surgery determine what functional problems a person will have afterward.

Some people require joint movement to prevent or relieve contractures. Others need coordination exercises. Because stroke often causes one-sided paralysis, exercise of the unaffected arm or leg is usually encouraged. The person is expected to practice other activities as well, such as moving in bed, turning, changing position, and sitting up. Regaining the ability to get out of bed and to transfer to a chair or wheelchair safely and independently is important to a person's physical and mental health.

Rehabilitation therapists treat problems with walking, lack of coordination, spastic muscles, vision problems (including partial or complete blindness in one or both eyes), and speech problems with specific therapies. For example, an ambulation exercise program is begun for people who are having trouble walking; this program may include learning how to prevent falls. Heat or cold therapy may temporarily decrease spasticity in muscles and allow muscles to be stretched. People with one-sided blindness are given special training to avoid bumping into door frames or other obstacles. Fine motor coordination may be improved with occupational therapy.

Cognitive impairment can also occur with stroke and other brain injury, especially concussion.▲ Cognitive impairment can include problems with orientation, attention and concentration, perception, comprehension, learning, organization of thought, problem solving, and memory. However, not every person has all of these symptoms.

Cognitive rehabilitation is a very slow process, has to be tailor-made to each person's situation, and requires one-on-one treatment. It encourages desirable behavior and discourages undesirable action through conditioning and repetition.

Spinal Injuries

Recovery from spinal cord injury depends on the location and degree of damage. The higher up the level of injury, the greater the physical

▲ see page 517

Just the Right Height

For people who are recovering from a leg injury or surgery, using a cane that is the correct height is important. A cane that is too long or too short can cause low back pain, poor posture, and instability. The cane should be held on the side opposite the injured leg.

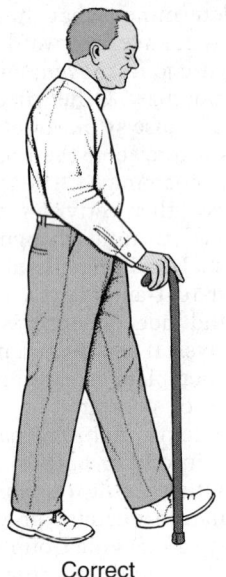   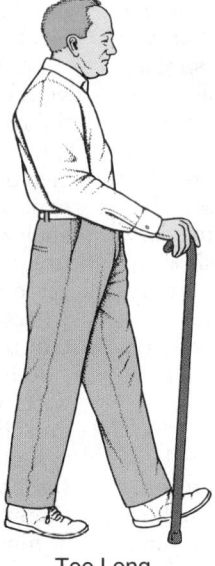   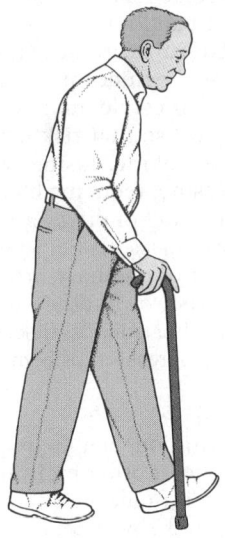

Correct   Too Long   Too Short

impairment. Injury at the level of the chest or below usually involves weakness or paralysis of the legs (paraplegia). Injury at the level of the neck usually involves weakness or paralysis of all four limbs (quadriplegia). If the level of injury is very high in the neck, the muscles that control breathing may be paralyzed, and a ventilator may be needed to assist breathing.

If the spinal cord is completely severed or destroyed, the body below that level becomes paralyzed. If the spinal cord is partly severed or damaged, the body below that level becomes spastic. There is little or no skin sensation in the affected area. In almost all cases of spinal cord damage, bowel and bladder control are lost (incontinence).

The two most important aspects of caring for people with quadriplegia or paraplegia are preventing bedsores and maintaining joint mobility. To prevent bedsores, the person moves or is turned frequently, and a special bed or bedding material is used.▲ When the person is seated in a wheelchair, a special cushion is used. To maintain joint mobility and prevent spasticity, heat, massage, and some medications are used.

A paraplegic person can live an independent life. Range-of-motion and strengthening exercises of the arms and hands enable the paraplegic person to use a wheelchair and to transfer from bed to a wheelchair and from a wheelchair to a toilet or to a car seat. A paraplegic person can be very independent in activities of daily living, and many engage in gainful employment. Some paraplegics are able to drive a car with the help of assistive devices.

A quadriplegic person can use a motorized wheelchair for independent mobility, but the person must be lifted into the wheelchair manually or mechanically. Some quadriplegics can move their hands or fingers slightly, in which case they can operate the motorized wheelchair with a hand switch. For quadriplegics whose hands and arms are completely motionless, a special device on the motorized wheelchair allows it to be controlled by chin movements or

▲ see page 1209

even by the person's breath, but this requires very intensive training. People with quadriplegia generally need support 24 hours a day.

Hip Fracture

Rehabilitation therapy is begun as soon as possible after hip fracture surgery, often within a day. The initial goals of therapy are to maintain the level of strength the person had before the fracture occurred by preventing loss of motion and atrophy of muscle and to prevent problems that result from bedrest. An additional goal is to restore the person's ability to walk as well as he was able to before the fracture occurred.

As soon as possible, sometimes within hours of surgery, the person is encouraged to sit in a chair, which reduces the risk of bedsores and blood clots and eases the transition to standing. The person is taught to perform daily exercises to strengthen the trunk and arm muscles and is sometimes taught exercises to strengthen the large muscles of both legs as well. Usually within the first day after surgery, the person is encouraged to stand up on the uninjured leg, often with the assistance of another person or while holding onto a chair or a bed rail. While performing these exercises, the person is directed to touch only the tips of toes of the injured leg on the floor. Full weight bearing on the injured leg is often encouraged on the second day after surgery but depends on the kind of fracture and repair.

Ambulation (walking) exercises are started after 4 to 8 days as long as the person can bear full weight on the injured leg without discomfort and has sufficient balance. Stair-climbing exercises are started soon after walking is resumed. In addition, the person may be taught how to use a cane or other assistive device and how to reduce the risk of falls.

Arm and Leg Amputation

Most **arm amputations** result from accidents. A small number are performed surgically to treat a medical condition (for example, to remove a cancerous tumor). The arm can be amputated below the elbow, above the elbow, or at the shoulder.

After amputation, a person is usually fitted for an artifical arm (an upper extremity prosthesis). The prosthesis consists of a terminal device (a hook or hand), a wrist unit, an elbow unit for an above-the-elbow amputation, and a socket. Movement of the hook or hand is controlled by movement of the shoulder muscles.

A hook may be more functional, although most people prefer the appearance of a hand. Control of an above-the-elbow prosthesis is more complicated than that of a below-the-elbow prosthesis. Recently, battery-operated and microcomputer-controlled prostheses have been developed, allowing a person more precisely controlled movements.

Rehabilitation after arm amputation includes general conditioning exercises, stretching of the shoulder and elbow, and strengthening of the arm muscles. Endurance exercises may also be necessary. The specific exercise program prescribed depends on whether one or both arms were amputated and whether the amputation was above or below the elbow.

Leg amputations occur almost equally as the result of an accident or as a surgical procedure performed to treat a consequence of a medical condition (for example, as the result of poor blood supply due to diabetes). The leg can be amputated below the knee, above the knee, or at the hip.

An artificial leg (a lower extremity prosthesis) consists of the terminal device (foot), a knee unit for an above-the-knee amputation, and a socket. Newer prostheses, which are battery operated or microcomputer controlled, allow a person to control movements with more precision.

Rehabilitation after leg amputation includes exercises for general conditioning, stretching of the hip and knee, and strengthening of all arm and leg muscles. The person is encouraged to begin standing and balancing exercises with parallel bars as soon as possible. Endurance exercises may be needed. The specific program prescribed depends on whether one or both legs were amputated and whether the amputation was above or below the knee.

Contracture (a shortening of muscle, producing limited range of motion) develops easily at the amputated limb, hip, or knee joint and usually results from prolonged sitting in a chair or wheelchair or improper body positioning in bed. If contracture is severe, a prosthesis may not fit properly, or the person may lose the ability to use a prosthesis. Therapists or nurses must teach methods of preventing contracture.

Therapists help people learn how to condition the stump, which promotes the natural process of stump shrinking (which must occur before a prosthesis is fitted). An elastic stump shrinker or bandages worn 24 hours a day can help taper the stump and prevent fluid buildup in the tissues. Early walking with a temporary prosthesis helps shrink the stump as well. Various temporary prostheses with adjustable sockets are available. A person with a temporary prosthesis can start ambulation exercises on parallel bars and progress to walking with crutches or a cane until a permanent prosthesis is made.

If the prosthesis is made before the stump stops shrinking, adjustments may be needed for comfort and to allow a good gait pattern. Manufacture of a permanent prosthesis is generally delayed for several weeks to allow the stump time to shrink completely.

Therapists teach amputees how to walk with a prosthesis. Strength and balance training are included in the program. Walking begins with direct assistance and progresses to walking with a walker, then with a cane. Within a few weeks, many amputees walk without a cane. The therapist teaches the amputee to use stairs, walk up and down hills, and traverse other uneven surfaces. Younger amputees may be taught to run and indeed participate in many athletic activities. Progress is slower and more limited for those who have above-the-knee amputation, for older people, and for those who are weak or poorly motivated.

The prosthesis needed for an above-the-knee amputation weighs much more than that for a below-the-knee amputation, and controlling a prosthetic knee joint requires skill. Walking requires 10 to 40% more energy after below-the-knee amputation and 60 to 100% more energy after above-the-knee amputation.

After **arm or leg amputation,** a sensation called "phantom limb" may be experienced, in which the person feels as if he still has the amputated limb. When this sensation occurs in the case of an amputated leg, for example, the person may stand up and thus fall back down. This kind of accident usually occurs at night when the person wakes to use the bathroom. Phantom limb can be extremely painful (phantom limb pain). Use of a prosthesis seems to accelerate the disappearance of a phantom limb. Massaging the stump also often helps.

Speech Disorders

Aphasia: Aphasia is a defect or loss in the ability to comprehend or express words, often resulting from a stroke or another type of brain injury that affects the language center in the brain.▲

▲ see art on page 476

The goal of therapy for people with aphasia is to establish the most effective means of communication. For people with mild impairment, the speech therapist uses an approach that emphasizes ideas and thoughts rather than words. Pointing to an object or picture, gesturing, nodding, and relying on facial expressions are often sufficient for rudimentary communication. For people with more severe impairment, a stimulation approach (in which words are repeatedly spoken to the person) and a programmed stimulation approach (in which words are spoken and objects are presented that can be touched and seen) help the person reacquire language ability. Caregivers of an aphasic person need to be very patient and appreciate the person's frustration. Caregivers must also realize that an aphasic person is not demented and should not be spoken to in baby language, which is insulting. Instead, the caregiver must speak normally and, if necessary, use gestures or point to objects.

Dysarthria: Dysarthria is an inability to articulate words properly because of problems in muscular control caused by damage to the nervous system. Rehabilitation goals depend on the cause of the dysarthria.

If the cause of dysarthria is stroke, head trauma, or brain surgery, the goal is to restore and preserve speech. For mild cases of dysarthria, repetition of words or sentences may sufficiently allow the person to relearn how to use facial muscles and the tongue for proper pronunciation. For severe cases of dysarthria, a letter or picture board or electronic communication device may be helpful.

If the dysarthria is caused by a progressive problem with the nervous system, such as amyotrophic lateral sclerosis (Lou Gehrig's disease) or multiple sclerosis, the goal of therapy is to maintain speech function for as long as possible. The person exercises to increase control of the mouth, tongue, and lips and is taught more appropriate speech rate and proper phrase length. Poor control of breathing muscles may force the person to take a breath in the middle of a sentence. Breathing exercises and planning punctuation within a sentence are helpful.

Verbal Apraxia: A person with verbal apraxia cannot produce the basic sound units of speech because of an abnormality in initiating, coordinating, or sequencing the muscle movements needed to talk. Verbal apraxia is often caused by brain injury, such as occurs with stroke or head trauma. In one therapeutic approach, the therapist has the person practice making sound patterns over and over again. In another approach, the therapist teaches the person to use natural melodic patterns for common phrases. Every phrase has its own melodic rhythm depending on the mood of the speaker. For example, "Good morning! How are you?" can be said in a flat melodic patter if the speaker is not up in the mood. However, when these phrases are said in a very cheerful manner, there is almost musical melodic rhythm. In treatment of verbal apraxia, the practitioner encourages the patient to repeat very exaggerated natural melody and rhythm patter. As the patient progresses, melody and rhythm cues are gradually faded.

Blindness

For rehabilitative purposes, blindness is classified into two groups: blindness present at birth (congenital) or at a very young age and blindness that develops later in life. Children who are born blind or who become blind at a very young age usually receive special education and become well adjusted. People who become blind later in life, however, must learn new ways of dealing with daily living. One ac-

tivity of daily living, feeding oneself, is commonly taught to blind people with use of the clock method, in which, for example, the dinner plate is located at 6 o'clock, the salad plate at 3 o'clock, and the beverage at 9 o'clock. The person also has to learn how to use a cane, and family members and other caregivers must learn how to walk with the blind person. The family is also instructed not to change the location of furniture or other objects without telling the blind person. Use of a seeing eye dog and learning Braille come much later. In the interim, audio books help the blind participate in reading.

Hearing Loss

Aural rehabilitation is used for people who became deaf in adulthood. Those deaf at a young age receive training in school. Rehabilitation teaches lip reading and how to optimally use a hearing aid.▲ Training also teaches the deaf person how to modulate his speaking volume, since without training a deaf person tends to speak loudly. Therapists can also recommend other assistive devices, such as door bells, phones, and alarms that display a flashing light when they ring.

CHAPTER 8

Death and Dying

A century ago, most people who suffered traumatic injuries or contracted serious infections died soon afterward. Even those who developed heart disease or cancer had little expectation of a long life after the disease was diagnosed. Most people expected little more than comfort measures from doctors.

Today, death is often seen as an event that can be deferred indefinitely rather than as an intrinsic part of life. Medical procedures commonly extend the lives of people who have such diseases as heart disease, cancer, stroke, chronic obstructive pulmonary disease, pneumonia, and dementia, often giving them many years in which quality of life and function are

quite good. Other times, procedures extend life, but the quality of life and function decline.

Talking about the likely outcomes of illness, including death and dying, is an important part of health care. Doctors and patients vary in the language they use and their comfort regarding such discussions. People should generally try to understand their situation and likely future course and to make any preferences about treatment and family support known.■ People who do not wish to talk about death and dying with their doctor

---

▲ see box on page 1251   ■ see page 54

should understand that major decisions may be made without their input.

Time Course of Dying

People often think that the doctor knows how long a person will live but is withholding this information from them. However, no one knows when an ill person will die. Families are advised not to press for exact predictions or to rely on those that are offered. Sometimes very sick people live a few months or years, well past what seemed possible. Other people die quickly. If a patient wants a particular person there at the time of death, arrangements may have to be made to accommodate that person for an indefinite time. Yet, predicting when a person will die of a disease is sometimes necessary. Health insurance often does not cover comfort measures for chronic disease, except for hospice care, which usually requires a prognosis of less than 6 months to live—an arbitrary time that may be difficult to predict accurately.

Doctors can make a fairly accurate short-term prognosis for an average person with certain conditions, based on statistical analyses of large groups of people with similar conditions. For example, they may accurately estimate that 5 out of 100 people with similar critical conditions will survive and leave the hospital. But predicting how long a particular person will survive is much more difficult. The best prediction a doctor can make is based on odds and the degree to which the doctor is confident in those odds. If the odds of survival for 6 months are 10%, people should acknowledge the 90% likelihood of dying and should make plans accordingly.

When statistical information is not available, a doctor may be unable to predict a prognosis or may make one on the basis of personal experience, which may be less accurate. Some doctors prefer to offer hope by describing remarkable recoveries without also mentioning the high likelihood that most people who have certain serious conditions will die. Gravely ill people and their families are entitled to the most complete information available and the most realistic prognosis possible. However, it may sometimes be necessary for them to express their desire for such information, rather than only for optimistic accounts.

Dying may be marked by deterioration over a long period of time, punctuated with bouts of complications and side effects. For people dying of cancer, energy, function, and comfort usually decrease substantially only in the last month or two before death. The person then is visibly failing, and the fact that death is near becomes obvious to all. However, dying usually follows other time courses. Sometimes, a person being treated aggressively for a serious illness in a hospital abruptly worsens and is known to be dying only a few hours or days before death.

Increasingly common, however, is dying with a slow decline in capabilities over a long period of time, perhaps with episodes of serious complications. Neurologic diseases, such as Alzheimer's disease, follow this pattern, as do emphysema, liver failure, kidney failure, and other chronic conditions. Severe heart disease disables people over time and causes severe symptoms intermittently, but it usually

Communicating With a Dying Person

Many people find it difficult to openly discuss death with a dying person, mistakenly believing that the dying person does not want to discuss his condition or will be hurt by such a discussion. However, family members should continue to speak with the dying person and include him in decision making. The following suggestions can help people to feel more comfortable in communicating with a dying person:

- Listen to what the person is saying. One might ask, "What are you thinking?" rather than shutting down communication with such comments as "Don't talk that way."
- Talk about what the person would envision for his family at a time long after his death and work back toward events nearer to death. This allows for easier discussion of more immediate concerns, such as the person's preferences regarding funeral arrangements and support for loved ones.
- Reminisce with the dying person; this is a way of honoring the person's life.
- Continue to speak with the dying person, even if he is unable to speak. Other ways of communicating, such as holding the person's hand, giving the person a massage, or just being near the person, can be very comforting.

kills suddenly with a disturbance in the heart's rhythm (arrhythmia).

Making Health Care Choices

Sick people and their families may feel swept along by the fatal illness and medical treatments, as if they have no control over the events. Sometimes, this sense of having no control is preferable to taking responsibility for thinking about what else might be done. People vary in the amount of information and involvement in decision making that they want and should usually be able to be as engaged as they want. Loved ones need to be satisfied that everything was done to enable the dying person to live as well and with as much dignity as possible while dying.

Honest, open communication between patient and doctor about the person's preferences for care at the end of life helps to ensure the best possible quality of life during a fatal illness. The doctor provides a candid assessment of the likelihood of recovery and disability during and after various treatment options, and the person tells the doctor and his family what he wants and does not want to experience. The person's health care decisions may include choosing a doctor and a system of care, stating his preferences for treatment and the limits he wants placed on that treatment, expressing wishes concerning where he wants to die and what he wants done when death is expected, and stating whether he wants to donate his organs after death.

Choosing a Doctor: When choosing a doctor, a person should ask about care at the end of life: Does the doctor have substantial experience caring for dying people? Does the doctor care for the person until death in all settings—hospital, nursing home, or home? Does the doctor treat symptoms fully (palliative care) at the end of life? Is the doctor familiar with the home health, physical therapy, and occupational therapy services in the community—who qualifies for them, how they are paid for, and how to help people and families get more intensive services when needed? In some cases, what a doctor may lack in experience is offset by a trusting, long-standing relationship that exists between the doctor and a patient and family and by the doctor's willingness to consult other experts.

Choosing a System of Care: A system of care includes a financing system, such as insurance

Services to Know About _____

- **Home care** is medically supervised care in a person's home by professional caregivers, who may help with administration of drugs, assess the person's condition, and provide baths and other personal services.

- **Hospice care** is care at the end of life that emphasizes relief of symptoms and provides psychologic and social support for a dying person and family members. The setting may be the person's home, a hospice facility, or a hospital. To obtain hospice care, a person usually has to have a prognosis of less than 6 months.

- **Nursing home care** is residential care in a licensed facility with nurses and support workers.

- **Respite care** is temporary care at home, in a nursing home, or in a hospice facility that enables family members or other caregivers to travel, rest, or attend to other matters. It may last days or weeks, depending on the care delivery system and funding.

- **Voluntary organizations** provide a variety of financial and support services to people who are ill and their families. Such organizations usually focus on people who have a certain disease.

policies and managed care, and a care delivery system, such as doctors, a hospital, a nursing home, and home health care agencies. Asking questions of doctors, nurses, other patients and families, social workers, and case managers can help a person find a good system of care: What treatments are available in the system? What information is available about the merits of possible treatments? How can a person talk to other patients and families who have been treated there? What experimental treatments are available? How have other patients done with these treatments? How are these treatments paid for?

Choosing Treatment Options: Often, the available choices are between dying sooner but remaining comfortable and attempting to live slightly longer by receiving aggressive therapy, which may increase discomfort and dependence. Nevertheless, dying people and their families may feel that they must try such therapies if any chance of prolonged survival exists, even when hope for a cure is unrealistic. Questions of philosophy, values, and religious beliefs come into play when such decisions are made by and for a dying person. People should discuss their wishes for end-of-life care well in advance of a crisis that makes such information critical.

A person nearing death is sometimes persuaded to try one last treatment, which often sacrifices the person's last few days to side effects without gaining quality time. The person and family should be skeptical of such treatments. In many cases, as a person nears death, the focus of care should shift entirely to providing comfort measures to ensure that the dying person does not suffer.

Some decisions, such as whether to allow resuscitation—the only treatment provided automatically in the hospital (unless specifically predecided otherwise)—are less significant than they seem. An order against attempting resuscitation makes sense for most people expected to die, and such a decision need not weigh heavily on the family. The person who is near death before the moment when the heart stops beating and breathing ceases (cardiopulmonary arrest) is not likely to benefit from a resuscitation attempt. Resuscitation efforts can be prohibited in advance directives▲ or through discussion between a patient and doctor, with the doctor writing the needed order. Food and water given through tubes (artificial nutrition and hydration) are not often useful to a dying person and can also be prohibited in advance.

Other decisions may include the setting in which the dying person will spend his final days. For instance, the family may want to have the person at home—a familiar, supportive setting—and not in a hospital. Family members should insist that doctors and other caregivers help make specific plans for these preferences and honor them. In some cases, hospitalization may be explicitly declined.

Choosing to Donate Organs: The dying person may wish to donate his organs after death. This decision is best made with the family in accord, if possible. In general, people dying of a chronic illness can donate only corneas, skin, and bone. People who die more suddenly can donate more organs, such as kidneys, liver, heart, and lungs. To become an organ donor,

the person usually needs only to sign a standard organ donor card and to let the doctor know of his wishes. Common concerns that may prevent some people from becoming organ donors can be allayed: Organ donation usually does not affect the appearance of the body at the funeral and does not cost the person or family any money. Also, organs are never taken until after death.

Symptoms During a Fatal Illness

Many fatal illnesses produce similar symptoms, including pain, shortness of breath, digestive problems, incontinence, skin breakdown, and fatigue. Depression, anxiety, confusion, unconsciousness, and disability may also occur.

Pain

Most people fear pain as they confront dying. However, pain can usually be controlled while allowing the person to remain awake, involved in the world, and comfortable.

Radiation can control certain types of cancer pain by reducing tumor size and growth. Physical therapy or analgesics, such as acetaminophen and aspirin, are used to control mild pain. For some people, hypnosis or biofeedback■—approaches that have no notable adverse effects—effectively relieves pain. However, opioids such as codeine and morphine are often needed.★ Opioids given by mouth can relieve pain effectively for many hours, and stronger opioids can be given by skin patch, injection, or continuous infusion into a vein. Drug addiction should not be a concern, and adequate medication should be given early, rather than held off until the pain is intolerable. There is no usual dose; some people need small doses, whereas others need much larger doses.

Shortness of Breath

The sensation of struggling to breathe is one of the worst ways to live or die; it is also usually controllable. Various methods can usually ease breathing—for example, relieving fluid buildup, changing the person's position, providing supplemental oxygen, or shrinking a tumor that obstructs the airways with radiation or corticosteroids. Opioids may help people who have mild, persistent shortness of breath breathe more easily, even if they do not have pain. Taking opioids at bedtime can promote

▲ see page 54   ■ see page 455
★ see page 450

comfortable sleep by preventing the person from waking up frequently, fighting to breathe.

When these treatments are not effective, most doctors who work in hospices agree that a person suffering in this way should be given an opioid in a dose that is high enough to relieve the perception of shortness of breath, even if the person might become unconscious. A person who wants to avoid shortness of breath at the end of life should make sure that the doctor will treat this symptom fully, even if such a treatment leads to unconsciousness or hastens death somewhat.

Digestive Problems

Digestive problems, including a dry mouth, nausea, constipation, an intestinal obstruction, and loss of appetite, are common in people who are very sick. Some of these problems are caused by the disease. Others, such as constipation, can be side effects of drugs.

A **dry mouth** can be relieved with wet mouth swabs or hard candy. Various commercially available products can soothe chapped lips. To prevent dental problems, a person should brush the teeth or use mouth sponges frequently to clean the teeth, gums, inside of the cheeks, and tongue.

Nausea and vomiting may be caused by drugs, an intestinal obstruction, or advanced disease. A doctor may have to change drugs or prescribe an antiemetic (antinausea) drug. Nausea caused by an intestinal obstruction may also be treated with antiemetics, and other comfort measures can be taken.

Constipation is very uncomfortable. A limited intake of food, a lack of physical activity, and certain drugs cause the intestine to be sluggish. Abdominal cramping may occur. A regimen of stool softeners, laxatives, and enemas may be needed to relieve constipation, especially when caused by opioids. Relief of constipation is usually beneficial, even at late stages of a disease.

An **intestinal obstruction** may require surgery. However, depending on the person's overall condition, likely life expectancy, and reason for the obstruction, the use of drugs to paralyze the intestine and decrease stomach secretions, sometimes with nasogastric suction to keep the stomach clear, may be preferable. Opioids are useful for pain relief.

Difficulty swallowing (dysphagia) occurs in some people, especially after a stroke, with advanced dementia, or from an obstruction with cancer. Sometimes the person can regain the ability to swallow by maintaining a certain body position while eating or by choosing foods that are easy to swallow. If the problem cannot be resolved, a decision must be made as to whether to allow tube feeding.

Loss of appetite eventually occurs in most people who are dying. A decrease in appetite is natural, does not cause additional physical problems, and probably plays a role in dying comfortably, although it may distress family members. People who are dying will not keep their strength up by forcing themselves to eat, but they may enjoy eating small amounts of favorite home-cooked dishes.

If death is not expected to occur within hours or days, nutrition or hydration—given intravenously or via a tube inserted through the nose into the stomach—may be tried for a limited time to see if it improves the person's comfort, mental clarity, or energy. Nonetheless, many people opt not to undergo such feedings. Either way, the dying person and family members should have an explicit agreement with the doctor about what they are trying to accomplish with these measures and when the measures should be stopped if they are not helping.

Reduced food or liquid intake does not cause suffering. In fact, as the heart and kidneys fail, a normal intake of liquids often causes shortness of breath, because fluid accumulates in the lungs. A reduced food and liquid intake may lessen the need for suctioning because of less fluid in the throat and may reduce pain in people with cancer because of reduced swelling around tumors. It may even help the body release larger amounts of the body's natural pain-relieving chemicals (endorphins). Therefore, people who are dying should not be forced to eat or drink, especially if doing so requires restraints, intravenous tubes, or hospitalization.

Incontinence

Many dying people lose the ability to control bowel and bladder function (incontinence), attributable either to the disease or to general weakness. Disposable diapers and attentive hygiene measures usually address the problem.

Bedsores

Dying people are susceptible to bedsores, which cause discomfort and can lead to infections. Those who move very little, are confined to bed, or sit much of the time are at greatest risk. Ordinary pressure on the skin from sitting or moving across sheets may tear or damage the skin. Every effort should be made to protect the skin, and reddened or broken skin should be reported to the doctor promptly. ▲ Frequent position changes decrease the likelihood of bedsores.

Fatigue

Most fatal illnesses produce fatigue. A person who is dying can try to save energy for activities that really matter. Often, making a trip to the doctor's office or continuing an exercise that is no longer helping is not essential, especially if doing so saps the energy needed for more satisfying activities. Sometimes, stimulant drugs help.

Depression and Anxiety

Feeling sad when contemplating the end of life is a natural response, but this sadness is not depression. A person who is depressed may lack interest in what is going on, see only the bleak side of life, or feel no emotions. ■ A dying person and his family should talk to the doctor about such feelings so that depression can be diagnosed and treated. Treatment, usually combining drugs and counseling, is often effective, even in the last weeks of life, by improving the quality of the time remaining.

Anxiety is more than normal worry: Anxiety is feeling so worried and fearful that it interferes with daily activities. ★ Feeling uninformed or overwhelmed can cause anxiety, which may be relieved by asking caregivers for more information or help. A person who typically feels anxiety during periods of stress may be more likely to feel anxiety when dying. Strategies that have helped the person in the past—including reassurance, drugs, and channeling worry into productive endeavors—will probably help him when dying. A dying person troubled by anxiety should get help from counselors and may need antianxiety drugs.

Confusion and Unconsciousness

People who are very sick become confused easily. Confusion may be precipitated by a drug, a minor infection, or even a change in living arrangements. Reassurance and reorientation may relieve the confusion, but the doctor should be notified so that treatable causes can be sought. A person who is very confused may need to be mildly sedated or constantly attended by a caregiver.

A dying person who is confused will not understand dying. Near death, a confused person sometimes has surprising periods of clear thinking. These episodes may be very meaningful to family members but can be misunderstood as improvement. The family should be prepared for such episodes but should not expect them.

Almost half of the people who are dying are unconscious most of the time during their last few days. If family members believe that a dying person who is unconscious is still able to hear, they can say their good-byes as if the person hears them. Drifting off while unconscious is a peaceful way to die, especially if the person and family are at peace and all plans have been made.

Disability

Progressive disability often accompanies fatal illnesses. People may gradually become unable to tend to a house or an apartment, prepare food, handle financial matters, walk, or care for themselves. Most people who are dying need help in their last weeks. Such disability should be anticipated, perhaps by choosing housing that is accessible to wheelchairs and close to family caregivers. Services such as occupational or physical therapy and home health nursing may help a person remain at home, even when the disability progresses.

Financial Concerns

Obtaining adequate financial coverage for care of a dying person can be difficult. Medicare regulations exclude supportive care except in a hospice program, which mostly provides services in the home. People with a prognosis of less than a few months to live may not be readily admitted to a nursing home. Information about coverage and regulations can be obtained from the doctor or from another health care professional, such as a medical social worker.

The family should investigate the cost of a family member's impending death. Family members often provide most of the care at the end of life for free, but they should explore how professional caregivers can help them so that the burdens are tolerable. There may be costs of giving up employment as well as expenses of drugs, home care, and travel. One study has shown that one third of families de-

---

▲ see page 1208   ■ see page 614

★ see page 605

plete most of their savings in caring for a dying relative. The family should talk openly about costs with the doctor, insisting on reasonable attention to costs and planning ahead to limit or prepare for them.

The planning of the dying person's estate is advisable. Although discussing property and financial issues is hard to do when death is impending, it is usually a good idea. Doing so often reveals things that could be signed or arranged by the dying person, easing the burden on the family.

Legal and Ethical Concerns

Advance Directives: A person can give directions in the form of advance directives▲ about the type of care he wants before he needs it. Advance directives are legal written agreements that allow a person to establish values and treatment preferences to be honored in the future when competency or capacity has lapsed. For example, advance directives can prohibit resuscitation or tube feeding, if this is the person's wish. Advance directives may be in the form of a living will, which expresses the person's preferences for medical care, or a durable power of attorney, in which the patient designates another person to make health care decisions, or both.■

Suicide: Many dying people consider suicide—even more so as the public debate about assisted suicide grows. Discussing suicide with a doctor may help; the doctor can increase efforts to control pain, assure the person and family that they are cherished, and help them find meaning. Nevertheless, some people opt for suicide to relieve an intolerable situation or to retain control of when and how they wish to die. However, people can ordinarily exert control by refusing treatments that might prolong life, including feeding tubes and ventilators. Making such decisions is not considered suicide.

The Death With Dignity Act was passed in Oregon in 1998, and similar measures are being considered in other states. This law made it legal for doctors in Oregon to prescribe drugs to assist terminally ill people who want to die. Included in this law are several measures to prevent potential abuses. Among these are a mandatory waiting period, counseling, and a second medical opinion following a request for assistance in dying.

Coming to Terms

Preparing for death often means finishing a life's work, setting things right with family and friends, and making peace with the inevitable. Spiritual and religious issues are important to many dying people and their families. Members of the clergy are part of the care team in some hospice and hospital facilities, and professional caregivers can help people and their families find appropriate spiritual assistance if they do not have a relationship with a minister or other spiritual leader.

Grieving is a normal process that usually begins before an anticipated death. According to Elisabeth Kubler-Ross, a pioneer in death and dying, the dying person typically experiences five emotional stages, often in the following order: denial, anger, bargaining, depression, and acceptance. A person in denial may act as if, talk as if, or think that he is not dying. Denial is caused by fears about loss of control, separation from loved ones, an uncertain future, and suffering. Talking to a doctor or other health care member can help the dying person understand that he can remain in control and that his pain and other symptoms will be controlled. Anger may be expressed as a sense of injustice: "Why me?". Bargaining can be a sign of reasoning with death, that is, seeking more time. When the person realizes that bargaining and other strategies are not working, depression may develop. Acceptance, sometimes described as facing the inevitable, may come after discussions with family, friends, and care providers.

Preparing for death is hard work, with many emotional ups and downs. However, for most people, it is a time of new understanding and growth. By dealing with past hurts and mending relationships, a dying person and family members can achieve a profound sense of peace.

When Death Is Near

The prospect of dying raises questions about the nature and meaning of life and the reasons for suffering and dying. No easy answers to these fundamental questions exist. In their pursuit of answers, seriously ill people and their families can use their own resources, religion, counselors, friends, and research. They can talk, participate in religious or family rituals, or

---

▲ see page 54   ■ see page 55

engage in meaningful activities. The most important antidote to despair is often feeling cherished by another person. The torrents of medical diagnoses and treatments should not be allowed to obliterate the larger questions and the importance of human relationships.

Often, there are characteristic signs that death is near. Consciousness may decrease. The limbs may become cool and perhaps bluish or mottled. Breathing may become irregular.

Secretions in the throat or the relaxing of the throat muscles can lead to noisy breathing, sometimes called the death rattle. Repositioning the person or using drugs to dry secretions can minimize the noise. Such treatment is aimed at the comfort of the family or caregivers, because noisy breathing occurs at a time when the dying person is unaware of it. This breathing can continue for hours.

At the time of death, a few muscle contractions may occur, and the chest may heave as if to breathe. The heart may beat a few minutes after breathing stops, and a brief seizure may occur. Unless the dying person has a contagious infectious disease that poses a risk to others, family members should be assured that touching, caressing, and holding the body of a dying person, even for a while after the death, are acceptable. Generally, seeing the body after death is helpful to those close to the person. Doing so seems to counter the irrational idea that the person really did not die.

When Death Occurs

Death must be pronounced by an authorized person (such as a doctor), and the cause and circumstances of death must be certified. Fulfilling these requirements varies substantially in different parts of the country. If a person plans to die at home, the family should know ahead of time what to expect and to do. When a person has hospice care, the hospice nurse generally explains all of this. If police or other public officials must be called, they should be notified in advance that the person is dying at home. Hospices and home care programs often have routines for notifying officials so as to spare the family uncomfortable encounters. If no hospice or home care agency is involved, the family should contact the medical examiner or funeral home director to learn what to expect. A death certificate is necessary for making insurance claims, getting access to financial accounts, conveying real property titled to the deceased, and settling the estate. The family should obtain enough copies.

The family may be reluctant to ask for or approve an autopsy. Although it will not help the deceased, an autopsy may help the family and other people who have the same disease by revealing more about the disease process. After the autopsy, the body can be prepared by the funeral home or family for burial or cremation. Incisions made during the autopsy are usually hidden by clothing.

Prearranging and even prepaying for funeral services can be very helpful to the family, as can knowing the dying person's preferences for the handling of his body after death. The options can range from burial to cremation to donating the body to research. Many families have some sort of reception to honor the memory of the loved one. Some choose to have a small service soon after the person has died, whereas others choose to have a large memorial service a few weeks or even months later.

Getting on with life after a loved one has died depends on the nature of the relationship with the deceased, the age of the deceased, the kind of dying that was experienced, and the emotional and financial resources available. Also, the family needs to feel sure that they did what they should. Having a talk with the doctor a few weeks after the death can help answer lingering questions. The loneliness, disorientation, and feeling of unreality experienced during the period near the death improve with time, but the sense of loss persists. People do not "get over" a death as much as they make sense of it and go on with life.

CHAPTER 9

Legal and Ethical Issues

Poor health can jeopardize a person's ability to defend his legal rights. Safeguarding those rights requires advance thinking and planning. Sudden illness can cause profound weakness and confusion, while chronic illness can affect the ability to think clearly, making a person vulnerable and perhaps leading to the unwilling forfeiture of control. Conducting personal or business affairs, making wishes known, and making sure those wishes are respected may be impossible for a person who is physically or mentally impaired. Nevertheless, adults of any age can take steps to protect themselves against losing control over their lives, and such steps are especially important for older people. A durable power of attorney, a living will, or a revocable trust in combination with a living will can help direct the legal system so that decisions affecting health care and property management and distribution are made in accordance with a person's wishes.

The legal system in the United States operates on federal, state, and local levels. In general, federal law affects how property is taxed when it is given away, either while the owner is alive or after death. Federal law also controls Medicare, a program that provides health care coverage for most people aged 65 and older. In general, state laws determine how people can direct their own care if they become incapacitated. State laws also determine who is qualified for benefits under Medicaid, a program that provides health care coverage for some of the poor and disabled. In addition, state laws control property distribution if a person dies without a will or trust. Because state laws differ significantly, seeking an attorney's advice is important, particularly concerning property matters. Regarding health care matters, people can take many steps on their own and can enlist the help of their doctor and a social worker. Preparation of a living will document or a durable power of attorney agreement does not require an attorney. Complex financial documents should be written by an attorney.

Competency and Capacity

Laws recognize that adults—in most states, people over age 18—have the right to manage their own affairs, conduct business, and make health care decisions. This legal status is called **competency.** Competency and all the rights that go with it remain in effect until death, unless a court of law determines that a person can no longer manage personal affairs in his own best interest (a status called **incompetency**) or unless the person willingly transfers those rights to someone else.

Only a court of law can declare a person incompetent and, in doing so, take away a person's right to make decisions. If a person is declared incompetent, then the court must find someone else to act in the person's best interests, unless the person has already named someone by preparing the proper documentation (for example, a durable power of attorney for health care or a living will).

Capacity is a medical judgment, rather than a legal judgment, regarding a person's ability to make decisions about treatment interventions and other health-related matters. **Inca-**

Legal Terms Related to Health Care

Competency: The right to manage one's own affairs (bestowed at age 18 in most states).

Incompetency: The inability to manage one's own affairs because of injury or disability; declared by a court of law.

Incapacity: The inability to make appropriate decisions or to carry them out, as determined by a doctor or other health care professional.

Advance directives: Documents in the form of either a living will or a durable power of attorney for health care.

Living will: A document, sometimes called a directive to doctors, that expresses a person's wishes regarding future medical interventions when the person can no longer communicate those decisions.

Durable power of attorney for health care: A document that allows a person to designate someone else to make medical treatment decisions on his behalf. Also called a proxy.

pacity is a medical judgment in which a doctor or other health care professional deems a person physically or mentally unable to make appropriate medical decisions or to carry them out. A person in a coma cannot make *any* decisions, whereas a person with a broken leg may be able to make decisions but be unable to carry them out. People with mild dementia may think clearly enough to understand discussions with their doctors and make decisions about their medical care but may be unable to make decisions about their business affairs. People with dementia must depend on their doctors, lawyers, and accountants to evaluate their level of cognition, memory, or judgment before proceeding with medical care or conducting major legal and business transactions. If a doctor finds that a patient is incapable of making medical decisions, he will turn to someone appointed by the patient or to a friend or relative to participate on the patient's behalf. This process of making health care decisions for people who cannot do so is rarely litigated in court.

The issues of incompetency and incapacity come up frequently when older people become ill. Before performing any invasive tests or providing medical treatment, doctors must obtain permission from a person who is able to understand the risks and benefits involved. If a person is not capable of understanding those risks, the doctor will turn to the person named in a durable power of attorney for health care agreement (also called a proxy); if none exists, the doctor may simply turn to the next of kin. A durable power of attorney for health care ensures that health care decisions will be made by the person selected by the patient.

Informed Consent

Self-determination, the concept that "every adult of sound mind has the right to decide what shall be done with his own body," is the foundation of the legal and ethical doctrine of informed consent. The process of informed consent should grow out of discussion between the patient and doctor. The patient asks questions about his condition and treatment options, and the doctor shares facts and insights along with support and advice. When a person's decision regarding treatment is based on information about risks, benefits, and alternative treatments gained from discussion with a doctor and incorporates the person's preferences, consent or refusal is said to be in-

formed and is ethically valid and legally binding. All states require that such consent precede medical intervention.

Along with the right of informed consent comes the right of informed refusal. A decision to refuse treatment—even if puzzling—does not mean that a person is incompetent. In many cases, however, a person refuses treatment based on misunderstanding or lack of trust. A refusal of care should prompt the doctor to initiate further discussion. Doctors are ethically bound to encourage acceptance of the therapeutic recommendation judged to be in the person's best interest. Nevertheless, a person's refusal of treatment is not considered to be attempted suicide, nor is the doctor's compliance with the person's wishes considered physician-assisted suicide. Rather, the subsequent death is considered to be a natural consequence of the disease process itself.

Confidentiality and Disclosure

Communication between the patient and doctor is strictly confidential. Even well-meaning family members are not automatically privy to such information. All people are entitled to confidentiality unless they give permission for disclosure or they clearly can no longer express a preference (for example, if they are severely confused or comatose).

Health care professionals are sometimes required by law to disclose certain information, usually because the condition may present a danger to others. For example, certain infectious diseases, such as syphilis and tuberculosis, must be reported to state agencies. Conditions that might seriously impair a person's ability to drive, such as dementia, must be reported to the Department of Motor Vehicles in some states.

Advance Directives

Two types of legal documents extend personal control over medical care when a person becomes incapacitated: a living will and a durable power of attorney for health care. Both documents are called advance directives because they direct, in advance (when the person is capacitated), decisions about aspects of medical care to be carried out during any period when the person can no longer effectively communicate those decisions. An advance directive becomes effective only after incapacity has been determined.

If no advance directive has been prepared, someone must be appointed to take control of medical care decisions. In such cases, doctors and hospitals usually turn to the next of kin. In the rare event that the issue is referred to a court, control is usually given to a family member. If no appropriate family member can be found, the court appoints a guardian or conservator, who may be a friend or a stranger, to oversee care. An advance directive eliminates almost any need for the courts to get involved and helps ensure that the person's health care decisions will be respected.

Living Will

A living will expresses a person's preferences for medical care (it is called a living will because it is in effect while the person is alive). In some states, the document is called a directive to doctors. State laws vary greatly regarding living wills. For example, in some states, only a terminally ill person can create a legally effective living will.

Many people believe that extreme heroic measures and technology should be used to extend life as long as possible, regardless of the degree of medical intervention required or the quality of life that results. Others feel just as strongly that death is preferable to being perpetually dependent on medical equipment or having no hope of returning to a certain quality of life. A living will allows a person to express either of these preferences (or any intermediate measure that the person finds acceptable).

To be valid, a living will must comply with state law. Some states require that living wills be written in a standardized way. Others are more flexible, permitting any language as long as the document is appropriately signed and witnessed.

To indicate preferences for aggressive medical treatment, the document might state: "I want my life to be prolonged to the greatest extent possible without regard to my condition, the chances I have for recovery, the burdens of the treatment, or the cost of the procedures."

To prevent heroic attempts to extend life, the document might state: "I do not want my life to be prolonged, and I do not want life-sustaining treatment (including artificial feeding and hydration) to be provided or continued if I can no longer recognize friends and loved ones and am not expected to resume an independent lifestyle." However, most living wills stipulate that comfort measures should always be taken.

To express a preference for an intermediate position, the document might state: "I want my life to be prolonged, and I want life-sustaining treatment to be provided unless I am in a coma or in a persistent vegetative state that my doctors reasonably believe to be irreversible. After my doctors have reasonably concluded that I am in an irreversible condition, I do not want life-sustaining treatment (including artificial feeding and hydration) to be provided or continued."

Durable Power of Attorney for Health Care

A power of attorney for health care for decision making is a document in which one person (the principal) names another person (the agent, or the attorney-in-fact) to make decisions about health care and *only* health care. A power is *durable* if it remains legally in force, even when the principal becomes incapacitated.

A durable power of attorney for health care differs from a living will. A living will states a person's specific preferences regarding medical treatment; it provides guidance as to what care should be provided under various circumstances. A durable power of attorney for health care designates an agent to make health care decisions. The agent is granted the power to discuss medical alternatives with the doctors and make a decision if an accident or illness incapacitates the person. The durable power of attorney for health care can include a living will provision—a description of health care preferences—but should do so only as guidance for the agent, rather than as a binding selection.

Selecting an agent should be done with great care. For example, a person who strongly wishes to avoid aggressive medical treatment should not designate as agent anyone who believes, based on personal philosophy or religious doctrine, that every possible medical intervention should be used to prolong life. Similarly, a spouse who is under enormous emotional stress may be unable to carry out the person's preferences, especially if these include limiting or terminating care. A better choice for a person who has strong preferences but who does not want the rigidity of a living will might be a trusted business associate or a longtime friend. Discussing the details of possible future medical choices with the person named as agent is important, since the agent should be guided by the person's preferences. In addition, the person should also ensure that the agent is willing to act in this role.

The durable power of attorney for health care should name an alternate or successor in case the first-named person is unable or unwilling to serve as agent. Two or more people may be named to serve together (jointly) or alone (severally). A **jointly held power** requires that all agents agree and act together. In this arrangement, all named agents must be contacted and must agree on every decision. However, this arrangement can lead to chaos and should probably be avoided unless there are special circumstances that warrant its use. A **severally held power** is usually preferable, because it allows any named agent to act alone.

A person who is competent can cancel a durable power of attorney at any time. The choice of agent does not have to be permanent. If circumstances change, the person can create a new durable power of attorney naming a new agent.

Special circumstances may have to be addressed in drawing up a durable power of attorney for health care. For instance, family members have priority as visitors in a hospital under most circumstances. Unmarried couples and same-sex partners may need special protection to preserve such privileges. A durable power of attorney for health care is critical if the patient wants special status and decision-making power for a person who is legally unrelated.

Ideally, a person should give copies of his living will and durable power of attorney for health care to every doctor providing care for him and to the hospital upon admission. Copies should also be placed in the person's permanent medical record. A copy of the durable power of attorney for health care should also be given to the person's appointed agent and another copy placed with important papers. The person's lawyer should hold a copy of all documents.

Some advance directive documents are overly complicated or unfamiliar to doctors and hospitals and create confusion. It is especially important if the person has both a living will and a durable power of attorney to stipulate which should be followed if they appear to be in conflict. In general, a durable power of attorney is preferable if the patient has a trusted person to appoint. This appointed person can then act as an advocate, question the medical staff, and help decide what the patient would want or what is in the best interest of the patient.

Medical Terms Related to Life-sustaining Treatment

> **Cardiopulmonary resuscitation (CPR):** An action taken to revive a person in cardiac or respiratory arrest.
>
> **Code:** The summoning of professionals trained in cardiopulmonary resuscitation to revive a person in cardiac or respiratory arrest.
>
> **No code:** An order signed by a patient's doctor stating that cardiopulmonary resuscitation should not be performed if cardiac or pulmonary arrest occurs. Also called a do-not-resuscitate (DNR) order.
>
> **Irreversibly ill:** The state of debilitation (coma or persistent vegetative state) from which the patient will not recover.
>
> **Terminally ill:** The medical state of being near death where there is no hope of cure.
>
> **Life-sustaining treatment:** Any treatment given to postpone the death of a terminally ill person.
>
> **Palliative care:** Measures taken to keep a terminally ill person as comfortable as possible.

Surrogate Decision Making

If a person is incapacitated and no advance directive exists, some other person or persons must provide direction in decision making. A surrogate can be a person designated by state law as a health care decision maker or an informally identified person, such as a close family member or close friend who happens to be available.

Most hospitals and doctors accept consent to provide care from a spouse, a sibling, or an adult child, or even from a distant or uninvolved relative who can be reached in a crisis, although in many states none of these people has the legal right to consent on a person's behalf without being appointed by a court. Many hospitals will limit these selections to relatives and will ignore or exclude close friends. Accepting the judgment of a close relative or friend over that of a distant relative or total stranger, however, makes practical and ethical sense. People without family or close friends who are alone in the hospital are far more likely to receive a court-appointed guardian.

The surrogate, once identified, much like the agent named in a durable power of attorney for health care, bases a decision on one of three standards, in the following order of importance:

• The instructions expressed by the person such as in a living will or orally when the person was still capable of making decisions

• Inferences about what the person would likely want in a particular situation based on what is known about his prior behavior and his patterns of decision making

• What the surrogate and health care team believe is in the person's best interest (which is resorted to when the person's wishes and values are not known).

Do-Not-Resuscitate Orders

The do-not-resuscitate (DNR) order placed in a person's medical record by his doctor informs the medical staff that cardiopulmonary resuscitation (CPR)▲ should not be performed. This order has been particularly useful in preventing unnecessary and unwanted invasive treatment at the end of life.

Doctors discuss with patients the possibility of cardiopulmonary arrest, describe CPR procedures, and ask patients about treatment preferences. If a person is incapable of making a decision about CPR, a surrogate may make the decision based on the person's previously expressed preferences or, if such preferences are unknown, in accordance with the person's best interests.

A DNR order does not mean "do not treat." Rather, it means only that CPR will not be performed. Other treatments (for example, antibiotic therapy, treatment for discomfort or pain, transfusions, dialysis, use of a ventilator) may still be provided if needed.

Management of Property

People should have contingency plans to deal with injury or illness. Even if an accident or illness does not affect a person's ability (capacity) to control assets, serious illness or injury may make it difficult to pay bills, manage finances, take care of property, and handle business affairs. Having plans to turn over legal authority to a trusted decision maker can minimize disruption and expenses.

Three principal mechanisms allow a person to arrange in advance for property and business to be overseen by someone else: a power of attorney, a revocable trust, and joint tenancy. These arrangements are best made with the help of an attorney.

A **power of attorney** is a document in which one person (the principal) appoints another person (the agent or attorney-in-fact) to perform specific actions—such as handling bank accounts, investments, or other property—if the principal is too ill or too severely injured to handle them personally. Usually it is wise to draw up separate powers of attorney for health care and business matters, even if the same person is named as agent. Many general powers of attorney do not empower the agent to make health care decisions.

A **revocable trust (living trust)** places legal title to property in the hands of a trustee, who holds the property for the use and benefit of the beneficiary. The trustee cannot legally use the trust property for any purpose not specifically described in the trust document.

Joint tenancy is a form of ownership that gives all named owners the right to manage the property. Many people hold their bank accounts and homes in joint tenancy. In joint tenancy, an owner's share passes automatically after death to the other joint tenants. For example, if a parent has a checking account in joint tenancy with an adult child, both parent and child can write checks from the account. If the parent dies, the child then owns the account. A house owned in joint tenancy becomes fully owned by the surviving joint tenants.

▲ see page 1688

SECTION 2

DRUGS

10 **Overview of Drugs** **60**

Drug Design and Development ▪ Placebos ▪ Effectiveness and
Safety

11 **Drug Administration and Kinetics** **64**

Drug Administration ▪ Drug Absorption ▪ Drug Distribution ▪
Drug Metabolism ▪ Drug Elimination

12 **Drug Dynamics** **69**

Site Selectivity ▪ Drug Action

13 **Factors Affecting Response to Drugs** **73**

Genetic Makeup ▪ Drug-Drug Interactions ▪ Dietary
Supplement–Drug Interactions ▪ Drug-Food Interactions ▪
Drug-Disease Interactions ▪ Tolerance and Resistance

14 **Drugs and Aging** **79**

15 **Adverse Drug Reactions** **82**

Types of Adverse Drug Reactions ▪ Severity of Adverse Drug
Reactions ▪ Benefits Versus Risks ▪ Risk Factors ▪ Drug
Allergies ▪ Overdose Toxicity

16 **Compliance With Drug Treatment**......................................**86**

Results of Not Complying ▪ Compliance Among Children ▪
Compliance Among Older People ▪ Ways to Improve Compliance

17 **Trade-Name and Generic Drugs** **88**

Patent Protection ▪ Generic Drug Development ▪
Bioequivalence and Interchangeability ▪ Trade-Name or Generic
Drug? ▪ Generic Nonprescription Drugs

18 **Over-the-Counter Drugs** **93**

Historical Background ▪ Safety Considerations ▪ Analgesics and
Anti-Inflammatory Drugs ▪ Cold Remedies ▪ Drugs to Treat
Allergies ▪ Antacids and Indigestion Remedies ▪ Motion
Sickness Drugs ▪ Sleep Aids ▪ Special Precautions

19 **Medicinal Herbs and Nutraceuticals** **103**

Chamomile ▪ Chromium Picolinate ▪ Cranberry ▪ Creatine ▪
Dehydroepiandrosterone ▪ Echinacea ▪ Feverfew ▪ Garlic ▪
Ginger ▪ Ginkgo ▪ Ginseng ▪ Goldenseal ▪ Licorice ▪
Melatonin ▪ Milk Thistle ▪ Saw Palmetto ▪ St. John's Wort ▪
Valerian

CHAPTER 10

Overview of Drugs

A drug is defined by United States law as any substance (other than a food or device) intended for use in the diagnosis, cure, relief, treatment, or prevention of disease or intended to affect the structure or function of the body. (Oral contraceptives are an example of drugs that affect the function of the body rather than a disease.) This comprehensive definition of a drug, although important for legal purposes, is rather complex for everyday use. A simpler but workable definition of a drug is any chemical substance that affects the body and its processes.

By law, drugs are divided into two categories: prescription drugs and nonprescription drugs. Prescription drugs—those considered safe for use only under medical supervision—may be dispensed only with a prescription from a licensed professional with governmental privileges to prescribe (for example, a physician, dentist, podiatrist, nurse practitioner, physician's assistant, or veterinarian). Nonprescription drugs—those considered safe for use without medical supervision (such as aspirin)—are sold over-the-counter.▲ In the United States, the Food and Drug Administration (FDA) is the government agency that decides which drugs require a prescription and which may be sold over-the-counter. (Alternative medicines, such as nutraceuticals and medicinal herbs,■ are not covered by this law; they have not undergone the stringent testing required by the FDA.)

To some people, the word *drug* means a substance that alters the brain's function in ways considered pleasurable—a mind-altering substance. Drug abuse—the excessive and persistent use of mind-altering substances without medical need—has accompanied the appropriate medical use of drugs throughout recorded history. Some drugs with potential for abuse have legitimate medical purposes, and others do not.★

Some knowledge of drug names can help in understanding drug product labels. Every drug has at least three names—a chemical name, a generic (nonproprietary or official) name, and a trade (proprietary or brand) name.

The chemical name describes the atomic or molecular structure of the drug. This name is usually too complex and cumbersome for general use. So usually, an official body assigns a generic name to a drug. The generic names for drugs of a particular type (class) usually have the same ending. For example, the names of all beta-blockers, which are used to treat such disorders as high blood pressure, end in "olol."

The trade name is chosen by the pharmaceutical company that manufactures or distributes the drug. Patented drugs are usually sold under a trade name. Generic versions of trade-name drugs—manufactured after expiration of the patent—may be sold under the generic name (for example, ibuprofen) or under their own trade name (for example, Advil).

Understanding what group a drug belongs to is also useful. Broadly, drugs are classified by therapeutic group—that is, by what disorder or symptom they are used to treat. For example, drugs used to treat high blood pressure are called antihypertensives, and drugs used to treat nausea are called antiemetic drugs (emesis is the technical term for vomiting). Within each therapeutic group, drugs are categorized by classes. Some classes are based on how the drugs work in the body to produce their effect. For example, calcium channel blockers, one class of antihypertensives, lower blood pressure by preventing calcium from entering certain cells. Calcium is necessary for the contraction of muscles, including those in the walls of arteries. So calcium channel blockers hinder the contraction of muscles in artery walls and thus cause arteries to widen, so that blood can flow through them more easily. Calcium channel blockers affect the contraction of heart muscle less, and they do not interfere with the contraction of muscles under conscious control (skeletal muscle).

Drug Design and Development

Many of the drugs in current use were discovered by experiments conducted in animals and humans. However, many drugs are now being designed with the specific disorder in

---

▲ see page 93   ■ see page 103

★ see page 646

60

view: Abnormal biochemical and cellular changes caused by disease are identified; then compounds that may specifically prevent or correct these abnormalities (by interacting with specific sites in the body) can be designed. When a new compound shows promise, its structure is usually modified many times to optimize its ability to target the intended site (selectivity) and remain attached to the site (affinity) and to optimize its strength (potency), effectiveness (efficacy), and safety. Other factors, such as whether the compound is absorbed through the intestinal wall and whether it is stable in body tissues and fluids, are also considered. These factors involve what the body does to the drug (drug kinetics)▲ and what the drug does to the body (drug dynamics).■

Ideally, a drug is highly selective for its target site, so that it has little or no effect on other body systems; that is, it has minimal or no side effects.★ The drug should also be very potent and effective, so that low doses can be used, even for disorders that are difficult to treat. The drug should be effective when taken by mouth (for convenient administration), absorbed well from the digestive tract, and reasonably stable in body tissues and fluids so that, ideally, one dose a day is adequate.

During drug development, standard or average doses are determined. However, people respond to drugs differently. Many factors, including age,● weight, genetic make-up, and the presence of other disorders, affect drug response.◆ These factors must be considered when doctors determine the dose for a particular patient.

Placebos

Placebos are substances that are made to resemble drugs but do not contain an active drug.

A placebo is made to look exactly like a real drug but is made of an inactive substance such as a starch or sugar. Placebos are usually used in research studies.

Placebos can result in or be coincidentally associated with many changes, both desirable and undesirable. This phenomenon, called the placebo effect, appears to have two components: anticipation of results, usually optimistic, from taking a drug (sometimes called suggestibility); and spontaneous change. Sometimes people improve spontaneously, without

Placebo: I Shall Please

In Latin, *placebo* means "I shall please." In 1785, the word placebo first appeared in a medical dictionary as "a commonplace method or medicine." Two editions later, the placebo had become "a make-believe medicine," allegedly inert and harmless. Now, the profound effects of placebos, both good and bad, are well known.

treatment. If spontaneous change—whether positive or negative—occurs after a placebo is taken, the placebo may incorrectly be credited with or blamed for the result.

Some people seem more susceptible to the placebo effect than others. People who have a positive opinion of drugs, doctors, nurses, and hospitals are more likely to respond favorably to placebos than are people who have a negative opinion. Some people who are particularly susceptible to placebos tend to become compulsive about using the drug; they tend to increase the dose, and they develop withdrawal symptoms when they are deprived of the placebo.

When a new drug is being developed, investigators conduct studies to compare the effect of the drug with that of a placebo because any drug can have a placebo effect, unrelated to its action. The true drug effect must be distinguished from a placebo effect. Half the study's participants are given the drug, and half are given an identical-looking placebo. Ideally, neither the participants nor the investigators know who received the drug and who received the placebo (this type of study is called a double-blind study).

When the study is completed, all changes observed in participants taking the active drug are compared with those in participants taking the placebo. The drug must perform significantly better than the placebo to justify its use. In some studies, as many as 50% of participants taking the placebo improve (an example of the placebo effect), making it difficult to show the effectiveness of the drug being tested.

▲ see page 64   ■ see page 69
★ see page 82   ● see page 79
◆ see page 73

FROM LABORATORY TO MEDICINE CABINET

After a drug that may be useful in treating a disorder is identified or designed, it is studied in laboratory settings (called preclinical testing), including studies in animals. Preclinical testing gathers information about how the drug works, how effectively it works, and what toxic effects it produces, including possible effects on reproductive capacity and the health of offspring. Many drugs are rejected at this stage because they are shown to be too toxic or not to be effective.

If a drug seems promising after preclinical testing, an investigational new drug application is filed with the Food and Drug Administration (FDA). The drug undergoes many more rounds, or phases, of study in people (called clinical studies). In addition to determining a drug's effectiveness, studies in humans focus on the type and frequency of side effects and on factors that make people susceptible to these reactions (such as age, sex, other disorders, and the use of other drugs).

If these studies indicate that the drug is effective and safe, a new drug application (including data from the animal and human tests, intended drug manufacturing procedures, package insert information, and product labeling) is filed with the FDA, which reviews all the information and decides whether the drug is sufficiently effective and safe to be marketed. If the FDA approves, the drug becomes available for treatment of patients. The whole process usually takes about 10 years. On average, only about 5 of 4,000 drugs studied in the laboratory are studied in people, and only about 1 of 5 drugs studied in people is approved and makes it to the medicine cabinet.

After a new drug is approved, the manufacturer must monitor the use of the drug and promptly report any additional, previously undetected side effects to the FDA. Doctors and pharmacists are encouraged to participate in the ongoing monitoring of the drug. Such monitoring is important because before the drug is marketed, even comprehensive studies can detect only relatively common side effects (that occur about once in every 1,000 doses). Important side effects that occur once in every 10,000 (or more) doses can be detected only when a large number of people use the drug, that is, after it is on the market. The FDA may withdraw approval if new evidence indicates that a drug may cause severe side effects. For example, the diet aid fenfluramine was withdrawn from the market because some people who took it developed serious heart disorders.

PHASE	TEST GROUP	PURPOSE	LENGTH
Preclinical testing	Laboratory settings (such as cell cultures and animals)	To determine the chemical and physical characteristics of the drug and to assess the safety and effects of the drug in living organisms	2–6.5 years
Clinical studies			
Phase I	10–100 healthy volunteers	To establish basic safety and blood levels achieved with different doses of the drug	1.5 years
Phase II	50–500 people who have the disorder being studied	To establish the drug's effectiveness and dosage range, to determine drug kinetics, and to identify side effects	2 years
Phase III	300–30,000 people who have the disorder being studied	To confirm the most effective dosage regimen and to obtain more information about the drug's effectiveness and side effects	3.5 years
FDA review	All information from preclinical and clinical studies	To determine whether the drug has been proved to be effective and safe	0.5–1 years
Postmarketing surveillance	All people taking the drug	To identify any problems that did not occur in phase I, II, or III, including other side effects, such as those that take a long time to appear and those that occur rarely	Ongoing

Effectiveness and Safety

The main goals of drug development are effectiveness (efficacy) and safety. Because all drugs can harm as well as help, safety is relative. The difference between the usual effective dose and the dose that produces severe or life-threatening side effects is called the margin of safety. The wider the margin of safety, the more useful the drug. If a drug's usual effective dose is also toxic, doctors do not use the drug unless the situation is serious and there is no safer alternative.

The most useful drugs are effective and, for the most part, safe. Penicillin is such a drug. Except for people who are allergic to it, penicillin is virtually nontoxic, even in large doses. On the other hand, barbiturates, which were once commonly used as sleep aids, can interfere with breathing, lower blood pressure, and even cause death if they are taken in excess. Newer sleep aids such as temazepam and zolpidem have a wider margin of safety than barbiturates do.

Designing effective drugs with a wide margin of safety and few side effects cannot always be achieved. Consequently, some drugs must be used even though they have a very narrow margin of safety. For example, warfarin, which is taken to prevent blood clotting, can cause bleeding, but it is used when the need is so great that the risk must be tolerated. People who take warfarin need frequent checkups to see whether the drug is causing the blood to clot too much, too little, or appropriately.

Clozapine is another example. This drug often helps people with schizophrenia when all other drugs have proved ineffective. But clozapine has a serious side effect: It can decrease the production of white blood cells, which are needed to protect against infection. Because of this risk, people who take clozapine must have their blood tested frequently as long as they take the drug.

To help ensure that their treatment plan is as safe and effective as possible, people should keep their health care practitioners well informed about their medical history, drugs (including over-the-counter drugs) and dietary supplements (including medicinal herbs▲) that they are currently taking, and any other relevant health information. In addition, they

Making the Most of Drug Treatment

People can help make their treatment plan as safe and effective as possible by doing the following:

- Seeking medical care promptly when a problem develops
- Telling their doctor, nurse, or pharmacist

  What medical problems they have

  What drugs (prescription and nonprescription) and dietary supplements (including medicinal herbs) they have taken in the previous few weeks

  Whether they are allergic to or have had an unusual reaction to any drug, food, or other substance

  Whether they follow special diets or have food restrictions

  Whether they are pregnant, plan to become pregnant, or are breastfeeding
- Obtaining prescriptions and taking drugs as directed
- Understanding what a drug is being taken for and what side effects are possible
- Reading the label on drug containers carefully before taking a drug whether it is prescription or nonprescription
- Reporting any side effects to the doctor or pharmacist
- Not drinking alcohol if so advised
- Never taking someone else's prescription drug
- Discarding drugs that have expired
- Keeping appointments
- Taking recommended preventive steps and participating in recommended health programs

should not hesitate to ask a doctor, nurse, or pharmacist to explain the goals of treatment, the types of side effects and other problems that may develop, and the extent to which they can participate in the treatment plan.

▲ see page 103

CHAPTER 11

Drug Administration and Kinetics

Drug administration is the giving of a drug by one of several means (routes). Drug kinetics (pharmacokinetics) involves what the body does to a drug, including the processes of absorption, distribution, metabolism, and elimination, and how long these processes take.

Drug treatment requires getting a drug to its target site or sites—specific sites in tissues where the drug performs its action. Typically, the drug is introduced (the process of administration) into the body far from this site. The drug must move into the bloodstream (the process of absorption) and be transported to the target sites where the drug is needed (the process of distribution). Some drugs are chemically altered (the process of metabolism) by the body before they perform their action; others are metabolized afterward; and still others are not metabolized at all. The final step is the removal of the drug and its metabolites from the body (the process of elimination). Many factors including a person's age and genetic makeup, can influence these processes.▲

Drug Administration

Drugs are introduced into the body by several routes. They may be taken by mouth (orally); given by injection into a vein (intravenously), into a muscle (intramuscularly), into the space around the spinal cord (intrathecally), or beneath the skin (subcutaneously); placed under the tongue (sublingually); inserted in the rectum (rectally) or vagina (vaginally); instilled in the eye (by the ocular route); sprayed into the nose and absorbed through the nasal membranes (nasally); breathed into the lungs, usually through the mouth (by inhalation); applied to the skin (cutaneously) for a local (topical) or bodywide (systemic) effect; or delivered through the skin by a patch (transdermally) for a systemic effect. Each route has specific purposes, advantages, and disadvantages.

Oral Route: Because the oral route is the most convenient and usually the safest and least expensive, it is the one most often used.

However, it has limitations because of the way a drug typically moves through the digestive tract. For drugs administered orally, absorption may begin in the mouth and stomach, but usually, most of the drug is absorbed from the small intestine. The drug passes through the intestinal wall and then the liver before it is transported via the bloodstream to its target site. The intestinal wall and liver chemically alter (metabolize) many drugs, decreasing the amount reaching the bloodstream. Consequently, for the same effect, such drugs are often given in smaller doses when they are injected directly into the bloodstream (intravenously).

When a drug is taken orally, food and other drugs in the digestive tract may affect how much of and how fast the drug is absorbed. Thus, some drugs should be taken on an empty stomach, others should be taken with food, others should not be taken with certain other drugs, and still others cannot be taken orally at all.

Some orally administered drugs irritate the digestive tract; for example, aspirin and most other nonsteroidal anti-inflammatory drugs■ can harm the lining of the stomach and small intestine and can cause or aggravate preexisting ulcers.★ Other drugs are absorbed poorly or erratically in the digestive tract or are destroyed by the acid and digestive enzymes in the stomach.

Other routes are usually used only when the oral route cannot be used: for example, when a person cannot take anything by mouth, when a drug must be administered rapidly or in a precise or very high dose, or when a drug is poorly or erratically absorbed from the digestive tract.

Injection Routes: Administration by injection (parenteral administration) includes the subcutaneous, intramuscular, intravenous, and intrathecal routes. A drug product can be prepared or manufactured in ways that prolong drug absorption from the injection site for hours, days, or longer; such products do not need to be administered as often as drug products with more rapid absorption.

For the subcutaneous route, a needle is inserted into fatty tissue just beneath the skin.

▲ see page 73   ■ see page 452
★ see page 714

Through the Skin

Sometimes a drug is given through the skin—by needle (subcutaneous, intramuscular, or intravenous route), by patch (transdermal route), or by implantation.

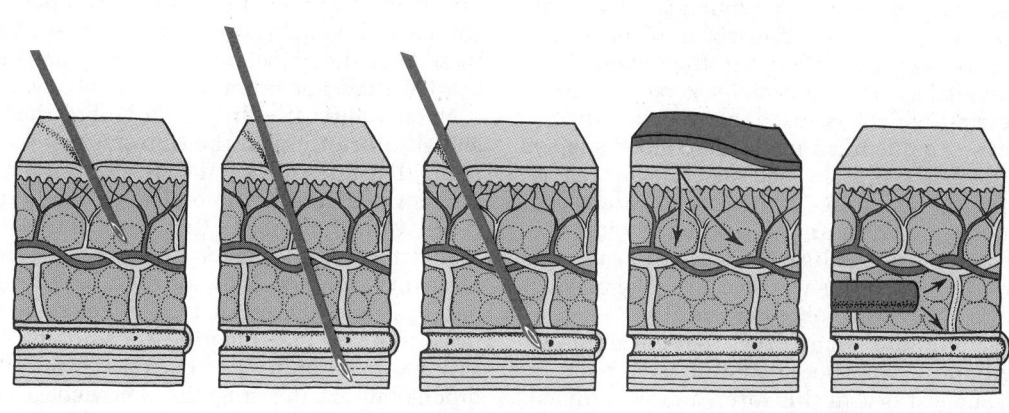

The drug is injected, then moves into small blood vessels (capillaries) and is carried away by the bloodstream or reaches the bloodstream through the lymphatic vessels. Protein drugs that are large in size, such as insulin, usually reach the bloodstream through the lymphatic vessels because these drugs move slowly from the tissues into capillaries. The subcutaneous route is used for many protein drugs because such drugs would be digested in the digestive tract if they were taken orally.

Certain drugs (such as progestin, used for birth control)▲ may be given by inserting plastic capsules under the skin (subcutaneously). This route is rarely used.

The intramuscular route is preferred to the subcutaneous route when larger volumes of a drug product are needed. Because the muscles lie below the skin and fatty tissues, a longer needle is used. Drugs are usually injected into muscle in the upper arm, thigh, or buttock. How quickly the drug is absorbed into the bloodstream depends, in part, on the blood supply to the muscle: The sparser the blood supply, the longer the drug takes to be absorbed. The blood supply is increased during physical activity.

For the intravenous route, a needle is inserted directly into a vein. A solution containing the drug may be given in a single dose or by continuous infusion. For infusion, the solution is moved by gravity (from a collapsible plastic bag) or by an infusion pump through thin flexible tubing to a tube (catheter) inserted in a vein, usually in the forearm. Intravenous administration is the best way to deliver a precise dose quickly and in a well-controlled manner throughout the body. It is also used for irritating solutions, which, if given by subcutaneous or intramuscular injection, would cause pain and tissue damage. An intravenous injection can be more difficult to administer than a subcutaneous or intramuscular injection, because inserting a needle or catheter into a vein may be difficult, especially if people are obese.

When given intravenously, a drug is immediately delivered to the bloodstream and tends to take effect more quickly than when given by any other route. Consequently, doctors closely monitor patients who receive an intravenous injection for signs that the drug is working or is causing undesired side effects. Also, the effect of a drug given by this route tends to last for a shorter time.

For the intrathecal route, a needle is inserted between two vertebrae in the lower spine and into the space around the spinal cord. The drug is then injected into the spinal canal. A small amount of local anesthetic is often used to numb the injection site. This route is used when a drug is needed to produce

▲ see page 1422

rapid or local effects on the brain, spinal cord, or the layers of tissue covering them (meninges)—for example, to treat infections of these structures. Anesthetics are sometimes given this way.

Sublingual Route: A few drugs are placed under the tongue (taken sublingually) so that they can be absorbed directly into the small blood vessels that lie beneath the tongue. The sublingual route is especially good for nitroglycerin—which is used to relieve angina (chest pain due to an inadequate blood supply to the heart muscle)—because absorption is rapid and the drug immediately enters the bloodstream without first passing through the intestinal wall and liver. However, most drugs cannot be taken this way because they may be absorbed incompletely or erratically.

Rectal Route: Many drugs that are administered orally can also be administered rectally as a suppository. In this form, a drug is mixed with a waxy substance that dissolves or liquefies after it is inserted into the rectum. Because the rectum's wall is thin and its blood supply rich, the drug is readily absorbed. A suppository is prescribed for people who cannot take a drug orally because they have nausea, cannot swallow, or have restrictions on eating, as is required after many surgical operations. Drugs that are irritating in suppository form may have to be given by injection.

Vaginal Route: Some drugs may be administered vaginally to women as a solution, tablet, cream, gel, or suppository. The drug is slowly absorbed through the vaginal wall. This route is often used to give estrogen to women at menopause, because the drug helps prevent thinning of the vaginal wall, an effect of menopause.▲

Ocular Route: Drugs used to treat eye disorders (such as glaucoma, conjunctivitis, herpes simplex infection, and injuries) can be mixed with inactive substances to make a liquid, gel, or ointment, so that they can be applied to the eye. Liquid eye drops are relatively easy to use but may run off the eye too quickly to be absorbed well. Gel and ointment formulations keep the drug in contact with the eye surface longer. Solid inserts, which release the drug continuously and in slow amounts, are also available, but they may be hard to put and keep in place. Ocular drugs are almost always

used for their local effects. For example, artificial tears are used to relieve dry eyes. Other drugs (for example, those used to treat glaucoma,■ such as acetazolamide and betaxolol and those used to dilate pupils, such as phenylephrine and tropicamide) produce a local effect after they are absorbed through the cornea and conjunctiva. Some of these drugs then enter the bloodstream and may have unwanted effects on other parts of the body.

Nasal Route: If a drug is to be breathed in and absorbed through the thin mucous membrane that lines the nasal passages, it must be transformed into tiny droplets in air (atomized). Once absorbed, the drug enters the bloodstream. Drugs taken by this route generally work quickly. Some of them irritate the nasal passages. Drugs that can be taken by the nasal route include nicotine (for smoking cessation), calcitonin (for osteoporosis), dihydroergotamine (for migraine headaches), and corticosteroids (for allergies and asthma).

Inhalation: Gases used for general anesthesia, such as nitrous oxide, are given by inhalation. Drugs given by inhalation through the mouth must be atomized into smaller particles than those given by the nasal route, so that the drug can pass through the windpipe (trachea) and into the lungs. How deeply into the lungs they go depends on the size of the droplets; smaller droplets go deeper. Inside the lungs, they are absorbed into the bloodstream. Relatively few drugs are taken this way because inhalation must be carefully monitored to ensure that a person receives the right amount of drug within a specified time. Usually, this method is used to administer drugs that act on the lungs, such as aerosolized antiasthmatic drugs in metered-dose containers.

Cutaneous Route: Drugs applied to the skin are usually used for their local effects and thus are most commonly used to treat superficial skin disorders, such as psoriasis, eczema, skin infections (viral, bacterial, and fungal), itching, and dry skin. The drug is mixed with inactive substances. Depending on the consistency of the inactive substances, the formulation may be an ointment, a cream, a lotion, a solution, a powder, or a gel.★

Transdermal Route: Some drugs are delivered bodywide through a patch on the skin. These drugs, sometimes mixed with a chemical (such as alcohol) that enhances penetration of the skin, pass through the skin to the bloodstream without injection. Through a patch, the drug can be delivered slowly and continu-

---

▲ see page 1359   ■ see table on page 1308
★ see page 1188

ously for many hours or days or even longer. As a result, levels of a drug in the blood can be kept relatively constant. Patches are particular useful for drugs that are quickly eliminated from the body, because such drugs, if taken in other forms, would have to be taken frequently. However, patches may irritate the skin of some people. In addition, patches are limited by how quickly the drug can penetrate the skin. Only drugs to be given in relatively small daily doses can be given through patches. Examples of such drugs include nitroglycerin (for angina), scopolamine (for motion sickness), nicotine (for smoking cessation), clonidine (for high blood pressure), and fentanyl (for pain relief).

Drug Absorption

Drug absorption is the movement of a drug into the bloodstream.

Absorption affects bioavailability—how quickly and how much of a drug reaches its intended (target) site of action. Factors that affect absorption (and therefore bioavailability) include the way a drug product is designed and manufactured, its physical and chemical properties, and the physiologic characteristics of the person taking the drug. Physiologic characteristics that may affect the absorption of drugs taken by mouth include how long the stomach takes to empty, what the acidity (pH) of the stomach is, and how quickly the drug is moved through the digestive tract.

A drug product is the actual dosage form of a drug—a tablet, capsule, suppository, transdermal patch, or solution. It consists of the drug (active ingredient) and additives (inactive ingredients). For example, tablets are a mixture of drug and diluents, stabilizers, disintegrants, and lubricants. The mixture is granulated and compressed into a tablet. The type and amount of additives and the degree of compression affect how quickly the tablet disintegrates and the drug is absorbed. Drug manufacturers adjust these variables to optimize absorption.

If a tablet releases the drug too quickly, the blood level of the drug may become too high, causing an excessive response. If the tablet does not release the drug quickly enough, much of the drug may be eliminated in the feces without being absorbed. Drug manufacturers formulate the tablet to release the drug at the desired speed.

Capsules consist of drugs and additives within a gelatin shell. The shell swells and releases its contents when it becomes wet, usually eroding quickly. The size of the drug particles and the properties of the additives affect how quickly the drug dissolves and is absorbed. Drugs tend to be absorbed more quickly from capsules filled with liquid than from those filled with solid particles.

Because drug products that contain the same drug (active ingredient) may have different inactive ingredients, absorption of the drug from different products may vary. Thus, a drug's effects, even at the same dose, may vary from one drug product to another. Drug products that not only contain the same active ingredient but also produce virtually the same blood levels over time are considered bioequivalent. Bioequivalence ensures therapeutic equivalence (that is, production of the same medicinal effect), and bioequivalent products are interchangeable.

If an orally administered drug can harm the stomach lining or decomposes in the acidic environment of the stomach, a tablet or capsule of the drug can be coated with a substance intended to prevent it from dissolving until it reaches the small intestine. These protective coatings are described as enteric, which refers to the small intestine. For the coatings to dissolve, they must come in contact with the less acidic environment of the small intestine or with the digestive enzymes there. However, the coatings do not always dissolve as intended; the tablet or capsule may be passed intact in the feces, especially in older people.

Some drug products are specially formulated to release their active ingredients slowly or in repeated small amounts over time—usually for a period of 12 hours or more. This dosage form is called modified-release, controlled-release, sustained-release, or extended-release.

Food, other drugs, and digestive disorders can affect drug absorption and bioavailability. For example, high-fiber foods may bind with a drug and prevent it from being absorbed. Laxatives and diarrhea, which speed up the passage of substances through the digestive tract, may reduce drug absorption. Surgical removal of parts of the digestive tract (such as the stomach or colon) may also affect drug absorption.

How and how long a drug product is stored can affect drug bioavailability. The drug in some products deteriorates and becomes ineffective or harmful if stored improperly or kept too long. Some products must be stored in the refrigerator or in a cool, dry, or dark place. Storage directions should be followed, and expiration dates observed.

Drug Distribution

Drug distribution refers to the movement of drug to and from the blood and various tissues of the body (for example, fat, muscle, and brain tissue) and the relative proportions of drug in the tissues.

After a drug is absorbed into the bloodstream, it rapidly circulates through the body; the average circulation time of blood is 1 minute. As the blood recirculates, the drug moves from the bloodstream into the body's tissues.

Once absorbed, most drugs do not spread evenly throughout the body. Drugs that dissolve in water (water-soluble drugs), such as the antihypertensive drug atenolol, tend to stay within the blood and the fluid that surrounds cells (interstitial space). Drugs that dissolve in fat (fat-soluble drugs), such as the anesthetic drug halothane, tend to concentrate in fatty tissues. Other drugs concentrate mainly in only one small part of the body (for example, iodine concentrates mainly in the thyroid gland), because the tissues there have a special attraction for and ability to retain (affinity) the drug.

Drugs penetrate different tissues at different speeds, depending on the drug's ability to cross membranes. For example, the anesthetic thiopental, a highly fat-soluble drug, rapidly enters the brain, but the antibiotic penicillin, a water-soluble drug, does not. In general, fat-soluble drugs can cross cell membranes more quickly than water-soluble drugs can. For some drugs, transport mechanisms aid movement into or out of the tissues.

Some drugs leave the bloodstream very slowly, because they bind tightly to proteins circulating in the blood. Others quickly leave the bloodstream and enter other tissues, because they are less tightly bound to blood proteins. Some or virtually all molecules of a drug in the blood may be bound to blood proteins. The protein-bound part is generally inactive. As unbound drug is distributed to tissues and its level in the bloodstream decreases, blood proteins gradually release the drug bound to them. Thus, the bound drug in the bloodstream may act as a reservoir for the drug.

Some drugs accumulate in certain tissues, which can also act as reservoirs of extra drug. These tissues slowly release the drug into the bloodstream, keeping blood levels of the drug from decreasing rapidly and thereby prolonging the effect of the drug. Some drugs, such as those that accumulate in fatty tissues, leave the tissues so slowly that they circulate in the bloodstream for days after a person has stopped taking the drug.

Distribution of a given drug may also vary from person to person. For instance, obese people may store large amounts of fat-soluble drugs, whereas very thin people may store relatively little. Older people, even when thin, may store large amounts of fat-soluble drugs because the proportion of body fat increases with age.

Drug Metabolism

Drug metabolism is the chemical alteration of a drug by the body.

Some drugs are chemically altered by the body (metabolized). The substances that result from metabolism (metabolites) may be inactive, or they may be similar to or different from the original drug in therapeutic activity or toxicity. Some drugs, called prodrugs, are administered in an inactive form, which is metabolized into an active form; the resulting metabolites produce the desired therapeutic effects. Metabolites may be metabolized further instead of being excreted from the body. The subsequent metabolites are then excreted.

Most drugs must pass through the liver, which is the site of most drug metabolism. Liver enzymes convert prodrugs to active metabolites or inactivate drugs. The group of P-450 enzymes is the liver's primary mechanism for chemically altering drugs. The levels of P-450 enzymes control the rate at which many drugs are metabolized. The capacity of the enzymes to metabolize is limited, so they can become overloaded when blood levels of a drug are high.▲

Because metabolic enzyme systems are only partially developed at birth, newborns have difficulty metabolizing certain drugs. As people age, enzymatic activity decreases, so that older people, like newborns, cannot metabolize drugs as well as younger adults and children

▲ see page 75

do. Consequently, newborns and older people often need smaller doses per pound of body weight than young or middle-aged adults do.

Drug Elimination

Drug elimination is the removal of drugs from the body.

All drugs are eliminated from the body in a chemically altered (metabolized) form or by excretion. Most drugs, particularly water-soluble drugs and their metabolites, are eliminated largely by the kidneys in urine.

Several factors, including certain characteristics of the drug, affect the kidneys' ability to excrete drugs. To be extensively excreted in urine, a drug or metabolite must be water soluble and must not be bound too tightly to proteins in the bloodstream. The acidity of urine, which is affected by diet, drugs, and kidney disorders, can affect the rate at which the kidneys excrete some drugs. In the treatment of poisoning with some drugs, the acidity of the urine is changed by giving antacids (such as sodium bicarbonate) or acidic substances (such as ammonium chloride) orally to speed up the excretion of the drug.

The kidneys' ability to excrete drugs also depends on urine flow, blood flow through the kidneys, and the condition of the kidneys. Kidney function can be impaired by many disorders (especially high blood pressure, diabetes, and recurring kidney infections), by exposure to high levels of toxic chemicals, and by age-related changes. As people age, kidney function decreases. The kidney of an 85-year-old person excretes drugs only about half as efficiently as that of a 35-year-old.

Doctors may adjust the dosage of a drug that is eliminated primarily through the kidneys. The normal age-related decrease in kidney function can help doctors determine an appropriate dosage based solely on a person's age. However, appropriate dosage can be determined more accurately by determining how well the kidneys are functioning: A blood test can be performed to measure the level of creatinine (a waste product) in the blood, or a urine test may be performed so that the amount of creatinine in urine collected for 12 to 24 hours relative to the level of creatinine in the blood—called creatinine clearance—can be estimated.

Some drugs pass through the liver and are excreted unchanged in the bile. The bile then enters the digestive tract. From there, drugs are eliminated in feces or reabsorbed into the bloodstream and thus recycled. Other drugs are converted to metabolites that are excreted in the bile. The metabolites may be excreted in the feces or converted back to the drug, which is then reabsorbed into the bloodstream and recycled.

If the liver is not functioning normally, doctors may adjust the dosage of a drug that is eliminated primarily by metabolism in the liver. However, there are no simple ways to assess liver function quantitatively for drug metabolism comparable to those for kidney function.

Some drugs are excreted in saliva, sweat, breast milk, and even exhaled air. Most are excreted in small amounts. The excretion of drugs in breast milk is significant only because the drug may affect the breastfeeding infant. Excretion in exhaled air is the main way that inhaled anesthetics are eliminated.

CHAPTER 12

Drug Dynamics

Drug dynamics (pharmacodynamics) involves what a drug does to the body.

Drug dynamics describes the therapeutic effects of drugs (such as relief of pain and reduction of blood pressure) and their side effects. But drug dynamics also describes where (the site) and how (the mechanism) a drug acts on the body. A drug's effects on the body may be influenced by many factors, such as a person's age▲ and genetic makeup and disorders the person has other than the one being treated.■

▲ see page 79   ■ see page 73

Site Selectivity

After being swallowed, injected, inhaled, or absorbed through the skin, most drugs enter the bloodstream and circulate throughout the body. Some drugs are administered directly to the area where they are wanted—for example, to the eyes in eyedrops. The drugs then interact with cells or tissues where they produce their intended effects (target sites). Some drugs are relatively nonselective; they affect many different tissues or organs. For example, atropine, a drug given to relax muscles in the digestive tract, may also relax muscles in the eyes and in the respiratory tract. Other drugs are relatively selective. For example, nonsteroidal anti-inflammatory drugs, such as aspirin and ibuprofen,▲ target any area where inflammation is present. Still other drugs are highly selective; they affect mainly a single organ or system. For example, digoxin, a drug given to manage heart failure, affects mainly the heart, increasing its pumping efficiency. Sleep aids target certain nerve cells of the brain.

How do drugs know where to exert their effects? The answer involves how they interact with cells or substances such as enzymes.

Receptors on Cells

On their surface, most cells have many different types of receptors. A receptor is a molecule with a specific three-dimensional structure, which allows only substances that fit precisely to attach to it—as a key fits in its lock. Receptors enable natural (originating in the body) substances outside the cell, such as neurotransmitters and hormones, to influence the activity of the cell. Drugs tend to mimic these natural substances and thus use receptors in the same way. For example, morphine and related pain-relieving drugs use the same receptors in the brain used by endorphins, which are substances produced by the body to help control pain. Some drugs attach to only one type of receptor; others, like a master key, can attach to several types of receptors throughout the body. A drug's selectivity can often be explained by how selectively it attaches to receptors.

Drugs that target receptors are classified as agonists or antagonists. Agonist drugs activate, or stimulate, their receptors, triggering a response that increases or decreases the cell's

▲ see page 452

A Perfect Fit

A receptor on the cell's surface has a three-dimensional structure that allows a specific substance, such as a drug, hormone, or neurotransmitter, to bind to it because the substance has a three-dimensional structure that perfectly fits the receptor, as a key fits a lock.

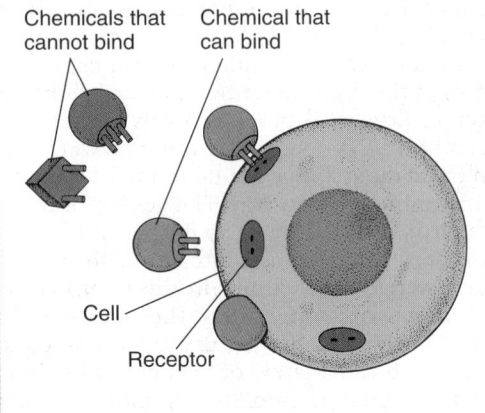

Chemicals that cannot bind

Chemical that can bind

Cell

Receptor

activity. Antagonist drugs block the access or attachment of the body's natural agonists, usually neurotransmitters, to their receptors and thereby prevent or reduce cell responses to natural agonists.

Agonist and antagonist drugs can be used together in patients with asthma. For example, albuterol can be used with ipratropium. Albuterol, an agonist, attaches to specific (adrenergic) receptors on cells in the respiratory tract, causing relaxation of smooth muscle cells and thus widening of the airways (bronchodilation). Ipratropium, an antagonist, attaches to other (cholinergic) receptors, blocking the attachment of acetylcholine, a neurotransmitter that causes contraction of smooth muscle cells and thus narrowing of the airways (bronchoconstriction). Both drugs widen the airways (and make breathing easier) but in different ways.

Beta-blockers, such as propranolol, are a widely used group of antagonists. These drugs are used to treat high blood pressure, angina (chest pain due to an inadequate blood supply to the heart muscle), and certain abnormal heart rhythms. They block or reduce stimulation of the heart by the agonist hormones epinephrine (adrenaline) and norepinephrine

TARGETS IN THE BODY: CELL RECEPTORS

Certain natural substances in the body, such as neurotransmitters and hormones, target specific receptors on the surface of cells. When these substances bind with the receptor on a cell, they stimulate that receptor to produce or to inhibit a specific action in the cell; that is, these substances are agonists. Drugs can also target and bind with these receptors.

Some drugs act as agonists, stimulating the receptor in the same way that the body's natural agonists do; others act as antagonists, blocking the action of the natural agonist on the receptor. Each type of receptor has many subtypes, and agonists may act on several types of receptors.

TYPE OF RECEPTOR	BODY'S NATURAL AGONIST	RESULTING ACTION	DRUGS THAT TARGET THE RECEPTOR
Adrenergic			
Alpha$_1$	Epinephrine and norepinephrine	"Fight-or-flight" reactions: constriction of the blood vessels in the skin, digestive tract, and urinary tract; breakdown of glucose in the liver (releasing energy); a decrease in activity of the stomach and intestines; and contraction of smooth muscle in the genital and urinary organs	Agonist: methoxamine, and phenylephrine Antagonist: doxazosin, prazosin, tamsulosin, and terazosin
Alpha$_2$	Epinephrine and norepinephrine	A decrease in insulin secretion, in the clumping of platelets, in the constriction of blood vessels in the skin and intestines, and in the release of norepinephrine from nerves	Agonist: clonidine Antagonist: yohimbine
Beta$_1$	Epinephrine and norepinephrine	An increase in heart rate, in the force of heart contraction, and in secretion of renin (a hormone involved in controlling blood pressure)	Agonist: dobutamine and isoproterenol Antagonist: beta-blockers (used to treat hypertension and heart disease), such as atenolol and metoprolol
Beta$_2$	Epinephrine and norepinephrine	Dilation of smooth muscle in the blood vessels, airways, digestive tract, and urinary tract; breakdown of glycogen in skeletal muscles (releasing glucose for energy)	Agonist: albuterol, isoetharine, and terbutaline Antagonist: propranolol
Cholinergic			
Muscarinic	Acetylcholine	A decrease in heart rate and the force of the heart's contraction; constriction of airways; dilation of blood vessels throughout the body; and an increase in activity of the stomach, intestines, bladder, and salivary, lacrimal, and sweat glands	Agonist: bethanechol and carbachol Antagonist: atropine, ipratropium, and scopolamine

Table continues on the following page.

TARGETS IN THE BODY: CELL RECEPTORS (Continued)

TYPE OF RECEPTOR	BODY'S NATURAL AGONIST	RESULTING ACTION	DRUGS THAT TARGET THE RECEPTOR
Cholinergic (continued)			
Nicotinic	Acetylcholine	Contraction of skeletal muscles	Agonist: none commonly used
			Antagonist: atracurium, pancuronium, and tubocurarine
Histaminergic			
H_1	Histamine	Production of an allergic response, contraction of muscles in the airways and digestive tract, dilation of small blood vessels, and drowsiness (sedation)	Agonist: none commonly used
			Antagonist: cetirizine, chlorpheniramine, clemastine, diphenhydramine, fexofenadine, and loratadine
H_2	Histamine	Stimulation of stomach secretions	Agonist: none commonly used
			Antagonist: cimetidine, famotidine, nizatidine, and ranitidine

(noradrenaline), which are released during stress. Antagonists such as beta-blockers are most effective when the local concentration of the agonist is high. Similar to the way a roadblock stops more vehicles during the 5:00 PM rush hour than at 3:00 AM, beta-blockers, given in doses that have little effect on normal heart function, may have a greater effect during sudden surges of hormones released during stress and thereby protect the heart from excess stimulation.

Enzymes

Instead of receptors, some drugs target enzymes, which regulate the rate of chemical reactions. Drugs that target enzymes are classified as inhibitors or activators (inducers). For example, the cholesterol-lowering drug lovastatin inhibits an enzyme called HMG-CoA reductase, which is critical in the body's production of cholesterol. A side effect of the antibiotic rifampin is the activation of the enzymes involved in metabolizing oral contraceptives. When women who are taking an oral contraceptive also take rifampin, the contraceptive is metabolized and removed from the body more quickly than usual and may therefore be ineffective.

Drug Action

Drugs affect only the rate at which existing biologic functions proceed; they do not change the basic nature of these functions or create new functions. For example, drugs can speed up or slow down the biochemical reactions that cause muscles to contract, kidney cells to regulate the volume of water and salts retained or eliminated by the body, glands to secrete substances (such as mucus, stomach acid, or insulin), and nerves to transmit messages.

Drugs cannot restore structures or function already damaged beyond repair by the body. This fundamental limitation of drug action underlies much of the current frustration in trying to treat tissue-destroying or degenerative diseases such as heart failure, arthritis, muscular dystrophy, multiple sclerosis, and Alzheimer's disease. Nonetheless, some drugs can help the body repair itself. For example, by stopping an infection, antibiotics can allow the body to repair damage caused by the infection.

Some drugs are hormones, such as insulin, thyroid hormones, or cortisol. They can be used to replace hormones that are missing from the body.

Reversibility

Most interactions between a drug and a receptor or between a drug and an enzyme are reversible: After a while, the drug disengages, and the receptor or enzyme resumes normal function. Sometimes an interaction is largely irreversible, and the drug's effect persists until the body manufactures more enzyme. For example, omeprazole, a drug used in the management of gastroesophageal reflux and ulcers, irreversibly inhibits an enzyme involved in the secretion of stomach acid.

Affinity and Intrinsic Activity

A drug's action is affected by the degree of attraction (affinity) between it and its receptor on the cell's surface and, once it is bound to its receptor, by its ability to produce an effect (intrinsic activity). Drugs vary in their affinity and intrinsic activity.

Drugs that activate receptors (agonists) must have both great affinity and intrinsic activity: They must bind effectively to their receptors, and the drug bound to its receptor (drug-receptor complex) must be capable of producing an effect in the targeted area. In contrast, drugs that block receptors (antagonists) must bind effectively, but they have little or no intrinsic activity, because their function is to prevent an agonist from interacting with its receptors.

Potency and Efficacy

A drug's effects can be evaluated in terms of strength (potency) or effectiveness (efficacy).

Potency refers to the amount of drug (usually expressed in milligrams) needed to produce an effect, such as relief of pain or reduction of blood pressure. For instance, if 5 milligrams of drug A relieves pain as effectively as 10 milligrams of drug B, drug A is twice as potent as drug B.

Efficacy refers to the potential maximum therapeutic response that a drug can produce. For example, the diuretic furosemide eliminates much more salt and water through urine than does the diuretic chlorothiazide. Thus, furosemide has greater efficacy than chlorothiazide. However, greater potency or efficacy does not necessarily mean that one drug is preferable to another. When judging the relative merits of drugs for a patient, doctors consider many factors, such as side effects, potential toxicity, duration of effect (which determines the number of doses needed each day), and cost.

Factors Affecting Response to Drugs

Everyone responds to drugs differently. The way a person responds to a drug is affected by many factors, including genetic makeup, age, body size, the use of other drugs and dietary supplements (such as medicinal herbs▲), the consumption of food (including beverages), the presence of diseases (such as kidney or liver disease), and the development of tolerance and resistance. For example, a large person generally needs more of a drug than a smaller person needs for the same effect. Whether people take a drug as instructed■ also affects their response to it. These factors may affect what the body does to the drug (pharmacokinetics★), what the drug does to the body (pharmacodynamics●), or both.

Because so many factors affect drug response, doctors must choose a drug appropriate for an individual patient and must adjust the dose carefully. This process is more complex if the patient takes other drugs and has other diseases, because drug-drug and drug-disease interactions are possible.

A standard or average dose is determined for every new drug. But the concept of an average

---

▲ see page 103   ■ see page 86

★ see page 64   ● see page 69

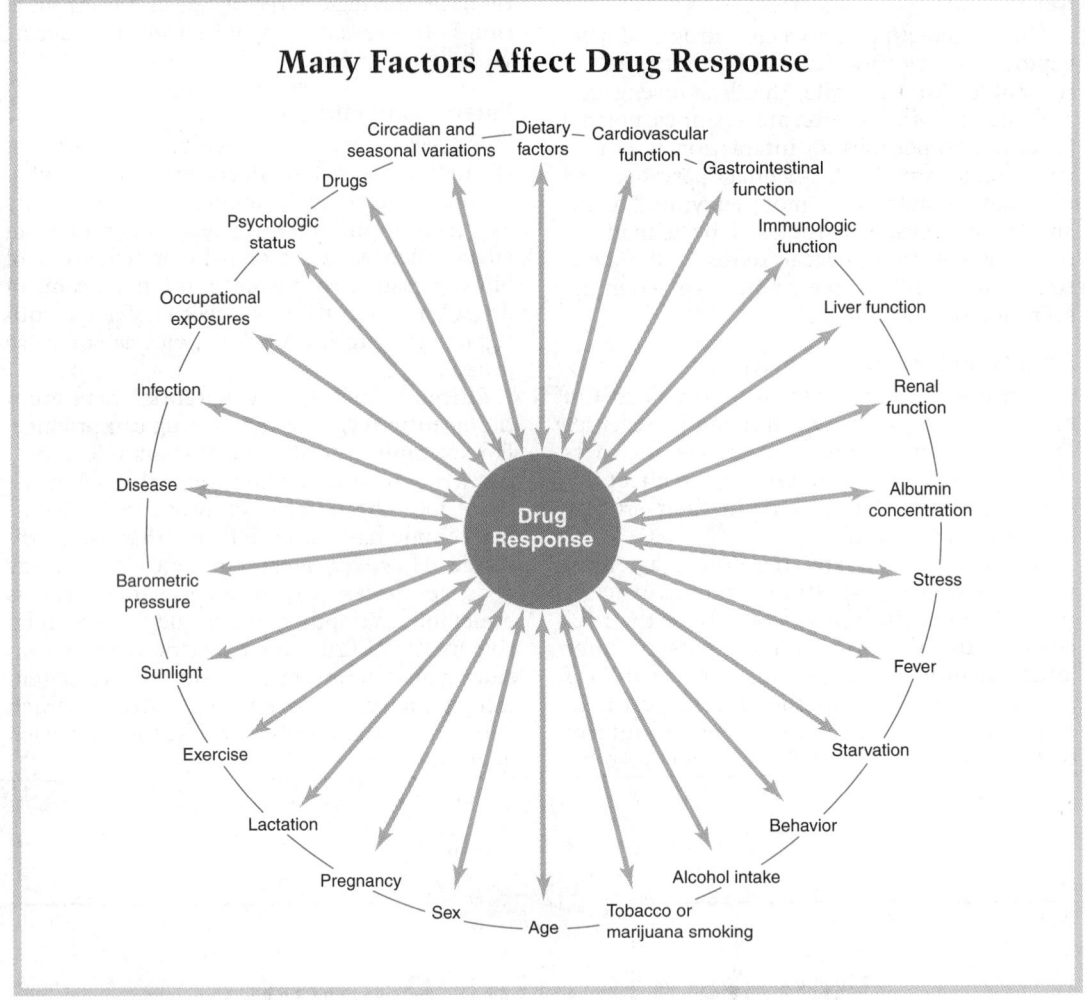

Many Factors Affect Drug Response

dose can be like "one size fits all" in clothing: It may fit a range of people well enough, but it may fit almost no one perfectly. For some drugs, the dose does not have to be adjusted, because the same dose works well in virtually everyone.

Genetic Makeup

Differences in genetic (inherited) makeup among individuals affect what the body does to a drug and what the drug does to the body. The study of genetic differences in the response to drugs is called pharmacogenetics.

Because of their genetic makeup, some people process (metabolize) drugs slowly; as a result, a drug may accumulate in the body, causing toxicity. Other people metabolize drugs so quickly that after they take a usual dose, drug levels in the blood never become high enough for the drug to be effective. Still others metabolize a drug given at the usual dose normally, but if the drug is given at a high dose or with another drug metabolized by the same enzyme system, the system may be overloaded, resulting in toxic levels of the first drug.

In about half of the people in the United States, N-acetyltransferase, a liver enzyme that metabolizes certain drugs, works slowly. In such people (called slow acetylators), drugs that are metabolized by this enzyme tend to reach higher blood levels and remain in the body longer than they do in people in whom this enzyme metabolizes drugs rapidly (fast acetylators).

About 1 of 1,500 people have low levels of pseudocholinesterase, a blood enzyme that inactivates drugs such as succinylcholine, which is given with an anesthetic during many surgical procedures to temporarily relax muscles. If succinylcholine is not rapidly inactivated, muscle relaxation may be prolonged, and people may not be able to breathe on their own as soon after surgery as is usual. They may need a ventilator for an extended time.

About 10% of black men and fewer black women have a deficiency of glucose-6-phosphate dehydrogenase (G6PD), an enzyme that protects red blood cells from certain toxic chemicals. For example, in people with G6PD deficiency, some drugs (such as chloroquine and primaquine, which are used to treat malaria) destroy red blood cells and cause hemolytic anemia.▲

About 1 of 20,000 people have a genetic defect that makes muscles overly sensitive to anesthetics such as halothane, isoflurane, and sevoflurane. When such people are given one of these anesthetics with a muscle relaxant (usually succinylcholine), a life-threatening disorder called malignant hyperthermia may develop. It produces a very high fever. Muscles stiffen, the heart races, and blood pressure falls.

Some people have low levels of P-450 liver enzymes, which inactivate many drugs.■ In such people, a drug's effects may be increased and prolonged. For example, the sedative effects of the sleep aid flurazepam can last much longer than usual and can cause drowsiness during the day.

Drug-Drug Interactions

Drug-drug interactions are changes in a drug's effects caused by another drug taken during the same time period.

Drug-drug interactions usually involve prescription drugs but can involve nonprescription (over-the-counter) drugs★—most commonly, aspirin, antacids, and decongestants. Although many people do not consider alcohol a drug, it affects body processes and interacts with many drugs. Doctors or pharmacists can answer questions about possible alcohol and drug interactions.

The effects of drugs given during the same time period are sometimes beneficial but more often are unwanted and harmful. Types of drug-drug interactions include duplication, opposition (antagonism), and alteration of what the body does to one or both drugs.

Duplication: When two drugs with the same effect are taken, their therapeutic effects and their side effects may be intensified. Duplication may occur when a person inadvertently takes two drugs, usually over-the-counter drugs, that have the same active ingredient. For example, a person may take a cold remedy and a sleep aid, both of which contain diphenhydramine, or a cold remedy and a pain reliever, both of which contain acetaminophen.

More often, duplication occurs when doctors prescribe two similar but not identical drugs. Sometimes, doctors deliberately prescribe such drugs to treat a disorder more effectively. For example, doctors may prescribe two antihypertensive drugs for a person whose high blood pressure is difficult to control. With this approach, blood pressure can be effectively lowered with fewer side effects than if one drug is prescribed at a higher dose. When treating cancer, doctors sometimes give several drugs (combination chemotherapy) to produce a better effect with fewer side effects. However, problems, sometimes severe, can develop when doctors inadvertently prescribe similar drugs. For example, excessive sedation and dizziness can occur when two doctors prescribe a sleep aid or when one prescribes a sleep aid and the other prescribes another drug that has sedative effects.

Opposition (Antagonism): Two drugs with opposing actions can interact, thereby reducing the effectiveness of one or both. For example, nonsteroidal anti-inflammatory drugs, (NSAIDs),● such as ibuprofen, which are taken to relieve pain, may cause the body to retain salt and fluid; diuretics, such as hydrochlorothiazide and furosemide, help rid the body of excess salt and fluid. If a person takes both types of drug, the NSAID may reduce the diuretic's effectiveness. Certain beta-blockers (such as propranolol), taken to control high blood pressure and heart disease, counteract beta-adrenergic stimulants, such as albuterol, taken to manage asthma. Both types of drugs target the same cell receptors—beta-2 receptors;◆ one type blocks them, and the other stimulates them.

Alteration: One drug may alter how the body absorbs, distributes, metabolizes, or excretes another drug. Some drugs affect the P-

---

▲ see page 987   ■ see page 68

★ see page 93   ● see page 452

◆ see table on page 71

How to Reduce the Risk of Drug-Drug Interactions

- Consult the primary care doctor before taking any new drugs, including over-the-counter drugs and dietary supplements, such as medicinal herbs.
- Keep a list of all drugs being taken, and periodically discuss this list with the doctor or pharmacist.
- Keep a list of all disorders, and periodically discuss this list with the doctor.
- Select a pharmacist who provides comprehensive services (including checking for possible interactions) and who maintains a complete drug profile for each patient, and have all prescriptions dispensed by this pharmacist.
- Learn about the purpose and actions of all drugs prescribed.
- Learn about the possible side effects of the drugs.
- Learn how to take the drugs, what time of day they should be taken, and whether they can be taken during the same time period as other drugs.
- Review the use of over-the-counter drugs with the pharmacist, and discuss any disorders present and any prescription drugs being taken.
- Take drugs as instructed.
- Report to the doctor or pharmacist any symptoms that might be related to the use of a drug.
- If seeing more than one doctor, make sure each doctor knows all the drugs being taken.

450 enzyme system in the liver (which inactivates many drugs) and may cause another drug to be inactivated more quickly or more slowly than usual. For example, by increasing the activity of P-450 enzymes, barbiturates such as phenobarbital cause the anticoagulant warfarin to be inactivated more quickly and thus to be less effective when taken during the same time period. Doctors may need to increase the dose of warfarin to compensate for this effect. If phenobarbital is later discontinued, the level of warfarin may increase dramatically, increasing the risk of bleeding. In such cases, doctors monitor the person closely and adjust the dose of warfarin as needed.

Chemicals in cigarette smoke can increase the activity of some liver enzymes. As a result, smoking decreases the effectiveness of some drugs, including propoxyphene (an analgesic) and theophylline (a drug that widens the airways called a bronchodilator).

The histamine-2 (H_2) blocker cimetidine (used to treat ulcers, heartburn, and gastroesophageal reflux) and the antibiotics ciprofloxacin and erythromycin may slow liver enzyme activity, prolonging the action of theophylline.

Some drugs affect the rate at which the kidneys excrete another drug. For example, large doses of vitamin C supplements increase the urine's acidity and thus may change the rate of excretion and activity of certain drugs. For example, the rate of excretion may be decreased for acidic drugs such as aspirin but may be increased for basic drugs such as pseudoephedrine.

Prevention

The risk of a drug-drug interaction depends on the number of drugs used, the tendency of particular drugs to interact, and the amount of drug taken. Many drug-drug interactions are discovered during drug development and testing. They are listed in the prescribing information, in the patient information insert, or on the container for each drug. However, many interactions are not discovered until drugs are used by more people and for longer periods of time. Doctors, nurses, and pharmacists can help reduce the risk of serious problems by keeping informed about potential drug-drug interactions and adjusting drug therapy accordingly. Reference books and computer software programs can help people learn about drug-drug interactions. People can help reduce their risk of interactions by being actively involved in their health care.

People being cared for by several doctors are at highest risk of drug-drug interactions because each doctor may not know all of the drugs being taken. People can reduce this risk by keeping each doctor informed about all drugs being taken and by using one pharmacy to obtain all prescriptions.

Dietary Supplement–Drug Interactions

Dietary supplement–drug interactions are changes in a drug's effects caused by a dietary supplement taken during the same time period.

SOME DRUG-FOOD INTERACTIONS

AFFECTED DRUG	INTERACTING FOOD	INTERACTION
Alendronate	Any food	Food, even orange juice, coffee, or mineral water, may markedly reduce the absorption and effectiveness of alendronate. Alendronate must be taken with plain water at least 1/2 hour before the first food, beverage, or drug of the day is taken
Anticoagulants	Foods high in vitamin K (such as broccoli, brussels sprouts, spinach, and kale)	Such foods may reduce the effectiveness of anticoagulants (such as warfarin), increasing the risk of clotting. Intake of such foods should be limited, and the amount consumed daily should remain constant
Certain benzodiazepines (such as triazolam) Calcium channel blockers (such as felodipine, nifedipine, and nisoldipine) Cyclosporine Estrogen and oral contraceptives Certain HMG-CoA reductase inhibitors (such as atorvastatin, lovastatin, and simvastatin)	Grapefruit juice	Grapefruit juice inhibits enzymes involved in drug metabolism and thereby intensifies the effect of certain drugs, many of which are not listed here
Digoxin	Oatmeal	The fiber in oatmeal and other cereals, when consumed in large amounts, can interfere with the absorption of digoxin
MAO inhibitors (such as phenelzine and tranylcypromine)	Foods high in tyramine, including many cheeses (such as American processed, cheddar, blue, brie, mozzarella, and Parmesan), yogurt, sour cream, cured meats (such as sausage and salami), liver, dried fish, caviar, avocados, bananas, yeast extracts, raisins, sauerkraut, soy sauce, fava beans, red wine, beer, and products containing caffeine	Severe headache and a potentially fatal increase in blood pressure (hypertensive crisis) can occur if people taking an MAO inhibitor (used most often to treat depression) consume these foods. These foods must be avoided
Tetracycline	Calcium or foods containing calcium, such as milk and other dairy products	These foods can reduce the absorption of tetracycline, which should be taken 1 hour before or 2 hours after eating

Dietary supplements, including medicinal herbs, are products (besides tobacco) that contain a vitamin, mineral, herb, or amino acid and that are intended as a supplement to the normal diet.▲ They are regulated as foods. However, they may interact with prescription or over-the-counter drugs.■ People who take dietary supplements should tell their doctors and pharmacists, so that interactions can be avoided.

Drug-Food Interactions

Drug-food interactions are changes in a drug's effects caused by food (including beverages) consumed during the same time period.

Like food, drugs taken by mouth must be absorbed through the lining of the stomach or the small intestine. Consequently, the presence of food in the digestive tract may reduce absorption of a drug. Often, such interactions can be avoided by taking the drug 1 hour before or 2 hours after eating.

Drug-Disease Interactions

Drug-disease interactions refer to the worsening of a disease by a drug.

Most drugs exert most of their effects on a specific organ or system; however, because most drugs circulate throughout the body, they may also affect other organs and systems. A drug taken for a lung disease may affect the heart, and a drug taken to treat a cold may affect the eyes. Because drugs can affect diseases other than the one being treated, people should tell their doctor all of the diseases they have before the doctor prescribes a new drug. Diabetes, high or low blood pressure, glaucoma, an enlarged prostate, poor bladder control, and insomnia are particularly important, because people with such diseases are more likely to have a drug-disease interaction.

Drug-disease interactions can occur in any age group but are common among older people, who tend to have more diseases.★

Tolerance and Resistance

Tolerance is a person's diminished response to a drug, which occurs when the drug is used repeatedly and the body adapts to the continued presence of the drug. Resistance refers to the ability of microorganisms or cancer cells to withstand the effects of a drug usually effective against them.

A person may develop tolerance to a drug when the drug is used repeatedly. For instance, when morphine or alcohol is used for a long time, larger and larger doses must be taken to produce the same effect. Usually, tolerance develops because metabolism of the drug speeds up (often because the liver enzymes involved in metabolizing drugs become more active) and because the number of sites (cell receptors) that the drug attaches to or the strength of the bond (affinity) between the receptor and drug decreases.●

Strains of microorganisms (bacteria or viruses) are said to develop resistance when they are no longer killed or inhibited by the drugs that are usually effective against them. In bacteria, these strains develop when bacteria mutate or when resistant genes are transferred from one bacterium to another.◆ Cancer cells may develop resistance when they mutate.

Depending on the degree of tolerance or resistance that develops, doctors may increase the dose or use a different drug.

▲ see page 103   ■ see table on page 104

★ see page 79   ● see page 70

◆ see page 1121

CHAPTER 14

Drugs and Aging

Older people tend to take more drugs than younger people because they are more likely to have several, often chronic disorders. On average, an older person takes four or five prescription drugs and two over-the-counter drugs each day. Also, older people are more than twice as susceptible to side effects of drugs as younger people.▲ Side effects are also likely to be more severe, affecting quality of life and resulting in visits to the doctor and in hospitalization.

As people age, the amount of water in the body decreases and the amount of fat tissue relative to water increases. Thus, in older people, drugs that dissolve in water reach higher concentrations because there is less water to dilute them, and drugs that dissolve in fat accumulate more because there is relatively

Anticholinergic: What Does It Mean?

Anticholinergic effects are caused by drugs that block the action of acetylcholine. Acetylcholine is a neurotransmitter—a chemical messenger released by a nerve cell to transmit a nerve signal to a neighboring nerve cell or a target cell in a muscle or gland. Acetylcholine stimulates smooth (involuntary) muscle cells, such as those in the heart or airways, to contract. Many commonly used drugs have anticholinergic effects. Most of these drugs were not designed to produce these effects, which are therefore usually considered undesirable side effects. Anticholinergic effects include confusion, blurred vision, constipation, dry mouth, light-headedness, and difficulty with urination or loss of bladder control. However, anticholinergic drugs can also, for example, reduce tremors and nausea—both useful effects.

Older people are more likely to experience anticholinergic effects because the amount of acetylcholine in the body decreases with age. Consequently, anticholinergic drugs block a higher percentage of acetylcholine. Also, the aging body is less able to use what little acetylcholine is present.

more fat tissue to store them. Also, as people age, the kidneys are less able to excrete drugs into the urine, and the liver is less able to metabolize many drugs.■ Because of all these age-related changes, many drugs tend to stay in an older person's body much longer than they would in a younger person's body, prolonging the drug's effect and increasing the risk of side effects. For these reasons, older people need to take smaller doses of certain drugs or perhaps fewer daily doses. Also, other, safer drugs can often be substituted.

Older people are more sensitive to the effects of many drugs. For example, older people tend to become sleepier and are more likely to become confused when using sleep aids or antianxiety drugs. Drugs that lower blood pressure by widening (dilating) arteries and reducing the amount of work the heart has to do tend to lower the pressure much more dramatically in older people than in the young.

Many commonly used drugs, such as some antidepressants and diphenhydramine (used in the treatment of insomnia), have anticholinergic effects. Older people are particularly susceptible to these effects, which include confusion, blurred vision, constipation, dry mouth, light-headedness, and difficulty with urination or loss of bladder control. Some anticholinergic effects, such as reduction of tremor (as in the treatment of Parkinson's disease) and reduction of nausea, are desirable, but most are not.

Drugs may produce a side effect because of interaction between the drug and a disease other than the one for which the drug is being taken (drug-disease interaction) or between the drug and another drug (drug-drug interaction), food (drug-food interaction), or a medicinal herb (drug–medicinal herb interaction).★ Because older people tend to have more diseases and to take more drugs than younger people, they are more likely to have drug-disease and drug-drug interactions. Patients, doctors, and pharmacists can take steps to reduce the risk of these interactions.●

▲ see page 82   ■ see page 68

★ see table on page 104   ● see box on page 76

SOME DRUGS WITH INCREASED RISK FOR OLDER PEOPLE

TYPE	DRUG	PROBLEM
Analgesics	Indomethacin	Of all the nonsteroidal anti-inflammatory drugs, indomethacin affects the brain the most. It sometimes causes confusion or dizziness.
	Meperidine	Meperidine, an opioid, is a strong analgesic when injected. But it is not very effective when taken orally and often causes confusion.
	Pentazocine	Pentazocine, an opioid, is more likely to cause confusion and hallucinations than are other opioids.
	Propoxyphene	Propoxyphene, an opioid, offers no more pain relief than acetaminophen. Like other opioids, it may be addictive and has such side effects as constipation, drowsiness, confusion, and (rarely) slowed breathing.
Antidepressants	Amitriptyline Doxepin	Because amitriptyline and doxepin have strong anticholinergic and sedating effects, they are usually not good choices for older people.
Antidiabetic drugs	Chlorpropamide	This drug has long-lasting effects, which are exaggerated in older people. It can lower blood sugar levels (hypoglycemia) for several hours. Chlorpropamide can also lower the level of sodium in the blood.
Antiemetic drugs (drugs used to manage nausea)	Trimethobenzamide	This drug is one of the least effective drugs for managing nausea. It can produce side effects, including abnormal movements of the arms, legs, and other parts of the body.
Antihistamines	Chlorpheniramine Cyroheptadine Dexchlorpheni- ramine Diphenhydramine Hydroxyzine Promethazine Tripelennamine Some combination cold remedies	All nonprescription and many prescription antihistamines have strong anticholinergic effects. Although sometimes helpful for managing allergic reactions and seasonal allergies, antihistamines are generally not appropriate for a runny nose and other symptoms of a viral infection in older people. When antihistamines are needed, those without anticholinergic effects (such as loratadine and astemizole) are preferable. Cough and cold remedies that do not include antihistamines are generally safer for older people. Older people should avoid taking sleep aids containing diphenhydramine.
Antihyperten- sives	Methyldopa	Methyldopa, alone or in combination with other drugs, may slow the heart rate and worsen depression.
	Reserpine	Most experts in geriatric medicine believe that reserpine is risky because it can produce dizziness when a person stands up, depression, erectile dysfunction, and drowsiness.
Antipsychotic drugs	Chlorpromazine Haloperidol Thioridazine Thiothixene	Although antipsychotics are effective in treating psychotic disorders, their effectiveness in treating behavioral disturbances associated with dementia (such as agitation, wandering, repeated questioning, noisiness, throwing, and hitting) has not been established. These drugs are commonly toxic, producing drowsiness, movement disorders, and anticholinergic effects. Generally, older people should take antipsychotics in small doses, if at all. The need for treatment should be reassessed often, and the drugs should be discontinued as soon as possible.

SOME DRUGS WITH INCREASED RISK FOR OLDER PEOPLE *(Cont'd)*

TYPE	DRUG	PROBLEM
Gastrointestinal antispasmodic drugs (drugs used to manage stomach cramps and pain)	Belladonna alkaloids Clidinium-chlordiazepoxide Dicyclomine Hyoscyamine Propantheline	Gastrointestinal antispasmodics are highly anticholinergic, and their usefulness—especially at the low doses tolerated by older people—is questionable.
Heart drugs	Digoxin	Small doses should be used because as people age, the kidneys are less able to excrete digoxin.
	Disopyramide	Disopyramide, a drug used to treat abnormal heart rhythms (antiarrhythmic drug), has strong anticholinergic effects and may cause heart failure in older people.
Histamine-2 (H_2) blockers	Cimetidine Famotidine Nizatidine Ranitidine	Typical doses of some H_2 blockers—especially cimetidine but, to some extent, famotidine, nizatidine, and ranitidine—may produce side effects, especially confusion.
Iron supplements	Ferrous sulfate	Doses greater than 325 milligrams daily do not greatly improve absorption of iron and are much more likely to cause constipation.
Muscle relaxants–antispasmodics	Carisoprodol Chlorzoxazone Cyclobenzaprine Metaxalone Methocarbamol Oxybutynin	Most muscle relaxant–antispasmodics have anticholinergic effects and cause drowsiness and weakness. The usefulness of all muscle relaxant–antispasmodics at the low doses tolerated by older people is questionable.
Sedatives, antianxiety drugs, and sleep aids	Barbiturates, such as phenobarbital and secobarbital	Barbiturates have more side effects than other drugs used to treat anxiety and insomnia. They also interact with many other drugs. Generally, older people should not take barbiturates, except to treat seizure disorders.
	Chlordiazepoxide Diazepam Flurazepam Nitrazepam	These drugs are benzodiazepines used to treat anxiety and insomnia. They have very long-lasting effects (often more than 96 hours) in older people. Alone or in combination with other drugs, these drugs can cause prolonged drowsiness and increase the risk of falls and fractures. Shorter-acting benzodiazepines, such as alprazolam and lorazepam, are generally much more appropriate for older people.
	Meprobamate	This drug offers no advantages over benzodiazepines and has many disadvantages. It is very addictive and sedating.

Not following a doctor's directions for taking a drug (noncompliance or nonadherence) can be risky.▲ Old age alone does not make a person less likely to take drugs as directed; however, 40% of older people do not do so. Not taking a drug, taking too little, or taking too much can cause problems. Taking less of a drug because it causes side effects may seem reasonable, but people should talk to a doctor before they make any changes in the way they take a drug.

▲ see page 86

CHAPTER 15

Adverse Drug Reactions

In the early 1900s, the German scientist Paul Ehrlich described an ideal drug as a "magic bullet"; such a drug would be aimed precisely at a disease site and would not harm healthy tissues. Although many new drugs are aimed more accurately than their predecessors, none of them, as of yet, hit the target precisely.

Most drugs produce several effects, but usually only one effect—the therapeutic effect—is wanted for the treatment of a disorder. The other effects may be regarded as unwanted, whether they are intrinsically harmful or not. For example, certain antihistamines cause drowsiness as well as control the symptoms of allergies. When an over-the-counter sleep aid containing an antihistamine is taken, drowsiness is considered a therapeutic effect. But when an antihistamine is taken to control allergy symptoms during the daytime, drowsiness is considered an annoying, unwanted effect.

Most people, including health care practitioners, refer to unwanted effects as side effects; another term used is adverse drug event. However, the term *adverse drug reaction* is technically more appropriate for drug effects that are unwanted, unpleasant, noxious, or potentially harmful.

Not surprisingly, adverse drug reactions are common. Most adverse drug reactions are relatively mild, and many disappear when the drug is stopped or the dose is changed. Some gradually subside as the body adjusts to the drug. Other adverse drug reactions are more serious and last longer. Between 3% and 7% of hospital admissions in the United States are estimated to be for treatment of adverse drug reactions. Each time a person is hospitalized, the risk of having at least one adverse drug reaction is 10 to 20%.

Digestive disturbances—loss of appetite, nausea, a bloating sensation, constipation, and diarrhea—are particularly common adverse drug reactions, because most drugs are taken by mouth and pass through the digestive tract.

However, almost any organ system can be affected. In older people, the brain is commonly affected, often resulting in drowsiness and confusion.

Types of Adverse Drug Reactions

Many adverse drug reactions represent an exaggeration of the drug's therapeutic effects (called type 1 or overdose reactions). For example, a person taking a drug to reduce high blood pressure may feel dizzy or light-headed if the drug reduces blood pressure too much. A person with diabetes may develop weakness, sweating, nausea, and palpitations if insulin or an oral antidiabetic drug reduces the blood sugar level too much. This type of adverse drug reaction is usually predictable but sometimes unavoidable. It may occur if a drug dose is too high, if the person is unusually sensitive to the drug, or if another drug slows the metabolism of the first drug and thus increases its level in the blood.▲ Type 1 reactions are usually not serious but are relatively common.

Some adverse drug reactions result from mechanisms that are not currently understood (called type 2 or idiosyncratic reactions). This type of adverse drug reaction is largely unpredictable. Examples of such adverse drug reactions include skin rashes, jaundice, anemia, a decrease in the white blood cell count, kidney damage, and nerve injury that may impair vision or hearing. These reactions tend to be more serious but typically occur in a very small number of people. Such people may be allergic or hypersensitive to the drug because of genetic differences in the way their body metabolizes or responds to drugs.

Some adverse drug reactions are not related to the drug's therapeutic effect but are usually predictable, because the mechanisms involved are largely understood. For example, stomach irritation and bleeding often occur in people who regularly use aspirin or other nonsteroidal anti-inflammatory drugs (NSAIDs).■ The reason is that these drugs reduce the production of prostaglandins, which help protect the digestive tract from stomach acid.

▲ see page 75   ■ see page 452

Severity of Adverse Drug Reactions

There is no universal scale for describing or measuring the severity of an adverse drug reaction. Assessment is largely subjective. Reactions can be described as mild, moderate, or severe.

Reactions usually described as mild and of minor significance include digestive disturbances, headaches, fatigue, vague muscle aches, malaise (a general feeling of illness or discomfort), and changes in sleep patterns.

However, such reactions can be very distressing to people who experience them. As a result, people may be less willing to take their drug as instructed, and the goals of treatment may not be achieved.

Reactions that are usually described as mild are considered moderate if the person experiencing them considers them distinctly annoying, distressing, or intolerable. Other moderate reactions include skin rashes (especially if they are extensive and persistent), visual disturbances (especially in people who wear correc-

SOME SERIOUS ADVERSE DRUG REACTIONS

ADVERSE DRUG REACTION	TYPES OF DRUGS	EXAMPLES
Peptic ulcers or bleeding from the stomach	Corticosteroids taken by mouth or by injection (not those applied to the skin in creams or lotions)	Hydrocortisone Prednisone
	Nonsteroidal anti-inflammatory drugs	Aspirin Ibuprofen Ketoprofen Naproxen
	Anticoagulants	Heparin Warfarin
Anemia (resulting from a decreased production or increased destruction of red blood cells)	Certain antibiotics	Chloramphenicol
	Some nonsteroidal anti-inflammatory drugs	Phenylbutazone (not available in the United States)
	Antimalarial and antituberculous drugs in people with G6PD enzyme deficiency	Chloroquine Isoniazid Primaquine
Decreased production of white blood cells, with increased risk of infection	Certain antipsychotic drugs	Clozapine
	Chemotherapy drugs	Cyclophosphamide Mercaptopurine Methotrexate Vinblastine
	Some drugs used to treat thyroid disorders	Propylthiouracil
Liver damage	Some analgesics	Acetaminophen (use of excessive doses)
	Some antituberculous drugs	Isoniazid
	Iron supplements (in excessive amounts)	
Kidney damage	Nonsteroidal anti-inflammatory drugs (repeated use of excessive doses)	Ibuprofen Ketoprofen Naproxen
	Aminoglycoside antibiotics	Gentamicin Kanamycin
	Some chemotherapy drugs	Cisplatin
Confusion and drowsiness	Sedatives, including many antihistamines	Diphenhydramine
	Antidepressants (especially in older people)	Amitriptyline Imipramine

tive lenses), muscle tremor, difficulty with urination (a common effect of many drugs in older men), any perceptible change in mood or mental function, and certain changes in blood components, such as a temporary, reversible decrease in the white blood cell count or in blood levels of some substances, such as glucose.

Mild or moderate adverse drug reactions do not necessarily mean that a drug must be discontinued, especially if no suitable alternative is available. However, doctors are likely to reevaluate the dose, frequency of administration (number of doses a day), and timing of doses (for example, before or after meals; in the morning or at bedtime). Other drugs may be used to control the adverse drug reaction (for example, a stool softener to relieve constipation).

Severe reactions include those that may be life threatening (such as liver failure or abnormal heart rhythms), that result in persistent or significant disability or hospitalization, and that cause a birth defect. Severe reactions are relatively rare. People who develop a severe reaction usually must stop using the drug and must be treated. However, doctors must sometimes continue administering high-risk drugs (for example, chemotherapy to patients with cancer or immunosuppressants to patients undergoing organ transplantation). Doctors use every possible means to control a severe adverse drug reaction.

Benefits Versus Risks

Every drug has the potential to do harm as well as good. When doctors consider prescribing a drug, they must weigh the possible risks against the expected benefits. Use of a drug is not justified unless the expected benefits outweigh the possible risks. Doctors must also consider the likely outcome of withholding the drug. Potential benefits and risks can never be determined with mathematical precision.

When assessing the benefits and risks of prescribing a drug, doctors consider the severity of the disorder being treated and the effect it is having on the patient's quality of life. For example, for relatively minor disorders—such as coughs and colds, muscle strains, or infrequent headaches—only a very low risk of adverse drug reactions is acceptable. For such symptoms, over-the-counter drugs are usually

effective and well tolerated. When used according to directions, over-the-counter drugs for treating minor disorders have a wide safety margin (the difference between the usual effective dose and the dose that produces severe adverse drug reactions). In contrast, for serious or life-threatening disorders (such as a heart attack, stroke, cancer, or organ transplant rejection), a higher risk of a severe adverse drug reaction is usually acceptable.

Risk Factors

Many factors can increase the likelihood of an adverse drug reaction. They include the simultaneous use of several drugs, very young or old age, pregnancy, and breastfeeding. Hereditary factors make some people more susceptible to the toxic effects of certain drugs. Certain diseases can alter drug absorption, metabolism, and elimination and the body's response to drugs,▲ increasing the risk of adverse drug reactions. How mind-body interactions, such as mental attitude, outlook, belief in self, and confidence in health care practitioners, influence adverse drug reactions remains largely unexplored.

Use of Several Drugs

Taking several drugs, whether prescription or over-the-counter, contributes to the risk of having an adverse drug reaction. The number and severity of adverse drug reactions increase disproportionately as the number of drugs taken increases. The use of alcohol, which is technically a drug, also increases the risk. Asking a doctor or pharmacist to periodically review all the drugs a person is taking and to make appropriate adjustments can reduce the risk of an adverse drug reaction.

Age

Infants and very young children are at high risk of adverse drug reactions because their capacity to metabolize drugs is not fully developed. For example, newborns cannot metabolize and eliminate the antibiotic chloramphenicol; newborns who are given the drug may develop gray baby syndrome, a serious and often fatal reaction. If tetracycline, another antibiotic, is given to infants and young children during the period when their teeth are being formed (up to about age 8), it may permanently discolor tooth enamel. Children under age 18 are at risk of Reye's syndrome if they are given aspirin while they have influenza or chickenpox.

▲ see page 78

Older people are at high risk of having an adverse drug reaction for several reasons.▲ They are likely to have many health problems and thus to be taking several prescription and over-the-counter drugs. Also, as people age, the liver is less able to metabolize many drugs,■ and the kidneys are less able to eliminate drugs from the body, increasing the risk of kidney damage by a drug and other adverse drug reactions. These age-related problems are often made worse by malnourishment and dehydration, which tend to become more common as people age.

Older people are also more sensitive to the effects of many drugs. For example, older people are more likely to experience light-headedness, confusion, and impaired coordination, putting them at risk of falling and fracturing a bone. Drugs that can cause these reactions include many antihistamines, sleep aids, antianxiety drugs, antihypertensives, and antidepressants.★

Pregnancy and Breastfeeding

Many drugs—for example, antihypertensive drugs such as angiotensin-converting enzyme (ACE) inhibitors and angiotensin II receptor blockers—pose a risk to the health and normal development of a fetus. To the extent possible, pregnant women should not take any drugs, especially during the first trimester.● However, for some drugs, including ACE inhibitors and angiotensin II receptor blockers, risk is greatest during the last trimester of pregnancy. Use of any prescription drugs, over-the-counter drugs, and dietary supplements (including medicinal herbs) during pregnancy requires a doctor's supervision. Social drugs (alcohol and nicotine) and illicit drugs (cocaine and opioids such as heroin) also pose risks to the pregnancy and the fetus.

Drugs and medicinal herbs may be transmitted through breast milk to a baby.◆ Some drugs should not be taken by women who are breastfeeding; others can be taken but require a doctor's supervision. Some drugs do not usually harm the breastfed baby. However, women who are breastfeeding should consult with a health care practitioner before they take any drugs. Social and illicit drugs may harm a breastfeeding baby.

Drug Allergies

Allergic (hypersensitivity) reactions to a drug are relatively uncommon. In contrast to other types of adverse drug reactions, the number and severity of allergic reactions do not usually correlate with the amount of drug taken. For people who are allergic to a drug, even a small amount of the drug can trigger an allergic reaction. These reactions range from minor and simply annoying to severe and life threatening.▼ Examples are skin rashes and itching; fever; constriction of the airways and wheezing; swelling of tissues (such as the larynx and glottis), which impairs breathing; and a fall in blood pressure, sometimes to dangerously low levels.

Drug allergies cannot be anticipated, because reactions occur after a person has been previously exposed to the drug (whether it was applied to the skin, taken by mouth, or injected) one or more times without any allergic reaction. A mild reaction may be treated with an antihistamine; a severe or life-threatening reaction may require an injection of epinephrine (also called adrenaline) or a corticosteroid, such as hydrocortisone.

Before prescribing a new drug, doctors usually ask if a person has any known drug allergies. People who have had severe allergic reactions should wear a Medic Alert necklace or bracelet inscribed with their drug allergies. This information (for example, penicillin allergy) can alert medical and paramedical personnel in case of an emergency.

Overdose Toxicity

Overdose toxicity refers to serious, often harmful, and sometimes fatal toxic reactions to an accidental overdose of a drug (because of a doctor's, pharmacist's, or patient's error) or to an intentional overdose (homicide or suicide).

A lower risk of overdose toxicity is often the reason doctors prefer one drug to another when both drugs are equally effective. For example, if a sedative, antianxiety drug, or sleep aid is needed, doctors usually prescribe benzodiazepines, such as diazepam and temazepam, rather than barbiturates, such as pentobarbital. Benzodiazepines are not more effective than barbiturates, but they have a wider margin of safety and are much less likely to cause severe toxicity in case of an accidental or intentional overdose. Safety is also the reason that newer

---

▲ see also page 79	■ see page 68
★ see table on page 80	● see table on page 1460
◆ see box on page 1462	
▼ see page 1063	

antidepressants, such as fluoxetine and paroxetine, have largely replaced older but equally effective antidepressants, such as imipramine and amitriptyline.▲

Young children are at high risk of overdose toxicity. Brightly colored tablets and capsules, most of which are adult-dose formulations, can attract the attention of toddlers and young children. In the United States, federal regulations require that all prescription drugs taken by mouth be dispensed in childproof containers unless a person signs a waiver to the effect that such a container presents a handicap.

Most metropolitan areas in the United States have poison control centers that provide information about chemical and drug poisoning, and most telephone directories list the number of the local center. This number should be copied and placed near a telephone or programmed into an automatic dialing telephone.

CHAPTER 16

Compliance With Drug Treatment

Compliance is the degree to which a person takes prescribed drugs as directed.

Compliance with (adherence to) drug treatment is important. However, only about half the people who leave a doctor's office with a prescription take the drug as directed. Among the many reasons people give for not complying with drug treatment, forgetfulness is the most common. The key question then is: Why do people forget? Often, the psychologic mechanism of denial is at work. Having a disorder causes concern, and having to take a drug is a constant reminder of the disorder. Or, something about the treatment, such as possible side effects, may greatly concern the person, resulting in a reluctance to follow the plan.

Results of Not Complying

Most obviously, if a person does not comply, symptoms may not be relieved or the disorder may not be cured. However, not complying may have other serious or costly consequences. It is estimated to result in 125,000 deaths due to cardiovascular disease (such as heart attack and stroke) each year. In addition, up to 23% of nursing home admissions, 10% of hospital admissions, and many doctor visits, diagnostic tests, and unnecessary treatments could be avoided if people took their drugs as directed.

Not only does not complying add to the cost of medical care, but it can also worsen the quality of life. For example, missed doses can lead to optic nerve damage and blindness in people with glaucoma, to an erratic heart rhythm and cardiac arrest in people with heart disease, and to stroke in people with high blood pressure. Not taking all prescribed doses of an antibiotic can cause an infection to flare up again and may contribute to the emergence of drug-resistant bacteria.

Compliance Among Children

Children are less likely than adults to take or be given drugs as directed. In a study of children who had streptococcal infections and for whom a 10-day course of penicillin was prescribed, 56% were not taking the drug by the third day, 71% by the sixth day, and 82% by the ninth day. For children with chronic diseases such as type 1 diabetes or asthma, compliance is difficult to achieve because their treatment plan is complex and must be continued for a long time.

Sometimes parents do not understand a doctor's instructions. Also, parents (and patients) forget, on average, about half the information 15 minutes after meeting with a doctor. They remember the first third of the discussion best and remember more about diagnosis than about the details of treatment. That is why pediatricians try to keep the treatment plan simple and often provide written instructions.

▲ see table on page 618

Compliance Among Older People

Although compliance is probably not affected by old age itself, it is affected by several factors that are common among older people, such as physical or mental impairments, the use of more drugs, and an increased risk of drug-drug interactions and side effects. Taking several drugs makes remembering when to take each drug harder and increases the risk of adverse drug-drug interactions,▲ particularly when over-the-counter drugs are also being taken. Doctors may be able to simplify the drug regimen—by using one drug that serves two purposes or by reducing the number of times a drug must be taken—to improve compliance and to reduce the risk of interactions.

Because older people are generally more sensitive to drugs than younger people, they are more likely to have adverse drug reactions and may require a lower dose of certain drugs.■

Ways to Improve Compliance

People are more likely to comply if they have a good relationship with their doctor and pharmacist. Such relationships involve two-way communication.

Communication can start with an information exchange. By asking questions, people can come to terms with the severity of their disorder, intelligently weigh the advantages and disadvantages of a treatment plan, and ensure that they understand their situation correctly. By discussing concerns, people can learn that denial of their disorder and misconceptions about their treatment can lead to forgetting to take drugs as directed, resulting in unwanted effects. Doctors and pharmacists can encourage compliance by providing clear explanations about how to take the drugs, why the drugs are necessary, and what to expect during treatment. When people know what to expect from a drug, good and bad, they and the health care practitioners involved in their care can better judge how well the drug is working and whether potentially serious problems are developing. Written instructions help people avoid mistakes caused by poor recall of their discussions with the doctor and pharmacist.

Good communication is important when people have more than one health care practitioner because it ensures that all practitioners know all the drugs prescribed by the others, and an integrated treatment plan can be devel-

Reasons for Not Complying with Drug Treatment

- Forgetting to take the drug
- Not understanding or misinterpreting the instructions
- Experiencing side effects (the treatment may be perceived as worse than the disorder)
- Denying the disorder (repressing the diagnosis or its significance)
- Not believing that the drug can help
- Mistakenly believing that the disorder has been sufficiently treated (for example, thinking an infection is over just because the fever disappears)
- Fearing adverse consequences from or dependence on the drug
- Worrying about the expense
- Not caring (being apathetic) about getting better
- Encountering obstacles (for example, having difficulty swallowing tablets or capsules, having problems opening bottles, considering treatment inconvenient, and being unable to obtain the drug)

oped. Such a plan can help reduce the number of side effects and drug-drug interactions and possibly result in a simpler drug regimen.

When people participate in decisions about their treatment plan, they are more likely to comply. By participating, people take responsibility for the plan and are therefore more likely to follow it. Taking responsibility includes helping monitor the good and bad effects of treatment and discussing concerns with at least one of their health care practitioners—doctor, physician assistant, pharmacist, or nurse. People should report unwanted or unexpected effects to a health care practitioner rather than adjust a drug dose or discontinue a drug on their own. When a person has good reasons for not following a plan and explains them, the doctor or other health care practitioner can usually make an appropriate adjustment.

People are also more likely to comply if they believe that their health care practitioner cares whether or not they follow the plan. People who receive explanations from a concerned practitioner are more likely to be satis-

---

▲ see page 75   ■ see page 79

fied with the care they receive and to like the practitioner more; the more they like the practitioner, the more likely they are to comply.

Obtaining all drugs from one pharmacist can also help, because pharmacists keep computerized records of the drugs a person is taking and can monitor them for possible duplication and for drug-drug interactions. People taking prescription drugs should inform their pharmacist about what over-the-counter drugs and dietary supplements (such as medicinal herbs) they are taking. Also, people can ask the pharmacist about what to expect from a drug, how to take it correctly, and which drugs interact with each other.

Support groups for people with particular disorders are often available. These groups can often reinforce the importance of following a treatment plan and provide suggestions for coping with problems. Names and telephone numbers of support groups can be obtained through local hospitals and community councils.▲

Memory aids can help people remember to take their drugs. For example, reminder cards can be placed in different areas of the home, or taking a drug can be associated with a specific daily task, such as brushing the teeth. A wristwatch that beeps can be used as a reminder of when to take a drug. A health care practitioner or the person can mark the drug dose and the time of day to take it on a calendar; when the drug is taken, the person checks the appropriate space.

A pharmacist can provide containers that help people take drugs as instructed. Daily doses for a month may be packaged in a blister pack marked with calendar days, so that people can keep track of doses taken by noting the empty spaces. Caps or stickers the same color as the tablet or capsule can be placed on each container to help people match the drug to the instructions on the container. Multicompartment boxes or trays that contain compartments for each day of the week and/or for different times of each day can be used. The person or caregiver fills the compartments on a regular basis, such as at the beginning of each week. By looking at the box, the person can determine whether the pills have been taken.

Containers with a computerized cap are available. These caps beep or flash at dosing time and can record how many times a container is opened each day and how many hours since the container was last opened. Another alternative is a paging service with a beeper (available from subscriber-based telecommunications companies).

CHAPTER 17

Trade-Name and Generic Drugs

Drugs often have several names. When a drug is first discovered, it is given a chemical name, which describes the atomic or molecular structure of the drug. The chemical name is thus usually too complex and cumbersome for general use. Next, a shorthand version of the chemical name or a code name (such as RU 486) is developed for easy reference among researchers.

When a drug is approved by the Food and Drug Administration (FDA—the government agency responsible for ensuring that drugs marketed in the United States are safe and effective), it is given a generic (official) name and a trade (proprietary or brand) name. The trade name identifies it as the exclusive property of a particular company. For example, phenytoin is the generic name and Dilantin is the trade name for the same drug.

In the United States, an official body—the United States Adopted Names (USAN) Council assigns the generic name. The company that manufactures the drug chooses the trade name. Generic and trade names must be unique to prevent one drug from being mistaken for another when drugs are prescribed and prescriptions are filled. To prevent this

---

▲ see also page 1732

WHAT'S IN A NAME?

CHEMICAL NAME	GENERIC NAME	TRADE NAME
N-(4-hydroxyphenyl) acetamide	Acetaminophen	Tylenol
7-chloro-1,3-dihydro-1-methyl-5-phenyl-2H-1,4-benzodi-azepin-2-one	Diazepam	Valium
4-[4-(p-chlorophenyl)-4-hydroxypiperidino]-4'-fluorobuty-rophenone	Haloperidol	Haldol
5-thia-1-azabicyclo [4.2.0]-oct-2-ene-2 carboxylic acid, 7-[(aminophenylacetyl)amino]-3-methyl-8-oxo-, mono-hydrate	Cephalexin	Keflex, Keforal, Keftabs
DL-threo-2-(methylamino)-1-phenylpropan-1-ol	Pseudoephedrine	Sudafed
N''-cyano-N-methyl-N'-[2-[[(5-methyl-1H-imidazol-4-yl) methyl]thio]ethyl]guanidine	Cimetidine	Tagamet

possible confusion, the FDA must agree to every proposed trade name.

Government officials, doctors, researchers, and others who write about the new compound use the drug's generic name because it refers to the drug itself, not to a particular company's brand of the drug or a specific product. However, doctors usually use the trade name on prescriptions, because it is easier to remember and doctors usually learn about new drugs by the trade name.

Generic names are usually more complicated and harder to remember than trade names. Many generic names are a shorthand for the drug's chemical name, structure, or formula. In contrast, trade names are usually catchy, often related to their intended use, and relatively easy to remember, so that doctors will prescribe the drug and consumers will look for it by name. Trade names often suggest a characteristic of the drug. For example, Lopressor lowers blood pressure, Vivactil is an antidepressant that might make a person more vivacious, Glucotrol lowers high blood sugar (glucose) levels, and Skelaxin relaxes skeletal muscles. Sometimes, the trade name is simply a shortened version of the drug's generic name—for example, Minocin for minocycline.

The term *generic*, when applied to such items as foods and household products, is used to describe a less expensive, sometimes less effective or lower-quality copycat version of a brand-name product. However, most generic drugs, although usually less expensive, are generally as effective and of the same quality as the brand-name drug.

Patent Protection

In the United States, a company that develops a new drug can be granted a patent for the drug itself, for the way the drug is made, for the way the drug is to be used, and even for the method of delivering and releasing the drug into the bloodstream. Thus, a company often owns more than one patent for a drug. Patents grant the company exclusive rights to a drug for 20 years. Additional patents can sometimes be filed to extend the patent life. Usually, about 10 years elapse between the time a drug is discovered (when the patent is obtained) and the time the drug is approved for human or veterinary use, leaving the company only about half of the patent time to exclusively market a new drug. (The FDA often accelerates the approval of drugs to treat AIDS, cancer, and other life-threatening disorders for which no current treatment exists.)

After a patent has expired, other companies may produce and sell a generic version of the drug, typically at a much lower price than the original trade-name drug. (However, before generic drugs can be marketed, they must be approved by the FDA.) A generic drug may be sold under its generic name or under a trade name (a branded generic drug) but not under the trade name used by the original patentholder.

Not all off-patent drugs have generic versions; sometimes a drug is too hard to duplicate, or adequate tests are not available to prove that the generic drug acts the same as the trade-name drug. Sometimes the market

WHEN GENERIC SUBSTITUTION MAY NOT BE APPROPRIATE

DRUG CATEGORY	EXAMPLES	COMMENTS
Drugs on the market before the 1938 Federal Food, Drug, and Cosmetic Act	Digoxin and other digitalis derivatives (for heart failure); thyroid hormone replacement products	Pre-1938 drugs are exempt from generic drug requirements, but only a few of these drugs are still prescribed. Switching among different versions is unwise because no standards are available by which to compare these drugs.
Drugs with little difference between a toxic dose and an effective dose (a narrow margin of safety)	Anticonvulsants such as phenytoin, carbamazepine, and valproate; digoxin (for heart failure); and the anticoagulant warfarin	The margin of safety is relatively small; too little drug may not work, and too much drug may cause side effects.
Antihypertensive drugs	Hydralazine, reserpine, reserpine plus hydrochlorothiazide, and reserpine plus hydroflumethiazide	Generic versions are not bioequivalent to trade-name drugs.
Antiasthmatic drugs taken by mouth	Theophylline, dyphylline, and some brands of aminophylline	Versions are generally not bioequivalent. If one version is effective, it should not be interchanged for another unless absolutely necessary.
Aerosol drugs, especially antiasthmatic drugs	Metaproterenol and terbutaline (widely used bronchodilators) and some aerosol corticosteroid preparations	Any of the versions may be effective, but standards for comparing them are still under development.
Corticosteroid creams, lotions, and ointments	Alclometasone, amcinonide, betamethasone, clocortolone, desonide, desoximetasone, dexamethasone, diflorasone, fluocinolone, fluocinonide, flurandrenolide, fluticasone, halcinonide, halobetasol, hydrocortisone, mometasone, and triamcinolone	These products are standardized by tests of skin response, and many have been rated as bioequivalent by the FDA. But response can vary, and different drug vehicles (creams, ointments, gels) can have different effects. Response is so unpredictable that if one version is effective, it should not be interchanged for another.
Corticosteroid tablets	Dexamethasone and some brands of prednisone	Many generic versions are not bioequivalent to trade-name drugs and should not be freely interchanged for them.
Hormones	Esterified estrogen (estrogen replacement therapy in postmenopausal women), some brands of medroxyprogesterone, and most generic brands of methyltestosterone	The two brands of esterified estrogen are not bioequivalent. Hormones are usually taken in small doses, so differences in brands could produce major swings in response.
Antidiabetic drugs	Glyburide (for adult-onset diabetes)	One version of glyburide, Glynase, may not be interchanged for the other.
Drugs to control gout	Probenecid and colchicine	Generic versions are not bioequivalent to the trade-name version.
Antipsychotic drugs	Chlorpromazine tablets	Generic versions are not bioequivalent to the trade-name version.
Antidepressants	A few brands of amitriptyline and one brand of amitriptyline plus perphenazine	Not all versions are interchangeable. A pharmacist can advise whether the FDA considers a particular generic drug bioequivalent to the trade-name drug.

WHEN GENERIC SUBSTITUTION MAY NOT BE APPROPRIATE (Cont'd)

DRUG CATEGORY	EXAMPLES	COMMENTS
Potassium	Most long-acting potassium replacement products in tablet form	Long-acting potassium products in capsule (not tablet) form are considered bioequivalent and may be interchanged.
Other drugs	Disulfiram, fluoxymesterone, mazindol, nicotine patches, phenytoin (prompt), promethazine tablets and suppositories, rauwolfia serpentina, and trichlormethiazide	Generic versions are not bioequivalent. Although any version can be effective, versions should not be interchanged.

for the drug is so small that producing another version does not make good business sense.

Generic Drug Development

When a company decides to develop a generic version of a trade-name drug, the company's experts in drug formulation figure out how to design it. They must ensure that the generic version is bioequivalent (within a few percentage points) to the original drug, that appropriate inactive ingredients are used, and that the generic version differs from its trade-name counterpart in size, color, and shape—a legal requirement. The company must then seek the FDA's approval of the generic version.

Bioequivalence Studies: The company must conduct studies to determine whether the generic version is bioequivalent to the original drug—that is, whether the two drugs have virtually the same effect in humans. Bioequivalence testing involves determining whether the generic version releases its active ingredient (the drug) into the bloodstream at virtually the same speed and in virtually the same amounts as the original drug and whether the generic version produces virtually the same levels of drug in the blood over time. For bioequivalence testing, a relatively small number (24 to 36) of healthy volunteers can be used. In contrast, studies of new drugs are more complex and require a large number of participants (and thus are much more expensive), because these studies must prove that the drugs are safe and effective.▲

Inactive Ingredients: A generic version is likely to have some inactive ingredients that are different from those of the original drug. Inactive ingredients are added for specific rea-sons—for example, to provide bulk so that a tablet is large enough to handle, to keep a tablet from crumbling between the time it is manufactured and the time it is used, to help a tablet dissolve in the stomach or intestine, or to provide a pleasant taste and color. Usually, inactive ingredients are harmless substances that do not affect the body. However, because inactive ingredients can cause unusual and sometimes severe allergic reactions in a few people, one version, or brand, of a drug may be preferable to another. For example, bisulfites (such as sodium metabisulfite), which are used as preservatives in many products, cause asthmatic allergic reactions in many people. Consequently, drug products containing bisulfites are now prominently labeled as such.

Evaluation and Approval Procedures: The FDA evaluates every generic version of a drug. The FDA approves a generic drug if studies indicate that the original trade-name drug and the generic version are essentially bioequivalent. The FDA also makes sure that a new generic drug contains the appropriate amount of the active (drug) ingredient and that it is manufactured according to federal standards (Good Manufacturing Practices).

Bioequivalence and Interchangeability

Legally, bioequivalence of different versions of a drug can vary by up to 20%, because for most drugs, such variation does not noticeably alter effectiveness or safety. However, actual differences between FDA-approved generic

▲ see box on page 62

and trade-name drugs are generally much smaller than the allowable 20%. Actual differences are typically only about 3.5% on average and rarely exceed 10% in any single study of bioequivalence.

Bioequivalence must be proved for any new form of a drug. New forms include new dosage forms or strengths of an existing trade-name drug product and any other modified form that is developed, as well as new generic drugs. Sometimes the form that was originally tested is modified for commercial reasons. For example, tablets may need to be made sturdier, flavoring or coloring may be added or changed, or inactive ingredients may be changed to increase consumer acceptance.

Sometimes generic substitution is not appropriate. For example, some generic versions cannot be determined to be bioequivalent to the original drug because no standards for comparison have been established. These versions may not be interchanged freely for the original drug.

Drugs that must be given in very precise amounts are less likely to be interchangeable, because the difference between an effective dose and a harmful or an ineffective dose (the margin of safety) is small. Digoxin, used to treat people with heart failure, is an example. Switching from a trade-name version of digoxin to a generic version may cause problems, because the two versions may not be sufficiently bioequivalent. Pharmacists and doctors can answer questions about which generic drugs are interchangeable for their trade-name counterparts and which are not.

A book published by the FDA each year and updated periodically also provides guidance about which drugs are interchangeable. This book, *Approved Drug Products With Therapeutic Equivalence Evaluations* (also known as "the orange book" because it has a bright orange cover), is available to anyone but is intended for use by doctors and pharmacists.▲

Trade-Name or Generic Drug?

Theoretically, a generic drug that is bioequivalent to its trade-name counterpart may be interchanged for it in any prescription. At the pharmacy, a consumer can usually choose

between a trade-name drug and a bioequivalent generic version unless the doctor has written on the prescription that no substitution can be made. However, a consumer may have to take whichever generic version the pharmacist has decided to stock. If a doctor specifies a trade-name drug on the prescription and the consumer wants an equivalent generic version, the consumer or pharmacist can discuss the matter with the doctor, who may then authorize the dispensing of a generic product.

The consumer's choice may be limited by an insurance plan or a managed care organization, which may require that generic drugs be prescribed and dispensed whenever possible to save money. Most plans allow a consumer to select a more expensive trade-name product, but the consumer must pay the difference in cost.

State law may also limit the consumer's choice. In some states, the consumer has no say; if the doctor prescribes a generic drug, the pharmacist must dispense a generic drug. In other states, the consumer may insist on a trade-name drug even if the doctor and pharmacist recommend a generic drug.

The substitution of a generic drug can sometimes cause other problems for the consumer. A doctor may write a prescription for a trade-name product and discuss the trade-name product with the consumer. If a pharmacist dispenses an equivalent generic product and its label does not also list the trade-name product, the consumer may not know how the generic product relates to what the doctor prescribed. To prevent this confusion, many pharmacists also include the trade name on the label when a generic product is substituted.

Generic Nonprescription Drugs

Generic versions of some nonprescription (over-the-counter) drugs are often sold as house brands by drug chains or cooperatives, usually at a lower cost. These drugs are evaluated in the same way that generic prescription drugs are evaluated and must meet the same requirements.

Pharmacists can advise which generic over-the-counter drug products should be as effective as the original. However, a consumer may prefer one product to another because of appearance, taste, consistency, or other characteristics.

▲ see page 1732

CHAPTER 18

Over-the-Counter Drugs

Over-the-counter (OTC) drugs are drugs that are available without a prescription.

OTC drugs enable people to relieve many annoying symptoms and to cure some diseases simply and without the cost of seeing a doctor. However, safe use of these drugs requires knowledge, common sense, and responsibility.

Most OTC drugs—unlike health foods, dietary supplements (including medicinal herbs),▲ and complementary therapies■—have been studied scientifically and extensively. Also, some OTC drugs were originally available only by prescription. (Some OTC drugs, such as aspirin, have always been available without prescription.) After many years of use under prescription regulation, drugs with excellent safety records may be approved by the FDA for over-the-counter sale. The analgesic ibuprofen and the indigestion remedy famotidine are examples of such drugs. Often, the OTC version has a substantially lower amount of active ingredient in each tablet, capsule, or caplet than does the prescription drug. When establishing appropriate doses of OTC drugs, manufacturers and the FDA try to balance safety and effectiveness.

OTC drugs are not always better tolerated than similar prescription drugs. For example, the OTC sleep aid diphenhydramine is neither as effective nor as safe, especially for older people, as many prescription sleep aids.

Historical Background

At one time, most drugs were available without a prescription. Before the federal Food and Drug Administration (FDA) existed, just about anything could be put in a bottle and sold as a sure-fire cure. Alcohol, cocaine, marijuana, and opium were included in some OTC products without notification to users. The Food, Drug, and Cosmetic (FD&C) Act, enacted in 1938, gave the FDA some authority to issue regulations, but the act did not provide clear guidelines as to which drugs could be sold by prescription only and which could be sold over the counter.

An amendment to the FD&C Act in 1951 attempted to clarify the difference between OTC and prescription drugs and to deal with issues of drug safety. Prescription drugs were defined as compounds that could be habit forming, toxic, or unsafe for use except under a doctor's supervision. Anything else could be sold over the counter.

As noted by the FD&C Act of 1962, OTC drugs were required to be both effective and safe.★ However, determining effectiveness and safety can be difficult. What is effective for one person may not be for another, and any drug may cause unwanted side effects (also called adverse effects or adverse drug reactions).● There is no organized system for reporting the side effects of OTC drugs. Consequently, the FDA and drug manufacturers have virtually no way of knowing how common or serious the side effects are.

Safety Considerations

Safety is a major concern when the FDA considers reclassifying a prescription drug as OTC. All drugs have benefits and risks; some degree of risk has to be tolerated if people are to receive a drug's benefits. Defining an acceptable degree of risk is a judgment call.

Safety depends on using a drug properly. For OTC drugs, proper use often relies on consumer self-diagnosis, which leaves room for error. For example, most headaches are not dangerous, but in rare cases, a headache is an early warning of a brain tumor or hemorrhage. Similarly, what seems like severe heartburn may signal an impending heart attack. Ultimately, people must use common sense in determining when a symptom or ailment is minor and when it requires medical attention.

People who purchase OTC drugs should read and follow the instructions carefully. Because different formulations—such as immediate-release and controlled-release (slow-release) formulations—may have the same brand name, the label should be checked each

▲ see page 103   ■ see page 1704

★ see page 63   ● see page 82

Guidelines for Choosing and Using Over-the-Counter Drugs

- Make sure that the self-diagnosis is as accurate as possible. Do not assume the problem is "something that is going around."
- Choose a product because the ingredients are appropriate for the condition, not because the product has a familiar brand name.
- Choose a product with the fewest appropriate ingredients. Products that attempt to relieve every possible symptom are likely to expose people to unnecessary drugs, pose additional risks, and cost more.
- Read the label carefully to determine the correct dose and precautions, including what conditions would make the drug a poor choice.
- When in doubt, ask a pharmacist or doctor what the most appropriate ingredient or product is.
- Ask a pharmacist to check for potential interactions with other drugs being used.
- Ask a pharmacist to identify possible side effects.
- Do not take more than the recommended dose.
- Do not take an OTC drug longer than the maximum time suggested on the label. Stop taking the drug if symptoms worsen.
- Keep all drugs, including OTC drugs, out of the reach of children.

time a product is purchased, and the dosage should be noted. Assuming that the dosage is the same is not safe. Also, different formulations with the same brand name may have different ingredients, so checking the ingredients on the label is important. For example, there are more than a dozen different Tylenol formulations with a vast array of ingredients. Some Maalox products contain aluminum and magnesium hydroxides; others contain calcium carbonate. When selecting a product, people should read the label carefully to determine which product is most appropriate for their particular problem. Labels on OTC drugs, which are required by the FDA, can

help people understand what a drug's benefits and risks are as well as how to use the drug correctly.

Often, the labels of OTC drugs do not list the full range of possible side effects. As a result, many people assume that these drugs have few, if any, side effects. For example, the package insert for one analgesic cautions people not to take the drug for more than 10 days for pain. However, the possible serious side effects that can occur with long-term use (such as life-threatening bleeding from the digestive tract) are not mentioned—not on the box, bottle, or package insert. Consequently, people with chronic pain or inflammation may take the drug for a long time without realizing that such use could lead to serious problems.

Analgesics and Anti-Inflammatory Drugs

OTC pain relievers (analgesics) include aspirin and other salicylates (such as choline or magnesium salicylate), ibuprofen, ketoprofen, naproxen sodium, and acetaminophen.▲ These drugs are used to reduce fever as well as relieve various types and degrees of pain, including headaches, menstrual cramps, and arthritis pain. OTC analgesics are reasonably safe to take for short periods of time, but their labels caution against using them for more than 7 to 10 days to treat pain. A doctor should be consulted if symptoms worsen or do not go away.

All OTC nonsteroidal anti-inflammatory drugs (NSAIDs), which encompass all OTC analgesics except acetaminophen, may irritate the stomach's lining and cause digestive upset, ulcers, and bleeding in the digestive tract. Other side effects include damage to the kidneys. A few people have a severe allergic reaction (anaphylaxis) to NSAIDs, leading to hives, itching, and severe breathing problems. Shock■ may occur. Such a reaction requires immediate medical attention. People who are allergic to aspirin or another NSAID must not use any NSAID because severe reactions are possible.

ASPIRIN

The oldest and least expensive OTC analgesic is aspirin (acetylsalicylic acid). Aspirin may be combined with an antacid (in a buffered product) to diminish the direct irritating effects on the stomach. The antacid creates an alka-

▲ see also page 452   ■ see page 148

line environment that helps aspirin dissolve and may reduce the time aspirin is in contact with the stomach lining. However, buffered aspirin can also irritate the stomach, because aspirin reduces the production of prostaglandins, which help protect the stomach's lining, and buffering does not prevent this effect.

Enteric-coated aspirin is designed to pass through the stomach intact and dissolve in the small intestine, thus minimizing direct irritation. (Enteric refers to the small intestine.) However, coated aspirin may be absorbed erratically. Eating food is likely to delay stomach emptying, the absorption of enteric-coated aspirin, and therefore pain relief.

Children and teenagers who have or may have influenza or chickenpox must not take aspirin because they could develop Reye's syndrome.▲ Although rare, Reye's syndrome can have serious consequences, including death.

IBUPROFEN, KETOPROFEN, AND NAPROXEN SODIUM

Ibuprofen, ketoprofen, and naproxen sodium are all NSAIDs. Ibuprofen was reclassified from prescription to OTC in 1984, ketoprofen in 1995, and naproxen sodium in 1994. Prescription-strength formulations of these drugs contain a larger amount of active ingredient per dose than the OTC formulations and are thus generally more effective. For OTC naproxen sodium, dosing instructions caution people not to take more than 3 caplets (or tablets) in 24 hours unless a doctor directs them to do so. People older than 65 years are cautioned not to take more than 1 caplet every 12 hours unless a doctor directs them to do so.

ACETAMINOPHEN

Originally introduced in 1955 for children's fever and pain, acetaminophen (known in some countries as paracetamol) became available over the counter in 1960. Acetaminophen, which is not an NSAID, is roughly comparable to aspirin in its pain-relieving potential and fever-lowering action.

Although acetaminophen has almost no adverse effects on the stomach, taking large doses of acetaminophen for a long time may have some risks, including risk of liver damage.

Many OTC products, such as those for allergies, colds, cough, influenza, pain, and sinus problems, contain acetaminophen. To avoid overdosing, people should check drug labels carefully and not take several products containing acetaminophen simultaneously.

Considerations in Reclassifying a Drug as Over-the-Counter

Safety
- What harmful effects (including those from misuse) may the drug produce?
- Is the drug habit forming?
- Do the benefits of OTC status outweigh the risks?

Ease of diagnosis and treatment
- Can the average person self-diagnose the condition that calls for the drug?
- Can the average person treat the condition without the help of a doctor or other health care practitioner?

Labeling
- Can adequate directions for use be written?
- Can warnings against unsafe use be written?
- Can the average person understand the information on the label?

Adapted from Gilbertson, WE: "FDA's Review of OTC Drugs," in *Handbook of Nonprescription Drugs*, 10th edition, Washington, DC, American Pharmaceutical Association, 1993, page 29.

Cold Remedies

More than 100 viruses can cause the misery attributed to the common cold, and a cure remains elusive. Some experts say that a person can take nothing and the cold will disappear in about a week, or a person can take a drug and feel better in about 7 days. However, people spend billions of dollars every year trying to relieve cold symptoms. Children are especially likely to get colds and be given cold remedies, even though the effectiveness of such drugs for preschool children has not been proved.

Ideally, each cold symptom should be treated with a single drug. However, most remedies contain a variety of drugs—antihistamines, decongestants, analgesics, expectorants (drugs that make phlegm easier to cough up), and cough suppressants—and are designed to treat a wide range of symptoms. If a congested nose is the problem, neither a cough suppressant, an expectorant, nor an analgesic is needed. If a cough is the problem, neither an antihistamine nor a decongestant is needed. If

▲ see box on page 1572

Reading a Drug Label

Nonprescription drugs are required to have labels that explain what a drug's benefits and risks are and how to use the drug correctly. The label is entitled "Drug Facts." Active ingredients are listed at the top, followed by uses, warnings, directions, other information, and inactive ingredients.

Active ingredient: The drug itself is the active ingredient. Combination products have more than one active ingredient. The drug's generic name is listed with the amount of drug in each tablet, capsule, or dose unit. The same generic drug may be sold under several different trade (brand) names.

Uses: Symptoms or disorders for which the drug product is recommended are listed.

Warnings: Factors that can alter the expected response to the drug are listed, usually in four sections.

■ "Ask a doctor before use if you have" lists conditions that can make taking the drug more problematic or unsafe. This section refers to drug-disease interactions.

■ "Ask a doctor or a pharmacist before use if you are taking" lists other drugs that can interfere with the drug's effectiveness or safety. This section refers to drug-drug interactions.

■ "When using this product" includes common side effects, foods that may interfere with the drug's effectiveness or safety (drug-food interactions), and special precautions to take (for example, not driving while taking the drug).

■ The last section lists special warnings for women who are pregnant or breastfeeding and for children, with instructions about what to do in case of an overdose.

Directions: How much of the drug and how often to take the drug are given for different age groups, because size and age, among other factors, affect how a person responds to a drug.

Other information: Special instructions, such as how to store the drug so that it does not deteriorate, are listed.

Inactive ingredients: In addition to the drug, drug products—the tablets, capsules, or other formulations that consumers buy—contain substances added to facilitate the administration of the drug, such as ingredients that provide bulk or a pleasant taste and color. Products with the same active ingredient may contain different inactive ingredients. Inactive ingredients are usually harmless, but some of them cause an allergic reaction in a few people, who should look for products made without those ingredients.

---

a sore throat is the only symptom, an analgesic (such as acetaminophen, aspirin, ibuprofen, or naproxen sodium) is likely to work. Throat lozenges, especially those with a local anesthetic such as dyclonine or benzocaine, or a saltwater gargle (half a teaspoon of salt in 8 ounces of warm water) may also help. Finding an appropriate treatment for each symptom can be a challenge. Reading the labels or consulting a pharmacist can help.

Occasionally, a cold or cough may be a sign of a more serious disorder. A doctor should be consulted if symptoms last more than a week, especially if chest pain occurs or a cough produces dark phlegm. Fever and pain are unlikely to accompany a common cold and may indicate influenza or a bacterial infection.

ANTIHISTAMINES

Many experts believe that antihistamines should not be included in OTC cold remedies.

The concern is that most antihistamines can cause drowsiness, making people feel less alert. Anyone who drives, operates heavy equipment, or performs other activities that require alertness should not take the antihistamines included in OTC products. However, not everyone reacts the same way to antihistamines. For example, Asians seem to be less susceptible to the sedative effects of diphenhydramine than are people of Western European origin. Also, antihistamines cause the opposite (paradoxical) reaction in some people, making them feel nervous, restless, and agitated. Children, older people, and people with brain damage are more likely to react this way.

Other side effects of antihistamines are less common. They include blurred vision, lightheadedness, headache, stomachache, noise in the ears (tinnitus), palpitations, dry mouth, difficulty with urination, constipation, and confusion. Older people are particularly susceptible to the side effects of antihistamines.▲

Older people, pregnant women, and breastfeeding women should consult a doctor before

▲ see page 79

they take any drug that contains an antihistamine. This precaution also applies to people with angle-closure (narrow-angle) glaucoma, heart disease (such as angina and abnormal heart rhythms), constipation, or an enlarged prostate gland. Despite widespread concern about these risks, most cold remedies contain antihistamines. Reading labels or consulting a pharmacist can help people identify cold remedies containing antihistamines.

Cold remedies containing antihistamines should not be taken with alcohol, sleep aids, tranquilizers, or other drugs that also cause drowsiness and decrease alertness. Such a combination may intensify the sedating effects of the drugs.

DECONGESTANTS

When viruses invade mucous membranes (especially in the nose), blood vessels dilate, causing swelling. Decongestants constrict vessels and thus provide some relief. Active ingredients in oral decongestants include pseudoephedrine and phenylephrine.

Side effects of decongestants may include nervousness, agitation, palpitations, and insomnia. Because these drugs circulate throughout the body, they constrict other blood vessels—not just those in the nose—possibly raising blood pressure. For this reason, people with high blood pressure or heart disease should take decongestants only under a doctor's supervision or not at all. People with diabetes or hyperthyroidism also require a doctor's supervision if they take decongestants.

In an attempt to avoid these side effects, people often use nasal spray formulations, which temporarily reduce swelling in nasal tissues without affecting other organ systems. However, nasal sprays work so fast and so well that many people are tempted to use them longer than the 3-day limit listed on the label. Overuse can lead to the vicious circle of rebound nasal congestion: As the spray's effect wears off, small blood vessels in the nose can expand, causing congestion and stuffiness. This feeling may be so uncomfortable that use of the nasal spray is continued. Such use may

PAIN RELIEVERS: OVER-THE-COUNTER VERSUS PRESCRIPTION*

DRUG	AMOUNT OF ACTIVE INGREDIENT IN OTC TABLETS (mg)	AMOUNT OF MAXIMUM DAILY OTC DOSE FOR ADULTS (mg)	ACTIVE INGREDIENT IN PRESCRIPTION TABLETS (mg)	MAXIMUM DAILY PRESCRIPTION DOSE FOR ADULTS (mg)
Acetaminophen	80 160 325 500	4,000		
Ibuprofen	50 100 200	1,200	300 400 600 800	3,200
Ketoprofen	12.5	75	25 50 75 100 (controlled-release) 150 (controlled-release) 200 (controlled-release)	300
Naproxen	220 naproxen sodium (equivalent to 200 mg naproxen)	660 naproxen sodium	250 375 500	1,500

*The directions for use on the label of OTC drugs should be followed closely; the maximum daily dose on the label should not be exceeded. Taking larger amounts requires a doctor's supervision.

Recognizing Antihistamines

Many different types of over-the-counter products (such as cold and allergy remedies, motion sickness drugs, and sleep aids) contain antihistamines. Most antihistamines decrease alertness and have many other side effects, and they may be dangerous for people with certain disorders. Consequently, being able to identify which products contain these antihistamines is useful. OTC antihistamines, which are listed under active ingredients on the package, that cause such side effects include the following:

Brompheniramine
Chlorpheniramine
Dexbrompheniramine
Diphenhydramine
Doxylamine
Phenindamine
Pheniramine
Pyrilamine
Triprolidine

lead to drug dependency that lasts months or years. Sometimes withdrawal has to be supervised by a doctor specializing in ear, nose, and throat disorders.

Long-acting nasal sprays contain oxymetazoline or xylometazoline, which may provide relief for as long as 12 hours. Long-acting nasal sprays can be identified by reading the label. They also should be used for no more than 3 days at a time.

COUGH REMEDIES

Coughing is a natural response to lung irritation; it rids the lungs of excess secretions or mucus as phlegm.▲ If a person is congested and can cough up phlegm, suppression of such a productive cough is unwise. Expectorants make phlegm easier to cough up. Guaifenesin, the only approved expectorant on the market, is supposed to help loosen lung secretions and make them easier to cough up, but the drug's actual benefit has been hard to establish.

An unproductive, or dry, cough can be very irritating, especially at night. A cough suppressant can provide relief and contribute to restful sleep. Dextromethorphan, a very effective cough suppressant, is the most common ingredient in OTC cough remedies. It is not an

opioid (narcotic), and it rarely causes side effects, although an upset stomach or drowsiness can occur.

Codeine, also a very effective cough suppressant, is available only by prescription in many states. However, other states permit pharmacists to sell cough remedies containing codeine without a prescription if the customer signs for it. Because codeine is an opioid, some people fear it may be addicting. In reality, addiction is uncommon. Codeine can be helpful at bedtime because of its slight sedative effect.

Codeine causes nausea, vomiting, and constipation in some people. Because codeine may also produce light-headedness, drowsiness, or dizziness, cough remedies containing codeine should not be taken by anyone who is about to drive a vehicle or perform a task that requires concentration. Allergy to codeine is uncommon. Side effects may be more likely and more pronounced when other drugs that also reduce concentration (such as alcohol, sedatives, sleep aids, antidepressants, and certain antihistamines) are taken at the same time as codeine. Consequently, such a combination should not be taken except under a doctor's supervision.

To choose a cough remedy suitable for their symptoms, people should check the list of active ingredients on the package and talk with their pharmacist. They may need a product to help them cough up phlegm (a product containing guaifenesin), to suppress the cough (a product containing codeine or dextromethorphan), or to do both. A remedy containing codeine may be useful when a cough interferes with sleep.

Drugs to Treat Allergies

For allergies affecting the nose and respiratory tract (such as hay fever), OTC antihistamines that can be taken by mouth are available.■ Examples are chlorpheniramine and diphenhydramine. Taking an antihistamine to treat allergies requires the same precautions as taking a cold remedy containing an antihistamine.★ (Several new antihistamines that have fewer side effects are available, but most require a prescription.)

For allergies affecting the skin (such as poison ivy), creams or lotions that contain an antihistamine, such as diphenhydramine, can be applied to the skin.● Lotions, creams, and ointments that contain hydrocortisone, a corticosteroid, are effective in relieving itching

---

▲ see page 249   ■ see also page 1064
★ see page 96   ● see page 1188

associated with allergies, minor skin irritations, and inflammation. Long-term use of corticosteroid products can cause side effects, such as irreversible thinning and redness of the skin, but the risk with hydrocortisone is minimal.

Antacids and Indigestion Remedies

Heartburn, indigestion, and sour stomach are a few of the many terms used to describe digestive upset. Self-diagnosis of indigestion is risky because its causes vary from a minor dietary indiscretion to peptic ulcer disease or even stomach cancer. Sometimes symptoms of heart disease resemble acute indigestion. If symptoms last longer than 2 weeks, people should see their doctor.

The goal of treatment for indigestion is to prevent the production of stomach acid or to neutralize the acid. Histamine-2 (H_2) blockers, including cimetidine, famotidine, nizatidine, and ranitidine, help prevent heartburn by reducing the amount of acid produced in the stomach. Antacids neutralize stomach acid. Although antacids cannot completely neutralize stomach acid, they can raise the pH level in the stomach from 2 (very acidic) to between 3 and 4. This increase neutralizes almost 99% of stomach acid and significantly relieves symptoms for most people. Antacids provide relief more quickly than H_2 blockers, but H_2 blockers provide longer-lasting relief.

Most antacid products contain one or more of four active ingredients: aluminum salts, magnesium salts, calcium carbonate, and sodium bicarbonate. All products provide relief in a minute or less, but products vary in how long they provide relief—from only about 10 minutes to more than an hour and a half.

Antacids can interact with many different prescription drugs, so a pharmacist should be consulted about possible drug-drug interactions before antacids are taken. Anyone who has heart disease, high blood pressure, or a kidney disorder should consult a doctor before selecting an antacid. The H_2 blocker cimetidine may also interact with some prescription drugs. Therefore, its use should be monitored by a doctor or pharmacist.

ALUMINUM AND MAGNESIUM

Antacids that contain both aluminum and magnesium salts once seemed ideal because one ingredient complemented the other. Aluminum salts, which dissolve slowly in the stomach, start to work gradually but provide long-lasting relief. They also cause constipation. Magnesium salts act fast and neutralize acids effectively. They can also act as a laxative. Antacids containing both ingredients should provide quick, long-lasting relief with less risk of diarrhea or constipation. However, the long-term safety of antacids containing aluminum has been questioned. Prolonged use may weaken bones by depleting the body of phosphorus and calcium.

CALCIUM CARBONATE

Calcium carbonate, or chalk, has been a mainstay of antacids for a long time. Calcium carbonate acts fast and neutralizes acids for a relatively long time. Also, it is an inexpensive source of calcium; amounts range from 500 to 1000 milligrams per tablet or dose. However, people can overdose on calcium.▲ The maximum daily amount should not exceed 2000 milligrams unless a doctor has directed otherwise.

SODIUM BICARBONATE

One of the least expensive and most readily available antacids is no farther away than the kitchen cabinet. Sodium bicarbonate, or baking soda, neutralizes acid quickly. The baking soda burp is a sign that this antacid is working; the burp is caused by release of carbon dioxide gas, which occurs when the antacid neutralizes the acid.

Although sodium bicarbonate may provide a short-term solution to indigestion, too much bicarbonate can wreak havoc with the body's acid-base balance and lead to metabolic alkalosis.■ The high sodium content may also cause problems for people with heart failure or high blood pressure.

Motion Sickness Drugs

Many of the drugs used to prevent motion sickness are antihistamines.★ They are occasionally prescribed but are also available over the counter. Motion sickness drugs are most likely to be effective if taken 30 to 60 minutes before a trip.

Motion sickness drugs often make a person drowsy and less alert. In fact, one motion sickness drug, the antihistamine diphenhydra-

---

▲ see page 901   ■ see page 932

★ see page 96

MOTION SICKNESS DRUGS: PRECAUTIONS FOR CHILDREN

Active Ingredient	Children Who Should Not Be Given the Drug (unless a doctor so directs)
Cyclizine	Under 6 years old
Dimenhydrinate	Under 2 years old
Diphenhydramine	Under 6 years old
Meclizine	Under 12 years old

mine, is the active ingredient in most OTC sleep aids. Anyone who performs an activity that requires alertness or concentration, including driving, should not take a motion sickness drug. A motion sickness drug should not be taken with alcohol, sleep aids, tranquilizers, or other drugs that also cause drowsiness and decrease alertness.

Other side effects of antihistamines are less common.▲ Infants and very young children may become agitated and should not be given a motion sickness drug except under a doctor's supervision. Too high a dose in a young child could lead to hallucinations or even seizures, which may be fatal.

Older people, pregnant women, and breast-feeding women should consult a doctor before they take any drug that contains an antihistamine, as should people with angle-closure glaucoma, heart disease, constipation, or an enlarged prostate gland.

Sleep Aids

Over-the-counter sleep aids are intended to manage an occasional sleepless night, not chronic insomnia, which could signal a serious underlying problem.■ Taking an OTC sleep aid for more than 7 to 10 days is not recommended. (Many prescription sleep aids may be safer than OTC sleep aids, especially for older people.)

OTC sleep aids contain diphenhydramine or doxylamine, both antihistamines.★ These drugs tend to make people drowsy or less alert, although not everyone reacts that way. Asians seem to be less sensitive to the sedative effects of diphenhydramine than are peo-

▲ see page 96   ■ see page 468
★ see page 96

ple of Western European origin. Sleep aids should not be taken with alcohol, tranquilizers, or other drugs that also cause drowsiness and decrease alertness.

Diphenhydramine or doxylamine causes the opposite (paradoxical) reaction in some people, making them feel nervous, restless, and agitated. Older people, people with brain damage, and young children are apparently more likely to react this way.

Older people, pregnant women, and breast-feeding women should consult a doctor before they take any product that contains an antihistamine. This precaution also applies to people with angle-closure glaucoma, heart disease, constipation, or an enlarged prostate gland.

Special Precautions

Certain groups of people, such as the very young, the very old, the very sick, and pregnant and breastfeeding women, are more vulnerable to harm from drugs, including OTC drugs. When such people use drugs, special precautions, which may include a doctor's supervision, should be taken.

To avoid dangerous drug-drug interactions, people should consult a pharmacist or doctor before they take prescription drugs and OTC drugs at the same time. People who have chronic disorders should also consult a pharmacist or doctor. OTC drugs are not designed to treat serious disorders and can make some disorders worse. An unanticipated reaction, such as a rash or insomnia, is a signal to stop taking the drug immediately and obtain medical advice.

CHILDREN

Children's bodies metabolize and react to drugs differently from the way adults' bodies do. A drug may be used by many people for many years before its hazards to children are discovered. For example, many years passed before researchers confirmed that the risk of Reye's syndrome was linked to the use of aspirin in children who had chickenpox or influenza. Doctors and parents alike are often surprised to learn that most OTC drugs, even those with recommended dosages for children, have not been thoroughly tested in children. The effectiveness of cough and cold remedies is unproved, especially in children, so that giving these drugs to children may unnecessarily expose the children to harmful effects of a drug and may be a waste of money.

Giving a child a correct drug dose can be tricky. Although children's doses are often expressed in terms of age ranges (for example, children aged 2 to 6 or 6 to 12), age is not the best criterion. Children can vary greatly in size within any age range, and experts do not agree on whether the best measurement for determining drug dose is weight, height, or total body surface. A recommended dose expressed in terms of the child's weight may be the easiest to interpret.

If the label does not give instructions on how much drug to give the child, a parent should not guess. When in doubt, a parent should consult a pharmacist or doctor. Such consultation may prevent a child from receiving a dangerous drug or a dangerously high dose of a potentially helpful drug.

Many drugs for treating children come in liquid form. Even though the label should give clear guidelines about the dose, a child may be given the wrong dose because the adult in charge uses an ordinary teaspoon. The only kitchen spoons accurate enough to measure liquid drugs are measuring spoons. However, a cylindrical measuring spoon is far better for measuring a child's dose, and an oral syringe is preferred for squirting a precise amount of drug into an infant's mouth. The cap should always be removed from the tip of an oral syringe before use. A child can choke if the cap is accidentally propelled into the windpipe.

Several children's drugs are available in more than one form. Adults must read labels carefully every time a new children's drug is used.

OLDER PEOPLE

Normal aging changes the speed and ways in which the body handles drugs,▲ and older people tend to have more diseases and to take more than one drug at a time. For these reasons, older people may be more likely than younger ones to experience side effects or drug interactions. More and more prescription drug labels specify whether different doses are needed for older people, but such information is rarely included on OTC drug labels.

Many OTC drugs are potentially hazardous for older people. The risk increases when drugs are taken regularly at the maximum dose. For example, an older person who has arthritis may frequently use an analgesic or anti-inflammatory drug, with potentially serious consequences, such as a bleeding peptic ulcer. Such an ulcer is life threatening for an older person and can occur without warning.

Antihistamines, such as diphenhydramine, also pose special risks for older people. Many nighttime pain relief formulas, cough and cold remedies, allergy drugs, and sleep aids contain antihistamines. Antihistamines may worsen some disorders common among older people, such as angle-closure glaucoma and an enlarged prostate gland. They can also make a person dizzy or unsteady, leading to falls and broken bones. Antihistamines, particularly at a high dose or in combination with other drugs, can sometimes cause blurred vision, light-headedness, dry mouth, difficulty with urination, constipation, and confusion in older people.

Older people may be more susceptible to the possible side effects of antacids. Those that contain aluminum are more likely to cause constipation, and those that contain magnesium are more likely to cause diarrhea and dehydration.

During visits to the doctor, older people should mention all OTC products they are taking, including vitamins, minerals, and medicinal herbs. This information helps the doctor evaluate the entire drug regimen and determine whether or not an OTC drug may be responsible for certain symptoms.

PREGNANT AND BREASTFEEDING WOMEN

Drugs can move from a pregnant woman to her fetus (primarily through the placenta),■ and drugs can be transmitted through breast milk to the baby. Such drugs can affect or harm the fetus or baby. During pregnancy, avoiding all drugs, including aspirin and nonprenatal vitamins, is best. Women who are breastfeeding can take most OTC drugs without harming the baby. However, women who are pregnant or breastfeeding should consult a health care practitioner before taking any drug, even an OTC drug, or medicinal herb. OTC drug labels should be checked because they contain warnings against use during pregnancy and breastfeeding, if applicable.

Certain types of drugs are particularly problematic. They include antihistamines (commonly contained in cough and cold remedies, allergy drugs, motion sickness drugs, and sleep aids) and nonsteroidal anti-inflammatory drugs (NSAIDs). NSAIDs should not be used during the last 3 months of pregnancy unless specified by a doctor, because they may

---

▲ see page 79   ■ see also page 1458

CHRONIC DISORDERS AND OVER-THE-COUNTER DRUGS

DISORDER	OTC DRUGS	PRECAUTIONS
Alcoholism	Cold remedies	Recovering alcoholics need to be vigilant about avoiding cold remedies that contain alcohol; some products contain as much as 25% alcohol.
Diabetes	Antihistamines Decongestants	People with diabetes should consult a doctor before they take antihistamines and decongestants because these drugs can worsen diabetes and cause dangerous side effects.
	Cough syrups	People with diabetes may need help locating a cough syrup that does not contain sugar.
Enlarged prostate	Antihistamines Decongestants	People with an enlarged prostate should consult a doctor before they take antihistamines and decongestants because side effects can be dangerous.
Glaucoma	Antihistamines	Taking an antihistamine can complicate glaucoma.
Heart disease	Antacids Cold remedies	People with heart disease should consult a doctor or pharmacist to help them select an antacid or cold remedy that does not interact with their prescription drugs.
	Antihistamines Decongestants	People with heart disease should consult a doctor before they take antihistamines and decongestants because side effects can be dangerous.
High blood pressure (hypertension)	Antacids	People with high blood pressure should consult a doctor before they select an antacid.
	Antihistamines Decongestants	People with high blood pressure should consult a doctor before they take antihistamines and decongestants because side effects can be dangerous.
Hyperthyroidism	Antihistamines Decongestants	People with hyperthyroidism should consult a doctor before they take antihistamines and decongestants because side effects can be dangerous.
Kidney disorders	Antacids	People with kidney disorders should consult a doctor before they select an antacid.
Lung disorders, such as asthma and emphysema	Antihistamines	Antihistamines, which are found in sleep aids, allergy products, and cough and cold remedies, should not be taken by anyone with asthma, emphysema, or a chronic lung disorder unless a doctor directs them to do so.

cause problems in the fetus or complications during delivery.

CHRONIC DISORDERS

A number of chronic disorders can become worse if an OTC drug is taken inappropriately. Because OTC drugs are intended primarily for occasional use by people who are essentially healthy, people who have a chronic or serious disorder or who plan to take an OTC drug every day should consult a health care practitioner before they purchase OTC products. In such cases, drug use is beyond the normal boundaries of self-care and requires the advice of an expert.

DRUG-DRUG INTERACTIONS

Many people neglect to mention their use of OTC drugs to their doctor or pharmacist. Drugs taken intermittently, such as those for colds, constipation, or an occasional headache, are mentioned even less often. Health care practitioners may not think of asking about use of OTC drugs or medicinal herbs when they are prescribing or dispensing a prescription. Yet many OTC drugs and medicinal herbs can interact adversely with a wide range of drugs.▲

▲   see also page 75

Some of these interactions can be serious, interfering with the effectiveness of a drug or causing side effects. For example, as little as one aspirin tablet can reduce the effectiveness of an angiotensin-converting enzyme (ACE) inhibitor, such as enalapril, in the treatment of severe heart failure. Taking aspirin with the anticoagulant warfarin can increase the risk of abnormal bleeding. An antacid containing aluminum or magnesium can reduce the absorption of digoxin, taken for heart disease. Taking a multiple vitamin and mineral supplement can interfere with the action of some prescription drugs. For example, the antibiotic tetracycline may be ineffective if swallowed with milk or other products containing calcium, magnesium, or iron.

OTC drug-drug interactions have not been studied systematically. Many serious problems have been discovered accidentally, after side effects or deaths were reported. Even when interaction warnings are printed on the label for OTC drugs, the language may be meaningless to most people. For example, the labels of some cold remedies that contain pseudoephedrine caution against using the product with a monoamine oxidase inhibitor (MAOI—given for depression)▲ or during the 2 weeks after discontinuing the MAOI. For the many people who do not know that the antidepressant they are taking is an MAOI (such as phenelzine and tranylcypromine), this important warning is not helpful.

The best way to reduce the risk of drug-drug interactions is to ask the pharmacist to check for them. Additionally, the doctor should be told about all drugs being taken, both prescription and OTC.■

DRUG OVERLAP

Another potential problem is drug overlap. OTC products used to treat different problems may contain the same active ingredient. Unless people read the labels on everything they take, they can accidentally overdose themselves. For example, a person who takes a sleep aid and a cold remedy, both of which contain diphenhydramine, may take double the dose considered safe. Many products contain acetaminophen. A person who simultaneously takes two different products that contain acetaminophen—one for a headache and another for allergies or sinus problems—may exceed the recommended dose.

CHAPTER 19

Medicinal Herbs and Nutraceuticals

Medicinal herbs generally refer to plant parts, sometimes ground, extracted, or otherwise prepared, used for health benefits. **Nutraceuticals,** *a more recent and more general term, refer to a group of natural substances that includes certain herbs and such products as cholesterol-lowering margarines and psyllium-fortified products that are used as dietary supplements and regulated as foods.*

Traditional systems of medicine have been used throughout the world for centuries. Certain ancient systems, such as traditional Chinese medicine, Ayurveda (the holistic system of medicine from India), and Tibetan medicine, are still used extensively, particularly in their country of origin. In the United States, interest in the therapies of such systems, particularly for the treatment of chronic illness, is growing. These therapies, usually referred to as complementary or alternative medicine,★ range from medicinal herbs to acupuncture to massage. Most of them have not been studied scientifically, and nearly all are unregulated.

The most commonly used alternative therapy is **dietary supplements,** which include medicinal herbs and nutraceuticals. Because the use of dietary supplements is widespread, the

---

▲ see page 617   ■ see box on page 76
★ see also page 1704

SOME POSSIBLE MEDICINAL HERB–DRUG INTERACTIONS

MEDICINAL HERB	AFFECTED DRUGS	INTERACTION
Chamomile	Anticoagulants (such as warfarin)	Chamomile taken with anticoagulants may increase the risk of bleeding
	Barbiturates (such as phenobarbital) and other sedatives	Chamomile may intensify or prolong the effects of sedatives
	Iron	Chamomile may reduce iron absorption
Echinacea	Drugs that can damage the liver (such as anabolic steroids, amiodarone, methotrexate, and ketoconazole)	Echinacea taken for more than 8 weeks may damage the liver. When echinacea is taken with another drug that can damage the liver, the risk of liver damage may be increased
	Immunosuppressants (such as corticosteroids and cyclosporine)	By stimulating the immune system, echinacea may negate the effects of immunosuppressants
Feverfew	Anticoagulants (such as warfarin)	Feverfew taken with anticoagulants may increase the risk of bleeding
	Iron	Feverfew may reduce iron absorption
	Drugs used to manage migraine headaches (such as ergotamine)	Feverfew may increase heart rate and blood pressure when it is taken with drugs used to manage migraine headaches
	Nonsteroidal anti-inflammatory drugs (NSAIDs)	NSAIDs reduce the effectiveness of feverfew in preventing and managing migraine headaches
Garlic	Anticoagulants (such as warfarin)	Garlic taken with anticoagulants may increase the risk of bleeding
	Drugs that decrease blood sugar levels (hypoglycemic drugs, such as insulin and glipizide)	Garlic may intensify the effects of these drugs, causing an excessive decrease in blood sugar levels (hypoglycemia)
	Saquinavir (used to treat HIV infection)	Garlic decreases blood levels of saquinavir, making it less effective
Ginger	Anticoagulants (such as warfarin)	Ginger taken with anticoagulants may increase the risk of bleeding
Ginkgo	Anticoagulants (such as warfarin), aspirin and other NSAIDs	Ginkgo taken with anticoagulants or with aspirin or other NSAIDs may increase the risk of bleeding
	Anticonvulsants (such as phenytoin)	Ginkgo may reduce the effectiveness of anticonvulsants in preventing seizures
	Monoamine oxidase inhibitors (MAOIs, a type of antidepressant)	Ginkgo may intensify the effects of these drugs and increase the risk of side effects, such as headache, tremors, and manic episodes
Ginseng	Anticoagulants (such as warfarin), aspirin and other NSAIDs	Ginseng taken with anticoagulants or with aspirin or other NSAIDs may increase the risk of bleeding
	Drugs that decrease blood sugar levels (hypoglycemic drugs)	Ginseng may intensify the effects of these drugs, causing an excessive decrease in blood sugar levels (hypoglycemia)
	Corticosteroids	Ginseng may intensify the side effects of corticosteroids

SOME POSSIBLE MEDICINAL HERB–DRUG INTERACTIONS (*Cont'd*)

MEDICINAL HERB	AFFECTED DRUGS	INTERACTION
Ginseng (*cont'd*)	Digoxin	Ginseng may increase digoxin levels
	Estrogen replacement therapy	Ginseng may intensify the side effects of estrogen
	MAOIs	Ginseng can cause headache, tremors, and manic episodes when it is taken with MAOIs
	Opioids (narcotics)	Ginseng may reduce the effectiveness of opioids
Goldenseal	Anticoagulants (such as warfarin)	Goldenseal may oppose the effects of anticoagulants and may increase the risk of blood clots
Licorice	Antihypertensives	Licorice may increase salt and water retention and increase blood pressure, making antihypertensives less effective
	Antiarrhythmics	Licorice may increase the risk of an abnormal heart rhythm, making antiarrhythmic therapy less effective
	Digoxin	Because licorice increases urine formation, it can result in low levels of potassium, which is excreted in urine. When licorice is taken with digoxin, the low potassium levels increase the risk of digoxin toxicity
	Diuretics	Licorice may intensify the effects of most diuretics, causing increased, rapid loss of potassium. Licorice may interfere with the effectiveness of potassium-sparing diuretics, such as spironolactone, making these diuretics less effective
	MAOIs	Licorice may intensify the effects of these drugs and increase the risk of side effects, such as headache, tremors, and manic episodes
Milk thistle	Drugs that decrease blood sugar levels (hypoglycemic drugs)	Milk thistle may intensify the effects of these drugs, causing an excessive decrease in blood sugar levels
	Saquinavir	Milk thistle decreases blood levels of saquinavir, making it less effective
Saw palmetto	Estrogen replacement therapy and oral contraceptives	Saw palmetto may intensify the effects of these drugs
St. John's wort	Benzodiazepines	St. John's wort may reduce the effectiveness of these drugs in reducing anxiety and may increase drowsiness and the risk of side effects such as drowsiness
	Cyclosporine	St. John's wort may reduce blood levels of cyclosporine, making it less effective, with potentially dangerous results (such as rejection of an organ transplant)
	Digoxin	St. John's wort may reduce blood levels of digoxin, making it less effective, with potentially dangerous results

Table continues on the following page

SOME POSSIBLE MEDICINAL HERB–DRUG INTERACTIONS (Cont'd)

Medicinal Herb	Affected Drugs	Interaction
St. John's wort (cont'd)	Indinavir (a drug used to treat AIDS)	St. John's wort may reduce blood levels of indinavir, making it less effective
	Iron	St. John's wort may reduce iron absorption
	MAOIs	St. John's wort may intensify the effects of MAOIs, possibly causing very high blood pressure that requires emergency treatment
	Photosensitizing drugs (such as lansoprazole, omeprazole, piroxicam, and sulfonamide antibiotics)	When taken with these drugs, St. John's wort may increase the risk of sun sensitivity
	Selective serotonin reuptake inhibitors (such as fluoxetine, paroxetine, and sertraline)	St. John's wort may intensify the effects of these drugs
	Warfarin	St. John's wort may reduce blood levels of warfarin, making it less effective and clot formation more likely
Valerian	Anesthetics	Valerian may prolong sedation time
	Barbiturates	Valerian may intensify the effects of barbiturates, causing excessive sedation

United States government passed the Dietary Supplement Health Education Act (DSHEA) in 1994. It defines a dietary supplement as any product (besides tobacco) that contains a vitamin, mineral, herb, or amino acid and that is intended as a supplement to the normal diet. The act requires that the label of a dietary supplement identify it as such. The label must state that the claims for the dietary supplement have not been evaluated by the Food and Drug Administration (FDA). The label must also list each ingredient by name, quantity, and total weight and must identify the plant parts from which each ingredient is derived.

Most dietary supplements used in alternative medicine are derived from plants; some are derived from animals. Because such dietary supplements are natural, some people assume that they are safe to use. However, a substance is not necessarily safe just because it is natural. For example, many potent poisons, such as hemlock, are derived from plants, and some, such as snake venoms, are derived from animals. Furthermore, almost all substances that affect the body—whether dietary supplements or drugs approved for medical use by the FDA▲ have both wanted and unwanted effects (side effects).

Safety and Effectiveness: Because dietary supplements are not regulated as drugs by the FDA, their manufacturers are not required to prove that dietary supplements are safe and effective (although they must have a history of safety). Consequently, few supplements have been rigorously studied for safety and effectiveness (although some may eventually be shown to be safe and effective). Furthermore, because the need to evaluate supplements in humans has only recently been recognized, much of the available information has not been gathered systematically or scientifically and so is difficult to evaluate. In contrast, both prescription and over-the-counter drugs have been extensively and systematically studied by researchers and reviewed for safety and effectiveness by the FDA.■ These studies include those in animals to detect the development of cancer and organ damage and those in humans to detect any signs of toxicity.

The amount and quality of evidence supporting the effectiveness of supplements varies greatly. For some supplements, evidence supporting their effectiveness is convincing. However, for most, scientific studies have not been designed well enough to provide the desired information. For some supplements, the only evidence suggesting effectiveness are reports about individual people or studies conducted in animals.

▲ see page 60   ■ see page 63

Purity and Standardization: Other areas of concern are the purity and standardization of supplements. Supplements, unlike drugs, are not regulated to ensure that they are pure or that they contain the ingredients or the amount of active ingredient they claim to contain. As a result, the supplement may not be pure. Or, the amount of active ingredient in a dose of a supplement may vary, especially when whole herbs are ground or made into extracts to produce a tablet, capsule, or solution. The buyer is at risk of getting less, more, or, in some cases, none of the active ingredient in a supplement. Standardization requires that each individual dosage form of the product contain a precise amount of its active ingredient or ingredients. However, most herbal products are mixtures of several substances, and which ingredient is the most active is not always known. Therefore, determining which ingredient or ingredients should be considered active and thus would be subject to standardization can be difficult. Some supplements have been standardized and may include a designation of standardization on the label.

Advice on how to choose a pure, standardized product varies from expert to expert. Most experts recommend buying from a well-known manufacturer, and many recommend buying products made in Germany, because oversight of supplements is stricter there than in the United States.

Interactions with Drugs: Supplements can interact with prescription and over-the-counter drugs. Such interactions may intensify or reduce the effectiveness of a drug or cause a serious side effect. Before taking supplements, people should consult their doctor, so that such interactions can be avoided. Few well-designed studies have been conducted to investigate supplement-drug interactions, so most information about these interactions comes from sporadic individual reports of interactions.

SOME DIETARY SUPPLEMENTS

The following substances are some of the more widely known supplements. They may or may not be useful in maintaining or restoring health.

Chamomile

Background: The daisy-like flower of this herb is dried and used as tea or in extracts.
Medicinal Claims: Various substances in chamomile reduce inflammation and fever. Chamomile, which has a soothing effect, is used as a mild sedative. Chamomile may be used to relieve stomach cramps and indigestion. It is also claimed to help gastric ulcers heal. Chamomile extract applied in a compress may soothe irritated skin.

Studies in animals suggest that substances in chamomile inhibit *Helicobacter pylori*, the bacteria that can contribute to stomach ulcers. However, few studies in humans have evaluated chamomile's effects, and there is no evidence that it speeds the healing of gastric ulcers. Chamomile is generally considered safe.
Possible Side Effects: Chamomile may reduce the absorption of drugs taken by mouth. Chamomile may also interact with drugs such as anticoagulants, sedatives (such as barbiturates), alcohol, and iron supplements. Some people are allergic to the pollen in chamomile products.

Chromium Picolinate

Background: Chromium is a mineral required in small quantities by the body. It enables insulin to function normally and helps the body process (metabolize) carbohydrates and fats. Good sources of chromium include carrots, potatoes, broccoli, whole-grain products, and molasses. Picolinate, a by-product of the amino acid tryptophan, is paired with chromium in supplements because it is claimed to help the body absorb chromium more efficiently.
Medicinal Claims: As a dietary supplement, chromium picolinate is used to promote weight loss, build muscle, reduce body fat, and enhance the function of insulin, but these effects have not been proved. It may lower levels of cholesterol and triglycerides.
Possible Side Effects: Some evidence suggests that chromium picolinate damages chromosomes and consequently may cause cancer.

Cranberry

Background: Cranberries can be consumed whole or made into food products such as jellies and juices.
Medicinal Claims: Consuming cranberries whole or as juices helps prevent urinary tract infections and relieve their symptoms. The effectiveness of cranberries in preventing urinary tract infections has been documented. In one study, researchers identified one way that cranberries may prevent infections: Natural unprocessed cranberry juice contains antho-

cyanidins, which prevent *Escherichia coli*, the bacteria that usually cause urinary tract infections, from attaching to the urinary tract wall.

Some people use cranberry juice to reduce fever and treat certain cancers; however, there is no scientific proof that it is effective for these uses.

Possible Side Effects: No side effects are known. However, because most cranberry juice is highly sweetened to offset its tart taste, people with diabetes should not consume cranberry juice unless it is unsweetened.

Creatine

Background: Creatine is an amino acid made in the liver and stored in muscles. It is a readily available source of energy in the body. In the diet, creatine is found in milk, red meat, and some fish.

Medicinal Claims: Creatine is used to improve physical or athletic performance and to decrease fatigue. A few studies indicate that creatine can increase the amount of work performed with a short maximal effort (for example, in sprinting). However, a few others indicate no improvement in this type of activity.

Possible Side Effects: Creatine can cause dehydration and may cause kidney dysfunction.

Dehydroepiandrosterone

Background: Dehydroepiandrosterone (DHEA) is a steroid produced in the adrenal glands and converted into sex hormones (estrogens and androgens). DHEA's effects on the body are similar to those of testosterone. DHEA can be extracted from the Mexican yam.

Medicinal Claims: DHEA supplements may stimulate the immune system. They are used to improve mood, energy, sense of well-being, and the ability to function well under stress. Other uses include deepening nightly sleep, lowering cholesterol levels, and decreasing body fat. Many athletes claim that DHEA builds muscles. It is also claimed to reverse aging and improve brain function in people with Alzheimer's disease. The medicinal claims of DHEA have not been proved.

Possible Side Effects: Theoretically, DHEA may result in breast enlargement in men and hairiness in women and may stimulate the growth of certain prostate and breast cancers, but these effects have not been substantiated. DHEA should not be used by children attempting to build muscle or enhance athletic performance.

Echinacea

Background: Echinacea is a perennial herb, which contains echinoside and several other active substances. Various parts of the plant are used medicinally.

Medicinal Claims: Several substances in echinacea may stimulate the immune system. Echinacea is used to help treat viral infections in the upper respiratory tract, such as the common cold. Applied as a cream or ointment, echinacea has been used to promote healing of wounds.

Many studies have evaluated the effects of echinacea, but none were designed well enough to provide conclusive results. Also, most of these studies evaluated products in which echinacea was combined with other herbs, making evaluation of echinacea's effects difficult. At least two relatively well-designed studies evaluated echinacea's effectiveness in upper respiratory tract infections: In one, echinacea reduced the duration of colds and the severity of symptoms; in the other, it reduced the frequency and number of recurrences.

Possible Side Effects: No significant side effects have been identified. Echinacea may interact with drugs that can cause liver damage, thereby increasing the risk of liver damage. Echinacea may negate the effects of immunosuppressants, which are used, for example, to prevent rejection of organ transplants. People who have type 1 diabetes, autoimmune diseases (such as rheumatoid arthritis and multiple sclerosis), or an impaired immune system (for example, as impaired by AIDS or tuberculosis) should consult their doctor before they take echinacea.

Feverfew

Background: Feverfew is a bushy perennial herb. Parthenolide and glycosides are thought to be its active components.

Medicinal Claims: Feverfew is used to prevent migraine headaches. It may reduce inflammation. Feverfew reduces the clotting tendency of platelets (cell-like particles in the blood that help stop bleeding by forming clots). Evidence from two of three relatively small but well-designed studies supports these effects. Differences in study findings may reflect the different formulations of feverfew used. In studies of people with arthritis, feverfew did not relieve symptoms.

Possible Side Effects: Mouth ulcers and skin inflammation (dermatitis) may occur. Taste may be altered, and heart rate increased. Feverfew may interact with anticoagulants, drugs used to manage migraine headaches, and nonsteroidal anti-inflammatory drugs (NSAIDs). It may reduce the absorption of iron. Feverfew is not recommended for children or for women who are pregnant or breast-feeding.

Garlic

Background: Garlic has long been used in cooking and in medicine. When a garlic bulb is cut or crushed, an amino acid by-product called allicin is released. Allicin is responsible for garlic's strong odor and medicinal properties.

Medicinal Claims: Garlic reduces the clotting tendency of platelets. Because garlic stops microorganisms (such as bacteria) from reproducing, it can be used as an antiseptic and antibacterial. In large doses, garlic can reduce blood pressure, overactivity of the intestine, and blood sugar levels (slightly). Advocates suggest that garlic lowers levels of low-density lipoprotein (LDL) cholesterol—the "bad" cholesterol. However, at least one well-designed study did not support this beneficial effect. Most studies have used aged garlic extracts. Preparations formulated to have little or no odor may be inactive and need to be studied.

Possible Side Effects: Garlic usually has no harmful effects other than making the breath or body smell like garlic. However, consuming large amounts can cause nausea and burning in the mouth, esophagus, and stomach. Garlic may interact with anticoagulants.

Ginger

Background: Like garlic, ginger has long been used in cooking and in medicine. The stem of this herb contains substances called gingerols, which give ginger its flavor and odor.

Medicinal Claims: Ginger appears to soothe the stomach, relieve intestinal cramps, and reduce inflammation and pain. Ginger may prevent nausea, vomiting, motion sickness, and dizziness (including vertigo). Ginger may be helpful in treating excessive vomiting during pregnancy. Some well-designed studies indicate that ginger is effective in preventing and lessening nausea, but others do not.

Possible Side Effects: Ginger is usually not harmful, although some people experience a burning sensation when they eat it. It may also cause digestive discomfort and produce a disagreeable taste in the mouth. Ginger may interact with anticoagulants.

Ginkgo

Background: Ginkgo is derived from the leaves of the ginkgo tree. The leaves contain several substances called ginkgolides.

Medicinal Claims: Ginkgo reduces the clotting tendency of platelets, dilates blood vessels (thereby improving blood flow), and reduces inflammation. Ginkgo is used to improve blood flow to the brain and in the lower legs. It may be useful in treating dizziness, headache, noise in the ears (tinnitus), memory loss for recent events, and mood disturbance. It may prevent damage to the kidneys caused by the immunosuppressant cyclosporine.

Evidence supports some of these claims. Many European studies have shown that a standardized preparation of ginkgo reduces symptoms in people with reduced blood flow to the brain or in the legs. For example, in people with peripheral arterial disease, it increased the distance that could be walked without pain. One large well-designed study in the United States indicated that ginkgo can stabilize or improve mental and social function in people with mild to moderate dementia, including Alzheimer's disease. Another study indicated that it can improve mental function in healthy older people.

Possible Side Effects: Although ginkgo leaf extracts usually have no side effects except mild digestive upset, the use of ginkgo should be supervised by a doctor; it is not suitable for self-medication. Ginkgo may interact with anticoagulants, aspirin, and other nonsteroidal anti-inflammatory drugs (NSAIDs), and it may reduce the effectiveness of anticonvulsants. Contact with the fruit pulp, which may be encountered under ginkgo trees (planted for ornamental purposes), can cause severe skin inflammation (dermatitis). The fruit is not used in ginkgo products.

Ginseng

Background: Ginseng is usually derived from two different species of plant: American and Asian ginseng. American ginseng is milder than Asian ginseng. Ginseng is available in many forms, such as fresh and dried roots, extracts, solutions, capsules, tablets, cosmetics, sodas, and teas. The active components are panaxosides in American ginseng and ginsenosides in Asian ginseng.

Siberian ginseng is not really ginseng and contains different active components, but it has antistress effects similar to those of American and Asian ginseng.

Ginseng products vary considerably in quality; many contain little or no detectable active ingredient. In a very few cases, some ginseng products from Asia have been purposefully mixed with mandrake root, which has been used to induce vomiting, or with phenylbutazone or aminopyrine—drugs that were removed from the market in the United States because of unacceptable side effects.

Medicinal Claims: Ginseng is used to enhance physical (including sexual) and mental performance and to increase energy and resistance to the harmful effects of stress and aging. Ginseng appears to reduce blood sugar levels and increase levels of high-density lipoprotein (HDL) cholesterol—the "good" cholesterol. It may also increase hemoglobin and protein levels in the blood.

Evaluating some of ginseng's effects is difficult because measuring an increase in energy and other quality-of-life effects is difficult. In one small study of people with diabetes, ginseng reduced blood sugar levels and, according to subjective report, improved mood and energy. In one large but short study, ginseng improved quality of life, according to subjective report.

Possible Side Effects: Ginseng has a reasonably good safety record. The most common side effects are nervousness and excitability, which usually decrease after the first few days. The ability to concentrate may be decreased, and blood sugar may decrease to abnormally low levels (causing hypoglycemia). Because ginseng has an estrogen-like effect, women who are pregnant or breastfeeding should not take it, nor should children. Occasionally, there have been reports of more serious side effects, such as asthma attacks, increased blood pressure, palpitations, and, in postmenopausal women, uterine bleeding. To many people, ginseng tastes unpleasant.

Ginseng can interact with anticoagulants, aspirin, other nonsteroidal anti-inflammatory drugs (NSAIDs), corticosteroids, digoxin, estrogen replacement therapy, monoamine oxidase inhibitors (MAOIs—used to treat depression), and drugs that decrease blood sugar levels (hypoglycemic drugs, used to treat diabetes).

Goldenseal

Background: Goldenseal, an endangered plant, is related to the buttercup. Its active components are hydrastine and berberine, which have antiseptic activity. Berberine is also active against diarrhea.

Medicinal Claims: Goldenseal is used as an antiseptic wash for mouth sores, inflamed and sore eyes, and irritated skin and as a douche for vaginal infections. It has been combined with echinacea as a cold remedy, but the effectiveness of goldenseal as a cold remedy has not been proved. Goldenseal is also used as a remedy for indigestion and diarrhea. In two relatively well-designed studies, berberine isolated from goldenseal reduced diarrhea.

Possible Side Effects: Goldenseal can produce many side effects, including digestive irritation and upset, contractions of the uterus, jaundice in newborns, and worsening of high blood pressure (hypertension). If taken in large amounts, goldenseal can cause seizures and respiratory failure and may affect contraction of the heart. Goldenseal may interact with anticoagulants. Women who are pregnant or breastfeeding, newborns, and people who have heart disease, epilepsy, or problems with blood clotting should not take goldenseal.

Licorice

Background: Natural licorice, which has a very sweet taste, is extracted from the root of a shrub and used medicinally. Most licorice candy made in the United States is artificially flavored and does not contain true licorice.

Medicinal Claims: Licorice is used to suppress coughs, to soothe a sore throat, and to relieve stomach upset. Applied externally, it is thought to soothe skin irritation (for example, eczema).

Possible Side Effects: Licorice may cause fluid retention. Frequently taking large amounts of licorice can result in high blood pressure (hypertension).

Melatonin

Background: Melatonin is a hormone produced by the pineal gland, located in the middle of the brain; it regulates the sleep-wake cycle. Melatonin used in supplements is derived from animals or produced artificially.

Medicinal Claims: Melatonin is used to treat insomnia and to help minimize the effects of jet lag. People who are traveling across time zones may benefit from melatonin given on the day or night of departure and for 2 or 3 nights after arrival. Melatonin has been used to prevent pregnancy, to enhance the immune system, and to prevent cancer.

Evidence suggests that melatonin supplements can affect the sleep-wake cycle. However, in one large well-designed study, melatonin supplements did not relieve symptoms of jet lag, and only a few small studies suggest that these supplements can treat insomnia. There is no evidence that melatonin can prevent pregnancy or cancer.

Possible Side Effects: Drowsiness may occur 30 minutes after taking melatonin and lasts for about 1 hour. Whether melatonin is safe when used long-term is unknown. Theoretically, a viral or prion infection▲ could result from taking melatonin derived from animal brains but not from taking artificially produced melatonin. Headache and transient depression have been reported. In people who are depressed, melatonin may worsen symptoms. Melatonin is best taken under medical supervision.

Milk Thistle

Background: The main active ingredient, silymarin, is found in the seeds of this prickly leafed, purple-flowered plant.

Medicinal Claims: Milk thistle affects primarily the liver, spleen, and kidneys. It increases production of protein by the liver and stimulates regeneration of liver tissue. It is claimed to protect the liver from toxic substances (such as viruses, alcohol, and the toxin from death cap mushrooms) and from certain drugs (such as the analgesic acetaminophen, the antidepressant amitriptyline, and the antibiotic erythromycin). Thus, milk thistle is used to prevent and treat mushroom poisoning and other liver disorders, such as cirrhosis and hepatitis C.

Two well-controlled studies of milk thistle in people with cirrhosis had mixed results. In reports that have collected information about many individual patients with mushroom poisoning, milk thistle reduced the death rate.

Possible Side Effects: Brief stomach upset and mild allergies, but no serious side effects, have been reported. Milk thistle may intensify the effects of drugs that decrease blood sugar levels (hypoglycemic drugs).

Saw Palmetto

Background: The plant's berries can be made into tea. Saw palmetto is also available as tablets, capsules, and a liquid extract.

Medicinal Claims: Saw palmetto opposes the actions of testosterone. It is used to treat benign enlargement of the prostate gland (benign prostatic hyperplasia). In seven of eight relatively well-designed studies, saw palmetto relieved the symptoms of an enlarged prostate gland, such as the frequent urge to urinate.

Claims that it increases sperm production, breast size, or sexual vigor are unproved.

Possible Side Effects: Headache and diarrhea occasionally occur. Because saw palmetto may have hormonal effects, women who are pregnant or who may become pregnant should not take it. Women taking hormone replacement therapy should consult their doctor before they take saw palmetto. Saw palmetto may interact with estrogen replacement therapy and oral contraceptives.

St. John's Wort

Background: The reddish substance in the plant's flowers contains hypericin, which is the main active component.

Medicinal Claims: In many small, mostly short-term, moderately well-designed studies, St. John's wort relieved symptoms in people with mild to moderate depression. However, in a recent large, well-designed study, St. John's wort was found to be ineffective in treating major depression.

St. John's wort has been used in the treatment of HIV infection and vitiligo, but its effectiveness in treating these disorders is unproved.

Possible Side Effects: When used as directed, St. John's wort does not seem to have the side effects or interactions with foods containing tyramine that can occur with other monoamine oxidase inhibitors (MAOIs).■ It can make the skin very sensitive to sunlight (photosensitive). Pregnant women should not take this supplement because it increases muscle tone in the uterus and thus may increase the risk of a miscarriage. St. John's wort may interact with oral contraceptives; protease inhibitors (such as indinavir and ritonavir), which are used to treat HIV infection; MAOIs and other antidepres-

▲ see page 1711   ■ see page 617

sants; the immunosuppressant cyclosporine; digoxin; iron supplements; and the anticoagulant warfarin.

Valerian

Background: The plant's dried root contains valepotriates, which may have calming effects.

Medicinal Claims: Valerian is used as a sedative and sleep aid, especially in parts of Europe. In two relatively well-designed studies, valerian improved sleep quality and shortened the time needed to fall asleep.

Possible Side Effects: Headaches, excitability, uneasiness, and heart disturbances have been reported. Valerian may prolong the effect of other sedatives (such as barbiturates) when it is taken with them. People who are driving or performing other activities requiring alertness should not take it.

HEART AND BLOOD VESSEL DISORDERS

20 **Biology of the Heart and Blood Vessels** 114

The Heart ▪ Blood Vessels ▪ Effects of Aging

21 **Symptoms and Diagnosis of Heart and Blood Vessel Disorders** 118

Pain ▪ Shortness of Breath ▪ Fatigue ▪ Limitation of Physical Activity ▪ Palpitations ▪ Light-Headedness and Fainting ▪ Swelling, Numbness, and Changes in Skin Color ▪ Medical History and Physical Examination ▪ Diagnostic Procedures

22 **High Blood Pressure** 131

23 **Low Blood Pressure** 141

Fainting ▪ Orthostatic Hypotension ▪ Postprandial Hypotension

24 **Shock** 148

25 **Heart Failure** 150

26 **Cardiomyopathy** 158

Dilated Cardiomyopathy ▪ Hypertrophic Cardiomyopathy ▪ Restrictive Cardiomyopathy

27 **Abnormal Heart Rhythms** 163

Atrial Premature Beats ▪ Atrial Fibrillation and Atrial Flutter ▪ Paroxysmal Supraventricular Tachycardia ▪ Wolff-Parkinson-White Syndrome ▪ Ventricular Premature Beats ▪ Ventricular Tachycardia ▪ Ventricular Fibrillation ▪ Pacemaker Dysfunction ▪ Heart Block ▪ Bundle Branch Block

28 **Heart Valve Disorders** 175

Mitral Regurgitation ▪ Mitral Valve Prolapse ▪ Mitral Stenosis ▪ Aortic Regurgitation ▪ Aortic Stenosis ▪ Tricuspid Regurgitation ▪ Tricuspid Stenosis ▪ Pulmonary Stenosis

29 **Infective Endocarditis** 184

30 **Pericardial Disease** 187

Acute Pericarditis ▪ Chronic Pericarditis

31   Heart Tumors..191

Myxomas ▪ Cancerous Tumors

32   Atherosclerosis 194

33   Coronary Artery Disease...199

Angina ▪ Heart Attack

34   Peripheral Arterial Disease...216

Occlusive Peripheral Arterial Disease ▪ Buerger's Disease ▪
Functional Peripheral Arterial Disease ▪ Raynaud's Disease and
Raynaud's Phenomenon ▪ Acrocyanosis ▪ Erythromelalgia

35   Aneurysms and Aortic Dissection 226

Abdominal Aortic Aneurysms ▪ Thoracic Aortic Aneurysms ▪
Aneurysms in Other Arteries ▪ Aortic Dissection

36   Venous Disorders 231

Deep Vein Thrombosis ▪ Superficial Thrombophlebitis ▪
Varicose Veins ▪ Arteriovenous Fistula

37   Lymphatic Disorders 239

Lymphedema ▪ Lymphadenitis ▪ Acute Lymphangitis

CHAPTER 20

Biology of the Heart and Blood Vessels

The heart and blood vessels constitute the cardiovascular (circulatory) system. The blood circulating in this system delivers oxygen and nutrients to the tissues of the body and removes waste products from the tissues.

The Heart

The heart, a hollow muscular organ, is located in the center of the chest. The right and left sides of the heart each have an upper chamber (atrium), which collects blood and pumps it into a lower chamber (ventricle), which pumps blood out.

To ensure that blood flows in only one direction, each ventricle has an "in" (inlet) valve and an "out" (outlet) valve. In the left ventri-cle, the inlet valve is the mitral valve, and the outlet valve is the aortic valve. In the right ventricle, the inlet valve is the tricuspid valve, and the outlet valve is the pulmonary (pulmonic) valve. Each valve consists of flaps (cusps or leaflets), which open and close like one-way swinging doors. The mitral valve has two cusps; the others (tricuspid, aortic, and pulmonary) have three. The large inlet valves (mitral and tricuspid) have tethers—consisting of the papillary muscles and cords of tissue—which prevent the valves from swinging backward into the atria. If a papillary muscle is damaged (for example, by a heart attack), the valve may then swing backwards and start leaking. If a valve opening is narrowed, blood flow through the valve is reduced. A valve may have both problems.

A Look Into the Heart

This cross-sectional view of the heart shows the direction of normal blood flow.

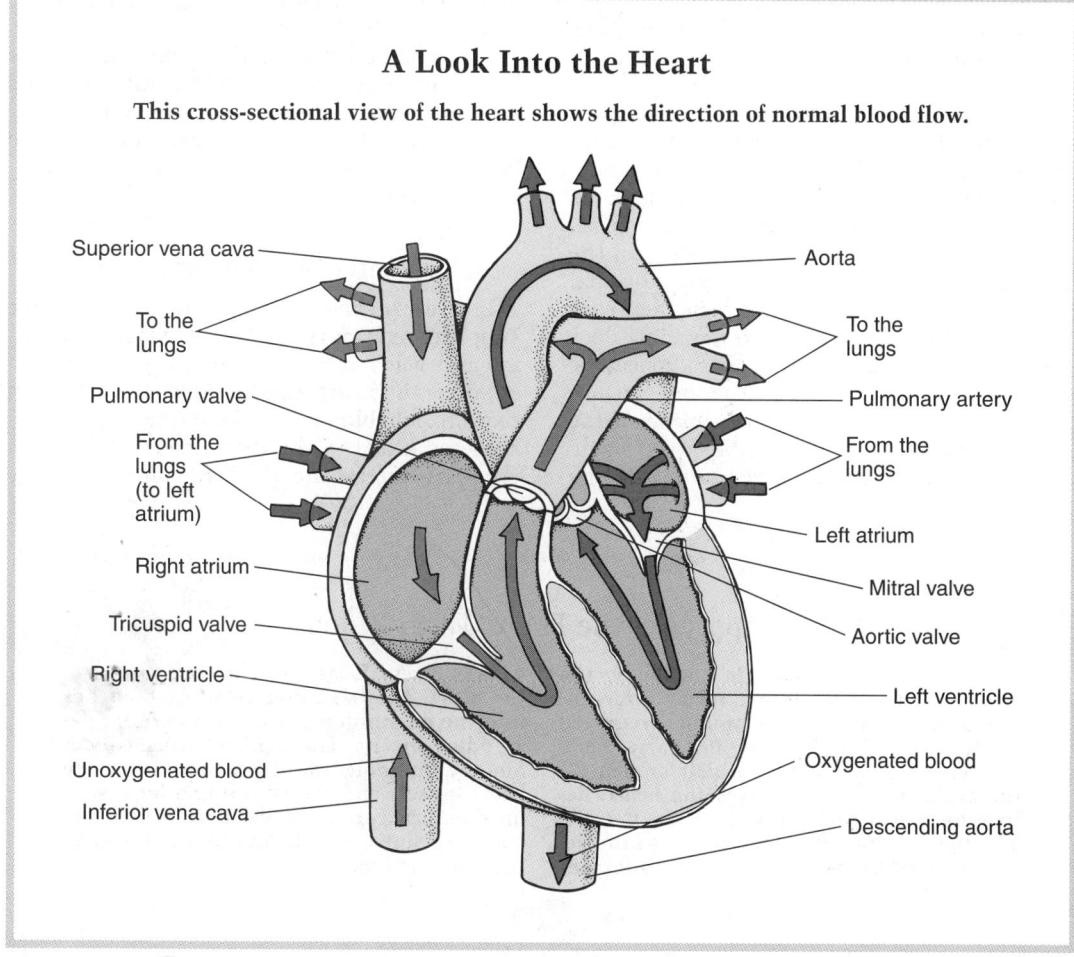

The heartbeats are evidence that the heart is pumping. The first sound (the lub of lub-dub) is the sound of the mitral and tricuspid valves closing. The second sound (the dub) is the sound of the aortic and pulmonary valves closing. Each heartbeat has two parts: diastole and systole. During diastole, the ventricles relax and fill with blood; then the atria contract, forcing more blood into the ventricles. During systole, the ventricles contract and pump blood, and the atria relax and begin filling with blood again.

FUNCTION OF THE HEART

The heart's only function is to pump blood. The right side of the heart pumps blood to the lungs, where oxygen is added to the blood and carbon dioxide is removed from it. The left side pumps blood to the rest of the body, where oxygen and nutrients are delivered to tissues and waste products (such as carbon dioxide) are transferred to the blood for removal by other organs (such as the lungs and kidneys).

Blood travels the following circuit: Blood from the body, which is depleted of oxygen and laden with carbon dioxide, flows through the two largest veins (the venae cavae) into the right atrium. When the right ventricle relaxes, blood in the right atrium pours through the tricuspid valve into the right ventricle. When the right ventricle is nearly full, the right atrium contracts, propelling additional blood into the right ventricle, which then contracts. This contraction propels blood through the pulmonary valve into the pulmonary arteries, which supply the lungs. In the lungs, blood flows through the tiny capillaries that surround the air sacs. Here, the blood absorbs oxygen and gives up carbon dioxide, which is then exhaled.

Blood from the lungs, which is now oxygen-rich, flows through the pulmonary veins into the left atrium. When the left ventricle relaxes, the blood in the left atrium pours through the mitral valve into the left ventricle. When the left ventricle is nearly full, the left atrium contracts, propelling additional blood into the left ventricle, which then contracts. (In older people, the left ventricle does not fill well before the left atrium contracts, making this contraction of the left atrium especially important.) The contraction of the left ventricle propels blood through the aortic valve into the aorta, the largest artery in the body. This blood carries oxygen to all of the body except to the lungs.

The circuit between the right side of the heart, the lungs, and the left atrium is called the pulmonary circulation. The circuit between the left side of the heart, most of the body, and the right atrium is called the systemic circulation.

BLOOD SUPPLY OF THE HEART

Like all organs, the heart needs a constant supply of oxygen-rich blood. A system of arteries and veins called the coronary circulation supplies the heart muscle (myocardium) with oxygen-rich blood and then returns oxygen-depleted blood to the right atrium. The right coronary artery and the left coronary artery

Supplying the Heart With Blood

Like any other tissue in the body, the muscle of the heart must receive oxygen-rich blood and have waste products removed by the blood. The right coronary artery and the left coronary artery, which branch off the aorta just after it leaves the heart, deliver oxygen-rich blood to the heart muscle. The right coronary artery branches into the marginal artery and the posterior interventricular artery, located on the back surface of the heart. The left coronary artery branches into the circumflex and the left anterior descending artery. The cardiac veins collect blood containing waste products from the heart muscle and empty it into a large vein on the back surface of the heart called the coronary sinus, which returns the blood to the right atrium.

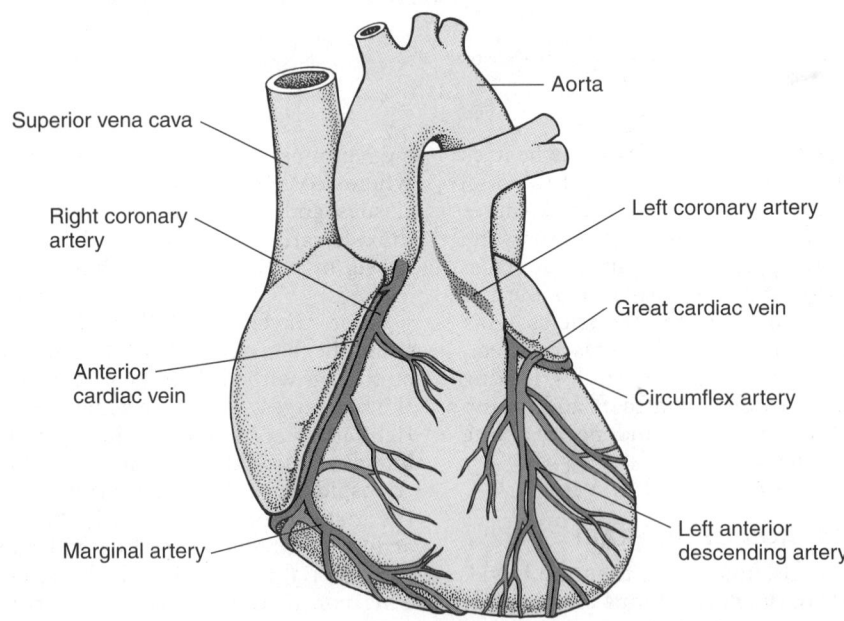

Superior vena cava

Right coronary artery

Anterior cardiac vein

Marginal artery

Aorta

Left coronary artery

Great cardiac vein

Circumflex artery

Left anterior descending artery

branch off the aorta (just after it leaves the heart) to deliver oxygen-rich blood to the heart muscle. These two arteries branch into other arteries, including the circumflex artery, that also supply blood to the heart. The cardiac veins collect blood from the heart muscle and empty it into a large vein on the back surface of the heart called the coronary sinus, which returns the blood to the right atrium. Because of the great pressure exerted in the heart as it contracts, most blood flows through the coronary circulation only while the heart is relaxing between beats (during diastole).

REGULATION OF THE HEART

The contraction of the muscle fibers in the heart is very organized and highly controlled. Rhythmic electrical impulses (discharges) flow through the heart in a precise manner along distinct pathways and at a controlled speed. The impulses originate in the heart's pacemaker (the sinus or sinoatrial node—a small mass of tissue in the wall of the right atrium), which generates a tiny electrical current.▲

The rate at which the pacemaker sends out its impulses (and thus governs the heart rate) is determined by two opposing systems—one to speed the heart rate up (the sympathetic division of the nervous system) and one to slow it down (the parasympathetic division).■ The sympathetic division works through a network of nerves called the sympathetic plexus and through the hormones epinephrine (adrenaline) and norepinephrine (noradrenaline), which are released by the adrenal glands and the nerve endings. The parasympathetic division works through a single nerve—the vagus nerve—which releases the neurotransmitter acetylcholine.

Blood Vessels

The blood vessels consist of arteries, arterioles, capillaries, venules, and veins. All blood is carried in these vessels. The arteries, which are strong, flexible, and resilient, carry blood away from the heart and bear the highest blood pressures. Because arteries are elastic, they narrow (recoil) passively when the heart is relaxing between beats and thus help maintain blood pressure. The arteries branch into smaller and smaller vessels, eventually becoming very small vessels called arterioles. Arteries and arterioles have muscular walls that can

adjust their diameter to increase or decrease blood flow to a particular part of the body.

Capillaries are tiny, extremely thin-walled vessels that act as a bridge between arteries (which carry blood away from the heart) and veins (which carry blood back to the heart). The thin walls of the capillaries allow oxygen and nutrients to pass from the blood into tissues and allow waste products to pass from tissues into the blood.

Blood flows from the capillaries into very small veins called venules, then into the veins that lead back to the heart. Veins have much thinner walls than do arteries, largely because the pressure in veins is so much lower. Veins can widen (dilate) as the amount of fluid in them increases. Some veins, particularly veins in the legs, have valves in them, to prevent blood from flowing backward. When these valves leak, the backflow of blood can cause the veins to stretch and become elongated and convoluted (tortuous). Stretched, tortuous veins near the body's surface are called varicose veins.★

If a blood vessel breaks, tears, or is cut, blood leaks out, causing bleeding. Blood may flow out of the body, as external bleeding, or it may flow into the spaces around organs or directly into organs, as internal bleeding.

Effects of Aging

As people age, the heart tends to enlarge slightly, developing thicker walls and slightly larger chambers. The increase in size is mainly due to an increase in the size of individual heart muscle cells.

During rest, the older heart functions in almost the same way as a younger heart except the heart rate is slightly lower. However, during exercise, the older heart cannot increase the amount of blood pumped out as much as a younger heart can.

The walls of the arteries and arterioles become thicker, and the space within the arteries expands slightly. Elastic tissue within the walls of the arteries and arterioles is lost. Together, these changes make the vessels stiffer and less resilient.

Because arteries and arterioles become less elastic as people age, they cannot relax as quickly during the rhythmic pumping of the heart. As a result, blood pressure increases

▲ see also page 163   ■ see also page 437

★ see page 236

more when the heart contracts (during systole)—sometimes above normal—than it does in younger people. Abnormally high blood pressure during systole with normal blood pressure during diastole is very common among older people; this disorder is called isolated systolic hypertension.▲

Many of the effects of aging on the heart and blood vessels can be reduced by regular exercise. Exercise helps people maintain cardiovascular fitness as well as muscular fitness as they age. Also, exercise is beneficial regardless of the age at which it is started.

CHAPTER 21

Symptoms and Diagnosis of Heart and Blood Vessel Disorders

Disorders that affect the heart or blood vessels are called cardiovascular disorders. These disorders are usually divided into heart disease and peripheral blood vessel disorders. Heart disease affects the heart and the blood vessels that supply the heart muscle. Peripheral blood vessel disorders affect the blood vessels of the arms, legs, and trunk (except those supplying the heart). Disorders that affect the blood vessels that supply the brain are called cerebrovascular disorders. Stroke is an example.■

Symptoms

No single symptom unmistakably indicates heart (cardiac) disease, but certain symptoms suggest the possibility, and several symptoms together may make the diagnosis almost certain. Doctors identify symptoms by interviewing the person to obtain the medical history and by performing a physical examination. Often, diagnostic procedures are performed to confirm the diagnosis. However, sometimes heart disease, even when serious, may produce no symptoms until it reaches a late stage. Routine health checkups or a visit to the doctor for another reason may uncover heart disease that has caused no symptoms. Sometimes doctors perform procedures to screen for heart disease even when there is no evidence of it.

The symptoms of heart disease include certain types of pain, shortness of breath, fatigue, palpitations (awareness of slow, fast, or irregular heartbeats), light-headedness, fainting, and swelling in the legs, ankles, and feet. However, these symptoms do not necessarily indicate heart disease. For example, chest pain may be due to a respiratory or digestive disorder rather than to heart disease.

Symptoms of peripheral blood vessel disorders vary depending on where the affected blood vessels are located. Symptoms may include pain, shortness of breath, muscle cramps, muscle fatigue, light-headedness, swelling, numbness, and a change in skin color of the affected part of the body.

Pain

When muscles do not get enough blood (a condition called ischemia), they do not get enough oxygen, which is carried to tissues by the blood. In addition, waste products, which are carried away from tissues by the blood, accumulate. As a result, cramps occur.

An inadequate blood supply to the heart can cause a tightness or squeezing sensation in the chest (angina). However, the type, location, and severity of pain or discomfort vary greatly from person to person. Some people with an inadequate blood supply have no pain at all. This condition is called silent ischemia.

An inadequate blood supply to other muscles, particularly to the calf muscles, usually causes a tightening and fatiguing pain in the muscle during exercise (claudication).

An inflammation of the sac that envelops the heart (pericarditis) causes pain that worsens when the person lies down and decreases when the person sits up and leans forward. Exertion does not increase the pain, but inhaling deeply does. Pain increased by inhaling deeply

▲ see page 131   ■ see page 502

can also be caused by an inflammation of the membranes covering the lungs (pleurisy).

Disorders affecting arteries can cause a sharp pain that comes and goes fairly quickly; the pain may be unrelated to physical activity. Pain due to an aneurysm (a bulge in a weakened area of an artery's wall) or a dissection (separation of the layers of an artery's wall) is sudden and excruciating. The pain is often felt in the back of the neck, between the shoulder blades, down the back, or in the abdomen, depending on the location of the damage.

The valve between the left atrium and left ventricle (mitral valve) may bulge back into the left atrium when the left ventricle contracts. This disorder, called mitral valve prolapse, sometimes causes brief episodes of stabbing or needle-like pain. Usually, the pain is centered below the left breast regardless of the person's position or physical activity.

Shortness of Breath

Shortness of breath (dyspnea)▲ is a common symptom of heart failure. It results from fluid seeping into the air spaces of the lungs—a condition called pulmonary congestion or pulmonary edema. Ultimately, this process is similar to drowning. In the early stages of heart failure, shortness of breath may occur only during physical activity. As heart failure worsens, shortness of breath occurs with less and less activity and eventually occurs at rest. Shortness of breath at rest occurs mostly when people lie down because fluid seeps throughout the lung tissue. When they sit up, gravity causes fluid to collect at the base of the lungs, causing less difficulty. Nocturnal dyspnea is shortness of breath that occurs when the person is lying down at night; it is relieved by sitting up and dangling the legs. Consequently, people with nocturnal dyspnea usually sleep propped up by pillows to avoid lying flat.

Shortness of breath occurs in people who have coronary artery disease. It usually occurs during physical activity, but in people with severe disease, it may occur during minimal activity or during rest.

Shortness of breath also occurs in people who have other disorders, such as a lung disorder, a disorder of the respiratory muscles, or a disorder of the nervous system that interferes with breathing. Any disorder that upsets the normal, delicate balance between oxygen supply and oxygen requirement can cause shortness of breath. For example, in anemia, the blood may not be able to carry enough oxygen because there are too few red blood cells.

Fatigue

When the heart pumps inefficiently as it does in heart failure, blood flow to the muscles may be inadequate during physical activity, causing feelings of weakness and fatigue. Symptoms are often subtle. People usually compensate by gradually reducing their activity level, or they may blame the symptoms on increasing age.

Limitation of Physical Activity

Heart disease can limit a person's ability to perform physical activities. One way to evaluate the severity of heart disease is to determine how limited this ability is. Doctors may use the New York Heart Association (NYHA) functional class system to make this evaluation. In mild disease (class I), ordinary physical activity may not be limited. In moderate disease (class II), ordinary activity causes symptoms, and in moderately severe disease (class III), less-than-ordinary activity causes symptoms. In severe disease (class IV), symptoms occur during rest, and any physical activity makes them worse. However, this system is not foolproof, because even serious heart disease may produce no symptoms if people reduce their activity level to compensate for the disease.

Palpitations

Ordinarily, people do not notice the beating of their heart. However, most people can feel heartbeats when they lie on their left side. Also, under certain circumstances—for example, when exercising strenuously or having a dramatic emotional experience—healthy people may become aware of their heartbeat. They may feel the heart beating very forcefully or rapidly or sense an irregular heartbeat.

Determining whether palpitations are abnormal depends on answers to a number of questions, such as whether they started suddenly or gradually, whether something seems to trigger them, how fast the heart beats, and whether and to what extent the beat seems to be irregular. Palpitations that occur with other symptoms, such as shortness of breath, pain, weakness, fatigue, or fainting, are more likely to result from an abnormal heart rhythm or a serious disorder. Doctors also listen to the heart with a stethoscope and may suggest

▲ see also page 250

other procedures, such as electrocardiography (ECG).

Light-Headedness and Fainting

If blood flow is inadequate because the heart rate or rhythm is abnormal or because the heart cannot pump adequately, light-headedness, faintness, or fainting (syncope) may result. These symptoms can also result from brain or spinal cord disorders, or they may have no serious cause. For example, healthy soldiers may feel faint or may faint when standing still for long periods (a phenomenon called parade ground syncope), because the leg muscles have to be active to help return blood to the heart. Strong emotion or pain, which activates part of the nervous system, also can cause fainting. Sitting or standing up too quickly can cause a feeling of faintness or fainting, because the change in position causes blood to pool in the legs, resulting in a fall in blood pressure. Normally, the body quickly adjusts to maintain blood pressure. Inability to adjust quickly is called orthostatic hypotension. This disorder is particularly common among older people.

People are more likely to feel faint or to faint when they are standing up. When they lie or fall down, blood flow to the brain is increased, generally ending the faint.

Doctors must distinguish fainting caused by heart disease from a seizure disorder, in which a loss of consciousness results from a brain disorder.

Swelling, Numbness, and Changes in Skin Color

Swelling is due to the accumulation of fluid (edema) in tissues. It occurs when blood pools in the leg veins, increasing pressure in the leg veins and forcing fluids out of the veins into tissues. Blood may pool because the heart cannot pump out all of the blood it receives from the rest of the body (in heart failure) or because a deep vein in the leg is blocked (in deep vein thrombosis).

Swelling in the legs, ankles, and feet or in the abdomen may indicate heart failure or a venous disorder, such as deep vein thrombosis. However, such swelling is most commonly caused by standing or sitting in one position too long or by age-related changes in leg veins. Swelling of the legs is also common during pregnancy. Swelling may also be due to liver or kidney disorders.

If the blood supply is inadequate, the affected part of the body may feel numb.

If the blood supply is inadequate, if anemia is present, or if the veins do not drain adequately, the skin may appear pale or bluish (or purplish).

Diagnosis

Usually, doctors can tell whether a person has a heart or blood vessel disorder on the basis of the medical history and the physical examination. Diagnostic procedures are used to confirm the diagnosis, determine the extent and severity of the disease, and help in planning treatment.

MEDICAL HISTORY AND PHYSICAL EXAMINATION

A doctor first asks about symptoms. Chest pain, shortness of breath, palpitations, and swelling in the legs, ankles, and feet or abdomen suggest heart disease. Other, more general symptoms, such as fever, weakness, fatigue, lack of appetite, and a general feeling of illness or discomfort (malaise), may suggest heart disease. Pain, numbness, or muscle cramps in a leg may suggest peripheral arterial disease, which affects the arteries of the arms, legs, and trunk (except those supplying the heart).

Next, the doctor asks about past infections; previous exposure to chemicals; use of drugs, alcohol, and tobacco; home and work environments; and recreational activity. The doctor also asks whether family members have had heart disease or any other disorders that may affect the heart or blood vessels.

During the physical examination, the doctor notes the person's weight and overall appearance and looks for paleness (pallor), sweating, or drowsiness, which may be subtle indicators of heart disease. The person's general mood and feeling of well-being, which also may be affected by heart disease, are noted.

Assessing skin color is important because pallor or a bluish or purplish coloration (cyanosis) may indicate anemia or inadequate blood flow. These findings may indicate that the skin is not receiving enough oxygen from the blood because of a lung disorder, heart failure, or various circulatory problems.

The doctor feels the pulse in arteries in the neck, beneath the arms, at the elbows and wrists, in the abdomen, in the groin, at the knees, and in the ankles and feet to assess whether blood flow is adequate and equal on both sides of the body. The blood pressure and body temperature are also checked. An abnormality may suggest a heart or blood vessel disorder.

The doctor inspects the veins in the neck while the person is lying down with the upper part of the body elevated at a 45° angle. These veins are inspected because they are directly connected to the right atrium (the upper chamber of the heart that receives oxygen-depleted blood from the body) and thus give an indication of the volume and pressure of blood entering the right side of the heart.

The doctor presses the skin over the ankles and legs and sometimes over the lower back to check for fluid accumulation (edema) in the tissues beneath the skin.

An ophthalmoscope▲ is used to view the blood vessels of the retina (the light-sensitive membrane on the inner surface of the back of the eye). The retina is the only place a doctor can directly view veins and arteries. Visible abnormalities in the retina are common among people with high blood pressure, diabetes, arteriosclerosis, and bacterial infections of the heart valves.

The doctor observes the chest to determine if the breathing rate and movements are normal. By tapping (percussing) the chest with the fingers, the doctor can determine if the lungs are filled with air, which is normal, or if they contain fluid, which is abnormal. Percussion also helps determine whether the sac surrounding the heart (pericardium) or the layers of membranes covering the lungs (pleura) contain fluid. Using a stethoscope, the doctor also listens to the breathing sounds to determine whether airflow is normal or obstructed and whether the lungs contain fluid as a result of heart failure.

By placing a hand on the person's chest, the doctor can feel (palpate) where the heartbeat is strongest and thus determine heart size. The quality and force of contractions during each heartbeat can also be determined. Sometimes abnormal, turbulent blood flow within vessels or between heart chambers causes a vibration (called a thrill) that can be felt with the fingertips or palm.

By listening to (auscultating) the heart with a stethoscope, the doctor can hear the distinctive sounds caused by the opening and closing of the heart valves. Abnormalities of the valves and heart structures create turbulent blood flow that causes characteristic sounds called murmurs. Turbulent blood flow typi-

cally occurs as blood moves through narrowed or leaking valves. However, not all heart diseases cause murmurs, and not all murmurs indicate heart disease. For example, pregnant women usually have heart murmurs because of a normal increase in blood flow. Harmless heart murmurs also are common among infants and children because of the rapid flow of blood through small structures in the heart. As blood vessel walls, valves, and other tissues gradually stiffen in older people, blood may flow turbulently, even when no serious heart disease is present. Also, the doctor may hear clicks and opening snaps when an abnormal valve opens. A gallop rhythm (a sound resembling that of a galloping horse), due to one or two extra heart sounds, is often heard in people who have heart failure.

By placing the stethoscope over arteries and veins elsewhere in the body, the doctor can listen for sounds of turbulent blood flow (bruits). Bruits may be caused by narrowing of blood vessels, increased blood flow, or an abnormal connection between an artery and a vein (arteriovenous fistula).

The doctor feels the abdomen to determine if the liver is enlarged. Enlargement may indicate that blood is pooled in the major veins leading to the heart. Swelling of the abdomen due to fluid accumulation may indicate heart failure. By pressing gently on the abdomen, the doctor checks the pulse and determines the width of the abdominal aorta.

DIAGNOSTIC PROCEDURES

There are many diagnostic procedures that can help doctors make a rapid, precise diagnosis. They include electrocardiography (ECG), stress testing, electrophysiologic testing, tilt table testing, radiologic procedures (x-rays), ultrasonography (including echocardiography), magnetic resonance imaging (MRI), radionuclide imaging, positron emission tomography (PET), cardiac catheterization, central venous catheterization, and angiography. Computed tomography (CT) and fluoroscopy are used infrequently. Blood tests to measure levels of sugar (to test for diabetes), cholesterol, and other substances are often performed.

Most of these procedures carry very small risk, but the risk increases with the complexity of the procedure and the severity of the heart disease.

▲ see art on page 1284

Electrocardiography

Electrocardiography (ECG) is a quick, simple, painless procedure in which electrical impulses flowing through the heart are amplified and recorded on a moving strip of paper. This record, the electrocardiogram (the ECG), provides information about the part of the heart that triggers each heartbeat (the pacemaker), the nerve conduction pathways of the heart, and the rate and rhythm of the heart.

Usually, ECG is performed if a heart disorder is suspected. It is also performed as part of a routine physical examination for most middle-aged and older people, even if they have no evidence of a heart disorder. It can be used as a basis of comparison with later ECGs if a heart disorder develops. This procedure can help doctors identify such heart disorders as a previous heart attack (myocardial infarction), abnormal heart rhythms (arrhythmias), an inadequate blood and oxygen supply to the heart (ischemia), and excessive thickening (hypertrophy) of heart muscle, which can result from high blood pressure. ECG can also detect bulges (aneurysms) in the heart's walls, which

ECG: Reading the Waves

An electrocardiogram (ECG) represents the electrical current moving through the heart during a heartbeat. The current's movement is divided into parts, and each part is given an alphabetic designation in the ECG.

Each heartbeat begins with an impulse from the heart's pacemaker (sinus or sinoatrial node). This impulse activates the upper chambers of the heart (atria). The P wave represents activation of the atria.

Next, the electrical current flows down to the lower chambers of the heart (ventricles).

The QRS complex represents activation of the ventricles.

The electrical current then spreads back over the ventricles in the opposite direction. This activity is called the recovery wave, which is represented by the T wave.

Many kinds of abnormalities can be seen on an ECG. For example, the heart rhythm may be abnormal: too fast, too slow, or irregular. By reading an ECG, doctors can usually determine where in the heart the abnormal rhythm starts and can begin to determine its cause.

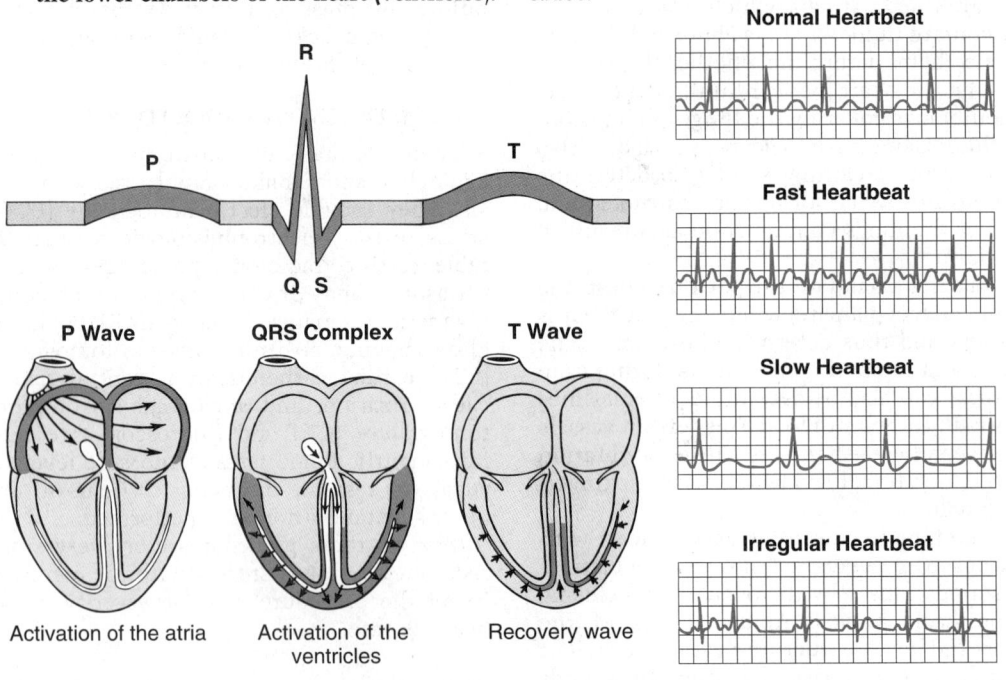

P Wave — Activation of the atria

QRS Complex — Activation of the ventricles

T Wave — Recovery wave

Normal Heartbeat

Fast Heartbeat

Slow Heartbeat

Irregular Heartbeat

develop in a weak area; aneurysms may result from a heart attack.

To obtain an ECG, an examiner places electrodes (small round sensors that stick to the skin) on the person's arms, legs, and chest. These electrodes measure the magnitude and direction of electrical currents in the heart during each heartbeat. The electrodes are connected by wires to a machine, which produces a record (tracing) for each electrode. Each tracing shows the electrical activity of the heart from different angles. The tracings constitute the ECG. ECG takes about 3 minutes, is painless, and has no risks.

Exercise Stress Testing

How well a person tolerates exercise is related to the existence and severity of coronary artery disease, other heart disorders, some other disorders (such as a lung disorder and anemia), and general fitness. An exercise stress test, which consists of ECG and blood pressure measurement during exercise, can detect problems that would not appear at rest. If the coronary arteries are only partially blocked, the heart may have an adequate blood supply when the person is resting but not when the person exercises. Because an exercise stress test specifically monitors how the heart is functioning, the test helps doctors distinguish between problems due to a heart disorder and those due to other disorders.

Electrodes are attached to the chest to record the ECG. During the test, the person walks on a treadmill or pedals an exercise bicycle. People who cannot use their legs can use an arm crank. Gradually, the pace of the exercise and the force required to do it (workload) are increased. The ECG is monitored continuously, and blood pressure is measured at intervals. Usually, the person being tested is asked to keep going until the heart rate reaches between 80% and 90% of the maximum for age and sex. If symptoms, such as shortness of breath or chest pain, become too uncomfortable or if significant abnormalities appear on the ECG or blood pressure recordings, the test is stopped sooner. Testing takes about 30 minutes. Exercise stress testing has a small risk; the chance of its causing a heart attack or death is 1 in 5,000.

People who cannot exercise can be evaluated using pharmacologic stress testing with ECG. This procedure provides information similar to that from an exercise stress test but does not involve exercise. Instead, a drug, such as dipyridamole, dobutamine, or adenosine, is injected to simulate the effects of exercise on blood flow.

Exercise or pharmacologic stress testing suggests coronary artery disease when certain ECG abnormalities appear, chest pain develops, or blood pressure decreases.

No test is perfect. Sometimes, these tests show abnormalities in people who do not have coronary artery disease (a false-positive result), and sometimes tests do not show any abnormalities in people who have the disease (a false-negative result). In people without symptoms, especially younger people, the likelihood of coronary artery disease is low, despite an abnormal test result. Nevertheless, exercise stress testing is often used for screening purposes in apparently healthy people—for example, before an exercise program is begun or during an evaluation for life insurance. However, in such cases, a positive result is usually more likely to be false than true. These false-positive results may cause considerable worry and medical expense. For these reasons, most experts discourage routine exercise stress testing in people who do not have symptoms.

The accuracy of exercise stress testing can be greatly increased by injecting a tiny amount of a radioactive substance (tracer), such as thallium.▲ However, the added expense of this procedure makes it inappropriate for routine screening.

Continuous Ambulatory Electrocardiography

Abnormal heart rhythms and inadequate blood flow to the heart muscle may occur only briefly or unpredictably. To detect such problems, doctors may use continuous ambulatory ECG, in which the ECG is recorded continuously for 24 hours while the person engages in normal daily activities.

For this procedure, the person wears a small battery-powered device (Holter monitor) held on with a shoulder strap. The monitor detects the heart's electrical activity through electrodes attached to the chest and records the ECG. While wearing the monitor, the person notes in a diary the time and type of any symptoms. Subsequently, the ECG is run through a computer, which analyzes the rate and rhythm of the heart, looks for changes in electrical activity that could indicate inadequate blood flow to the heart muscle, and produces a record of every heartbeat during the 24

▲ see page 127

hours. Symptoms recorded in the diary can then be correlated with changes in the ECG.

If necessary, the ECG can be transmitted by telephone to a computer at the hospital or doctor's office for an immediate reading as soon as symptoms occur.

An event monitor is used when a person must be monitored longer than 24 hours. It is similar to a Holter monitor, but it records only when the user activates it—that is, when symptoms occur.

Continuous Ambulatory Blood Pressure Monitoring

If the diagnosis of high blood pressure is in doubt (for example, if the measurements taken in the office vary too much), a 24-hour

blood pressure monitor may be used. The monitor is a portable battery-operated device, worn on the hip, connected to a blood pressure cuff, worn on the arm. This monitor repeatedly records blood pressure throughout the day and night over a 24- or 48-hour period. The readings determine not only whether high blood pressure is present but also how severe it is.

Electrophysiologic Testing

Electrophysiologic testing is used to evaluate serious abnormalities in heart rhythm or electrical conduction. Testing is performed in the hospital. After injecting a local anesthetic, a doctor inserts a catheter with tiny electrodes at its tip through an incision, usually in the groin, into a vein or sometimes an artery. The catheter is threaded through the major blood vessels into the heart chambers, using fluoroscopy (a continuous x-ray procedure) for guidance. The catheter is used to record the ECG from within the heart and to identify the precise location of the electrical conduction pathways.

Usually, a doctor intentionally provokes an abnormal heart rhythm during testing to find out whether a particular drug can stop the disturbance or whether an operation will help by eliminating abnormal electrical connections within the heart. If necessary, a doctor can quickly restore a normal rhythm with a brief electrical shock to the heart (cardioversion). Although electrophysiologic testing is an invasive procedure and an anesthetic is required, the procedure is very safe: The risk of death is 1 in 5,000. This procedure usually takes 1 to 2 hours.

Tilt Table Testing

Tilt table testing is usually recommended for people who experience fainting (syncope) for an unknown reason and who do not have structural heart disease (such as aortic valve stenosis). Typically, a person is tilted at a 60° to 80° angle on a motorized table for 15 to 20 minutes while blood pressure and heart rate are continuously monitored. If blood pressure does not decrease, the person is given isoproterenol (a drug that stimulates the heart) intravenously in a dose large enough to accelerate the heart rate by 20 beats per minute, and the test is repeated. The procedure produces many false-positive results; that is, it often appears to indicate heart disease when none is present. This procedure takes 30 to 60 minutes and is very safe.

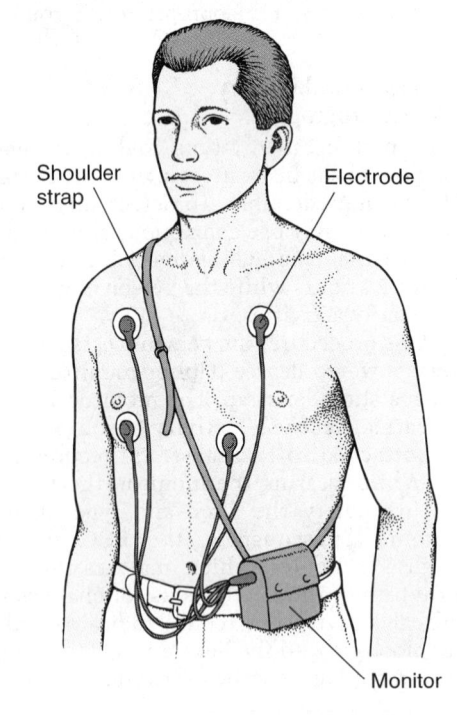

Holter Monitor: Continuous ECG Readings

The small monitor is attached to a strap worn over one shoulder. Through electrodes attached to the chest, the monitor continuously records the electrical activity of the heart.

Shoulder strap

Electrode

Monitor

Radiologic Procedures

Anyone thought to have heart disease has chest x-rays taken from the front and the side. The x-rays show the shape and size of the heart and outline blood vessels in the lungs and chest. Abnormal heart shape or size and abnormalities such as calcium deposits within heart tissue are readily seen. Chest x-rays also can detect information about the condition of the lungs, particularly whether blood vessels in the lungs are abnormal and whether there is fluid in or around the lungs.

X-rays can detect enlargement of the heart, which is often due to heart failure or a heart valve disorder. The heart does not enlarge when heart failure results from constrictive pericarditis, in which scar tissue forms throughout the sac that envelops the heart (pericardium).

The appearance of blood vessels in the lungs is often more useful in making a diagnosis than the appearance of the heart itself. For instance, enlargement of the pulmonary arteries (the arteries that carry blood from the heart to the lungs) and narrowing of the arteries within the lung tissue suggest thickening of the muscle of the right ventricle (the lower heart chamber that pumps blood through the pulmonary arteries to the lungs) due to high blood pressure in the pulmonary arteries.

X-rays of other parts of the body may be taken to detect blockages in other blood vessels.

The x-ray machine is positioned so that x-rays are beamed at the area to be examined. Exposure to x-rays lasts only a fraction of a second.

Radiation from x-rays causes no immediate problems. There is a very small risk that radiation may damage cells, leading to cancer later in life. The greater the exposure, the greater the risk. For this reason, a very low dose is used, and lead shields may be used to protect areas that are not being x-rayed from exposure. Shielding is particularly important for pregnant women.

Computed Tomography

Ordinary computed tomography (CT) is not often used in diagnosing heart disease. However, CT can detect structural abnormalities of the heart, the sac that envelops the heart (pericardium), major blood vessels, lungs, and supporting structures in the chest.

For this procedure, a person lies on a motorized bed inside a CT scanner, which takes a se-ries of x-rays from different angles. When one series, or scan, is completed, the bed is moved forward, and another scan is taken. The person may be asked not to breathe during a scan so that the image will not be blurred. CT scans differ from ordinary x-rays because they show different levels of tissue density and so produce more detailed images. From these scans, a computer creates cross-sectional images of the whole chest (or other body parts) and displays them on a monitor. These images enable doctors to precisely locate abnormalities. A set of scans can be taken in about 30 minutes.

Newer ultrafast computed tomography, also called cine-computed tomography, provides a three-dimensional moving image of the heart. This procedure may be used to assess abnormalities in the structure and motion of the heart wall but is not widely available.

Computed tomography angiography (CTA) is a type of computed tomography that is used to produce three-dimensional images of the major arteries of the body, except those that supply the heart (coronary arteries). The images are similar in quality to those produced by coronary angiography.▲ It can be used to detect narrowing of the arteries supplying the kidneys (renal stenosis) and clots that have broken off within an artery, traveled through the bloodstream, and lodged in the small arteries of the lungs (pulmonary emboli).

Unlike angiography, CTA is not an invasive procedure. Usually, a dye that can be seen on x-rays (radiopaque dye or contrast agent) is injected into a vein rather than into an artery as in angiography. CTA usually takes less than 30 minutes.

Fluoroscopy

Fluoroscopy is a continuous x-ray procedure that shows the heart beating and the lungs inflating and deflating on a screen. However, fluoroscopy, which involves a relatively high dose of radiation, has been largely replaced by echocardiography and other procedures. Fluoroscopy is still used as a component of cardiac catheterization and electrophysiologic testing.

Echocardiography and Other Ultrasound Procedures

Ultrasonography uses high-frequency (ultrasound) waves bounced off internal structures to produce a moving image. It uses no x-rays. Ultrasonography of the heart (echocardiogra-

▲ see page 129

phy) is one of the most widely used procedures for diagnosing heart disorders because it is noninvasive, harmless, relatively inexpensive, and widely available and because it provides excellent images. Ultrasonography is also used in the diagnosis of disorders affecting blood vessels in other parts of the body.

Echocardiography can be used to detect abnormalities in heart wall motion and to measure the volume of blood being pumped from the heart with each beat. This procedure can also detect abnormalities in the heart's structure, such as defective heart valves, birth defects, and enlargement of the heart's walls or chambers, as occurs in people with heart failure or cardiomyopathy. Echocardiography can also be used to detect pericardial effusion, in which fluid accumulates between the two layers of the sac that envelops the heart (pericardium), and constrictive pericarditis, in which scar tissue forms throughout the pericardium.

The main types of ultrasonography are M-mode, two-dimensional, Doppler, and color Doppler. In M-mode ultrasonography, the simplest technique, a single beam of ultrasound is aimed at the part of the heart being studied. Two-dimensional ultrasonography, the most widely used technique, produces realistic two-dimensional images in computer-generated "slices." Stacking the slices together can recreate a three-dimensional structure.

Doppler ultrasonography shows the direction and velocity of blood flow and thus can detect turbulent flow due to narrowing or blockage of blood vessels. Color Doppler ultrasonography shows the different rates of blood flow in different colors. Doppler ultrasonography and color Doppler ultrasonography are commonly used to help diagnose disorders affecting the heart and the arteries and veins in the trunk, legs, and arms. Because these procedures can show the direction and rate of blood flow in the chambers and blood vessels of the heart, they enable doctors to evaluate the structure and function of these structures. For example, doctors can determine if the heart valves open and close properly, if and how much they leak when closed, and if blood flows normally. Abnormal connections between an artery and a vein or between heart chambers can also be detected.

The ultrasound waves are emitted by a handheld recording probe (transducer). For echocardiography, the examiner places gel on the chest over the heart and moves the probe over that area. The probe is connected to a monitor that displays an image. The image is recorded on a videocassette, a computer disk, or paper. By varying the placement and angle of the probe, doctors can view the heart and nearby major blood vessels from various angles and thus get an accurate picture of heart structure and function. Echocardiography is painless and takes 20 to 30 minutes.

If doctors need to obtain greater clarity or to analyze the aorta or structures at the back of the heart (particularly the left atrium or left ventricle), transesophageal echocardiography can be used. For this procedure, a probe is passed down the person's throat into the esophagus. The probe records signals from just behind the heart. Transesophageal echocardiography is also used when regular echocardiography is difficult to perform because of obesity, lung disorders, or other technical problems.

Magnetic Resonance Imaging

With magnetic resonance imaging (MRI), a powerful magnetic field and radio waves are used to produce detailed images of the heart and chest. This expensive and sophisticated procedure is used predominantly for the diagnosis of complex heart disease that is present at birth (congenital).

The person is placed inside a large electromagnetic chamber that causes the nuclei of atoms in the body to line up parallel to each other. (Normally, nuclei randomly point in different directions.) Then a pulse of radio waves is emitted, making the nuclei vibrate out of alignment. As the nuclei line up again, they give out characteristic signals, which are converted into two- and three-dimensional images of heart structures. Usually, an injection of a substance that can be seen on scans (contrast agent) to enhance the image is not needed. Occasionally, however, a paramagnetic contrast agent (a substance that is weakly attracted by strong magnetic fields) is given intravenously to help identify areas of inadequate blood flow in the heart muscle.

MRI has some disadvantages. It takes longer to produce MRI images than computed tomography (CT) images. Because of the movement of the heart, the images obtained with MRI are fuzzier than those obtained with CT. In addition, some people become claustrophobic during MRI because they must lie very still in a narrow space in a giant machine. A new MRI scanner that has one open side can be used for people who have claustrophobia or who are obese. However, the images produced by this type of scanner are inferior to those produced by the traditional scanner.

Magnetic resonance angiography (MRA) is a type of magnetic resonance imaging (MRI) that focuses on blood vessels rather than organs. MRA produces images of blood vessels and blood flow similar in quality to those produced by coronary angiography.▲ MRA can be used to detect aneurysms (bulges) in the aorta, narrowing of the arteries supplying the kidneys (renal stenosis), and a narrowing or blockage in the arteries supplying the heart (coronary arteries) or the arms and legs (peripheral arteries).

Unlike angiography, MRA is not an invasive procedure. Sometimes a paramagnetic contrast agent is injected into a blood vessel. MRA uses the same scanner as is used for MRI and thus also requires that the person lie still in a narrow space. MRA usually takes less than 1 hour.

Radionuclide Imaging

In radionuclide imaging, a tiny amount of a radioactive substance (radionuclide), called a tracer, is injected into any vein. The amount of radiation the person receives is tiny—less than that produced by most x-rays.

The tracer is quickly distributed throughout the body. How much of the tracer a tissue takes up indicates how active that tissue is. The tracer emits gamma rays, which are detected by a gamma camera. A computer analyzes this information and constructs an image, which is displayed on a screen and stored on a computer disk for further analysis. Each scan produces a single image. The different colors in the image indicate different amounts of tracer taken up by tissues.

Radionuclide imaging is particularly useful in the diagnosis of chest pain when the cause is unknown. If the coronary arteries are narrowed, radionuclide imaging is used to learn how the narrowing is affecting the heart's blood supply and function. Radionuclide imaging is also used to assess improvement in blood supply to the heart muscle after bypass surgery or similar procedures and may be used to determine a person's prognosis after a heart attack.

Different tracers are used depending on what disorder is suspected. For evaluating blood flow through heart muscle, the tracer typically used is technetium-99 sestamibi or thallium-201, and images are obtained while the person performs an exercise stress test.■

The amount of tracer absorbed by the heart muscle cells depends on the blood flow. At peak exercise, an area of heart muscle that has an inadequate blood supply (ischemia) absorbs less tracer—and produces a fainter image—than neighboring muscle with a normal supply. In people unable to exercise, an intravenous injection of a drug, such as dipyridamole, dobutamine, or adenosine, may be used to simulate the effects of exercise on blood flow. These drugs divert the blood supply from abnormal to normal blood vessels, depriving the area with inadequate blood flow even further.

After the person rests for a few hours, a second scan is performed, and the resulting image is compared with that obtained during exercise. Doctors can then distinguish areas of the heart where inadequate blood flow is reversible (usually caused by narrowing of the coronary arteries) from areas where it is irreversible (usually caused by scarring due to a previous heart attack).

If a heart attack may have occurred very recently, technetium 99m is used instead of thallium-201. With technetium, damage due to a heart attack can be detected after 12 to 24 hours and up to about 1 week. Unlike thallium, which accumulates primarily in normal tissue, technetium accumulates primarily in abnormal tissue. However, because technetium also accumulates in bone, the ribs somewhat obscure the image of the heart.

A specialized type of radionuclide imaging called single photon emission computed tomography (SPECT) can produce a series of computer-enhanced cross-sectional images. A three-dimensional image can also be produced. SPECT provides more information about function, blood flow, and abnormalities than does conventional radionuclide imaging.

Positron Emission Tomography

In positron emission tomography (PET), a substance necessary for heart cell function (such as oxygen or sugar) is labeled with a radioactive substance (radionuclide) that gives off positrons (electrons with a positive charge). The labeled nutrient is injected into a vein and reaches the heart in a few minutes. PET is used to determine how much blood is reaching different parts of the heart muscle and how different parts of the heart muscle pro-

▲ see page 129   ■ see page 123

cess (metabolize) various substances. For example, when labeled sugar is injected, doctors can determine which parts of the heart muscle have an inadequate blood supply because those parts use more sugar than normal.

PET scans produce clearer images than do other radionuclide procedures. However, the procedure is very expensive and not widely available. It is used in research and in cases in which simpler, less expensive procedures are inconclusive.

The person is placed inside a ring-shaped PET scanner, which detects radiation all around the person and records sites of high activity. The more active an area of the heart muscle, the more positrons it takes up and the more radiation it gives off. Different colors in the resulting scan indicate how active different areas of heart muscle are. A computer constructs a three-dimensional image of the area.

Cardiac Catheterization and Coronary Angiography

Cardiac catheterization used with coronary angiography is the most accurate method of diagnosing coronary artery disease. Used together, the two procedures are the only way to directly measure the pressure of blood in each chamber of the heart and to obtain an image of the interior of coronary arteries. These procedures are performed to determine whether angioplasty or coronary artery bypass surgery is technically feasible. They may be performed to confirm the diagnosis of other heart disorders, to determine the severity of a heart disorder, or to detect the cause of worsening symptoms.

More than a million cardiac catheterizations and angiographic procedures are performed every year. They are relatively safe, and complications are rare. With cardiac catheterization and angiography, the chance of a serious complication—such as stroke, heart attack, or death—is 1 in 1,000. Fewer than 0.01% of people undergoing these procedures die; most of those who die already have a severe heart disorder or other disorder. The risk of complications and death is increased for older people.

Cardiac Catheterization: Cardiac catheterization is used extensively for the diagnosis and treatment of heart disease that is not due to disease of the coronary arteries. Cardiac catheterization can be used to measure how much blood the heart pumps out per minute

(cardiac output) and to detect birth defects of the heart and tumors, such as a myxoma.

In cardiac catheterization, a thin catheter (a tubular, flexible surgical instrument) is inserted into an artery or vein through a puncture made with a needle or a tiny incision. A local anesthetic is given to numb the insertion site. The catheter is then threaded through the major blood vessels and into the heart chambers. The procedure is performed in the hospital and takes 40 to 60 minutes.

Various instruments may be placed at the tip of the catheter. They include instruments to measure the pressure of blood in each heart chamber and in blood vessels connected to the heart, view the interior of blood vessels, take blood samples from different parts of the heart, or remove a tissue sample from inside the heart for examination under a microscope (biopsy). Pressure in the heart chambers is measured in an intensive care or coronary care unit with a catheter that is designed for that purpose and that has a balloon at its tip (Swan-Ganz catheter).

When a catheter is used to inject a dye that can be seen on x-rays, the procedure is called **angiography.** When a catheter is used to widen a narrowed heart valve opening, the procedure is called **valvuloplasty.** When a catheter is used to clear a narrowed or blocked artery, the procedure is called **angioplasty.**▲

If an artery is used for catheter insertion, the puncture or incision site must be steadily compressed for 10 to 20 minutes after all the instruments are removed. Compression prevents bleeding and bruise formation. However, bleeding occasionally occurs at the incision site, leaving a large bruise that can persist for weeks but that almost always goes away on its own.

Because inserting a catheter into the heart may cause abnormal heart rhythms, the heart is monitored with electrocardiography (ECG). Usually, doctors can correct an abnormal rhythm by moving the catheter to another position. If this maneuver does not help, the catheter is removed. Very rarely, the heart wall is damaged or punctured when a catheter is inserted; immediate surgical repair may be required.

Cardiac catheterization may be performed on the right or left side of the heart.

Catheterization of the right side of the heart is performed to obtain information about the heart chambers on the right side (right atrium and right ventricle) and the tricuspid valve (located between these two chambers). The right atrium receives oxygen-depleted blood from the body, and the right ventricle pumps the blood into the lungs, where blood takes up oxygen and drops off carbon dioxide. In this procedure, the catheter is inserted into a vein, usually in an arm or the groin. Pulmonary artery catheterization, in which the balloon at the catheter's tip is passed through the right atrium and ventricle and lodged in the pulmonary artery, is usually performed as part of right heart catheterization.

Catheterization of the left side is performed to obtain information about the heart chambers on the left side (left atrium and left ventricle), the mitral valve (located between the left atrium and left ventricle), and the aortic valve (located between the left ventricle and the aorta). The left atrium receives oxygen-rich blood from the lungs, and the left ventricle pumps the blood into the rest of the body. The left side is catheterized more often than the right. For example, catheterization of the left side is performed when coronary artery disease has been detected (to determine the extent of the disease) or is suspected (to confirm the diagnosis). This procedure is usually combined with coronary angiography to obtain information about the coronary arteries.

For catheterization of the left side of the heart, the catheter is inserted into an artery, usually in an arm or the groin. Less commonly, the catheter is inserted into a vein in the groin and threaded into the right side of the heart (as in catheterization of the right side). The catheter is then threaded into the left side by puncturing the wall (septum) separating the right atrium from the left.

Coronary Angiography: This procedure provides information about the coronary arteries, which supply the heart with oxygen-rich blood. Coronary angiography is similar to catheterization of the left side of the heart, and the two procedures are almost always performed at the same time. After injecting a local anesthetic, a doctor inserts a thin catheter into an artery through an incision in an arm or the groin. The catheter is threaded toward the heart, then into the coronary arteries. During insertion, the doctor uses fluoroscopy (a continuous x-ray procedure) to observe the progress of the catheter as it is threaded into place. After the catheter tip is in place, a radiopaque dye, which can be seen on x-rays, is injected through the catheter into the coronary arteries, and the outline of

the arteries appears on a video screen and is recorded on a tape or disk. Usually, motion picture techniques that produce continuous images are used; this procedure is then called **cineangiography.** It provides clear pictures of the heart chambers and coronary arteries as they move.

Coronary angiography is seldom uncomfortable and usually takes 30 to 50 minutes. It is performed as an outpatient procedure unless the person is very ill.

When the radiopaque dye is injected into the aorta or heart chambers, the person has a temporary feeling of warmth throughout the body as the dye spreads through the bloodstream. The heart rate may increase, and blood pressure may fall slightly. Rarely, the dye causes the heart to slow briefly or even stop. The person may be asked to cough vigorously during the procedure to help correct such problems, which are rarely serious. Rarely, mild complications, such as nausea, vomiting, and coughing, occur. Serious complications, such as shock,▲ seizures, kidney problems, and sudden cessation of the heart's pumping (cardiac arrest), are very rare. Allergic reactions to the dye range from skin rashes to a rare life-threatening reaction called anaphylaxis.■ The team performing the procedure is prepared to treat the complications of coronary angiography immediately.

Risk of complications is higher in older people, although it is still low. Coronary angiography is essential when angioplasty or coronary artery bypass surgery is being considered.★

Ventriculography is a type of angiography in which x-rays are taken as a radiopaque dye is injected into the left or right ventricle of the heart through a catheter. It is performed during cardiac catheterization. With this procedure, doctors can see the motion of the left or right ventricle and can thus evaluate the pumping ability of the heart. Based on the heart's pumping ability, doctors can calculate the ejection fraction (the percentage of blood pumped out by the left ventricle with each heartbeat). Evaluation of the heart's pumping helps determine how much of the heart has been damaged.

Pulmonary Artery Catheterization

Pulmonary artery catheterization is a useful measure of overall heart function in people

---

▲ see page 148   ■ see page 1072
★ see pages 208 and 209

who are critically ill, particularly when fluids are being given intravenously. Such people include those who have severe heart or pulmonary disorders (such as heart failure, heart attack, abnormal heart rhythms, or pulmonary embolism when these disorders are accompanied by complications), those who have just undergone heart surgery, those who are in shock,▲ and those who have severe burns.

Pulmonary artery catheterization is also performed to measure pressure in the right heart chambers and to estimate pressure in the left heart chambers, the amount of blood the heart pumps per minute (cardiac output), resistance to blood flow in the arteries that carry blood from the heart (peripheral resistance), and the volume of blood. This procedure can provide useful information about cardiac tamponade■ and pulmonary embolism.★

As in right heart catheterization, a catheter with a balloon at its tip is inserted into a vein, usually in the neck (under the collarbone) or an arm, and is threaded toward the heart. The tip of the catheter may be passed through the superior vena cava or inferior vena cava (the large vein that returns blood to the heart from the lower part of the body), through the right atrium and right ventricle to the pulmonary artery. The balloon at the catheter's tip is lodged in the pulmonary artery. A chest x-ray is taken or fluoroscopy may be used to make sure the tip is placed correctly.

The balloon is inflated to temporarily block the pulmonary artery, so that pressure in the capillaries of the lungs (pulmonary capillary wedge pressure) can be measured. This measurement is an indirect way to determine pressure in the left atrium. Blood samples can be taken through the catheter, so that the oxygen and carbon dioxide levels in the blood can be measured.

The procedure may cause many complications, but they are usually rare. They include an air pocket between the layers of membranes covering the lungs (pneumothorax), abnormal heart rhythms (arrhythmias), infection, damage or clotting in the pulmonary artery, and injury to an artery or vein.

▲ see page 148
■ see box on page 189
★ see page 285
● see art on pages 208 and 210

Central Venous Catheterization

Central venous catheterization can be used to monitor central venous pressure (pressure in the superior vena cava, the large vein that returns blood to the heart from the upper part of the body). Central venous pressure reflects the pressure in the right atrium when it is filled with blood. This measurement helps doctors estimate whether the person is dehydrated and how well the heart is functioning. This procedure has largely been replaced by pulmonary artery catheterization.

Angiography of Peripheral Blood Vessels

Angiography of the peripheral arteries (those of the arms, legs, and trunk—except those supplying the heart) is similar to coronary angiography, except the catheter is threaded to the artery being investigated. Angiography may be performed to detect an abnormal channel between an artery and a vein (arteriovenous fistula).

If Doppler ultrasonography or x-rays detect a problem in a peripheral artery, **selective angiography** is performed to determine whether angioplasty or bypass surgery● is needed. In selective angiography, the radiopaque dye is injected through a catheter into an artery in the area to be studied and thus is concentrated in that area.

Angiography of the aorta (**aortography**) can be used to detect abnormalities (such as an aneurysm or a dissection) in the aorta. It can also be used to detect leakage of the valve between the left ventricle and the aorta (aortic regurgitation).

Digital subtraction angiography may be performed before selective angiography to detect and visualize problems such as narrowing or blockage of an artery. However, this type of angiography is seldom adequate to determine whether surgery (with or without angioplasty) is needed. Digital subtraction angiography is not used for coronary arteries because it is unnecessary; clear images of these arteries can be obtained when a radiopaque dye is injected directly into a coronary artery.

In digital subtraction angiography, images of arteries are obtained before and after a radiopaque dye is injected, and a computer subtracts one image from the other. Images of tissues other than the arteries (such as bones) are thus eliminated. As a result, the arteries can be seen more clearly, much less dye is required, and the procedure may be safer than standard angiography.

CHAPTER 22

High Blood Pressure

High blood pressure (hypertension) is abnormally high pressure in the arteries.

To many people, the word hypertension suggests excessive tension, nervousness, or stress. In medical terms, hypertension refers to high blood pressure, regardless of the cause. Because it usually does not cause symptoms for many years—until a vital organ is damaged—it has been called "the silent killer." Uncontrolled high blood pressure increases the risk of problems such as stroke, aneurysm, heart failure, heart attack, and kidney damage.

More than 50 million Americans are estimated to have high blood pressure. High blood pressure occurs more often in blacks—in 32% of black adults compared with 23% of whites and 23% of Mexican Americans. Also, the consequences of high blood pressure are worse for blacks. High blood pressure occurs more often in older people—in about three fourths of women and almost two thirds of men aged 75 or older, compared with only about one fourth of people aged 20 to 74. High blood pressure is twice as common among people who are obese as among those who are not.

In the United States, only an estimated two of three people with high blood pressure have been diagnosed. Of these people, about 75% receive drug treatment, and of these, about 45% receive adequate treatment.

When blood pressure is checked, two values are recorded. The higher value reflects the highest pressure in the arteries, which is reached when the heart contracts (during systole). The lower value reflects the lowest pressure in the arteries, which is reached just before the heart begins to contract again (during diastole). Blood pressure is written as systolic pressure/diastolic pressure—for example, 120/80 mm Hg (millimeters of mercury). This reading is referred to as "120 over 80."

High blood pressure is defined as a systolic pressure at rest that averages 140 mm Hg or more, a diastolic pressure at rest that averages 90 mm Hg or more, or both. However, the higher the blood pressure, the greater the risks—even within the normal blood pressure range—so these limits are somewhat arbitrary. The limits were established because people with blood pressure above these levels are at increasing risk of complications. In most people with high blood pressure, both systolic and diastolic pressures are high. The exception is older people who commonly have high systolic pressure (140 mm Hg or more) with normal or low diastolic pressure (less than 90 mm Hg). This disorder is called **isolated systolic hypertension.**

Blood pressure that is more than 180/110 mm Hg and does not produce any symptoms is a hypertensive urgency.

Malignant hypertension, a particularly severe form of high blood pressure, is a hypertensive emergency. Blood pressure is at least 210/120 mm Hg. It occurs in only about 1 of 200 people who have high blood pressure. However, it is several times more common among blacks than among whites, among men than among women, and among people in lower socioeconomic groups than among those in higher socioeconomic groups. Unlike a hypertensive urgency, malignant hypertension may produce a variety of severe symptoms. If untreated, malignant hypertension usually leads to death in 3 to 6 months.

The Body's Control of Blood Pressure

The body has many mechanisms that control blood pressure: The body can change the amount of blood the heart pumps, the diameter of arteries, and the volume of blood in the bloodstream. To increase blood pressure, the heart can pump more blood by pumping more forcefully or more rapidly. Small arteries (arterioles) can narrow (constrict), forcing the blood from each heartbeat through a narrower space than normal. Because the space in the arteries is narrower, the same amount of blood passing through them increases the blood pressure. Veins can constrict to reduce their capacity to hold blood, forcing more blood into the arteries. As a result, blood pressure increases. Fluid can be added to the bloodstream to increase blood volume and thus increase blood pressure. Conversely, to decrease blood pressure, the heart can pump less forcefully or rapidly, arterioles and veins can widen (dilate), and fluid can be removed from the bloodstream.

Ups and Downs of Blood Pressure

Blood pressure varies naturally over a person's life. Infants and children normally have much lower blood pressure than adults. For almost everyone living in industrialized countries such as the United States, blood pressure increases with age. Systolic pressure increases until at least age 80, and diastolic pressure increases until age 55 to 60, then levels off or even decreases. However, for people living in some developing countries, neither systolic nor diastolic pressure increases with age, and high blood pressure is practically nonexistent, possibly because salt (sodium) intake is low and the physical activity level is higher.

Activity temporarily affects blood pressure, which is higher when a person is active and lower when a person rests. Blood pressure also varies with the time of day: It is highest in the morning and lowest at night during sleep. These variations are normal.

These mechanisms are controlled by the sympathetic division of the autonomic nervous system (the part of the nervous system that regulates internal body processes requiring no conscious effort) and by the kidneys. The sympathetic division uses several means to temporarily increase blood pressure during the fight-or-flight response (the body's physical reaction to a threat). The sympathetic division stimulates the adrenal glands to release the hormones epinephrine (adrenaline) and norepinephrine (noradrenaline). These hormones stimulate the heart to beat faster and more forcefully, most arterioles to constrict, and some arterioles to dilate. The arterioles that dilate are those in areas where an increased blood supply is needed (such as in skeletal muscle—the muscles controlled by conscious effort). The sympathetic division also stimulates the kidneys to decrease their excretion of salt and water, thereby increasing blood volume.

The kidneys also respond directly to changes in blood pressure. If blood pressure increases, the kidneys increase their excretion of salt and water, so that blood volume decreases and blood pressure returns to normal. Conversely, if blood pressure decreases, the kidneys decrease their excretion of salt and water, so that blood volume increases and blood pressure returns to normal. The kidneys can increase blood pressure by secreting the enzyme renin, which eventually results in the production of the hormone angiotensin II. Angiotensin II helps increase blood pressure by causing the arterioles to constrict and by triggering the release of another hormone, aldosterone, which causes the kidneys to increase the retention of salt and water.

Normally, whenever a change (for example, increased activity or a strong emotion) causes a transient increase in blood pressure, one of the body's compensatory mechanisms is triggered to counteract the change and keep blood pressure at normal levels. For example, an increase in the amount of blood pumped out by the heart—which tends to increase blood pressure—causes dilation of blood vessels and an increase in the kidneys' excretion of salt and water—which tend to reduce blood pressure.

Causes

High blood pressure with no known cause is called primary or essential hypertension. Between 85% and 90% of people with high blood pressure have primary hypertension. Several changes in the heart and blood vessels probably combine to increase blood pressure. For instance, the amount of blood pumped per minute (cardiac output) may be increased, and the resistance to blood flow may be increased because blood vessels are constricted. Blood volume may be increased also. The reasons for such changes are not fully understood but appear to involve an inherited abnormality affecting the constriction of arterioles, which help control blood pressure.

High blood pressure with a known cause is called secondary hypertension. Between 10% and 15% of people with high blood pressure have secondary hypertension. Many kidney disorders can cause high blood pressure, because the kidneys are important in controlling blood pressure. For example, damage to the kidneys may impair their ability to remove enough salt and water from the body, increasing blood volume and blood pressure. In 5 to 10% of people with high blood pressure, the cause is a kidney disorder. Such disorders include renal artery stenosis (narrowing of the artery supplying one of the kidneys), kidney inflammation, and injury.

In 1 to 2%, secondary hypertension is caused by another disorder, such as a hormonal disor-

Regulating Blood Pressure:
The Renin-Angiotensin-Aldosterone System

The renin-angiotensin-aldosterone system is a series of reactions designed to help regulate blood pressure.

1. When blood pressure falls (for systolic, to 100 mm Hg or lower), the kidneys release the enzyme renin into the bloodstream.

2. Renin splits angiotensinogen, a large protein that circulates in the bloodstream, into pieces. One piece is angiotensin I.

3. Angiotensin I, which is relatively inactive, is split into pieces by angiotensin-converting enzyme (ACE). One piece is angiotensin II, which is very active.

4. Angiotensin II, a hormone, causes the muscular walls of small arteries (arterioles) to constrict, increasing blood pressure. Angiotensin II also triggers the release of the hormone aldosterone from the adrenal glands.

5. Aldosterone causes the kidneys to retain salt (sodium) and excrete potassium. The sodium causes water to be retained, thus increasing blood volume and blood pressure.

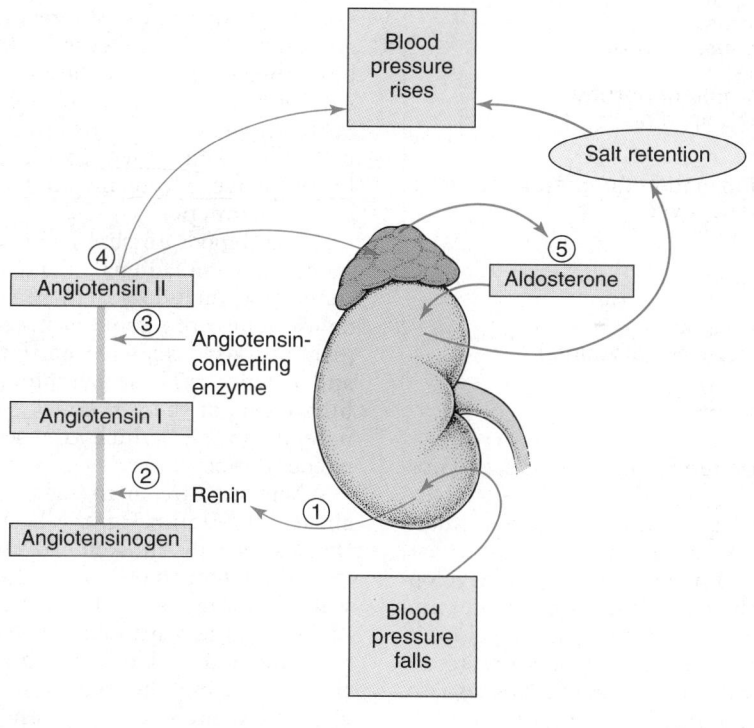

der, or by the use of certain drugs, such as birth control pills (oral contraceptives). Hormonal disorders that cause high blood pressure include Cushing's syndrome (a disorder characterized by high levels of cortisol); hyperthyroidism (an overactive thyroid gland); hyperaldosteronism (overproduction of aldosterone, often by a tumor in one of the adrenal glands); and, rarely, a pheochromocytoma (a tumor that is located in an adrenal gland and that produces the hormones epinephrine and norepinephrine).

Arteriosclerosis interferes with the body's control of blood pressure, increasing the risk of high blood pressure. Arteriosclerosis makes arteries stiff, preventing the dilation that

Some Causes of Secondary Hypertension

Kidney disorders
  Renal artery stenosis
  Pyelonephritis
  Glomerulonephritis
  Kidney tumors
  Polycystic kidney disease (usually
    inherited)
  Injury to a kidney
  Radiation therapy affecting the kidneys

Hormonal disorders
  Hyperthyroidism
  Hyperaldosteronism
  Cushing's syndrome
  Pheochromocytoma
  Acromegaly

Other disorders
  Coarctation of the aorta
  Arteriosclerosis
  Preeclampsia (a complication of
    pregnancy)
  Acute intermittent porphyria
  Acute lead poisoning

Drugs
  Nonsteroidal anti-inflammatory drugs
  Oral contraceptives
  Corticosteroids
  Cyclosporine
  Erythropoietin
  Cocaine
  Alcohol abuse
  Licorice (excessive amounts)

would otherwise return blood pressure to normal.▲

Obesity, a sedentary lifestyle, stress, smoking, and excessive amounts of alcohol or salt in the diet all can play a role in the development of high blood pressure in people who have an inherited tendency to develop it. Stress tends to cause blood pressure to increase temporarily, but blood pressure usually returns to normal once the stress is over. An example is "white coat hypertension," in which the stress of visiting a doctor's office causes blood pressure to increase enough to be diagnosed as high blood pressure in someone who has normal blood pressure at other times. In susceptible people, these brief increases in blood pressure are thought to cause damage

---

▲ see box on page 195   ■ see page 163
★ see page 150

that eventually results in permanent high blood pressure, even when no stress is present. This theory has not been proved.

Symptoms

In most people, high blood pressure causes no symptoms, despite the coincidental occurrence of certain symptoms that are widely, but erroneously, associated with high blood pressure: headaches, nosebleeds, dizziness, a flushed face, and fatigue. People with high blood pressure may have these symptoms, but the symptoms occur just as frequently in people with normal blood pressure.

Severe or long-standing high blood pressure that is untreated (especially malignant hypertension) can produce symptoms because it can damage the brain, eyes, heart, and kidneys. Symptoms include headache, fatigue, nausea, vomiting, shortness of breath, restlessness, and blurred vision. Occasionally, severe high blood pressure causes the brain to swell, resulting in nausea, vomiting, worsening headache, drowsiness, confusion, seizures, sleepiness, and even coma. This condition, called hypertensive encephalopathy, requires emergency treatment.

If high blood pressure is due to a pheochromocytoma (an adrenal gland tumor), symptoms may include severe headache, anxiety, an awareness of a rapid or irregular heart rate (palpitations), excessive perspiration, tremor, and paleness. These symptoms result from high levels of the hormones epinephrine and norepinephrine, which are secreted by the pheochromocytoma.

When pressure in the arteries is increased above 140/90 mm Hg, the heart enlarges and the heart's walls thicken because the heart has to work harder to pump blood. The thickened walls are stiffer than they normally are. Consequently, the heart's chambers do not expand normally and are harder to fill with blood, further increasing the heart's workload. These changes in the heart may result in abnormal heart rhythms■ and heart failure.★

Diagnosis

Blood pressure is measured after a person sits or lies down for 5 minutes. It should be measured again after the person stands for a few minutes, especially if the person is older or has diabetes. A reading of 140/90 mm Hg or more is considered high, but a diagnosis cannot be based on a single high reading. Sometimes, even several high readings are not

Measuring Blood Pressure

Several instruments can measure blood pressure quickly and with little discomfort. A sphygmomanometer is commonly used. It consists of a soft rubber cuff connected to a rubber bulb that is used to inflate the cuff and a meter that registers the pressure of the cuff. The meter may be a dial or a glass column filled with mercury. Blood pressure is measured in millimeters of mercury (mm Hg) because the first instrument used to measure it was a mercury column.

When a sphygmomanometer is used, a person sits with an arm bared (sleeves rolled up), bent, and resting on a table, so that the arm is about the same level as the heart. The cuff is wrapped around the arm. Using a cuff that is proportional to the size of the arm is important because if the cuff is too small, the blood pressure reading is too high, and if the cuff is too large, the reading is too low.

Listening with a stethoscope placed over the artery below the cuff, a health care practitioner inflates the cuff by squeezing the bulb until the cuff compresses the artery tightly enough to temporarily stop blood flow, usu-ally to a pressure that is about 30 mm Hg higher than the person's usual systolic pressure (the pressure exerted when the heart beats). Then the cuff is gradually deflated. The pressure at which the practitioner first hears a pulse in the artery is the systolic pressure. The cuff continues to be deflated, and at some point, the sound of blood flowing stops. The pressure at this point is the diastolic pressure (the pressure exerted when the heart relaxes, between beats).

Some instruments can measure blood pressure automatically, without use of a stethoscope or rubber bulb. These devices may fit around the upper arm, finger, or wrist. For people older than 50, blood pressure measured at the upper arm is the most accurate. Sometimes a precise measurement of blood pressure is needed—for example, for a person in an intensive care unit. In such cases, a catheter can be inserted inside an artery to measure blood pressure directly.

Instruments to measure blood pressure are available for home use by people who have high blood pressure.

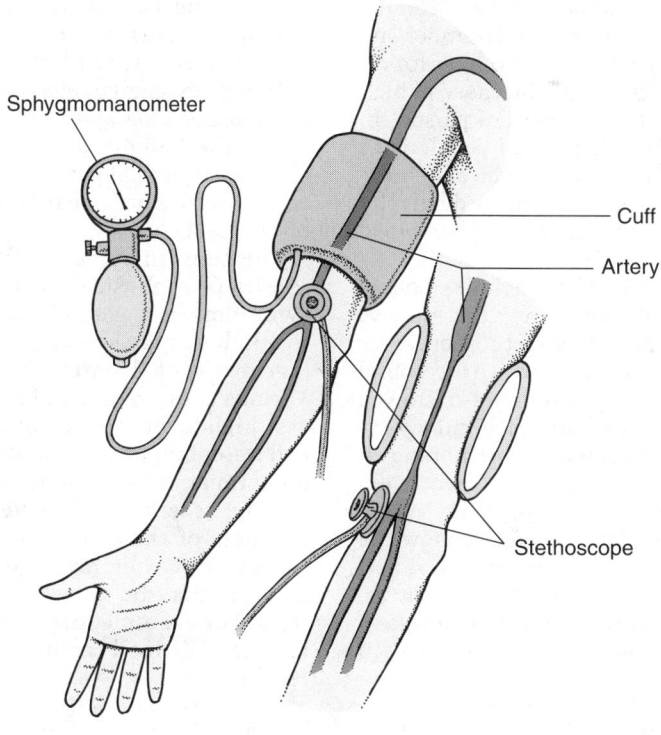

Sphygmomanometer

Cuff

Artery

Stethoscope

enough to make the diagnosis—because for example, the readings may vary too much. If a person has an initial high reading, blood pressure is measured again during the same visit and then measured twice on at least two other days to make sure that the high blood pressure persists.

If there is still doubt, a 24-hour blood pressure monitor may be used. It is a portable battery-operated device, worn on the hip, connected to a blood pressure cuff, worn on the arm. This monitor repeatedly records blood pressure throughout the day and night over a 24-hour or 48-hour period. The readings determine not only whether high blood pressure is present but also how severe it is.

In people with very stiff arteries (most commonly, in older people), blood pressure may be measured as high when it is not. This phenomenon is called **pseudohypertension.** It occurs when the artery in the arm is too stiff to be compressed by the blood pressure cuff, and as a result, blood pressure cannot be measured accurately.

After high blood pressure has been diagnosed, its effects on key organs, especially the blood vessels, heart, brain, and kidneys, are usually evaluated. Doctors also look for the cause of high blood pressure. The number and type of tests that are performed to look for organ damage and to determine the cause of high blood pressure vary from person to person. In general, routine evaluation for all people with high blood pressure involves a medical history, a physical examination, electrocardiography (ECG), blood tests (including a complete blood cell count), and urine tests.

The physical examination includes checking the area of the abdomen over the kidneys for tenderness and placing a stethoscope over the abdomen to listen for a bruit (the sound caused by blood rushing through a narrowed artery) in the artery supplying each kidney.

The retina (the light-sensitive membrane on the inner surface of the back of the eye) is examined with an ophthalmoscope.▲ The retina is the only place doctors can directly view the effects of high blood pressure on arterioles. The assumption is that the changes in the arterioles of the retina are similar to changes in arterioles and other blood vessels elsewhere in the body, such as in the kidneys. By determining the degree of damage to the retina (retinopathy),■ doctors can classify the severity of high blood pressure.

A stethoscope is used to detect heart sounds. An abnormal heart sound, called the fourth heart sound, is one of the earliest changes in the heart caused by high blood pressure. This sound develops because the left atrium of the heart has to contract harder to fill the enlarged, stiff left ventricle, which pumps blood to all of the body except the lungs.

Electrocardiography (ECG)★ can detect changes in the heart—particularly enlargement. However, in the early stages, such changes are best detected by echocardiography.●

Kidney damage can be detected by urine and blood tests. Urine tests can detect early evidence of kidney damage. The presence of blood cells and albumin (the most abundant protein in blood) in the urine may indicate such damage. Symptoms of kidney damage (such as lethargy, poor appetite, and fatigue) do not usually develop until 70 to 80% of kidney function is lost.

The higher the blood pressure and the younger the person, the more extensive the search for a cause is likely to be, even though a cause is identified in less than 10% of people. A more extensive evaluation may include x-ray, ultrasonography, and radionuclide imaging of the kidneys and their blood supply; a chest x-ray; and blood and urine tests to detect certain hormones, such as epinephrine, aldosterone, and cortisol.

The cause may be suggested by abnormal results of a physical examination or by the symptoms. For example, a bruit in the artery to a kidney may suggest renal artery stenosis (narrowing of the artery supplying a kidney). Various combinations of symptoms may suggest high levels of the hormones epinephrine and norepinephrine, produced by a pheochromocytoma. The presence of a pheochromocytoma is confirmed when the breakdown products of these hormones are detected in the urine. Other rare causes of high blood pressure may be detected by certain routine tests. For example, measuring the potassium level in the blood can help detect hyperaldosteronism.◆

▲ see art on page 1284   ■ see page 1312

★ see page 122   ● see page 125

◆ see page 960

Treatment

Primary hypertension cannot be cured, but it can be controlled to prevent complications.

CLASSIFYING BLOOD PRESSURE IN ADULTS

Blood pressure is classified by its severity because treatment is based, in part, on severity. When a person's systolic and diastolic pressures fall into different categories, the higher category is used to classify blood pressure. For instance, 160/92 is classified as stage 2 hypertension, and 150/115 is classified as stage 3 hypertension.

The optimal blood pressure for minimizing the risk of cardiovascular problems (such as heart attack and heart failure) and stroke is below 120/80 mm Hg.

CATEGORY	SYSTOLIC BLOOD PRESSURE (MM HG)	DIASTOLIC BLOOD PRESSURE (MM HG)	RECOMMENDED FOLLOW-UP
Normal blood pressure	Below 130	Below 85	Blood pressure is rechecked in 2 years
High-normal blood pressure	130–139	85–89	Blood pressure is rechecked in 1 year, and advice about lifestyle changes is provided
Stage 1 (mild) hypertension	140–159	90–99	The high blood pressure is confirmed within 1 month, and advice about lifestyle changes is provided
Stage 2 (moderate) hypertension	160–179	100–109	The person is evaluated or referred to a source of care within 1 month
Stage 3 (severe) hypertension	180 or higher	110 or higher	The person is evaluated or referred to a source of care immediately or within 1 week, depending on the person's condition

Because high blood pressure itself has no symptoms, doctors try to avoid treatments that cause side effects or interfere with a person's lifestyle. Before any drugs are prescribed, alternative measures are usually tried.

Overweight people with high blood pressure are advised to lose weight. Losing as few as 10 pounds can lower blood pressure. For people who are obese or who have diabetes or high cholesterol levels, changes in diet are important for reducing the risk of heart and blood vessel disease. Smokers should stop smoking.

Reducing the intake of alcohol and sodium (while maintaining an adequate intake of calcium, magnesium, and potassium) may make drug therapy for high blood pressure unnecessary. Daily alcohol intake should be reduced to no more than 2 drinks (a daily total of 24 ounces of beer, 8 ounces of wine, or 2 ounces of 100-proof whiskey or other liquor). Daily sodium intake should be reduced to less than 2 grams, or sodium chloride intake, to 5 grams.

Moderate aerobic exercise is helpful. People with primary hypertension do not have to restrict their physical activity as long as their blood pressure is controlled. Regular exercise helps reduce blood pressure and weight and improves the functioning of the heart and overall health.▲

Doctors often recommend that people with high blood pressure monitor their blood pressure at home. Monitoring their own blood pressure probably helps motivate people to follow a doctor's recommendations regarding treatment.

▲ see page 31

℞ ANTIHYPERTENSIVE DRUGS

TYPE	EXAMPLES	SELECTED SIDE EFFECTS
Diuretics		
Loop diuretics	Bumetanide Ethacrynic acid Furosemide Torsemide	Decreased levels of potassium and magnesium, temporarily increased levels of blood sugar and cholesterol, an increased level of uric acid, sexual dysfunction in men, and digestive upset
Potassium-sparing diuretics	Amiloride Spironolactone Triamterene	With all, a high potassium level and digestive upset With spironolactone, breast enlargement in men (gynecomastia) and menstrual irregularities in women
Thiazide and thiazide-like diuretics	Chlorhalidone Hydrochlorothiazide Indapamide Metolazone	Decreased levels of potassium and magnesium, increased levels of calcium and uric acid, sexual dysfunction in men, and digestive upset
Adrenergic blockers		
Alpha-blockers	Doxazosin Prazosin Terazosin	Fainting (syncope) with the first dose, awareness of rapid heartbeats (palpitations), dizziness, low blood pressure when the person stands (orthostatic hypotension), and fluid retention (edema)
Beta-blockers	Acebutolol Atenolol Betaxolol Bisoprolol Carteolol Metoprolol Nadolol Penbutolol Pindolol Propranolol Timolol	Spasm of the airways (bronchospasm), an abnormally slow heart rate (bradycardia), heart failure, possible masking of low blood sugar levels after insulin injections, impaired peripheral circulation, insomnia, fatigue, shortness of breath, depression, Raynaud's phenomenon, vivid dreams, hallucinations, and sexual dysfunction With some beta-blockers, an increased triglyceride level
Alpha-beta blockers	Carvedilol Labetalol	Low blood pressure when the person stands and spasm of the airways
Peripherally acting adrenergic blockers	Guanadrel Guanethidine Reserpine	With guanadrel and guanethidine, diarrhea, sexual dysfunction, low blood pressure when the person stands, and fluid retention With reserpine, depression, nasal congestion, lethargy, and bleeding of a peptic ulcer
Centrally acting alpha-agonists		
	Clonidine Guanabenz Guanfacine Methyldopa	Drowsiness, dry mouth, fatigue, an abnormally slow heart rate, rebound high blood pressure when the drug is withdrawn (except with methyldopa), and sexual dysfunction With methyldopa, depression, low blood pressure when the person stands, and liver and autoimmune disorders

R_x ANTIHYPERTENSIVE DRUGS (Continued)

TYPE	EXAMPLES	SELECTED SIDE EFFECTS
Angiotensin-converting enzyme (ACE) inhibitors	Benazepril Captopril Enalapril Fosinopril Lisinopril Moexipril Perindopril Quinapril Ramipril Trandolapril	Cough (in up to 20% of people), low blood pressure, an increased potassium level, rash, angioedema (allergic swelling that affects the face, lips, and windpipe and may interfere with breathing), and, in pregnant women, serious injury to the fetus
Angiotensin II blockers	Candesartan Eprosartan Irbesartan Losartan Telmisartan Valsartan	Dizziness, an increased potassium level, angioedema (rare), and, in pregnant women, serious injury to the fetus
Calcium channel blockers Dihydropyridines	Amlodipine Felodipine Isradipine Nicardipine Nifedipine (sustained-release only) Nisoldipine	Dizziness, fluid retention in the ankles, flushing, headache, heartburn, enlarged gums, and an abnormally fast heart rate (tachycardia)
Nondihydropyridines	Diltiazem (sustained-release only) Verapamil	Headache, dizziness, flushing, fluid retention, problems in the heart's electrical conduction system (including heart block), an abnormally slow heart rate (bradycardia), heart failure, and enlarged gums With verapamil, constipation
Direct vasodilators	Hydralazine Minoxidil	Headache, an abnormally fast heart rate (tachycardia), and fluid retention

Drug Therapy: Drugs that are used in the treatment of high blood pressure are called antihypertensives. With the wide variety of antihypertensives available, high blood pressure can be controlled in almost anyone, but treatment has to be tailored to the individual. Treatment is most effective when patient and doctor communicate well and collaborate on the treatment program.

The blood pressure goals for antihypertensive therapy vary depending on what other disorders are present. For most people, lowering diastolic blood pressure to 70 mm Hg is safe. For people with coronary artery disease or angina, diastolic blood pressure should not go below 80 mm Hg. For people with diabetes, the target is below 130/80 mm Hg. For older people, the target is below 140/90 mm Hg.

Different types of antihypertensives reduce blood pressure by different mechanisms; therefore, many different treatment strategies are possible. For some people, doctors use a stepped approach to drug therapy: They start with one type of antihypertensive and add others as necessary. For other people, doctors find a sequential approach is preferable: They prescribe one antihypertensive; if it is ineffective, they discontinue it and prescribe another type. In choosing an antihypertensive, doctors consider such factors as the person's age, sex, and race; the severity of high blood pressure; the presence of other conditions, such as diabetes or high blood cholesterol levels; potential side effects, which vary from drug to drug; and the costs of the drugs and of tests needed to check for certain side effects.

Most people tolerate their prescribed antihypertensive drugs without problems. But any antihypertensive drug can cause side effects. So if side effects develop, a person should tell the doctor, who can adjust the dose or substitute another drug. Usually, an antihypertensive drug must be taken indefinitely to control blood pressure.

A **thiazide diuretic** is often the first drug given to treat high blood pressure. Diuretics cause blood vessels to dilate. Diuretics also help the kidneys eliminate salt and water, decreasing fluid volume throughout the body and thus lowering blood pressure. Because thiazide diuretics cause potassium to be excreted in the urine, potassium supplements or a diuretic that does not cause potassium loss or that causes potassium levels to increase (a potassium-sparing diuretic) sometimes must be taken with a thiazide diuretic. Usually, potassium-sparing diuretics are not used alone because they do not control blood pressure as well as thiazide diuretics do; however, the potassium-sparing diuretic spironolactone is sometimes used alone. Diuretics are particularly useful for blacks, older people, obese people, and people with heart failure or chronic kidney failure.

Adrenergic blockers include alpha-blockers, beta-blockers, alpha-beta blockers, and peripherally acting adrenergic blockers. These drugs block the effects of the sympathetic division, the part of the nervous system that can rapidly respond to stress by increasing blood pressure. The most commonly used adrenergic blockers, the beta-blockers, are particularly useful for whites, young people, people who have had a heart attack, and people who have a rapid heart rate, angina pectoris (chest pain due to inadequate blood supply to the heart muscle), or migraine headaches. The risk of side effects is higher for older people.

Centrally acting alpha-agonists lower blood pressure through a mechanism that somewhat resembles that of adrenergic blockers. By stimulating certain receptors in the brain stem, these agonists inhibit the effects of the sympathetic division of the nervous system. These drugs are rarely used now.

Angiotensin-converting enzyme (ACE) inhibitors lower blood pressure in part by dilating arterioles. They dilate arterioles by preventing the formation of angiotensin II, which causes arterioles to constrict; specifically, they block the action of angiotensin-converting enzyme, which converts angiotensin I to angiotensin II.▲ These drugs are particularly useful for people with coronary artery disease or heart failure, whites, young people, people with protein in their urine because of chronic kidney disease or diabetic kidney disease, and men who develop sexual dysfunction as a side effect of another antihypertensive drug.

Angiotensin II blockers lower blood pressure by a mechanism similar to the one used by angiotensin-converting enzyme inhibitors: They directly block the action of angiotensin II, which causes arterioles to constrict. Because the mechanism is more direct, angiotensin II blockers may cause fewer side effects.

Calcium channel blockers cause arterioles to dilate by a completely different mechanism. They are particularly useful for blacks; older people; and people who have angina pectoris, certain types of rapid heart rate, or migraine headaches. Calcium channel blockers may be short-acting or long-acting. Reports suggest that people using short-acting calcium channel blockers may have an increased risk of death due to heart attack, but no reports suggest such effects for long-acting calcium channel blockers.

Direct vasodilators dilate blood vessels by another mechanism. A drug of this type is almost never used alone; rather, it is added as a second drug when another drug alone does not lower blood pressure sufficiently.

Treatment of Secondary Hypertension

The cause of the high blood pressure is treated if possible. Treating kidney disease can sometimes return blood pressure to normal or at least lower it, so that antihypertensive therapy is more effective. A narrowed artery to the kidney may be dilated by inserting a balloon-tipped catheter and inflating the balloon (angioplasty).■ Or the narrowed part of the artery supplying the kidney can be bypassed; often

---

▲ see art on page 133   ■ see art on page 208

such surgery cures high blood pressure. Tumors that cause high blood pressure, such as a pheochromocytoma, usually can be removed surgically.▲

Treatment of Hypertensive Urgencies and Emergencies

Hypertensive urgencies are treated with clonidine, an adrenergic blocker, given by mouth. The calcium channel blocker nifedipine, given under the tongue (sublingually), has been used but is less safe.

In hypertensive emergencies, such as malignant hypertension and hypertensive encephalopathy, blood pressure must be lowered rapidly. Most drugs used to rapidly lower blood pressure, such as nitroprusside or labetalol, are given intravenously. If an aneurysm is suspected, labetalol is preferred.

Prognosis

Untreated high blood pressure increases a person's risk of developing heart disease (such as heart failure, heart attack, or sudden cardiac death), kidney failure, or stroke at an early age. High blood pressure is the most important risk factor for stroke. It is also one of the three most important risk factors for heart attack that a person can modify (the other two are smoking and high cholesterol levels in the blood). Treatment that lowers high blood pressure greatly decreases the risk of stroke and heart failure. Such treatment may also decrease the risk of a heart attack, although not as dramatically. Without treatment, fewer than 5% of people with malignant hypertension survive for a year.

CHAPTER 23

Low Blood Pressure

Low blood pressure (hypotension) is blood pressure low enough to cause symptoms such as dizziness and fainting.

Normally, the body maintains the pressure of blood in the arteries within a narrow range. If blood pressure is too high, it can damage a blood vessel and even rupture it, causing bleeding or other complications. If blood pressure is too low, not enough blood reaches all parts of the body; as a result, cells do not receive enough oxygen and nutrients, and waste products are not adequately removed. Even so, having low blood pressure is generally better than having high blood pressure. Healthy people who have blood pressure that is low but still in the normal range (when measured at rest) tend to live longer than those who have higher normal blood pressure.

The body has several compensatory mechanisms that control blood pressure.■ They involve changing the diameter of veins and small arteries (arterioles), the amount of blood pumped from the heart (cardiac output), and the volume of blood in the blood vessels. These mechanisms return blood pressure to

normal after it increases or decreases during normal activities, such as exercise or sleep.

Veins can widen (dilate) and narrow (constrict) to change how much blood they can hold (capacity). When veins constrict, their capacity to hold blood is reduced, forcing more blood into the arteries. As a result, blood pressure increases. Conversely, when veins dilate, their capacity to hold blood is increased, forcing less blood into the arteries. As a result, blood pressure decreases.

Arterioles can also dilate and constrict. The more constricted arterioles are, the greater their resistance to blood flow and the higher the blood pressure. Constriction of arterioles (decreasing their diameter) increases blood pressure because more pressure is needed to force blood through the narrower space. Conversely, dilation of arterioles reduces resistance to blood flow, thus reducing blood pressure.

▲ see page 960

■ see also page 131

SOME CAUSES OF LOW BLOOD PRESSURE

Change in Compensatory Mechanism	Causes
Decrease in cardiac output	Abnormal heart rhythms
	Heart muscle damage or malfunction (such as that due to a heart attack or viral infection)
	Heart valve disorders
	Pulmonary embolism
Dilation of blood vessels	Alcohol
	Some antidepressants, such as amitriptyline
	Antihypertensive drugs that dilate blood vessels (such as calcium channel blockers, angiotensin-converting enzyme inhibitors, and angiotensin II receptor blockers)
	Nitrates
	Bacterial infections
	Exposure to heat
	Nerve damage (such as that due to diabetes, amyloidosis, or spinal cord injuries)
Decrease in blood volume	Diarrhea
	Diuretics (such as furosemide and hydrochlorothiazide)
	Excessive bleeding
	Excessive sweating
	Excessive urination (a common symptom of untreated diabetes or Addison's disease)
Inhibition of the brain centers that control blood pressure	Alcohol
	Antidepressants
	Antihypertensives such as methyldopa and clonidine
	Barbiturates
Impairment of the autonomic nervous system	Amyloidosis
	Diabetes
	Multiple systems atrophy (Shy-Drager syndrome)
	Parkinson's disease

The more blood pumped from the heart per minute (that is, the larger the cardiac output), the higher the blood pressure—as long as resistance to blood flow in the arteries remains constant. The body can change the amount of blood pumped during each heartbeat by making the heart rate slower or faster or by making each contraction weaker or stronger.

The higher the volume of blood in the blood vessels, the higher the blood pressure—as long as resistance to blood flow in the arteries remains constant. To increase or decrease blood volume, the kidneys can vary the amount of fluid excreted in urine.

The compensatory mechanisms are activated by specialized cells that act as sensors, called baroreceptors. Located within arteries, these sensors constantly monitor blood pressure. Those in the neck and chest are particularly important. When sensors detect a change in blood pressure, they trigger a change in one of the compensatory mechanisms and so maintain a steady blood pressure. Nerves carry signals from these sensors and the brain to several key organs, which control the compensatory mechanisms:

• The heart is signaled to change the rate and force of heartbeats (thus changing the amount of blood pumped). This change is one of the first; it corrects blood pressure quickly.

• The arterioles are signaled to constrict or dilate (thus changing the resistance of blood vessels).

• The veins are signaled to constrict or dilate (thus changing their capacity to hold blood).

• The kidneys are signaled to change the amount of fluid excreted (thus changing the volume of blood in blood vessels). This change takes a long time to produce results and thus is the slowest mechanism for blood pressure control.

For example, when a person is bleeding, blood volume and thus blood pressure decrease. In such cases, sensors activate the compensatory mechanisms to prevent blood pressure from decreasing too much: The heart rate increases, increasing the amount of blood pumped; the veins constrict, reducing their capacity to hold blood; and the arterioles constrict, increasing their resistance to blood flow. If the bleeding is stopped, fluids from the rest of the body move into the blood vessels to begin restoring blood volume and thus blood pressure. The kidneys decrease their production of urine. Thus, they help the body retain as much fluid as possible to return to the blood vessels. Eventually, the bone marrow and spleen produce new blood cells, and blood volume is fully restored.

Nonetheless, these compensatory mechanisms have limitations. For example, if a person loses a lot of blood quickly, these mechanisms cannot compensate quickly enough, and blood pressure falls.

Causes

Various disorders and drugs can cause the compensatory mechanisms to malfunction, and low blood pressure may result. For example, cardiac output may be reduced as a result of heart disease, such as a heart attack (myocardial infarction), a heart valve disorder, an extremely rapid heartbeat (tachycardia), a very slow heartbeat (bradycardia), or another abnormal heart rhythm (arrhythmia). These disorders impair the heart's pumping ability. Arterioles may be dilated by toxins produced by bacteria during a bacterial infection. Blood volume can be reduced as a result of dehydration, bleeding, or kidney disorders. Some kidney disorders impair the kidneys' ability to return fluid to the blood vessels, resulting in the loss of large amounts of fluid in the urine. (Conversely, kidney failure, in which the kidneys cannot remove fluid from the blood, may result in overhydration leading to high blood pressure.) The ability of the nerves to conduct signals between sensors and the organs that control the compensatory mechanisms may be impaired by neurologic disorders (a condition called autonomic nervous system failure). In addition, as people age, compensatory mechanisms respond to changes in blood pressure more slowly.

Symptoms

When blood pressure is too low, the first organ to malfunction is usually the brain. The brain malfunctions first because it is located at the top of the body and blood has to fight gravity to reach the brain. Consequently, most people with low blood pressure feel dizzy or light-headed when they stand, and some may even faint. People who faint fall to the floor, usually bringing the brain to the level of the heart. As a result, blood can flow to the brain without having to fight gravity, and blood flow to the brain increases, helping protect it from injury. However, if blood pressure is low enough, brain damage can still occur.

Low blood pressure occasionally causes shortness of breath or chest pain due to an inadequate blood supply to the heart muscle (angina).

All organs begin to malfunction if blood pressure becomes sufficiently low and remains low; this condition is called shock.▲

The disorder causing low blood pressure may produce many other symptoms, which are not due to low blood pressure itself. For example, an infection may produce a fever.

Some symptoms occur when the body's compensatory mechanisms try to increase blood pressure that is low. For example, when arterioles constrict, blood flow to the skin, feet, and hands decreases. These areas may become cold and turn blue. When the heart beats more quickly and more forcefully, a person may feel palpitations (awareness of heartbeats).

Fainting

Fainting (syncope) is a sudden, brief loss of consciousness.

Fainting is a symptom of an inadequate supply of oxygen and other nutrients to the brain, usually caused by a temporary decrease in blood flow. Blood flow to the brain can decrease whenever the body cannot quickly compensate for a fall in blood pressure.

Causes

Fainting may occur if the heart cannot pump enough blood to maintain a normal blood pressure. For example, an abnormal heart rhythm or a heart valve disorder may impair the heart's pumping ability. People with such disorders may feel fine when resting. However, they feel faint or actually faint when exercising because the heart cannot pump enough blood to meet the body's increased demand for oxygen. This type of fainting is called exertional or effort syncope. People with these disorders may also faint *after* exercising. During exercise, the increase in heart rate may enable the heart to pump enough blood to maintain adequate blood pressure, although just barely. When exercise stops, the heart rate (and the amount of blood pumped) begins to decrease. However, the blood vessels in muscles, which dilate (widen) during exercise to move more blood to and from the muscles, remain dilated. (The arterioles in muscles remain dilated to help supply oxygen and nutrients to muscle tissue, and the

▲ see page 148

veins remain dilated to remove metabolic waste products produced during exercise.) The decrease in the amount of blood pumped out combined with dilation of the arterioles and veins causes blood pressure to fall, and fainting results.

An abnormality of the heart called hypertrophic cardiomyopathy▲ can also cause fainting that usually occurs during exercise. This disorder may occur in younger people as well as older people, particularly those who have high blood pressure. If untreated, it can lead to death.

Fainting may occur if blood volume is too low. An obvious cause of low blood volume is bleeding. Another cause is dehydration, which may be due to diarrhea, excessive sweating, inadequate intake of fluids, or excessive urination (which is a common symptom of untreated diabetes■ or Addison's disease★). In older people, the use of diuretics is a common cause of dehydration, particularly during warm weather or during an illness when obtaining or drinking enough fluids may be difficult. (Diuretics help the kidneys eliminate salt and water by increasing urine formation and thus decrease fluid volume in the body.)

Fainting may occur if the vagus nerve, which supplies the neck, chest, and intestine, is stimulated. When stimulated, the vagus nerve slows the heart. Such stimulation also causes nausea and cool, clammy skin. This type of fainting is called vasovagal (vasomotor) syncope. The vagus nerve is stimulated by pain (such as intestinal cramps), fear, other distress (such as that due to the sight of blood), vomiting, a large bowel movement, and urination. Fainting during or immediately after urination is called micturition syncope. Rarely, vigorous swallowing causes fainting due to stimulation of the vagus nerve.

Fainting may also occur if straining reduces the amount of blood flowing back to the heart. Fainting due to coughing (cough syncope) usually results from such straining. Fainting after urination (micturition syncope) or after a bowel movement is partly due to straining (in addition to stimulation of the vagus nerve). Older men who must strain to empty their bladder because of a large prostate gland are particularly susceptible. Fainting when lifting

weights (weight lifter's syncope) results from the strain of trying to lift or push heavy weights without breathing adequately during the exercise.

Fainting that occurs when a person sits or stands up too quickly is called orthostatic (postural) syncope. It is particularly common among older people. It is caused by orthostatic hypotension.● In orthostatic hypotension, the compensatory mechanisms, particularly the constriction of blood vessels and the increase in heart rate, do not adequately restore blood pressure when a person stands and gravity causes blood to pool in the leg veins. A related form of fainting, called parade ground syncope, occurs when people stand still for a long time on a hot day. If the leg muscles are not used, blood is not pumped back to the heart. As a result, blood pools in the leg veins, and blood pressure falls.

In older people, an excessive decrease in blood pressure after eating a meal (postprandial hypotension)◆ may cause fainting.

Fainting may result from very rapid breathing (overbreathing, or hyperventilation), which may be due to anxiety. This type of fainting is called hyperventilation syncope. Overbreathing removes large amounts of carbon dioxide from the body. The decreased level of carbon dioxide causes blood vessels in the brain to constrict, and the person may feel faint or actually faint.

Rarely, fainting results from a mild stroke in which blood flow to a part of the brain suddenly decreases. Fainting due to a stroke is more common among older people. Many other disorders, such as a deficiency of red blood cells (anemia), lung disorders, a decreased blood sugar level (hypoglycemia), and diabetes can cause fainting, especially if the compensatory mechanisms are also impaired.

Certain drugs may cause fainting. They include many of those used to treat high blood pressure, angina, and heart failure. Doses of these drugs must be carefully adjusted to prevent blood pressure from decreasing too much.

Symptoms

Dizziness or light-headedness may precede fainting, especially if the person is standing. After the person falls, blood pressure increases, partly because the person is lying down (and blood can flow to the brain without having to fight gravity) and often because the cause of fainting has passed. However, getting

---

▲ see page 161   ■ see page 962

★ see page 956   ● see page 146

◆ see page 147

up too quickly may make the person faint again.

When the cause is an abnormal heart rhythm (arrhythmia), fainting usually begins and ends suddenly. Sometimes the person feels palpitations (awareness of heartbeats) just before fainting.

Vasovagal syncope may occur when a person is sitting or standing. It is often preceded by nausea, weakness, yawning, blurring of vision, and sweating. The skin may become cool and clammy. The person becomes ghostly pale, the pulse becomes very slow, and the person faints.

Fainting that begins gradually with warning symptoms and also disappears gradually suggests changes in the blood, such as a decreased level of sugar (hypoglycemia) or carbon dioxide (hypocapnia). Hypocapnia is often preceded by a pins-and-needles sensation in the fingertips and around the lips.

Diagnosis

Doctors try to determine the cause of fainting because some causes are more serious than others. Heart disease, such as an abnormal heart rhythm or narrowing (stenosis) of the aortic valve, can be fatal. Other causes are much less worrisome.

Factors that help doctors make a diagnosis include the circumstances under which fainting occurs, any warning signs before a fainting episode, and the speed of recovery. Descriptions from witnesses of the fainting episode may be helpful. Doctors also need to know whether the person has any disorders and whether the person is taking any prescription or over-the-counter drugs.

If the cause of fainting occurs during stressful situations or is preceded by symptoms of vasovagal syncope (such as nausea, sweating, cool and clammy skin, and paleness), fainting usually is not serious, and extensive diagnostic procedures and treatment are rarely necessary.

Doctors rule out hysterical fainting, which is not true fainting. In hysterical fainting, the person only appears to be unconscious. Heart rate and blood pressure are normal, and the person does not sweat or turn pale.

Electrocardiography (ECG), which records the electrical activity of the heart, can detect an underlying heart disorder. Continuous ECG may be required to determine the cause of fainting. For this procedure, the person wears a small battery-powered device (Holter monitor). It records the heart's electrical activity for 24 hours or more as the person engages in normal daily activities.▲ If an irregular heart rhythm coincides with a fainting episode, it is probably—but not necessarily—the cause.

Other procedures, such as echocardiography (which uses ultrasound waves to produce an image of the heart),■ can detect whether the heart has a structural or functional abnormality. Blood tests may show that the person has hypoglycemia or anemia.

Loss of consciousness due to a seizure★ is distinguished from fainting because the causes and treatment are different. To distinguish between the two, doctors may use electroencephalography (EEG), which records the brain's electrical activity.● Also, after a seizure, recovery from unconsciousness is much slower, causing drowsiness that usually lasts for at least 10 minutes.

To confirm a suspected cause, doctors may attempt to re-create a fainting episode under safe conditions. For example, the person may be asked to breathe quickly and deeply. Or, while monitoring the heartbeat with electrocardiography (ECG), a doctor may press gently over the carotid sinus (a part of the internal carotid artery containing sensors that monitor blood pressure). This pressure temporarily increases blood pressure inside the carotid sinus, tricking the body into thinking that blood pressure has increased throughout the body. The sinus then sends signals to the brain to reduce blood pressure, and faintness or fainting may result.

Tilt table testing◆ is commonly performed to determine the cause of fainting. The person is strapped to a motorized table, which tilts the person from a supine to an almost standing position. This position is held for up to 45 minutes. Blood pressure and heart rate are continuously monitored during the test. If blood pressure does not decrease, the person is given isoproterenol (a drug that stimulates the heart), and the test is repeated. Use of this drug makes the test more sensitive.

Treatment

Usually, lying flat restores consciousness. Raising the legs can speed recovery by increas-

---

▲ see art on page 124   ■ see page 125

★ see page 495   ● see page 445

◆ see page 124

ing blood flow to the heart and brain. If the person sits up too rapidly or is propped up or carried in an upright position, another fainting episode may occur. Therefore, the person should remain lying down until fully recovered.

A heart rate that is too slow can be corrected by surgically implanting a pacemaker, an electronic device that stimulates heartbeats.▲ A heart rate that is too rapid can be slowed by using drugs, particularly a beta-blocker (such as atenolol or metoprolol). A defibrillator can be implanted to restore normal rhythm if the heart beats irregularly.■ Other causes of fainting—such as hypoglycemia and anemia—can be treated. If blood volume is very low, fluids may be given intravenously. Surgery may be considered for heart valve disorders.

Orthostatic Hypotension

Orthostatic hypotension is an excessive decrease in blood pressure that occurs when a person stands up, resulting in reduced blood flow to the brain and dizziness or fainting.

Orthostatic hypotension is particularly common among older people.

Orthostatic hypotension is not a specific disease but an inability to compensate quickly for changes in blood pressure. When a person stands up suddenly, gravity causes about a pint of blood to pool in the veins of the legs and lower body. As a result, the amount of blood returned to the heart and pumped out by the heart is reduced, and blood pressure falls. Normally, the body quickly responds to a decrease in blood pressure: The heart beats faster and more forcefully to increase its output of blood and the arterioles constrict to increase resistance to blood flow.★ If these compensatory mechanisms malfunction or function too slowly—both of which commonly occur in older people—orthostatic hypotension may occur.

Causes

Orthostatic hypotension is caused by conditions that interfere with the compensatory mechanisms that control blood pressure. These conditions include many disorders and drugs as well as normal age-related changes.

Some conditions cause orthostatic hypotension by affecting the heart's ability to increase its output enough when a person stands. This problem can be caused by heart disease, such as abnormal heart rhythms and heart valve disorders. Also, with aging, the body becomes less able to increase the heart rate (and thus the heart's output) when a person stands.

Some conditions cause orthostatic hypotension by reducing blood volume. Diuretics, which are used to treat high blood pressure, can reduce blood volume by removing fluid from the body. Diuretics, especially potent ones given in high doses, are a common cause of orthostatic hypotension. Other causes of reduced blood volume include bleeding and an excessive loss of fluid due to severe vomiting, diarrhea, excessive sweating, or excessive urination (which is a common symptom of untreated diabetes or Addison's disease). Among older people, dehydration during an illness is a common cause of low blood volume leading to orthostatic hypotension. People who are ill may not be able to obtain fluids without assistance. Also, during an illness, the leg muscles are not used regularly. As a result, blood pools in the leg veins and is not pumped back to the heart.● Because this pooling reduces the amount of blood returning to the heart, it, in effect, reduces blood volume and thus reduces blood pressure.

Some conditions cause orthostatic hypotension by dilating arterioles and veins. Drugs that dilate arterioles (vasodilators) can cause orthostatic hypotension. They include nitrates, calcium channel blockers, angiotensin-converting enzyme (ACE) inhibitors, angiotensin II receptor blockers, alpha blockers, alcohol, and antidepressants. Disorders such as diabetes, amyloidosis, and spinal cord injuries may damage the nerves that regulate blood vessel diameter. In addition, veins dilate when body temperature increases, for example because of a warm day, a warm room, or too much clothing. Fever also has this effect.

Fatigue, exercise (which causes blood vessels to dilate), or consumption of a heavy meal (which requires increased blood flow to the intestines) can contribute to orthostatic hypotension.

Symptoms and Diagnosis

Most people with orthostatic hypotension experience some faintness, light-headedness, dizziness, confusion, or blurred vision when they get out of bed abruptly or stand up after

---

▲ see art on page 168   ■ see page 167
★ see page 141   ● see page 232

sitting for a long time. Symptoms are worse if people are tired, have been exercising, have consumed alcohol, or have eaten a heavy meal. A severe decrease in blood flow to the brain can cause the person to faint and even to have convulsions.

These symptoms suggest orthostatic hypotension. The diagnosis can be confirmed if the blood pressure falls significantly when the person stands and returns to normal when the person lies down. Doctors then look for the cause of orthostatic hypotension, because treatment and prognosis depend on the cause.

Treatment

Even when the cause of orthostatic hypotension cannot be treated, certain measures can often reduce or eliminate symptoms. For example, susceptible people should not sit or stand up rapidly or remain standing still for long periods. They should sit or stand up slowly. Wearing fitted elastic stockings up to the waist may help reduce pooling of blood in the leg veins. If orthostatic hypotension results from prolonged bed rest, gradually increasing the time spent sitting up each day may help.

Several measures help maintain blood volume. People with orthostatic hypotension should drink plenty of fluids and little or no alcohol. People who do not have heart failure or high blood pressure are often told to salt their food liberally or to take salt tablets. However, a doctor's supervision is necessary, because a high-salt diet can lead to heart failure,▲ particularly in older people. For people who have severe symptoms, taking hormones that cause salt to be retained, such as fludrocortisone, can increase blood volume. However, use of such hormones increases the risk of heart failure, particularly for older people and for people who have heart disease. Use of fludrocortisone can also cause a loss of potassium, so taking a potassium supplement may be necessary. Midodrine may be taken with fludrocortisone to help prevent blood pressure from falling. Midodrine constricts arterioles, thereby reducing their capacity to hold blood and increasing resistance to blood flow.

If these measures are ineffective, other drugs (such as pindolol, dihydroergotamine, ibuprofen, and clonidine), which work in various ways, may help relieve orthostatic hypotension. However, the risk of side effects from these drugs may make their use undesirable, particularly by older people.

Postprandial Hypotension

Postprandial hypotension is an excessive decrease in blood pressure that occurs after a meal.

Postprandial hypotension occurs in up to one third of older people but virtually never occurs in younger people. It is more likely to occur in people who have high blood pressure or disorders that impair the brain centers controlling the autonomic nervous system (which regulates internal body processes). Examples of such disorders are Parkinson's disease, multiple systems atrophy (Shy-Drager syndrome), and diabetes.

The intestines require a large amount of blood for digestion. When blood flows to the intestines after a meal, the heart rate increases and blood vessels in other parts of the body constrict to help maintain blood pressure. However, in some older people, such mechanisms may be inadequate. Blood flows normally to the intestines, but the heart rate does not increase adequately and blood vessels do not constrict enough to maintain blood pressure. As a result, blood pressure falls.

Postprandial hypotension can cause dizziness, light-headedness, faintness, and falls. If an older person experiences these symptoms after eating, doctors measure blood pressure before and after meals to determine if postprandial hypotension is the cause.

People who have symptoms of postprandial hypotension should not take antihypertensive drugs before meals and should lie down after meals. Taking a smaller dose of the antihypertensive drugs and eating small, low-carbohydrate meals more frequently may help reduce the effects of this disorder. For some people, walking after a meal helps improve blood flow, but blood pressure may fall when they stop walking.

Taking certain drugs before a meal may help. For example, nonsteroidal anti-inflammatory drugs (NSAIDs)■ cause salt to be retained and thus increase blood volume. Octreotide reduces the amount of blood flowing to the intestines. Caffeine, with or without dihydroergotamine, causes blood vessels to constrict. Caffeine should be taken only before breakfast so that sleep is not affected and the person does not become tolerant of caffeine's effects.

▲ see page 150   ■ see page 452

CHAPTER 24

Shock

Shock is a life-threatening condition in which blood pressure is too low to sustain life.

In the United States, hospital emergency departments report more than 1 million cases of shock each year. People go into shock when their blood pressure becomes very low—much lower and for a longer time than the low blood pressure that causes fainting (syncope).▲ When blood pressure is very low, the body's cells do not receive enough blood and therefore do not receive enough oxygen. As a result, cells can be quickly and irreversibly damaged and die; organs, including the brain, kidneys, liver, and heart, may cease to function normally. People in shock require immediate emergency treatment.

Shock has several causes: a low blood volume, which causes hypovolemic shock; inadequate pumping action of the heart, which causes cardiogenic shock; or excessive widening of blood vessels, which causes vasodilatory shock. These types of shock are unrelated to another condition called shock that is caused by emotional stress.

Low blood volume results in less-than-normal amounts of blood entering the heart with every heartbeat and therefore less-than-normal amounts of blood being pumped out to the body. Blood volume may be low because of severe bleeding, an excessive loss of body fluids, or inadequate fluid intake. Blood may be rapidly lost because of external bleeding, such as that caused by an accident, or internal bleeding, such as that caused by an ulcer in the stomach or intestine, a ruptured blood vessel, or a ruptured ectopic pregnancy (a pregnancy outside the uterus). An excessive loss of body fluids other than blood can result from major burns, inflammation of the pancreas (pancreatitis), perforation of the intestinal wall, severe diarrhea, kidney disease, or excessive use of loop diuretics, which increase the output of urine.■ Fluid intake may be inadequate because a physical disability (such as severe joint disease) or a mental disability (such as Alzheimer's disease) prevents people from obtaining enough fluids even though they feel thirsty.

Inadequate pumping action of the heart can also result in less-than-normal amounts of blood being pumped out with every heartbeat. The inadequate pumping action may result from a heart attack, pulmonary embolism, malfunction of a heart valve (particularly an artificial valve), rupture of the wall between the two sides of the heart (septum),★ or an abnormal heart rhythm (arrhythmia).

Excessive dilation of blood vessels (vasodilation) increases the capacity of blood vessels, so that blood meets with less resistance as it flows through them. Blood vessels may be excessively dilated because of a head injury, liver failure, poisoning, overdoses of drugs that dilate blood vessels, or a severe bacterial infection (shock caused by such an infection is called septic shock●). The mechanisms by which these conditions cause vasodilation vary. For example, a head injury may affect the area in the brain that maintains the tone of arteries; poisons or toxins released by bacteria can cause the blood vessels to dilate.

Symptoms and Diagnosis

Symptoms of shock are similar when the cause is low blood volume or inadequate pumping action of the heart. The condition may begin with lethargy, sleepiness, and confusion. The skin becomes cold and sweaty and often bluish and pale. If the skin is pressed, color returns much more slowly than normal. A bluish network of lines may appear under the skin. The pulse is weak and rapid, unless a slow heartbeat is causing the shock. Usually, breathing is rapid, but breathing and the pulse may both slow down if death is imminent. Blood pressure drops so low that it often cannot be measured with a blood pressure cuff. Eventually, the person cannot sit up without passing out and may die.

When shock results from excessive dilation of blood vessels, the symptoms are somewhat different. The skin may be warm and flushed, particularly at first. However, later on, shock due to excessive dilation of blood vessels also produces cold, clammy skin and lethargy.

▲ see page 143   ■ see table on page 138
★ see box on page 212   ● see page 1119

In the earliest stages of shock, especially septic shock, many symptoms may be absent or may be undetected unless they are specifically looked for. In older people, the only symptom may be confusion. The blood pressure is very low. Urine flow is very reduced (because blood supply to the kidneys is reduced), and waste products build up in the blood.

Prognosis and Treatment

If untreated, shock is usually fatal. If shock is treated, the outlook depends on the cause, the other disorders the person has, the amount of time that passes before treatment begins, and the type of treatment given. Regardless of treatment, the likelihood of death due to shock after a massive heart attack or due to septic shock, especially in older people, is great.

The first person to arrive on the scene can take several measures that help, including calling for additional help. A person who is in shock should be laid down and kept warm, with the legs elevated about 12 to 24 inches to facilitate the return of blood to the heart. Any bleeding should be stopped, and breathing should be checked. The head should be turned to the side to prevent inhalation of vomit. Nothing should be given by mouth.

When emergency medical personnel arrive, they may provide oxygen given through a face mask or a mechanical device to assist breathing. Drugs, if needed, are given intravenously. Opioids (narcotics) and sedatives are usually not used because they tend to decrease blood pressure. Attempts may be made to increase blood pressure with military (or medical) anti-shock trousers (MAST). These pants apply pressure to the lower body, thus driving blood from the legs to the heart and brain. Fluids are given intravenously at a fast rate and in large volumes. Usually, blood is cross-matched before a blood transfusion is given, but in an emergency when there is no time for cross-matching, type O negative blood can be given to anyone.

The intravenous fluid and blood transfusion may not be enough to counteract the shock if bleeding or fluid loss continues or if the shock is caused by a heart attack or another problem unrelated to blood volume. Drugs that constrict the blood vessels may be given to boost blood flow to the brain or heart. However, such drugs should be used as briefly as possible because they can reduce blood flow to other tissues in the body.

When shock is caused by an inadequate pumping action of the heart, efforts are made to improve the heart's performance. The rate and rhythm abnormalities of the heartbeat are corrected, and blood volume is increased if necessary. Atropine may be used to increase a slow heart rate, and other drugs may be given to improve the ability of the heart muscle to contract.

If the cause is a heart attack and shock persists after emergency treatment, a balloon pump may be inserted into the aorta to reverse shock temporarily. After this procedure, emergency percutaneous transluminal coronary angioplasty (PTCA) or coronary artery bypass surgery▲ may be needed. By opening a blocked coronary artery (one of the arteries supplying the heart muscle), emergency PTCA can improve the heart's pumping action and can reverse the shock. If emergency PTCA or bypass surgery is not performed, a drug that helps break up clots (thrombolytic drug) is given as soon as possible, unless it could worsen problems in people who have another disorder, such as a bleeding ulcer, or who have had a stroke recently.

If the cause is a malfunctioning heart valve or rupture of the septum, surgery may also be needed.

Shock caused by excessive dilation of the blood vessels is treated primarily with drugs that constrict the vessels. The cause of the excessive dilation is also treated. For example, a bacterial infection is treated with antibiotics.

▲ see pages 208 and 209

CHAPTER 25

Heart Failure

Heart failure is a disorder in which the heart pumps blood inadequately, leading to reduced blood flow, back-up (congestion) of blood in the veins and lungs, and other changes that may further weaken the heart.

Heart failure can occur in people of any age, even in young children (especially those born with a heart defect). However, it is much more common among older people, because older people are more likely to have disorders that damage the heart muscle and because age-related changes in the heart tend to make the heart pump less efficiently. Heart failure develops in about 1 of 100 people. The disorder is likely to become more common because people are living longer and because, in some countries, certain risk factors for heart disease (such as smoking, high blood pressure, and a high-fat diet) are affecting more people.

Heart failure does not mean that the heart has stopped, as some people mistakenly believe; it means that the heart cannot keep up with the work required of it (its workload). However, this definition is remarkably simplified. Heart failure is extremely complex, and no simple definition can encompass its many causes, aspects, forms, and consequences.

The function of the heart is to pump blood. Pumping has two aspects: to move a fluid into something (the heart pumps blood into the arteries) and to move a fluid out of something (the heart moves blood out of the veins, as a sump pump moves water out of a basement). Heart failure develops when the pumping action of the heart is inadequate. As a result, blood flow to body tissues is reduced and blood returning to the heart accumulates, causing congestion in the veins. That is why heart failure is also known as congestive heart failure.

Accumulation of blood coming into the left side of the heart (from the lungs)▲ causes congestion in the lungs, impairing lung function and making breathing difficult. Accumulation of blood coming into the right side of the heart (from the rest of the body) causes congestion

in other parts of the body, including fluid accumulation (edema) in the legs and enlargement of organs such as the liver. Heart failure usually affects both the right and left sides of the heart to some degree. However, one side may be affected more than the other. In such cases, heart failure may be described as right-sided heart failure or left-sided heart failure.

In heart failure, the heart cannot pump enough blood to meet the body's need for oxygen and nutrients, which are supplied by the blood. As a result, arm and leg muscles may tire more quickly, and the kidneys may not function normally. Blood pressure in the arteries normally enables the kidneys to filter fluid and waste products from the blood into the urine. When the heart cannot pump adequately, blood pressure falls and the kidneys malfunction: The kidneys cannot remove excess fluid from the blood. As a result, the amount of fluid in the bloodstream increases, and the workload of the failing heart increases, creating a vicious circle. Thus, heart failure becomes even worse.

Heart failure has two main forms: systolic dysfunction (which is more common) and diastolic dysfunction. In systolic dysfunction, the heart contracts less forcefully and cannot pump out as much of the blood that is returned to it as it normally does. As a result, more blood remains in the lower chambers of the heart (ventricles). Blood then accumulates in the veins. In diastolic dysfunction, the heart is stiff and does not relax normally after contracting. Even though it may be able to pump a normal amount of blood out of the ventricles, the stiff heart does not allow as much blood to enter its chambers from the veins. As in systolic dysfunction, the blood returning to the heart then accumulates in the veins. Often, both forms of heart failure occur together.

Causes

Any disorder that directly affects the heart can lead to heart failure, as can some disorders that indirectly affect the heart. Some disorders cause heart failure quickly; others do so only after many years. Some disorders cause systolic dysfunction, impairing the heart's ability

---

▲ see art on page 115

Heart Failure: Pumping and Filling Problems

Normally, the heart stretches as it fills with blood (during diastole), then contracts to pump out the blood (during systole).

Heart failure due to systolic dysfunction usually develops because the heart cannot contract normally. It may fill with blood, but it cannot pump out as much of the blood it contains because the muscle is weaker. As a result, the amount of blood pumped to the body and to the lungs is reduced, and the heart, particularly the left ventricle, usually enlarges.

Heart failure due to diastolic dysfunction develops because the heart's walls stiffen and may thicken so that the heart cannot fill normally with blood. Consequently, blood backs up in the left atrium and lung (pulmonary) blood vessels and causes congestion. Nonetheless, the heart may be able to pump out a normal percentage of the blood it receives.

Because the heart contracts to enclose the amount of blood it contains, there is never any empty space in its chambers. The different amounts of blood entering or leaving the chambers is indicated by the thickness of the arrows.

	Normal	**Systolic Dysfunction**	**Diastolic Dysfunction**

Diastole
(filling)

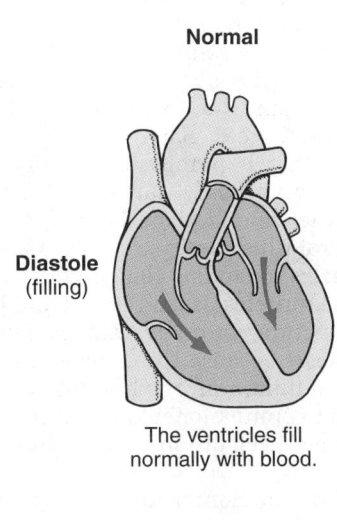

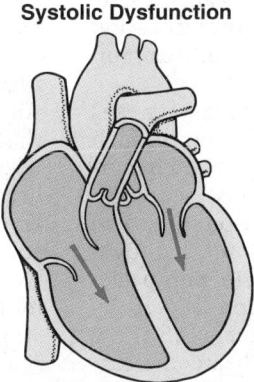

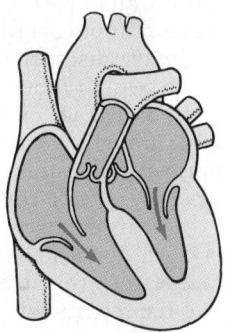

The ventricles fill normally with blood.

The enlarged ventricles fill with blood.

The stiff ventricles fill with less blood than normal.

Systole
(pumping)

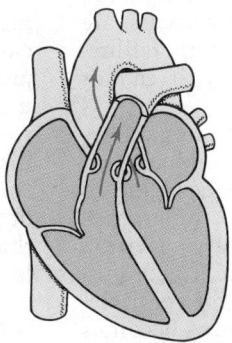

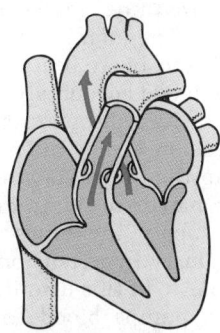

The ventricles pump out about 60% of the blood.

The ventricles pump out less than 40 to 50% of the blood.

The ventricles pump out about 60% of the blood, but the amount may be lower than normal.

to pump out blood, and others cause diastolic dysfunction, impairing the heart's ability to fill with blood. Some disorders, such as high blood pressure and heart valve disorders, can cause both types of dysfunction.

Systolic Dysfunction: Disorders that cause systolic dysfunction may impair the entire heart or one area of the heart. As a result, the heart does not contract normally.

Coronary artery disease is a common cause of systolic dysfunction. It can impair large areas of heart muscle because it reduces the flow of oxygen-rich blood to the heart muscle, which needs oxygen for normal contraction. Blockage of a coronary artery can cause a heart attack, which destroys an area of heart muscle. As a result, that area can no longer contract normally.

Myocarditis (inflammation of heart muscle) caused by a bacterial, viral, or other infection can damage all or part of the heart muscle, impairing its pumping ability.

Heart valve disorders—narrowing (stenosis) of a valve, which hinders blood flow through the heart, or leakage of blood backward (regurgitation) through a valve—can cause heart failure. Both stenosis and regurgitation of a valve can severely stress the heart, so that over time, the heart enlarges and cannot pump adequately. An abnormal connection (septal defects)▲ between the heart chambers can allow blood to recirculate within the heart, increasing the workload of the heart, and thus can cause heart failure.

Disorders that affect the heart's electrical conduction system, producing changes in heart rhythms, (especially if heartbeats are fast or irregular), can cause heart failure. When the heart beats abnormally, it cannot pump blood adequately.

Some lung disorders, such as pulmonary hypertension,■ may alter or damage blood vessels in the lungs. As a result, the heart has to work harder to pump blood into the arteries that supply the lungs (pulmonary arteries). Pulmonary hypertension may lead to cor pulmonale.★ In this disorder, the right ventricle, which pumps blood to the lungs, becomes enlarged, eventually resulting in right-sided heart failure.

Sudden, usually complete blockage of a pulmonary artery by several small blood clots or one very large clot (pulmonary embolism) also makes pumping blood into the pulmonary arteries difficult. A very large clot can be immediately life threatening. The increased effort required to pump blood into the blocked pulmonary arteries can cause the right side of the heart to enlarge and may cause the walls of the right ventricle to thicken, resulting in right-sided heart failure.

Disorders that indirectly affect the heart's pumping ability include a deficiency of red blood cells or hemoglobin (anemia), an overactive thyroid gland (hyperthyroidism), an underactive thyroid gland (hypothyroidism), and kidney failure. Red blood cells contain hemoglobin, which enables them to carry oxygen from the lungs and deliver it to body tissues. Anemia reduces the amount of oxygen the blood carries, so that the heart must work harder to provide the same amount of oxygen to tissues. (Anemia has many causes, including chronic bleeding due to a stomach ulcer). An overactive thyroid gland overstimulates the heart, so that it pumps too rapidly and does not empty normally during each heartbeat. When the thyroid gland is underactive, levels of thyroid hormones are low. As a result, all muscles, including the heart, become weak because muscles depend on thyroid hormones to function normally. Kidney failure strains the heart because the kidneys cannot remove excess fluid from the bloodstream, so the heart has to pump more blood. Eventually, the heart cannot keep up, and heart failure develops.

Diastolic Dysfunction: Inadequately treated high blood pressure is the most common cause of diastolic dysfunction. High blood pressure stresses the heart because the heart must pump blood more forcefully than normal to force blood into the arteries against the higher pressure. Eventually, the heart's walls thicken (hypertrophy), then stiffen. The stiff heart does not fill quickly or adequately, so that with each contraction, the heart pumps less blood than it normally does.

As people age, the heart's walls also tend to stiffen. The combination of high blood pressure, which is common among older people, and age-related stiffening makes heart failure particularly common among older people.

Heart failure may result from disorders that cause the heart's walls to stiffen, such as infiltrations and infections. For example, in amyloidosis, amyloid, an unusual protein not normally present in the body, infiltrates many

▲ see page 1514 and box on page 1516

■ see page 322   ★ see box on page 323

tissues in the body. If amyloid infiltrates the heart's walls, they stiffen, and heart failure results. In tropical countries, infiltration by certain parasites into heart muscle can cause heart failure, even in young people. Some heart valve disorders, such as aortic valve stenosis, hinder blood flow out of the heart. As a result, the heart muscle has to work harder and thickens, and diastolic dysfunction develops initially. Eventually, systolic dysfunction also develops.

In constrictive pericarditis, the sac that envelops the heart (pericardium) stiffens, preventing even a healthy heart from pumping and filling normally.

Compensatory Mechanisms

The body has several mechanisms to compensate for heart failure. The body's first response to stress, including that due to heart failure, is to release the fight-or-flight hormones, epinephrine (adrenaline) and norepinephrine (noradrenaline). For example, these hormones may be released immediately after a heart attack damages the heart. Epinephrine and norepinephrine cause the heart to pump faster and more forcefully. They help the heart increase the amount of blood pumped out (cardiac output), sometimes to a normal amount, and thus help compensate partially and temporarily for the heart's impaired pumping ability.

People who do not have heart disease usually benefit from release of these hormones when more work is temporarily required of the heart. However, for people who have chronic heart failure, this response results in increased demands on an already damaged heart. Over time, the increased demands lead to further deterioration of heart function.

Another of the body's main compensatory mechanisms for heart failure is to decrease the amount of salt and water excreted by the kidneys. Retaining salt and water instead of excreting it into urine increases the volume of blood in the bloodstream and helps maintain blood pressure. The larger volume of blood also stretches the heart muscle, enlarging the heart chambers, particularly the ventricles, which pump blood out of the heart. The more the heart muscle is stretched, the more forcefully it contracts. At first, this mechanism improves heart function, but after a point, stretching no longer helps but instead weakens the heart's contractions (as when a rubber band is overstretched). Consequently, heart failure worsens.

Another important compensatory mechanism is enlargement of the muscular walls of the ventricles (ventricular hypertrophy). When the heart must work harder, the heart's walls enlarge and thicken, as biceps muscles enlarge after months of weight training. At first, the thickened heart walls can contract more forcefully. However, the thickened heart walls eventually become stiff, worsening diastolic dysfunction. Eventually, the contractions become weaker, causing systolic dysfunction.

Symptoms

Symptoms of heart failure may begin suddenly, especially if the cause is a heart attack. However, in most people, symptoms develop over days to months. The disorder may stabilize for periods of time but often progresses slowly and insidiously.

People with heart failure feel tired and weak when performing physical activities, because their muscles are not receiving enough blood. In older people, heart failure sometimes causes vague symptoms such as sleepiness, confusion, and disorientation, as well as weakness and fatigue.

Right-sided heart failure and left-sided heart failure produce different symptoms. Although both types of heart failure may be present, the symptoms of failure of one side often predominate. The main symptoms of right-sided heart failure are fluid accumulation and swelling (edema) in the feet, ankles, legs, liver, and abdomen. Where the fluid accumulates depends on the amount of excess fluid and the effects of gravity. If a person is standing, fluid accumulates in the legs and feet. If a person is lying down, fluid usually accumulates in the lower back. If the amount of fluid is large, fluid also accumulates in the abdomen. Fluid accumulation in the liver or stomach can cause nausea and loss of appetite. Eventually, food is not absorbed well, resulting in loss of weight and muscle. This condition is called cardiac cachexia.

Left-sided heart failure leads to fluid accumulation in the lungs, which causes shortness of breath. At first, shortness of breath occurs only during exertion, but as heart failure progresses, it occurs with less and less exertion and eventually occurs even at rest. People with severe left-sided heart failure may be short of breath when lying down (a condition called orthopnea▲), because gravity causes

---

▲ see page 251

more fluid to move into the lungs. Such people often wake up, gasping for breath or wheezing (a condition called paroxysmal nocturnal dyspnea). Sitting up causes some of the fluid to drain to the bottom of the lungs, making breathing easier. Eventually, left-sided heart failure causes right-sided heart failure.

A sudden accumulation of a large amount of fluid in the lungs (acute pulmonary edema) causes extreme difficulty breathing, rapid breathing, bluish skin, and feelings of restlessness, anxiety, and suffocation. Some people have severe spasms of the airways (bronchospasms) and wheezing; this condition is called **cardiac asthma,** which resembles asthma but has a different cause. Acute pulmonary edema is a life-threatening emergency.

When heart failure is advanced, Cheyne-Stokes respiration (periodic breathing) may develop. In this unusual pattern of breathing, a person breathes rapidly and deeply, then more slowly, then not at all for several seconds. Cheyne-Stokes respiration develops because blood flow to the brain is reduced and the areas of the brain that control breathing therefore do not receive enough oxygen.

When the heart cannot pump a normal amount of blood out of its chambers, blood clots can form because blood flow within the chambers is sluggish. Clots may break loose (becoming emboli), travel through the bloodstream, and partially or completely block an artery elsewhere in the body. If a clot blocks an artery to the brain, a stroke may result.

Diagnosis

Doctors usually suspect heart failure on the basis of symptoms alone. The diagnosis is supported by the results of a physical examination, including a weak, often rapid pulse, reduced blood pressure, abnormal heart sounds and fluid accumulation in the lungs (both heard through a stethoscope), an enlarged heart, swollen neck veins, an enlarged liver, and swelling in the abdomen or legs. A chest x-ray can show an enlarged heart and fluid accumulation in the lungs.

Procedures to evaluate heart function are usually performed. Electrocardiography (ECG)▲ is almost always performed to determine whether the heart rhythm is normal, whether the walls of the ventricles are thickened, and whether the person has had a heart attack.

▲ see page 122   ■ see page 125
★ see page 128   ● see pages 205 to 210

Echocardiography,■ which uses sound waves to produce an image of the heart, is one of the best procedures for evaluating heart function, including the pumping ability of the heart and the functioning of heart valves. It can show whether the heart walls are thickened, whether the valves are functioning normally, whether contractions are normal, and whether any area of the heart is contracting abnormally. Echocardiography may help determine whether heart failure is due to systolic or diastolic dysfunction by enabling doctors to estimate the thickness of the heart walls and the ejection fraction. The ejection fraction, an important measure of heart function, is the percentage of blood pumped out by the heart with each beat. A normal left ventricle ejects about 60% of the blood in it. If the ejection fraction is low, systolic dysfunction is likely; if it is normal or high, diastolic dysfunction is likely.

Other procedures, such as radionuclide imaging and cardiac catheterization with angiography,★ may be performed to identify the cause of heart failure. Rarely, a biopsy is needed, usually when doctors suspect infiltration of the heart (as occurs in amyloidosis) or myocarditis due to a bacterial, viral, or other infection.

Prevention and Treatment

Some disorders that cause heart failure, such as high blood pressure, severe anemia, and an overactive or underactive thyroid gland, can be treated before they lead to heart failure. Preventing heart attacks by treating coronary artery disease can also prevent heart failure.

Although heart failure is a chronic disorder for most people, much can be done to make physical activity more comfortable, improve the quality of life, and prolong life. Treatment focuses on treating the disorder causing heart failure, controlling factors that can worsen heart failure (contributing factors), and treating heart failure itself.

Treatment of the Cause: If the cause of heart failure is a narrowed or leaking heart valve or an abnormal connection between heart chambers, surgery can often correct the problem. Blockage of a coronary artery may require treatment with drugs, surgery, or angioplasty.● Antihypertensive drugs can reduce and control high blood pressure. Antibiotics can eliminate some infections. Treatment of a stomach ulcer or use of an iron supplement may correct anemia. Drugs, surgery, or radiation therapy can be used to manage an overactive thyroid gland, and thyroid hormones can be given to manage an underactive thyroid gland.

Control of Contributing Factors: Several factors that contribute to heart failure can be minimized or eliminated by changes in lifestyle. People who have heart failure should stay as physically fit as possible, even if they cannot exercise vigorously. People who have mild heart failure should follow an exercise program as described by a doctor. Those with more severe heart failure may need to exercise in a cardiovascular rehabilitation facility under the supervision of a trained attendant.

In people who have heart failure and are overweight, the heart must work harder during activity, worsening heart failure. Such people should follow a weight loss diet.▲

Smoking damages blood vessels, increasing the risk of a heart attack. Large amounts of alcohol can act as a direct toxin to the heart. Thus, smoking and drinking alcohol can worsen heart failure and should be stopped.

Exercise, weight loss, and stopping smoking help reduce the risk of coronary artery disease, as do good control of diabetes and lowering of cholesterol levels.

Excess salt (sodium) in the diet can cause fluid retention, which counteracts drugs given to increase the excretion of water (such as diuretics) and relieve fluid accumulation. Thus, consuming excess salt worsens symptoms. Almost everyone with heart failure should limit their intake of table salt and salty foods and their use of salt in cooking. The sodium content of packaged foods can be determined by reading the label. People with severe heart failure are usually given detailed information about how to limit salt intake. People who limit their salt intake can usually consume a normal amount of water unless fluid retention is severe. Drinking extra amounts of water is not recommended.

A simple, reliable way to check whether the body is retaining fluid is to check body weight daily. Doctors often ask people with heart failure to weigh themselves as accurately as possible every day, typically once in the morning, after they arise and urinate and before they eat breakfast. Trends are easier to spot when people weigh themselves at the same time every day, use the same scale, wear a similar amount of clothing, and keep a written record of their daily weight. Increases of more than 2 pounds

(about 1 kilogram) per day are early warning signs of fluid retention. A consistent, rapid weight gain (such as 2 pounds per day) is a clue that heart failure is worsening.

Many people who limit their salt intake still have swelling. Swollen legs should be kept elevated on a stool when sitting. This position helps the body reabsorb and eliminate the excess fluid. Some people also need to wear full-length supportive stockings that help prevent accumulation of fluid. If fluid accumulates in the lungs, sleeping with several pillows or elevating the head of the bed makes sleeping easier.

Treatment of Heart Failure: Heart failure can be treated with several different types of drugs. Regular communication with and examinations by doctors and other health care practitioners who are trained in the treatment of heart failure are critical, because heart failure can worsen suddenly. For example, nurses often call a person who has heart failure regularly to ask about changes in weight and in symptoms. Thus, they can gauge whether the person needs to see a doctor.

When salt restriction alone does not reduce fluid retention, doctors often prescribe diuretics.■ These drugs help the kidneys eliminate salt and water by increasing urine formation and thus decrease fluid volume throughout the body. The diuretics most commonly used for heart failure are furosemide and bumetanide, which are loop diuretics. These diuretics are most commonly taken by mouth on a long-term basis, but in an emergency, they are very effective when given intravenously. Loop diuretics are preferred for moderate to severe heart failure; thiazide diuretics, which have milder effects, may be prescribed for mild heart failure. Because loop and thiazide diuretics can cause potassium to be lost in the urine, a potassium supplement or a diuretic that does not cause potassium loss or that causes potassium levels to increase (a potassium-sparing diuretic) may be given as well. For people with severe heart failure due to systolic dysfunction, spironolactone is the preferred potassium-sparing diuretic to be added. It can prolong life in people with heart failure. Taking diuretics can worsen urinary incontinence. However, a dose of a diuretic can usually be timed so that episodes of incontinence do not

---

▲ see page 884

■ see table on page 138

℞ SOME DRUGS USED TO TREAT HEART FAILURE*

TYPE	DRUG	COMMENTS

Angiotensin-converting enzyme (ACE) inhibitors

	Benazepril Captopril Enalapril Fosinopril Lisinopril Moexipril Perindopril Quinapril Ramipril Trandolapril	ACE inhibitors cause blood vessels to widen (dilate), thus decreasing the amount of work the heart has to do; they may also have direct beneficial effects on the heart. These drugs are the mainstay of heart failure treatment. They reduce symptoms and the need for hospitalization, and they prolong life.

Angiotensin II receptor blockers

	Candesartan Eprosartan Irbesartan Losartan Telmisartan Valsartan	Angiotensin II receptor blockers have effects similar to those of ACE inhibitors and may be tolerated better. However, their effects are still being evaluated in people with heart failure. They may be used with an ACE inhibitor or used alone in people who cannot take an ACE inhibitor.

Beta-blockers

	Bisoprolol Carvedilol Metoprolol	Beta-blockers drugs slow the heart rate and block excessive stimulation of the heart. They are appropriate for some people with heart failure. These drugs are usually used with ACE inhibitors and provide an added benefit. They may temporarily worsen symptoms but result in long-term improvement in heart function.

Other vasodilators

	Hydralazine Isosorbide dinitrate Nitroglycerin	Vasodilators cause blood vessels to dilate. These vasodilators are usually given to people who cannot take an ACE inhibitor or angiotensin II receptor blocker. Nitroglycerin is particularly useful in people who have heart failure and angina.

Cardiac glycosides

	Digitoxin Digoxin	Cardiac glycosides increase the force of each heartbeat and slow a heart rate that is too fast.

Loop diuretics

	Bumetanide Ethacrynic acid Furosemide	These diuretics help the kidneys eliminate salt and water, thus decreasing the volume of fluid in the bloodstream.

Potassium-sparing diuretics

	Amiloride Spironolactone Triamterene	Because these diuretics prevent potassium loss, they may be given in addition to thiazide or loop diuretics, which cause potassium to be lost. Spironolactone is particularly useful in the treatment of severe heart failure.

Thiazide and thiazide-like diuretics

	Chlorthalidone Hydrochlorothiazide Indapamide Metolazone	The effects of these diuretics are similar to but milder than those of loop diuretics. The two types of diuretics are particularly effective when used together.

℞ SOME DRUGS USED TO TREAT HEART FAILURE* (Continued)

TYPE	DRUG	COMMENTS
Anticoagulants		
	Heparin Warfarin	Anticoagulants may be given to prevent clots from forming in the heart chambers.
Opioids		
	Morphine	Morphine is given to relieve the anxiety that usually accompanies acute pulmonary edema, which is a medical emergency.
Positive inotropic drugs (drugs that make muscle contract more forcefully)		
	Inamrinone Dobutamine Dopamine Milrinone	For people who have severe symptoms, these drugs may be given intravenously to stimulate heart contractions and help keep blood circulating.

*Selected side effects for ACE inhibitors, angiotensin II receptor blockers, diuretics, and beta-blockers are listed in the table on pages 138 and 139.

occur when a bathroom is unavailable or when access to one is inconvenient.

The mainstay of heart failure treatment is a group of drugs called angiotensin-converting enzyme (ACE) inhibitors.▲ These drugs not only reduce symptoms and the need for hospitalization but also prolong life. ACE inhibitors reduce the blood levels of the hormones angiotensin II and aldosterone (which normally help increase blood pressure).■ By doing so, ACE inhibitors cause arteries and veins to widen (dilate) and help the kidneys excrete excess water, thus decreasing the amount of work the heart has to perform. These drugs also may have direct beneficial effects on the heart and blood vessel walls.

Angiotensin II receptor blockers★ have effects similar to those of ACE inhibitors. Angiotensin II receptor blockers are used with ACE inhibitors in some people or are used alone in people who cannot tolerate ACE inhibitors because of cough, a side effect of ACE inhibitors. However, the role of angiotensin II receptor blockers is still being evaluated in the treatment of heart failure.

Other drugs that dilate blood vessels (vasodilators) are not used as often as ACE inhibitors, which are more effective. Nonetheless, people who do not respond to or cannot take ACE inhibitors can benefit from vasodilators, such as hydralazine, isosorbide dinitrate, and nitroglycerin patches or spray.

Beta-blockers, a group of drugs that used to be avoided in the treatment of heart failure, are now being used with ACE inhibitors to treat heart failure. Because these drugs slow the heart rate and reduce the force of the heart's contractions, they may initially worsen symptoms. However, by blocking the action of the hormone norepinephrine (which causes the heart to pump faster and more forcefully), these drugs produce long-term improvement in heart function and survival.

Digoxin, one of the oldest treatments for heart failure, increases the force of each heartbeat and slows a heart rate that is too rapid. Digoxin helps relieve symptoms for some people with systolic dysfunction, especially if atrial fibrillation is present, but it does not prolong life.

Anticoagulants, such as warfarin, may be given to prevent clots from forming in the heart chambers. If the heart rhythm is abnormal, antiarrhythmic drugs● may be given, or an implantable defibrillator◆ may be recommended.

Heart transplantation may be an option for a few otherwise healthy people who have very

---

▲ see table on page 139   ■ see art on page 133
★ see table on page 139
● see table on page 166
◆ see page 167

severe, worsening heart failure and who have not responded to drug therapy. Temporary partial or complete mechanical hearts are still largely experimental. Problems of effectiveness, infection, and blood clots are still being worked out.

Several experimental operations are under study; their benefits are doubtful and they are performed only at some research centers. One operation consists of surgically removing the flabby, nonfunctioning heart muscle. In another operation, tiny pumps that boost the pumping action of the heart are inserted in the body, often in the abdomen near the heart. These pumps can help prolong the life of people who are waiting for a heart transplantation. Other experimental procedures include implantation of a pacemaker in each ventricle and delivery of room air or oxygen that is under pressure through a face mask (continuous positive airway pressure).

Treatment of Acute Heart Failure: Heart failure that develops or worsens quickly requires emergency treatment in a hospital.

If acute pulmonary edema develops,▲ oxygen is given through a face mask. Diuretics given intravenously and other drugs such as nitroglycerin given intravenously or under the tongue can produce rapid, dramatic improvement. Morphine relieves the anxiety that usually accompanies acute pulmonary edema. It also decreases the rate of breathing, slows the heart rate, dilates blood vessels, and thereby reduces the amount of work the heart has to do. If these measures do not adequately improve breathing, a tube may be inserted into the person's airway so that a mechanical ventilator can assist breathing.

For people who have severe symptoms and have not responded well to treatments, drugs that are similar to epinephrine and norepinephrine (such as dopamine or dobutamine) or other drugs that make muscle contract more forcefully (such as milrinone or amrinone) are sometimes used for a short time to stimulate heart contractions. These drugs are not useful for long-term treatment.

End-of-Life Issues: Although many people with heart failure live for many years, up to 70% of people die of the disorder within 10 years. Life expectancy depends on how severe the heart failure is, whether its cause can be corrected, and which treatment is used. About half of people who have mild heart failure live at least 10 years, and about half of those who have severe heart failure live at least 2 years. Eventually, for a person with chronic heart failure, quality of life may deteriorate and the possibilities for further treatment may become limited, especially for an older person for whom heart transplantation may not be feasible. Keeping the person comfortable may eventually become more important than trying to prolong life. The person and the family members should be involved in these decisions. Much can be done to provide compassionate care, relieve symptoms, and maintain the person's dignity.■

Heart failure can cause death suddenly and unexpectedly, without symptoms worsening. Consequently, when possible, people who have heart failure should prepare advance directives about the type of care desired in case they are no longer able to make decisions about their care.★ Also, making or updating a will is important.

CHAPTER 26

Cardiomyopathy

Cardiomyopathy refers to progressive impairment of the structure and function of the muscular walls of the heart chambers.

Cardiomyopathy can be caused by many disorders, or it may have no identifiable cause.

The main types of cardiomyopathy—which may overlap—are dilated, hypertrophic, and restrictive.

Dilated Cardiomyopathy

Dilated (congestive) cardiomyopathy is a group of heart muscle disorders in which the ventricles enlarge but are not able to pump

▲ see page 154   ■ see page 48
★ see page 54

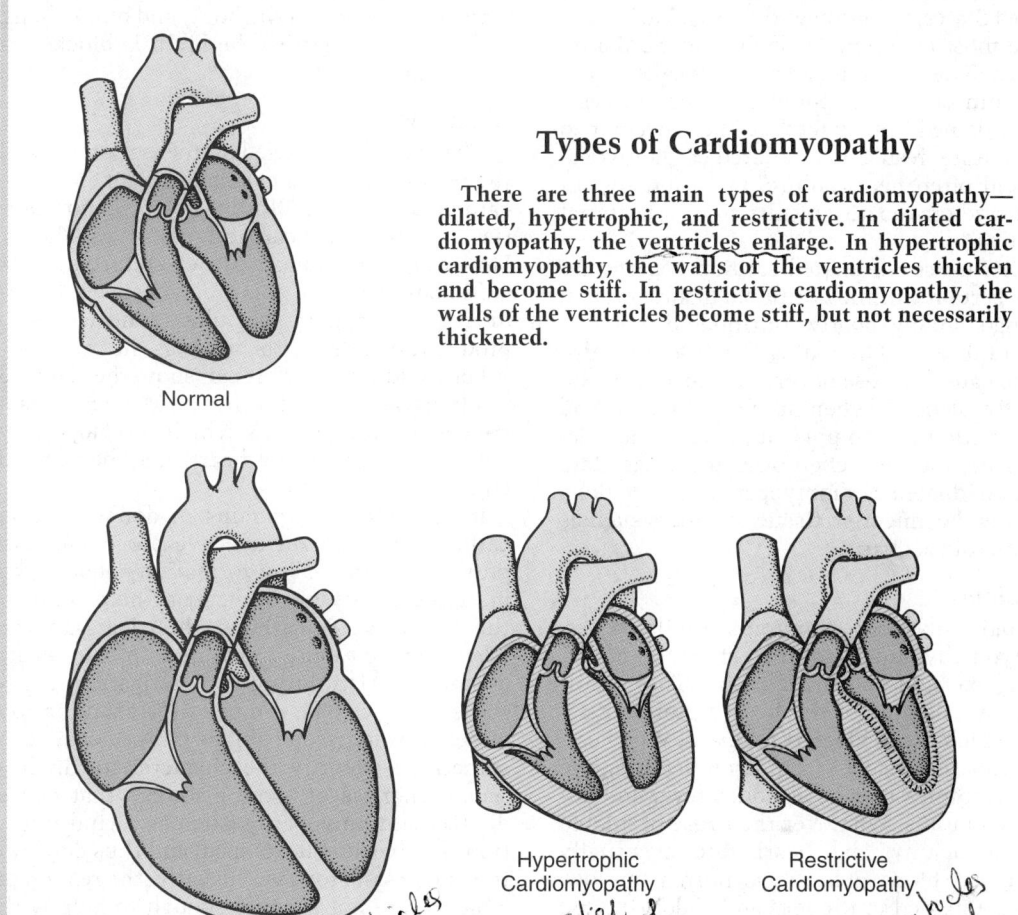

Types of Cardiomyopathy

There are three main types of cardiomyopathy—dilated, hypertrophic, and restrictive. In dilated cardiomyopathy, the ventricles enlarge. In hypertrophic cardiomyopathy, the walls of the ventricles thicken and become stiff. In restrictive cardiomyopathy, the walls of the ventricles become stiff, but not necessarily thickened.

Normal

Dilated
Cardiomyopathy

ventricles enlarge

Hypertrophic
Cardiomyopathy

walls stiff & thick

Restrictive
Cardiomyopathy

ventricles stiff

enough blood for the body's needs, resulting in heart failure.

Dilated cardiomyopathy can develop at any age but is more common among people aged 20 to 60 years. About 10% of people who develop dilated cardiomyopathy are older than 65. The disorder occurs in about 3 times as many men as women and 3 times as many blacks as whites. About 5 to 8 of every 100,000 people develop the disorder each year.

In the United States, the most common identifiable cause of dilated cardiomyopathy is extensive coronary artery disease. Such coronary artery disease results in an inadequate blood supply to the heart muscle, which leads to permanent injury and death of heart muscle. As a result, the heart cannot pump as forcefully. The dead heart muscle is replaced by fibrous (scar) tissue. The remaining uninjured heart muscle then stretches and thickens (hypertrophies) to compensate for the lost pumping action. The more the heart muscle is stretched, the more forcefully it contracts or pumps but only up to a point. After that point, the stretching and thickening do not adequately compensate, and dilated cardiomyopathy with heart failure develops.

Dilated cardiomyopathy may be caused by an acute inflammation of the heart muscle (myocarditis) due to a viral infection. This disorder is called viral cardiomyopathy. In the United States, infection with coxsackie B virus is the most common cause of viral cardiomyopathy. The virus infects and weakens the heart muscle. As in coronary artery disease, the weakened heart stretches in an attempt to compensate, resulting in dilated cardiomyopathy and often heart failure. Occasionally, dilated cardiomyopathy results from a bacterial infection.

Other causes of dilated cardiomyopathy include certain chronic hormonal disorders such as long-standing, poorly controlled diabetes or thyroid disease. Dilated cardiomyopathy also can be caused by use of certain substances, especially alcohol (when intake is heavy and malnutrition is also present), cocaine, antidepressants, and a few chemotherapy drugs. Rare causes of dilated cardiomyopathy include pregnancy and connective tissue disorders such as rheumatoid arthritis.

Symptoms

Usually, the first symptoms of dilated cardiomyopathy are becoming short of breath during exertion and tiring easily. They result from a weakening of the heart's pumping action, which is called heart failure.▲ When cardiomyopathy results from an infection, the first symptoms may be a sudden fever and flu-like symptoms. Whatever the cause of dilated cardiomyopathy, the heart rate eventually speeds up, blood pressure is normal or low, fluid is retained in the legs and abdomen, and the lungs fill with fluid.

Because the heart is enlarged, the heart valves may be unable to close normally. The mitral valve, which opens from the left atrium (upper heart chamber) into the left ventricle (lower heart chamber), and the tricuspid valve, which opens from the right atrium into the right ventricle, often leak. Leakage causes murmurs, which doctors can hear with a stethoscope. Damage to and stretching of the heart muscle may result in abnormal heart rhythms (arrhythmias). The leakage of the valves and the abnormal heart rhythms may interfere further with the heart's pumping action.

Blood pools in the enlarged heart, increasing the risk of blood clots forming on heart chamber walls. The clots can break into pieces (be-

coming emboli), travel from the heart to blood vessels elsewhere in the body, and block them. If the blood supply to the brain is blocked, a stroke can result.

Diagnosis

The diagnosis is based on the symptoms and the results of a physical examination. Electrocardiography (ECG)■ may detect abnormalities in the electrical activity of the heart. However, these abnormalities are usually not sufficient evidence for a diagnosis. Echocardiography,★ which uses ultrasound waves to produce an image of the heart, is the most useful procedure because it can show the size and pumping action of the heart. Magnetic resonance imaging (MRI),● which produces very detailed images of the heart, may be used to confirm the diagnosis.

If the diagnosis remains in doubt, cardiac catheterization,◆ an invasive procedure, can provide additional information about the pumping ability of the heart or help confirm the diagnosis. A catheter threaded into the heart can measure pressures in the heart chambers. Also during catheterization, a tissue sample can be removed for examination under a microscope (biopsy). A biopsy can sometimes identify the characteristic microscopic changes of some disorders that cause dilated cardiomyopathy (such as a viral infection that has just developed) and thus confirm the diagnosis. However, usually, the results of a biopsy are not specific enough to help with the diagnosis.

Prognosis and Treatment

About 70% of people with dilated cardiomyopathy die within 5 years of when their symptoms begin, and the prognosis worsens as the heart walls become thinner and the heart functions less well. Abnormal heart rhythms also indicate a worse prognosis. Overall, men survive only half as long as women, and blacks survive half as long as whites. About 50% of deaths are sudden, probably resulting from an abnormal heart rhythm.

Treating the cause, such as alcohol abuse (by abstaining from alcohol) or a bacterial infection (by using antibiotics), can prolong life.

People who also have coronary artery disease may require treatment for it. Such treatment may include a nitrate, a beta-blocker, or a calcium channel blocker.▼ However, calcium channel blockers may reduce the force of heart contractions and thus may

---

▲ see page 150   ■ see page 122
★ see page 125   ● see page 126
◆ see page 128   ▼ see table on page 206

worsen the heart failure that accompanies dilated cardiomyopathy. Getting enough rest and avoiding stress help reduce strain on the heart.

Antiarrhythmic drugs may be given to prevent abnormal heart rhythms.▲ Most of these drugs are prescribed in small doses. They are increased in small increments, because if the dose is too large, an antiarrhythmic drug may reduce the force of heart contractions and thereby worsen heart failure.

Heart failure is treated with an angiotensin-converting enzyme (ACE) inhibitor, a beta-blocker, digoxin, and often a diuretic.■ However, unless a specific cause of dilated cardiomyopathy can be treated, the heart failure is likely to eventually be fatal. Because of this poor prognosis, dilated cardiomyopathy is the most common reason for heart transplantation.★ Successful heart transplantation cures the disorder, but it has its own complications and limitations.

Regardless of the cause of dilated cardiomyopathy, anticoagulants, such as warfarin, are usually given to prevent blood clots, which may form on the heart chamber walls.

Hypertrophic Cardiomyopathy

Hypertrophic cardiomyopathy includes a group of heart disorders in which the walls of the ventricles thicken (hypertrophy) and become stiff, even though the workload of the heart is not increased.

Generally, hypertrophic cardiomyopathy affects men and women equally. But among older people, it is more common among women than among men, mainly because women live longer than men. It occurs in about 4% of older people.

Hypertrophic cardiomyopathy may be present at birth (congenital) or acquired later in life. Congenital hypertrophic cardiomyopathy is caused by an inherited genetic defect. Acquired hypertrophic cardiomyopathy may be caused by such disorders as acromegaly (excessive growth due to overproduction of growth hormone, usually by a benign pituitary tumor) and a pheochromocytoma (a tumor that overproduces the hormone epinephrine). Neurofibromatosis, a hereditary disorder, may also cause hypertrophic cardiomyopathy.

Symptoms and Diagnosis

Symptoms include fainting (syncope), chest pain, shortness of breath, and awareness of irregular heartbeats (palpitations) produced by an abnormal heart rhythm (arrhythmia). Fainting, usually after exertion, occurs because the heart does not supply the brain with enough blood. The heart cannot supply enough blood, for example, because the heart rhythm is irregular or because the stiff, thickened ventricle does not fill with blood adequately and impedes blood flow from the heart. Fainting is more likely to occur after exertion because during exertion, the heart rate increases and more blood is pumped out, thus overcoming, to some extent, the impediment to blood flow. After exertion, the heart rate slows and the amount of blood pumped out is no longer enough to overcome the impediment.

Shortness of breath develops because fluid accumulates in the lungs. Fluid accumulates because the thickened, stiff heart resists filling with blood from the lungs and blood consequently pools in the lung (pulmonary) veins.

Because the ventricle walls thicken, the mitral valve (the valve that opens from the left atrium into the left ventricle) may be unable to close normally, resulting in a small amount of leakage. This abnormality increases the risk of infective endocarditis● for people with hypertrophic cardiomyopathy. In some people, the thickened muscle blocks the flow of blood out of the heart below the aortic valve; this variation is called hypertrophic obstructive cardiomyopathy.

Doctors can usually make a preliminary diagnosis of hypertrophic cardiomyopathy based on the results of a physical examination. For example, the heart sounds heard through a stethoscope are usually characteristic. Echocardiography◆ is the best way to confirm the diagnosis. Electrocardiography (ECG)▼ and a chest x-ray are also helpful. Cardiac catheterization,► an invasive procedure, is performed to measure pressures in the heart chambers only if surgery is being considered.

Prognosis and Treatment

About 4% of people with hypertrophic cardiomyopathy die each year. Death is usually sudden, presumably due to an abnormal heart rhythm. Death due to chronic heart failure is less common. People who learn that they have

---

▲ see table on page 166

■ see table on page 156   ★ see page 1079

● see page 184   ◆ see page 125

▼ see page 122   ► see page 128

inherited this disorder may wish to obtain genetic counseling when they plan a family.

If acromegaly is the cause, octreotide, a synthetic hormone, may be given to block the production of growth hormone. If a pheochromocytoma is the cause, an alpha- or beta-blocker▲ may be given to block the effects of epinephrine. Alternatively, the tumor that is producing the hormone may be removed surgically or destroyed by radiation therapy.

Treatment of hypertrophic cardiomyopathy is aimed primarily at reducing the heart's resistance to filling with blood between heartbeats. Beta-blockers and calcium channel blockers—taken separately or together—are the main treatment. Both reduce the extent to which heart muscle contracts, so that the heart contracts less forcefully. As a result, the heart can fill better and, if the thickened muscle was blocking blood flow, blood can flow out of the heart more easily. Also, beta-blockers and some calcium channel blockers slow the heart rate, so that the heart has more time to fill. Sometimes disopyramide, a drug that decreases the strength of heart contractions, is also used.

Surgery to remove some of the thickened heart muscle (myectomy) can improve the flow of blood from the heart, but it is performed only when symptoms are incapacitating despite drug therapy. Surgery can relieve symptoms, but it does not reduce the risk of death.

Before a dental or surgical procedure,■ antibiotics are usually given to reduce the risk of infective endocarditis.

Restrictive Cardiomyopathy

Restrictive (infiltrative) cardiomyopathy includes a group of heart disorders in which the walls of the ventricles become stiff, but not necessarily thickened, and resist normal filling with blood between heartbeats.

The least common form of cardiomyopathy, restrictive cardiomyopathy, shares many features with hypertrophic cardiomyopathy. Its cause is usually unknown.

There are two basic types of restrictive cardiomyopathy. In one type, the heart muscle is

gradually replaced by scar tissue. Scarring may result from injury due to radiation therapy for cancer. In the other type, abnormal substances accumulate in or infiltrate the heart muscle. For example, if the body contains too much iron, iron may accumulate in the heart muscle, as it does in people who have iron overload (hemochromatosis★). Amyloid, an unusual protein not normally present in the body, may accumulate in heart muscle and other tissues, causing amyloidosis●. Amyloidosis is more common among older people. Other examples are tumors and granuloma tissue (abnormal collections of certain white blood cells that form in response to chronic inflammation), which, for example, develops in people who have sarcoidosis.◆

Symptoms and Diagnosis

Restrictive cardiomyopathy causes heart failure▼ with shortness of breath and fluid accumulation in tissues (edema). Chest pain and fainting (syncope) are less likely than in hypertrophic cardiomyopathy, but abnormal heart rhythms (arrhythmias) and awareness of heartbeats (palpitations) are common. Usually, symptoms do not occur during rest, because in restrictive cardiomyopathy, the heart can supply the body with enough blood and oxygen during rest, even though the stiff heart resists filling with blood. Symptoms occur during exercise, when the stiff heart cannot pump enough blood to meet the body's increased need for blood and oxygen.

Restrictive cardiomyopathy is one of the possible causes investigated when a person has heart failure. The diagnosis is based largely on the results of a physical examination, electrocardiography (ECG), and echocardiography. ECG can typically detect abnormalities in the heart's electrical activity, but they are not specific enough for a diagnosis. Echocardiography shows that the atria are enlarged and that the heart is functioning normally only when the heart contracts (during systole). Magnetic resonance imaging (MRI) can detect abnormal texture in heart muscle due to accumulation of or infiltration with abnormal substances, such as iron and amyloid. A precise diagnosis usually requires cardiac catheterization to measure pressures in the heart chambers and removal of a sample of heart muscle for examination under a microscope (biopsy), which may enable doctors to identify the infiltrating substance.

▲ see table on page 138

■ see box on page 187   ★ see box on page 909

● see page 1715   ◆ see page 304

▼ see page 150

Prognosis and Treatment

About 70% of people with restrictive cardiomyopathy die within 5 years of when symptoms begin. For most people, treatment is not very helpful. For example, diuretics, which are usually taken to treat heart failure, may reduce the amount of blood entering the heart, worsening the disorder instead of improving it. Drugs commonly used in heart failure to reduce the heart's workload, such as ACE inhibitors, are usually not helpful because they reduce blood pressure too much. As a result, not enough blood reaches the rest of the body. Similarly, digoxin is usually not helpful and is sometimes harmful.

Sometimes, the disorder causing restrictive cardiomyopathy can be treated to prevent heart damage from worsening or even to partially reverse it. For example, removing blood at regular intervals reduces the amount of stored iron in people with iron overload. People who have sarcoidosis may take corticosteroids, which cause the granuloma tissue to disappear.

CHAPTER 27

Abnormal Heart Rhythms

Abnormal heart rhythms (arrhythmias) are sequences of heartbeats that are irregular, too fast, too slow, or conducted via an abnormal electrical pathway through the heart.

The heart is a muscular organ with four chambers designed to work efficiently, reliably, and continuously over a lifetime. The muscular walls of each chamber contract in a regulated sequence, pumping blood as required by the body while expending as little energy as possible during each heartbeat.

Contraction of the muscle fibers in the heart is controlled by electricity that flows through the heart in a precise manner along distinct pathways and at a controlled speed. The electrical current that begins each heartbeat originates in the heart's pacemaker (sinus or sinoatrial node), located in the top of the upper right heart chamber (right atrium). The rate at which the pacemaker discharges the electrical current determines the heart rate. This rate is influenced by nerve impulses and by levels of certain hormones in the bloodstream.

The heart rate is regulated automatically by the autonomic nervous system,▲ which consists of the sympathetic and parasympathetic divisions. The sympathetic division increases the heart rate through a network of nerves called the sympathetic plexus. The parasympathetic division decreases the heart rate through a single nerve, the vagus nerve.

Heart rate is also influenced by hormones released into the bloodstream by the sympathetic division: epinephrine (adrenaline) and norepinephrine (noradrenaline), which increase the heart rate. Thyroid hormone, which is released into the bloodstream by the thyroid gland, also increases the heart rate.

In an adult at rest, the normal heart rate is usually between 60 and 100 beats per minute. However, lower rates may be normal in young adults, particularly those who are physically fit. A person's heart rate varies normally in response to exercise and such stimuli as pain and anger. Heart rhythm is considered abnormal only when the heart rate is inappropriately fast (called tachycardia) or slow (called bradycardia), or is irregular or when electrical impulses travel along abnormal pathways.

Normal Electrical Pathway

The electrical current from the pacemaker flows first through the right atrium and then through the left atrium, causing the muscles of these chambers to contract and blood to be pumped from the atria into the lower heart chambers (ventricles). The electrical current then reaches the atrioventricular node, located in the lower part of the wall between the atria near the ventricles. The atrioventricular node provides the only electrical connection

▲ see page 437

Tracing the Heart's Electrical Pathway

The sinoatrial node (1) initiates an electrical impulse that flows through the right and left atria (2), making them contract. When the electrical impulse reaches the atrioventricular node (3), it is delayed slightly. The impulse then travels down the bundle of His (4), which divides into the right bundle branch for the right ventricle (5) and the left bundle branch for the left ventricle (5). The impulse then spreads through the ventricles, making them contract.

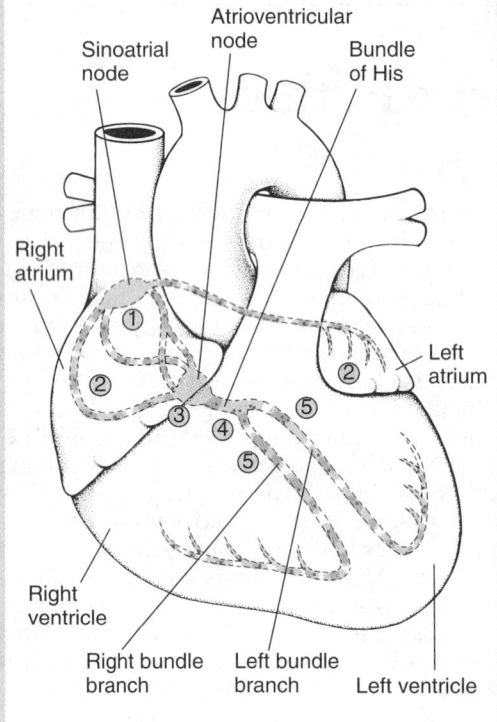

Sinoatrial node

Atrioventricular node

Bundle of His

Right atrium

Left atrium

Right ventricle

Right bundle branch

Left bundle branch

Left ventricle

between the atria and ventricles; otherwise, the atria are insulated from the ventricles by tissue that does not conduct electricity. The atrioventricular node delays transmission of the electrical current so that the atria can contract completely and the ventricles can fill with as much blood as possible before the ventricles are electrically signaled to contract.

After passing through the atrioventricular node, the electrical current travels down the bundle of His, a group of fibers that divide into a left bundle branch for the left ventricle and a right bundle branch for the right ventricle. The electrical current then spreads in a regulated manner over the surface of the ventricles, from the bottom up, initiating contraction of the ventricles, which ejects blood from the heart.

Causes

The most common cause of arrhythmias is heart disease, particularly coronary artery disease, heart valve disorders, and heart failure. Many drugs, prescription or nonprescription, can lead to arrhythmias. Some arrhythmias are caused by anatomic abnormalities present at birth (congenital birth defects). Age-related changes in the heart's electrical system make some arrhythmias more likely. An overactive thyroid gland (hyperthyroidism), producing high levels of thyroid hormone, may cause fast arrhythmias. An underactive thyroid gland (hypothyroidism), producing low levels of thyroid hormone, may cause slow arrhythmias. Sometimes no cause for an arrhythmia can be identified.

Fast arrhythmias (tachyarrhythmias) may be triggered by exercise, emotional stress, excessive alcohol consumption, smoking, or use of drugs that contain stimulants, such as cold and hay fever remedies. Slow arrhythmias (bradyarrhythmias) may be triggered by pain, hunger, fatigue, digestive disorders (such as diarrhea and vomiting), or swallowing, which can stimulate the vagus nerve excessively. (With enough stimulation, which is rare, the vagus nerve can cause the heart to stop.) In most of these circumstances, the arrhythmia tends to resolve on its own.

Symptoms

Some people who have abnormal heartbeats may be aware of them. However, awareness of heartbeats (called palpitations) varies widely among people. Some people can feel normal heartbeats, and most people can feel heartbeats when they lie on their left side.

Arrhythmias have consequences that range from harmless to life threatening. The seriousness of an arrhythmia may not be closely linked with the severity of the symptoms it causes. Some life-threatening arrhythmias cause no symptoms, and some otherwise inconsequential arrhythmias cause severe symptoms. Often, the nature and severity of the underlying heart disease are more important than the arrhythmia itself.

When arrhythmias impair the heart's ability to pump blood, they can produce weakness, a reduced capacity for exercise, light-headedness, dizziness, and fainting (syncope).▲ Fainting occurs when the heart is pumping so inefficiently that it can no longer maintain adequate blood pressure. If such an arrhythmia persists, death may result. Arrhythmias may also aggravate the symptoms of underlying heart disease, including chest pain and shortness of breath. Arrhythmias that produce symptoms require prompt attention.

Diagnosis

Often, a person's description of symptoms can help doctors make a preliminary diagnosis and determine the severity of the arrhythmia. The most important considerations are whether the palpitations are fast or slow, regular or irregular, or brief or prolonged and whether the arrhythmia produces symptoms. Doctors also need to know whether the palpitations occur at rest or only during strenuous or unusual activity and whether they start and stop suddenly or gradually. However, certain diagnostic procedures are often needed to determine the exact nature of the arrhythmia and its cause.

Electrocardiography (ECG)■ is the main diagnostic procedure for detecting arrhythmias and determining their cause. This procedure provides a graphic representation of the electrical current producing each heartbeat. Usually, ECG records the heart rhythm for only a very short time. Because arrhythmias are often intermittent, a portable ECG monitor (Holter monitor)★ may be used to record heart rhythm continuously or when the wearer senses an abnormal heart rhythm and activates the monitor. This monitor, usually worn for 24 hours, can record sporadic arrhythmias as the person engages in normal daily activities. During the 24-hour period, the person also keeps a diary of symptoms and activities, which are correlated with the arrhythmias.

People with suspected life-threatening arrhythmias are usually hospitalized. Their heart rhythm is continuously recorded and displayed on a television-type monitor by the bedside or nursing station. Thus, any problems can be identified promptly.

Other diagnostic procedures include exercise stress testing (ECG and blood pressure measurement during exercise)● and electrophysiologic testing.◆ During electrophysiologic testing, catheters with tiny electrodes at their tip are inserted through a vein and threaded into the heart. The electrodes are used to stimulate the heart, and the heart's response is monitored, so that the type of arrhythmia and the preferred treatment options can be determined.

Prognosis and Treatment

Most arrhythmias neither cause symptoms nor interfere with the heart's ability to pump blood. Thus, they usually pose little or no risk, although they can cause considerable anxiety if a person becomes aware of them. However, some arrhythmias, harmless in themselves, can lead to more serious arrhythmias. Any arrhythmia that impairs the heart's ability to pump blood adequately is serious. How serious depends in part on whether the arrhythmia originates in the heart's normal pacemaker, in the atria, or in the ventricles. Generally, arrhythmias that originate in the ventricles are more serious than those that originate in the atria, which are more serious than those that originate in the pacemaker. However, there are many exceptions.

For people who have a harmless yet worrisome arrhythmia, reassurance that the arrhythmia is harmless may be treatment enough. Sometimes arrhythmias occur less often or even stop when doctors change a person's drugs or adjust the dosages. Avoiding alcohol, caffeine (in beverages and foods), smoking, or strenuous exercise may also help.

Antiarrhythmic drugs are useful for suppressing fast arrhythmias that cause intolerable symptoms or pose a risk. No single drug cures all arrhythmias in all people. Sometimes several drugs must be tried until the response is satisfactory. Sometimes antiarrhythmic drugs can worsen or even cause arrhythmias; this effect is called proarrhythmia. Antiarrhythmic drugs also produce other side effects.

Artificial pacemakers are electronic devices that act in place of the heart's own pacemaker. These devices are implanted surgically under the skin, usually below the left or right collarbone. They are connected to the heart by wires running inside a vein. Because of new low-energy circuitry and battery designs, these units now last about 10 to 15 years. New

---

▲ see page 143   ■ see page 122
★ see art on page 124   ● see page 123
◆ see page 124

℞ SOME DRUGS USED TO TREAT ARRHYTHMIAS

TYPE	EXAMPLES	SELECTED SIDE EFFECTS	COMMENTS
Sodium channel blockers	Disopyramide Flecainide Lidocaine Mexiletine Moricizine Phenytoin Procainamide Propafenone Quinidine Tocainide	Arrhythmias (which can be fatal, particularly in people who have heart disease), digestive upset, dizziness, light-headedness, tremor, retention of urine, increased intraocular pressure in people who have glaucoma, and dry mouth	These drugs slow the conduction of electrical impulses through the heart. These drugs are used to treat ventricular premature beats, ventricular tachycardia, and ventricular fibrillation and to convert atrial fibrillation to normal rhythm (cardioversion).
Beta-blockers	Atenolol Metoprolol Nadolol Propranolol	An abnormally slow heart rate (bradycardia); heart failure; spasm of the airways (bronchospasm); possible masking of low blood sugar levels; impaired circulation in the trunk, arms and legs; insomnia; shortness of breath; depression; Raynaud's phenomenon; hallucinations; sexual dysfunction; fatigue; and, with some beta-blockers, an increase in the triglyceride level	These drugs are used to treat ventricular premature beats, ventricular tachycardia, ventricular fibrillation, and paroxysmal supraventricular tachycardia. They are also used to slow the ventricular rate in people with atrial fibrillation or atrial flutter. People who have asthma should not take these drugs.
Potassium channel blockers	Amiodarone Bretylium Ibutilide Sotalol	Arrhythmias, scarring in the lungs (pulmonary fibrosis), and low blood pressure For sotalol, which is also a beta-blocker, see above	These drugs are used to treat ventricular premature beats, ventricular tachycardia, ventricular fibrillation, atrial fibrillation, and atrial flutter. Because amiodarone can be toxic, it is used for long-term treatment only in some people who have serious arrhythmias. Bretylium is used only for short-term treatment of life-threatening ventricular tachycardias.
Calcium channel blockers	Diltiazem Verapamil	Constipation, diarrhea, low blood pressure, and swollen feet	Only certain calcium channel blockers, such as diltiazem and verapamil, are useful. They are used to slow the ventricular rate in people who have atrial fibrillation or atrial flutter and to treat paroxysmal supraventricular tachycardia. Diltiazem and verapamil slow the conduction of electrical impulses through the atrioventricular node. Certain people with Wolff-Parkinson-White syndrome should not take verapamil or diltiazem.

R_x SOME DRUGS USED TO TREAT ARRHYTHMIAS (Continued)

TYPE	EXAMPLES	SELECTED SIDE EFFECTS	COMMENTS
Digoxin			
		Rarely, weight loss, nausea, vomiting, and serious arrhythmias; if the dose is too high, xanthopsia (a condition in which objects appear greenish yellow)	Digoxin slows conduction of electrical impulses through the atrioventricular node. Digoxin is used to decrease the ventricular rate in people who have atrial fibrillation or atrial flutter and to treat paroxysmal supraventricular tachycardia. The drug is given to infants and children younger than 10 years who have Wolff-Parkinson-White syndrome, but older people with the syndrome should not take digoxin.
Purine nucleoside			
	Adenosine	Spasm of the airways (bronchospasm) and flushing (for a short time)	Adenosine slows conduction of electrical impulses through the atrioventricular node. Adenosine is used to end episodes of paroxysmal supraventricular tachycardia. People who have asthma are not given this drug.

circuitry has almost completely eliminated the risk of interference from automobile distributors, radar, microwaves, and airport security detectors. However, some equipment may interfere with pacemakers. Examples are machines used in magnetic resonance imaging (MRI) and in diathermy (physical therapy in which heat is applied to muscles).

The most common use of pacemakers is to treat slow arrhythmias. When the heart slows below a set threshold, the artificial pacemaker begins to fire off electrical impulses. Less commonly, pacemakers are used to treat fast arrhythmias by delivering a series of impulses to decrease the heart rate.

Sometimes an electrical shock to the heart can stop a fast arrhythmia and restore normal rhythm. Using an electrical shock for this purpose is called cardioversion, defibrillation, or electroversion. Cardioversion may be used for arrhythmias starting in the atria or the ventricles. The machine that delivers the shock (a defibrillator) is used by a team of doctors and nurses, by paramedics, or by firefighters. Also, an implantable defibrillator, which is about one half the size of a deck of cards, can be sur-

gically implanted just as a pacemaker is. The implantable defibrillator automatically senses fast arrhythmias and delivers a shock to convert the arrhythmia back to a normal rhythm. Most commonly, these devices are used in people who would otherwise die of the arrhythmia. Because implantable defibrillators do not prevent arrhythmias, drugs often must be taken as well.

A new type of defibrillator, called an automated external defibrillator (AED), requires only minimal training for its use. For example, AEDs can be used by people who receive first-aid instruction in its use.▲ AEDs can detect the presence of an arrhythmia, determine if a shock is advisable, and deliver the shock automatically. They are being placed in many public places, such as airports, sports arenas, hotels, and shopping malls.

Certain types of arrhythmias can be controlled by performing surgical and other invasive procedures. For example, performing angioplasty or coronary artery bypass surgery■

▲ see box on page 1689 ■ see pages 208 and 209

Keeping the Beat: Artificial Pacemakers

Artificial pacemakers are electronic devices that act in place of the heart's natural pacemaker (the sinus or sinoatrial node); that is, they generate electrical impulses that initiate each heartbeat. Pacemakers consist of a battery, an impulse generator, and wires that connect the pacemaker to the heart.

An artificial pacemaker is implanted surgically. After a local anesthetic is used to numb the insertion site, the wires that connect the pacemaker are usually inserted into a vein near the collarbone and threaded toward the heart. Through a small incision, the impulse generator, which is about the size of a silver dollar, is inserted just under the skin near the collarbone and connected to the wires. The incision is stitched closed. Usually, the procedure takes about 30 to 60 minutes. The person may be able to go home shortly afterward or may stay in the hospital for a few days. The battery for a pacemaker usually lasts 10 to 15 years. Nevertheless, the battery should be checked regularly. Battery replacement is a quick procedure.

There are different types of pacemakers. Some take over the control of the heart rate, overriding the electrical impulses generated by the heart. Others, called demand pacemakers, allow the heart to beat naturally unless it skips a beat or begins to beat at an abnormal rate. Still others, called programmable pacemakers, can do either. Some pacemakers can adjust their rate depending on the wearer's activity, increasing the heart rate during exercise and decreasing it during rest.

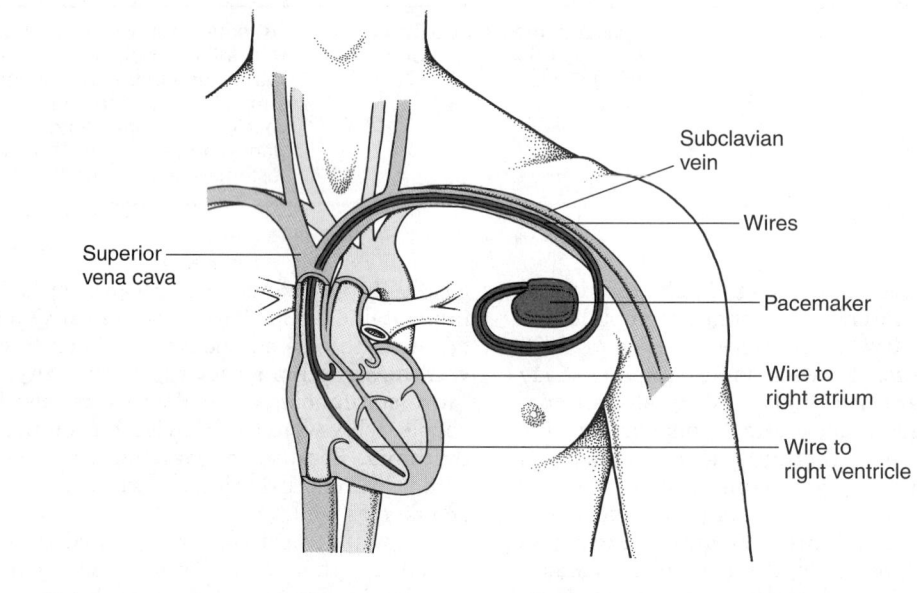

Superior vena cava

Subclavian vein

Wires

Pacemaker

Wire to right atrium

Wire to right ventricle

may control arrhythmias due to coronary artery disease. An arrhythmia due to a localized abnormal area in the heart's electrical system can be controlled by destroying or removing that area. Most often, the abnormal area is destroyed by radiofrequency ablation (delivery of energy of a specific frequency through an electrode catheter inserted in the heart). This procedure is successful in 90 to 95% of people, takes 2 to 4 hours, and requires only 1 to 2 days in the hospital. Less commonly, the area is destroyed or removed during open-heart surgery.

Atrial Premature Beats

An atrial premature beat (atrial ectopic beat, premature atrial contraction) is an extra heartbeat caused by electrical activation of the atria from an abnormal site before a normal heartbeat would occur.

Atrial premature beats occur in many healthy people and rarely cause symptoms. Atrial premature beats are common among people who have lung disorders and are more common among older people than among younger people. These beats may be caused or worsened by consuming coffee, tea, or alcohol and by using some cold, hay fever, and asthma remedies.

Diagnosis and Treatment

Atrial premature beats may be detected during a physical examination and are confirmed by electrocardiography (ECG). Rarely, when these beats occur frequently and cause intolerable palpitations, treatment is necessary. Antiarrhythmic drugs are usually effective.

Atrial Fibrillation and Atrial Flutter

Atrial fibrillation and atrial flutter are very fast electrical discharge patterns that make the atria contract very rapidly, with some of the electrical impulses reaching the ventricles and causing them to contract faster and less efficiently than normal.

Atrial fibrillation and atrial flutter are more common among older people.

Atrial fibrillation and atrial flutter may be intermittent or sustained. During atrial fibrillation or flutter, the contractions of the atria are so fast that the atrial walls quiver. As a result, blood is not pumped effectively to the ventricles. During atrial fibrillation, the atrial rhythm is irregular, so the ventricular rhythm is also irregular. During atrial flutter, the atrial rhythm is regular, and the ventricular rhythm may be regular or irregular. In both cases, the ventricles beat more slowly than the atria because the atrioventricular node cannot conduct electrical impulses at such a fast rate. As a result, only some impulses get through. Even though the ventricles beat more slowly than the atria, the ventricles often still beat too fast to fill completely. Therefore, the heart pumps inefficiently, blood pressure may fall, and heart failure may occur.

In atrial fibrillation or flutter, the atria do not empty completely into the ventricles with each beat. Over time, some blood inside the atria may stagnate, and clots may form. Pieces of the clot may break off, often shortly after atrial fibrillation converts back to normal rhythm—whether spontaneously or because of treatment. These pieces may pass into the left ventricle, travel through the bloodstream

(becoming emboli), and block a smaller artery. If pieces of a clot block an artery in the brain, a stroke results. Rarely, a stroke is the first sign of atrial fibrillation or flutter.

Atrial fibrillation or flutter may occur even when there is no other sign of heart disease. However, more often, these arrhythmias are caused by such conditions as rheumatic fever, high blood pressure, coronary artery disease, alcohol abuse, an overactive thyroid gland (hyperthyroidism), or a birth defect of the heart. Rheumatic fever (which leads to heart valve disorders) and high blood pressure cause the atria to enlarge, making atrial fibrillation or flutter more likely.

Symptoms and Diagnosis

Symptoms of atrial fibrillation or flutter depend largely on how fast the ventricles beat. A modest increase in the ventricular rate—to less than about 120 beats per minute—may produce no symptoms. Higher rates cause unpleasant palpitations or chest discomfort.

In people with atrial fibrillation, the pulse is irregular and usually fast. In people with atrial flutter, the pulse is more likely to be regular and fast.

The reduced pumping ability of the heart may cause weakness, faintness, and shortness of breath. Some people, especially older people, develop heart failure or chest pain. Very rarely, shock (very low blood pressure)▲ occurs in people who have atrial fibrillation or flutter and very severe heart disease.

Symptoms suggest the diagnosis of atrial fibrillation or flutter, and electrocardiography (ECG) confirms it.

Treatment

Treatment of atrial fibrillation or flutter is designed to control the rate at which the ventricles contract, to restore the normal rhythm of the heart, and to treat the disorder causing the arrhythmia. Drugs to prevent the formation of clots and emboli (anticoagulants) may also be given.

Usually, the first step in treating atrial fibrillation or flutter is to slow the beating of the ventricles so that the heart pumps blood more efficiently. Often, the first drug tried is digoxin, which may slow the conduction of impulses to the ventricles. However, digoxin is often insufficient and another drug may be required. A beta-blocker, such as propranolol

▲ see page 148

or atenolol, or a calcium channel blocker, such as verapamil or diltiazem, may be used.

Atrial fibrillation or flutter may spontaneously convert to a normal rhythm. However, these arrhythmias must often be actively converted to normal. Certain antiarrhythmic drugs (most commonly, amiodarone, propafenone, or sotalol) may be effective, but cardioversion, or defibrillation (delivery of an electrical shock to the heart), is the most effective approach. Conversion to a normal rhythm by any means becomes less likely the longer the arrhythmia has been present (especially after 6 months or more), the larger the atria become, and the more severe the underlying heart disease becomes. When conversion is successful, the risk of recurrence is high, even if people are taking a drug to prevent recurrence (that is, one of the drugs used to convert the arrhythmia to a normal rhythm).

Rarely, when all other treatments of atrial fibrillation are ineffective, parts of the atrioventricular node can be destroyed by radiofrequency ablation (delivery of energy of a specific frequency through an electrode catheter inserted in the heart). This procedure slows the ventricular rate in some people who have atrial fibrillation or flutter. If this procedure is not successful, radiofrequency ablation is used to destroy the entire atrioventricular node, completely stopping conduction from the atria to the ventricles. In such cases, a permanent artificial pacemaker is required to activate the ventricles afterward. For people who have atrial flutter, radiofrequency ablation may be used to interrupt the flutter circuit and permanently re-establish normal rhythm. This procedure is successful in about 85% of people.

Usually, treatment of the underlying disorder does not alleviate atrial arrhythmias. However, treatment of an overactive thyroid gland or surgery to correct a heart valve disorder or a birth defect of the heart may help.

When atrial fibrillation or flutter is converted back to normal rhythm, the risk that a clot will be dislodged and cause a stroke is particularly high. Most people with atrial fibrillation or flutter and one or more risk factors for developing clots are given an anticoagulant to prevent clots, because they are at risk of a stroke. (Risk factors for developing blood clots include advancing age, high blood pressure, diabetes, an enlarged left atrium, and structural heart disease, especially mitral valve disorders.)▲ Unless conversion to a normal rhythm is needed immediately, doctors recommend that most people take an anticoagulant for 4 weeks before cardioversion of established atrial fibrillation or flutter is attempted. However, sometimes there is a specific reason not to use an anticoagulant. For example, people who have uncontrolled high blood pressure or a bleeding disorder should not be given anticoagulants. Anticoagulant therapy can cause bleeding, which can lead to hemorrhagic stroke and other bleeding complications, such as excessive bleeding after surgery. Therefore, doctors balance the potential benefits and risks for each person.

Paroxysmal Supraventricular Tachycardia

Paroxysmal supraventricular (atrial) tachycardia is a regular, fast (160 to 200 beats per minute) heart rate that begins and ends suddenly and originates in heart tissue other than that in the ventricles.

Paroxysmal supraventricular tachycardia is most common among young people and is more unpleasant than dangerous. It may occur during vigorous exercise.

Paroxysmal supraventricular tachycardia may be triggered by a premature heartbeat that repeatedly activates the heart at a fast rate. This repeated, rapid activation may be caused by several abnormalities. There may be two electrical pathways in the atrioventricular node (an arrhythmia called atrioventricular nodal reentrant supraventricular tachycardia). There may be an abnormal electrical pathway between the atria and the ventricles (an arrhythmia called atrioventricular reciprocating supraventricular tachycardia). Much less commonly, the atria may generate abnormal rapid or circling impulses (an arrhythmia called true paroxysmal atrial tachycardia).

The fast heart rate tends to begin and end suddenly and may last from a few minutes to many hours. It is almost always experienced as an uncomfortable palpitation. It is often associated with other symptoms, such as weakness, light-headedness, shortness of breath, and chest pain. Usually, the heart is otherwise normal.

Treatment

Episodes of paroxysmal supraventricular tachycardia often can be stopped by one of

---

▲ see page 175

several maneuvers that stimulate the vagus nerve and thus decrease the heart rate. These maneuvers are usually conducted or supervised by a doctor, but people who repeatedly experience the arrhythmia often learn to perform the maneuvers themselves. Maneuvers include straining as if having a difficult bowel movement, rubbing the neck just below the angle of the jaw (which stimulates a sensitive area on the carotid artery called the carotid sinus), and plunging the face into a bowl of ice-cold water. These maneuvers are most effective when they are used shortly after the arrhythmia starts.

If these maneuvers are not effective, if the arrhythmia produces severe symptoms, or if the episode lasts more than 20 minutes, people are advised to seek medical intervention to stop the episode. Doctors can usually stop an episode promptly by giving an intravenous injection of a drug, usually adenosine or verapamil. Rarely, drugs are ineffective, and cardioversion (delivery of an electrical shock to the heart) may be necessary.

Prevention is more difficult than treatment, but almost any antiarrhythmic drug may be effective. Drugs commonly used include beta-blockers, digoxin, diltiazem, verapamil, propafenone, and flecainide. Increasingly, radio-frequency ablation (delivery of energy of a specific frequency through an electrode catheter inserted in the heart) is being used to destroy the tissue in which paroxysmal supraventricular tachycardia originates.

Wolff-Parkinson-White Syndrome

Wolff-Parkinson-White syndrome is a disorder in which an extra electrical connection between the atria and the ventricles is present at birth.

Wolff-Parkinson-White syndrome is the most common of several disorders that involve an extra (accessory) pathway between the atria and the ventricles. (Such disorders are called atrioventricular reciprocating supraventricular tachycardias.) This extra pathway makes fast arrhythmias more likely to occur. Wolff-Parkinson-White syndrome is present at birth, but the arrhythmias it causes usually become apparent during the teens or early twenties. However, arrhythmias may occur during the first year of life or after age 60.

Symptoms and Diagnosis

Wolff-Parkinson-White syndrome is a common cause of paroxysmal supraventricular tachycardia. Very rarely, this syndrome results in a very fast, life-threatening heart rate during atrial fibrillation.

When infants develop arrhythmias due to this syndrome, they may become short of breath or lethargic, stop eating well, or have rapid, visible pulsations of the chest. Heart failure may develop.

Typically, when teenagers or people in their early 20s first experience an arrhythmia due to this syndrome, it is an episode of paroxysmal supraventricular tachycardia that begins suddenly, often during exercise. It may last for only a few seconds or may persist for several hours. In a young and otherwise physically fit person, the episodes usually cause few symptoms. Nonetheless, a very fast heart rate is uncomfortable and distressing and can cause fainting.

When episodes of paroxysmal supraventricular tachycardia due to Wolff-Parkinson-White syndrome occur later in life, they tend to produce more symptoms, such as fainting, shortness of breath, and chest pain.

Atrial fibrillation may be particularly dangerous for people with Wolff-Parkinson-White syndrome. The extra pathway can conduct the rapid impulses to the ventricles at a much faster rate than the normal pathway (through the atrioventricular node) can. The result is an extremely fast ventricular rate that may be life threatening. Not only is the heart very inefficient when it beats so rapidly, but this extremely fast heart rate may also progress to ventricular fibrillation, which is fatal unless treated immediately.

Because Wolff-Parkinson-White syndrome changes the pattern of electrical activation in the heart, it can be diagnosed using electrocardiography (ECG),▲ which records the electrical activity of the heart.

Treatment

Episodes of paroxysmal supraventricular tachycardia due to Wolff-Parkinson-White syndrome can often be stopped by one of several maneuvers that stimulate the vagus nerve and thus slow the heart rate.■ The maneuvers are

---

▲ see page 122   ■ page 170

most effective when they are used shortly after the arrhythmia starts. When these maneuvers are ineffective, drugs such as verapamil or adenosine are usually given intravenously to stop the arrhythmia. Antiarrhythmic drugs may then be continued indefinitely to prevent episodes of a fast heart rate.

In infants and children younger than 10 years, digoxin may be given to suppress episodes of paroxysmal supraventricular tachycardia due to Wolff-Parkinson-White syndrome. However, adults with the syndrome should not take digoxin because it can facilitate conduction by the extra pathway and increase the risk that atrial fibrillation will degenerate into ventricular fibrillation. For this reason, digoxin is usually stopped before people with this syndrome reach puberty.

Destruction of the extra conduction pathway by radiofrequency ablation (delivery of energy of a specific frequency through an electrode catheter inserted in the heart) is successful in more than 95% of people. The risk of death during the procedure is less than 1 in 1,000. Radiofrequency ablation is particularly useful for young people who might otherwise have to take antiarrhythmic drugs for a lifetime.

Ventricular Premature Beats

A ventricular premature beat (ventricular ectopic beat, premature ventricular contraction) is an extra heartbeat resulting from abnormal electrical activation originating in the ventricles before a normal heartbeat would occur.

Ventricular premature beats are common, particularly among older people. This arrhythmia may be caused by physical or emotional stress, intake of caffeine (in beverages and foods) or alcohol, or use of cold or hay fever remedies containing drugs that stimulate the heart, such as pseudoephedrine. Other causes include coronary artery disease (especially during or shortly after a heart attack) and disorders that cause ventricles to enlarge, such as heart failure and heart valve disorders.

Symptoms and Diagnosis

Isolated ventricular premature beats have little effect on the pumping action of the heart and usually do not cause symptoms, unless they are extremely frequent. The main symptom is the perception of a strong or skipped

beat. Ventricular premature beats are not dangerous for people who do not have heart disease. However, when they occur frequently in people who have structural heart disease, they may be followed by more dangerous arrhythmias such as ventricular tachycardia or ventricular fibrillation, which can cause sudden death.

Electrocardiography (ECG)▲ is used to diagnose ventricular premature beats.

Treatment

In an otherwise healthy person, no treatment is needed other than decreasing stress and avoiding caffeine, alcohol, and over-the-counter cold or hay fever remedies containing drugs that stimulate the heart. Drug therapy is usually prescribed only if symptoms are intolerable or if the pattern of ventricular premature beats suggests a risk of progression to ventricular tachycardia or ventricular fibrillation. For example, the presence of structural heart disease or runs of consecutive ventricular beats suggest this risk. Beta-blockers are usually tried first because they are relatively safe drugs. However, some people do not want to take them because they can cause sluggishness.

After a heart attack, people who have frequent ventricular premature beats may reduce the risk of sudden death due to ventricular tachycardia or ventricular fibrillation by taking beta-blockers or undergoing angioplasty or coronary artery bypass surgery to treat coronary artery disease.■ Antiarrhythmic drugs can suppress ventricular premature beats, but they also may increase the risk of a fatal arrhythmia. Therefore, doctors prescribe them only for carefully selected people who have been evaluated for risk of developing serious arrhythmias.

Ventricular Tachycardia

Ventricular tachycardia is a heart rhythm that originates in the ventricles and produces a heart rate of at least 120 beats per minute.

Ventricular tachycardia may be thought of as a sequence of consecutive ventricular premature beats. Sometimes only a few such beats occur together, and then the heart returns to a normal rhythm. Ventricular tachycardia that lasts more than 30 seconds is called sustained ventricular tachycardia. Sustained ventricular tachycardia usually occurs in people with structural heart disease that damages the ventricles. Most commonly, it

---

▲ see page 122   ■ see pages 208 and 209

occurs weeks or months after a heart attack. It is more common among older people. However, rarely, ventricular tachycardia develops in young people who do not have structural heart disease.

Symptoms and Diagnosis

People with ventricular tachycardia almost always have palpitations. Sustained ventricular tachycardia can be dangerous because the ventricles cannot fill adequately or pump blood normally. Blood pressure tends to fall, and heart failure follows. Sustained ventricular tachycardia is also dangerous because it can worsen until it becomes ventricular fibrillation—a form of cardiac arrest. Sometimes ventricular tachycardia causes few symptoms, even at rates of up to 200 beats per minute, but it may still be extremely dangerous.

Electrocardiography (ECG)▲ is used to diagnose ventricular tachycardia and to help determine whether treatment is required. A portable ECG (Holter) monitor may be used to record heart rhythm over a 24-hour period.

Treatment

Ventricular tachycardia is treated when it causes symptoms or when episodes last more than 30 seconds even without causing symptoms. Sustained ventricular tachycardia often requires emergency treatment. If episodes cause blood pressure to fall to a low level, cardioversion is needed immediately. Drugs may be given intravenously to end or suppress ventricular tachycardia. The most commonly used drugs are lidocaine, procainamide, and amiodarone.

Certain procedures may be performed to destroy the small abnormal area in the ventricles, identified by ECG, that is usually responsible for sustained ventricular tachycardia. They include radiofrequency ablation (delivery of energy of a specific frequency through an electrode catheter inserted in the heart) and open-heart surgery.

If other therapy is ineffective, an automatic defibrillator (a small device that can detect an arrhythmia and deliver a shock to correct it) may be implanted. This procedure is similar to implantation of an artificial pacemaker.

Ventricular Fibrillation

Ventricular fibrillation is a potentially fatal, uncoordinated series of very rapid, ineffective contractions of the ventricles caused by many chaotic electrical impulses.

In ventricular fibrillation, the ventricles merely quiver and do not contract in a coordinated way. No blood is pumped from the heart, so ventricular fibrillation is a form of cardiac arrest. It is fatal unless treated immediately.

The most common cause of ventricular fibrillation is inadequate blood flow to the heart muscle due to coronary artery disease, as occurs during a heart attack. Other causes include shock (very low blood pressure),■ which can result from coronary artery disease and other disorders; electrical shock; drowning; very low levels of potassium in the blood (hypokalemia); and drugs that affect electrical currents in the heart (such as sodium or potassium channel blockers).★

Symptoms and Diagnosis

Ventricular fibrillation causes unconsciousness in seconds. If untreated, the person usually has seizures and develops irreversible brain damage after about 5 minutes because oxygen no longer reaches the brain. Death soon follows.

Cardiac arrest is diagnosed when a person suddenly collapses, turns deadly white, has very dilated pupils, and has no detectable pulse, heartbeat, or blood pressure. Ventricular fibrillation is diagnosed as the cause of the cardiac arrest by electrocardiography (ECG).

Treatment

Ventricular fibrillation must be treated as an extreme emergency. Cardiopulmonary resuscitation (CPR) must be started as soon as possible—within a few minutes. It must be followed by cardioversion, or defibrillation (an electrical shock delivered to the chest), as soon as the defibrillator is available. Antiarrhythmic drugs may then be given to help maintain the normal heart rhythm.

When ventricular fibrillation occurs within a few hours of a heart attack in people who are not in shock and who do not have heart failure, prompt cardioversion restores normal rhythm in 95% of people, and the prognosis is good. Shock and heart failure suggest major damage to the ventricles. If they are present, even prompt cardioversion has only a 30% success rate, and 70% of resuscitated survivors die without regaining normal function.

People who are successfully resuscitated from ventricular fibrillation and survive are at

---

▲ see page 122   ■ see page 148

★ see table on page 166

high risk of another episode. If ventricular fibrillation is caused by a reversible disorder, that disorder is treated. Otherwise, drugs are given to prevent recurrences, or a defibrillator is surgically implanted to correct the problem, if it recurs, by delivering a shock.

Pacemaker Dysfunction

Dysfunction of the heart's pacemaker (sinus or sinoatrial node) may result in a persistently slow heartbeat (sinus bradycardia) or complete cessation of normal pacemaker activity (sinus arrest). When activity ceases, another area of the heart usually takes over the function of the pacemaker. This area, called an escape pacemaker, may be located lower in the atrium, in the atrioventricular node, in the conduction system, or even in the ventricle.

All types of pacemaker dysfunction are more common among older people. Some drugs and an underactive thyroid gland (hypothyroidism) can cause pacemaker dysfunction. However, the cause is usually unknown. When the cause is unknown, the disorder is called **sick sinus syndrome.**

An important subtype of the sick sinus syndrome is the bradycardia-tachycardia syndrome, in which periods of slow heart rhythms (bradycardia) alternate with periods of fast atrial arrhythmias (tachycardia), such as atrial fibrillation and atrial flutter.

Symptoms and Diagnosis

Many types of pacemaker dysfunction cause no symptoms. A persistent slow heart rate commonly causes weakness and tiredness. Fainting may occur if the rate becomes very slow. A fast heart rate is often perceived by the person as palpitations. When the fast heart rate stops, fainting may occur if the pacemaker is slow in restarting normal heart rhythm.

A slow pulse (especially an irregular one), a pulse that varies greatly without any change in the person's activity, or a pulse that does not increase during exercise suggests pacemaker dysfunction. Doctors can usually diagnose pacemaker dysfunction based on symptoms and the results of electrocardiography (ECG),▲ particularly when heart rhythm is recorded over a 24-hour period with a Holter monitor.

Treatment

People with symptoms are usually given a permanent artificial pacemaker to accelerate the heart rate. If they also sometimes have a fast rate, they may also need drugs to slow the heart rate (such as a beta-blocker or a calcium channel blocker).■

Heart Block

Heart block is a delay in the conduction of electrical current as it passes through the atrioventricular node, bundle of His, or both bundle branches, all of which are located between the atria and the ventricles.

Heart block is classified as first-degree when electrical conduction to the ventricles is slightly delayed, second-degree when conduction is intermittently blocked, or third-degree (complete) when conduction is completely blocked. Most types of heart block are more common among older people.

In first-degree heart block, every electrical impulse from the atria reaches the ventricles, but each is slowed for a fraction of a second as it moves through the atrioventricular node. First-degree heart block is common among well-trained athletes, teenagers, young adults, and people with a highly active vagus nerve. However, the disorder also occurs in people with rheumatic fever, sarcoidosis that affects the heart,★ or other structural heart diseases. It may be caused by drugs, particularly those that slow conduction of electrical impulses through the atrioventricular node (such as beta-blockers, diltiazem, verapamil, and amiodarone). This disorder produces no symptoms and can be detected only by electrocardiography (ECG), which shows the conduction delay.

In second-degree heart block, only some electrical impulses reach the ventricles. The heart may beat slowly, irregularly, or both. Some forms of second-degree heart block progress to third-degree heart block.

In third-degree heart block, no impulses from the atria reach the ventricles, and the ventricular rate and rhythm are controlled by the atrioventricular node, bundle of His, or the ventricles themselves. These substitute pacemakers are slower than the heart's normal pacemaker (sinus or sinoatrial node) and are often irregular and unreliable. Thus, the ventricles beat very slowly—less than 50 beats per minute and sometimes as slowly as 30 beats per minute. Third-degree heart block is a seri-

---

▲ see page 122   ■ see table on page 138
★ see page 304

ous arrhythmia that can affect the heart's pumping ability. Fatigue, dizziness, and fainting are common. When the ventricles beat faster than 40 beats per minute, symptoms are less severe.

Treatment

First-degree heart block requires no treatment even when it is caused by heart disease. Some people with second-degree heart block require an artificial pacemaker. Almost all people with third-degree heart block require an artificial pacemaker. A temporary pacemaker may be used in an emergency until a permanent one can be implanted. Most people need an artificial pacemaker for the rest of their lives, although heart rhythm may return to normal if the cause of the heart block resolves—for example, after recovery from a heart attack.

Bundle Branch Block

Bundle branch block is a type of conduction block involving partial or complete interruption of the flow of electrical impulses through the right or left bundle branches.

The bundle of His is a group of fibers that conducts electrical impulses from the atrioventricular node. The bundle of His divides into two bundle branches.▲ The left bundle branch conducts impulses to the left ventricle, and the right bundle branch conducts impulses to the right ventricle. Conduction may be blocked in the left or right bundle branch.

Bundle branch block usually causes no symptoms. Right bundle branch block is not serious in itself and may occur in apparently healthy people. However, it may also indicate significant heart damage due to, for example, a previous heart attack. Left bundle branch block tends to be more serious. In older people, it often indicates heart disease due to high blood pressure or atherosclerosis.

Bundle branch block can be detected by electrocardiography (ECG).■ Each type of block produces a characteristic pattern. Usually, no treatment is needed for either type. However, an artificial pacemaker★ may be implanted in people who are at high risk of complete heart block (such as people with second-degree heart block) to maintain the heart rate if complete heart block occurs.

CHAPTER 28

Heart Valve Disorders

Heart valves regulate the flow of blood through the heart's four chambers—two small, round upper chambers (atria) and two larger, cone-shaped lower chambers (ventricles).● Each ventricle has a one-way "in" (inlet) valve and a one-way "out" (outlet) valve. In the right ventricle, the inlet valve is the tricuspid valve, which opens from the right atrium, and the outlet valve is the pulmonary (pulmonic) valve, which opens into the pulmonary arteries. In the left ventricle, the inlet valve is the mitral valve, which opens from the left atrium, and the outlet valve is the aortic valve, which opens into the aorta. Each valve consists of flaps (cusps or leaflets), which open and close like one-way swinging doors.

The heart valves can malfunction either by leaking (causing regurgitation) or by not opening adequately and thus partially blocking the flow of blood through the valve (causing stenosis). Either problem can greatly interfere with the heart's ability to pump blood. Sometimes a valve has both problems.

Mitral Regurgitation

Mitral regurgitation (mitral valve regurgitation, mitral incompetence, mitral insuffi-

---

▲ see art on page 115   ■ see page 122

★ see art on page 168   ● see art on page 115

Understanding Stenosis and Regurgitation

The heart valves can malfunction either by leaking (causing regurgitation) or by not opening adequately and thus partially blocking the flow of blood through the valve (causing stenosis). Stenosis and regurgitation can affect any of the heart valves. These two disorders are shown below at the mitral valve.

Normal Valve Mechanisms

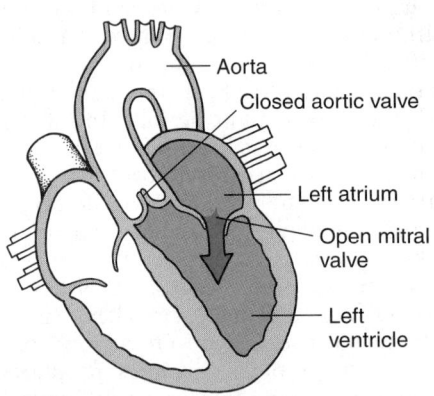

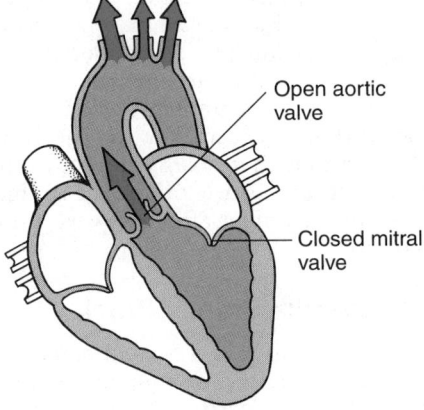

Normally, just after the left ventricle finishes contracting (during diastole), the aortic valve closes, the mitral valve opens, and some blood flows from the left atrium into the left ventricle. Then the left atrium contracts, ejecting more blood into the left ventricle.

As the left ventricle begins to contract (during systole), the mitral valve closes, the aortic valve opens, and blood is ejected into the aorta.

Mitral Stenosis

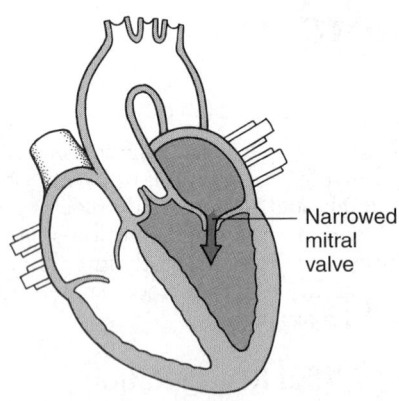

Mitral Regurgitation

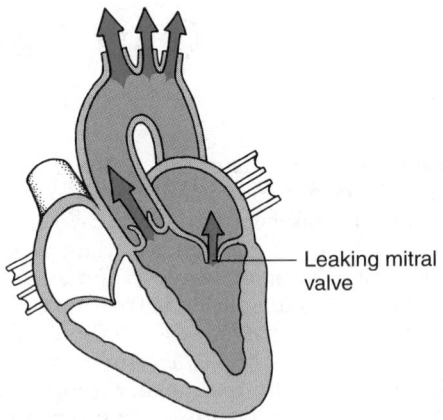

In mitral stenosis, the mitral valve opening is narrowed, and blood flow from the left atrium into the left ventricle during diastole is reduced.

In mitral regurgitation, the mitral valve leaks when the left ventricle contracts (during systole), and some blood flows backward into the left atrium.

ciency) is leakage of blood backward through the mitral valve each time the left ventricle contracts.

As the left ventricle pumps blood into the aorta, some blood leaks backward into the left atrium, increasing blood volume and pressure there. The increased blood pressure in the left atrium increases blood pressure in the veins leading from the lungs to the heart (pulmonary veins). If regurgitation is severe, the increased pressure may result in fluid accumulation (congestion) in the lungs.

Rheumatic fever▲—a childhood illness that sometimes occurs after untreated strep throat—used to be the most common cause of mitral regurgitation. But today, rheumatic fever is rare in North America, Australasia, Western Europe, and other regions where antibiotics are widely used to prevent infections such as strep throat. In these regions, rheumatic fever is a common cause of mitral regurgitation only among older people who did not have the benefit of antibiotics during their youth. However, in regions in which antibiotics are not widely used, rheumatic fever is still common and still commonly causes mitral stenosis or regurgitation among all age groups.

In North America, Western Europe, and Australasia, a more common cause of mitral regurgitation is a heart attack, which can damage the supporting structures of the mitral valve. Another common cause is myxomatous degeneration, a hereditary connective tissue disorder that causes a jellylike deterioration of tissue. As a result, the heart valve gradually becomes floppy; rarely, the valve tears.

Symptoms

Mild mitral regurgitation may not produce any symptoms. When regurgitation is more severe, people, particularly when lying on their left side, may have palpitations; that is, they become aware of their heartbeats, which are more forceful. Heartbeats are more forceful because the left ventricle has to pump more blood, to compensate for the leakage back into the left atrium. The left ventricle gradually enlarges and thickens to increase the force of each heartbeat.

Similarly, the left atrium also tends to enlarge because it must accommodate the extra blood leaking back from the ventricle. A very enlarged atrium often beats rapidly in an irregular pattern (a disorder called atrial fibrillation), which reduces the heart's pumping effi-

ciency. A fibrillating atrium is just quivering, not pumping. Consequently, blood does not flow through it normally, allowing blood clots to form. If a clot breaks loose (becoming an embolus), it is pumped out of the heart and may block an artery, possibly causing a stroke or other damage.

If regurgitation is severe, the forward flow of blood is reduced enough to cause heart failure, which may produce coughing, shortness of breath during exertion, and swelling in the legs.

Diagnosis

Mitral regurgitation is usually diagnosed based on the characteristic heart murmur heard through a stethoscope. The murmur is a distinctive sound produced by blood leaking backward into the left atrium when the left ventricle contracts. The disorder is sometimes diagnosed when doctors hear this murmur during a routine physical examination.

Electrocardiography (ECG) and chest x-rays show that the left ventricle is enlarged. If mitral regurgitation is severe, the chest x-ray may also show fluid accumulation in the lungs. The most informative procedure is echocardiography,■ which uses ultrasound waves to produce an image of the faulty valve. This procedure can show the size of the atrium and ventricle and the amount of blood leaking, so that the severity of the regurgitation can be determined.

Treatment

Atrial fibrillation, if present, may require treatment,★ including use of anticoagulants to prevent clots.

If regurgitation is mild, mild heart failure can be treated with an angiotensin-converting inhibitor (ACE inhibitor), such as enalapril or lisinopril, with or without digoxin. However, in people with moderate regurgitation, surgery increases the chance of a good outcome and reduces the risk of worsening heart failure.

If regurgitation is severe, surgery is needed. Surgery must be performed before the left ventricle becomes so abnormal that the problem cannot be corrected. So, echocardiography is usually performed periodically to determine how rapidly the left ventricle is enlarging. Surgery may involve repairing the valve (valvuloplasty) or replacing it with an artificial

▲ see page 1565   ■ see page 125
★ see page 169

(prosthetic) valve. Repairing the valve eliminates regurgitation or reduces it enough to make the symptoms tolerable and prevent damage to the heart. Replacing the valve eliminates regurgitation. The damaged valve can be replaced with a mechanical valve or a biologic one made partly from a pig's valve. Each type has advantages and disadvantages. Mechanical valves are usually effective and last a long time. However, they increase the risk of blood clots, so anticoagulants are usually taken indefinitely to reduce this risk. Biologic valves are effective and do not pose a risk of blood clots, but they do not last as long as mechanical valves. If an artificial valve malfunctions, it must be replaced immediately.

Damaged heart valves are susceptible to a serious infection by bacteria (infective endocarditis). People with a damaged or an artificial valve should take antibiotics before surgical, dental, or medical procedures▲ to reduce the risk of an infection on a valve, even though this risk is small.

Mitral Valve Prolapse

Mitral valve prolapse is a disorder in which the valve cusps bulge into the left atrium when the left ventricle contracts, sometimes allowing leakage (regurgitation) of small amounts of blood into the atrium.

About 2 to 5% of people have mitral valve prolapse. It rarely causes serious heart problems.

Symptoms and Diagnosis

Most people with mitral valve prolapse have no symptoms. Others have symptoms that are difficult to explain on the basis of the mechanical problem alone; these symptoms include chest pain, a rapid pulse, palpitations (awareness of heartbeats), migraine headaches, fatigue, and dizziness. In some people, blood pressure may fall below normal when they stand up (a disorder called orthostatic hypotension).

Doctors diagnose mitral valve prolapse after hearing the characteristic clicking sound through a stethoscope. Regurgitation is diagnosed if a murmur is heard when the left ventricle contracts. Echocardiography■ enables

doctors to view the prolapse and determine the severity of regurgitation if present.

Treatment

Most people with mitral valve prolapse do not need treatment. If the heart is beating too fast, a beta-blocker may be taken to slow the heart rate and to reduce palpitations and other symptoms.

If regurgitation is also present, antibiotics should be taken before surgical, dental, or medical procedures★ because bacterial infection of the heart valve (infective endocarditis) is a risk, although a small one.

Mitral Stenosis

Mitral stenosis (mitral valve stenosis) is a narrowing of the mitral valve opening that increases resistance to blood flow from the left atrium to the left ventricle.

In mitral stenosis, blood flow through the narrowed valve opening is reduced. As a result, the volume and pressure of blood in the left atrium increases, and the left atrium enlarges.

Mitral stenosis almost always results from rheumatic fever, a childhood illness that sometimes occurs after untreated strep throat or scarlet fever.● Rheumatic fever is now rare in North America, Australasia, and Western Europe because antibiotics are widely used to prevent infection. Thus, in these regions, mitral stenosis occurs mostly in older people who had rheumatic fever and who did not have the benefit of antibiotics during their youth or in immigrants. In regions where antibiotics are not widely used, rheumatic fever is common, and it leads to mitral stenosis in adults, teenagers, and sometimes even children. Typically, when rheumatic fever is the cause of mitral stenosis, the mitral valve cusps are partially fused together.

Mitral stenosis can also be present at birth (congenital). Infants born with the disorder rarely live beyond age 2, unless they have surgery.

Two conditions unrelated to mitral stenosis can produce the same effects as the stenosis. They include a myxoma (a noncancerous tumor in the left atrium) and a blood clot that reduces blood flow through the mitral valve.

Symptoms and Diagnosis

If mitral stenosis is severe, pressure increases in the left atrium and in the veins of the lungs, resulting in heart failure with fluid

---

▲ see box on page 187   ■ see page 125
★ see box on page 187   ● see page 1565

Replacing a Heart Valve

A damaged heart valve may be replaced with a mechanical valve made of plastic and metal or with a biologic valve made of tissue, usually from pigs, placed in a synthetic ring. There are many types of mechanical valves; a St. Jude valve is commonly used.

Choice of a valve depends on many factors, including characteristics of the valve. A mechanical valve lasts longer than a biologic valve but requires that anticoagulants be taken indefinitely to prevent the formation of blood clots on the valve. A biologic valve rarely requires the use of anticoagulants. So whether a person can take anticoagulants is an important factor. For example, anticoagulants may not be appropriate for women of childbearing age because anticoagulants cross the placenta and may affect the fetus. Also considered are how old the person is, what the person's activity level is, how well the heart is

working, and which heart valve is damaged. Mechanical valves are usually preferred in younger people.

For heart valve replacement, a general anesthetic is given. The heart must be still to be operated on, so a heart-lung machine is used to pump blood through the bloodstream. The damaged valve is removed, and the replacement valve is sewn in place. The incisions are closed, the heart-lung machine is disconnected, and the heart is restarted. The operation takes from 2 to 5 hours. For some people, a heart valve can be replaced using a less invasive procedure, available at some medical centers.

After surgery, the person is monitored in an intensive care unit for a day or two, before being moved to a regular unit. The length of the hospital stay varies from person to person. Full recovery may take 6 to 8 weeks.

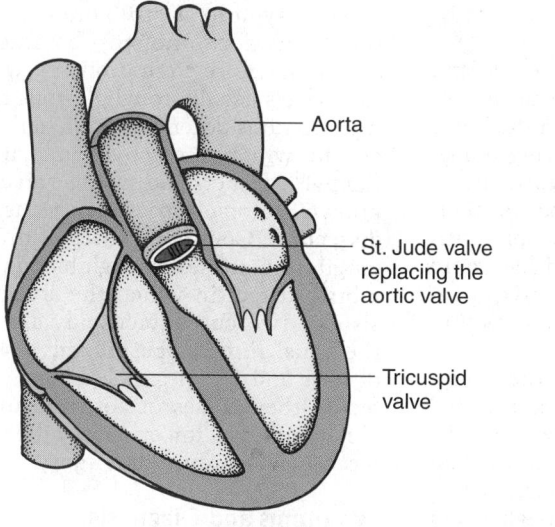

Aorta

St. Jude valve replacing the aortic valve

Tricuspid valve

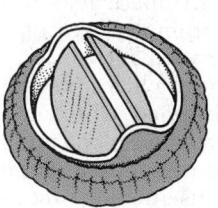

St. Jude valve

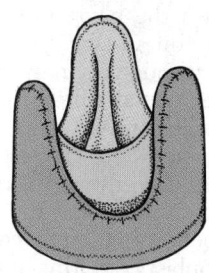

Tissue valve

accumulation in the lungs. If a woman with severe mitral stenosis becomes pregnant, heart failure may develop rapidly. People with heart failure become easily fatigued and short of breath. Shortness of breath may occur only during physical activity at first, but later, it may occur even during rest. Some people can breathe comfortably only when they are propped up with pillows or sitting upright.

Severe mitral stenosis may result in high blood pressure in the lungs (pulmonary hypertension) and a low level of oxygen in the blood. This combination of problems produces a plum-colored flush in the cheeks (called mitral facies). People may cough up blood if the high pressure causes a vein or capillaries in the lungs to burst. The resulting bleeding into the lungs is usually slight and rarely massive.

The enlarged left atrium often beats rapidly in an irregular pattern (a disorder called atrial fibrillation). As a result, the heart's pumping efficiency is reduced.

With a stethoscope, doctors can hear the characteristic heart murmur as blood tries to pass through the narrowed valve opening from the left atrium into the left ventricle. Unlike a normal valve, which opens silently, the abnormal valve often makes a snapping sound as it opens to allow blood into the left ventricle. The diagnosis is usually confirmed by electrocardiography (ECG), a chest x-ray showing an enlarged atrium, or echocardiography, which uses ultrasound waves to produce an image of blood passing through the narrowed valve opening. If surgery is being considered, cardiac catheterization▲ is necessary to further define the extent and characteristics of the blockage.

Prevention and Treatment

Mitral stenosis can be prevented only by preventing rheumatic fever, which can be prevented by promptly treating strep throat or scarlet fever with antibiotics.

Treatment includes use of diuretics and digoxin. Diuretics, which increase urine formation, can reduce blood pressure in the lungs by reducing the volume of circulating blood. Digoxin is useful only in the treatment of atrial fibrillation, which may be present. Digoxin slows the heart rate in people with atrial fibrillation so that the blood has more time to flow through the narrowed valve opening. However, atrial fibrillation may require additional treatment.■

If drug therapy does not reduce the symptoms satisfactorily, the valve may be repaired or replaced. Sometimes the valve can be stretched open using a procedure called balloon valvuloplasty. In this procedure, a balloon-tipped catheter is threaded through a vein and eventually into the heart.★ Once inside the valve, the balloon is inflated, separating the valve leaflets. Alternatively, heart surgery may be performed to separate the fused cusps. If the valve is too badly damaged, it may be surgically replaced with an artificial valve.

People with mitral stenosis are given antibiotics before a surgical, dental, or medical procedure● to reduce the small risk of developing a heart valve infection (infective endocarditis).

▲ see page 128   ■ see page 169

★ see page 128   ● see box on page 187

◆ see page 1517

Aortic Regurgitation

Aortic regurgitation (aortic incompetence, aortic insufficiency) is leakage of the aortic valve each time the left ventricle relaxes.

As the left ventricle relaxes to fill with blood from the left atrium, blood leaks backward from the aorta, increasing the volume and pressure of blood in the left ventricle. As a result, the amount of work the heart has to do increases. To compensate, the muscular walls of the ventricles thicken (hypertrophy), and the chambers of the ventricles enlarge (dilate). Eventually, despite this compensation, the heart may be unable to meet the body's need for blood, leading to heart failure.

Rheumatic fever and syphilis used to be the most common causes of aortic regurgitation in North America, Australasia, and Western Europe, where both disorders are now rare because of the widespread use of antibiotics. In regions in which antibiotics are not widely used, aortic regurgitation due to rheumatic fever or syphilis is still common. Aside from these infections, the most common causes of severe aortic regurgitation are weakening of the valve's usually tough, fibrous tissue due to myxomatous degeneration (a hereditary disorder in which the valve gradually becomes floppy); degeneration of the valve due to unknown factors; aortic aneurysms; and aortic dissection. Common causes of mild aortic regurgitation are severe high blood pressure and a birth defect in which the aortic valve consists of two cusps (bicuspid valve) instead of the usual three (tricuspid valve).◆ About 2% of boys and 1% of girls are born with this defect. Other causes of aortic regurgitation include bacterial infection of a heart valve (infective endocarditis) and injury.

Symptoms and Diagnosis

Mild aortic regurgitation produces no symptoms other than a characteristic heart murmur that can be heard with a stethoscope each time the left ventricle relaxes. People with severe regurgitation may have palpitations (awareness of heartbeats) because the left ventricle enlarges and contracts more forcefully. It enlarges as the volume of blood it contains increases. Eventually, heart failure with fluid accumulation in the lungs results. Heart failure causes shortness of breath during exertion. Lying flat, especially at night, makes breathing difficult. Sitting up allows backed-up fluid to drain out of the upper part of the lungs, restoring normal breathing. About 5% of people with aortic regurgitation have chest pain due to an inadequate blood supply to the heart muscle (angina), especially at night.

The pulse, sometimes called a collapsing pulse, is momentarily strong, then disappears quickly because the blood leaks backward through the aortic valve, causing blood pressure to decrease sharply.

Doctors usually suspect the diagnosis based on the results of a physical examination (such as the collapsing pulse and characteristic heart murmur) and an enlarged heart seen on an x-ray. Electrocardiography (ECG) may show signs of an enlarged left ventricle. Echocardiography can show the faulty valve and help doctors determine how severe regurgitation is and whether heart valve replacement surgery is needed. Coronary angiography is performed before surgery because about 20% of people with aortic regurgitation also have coronary artery disease.

Treatment

Heart failure due to aortic regurgitation can initially be treated with drugs. Unless aortic regurgitation is mild, surgery is ultimately almost always required. In the weeks before surgery, heart failure is treated with digoxin, diuretics, and a drug that dilates blood vessels and thus reduces the work of the heart, such as a calcium blocker, an angiotensin-converting enzyme (ACE) inhibitor, or hydralazine plus a nitrate.▲ An angiotensin II receptor blocker may be used when an ACE inhibitor cannot be used. Use of a pacemaker■ to increase the heart rate can sometimes help reduce the severity of heart failure.

The damaged valve should be surgically replaced with an artificial valve before the left ventricle becomes irreversibly damaged and heart failure becomes too severe. Usually, echocardiography is performed periodically to determine how rapidly the left ventricle is enlarging, so that surgery can be scheduled at an appropriate time.

People with aortic regurgitation, even when mild, are given antibiotics before surgical, dental, or medical procedures★ to reduce the risk of infection of the damaged heart valve.

Aortic Stenosis

Aortic stenosis is a narrowing of the aortic valve opening that increases resistance to blood flow from the left ventricle to the aorta.

In aortic stenosis, the wall of the left ventricle usually thickens because the ventricle must work harder to pump the blood through the narrowed valve opening into the aorta. The thickened wall occupies space inside the ventricle and thus makes the interior of the left ventricle smaller. The thickened heart muscle requires an increasing supply of blood from the coronary arteries, and eventually, the blood supply becomes inadequate. The heart muscle can be damaged when it does not receive enough blood. A damaged heart cannot pump enough blood for the body's needs, leading to heart failure.

In North America and Western Europe, aortic stenosis is mainly a disease of older people—the result of scarring and calcium accumulation (calcification) in the valve cusps. In such cases, aortic stenosis begins after age 60 but does not usually produce symptoms until age 70 or 80. Aortic stenosis may also result from rheumatic fever contracted in childhood. When rheumatic fever is the cause, aortic stenosis is usually accompanied by mitral stenosis, leakage (regurgitation), or both.

In younger people, the most common cause is a birth defect, such as a valve with only two cusps instead of the usual three or a valve with an abnormal funnel shape.● The narrowed aortic valve opening may not be a problem in infancy but becomes one as a person grows. The valve opening remains the same size, but the heart grows and enlarges further as it tries to pump increasing amounts of blood through the small valve opening. Over the years, the opening of a defective valve often becomes stiff and narrow because calcium accumulates.

Symptoms and Diagnosis

Chest pain (angina) occurs during exertion because the blood supply to the enlarged heart muscle is inadequate. Eventually, heart failure develops, causing fatigue and shortness of breath during exertion.

People who have severe aortic stenosis may faint during exertion because blood pressure may fall suddenly. This sudden fall in blood pressure occurs because the arteries in skeletal muscles dilate during exercise to receive more oxygen-rich blood, but the narrowed valve opening prevents the left ventricle from

---

▲ see table on page 156   ■ see art on page 168
★ see box on page 187   ● see page 1517

pumping enough blood to compensate. People who have severe aortic stenosis can die suddenly, so treatment should not be delayed.

The damaged aortic valve can become infected by bacteria, resulting in infective endocarditis.

Doctors usually base the diagnosis on a characteristic heart murmur heard through a stethoscope, on pulse abnormalities, and on results of electrocardiography indicating thickening of the heart wall. For people who experience angina, shortness of breath, or faintness, echocardiography▲ is the best procedure for measuring the thickness of the left ventricle wall. Echocardiography is used to monitor how quickly the left ventricle wall is thickening. Color Doppler echocardiography shows different rates of blood flow through the narrowed valve opening in different colors and can indicate how narrow the valve opening is. Cardiac catheterization■ shows exactly how narrow the opening is and can show whether the coronary arteries are also narrowed because of coronary artery disease.

Treatment

Adults who have aortic stenosis but no symptoms should see their doctor regularly and should avoid overly stressful exercise. Echocardiography is performed periodically to monitor heart size and valve function. If heart size increases significantly or valve function worsens, the doctor may recommend surgery.

In adults who have aortic stenosis that causes fainting, angina, or shortness of breath during exertion, the aortic valve is surgically replaced, preferably before the left ventricle is irreversibly damaged. Echocardiography, usually performed periodically, can help doctors determine when to schedule surgery. Before surgery, heart failure (indicated by shortness of breath) is treated with diuretics.★ Surgical replacement of the abnormal valve is the best treatment for adults of all ages, and the prognosis after valve replacement is excellent. People with an artificial valve must take antibiotics before a surgical, dental, or medical procedure● to reduce the risk of an infection on the valve (infective endocarditis).

For children who have severe stenosis, surgery may be performed even before symp-

toms develop, because sudden death may occur before symptoms develop. Safe, effective alternatives to valve replacement are surgical repair of the valve and balloon valvuloplasty. In balloon valvuloplasty, a balloon-tipped catheter is threaded through a vein and eventually into the heart.◆ Once inside the valve, the balloon is inflated to expand the valve opening. However, later, when children are fully grown, the valve usually must be replaced. In adults, stenosis always recurs after balloon valvuloplasty; so among adults, this procedure is used only for frail older people who cannot tolerate surgery.

Tricuspid Regurgitation

Tricuspid regurgitation (tricuspid incompetence, tricuspid insufficiency) is leakage of blood backward through the tricuspid valve each time the right ventricle contracts.

As the right ventricle contracts to pump blood forward to the lungs, some blood leaks backward into the right atrium, increasing the volume of blood there. As a result, the right atrium enlarges, and pressure in the veins that enter the right atrium is increased, creating resistance to blood flow from the body to the heart.

Tricuspid regurgitation usually results when the right ventricle enlarges and resistance to blood flow from the right ventricle to the lungs is increased. Resistance may be increased by a severe, long-standing lung disorder, such as emphysema or pulmonary hypertension, or by narrowing of the pulmonary valve (pulmonary stenosis). To compensate, the right ventricle enlarges and thickens so that it can pump harder, and the valve opening stretches.

Other, less common causes are infection of the heart valves (infective endocarditis), use of fenfluramine, birth defects of the tricuspid valve, injury, and myxomatous degeneration (a hereditary disorder in which the valve gradually becomes floppy).

Symptoms and Diagnosis

Tricuspid regurgitation can cause vague symptoms, such as weakness and fatigue. They develop because the heart is pumping a smaller amount of blood. Usually, the only other symptoms are pulsations in the neck and discomfort in the right upper part of the abdomen due to an enlarged liver. These symptoms develop because blood flows backward from the heart into the veins. Enlargement of

---

▲ see page 125   ■ see page 128

★ see table on page 156

● see box on page 187   ◆ see page 128

the right atrium can result in a rapid, irregular heartbeat (atrial fibrillation). Eventually, heart failure develops, resulting in accumulation of fluid in the body, mainly in the legs.

The diagnosis is based on the person's medical history and results of a physical examination, electrocardiography (ECG), and chest x-ray. Through a stethoscope, doctors can hear a characteristic murmur produced by the blood leaking backward through the tricuspid valve. Echocardiography▲ can produce an image of the leaky valve and the amount of blood leaking, so that the severity of the regurgitation can be determined.

Treatment

Usually, tricuspid regurgitation requires little or no treatment. However, the underlying disorder, such as emphysema, pulmonary hypertension, or pulmonary stenosis may require treatment. Usually, treatment of the resulting atrial fibrillation and heart failure does not include surgery on the tricuspid valve.

Tricuspid Stenosis

Tricuspid stenosis is a narrowing of the tricuspid valve opening that increases resistance to blood flow from the right atrium to the right ventricle.

Over many years, the right atrium enlarges because blood flow through the narrowed valve opening is partially blocked, increasing the volume of blood in the atrium. In turn, this increased volume causes an increase in pressure in the veins bringing blood back to the heart from the body (except the lungs). However, the right ventricle shrinks, because the amount of blood entering it from the right atrium is reduced. Tricuspid regurgitation rarely occurs.

Nearly all cases are caused by rheumatic fever, which has become rare in North America, Australasia, and Western Europe. Rarely, the cause is a tumor in the right atrium, a connective tissue disorder, or, even more rarely, a birth defect of the heart.

Symptoms are usually mild. They include palpitations (awareness of heartbeats), a fluttering discomfort in the neck, cold skin, and fatigue. Abdominal discomfort may result if the increased pressure in the veins causes the liver to enlarge.

Through a stethoscope, doctors may hear the characteristic murmur of tricuspid stenosis. A chest x-ray shows that the right atrium is enlarged. Echocardiography■ can produce an image of the narrowed valve opening and show the amount of blood passing through the valve, so that the severity of the stenosis can be determined. Electrocardiography (ECG)★ shows changes indicating that the right atrium is strained.

Tricuspid stenosis is rarely severe enough to require surgical repair.

Pulmonary Stenosis

Pulmonary stenosis is a narrowing of the pulmonary valve opening that increases resistance to blood flow from the right ventricle to the pulmonary arteries.

Pulmonary stenosis, which is rare among adults, is usually due to a birth defect.● When significant, it is usually diagnosed during childhood, because it produces a loud heart murmur. Severe pulmonary stenosis occasionally causes heart failure in children but often does not produce symptoms until adulthood.

Young children with this disorder often require heart surgery. In adults and older children, balloon valvuloplasty may be performed. In this procedure, the valve is stretched open using a balloon-tipped catheter threaded through a vein and eventually into the heart. Once inside the valve, the balloon is inflated, separating the valve leaflets.

▲ see page 125   ■ see page 125
★ see page 122   ● see page 1518

CHAPTER 29

Infective Endocarditis

Infective endocarditis is an infection of the lining of the heart (endocardium) and usually also of the heart valves.

Infective endocarditis affects twice as many men as women of all ages but 8 times as many older men as older women. It has become more common among older people: More than one fourth of all cases occur in people older than 60.

Infective endocarditis refers specifically to infection of the lining of the heart, but the infection usually also affects the heart valves and often affects the muscle of the heart. There are two forms of infective endocarditis. One form, called acute infective endocarditis, develops suddenly and may become life threatening within days. The other form, called subacute infective endocarditis or subacute bacterial endocarditis, develops gradually and subtly over a period of weeks to several months.

Bacteria (or, less often, fungi) may be introduced into the bloodstream. These organisms can then lodge on heart valves and infect the endocardium. Abnormal or damaged valves are more susceptible to infection than normal valves. The bacteria that cause subacute bacterial endocarditis nearly always infect abnormal or damaged valves. However, normal valves can be infected by some aggressive bacteria, especially if many bacteria are present.

Risk factors for children and young adults include birth defects, particularly a defect that allows blood to leak from one part of the heart to another. One risk factor for older people is calcium deposits in the mitral valve (which opens from the left atrium into the left ventricle) or in the aortic valve (which opens from the left ventricle into the aorta). Damage to the heart by rheumatic fever as a child (rheumatic heart disease)▲ is also a risk factor. Rheumatic fever has become a less common risk factor in countries where antibiotics have become widely available. In such countries, rheumatic fever is a risk factor for people who did not have the benefit of antibiotics during their childhood (such as immigrants).

People who inject illicit drugs are at high risk of endocarditis because they are likely to inject bacteria directly into their bloodstream through dirty needles, syringes, or drug solutions. People who have an artificial (prosthetic) heart valve are also at high risk. For them, the risk of infective endocarditis is greatest during the first year after heart valve surgery; after that, the risk decreases but remains slightly higher than normal. For unknown reasons, the risk is always greater with an artificial aortic valve than with an artificial mitral valve and with a mechanical valve rather than with a valve transplanted from a pig.

Causes

Although bacteria are not normally found in the blood, an injury to the skin, lining of the mouth, or gums (even an injury from a normal activity such as chewing or brushing the teeth) can allow a small number of bacteria to enter the bloodstream. Gingivitis (inflammation of the gums) with infection, minor skin infections, and infections elsewhere in the body may introduce bacteria into the bloodstream.

Certain surgical, dental, and medical procedures may also introduce bacteria into the bloodstream. Rarely, bacteria are introduced into the heart during open-heart surgery or heart valve replacement surgery. In people with normal heart valves, usually no harm is done, and the body's white blood cells rapidly destroy these bacteria. However, damaged heart valves may trap the bacteria, which can then lodge on the endocardium and start to multiply. Sepsis,■ a severe blood infection, introduces a large number of bacteria into the bloodstream. When the number of bacteria in the bloodstream is large enough, endocarditis can develop, even in people who have normal heart valves.

If the cause of infective endocarditis is injection of illicit drugs or prolonged use of intravenous lines, the tricuspid valve (which opens from the right atrium into the right ventricle) is most often infected. In most other cases of endocarditis, the mitral valve or the aortic valve is infected.

▲ see page 1565   ■ see page 1118

Symptoms

Acute bacterial endocarditis usually begins suddenly with a high fever (102° to 104° F [38.9° to 40° C]), fast heart rate, fatigue, and rapid and extensive heart valve damage.

Subacute bacterial endocarditis may produce such symptoms as fatigue, mild fever (99° to 101° F [37.2° to 38.3° C]), a moderately fast heart rate, weight loss, sweating, and a low red blood cell count (anemia). These symptoms may occur for months before the endocarditis results in blockage of an artery or damages heart valves and thus makes the diagnosis clear to doctors.

Arteries may become blocked if accumulations of bacteria and blood clots on the valves (called vegetations) break loose (becoming emboli), travel through the bloodstream to other parts of the body, and lodge in an artery, blocking it. Sometimes blockage can have serious consequences. Blockage of an artery to the brain can cause a stroke, and blockage of an artery to the heart can cause a heart attack. Emboli can also cause an infection in the area in which they lodge. Collections of pus (abscesses) may develop at the base of infected heart valves or wherever infected emboli settle.

Heart valves may become perforated and may start to leak (causing regurgitation▲) significantly within a few days. Some people go into shock, and their kidneys and other organs stop functioning (a condition called septic shock■). Infections in arteries can weaken artery walls, causing them to bulge or rupture. A rupture can be fatal, particularly if it occurs in the brain or near the heart.

Other symptoms of acute and subacute bacterial endocarditis may include chills, joint pain, paleness (pallor), painful nodules under the skin, and confusion. Tiny reddish spots that resemble freckles may appear on the skin and in the whites of the eyes. Small streaks of red (called splinter hemorrhages) may appear under the fingernails. These spots and streaks are caused by tiny emboli that have broken off the heart valves. Larger emboli may cause stomach pain, blood in the urine, or pain or numbness in an arm or a leg as well as a heart attack, or a stroke. Heart murmurs may develop, or preexisting ones may change. The spleen may enlarge.

Endocarditis of an artificial heart valve may be an acute or subacute infection. Compared with infection of a natural valve, infection of an artificial valve is more likely to spread to the heart muscle at the base of the valve and

Endocarditis Without Infection

Another form of endocarditis is non-infective endocarditis. It develops when blood clots form on damaged heart valves. Damage may be due to a birth defect, rheumatic fever, or an autoimmune disorder (in which antibodies attack the heart valves). Rarely, damage results from insertion of a catheter into the heart. People most at risk include those with systemic lupus erythematosus (an autoimmune disorder); lung, stomach, or pancreatic cancer; tuberculosis; pneumonia; sepsis (a severe blood infection); uremia (the buildup of wastes in the blood); and burns. Noninfective endocarditis, like infective endocarditis, may cause heart valves to leak or not open normally. The risk of a blood clot breaking off (becoming an embolus) and causing a stroke or heart attack is high.

Distinguishing between noninfective and infective endocarditis is difficult but important, because treatment differs. Noninfective endocarditis may be diagnosed when echocardiography detects vegetations on heart valves, but no bacteria are detected in blood samples. Anticoagulants may be used to prevent clotting, but their benefits have not been confirmed.

can loosen the valve. Alternatively, the heart's electrical conduction system may be interrupted, resulting in slowing of the heartbeat, which may lead to a sudden loss of consciousness or even death.

Diagnosis

Because many of the symptoms are vague and general, doctors may have difficulty making a diagnosis. Usually, people suspected of having acute or subacute infective endocarditis are hospitalized promptly for diagnosis as well as treatment.

Doctors may suspect endocarditis in people with a fever and no obvious source of infection, especially if they have characteristic symptoms; have a heart valve disorder; have recently had certain surgical, dental, or medical procedures; or inject illicit drugs. Development of a heart murmur or a change in a preexisting heart murmur further supports the diagnosis.

▲ see art on page 176   ■ see page 1119

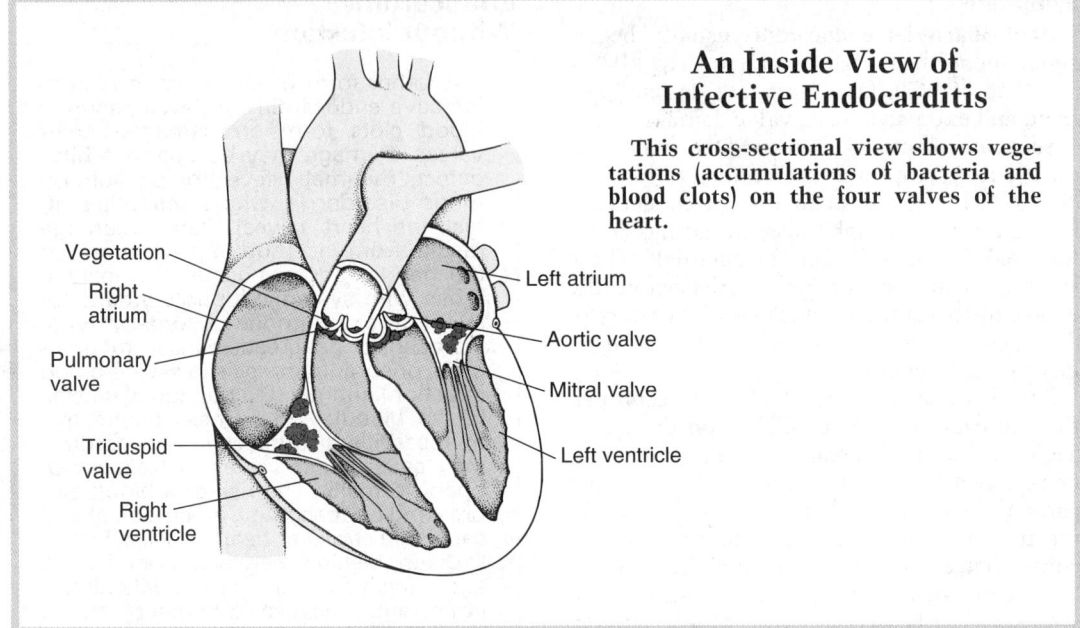

An Inside View of Infective Endocarditis

This cross-sectional view shows vegetations (accumulations of bacteria and blood clots) on the four valves of the heart.

Vegetation

Right atrium

Pulmonary valve

Tricuspid valve

Right ventricle

Left atrium

Aortic valve

Mitral valve

Left ventricle

A blood sample is drawn to test for the presence of bacteria. Detecting bacteria in the blood helps doctors make the diagnosis.

To identify the disease-causing bacteria (so that a suitable antibiotic can be chosen), doctors send blood samples to be cultured. Because bacteria are continuously released from heart valve vegetations into the bloodstream, three or more blood samples are taken at different times to determine whether bacteria continue to be present in the bloodstream. Various antibiotics are tested against the bacteria to determine the best one to use. If endocarditis develops after a heart valve is replaced with an artificial one, the bacteria that caused the endocarditis may be resistant to antibiotics. Antibiotics are given before heart valve replacement surgery to prevent infection. If antibiotics do not prevent infection, the bacteria causing the resulting infection are probably resistant.

Sometimes bacteria cannot be cultured from blood samples. Special techniques may be needed to grow the particular bacteria, or the person may have taken antibiotics that did not cure the infection but did reduce the number of bacteria enough to be undetectable. Another possible explanation is that the person does not have endocarditis but has a disorder, such as a heart tumor,▲ that produces symptoms very similar to those of endocarditis.

Echocardiography, which uses ultrasound waves,■ can produce images showing heart valve vegetations and damage to the heart. Transesophageal echocardiography (a procedure in which the ultrasound probe is passed down the throat into the esophagus just behind the heart) can detect endocarditis in more than 90% of affected people.

Prevention

As a preventive measure, people with heart valve abnormalities, artificial valves, or congenital heart defects are given antibiotics before certain surgical, dental, and medical procedures. Consequently, surgeons, dentists, and other health care practitioners need to know if a person has had a heart valve disorder. Although the risk of endocarditis is not very high for these procedures and preventive antibiotics are not always effective, the consequences of endocarditis are so severe that most doctors believe that giving antibiotics before these procedures is a reasonable precaution.

Treatment and Prognosis

Treatment usually consists of at least 2 weeks and often up to 6 weeks of antibiotics given intravenously in high doses. Antibiotic

▲ see page 191   ■ see page 125

WHICH PROCEDURES REQUIRE PREVENTIVE ANTIBIOTICS?

As a preventive measure before certain procedures, antibiotics are given to people at risk of developing infective endocarditis.

SURGICAL PROCEDURES	DENTAL PROCEDURES	MEDICAL PROCEDURES
Heart valve replacement	Tooth extraction	Use of catheters or intravenous lines to provide fluids, nutrition, or drugs
Open-heart surgery	Periodontal procedures such as gum surgery, scaling, root planing, and probing	Bronchoscopy
Removal of tonsils or adenoids	Placement of dental implants	Cystoscopy
Lung surgery	Replacement of a tooth that was knocked out	Dilation of the esophagus
Surgery on the intestines or bile ducts	Root canal surgery beyond the end of the root	Dilation of the urethra
Prostate surgery	Placement of orthodontic bands beneath the gums	Endoscopic retrograde cholangiopancreatography (endoscopy, with injection of a dye that can be seen on x-rays, to remove gallstones in the bile duct)
	Injection of an anesthetic into a ligament	Sclerotherapy for varicose veins in the esophagus
	Cleanings if bleeding is expected to result	

therapy is almost always started in the hospital but may be finished at home with the help of a home nurse.

Antibiotics alone do not always cure an infection, particularly if the valve is artificial. Heart surgery may be needed to repair or replace damaged valves and remove vegetations. For example, if infection of an artificial heart valve loosens the valve, emergency surgery to replace the valve is needed, because heart failure from significant valvular leaks can be fatal.

If untreated, infective endocarditis is always fatal. When treatment is given, risk of death depends on factors such as the person's age, duration of the infection, the presence of an artificial heart valve, and the type of infecting organism. Nonetheless, with aggressive antibiotic treatment, most people survive.

CHAPTER 30

Pericardial Disease

Pericardial disease affects the pericardium, which is the flexible two-layered sac that envelops the heart.

The pericardium helps keep the heart in position, prevent the heart from overfilling with blood, and protect the heart from being damaged by chest infections. However, the pericardium is not essential to life; if the pericardium is removed, there is little measurable effect on the heart's performance.

Normally, the pericardium contains just enough lubricating fluid between its two layers for them to slide easily over one another. There is very little space between the two layers. However, in some disorders, extra fluid accumulates in this space (called the pericardial space), causing it to expand.

Rarely, the pericardium is missing at birth or has defects, such as weak spots or holes. These defects can be dangerous because the heart or a major blood vessel may bulge (herniate) through a hole in the pericardium and become trapped. In such cases, death can occur in minutes. Therefore, these defects are usually surgically repaired; if repair is not feasible, the whole pericardium may be removed. Other diseases of the pericardium may result from infections, injuries, or spread of cancer.

Acute Pericarditis

Acute pericarditis is inflammation of the pericardium that begins suddenly, is often painful, and causes fluid and blood components such as fibrin, red blood cells, and white blood cells to pour into the pericardial space.

Acute pericarditis usually results from infection or other conditions that irritate the pericardium. Infection is usually due to a virus but may be caused by bacteria, parasites (including protozoa), or fungi.

In some inner city hospitals, AIDS is the most common cause of pericarditis with extra fluid in the pericardial space (pericardial effusion). In people who have AIDS, a number of infections, including tuberculosis, may result in pericarditis. Pericarditis due to tuberculosis (tuberculous pericarditis) accounts for less than 5% of cases of acute pericarditis in the United States but accounts for the majority of cases in some areas of India and Africa.

Other conditions can irritate the pericardium and thus can cause acute pericarditis. These conditions include a heart attack, heart surgery, systemic lupus erythematosus, rheumatoid arthritis, kidney failure, injury, cancer (such as leukemia and, in people with AIDS, Kaposi's sarcoma), rheumatic fever, an underactive thyroid gland (hypothyroidism), radiation therapy, and leakage of blood from an aortic aneurysm (a bulge in the wall of the aorta). After a heart attack, acute pericarditis develops during the first day or two in 10 to 15% of people and after about 10 days to 2 months in 1 to 3%. Acute pericarditis may occur as a side effect of certain drugs, including anticoagulants (such as warfarin and heparin), penicillin, procainamide (an antiarrhythmic drug), phenytoin (an anticonvulsant), and phenylbutazone (a nonsteroidal anti-inflammatory drug).

▲ see page 210   ■ see page 125
★ see page 122

Symptoms

Usually, acute pericarditis causes fever and chest pain, which typically extends to the left shoulder and sometimes down the left arm. The pain may be similar to that of a heart attack, except that it tends to be made worse by lying down, swallowing food, coughing, or even deep breathing. The accumulating fluid or blood in the pericardial space puts pressure on the heart, interfering with its ability to pump blood. If the pressure is too high, cardiac tamponade—a potentially fatal condition—may occur.

Acute pericarditis due to tuberculosis begins insidiously, sometimes without obvious symptoms of lung infection. It may produce fever and symptoms of heart failure. Cardiac tamponade may occur.

Acute pericarditis due to a viral infection is usually painful but short-lived and has no lasting effects.

When acute pericarditis develops in the first day or two after a heart attack, symptoms of pericarditis are seldom noticed, because symptoms of the heart attack are the main concern.▲ Pericarditis that develops about 10 days to 2 months after a heart attack is usually accompanied by Dressler's syndrome (post–myocardial infarction syndrome), which includes fever, pericardial effusion (extra fluid in the pericardial space), pleurisy (inflammation of the pleura, which are the membranes covering the lungs), pleural effusion (fluid between the two layers of the pleura), and joint pain.

Diagnosis

Doctors can diagnose acute pericarditis based on the person's description of the pain and the sounds heard by listening through a stethoscope placed on the person's chest. Pericarditis can produce a crunching sound similar to the creaking of a leather shoe or a scratchy sound similar to the rustling of dry leaves (pericardial rub). Doctors can often diagnose pericarditis a few hours to a few days after a heart attack based on hearing these sounds.

A chest x-ray and echocardiography (a procedure that uses ultrasound waves to produce an image of the heart)■ may be useful because they can usually detect too much fluid in the pericardial space. Echocardiography may suggest the cause—for example, cancer. Electrocardiography (ECG) may be performed.★ ECG results may suggest pericarditis, but distinguishing pericarditis from a heart attack based

Cardiac Tamponade: The Most Serious Complication of Pericarditis

Cardiac tamponade is most commonly caused by accumulation of fluid or blood between the two layers of the pericardium as a result of cancer, injury, or surgery. Viral and bacterial infections and kidney failure are other common causes. The accumulating fluid or blood puts pressure on the heart, interfering with its ability to pump blood. As a result, when a person breathes in, blood pressure may fall rapidly to abnormally low levels and the pulse may correspondingly weaken. When a person breathes out, blood pressure increases and the pulse becomes stronger. This exaggeration in the variation in blood pressure and pulse that occurs with breathing is called a paradoxical pulse. Echocardiography (which uses ultrasound waves to produce an image of the heart) may be used to confirm the diagnosis. This procedure can detect characteristic changes, such as compression of the heart and the variations in blood flow in the heart that occur with breathing.

Cardiac tamponade is usually a medical emergency. Doctors treat it immediately by removing fluid from the pericardium using a needle or catheter to relieve the pressure in a procedure called pericardiocentesis. When time permits, fluid removal is closely monitored using echocardiography. Fluid may be surgically drained using a balloon-tipped catheter inserted through the skin (a procedure called percutaneous balloon pericardiotomy) or using a tube inserted through a small incision in the chest (a procedure called subxiphoid limited pericardiotomy). If the cause of pericarditis is unknown, doctors may send a sample of the fluid removed from the pericardium for examination under a microscope. This examination may provide information that helps identify the cause.

After the pressure is relieved, the person is usually kept in the hospital in case cardiac

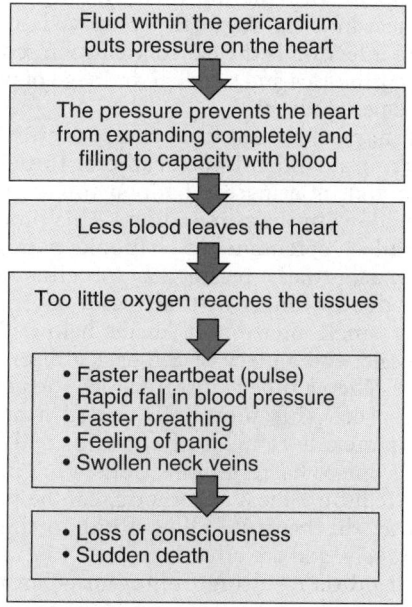

Fluid within the pericardium puts pressure on the heart

⬇

The pressure prevents the heart from expanding completely and filling to capacity with blood

⬇

Less blood leaves the heart

⬇

Too little oxygen reaches the tissues

⬇

- Faster heartbeat (pulse)
- Rapid fall in blood pressure
- Faster breathing
- Feeling of panic
- Swollen neck veins

⬇

- Loss of consciousness
- Sudden death

tamponade recurs. The person is usually monitored for 24 hours. The length of the hospital stay depends on the cause of tamponade. If a drain is in place, the person stays in the hospital until no more drainage occurs and the drain is removed.

If cardiac tamponade recurs, the same procedures may be performed again, or a different procedure may be tried. Other procedures include injection of a solution that obliterates the pericardium by causing scar tissue to form (sclerotherapy) and removal of the pericardium (pericardiectomy).

---

on ECG results may be difficult. Blood tests can detect some of the conditions that cause pericarditis—for example, leukemia, AIDS, other infections, rheumatic fever, and increased levels of urea in the blood resulting from kidney failure.

Treatment and Prognosis

Regardless of the cause, doctors usually hospitalize people with pericarditis, give them drugs that reduce inflammation and pain (such as aspirin, ibuprofen, or another nonsteroidal anti-inflammatory drug▲), and watch for complications, particularly cardiac tamponade. Intense pain may require an opioid, such as morphine, or a corticosteroid, such as prednisone. Prednisone does not directly reduce pain but relieves it by reducing inflammation. Drugs that may cause pericarditis are discontinued whenever possible.

▲ see page 452

Further treatment of acute pericarditis varies, depending on the cause. For people who have kidney failure, increasing the frequency of dialysis usually results in improvement. People who have cancer may respond to chemotherapy or radiation therapy, but often, the pericardium is surgically removed. If a bacterial infection is the cause, treatment consists of antibiotics and surgical drainage of pus from the pericardium.

Fluid may be drained from the pericardium by inserting a balloon-tipped catheter through the skin and inflating the balloon to create a hole (window) in the pericardium. This procedure, called percutaneous balloon pericardiotomy, is usually performed for effusions that are due to cancer or that recur. Alternatively, a small incision is made below the breast bone, and a piece of the pericardium is removed. Then a tube is inserted into the pericardial space. This procedure, called a subxiphoid pericardiotomy, is often performed for effusions due to bacterial infections. Both procedures require a local anesthetic, can be performed at the bedside, allow fluid to drain continuously, and are effective.

If pericarditis resulting from a virus, an injury, or an unidentified disorder recurs, aspirin, ibuprofen, or corticosteroids may provide relief. For some people, colchicine is effective. If drug treatment is ineffective, the pericardium is usually removed surgically.

When acute pericarditis occurs within the first few hours or days of a heart attack, treatment for the heart attack, including aspirin and stronger analgesics such as morphine, can usually reduce any discomfort due to pericarditis.

The prognosis for people who have pericarditis depends on the cause. When pericarditis is caused by a virus or when the cause is not apparent, recovery usually takes 1 to 3 weeks. Complications or recurrences can slow recovery. People with cancer that has invaded the pericardium rarely survive beyond 12 to 18 months.

Chronic Pericarditis

Chronic pericarditis is inflammation that begins gradually, is long-lasting, and results in fluid accumulation in the pericardial space or thickening of the pericardium.

There are two main types of chronic pericarditis. In **chronic effusive pericarditis,** fluid slowly accumulates in the pericardial space, between the two layers of the pericardium.

Chronic constrictive pericarditis is a rare disease that usually results when scarlike (fibrous) tissue forms throughout the pericardium. The fibrous tissue tends to contract over the years, compressing the heart. Thus, the heart does not enlarge as it does in most types of heart disease. Because higher pressure is needed to fill the compressed heart, pressure in the veins that return blood to the heart increases. Fluid accumulates in the veins, then leaks out, and accumulates in other areas of the body, such as under the skin.

Causes

Usually, the cause of chronic effusive pericarditis is unknown, but it may be cancer, tuberculosis, or an underactive thyroid gland (hypothyroidism).

Usually, the cause of chronic constrictive pericarditis is also unknown. The most common known causes are viral infections and radiation therapy for breast cancer or lymphoma. Chronic constrictive pericarditis may also result from any condition that causes acute pericarditis, such as rheumatoid arthritis, systemic lupus erythematosus, a previous injury, heart surgery, or a bacterial infection. Previously, tuberculosis was the most common cause of chronic pericarditis in the United States, but today tuberculosis accounts for only 2% of cases. In Africa and India, tuberculosis is still the most common cause of all forms of pericarditis.

Symptoms and Diagnosis

Symptoms of pericarditis include shortness of breath, coughing, and fatigue. Coughing occurs because the high pressure in the veins of the lungs forces fluid into the air sacs. Fatigue occurs because the abnormal pericardium interferes with the heart's pumping action, so that the heart cannot pump enough blood to meet the body's needs. Other common symptoms are accumulation of fluid in the abdomen (ascites) and in the legs (edema). Sometimes fluid accumulates in the space between the two layers of the pleura, the membranes covering the lungs (a condition called pleural effusion)▲. However, chronic pericarditis does not cause pain.

Chronic effusive pericarditis may produce few symptoms if fluid accumulates slowly.

▲ see page 314

The reason is that the pericardium can stretch gradually, so that cardiac tamponade may not occur. However, if fluid accumulates rapidly, the heart can become compressed and cardiac tamponade may occur.

Symptoms provide important clues that a person has chronic pericarditis, particularly if there is no other reason for reduced heart performance—such as high blood pressure, coronary artery disease, or a heart valve disorder.

Echocardiography▲ is often performed to confirm the diagnosis. It can detect the amount of fluid in the pericardial space and the formation of fibrous tissue around the heart. It can confirm the presence of cardiac tamponade. Chest x-rays may detect calcium deposits in the pericardium. These deposits develop in nearly half of the people who have chronic constrictive pericarditis.

The diagnosis can be confirmed in one of two ways. Cardiac catheterization can be used to measure blood pressure in the heart chambers and major blood vessels. These measurements help doctors distinguish pericarditis from similar disorders. Alternatively, magnetic resonance imaging (MRI) or computed tomography (CT) can be used to determine the thickness of the pericardium. Normally, the pericardium is less than $1/8$ inch thick, but in chronic constrictive pericarditis, it is usually $1/4$ inch thick or more.

A biopsy may be performed to help determine the cause of chronic pericarditis—for example, tuberculosis. A small sample of the pericardium is removed during exploratory surgery and examined under a microscope. Alternatively, a sample can be removed using a pericardioscope (a fiber-optic tube used to view the pericardium and to obtain tissue samples) inserted through an incision in the chest.

Treatment

Known causes of chronic effusive pericarditis are treated when possible. If heart function is normal, doctors take a wait-and-see approach. If the disorder causes symptoms or if an infection is suspected, surgical drainage may be performed.■

For people with chronic constrictive pericarditis, bed rest, restriction of salt in the diet, and diuretics (drugs that increase the excretion of fluid) may relieve symptoms. However, the only possible cure is surgical removal of the pericardium. Surgery cures about 85% of people. However, because the risk of death from surgery is 5 to 15%, most people do not have surgery unless the disease substantially interferes with daily activities. Surgery is not performed in the early stages of the disorder (before significant symptoms appear) or in the late stages (when symptoms occur at rest).

CHAPTER 31

Heart Tumors

A tumor is any type of abnormal growth, whether cancerous (malignant) or noncancerous (benign). Tumors that originate in the heart are called primary tumors. They may develop in any of the heart tissues and may be cancerous or noncancerous. Primary heart tumors are rare, occurring in fewer than 1 of 2,000 people. In adults, the most common type of noncancerous primary heart tumor is a myxoma, which accounts for about 50% of such tumors. In infants and children, the most common type of noncancerous primary heart tumor is a rhabdomyoma, which accounts for

about 40% of such tumors. Fibromas are the second most common noncancerous primary tumors in infants and children. Other tumors are extremely rare.

Myxomas usually develop in the heart's left upper chamber (atrium). They may develop from embryonic cells located in the inner layer (lining) of the heart's wall. Rhabdomyomas, which typically occur in groups, usually grow within the heart wall and develop di-

---

▲ see page 125   ■ see page 190

rectly from the heart's muscle cells. Rhabdomyomas commonly develop during infancy or childhood, often as part of a rare disease called tuberous sclerosis. Fibromas, which typically occur as a single tumor, usually grow on heart valves and develop from the heart's fibrous tissue cells.

Tumors that originate in some other part of the body—usually the lung, breast, blood, or skin—and then spread (metastasize) to the heart are called secondary tumors. They are always cancerous. Secondary heart tumors of the heart are 30 to 40 times more common than primary heart tumors but are still uncommon. About 10% of people who have lung or breast cancer—two of the most common cancers—and about 75% of people with malignant melanoma (which is becoming increasingly common) have metastases to the heart.

Symptoms

Heart tumors may cause no symptoms, minor symptoms, or symptoms of life-threatening heart malfunction, which resemble those of other heart diseases but which develop suddenly. For example, tumors may cause heart failure, abnormal heart rhythms (arrhythmias), or a decrease in blood pressure caused by bleeding into the pericardium, the sac that envelops the heart. Heart murmurs develop in about half of the people who have tumors that develop near or on a heart valve (such as myxomas and fibromas), because blood does not flow through the valve normally. Noncancerous tumors can be as deadly as cancerous ones if they interfere with the function of the heart.

Heart tumors, especially myxomas, may degenerate so that pieces of them break off and travel through the bloodstream (becoming emboli). Emboli may lodge in small arteries and block blood flow. Also, blood clots that form on the surface of tumors, such as myxomas, may break off as emboli and block arteries. Symptoms due to emboli depend on which tissues or organ is supplied by the blocked artery.

Diagnosis

Primary heart tumors are difficult to diagnose because they are relatively uncommon and because their symptoms resemble those of

many other disorders. Doctors may suspect a primary heart tumor in people who have heart murmurs, abnormal heart rhythms, unexplained symptoms of heart failure, or unexplained fever (which may be due to a myxoma). Secondary heart tumors are suspected when people who have cancer elsewhere in the body come to a doctor with symptoms of heart malfunction.

If a tumor is suspected, echocardiography▲ is usually performed to confirm the diagnosis. For this procedure, a probe that emits ultrasound waves is passed over the chest, producing an image of heart structures. If another view of the heart is needed, the probe can be passed down the throat into the esophagus to record signals from just behind the heart. This procedure is called transesophageal echocardiography. Computed tomography (CT)■ or magnetic resonance imaging (MRI) can provide additional information.★ Coronary angiography● can produce an outline of a heart tumor that can be seen on x-rays, but this procedure is rarely needed.

If a tumor is detected in the right side of the heart, a small sample may be removed for examination under a microscope (biopsy). The sample is removed with a catheter that is inserted into a vein, usually in the leg, and threaded toward the heart in a procedure called cardiac catheterization.◆ This procedure helps doctors identify the type of tumor and select the appropriate treatment. Biopsy of tumors on the left side is rarely performed, because the risks of the procedure outweigh the benefits.

Treatment

A single small noncancerous primary heart tumor can be surgically removed, usually resulting in a cure. If a large noncancerous primary tumor is significantly reducing blood flow through the heart, removal of the part of the tumor that does not grow into the heart wall may improve heart function. However, if a large part of the heart wall is involved, surgery may be impossible.

In about half of newborns who have noncancerous rhabdomyomas, tumors regress without treatment; in the other half, the tumors do not grow any larger and do not require treatment. In infants and children, a fibroma may be successfully removed if it does not affect the wall between the ventricles (septum). Tumors that affect this wall usually also affect the electrical conduction system of the heart

---

▲ see page 125   ■ see page 125
★ see page 126   ● see page 128
◆ see page 128

and cannot be surgically removed. Children with this type of tumor usually die of an abnormal heart rhythm at an early age. If a fibroma is large, blocks blood flow, and has grown into the surrounding tissue, heart transplantation may be required.

Primary cancerous tumors cannot be surgically removed and are usually fatal.

Myxomas

A myxoma is a noncancerous primary tumor, usually irregular in shape and jellylike in consistency.

Half of all primary heart tumors are myxomas. Three fourths of myxomas occur in the left atrium, the chamber of the heart that receives oxygen-rich blood from the lungs. Some types of myxomas tend to run in families. These hereditary myxomas usually develop in young men in their mid-20s. Myxomas that are not hereditary usually develop in women, typically between the ages of 40 and 60. These myxomas are more likely to occur in the left atrium than are hereditary myxomas.

Myxomas in the left atrium often grow from a stalk and swing freely with the flow of blood, as a tetherball does. As they swing, they may move in and out of the nearby mitral valve, the valve that opens from the left atrium into the left ventricle. This swinging motion may plug and unplug the valve over and over again, so that blood flow stops and starts intermittently.

Symptoms

When they stand, people with a myxoma in the left atrium may feel short of breath or may faint. With standing, the force of gravity pulls the myxoma into the opening of the mitral valve, blocking blood flow through the heart. This blockage causes transient heart failure. Lying down typically causes the myxoma to move away from the valve and relieves the symptoms.

Pieces of a myxoma or blood clots that form on the surface of the myxoma may break off (becoming emboli), travel through the bloodstream to other organs, and block arteries there. The resulting symptoms depend on which artery is blocked. For example, a blocked artery in the brain may cause a stroke; a blocked artery in the lung may cause pain and coughing up of blood.

How a Myxoma Can Block Blood Flow in the Heart

A myxoma in the left atrium often grows from a stalk and swings freely with the flow of blood. As it swings, the myxoma may move in and out of the nearby mitral valve, which opens from the left atrium into the left ventricle. This swinging motion may plug and unplug the valve over and over again, so that blood flow stops and starts intermittently.

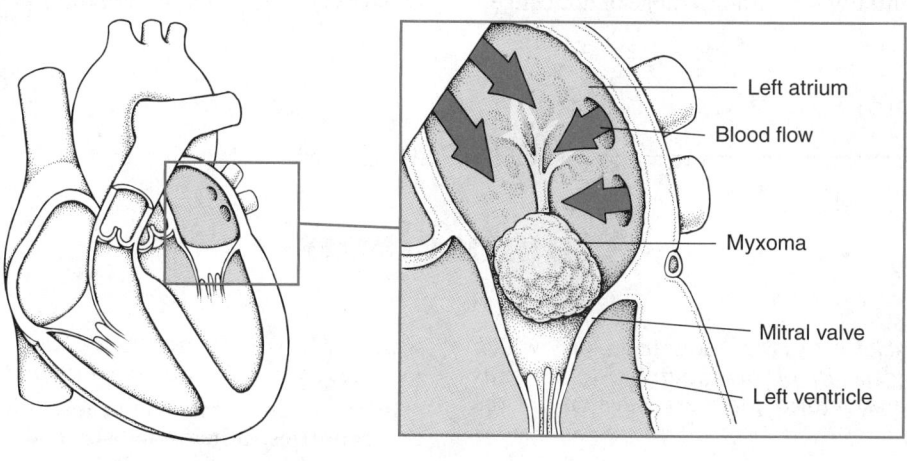

Left atrium
Blood flow
Myxoma
Mitral valve
Left ventricle

Other symptoms of myxomas include fever, weight loss, Raynaud's phenomenon (the fingers and toes become cold and painful when exposed to cold), a low red blood cell count (anemia), a high white blood cell count, and a low platelet count.

Diagnosis and Treatment

Myxomas are suspected based on the symptoms. With a stethoscope, doctors may hear a sound (heart murmur) produced by leakage of blood back through the mitral valve (mitral regurgitation▲). The cause may be damage to the mitral valve by a myxoma (a very rare cause) or damage by rheumatic fever (a relatively more common cause). Doctors can usually distinguish between a tumor and rheumatic fever based on the heart sounds and the person's medical history.

The diagnosis is confirmed by echocardiography. Other procedures, including angiography, computed tomography (CT), magnetic resonance imaging (MRI), and biopsy are sometimes necessary.

Surgical removal of the myxoma usually cures the person.

Cancerous Tumors

Cancerous primary heart tumors are extremely rare, accounting for about one fourth of primary heart tumors. The most common are sarcomas that develop from blood vessel tissue. Secondary heart tumors are far more common, but how common is difficult to determine.

Symptoms

The symptoms of cancerous heart tumors are essentially the same as those of noncancer-ous heart tumors and vary depending on the tumor's location. However, the symptoms of cancerous tumors tend to worsen more quickly than those of noncancerous tumors, because the cancerous tumor grows much faster. Other symptoms include sudden development of heart failure, abnormal heart rhythms, and bleeding into the pericardium, which may interfere with the heart's functioning and cause cardiac tamponade.■ Cancerous primary heart tumors may spread (metastasize) to the spine, nearby tissues, or organs such as the lungs and brain.

Symptoms of a secondary heart tumor often include those caused by the original tumor and may include those caused by metastases elsewhere in the body. Cancers, such as lung or breast cancer, may spread to the heart by direct invasion, often into the pericardium; the heart may be compressed because cancers cause blood and fluid to accumulate. Cancers may also spread to heart muscle and chambers through the bloodstream or through the lymph system; these cancers may produce symptoms of heart failure.

Diagnosis and Treatment

The procedures used to diagnose cancerous heart tumors are the same as those used for noncancerous heart tumors. For secondary tumors, procedures are performed to find the original tumor, unless its location is already known.

Because cancerous heart tumors—both primary and secondary—are almost always incurable, treatment is designed to reduce symptoms. Depending on the type of tumor, radiation therapy or chemotherapy is used.

CHAPTER 32

Atherosclerosis

Atherosclerosis is a condition in which patchy deposits of fatty material (atheromas or atherosclerotic plaques) develop in the walls of medium-sized and large arteries, leading to reduced or blocked blood flow.

In the United States and most other Western countries, atherosclerosis is the leading cause of illness and death. In the United States alone, it caused almost 1 million deaths in

---

▲ see page 175   ■ see box on page 189

1996—twice as many as cancer caused and 10 times as many as accidents caused. Despite significant medical advances, heart attacks due to coronary artery disease (atherosclerosis that affects the arteries supplying blood to the heart▲) and strokes (due to atherosclerosis that affects the arteries to the brain■) are responsible for more deaths than all other causes combined.

Atherosclerosis can affect the medium-sized and large arteries of the brain, heart, kidneys, other vital organs, and legs. It is the most important and most common type of **arteriosclerosis,** a general term for several diseases in which the wall of an artery becomes thicker and less elastic.

There are two main theories about why atherosclerosis develops: High levels of cholesterol in the blood injure the artery's lining, causing an inflammatory reaction and enabling cholesterol and other fatty materials to accumulate there. Or, repeated injury to the artery's wall may occur through various mechanisms involving the immune system or through direct toxicity. In both cases, there are changes that can lead to the formation of atheromas. The two theories are probably interrelated and are not mutually exclusive.

Atherosclerosis is thought to also involve inflammation, because certain white blood cells—lymphocytes, monocytes, and macrophages—are present throughout the development of atherosclerosis. These cells usually gather only when inflammation develops. Atherosclerosis begins when monocytes are activated and move out of the bloodstream into the wall of an artery. There, they are transformed into foam cells, which collect cholesterol and other fatty materials. In time, these fat-laden foam cells accumulate. They form patchy deposits (atheromas) in the lining of the artery's wall, causing a thickening there.

Infection may have a role in the development of atherosclerosis. The infection may be due to bacteria (*Chlamydia pneumoniae,* which can cause pneumonia, or *Helicobacter pylori,* which can contribute to stomach ulcers) or to a virus (as yet unidentified). Infection may damage the lining of the artery's wall, enabling atherosclerosis to begin.

Atheromas may be scattered throughout medium-sized and large arteries, but they usually form where the arteries branch—presumably because the constant turbulent blood flow at these areas injures the artery's wall,

What Is Arteriosclerosis?

Arteriosclerosis, which means hardening (sclerosis) of the arteries (arterio-), is a general term for several diseases in which the wall of an artery becomes thicker and less elastic. There are three types: atherosclerosis, arteriolosclerosis, and Mönckeberg's arteriosclerosis.

Atherosclerosis, the most common type, means hardening related to atheromas, which are deposits of fatty materials. It affects medium-sized and large arteries.

Arteriolosclerosis means hardening of the arterioles, which are small arteries. It affects primarily the inner and middle layers of the walls of arterioles. The walls thicken, narrowing the arterioles. As a result, organs supplied by the affected arterioles do not receive enough blood. The kidneys are often affected. This disorder occurs mainly in people who have high blood pressure or diabetes. Either of these disorders may stress the walls of arterioles, resulting in thickening.

Mönckeberg's arteriosclerosis affects small to medium-sized arteries. Calcium accumulates within the walls of arteries, making them stiff but not narrow. This essentially harmless disorder usually affects men and women older than 50.

making these areas more susceptible to atheroma formation.

Arteries affected by atherosclerosis also lose their elasticity, possibly contributing to high blood pressure. As the atheromas grow, the interior (lumen) of the arteries narrows. With time, calcium accumulates in the atheromas, which may become brittle and rupture. Blood may enter a ruptured atheroma, making it larger, so that it narrows the artery even more. A ruptured atheroma also may spill its fatty contents into the bloodstream. This fatty mass (fat embolus) may travel through the bloodstream and block an artery elsewhere in the body. More often, the rupture of an atheroma triggers the formation of a blood clot (thrombus), which is the main cause of a heart attack or stroke. The clot may further narrow or even block the artery, or the clot may detach (becoming an embolus), travel through the bloodstream, and block another artery downstream.

▲ see page 199   ■ see art on page 503

How Atherosclerosis Develops

The wall of an artery is composed of several layers. The lining or inner layer (endothelium) is usually smooth and unbroken. Atherosclerosis begins when the lining is injured or diseased. Then certain white blood cells called monocytes are activated and move out of the bloodstream and through the lining of an artery into the artery's wall. Inside the lining, they are transformed into foam cells, which are cells that collect fatty materials, mainly cholesterol. In time, smooth muscle cells move from the middle layer into the lining of the artery's wall and multiply there. Connective and elastic tissue materials also accumulate there, as may cell debris, cholesterol crystals, and calcium. This accumulation of fat-laden cells, smooth muscle cells, and other materials forms a patchy deposit called an atheroma or atherosclerotic plaque. As they grow, atheromas thicken the artery's wall and bulge into the channel of the artery. They may narrow or block an artery, reducing or stopping blood flow.

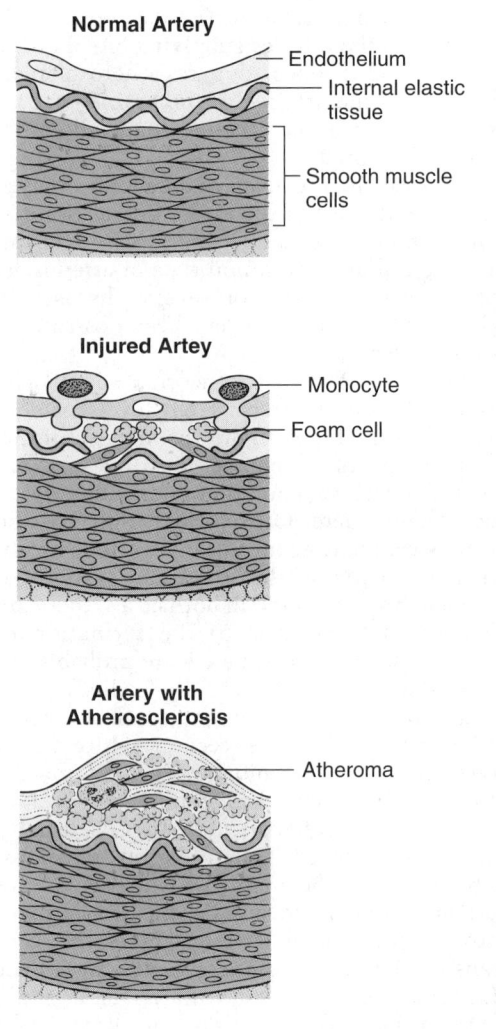

Normal Artery
— Endothelium
— Internal elastic tissue
— Smooth muscle cells

Injured Artey
— Monocyte
— Foam cell

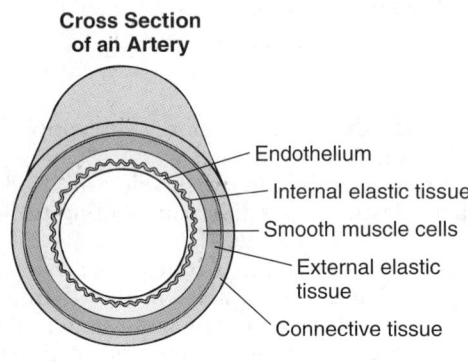

Cross Section of an Artery
— Endothelium
— Internal elastic tissue
— Smooth muscle cells
— External elastic tissue
— Connective tissue

Artery with Atherosclerosis
— Atheroma

Risk Factors

Risk factors for atherosclerosis include smoking, high levels of cholesterol in the blood, high blood pressure, diabetes, obesity, physical inactivity, and high blood levels of homocysteine (an amino acid). These risk factors can usually be modified.▲ Risk factors that cannot be modified include having a fam-

ily history of early atherosclerosis (that is, having a close relative who developed the disease at a young age), advancing age, and male sex. Men have a higher risk than women, although women who have coronary artery disease are more likely to die than men who have the disease.

Smoking: One of the most important modifiable risk factors is smoking. A smoker's risk of developing coronary artery disease is directly related to the number of cigarettes smoked daily. In people who already have a

▲ see also page 200

high risk of heart disease, smoking is particularly dangerous.

Smoking decreases the level of high-density lipoprotein (HDL) cholesterol—the "good" cholesterol—and increases the level of low-density lipoprotein (LDL) cholesterol—the "bad" cholesterol. Smoking increases the level of carbon monoxide in the blood, which may increase the risk of injury to the lining of the artery's wall. Smoking causes arteries already narrowed by atherosclerosis to constrict, further decreasing the amount of blood reaching the tissues. In addition, smoking increases the blood's tendency to clot (by making platelets stickier), so that it increases the risk of peripheral arterial disease (atherosclerosis affecting arteries other than those that supply the heart and brain),▲ coronary artery disease,■ stroke,★ and blockage of an arterial graft placed during bypass surgery.●

People who quit smoking have only half the risk of those who continue to smoke—regardless of how long they smoked before quitting. Quitting also decreases the risk of death after coronary artery bypass surgery or a heart attack and the risk of illness and death in people who have peripheral arterial disease. The benefits of quitting smoking begin immediately and increase with time.

Secondhand smoke (smoke breathed in from someone else's smoking) appears to increase risk also. It should be avoided.

High Cholesterol Levels: A high cholesterol level is another important modifiable risk factor. Lowering high cholesterol levels through the use of statins◆ can significantly reduce the risk of heart attacks, strokes, and death. Many of the risk factors for high cholesterol levels are also risk factors for atherosclerosis. They include smoking, diabetes, obesity, and physical inactivity. A high-fat diet causes cholesterol levels to increase in susceptible people. Cholesterol levels increase as people age and are normally higher in men than in women, although levels increase in women after menopause.

However, not all types of cholesterol increase the risk of atherosclerosis. A high level of LDL (bad) cholesterol increases the risk. A high level of HDL (good) cholesterol decreases the risk, and a low level increases the risk. Ideally, the level of total cholesterol, which includes LDL and HDL cholesterol and triglycerides, is 140 to 200 mg/dL. Risk of a heart attack more than doubles when the total cholesterol level approaches 300 mg/dL. The risk is decreased when the LDL cholesterol level is below 130 mg/dL, and the HDL cholesterol level is above 40 mg/dL.▼ However, the percentage of HDL cholesterol in relation to total cholesterol is a more reliable measure of risk than is the total or LDL cholesterol level. HDL cholesterol should account for more than 25% of total cholesterol. High triglyceride levels are often associated with low HDL cholesterol levels. However, evidence suggests that high triglyceride levels alone may also increase the risk of atherosclerosis.

Several hereditary disorders that result in high levels of cholesterol or other fats also increase the risk of atherosclerosis. For example, familial hypercholesterolemia, which can result in extremely high levels of cholesterol, causes atheromas to form, primarily in the coronary arteries. People who have this disease and are untreated die of coronary artery disease at an early age.

High Blood Pressure: Uncontrolled high diastolic or systolic blood pressure is a risk factor for heart attack and stroke, which are caused by atherosclerosis.

Diabetes Mellitus: People who have type I diabetes► tend to develop atherosclerosis that affects small arteries, such as those in the eyes and kidneys. Some people with type I diabetes and most people with type II diabetes tend to develop atherosclerosis in large arteries. These people also tend to develop atherosclerosis at an earlier age and more extensively than do people who do not have diabetes. The risk of developing atherosclerosis is 2 to 6 times higher for people with diabetes, particularly women. Women who have diabetes, unlike those who do not, are not protected from atherosclerosis before menopause.

Obesity: Obesity, particularly abdominal (truncal) obesity, increases the risk of coronary artery disease (atherosclerosis of the arteries that supply blood to the heart). Abdominal obesity increases the risk of other risk factors for atherosclerosis: high blood pressure, type 2 diabetes, and high cholesterol levels. Losing weight reduces the risk of all these disorders.

Physical Inactivity: Physical inactivity appears to increase the risk of developing coro-

---

▲ see page 216   ■ see page 199

★ see page 502   ● see pages 209 and 220

◆ see table on page 925

▼ see table on page 922   ► see page 962

nary artery disease, and much evidence suggests that regular exercise reduces this risk. Exercise can also help modify other risk factors for atherosclerosis—by lowering blood pressure and cholesterol levels and by helping with weight loss.

High Blood Levels of Homocysteine (Hyperhomocysteinemia): High levels of homocysteine (an amino acid) in the blood may directly injure the lining of arteries, making the formation of atheromas more likely. High homocysteine levels may also promote the formation of blood clots. Homocysteine levels increase with age, particularly after menopause. High homocysteine levels in the blood may be caused by homocystinuria (a hereditary disorder that causes excessive excretion of homocysteine in the urine). People who have this disorder develop extensive atherosclerosis, often at a young age. Atheromas form in many arteries, but not primarily in the coronary arteries, which supply the heart.

If hyperhomocysteinemia is due to a condition other than hereditary homocystinuria, the risk of atherosclerosis affecting the coronary arteries (as well as the arteries to the brain and the peripheral arteries) is increased. Conditions that may increase homocysteine levels in the blood include a deficiency of folic acid or of vitamin B_6 or B_{12}, kidney failure, some cancers (such as breast cancer), psoriasis, heavy smoking, and use of certain drugs. These drugs include those that interact with folic acid or vitamin B_6 or B_{12}, such as methotrexate (used to treat cancer) and the anticonvulsants phenytoin and carbamazepine; drugs that interfere with the absorption of homocysteine, such as the cholesterol-lowering drugs colestipol, cholestyramine, and niacin; and drugs that interfere with the metabolism of homocysteine, such as the antibiotic isoniazid.

Symptoms

Usually, atherosclerosis does not produce symptoms until it narrows the interior of an artery by more than 70%. Symptoms depend on where the narrowing or blockage, which can occur almost anywhere in the body, is. If the arteries supplying the heart (coronary arteries) are narrowed, chest pain (angina) can result; if they are blocked, a heart attack can result. Abnormal heart rhythms and heart failure may also develop. Blockage in the arteries supplying the brain (carotid arteries) can cause a stroke. Narrowing of the arteries in the legs can cause leg cramps (intermittent claudication▲). In people older than 55, the arteries supplying one or both kidneys may become narrowed or blocked, sometimes causing kidney failure or dangerously high blood pressure (malignant hypertension■).

Symptoms occur because as atherosclerosis narrows an artery more and more, tissues supplied by the artery may not receive enough blood and oxygen. The first symptom of a narrowing artery may be pain or cramps at times when blood flow cannot keep up with the tissues' need for oxygen. For instance, during exercise, a person may feel chest pain because the oxygen supply to the heart is inadequate; while walking, a person may feel leg cramps because the oxygen supply to the legs is inadequate.

Typically, symptoms develop gradually as the atheroma slowly narrows an artery. However, sometimes the first symptoms occur suddenly because the blockage occurs suddenly—for example, when a blood clot lodges in an artery narrowed by an atheroma, causing a heart attack or stroke.

Prevention and Treatment

To help prevent atherosclerosis, a person needs to be aware of the risk factors that can be modified—for example, smoking, high blood cholesterol levels, high blood pressure, obesity, and physical inactivity. So depending on a person's risk factors, prevention may consist of quitting smoking,★ lowering cholesterol levels,● lowering blood pressure,◆ losing weight,▼ and beginning an exercise program.▶

When atherosclerosis becomes severe enough to cause complications, the complications themselves must be treated. Complications include angina, heart attack, abnormal heart rhythms, heart failure, kidney failure, stroke, and leg cramps (intermittent claudication).

▲ see page 217   ■ see page 131

★ see page 200   ● see page 922

◆ see page 139   ▼ see page 918

▶ see page 32

CHAPTER 33

Coronary Artery Disease

Coronary artery disease is a condition in which the blood supply to the heart muscle is partially or completely blocked.

Coronary artery disease was once widely thought to be a man's disease. On average, men develop it about 10 years earlier than women, because until menopause, women are protected from the disease by high levels of estrogen. However, after menopause, the disease becomes more common among women. Among people aged 75 and older, a higher proportion of women have the disease, because women live longer.

In the United States, cardiovascular disease is the leading cause of death among both sexes, and coronary artery disease is the most common type of cardiovascular disease, occurring in about 5 to 9% (depending on sex and race) of people aged 20 and older. The death rate increases with age and overall is higher for men than for women, particularly between the ages of 35 and 55. After age 55, the death rate for men declines, and the rate for women continues to climb. After age 70 to 75, the death rate for women exceeds that for men who are the same age.

Coronary artery disease affects people of all races, but the incidence is extremely high among blacks and southeast Asians. The death rate is higher for black men than for white men until age 60 and is higher for black women than for white women until age 75.

Coronary artery disease is almost always due to the buildup of cholesterol and other fatty materials (called atheromas or atherosclerotic plaques) in the wall of a coronary artery. However, occasionally, the cause is spasm of an artery, and rarely, the cause is a birth defect, a viral infection (such as Kawasaki syndrome), lupus erythematosus, inflammation of the arteries (arteritis), or physical damage (from an injury or radiation therapy).

Fatty materials can build up gradually in arteries; this process, called atherosclerosis,▲ can affect different arteries. Coronary artery disease is due to atherosclerosis that develops in the arteries that encircle the heart and supply it with blood—the coronary arteries and their branches. As the atheromas grow, they bulge into the arteries, narrowing the interior (lumen) of the arteries and partially blocking blood flow. With time, calcium accumulates in the atheromas. An atheroma may rupture. Blood may enter a ruptured atheroma, making it larger, so that it narrows the artery even more. The rupture of an atheroma triggers the formation of a blood clot (thrombus). The clot may further narrow or even block the artery, or the clot may detach (becoming an embolus) and block another artery further downstream.

As an atheroma blocks more and more of a coronary artery, the supply of oxygen-rich blood to the heart muscle (myocardium) can become inadequate. An inadequate blood supply to the heart muscle is called myocardial ischemia. If the heart does not receive enough blood, it can no longer contract and pump blood normally. If an atheroma blocks an artery completely, the area of the heart muscle supplied by the artery dies, and a heart attack results.

Coronary artery disease is the most common cause of myocardial ischemia. The major complications of coronary artery disease are chest pain due to myocardial ischemia (angina) and heart attack (myocardial infarction).

Risk Factors

Some factors that affect whether a person develops coronary artery disease cannot be modified. They include advancing age, male sex, and a family history of early coronary artery disease (that is, having a close relative who developed the disease before age 50 to 55).

Other risk factors for coronary artery disease involve a person's lifestyle, which can be modified to reduce risk. These factors include high cholesterol levels, high blood pressure, smoking (the most important modifiable risk factor), a high-fat diet, physical inactivity, and obesity.

Reducing high levels of total and low-density lipoprotein (LDL) cholesterol■ and high blood pressure (hypertension)★ is important

---

▲ see page 194   ■ see pages 197 and 920
★ see page 131

because these disorders increase the risk of coronary artery disease. Changes in lifestyle or use of drugs can modify both disorders.

Smoking more than doubles the risk of developing coronary artery disease and having a heart attack. Secondhand smoke appears also to increase risk and should be avoided. Obesity,▲ which is becoming more common (especially in North America and Europe), also contributes greatly to the risk of coronary artery disease, particularly when fat is stored in the abdomen.

High levels of lipoprotein(a)—another type of cholesterol—and of triglycerides—another fat in the blood—may also increase risk. But high levels of high-density lipoprotein (HDL) cholesterol—the good cholesterol—may reduce risk. It may be increased by lifestyle changes.

Risk is also increased by a diet that is low in fiber, vitamins C and E, and phytochemicals (which are present in fruits and vegetables and which are thought to promote health). For some people, a diet low in fish oils (omega-3 polyunsaturated fatty acids) increases risk.

Having one or two drinks of alcohol a day appears to slightly reduce the risk of coronary artery disease (while slightly increasing that of stroke). However, having more than two drinks a day increases the risk, and the larger the amount, the greater the risk.

Certain disorders increase the risk of coronary artery disease. They include high levels of the amino acid homocysteine in the blood (hyperhomocysteinemia),■ diabetes, and low levels of thyroid hormones (hypothyroidism). Diabetes greatly increases the risk. Many people with diabetes have high blood pressure, have high cholesterol levels, are obese, and tend to be physically inactive. The cause of death in more than 80% of people with diabetes is a heart or blood vessel disorder.

Whether infection with certain organisms contributes to the development of coronary artery disease is uncertain. The organisms suspected include *Chlamydia pneumoniae* (which can cause pneumonia), *Helicobacter pylori* (which can contribute to stomach ulcers), and a virus (as yet unidentified). Nonetheless, inflammation, whether caused by infection or not, appears to contribute to the development of coronary artery disease. If an atheroma becomes inflamed, it softens and is more likely to rupture, and blood clots are more likely to form.

For men and women, the use of male steroids (androgens)—either the hormone testosterone or the synthetic anabolic steroids★—may also increase the risk of coronary artery disease. These drugs lower HDL (the good) cholesterol levels, increase LDL (the bad) cholesterol levels, and cause high blood pressure. All of these effects may contribute to having a heart attack at an early age or to having a stroke. What effects the use of anabolic steroids early in life have later in life are unclear.

Prevention

Modifying risk factors can help prevent coronary artery disease. Some of these factors are interrelated, so that modifying one also modifies another.

Smoking: Quitting smoking is most important. People who quit smoking decrease their risk of developing coronary artery disease by half compared with those who continue to smoke. How long people smoked before quitting does not matter. Quitting also decreases the risk of death after coronary artery bypass surgery or after a heart attack.

Diet: Limiting the amount of fat to no more than 25 to 35% of daily calories is recommended to promote good health. However, some experts believe that fat must be limited to 10% of daily calories to reduce the risk of coronary artery disease. A low-fat diet also helps lower high total and LDL (the bad) cholesterol levels, another risk factor for coronary artery disease.

The type of fat consumed is important. There are three types: saturated, monounsaturated, and polyunsaturated. Saturated fats are found in meats, non-skim dairy products, and artificially hydrogenated vegetable oils. The more solid the product, the higher the proportion of saturated fats. Monounsaturated fats are found in olive oil and canola oil. Polyunsaturated fats include omega-3 fats, contained in deep-sea fatty fish (such as mackerel, salmon, and tuna), and omega-6 fats, contained in vegetable oils. The ideal combination of types of fats is unknown. However, a diet high in saturated fats is known to promote coronary artery disease, and a diet high in monounsaturated or omega-3 fats is less likely to do so. Thus, eating fish regularly is recommended.

Eating at least five servings of fruits and vegetables daily can decrease the risk of coro-

▲ see page 914   ■ see page 198
★ see box on page 648

nary artery disease. Such foods contain many phytochemicals. Whether the phytochemicals are responsible for the risk reduction is unclear because people who consume such diets also tend to eat less fat, more fiber, and more foods containing vitamins C and E. One group of phytochemicals called flavonoids (found in red and purple grapes, red wine, and black teas) appears to be particularly protective.

A high-fiber diet is also recommended. There are two kinds of fiber. Soluble fiber (which dissolves in liquid) is found in oat bran, oatmeal, beans, peas, rice bran, barley, citrus fruits, strawberries, and apple pulp. It helps lower high cholesterol levels. It may decrease or sta-

bilize high blood sugar levels and increase low insulin levels. Thus, soluble fiber may help people with diabetes reduce their risk of coronary artery disease. Insoluble fiber (which does not dissolve in liquid) is found in most grains and grain products and in fruits and vegetables such as apple skin, cabbage, beets, carrots, brussels sprouts, turnips, and cauliflower. It helps with digestive function. However, eating too much fiber can interfere with the absorption of certain vitamins and minerals.

Eating soy products, such as tofu and tempeh, also seems to reduce the risk of coronary artery disease. Eating foods high in folic acid, such as citrus fruits, tomatoes, vegetables, and

Butter, Margarine, or Cholesterol-Lowering Margarine?

Substituting margarine for butter has been recommended as a way to help lower cholesterol levels and reduce the risk of coronary artery disease. Butter contains saturated fat, which is known to increase cholesterol levels, and margarine contains unsaturated fat, which has been thought to help lower cholesterol levels. However, some evidence suggests that margarines containing trans fatty acids increase LDL (the bad) cholesterol levels and lower HDL (the good) cholesterol levels. Whether these effects increase the risk of coronary artery disease is not known. Nonetheless, these effects suggest that avoiding such products is wise.

"Saturated" refers to the number of hydrogen atoms in a molecule of fat. Saturated fats contain as many hydrogen atoms as they can. They are usually solid at room temperature. Unsaturated fats (monounsaturated and polyunsaturated) do not contain as many hydrogen atoms as they could. Monounsaturated fats could contain one more hydrogen atom. They are usually liquid at room temperature but

start to solidify in the refrigerator. Olive oil and canola oil are examples. Polyunsaturated fats could contain more than one hydrogen atom. These fats are usually liquid at room and refrigerator temperatures. They tend to become rancid at room temperature. Corn oil is an example. Thus, liquid vegetable oils, such as olive or canola oil, contain less saturated fat than solid margarines or butter.

In a process called hydrogenation, hydrogen atoms are artificially added to polyunsaturated oils so that these oils may be used to make food products that do not become rancid and to make solid fat products, such as margarine. Trans fatty acids result from this process. ("Trans" refers to where the hydrogen atoms are added to the fat molecule.) Trans fatty acids are also found in prepared foods, such as cookies, crackers, doughnuts, french fries, and other fried foods.

Some evidence suggests that reducing the consumption of foods containing trans fatty acids can help lower cholesterol levels and thus reduce the risk of coronary artery disease. Identify-

ing foods containing trans fatty acids may be difficult because trans fatty acids are not listed on food labels. However, if hydrogenated fat or partially hydrogenated fat is the first fat on the list of ingredients, the product contains trans fatty acids. The appearance of a margarine or oil can also help identify foods containing these fatty acids—the softer or more liquidy, the smaller the trans fatty acid content. For example, the trans fatty acid content of tub margarines is smaller than that of stick margarines.

Some margarine products contain a plant sterol or stanol, which can lower total and LDL cholesterol levels. Plant sterols and stanols may have this effect because they are not absorbed well in the digestive tract and they interfere with the absorption of cholesterol. These margarine products have been approved as heart healthy foods when they are used as part of a healthy diet. These products are made from unsaturated fat, contain less saturated fat than butter, and do not contain trans fatty acids. However, they are expensive.

grain products, may lower homocysteine levels and thus help reduce risk. However, this effect has not been proved.

Overall, a person should maintain a healthy weight and eat a variety of foods. The Mediterranean diet, which consists of large portions of fruits, vegetables, nuts, and olive oil, appears to reduce the risk of coronary artery disease.

The diet should contain the recommended daily requirements of vitamins and minerals. Vitamin supplements are not considered an acceptable substitute for a healthy diet. The role of supplements in reducing the risk of coronary artery disease is somewhat controversial. There is no proof that taking supplements of vitamin E or vitamin C prevents coronary artery disease. Taking folic acid or vitamins B_6 and B_{12} may lower homocysteine levels, but evidence supporting their use by the general population is scanty.

Physical Inactivity: People who are physically active are less likely to develop coronary artery disease and high blood pressure. Exercise that promotes endurance (aerobic exercise such as brisk walking, bicycling, and jogging) or muscle strength (resistance training with free weights or weight machines) helps prevent coronary artery disease.▲ People who are out of shape or who have not exercised in a long time should consult their doctor before they start an exercise program.

Obesity: Modifying the diet and engaging in physical activity can help control obesity. Decreasing alcohol consumption can also help because alcohol is high in calories. A loss of even 10 to 20 pounds can reduce the risk of coronary artery disease.

High Cholesterol Levels: High total and LDL (the bad) cholesterol levels can be lowered by exercising and by quitting smoking as well as by reducing the amount of fat in the diet. Drugs that lower levels of total and LDL cholesterol in the blood (lipid-lowering drugs) may be used.■ The benefits of lowering cholesterol levels are greatest in people with other risk factors, such as smoking, high blood pressure, obesity, and physical inactivity.

Increasing the level of HDL (the good) cholesterol also helps reduce the risk of coronary artery disease. The same lifestyle changes that lower total and LDL cholesterol levels can help increase HDL cholesterol lev-

els. For people who are overweight, losing weight can also help.

High Blood Pressure: Lowering high blood pressure reduces the risk of coronary artery disease. Treatment of high blood pressure begins with lifestyle changes: eating a healthy diet that is low in salt and, if needed, losing weight and increasing physical activity. Drug therapy★ may also be necessary.

Diabetes Mellitus: Good control of diabetes reduces the risk of some complications of diabetes, but the effects of such control on the development of coronary artery disease are less clear. Good control of diabetes may also reduce the risk of complications of coronary artery disease.

Angina

Angina, also called angina pectoris, is temporary chest pain or a sensation of pressure that occurs while the heart muscle is not receiving enough oxygen.

In the United States, almost 6.5 million people have angina, and it is newly diagnosed in about 350,000 people each year. Angina tends to develop in women at a later age than in men. On average, angina occurs in about 3.9% of white women, 6.2% of black women, and 5.5% of Hispanic women and in about 2.6% of white men, 3.1% of black men, and 4.1% of Hispanic men.

Narrowing of the arteries due to fatty deposits (atheroma) or occasionally due to another abnormality may interfere with blood flow to the heart muscle and prevent it from receiving enough blood and oxygen. An inadequate blood supply (ischemia) to the heart sometimes causes angina. Angina usually first occurs during physical exertion or emotional distress, which make the heart work harder and increase its need for oxygen. The reduced blood flow through narrowed arteries cannot meet this increased need. If the artery is narrowed enough (usually by more than 70%), angina can occur even at rest, when the demands on the heart are at their minimum.

Not everyone with ischemia experiences angina. Ischemia without angina is called **silent ischemia.** Doctors do not understand why ischemia is sometimes silent, and some debate its significance. However, most experts consider silent ischemia as serious as ischemia with angina.

Nocturnal angina is angina that occurs at night, during sleep.

▲ see page 33   ■ see table on page 925
★ see table on page 138

Angina decubitus is angina that occurs when a person is lying down (not necessarily only at night) without any apparent cause. Angina decubitus occurs because gravity redistributes fluids in the body. This redistribution makes the heart work harder.

Variant angina results from a spasm of one of the large coronary arteries on the surface of the heart. It is called variant because it is characterized by pain during rest, not during exertion, and by specific changes detected with electrocardiography (ECG) during an episode of angina.

Unstable angina refers to angina in which the pattern of symptoms changes. Because the characteristics of angina in a particular person usually remain constant, any change—such as more severe pain, more frequent attacks, or attacks occurring with less exertion or during rest—is serious. Such change usually reflects a rapid progression of coronary artery disease, with an increasing narrowing of a coronary artery because an atheroma has ruptured or a clot has formed. The risk of a heart attack is high. Unstable angina is a medical emergency.

Causes

Usually, angina results from coronary artery disease.

A sudden temporary constriction of an artery (arterial spasm) may cause angina by abruptly decreasing the supply of blood and thus oxygen. Severe anemia may also cause angina. In anemia, the number of red blood cells (which contain hemoglobin—the molecule that carries oxygen) or the amount of hemoglobin in the cells is below normal. As a result, the oxygen supply to the heart muscle is reduced.

Syndrome X is a form of angina caused neither by spasm nor by any apparent blockage in the large coronary arteries. Temporary narrowing of much smaller coronary arteries may be responsible, at least in some people. The reasons for the temporary narrowing are unknown but may involve a chemical imbalance in the heart or abnormalities in the functioning of small arteries (arterioles). This syndrome is sometimes called cardiac syndrome X to distinguish it from another disorder also called syndrome X (metabolic syndrome X or the syndrome of insulin resistance▲).

Unusual causes of angina include severe high blood pressure; narrowing of the aortic valve (aortic valve stenosis); leakage of the aortic valve (aortic valve regurgitation); and thickening of the walls of the ventricles (hy-

pertrophic cardiomyopathy), especially thickening of the wall separating the ventricles (hypertrophic obstructive cardiomyopathy). These conditions increase the amount of work (workload) for the heart and thus the amount of oxygen needed by the heart muscle. When the need for oxygen exceeds the supply, angina results. Abnormalities of the aortic valve may reduce blood flow through the coronary arteries, because the openings of the coronary arteries are located just beyond this valve.

Symptoms

Most commonly, a person feels angina as pressure or an ache beneath the breastbone (sternum). Pain also may occur in either shoulder or down the inside of either arm; through the back; and in the throat, jaw, or teeth. Many people describe the feeling as discomfort or heaviness rather than pain.

In older people, symptoms may be different and therefore easily misdiagnosed. For instance, the pain is less likely to occur beneath the breastbone. Pain may occur in the back and shoulders and may be incorrectly blamed on arthritis. Pain may occur in the stomach area, particularly after meals (because extra blood is needed to help in digestion). Such pain may be called indigestion and blamed on a stomach ulcer. Also, older people who have confusion or dementia may have difficulty in communicating that they have pain.

Symptoms may also be different in women. Women are more likely to have unusual types of chest discomfort.

Typically, angina is triggered by exertion, lasts no more than a few minutes, and subsides with rest. Some people experience angina predictably with a specific degree of exertion. In other people, episodes occur unpredictably. Often, angina is worse when exertion follows a meal. It is usually worse in cold weather. Walking into the wind or moving from a warm room into the cold air may trigger angina. Emotional stress may also cause or worsen angina. Sometimes, experiencing a strong emotion while resting or having a bad dream during sleep can cause angina.

Diagnosis

Doctors diagnose angina largely based on a person's description of the symptoms. A physical examination and electrocardiography

---

▲ see box on page 922

(ECG)▲ may detect little, if anything, abnormal between and sometimes even during attacks of angina, even in people with extensive coronary artery disease. During an attack, the heart rate may increase slightly, blood pressure may go up, and with a stethoscope, doctors may hear a change in the heartbeat. ECG may detect changes in the heart's electrical activity.

When symptoms are typical, the diagnosis is usually easy for doctors. The kind of pain, its location, and its association with exertion, meals, weather, and other factors help doctors make the diagnosis. The presence of risk factors for coronary artery disease also helps establish the diagnosis. If a person experiences chest pain during the examination, a doctor may place a dose of nitroglycerin (a drug that dilates blood vessels) under the person's tongue as a test; if the pain is due to angina, relief should occur in less than 3 minutes.

The following procedures may help evaluate the inadequate blood supply (ischemia) to the heart muscle and determine whether coronary artery disease is present and how extensive it is.

For **exercise stress testing,**■ the person walks on a treadmill or rides a stationary bicycle while being monitored by ECG. This procedure can help doctors determine whether coronary angiography or coronary artery bypass surgery is needed. If people cannot exercise, testing is performed after a drug that makes the heart work harder is injected.

For **radionuclide imaging,**★ a tiny amount of a radioactive substance is injected into a vein. Radionuclide imaging can identify the location and extent of ischemia and show the amount of blood reaching the heart muscle. This procedure may be combined with stress testing.

Echocardiography● uses ultrasound waves to produce images of the heart (echocardiograms). This procedure shows heart size, movement of the heart muscle, blood flow through the heart valves, and valve function. Echocardiography is performed during rest and exercise. When ischemia is present, the pumping motion of the left ventricle is abnormal.

For **coronary angiography,**◆ x-rays of arteries are taken after a radiopaque dye is injected. Coronary angiography, the most accurate procedure for diagnosing coronary artery disease, may be performed when a diagnosis is uncertain. Coronary angiography is commonly used to help evaluate whether coronary artery bypass surgery or angioplasty is appropriate. Angiography can also detect spasm of an artery. A drug that can produce a spasm may be used during angiography if a spasm does not occur.

In a few people who have typical symptoms of angina and abnormal results on an exercise stress test, coronary angiography does not confirm the presence of coronary artery disease. Some of these people have syndrome X, but for most, the source of the symptoms does not involve the heart.

Continuous ECG monitoring with a Holter monitor▼ may detect abnormalities indicating symptomatic or silent ischemia or variant angina (which typically occurs during rest).

Prognosis

Key factors that can worsen the outcome (prognosis) for people who have angina include advancing age, extensive coronary artery disease, diabetes, the presence of other risk factors (particularly smoking), severe pain, and, most important, reduced pumping ability of the heart (ventricular function). For example, the more coronary arteries affected or the larger the blockage of the arteries, the worse the prognosis. The prognosis is surprisingly good for people with stable angina and normal pumping ability. Reduced pumping ability dramatically worsens the prognosis. The prognosis for people with syndrome X does not differ from that for people without coronary artery disease.

The death rate each year for people with angina and no other risk factors is about 1.4%. The rate is higher for people with risk factors such as high blood pressure, abnormal ECG results, or a previous heart attack.

Treatment

Treatment begins with attempts to slow the progression of coronary artery disease or to reverse it by dealing with risk factors. Risk factors, such as high blood pressure and high cholesterol levels, are treated promptly. Quitting smoking is crucial. A low-fat, varied diet and exercise (for most people) are recommended. Weight loss, if needed, is also recommended.

Treatment of angina depends partly on the stability and severity of the symptoms. When symptoms are stable and mild to moderate,

---

▲ see page 122   ■ see page 123
★ see page 127   ● see page 125
◆ see page 128   ▼ see art on page 124

the most effective treatment may be modification of risk factors and the use of certain drugs. When symptoms worsen rapidly, immediate hospitalization is usually also required. If lifestyle changes (including a change in diet) to modify risk factors and drug therapy do not cause symptoms to subside markedly, angiography may be used to determine if coronary artery bypass surgery or angioplasty is needed and feasible. However, surgical techniques are only mechanical measures for correcting the immediate problem. They do not cure the underlying disease. To improve their overall prognosis, people still need to modify risk factors. For example, lowering LDL cholesterol levels as much as possible using drugs may reduce angina as effectively as angioplasty over a period of 6 months or more.

Treatment of stable angina is designed to prevent or reduce ischemia and to minimize symptoms. Five types of drugs are available: beta-blockers, nitrates, calcium channel blockers, angiotensin-converting enzyme (ACE) inhibitors, and antiplatelet drugs.

People with syndrome X are usually given nitrates or beta-blockers to relieve symptoms.

People with unstable angina should usually be hospitalized, so that doctors can closely monitor drug therapy and use other therapies if necessary. These people are given drugs that reduce the clotting tendency of blood. These drugs include heparin (an anticoagulant given intravenously) and aspirin (an antiplatelet drug). People with an allergy to aspirin may be given ticlopidine or clopidogrel instead. A glycoprotein IIb/IIIa inhibitor (another type of antiplatelet drug), such as abciximab and tirofiban, may also be given. Beta-blockers and intravenous nitroglycerin are given to reduce the workload of the heart. If drug therapy is not effective, coronary angiography followed, if possible, by angioplasty or coronary artery bypass surgery may be necessary. Doctors may decide to perform angioplasty or coronary artery bypass surgery after they consider many factors, including the severity of disease and the characteristics of the person (including age).

Drug Therapy

Beta-blockers interfere with the effects of the hormones epinephrine (adrenaline) and norepinephrine (noradrenaline) on the heart and other organs. These hormones stimulate the heart to beat faster and more forcefully and most arterioles to constrict (causing blood pressure to increase▲). Thus, beta-blockers reduce the resting heart rate and blood pressure. During exercise, they limit the increase in heart rate and in blood pressure and so reduce the demand for oxygen. Beta-blockers reduce the risk of heart attacks and sudden death, improving the long-term outcome for people with coronary artery disease.

Nitrates, such as nitroglycerin, dilate blood vessels. Either short-acting or long-acting nitrates can be taken. Taking nitroglycerin, a short-acting nitrate, usually relieves an episode of angina in 1 to 3 minutes; the effects last 30 minutes. Nitroglycerin is usually taken as a tablet placed under the tongue (sublingual administration) or as a spray inhaled through the mouth. Alternatively, the tablet may be placed next to the gum. People with chronic stable angina should keep nitroglycerin tablets or spray with them at all times. Taking nitroglycerin just before reaching a level of exertion known to induce angina may be useful.

Long-acting nitrates (such as isosorbide) are taken by mouth 1 to 4 times a day. Nitrate skin patches and paste, in which the drug is absorbed through the skin over many hours, are also effective. Long-acting nitrates taken regularly can soon lose their ability to provide relief. Most experts recommend that people not take the drug for an 8- to 12-hour period each day, usually at night unless that is when angina occurs. This approach helps maintain the long-term effectiveness of the drug. Unlike beta-blockers, nitrates do not reduce the risk of heart attacks and sudden death, but they greatly reduce symptoms in people with coronary artery disease.

Calcium channel blockers prevent blood vessels from narrowing (constricting) and can counter coronary artery spasm. These drugs are also effective in treating variant angina. All calcium channel blockers reduce blood pressure. Some of these drugs, such as verapamil and diltiazem, may also reduce the heart rate. This effect can be useful to many people, especially those who cannot take beta-blockers.

ACE inhibitors, such as ramipril, are often given to people who have evidence of coronary artery disease, including angina. These drugs can reduce the risk of heart attack and of death due to coronary artery disease.

▲ see page 140

TYPE	EXAMPLES	SIDE EFFECTS	COMMENTS
Anticoagulants	Enoxaparin Heparin Hirudin Warfarin	Bleeding, especially when used with other drugs that have a similar effect (such as aspirin and other non-steroidal anti-inflammatory drugs)	These drugs prevent blood from clotting. They are used to treat people who have unstable angina or who have had a heart attack.
Antiplatelet drugs	Aspirin Clopidogrel Ticlopidine	Bleeding, especially when used with other drugs that have a similar effect (such as anticoagulants) With aspirin, stomach irritation With ticlopidine and less so with clopidogrel, a small risk of reducing the white blood cell count	These drugs prevent platelets from clumping and blood clots from forming. They also reduce the risk of a heart attack. They are used to treat people who have stable or unstable angina or who have had a heart attack. Aspirin is taken as soon as a heart attack is suspected. People with an allergy to aspirin may take clopidogrel or ticlopidine as an alternative.
Glycoprotein IIb/IIIa inhibitors (a type of antiplatelet drug)	Abciximab Eptifibatide Tirofiban	Bleeding, especially when used with other drugs that have a similar effect (such as anticoagulants or thrombolytic drugs); reduction of the platelet count	These drugs prevent platelets from clumping and blood clots from forming. They are used to treat people who have unstable angina or who are undergoing percutaneous transluminal coronary angioplasty after a heart attack.
Beta-blockers	Acebutolol Atenolol Betaxolol Bisoprolol Carteolol Metoprolol Nadolol Penbutolol Propranolol Timolol	Spasm of airways (bronchospasm), an abnormally slow heart rate (bradycardia), heart failure, cold hands and feet, insomnia, fatigue, shortness of breath, depression, Raynaud's phenomenon, vivid dreams, hallucinations, and sexual dysfunction With some beta-blockers, an increased triglyceride level	These drugs reduce the workload of the heart and the risk of a heart attack and sudden death. They are used to treat people who have stable or unstable angina or syndrome X or who have had a heart attack.
Calcium channel blockers	Amlodipine Diltiazem Felodipine Isradipine Nicardipine Nifedipine (sustained-release only) Nisoldipine Verapamil	Dizziness, fluid accumulation (edema) in the ankles, flushing, headache, heartburn, enlarged gums, and abnormal heart rhythms (arrhythmias) With verapamil, constipation	These drugs prevent blood vessels from narrowing and can counter artery spasm. Diltiazem and verapamil reduce the heart rate. Calcium channel blockers are used to treat people who have stable angina.

206

TYPE	EXAMPLES	SIDE EFFECTS	COMMENTS
Calcium channel blockers (*continued*)			
		With short-acting, but not long-acting, calcium channel blockers, possible increased risk of death due to heart attack, especially in people who have unstable angina or who have had a heart attack recently	
Nitrates			
	Isosorbide dinitrate Isosorbide mononitrate Nitroglycerin	Flushing, headache, and a temporarily fast heart rate (tachycardia)	These drugs relieve angina, prevent episodes of angina, and reduce the risk of a heart attack and sudden death. (However, risk reduction is much less than that with beta-blockers.) They are used to treat people who have stable or unstable angina or syndrome X. 8- to 12-hour periods without taking the drug are needed daily to maintain the long-term effectiveness of the drug.
Opioids			
	Morphine	Low blood pressure when a person stands, constipation, nausea, vomiting, and confusion (especially in older people)	In people who have had a heart attack, these drugs are used to relieve anxiety and pain if the pain persists despite use of other drugs.
Thrombolytic drugs			
	Anistreplase Recombinant tissue plasminogen activator (alteplase) Reteplase Streptokinase Tenecteplase	Bleeding after injuries and, rarely, bleeding within the brain (intracerebral hemorrhage)	These drugs dissolve blood clots. They are used to treat people who have had a heart attack.

Antiplatelet drugs, such as aspirin, ticlopidine, and clopidogrel, modify platelets so that they do not clump on blood vessel walls. Platelets, which circulate in the blood, promote clot formation (thrombosis) when a blood vessel is injured. However, when platelets collect on atheromas in an artery's walls, the resulting clot can narrow or block the artery and result in a heart attack. Aspirin modifies platelets irreversibly and thus reduces the risk of death from coronary artery disease. Doctors recommend that most people who have coronary artery disease take one baby aspirin, one half of an adult aspirin, or one full adult aspirin daily to reduce the risk of a heart attack. People with an allergy to aspirin may take ticlopidine or clopidogrel as an alternative. Antiplatelet drugs are given to people with angina unless there is a reason not to; for example, they are not given to people who have a bleeding disorder.

Coronary Angioplasty

Generally, angioplasty (also called percutaneous transluminal coronary angioplasty—PTCA) is preferred to bypass surgery because it is a less invasive procedure. However, the affected area of the coronary artery may not be suited to angioplasty because of its location, its length, the amount of calcium that accumulates, or other conditions. Thus, doctors carefully determine whether a person is a good candidate for the procedure. When the affected area is clearly defined or the person is critically ill, angioplasty may be performed during angiography. The person is usually awake during the procedure.

Less than 1 to 2% of people die during angioplasty, and 3 to 5% have nonfatal heart attacks. Coronary artery bypass surgery becomes necessary immediately after angioplasty for 2 to 4% of people.

For the procedure, a large needle is inserted into a large peripheral artery, usually the main artery of the thigh (femoral artery). Then a long guide wire is threaded through the nee-

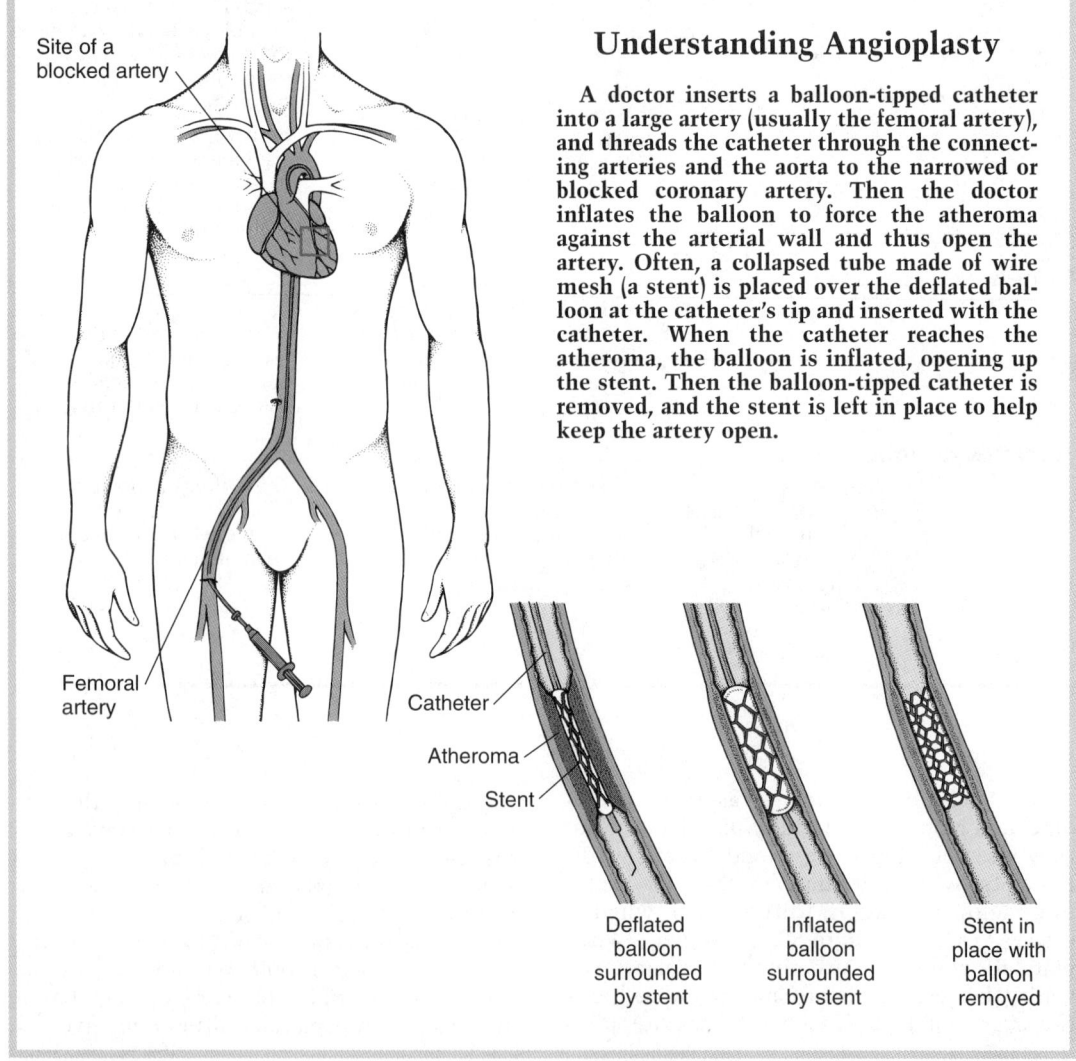

Site of a blocked artery

Femoral artery

Catheter

Atheroma

Stent

Understanding Angioplasty

A doctor inserts a balloon-tipped catheter into a large artery (usually the femoral artery), and threads the catheter through the connecting arteries and the aorta to the narrowed or blocked coronary artery. Then the doctor inflates the balloon to force the atheroma against the arterial wall and thus open the artery. Often, a collapsed tube made of wire mesh (a stent) is placed over the deflated balloon at the catheter's tip and inserted with the catheter. When the catheter reaches the atheroma, the balloon is inflated, opening up the stent. Then the balloon-tipped catheter is removed, and the stent is left in place to help keep the artery open.

Deflated balloon surrounded by stent

Inflated balloon surrounded by stent

Stent in place with balloon removed

dle, into the artery, and eventually through the aorta into the narrowed coronary artery. A catheter with a balloon attached to the tip is threaded over the guide wire and into the narrowed coronary artery. The catheter is positioned so that the balloon is at the level of the narrowing. The balloon is then inflated for several seconds. Inflation and deflation may be repeated several times.

The person is closely monitored during the procedure because balloon inflation momentarily blocks blood flow in the affected coronary artery. This blockage can produce chest pain and changes in the heart's electrical activity (detected by ECG) in some people. The inflated balloon compresses the atheroma that is narrowing the artery and widens the artery. When angioplasty is successful, the narrowing is greatly reduced. In 80 to 90% of people, the narrowed arteries that are reached are opened.

In about 20 to 30% of people, the coronary artery becomes blocked again within 6 months—often within the first few weeks after the procedure. A second angioplasty is often performed and may successfully control coronary artery disease over the long term. To keep the artery open, doctors may insert a tube made of wire mesh (a stent) into the artery. This procedure appears to reduce the risk of a subsequent narrowing in the same place by half. Stents are used in 60 to 85% of people who undergo angioplasty.

Few studies have compared the results of angioplasty with drug therapy. Success rates of angioplasty are thought to be similar to those of bypass surgery. In a study comparing bypass surgery with angioplasty, recovery time was shorter after angioplasty, and the risk of death and heart attack remained about the same over the 2½ years of the study. People who have diabetes appear to have a better outcome with bypass surgery than with angioplasty.

Coronary Artery Bypass Surgery

This surgery, commonly called bypass surgery, is highly effective for people who have angina and coronary artery disease. It can improve exercise tolerance, relieve symptoms, and decrease the number or dose of drugs needed. Bypass surgery is most likely to benefit people who have severe angina that is not relieved by drug therapy, a normally functioning heart, no previous heart attacks, and no other conditions that would make surgery hazardous (such as chronic obstructive pulmonary disease). For such people, bypass

surgery that is not performed on an emergency basis carries a risk of death of 1% or less and a risk of heart damage (such as a heart attack) during surgery of less than 5%. About 85% of people have complete or dramatic relief of symptoms after surgery.

The risks from surgery are somewhat higher for people with reduced pumping ability of the heart (poor left ventricular function), damaged heart muscle from a previous heart attack, or other cardiovascular problems. However, if these people survive the surgery, their prospects for long-term survival are improved.

Bypass surgery consists of grafting veins or arteries from another part of the body to a coronary artery and to the aorta (the major artery that takes blood from the heart to the rest of the body). Blood flow is thus rerouted, skipping over (bypassing) the narrowed or blocked area. Veins are usually taken from the leg. Arteries are usually taken from beneath the breastbone (sternum) or from the forearm. Artery grafts rarely develop coronary artery disease, and more than 90% of them still work properly 10 years after the bypass surgery. However, vein grafts may gradually become narrowed by atheromas, and after 5 years, one third or more may be completely blocked.

The operation takes 2 to 4 hours, depending on the number of blood vessels to be grafted. A numeric modifier (for example, triple or quadruple) before bypass refers to the number (3 or 4) of arteries that are bypassed. The person is given a general anesthetic. Then, an incision is made down the center of the chest from the neck to the top of the stomach, and the breastbone is parted. This type of surgery is called open-heart surgery. Usually, the heart is stopped so that it is not moving and thus easier to operate on. A heart-lung machine is then used to pump blood through the bloodstream. When only one or two blood vessels require grafting, the heart may be left pumping. The hospital stay is typically 5 to 7 days, usually less if a heart-lung machine was not used during surgery.

With new techniques, chest incisions can be much smaller, resulting in minimally invasive coronary artery bypass surgery. One technique involves robotics. While sitting at a computer console, a surgeon uses pencil-sized robotic arms to perform the operation. The arms hold specially designed surgical instruments that can perform intricate movements, mimicking those of the surgeon's hands. Through a viewing scope, the surgeon watches a magnified

Coronary Artery Bypass Surgery

Coronary artery bypass surgery consists of attaching an artery or part of a vein to a coronary artery, so that the blood has an alternate route to the aorta. As a result, the narrowed or blocked area is bypassed. An artery is preferred to a vein because arteries are less likely to become blocked later. In one type of bypass surgery, one of the two internal mammary arteries is cut, and one of the cut ends is attached to a coronary artery beyond the blocked area. The other end of this artery is tied off. If an artery cannot be used or if there is more than one blockage, a section of a vein—usually, from the saphenous vein, which runs from the groin to the ankle—is used. One end of the section (graft) is attached to the aorta, and the other to a coronary artery beyond the blocked area. Sometimes a vein graft is used in addition to the mammary artery graft.

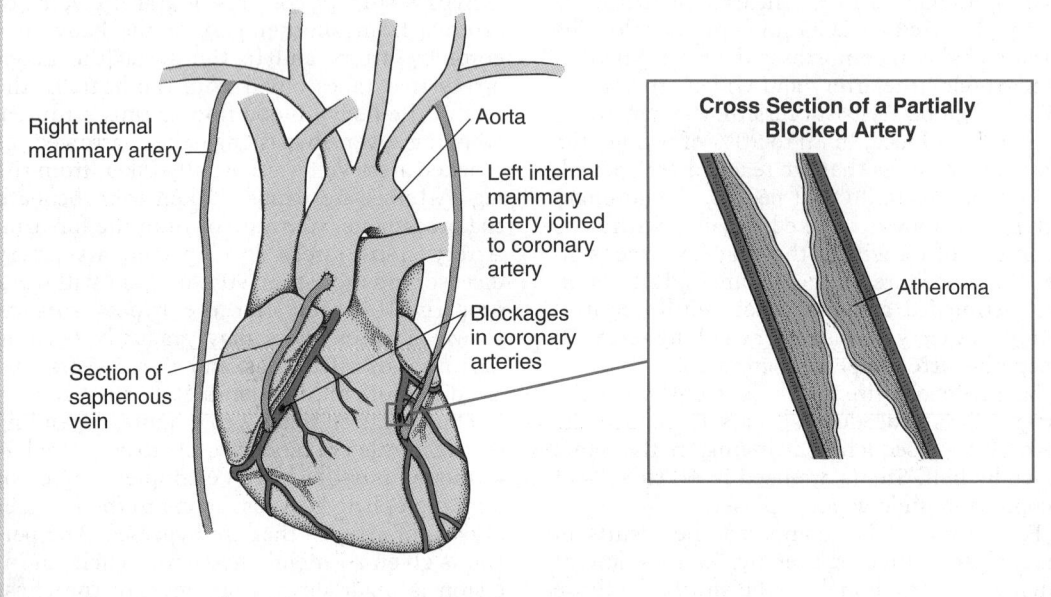

Right internal mammary artery

Aorta

Left internal mammary artery joined to coronary artery

Blockages in coronary arteries

Section of saphenous vein

Cross Section of a Partially Blocked Artery

Atheroma

three-dimensional image of the operation. Thus, the surgeon does not need to be in the same room as the patient. The operation requires three 1-inch incisions—one for each of the two robotic arms and one for a camera, which is connected to the scope. The operating time and hospital stay are usually shorter with the new procedures than with open-heart surgery.

In an experimental technique (called percutaneous in situ coronary venous arterialization), bypass is performed without surgery. A catheter is threaded to the blocked or narrowed coronary artery and used to make a connection between the artery and a nearby coronary vein. The vein then functions as an artery, supplying blood to the heart.

Other Techniques

New techniques to remove atheromas include the use of tiny blades, burrs, or lasers to remove thick, fibrous, and calcified atheromas by cutting, shaving, crushing, or dissolving them. Some of these techniques are still being evaluated, but so far, the results, especially over the long term, have been disappointing.

Heart Attack

Heart attack (myocardial infarction) is a medical emergency in which some of the heart's blood supply is suddenly and severely reduced or cut off, causing the heart muscle (myocardium) to die because it is deprived of its oxygen supply.

In the United States, more than 1.1 million people have a heart attack each year; about two thirds of them are men. Almost all of them have underlying coronary artery disease.

A heart attack usually occurs when a blockage in a coronary artery greatly reduces or cuts off the blood supply to an area of the heart. If the supply is greatly reduced or cut off for more than a few minutes, heart tissue dies.

Causes

A blood clot is the most common cause of a blocked coronary artery. Usually, the artery is already partially narrowed by atheromas. An atheroma may rupture or tear, narrowing the artery further and making blockage by a clot more likely. The ruptured atheroma not only reduces the flow of blood through an artery but also releases substances that make platelets stickier, further encouraging clots to form.

Uncommonly, a heart attack results when a clot forms in the heart itself, breaks away, and lodges in a coronary artery. Another uncommon cause is a spasm of a coronary artery that stops blood flow. Spasms may be caused by drugs. Sometimes the cause is unknown.

Symptoms

About two of three people who have heart attacks experience intermittent chest pain (angina▲), shortness of breath, or fatigue a few days or weeks beforehand. The episodes of pain may become more frequent and occur after less and less physical exertion. Such a change in the pattern of chest pain (unstable angina■) may culminate in a heart attack.

Usually, the most recognizable symptom of a heart attack is pain in the middle of the chest that may spread to the back, jaw, or left arm. Less often, the pain spreads to the right arm. The pain may occur in one or more of these places and not in the chest at all. The pain of a heart attack is similar to the pain of angina but is generally more severe, lasts longer, and is not relieved by rest or nitroglycerin. Less often, pain is felt in the abdomen, where it may be mistaken for indigestion, especially because belching may bring partial or temporary relief.

About one third of people who have a heart attack do not have chest pain. Such people are more likely to be women, people who are not white, those who are older than 75, those who have heart failure or diabetes, or those who have had a stroke.

Other symptoms include a feeling of faintness, sudden heavy sweating, nausea, shortness of breath, and a heavy pounding of the heart.

Abnormal heart rhythms (arrhythmias) occur in more than 90% of people who have had a heart attack. Immediately and up to a few days after a heart attack, abnormal heart rhythms are a common reason that the heart cannot pump adequately. Abnormal heart rhythms originating in the ventricles (ventricular arrhythmias) may greatly interfere with the heart's pumping ability or may cause the heart to stop pumping effectively (cardiac arrest). A loss of consciousness or death can result. Sometimes loss of consciousness is the first symptom of a heart attack.

During a heart attack, a person may become restless, sweaty, and anxious and may experience a sense of impending doom. The lips, hands, or feet may turn slightly blue.

Older people may have unusual symptoms. In many, the most obvious symptom is breathlessness. Symptoms may resemble those of a stomach upset or a stroke. Older people may become disoriented. Nonetheless, about two thirds of older people have chest pain as do younger people. Older people, especially women, often take longer than younger people to admit they are ill or to seek medical help.

Despite all the possible symptoms, as many as one of five people who have a heart attack have only mild symptoms or none at all. Such a silent heart attack may be recognized only when electrocardiography (ECG) is routinely performed some time afterward.

During the early hours of a heart attack, heart murmurs and other abnormal heart sounds may be heard through a stethoscope.

Complications

The heart's ability to keep pumping after a heart attack is directly related to the extent and location of the damaged or dead tissue. Dead tissue is eventually replaced by scar tissue, which does not contract. Because each coronary artery supplies a specific area of the heart, the location of the damage is determined by which artery is blocked. If more than half of the heart tissue is damaged or dies, the heart generally cannot function, and severe disability or death is likely. Even when damage is less extensive, the heart may be unable to pump adequately, resulting in heart

▲ see page 202   ■ see page 203

Complications of a Heart Attack

A person who has a heart attack may experience any of the following complications: rupture of the heart muscle (myocardial rupture); formation of scar tissue; a bulge in the wall of the ventricle (ventricular aneurysm); blood clots; heart failure; low blood pressure (hypotension);▲ abnormal heart rhythms,■ particularly originating in the ventricles (ventricular arrhythmias); shock;★ or inflammation of the two-layered sac that envelops the heart (pericarditis).●

Myocardial Rupture

Rarely, the heart muscle ruptures under the pressure of the heart's pumping action because the damaged heart muscle is weak. Rupture usually occurs 1 to 10 days after a heart attack and is more common among women. Parts of the heart that are particularly susceptible to rupture during or after a heart attack are the wall separating the two ventricles (septum), the external heart wall, and the muscles that open and close the mitral valve. Rupture of the septum results in too much blood being diverted to the lungs, causing accumulation of fluid (pulmonary edema). Rupture of the external wall results in massive amounts of blood between the two layers of the pericardium. This condition is called hemopericardium. Cardiac tamponade usually follows.◆ A rupture of the septum can sometimes be repaired surgically, but a rupture of the external heart wall almost always leads to rapid death. If the mitral valve muscles rupture, the valve cannot function—the result is sudden and severe heart failure.

Scar Tissue

Often, the heart muscle damaged by a heart attack does not contract properly even if it is not torn or ruptured. The dead muscle cells are replaced by tough, fibrous scar tissue that does not contract at all. Sometimes part of the heart wall expands or bulges when it should contract. Beta-blockers and especially angiotensin-converting enzyme (ACE) inhibitors can reduce the extent of these abnormal areas by reducing the workload of and the stress on the heart. Thus, these drugs help the heart maintain its shape and function more normally.

Ventricular Aneurysm

The damaged muscle may form a thin bulge (aneurysm) on the wall of the ventricle. Doctors may suspect an aneurysm based on abnormal results of electrocardiography (ECG), but echocardiography is performed to be sure. These aneurysms may cause episodes of abnormal heart rhythms and may reduce the heart's pumping ability. Because blood flows more slowly through aneurysms, blood clots can form in the heart's chambers. If heart failure or abnormal heart rhythms develop, the aneurysm may be removed surgically.

Blood Clots

In about 40 to 50% of people who have had a heart attack, clots form in arteries supplying the heart, over the area of dead heart muscle. In up to 5% of these people, parts of the clots break off, travel through the bloodstream, and lodge in smaller blood vessels throughout the body. They may block the blood supply to part of the brain (causing a stroke) or to other organs. Echocardiography may be performed to detect clots forming in the heart or to determine whether a person has factors that make clots more likely to form. For example, an area of the left ventricle may not be beating as well as it should. Doctors often prescribe anticoagulants such as heparin and warfarin to help prevent clot formation. Heparin is given intravenously in the hospital for at least 2 days. Then, if the heart attack was massive or if areas of the heart are not beating well, warfarin is given by mouth. It is usually taken for 3 to 6 months after a heart attack. Aspirin, once started, should be taken indefinitely if possible.

Heart Failure

In a heart attack, part of the heart muscle dies. Consequently, there is less muscle to pump blood. If enough muscle dies, the heart's pumping ability may be so reduced that the heart cannot meet the body's need for blood and oxygen, and heart failure develops.

▲ see page 141

■ see page 163

★ see page 148

● see page 187

◆ see box on page 189

failure or shock. The damaged heart may enlarge, partly to compensate for the decrease in pumping ability (a larger heart beats more forcefully). Enlargement of the heart makes abnormal heart rhythms more likely.

Pericarditis (inflammation of the membranes enveloping the heart) may develop in the first day or two after a heart attack or about 10 days to 2 months later. Symptoms of early developing pericarditis are seldom noticed, because symptoms of the heart attack are more prominent. However, pericarditis produces a scratchy rhythmic sound that can sometimes be heard through a stethoscope 2 to 3 days after a heart attack. Later developing pericarditis is usually called Dressler's (post–myocardial infarction) syndrome. This syndrome causes fever, pericardial effusion (extra fluid in the space between the two layers of the pericardium), pleurisy (inflammation of the pleura, which are the membranes covering the lungs), pleural effusion (extra fluid in the space between the two layers of the pleura), and joint pain.

Other complications after a heart attack include rupture of the heart muscle, a bulge in the wall of the ventricle (ventricular aneurysm), blood clots (emboli), and low blood pressure (hypotension). Nervousness and depression are common after a heart attack. Depression after a heart attack may be significant and may persist.

Diagnosis

Whenever a man over age 35 or a woman over age 50 reports chest pain, doctors usually consider the possibility of a heart attack. But several other conditions can produce similar pain: pneumonia, a blood clot in the lung (pulmonary embolism), pericarditis, a rib fracture, spasm of the esophagus, indigestion, or chest muscle tenderness after injury or exertion.

Electrocardiography (ECG)▲ and certain blood tests can usually confirm the diagnosis of a heart attack within a few hours.

ECG is the most important initial diagnostic procedure when doctors suspect a heart attack. This procedure provides a graphic representation of the electrical current producing each heartbeat—the electrocardiogram (the ECG). In many instances, it immediately shows that a person is having a heart attack. Several abnormalities may be detected by ECG, depending mainly on the size and location of the heart muscle damage. If a person has had previous heart problems, which can

alter the ECG, the current muscle damage may be harder for doctors to detect. Such people should carry a small copy of their ECG in their wallets, so that if they have symptoms of a heart attack, doctors can compare the previous ECG with the current ECG. If a few ECGs recorded over several hours are normal, doctors consider a heart attack unlikely.

Measuring levels of certain substances (called serum markers) in the blood also helps doctors diagnose a heart attack. The presence of these substances in the blood indicates damage to or death of heart muscle. These substances are normally found in heart muscle but are released into the bloodstream when heart muscle is damaged. Most commonly measured is an enzyme called CK-MB. Levels in the blood are elevated within 6 hours of a heart attack and remain elevated for 36 to 48 hours. Levels of CK-MB are usually checked when the person is admitted to the hospital and at 6- to 8-hour intervals for the next 24 hours. However, two proteins called troponin T and troponin I may be more specific markers for damage to the heart. These proteins are involved in muscle contraction and are released into the bloodstream when cells are damaged.

When ECG and serum marker measurements do not provide enough information, echocardiography or radionuclide imaging may be performed. Echocardiography may show reduced motion in part of the wall of the left ventricle (the heart chamber that pumps blood to the body). This finding suggests damage due to a heart attack. Radionuclide imaging may show a persistent reduction in blood flow to an area of the heart muscle, suggesting scar tissue due to a heart attack.

Dressler's syndrome (pericarditis that develops 10 days to 2 months after a heart attack) is diagnosed based on the symptoms it produces and on the time it occurs.

Treatment

A heart attack is a medical emergency. Half of deaths due to a heart attack occur in the first 3 or 4 hours after symptoms begin. The sooner treatment begins, the better the chances of survival. Anyone having symptoms that might indicate a heart attack should obtain prompt medical attention. Prompt transportation to a hospital's emergency department by an ambulance with trained personnel may save the person's life. Trying to contact

▲ see page 122

the person's doctor, relatives, friends, or neighbors is a dangerous waste of time.

People who may be having a heart attack are usually admitted to a hospital that has a cardiac care unit. Heart rhythm, blood pressure, and the amount of oxygen in the blood are closely monitored so that heart damage can be assessed. Nurses in these units are specially trained to care for people with heart problems and to handle cardiac emergencies.

If no complications occur during the first few days, most people can safely leave the hospital within a few more days. If complications such as abnormal heart rhythms develop or the heart can no longer pump adequately, hospitalization can be prolonged.

Initial Treatment: People who think they may be having a heart attack should call an ambulance, then chew an aspirin tablet. If aspirin is not taken at home or given by emergency personnel, it is usually immediately given at the hospital. This therapy improves the chances of survival by reducing the size of the clot (if present) in the coronary artery. People with an allergy to aspirin may be given clopidogrel or ticlopidine instead. Because decreasing the heart's workload also helps limit tissue damage, a beta-blocker is usually given to slow the heart rate, to enable the heart to work less hard, and to reduce the area of damaged tissue.

Often, oxygen is given through nasal prongs or a face mask. By increasing oxygen pressure in the blood, this therapy provides more oxygen to the heart and helps keep heart tissue damage to a minimum.

If a blocked coronary artery can be cleared quickly, heart tissue may be saved. Often, blood clots in an artery can be dissolved by a thrombolytic drug such as streptokinase, recombinant tissue plasminogen activator (alteplase), or reteplase. To be effective, a thrombolytic drug must be given intravenously within 6 hours of the start of heart attack symptoms. After 6 hours, most damage is permanent, and removing the blockage may not help. Early treatment increases blood flow in 60 to 80% of people and helps keeps heart tissue damage to a minimum. Aspirin, which prevents platelets from forming blood clots, or heparin, which stops clotting, may enhance the effectiveness of a thrombolytic drug.

Because thrombolytic drugs can cause bleeding, they are not usually given to people who have bleeding in the digestive tract, who have severe high blood pressure, who have recently had a stroke, or who have had surgery during the month before the heart attack. Older people who do not have any of these conditions can be safely given a thrombolytic drug.

In some cardiovascular treatment centers, angioplasty or coronary artery bypass surgery▲ is performed immediately after the heart attack to clear the arteries instead of using a thrombolytic drug. This approach is preferred for people who cannot take thrombolytic drugs and for those who are very ill after having a massive heart attack. For some people, a thrombolytic drug is used with angioplasty or with an antiplatelet drug, such as a glycoprotein IIb/IIIa inhibitor (for example, abciximab or tirofiban).

Because most people who have had a heart attack are experiencing severe discomfort and anxiety, morphine is often used. This drug has a calming effect and reduces the workload of the heart. Most people are given nitroglycerin, which relieves pain by reducing the workload of the heart and possibly by dilating arteries. Usually, it is first given under the tongue, then intravenously.

Angiotensin-converting enzyme (ACE) inhibitors■ can reduce heart enlargement and increase the chance of survival for many people. Therefore, these drugs are usually given in the first few days after a heart attack and prescribed indefinitely.

Subsequent Treatment: Because physical exertion, emotional distress, and excitement stress the heart and make it work harder, a person who has just had a heart attack should stay in bed in a quiet room for a few days. Visitors are usually limited to family members and close friends. Watching television may be permitted if the programs do not cause stress.

Smoking, a major risk factor for coronary artery disease and heart attack, is prohibited in hospitals and in cardiac care units. Moreover, a heart attack is a compelling reason to stop smoking.

Stool softeners and gentle laxatives may be used to prevent constipation, so that the person does not have to strain. If the person cannot pass urine or if the doctors and nurses must keep track of the precise amount of urine produced, a urinary catheter is used.

For severe nervousness (which can stress the heart), a mild antianxiety drug (for example, a benzodiazepine such as lorazepam) may be prescribed. To deal with mild depression and de-

---

▲ see page 209   ■ see page 140

nial of illness, which are common after a heart attack, patients and their family members and friends are encouraged to talk about their feelings with doctors, nurses, and social workers. Some patients require an antidepressant.

After about 5 to 7 days in the hospital, people who have had a heart attack are usually discharged. Nitroglycerin, aspirin, a beta-blocker, an ACE inhibitor, and a lipid-lowering drug (most often, a statin)▲ are usually prescribed. Soon after discharge, people should see their primary care doctor, who can refer them to a cardiologist or to a cardiac rehabilitation program if needed.

People who develop Dressler's syndrome are usually given aspirin. Even with treatment, the syndrome can recur. If the syndrome is severe, a corticosteroid or a nonsteroidal anti-inflammatory drug other than aspirin (such as ibuprofen) may be needed for a short time.

Prognosis and Prevention

Most people who survive for a few days after a heart attack can expect a full recovery, but about 10% die within a year. Most deaths occur in the first 3 or 4 months, typically in people who continue to have angina, abnormal heart rhythms originating in the ventricles (ventricular arrhythmias), and heart failure. All of these disorders may result from a heart attack. The prognosis is worse if the heart has enlarged after a heart attack than if heart size remains normal. Older people are more likely to die after a heart attack and to have complications, such as heart failure. The prognosis for smaller people is worse than that for larger people. This finding may help explain why the prognosis for women who have had a heart attack is, on average, worse than that for men. Women also tend to be older and to have more serious disorders when they have a heart attack. Also, they tend to wait longer after a heart attack to go to the hospital than do men.

Other procedures may be performed to determine whether a person needs additional treatment or is likely to have more heart problems. For instance, a person may have to wear a Holter monitor, which records the heart's electrical activity for 24 hours.■ This procedure enables doctors to detect whether the person has abnormal heart rhythms (arrhythmias) or episodes of inadequate blood supply without symptoms (silent ischemia). An exer-

cise stress test (electrocardiography performed during exercise)★ before or shortly after discharge can help determine how well the person is doing after the heart attack and whether ischemia is continuing. If these procedures detect abnormal heart rhythms or ischemia, drug therapy may be recommended. If ischemia persists, doctors may recommend coronary angiography to evaluate the possibility of performing angioplasty or bypass surgery to restore blood flow to the heart.

Taking one baby aspirin, one half of an adult aspirin, or one full adult aspirin daily after a heart attack is recommended. Because aspirin prevents platelets from forming clots, it reduces the risk of death and the risk of a second heart attack by 15 to 30%. People with an allergy to aspirin may take clopidogrel or ticlopidine instead. Usually, doctors also prescribe a beta-blocker (such as metoprolol, propranolol, or timolol) because they reduce the risk of death by about 25%. The more serious the heart attack, the more benefit beta-blockers provide. However, some people cannot tolerate the side effects (such as wheezing, tiredness, and cold limbs), and not everyone benefits.

Taking lipid-lowering drugs may reduce the risk of death after a heart attack.

ACE inhibitors, such as captopril, enalapril, lisinopril, and ramipril, are often prescribed after a heart attack. They help prevent death and the development of heart failure, particularly in people who have had a massive heart attack or who have heart failure.

Rehabilitation

Cardiac rehabilitation, an important part of recovery, begins in the hospital. Remaining in bed for longer than 2 or 3 days leads to physical deconditioning and sometimes to depression and a sense of helplessness. Barring complications, people who have had a heart attack can usually progress to sitting in a chair, passive exercise, use of a commode chair, and reading on the first day. By the second or third day, people are encouraged to walk to the bathroom and engage in nonstressful activities, and they can perform more activities each day.●

▲ see table on page 925   ■ see art on page 124
★ see page 123   ● see also page 40

CHAPTER 34

Peripheral Arterial Disease

Peripheral arterial disease results in reduced blood flow in the arteries of the trunk, arms, and legs.

Most often, doctors use the term peripheral arterial disease to describe poor circulation in the arteries of the legs that results from atherosclerosis. However, peripheral arterial disease can affect other arteries and can have other causes. Disorders affecting arteries that supply the brain are considered separately as cerebrovascular disease.

Peripheral arterial disease may be described as occlusive or functional. Occlusive peripheral arterial disease is due to structural changes that narrow or block arteries. Functional peripheral arterial disease is usually due to a sudden temporary narrowing (spasm) or, rarely, to a widening (vasodilation) of arteries.

Occlusive Peripheral Arterial Disease

Occlusive peripheral arterial disease is common among older people because it often results from atherosclerosis, which becomes more common with age. Occlusive peripheral arterial disease may affect 15 to 20% of people older than 70. The disease is particularly common among people who have ever smoked regularly and among those who have diabetes, whether type 1 or type 2.▲

Occlusive peripheral arterial disease is also common among people who have a family history of atherosclerosis, high blood pressure, high cholesterol levels, or high homocysteine levels; people who are obese; and people who are physically inactive. Each of these conditions contributes not only to the development of occlusive peripheral arterial disease but also to the worsening of the disease.

Occlusive peripheral arterial disease may result from gradual narrowing or sudden blockage of an artery. When an artery narrows, the parts of the body it supplies may not receive enough blood. An inadequate blood supply is called ischemia. Ischemia may develop suddenly or gradually. When an artery is suddenly and completely blocked, the tissue it supplies may die.

Gradual narrowing of arteries is usually due to atherosclerosis, in which deposits of cholesterol and other fatty materials (atheromas or atherosclerotic plaques) develop in the walls of arteries. Atheromas may gradually narrow the interior (lumen) of the artery and reduce blood flow.■ Also, calcium may accumulate in the atheromas, making the arteries stiff.

Less commonly, arteries are gradually narrowed by an abnormal growth of muscle in the artery's wall (fibromuscular dysplasia) or pressure from an expanding mass, such as a tumor or fluid-filled sac (cyst), outside the artery.

Sudden, complete blockage may result when a blood clot (thrombus) forms in an artery that is already narrowed. A sudden blockage may also result when a clot breaks off (becoming an embolus) from a site such as the heart or aorta, travels through the bloodstream, and lodges in an artery downstream. Some disorders increase the risk of blood clot formation. They include atrial fibrillation, other heart disorders, clotting disorders, and inflammation of blood vessels (vasculitis), which may be due to an autoimmune disorder.

Sometimes a piece of fatty material breaks off from an atheroma and suddenly blocks an artery. Sudden blockage may also result from an aortic dissection,★ in which the inner layer of the aorta tears, allowing blood to surge through the tear into the middle layer. As the dissection enlarges, it can block one or more arteries connected to the aorta.

Obstructive peripheral arterial disease may also be caused by the thoracic outlet syndrome.● In this syndrome, blood vessels (as well as nerves) in the passageway between the neck and the chest become compressed.

Obstructive peripheral arterial disease can affect arteries in different parts of the body. It commonly develops in the arteries of the legs, including the main arteries of the thighs (femoral arteries), of the knees (popliteal arteries), and of the calves (tibial and peroneal arteries). Much less commonly, the disease develops in the arteries of the shoulders or arms.

▲ see page 962   ■ see art on page 196
★ see page 229   ● see page 582

It may develop in the part of the aorta that passes through the abdomen (abdominal aorta) or in its branches, including the lower aorta where it divides into two branches that supply blood to the legs (common iliac arteries). The branches that supply the kidneys (renal arteries) are a relatively common site of gradual narrowing due to atherosclerosis. But sudden, complete blockage of one of the renal arteries is relatively rare. The branch that supplies the intestines (superior mesenteric artery) is also blocked less commonly. Blockage of the branches that supply the liver (hepatic artery) and spleen (splenic artery) is very rare.

Symptoms

Symptoms vary depending on which artery is affected, how completely the artery is blocked, and whether the artery is gradually narrowed or suddenly blocked. Usually, about 70% of the artery's interior has to be blocked before symptoms occur. Gradual narrowing of an artery may result in less severe symptoms than sudden blockage—even if the artery eventually becomes completely blocked. Symptoms may be less severe because gradual narrowing allows time for nearby blood vessels to expand or new blood vessels (called collateral vessels) to grow. Thus, the affected tissue can still be supplied with blood. If an artery is suddenly blocked, there is no time for collateral vessels to develop, so symptoms are usually severe.

Arteries of the Legs and Arms: Sudden, complete blockage of an artery in a leg or an arm may cause severe pain, coldness, and numbness in the affected limb. The person's leg or arm is either pale or bluish (cyanotic). No pulse can be felt below the blockage. The sudden, drastic decrease in blood flow to the limb is a medical emergency. The absence of blood flow can quickly result in loss of sensation in or paralysis of a limb.

Intermittent claudication, the most common symptom of peripheral arterial disease, results from gradual narrowing of a leg artery. It is a painful, aching, cramping, or tired feeling in the muscles of the leg—not in the joints. Intermittent claudication occurs regularly and predictably during physical activity but is always relieved promptly by rest. The muscles ache when a person walks, and the pain begins more quickly and is more severe when the person walks quickly or uphill. Usually, after 1 to 5 minutes of rest (sitting is not necessary), the person can walk the same distance already covered, although continued walking will again provoke the pain at a comparable distance. Most commonly, the pain occurs in the calf, but it can also occur in the thigh, hip, or buttock, depending on the location of the blockage. Very rarely, pain occurs in the foot.

As a leg artery is narrowed further, the distance a person can walk without pain decreases. Eventually, as the disease becomes very severe, leg muscles may ache even at rest, especially when the person is lying down. Such pain usually begins in the lower leg or front of the foot, is severe and unrelenting, and worsens when the leg is elevated. The pain often interferes with sleep. For relief, the person may hang the feet over the side of the bed or rest sitting up with the legs hanging down.

Large blockages of the arm arteries, which are rare, may cause fatigue, cramping, or pain felt in the arm muscles when the arm is used repeatedly.

When the blood supply is only mildly or moderately reduced, the leg or arm may look almost normal. When the blood supply to a foot is severely reduced, the foot may be cold. The skin of the foot or leg may be dry, scaly, shiny, or cracked. Nails may not grow normally, and the hair on the limb may not grow. As the artery is narrowed further, a person may develop sores that do not easily heal, typically on the toes or heel and occasionally on the lower leg, especially after an injury. Infections occur easily and become serious quickly. In people with severe occlusive peripheral arterial disease, wounds in the skin may take weeks or months to heal or may not heal. Foot ulcers may develop. Leg muscles usually shrink (atrophy). A large blockage may cause gangrene.

In some people who have had predictable, stable claudication, claudication can suddenly worsen. For example, calf pain that occurs after walking 10 blocks may suddenly occur after walking one block. This change may indicate that a new clot has formed in a leg artery. Such people should be evaluated by a specialist as soon as possible.

Lower Aorta and Common Iliac Arteries: Sudden blockage of the lower aorta where it divides into the common iliac arteries causes both legs to suddenly become painful, pale, and cold. No pulse can be felt in the legs, which may become numb.

Gradual narrowing of the lower aorta or of both common iliac arteries can cause intermittent claudication that affects the buttocks and thighs of both legs. The legs may also feel cold or appear pale, although they usually appear normal. This combination of symptoms is sometimes called Leriche's syndrome. Leriche's syndrome usually occurs in men and commonly also causes impotence (erectile dysfunction).

Renal Arteries: Sudden, complete blockage of one of the renal arteries, which supply the kidneys, may cause a sudden pain in the side, and the urine may become bloody. These symptoms indicate a medical emergency.

Gradual, moderate narrowing of one or both renal arteries may not cause symptoms or affect kidney function. More rarely, more complete narrowing of one or both renal arteries contributes to the development of kidney failure or high blood pressure (a disorder called renovascular hypertension). Less than 5% of people with high blood pressure have renovascular hypertension.

Superior Mesenteric Artery: Sudden, complete blockage of the superior mesenteric artery is a medical emergency. Initially, most people with such a blockage vomit and feel an urgent need to have a bowel movement. They may become seriously ill and have severe abdominal pain because the superior mesenteric artery supplies a large part of the intestine. The abdomen may feel tender when a doctor presses on it, but the severe abdominal pain is usually more prominent than the tenderness, which is widespread and vague. The abdomen may be slightly swollen (distended). Through a stethoscope, a doctor initially hears fewer bowel sounds in the abdomen than normal. Later, no bowel sounds can be heard. The stool initially contains small amounts of blood but soon looks bloody. Blood pressure falls, and shock may result as gangrene develops in the intestine.

Gradual narrowing of the superior mesenteric artery typically causes pain about 30 to 60 minutes after each meal, because the intestine requires more blood during digestion. The pain is steady, severe, and usually centered at the navel. This pain makes people afraid to eat, so they may lose considerable weight. Because the blood supply to the intestine is reduced, nutrients may be poorly absorbed into the bloodstream, contributing to the weight loss.

Hepatic and Splenic Arteries: Blockage of the hepatic artery, which supplies the liver, or the splenic artery, which supplies the spleen, is usually not as dangerous as blockage of the major arteries that supply the intestine. However, parts of the liver or spleen may be damaged.

Diagnosis

The diagnosis of occlusive peripheral arterial disease is based on the symptoms and the results of a physical examination. Procedures that directly measure blood pressure or blood flow are also performed.

A doctor or nurse assesses each pulse, including those at the armpits, elbows, wrists, groin, and ankles and those behind the knees. The pulse in arteries beyond the blockage may be weak or absent. For example, if doctors suspect a blockage in a leg artery, they check the pulse below a certain point in the leg. (For arteries in which the pulse is inaccessible, such as the renal arteries, procedures that provide images of blood flow are performed.) A stethoscope is used to listen for abnormal sounds caused by turbulent blood flow through a narrowed artery (bruits). Doctors examine the skin of the limbs, noting the color and temperature and pressing gently to see how quickly color returns after pressure is removed. These observations can help doctors determine whether circulation is adequate.

Most of the procedures used in the diagnosis of peripheral arterial disease are noninvasive and can be performed in a doctor's office or in a hospital on an outpatient basis. Most commonly, a standard blood pressure cuff and a special electronic stethoscope are used to measure the systolic blood pressure in both arms and both legs. If blood pressure in the ankle is lower than that in the arms by a certain amount, blood flow to the legs is inadequate, and occlusive peripheral arterial disease is diagnosed. If doctors suspect a blockage in an arm artery, they measure systolic blood pressure in both arms. Pressure that is consistently higher in one arm suggests a blockage in the arm with lower blood pressure, and occlusive peripheral arterial disease is diagnosed. However, the blood pressure measurement is not always accurate in people who have arteries stiffened by calcium deposits or in those who have had diabetes for a long time.

Doppler ultrasonography▲ can be used to directly measure blood flow and can confirm the diagnosis of occlusive peripheral arterial disease. This procedure can accurately detect narrowing or blockage of blood vessels. Color Doppler is useful because it shows different

▲ see page 126

When the Blood Supply to the Intestine Is Blocked

The superior mesenteric artery supplies a large part of the intestine with blood. When this artery is blocked, intestinal tissue begins to die.

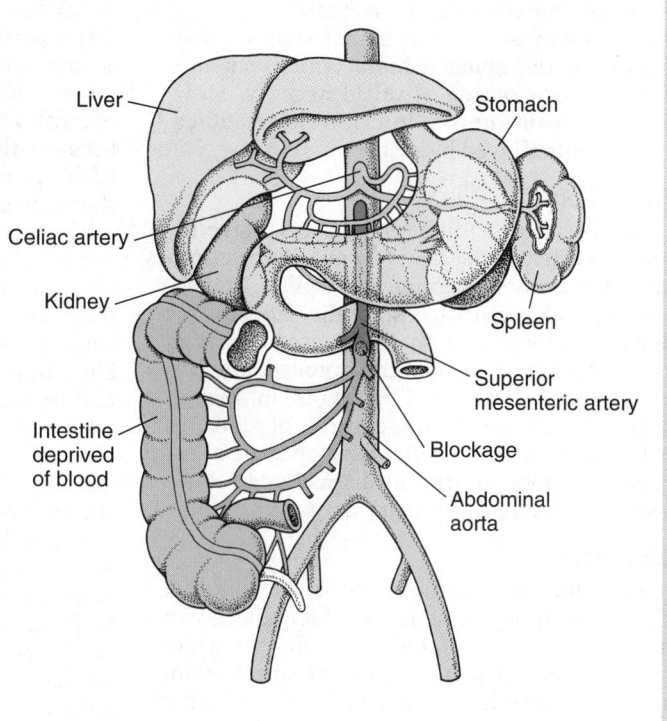

Liver

Stomach

Celiac artery

Kidney

Spleen

Superior mesenteric artery

Intestine deprived of blood

Blockage

Abdominal aorta

rates of blood flow in different colors. Doppler ultrasonography to measure blood flow may be performed during exercise stress testing,▲ because some problems appear only during exercise. X-rays and other noninvasive procedures (for example, procedures to evaluate blood flow or to measure the amount of oxygen in the blood) may be performed.

Usually, angiography,■ an invasive procedure, is performed only after the need for surgery or angioplasty has been established. In such cases, its purpose is to provide doctors with clear images of the affected arteries before surgery or angioplasty is performed. Rarely, angiography is needed to determine whether surgery or angioplasty is possible. In angiography, a radiopaque dye, which can be seen on x-rays, is injected into an artery. The dye outlines the artery. Thus angiography can show the precise diameter of the artery and is more accurate than Doppler ultrasonography in detecting some blockages. Alternatively, digital subtraction angiography may be used. It uses a computer to enhance images, so that less dye is needed. Thus, the procedure may be safer and cause less discomfort than standard angiography. At some medical centers, a less invasive type of angiography can be performed with spiral computed tomography (called CT angiography) or with a type of magnetic resonance imaging (called magnetic resonance angiography, or MRA★).

For people with atherosclerosis, doctors try to identify risk factors, such as high levels of cholesterol, sugar, and homocysteine and high blood pressure. Blood tests are performed to measure levels of cholesterol, sugar, and, occasionally, homocysteine. Blood pressure is measured on more than one occasion to determine if it is consistently high.

Blood tests may be performed to identify other causes of narrowed or blocked arteries, such as inflammation of blood vessels due to an autoimmune disorder. Such procedures include the erythrocyte sedimentation rate (ESR) and tests for C-reactive protein, which is produced only when inflammation is present. For blockage of an arm artery, doctors try to

▲ see page 123   ■ see page 130
★ see page 127

determine if the cause is atherosclerosis, thoracic outlet syndrome, or arteritis.

Doctors must rule out spinal stenosis (narrowing of the spinal canal), which can also produce pain during physical activity. However, this pain, unlike intermittent claudication, is not relieved by rest.

Prevention

The best way to help prevent occlusive peripheral arterial disease is to modify or eliminate risk factors for atherosclerosis. ▲ Prevention includes quitting smoking; controlling diabetes; lowering high blood pressure, high cholesterol levels, and high homocysteine levels; losing weight; and engaging in regular physical activity. Good control of diabetes helps delay or prevent the development of occlusive peripheral arterial disease and reduce the risk of other complications. ■

Treatment

The aims of treatment are to prevent the disease from progressing; to reduce the risk of heart attack, stroke, and death due to widespread atherosclerosis; to prevent amputation; and to improve the quality of life by relieving symptoms (such as intermittent claudication). Treatments include drugs such as those that relieve claudication and those that cause clots to dissolve (thrombolytic drugs ★), angioplasty, surgery, and other measures, such as exercise and foot care. Which treatments are used depends on the severity of the symptoms, the severity and location of the blockage, the risks related to the treatment (particularly for surgery), and the overall health of the person. Regardless of the specific treatments used, people still need to modify risk factors for atherosclerosis to improve their overall prognosis. Angioplasty and surgery are only mechanical measures for correcting the immediate problem. They do not cure the underlying disease.

Angioplasty is often performed immediately after angiography. Angioplasty may be performed to relieve symptoms and thus postpone or avoid surgery. Sometimes it is used in combination with surgery. Angioplasty consists of inserting a catheter with a balloon at its tip into the narrowed part of the artery and then inflating the balloon to clear the blockage. ● To keep the artery open, doctors may insert a permanent wire mesh (a stent) into the artery. Angioplasty is usually performed as an outpatient procedure. Angioplasty is rarely painful but may be somewhat uncomfortable because the person has to lie still on a hard table. A mild sedative, but no general anesthetic, is given.

The success of angioplasty varies, depending on the location of the blockage and the severity of peripheral arterial disease. Afterward, the person is given an antiplatelet drug (such as aspirin or clopidogrel) to help prevent clots from forming in the arteries of the limb and to prevent a subsequent heart attack and stroke. Also, Doppler ultrasonography is performed regularly to monitor blood flow through the artery and thus detect whether the artery is narrowing again.

Angioplasty cannot be performed successfully if too many areas of an artery are narrowed, if the narrowed section is too long, or if the artery is severely and extensively hardened. After angioplasty, surgery may be needed if a blood clot (thrombus) forms in the narrowed area, if a piece of the clot (embolus) breaks off and blocks an artery downstream, if blood seeps into the lining of the artery causing a bulge inward that blocks blood flow (a disorder called dissection), or if severe bleeding occurs.

Other devices—including lasers, mechanical cutters, ultrasonic catheters, and rotational sanders—can be used instead of a balloon catheter during angioplasty, but none appear to be more effective.

Surgery to remove blood clots (thromboendarterectomy) can be performed when thrombolytic drugs are ineffective or too dangerous. Surgery to remove atheromas (endarterectomy) or other blockages may also be performed. Alternatively, bypass surgery may be performed. In bypass surgery, a graft consisting of a tube made of a synthetic material or a part of a vein from another part of the body is joined to the blocked artery above and below the blockage. Thus, blood is rerouted around the blocked artery. Another approach is to remove the narrowed or blocked section and insert a graft in its place. Usually before surgery, doctors assess heart function and blood flow through the heart to determine the relative safety of surgery, because many people with occlusive peripheral arterial disease also have coronary artery disease.

▲ see pages 196 and 200   ■ see page 964

★ see page 214

● see art on page 208

Arteries of the Legs and Arms: For sudden, complete blockage of these arteries, surgery is performed as soon as possible to prevent irreversible loss of limb function or amputation.

For most people with intermittent claudication, exercise or drugs can relieve the pain. Exercise is the most effective treatment and may be appropriate for motivated people who can follow a prescribed daily exercise program. Exactly how exercise relieves claudication is not well understood, but exercise probably improves muscle function. There is no evidence that exercise improves blood flow or causes new (collateral) blood vessels to grow. People with claudication should walk at least 30 minutes a day at least 3 times a week, if possible. For most people, following this routine increases the distance they can walk comfortably. Discomfort felt during walking is not dangerous. When discomfort is felt, a person should stop walking until the discomfort subsides and then walk again. The total walking time (excluding rest periods) must be at least 30 minutes to improve walking distance.

Exercise is usually most effective when it is supervised by a trained therapist in a rehabilitation program. Doctors recommend that people with claudication undergo an exercise stress test▲ before they begin a rehabilitation program to make sure that the blood supply to heart muscle is adequate.

People with very severe occlusive peripheral arterial disease (that is, who have pain during rest, gangrene, or wounds that do not heal) should avoid exposure to cold, which causes blood vessels to narrow (constrict), and the use of drugs that cause blood vessels to constrict. These drugs include ephedrine or pseudoephedrine, which are components of some headache and cold remedies.

Pentoxifylline or cilostazol may be used to treat claudication. These drugs may increase blood flow and thus the oxygen supply to muscles. Both drugs must be taken for 2 to 3 months to determine whether they are effective. However, the usefulness of pentoxifylline is now in doubt, and many experts no longer recommend its use. In contrast, cilostazol may result in a 50 to 100% increase in the distance that can be walked without pain. Cilostazol should not be used by people with heart failure. Drugs that cause the arteries to widen (dilate), such as calcium channel blockers, may be used, but they have not been shown to relieve claudication. The dietary supplements carnitine and ginkgo■ have been reported to

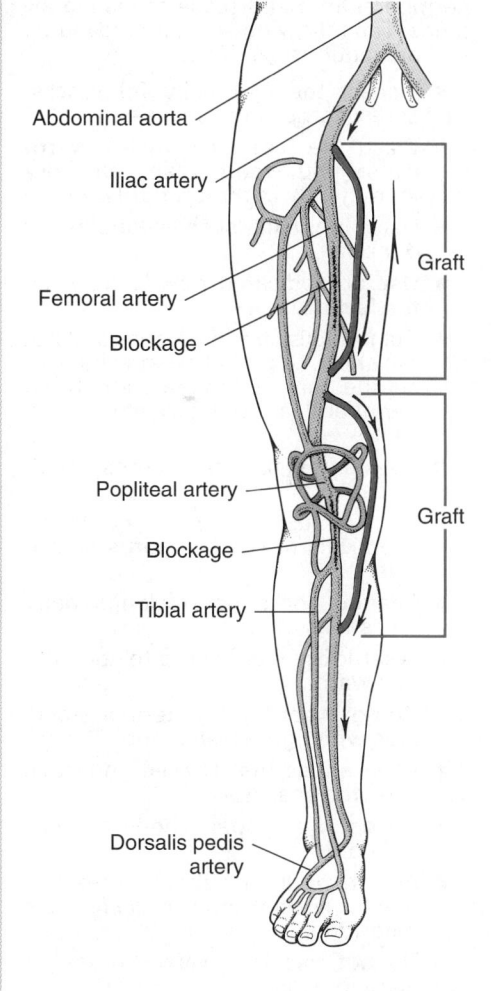

Bypass Surgery in the Leg

Bypass surgery may be performed to treat arteries that are narrowed or blocked. In this procedure, blood is rerouted around the affected artery—for example, around part of the femoral artery in the thigh or part of the popliteal artery in the knee. A graft consisting of a tube made of a synthetic material or part of a vein from another part of the body is joined to the blocked artery above and below the blockage. If a vein is used, its ends are tied, and the blood is diverted to other veins in the leg.

Abdominal aorta

Iliac artery

Graft

Femoral artery

Blockage

Popliteal artery

Graft

Blockage

Tibial artery

Dorsalis pedis artery

▲ see page 123   ■ see page 109

relieve claudication. However, compared with prescribed drugs, these supplements have only a small effect.

Aspirin or clopidogrel is usually given because these drugs help prevent clot formation and reduce the risk of heart attack or stroke. They modify platelets so that they do not adhere to blood vessel walls. Normally, platelets, which circulate in the blood, gather and form a clot to stop bleeding when a blood vessel is injured.

Performing Foot Care

> Foot care is essential for people with peripheral arterial disease of the leg arteries. The following self-care measures and precautions can help:
>
> - Inspect the feet daily for cracks, sores, corns, and calluses.
> - Wash the feet daily in lukewarm water with mild soap, and dry them gently and thoroughly.
> - Use a lubricant, such as lanolin, for dry skin.
> - Use unmedicated powder to keep the feet dry.
> - Cut toenails straight across and not too short. (A podiatrist may have to cut the nails; tell the podiatrist that peripheral arterial disease is present.)
> - Have a podiatrist treat corns or calluses.
> - Do not use adhesive or harsh chemicals to remove corns or calluses.
> - Change socks or stockings daily and shoes often.
> - Wear loose wool socks to keep the feet warm.
> - Do not wear tight garters or stockings with tight elastic tops.
> - Wear shoes that fit well and have wide toe spaces.
> - Do not wear open shoes or walk barefoot.
> - Ask the podiatrist about a prescription for special shoes if the feet are deformed.
> - Do not use hot water bottles or heating pads.

Surgery to remove the blockage or bypass surgery may be performed if other treatments do not relieve claudication. Surgery is usually performed to avoid amputation of a leg when blood flow is greatly reduced—that is, when claudication is incapacitating or occurs during rest, when wounds do not heal, or when gangrene develops.

Good foot care is important. It helps prevent wounds or foot ulcers from becoming infected and painful or resulting in gangrene. Good foot care also helps prevent amputation. Foot ulcers require meticulous care. Such care is needed to treat infection, to protect the skin from further damage, and to enable the person to continue to walk.

A foot ulcer must be kept clean: It should be washed daily with a mild soap or antibacterial solution and covered daily with clean, dry dressings. The legs should be kept below the level of the heart to help improve blood flow. People with diabetes must control blood sugar levels as well as possible. As a rule, anyone with poor circulation to the feet or with diabetes should have a doctor check a foot ulcer that is not healing after about 7 days. Often, a doctor prescribes an antibiotic ointment.

If foot ulcers are not healing, a person may need complete bed rest. If bed rest is required, bandages with heel pads or foam-rubber booties should be worn to prevent bedsores (pressure sores) from developing on the feet. The head of the bed should be raised 6 to 8 inches and the legs kept at or below heart level, so that gravity helps blood flow through the arteries. If the ulcer is infected, doctors usually prescribe antibiotics to be taken by mouth, and the person may need to be hospitalized.

Rarely, amputation of the leg is required to remove infected tissue, relieve unrelenting pain, or stop worsening gangrene. Surgeons remove as little of the leg as possible. Preserving the knee is particularly important if the person plans to wear an artificial leg. Rehabilitation after leg amputation is important.▲

Lower Aorta and Common Iliac Arteries: For sudden, complete blockage of the lower aorta and common iliac arteries, surgery is performed immediately.

Renal Arteries: For sudden, complete blockage of a renal artery, angioplasty or surgery, if performed promptly, can restore blood flow and kidney function.

For gradual, moderate blockage of a renal artery, no specific treatment is required as long as blood pressure is controlled and blood

▲ see page 43

tests indicate that the kidneys are functioning adequately. If renovascular hypertension develops, antihypertensives▲ are used. Often, at least three antihypertensives are needed. Angiotensin-converting enzyme (ACE) inhibitors are particularly useful; however, kidney function must be monitored when these drugs are used. If renovascular hypertension persists and is severe or if kidney function is deteriorating, doctors may perform angioplasty or bypass surgery to restore blood flow to the kidney.

Superior Mesenteric Artery: If the superior mesenteric artery is suddenly and completely blocked, only immediate surgery can restore the blood supply fast enough to save the person's life. Whether a person survives and whether the intestine can be saved depends on how fast the blood supply is restored. To save precious time, doctors may send a person for surgery without even taking x-rays.

If the superior mesenteric artery has gradually narrowed, nitroglycerin may relieve the abdominal pain, but angioplasty or surgery is needed to widen the artery. Doppler ultrasonography and angiography can determine how narrow the artery is and help doctors decide whether to operate.

Hepatic and Splenic Arteries: Surgery is needed to clear a blockage of the hepatic or splenic artery.

BUERGER'S DISEASE

Buerger's disease (thromboangiitis obliterans) is inflammation and subsequent blockage of small and medium-sized arteries of the legs or arms.

Buerger's disease is a rare disease that usually develops in smokers, most commonly in men aged 20 to 40. Buerger's disease was once considered a man's disease, but it is becoming increasingly common among women. Now, about one third of people with the disease are women, perhaps because more women are smoking.

How cigarette smoking relates to Buerger's disease is poorly understood, and what causes the disease is unknown. One theory is that smoking triggers inflammation and constriction of arteries. However, only a small number of smokers develop Buerger's disease; some people may be more susceptible than others for as yet unknown reasons. Nonetheless, Buerger's disease invariably worsens in people who continue to smoke, and amputation is commonly required. In contrast, if people with Buerger's disease quit smoking, amputation is rarely required.

Symptoms

Usually, symptoms of a reduced blood supply to the arms or legs—coldness, numbness, tingling, a burning sensation, or pain—develop gradually. These abnormal sensations start at the fingertips or toes and progress up the legs or arms. The legs are affected more often than the arms. People with Buerger's disease may feel abnormal sensations before their doctor sees any skin changes indicating an inadequate blood supply (ischemia) or gangrene. Raynaud's phenomenon■ and muscle discomfort during exertion (intermittent claudication)★ may develop. Cramps occur in the calf muscles or feet if the legs are affected and in the hands or forearms if the arms are affected.

As the disease progresses, cramps become more painful and last longer. Late in the disease, skin ulcers, gangrene, or both may appear, usually on one or more toes or fingers. The foot or hand feels cold and may turn bluish, probably because blood flow is greatly reduced.

A small percentage of people with this disease also have episodes of inflammation in the veins (migratory phlebitis), usually in the superficial veins.

Diagnosis

Usually, doctors suspect Buerger's disease on the basis of symptoms and results of the physical examination. In most people with Buerger's disease, the pulse is weak or absent in one or more arteries of the feet or wrists. Often, the affected hands, feet, fingers, or toes become pale when raised above the heart and red when lowered.

Ultrasonography detects a substantial decrease in blood pressure and blood flow in the affected feet, toes, hands, and fingers. Angiography● can detect specific patterns of narrowing and thus can help confirm the diagnosis of Buerger's disease. Sometimes a biopsy (removal of a tissue sample for examination under a microscope) of the affected artery or referral to a specialist is needed to confirm the diagnosis.

Treatment

A person with Buerger's disease must stop smoking immediately, or symptoms will re-

▲ see table on page 138   ■ see page 224
★ see page 217   ● see page 130

lentlessly worsen. Amputation is then likely to become necessary. Exposure to cold, which causes blood vessels to narrow (constrict), and use of certain drugs should be avoided. These drugs include those that cause blood vessels to constrict (such as ephedrine or pseudoephedrine, which are components of some headache and cold remedies) and those that increase the tendency of blood to clot (such as estrogen). Care should be taken to prevent any injury to the affected limb, including burns and injuries from cold or minor surgery (such as trimming calluses). Corns and calluses should be treated by a podiatrist. Wearing shoes that fit well and have wide toe spaces can help prevent injury to the feet.

For people who quit smoking but still have blocked arteries, surgeons may perform bypass surgery in an attempt to avoid amputation. Alternatively, they may cut certain nearby nerves (a procedure called sympathectomy) to prevent blood vessels from constricting. These procedures are seldom performed, because they usually improve blood flow only temporarily.

Functional Peripheral Arterial Disease

Functional peripheral arterial disease is much less common than occlusive peripheral arterial disease. Normally, the arteries of the arms and legs widen (dilate) and narrow (constrict) in response to changes in the environment, such as a change in temperature. Functional peripheral arterial disease usually occurs when the normal mechanisms that dilate and constrict these arteries are exaggerated. The affected arteries constrict more tightly and more often. These changes in constriction can be caused by an inherited defect in the blood vessels, by disturbances of the nerves that control the dilation and constriction of arteries (sympathetic nervous system), by injuries, or by drugs.

RAYNAUD'S DISEASE AND RAYNAUD'S PHENOMENON

Raynaud's disease and Raynaud's phenomenon are conditions in which small arteries (arterioles), usually in the fingers or toes, constrict more tightly in response to exposure to cold.

Doctors use the term Raynaud's disease when no cause is apparent. They use the term Raynaud's phenomenon when a cause is known. Raynaud's disease is much more common than Raynaud's phenomenon. Between 60% and 90% of cases of Raynaud's disease occur in young women aged 15 to 40.

Anything that stimulates the sympathetic nervous system, particularly exposure to cold but also strong emotion, can cause arteries to constrict and thus trigger Raynaud's disease.

Raynaud's phenomenon may be caused by scleroderma, rheumatoid arthritis, atherosclerosis, cryoglobulinemia, an underactive thyroid gland (hypothyroidism), injury, or reactions to certain drugs, such as beta-blockers, clonidine, and the antimigraine drugs ergotamine and methysergide. Use of such drugs, which constrict blood vessels, can also make Raynaud's phenomenon worse. Some people with Raynaud's phenomenon also have other disorders that occur when arteries are prone to constrict. These disorders include migraine headaches, variant angina, and high blood pressure in the lungs (pulmonary hypertension). The association of Raynaud's phenomenon with these disorders suggests that the cause of arterial constriction may be the same in all of them.

Symptoms and Diagnosis

Constriction of small arteries in the fingers and toes begins quickly, most often triggered by exposure to cold. It may last minutes or hours. The fingers and toes become pale or bluish, usually in patches. Only one finger or toe or parts of one or more may be affected. The fingers or toes usually do not hurt, but numbness, tingling, a pins-and-needles sensation, and a burning sensation are common. As the episode ends, the affected areas may be redder than usual or bluish. Rewarming the hands or feet restores normal color and sensation. However, if episodes of Raynaud's phenomenon recur and are prolonged (especially in people with scleroderma), the skin of the fingers or toes may become smooth, shiny, and tight. Small painful sores may appear on the tips of the fingers or toes.

Often, no procedures are needed to make the diagnosis. If doctors suspect an artery is blocked, color Doppler ultrasonography▲ may be performed before and after the person is exposed to cold. Doctors may also order blood tests to check for conditions that can cause Raynaud's phenomenon.

▲ see page 126

Treatment

People can control mild Raynaud's disease by protecting their head, trunk, arms, and legs from cold. For those who experience symptoms when they get excited, mild sedatives or biofeedback may help. People who have the disorder must stop smoking because nicotine constricts blood vessels.

Raynaud's disease is commonly treated with a calcium channel blocker,▲ such as nifedipine, amlodipine, diltiazem, or verapamil. Other antihypertensives, such as doxazosin, phenoxybenzamine, prazosin, reserpine, and terazosin, may be effective. They may be used alone or in combination.

If the disorder becomes progressively disabling and other treatments do not work, certain sympathetic nerves may be temporarily blocked or even cut to relieve the symptoms in a procedure called sympathectomy. However, even when this procedure is effective, relief may last only 1 to 2 years. This procedure is usually more effective for people with Raynaud's disease than for those with Raynaud's phenomenon. For people with Raynaud's phenomenon, the disorder causing it is treated.

ACROCYANOSIS

Acrocyanosis is a persistent, painless bluish discoloration of both hands and, less commonly, of both feet, caused by unexplained spasm of the small blood vessels within the skin.

The disorder usually occurs in women. The fingers and hands or toes and feet tend to feel cold and to be bluish. They sometimes sweat profusely and may swell. Exposure to cold usually intensifies the bluish discoloration, and warming reduces it. The disorder is not painful and does not damage the skin.

Doctors diagnose the disorder based on symptoms that are limited to the person's hands or feet and that persist even though pulses are normal. Treatment is usually unnecessary. Doctors may prescribe drugs that dilate the arteries (such as calcium channel blockers■), but these drugs usually do not help. Very rarely, an operation to cut certain sympathetic nerves (sympathectomy) is performed to relieve symptoms. Usually, reassurance that the bluish skin discoloration does not indicate a serious disorder is all that is necessary.

ERYTHROMELALGIA

Erythromelalgia (erythermalgia) is a rare syndrome in which arterioles of the skin dilate periodically, causing a burning pain, making the skin feel hot, and making the feet and, less often, the hands turn red.

Usually, the cause of erythromelalgia is unknown. In such cases, the disorder tends to start when people are in their 20s or older. A rare hereditary form of erythromelalgia starts at birth or during childhood. Less commonly, the disorder is related to the use of some drugs, such as nifedipine (an antihypertensive) or bromocriptine (a drug used to treat Parkinson's disease). It also occurs in people who have certain blood disorders (myeloproliferative disorders), high blood pressure, venous insufficiency, diabetes mellitus, rheumatoid arthritis, lichen sclerosis, gout, spinal cord disorders, or multiple sclerosis. Erythromelalgia usually develops 2 to 3 years before the underlying disorder is diagnosed.

Symptoms include burning pain in the feet or hands, which feel hot and appear red. Attacks are usually triggered by environmental temperatures of over 84° F (over about 29° C). Symptoms may remain mild for years or may progress and become completely incapacitating.

Diagnosis is based on the symptoms and the increase in skin temperature. Tests, such as blood cell counts, are usually performed to help identify a cause.

Treatment includes resting, elevating the legs or arms, and applying cold packs to the legs or arms or immersing them in cold water. These measures sometimes relieve symptoms or prevent attacks. If no underlying disorder is identified, aspirin may relieve symptoms, and drugs that constrict blood vessels (such as ephedrine, methysergide, and propranolol) may help. However, aspirin does not relieve symptoms for the form that starts at birth or during childhood. If an underlying disorder is identified, treating that disorder may relieve symptoms.

▲ see table on page 139

■ see table on page 139

CHAPTER 35

Aneurysms and Aortic Dissection

The aorta, which is about 1 inch in diameter, is the largest artery of the body. It receives oxygen-rich blood from the left ventricle and distributes it to all of the body except the lungs (which receive blood from the right ventricle). Just after the aorta leaves the heart, smaller arteries that carry blood to the head and arms branch off. The aorta then arches down, with additional smaller arteries branching off along its route from the left ventricle to the lower abdomen at the top of the hipbone (pelvis). At this point, the aorta divides into the two iliac arteries, which supply blood to the legs.

Disorders of the aorta include bulges (aneurysms) in weak areas of its walls and separation of the layers of its wall (dissection). These disorders can be immediately fatal, but they usually take years to develop. Aneurysms may also develop in other arteries.

Aneurysms

An aneurysm is a bulge (dilation) in the wall of an artery, usually the aorta.

The bulge usually occurs in a weak area of the artery's wall. The pressure of blood inside the artery forces the weak area to balloon outward. If untreated, an aneurysm may rupture, resulting in internal bleeding.

Aneurysms can develop anywhere along the aorta. Three fourths of aortic aneurysms develop in the part that passes through the abdomen (the abdominal aorta), and the rest develop in the part that passes through the chest (thoracic aorta). Aneurysms can also develop in the arteries at the back of the knee (popliteal arteries), the main arteries of the thighs (femoral arteries), the arteries supplying the head (carotid arteries), the arteries supplying the brain (cerebral arteries), and the arteries supplying the heart muscle (coronary arteries). In older people, aneurysms are most likely to occur in areas where arteries branch (for example, where the abdominal aorta branches into the iliac arteries) or in areas of stress (for example, in the popliteal artery). Aneurysms may be round (saccular) or tube-like (fusiform). Most are fusiform.

The most common cause of aortic aneurysms is atherosclerosis, which weakens the wall of the aorta. Less common causes include injuries, inflammatory diseases of the aorta (aortitis), hereditary connective-tissue disorders such as Marfan syndrome, and some infectious diseases such as syphilis. In people with Marfan syndrome, an aneurysm is most likely to develop in the first part of the aorta, where it emerges from the heart (the ascending aorta). In older people, almost all aneurysms are associated with atherosclerosis. High blood pressure, which is common among older people, and cigarette smoking increase the risk of an aneurysm.

A blood clot (thrombus) often develops in the aneurysm because blood flow inside the aneurysm is sluggish. The clot may extend along the entire wall of the aneurysm. A blood clot may break loose (becoming an embolus), travel through the bloodstream, and block arteries. Aneurysms in the popliteal arteries are more likely to produce emboli than aneurysms in other arteries. Occasionally, calcium is gradually deposited in the wall of an aneurysm.

ABDOMINAL AORTIC ANEURYSMS

Abdominal aortic aneurysms are aneurysms that occur in the part of the aorta that passes through the abdomen (abdominal aorta).

Abdominal aortic aneurysms may occur at any age but are most common among men aged 50 to 80 years. Abdominal aortic aneurysms tend to run in families and to occur in people who have high blood pressure, especially those who also smoke. About 20% of abdominal aneurysms eventually rupture.

Symptoms

People who have an abdominal aortic aneurysm often become aware of a pulsing sensation in their abdomen. The aneurysm may cause pain, typically a deep, penetrating pain mainly in the back. The pain can be severe and is usually unrelenting if the aneurysm is leaking.

When an aneurysm ruptures, the first symptom is usually excruciating pain in the lower

Where Do Aortic Aneurysms Occur?

Aneurysms can develop anywhere along the aorta. Most develop in the abdominal aorta. The rest develop in the thoracic aorta, most commonly in the ascending aorta.

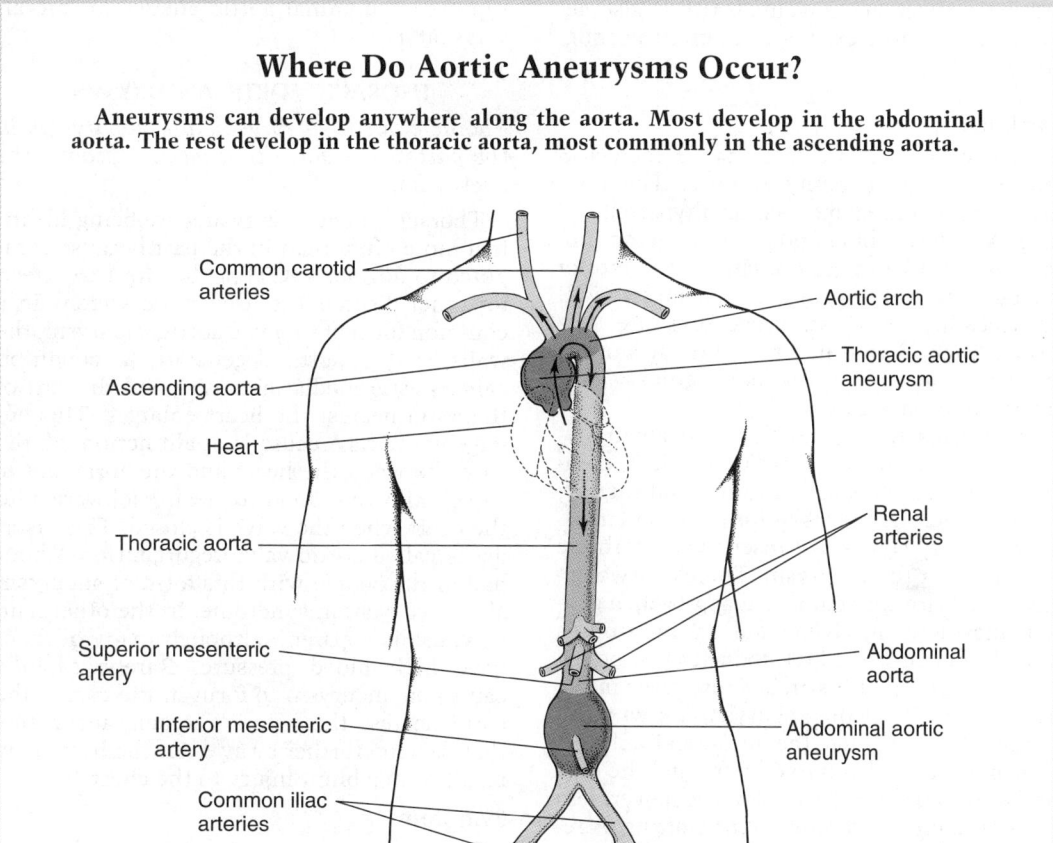

Common carotid arteries
Ascending aorta
Heart
Thoracic aorta
Superior mesenteric artery
Inferior mesenteric artery
Common iliac arteries

Aortic arch
Thoracic aortic aneurysm
Renal arteries
Abdominal aorta
Abdominal aortic aneurysm

abdomen and back and tenderness in the area over the aneurysm. If the resulting internal bleeding is severe, a person may rapidly go into shock.▲ A ruptured abdominal aneurysm is often fatal.

Diagnosis

Pain is a useful but late clue. However, many people with aneurysms have no symptoms and are diagnosed by chance when a routine physical examination or an imaging procedure (such as x-rays or ultrasonography) is performed for another reason. Doctors may feel a pulsating mass in the midline of the abdomen. With a stethoscope placed on the middle of the abdomen, doctors can usually hear a whooshing sound (bruit) caused by turbulence as blood rushes past the aneurysm. However, in obese people, even large aneurysms may not be detected. Rapidly enlarging aneurysms

that are about to rupture commonly hurt or feel tender when pressed during an abdominal examination.

Occasionally, an abdominal x-ray detects an aneurysm that has calcium deposits in its wall, but this procedure provides little other information. Other procedures are more useful for detecting aneurysms and determining their size. Usually, ultrasonography can clearly show the size of an aneurysm. If an aneurysm is detected, ultrasonography may be repeated every few months to determine if and how quickly the aneurysm is enlarging. Computed tomography (CT) of the abdomen, particularly if performed after a radiopaque dye is injected intravenously, can determine the size and shape of an aneurysm more accurately than ultrasonography but is more expensive.

▲ see page 148

Magnetic resonance imaging (MRI) is also accurate but is more expensive than ultrasonography or CT.

Treatment

Aneurysms that are less than 2 inches (5 centimeters) wide rarely rupture. The only treatment required may be antihypertensive drugs ▲ to lower blood pressure. Imaging procedures are performed to estimate the rate of enlargement and determine when surgery will be necessary. At first, procedures are performed every 3 to 6 months, then at various intervals, depending on how quickly the aneurysm is enlarging.

Aneurysms that are wider than about $2\frac{1}{2}$ inches (6 centimeters) rupture fairly commonly, so doctors usually recommend surgery, unless surgery is too risky for a particular patient. Surgery consists of inserting a synthetic graft to repair the aneurysm. There are two approaches. With the traditional approach, a general anesthetic is given, and an incision is made from below the breastbone to just below the navel. The graft is stitched into place in the aorta, the walls of the aneurysm are wrapped around the graft, and the incision is closed. This procedure takes 3 to 6 hours, and the hospital stay is usually 5 to 8 days. A newer, less invasive approach is called stent grafting. A regional (epidural) anesthetic, which causes loss of sensation only from the waist down, is used. Through a small incision made in the groin, a long, thin guide wire is threaded into the aorta to the aneurysm. A tube (catheter) containing the stent-graft (which resembles a meshed, collapsible straw) is guided over the wire and positioned inside the aneurysm. Then the stent-graft is opened, forming a stable channel for blood flow. This procedure takes 2 to 5 hours, and the hospital stay is usually 2 to 5 days. The risk of death during surgery to insert a graft is about 2 to 5%.

Rupture or threatened rupture of an abdominal aortic aneurysm requires emergency surgery. The risk of death during an operation for a ruptured aneurysm is about 50%. When an aneurysm ruptures, the kidneys may be injured because their blood supply is disrupted or because blood loss results in shock. If kidney failure develops after the operation, the chances of survival are very poor. Untreated ruptured abdominal aortic aneurysms are always fatal.

THORACIC AORTIC ANEURYSMS

Thoracic aortic aneurysms are aneurysms in the part of the aorta that passes through the chest (thorax).

Thoracic aortic aneurysms are being identified more often than in the past because computed tomography (CT) of the chest to screen for other disorders is used more widely. In a common form of thoracic aortic aneurysm, the walls of the aorta degenerate (a condition called cystic medial necrosis), and the part of the aorta nearest the heart enlarges. This enlargement may cause a malfunction of the valve between the heart and the aorta (aortic valve), allowing blood to leak backward into the heart when the valve is closed. This disorder is called aortic valve regurgitation. About half of the people with this form of aneurysm also have Marfan syndrome. In the other half, no cause is apparent, although many of them have high blood pressure. Rarely, syphilis causes an aneurysm to form in the part of the aorta nearest the heart. Thoracic aneurysms that develop further away from the heart may result from a blunt injury to the chest.

Symptoms

Thoracic aortic aneurysms may become huge without causing symptoms. Symptoms result from the pressure of the enlarging aorta against nearby structures and thus depend on where the aneurysm develops. Typical symptoms are pain (usually high in the back), coughing, and wheezing. Rarely, a person coughs up blood because of pressure on or erosion of the windpipe (trachea) or nearby airways. Swallowing may be difficult if an aneurysm puts pressure on the esophagus, which carries food to the stomach. Hoarseness may result from pressure on the nerve to the voice box (larynx). A group of symptoms called Horner's syndrome ■ may result from pressure on certain nerves in the chest. Symptoms include a constricted pupil, drooping eyelid, and sweating on one side of the face. Abnormal pulsations felt in the chest may indicate a thoracic aortic aneurysm. A displaced windpipe may be seen on chest x-rays.

When a thoracic aortic aneurysm ruptures, excruciating pain usually begins high in the back. It may radiate down the back and into the abdomen as the rupture progresses. The pain may also be felt in the chest and arms, as

---

▲ see table on page 138

■ see box on page 592

it is during a heart attack. A person can quickly go into shock▲ and die because of internal bleeding.

Diagnosis

Doctors may diagnose a thoracic aortic aneurysm based on symptoms, or they may discover the aneurysm by chance during a routine physical examination.   A chest x-ray taken for another reason may detect an aneurysm. Computed tomography (CT), magnetic resonance imaging (MRI), or transesophageal ultrasonography (in which the ultrasound probe is passed down the throat into the esophagus) is used to determine the precise size of the aneurysm. Aortography (an x-ray procedure performed after injection of a radiopaque dye that outlines the aneurysm) is usually performed to help doctors determine what type of surgery, if any, is needed. Magnetic resonance angiography or computed tomography angiography may be performed.

Treatment

If a thoracic aortic aneurysm is $2\frac{1}{2}$ inches (6 centimeters) wide or larger, surgical repair using a synthetic graft is usually performed, as for an abdominal aortic aneurysm. Before surgery, a beta-blocker, calcium channel blocker, or another antihypertensive drug■ may be given to reduce the heart rate and blood pressure and thus reduce the risk of a rupture. The hospital stay is 5 to 8 days for traditional surgery (in which the chest in opened) and 2 to 5 days for stent-grafting (in which a collapsible graft is threaded to the aorta through a small incision, usually in the groin). In people who have Marfan syndrome, a rupture is more likely, so doctors may recommend surgical repair even for smaller aneurysms.

The risk of death is about 5 to 15% during repair of thoracic aortic aneurysms but is about 50% during an operation for a ruptured thoracic aneurysm. Untreated ruptured thoracic aortic aneurysms are always fatal.

ANEURYSMS IN OTHER ARTERIES

Aneurysms may occur in arteries other than the aorta, such as the popliteal arteries (at the back of the knees), the femoral arteries (in the thighs), the coronary arteries (around the heart), and, rarely, the carotid arteries (in the neck). Older people are more likely to have aneurysms in these arteries than are younger people.

Many of these aneurysms result from a weakness present at birth (congenital) or arteriosclerosis.   Others result from injuries caused by stab or gunshot wounds or from bacterial or fungal infections in the wall of the artery. Such infections usually start elsewhere in the body, typically in a heart valve.★

Most popliteal and femoral aneurysms do not produce symptoms. However, blood clots can form within the aneurysm, break loose (becoming emboli), and block an artery in the lower leg or foot. Emboli from carotid aneurysms can block an artery in the brain and cause a stroke. Popliteal, femoral, coronary, and carotid aneurysms rarely rupture.

Doctors may feel a pulsating mass in the affected artery. Ultrasonography or computed tomography (CT) can confirm the diagnosis. For popliteal aneurysms larger than 1 inch (2.5 centimeters) in diameter, surgery to repair the aneurysm is usually performed. Usually, femoral and carotid aneurysms are surgically repaired.

Aneurysms may also occur in the arteries of the brain (cerebral arteries). Rupture of a cerebral aneurysm may cause bleeding into the brain tissue (intracerebral hemorrhage), resulting in a stroke. Because cerebral aneurysms are near the brain and are usually small, their diagnosis and treatment differ from those of other aneurysms.● Infected aneurysms of the cerebral arteries are particularly dangerous, making early treatment important. Treatment often involves surgical repair, which is very risky.

Aortic Dissection

An aortic dissection (dissecting aneurysm, dissecting hematoma) is an often fatal disorder in which the inner layer (lining) of the aortic wall tears.

When the lining of the aorta tears, blood can surge through, separating (dissecting) the middle layer of the wall from the still intact outer layer. As a result, a new, false channel forms in the wall of the aorta. Aortic dissections are 3 times more common among men and are more common among blacks and less common among Asians. About three fourths of aortic dissections occur in people aged 40 to 70.

▲ see page 148   ■ see table on page 138

★ see page 184   ● see page 512

Understanding Aortic Dissection

In an aortic dissection, the inner layer (lining) of the aortic wall tears, and blood surges through the tear, separating (dissecting) the middle layer from the outer layer of the wall. As a result, a new, false channel forms in the wall.

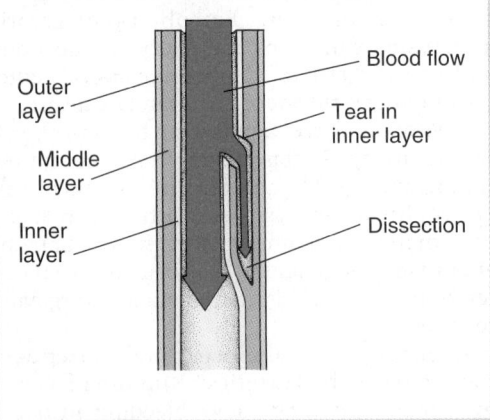

Outer layer

Middle layer

Inner layer

Blood flow

Tear in inner layer

Dissection

Most aortic dissections occur because the artery's wall deteriorates. Most commonly, such deterioration is associated with high blood pressure, which is present in more than two thirds of people who have an aortic dissection. Aortic dissection may be caused by hereditary connective-tissue disorders, especially Marfan syndrome▲ and Ehlers-Danlos syndrome.■ It may also be caused by birth defects of the heart and blood vessels,★ such as coarctation of the aorta, patent ductus arteriosus (a connection between the aorta and the pulmonary artery), and defects of the aortic valve. Other causes include arteriosclerosis and injury. Rarely, a dissection occurs accidentally when doctors are inserting a catheter into an artery (for example, during aortography or angiography) or performing surgery on the heart or blood vessels.

Symptoms

Virtually everyone who has an aortic dissection experiences pain—typically sudden, ex-

---

▲ see page 1608
★ see page 1513
◆ see page 125

■ see page 1608
● see box on page 189

---

cruciating pain, often described as tearing or ripping. Most commonly, the pain is felt across the chest but is often also felt in the back between the shoulder blades. The pain frequently travels along the path of the dissection as it advances along the aorta.

As the dissection advances, it can close off the points at which one or more arteries branch off from the aorta, blocking blood flow. The consequences vary depending on which arteries are blocked. Consequences include stroke (if the cerebral arteries, which supply the brain, are blocked), heart attack (if the coronary arteries, which supply the heart muscle, are blocked), sudden abdominal pain (if the mesentery arteries, which supply the intestines, are blocked), lower back pain (if the renal arteries, which supply the kidneys, are blocked) and nerve damage that causes tingling or an inability to move a limb (if the spinal arteries are blocked).

Blood may leak from the dissection and accumulate in the chest. Blood leaking from a dissection near the heart may enter the pericardial space (between the two layers of membranes that surround the heart), preventing the heart from filling properly and causing cardiac tamponade—a life-threatening disorder.●

Diagnosis

The distinctive symptoms of an aortic dissection usually make the diagnosis obvious to doctors, although the disorder produces a variety of symptoms that sometimes resemble those of other disorders. In about two thirds of people with aortic dissection, pulses in the arms and legs are diminished or absent. A dissection that is moving backward toward the heart may cause a murmur that can be heard through a stethoscope.

Chest x-rays are the first step in detecting aortic dissection; they show a widened aorta in 90% of people with symptoms. However, this finding may be due to other disorders. Computed tomography (CT) performed after injecting a radiopaque dye can quickly and reliably detect aortic dissection and thus is useful in an emergency. Standard or transesophageal echocardiography◆ can also reliably detect aortic dissections, even very small ones.

Treatment and Prognosis

People with an aortic dissection are admitted to intensive care units, where their vital signs (pulse, blood pressure, and rate of breathing) are closely monitored. Death can occur a few hours after an aortic dissection begins. Therefore, as soon as possible, drugs, usually sodium nitroprusside plus a beta-blocker, are given intravenously to reduce the heart rate and blood pressure to the lowest level that can maintain a sufficient blood supply to the brain, heart, and kidneys. Soon after drug therapy begins, doctors must decide whether to recommend surgery or to continue drug therapy without surgery.

Doctors almost always recommend surgery for dissections that involve the first few inches of the aorta closest to the heart, unless complications of the dissection make the risk of surgery too high. For dissections farther from the heart, doctors usually continue drug therapy without surgery. However, surgery is necessary if the dissection causes the artery to leak blood, blocks the blood supply to the legs or to vital organs in the abdomen, causes symptoms, is enlarging, or occurs in a person with Marfan syndrome. In specialized major medical centers, the risk of death during surgery is about 15% for aortic dissections close to the heart and is somewhat higher for those farther away (because the risk of complications is higher).

During surgery, the surgeon removes the largest possible area of dissected aorta, closes the false channel between the middle and outer layers of the aorta's wall, and rebuilds the aorta with a synthetic graft. If the aortic valve is leaking, the surgeon repairs or replaces it. Removal and repair of a dissected aorta usually takes 3 to 6 hours, and the hospital stay is usually 7 to 10 days.

All people who have an aortic dissection, including those treated surgically, have to take drug therapy to keep their blood pressure down, usually for the rest of their lives. Such therapy helps reduce stress on the aorta. Drug therapy usually consists of a beta-blocker or calcium channel blocker plus another antihypertensive drug such as an angiotensin-converting enzyme (ACE) inhibitor.▲

Doctors watch closely for late complications. The most important are another dissection, development of aneurysms in the weakened aorta, and increasing leakage backward through the aortic valve. Any of these complications may require surgical repair.

Without treatment, about 75% of people who have an aortic dissection die within the first 2 weeks. With treatment, 60% of people who survive the first 2 weeks are still alive 5 years after treatment; 40% live at least 10 years. Of people who die after the first 2 weeks, about one third die of complications of the dissection; the other two thirds die of other disorders.

CHAPTER 36

Venous Disorders

Veins return blood to the heart from all the organs of the body. The large veins parallel the large arteries and often share the same name, but the pathways of the venous system are more difficult to trace than those of the arteries. Many unnamed small veins form irregular networks and connect with the large veins.

Many veins, particularly those in the arms and legs, have one-way valves. Each valve consists of two flaps (cusps or leaflets) with edges that meet. Blood, as it moves toward the heart, pushes the cusps open like a pair of one-way swinging doors. If gravity or muscle contractions try to pull the blood backward or if blood begins to back up in a vein, the cusps are pushed closed, preventing backward flow. Thus, valves help return blood to the heart—by opening when the blood flows toward the heart and closing when it tries to flow backward.

The main problems that affect the veins include inflammation, clotting, and defects that lead to distention and varicose veins. The veins in the legs are particularly affected because when a person is standing, blood must flow upward from the leg veins, against gravity, to reach the heart.

▲ see table on page 139

One-Way Valves in the Veins

One-way valves consist of two flaps (cusps or leaflets) with edges that meet. These valves help veins return blood to the heart. Blood, as it moves toward the heart, pushes the cusps open like a pair of one-way swinging doors (shown on the left). If gravity momentarily pulls the blood backward or if blood begins to back up in a vein, the cusps are immediately pushed closed, preventing backward flow (shown on the right).

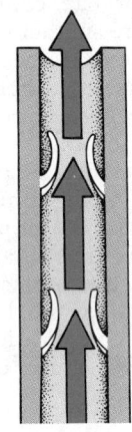   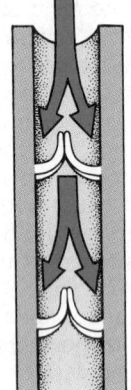

Valves Open   Valves Closed

The legs contain superficial veins, located in the fatty layer under the skin, and deep veins, located in the muscles. Short veins, called connecting veins, link the superficial and deep veins.

The deep veins play a major role in propelling blood upward. The one-way valves in deep veins prevent blood from flowing backward, and the muscles surrounding the deep veins compress them, helping force the blood upward, just as squeezing a toothpaste tube ejects toothpaste. The powerful calf muscles are particularly important, forcefully compressing the deep veins with every step. The deep veins carry 90% or more of the blood from the legs toward the heart.

▲ see page 236   ■ see page 285

Superficial veins play only a minor role in carrying blood to the heart. They have the same type of valves as deep veins, but they are not surrounded by muscle. Thus, blood in the superficial veins is not forced upward by the squeezing action of muscles, and it flows more slowly than blood in the deep veins. Much of the blood that flows up the superficial veins is diverted into the deep veins through the many connecting veins between the deep and superficial veins. Valves in the connecting veins allow blood to flow from the superficial veins into the deep veins but not vice versa.

Deep Vein Thrombosis

Deep vein thrombosis is the formation of blood clots (thrombi) in the deep veins.

Thrombi can occur either in the deep leg veins, causing deep vein thrombosis, or in the superficial leg veins, causing superficial thrombophlebitis.▲

Thrombophlebitis is a disorder in which the formation of blood clots (thrombosis) and inflammation of the vein (phlebitis) occur together. Because thrombosis is almost always accompanied by phlebitis, some doctors use thrombosis and thrombophlebitis interchangeably. However, there is an important distinction between deep vein thrombosis and thrombophlebitis. Deep vein thrombosis causes only a little inflammation. The less inflammation around a thrombus, the less tightly the thrombus adheres to the vein wall and the more likely it will break loose (becoming an embolus), travel through the bloodstream, and lodge in an artery downstream, blocking blood flow. In addition, the squeezing action of the calf muscles can dislodge a thrombus in a deep vein, especially when a convalescing person becomes more active. Thus, only thrombi in the deep veins are potentially dangerous. Superficial thrombophlebitis is painful but comparatively harmless, because thrombi in small, superficial veins usually do not become emboli.

Because blood in the leg veins travels to the heart and then to the lungs, emboli originating in the leg veins usually pass through the heart and block one or more arteries in the lungs, a condition called **pulmonary embolism.**■ The seriousness of pulmonary embolism depends on the size and number of emboli. A small embolus may block a small artery in the lungs, causing the death of a small piece of lung tissue (pulmonary infarction). However, a large pulmonary embolus can block all or nearly all of the blood traveling from the right side of the heart to the lungs, quickly causing death. Such massive emboli are not common, but no one can predict which case of deep vein thrombosis, if untreated, will lead to a massive embolus. Thus, doctors are greatly concerned about every person who has deep vein thrombosis.

Causes

Three main factors (known as Virchow's triad) can contribute to deep vein thrombosis: injury to the vein's lining, an increased tendency for blood to clot, and slowing of blood flow.

Veins may be injured during surgery, by injection of irritating substances, or by certain disorders, such as Buerger's disease. They may also be injured by a clot, making formation of a second clot more likely.

Some disorders, such as disseminated intravascular coagulation, cause blood to clot when it should not. Some cancers and, rarely, use of oral contraceptives can cause blood to clot more readily. Sometimes blood clots more readily after childbirth or surgery. Among older people, dehydration and smoking are common causes of this tendency and can therefore contribute to deep vein thrombosis.

During prolonged bed rest, blood flow slows, because the calf muscles are not contracting and squeezing the blood toward the heart. For example, deep vein thrombosis may develop in people who have had a heart attack and lie in hospital beds for several days without sufficiently moving their legs or in people whose legs and lower body are paralyzed (paraplegics). Deep vein thrombosis can develop after hip repair or replacement. Thrombosis can even occur in healthy people who sit for long periods, for example, during long drives or airplane flights.

Symptoms

Because deep vein thrombosis usually causes little inflammation, pain and redness of the skin over the vein are usually minimal. About half of the people with deep vein thrombosis have no symptoms at all. In these people, chest pain caused by pulmonary embolism may be the first indication that something is wrong. When deep vein thrombosis blocks blood flow in a large leg vein, the calf swells and may be painful, tender to the touch, and warm. The ankle, foot, or thigh may also swell, depending on which veins are involved.

Some thrombi heal by being converted to scar tissue, which may damage the valves in the veins. Because the damaged valves prevent the veins from functioning normally, fluid accumulates (a condition called edema) and the ankle swells. The edema can extend up the leg and even affect the thigh if the blockage is high enough in the vein. Edema is worse toward the end of the day, because blood must flow upward, against gravity, to reach the heart when a person is standing or sitting. Overnight, edema subsides because the veins empty well when the legs are horizontal.

Chronic Deep Vein Insufficiency: This complication occurs late in the course of deep vein thrombosis. The valves in the deep veins and connecting veins of the legs are destroyed. Consequently, blood is not adequately returned to the heart from the legs. Eventually, the affected veins may be obliterated.

Edema in the legs is always present, generally worsening at the end of the day. The skin on the inside of the ankle becomes scaly and itchy and may turn a reddish brown. The discoloration is caused by red blood cells that escape from swollen (distended) veins into the skin. The discolored skin is vulnerable, and even a minor injury, such as that from scratching or a bump, can break it open, resulting in an ulcer. Varicose veins may be present. In addition to ulcer pain, there may be throbbing pain when standing or walking.

If edema is severe and persistent, scar tissue develops and traps fluid in the tissues. As a result, the calf permanently enlarges and feels hard. In such cases, ulcers are more likely to develop, and they heal less easily.

Diagnosis

Deep vein thrombosis may be difficult for doctors to detect, especially when pain and swelling are absent or very slight. When this disorder is suspected, color Doppler ultrasonography▲ can confirm the diagnosis. If the person has symptoms of pulmonary embolism, chest scanning using a radioactive marker■ is performed to confirm the diagnosis of pulmonary embolism, and color Doppler ultrasonography is performed to check the legs for clots. These procedures are performed except when a person collapses. Collapse suggests massive pulmonary embolism and requires immediate treatment.

▲ see page 126   ■ see page 255

Prevention

Although the risk of deep vein thrombosis cannot be entirely eliminated, it can be reduced in several ways. People at risk of deep vein thrombosis should flex and extend the ankles about 10 times every 30 minutes. Such people include those who have just had major surgery and those taking long trips. During long flights, everyone should walk and stretch every 2 hours.

Continuously wearing elastic stockings (support hose) makes the veins narrow slightly and the blood flow more rapidly. As a result, clotting is less likely. However, elastic stockings are not sufficient protection against developing deep vein thrombosis. Also, they may give a false sense of security and discourage more effective methods of prevention. If not worn correctly, they may bunch up and aggravate the problem by blocking blood flow in the legs.

Pneumatic stockings are an effective way to prevent clots. Usually made of plastic, these stockings are automatically pumped up and emptied by an electric pump. They repeatedly squeeze the calves and empty the veins. The stockings are put on before surgery and kept on during and after surgery, until the person can walk again.

An anticoagulant,▲ such as heparin or warfarin, is given to people at high risk of developing deep vein thrombosis before, during, and sometimes after surgery. Such people include those who have clotting disorders■ and those who have recently had one or more episodes of deep vein thrombosis. For certain types of surgery (such as hip replacement surgery), the risk is particularly high. People who are at particularly high risk may be given an anticoagulant when they are hospitalized even though they are not undergoing surgery. Anticoagulants reduce blood clotting much more effectively than wearing elastic stockings.

Treatment

For deep vein thrombosis, treatment involves prevention of pulmonary embolism. Hospitalization may be necessary at first, but because of the advances in treatment, some people with deep vein thrombosis can be treated at home. Bed rest with the foot of the bed raised 6 inches is usually required to help prevent the thrombus from enlarging, as are

anticoagulants. Usually, anticoagulant therapy consists of low-molecular-weight heparin given by injection under the skin (subcutaneously), followed by warfarin taken by mouth. How long warfarin must be taken varies. Young, active people who have had only one episode of deep vein thrombosis may need to continue the drug for only 2 months. People who have had deep vein thrombosis followed by pulmonary embolism continue to be at increased risk of deep vein thrombosis. They may need to continue the drug for 6 months. People who have had two or more episodes of deep vein thrombosis should continue warfarin indefinitely.

Use of warfarin increases the risk of bleeding, both internally and externally. To keep this risk as low as possible, doctors periodically perform blood tests to measure clotting time and adjust the dose of warfarin on the basis of test results.

Drugs to dissolve the thrombus (thrombolytic drugs), such as tissue plasminogen activator, may also be given intravenously, particularly if the thrombus has been present for less than 48 hours. After 48 hours, scar tissue begins to develop in the thrombus, making the thrombus less likely to dissolve.

Sometimes, a filter (umbrella) is placed inside a large vein between the heart and the area affected by deep vein thrombosis, usually the inferior vena cava, which returns blood to the heart from the lower part of the body. A filter can trap emboli, preventing them from reaching the lungs.

If pulmonary embolism occurs, treatment usually includes oxygen (usually given by a face mask or nasal prongs), analgesics to relieve pain, and heparin followed by warfarin. If pulmonary embolism is life threatening, thrombolytic drugs are given or surgery is performed to remove the embolus.

Swelling of the legs can be reduced by resting in bed and elevating the legs or by wearing compression bandages from the base of the toes to the knee. Improperly applied, the bandages may be wrapped more tightly around the upper calf than around the foot and ankle, resulting in a tourniquet effect. Therefore, only a trained doctor or nurse should apply compression bandages. During this time, walking is important. If the swelling does not completely subside, the bandages must be reapplied. The veins never completely recover after deep vein thrombosis develops, and surgery to repair the valves of the veins is ex-

▲ see page 288   ■ see page 995

Umbrellas: Preventing Pulmonary Embolism

In people who have deep vein thrombosis, a blood clot may break loose from an affected vein in the leg and travel through the bloodstream. A clot that breaks loose is called an embolus.

The embolus travels toward the heart and passes through the right atrium and ventricle and into one of the pulmonary arteries, which carry blood to the lungs. The clot may lodge in an artery in a lung and block blood flow,

resulting in pulmonary embolism. Pulmonary embolism may be life threatening, depending on the size of the blocked artery.

To prevent pulmonary embolism, doctors may recommend that a filter, called an umbrella, be permanently placed in the inferior vena cava. The filter traps emboli before they reach the heart but allows blood to flow through freely. Emboli that are trapped sometimes dissolve on their own.

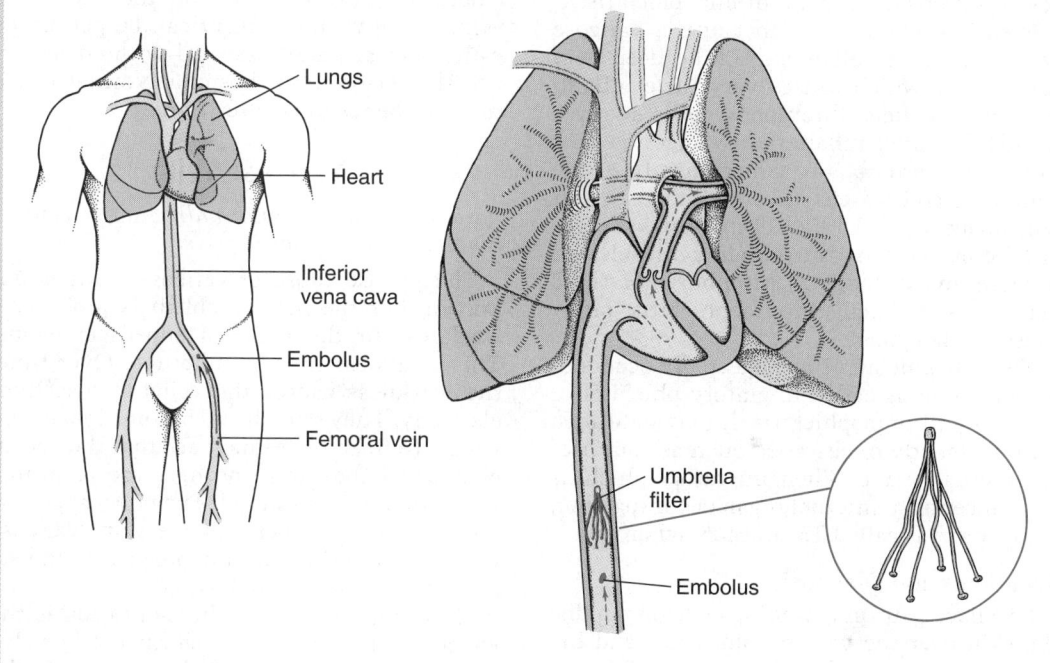

perimental. After the compression bandages are removed, elastic stockings are worn every day to prevent swelling from recurring. The stockings do not have to be worn above the knee; swelling above the knee is of little concern and causes no complications. Usually, thick elastic stockings or strong elastic pantyhose is not needed.

If painful skin ulcers develop, properly applied compression bandages can help. When these bandages are applied once or twice a week, the ulcer almost always heals because blood flow in the veins improves. The ulcers are almost always infected, and pus and a foul-

smelling discharge appear on the bandage each time it is changed. The pus and discharge can be washed off the skin with soap and water. Skin creams, balms, and skin medications of any kind have little effect.

Once blood flow in the veins has improved, the ulcer heals by itself. After it has healed, wearing an elastic stocking daily can prevent a recurrence. The stocking must be replaced as soon as it becomes too loose. If possible, the person should purchase seven stockings or pairs of stockings (if both legs are involved)— one for each day of the week. This way, stockings remain effective considerably longer.

Rarely, ulcers that do not heal require skin grafting. After grafting, an elastic stocking must be worn to prevent ulcers from returning.

Superficial Thrombophlebitis

Superficial thrombophlebitis (superficial phlebitis) is inflammation and clotting in a superficial vein.

Superficial thrombophlebitis most often affects the superficial veins in the legs but may also affect superficial veins in the groin. Often, thrombophlebitis occurs in people with varicose veins; however, most people with varicose veins do not develop thrombophlebitis.

Even a slight injury can cause a varicose vein to become inflamed. Unlike deep vein thrombosis, which causes very little inflammation, superficial thrombophlebitis involves a sudden (acute) inflammatory reaction that causes the thrombus to adhere firmly to the vein wall and lessens the likelihood that it will break loose. Unlike deep veins, superficial veins have no surrounding muscles to squeeze and dislodge a thrombus. For these reasons, superficial thrombophlebitis rarely causes embolism.

Thrombophlebitis that repeatedly occurs in normal veins is called migratory phlebitis or migratory thrombophlebitis. It may indicate a serious underlying disorder, such as cancer of an internal organ. When migratory phlebitis and cancer of an internal organ occur together, the disorder is called Trousseau's syndrome.

Symptoms and Diagnosis

Localized pain and swelling develop rapidly, the skin over the vein becomes red, and the area feels warm and is very tender. Because blood in the vein is clotted, the vein feels like a hard cord under the skin, not soft like a normal or varicose vein. The vein may feel hard along its entire length. The diagnosis is usually obvious to doctors just from examining the painful area. However, doctors must distinguish superficial thrombophlebitis from cellulitis, which is treated differently.

Treatment

Most often, superficial thrombophlebitis subsides by itself. Taking an analgesic, such as aspirin or another nonsteroidal anti-inflammatory drug (NSAIDs),▲ usually helps relieve

the pain. Although the inflammation generally subsides in a matter of days, several weeks may pass before the lumps and tenderness subside completely. To provide early relief, doctors may inject a local anesthetic, remove the thrombus, and then apply a compression bandage, which the person wears for several days.

When superficial thrombophlebitis occurs in the groin, where the main superficial vein joins the main deep vein, a thrombus may extend into the deep vein. Such a thrombus may break loose to become an embolus. To prevent this extension, some surgeons recommend emergency surgery to tie off the superficial vein. Usually, this surgery can be performed using a local anesthetic and without admitting the person to the hospital. Normal activities may be resumed afterward.

Varicose Veins

Varicose veins are abnormally enlarged superficial veins in the legs.

The precise cause of varicose veins is unknown, but the main problem is probably a weakness in the walls of superficial veins. This weakness may be inherited. Over time, the weakness causes the veins to lose their elasticity. They stretch and become longer and wider. To fit in the same space that they occupied when they were normal, the elongated veins become convoluted. They may appear as a snakelike bulge beneath the skin. Varicose veins often develop during pregnancy and resolve shortly after childbirth.

More important than the elongation is the widening of the veins, which causes the valve cusps to separate. When the person stands, the blood is pulled backward by gravity and is not stopped because the valve cusps are separated. Thus, blood flows backward, rapidly filling the veins. The backward flow of blood causes the thin-walled, convoluted veins to enlarge even more. Some of the connecting veins, which normally allow blood to flow only from the superficial veins into the deep veins, also enlarge. If they enlarge, their valve cusps also separate. Consequently, blood squirts backward into the superficial veins when the muscles squeeze the deep veins, causing the superficial veins to stretch further.

Many people with varicose veins also have spider veins, which are enlarged capillaries. Spider veins may be caused by the pressure from blood in varicose veins, but the cause is

▲ see page 452

generally thought to be hormonal factors that are not yet understood. A hormonal cause would explain why spider veins most commonly occur in women, particularly during pregnancy.

Symptoms and Complications

Besides being unsightly, varicose veins commonly ache and make the legs feel tired. However, many people, even some with very large veins, have no pain. The lower part of the leg and ankle may itch, especially if the leg is warm after a person has been wearing socks or stockings. Itching can lead to scratching and can cause redness or a rash, which is often incorrectly attributed to dry skin. The pain is sometimes worse when varicose veins are developing than when they are fully stretched.

Only a small percentage of people with varicose veins have complications, such as dermatitis, inflammation of the veins (phlebitis), or bleeding. Dermatitis produces a red, scaling, itchy rash or a brown area, usually on the inside of the leg above the ankle. Scratching or a minor injury, particularly from shaving, can cause bleeding or development of a painful ulcer that does not heal. Ulcers may also bleed. Phlebitis may occur spontaneously or result from an injury. Although usually painful, phlebitis that occurs with varicose veins is rarely harmful.

Diagnosis

Varicose veins can usually be seen bulging under the skin, but symptoms may develop before the veins become visible. When varicose veins are not visible, doctors experienced in checking for them can palpate the leg to determine the extent of the problem.

X-rays or ultrasonography may be performed to assess the functioning of the deep veins. Usually, such procedures are necessary only if malfunction of the deep veins is suggested by changes in the skin or by swollen ankles. The ankles swell because fluid accumulates in the tissue under the skin—a condition called edema. Varicose veins alone do not cause edema.

Treatment

Although individual varicose veins can be removed or eliminated by surgery or injection therapy, the disorder cannot be cured. Thus, treatment mainly relieves symptoms, improves appearance, and prevents complications. Elevating the legs—by lying down or

Valves in Varicose Veins

In a normal vein, the cusps of the valves close to prevent backward flow of blood. In a varicose vein, the cusps cannot close because the vein is abnormally widened. Consequently, blood can flow in the wrong direction.

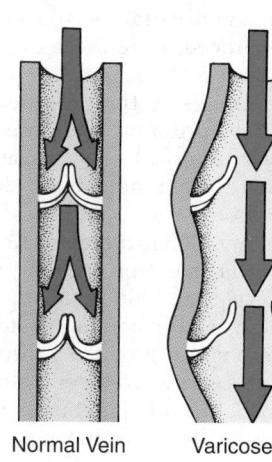

Normal Vein   Varicose Vein

using a footstool when sitting—relieves the symptoms of varicose veins but does not prevent new varicose veins from forming. Usually, varicose veins that appear during pregnancy largely subside during the 2 or 3 weeks after delivery. During this time, they should not be treated.

Elastic stockings (support hose) compress the veins and prevent them from stretching and hurting. People who do not want surgery or injection therapy or who have a medical condition that prevents them from having these treatments may choose to wear elastic stockings.

Surgery: Surgery aims to remove as many of the varicose veins as possible. However, surgeons try to preserve the saphenous vein because it can be used as a bypass graft if coronary artery or peripheral artery disease develops. This vein is the longest superficial vein in the body, extending from the ankle to the groin, where it joins the femoral vein (the main deep vein in the leg). If the saphenous vein must be removed, a procedure called stripping is performed. The surgeon makes two incisions, one at the groin and one at the ankle, and opens the vein at each end. A flexible wire is threaded through the entire vein and then pulled out to remove the vein.

To remove other varicose veins, the surgeon makes incisions in other areas. Because the superficial veins play a less significant role than the deep veins in returning blood to the heart, their removal does not impair circulation if the deep veins are functioning normally.

Removal of varicose veins is a lengthy procedure, so the person is usually given a general anesthetic. This procedure relieves the symptoms and prevents complications, but it leaves scars. The more extensive the procedure, the longer the time before new varicose veins develop. However, removal of varicose veins does not eliminate the tendency to develop new varicose veins.

Injection Therapy (Sclerotherapy): An alternative to surgery is injection therapy, which seals the veins, so that blood can no longer flow through them. A solution is injected into the vein to irritate it and produce a thrombus. In essence, this procedure produces a harmless kind of superficial thrombophlebitis. Healing of the thrombus leads to formation of scar tissue, which blocks the vein. However, the thrombus may dissolve instead of becoming scar tissue, and the varicose vein then reopens.

Injection therapy was common in the United States between the 1930s and 1950s but fell out of favor because of poor results and complications. Current techniques are more likely to be successful and are safe for varicose veins of all sizes.

Current techniques include special bandaging that reduces the size of the thrombus by compressing the diameter of the injected vein. A smaller thrombus is more likely to form scar tissue, as desired. A further advantage of this technique is that adequate compression virtually eliminates the pain usually associated with superficial phlebitis.

Although injection therapy is more time-consuming than surgery, it has several advantages: Anesthesia is not necessary, new varicose veins can be treated as they develop, and people can go about their normal daily activities between treatments. However, even with current techniques, some doctors consider injection therapy only when varicose veins return after surgery or when a person desires cosmetic improvement.

If spider veins cause pain or a burning sensation or are unsightly, they also may be treated with injection therapy.

Laser Therapies: Laser therapy is being used experimentally by some surgeons for the treatment of varicose veins. This therapy uses a highly focused, continuous stream of high-intensity light to cut or destroy tissue. However, the usefulness of this therapy has not yet been determined. Intense pulsed light therapy can be used to treat small spider veins. This therapy is similar to laser therapy except that the light is applied in pulses.

Arteriovenous Fistula

An arteriovenous fistula is an abnormal channel between an artery and a vein.

Normally, blood flows from arteries into capillaries and then into veins. When an arteriovenous fistula is present, blood flows directly from an artery into a vein, bypassing the capillaries. A person may be born with an arteriovenous fistula (congenital fistula), or a fistula may develop after birth (acquired fistula).

Congenital arteriovenous fistulas are uncommon. Acquired arteriovenous fistulas can be caused by any injury that damages an artery and a vein that lie side by side. Typically, the injury is a piercing wound, as from a knife or bullet. The fistula may appear immediately or may develop after a few hours. The area can swell quickly if blood escapes into the surrounding tissues.

Some medical treatments, such as kidney dialysis, require that a vein be pierced for each treatment. With repeated piercing, the vein becomes inflamed and clotting can develop. Eventually, scar tissue may develop and destroy the vein. To avoid this problem, doctors may deliberately create an arteriovenous fistula, usually between an adjoining vein and artery in the arm. This procedure widens the vein, making needle insertion easier and enabling the blood to flow faster. Faster flowing blood is less likely to clot. Unlike some large arteriovenous fistulas, these small, intentionally created fistulas do not lead to heart problems, and they can be closed when no longer needed.

Symptoms and Diagnosis

When congenital arteriovenous fistulas are near the surface of the skin, they may appear swollen and reddish blue. In conspicuous places, such as the face, they appear purplish and may be unsightly.

If a large acquired arteriovenous fistula is not treated, a large volume of blood flows under high pressure from the artery into the vein network. Vein walls are not strong enough to withstand such high pressure, so the walls stretch and the veins enlarge and bulge (sometimes resembling varicose veins). In addition, blood flows more freely into the enlarged veins than it would if it continued its normal course through the arteries. As a result, blood pressure falls. To compensate for this fall in blood pressure, the heart pumps more forcefully and more rapidly, thus greatly increasing its output of blood. Eventually, the increased effort may strain the heart, causing heart failure. The larger the fistula, the more quickly heart failure can develop.

With a stethoscope placed over a large acquired arteriovenous fistula, doctors can hear a distinctive "to-and-fro" sound, like that of moving machinery. This sound is called a machinery murmur. Doppler ultrasonography is used to confirm the diagnosis and to determine the extent of the problem. For fistulas between deeper blood vessels (such as the aorta and vena cava), magnetic resonance imaging (MRI) is more useful.

Treatment

Small congenital arteriovenous fistulas can be cut out or eliminated with laser coagulation therapy. This procedure must be performed by a skilled vascular surgeon, because the fistulas are sometimes more extensive than they appear to be on the surface. Arteriovenous fistulas near the eye, brain, or other major structures can be especially difficult to treat.

Acquired arteriovenous fistulas are corrected by a surgeon as soon as possible after diagnosis. Before the surgery, a radiopaque dye, which can be seen on x-rays, may be injected to outline the fistula more clearly in a procedure called angiography.▲ If the surgeon cannot reach the fistula easily (for example, if it is in the brain), complex injection techniques that cause clots to form may be used to block blood flow through the fistula. For example, coils or plugs may be inserted into the fistula at the various points where the vein and the artery meet. This procedure is performed using x-rays for guidance and does not require open surgery.

CHAPTER 37

Lymphatic Disorders

Like the venous system, the lymphatic system transports fluids throughout the body. The lymphatic system consists of thin-walled lymphatic vessels, lymph nodes, and two collecting ducts.■ Lymphatic vessels, located throughout the body, are larger than capillaries, and most are smaller than the smallest veins. Most of the lymphatic vessels have valves like those in veins to keep the lymph, which can clot, flowing in the one direction. Lymphatic vessels drain fluids that have diffused through the very thin walls of capillaries. The fluids contain proteins, minerals, nutrients, and other substances, which provide nourishment to tissues. However, most of the fluid is reabsorbed into the capillaries. The rest of the fluid (lymph) is drained from the spaces surrounding the cells into the lymphatic vessels, which eventually return it to the veins. Lymphatic vessels also collect and transport damaged cells, cancer cells, and foreign particles (such as bacteria

and viruses) that may have entered the tissue fluids.

All of lymph passes through strategically placed lymph nodes, which filter damaged cells, cancer cells, and foreign particles out of the lymph. Lymph nodes also produce specialized blood cells designed to engulf and destroy damaged cells, cancer cells, and foreign particles. Thus, important functions of the lymphatic system are to remove damaged cells from the body and to provide protection against the spread of infection and cancer.

The lymph vessels drain into collecting ducts, which empty their contents into the two subclavian veins, located under the collarbones. These veins join to form the superior vena cava, the large vein that drains blood from the upper body into the heart.

The lymphatic system may not perform its function adequately when the quantity of

▲ see page 130   ■ see art on page 1053

fluid is excessive or when the lymph vessels or nodes become blocked by a tumor or become inflamed.

Lymphedema

Lymphedema is the accumulation of lymph resulting in swelling.

Lymphedema differs from accumulation of fluid (edema) due to venous insufficiency, which develops when blood that is backed up in veins causes fluid to leak from blood vessels into tissues. Edema may be caused by heart failure,▲ but lymphedema is not. Lymphedema results when an abnormality prevents lymph from being reabsorbed into the capillaries as it normally is. As a result, the lymphatic system cannot adequately drain lymph from the tissues.

Lymphedema may be due to conditions present at birth (congenital) or to conditions that develop later (acquired).

Congenital lymphedema results from having so few lymphatic vessels that they cannot handle all the lymph. The problem almost always affects the legs; rarely, it affects the arms. Women are much more likely than men to have congenital lymphedema.

Rarely, the swelling is obvious at birth, but usually, the lymphatic vessels can handle the small amount of lymph produced in an infant. More often, the swelling appears later in life, as the volume of lymph increases and overwhelms the small number of lymph vessels. The swelling starts gradually in one or both legs. The first sign of lymphedema may be puffiness of the foot, making the shoe feel tight at the end of the day. The shoe may leave indentations in the skin of the foot. (Many people who do not have lymphedema experience swelling after they stand for prolonged periods. They may have indentations around their ankles after they wear ankle socks, but the indentations are much less deep than those of lymphedema, and the surrounding area is not puffy.)

In the early stages of congenital lymphedema, the swelling goes away when the leg is elevated. This disorder worsens with time: The swelling becomes more obvious and does not disappear completely, even after a night's rest.

Acquired lymphedema is more common than congenital lymphedema. It typically appears after major surgical treatment, especially after cancer treatment in which lymph nodes and lymphatic vessels are removed or treated with radiation. For example, the arm tends to swell after removal of a cancerous breast and the associated lymph nodes. Scarring of repeatedly infected lymphatic vessels may also cause lymphedema, but this type of scarring is very uncommon except among people who have an infection due to the tropical parasite *Filaria* (filariasis).

In acquired lymphedema, the skin looks healthy but is puffy or swollen. Pressing the area with a finger does not leave a significant indentation, as it does when edema results from inadequate blood flow in the veins. Rarely, especially in filariasis, the swollen limb becomes extremely large and the skin is so thick and ridged that it looks almost like elephant skin. This disorder is called **elephantiasis.**

Treatment

Lymphedema has no cure. For people with mild lymphedema, compression bandages can reduce the swelling. People who are more severely affected may wear pneumatic stockings■ every day for an hour or two to reduce the swelling. Once the swelling has been reduced, the person must wear elastic stockings up to the knee every day from the moment of rising until bedtime. This measure controls the swelling to some degree. For lymphedema in the arm, pneumatic sleeves—like pneumatic stockings—can be used every day to reduce the swelling; elastic sleeves are also available. For elephantiasis, an extensive operation may be performed to remove most of the swollen tissues under the skin.

Lymphadenitis

Lymphadenitis is inflammation of one or more lymph nodes, which usually become swollen and tender.

Lymphadenitis is almost always caused by an infection, which may be due to bacteria, viruses, protozoa, rickettsiae, or fungi. Typically, the infection spreads to a lymph node from a skin, ear, nose, or eye infection or from such infections as infectious mononucleosis, cytomegalovirus infection, streptococcal infection, tuberculosis, or syphilis. The infection may affect many lymph nodes or only those in one area of the body.

Symptoms and Diagnosis

Infected lymph nodes enlarge and are usually tender and painful. Sometimes, the skin over

---

▲ see page 150   ■ see page 234

the infected nodes looks red and feels warm. Occasionally, pockets of pus (abscesses) develop. Enlarged lymph nodes that do not produce pain, tenderness, or redness may indicate a serious disorder, such as lymphoma, tuberculosis, or Hodgkin's disease. Such lymph nodes require a doctor's attention.

Usually, lymphadenitis can be diagnosed on the basis of symptoms, and its cause is an obvious nearby infection. When the cause cannot be identified easily, a biopsy (removal and examination of a tissue sample under a microscope) and culture may be needed to confirm the diagnosis and to identify the organism causing the infection.

Treatment and Prognosis

Treatment depends on the organism causing the infection. For a bacterial infection, an antibiotic is usually given intravenously or orally. Warm compresses may help relieve the pain in inflamed lymph nodes. Usually, once the infection has been treated, the lymph nodes slowly shrink, and the pain subsides. Sometimes the enlarged nodes remain firm but no longer feel tender. Abscesses must be drained surgically.

Acute Lymphangitis

Acute lymphangitis is inflammation of one or more lymphatic vessels, usually caused by a streptococcal infection.

Streptococci bacteria usually enter the lymphatic vessels from a scrape or wound in an arm or a leg. Often, a streptococcal infection in the skin and the tissues just beneath the skin (cellulitis)▲ spreads to the lymph vessels. Occasionally, staphylococci or other bacteria are the cause.

Red, irregular, warm, tender streaks develop under the skin in the affected arm or leg. The streaks usually stretch from the infected area toward a group of lymph nodes, such as those in the groin or armpit. The lymph nodes become enlarged and feel tender.

Common symptoms include a fever, chills, a rapid heart rate, and a headache. Sometimes these symptoms occur before the red streaks appear. The spread of the infection from the lymph system into the bloodstream can cause infection throughout the body, often with startling speed. The skin or tissues over the infected lymph vessel becomes inflamed. Rarely, skin ulcers develop.

The diagnosis of acute lymphangitis is based on symptoms. A blood test usually shows that the number of white blood cells has increased to fight the infection. Doctors have difficulty identifying the organisms causing the infection unless the organisms have spread through the bloodstream or pus can be taken from a wound in the affected area.

Most people are cured quickly with antibiotics that kill staphylococci and streptococci, such as dicloxacillin, nafcillin, or oxacillin.

▲ see page 1220

LUNG AND AIRWAY DISORDERS

38 Biology of the Lungs and Airways 244

The Respiratory System ▪ The Chest Cavity ▪ Exchanging
Oxygen and Carbon Dioxide ▪ Control of Breathing ▪ Defense
Mechanisms ▪ Effects of Aging

39 Symptoms and Diagnosis of Lung Disorders 248

Cough ▪ Dyspnea ▪ Chest Pain ▪ Wheezing ▪ Stridor ▪
Hemoptysis ▪ Cyanosis ▪ Finger Clubbing ▪ Medical History
and Physical Examination ▪ Pulmonary Function Testing ▪ Sleep
Studies ▪ Arterial Blood Gas Analysis ▪ Chest Imaging ▪
Positron Emission Tomography ▪ Thoracentesis ▪ Needle Biopsy
of the Pleura or Lung ▪ Bronchoscopy ▪ Thoracoscopy ▪
Mediastinoscopy ▪ Thoracotomy ▪ Suctioning

40 Pulmonary Rehabilitation 259

Enrollment and Goal Setting ▪ Exercise Training ▪ Psychosocial
Counseling ▪ Nutritional Evaluation and Counseling ▪ Drug
Use and Education ▪ Oxygen Therapy ▪ Chest Physical
Therapy ▪ Postural Drainage ▪ Suctioning ▪ Breathing
Exercises

41 Bronchitis 262

42 Pneumonia 264

Community-Acquired Pneumonia ▪ Hospital-Acquired and
Institutional-Acquired Pneumonia ▪ Fungal Pneumonia ▪
Pneumocystis Pneumonia ▪ Aspiration Pneumonia

43 Lung Abscess 272

44 Asthma 274

45 Chronic Obstructive Pulmonary Disease 281

46 Pulmonary Embolism 285

47 Bronchiectasis 289

48 Atelectasis 292

49 Occupational Lung Diseases 294

Silicosis ▪ Black Lung ▪ Asbestosis ▪ Beryllium Disease ▪
Flock Worker's Lung ▪ Occupational Asthma ▪ Byssinosis ▪
Benign Pneumoconioses ▪ Gas and Chemical Exposure

50   Infiltrative Lung Diseases...301

Idiopathic Pulmonary Fibrosis ▪ Desquamative Interstitial
Pneumonia ▪ Lymphoid Interstitial Pneumonia ▪ Cryptogenic
Organizing Pneumonitis ▪ Langerhans' Cell Granulomatosis ▪
Sarcoidosis ▪ Pulmonary Alveolar Proteinosis

51   Allergic Diseases of the Lungs...308

Hypersensitivity Pneumonitis ▪ Eosinophilic Pneumonia ▪
Allergic Bronchopulmonary Aspergillosis ▪ Goodpasture's
Syndrome

52   Pleural Disorders..312

Pleurisy ▪ Pleural Effusion ▪ Pneumothorax

53   Cystic Fibrosis...317

54   Pulmonary Hypertension..322

55   Respiratory Failure..325

56   Acute Respiratory Distress Syndrome...326

57   Lung Cancer..328

CHAPTER 38

Biology of the Lungs and Airways

To sustain life, the body must produce sufficient energy. Energy is produced by burning molecules in food, which is done by the process of oxidation (whereby food molecules are combined with oxygen). Oxidation results in carbon and hydrogen being combined with oxygen to form carbon dioxide and water. The consumption of oxygen and the production of carbon dioxide are thus indispensable to life. It follows that the human body must have an organ system designed to exchange carbon dioxide and oxygen between the circulating blood and the atmosphere at a rate rapid enough to sustain life. The respiratory system enables oxygen to enter the body and carbon dioxide to leave the body.

The Respiratory System

The respiratory system starts at the nose and mouth and continues through the airways to the lungs. Air enters the respiratory system through the nose and mouth and passes down the throat (pharynx) and through the voice box, or Adam's apple (larynx). The entrance to the larynx is covered by a small flap of tissue (epiglottis) that automatically closes when swallowing, thus preventing food or drink from entering the airways.

The largest airway is the windpipe (trachea), which branches into two smaller airways: the left and right bronchi, which lead to the two lungs. The left lung is a little smaller than the right lung because it shares space in the left side of the chest with the heart. Each lung is divided into sections (lobes): three in the right lung and two in the left lung.

The bronchi themselves divide many times before branching into smaller airways (bronchioles). These are the narrowest airways—as small as one half of a millimeter across. The larger airways resemble an upside-down tree, which is why this part of the respiratory system is often called the bronchial tree. The airways are held open by flexible, fibrous connective tissue called cartilage. Circular airway muscles can dilate or constrict the airways, thus changing the size of the airway.

At the end of each bronchiole are thousands of small air sacs (alveoli). Together, the millions of alveoli of the lungs form a surface of more than 100 square meters. Within the alveolar walls is a dense network of tiny blood vessels called capillaries. The extremely thin barrier between air and capillaries allows oxygen to move from the alveoli into the blood and allows carbon dioxide to move from the blood in the capillaries into the alveoli.

The pleura is a slippery membrane that covers the lungs as well as the inside of the chest wall. It allows the lungs to move smoothly during breathing and as the person moves around. Normally, the two layers of the pleura have only a small amount of lubricating fluid between them. The two layers glide smoothly over each other as the lungs change size and shape.

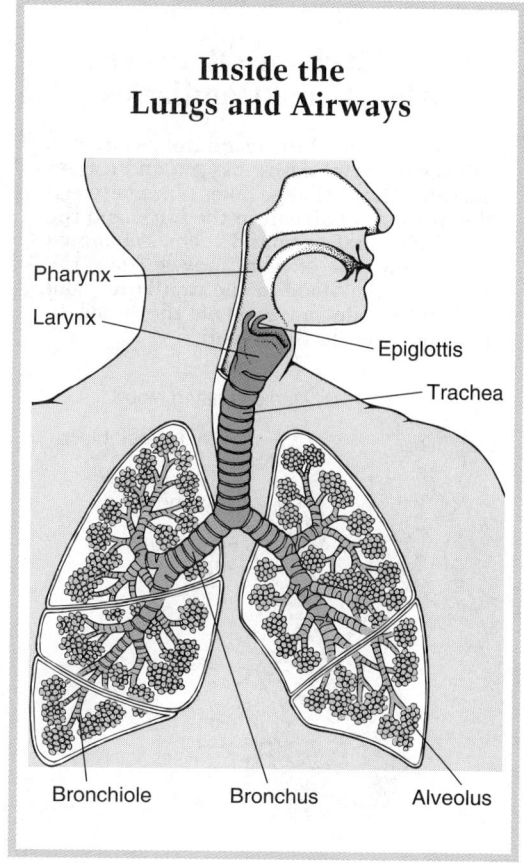

Inside the Lungs and Airways

Pharynx

Larynx

Epiglottis

Trachea

Bronchiole   Bronchus   Alveolus

The Chest Cavity

The lungs are housed in the chest cavity, a space that also includes the mediastinum. The mediastinum contains the heart, thymus, and lymph nodes, along with portions of the aorta, vena cava, trachea, esophagus, and various nerves. It encompasses the area bordered by the sternum in front, the spinal column in back, the entrance to the chest cavity above, and the diaphragm below. Functionally, the mediastinum isolates the left and right lung from each other. For example, if the chest wall is punctured on one side, causing that lung to collapse, the other lung remains inflated and functioning, because the two lungs are separated.

The lungs and other organs in the chest are protected by a bony cage, which is formed by the breastbone (sternum), ribs, and spine. The 12 pairs of ribs curve around the chest from the back. Each pair is joined to the bones (vertebrae) of the spine. In the front of the body, the upper seven pairs of ribs are attached to the sternum by cartilage. The eighth, ninth, and tenth pairs of ribs join the cartilage of the pair above; the last two pairs (floating ribs) are shorter and do not join in the front.

Exchanging Oxygen and Carbon Dioxide

The primary function of the respiratory system is to exchange oxygen and carbon dioxide. Inhaled oxygen enters the lungs and reaches the alveoli. The cells lining the alveoli and the surrounding capillaries are each only one cell thick and are in very close contact with each other. This barrier averages about 1 micron (1/10,000 of a centimeter) in thickness. Oxygen passes through this air-blood barrier quickly and into the blood in the capillaries. Similarly, carbon dioxide passes from the blood into the alveoli and is then exhaled.

Gas Exchange Between Alveoli and Capillaries

The function of the respiratory system is to exchange two gases: oxygen and carbon dioxide. The exchange takes place between the millions of alveoli in the lungs and the capillaries that surround them. As shown below, inhaled oxygen moves from the alveoli to the blood in the capillaries, and carbon dioxide moves from the blood in the capillaries to the alveoli.

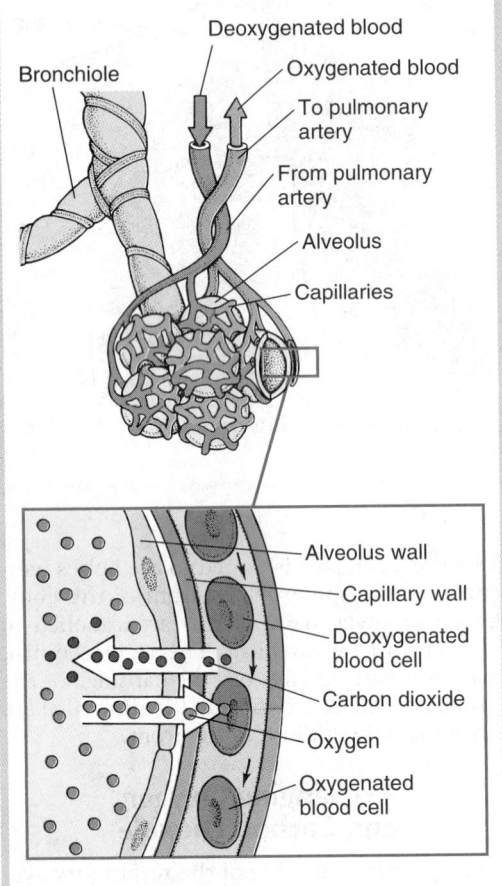

Bronchiole

Deoxygenated blood

Oxygenated blood

To pulmonary artery

From pulmonary artery

Alveolus

Capillaries

Alveolus wall

Capillary wall

Deoxygenated blood cell

Carbon dioxide

Oxygen

Oxygenated blood cell

Oxygenated blood travels from the lungs through the pulmonary veins and into the left side of the heart, which pumps the blood to the rest of the body.▲ Oxygen-depleted, carbon dioxide–rich blood returns to the right side of the heart through two large veins, the

superior vena cava and the inferior vena cava. Then the blood is pumped through the pulmonary artery to the lungs, where it picks up oxygen and releases carbon dioxide.■

To support the exchange of oxygen and carbon dioxide, about 6 to 10 liters of fresh air per minute are brought into the lungs, and about three tenths of a liter of oxygen is transferred from the alveoli to the blood each minute, even when the person is at rest. At the same time, a similar volume of carbon dioxide moves from the blood to the alveoli and is exhaled. During exercise, it is possible to breathe in as much as 100 liters of air per minute and extract 3 liters of oxygen from this air per minute. The rate at which oxygen enters the body is one useful measure of the total amount of energy expended by the body.

Three processes are essential for the transfer of oxygen from the outside air to the blood flowing through the lungs: ventilation, diffusion, and perfusion. Ventilation is the process by which air moves in and out of the lungs. Diffusion is the spontaneous movement of gases, without the use of any energy or effort by the body, between the gas in the alveoli and the blood in the pulmonary capillaries. Perfusion is the action by which the cardiovascular system pumps blood throughout the lungs. The body's circulation is an essential link between the atmosphere, which contains oxygen, and the cells of the body, which consume oxygen. For example, the delivery of oxygen to the muscle cells throughout the body depends not only on the lungs but also on the ability of the blood to carry oxygen and on the ability of the circulation to transport it.

Control of Breathing

Breathing is usually automatic, controlled subconsciously by the respiratory center at the base of the brain. Breathing continues during sleep and usually even when the person is unconscious. Small sensory organs in the brain and in the aorta and carotid arteries monitor the blood and sense when oxygen levels are too low or carbon dioxide levels are too high. In healthy people, an increased concentration of carbon dioxide is the strongest stimulus to breathe more deeply and more quickly. Conversely, when the carbon dioxide concentration in the blood is low, breathing is reduced. Then, the brain decreases the frequency and size of breaths. In quiet breathing,

▲ see page 115   ■ see page 116

Diaphragm's Role in Breathing

When the diaphragm contracts, the chest cavity enlarges, reducing the pressure inside. To equalize the pressure, air rushes into the lungs. When the diaphragm relaxes, the elasticity of the lungs and chest wall pushes air out of the lungs.

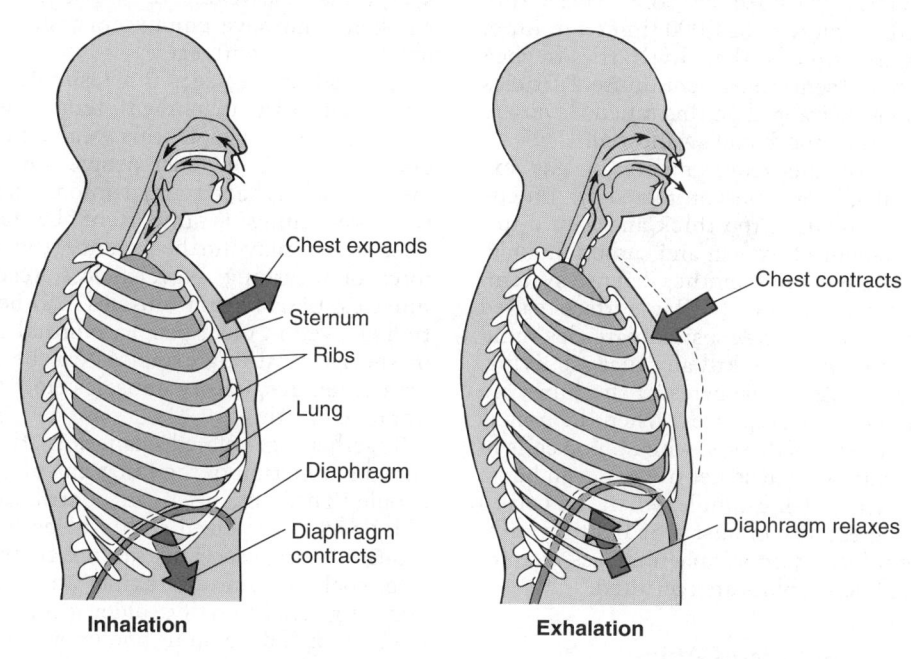

Chest expands

Sternum

Ribs

Lung

Diaphragm

Diaphragm contracts

Inhalation

Chest contracts

Diaphragm relaxes

Exhalation

the average adult inhales and exhales about 15 times a minute.

Because the lungs have no skeletal muscles of their own, the work of breathing is done by the diaphragm, the muscles between the ribs (intercostal muscles), the muscles in the neck, and the abdominal muscles. The diaphragm, a bell-shaped sheet of muscle that separates the lungs from the abdomen, is the most important muscle used for breathing in (called inhalation or inspiration). The diaphragm is attached to the base of the sternum, the lower parts of the rib cage, and the spine. When the diaphragm contracts, it increases the length and diameter of the chest cavity and thus expands the lungs. The intercostal muscles help move the rib cage and thus assist in breathing. All the muscles used in breathing contract only if the nerves connecting them to the brain are intact. In some neck and back injuries, the spinal cord can be severed, and the person will die unless he is artificially ventilated.

The process of breathing out (called exhalation or expiration) is usually passive when a person is not exercising. Energy stored in the elasticity of the lungs and chest wall can be used to expel air out of the lungs. Therefore, when a person is at rest, no effort is needed by the respiratory muscles. During vigorous exercise, however, a number of muscles assist in exhalation. The abdominal muscles are the most important of these. Abdominal muscles contract, raise abdominal pressure, and push a relaxed diaphragm against the lungs, causing air to be expelled.

Defense Mechanisms

The average person who is moderately active during the daytime breathes about 20,000 liters of air every 24 hours. Inevitably, this air (which would weigh more than 20 kilograms) contains toxic particles and gases. Particles, such as dust and soot, mold, fungi, bacteria, and viruses, all deposit on airway and alveolar surfaces. Fortunately, the respiratory system has defense mechanisms to protect it.

One such defense mechanism involves tiny muscular projections (cilia), which line the airways. The airways are covered by a liquid layer that is propelled by cilia. These tiny muscles beat more than 1,000 times a minute, moving the mucus that lines the trachea about 0.5 to 1 centimeter per minute. Particles and pathogens trapped on this mucus layer are cleared to the mouth and swallowed.

Because of the requirements of gas exchange, alveoli are not protected by mucus and cilia—mucus is too thick and would impair movement of oxygen and carbon dioxide. Instead, the body has another defense system. Mobile cells on the alveolar surface called phagocytes seek out deposited particles, bind to them, ingest them, kill any that are living, and digest them. Phagocytes in the lungs are called alveolar macrophages. When the lung is exposed to serious threats, white blood cells in the circulation, such as neutrophils, can be recruited to help. For example, when the person inhales a great deal of dust or is fighting a respiratory infection, more macrophages are produced and neutrophils are recruited.

Effects of Aging

The effects of aging on the respiratory system are similar to those that occur in other organs: maximum function gradually declines. Age-related changes in the lungs include a decrease in the peak airflow, gas exchange, and vital capacity (the amount of air that can be breathed out following a maximum inhalation), as well as a decrease in the defense mechanisms of the lungs. In the nonsmoker, these age-related changes seldom lead to symptoms. However, in smokers and ex-smokers who have emphysema, shortness of breath worsens with age.

With advancing age, the respiratory muscles, such as the diaphragm, tend to weaken. In healthy older people, this weakening is seldom important. In older people who have a disease such as bacterial pneumonia, however, this weakening is important because the pneumonia may further reduce the muscle force of breathing. Nevertheless, respiratory muscles, like skeletal muscles, can be conditioned, even in older people. Normal exercise or special breathing exercises can be used to strengthen respiratory muscles and thus to improve breathing.

Together, age-related changes in the structure and function of the lungs can affect older people. These changes can contribute to an older person's reduced ability to perform vigorous exercise, especially intense aerobic exercise, such as running, biking, and mountain climbing. Additionally, older people are at higher risk of developing pneumonia after bacterial or viral infections. Most importantly, age-related changes in the lungs compound the effects of any other heart and lung diseases the person may have, especially those caused by the destructive effects of smoking.

CHAPTER 39

Symptoms and Diagnosis of Lung Disorders

Disorders that affect the lungs and airways are called lung or pulmonary disorders. Depending on the person's symptoms, a doctor usually recommends a variety of tests to help determine the person's exact disorder.

Symptoms

Among the most common symptoms of lung disorders are cough, shortness of breath (dyspnea), wheezing, and a crowing sound when breathing (stridor). Problems in the lungs can also lead to coughing up of blood (hemoptysis), a bluish discoloration of the skin due to a lack of oxygen in the blood (cyanosis), and chest pain. Prolonged lung disease can even produce changes in other parts of the body, including finger clubbing. Some of these symptoms do not always indicate a respiratory problem. Chest pain, for example, may also result from a heart or gastrointestinal disorder, and shortness of breath can be caused by a heart problem.

COUGH

A cough is a sudden, explosive movement of air; the function of a cough is to clear material from the airways.

Coughing, a familiar but complicated reflex, is one way in which the lungs and airways are protected. Along with other mechanisms, coughing helps to protect the lungs from particles that have been inhaled (aspirated). Coughing sometimes brings up sputum (also called phlegm)—a mixture of mucus, debris, and cells expelled by the lungs.

Coughing occurs when the airways are irritated. Respiratory infections—either bacterial or viral—irritate the airways and are a common cause of coughing. Allergies can irritate the airways as well. People who smoke cough because of the irritating effects of the smoke and because of the damage smoking causes to the cells that line the airways, including the hairlike projections that normally cleanse the airways of debris (cilia).

Coughs vary considerably. A cough may be distressing, especially if coughing episodes are accompanied by chest pain, shortness of breath, or unusually large amounts of or very sticky sputum. However, if coughing develops over decades, as it may in a smoker, the person may hardly be aware of it.

Information about a cough helps a doctor determine its cause. Therefore, a doctor may ask:

- How long the cough has been present
- What time of day the cough occurs
- Which factors—such as cold air, posture, talking, eating, or drinking—influence the cough
- Whether the cough is accompanied by chest pain, shortness of breath, hoarseness, dizziness, or wheezing
- Whether the cough brings up sputum or blood
- The color of the sputum

The appearance of the sputum may help the doctor identify the cause. A yellowish, greenish, or brownish appearance usually indicates a bacterial infection. Clear but very sticky (mucoid) sputum is characteristic of asthma. A doctor may examine the sputum microscopically; bacteria and white blood cells seen under the microscope are additional indications of infection. The presence of a specific type of white blood cell (eosinophil) suggests asthma. A cough may also produce blood, which commonly suggests bronchitis, but may also suggest more serious disorders.

Treatment

Because coughing plays an important role in bringing up sputum and clearing the airways, a cough that produces a lot of sputum generally should not be suppressed. Treating the underlying cause—such as an infection, fluid in the lungs, or asthma—is more important. For example, antibiotics can be given for an infection, or inhalers can be used for asthma. Depending on the severity of the cough and its cause, a variety of drugs may be needed for treatment. Many people need to have their coughs suppressed somewhat at night to allow them to sleep.

Antitussive Therapy: Antitussive drugs suppress a cough. All **opioids** are antitussives because they suppress the cough center in the brain. Codeine is the opioid used most often for cough. Codeine may cause nausea, vomiting, and constipation; it may also be addictive. If codeine is taken for a prolonged period, the dose needed to suppress a cough may need to be increased. Opioid cough suppressants can make people drowsy and are not always safe, and doctors reserve them for special situations.

Several **non-opioid cough suppressants,** such as dextromethorphan and benzonatate, are effective antitussives that also work by suppressing the cough center in the brain. These drugs, and others, are the active ingredients in many over-the-counter and prescription cough medications.▲ They are not addictive and produce little drowsiness. In certain people, especially those who are coughing up an abundant amount of sputum, frequent use of these cough suppressants is not recommended.

Steam inhalation, for example from a vaporizer, can help stop a cough by reducing irritation in the throat (pharynx) and airways. The moisture from the steam also loosens secretions, making them easier to cough up. A cool-mist humidifier can achieve the same result. Many doctors believe that drinking sufficient water can produce good hydration and is as effective as steam inhalation for loosening secretions.

▲ see page 98

Expectorants and Mucolytics: Expectorants help loosen mucus by making bronchial secretions thinner and easier to cough up, although these drugs do not suppress a cough. Over-the-counter preparations containing guaifenesin or terpin hydrate are the most common.▲ A small dose of syrup of ipecac may help in children, especially in those who have croup.

Drugs that reduce the thickness of mucus (called mucolytics), such as acetylcysteine, are sometimes used when thick, sticky bronchial secretions are a major problem. In cystic fibrosis, dornase alfa (inhaled recombinant human deoxyribonuclease I) is used to help thin the pus-filled mucus that results from chronic respiratory tract infections.

Antihistamines, Decongestants, and Bronchodilators: Antihistamines, which dry the respiratory tract, have little or no value in treating a cough, except when it is caused by an upper airway allergy. With coughs from other causes, such as bronchitis, the drying action of antihistamines can be harmful, thickening respiratory secretions and making them difficult to cough up.

Decongestants such as phenylephrine that relieve a stuffy nose are not useful in relieving a cough, unless the cough is caused by postnasal drip.

Bronchodilators such as inhaled sympathomimetic agents or oral theophylline may be prescribed if a cough occurs with airway narrowing (bronchoconstriction), as happens in asthma and emphysema. They are rarely useful for people who do not have an underlying lung disease. However, some people who develop wheezing and prolonged cough after viral lung infections appear to benefit from short-term use of bronchodilators.

DYSPNEA

Dyspnea (also referred to as shortness of breath) is the unpleasant sensation of difficulty in breathing.

An increase in breathing occurs normally during exercise and at high altitudes, but the increase seldom causes discomfort. Breathing is also increased at rest in people with many illnesses, whether of the lungs or of other parts of the body. For example, people with a fever generally breathe faster.

With dyspnea, faster breathing is accompanied by the sensation of running out of air. The person feels a sensation of not being able to breathe fast enough or deeply enough. Other sensations include an awareness of increased muscular effort to expand the chest when breathing in or to expel air when breathing out, the uncomfortable sensation that inhaling (inspiration) is urgently needed before exhaling (expiration) is completed, and various sensations most often described as tightness in the chest.

Types of Dyspnea

People who have lung disease often experience dyspnea when they physically exert themselves. During exercise, the body makes more carbon dioxide and uses more oxygen. The respiratory center in the brain accelerates breathing when blood levels of oxygen are low or blood levels of carbon dioxide are high. If the heart or lungs are not functioning properly, even a little exertion can lead to dramatic increases in breathing rates and dyspnea. As lung disease becomes more severe, dyspnea may even occur at rest.

Dyspnea may result from restrictive or obstructive lung disorders. Restrictive lung disorders (such as idiopathic pulmonary fibrosis■) cause stiff lungs (lungs that do not expand well during inhalation). Severe curvature of the spine (scoliosis) causes restriction by reducing the movement of the rib cage. In restrictive disorders, dyspnea occurs because of increased effort and a high rate of breathing due to this stiffness. In obstructive disorders (such as chronic bronchitis, emphysema, asthma), resistance to airflow is increased because the airways are narrowed. Because the airways widen when the person inhales, air can usually be pulled in, but that air cannot be exhaled from the lungs as fast as normal, because the airways narrow on exhalation and breathing becomes more labored.

Pulmonary function testing★ can measure the degree of restriction and obstruction. A respiratory problem may include both restrictive and obstructive defects.

Because the heart pumps blood through the lungs, the heart must function properly for the lungs to function normally. If the heart is pumping inadequately, fluid may accumulate in the lungs, a condition called pulmonary edema. This condition causes dyspnea that is often accompanied by a feeling of smothering or heaviness in the chest. The fluid accumula-

---

▲ see page 98   ■ see page 301

★ see page 254

tion in the lungs may also lead to airway narrowing and wheezing—a condition called cardiac asthma.▲

Orthopnea is shortness of breath when a person lies down that is relieved by sitting up. Some people whose heart pumps inadequately experience this condition. Paroxysmal nocturnal dyspnea is a sudden, often terrifying, attack of shortness of breath during sleep. The person awakens gasping and must sit or stand to take a breath. This condition is an extreme form of orthopnea and a sign of severe heart failure.■

Dyspnea can also occur in people who have anemia or blood loss because of a decreased number of red blood cells, which carry oxygen to the tissues. The person breathes rapidly and deeply, in a reflex effort to try to increase the amount of oxygen in the blood.

Someone with severe kidney failure feels out of breath and may begin to pant quickly because of a combination of metabolic acidosis, heart failure, and anemia.

Hyperventilation syndrome causes people to feel that they cannot get enough air, and they breathe heavily and rapidly. This condition is commonly caused by anxiety rather than a physical problem. Many people who experience this syndrome are frightened and may believe they are having a heart attack. The symptoms result from changes in the blood gas levels (mostly from a lowering of the carbon dioxide level) caused by the overbreathing. People may experience a change in consciousness usually described as a feeling that events occurring around them are far away, and they may experience a tingling feeling in the hands and feet and around the mouth.

CHEST PAIN

Chest pain may arise from the pleura (the two-layered membrane covering the lungs), the lungs, or chest wall. Alternatively, chest pain may arise from internal structures that are not part of the respiratory system, especially the heart. In these cases, the chest pain does not indicate a lung disorder.

Pleuritic pain, a sharp pain arising from an inflammation of the pleura (pleurisy), is made worse by deep breathing and coughing. The pain can be reduced by keeping the chest wall still—for example, by holding the side that hurts and avoiding deep breathing or coughing. Usually, the site of the pain can be pinpointed, although it may move over time.

Pleurisy at the base of a lung may be felt as pain in the shoulder of the affected side. Pleural effusion, a fluid buildup in the space between the two layers of pleura,★ may produce pleuritic pain at first, but the pain often subsides as the two layers are separated by accumulating fluid. There are many causes of pleuritic pain, including viral and bacterial infections, cancer, and blood clots that travel through the bloodstream to the lungs (pulmonary embolism●) lodging in the pulmonary arteries.

Pain arising from other lung disorders (such as a lung abscess or tumor) is usually more difficult to describe than pleuritic pain. The pain is often described as a vague, deep-seated ache in the chest. Almost any injury to the lungs or airways can cause such pain.

Pain can also originate in the chest wall itself. This pain may worsen with deep breathing or coughing and often is confined to one area in the chest wall, which also feels sore when pressed. The most common causes are chest wall injuries, such as broken ribs and torn or injured muscles located between the ribs (intercostal muscles). Even hard coughing can injure these muscles, causing days or weeks of pain. A tumor growing into the chest wall may cause pain in a small spot or, if it grows into an intercostal nerve, may cause pain along the whole area supplied by that nerve (referred pain◆). Shingles, caused by the varicella-zoster virus, sometimes causes chest pain during each breath before the telltale rash appears.▼

WHEEZING

Wheezing is a whistling, musical sound during breathing resulting from partially obstructed airways.

Wheezing results from an obstruction somewhere in the airways. It may be caused by a general narrowing of the airways (as in asthma or chronic obstructive pulmonary disease), by a local narrowing (as with a tumor), or by a foreign particle lodged in an airway. The most common cause of recurrent wheezing is asthma, although many people who have never had asthma wheeze at some time in their lives.

▲ see page 154   ■ see page 153

★ see page 314   ● see page 285

◆ see art on page 448   ▼ see page 1162

A doctor usually is able to detect wheezing by listening with a stethoscope as the person breathes. Loud wheezing can be heard easily without a stethoscope. When wheezing is caused by a local narrowing, the doctor may detect a vibration that accompanies the wheezing by palpating the chest wall over the area of obstruction (such as a tumor or a foreign object) when the person breathes forcefully. A persistent wheeze that occurs in one location in a smoker may be due to lung cancer, and even if a chest x-ray is unrevealing, doctors may perform bronchoscopy.▲ Pulmonary function testing■ may be needed to help measure the extent of airway narrowing and to assess the benefits of treatment.

STRIDOR

Stridor is a crowing sound during breathing resulting from a partial blockage of the throat (pharynx), voice box (larynx), or windpipe (trachea); stridor is often more evident when the person inhales.

Stridor is usually loud enough to be heard at some distance, but it may be audible only during a deep breath. The sound is caused by turbulent airflow through a narrowed upper airway. In children, the cause may be an infection of the epiglottis★ or an inhaled foreign object. In adults, the cause may be a tumor, an abscess, swelling (edema) in the upper airway, or a malfunction of the vocal cords.

Stridor causing dyspnea when the person is at rest is a medical emergency. In such cases, a tube may be inserted through the person's mouth or nose (tracheal intubation) or by a small surgical incision directly into the trachea (tracheostomy) to allow air to get past the blockage and avoid suffocation.

HEMOPTYSIS

Hemoptysis is the coughing up of blood from the respiratory tract.

Although hemoptysis can often be frightening, most causes turn out not to be serious. Infection is the most common cause. Unexplained or large amounts of blood in the sputum require evaluation by a doctor.

Tumors, especially those due to lung cancer, account for up to 20% of cases of hemoptysis.

Doctors check for lung cancer in smokers older than 40 (and even in younger smokers if the person started smoking in adolescence) who develop hemoptysis, even if the sputum is only blood streaked. Death of lung tissue (pulmonary infarction●) from blockage of an artery by a blood clot (pulmonary embolism) may also cause hemoptysis.

Sometimes, especially in people who are critically ill, a catheter is placed into the pulmonary artery to measure the blood pressure in the heart and in the blood vessels of the lungs. If the balloon on the catheter ruptures the vessel, bleeding can become very severe. High blood pressure in the pulmonary veins, as may occur in heart failure and mitral valve stenosis, may also cause hemoptysis. Other lung circulation problems, including arteriovenous malformations, may cause hemoptysis.

Diagnosis

If hemoptysis is severe or unexplained, a diagnostic evaluation is necessary. Bronchoscopy may be needed to identify the bleeding site. A scan using a radioactive marker (lung perfusion scan◆) may reveal a pulmonary embolism. Despite testing, the cause of hemoptysis is not found in 30 to 40% of cases; however, when hemoptysis is severe, the cause is usually found.

Treatment

Mild hemoptysis may require no treatment or only antibiotics to treat an infection. Bleeding may produce clots that block the airways and lead to further breathing problems; therefore, coughing is important to keep the airways clear and should not be suppressed with antitussive drugs. If a large clot blocks a major airway, doctors may have to remove the clot using bronchoscopy.

Bleeding from smaller vessels usually stops by itself. However, bleeding from a major vessel usually requires treatment. A doctor may try to close off the bleeding vessel using a procedure called bronchial artery embolization. Using x-rays for guidance, the doctor passes a catheter into the vessel and then injects a chemical, fragments of a gelatin sponge, or a wire coil to block the blood vessel and thereby stop the bleeding. Bleeding caused by an infection or heart failure usually subsides if the underlying disorder is treated successfully. Sometimes bronchoscopy or surgery may be needed to stop the bleeding, or surgery may be needed to remove a diseased portion of the

▲ see page 256   ■ see page 254

★ see page 1564   ● see page 285

◆ see page 287

lung. These high-risk procedures are used only as last resorts. If clotting abnormalities are contributing to the bleeding, a transfusion of plasma, clotting factors, or platelets may be needed.

CYANOSIS

Cyanosis is a bluish discoloration of the skin resulting from an inadequate amount of oxygen in the blood.

Cyanosis occurs when oxygen-depleted blood, which is bluish rather than red, circulates through the skin. Cyanosis can be caused by many types of severe lung or heart disease that produce low levels of oxygen in the blood. It can also result from certain blood vessel and heart malformations that allow blood to flow directly into veins returning blood from the lungs to the heart or into the left side of the heart. A bypass (shunt) exists if a malformation returns blood directly to the heart without ever flowing past the air sacs of the lung (alveoli) where oxygen is extracted from the air.

The amount of oxygen in the blood can be determined by arterial blood gas analysis.▲ Chest x-rays, blood flow studies, and lung and heart function tests may be needed to determine the cause of decreased oxygen in the blood and the resulting cyanosis. Pulse oximetry, which utilizes an electrode clipped on a finger or an earlobe, allows the doctor to continuously monitor the oxygen concentration in a person who is critically ill. Oxygen therapy is often the first treatment given.

FINGER CLUBBING

Finger clubbing is an enlargement of the tips of the fingers or toes and a loss of the angle where the nails emerge.

Finger clubbing occurs when the amount of soft tissue beneath the nailbeds increases. The reason this increase occurs is not clear, but clubbing seems to occur with some pulmonary disorders (lung cancer, lung abscess, bronchiectasis), but not with others (pneumonia, asthma, emphysema). Finger clubbing also occurs with some congenital heart diseases or, in some cases, may be inherited and not indicate any disease.

Diagnosis

A doctor usually can tell whether a person has a lung or airway disorder based on the medical history and physical examination. Di-

Recognizing Finger Clubbing

Finger clubbing is characterized by enlarged fingertips and a loss of the normal angle at the nail bed.

Normal Finger   Clubbed Finger

agnostic procedures are used to confirm the diagnosis, determine the extent and severity of the disease, and help in planning treatment.

MEDICAL HISTORY AND PHYSICAL EXAMINATION

A doctor first asks the person about symptoms. Chest pain, shortness of breath (dyspnea), cough, coughing up of blood (hemoptysis), wheezing, and a crowing sound while breathing (stridor) suggest lung or airway disease. Other, more general symptoms, such as fever, weakness, fatigue, and a general feeling of illness or discomfort (malaise), may also point to lung or airway disease.

Next, the doctor asks the person about past infections; previous exposure to chemicals; use of drugs, alcohol, and tobacco; home and work environments; travels; and recreational activities. A doctor also asks the person about whether family members have had lung or airway disease and any other diseases that may affect the lungs or airways.

During the physical examination, a doctor notes the person's weight and overall appearance. The person's general mood and feeling of well-being, which also may be affected by lung or airway disease, are also noted. A doctor may ask a person to walk around or climb a flight of stairs to see if either activity causes shortness of breath.

Assessing skin color is important because pallor or cyanosis may indicate anemia or poor blood flow. These findings can indicate that the skin is receiving inadequate oxygen from

▲ see page 255

Using a Spirometer

A spirometer consists of a mouthpiece, tubing, and a recording device. To use a spirometer, a person inhales deeply, then exhales vigorously and as quickly as possible through the tubing. The recording device measures the volume of air inhaled or exhaled and the length of time each breath takes.

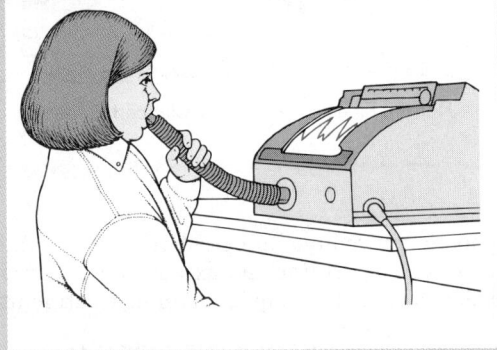

the blood because of lung or airway disease. Fingers are examined for evidence of clubbing.

A doctor observes the chest to determine if the breathing rate and movements are normal. By tapping (percussing) the chest, a doctor can determine if the lungs are filled with air, which is normal, or if they contain fluid, which is abnormal. Using a stethoscope, a doctor also listens to the breath sounds to determine whether airflow is normal or obstructed and whether the lungs contain fluid as a result of respiratory failure or pneumonia. In addition to examination of the chest, a complete physical examination may be needed, because many disorders not related to the lungs first present with evidence of lung problems (for example, the presence of pleural fluid, which may represent metastasis from an abdominal tumor).

PULMONARY FUNCTION TESTING

Tests for lung disease are designed to give an accurate assessment of how well the lungs are working. Each test assesses a different aspect of lung function.

One group of tests, called pulmonary function tests, measure the lungs' capacity to hold air, to move air in and out, and to exchange

oxygen and carbon dioxide. These tests are better at detecting the type and severity of lung disorders than at defining the specific cause of problems. The tests are used to diagnose some diseases, however, including asthma. Pulmonary function tests include lung volumes and flow rate measurements, flow volume testing, muscle strength assessment, and diffusing capacity measurement.

Lung Volume and Flow Rate Measurements: The assessment of lung disease often involves testing how much air the lungs can hold as well as how much and how quickly air can be exhaled. These measurements are made with a spirometer, which consists of a mouthpiece and tubing connected to a recording device. A person inhales deeply, then exhales forcefully as quickly as possible through the tubing while measurements are taken. The volume of air inhaled or exhaled and the length of time each breath takes are recorded and analyzed. Often, the tests are repeated after a person takes a drug that opens the airways of the lungs (bronchodilator).

A simpler device for measuring how quickly air can be exhaled is the peak flow meter. After inhaling deeply, a person blows into a small, handheld device as hard as possible. This inexpensive device helps people who have asthma or other lung diseases monitor the severity of their disease and the effectiveness of treatment at home.

Lung volume measurements reflect the stiffness or elasticity of the lungs and rib cage as well as the strength of respiratory muscles. The measurements are abnormally low in disorders such as pulmonary fibrosis, curvature of the spine (scoliosis), and a variety of neuromuscular disorders that cause weakness of the diaphragm and other respiratory muscles, such as myasthenia gravis▲ and Guillain-Barré syndrome.■

Flow rate measurements reflect the degree of narrowing or obstruction of the airways. The measurements are abnormal in obstructive disorders, such as bronchitis, emphysema, and asthma.

Flow Volume Testing: Most newer spirometers can continuously display lung volumes and flow rates during a forced breathing maneuver. These flow rates can be particularly helpful in detecting abnormalities that partially block the voice box (larynx) and windpipe (trachea).

Muscle Strength Assessment: The strength of the respiratory muscles can be measured by

▲ see page 577   ■ see page 585

having the person forcibly inhale and exhale against a pressure gauge. A disease that weakens the muscles, such as muscular dystrophy, makes breathing more difficult and results in low pressures during inhalation and exhalation. This test also helps predict whether a person on a ventilator will be able to breathe independently after being taken off it.

Diffusing Capacity Measurement: A diffusing capacity test can estimate how efficiently oxygen is transferred from the air sacs of the lungs (alveoli) to the bloodstream. Because the diffusing capacity of oxygen is difficult to measure directly, a person inhales a small amount of carbon monoxide, holds the breath for 10 seconds, and then exhales into a carbon monoxide detector.

If the test shows that carbon monoxide is not well absorbed, oxygen will not be exchanged normally between the lungs and the bloodstream either. The diffusing capacity is characteristically abnormal in people with pulmonary fibrosis, emphysema, and disorders affecting the blood vessels of the lungs.

SLEEP STUDIES

Breathing is usually automatic and controlled by centers in the brain that respond to the levels of oxygen and carbon dioxide in the blood. If this control is abnormal, breathing may stop for prolonged periods, especially during sleep—a condition called sleep apnea.▲ The test for sleep apnea consists of monitoring brain wave activity (with an electroencephalogram, also called an EEG), the oxygen concentration in the blood (with pulse oximetry, which utilizes an electrode clipped on a finger or an earlobe), the movement of air during breathing (using a device placed in one nostril), and chest wall motion. Combining all these measurements as part of a single test is called a polysomnogram.

ARTERIAL BLOOD GAS ANALYSIS

Arterial blood gas tests measure the levels of oxygen and carbon dioxide in the arterial blood. A sample from a vein cannot be used. Taking a sample from an artery requires skill and may cause a few minutes of discomfort for the person. Usually the sample is taken from an artery in the wrist (radial artery). Oxygen and carbon dioxide levels are important indicators of lung function because they reflect how well the lungs are getting oxygen into the blood and getting carbon dioxide out of it.

Oxygen concentrations can be monitored using an electrode placed on a finger or an earlobe—a procedure called oximetry. When a person is seriously ill or a doctor also needs a carbon dioxide and blood acidity measurement, an arterial sample is needed.

CHEST IMAGING

Routinely, chest x-rays are taken from the back to front, but sometimes doctors supplement this view with a side view. Chest x-rays provide a good outline of the heart and major blood vessels and usually can reveal a serious disease in the lungs, the adjacent spaces, and the chest wall, including the ribs. For example, chest x-rays can clearly show pneumonia, lung tumors, emphysema, a collapsed lung (atelectasis), and air (pneumothorax) or fluid (pleural effusion) in the pleural space. Although chest x-rays seldom give enough information to determine the exact cause of the abnormality, they can help a doctor determine which other tests are needed to make a diagnosis.

Computed tomography (CT) of the chest provides more detail than a plain x-ray. With CT, a series of x-rays is analyzed by a computer, which then provides several cross-sectional views. During CT, a radiopaque dye may be injected into the bloodstream or given by mouth to help clarify certain abnormalities in the chest.

Magnetic resonance imaging (MRI) also produces highly detailed pictures that are especially useful when a doctor suspects blood vessel abnormalities in the chest, such as an aortic aneurysm. Unlike CT, MRI does not use radiation.

Ultrasound creates a picture on a monitor from the reflection of sound waves in the body. Ultrasound is often used to detect fluid in the pleural space (the space between the two layers of pleura covering the lung and inner chest wall). Ultrasound can also be used for guidance when using a needle to aspirate the fluid.

Nuclear lung scanning uses minute amounts of short-lived radioactive materials to depict the flow of air and blood through the lungs. Usually, the test is done in two stages. In the first stage (lung ventilation scan), a person inhales a radioactive gas, and a scanner creates a picture of how the gas is distributed throughout the airways and the alveoli. In the second

▲ see page 472

stage (lung perfusion scan), a radioactive substance is injected into a vein, and a scanner creates a picture of how it is distributed throughout the blood vessels of the lung. This type of imaging is particularly useful in detecting blood clots in the lungs (pulmonary emboli); it also may be used during the preoperative assessment of people who have lung cancer.

Angiography accurately shows the blood supply to the lungs. Radiopaque dye, which can be seen on x-rays, is injected into a blood vessel, and pictures are taken of the arteries and veins in the lungs. Angiography is used most often when pulmonary embolism is suspected, usually on the basis of abnormal lung scan results. Pulmonary artery angiography is considered the definitive test for diagnosing and for ruling out pulmonary embolism.

POSITRON EMISSION TOMOGRAPHY

Positron emission tomography (PET) scanning is a radiographic imaging technique that relies on the different metabolic rates of malignant (cancerous) versus benign (noncancerous) tissues. This procedure may be used when a cancer is suspected. Glucose molecules that are tagged with a tracer are injected intravenously; these molecules accumulate in rapidly metabolizing tissue (such as in malignant lymph nodes) and can be detected using PET. Benign growths usually do not accumulate enough activity to be detected.

THORACENTESIS

In thoracentesis, fluid that has collected abnormally in the pleural space (pleural effusion▲) is removed with a needle and syringe, so it can be analyzed. The two principal reasons to perform thoracentesis are to relieve shortness of breath caused by lung tissue compression or to obtain a fluid sample for diagnostic testing.

During the procedure, the person sits comfortably and leans forward, resting the arms on supports. A small area of skin on the back is cleaned and numbed with a local anesthetic. Then a doctor inserts a needle between two ribs and withdraws some fluid into a syringe. Sometimes the doctor uses ultrasound for guidance while inserting the needle. The collected fluid is analyzed to assess its chemical makeup and to determine whether bacteria or cancerous cells are present.

If a large volume of fluid has accumulated, it may need to be removed through a plastic catheter. During thoracentesis, a doctor can also instill substances, such as doxycycline (an antibiotic derived from tetracycline) into the pleural space to prevent a reaccumulation of fluid.

The risk of complications during and after thoracentesis is low. Occasionally, a person may feel some pain as the lung fills with air and expands against the chest wall. Also, a person may briefly feel light-headed and short of breath. Other possible complications include puncture of the lung with leakage of air into the pleural space (pneumothorax), bleeding into the pleural space or chest wall, fainting, infection, puncture of the spleen or liver, and very rarely, accidental entry of air bubbles into the bloodstream (air emboli). A chest x-ray may be performed after the procedure to ensure that none has occurred.

NEEDLE BIOPSY OF THE PLEURA OR LUNG

If thoracentesis does not uncover the cause of a pleural effusion (a fluid buildup in the space between the two layers of the pleura), a doctor may perform a pleural biopsy. First, the skin is anesthetized as for thoracentesis. Then using a larger cutting needle, a doctor takes a small sample of tissue from the pleura and sends it to a laboratory to be examined for signs of cancer or tuberculosis. About 85 to 90% of the time, a pleural biopsy is accurate in diagnosing these diseases.

If a tissue specimen needs to be obtained from a lung tumor, a doctor may perform a needle biopsy. After anesthetizing the skin, a doctor, often using chest computed tomography (CT) for guidance, directs a biopsy needle into a tumor and obtains cells or a small piece of tissue to be sent to the laboratory for analysis. Tissue can also be sent for culture if a lung infection is suspected. Complications of pleural and lung biopsies are similar to those for thoracentesis.

BRONCHOSCOPY

Bronchoscopy is a direct visual examination of the voice box (larynx) and airways through a flexible viewing tube (a bronchoscope). A bronchoscope has a light at the end that allows a doctor to look down through the larger airways (bronchi) into the lungs.

Bronchoscopy can help a doctor make a diagnosis and treat certain conditions. A flexible bronchoscope can be used to remove secre-

▲ see page 314

tions, blood, pus, and foreign bodies; to place drugs in specific areas of the lung; and to investigate the source of bleeding. If a doctor suspects lung cancer, the airways can be examined and specimens can be taken from any suspicious areas. Bronchoscopy is used for collecting the organisms causing pneumonia and that are difficult to collect and identify in other ways. Bronchoscopy is especially helpful for obtaining specimens from the lungs in people who have AIDS and other immune deficiencies. When people have been burned or have inhaled smoke, bronchoscopy helps doctors assess for burns and smoke injury of the larynx and airways.

For at least 4 hours before bronchoscopy, the person should not eat or drink. A sedative is often given to ease anxiety, and atropine may be given to reduce the risks of spasm of the voice box and slowing of the heart rate, which sometimes occur during the procedure. The throat and nasal passage are sprayed with an anesthetic, and the flexible bronchoscope is passed through a nostril and into the airways of the lungs.

Bronchoalveolar lavage is a procedure doctors can use to collect specimens from the smaller airways and alveoli that cannot be seen through the bronchoscope. After wedging the bronchoscope into a small airway, a doctor instills salt water (saline) through the instrument. The fluid is then suctioned back into the bronchoscope, bringing cells and any bacteria with it. Examination of the material under the microscope helps in diagnosing infections and cancers; culturing the fluid is a better way to diagnose infections. Bronchoalveolar lavage can also be used to treat pulmonary alveolar proteinosis▲ and other conditions.

Transbronchial lung biopsy involves obtaining a specimen of lung tissue through the bronchial wall. A doctor removes pieces of tissue from a suspicious area by passing a biopsy instrument through a channel in the bronchoscope and then through the wall of a small airway and into the suspicious area of lung. A doctor may use a fluoroscope for guidance in identifying the suspicious area. Such guidance can also decrease the risk of accidentally perforating the lung and causing leakage of air into the pleural space (pneumothorax■). Although transbronchial lung biopsy increases the risk of complications, it often provides additional diagnostic information and may make major surgery unnecessary.

Understanding Bronchoscopy

To view the airways directly, a doctor passes a flexible bronchoscope through a person's nostril and down into the airways. The circular inset shows the doctor's view.

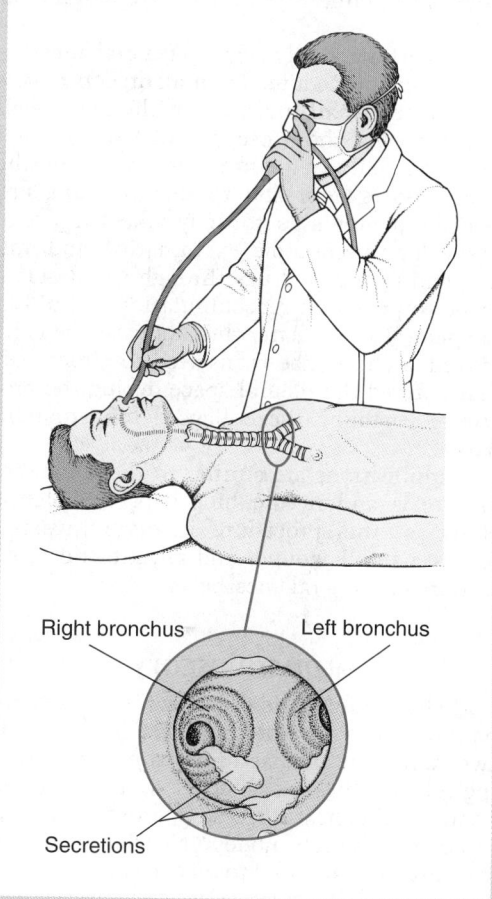

Right bronchus
Left bronchus
Secretions

Transbronchial needle aspiration is sometimes performed. In this procedure, a needle is passed through the bronchoscope into the bronchial wall. A doctor may be able to extract cells from suspicious lymph nodes to sample.

After bronchoscopy, the person is observed for several hours. If a tissue specimen was removed, the doctor takes chest x-rays to check for complications, such as bleeding.

▲ see page 306   ■ see page 316

THORACOSCOPY

Thoracoscopy is the visual examination of the lung surfaces and pleural space through a viewing tube (a thoracoscope). Thoracoscopy is the most common means for obtaining a sample of lung tissue for a biopsy. A thoracoscope also may be used in treating accumulations of fluid in the pleural space (pleural effusions).

The person usually is given general anesthesia for this procedure. Then a surgeon makes up to three small incisions in the chest wall and passes a thoracoscope into the pleural space; this allows air to enter, collapsing the lung. Besides being able to view the lung surface and pleura, a doctor may take samples of tissue for microscopic examination and culture and may give drugs through the thoracoscope to prevent a reaccumulation of fluid in the pleural space. After the thoracoscope is removed, a chest tube is inserted to remove air that entered the pleural space during the procedure, enabling the collapsed lung to reinflate.

Complications are similar to those for thoracentesis and needle biopsy of the pleura. However, this procedure is more invasive, leaves a small wound, and requires hospitalization and general anesthesia.

MEDIASTINOSCOPY

Mediastinoscopy is the direct visual examination of the area of the chest between the two lungs (the mediastinum) through a viewing tube (mediastinoscope). The mediastinum contains the heart, trachea, esophagus, thymus, and lymph nodes. Nearly all mediastinoscopies are used to diagnose the cause of enlarged lymph nodes or to evaluate how far lung cancer has spread before chest surgery (thoracotomy) is performed.

Mediastinoscopy is performed in an operating room with the person under general anesthesia. A small incision is made in the notch just above the breastbone (sternum). The instrument then is passed down into the chest, allowing the doctor to observe all the contents of the mediastinum and to obtain specimens for diagnostic tests if necessary. Complications are similar to those for thoracentesis and needle biopsy of the pleura.

THORACOTOMY

Thoracotomy is an operation in which the chest wall is opened to view the internal chest organs, to obtain samples of tissue for laboratory examination, and to treat diseases of the lungs, heart, or major arteries.

Although thoracotomy is the most accurate means of assessing lung diseases, it is a major operation and therefore is used less often than other diagnostic techniques. Thoracotomy is used when procedures such as thoracentesis, bronchoscopy, or mediastinoscopy fail to provide adequate information. The lung problem is identified in more than 90% of people who undergo this operation because the sample site can be seen and selected and because large tissue samples can be taken.

Thoracotomy requires general anesthesia in an operating room. An incision is made in the chest wall, and tissue samples of the lung are removed for microscopic examination. If specimens are to be taken from areas in both lungs, the breastbone is often split. If necessary, a lung segment, a lung lobe, or an entire lung can be removed.

A chest tube is inserted and left in place for 24 to 48 hours afterward. The person usually stays in the hospital for several days. Complications include infection, persistent bleeding, and a persistent air leak.

SUCTIONING

Suctioning is used to obtain secretions and cells from the trachea and large bronchi. It is used to obtain specimens for microscopic examination or a sputum culture and to help clear secretions from the airways when cough is inadequate.

One end of a long, flexible, clear plastic tube is attached to a suction pump; the other end is passed through a nostril or the mouth and into the trachea. When the tube is in position, suction is applied in intermittent bursts lasting 2 to 5 seconds. With people who have an artificial opening directly into the trachea (tracheostomy), the tube can be inserted directly into the trachea.

CHAPTER 40

Pulmonary Rehabilitation

Pulmonary rehabilitation is a program designed for people who have chronic lung disease; the primary goal for the person enrolled is to achieve and maintain the maximum level of independence and functioning. Although most pulmonary rehabilitation programs focus on the needs of people who have chronic obstructive pulmonary disease, people with other types of lung disease may benefit as well. All age groups can benefit, including people older than 70.

Pulmonary rehabilitation programs are effective for people who have severe shortness of breath, which impairs quality of life; an inability to exercise, which may affect daily activities; and multiple hospitalizations or emergency room visits because of lung disease. A successful rehabilitation program may significantly improve the person's quality of life by reducing shortness of breath, increasing exercise tolerance, promoting a sense of well-being, and, to a lesser extent, decreasing the number of hospitalizations. However, these programs do not significantly improve survival.

These programs are usually conducted in an outpatient setting or in the person's home. Inpatient services often take place in special rehabilitation centers. Inpatient services are used mainly for people who are recovering from hospitalization, often because of a severe respiratory problem. These people are often not stable enough to go home but no longer require care in an intensive care unit. The most successful rehabilitation programs are those in which services are provided by a variety of health care professionals (called a pulmonary rehabilitation team) to coordinate complex medical services. For example, a respiratory or physical therapist, a nurse, a doctor, a psychologist or social worker, and a dietitian are often needed. Most people are enrolled in these programs for about 8 to 12 weeks.

Supportive lung therapy, which includes oxygen therapy and chest physical therapy, can be used in conjunction with pulmonary rehabilitation. Supportive therapy can also be used for people not enrolled in these programs but who have chronic lung disorders (such as cystic fibrosis or bronchiectasis) or acute lung conditions (such as pneumonia).

Enrollment and Goal Setting

The first step for the team members is to determine the person's short-term and long-term goals. For example, an older person may desire to travel by air to visit a grandchild. If the person can walk only 300 feet because of shortness of breath but must be able to walk 1,000 feet to board the airplane, the initial short-term goal may be to increase the walking distance by small increments. Team members must encourage the person while also setting realistic goals. Periodic reevaluation (weekly) is important to ensure that these goals are being met.

It is also important for the team members to identify factors that may limit the program's effectiveness for a particular person; these factors may include problems with financial resources, transportation to the rehabilitation center, cognition, and family dynamics. An example of a problem with cognition would be when a person who has lung problems also has dementia. Such a person may need a specific approach to enhance comprehension. An example of a problem with family dynamics would be when a person who is enrolled in a program is dependent on a caretaker who is mentally or physically abusive. It is important for team members to recognize such problems and plan ways to help the person.

Long-term goals are also established, and team members teach people to recognize changes in their lung condition, so that they will contact their doctor promptly. Treatment may need to be modified in response to changes in symptoms.

Exercise Training

Exercise training is probably the most important component of pulmonary rehabilitation. It reduces the effects of inactivity and deconditioning, resulting in less shortness of breath and an increased ability to exercise. However, physical limitations may restrict the types of exercise training that can be used.

In some people who are dependent on ventilators, exercise training may help them to be weaned off the use of ventilators.

Exercise of the lower extremities is the cornerstone of training. Because walking is necessary for most activities of daily living, many rehabilitation programs use walking as the preferred mode of training. Some people may prefer exercising on a stationary bicycle. Choosing an exercise that is comfortable and satisfying for the person enhances long-term compliance.

Exercise training of the arms is also beneficial for people with chronic respiratory diseases who complain of symptoms during their normal activities of daily living, such as washing the hair and shaving. Such training is needed because some of the shoulder muscles are used in breathing as well as in moving the arms; arm work can quickly overexert these muscles.

Psychosocial Counseling

Because strong emotions tend to worsen shortness of breath, some people suppress their emotions and thus may be caught in an emotional straitjacket. Yet, depression and anxiety are common. In addition, shortness of breath may cause anxiety and depression and interfere with sexual activity. Furthermore, a person may be unable to manage stress and relax. Through counseling, group therapy, and, when needed, drug treatment, the person may be able to better cope with these psychosocial problems.

Nutritional Evaluation and Counseling

People who have lung disease often need nutritional evaluation and counseling. For example, those with the most severe chronic obstructive pulmonary disease often experience weight loss. Pulmonary rehabilitation programs help people avoid weight loss and maintain muscle mass. People must be taught to eat in such a way that they maintain adequate caloric intake while avoiding becoming too full, which can interfere with breathing. Alternatively, some people gain weight because of a reduced activity level. In this case, breathing becomes even more difficult, and a weight-loss program is needed.

Drug Use and Education

People with advanced lung disease usually take multiple drugs on complex schedules that require precise dosing. Through a rehabilitation program, people can learn about the appropriate timing and doses of all drugs they need to take. Education often includes information about the nature of the lung disease and the role of drug therapy, including expected benefits, potential side effects, and the proper technique for use of inhaled drugs. Programs closely monitor compliance and teach people and families about the importance of appropriate drug use.

Oxygen Therapy

Oxygen therapy is used either short-term for people who are recovering from acute lung disorders or longer for people with chronic lung disorders in whom oxygen levels are consistently low. Oxygen therapy is used in the hospital not only for people with chronic lung disorders, but also for people with acute lung disorders, such as pneumonia, or conditions that temporarily benefit from maintaining a higher level of oxygen in the blood, such as angina (a condition in which the heart muscle is not receiving enough oxygen).▲

The use of therapeutic oxygen improves survival in people with chronic lung disease who consistently have low levels of oxygen in their blood. The more hours a day the oxygen is used, the better the result. Survival is better when 12 hours of oxygen are used than when no oxygen is used; survival is even better when oxygen is used continuously (24 hours per day). Other benefits of long-term oxygen use include a reduction on the strain of the heart that lung disease causes and less shortness of breath. Both sleep and the ability to exercise tend to improve.

Some people with chronic lung disease have low levels of oxygen only when they physically exert themselves. These people can limit their oxygen use to periods of exertion. Other people have low levels only when they are sleeping. These people can limit their oxygen use to overnight hours.

Once the critical level of oxygen is determined, oximetry may be used to adjust oxygen flow settings over time.■ Oximetry is painless and uses a simple finger or ear device to measure the amount of oxygen in the blood.

Long-term home oxygen is available from three different delivery systems: electrically

---

▲ see page 202   ■ see also page 255

driven oxygen concentrators, liquid systems, and compressed gas. Inside the home, liquid and compressed gas systems use large tanks to store oxygen. Small, portable tanks of compressed oxygen also may be needed for brief periods—a few hours—outside the home. Each system has advantages and disadvantages. Oxygen is typically administered with continuous flow through a 2-pronged nasal tube (cannula), even though this system is highly wasteful of oxygen. To improve efficiency and increase the person's mobility, several devices, including reservoir cannulas, demand-type systems, and transtracheal catheters, can be used. Usually, a respiratory therapist or physician instructs the person about proper oxygen use.

While using oxygen therapy at home, it is important to stabilize the tank (possibly using a stand) and store it in an area that is out of the way so it will not fall. The tank should be closed tightly when not in use. Because oxygen can cause an explosion, it is also important to be careful to keep the tank away from any flammable source, such as matches, heaters, or hair dryers. No one in the house should smoke when oxygen is in use.

Chest Physical Therapy

Respiratory therapists use several different techniques to help treat lung disease, including postural drainage, suctioning, and breathing exercises. The choice of therapy is based on the underlying disease and the person's overall condition.

Postural Drainage

In postural drainage, the person is tilted or propped at an angle to help drain secretions from the lungs. Also, the chest or back may be clapped with a cupped hand to help loosen secretions—a technique called chest percussion. Alternatively, the therapist or a trained family member may use a mechanical vibrator.

These techniques are used at intervals on people who have conditions that produce a great deal of sputum, such as cystic fibrosis, bronchiectasis, and lung abscess. The techniques may also be used when a person cannot cough up sputum effectively, as may happen with older people, people who have muscle weakness, and people recovering from surgery, an injury, or a severe illness.

Postural drainage cannot be used for people who are unable to tolerate the position required, are taking anticoagulation drugs, have recently vomited up blood, have had a recent rib or vertebral fracture, or have severe osteoporosis. Postural drainage also cannot be used for people who are unable to produce any secretions (because when this happens, further attempts at postural drainage may lower the level of oxygen in the blood).

Suctioning

Respiratory therapists and nurses may use suctioning to help remove secretions from the airways. To perform suctioning, they usually introduce a small plastic tube through the nose and a few inches into the windpipe (trachea). A gentle vacuum sucks out the secretions that cannot be coughed up. Suctioning is also used to clear secretions in someone who has a tracheostomy (a surgical opening in the trachea to allow breathing) or who has a breathing tube inserted through the nose or mouth and into the trachea (intubation) while on a ventilator.

Breathing Exercises

Breathing exercises may help strengthen the muscles that inflate and deflate the lungs, but they do not directly improve lung function. Still, breathing exercises decrease the likelihood of lung complications after surgery in heavy smokers and others with lung disease. Such exercises are particularly helpful for sedentary people who have chronic obstructive pulmonary disease or those who have been put on a ventilator.

Often, these exercises involve using an instrument called an incentive spirometer.▲ A person breathes in as hard as possible on a tube attached to a hand-held plastic chamber. The chamber houses a ball, and each breath lifts the ball. Ideally, this maneuver is done 5 to 10 consecutive times each hour while the person is awake. This device is used routinely in hospitals before and after surgery. However, deep breathing exercises encouraged by nurses and respiratory therapists may be more effective than breathing exercises using an incentive spirometer.

Pursed-lip breathing is a type of exercise that may be helpful when people who have chronic obstructive pulmonary disease overinflate their lungs during attacks of airway nar-

▲ see page 254

rowing, panic, or exercise. It also can function as an additional breathing exercise for people undergoing respiratory training. The person is taught—or often discovers by himself—to exhale against partially closed (pursed) lips, as if preparing to whistle. This measure increases pressure in the airways and helps prevent them from collapsing. The exercise causes no ill effects, and some people adopt the habit without instruction. People may also benefit from bending forward while performing pursed-lip breathing. In this position, the person stands with the arms and hands outstretched and supports the body on a table or similar structure. This position improves functioning of the diaphragm (the most important breathing muscle) and reduces shortness of breath.

CHAPTER 41

Bronchitis

Bronchitis is inflammation of the large airways that branch off the trachea (bronchi), usually caused by infection but sometimes caused by irritation from a gas or particle.

Symptoms lasting up to 90 days are usually classified as acute bronchitis; symptoms lasting longer, sometimes for months or years, are usually classified as chronic bronchitis. When chronic bronchitis also decreases airflow, it is considered a defining characteristic of chronic obstructive pulmonary disease.▲ This chapter discusses acute bronchitis only.

Causes

Acute bronchitis can be caused by infection or by exposure to irritants.

Infectious bronchitis occurs most often during the winter and is most often caused by viruses. Even after a viral infection has resolved, the irritation it causes can continue to cause symptoms for weeks. Infectious bronchitis may also be caused by bacteria, and it often follows an upper respiratory viral infection. *Mycoplasma pneumoniae* and *Chlamydia pneumoniae* often cause bacterial bronchitis in young adults. Among middle-aged and older people, *Streptococcus pneumoniae*, *Haemophilus influenzae*, and *Moraxella catarrhalis* are the most common organisms causing bacterial bronchitis. Viral bronchitis may be caused by a number of common viruses, including the influenza virus. A person often has a combination of bacterial and viral bronchitis.

Smokers and people who have chronic lung diseases may have repeated attacks of acute bronchitis because mucus is less able to drain from their airways. Malnutrition increases the risk of upper respiratory tract infections and subsequent acute bronchitis, especially in children and older people. Chronic sinus infection, bronchiectasis,■ and allergies also increase the risk of repeated episodes of acute bronchitis. Children with enlarged tonsils and adenoids may have repeated episodes of bronchitis.

Irritative bronchitis (also called industrial or environmental bronchitis) may be caused by exposure to various mineral and vegetable dusts. Exposure to fumes from strong acids, ammonia, some organic solvents, chlorine, hydrogen sulfide, sulfur dioxide, and bromine can also cause irritative bronchitis.

Symptoms

Infectious bronchitis generally begins with the symptoms of a common cold: runny nose, sore throat, fatigue, chilliness, and back and muscle aches. A slight fever (100° to 101° F) may be present. The onset of cough (usually dry at first) signals the beginning of acute bronchitis. With viral bronchitis, small amounts of white mucus are often coughed up. When the coughed-up mucus changes from white to green or yellow, the condition may have been complicated by a bacterial infection.

With severe bronchitis, fever may be as high as 101° to 102° F and may last for 3 to 5 days even with antibiotic treatment. The cough is the last symptom to subside and often takes several weeks or even longer to resolve. Vi-

▲ see page 281   ■ see page 289

Understanding Bronchitis

In bronchitis, areas of the bronchial wall become inflamed and swollen, and mucus increases. As a result, the air passageway is narrowed. Bacteria and viruses are usually present.

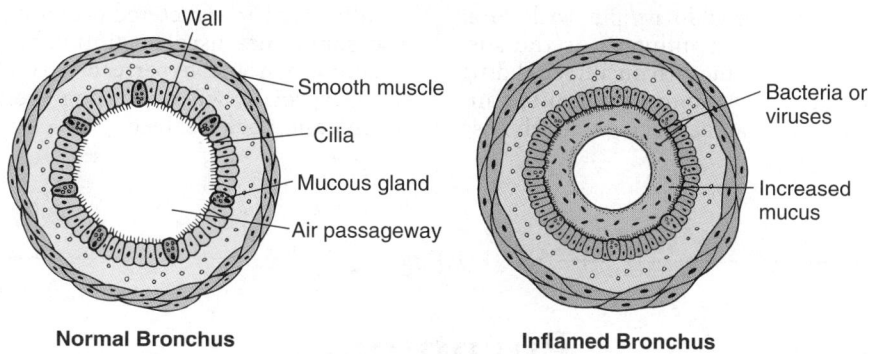

Wall
Smooth muscle
Cilia
Mucous gland
Air passageway

Bacteria or viruses
Increased mucus

Normal Bronchus   **Inflamed Bronchus**

ruses can damage the epithelial cells lining the bronchi, and the body needs time to repair the damage. Airway hyperreactivity, which is a short-term narrowing of the airways with impairment or limitation of the amount of air flowing into the lungs, is common with acute bronchitis. The impairment of airflow may be triggered by common stimuli, such as inhaling mild irritants, inhaling cold, outdoor air, or smelling strong odors. If the impairment of airflow is severe, the person may be short of breath. Wheezing, especially after coughing, is common.

Serious complications, such as acute respiratory failure▲ or pneumonia,■ usually occur only in people who have an underlying chronic lung disease, such as chronic obstructive pulmonary disease or asthma.

Diagnosis

A doctor usually makes a diagnosis of bronchitis based on the symptoms and the lack of evidence of pneumonia. The doctor may hear wheezing during the physical examination.

The doctor may inspect a sample of sputum: clear or white sputum suggests a viral infection; yellow or green sputum suggests a bacterial infection. If symptoms are severe, the doctor may order a chest x-ray to exclude pneumonia. If a cough persists for more than two months, a chest x-ray is performed to exclude an underlying lung disease, such as lung cancer.

Treatment

Cough medicines can be used to suppress a dry, disturbing cough.★ However, a cough that produces a lot of sputum usually should not be suppressed. Expectorants may help to thin secretions and make them easier to cough up. Adults may take aspirin, acetaminophen, or ibuprofen to reduce fever and general feelings of illness, but children should take only acetaminophen or ibuprofen, not aspirin. People with acute bronchitis, especially those who have a fever, should rest and drink enough fluid to keep their urine pale (except on arising from sleep, when urine is usually darker).

Antibiotics are used to treat acute bronchitis that appears to be caused by a bacterial infection and may be given as a precaution to people with underlying lung disease, even when there is no evidence of bacterial infection. Adults may be given amoxicillin, tetracycline, doxycycline, or trimethoprim-sulfamethoxazole. When *Mycoplasma pneumoniae* or *Chlamydia pneumoniae* is the suspected cause, erythromycin or doxycycline is usually given. Newer antibiotics, such as several oral cephalosporins (cefaclor, cefuroxime), azithromycin, clarithromycin, and the newer fluoroquinolones (levofloxacin, gatifloxacin) are

▲ see page 325   ■ see page 264

★ see page 249

highly effective, but because of their high cost, they are generally used for more serious lung infections. For children, amoxicillin is usually given. When symptoms persist or recur or when bronchitis is unusually severe, a laboratory culture of coughed-up sputum may show whether a different antibiotic is needed.

Antibiotics do not help people with viral bronchitis. However, if influenza is the suspected cause, treatment with an antiviral drug may be helpful. The symptoms of limited airflow and wheezing can be treated with the use of cool-mist humidifiers or steam vaporizers. The person can also inhale warm water vapor while leaning over a bathroom sink filled with hot water with a towel loosely draped over the head. Bronchodilators, which dilate the bronchi, can be used to temporarily open the airways and reduce wheezing. Corticosteroids, usually given in a metered-dose inhaler,▲ are also sometimes used to diminish cough and inflammation and hyperreactivity of the airways, especially when the cough persists after the infection has resolved.

CHAPTER 42

Pneumonia

Pneumonia is an infection of the small air sacs of the lungs (alveoli) and the tissues around them.

In the United States, about 2 million people develop pneumonia each year, and 40,000 to 70,000 of them die. Often, pneumonia is the final illness in people who have other serious, chronic diseases. It is the sixth most common cause of death overall, and the most common fatal infection acquired in hospitals. In developing countries, pneumonia is either the leading cause of death or second only to dehydration from severe diarrhea.

The setting in which pneumonia develops is one of the most important features to doctors. Pneumonia may develop in people living in the community (community-acquired pneumonia), in the hospital (hospital-acquired pneumonia), or in some other institutional setting, such as a nursing home (institution-acquired pneumonia). The setting often helps determine what infecting organism is responsible for the pneumonia. For example, community-acquired pneumonia is more likely to stem from infection with the gram-positive bacterium *Streptococcus pneumoniae*. Hospital-acquired pneumonia is more likely to be caused by *Staphylococcus aureus* or a gram-negative bacterium, such as *Klebsiella pneumoniae* or *Pseudomonas aeruginosa*. Depending on the infecting organism, there is usually a difference in the severity of pneumonia and the way it is treated (for example, whether with oral drugs at home or with intravenous drugs in the hospital).

Another critical feature is whether the pneumonia occurs in a healthy person or in someone who has an impaired immune system. Certain drugs (such as corticosteroids) can impair the immune system, as can the presence of diseases, such as AIDS. Sometimes the immune system can be worn down by a severe acute or chronic illness, as is often the case with older people. A person who has an impaired immune system is far more likely to contract pneumonia, including pneumonia caused by unusual organisms; this person may not respond as well to treatment as someone whose immune system is healthy. Other conditions that predispose certain people to pneumonia include alcoholism, cigarette smoking, diabetes, heart failure, and chronic obstructive pulmonary disease. The very young and very old are at higher-than-average risk. Also at risk are people who are debilitated, bedridden, paralyzed, or unconscious.

Causes

Pneumonia is not a single illness but rather many different ones, each caused by a different microscopic organism—whether it is a bacterium, virus, or fungus. Usually pneumonia starts after organisms are inhaled into the lungs, but sometimes the infection is carried to the lungs by the bloodstream or it migrates

▲ see art on page 279

Preventing Certain Pneumonias With Vaccines

Although not all pneumonias can be prevented, certain pneumonias can be prevented with immunizations. For example, pneumococcal pneumonia, which is caused by *Streptococcus pneumoniae*, can be prevented with the **pneumococcal pneumonia vaccine**. This vaccine protects people from serious pneumococcal infections. Vaccination is recommended for people at high risk of pneumococcal pneumonia—such as all those older than 65 and younger adults who have lung or heart disease, weakened immune systems, or diabetes. The protection from vaccination may last a lifetime, although it is recommended that people at highest risk be revaccinated after 5 years. Although temporary soreness at the site of injection is common, only 1% of people develop a fever and muscle pain after vaccination. Even fewer people have a severe allergic reaction. Pregnant women should not receive this vaccine.

Pneumonia caused by *Haemophilus influenzae* type b strain can be prevented with the **Haemophilus influenzae type b vaccine**. This vaccine is recommended for all children. The vaccine is given in three doses—at ages 2 months, 4 months, and 6 months.

Pneumonia caused by the influenza virus can be prevented with the **influenza vaccine**. Annual influenza vaccinations are recommended for health care workers, older people, and people with chronic conditions such as emphysema, diabetes, heart disease, and kidney disease. Vaccination should take place every year during the fall (September through November), so that levels of antibodies will be highest during the peak influenza months—November through March. A different vaccine is introduced every year based on predictions of which strains are most likely to cause influenza.

Pneumonia caused by the chickenpox virus may be prevented with the **chickenpox vaccine**. Pneumonia caused by this virus is very rare. Vaccination in children is with one dose. All children aged 12 to 18 months of age should be routinely vaccinated. Children between 18 months and 12 years should be vaccinated, unless testing indicates a natural immunity from a previous infection. Vaccination without testing is acceptable, because vaccination appears to be safe even if a person has had chickenpox. In people 13 years and older, vaccination should be given only if testing does not indicate natural immunity. For these people, two doses are given 4 to 8 weeks apart.

---

to the lungs directly from a nearby infection. Pneumonia may follow surgery, particularly abdominal surgery, or an injury (trauma), particularly a chest injury, because of the resulting shallow breathing, impaired ability to cough, and retention of mucus. Sometimes pneumonia occurs when particles from the mouth are inhaled and are not cleared, or when an obstruction (such as a tumor) causes bacteria to become trapped. The former type is called aspiration pneumonia; the latter type is called obstructive pneumonia.

Symptoms and Diagnosis

The most common symptom of pneumonia is a cough that produces sputum. Other common symptoms include chest pain, chills, fever, and shortness of breath. These symptoms may vary, however, depending on how extensive the disease is and which organism is causing it.

A doctor or nurse checks for pneumonia by listening to the chest with a stethoscope. Pneumonia usually produces distinctive sounds; these abnormal sounds are caused by narrowing of airways or filling of the normally air-filled parts of the lung with inflammatory cells and fluid, a process called consolidation.

In most cases, the diagnosis of pneumonia is confirmed with a chest x-ray. For most bacterial pneumonias, the involved tissue of the lung appears on the x-ray as a dense white patch (because the x-ray beam does not get through), compared with nearby healthy lung tissue that appears black (because the x-rays get through easily, exposing the film). Viral pneumonias typically produce faint, widely scattered white streaks or patches. Some pneumonias can lead to a lung abscess,▲ which appears on the x-ray as a space filled with fluid (pus). There may be changes at the top of the lung, suggesting tuberculosis.■ Thus, the x-ray may (but not always) help a doctor determine which organism is causing the disease.

▲ see page 272   ■ see page 1125

Antibiotics Used for Bacterial Pneumonias

Streptococcus pneumoniae (pneumococcus)
  Penicillin
  Amoxicillin
  Cephalosporins
  Erythromycin
  Azithromycin
  Clarithromycin
  Fluoroquinolones

Haemophilus influenzae
  Cephalosporins (2nd and 3rd generation)
  Amoxicillin-clavulanate
  Azithromycin
  Fluoroquinolones
  Trimethoprim-sulfamethoxazole

Legionella pneumophila
  Erythromycin (with or without rifampin)
  Azithromycin
  Fluoroquinolones

Mycoplasma pneumoniae
  Erythromycin
  Doxycycline
  Azithromycin
  Clarithromycin
  Fluoroquinolones

Chlamydia pneumoniae
  Erythromycin
  Doxycycline
  Azithromycin
  Clarithromycin
  Fluoroquinolones

Staphylococcus aureus
  Cephalosporins (1st generation)
  Nafcillin
  Oxacillin
  Vancomycin

Anaerobic bacteria
  Clindamycin
  Metronidazole

Gram-negative bacteria
  Imipenem
  Cephalosporins (3rd and 4th generation)
  Aminoglycosides
  Fluoroquinolones

Newer fluoroquinolones = levofloxacin, moxifloxacin, gatifloxacin.

Doctors culture sputum and blood specimens in an attempt to identify the organism causing pneumonia. However, despite these tests, the precise organism cannot be identified in up to half of people who have pneumonia. When it is necessary to identify the organism, such as when the person is severely ill and is not responding well to therapy, doctors can try to obtain better specimens by inserting a bronchoscope into the airways (bronchoscopy).▲

Prevention and Treatment

Several types of pneumonia can be prevented with the use of vaccines. Vaccines are available to protect against pneumococcal pneumonia, pneumonia caused by the bacterium *Haemophilus influenzae*, and pneumonia caused by the influenza virus, which also often leads to a secondary bacterial pneumonia.

Deep-breathing exercises and therapy to clear secretions help prevent pneumonia in people at high risk, such as those who have had chest or abdominal surgery and those who are debilitated.

People with pneumonia also need to clear secretions and benefit from deep-breathing exercises and therapy as well. If people with pneumonia are short of breath or their blood is low in oxygen, supplemental oxygen is provided. Although rest is an important part of treatment, moving often and getting out of bed and into a chair are encouraged.

Usually antibiotics are started whenever bacterial pneumonia is suspected (including obstructive pneumonia), even before the bacteria is identified. The prompt use of antibiotics likely reduces the severity of pneumonia and the chance of developing complications, some of which can lead to death.

When choosing an antibiotic, doctors consider which bacteria is likely to be the cause. The doctor can change the choice of antibiotic later, after the bacteria has been identified and its susceptibility to various antibiotics known. Often, people who have pneumonia but are not very sick can take oral antibiotics and remain at home. Older people and those who are short of breath or have preexisting heart or lung disease are generally hospitalized and given intravenous antibiotics to start. Those antibiotics are usually switched to oral ones after a few days. These people may also need

▲ see page 256

supplemental oxygen, intravenous fluids, and mechanical respiratory support.▲

Antibiotics are not helpful for viral pneumonias. However, antibiotics are given for viral pneumonias that are likely to be followed by bacterial infections, such as those caused by respiratory syncytial virus infection in infants and sometimes those caused by the influenza virus, at least in some people who are very susceptible to pneumonia.

Community-Acquired Pneumonia

Streptococcus is the most common bacterial cause of community-acquired pneumonia. Other causes of community-acquired pneumonia include *Haemophilus influenzae, Legionella,* mycoplasma, chlamydia, and viruses. *Staphylococcus* may rarely cause community-acquired pneumonia, but this organism is more often a cause of hospital-acquired pneumonia. Community-acquired pneumonia occurs most commonly in very young and very old people.

Pneumococcal Pneumonia: Pneumococcal pneumonia is caused by *Streptococcus pneumoniae* (pneumococcus). It usually starts after an upper respiratory tract viral infection (a cold or influenza) damages the defenses of the airways enough to allow bacteria to infect the area. Shaking and chills are followed by a fever, a cough that produces sputum, shortness of breath, and chest pain on the side of the affected lung when breathing. Nausea, vomiting, fatigue, and muscle aches are also common. The sputum is often rust-colored from blood.

Pneumococcal pneumonia, although usually treatable, can be fatal, especially in the very young, the very old, and those people who have other severe illnesses. Pneumococcal pneumonia can lead to a life-threatening infection of the blood (pneumococcal septicemia). Many people develop fluid in the pleural space (the space between the two layers of the membranes covering the lungs [pleura]); this condition is called pleural effusion.■ Rarely, pneumococcal infection can spread to the coverings of the brain (meninges), causing pneumococcal meningitis and leading to confusion, a stiff neck, seizures, and possibly coma.

A person who has been infected with one of the 80 known types of pneumococcus develops partial immunity to reinfection with that type but no immunity to the others. A vaccine is available that protects against 23 of the most prevalent and serious types of pneumococci that cause infection.★

Pneumococcal pneumonia may be treated with any of several types of antibiotics, including penicillins and cephalosporins, but the organism that causes pneumococcal pneumonia has developed increasing resistance to these drugs in the last decade. People who are infected with resistant strains of pneumococcus or who are allergic to penicillin are given erythromycin, a fluoroquinolone, or another antibiotic instead.

Pneumonia Caused by *Haemophilus influenzae:* *Haemophilus influenzae* is a bacterium; despite its name, it is not the influenza virus that causes the flu. *Haemophilus influenzae* type b strains are the most virulent and cause serious diseases, including meningitis, epiglottitis, and pneumonia, usually in children younger than 5 years. However, because of the widespread use of the *Haemophilus influenzae* type b vaccine, serious disease from this organism is becoming less common. This type of pneumonia is more common among Native Americans, Eskimos, blacks, people with sickle cell disease, and people with immune system disorders. Most such cases are caused by strains other than those used in the *Haemophilus influenzae* type b vaccine.

Signs of the infection include typical pneumonia symptoms, such as a fever, a cough that produces sputum, and shortness of breath.

Vaccination for type b strains of *Haemophilus influenzae* is recommended for all children. The vaccine is given in three doses—at ages 2 months, 4 months, and 6 months.

Antibiotics are used to treat *Haemophilus influenzae* type b pneumonia. Trimethoprim-sulfamethoxazole is commonly used and can be taken by mouth. Many other antibiotics work as well.

Legionnaires' Disease: Legionnaires' disease is caused by the bacterium *Legionella pneumophila* and other species of *Legionella.* It accounts for about 1 to 8% of all pneumonias and about 4% of fatal pneumonias acquired in hospitals. *Legionella* bacteria live in water, and outbreaks have occurred primarily in hotels and hospitals when the organism has spread through the air conditioning systems or water supplies, such as showers. No cases

---

▲ see page 326   ■ see page 314
★ see page 1094

have been identified in which one person directly infected another.

Although Legionnaires' disease may occur at any age, people who are middle-aged and older have been affected most often. People who smoke tobacco, take corticosteroids, have chronic kidney failure, or have undergone organ transplantation seem to be at greater risk. Legionnaires' disease can be life threatening.

The first symptoms, appearing 2 to 10 days after the infection is transmitted, include fatigue, fever, headache, and muscle aches. A dry cough later becomes productive of sputum. People with serious infections can become extremely short of breath and may have diarrhea or mental disturbances.

Laboratory tests are performed on sputum, blood, and urine samples to confirm the diagnosis. Because people infected with *Legionella pneumophila* produce antibodies to fight the disease, blood tests show an increasing concentration of these antibodies. However, the results of antibody tests usually are not available until after the pneumonia has run its course.

Antibiotics, such as the fluoroquinolones, erythromycin (with or without rifampin), or azithromycin, are used for treatment. About 20% of the people who develop the disease die. The death rate is much higher among those who contract the disease in the hospital or who have an impaired immune system.

Mycoplasmal Pneumonia: *Mycoplasma pneumoniae* is the most common cause of pneumonia in people aged 5 to 35, but it is an uncommon cause in other people. Epidemics occur especially in confined groups such as students, military personnel, and families. The epidemics tend to spread slowly because the incubation period lasts 10 to 14 days. Most commonly, this type of pneumonia strikes in the spring.

Mycoplasmal pneumonia often starts with fatigue, a sore throat, and a dry cough and thus resembles influenza. The symptoms slowly worsen. Attacks of severe coughing may eventually produce sputum. About 10 to 20% of people develop a rash. Occasionally, anemia, joint pains, or neurologic problems (such as meningitis) develop. Symptoms often persist for 1 to 2 weeks, followed by slow improvement. Some people still feel weak and tired after several weeks. Although mycoplasmal pneumonia is usually mild and most people recover without treatment, severe cases do occur occasionally.

An x-ray shows that the person has pneumonia. Most laboratories do not offer blood tests that accurately identify mycoplasma.

When the symptoms and x-ray results lead a doctor to suspect mycoplasmal pneumonia, treatment is often started, even if mycoplasma has not been accurately identified. Erythromycin and doxycycline are the preferred antibiotics for treating mycoplasmal pneumonia. Clarithromycin, azithromycin, and the fluoroquinolones are also effective. Antibiotic treatment reduces the period of fever and lung involvement and promotes recovery. However,

Psittacosis: An Unusual Type of Pneumonia

Psittacosis (parrot fever) is a rare pneumonia caused by *Chlamydia psittaci*, a bacterium found mainly in birds such as parrots, parakeets, and lovebirds. It is also found in other birds, such as pigeons, finches, chickens, and turkeys. Usually, people are infected by inhaling dust from the feathers or the waste of infected birds. The organism also may be transmitted by a bite from an infected bird and, rarely, from person to person in cough droplets. Psittacosis is mainly an occupational disease of people who work in pet shops or on poultry farms.

About 1 to 3 weeks after being infected, a person develops a fever, chills, fatigue, and loss of appetite. A cough develops, which is initially dry but later brings up greenish sputum. The fever persists for 2 to 3 weeks and then slowly subsides. The disease may be mild or severe, depending on the person's age and the extent of lung tissue involved. Blood antibody tests are the most reliable method for confirming the diagnosis.

Bird breeders and owners can protect themselves by avoiding the dust from the feathers and the cages of sick birds. Importers are required to treat susceptible birds with a 45-day course of tetracycline, which generally gets rid of the organism. Psittacosis is treated with tetracycline taken by mouth for at least 10 days. Recovery may take a long time, especially in severe cases. The death rate may reach 30% in severe untreated cases.

antibiotics do not cure mycoplasmal pneumonia immediately, because people treated with antibiotics continue to carry and spread the organism for several weeks.

Pneumonia Caused by *Chlamydia pneumoniae*: *Chlamydia* is another common cause of pneumonia in people aged 5 to 35. It also affects some older people. The disease is transmitted from person to person in tiny airborne droplets spread by coughing. The symptoms are similar to those of mycoplasmal pneumonia. Most people do not become seriously ill. X-rays show evidence of pneumonia, but the diagnosis of *Chlamydia* as the cause can only be established by blood tests and tests of sputum samples that are performed in research laboratories.

The antibiotics erythromycin, doxycycline, clarithromycin, azithromycin, and the fluoroquinolones are effective. If treatment is stopped too early, symptoms tend to return.

Viral Pneumonia: Many viruses can infect the lungs, causing viral pneumonia. Two types of influenza virus, called types A and B, cause pneumonia.▲ The chickenpox virus can also cause pneumonia in adults. Parainfluenza, respiratory syncytial virus, and adenovirus can cause pneumonia, sometimes more commonly in children and people who are very old. The measles virus also may cause pneumonia, especially in malnourished children. People of any age who have an impaired immune system may develop severe pneumonia from cytomegalovirus.

Viral pneumonias cause cough, which may be non-productive of sputum or productive of whitish sputum. Many people develop headache, fever, and muscle aches.

X-rays show a less dense pattern of infection than that seen with bacterial pneumonias. Stains of respiratory secretions can be used to detect some viruses, such as respiratory syncytial virus and influenza. Many viruses can be cultured, but culturing is time-consuming, expensive, and usually not helpful. It is also possible to show elevations of antibodies to specific viruses, but usually the person has recovered by the time the results are positive.

Annual influenza vaccinations are recommended for health care workers, older people, and people with chronic conditions such as emphysema, diabetes, heart disease, and kidney disease. Many viral pneumonias can be treated with drugs to kill the virus.

Viral pneumonia can cause a cough that lingers long after the infection has resolved.

Drugs Used for Viral Pneumonias

Influenza type A
Amantadine, rimantadine, oseltamivir, zanimavir

Influenza type B
Oseltamivir, zanimavir

Respiratory syncytial virus
Ribavirin

Chickenpox
Acyclovir

Herpes simplex
Acyclovir

Cytomegalovirus
Ganciclovir, foscarnet, cidofovir

Additionally, many people develop secondary bacterial pneumonia after a viral infection because of the damage the viruses wreak on the lining of the airways; antibiotics may be needed when such a bacterial superinfection (an infection that develops while a person is being treated for another infection) occurs.

Hospital-Acquired and Institutional-Acquired Pneumonia

Pneumonia that is acquired in the hospital or another type of institution tends to be far more severe than pneumonia acquired in the community. The organisms in these institutions tend to be more aggressive and harder to treat. Additionally, people in hospitals and nursing homes tend to be sicker even without pneumonia than those living in the community and therefore are not as able to fight the infection.

Staphylococcal Pneumonia: *Staphylococcus aureus* causes only 2% of community-acquired pneumonias, but it causes 10 to 15% of hospital-acquired pneumonias. This type of pneumonia is most likely to occur while people are hospitalized for another disorder, and it tends to develop in the very young, the very old, and people who are already debilitated by other illnesses. It also tends to occur in alcoholics. Although uncommon, it is serious—the death rate is about 15 to 40%—in part because those who develop staphylococcal pneumonia are usually already seriously ill.

▲ see page 1159

Staphylococcus causes typical pneumonia symptoms, but the chills and fever are more persistent in staphylococcal pneumonia than in pneumococcal pneumonia. Sometimes the symptoms worsen rapidly, with severe and potentially fatal deterioration in lung function. *Staphylococcus* may occasionally cause collections of pus (abscesses) in the lungs and, in children, may produce lung cysts that contain air (pneumatoceles). Bacteria may be carried from the lung by the bloodstream and produce pus elsewhere. Collections of pus in the pleural space (empyema) are relatively common.▲ These collections are drained using a needle or a chest tube.

Antibiotics that are active against *Staphylococcus*, usually a type of penicillin called oxacillin or nafcillin or the equivalent, are started as soon as possible. However, more and more strains of *Staphylococcus* are becoming resistant to these penicillins, requiring the use of other antibiotics, such as vancomycin.

Gram-negative Bacterial Pneumonia: Gram-negative bacteria, such as *Klebsiella* (Friedländer's pneumonia), *Pseudomonas*, *Enterobacter*, *Proteus*, *Serratia*, and *Acinetobacter*, cause pneumonia that tends to be serious.

Gram-negative bacterial pneumonias almost always occur only in people who are hospitalized or who live in nursing homes; they rarely infect the lungs of healthy adults. Gram-negative bacteria are particularly common causes of pneumonia in people who are on ventilators (breathing machines used in intensive care units). Other people at risk are infants, older people, alcoholics, and people with chronic diseases, especially immune system disorders.

The symptoms of gram-negative bacterial pneumonia are the same as for gram-positive pneumonia, except that people tend to be sicker and worsen quickly. Gram-negative bacteria may rapidly destroy lung tissue, so gram-negative pneumonia tends to become serious quickly. Fever, coughing, and shortness of breath are common. The coughed-up sputum may be thick and red—the color and consistency of currant jelly.

Because of the seriousness of the infection, the person is treated intensively in the hospital with antibiotics, supplemental oxygen, and intravenous fluids. Sometimes the person must be put on a ventilator. Despite receiving excellent treatment, about 25 to 50% of people with gram-negative pneumonia die.

Fungal Pneumonia

Three types of fungi commonly cause pneumonia: *Histoplasma capsulatum*, which causes histoplasmosis, *Coccidioides immitis*, which causes coccidioidomycosis, and *Blastomyces dermatitidis*, which causes blastomycosis. Most people who become infected have only minor symptoms and do not know that they are infected. Some people become gravely ill. Infections caused by other fungi occur primarily in people with a severely weakened immune system.

Histoplasmosis: Histoplasmosis occurs worldwide but is prevalent in river valleys in temperate and tropical climates. In the United States, the fungus occurs most commonly in the Mississippi and Ohio river valleys and in the river valleys of the East. More than 80% of people living in the Mississippi and Ohio river valleys have been exposed to the fungus.

After being inhaled, the fungus causes no symptoms in many people. In fact, many people learn that they have been exposed only after having a skin test or a chest x-ray that shows a nodule or enlarged lymph nodes. Calcium deposits can often be seen in these areas also. Other people may have a cough, fever, muscle aches, and chest pain. The infection may cause acute pneumonia, or it may develop into chronic pneumonia with symptoms that persist for months. Rarely, the infection spreads to other areas of the body, especially the bone marrow, liver, spleen, and digestive tract. This disseminated form of the disease tends to occur in people who have AIDS or other immune system disorders.■

Usually, the diagnosis is made by identifying the fungus in a sputum sample, by performing a blood or urine test that detects the organism, or by performing a blood test that identifies certain antibodies. Treatment typically consists of taking an antifungal drug, such as itraconazole or amphotericin B.

Coccidioidomycosis: Coccidioidomycosis (also called valley fever) occurs primarily in semiarid climates, especially the southwestern United States and certain parts of South America and Central America. After being inhaled, the fungus may cause no symptoms, or it may cause either acute or chronic pneumonia. In some cases, the infection spreads beyond the respiratory system—typically to the

---

▲ see page 314   ■ see page 1152

skin, bones, joints, and tissues covering the brain (meninges). This complication is more common in men, especially Filipinos and blacks, and in people who have AIDS or other immune system disorders.▲

The diagnosis is made by identifying the fungus in a sputum sample or a sample taken from another infected area or by performing a blood test that identifies certain antibodies. Treatment typically consists of giving an antifungal drug, such as fluconazole or amphotericin B.

Blastomycosis: Blastomycosis occurs primarily in the southeastern, south central, and midwestern United States and in areas around the Great Lakes. After being inhaled, the fungus causes infection primarily in the lungs; however, the infection usually produces no symptoms. Some people have a flu-like illness. Occasionally, symptoms of a chronic lung infection last for months. The disease may spread to other parts of the body, especially the skin, bones, joints, and prostate gland.■

Usually, the diagnosis is made by identifying the fungus in sputum or in another specimen. There is no blood test for this fungus. Treatment typically consists of an antifungal drug, such as itraconazole or amphotericin B. However, many people do not require treatment.

Other Fungal Infections: These infections include cryptococcosis, caused by *Cryptococcus neoformans*; aspergillosis, caused by *Aspergillus*; and mucormycosis, caused by fungi of the order Mucorales. All these infections occur throughout the world. Cryptococcosis, the most common one, may occur in an otherwise healthy person but usually is severe only in people with underlying immune system disorders, such as AIDS.★ Cryptococcosis may spread, especially to the meninges, where the resulting disease is called cryptococcal meningitis. Aspergillosis is a common and important cause of pulmonary infections in people who have acute leukemia or AIDS, have undergone organ transplantation, or are receiving long-term treatment with corticosteroids.● Mucormycosis, a relatively rare fungal infection,◆ occurs most often in people who have severe diabetes or leukemia. The three infections are treated with antifungal drugs, such as itraconazole, fluconazole, and amphotericin B. However, people who have AIDS or other immune system disorders may not recover from these infections.

Pneumocystis Pneumonia

Pneumocystis carinii is a common organism that may reside harmlessly in normal lungs. It generally causes pneumonia only when the body's defenses are weakened because of cancer, cancer treatment, or AIDS. Often, it is the first indication that a person with human immunodeficiency virus (HIV) infection has developed AIDS.

Most people develop a fever, shortness of breath, and a dry cough. These symptoms usually arise over several weeks. The lungs may not be able to deliver sufficient oxygen to the blood, leading to severe shortness of breath.

X-rays show either no abnormality or patchy infection, similar to what is seen in some viral infections. The diagnosis is made by microscopic examination of a sputum specimen obtained by one of two techniques—sputum induction (in which a vapor is used to stimulate coughing) or bronchoscopy (in which an instrument is inserted into the airways to collect a specimen).▼

The combination antibiotic trimethoprim-sulfamethoxazole can be used to help prevent pneumocystis pneumonia in people at risk. This drug's side effects, which are particularly common in people who have AIDS, include rashes, a reduced number of infection-fighting white blood cells, and fever. Alternative preventive drug treatments are dapsone, atovaquone, and pentamidine (which can be taken as an aerosol, inhaled directly into the lungs).

Drugs used to treat pneumocystis pneumonia are trimethoprim-sulfamethoxazole, dapsone combined with trimethoprim, clindamycin and primaquine, atovaquone, or intravenous pentamidine. When blood oxygen pressure falls below a certain level, corticosteroids may also be given.

Even when the pneumonia is treated, the overall death rate is 15 to 20%.

Aspiration Pneumonia

Tiny particles from the mouth frequently dribble or are inhaled (aspirated) into the airways, but usually they are cleared out by normal defense mechanisms before they can get into the lungs and cause inflammation or in-

---

▲ see page 1151   ■ see page 1149
★ see page 1151   ● see page 1149
◆ see page 1153   ▼ see page 256

fection. When such particles are not cleared, they can cause aspiration pneumonia. Older people and people who are debilitated, intoxicated by alcohol or drugs, or unconscious from anesthesia or a medical condition are especially at risk for this type of pneumonia. Even a healthy person who inhales a large amount of material, as may happen during vomiting, can develop aspiration pneumonia.

Symptoms of pneumonia do not begin for at least a day or two. Treatment requires antibiotics. Many antibiotics can be used, but treatment often begins with clindamycin or metronidazole plus penicillin. If a solid particle was inhaled, a bronchoscopy may be needed to remove it.▲

Chemical pneumonitis occurs when a person inhales (aspirates) material that is toxic to the lungs; the problem is more the result of irritation than infection. A commonly inhaled toxic material is stomach acid, so that chemical pneumonitis may result whenever a person inhales what has been vomited up. Sudden shortness of breath and a cough develop within minutes or hours. Other symptoms may include fever and pink frothy sputum. In less severe cases, the symptoms of aspiration pneumonia may follow a day or two later.

The diagnosis of chemical pneumonitis is usually obvious from the sequence of events. Chest x-rays and measurements of oxygen concentrations in arterial blood may help. When the diagnosis remains unclear, a bronchoscopy is sometimes performed.

Treatment consists of oxygen therapy ■ and mechanical ventilation★ if necessary. The trachea may be suctioned to clear secretions and aspirated food particles out of the airways. Bronchoscopy may also be used for this purpose.

Antibiotics are usually given because doctors cannot easily distinguish this form of aspiration pneumonia from a bacterial infection. Generally, people with chemical pneumonitis either recover rapidly, progress to acute respiratory distress syndrome, or develop a bacterial infection. Up to 30 to 50% of people with serious chemical pneumonitis die.

CHAPTER 43

Lung Abscess

A lung abscess is a pus-filled cavity in the lung surrounded by inflamed tissue and caused by an infection.

Causes

A lung abscess is usually caused by bacteria that normally live in the mouth or throat and that are inhaled into the lungs, resulting in an infection. Often, gum (periodontal) disease is the source of the bacteria that cause a lung abscess. The body has many defenses (such as a cough) to help prevent bacteria from getting into the lungs. Infection occurs primarily when these defenses are impaired—for example, when a person is unconscious or very drowsy because of sedation, anesthesia, alcohol or drug abuse, or a disease of the nervous system.

In some people, particularly those older than age 40 who smoke, a lung tumor may lead to the formation of a lung abscess by blocking an airway (a bronchus). An abscess can form because secretions (mucus) can accumulate behind the tumor. Bacteria are able to accumulate in the secretions, and the obstruction prevents the bacteria-laden secretions from being brought back up through the airway where they would normally be coughed up; thus, the right conditions for bacterial infection are formed. Foreign objects that are inhaled (aspirated) may block an airway and also form the right conditions for bacterial infection.

Pneumonia caused by certain bacteria, such as *Staphylococcus aureus* or *Legionella pneumophila,* or fungi may lead to a lung abscess. Less common organisms may cause a lung abscess in a person who has a poorly functioning

▲ see page 256   ■ see page 260
★ see page 326

immune system. Rarely, bacteria or infected blood clots that travel through the bloodstream to the lung from another infected site in the body (septic pulmonary emboli) may cause a lung abscess.

Usually, a person develops only one lung abscess, but when several develop, they are typically in the same lung. If an infection reaches the lung through the bloodstream, many scattered abscesses may develop in both lungs. This problem is most common among addicts who inject drugs using dirty needles, which can also cause infection of the lining of the right side of the heart (endocarditis).▲

Eventually, most abscesses rupture into an airway, producing a lot of sputum that gets coughed up. A ruptured abscess leaves a cavity in the lung that is filled with fluid and air. When a large abscess ruptures into an airway, pus may spread throughout the lung, causing widespread pneumonia and acute respiratory distress syndrome.■ Sometimes an abscess ruptures into the pleural space (the space between the membrane layers covering the lungs and the chest wall), filling the space with pus, a condition called empyema. If an abscess destroys a blood vessel wall, serious bleeding may result, sometimes leading to death.

Symptoms and Diagnosis

The symptoms may start slowly or suddenly. Early symptoms resemble those of pneumonia: fatigue, loss of appetite, sweating, fever, and a cough that brings up sputum. The sputum may be foul smelling (because certain bacteria from the mouth or throat tend to produce foul odors) or streaked with blood. The person also may feel chest pain with breathing, especially if the pleura is inflamed (pleurisy).★ Many people have these symptoms for weeks or months before seeking medical attention. These people have chronic abscesses and, in addition to the other symptoms, lose a substantial amount of weight, have a fever every day, and also have night sweats.

Chest x-rays nearly always reveal a lung abscess. However, when an x-ray only suggests an abscess, computed tomography (CT) of the chest can confirm the presence of a lung abscess and possibly determine its cause. Cultures of sputum from the lungs may help identify the organism causing the abscess, but this test is not always useful.

Treatment

Prompt, complete healing of a lung abscess requires the administration of antibiotics. These are initially given intravenously in most cases and later by mouth when the person has improved and the fever has resolved. Antibiotic treatment continues until the symptoms disappear and a chest x-ray shows that the abscess has disappeared. Such improvement usually requires several weeks or months of antibiotic therapy. Postural drainage may be used to help drain the abscess.●

Bronchoscopy◆ is performed to confirm the presence of an obstruction when the cause is thought to be a blocked airway due to a tumor or a foreign object. Bronchoscopy may also be used to remove a foreign object or to help drain a lung abscess that does not respond to antibiotics.

About 5% of people with lung abscesses need additional treatment. Occasionally, an abscess requires drainage through a tube inserted through the chest wall and into the abscess. More often, infected lung tissue may have to be removed surgically. Sometimes an entire lobe of a lung or even an entire lung has to be removed.

The death rate for people with lung abscesses is about 5%. The rate is higher when the person is debilitated or has an impaired immune system, lung cancer, or a very large abscess.

▲ see page 184   ■ see page 326
★ see page 313   ● see page 261
◆ see page 256

CHAPTER 44

Asthma

Asthma is a condition in which the airways narrow—usually reversibly—in response to certain stimuli.

Asthma affects about 17 to 18 million people in the United States and is becoming more common. Between 1982 and 1992, the number of people with asthma increased by 42%. Asthma is particularly common in blacks living in urban environments (affecting about 7%) and even more so in Hispanic populations living in urban environments (affecting about 11%). The condition also seems to be becoming more serious, requiring more people to be hospitalized. Between 1982 and 1992, the death rate from asthma in the United States increased by 35%. The condition usually begins in childhood, although some adults develop asthma, even at an old age. Asthma in children can interfere with normal growth and development.▲

The reason for the increase in the prevalence of asthma among children is not known, but it may relate to one or both of the following theories. One theory is that the widespread use of vaccines and antibiotics in children has shifted the activity of a special subgroup of white blood cells (called lymphocytes) in the body from fighting infection to releasing chemical substances that inadvertently promote the development of allergies. Another theory is that, because children are spending more time indoors and living in better-insulated homes than they were in the past, the exposure to potentially allergic substances is increased. There are few data to support either theory.

The most important characteristic of asthma is airway obstruction. The airways of the lungs (the bronchi) are basically tubes with muscular walls.■ Cells lining the bronchi have microscopic structures, called receptors. There are three main types of receptors: beta-adrenergic, cholinergic, and peptidergic. These receptors sense the presence of specific substances and stimulate the underlying muscles to contract and relax, thus altering the flow of air. Beta-adrenergic receptors respond to chemicals such as epinephrine and make the muscles relax, thereby widening (dilating) the airways and increasing airflow. Cholinergic receptors respond to a chemical called acetylcholine, making the muscles contract and decreasing airflow. Peptidergic receptors respond to substances called neurokinins, also making the underlying muscles of the airways contract.

Causes

Airway obstruction is often caused by abnormal sensitivity of cholinergic and peptidergic receptors, which cause the muscles of the airways to contract when they should not. Certain cells in the airways, particularly mast cells, are thought to be responsible for initiating the airway narrowing. Mast cells throughout the bronchi release substances such as histamine and leukotrienes, which cause smooth muscle to contract, mucus secretion to increase, and certain white blood cells to migrate to the area. Eosinophils, a type of white blood cell found in the airways of people with asthma, release additional substances, contributing to airway narrowing.

In an asthma attack, the smooth muscles of the bronchi narrow (called bronchoconstriction), and the tissues lining the airways swell from inflammation and secrete mucus into the airways. The top layer of the lining of the airways can become damaged and shed cells. These actions further narrow the diameter of the airways; the narrowing requires the person to exert more effort to move air in and out of the lungs. In asthma, airway obstruction is reversible, meaning that with appropriate treatment or on their own, the muscular contractions of the airways stop, the airway obstruction ends, and the airflow into and out of the lungs returns to normal.

In a person who has asthma, the airways narrow in response to stimuli that usually do not affect the airways in normal lungs. The narrowing can be triggered by many inhaled allergens, such as pollens, particles from dust mites, body secretions from cockroaches, particles from feathers, and animal dander. These allergens combine with immunoglobulin E (a type of antibody) on the surface of mast cells to trigger

---

▲ see page 1583   ■ see page 245

How Airways Narrow

During an asthma attack, the smooth muscle layer goes into spasm, narrowing the airway. The middle layer swells because of inflammation, and more mucus is produced. In some segments of the airway, the mucus forms clumps that nearly or completely block the airway. These clumps are called mucus plugs.

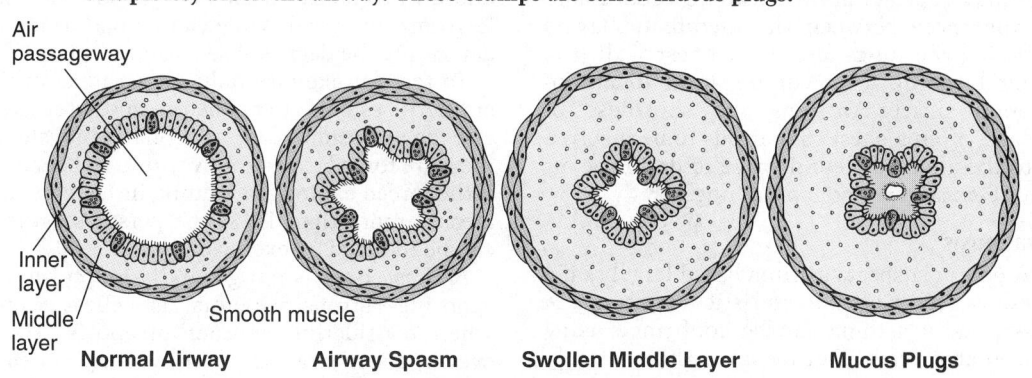

Air passageway

Inner layer

Middle layer

Smooth muscle

Normal Airway   **Airway Spasm**   **Swollen Middle Layer**   **Mucus Plugs**

the release of asthma-causing chemicals from these cells. (This type of asthma is called allergic asthma.) Although food allergies induce asthma only rarely, certain foods (such as shellfish and peanuts) can induce severe attacks in people who are sensitive to these foods.

Cigarette smoke, cold air, and viral infections can also provoke asthma attacks. Additionally, a person who has asthma can develop bronchoconstriction when exercising. Stress and anxiety can trigger mast cells to release histamine and leukotrienes and stimulate the vagus nerve (which connects to the airway smooth muscle), which then contracts and narrows the bronchi.

Symptoms and Complications

Asthma attacks vary in frequency and severity. Some people who have asthma are symptom-free most of the time, with only an occasional, brief, mild episode of shortness of breath. Other people cough and wheeze most of the time and have severe attacks after viral infections, exercise, or exposure to allergens or irritants, including cigarette smoke. Crying or hearty laughing may bring on symptoms in some people. Some people with asthma produce a clear and at times sticky (mucoid) phlegm (sputum). Asthma attacks occur most often in the early morning hours when the effects of protective medications wear off and the body is least able to prevent bronchoconstriction.

An asthma attack may begin suddenly with wheezing, coughing, and shortness of breath. Wheezing is particularly noticeable when the person breathes out. At other times, an asthma attack may come on slowly with gradually worsening symptoms. In either case, people with asthma usually first notice shortness of breath, coughing, or chest tightness. The attack may be over in minutes, or it may last for hours or days. Itching on the chest or neck may be an early symptom, especially in children. A dry cough at night or while exercising may be the only symptom.

During an asthma attack, shortness of breath may become severe, creating a feeling of severe anxiety. The person instinctively sits upright and leans forward, using the neck and chest muscles to help in breathing, but still struggles for air. Sweating is a common reaction to the effort and anxiety. The pulse usually quickens, and the person may feel a pounding in the chest.

In a very severe asthma attack, a person is able to say only a few words without stopping to take a breath. However, wheezing may diminish, because hardly any air is moving in and out of the lungs. Confusion, lethargy, and a blue skin color (cyanosis) are signs that the person's oxygen supply is severely limited, and emergency treatment is needed. Usually, a person recovers completely with appropriate treatment, even from a severe asthma attack. Rarely, some people develop attacks so quickly that they may lose consciousness before they can give themselves effective therapy. Such people should wear a medical alert bracelet and perhaps carry a cellular phone to call 911.

Rarely, the small air sacs of the lung (alveoli) may rupture, allowing air to accumulate in the space between the membrane layers covering the lungs and inner chest wall (the pleural space). This complication (pneumothorax) greatly worsens the shortness of breath; often a chest tube needs to be inserted into the affected pleural space to drain the air and re-expand the collapsed lung. ▲

Diagnosis

A doctor suspects asthma based largely on a person's report of characteristic symptoms. A diagnosis of asthma can be confirmed using spirometry tests. During an asthma attack, the test reveals decreased air flow, but over hours or days, narrowing improves and is therefore reversible. More commonly, the doctor performs spirometry or pulmonary function tests ■ before and after giving the person an inhaled beta-adrenergic agonist. If results are significantly better after the person receives the beta-adrenergic agonist, asthma is thought to be present. If the airways are not narrowed at the time of the first test, a diagnosis can be confirmed by a test in which the person inhales a chemical (usually methacholine but histamine may be used also) in doses too low to affect a normal person but which causes airway narrowing in a person who has asthma.

Spirometry is also used to assess the severity of the airway obstruction and to monitor treatment. Peak expiratory flow (the fastest rate at which air can be exhaled) can be measured using a small handheld peak flow meter. Often, this test is used at home to monitor the severity of asthma. Usually, peak flow rates are lowest between 4:00 and 6:00 A.M. and highest at 4:00 P.M. However, more than a 30% difference in rates at these times is considered evidence of moderate to severe asthma.

Determining what triggers a person's asthma is often difficult. Allergy testing is appropriate when there is a suspicion that some avoidable substance is stimulating attacks. Skin testing can help identify allergens that may trigger asthma symptoms. However, an allergic response to a skin test does not necessarily mean that the allergen being tested is causing the asthma. The person still has to note whether attacks occur after exposure to this allergen. If a doctor suspects a particular allergen, a blood test that measures the level of antibody produced in response to the allergen (the radioallergosorbent test [RAST]) can be performed to determine the degree of sensitivity.

To test for exercise-induced asthma, an examiner uses spirometry before and after exercise on a treadmill or stationary bicycle to measure forced expiratory volume in 1 second. If the forced expiratory volume in 1 second decreases more than 15%, the person's asthma can be induced by exercise.

A chest x-ray is not generally helpful in diagnosing asthma. Doctors use chest x-rays when considering another diagnosis. However, a chest x-ray is often obtained when a person with asthma needs to be hospitalized or is treated in the emergency department with severe asthma.

Prevention and Treatment

There is an array of drugs that can be used to prevent and treat asthma attacks. Most of the drugs used to prevent asthma are also used to treat an asthma attack but in higher doses or in different forms. Some people need to use more than one drug to prevent and treat their symptoms.

Therapy is based on two classes of antiasthmatic drugs. The first are anti-inflammatory drugs, which suppress the inflammation that triggers the airways to narrow. The second are bronchodilators, which help to relax and widen (dilate) the airways. Within each of these two classes, several drugs are available. Anti-inflammatory drugs include corticosteroids (which are inhaled, taken by mouth, or given intravenously), leukotriene modifiers, and cromolyn. Bronchodilators include beta-adrenergic agonists and theophylline.

Education about how to prevent and treat asthma attacks is beneficial for all people who have asthma and often for their family members. Proper use of inhalers is essential for effective treatment. People should know what can stimulate an attack, what helps to prevent an attack, how to use drugs properly, and when to seek medical care. Many people use a hand-held peak flow meter to evaluate their breathing and determine when they need intervention, before their symptoms get extreme. A person who experiences frequent,

---

▲ see page 317   ■ see page 254

Avoiding Common Causes of Asthma Attacks

The most common indoor allergens are house dust mites, feathers, cockroaches, and animal dander. Anything that can be done to reduce exposure to these allergens may reduce the number or severity of attacks. Exposure to house dust mites can be reduced by removing wall-to-wall carpets and using air conditioning to keep the relative humidity low (preferably below 50%) in the summer.

Also, special pillow and mattress covers can help reduce exposure to these dust mites. Cats and dogs must be removed to significantly decrease animal dander.

Irritating fumes such as cigarette smoke should also be avoided. In some people with asthma, aspirin and other nonsteroidal anti-inflammatory drugs trigger attacks. Tartrazine, a yellow coloring used in some drug tablets and

food, may also bring on an attack. Sulfites—commonly added to foods as a preservative—may trigger attacks after a susceptible person eats a certain food or drinks beer or red wine.

For outdoor activity in cold weather, the person with asthma can wear a ski mask or scarf that covers the nose and mouth to help keep the air being breathed in warm and moist.

---

severe asthma attacks should know how to reach help quickly.

Many people have a written treatment plan that was devised in collaboration with their doctor. Such a plan allows them to take control of their own treatment and has been shown to decrease the number of times people need to seek care for asthma in the emergency department.

Preventing Attacks

Asthma is a chronic condition that cannot be prevented or cured; however, individual attacks can often be prevented. Asthma attacks may commonly be prevented if the factors that trigger them are identified and treated or avoided. People who have asthma should avoid cigarette smoke. Often, attacks triggered by exercise can be blocked by taking medication beforehand. When dust and allergens are the problem, air filters, air conditioners, and other types of barriers (such as mattress covers, which reduce the amount of particles from dust mites that are in the air) can help considerably. For people whose asthma is stimulated by allergies, desensitization through the use of allergy shots may prevent attacks.

Some people who have asthma may have a sensitivity to aspirin or other nonsteroidal anti-inflammatory drugs (NSAIDs); if this is the case, these drugs must be avoided. Drugs that block the beneficial effects of beta-adrenergic agonists (called beta-blockers) usually worsen asthma.

Most people with asthma take drugs, such as inhaled or oral corticosteroids, leukotriene modifiers, long-acting beta-adrenergic agonists, theophylline, antihistamines, or cromolyn to prevent attacks. Prevention efforts

are individualized according to the frequency of attacks and the stimuli that trigger the attacks.

A new treatment for asthma is being studied and developed based on use of a special antibody (given intravenously or injected just under the skin) that binds immunoglobulin E, blocking its attachment to mast cells. By preventing immunoglobulin E from attaching to mast cells, these cells can no longer release the substances that cause allergic asthma.

Treating Attacks

An asthma attack can be frightening, both to the person experiencing it and to others around. Even when relatively mild, the symptoms provoke anxiety and alarm. A severe asthma attack is a life-threatening emergency that requires immediate, skilled, professional care. If not treated adequately and quickly, a severe asthma attack can cause death.

People who have asthma are generally able to treat most attacks without assistance from a health care professional. Typically, they use an inhaler to deliver a dose of a short-acting beta-adrenergic agonist, move into fresh air (away from cigarette smoke or other irritants), and sit down and rest. Some people may inhale a corticosteroid in addition to a beta-adrenergic agonist. An attack usually subsides in 5 to 10 minutes. An attack that does not subside in 15 minutes or that gets worse is likely to require additional treatment supervised by a doctor.

Because people with severe asthma commonly have low blood oxygen levels, a doctor may check the level of oxygen either by using a sensing monitor on a finger or ear or by tak-

Rx DRUGS USED TO TREAT ASTHMA

TYPE	DRUG	SOME SIDE EFFECTS	COMMENTS
Beta-adrenergic agonists			
	Albuterol (short-acting) Salmeterol (long-acting)	Increased heart rate; shakiness	Albuterol may be taken by mouth or inhaled through a metered-dose inhaler or by using a nebulizer; salmeterol is only taken by inhalation
Methylxanthines			
	Theophylline	Increased heart rate; shakiness; stomach upset. Seizures and serious heartbeat irregularities (if blood level is high)	Can be used for prevention and treatment, taken by mouth but can be administered intravenously in a hospital
Anticholinergic drugs			
	Ipratropium	Dry mouth; rapid heart rate	Used in combination with beta-adrenergic blockers mainly in the emergency department
Mast cell stabilizers			
	Cromolyn Nedocromil	Coughing or wheezing	Useful for preventing attacks but not for treatment
Corticosteroids (inhaled)			
	Beclomethasone Budesonide Flunisolide Fluticasone Triamcinolone	Fungal infection of the mouth (thrush); a change in voice	Inhaled use is for prevention (long-term control) of asthma
Leukotriene modifiers			
	Montelukast Zafirlukast Zileuton	Churg-Strauss syndrome; zileuton causes an elevation in liver function test results	Used more for prevention (long-term control) than for treatment

ing a sample of blood from an artery.▲ Supplemental oxygen may be given during attacks. However, in severe attacks, a doctor also needs to monitor carbon dioxide levels, and this test requires a sample of blood from an artery. A doctor may also check pulmonary function, usually with a spirometer or a peak flow meter. Usually, a chest x-ray is needed only in severe asthma attacks. People experiencing very severe asthma attacks may need to have an artificial airway passed through their mouth and throat (intubation) and be placed on a mechanical ventilator.■

Generally, people who have severe asthma are admitted to the hospital if their lung function does not improve after receiving a beta-adrenergic agonist and corticosteroids or if they have a seriously low blood oxygen level or a high blood carbon dioxide level.

Intravenous fluids may be needed if the person is dehydrated. Antibiotics also may be needed if a doctor suspects a lung infection; however, most such infections are due to viruses for which (with a few exceptions) no treatment exists.

Drugs for Preventing or Treating Attacks

Drugs allow most people with asthma to lead relatively normal lives. Most of the drugs

▲ see page 255   ■ see page 326

used to treat an asthma attack can be used (often in lower doses) to prevent attacks.

Short-acting Beta-adrenergic Agonists: Short-acting beta-adrenergic agonists are usually the best drugs for relieving asthma attacks. They can prevent certain attacks, such as exercise-induced asthma. These drugs are also referred to as bronchodilators because they stimulate beta-adrenergic receptors to widen (dilate) the airways. Bronchodilators that act on all beta-adrenergic receptors throughout the body, such as epinephrine, cause side effects such as rapid heartbeat, restlessness, headache, and muscle tremors. Bronchodilators (such as albuterol) that act mainly on $beta_2$-adrenergic receptors, which are found primarily on cells in the lungs, have little effect on other organs and thus cause fewer side effects. Most beta-receptor agonists, especially the inhaled ones, act within minutes, but the effects last only

2 to 6 hours. New, longer-acting bronchodilators are available, but because they do not begin to act as quickly, they are used for prevention rather than for attacks of asthma. When the long-acting beta-adrenergic agonists are used together with inhaled corticosteroids, better results are obtained. A combination of salmeterol (a long-acting beta-adrenergic agonist) with a corticosteroid in an inhaler is also available.

Most often, beta-adrenergic agonists are inhaled using metered-dose inhalers (handheld cartridges containing gas under pressure). The pressure turns the drug into a fine spray containing a measured dose of drug. Inhalation deposits the drug directly in the airways, so that it acts quickly, but the drug may not reach the airways that are severely obstructed. For people who have difficulty using a metered-dose inhaler, spacers or holding chambers can be

How to Use a Metered-Dose Inhaler

- **Shake the inhaler after removing the cap.**
- **Breathe out for 1 or 2 seconds.**
- **Put the inhaler in your mouth or 1 to 2 inches from it and start to breathe in slowly, like sipping hot soup.**
- **While starting to breathe in, press the top of the inhaler.**
- **Breathe in slowly until your lungs are full. (This should take about 5 or 6 seconds.)**
- **Hold your breath for 4 to 6 seconds.**
- **Breathe out and repeat the procedure.**
- **If this method is difficult, a spacer can be used.**

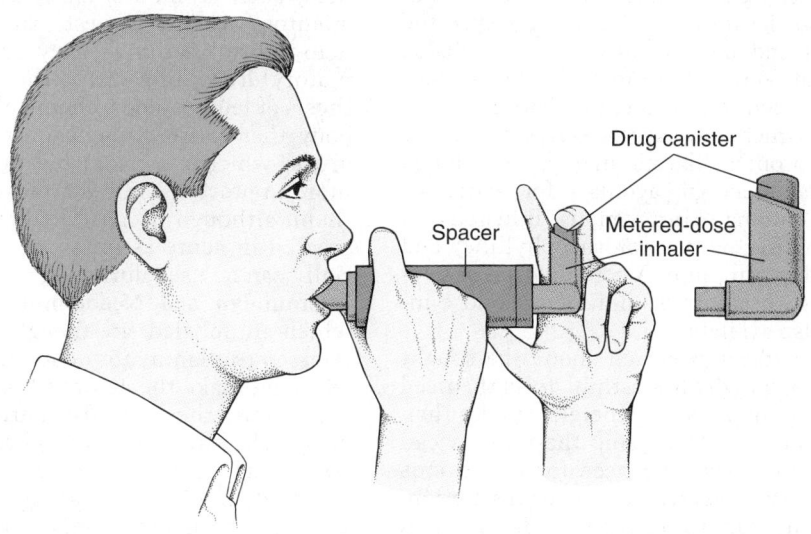

Status Asthmaticus

The most severe form of asthma is called status asthmaticus. In this condition, the lungs are no longer able to provide the body with adequate oxygen or adequately remove carbon dioxide. Without oxygen, many organs begin to malfunction. The buildup of carbon dioxide leads to acidosis, an acidic state of the blood that affects the function of almost every organ. Blood pressure may fall to low levels. The airways are so narrowed that it is difficult to move air in and out of the lungs.

Status asthmaticus requires intubation and ventilator support as well as maximum doses of several medications. Support is also given to correct acidosis.

used. With any type of inhaler, proper technique is vital; if the device is not used properly, the drug will not reach the airways. A dry powder drug formulation is also available. The powder formulation is easier for some people to use, in part because it requires less coordination with breathing.

Beta-adrenergic agonists can also be delivered directly to the lungs using a nebulizer. A nebulizer creates a mist of drug, and its use does not have to be coordinated with breathing. Nebulizers are more portable than they were in the past; some units can even be plugged into a cigarette lighter in a car.

Beta-adrenergic agonists can also be taken in liquid or tablet form or injected. However, the oral drugs tend to work slower than the inhaled or injected ones and are more likely to cause side effects. Side effects include abnormal heart rhythms, which may suggest excessive use.

Other bronchodilators may be combined with beta-adrenergic agonists for acute attacks, including intravenous infusions of aminophylline (a type of theophylline) and nebulized ipratropium. A combination of ipratropium with albuterol in a metered-dose inhaler is also available.

Quick medical attention should be sought when a person who has asthma feels the need to use more of a beta-adrenergic agonist than is recommended. Overusing these drugs can be very dangerous. The need for continuous use indicates severe bronchoconstriction, which can lead to respiratory failure and death.

Theophylline: Theophylline is another drug that produces bronchodilation. It is usually taken by mouth but can be given intravenously in the hospital. Oral theophylline comes in many forms, from short-acting tablets and syrups to longer-acting sustained release capsules and tablets. Theophylline is used for both prevention and treatment of asthma.

The amount of theophylline in the blood can be measured in a laboratory and must be closely monitored by a doctor. Too little drug in the blood may provide little benefit, and too much drug may cause life-threatening abnormal heart rhythms or seizures. When first taking theophylline, a person who has asthma may feel slightly jittery and may develop headaches. These side effects usually disappear as the body adjusts to the drug. Larger doses may cause a rapid heartbeat, nausea, or palpitations. A person may also experience insomnia, agitation, vomiting, and seizures.

Anticholinergic Drugs: Anticholinergic drugs, such as ipratropium, block acetylcholine from causing smooth muscle contraction and from producing excess mucus in the bronchi. These drugs are usually inhaled but can be given intravenously in the hospital. These drugs further widen (dilate) the airways in people who have already been given beta-adrenergic agonists. However, doctors use anticholinergic drugs mainly in the emergency department in combination with a beta-adrenergic agonist. When used alone, anticholinergics are only marginally effective.

Leukotriene Modifiers: Leukotriene modifiers, such as montelukast, zafirlukast, and zileuton, are the newest drugs available to help control asthma. They are anti-inflammatory drugs, preventing the action or synthesis of leukotrienes, chemicals made by the body that cause bronchoconstriction. These drugs, which are taken by mouth, are used more to prevent asthma attacks than to treat them, although because leukotrienes are increased in acute asthma, these drugs potentially can be used during an attack as well.

Cromolyn and Nedocromil: These drugs, which are inhaled, are thought to inhibit the release of inflammatory chemicals from mast cells and make the airways less likely to narrow. Thus, they are also anti-inflammatory drugs. They are useful for preventing but not treating an attack. These drugs may be helpful for children who have asthma and for people who develop asthma from exercise. Cromolyn and nedocromil are very safe and must be taken regularly even when a person is free of symptoms.

Corticosteroids: These drugs block the body's inflammatory response and are exceptionally effective at reducing asthma symptoms. They are the most potent form of anti-inflammatory drugs and have been an important part of asthma treatment for decades. They are given in the inhaled form to prevent attacks and improve lung function. They are given by mouth in higher doses for people experiencing severe attacks. Corticosteroids given by mouth are generally continued for at least several days after a severe attack. Corticosteroids can be taken in several different forms. Often, inhaled versions are best because they deliver the drug directly to the airways and minimize the amount sent throughout the body. They come in several strengths and are generally used twice a day. The person should rinse the mouth after use to decrease the likelihood that an infection of the mouth (thrush) develops.▲ Oral or injected corticosteroids may be used in high doses to relieve a severe asthma attack and are generally continued for 1 to 2 weeks. Oral corticosteroids are prescribed on a long-term basis only when no other treatments can control the symptoms.

If taken for long periods, corticosteroids gradually reduce the likelihood of an asthma attack by making the airways less sensitive to a number of provocative stimuli. Long-term use of corticosteroids, especially larger doses taken by mouth, can produce side effects.

CHAPTER 45

Chronic Obstructive Pulmonary Disease

Chronic obstructive pulmonary disease is persistent obstruction of the airways occurring with emphysema, chronic bronchitis, or both disorders.

In the United States, about 16 million people suffer from chronic obstructive pulmonary disease (COPD). It is second only to heart disease as a cause of disability that forces people to stop working. It is the fourth most common cause of death, accounting for more than 100,000 deaths per year in the United States; the number of deaths from COPD has increased by 40% over the last 20 years. More than 95% of all deaths from COPD occur in people older than age 55. COPD affects men more often than women and is more often fatal in men, although there has been a recent increase in the rate of deaths in women. COPD is also more often fatal in whites than in nonwhites and in blue-collar workers than in white-collar workers.

COPD leads to chronic airflow obstruction, which is defined as a persistent decrease in the rate of airflow through the lungs when the person breathes out (exhales). Both emphy- sema and chronic bronchitis contribute to the airflow obstruction of COPD. Emphysema is irreversible enlargement of many of the 300 million air sacs (alveoli) that make up the lungs and destruction of the air sac walls. Chronic bronchitis is characterized by a cough that produces sputum for 3 months or more during 2 successive years; the cough is not due to another lung disease.

The small airways of the lungs are normally held open by their alveolar wall attachments. In emphysema, the destruction of alveolar wall attachments results in collapse of the small airways, causing permanent airflow obstruction. In chronic bronchitis, the glands lining the bronchi enlarge, causing increased secretion of mucus. Inflammation of the small airways (bronchioles) develops and causes smooth muscle spasm and blockage by secretions. Asthma is also characterized by airflow obstruction.■ However, in contrast with the airflow obstruc-

▲ see page 1150   ■ see page 274

tion of COPD, the airflow obstruction of asthma is completely reversible in most people, either spontaneously or with treatment.

The airflow obstruction of COPD leads to an increase in the effort required for a person to breathe. The obstruction causes air to become trapped in the lungs, so that the amount of air remaining in the lungs after a full exhalation is increased. The number of capillaries in the walls of the alveoli decreases. These abnormalities impair the exchange of oxygen and carbon dioxide between the alveoli and the blood. In the earlier stages of COPD, oxygen levels in the blood are decreased, but carbon dioxide levels remain normal. In the later stages, carbon dioxide levels increase and oxygen levels fall even further. The decrease in oxygen levels in the blood stimulates the bone marrow to send more red blood cells into the bloodstream, a condition known as secondary polycythemia.▲

Causes

Cigarette smoking is the most important cause of COPD, although only about 15 to 20% of smokers develop the disease. Pipe and cigar smokers develop COPD more often than nonsmokers but not as often as cigarette smokers. With age, susceptible cigarette smokers lose lung function more rapidly than nonsmokers. If a person stops smoking, there is little improvement in lung function. However, the rate of decline of lung function does return to that of nonsmokers when the person stops smoking, thus delaying the progression of symptoms.

COPD tends to occur more often in some families, so there may be an inherited tendency. Working in an environment polluted by chemical fumes or dust may increase the risk of COPD.■ Exposure to air pollution and to smoke from nearby cigarette smokers (secondhand or passive smoke exposure) worsens a person's COPD and may cause COPD.

A rare cause of COPD is a hereditary condition in which the body produces a markedly decreased amount of the protein alpha₁-antitrypsin. The main role of this protein is to prevent neutrophil elastase from damaging the alveoli. Consequently, emphysema develops by early middle age in people with severe

---

▲ see box on page 1024   ■ see page 294

★ see page 801   ● see box on page 323

◆ see page 253   ▼ see page 316

alpha₁-antitrypsin deficiency,★ especially in those who also smoke.

Symptoms

In a person with COPD, a mild cough that produces clear sputum develops by around age 45, usually when the person first gets out of bed in the morning. Cough and sputum production persist for the next 10 years; shortness of breath may be noted with exertion. Sometimes, shortness of breath is first noted only with a lung infection, during which time the person coughs more and has an increased amount of sputum. The color of the sputum changes from clear to yellow or green.

By the time the person reaches his middle to late 60s, especially with continued smoking, shortness of breath with exertion becomes more troublesome. A lung infection may result in severe shortness of breath even when the person is at rest and may require hospitalization. Shortness of breath during activities of daily living, such as toileting, washing, dressing and sexual activity, may persist after the person has recovered from the lung infection.

About one third of people with severe COPD experience severe weight loss, in part because shortness of breath makes eating difficult and in part because of increased levels in the blood of a substance called tumor necrosis factor. Swelling of the legs often develops, which may be due to cor pulmonale.● People with COPD may intermittently cough up blood, which is usually due to inflammation of the bronchi, but which always raises the concern of lung cancer. Morning headaches may occur because breathing decreases during sleep, which causes increased retention of carbon dioxide.

As COPD progresses, some people, especially those who have emphysema, develop unusual breathing patterns. Some people breathe out through pursed lips. Others find it more comfortable to stand over a table with their arms outstretched and weight on their palms, a maneuver that improves the function of the diaphragm. Over time, many people develop a barrel chest as the size of the lungs increases because of trapped air. Low oxygen levels in the blood can give a blue tint to the skin (cyanosis). Clubbing of the fingers is rare◆ and raises the suspicion of lung cancer.

Fragile areas in the lungs may rupture, permitting air to leak from the lung into the pleural space, a condition called pneumothorax.▼ This condition often causes sudden pain and shortness of breath and requires immediate intervention by a doctor to evacuate the air from the pleural space.

Symptoms may suddenly worsen during flare-ups of COPD. A flare-up is a worsening of symptoms of cough, increased sputum, and shortness of breath. Sputum color often changes from white to yellow or green, and fever and body aches sometimes occur. Shortness of breath may be present when the person is at rest and may be severe enough to require hospitalization. Severe air pollution, common allergens, and viral or bacterial infections may cause flare-ups.

Diagnosis

Chronic bronchitis is diagnosed by the history of a prolonged productive cough. Emphysema is diagnosed by a constellation of findings observed during a physical examination and on pulmonary function test results; however, by the time the doctor notices these abnormalities, emphysema is moderately severe. It is not important for doctors to differentiate between chronic bronchitis and emphysema; the most important determinant of how the person feels and functions is the severity of airflow obstruction.

In mild COPD, a doctor may find nothing during a physical examination. As the disease progresses, wheezes may be heard through the stethoscope, and prolonged expiration and decreased breathing sounds become apparent. Chest movement diminishes during breathing, and use of the neck and shoulder muscles in breathing may be noted.

In mild COPD, results of a chest x-ray are usually normal. As COPD worsens, the chest x-ray shows over-inflation of the lungs; decreased shadows of blood vessels denote the presence of emphysema.

Doctors can evaluate airflow obstruction with forced expiratory spirometry.▲ Decrease in the forced expiratory volume in 1 second (FEV_1) and the ratio of the FEV_1 to the forced vital capacity (FVC) are required to demonstrate airflow obstruction and to make the diagnosis.

A blood test may show an abnormally high level of red blood cells (polycythemia). Pulse oximetry or a sample of blood taken from an artery often shows low levels of oxygen. High levels of carbon dioxide in the arteries are seen late in the course of the disease.

If a person develops COPD at a young age, especially when the person has a family history of COPD, the alpha$_1$-antitrypsin blood level is measured to determine whether the person has alpha$_1$-antitrypsin deficiency. This genetic disorder is also suspected when COPD develops in someone who has never smoked.

Treatment

The most important treatment for COPD is to stop smoking. Stopping smoking when the airflow obstruction is mild or moderate often improves cough, reduces the amount of sputum, and slows the development of shortness of breath. Stopping smoking at any point in the disease process provides some benefit. The person should also try to avoid exposure to other airborne irritants, including secondhand smoke and air pollution.

If the person contracts influenza or pneumonia, COPD may worsen markedly. Therefore, a person with COPD should receive an influenza vaccination every year and a pneumococcal vaccination 5 years after an initial pneumococcal vaccination.

Treatment of Symptoms: Wheezing and shortness of breath are relieved when airflow obstruction improves. Although the airflow obstruction due to emphysema is not reversible, bronchial smooth muscle spasm, inflammation, and increased secretions are potentially reversible.

The anticholinergic drug ipratropium given by metered-dose inhaler 4 times daily is the drug of choice to help relieve shortness of breath. When symptoms are more severe, inhaled short-acting beta-adrenergic agonists, such as albuterol, more rapidly relieve shortness of breath than ipratropium. Salmeterol, a long-acting beta-adrenergic agonist with a delayed onset of action, can be given by inhalation every 12 hours. This drug is useful for prolonged relief of symptoms in some people, especially at night.

The combination of ipratropium and albuterol in a metered-dose inhaler has the advantage of decreasing the number of inhalers the person must use. People who have difficulty using metered dose inhalers benefit by inhaling the drug from a delivery device called a spacer.■ Solutions of ipratropium and the beta-adrenergic agonists may also be given using nebulizers; this mode of therapy is reserved for people who have severe disease. A nebulizer creates a mist of drug, and its use

---

▲ see page 254   ■ see art on page 279

does not have to be coordinated with breathing. Nebulizers are more portable than they were in the past; some units can even be plugged into a cigarette lighter in a car. Beta-adrenergic agonists are rarely given by mouth for people with COPD because they tend to work slower than the inhaled form and are more likely to cause side effects, including abnormal heart rhythms.

Theophylline acts by different mechanisms than ipratropium or the beta-adrenergic agonists. It is given only to people who do not respond to other drugs. The dose must be carefully controlled by the doctor, and levels of the drug in the blood must be measured periodically. A long-acting form of the drug permits twice-daily dosing in many people and helps to control shortness of breath at night.

Corticosteroids are helpful for many people with moderate and severe COPD whose symptoms cannot be controlled by the other drugs. Inhaled corticosteroids do not prevent decline of lung function over time. However, their use improves symptoms and results in decreased frequency of COPD flare-ups. Because of local delivery of drug to the lungs, inhaled corticosteroids produce fewer side effects than treatment given by mouth. However, high doses of inhaled corticosteroids can have effects throughout the body, such as worsening of osteoporosis. Corticosteroids given by mouth are largely restricted to treatment of COPD flare-ups or are given to people who continue to have symptoms from airflow obstruction and who are not responding to a simpler regimen.

There is no reliable therapy for thinning secretions so they can be coughed up more easily. However, avoiding dehydration may prevent thick secretions. A rule of thumb is to drink enough fluids to keep the urine pale except for that passed first in the morning. In severe COPD, respiratory therapy may help loosen secretions in the chest.

A doctor often uses spirometry and pulse oximetry during treatment to monitor the person's symptoms. Arterial blood gas measurements add information that is useful in severe disease.

Treatment of Flare-ups: Flare-ups should be treated by the doctor as soon as possible. If treatment fails, hospitalization may be needed. When bacterial infection is suspected by the doctor, a 7- to 10-day course of antibi-

otic treatment is often prescribed. Many doctors give people who have COPD a supply of an antibiotic and advise them to start taking the drug early in a flare-up. A number of antibiotics can be taken by mouth, including trimethoprim-sulfamethoxazole, doxycycline, amoxicillin-clavulanate, and ampicillin. Many doctors reserve the newer antibiotics, such as azithromycin, clarithromycin, and levofloxacin, for more severe lung infections or for people in whom treatment with the older and less expensive drugs has not worked. Although many people with COPD think they should take antibiotics to prevent flare-ups, there is no indication that these drugs do prevent flare-ups. Sometimes corticosteroids are given by mouth for 10 to 14 days to help reduce the severity and length of flare-ups.

Oxygen Therapy: Long-term oxygen therapy▲ prolongs the life of people who have advanced COPD and severely reduced oxygen levels in the blood. Although round-the-clock therapy is best, using oxygen 12 hours a day also has some benefits. This therapy reduces the excess of red blood cells caused by low blood oxygen levels, improves mental functioning, and helps to relieve heart failure caused by COPD. Oxygen therapy may also improve shortness of breath during exercise.

Different devices are available for oxygen therapy. Electrically driven oxygen concentrators are used for people who are mainly homebound. The use of compressed oxygen in small tanks permits short periods outside the home for such people. Liquid oxygen systems are more expensive but are preferable for active people. They permit several hours away from the source reservoir by use of portable liquid oxygen containers. People must never use oxygen therapy near open flames or while smoking.

Pulmonary Rehabilitation: Pulmonary rehabilitation can help people who have COPD.■ However, lung function does not improve with pulmonary rehabilitation. Programs encompass education about the disease, exercise, and nutritional and psychosocial counseling. These programs can improve the person's independence and quality of life, decrease the frequency and length of hospital stays, and improve the person's ability to exercise. Exercise programs can be carried out in the clinic and at home. Stationary bicycling, stair climbing, and walking are used to exercise the legs. Weight lifting is used for the arms. Often, oxygen is recommended during

▲ see also page 260   ■ see also page 259

exercise. As with any exercise program, gains in conditioning are quickly lost if the person stops exercising. Special techniques are taught for decreasing shortness of breath during activities, such as cooking, engaging in hobbies, and sexual activity.

Other Treatments: For people with a severe alpha$_1$-antitrypsin deficiency, the missing protein can be replaced. The treatment, which requires weekly intravenous infusions of the protein, is expensive. Single lung transplantation may be used in certain people who are usually younger than 55.

An experimental operation known as lung volume reduction surgery can be carried out in people who have severe emphysema in the upper portions of their lungs. In this operation, the most severely diseased portions of the lungs are removed, thus permitting the remaining portions of the lungs and the diaphragm to function better. It is not known how long the improvement lasts. People are required to stop smoking for at least 6 months before surgery, and they should undergo an intense rehabilitation program to be certain lung function has improved significantly before undertaking this operation, which carries a mortality rate of about 5 to 8%.

Prognosis and End-of-Life Issues

The prognosis for people with mild COPD is favorable, little worse than the prognosis for smokers without COPD; continued smoking, however, virtually assures that symptoms will worsen. With moderate and severe airway obstruction, the prognosis becomes progressively worse. People with an FEV$_1$ between 35% and 50% of normal are still only slightly more likely to die within 10 years than a normal person. However, about 30% of people with more severe airway obstruction die in 1 year; 95% die in 10 years. Death may result from respiratory failure, pneumonia, pneumothorax, heart rhythm abnormalities (arrhythmias), or blockage of the arteries leading to the lungs (pulmonary embolism). People with COPD have a risk of lung cancer beyond that due to their use of cigarettes.

People in advanced stages of COPD are likely to need considerable help with medical care and with activities of daily living. People with end-stage disease who develop flare-ups may need an endotracheal tube and mechanical ventilation.▲ The period of mechanical ventilation may be prolonged and some people remain ventilator-dependent. It is important for people to consider with their doctors and loved ones whether or not they wish this kind of supportive therapy. The best way of assuring that the person's wishes are carried out is to have completed an advanced directive, preferably by the appointment of a health care proxy.■

CHAPTER 46

Pulmonary Embolism

Pulmonary embolism is the sudden blocking of an artery of the lung (pulmonary artery) by an embolus—usually a blood clot (thrombus).

The functions of the arteries of the lungs are to carry enough blood containing oxygen and nutrients to keep the lung tissue healthy and to carry carbon dioxide to the lungs for removal from the body.★ However, when a large artery to the lung is blocked by an embolus, the amount of blood supplied may be insufficient, eventually causing lung tissue to die.

About 10% of people with pulmonary embolism suffer some lung tissue death (called **pulmonary infarction**). Sometimes the body breaks up small clots quickly, keeping damage to a minimum. Large clots take much longer to disintegrate, so more damage is done. Large clots may cause sudden death by blocking so

▲ see page 326   ■ see page 54
★ see page 245

much of the lung arteries that the oxygen supply to the body is inadequate to sustain life or by placing an excessive strain on the heart.

The prevalence of pulmonary embolism in people admitted to the hospital is about 1%. When an autopsy is performed, pulmonary embolism is often unexpectedly found to be the cause of death in about 5% of people.

Causes

The most common type of embolus that travels to the lungs is a blood clot, usually one that forms in a leg or pelvic vein▲ when blood flow slows down or stops, as may occur in the leg veins when a person stays in one position for a long time. People who have been on prolonged bed rest and those sitting for long time periods without moving around (as may happen during air travel) are at particular risk. When the person starts moving again, the clot can break loose. Far less often, blood clots form in the veins of the arms or in the right side of the heart. Once a clot breaks free into the bloodstream, it usually travels to the lungs.

Another type of embolus may form from fat, which can escape into the blood from the bone marrow when a bone is fractured. An embolus also may form from amniotic fluid being forced into the pelvic veins during childbirth. However, both fat and amniotic fluid emboli are rare. If they form, they usually lodge in small vessels such as the arterioles and capillaries of the lung, where they generally cause less damage than blood clots. However, if many of these smaller vessels become obstructed, acute respiratory distress syndrome■ or pulmonary hypertension★ may develop; both of these conditions can lead to respiratory failure, heart failure, and shock.

Cancerous tumor fragments may break free into the circulation to form emboli, which, if they are numerous, can cause pulmonary hypertension as the cancer spreads throughout the lungs.

Air bubbles may form an emboli and cause pulmonary embolism after a vein has been exposed to large amounts of air, as may occur during intravenous infusion of drugs, nutrients, or fluid. Air emboli may also form when a vein is being operated on (such as when a blood clot is being removed) or when a person is being resuscitated (because of the force of chest compressions). An additional risk is when a person dives underwater; the risk depends on how deep the person dives and how fast he ascends to the surface of the water.●

Symptoms

Symptoms depend on the extent that the pulmonary artery is blocked and on the person's overall health. For example, people who have another disease such as chronic obstructive pulmonary disease or coronary artery disease may have more disabling symptoms.

Small emboli may not cause any symptoms, but most emboli cause shortness of breath, which comes on very quickly. Shortness of breath may be the only symptom, especially if pulmonary infarction does not develop. Often, the breathing is very rapid, and the person may feel anxious or restless and appear to have an anxiety attack. Larger emboli commonly cause sharp pain in the chest, especially when the person inhales; the pain is called pleuritic chest pain.

In some people, the first symptoms of pulmonary embolism may be light-headedness, fainting, or seizures. These symptoms usually result from a sudden decrease in the heart's ability to deliver enough oxygen-rich blood to the brain and other organs. Irregular heartbeats may also occur. People with obstruction of one or more large pulmonary arteries may have a blue skin color (cyanosis) and can die suddenly.

The symptoms of pulmonary embolism usually develop abruptly, whereas the symptoms of pulmonary infarction develop over the following hours. If pulmonary infarction occurs, the person experiences coughing that may produce blood-stained sputum, sharp chest pain when the person breathes in, and in some cases, fever. Symptoms of infarction often last several days but usually become milder every day.

In people who have recurring episodes of small pulmonary emboli, symptoms such as chronic shortness of breath, swelling of the ankles or legs, and weakness tend to develop progressively over weeks, months, or years.

Diagnosis

A doctor suspects pulmonary embolism based on the person's symptoms and predisposing factors, such as a recent surgery or a prolonged period of bed rest. A large pulmonary embolism may be relatively easy for a

---

▲ see page 232   ■ see page 326
★ see page 322   ● see page 1668

doctor to diagnose, especially when there are obvious preconditions, such as signs of a blood clot in a leg. Certain procedures are often needed to confirm the diagnosis. Even with these procedures, however, many emboli can be quite subtle and difficult for doctors to diagnose conclusively.

A chest x-ray may reveal subtle changes in the blood vessel patterns after embolism and signs of pulmonary infarction. However, the results are often normal, and even when they are abnormal, they rarely enable the doctor to establish the diagnosis with certainty.

An electrocardiogram may show abnormalities, but often these abnormalities are transient and can only support the possibility of pulmonary embolism.

A lung perfusion scan is one of the best tests for diagnosing pulmonary embolism. A tiny amount of radioactive substance is injected into a vein and travels to the lungs, where it outlines the blood supply (perfusion) of the lung. Areas without normal blood supply appear dark on the scan because no radioactive particles can reach them. Normal scan results indicate that the person does not have a significant blood vessel obstruction. Abnormal scan results support the possibility of pulmonary embolism but may also reflect conditions other than pulmonary embolism, such as obstructive lung disease (for example, emphysema, which can result in decreased blood flow to areas where lung tissue has been damaged).

Usually, the perfusion scan is coupled with a lung ventilation scan. The person inhales a harmless gas containing a trace amount of radioactive material, which is distributed throughout the small air sacs of the lungs (alveoli). The areas where carbon dioxide is being released and oxygen taken up can then be seen on a scanner. By comparing this scan to the pattern of blood supply shown on the perfusion scan, a doctor can usually determine whether a person has had a pulmonary embolism by a mismatch between ventilation and blood perfusion.

Pulmonary angiography▲ is an accurate means of diagnosing pulmonary embolism, but it poses some risk and is more uncomfortable than the other tests. It is usually performed only if the other tests fail to demonstrate a conclusive diagnosis of a pulmonary embolism. In an x-ray procedure, a radiopaque dye is injected into the pulmonary arteries. A pulmonary embolism shows up as blockage in

What Predisposes Someone to Blood Clots?

The cause of blood clots in the veins may not be discernible, but many times predisposing conditions are obvious. These conditions include:

- Advanced age
- Blood clotting disorder (increased risk of clotting, called hypercoagulable state)
- Cancer
- Heart attack
- Heart failure
- Irregular heartbeat (atrial fibrillation)
- Major surgery
- Obesity
- Paralysis
- Pelvis, hip, or leg fracture
- Prior blood clot
- Prolonged bed rest or inactivity (such as sitting during a long car or plane trip)
- Stroke
- Use of oral contraceptives—especially after age 35 and in someone who smokes

an artery. A certain type of computed tomography (CT) called CT angiography is another accurate test. CT angiography can be used if pulmonary angiography is not available or if the person should not undergo this test for some reason.

Additional tests, such as an ultrasound to examine the legs for blood clots in the veins, may be performed to find out where the embolus originally developed. A blood test (D-dimer test) can provide additional support of the diagnosis. A normal test result can help to exclude pulmonary embolism as the cause of a person's symptoms.

Prevention

Given the danger of pulmonary embolism and the limitations of treatment, doctors try to prevent blood clots from forming in the veins of people at risk of pulmonary embolism. In general, a person who is prone to clotting should try to be active and move around as much as possible. For example, when traveling on an airplane for a long pe-

▲ see page 256

riod, the person should try to get up and move around every two hours.

For people who have undergone surgery—especially older people—the risk of clot formation can be reduced by the following measures: wearing compression elastic stockings, doing leg exercises, and getting out of bed and becoming active as soon as possible. For people who cannot move their legs, intermittent air compression devices can provide rhythmic external pressure to keep blood moving in the legs and thighs. However, these devices alone are inadequate to prevent clot formation in people who have undergone hip or knee surgery.

Anticoagulant drugs are given. Heparin is the most widely used therapy for reducing the likelihood of clots forming in calf veins after any type of major surgery, especially surgery for the legs.▲ Hospitalized people at high risk of developing pulmonary embolism (such as those with heart failure, an acute myocardial infarction, chronic lung disease, obesity, a stroke or other neurologic problem or who have had clots in the past) benefit from small doses of heparin even if they are not undergoing surgery. Small doses are injected just under the skin shortly before the operation and ideally until the person is up and walking again. Low-dose heparin does not increase the frequency of major bleeding complications, but heparin can increase minor oozing of blood from wounds. Low-dose heparin can also be used for operations involving the spine or brain.

A different form of heparin, called low-molecular–weight heparin, is equally or even more effective in preventing clots than the use of traditional heparin. Low-molecular–weight heparin is also injected just under the skin and is usually continued until the risk of developing clots has passed.

Warfarin, an anticoagulant given by mouth, may be given when a person has undergone certain kinds of surgery that are particularly likely to result in clots, such as surgery for a hip fracture or a joint replacement. Warfarin therapy may need to be continued for several weeks or months. Low-molecular–weight heparin is also effective for people in this situation.

Treatment

Treatment of pulmonary embolism begins with the administration of oxygen and, if nec-

essary, analgesics to relieve pain. Anticoagulant drugs such as heparin are given to prevent existing blood clots from enlarging and additional clots from forming. Heparin is given intravenously to achieve a rapid effect, and doctors carefully regulate the dose. Doctors strive to achieve a full effect within the first 24 hours of treatment. Otherwise, the person is at high risk of more pulmonary emboli, and new clots or enlargement of existing clots in leg and pelvic veins. Low-molecular–weight heparin is probably equally effective to traditional heparin and does not require the blood test monitoring that conventional heparin requires. Warfarin, which also inhibits clotting but takes longer to start working, is given next. Because warfarin is taken by mouth, it can be used long-term. Heparin and warfarin are given together for 5 to 7 days, until blood tests show that the warfarin is effectively preventing clotting. Then, the heparin is discontinued.

How long anticoagulants are given depends on the person's situation. If pulmonary embolism is caused by a temporary predisposing factor, such as surgery, treatment is given for 2 to 3 months. If the cause is some longer-term problem, such as prolonged bed rest, treatment usually is given for 3 to 6 months, but sometimes it must continue indefinitely. For example, people who have recurrent pulmonary embolism, often due to a hereditary predisposition to clotting, usually take anticoagulants indefinitely. While taking warfarin, the person periodically has to have a blood test to determine if the dose needs to be adjusted. Changes in diet and many other drugs may affect the magnitude of anticoagulation by this drug. If excessive anticoagulation occurs, severe bleeding in a number of body organs can develop.

Thrombolytic therapy is used for people who appear to be in danger of dying of pulmonary embolism. Thrombolytic drugs such as streptokinase or tissue plasminogen activator (TPA) break up and dissolve the clot. However, these drugs cannot be given to people who have had surgery in the preceding 2 weeks, are pregnant, have had a recent stroke, or tend to bleed excessively. Surgery may be needed to save someone with severe embolism; removal of the embolus from the pulmonary artery may be lifesaving. Surgery is also used to remove long-standing pulmonary artery clots that cause persistent shortness of breath and pulmonary hypertension.

▲ see also box on page 996

A filter can be surgically placed in the main vein in the abdomen that drains blood from the legs and pelvis to the right side of the heart.▲ Such a filter can be used if emboli recur despite anticoagulant treatment or if anticoagulants cannot be used or cause significant bleeding. Because clots generally originate in the legs or pelvis, this filter usually prevents them from being carried into the pulmonary artery.

For emboli that form from fat or amniotic fluid, oxygen therapy and use of a ventilator may be needed. In addition, because emboli that develop from amniotic fluid may stimulate the formation of blood clots (coagulation), agents such as cryoprecipitate are sometimes needed to block certain key steps in the formation of these clots (such as the development of fibrin deposits in the circulation).

Prognosis

About half of the people with untreated pulmonary embolism will have another embolism. As many as half of these recurrences may be fatal. Anticoagulant treatment can reduce the rate of recurrence to about 1 in 20 people; only about 1 in 5 of these people will die of pulmonary embolism. The likelihood of dying depends on the size of the embolus, the size and number of pulmonary arteries blocked, and the person's overall health status. Anyone with a serious heart or lung problem is at greater risk of dying from pulmonary embolism. A person with normal heart and lung function usually survives unless the embolus blocks half or more of the pulmonary vessels. If death occurs from pulmonary embolism, it usually occurs rapidly, often within 1 to 2 hours.

An air embolism can cause death, but only if the amount of air that reaches the heart and pulmonary arteries is large. Death occurs with a large air embolus not only because blood flow to much of the lungs is blocked but also because the heart cannot effectively pump blood.

Bronchiectasis

Bronchiectasis is an irreversible widening (dilation) of portions of the airways (bronchi) resulting from damage to the bronchial wall.

Bronchiectasis can result from several conditions that injure the bronchial wall directly or indirectly by interfering with its normal defenses against potentially harmful substances.■ The most common cause is severe respiratory infections. Immune deficiency disorders, hereditary disorders (such as cystic fibrosis, in which abnormal mucus impairs the ability of cilia to clear the bronchi of organisms that cause infections★), and mechanical factors (such as bronchial obstruction caused by an inhaled object, a lung tumor, or other disorders) may predispose a person to infections that lead to bronchiectasis. A small number of cases probably result from inhaling toxic substances that injure the bronchi, such as noxious fumes, gases, smoke (including tobacco smoke), and injurious dust (silica, coal dust).

In bronchiectasis, areas of the bronchial wall are destroyed and become chronically inflamed, ciliated cells are damaged or destroyed, and secretions (mucus) accumulate. Also, the bronchial wall becomes less elastic—the affected airways become wider and flabby and may develop outpouchings or sacs that resemble tiny balloons. The increased mucus production promotes the growth of bacteria, often obstructs the bronchi, and leads to pooling of infected secretions and further damage to the bronchial wall. The inflammation and infection can extend to the small air sacs of the lungs (alveoli) and produce pneumonia, scarring, and a loss of functioning lung tissue.

In severe cases, scarring and a loss of blood vessels in the lung can ultimately strain the right side of the heart as the heart tries to pump blood through the altered vessels. Also, inflammation and an increased number of

---

▲ see art on page 235   ■ see page 247
★ see page 317

Understanding Bronchiectasis

In bronchiectasis, mucus production increases, the cilia are destroyed or damaged, and areas of the bronchial wall become chronically inflamed and are destroyed.

Normal Bronchus — Wall, Mucous gland, Cilia, Air passageway, Mucus

Bronchiectasis — Loss of cilia, Increased mucus, Destruction of wall

blood vessels in the bronchial wall (which are fragile) can result in a person coughing up blood. Blockage of the damaged airways can lead to abnormally low levels of oxygen in the blood.

Bronchiectasis may affect many areas of the lung, or it may appear in only one or two areas. Typically, bronchiectasis causes widening of medium-sized bronchi, but often smaller bronchi become scarred and destroyed. Occasionally, a form of bronchiectasis affecting larger bronchi occurs in allergic bronchopulmonary aspergillosis, a condition caused by an allergic response to the *Aspergillus* fungus.▲

Symptoms

Bronchiectasis can develop at any age; often, the process begins in early childhood. However, symptoms may not appear until much later. In most people, symptoms begin gradually, usually after a respiratory infection, and tend to worsen over the years. Most people develop a chronic cough that produces sputum; the amount and type of sputum depend on how extensive the disease is and whether there is a complicating infection. Often, the person has coughing spells only early in the morning and late in the day. Coughing up of blood is common and may be the first or only symptom.

Recurrent fever or chest pain, with or without frequent bouts of pneumonia, may also occur. People with widespread bronchiectasis may develop wheezing or shortness of breath; they may also have chronic bronchitis, emphysema, or asthma. Very severe cases of bronchiectasis, which occur more commonly in underdeveloped countries and in people who have advanced cystic fibrosis, may impair breathing and the lung's ability to oxygenate the blood and rid the body of carbon dioxide, a condition called respiratory failure.■ Very severe bronchiectasis may also strain the right side of the heart and lead to cor pulmonale.★

Diagnosis

Doctors may suspect bronchiectasis because of a person's symptoms or the presence of a condition thought to cause bronchiectasis. Tests are performed to confirm the diagnosis and assess the extent and location of the disease. Chest x-rays can often detect the lung changes caused by bronchiectasis; however, occasionally, results are normal. Computed tomography (CT) is usually the most sensitive test to identify and confirm the diagnosis and to determine the extent and severity of the disease; these are important factors when surgical treatment is being considered.

After bronchiectasis is diagnosed, tests are often performed to check for diseases that

▲ see page 311

■ see page 325

★ see box on page 323

may be causing or contributing to it if they were previously not identified. Such tests may include measuring the immunoglobulin levels in blood, testing for HIV infection and other immune system disorders, measuring the salt levels in sweat (which are abnormal in people with cystic fibrosis), and examining nasal, bronchial, or sperm specimens with a special microscope and other tests to determine if the cilia are structurally or functionally defective. When bronchiectasis is limited to one area—for example, a lung lobe or segment—doctors may perform bronchoscopy▲ to determine whether an inhaled foreign object or lung tumor is the cause. Other tests may be performed to identify underlying diseases, such as allergic bronchopulmonary aspergillosis or tuberculosis.

Genetic testing for cystic fibrosis may be needed when there is a family history, repeated respiratory infections, or other suspicious findings in a child or young adult, even when other typical features of cystic fibrosis are absent.

Prevention

Early identification and treatment of conditions that tend to cause bronchiectasis may prevent the development of bronchiectasis or reduce its severity. More than half the cases of bronchiectasis in children can be accurately diagnosed and promptly treated.

Childhood immunizations against measles and whooping cough, appropriate use of antibiotics, and improved living conditions and nutrition have significantly reduced the number of people who develop bronchiectasis. Annual influenza vaccines, use of the pneumococcal vaccine, and use of appropriate drugs early in the course of infections (such as pneumonia and tuberculosis) help to prevent bronchiectasis or reduce its severity. Receiving immunoglobulin for an immunoglobulin deficiency syndrome may prevent recurring infections. In people who have allergic bronchopulmonary aspergillosis, the appropriate use of corticosteroids and perhaps the antifungal drug itraconazole may reduce the bronchial damage that results in bronchiectasis.

Avoiding toxic fumes, gases, smoke, and injurious dusts also helps prevent bronchiectasis or reduce its severity. Inhalation of foreign objects into the airways by children may be prevented by carefully watching what they put in their mouth. Additionally, avoiding oversedation from drugs or alcohol and seek-

Selected Causes of Bronchiectasis

Respiratory infections
- Bacterial infection, such as whooping cough or infections caused by *Klebsiella, Staphylococcus,* or *Pseudomonas*
- Fungal infection, such as aspergillosis
- Mycobacterial infection, such as tuberculosis
- Viral infection, such as influenza, adenoviral infection, respiratory syncytial virus infection, or measles
- Mycoplasma infection

Bronchial obstruction
- Inhaled object
- Enlarged lymph glands
- Lung tumor
- Mucus plug

Inhalation injuries
- Injury from noxious fumes, gases, or particles
- Inhalation of stomach acid and food particles

Hereditary conditions
- Cystic fibrosis
- Primary ciliary dyskinesia, including Kartagener's syndrome
- Marfan syndrome

Immunologic abnormalities
- Immunoglobulin deficiency syndromes
- White blood cell dysfunction
- Complement deficiencies
- Certain autoimmune or hyperimmune disorders, such as rheumatoid arthritis and ulcerative colitis

Other conditions
- Drug abuse, such as heroin abuse
- Human immunodeficiency virus (HIV) infection
- Young's syndrome (obstructive azoospermia)
- Yellow nail syndrome (with lymphedema)

ing medical care for neurologic symptoms (such as impaired consciousness) or gastrointestinal symptoms (such as difficulty in swallowing and regurgitation or coughing after

▲ see page 256

eating) may help to prevent aspiration. Also, drops of mineral oil or other oils should never be placed in the mouth or nose because they can be inhaled into the lungs.

Treatment and Prognosis

Treatment of bronchiectasis is directed against eradicating infections, decreasing the build up of mucus and inflammation, relieving airway obstruction, and reducing complications (such as coughing up of blood, low oxygen levels in the blood, respiratory failure, and cor pulmonale). Drugs that suppress coughing may worsen the condition and generally should not be used.

Infections are treated with antibiotics, bronchodilators, and physical therapy to promote drainage of secretions. Sometimes antibiotics are prescribed for a long period to prevent recurring infections, especially in people who have cystic fibrosis.

For inflammation and the buildup of mucus, anti-inflammatory drugs such as inhaled corticosteroids and drugs that thin the pus and mucus (mucolytics) may also be given, although the effectiveness of mucolytics is uncertain. To help drain the mucus, postural drainage and chest percussion▲ are used.

To detect and treat a bronchial obstruction, bronchoscopy can be used before severe damage occurs.■ Rarely, part of a lung needs to be surgically removed. Such surgery usually is an option only if the disease is confined to one lung, or preferably to one lung lobe or segment. Surgery may be considered for people

who have recurrent infections despite treatment or who cough up large amounts of blood. Alternatively, a doctor may deliberately block a bleeding bronchial vessel by using a procedure called bronchial arterial embolization.

If the person's blood oxygen level is low, oxygen therapy★ may help prevent complications such as cor pulmonale. If the person has wheezing or shortness of breath, corticosteroids taken with or without bronchodilators often help. Respiratory failure, if present, should be treated.●

Lung transplantation can be performed in certain people who have advanced bronchiectasis, mostly those who also have advanced cystic fibrosis. Five-year survival rates as high as 65 to 75% have been reported when a heart-lung or a double lung transplantation is used. Pulmonary function (as measured by the amount of air in the lungs and the rate and amount of air moving in and out of the lungs with each breath) usually improves within 6 months, and the improvement may be sustained for at least 5 years.

Overall prognosis for people with bronchiectasis depends on how well infection and other complications are prevented or controlled. Because other conditions (such as chronic bronchitis, emphysema, pulmonary hypertension, cor pulmonale, or other serious diseases that affect the whole body [systemic diseases]) diminish the effectiveness of prevention and treatment, people with these conditions tend to have a worse prognosis.

CHAPTER 48

Atelectasis

Atelectasis is a condition in which all or part of a lung becomes airless and contracts.

Atelectasis may be an acute or chronic condition. In acute atelectasis, the lung has recently collapsed and is primarily notable only

for airlessness. In chronic atelectasis, the affected area is often characterized by a complex mixture of airlessness, infection, widening of the bronchi (bronchiectasis◆), destruction, and scarring (fibrosis). People who smoke have a greater risk of developing atelectasis.

Causes

The most common cause of atelectasis is an obstruction of a large bronchus (one of the two main branches of the trachea leading directly

▲ see page 261   ■ see page 256
★ see page 260   ● see page 325
◆ see page 289

to the lungs). Smaller airways can also become blocked. The obstruction may be caused by a plug of mucus, a tumor, or an inhaled foreign object inside the bronchus. Alternatively, the bronchus may be blocked by something pressing from the outside, such as a tumor, enlarged lymph nodes, or a significant amount of fluid (pleural effusion) or air (pneumothorax) in the pleural space.▲ When an airway becomes blocked, the air in the small air sacs of the lung (alveoli) beyond the blockage is absorbed into the bloodstream, causing the alveoli to shrink and retract. The collapsed lung tissue commonly fills with blood cells, serum, and mucus and becomes infected.

Atelectasis can occur in jet fighter pilots when the high forces generated by high-speed flying close small airways. Atelectasis under these circumstances, sometimes described as acceleration atelectasis, leads to collapse of the alveoli in much of both lungs.

Additionally, atelectasis can result if there is a deficiency in the amount or effectiveness of the liquid substance (surfactant) that coats the lining of the alveoli. Normally, this liquid prevents the alveoli from collapsing.

Acute Atelectasis: Acute atelectasis is a common postoperative complication, especially after chest or abdominal surgery. Acute atelectasis may also occur with an injury, usually to the chest (such as that caused by a car accident, a fall, or a stabbing). Atelectasis following surgery or injury, sometimes described as massive, involves most alveoli in one or more regions of the lungs. In these circumstances, the degree of collapse among alveoli tends to be quite consistent and complete. Large doses of opioids or sedatives, tight bandages, chest or abdominal pain, abdominal swelling (distention), and immobility of the body increase the risk of acute atelectasis following surgery or injury, or even spontaneously. Certain neurologic conditions and chest deformities are additional factors that can limit chest movement, lead to shallow breathing, cause bronchial secretions to accumulate, preclude the lung from expanding fully, and suppress the cough reflex.

In acute atelectasis that occurs because of a deficiency in the amount or effectiveness of surfactant, many but not all alveoli collapse, and the degree of collapse is not uniform. Atelectasis in these circumstances may be limited to only a portion of one lung, or it may be present throughout both lungs. When premature babies are born with surfactant defi-

ciency, they always develop acute atelectasis that progresses to neonatal respiratory distress syndrome■ unless they are treated with replacement surfactant. Adults can also develop acute atelectasis from excessive oxygen therapy and from mechanical ventilation, because of decreased effectiveness of surfactant. Another cause of acute atelectasis resulting from decreased effectiveness of surfactant is acute respiratory distress syndrome. ★

Chronic Atelectasis: Chronic atelectasis may take one of two forms—middle lobe syndrome or rounded atelectasis. In middle lobe syndrome, the middle lobe of the right lung contracts, usually because of pressure on the bronchus from enlarged lymph glands and occasionally a tumor. The blocked, contracted lung may develop pneumonia that fails to resolve completely and leads to chronic inflammation, scarring, and bronchiectasis.

In rounded atelectasis (folded lung syndrome), an outer portion of the lung slowly collapses as a result of scarring and shrinkage of the membrane layers covering the lungs (pleura). This produces a rounded appearance on x-ray that doctors may mistake for a tumor. Rounded atelectasis is usually a complication of asbestos-induced disease of the pleura, but it may also result from other types of chronic scarring and thickening of the pleura.

Symptoms

The loss of functioning lung tissue leads to shortness of breath. The persistence of blood flow through the collapsed area leads to a decrease in the blood oxygen level—the heart rate increases, and sometimes the person may look bluish (a condition called cyanosis).

The severity of symptoms depends on how rapidly the bronchus is blocked, how much of the lung is affected, what the precipitating factor was, and whether infection is present. When blockage happens quickly and a lot of lung tissue is affected, a person may become blue or ashen in color, have sharp pain on the affected side, and have sudden and extreme shortness of breath. The person may also experience shock● with a severe drop in blood pressure; a rapid heart rate; and fever if infection develops.

Widespread atelectasis resulting from deficient or ineffective surfactant produces short-

---

▲ see page 316   ■ see page 1499
★ see page 326   ● see page 148

ness of breath; rapid, shallow breathing; a low blood oxygen level; and other symptoms depending on the cause of the acute lung injury (for example, fever and low blood pressure from sepsis) and any accompanying effects of low blood oxygen (such as abnormal heart rhythms) on organs other than the lung.

Slowly developing atelectasis may cause no symptoms or only minor ones, such as shortness of breath or an increased heart rate. People with middle lobe syndrome and rounded atelectasis may have no symptoms, although some people with middle lobe syndrome have a hacking cough or develop pneumonia that resolves slowly or incompletely.

Diagnosis

Doctors suspect atelectasis based on a person's symptoms, the physical examination findings, and the setting in which the symptoms occurred. A chest x-ray that shows the airless area confirms the diagnosis, but the x-ray may appear normal even when the person is feeling breathless. When bronchial obstruction is suspected, computed tomography (CT), bronchoscopy, or both these tests may be performed to find the cause, especially when the collapse persists despite usual treatment measures.

Prevention and Treatment

People who smoke can decrease their risk of atelectasis after surgery by stopping smoking 6 to 8 weeks before an operation. After an operation, all people should be encouraged to breathe deeply, cough regularly, and move about as soon as possible. The use of breathing devices to encourage voluntary deep breathing (incentive spirometry) and certain exercises, including changing position to increase the drainage of lung secretions, may help to prevent atelectasis.

People with chest deformities or neurologic conditions that cause shallow breathing for long periods may benefit from mechanical devices that assist their breathing. One method is continuous positive airway pressure, which delivers oxygen through a nose or face mask to help ensure that the airways do not collapse, even at the end of a breath. Sometimes additional respiratory support is needed with a mechanical ventilator.▲

The primary treatment for acute massive atelectasis is correction of the underlying cause. A blockage that cannot be removed by coughing or by suctioning the airways often can be removed by bronchoscopy.■ Antibiotics are given for an infection. Chronic atelectasis often is treated with antibiotics because infection is almost inevitable. In certain cases, the affected part of the lung may be surgically removed when recurring or chronic infections become disabling or bleeding is significant. If a tumor is blocking the airway, relieving the obstruction by surgery, radiation therapy, chemotherapy, or laser therapy may prevent atelectasis from progressing and recurrent obstructive pneumonia from developing.

In treatment of atelectasis due to deficient or ineffective surfactant, attention is directed at treating the low blood oxygen (often with mechanical ventilation or positive end expiratory pressure) and its effects promptly and at identifying and treating the underlying condition. Treatment with a surfactant drug is lifesaving for premature babies with a surfactant deficiency. Such therapy is experimental in adults with the acute respiratory distress syndrome who have reduced surfactant activity.

CHAPTER 49

Occupational Lung Diseases

Occupational lung diseases are caused by harmful particles, mists, vapors, or gases that are inhaled, usually while a person works. If the lung disease is due to inhaled particles, the term pneumoconiosis is often used. Where in the airways or lungs an inhaled substance ends up and what type of lung disease develops depend on the size and kind of particles inhaled. Large particles may get trapped in the nose or large airways, but very small ones may

---

▲ see page 326   ■ see page 256

reach the lungs. There, some particles dissolve and may be absorbed into the bloodstream; most solid particles that do not dissolve are removed by the body's defenses.

The body has several means of getting rid of inhaled particles. In the airways, an accumulation of secretions (mucus) coats particles so that they can be coughed up more easily. Additionally, tiny cells lining the airways (cilia) are able to brush inhaled particles upward, out of the lungs. In the small air sacs of the lungs (alveoli), special scavenger cells (macrophages) engulf most particles and render them harmless.

Many different kinds of particles can harm the lungs. Some are organic, meaning that they are made of materials that contain carbon and are parts of the building blocks of living organisms (such as grain dusts, cotton dust, or animal dander). Some are inorganic, meaning that they are usually salts of metals (such as asbestos).

Different types of particles produce different reactions in the body. Some particles—animal dander, for example—can cause allergic reactions, such as hay fever–like symptoms or a type of asthma. Other particles cause harm not by triggering allergic reactions but by being toxic to the cells of the airways and air sacs in the lung. Some particles, such as quartz dust and asbestos, may cause chronic irritation that can lead to scarring of lung tissue (pulmonary fibrosis▲). Certain toxic particles, such as asbestos, can cause lung cancer, especially in smokers, or cancer of the lining of the chest and lung (mesothelioma), regardless of the person's smoking history.

Silicosis

Silicosis is permanent scarring of the lungs caused by inhaling silica (quartz) dust.

Silicosis, the oldest known occupational lung disease, develops in people who have inhaled silica dust for many years. Silica is the main constituent of sand, so exposure is common among metal miners, sandstone and granite cutters, foundry workers, and potters.

When inhaled, silica dust passes into the lungs, and scavenger cells such as macrophages engulf it.■ Enzymes released by the scavenger cells cause the lung tissue to scar. At first, the scarred areas are tiny round lumps (simple nodular silicosis), but eventually they may combine into larger masses (complicated silicosis). These scarred areas cannot transfer

oxygen into the blood normally. The lungs become less flexible, and breathing takes more effort.

Symptoms and Diagnosis

Usually, symptoms appear only after 20 or more years of exposure to the dust. However, in occupations such as sandblasting, tunneling, and manufacturing abrasive soaps, in which high levels of silica dust are produced, symptoms may appear in less than 10 years.

The least serious type of lung disease from silica is simple nodular silicosis. People with simple nodular silicosis usually have no trouble breathing, but they may cough and produce sputum (also called phlegm) because their large airways are inflamed (a condition called chronic bronchitis★).

People who have the more serious type, complicated silicosis, may cough, produce sputum, and have severe shortness of breath. At first, the shortness of breath may occur only during exercise, but eventually it occurs even during rest. Breathing may worsen for years after the person stops working with silica. The lung damage strains the right side of the heart and can lead to a type of heart failure (called cor pulmonale●), which can be fatal. Also, when exposed to the organism that causes tuberculosis, people with silicosis are many times more likely to develop tuberculosis than people without silicosis.

Silicosis is diagnosed when someone who has worked with silica has a chest x-ray that shows the distinctive patterns of scarring and nodules. Breathing tests are often performed to determine if lung function is impaired.

Prevention

Controlling silica dust in the workplace is key to preventing silicosis. When dust cannot be controlled, as may be true in the sandblasting industry, workers should wear protective gear, such as hoods that supply clean external air or special masks that efficiently filter out the tiny particles. Such protection may not be available to all people working in a dusty area (for example, painters and welders), so whenever possible, abrasives other than sand should be used.

Workers exposed to silica dust should have regular chest x-rays—every 6 months for sand-

---

▲ see page 301   ■ see box on page 1052
★ see page 262   ● see box on page 323

blasters and every 2 to 5 years for other workers—so that problems can be detected early. If the x-rays show silicosis, a doctor will probably advise the worker to avoid continued exposure to silica.

Treatment

Silicosis cannot be cured, but its progression can be slowed if exposure to silica is avoided, especially at an early stage of the disease. A person who has difficulty breathing may benefit from the treatments used for chronic obstructive pulmonary disease, such as drug therapy to keep the airways open and free of mucus.▲ Because people with silicosis have a high risk of developing tuberculosis, they should have regular checkups that include a tuberculosis skin test.

Black Lung

Black lung (coal workers' pneumoconiosis) is a lung disease caused by deposits of coal dust in the lungs.

Black lung results from inhaling coal dust over a long time. Although coal dust is relatively inert and does not provoke much reaction, it spreads throughout the lungs and shows up as tiny spots on an x-ray. Coal dust may block the airways. In simple black lung, coal dust collects around the small airways (bronchioles) of the lungs. Every year, 1 to 2% of people with simple black lung develop a more serious form of the disease called progressive massive fibrosis, in which large scars (at least ½ inch in diameter) develop in the lungs as a reaction to the dust. Progressive massive fibrosis may worsen even after exposure to coal dust stops. Lung tissue and the blood vessels in the lungs can be destroyed by the scarring.

In Caplan's syndrome, a rare disorder that can affect coal miners who also have rheumatoid arthritis, large round nodules of scarring develop quickly in the lung. Such nodules may form in people who have had significant exposure to coal dust, even if they do not have black lung.

Symptoms and Diagnosis

Simple black lung usually does not cause symptoms. However, many people with this disease cough and easily become short of breath because they also have an airway dis-

ease, such as bronchitis or emphysema, and these are more likely to occur in smokers. The severe stages of progressive massive fibrosis, on the other hand, cause coughing and often disabling shortness of breath.

A doctor makes the diagnosis after noting characteristic spots on the chest x-ray of a person who has been exposed to coal dust for a long time—usually someone who has worked in a coal mine for at least 10 years.

Prevention and Treatment

Prevention is crucial because there is no cure for black lung. Black lung can be prevented by adequately suppressing coal dust at a work site; ventilation systems may help. Face pieces (masks) that filter and purify the air may provide some additional preventive benefit.

Coal workers should have chest x-rays every year, so that the disease can be detected at a relatively early stage. If the disease is detected, the worker should be transferred to an area where coal dust levels are low to help prevent progressive massive fibrosis.

A person who is short of breath may benefit from the treatments used for chronic obstructive pulmonary disease, such as drug therapy to keep the airways open and free of mucus.■

Asbestosis

Asbestosis is widespread scarring of lung tissue caused by breathing asbestos dust.

Asbestos is composed of fibrous mineral silicates of different chemical compositions. When inhaled, asbestos fibers settle deep in the lungs, causing scars. Asbestos inhalation also can cause the two layers of membrane covering the lungs (the pleura) to thicken; these thickenings are called pleural plaques. These plaques do not become cancerous.

Inhaling asbestos fibers can occasionally cause fluid to accumulate in the space between the two pleural layers of the lungs (pleural space); this is called a noncancerous (benign) asbestos effusion.

Asbestos also causes cancer in the pleura, called mesothelioma, or in the membranes of the abdomen, called peritoneal mesothelioma. In the United States, asbestos is the only known cause of cancerous (malignant) mesothelioma. Smoking is not a cause of cancerous mesothelioma. Mesotheliomas most commonly appear after exposure to crocidolite, one of four types of asbestos. Amosite, another type,

---

▲ see page 283   ■ see page 283

Who Is at Risk for Occupational Lung Diseases?

Silicosis
- Lead, copper, silver, and gold miners
- Certain coal miners (for example, roof bolters)
- Foundry workers
- Potters
- Sandstone or granite cutters
- Tunnel workers
- Workers who make abrasive soaps
- Sandblasters
- Tombstone makers

Black lung
- Coal workers

Asbestosis
- Workers who mine, mill, or manufacture asbestos
- Construction workers who install or remove materials (including insulation) that contain asbestos
- Shipyard workers

Beryllium disease
- Aerospace workers
- Metallurgical (castings) workers

Flock worker's lung
- Synthetic fiber flocking workers

Benign pneumoconiosis
- Welders
- Iron miners
- Barium workers
- Tin workers

Occupational asthma
- People who work with grains, western red cedar wood, castor beans, isocyanates (urethanes), dyes, antibiotics, epoxy resins, tea, and enzymes used in manufacturing detergent, malt, leather goods, latex, jewelry, abrasives and paints used in automobile body repairs, animals, shellfish, irritating gases, vapors, and mists

Byssinosis
- Cotton, hemp, jute, and flax workers

Silo filler's disease
- Farmers

Hypersensitivity pneumonitis
- Office workers (because of air-conditioning systems contaminated by certain fungi and bacteria)
- Swimming pool/spa workers (because of contaminated sprays)
- Farmers, mushroom workers, bird keepers, workers exposed to isocyanates

also causes mesotheliomas. Chrysotile probably causes fewer cases of mesotheliomas than other types, but chrysotile is often contaminated with tremolite, which does. Mesotheliomas usually develop 30 to 40 years after exposure and can occur after low exposure.

Asbestos can also cause lung cancer. Lung cancer from asbestos is related in part to the level of exposure to asbestos fibers; however, among people with asbestosis, lung cancer occurs most commonly in those who also smoke cigarettes, particularly those who smoke more than a pack a day.▲

Although the general public has become alarmed about the risks of asbestos, most nonoccupationally exposed people are at extremely low risk of developing asbestos-related lung disease. The asbestos must be broken into tiny pieces to be inhaled into the lungs. Workers who demolish buildings that have insulation containing asbestos are at increased risk. People who regularly work with asbestos are at greatest risk of developing lung disease. The more a person is exposed to asbestos fibers, the greater the risk of developing an asbestos-related disease.

Symptoms

Symptoms of asbestosis appear gradually only after large areas of the lung become scarred. The scarring causes the lungs to lose their elasticity. The first symptoms are a mild shortness of breath and a decreased ability to exercise. Smokers who have chronic bronchitis along with asbestosis may cough and wheeze. Gradually, breathing becomes more and more difficult. In about 15% of people with asbestosis, severe shortness of breath and respiratory failure develop.

A person with noncancerous asbestos effusion may have difficulty in breathing because of fluid accumulation. Pleural plaques cause only a mild breathing difficulty that results from stiffness of the chest wall. Persistent pain in the

▲ see also page 328

chest and shortness of breath are the most common symptoms caused by mesothelioma.

Diagnosis

Usually, the person with asbestosis has abnormal lung function, and a doctor listening with a stethoscope placed over the lungs can hear abnormal sounds called crackles. In a person who has a history of exposure to asbestos, a doctor sometimes can diagnose asbestosis with a chest x-ray or a chest computed tomography (CT) that shows characteristic changes. Pleural plaques that develop in many people with exposure to asbestos often contain calcium, which makes them easy to see on chest x-rays and CT. A lung biopsy is rarely needed to make the diagnosis.

If a tumor of the pleura is found on x-ray, a doctor must perform a biopsy (remove a small piece of pleura and examine it under a microscope) to determine if it is cancerous. Fluid around the lungs may be removed with a needle and analyzed for cancer cells (a procedure called thoracentesis). However, thoracentesis is not usually as accurate as performing a pleural biopsy. If a chest x-ray reveals something that looks like a tumor, there is a good possibility that the area is a primary lung cancer and should be evaluated fully.

Prevention and Treatment

Diseases caused by asbestos inhalation can be prevented by minimizing asbestos dust and fibers in the workplace. Because industries that use asbestos have improved dust control, fewer people develop asbestosis today, but mesotheliomas are still occurring in people who were exposed as many as 40 years ago. Asbestos in the home should be removed by workers trained in safe removal techniques. Smokers who have been in contact with asbestos can reduce their risk of lung cancer by giving up smoking and should probably have a chest x-ray annually.

Most treatments for asbestosis ease symptoms—for example, oxygen therapy relieves shortness of breath. Draining fluid from around the lungs using a procedure called thoracentesis also may make breathing easier. Occasionally, lung transplantation has been successful in treating asbestosis.

Mesotheliomas are invariably fatal; most people with mesotheliomas die within 1 to 4 years of diagnosis. Chemotherapy and radia-

tion therapy do not work well, and surgical removal of the tumor does not cure the cancer. Other treatment is focused on controlling pain and shortness of breath, in an effort to preserve as much quality-of-life as possible.▲

Beryllium Disease

Beryllium disease (sometimes called berylliosis) is a lung inflammation caused by inhaling dust or fumes that contain beryllium.

In the past, beryllium was commonly mined and extracted for use in the electronics and chemical industries and in the manufacture of fluorescent light bulbs. Today, it is used mainly in the aerospace industry and in beryllium-aluminum castings. Besides workers in these industries, a few people living near beryllium refineries also have developed beryllium disease.

Beryllium disease differs from other occupational lung diseases in that at low levels of exposure, lung problems seem to occur only in people who are sensitive to beryllium—about 2% of those who come in contact with it. The disease can occur in such people even with a relatively brief exposure to beryllium.

Symptoms and Diagnosis

In some people, beryllium disease develops suddenly (acute beryllium disease), mainly as an inflammation of the lungs (pneumonitis). In these people, the lungs are stiff and function poorly. People with acute disease have an abrupt onset of coughing, difficulty in breathing, and weight loss. Acute beryllium disease also can affect the skin and eyes.

Other people develop chronic beryllium disease, in which abnormal tissue forms in the lungs and the lymph nodes enlarge. In these people, coughing, difficulty in breathing, and weight loss develop gradually, often 10 to 20 years after exposure.

The diagnosis is based on the person's history of exposure to beryllium, the symptoms, and characteristic changes on a chest x-ray. However, x-rays of people with beryllium disease resemble those of another lung disease, sarcoidosis,■ and additional immunologic tests (such as the beryllium lymphocyte transformation test) may be needed.

Prognosis, Prevention, and Treatment

Acute beryllium disease may be severe. Most people recover in 7 to 10 days, with appropriate treatment, such as ventilator sup-

▲ see page 48   ■ see page 304

port and corticosteroid drugs. However, some people with severe disease die.

The course of people who develop symptoms late is completely different. People with chronic beryllium disease continue to have symptoms, which tend to progress. If the lungs are severely damaged, the heart may become strained, causing a type of heart failure (cor pulmonale▲) and death. Sometimes corticosteroids, such as oral prednisone, are prescribed for chronic beryllium disease, although they generally are not very helpful. Beryllium disease can be prevented by strictly limiting exposure to beryllium.

Flock Worker's Lung

Flock worker's lung is a chronic lung disease occurring because of inhalation of certain synthetic fibers.

Workers in the nylon flocking industry worldwide are at increased risk of chronic inflammation and scarring of the walls of small airways and spaces between the airways and air sacs (interstitium) in the lung. Flocking, widely used in the production of industrial synthetic textiles, is a process whereby short lengths of fibers are applied to backing fabric to produce plush "fleece" material. The risk of disease seems to be concentrated in areas of nylon flocking only, not in all nylon processing.

Affected workers develop shortness of breath, and abnormalities can be seen on chest x-rays. Symptoms improve, but do not always resolve completely, when exposure stops. Corticosteroids may help to further reduce symptoms.

Occupational Asthma

Occupational asthma is a reversible narrowing of the airways caused by inhaling work-related particles or vapors that act as irritants or cause an allergic reaction.

Many substances in the workplace can cause narrowing of the airways, which makes breathing difficult. Some people are particularly sensitive to airborne irritants, and some develop sick building syndrome.■ Examples of workers at risk for occupational asthma from exposure to allergens include animal handlers and bakers.

Symptoms

Occupational asthma may cause shortness of breath, a tightness in the chest, wheezing, coughing, sneezing, runny nose, and watery eyes. For some people, wheezing at night is the only symptom. Symptoms may develop during work hours but often do not start until a few hours after work. In some people, symptoms begin as much as 24 hours after exposure. Also, symptoms may come and go for a week or more after exposure. Thus, the link between the workplace and the symptoms is often obscured. Symptoms often become milder or disappear on weekends or over holidays. They worsen with repeated exposure.

Diagnosis

To make a diagnosis, a doctor asks the person about the symptoms and exposure to a substance known to cause asthma. Occasionally, the allergic reaction can be detected with a skin test (patch test), in which a small amount of a suspected substance is placed on the skin. When making the diagnosis is more difficult, doctors in specialized centers use an inhalation challenge test, in which the person inhales small amounts of the suspected substance and is observed for wheezing and shortness of breath and tested for decreasing lung function.

Because the airways may begin to narrow before symptoms appear, a person with delayed symptoms may use a device to monitor the airways while at work. This device, a portable peak flow meter, measures the speed at which a person can blow air out of the lungs. When the airways narrow, the rate slows significantly, suggesting occupational asthma.

Prevention and Treatment

Industries using substances that can cause asthma must have dust and vapor control measures, but sometimes eliminating the dusts and vapors may be impossible. Workers with occupational asthma should change jobs, if possible. Continued exposure often leads to more severe and persistent asthma.

Treatments are the same as for other types of asthma.★ Drugs that open the airways (bronchodilators) may be given, preferably in an inhaler (for example, albuterol) or as a tablet (for example, theophylline). Drugs that reduce inflammation may be given, either in an inhaler (for example, triamcinolone) or as a tablet (for example, montelukast). For severe attacks, corticosteroids (such as prednisone) may be taken by mouth for a short time. For

▲ see box on page 323   ■ see page 1720
★ see page 276

long-term management, inhaled corticosteroids are preferred.

Byssinosis

Byssinosis is a narrowing of the airways caused by inhaling cotton, flax, or hemp particles.

In the United States and Great Britain, byssinosis occurs almost exclusively in people who work with unprocessed cotton. Those who work with flax and hemp may also develop the condition. People who open bales of raw cotton or who work in the first stages of cotton processing seem to be most affected. Apparently, something in the raw cotton causes the airways of susceptible people to narrow. Variations of this condition may occur in people exposed to grain dusts in agricultural environments (grain worker's lung).

Symptoms and Diagnosis

Byssinosis may cause wheezing and tightness in the chest, usually on the first day of work after a break. Unlike with asthma, the symptoms tend to diminish after repeated exposure, and the chest tightness may disappear by the end of the workweek. However, after a person has worked with cotton for many years, the chest tightness may last for 2 or 3 workdays or even the whole week. Prolonged exposure to cotton dust increases the frequency of symptoms (cough, chest tightness) and leads to permanent lung disease, which can sometimes be disabling.

The diagnosis is made by using a test that shows decreasing lung capacity over the course of a workday; usually, this decrease is greatest on the first day of the workweek.

Prevention and Treatment

Controlling dust is the best way to prevent byssinosis. Workers with symptoms who also experience sudden drops in lung function on the first day of the workweek should be removed from exposure. Wheezing and chest tightness can be treated with the drugs used for asthma. Drugs that open the airways (bronchodilators) may be given.

Benign Pneumoconioses

Certain substances occasionally cause the lungs to appear abnormal on x-rays. However, these substances do not cause much of a reaction in the lungs, so people exposed to them do not have symptoms or impaired function. Siderosis results from inhalation of iron oxide, baritosis from inhalation of barium, and stannosis from inhalation of tin particles.

Gas and Chemical Exposure

Many types of gases—such as chlorine, phosgene, sulfur dioxide, hydrogen sulfide, nitrogen dioxide, and ammonia—may suddenly be released during industrial accidents and may severely irritate the lungs. Gases such as chlorine and ammonia easily dissolve and immediately irritate the mouth, nose, and throat. The lower parts of the lungs are affected only when the gas is inhaled deeply. Radioactive gases, which may be released in a nuclear reactor accident, may cause lung and other cancers many years after the exposure.

Some gases—for instance, nitrogen dioxide—do not dissolve easily. Therefore, they do not produce early warning signs of exposure, such as irritation of the nose and eyes, and they are more likely to be inhaled deeply into the lungs. Such gases can cause inflammation of the small airways (bronchiolitis) or lead to fluid accumulation in the lungs (pulmonary edema).

Silo filler's disease (which mostly affects farmers) results from inhaling fumes that contain nitrogen dioxide given off by moist silage. Fluid may develop in the lungs as late as 12 hours after exposure; the condition may temporarily improve and then recur 10 to 14 days later, even without further contact with the gas. A recurrence tends to affect the bronchioles.

Inhalation of some gases and chemicals may also trigger an allergic response that leads to inflammation, and in some cases, scarring in and around the tiny air sacs (alveoli) and smallest airways (bronchioles) of the lung; this condition is called hypersensitivity pneumonitis.▲

In some people, inhalation of small amounts of gas or other chemicals over a long period may result in chronic bronchitis. Also, inhalation of some chemicals, such as arsenic compounds and hydrocarbons, can cause cancer. Cancer may develop in the lungs or elsewhere in the body, depending on the substance inhaled.

Symptoms and Diagnosis

Soluble gases such as chlorine, ammonia, and hydrofluoric acid cause severe burning in

▲ see page 308

the eyes, nose, throat, windpipe, and large airways within minutes of exposure to them. In addition, they often produce a cough and blood in the sputum (hemoptysis). Retching and shortness of breath also are common. Less soluble gases such as nitrogen dioxide and ozone produce shortness of breath, which may be severe, after a delay of 3 to 4 hours and sometimes up to 12 hours after exposure.

A chest x-ray can show whether pulmonary edema or bronchiolitis has developed.

Prognosis, Prevention, and Treatment

Most people recover completely from accidental exposure to gases. The most serious complications are lung infection or severe damage with scarring of the small airways (bronchiolitis obliterans). Recent studies, however, have shown long-term impairment of the lungs years after episodes of exposure to gases.

The best way to prevent exposure is to use extreme care when handling gases and chemicals. Gas masks with their own air supply should be available in case of accidental spillage. Farmers need to know that accidental exposure to toxic gases in silos is dangerous, even fatal.

Oxygen is the mainstay of treatment for people who are exposed to gases. If lung damage is severe, a person may need mechanical ventilation.▲ Drugs that open the airways (bronchodilators), intravenous fluids, and antibiotics may be helpful. Corticosteroids such as prednisone are often prescribed to reduce inflammation in the lungs.

CHAPTER 50

Infiltrative Lung Diseases

Several diseases with similar symptoms result from abnormal infiltration of inflammatory cells into lung tissue. Early in the course of these infiltrative lung diseases, inflammatory cells (white blood cells and macrophages) and protein-rich fluid accumulate in the air sacs of the lungs (alveoli), in the walls of alveoli, and in the spaces between the alveoli (the interstitial space), causing inflammation (alveolitis). If the inflammation persists, the fluid may solidify and scarring (fibrosis) may replace lung tissue.

As alveoli are progressively destroyed, thick-walled cysts (called honeycombing because they resemble the hexagonal cells of a beehive) are left in their place. The condition resulting from these changes is called pulmonary fibrosis. Many diseases can cause pulmonary fibrosis, especially those that involve abnormalities of the immune system.

Although experts in pulmonary medicine think of infiltrative lung diseases separately, they often have similar features. All lead to a decreased ability to transfer oxygen to the blood and all cause stiffening and shrinkage of the lungs, which makes breathing difficult.

However, the elimination of carbon dioxide from the blood is usually not a problem.

Idiopathic Pulmonary Fibrosis

Idiopathic pulmonary fibrosis is a specific form of pulmonary fibrosis; the cause is unknown.

In about half of the people who have pulmonary fibrosis, the cause is never identified. These people are said to have idiopathic pulmonary fibrosis. The word *idiopathic* means "of unknown cause."

In idiopathic pulmonary fibrosis, the lungs suffer repeated episodes of injury for a long period of time. The injury causes chronic inflammation that eventually leads to pulmonary fibrosis.

Symptoms and Diagnosis

Symptoms depend on the extent of the lung damage, the rate at which the disease progresses, and the development of complications, such as lung infections and cor pul-

▲ see page 326

Causes of Infiltrative Lung Disease

- Autoimmune diseases (rheumatoid arthritis, scleroderma, polymyositis and dermatomyositis, mixed connective tissue disease, relapsing polychondritis, systemic lupus erythematosus)
- Infection (viruses, rickettsias, mycoplasmas, fungi, disseminated tuberculosis)
- Mineral dust (silica, carbon, metal dusts, asbestos)
- Organic dust (molds, bird droppings)
- Gases, fumes, and vapors (chlorine, sulfur dioxide)
- Therapeutic or industrial radiation
- Drugs and poisons (methotrexate, busulfan, cyclophosphamide, gold, penicillamine, nitrofurantoin, sulfonamides, amiodarone, paraquat)

monale.▲ The main symptoms start insidiously as shortness of breath on exertion, cough, and diminished stamina. Common symptoms include weight loss and fatigue. In most people, symptoms worsen over several years.

Late in the disease, as the level of oxygen in the blood decreases, the skin may take on a bluish tinge (called cyanosis), and the ends of the fingers may become thick or club-shaped.■ Strain on the heart may cause the right ventricle to enlarge, eventually resulting in cor pulmonale. Through a stethoscope, a doctor often hears crackling sounds. These sounds are called Velcro crackles or rales, described as such because the sound is similar to that of Velcro when it is pulled apart.

A chest x-ray may show widespread tiny white lines, often in a netlike pattern, most profuse in the lower parts of both lungs. Computed tomography (CT) is more sensitive than a chest x-ray for detecting disease early and helps the doctor make a more specific diagnosis. Typically the CT shows a pattern of patchy, white lines in the lower lungs. In areas of more severe involvement, the thick scarring often creates a honeycombing appearance. Pulmonary function tests ★ show that the amount of air the lungs can hold is below normal. Analysis of a blood sample shows a

low level of oxygen with minimal exercise (walking at a normal pace) and, as the disease progresses, even when the person is resting.

To confirm the diagnosis, a doctor may perform a lung biopsy (removal of a small piece of lung tissue for microscopic examination) using a procedure called bronchoscopy.● Many times, a larger tissue specimen is needed and must be removed surgically, sometimes with use of a thoracoscope.◆

Blood tests cannot confirm the diagnosis but are performed as part of the search for other diseases that may cause a similar pattern of inflammation and scarring. Doctors perform other blood tests to screen for certain autoimmune disorders.

Doctors may also perform other tests (for example, an electrocardiogram or echocardiogram) to identify if any changes in the heart have resulted from the lung disease.

Treatment and Prognosis

If a chest x-ray or lung biopsy shows that scarring is not extensive, the usual treatment is a corticosteroid, such as prednisone. A doctor evaluates the person's response using chest x-rays, CT, and pulmonary function tests. High doses of prednisone are usually given for about 3 months; then the dose is gradually reduced for another 3 months. Much lower doses are then continued for 6 more months. A few people who are not helped by prednisone may improve with azathioprine or cyclophosphamide. Unfortunately, treatment with corticosteroids fails to help most people. One promising treatment is interferon gamma-1b, which appears to block scar formation in the lungs.

Other treatments are aimed at relieving symptoms: oxygen therapy for low blood oxygen levels, antibiotics for infection, and drugs for the heart failure that is produced by cor pulmonale. Lung transplantation (often with a single lung) has been successful in some people with severe idiopathic pulmonary fibrosis.

The prognosis varies greatly. Most people continue to get worse. On average, people live 4 to 6 years after diagnosis. Some survive for many years; a few die within several months.

Desquamative Interstitial Pneumonia

Desquamative interstitial pneumonia is chronic lung inflammation that occurs in current or former cigarette smokers.

▲ see box on page 323   ■ see art on page 253

★ see page 254   ● see page 257

◆ see page 258

Although the word "pneumonia" is used, there is no evidence that an infection causes the inflammation. The condition affects cigarette smokers in their 30s and 40s, with most people developing breathlessness with even minimal exertion.

A chest x-ray shows less severe changes than in idiopathic pulmonary fibrosis and may show no changes in up to 10% of people. Pulmonary function tests show a decline in the amount of air contained in the lungs at the end of a person's strongest effort to breathe in (maximal inspiration). The amount of oxygen in a blood sample is low.

A lung biopsy is often needed to confirm the diagnosis and usually shows a distinctive pattern of diffuse and uniform lung inflammation. The most striking feature is the presence of numerous macrophages (cells that clear the alveoli of small inhaled particles and bacteria) within most of the smallest airways (bronchioles) and the alveoli.

About 70% of people who have desquamative interstitial pneumonia survive for 10 years or longer; the response is even better when the person stops smoking and takes corticosteroids.

Lymphoid Interstitial Pneumonia

Lymphoid interstitial pneumonia is an uncommon lung disease in which mature lymphocytes (a type of white blood cell) accumulate in the alveoli and in the spaces between alveoli.

Lymphoid interstitial pneumonia occurs in children but rarely in adults. About one fourth of cases occur in people with Sjögren's syndrome.▲ Lymphoid interstitial pneumonia also may develop in children and adults with HIV infection. The disease progresses slowly but may lead to the formation of cysts in the lungs and to lymphoma. Lymphoid interstitial pneumonia is sometimes relieved by corticosteroids.

Cryptogenic Organizing Pneumonitis

Cryptogenic organizing pneumonitis (also called idiopathic bronchiolitis obliterans with organizing pneumonia) is a rapidly developing pneumonia-like illness characterized by lung inflammation and scarring that obstruct the small airways and air sacs of the lungs (alveoli).

The cause of cryptogenic organizing pneumonitis is unknown. The disease usually begins between the ages of 40 and 60 and affects men and women equally.

Almost 75% of people have symptoms for less than two months before seeking medical attention. A flu-like illness, with a cough, fever, a feeling of illness (malaise), fatigue, and weight loss heralds the onset in about 40% of people.

Doctors do not find any specific abnormalities on routine laboratory tests or on a physical examination, except for the frequent presence of crackling sounds (called Velcro crackles) when the doctor listens with a stethoscope. Pulmonary function tests usually show that the amount of air the lungs can hold is below normal. The amount of oxygen in the blood is often low at rest and is even lower with exercise.

The chest x-ray is distinctive with features that appear similar to an extensive pneumonia, with both lungs showing widespread white patches. The white patches may seem to migrate from one area of the lung to another as the disease persists or progresses. Computed tomography (CT) may be used to confirm the diagnosis. Often, the findings are typical enough to allow the doctor to make a diagnosis without ordering additional tests.

To confirm the diagnosis, a doctor may perform a lung biopsy using a bronchoscope.■ Many times, a larger specimen is needed and must be removed surgically. About two thirds of people recover with corticosteroid therapy.

Langerhans' Cell Granulomatosis

Langerhans' cell granulomatosis (histiocytosis X) is a group of disorders (Letterer-Siwe disease, Hand-Schüller-Christian disease, pulmonary histiocytosis X) in which cells called histiocytes and eosinophils proliferate, especially in the bone and lung, often causing scarring.

The cause of these disorders is not known. They all start with infiltration of the lung (and other tissues) by histiocytes, which are cells that scavenge for foreign materials, and to a lesser extent by eosinophils, which are cells that are normally involved in allergic reactions.

▲ see page 382   ■ see page 257

Letterer-Siwe disease starts before age 3 and is usually fatal without treatment. The histiocytes damage not only the lungs but also the skin, lymph glands, bones, liver, and spleen. A small portion of the lung may rupture into the pleural space (a condition called pneumothorax).▲

Hand-Schüller-Christian disease usually begins in early childhood but can start in late middle age. The lungs and bones are most frequently affected. Rarely, damage to the pituitary gland causes diabetes insipidus,■ a condition in which large quantities of urine are produced, leading to dehydration. Some people develop bulging eyes (exophthalmos) because the bones of the eye sockets are affected.

Pulmonary histiocytosis X (eosinophilic granuloma) is a rare, smoking-related lung disease. The disease occurs more often in men than in women. Symptoms usually start between the ages of 20 and 40. About 16% of people have no symptoms, but the rest develop coughing, shortness of breath, fever, chest pain, and weight loss. Pneumothorax is a common complication due to rupture of a lung cyst. Scarring makes the lungs stiff and impairs their ability to transfer oxygen into and out of the blood.

Diagnosis

Chest x-rays show nodules, small lung cysts (honeycombing), and other changes that are typical of these diseases. X-rays may also show that the bones are affected. Pulmonary function tests show reduced function. Coughing up of blood (hemoptysis) and diabetes insipidus are rare complications.

Prognosis and Treatment

People with Hand-Schüller-Christian disease may recover spontaneously. Most people with pulmonary histiocytosis X have persistent or progressive disease. Death usually results from respiratory failure or cor pulmonale,★ although when people with pulmonary histiocytosis X stop smoking, improvement occurs in about one third of cases.

All three disorders may be treated with corticosteroids and immunosuppressant drugs such as cyclophosphamide, although no therapy is

clearly beneficial. The treatment for affected bones is similar to that for bone tumors.●

Sarcoidosis

Sarcoidosis is a disease in which abnormal collections of inflammatory cells (granulomas) form in many organs of the body.

The cause of sarcoidosis is unknown. It may result from an infection or from an abnormal response of the immune system. Inherited factors may be important. Sarcoidosis develops predominantly between the ages of 20 and 40 and is most common among Swedes and American blacks, although it can occur in anyone.

Sarcoidosis is characterized by the presence of collections of inflammatory cells (granulomas). The disease is primarily one of the lungs, but granulomas also form in the lymph nodes, lungs, liver, eyes, and skin, and less often in the spleen, bones, joints, skeletal muscles, kidneys, heart, and nervous system. The granulomas may eventually disappear completely or become scar tissue.

Symptoms

Many people with sarcoidosis have no symptoms, and the disease is discovered during a chest x-ray that is taken for other reasons. Most people develop minor symptoms that do not progress. Serious symptoms are rare.

The symptoms of sarcoidosis vary greatly according to the site and extent of the disease. Fever, fatigue, vague chest pain, a feeling of illness (malaise), weight loss, and aching joints may be the first indications of a problem in about one third of people. Enlarged lymph nodes are common but do not often cause symptoms. Fever and night sweats may recur throughout the illness.

The organ most affected by sarcoidosis is the lung. Enlarged lymph nodes at the place where the lungs meet the heart or to the right of the windpipe (trachea) may be seen on a chest x-ray. Sarcoidosis produces inflammation in the lungs that may eventually lead to scarring and the formation of cysts, which can cause coughing and shortness of breath. Fortunately, such progressive scarring occurs infrequently. Severe lung disease can eventually weaken the right side of the heart (cor pulmonale◆).

The skin is frequently affected by sarcoidosis. In Europeans, sarcoidosis often starts as raised, tender, red lumps, usually on the shins

---

▲ see page 316 ■ see page 944

★ see box on page 323 ● see page 359

◆ see box on page 323

(erythema nodosum▲), accompanied by a fever and joint pain, but this is less common in the United States. Prolonged sarcoidosis may lead to the formation of flat patches (plaques), raised patches, or lumps just under the skin with discoloration of the nose, cheeks, lips, and ears (lupus pernio). Lupus pernio is most common in black women.

About 70% of people with sarcoidosis have granulomas in their liver. These granulomas often produce no symptoms, and the liver seems to function normally. Fewer than 10% of people with sarcoidosis have an enlarged liver. Jaundice caused by liver malfunction is rare. The spleen also enlarges.

The eyes are affected in 15% of people with sarcoidosis. Inflammation of certain internal eye structures (uveitis) makes the eyes red and painful and interferes with vision. Inflammation that persists for a long time may block fluid from draining from the eye, causing glaucoma,■ which can lead to blindness. Granulomas may form in the conjunctiva (the membrane over the eyeball and inside the eyelids). Such granulomas often do not cause symptoms, but the conjunctiva is an accessible site from which a doctor can take tissue samples for examination. Some people with sarcoidosis complain of dry, sore, and red eyes, probably caused by sluggish tear glands that have been affected by the disease and no longer produce enough tears to keep the eyes lubricated.

Granulomas that form in the heart may cause chest pain (angina) or heart failure. Those granulomas that form near the heart's electrical conducting system can trigger potentially fatal irregularities in the heartbeat.

Inflammation can cause widespread pain in the joints. The joints in the hands and feet are most commonly affected. Cysts form in the bones and can make nearby joints swollen and tender.

Sarcoidosis can affect the cranial nerves (nerves of the head), causing double vision and making one side of the face droop. If the pituitary gland or the bones surrounding it are affected, diabetes insipidus★ may result. The pituitary gland stops producing vasopressin, a hormone needed by the kidney to concentrate urine, causing frequent urination and excessive amounts of urine.

Sarcoidosis can cause high levels of calcium to accumulate in the blood and urine. These high levels occur because sarcoid granulomas produce activated vitamin D, which enhances calcium absorption from the intestine. High blood calcium levels lead to a loss of appetite, nausea, vomiting, thirst, and excessive urine production. If present for a long time, high blood calcium levels may lead to the formation of kidney stones or calcium deposits in the kidney and, eventually, to kidney failure.

Diagnosis

Doctors most often diagnose sarcoidosis by observing its distinctive changes, including enlarged lymph nodes and a hazy, ground-glass appearance of lung tissue on a chest x-ray or on computed tomography (CT). When further testing is necessary, microscopic examination of a tissue specimen showing inflammation and granulomas confirms the diagnosis. Bronchoscopy with transbronchial lung biopsy is the best procedure for most people. Other possible sources of tissue specimens are skin abnormalities, enlarged lymph nodes close to the skin, and granulomas on the conjunctiva. Examination of a specimen from one of these tissues is accurate in 87% of cases. A liver biopsy is rarely needed even if there is evidence that the liver is affected.

Tuberculosis can cause many changes similar to those caused by sarcoidosis. Therefore, a doctor also performs a tuberculin skin test (and sometimes a lung biopsy) to make sure the problem is not tuberculosis.

Other methods that can help a doctor diagnose sarcoidosis or assess its severity include measuring the level of angiotensin-converting enzyme (ACE) in the blood, irrigating the lungs and examining the fluid, and using a whole-body gallium scan. In many people with sarcoidosis, the level of angiotensin-converting enzyme in the blood is high. The washings from a lung with active sarcoidosis contain a large number of lymphocytes, but this is not unique to sarcoidosis. Because gallium scanning shows abnormal patterns in the lungs or lymph nodes of a person with sarcoidosis in those places, this test is sometimes used when the diagnosis is uncertain.

In people with lung scarring, pulmonary function tests may show that the amount of air the lung can hold is below normal. Blood tests may reveal a low number of white blood cells or platelets. Immunoglobulin levels are often high, especially in blacks. The levels of

▲ see page 1200   ■ see page 1306

★ see page 944

liver enzymes, particularly alkaline phosphatase, may be high if the liver is affected.

Prognosis

Sarcoidosis improves or clears up spontaneously in nearly two thirds of people with lung sarcoidosis. Even enlarged lymph nodes in the chest and extensive lung inflammation may disappear in a few months or years. The course can be chronic or progressive in 10 to 30% of people. Serious involvement outside of the chest (for example, of the heart, nervous system, eyes, or liver) occurs in 4 to 7% of people at the beginning of their illness; the chance of involvement outside of the chest increases if lung disease persists.

People who have sarcoidosis that has not spread beyond the chest do better than those who also have sarcoidosis elsewhere in the body. People with enlarged lymph nodes in the chest but no sign of lung disease have a very good prognosis. Those whose disease began with erythema nodosum have the best prognosis. About 50% of people who once had sarcoidosis have relapses.

About 10% of people with sarcoidosis develop a serious disability from damage to the eyes, respiratory system, or elsewhere. Lung scarring leading to respiratory failure, and cor pulmonale is the most common cause of death, followed by bleeding from lung infection caused by the fungus *Aspergillus*. This fungus tends to grow in the lung cysts that develop in patients with progressive, chronic lung sarcoidosis.

Treatment

Most people with sarcoidosis do not need treatment. Corticosteroids are given to suppress severe symptoms such as shortness of breath, joint pain, and fever. These drugs also are given if tests show high levels of calcium in the blood; if the heart, liver, or nervous system is affected; if the sarcoidosis causes disfiguring skin lesions or eye disease that corticosteroid eyedrops fail to cure; or if lung disease continues to worsen. People who have no symptoms should not take corticosteroids. Although corticosteroids control symptoms well, they do not prevent lung scarring over the years. About 10% of those who need treatment fail to respond to corticosteroids and are

switched to chlorambucil or methotrexate, which may be very effective. Hydroxychloroquine is sometimes helpful in eliminating disfiguring skin lesions.

The success of treatment can be monitored with chest x-rays, CT, pulmonary function tests, and measurements of calcium or angiotensin-converting enzyme levels in the blood. These tests are repeated regularly to detect relapses after treatment stops.

Pulmonary Alveolar Proteinosis

Pulmonary alveolar proteinosis is a rare disease in which the air sacs of the lungs (alveoli) become plugged with a protein-rich fluid.

The disease generally affects people between the ages of 20 and 60 who have not previously had lung disease. The cause of pulmonary alveolar proteinosis is unknown. Occasionally, it is related to exposure to toxic substances, such as inorganic dusts, infection with *Pneumocystis carinii*,▲ certain cancers, and immunosuppressant drugs.

The protein in the lungs plugs up the alveoli and small airways. In rare instances, lung tissue becomes scarred. The disease may progress, remain stable, or disappear spontaneously.

Symptoms and Diagnosis

When the alveoli are plugged up, the transfer of oxygen to the blood from the lungs is severely impaired. Consequently, most people with pulmonary alveolar proteinosis experience shortness of breath when they exert themselves. Some have severe difficulty breathing, even at rest. Most also have a cough that does not usually produce sputum unless they are smokers. People often have severe disability from inadequate lung function. Lung infections may quickly worsen symptoms of shortness of breath and produce fever.

A chest x-ray shows extensive dense white patches in both lungs, usually located centrally near the heart. Computed tomography (CT) shows similar and other changes that suggest the disease. Pulmonary function tests■ reveal that the volume of air that the lungs can hold is abnormally small. Tests show low levels of oxygen in the blood, at first only during exercise but later also at rest. Even breathing pure oxygen results in well below the expected level of oxygen in the blood. Blood test results are not specific, although levels of some substances (for example, lactic

---

▲ see page 271   ■ see page 254

UNUSUAL INFILTRATIVE LUNG DISEASES

CONDITION	SYMPTOMS	TREATMENT	COMMENTS
Drug-induced interstitial lung disease	The onset of illness may be slow, over weeks to months, or may be abrupt and severe Shortness of breath, cough	Discontinuation of the offending drug (eg, a chemotherapeutic agent, antibiotic, amiodarone, over-the-counter medications, oily nose drops or petroleum products, and supplements) The addition of corticosteroids is effective in some cases	Many classes of drugs may cause disease Lung disease may occur weeks to years after the drug has been discontinued The disease is often more severe in older people A syndrome of drug-induced lupus (manifested in the lung) can be seen The extent and severity of the disease is sometimes related to the dose of the drug, but not always
Alveolar hemorrhage syndromes (iron in the lungs)	Most common symptom is the coughing up of blood (hemoptysis)	Corticosteroids and cytotoxic drugs, such as azathioprine may help during flare-ups Blood transfusions may be needed for blood loss Oxygen therapy may be needed for a low level of oxygen in the blood	Rare disease in which blood leaks from the capillaries into the lungs for unknown reasons The condition is associated with Goodpasture's syndrome; Wegener's granulomatosis; systemic lupus erythematosus; idiopathic pulmonary hemosiderosis; drug reactions Excessive blood loss leads to anemia; massive bleeding can cause death Kidney failure may occur because of glomerulonephritis
Chronic, recurrent aspiration pneumonitis	Difficulty swallowing, cough, especially at night	Discontinuation of the offending agent (eg, mineral oil); corticosteroids; tube feedings	Associated with gastroesophageal disorders, neurologic disease, use of sedatives Use of mineral oil at bedtime to prevent constipation or use of petroleum-based products (eg, Vaseline) to lubricate nasal passages increases the risk
Respiratory bronchiolitis-associated interstitial lung disease	Similar to those of desquamative interstitial pneumonia (see text)	Quitting smoking is important	Most often occurs in current or former cigarette smokers

dehydrogenase [LDH] and gamma globulin levels) are often elevated.

To make a definitive diagnosis, a doctor examines a sample of the fluid from the alveoli. To obtain a sample, a doctor uses a bronchoscope▲ to wash segments of the lung with a salt solution and then collects the washings. Sometimes a doctor performs a lung biopsy (obtains a lung tissue sample for microscopic examination) during bronchoscopy. Occasionally, a larger specimen is needed, which must be removed surgically.

Treatment

People who have few or no symptoms do not require treatment. For those with disabling symptoms, the protein-rich fluid in the alveoli can be washed out with a salt solution during bronchoscopy or through a special tube inserted through the mouth into or through the windpipe (trachea). Sometimes only a small section of the lung must be washed, but if symptoms are severe and the levels of oxygen in the blood are very low, the person is given general anesthesia, so that one entire lung can be washed. About 3 to 5 days later, the other lung is washed, again with the person under general anesthesia. One washing is enough for some people, while others need washings every 6 to 12 months for many years.

The usefulness of other treatments, such as potassium iodide and enzymes that break up proteins, is unclear. Corticosteroids, such as prednisone, are not effective and may actually increase the chance of infection. Bacterial infections are treated with antibiotics, usually taken by mouth.

Some people with pulmonary alveolar proteinosis are short of breath indefinitely, but the disease is rarely fatal as long as they have regular lung washings.

CHAPTER 51

Allergic Diseases of the Lungs

The lungs are particularly prone to allergic reactions because they are exposed to large quantities of airborne substances that commonly cause allergic reactions (called antigens), including dusts, pollens, fungi, and chemicals. Exposure to irritating dusts or airborne substances, often when a person is at work, may increase the likelihood of an allergic respiratory reaction. Allergic reactions involving the lungs may also occur from eating a certain food or taking a certain drug.

The body reacts to an antigen by forming proteins that react with antigens (antibodies). Antibodies typically bind to an antigen (such as a fungus), thereby rendering it harmless in an immune response.■ Sometimes, however, when the antibody and antigen interact, inflammation and tissue damage occur; this is called an allergic reaction. Allergic reactions are classified by the mechanisms that are involved in causing the tissue damage. Many allergic reactions involve a combination of more than one type of tissue damage. Some allergic reactions depend on antigen-specific lymphocytes (a type of white blood cell) rather than on antibodies. Reactions are typically categorized as type I, II, III, or IV.

Hypersensitivity Pneumonitis

Hypersensitivity pneumonitis (extrinsic allergic alveolitis, allergic interstitial pneumonitis, organic dust pneumoconiosis) is inflammation in and around the tiny air sacs (alveoli) and smallest airways (bronchioles) of the lung caused by an allergic reaction to inhaled organic dusts or, less commonly, chemicals.

Causes

Many types of dust can cause allergic reactions in the lungs. Organic dusts that contain

---

▲ see page 256   ■ see also page 1049

microorganisms or proteins and chemicals, such as isocyanates, may cause hypersensitivity pneumonitis. Farmer's lung, which results from repeated inhalation of heat-loving (thermophilic) bacteria in moldy hay, is a well-known example of hypersensitivity pneumonitis. Air conditioner lung is another example; it occurs when contaminated humidifiers or air conditioners (especially large systems in office buildings) circulate antigens that are capable of causing a hypersensitivity reaction.

Only a small number of people who inhale these common dusts develop allergic reactions, and only a small percentage of those people who develop allergic reactions suffer irreversible damage to the lungs. Generally, a person must be exposed to large amounts of these antigens continuously or frequently over time before sensitivity and resultant disease develop.

Lung damage appears to result from a combination of immune complex reactions and cell-mediated allergic reactions. Initial exposures to the dusts sensitize lymphocytes. Some lymphocytes then help to produce antibodies that play a role in tissue damage. Other lymphocytes participate directly in inflammation after subsequent antigen exposure. Recurrent exposure to the antigen results in a chronic inflammatory response, which is manifested by a buildup of white blood cells in the walls of the alveoli and small airways. This buildup leads progressively to symptoms and disease.

Symptoms and Diagnosis

If a person has developed hypersensitivity to an organic dust, then fever, cough, chills, and shortness of breath typically appear 4 to 8 hours after reexposure to it. Wheezing is unusual. If the person has no further contact with the antigen, symptoms usually improve over a day or two, but complete recovery may take weeks.

In a slower form of hypersensitivity pneumonitis (subacute form), cough and shortness of breath may develop over days or weeks and sometimes may be so severe that the person needs to be hospitalized.

With chronic hypersensitivity pneumonitis, a person repeatedly comes in contact with an allergen over months to years, and lung scarring (fibrosis) may result. Shortness of breath during exercise, coughing up of sputum, fatigue, and weight loss may gradually progress

WHAT CAUSES HYPERSENSITIVITY PNEUMONITIS?

DISEASE	SOURCE OF DUST PARTICLES OR ANTIGENS
Farmer's lung	Moldy hay
Bird fancier's lung, pigeon breeder's lung, hen worker's lung	Droppings from parakeets, pigeons, chickens
Air conditioner lung	Humidifiers, air conditioners
Bagassosis	Sugarcane
Mushroom worker's lung	Mushroom compost
Cork worker's lung (suberosis)	Moldy cork
Maple bark stripper's lung	Infected maple bark
Malt worker's lung	Moldy barley or malt
Sequoiosis	Moldy sawdust from redwoods
Cheese washer's lung	Cheese mold
Miller's lung	Weevil-infested wheat flour
Coffee worker's lung	Unroasted coffee beans
Woodworker's lung	Wood dust
Chemical worker's lung	Chemicals used in manufacturing polyurethane foam, molding, insulation, synthetic rubber, and packaging materials

over months or years. Eventually, the disease may lead to respiratory failure.▲

The diagnosis of hypersensitivity pneumonitis depends on the clinical features, identification (if possible) of the dust or other substance causing the problem, and evidence of the person's exposure to the suspected agent, as determined by the presence of antibodies on a blood test.

Doctors may suspect the diagnosis based on finding something abnormal on a chest x-ray. Results of pulmonary function tests■—which measure the lungs' capacity to hold air and their ability to move air in and out and to ex-

▲ see page 325　　■ see page 254

change oxygen and carbon dioxide—may help support a diagnosis of hypersensitivity pneumonitis. Blood tests for antibodies may show that the person has been exposed to the suspected antigen. When the antigen cannot be identified and the diagnosis is in doubt, re-exposing the recovered person to the allergen and observing the person for symptoms or changes in lung function may occasionally be useful to confirm the diagnosis. Lung function can be determined using pulmonary function testing.

In cases that are not clear, especially when an infection is suspected, doctors may remove a small piece of lung tissue for examination under a microscope (lung biopsy). They may remove the tissue while examining the airways using a viewing tube (bronchoscopy▲). Sometimes, rather than (or in addition to) removing tissue using a sharp instrument, the person performing bronchoscopy may wash out the lung with fluid (bronchoalveolar lavage) to extract cells for examination. Rarely, an examination of the lung surface and pleural space using a viewing tube (thoracoscopy) or an operation in which the chest wall is opened (thoracotomy) may be needed.■

Prevention and Treatment

The best prevention is to avoid exposure to the antigen, but this may be impractical if the person cannot change jobs. Eliminating or reducing dust or wearing protective masks may help prevent a recurrence. Chemically treating hay or sugarcane waste and using good ventilation systems help to minimize exposure to the antigen, which may prevent workers from initially becoming sensitized to these materials.

People who have an acute episode of hypersensitivity pneumonitis usually recover if further contact with the substance is avoided. If the episode is severe, corticosteroids, such as prednisone, reduce symptoms and may help reduce severe inflammation. Prolonged or recurring episodes may lead to irreversible disease and progressive disability.

Eosinophilic Pneumonia

Eosinophilic pneumonia (also called pulmonary infiltrates with eosinophilia syndrome) comprises a group of lung diseases in which eosinophils (a type of white blood cell) appear in increased numbers in the lungs and usually in the bloodstream.

Eosinophils participate in the immune response of the lung. The number of eosinophils increases during many inflammatory and allergic reactions, including asthma, which frequently accompanies certain types of eosinophilic pneumonia. Unlike typical pneumonias caused by bacteria, viruses, and most fungi, the tiny air sacs of the lungs (alveoli) are not infected in people with eosinophilic pneumonia. However, the alveoli and often the airways do fill with eosinophils. Even the blood vessel walls may be invaded by eosinophils, and the narrowed airways may become plugged with an accumulation of secretions (mucus) if asthma develops.

The exact reason that eosinophils build up in the lungs is not well understood, and often it is not possible to identify the substance that is causing the allergic reaction. However, there are some known causes of eosinophilic pneumonia, including certain drugs (penicillin, aminosalicylic acid, carbamazepine, naproxen, isoniazid, nitrofurantoin, chlorpropamide, and sulfonamides [such as trimethoprim-sulfamethoxazole]); chemical fumes (nickel inhaled as a vapor); fungi (*Aspergillus fumigatus*); and parasites (roundworms, including nematodes).

Symptoms and Diagnosis

Symptoms may be mild or life threatening. Simple eosinophilic pneumonia (Löffler's syndrome) and similar pneumonias (such as tropical eosinophilia, which is due to infestation by several species of filariae—types of nematode worms) may produce a slight fever and mild respiratory symptoms, if any. A person may cough, wheeze, and feel short of breath but usually recovers quickly. Another disease known as acute eosinophilic pneumonia may cause the level of oxygen in the blood to decrease severely; it can progress to acute respiratory failure in a few hours or days if not treated.

Chronic eosinophilic pneumonia, which slowly progresses over weeks to months, is a distinct disorder that may also become severe. Life-threatening shortness of breath can develop if the condition is not treated.

With acute eosinophilic pneumonia, tests show large numbers of eosinophils in the blood, sometimes as many as 10 to 15 times the normal number. However, with chronic

▲ see page 256   ■ see page 258

eosinophilic pneumonia, the numbers of eosinophils in the blood may be normal.

A chest x-ray usually shows white patches in the lungs that are characteristic of pneumonia. However, unlike pneumonia caused by bacteria or viruses, acute eosinophilic pneumonias typically show rapidly appearing and disappearing patches when x-rays are repeated. In contrast, the chest x-ray in chronic eosinophilic pneumonia shows persistent patches located mainly in the outer zones of the lungs.

Microscopic examination of coughed-up sputum or washings of the alveoli obtained during bronchoscopy typically shows clumps of eosinophils. Other laboratory tests may be performed to search for an infection with fungi or parasites; these tests may include microscopic examination of stool specimens. A doctor also considers whether any drug the person is taking may be the cause.

Prognosis and Treatment

Eosinophilic pneumonia may be mild, and people with the disease may get better without treatment. For acute cases, a corticosteroid such as prednisone is usually needed. In chronic eosinophilic pneumonia, prednisone may be needed for many months or even years. If a person develops wheezing, the same treatments used for asthma are given as well.▲ If worms or other parasites are the cause, the person is treated with appropriate drugs. Ordinarily, drugs that may be causing the illness are discontinued.

Allergic Bronchopulmonary Aspergillosis

Allergic bronchopulmonary aspergillosis is an allergic lung disorder that often mimics pneumonia and is characterized by asthma, airway and lung inflammation with eosinophils (a type of white blood cell), and increased numbers of eosinophils in the blood.

Allergic bronchopulmonary aspergillosis is caused by an allergic reaction to a fungus, most commonly *Aspergillus fumigatus*. This fungus flourishes in soil, decaying vegetation, foods, dusts, and water. A person who inhales the fungus may become sensitized and develop allergic asthma. Other fungi, including *Penicillium, Candida, Curvularia,* and *Helminthosporium,* can cause an identical illness. In some people, a more complex allergic reaction can develop in the airways and lungs.

The disorder differs from typical pneumonias caused by bacteria, viruses, and most fungi, in that the fungus does not actually invade the lungs or directly destroy tissue. The fungus does colonize the asthmatic mucus in the airways and causes recurrent allergic inflammation in the lung. The tiny air sacs of the lungs (alveoli) become packed primarily with eosinophils. Increased numbers of mucus-producing cells may also appear. In advanced cases, inflammation may cause the central airways to widen permanently, a condition called bronchiectasis.■ Eventually, the lungs are likely to become scarred.

Other forms of aspergillosis can occur. *Aspergillus* can invade the lungs and cause serious pneumonia in people with an impaired immune system. This condition is an infection, not an allergic reaction. The fungus can also form a fungus ball, called an aspergilloma, in cavities and cysts of lungs already damaged by another disease, such as tuberculosis. The major consequence of such fungus balls is lung bleeding, often severe, which becomes apparent when the person coughs up blood and is short of breath.

Symptoms and Diagnosis

The first indications of allergic bronchopulmonary aspergillosis are usually progressive symptoms of asthma, such as wheezing and shortness of breath, and a mild fever. The person usually does not feel well. Brownish flecks or plugs may appear in coughed-up sputum.

Repeated chest x-rays show areas that look like pneumonia, but they move around, most often in the upper parts of the lungs. With long-standing disease, chest x-rays or computed tomography (CT) may show widened airways often plugged with mucus. The fungus itself, along with excess eosinophils, may be seen when the sputum is examined under the microscope. Blood tests reveal high levels of eosinophils and antibodies to *Aspergillus.* Skin testing can determine if the person is allergic to *Aspergillus,* but the test does not distinguish between allergic bronchopulmonary aspergillosis and a simple allergy to *Aspergillus,* which may occur in people who have allergic asthma without aspergillosis.

Treatment

Because *Aspergillus* appears in many places in the environment, the fungus is difficult to

▲ see page 276   ■ see page 289

avoid. Antiasthma drugs, especially corticosteroids, are used to treat allergic bronchopulmonary aspergillosis.▲ Antiasthma drugs also open up the airways, making it easier to cough up mucus plugs and clear out the fungus. The corticosteroid prednisone taken initially in high doses and over a long period of time in lower doses may prevent progressive lung damage. Most specialists recommend oral corticosteroids; the inhaled kind has not been shown to work well for this condition. The antifungal drug itraconazole may be helpful. Allergy shots (desensitization) may cause complications and are not recommended.

Because the lung damage may worsen without causing any noticeable symptoms, a doctor regularly monitors the person using chest x-rays, pulmonary function tests,■ and antibody measurements of immunoglobulin E (IgE) and other immunoglobulins. As the disease is controlled, the antibody levels usually fall, but they may rise again as an early sign of flare-ups.

Goodpasture's Syndrome

Goodpasture's syndrome is an uncommon autoimmune disorder in which bleeding into the lungs and progressive kidney failure occur.

This disease usually affects young men. For unknown reasons, people with Goodpasture's syndrome produce antibodies against certain parts of their own bodies, especially certain structures in the filtering apparatus of the kidneys and in the walls of the tiny air sacs (alveoli) and capillaries of the lungs. These antibodies trigger inflammation that interferes with kidney and lung function. Presumably, they are the direct cause of the disease.

Symptoms and Diagnosis

A person with this disease typically develops shortness of breath and coughs up blood. Symptoms can quickly become severe: Breathing can fail, and large amounts of blood can be lost. At the same time, the kidneys can rapidly fail. There may be small amounts of blood in the urine.

Laboratory tests reveal the characteristic antibodies in the blood. Urine examination reveals blood and protein in the urine. Anemia is often present. A chest x-ray shows abnormal white patches (due to lung bleeding) in both lungs. A kidney tissue needle biopsy shows microscopic deposits of antibodies in a specific pattern.

Treatment

The disease may very rapidly lead to a complete loss of kidney function or death. High doses of corticosteroids (such as prednisone) and cyclophosphamide may be given intravenously to suppress the activity of the immune system. The person may also undergo plasmapheresis—a procedure in which blood is removed from the circulation, the unwanted antibodies are removed from the blood, and the blood cells are returned to the circulation.★ The early use of this combination of treatments may help save kidney and lung function. Once damage occurs to the kidneys, it is usually permanent.

Many people may need supportive care until the disease runs its course. Treatment may require supplemental oxygen or being on a ventilator for a period of time. Blood transfusions may also be needed. If the kidneys fail, kidney dialysis or a kidney transplant may be required.

CHAPTER 52

Pleural Disorders

The pleura is a thin, transparent, two-layered membrane that covers the lungs and also lines the inside of the chest wall. The layer that covers the lungs lies in close contact with the layer that lines the chest wall. Between the two thin flexible layers is a small amount of fluid that lubricates them as they slide smoothly over one another with each breath.

In abnormal circumstances, air, blood, plasma (the liquid component of blood without cells), or lymph (a fluid containing white blood cells and fat) can get between the pleural

---

▲ see table on page 278   ■ see page 254
★ see box on page 986

Two Views of the Pleura

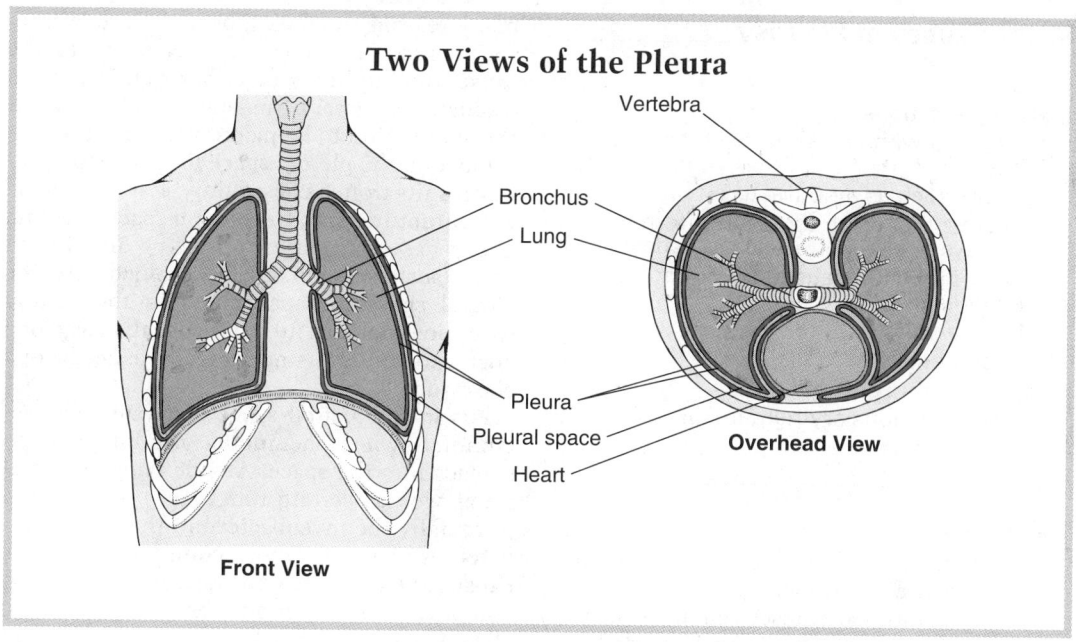

Vertebra

Bronchus

Lung

Pleura

Pleural space

Heart

Overhead View

Front View

surfaces, creating a space. If too much fluid accumulates (called pleural effusion), one or both lungs may not be able to expand normally with breathing, resulting in the collapse of lung tissue. Air in the pleural space (pneumothorax) can do the same.

Pleurisy

Pleurisy is inflammation of the pleura.

Pleurisy develops when something (usually a virus or bacterium) irritates the pleura, resulting in inflammation. Certain autoimmune diseases (such as systemic lupus erythematosus) can irritate the pleura. Pleurisy may also develop when cancer spreads from the lung or another part of the body to the pleura, irritating it. Inhalation of asbestos can also cause pleurisy, as can (rarely) the use of certain drugs, such as nitrofurantoin or procainamide. Fluid may accumulate in the pleural space (a condition called pleural effusion), or fluid may not accumulate (a condition called dry pleurisy). After the inflammation subsides, the pleura may return to normal, or adhesions may form that make the pleural layers stick together.

Symptoms and Diagnosis

The most common symptom of pleurisy is chest pain (pleuritic pain), which may begin

suddenly. The pain varies from vague discomfort to an intense stabbing pain. It may be felt only when the person breathes deeply or coughs, or it may be felt continuously but may be worsened by deep breathing and coughing. The pain results from inflammation of the outer layer of pleura and is usually felt in the chest wall right over the site of the inflammation. However, the pain may be felt also or only in the upper abdominal region or neck and shoulder as referred pain.▲

Breathing may be rapid and shallow because deep breathing induces pain; the muscles on the painful side move less than those on the other side. If a large amount of fluid accumulates, it may separate the pleural layers, so the chest pain disappears. Large amounts of fluid can cause difficulty in expanding one or both lungs when breathing, causing respiratory distress.

Pleurisy is often easy for doctors to diagnose because pleuritic pain is so distinctive. Using a stethoscope, a doctor may hear a squeaky to-and-fro rubbing sound, called a pleural rub. Even though a chest x-ray will not show pleurisy, it may reveal a small accumulation of fluid in the pleural space or give clues to a cause.

▲ see art on page 448

Major Causes of Pleurisy

- Cancer
- Drug reactions
- Infection with parasites, such as amebas
- Injury, such as a rib fracture
- Irritants that reach the pleura from the airways or elsewhere, such as asbestos
- Lung infarction caused by pulmonary embolism
- Pancreatitis
- Pneumonia
- Rheumatoid arthritis
- Systemic lupus erythematosus
- Tuberculosis

Treatment

The treatment of pleurisy depends on the particular cause. If the cause is a bacterial infection, antibiotics are prescribed. If the cause is a viral infection, no treatment is needed for the infection. If the cause is an autoimmune disease, such as systemic lupus erythematosus, treatment with corticosteroids often quickly cures the pleurisy.

A nonsteroidal anti-inflammatory drug (NSAID)▲ usually helps relieve the chest pain of pleurisy, regardless of its cause. Codeine and other opioids are stronger pain relievers, but they tend to suppress coughing, which is not a good idea because deep breathing and coughing help prevent lung collapse and subsequent pneumonia. Thus, a person with pleurisy is encouraged to breathe deeply and cough as soon as breathing becomes less painful. Coughing may be less painful if the person or a helper holds a pillow firmly against the part of the chest that hurts. Wrapping the entire chest in wide, nonadhesive elastic bandages may help relieve severe chest pain. However, binding the chest to reduce expansion during breathing increases the risk of lung collapse (atelectasis) and pneumonia.

Pleural Effusion

Pleural effusion is the abnormal accumulation of fluid in the pleural space.

Normally, only a thin layer of fluid separates the two layers of the pleura. An excessive amount of fluid may accumulate for many reasons, including heart failure, cirrhosis, pneumonia, and cancer. Depending on the cause, the fluid may be either rich in protein (exudate) or watery (transudate). Doctors use this distinction to help determine the cause.

Blood in the pleural space (**hemothorax**) usually results from a chest injury. Rarely, a blood vessel ruptures into the pleural space when no injury has occurred, or a bulging area in the aorta (aortic aneurysm) leaks blood into the pleural space. Because blood in the pleural space does not clot fully, it is usually easy for a doctor to remove using a large-bore needle or a chest tube.

Pus in the pleural space (**empyema**) can accumulate when pneumonia or a lung abscess spreads into the space. A wide range of bacteria as well as certain fungi and mycobacteria (especially the mycobacterium that causes tuberculosis) are the most common organisms causing pleural effusion. Empyema may also complicate an infection from chest wounds, chest surgery, rupture of the esophagus, or an abscess in the abdomen.

Milky fluid in the pleural space (**chylothorax**) is caused by an injury to the main lymphatic duct in the chest (thoracic duct) or by a blockage of the duct by a tumor.

High-cholesterol fluid in the pleural space results from a long-standing pleural effusion caused by a condition such as tuberculosis or rheumatoid arthritis.

Symptoms and Diagnosis

The most common symptoms, regardless of the type of fluid in the pleural space or its cause, are shortness of breath and chest pain. However, many people with pleural effusion have no symptoms at all.

A chest x-ray, which shows fluid in the pleural space, is usually the first step in making the diagnosis. Computed tomography (CT) more clearly shows the lung and the fluid and may show evidence of pneumonia, a lung abscess, or a tumor. An ultrasound may help a doctor determine the position of a small accumulation of fluid.

A specimen of the fluid is almost always removed for examination using a needle, a procedure called thoracentesis.■ The appearance of the fluid may help a doctor determine its cause. Certain laboratory tests evaluate the chemical composition of the fluid and determine the presence of bacteria, including the bacteria that cause tuberculosis. The fluid specimen is also examined for the number and

▲ see page 452   ■ see page 256

types of cells and for the presence of cancerous cells.

If these tests cannot identify the cause of the pleural effusion, a biopsy of the pleura may be needed,▲ which can detect cancer and tuberculosis. Using a biopsy needle, a doctor removes a sample of the outer layer of the pleura for analysis. If the specimen is too small for an accurate diagnosis, a tissue sample must be taken through a small incision in the chest wall, a procedure called an open pleural biopsy. Sometimes, a sample is obtained using a thoracoscope (a viewing tube that allows a doctor to examine the pleural space and obtain samples■).

Occasionally, bronchoscopy (a direct visual examination of the airways through a viewing tube) helps the doctor find the cause of the fluid. In about 20% of people with pleural effusion, the cause is not obvious after initial testing, and in some people a cause is never found, even after extensive testing.

Treatment

Small pleural effusions may require treatment of only the underlying cause. Larger pleural effusions, especially those that cause shortness of breath, may require drainage of the fluid. Usually, drainage dramatically relieves shortness of breath. Often, fluid can be drained using thoracentesis. An area of skin between two lower ribs is anesthetized, then a small needle is inserted and gently pushed deeper until it reaches the fluid. A thin plastic catheter is often guided over the needle into the fluid to lessen the chance of puncturing the lung and causing a pneumothorax. Although thoracentesis is usually performed for diagnostic purposes, a doctor can safely remove as much as 1.5 liters of fluid at a time using this procedure.

When larger amounts of fluid must be removed, a tube (chest tube) may be inserted through the chest wall. After numbing the area by injecting a local anesthetic, a doctor inserts a plastic tube into the chest between two ribs. Then the doctor connects the tube to a water-sealed drainage system that prevents air from leaking into the pleural space. A chest x-ray is taken to check the tube's position. Drainage can be blocked if the chest tube is incorrectly positioned or becomes kinked. If the fluid is very thick or full of clots, it may not flow out.

An accumulation of pus from an infection (empyema) requires intravenous antibiotics

Common Causes of Pleural Effusion

- Abscess under the diaphragm
- Cirrhosis
- Coccidioidomycosis and other fungal infections
- Drugs such as hydralazine, procainamide, isoniazid, phenytoin, chlorpromazine, nitrofurantoin, bromocriptine, dantrolene, procarbazine
- Heart failure
- Heart surgery
- Improper placement of feeding tubes or intravenous catheters
- Injury to the chest
- Low protein levels in the blood
- Pancreatitis
- Pneumonia
- Pulmonary embolus
- Rheumatoid arthritis
- Systemic lupus erythematosus
- Tuberculosis
- Tumors

and drainage of the fluid. Tuberculosis or fungal infections such as coccidioidomycosis require prolonged treatment with antibiotics or antifungal drugs. If the pus is very thick or if it has formed within fibrous compartments, drainage is more difficult. Sometimes drugs called fibrinolytics are instilled into the pleura space to help drainage, which may avoid the need for surgery. If surgery is needed, it can be performed by a procedure called video-assisted thorascopic debridement or by thoracotomy. During surgery, a thick peel of fibrous material is removed from the lung surface to allow the lung to expand normally.

Fluid accumulation caused by tumors of the pleura may be difficult to treat because fluid tends to reaccumulate rapidly. Draining the fluid and giving antitumor drugs sometimes prevents further fluid accumulation. But if fluid continues to accumulate, sealing the pleural space (pleurodesis) may be helpful. All fluid is drained through a tube, which is then used to administer a pleural irritant, such as a doxycycline solution or a talc mixture, into the space. The irritant seals the two layers of

▲ see page 256   ■ see page 256

What Is
Tension Pneumothorax?

Tension pneumothorax is a serious and potentially life-threatening form of pneumothorax. In this condition, the tissues surrounding the area where air is entering the pleural space act as a one-way valve, allowing air to enter but not to exit. This situation causes such high pressure in the pleural cavity that the lung completely collapses, and the heart and other structures in the chest cavity are pushed over to the opposite side of the chest.

If not relieved quickly, tension pneumothorax can cause death in minutes. A doctor immediately suctions out air through a large syringe attached to a needle inserted into the chest. Then, a tube is inserted separately to drain the air continuously.

pleura together, so that no room remains for additional fluid to accumulate.

If blood has entered the pleural space, usually drainage through a tube is all that is needed—as long as the bleeding has stopped. Drugs that help break up blood clots, such as streptokinase and urokinase, are occasionally administered through the drainage tube if a substantial portion of the clot remains in the pleural space. Caution should be taken because these drugs can trigger rebleeding. If the bleeding continues or if the accumulation of fluid cannot be removed adequately with a tube, surgery may be needed.

Treatment of chylothorax focuses on repairing the damage to the lymphatic duct. Such treatment may consist of surgery, chemotherapy, or radiation treatment for a cancer that is blocking lymph flow.

Pneumothorax

A pneumothorax is a pocket of air between the two layers of pleura, resulting in collapse of the lung.

Normally, the pressure in the pleural space is lower than that inside the lungs. If air enters the pleural space, the pressure in the pleural space becomes greater than that in the lungs, and the lung collapses partially or completely. Sometimes most or all of the lung collapses,

▲ see page 326

leading to immediate and severe shortness of breath.

A pneumothorax may occur for no identifiable reason; doctors call this a spontaneous pneumothorax. Spontaneous pneumothorax usually occurs when a small weakened area of lung (bulla) ruptures (primary spontaneous pneumothorax). The condition is most common in tall men younger than age 40. Most incidents of primary spontaneous pneumothorax do not occur during exertion. Some occur during diving or high-altitude flying, apparently because of pressure changes in the lungs. Most people recover fully; however, primary spontaneous pneumothorax recurs in about 30 to 50% of people regardless of the person's relation to sea level.

Spontaneous pneumothorax also occurs in people with extensive lung disease (secondary spontaneous pneumothorax). This type of pneumothorax most often results from the rupture of a bulla in older people who have emphysema, but it also occurs in people with other lung conditions, such as cystic fibrosis, Langerhans' cell granulomatosis, sarcoidosis, lung abscess, tuberculosis, and pneumocystis pneumonia. Because of the underlying lung disease, the symptoms and outcome are generally worse in secondary spontaneous pneumothorax; the recurrence rate is similar to that of primary spontaneous pneumothorax.

A pneumothorax may also follow an injury or a medical procedure that introduces air into the pleural space, such as thoracentesis. Ventilators can cause pressure damage to the lungs (barotrauma) that leads to a pneumothorax—most often in people with severe acute respiratory distress syndrome.▲

Symptoms and Diagnosis

Symptoms vary greatly depending on how much air enters the pleural space, how much of the lung collapses, and the person's lung function before the pneumothorax occurred. They range from a little shortness of breath or chest pain to severe shortness of breath, shock, and life-threatening cardiac arrest. Most often, sharp chest pain and shortness of breath and occasionally a dry hacking cough begin suddenly. Pain may also be felt in the shoulder, neck, or abdomen. Symptoms tend to be less severe in a slowly developing pneumothorax than in a rapidly developing one. Except with a very large pneumothorax or a tension pneumothorax, symptoms usually subside as the body adapts to the lung collapse, and the lung slowly begins to reinflate as the air is reabsorbed from the pleural space.

A physical examination can usually confirm the diagnosis if the pneumothorax is large. Using a stethoscope, a doctor may note that one part of the chest does not transmit the normal sounds of breathing, while tapping (percussing) the chest produces a hollow, drumlike sound. A chest x-ray shows the air pocket and the collapsed lung outlined by the thin inner pleural layer. A chest x-ray can also show if the trachea (the large airway that passes through the front of the neck) is being pushed to one side because of a collapsed lung.

Treatment

A small primary spontaneous pneumothorax usually requires no treatment. It usually does not cause serious breathing problems, and the air is absorbed in several days. The full absorption of air in a larger pneumothorax may take 2 to 4 weeks; however, the air can be removed more quickly by inserting a chest tube into the pneumothorax.

A chest tube is needed if the pneumothorax is large enough to impair breathing. The chest tube is inserted through an incision in the chest wall and is connected to a water-sealed drainage system or a one-way valve that al-

lows the air to exit without allowing any air to get back in. A suction pump may have to be attached to the chest tube if air keeps leaking in from an abnormal connection (fistula) between an airway and the pleural space. Occasionally, surgery is necessary. Often the surgery is performed using a thoracoscope inserted through the chest wall and into the pleural space.

A recurring pneumothorax can cause considerable disability. For people at high risk—for example, divers and airplane pilots—surgery is considered after the first episode of pneumothorax. Usually surgery involves repairing leaking areas of the lung and firmly attaching the inner layer of pleura to the outer layer. For people who have a pneumothorax that will not heal or a pneumothorax that has occurred twice on the same side, surgery, often using a thoracoscope, is performed to eliminate the cause of the problem. In secondary spontaneous pneumothorax with a persistent air leak into the pleural space or with a recurring pneumothorax, the underlying lung disease may make surgery hazardous. Often, the pleural space can be sealed by administering a talc mixture into the space or by giving the drug doxycycline through a chest tube that is draining air from the space.

CHAPTER 53

Cystic Fibrosis

Cystic fibrosis is a hereditary disease that causes certain glands to produce abnormal secretions, resulting in tissue and organ damage, especially in the lungs and the digestive tract.

Cystic fibrosis is the most common inherited disease leading to a shortened life span among white people in the United States. It occurs in about 1 of 3,300 white infants and in 1 of 15,300 black infants. It is rare in Asians. Cystic fibrosis is equally common in boys and girls.

Cystic fibrosis results when a person inherits two defective copies (mutations) of a particular gene. This gene controls the production of a protein that regulates the transport of

chloride and sodium (salt) across cell membranes. Worldwide, about 3 of 100 white people carry one defective copy of the gene; thus, they are carriers but they themselves do not get sick. About 3 of 10,000 white people inherit two defective copies of the gene; thus, they develop cystic fibrosis. In these people, chloride and sodium transport is disrupted and dehydration and increased stickiness of secretions occur.

Cystic fibrosis affects many organs throughout the body and nearly all the glands that secrete fluids into a duct (exocrine glands). The secretions are abnormal in different ways, and they affect gland function differently. In some glands, such as the pancreas, the secretions are

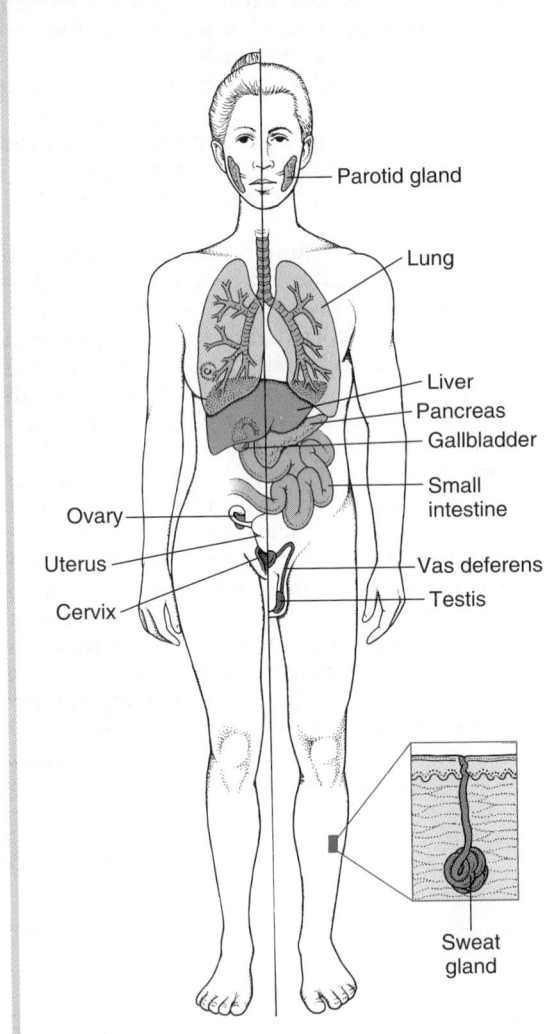

Parotid gland

Lung

Liver

Pancreas

Gallbladder

Small intestine

Ovary

Uterus

Vas deferens

Cervix

Testis

Sweat gland

Cystic Fibrosis: Not Just a Lung Disease

In the lungs, thick bronchial secretions block the small airways, which become inflamed. As the disease progresses, the bronchial walls thicken, the airways fill with infected secretions, areas of the lung contract, and lymph nodes enlarge. In the liver, thick secretions block the bile ducts. Obstruction may also occur in the gallbladder. In the pancreas, thick secretions may block the gland completely. In the small intestine, intestinal obstruction (meconium ileus) can result from thick secretions and requires surgery in some newborns. The reproductive organs are affected by cystic fibrosis in various ways, often resulting in infertility. The sweat glands in the skin and small salivary glands in the cheek (parotid glands) secrete fluids containing more salt than normal.

---

thick or solid and may block the gland completely. Eventually, the pancreas can become scarred. The mucus-producing glands in the airways of the lungs produce abnormal secretions that clog the airways and allow bacteria to multiply. The sweat glands and small salivary glands in the cheek (parotid glands) secrete fluids containing more salt than normal.

Symptoms

The lungs are normal at birth, but breathing problems can develop at any time afterward. Thick secretions eventually block the small

▲ see page 292

airways, which leads to inflammation and thickening of their walls. As larger airways fill with secretions, areas of the lung collapse and contract (a condition called atelectasis▲), and the lymph nodes enlarge. All these changes make breathing increasingly difficult and reduce the lungs' ability to transfer oxygen to the blood. Respiratory tract infections occur because of bacterial growth in the bronchial secretions and walls of the airways.

The blockage of pancreatic ducts and intestinal glands leads to digestive problems, including poor absorption of fats, proteins, and vitamins. This, in turn, can lead to nutritional deficiencies, and slower than expected growth.

Some people may have episodes of intestinal obstruction when abnormal stool contents block the bowel.

About 15 to 20% of newborns who have cystic fibrosis have meconium ileus, a serious obstruction of the small intestine.▲ Meconium ileus is sometimes complicated by a twisting of the intestine on itself (volvulus) or incomplete development of the intestine. Newborns who have meconium ileus almost always develop other symptoms of cystic fibrosis later. Meconium can also temporarily obstruct the large intestine in some newborns with cystic fibrosis, so that a bowel movement may not occur in these newborns until 1 to 2 days after birth.

The first symptom of cystic fibrosis in an infant who does not have meconium ileus is often a delay in regaining birth weight or poor weight gain at 4 to 6 weeks of age. Inadequate amounts of pancreatic enzymes, which are essential for proper digestion of fats and proteins, lead to poor digestion in most infants with cystic fibrosis. The infant has frequent, bulky, foul-smelling, oily stools and may have a distended abdomen and small muscles. Weight gain is slow despite a normal or large appetite.

About half the children with cystic fibrosis are first taken to the doctor because of frequent coughing, wheezing, and respiratory tract infections. Coughing, the most noticeable symptom, is often accompanied by gagging, vomiting, and disturbed sleep. As the disease progresses, the chest becomes barrel-shaped, and insufficient oxygen may make the fingers clubbed■ and the nail beds bluish. Polyps may form in the nose. The sinuses may fill with thick secretions, leading to chronic or recurrent sinus infections.

When a child or adult with cystic fibrosis sweats excessively in hot weather or because of a fever, dehydration may result because of the increased loss of salt and water. A parent may notice the formation of salt crystals or even a salty taste on the child's skin.

Adolescents often have slowed growth, delayed puberty, and declining physical endurance. As the disease progresses, lung infection becomes a major problem. Recurrent bronchitis and pneumonia gradually destroy the lungs.

Complications

Inadequate absorption of the fat-soluble vitamins—A, D, E, and K—may lead to night blindness, rickets, anemia, and bleeding disorders. In about 20% of untreated infants and toddlers, the lining of the rectum protrudes through the anus, a condition called rectal prolapse. Infants with cystic fibrosis who have been fed soy protein formula or breast milk may develop anemia and swelling of the extremities, because they are not absorbing enough protein.

Complications in adolescents and adults with cystic fibrosis include a rupture of the small air sacs of the lung (alveoli) into the pleural space (the space between the lung and chest wall). This rupture can allow air to enter into this space (pneumothorax), which collapses the lung.★ Other complications include heart failure and massive or recurrent bleeding in the lungs.

About 15% of adults with cystic fibrosis develop insulin-dependent diabetes because the scarred pancreas can no longer produce enough insulin. The blockage of bile ducts by thick secretions can lead to inflammation of the liver and eventually to scarring of the liver (cirrhosis) in about 5% of adults with cystic fibrosis.● Cirrhosis may increase the pressure in the veins entering the liver (portal hypertension◆), leading to enlarged, fragile veins at the lower end of the esophagus (esophageal varices), which can rupture and bleed profusely. In almost all people with cystic fibrosis, the gallbladder is small and filled with thick bile and does not function well. About 10% of people develop gallstones, but only a small percentage develop symptoms. Surgical removal of the gallbladder is rarely needed.

People with cystic fibrosis often have impaired reproductive function. Almost all men have a low sperm count (which makes them sterile) because one of the ducts of the testis (the vas deferens) has developed abnormally and blocks the passage of sperm. In women, cervical secretions are too thick, causing decreased fertility. Otherwise, sexual function is not affected. Women with cystic fibrosis have a higher likelihood of complications during pregnancy (such as developing a lung infection or diabetes), but many women with cystic fibrosis have given birth.

▲ see also page 1521 ■ see page 253

★ see page 316 ● see also page 797

◆ see page 793

Other complications may include arthritis, kidney stones, and inflammation of the blood vessels (vasculitis).

Diagnosis

The diagnosis of cystic fibrosis is usually confirmed in infancy or early childhood, but cystic fibrosis goes undetected until adolescence or early adulthood in about 10% of people with the disease.

The diagnosis is suggested by one or more of the typical symptoms and is confirmed by a sweat test. This test measures the amount of salt in sweat. The drug pilocarpine is placed on the skin to stimulate sweating, and filter paper or thin tubing is placed against the skin to collect the sweat. The concentration of salt in the sweat is then measured. A salt concentration higher than normal confirms the diagnosis in people who have symptoms of cystic fibrosis or who have a sibling with cystic fibrosis. Although the results of this test are valid any time after a newborn is 48 hours old, collecting a large enough sweat sample from a newborn younger than 3 or 4 weeks old may be difficult. The sweat test, which can be performed on an outpatient basis, can also confirm the diagnosis in older children and young adults.

In newborns with cystic fibrosis, the level of the digestive enzyme, trypsin, in the blood is high. This enzyme level can be measured in a small drop of blood collected on a piece of filter paper. Measurement of this enzyme in addition to sweat testing and genetic testing is the basis of cystic fibrosis newborn screening programs performed in many parts of the world. However, this test is not yet routinely performed in the United States.

The diagnosis of cystic fibrosis can also be confirmed by genetic testing in a person who exhibits one or more typical symptoms or has a history of cystic fibrosis in a sibling. Finding two abnormal cystic fibrosis genes (mutations) confirms the diagnosis. However, because genetic testing can confirm only a small percentage of the more than 1000 different kinds of cystic fibrosis mutations, failure to detect two mutations does not exclude a diagnosis of cystic fibrosis. The disease can be diagnosed prenatally by performing genetic testing on the fetus using chorionic villus sampling or amniocentesis.▲

▲ see page 1429   ■ see page 254
★ see page 1093

Because cystic fibrosis can affect several organs, other tests may be helpful. If pancreatic enzyme levels are reduced, an analysis of the person's stool may reveal low or undetectable levels of the digestive enzymes trypsin and chymotrypsin (both secreted by the pancreas) or high levels of fat. If insulin secretion is reduced, blood sugar levels are high. Pulmonary function tests■ may show that breathing is compromised and are good indicators of how well the lungs are functioning. Also, chest x-rays and computed tomography may be helpful to document lung infection and the extent of lung damage.

Carrier testing can be performed for prospective parents. In particular, relatives of a child with cystic fibrosis may want to know if they are likely to have children with the disease, and they should be offered genetic testing and counseling. A small blood sample is taken to help determine if a person has a defective cystic fibrosis gene. Unless both prospective parents have at least one such gene, their children will not have cystic fibrosis. If both parents carry a defective cystic fibrosis gene, each pregnancy has a 25% chance of producing a child with cystic fibrosis.

Treatment

A person with cystic fibrosis should have a comprehensive program of therapy directed by an experienced doctor—usually a pediatrician or an internist—along with a team of other doctors, nurses, a dietitian, social worker, genetics counselor, psychologist, and physical and respiratory therapists. The goals of therapy include long-term prevention and treatment of lung and digestive problems and other complications, maintenance of good nutrition, and encouragement of physical activity.

Children with cystic fibrosis need psychologic and social support because they may be unable to participate in normal childhood activities and may feel isolated. Much of the burden of treating a child with cystic fibrosis falls on the parents, who should receive adequate information and training so they can understand the condition and the reasons for the treatments.

The treatment of lung problems focuses on preventing airway blockage and controlling infection. The person should receive all routine immunizations★ and the influenza vaccine, because viral infections can further damage the lungs. Infants and toddlers should receive pneumococcal immunization as part of their routine care.

Respiratory therapy—consisting of postural drainage, percussion, hand vibration over the chest wall, and encouragement of coughing—is started at the first sign of lung problems.▲ Parents of a young child can learn these techniques and carry them out at home every day. Older children and adults can carry out respiratory therapy independently, using special breathing devices or a compression vest.

Often, people are given drugs that help prevent their airways from narrowing (bronchodilators). People with severe lung problems and a low level of oxygen in the blood may need supplemental oxygen therapy. In general, people with respiratory failure do not benefit from using a ventilator; however, occasional, short periods of mechanical ventilation in the hospital may help during an acute infection, after a surgical procedure, or while waiting for a lung transplant.

An aerosol drug, such as dornase alfa (recombinant human deoxyribonuclease I) is widely used to help thin the pus-filled mucus; such a drug makes it easier to cough up sputum, improves lung function, and may also decrease the frequency of serious respiratory tract infections. Mist tents have no proven benefit. Corticosteroids can relieve symptoms in infants with severe bronchial inflammation and in people who have narrowed airways that cannot be opened with bronchodilators. Sometimes, a nonsteroidal anti-inflammatory drug (NSAID)■ is used to slow the deterioration of lung function.

Respiratory tract infections must be treated as early as possible with antibiotics. At the first sign of a respiratory tract infection, a sample of coughed-up sputum or a throat culture is collected and tested, so that the infecting organism can be identified and the doctor can choose the drugs most likely to control it. *Staphylococcus aureus* and *Pseudomonas* species are commonly found. An antibiotic often can be given by mouth, or an antibiotic such as tobramycin can be given in an aerosol mist. However, if the infection is severe, intravenous antibiotics may be needed. This treatment often requires hospitalization but may be given at home. Taking oral or aerosol antibiotics intermittently or continuously may help prevent recurrences of infection and slow the decline in lung function.

People who have pancreatic problems must take pancreatic enzyme replacements with each meal; a powder (for infants) and capsules are available. Special milk formulas containing protein and fats that are easy to digest may help infants who have pancreatic problems and poor growth.

The diet should provide enough calories and protein for normal growth. The proportion of fat should be normal to high. Because people with cystic fibrosis need more calories, they need to consume higher than normal amounts of fat to ensure adequate growth. People with cystic fibrosis should take double the usual recommended daily amount of fat-soluble vitamins (A, D, E, and K) in a special formulation that is more easily absorbed. When they exercise, have a fever, or are exposed to hot weather, people who have cystic fibrosis should increase their salt intake. Children who cannot absorb enough nutrients from food may need supplementary feedings through a tube inserted into the stomach or small intestine.

At some time, surgery may be needed to treat a pneumothorax, chronic sinus infection, severe chronic infection restricted to one area of the lung, bleeding from blood vessels in the esophagus, gallbladder disease, or obstruction of the intestine. Massive or recurrent bleeding in the lung can be treated by a procedure called embolization, which blocks off the bleeding artery.

Liver transplantation has been successful for severe liver damage. Double lung transplantation for severe lung disease is becoming more routine and more successful with experience and improved techniques. One year after transplantation of both the right and the left lungs, about 75% of people are alive, and their condition is much improved.

Gene therapy, in which normal cystic fibrosis genes are delivered directly to the airways, holds great promise for treating cystic fibrosis. However, this therapy is only available in research trials. A number of new drugs, delivered by mouth or aerosol, are under investigation.

Prognosis

The severity of cystic fibrosis varies greatly from person to person regardless of age; the severity is determined largely by how much the lungs are affected. In the United States, half of the people with cystic fibrosis live

---

▲ see page 261   ■ see page 452

about 33 years or longer. The outlook for longer survival has improved steadily over the past 50 years, mainly because treatments can now postpone some of the changes that occur in the lungs. Long-term survival is somewhat better in males and in people whose initial symptoms were restricted to the digestive tract; however, long-term survival is also significantly better in people who do not develop pancreatic problems.

However, deterioration is inevitable, leading to loss of lung function and eventually death. People with cystic fibrosis usually die of respiratory failure after many years of deteriorating lung function. A small number, however, die of heart failure, liver disease, bleeding into the airways, or complications of surgery. Despite their many problems, people with cystic fibrosis usually attend school or work until shortly before death.

CHAPTER 54

Pulmonary Hypertension

A condition in which blood pressure in the arteries of the lungs (pulmonary arteries) is abnormally high.

Blood travels from the right side of the heart through the pulmonary arteries into the lungs. There, carbon dioxide is removed from the blood and oxygen is added to it. Normally, the right side of the heart is weaker than the left side, because relatively little muscle and effort are needed to push the blood through the pulmonary arteries. In contrast, the left side of the heart is stronger and more muscular because it has to push blood through the entire body. Likewise, blood pressure through the pulmonary arteries is lower than that of the general circulation. While the pressure in the general circulation is normally about 120/80 mm Hg, in the pulmonary arteries it is only 25/15 mm Hg.

If the pressure of the blood in the pulmonary arteries is abnormally high, the condition is called pulmonary hypertension. Over time, the increased pressure damages both the large and small pulmonary arteries. The walls of the smallest blood vessels thicken and are no longer able to transfer oxygen and carbon dioxide normally between the blood and the lungs. Thus, the levels of oxygen in the blood may fall. The low oxygen level can cause narrowing (constriction) of the pulmonary arteries. These

changes contribute further to the increased pressure in the pulmonary circulation.

With pulmonary hypertension, the right side of the heart must work harder to push the blood through the pulmonary arteries into the lungs. Over time, the right ventricle becomes thickened and enlarged, leading to a condition called cor pulmonale. Heart failure develops.▲

In some people, the bone marrow produces more red blood cells to compensate for less oxygen in the blood, leading to a condition called polycythemia.■ The extra red blood cells cause the blood to become thicker and stickier, further increasing the load on the heart. These changes also put a person with cor pulmonale at increased risk of pulmonary embolism,★ because the thickened blood may clump and form clots, mainly in the veins of the legs. These clots can dislodge and travel to the lungs.

Cor pulmonale and pulmonary hypertension are sometimes thought of as synonymous, but they are not. Pulmonary hypertension is the underlying cause of cor pulmonale. Everyone who has cor pulmonale has pulmonary hypertension. However, a person can have pulmonary hypertension and not have cor pulmonale, although pulmonary hypertension often eventually leads to cor pulmonale.

Causes

There are two types of pulmonary hypertension: primary and secondary. Primary pulmonary hypertension is much less common than secondary pulmonary hypertension. In pri-

▲ see page 150   ■ see page 1023
★ see page 285

Cor Pulmonale: A Disorder Stemming From Pulmonary Hypertension

Cor pulmonale is a disorder in which the right ventricle of the heart becomes enlarged and thickened, eventually resulting in heart failure.

Cor pulmonale has only one cause: pulmonary hypertension. In time, pulmonary hypertension leads to thickening of the pulmonary arteries and narrowing of the passageways through which blood flows. Once pulmonary hypertension develops, the right side of the heart works harder to compensate, but the increased effort causes it to become enlarged and thickened. These changes can lead to right-sided heart failure (usually heart failure stems from problems with the left side of the heart). The enlarged right ventricle places a person at risk for pulmonary embolism because blood tends to pool in the ventricle and in the legs. If clots form in the pooled blood, they may eventually travel and lodge in the lungs, with disastrous consequences.

There are often no symptoms until cor pulmonale is quite advanced. Then the symptoms are still those of pulmonary hypertension: shortness of breath upon exertion, lightheadedness, fatigue, and chest pain. Symptoms of heart failure, such as swelling (edema) in the legs and progressively worse shortness of breath, develop.

A number of tests are available to help a doctor diagnose cor pulmonale, but the diagnosis is often suspected on the basis of the physical examination. By listening through a stethoscope, a doctor can hear certain characteristic heart sounds that occur when the right ventricle becomes enlarged. Chest x-rays can show the enlarged right ventricle and pulmonary arteries. The doctor evaluates the function of the left and right ventricle with echocardiography, radionuclide studies, and cardiac catheterization.

Treatment is usually directed at the underlying lung disease. Measures to relieve right-sided heart failure are also taken. Because people with cor pulmonale are at increased risk of pulmonary embolism, a doctor may prescribe an anticoagulant to be taken long-term.

mary pulmonary hypertension, the cause is not known, but likely begins with spasm (contraction) of the muscle layer in the pulmonary arteries. Women are affected by primary pulmonary hypertension twice as often as men, and half of the people are 35 or older at the time of diagnosis. Secondary pulmonary hypertension means that the condition occurred because of another disorder that affects lung structure or function.

Secondary pulmonary hypertension can be caused by any disease that impedes the flow of blood through the lungs or that causes sustained periods of low oxygen in the blood. One of the most common causes is chronic obstructive pulmonary disease.▲ When the lungs are impaired by disease, it takes more effort to pump blood through them. Over time, chronic obstructive pulmonary disease destroys the small air sacs (alveoli) together with their small vessels (capillaries) in the lungs. The single most important cause of pulmonary hypertension in chronic obstructive pulmonary disease is the narrowing of the pulmonary artery that occurs as a result of low blood oxygen levels.

Another disease that can cause pulmonary hypertension is pulmonary fibrosis,■ which causes extensive scar tissue to form in the lungs. The scar tissue destroys the pulmonary circulation and makes blood flow more difficult. Other lung diseases that may cause pulmonary hypertension include cystic fibrosis★ and certain occupational lung diseases, such as asbestosis● and silicosis.◆

Less often, pulmonary hypertension is caused by extensive loss of lung tissue from surgery or trauma, or by heart failure, scleroderma, obesity with reduced ability to breathe (Pickwickian syndrome), neurologic diseases involving the respiratory muscles, chronic liver disease, HIV infection, and diet drugs (for example, dexfenfluramine-phentermine [fenphen]). A sudden cause of pulmonary hypertension is pulmonary embolism,▼ a condition in which blood clots become lodged in the arteries of the lung, causing serious problems.

Symptoms

Shortness of breath upon exertion is the most common symptom of pulmonary hypertension, and virtually everyone who has the

▲ see page 281   ■ see page 301
★ see page 317   ● see page 296
◆ see page 295   ▼ see page 285

condition develops it. Some people feel light-headed or fatigued upon exertion, and an angina-like chest pain is common. The person is likely to feel weak because body tissues are not receiving enough oxygen. Other symptoms, such as coughing and wheezing, are usually caused by the underlying lung disease. Swelling (edema), particularly of the legs, may occur because fluid may leak out of the veins and into the tissues, but this is usually a sign that cor pulmonale has developed.

Some people with pulmonary hypertension have connective tissue disorders, especially scleroderma;▲ when people have both conditions, Raynaud's phenomenon often develops before symptoms of pulmonary hypertension appear, sometimes as long as years earlier.■

For unknown reasons, some people with primary pulmonary hypertension develop achy joints, often years before the apparent onset of the disorder.

Diagnosis

Based on the symptoms, a doctor may suspect pulmonary hypertension in people who have an underlying lung disorder. A chest x-ray may show that the pulmonary arteries are enlarged. An electrocardiogram and an echocardiogram enable the doctor to look for certain problems with the right side of the heart even before cor pulmonale develops. For example, thickening of the right ventricle or a partial reversal (back flow) of blood through the tricuspid valve between the right atrium and right ventricle may be detected on an echocardiogram. Pulmonary function tests help the doctor assess the extent of lung damage. A sample of blood may be taken from an artery in an arm to measure the level of oxygen in the blood.

A definite diagnosis of pulmonary hypertension usually requires passing a tube through a vein in an arm or a leg into the right side of the heart to measure the blood pressure in the right ventricle and the pulmonary artery.

Treatment

Treatment of secondary pulmonary hypertension is often directed at the underlying lung disease. Vasodilators (drugs to dilate blood vessels), such as calcium channel blockers, nitric oxide, and prostacyclin, are often helpful for secondary pulmonary hypertension associated with scleroderma, chronic liver disease, and HIV infection. In contrast, these drugs have not been proven effective for people with secondary pulmonary hypertension due to an underlying lung disease. For most people with primary pulmonary hypertension, vasodilators, such as prostacyclin, drastically reduce blood pressure in the pulmonary arteries. Prostacyclin given intravenously through a catheter surgically implanted in the skin improves the quality of life, increases survival, and reduces the urgency of lung transplantation. However, a doctor will first test the effectiveness of vasodilators in a given person in a cardiac catheterization laboratory, because their use may be dangerous in some people. A subcutaneous (under the skin) form of prostacyclin is now available and has been effective in some people.

Bosentan, a new drug given by mouth, has been effective in some people. A drug similar to prostacyclin, called iloprost, can be administered by inhalation and, as a result, has a much lower risk of complications than prostacyclin. However, this drug is not available in the United States.

If a person with pulmonary hypertension has a low oxygen level in the blood, the continuous use of oxygen through nasal prongs or an oxygen mask may reduce blood pressure in his pulmonary arteries and may help relieve his shortness of breath. A diuretic drug may improve the exchange of gases in the lungs, presumably by relieving the buildup of fluid as well as diminishing the buildup of fluid in the rest of the body. An anticoagulant may be prescribed to reduce the risk of blood clots and subsequent pulmonary embolism.★

Single or double lung transplantation is an established procedure for treating primary pulmonary hypertension. Without a transplant, most people die 2 to 5 years after the disease is diagnosed. Transplantation may be a possible treatment for severe secondary pulmonary hypertension if treatment of the underlying disorder fails.

▲ see page 380   ■ see page 224

★ see page 285

CHAPTER 55

Respiratory Failure

Respiratory failure is a condition in which the level of oxygen in the blood becomes dangerously low or the level of carbon dioxide becomes dangerously high.

Respiratory failure, which is a medical emergency, is often the final stage of chronic lung disease. Respiratory failure can also result from severe, sudden lung disease (such as acute respiratory distress syndrome▲) in otherwise healthy people. Almost any condition that affects breathing or the lungs can lead to respiratory failure. An overdose of opioids or alcohol can cause such profound sedation that a person stops breathing and suffers respiratory failure. Obstruction of the airways, injury to the lung tissues, damage to the bones and tissues around the lungs, and weakness of the muscles that normally inflate the lungs are also common causes. Respiratory failure can occur if blood flow through the lungs becomes abnormal, as happens in pulmonary embolism.■ This disorder does not stop air from moving in and out of the lungs, but without blood flow to a portion of the lungs, oxygen is not properly extracted from the air.

Symptoms and Diagnosis

Low oxygen levels in the blood cause a bluish coloration (cyanosis), and high carbon dioxide levels and increasing acidity of the blood cause confusion and sleepiness. The body tries to rid itself of carbon dioxide by deep, rapid breathing, but if the lungs cannot function normally, this breathing pattern may not help. Eventually low levels of oxygen make the brain and heart malfunction, resulting in deteriorating consciousness or unconsciousness and abnormal heart rhythms (arrhythmias), which can lead to death.

Some symptoms of respiratory failure vary with the cause. A child with an obstructed airway due to the inhalation (aspiration) of a foreign object may gasp and struggle for breath;★ someone who is intoxicated or weak may quietly slip into a coma.

A doctor may suspect respiratory failure from the symptoms and examination. A blood test confirms the diagnosis when it shows a dangerously low level of oxygen or a dangerously high level of carbon dioxide.

If respiratory failure develops slowly, pressure in the blood vessels of the lungs increases, a condition called pulmonary hypertension.● If left untreated, this condition damages the blood vessels, further impairs the transfer of oxygen to the blood, and stresses the heart, causing heart failure.

Treatment

Almost always, oxygen is given initially. Usually, the amount given is more than is needed, but this can be readjusted at a later time. In people with chronically high carbon

WHAT CAUSES RESPIRATORY FAILURE?

Underlying Problem	Cause
Airway obstruction	Chronic bronchitis, emphysema, bronchiectasis, cystic fibrosis, asthma, bronchiolitis, inhaled particles
Poor breathing	Obesity, sleep apnea, drug intoxication
Muscle weakness	Myasthenia gravis, muscular dystrophy, polio, Guillain-Barré syndrome, polymyositis, stroke, amyotrophic lateral sclerosis, spinal cord injury
Abnormality of lung tissue	Acute respiratory distress syndrome, drug reaction, pulmonary fibrosis, fibrosing alveolitis, widespread tumors, radiation, sarcoidosis, burns
Abnormality of chest wall	Scoliosis, chest wound, extreme obesity, thoracoplasty (an operation to remove part of the ribs to collapse a diseased lung)

▲ see page 326   ■ see page 285
★ see page 1583   ● see page 132

dioxide levels, excess oxygen can result in slowing of the movement of air (ventilation) in and out of the lungs and a dangerous further increase in the carbon dioxide level. In such people, the dosage of oxygen needs to be more carefully regulated.

The underlying cause of the respiratory failure must also be treated. Antibiotics are used to fight infection, and bronchodilators are used to open the airways. Other drugs may be given to decrease inflammation or prevent blood clots.

Mechanical Ventilation: Some very ill people need mechanical ventilation to aid breathing. Mechanical ventilation can be lifesaving whenever people are not able to move enough air in and out of their lungs. A plastic tube is inserted through the nose or mouth into the trachea; this tube is attached to a machine that forces air into the lungs. Exhalation occurs passively because of the elastic recoil of the lungs. Many types of ventilators and modes of operation may be used, depending on the underlying disorder. If the lungs are not functioning well, additional oxygen may be delivered through the ventilator. In people who do not require complete support of their breathing, a

mask may be placed over the nose or face, which permits the delivery of positive pressure, thus assisting the person's own breathing efforts and preventing fatigue of the respiratory muscles. In about half of the people with respiratory failure, use of these techniques (called bi-level positive airway pressure or continuous positive airway pressure) can avoid the need to intubate the trachea. Use of bi-level positive airway pressure at night can help people whose respiratory failure was caused by muscle weakness, because after resting at night, the respiratory muscles are able to function more effectively during the day.

The amount of fluid in the body must be carefully monitored and adjusted to maximize lung and heart function. The acidity of the blood must be kept in balance by adjusting the frequency and size of breaths delivered by the ventilator. A person undergoing mechanical ventilation may experience agitation, which can be controlled with sedating drugs such as lorazepam and midazolam or opioids such as morphine or fentanyl. Bacterial infections that may develop while the person undergoes mechanical ventilation must be diagnosed as quickly as possible and treated.

CHAPTER 56

Acute Respiratory Distress Syndrome

Acute respiratory distress syndrome is a type of lung failure resulting from many different disorders that cause fluid to accumulate in the lungs and oxygen levels in the blood to be too low.

Acute respiratory distress syndrome (ARDS) is a medical emergency that often occurs in people who have severe lung disease. However, even people who previously had normal lungs can develop ARDS. This syndrome is sometimes called *adult* respiratory distress syndrome, although it can occur in children. The less severe form of this syndrome is called acute lung injury.

Causes

Any disease or condition that injures the lungs can cause ARDS. About one third of the people with the syndrome develop it as a consequence of a severe, widespread infection (sepsis). Other people develop ARDS because of significant damage at first to another organ, such as the pancreas. Damage to the pancreas can release proteins such as enzymes and cytokines, which are capable of injuring other organs and tissues in the body, including the lungs.

When the small air sacs (alveoli) and tiny blood vessels (capillaries) of the lungs are injured, blood and fluid leak into the spaces between the air sacs and eventually into the sacs themselves. Collapse of many alveoli (a condition called atelectasis▲) may also result because of a reduction in surfactant activity. Surfactant is the liquid that coats the inside surface of the alveoli, helping to hold them open. Fluid in the alveoli and the collapse of many alveoli interfere with the movement of oxygen from inhaled air into the blood, causing oxygen levels in the blood to decrease sharply. Movement of carbon dioxide from the blood to air that is exhaled is affected less, and levels of carbon dioxide in the blood change very little.

Symptoms and Diagnosis

ARDS usually develops within 24 to 48 hours of the original injury or disease. The person first experiences shortness of breath, usually with rapid, shallow breathing. Through a stethoscope, a doctor may hear crackling or wheezing sounds in the lungs, or the doctor may hear nothing abnormal. Because of low oxygen levels in the blood, the skin may become mottled or blue (cyanosis), and other organs such as the heart and brain may malfunction, resulting in a rapid heart rate, confusion, and lethargy.

The oxygen deprivation caused by ARDS and the leakage into the bloodstream of certain proteins (cytokines) produced by lung cells and white blood cells can lead to inflammation and complications in other organs; failure of several organs (a condition called multiple organ system failure) may also result. Organ failure can begin soon after the onset of ARDS or days or weeks later. Additionally, people with ARDS are less able to fight lung infections, and they tend to develop bacterial pneumonia.

Analysis of a blood sample taken from an artery indicates low levels of oxygen in the blood,■ and chest x-rays show fluid in spaces that should be filled with air. Further tests may be needed to ensure that heart failure is not the cause of the problem.★

Treatment and Prognosis

People with ARDS are treated in an intensive care unit. Successful treatment depends on correcting the underlying cause; oxygen therapy, which is vital to correcting low oxygen levels, is combined with treatment of the underlying cause.

Causes of Acute Respiratory Distress Syndrome

- Aspiration (inhalation) of food into the lung
- Burns
- Cardiopulmonary bypass surgery
- Chest injury
- Inflammation of the pancreas (pancreatitis)
- Inhalation of large amounts of smoke
- Inhalation of other toxic gas
- Injury to the lungs from inhaling high concentrations of oxygen
- Massive blood transfusions
- Near drowning
- Overdose of a drug, such as heroin, methadone, propoxyphene, and aspirin
- Pneumonia
- Prolonged or severe low blood pressure (shock)
- Pulmonary embolism
- Severe, widespread infection (sepsis)

If oxygen delivered by a face mask or nasal prongs does not correct the low blood oxygen levels, or if excessively high doses of inhaled oxygen are required, a ventilator must be used; this treatment is called mechanical ventilation.● A ventilator delivers oxygen-rich air under pressure using a tube inserted through the mouth into the trachea. For people who have ARDS, the ventilator pressure is delivered both during the inhaled breath and at a lower pressure during exhalation (called positive end-expiratory pressure). The pressure supplied by the ventilator during and after a breath opens collapsed (atelectatic) regions of the lung and allows oxygen to move through the walls of the injured lungs into the blood.

The pressure and volume of air that the ventilator delivers to the lungs with each breath must be adjusted to help keep the small airways and alveoli open while avoiding rupturing the fragile air sacs, which can lead to air accumulating around the lung and collapsing it (called pneumothorax◆). Monitoring and adjusting the pressure also ensures that the

▲ see page 292   ■ see page 255
★ see page 150   ● see page 326
◆ see page 316

lungs do not receive an excessive concentration of oxygen, which can damage the lungs and worsen ARDS. Limiting the volume of air with each breath also ensures that the lungs are not further damaged from overstretching. Sedating drugs such as midazolam are often given to calm the person and reduce their sense of being short of breath.

In some cases, diuretic drugs may be needed to help remove fluid from the lungs. Antibiotics are usually needed for people who develop bacterial pneumonia. Some people may benefit from the use of intravenous corticosteroids in the later stages of ARDS. Other supportive treatment, such as providing liquid nutritional supplements through a small feeding tube placed in the stomach or small intestine,▲ is also important because dehydration or malnutrition may increase the likelihood of multiple organ system failure. If a person cannot be adequately fed in this way, food may need to be delivered intravenously.

Without prompt treatment, the severe oxygen deprivation resulting from ARDS causes death in 90% of people with the disorder. However, with appropriate treatment, about half of all people with severe ARDS survive.

People who respond promptly to treatment usually recover completely with few or no long-term lung abnormalities. Those whose treatment involves long periods on a ventilator are more likely to develop lung scarring. Such scarring may improve over a few months after the person is taken off the ventilator.

CHAPTER 57

Lung Cancer

Lung cancer is the most common cause of death from cancer in both men and women. It occurs most commonly between the ages of 45 and 70. Lung cancer is more common in women now than in the past because more women are smoking cigarettes.

Lung cancer that originates in the cells of the lungs is called primary lung cancer; however, cancer may also spread (metastasize) to the lung from other parts of the body. Metastatic cancers spread to the lungs most commonly from the breast, colon, prostate, kidney, thyroid gland, stomach, cervix, rectum, testis, bone, and skin (melanoma).

More than 90% of primary lung cancers start in the bronchi (the large airways that branch off the trachea to supply the lungs); such lung cancer is called bronchogenic carcinoma. The specific types of lung cancer are small cell (oat cell) carcinoma, squamous cell carcinoma, large cell carcinoma, and adenocarcinoma. The last three types of lung cancer are often referred to as nonsmall cell lung cancers.

Alveolar cell carcinoma (a subtype of adenocarcinoma) originates in the small air sacs of the lung (alveoli). Although alveolar cell carcinoma can occur at a single site, it often develops simultaneously in more than one area of the lung.

Less common lung tumors are bronchial carcinoid (which may be cancerous or noncancerous), chondromatous hamartoma (noncancerous), and sarcoma (cancerous). Lymphoma is a cancer of the lymphatic system; it may start in the lungs or spread to them.

Causes

Cigarette smoking is the cause of about 90% of lung cancer cases in men and about 80% of cases in women. The greater the quantity and duration of smoking, the greater the risk of developing lung cancer. About 10 to 12% of all smokers eventually develop lung cancer.

A small proportion of lung cancers (about 10% in men and about 5% in women) are caused by substances encountered or breathed in at work. Working with asbestos, radiation, arsenic, chromates, nickel, chloromethyl ethers, mustard gas, and coke-oven emissions has been linked with lung cancer. The risk of contracting lung cancer is greater in people who are exposed to these substances and who also smoke cigarettes. Air pollution causes

---

▲ see page 889

about 1% of lung cancer cases. Exposure to radon gas in the home causes lung cancer in less than 1% of cases. Occasionally, lung cancers, especially adenocarcinoma and alveolar cell carcinoma, develop in people whose lungs have been scarred by other lung diseases, such as tuberculosis and fibrosis.

Symptoms and Complications

The symptoms of lung cancer depend on its type, its location, and the way it spreads. Usually, the first and most common symptom is a persistent cough. People with chronic bronchitis who develop lung cancer often notice that their coughing becomes worse. If sputum can be coughed up, it may be streaked with blood (called hemoptysis▲). If a lung cancer grows into underlying blood vessels, it may cause severe bleeding.

Lung cancer may cause wheezing by narrowing the bronchus in or around which it is growing. Blockage of a bronchus may lead to the collapse of the part of the lung that the bronchus supplies, a condition called atelectasis.■ Other consequences of a blocked bronchus are shortness of breath, and pneumonia, with coughing, fever, and chest pain. If the tumor grows into the chest wall, it may produce persistent chest pain.

Lung cancer may grow into certain nerves in the neck, causing a droopy eyelid, small pupil, sunken eye, and reduced perspiration on one side of the face—together these symptoms are called **Horner's syndrome.**★ Cancers at the top of the lung may grow into the nerves that supply the arm, making the arm painful, numb, and weak—this condition is called **Pancoast syndrome.** Nerves to the voice box may also be damaged, making the voice hoarse. This damage happens mainly in people whose cancers involve the left lung.

Lung cancer may grow directly into the esophagus, or it may grow near it and put pressure on it, leading to difficulty in swallowing. Occasionally, an abnormal channel (fistula) between the esophagus and bronchi develops because of invasion by the cancer, causing severe coughing during swallowing because food and fluid enter the lungs.

A lung cancer may grow into the heart, causing abnormal heart rhythms, blockage of blood flow through the heart, or fluid in the pericardial sac surrounding the heart. The cancer may grow into or compress the superior vena cava (one of the large veins in the chest); this condition is called **superior vena cava syndrome.**

Deaths Due to Lung Cancer

Among cancers, lung cancer is the most common cause of death in men and women. The number of deaths due to lung cancer has been increasing because the number of smokers has been increasing. In 2001, more than 157,000 are expected to die of lung cancer—about 90,000 men and 67,000 women. This number represents about 28% of all deaths due to cancer.

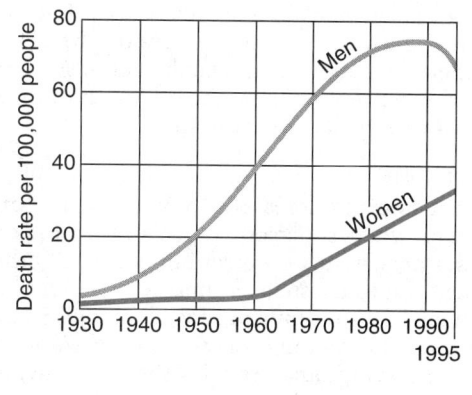

Obstruction of this vein causes blood to back up in other veins of the upper body. The veins in the chest wall enlarge. The face, neck, and upper chest wall—including the breasts—swell and become tinged with purple. The condition also produces shortness of breath, headache, distorted vision, dizziness, and drowsiness. These symptoms usually worsen when the person bends forward or lies down.

Symptoms of lung cancer that usually arise later include loss of appetite, weight loss, fatigue, and weakness. Fluid accumulations around the lung (pleural effusions●) occur when the cancer has spread into the pleural space. They can lead to shortness of breath. Severe shortness of breath, low levels of oxygen in the blood, and cor pulmonale◆ may develop if cancer spreads within the lungs.

Lung cancer may also spread through the bloodstream to the liver, brain, adrenal glands,

---

▲ see page 252   ■ see page 292
★ see box on page 592   ● see page 314
◆ see box on page 323

spinal cord, and bone; less commonly lung cancer may spread to other parts of the body. The spread of lung cancer may occur early in the disease, especially with small cell carcinoma. Symptoms—such as headache, confusion, seizures, and bone pain—may develop before any lung problems become evident, making an early diagnosis difficult.

Paraneoplastic syndromes▲ consist of effects that are caused by lung cancer but occur far from the lungs, such as in the metabolic system, nerves, and muscles. These syndromes are not related to the size or location of the lung cancer and do not necessarily indicate that the cancer has spread outside the chest; rather, they are caused by substances secreted by the cancer (such as hormones, cytokines, and a variety of other proteins).

Diagnosis

A doctor explores the possibility of lung cancer when a person, especially a smoker, has a persistent or worsening cough or other lung symptoms (such as shortness of breath or coughed-up sputum tinged with blood). Sometimes a shadow on a chest x-ray of someone with no symptoms provides the first clue, although a shadow on an x-ray is not proof of cancer. A chest x-ray can detect most lung tumors, although it may miss small ones.

A computed tomography (CT) may show small nodules that do not appear on chest x-rays. CT can also reveal whether the lymph nodes are enlarged; a biopsy of enlarged lymph nodes is often needed to determine if inflammation or cancer is responsible for the enlargement.

A microscopic examination of lung tissue is usually needed to confirm the diagnosis. Sometimes a sample of coughed-up sputum can provide enough material for an examination (called sputum cytology). Bronchoscopy may be performed to obtain that tissue.■ If the cancer is too deep in the lung to be reached with a bronchoscope, a doctor can usually obtain a specimen by inserting a needle through the skin while using CT for guidance; this procedure is called a needle biopsy.★ Sometimes, a specimen can be obtained only by a surgical procedure called a thoracotomy.●

CT of the abdomen or head may be performed to determine if lung cancer has spread, especially to the liver, adrenal glands, or brain. A bone scan may show that it has spread to the bones. Because small cell carcinoma tends to spread to the bone marrow, a doctor sometimes performs a bone marrow biopsy. New techniques, such as positron emission tomography (PET)◆ and a certain type of CT called spiral CT, show promise for improving the ability to detect small cancers.

Cancers are categorized based on how large the tumor is, whether it has spread to nearby lymph nodes, and whether it has spread to distant organs. The different categories are called stages.▼ The stage of a cancer suggests the most appropriate treatment and enables a doctor to estimate the person's prognosis.

Screening and Prevention

Screening for lung cancer using chest x-rays and sputum examination is not recommended for everyone at this time. However, for people at high risk of lung cancer, a chest x-ray or CT performed yearly may help to detect lung cancer before it has spread.

Prevention of lung cancer includes quitting smoking and avoiding exposure to potentially cancer-causing substances in the work environment.

Treatment

Noncancerous bronchial tumors (including carcinoid tumors and chondromatous hamartomas) are usually removed surgically because they may block the bronchi and some may become cancerous over time. Often, a doctor cannot be sure if such a tumor is cancerous until it has been removed and examined microscopically.

Surgery: Surgery is the treatment of choice for lung cancer that has not spread beyond the lung. However, surgery is not useful for small cell carcinoma. Older people should not be excluded from surgery based solely on their age. Surgery may not be possible if the cancer has spread beyond the lungs, if the cancer is too close to the trachea, or if the person has other serious conditions (such as severe heart or lung disease).

Before surgery, a doctor performs pulmonary function tests► to determine if the amount of lung remaining after surgery will be able to provide enough breathing function. If the test results indicate that removing the cancerous part of the lung will result in inade-

▲ see box on page 1037   ■ see page 256

★ see page 256   ● see page 258

◆ see page 256   ▼ see page 1041

► see page 254

quate lung function, surgery is not possible. The amount of lung to be removed is decided during surgery, with the amount varying from a small part of a lung segment to an entire lung.

Although 10 to 35% of cancers can be removed surgically, removal does not always result in a cure. Among people who have an isolated, slow-growing tumor removed, 25 to 40% survive at least 5 years after the diagnosis. A few people with small, early-stage nonsmall cell lung cancers have up to a 60 to 70% 5-year survival rate. People die mostly from recurrence of their cancer, either in the lung or at another site. Some people die because of another disorder, such as chronic obstructive pulmonary disease or coronary heart disease, or from the development of a new cancer. Survivors must have regular checkups, including periodic chest x-rays and CT scans.

Occasionally, cancer that begins elsewhere (for example, in the colon) and spreads to the lungs is removed from the lungs after being removed at the source. This procedure is recommended rarely, and tests must show that the cancer has not spread to any site outside of the lungs. Only about 10% of people who undergo this type of surgery survive 5 years or more.

Recent advances in the treatment of nonsmall cell lung cancer include using chemotherapy and radiation therapy before, after, or instead of the surgical removal of a cancer in some people who have cancer that has not spread beyond the lung.

Radiation Therapy: Radiation therapy may be given to people who refuse surgery, who cannot undergo surgery because they have another condition (such as severe coronary artery disease), or whose cancer has spread to the nearby structures, such as the lymph nodes. Although radiation therapy only partially shrinks the cancer or slows its growth in most of these people, it results in a long-term remission in 10 to 15% of them. Combining chemotherapy with radiation therapy further improves survival in this group. Radiation therapy is also useful for controlling the complications of lung cancer, such as coughing up of blood, bone pain, superior vena cava syndrome, and spinal cord compression.

Chemotherapy: Chemotherapy, sometimes coupled with radiation therapy, is the treatment of choice for small cell carcinoma of the lung. This is because the cancer has almost always spread to distant parts of the body by the time of diagnosis. In about 25% of people, chemotherapy substantially prolongs survival. Without chemotherapy, only half of the people with small cell carcinoma survive 4 months. With chemotherapy, there is a four- to fivefold increase in survival. People with small cell carcinoma of the lung who have been responding well to chemotherapy may benefit from radiation therapy to the head to treat cancer that has spread to the brain, even though the spread is early enough that no symptoms are apparent and nothing abnormal can be seen on a CT or MRI of the head.

The effectiveness of chemotherapy alone is very limited for nonsmall cell lung cancer. In metastatic nonsmall cell lung cancer, some people survive significantly longer when given chemotherapy than if they had not received it.

Other Treatments: Other treatments are often needed for people who have lung cancer. Because many people who have lung cancer experience a substantial decrease in lung function, whether or not they undergo treatment, oxygen therapy▲ and bronchodilators (drugs that widen the airways) may aid breathing. Many people with advanced lung cancer develop such extreme pain and difficulty in breathing that they require large doses of opioids in the weeks or months before their death. Fortunately, opioids can help substantially if adequate doses are used.

Prognosis

Lung cancer has a poor prognosis. On average, people with untreated lung cancer survive 8 months. Overall, even with therapy, the 5-year survival rate is only 13%. Because small cell carcinoma has almost always spread beyond the lung at the time of diagnosis, its prognosis is generally worse than for other types of lung cancer. People who survive lung cancer but continue to smoke are at high risk of another cancer.

Because many people die from lung cancer, terminal care is usually necessary. Advances in end-of-life care, particularly the recognition that anxiety and pain are common in people with incurable lung cancer and that they can be alleviated by appropriate drugs, have led to an increasing number of people being able to die comfortably at home.■

▲ see page 260   ■ see also page 48

BONE, JOINT, AND MUSCLE DISORDERS

58 Biology of the Musculoskeletal System 334

Bones ▪ Muscles ▪ Tendons and Bursas ▪ Ligaments ▪ Joints ▪ Effects of Aging

59 Symptoms and Diagnosis of Musculoskeletal Disorders 339

Pain ▪ Inflammation ▪ Muscle Weakness ▪ Joint Stiffness ▪ Joint Noises ▪ Joint Range of Motion ▪ Physical Examination ▪ Laboratory Tests ▪ Nerve Tests ▪ X-rays ▪ Dual-Energy X-ray Absorptiometry ▪ Computed Tomography and Magnetic Resonance Imaging ▪ Bone Scanning ▪ Joint Aspiration ▪ Arthroscopy ▪ Biopsy

60 Osteoporosis..343

61 Paget's Disease of Bone 346

62 Fractures 348

Foot Fractures ▪ Leg Fractures ▪ Hip Fractures ▪ Fractures of the Pelvis ▪ Fractures of the Spinal Column ▪ Shoulder Fractures ▪ Arm Fractures ▪ Hand Fractures

63 Bone Tumors 359

Noncancerous Bone Tumors ▪ Primary Cancerous Bone Tumors ▪ Metastatic Bone Tumors

64 Avascular Necrosis of the Bone..362

65 Bone and Joint Infections 364

Osteomyelitis ▪ Infectious Arthritis

66 Osteoarthritis..367

67 Rheumatoid Arthritis and Other Types of Inflammatory Arthritis 370

Rheumatoid Arthritis ▪ Psoriatic Arthritis ▪ Reiter's Syndrome ▪ Ankylosing Spondylitis

68 Autoimmune Disorders of Connective Tissue 378

Systemic Lupus Erythematosus ▪ Scleroderma ▪ Sjögren's Syndrome ▪ Polymyositis and Dermatomyositis ▪ Mixed Connective Tissue Disease ▪ Relapsing Polychondritis ▪ Eosinophilic Fasciitis

69   Vasculitic Disorders of Connective Tissue.....................**386**

Polyarteritis Nodosa ▪ Temporal Arteritis ▪ Polymyalgia
Rheumatica ▪ Wegener's Granulomatosis ▪ Behçet's Syndrome

70   Gout and Pseudogout..**391**

71   Hand Disorders **395**

Ganglia ▪ Deformities ▪ Carpal Tunnel Syndrome ▪ Cubital
Tunnel Syndrome ▪ Radial Tunnel Syndrome ▪ Kienböck's
Disease ▪ Shoulder-Hand Syndrome ▪ Infections

72   Foot Problems **403**

Foot Pain ▪ Ankle Sprain ▪ Tarsal Tunnel Syndrome ▪ Plantar
Fasciitis ▪ Achilles Tendon Bursitis ▪ Ingrown Toenail ▪
Onychomycosis ▪ Onychia ▪ Corns and Calluses ▪
Onychauxis and Onychogryphosis ▪ Hallux Valgus and Bunion ▪
Hammer Toe ▪ Sesamoiditis

73   Muscular Dystrophy and Related Disorders..................**412**

Duchenne and Becker Muscular Dystrophies ▪ Other Muscular
Dystrophies ▪ Myotonic Myopathies ▪ Periodic Paralysis

74   Disorders of Muscles, Bursas, and Tendons **415**

Muscle Cramps ▪ Fibromyalgia ▪ Bursitis ▪ Tendinitis and
Tenosynovitis ▪ De Quervain's Syndrome ▪ Baker's Cysts

75   Sports Injuries **419**

Stress Fractures of the Foot ▪ Shin Splints ▪ Popliteus
Tendinitis ▪ Achilles Tendinitis ▪ Runner's Knee ▪ Hamstring
Injury ▪ Lateral Epicondylitis ▪ Medial Epicondylitis ▪
Rotator Cuff Tendinitis

CHAPTER 58

Biology of the Musculoskeletal System

The musculoskeletal system provides form, stability, and movement to the human body. It consists of the body's bones (which make up the skeleton), muscles, tendons, ligaments, joints, cartilage, and other connective tissue. The term "connective tissue" is used to describe the tissue that binds other tissues and organs together. Its chief components are elastic fibers and collagen, a protein substance.

Connective tissue provides support to the various structures of the body—it holds organs in place and provides the underlying structure for all tissues.

Bones

Bone is a constantly changing tissue that has several functions. Bones serve as rigid structures to the body and as shields to protect delicate internal organs. They provide housing for the bone marrow, where the blood cells are formed. Bones also maintain the body's reservoir of calcium. In children, some bones have areas called growth plates. Bones lengthen in these areas until the person reaches full height, at which time the growth plates close. Thereafter, bones grow very slowly—in thickness far more than in length.

Bones have two shapes: flat (such as the plates of the skull and the vertebrae) and tubular (such as the thighbones and arm bones, which are called long bones). All bones have essentially the same structure. The hard outer part consists largely of proteins, such as collagen, and a substance called hydroxyapatite. Composed mainly of calcium and other minerals, hydroxyapatite stores much of the body's calcium and is largely responsible for the strength and density of bones. The marrow in the center of bones is softer and less dense than the rest of the bone and contains specialized cells that produce blood cells. Blood vessels supply blood to the bone, and nerves surround the bone. Bones have a unique way of healing.▲

Bones undergo a continuous process known as remodeling.■ In this process, old bone tissue is gradually replaced by new bone tissue. Every bone in the body is completely reformed about every 10 years. To maintain bone density, the body requires an adequate supply of calcium and other minerals and must produce the proper amounts of several hormones, such as parathyroid hormone, growth hormone, calcitonin, estrogen, and testosterone.

Bones are surrounded by a thin membrane called the periosteum. Bones can feel pain because of nerves located mostly in the periosteum and receive blood through blood vessels that enter through it.

Muscles

There are three types of muscles: skeletal, smooth, and cardiac (heart). Two of these kinds—skeletal and smooth—are part of the musculoskeletal system.

Skeletal muscle is what most people think of as muscle, the type that can be contracted to move the various parts of the body. Skeletal muscles are bundles of contractile fibers that are organized in a regular pattern, so that under a microscope they appear as stripes (hence, they are also called striped or striated muscles). Skeletal muscles, which are responsible

for posture and movement, are attached to bones and arranged in opposing groups around joints. For example, muscles that bend the elbow (biceps) are countered by muscles that straighten it (triceps). Skeletal muscles are controlled by the brain and are called voluntary muscles because they operate with a person's awareness. The size and strength of skeletal muscles are maintained or increased by regular exercise. In addition, growth hormone and testosterone help muscles grow in childhood and maintain their size in adulthood.

Smooth muscle controls certain bodily functions that are not readily noticeable. Smooth muscle surrounds many arteries and contracts to adjust blood flow. It surrounds the intestines and contracts to move food and feces along the digestive tract. Smooth muscle is controlled by the brain also, but not voluntarily. The triggers for contracting and relaxing smooth muscle are controlled by the body's needs, so smooth muscle operates without a person's awareness. Smooth muscles are also called involuntary muscles.

Cardiac (heart) muscle is the type of muscle that forms the heart; it is not part of the musculoskeletal system. Like skeletal muscle, cardiac muscle has a regular pattern of fibers that also appear as stripes under the microscope. However, cardiac muscle contracts and relaxes rhythmically without a person's awareness.

Tendons and Bursas

Tendons are tough bands of connective tissue made up mostly of a tough protein called collagen. They do not stretch. Tendons firmly attach each end of a muscle to a bone. They are located within sheaths, which are lubricated to allow the tendons to move without disturbing surrounding tissue.

Bursas are small fluid-filled sacs that lie under a tendon, cushioning the tendon and protecting it from injury. Bursas also provide extra cushioning to adjacent structures that otherwise might rub against each other, causing wear and tear—for example, between a bone and a ligament.

Ligaments

Ligaments are tough fibrous cords, composed of connective tissue that contains both

---

▲ see box on page 349   ■ see also page 343

Musculoskeletal System

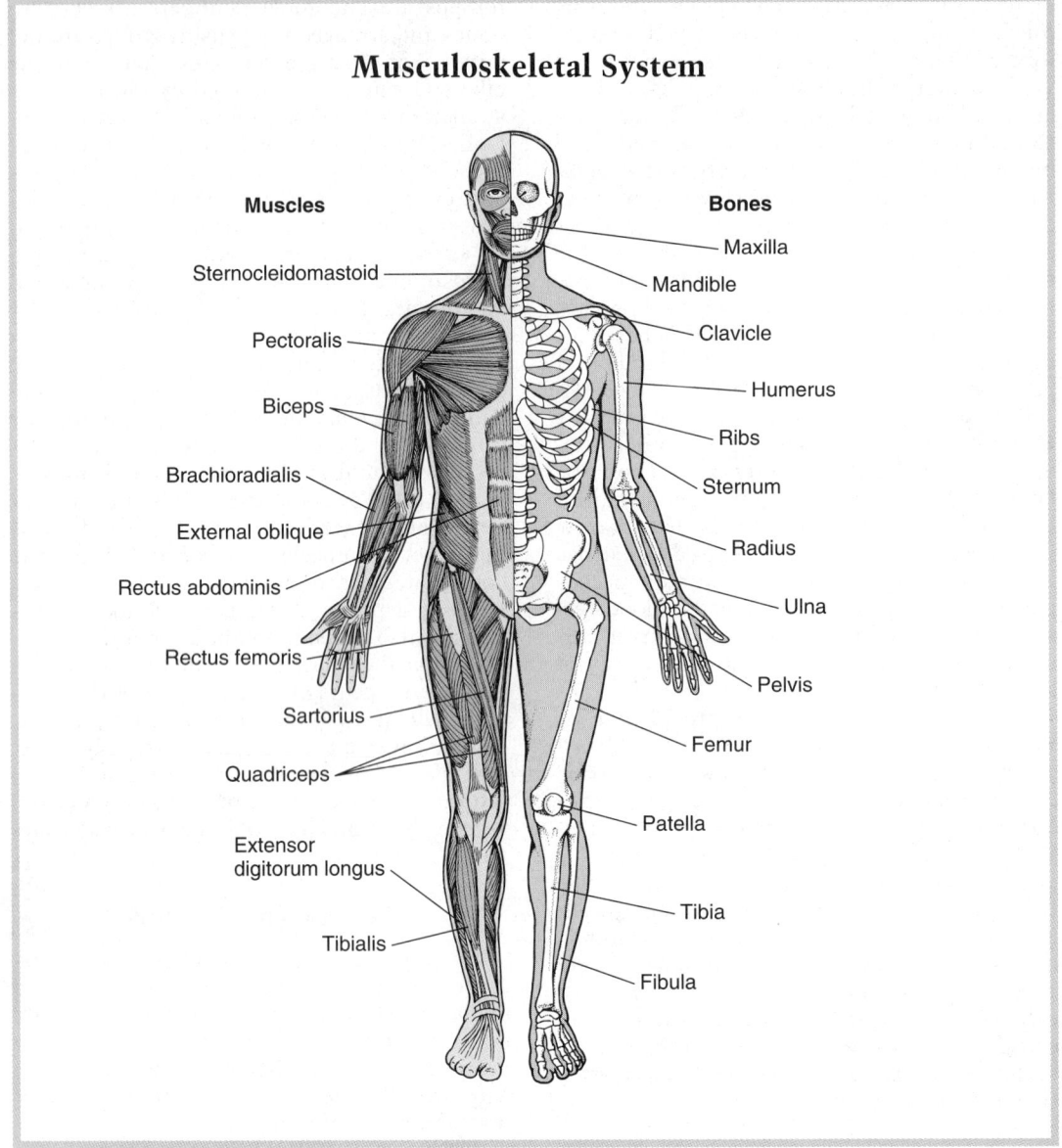

Muscles

Sternocleidomastoid

Pectoralis

Biceps

Brachioradialis

External oblique

Rectus abdominis

Rectus femoris

Sartorius

Quadriceps

Extensor digitorum longus

Tibialis

Bones

Maxilla

Mandible

Clavicle

Humerus

Ribs

Sternum

Radius

Ulna

Pelvis

Femur

Patella

Tibia

Fibula

collagen and some elastic fibers. The elastic fibers allow the ligaments to stretch to some extent. Ligaments surround joints and bind them together; they help strengthen and stabilize joints, permitting movement only in certain directions. Ligaments also connect one bone to another.

Joints

Bones come together to form joints. The configuration of a joint determines the degree and direction of possible motion. Some joints do not move, except in very young children (during and for a short time after birth). Examples of such joints are those located between the plates of the skull. Other joints allow a large and complex range of motion. For example, the shoulder joints, which have a ball-and-socket design, allow inward and outward rotation as well as forward, backward, and sideways motion of the arms. Hinge joints in the elbows, fingers, and toes allow only bending (flexion) and straightening (extension).

Musculoskeletal System

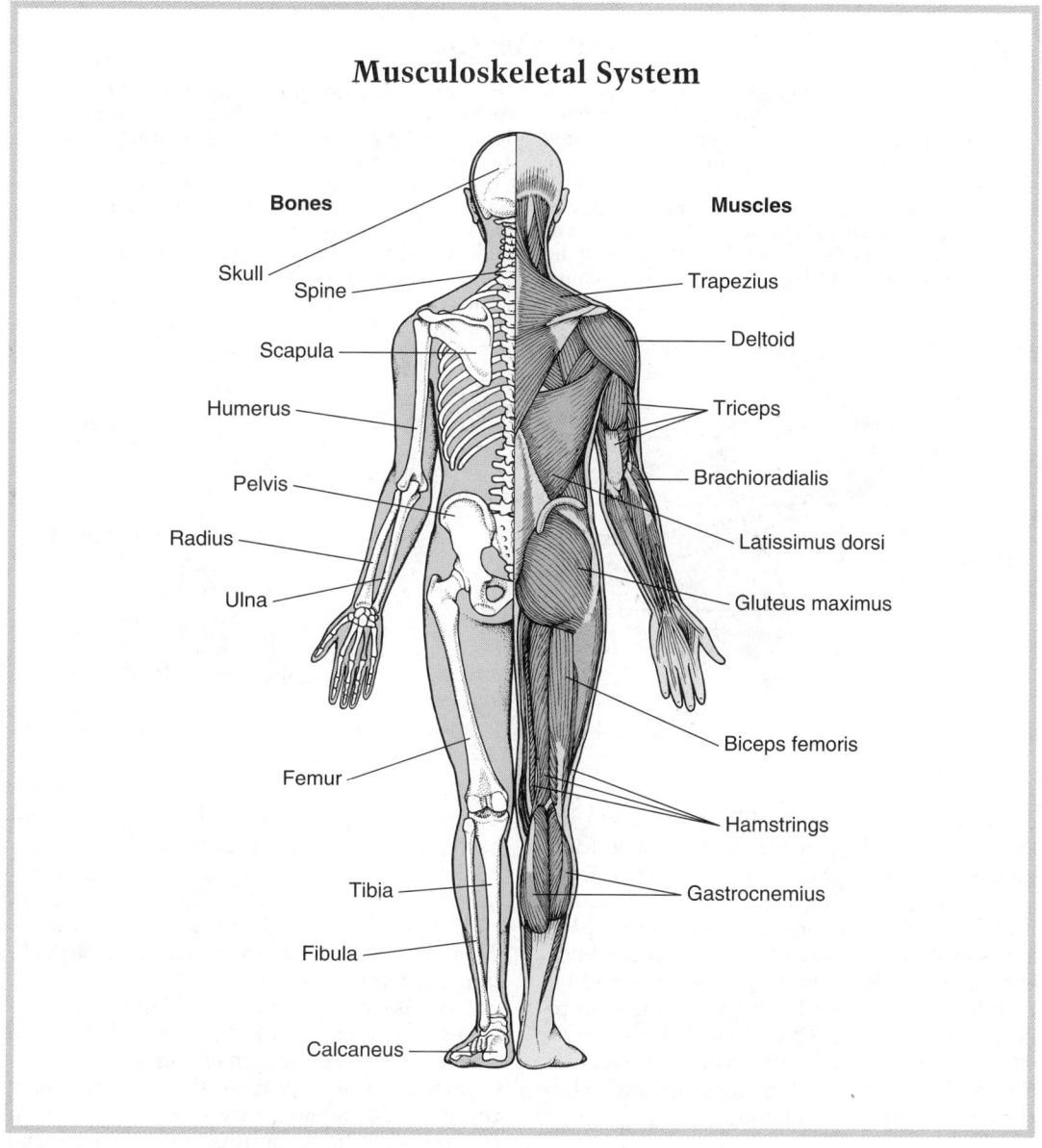

Bones

- Skull
- Spine
- Scapula
- Humerus
- Pelvis
- Radius
- Ulna
- Femur
- Tibia
- Fibula
- Calcaneus

Muscles

- Trapezius
- Deltoid
- Triceps
- Brachioradialis
- Latissimus dorsi
- Gluteus maximus
- Biceps femoris
- Hamstrings
- Gastrocnemius

The components of joints provide stability and reduce the risk of damage from constant use. In a joint, the ends of the bones are covered with cartilage—a smooth, tough, resilient protective tissue composed of collagen, water, and proteoglycans that reduces friction as joints move. (Collagen is a tough fibrous tissue; proteoglycans are substances that provide the cartilage's resilience.) Joints also have a lining (synovial tissue) that encloses them to form the joint capsule. Cells in the synovial tissue produce a small amount of clear fluid (synovial fluid), which provides nourishment to the cartilage and further reduces friction while facilitating movement.

The components of a joint work together to facilitate movement that is balanced and causes no damage to any component of the musculoskeletal system. For example, when the knee joint is bent to take a step, the hamstring muscles on the back of the thigh contract and shorten, pulling the lower leg in and bending the knee. At the same time, the quadriceps muscles on the front of the thigh

Inside the Knee

The knee is designed for its own protection. It is completely surrounded by a joint capsule that is flexible enough to allow movement but strong enough to hold the joint together. The capsule is lined with synovial tissue, which secretes synovial fluid to lubricate the joint. Wear-resistant cartilage covering the ends of the thighbone (femur) and shinbone (tibia) helps reduce friction during movement. Pads of cartilage (menisci) act as cushions between the two bones and help distribute body weight in the joint. Fluid-filled sacs (bursas) provide cushioning as skin or tendons move across bone. Ligaments along the sides and the back of the knee reinforce the joint capsule, adding stability. The kneecap (patella) protects the front of the joint.

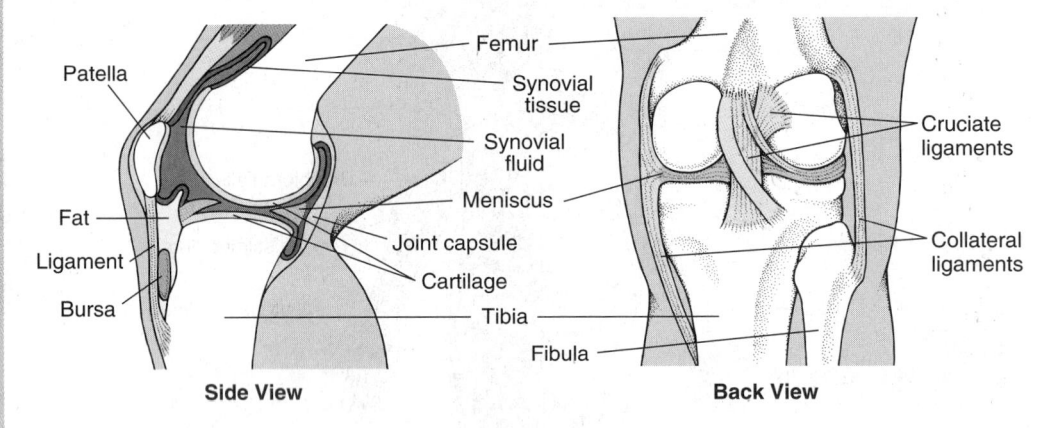

Side View   Back View

relax, so that the knee is able to bend. Within the knee joint, the cartilage and synovial fluid minimize friction. Also within the knee joint lie two pads of cartilage, called the medial meniscus and the lateral meniscus; these pads act as cushions between the bones at the knee and give the knee joint increased stability. Five ligaments around the knee joint help to keep the bones properly aligned. Bursas provide cushioning between structures such as the shinbone (tibia) and the tendon attached to the kneecap (patellar tendon).

Effects of Aging

From about age 30, the density of bones begins to diminish in men and women; this loss of density accelerates in women after menopause. As a result, the bones become more fragile and are more likely to break,▲ especially in old age.

As people age, their joints are affected by changes in cartilage and in connective tissue. The cartilage inside a joint becomes thinner;

components of the cartilage (the proteoglycans) become altered, which may make the joint less resilient and more susceptible to damage. Thus, in some people, the surfaces of the joint do not slide as well over each other as they used to. This process may lead to osteoarthritis.■ Additionally, joints become stiffer because the connective tissue within ligaments and tendons becomes more rigid and brittle. This change also limits the range of motion of joints.

Sarcopenia is a process that starts around the age of 30 and progresses throughout life. In this process, the amount of muscle tissue and the number and size of muscle fibers gradually decrease. The result of sarcopenia is a gradual loss of muscle mass and muscle strength. Fortunately, the loss in muscle mass and strength can partially be overcome or at least significantly delayed by regular exercise. The types of muscle fibers are affected by aging as well. Certain muscle fibers contract faster than others, and with age the number of these fibers decreases much more so than the number of the slower type. Thus, muscles are not able to contract as quickly in old age.

▲ see page 343   ■ see page 367

CHAPTER 59

Symptoms and Diagnosis
of Musculoskeletal Disorders

The musculoskeletal system comprises muscles, joints, ligaments, tendons, and bursas. Any of these components can be injured by trauma or a number of diseases. Different diagnostic tests are available to diagnose musculoskeletal disorders.

Symptoms

Pain

Pain is the chief symptom of most musculoskeletal disorders. The pain may be mild or severe, local or diffuse, according to where the injury occurred. Although pain may be acute and short-lived, as is the case with most injuries, pain may be ongoing with chronic illnesses, such as arthritis.

Bone pain is usually a deep, penetrating, or dull pain. It commonly results from injury. Other causes of bone pain include infection and tumors.

Muscle pain is often less intense than that of bone pain but can be very unpleasant. For example, a muscle spasm or cramp (a sustained painful muscle contraction) in the calf is an intense pain that is commonly called a charleyhorse. Pain can occur when a muscle is injured as a result of a sports injury, an autoimmune reaction,▲ loss of blood flow to the muscle, infection, or invasion by a tumor.

Virtually all joint injuries and diseases produce a stiff, aching pain, often referred to as "arthritic" pain. However, because joint pain is so common, doctors usually base a specific diagnosis on the presence of other symptoms and results of laboratory tests. For example, Lyme disease is characterized by joint pain and a bull's eye skin rash; blood tests show antibodies to the bacteria that cause Lyme disease. Gout is characterized by a sudden attack of pain in the joint at the base of the big toe; blood tests generally show high levels of uric acid.

Sometimes pain can affect the tendons of the palm; this condition is called trigger finger.■

Inflammation

Inflammation causes swelling, warmth, and tenderness, along with pain, and impairment of function. If a large part of the musculoskeletal system is inflamed, a low-grade fever may be present. Inflammation is a very common reaction of joints to a variety of abnormal circumstances, such as infection or autoimmune disease. Rheumatoid arthritis is one of many autoimmune diseases that cause joint inflammation. For joints, the swelling is often the result of fluid inside the joint. Loss of function occurs as a reduced range of motion.

Muscle inflammation (myositis) can result from a number of diseases, including a viral infection. Like any inflammation, muscle inflammation can cause pain and tenderness, swelling, warmth, and impairment of function, occurring as muscle weakness.

Muscle Weakness

Weakness can occur when any part of the musculoskeletal system is abnormal. If the muscle itself cannot contract, weakness occurs. If a nerve does not adequately stimulate the muscle, the muscle contractions are weak. If a joint is frozen and unable to move normally, the muscle may not be adequately able to cause movement. Even pain, due to inflammation, prevents normal movement, causing weakness. Weakness may be limited to one joint or limb, as is typically the case when a nerve, joint, or single muscle is diseased, or diffuse, as occurs in widespread neurologic or muscular diseases. Muscle strength may also be limited by pain in the muscles, tendons, bones, or joints, giving the impression of weakness.

Weakness is a common symptom of muscle injury or disease. Muscle weakness can also result from many diseases affecting the whole body. Although many people complain of muscle weakness when they feel tired or run down, true muscle weakness means that full effort does not generate normal strength. True muscle weakness can be caused by problems in the muscle itself (such as in muscular dystrophy★ or polymyositis●); by problems in the nervous system, which helps to con-

---

▲ see page 1073   ■ see art on page 398
★ see page 412   ● see page 383

CLASSIFYING MUSCLE WEAKNESS

Underlying Problem	Example	Description
Muscle disease	Muscular dystrophies	A group of inherited muscle disorders that lead to muscle weakness of varying severity
	Infections or inflammatory disorders (acute viral myositis, polymyositis)	Muscles tender or painful and weak
Disease of the neuromuscular junction	Myasthenia gravis, curare toxicity, Eaton-Lambert syndrome, insecticide poisoning, botulism, diphtheria	Weakness or paralysis of many muscles
Spinal cord damage	Trauma to the neck or back, spinal cord tumors, spinal stenosis, multiple sclerosis, transverse myelitis, vitamin B_{12} deficiency	Weakness or paralysis of the arms and legs below the level of injury, progressive loss of sensation below the level of injury, back pain. Bowel, bladder, and sexual function may be affected
Degeneration of nerve cell bodies in the spinal cord	Amyotrophic lateral sclerosis	Progressive loss of muscle bulk and strength, but no loss of sensation
Spinal nerve root damage	Ruptured disk in the neck or lower spine	Pain in the neck and weakness or numbness in an arm, low back pain shooting down the leg (sciatica), and leg weakness or numbness
Damage to a single nerve (mononeuropathy)	Diabetic neuropathy, local pressure	Weakness or paralysis of muscles and loss of sensation in the area served by the injured nerve
Damage to many nerves (polyneuropathy)	Diabetes, Guillain-Barré syndrome, folate deficiency, other metabolic diseases	Weakness or paralysis of muscles and loss of sensation in the areas served by the affected nerves
Use of corticosteroid drugs	Corticosteroid myopathy	Weakness usually begins at the hips and gradually spreads to all muscles
Low blood levels of potassium	Hypokalemic myopathy	The person experiences periods of weakness throughout the body that begin rapidly
Abnormal levels of thyroid hormone	High levels of thyroid hormone (hyperthyroidism) or low levels of thyroid hormone (hypothyroidism)	High levels of thyroid hormone produce weakness that is usually more pronounced in the shoulders than in the legs. Low levels of thyroid hormone produce weakness that is usually more pronounced in the legs
Low levels of vitamin D	Osteomalacia	Pain in the back, with weakness in the legs; rarely pain throughout the body
Psychologic problems	Depression, imagined symptoms, hysteria (conversion reaction)	Complaint of whole body weakness, paralysis with no evidence of nerve damage

trol movement (such as following a stroke or after a spinal cord injury; or by disease affecting the connection between the nerve and the muscles, called the neuromuscular junction (such as myasthenia gravis). Muscle weakness can occur in old age because of an age-related reduction in muscle mass called sarcopenia.▲ The word "asthenia" is sometimes used by doctors to describe weakness, but in the sense of feebleness or infirmity (debility) rather than simply muscle weakness.

Joint Stiffness

Joint stiffness is common with arthritis. Disorders of joints often interfere with joint movement sufficiently to produce stiffness. A common example is the morning stiffness that occurs with rheumatoid arthritis, in which stiffness typically occurs on arising and gradually improves with activity only after an hour or two. Some conditions, such as injuries that stretch or tear ligaments, may increase joint looseness (laxity), usually allowing excessive or abnormal bending of joints and thereby making the joints unstable. Joint looseness may occur in a connective tissue disease called cutis laxa.■

Joint Noises

Joint noises, such as creaks and clicks, are common in many people, but they can also occur with specific problems of the joints. For example, the base of the knee cap may creak when it is damaged by osteoarthritis, and the jaw may click in a person who has temporomandibular joint disorder.

Joint Range of Motion

The range of motion in a joint may be reduced because it hurts to move the joint (such as when the joint is inflamed), because the joint itself has been damaged by disease, or because long-term lack of movement has allowed the joint to become fixed. For example, when a person's arm is paralyzed by a stroke, the joints in the shoulder and elbow may freeze in place if the arm is not regularly flexed and stretched.

Diagnosis

A doctor can often diagnose a musculoskeletal disorder based on the symptoms and on the results of a physical examination. Laboratory tests, imaging tests, or other diagnostic procedures are sometimes necessary to help the doctor make or confirm a diagnosis.

Physical Examination

A doctor looks for certain things during a physical examination depending on what disorder is suspected. When evaluating bones, if a fracture is suspected,★ the doctor may notice that the affected part (such as an arm or a leg) is abnormally shaped, suggesting that the segments of bone are out of alignment. If a bone infection (osteomyelitis) is suspected, the doctor looks for tenderness over the infected bone, together with an elevated body temperature. The doctor may feel (palpate) the surfaces of the bones, to detect any abnormal bumps, which may indicate a tumor.

When a person complains of muscle weakness, the doctor checks muscles for bulk and texture and for tenderness. Muscles are also checked for abnormal movements, which may indicate a nerve disease rather than a muscle disease. Doctors look for wasting away of muscle (atrophy), which can result from damage to the muscle or its nerves or from lack of use (disuse atrophy), as sometimes occurs from prolonged bed rest. Doctors also look for muscle enlargement (hypertrophy), which normally occurs with an exercise such as weight lifting. However, when a person is ill, hypertrophy may result from one muscle working harder to compensate for the weakness of another. Muscles can also enlarge when normal muscle tissue is replaced by abnormal tissue (increasing the size but not the strength of the muscle), which occurs in amyloidosis and in certain inherited muscle disorders, such as Duchenne muscular dystrophy.

Doctors try to establish which (if any) muscles are weak and how weak they are. The muscles are tested systematically, usually beginning with the face and neck, then the arms, and finally the legs. Normally, a person should be able to hold the arms extended for one minute without their sagging, turning, or shaking. Downward drift of the arm with palms turned inward is a sign of weakness. Strength against resistance is tested by pushing or pulling while the doctor pushes and pulls in the opposite direction.

When examining joints, the doctor tests a joint's range of motion and muscle tone by moving the limb around a joint while the person is completely relaxed (passive movement). Resistance to such movement (passive resis-

---

▲ see also page 338   ■ see page 1610

★ see page 348

tance) may be decreased when the nerve leading to the muscle is injured or severed; resistance may be increased when the spinal cord or brain is injured.

Laboratory Tests

Laboratory tests are often helpful in making the diagnosis of a musculoskeletal disorder. For example, the erythrocyte sedimentation rate (ESR—a test that measures the rate at which red blood cells settle to the bottom of a test tube containing blood) is increased when inflammation is present. The level of creatine kinase (a normal muscle enzyme that leaks out and is released into the bloodstream when muscle is damaged) may also be tested. In rheumatoid arthritis, a blood test to identify rheumatoid factor is helpful to diagnosis. In gout, a blood test often shows a high level of uric acid.

Laboratory tests are also often useful to help monitor the progress of treatment (for example, the ESR can be particularly useful in monitoring the progress of treatment in rheumatoid arthritis or polymyalgia rheumatica and in confirming the diagnosis of osteomyelitis).

Nerve Tests

Nerve conduction studies▲ help determine if the nerves supplying the muscles are functioning normally; they are used in the diagnosis of such disorders as polyarteritis nodosa and ulnar nerve palsy. Electromyography,■ often conducted at the same time as nerve conduction studies, is a test in which electrical impulses reaching muscles from the nerves are recorded to help determine whether the muscles and the connection between nerves and muscles (neuromuscular junction) are normal. The test helps determine whether there is a problem primarily in the muscles or in the nerves supplying those muscles. It is also useful in diagnosing such disorders as amyotrophic lateral sclerosis and dermatomyositis.

X-rays

X-rays are taken to evaluate painful areas of bone; often, x-rays can help to detect fractures, tumors, injuries, infections, and deformities (such as congenial hip dysplasia). To help determine whether the joint has been damaged, a doctor may use an ordinary (plain) x-ray or

one taken with the joint under stress (stress x-ray).

Arthrography is an x-ray procedure in which a radiopaque dye is injected into a joint space to outline the structures, such as ligaments inside the joint. Arthrography can be used to view torn ligaments and fragmented cartilage in the joint. However, MRI is now generally used in preference to arthrography.

Dual-Energy X-ray Absorptiometry

The most accurate way to evaluate bone density, which is necessary when screening for or diagnosing osteoporosis, is with dual-energy x-ray absorptiometry (DEXA). In this test, low-dose x-rays are used to examine bone at two sites: the spine and hip. Two different energies are used to distinguish between bone and soft tissue, giving a very accurate measurement of bone density at these sites.

Computed Tomography and Magnetic Resonance Imaging

Computed tomography (CT) and magnetic resonance imaging (MRI) give much more detail than conventional x-rays and may be performed to determine the extent and exact location of damage. MRI is especially valuable for imaging muscles, ligaments, and tendons; CT is best for imaging the bone. The amount of time a person spends undergoing CT is much less than for MRI. MRI is more expensive than CT and, with the exception of when the open-sided units are used, many people feel claustrophobic inside the MRI unit.

Bone Scanning

Bone scanning is an imaging procedure that is sometimes used to diagnose a fracture, particularly if other tests do not reveal the fracture. Bone scanning involves use of a radioactive substance (technetium-99m–labeled pyrophosphate) that is taken up by any healing bone. The technique can also be used when a bone infection or a metastasis (from a cancer elsewhere in the body) is suspected. The radioactive substance is given intravenously and is detected by a bone-scanning device, creating an image of the bone that can be viewed on a computer screen.

Joint Aspiration

Joint aspiration is used to diagnose joint problems. A needle is inserted into a joint space, and fluid (synovial fluid) is sucked out (aspirated) and examined under a microscope. A doctor can often make a diagnosis after ana-

---

▲ see also page 446   ■ see also page 446

lyzing the fluid. For example, a sample of synovial fluid may contain bacteria, which confirms a diagnosis of infection. Or, it may contain urate crystals, which confirms a diagnosis of gout or pseudogout.▲ Usually performed in the doctor's office, this procedure is generally quick, easy, and almost painless. The risk of joint infection is minimal.

Arthroscopy

Arthroscopy is a procedure in which a small fiber-optic scope is inserted into a joint space, allowing the doctor to look inside the joint, take a piece of tissue for analysis (biopsy), and, if necessary, perform surgery to correct the condition.

Disorders commonly found during arthroscopy include inflammation of the synovium lining the joint (synovitis); ligament, tendon, or cartilage tears; loose pieces of bone or cartilage. All of these conditions can be repaired or removed during arthroscopy. There is a very small risk of joint infection with this procedure.

Biopsy

A biopsy is a procedure in which a small piece of tissue is taken, usually with a needle (needle biopsy), and examined under a microscope. Biopsy samples may be taken from virtually any tissue, including muscle, bone, and joints. The risk of infection is minimal.

CHAPTER 60

Osteoporosis

Osteoporosis is a condition in which a progressive decrease in the density of bones weakens the bones, making fractures likely.

Bones contain minerals, such as calcium and phosphorus, which make them hard and dense. To maintain bone density, the body requires an adequate supply of calcium and other minerals and must produce the proper amounts of several hormones, such as parathyroid hormone, growth hormone, calcitonin, estrogen, and testosterone. An adequate supply of vitamin D is also needed to absorb calcium from food and incorporate it into bones. Vitamin D is absorbed from the diet and also manufactured in the skin by sunlight.■

So that bones can adjust to the changing demands placed on them, they are continuously broken down and reformed, or remodeled.★ In this process, small areas of bone tissue are removed and new bone tissue is deposited. This process is continuous and moves through healthy bone. Remodeling affects the shape and density of the bones. In youth, the bones grow in width and length as the body grows. In later life, bones may sometimes enlarge in width but do not continue to grow longer.

Because more bone is formed than is broken down in the young adult years, bones progressively increase in density until about age 30,

when they are at their strongest. After that, as breakdown outstrips formation, bones slowly decrease in density. If the body is unable to maintain an adequate amount of bone formation, bones continue to lose density and become increasingly fragile, eventually resulting in osteoporosis.

Types

About 8 million women and 2 million men in the United States have osteoporosis. There are two main types of osteoporosis: primary osteoporosis, which occurs spontaneously, and secondary osteoporosis, which is caused by another disease and occurs in fewer than 5% of people who have osteoporosis. Examples of diseases that may cause secondary osteoporosis are chronic kidney failure and hormonal disorders (especially Cushing's disease, hyperparathyroidism, hyperthyroidism, hypogonadism, and diabetes mellitus). Examples of drugs that may cause secondary osteoporosis are corticosteroids, barbiturates, and anticonvulsants. Excessive alcohol consumption and cigarette smoking may worsen preexisting osteoporosis but are unlikely to cause it on their own.

▲ see page 391   ■ see page 894

★ see also page 335

Loss of Bone Density in Women

In women, bone density (or mass) progressively increases until about age 30, when bones are at their strongest. After that, bone density gradually decreases. The decrease in bone loss accelerates after menopause, which occurs on average around age 51.

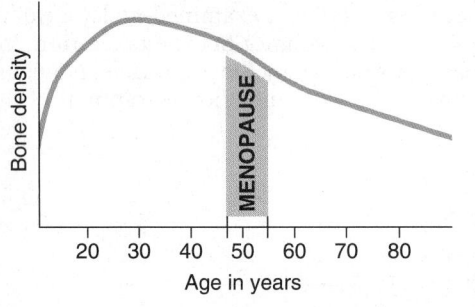

Primary osteoporosis has three subtypes: postmenopausal osteoporosis, senile osteoporosis, and idiopathic osteoporosis. Most older women who have osteoporosis have a combination of postmenopausal and senile osteoporosis.

Postmenopausal Osteoporosis: Postmenopausal osteoporosis (type I osteoporosis) is caused by a lack of estrogen, the main female hormone, which helps to regulate the incorporation of calcium into bone in women. (Type I osteoporosis also occurs in men who are castrated or in men with low testosterone levels, as may occur in older men; however, it is 6 times more common in women.) Usually, postmenopausal osteoporosis develops in women after menopause, between the ages of 51 and 75, but it can begin earlier or later. Although bone loss is gradual in women leading up to menopause, it accelerates at menopause. Indeed, women can lose up to 20% of their bone mass in the 5 to 7 years after menopause. Not all women are at equal risk of developing postmenopausal osteoporosis. For example, low body weight increases the risk of postmenopausal osteoporosis, probably for two reasons:

• Thin women have smaller bones than do heavier women, even at about age 30 when their bones are at their strongest.

• Thin women usually have lower body fat than do heavier women; estrogen levels are

lower in thin women because fat tissue activates certain forms of estrogen.

Women most at risk for osteoporosis are white, fair-skinned, and thin and/or with a light frame. Black and Hispanic women are less prone to osteoporosis than are white and Asian women. The main reason appears to be that, because black and Hispanic women have stronger bones in young adulthood, they can tolerate the bone loss that occurs with age and menopause better than other women can. Other risk factors include advanced age, menopause that occurred early or was surgically induced, abnormal absence of menstrual periods (amenorrhea), and anorexia nervosa.

Senile Osteoporosis: Senile osteoporosis (type II osteoporosis) probably results from an age-related calcium deficiency or a vitamin D deficiency and an imbalance between the rate of bone breakdown and new bone formation. Senile means only that the condition occurs in older people. It usually affects people older than 70 and is twice as common in women as in men. Women often have both senile and postmenopausal osteoporosis.

Idiopathic Osteoporosis: Idiopathic osteoporosis is a rare type of osteoporosis; the word *idiopathic* simply means that the cause is unknown. This type of osteoporosis occurs in children and young adults who have normal hormone levels, normal vitamin levels, and no obvious reason to have weak bones.

Symptoms

At first, osteoporosis produces no symptoms because bone density loss occurs very gradually. Some people never develop symptoms.

Eventually, however, bone density may decrease enough for bones to collapse or fracture, producing severe sudden pain or gradually developing aching bone pain and deformities. In long bones, such as the bones of the arms and legs, the fracture usually occurs at the ends of the bones rather than in the middle. In the bones of the spinal column (vertebrae), the fracture usually occurs in the middle to lower back; this type of bone is particularly at risk for fracture due to osteoporosis.

Vertebral crush fractures (fractures of spinal vertebrae) may occur in people who have any type of osteoporosis; these fractures are called osteoporotic fractures. The weakened vertebrae may collapse spontaneously or after a slight injury. Chronic back pain may occur because of these fractures. Usually, pain starts suddenly, stays in a particular area of the back, and worsens when a person stands or walks. The area may be tender. Usually the pain and tenderness go away gradually after a few weeks or months. If several vertebrae break, an abnormal curvature of the spine (a "dowager's hump") may develop, causing muscle strain and soreness as well as deformity.

Bones in other parts of the body may fracture, often because of a minor strain or fall. One of the most serious fractures is a hip fracture, a major cause of disability and loss of independence in older people.▲ Wrist fractures, called Colles' fractures,■ occur commonly, especially in people with postmenopausal osteoporosis. In addition, fractures tend to heal slowly in people who have osteoporosis.

Diagnosis

A doctor may suspect osteoporosis in anyone, especially an older woman, who breaks a bone with little or no force. Bone mineral density testing can be used to detect or confirm suspected osteoporosis, even before a fracture occurs. A number of rapid screening techniques are available to measure density at the wrist or the heel; however, the most useful test is the dual-energy x-ray absorptiometry (DEXA), which measures bone density at the sites at which major fractures are likely to occur: the spine and hip. This test is painless and can be performed in about 5 to 15 minutes. It is useful for people at high risk of developing osteoporosis and for those in whom the diagnosis is uncertain. It is also useful for monitoring the response to treatment.

Blood tests may be performed to measure calcium and phosphorus. Further testing may be needed to rule out treatable conditions that might lead to osteoporosis. If such a condition is found, the diagnosis is secondary osteoporosis.

Prevention

Prevention is generally more successful than treatment—it is easier to prevent loss of bone density than to restore density once it has been lost. Prevention involves maintaining or increasing bone density by consuming adequate amounts of calcium and vitamin D, engaging in weight-bearing exercise, and, for some people, taking certain drugs.

Consuming an adequate amount of calcium and vitamin D is effective, especially before maximum bone density is reached (around age 30) but also after this time. About 1500 milligrams of calcium and 400 to 800 units of vitamin D daily are recommended. Drinking two 8-ounce glasses of vitamin D–fortified milk,

Risk Factors for Osteoporosis in Women

- Family members with osteoporosis
- Insufficient calcium in the diet
- Sedentary lifestyle
- White or Asian race
- Thin build
- Use of certain drugs, such as corticosteroids and excessive amounts of thyroid hormones
- Early menopause
- Cigarette smoking
- Excessive alcohol consumption

eating a balanced diet, and taking a vitamin D supplement are important, but many women may also need to take a calcium supplement. Many calcium preparations are available; some include supplemental vitamin D.

Weight-bearing exercise, such as walking and stair-climbing, increases bone density. Exercises that do not involve weight bearing, such as swimming, do not increase bone density. Exercise is also important to improve balance, which can help to prevent a fracture that may occur from falling. Curiously, in premenopausal women, high degrees of exercise, such as occurs in athletes, can actually cause a small reduction in bone density because such exercise suppresses the production of estrogen by the ovaries.

Drugs called bisphosphonates, such as alendronate or risedronate, may be used alone as preventive therapy or, in women, combined with estrogen replacement therapy.

Estrogen replacement therapy helps maintain bone density in women. This therapy is most effective when started within 4 to 6 years after menopause, but starting it later can still slow bone loss and reduce the risk of fractures. Decisions about using estrogen replacement therapy after menopause are complex,★ because the treatment may have side effects and risks, including an increased risk of uterine cancer and a slightly increased risk of breast cancer. Taking progesterone with the estrogen reduces the risk of uterine cancer but not of breast cancer.

Raloxifene is an estrogen-like drug that may be less effective than estrogen in preventing

▲ see page 355   ■ see page 358
★ see page 1358

bone loss, but it does not have estrogen's typical side effects on the breast and uterus. Raloxifene is used in people who cannot or prefer not to take estrogen.

Treatment

Treatment is aimed at increasing bone density. The first step is to consume or take an adequate daily amount of calcium and vitamin D.

The bisphosphonates (alendronate and risedronate) are useful in preventing and treating all types of osteoporosis. These bisphosphonates have been shown to increase bone mass in the spine and hips and reduce the incidence of fractures. A bisphosphonate must be swallowed with a full glass of water (6 to 8 ounces) on arising for the day, and no other food, drink, or drug should be consumed for the next 30 minutes. Because bisphosphonates can irritate the lining of the esophagus, the person must not lie down after taking a dose for at least 30 minutes, and then must not lie down until after something has been eaten.

Certain people, including those who have difficulty in swallowing, cannot take the bisphosphonates by mouth. In these people, another bisphosphonate, pamidronate, can be given intravenously. In addition, the following people should not take bisphosphonates: people who have certain disorders of the esophagus or stomach, women who are pregnant or nursing, people who have low levels of calcium in the blood, and people who have severe kidney disease.

Calcium and vitamin D supplements are usually recommended for women and men, especially if tests show that their body is not absorbing adequate amounts of calcium. Men do not benefit from estrogen but may benefit from testosterone replacement therapy if their testosterone level is low. Men may also benefit from taking a bisphosphonate.

Calcitonin, which inhibits the breakdown of bone, is also used for treatment, particularly for people who have painful fractures of the vertebrae. Calcitonin can be taken by injection or nasal spray. Its use can decrease blood levels of calcium; these levels must be monitored.

Parathyroid hormone injected daily in small amounts can increase the formation of new bone, increase bone density, and decrease the likelihood of fractures. Although this medication is promising, it is not yet available.

Fluoride supplements can increase bone density. However, because the resulting bone may be abnormal and fragile, fluoride supplements are not generally recommended. New forms of fluoride, which may not have side effects on bone quality, are being tested.

Fractures resulting from osteoporosis must be treated. For hip fractures, usually part or all of the hip is replaced surgically.▲ Surgery may be needed for a wrist fracture, or the wrist may need to be placed in a cast. Supportive back braces are used temporarily for people with painful vertebral crush fractures.

A collapsed vertebra can be repaired by a procedure called vertebroplasty. In this procedure, which takes about an hour for each vertebra, a material called polymethylmethacrylate (PMMA)—an acrylic "bone cement"—is injected into the collapsed vertebra, helping to relieve pain and reduce deformity. Kyphoplasty is a similar procedure, in which an orthopedic balloon is used to expand the vertebra back to its normal shape, prior to the injection of the acrylic bone cement.

CHAPTER 61

Paget's Disease of Bone

Paget's disease of bone is a chronic disorder of the skeleton in which areas of bone undergo abnormal turnover, resulting in areas of enlarged and softened bone.

Paget's disease can affect any bone, but the most commonly affected bones are the pelvis, thighbone (femur), skull, shin (tibia), spine (vertebrae), collarbone (clavicle), and upper arm bone (humerus).

Paget's disease rarely occurs in people younger than 40. In the United States, about

▲ see page 355

1% of people older than 40 have the disorder; the prevalence increases with age. Men are 50% more likely than women to develop it. Paget's disease is more common in Europe (excluding Scandinavia), Australia, and New Zealand than in the Americas, Africa, and Asia. It is particularly common in England.

Normally, cells that break down old bone (osteoclasts) and cells that form new bone (osteoblasts) work in balance to maintain bone structure and integrity. In Paget's disease, both osteoclasts and osteoblasts become overactive in some areas of bone, and the rate at which bone is broken down and rebuilt (bone remodeling▲) in these areas increases tremendously. The overactive areas enlarge but are structurally abnormal and therefore weaker than normal areas.

The cause of Paget's disease is unknown. Although the disorder tends to run in families, no specific genetic pattern has been discovered. Some evidence suggests that a virus (the paramyxovirus) is involved. Even if it is, there is no evidence that the disorder is contagious.

Symptoms

Paget's disease usually produces no symptoms, although bone pain, bone enlargement, or bone deformity may occur. Bone pain may be deep, aching, and occasionally severe and may worsen at night. The enlarging bones may compress nerves, adding to the pain. Sometimes Paget's disease distorts the adjacent joint structure and leads to the development of painful osteoarthritis.■ Stiff joints and fatigue may develop slowly and subtly.

Symptoms vary, depending on which bones are affected. The skull may enlarge, and the brow and forehead may look more prominent. A person may notice this enlargement when a larger-size hat is needed. Enlarged skull bones can cause hearing loss and dizziness, by damaging the inner ear (cochlea) or compressing the nerve that connects the ear to the brain. The enlarged skull bones can also cause headaches, by compressing nerves. The veins on the scalp may bulge, possibly because of the increased blood flow through the skull bones. The vertebrae may enlarge, weaken, and buckle, resulting in a loss of height. Damaged vertebrae may pinch the nerves of the spinal cord, causing pain, numbness, tingling, weakness, or even paralysis in the legs. People whose hip or leg bones are affected may have bowed legs and take short, unsteady steps. Affected bones are more likely to break.

Rarely, heart failure develops because the increased blood flow through the affected bone puts extra stress on the heart. In fewer than 1% of people who have Paget's disease, the affected bone becomes cancerous.

High blood levels of calcium (hypercalcemia)★ occasionally occur in bedridden older people with Paget's disease or in anyone with severe Paget's disease who becomes immobilized or dehydrated. These high levels of calcium can result in many symptoms, such as high blood pressure, muscle weakness, mild bowel disturbances, and stones in the urine.

Diagnosis and Treatment

Paget's disease is often discovered accidentally when x-rays or laboratory tests are performed for other reasons. Otherwise, the diagnosis may be suspected on the basis of the symptoms and physical examination. The diagnosis can be confirmed by x-rays showing abnormalities characteristic of Paget's disease and by a laboratory test measuring blood levels of alkaline phosphatase, an enzyme involved in bone cell formation. A bone scan (a radionuclide test using technetium) shows which bones are affected.

A person who has Paget's disease needs treatment if the symptoms cause discomfort or if there is a significant risk or suggestion of complications, such as hearing loss, osteoarthritis, and deformity.

Aspirin, other nonsteroidal anti-inflammatory drugs, and commonly used analgesics such as acetaminophen may reduce bone pain. If one leg becomes bowed, heel lifts can help make walking easier. Sometimes surgery is needed to relieve pinched nerves or to replace a joint that has become arthritic from Paget's disease.

One of several bisphosphonates—alendronate, etidronate, pamidronate, risedronate, or tiludronate—can be used to slow the progression of Paget's disease. Except for pamidronate, which is usually given intravenously, these drugs are given by mouth. These drugs are given before surgery to prevent or reduce bleeding during surgery; they are also given to treat pain caused by Paget's disease, to prevent or slow the progression of weakness or paralysis in people who cannot have surgery, and to

---

▲ see also page 343   ■ see page 367

★ see also page 904

attempt to prevent arthritis, further hearing loss, or further bone deformity.

Calcitonin is occasionally used as an injection under the skin or in muscle. It is not as effective as the bisphosphonates and is used only when the other drugs cannot be given.

Bed rest (except for sleeping at night) should be avoided, if possible, to prevent hypercalcemia. If hypercalcemia does develop, intravenous fluids and diuretics such as furosemide are given.

Dietary intake of calcium and vitamin D (necessary for calcium uptake) should be sufficient to ensure that the incorporation of calcium into bone (bone mineralization) is ade-quate in bone that is being remodeled rapidly.▲ Otherwise, poor mineralization (osteomalacia■) may occur.

Prognosis

The prognosis for people with Paget's disease is most often very good. However, the few people who develop bone cancer (osteosarcoma, fibrosarcoma, or chondrosarcoma★) have a poor prognosis. People who develop other complications, such as heart failure, compression of the spinal cord, or hypercalcemia may also have a poor prognosis, unless treatment of these complications is timely and successful.

CHAPTER 62

Fractures

A fracture is a break in a bone, usually accompanied by injury to the surrounding tissues.

Fractures vary greatly in size, severity, and the treatment needed. They can range from a small, easily missed crack in a hand bone to a massive, life-threatening break of the pelvis. Serious injuries, including injuries to the skin, nerves, blood vessels, muscles, and organs, may occur at the same time as the fracture. These injuries can complicate treatment of the fracture.

Trauma is the most common cause of fractures. Low-energy trauma, such as a fall on level ground, usually causes minor fractures. High-energy trauma, such as high-speed motor vehicle accidents and falls from buildings, can cause severe fractures that involve several bones.

Certain underlying disorders can weaken parts of the skeleton so that breaks are more likely to occur. Such disorders include certain infections, benign bone tumors, cancer, and osteoporosis.

Symptoms and Complications

Pain is the most obvious symptom. Fractures hurt, especially when force is applied, such as when a person tries to put weight on an injured limb. The area around the broken bone is also tender to touch. Swelling of soft tissue around the fracture begins within a few hours. The limb may not function properly, so that moving an arm, standing on a leg, or gripping with a hand is very painful. For a person who cannot speak (for example, a very young child, a person with a head injury, or an older person with dementia), refusal to move an extremity may be the only sign of a fracture. People with pathologic fractures often experience steadily increasing pain beginning weeks before the fracture actually occurs.

Internal bleeding may occur with a closed fracture (one in which the skin is not torn). The bleeding may occur from the bone itself or from surrounding soft tissues. The blood eventually works its way to the surface, forming a bruise, which at first is purplish-black then slowly turns to green and yellow as the blood is broken down and reabsorbed back into the body. The blood can move quite a distance from the fracture, and the entire process takes a few weeks to complete. The blood can

---

▲ see page 335   ■ see page 894
★ see page 360

How Bones Heal

When tissues, such as those of the skin, muscles, and internal organs, become injured, they tend to mend by having scar tissue take the place of healthy tissue. The scar tissue often compromises the tissue's appearance or function in some way. In contrast, bone is unique in that it heals with its own tissue—bone—rather than with scar tissue. This unusual capacity for regeneration enables a mending bone to heal itself after a fracture. Even shattered fragments of bone, with proper treatment, can often be restored to their normal function.

Fractures heal in three overlapping phases: inflammation, repair, and remodeling. Healing begins immediately with the **inflammatory phase.** In this phase, damaged soft tissue, bone fragments, and lost blood caused by the injury are removed by cells of the immune system. The region around the fracture becomes swollen and tender as cell activity and blood flow increase. The inflammatory phase reaches peak activity in a couple of days, but takes weeks to subside. This process accounts for most of the early pain people experience with fractures.

The **repair phase** begins within days of the injury and lasts for weeks to months. New repaired bone, called the external callus, is formed during this phase. When first produced, the callus has no calcium; it is soft and rubbery and cannot be seen on an x-ray. This new bone is neither strong nor stable, so that during this period the fractured bone can easily collapse and become displaced (that is, slip out of its proper place). At 3 to 6 weeks, the callus calcifies and becomes much stiffer and stronger and becomes visible on x-rays.

The **remodeling phase** (in which the bone is built back to its normal state) lasts many months. The bulky external callus is slowly resorbed and replaced by stronger bone; in this phase, the normal contours and architecture of the bone are restored. It is not likely that the bone will fracture again during this phase; however, people may experience mild pain with exertion.

---

cause temporary pain and stiffness in surrounding structures. Shoulder fractures, for instance, can bruise the entire arm and cause pain in the elbow and wrist. Some fractures, especially hip fractures, can lose quite a lot of blood into the surrounding tissues, causing low blood pressure.

The person usually feels some discomfort with activities even after fractures have healed sufficiently to allow full weight bearing. For example, although a fractured wrist may be strong enough to allow some use in about 2 months, the wrist will not have completely undergone remodeling, and it will be painful with forceful gripping for up to 1 year. The person may also notice increased pain and stiffness when the weather is damp, cold, or stormy.

Most fractures heal with few problems. However, sometimes even with proper treatment, fractures can cause serious complications.

Compartment Syndrome: Compartment syndrome is a serious limb-threatening condition caused by excessive swelling of injured muscles, which may occur as a result of a fracture or crush injury to a limb. Muscles are surrounded by a fibrous covering that forms a closed space (compartment). An injured muscle swells; when the swelling is significantly confined by the muscle's compartment, and particularly when it is further confined by a cast, the pressure within the muscle tissue may increase. This increase in pressure decreases the normal blood flow that provides oxygen to the muscle. When the muscle is deprived of oxygen for too long, further injury to the muscle occurs, which leads to further swelling and higher tissue pressures. After only a few hours, irreversible injury and death of muscle and nearby soft tissues may result.

A doctor becomes concerned about compartment syndrome when the person feels increasing pain in an immobilized limb after a fracture, pain when the fingers of an immobilized arm or toes of an immobilized leg are moved gently, or numbness in the limb. The diagnosis of compartment syndrome can be confirmed using a device that measures pressure in the muscles.

Pulmonary Embolism: Pulmonary embolism is the sudden blocking of a lung artery by an embolus, nearly always resulting from a blood clot that can travel to the lungs, especially from the deep veins of the leg.▲ Pulmonary embolism is the most common fatal complication of serious hip and pelvic fractures. People

---

▲ see also page 285

TYPES OF FRACTURES

Type	Description	Type	Description
Open	The skin and soft tissue covering the bone are torn; dirt, debris, or bacteria can easily contaminate the wound	Occult	Fractures that are difficult or impossible for a doctor to see on an initial x-ray; may appear as dark or white lines days to weeks after injury
Closed	The skin is not torn		
Avulsion	Small fragments of bone detach from where tendons or ligaments attach to bones; usually affect hand, foot, ankle, knee, shoulder	Greenstick	A partial crack and a bend in the bone but not a break through the bone completely; occur in children only
Osteoporotic	Certain areas of the skeleton are selectively weakened by osteoporosis, making them more likely to break; occur in older people, usually in the hip, wrist, spine, shoulder, pelvis	Growth plate	A break through part of the bone that allows bones to lengthen (growth plate); may cause a bone to stop growing or to grow crookedly; occur only in children
Compression	The bone collapses into itself; occur in older people, most commonly affecting the spine	Simple transverse	A clean square break that divides a bone cleanly across
Joint (intra-articular)	Occur within a joint; lead to a loss of motion and gradually developing osteoarthritis	Displaced	The broken ends of the bones are separated or bent at an angle
Pathologic	An underlying disorder (such as infection, a noncancerous bone tumor, cancer) weakens a bone, leading to a fracture	Nondisplaced	The normal shape and alignment of a bone are maintained despite cracks completely through the bone
Stress	A bone becomes stressed repeatedly over time because of certain activities, such as walking with a heavy pack or running	Spiral	Sharp, triangular bone ends
		Comminuted	The bone is broken into multiple pieces, often because of high-energy trauma or weakening by osteoporosis

with hip fractures are at high risk of pulmonary embolism because of the combination of trauma to the leg, forced immobilization for hours or days, and swelling around the fracture site blocking blood flow in the veins. Of people with a hip fracture who die, about one third die of pulmonary embolism. Pulmonary embolism occurs much less commonly with fractures of the lower leg and very rarely with fractures of the upper body.

Doctors may suspect pulmonary embolism based on a range of symptoms, including chest pain, cough, and shortness of breath. Confirmation may involve chest x-ray, electrocardiogram, and one or more of a variety of imaging studies.

Diagnosis

X-rays are the most important tool for diagnosing a fracture. They not only show the frac-

ture but also help a doctor understand how the fragments of bone are misaligned. Small or nondisplaced fractures can be difficult to see on routine x-rays, and sometimes additional x-rays are taken at special angles. Occult or stress fractures may take days or weeks to show clearly on x-rays. Pathologic fractures are diagnosed by x-rays that show bone abnormalities, such as punched-out (lytic) areas caused by infection, benign tumors, or cancer.

Computed tomography (CT) and magnetic resonance imaging (MRI) can show features not seen on routine x-rays. CT can show the fine details of a fractured joint surface or can reveal areas of a fracture hidden by overlying bone. MRI shows the soft tissue around the bone, which helps to detect injury to nearby tendons and ligaments, and can show evidence of cancer. MRI also shows injury (swelling or bruising) within the bone and can thus reveal occult fractures before they appear on x-rays.

Bone scanning▲ is an imaging procedure that involves use of a radioactive substance (technetium-99m–labeled pyrophosphate) that is taken up by any healing bone. Occult fractures can be detected on bone scans 3 to 5 days after the injury. If a pathologic fracture is suspected, bone scans help to check for problems in other bones—ones that might not yet be producing symptoms.

Treatment

Fractures require immediate attention because they cause pain and loss of function for the person. After initial emergency care, fractures usually require further treatment, including immobilization with casts or traction, or fixation with surgery.

Fractures in children are often treated differently than those in adults because bones in children are smaller, more flexible and less brittle, and most importantly, still growing. Treatment with casts or traction is often preferred over surgery to avoid damage to the growth plate.

Initial Treatment: When a fracture is suspected, the person should call his or her doctor, who will determine the appropriate facility for treatment. The choice of a facility depends on the severity of the injury. For example, people with minor wrist and shoulder fractures can be treated in medical offices. Because people with hip fractures are in severe pain and are unable to move, they must be transported by ambulance to a hospital with surgical facilities.

Open fractures need to be treated immediately with surgery to carefully clean and close the wound. Massive open fractures with great losses of the skin, muscle, and blood supply to the bone are the most serious and difficult to treat.

For most closed fractures, treatment with casts or surgery can be delayed up to 1 week without affecting the long-term result. However, there is usually no advantage to waiting, because until they are treated, people are troubled by pain and loss of function. Before seeing a doctor, the person should immobilize and support the injured limb with a makeshift splint, sling, or a pillow; elevate the limb to the level of the heart to limit swelling; apply ice to control pain and swelling; and take only acetaminophen to relieve pain. Aspirin and other nonsteroidal anti-inflammatory drugs (NSAIDs) should not be taken because they may worsen bleeding.■

The doctor may recommend the person continue to keep an injured arm or leg elevated to control swelling. For arm fractures, pillows are used for elevation. For leg fractures, the person should periodically lie flat with the leg on a pillow. The doctor compares the swelling of the injured limb with the normal appearance of the uninjured limb to help determine how long or often elevation is needed. During the later stages of healing, elastic stockings may be used during the daytime to help control swelling when the person is sitting or standing.

Immobilization: Most fractures can be treated without surgery. They are immobilized with a splint, sling, or cast until they heal sufficiently. Displaced fractures must be aligned (by a procedure called reduction) before being immobilized. When minor fractures (such as those of the fingers or wrist) are aligned, the person may need an injection of a local anesthetic, such as lidocaine, to prevent pain. When major fractures of the arm, shoulder, or lower leg are aligned, the person may need general or spinal anesthesia; this procedure is called closed reduction.

A **splint** is a long, narrow slab of plaster or fiberglass applied with elastic wrap or tape. The slab does not completely encircle the limb, which allows for some expansion due to tissue swelling. For this reason, splints are often used for initial treatment of fractures. For finger fractures, aluminum splints covered with foam are commonly used.

A **sling** by itself provides sufficient support for many shoulder and elbow fractures. The weight of the arm pulling downward helps to keep many shoulder fractures well aligned. A strap passing around behind the back can be added to keep the arm from swinging outward, especially at night. Slings permit some use of the hand.

A **cast** is made by wrapping rolls of plaster or fiberglass strips that harden once wetted. Plaster is often chosen for the initial cast when a displaced fracture is being treated. It molds well and has less of a tendency to cause painful contact points between the body and cast. Otherwise, fiberglass has the advantage of being stronger, lighter, and more durable. In

▲ see also page 342   ■ see page 452

Taking Care of a Cast

- When bathing, enclose the cast in a plastic bag and carefully seal the top with rubber bands or tape. Commercially available waterproof covers are convenient to use and are more fail-safe. If a cast becomes wet, the underlying padding may retain moisture. A hair dryer can remove some dampness. Otherwise, the cast must be changed to prevent the breakdown of skin.

- Never push a sharp or pointed object down inside the cast (for example, to scratch the skin).

- Check the skin around the cast every day, and apply lotion to any red or sore area.

- When resting, position the cast carefully, possibly using a small pillow or pad, to prevent the edge from pinching or digging into the skin. Chafing or pressure sores may develop where the skin is in contact with the edge of the cast. If the edge of the cast feels rough, it can be padded with soft adhesive tape, moleskin, tissues, or cloth.

- Elevate the cast regularly, as directed by the doctor, to control swelling.

- Contact a doctor immediately if the cast causes persistent pain or excessive tightness. Pressure sores or unexpected swelling may require immediate removal of the cast.

either case, the cast is lined with soft cottony material to protect the skin from pressure and rubbing. If the cast becomes wet, it is often impossible to completely dry the lining; this can lead to skin softening and breakdown (maceration). For partially healed fractures, a special, more expensive and less protective waterproof lining is sometimes substituted.

After a cast is applied (especially for the first 24 to 48 hours), it should be kept elevated when possible to the level of the heart to combat swelling. Regular flexion and extension of the fingers or wiggling of the toes helps the blood to drain from the limb and also helps to prevent swelling. Pain, pressure, or numbness that remains constant or worsens over time should be reported to a doctor immediately. These conditions may be due to a developing bedsore or compartment syndrome.

Traction: Traction is sometimes used to keep the bones aligned while a fracture heals.

An array of ropes, pulleys, and weights are used to continuously pull on the limb. In adults, traction is used only until the fracture can be safely treated with a cast or surgery. In children, certain fractures are best treated with traction because the healing time is shorter than in adults. Also, traction does not injure the growth plate, whereas surgery may do so.

Surgical Treatment: Fractures sometimes require surgical treatment. For instance, the doctor must explore and carefully clean open fractures to ensure that no foreign material has contaminated the bone ends. When a bone fragment or a tendon is trapped in the bone ends, a doctor may not be able to align a displaced fracture and surgery is needed. Comminuted fractures are often too unstable for a cast to maintain alignment against the forces of muscle contraction, which can cause the bone to shorten or angle. Joint fractures require a near-perfect alignment of the joint surfaces or the person will later develop arthritis. If possible, pathologic fractures are stabilized surgically before they break through completely. This approach avoids the pain, disability, and the more complex surgery involved with a displaced fracture. Finally, if fractures of the femur (thighbone), which includes most hip fractures, are not treated surgically, they would require months of immobilization in bed before the person is strong enough to bear weight. In contrast, surgical stabilization usually permits the person to walk with crutches or a walker within days.

Surgical stabilization involves first accurately reducing the fracture to restore the bone's original shape and length. The surgeon uses anesthesia to relax the muscles and x-ray equipment to help align the bones. A surgeon exposes the fracture to see and manipulate the fragments with special instruments. Then, the bone fragments are securely fixed using some combination of metal wires, pins, screws, rods, and plates. Metal plates are contoured and fixed to the outside of the bone with screws. Metal rods are inserted from one end of the bone into the marrow cavity. These implants are made of stainless steel, high-strength alloy metal, or titanium. All such implants made in the last 15 years are compatible with the strong magnets that are used for magnetic resonance imaging (MRI). Most will not set off security devices at airports.

A **joint replacement procedure** (arthroplasty) may need to be performed when fractures severely damage the upper end of the femur (thighbone) or humerus (armbone) that form the outer half of the hip and shoulder joints.

Bone grafting may be used to assist healing of fractures initially, if the gap between fragments is too large, or later, if the healing process has slowed (delayed union) or stopped (nonunion).

Treatment of Complications: For compartment syndrome, initial treatment consists of immediately removing or loosening anything that may be confining the limb, such as a splint or a cast. When the muscle compartment continues to cause increased pressure, an emergency surgery called fasciotomy must be performed to open this constricting tissue. Otherwise, the muscles and nerves could die because of a lack of oxygen. If this occurs, it may be necessary to amputate the limb.

Pulmonary embolism can be prevented with drugs such as heparin, low-molecular-weight heparin, warfarin, and fondaparinux (a new drug similar to heparin). These drugs reduce the tendency of the blood to clot, and are given to people with fractures that put them at risk of forming a pulmonary embolism. If an embolus occurs, emergency treatment is needed.▲

Rehabilitation and Prognosis

Children's fractures heal much faster and more perfectly than adult fractures do. Several years after most fractures in children, the bone can look almost normal on x-ray. In addition, children develop less stiffness with cast treatment and are more likely to regain normal motion if a fracture involves a joint.

Healing in older people is often slower than in younger adults. Fractures significantly impair an older person's ability to perform normal daily activities. Diminished strength, flexibility, and balance can impair a person's independence in eating, dressing, bathing, and even walking (if the person is dependent on a walker). Nonuse of muscles can lead to stiffness, weakness, and further impairment. Nurses and caregivers must assist older people in regaining their ability to perform normal daily activities.

Older people with poor circulation are at risk for bedsores when an injured limb rests on the cast.■ The areas in which the skin is in contact with the cast (contact points)—especially the heels—should be padded and inspected diligently for any sign of skin breakdown. Nurses and caregivers should be sure an older person periodically changes position to

avoid stiffness. For example, prolonged sitting can lead to the hip and knee becoming fixed in a bent position. Periods of standing and walking or, in someone who is bedridden, lying down supine with the legs straight, alternating with periods of sitting with the knees bent, can help to prevent stiffness.

After surgery, people with leg fractures usually start walking with crutches or a walker for a time. Sometimes supplemental casting is needed as well. Healing time varies from days to weeks to months, depending on the nature of the fracture. People with arm fractures have similar initial activity restrictions.

Stiffness and loss of strength are natural consequences of immobilization. A joint of a fractured limb immobilized in a cast becomes progressively stiffer each week, eventually losing its ability to fully extend and flex. Wasting away of muscle (atrophy) also can be severe. For instance, after wearing a long leg cast for a few weeks, most people can insert their hand into the formerly tight space between the cast and their thigh. When the cast is removed, the weakness resulting from muscle atrophy is very apparent.

Daily exercise using range-of-motion and muscle-strengthening exercises★ helps to combat stiffness and regain strength. While the fracture is healing, the joints outside the cast can be exercised. The joints within the cast cannot be exercised until the fracture has healed sufficiently and the cast can be removed. When exercising, the person should pay attention to how the injured limb feels and avoid exercising too forcefully. Passive exercises (in which a therapist applies external force)● must be used when muscles are too weak for effective motion and when strong muscle contractions might displace a fracture. Ultimately, active exercise (in which the person uses his own muscle force) against gravity or weight resistance is necessary to regain full strength of an injured limb.

Foot Fractures

Fractures of the foot bones occur commonly, caused by falls, twisting injuries, or direct impact of the foot against hard objects. Foot fractures cause considerable pain, which is almost always made worse by attempting to walk or put weight on the foot.

▲ see page 288   ■ see also page 218
★ see page 39   ● see art on page 38

Foot Fractures

Foot fractures are common. They may occur in the toes, the middle bones of the foot (metatarsals), the two small round bones just below the big toe (sesamoids), or the ankle bones. The big toe (hallux) is the toe most often fractured.

Phalanges

Fracture of the hallux

Metatarsal bones

Sesamoid bones

Cuneiform bones

Navicular bone

Cuboid

Talus

Calcaneus

Diagnosis is usually made by x-ray. Sometimes computed tomography (CT) or magnetic resonance imaging (MRI) is required. Treatment varies with the bone involved and the type of fracture but generally involves placing the foot and ankle in a cast.

Toe (phalanges) fractures can occur when an unprotected foot strikes a hard object. If the toe is abnormally bent, it may need to be realigned. Simple fractures of the four smaller toes heal without a cast. Certain measures, including splinting the toe with tape or nylon fastening (Velcro) to the adjacent toes for several weeks and wearing comfortable shoes, can provide comfort and protect the toe. Stiff-soled shoes support the fracture, and wide, soft shoes place less pressure on the swollen toe. If walking in normal shoes is too painful, the doctor can prescribe specially fabricated boots.

A fracture of the **big toe** (hallux) tends to be more severe than that of the other toes, causing more intense pain, swelling, and bleeding

▲ see also page 422

under the skin. A big toe can break when a person stubs it or drops a heavy object onto it. Fractures that affect the joint of the big toe may require surgery.

The **sesamoids** are two small round bones located within the flexor tendon under the big toe. These bones may fracture from running, hiking, and sports involving coming down too hard on the ball of the foot (such as basketball and tennis). Using padding or specially constructed orthoses (insoles) for the shoe helps relieve the pain. If pain continues, a sesamoid bone may need to be removed surgically.

A stress fracture of the **metatarsals** (the bones in the middle of the foot) can occur when a person walks or runs excessively.▲ Putting full weight on the foot causes increased pain. The affected area on the metatarsal bone is tender to touch. When a developing stress fracture is recognized early, the person can stop activities that aggravate the fracture. In more advanced and severe cases, crutches and a cast are necessary.

An avulsion fracture of the 5th metatarsal (a bone in the outside edge of the middle of the foot) occurs commonly after the foot is injured by turning inward. The outside edge of the foot develops tenderness and a swollen bruise. A cast is not usually necessary but can make walking easier. Crutches may be needed for a few days.

The **ankle** may fracture when the foot rolls inward or outward during a fall. Small avulsion fractures of the ligament attachments are similar to a severe sprain. This type of fracture is treated with a brace or cast for 3 to 6 weeks and generally heals well. Fractures through the bony bumps (malleoli) on the inside and outside of the ankle are more serious. When the malleoli are broken, standing and walking are very painful. Nondisplaced fractures of the malleoli can be treated with a cast. Displaced fractures require surgical fixation.

Leg Fractures

Fractures of the **shaft of the tibia** (situated between the knee and the ankle) generally result from high-energy injuries, such as motor vehicle accidents, collisions, and falls during skiing, and when pedestrians are struck by a car. This type of fracture can be very serious, particularly if the skin, muscle, nerves, or blood vessels are damaged.

For closed fractures of the tibia, an above-the-knee cast is needed until healing is under way, and then changed to a below-the-knee cast. The total time the person needs to wear these casts is usually about 3 months, but healing can take much longer. Many of these closed fractures are treated surgically with metal rods or plates. After surgery, usually no cast is required, and rehabilitation can begin sooner. If the skin is severely damaged and bare bone is exposed, an external fixator (a frame of rods clamped to stainless steel pins that pass through the skin into the bone) is used.

Fractures of the **shaft of the femur** (the large bone above the knee) are serious injuries usually caused by falls from a height or high-speed motor vehicle accidents. Special traction equipment is needed for transport to the hospital. In adults, these fractures are treated with urgent surgery to align and fixate the fracture with metal rods or plates. After surgery, most people begin to walk with crutches immediately.

Hip Fractures

More than 270,000 hip fractures occur in the United States each year, with about 90% of them occurring in people older than 60. Hip fractures are more common in older people because of osteoporosis and because older people are more likely to fall. Use of some drugs increases the risk of hip fractures in older people.▲ One in three women and one in six men who reach age 90 will fracture a hip during his or her lifetime.

The upper end of the femur (thighbone) has large bony bumps (trochanters) where powerful muscles attach, then a short neck, and finally a spherical head that forms the outer half of the hip joint. Most hip fractures occur just below the spherical head (femoral neck or subcapital hip fractures) or through the trochanters (intertrochanteric hip fractures).

Femoral neck hip fractures are particularly problematic because the fracture often disrupts the blood supply to the femoral head, which forms the hip joint. Without a good blood supply, the bone cannot heal and eventually collapses and dies. Intertrochanteric hip fractures tend to create large broken bone surfaces that cause internal bleeding.

Symptoms and Diagnosis

Most older people fracture their hips by falling while walking on level ground, often when indoors. They usually cannot move their leg, much less stand or walk. When a doctor examines the person, the leg appears shortened and turned outward because of the unbalanced pull of muscles and gravity. Swelling and a purplish bruise develop because of blood leaking from the fracture.

An x-ray usually shows an obvious fracture and can help a doctor confirm the diagnosis. However, faint fracture lines may not be seen initially on x-ray. Thus, when a person continues to have pain and is unable to stand a day or more after a fall, the x-ray may have to be repeated or a magnetic resonance imaging (MRI) or bone scan obtained.

Treatment

Most people with a hip fracture are treated with surgery. The type of surgery depends on the type of fracture.

Treatment of severe femoral neck hip fractures involves removing the broken pieces surgically because the blood supply to the femoral head has been damaged. If damage to the femoral neck is incomplete (the break does not go all the way through), metal pins can be inserted surgically to support the femoral head (internal fixation). This is a smaller surgical procedure and the person's own hip joint is preserved.

Intertrochanteric hip fractures are treated with an implant, such as a sliding compression screw and side plate. This implant securely holds the bone fragments in their proper position while the fracture heals. The fixation is usually strong enough to permit the person to bear weight as tolerated. While the bone fragments generally heal in a couple of months, most people continue to improve in terms of comfort, strength, and walking ability for at least 6 months.

If partial hip replacement is needed, special metallic implants are used that have a polished spherical surface to match with the joint socket and a strong stem to fit within the central marrow canal of the thighbone. Some prosthetic implants are secured to the bone with a rapid-setting plastic cement. Others have special porous or ceramic coatings into which the surrounding living bone can grow and bond directly.

After joint replacement surgery, the person usually begins walking with crutches or a walker immediately and switches to a cane in 6 weeks. However, artificial joints do not last

▲ see page 79

Repairing a Fractured Hip

There are two common types of hip fractures. Femoral neck or subcapital hip fractures occur in the neck of the femur. Intertrochanteric fractures occur in the large bony bumps (trochanters) where the powerful muscles of the buttocks and legs attach. When the fracture is not too severe, metal pins can be inserted surgically to support the femoral head. This surgical procedure preserves the person's own hip joint.

| Femoral Neck Fracture | Repair | Intertrochanteric Fracture | Repair |

forever. The person, especially someone who is active or heavy, may need to undergo another operation 10 to 20 years later. Joint replacement is often advantageous for older people, because the likelihood that additional surgery will be needed is very low. In addition, older people benefit greatly from being able to walk almost immediately after surgery.

Sometimes the whole joint needs to be replaced. This procedure is performed rarely for fractures, but most commonly for osteoarthritis.▲

If people with hip fractures are forced by their illness to stay in bed, they are at increased risk for serious complications, such as bedsores, blood colts leading to pulmonary embolism, mental confusion, and pneumonia. A great benefit of surgical fixation is that it allows the person to get out of bed and begin walking as soon as possible. Usually, the person can take a few steps with a walker 1 to 2 days after the operation. Physical rehabilitation is started as soon as possible.■

▲ see page 367   ■ see also page 43

Fractures of the Pelvis

The pelvis is made up of pairs of large broad (iliac) bones in the back joined by two smaller connecting bone struts (the pubic and ischial rami) in the front. In young adults, major fractures of the entire pelvis can occur as a result of high-speed motor vehicle accidents or falls from a height. These fractures can cause life-threatening bleeding and injury to internal organs. In older people, the rami, often weakened by osteoporosis, can fracture from even a minor fall on level ground.

Symptoms and Diagnosis

With fractures of the pelvic rami in older people, most people feel considerable pain in the groin even when lying down or sitting; this pain becomes much worse when the person tries to walk. The person may need to be admitted to a hospital or rehabilitation center.

Doctors suspect a pelvic fracture based on the symptoms and confirm the diagnosis using x-rays. Sometimes, computed tomography (CT) or magnetic resonance imaging (MRI) is required.

Prognosis and Treatment

Fractures of the pelvic rami in older people typically heal without causing permanent disabilities and rarely require surgical treatment. Analgesics and nonsteroidal anti-inflammatory drugs (NSAIDs)▲ help relieve pain and inflammation. To avoid the weakness, stiffness, and other complications that occur with bed rest, walking and bearing weight fully should begin as soon as possible. Because the iliac arches rather than the rami are used for structural support while walking, people can try to walk without injuring the area further. Most people can walk short distances with a walker by 1 week and are moderately comfortable in 1 to 2 months.

In young adults, a pelvic fracture due to trauma often requires emergency surgical treatment, and permanent disability often results if the socket of the hip joint has been damaged.

Fractures of the Spinal Column

In young adults, fractures of the spinal column result from forceful injuries, such as falls from a height, and from motor vehicle and sports accidents. In older people with osteoporosis, compression fractures of the spine can occur with minor trauma or even with lifting, bending forward, or taking a misstep. The cylindrical shaped vertebral body that makes up the forward weight-bearing column of the spine becomes compressed into a wedge shape.

Symptoms and Diagnosis

Spinal fractures cause pain that may worsen with standing, walking, or prolonged sitting. When the doctor gently taps over the spine, the person feels discomfort. Doctors use x-rays to confirm the diagnosis, check the spine for stability, and exclude the possibility of cancer. Because the spinal cord and nerve roots are contained within the spine, the cord or nerve roots may be injured, which may result in a loss of sensation and paralysis. Signs of nerve injury include pain radiating into the leg, weakness of the leg muscles, and involuntary wetting or soiling of clothing.

In older people, compression fractures of the spine sometimes occur suddenly and painfully, and sometimes they occur without symptoms. The result in both cases is a bending forward of the spine (kyphosis) and loss of height. If compression fractures occur over time at several levels of the spine, a person can lose several

Replacing a Hip

When the topmost part (head) of the thighbone (femur) is badly damaged, it may be replaced with an artificial part (prosthesis), made of metal. This procedure is called partial hip replacement. Very rarely, the socket into which the femoral head fits (forming the hip joint) must also be replaced. The part used is a metal shell lined with durable plastic. This procedure is called total hip replacement.

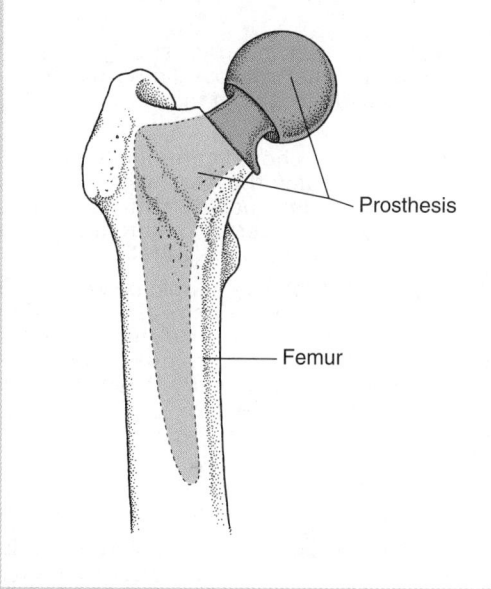

Prosthesis

Femur

inches of stature, develop a humpback deformity, and be unable to stand up straight.

Prognosis and Treatment

Great caution is taken with anyone with a possible spinal injury. Accident victims attended by emergency medical technicians are transported using special neck braces and spine boards.

Braces are most effective for fractures located in the lower part of the spine; they can relieve pain and enable the person to more rapidly return to daily activities. Initially, bed rest may be required for a few days, but sitting up and walking for short periods as soon as possible can help prevent loss of function and further loss of bone density.

▲ see page 452

Preventing Falls

Because falling is the most common reason for a fracture, especially in older people, preventing falls is important. Certain measures may help to reduce the likelihood of a fall or minimize an injury related to a fall:

- The person's home should be assessed for safety hazards, including poor lighting, torn carpets, area rugs, unstable chairs, slippery surfaces in bathrooms and kitchens, and missing steps.
- Any visual impairment should be corrected.
- Exercise can improve strength and muscle tone; improved fitness helps to speed recovery if the person does fall.
- The doctor should continually monitor the drugs the person is taking. Certain drugs, including analgesics, antihypertensives, and diuretics, can contribute to the risk of falls.
- Sensible footwear should be worn. If necessary, appropriate aids should be used, including wheelchairs, walkers, and padding worn over the hip if the person has already fallen and is at risk for a hip injury.

In older people, compression fractures of the spine that are not complicated by instability, nerve injury, or cancer, heal on their own but slowly. Treatment consists of comfort measures.

Shoulder Fractures

Shoulder fractures include fractures of the clavicle (collar bone), scapula (shoulder blade) and proximal humerus (upper arm bone). Trauma can also produce disruptions of the joints connecting these bones.

Clavicle fractures occur commonly after a fall, such as from a bicycle or jungle gym. Because the clavicle lies just under the skin with little muscle covering, swelling and deformity are easily visible after a fracture. Fractures of the inner and middle part of the clavicle are usually treated with a brace that helps to align the clavicle by pulling the shoulders backward. Fractures of the outer clavicle are treated with a regular sling. A strap passing around behind the back can be added to keep the arm from swinging outward, especially at night. Surgery is rarely needed.

Fractures of the **proximal humerus** (upper arm bone) are common after a fall on an outstretched arm. Symptoms include pain and an inability to raise the arm. Most breaks can be treated with a sling. Surgery is needed if the fracture pieces are widely separated. If the joint fragment is badly damaged, a prosthetic implant (or a partial shoulder replacement) may be needed.

Fractures of the shaft of the humerus occur with high-energy injuries, such as high-speed motor vehicle accidents, including when pedestrians are struck by a car, falls during skiing, and falls from buildings. Most are treated with a sling and bracing.

Arm Fractures

Elbow fractures can involve any of the three bones that make up the joint (radius, ulna, and humerus). Radial neck fractures (the upper end of the radius) occur commonly in active adults after a fall on an outstretched arm. A tender spot develops on the outer side of the elbow and becomes painful when the arm is straightened. X-rays may just show a faint crack in less severe cases. Most people are treated with a sling. After 3 to 10 days, gentle stretching exercises are begun and are gradually increased, as tolerated by the person, to regain normal range of motion. Severe fractures may require cast or surgical treatment.

Colles' fractures (fractures of the radius at the wrist) occur commonly in older people, following a fall on an outstretched arm. People have pain, swelling, tenderness, and often the fracture causes the wrist to rest in an unnatural position. If the fracture is not badly displaced, a splint or cast is applied. Otherwise, reduction may be needed first. A cast may be worn for 3 to 6 weeks. Daily motion of the fingers, elbow (if free), and shoulder helps to avoid stiffness. Elevation of the hand is important to control swelling. Comfort, flexibility, and strength of the wrist continue to improve for 6 to 12 months after the fracture. These fractures require surgical treatment if the joint surface is out of place, especially in active adults who need to be able to fully use their wrist. An external fixator (a frame of rods clamped to stainless steel pins that pass through the skin into the bone) is often applied.

Hand Fractures

Hand fractures involve the bones of the wrist (carpals), palm (metacarpals), or fingers and thumb (phalanges). However, normal hand function is the result of a complex interaction of an intricate arrangement of muscles, tendons, ligaments, and joints, as well as bones. Thus, seemingly minor fractures can cause serious soft tissue injuries that, if not treated properly, can lead to disabling stiffness, weakness, or deformity.

Fractures of the ends of the 4th and 5th metacarpals commonly occur from punching a hard object. This type of fracture, called a boxer's fracture, causes swelling and tenderness of the knuckle. Most of these fractures are treated with a cast, after a reduction if the fracture is badly angled. Typically good function of the finger returns.

Avulsion fractures at the site of tendon and joint capsule attachments occur commonly in the fingers. A mallet finger injury refers to the drooping of the fingertip that occurs when the tendon that extends the finger becomes detached.▲ Simple mallet finger injuries can respond to splinting the finger straight for 6 weeks, but those with serious tendon or bone injuries may require surgery. Other less common fractures of the hand include fractures of the scaphoid bone■ and the tuft of the fingertip.

CHAPTER 63

Bone Tumors

Bone tumors are growths of abnormal cells in bones.

Bone tumors may be noncancerous (benign) or cancerous (malignant). Noncancerous bone tumors are relatively common, but cancerous ones are rare. Also, bone tumors may be primary—noncancerous or cancerous tumors that originate in the bone itself—or metastatic—cancerous tumors that originate elsewhere in the body (for example, in the breast or prostate gland) and then spread to bone. In children, most cancerous bone tumors are primary; in adults, most are metastatic.

Bone pain is the most common symptom of bone tumors. The pain can be severe (somewhat like a toothache, which is also a form of bone pain). In addition, a lump may be noticeable. Sometimes a tumor, especially if cancerous, weakens a bone, causing it to fracture with little or no stress (pathologic fracture).

A persistently painful joint or limb should be x-rayed. However, x-rays tend to show only that there is an abnormality suggestive of an abnormal growth, usually without indicating whether a tumor is noncancerous or cancerous. Computed tomography (CT) and magnetic resonance imaging (MRI) often help determine the exact location and size of the tumor and give additional information as to the nature of the tumor, but these tests rarely provide a specific diagnosis.

Usually, removing a tissue sample of the tumor for examination under a microscope (biopsy) is necessary for diagnosis. For many tumors, a sample may be taken by inserting a needle into the tumor and withdrawing some cells (aspiration biopsy); however, because the needle used is very small, sometimes normal cells may be sampled and cancer cells missed, even when cancer cells are lying right beside the normal cells. Sometimes, a surgical procedure called open biopsy is necessary to obtain an adequate sample for diagnosis.

Noncancerous Bone Tumors

Osteochondromas (osteocartilaginous exostoses), the most common type of noncancerous bone tumors, usually occur in people aged 10 to 20 years. These tumors are growths on the surface of a bone, which protrude as hard lumps. A person may have one or several

---

▲ see page 396   ■ see art on page 401

tumors. The tendency to develop several tumors may run in families.

At some point in their lives, about 10% of the people who have more than one osteochondroma develop a cancerous bone tumor called a chondrosarcoma (presumably formed from an existing osteochondroma); surgical removal is generally appropriate if one of the tumors enlarges or causes new symptoms. Such people should also visit their doctor for regular examinations. However, people who have only one osteochondroma are unlikely to develop a chondrosarcoma; therefore, a single osteochondroma usually does not need to be removed unless it causes problems, such as increased swelling.

Chondromas, which usually occur in people aged 10 to 30 years, develop in the central part of a bone. These tumors often are discovered when x-rays are taken for other reasons and often can be diagnosed by their appearance on the x-ray. Some chondromas cause pain. If a chondroma does not cause pain, it does not have to be removed or treated. However, follow-up x-rays may be taken to monitor its size. If the tumor cannot be diagnosed with certainty on x-rays or if it causes pain, a biopsy may be needed, usually consisting of the entire tumor (excisional biopsy), to determine whether it is noncancerous or cancerous.

Chondroblastomas are rare tumors that grow in the ends of bones. They usually occur in people aged 10 to 20 years. These tumors may cause pain, leading to their discovery. If untreated, these tumors may continue to grow and destroy bone; therefore, treatment consists of surgical removal. Occasionally, these tumors recur after surgery.

Chondromyxoid fibromas (chondromyxofibromas) are very rare tumors that occur in people younger than 30; they are usually located near the ends of long bones. Pain is the usual symptom. These tumors have a distinctive appearance on x-rays. Treatment consists of surgical removal, which usually provides a cure, although tumors sometimes recur.

Osteoid osteomas are very small tumors that commonly develop in people aged 20 to 40. They are most common in the arms or legs but can occur in any bone. They usually cause pain that worsens at night and is relieved by low doses of aspirin. Sometimes the muscles surrounding the tumor waste away (atrophy); this condition may improve after the tumor is removed. Bone scans using radioactive tracers help determine the exact location of the tumor. Sometimes the tumor is difficult to locate, and additional tests, such as CT, may be needed. Surgically removing the tumor is one way to eliminate the pain permanently. However, some people prefer to take aspirin indefinitely rather than undergo surgery. Another procedure is less invasive than surgery. In this procedure, a doctor inserts a needlelike probe into the tumor, using CT as guidance for placement. A radio frequency pulse is then applied to destroy the tumor. Apart from the pain, the prognosis is good.

Giant cell tumors usually occur in people in their 20s and 30s. These tumors most commonly originate in the ends of bones and may extend into adjacent tissue. They usually cause pain. Treatment depends on the tumor's size. A tumor can be surgically removed, and the hole can be filled with a bone graft or a synthetic bone cement to preserve the bone's structure. Occasionally, very extensive tumors may require removal of the affected segment of bone. About 10% of the tumors recur after surgery. These tumors rarely become cancerous.

Primary Cancerous Bone Tumors

Multiple myeloma, the most common type of primary cancerous bone tumor, originates in the bone marrow cells that produce blood cells.▲ This tumor may affect one or more bones, so pain may occur in one location or in several. If only one bone is involved, the condition is called plasmacytoma; if more than one bone is involved, the condition is called multiple myeloma. Treatment is complex and may include chemotherapy, radiation therapy, and surgery.

Osteosarcoma (osteogenic sarcoma) is the second most common type of primary cancerous bone tumor. Although most common in people aged 10 to 20 years, osteosarcomas can occur at any age. Older people who have Paget's disease ■ sometimes develop this type of tumor. About half these tumors occur in or around the knee, but they can originate in any bone. They tend to spread (metastasize) to the lungs. Usually, these tumors cause pain and swelling. A biopsy is needed for diagnosis.

▲ see also page 1007   ■ see page 346

Osteosarcomas are usually treated with a combination of chemotherapy and surgery. Usually, chemotherapy is given first; pain often subsides during this phase of treatment. Then the tumor is surgically removed. About 75% of people who have this type of tumor survive for at least 5 years after diagnosis. Because surgical procedures have improved, the affected arm or leg can usually be saved; in the past, the affected limb often had to be amputated.

Fibrosarcomas and **malignant fibrous histiocytomas** are similar to osteosarcomas in appearance, location, symptoms, and prognosis. Treatment is the same as for osteosarcoma.

Chondrosarcomas are tumors composed of cancerous cartilage cells. Many chondrosarcomas are slow-growing or low-grade tumors, meaning that they are less likely to spread than some other tumors; they often can be cured with surgery. However, some chondrosarcomas are high-grade tumors, which tend to spread. A biopsy is needed for diagnosis. During treatment, a chondrosarcoma must be completely removed surgically, because it does not respond to chemotherapy or radiation therapy. Amputation of the arm or leg is rarely necessary. More than 75% of people who have a chondrosarcoma survive if the entire tumor is removed.

Ewing's tumor (Ewing's sarcoma) is a cancerous tumor that affects males more often than females and appears most commonly in people aged 10 to 20 years. Most of these tumors develop in the arms or legs, but they may develop in any bone. Pain and swelling are the most common symptoms. Tumors may become quite large, sometimes affecting the entire length of a bone. Although CT and MRI can help determine the exact size of the tumor, a biopsy is needed for diagnosis. Treatment consists of a combination of surgery, chemotherapy, and radiation therapy, which can cure more than 60% of people who have Ewing's tumor.

Malignant lymphoma of bone (reticulum cell sarcoma) is a cancerous tumor that usually affects people in their 40s and 50s. It can originate in any bone or elsewhere in the body and then spread to bone. Usually, this tumor causes pain and swelling, and the damaged bone is prone to fractures. Treatment usually consists of a combination of chemotherapy and radiation therapy, which appears to be as effective as surgical removal of the tumor. Amputation is rarely necessary.

Metastatic Bone Tumors

Metastatic bone tumors are cancers that have spread to the bone from their original site elsewhere in the body.▲ Cancers most likely to spread to the bone include those of the breast, lung, prostate gland, kidney, and thyroid gland. Cancer may spread to any bone but usually does not spread beyond the elbow and knee.

A person who has or has had cancer and develops bone pain or swelling usually is examined for metastatic bone tumors. Bone scans using radioactive tracers and x-rays can help locate these tumors. Occasionally, a metastatic bone tumor produces symptoms before the original cancer has been detected. Symptoms may consist of pain or a fracture where the tumor has weakened the bone (a pathologic fracture). In these situations, a biopsy usually gives clues as to the location of the original cancer, because the type of tissue from which the cancer derived can often be recognized under the microscope.

Treatment depends on the type of cancer that has spread to the bone. Some types respond to chemotherapy, some to radiation therapy, some to both, and some to neither. Surgery to stabilize the bone can sometimes prevent fractures. When the original (primary) cancer has been removed and only a single metastasis in the bone remains, surgical removal combined with radiation therapy, chemotherapy, or both is sometimes curative.

▲ see page 1031

CHAPTER 64

Avascular Necrosis of the Bone

Avascular necrosis of the bone (osteonecrosis, aseptic necrosis, osteochondritis dissecans) is the death of bone tissue due to an impaired blood supply.

Avascular necrosis most commonly occurs in people between the ages of 30 and 60. It most commonly affects the thigh bone (femur) at the hip (the head of the femur). Often, both hips are affected. In people older than 50, avascular necrosis is usually caused by a hip fracture but may be caused by a disease that blocks the small blood vessels that supply to the ends of the long bones. For instance, emboli consisting of fatty material may block these blood vessels in people with alcohol-induced liver damage. The thigh bone at the knee is also commonly affected; the arm bone at the shoulder is sometimes affected.

Doctors classify avascular necrosis according to whether or not it is caused by an injury. Only serious injuries can cause the disorder; minor ones do not. Commonly, displaced fractures or dislocations, in which the blood vessels to part of the bone have been torn or physically damaged, are the types of injuries that can cause avascular necrosis. Nontraumatic causes include alcohol abuse, high doses of corticosteroids (especially when given for prolonged periods of time), decompression sickness (which occurs in divers who surface too quickly),▲ and sickle cell disease.■ Less commonly, Gaucher's disease, tumors (for example, lymphomas), and radiation therapy can cause avascular necrosis. Certain blood clotting disorders can also cause it. In about 25% of people with the disorder, the cause is unknown. Avascular necrosis of the knee can occur spontaneously, primarily in women older than 55 who have no risk factors for the disorder. Some experts dispute whether spontaneous avascular necrosis of the knee is really avascular necrosis or some other unknown disorder.

Symptoms

In some people, severe incapacitating pain starts suddenly—these people can often re-member the precise day and hour when the pain started. This sudden onset of pain probably occurs when the blood supply is cut off. However, most people have avascular necrosis for some time before symptoms appear. Pain occurs when the dead bone finally collapses. Such pain is brought on by standing, walking, or moving the affected bone and generally improves when the person is resting.

In avascular necrosis of the hip, groin pain may extend down the front and inner portions of the thigh or be felt in the buttocks. The person limps, trying to minimize all hip movements. As the disorder progresses, more and more tiny fractures of the hip occur, and the bone eventually collapses. The pain also increases, and the hip joint feels stiff and loses some of its range of motion.

Avascular necrosis of the knee often begins suddenly as severe constant pain and tenderness, usually over the inner part of the knee. In about one third of people, the knee joint is swollen because it contains excess fluid.

Avascular necrosis of the shoulder may produce mild or temporary symptoms and may be hardly noticeable. The person usually minimizes shoulder movements to avoid pain.

Diagnosis

Because avascular necrosis is often painless at first, it is often not diagnosed in its early stages. When avascular necrosis occurs because of a serious injury, the disorder cannot be detected microscopically for days to weeks and cannot be detected on x-ray until some months later.

Magnetic resonance imaging (MRI) is the best test to detect avascular necrosis early, so that complications (such as collapse of the head of the femur) can be avoided. X-rays or computed tomography (CT) is used to determine whether the bone has collapsed, how advanced the disorder is, and whether the person has osteoarthritis involving the unaffected side of the joint.

Treatment

Simple treatment measures include use of nonsteroidal anti-inflammatory drugs (NSAIDs)

▲ see page 1669   ■ see page 992

or other analgesics for pain,▲ and avoidance of weight-bearing or strain on affected bones and joints. Often, these treatments must be maintained for 6 months or more. Exercises to increase a joint's range of motion are useful. However, these treatments are rarely adequate by themselves and do not cure the disorder.

The simplest surgical procedure is called core decompression, which involves taking a plug of bone out of the involved area. This procedure is very effective for early disease that has not yet progressed to bone collapse; it may even prevent collapse. Core decompression may also be used for someone younger than 50 whose bone has collapsed; this treatment may delay the need for a total joint replacement by several years because the person's pain is relieved or decreased. The procedure takes less than an hour to perform. The person must use crutches for 4 to 6 weeks afterward.

Another procedure is bone grafting. For avascular necrosis at the hip, bone grafting consists of taking bone tissue with the blood vessels intact from elsewhere in the body and attaching the bone tissue and blood vessels near the hip. The graft serves as an infrastructure from which the body forms new bone; however, for the operation to be successful, the body also has to form a new blood supply. This operation takes several hours to perform. The person must spend several months on crutches afterward.

If core decompression or bone grafting is performed before the bone collapses, it can help to prevent serious joint damage, particularly when the hip or knee is affected. Early surgery is less often needed when the shoulder is affected because the shoulder does not bear weight and often does well without surgery.

A procedure by which the bone is cut (called osteotomy) is used to delay the need for joint replacement in people who are younger than 50, in whom collapse of the bone has occurred. People who undergo an osteotomy are those who are not eligible for core decompression or bone grafting because too much damage has occurred. Usually, the location of the avascular necrosis is in a weight-bearing area of the bone. In some cases, the bone can be cut below the area that is involved and rotated or

Causes of Avascular Necrosis

Definite causes
- Alcohol abuse
- Atherosclerosis
- Decompression sickness
- Gaucher's disease
- High doses of corticosteroids
- Hip dislocation
- Hip fracture of the femoral neck
- Radiotherapy
- Sickle cell disease
- Tumors

Possible causes
- Blood clotting disorders
- Cushing's syndrome
- Diabetes mellitus
- Fatty liver
- Gout
- Lipid disturbances
- Pancreatic cancer
- Pancreatitis
- Smoking
- Systemic lupus erythematosus

turned so that an uninvolved portion of the bone can become the new weight-bearing area.

A total joint replacement■ is the only effective procedure when avascular necrosis has caused significant osteoarthritis on the other side of the joint. Although the success rate for this procedure is higher than 95%, doctors must carefully consider the decision to recommend a joint replacement because artificial joints do not last forever and in young people may have to be replaced at some later time. Therefore, for some younger people, many surgeons use a procedure called femoral head resurfacing if the socket of the hip joint is not involved. This procedure involves implanting a metal cap over the femoral head (similar to capping a tooth rather than pulling the tooth and putting in a false tooth). Some people undergo the femoral head resurfacing procedure followed later by total hip replacement.

▲ see page 452   ■ see page 352

CHAPTER 65

Bone and Joint Infections

Bones and the fluid and tissues of joints can become infected. Such infections include osteomyelitis and infectious arthritis.

Osteomyelitis

Osteomyelitis is a bone infection usually caused by bacteria, including mycobacteria, but sometimes caused by fungi.

Osteomyelitis occurs most commonly in young children and in older people, but all age groups are at risk. Osteomyelitis is also more likely to occur in people with serious medical conditions.

When a bone becomes infected, the soft, inner part (bone marrow) often swells. As the swollen tissue presses against the rigid outer wall of the bone, the blood vessels in the bone marrow may become compressed, which reduces or cuts off the blood supply to the bone. Without an adequate blood supply, parts of the bone may die. The infection can also spread outward from the bone to form collections of pus (abscesses) in adjacent soft tissues, such as the muscle.

Causes

Bones, which usually are well protected from infection, can become infected through three routes: the bloodstream (which may carry an infection from another part of the body to the bones), direct invasion (infection), and infections in adjacent bone or soft tissues.

Osteomyelitis usually occurs in the ends of leg and arm bones in children and in the spine (vertebrae) in adults, particularly in older people. Infections of the leg and arm bones and those of the vertebrae are usually acquired through the bloodstream. Infections of the vertebrae are referred to as vertebral osteomyelitis. People who undergo kidney dialysis and those who inject illegal drugs are particularly susceptible to vertebral osteomyelitis.

Bacteria or fungal spores may infect the bone directly through open fractures, during bone surgery, or from contaminated objects that pierce the bone. *Staphylococcus aureus* is the bacteria most commonly responsible. *Mycobacterium tuberculosis* (one of the bacteria that cause tuberculosis) can infect the vertebrae to cause osteomyelitis.

Osteomyelitis may also occur where a piece of metal has been surgically attached to a bone, as is done to repair hip or other fractures. For instance, bacteria or fungal spores may also infect the space around an artificial joint; the organisms may be carried into the area of bone surrounding the artificial joint during the operation in which the joint is installed, or the infection may occur later. Any artificial device in the body may serve as a focus for infection.

Osteomyelitis may also result from an infection in an adjacent soft tissue; the infection spreads to the bone after several days or weeks. This type of spread is particularly likely to occur in older people. Such an infection may start in an area damaged by an injury, radiation therapy, or cancer, or in a skin ulcer (particularly a foot ulcer) caused by poor circulation or diabetes. A sinus, gum, or tooth infection may spread to the skull.

Symptoms

Infections of the leg and arm bones cause fever and, sometimes days later, pain in the infected bone. The area over the bone may be sore, warm, and swollen, and movement may be painful. The person may lose weight and feel tired.

Infections of the vertebrae usually develop gradually, producing persistent back pain and tenderness when touched. Pain worsens with movement and is not relieved by resting, applying heat, or taking analgesics. Fever, usually the most obvious sign of an infection, is often absent.

When osteomyelitis results from infections in adjacent soft tissues or direct invasion by an organism, the area over the bone swells and becomes painful; abscesses may form in the surrounding tissue. These infections may not cause fever, and blood test results may be normal. Infection around an infected artificial joint or limb typically causes persistent pain in that area.

Chronic osteomyelitis may develop if osteomyelitis is not treated successfully. It is a persistent infection that is very difficult to eradicate. Sometimes, chronic osteomyelitis is undetectable for a long time, producing no symptoms for months or years. More commonly, chronic osteomyelitis causes bone pain, recurring infections in the soft tissue over the bone, and constant or intermittent drainage of pus through the skin. This drainage occurs when a passage (sinus tract) forms from the infected bone to the skin surface and pus drains through the sinus tract.

Diagnosis

Symptoms and findings during a physical examination may suggest osteomyelitis. For example, doctors may suspect osteomyelitis in a person who has persistent bone pain with or without a fever and feels tired much of the time.

As with any chronic infection, blood tests usually indicate elevated levels of white blood cells, an elevated erythrocyte sedimentation rate (ESR—a test that measures the rate at which red blood cells settle to the bottom of a test tube containing blood), and an elevated level of C-reactive protein (a protein that circulates in the blood and dramatically increases in level when there is inflammation).

An x-ray may show changes suspicious of osteomyelitis. However, the abnormal area may not be detected on an x-ray until more than 3 weeks after the first symptoms occur. The infected area almost always appears abnormal on bone scans (images of bone made by injection of radioactive technetium), except in infants, because scans do not reliably indicate abnormalities in growing bones. Computed tomography (CT) and magnetic resonance imaging (MRI) can also identify the infected area. However, these tests cannot always distinguish infections from other bone disorders.

To diagnose a bone infection and identify the organisms causing it, doctors may take samples of blood, pus, joint fluid, or the bone itself to test. Usually, for vertebral osteomyelitis, samples of bone tissue are removed with a needle or during surgery.

Prevention and Prognosis

People who have artificial joints or metal components attached to a bone should take preventive antibiotics before surgery, including dental surgery, because these people have an increased risk of infection from bacteria normally found in the mouth and other parts of the body.

The prognosis for people with osteomyelitis is usually good with early and proper treatment. However, sometimes, chronic osteomyelitis develops, and a bone abscess may recur weeks to months or even years later.

Treatment

For children and adults who have recently developed bone infections through the bloodstream, antibiotics are the most effective treatment. If the bacteria causing the infection cannot be identified, then antibiotics that are effective against *Staphylococcus aureus* or, in some cases, broad-spectrum antibiotics (antibiotics effective against many types of bacteria) are used. Depending on the severity of the infection, antibiotics may be given intravenously at first, but they may be given by mouth later during a 4-week to 6-week course of treatment. Some people need months of antibiotic treatment.

If a fungal infection is identified or suspected, antifungal drugs are required for several months. If the infection is detected at an early stage, surgery is usually not necessary. Occasionally, however, an abscess forms, which may be drained surgically.

For adults who have bacterial osteomyelitis of the vertebrae, the usual treatment is antibiotics for 6 to 8 weeks. Sometimes bed rest is needed, and the person may need to wear a brace. Surgery may be needed to drain abscesses or to stabilize affected vertebrae (to prevent the vertebrae from collapsing and thereby damaging nearby nerves or blood vessels).

When osteomyelitis results from an adjacent soft tissue infection (such as in a foot ulcer caused by poor circulation or diabetes), treatment is more complex. Usually, all the dead tissue and bone are removed surgically, and the resulting empty space is packed with healthy bone, muscle, or skin. Then the infection is treated with antibiotics.

Usually, an artificial joint that has an infection around it is removed and replaced. Antibiotics may be given several weeks before surgery to try to eradicate the infection, so that the contaminated artificial joint can be removed and a new one can be implanted at the same time. Rarely, treatment is not successful and the infection continues, requiring surgery to fuse the joint or amputate the limb.

Infectious Arthritis

Infectious arthritis (septic arthritis) is infection in the fluid and tissues of a joint usually caused by bacteria, but sometimes caused by viruses or fungi.

People at risk for infectious arthritis include those who have abnormal joints because of rheumatoid arthritis, osteoarthritis, or injury (traumatic arthritis) who develop an infection that reaches the bloodstream. For example, an older person with pneumonia and sepsis (a bloodstream infection) may fall and injure a wrist. Bleeding into the injured wrist may then result in infectious arthritis.

Infecting organisms, mainly bacteria, usually reach the joint through the bloodstream, but a joint can be infected directly if it is contaminated by surgery, an injection, or an injury. Different bacteria can infect a joint, but the bacteria most likely to cause infection depend on a person's age. Staphylococci and bacteria known as gram-negative bacilli most often infect infants and young children, whereas gonococci (bacteria that cause gonorrhea), staphylococci, and streptococci most often infect older children and adults. Occasionally, spirochetes (a type of bacteria), such as those that cause Lyme disease and syphilis, can infect joints.

Viruses—such as the human immunodeficiency virus (HIV), parvoviruses, and those that cause rubella, mumps, and hepatitis B—can infect joints in people of any age. A slowly developing chronic infectious arthritis is most often caused by *Mycobacterium tuberculosis* (one of the bacteria that cause tuberculosis) or fungi.

Symptoms

Infants usually have fever and pain and tend to be fussy. Generally, infants do not move the infected joint because moving or touching it is painful. Young children with knee or hip infections may refuse to walk. In older children and adults, symptoms usually begin very suddenly. The infected joint usually becomes red and warm, and moving or touching it is very painful. Fluid collects in the infected joint, causing it to swell and stiffen. Symptoms also include fever and chills. Less dramatic symptoms (less pain, lower fever) usually occur in people with chronic infectious arthritis that is caused by mycobacteria or fungi.

The joints most commonly infected are the knee, shoulder, wrist, hip, elbow, and the joints of the fingers. Most bacterial, fungal, and mycobacterial infections affect only one joint or, occasionally, several joints. For example, the bacteria that cause Lyme disease most often infect knee joints. Gonococcal bacteria and viruses can infect a few or many joints at the same time.

Diagnosis

Several tests need to be performed immediately if infectious arthritis is suspected. Usually, a sample of joint fluid is removed with a needle. It is examined for white blood cells and tested for bacteria and other organisms. The laboratory can almost always grow and identify the infecting bacteria from the joint fluid, unless the person has recently taken antibiotics. However, the bacteria that cause gonorrhea, Lyme disease, and syphilis are difficult to recover from joint fluid. If bacteria do grow in culture, the laboratory then tests which antibiotics would be effective.

A doctor usually orders blood tests because bacteria from joint infections often appear in the bloodstream. Sputum, spinal fluid, and urine may also be tested for bacteria to help determine the source of infection.

Prognosis and Treatment

Because an infected joint can be destroyed within days without prompt treatment, antibiotics must be started as soon as an infection is suspected, even before the laboratory has identified the infecting organism. Antibiotics that kill the most likely bacteria are given first, then other antibiotics are given later, if necessary. Antibiotics are often given intravenously at first, to ensure that enough of the drug reaches the infected joint. If the antibiotics are effective against the infecting bacteria, improvement usually occurs within 48 hours. As soon as the doctor receives the laboratory results, the choice of antibiotic may be adjusted depending on the sensitivity of the particular bacteria to specific antibiotics.

The doctor removes pus with a needle to prevent its accumulation; accumulated pus may damage a joint. If drainage with a needle is difficult (as with a hip joint) or unsuccessful, arthroscopy (a procedure using a small scope to view the interior of the joint directly)▲ or surgery may be needed to drain the joint. Sometimes a tube is left in place to drain the pus. Splinting the joint (to keep it from moving) can help ease pain at first, but physical therapy is also needed to prevent stiffness and permanent loss of function.

Infections caused by fungi are treated with antifungal drugs; infections caused by mycobacteria are treated with a combination of antibiotics.■ Viral infections usually get better on their own—only acetaminophen or a nonsteroidal anti-inflammatory drug (NSAID) is needed for pain and fever.

▲ see page 343   ■ see page 1129

CHAPTER 66

Osteoarthritis

Osteoarthritis (previously called degenerative arthritis, degenerative joint disease) is a chronic disorder of joint cartilage and surrounding tissues that is characterized by pain, stiffness, and loss of function.

Osteoarthritis, the most common joint disorder, affects most people to some degree by age 70. Before the age of 40, men develop osteoarthritis more often than do women, because of injury. From age 40 to 70, women develop the disorder more often than do men. After age 70, the disorder develops in both sexes equally. Osteoarthritis also occurs in almost all animals with a backbone—including fish, amphibians, and birds. Because the disorder is so widespread in the animal kingdom, some authorities believe that osteoarthritis may have evolved from an ancient method of cartilage repair.

Many myths about osteoarthritis persist—for example, that it is an inevitable part of aging, like gray hair and skin changes; that it results in little disability; and that treatment is not effective. Although osteoarthritis is more common in older people, it is not caused simply by the wear and tear that occurs with years of use. Instead, microscopic changes in the structure and composition of cartilage appear to be responsible. Most people who have the disorder, especially younger people, have few if any symptoms; however, some older people develop significant disabilities.

Causes

Normally, joints have such a low friction level that they are protected from wearing out, even after years of use. Osteoarthritis probably begins most often with an abnormality of the cells that synthesize the components of cartilage, such as collagen (a tough, fibrous protein in connective tissue) and proteoglycans (substances that provide resilience). Next, the cartilage may swell because of water retention, become soft, and then develop cracks on the surface. Tiny cavities form in the bone beneath the cartilage, weakening the bone. Bone can overgrow at the edges of the joint, producing bumps (osteophytes) that can be seen and felt. Ultimately, the smooth, slippery surface of the cartilage becomes rough and pitted, so that the joint can no longer move smoothly and absorb impact. All the components of the joint—bone, joint capsule (tissues that enclose most joints), synovial tissue (tissue lining the joint), tendons, ligaments, and cartilage—fail in various ways, thus altering the joint.

Osteoarthritis is classified as primary (or idiopathic) when the cause is not known (the large majority of cases). It is classified as secondary when the cause is another disease or condition, such as Paget's disease,▲ an infection, deformity, injury, or overuse of a joint. Some people who repetitively stress one joint or a group of joints, such as foundry workers, coal miners, and bus drivers, are particularly at risk. Much of the risk for osteoarthritis of the knee comes from occupations that involve bending of the joint. Curiously, long-distance running champions appear not to be at higher risk of developing the disorder. However, once osteoarthritis develops, this type of exercise often makes the disorder worse. Obesity may be a major factor in the development of osteoarthritis, particularly of the knee and especially in women.

Symptoms

Usually, symptoms develop gradually and affect only one or a few joints at first. Joints of the fingers, base of the thumbs, neck, lower back, big toes, hips, and knees are commonly affected. Pain, usually made worse by activities that involve weight bearing (such as standing), is the first symptom. In some people, the joint may be stiff after sleep or some other inactivity, but the stiffness usually subsides within 30 minutes of moving the joint.

As the condition causes more symptoms, the joint may become less movable and eventually may not be able to fully straighten or bend. The attempt of the tissues to repair may lead to new growth of cartilage, bone, and other tissue, which can enlarge the joints. The irregular cartilage surfaces cause joints to grind, grate, or crackle when they are moved.

▲ see page 346

How to Live
With Osteoarthritis

- Exercise affected joints gently (in a pool, if possible)
- Massage at and around affected joints (this measure should preferably be performed by a trained therapist)
- Apply a heating pad or a damp and warm towel to affected joints
- Maintain an appropriate weight (so as not to place extra stress on joints)
- Use special equipment as necessary (for example, cane, crutches, walker, neck collar, or elastic knee support to protect joints from overuse; a fixed seat placed in a bathtub to enable less stretching while washing)
- Wear well-supported shoes or athletic shoes

Bony growths commonly develop in the joints at the ends or middle of the fingers (called Heberden's or Bouchard's nodes).

In some joints (such as the knee), the ligaments, which surround and support the joint, stretch so that the joint becomes unstable. Alternatively, the hip or knee may become stiff, losing its range of motion. Touching or moving the joint (particularly when standing, climbing stairs, or walking) can be very painful.

Osteoarthritis often affects the spine. Back pain is the most common symptom. Usually, damaged disks or joints in the spine cause only mild pain and stiffness. However, osteoarthritis in the neck or lower back can cause numbness, pain, and weakness in an arm or leg if the overgrowth of bone presses on nerves. The overgrowth of bone may be within the spinal canal, pressing on nerves before they exit the canal to go to the legs. This may cause leg pain after walking, suggesting incorrectly that the person has a reduced blood supply to the legs (intermittent claudication▲). Rarely, bony growths compress the esophagus, making swallowing difficult.

Osteoarthritis may be stable for many years or may progress very rapidly, but most often it progresses slowly after symptoms develop. Many people develop some degree of disability.

▲ see page 217   ■ see page 370

Diagnosis

The doctor makes the diagnosis based on the characteristic symptoms, physical examination, and the x-ray appearance of joints (such as bone enlargement and narrowing of the joint space). By age 40, many people have some evidence of osteoarthritis on x-rays, especially in weight-bearing joints such as the hip and knee, but only half of these people have symptoms. However, x-rays are not very useful for detecting osteoarthritis early because they do not show changes in cartilage, which is where the earliest abnormalities occur. Also, changes on the x-ray correlate poorly with symptoms. For example, an x-ray may show only a minor change while the person is having severe symptoms, or an x-ray may show numerous changes while the person is having very few, if any, symptoms.

Magnetic resonance imaging (MRI) can reveal early changes in cartilage, but it is rarely needed for the diagnosis. Also, MRI is too expensive to justify routine use. There are no blood tests for the diagnosis of osteoarthritis, although blood tests may help rule out other disorders (such as rheumatoid arthritis■).

Treatment

Appropriate exercises—including stretching, strengthening, and postural exercises—help maintain healthy cartilage, increase a joint's range of motion, and strengthen surrounding muscles so that they can absorb shock better. Exercise must be balanced with rest of painful joints, but immobilizing a joint is more likely to worsen osteoarthritis than to improve it. Using excessively soft chairs, recliners, mattresses, and car seats may worsen symptoms; using car seats moved forward, straight-backed chairs with relatively high seats (such as kitchen or dining room chairs), firm mattresses, and bed boards (available at many lumber yards) is often recommended.

For osteoarthritis of the spine, specific exercises sometimes help, and back supports or braces may be needed when pain is severe. Exercises should include both muscle strengthening as well as low impact aerobic exercises (such as walking, swimming, and bicycle riding). If possible, the person should maintain ordinary daily activities and continue to perform his or her normal activities, such as a hobby or job. However, physical activities may have to be adjusted to avoid bending and thus aggravating the pain of osteoarthritis.

Replacing a Knee

A knee joint damaged by osteoarthritis may be replaced with an artificial joint. After a general anesthetic is given, the surgeon makes an incision over the damaged knee. The knee cap (patella) is removed, and the ends of the thigh bone (femur) and shinbone (tibia) are smoothed so that the parts of the artificial joint (prothesis) can be attached more easily. One part of the artificial joint is inserted into the thigh bone, and the other part into the shinbone, and the parts are cemented in place.

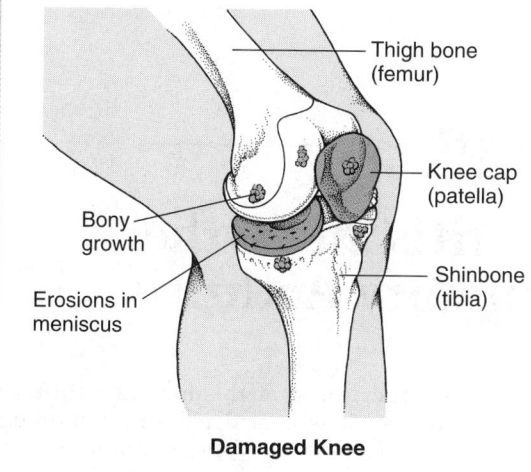

Thigh bone (femur)

Knee cap (patella)

Bony growth

Shinbone (tibia)

Erosions in meniscus

Damaged Knee

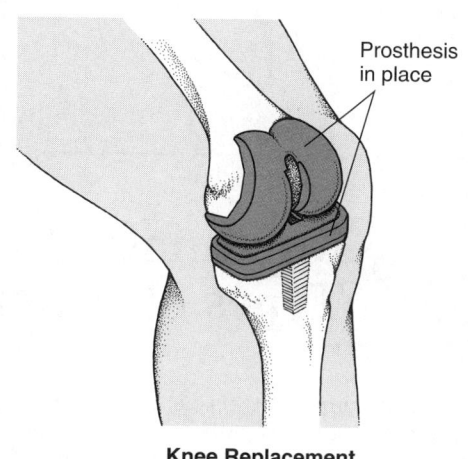

Prosthesis in place

Knee Replacement

Physical therapy, often with heat therapy,▲ can be helpful. Heat improves muscle function by reducing stiffness and muscle spasm. Cold may be applied to reduce pain. Splints or supports (such as a cane, crutch, brace, or even a walker) can protect specific joints during painful activities. Shoe inserts (orthotics) may help reduce pain from walking. Massage by trained therapists, traction,■ and deep heat treatment with diathermy or ultrasound may be useful.

Drugs are used to supplement exercise and physical therapy. Drugs, which may be used in combination or individually, do not directly alter the course of osteoarthritis; they are used to reduce symptoms and thus allow more appropriate exercise. A simple pain medicine (analgesic), such as acetaminophen, may be all that is needed. Alternatively, a nonsteroidal anti-inflammatory drug (NSAID) may be taken to lessen pain and swelling. NSAIDs reduce pain and inflammation in joints.★ The cyclooxygenase-2 (COX-2) inhibitors (coxibs) provide relief equivalent to the other NSAIDs but may have fewer gastrointestinal side effects.● People at risk for gastrointestinal problems may prefer them. Sometimes other types of pain medicine may be needed, such as a skin cream derived from cayenne pepper—the active ingredient is capsaicin—which is applied directly to the skin over the joint.

If a joint suddenly becomes inflamed, swollen, and painful, most of the fluid inside the joint may need to be removed and a special form of cortisone may be injected directly into the joint. This treatment may provide only short-term relief, and a joint treated with cortisone should not be used too often or damage may result. A series of injections of hyaluronate (a component of normal joint fluid) into the joint may provide significant pain relief in some people for prolonged periods of

▲ see page 37   ■ see page 352
★ see page 452   ● see page 454

time. Several nutritional supplements (such as glucosamine and chondroitin sulfate) are being tested for potential benefit in osteoarthritis.

Surgery may help when all other treatments fail to relieve pain. Some joints, most commonly the hip and knee, can be replaced with an artificial joint;▲ replacement is usually very successful, almost always improving motion and function and dramatically decreasing pain. Therefore, joint replacement should be considered when function becomes limited.

Because the artificial joint does not last forever, such surgery is often delayed as long as possible in young people so the need for repeated replacements can be minimized.

A variety of methods that restore cells inside cartilage have been used in younger people with osteoarthritis to help heal small defects in cartilage. However, such methods have not yet been proven valuable when cartilage defects are extensive, as commonly occurs in older people.

CHAPTER 67

Rheumatoid Arthritis and Other Types of Inflammatory Arthritis

Several connective tissue diseases produce prominent joint inflammation. These include rheumatoid arthritis, psoriatic arthritis, Reiter's syndrome (reactive arthritis), and ankylosing spondylitis. Although many other conditions may also cause inflammation of the joints, these four disorders are often discussed together as inflammatory arthritic disorders.

Rheumatoid Arthritis

Rheumatoid arthritis is an inflammatory arthritis in which joints, usually including those of the hands and feet, are inflamed, resulting in swelling, pain, and often the destruction of joints.

Worldwide, rheumatoid arthritis develops in about 1% of the population, regardless of race or country of origin, affecting women 2 to 3 times more often than men. Usually, rheumatoid arthritis first appears between 25 and 50 years of age, but it may occur at any age. Rheumatoid arthritis can occur in children—the disease is then called juvenile rheumatoid arthritis, and the symptoms and prognosis are somewhat different).■

The exact cause of rheumatoid arthritis is not known. It is considered an autoimmune disease.★ Components of the immune system attack the soft tissue that lines the joints and can also attack connective tissue in many other parts of the body, such as the blood vessels and lungs. Eventually, the cartilage, bone, and ligaments of the joint erode, causing deformity, instability, and scarring within the joint. The joints deteriorate at a highly variable rate. Many factors, including genetic predisposition, may influence the pattern of the disease.

Symptoms

People with rheumatoid arthritis may have a mild course, occasional flare-ups with long periods of remission without disease, or a steadily progressive disease, which may be slow or rapid. Rheumatoid arthritis may start suddenly, with many joints becoming inflamed at the same time. More often, it starts subtly, gradually affecting different joints. Usually, the inflammation is symmetric, with joints on both sides of the body affected. Typically, the small joints in the fingers, toes, hands, feet, wrists, elbows, and ankles become inflamed first. The inflamed joints are usually painful and often stiff, especially just after awakening (such stiffness generally lasts for at least 30 minutes and often much longer) or after prolonged inactivity. Some people feel

▲ see art on pages 357 and 369
■ see page 1612   ★ see page 1073

tired and weak, especially in the early afternoon. Rheumatoid arthritis may produce a low-grade fever.

Affected joints enlarge because of swelling of the soft tissue and can quickly become deformed. Joints may freeze in one position so that they cannot bend or open fully. The fingers may tend to dislocate slightly from their normal position toward the little finger on each hand, causing tendons in the fingers to slip out of place.

Swollen wrists can pinch a nerve and result in numbness or tingling due to carpal tunnel syndrome.▲ Cysts, which may develop behind affected knees, can rupture, causing pain and swelling in the lower legs. Up to 30% of people with rheumatoid arthritis have hard bumps (called rheumatoid nodules) just under the skin, usually near sites of pressure (such as the back of the forearm near the elbow).

Rarely, rheumatoid arthritis causes an inflammation of blood vessels (vasculitis■); this condition reduces the blood supply to tissues and may cause nerve damage or leg sores (ulcers). Inflammation of the membranes that cover the lungs (pleura) or of the sac surrounding the heart (pericardium) or inflammation and scarring of the lungs can lead to chest pain or shortness of breath. Some people develop swollen lymph nodes; Sjögren's syndrome, which consists of dry eyes or mouth; ★ or red, painful eyes due to inflammation.

Diagnosis

In addition to the important characteristic pattern of symptoms, the doctor may use the following to support the diagnosis: laboratory tests, an examination of a joint fluid sample obtained with a needle, and even a biopsy (removal of a tissue sample for examination under a microscope) of rheumatoid nodules. Characteristic changes in the joints may be seen on x-rays.

In 9 of 10 people who have rheumatoid arthritis, the erythrocyte sedimentation rate (ESR—a test that measures the rate at which red blood cells settle to the bottom of a test tube containing blood) is increased, which suggests that active inflammation is present. However, this test alone cannot identify the cause of the inflammation. Doctors may monitor the ESR when symptoms are mild to help determine whether the disease is still active.

Many people with rheumatoid arthritis have distinctive antibodies in their blood, such as rheumatoid factor, which is present in 70% of people with rheumatoid arthritis. (Rheumatoid factor also occurs in several other diseases, such as hepatitis and some other infections; some people even have rheumatoid factor in their blood without any evidence of disease.) Usually, the higher the level of rheumatoid factor in the blood, the more severe the rheumatoid arthritis and the poorer the prognosis. The rheumatoid factor level may decrease when joints are less inflamed.

Most people have mild anemia (an insufficient number of red blood cells●). Rarely, the white blood cell count becomes abnormally low. When a person with rheumatoid arthritis has a low white blood cell count and an enlarged spleen, the disorder is called Felty's syndrome.

Prognosis and Treatment

Rarely, rheumatoid arthritis resolves spontaneously. Treatment alleviates symptoms in 3 of 4 people. However, at least 1 of 10 people eventually becomes severely disabled.

Treatments range from simple, conservative measures to drugs and even surgery. Simple measures are meant to help the person's symptoms and include rest and adequate nutrition. Certain drugs—the slow-acting drugs—may actually improve the disease rather than just the symptoms. Treatment starts with the least aggressive measures; however, drugs that can slow disease progression should generally be added during the first several months.

Severely inflamed joints should be rested, because using them can aggravate the inflammation. Regular rest periods often help relieve pain, and sometimes a short period of bed rest helps relieve a severe flare-up in its most active, painful stage. Splints can be used to immobilize and rest one or several joints, but some systematic movement of the joints is needed to prevent adjacent muscles from weakening and joints from freezing in place.

A regular, healthy diet is generally appropriate. A diet rich in fish and plant oils but low in red meat can have small beneficial effects on the inflammation. Rarely, people have flare-ups after eating certain foods, and if so, these foods should be avoided.

The main categories of drugs used to treat rheumatoid arthritis are the nonsteroidal anti-

---

▲ see page 398   ■ see also page 386

★ see page 382   ● see page 987

℞ DRUGS USED TO TREAT RHEUMATOID ARTHRITIS

TYPE	DRUG	SELECTED SIDE EFFECTS	COMMENTS
Nonsteroidal anti-inflammatory drugs (NSAIDs)			
	Aspirin, ibuprofen, naproxen, diclofenac, many others (see box on page 454)	Upset stomach, stomach ulcers, increased blood pressure, adverse effects on the kidneys	All NSAIDs treat the symptoms and decrease inflammation but do not alter the course of the disease
	Cyclooxygenase-2 (COX-2) inhibitors (coxibs): celecoxib, rofecoxib, valdecoxib	Risk of adverse effects on the kidneys, increased blood pressure; less risk of stomach ulcer than other NSAIDs	
Slow-acting drugs			
	Gold compounds	Adverse effects on the kidneys; rashes, itchy skin, decreased numbers of blood cells	All slow-acting drugs can slow progression of joint damage as well as gradually decrease pain and swelling
	Penicillamine	Suppression of blood cell production in the bone marrow, kidney problems, muscle disease, rash, bad taste in the mouth	
	Hydroxychloroquine	Usually mild—rashes, muscle aches, eye problems	
	Sulfasalazine	Stomach upset, liver problems, blood cell disorders, and rashes	
Corticosteroids			
	Prednisone	Numerous side effects throughout the body with long-term use	Can reduce inflammation quickly; may not be useful long term because of side effects
Immunosuppressive drugs			
	Methotrexate, leflunomide, azathioprine, cyclophosphamide, cyclosporine	Liver disease, lung inflammation, an increased susceptibility to infection, suppression of blood cell production in the bone marrow	Methotrexate or leflunomide can be used early for severe rheumatoid arthritis; can slow joint damage
	Etanercept, infliximab	Potential risk of infection or malignancy	Dramatic, prompt response in most people; can slow joint damage

inflammatory drugs (NSAIDs), slow-acting drugs, corticosteroids, and methotrexate or other immunosuppressive drugs, including the tumor necrosis factor (TNF) inhibitors. A newer biologic therapy, involving the use of interleukin-1 receptor antagonists, is available. Generally, the stronger drugs have important side effects that must be looked for during treatment.

▲ see also page 452

Nonsteroidal Anti-Inflammatory Drugs: The nonsteroidal anti-inflammatory drugs (NSAIDs)▲ are the most widely used drugs to treat the symptoms of rheumatoid arthritis. They can reduce the swelling in affected joints and relieve pain. However, all NSAIDs (including aspirin) can upset the stomach and cannot be taken by anyone who has active digestive tract (peptic) ulcers—including stomach ulcers or duodenal ulcers.

Symptoms of upset stomach may be reduced by eating food while taking an NSAID or taking antacids or other drugs such as the histamine-2 blockers (ranitidine, famotidine, or cimetidine) at the same time. Misoprostol or proton pump inhibitors are sometimes given in conjunction with an NSAID and can reduce the risk of stomach ulcers in people who need long-term treatment with an NSAID for rheumatoid arthritis. Misoprostol may cause diarrhea and does not prevent the nausea or abdominal pain that can result from taking aspirin or other NSAIDs.

Aspirin has been the traditional cornerstone of treatment for rheumatoid arthritis for many years. Ringing in the ears is a side effect that suggests the dose is too high. Other NSAIDs, including ibuprofen, naproxen, and diclofenac, are more often prescribed than is aspirin. Fewer pills are required (sometimes just 1 or 2 a day); these drugs may also have fewer side effects than high doses of aspirin.

A new type of NSAID, the cyclooxygenase (COX-2) inhibitors (coxibs), are similar in action to the other NSAIDs but are much less likely to cause damage to the stomach. These drugs do not inhibit the function of platelets, and thus are safer to use than the traditional NSAIDs for people who are at risk of bleeding. Two examples are celecoxib and rofecoxib.

Slow-Acting Drugs: Slow-acting drugs, such as gold compounds, penicillamine, hydroxy-chloroquine, and sulfasalazine, sometimes can improve the course of rheumatoid arthritis, although improvement may take several months. These drugs are usually added promptly if the disease persists (as it usually does) in people taking NSAIDs, including the coxibs. Even if pain is decreased, a doctor will likely prescribe a slow-acting drug within the first 2 months if joint swelling persists.

Gold compounds, which can slow the formation of bone deformities, may cause a temporary remission of the disease. Usually, a gold compound is given as a weekly injection. A preparation given by mouth is available but is not as effective. The weekly injections are continued until a total of 1 gram has been given or until side effects preclude their use or significant improvement occurs, whichever comes first. If the drug is effective, the frequency of the injections can be gradually decreased. Sometimes improvement is sustained for years on maintenance doses.

Gold compounds can adversely affect several organs, and people who have severe liver or kidney disease or certain blood disorders cannot take these drugs. Consequently, blood and urine samples are tested before treatment begins and frequently—up to once a week—during treatment. Side effects of these drugs include potentially dangerous rashes, itchy skin, and decreased numbers of blood cells. Less commonly, gold compounds can affect the liver and lungs, and rarely, they cause diarrhea. The gold compound is usually discontinued if any of these severe side effects occur, although the compound may be started again after a mild rash resolves.

Penicillamine is taken by mouth and has beneficial effects similar to those of gold compounds and may be used when gold compounds are not effective or when they cause intolerable side effects. The dose of penicillamine is gradually increased until a person shows some improvement. Side effects include suppression of blood cell production in the bone marrow, kidney problems, muscle disease, rash, and a bad taste in the mouth. Penicillamine can also cause disorders such as myasthenia gravis, Goodpasture's syndrome, and a lupus-like syndrome. If any of these side effects occur, the drug must be discontinued. Because of these side effects, penicillamine is not usually an early choice. Blood and urine samples are tested as often as every 2 to 4 weeks during treatment.

Hydroxychloroquine is given daily by mouth and is often used rather than gold compounds or penicillamine to treat less severe rheumatoid arthritis; it may be added to other slow-acting drugs or methotrexate and seems to provide an additive effect. Side effects, which are usually mild, include rashes, muscle aches, and eye problems. However, some eye problems can be permanent, so people taking hydroxychloroquine must have their eyes checked by an ophthalmologist before treatment begins and every 6 months during treatment. If the drug has not helped after 6 months, it is discontinued. Otherwise, hydroxychloroquine can be continued as long as necessary.

Sulfasalazine tablets can also be used in people who have less severe rheumatoid arthritis or added to other drugs to boost their effectiveness. The dose is increased gradually, and improvement usually occurs within 3 months. Like the other slow-acting drugs, it can cause stomach upset, liver problems, blood cell disorders, and rashes.

Corticosteroids: Corticosteroids, such as prednisone, are the most dramatically effective drugs for reducing inflammation anywhere in the body. Although corticosteroids are effective for short-term use, they tend to become less effective over time, and rheumatoid arthritis is usually active for years.

There is some controversy as to whether corticosteroids can slow the progression of rheumatoid arthritis. Furthermore, the long-term use of corticosteroids almost invariably leads to side effects, involving almost every organ in the body. Consequently, doctors usually reserve corticosteroids for the short-term use in severe flare-ups when many joints are affected or when all other drugs have been ineffective. They are also useful in treating inflammation outside of joints, for example, in the membranes covering the lungs (pleura) or in the sac surrounding the heart (pericardium). Because of the risk of side effects, the lowest effective dose is almost always used. Corticosteroids can be

injected directly into the affected joints for fast, short-term relief. However, they can actually contribute to long-term damage, especially when a person who receives frequent injections overuses the temporarily pain-free joint, hastening its destruction.

Immunosuppressive Drugs: Although corticosteroids suppress the immune system, other drugs do so even more potently and are referred to as immunosuppressive drugs. Each of these drugs can slow the progression of disease and decrease the damage to bones adjacent to joints. Such drugs include methotrexate (which is often the first drug used after NSAIDs), leflunomide, azathioprine, cyclophosphamide, cyclosporine, and tumor necrosis factor (TNF) inhibitors.

Immunosuppressive drugs are effective in treating severe rheumatoid arthritis. They

Corticosteroids: Uses and Side Effects

Corticosteroids are the strongest drugs available for reducing inflammation in the body. They are useful in any condition in which inflammation occurs, including rheumatoid arthritis and other connective tissue disorders, multiple sclerosis, and in emergencies such as brain swelling, asthma attacks, and severe allergic reactions. They are important in the treatment of severe chronic obstructive pulmonary disease. They may even be applied directly to the affected area for certain skin conditions, such as eczema and psoriasis. When inflammation is severe, use of these drugs is often life-saving.

Corticosteroids are prepared synthetically to have the same action as cortisol, a steroid hormone produced by the outer layer (cortex) of the adrenal glands—hence the name "corticosteroid." Many synthetic corticosteroids are, however, more powerful than cortisol, and most are longer acting.

Examples of corticosteroids include prednisone, dexamethasone, triamcino-

lone, betamethasone, beclomethasone, flunisolide, and fluticasone. All of these drugs are very strong. Hydrocortisone is a milder corticosteroid that is available in over-the-counter skin creams. Corticosteroids can be given intravenously (especially in emergency situations), by mouth, or directly applied to the inflamed organ (as in inhaled versions for the lungs, in eye drops, and in a skin cream).

Because corticosteroids reduce the body's ability to fight infections by suppressing inflammation, they are used with extreme care when infections are present. Their use may worsen high blood pressure, heart failure, diabetes, peptic ulcer, kidney failure, and osteoporosis and are used in such conditions only when necessary.

When they are taken by mouth or by injection, corticosteroids should not be discontinued abruptly. This is because corticosteroids inhibit production of cortisol by the adrenal glands, and this production must be given time to recover. Thus, at the end of a course of

corticosteroids, the dose is gradually reduced. It is important for a person who takes corticosteroids to follow the doctor's instructions on dosage very carefully.

The long-term use of corticosteroids, particularly at higher doses and particularly when given intravenously or by mouth, invariably leads to many side effects, involving almost every organ in the body. Common side effects include thinning of the skin with stretch marks and bruising, high blood pressure, elevated blood sugar levels, cataracts, puffiness in the face (moon face) and abdomen, and thinning of the arms and legs, poor wound healing, stunted growth in children, loss of calcium from the bones (which can lead to osteoporosis), stomach bleeding, hunger, weight gain, and mental problems. Because most of their effects are produced locally, inhaled corticosteroids and those that are applied directly to the skin cause far fewer symptoms than the intravenous version or that given by mouth.

suppress the inflammation so that cortico-steroids can be avoided or given in lower doses. But immunosuppressive drugs have their own potentially serious side effects, including liver disease, lung inflammation, an increased susceptibility to infection, the suppression of blood cell production in the bone marrow, and, with cyclophosphamide, bleeding from the bladder. In addition, azathioprine and cyclophosphamide may increase the risk of developing cancer. In women who are considering pregnancy, immunosuppressive drugs should be used only after discussion with a doctor.

Methotrexate, given by mouth once a week in gradually increasing doses, is the drug used increasingly to treat rheumatoid arthritis in its early stages. This drug can take effect quickly—sometimes after several weeks. Methotrexate may be given before slow-acting drugs when the joint inflammation is severe. Most people tolerate methotrexate well but must be closely monitored and their white blood cell counts tested about every 2 months. They must refrain from drinking alcohol to minimize the risk of liver damage. Folic acid tablets may decrease some of the side effects, such as mouth ulcers.

Leflunomide is a drug with benefits and risks that are similar to those of methotrexate. It is given daily by mouth, sometimes with the first three doses (loading doses) being higher to speed the onset of action.

Etanercept or infliximab, which are tumor necrosis factor (TNF) inhibitors, can be dramatically effective for people who do not respond sufficiently to methotrexate alone. Etanercept is given twice weekly by injection under the skin, and infliximab is given intravenously every 8 weeks after loading doses. These drugs should be avoided in people who have active infections or malignancies because TNF may make such conditions worse.

Other Treatments: Along with drugs to reduce joint inflammation, a treatment plan for rheumatoid arthritis should include non-drug therapies, such as exercise, physical or occupational therapy, and sometimes surgery. Inflamed joints should be exercised gently so they do not freeze in one position. As the inflammation subsides, regular, active exercises can help, although a person should not exercise to the point of fatigue. For many people, exercise in water may be easier.

Treatment of tight joints consists of intensive exercises and occasionally the use of splints to gradually extend the joint. If drugs have not helped, surgery may be needed. Surgically replacing knee or hip joints is the most effective way to restore mobility and function when the joint disease is advanced. Joints can also be removed or fused together, especially in the foot, to make walking less painful. The thumb can be fused to enable a person to grasp, and unstable vertebrae at the top of the neck can be fused to prevent them from compressing the spinal cord.

People who are disabled by rheumatoid arthritis can use several aids to accomplish daily tasks. For example, specially modified orthopedic or athletic shoes can make walking less painful, and devices such as grippers reduce the need to squeeze the hand forcefully.

Psoriatic Arthritis

Psoriatic arthritis is a form of joint inflammation that occurs in some people who have psoriasis of the skin or nails.

The disease resembles rheumatoid arthritis but does not produce the antibodies characteristic of rheumatoid arthritis. Psoriatic arthritis occurs in about 7% of people with psoriasis (a skin condition causing flare-ups of red, scaly rashes and thickened, pitted nails▲). A severe form of psoriatic arthritis can occur in some people with AIDS.■

Symptoms and Diagnosis

Inflammation usually affects joints of the fingers and toes, although other joints, including the hips and spine, are often affected as well. The joints may become swollen and deformed when inflammation is chronic. Arthritis often involves joints less symmetrically than in rheumatoid arthritis and involves fewer joints. The joints at the end of the fingers adjacent to the diseased nails may be involved. The skin and joint symptoms sometimes appear and disappear together.

The diagnosis is made by identifying the characteristic joint inflammation in a person who has psoriasis or a family history of psoriasis. There are no tests to confirm the diagnosis, but x-rays help show the extent of joint damage.

Prognosis and Treatment

The prognosis for psoriatic arthritis is usually better than that for rheumatoid arthritis

---

▲ see page 1201   ■ see page 1168

because fewer joints are affected. Nonetheless, the joints can be severely damaged.

Treatment is aimed at controlling the skin rash and relieving the joint inflammation. Several drugs that are effective in treating rheumatoid arthritis are also used to treat psoriatic arthritis. They include gold compounds, methotrexate, cyclosporine, sulfasalazine, and tumor necrosis factor (TNF) inhibitors. Another drug, etretinate (which is used for severe acne), is usually effective in severe cases, but its side effects may be serious. Because etretinate can cause birth defects, it should not be taken by pregnant women. Moreover, etretinate remains in the body for a long time, so women should not become pregnant while taking the drug or for at least 1 year after discontinuing it.

Some people take methoxsalen (psoralen) by mouth and undergo ultraviolet A light (PUVA—ultraviolet light with psoralen) treatments. This combination relieves the skin symptoms and most of the joint inflammation but may not help inflammation of the spine.

Reiter's Syndrome

Reiter's syndrome (reactive arthritis) is inflammation of the joints and tendon attachments at the joints, often accompanied by inflammation of the eye's conjunctiva▲ and the mucous membranes, such as those of the mouth and genitourinary tract, and by a distinctive rash.

Reiter's syndrome is also called reactive arthritis because the joint inflammation appears to be a reaction to an infection originating in the intestine or genital tract. This syndrome is most common in men aged 20 to 40.

There are two forms of Reiter's syndrome. One occurs with sexually transmitted diseases such as a chlamydial infection and occurs most often in young men; the other usually follows an intestinal infection such as shigellosis or salmonellosis. Most people who have these infections do not develop Reiter's syndrome. People who develop Reiter's syndrome after exposure to these infections appear to have a genetic predisposition to this type of reaction, related in part to the same gene found in people who have ankylosing spondylitis. There is some evidence that the chlamydia and possibly other bacteria actually spread to the joints, but the roles of the infection and the immune reaction to it are not clear.

▲ see page 1296

Symptoms

Typically, symptoms begin 7 to 14 days after the infection. Inflammation of the urethra (the channel that carries urine from the bladder to the outside of the body) can result either directly from infection of the urethra or even from a reaction to the intestinal infection. In men, inflammation of the urethra causes moderate pain and a discharge from the penis or a rash on the glans of the penis (balanitis circinata). The prostate gland may be inflamed and painful. The genital and urinary symptoms in women, if any occur, are usually mild, consisting of a slight vaginal discharge or uncomfortable urination.

The conjunctiva (the membrane that lines the eyelid and covers the eyeball) can become red and inflamed, causing itching or burning and excessive tearing. Joint pain and inflammation may be mild or severe. Several joints are usually affected at once—especially the knees, toe joints, and areas where tendons are attached to bones, such as at the heels.

Small, painless or tender sores can develop in the mouth. Occasionally, a distinctive rash of hard, thickened spots may develop on the skin, especially of the palms and soles (keratoderma blennorrhagicum). Yellow deposits may develop under the fingernails and toenails.

In most people, the initial symptoms disappear in 3 or 4 months. In half of the people, however, joint inflammation or other symptoms recur over several years. Joint and spinal deformities may develop if the symptoms persist or recur frequently. Very few people who have Reiter's syndrome become permanently disabled.

Diagnosis and Treatment

The combination of joint, genital, urinary, skin, and eye symptoms leads a doctor to suspect Reiter's syndrome. Because these symptoms may not appear simultaneously, the disease may not be diagnosed for several months. No simple laboratory tests are available to confirm the diagnosis, but x-rays are often performed to assess the status of joints. A sample taken from the urethra with a swab or a sample of joint fluid may be tested, or a biopsy (removal of tissue for examination under a microscope) of the joint may be performed to try to identify the infectious organism that triggered the syndrome.

When the disease affects the genitals and urinary tract, antibiotics are given to treat the infection, but treatment is not always successful and its optimal duration is not known.

Joint inflammation is usually treated with a nonsteroidal anti-inflammatory drug (NSAID).▲ Sulfasalazine or methotrexate, an immunosuppressive drug, may be used, as in rheumatoid arthritis. Corticosteroids are generally not given by mouth but by direct injection into an inflamed joint, which sometimes helps.

Conjunctivitis and skin sores do not usually need treatment, although severe eye inflammation may require a corticosteroid ointment or eyedrops.

Ankylosing Spondylitis

Ankylosing spondylitis is inflammation of the spine and large joints, resulting in stiffness and pain.

The disease is 3 times more common in men than in women, developing most commonly between the ages of 20 and 40. Its cause is not known, but the disease tends to run in families, indicating that genetics plays a role. Ankylosing spondylitis is 10 to 20 times more common in people whose parents or siblings have it.

Symptoms

Mild to moderate flare-ups of inflammation generally alternate with periods of almost no symptoms.

The most common symptom is back pain, which varies in intensity from one episode to another and from one person to another. Pain is often worse at night and in the morning. Early morning stiffness that is relieved by activity is also very common. Pain in the lower back and the associated muscle spasms are often relieved by bending forward. Therefore, people often assume a stooped posture, which can lead to a permanent bent-over position. In others, the spine becomes noticeably straight and stiff.

Loss of appetite, weight loss, fatigue, and anemia can accompany the back pain. If the joints connecting the ribs to the spine are inflamed, the pain may limit the ability to expand the chest to take a deep breath. Occasionally, pain starts in large joints, such as the hips, knees, and shoulders.

One third of the people have recurring attacks of mild eye inflammation, which usually does not impair vision. In a few people, inflammation of a heart valve results in a permanently damaged valve. If the damaged vertebrae press against nerves or the spinal cord, numbness, weakness, or pain can develop in the area supplied by the affected nerves. The

cauda equina (horse's tail) syndrome is a rare complication.■

Diagnosis

The diagnosis is based on the pattern of symptoms and on x-rays of the spine and affected joints, which show a wearing away (erosion) of the joint between the spine and the hip bone (sacroiliac joint) and the formation of bony bridges between the vertebrae, making the spine stiff. The erythrocyte sedimentation rate (ESR), a test that measures the rate at which red blood cells settle to the bottom of a test tube containing blood, tends to be high, indicating inflammation. In addition, a specific gene, HLA-B27, is found in about 90% of people who have this disease; however, because this gene is also found in about 6 to 7% of healthy white people, its presence is of limited value in diagnosis.

Prognosis and Treatment

Most people develop some disabilities but can still lead normal, productive lives. In some people, the disease is more progressive, causing severe deformities.

Treatment focuses on relieving back and joint pain and preventing or correcting spinal deformities. Nonsteroidal anti-inflammatory drugs (NSAIDs)★ can reduce the pain and inflammation, thus enabling people to do important exercises to retain posture, including stretching and deep breathing. Sulfasalazine may help the pain in joints other than those of the back. The tumor necrosis factor (TNF) inhibitors etanercept or infliximab can relieve the pain and inflammation.

Corticosteroids help only in the short-term treatment of inflammation of the eyes and of joints other than the spine. Muscle relaxants and opioid analgesics are usually used for only brief periods to relieve severe pain and muscle spasms. If hips or knees become eroded or fixed in a bent position, surgery to replace the joint can relieve pain and restore function.

The long-range goals of treatment are to maintain proper posture and develop strong back muscles. Daily exercises strengthen the muscles that oppose the tendency to bend and stoop. It has been suggested that people spend some time each day—often while reading—lying on their stomach propped up on their elbows; this position extends the back and helps to prevent too much flexion.

▲ see page 452   ■ see box on page 565

★ see pages 372 and 452

CHAPTER 68

Autoimmune Disorders of Connective Tissue

In an autoimmune disorder, antibodies or cells produced by the body attack the body's own tissues.▲ Many autoimmune disorders affect connective tissue in a variety of organs. Connective tissue is the structural tissue that gives strength to joints, tendons, ligaments, and blood vessels.■

In autoimmune disorders, inflammation and the immune response may result in connective tissue damage, not only in and around joints but also in other tissues, including vital organs, such as the kidneys and brain. The sac that surrounds the heart (pericardium), the membrane that covers the lungs (pleura), and even the brain can be affected. The type and severity of symptoms depend on which organs are affected.

An autoimmune disorder of connective tissue is diagnosed on the basis of its particular symptom pattern, the findings during a physical examination, and the results of laboratory tests. Sometimes the symptoms of one disease overlap with those of another so much that doctors cannot make a distinction; in this case, the disorder may be called undifferentiated connective tissue disease or overlap disease.

Systemic Lupus Erythematosus

Systemic lupus erythematosus (lupus) is a chronic inflammatory connective tissue disorder that can involve joints, kidneys, mucous membranes, and blood vessel walls.

About 90% of people who have lupus are young women in their late teens to 30s, but children (mostly girls) and older men and women can also be affected. Lupus occurs in all parts of the world but may be more common in blacks and in Asians.

The cause of lupus is usually not known. Occasionally, the use of certain drugs (such as hydralazine and procainamide, which are used to treat heart conditions, and isoniazid, which is used to treat tuberculosis) can cause lupus. Drug-induced lupus usually disappears after the drug is discontinued.

The number and variety of antibodies that can appear in lupus are greater than those in any other disorder. These antibodies, which are the underlying physiologic problem in lupus, along with other unknown factors, determine which symptoms develop. However, the levels of these antibodies may not always be proportional to the person's symptoms.

Discoid lupus erythematosus is a form of lupus that affects only the skin. In this condition, raised round bumps occur, with scaling and sometimes with scarring and hair loss in affected areas. In 10% of people, manifestations of lupus—for example, those affecting the joints, kidneys, and brain—may occur but are generally mild.

Symptoms

Symptoms vary greatly from person to person. Symptoms may begin suddenly with fever, resembling an acute infection, or may develop gradually over months or years with episodes (called flare-ups) of fever, feeling unwell, or any of the symptoms discussed below alternating with periods when symptoms are absent or minimal. For many women, lupus flare-ups occur during the second half of the menstrual cycle, with symptoms disappearing when menstruation starts.

Migraine-type headaches, epilepsy, or severe mental disorders (psychoses) may be the first abnormalities that are noticed. Eventually, however, symptoms may affect any organ system. Joint symptoms, ranging from intermittent joint pains (arthralgias) to sudden inflammation of multiple joints (acute polyarthritis), occur in about 90% of people and may exist for years before other symptoms appear. In long-standing disease, marked joint deformity may occur (Jaccoud's arthropathy). However, joint inflammation is generally intermittent and usually does not damage the joints.

Skin rashes include a butterfly-like redness across the nose and cheeks (malar butterfly erythema); raised bumps or patches of thin skin; and red, flat or raised areas on the face and sun-exposed areas of the neck, upper chest, and elbows. Blisters and skin ulcers are

▲ see page 1073   ■ see page 334

rare, although ulcers do commonly occur on mucous membranes, particularly on the roof of the mouth, on the inside of the cheeks, on the gums, and inside the nose. Generalized or patchy loss of hair (alopecia) is common during flare-ups. Mottled red areas on the sides of the palms and up the fingers, redness and swelling around the nails, and flat, reddish-purple blotches between the knuckles on the inner surfaces of the fingers also may occur. Purplish spots (petechiae) may occur because of bleeding in the skin as a result of low platelet levels in the blood. Sensitivity to sunlight (photosensitivity) occurs in 40% of people, particularly in whites.

It is common for the person to feel pain when breathing deeply. The pain is due to recurring inflammation of the sac around the lungs (pleurisy), with or without fluid (effusion) inside this sac. Inflammation of the lungs (lupus pneumonitis), resulting in breathlessness, is rare, although minor abnormalities in lung function are common. Life-threatening bleeding into the lungs may rarely occur.

Chest pain due to inflammation of the sac around the heart (pericarditis) is often present. More serious but rare effects on the heart are inflammation of the walls of the coronary arteries (coronary artery vasculitis), which can lead to angina▲ or inflammation of the heart muscle with scarring (fibrosing myocarditis), which can lead to heart failure.■

Widespread enlargement of the lymph nodes is common, particularly in children, young adults, and in blacks of all ages. Enlargement of the spleen (splenomegaly) occurs in about 10% of people. The person may experience nausea, diarrhea, and vague abdominal discomfort. The occurrence of these symptoms may be the forewarning of a flare-up.

Involvement of the brain (neuropsychiatric lupus) can cause headaches, mild impairment of thinking, personality changes, stroke, epilepsy, severe mental disorders (psychoses), or a condition in which a number of physical changes may occur in the brain, resulting in disorders such as dementia.

Blockage of arteries in the brain or lung due to thrombosis or embolism can also occur.

Kidney involvement may be minor and without symptoms or relentlessly progressive and fatal. The most common result of this impairment is protein in the urine.

Rarely, the blood vessels at the back of the eye become inflamed (retinitis). Blindness can develop over a few days.

Characteristics of Lupus

At least four of the following symptoms are generally present for a diagnosis to be made:
- Red, butterfly-shaped rash on the face, affecting the cheeks
- Typical skin rash on other parts of the body
- Sensitivity to sunlight
- Mouth sores
- Joint inflammation (arthritis)
- Fluid around the lungs, heart, or other organs (serositis)
- Kidney dysfunction
- Low white blood cell count, low red blood cell count due to hemolytic anemia, or low platelet count
- Nerve or brain dysfunction
- Positive results of a blood test for antinuclear antibodies
- Positive results of a blood test for antibodies to double-stranded DNA

Diagnosis

Doctors suspect lupus mainly on the basis of its symptoms and findings on a careful physical examination, particularly if they occur in a young woman. Nonetheless, because of the wide range of symptoms, distinguishing lupus from similar diseases can be difficult for a doctor at first.

Laboratory tests can help doctors confirm the diagnosis. A blood test can detect antinuclear antibodies, which are present in almost all people who have lupus. However, these antibodies also occur in other diseases. Therefore, if antinuclear antibodies are detected, a test for antibodies to double-stranded DNA is also performed. A high level of these antibodies almost definitely means the person has lupus, but not all people who have lupus have these antibodies. Other blood tests may be performed to predict the activity and course of the disease. A blood test to detect antibodies to phospholipids can help identify people at risk for thrombosis. Blood tests can also indicate anemia, a low white blood cell count, or a low platelet count.

Laboratory tests can detect the presence of protein or red blood cells in the urine or an elevation of creatinine in the blood; these find-

▲ see page 202   ■ see page 150

ings indicate kidney damage caused by glomerulonephritis. Sometimes a biopsy of kidney tissue must be performed to help the doctor plan treatment.

Prognosis and Treatment

Lupus tends to be chronic and relapsing, often with symptom-free periods that can last for years. Flare-ups occur less often after menopause. Because many people are being diagnosed earlier than in the past and because better treatment is available, the prognosis has improved markedly over the last two decades. However, because the course of lupus is unpredictable, the prognosis varies widely. Usually, if the initial inflammation is controlled, the long-term prognosis is good. Early detection and treatment of kidney damage reduces the incidence of severe kidney disease.

Treatment depends on which organs are affected and whether the lupus is mild or severe.

Mild lupus may require little or no treatment. Aspirin or other nonsteroidal anti-inflammatory drugs (NSAIDs)▲ often can relieve joint pain. Aspirin is used in low doses if the person's blood has a tendency to clot, as happens in some people with lupus (aspirin reduces the tendency of blood to clot by reducing the tendency of blood platelets to stick together); aspirin or NSAID doses that are too high can harm the liver and kidney. Hydroxychloroquine, chloroquine, or quinacrine, sometimes taken in combination, helps relieve joint and skin symptoms. Sunscreen lotions (with a sun protection factor of at least 30) should be used, especially by people who have skin rashes.

Severe lupus is treated immediately with a corticosteroid such as prednisone.■ The dose and duration of treatment depend on which organs are affected. Sometimes an immunosuppressive drug such as azathioprine or cyclophosphamide is given to suppress the body's autoimmune attack. Mycophenylate mofetil is another new alternative immunosuppressive drug. The combination of a corticosteroid and an immunosuppressive drug is most often used for severe kidney disease or nervous system disease and for vasculitis.

Once the initial inflammation is controlled, a doctor determines the dose that most effectively suppresses inflammation over the long term. Usually, the dose of prednisone is gradu-

ally decreased when symptoms are controlled and laboratory test results improve. Relapses or flare-ups can occur during this process. For most people who have lupus, the dose of prednisone can eventually be decreased or occasionally discontinued.

Surgical procedures and pregnancy are more complicated for people who have lupus, and they require close medical supervision. Miscarriages and flare-ups after childbirth are common, but pregnancy need not be avoided if conception is delayed until after flare-ups subside.

If inflammation of the blood vessels at the back of the eye occurs, doctors give prompt treatment with an immunosuppressive drug because of the high risk of blindness.

Scleroderma

Scleroderma (systemic sclerosis) is a chronic disorder characterized by degenerative changes and scarring in the skin, joints, and internal organs and by blood vessel abnormalities.

The cause of scleroderma is not known. The disorder is 4 times more common in women than in men and is rare in children. Symptoms of scleroderma may occur as part of mixed connective tissue disease, and some people with mixed connective tissue disease develop severe scleroderma.

Symptoms

The usual initial symptom of scleroderma is swelling, then thickening and tightening of the skin at the ends of the fingers. Raynaud's phenomenon, in which the fingers suddenly become very pale and tingle or become numb and/or painful in response to cold or emotional upset★ is also common. Fingers typically become bluish as they warm up. Heartburn, difficulty in swallowing, and shortness of breath are occasionally the first symptoms of scleroderma. Aches and pains in several joints often accompany early symptoms. Sometimes polymyositis, with its accompanying muscle pain and weakness, develops.

Scleroderma can damage large areas of skin or only the fingers (sclerodactyly). One form of scleroderma, called limited scleroderma, tends to stay restricted to the skin of the hands. In another form, called diffuse scleroderma, the disorder progresses; the skin becomes more widely taut, shiny, and darker than usual. The skin on the face tightens, sometimes resulting in an inability to change

---

▲ see page 452   ■ see box on page 374

★ see also page 224

facial expressions. Especially in the limited form, spider veins (telangiectasia) can appear on the fingers, chest, face, lips, and tongue; bumps composed of calcium can develop on the fingers, on other bony areas, or at the joints.

Sometimes, a grating sound can be felt or heard as inflamed tissues move over each other, particularly at and below the knees. The fingers, wrists, and elbows may freeze (forming a contracture) in flexed positions because of scarring in the skin. Sores can develop on the fingertips and knuckles.

Scarring commonly damages the lower end of the esophagus (the tube connecting the mouth and stomach). The damaged esophagus can no longer propel food to the stomach efficiently. Swallowing difficulties and heartburn eventually develop in most people who have scleroderma. Abnormal cell growth in the esophagus (Barrett's esophagus▲) occurs in about one third of the people, increasing their risk of esophageal blockage (stricture) due to a fibrous band or to cancer. Damage to the intestines can interfere with food absorption (malabsorption) and cause weight loss. The drainage system from the liver may become blocked by scar tissue (biliary cirrhosis), resulting in liver damage and jaundice.

Scleroderma can cause scar tissue to accumulate in the lungs, resulting in abnormal shortness of breath during exercise. It can also cause several life-threatening heart abnormalities, including heart failure and abnormal rhythms.

Severe kidney disease can result from scleroderma. The first symptom of kidney damage may be an abrupt, progressive rise in blood pressure. High blood pressure is an ominous sign, although treatment usually controls it.

The **CREST syndrome,** also called limited cutaneous scleroderma (sclerosis) is usually a less severe form of the disorder that is less likely to cause serious internal organ damage. It is named for its symptoms: *C*alcium deposits in the skin and throughout the body, *R*aynaud's phenomenon, *E*sophageal dysfunction, *S*clerodactyly (skin damage on the fingers), and *T*elangiectasia (spider veins). Skin damage is limited to the fingers. People who have the CREST syndrome can develop pulmonary hypertension,■ which can cause heart and lung failure.

Sometimes scleroderma worsens rapidly and becomes fatal. At other times, it affects only the skin for decades before affecting internal organs, although some damage to internal organs (such as the esophagus) is almost inevitable, even in the CREST syndrome.

Diagnosis

A doctor diagnoses scleroderma by the characteristic changes in the skin and internal organs. The symptoms may overlap with those of several other connective tissue disorders, but the whole pattern is usually distinctive. Laboratory tests alone cannot identify scleroderma because test results, like the symptoms, vary greatly. However, tests for an antibody to centromeres (part of a chromosome) may help distinguish limited cutaneous scleroderma from the more generalized form; the more generalized form may contain a different antibody (called anti-topoisomerase).

Prognosis and Treatment

The course of scleroderma varies and is unpredictable, sometimes being fatal. The prognosis is worst for those who have early symptoms of heart, lung, or kidney damage.

No drug can stop the progression of scleroderma. However, drugs can relieve some symptoms and reduce organ damage. Nonsteroidal anti-inflammatory drugs (NSAIDs)★ help relieve severe muscle and joint pain. If the person has weakness because of polymyositis, corticosteroids may be needed. Penicillamine is thought by some experts to slow the rate of skin thickening and may delay the involvement of additional internal organs, but this use is controversial and some people cannot tolerate the side effects of this drug. Drugs that suppress the immune system, such as cyclophosphamide and methotrexate, may help some people whose lungs are affected.

Heartburn can be relieved by eating small meals and taking antacids, histamine-blocking drugs, and proton pump inhibitors, which block stomach acid production. Sleeping with the head of the bed elevated often helps. Surgery can sometimes correct severe reflux of stomach acid. Areas of the esophagus narrowed by scar tissue can be surgically widened (dilated). Tetracycline or other antibiotics can help prevent malabsorption of food caused by excessive growth (overgrowth) of bacteria in the damaged intestine. Nifedipine or an angiotensin II receptor blocker may relieve the symptoms of Raynaud's phenomenon● but

---

▲ see page 765   ■ see page 322
★ see page 452   ● see page 224

may also increase the reflux of stomach acid. Drugs for high blood pressure, particularly angiotensin-converting enzyme (ACE) inhibitors, are useful in treating kidney disease and the rise in blood pressure.

Physical therapy and exercise can help to maintain muscle strength but cannot totally prevent joints from freezing in permanent (usually flexed) positions (contractures).

Sjögren's Syndrome

Sjögren's syndrome is characterized by excessive dryness of the eyes, mouth, and other mucous membranes.

Sjögren's syndrome is thought to be an autoimmune disorder, but its cause is not known. It is more common in women than in men.

White blood cells infiltrate the glands that secrete fluids, such as the salivary glands in the mouth and the tear glands in the eyes. The white blood cells injure the glands, resulting in a dry mouth and dry eyes—the hallmark symptoms of this syndrome.

Symptoms

In some people, only the mouth or eyes are dry (a condition called sicca complex or sicca syndrome). Dryness of the eyes may severely damage the cornea, resulting in a scratchy or irritated sensation, and a lack of tears can cause permanent eye damage. Insufficient saliva in the mouth can dull taste and smell, make eating and swallowing painful, and cause cavities. The salivary glands in the cheeks (parotids) become enlarged and slightly tender in about one third of people. The mouth may also burn, which may sometimes indicate a complicating yeast infection.

In other people, many organs are affected. Sjögren's syndrome can dry out the mucous membranes lining the digestive tract, windpipe (trachea), vulva, and vagina. Dryness of the trachea and lungs can make these organs more susceptible to infection, leading to pneumonia. Dryness of the vulva and vagina can make sexual intercourse difficult. The protective sac surrounding the heart (pericardium) may be inflamed—a condition called pericarditis. Nerve, lung tissue, and other tissues may be damaged by the inflammation.

Joint inflammation (arthritis) occurs in about one third of people, affecting the same joints that rheumatoid arthritis affects, but the joint inflammation of Sjögren's syndrome tends to be milder and is usually not destructive. Some people also have severe rheumatoid arthritis or systemic lupus erythematosus.

Lymphoma, a cancer of the lymphatic system, is much more common in people who have Sjögren's syndrome than in the general population.

Diagnosis

Although a sensation of dry mouth or dry eyes is fairly common, a sensation of dry mouth and dry eyes accompanied by joint inflammation probably indicates that the person has Sjögren's syndrome. Various tests can help a doctor diagnose this disorder and differentiate it from other connective tissue disorders that can produce similar symptoms.

The amount of tears produced can be estimated by placing a filter paper strip under each lower eyelid and observing how much of the strip is moistened (Schirmer test). A person who has Sjögren's syndrome may produce less than one third of the normal amount. An ophthalmologist can test for damage to the eye's surface. More sophisticated tests to evaluate salivary gland secretion may be performed, and a doctor may order scans or a biopsy of the salivary glands.

Blood tests can detect abnormal antibodies, including SS-B, an antibody that is highly specific for Sjögren's syndrome. Often, people with Sjögren's syndrome also have antibodies that are more characteristic of rheumatoid arthritis or lupus. The erythrocyte sedimentation rate (ESR), a test that measures the rate at which red blood cells settle to the bottom of a test tube containing blood, is elevated in about 7 of 10 people. About 1 of 3 people has a decreased number of red blood cells (anemia) or of certain types of white blood cells (leukopenia).

Prognosis and Treatment

The prognosis is generally good. However, if the lungs, kidneys, or lymph nodes are damaged by the antibodies, pneumonia, kidney failure, or lymphoma may result.

No cure for Sjögren's syndrome is available, but symptoms can be relieved. Dry eyes can be treated with artificial tear drops. A dry mouth can be moistened by continuously sipping liquids, chewing sugarless gum, or using a mouth rinse. Drugs that reduce the amount of saliva, such as decongestants, antidepressants, and antihistamines, should be avoided because they can worsen the dryness. The drug pilocarpine may help stimulate the production of saliva if the salivary glands are not too severely damaged.

Fastidious dental hygiene and frequent dental visits can minimize tooth decay and loss. Painful, swollen salivary glands can be treated with analgesics. Because joint symptoms are usually mild, treatment with nonsteroidal anti-inflammatory drugs (NSAIDs) and rest is often sufficient. When symptoms resulting from damage to internal organs are severe, corticosteroids such as prednisone given by mouth can be useful.

Polymyositis and Dermatomyositis

*Polymyositis is characterized by inflammation and degeneration of the muscles; **dermatomyositis** is polymyositis accompanied by skin inflammation.*

These disorders result in disabling muscle weakness. The weakness typically occurs in the shoulders and hips but can affect muscles symmetrically throughout the body.

Polymyositis and dermatomyositis usually occur in adults from ages 40 to 60 or in children from ages 5 to 15 years. Women are twice as likely as men to develop either disorder. In adults, these disorders may occur alone or as part of other connective tissue disorders, such as mixed connective tissue disease.

The cause of polymyositis and dermatomyositis is unknown. Viruses or autoimmune reactions may play a role. Cancer may also trigger polymyositis and dermatomyositis—it is possible that an immune reaction against cancer may be directed against a substance in the muscles.

Symptoms

In **polymyositis,** the symptoms are similar for people of all ages, but the disorder usually develops more abruptly in children than in adults. Symptoms, which may begin during or just after an infection, include symmetrical muscle weakness (particularly in the upper arms, hips, and thighs), joint pain (but often little muscle pain), difficulty in swallowing, fever, fatigue, and weight loss. Raynaud's phenomenon (in which the fingers suddenly become very pale and tingle or become numb in response to cold or emotional upset▲) occurs more in people who have polymyositis along with other connective tissue disorders.

Muscle weakness may start slowly or suddenly and may worsen for weeks or months.

Because muscles close to the center of the body are affected most, tasks such as lifting the arms above the shoulders, climbing stairs, and getting out of a chair can become very difficult. If the neck muscles are affected, even raising the head from a pillow may be impossible. Weakness in the shoulders or hips can confine a person to a wheelchair or bed. Muscle damage in the upper part of the esophagus can cause swallowing difficulties and regurgitation of food. The muscles of the hands, feet, and face, however, are not affected.

Joint aches and inflammation occur in about one third of the people. The pain and swelling tend to be mild.

Polymyositis usually does not affect internal organs other than the throat and esophagus. However, the lungs and heart may be affected, causing shortness of breath and a cough.

In **dermatomyositis,** all the symptoms of polymyositis occur. In addition, rashes tend to appear at the same time as muscle weakness and other symptoms. A shadowy-red or purplish rash (heliotrope rash) can appear on the face. A reddish-purple swelling around the eyes is characteristic. Another rash, which may be scaly, smooth, or raised, may appear almost anywhere on the body but is especially common on the knuckles and sides of the hands. The nail beds may redden. When the rashes fade, brownish pigmentation, scarring, shriveling, or pale depigmented patches may develop on the skin.

Diagnosis

Doctors use the following criteria to make the diagnosis of polymyositis or dermatomyositis: muscle weakness at the shoulders or hips, a characteristic rash, increased blood levels of certain muscle enzymes (especially creatine kinase), characteristic changes in muscle tissue obtained by biopsy and observed under a microscope, and abnormalities in the electrical activity of muscles measured by electromyography.■ Laboratory tests are helpful but cannot specifically identify polymyositis or dermatomyositis. Blood levels of creatine kinase are often much higher than normal, indicating muscle damage. These enzymes are measured repeatedly in blood samples to monitor the disorder; the levels usually fall to normal or near normal with effective treatment.

▲ see also page 224   ■ see page 446

Magnetic resonance imaging (MRI) may also show areas of inflammation and help the doctor select a site for biopsy. Special tests performed on muscle tissue samples may be needed to rule out other muscle disorders.

Treatment and Prognosis

Restricting activities when the inflammation is most intense often helps. Generally, a corticosteroid, usually prednisone, given by mouth in high doses slowly improves strength and relieves pain and swelling, controlling the disease. After about 6 to 12 weeks, when the muscle enzyme levels have returned to normal and muscle strength has returned, the dose is gradually decreased. Most adults must continue taking a low dose of prednisone for many years or even indefinitely to prevent a relapse. After about a year, children may be able to stop taking the drug and stay symptom-free.

Occasionally, the side effects of prednisone actually worsen the symptoms.▲ In these cases, an immunosuppressive drug (methotrexate, cyclophosphamide, chlorambucil, azathioprine, or cyclosporine) is used instead of or in addition to prednisone. When other drugs are ineffective, gamma globulin (a substance that contains large quantities of many antibodies) may be given intravenously.

When polymyositis is associated with cancer, it usually does not respond well to prednisone. However, the condition usually improves if the cancer can be successfully treated.

Adults with severe, progressive disease who develop difficulty in swallowing, malnutrition, pneumonia, or respiratory failure may die from the disease.

Mixed Connective Tissue Disease

Mixed connective tissue disease is a term used by some experts to describe a collection of symptoms similar to those of systemic lupus erythematosus, scleroderma, polymyositis, and dermatomyositis.

About 80% of people who have this disease are women. Mixed connective tissue disease affects people from ages 5 to 80. Its cause is unknown, but it appears to be an autoimmune disorder.

Symptoms

The typical symptoms are Raynaud's phenomenon (in which the fingers suddenly become very pale and tingle or become numb in response to cold or emotional upset),■ joint inflammation (arthritis), swollen hands, muscle weakness, difficulty in swallowing, heartburn, and shortness of breath. Raynaud's phenomenon may precede other symptoms by many years. Regardless of how mixed connective tissue disease starts, it tends to worsen, and symptoms spread to several parts of the body.

The hands are frequently so swollen that the fingers look like sausages. A purplish butterfly-shaped rash on the cheeks and bridge of the nose, red patches on the knuckles, a violet discoloration of the eyelids, and red spider veins on the face and hands all may appear. Skin changes similar to those in scleroderma also may occur. The hair may thin.

Almost everyone with mixed connective tissue disease has aching joints; about 75% develop the swelling and pain typical of joint inflammation (arthritis). Mixed connective tissue disease damages the muscle fibers, so the muscles may feel weak and sore, especially in the shoulders and hips.

Although the esophagus is often affected, it seldom causes difficulty in swallowing and is not painful. Fluid may collect in or around the lungs. In some people, abnormal lung function is the most serious problem, causing shortness of breath during exertion.

Occasionally, the heart is weakened, leading to heart failure.★ Symptoms of heart failure may include fluid retention, shortness of breath, and fatigue. The kidneys and nerves are affected in only 10% of people, and the damage is usually mild compared to the damage caused by lupus. Other symptoms may include a fever, swollen lymph nodes, abdominal pain, and persistent hoarseness. Sjögren's syndrome may develop. Over time, most people develop symptoms that are more typical of lupus or scleroderma.

Diagnosis and Treatment

Doctors suspect mixed connective tissue disease when some symptoms from lupus, scleroderma, polymyositis, or rheumatoid arthritis overlap.

Blood tests are performed to detect an antibody to ribonucleoprotein, which is present in almost all people who have mixed connective tissue disease. A high level of this antibody

▲ see box on page 374   ■ see also page 224

★ see page 150

without the other antibodies present in lupus is reasonably specific for mixed connective tissue disease.

The treatment is similar to that of lupus. Corticosteroids are usually effective, especially when the disease is diagnosed early. Mild cases can be treated with aspirin or other non-steroidal anti-inflammatory drugs (NSAIDs), quinacrine or similar drugs, or very low doses of corticosteroids. The more severe the disease, the higher the dose of corticosteroid needed. In severe cases, immunosuppressive drugs may also be needed.

In general, the more advanced the disease and the greater the organ damage, the less effective the treatment. Scleroderma-like damage to the skin and esophagus is least likely to respond to treatment. Symptom-free periods can last for many years with little or no continuing treatment with a corticosteroid. Despite treatment, mixed connective tissue disease progresses in about 13% of the people, producing potentially fatal complications in 6 to 12 years.

Relapsing Polychondritis

Relapsing polychondritis is characterized by episodes of painful, destructive inflammation of the cartilage and other connective tissues in many organs.

This disorder affects men and women equally, usually in middle age. The cause is unknown, but autoimmune reactions to cartilage are suspected.

Symptoms

Typically, one or both ears become red, swollen, and very painful. At the same time or later, a person can develop joint inflammation (arthritis), which may be mild or severe. Cartilage in any joint may be affected, and the cartilage that connects the ribs to the breastbone may become inflamed. Cartilage in the nose is also a common site of inflammation; the nose may become tender and cartilage can collapse.

Other affected sites include the eyes (resulting in conjunctivitis; rarely the cornea may become perforated, resulting in blindness; voice box (larynx) and windpipe (trachea), resulting in hoarseness, a nonproductive cough, and tenderness over the Adam's apple; and bronchi, sometimes resulting in pneumonia. Less often, the heart is involved, leading to heart murmurs and occasionally to heart failure. Blood vessels may become inflamed;

when blood vessels in the brain are involved, seizures and strokes may occur. The kidneys may become inflamed, sometimes leading to kidney failure. The skin may become inflamed, resulting in a variety of rashes.

Flare-ups of inflammation and pain last a few weeks, subside, then recur over a period of several years. Eventually, the supporting cartilage can be damaged, resulting in floppy ears, a sloping saddle nose, and vision, hearing, and balance problems.

People who have this disorder may die if the cartilage in their airways collapses, blocking the flow of air, or if their heart and blood vessels are severely damaged.

Diagnosis and Treatment

Relapsing polychondritis is diagnosed when a doctor observes at least three of the following symptoms developing over time: inflammation of both ears, painful swelling in several joints, inflammation of the cartilage in the nose, inflammation of the eye, cartilage damage in the respiratory tract, and hearing or balance problems.

A biopsy of the affected cartilage may show characteristic abnormalities. Blood tests, such as the erythrocyte sedimentation rate (ESR), which measures the rate at which red blood cells settle to the bottom of a test tube containing blood, can detect evidence of chronic inflammation.

Mild relapsing polychondritis can be treated with aspirin or other nonsteroidal anti-inflammatory drugs (NSAIDs).▲ In more severe cases, daily doses of prednisone are given, then tapered off as the symptoms begin to improve. Sometimes very severe cases are treated with immunosuppressive drugs such as methotrexate or cyclophosphamide. These drugs treat the symptoms but have not been shown to alter the ultimate course of the disorder.

Eosinophilic Fasciitis

Eosinophilic fasciitis is a disorder in which the skin of the arms and legs becomes painfully inflamed and swollen and gradually hardens.

The name eosinophilic refers to the initially high blood levels of a type of white blood cell called eosinophils. Fasciitis refers to inflam-

▲ see page 452

mation of the fascia, which is the tough fibrous tissue that lies beneath the skin.

The cause of eosinophilic fasciitis is unknown. The disorder occurs mainly in men aged 40 to 50, but it may occur in women and children.

Symptoms

The usual initial symptoms are pain, swelling, and inflammation of the skin, particularly over the inside of the arms and the front of the legs. The skin of the face, chest, and abdomen may occasionally be affected also. In contrast to scleroderma, the skin of the feet and hands is not affected and Raynaud's phenomenon does not occur.

Symptoms may first be noticed after strenuous physical activity, particularly in a person who usually does not exercise very much. Symptoms usually progress gradually. After weeks, the inflamed skin begins to harden, eventually acquiring a texture similar to an orange peel.

As the skin gradually hardens, the arms and legs become difficult to move. Eventually, the arms and legs may become stuck in unusual positions. Weight loss and fatigue are common. Muscle strength does not usually decrease, but muscle and joint pain may occur. Rarely, if the arms are involved, the person may develop carpal tunnel syndrome.▲

Sometimes, the numbers of red blood cells and platelets in the bloodstream become very low, resulting in anemia and a tendency to bleed easily.

Diagnosis

A doctor suspects eosinophilic fasciitis because of its typical symptoms. Blood tests are performed to detect increased proteins called globulins. The number of eosinophils (a type of white blood cell) is increased as is the erythrocyte sedimentation rate (ESR); this increase indicates inflammation.

The diagnosis is confirmed by taking and examining under a microscope a small sample (biopsy) of affected skin and the tissues underneath it (the fascia). The biopsy sample must include all skin layers down to the muscle. Magnetic resonance imaging (MRI) can help confirm the diagnosis but is usually unnecessary because the biopsy and other tests are typically sufficient.

Treatment and Prognosis

Most people respond rapidly to high doses of corticosteroids. Treatment should be started as early as possible to prevent scarring, tissue loss (atrophy), and contractures. Corticosteroids may not reverse atrophied and scarred tissue. Doses are gradually reduced, but corticosteroids may need to be continued at low levels for 2 to 5 years. The use of other drugs is experimental for people who cannot use or do not fully respond to corticosteroids.

Although the long-term outlook is unknown, eventually, with or without treatment, the inflammation of eosinophilic fasciitis generally resolves on its own, leaving the scars that appeared before treatment.

CHAPTER 69

Vasculitic Disorders of Connective Tissue

Vasculitic disorders develop from inflammation of the blood vessels (vasculitis). Vasculitis commonly occurs in disorders that affect connective tissue, but it can also occur in conditions that do not affect connective tissue. Vasculitis is not a disease but rather a disease process.

Usually the triggers of vasculitis are not known. However, certain viruses, especially hepatitis viruses, can initiate it. Other triggers appear to be certain infections and reactions to certain drugs and vaccines. Presumably, the inflammation occurs when the immune system mistakenly identifies blood vessels or parts of a blood vessel as foreign and attacks them. Cells of the immune system, which

▲ see page 398

cause inflammation, surround and infiltrate the affected blood vessels, damaging them and possibly damaging the tissues they supply. The damaged blood vessels may become leaky or clogged; either way, blood flow to the areas supplied by the damaged vessels is disrupted. The areas deprived of blood (ischemic areas) can be damaged permanently. Symptoms may result from direct damage to the blood vessels or from indirect damage to tissues (such as nerves or organs) whose blood supply has been disrupted.

Any blood vessel may be affected. Vasculitis may be limited to veins, large arteries, small arteries, or capillaries, or it may be limited to vessels in one part of the body, such as the head, leg, or kidney. Disorders such as Henoch-Schönlein purpura, erythema nodosum, polyarteritis nodosa, temporal (giant cell) arteritis, and Takayasu's arteritis are characterized by vasculitis that is limited to blood vessels of a particular size or depth.

Polyarteritis Nodosa

Polyarteritis nodosa is a disorder in which segments of medium-sized arteries become inflamed and damaged, reducing the blood supply to certain organs and tissues.

Polyarteritis nodosa most often develops at 40 to 50 years of age but can occur at any age. Men are 3 times more likely than women to develop this type of vasculitis.

Its cause is unknown but sometimes appears to be a reaction to certain drugs and vaccines. Viral infections (such as hepatitis B infection) and bacterial infections (such as streptococcal or staphylococcal infections) sometimes appear to trigger the inflammation, but most often no initiating event or substance can be found.

Symptoms

The disorder can be mild at first but can worsen rapidly and be fatal within several months, or it can develop subtly as a chronic debilitating disease. Any organ or combination of organs in the body can be affected (except the lungs); the symptoms depend on which organs are affected. Because vasculitis is often associated with inflammation of connective tissue, joints are often affected. Muscle and joint pain is common, and joint inflammation (arthritis) may occur.

A fever is a common early symptom. Abdominal pain, numbness and tingling in the

SELECTED DISORDERS CHARACTERIZED BY VASCULITIS

DISORDER	DESCRIPTION
Henoch-Schönlein purpura	Inflammation of small blood vessels, causing hard, purple blotches on the skin and bleeding from the intestine or kidneys; most common in children
Erythema nodosum	Inflammation of blood vessels in the deep layers of the skin, causing deep, tender red bumps on the arms and legs
Polyarteritis nodosa	Inflammation of medium-sized arteries, impairing blood flow through vessels and to the surrounding tissues of several organs
Temporal (giant cell) arteritis	Inflammation of arteries in the brain and head, sometimes causing headaches and blindness; most common in older people
Takayasu's arteritis	Inflammation of large arteries, such as the aorta and its branches, causing blockages and loss of pulse; most common in children
Hypersensitivity vasculitis	Inflammation limited to small blood vessels in the skin, producing tender, red superficial lumps most often on the legs

hands and feet, weakness, and weight loss can also develop early. Three fourths of people who have polyarteritis nodosa develop kidney damage (because blood vessels supplying the kidneys are affected), which can cause high blood pressure, swelling from water retention, and decreased production of urine.

When blood vessels in the digestive tract are affected, areas of this tract can become perforated, causing an abdominal infection (peritonitis), severe pain, bloody diarrhea, and a high fever. When blood vessels to the heart are affected, chest pain and heart attacks can result. Damaged blood vessels in the brain can cause headaches, seizures, and hallucinations. Damaged blood vessels in the liver can cause extensive liver damage. Blood vessels near the skin may feel bumpy and irregular to the touch, and occasionally ulcers form on the skin over the blood vessels.

Diagnosis and Treatment

No blood test can confirm the diagnosis of polyarteritis nodosa. Doctors suspect the disease when the combination of symptoms and laboratory test results cannot be explained any other way. For instance, they may suspect it when fever and evidence of nerve damage, such as patchy numbness, tingling, or paralysis, develop in a previously healthy middle-aged man. The diagnosis can be confirmed by a biopsy of an affected blood vessel. A biopsy of the liver or kidney may also be needed. X-rays taken after a radiopaque dye, which is visible on x-rays, is injected into the arteries may show bulges (aneurysms) in the walls of affected arteries.

Without treatment, only 33% of affected people survive for 1 year; 88% die within 5 years. Aggressive treatment can delay or prevent death from this disorder.

Any drugs that may have precipitated the disease are discontinued. Any other possible triggering factors, such as an infection, are treated.

High doses of a corticosteroid, such as prednisone, can prevent the disease from worsening and induce a symptom-free period in about one third of the people. Because long-term treatment with a corticosteroid is usually needed and because such long-term treatment can produce significant side effects, doctors reduce the dose once symptoms have subsided. If corticosteroids do not reduce the inflammation adequately, they may be replaced with or accompanied by drugs that suppress the immune system, such as cyclophosphamide. Other treatments, such as those used to control high blood pressure, are often needed to prevent damage to internal organs.

Even with treatment, several vital organs may fail or a weakened blood vessel may rupture. Kidney failure is a common cause of death. Potentially fatal infections may occur because the long-term use of corticosteroids and immunosuppressive drugs reduces the body's ability to fight infections.

Temporal Arteritis

Temporal (giant cell) arteritis is chronic inflammation of large arteries, typically of the temporal artery, an artery on the side of the scalp.

This disorder affects about 1 of 1,000 people older than 50 and slightly more women than men. Its cause is unknown. Temporal arteritis often occurs with polymyalgia rheumatica.

Symptoms

The symptoms vary, depending on which arteries are affected. Typically, the large arteries to the head are affected, and a severe headache usually develops suddenly at the temples or back of the head. The blood vessels in the temple may feel swollen and bumpy. The scalp may feel painful when the hair is brushed. Double vision, blurred vision, large blind spots, blindness of one eye, or other eye problems may develop. The greatest danger is permanent blindness, which can occur suddenly if the blood supply to the optic nerve is blocked.

Characteristically, the jaw, chewing muscles, and tongue may hurt when eating or speaking. Other symptoms may include severe pain in the neck, shoulders, and hip, which also occurs in polymyalgia rheumatica.

Diagnosis and Treatment

Doctors base their diagnosis on the symptoms and a physical examination and confirm it by performing a biopsy of the temporal artery, located in the temple. Blood tests are also helpful, usually detecting anemia and a very high erythrocyte sedimentation rate (ESR), which indicates inflammation.

Because temporal arteritis causes blindness in 20% of untreated people, treatment must begin as soon as the disease is suspected. Treatment is usually started even before a biopsy is performed; treatment does not affect the biopsy results as long as the biopsy is performed within several days of starting treatment. Prednisone, a corticosteroid, is highly effective. Initially, the dose is high—to stop the inflammation in the blood vessels; after several weeks, doctors slowly taper the dose if the person is improving. Some people can stop taking prednisone within a few years, but many need very low doses for many years to control symptoms and prevent blindness.

Polymyalgia Rheumatica

Polymyalgia rheumatica causes severe pain and stiffness in the muscles of the neck, shoulders, and hips.

Polymyalgia rheumatica occurs in people older than 50 and is twice as common in women as in men. Its cause is not known. Because polymyalgia rheumatica may occur with temporal (giant cell) arteritis, it is suggested that the two disorders may develop in the same way.

Symptoms and Diagnosis

Polymyalgia rheumatica causes severe pain and stiffness in the neck, shoulders, and hips. The stiffness is worse in the morning and after periods of inactivity. A fever, vague discomfort, weight loss, and depression may accompany the muscle symptoms. All these symptoms may develop suddenly or gradually. Muscle damage or weakness does not occur. Some people with polymyalgia rheumatica also develop symptoms of temporal arteritis, which can lead to blindness. Some people may have mild arthritis, but if the arthritis is prominent, rheumatoid arthritis▲ is more likely to be the diagnosis.

A doctor makes the diagnosis on the basis of the person's symptoms, physical examination, and test results. Blood test results, such as the erythrocyte sedimentation rate (ESR) and C-reactive protein, are usually very high, indicating active inflammation. Biopsies of muscle tissue are usually not needed but, if performed, show no evidence of muscle damage; electromyography■ shows no abnormalities. Blood tests may detect anemia.

Treatment

Polymyalgia rheumatica usually improves dramatically with low doses of prednisone, a corticosteroid. When temporal arteritis also occurs, higher doses of a corticosteroid are needed, particularly to reduce the risk of blindness. As the symptoms subside, the dose is gradually reduced to the lowest effective one. Many people can stop taking prednisone in 2 to 4 years, although some people need low doses for an even longer time. Aspirin or other nonsteroidal anti-inflammatory drugs may provide less relief.

Wegener's Granulomatosis

Wegener's granulomatosis is vasculitis that often begins with inflammation of the lining of the nose, sinuses, throat, or lungs and may progress to inflammation of blood vessels throughout the body (generalized vasculitis) with potentially fatal kidney failure.

Wegener's granulomatosis can occur at any age and is twice as common in men as in

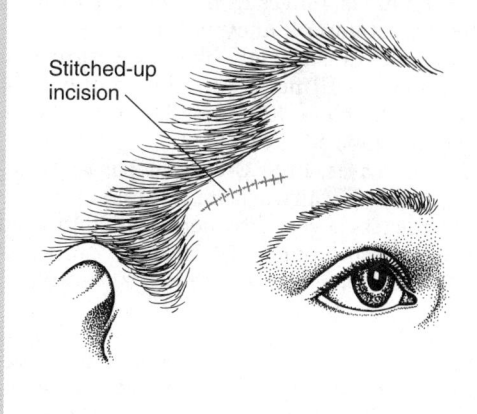

Biopsy of the Temporal Artery

A biopsy of the temporal artery is the definitive procedure for diagnosing temporal arteritis. Doppler ultrasonography is occasionally used to locate the part of the temporal artery to be biopsied. After a local anesthetic is injected, a shallow incision is made directly over the artery, and at least a 1-inch segment of the artery is removed. The incision is then stitched up.

Stitched-up incision

women. Its cause is unknown. It resembles an infection, but no infecting organism has been found. Wegener's granulomatosis is thought to be caused by an allergic response to a trigger that has not yet been identified. The result is a potent, inappropriate immune reaction that damages many tissues in the body.

The disorder produces inflammation of blood vessels (vasculitis) and an unusual type of inflammatory tissue called a granuloma, which ultimately destroys normal tissue.

Symptoms

The disorder may begin suddenly or gradually. The first symptoms usually affect the upper respiratory tract—the nose, sinuses, ears, and windpipe (trachea)—and may include severe nosebleeds, sinusitis, middle ear infections (otitis media), coughing, coughing up of blood, and shortness of breath. The lining of the nose may become red and rough, bleeding

▲ see page 370   ■ see page 446

easily. A fever, a generally sick feeling (malaise), loss of appetite, joint aches and swelling, and inflammation of the eye or ear may develop. The disease may affect arteries to the heart, causing chest pain or a heart attack, or it may affect the brain or spinal cord, producing symptoms that resemble those of several neurologic diseases.

The disorder may progress to a generalized (disseminated) phase, with inflammation of blood vessels throughout the body. As a result, sores appear on the skin and spread extensively; they can severely scar the skin. Kidney damage, common at this stage of Wegener's granulomatosis, ranges from mild impairment to life-threatening kidney failure. Severe kidney disease causes high blood pressure and symptoms resulting from the buildup of wastes in the blood (uremia). Anemia is common and can be severe.

In some cases, only the nasal passages, sinuses, and upper airways are affected for many years; this less severe disorder is called limited Wegener's granulomatosis. However, progression to the more serious disorder is possible.

Diagnosis

Wegener's granulomatosis must be diagnosed and treated early to prevent complications, including kidney disease, lung disease, heart attacks, and brain damage.

A doctor usually recognizes the distinctive pattern of symptoms. Although blood test results cannot specifically identify Wegener's granulomatosis, they can strongly support the diagnosis. A blood test can detect antineutrophil cytoplasmic antibodies in the blood, which strongly suggest this disease. If the nose, throat, or skin is not affected, diagnosis can be difficult because the symptoms and x-rays can resemble those of several lung diseases.

A chest x-ray may show cavities or dense areas in the lungs that look like cancer. Doctors can make a definite diagnosis only by examining a small piece of tissue under a microscope (a biopsy); the tissue sample may be taken from an affected area, such as the nasal passages, airways, or lungs. Skin and kidney biopsies may be less helpful.

Treatment

Corticosteroids may be used alone to treat the early symptoms of Wegener's granulomatosis. However, most people also need an other immunosuppressive drug, such as cyclophosphamide.

The generalized form of Wegener's granulomatosis is treated with immunosuppressive drugs, such as cyclophosphamide and azathioprine, which control the disease by reducing the body's inappropriate immune reaction. Such use significantly improves the prognosis because, without treatment, this form of the disorder is fatal. Treatment is usually continued for at least a year after the symptoms disappear. Corticosteroids, given at the same time to suppress inflammation, can usually be tapered off and discontinued.

For people who are receiving immunosuppressive drugs, a doctor treats any suspected infection as early as possible because of the body's decreased ability to fight infections. Pneumonia is particularly common when the lungs are damaged. An antibiotic may be used to prevent infections in people who have been taking immunosuppressive drugs for years.

Behçet's Syndrome

Behçet's syndrome is a chronic, relapsing inflammatory disorder that can produce recurring, painful mouth sores, skin blisters, genital sores, and swollen joints; the eyes, blood vessels, nervous system, and digestive tract may also become inflamed.

This syndrome affects men twice as often as women. It usually appears in people during their 20s, but sometimes it develops in childhood. Behçet's syndrome is uncommon in the United States. People from Mediterranean countries, Japan, Korea, and the area along the silk route through China are at highest risk. The cause of Behçet's syndrome is unknown, but viruses and autoimmune disorders may play a role.

Symptoms

Almost everyone with this syndrome has recurring, painful mouth sores, similar to canker sores. Sores may also appear on the penis, scrotum, and vulva and tend to be painful; those in the vagina may be painless.

Other symptoms appear days to years later. A recurring inflammation of part of the eye (relapsing iridocyclitis) produces eye pain, sensitivity to light, and hazy vision. Several other eye problems can occur; one of them, uveitis,▲ can cause blindness if untreated.

Skin blisters and pus-filled pimples develop in about 80% of people. A minor injury, even a puncture from a hypodermic needle, can cause

▲ see page 1305

the area to become swollen and inflamed. About half of the people develop a relatively mild, nonprogressive joint inflammation (arthritis) in the knees and other large joints. Vasculitis throughout the body can cause blood clot formation, aneurysms (bulges in weakened blood vessel walls), strokes, and kidney damage. When the digestive tract is affected, symptoms may range from mild discomfort to severe cramping and diarrhea.

The recurring symptoms of Behçet's syndrome can be very disruptive. The symptoms or the symptom-free periods (remissions) may last weeks, years, or decades. Occasionally, damage to the nervous system, digestive tract, or blood vessels is fatal.

Diagnosis and Treatment

The diagnosis is based on the physical examination because no laboratory tests can detect Behçet's syndrome. However, symptoms resemble those of many other diseases, including Reiter's syndrome (reactive arthritis), Stevens-Johnson syndrome, systemic lupus erythematosus, Crohn's disease, herpes infection, and ulcerative colitis.

Although there is no cure, specific symptoms can usually be relieved by treatment. For example, a corticosteroid applied externally (rather than by mouth) can help heal inflamed eyes and skin sores. People who develop a severe inflammation of the eyes or the nervous system may need to be treated with prednisone or another corticosteroid. Cyclosporine, an immunosuppressive drug, may be given when the eye problems are severe or when prednisone does not adequately control symptoms. Colchicine given by mouth in low doses may help prevent oral and genital ulcers. Thalidomide is being investigated for use. Needle punctures should be avoided because the skin may become inflamed.

CHAPTER 70

Gout and Pseudogout

Gout and pseudogout are characterized by joint inflammation (arthritis) and pain. Both disorders are caused by deposits of crystals in the joints, although the type of crystal differs.

Gout

Gout is a disorder that results from deposits of sodium urate crystals, which accumulate in the joints because of high blood levels of uric acid (hyperuricemia), leading to attacks of painful joint inflammation.

Gout is more common in men than in women. Usually, gout develops during middle age in men and after menopause in women. Gout is rare in younger people but is often more severe in people who develop the disorder before age 30. Gout often runs in families.

Gout most often affects the joints in the feet, particularly at the base of the big toe (podagra). However, it also commonly affects other joints: the ankle, knee, wrist, and elbow. Urate crystals may form in these joints because the joints are cooler than the central part of the body, and urate crystals form readily at cooler temperatures. Gout rarely affects the joints of the spine, hips, or shoulders.

Causes

Normally, uric acid, a by-product of cell nucleic acid breakdown, is present in small amounts in the blood because the body continually breaks down cells and forms new cells. Also, the body readily transforms substances in foods called purines into uric acid. Foods high in purines include anchovies, asparagus, consommé, herring, meat gravies and broths, mushrooms, mussels, all organ meats, sardines, and sweetbreads. Most often, the uric acid level in the blood becomes abnormally high when the kidneys cannot eliminate enough uric acid in the urine. Too much uric acid in the blood can result in urate crystals being formed and deposited in joints. Additionally, combining a high-purine diet with alcohol can worsen matters, because alcohol both increases the production of uric acid and interferes with its elimination by the kidneys.

Risk Factors for the Development of Gout

- Certain cancers and blood disorders
- Certain drugs (such as thiazide diuretics, cyclosporine, pyrazinamide, ethambutol, nicotinic acid, warfarin, and low doses of salicylates)
- Certain foods (such as anchovies, asparagus, consommé, herring, meat gravies and broths, mushrooms, mussels, all organ meats, sardines, and sweetbreads)
- Hypothyroidism
- Lead poisoning (from "moonshine" whiskey)
- Obesity
- Radiation treatment
- Renal failure
- Starvation

Less commonly, gout may be due to an identifiable underlying disorder; this is called secondary gout. For instance, large amounts of uric acid may be produced because of an inherited enzyme abnormality or a disease such as leukemia, in which cells multiply and are rapidly destroyed. Some types of kidney disease and certain drugs (eg, thiazide diuretics) impair the kidneys' ability to eliminate uric acid, so levels of uric acid rise. High levels of uric acid in the blood lead to high levels of uric acid in the joints; this process may then result in the formation of urate crystals in the joint tissue and the fluid within the joints (synovial fluid).

Symptoms

Attacks of gout (acute gouty arthritis) can occur without warning. They may be triggered by an injury, surgery, consumption of large quantities of alcohol or purine-rich food, fatigue, emotional stress, or illness. Typically, severe pain occurs suddenly in one or more joints, often at night (probably because of the metabolic changes that occur when a person lies down). The pain becomes progressively worse and is often excruciating, particularly when the joint is moved or touched. The joint becomes inflamed—it swells and feels warm, and the skin over the joint appears red or purplish, tight, and shiny.

Other symptoms of an attack can include fever (which may reach 102° F [38.9° C]), chills, a general sick feeling, and a rapid heartbeat. The first few attacks usually affect only one joint and last for a few days. The symptoms gradually disappear, joint function returns, and no symptoms appear until the next attack. However, if the disorder progresses, untreated attacks last longer, occur more frequently, and affect several joints.

After repeated attacks, gout can become severe and chronic and may lead to the destruction of tissue and a joint deformity.

Over time, joint motion becomes progressively restricted by damage caused by deposits of urate crystals in the joints and tendons. Hard lumps of urate crystals (tophi) are first deposited in the joint (synovial) lining or cartilage or in bone near the joints and then under the skin around joints. Tophi can also develop in the kidney and other organs, under the skin on the ears, in the tough band extending from the calf muscles to the heel (Achilles tendon), or around the elbows. If untreated, tophi can burst and discharge chalky masses of urate crystals through the skin.

About one fifth of people who have gout develop kidney stones (urolithiasis), which are composed of uric acid.▲ The stones may block the urinary tract, resulting in excruciating pain and, if untreated, infection and kidney damage. In people with gout who also have another disorder that damages the kidneys (such as diabetes or high blood pressure), increasingly poor kidney function reduces the excretion of uric acid and makes the gout and its joint damage progressively worse.

Diagnosis

Doctors often diagnose gout on the basis of its distinctive symptoms and an examination of the affected joints. A high uric acid level in the blood supports the diagnosis; however, this level is often normal, especially during an acute attack. A blood test may show increased numbers of white blood cells due to the inflammation caused by the urate crystals. The diagnosis is confirmed when needle-shaped urate crystals are identified in a sample of a tophus or in joint fluid removed (joint aspiration) with a needle and viewed under a microscope with polarized light. X-rays may show joint damage and the presence of tophi (urate crystal tophi that displace bone and produce cysts). Gout is often misdiagnosed as another type of arthritis.

▲ see page 864

R̲x̲ DRUGS USED TO TREAT GOUT

TYPE	DRUG	SELECTED SIDE EFFECTS	COMMENTS
Nonsteroidal anti-inflammatory drugs (NSAIDs)			
	All NSAIDs including cyclooxygenase-2 (COX-2) inhibitors (coxibs)	Upset stomach, bleeding, kidney damage, high potassium levels, retention of sodium and potassium	Used to treat an acute attack or to prevent an attack
Antigout drug			
	Colchicine	Diarrhea (occurs often), suppression of blood cell production in the bone marrow (occurs very rarely if the drug is used properly), skin irritation	Used for prevention and for treatment of attacks
Corticosteroids			
	Prednisone (taken by mouth)	Retention of sodium, with swelling or high blood pressure	Used only if other treatments cannot be used, but the benefit is dramatic
	Prednisolone tebutate or triamcinolone hexacetonide (taken by injection)	Pain, discomfort, joint damage with overuse, inflammation (occasionally), infection (rarely)	Injected into the joint if only one or two joints are affected
Uricosuric drugs			
	Probenecid, sulfinpyrazone	Headache, nausea, vomiting, kidney stones	Can be used long-term to lower blood levels of uric acid for prevention of attacks; aspirin should not be used at the same time
	Allopurinol	Upset stomach, skin rash, decrease in the number of white blood cells, liver or kidney damage, inflammation of blood vessels (vasculitis)	Can be used long-term to lower blood levels of uric acid for prevention of attacks; may also remove crystals or stones already in the kidney

Treatment

The first step is to relieve pain by controlling the inflammation.

Nonsteroidal anti-inflammatory drugs (NSAIDs), including the cyclooxygenase-2 (COX-2) inhibitors (coxibs), are often effective in relieving pain and swelling in the joint.▲ Rarely, additional analgesics such as codeine and meperidine are needed to control pain. The inflamed joint may be immobilized with a splint to reduce pain.

Colchicine is the traditional, but no longer the most common, first-step treatment. Usually, joint pain begins to subside after 12 hours of treatment with colchicine and is gone within 36 to 48 hours. Colchicine is usually taken in tablet form each hour until symptoms are relieved, but it can be given intra-venously if the person cannot take drugs by mouth. Colchicine can cause abdominal pain and diarrhea. It can occasionally cause more serious side effects, including damage to the bone marrow.

Corticosteroids, such as prednisone, are sometimes useful to reduce joint inflammation (including the swelling) in people who cannot tolerate the other drugs. If only one or two joints are affected, a corticosteroid suspension, such as prednisolone tebutate, can be injected using the same needle that is used to remove fluid from the joint.

The second step is to prevent recurrences of gout attacks. Avoiding alcoholic beverages,

---

▲ see pages 452 to 454

losing weight, stopping drugs that cause elevated blood levels of uric acid, and eating smaller amounts of purine-rich foods may be all that is needed. Most people who have primary gout are overweight. As they gradually lose weight, their blood urate levels often return to normal or near normal, and gout attacks subsequently cease.

Preventive daily drug treatment may be needed for people who experience repeated, severe attacks. Colchicine may be taken daily to prevent attacks or to greatly reduce their frequency. Nonsteroidal anti-inflammatory drugs (NSAIDs) taken daily can also prevent attacks. However, preventing attacks does not prevent or heal existing joint damage caused by urate crystals because the crystals still persist in the joints, and the drugs do pose some risks for people who have kidney or liver disease.

Drugs that cause excretion of uric acid in the urine (uricosuric drugs), such as probenecid or sulfinpyrazone, can be used to lower the uric acid level in the blood (in people who have normal kidney function) by increasing the kidney's excretion of uric acid. Aspirin blocks the effects of probenecid and of sulfinpyrazone and should not be used at the same time as either of these drugs. If pain medication is needed, acetaminophen or other analgesics can be safely used instead.

Although uricosuric drugs lower the concentration of uric acid in the blood, they can increase the concentration of uric acid in the urine; drinking plenty of fluids—at least 3 quarts a day—may help reduce the risk of urate stones developing in the urinary tract. Making the urine alkaline▲ by taking sodium bicarbonate or trisodium citrate (which increases the solubility of uric acid in the urine) can further help reduce the risk of urate stones forming in the urinary tract. However, if the urine becomes too alkaline, crystals or stones of another and more dangerous kind—calcium oxalate—may form. When starting a uricosuric drug, there is a risk of causing a gout attack. Because low-dose colchicine or an NSAID can decrease this risk, one of these drugs is usually given for a few months as well.

Allopurinol is another drug that is used to lower the blood level of uric acid. This drug blocks the production of uric acid in the body and is especially helpful for people who have a high blood uric acid level and urate stones or kidney damage. However, allopurinol can upset the stomach, cause a skin rash, decrease the number of white blood cells, or cause liver damage. As with uricosuric drugs, allopurinol can cause a gout attack when it is first taken. Low-dose colchicine or an NSAID is usually given at the same time, for a few months, to decrease this risk.

Most tophi on the ears, hands, or feet shrink slowly when the uric acid level becomes sufficiently low. However, extremely large tophi may have to be removed surgically.

Urate stones in the urinary tract can be broken up, and thereby washed out in the urine, using ultrasound directed at the stones from outside the body (extracorporeal shock wave lithotripsy ■).

Pseudogout

Pseudogout (calcium pyrophosphate dihydrate crystal deposition disease) is a disorder caused by deposits of calcium pyrophosphate crystals in the cartilage and then in the fluid of the joints, leading to intermittent attacks of painful joint inflammation.

Pseudogout usually occurs in older people and affects men and women equally.

Causes and Symptoms

The reason that calcium pyrophosphate crystals deposit in the joints of some people is unknown. It may occur in people who have other diseases, such as an abnormally high calcium level in the blood caused by a high level of parathyroid hormone (hyperparathyroidism), an abnormally high iron level in the tissues (hemochromatosis), or an abnormally low magnesium level in the blood (hypomagnesemia). However, most people with pseudogout have none of these conditions. The disorder can be hereditary.

Symptoms vary widely. Some people have attacks of painful joint inflammation, usually in the knees, wrists, or other relatively large joints. Other people have lingering, chronic pain and stiffness in joints of the arms and legs, which doctors may confuse with rheumatoid arthritis. Acute attacks are usually less severe than those of gout, but as in gout, attacks in pseudogout can cause fever. Some people have no pain between attacks, and some have no pain at any time, despite large deposits of crystals. Unlike in gout, people with pseudogout do not develop tophi.

▲ see page 930   ■ see art on page 865

Diagnosis

Doctors make the diagnosis by taking fluid from an inflamed joint through a needle (joint aspiration). Calcium pyrophosphate crystals (rather than urate crystals) are found in the joint fluid. They can be distinguished from urate crystals using a polar light microscope. Masses of calcium pyrophosphate crystals, unlike urate crystals, are radiopaque and can therefore be seen on x-ray.

Prognosis and Treatment

Often, the inflamed joints heal without any residual problems, but in many people, permanent joint damage can occur, with some joints so severely destroyed that they can be confused with Charcot's joints.▲

Usually, treatment can stop acute attacks and prevent new attacks but cannot prevent damage to the affected joints. Most often, nonsteroidal anti-inflammatory drugs (NSAIDs), including the COX-2 inhibitors (coxibs), are used to reduce the pain and inflammation.■ Occasionally, colchicine may be given intravenously to relieve the inflammation and pain during attacks and can be given by mouth in low doses daily to prevent attacks. Sometimes, excess joint fluid is drained and a corticosteroid suspension is injected into the joint to reduce the inflammation. No effective long-term treatment is available; however, physical therapy (such as muscle-strengthening and range-of-motion exercises) may be helpful.

CHAPTER 71

Hand Disorders

A number of different disorders may affect the hands, including ganglia, deformities, disorders related to nerves or blood vessels, injuries, and infections. Some other disorders that affect the hands are covered elsewhere in the book, including fractures, osteoarthritis, tendinitis and tenosynovitis, de Quervain's syndrome, Raynaud's phenomenon, finger clubbing, and certain birth defects.

Ganglia

Ganglia (ganglion cysts) are gelatinous swellings on the hands and wrists.

Ganglia typically occur in people between the ages of 20 and 50. Women are affected 3 times more often than are men. The most usual place for ganglia to develop is the back (dorsal aspect) of the wrist. Ganglia also develop on the front of the wrist (palmar aspect) and on the back of the finger, a few millimeters behind the cuticle (where they are also called mucous cysts).

Why ganglia develop on the wrist is not known, although they may be related to a previous injury. Ganglia on the back of the finger usually are related to arthritis of the last joint of the finger.

Ganglia are firm, round or elliptical sac-like swellings that rise from the skin surface; they contain a clear, gelatinous and usually sticky material. They are usually painless but occasionally cause discomfort. A doctor can readily make the diagnosis by examining the hand.

Some ganglia disappear on their own, so treatment may not be necessary. However, if they are unsightly, cause discomfort, or continue to increase in size, the gelatinous material inside them can (in 50% of people) be removed successfully by a doctor using a needle and a syringe. Sometimes a corticosteroid suspension is injected afterward to further ease any discomfort. The traditional method of removing a ganglion—placing the hand on a firm surface (such as a table) and hitting the ganglion with a large book—is not advisable; this method may cause injury and is unreliable. In about 50% of people, surgical removal may be necessary. After surgical removal, ganglia recur in about 5% of people.

Deformities

Hand deformities may be caused by an injury or may result from another disorder (for example, rheumatoid arthritis★). Deformities

---

▲ see box on page 585   ■ see pages 452 to 454
★ see page 370

should be treated promptly, if possible. Otherwise, they tend not to respond to simple treatments, such as splinting or exercises, and often require surgery.

MALLET FINGER

Mallet finger is a deformity in which the fingertip is curled in and cannot straighten itself.

This deformity usually results from injury, which either damages the tendon or tears the tendon from the bone. It can affect one or more fingers. A doctor can make the diagnosis by examining the finger. An x-ray is usually taken to be sure that there is no fracture. The usual treatment is placing a splint on the finger with the finger straightened. The tendon may take 6 to 8 weeks to heal. Mallet finger rarely requires surgery, unless a large fragment of bone has broken off or the joint is partially dislocated, even in the splint.

SWAN-NECK DEFORMITY

Swan-neck deformity is a bending in (flexion) of the base of the finger, a straightening out (extension) of the middle joint, and a bending in (flexion) of the outermost joint.

The most common cause is rheumatoid arthritis. Other causes include untreated mallet finger, looseness (laxity) of the fibrous plate inside the hand at the base of the fingers or of the finger ligaments, muscle spasm affecting the hands, and a misalignment in the healing of a fracture of the middle bone of the finger. Closing the finger may become impossible; the deformity can therefore result in considerable disability.

True swan-neck deformity does not affect the thumb, which has one less joint than the other fingers. However, in a variant of swan-neck deformity, called duck-bill deformity, the top joint of the thumb is severely over-

---

When the Fingers Are Abnormally Bent

Some disorders, such as rheumatoid arthritis, and injury can cause the fingers to bend abnormally. In mallet finger, the fingertip is curled in and cannot straighten. In swan-neck deformity, the joint at the base of the finger bends in (flexes), the middle joint straightens out (extends), and the outermost joint bends in. In Boutonnière deformity, the middle finger joint is bent inward (toward the palm) and the outermost finger joint is bent outward (away from the palm).

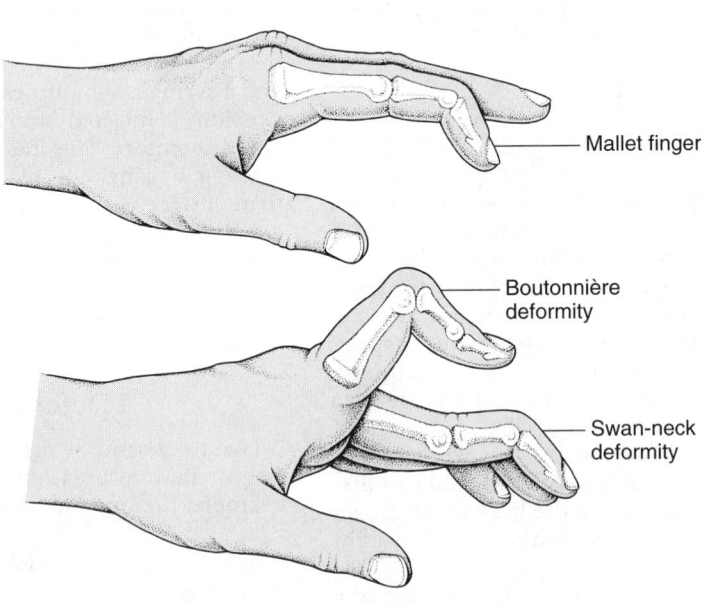

Mallet finger

Boutonnière deformity

Swan-neck deformity

straightened with a bending in of the joint at the base of the thumb to form a 90° angle. If duck-bill deformity and swan-neck deformity of one or more fingers occur together, the ability to pinch can be seriously reduced.

A doctor makes the diagnosis by examining the hand and finger. Treatment is aimed at correcting the underlying cause when possible. Mild deformities may be treated with finger splints (ring splints), which correct the deformity while still allowing a person to use the hand. Problems with the ability to pinch can be greatly improved by surgically realigning the joints or by fusing the thumb or finger joints together (called interphalangeal arthrodesis) into positions that allow for optimal function.

BOUTONNIÈRE DEFORMITY

Boutonnière deformity (buttonhole deformity) is a deformity in which the middle finger joint is bent in a fixed position inward (toward the palm) and the outermost finger joint is bent excessively outward (away from the palm).

This disorder most often results from rheumatoid arthritis▲ but can also occur from injury (deep cuts, joint dislocation, fractures) or osteoarthritis.■ People with rheumatoid arthritis can develop the disorder because they have long-standing inflammation of the middle joint of a finger. If the deformity is due to an injury, the injury usually occurs at the base of a tendon (called the middle phalanx extensor tendon). As a result, the middle joint (called the proximal interphalangeal joint) becomes "buttonholed" between the outer bands of the tendon that runs to the end of the finger. The deformity can, but need not, interfere with hand function. The doctor makes the diagnosis by examining the finger.

A boutonnière deformity caused by an extensor tendon injury can usually be corrected with a splint that keeps the middle joint fully extended for 6 weeks. When splinting is ineffective, or when buttonhole deformity is due to rheumatoid arthritis, surgery may be needed.

EROSIVE (INFLAMMATORY) OSTEOARTHRITIS

Erosive (inflammatory) osteoarthritis is a form of hereditary osteoarthritis that, in the hand, causes swelling, pain, and formation of cysts on the finger joints (particularly the outermost ones).

Osteoarthritis of the hand is apparent by enlargement of bones over the outermost joints of the fingers (Heberden's nodes) and overgrowth of bones over the middle joints of the fingers (Bouchard's nodules). With erosive osteoarthritis, there is also swelling of surrounding tissues. The joints between the fingers and hand and the wrists are usually not affected. The involved joints can become misaligned.

The deformity can be seen on x-rays. Unlike in rheumatoid arthritis, results of blood tests that indicate inflammation (such as the erythrocyte sedimentation rate [ESR] and the numbers of white blood cells) are usually normal, regardless of how severe the disorder is.

Treatment includes range-of-motion exercises in warm water to relieve pain during the exercises and to keep the joints as flexible as possible, splinting intermittently to prevent deformity, and use of analgesics or nonsteroidal anti-inflammatory drugs (NSAIDs) to relieve pain and swelling. Occasionally, a corticosteroid suspension may need to be injected into severely affected joints to relieve pain and increase range of motion. Rarely, when osteoarthritis is advanced and other treatments are not effective, the joint may need to be reconstructed or fused surgically.

DUPUYTREN'S CONTRACTURE

Dupuytren's contracture (palmar fibromatosis) is a progressive shrinking of the bands of fibrous tissue (called fascia) inside the palms, producing a curling in of the fingers that eventually can result in a clawlike hand.

Dupuytren's contracture is a common hereditary disorder that occurs particularly in men and especially after age 45. However, having the abnormal gene does not guarantee that someone will have the disorder. The prevalence of Dupuytren's contracture in the United States is about 5%; the prevalence worldwide ranges from 2 to 42%. The disorder affects both hands in 50% of people; when only one hand is affected, the right hand is involved twice as often as the left.

Dupuytren's contracture is more common in people with diabetes, alcoholism, or epilepsy. The disorder is occasionally associated with other disorders, including thickening of fibrous tissue above the knuckles (Garrod's pads), shrinking of fascia inside the penis that

---

▲ see page 370   ■ see page 367

What Is Trigger Finger?

In trigger finger (flexor digital tenosynovitis), a finger becomes locked in a bent position. The finger locks when one of the tendons that flex the finger becomes inflamed and swollen. Normally, the tendon moves smoothly in and out of its surrounding sheath as the finger straightens and bends. In trigger finger, the inflamed tendon can move out of the sheath as the finger bends. However, when the tendon is very swollen, it cannot easily move back in as the finger straightens, and therefore the finger locks.

Trigger finger can result from repetitive use of the hands (as may occur from using heavy gardening shears) or from inflammation (as occurs in rheumatoid arthritis). To straighten the finger, a person must force the swollen area into the sheath—producing a popping sensation similar to that felt when pulling a trigger. Sometimes a corticosteroid and a local anesthetic are injected into the tendon sheath. Surgery is commonly needed to treat chronic trigger finger.

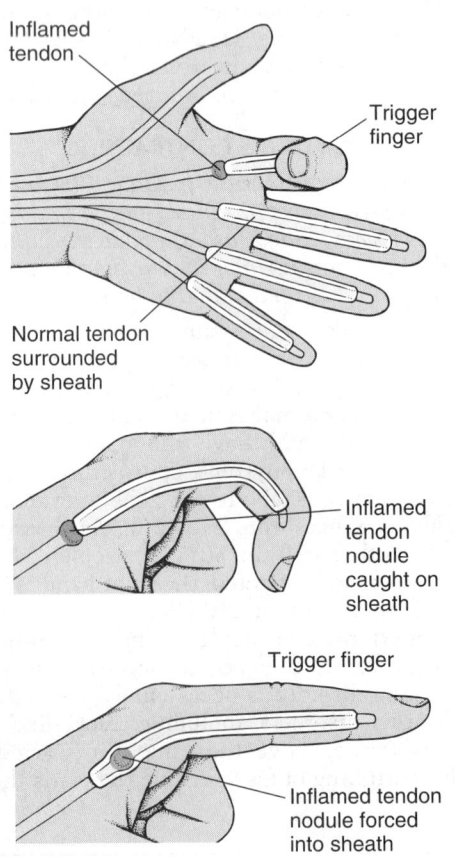

Inflamed tendon

Trigger finger

Normal tendon surrounded by sheath

Inflamed tendon nodule caught on sheath

Trigger finger

Inflamed tendon nodule forced into sheath

leads to deviated and painful erections (penile fibromatosis [Peyronie's disease]▲), and nodules on the soles of the feet (plantar fibromatosis). However, the precise mechanism that causes the fascia of the palm to thicken and curl in is unknown.

The first symptom is usually a tender nodule in the palm (most often at the third or fourth finger). The nodule may initially cause discomfort but gradually becomes painless. Gradually, the fingers begin to curl. Eventually, the curling worsens, and the hand can become arched (clawlike). The doctor makes the diagnosis by examining the hand.

An injection of a corticosteroid suspension into the nodule may help decrease the tenderness in the area but will not delay progression of the disorder. Surgery is usually needed when the hand cannot be placed flat on a table or when the fingers curl so much that hand function is limited. Surgery to remove the diseased fascia is difficult, because the fascia surrounds nerves, blood vessels, and tendons. Dupuytren's contracture may recur after surgery if removal of the fascia was incomplete. It may also recur spontaneously, especially in people in whom the disorder appeared at a young age, those with the disorder running in the family, and those with Garrod's pads, Peyronie's disease, or nodules on the soles of the feet.

Carpal Tunnel Syndrome

Carpal tunnel syndrome is a painful compression of the median nerve as it passes through the wrist.

Carpal tunnel syndrome results from compression of the median nerve, which is located at the palm side of the wrist (an area called the carpal tunnel). The median nerve serves the thumb side of the hand. The compression results when swelling or bands of fibrous tissue form for a variety of reasons on the palm side of the wrist.

Carpal tunnel syndrome is common—especially in women—and may affect one or both hands. Particularly at risk are people whose work requires repeated forceful movements with the wrist extended, such as using a screwdriver. Another cause is use of a computer keyboard that is not positioned properly. Prolonged exposure to vibrations (for example,

▲ see page 1326

by using certain tools) has also been claimed to cause carpal tunnel syndrome. Pregnant women and people who have diabetes, an underactive thyroid gland, gout, or rheumatoid arthritis are at increased risk of developing carpal tunnel syndrome.

The symptoms, due to the nerve compression, are odd sensations, numbness, tingling, and pain in the first three fingers on the thumb side of the hand. Occasionally, there is also pain and a burning or tingling sensation in the arm and shoulder. The pain may be more severe while the person is sleeping because of the way the hand is positioned. With time, the muscles in the hand on the thumb side can weaken and shrink through lack of use (atrophy).

Diagnosis is made largely by examining the affected hand and wrist. Before surgery, a doctor may first perform nerve conduction studies▲ to be certain that the problem is carpal tunnel syndrome.

The disorder is best treated by avoiding positions that overextend the wrist or put extra pressure on the median nerve. Wrist splints that hold the hand in a neutral position (especially at night) and such measures as adjusting the angle of a computer keyboard may help. Treating underlying disorders (such as rheumatoid arthritis or an underactive thyroid gland) can help to relieve symptoms.

Injections of a corticosteroid suspension into the carpal tunnel occasionally bring long-lasting relief. If pain is severe or if the muscle atrophies or weakens, surgery is the best way to relieve pressure on the median nerve. A surgeon can cut away the bands of fibrous tissue that place pressure on the nerve.

Cubital Tunnel Syndrome

Cubital tunnel syndrome (ulnar nerve palsy) is a disorder caused by compression of the ulnar nerve at the elbow.

The ulnar nerve passes close to the surface of the skin at the elbow ("funny bone") and is easily damaged by repeatedly leaning on the elbow, by bending the elbow for prolonged periods, or sometimes by abnormal bone growth in the area. Baseball pitchers are prone to cubital tunnel syndrome because of the extra twist of the arm required to throw a slider.

The symptoms include pain and numbness of the elbow and a pins-and-needles sensation of the ring and little fingers. Eventually, weak-

Proper Keyboard Position

Using a computer keyboard that is positioned improperly can result in carpal tunnel syndrome. To prevent injury, the user should keep the wrist in a neutral position. That is, the line from the hand to the forearm should be straight. The hand may be slightly lower than the forearm. But the hand should never be higher, and the wrist should not be cocked. The keyboard should be positioned relatively low, keeping the hand slightly lower than the elbow. A wrist pad can be used to support the wrist.

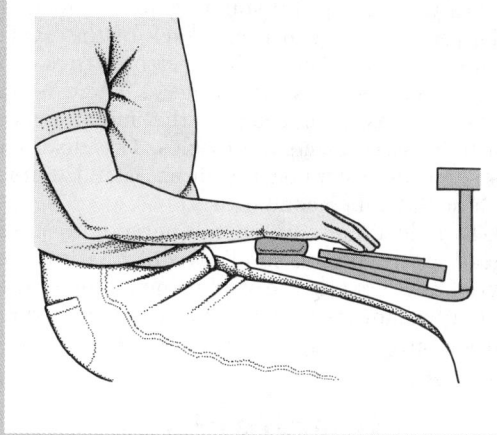

ness of the ring and little fingers may develop. Weakness may also interfere with the ability to pinch using the thumb and index finger, because most of the small muscles in the hand are controlled by the ulnar nerve. Severe, chronic cubital tunnel syndrome can lead to muscle wasting (atrophy) and a clawlike deformity of the hand.

Nerve conduction studies■ can help pinpoint the exact area of nerve damage. Mild cases of cubital tunnel syndrome are usually treated with physical therapy (including a splint at night to avoid overbending the elbow) and by avoiding pressure over the elbow; an elbow pad can be helpful. People who do not respond to splinting or who have more severe cases of nerve compression may benefit from surgery, which usually consists of releasing pressure on the nerve and moving the nerve

▲ see page 446   ■ see page 446

from the back to the front of the elbow. Surgery is successful in about 85% of people.

Radial Tunnel Syndrome

Radial tunnel syndrome is a disorder resulting from compression of a branch of the radial nerve in the forearm or back of the arm, or at the elbow.

Causes of compression of the radial nerve at the elbow include injury, ganglia, lipomas (noncancerous fatty tumors), bone tumors, and inflammation of the surrounding bursa or muscles.

Compression of the radial nerve results in cutting, piercing, or stabbing pain affecting the top of the forearm and back of the hand. Pain results when the person tries to straighten the wrist and fingers. There is no loss of sensation, because the radial nerve principally connects to muscles. This disorder is sometimes confused with backhand tennis elbow (lateral epicondylitis▲).

To reduce pressure on the nerve and speed healing, the person should avoid rotating the wrist and bending the arm at the elbow. If the wrist becomes weak and tends to droop (wrist-drop), surgery may be needed to relieve pressure on the nerve.

Kienböck's Disease

Kienböck's disease is the death of bone tissue due to an impaired blood supply (avascular necrosis■) affecting the lunate bone in the hand.

The cause of this relatively unusual disease is unknown. It occurs most commonly in the dominant hand of men aged 20 to 45 years of age.

Symptoms generally start with wrist pain that begins gradually, in the area of the lunate bone, which is in the middle of the wrist at the base. Eventually, swelling occurs on top of the wrist, which may become stiff. The person has no recollection of injury. The disorder occurs in both hands in 10% of cases and most often occurs in workers doing heavy manual labor. Diagnosis is possible at an early stage by magnetic resonance imaging (MRI) or computed tomography (CT) and is later confirmed by x-ray.

Surgery is performed to relieve pressure on the lunate bone. Alternative treatments attempt to reestablish the blood supply to the bone. If the lunate bone has collapsed, the wrist bones may be removed or surgically fused together as a last resort to relieve pain. Attempts to treat this disease with methods other than surgery have not been successful.

Shoulder-Hand Syndrome

Shoulder-hand syndrome is a type of reflex sympathetic dystrophy★ characterized by pain and limited motion of the shoulder and hand of the affected arm.

Causes include injury (such as falling on the hand, breaking the wrist bone [Colles' fracture]), heart attack, stroke, and possibly use of certain drugs (such as barbiturates). The precise way that shoulder-hand syndrome develops is not known, although some people seem more likely to develop the disorder than others.

Symptoms occur in three stages: stage 1 begins with sudden onset of widespread swelling (edema) and tenderness of the top of the hand and paleness of the hand due to narrowing (constriction) of the blood vessels in the hand. Pain in the shoulder and hand occurs, especially during movement. X-rays of the hands commonly show patchy areas of bone loss (osteoporosis●). Stage 2 is characterized by a reduction in the swelling and tenderness; hand pain is less severe. Stage 3 is characterized by the disappearance of swelling, tenderness, and pain, but hand motion is limited because the fingers may be stiff or clawlike, resembling Dupuytren's contractures. X-rays at this stage often show a widespread loss in the density of bones.

Causes should be treated or eliminated. Permanent curling in of the fingers can usually be prevented with hand exercises if the disorder is diagnosed and treated early enough. Repeated injections of a local anesthetic to block the sympathetic nerves are also usually needed. This approach usually relieves pain, permitting the person to resume normal activity, but repeated injections over weeks or months may be required. Alternatively, high doses of corticosteroids taken by mouth may help. This approach is only recommended by some doctors for short durations, because long-term use of corticosteroids can cause serious and potentially permanent problems.◆

▲ see page 427   ■ see page 362

★ see page 449   ● see page 343

◆ see box on page 374

Common Hand Injuries

Gamekeeper's thumb is a rupture of the ligament on the palm side of the thumb, which is responsible for pinching movements. It usually results from a fall that jams the thumb backward onto a hard surface. This injury is so named because it used to be an occupational hazard of gamekeepers in England, who broke the necks of rabbits with their hands. Treatment usually consists of a splint, but surgery is sometimes necessary.

Rupture of the scapholunate ligament may result from falling on an outstretched hand. Pain is felt mostly on top of the wrist. Treatment consists of surgical repair of the ligament and pinning of the bones.

Scaphoid fractures are a common type of wrist fracture. Tenderness is felt in the wrist below the thumb. Untreated scaphoid fractures often do not heal, eventually leading to arthritis of the wrist. Treatment consists of a cast or surgery. The bone may take 3 to 4 months to heal.

Dislocations may occur at the joint at the base of the thumb or other fingers or at the middle joints of the fingers. Dislocations usually result when the thumb is bent too far out or the fingers are bent too far back. Surgery is often required to correct dislocations at the base of the thumb or fingers. Dislocations of the middle joints may be treated by taping the dislocated finger to an adjacent finger. If the ligament is badly torn, a splint is used, usually for 3 weeks.

Fractures of the hook of hamate may result from striking the ground with a stick or making a divot playing golf. The lower part of the palm below the little finger is tender. The hand is put in a cast for 4 to 6 weeks, but the fracture may not fully heal. If unhealed fracture causes pain, weakness, or numbness of the little finger, surgery to remove the unattached part of the bone may be necessary.

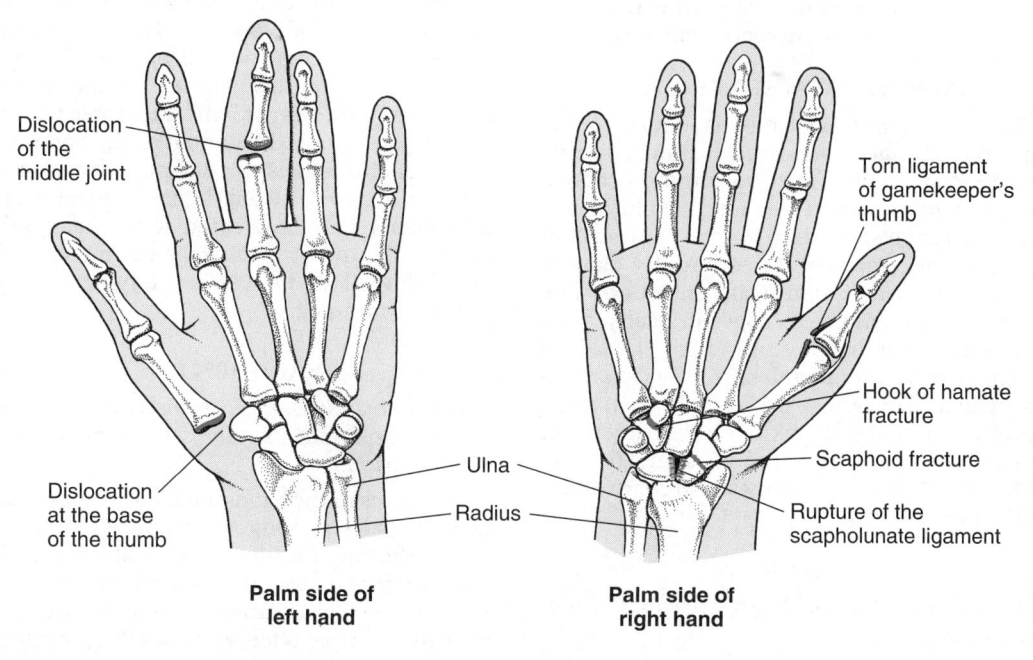

Dislocation of the middle joint

Torn ligament of gamekeeper's thumb

Hook of hamate fracture

Scaphoid fracture

Ulna

Radius

Dislocation at the base of the thumb

Rupture of the scapholunate ligament

Palm side of left hand

Palm side of right hand

Injuries

Hand injuries cause swelling, pain, stiffness, and sometimes limited movement. The most common injuries are tears (ruptures) of ligaments or fractures of bone. When a ligament is ruptured, bones can move out of position, resulting in a dislocated joint.

Sometimes doctors can diagnose a hand injury by examining the hand. A local anesthetic may be given before the examination, which otherwise might be too painful. However, x-rays may be needed to determine whether the joint is unstable and to detect fractures. Occasionally, computed tomography (CT) or magnetic resonance imaging (MRI) is needed. Often, an untreated injury can result in a permanent deformity of the hand. Therefore, an injured hand should be immobilized so that it can heal normally. A bandage, splint, or cast may be used, depending on the injury. Surgery is sometimes necessary if bones are out of position or a joint is unstable. Hand exercises are begun as soon as possible to prevent loss of function.

Infections

Human and animal bites can cause an infection of the hands; some other infections are felon, paronychia, and herpetic whitlow.

INFECTIONS CAUSED BY BITES

The most common cause is injury to the knuckles by the teeth from a punch to the mouth. Animal bites are also common causes. Wound contamination by a number of types of bacteria can result from human and animal bites. All bite injuries are potentially dangerous and can cause significant infection. The injured area should be cleaned surgically, with the wound left open. Antibiotics should be given to prevent joint infection (septic arthritis), which can otherwise lead to permanent destruction of the knuckle joints. Bacteria in human and animal bites are resistant to many antibiotics but are generally sensitive to ampicillin and penicillin.

FELON

A felon is infection of the soft tissue (pulp) at the fingertip.

An infection of the fingertip can lead to an abscess, which creates pressure and death of nearby tissues. The fingertip becomes very swollen and firm with intense throbbing pain. The doctor makes the diagnosis by examining the affected finger. If a felon is not treated promptly, the underlying bone, joint, or tendons may become infected. Minor felons may be treated with warm soaks several times a day to increase blood flow. An antibiotic is usually needed. Treatment may require prompt surgical drainage of the abscess as well.

HERPETIC WHITLOW

Herpetic whitlow is a viral infection of the fingertip.

Herpes simplex virus may cause an intense, painful skin infection. The fingertip is sore and swollen but is not as firm as in a felon. The appearance of tiny fluid-filled blebs (vesicles) on the fingers is diagnostic. A herpetic whitlow is often mistaken for a felon. The disorder eventually goes away on its own. Surgery is not needed.

PARONYCHIA

Paronychia is infection of the cuticle.

This very common hand infection can be caused by an injury to the nail and cuticle, nail biting, or aggressive manipulation of the cuticle during a manicure. Paronychia can be caused by many different bacteria, including *Pseudomonas* and *Proteus.* The cuticle and tissue at the margin of the nail become red, swollen, and intensely painful. If left untreated, an abscess will develop and can spread to the fingertip (leading to a felon) or to the bone.

The doctor makes the diagnosis by examining the affected finger. In its earliest stage, paronychia may be treated with oral antibiotics and frequent warm soaks to increase the blood flow. If an abscess develops, it must be surgically drained.

HAND ABSCESS

A hand abscess is an accumulation of pus affecting the hand, usually caused by a bacterial infection.

Abscesses in the hands are fairly common and usually result from injury. An abscess in the soft pad at the tip of a finger nearly always results from a minor injury, such as a splinter or needle prick. Severe pain, warmth, and redness develop over the abscess, often with swelling of nearby lymph nodes in the arm. Infection of the bone underneath the abscess may cause more pain.

Abscesses may occur around the tendons that run along the inside of the fingers. This type of abscess is caused by an injury that penetrates one of the creases on the palm side of a finger. Infection and pus form around the tendon and rapidly destroy tissue. The gliding mechanism of the tendon becomes damaged, so the finger can barely move. Symptoms include swelling and inflammation of the finger, tenderness over the tendon sheath, and extreme pain when trying to move the finger. Swollen lymph nodes near the abscess are common. Fever is also common.

An abscess may occur in any part of the palm and spread between the metacarpal bones (the hand bones between the wrist and fingers). Such an infection may occur after the skin is ripped or the hand is punctured by something sharp. Palm abscesses (also called collar-button abscesses) may develop from an infected callus. Palm abscesses begin as in-

tense throbbing pain with swelling and severe tenderness to touch.

Treatment involves surgically draining the pus. Laboratory cultures of the pus are carried out to determine which antibiotic is best for treatment (usually a cephalosporin).

INFECTION OF THE TENDON SHEATH

An infection of the flexor tendon sheath is characterized by pain and swelling, with tenderness along the length of the tendon sheath and pain when straightening the finger. Pus may spread inside the hand to form a horseshoe-shaped abscess. Surgical drainage of the abscess is required. Antibiotic therapy is also required (the choice depending on the results of laboratory cultures of the pus).

CHAPTER 72

Foot Problems

Some foot problems start in the foot itself, for example, from a foot injury; others result from diseases that affect many parts of the body, such as diabetes. Problems can occur in any bone, joint, muscle, tendon, or ligament of the foot. Foot fractures are fairly common.▲ Nail discoloration of the foot should always be looked into because it may be caused by certain disorders, including a fungal infection.

With age, many changes occur in the feet. For instance, there is typically less hair; brown coloration (pigmentation) may occur in spots or patches; and the skin may become dry. The toenails often become thicker and curved, and fungal infections of the nails occur commonly. The feet may actually enlarge in length and width because of changes in the ligaments and joints. A person with these types of changes may need to wear larger shoes. Elderly feet have often been damaged by a lifetime of ill-fitting shoes.

Foot Pain

Although any foot problem can cause pain, this chapter focuses on the most common locations for pain—the ball of the foot (the underside of the front end of the metatarsal

bones—the metatarsal heads), the toe joint, and at a heel spur.

PAIN IN THE BALL OF THE FOOT

Pain in the ball of the foot may have many different causes (including arthritis, poor circulation, pinching of the nerves between the toes, abnormal metatarsal length and posture problems, and various diseases). However, most often the pain is caused by nerve damage or by an age-related change that affects the foot, called metatarsalgia.

Pain Caused by Damage to the Nerves in the Foot: The nerves that supply the bottom of the foot and toes travel between the bones of the toes. Pain in the ball of the foot may be caused by noncancerous (benign) growths of tissue (neuromas) wrapped around nerves, usually between the base of the third and fourth toes (Morton's neuroma), although these growths may occur between any of the toes. Neuromas usually develop in only one foot and are more common in women than in men.

▲ see page 353

In the early stages, a neuroma may cause only a mild ache around the third or fourth toe, occasionally accompanied by a burning or tingling sensation in the toes. These symptoms are generally more pronounced when a person wears certain types of shoes, especially those that are too narrow for the front part of the foot, including those that are pointed. As the condition progresses, a constant burning sensation may radiate to the tips of the toes, regardless of what shoes are worn. A person may also feel as if a marble or pebble were inside the ball of the foot.

Doctors diagnose the condition by considering the history of the problem and examining the foot. X-rays, magnetic resonance imaging (MRI), and ultrasound cannot accurately identify this disorder.

Injecting the tender spot in the foot with corticosteroids mixed with a local anesthetic and wearing orthotics may relieve the symptoms. Repeating the injections two or three times at intervals of 1 or 2 weeks may be necessary. If these treatments do not help, surgical removal of the neuroma often relieves the discomfort completely but may cause permanent numbness in the area.

Pain Caused by Metatarsalgia: With age, there is a loss of the protective pad of fat that cushions the metatarsal heads. Pain at this location is called metatarsalgia. If untreated, the condition can cause inflammation to develop in the bursas that are situated below each metatarsal head (metatarsal bursitis). Rheumatoid arthritis can also cause pain and swelling at this location.

Treatment is by means of special shoes, cushioning, or orthotic devices that shift weight from the ball of the foot to more evenly distribute weight across the entire foot.

TOE JOINT PAIN

Pain involving the joints of the four smaller toes is a very common problem, usually caused by misalignment of the joints. This misalignment may result from high or low arched feet that cause the toes to stay in a bent position (hammer toes). Constant friction against the bent toes causes the skin over the joint to thicken, resulting in a corn. Treatment is directed at relieving the pressure caused by toe misalignment: Making the shoes deeper, applying protective sleeves or shields on the toes, placing pads in the shoes, surgically straightening the toes, and paring down the corn may help.

Chronic arthritis (osteoarthritis▲) at the base of the big toe (also called hallux rigidus) is extremely common. Certain factors, such as flat feet, a long big toe and a foot that rolls inward, are thought to predispose a person to hallux rigidus. When a person stands and walks with a foot position that lowers the arch, it may cause the foot to roll inward. This abnormal foot alignment is called pronation and is often responsible for the increased stress at the big toe joint that produces pain and osteoarthritis with limited motion in that joint. Occasionally, an injury to the big toe may also cause painful arthritis. Joint pain in the big toe is usually aggravated by wearing poor-fitting shoes or shoes that are too flexible, causing increased motion with pain at the big toe joint. Shoes with increased support and rigid soles may help. Later, a person may become unable to bend the big toe during walking. The area is not warm to the touch. This osteoarthritis is different from that occurring in gout, which can develop as severe pain at the same location, but the area is warm to the touch.■

Fitting the shoe with orthotic devices to correct improper foot motion and relieve pressure on the affected joints is the mainstay of treatment. Pain in the big toe that started recently may be relieved by toe traction and exercises that move and extend the joint. Injections of a local anesthetic can relieve pain and decrease muscle spasm so that the joint can move more easily, and a corticosteroid may also be injected to decrease inflammation. If these treatments are not successful, surgery to improve joint alignment and function may relieve the pain.

HEEL SPUR PAIN

Heel spurs are growths of extra bones at the heel. They can result from excessive pulling on the heel bone by tendons or the connective tissue attached to the bone (fascia).

Heel spurs are common but typically do not cause pain. They cause pain when inflammation develops in adjacent tissues. Heel spur pain is also called plantar heel pain syndrome. The first symptoms of heel spurs are typically noticed when the person arises and puts the foot down first thing in the morning. They may also occur with the first few steps after sitting for a long time.

▲ see page 367   ■ see page 391

Usually, heel spur pain can be diagnosed during a physical examination. Pressing on the bottom of the heel where the arch begins usually causes pain. Pain with pressure to the center of the heel indicates that an inflamed bursa may also be present. X-rays may be taken to confirm the diagnosis, but results may be normal at first.

Treatment is aimed at relieving pain. Wrapping the foot and arch with padding and tape or using orthotics, which help to stabilize the heel, can minimize stretching of the fascia and reduce pain. Heel cushion pads and supportive shoes with soft soles may also help. Calf stretching exercises and ice massage are also effective. Ice massage consists of massaging an area of skin, using ice. One way to do this is to freeze water in a paper cup, then turn the cup upside down and rub the ice against the skin. As the ice melts, the paper is progressively peeled away. A mixture of corticosteroids and a local anesthetic can be injected into the painful area of the heel. Most painful heels spurs resolve without surgery.

Surgery to remove the spur or the dense band of tissue that extends from the spur at the bottom of the heel bone to the base of the toes (plantar fascia) should be performed only when constant pain is not relieved by other treatment measures. Surgery should be considered only as a last resort because the results are not predictable. Occasionally, pain persists after surgery.

Ankle Sprain

An ankle sprain is an injury to the ligaments (the tough elastic tissue that connects bones to one another) in the ankle.

Any of the ligaments in the ankle can be injured. Sprains usually occur when the ankle rolls outward, causing the sole of the foot to face the other foot (invert). This kind of injury usually occurs when a person steps on uneven ground, especially when stepping on a rock or off the edge of a curb. Loose ligaments in the ankle, weak or nerve-damaged leg muscles, certain types of shoes such as spiked heels, and certain walking patterns (such as an in-toed pattern) tend to cause the ankle to roll outward, increasing the risk of a sprain. People with specific foot types, such as a high arch, may also be more prone to ankle sprains.

Symptoms

The severity of the sprain depends on the degree of stretching or tearing of the liga-

What Is a Heel Spur?

A heel spur is a growth of extra bone on the heel bone (calcaneus). It may form when the plantar fascia, the connective tissue extending from the bottom of the heel bone to the base of the toes, pulls excessively on the heel. Usually the spur is painful as it develops, but it may become less painful as the foot adjusts to it. Most spurs can be treated without surgery.

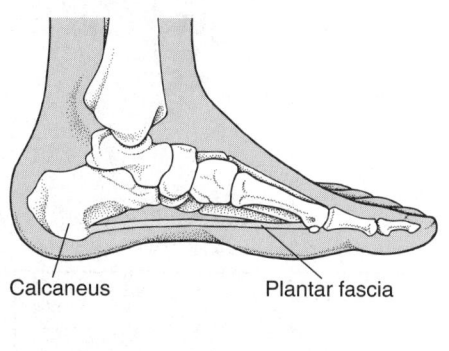

Calcaneus   Plantar fascia

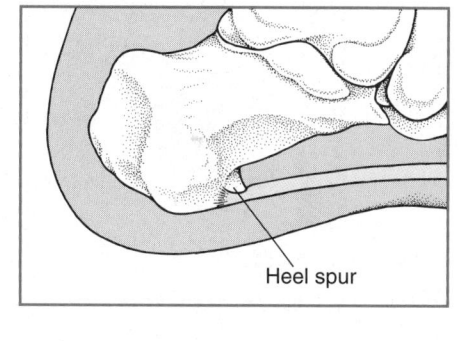

Heel spur

ments. In a mild sprain, the ligaments may stretch, but they do not actually tear. The ankle usually does not hurt or swell very much, but a mild sprain increases the risk of a repeat injury. In a moderate sprain, a ligament tears partially. Obvious swelling and bruising are common, and walking is usually painful and difficult. In a severe sprain, a ligament tears completely, causing swelling and sometimes bleeding under the skin. As a result, the ankle is unstable and unable to bear weight.

Diagnosis and Treatment

Physical examination of the ankle can give clues as to the extent of ligament damage. X-

Spraining an Ankle

An ankle sprain may occur when the ankle rolls outward (inverts), tearing the ligament along the outside of the ankle.

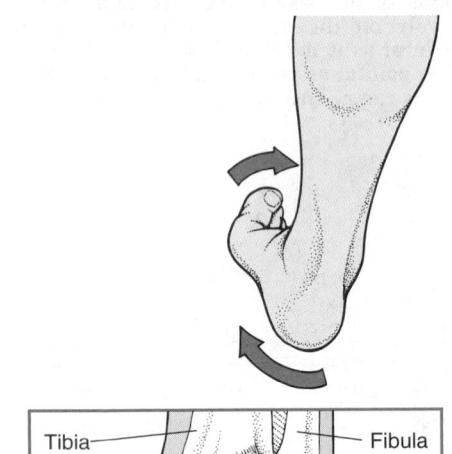

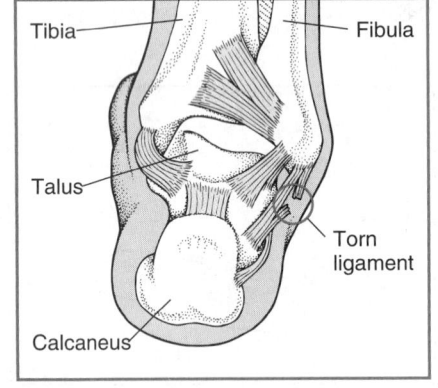

Tibia — Fibula

Talus

Torn ligament

Calcaneus

---

compression, elevation (RICE). For moderate sprains, a walking cast or a removable cast boot can be applied and left in place for up to 3 weeks. It immobilizes the lower leg but allows a person to walk on the injured ankle.

A severe ankle sprain requires immediate medical attention; if left untreated, it may result in long-term instability of the ankle, pain, and osteoarthritis of the ankle. Surgery may be needed. However, physical therapy is usually tried first. Whether to perform surgery is controversial; some surgeons believe that surgically reconstructing badly damaged and torn ligaments is no better than treatment without surgery. Physical therapy to restore movement, strengthen muscles, and improve balance and response time is very important before a person resumes strenuous activity.

For people who sprain their ankles easily, subsequent injuries may be prevented by wearing soft or rigid ankle supports (depending on the type and degree of injury). High-top shoes and the use of padding or inserts (orthotics) in the shoe can help to stabilize the foot and ankle.

Complications

Sometimes a moderate or severe sprain causes problems even after the ligament has healed. A small nodule (meniscoid body) can develop in one of the ankle's ligaments and cause constant friction in the joint, leading to chronic inflammation and eventually permanent damage. Relief from the pain and inflammation is usually possible by having the doctor inject the ankle with a mixture of corticosteroids (usually two different formulations to provide short- and longer-lasting effects) along with a local anesthetic (such as lidocaine). Surgery is rarely needed.

A nerve that travels over one of the ankle's ligaments may also be damaged in a sprain. The resulting pain (neuralgia) and tingling are often relieved, sometimes permanently, by an injection of a mixture of a local anesthetic and a corticosteroid.

People who have a sprained ankle may walk in a way that overuses the tendons on the outside of the ankle, resulting in inflammation. This condition, called peroneal tenosynovitis, can cause chronic swelling and tenderness of the outer ankle. Treatment consists of wearing ankle supports that limit movement of the ankle joint. Cortisone injections into the sheath of the tendon may also be effective but must not be overused.

---

rays are often taken to determine whether a bone is broken, but they cannot assess the ligaments. Stress x-rays (taken with the ankle in different positions) may indicate the extent of ligament damage, as can magnetic resonance imaging (MRI). Arthroscopy, in which a fiberoptic scope is used to view inside the joint, is used only if surgery to repair a torn ligament is being considered.

Treatment depends on how severe the sprain is. Usually, mild sprains are treated by wrapping the ankle and foot with an elastic bandage or tape, applying ice packs to the area, elevating the ankle, and, as the sprain heals, gradually increasing the amount of walking and exercise. Treatment consists of rest, ice,

Occasionally, the shock of a severe sprain causes blood vessels in the ankle to go into prolonged spasm, thereby reducing blood flow. As a result, areas of bone and other tissues may be damaged because they are deprived of blood and may begin to waste away. This condition, called reflex sympathetic dystrophy▲ or Sudeck's atrophy, is a rare complication of an ankle sprain. It can cause the foot to swell painfully. Pain, often severe, can move from one location to another in the ankle and foot. Despite the pain, a person usually should continue to walk. Physical therapy and analgesics taken by mouth may help. A local anesthetic injected into or around the nerve (a nerve block) supplying the ankle, corticosteroids, and psychologic counseling can help people cope with the chronic, intense pain.

Sinus tarsi syndrome is persistent pain in the area between the heel bone (calcaneus) and the ankle bone (talus) after a sprain. It may be related to partial tearing of ligaments deep in the foot. Injections of corticosteroids and local anesthetics often help.

Tarsal Tunnel Syndrome

Tarsal tunnel syndrome (posterior tibial neuralgia) is pain in the ankle, foot, and toes caused by compression of or damage to the nerve supplying the heel and sole (posterior tibial nerve).

The posterior tibial nerve runs along the back of the calf, through a fibrous canal near the heel, and into the sole of the foot. When tissues around this nerve become inflamed, they can press on the nerve, causing pain.

Pain, the most common symptom of tarsal tunnel syndrome, usually has a burning or tingling quality. It may occur when a person stands, walks, or wears a particular type of shoe. Pain located around the ankle and extending to the toes usually worsens during walking and is relieved by rest. Occasionally, pain also occurs during rest.

To diagnose this condition, a doctor manipulates the affected foot during a physical examination. For example, tapping the injured or compressed area often causes tingling, which may extend to the heel, arch, or toes. Extensive tests may be needed to determine the cause of the injury, especially if foot surgery is being considered.

Injections of a mixture of corticosteroids and local anesthetics into the area may relieve pain. Other treatments include wrapping the foot and placing specially constructed orthotic devices in the shoe to reduce pressure on the nerve. When other treatments do not relieve the pain, surgery to relieve pressure on the nerve may be necessary.

Plantar Fasciitis

Plantar fasciitis is inflammation of the dense band of tissue called the plantar fascia that extends from the bottom of the heel bone to the base of the toes (ball of the foot).

The plantar fascia connects the bottom of the heel bones to the ball of the foot and is involved in walking and running, giving spring to the step. Although the term fasciitis means "inflammation" of the fascia, the disorder is primarily one of repeated stress to the fascia rather than one of inflammation. Often a small tear results from excessive strain placed on the plantar fascia. Plantar fasciitis is one of the most common causes of heel pain. Pain may occur anywhere along the course of the plantar fascia but most commonly is located where the fascia joins the bottom of the heel bone. Many people who develop the disorder have very high or very low arches in their feet. Tight calf muscles or a tight Achilles tendon (which attaches the calf muscles to the heel bone) may cause the foot to flatten, which can lead to a painful "bowstringing" of the fascia.

The disorder is common in runners and in dancers and may occur in people whose occupations involve standing for prolonged periods. A change in shoe style can also lead to plantar fasciitis. Disorders that may cause or aggravate plantar fasciitis are obesity, rheumatoid arthritis, Reiter's syndrome (reactive arthritis), psoriasis, and fibromyalgia.

Symptoms and Diagnosis

A person with plantar fasciitis often feels a great deal of pain after resting, particularly when placing weight on the foot first thing in the morning. The pain temporarily diminishes after the person first walks. It may also begin when the person walks or runs; in this case, the pain radiates from the bottom of the heel toward the toes.

The doctor may make the diagnosis after examining the foot. Tenderness is evident where the plantar fascia enters the heel bone or at the bottom of the ball of the foot.

▲ see page 449

Bursitis in the Heel

Normally, only one bursa is found in the heel, between the Achilles tendon and the heel bone (calcaneus). This bursa may become inflamed, swollen, and painful, resulting in anterior Achilles tendon bursitis.

Abnormal pressure and foot dysfunction can cause a protective bursa to form between the Achilles tendon and the skin. This bursa may also become inflamed, swollen, and painful, resulting in posterior Achilles tendon bursitis.

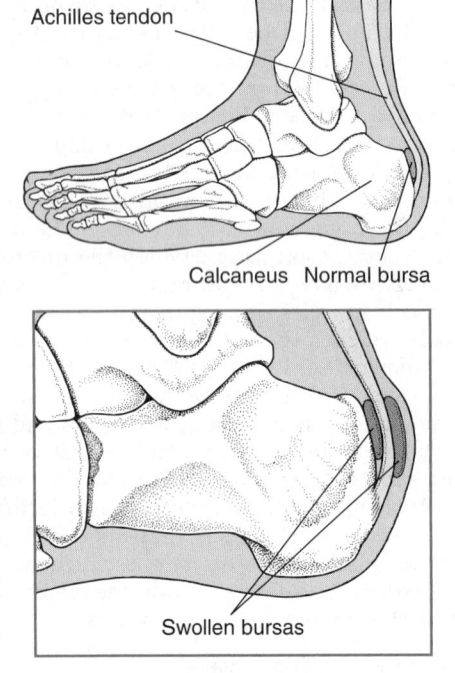

Achilles tendon

Calcaneus   Normal bursa

Swollen bursas

X-rays may reveal the presence of a heel spur protruding from the bottom front edge of the heel bone. This heel spur is a growth of extra bone produced over time because of a combination of the increased strain on the fascia and foot dysfunction. Other diagnostic tests, such as a bone scan, magnetic resonance imaging (MRI), and ultrasound, are rarely needed.

Treatment

To alleviate the stress and pain on the fascia, the person can take shorter steps and avoid walking barefoot. Activities that involve leg impact, such as jogging, should be avoided. The person may need to lose weight. Stretching the calf muscles often accelerates healing. Orthotics placed into well-fitting supportive shoes can help to cushion, elevate, and support the heel.

Other measures that may be needed include use of adhesive strapping or arch-supporting wraps, ice massage, use of nonsteroidal anti-inflammatory drugs (NSAIDs), corticosteroid injections into the heel, physical therapy, use of orthotics, and splinting at night to stretch the calf muscles and fascia during sleep. If these measures do not help sufficiently, surgery is occasionally required to attempt to partially release pressure on the fascia and remove any heel spurs.

Achilles Tendon Bursitis

Achilles tendon bursitis is inflammation of the fluid-filled sac (bursa) located either between the skin of the heel and the Achilles tendon (posterior Achilles tendon bursitis) or in front of the attachment of the Achilles tendon to the heel bone (anterior Achilles tendon bursitis, retrocalcaneal bursitis).

The Achilles tendon is the tendon that attaches the calf muscles to the heel bone. Posterior Achilles tendon bursitis is often associated with formation of a spur called Haglund's deformity or "pump bump" on the heel bone. Anterior Achilles tendon bursitis is also called Albert's disease.

Posterior Achilles tendon bursitis occurs mainly in young women but can develop in men. Walking in a way that repeatedly presses the soft tissue behind the heel against the stiff back support of a shoe can cause or aggravate the bursitis. Shoes that taper sharply inward toward the posterior heel (such as high-heeled shoes) can lead to the development of this bursitis.

Any condition that puts extra strain on the Achilles tendon can cause anterior Achilles tendon bursitis. Injuries to the heel and diseases such as rheumatoid arthritis can also cause it.

Symptoms

When the bursa becomes inflamed after an injury, symptoms usually develop suddenly; when it develops without an injury, symptoms may develop gradually. With both posterior and anterior Achilles tendon bursitis, symptoms usually include swelling and warmth at the back of the heel. A mildly red, swollen, tender spot develops on the back of the heel. When the inflamed bursa enlarges, it appears as a red lump under the skin of the heel and causes pain at and above the heel. If the condition becomes chronic, the swelling may harden.

Diagnosis and Treatment

Diagnosis is suspected on the basis of the symptoms and the clinical examination. For anterior and posterior Achilles tendon bursitis, x-rays are needed to rule out a fracture of the heel bone or damage to the heel bone due to rheumatoid arthritis or another inflammatory arthritis.

With posterior Achilles tendon bursitis, treatment is aimed at reducing the inflammation and adjusting the foot's position in the shoe to relieve pressure on the heel. Foam rubber or felt heel pads can be placed in the shoe to eliminate pressure by elevating the heel. Stretching the back part of the shoe or placing padding around the inflamed bursa may help. Sometimes a special shoe, such as a running shoe designed to stabilize the midsole heel, can help to control abnormal heel motion. Other shoes have padding that reduces irritation to the posterior heel and Achilles tendon.

With anterior and posterior Achilles tendon bursitis, applying warm or cool compresses to the area and using nonsteroidal anti-inflammatory drugs (NSAIDs) can temporarily relieve the pain and inflammation, as can injections of a mixture of corticosteroids and local anesthetics into the inflamed bursa; the doctor is careful not to inject the mixture into the tendon. After this treatment, the person must rest. When these treatments are not effective, part of the heel bone may need to be surgically removed.

Ingrown Toenail

An ingrown toenail is a condition in which the edges of the nail grow into the surrounding skin.

An ingrown nail can result when a deformed toenail grows improperly into the skin or when the skin around the nail grows abnormally fast and engulfs part of the nail. Wearing narrow, ill-fitting shoes and trimming the nail into a curve with short edges rather than trimming it straight across can cause or worsen ingrown toenails.

Ingrown nails may produce no symptoms at first but eventually may become painful, especially when pressure is applied to the ingrown area. The area is usually red and may be warm; if not treated, it is prone to infection. If infected, the area becomes painful, red, and swollen, and pus-filled blisters (paronychia) may develop and drain.

Mildly ingrown toenails can be trimmed away, the free edge gently lifted, and sterile cotton placed under the nail until the swelling goes away. If an ingrown nail requires medical attention, a doctor usually numbs the area with a local anesthetic (eg, lidocaine), then cuts away and removes the ingrown section of nail. The inflammation can then subside, and the ingrown nail usually does not recur.

Onychomycosis

Onychomycosis is a fungal infection of the nails.

The fungus can be acquired by walking barefoot in public places or, most commonly, as part of an infection called athlete's foot.▲ Older people, people who have diabetes, and people with poor circulation to the feet are particularly prone to this type of fungal infection.

Mild infections may produce few or no symptoms; in more severe infections, the nails turn white to yellow-brown in color, thicken, and detach from the nail bed. Usually, debris from the infected nail collects under its free edge. A doctor may confirm the diagnosis by examining a sample of the nail debris under a microscope and culturing it to determine which fungus is causing the infection.

Fungal infections are difficult to cure, so treatment depends on how severe or bothersome the symptoms are. The nails should be kept trimmed very short to minimize discomfort. For mild to moderate infections of the nails, ciclopirox, an antifungal drug that is placed in a nail lacquer, may be effective. The person applies the lacquer directly to the nail; the drug penetrates the nail plate to reach the infected nail bed below. Because ciclopirox has minimal to no side effects, it may even be preferred to antifungal drugs that are given by mouth.

Other antifungal drugs, such as griseofulvin or terbinafine, are taken by mouth and may

▲ see page 1225

improve the condition; occasionally, these drugs completely cure it. Terbinafine acts more quickly than griseofulvin, is more effective, and causes fewer side effects. Alternative antifungal drugs include triaconazole and fluconazole.

Onychia

Onychia is inflammation and infection of the nail and nail bed (matrix).

The most usual cause is injury—either direct injury or pressure from ill-fitting shoes. Skin diseases, such as psoriasis or eczema, may also cause it. Diabetes is a common contributing cause, because of poor blood circulation in the foot and reduced resistance to infection. Insufficient intake of nutrients in the diet (nutritional deficiency) may also be responsible.

The affected toe becomes inflamed, swollen, and painful. Infected material (pus) may drain from the toe into surrounding tissue areas, spreading the infection.

Treatment consists of removing the affected portion of the nail. Often when the nail is removed, the pus drains out. If it does not drain out on its own, a small incision with a scalpel blade helps to drain the pus. The nail is usually partially removed to further help healing. Antibiotics can be taken by mouth or an antibiotic ointment is applied to help cure the infection and astringent soaks, such as with Epsom salts, help to drain the pus and heal the nail. In cases that are not cured with treatment, permanent removal of a portion of or all of the nail growth (surgical matrixectomy) may be necessary.

Corns and Calluses

Corns are hard cone-shaped bumps commonly found on the upper surface of the smaller toes, particularly over a joint. Calluses are somewhat rounded flat thickenings of the skin located on the under-surface of the foot.

Corns and calluses are usually caused by friction and pressure, particularly from tight or ill-fitting shoes. Hammer toe and other toe deformities are often responsible for the development of corns. Calluses often develop under the ball of the foot because of faulty foot positioning and poor weight distribution. Symptoms include a generalized burning sensation or (at times) severe pain in a specific area. If

not properly treated, underlying tissues can become inflamed and infected.

Treatment usually requires removal through scraping with a scalpel. After this procedure, padding of various sorts (for example, felt or moleskin) may be applied, to remove pressure from the healing area. Orthotics or other inserts that have padding can help.

If the blood supply to the affected area is poor, debridement may not be possible. In this case, special shoes that reduce pressure over the affected area may be necessary.

Onychauxis and Onychogryphosis

Onychauxis is a thickening (hypertrophy) of the base of the nail (nail bed). Onychogryphosis is long-standing thickening, in which typically a curved hooked nail (ram's horn nail) occurs.

The thickening of a nail, which is common in older people, may be caused by several factors, including injury (such as that caused by ill-fitting shoes), infection, poor blood supply, diabetes, or inadequate intake of nutrients.

Pressure on an affected nail (even from bedsheets) may produce severe pain. Onychogryphosis may occur at the same time, almost always resulting from damage to the nail bed. In onychogryphosis, the curved hooked nail may injure an adjoining toe.

The nails should be kept trimmed, and injury to nearby toes can be prevented by placing lambswool between the toes. Footwear or stockings that gather at the toes should be avoided.

Hallux Valgus and Bunion

Hallux valgus is an abnormally positioned big toe, in which the joint at the base of the toe bulges outward from the inner side of the foot and the big toe points inward (toward the smaller toes). A bunion is a painful swelling of the fluid-filled sac (bursa) at the base of the big toe that occurs because of the hallux valgus.

The cause of hallux valgus is usually ill-fitting footwear, but vulnerability to this disorder seems to run in families. Because women's fashions often dictate shoes that fit poorly, women are more prone to developing these deformities.

The hallux valgus actually creates a widening of the foot because the base of the big toe bulges outward from the foot. Deviation of the big toe also occurs, so that the big toe points toward the smaller toes. The result is a bump

Hallux Valgus With a Bunion

A **hallux valgus** is a bulging out of the base of the big toe sideways, away from the foot. The end of the big toe tilts in toward the second toe. A **bunion** is a painful swelling of the fluid-filled sac (bursa) at the base of the big toe. A bunion is caused by hallux valgus.

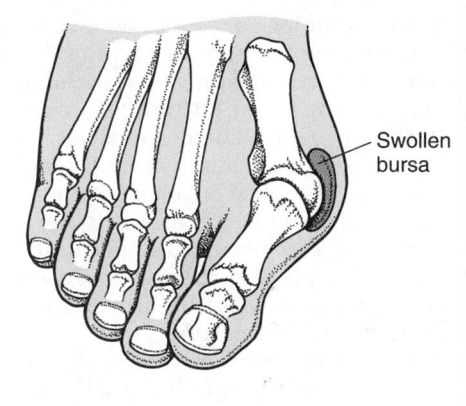

Swollen bursa

on the inside edge of the foot, where the metatarsal head meets the base of the big toe. Under this bump is a bursa (a fluid-filled sac). The bursa becomes irritated by friction with the shoe, resulting in swelling of the bursa underneath the bump, thus increasing the size of the bump—this is called a bunion. Continued irritation of the bunion by friction with the shoe leads to increased bone growth and further swelling of the bursa, enlarging the bunion and further widening the foot.

A doctor can usually make the diagnosis of hallux valgus and bunion by directly examining the foot. X-rays may help to determine the degree of the hallux valgus.

Pain can be treated by injecting a corticosteroid mixed with a local anesthetic into the bunion. Bunion shield pads or modified shoes may also help relieve painful pressure over the bunion. Severely painful bunions or a severe degree of hallux valgus may require surgical correction of the toe's position.

Hammer Toe

A toe that is in a fixed (rigid) contracted position.

The most usual cause of a hammer toe is years of wearing ill-fitting shoes. Because part of the toe is higher than normal, excessive friction may result, sometimes leading to ulcers on the top of the toe. Treatment is first attempted by ensuring that shoes are comfortable and do not further irritate the toe. Any ulcer or other skin irritation is treated. Surgery to straighten the hammer toe may be needed when the toe has become fixed. Rarely, surgery is necessary to straighten the toe.

Sesamoiditis

Inflammation or irritation of the tendon and surrounding structures around a small bone (the sesamoid) below the metatarsal head where it adjoins the big toe (first metatarsal head).

The cause of sesamoiditis is usually repeated injury. Sesamoiditis is particularly common among dancers, joggers, and those who wear high heels. The area may be swollen and is painful when walking and when pressure is applied to it. The doctor makes the diagnosis by examining the foot and confirms the diagnosis by x-rays to exclude a fracture of the sesamoid bone.

Treatment consists of placing a special pad ("dancer's pad") inside the shoe to reduce pressure on the area. A nonsteroidal anti-inflammatory drug (NSAID) taken by mouth and injections of corticosteroids and local anesthetic into the affected area can be helpful.

What Is Hammer Toe?

In hammer toe, the second, third, or fourth toe becomes bent and cannot be straightened.

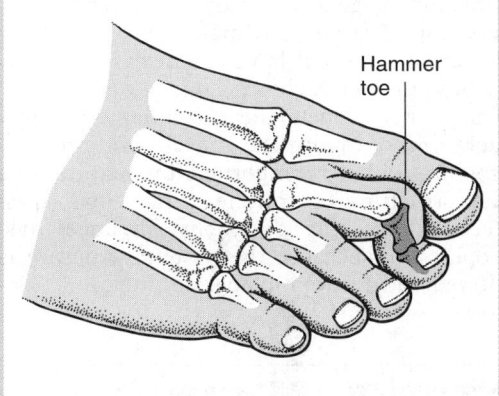

Hammer toe

CHAPTER 73

Muscular Dystrophy and Related Disorders

Muscular dystrophies are a group of inherited muscle disorders that lead to muscle weakness▲ of varying severity. Other inherited muscle disorders include myotonic myopathies, periodic paralysis, and glycogen-storage diseases. Glycogen-storage diseases are a group of rare inherited disorders in which muscles cannot metabolize sugars normally,■ so they build up large stores of glycogen (a starch that is formed from sugars).

Duchenne and Becker Muscular Dystrophies

Duchenne and Becker muscular dystrophies cause weakness in the muscles closest to the torso.

These dystrophies are the most common muscular dystrophies and nearly always occur in boys. On average, 1 of 3,300 boys born has Duchenne dystrophy, whereas on average 1 of 18,000 boys born has Becker muscular dystrophy.

The gene defect that causes Duchenne muscular dystrophy is different from the gene defect that causes Becker muscular dystrophy, but both defects involve the same gene. The gene for either of these traits is recessive and is carried on the X chromosome. Therefore, although a female can carry the defective gene, she will not develop the disease because the normal gene on one X chromosome compensates for the gene defect on the other X chromosome. However, any male who receives the defective gene will have the disease, because he has only one X chromosome.

Boys with Duchenne muscular dystrophy lack almost totally the muscle protein, dystrophin, which is important for maintaining the structure of muscle cells. Boys with Becker muscular dystrophy produce dystrophin, but because the protein structure is altered, the dystrophin does not function properly.

Symptoms

In boys with Duchenne muscular dystrophy, the first symptoms are developmental delay (particularly a delay in starting to walk), difficulty walking or climbing stairs, and falling. Starting between the ages of 3 and 7, the gait becomes waddling, and the child has difficulty rising from a sitting position.

Weakness in the shoulder muscles usually follows and gets steadily worse. As the muscles weaken they also enlarge, but the abnormal muscle tissue is not strong. In over 80% of boys with Duchenne muscular dystrophy, the heart muscle also enlarges and weakens, causing problems with the heartbeat, which show up on an electrocardiogram.

In boys with Duchenne muscular dystrophy, the arm and leg muscles usually contract around the joints, so that the elbows and knees cannot fully extend. Eventually, an abnormally curved spine (scoliosis) develops. By age 10 or 12, most children with the disease are confined to a wheelchair. The increasing weakness also makes them susceptible to pneumonia and other illnesses, and most die by the age of 20.

In boys with Becker muscular dystrophy, weakness is less severe and first appears a little later, at about age 12. The pattern of weakness resembles that of Duchenne muscular dystrophy. However, very few adolescents become confined to a wheelchair. The average age of death is 42 years.

Diagnosis

Doctors suspect muscular dystrophy when a young boy becomes weak and grows weaker. An enzyme (creatine kinase) leaks out of muscle cells, causing levels of creatine kinase in the blood to be abnormally high. However, high blood levels of creatine kinase do not necessarily mean that a person has muscular dystrophy; other muscle diseases may also cause elevated levels of this enzyme. Duchenne muscular dystrophy is diagnosed when blood tests show the gene for the protein dystrophin to be absent or abnormal and a muscle

---

▲ see page 339   ■ see page 1616

biopsy▲ shows extremely low levels of dystrophin in the muscle. Under the microscope, the muscle generally shows dead tissue and abnormally large muscle fibers. In the late stages of muscular dystrophy, fat and other tissues replace the dead muscle tissue. Similarly, Becker muscular dystrophy is diagnosed when blood tests show the gene for the protein dystrophin to be abnormal and a muscle biopsy shows low levels of dystrophin in the muscle, but not as low as in Duchenne muscular dystrophy.

Other tests to support the diagnosis include electrical studies of muscle function (electromyography) and nerve conduction studies.■

Families with members who have either Duchenne or Becker muscular dystrophy are advised to consult a genetic counselor for help in evaluating the risk of passing the muscular dystrophy trait on to their children. In families with a history of these disorders, doctors can perform prenatal tests on the fetus to determine if the child is likely to be affected.

Treatment

Neither Duchenne nor Becker muscular dystrophy can be cured. Physical therapy and exercise help prevent the muscles from contracting permanently around joints. Sometimes surgery is needed to release tight, painful muscles.

Prednisone, a corticosteroid, taken by mouth daily, improves the person's strength. However, long-term use causes many side effects,★ so it is not given to every child with muscular dystrophy. Use of prednisone is generally reserved for people whose muscle weakness has severely interfered with the normal activities of daily living. Creatine, a supplement taken by mouth, has recently been shown to improve strength. Gene therapy that would enable muscles to produce dystrophin and thereby relieve the weakness is under investigation but has so far not proved successful.

Other Muscular Dystrophies

Several much less common forms of muscular dystrophy, all inherited, also cause progressive muscle weakness.

Facioscapulohumeral (Landouzy-Dejerine) muscular dystrophy is transmitted by an autosomal dominant gene; therefore, a single abnormal gene is sufficient to cause the disorder, and the disorder can appear in either males or females. Symptoms usually begin between the ages of 7 and 20. The facial and shoulder mus-

cles are always affected, so that a child has difficulty whistling, closing the eyes tightly, or raising the arms. Some people with the disease also develop a footdrop (the foot flops down). The weakness is rarely severe, and people who have Landouzy-Dejerine muscular dystrophy have a normal life expectancy.

Limb-girdle muscular dystrophies cause weakness in the muscles of either the pelvis (Leyden-Möbius muscular dystrophy) or the shoulder (Erb's muscular dystrophy). These inherited disorders usually do not appear until adulthood and rarely produce serious weakness.

Mitochondrial myopathies are muscle disorders inherited through faulty genes in mitochondria (the energy factories of cells; they carry their own genes). Because sperm do not contribute mitochondria during fertilization, all mitochondrial genes come from the mother.● Therefore, although they are equally likely in males and females, these disorders can never be inherited from the father. These rare disorders sometimes cause increasing weakness in one or a few muscle groups, such as the eye muscles (ophthalmoplegia). One mitochondrial myopathy is called the Kearns-Sayre syndrome.

Diagnosis and Treatment

Diagnosis requires taking a sample of the weak muscle tissue for biopsy and either examining it under a microscope or performing chemical tests on it. Specific treatments are not available, but gene therapy holds promise for the future.

Myotonic Myopathies

Myotonic myopathies are inherited disorders in which the muscles are not able to relax normally after contraction; muscle weakness and spasms may also occur.

Myotonia congenita (Thomsen's disease) is a rare autosomal dominant disorder that affects males and females. Symptoms usually start in infancy. The hands, legs, and eyelids become very stiff because of an inability to relax the muscles. Muscle weakness, however, is usually minimal. The diagnosis is made from the child's characteristic appearance, inability to relax the grip of the hand rapidly after closing the hand, and prolonged contrac-

---

▲ see also page 343   ■ see page 446
★ see box on page 374   ● see page 14

tion after the doctor taps a muscle. An electromyogram (a test in which electrical impulses from muscles are recorded▲) is needed to confirm the diagnosis. Myotonic congenita is treated with phenytoin, quinine, procainamide, or mexiletine to relieve muscle stiffness and cramping; however, each of these drugs has undesirable side effects. Regular exercise may be beneficial. People with myotonic congenita have a normal life expectancy.

Myotonic dystrophy (Steinert's disease) is an autosomal dominant disorder affecting males and females. The disorder produces weakness and stiff muscles, especially in the hands. Drooping eyelids are also common. Symptoms can appear at any age and can range from mild to severe. People with the most severe form of the disorder have extreme muscle weakness and many other symptoms, including cataracts, small testes (in men), premature balding in the front (in men), irregular heartbeats, diabetes, and mental retardation. They usually die by age 50. Treatment with quinine, phenytoin, procainamide, and other drugs has been used, but these drugs do not improve the weakness, which is the most bothersome symptom to the person. Also, each of these drugs has undesirable side effects. The only treatment for muscle weakness is supportive measures, such as ankle braces and other devices.

Periodic Paralysis

Periodic paralysis is an autosomal dominant inherited disorder that causes sudden attacks of weakness and paralysis; there are several variants.

During an attack of periodic paralysis, muscles do not respond to normal nerve impulses or even to artificial stimulation with an electronic instrument. The person remains completely awake and alert. The precise form that the disorder takes varies in different families. In some families, the paralysis is related to high levels of potassium in the blood (hyper-

kalemia); in others, the paralysis is related to low levels of potassium in the blood (hypokalemia) or, rarely, to normal levels.

Symptoms and Diagnosis

In the hyperkalemic form of the disorder, attacks often begin by age 10. The attacks last 15 minutes to 1 hour. In the hypokalemic form, attacks generally first appear before age 16 but may appear during the 20s and always by age 30. The attacks last longer (occasionally for 2 to 3 days) and are more severe. Fasting, strenuous work, and exposure to cold may precipitate attacks in people who have the hyperkalemic form. Some people with the hypokalemic form are prone to attacks of paralysis after eating meals rich in carbohydrates (sometimes hours or even the day after), but exercise also precipitates attacks. Eating carbohydrates and exercising vigorously drive sugar into cells; potassium moves with the sugar and the result is lowered potassium levels in the blood. On awakening the day after engaging in vigorous exercise, a person with either the hyperkalemic form or the hypokalemic form may feel some weakness or even paralysis in certain muscle groups or in the arms and legs. The weakness generally lasts 1 or 2 days.

A doctor's best clue to the diagnosis is a person's description of a typical attack. If possible, the doctor draws blood while an attack is in progress to check the level of potassium. Doctors usually perform additional tests to be sure abnormal potassium levels in the blood are not from other causes.

Prevention and Treatment

Acetazolamide, a drug that alters the blood's acidity, may prevent attacks in all types of periodic paralysis. People with the hypokalemic form can take potassium chloride in an unsweetened solution while the attack is in progress. Usually symptoms improve considerably within an hour. People with the hypokalemic form should also avoid meals rich in carbohydrates and strenuous exercise. People with the hyperkalemic form can prevent attacks by eating frequent meals rich in carbohydrates and low in potassium.

▲ see page 446

CHAPTER 74

Disorders of Muscles, Bursas, and Tendons

The muscles, bursas, tendons, and bones must be healthy and functioning properly for the body to move normally. Muscles, which contract to produce movement, are connected to the bones by tendons. Bursas are flat sacs containing joint (synovial) fluid that reduce friction in areas where skin, muscles, tendons, and ligaments rub over bones.

Often, muscles, bursas, and tendons are injured in sports activities.▲ Injury, overuse, infection, and occasionally disease can temporarily or permanently damage muscles, bursas, and tendons. Damage can cause pain, limit control over movement, and reduce the normal range of motion.

Muscle Cramps

A cramp is a sudden, brief, usually painful contraction of a muscle or group of muscles.

Cramps are common among healthy people, especially during or after vigorous exercise. Middle-aged and older people commonly have cramps after light exercise or during rest. Some people have leg cramps during sleep. These painful cramps usually affect the calf and foot muscles, causing the foot and toes to curl downward.

Cramps may be caused by inadequate blood flow to the muscles. For example, they may occur after eating, when blood flows primarily to the digestive tract rather than to the muscles. Low blood levels of electrolytes, such as potassium, can also cause cramps. Low potassium levels■ may result from use of some diuretics or from dehydration.

Cramps can usually be prevented by not exercising immediately after eating and by gently stretching the muscles before exercising or going to bed. Stretching makes the muscles and tendons more flexible and less likely to contract spontaneously. Not consuming caffeine (for example, in coffee or chocolate) and not smoking also help to prevent cramps. Drugs that are stimulants, such as ephedrine or pseudoephedrine (a decongestant contained in many over-the-counter products), should not be used if cramps are a problem. Drinking plenty of fluids (particularly beverages that contain potassium) after exercise also helps to prevent cramps.

Most of the drugs prescribed to relieve cramps (including quinine sulfate, magnesium carbonate, and benzodiazepines such as diazepam) have not proven to be effective and can cause side effects. Calcium supplements are well tolerated, but they also have not proven to be effective. Mexiletine sometimes helps but has many side effects.

Fibromyalgia

Fibromyalgia describes several disorders, all characterized by achy pain and stiffness in soft tissues, including muscles, tendons, and ligaments.

The term fibromyalgia is used to describe several related disorders. Various alternative terms for these disorders have been used, including generalized fibromyalgia, primary fibromyalgia syndrome, secondary fibromyalgia syndrome, localized fibromyalgia, and myofascial pain syndrome, each having different connotations. Previously, these disorders were collectively called fibrositis or fibromyositis syndromes, but because inflammation is not present, the "itis" suffix was dropped.

In generalized fibromyalgia, which is about 7 times more common in women than in men, the pain and stiffness are widespread, occurring throughout the body. Primary fibromyalgia syndrome is the most common variation of generalized fibromyalgia; it usually occurs in young or middle-aged women who have no associated or contributing underlying disorder.

Secondary fibromyalgia syndrome is a type of generalized fibromyalgia and refers to fibromyalgia symptoms in a person who has another underlying disorder that is causing the fibromyalgia symptoms, such as hypothyroidism. Other disorders, such as systemic lupus erythematosus or rheumatoid arthritis, may be associated with fibromyalgia, but not be the underlying cause.

▲ see page 419   ■ see page 910

Fibromyalgia: Finding the Tender Points

Tender points are areas of tenderness that develop in people with fibromyalgia. For a diagnosis of fibromyalgia, a person must feel pain in at least 11 of the 18 tender points.

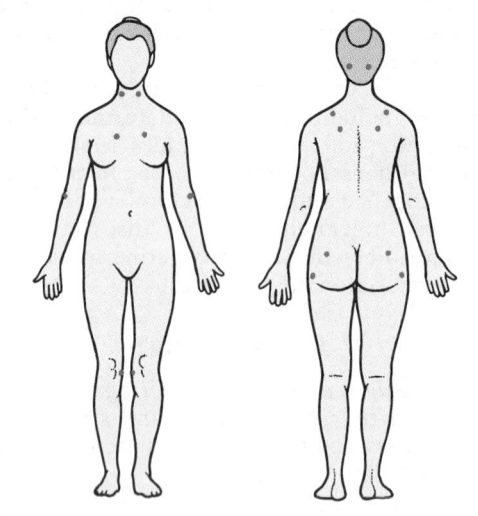

In localized fibromyalgia, pain and stiffness occur in a particular area, or at a few sites, such as the jaw, neck, and/or shoulder muscles. Localized fibromyalgia is somewhat more likely to occur in men, possibly because they are more likely to engage in more physically muscular activities in occupational or sports situations. Sometimes, localized fibromyalgia gradually spreads to become generalized fibromyalgia. Myofascial pain syndrome is a type of localized or regional fibromyalgia which may occur in various sites. In the temporomandibular type,▲ the chewing muscles on the side of the face are commonly involved and may become painful and tender.

Fibromyalgia is not dangerous or life threatening. Nonetheless, persistent symptoms can be very disruptive.

Causes

Usually, the cause of generalized fibromyalgia is unknown; in primary fibromyalgia syn-

---

▲ see also page 686

■ see page 756

drome, the cause is always unknown. However, generalized fibromyalgia may be worsened by physical or mental stress, poor sleep, repetitive strains, an injury, or chronic exposure to dampness and cold. In secondary fibromyalgia syndrome, an underlying cause is known. The syndrome may occur as a complication of certain infections (for example, Lyme disease), or hypothyroidism. Another associated disorder, such as rheumatoid arthritis or systemic lupus erythematosus, may be coincidental or may sometimes increase the symptoms of fibromyalgia.

Localized fibromyalgia often results from an occupational or recreational muscle strain. The temporomandibular type of myofascial pain syndrome can be caused by clenching and grinding of the teeth, especially while the person is asleep.

Symptoms

Aching stiffness and pain usually develop gradually in generalized fibromyalgia. In localized fibromyalgia, the pain may begin more suddenly after muscle strains, and be sharp. In both syndromes, the pain usually worsens with fatigue, straining, or overuse. Specific discrete areas of muscle may be tender when firm fingertip pressure is applied; these areas are called either tender or trigger points. (Both points are tender, but "trigger" points radiate the pain to a distant site.) During flare-ups, muscle tightness or even spasms may occur. Any soft tissue (muscles, tendons, and ligaments) may be affected. Soft tissue of the neck, shoulders, chest and rib cage, lower back, and thighs as well as joints are especially likely to be painful.

In primary fibromyalgia syndrome, widespread pain typically occurs and is often accompanied by other symptoms, such as poor sleep, anxiety, depression, fatigue, and irritable bowel syndrome.■

In the temporomandibular type of myofascial pain syndrome, the mouth often cannot be opened fully, and opening the mouth may be painful. Clenching or grinding of the teeth during sleep can lead to a headache on awakening that improves over the course of the day. Sometimes the teeth clenching or grinding continues throughout the day.

Diagnosis and Treatment

The diagnosis of fibromyalgia is based on the pattern and location of the pain as well as the presence of tender points. Doctors firmly press designated areas of the body to determine whether the person feels pain in one spot (a tender point) or whether the pain seems to travel (refer) to another area (a trigger point). Diagnosis requires tenderness at 11 or more of the 18 designated tender points.

Nondrug treatments are usually the most helpful. Reducing stress can alleviate some mild cases of fibromyalgia. Stretching and conditioning exercises of gradually increasing intensity, improvements in the quality of sleep, application of heat to the affected area, gentle massage, and keeping warm are usually beneficial.

Aspirin or other nonsteroidal anti-inflammatory drugs (NSAIDs) are generally of limited benefit. Occasionally, local anesthetics (eg, lidocaine, alone or with corticosteroids [eg, hydrocortisone]) are injected directly into a particularly tender area or trigger point, but these injections should not be relied on for repetitive use. Doctors may prescribe low doses of tricyclic antidepressants▲ 1 or 2 hours before bedtime, which are prescribed to improve sleep rather than to relieve depression.

For people who have the temporomandibular type of myofascial pain syndrome, using a plastic mouth guard can keep the teeth from touching each other and thereby prevent them from clenching and grinding. A benzodiazepine or tricyclic antidepressant at bedtime is sometimes used to relieve symptoms until a mouth guard can be obtained. Nonsteroidal anti-inflammatory drugs (NSAIDs) or acetaminophen is useful. Because the condition tends to persist, opioids should not be used, except possibly for short times. The person should be taught to stop clenching the jaw and grinding the teeth. Foods that are hard to chew and chewing gum should be avoided. Physical therapy, biofeedback to encourage relaxation, and psychologic counseling help some people. Most people, even if untreated, stop having significant symptoms within 2 to 3 years.

Bursitis

Bursitis is painful inflammation of a bursa (a flat sac containing joint [synovial] fluid that reduces friction in areas where skin, muscles, tendons, and ligaments rub over bones).

A bursa normally contains very little fluid. If injured or overused, however, the bursa may become inflamed and fill with fluid.

Bursitis is usually caused by irritation from unusual uses or overuses. It may also be caused by injury, gout, pseudogout, rheumatoid arthritis, or certain infections, especially those caused by *Staphylococcus aureus*; often, the cause is unknown. Although the shoulder is most susceptible to bursitis, bursas in the elbows, hips (trochanteric bursitis), pelvis, knees, toes, and heels (Achilles tendon bursitis■) commonly become inflamed.

Symptoms

Bursitis causes pain and tends to limit movement, but the specific symptoms depend on the location of the inflamed bursa. For example, when a bursa in the shoulder becomes inflamed, raising the arm out from the side of the body (as when putting on a jacket) is painful and difficult.

Acute bursitis occurs suddenly. The inflamed area is painful when moved or touched. The skin over bursas located close to the surface, such as near the knee and elbow, may appear red and swollen. Acute bursitis caused by an infection or gout★ is particularly painful, and the affected area is red and feels warm when touched.

Chronic bursitis may result from previous bouts of acute bursitis or repeated injuries. In some cases, the walls of the bursa thicken, and abnormal material with solid, chalky calcium deposits may accumulate. Damaged bursas are susceptible to additional inflammation when subjected to unusual exercise or strain. Long-standing pain and swelling can limit movement, causing muscles to waste away (atrophy) and become weak. Flare-ups of chronic bursitis may last a few days to several weeks and frequently recur.

Diagnosis and Treatment

A doctor suspects bursitis if the area around a bursa is sore when touched and specific joint movements are painful. If the bursa is noticeably swollen, the doctor may remove a sample of fluid from the bursa with a needle to test for causes of the inflammation, such as an infection or gout. X-rays are usually not helpful; however, they may be able to detect the calcium deposits of chronic bursitis.

Acute bursitis not caused by an infection is usually treated with rest, temporary immobilization of the affected joint, ice applied to the

---

▲ see table on page 618   ■ see page 408

★ see page 391

painful area, and a nonsteroidal anti-inflammatory drug (NSAID).▲ Occasionally, stronger analgesics (such as an opioid) are needed. Often, when the bursa is not infected, a doctor may inject a mixture of a local anesthetic and a corticosteroid directly into the bursa. This treatment provides relief immediately or within a few hours to days. The injection may have to be repeated after a few months.

People who have severe acute bursitis may occasionally be given a corticosteroid, such as prednisone, by mouth for a few days. As the pain subsides, the person can perform specific exercises to increase the joint's range of motion.

Chronic, noninfected bursitis is treated in a similar way, although rest and immobilization are less likely to help. Rarely, when large calcium deposits occur in the shoulder, they may be irrigated through a wide-gauge needle (after being loosened, the sediment can be drawn out through the needle). This procedure may be performed in the doctor's office. Large deposits may need to be removed surgically.

Disabling bursitis in the shoulder may be relieved by several repeated injections of corticosteroids along with intensive physical therapy to restore the joint's function. Exercises can help strengthen weakened muscles and reestablish the joint's full range of motion. Bursitis often recurs if the underlying cause, such as gout, rheumatoid arthritis, or chronic overuse, is not corrected.

Infected bursas must be drained, and appropriate antibiotics given, often against *Staphylococcus aureus.*

Tendinitis and Tenosynovitis

Tendinitis is inflammation of a tendon; tenosynovitis is tendinitis accompanied by inflammation of the protective sheath around the tendon (tendon sheath).

Tendons are fibrous cords of tough tissue that connect muscles to bones. Tendon sheaths surround some tendons.

Tendinitis usually occurs in middle or old age, as the tendons become more susceptible to injury. However, it also occurs in younger people who exercise vigorously (who may develop rotator cuff tendinitis■) and in people who perform repetitive tasks.

Certain tendons, especially those of the hand and forearm, are particularly susceptible

---

▲ see page 452   ■ see page 429

★ see art on page 398   ● see page 424

to inflammation. Inflammation in the tendon that extends the thumb away from the hand is called de Quervain's syndrome. Also, inflammation can cause the flexor tendons that control clenching of the fingers to get caught in their sheaths, producing a popping feeling (trigger finger★). Tendinitis above the biceps muscle in the upper arm (bicipital tendon) causes pain when the elbow is bent or the arm is elevated or rotated. The Achilles tendon in the heel● and a tendon that runs over the top of the foot also commonly become inflamed.

Certain joint diseases, such as rheumatoid arthritis, scleroderma, gout, and Reiter's syndrome, can cause tenosynovitis. In people who contract gonorrhea, especially women, gonococcal bacteria can spread during menstruation or pregnancy and cause tenosynovitis, usually affecting the tissues of the shoulders, wrists, fingers, hips, ankles, and feet.

Symptoms and Diagnosis

The inflamed tendons are usually painful when moved or touched. Moving the joints near the tendon, even a little, may cause severe pain. The tendon sheaths may be visibly swollen from the accumulation of fluid and inflammation. In chronic tenosynovitis, as may occur in scleroderma, the tendon sheaths may remain dry and rub against other tissues, causing a grating sensation that may be felt or a sound that may be heard with a stethoscope when the joint is moved; this is called a "tendon friction rub."

Treatment

Several forms of treatment may relieve the symptoms of tendinitis. Rest, immobilization with a splint or cast, and application of heat or cold—whichever works—are often helpful. Nonsteroidal anti-inflammatory drugs (NSAIDs) can reduce the pain and inflammation when used for 7 to 10 days.

Sometimes corticosteroids (for example, dexamethasone, methylprednisolone, or triamcinolone) and local anesthetics (for example, lidocaine) are injected into the tendon sheath. Rarely, the injection causes pain because crystals of the corticosteroid temporarily form inside the joint or sheath; this flare-up lasts for less than 24 hours and can be treated with cold compresses and analgesics.

Treatments may have to be repeated every 2 or 3 weeks for a month or two before the inflammation subsides completely. Chronic, persistent tendinitis, as may occur in rheumatoid arthritis, may have to be treated surgically to remove inflamed tissues, and physical therapy may be needed after surgery. Surgery is occasionally needed to remove calcium deposits from areas of long-standing tendinitis, such as the area around the shoulder joint.

De Quervain's Syndrome

De Quervain's syndrome (also called washerwoman's sprain) is swelling and inflammation of the tendons or tendon sheaths that move the thumb outward.

This disorder usually occurs after repetitive use of the wrist. The main symptom is aching pain on the thumb side of the wrist and at the base of the thumb, which becomes worse with movement. The area at the base of the thumb at the wrist is also tender.

To diagnose the disorder, a doctor performs a Finkelstein test. The person bends the affected thumb into the palm and wraps the fingers over the thumb. With the palm facing up, the doctor rotates the palm toward the middle of the body. If this movement causes pain, the test is positive for de Quervain's syndrome.

Rest, warm soaks, and nonsteroidal anti-inflammatory drugs (NSAIDs) are effective only for very mild cases. Injections of corticosteroids into the tendon sheath are helpful in 80 to 90% of cases; surgery is needed occasionally.

Baker's Cysts

Baker's cysts (popliteal cysts) are tiny sacs filled with joint (synovial) fluid that form in an extension of the joint capsule behind the knee.

A Baker's cyst results from an accumulation of trapped joint fluid, which bulges from the joint capsule behind the knee as a protruding sac. Causes of the joint fluid accumulation include rheumatoid arthritis, osteoarthritis, and overuse of the knees. Baker's cysts produce discomfort at the back of the knee. The cysts may enlarge and extend downward into the calf muscles.

A rapid increase in the amount and pressure of fluid within the cyst can cause it to rupture. The fluid released from the cyst can cause the surrounding tissues to become inflamed, resulting in symptoms that may mimic those of thrombophlebitis.▲ Moreover, a bulging or ruptured Baker's cyst can cause thrombophlebitis in the popliteal vein (which is located behind the knee) by pressing on the vein.

The doctor can usually make a diagnosis by asking the person specific questions about symptoms and feeling a swelling behind the knee or in the calf. Ultrasound, magnetic resonance imaging (MRI), or arthrography, can sometimes aid in the diagnosis and document how far the cyst extends.

When arthritis causes chronic knee swelling, the doctor may need to remove the fluid with a needle (a procedure called joint aspiration) and inject a long-acting corticosteroid (such as triamcinolone acetonide) to prevent the formation of a Baker's cyst. Removing the cyst surgically is an alternative if other treatments are not effective.

If the cyst has ruptured, the pain is treated with a nonsteroidal anti-inflammatory drug (NSAID). If the ruptured cyst causes thrombophlebitis in the popliteal vein, this is treated with bed rest, elevation of the leg, warm compresses and anticoagulants. Occasionally, antibiotics are needed also.

CHAPTER 75

Sports Injuries

More than 10 million sports injuries are treated each year in the United States. Common sports injuries include stress fractures of the foot, shin splints, tendinitis, runner's knee, hamstring injuries, tennis elbow, head injuries,■ foot injuries,★ and myriad other sprains and pulled muscles. In addition, certain sports, including weight lifting, can cause low back pain.● The techniques used to treat sports injuries can be used to treat many other types of musculoskeletal injuries, which often

▲ see page 326   ■ see page 513
★ see page 403   ● see page 568

resemble sports injuries but have different causes. For example, tennis elbow can be caused by carrying a suitcase, turning a screw, or opening a stuck door. Runner's knee can be caused by rolling the feet onto the outside (pronation) excessively while walking.

Causes

The most common cause of sports injuries is overuse, which is generally due to faulty training methods: The exerciser does not allow for adequate recovery after a workout or does not stop exercising when pain develops. Every time muscles are stressed by an intensive workout, some muscle fibers are injured and others use up their available energy, which has been stored as the carbohydrate glycogen. More than 2 days are required for fibers to heal and glycogen to be replaced. Because only uninjured and adequately nourished fibers function properly, closely spaced, intensive workouts eventually require comparable work from fewer healthy fibers, increasing the likelihood of injury. Stopping exercise at the first sign of pain, which precedes most wear-and-tear injuries, limits the injury to these fibers, resulting in a quicker recovery. However, continuing to exercise with pain tears more fibers, extending the damage and delaying recovery.

Structural abnormalities can make a person susceptible to a sports injury by stressing parts of the body unevenly. For example, when the legs are unequal in length, unequal forces are placed on the hip and knee. Habitually running along the sides of banked roads has the same effect; repeatedly hitting the slightly higher surface increases the risk of pain or injury on that side and increases the forces acting on the other leg, exposing it to injury as well. A person who has an exaggerated curve in the lower spine (lordosis) may have back pain when swinging a baseball bat or golf club.

Excessive pronation—a rolling onto the outside of the feet after they strike the ground—is the cause of most foot, leg, and hip injuries. Some degree of pronation is normal and prevents injuries by helping distribute the foot's striking force throughout the foot. However, excessive pronation can cause foot, knee, and leg pain. In people with excessive pronation, the ankles are so flexible that the arches of the feet touch the ground during walking or running, giving the appearance of flatfeet. A runner with excessive pronation may have knee pain when running long distances.

The opposite problem—too little pronation—can occur in people who have rigid ankles. In these people, the foot appears to have a very high arch and does not absorb shock well, increasing the risk of developing small cracks in the bones (stress fractures) of the feet and legs.

The way in which the legs are aligned on the hip bone (pelvis) can produce pain in the legs, particularly in women with wide hips. Such women develop knocked knees, with a tendency for the knee caps to be pushed outward from the midline. This force on the knee caps causes pain. Wide hips also can result in increased tension on a structure called the iliotibial band, causing pain over the outer part of the pelvis and down the outer side of each thigh.

Muscles, tendons, and ligaments tear when subjected to forces greater than their inherent strength. For example, they may be injured if they are too weak or tight for the exercise being attempted. Joints are more prone to injury when the muscles and ligaments that support them are weak, as they are after a sprain. Bones weakened by osteoporosis may fracture easily.

Many injuries are caused by chronic wear and tear, which results from repetitive motion that stresses susceptible tissues. Such is particularly the case in people with structural abnormalities that stress certain parts of the body more than others. In addition, sports injuries are more likely when people do not warm up properly (exercising muscles at a relaxed pace) before an intense workout. Improper technique while exercising is a major contributor to sports injuries. Performing exercises in ways that place joints at unstable angles, increase the impact on tender structures, or overstress ligaments are common causes of sports injuries. Exercises performed too quickly or with an excessive load on the muscles can also lead to injury while the person is training.

Diagnosis

To diagnose a sports or other musculoskeletal injury, a doctor asks when and how the injury happened, what recreational and occupational activities the person has recently or routinely been engaged in, and whether there has been a change in the intensity of the activity. The doctor also examines the injured area. The person may be referred to a specialist for further testing. Diagnostic tests may include x-rays, computed tomography (CT), magnetic resonance imaging (MRI), ultrasound, bone scanning, dual-energy x-ray absorptiometry (DEXA),▲ arthroscopy,■ electromyography,★ and computer-aided testing of muscle and joint function.

Prevention

Allowing at least 2 days between intensive workouts or alternating workouts that stress different parts of the body can help prevent chronic injury. Some training programs alternate a hard workout one day with rest or an easy workout the next. The person can also change the type of exercise to stress different body parts. If an athlete trains twice a day, each hard workout should be followed by at least three easy ones (for instance, a hard morning workout should be followed by an easy workout in the afternoon and two easy workouts the next day). Only swimmers can perform both a hard and an easy workout every day without injury. The buoyancy of the water helps protect their muscles and joints.

Warming up before beginning strenuous exercise helps to prevent injuries. Exercising at a relaxed pace for 3 to 10 minutes warms the muscles enough to make them more pliable and resistant to injury. This active method of warming up prepares muscles for strenuous exercise more effectively than passive methods such as warm water, heating pads, ultrasound, or an infrared lamp. Passive methods do not increase blood circulation significantly.

Stretching exercises do not generally seem to prevent injuries, but they do lengthen muscles so they can contract more effectively and perform better. To avoid damaging muscles when stretching, a person should stretch after warming up or exercising, and each stretch should be comfortable enough to hold for a count of 10.

Cooling down—gradually slowing down before stopping exercise—prevents dizziness by keeping blood flowing. When strenuous exercise is stopped abruptly, blood may collect (pool) in the leg veins, temporarily reducing the flow of blood to the head. The result may be dizziness and even fainting. Cooling down also helps remove waste products, such as lactic acid, from the muscles, but it does not seem to prevent next-day muscle soreness, which is caused by damaged muscle fibers.

Strengthening exercises help prevent injuries. Regular endurance (aerobic) exercise neither enlarges nor strengthens muscles significantly. The only way to strengthen muscles is to exercise against progressively greater resistance, as in performing a sport more intensely, lifting progressively heavier weights, or using special strength training machines. Rehabilitation exercises to strengthen healed muscles and tendons are usually done by lifting or pressing against resistance, in sets of 8 to 12 repetitions, no more often than every other day.

Shoe inserts (orthotics) can often correct foot problems such as excessive pronation. The inserts, which may be flexible, semirigid, or rigid and may vary in length, should be fitted into appropriate running shoes. Orthotics are used in place of the inserts found in the shoes at the time they are purchased. Good running shoes have a rigid heel counter (the back part of the shoe that surrounds the heel) to control movement of the back of the foot, a support across the instep (saddle) to prevent excessive pronation, and a padded opening (collar) to support the ankle. The shoe must have adequate space for the insert. Orthotics usually reduce the shoe's width by one letter size; for example, a D width shoe with an orthotic becomes a C width shoe.

Treatment

Immediate treatment for almost all sports injuries consists of *r*est, *i*ce, *c*ompression, and *e*levation (RICE). The injured part is rested immediately to minimize internal bleeding and swelling and to prevent the injury from worsening. Ice helps to limit inflammation and reduce pain. Wrapping the injured part with tape or an elastic bandage (compression) and raising the injured part above the heart (elevation) help limit swelling. A commercial ice pack or a bag of crushed or chipped ice—which conforms to body contours better than ice cubes—can be placed on a towel over the injured part for 10 minutes. An elastic bandage can be wrapped loosely around the ice bag and the injured part. The injured part is kept elevated, but the ice is removed for 10 minutes, then reapplied for 10 minutes over a period of 1 to 1 1/2 hours. This process can be repeated several times during the first 24 hours.

Ice reduces pain and swelling in several ways. The injured part swells because fluid leaks from blood vessels. By causing the blood

▲ see page 342   ■ see page 343
★ see page 446

What Is a
Stress Fracture?

Stress fractures are small cracks in a bone caused by repetitive impact. They commonly occur in the bones of the midfoot—the metatarsals.

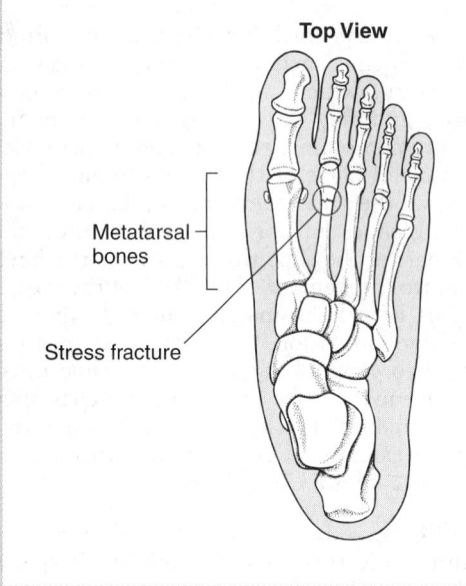

Top View

Metatarsal bones

Stress fracture

Dietary supplementation with glucosamine and chondroitin sulfate may be useful to help repair damage to an injured joint. However, such supplementation must be taken for 6 months or longer.

Physical therapists may incorporate heat, cold, electricity, sound waves, traction, or water exercise into a treatment plan in addition to therapeutic exercises.▲ How long physical therapy is needed depends on the severity and complexity of the injury.

The activity or sport that caused the injury should be avoided or modified until the injury has healed. Substituting activities that do not stress the injured part is preferable to abstaining from all physical activity because complete inactivity causes muscles to lose mass, strength, and endurance. For example, a week of rest requires at least 2 weeks of exercise to return to the level of fitness before the injury. Substitute activities include bicycling, swimming, skiing, and rowing when the lower leg or foot is injured; jogging in place or on a trampoline, swimming, and rowing when the upper leg is injured; bicycling and swimming when the lower back is injured; and jogging and skating when the shoulder or arm is injured.

Stress Fractures of the Foot

Stress fractures are small cracks in bones that often develop from chronic, excessive impact, bending, or twisting.

In runners, the bones of the midfoot (metatarsals) are especially prone to stress fractures. The bones most likely to fracture are the metatarsal bones that connect to the middle three toes. The metatarsal bone of the big toe is relatively immune to injury because of its strength and larger size, and the metatarsal bone of the little toe is usually protected because the greatest force from pushing off (toeing off) is exerted on the big toe and the toe next to it. However, when a stress fracture does affect the big or little toe, healing usually takes longer than with the other toes; the person may need to be immobile for a long time or may need surgery.

Risk factors for stress fractures in the foot include high arches, running shoes with inadequate shock absorption, and a sudden increase in the intensity or amount of exercise. People with narrow, thin bones are at an increased risk because these bones are not as strong. Postmenopausal women may be par-

vessels to constrict, cold reduces their tendency to leak, thus restricting the amount of fluid and swelling in the injured part. Lowering the temperature of the skin over the injury can reduce pain and muscle spasms. It also limits tissue destruction.

Applying ice for too long, however, can damage tissue. The skin reacts reflexively when it reaches a low temperature (around 59° F [15° C]) by widening blood vessels in the cold area. The skin turns red, feels hot and itchy, and may hurt.

Injections of corticosteroids into an injured joint or the surrounding tissue are sometimes used in addition to rest to relieve pain and reduce swelling. However, corticosteroid injections can delay healing, increase the risk of tendon and cartilage damage, and enable a person to use an injured joint before it is fully healed, perhaps worsening the injury.

▲ see page 37

ticularly susceptible to stress fractures because of osteoporosis.▲ Younger women athletes may also be susceptible to stress fractures, because the extreme exercise may suppress their ovaries, stop them from having periods, and cause osteoporosis.

The primary symptom is pain in the front part of the foot, usually during a long or intense workout. At first, the pain disappears within minutes of stopping exercise. If workouts are continued, however, the pain returns earlier in the workout and lasts longer after stopping exercise. Ultimately, severe pain may make running impossible, and pain may persist even during rest. The area around the fracture may swell.

A doctor can often make the diagnosis from a history of the symptoms and an examination of the foot. The fracture site hurts when touched. Stress fractures are so fine that they often cannot be seen on x-rays immediately, but doctors can use x-rays to detect the tissue (callus) that forms around the broken bone 2 or 3 weeks after the injury, as the bone heals. A bone scan can confirm the diagnosis earlier but is rarely needed.

Treatment requires that a person not run until the stress fracture has healed, but other exercises can be substituted. After the fracture has healed, wearing athletic shoes with adequate shock-absorbing support and running on grass or other soft surfaces can help prevent a recurrence. A cast is rarely needed. When used, it is removed after 3 weeks to prevent the muscles from becoming weak. Healing generally takes 3 to 12 weeks but may take longer in older people or in people who are bedridden. The smallest toe often takes a long time to heal and sometimes requires surgery.

Shin Splints

A shin splint is pain resulting from damage to the muscles along the shin.

The usual cause is long-standing, repeated stress to the lower leg. Two groups of muscles in the shin are susceptible to shin splints. The location of the pain depends on which group is affected.

Anterolateral shin splints affect the muscles in the front (anterior) and outside (lateral) parts of the shin. This type of injury results from a natural imbalance in the size of opposing muscles. The shin muscles pull the foot up, and the larger and much stronger calf muscles pull the foot down each time the heel

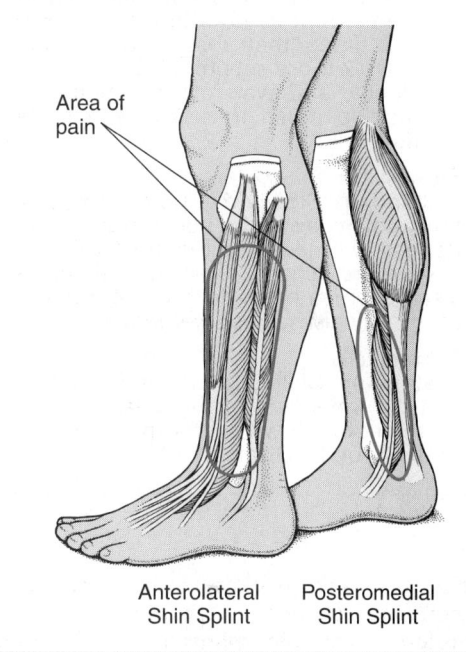

Shin Splints

Shin splints may develop in the muscles in the front and outer parts of the shin (anterolateral shin splints) or in the muscles in the back and inner parts (posteromedial shin splints). Pain is felt in different areas, depending on which muscles are affected.

Area of pain

Anterolateral
Shin Splint

Posteromedial
Shin Splint

touches the ground during walking or running. The calf muscles exert so much force that they can injure the shin muscles.

The main symptom of anterolateral shin splints is pain along the front and outside of the shin. At first, the pain is felt only immediately after the heel strikes the ground during running, walking, skiing, or other similar exercises. If the person continues to run, the pain occurs throughout each step, eventually becoming constant. Usually by the time the person sees a doctor, the shin hurts when touched.

To allow this type of shin splint to heal, the runner must stop running temporarily and do other kinds of exercise. Exercises to stretch the calf muscles are helpful. Once the shin muscles start to heal, exercises to strengthen

▲ see page 343

Strengthening the Shin Muscles

Bucket-handle exercise

Wrap a towel around the handle of an empty water bucket. Sit on a table or other surface high enough to prevent the feet from touching the floor. Place the bucket handle over the front part of one shoe. Slowly raise the front of the foot by flexing the ankle, then slowly extend the foot by pointing the toe. Repeat 10 times, then rest for a few seconds. Do 2 more sets of 10. To increase resistance, add water to the bucket—but not so much that the exercise is painful.

Toe raises

Stand up. Slowly rise up on the toes, then slowly lower the heels to the floor. Repeat 10 times, then rest for 1 minute. Do 2 more sets of 10. When this exercise becomes easy, do it while holding progressively heavier weights.

Outward rolls

Stand up. Slowly roll the ankle out so that the inner part of the sole is raised off the floor. Slowly lower the sole back to the floor. Do 3 sets of 10.

---

them, such as the bucket-handle exercise, can be done in 3 sets of 10 every other day.

Posteromedial shin splints affect the muscles in the back (posterior) and inner (medial) parts of the shin, which are responsible for lifting the heel just before the toes push off. This type of shin splint often results from running on banked tracks or crowned roads and can be worsened by rolling onto the outside of the feet (pronation) excessively or by wearing running shoes that do not adequately prevent such rolling.

The pain produced by this type of shin splint usually starts along the inside of the lower leg, about 1 to 8 inches above the ankle, and worsens when a runner rises up on the toes or rolls the ankle in. If the person continues to run, the pain moves forward, affecting the inner aspect of the ankle, and may extend up the shin to within 2 to 4 inches of the knee. The severity of the pain increases as the shin splint progresses. At first, only the muscle tendons are inflamed and painful, but if the person keeps running, the muscles themselves can be affected. Eventually, tension on the inflamed tendon can actually pull it from its at-

tachment to bone, causing bleeding and further inflammation.

The primary treatment is to stop running and do other types of exercise until running is no longer painful. Running shoes with a rigid heel counter (the back part of the shoe) and special arch supports can keep the foot from rolling onto the outside excessively. Avoiding running on banked surfaces can help prevent shin splints from recurring. Exercises to strengthen the injured muscles are useful.

An experimental treatment consists of calcitonin (a hormone that builds bone) injected daily or alendronate (a drug that slows bone loss) given by mouth; this treatment has healed some shin splints that were unresponsive to other measures. Sometimes none of the available treatments are effective, and the runner must abandon running permanently.

Popliteus Tendinitis

Popliteus tendinitis is inflammation in the popliteus tendon, which extends from the outer surface of the bottom of the thighbone (femur) diagonally across the back of the knee to the inner side of the top of the shinbone (tibia).

The popliteus tendon prevents the lower leg from twisting outward during running. Excessive rolling of the feet onto the outside (pronation), as well as running downhill, tends to put excessive stress on this tendon, which can tear it.

Pain and soreness, particularly when running downhill, develop along the outside of the knee. A person should not run until the area is free of pain and should not run downhill for at least 3 weeks after resuming running. Bicycling is a good alternative exercise during healing. Shoe inserts, especially a triangular wedge (varus wedge) placed in front of the heel, can help keep the foot from rolling inward.

Achilles Tendinitis

Achilles tendinitis is inflammation of the Achilles tendon, the tough band extending from the calf muscles to the heel.

The calf muscles and the Achilles tendon lower the forefoot after the heel touches the ground and raise the heel as the toes push off just before stepping to the other foot.

Achilles tendinitis occurs when stresses placed on the tendon are greater than the tendon's strength. Running downhill places extra stress on the Achilles tendon because the fore-foot has farther to go before touching the ground. Running uphill also stresses this tendon because the calf muscles must exert greater force to raise the heel as the toes push off. A soft heel counter (the back part of the shoe that surrounds the heel) allows excessive movement of the heel, stressing the Achilles tendon unevenly and increasing the likelihood that it will tear. Stiff-soled shoes that do not bend where the toes join the foot place great stress on the Achilles tendon just before the toes push off.

Various functional and structural abnormalities predispose the Achilles tendon to injury. These abnormalities include rolling the feet onto the outside (pronation) excessively, the habit of landing too far back on the heel (checking the sole of the running shoe can show where the heel is most worn), bowed legs, tight hamstring and calf muscles, high arches, tight Achilles tendons, and heel deformities. The Achilles tendon is enclosed in a protective sheath; between the tendon and its sheath is a thin layer of fat, which enables the tendon to move freely. When the tendon is injured, scars form between it and its sheath, causing the tendon to pull on the sheath with each movement.

Pain, the major symptom, is usually most severe when a person starts to move. It is often relieved by continuing to walk or run despite the pain and stiffness. Continuing to walk or run relieves the pain because it increases the temperature of the sheath, making it more pliable, so that the tendon can move more freely.

If the person ignores the pain and continues to run, rigid scar tissue replaces the elastic tendon, and the tendon will always hurt during exercise, with virtually no chance of a cure. Refraining from running and from pedaling a bicycle as long as the pain persists is an important part of treatment. Other measures depend on the probable cause or predisposing conditions and include wearing shoes with flexible soles and placing heel lifts in running shoes to reduce tension on the tendon and stabilize the heel. The blood flow to the Achilles tendon is reduced when the foot is bent upwards; a heel wedge reduces this effect. Exercises to stretch the hamstring muscles can be started as soon as they can be done without pain. Exercises to strengthen the Achilles tendon, such as toe raises, are helpful. After running is resumed, the person should not run up-

Strengthening the Vastus Medialis (Inner Thigh) Muscle

- Stand with both knees straight. Contract the quadriceps muscles (in the front of the thighs), raising the kneecaps. Hold this position for a count of 10, then relax.
  Repeat frequently throughout the day.
- Sit on the floor with both knees straight and the legs far apart. Rotate legs outward so that the toes point as far to the side as possible. Slowly raise the injured leg from the hip (with the knee straight), hold for 10 seconds 10 inches from the ground, and then lower it, keeping the knee straight. Do 3 sets of 10 every other day.
- Sit on the floor with two or more pillows under each knee so that it is flexed at a 135° angle. Place a 5-pound weight on the ankle. Slowly raise the foot by straightening the knee, then slowly lower the foot. Do 3 sets of 10. Progress by increasing the weight, not the number of repetitions.

hill or downhill at a fast pace until the tendon is fully healed—which can be weeks to years later. Surgery may be required; a procedure called lithotripsy is sometimes used as an alternative to surgery.

Runner's Knee

Runner's knee (patellofemoral stress syndrome) is a condition in which the kneecap (patella) rubs roughly against the end of the thighbone (femur) when the knee moves.

The kneecap is a circular bone that is attached to ligaments and tendons around the knee. The kneecap normally moves up or down slightly without touching the thighbone during running.

Runner's knee may be caused by a structural defect, such as a kneecap located too high or too low in the knee joint, off-center insertion of the muscles into the kneecap, tight hamstrings, tight Achilles tendons, and weak thigh muscles—which normally help stabilize the knee. Weak thigh muscles are the most common treatable cause of runner's knee; these weak muscles allow the kneecap to move sideways and rub against the thigh bone. A second common treatable cause is rolling of the feet onto the outside (pronation) exces-

Runner's Knee

Normally, the kneecap (patella) moves up or down slightly without touching the thighbone (femur) during running. If the feet roll in excessively (pronation), the lower leg twists inward, pulling the kneecap inward, while the quadriceps muscles pull the kneecap outward. These opposing forces cause the back of the kneecap to rub against the end of the thighbone, resulting in injury and pain.

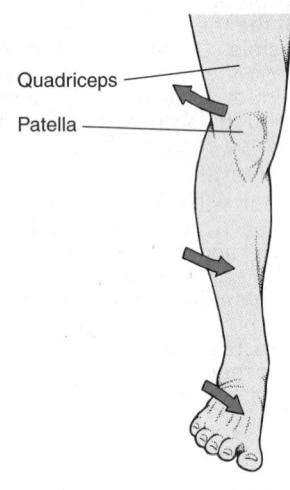

Quadriceps

Patella

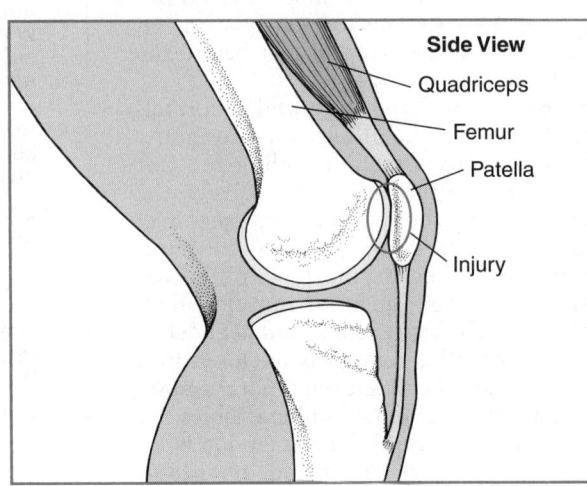

Side View

Quadriceps

Femur

Patella

Injury

sively when walking or running while the front thigh muscles (quadriceps) pull the kneecap outward. Together, these forces cause the kneecap to rub against the end of the thighbone.

Pain and sometimes swelling usually start during running and are concentrated on the undersurface of the kneecap. At first, only running downhill is painful, but later any running and eventually even other leg movements, particularly walking down steps, are painful.

Refraining from running until it can be done without pain is important. Other exercises, such as riding a bicycle (if not painful), rowing, and swimming, can be continued to maintain physical fitness. Exercises to stretch the muscles in the back (hamstrings) and front (quadriceps) of the thigh and to strengthen the vastus medialis, an inner thigh muscle that pulls the kneecap inward, are helpful. Commercially available arch supports placed in both exercise and street shoes may help. Sometimes, shoe inserts have to be custom-made.

Hamstring Injury

A hamstring injury (posterior femoral muscle strain, hamstring tear) is any injury to the hamstring muscles, the muscles in the back of the thigh.

The hamstrings, which extend the hip and bend the knee, are weaker than the opposing quadriceps (the muscles in the front of the thigh). If the hamstrings are not at least 60% as strong as the quadriceps, the quadriceps can overpower and injure them. A hamstring injury usually causes sudden pain in the back of the thigh when the hamstrings are contracted suddenly and violently, as can occur when a person sprints.

Immediate treatment includes *rest, ice, compression,* and *elevation* (RICE). A person should not run or jump but may jog in place, row, or swim—unless these activities cause pain—while the muscle heals. After healing begins, exercises to strengthen the hamstrings can help prevent a recurrence.

Strengthening the Hamstrings

- Attach a 5-pound weight to the foot on the injured side and lie face down on a bed with the lower part of the body (from the waist down) off the bed and the toes touching the floor. Keeping the knee straight, slowly raise and lower the leg. Do 3 sets of 10 every other day. As strength returns, use increasingly heavier weights. This exercise strengthens primarily the upper part of the hamstrings.
- Attach a 5-pound weight to the foot on the injured side. Stand on the other leg. Slowly raise the weighted foot toward the buttocks by bending the knee, and lower it toward the floor by straightening the knee. Do 3 sets of 10 every other day. As strength returns, use increasingly heavier weights. This exercise strengthens primarily the lower part of the hamstrings.

Lateral Epicondylitis

Lateral epicondylitis (backhand tennis elbow) is damage to the tendons that extend or bend the wrist away from the palm, causing pain in the elbow and on the outer, back side of the forearm.

The forearm muscles that are attached to the outer part of the elbow become sore when excessive stress is placed on the point of attachment. Lateral epicondylitis is most often felt during a backhand return, but can be felt during sports other than tennis. The force of the racket hitting the ball can damage the tendons where they are attached to the lower end of the upper arm bone. Factors that increase the chance of developing lateral epicondylitis include using improper backhand strokes (called leading elbow backhand), having weak shoulder and wrist muscles, playing with a racket that is too tightly strung or too short, hitting the ball off center on the racket, and hitting heavy, wet balls.

Tennis Elbow

The two types of tennis elbow—backhand and forehand tennis elbow—cause pain in different areas of the elbow and forearm.

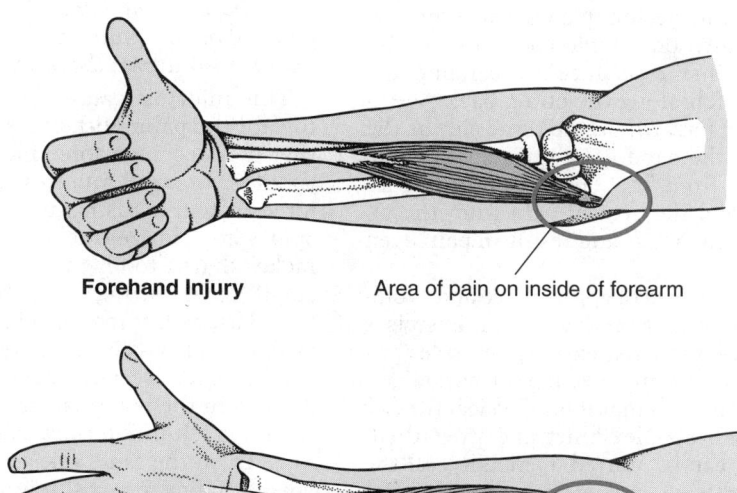

Forehand Injury   Area of pain on inside of forearm

Backhand Injury   Area of pain on outside of forearm

Strengthening the Wrist Muscles

For lateral epicondylitis (backhand tennis elbow)
- Sit on a chair next to a table. Place the injured forearm on the table, palm down, with the elbow straight and the wrist and hand hanging over the edge. Hold a 1-pound weight in the hand. Slowly raise and lower the hand by bending and straightening the wrist. Repeat 10 times. Rest 1 minute, then do 2 more sets of 10. If the exercise causes pain, stop immediately and try again the next day. Do this exercise every other day. Increase the weight as the exercise becomes easier.

- With the palm down, hold a piece of wood the diameter of a broomstick with a 1-pound weight attached to it by a rope. Wind the weight up. Repeat 10 times. Stop if any pain is felt. Do this exercise every other day. Gradually increase the weight but not the number of repetitions.

- Place back of hand on a table with fingers directed toward the body and the elbow bent. Slowly extend the elbow, keeping the hand in contact with the table and hold this position for 10 seconds. Repeat 10 times. Stretch only to the point that it causes pain.

For medial epicondylitis (forehand tennis elbow)
- Sit on a chair next to a table. Place the injured forearm on the table, palm up, with the wrist and hand hanging over the edge. Hold a 1-pound weight in the hand. Slowly raise and lower the hand by bending and straightening the wrist. Repeat 10 times. Rest 1 minute, then do 2 more sets of 10. If the exercise causes pain, stop and try again the next day. As the exercise becomes easier, increase the weight.

- With the palm up, hold a piece of wood the diameter of a broomstick with a 1-pound weight attached to it by a rope. Wind the weight up. Repeat 20 times. Stop if the exercise becomes painful. Gradually increase the weight but not the number of repetitions.

- Several times a day, gently squeeze a soft sponge ball, then relax.

The first symptom is pain during a backhand stroke or other similar repetitive movements. Pain may occur with any exercise that requires extension of the wrist. The elbow hurts when the person places the arm and hand palm down on a table and tries to raise the hand against resistance by bending the wrist. Pain is felt along the outer, back side of the elbow and forearm on the same side as the thumb when the hand is by the side with the thumb away from the body. Continuing to play can extend the area of pain from the elbow down to the wrist and result in pain even at rest.

Treatment consists of applying ice and avoiding any exercise that produces pain. Exercises that do not use the wrist extensor muscles primarily, such as jogging, cycling, or basketball, can be substituted to maintain physical fitness. As the injury heals, flexibility and strengthening exercises can be started. Generally, all the muscles that bend and straighten the wrist should be strengthened. When lateral epicondylitis occurs persistently, a corticosteroid may need to be injected at the tendon that bends the elbow (flexor tendon), but exercises and altered use of the elbow are still needed or the problem will recur. The use of a brace may be helpful.

Medial Epicondylitis

Medial epicondylitis (forehand tennis elbow, baseball elbow, suitcase elbow) is damage to the tendons that bend the wrist toward the palm, causing pain on the palm side of the forearm from the elbow toward the wrist.

This injury is caused by bending the wrist toward the palm with excessive force. Factors that produce such force include having weak shoulder or hand muscles; serving with great force in tennis; using an overhand and a top spin serve; hitting heavy, wet balls; using a racket that is too heavy, has a grip that is too small, or has strings that are too tight; pitching a baseball; throwing a javelin; certain golf swings, and carrying a heavy suitcase. Continuing to exercise with pain can pull the tendons from the bone, causing bleeding.

Pain is felt in the palm side of the elbow and forearm on the same side as the smallest finger when bending the wrist toward the palm against resistance or when squeezing a hard rubber ball. To confirm the diagnosis, a doctor asks the person to sit in a chair with the injured arm resting on a table, palm up. The doctor holds the wrist down and asks the person to raise the hand by bending the wrist. A person who has medial epicondylitis feels pain at the elbow.

Any activity that causes pain when the wrist is bent toward the palm or turned so that the little finger is next to the body should be avoided. After the injury has healed, the person should strengthen the wrist and shoulder muscles, as well as the injured muscles. Surgery is rarely needed. Surgery is more common on the lateral side; the Nirschl procedure removes scar tissue from the muscle to promote healing.

Rotator Cuff Tendinitis

Rotator cuff tendinitis (swimmer's shoulder, tennis shoulder, pitcher's shoulder, shoulder impingement syndrome) is a tearing and swelling of the rotator cuff (the muscles and tendons that hold the upper arm in the shoulder joint).

Rotator cuff tendinitis often occurs in sports that require the arm to be moved over the head repeatedly, such as pitching in baseball, lifting heavy weights over the shoulder, serving the ball in racket sports, and swimming freestyle, butterfly, or backstroke. Repeatedly moving the arm over the head causes the top of the arm bone to rub against part of the shoulder joint and its tendons, tearing individual fibers. If the movement is continued despite the pain, the tendon can tear or actually pull off part of the bone.

Shoulder pain is the main symptom. Initially, the pain occurs only during activities that require lifting the arm over the head and forcibly bringing it forward. Later, pain can occur even when the arm is moved forward to shake hands. Usually, pushing objects away is painful, but pulling them in toward the body is not. The involved shoulder may be particularly painful at night, disrupting the person's sleep.

The diagnosis is made when specific movements, especially raising the arm above the shoulder, cause pain and soreness. Magnetic resonance imaging (MRI) is the best diagnostic tool for this condition.

Strengthening the Shoulders

Four-Quadrant Theraband Exercise

Tie a therapeutic rubber band at waist height to a doorknob. Facing the door with the arm at the side and the forearm parallel to the floor, pull back on the rubber band 10 times. Rotate body 90 degrees, and with the arm parallel to the floor, rotate the arm away from the chest 10 times. Then turn 90 degrees facing away from the door; still holding the rubber band, push the arm out in front of the body with the forearm parallel to the floor 10 times. Then turn 90 degrees with the elbow against the chest, and rotate the arm across the body to the abdomen with the arm parallel to the floor. Repeat this movement 10 times. Repeat the entire set of movements 3 times. This exercise restores strength to the rotator cuff and helps with overhead reaching activities.

Treatment consists of resting the injured tendons and strengthening the shoulder. Exercises that involve pushing something away or raising the elbows over the shoulder should be avoided. Another exercise consists of the person using an elastic cord; the person places the arm at the side with the forearm parallel to the floor. The arm is then moved forward, backward, and rotated out away from the chest and then back in across the chest. This exercise program should restore balance to the rotator cuff and decrease impingement of the rotator cuff during activities that involve reaching overhead. Surgery is sometimes needed when the injury is particularly severe, the tendon is completely torn, or the injury does not heal within a year. Surgery removes excess bone from the shoulder to create a larger space for the rotator cuff. The rotator cuff is repaired at the same time.

BRAIN, SPINAL CORD, AND NERVE DISORDERS

76 Biology of the Nervous System **433**

Brain ▪ Spinal Cord ▪ Peripheral Nerves ▪ Effects of Aging

77 Diagnosis of Brain, Spinal Cord, and Nerve Disorders...............**439**

Medical History ▪ Physical Examination ▪ Diagnostic Procedures

78 Pain **447**

Evaluation of Pain ▪ Types of Pain ▪ Treatment of Pain

79 Headaches..**456**

Tension-Type Headaches ▪ Migraine Headaches ▪ Cluster Headaches

80 Dizziness and Vertigo **461**

Vertigo ▪ Motion Sickness ▪ Benign Paroxysmal Positional Vertigo

81 Sleep Disorders **467**

Insomnia ▪ Hypersomnia ▪ Narcolepsy ▪ Sleep Apnea Syndromes ▪ Parasomnias ▪ Sleep Disorders in People With Dementia

82 Brain Dysfunction **475**

Dysfunction by Location ▪ Aphasia ▪ Dysarthria ▪ Apraxia ▪ Agnosia ▪ Amnesia

83 Delirium and Dementia **480**

Delirium ▪ Alzheimer's Disease ▪ Lewy Body Dementia ▪ Vascular Dementia ▪ Other Dementias

84 Stupor and Coma **490**

85 Seizure Disorders **495**

86 Stroke..**502**

Transient Ischemic Attacks ▪ Ischemic Stroke ▪ Hemorrhagic Stroke

87   Head Injuries 513

Skull Fracture ▪ Concussion ▪ Cerebral Contusions and
Lacerations ▪ Intracranial Hematomas

88   Tumors of the Nervous System 519

Brain Tumors ▪ Spinal Cord Tumors ▪ Neurofibromatosis ▪
Radiation Damage to the Nervous System

89   Infections of the Brain and Spinal Cord 529

Acute Bacterial Meningitis ▪ Chronic Meningitis ▪ Rabies ▪
Arbovirus Encephalitis ▪ Lymphocytic Choriomeningitis ▪
Progressive Multifocal Leukoencephalopathy ▪ Tropical Spastic
Paraparesis ▪ Brain Abscess ▪ Subdural Empyema ▪ Parasitic
Infections

90   Prion Diseases 541

Creutzfeldt-Jakob Disease ▪ Fatal Familial Insomnia ▪
Gerstmann-Sträussler-Scheinker Disease ▪ Kuru

91   Movement Disorders 544

Myoclonus ▪ Tremor ▪ Parkinson's Disease ▪ Progressive
Supranuclear Palsy ▪ Shy-Drager Syndrome ▪ Tics ▪ Chorea
and Athetosis ▪ Huntington's Disease ▪ Dystonia ▪
Coordination Disorders

92   Multiple Sclerosis and Related Disorders 556

93   Spinal Cord Disorders 561

Accident-Related Injuries ▪ Spinal Cord Compression ▪
Cervical Spondylosis ▪ Spinal Hematoma ▪ Syrinx ▪
Hereditary Spastic Paraparesis ▪ Acute Transverse Myelitis ▪
Blockage of the Blood Supply ▪ Subacute Combined Degeneration
of the Spinal Cord

94   Low Back Pain 568

95   Peripheral Nerve Disorders 575

Disorders of Muscle Stimulation ▪ Myasthenia Gravis ▪
Botulism ▪ Eaton-Lambert Syndrome ▪ Plexus Disorders ▪
Thoracic Outlet Syndromes ▪ Mononeuropathy ▪ Mononeuritis
Multiplex ▪ Polyneuropathy ▪ Guillain-Barré Syndrome ▪
Hereditary Neuropathies ▪ Spinal Muscular Atrophies

96   Cranial Nerve Disorders 588

Internuclear Ophthalmoplegia ▪ Palsies of Cranial Nerves That
Control Eye Movement ▪ Trigeminal Neuralgia ▪ Bell's Palsy ▪
Hemifacial Spasm ▪ Glossopharyngeal Neuralgia ▪
Hypoglossal Nerve Disorders

97   Smell and Taste Disorders 594

CHAPTER 76

Biology of the Nervous System

The nervous system has two distinct parts: the central nervous system (the brain and spinal cord) and the peripheral nervous system (the nerves outside the brain and spinal cord).

The basic unit of the nervous system is the nerve cell (neuron). Nerve cells consist of a large cell body and nerve fibers—one elongated extension (axon) for sending impulses and usually many branches (dendrites) for receiving impulses. Normally, nerves transmit impulses electrically in one direction—from the impulse-sending axon of one nerve cell to the impulse-receiving dendrites of the next nerve cell. At contact points between nerve cells (synapses), the axon secretes tiny amounts of chemical messengers called neurotransmitters. Neurotransmitters trigger the receptors on the next nerve cell's dendrites to start up a new electrical current. Different types of nerves use different neurotransmitters to convey impulses across the synapses.

The nervous system is an extraordinarily complex communication system that can send and receive voluminous amounts of information simultaneously. However, the system is vulnerable to diseases and injuries. For example, nerves can degenerate, causing Alzheimer's disease or Parkinson's disease. Bacteria or viruses can infect the brain or spinal cord, causing encephalitis or meningitis. A blockage in the blood supply to the brain can cause a stroke. Injuries or tumors can cause structural damage to the brain or spinal cord.

Brain

The brain's functions are both mysterious and remarkable. From the brain come all thoughts, beliefs, memories, behaviors, and moods. The brain is the site of thinking and the control center for the rest of the body. The brain coordinates the abilities to move, touch, smell, taste, hear, and see. It enables people to form words, understand and manipulate numbers, compose and appreciate music, recognize and understand geometric shapes, communicate with others, plan ahead, and even fantasize.

The brain reviews all stimuli—from the internal organs, surface of the body, eyes, ears, nose, and mouth. It then reacts to these stimuli by correcting the position of the body, the movement of limbs, and the rate at which the internal organs function. The brain can also adjust mood and levels of consciousness and alertness.

No computer has yet come close to matching the capabilities of the human brain. However, this sophistication comes with a price. The brain needs constant nourishment; it demands an extremely high and continuous flow of blood and oxygen—about 20% of the blood flow from the heart. A loss of blood flow to the brain for more than about 10 seconds can cause loss of consciousness. Lack of oxygen, abnormally low sugar (glucose) levels in the blood, or toxic substances can cause the brain to malfunction within minutes. However, the brain is defended by several mechanisms that can usually prevent these problems. For example, if blood flow to the brain decreases, the brain immediately signals the heart to beat faster and more forcefully and thus to pump more blood. If the sugar level in the blood becomes too low, the brain signals the adrenal glands to release epinephrine (adrenaline), which stimulates the liver to release stored sugar.

In spite of its high demand for oxygen and nutrients supplied by the blood, the brain is separated from the blood by a thin barrier called the blood-brain barrier. In the brain, unlike in most of the body, the cells that form the walls of the capillaries are tightly sealed, forming the blood-brain barrier. (Capillaries are the smallest of the body's blood vessels, where the exchange of nutrients and oxygen between the blood and tissues of the body occurs.) The blood-brain barrier limits the types of substances that can pass into the brain and thus protects brain cells from some potentially toxic substances. For example, penicillin, many chemotherapy drugs, and most proteins (such as albumin—the most abundant protein in blood) cannot pass into the brain except in very tiny amounts. On the other hand, alcohol, caffeine, nicotine, and antidepressants can pass into the brain. Some substances needed by the brain, such as sugar and amino acids, do not readily pass through the barrier. However, the blood-brain barrier has transport systems that move substances the brain needs across the barrier to brain tissue.

The activity of the brain results from electrical impulses generated by nerve cells (neurons), which process and store information. The impulses pass along the nerve fibers within the brain. How much and what type of brain activity occurs and where in the brain it is initiated depend on a person's level of consciousness and the specific activity that the person is performing.

The brain has three main parts: the cerebrum, the brain stem, and the cerebellum.

The **cerebrum** consists of dense, convoluted masses of tissue. The outer layer is the cerebral cortex (gray matter). In adults, the cerebral cortex contains most of the nerve cells in the nervous system. Underneath the cortex is the white matter, which consists mainly of nerve fibers that connect the nerve cells in the cortex with other parts of the nervous system.

The cerebrum is divided into two halves—the left and right cerebral hemispheres. The hemispheres are connected in the middle by nerve fibers called the corpus callosum. Each hemisphere is further divided into a frontal, parietal, occipital, and temporal lobe.

The frontal lobes initiate many voluntary actions, ranging from looking toward an object of interest, to crossing a street, to relaxing the bladder to urinate. The frontal lobes control learned motor skills, such as writing, playing musical instruments, and tying shoelaces. They also control complex intellectual processes, such as speech, thought, concentration, problem-solving, and planning for the future. They control facial expressions and hand and arm gestures and coordinate expressions and gestures with mood and feelings. Particular areas of the frontal lobes control specific movements, typically of the opposite side of the body. In most people, the left frontal lobe controls most language functions.

The parietal lobes interpret sensory information from the rest of the body and control body movement. They combine impressions of form, texture, and weight into general perceptions. These lobes influence mathematical and language skills, which are controlled more specifically by adjacent areas of the temporal lobes. The parietal lobes store spatial memories that enable people to orient themselves in space (know where they are) and to maintain a sense of direction (know where they are going). The parietal lobes also process informa-

tion that helps people know the position of their body parts.

The occipital lobes process and interpret vision, enable people to form visual memories, and integrate visual perceptions with the spatial information provided by the adjacent parietal lobes.

The temporal lobes generate memory and emotions. They process immediate events into recent and long-term memory as well as store and retrieve long-term memories. They also comprehend sounds and images, enabling people to recognize other people and objects and to integrate hearing and speech.

Collections of nerve cells—the basal ganglia, thalamus, and hypothalamus—are located at the base of the cerebrum. The basal ganglia coordinate and smooth out movements. The thalamus generally organizes sensory messages to and from the highest levels of the brain (cerebral cortex), providing a general awareness of such sensations as pain, touch, and temperature. The hypothalamus coordinates some of the more automatic functions of the body, such as control of sleep and wakefulness, maintenance of body temperature, and regulation of appetite and the balance of water within the body.

A system of nerve fibers—called the limbic system—connects the hypothalamus with other areas of the frontal and temporal lobes, which include the hippocampus and amygdala. The limbic system controls the experience and expression of emotions, as well as automatic functions of the body. By producing emotions (such as fear, anger, pleasure, and sadness), the limbic system enables people to behave in ways that help them communicate and survive physical and psychologic upsets. The hippocampus is also involved in the formation and retrieval of memories. Through the limbic system, memories that are emotionally charged are easier to recall than those that are not.

The **brain stem** connects the cerebrum with the spinal cord. A system of nerve cells and fibers (called the reticular activating system) located deep within the upper part of the brain stem controls levels of consciousness and alertness. The brain stem also automatically regulates critical body functions, such as breathing, swallowing, blood pressure, and heartbeat, and it helps adjust posture. If the entire brain stem becomes severely damaged, consciousness is lost, and these automatic body functions cease. Death soon follows.

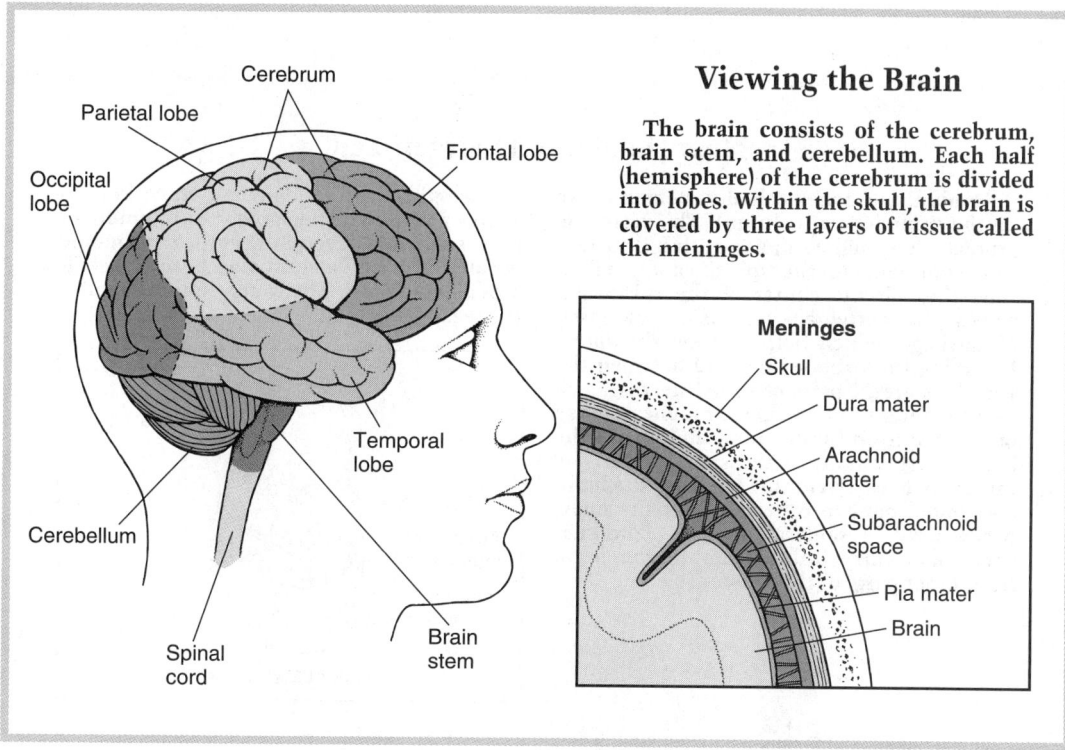

Viewing the Brain

The brain consists of the cerebrum, brain stem, and cerebellum. Each half (hemisphere) of the cerebrum is divided into lobes. Within the skull, the brain is covered by three layers of tissue called the meninges.

The **cerebellum,** which lies below the cerebrum just above the brain stem, coordinates the body's movements. With information it receives from the cerebral cortex and the basal ganglia about the position of the limbs, the cerebellum helps the limbs move smoothly and accurately. It does so by constantly adjusting muscle tone and posture. The cerebellum interacts with areas in the brain stem called vestibular nuclei, which are connected with the organs of balance (semicircular canals) in the inner ear. Together, these structures provide a sense of balance. The cerebellum also stores memories of practiced movements, enabling highly coordinated movements, such as a ballet dancer's pirouette, to be performed with speed and balance.

Both the brain and spinal cord are covered by three layers of tissue (meninges). The thin pia mater is the innermost layer, which adheres to the brain and spinal cord. The delicate, spider web–like arachnoid mater is the middle layer. The space between the arachnoid mater and the pia mater (the subarachnoid space) is a channel for cerebrospinal fluid, which helps protect the brain and spinal cord. Cerebrospinal fluid flows over the surface of

the brain between the meninges, fills internal spaces within the brain (the four ventricles), and cushions the brain against sudden jarring and minor injury. The leathery dura mater is the outermost and toughest layer. The brain and its meninges are contained in a tough, bony protective structure, the skull.

Spinal Cord

The spinal cord is a long, fragile tubelike structure that begins at the end of the brain stem and continues down almost to the bottom of the spine (spinal column). The spinal cord consists of nerves that carry both incoming and outgoing messages between the brain and the rest of the body. It is also the center for reflexes, such as the knee jerk reflex.▲ Like the brain, the spinal cord is covered by three layers of tissue (meninges). The spinal cord and meninges are contained in the spinal canal, which runs through the center of the spine. In most adults, the spine is composed of 26 vertebrae, which are the individual bones of the back. Just as the skull protects the

▲ see art on page 442

How the Spine Is Organized

A column of bones called vertebrae make up the spine (spinal column). The vertebrae protect the spinal cord, a long, fragile structure contained in the spinal canal, which runs through the center of the spine. Between the vertebrae are disks composed of cartilage, which help cushion the spine. Emerging from the spinal cord between the vertebrae are 31 pairs of spinal nerves. Each nerve emerges in two short branches (roots): one at the front (motor root) and one at the back (sensory root) of the spinal cord. The motor roots carry commands from the brain and spinal cord to other parts of the body, particularly to skeletal muscles. The sensory roots carry information to the brain from other parts of the body.

The spinal cord ends about three fourths of the way down the spine, but a bundle of nerves extends beyond the cord. This bundle is called the cauda equina because it resembles a horse's tail. The cauda equina supplies the legs.

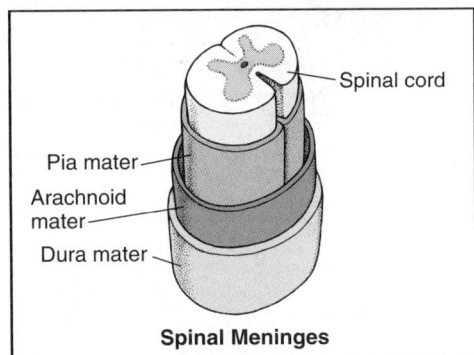

Spinal cord

Pia mater

Arachnoid mater

Dura mater

Spinal Meninges

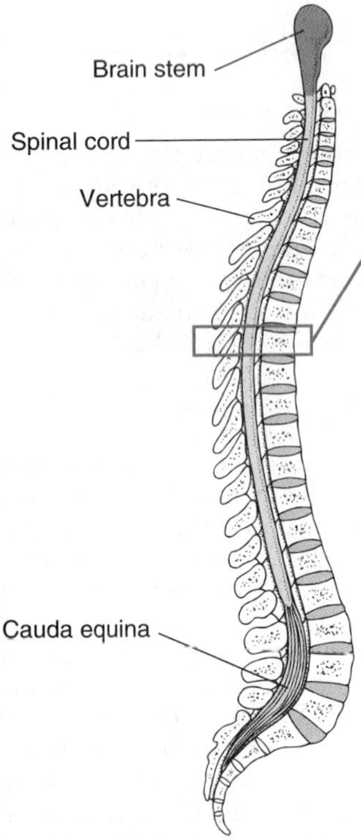

Brain stem

Spinal cord

Vertebra

Cauda equina

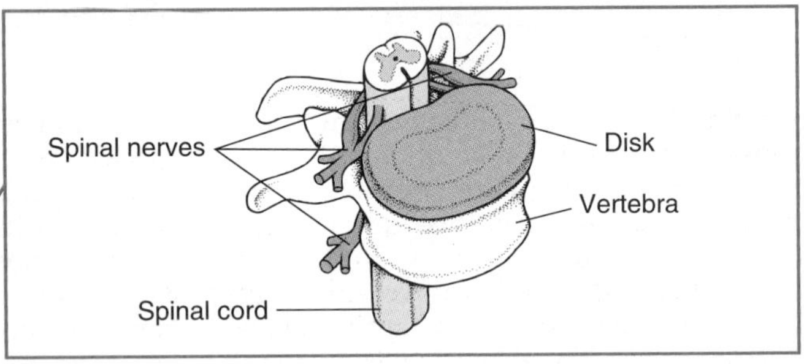

Spinal nerves

Disk

Vertebra

Spinal cord

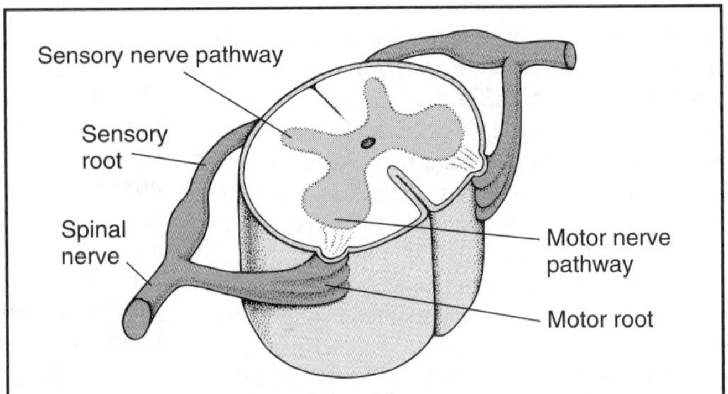

Sensory nerve pathway

Sensory root

Spinal nerve

Motor nerve pathway

Motor root

Spinal Cord Structure

brain, vertebrae protect the spinal cord. The vertebrae are separated by disks made of cartilage, which act as cushions, reducing the forces generated by movements such as walking and jumping.

Like the brain, the spinal cord consists of gray and white matter. The butterfly-shaped center of the cord consists of gray matter. The front "wings" (called horns) contain motor nerves, which transmit information from the brain or spinal cord to muscles, stimulating movement. The back horns contain sensory nerves, which transmit sensory information from other parts of the body through the spinal cord to the brain. The surrounding white matter contains columns of nerve fibers that carry sensory information to the brain from the rest of the body (ascending tracts) and columns that carry impulses from the brain to the muscles (descending tracts).

Peripheral Nerves

The peripheral nervous system consists of more than 100 billion nerve cells that run throughout the body like strings, making connections with the brain, other parts of the body, and often with each other. Peripheral nerves consist of bundles of nerve fibers. Nerves conduct impulses at different speeds depending on their diameter.

The peripheral nervous system has two parts: the somatic nervous system and the autonomic nervous system. The somatic nervous system consists of nerves that connect the brain and spinal cord with muscles controlled by conscious effort (voluntary or skeletal muscles) and with sensory receptors in the skin. (Sensory receptors are specialized endings of nerve fibers that detect information in and around the body.)

The autonomic nervous system connects the brain stem and spinal cord with internal organs and regulates internal body processes that require no conscious effort. Examples are the rate of heart contractions, blood pressure, the rate of breathing, the amount of stomach acid secreted, and the speed at which food passes through the digestive tract. The autonomic nervous system has two divisions: the sympathetic and the parasympathetic. These divisions work together, usually with one activating and the other inhibiting the actions of internal organs. The main function of the sympathetic division is to prepare the body for stressful or emergency situations—for fight or flight. The main function of the parasympathetic division is to prepare the body for ordinary situations. For example, the sympathetic division increases pulse, blood pressure, and breathing rates, and the parasympathetic system decreases each of them.

Cranial and Spinal Nerves: Nerves that connect the brain with the eyes, ears, nose, and

Typical Structure of a Nerve Cell

A nerve cell (neuron) consists of a large cell body and nerve fibers—one elongated extension (axon) for sending impulses and usually many branches (dendrites) for receiving impulses. Each large axon is surrounded by oligodendrocytes in the brain and spinal cord and by Schwann cells in the peripheral nervous system. The membranes of these cells consist of a fat (lipoprotein) called myelin. The membranes are wrapped tightly around the axon, forming a multilayered sheath. This myelin sheath resembles insulation, such as that around an electrical wire. Nerve impulses travel much faster in nerves with a myelin sheath than in those without one. If the myelin sheath of a nerve is damaged, nerve transmission slows or stops.

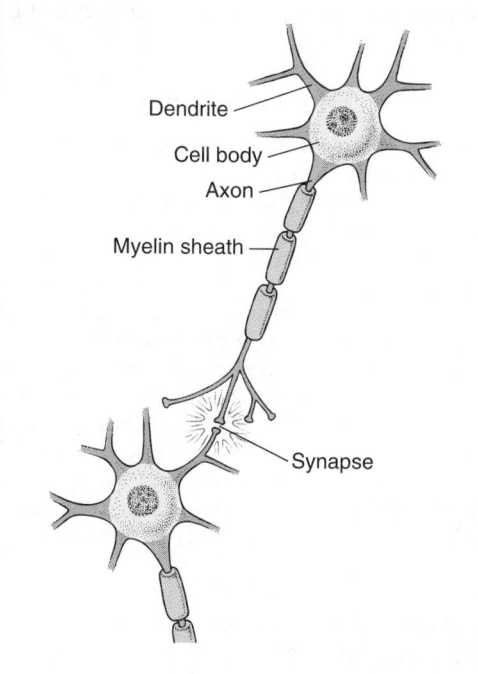

Dendrite

Cell body

Axon

Myelin sheath

Synapse

throat and with various parts of the head, neck, and trunk are called cranial nerves; there are 12 pairs of them.▲ Nerves that connect the spinal cord with other parts of the body are called spinal nerves. The brain communicates with most of the body through the spinal nerves. There are 31 pairs of them, located at intervals along the length of the spinal cord.■ Several cranial nerves and most spinal nerves are involved in both the somatic and autonomic parts of the peripheral nervous system.

Spinal nerves emerge from the spinal cord through spaces between the vertebrae. Each nerve emerges as two short branches (called spinal nerve roots): one at the front of the spinal cord and one at the back. Nerves at the front, which are motor nerves, carry commands from the brain and spinal cord to other parts of the body, particularly to skeletal muscles. Those at the back, which are sensory nerves, carry sensory information (about body position, light, touch, temperature, and pain) to the brain from other parts of the body. Each sensory nerve carries information from a specific area of the body, called a dermatome.★

After leaving the spinal cord, some spinal nerves form networks of interwoven nerves, called nerve plexuses. In a plexus, nerve fibers from different spinal nerves are sorted and recombined so that all fibers going to or coming from one area of a specific body part are put together in one nerve.●

Effects of Aging

Brain: Brain function varies normally as people pass from childhood through adulthood to old age. During childhood, the ability to think and reason steadily increases, enabling a child to learn increasingly complex skills. During most of adulthood, brain function is relatively stable. After a certain age, which varies from person to person, brain function declines. Different aspects of brain function are affected at different times. Short-term memory and the ability to learn new material tend to be affected relatively early. Verbal abilities, including vocabulary and word usage, may begin to decline at about age 70. Intellectual performance—the ability to process infor-

mation (regardless of speed)—is usually maintained until about age 80 if no neurologic disorders are present. Reaction time and performance of tasks may become slower because the brain processes nerve impulses more slowly. However, the effects of aging on brain function may be difficult to separate from the effects of various disorders that are common among older people. These disorders include depression, stroke, an underactive thyroid gland (hypothyroidism), and degenerative brain disorders such as Alzheimer's disease.

As people age, the number of nerve cells in the brain usually decreases, although the number lost varies greatly from person to person, depending on the person's health. As the number of nerve cells decreases, new connections are made between remaining nerve cells. These connections may help compensate for the loss of nerve cells. In addition, the brain has more cells than it needs to function normally—a characteristic called redundancy. Redundancy may also help compensate for the loss of nerve cells that occurs with aging and disease. Furthermore, new nerve cells may form in some areas of the brain, even during old age.

As people age, blood flow to the brain may decrease by an average of 20%. The decrease in blood flow is greater in people who have atherosclerosis affecting the arteries to the brain (cerebrovascular disease), which may be associated with smoking, high cholesterol levels, diabetes, or high blood pressure. The decreased blood flow that results from these conditions can cause nerve cells in the brain to be lost prematurely. Consequently, brain function may decline prematurely.

Spinal Cord: As people age, the bone of the spine may overgrow, putting pressure on the spinal cord. As a result, the number of axons in the spinal cord decreases, leading to a slight decrease in sensation.

Peripheral Nerves: As people age, peripheral nerves may conduct signals more slowly. Usually, this effect is so minimal that no change in function is noticeable. Also, the peripheral nervous system's response to injury is reduced. When the axon of a peripheral nerve is damaged in younger people, the nerve is able to repair itself as long as the cell body is undamaged. This self-reparation occurs more slowly and incompletely in older people than in younger people, making older people more vulnerable to injury and disease.

▲ see page 588   ■ see page 561
★ see art on page 563   ● see art on page 581

CHAPTER 77

Diagnosis of Brain, Spinal Cord, and Nerve Disorders

A neurologic examination can detect disorders of the brain, spinal cord, and nerves. This examination can also help detect muscle disorders because muscle contraction depends on stimulation by a nerve. The two main components of a neurologic examination are the medical history and the physical examination (including mental status evaluation). If necessary, diagnostic procedures are performed to confirm the diagnosis or exclude other possible disorders.

A neurologic examination differs from a psychiatric examination, which focuses on a person's behavior. However, the two examinations overlap somewhat because abnormal behavior often provides clues about the brain's physical condition.

Medical History

Before performing a physical examination, doctors interview the person. Doctors ask the person to describe current symptoms, telling precisely where and how often they occur, how severe they are, how long they last, and whether daily activities can still be performed. Many different symptoms can be caused by neurologic disorders, but such symptoms can be caused by other disorders.

The person is also asked about past or present illnesses and past operations, serious illnesses in close blood relatives, allergies, and drugs currently being taken. In addition, doctors may ask if the person has had work-related or home-related difficulties, such as loss of a loved one, because such circumstances may affect the person's health and ability to cope with illness.

Physical Examination

When a neurologic disorder is suspected, doctors usually evaluate all of the body systems during the physical examination but focus on the nervous system. The neurologic aspect includes evaluation of mental status, cranial nerves, motor and sensory nerves, reflexes, coordination, stance, gait, regulation of internal body processes (by the autonomic nervous system), and blood flow to the brain.

Mental Status: Doctors evaluate the person's attention; orientation to time, place, and person; memory; and various abilities, such as thinking abstractly, following commands, using language, and solving math problems. The evaluation consists of a series of questions and tasks, such as naming objects, recalling short lists, writing sentences, and copying shapes. The person's answers are recorded and scored for accuracy. Mood is also evaluated. If the person reports feeling depressed, doctors ask if there have been any thoughts of suicide.

Cranial Nerves: Doctors test the function of the 12 cranial nerves, which are connected directly to the brain.▲ How many nerves are tested depends on what type of disorder is suspected. For example, cranial nerve I (the nerve of smell) is not usually tested when a muscle disorder is suspected, but it is tested when a head injury has occurred. A cranial nerve may be damaged anywhere along its length as a result of an injury, a tumor, or an infection. The exact site of the damage must be identified.

Motor and Sensory Nerves: Motor nerves carry impulses from the brain to the voluntary muscles (muscles controlled by conscious effort), such as leg muscles. Weakness or paralysis of a muscle may indicate damage to a motor nerve. Doctors look for muscle wasting (atrophy), which results when a motor nerve is not stimulating the muscle, and then test for weakness in various muscles by asking the person to push or pull against resistance.

Sensory nerves carry information to the brain about such things as touch, pain, heat, cold, vibration, the position of body parts, and the shape of objects. Abnormal sensations or reduced perception of sensations may indicate damage to a sensory nerve. Doctors may be able to pinpoint the specific location (level) of damage to the spinal cord by evaluating sensory nerves. Sensory nerves carry information from specific areas on the body's surface, called

▲ see table on page 590

What Is a Neurologic Symptom?

Neurologic symptoms—symptoms caused by a disorder that affects part or all of the nervous system—can be almost anything, because the nervous sytem controls all body functions. However, many symptoms that can be neurologic, such as headache, are usually caused by other disorders. Neurologic disorders commonly cause pain. Muscles may malfunction because a nerve is damaged or compressed. Changes in sensation, including vision, may occur. Neurologic disorders can interfere with sleep or affect the level or content of consciousness. Neurologic symptoms may indicate a relatively minor disorder (such as a foot that has fallen asleep), a disorder that can be corrected or controlled with treatment (such as a herniated disk or diabetes), or a serious, life-threatening disorder (such as a brain tumor). Often, the characteristics and pattern of symptoms help doctors diagnose or exclude a neurologic disorder. The following are some relatively common neurologic symptoms:

Pain
- Back pain
- Neck pain
- Headache
- Pain along a nerve pathway (as in sciatica or shingles)

Muscle malfunction
- Weakness
- Tremor
- Paralysis
- Involuntary movements (such as tics)
- Abnormalities in walking
- Clumsiness or poor coordination
- Muscle spasms
- Rigidity
- Slowed movements

Changes in sensation
- Blurred vision
- Partial or complete loss of vision
- Deafness

- Tingling or a pins-and-needles sensation
- Vertigo
- Double vision
- Misinterpretation of visual images
- Loss of sensation for touch, cold, heat, or pain
- Loss of position sense

Sleep problems
- Difficulty falling or staying asleep
- Uncontrollable leg movements
- Sleeping too much (such as narcolepsy)

Changes in consciousness
- Dizziness
- Fainting
- Dissociation
- Confusion or delirium
- Dementia
- Seizures
- Coma
- Stupor
- Persistent vegetative state

dermatomes,▲ to a specific level of the spinal cord. Therefore, loss of sensation in areas on the body's surface supplied by a specific level of the spinal cord and the levels below it indicates damage to that level of the spinal cord.

The surface of the body is tested for loss of sensation. Usually, doctors concentrate on the area where the person feels numbness, tingling, or pain. A pin is used first, then a blunt object (such as the head of a safety pin) to see if the person can tell the difference between sharp and dull sensations. The person's ability to detect a gentle touch, heat, and vibration may be tested. To test position sense, doctors

tell the person to close the eyes; then they move the person's finger or toe up or down and ask the person to describe its position.

Reflexes: A reflex is an automatic response to a stimulus. For example, the lower leg jerks when the tendon below the kneecap is gently tapped with a small rubber hammer. The pathway that a reflex follows (reflex arc) is a complete circuit, without involvement of the brain. Doctors test reflexes to determine whether the sensory nerve to the spinal cord, the nerve connections in the spinal cord, and the motor nerves back to the muscle are all functioning. The reflexes most commonly tested are the knee jerk and similar reflexes at the elbow and ankle.

▲ see art on page 563

A test for Babinski's sign is performed by firmly stroking the outer border of the sole of the foot with a key or other object that causes minor discomfort. Normally, the toes curl downward, except in infants aged 6 months or younger. Having the big toe go upward and the other toes spread out is a sign of an abnormality in the brain or spinal cord.

Coordination, Stance, and Gait: To test coordination, doctors ask a person first to use the forefinger to reach out and touch their finger, then the person's own nose, and then to repeat these actions rapidly. The person may be asked to perform these actions first with the eyes open, then with the eyes closed. For the Romberg test, the person may be asked to stand still with both feet together and the eyes closed. Then the person may be asked to walk in a straight line, placing one foot in front of the other. These actions test the motor and sensory nerves as well as brain function. Other simple tests may also be performed.

Autonomic Nervous System: The autonomic (involuntary) nervous system regulates internal body processes that require no conscious effort. An abnormality of this system may cause such problems as a fall in blood pressure when a person stands (orthostatic hypotension), reduction or absence of sweating, or sexual problems such as difficulty initiating or maintaining an erection. Doctors may perform a variety of tests, such as measuring blood pressure while the person is sitting and after the person stands.

Blood Flow to the Brain: A severe narrowing of the arteries that carry blood to the brain reduces blood flow and puts a person at risk of stroke. The risk is higher for people who are

MENTAL STATUS TESTING

WHAT PEOPLE MAY BE ASKED TO DO	WHAT THIS TEST INDICATES
State the current date and place, and name specific people	Orientation to time, place, and person
Repeat a short list of objects	Attention
Recall the short list of objects after 3 to 5 minutes	Immediate recall
Describe an event that happened in the last day or two	Recent memory
Describe events from the distant past	Remote memory
Interpret a proverb (such as "a rolling stone gathers no moss"), or explain a particular analogy (such as "why the brain is like a computer")	Abstract thinking
Describe feelings and opinions about the illness	Insight into illness
Name the last five presidents and the state capital	Fund of knowledge
Tell how they feel on this day and how they usually feel	Mood
Follow a simple command that involves three different body parts and requires distinguishing right from left (such as "put your right thumb over your left ear and stick out your tongue")	Ability to follow simple commands
Name simple objects and body parts, and read, write, and repeat certain phrases	Ability to use language
Identify small objects held in the hand and numbers written on the palm, and discriminate between being touched in one or two places (for example, on the palm and on the fingers)	Ability of the brain to process information from sense organs
Copy simple and complex structures (for example, using building blocks) or finger positions, and draw a clock, cube, or house	Ability to understand spatial relationships
Brush the teeth or take a match out of a box and strike it	Ability to perform an action
Perform simple arithmetic	Ability to solve math problems

Reflex Arc: A No-Brainer

A reflex arc is the pathway that a nerve reflex, such as the knee jerk reflex, follows.

1. A tap on the knee stimulates sensory receptors, generating a nerve signal.
2. The signal travels along a nerve pathway to the spinal cord.
3. At the spinal cord, the signal is transmitted from the sensory nerve to a motor nerve.
4. The motor nerve sends the signal back to a muscle in the thigh.
5. The muscle contracts, causing the lower leg to jerk upward. The entire reflex occurs without involving the brain.

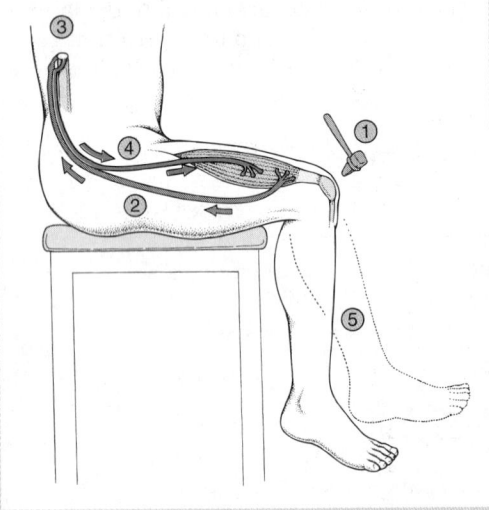

older or who have high blood pressure, diabetes, or disorders of the arteries or heart. To evaluate the arteries, doctors place a stethoscope on the neck and listen for characteristic sounds caused by turbulent blood flow through a narrowed area (bruits). However, procedures such as color Doppler ultrasonography, magnetic resonance angiography, or cerebral angiography are needed for an accurate evaluation of narrowed arteries.

Diagnostic Procedures

Diagnostic procedures may be needed to confirm a diagnosis suggested by the medical history and physical examination.

▲ see art on page 1284   ■ see art on page 515

Spinal Tap

For a spinal tap (lumbar puncture), a sample of the fluid that surrounds the brain and spinal cord (cerebrospinal fluid) is withdrawn with a needle and sent to a laboratory for examination.

Examination of the cerebrospinal fluid can detect evidence of infections, injuries, tumors, and bleeding in the brain and spinal cord. These disorders may change the appearance and content of the cerebrospinal fluid, which is normally clear and colorless. For example, white blood cells in the cerebrospinal fluid make it appear cloudy and suggest a bacterial infection of the layers of tissue covering the brain and spinal cord (bacterial meningitis).

High protein levels in the fluid indicate damage to the brain, the spinal cord, or a spinal nerve root, which is the part of a spinal nerve next to the spinal cord, but they do not indicate the cause of the damage. Abnormal antibodies in the fluid suggest multiple sclerosis. Low sugar (glucose) levels suggest meningitis or cancer. Blood in the fluid suggests a brain hemorrhage. Many disorders, including brain tumors and meningitis, can increase the fluid's pressure.

Before performing a spinal tap, doctors use an ophthalmoscope to examine the optic nerve,▲ which bulges when the pressure within the skull is increased. If the pressure is increased because of a mass (such as a tumor) within the skull, performing a spinal tap may result in herniation of the brain,■ a potentially fatal complication. Results of the neurologic examination may help doctors determine whether a mass is present. If doctors are still unsure, computed tomography (CT) of the head is performed.

For a spinal tap, a needle is inserted between two vertebrae in the lower spine below the end of the spinal cord. During a spinal tap, doctors can directly measure the pressure within the skull. Pressure is measured by attaching a gauge (manometer) to the needle used for the spinal tap and noting the height of the cerebrospinal fluid in the gauge.

A spinal tap usually takes no more than 15 minutes and is usually performed at the person's bedside. A local anesthetic is used to numb the insertion site.

About 1 of 10 people develop a headache when they stand up after a spinal tap. The headache usually disappears after a few days to weeks. Other problems are very rare.

How a Spinal Tap Is Performed

A small, hollow needle is inserted between two vertebrae in the lower spine, usually the third and fourth lumbar vertebrae, below the point where the spinal cord ends, and a sample of cerebrospinal fluid is withdrawn. (Cerebrospinal fluid is contained in the space between the middle and inner layers of tissue covering the spinal cord—the subarachnoid space.) Cerebrospinal fluid is allowed to drip into a test tube, and the sample is sent to a laboratory for examination.

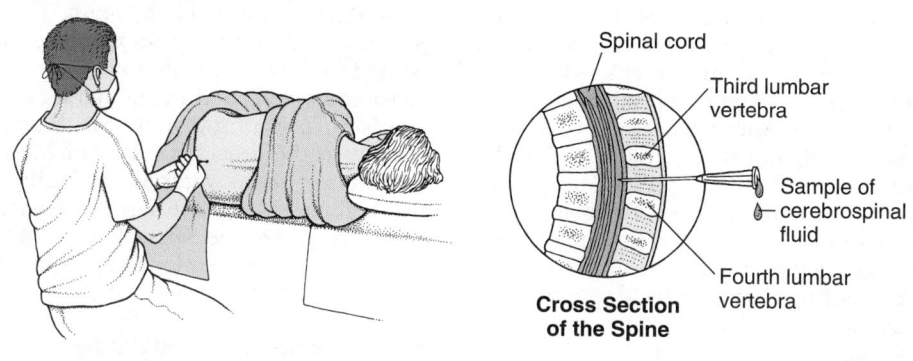

Spinal cord

Third lumbar vertebra

Sample of cerebrospinal fluid

Fourth lumbar vertebra

Cross Section of the Spine

Computed Tomography

Computed tomography (CT) is a computer-enhanced scanning technique for analyzing a series of x-rays taken from different angles. A computer generates two-dimensional, high-resolution images that resemble anatomic slices of the organ being imaged.

CT can precisely detect a wide range of brain and spinal cord disorders, such as hydrocephalus, birth defects, tumors, areas of dead brain tissue due to stroke, and a ruptured or herniated disk. CT is used not only to diagnose neurologic disorders but also to monitor the effectiveness of treatment—for example, treatment of a brain abscess with antibiotics and treatment of brain cancer with radiation therapy. CT provides clearer images of abnormalities affecting the skull and spine and of bleeding due to hemorrhagic stroke during the first 24 hours afterward than does magnetic resonance imaging (MRI).

A person must lie still during the procedure, so that the image will not be blurred. The procedure may take 15 minutes to 1 hour, depending on the part of the body being scanned and the degree of resolution needed. For example, after an injury, fast CT with low resolution may be performed to obtain results quickly.

For spiral (helical) CT, the scanner rapidly rotates around the person and takes many x-rays in sequence. This procedure can provide images of blood vessels that are almost as clear as those obtained with magnetic resonance angiography.▲

A radiopaque dye, which can be seen on x-rays, may be injected intravenously to enhance abnormalities in the images. When the dye is injected, the person may feel a warm sensation throughout the body. A few people have an allergic reaction to the dye.

Magnetic Resonance Imaging

Magnetic resonance imaging (MRI) of the brain or spinal cord uses a magnetic field and very high frequency radio waves to produce highly detailed anatomic images. MRI detects most neurologic disorders (including previous strokes, most brain tumors, abnormalities of the brain stem and cerebellum, and multiple sclerosis) better than CT.

For the procedure, the person is placed in a tubular electromagnetic chamber and pulsed with radio waves, causing tissues in the body to emit radio signals back. These signals are converted to images. In about one fourth of

▲ see page 444

the procedures, a substance that is weakly attracted by strong magnetic fields (paramagnetic contrast agent) is injected intravenously to enhance the images. No x-rays are involved, and MRI is usually very safe. As during CT, the person must lie still. A complete scan may take from 10 to 90 minutes, depending on the part of the body being scanned.

MRI can be used in different ways to investigate the brain. The same machine is used for all, but different software is used. Functional MRI can produce images of areas in the brain that are active in performing a task, whether it is reading, writing, remembering, calculating, or moving a limb. Another use involves identifying certain chemicals in small areas of the brain so that a brain tumor can be distinguished from a brain abscess. Perfusion MRI can be used to estimate blood flow in a particular area. Diffusion MRI can be used to detect the sudden accumulation of fluid (edema).

MRI cannot be used for people who have an artificial pacemaker, magnetic metallic clips (used to treat aneurysms), or other movable, magnetic devices in their body because the magnetic field may cause movement, overheating, or other dysfunction of the device. Other metal devices, such as an artificial hip and the rods used to straighten the spine, are not affected by MRI. CT is used when MRI cannot be. People who are dependent on ventilators can be attached to special ventilators that have no magnetic parts, or a technician can stay with them and manually supply them with oxygen using a bag and mask.

Giving people who are prone to severe claustrophobia a sedative may help. Alternatively, an MRI scanner that has one or more open sides (open MRI) can be used. This procedure eliminates the need for a person to be placed in a narrow tube. Open MRI is also useful for people who are overweight and cannot fit into the MRI tube. However, the images are somewhat less clear and less detailed than those produced by standard closed MRI.

Magnetic Resonance Angiography

Magnetic resonance angiography (MRA) is magnetic resonance imaging (MRI) that is used to produce images of blood vessels of the head and neck. MRA is often used with MRI to evaluate people who have had a stroke. MRA is also useful when the risks of cerebral angiography are too high for a particular person or when a person refuses cerebral angiography.

Unlike cerebral angiography, MRA is not an invasive procedure, does not require insertion of a catheter into an artery, and may not require an intravenous injection of a paramagnetic contrast agent. However, cerebral angiography provides more accurate images of blood vessels than MRA.

Echoencephalography

Echoencephalography uses ultrasound waves to produce an image of the brain. This simple, painless, and relatively inexpensive procedure is used mainly for children younger than 2 because their skull is thin enough for ultrasound waves to pass through. It can be performed quickly at the bedside to detect hydrocephalus (commonly called water on the brain) or bleeding. CT and MRI have largely replaced echoencephalography because they produce much better images, especially in older children and adults.

Positron Emission Tomography

In positron emission tomography (PET), a substance necessary for brain function (such as oxygen or sugar) is labeled with a radioactive molecule (radionuclide) that gives off positively charged signals (positrons) for a very short time. PET can provide information about seizure disorders, brain tumors, and strokes. However, functional MRI, which is less invasive and does not involve radioactivity, has replaced PET. PET is used mainly in research.

For the procedure, the labeled substance, called a tracer, is injected into a vein. It is distributed throughout the brain in about 1 minute. The person's head is placed within a ring-shaped PET scanner, which detects radiation from different angles and records sites of high activity. The more metabolically active an area of the brain, the larger the amount of tracer it takes up and the more radiation given off. The resulting scan shows the different levels of activity in different colors. For example, the procedure may show which part of the brain is most active during mathematical calculations. A computer can be used to construct a three-dimensional image of the area. The radioactivity is low level, does not injure the body, and disappears within hours.

Single Photon Emission Computed Tomography

Single photon emission computed tomography (SPECT) uses radionuclides to produce images of blood flow to the brain. The radionuclides are injected intravenously, reaching the brain through the bloodstream. How much of the radionuclide brain tissue takes up provides an estimate of how much blood is flowing through it. A rotating camera detects the energy (gamma-ray photons) given off by the radionuclide. A computer analyzes this information and constructs a cross-sectional or three-dimensional image. The procedure is not very accurate, and it is not as specific as positron emission tomography. It has been largely replaced by perfusion MRI.

Cerebral Angiography

Cerebral angiography (arteriography) is an invasive procedure used to detect abnormalities in the blood vessels of the brain. Cerebral angiography can detect a bulge in the weakened wall of an artery (aneurysm), inflammation of arteries (arteritis), a blood vessel (arteriovenous) malformation, or a blocked blood vessel, which can cause a stroke.

For the procedure, a catheter is inserted through an incision into an artery, usually in the groin. A local anesthetic is given to numb the insertion site. The catheter is then threaded through the aorta to an artery in the neck. After the catheter is in place, a radiopaque dye is injected through the catheter into the artery. The radiopaque dye outlines the blood vessels so that blood flow patterns in the brain can be seen on x-rays. The images of blood vessels produced by cerebral angiography are more detailed than those of MRA.

Color Doppler Ultrasonography

Color Doppler ultrasonography shows different rates of blood flow in different colors.▲ It is used mainly to measure blood flow through the arteries in the neck (carotid arteries) or through the arteries at the base of the brain (vertebral arteries, basilar arteries, circle of Willis, and middle cerebral arteries) and to identify and evaluate narrowing or blockage of these arteries. Thus, color Doppler ultrasonography can help assess the risk of stroke. The procedure is useful for evaluating people who have had a transient ischemic attack and people who have risk factors for atherosclerosis but no symptoms.

For this painless procedure, a handheld recording probe (transducer) that emits high-frequency (ultrasound) waves is used. The waves bounce off structures in the body and produce a moving image. After placing gel on the person's neck, the examiner moves the probe over that area. The probe is connected to a monitor that displays the image. Color Doppler ultrasonography can be performed at the person's bedside or in the doctor's office, is relatively inexpensive, and does not use x-rays.

Myelography

In myelography, x-rays of the spinal cord are taken after a radiopaque dye, usually iohexol, is injected into the cerebrospinal fluid via a spinal tap. Myelography has been largely replaced by MRI, which produces more detailed images, is simpler, and is safer. Myelography with CT is still used when additional detail of the spinal canal and surrounding bone, which MRI cannot provide, is needed. Myelography with CT is also used in emergencies when MRI is not available.

Electroencephalography

Electroencephalography (EEG) is a quick, simple, painless procedure in which the brain's electrical activity is recorded as wave patterns on a strip of moving paper or is collected in a database on a computer.■ EEG can help identify seizure disorders, sleep disturbances, and certain metabolic or structural disorders of the brain. For example, EEG can show the characteristic patterns of electrical activity associated with confusion due to liver failure and the reduced electrical activity produced by damage to the brain (such as that due to stroke).

For the procedure, an examiner places small, round adhesive sensors (electrodes) on the person's scalp. The electrodes are connected by wires to a machine, which produces a record (tracing) of small changes in voltage detected by each electrode. These tracings constitute the electroencephalogram.

For people who have a seizure disorder, EEG is performed after a long period without sleep because sleep deprivation tends to increase seizure activity. EEG is also performed after the person is asked to breathe deeply and rapidly (hyperventilate) and is exposed to a flashing light, because both can trigger abnormal electrical activity.

Sometimes (for example, when a behavior that resembles a seizure is difficult to distinguish from a psychiatric disorder), the brain's

---

▲ see also page 126

■ see art on page 498

electrical activity is recorded for 24 hours or longer while the person is monitored in the hospital by a television camera. The camera detects the seizure-like behavior, and examination of the EEG at that moment reveals either seizure activity or continued normal electrical activity, indicating a psychiatric disorder.

Evoked Responses

Stimuli for sight, sound, and touch are used to activate specific areas of the brain, that is, to evoke responses. For example, a flashing light stimulates the retina of the eye, the optic nerve, and the nerve pathway to the back part of the brain where vision is perceived and interpreted. Electroencephalography (EEG) is used to detect electrical activity evoked by the stimuli. Ordinarily, the brain's response to one stimulus is too slight to be detected by EEG. However, if many stimuli are used, the brain's responses to them can be averaged by a computer to produce a wave pattern.

Evoked responses provide information about how an area of the brain is functioning. This procedure is particularly useful in testing how well the senses are functioning in infants and children. For example, doctors can test an infant's hearing by checking for a response after a clicking sound is made at each ear. Evoked responses are also useful in identifying the effects of multiple sclerosis and other disorders on areas of the optic nerve, brain stem, and spinal cord. Such effects may or may not be detected by MRI.

Electromyography

In electromyography, small needles are inserted into a muscle to record the electrical activity of a muscle when the muscle is at rest and when it is contracting. Normally, resting muscle produces no electrical activity. A slight contraction produces some electrical activity, which increases as the contraction increases.

This procedure is used with nerve conduction studies to help doctors diagnose disorders of muscles, peripheral nerves, spinal nerve roots, and the neuromuscular junction. Disorders that weaken the nerve's connection to a muscle produce abnormal electrical activity in muscles. Examples of such disorders are carpal tunnel syndrome and diabetic neuropathy. Disorders of the muscle itself (the nerve is normal) produce a different kind of electrical activity. Polymyositis is an example of a muscle disorder.

Nerve Conduction Studies

Nerve conduction studies measure the speed at which motor or sensory nerves conduct impulses. Nerve conduction studies are used to determine whether symptoms such as muscle weakness are caused by a nerve disorder. If muscle weakness is caused by a nerve disorder (such as carpal tunnel syndrome, in which a nerve is pinched by ligaments in the wrist), the nerve conduction speed is usually slowed. If muscle weakness is caused by a muscle disorder, the nerve conduction speed remains normal. If muscle weakness is caused by a disorder of the brain or spinal cord, nerve conduction speed and electromyography results are normal. Weakness can also result when the connection between a normal nerve and a normal muscle (neuromuscular junction) malfunctions. Examples include myasthenia gravis, botulism, and diphtheria.

For the procedure, the nerve being tested is stimulated with a small charge of electricity to trigger an impulse. The charge may be delivered with several electrodes placed on the surface of the skin or with several needles inserted along the pathway of the nerve thought to be affected. The impulse moves along the nerve, eventually reaching the muscle and causing it to contract. By measuring the time the impulse takes to reach the muscle and the distance from the stimulating electrode or needle to the muscle, doctors can calculate the speed of the impulse.

A nerve may be stimulated repeatedly to determine how well the connection between the nerve and muscle is functioning. At this connection, the nerve impulse must cross from the nerve to the muscle. If this connection is malfunctioning (as in myasthenia gravis), nerve conduction studies using repeated stimulation of the nerve detect a progressively weaker response of the muscle.

CHAPTER 78

Pain

Pain may be sharp or dull, intermittent or constant, or throbbing or steady. Sometimes pain is very difficult to describe. Pain may be felt at a single site or over a large area. The intensity of pain can vary from minor to intolerable.

People differ remarkably in their ability to tolerate pain. One person cannot tolerate the pain of a small cut or bruise, but another person can tolerate pain caused by a major accident or knife wound with little complaint. The ability to withstand pain varies according to mood, personality, and circumstance. In a moment of excitement during an athletic match, an athlete may not notice a severe bruise but is likely to be very aware of the pain after the match, particularly if the team lost.

The ability to tolerate pain may change with age. As people age, they complain less of pain, perhaps because changes in the body decrease the sensation of pain. On the other hand, older people may simply be more stoic than younger people.

Pain Pathways: Pain due to injury begins at special pain receptors scattered throughout the body. These pain receptors transmit messages or signals as electrical impulses along nerves to the spinal cord and then upward to the brain. Sometimes the signal evokes a reflex response.▲ When the signal reaches the spinal cord, a signal is immediately sent back along motor nerves to the original site of the pain, triggering the muscles to contract without involving the brain. For example, when people inadvertently touch something very hot, they immediately pull away. This reflex reaction helps prevent permanent damage. The pain signal is also sent to the brain. Only when the brain processes the signal and interprets it as pain do people become conscious of the pain.

Pain receptors and their nerve pathways differ in different parts of the body. For this reason, pain sensation varies with the type and location of injury. For example, pain receptors in the skin are plentiful and capable of transmitting precise information, including where an injury is located and whether the source was sharp, such as a knife wound, or dull, such as pressure, heat, or cold. In contrast, pain receptors in the intestine are limited and imprecise. The intestine can be pinched, cut, or burned without generating a pain signal. However, stretching and pressure can cause severe intestinal pain, even from something as relatively harmless as a trapped gas bubble. The brain cannot identify the precise source of intestinal pain; the pain is difficult to locate and is likely to be felt over a large area.

Sometimes pain felt in one area of the body does not accurately represent where the problem is, because the pain is referred there from another area. Pain can be referred because signals from several areas of the body often travel through the same nerve pathways going to the spinal cord and brain. For example, pain from a heart attack may be felt in the neck, jaws, arms, or abdomen. Pain from a gallbladder attack may be felt in the back of the shoulder.

Evaluation of Pain

Doctors ask about the history and characteristics of pain, so that they can identify its cause and develop a treatment strategy. To evaluate the severity of pain, doctors sometimes use a scale of 0 (none) to 10 (severe) or ask the person to describe the pain as mild, moderate, severe, or excruciating. For children, drawings of faces in a series—from smiling to frowning and crying—can be used to determine the severity of pain. No laboratory test can document the presence or the severity of pain.

Doctors always try to determine whether a bodily injury or disease is causing the pain; they also consider psychologic causes. Many chronic disorders (such as cancer, arthritis, sickle cell anemia, and inflammatory bowel disease) cause pain, as do acute disorders (such as wounds, burns, torn muscles, broken bones, sprained ligaments, appendicitis, kidney stones, and a heart attack). Psychologic disorders (such as depression and anxiety) can worsen pain. Sometimes pain is determined to be caused mostly or completely by psychologic disorders; such pain is called psychogenic pain.

▲ see art on page 442

What Is Referred Pain?

Pain felt in one area of the body does not always represent where the problem is, because the pain may be referred there from another area. For example, pain produced by a heart attack may feel as if it is coming from the arm because sensory information from the heart and the arm converge on the same nerve cells in the spinal cord.

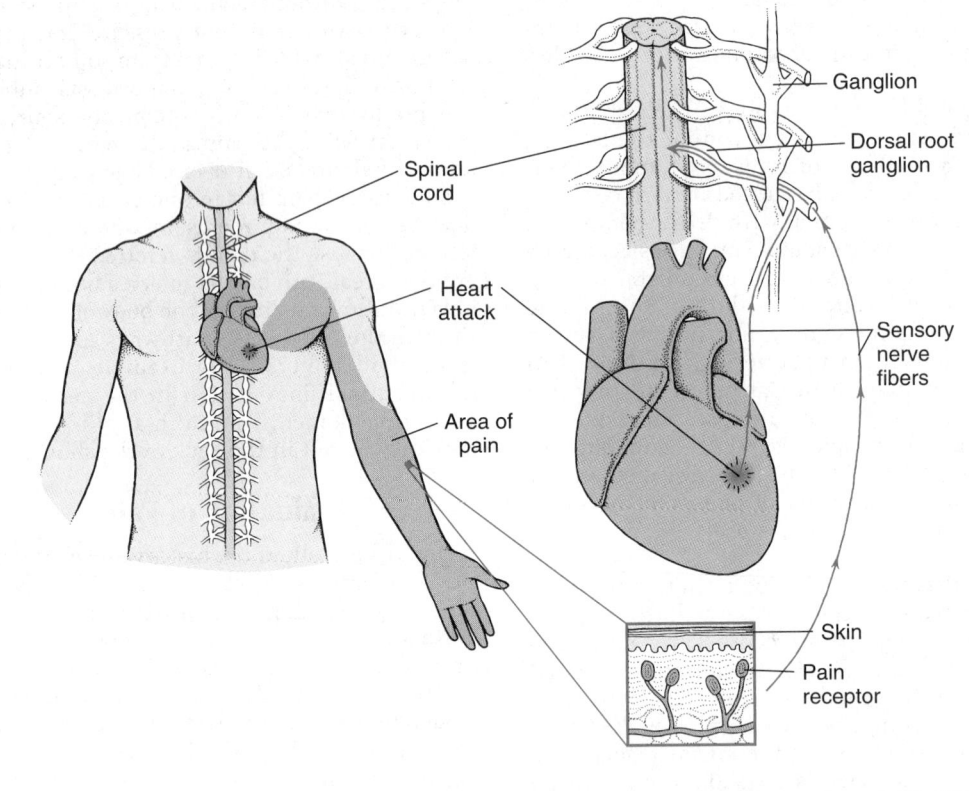

Doctors also consider whether pain is acute or chronic. Acute pain begins suddenly and usually does not last long. When severe, it may cause anxiety, a rapid heartbeat, an increased breathing rate, elevated blood pressure, sweating, and dilated pupils. Chronic pain persists for weeks or months. The term usually describes pain that persists for more than 1 month beyond the usual course of an illness or injury, pain that recurs off and on for months or years, or pain that is associated with a chronic disorder such as cancer. Usually, chronic pain does not affect the heartbeat, breathing rate, blood pressure, or pupils, but it may result in other problems, such as depression, disturbed sleep, decreased energy, loss of appetite, weight loss, and loss of interest in sexual activity.

Many people who are being treated for chronic pain may experience a brief, often severe flare-up of pain. It is called breakthrough pain because it breaks through the regularly scheduled pain treatment. Typically, breakthrough pain begins suddenly, lasts up to 1 hour, and feels much like the person's chronic pain except it is more severe. Breakthrough pain may differ from person to person and is often unpredictable.

Types of Pain

There are several types of pain, including nociceptive pain (such as pain after surgery and pain due to cancer), neuropathic pain (such as sciatica▲), and psychogenic pain.

NOCICEPTIVE PAIN

Nociceptive pain is caused by an injury to body tissues.

The injury may be a cut, bruise, bone fracture, crush injury, burn, or anything that damages tissues. This type of pain is typically aching, sharp, or throbbing. Most pain is nociceptive pain. Pain receptors for tissue injury (nociceptors) are located mostly in the skin or in the internal organs.

The pain almost universally experienced after surgery is nociceptive pain. The pain may be constant or intermittent, often worsening when a person moves, coughs, laughs, or breathes deeply or when the dressings over the surgical wound are changed.

Most of the pain due to cancer is nociceptive. When a tumor invades bones and organs, it may cause mild discomfort or severe, unrelenting pain. Some cancer treatments, such as surgery and radiation therapy, can also cause nociceptive pain.

NEUROPATHIC PAIN

Neuropathic pain is caused by abnormalities in the nerves, spinal cord, or brain.

Neuropathic pain may be felt as a burning or tingling sensation or as hypersensitivity to touch or cold. Neuropathic pain includes such syndromes as phantom limb pain, postherpetic neuralgia, reflex sympathetic dystrophy, and causalgia.

Phantom limb pain is seemingly felt in an amputated part of the body, usually a limb. It differs from phantom limb sensation—the feeling that the amputated part is still there—which is much more common. Phantom limb pain cannot be caused by a problem in the limb; rather, it must be caused by a change in the nervous system above the site where the limb was amputated. The brain misinterprets the nerve signals as coming from the amputated limb. Usually, the pain is felt in the toes, ankle, and foot of an amputated leg or the fingers and hand of an amputated arm. The pain may resemble squeezing, burning, or crushing sensations, but it often differs from any sensation previously experienced. For some people, phantom limb pain occurs less frequently as time passes, but for others, it persists. Massage can sometimes help, but drug therapy is sometimes necessary.

Postherpetic neuralgia results from herpes zoster (shingles), which causes inflammation of nerve tissue. The pain is felt as a constant deep aching or burning, as a sharp and intermittent pain, or as hypersensitivity to touch or cold. The pain may be debilitating.

Reflex sympathetic dystrophy (complex regional pain syndrome, type 1) and **causalgia** (complex regional pain syndrome, type 2) are chronic pain syndromes. They are defined as persistent burning pain accompanied by certain abnormalities that occur in the same area as the pain. Abnormalities include increased or decreased sweating, swelling, changes in skin color, and damage to the skin, hair, nails, muscle, and bone (including muscle wasting and bone loss). Both syndromes typically occur after an injury. Reflex sympathetic dystrophy results from injury to tissues other than nerve tissue (as in the shoulder-hand syndrome). Causalgia results from injury to nerve tissue.

Some types of reflex sympathetic dystrophy and causalgia are made worse by activity of the sympathetic nervous system, which normally prepares the body for stressful or emergency situations—for fight or flight. For this reason, doctors suggest treatment with a sympathetic nerve block.■

PSYCHOGENIC PAIN

Psychogenic pain is entirely or mostly related to a psychologic disorder.

When people have persistent pain with evidence of psychologic disturbances and without evidence of a disorder that could cause the pain, the pain may be described as psychogenic. Pain that is purely psychogenic is rare. More commonly, the pain has a physical cause, but the doctor's assessment indicates that the degree of pain and the disability experienced are out of proportion to what most people with a similar disorder experience. Sometimes this type of pain is described as a chronic pain syndrome. Psychologic factors often contribute to disability and to an exaggeration of pain complaints. Any kind of pain can be complicated by psychologic factors. Even when pain is suspected to be psychogenic, doctors still investigate whether a physical disorder is contributing to the pain.

The fact that the pain is caused or worsened by psychologic factors does not mean that it is

---

▲ see art on page 571   ■ see page 455

not real. Most people who report pain are really experiencing it, even if a physical cause cannot be identified. Pain complicated by psychologic factors still requires treatment, often by a team that includes a psychologist or psychiatrist. As with other kinds of treatment for chronic pain, the treatment for this type of pain varies from person to person, and doctors try to match the treatment with the person's needs. For most people who have chronic psychogenic pain, the goals of treatment are to improve comfort and physical and psychologic function. Doctors may make specific recommendations for gradually increasing physical and social activities. Drugs and nondrug treatments—such as biofeedback, relaxation training, distraction techniques, hypnosis, transcutaneous electrical nerve stimulation (TENS), and physical therapy—may be used. Psychologic counseling is often needed.

Treatment of Pain

In some cases, treating the underlying disorder eliminates or minimizes the pain. For example, setting a broken bone in a cast or giving antibiotics for an infected joint helps reduce pain. However, even if the underlying disorder can be treated, pain relievers (analgesics) may still be needed to quickly manage the pain. Doctors choose an analgesic based on the type and duration of pain and on the likely benefits and risks. Most analgesics are effective for nociceptive pain but are less effective for neuropathic pain, which often requires different drugs. For some types of pain, especially chronic pain, nondrug treatments are also important.

Analgesics fall into three categories: opioid (narcotic) analgesics, nonopioid analgesics, and adjuvant analgesics (drugs that are usually given for reasons other than pain but that sometimes relieve pain).

OPIOID ANALGESICS

Opioid analgesics (narcotics), the most powerful analgesics, are the mainstay for treatment of severe acute pain and chronic pain due to cancer and other serious disorders. Opioids are preferred because they are so effective in controlling pain. The use of opioids to treat chronic pain not due to cancer is becoming

more acceptable but is still relatively uncommon. Opioids are not appropriate for everyone.

Opioids are all chemically related to morphine, a natural substance extracted from poppies, although some opioids are extracted from other plants and other opioids are produced in a laboratory.

Opioids have many side effects. People who take opioids for acute pain often become drowsy. For some people, this drowsiness is welcome, but for others, it is not. Most people who take opioids become tolerant of this effect and do not continue to feel drowsy. Some people who continue to feel drowsy are given stimulant drugs, such as methylphenidate, to keep them awake and alert. Opioids may also cause confusion, especially in older people.

Opioids often cause constipation and retention of urine, especially in older people. Stimulant laxatives,▲ such as senna, help prevent or relieve the constipation. Increasing intake of fluids can also help.

Sometimes people with pain feel nauseated, and opioids can increase the nausea. Antiemetic drugs taken by mouth, suppository, or injection help prevent or relieve nausea. Some commonly used antiemetic drugs are metoclopramide, hydroxyzine, and prochlorperazine.

Taking too much of an opioid can have serious side effects, including a dangerous slowing of breathing and even coma. These effects can be reversed with naloxone, an antidote given intravenously. Nurses and family members should watch for side effects of opioids.

Doctors carefully weigh the benefits and side effects when they consider these drugs for the treatment of chronic pain. With repeated use of opioids over time, some people need higher doses because the body adapts to and thus responds less well to the drug; this phenomenon is called tolerance. For other people, the same dose remains effective for a long time.

People who take opioids for a long time usually become dependent on them; that is, they experience withdrawal symptoms if the drug is stopped. When opioids are stopped after long-term use, the dose must be gradually tapered to minimize the development of such symptoms. Dependence is not the same as addiction, which is the disruptive behavior or activity associated with obtaining and using the drug. Although addiction is possible, it appears to be rare among people who take opioids to control pain. Too often, exaggerated concern about the addiction potential of opioids■ leads to undertreatment of pain and

---

▲ see page 752

■ see page 652

DRUG	LENGTH OF EFFECTIVENESS	COMMENTS
Morphine	By intravenous or intramuscular injection: 2 to 3 hours Immediate release by mouth: 3 to 4 hours Sustained release by mouth: 8 to 24 hours	Morphine starts to work quickly. The oral form can be very effective for chronic pain
Codeine	By mouth: 3 to 4 hours	Codeine is less potent than morphine. It is usually taken with aspirin or acetaminophen
Fentanyl	By mouth: 3 to 4 hours By patch: up to 72 hours	Fentanyl is available as a lozenge that is dissolved in the mouth; it is used to treat breakthrough pain. The patch is often used to treat chronic pain
Meperidine	By intravenous or intramuscular injection: about 3 hours By mouth: not very effective	Although meperidine can be effective for short-term use, it is not preferred for long-term use because it causes side effects, such as psychosis, muscle spasms, tremors, and seizures
Methadone	By mouth: 4 to 6 hours, sometimes longer	Methadone is also used for treating addiction to heroin and other opioids
Propoxyphene	By mouth: 3 to 4 hours	Propoxyphene is usually taken with aspirin or acetaminophen to relieve mild pain
Levorphanol	By intravenous or intramuscular injection: 4 hours By mouth: about 4 hours	The oral form is strong. It can be used instead of morphine
Hydromorphone	By intravenous or intramuscular injection: 2 to 4 hours By mouth: 2 to 4 hours By rectal suppository: 4 hours	Hydromorphone begins to work quickly. It can be used instead of morphine and is useful for chronic pain
Oxycodone	By mouth: 3 to 4 hours	Oxycodone can be used instead of morphine to treat chronic pain. The short-acting formulation is usually combined with aspirin or acetaminophen
Oxymorphone	By intravenous or intramuscular injection: 3 to 4 hours By rectal suppository: 4 hours	Oxymorphone starts to work quickly
Pentazocine	By mouth: up to 4 hours	Pentazocine can block the pain-relieving action of other opioids. It is about as strong as codeine. Pentazocine can cause confusion and anxiety, especially in older people

needless suffering. People with severe pain should not avoid opioids, and adequate doses should be taken as needed.

When possible, opioids are taken by mouth. Opioids are given by injection when people cannot take them by mouth. For people who are helped by an opioid but cannot tolerate its side effects, an opioid can be administered directly into the space around the spinal cord through a pump, thus providing high concentrations of the drug to the brain. One opioid, fentanyl, is available as a skin patch. It provides pain relief for up to 72 hours.

Different opioid analgesics have different advantages and disadvantages. Morphine, the prototype of these drugs, can be taken by mouth (orally) or by injection. There are two oral forms: sustained-release and immediate-release. Different sustained-release forms provide relief for 8 to 24 hours. These drugs are widely used to treat chronic pain. The immediate-release form provides short-lived relief, usually for less than 3 hours. In injected forms, 2 to 6 times less morphine is required than in oral forms, because when morphine is taken by mouth, much of the drug is chemically altered (metabolized) by the liver before it reaches the bloodstream. Usually, the difference in the amount needed for the different routes does not change the effects of the drug. Pain relief with injected forms is quicker than that with oral forms, but relief does not last as long.

Morphine may be injected into a vein (intravenously), into a muscle (intramuscularly), or under the skin (subcutaneously). With the intravenous form of morphine, pain relief is almost immediate but does not last very long. With the intramuscular form, pain relief is less rapid but lasts somewhat longer. With the subcutaneous form, pain relief is the least rapid but lasts the longest.

Injections can be given every few hours, but repeated injections can become annoying. Alternatively, a catheter can be inserted in a vein or under the skin and connected to a continuous-infusion pump, which supplies morphine continuously. The continuous infusion can be supplemented with extra doses when needed. Sometimes a device that enables a person to control release of the drug by pressing a button is used. This technique is called patient-controlled analgesia. Usually, continuous infusion is used for people who have severe pain due to a serious disorder.

Opioids are essential to the management of acute pain. For example, opioid analgesics are usually prescribed after surgery. They are most effective when taken every few hours, before pain becomes severe. The dose may be increased, or another drug (such as a nonsteroidal anti-inflammatory drug) may be added if the pain temporarily worsens, if the person needs to exercise (movement can be more painful), or if the wound dressing is about to be changed. When the pain eases, doctors reduce the dose and prescribe nonopioid analgesics, such as acetaminophen.

NONOPIOID ANALGESICS

A variety of nonopioid analgesics are available. Several (such as aspirin, ibuprofen, ketoprofen, naproxen, and acetaminophen) are available in prescription and nonprescription (over-the-counter, or OTC) strengths.▲ Prescription-strength formulations contain more active ingredient per dose than OTC formulations. OTC analgesics are reasonably safe to take for short periods of time, but their labels caution against taking them for more than 7 to 10 days to treat pain. A doctor should be consulted if symptoms worsen or do not go away.

Nonsteroidal Anti-Inflammatory Drugs

Most nonopioid analgesics are classified as nonsteroidal anti-inflammatory drugs (NSAIDs). NSAIDs are used to treat mild to moderate pain and may be combined with opioids to treat moderate to severe pain. NSAIDs not only relieve pain, but they also reduce the inflammation that often accompanies and worsens pain.

NSAIDs tend to irritate the stomach's lining and cause digestive upset (such as heartburn, indigestion, nausea, bloating, diarrhea, and stomach pain), peptic ulcers, and bleeding in the digestive tract. Coxibs (COX-2 inhibitors), a new type of NSAIDs, are less likely to irritate the stomach and cause bleeding than other NSAIDs.

Taking NSAIDs with food and using antacids may help prevent stomach irritation. The drug misoprostol can help prevent stomach irritation and ulcers, but it can cause other problems, including diarrhea. Proton pump inhibitors (such as omeprazole) or histamine-2 (H_2) blockers (such as famotidine), which are used to treat peptic ulcers, can also help prevent stomach problems due to NSAIDs.

NSAIDs interfere with the clotting tendency of platelets (cell-like particles in the blood that

▲ see also page 94

How Nonsteroidal Anti-Inflammatory Drugs Work

Nonsteroidal anti-inflammatory drugs (NSAIDs) work in two ways: They reduce the sensation of pain, and they reduce the inflammation that often accompanies and worsens pain. NSAIDs produce these effects because they reduce the production of hormone-like substances called prostaglandins. Different prostaglandins have different functions, such as sensitizing pain receptors to mechanical and chemical stimulation and causing blood vessels to dilate.

Most NSAIDs reduce prostaglandin production by blocking both cyclooxygenase (COX) enzymes (COX-1 and COX-2), which are crucial to the formation of prostaglandins. A new group of NSAIDs, the coxibs (COX-2 inhibitors), tend to block only COX-2.

Prostaglandins that are formed through the action of the COX-2 enzymes are released in response to an injury—burn, break, sprain, strain, or invasion by a microorganism. The result is inflammation, which is a protective response: The blood supply to the injured area increases, bringing in fluids and white blood cells to wall off the damaged tissue and remove any invading microorganisms.

Prostaglandins that are formed through the action of COX-1 enzymes help protect the digestive tract from stomach acid and play a crucial role in blood clotting. All NSAIDs, even the coxibs, reduce the production of these prostaglandins. Consequently, NSAIDs may irritate the stomach's lining and cause digestive upset, peptic ulcers, and bleeding in the digestive tract.

---

help stop bleeding when blood vessels are injured). Consequently, NSAIDs increase the risk of bleeding, especially in the digestive tract if they also irritate the stomach's lining.

NSAIDs cause fluid retention and swelling in 1 to 2% of people. Regular use of NSAIDs may also increase the risk of developing a kidney disorder, sometimes resulting in renal failure (a disorder called analgesic nephropathy).

For older people, the risk of side effects due to NSAIDs is increased. For people who drink alcoholic beverages regularly and take NSAIDs, the risk of digestive upset, ulcers, and liver damage may be increased. People with heart failure, high blood pressure, or kidney or liver disorders require a doctor's supervision when they take NSAIDs. Some prescription heart and blood pressure drugs may not work as well when taken with these analgesics.

NSAIDs vary in how quickly they work and how long they relieve pain. Although NSAIDs are about equally effective, people respond to them differently; one person may find a particular drug to be more effective or to have fewer side effects than another.

Aspirin: Aspirin (acetylsalicylic acid) has been used for about 100 years. Aspirin is taken by mouth and provides 4 to 6 hours of moderate pain relief.

Because aspirin can irritate the stomach, it may be combined with an antacid (in a buffered product) to reduce this effect. The antacid creates an alkaline environment that helps aspirin dissolve and may reduce the time aspirin is in contact with the stomach lining. However, buffered aspirin can still irritate the stomach because aspirin also reduces the production of substances that help protect the stomach's lining (these substances are a type of prostaglandin).

Enteric-coated aspirin is designed to pass through the stomach intact and dissolve in the small intestine, thus minimizing direct irritation of the stomach. (Enteric refers to the small intestine.) However, enteric-coated aspirin may be absorbed erratically. If food and enteric-coated aspirin are ingested at about the same time, the aspirin is not absorbed as quickly because food delays the emptying of the stomach. Consequently, pain relief is delayed.

Aspirin also increases the risk of bleeding throughout the body because it reduces the clotting tendency of platelets. People who bruise easily may be especially vulnerable to this effect. Anyone who has ever had a bleeding disorder or uncontrolled high blood pressure should not take aspirin except under a doctor's supervision. People who take aspirin and anticoagulants (such as warfarin) are closely monitored to avoid life-threatening bleeding. Usually, aspirin should not be taken in the week before scheduled surgery.

Aspirin can aggravate asthma. People with nasal polyps are likely to develop wheezing if they take aspirin. A few people, who are sensitive (allergic) to aspirin, may have a severe al-

NONSTEROIDAL ANTI-INFLAMMATORY DRUGS

TYPE	DRUG
Salicylates	Aspirin
	Choline magnesium
	trisalicylate
	Diflunisal
	Salsalate
Coxibs	Celecoxib
	Rofecoxib
	Valdecoxib
Others	
	Diclofenac
	Etodolac
	Fenoprofen
	Flurbiprofen
	Ibuprofen
	Indomethacin
	Ketoprofen
	Ketorolac
	Meclofenamate
	Mefenamic acid
	Meloxicam
	Nabumetone
	Naproxen
	Oxaprozin
	Piroxicam
	Sulindac
	Tolmetin

lergic reaction (anaphylaxis), leading to a rash, itching, severe breathing problems, or shock.▲ Such a reaction requires immediate medical attention.

In very high doses, aspirin can cause serious side effects such as abnormal breathing. One of the first signs of an overdose is noise in the ears (tinnitus).

Children and teenagers who have or may have influenza or chickenpox must not take aspirin because they could develop Reye's syndrome. Although rare, Reye's syndrome can have serious consequences, including death.

Ibuprofen, Ketoprofen, and Naproxen: NSAIDs such as ibuprofen, ketoprofen, and naproxen are generally believed to be gentler on the stomach than aspirin, although few studies have compared the drugs. Like aspirin, these drugs can cause digestive upset, ulcers, and bleeding in the digestive tract.

Although ibuprofen, ketoprofen, and naproxen generally interfere with blood clotting less than aspirin does, people should not take

▲ see page 148

these drugs with anticoagulants (such as warfarin) except under a doctor's close supervision.

People who are allergic to aspirin may also be allergic to ibuprofen, ketoprofen, and naproxen. If a rash, itching, breathing problems, or shock develops, medical attention is required immediately.

Coxibs (COX-2 Inhibitors): Coxibs, such as celecoxib, rofecoxib, and valdecoxib, are a new type of NSAID. Other NSAIDs block two enzymes: COX-1, which is involved in the production of the prostaglandins that protect the stomach and play a crucial role in blood clotting; and COX-2, which is involved in the production of the prostaglandins that promote inflammation. Coxibs tend to block only COX-2 enzymes. Thus, coxibs are as effective as other NSAIDs in the treatment of pain and inflammation. But coxibs are less likely to damage the stomach; to cause nausea, bloating, heartburn, bleeding, and peptic ulcers; and to interfere with clotting than are other NSAIDs.

Because of these differences, coxibs are useful for people who cannot tolerate other NSAIDs and for people who are at high risk of complications from use of other NSAIDs. Such people include older people, people who are taking anticoagulants, those who have a history of ulcers, and those who must take an analgesic for a long time.

Acetaminophen

This drug is roughly comparable to aspirin in its potential to relieve pain and lower a fever. But unlike NSAIDs, acetaminophen has virtually no useful anti-inflammatory activity, does not affect the blood's ability to clot, and has almost no adverse effects on the stomach. How acetaminophen works is not clearly understood.

Acetaminophen is taken by mouth or suppository, and its effects generally last 4 to 6 hours. High doses can lead to liver damage, which may be irreversible. People with a liver disorder should use lower doses than usually taken. Whether lower doses taken for a long time can harm the liver is less certain. People who consume large amounts of alcohol are probably at highest risk of liver damage from overuse of acetaminophen. People who are taking acetaminophen and stop eating because of a bad cold, influenza, or another reason may be more vulnerable to liver damage. Taking high doses for a long time may lead to kidney damage.

ADJUVANT ANALGESICS

Adjuvant analgesics are drugs that are not usually used for pain relief but may relieve pain in certain circumstances and that, when used to relieve pain, are usually used with other analgesics or nondrug pain treatments.

The adjuvant analgesics most commonly used for pain are antidepressants (such as amitriptyline and desipramine),▲ anticonvulsants (such as gabapentin, carbamazepine, and phenytoin),■ and oral and topical local anesthetics.

Antidepressants can potentially relieve pain in people who do not have depression. There is some evidence that tricyclic antidepressants are more effective for this purpose than other antidepressants, but selective serotonin reuptake inhibitor (SSRI) antidepressants (such as fluoxetine) are tolerated better. People may respond to one antidepressant and not others.

Anticonvulsants may be used to relieve neuropathic pain. Gabapentin is used most often, but many others, including phenytoin, carbamazepine, clonazepam, divalproex, lamotrigine, topiramate, and oxcarbazepine, may be tried. Anticonvulsants, such as divalproex, can also prevent migraine headaches.

Mexiletine, a local anesthetic taken by mouth to treat abnormal heart rhythms, is sometimes used to treat neuropathic pain. Local anesthetics are more commonly placed directly on or near a sore area to help reduce pain. For example, doctors may inject a local anesthetic, such as lidocaine, into the skin to control pain due to an injury or even due to neuropathic pain syndromes. Local anesthetics are also used in nerve blocks. For example, a sympathetic nerve block involves injecting a local anesthetic into a group of nerves near the spine—in the neck for pain in the upper body or in the lower back for pain in the lower body.

Occasionally, pain related to nerve injury can be treated by injecting a caustic substance, such as phenol, into a nerve to destroy it, by freezing the nerve (in cryotherapy), or by burning the nerve with a radiofrequency probe. These techniques may be used to treat facial pain due to trigeminal neuralgia.

Topical anesthetics, such as lidocaine applied as a lotion, ointment, or skin patch, can be used to control pain due to some conditions. These anesthetics are usually used for a short period of time. For example, an anesthetic mouthwash can be used to relieve a sore throat. However, some people with chronic pain benefit from using topical anesthetics for a long time. For example, a lidocaine patch can be used to relieve postherpetic neuralgia.

A cream containing capsaicin, a substance found in hot peppers, sometimes helps reduce the pain caused by such disorders as herpes zoster and osteoarthritis. It is most often used by people with localized pain due to arthritis. This cream must be applied several times a day.

NONDRUG PAIN TREATMENTS

In addition to drugs, many other treatments can help relieve pain. Applying cold or warm compresses directly to a painful area often helps.★ Ultrasonography that provides deep heat (diathermy) may relieve the pain of osteoarthritis and muscle strain.

Some people benefit from transcutaneous electrical nerve stimulation (TENS). A gentle electric current is applied through electrodes placed on the skin's surface. TENS produces a tingling sensation without increasing muscle tension. It can be applied continuously or several times a day for 20 minutes to several hours. The timing and length of stimulation vary because each person responds differently. Often, people are taught to use the TENS device, so that they can use it as needed. TENS may be useful for chronic pain.

Acupuncture involves inserting tiny needles into specific areas of the body.● The mechanisms by which acupuncture works are poorly understood, and some experts still doubt the technique's effectiveness. Some people find substantial relief with acupuncture, at least for a time.

Biofeedback and other cognitive techniques (such as relaxation training, hypnosis, and distraction techniques) can help people control, reduce, or cope with pain by changing the way they focus their attention. In one distraction technique, people may learn to visualize themselves in a calm, comforting place (such as in a hammock or on a beach) when they feel pain.

The importance of psychologic support for people in pain should not be underestimated. Friends and family members should be aware that people in pain suffer, need support, and may develop depression and anxiety, which may require psychologic counseling.

▲ see table on page 618
■ see table on page 500
★ see page 37   ● see also page 1705

CHAPTER 79

Headaches

Headaches are a very common medical problem and a common cause of disability among men and women. Headaches interfere with the ability to work and to perform daily tasks. Some people have frequent headaches; other people hardly ever have them.

Causes

Although headaches can be painful and distressing, they rarely indicate a serious condition. Most headaches—tension-type, migraine, and cluster headaches—are not caused by another identifiable disorder. Tension-type headaches are the most common.

Less commonly, headaches result from another disorder. Usually, the disorder is not serious. Disorders that cause headaches are often minor or temporary ones that affect the eyes, nose, throat, sinuses, teeth, jaws, ears, or neck.

Rarely, headaches are caused by a serious disorder. Such disorders include a head injury, stroke, bulge in the wall of an artery supplying the brain (cerebral aneurysm), brain infection (brain abscess, meningitis, and encephalitis), and blood vessel (arteriovenous) malformation near the brain. Infections such as tuberculosis may affect the brain and cause headaches. Disorders that increase pressure within the skull can cause headaches by putting pressure on the brain. Examples are a brain tumor, bleeding (hemorrhage), an accumulation of blood (hematoma), and pseudotumor cerebri,▲ in which pressure within the skull increases but no cause can be identified.

Other serious diseases that may cause headache include very high blood pressure, which may produce a throbbing sensation in the head. (However, high blood pressure does not usually cause headaches.) Lung disorders (such as emphysema) that reduce the oxygen supply to the brain may cause headaches, as may sleep apnea, which temporarily increases levels of carbon dioxide in the blood. Inflammation of large arteries (temporal arteritis), usually in the neck and head, may cause headaches. Temporal arteritis affects older people primarily. Severe cases of influenza and high fever may cause headaches. Lyme disease in its early stages commonly causes headaches.

Headaches commonly result from withdrawal of caffeine, withdrawal of analgesics after long-term use, and use of certain drugs that widen blood vessels (such as nitroglycerin).

Diagnosis

Usually, doctors can determine the type or cause of headaches on the basis of the person's medical history, the characteristics of the headache, and results of a physical examination. Characteristics of the headache include its frequency, duration, location, severity, and associated symptoms.

The following characteristics may indicate that a serious disorder is the cause of headaches, and prompt medical attention is required.

• Frequent headaches in a person who rarely has headaches
• Mild headaches that become severe
• Headaches that awaken a person from sleep
• Any change in the pattern or nature of headaches
• Headaches associated with symptoms such as a fever and a stiff neck, changes in sensation or vision, weakness, loss of coordination, or fainting

For example, a severe headache with a fever and a stiff neck suggests meningitis—a life-threatening infection of the layers of tissue covering the brain and spinal cord (meninges). A headache that occurs suddenly and that is more severe than any others the person has experienced suggests a subarachnoid hemorrhage—often due to a ruptured aneurysm.

When doctors suspect a serious disorder, additional diagnostic procedures are usually performed. If meningitis is suspected, a spinal tap (lumbar puncture)■ is performed immediately. A spinal tap may also be performed if doctors suspect a ruptured aneurysm. Occasionally, blood tests are performed to check for a disorder such as Lyme disease. The erythrocyte sedimentation rate (ESR—the rate at which red blood cells settle to the bottom of a test tube containing blood) may be determined to check for temporal arteritis. A high ESR suggests inflammation.

▲ see box on page 523　　■ see art on page 443

If doctors suspect a tumor, stroke, hemorrhage, or another structural brain disorder, computed tomography (CT) or magnetic resonance imaging (MRI) of the head is performed.

Tension-Type Headaches

A tension-type headache is usually mild to moderate, band-like pain that affects the whole head.

The cause of tension-type headaches is not well understood but may be related to a lower-than-normal threshold for pain. Stress may be involved. However, its role is not clearly understood, and it is not the only explanation for the symptoms.

Symptoms and Diagnosis

The pain is usually mild to moderate, although it may be severe. It feels like tightening of a band around the head, making the whole head ache. The pain may last 30 minutes to 1 week. Unlike a migraine headache, a tension-type headache is not associated with nausea and vomiting and is not made worse by physical activity, light, sounds, or smells. Tension-type headaches typically start several hours after waking and rarely awaken a person from sleep.

The diagnosis is based on the person's description of the headache and the results of a physical examination. No specific procedures can confirm the diagnosis. Rarely, computed tomography (CT) or magnetic resonance imaging (MRI) of the head is performed to rule out other disorders that may be causing the headache, particularly if headaches have developed recently.

Treatment

For most mild to moderate tension-type headaches, almost any over-the-counter analgesic, such as aspirin, acetaminophen, or ibuprofen,▲ can provide fast, temporary relief. Massaging the affected area may help relieve the pain. Severe headaches may require stronger, prescription analgesics, some of which contain opioids (narcotics), such as codeine or oxycodone.■ For some people, caffeine, an ingredient of some headache preparations, enhances the effect of analgesics. However, overuse of analgesics or caffeine can lead to chronic daily headaches. Such headaches, called rebound headaches, occur when a dose of an analgesic is missed or late or when caffeine intake is reduced or stopped.

Migraine Headaches

A migraine headache is throbbing, moderate to severe pain, usually on one side of the head, that is worsened by physical activity, light, sounds, or smells and that is associated with nausea and vomiting.

Although migraines can start at any age, they usually begin between the ages of 10 and 40. In most people, migraines recur periodically, but they usually become significantly less severe or resolve entirely after age 50 or 60. Migraines are 3 times more common among women than among men. Migraines tend to run in families; more than half of the people who have migraines have close relatives who also have them.

The cause of migraines is not well understood. According to one theory, migraines occur when arteries to the brain become narrow (constrict) and then widen (dilate); dilation is thought to activate nearby pain receptors. However, this theory is too simple to explain the complex changes in blood flow that occur in the brain during a migraine. Furthermore, a series of changes in the nerve cells of the brain occur before the changes in blood flow. A rare subtype of migraine called familial hemiplegic migraine is associated with a genetic defect on chromosomes 1 and 19. The role of genes in the more common forms of migraine is under study.

Estrogen, the main female hormone, appears to trigger migraines, possibly explaining why migraines are more common among women. During puberty (when estrogen levels increase), migraines become much more common among girls than among boys. Some women have migraines just before, during, or just after menstrual periods. As menopause approaches (when estrogen levels are fluctuating), migraines become particularly difficult to control. Oral contraceptives (which contain estrogen) and estrogen replacement therapy often make migraines worse. Insomnia, changes in barometric pressure, and hunger may also trigger migraines.

Symptoms and Diagnosis

In a migraine, throbbing pain is typically felt on one side of the head. The pain may be moderate but is often severe and incapacitating. Physical activity, light, sounds, or smells may make the headache worse. The headache

▲ see pages 94 and 452

■ see table on page 451

HOW HEADACHES DIFFER

TYPE OR CAUSE	CHARACTERISTICS*	DIAGNOSTIC PROCEDURES
Tension-type	The pain is usually mild to moderate, feels like tightening of a band around the head, and affects the whole head. The pain lasts 30 minutes to 7 days. Headaches are not worsened by physical activity, light, sounds, or smells and are not associated with nausea and vomiting.	CT or MRI of the head is performed to rule out other disorders, particularly if the headaches have developed recently or if the symptom pattern has changed
Migraine	The pain is moderate to severe, throbbing, and usually felt on one side of the head. The pain lasts 4 hours to 3 days. Headaches may be worsened by physical activity, light, sounds, or smells and are associated with nausea and vomiting. Attacks can occur for a long period of time but then disappear for weeks, months, or years. Often, attacks are preceded by a sensation that a migraine is beginning (such as mood changes, loss of appetite, and nausea) and temporary disturbances in sensation, balance, muscle coordination, speech, or vision (such as flashing lights and blind spots).	Procedures are the same as those for tension-type headaches
Cluster	The pain is severe and piercing and is focused around the eye. The pain lasts 15 minutes to 3 hours. Because the pain is so severe, people with cluster headaches cannot lie down, frequently pace, and sometimes bang their heads. Headaches occur in clusters, separated by periods when no headaches occur. They are usually not worsened by light, sounds, or smells and are not associated with nausea and vomiting. On the same side as the pain, the nostril runs, the eye waters, the eye lid droops, and the area below the eye may swell.	Procedures are the same as those for tension-type headaches
High blood pressure (hypertension)	Severe high blood pressure that has been present a long time can cause headaches. The pain is throbbing, occurs in spasms, and is felt at the back or top of the head.	Blood pressure is measured, and blood tests and kidney function tests are performed
Eye disorders (iritis, glaucoma, and papillitis)	The pain is moderate or severe and is often worse after using the eyes. It is felt at the front of the head or in or over the eyes.	An eye examination is performed
Sinus disorders	The pain is severe and may be dull or sharp. It is felt at the front of the head. It may begin suddenly and last only a short time, or it may begin gradually and be persistent. It is usually worse in the morning and less severe in the afternoon. Cold, damp weather and lying down make the pain worse.	The sinuses are x-rayed, or CT is performed
Brain tumor	Pain is mild to severe and becomes progressively worse. It usually recurs more and more often and eventually becomes constant without relief. Headaches are often worse when the person lies down and may awaken the person from sleep. A gradually growing tumor causes a headache that is worse when the person first awakens. The new development of such headaches requires medical attention.	MRI or CT is performed

HOW HEADACHES DIFFER *(Continued)*

Type or Cause	Characteristics*	Diagnostic Procedures
Brain abscess	The pain is mild to severe and intermittent; it may be felt in one spot or over the whole head. The pain is similar to that caused by a brain tumor. However, if an abscess ruptures, acute meningitis results, causing an intense headache and a stiff neck.	MRI or CT is performed
Meningitis	The pain is severe and constant and is felt over the whole head; it travels down the neck, making bending the neck to rest the chin on the chest difficult. People with meningitis feel ill, have a fever, and vomit.	Blood tests and a spinal tap are performed
Subdural hematoma	The pain is mild to severe and intermittent or constant. It can be felt in one spot or over the whole head and travels down the neck.	MRI or CT is performed
Subarachnoid hemorrhage	The pain is severe, constant, and widespread. Occasionally, it is felt in and around one eye; the eyelid droops. People often describe the headache as the worst ever experienced.	MRI or CT is performed; if the results are negative, a spinal tap is performed
Temporal arteritis	The pain is felt on one side of the head at the temple. The arteries in the temples may be enlarged. The disorder may cause disturbances or loss of vision.	Biopsy of the temporal arteries is performed, and the erythrocyte sedimentation rate (ESR) is determined
Other disorders if they affect the brain (cancer, cryptococcosis, sarcoidosis, syphilis, tuberculosis)	The pain may be mild or severe and dull or sharp; it is felt over the whole head. People whose headache is caused by one of these disorders have a moderate fever and a history of the disorder.	A spinal tap and MRI or CT are performed

*One, some, or all of the characteristics listed may be present. CT = computed tomography; MRI = magnetic resonance imaging

is often accompanied by nausea, sometimes with vomiting.

A migraine attack often involves more than a headache. It may include a prodrome, an aura, and a postdrome. The prodrome is a change in mood or behavior, which can precede the rest of the migraine by 24 hours. People may become depressed, elated, irritable, or restless. Nausea or loss of appetite may also occur. About 25% of people experience an aura. The aura involves temporary, reversible disturbances in vision, sensation, balance, movement, or speech. Commonly, people see jagged, shimmering, or flashing lights or develop a blind spot with flickering edges. Less commonly, people experience tingling sensations, loss of balance, weakness in an arm or a leg, or difficulty talking. The aura occurs within the hour before the migraine and ends as the migraine begins. About 25% of people experience a postdrome, which involves changes in mood and behavior after the migraine.

Migraine attacks may occur frequently for a long period of time but then may disappear for many weeks, months, or even years.

Migraines are diagnosed on the basis of symptoms. No procedure can confirm the diagnosis. If headaches have developed recently or if the pattern of symptoms has changed, computed tomography (CT) or magnetic resonance imaging (MRI) of the head is performed to exclude other disorders.

℞ DRUGS USED TO TREAT MIGRAINES

USE	TYPE	EXAMPLES	SELECTED SIDE EFFECTS
Preventive			
	Anticonvulsants	Divalproex	See table on page 500
	Beta-blockers	Propranolol	See table on page 138
	Calcium channel blockers	Verapamil	See table on page 139
	Serotonin blockers	Methysergide	Formation of scar tissue deep within the abdomen (retroperitoneal fibrosis), which can block the blood supply to vital organs; diarrhea; nausea; vomiting; drowsiness; weakness; and weight gain or loss
	Tricyclic antidepressants	Amitriptyline Nortriptyline	See table on page 618
Abortive			
	Ergot derivatives	Dihydroergotamine Ergotamine	Nausea, vomiting, minor muscle cramping, and, rarely, chest pain due to an inadequate blood supply to the heart muscle (angina)
	Antiemetic drugs	Metoclopramide Prochlorperazine	Low blood pressure, drowsiness, and muscle spasms
	Triptans (5-hydroxytryptophan [5-HT] agonists)	Almotriptan Naratriptan Rizatriptan Sumatriptan Zolmitriptan	Flushing, dizziness, drowsiness, nausea, spasm of the esophagus, and, rarely, angina
Analgesic			
		Acetaminophen	Rebound headache if the dose is increased and, occasionally, skin rash
	Nonsteroidal anti-inflammatory drugs (NSAIDs)	Aspirin Indomethacin Naproxen	Rebound headache if the dose is increased. With indomethacin, worsening of depression, seizures, and tremors with decreased mobility and muscle stiffness; in older people, dizziness and confusion
	Opioids	Codeine Meperidine Oxycodone	See table on page 451

Prevention and Treatment

Treatment of migraine headaches involves three types of drugs: drugs to prevent migraines, drugs to stop (abort) a migraine as it is beginning, and drugs to relieve pain.

People who have more than one migraine a week often benefit from taking drugs every day to prevent migraine attacks. Beta-blockers, such as propranolol, are often given first.

Calcium channel blockers, antidepressants, and some anticonvulsants, particularly divalproex, are also effective. The choice of a preventive drug is based on the side effects of the drug and on other disorders present. For example, if weight gain could cause problems, divalproex is usually not prescribed. If the person has depression, a tricyclic antidepressant such as nortriptyline▲ may be prescribed.

To abort a migraine as it is beginning, most doctors prefer a relatively new group of drugs called triptans (5-hydroxytryptophan [5-HT]

▲ see table on page 618

agonists). Triptans specifically target the receptors that stimulate the nerves supplying the cerebral blood vessels. Thus, triptans may reverse the dilation of these blood vessels, which contributes to a migraine. As soon as people sense a migraine attack is beginning, they take one of these drugs to stop the attack from progressing. Other drugs used to abort migraines, such as ergotamine, are sometimes used, but they are not as safe or as effective as triptans. Because triptans and ergotamine cause blood vessels to narrow (constrict), they are not recommended for people who have angina or other heart disease or for people who have prodromal symptoms that resemble those of stroke (because constriction of arteries may trigger a stroke).

For less severe migraines, analgesics alone or analgesics that contain caffeine can be useful. They can be taken as needed during a migraine, with or instead of a triptan. As for tension-type headaches, overuse of analgesics or caffeine can make the migraine worse. For more severe migraines, opioids may be needed.▲

Cluster Headaches

A cluster headache is severe pain that is felt at the temple or around the eye on one side of the head, that lasts a relatively short time (less than 4 hours), and that usually occurs in groups for a 6- to 8-week period.

Cluster headaches are relatively rare, affecting about 1 to 4 of 1,000 people. Cluster headaches affect mostly men older than 30. Use of alcohol or nicotine may trigger attacks.

Symptoms

An attack almost always starts suddenly and lasts 15 minutes to 3 hours. It may begin with itching of or a watery discharge from one nostril. Intense pain on the same side of the head follows and spreads around the eye. The pain often awakens people from sleep. Because the pain is so severe, people with cluster headaches cannot lie down, frequently pace, and sometimes bang their heads. After the attack, the eyelid on the same side as the headache may droop, and the pupil often constricts. The headaches are usually not associated with nausea and vomiting and are not worsened by light, sounds, or smells.

Attacks may occur twice a week up to several times a day. They usually occur in groups or clusters for a 6- to 8-week period, occasionally longer, followed by a headache-free interval of several months before they recur. They may recur at the same time of day or night.

Diagnosis and Treatment

Diagnosis is based on the person's description of the headache and the accompanying symptoms. If the pattern of symptoms changes, computed tomography (CT) or magnetic resonance imaging (MRI) of the head is performed.

Most people with cluster headaches need to take drugs to prevent recurrences. Drugs include those used to prevent migraines, verapamil, lithium, indomethacin, and, occasionally, methysergide. Oxygen, given by nasal prongs, or the corticosteroid methylprednisolone, given by mouth, can stop (abort) a cluster headache as it is beginning.

CHAPTER 80

Dizziness and Vertigo

Dizziness is a vague term used to describe various sensations, including faintness, light-headedness, a loss of balance, a sense of spinning, a vague spaced-out feeling, and weakness. Vertigo is a specific sensation in which the person or the person's surroundings seem to be moving or spinning.

Doctors usually classify dizziness as faintness or light-headedness, in which the person feels about to lose consciousness; loss of balance, in which the person feels unsteady and about to fall; vertigo; a mixture of these types; or none of these types. Dizziness may be temporary or chronic. Chronic dizziness is more common among older people.

▲ see table on page 451

Dizziness accounts for about 5 to 6% of visits to the doctor. It may occur at any age but becomes more common as people age. It affects about 40% of people older than 40 at some time.

Although dizziness may be disturbing and even incapacitating, only about 5% of cases result from a serious disorder. Each type of dizziness tends to have characteristic causes. For example, faintness and light-headedness may result from a sudden fall in blood pressure▲ or other disorders that result in an inadequate blood supply to the brain. Such disorders include coronary artery disease, abnormal heart rhythms, and heart failure. Anxiety disorders and abnormally rapid breathing (hyperventilation) may also cause light-headedness.

Loss of balance may result from vision disorders, especially double vision, because the body depends on visual cues to maintain balance. Loss of balance may also result from musculoskeletal disorders, which cause muscle weakness and thus interfere with walking; use of certain drugs, such as anticonvulsants and sedatives; or disorders of the inner ear, which can also cause vertigo. Vertigo has many causes, including motion sickness, benign paroxysmal positional vertigo,■ and Meniere's disease.★ Chronic dizziness, especially in older people, may result from several disorders.

At any age, dizziness can cause problems, particularly when performing an exacting or a dangerous task. In older people, chronic dizziness increases the risk of falling and fractures and decreases the ability to perform daily activities.

Diagnosis and Treatment

People who have dizziness that persists or interferes with daily activities should see a doctor.

Before dizziness can be treated, doctors must determine its nature and its cause. Doctors ask the person to describe in detail the sensations felt: whether the feeling during the episode was faintness, light-headedness, loss of balance, spinning or movement of self or the surroundings (vertigo), or another sensation. The person is asked when the dizziness began, how long it lasted, what triggered or relieved it, and what other symptoms—headaches, deafness, noise in

the ears (tinnitus), impaired vision, weakness, or difficulty walking—were present. Such details help pinpoint the nature of the dizziness.

Balance is tested by asking the person to stand still and then to walk a straight line, first with the eyes open, then with the eyes closed. Vision tests are performed, and the eyes may be checked for abnormal movements (such as nystagmus●). Hearing tests are performed, because they can often detect inner ear disorders that affect both balance and hearing.

To determine whether the cause of the dizziness is a sudden fall in blood pressure, doctors measure blood pressure and pulse when the person is sitting or lying down, then after the person stands. Electrocardiography, echocardiography, and exercise stress testing may also be performed to evaluate heart function.

Additional diagnostic procedures may include computed tomography (CT) or magnetic resonance imaging (MRI) of the head and a spinal tap (lumbar puncture). If doctors suspect that the blood supply to the brain is inadequate, angiography, magnetic resonance angiography (MRA), or Doppler ultrasonography of the head may be performed. These procedures can show whether arteries to the brain are narrowed or blocked. Because MRA is not invasive, MRA with ultrasonography is generally preferred to angiography, which involves insertion of a catheter into an artery.

When no cause is identified, doctors can reassure the person that no serious disorder has been identified. When a cause is identified or suspected, treatment varies, depending on the cause. For example, if the cause is a drug, the drug is discontinued or the dose reduced. Drugs may be given to relieve accompanying symptoms (such as nausea) or to prevent blood pressure from falling. Anticoagulants may be given to prevent clot formation and stroke. Rarely, surgery is performed—for example, to remove a tumor. Benign paroxysmal positional vertigo can be relieved by a simple maneuver (Epley maneuver) performed in the doctor's office.

Vertigo

Vertigo is a false sensation that one's self or the surroundings are moving or spinning, usually accompanied by nausea and loss of balance.

Vertigo, a type of dizziness, resembles the feeling produced by the childhood game of spinning round and round, then suddenly stop-

▲ see page 141   ■ see page 465
★ see page 1259   ● see page 464

ping and watching the surroundings spin around. Most cases of dizziness are not vertigo.

Causes

Vertigo can be caused by disorders affecting the inner ear (including the semicircular canals), which enables the body to sense position and maintain balance. Vertigo may also be caused by disorders affecting the acoustic nerve (cranial nerve VIII), which connects the inner ear to the brain, or disorders affecting the connections in the brain stem and the cerebellum, which also help control balance.

Most commonly, vertigo results from motion sickness. Motion sickness may develop in people whose inner ear is sensitive to particular motions, such as swaying or sudden stopping and starting.

Another common cause of vertigo is the formation of sludge in the semicircular canals of the inner ear. The resulting disorder, called benign paroxysmal positional vertigo, is especially common among older people. It occurs when the head is moved in certain ways.

Meniere's disease, another disorder of the inner ear, produces attacks of vertigo. The cause of Meniere's disease is thought to involve swelling in the inner ear. Meniere's disease may result from a viral infection, an injury, or an allergy, but the cause is often unknown.

Other disorders that cause vertigo by affecting the inner ear or its nerve connections include bacterial or viral infections (such as viral labyrinthitis, herpes zoster, and mastoiditis), Paget's disease, tumors (such as an auditory nerve tumor), inflammation of nerves, or use of drugs that damage the inner ear (such as aminoglycoside antibiotics, aspirin, the chemotherapy drug cisplatin, and certain diuretics, including furosemide).

A transient ischemic attack commonly causes vertigo when the blood supply through arteries to the brain stem, cerebellum, and back of the brain is reduced. This disorder is called vertebrobasilar insufficiency. The arteries affected include the vertebral arteries and basilar artery, which is formed when the two vertebral arteries join together in the back of the head. Less common disorders that cause vertigo by affecting the brain stem or cerebellum include multiple sclerosis, skull fractures, seizures, infections, and tumors growing in or near the base of the brain.

Occasionally, vertigo is caused by disorders that suddenly increase pressure within the skull, putting pressure on the brain. These dis-

orders include benign intracranial hypertension, brain tumors, and bleeding (hemorrhage) within the skull.

Vertigo may be caused by damage to nerves in the neck. If these nerves are damaged, the brain has difficulty monitoring the relative position of the neck and trunk. This type of vertigo is called cervical vertigo. Whiplash injuries, blunt injuries to the top of the head, or severe arthritis in the neck (cervical spondylosis) may cause cervical vertigo.

Vertigo may be caused by drugs, including the sedative phenobarbital, the anticonvulsant phenytoin, and the antipsychotic chlorpromazine. Excessive use of alcohol can also cause temporary vertigo.

Symptoms

Vertigo is characterized by an unusual and uncomfortable sense of spinning: the person, the surroundings, or both seem to spin around. The resulting loss of balance makes walking and driving difficult. Nystagmus (the rapid movement of the eyes in one direction followed by a slower drift back to the original position) occurs repeatedly during an episode of vertigo. Nausea, sometimes with vomiting, often accompanies vertigo.

Vertigo may last for only a few moments or may continue for hours or even days. People who have vertigo sometimes feel better when lying down or sitting still; however, vertigo may continue even when they are not moving at all.

People with Meniere's disease may have sudden, episodic attacks of vertigo, with noise in the ears (tinnitus), progressive deafness, and a sense of fullness in the affected ear. Often, severe nausea and vomiting accompany the vertigo. Episodes usually last from several minutes to several hours.

In people with a viral infection of the inner ear (viral labyrinthitis), vertigo usually begins suddenly and worsens over several hours. Nausea may be intense. People with this disorder may sit very still, because moving the head or eyes may trigger vomiting. Labyrinthitis begins to subside over a period of days, but it may last weeks or even months.

Vertigo due to a brain disorder, including vertebrobasilar insufficiency, may be accompanied by headaches, slurred speech, double vision, weakness of an arm or a leg, uncoordinated movements, and loss of consciousness.

Vertigo due to a disorder that suddenly increases pressure within the skull may be accompanied by temporary blurring of vision and unsteadiness when walking.

Cervical vertigo occurs when the head is turned, especially if the chin is brought down to a shoulder. The neck's range of motion may be limited.

Diagnosis

Doctors ask the person to describe the nature and circumstances of the sensations felt. Balance and hearing are tested.

The eyes are checked for abnormal movements, such as nystagmus. Abnormal eye movements suggest a disorder affecting the inner ear or nerve connections in the brain stem. Doctors may deliberately induce nystagmus, because the direction in which the eyes move helps doctors make the diagnosis. Before nystagmus is induced, the person may be given thick magnifying glasses called Frenzel glasses to wear. Doctors can easily see the person's magnified eyes through the lenses, but the person sees a blur and cannot fix the eyes on an object. Fixing the eyes on a unmoving object can prevent nystagmus from occurring. During the maneuver, eye movements may be recorded using electrodes (small round sensors that stick to the skin) placed around each eye. This procedure is called electronystagmography.

Maneuvers to induce nystagmus include putting ice-cold water into the ear canal (caloric testing), rapidly shaking the person's head from side to side for 20 seconds, or rapidly changing the position of the person's head using the Dix-Hallpike maneuver. The Dix-Hallpike maneuver, which is used in diagnosis, resembles the Epley maneuver, which is used to treat benign paroxysmal positional vertigo.▲ In the Dix-Hallpike maneuver, the head is not turned as far.

If cervical vertigo is suspected, the person wears Frenzel glasses and is seated in a swivel chair. The doctor holds the person's head still while the person swivels from right to left. If nystagmus and vertigo occur, cervical vertigo is diagnosed.

Computed tomography (CT) or magnetic resonance imaging (MRI) of the head can detect some of the disorders that can cause vertigo. CT can show abnormalities in bone, such as an infection of the bone behind the ear (mastoiditis), fractures at the base of the skull, erosion of bone by tumors, and abnormal bone

formation as occurs in Paget's disease. MRI produces better images of the brain stem and cranial nerves than CT. If an ear infection is suspected, doctors may take a sample of pus or fluid from the ear with a needle or swab. If multiple sclerosis or a brain infection is suspected, a spinal tap (lumbar puncture) may be performed to obtain a sample of cerebrospinal fluid from the spine. If doctors suspect that the blood supply to the brain is inadequate, angiography, magnetic resonance angiography (MRA), or Doppler ultrasonography of the head may be performed.

Prevention and Treatment

Vertigo due to certain disorders can be prevented. For example, if vertigo is due to motion sickness, situations that cause it (such as a rocking boat) can be avoided, and fixing the eyes on an unmoving object can help avert an attack. Taking the drug scopolamine can help prevent as well as treat vertigo.

Drugs that relieve vertigo and the accompanying nausea include cyclizine, dimenhydrinate, diphenhydramine, hydroxyzine, meclizine, and promethazine. These drugs are taken by mouth. Scopolamine, taken through a skin patch worn behind the ear, may also be used. It is effective for several days and may be preferred if nausea is present. All of these drugs are antihistamines■ and may cause drowsiness, dry mouth, and other side effects, especially in older people. Scopolamine given through a patch tends to produce the fewest side effects. These drugs may cause agitation in infants and very young children and should not be given to them except under a doctor's supervision.

If the vertigo is severe and causes anxiety, sedatives may be needed. Most often, benzodiazepines, such as diazepam, are used. For older people, the benzodiazepines alprazolam and lorazepam are preferred, because they are shorter-acting.

If the cause is cervical vertigo, muscle relaxants such as cyclobenzaprine, given by mouth, may be used. Wearing a soft support (cervical) collar for several hours a day can help, and physical therapy may improve the range of motion in the neck. If the cause is viral labyrinthitis, sedatives (such as benzodiazepines) and drugs that relieve vertigo, nausea, and vomiting (such as meclizine, prochlorperazine, and promethazine) are used. Occasionally, when vertigo is disabling—as it sometimes is in Meniere's disease—surgery is recommended.

▲ see art on page 466   ■ see page 96

Motion Sickness

Motion sickness (also known as car, sea, train, or air sickness) involves a group of symptoms, particularly nausea, caused by movement during travel.

Motion sickness occurs when the brain receives contradictory information from its motion sensors—the eyes, the semicircular canals in the inner ear (which help control balance), and the muscle sensors that provide information about body position. Motion sickness commonly occurs during boat travel, when the boat rolls and rocks. It may also occur in a moving car, amusement park rides, or other moving vehicles. Some people are more susceptible than others. Fear, anxiety, and poor ventilation increase the likelihood of experiencing motion sickness.

Symptoms and Diagnosis

Symptoms begin relatively suddenly. Nausea, a feeling of general discomfort, vertigo, headache, and fatigue usually develop. The face becomes pale, and the person starts to sweat and feel unpleasantly warm. Vomiting often occurs. Other symptoms may include increased saliva production (often as a prelude to vomiting) and rapid, deep breathing (hyperventilation). Hyperventilation may produce faintness. Nausea and vomiting make the person feel weak. Prolonged vomiting can lead to low blood pressure and dehydration. However, symptoms tend to gradually subside when the motion stops or the person leaves the vehicle. Also, people who are on long trips, as on a ship, usually adapt to the motion (helped by the stabilizers used in modern ships to minimize motion) and gradually recover.

Motion sickness is diagnosed based on a description of the symptoms and the circumstances in which they occur.

Prevention and Treatment

Prevention is key. Measures include
• Choosing a seat where motion is felt least (such as the front seat of a car, a seat over the wings in an airplane, or the forward or middle cabin or upper deck of a ship)
• Keeping the head and body as still as possible
• Sitting face forward and in a reclining position
• Keeping the eyes on the horizon or another distant, unmoving object
• Not reading

• Getting fresh air by opening a window, opening an air vent, or going to a ship's top deck
• Not drinking alcoholic beverages and not smoking (both can aggravate nausea)
• Eating small amounts of low-fat, starchy foods and not eating strong-smelling or strong-tasting foods
• Avoiding food and drink on short airplane trips, especially on small airplanes

Before traveling, people who are susceptible to motion sickness can ask their doctor to recommend an over-the-counter drug or prescribe a drug to prevent the disorder. These drugs include cyclizine, dimenhydrinate, diphenhydramine, meclizine, perphenazine, and scopolamine. All of these drugs cause drowsiness but may cause agitation in infants and very young children and should not be given to them except under a doctor's supervision.▲

If motion sickness develops, eating soda crackers or drinking carbonated soda, such as ginger ale, may help. Because of the nausea, scopolamine, the only drug for motion sickness that is given through a skin patch, is often more useful than other drugs, which are taken by mouth. Drugs can also be given by injection if necessary.

Benign Paroxysmal Positional Vertigo

Benign paroxysmal positional vertigo is a common disorder in which vertigo is due to a change in head position.

A change in head position—typically occurring when a person lies down, gets up, turns over in bed, or tips the head backward to look up—triggers most episodes of this disorder. The disorder usually develops when calcium particles, which normally are distributed evenly in the three semicircular canals, form a sludge and clump together in one of the semicircular canals. (The semicircular canals are the part of the inner ear that helps with balance.)■ Normally, when the head moves, the calcium particles stimulate nerve receptors (hair cells) inside the canals. These cells send the brain a signal indicating the direction of the head movement. When the particles form a free-floating clump in one area, the signal is exaggerated: It suggests to the brain that the head has moved more than it has. This information does not

---

▲ see page 100   ■ see art on page 1245

A Cure for Vertigo?

Some people experience vertigo when they change the position of their head rapidly. This disorder is called benign paroxysmal positional vertigo. It is caused when calcium particles form sludge in one of the semicircular canals. Often, the disorder can be cured by the Epley maneuver, a simple maneuver in which the person is moved to a recumbent position and the person's head is rapidly turned several times. Each head position is held for about 20 to 30 seconds. Often, the rapid movements separate the particles, and gravity causes the pieces to be redistributed through the semicircular canals.

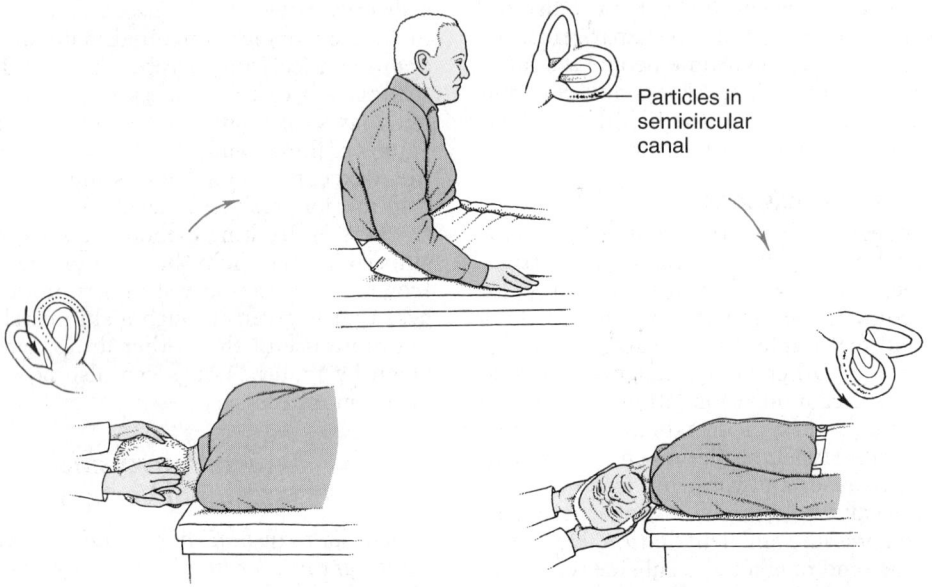

Particles in semicircular canal

The head is rapidly turned even further (so that the person nearly faces the floor). The person is returned to a seated position and should remain at least semiupright for the next 24 hours.

The doctor rapidly moves the person from a seated to a recumbent position with the head hanging over the table edge and turned at about a 45° angle to the same side as the affected ear. Gravity causes the particles in the semicircular canal to move.

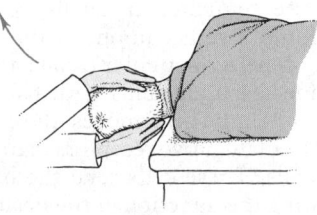

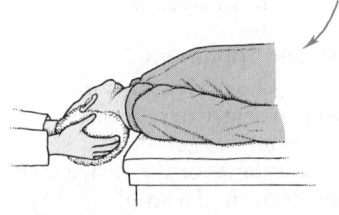

The head is rapidly turned another 45° (so that the ear is parallel to the floor).

The head is rapidly turned to the other side at the same angle.

match that from the eyes, and the mismatch results in a brief episode of vertigo. Sludging can be caused by damage to the lining of the semicircular canals. Such damage may be caused by ear infections, injury, surgery, or blockage of an artery to the inner ear.

This type of vertigo can be frightening, but it is harmless. An episode of vertigo begins 5 to 10 seconds after the head moves and lasts less than a minute. Episodes usually subside on their own in weeks. Occasionally, they persist for months and can cause dehydration due to nausea and vomiting. No hearing loss or noise in the ears (tinnitus) occurs.

Avoiding the positions that cause vertigo can help. People can learn to perform the Epley maneuver, which separates the calcium particles and redistributes them through the semicircular canals. As a result, the particles can be absorbed, then form again, as normally occurs. In about 90 to 95% of people, this maneuver provides immediate relief without the use of drugs. In some people, the vertigo recurs, and the maneuver must be repeated.

CHAPTER 81

Sleep Disorders

Sleep disorders are disturbances that affect the ability to fall asleep, stay asleep, or stay awake or that produce abnormal behaviors during sleep, such as night terrors or sleepwalking.

Sleep is necessary for survival and good health, but why sleep is needed and exactly how it benefits people are not fully understood. Individual requirements for sleep vary widely; healthy adults may need as few as 4 hours or as many as 10 hours of sleep every day. Most people sleep at night. However, many people must sleep during the day to accommodate work schedules—a situation that often leads to sleep disorders.

How long a person sleeps and how rested a person feels after waking can be influenced by many factors, including level of excitement or emotional distress, age, diet, and use of drugs. For example, some drugs make a person sleepy, and others make sleeping difficult. Some food components or additives, such as caffeine, strong spices, and monosodium glutamate (MSG), may affect sleep. Older people tend to fall asleep earlier, to awaken earlier, and to be less tolerant of changes in sleep patterns (for example, they may be more prone to jet lag). Compared with younger adults and children, older people are more easily aroused from sleep and awaken more often during the night. Whether older people need less sleep is unclear. Napping during the day may help compensate for poor sleep during the night, but it may also contribute to the problem.

All sleep is not the same. There are two main types of sleep: rapid eye movement (REM) sleep and nonrapid eye movement (non-REM) sleep, which has four stages. People normally cycle through the four stages of non-REM sleep, usually followed by a brief interval of REM sleep, 5 or 6 times every night.

Sleep progresses from stage 1 (the lightest level, during which the sleeper can be awakened easily) to stage 4 (the deepest level, during which the sleeper can be awakened only with difficulty). In stage 4, blood pressure is at its lowest, and heart and breathing rates are at their slowest.

During REM sleep, electrical activity in the brain is unusually high, somewhat resembling that during wakefulness. The eyes move rapidly, and muscles may jerk involuntarily. The rate and depth of breathing increase, but the muscles, except for the diaphragm, are greatly relaxed—more so than during the deepest levels of non-REM sleep.

Most dreaming occurs during REM sleep. Most talking during sleep, night terrors, and sleepwalking occur during stages 3 and 4.

Usually, sleep disorders can be diagnosed based on the medical history, including a description of the current problem, and the results of a physical examination. When the diagnosis is uncertain, doctors may recommend evaluation in a sleep laboratory. The evalua-

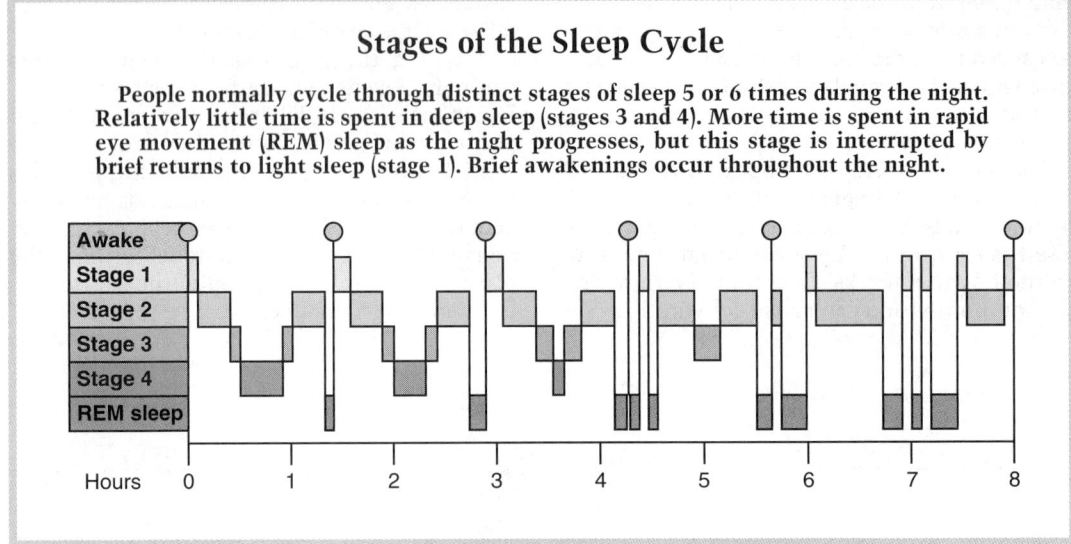

Stages of the Sleep Cycle

People normally cycle through distinct stages of sleep 5 or 6 times during the night. Relatively little time is spent in deep sleep (stages 3 and 4). More time is spent in rapid eye movement (REM) sleep as the night progresses, but this stage is interrupted by brief returns to light sleep (stage 1). Brief awakenings occur throughout the night.

tion consists of polysomnography and observation of unusual movements during an entire night's sleep. Polysomnography includes recording and monitoring of breathing, heart rate, and other functions; electroencephalography (EEG), which records the brain's electrical activity;▲ and electro-oculography, which records eye movement during REM sleep.

Insomnia

Insomnia is difficulty falling asleep or staying asleep or a disturbance in sleep that makes sleep seem inadequate or unrefreshing.

Insomnia is not a disease. It is a symptom that can have many different causes, including an irregular sleep-wake schedule, physical disorders, drug use or withdrawal, drinking large amounts of alcohol in the evening, emotional problems, and stress. Often, the cause is anxiety, nervousness, depression, or fear. Sometimes the cause is simply lack of fatigue. Some people have long-standing (chronic) insomnia that has little or no apparent relationship to a physical disorder, use or withdrawal of drugs, or any stress.

Difficulty falling asleep is common among young and old. About 10% of adults have chronic insomnia, and about 50% have insomnia sometimes.

Because sleep patterns change as people age, older people may think they have insomnia when they do not. As people age, they tend to sleep less at night and to nap during the day. Stage 4 sleep, the period of deep sleep, becomes shorter and eventually disappears. Also, older people awaken more during all stages of sleep. These changes are normal and usually do not indicate a sleep disorder.

There are several types of insomnia. Difficulty falling asleep, called sleep-onset insomnia, often occurs when people cannot let their minds relax and they continue to think and worry. Difficulty staying asleep, called sleep maintenance insomnia, is more common among older people than among younger people. People with this type of insomnia fall asleep normally but wake up several hours later and cannot fall asleep again easily. Sometimes they drift in and out of a restless, unsatisfactory sleep. Early morning awakening, another type of insomnia, may be a sign of depression in people of any age.

Sleep-wake schedule disorder may occur in people whose sleep patterns have been disrupted: They fall asleep at inappropriate times and then cannot sleep when they should. These sleep-wake reversals often result from jet lag (especially when traveling from east to west), working irregular night shifts, frequent changes in work hours, or excessive use of alcohol. Sometimes sleep-wake reversals are a side effect of drugs. Sleep-wake reversals are

▲ see page 445

common among people who are hospitalized because they are often awakened during the night. Damage to the brain's built-in biologic clock (caused by encephalitis, stroke, or Alzheimer's disease, for example) can also disrupt sleep patterns.

Symptoms and Diagnosis

Symptoms include irritability, fatigue during the day, and problems concentrating or performing under stress.

To diagnose insomnia, doctors evaluate a person's sleep pattern, use of drugs (including alcohol and illicit drugs), degree of psychologic stress, medical history, and level of physical activity. Some people need less sleep than others, so the diagnosis of insomnia is based on a person's individual needs.

Treatment

The treatment of insomnia depends on its cause and severity. If insomnia results from another disorder, treatment of that disorder may improve sleep. For most people who have insomnia, some simple changes in lifestyle, such as following a regular sleep schedule, can improve sleep.

Bright light therapy (which exposes a person to bright light at appropriate times) can help reset the biologic clock. This therapy is especially useful for people who have sleep-wake reversal due to jet lag, those who have sleep-onset insomnia, and those who go to sleep and wake too early.

When a sleep disorder interferes with a person's normal activities and sense of well-being, the intermittent use of sleep aids (also called hypnotics) for up to a week may be helpful. Most sleep aids require a prescription. Sleep aids available without a prescription (over-the-counter, or OTC)▲ contain diphenhydramine or doxylamine, both antihistamines. These drugs may have side effects, especially in older people.

Older people experiencing age-related sleep changes usually do not need to take sleep aids. Because total nighttime sleeping time tends to decrease with age, older people may sleep better if they go to bed later, get up earlier, or nap less during the day. Even when older people have insomnia, treatment with sleep aids often causes more problems (such as confusion, falls, and incontinence) than the insomnia.

If emotional stress is causing insomnia, treatment to relieve the stress is more useful than taking sleep aids. People who have insomnia

Science Wakes Up to Sleep Disorders

People with all types of sleep disorders are sent to sleep laboratories for evaluation, diagnosis, and treatment. The following symptoms may prompt a referral to a sleep laboratory:

- Excessive daytime sleepiness
- Insomnia
- Dependence on sleep aids
- Pauses in breathing
- Severe snoring or choking
- Nightmares
- Sleep abnormalities as witnessed by a sleep partner

An initial evaluation at a sleep laboratory may include the following:

- A sleep history, often including a sleep diary
- A general medical history
- A physical examination
- Blood tests
- A laboratory sleep evaluation

Two examples of laboratory sleep evaluations are overnight polysomnography and a multiple sleep latency test. In overnight polysomnography, a person spends the night in a sleep laboratory with electrodes attached to the head to record brain activity. With this information, sleep stages can be characterized. Other bodily functions, such as heart rate and breathing pattern, are also monitored and recorded. This procedure is used to detect sleep apnea and movement disorders during sleep (parasomnias). In a multiple sleep latency test, a person spends the day in a sleep laboratory, taking four or five naps at 2-hour intervals. This test is used to detect daytime sleepiness, especially that due to narcolepsy.

and depression should be evaluated by a doctor, and the depression should be treated. Treating depression often relieves the insomnia, but some antidepressants can improve sleep directly because they have sedating effects.

Melatonin■ is sometimes used to treat insomnia, especially in older people, who may have low levels of melatonin. The drug is also sometimes used to help minimize the effects

---

▲ see page 100   ■ see page 110

Ways to Improve Sleep

Follow a regular sleep schedule: People should go to bed at the same time each night and, more importantly, get up at the same time each morning, even on weekends.

Follow a bedtime routine: A regular pattern of activities—such as walking at a relaxed pace, listening to soft music, brushing the teeth, washing the face, and setting the alarm clock—can set the mood for sleep. This routine should be followed every night, at home or away.

Make the environment conducive to sleep: The bedroom should be kept dark and quiet and not too warm or too cold. If noises disturb sleep, wearing ear plugs, using a white-noise machine or a fan, or installing heavy curtains in the bedroom (to block out outside noises) may help.

Use the bedroom primarily for sleeping: The bedroom should not be used for eating, reading, watching television, paying bills, or other activities associated with wakefulness.

Avoid substances that interfere with sleep: Food and beverages that contain alcohol or caffeine (such as coffee, tea, cola drinks, and chocolate) can interfere with sleep, as can appetite suppressants and diuretics. These substances should not be consumed, especially near bedtime. Quitting smoking may help. Drinking a large amount of alcohol in the evening causes early morning awakenings.

Use pillows: Pillows between the knees or under the waist can make people more comfortable. For people with back problems, lying on the side with a large pillow between the knees may be helpful.

Get up: When falling asleep is difficult, getting up and doing something else in another room may be more effective than lying in bed and trying harder and harder to fall asleep.

Exercise regularly: Exercise can help people fall asleep naturally. However, exercise late in the evening can stimulate the heart and brain and keep people awake.

Relax: Stress and worry are major impediments to sleep. People who are not sleepy at bedtime can relax by reading or taking a warm bath. People can aim to leave their problems at the bedroom door. Avoiding too much mental stimulation during the hour or so before bedtime can help.

Eat a snack: Hunger can interfere with going to sleep. A light snack, especially if warm, can help.

of jet lag. However, its use is controversial. Melatonin appears to be safe for short-term use (up to a few weeks), but the effects of using it for a long time are unknown.

Hypersomnia

Hypersomnia is a substantial increase in total sleeping time.

Hypersomnia, which is less common than insomnia, refers to an increase of at least 25% in total sleeping time that continues for more than a few days. Hypersomnia does not refer to sleeping substantially more for a few nights or days after a period of sleep deprivation or unusual physical exertion. In such circumstances, extra sleep is a normal response.

Hypersomnia may indicate a serious disorder such as a neurologic disorder (for example, encephalitis, meningitis, or a brain tumor), a heart or lung disorder, or liver failure. Hypersomnia may also be a symptom of sleep apnea or a psychologic disorder (such as severe anxiety or depression). Chronic hypersomnia that begins during adolescence may be a symptom of narcolepsy. Hypersomnia may also result from overuse of sleep aids.

When evaluating a person who has become excessively sleepy, doctors ask about the person's mood, sleep-wake schedule, and use of drugs. Often, a sleep partner can describe the person's sleep abnormalities best. These abnormalities may include snoring and breathing pauses (which suggest obstructive sleep apnea) as well as grinding of teeth, kicking, and sleepwalking. Doctors may evaluate the heart, lungs, and liver to determine whether a disorder is causing hypersomnia. A neurologic examination may also be necessary.▲ It may detect impaired memory or other problems suggesting a neurologic disorder. If a neurologic disorder is suspected, computed tomography (CT) or magnetic resonance imaging (MRI) is performed, and the person is referred to a neurologist.

Narcolepsy

Narcolepsy is a sleep disorder marked by recurring, uncontrollable episodes of sleep during normal waking hours, as well as by sudden episodes of muscle weakness (cataplexy), sleep paralysis, and hallucinations.

▲ see page 439

Sleep Aids: Not to Be Taken Lightly

Among the most commonly used sleep aids are sedatives, minor tranquilizers, and antianxiety drugs. Most are quite safe, but all sleep aids can lose their effectiveness once a person becomes accustomed to them. Sleep aids may also produce withdrawal symptoms when they are discontinued. If a sleep aid is taken for more than a few days, discontinuing it can make the original sleep problem suddenly worse (causing rebound insomnia) and can increase anxiety. Doctors recommend reducing the dose slowly. Complete withdrawal can take several weeks.

Most sleep aids require a doctor's prescription because they may be habit-forming or addictive, and overdose is possible. Sleep aids are particularly risky for older people and for people with breathing problems because they tend to suppress areas of the brain that control breathing. They also reduce daytime alertness, making driving or operating machinery hazardous. Sleep aids are especially dangerous when taken with alcohol, opioids, antihistamines, or antidepressants. All of these drugs also cause drowsiness and can suppress breathing; the combined effects are more dangerous.

The most common and safest sleep aids are **benzodiazepines.** Because they do not decrease the total amount of REM sleep, they do not reduce dreaming. Some benzodiazepines remain in the body longer than others. Older people, who cannot metabolize and excrete drugs as well as younger people, may be more likely to experience daytime drowsiness, slurred speech, and falls. Therefore, doctors try to avoid prescribing long-acting benzodiazepines, such as chlordiazepoxide, diazepam, flurazepam, and nitrazepam, for older people.

Two useful sleep aids that are not benzodiazepines are zopiclone and zolpidem. They are short-acting. They help people with insomnia sleep better without changing the natural sleep pattern. Older people appear to tolerate these drugs well.

Barbiturates, once the most commonly used sleep aid, and **meprobamate** are not as safe as benzodiazepines. **Chloral hydrate** is relatively safe but relatively weak. It is used much less often than benzodiazepines.

Some **antidepressants,** amitriptyline for example, can relieve depression-associated insomnia and early morning awakening caused by panic attacks, but side effects can be a problem, especially for older people.

Diphenhydramine and **dimenhydrinate** are two inexpensive nonprescription (over-the-counter) drugs that can relieve occasional or mild sleeping problems. However, they are not used primarily as sleep aids, and they may have side effects, especially in older people.

Narcolepsy occurs in about 1 of 200,000 people. The disorder tends to run in families, but its cause is unknown. Although narcolepsy has no serious medical consequences, it can be disabling and may increase the risk of motor vehicle and other accidents.

Symptoms

Symptoms usually begin during adolescence or young adulthood and persist throughout life. Only about 10% of people with narcolepsy have all the symptoms; most people have only a few.

People with narcolepsy are overcome by sudden episodes of uncontrollable sleepiness that can occur at any time. Falling asleep can be resisted only temporarily. A person may have many episodes or only a few in a single day; each usually lasts half an hour or less. Episodes are most likely to occur in monotonous situations, such as during boring meetings or long periods of highway driving. When intentionally taking short naps, the person usually feels refreshed after awakening.

A sudden episode of muscle weakness without loss of consciousness—called cataplexy—may be triggered by a sudden emotional reaction such as anger, fear, joy, laughter, or surprise. The person may become limp, drop something being held, or fall to the ground. These episodes resemble the muscle relaxation that occurs during REM sleep and, to a lesser degree, the experience of being "weak with laughter."

Occasionally, when just falling asleep or immediately after awakening, the person tries to move but cannot. This experience, called sleep paralysis, can be terrifying. The touch of another person may relieve the paralysis. Otherwise, the paralysis disappears on its own after several minutes.

When just falling asleep or, less often, when awakening, the person may clearly see images or hear sounds that are not there. These extremely vivid hallucinations (called hypnagogic hallucinations) are similar to those of normal dreaming but are more intense.

Diagnosis and Treatment

The diagnosis is usually based on the symptoms, but the same symptoms can be caused by other disorders. Sleep paralysis and hallucinations occasionally occur in otherwise healthy adults. If the diagnosis is uncertain, electroencephalography (EEG), which records the brain's electrical activity,▲ is performed, usually in a sleep laboratory. If a person has narcolepsy, EEG typically shows that REM-type sleep activity occurs as the person falls asleep, rather than later in the sleep cycle as it normally does. Usually, narcolepsy does not result from abnormalities that can be detected by imaging procedures.

Stimulant drugs, such as amphetamine, dextroamphetamine, methylphenidate, modafinil, and pimoline, may help reduce the sleepiness. The dose may have to be adjusted to prevent side effects such as jitteriness, overactivity, or weight loss. Consequently, doctors monitor people closely when they begin drug treatment. Modafinil may have fewer side effects than the other drugs. An antidepressant such as imipramine usually helps relieve cataplexy. Frequent, short (15- to 20-minute) naps during the day often help.

Sleep Apnea Syndromes

Sleep apnea syndromes are a group of serious sleep disorders in which breathing repeatedly stops long enough during sleep to decrease the amount of oxygen and increase the amount of carbon dioxide in the blood and brain.

Sleep apnea occurs when breathing is temporarily interrupted during sleep. There are three types.

Obstructive sleep apnea, the most common type, is caused by a blockage in the throat or upper airway. It affects about 4 to 6% of middle-aged men and 1 to 2% of middle-aged women in the United States. Obstructive sleep apnea most commonly occurs in obese people, who tend to sleep on their back. Obesity, perhaps in combination with aging body tissues and other factors, leads to narrowing of the upper airway. Smoking and excessive use of alcohol worsen obstructive sleep apnea.

Lung disorders (such as emphysema) contribute to the lack of oxygen. Having a narrow throat and upper airway, which tend to run in families, increases the risk of sleep apnea. In children, enlarged tonsils or adenoids can cause obstructive sleep apnea.

Central sleep apnea, a much rarer type, is caused by dysfunction in the part of the brain that controls breathing (brain stem). Normally, the brain stem is very sensitive to changes in the blood level of carbon dioxide (a by-product of the metabolism of oxygen). When the level is high, the brain stem signals the respiratory muscles to breathe harder and faster to remove carbon dioxide through exhalation, and vice versa. In central sleep apnea, the brain stem is less sensitive to changes in the carbon dioxide level. Because the brain stem responds slowly to the buildup of carbon dioxide in the blood, the body's response is exaggerated, resulting in prolonged hyperventilation. Similarly, because the brain stem responds slowly to the removal of carbon dioxide from the blood, the body's response—a pause in breathing—is prolonged. Brain stem dysfunction that leads to central sleep apnea may be due to brain tumors. People who have heart failure may have central sleep apnea. In one form of central sleep apnea, called Ondine's curse, people may breathe inadequately or not at all except when they are fully awake. Central sleep apnea is not associated with obesity.

Mixed sleep apnea, the third type, is a combination of obstructive sleep apnea and central sleep apnea. For example, obstructive sleep apnea sometimes causes central sleep apnea—by decreasing oxygen levels and increasing carbon dioxide levels in the blood long enough to cause the brain stem to malfunction. Mixed sleep apnea is rare.

Symptoms

Because symptoms occur during sleep, they are usually first noticed by a sleep partner. In all types of sleep apnea, breathing may become abnormally slow and shallow, or breathing may suddenly stop for at least 10 seconds (sometimes up to 1 minute), then resume.

In obstructive sleep apnea, the most common symptom is snoring, with episodes of gasping, choking, pauses in breathing, and sudden awakenings. When obstructive sleep apnea is severe, repeated bouts of sleep-related obstructive choking occur at night and involuntary naps occur during the day. Eventually, these naps interfere with daytime work and

▲ see page 445

reduce the quality of life. Memory may be impaired, sex drive may be reduced, and personality may change. In people with obstructive sleep apnea, the risk of such complications as stroke, heart attack, and high blood pressure is increased. If episodes of obstructive sleep apnea are more frequent than 20 per hour, the risk of death is increased.

People who are extremely obese often have obesity-hypoventilation syndrome (pickwickian syndrome) as well as obstructive sleep apnea. Excess body fat interferes with the movement of the chest wall, reducing the amount of air that reaches the lungs. Excess body fat below the diaphragm compresses the lungs, making breathing shallow. Excess body fat around the throat compresses the upper airway, reducing air flow.

In central sleep apnea, snoring does not usually occur. However, patterns of breathing may be abnormal. Cheyne-Stokes respiration (periodic breathing) is an example. In Cheyne-Stokes respiration, breathing gradually becomes more rapid, gradually slows down, stops for a short period, then starts again. Then the cycle repeats. Each cycle lasts 30 seconds to 2 minutes.

In all types of sleep apnea, the disturbances in sleep can result in daytime sleepiness, fatigue, irritability, headaches in the mornings, slowness of thought, and difficulty concentrating. Because oxygen levels in the blood may decrease significantly, abnormal heart rhythms may develop, and blood pressure may increase.

Prolonged, severe sleep apnea of any type eventually leads to heart failure and malfunction of the lungs. Then the heart cannot pump enough blood to the body, and the lungs cannot provide enough oxygen to or remove enough carbon dioxide from the body.

Diagnosis

In its early stages, sleep apnea is often diagnosed on the basis of information provided by the person's sleep partner. The partner may report that the person snores loudly, periodically stops breathing, awakens choking and frightened from sleep, and is becoming increasingly tired during the day. For example, the person may fall asleep while watching television, while attending a meeting, or even while driving.

The diagnosis is best confirmed and severity is best determined in a sleep laboratory. Electroencephalography (EEG)▲ is used to monitor changes in levels of sleep. Eye movements can be recorded during REM sleep with electrodes placed near the eyes (a procedure called

electro-oculography). Also, the oxygen level in the blood is measured with an electrode placed on a finger or an earlobe (a procedure called oximetry). Airflow is measured with a device placed in front of the nostrils, and the motion and pattern of breathing are measured with an electrode or gauge placed on the chest. This evaluation can help doctors distinguish between obstructive and central sleep apnea.

Treatment

Obstructive Sleep Apnea: Losing weight, quitting smoking, and not using alcohol excessively can help. Heavy snorers and people who often choke in their sleep should not consume alcohol or take sleep aids, antihistamines, or other drugs that cause drowsiness. Nasal infections and allergies should be treated.

Sleeping on the side or elevating the head of the bed can help reduce snoring. Special anti-snoring pillows strapped on the back help prevent people from sleeping on their back. The various other devices marketed to reduce snoring usually help only when snoring is mild, and they do not relieve obstructive sleep apnea. If treatment is needed for heavy snoring, the small piece of tissue that hangs down at the back of the mouth (uvula) may be surgically removed in a procedure called uvulo-palatoplasty.

Removable oral appliances, fitted by dentists, can help relieve obstructive sleep apnea (and snoring) for many people. These appliances, which are worn only while sleeping, help keep the airway open. Most appliances separate the jaws and push the lower jaw forward so the tongue cannot move backward to block the throat. Others hold the tongue forward.

If the above measures do not eliminate or relieve sleep apnea, people may benefit from continuous positive airway pressure (CPAP). With CPAP, room air that is under pressure is delivered through a face mask. The pressure keeps the airways open as the person breathes in. For the first two weeks of use, wearing the mask may seem uncomfortable and the nasal passages may dry out. But with continued use, many people can adapt. Also using a humidifier helps some people adapt.

Surgery to enlarge the airway through the throat (uvulopalatopharyngoplasty) is occasionally performed, but it is usually successful only in people who have mild sleep apnea.

▲ see page 445

Central Sleep Apnea: The underlying disorder is treated if possible. For example, drugs may be given to reduce the severity of heart failure.▲ As in obstructive sleep apnea, people with central sleep apnea also often benefit from CPAP. Oxygen delivered by nasal prongs (not under pressure) may also be helpful. Acetazolamide and theophylline are used occasionally. These drugs can stimulate the drive to breathe.

Parasomnias

Parasomnias are unusual behaviors that occur during sleep.

Various unconscious and largely unremembered behaviors can occur during sleep, more often in children than in adults. Just before falling asleep, almost all people occasionally experience brief, involuntary jerks of the arms or the entire body. Occasionally, the legs jerk. Some people also experience sleep paralysis (attempting but being unable to move) or brief hallucinations when they are just falling asleep or awakening. People may clench or grind their teeth or have nightmares. Sleepwalking, head-banging, and night terrors are more common among children and can be very distressing for their parents. Usually, the children do not remember these episodes.

Restless legs syndrome is a relatively common disorder, probably affecting 1 to 5% of people. It is particularly common among people older than 50. The cause is unknown, but one third or more of people with the syndrome have family members with the syndrome. Risk factors include a sedentary lifestyle, smoking, and obesity. Use of alcohol, caffeine, and many drugs (mostly antidepressants) worsens the syndrome, as do iron deficiency and pregnancy.

Typically, people with restless leg syndrome feel vague but intense crawling sensations in their legs and have an urge to move their legs when sitting still or when lying in bed before falling asleep. Walking or moving the legs can relieve the sensations. During sleep, the legs move spontaneously and uncontrollably, often awakening the sleeper. Symptoms are more likely to occur when people are under stress. The resulting sleep loss and distress may be extreme.

Benzodiazepine drugs (such as clonazepam in low doses), taken at bedtime, sometimes relieve the symptoms of restless legs syndrome. People with severe symptoms may benefit from drugs used to treat Parkinson's disease, such as pergolide, levodopa-carbidopa, or pramipexole.■ The opioid oxycodone or the anticonvulsants gabapentin or carbamazepine★ are effective in some people.

Night terrors are frightening episodes during which a person sits up, screams, and flails about. The eyes are wide open, and the heart races. Episodes usually occur during non-REM stages of sleep. Night terrors are more common among children. Children should not be awakened. They usually stop having episodes when they become older. Episodes in adults are often associated with psychologic problems or alcoholism. Treatment with certain benzodiazepines, such as clonazepam, or tricyclic antidepressants, such as imipramine, may be helpful.

Nightmares are vivid, frightening dreams, followed by sudden awakening. Children and adults can have nightmares. Nightmares occur during REM sleep. They are more likely to occur when a person is under stress, has a fever, is excessively tired, or has consumed alcohol. Treatment, if necessary, focuses on the underlying problem.

Sleepwalking (somnambulism), most common in late childhood and adolescence, is walking in a semiconscious manner without being aware of it. It occurs during the deepest stages of sleep. People do not dream while sleepwalking—in fact, brain activity during sleepwalking, although abnormal, is more like that of a wakeful state than of a sleeping one. Sleepwalkers may mumble repetitiously and can hurt themselves by walking into obstacles. Most sleepwalkers have no memory of sleepwalking.

No specific treatment is available, but the sleepwalker can be gently led back to bed. Leaving a light on in the bedroom or adjacent hall sometimes reduces the tendency to sleepwalk. Forcibly awakening the sleepwalker may provoke an angry reaction and is not advised. Obstacles or breakable objects in the sleepwalker's potential path should be removed, and windows should be kept closed and locked. Benzodiazepines, particularly diazepam and alprazolam, may help. Selective serotonin reuptake inhibitors (SSRIs)● may be used if benzodiazepines are ineffective.

▲ see table on page 156   ■ see table on page 549
★ see table on page 500   ● see table on page 618

Sleep Disorders in People With Dementia

In people with dementia,▲ such as Alzheimer's disease, sleep patterns are often abnormal. As dementia progresses, the time spent in light sleep increases, so people are easily awakened.

People with dementia may have disorders that contribute to sleep problems. Disorders such as arthritis, dehydration, and infections may cause pain or discomfort, interfering with sleep. Use of certain drugs or interactions between drugs may also interfere with sleep.

Treatment of the underlying disorder may help improve sleep. Naps during the day are not helpful because they may make sleeping at night more difficult. Walking outside in the sunshine, keeping the temperature in the bedroom comfortable, and not consuming beverages or foods that contain caffeine during the evening may help.

CHAPTER 82

Brain Dysfunction

When the brain is damaged, it can malfunction in many ways. Such dysfunction ranges from complete loss of consciousness (as occurs in a coma), to disorientation and an inability to pay attention (as occurs in delirium), to impairment of one or several of the many specific functions that contribute to conscious experience. The type and severity of brain dysfunction depend on how extensive brain damage is, where the damage is, and how quickly the disorder causing it is progressing.

Brain dysfunction may be widespread (diffuse) or limited to a specific area (localized). Diffuse dysfunction is caused by disorders that affect large areas of the brain. These disorders include those that produce metabolic abnormalities, such as low levels of sugar in the blood (hypoglycemia) or low levels of oxygen in the blood (usually due to a lung or heart disorder); infections, such as meningitis and encephalitis; and very high or low blood pressure. Diffuse brain dysfunction may also result from disorders that cause swelling of or put pressure on a large area of the brain. These disorders include brain tumors, brain abscesses, and severe head injuries. Certain drugs, such as opioids (narcotics), some sedatives (for example, benzodiazepines and barbiturates), and antidepressants may cause diffuse brain dysfunction if people are sensitive to their effects (as older people are) or if the level of drug in the blood is too high.

Localized brain dysfunction is caused by disorders that affect a specific area of the brain. These disorders include structural abnormalities, such as a brain tumor; disorders that reduce the blood (and thus the oxygen) supply to a specific area, such as a stroke; and certain types of seizure disorders.

The extent and location of brain damage are interrelated in the way they affect the severity of brain dysfunction. Within a relatively large area of the brain such as the cerebral cortex, the degree of dysfunction is relative to the extent of the damage: The more extensive the damage, the more severe the dysfunction is likely to be. However, in a smaller area such as the brain stem (which regulates critical body functions and levels of consciousness), a relatively small amount of damage may cause complete loss of consciousness and even death.

Disorders that progress rapidly are more likely to cause noticeable symptoms of brain dysfunction than disorders that progress slowly—for example, a fast-growing brain tumor versus a slow-growing one. The brain compensates for gradual changes more easily than for rapid changes.

Three characteristics of the brain contribute to its ability to compensate and recover after it has been damaged:

• Redundancy (many brain functions can be performed by more than one area)

▲ see page 484

When Specific Areas of the Brain Are Damaged

Different areas of the brain control specific functions. Consequently, where the brain is damaged determines which function is lost.

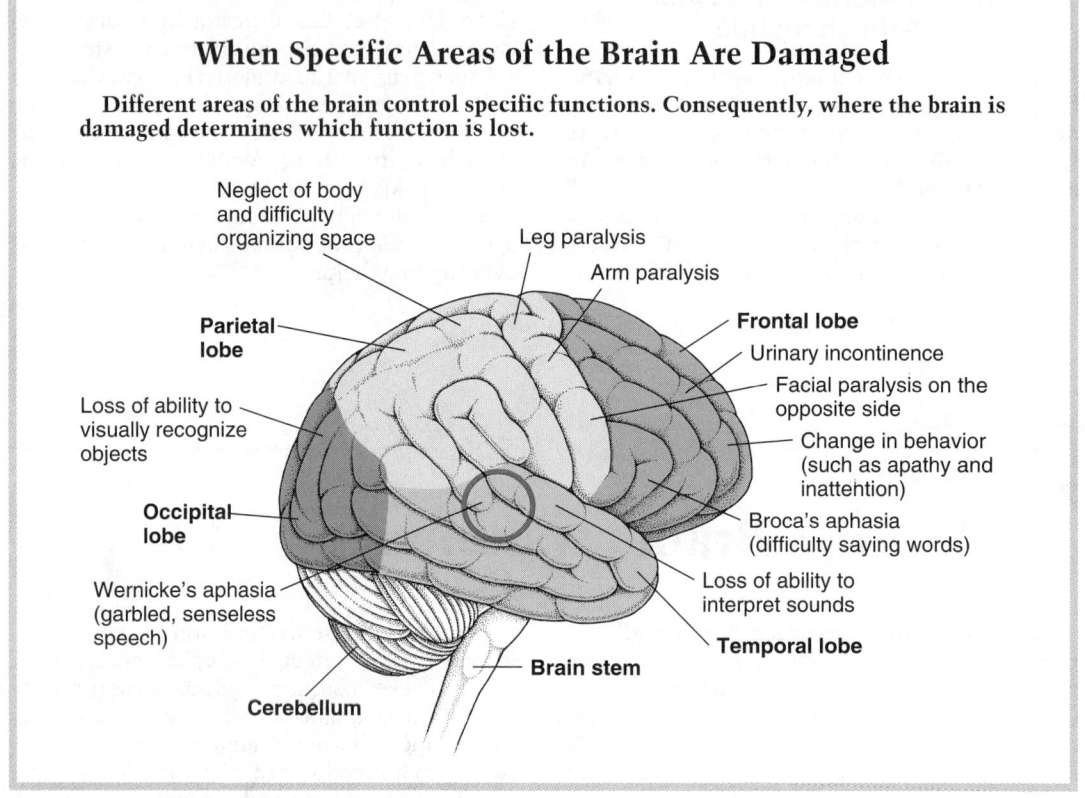

- Adaptation (areas with somewhat overlapping functions can sometimes compensate for lost functions)
- Plasticity (certain areas can shift to a different function)

Consequently, undamaged areas of the brain sometimes take over functions performed by a damaged area, contributing to recovery. However, as people age, the brain becomes less able to shift functions from one area to another. Some functions, such as vision, cannot be performed by other areas of the brain. Direct damage to areas that control such functions may have permanent effects.

Dysfunction by Location

Because different areas of the brain control specific functions,▲ the location of the brain damage determines the type of dysfunction that results. Which side of the brain is affected is also important because the functions of the

▲ see page 434

two halves of the cerebrum (cerebral hemispheres) are not identical. Some functions of the brain are performed exclusively by one hemisphere. For example, movement and sensation on one side of the body are controlled by the hemisphere on the opposite side. Other functions are performed predominantly by one hemisphere. For example, the left hemisphere is predominantly responsible for language. Damage to only one hemisphere of the brain may cause complete loss of such functions. However, other functions, such as memory, are performed by both hemispheres, so that complete loss of a function requires damage to both hemispheres.

Specific patterns of dysfunction can be related to the area of the brain that has been damaged.

Frontal Lobe Damage: Generally, damage to the frontal lobes causes loss of the ability to solve problems and to plan and initiate actions, such as crossing the street or answering a complex question.

If the back part of the frontal lobe (which controls voluntary movements) is damaged, weakness or paralysis can result. Because each side of the brain predominantly controls movement of the opposite side of the body, damage to the left hemisphere causes weakness on the right side of the body, and vice versa.

If the middle part of the frontal lobe is damaged, the ability to move the eyes, to perform complex movements in the correct sequence, or to say words may be impaired. Impairment of the ability to say words is called expressive aphasia.▲

If the front part of the frontal lobe is damaged, the result may be impaired concentration and reduced fluency of speech; apathy, inattentiveness, and delayed responses to questions; or a striking lack of inhibition, including socially inappropriate behavior. People who lose their inhibitions may be inappropriately euphoric or depressed, excessively argumentative or passive, and vulgar. They may show disregard for the consequences of their behavior. They may also repeat what they say.

Parietal Lobe Damage: Damage to the front part of the parietal lobe on one side causes numbness and impairs sensation on the opposite side of the body. Affected people have difficulty identifying a sensation's location and type (pain, heat, cold, or vibration). Damage to the back part of the parietal lobe causes right-left disorientation and problems with calculations and drawing. Damage to the right parietal lobe can cause apraxia—the inability to perform simple skilled tasks, such as brushing the hair or dressing. Sudden damage to the parietal lobe can cause people to ignore the serious nature of their disorder and even neglect or deny the existence of the side of the body opposite the injury. Such people may become confused or delirious and unable to dress themselves or to perform other ordinary tasks.

Temporal Lobe Damage: Damage to the right temporal lobe tends to impair memory for sounds and shapes. Damage to the left temporal lobe can drastically impair memory for words as well as the ability to understand language (causing receptive aphasia). Sometimes damage to a part of the temporal lobe can cause personality changes such as humorlessness, extreme religiosity, and loss of libido.

Occipital Lobe Damage: The occipital lobe contains the main center for processing visual information. When the occipital lobe on both sides of the brain is damaged, cortical blindness results. People with this disorder cannot see, even though the eyes themselves are func-

Testing a Person With Aphasia

Broca's aphasia: Answers to questions are given hesitantly but are sensible.
Question: "What is this a picture of?" (dog barking)
Answer: "D--d--d--dg, eh, no...d-d...damn...p-p-pet, yeah, yeah, pet, pet, pet...b--b--...makes noise."

Wernicke's aphasia: Answers to questions are given fluently but are nonsensical.
Question: "How are you today?"
Answer: "When? Easy for my river runs black boxes wizzel abata H on when boobles come."

Conduction aphasia: Language is understood and spontaneous speech is unaffected, but sentences spoken or written by others cannot be repeated.
Question: Repeat the following "No ifs, ands, or buts about it."
Answer: "No nifs nand nor but..."

Anomia: Naming things is difficult.
Question: "What is this?" (Point to a jacket lapel, watch band, or pen.)
Answer: "What you wear, thing for time, you write with it."

tioning normally. Some people with cortical blindness are unaware that they cannot see. Damage to the front part of the occipital lobe can impair the ability to recognize familiar objects and faces and to accurately interpret what is seen.

Specific Types of Dysfunction

Many functions of the brain are performed by several areas of the brain working together (networks), not by a single area in the brain. Damage to these networks can cause aphasia, apraxia, agnosia, or amnesia.

APHASIA

Aphasia is a partial or complete loss of the ability to express or understand spoken or written language because of damage to the language areas of the brain.

In most people, part of the left temporal lobe called Wernicke's area and part of the frontal lobe called Broca's area control language function. Damage to any part of these

▲ see page 478

small areas by a stroke, a tumor, a head injury, or an infection interferes with at least some aspect of language function.

Aphasia is loss of the ability to express or understand language, but it takes many forms and may be partial or complete. The variety reflects the complex nature of language function. Aphasia may involve loss of only the ability to comprehend written words (alexia) or the ability to recall or say the names of objects (anomia). Some people with anomia cannot remember the right word at all; others have a word in mind but cannot say it. People with conduction aphasia understand spoken and written words and can speak fluently but cannot repeat words, phrases, or sentences.

People with **Wernicke's aphasia,** which can result from damage to Wernicke's area, speak fluently, but the sentences come out as garbled, confused strings of words (sometimes referred to as word salad).

People with **Broca's aphasia** (expressive aphasia), which can result from damage to Broca's area, largely understand the meaning of words and know how they want to respond. However, they have trouble saying the words. Their words are forced out slowly and with great effort, sometimes interrupted by expletives. Usually, writing is affected the same way as speech.

Damage to the left temporal and frontal lobes may cause complete (global) aphasia, making a person almost entirely mute. The person may be able to utter expletives because the right side of the brain, which is more involved in emotions, is not damaged. During recovery, the person has impaired speech (dysphasia), writing (dysgraphia), and understanding of language (receptive aphasia).

Speech therapists can help people who develop aphasia after brain damage due to such disorders as a stroke or head injury.▲ Treatment is usually started as soon as the person is able to participate.

DYSARTHRIA

Dysarthria is loss of the ability to articulate words normally.

Although dysarthria seems to be a language problem, it is really a muscular (motor) problem. It may be caused by damage to the brain stem or to the nerve fibers that connect the

cerebral cortex to the brain stem. These parts of the brain control the muscles used to make sounds or to coordinate movements of the lips, tongue, palate, and vocal cords, which are used to produce speech.

People who have dysarthria produce sounds that approximate what they mean and that are in the correct order. Speech may be jerky, staccato, breathy, irregular, imprecise, or monotonous, depending on where the damage is. Because the ability to understand and use language is not usually affected, most people with dysarthria can read and write normally. Speech therapy helps some people with dysarthria.■

APRAXIA

Apraxia is loss of the ability to perform tasks that require remembering patterns or sequences of movements.

Apraxia, an uncommon disability, is usually caused by damage to the parietal or frontal lobes. In apraxia, the memory of the sequence of movements needed to complete simple skilled or complex tasks is impaired. For example, buttoning a button, which consists of a series of steps, may be impossible, even though the hands are physically capable of performing the task. People with verbal apraxia cannot produce the basic sound units of speech because they cannot initiate, coordinate, or sequence the muscle movements needed to talk.

Some forms of apraxia affect only particular tasks. For example, a person may lose the ability to do any one of the following: draw a picture, write a note, button a jacket, tie a shoelace, pick up a telephone receiver, or play a musical instrument.

Occupational therapy may help some people with apraxia learn to compensate for their losses.★

AGNOSIA

Agnosia is loss of the ability to associate objects with their usual role or function.

Agnosia is relatively rare. Agnosia is caused by dysfunction in the parietal, temporal, or occipital lobes of the brain, where memories of the uses and importance of familiar objects, sights, and sounds are stored. Agnosia often develops suddenly after a head injury or stroke. When one parietal lobe is damaged (usually the result of a stroke), people have difficulty identifying a familiar object, such as a key or safety pin, that is placed in the hand on the side of the body opposite the damage.

▲ see page 44   ■ see page 44
★ see page 44

However, when they look at the object, they immediately recognize and can identify it. When the occipital lobe is damaged, people have visual agnosia. They cannot recognize familiar faces or common objects, such as a spoon or a pencil, even though they can see these things. When the temporal lobe is damaged, people have auditory agnosia. They cannot recognize sounds even though they can hear sounds. Some people with agnosia improve or recover spontaneously; others must learn to cope with their strange disability. No specific treatment exists.

AMNESIA

Amnesia is total or partial loss of the ability to recall experiences or events that happened in the preceding few seconds (immediate memory), in the preceding few seconds to few days (intermediate memory), or further back in time (remote or long-term memory).

The causes of amnesia are only partly understood. Damage to the brain can produce memory loss of events that occurred just before (retrograde amnesia) or just after (posttraumatic amnesia) the damage occurred. Depending on the severity of the damage, most amnesias last for only minutes or hours and disappear without treatment. However, with severe brain damage, amnesia can be permanent.

Learning requires memory. The brain's mechanisms for storing information and recalling it from memory are located primarily in the temporal and frontal lobes. Emotions originating from the brain's limbic system can influence both the storing of memories and their retrieval. The limbic system is also closely connected to areas responsible for alertness and awareness. Because memory involves many interwoven brain functions, virtually any type of brain damage can result in memory loss.

Transient global amnesia is a sudden temporary loss of the ability to store new memories, resulting in forgetfulness and confusion about time, place, and sometimes the identity of other people. This type of amnesia may be caused by temporary blockage of the arteries that supply blood to the temporal lobe in people with atherosclerosis, especially older people. It may also be caused by a seizure originating in the temporal lobe. Often, the cause is unknown. In young adults, migraine headaches, which temporarily reduce blood flow to the brain, may cause transient global amnesia.

Most people with transient global amnesia have only one episode in a lifetime; about 10% have repeated episodes. Episodes can last from 30 minutes to about 12 hours. The amnesia may totally disorient a person and block recall of events that happened during the previous few years. After an episode, the confusion usually clears quickly, and total recovery is the rule.

The **Wernicke-Korsakoff syndrome,** an unusual form of amnesia, may develop in alcoholics and other malnourished people. The syndrome is a combination of two disorders: an acute confusional state (Wernicke's encephalopathy) and an amnesia (Korsakoff's syndrome). Korsakoff's syndrome accompanies Wernicke's encephalopathy in about 80% of people.

Both Wernicke's encephalopathy and Korsakoff's syndrome can be caused by a deficiency of thiamin (vitamin B_1), which is necessary for the body to process carbohydrates. Drinking large amounts of alcohol without eating foods that contain thiamin decreases the brain's supply of this vitamin. In malnourished people (who do not consume enough thiamin), Wernicke's encephalopathy can be suddenly triggered by eating a large carbohydrate-rich meal (such as spaghetti), drinking highly sweetened liquids, or receiving a large amount of glucose (a sugar) intravenously to treat dehydration.

The Wernicke-Korsakoff syndrome may also result from damage to the temporal lobe by an injury, a stroke, a tumor, or a brain infection (encephalitis).

In addition to confusion, symptoms of Wernicke's encephalopathy include loss of balance, drowsiness, a tendency to stagger, and eye movement problems, such as paralysis of eye movements, double vision, and a rapid movement of the eyes in one direction followed by a slower drift back to the original position (nystagmus). Memory loss is often severe initially.

Korsakoff's syndrome may be permanent if it follows severe or repeated episodes of encephalopathy or of severe symptoms after alcohol withdrawal (delirium tremens). Severe memory loss is often accompanied by agitation and delirium. In Korsakoff's syndrome, immediate memory is retained, but intermediate memory and memory for relatively remote events (of previous weeks or months) are lost. However, more remote memory sometimes survives. People with chronic Korsakoff's syndrome may be able to interact socially and converse coherently even though they cannot remember anything that happened in the preceding few days, months, or years or even in the preceding few minutes. Bewildered by the lack of memory, they tend to make things up (confabulate) rather than admit that they cannot remember. Then they cannot distinguish real memories from the ones they have made up. People with Korsakoff's syndrome are highly suggestible; for example, they can be led to say they see things that are not there. They can read the same magazine over and over as if for the first time.

For alcoholics, thiamin is given intravenously as soon as possible after symptoms be-

gin. Such treatment can correct Wernicke's encephalopathy. Untreated, Wernicke's encephalopathy can be fatal. For this reason, alcoholics who go to the hospital for any reason are promptly given thiamin. Prompt treatment with thiamin also prevents Korsakoff's syndrome, which develops if treatment is delayed. Thiamin does not correct Korsakoff's syndrome but is necessary because Korsakoff's syndrome can be fatal unless treated promptly. Sometimes Wernicke-Korsakoff syndrome gradually resolves if alcohol is avoided and a healthy diet is consumed. However, when Wernicke-Korsakoff syndrome is due to temporal lobe damage, recovery is gradual and may be incomplete.

CHAPTER 83

Delirium and Dementia

Delirium and dementia are the most common causes of mental (cognitive) dysfunction—the inability to acquire, retain, and use knowledge normally. Although delirium and dementia may occur together, they are quite different. Delirium begins suddenly, causes fluctuations in mental function, and is usually reversible. Dementia begins gradually, is slowly progressive, and is usually irreversible. Also, the two disorders affect mental function differently. Delirium impairs the ability to pay attention and to think clearly. Dementia causes loss of memory and a severe decline in all aspects of mental function. Both delirium and dementia may occur at any age but are much more common among older people, because of age-related changes in the brain.▲

Delirium

Delirium is a sudden, fluctuating, and usually reversible cognitive disorder characterized by disorientation, the inability to pay attention, the inability to think clearly, and a change in the level of consciousness.

Delirium is an abnormal mental state, not a disease. Although the term has a specific med-

ical definition, it is often used to describe any type of confusion.

Because delirium is a temporary condition, determining how many people have it is difficult. Delirium, which is usually a sign of a newly developed disorder, affects about one third of hospitalized people aged 70 or older.

Causes

Development or worsening of almost any disorder can cause delirium. Any person can become delirious when they are extremely ill or are taking drugs that affect brain function. However, delirium can result from less severe conditions in older people and in people whose brain has been affected by a stroke, dementia, or other disorders that cause nerve degeneration. In such people, delirium can result from a relatively minor illness, such as retention of urine or feces; sensory deprivation, such as that due to being socially isolated or not wearing glasses or hearing aids; or prolonged sleep deprivation. For example, the sensory and sleep deprivation that occurs in intensive care units (ICUs) may contribute to delirium. This disorder is sometimes called ICU psychosis.

Being in the hospital can also contribute to or trigger delirium. About 10 to 20% of older people develop delirium *while* they are in the

▲ see page 438

hospital. Delirium is also very common after surgery, probably because of the stress of surgery, the anesthetics used during surgery, and the analgesics used after surgery.

The most common reversible cause of delirium is drugs. Delirium may result from use of a drug or from withdrawal of a drug that has been taken for a long time. In younger people, ingestion of poisons (such as rubbing alcohol or antifreeze), use of illicit drugs, or acute intoxication with alcohol are common causes of delirium. In older people, prescription drugs are usually the cause. Psychoactive drugs, such as opioids (including morphine and meperidine), sedatives (including benzodiazepines), antipsychotics, and antidepressants, impair brain function by their direct effects on nerve cells. Delirium may result. Drugs with anticholinergic effects,▲ including many over-the-counter (OTC) antihistamines, may cause delirium. Amphetamines, which are stimulants, may also cause delirium. Sudden withdrawal of a sedative (such as a benzodiazepine or barbiturate) that has been taken for a long time frequently results in delirium. Delirium commonly occurs in alcoholics who suddenly stop drinking alcohol■ and in heroin users who suddenly stop using heroin.

Abnormal blood levels of electrolytes, such as calcium, sodium, or magnesium, can interfere with the metabolic activity of nerve cells and lead to delirium. Abnormal electrolyte levels may result from use of a diuretic, dehydration, or disorders such as kidney failure and widespread cancer. An underactive thyroid gland (hypothyroidism) causes delirium with lethargy; an overactive thyroid gland (hyperthyroidism) causes delirium with hyperactivity.

In younger people, the cause of delirium is usually a condition that directly affects the brain—for example a brain infection, such as meningitis or encephalitis. In older people, the cause is usually drugs or a disorder that affects other parts of the body—for example, an infection that affects the brain indirectly, such as a urinary tract infection, pneumonia, or influenza.

Symptoms

Delirium usually begins suddenly and progresses over hours or days. The actions of people with delirium vary but roughly resemble those of a person who is becoming progressively more intoxicated.

The hallmark of delirium is an inability to pay attention. People with delirium cannot

What Is Confusion?

Confusion means different things to different people, but doctors use the term to describe people who cannot process information normally. Confused people cannot

- follow a conversation
- answer questions appropriately
- understand where they are
- make critical judgments that affect safety
- remember important facts

Confusion has many different causes, including the use of certain drugs (prescription, over-the-counter, and illicit) and a wide variety of disorders. Delirium and dementia, though very different disorders, both cause confusion.

When a person is confused, doctors try to determine what the cause is, particularly if it is delirium or dementia. If confusion develops or worsens suddenly, the cause may be delirium. In such cases, medical attention is needed immediately, because delirium may be caused by a serious disorder. Also, treating the cause, once identified, can often reverse the delirium. If confusion develops slowly, the cause may be dementia. Medical attention is needed but not urgently. Treatment may slow the mental decline in people with dementia but cannot restore mental function and usually cannot stop the decline.

concentrate, so they have trouble processing new information and cannot recall recent events. Sudden confusion about time and, at least partially, about place (where they are) may be an early sign of delirium. If delirium is severe, people may not know who they are. Thinking is confused, and people with delirium ramble, sometimes becoming incoherent. The level of consciousness may fluctuate between increased wakefulness and drowsiness. Symptoms often change within minutes and tend to worsen late in the day (a phenomenon called sundowning). People with delirium often sleep restlessly or reverse their sleep-wake cycle, sleeping during the day and staying awake at night.

People with delirium may be frightened by bizarre visual hallucinations, seeing things or

▲ see box on page 79 ■ see page 649

IS IT DELIRIUM OR PSYCHOSIS?

COMMON SIGNS OF DELIRIUM	COMMON SIGNS OF PSYCHOSIS DUE TO A PSYCHIATRIC DISORDER
Confusion about current time, date, place, or identity	Usually, awareness of time, date, place, and identity
Difficulty paying attention	Retention of ability to pay attention
Loss of recent memory	Retention of recent memory
Inability to think logically	Inability to think logically
Inability to perform simple calculations	Retention of ability to calculate
Preoccupations commonly inconsistent	Preoccupations often fixed and consistent
Hallucinations (if any) mostly visual or involving touch	Hallucinations (if any) mostly auditory
Fever or other signs of infection	History of previous psychiatric disturbances
Evidence of recent drug use	Drug use not necessarily involved
Tremor	Usually, no tremor

people that are not there. Some people develop paranoia or have delusions (false beliefs usually involving a misinterpretation of perceptions or experiences).

Personality and mood may change. Some people become so quiet and withdrawn that no one notices that they are delirious. Others become agitated and restless and may pace. People who develop delirium after taking sedatives are likely to become very drowsy and withdrawn. Those who have taken amphetamines or who have stopped taking sedatives may become aggressive and hyperactive.

Delirium can last hours, days, or even longer, depending on the severity and the cause. If the cause of delirium is not quickly identified and treated, the person may become increasingly drowsy and unresponsive, requiring vigorous stimulation to be aroused (a condition called stupor▲). Stupor may lead to coma or death. Delirium is often the first sign of another, sometimes serious disorder, especially in older people.

▲ see page 490　　■ see page 439

Diagnosis

Mild delirium may be difficult to recognize. Doctors may miss up to 80% of all cases of delirium in hospitalized people.

Most people thought to have delirium are hospitalized for evaluation and protection. Diagnostic procedures can be performed quickly and safely in the hospital, and any disorders detected can be treated quickly.

Because delirium may be caused by a serious disorder (which could be rapidly fatal), doctors try to identify the cause as quickly as possible. Treating the cause, once identified, can often reverse the delirium.

Doctors first try to distinguish delirium from other disorders that affect mental function. Doctors collect as much information about the person's medical history as possible. Friends, family members, or other observers are asked how the confusion began, how quickly it progressed, and what they know about the person's physical and mental health and use of drugs (including alcohol and illicit drugs, especially for younger people). Information may come from medical records, the police, emergency medical personnel, or evidence such as pill bottles and certain documents. Documents such as a checkbook, recent letters, or notification of unpaid bills or missed appointments can indicate a change in mental function. In older people, doctors try to distinguish delirium from dementia by determining how quickly the confusion developed and what the person's usual mental function is. However, distinguishing the two disorders may be difficult, because people who have dementia can also develop delirium. Therefore, doctors usually treat people whose mental function suddenly worsens—even if they have dementia—as if they have delirium until proved otherwise.

If delirium is accompanied by agitation and hallucinations, delusions, or paranoia, it must be distinguished from a psychosis due to a psychiatric disorder, such as manic-depressive illness or schizophrenia. People with a psychosis due to a psychiatric disorder do not have confusion or memory loss, and the level of consciousness does not change. However, if a psychosis begins during old age, it usually results from delirium or dementia. Psychosis due to a psychiatric disorder rarely begins during old age.

Doctors perform a physical examination, which includes a neurologic examination.■ The examination includes blood and urine

COMPARING DELIRIUM AND DEMENTIA

FEATURE	DELIRIUM	DEMENTIA
Development	Sudden	Slow
Duration	Days to weeks	Months to years
Presence of other disorders or physical problems	Almost always present; may be a severe illness, drug use or withdrawal, or a problem with metabolism	Possibly none
Variation at night	Almost always worse	Often worse
Attention	Greatly impaired	Maintained until late stages
Level of consciousness	Fluctuates from lethargy to agitation	Normal until late stages
Orientation to surroundings	Varies	Impaired
Use of language	Slow, often incoherent, and inappropriate	Sometimes difficulty finding the right word
Memory	Jumbled and confused	Lost, especially for recent events
Mental function	Lost, variably and unpredictably	Lost, relatively consistently for all functions
Cause	Usually an acute illness or drugs; in older people, usually infection, dehydration, or drugs	Usually Alzheimer's disease, vascular dementia, or Lewy body dementia
Need for treatment	Emergency medical attention	Nonemergency medical attention

tests, such as cultures to look for signs of infection. Computed tomography (CT) or magnetic resonance imaging (MRI) may be performed. In younger and some older people, a spinal tap (lumbar puncture)▲ may be performed to obtain cerebrospinal fluid for analysis. Such analysis helps doctors rule out infection or bleeding.

Treatment and Prognosis

Most people who have delirium are hospitalized for treatment. However, when the cause of delirium is obvious and can be corrected readily (for example, when the cause is a drug) and when the person has family members who can provide care, a person with delirium may be cared for at home.

Treatment of delirium depends on its cause. For example, doctors treat infections with antibiotics, dehydration with fluids and electrolytes given intravenously, and delirium due to alcohol withdrawal with benzodiazepines (as well as with measures to stop the use of alcohol).

General measures are also important. The environment is kept as quiet and calm as possible. At every opportunity, staff and family members should reassure the person, help orient the person to time and place, and explain procedures and other proceedings. People who have delirium are prone to many problems, including dehydration, malnutrition, incontinence, falls, and bed sores. Preventing such problems requires meticulous care.

Measures may be needed to prevent people who are extremely agitated or who have hallucinations from injuring themselves or their caregivers. For example, family members are encouraged to stay with the person, or the person is put in a room near the nurses' station. However, sometimes during hospitalization, use of padded restraints is necessary—for example, to keep the person from pulling out intravenous lines. Restraints are applied carefully, released at frequent intervals, and dis-

▲ see art on page 443

continued as soon as possible, because they can upset the person and worsen the agitation.

For agitation, drugs are used only after all other measures have been ineffective. For most people who are agitated, the drugs of choice are antipsychotic drugs,▲ or sedatives, such as benzodiazepines.■ Sedatives are particularly useful when delirium is due to the sudden withdrawal of alcohol after heavy use for a long time. Doctors are careful when prescribing these drugs, particularly for older people. Drugs may worsen the agitation and confusion and may mask an underlying problem.

Most people recover fully if the condition causing delirium is rapidly identified and treated. Any delay greatly decreases the chance of a full recovery. Even when delirium is treated, some symptoms may persist for many weeks or months, and improvement may occur slowly. In some people, delirium evolves into chronic brain dysfunction similar to dementia.

Hospitalized people who have delirium are up to 10 times more likely to develop complications in the hospital (including death) than those who do not have delirium. Hospitalized people who have delirium, particularly older people, have a longer stay in the hospital, higher treatment costs, and a longer recovery time after they leave the hospital.

Dementia

Dementia is a slow, progressive decline in mental function in which memory, thinking, judgment, and the ability to learn are impaired.

In the United States, an estimated 6 million people have dementia. Dementia occurs primarily in people older than age 65, affecting about 6 to 8% of people in this age group. More than 30% of those aged 85 or older (the most rapidly growing segment of the population) may have dementia. Nevertheless, dementia is never a normal part of aging. More than 50% of people older than 100 do not have dementia.

As people age, changes in the brain cause some decline in short-term memory and slowing in learning ability. These normal age-related changes, unlike dementia, do not affect the ability to function. Such memory loss in older people (sometimes called benign senescent forgetfulness or age-associated memory impairment) is not necessarily a sign of dem-

entia or early Alzheimer's disease. Dementia is a much more serious decline in mental ability, and one that worsens with time. People who are aging normally may misplace things or forget details, but people who have dementia may forget entire events. People who have dementia have difficulty performing normal daily tasks such as driving, cooking, and handling finances.

Some older people develop a disorder that resembles dementia but is actually depression. It is called pseudodementia or the dementia of depression. People with pseudodementia eat and sleep little, and they complain bitterly about their memory loss, in contrast to people who have true dementia, who lack insight about their condition and often deny memory loss. People who have pseudodementia regain mental function after the depression is treated. Depression may also coexist with dementia. In such cases, treatment of depression may improve but not entirely restore mental function.

Causes

The most common cause of dementia is Alzheimer's disease. Other common causes are Lewy body dementia and destruction of brain tissue by strokes, which results in vascular dementia (multi-infarct dementia). Many people have more than one of these dementias (a condition called mixed dementia).

Less common causes include Parkinson's disease, infections such as AIDS, normal-pressure hydrocephalus, and drug or alcohol abuse. Rare causes of dementia are Pick's disease and Creutzfeldt-Jakob disease, including its variant form, which is thought to result from consuming contaminated meat. Dementia may also result from brain damage due to a head injury or from cardiac arrest (sudden stopping of the heart's pumping). Radiation therapy to the head as treatment for cancer (such as that for children with leukemia or for adults with a brain tumor) occasionally causes dementia that develops many months or years after treatment, as part of a condition called late radiation damage.

Sometimes dementia is worsened by disorders that can be modified. For example, diabetes, emphysema, or heart failure, if inadequately treated, can worsen dementia. Many people can be substantially helped when such disorders are treated or corrected. In about 10%, the symptoms of dementia can be completely reversed.

▲ see table on page 645

■ see box on page 471 and table on page 607

Many drugs may temporarily worsen the symptoms of dementia. Some of these drugs can be purchased without a prescription (over the counter). Sleep aids (which are sedatives), cold remedies, antianxiety drugs, and some antidepressants are common offenders. Drinking alcohol, even in moderate amounts, may also worsen dementia, and most experts recommend that people with dementia stop drinking alcohol.

Symptoms

In people with dementia, mental function typically deteriorates over a period of 2 to 10 years. However, dementia progresses at different rates depending on the cause. In people with vascular dementia, symptoms tend to worsen in steps, worsening suddenly with each new stroke, with some improvement in between. In people with Alzheimer's disease or Lewy body dementia, symptoms tend to worsen more steadily.

The rate of progression also varies from person to person. Looking back at how fast it worsened during the previous year often gives an indication about the coming year. Symptoms may worsen when people with dementia are moved to nursing homes or other institutions, because people with dementia have difficulty remembering and following rules and routines. Problems, such as pain, shortness of breath, retention of urine, and constipation, may cause delirium with rapidly worsening confusion in people who have dementia. If these problems are corrected, people usually return to the level of functioning they had before the problem.

Because dementia usually begins slowly and worsens over time, it may not be identified at first. Memory, especially for recent events, is one of the first mental functions to noticeably deteriorate. As dementia worsens, the ability to keep track of time and the ability to recognize people, places, and objects are reduced. People with dementia typically have problems finding and using the right word and have difficulty with abstract thinking (such as working with numbers). Emotions may be changeable, unpredictably and rapidly switching from happiness to sadness. Changes in personality are also common. Often, a particular personality trait becomes increasingly exaggerated: People who were always concerned with money become obsessed with it, or people who were often worried become constant worriers. Sleep patterns are often abnormal.

Some people with dementia hide their deficiencies well. They avoid complex activities such as balancing a checkbook, reading, and working. People who do not modify their lives may become frustrated with their inability to perform daily tasks. They may forget to do important tasks or may perform them incorrectly; for example, they may forget to pay bills or to turn off the lights or stove.

People with dementia may become withdrawn and less capable of controlling their behavior, sometimes acting disruptively (for example, by yelling, throwing, hitting, or wandering). Several effects of dementia contribute to these actions. Because people with dementia have difficulty understanding what they see and hear, they may misinterpret an offer of help as a threat and lash out. Because their short-term memory is impaired, they cannot remember what they are told or have done. They repeat questions and conversations, demand constant attention, or ask for things (such as meals) they have already received. Because they cannot express their needs clearly or at all, they may yell when in pain or wander when lonely or frightened. About 10% of people with dementia also have a psychosis, with hallucinations, delusions, or paranoia.

Eventually, people with dementia become unable to follow conversations and may become unable to speak. In its most advanced forms, dementia results in a near-complete destruction of the brain's ability to function. People become totally dependent on others, and many become bedridden. Eventually, people may have difficulty swallowing food without choking. Death often results from an infection, such as pneumonia.

Diagnosis

Forgetfulness is usually the first sign noticed by family members or doctors. Doctors and other health care practitioners can usually diagnose dementia by asking the person and family members a series of questions. The person is also given a mental status test, consisting of simple questions and tasks, such as naming objects, recalling short lists, writing sentences, and copying shapes.▲ More detailed testing (called neuropsychologic testing) is sometimes needed to clarify the degree of impairment or to determine whether the person is experiencing true mental decline. This

▲ see table on page 441

testing covers all the main areas of mental function, including mood, and usually takes 1 to 3 hours.

Doctors diagnose dementia based on the person's age and family history, the development and progression of symptoms, the results of a neurologic examination,▲ and the presence of other disorders, such as brain damage due to a stroke or, in alcoholics, undernutrition.

Doctors search for treatable disorders that may be causing or contributing to the dementia. Examples are thyroid disorders, abnormal levels of electrolytes in the blood, infections, vitamin deficiencies (especially vitamin B_{12}), toxicity due to a drug, and depression. Blood tests are performed, and doctors review all of the person's prescription drugs to see if one or more of them may be the cause. Doctors look for clues suggesting depression as a possible cause and ask questions about emotional health, especially with older people. Computed tomography (CT) or magnetic resonance imaging (MRI) is performed to rule out a brain tumor, normal-pressure hydrocephalus, and stroke.

Doctors also determine whether another, unrelated physical disorder or psychiatric disorder (such as schizophrenia) is also present, because treatment of these disorders may improve the general condition of people with dementia.

Treatment

For most dementias, no treatment can restore mental function. However, treating disorders that are worsening the dementia sometimes slows mental decline. For people who have dementia and depression, antidepressants (such as sertraline and paroxetine■) and counseling may help, at least temporarily. Abstaining from alcohol can result in long-term improvement.

Environmental Measures: Creating a supportive environment can be remarkably helpful. People who have mild to intermediate dementia usually function best in familiar surroundings and can usually remain at home. Homes can be evaluated for safety by a visiting nurse agency and modified accordingly. For example, dim light can cause safety hazards and worsen the tendency of people with dementia to misinterpret what they see, so lighting should be relatively bright.

Structure and routine help people with dementia stay oriented and give them a sense of security and stability. Low-stress activities scheduled on a regular basis can help people feel independent and needed by focusing their attention on pleasurable or useful tasks. Such activities can also help relieve depression. Physical activity is particularly important because it helps prevent disruptive behavior, such as agitation and wandering. Continued mental activity, including hobbies, interest in current events, and reading, should be encouraged. Excessive stimulation should be avoided, but people should not be socially isolated. Some improvement may occur if daily routines are simplified, if expectations for people with dementia are realistic, and if they are enabled to maintain some sense of dignity and self-esteem.

Because dementia is usually progressive, planning for the future is essential. Such planning usually involves the efforts of a doctor, a social worker, nurses, and a lawyer, but most of the responsibility falls on family members. Decisions about moving a person with dementia to a more supportive environment involve balancing the desire to keep the person safe with the desire to maintain the person's sense of independence as long as possible. Such decisions depend on many factors, including the severity of the dementia, the home environment, availability of family members and caregivers, financial resources, and the presence of other, unrelated disorders and physical problems.

Drugs: Donepezil, galantamine, rivastigmine, and tacrine may improve mental function temporarily, but they do not slow the progression of dementia.

Antipsychotic drugs, such as haloperidol, olanzapine, and risperidone,★ are often used to control the agitation and outbursts that may accompany advanced dementia. However, these drugs are not very effective for this purpose, and they can cause serious side effects. Antipsychotic drugs are most effective in people who have hallucinations, delusions, or paranoia in addition to dementia.

Many dietary supplements have been tried but have generally proved of little value in treating dementia. They include lecithin, ergoloid mesylates, and cyclandelate. Ginkgo biloba, a dietary supplement that is marketed as a memory enhancer, may modestly benefit some people with dementia.● Vitamin B_{12} supplements are effective only in people who have vitamin B_{12} deficiency, and thyroid hormone replacement is effective only in those

---

▲ see page 439   ■ see table on page 618

★ see table on page 645   ● see page 109

who have an underactive thyroid gland (hypothyroidism).

End-of-Life Issues: Before dementia becomes too severe, decisions should be made about medical care and finances. People with dementia, if sufficiently able, should appoint a health care proxy (who is legally authorized to make treatment decisions on their behalf), and they should discuss health care wishes with their surrogate (proxy) and doctor.▲

As dementia worsens, treatment tends to be directed at maintaining the person's comfort rather than at attempting to prolong life. For example, the proxy and family members may have to make decisions about whether to allow artificial feeding or to treat an acute illness such as pneumonia. Such issues are best discussed with all concerned long before decisions are necessary.

ALZHEIMER'S DISEASE

Alzheimer's disease is a progressive, relentless loss of mental function, characterized by degeneration of brain tissue, including loss of nerve cells and the development of senile plaques and neurofibrillary tangles.

The most common cause of dementia is Alzheimer's disease. In older people, it accounts for up to 65% of dementias. It is very rare among people younger than 60. It becomes more common with increasing age. It affects only about 1% of people aged 60 to 64, but up to 30% of those older than 85. In the United States, about 4 million people have Alzheimer's disease.

What causes Alzheimer's disease is unknown, but genetic factors play a role: The disease seems to run in some families and is caused or influenced by several specific gene abnormalities. One abnormality affects apolipoprotein E (apo E)—the protein part of certain lipoproteins, which transport cholesterol through the bloodstream. There are three types of apo E (ϵ2, ϵ3, and ϵ4). People with the ϵ4 type develop Alzheimer's disease more commonly and at an earlier age than other people. In contrast, people with the ϵ2 type seem to be protected against Alzheimer's disease. People with the ϵ3 type are neither protected nor more likely to develop the disease. (These associations have been studied primarily in whites and may not apply to other races.) Genetic testing for apo E type cannot determine whether a person will develop Alzheimer's disease. Therefore, this testing is not routinely recommended.

Creating a Beneficial Environment for People With Dementia

People with dementia can benefit from an environment that is

- **Safe:** Extra safety measures are usually needed. For example, large signs can be posted as safety reminders (such as "remember to turn the stove off"), or timers can be installed on stoves or electrical equipment. Hiding car keys and placing detectors on doors may help prevent accidents if wandering is a problem. Identification bracelets may also be helpful.

- **Familiar:** People with dementia usually function best in familiar surroundings. Moving to a new home or city, rearranging furniture, or even repainting can be disruptive.

- **Stable:** Establishing a regular routine for bathing, eating, sleeping, and other activities can give people with dementia a sense of stability. Regular contact with the same people can also help.

- **Planned to help with orientation:** A large daily calendar, a clock with large numbers, a radio, well-lit rooms, and a night-light can help with orientation. Also, family members or caregivers can make frequent comments that remind people with dementia of where they are and what is going on.

In Alzheimer's disease, parts of the brain degenerate, destroying nerve cells and reducing the responsiveness of the remaining ones to many of the chemical messengers that transmit signals in the brain (neurotransmitters). Abnormalities in brain tissue consist of senile or neuritic plaques (clumps of dead nerve cells containing an abnormal, insoluble protein called amyloid) and neurofibrillary tangles (twisted strands of insoluble proteins in the nerve cell). Such abnormalities develop to some degree in all people as they age but are much more numerous in people with Alzheimer's disease.

Symptoms

Dementia resulting from Alzheimer's disease usually begins subtly. People whose disease develops while they are still employed

---

▲ see pages 51 and 54

Caring for Caregivers

Caring for people with dementia is stressful and demanding, and caregivers may become depressed and exhausted, often neglecting their own mental and physical health. The following measures can help caregivers:

- **Learning about how to effectively meet the needs of people with dementia and what to expect from them:** For example, caregivers need to know that scolding about making mistakes or not remembering may only make behaviors worse. Such knowledge helps prevent unnecessary distress. Information about what to do on a daily basis may be obtained from nurses, social workers, and organizations, as well as from published materials.

- **Seeking help when it is needed:** Relief from the burdens of around-the-clock care of a person with dementia is often available, depending on the specific behavior and capabilities of the person and on family and community resources. Social agencies, including the social service department of the local community hospital, can help locate appropriate sources of help. Options include day-care programs, visits by home nurses, part-time or full-time housekeeping assistance, and live-in assistance. Transportation and meal services may be available. Full-time care can be very expensive, but many insurance plans cover some of the cost. Caregivers may benefit from counseling and support groups.

- **Caring for self:** Caregivers need to remember to take care of themselves. For example, engaging in physical activity can improve mood as well as health. Friends, hobbies, and activities should not be abandoned.

may not perform as well in their jobs. In those who are retired and not very active, the changes may not be as noticeable. The first sign may be forgetting recent events, although sometimes the disease begins with depression, fears, anxiety, decreased emotion, or other personality changes. In the early stages, judgment and abstract thinking may be impaired. Speech patterns may change slightly; the person may use simpler words, use words incorrectly, or be unable to find the appropriate word. An inability to interpret visual cues may make driving a car difficult. People with Alzheimer's disease may be able to function socially but may behave unusually. For example, they may forget the name of a recent visitor, and their emotions may change unpredictably and rapidly. They may get lost on their way to the store.

As Alzheimer's disease progresses, people have trouble remembering events in the past. They may require help with eating, dressing, bathing, or going to the toilet. Wandering, agitation, irritability, hostility, and physical aggression are common. All sense of time and place is lost: People with Alzheimer's disease may even get lost on their way to the bathroom at home. Their increasing confusion puts them at risk of falling. Psychoses, with hallucinations, delusions, and paranoia, develop at some point in about half of people with Alzheimer's disease.

Eventually, people with Alzheimer's disease cannot walk or take care of their personal needs. They may be incontinent and unable to swallow, eat, or speak. These changes put them at risk of undernutrition, pneumonia, and bedsores (pressure sores). Memory is completely lost. Because these people become totally dependent on others, a nursing home may become necessary. Ultimately, coma and death, often due to infections, result.

Progression is unpredictable. The expected survival from the time the disorder is diagnosed ranges from 2 to 10 years, but usually 3 to 5 years. On average, people with Alzheimer's disease who can no longer walk live no more than 6 months.

Diagnosis

Doctors suspect Alzheimer's disease as the most likely cause of dementia in older people whose memory gradually deteriorates. Although a diagnosis based on examination of the person can be correct most of the time, the diagnosis of Alzheimer's disease is proved only by microscopic examination of brain tissue obtained during an autopsy. When brain tissue is examined, the characteristic loss of nerve cells, neurofibrillary tangles, and senile plaques containing amyloid can be seen throughout the brain but particularly in the area of the temporal lobe that is involved in the formation of new memories. Analysis of spinal fluid and positron emission tomography (PET)▲ have been suggested as ways to diagnose Alzheimer's disease during life, but these procedures are not yet reliable in predicting who will develop Alzheimer's disease or in identifying people who already have it.

Treatment

General measures for treatment of Alzheimer's disease are the same as for all dementias.■

The use of certain drugs (such as nonsteroidal anti-inflammatory drugs [NSAIDs]) to prevent and slow the progression of Alzheimer's disease is under study. Estrogen and vitamin E may help prevent and slow progression of the disease, although study results are inconsistent. Before any of these substances are taken, their risks and benefits should be discussed with a doctor.

Donepezil, rivastigmine, tacrine, and galantamine increase the levels of the chemical messenger (neurotransmitter) acetylcholine, which may be low in many forms of dementia. These drugs may improve cognitive function temporarily, but they do not slow the progression of the disease. About half of the people who have Alzheimer's disease benefit from these drugs. For these people, the drugs effectively turn the clock back 6 to 9 months. These drugs are most effective in people with mild to moderate disease. Because the drugs are expensive and may have side effects, they should not be continued in people who do not benefit from them. The most common side effects include nausea, vomiting, weight loss, and abdominal pain or cramps. Side effects are usually mild and relatively uncommon with donepezil and galantamine.

An extract of ginkgo biloba (called EGb) has been claimed to have effects similar to those of the drugs described above.★ However, further study of this medicinal herb is needed.

LEWY BODY DEMENTIA

Lewy body dementia is progressive loss of mental function due to specific changes in brain tissue, including the development of Lewy bodies in nerve cells and degeneration of part of the brain stem.

Lewy body dementia is a common cause of dementia, but experts disagree about its prevalence and significance. It is more common among men than among women. Microscopic changes in the brain differ from those due to Alzheimer's disease in that nerve cells develop abnormal structures called Lewy bodies. Lewy bodies also occur in Parkinson's disease. In Parkinson's disease, they occur only in one part of the brain, but in Lewy body dementia, they occur throughout the brain.

The symptoms of Lewy body dementia are very similar to those of Alzheimer's disease. However, people with Lewy body dementia tend to have more hallucinations, usually visual ones that are often complex and detailed, and they often have severe adverse reactions to antipsychotic drugs.● Another distinguishing feature is that in the early stages of the dementia, mental function varies from day to day, often dramatically. One day, people may be able to converse coherently, and the next day, they may be inattentive, drowsy, and almost mute. Like people who have Parkinson's disease, people with Lewy body dementia move slowly and sluggishly, shuffle when they walk, and stoop over.

The expected survival from the time symptoms begin is 6 to 12 years. There is no specific treatment for Lewy body dementia, but the same drugs used to treat Alzheimer's disease may be helpful. General measures for treatment are the same as those for all dementias.

VASCULAR DEMENTIA

Vascular dementia (multi-infarct dementia) is mental dysfunction due to destruction of brain tissue by strokes, either a few large ones or many small ones.

A series of strokes may result in vascular dementia. These strokes are more common among men and usually begin after age 70. Risk factors for vascular dementia include high blood pressure and diabetes (both of which damage blood vessels in the brain). People who smoke or have smoked are also at risk.

The strokes gradually destroy brain tissue by blocking the blood supply to the brain. The areas destroyed are called infarcts. Small strokes cause little or no immediate weakness and seldom cause the paralysis that results from larger strokes.

Unlike dementia caused by Alzheimer's disease, vascular dementia may progress in steps, worsening suddenly but then improving somewhat, only to worsen again months or years later when another stroke occurs. Symptoms (memory loss, difficulty performing simple tasks, and a tendency to wander) are similar to those of other dementias, but judgment and personality may be affected less than in

---

▲ see page 444   ■ see page 486
★ see page 109   ● see table on page 645

people with Alzheimer's disease. Symptoms can vary depending on what part of the brain is destroyed. Usually, some aspects of mental function are not impaired, because the strokes destroy tissue in only part of the brain.

The presence of neurologic signs that usually result from small strokes can help doctors identify vascular dementia. Signs include partial loss of sight, slow and slurred speech, weakness or paralysis of one leg, and difficulty walking.

General measures for treatment of vascular dementia are the same as those for all dementias.▲ Treating diabetes and high blood pressure can help prevent and slow or stop the progression of vascular dementia. Stopping smoking is also recommended.

There is no specific treatment for vascular dementia. Anticoagulants, which inhibit blood clotting, are given to some people who have had strokes to prevent additional strokes. Warfarin, a strong anticoagulant, is given to people who have an irregular heart rhythm, which increases the risk of strokes due to blood clots from the heart. Aspirin is beneficial for people who have had strokes caused by narrowed blood vessels that supply the brain.

OTHER DEMENTIAS

Dementia develops in many disorders. About 15 to 20% of people with **Parkinson's disease** develop dementia sooner or later.

Pick's disease, a rare disorder, is much like Alzheimer's disease except that it affects only a small area of the brain and progresses more rapidly. Symptoms include apathy, memory loss, carelessness, and poor personal hygiene.

Normal-pressure hydrocephalus develops when the cerebrospinal fluid that normally surrounds the brain and protects it from injury is not reabsorbed normally. The increasing amount of fluid around the brain puts pressure on brain tissue, causing an unusual type of dementia. Normal-pressure hydrocephalus causes not only loss of mental function but also urinary incontinence and an abnormally slow, unsteady, wide-legged walk. If diagnosed early, normal-pressure hydrocephalus can sometimes be treated by removing the excess fluid within the brain through a drainage tube (shunt). However, after this procedure, walking and continence often improve more dramatically than does mental function.

Creutzfeldt-Jakob disease, an infectious disease, causes a rare, rapidly progressive dementia due to an infection with a prion, an abnormal protein.■ Usually Creutzfeldt-Jakob disease rapidly leads to severe dementia and death, often within a year. No treatment is available. Variant Creutzfeldt-Jakob disease, thought to be acquired from eating contaminated beef, causes a dementia similar to that due to Creutzfeldt-Jakob disease. It is also caused by a prion.

Dementia due to AIDS probably results from infection of the brain with the human immunodeficiency virus (HIV). This dementia usually begins subtly but progresses steadily over a few months or years. It usually develops after other symptoms of AIDS. Symptoms of this dementia include slowed thinking and expression, difficulty concentrating, and apathy. Movements are slow, and muscle weakness and lack of coordination may be present. Treatment with zidovudine and other drugs used to treat HIV infection sometimes produces dramatic improvement.

Dementia pugilistica (chronic progressive traumatic encephalopathy) may develop in people who have repeated head injuries—boxers, for example. They often develop symptoms similar to those of Parkinson's disease, and some of them also develop normal-pressure hydrocephalus.

CHAPTER 84

Stupor and Coma

Stupor is an unresponsive state from which a person can be aroused only briefly and with vigorous, repeated attempts. Coma is an unresponsive state from which a person cannot be aroused, even with vigorous, repeated attempts.

Normally, the brain can quickly adjust its own levels of activity and consciousness as

▲ see page 486   ■ see page 541

needed. The brain makes these adjustments based on information it receives from the eyes, ears, skin, and other sensory organs. For example, the brain can decrease its metabolic activity and induce sleep. The system of nerve cells and fibers that controls consciousness or arousal levels (the reticular activating system) is located deep within the brain stem.▲

The brain's ability to adjust its activity and consciousness levels can be impaired. Impairment may result when the nerve fibers connecting the brain and the sensory organs malfunction, when blood flow to the brain decreases, or when toxic substances damage the brain.

Periods of impaired consciousness can be short or long. Levels of impaired consciousness can range from reduced alertness or clouded consciousness (obtundation) to stupor to coma. Stupor (hypersomnia) is an excessively long or deep sleeplike state from which a person can be awakened only briefly by vigorous stimulation, such as repeated shaking, loud calling, pinching, or sticking with a pin. Coma is a state of complete unresponsiveness, from which a person cannot be aroused at all. A person in a deep coma lacks even the most basic responses, such as avoidance of pain, although reflexes may be present.

Causes

Stupor or coma can be caused by many disorders. A head injury can directly damage the areas of the brain stem that control consciousness levels or can cause bleeding (hemorrhage) in or around the brain. Blood can also directly damage these areas of the brain stem, or an accumulation of blood (hematoma) can put pressure on these areas. Brain tumors or collections of pus (abscesses) can also put pressure on these areas.

Alcohol intoxication and overdose of certain drugs (such as sedatives■—and opioids★) are common causes of stupor or coma. Occasionally, the use of certain antipsychotic drugs results in an unresponsive state called neuroleptic malignant syndrome. Abnormally low or high levels of substances (including sugar and electrolytes such as sodium) in the blood can interfere with brain function and impair consciousness. Brain infections (such as encephalitis and meningitis) and severe infections outside the brain can lead to coma. In older people, toxic reactions to drugs, dehydration (which results in a high sodium level), and infections are common causes of stupor.

Other causes of stupor or coma include the sudden stopping of the heart's pumping (cardiac arrest), aneurysms, severe lung disorders, inhalation of carbon monoxide, stroke, seizures, an underactive thyroid gland (hypothyroidism), liver or kidney failure, and low or high body temperature (hypothermia or hyperthermia).

Diagnosis

A person who becomes stuporous or comatose must be taken to the hospital immediately because either state may be caused by a life-threatening disorder. People with disorders that put them at risk of stupor or coma should carry medical identification or wear a Medic Alert identification bracelet or necklace. Thus, if they lose consciousness, medical personnel can quickly identify the probable cause.

Because a stuporous or comatose person cannot communicate, family members and friends must be honest with doctors about the person's use of drugs, alcohol, or other toxic substances. If a drug or toxic substance was ingested, family members or friends should give a sample of that substance or its container to the doctor.

When emergency medical personnel or doctors examine a stuporous or comatose person, they first check whether the airway is open, whether breathing is adequate, and whether blood pressure and pulse are normal. Body temperature is checked: An abnormally high temperature may indicate infection; an abnormally low temperature may indicate prolonged exposure to cold, an underactive thyroid gland, alcohol intoxication, or, in older people, infection. The skin is examined for signs of injury, drug injections, and allergic reactions, and the scalp is examined for cuts and bruises. Doctors also perform as thorough a neurologic examination as is possible with a stuporous or comatose person.

Doctors look for signs of brain damage or impaired brain function. One sign of brain damage is Cheyne-Stokes respiration (periodic breathing), an unusual pattern in which a person breathes rapidly, then more slowly, then not at all for several seconds. Unusual postures may be signs of significant brain damage. Such postures include decerebrate rigidity, in which the head is tilted back and the arms and legs are extended, and decorticate rigidity, in which the arms are flexed. General limpness of the entire body is of even greater concern, indicating widespread loss of activity in all

---

▲ see page 434 ■ see box on page 471
★ see table on page 451

SOME CAUSES OF STUPOR AND COMA

CAUSE	COMMENTS
Head injury	Head injuries, such as concussions, cuts, and bruises, can directly damage brain tissue or cause bleeding in or around the brain. Blood may directly damage brain tissue or may accumulate, producing a hematoma, which puts pressure on the brain. Coma may develop immediately or gradually over several hours. Depending on the severity of the injury, the coma may be short or may persist until death.
Cardiac arrest (sudden stopping of the heart's pumping)	In cardiac arrest, blood does not reach the brain, and brain tissue dies because it is deprived of oxygen. Complete oxygen deprivation for only a few minutes can damage the brain irreversibly. Coma results immediately and may soon become irreversible, depending on the how long the heart is stopped and how extensive the brain damage is.
Brain tumor or abscess	A large mass can push the brain against relatively rigid structures inside the skull, thereby causing dysfunction. Coma results when the part of the brain stem that controls levels of consciousness is damaged.
Aneurysm (a bulge in a weakened area of an artery wall)	An aneurysm near the brain can bleed. Blood may directly damage brain tissue or cause pressure within the skull to increase rapidly, reducing blood flow to the brain. Coma may result.
Infections	Infections of the brain, such as encephalitis and meningitis, and other infections that produce high fevers, such as sepsis, can affect brain function and lead to coma.
Severe lung disorders	Asthma, chronic obstructive pulmonary disease, pulmonary edema, and pulmonary embolism sometimes cause breathing to stop. Coma results because the brain does not receive enough oxygen.
Inhalation of large amounts of carbon monoxide	Carbon monoxide attaches to the hemoglobin of red blood cells and prevents them from carrying oxygen. Severe carbon monoxide poisoning can cause coma or irreversible brain damage due to oxygen deprivation.
Strokes affecting the brain stem	If blood flow to part of the brain stem is blocked, sudden loss of consciousness and coma can result. If blood flow to the entire brain stem is blocked, death results.
Seizures	Coma can result when a person has recurring seizures and does not regain consciousness between them. Such a coma is life-threatening.
Toxic effects of drugs	Many drugs (such as barbiturates and opioids including morphine) can cause coma. Overdose with drugs such as sedatives (for example, diazepam) can cause coma. If treated early, this type of coma is completely reversible. Use of illicit drugs can cause delirium, seizures, and coma.
Alcohol intoxication	Alcohol intoxication can cause stupor or coma, especially when the blood alcohol level exceeds 0.2%.
Hypothyroidism (an underactive thyroid gland)	Untreated hypothyroidism may cause mental confusion, which may progress to stupor and coma.
Liver encephalopathy or failure	These disorders can lead to the buildup of toxic waste products in the blood, resulting in coma. Coma that results from chronic liver failure is usually reversible. Coma that results from acute, severe liver failure causes fluid accumulation in the brain (cerebral edema) and is often fatal.
Kidney failure	Kidney failure can lead to the buildup of toxic waste products in the blood and results in coma unless dialysis is performed.

SOME CAUSES OF STUPOR AND COMA (*Continued*)

CAUSE	COMMENTS
Low or high blood sugar levels	An abnormally low blood sugar level (hypoglycemia) can cause coma. Immediate treatment with glucose, given intravenously, prevents permanent brain damage. An abnormally high blood sugar level (hyperglycemia) makes the blood syrupy and draws fluid from the brain, causing stupor or coma.
Low or high level of blood sodium	A low blood sodium level (hyponatremia), usually due to overhydration, or a high blood sodium level (hypernatremia), usually due to dehydration, interferes with the metabolic activity of the brain. Seizures and coma can result.
Low or high body temperature	A body temperature below 88° F (31.1° C) slows brain function to a level of stupor or coma. A very high fever (above 108° F [42.2° C]) can damage the brain and cause coma, as may occur in heatstroke.

parts of the central nervous system, including the brain stem and the nerve fibers that connect the upper part of the brain (cerebrum) to the spinal cord.

The eyes also provide important clues. The position of the pupils, their size, their reaction to bright light, their ability to follow a moving object (in people who are not comatose), and the appearance of the retina are checked. A widened (dilated) pupil that does not react to bright light may indicate pressure on cranial nerve III, which helps control eye movement, or on the brain stem. Doctors need to know if the person's pupils are normally different sizes or if the person takes a drug to treat glaucoma, which can affect pupil size.

Laboratory procedures provide further clues about the possible cause of stupor or coma. Blood levels of substances such as sugar, sodium, alcohol, oxygen, and carbon dioxide are measured. The red and white blood cell counts are determined. Urine is analyzed to determine whether sugar or toxic substances are present.

Additional procedures include computed tomography (CT) or magnetic resonance imaging (MRI) of the head to rule out the possibility of structural brain damage, such as that due to bleeding (hemorrhage), a tumor, or an abscess. If meningitis is remotely possible, a spinal tap (lumbar puncture) is performed to withdraw and examine a sample of cerebrospinal fluid.▲ Because a coma may also be due to a brain tumor or hemorrhage, emergency CT or MRI of the brain is often performed before the spinal tap to determine whether the increased pressure inside the skull has forced the brain downward in the

skull. If the pressure is high enough, the brain may be forced through the small natural opening in the relatively rigid sheets of tissue that separate the brain into compartments. This life-threatening disorder is called brain herniation.■ Performing a spinal tap reduces the pressure below the brain and thus may trigger or worsen a herniation.

Treatment

A rapidly deteriorating level of consciousness is a medical emergency requiring immediate treatment, sometimes even before a diagnosis is made.

The person is admitted to a hospital intensive care unit, where nurses can monitor heart rate, blood pressure, temperature, and the oxygen level in the blood. Oxygen is often given immediately, and an intravenous line is put in place so that drugs can be given quickly. If the person is bleeding, attempts are made to stop the bleeding, and if blood loss is significant, a blood transfusion is given. Antiarrhythmic drugs★ may be given to keep the heart beating normally. If blood pressure continues to fall, fluids and drugs that narrow (constrict) blood vessels are given to keep blood pressure normal.

Usually, glucose, a sugar, is given intravenously after blood has been drawn to measure the blood sugar level but before the blood sugar level has been determined. Giving glucose often results in instant recovery if the cause of the coma is a low blood sugar level (hypoglycemia).

▲ see art on page 443   ■ see art on page 515
★ see table on page 166

Thiamine is always given with glucose because in malnourished people such as alcoholics, glucose alone can trigger or worsen a brain disorder called Wernicke's encephalopathy.

If taking an opioid (narcotic) is the suspected cause, the antidote naloxone may be given while doctors wait for blood and urine test results. If ingestion of a toxic substance is suspected, the stomach may be pumped to identify its contents and to prevent more of the substance from being absorbed.

People in the deepest stages of coma need a ventilator, because the brain cannot perform essential body functions, including maintenance of breathing.

Prognosis

The likelihood of recovery from a deep coma that lasts more than a few hours depends on the cause. Recovery is likely when the cause is an overdose of a sedative. When the cause is a low blood sugar level, complete recovery is possible if the brain was not deprived of sugar for more than about 1 hour. When the cause is a head injury, substantial recovery may occur, even if the coma lasts several weeks (but not if it lasts more than 3 months). When the cause is cardiac arrest or oxygen deprivation, full recovery rarely occurs if after 1 week, the person cannot move the limbs when asked to do so.

For people who remain in a deep coma longer than a few weeks, decisions about continued use of a ventilator, feeding tube, and drugs should be made. Family members should discuss these issues with the doctors. If the person in a coma has advance medical directives, such as a living will or durable power of attorney for health care,▲ they should be reviewed.

A **vegetative state** occasionally results after severe brain damage due to a head injury, oxygen deprivation, or a severe disorder. This state results when the cerebrum, which controls thought and behavior, is destroyed, but the thalamus and brain stem, which control sleep cycles, body temperature, breathing, and heart rate, are spared. People in this state often open their eyes, and they have relatively normal sleeping and waking patterns, breathe and swallow spontaneously, and may even show a startle reaction to loud noises. However, they have lost all capacity for conscious thought and behavior, and their capacity for interacting with the environment is limited to reflex responses. Most people in a vegetative state have prominent abnormal reflexes, including stiffening or jerking of the arms and legs. If a vegetative state persists for more than a few months, recovery of consciousness is unlikely. Nevertheless, with skilled nursing care, such people can live for years.

The **locked-in state** is a rare condition in which people are conscious and able to think but are so severely paralyzed that they can communicate only by opening and closing the eyes in response to questions. The locked-in state can be caused by severe paralysis of peripheral nerves or by strokes that affect the brain stem but not the cerebrum.

Brain death is the most severe form of unconsciousness. In this condition, the brain has permanently lost the ability to perform all vital functions, including maintenance of breathing. The person is legally dead. A widely accepted legal definition of brain death is cessation of all brain functions, even though the heart continues to beat. Established criteria for brain death include no grimacing or moving in response to painful stimulation, no reaction of the eyes to light, and the inability to breathe without assistance. If these criteria are met, the person is declared brain dead.

However, doctors cannot declare brain death until they have corrected all treatable medical problems that could slow brain function and thus could be misdiagnosed as brain death. These problems include a low body temperature, severe abnormalities in levels of electrolytes (such as sodium) in the blood, overdose of a sedative, and ingestion of certain potentially toxic drugs.

After these medical problems are corrected, diagnostic procedures may be performed to confirm brain death. Electroencephalography (EEG—a recording of the brain's electrical activity■) shows no brain waves if a person is brain dead. Procedures such as angiography, single photon emission computed tomography (SPECT—a procedure that uses a radioactive molecule called a radionuclide to produce images of blood flow), and Doppler ultrasonography, can show that blood is not flowing to the brain. Such procedures enable doctors to declare brain death quickly after catastrophic head injuries, as may occur in motor vehicle accidents.

▲ see page 54   ■ see page 445

CHAPTER 85

Seizure Disorders

Seizure disorders involve periodic disturbances of the brain's electrical activity, resulting in some degree of temporary brain dysfunction.

Normal brain function requires an orderly, organized, coordinated discharge of electrical impulses. Electrical impulses enable the brain to communicate with the spinal cord, nerves, and muscles as well as within itself. When electrical impulses discharge abnormally, a seizure may occur.

About 2% of adults have a seizure at some time during their lifetime. Two thirds of these people never have another one. Most commonly, seizure disorders begin in early childhood or in late adulthood. The term "seizure disorder" is preferred to "epilepsy" because epilepsy is often incorrectly thought to include some degree of brain damage or a tendency to be violent.

Causes

Seizures starting before age 2 are usually caused by high fevers▲ or metabolic disorders, such as abnormal blood levels of sugar (glucose), calcium, magnesium, vitamin B_6, or sodium. If the seizures recur, the cause is likely to be a hereditary brain disorder (such as nocturnal frontal lobe epilepsy, which is inherited as an autosomal dominant trait■). Many seizures that begin between the ages of 2 and 14 years have no known cause. Seizures starting after age 25 may be caused by structural damage to the brain such as from a head injury, stroke, or tumor. However, in about half of people in this age group, the cause is unknown. When no cause can be identified, seizures are called idiopathic.

People with a seizure disorder are more likely to have a seizure when they are under excess physical or emotional stress or deprived of sleep. Strong stimuli that irritate the brain— such as injury, certain drugs, sleep deprivation, infections, fever, low levels of oxygen in the blood, or very low levels of sugar in the blood—can trigger a seizure whether a person has a seizure disorder or not. These seizures are known as "provoked seizures." Avoiding such stimuli can help prevent seizures.

Rarely, seizures are triggered by repetitive sounds, flashing lights, video games, or even touching certain parts of the body. This disorder is called reflex epilepsy.

Symptoms

In about 20% of people who have a seizure disorder, seizures are preceded by unusual sensations of smell, taste, or vision or an intense feeling that a seizure is about to begin (aura). Usually, an aura is associated with an unpleasant sensation, such as an odor of burning garbage or decaying flesh.

Almost all seizures are relatively brief, lasting from a few seconds to a few minutes. Most seizures last 2 to 5 minutes. When a seizure stops, the person may have a headache, sore muscles, unusual sensations, confusion, and profound fatigue. These after-effects are called the postictal state. In some people, one side of the body is weak, and the weakness lasts longer than the seizure (a condition called Todd's paralysis). Most people who have a seizure disorder look and behave normally between seizures and can live normal lives.

Symptoms vary depending on which area of the brain is affected by the abnormal electrical discharge.★ For example, if an abnormal electrical discharge occurs in the area that controls smell (located deep within temporal lobe), the person may sense an intensely pleasant or unpleasant smell. If it occurs in another area of the temporal lobe, the person may experience a sense of déjà vu, in which unfamiliar surroundings seem inexplicably familiar. If the abnormal discharge affects the frontal lobe, the person may be unable to speak. If the abnormal discharge affects large areas, it can cause a convulsion (jerking and spasms of muscles, usually throughout the body). Other symptoms include numbness or tingling in a specific body part, brief attacks of altered consciousness (such as drowsiness), loss of consciousness, confusion, and loss of muscle or bladder control.

Symptoms also vary depending on whether the seizure is partial (affecting only one side of the brain) or generalized (affecting large areas on both sides of the brain). Partial seizures

---

▲ see page 502　　■ see art on page 12
★ see pages 434 and 476

CAUSES OF SEIZURES

CAUSE	EXAMPLES	CAUSE	EXAMPLES
High fever	Heatstroke Infections	Structural damage to the brain (*continued*)	Head injury Intracranial hemorrhage Stroke
Brain infections	Abscess AIDS Malaria Meningitis Rabies Syphilis Tetanus Toxoplasmosis Viral encephalitis	Fluid accumulation in the brain (cerebral edema)	Eclampsia Hypertensive enceph- alopathy Lupus erythematosus
Metabolic disorders	High blood levels of sugar or sodium Kidney or liver failure Low blood levels of sugar, calcium, magnesium, or sodium Phenylketonuria Underactive parathyroid gland	Exposure to toxic drugs or substances	Amphetamines Camphor Chloroquine Cocaine overdose Lead Pentylenetetrazol Picrotoxin Strychnine
Inadequate oxygen supply to the brain	Abnormal heart rhythms Carbon monoxide poisoning Near drowning Near suffocation Stroke	Withdrawal after heavy use	Alcohol General anesthetics (used during surgery) Sedatives, including sleep aids
Structural damage to the brain	Brain tumor (non- cancerous or cancerous)	Prescription drugs	Ceftazidime Chlorpromazine Ciprofloxacin Imipenem Indomethacin Meperidine Phenytoin Theophylline

may be simple, in which a person is completely conscious and aware of the surroundings, or complex, in which consciousness is impaired but not completely lost. Partial seizures include simple partial seizures, Jacksonian seizures, complex partial seizures, and epilepsia partialis continua. Generalized seizures cause a loss of consciousness and abnormal movements, usually immediately. Loss of consciousness may be brief or prolonged. Generalized seizures include tonic-clonic seizures, primary generalized epilepsy, absence seizures, atonic seizures, myoclonic seizures, and status epilepticus.

About 70% of people have only one type of seizure. The rest have two or more types. For example, some children who have **juvenile myoclonic epilepsy** also have tonic-clonic seizures and absence seizures in addition to the myoclonic seizures, which usually involve the arms.

In **simple partial seizures,** electrical discharges begin in a small area of the brain and remain confined to that area. Because only a small area of the brain is affected, symptoms are related to the function controlled by that area. For example, if the small area of the brain that controls the right arm's movements (in the left frontal lobe) is affected, the right arm may begin to shake and jerk. A simple partial seizure may progress to a complex partial seizure.

Jacksonian seizures produce symptoms that start in one part of the body, then spread to another. Abnormal movements may occur in the hand or foot, then "march up" the limb as the electrical activity spreads in the brain. The person is completely aware of what is occurring during the seizure. Thus, Jacksonian seizures are simple partial seizures.

Complex partial (psychomotor) seizures usually begin with an aura that lasts 1 to 2 minutes. During the aura, the person starts to lose touch with the surroundings. During or immediately after the aura, some people stare, move the arms and legs in strange and purposeless ways, utter meaningless sounds, do not understand what other people are saying, and resist help. Other people are able to converse, but their conversation lacks spontaneity, and the content is somewhat sparse. This state may last for several minutes. People may then recover fully. Or, the abnormal electrical discharge may spread to adjacent areas and to the other side of the brain. The result is a generalized seizure, which includes jerking of limbs, frothing at the mouth, and loss of consciousness.

Epilepsia partialis continua is a rare type of continuous or frequently recurring partial seizure, usually affecting a hand or the face. Seizures occur every few seconds or minutes for days to years at a time. These seizures usually result from localized damage (such as scarring due to a stroke) in adults or from inflammation of the brain (such as encephalitis and measles) in children.

Tonic-clonic (grand mal) seizures usually begin with an abnormal electrical discharge in a small area of the brain, resulting in a complex partial seizure. However, the discharge quickly spreads to adjoining parts of the brain, causing the entire area to malfunction. **Primary generalized epilepsy** begins with abnormal discharges in a large area of the brain. The abnormal discharges quickly spread to even more areas. In tonic-clonic seizures and primary generalized epilepsy, abnormal discharges result in a temporary loss of consciousness and a convulsion, with severe muscle spasms and jerking throughout the body. The head may forcefully turn to one side, the teeth may clench, the tongue is often bitten, and bladder control may be lost. The seizures usually last 1 to 2 minutes. Afterward, the person may have a headache, be temporarily confused, and feel extremely tired. Usually, the person does not remember what happened during the seizure.

Absence (petit mal) seizures begin in childhood, usually between the ages of 5 and 15. They do not produce the convulsions and other dramatic symptoms of tonic-clonic seizures. A person does not fall down, collapse, or move jerkily. Instead, the person has episodes of staring with fluttering eyelids and sometimes twitching facial muscles. The person is completely unaware of the surround-

ings. These episodes last 2 to 3 seconds and, rarely, 10 to 30 seconds. The person abruptly stops activity and resumes it just as abruptly, experiencing no after-effects and not knowing that a seizure has occurred.

Atonic seizures, which occur primarily in children, are characterized by complete loss of muscle tone and consciousness. They are brief, but they cause the child to collapse to the ground, increasing the risk of injury.

Myoclonic seizures are characterized by quick jerks of one or several limbs or the trunk. The seizures are brief and do not cause loss of consciousness, but they may occur repetitively.

In **status epilepticus,** the most serious seizure disorder and a medical emergency, the seizure does not stop. Electrical discharges occur throughout the brain. The discharges produce a generalized seizure lasting more than 15 minutes or recurring seizures between which the person does not completely regain consciousness. The person has convulsions with intense muscle contractions and cannot breathe adequately. Without rapid treatment, the heart and brain can become overtaxed and permanently damaged, and the person may die.

Seizures may have serious consequences. Intense, rapid muscle contractions can cause injuries, including broken bones. Sudden loss of consciousness can cause serious injury due to falls and accidents. The turbulent electrical activity of convulsive seizures that recur without recovery between them can cause brain damage. Most people who have a seizure disorder experience dozens or more seizures in their lives without serious brain damage. A single seizure does not impair intelligence, but recurring convulsive seizures may eventually do so.

Diagnosis

People who have at least two unprovoked seizures that occur at different times have a seizure disorder. A diagnosis is made based on the person's history and the observations of eyewitnesses. Seizures may be suspected if symptoms such as loss of consciousness, muscle spasms that shake the body, loss of bladder control, sudden confusion, and an inability to pay attention occur. However, true seizures are much less common than most people think; most episodes of brief unconsciousness are more likely to be fainting (syncope▲).

▲ see page 143

Brain Activity During a Seizure

An electroencephalogram (EEG) is a recording of the brain's electrical activity. The procedure is simple and painless. About 20 small adhesive electrodes are placed on the scalp, and the brain's activity is recorded under normal conditions. Then the person is exposed to various stimuli, such as bright or flashing lights, to try to provoke a seizure. During a seizure, electrical activity in the brain accelerates, producing a jagged wave pattern. Such recordings of brain waves help identify a seizure disorder. Different types of seizures have different wave patterns.

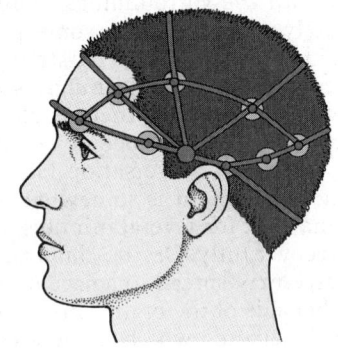

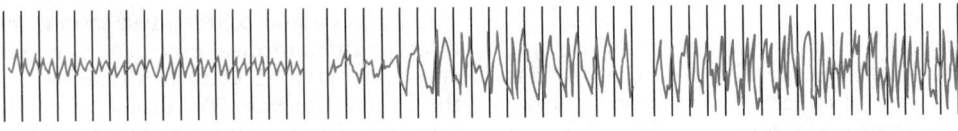

Normal Adult Brain Wave   **Absence Seizure**   **Tonic-Clonic Seizure**

An eyewitness report of the episode can be very helpful to doctors. An eyewitness can describe exactly what happened, whereas the person who had the episode usually cannot. An accurate description of the circumstances is needed: how fast the episode started; whether it involved abnormal muscle movements (such as spasms of the head, neck, or facial muscles), tongue biting, or loss of bladder control; how long it lasted; and how quickly the person recovered. Doctors also need to know what the person experienced before the episode: whether the person had a premonition or warning that something unusual was about to happen and whether anything, such as certain sounds or flashing lights, seemed to trigger the episode.

To help diagnose a seizure disorder, doctors use electroencephalography (EEG), a painless, safe procedure that records electrical activity in the brain.▲ Doctors examine the recording (electroencephalogram) for evidence of abnormal electrical discharges. Because abnormal discharges are more likely to occur after too little sleep, EEG is sometimes scheduled after a person has been deprived of sleep for 18 to 24 hours. Even if a seizure did not occur during

EEG, abnormalities may be present. Because of the limited recording time, EEG can miss abnormalities and the electroencephalogram may appear normal, even in people who have a seizure disorder.

Once a seizure disorder is diagnosed, more tests are usually needed to identify the cause. Routine blood tests are performed to measure the levels of sugar, calcium, and sodium in the blood and to determine whether the liver and kidneys are functioning properly. A complete blood count is performed to determine how many white and red blood cells are present. A high white blood cell count may indicate an infection. A low red blood cell count (anemia) may indicate an inadequate supply of oxygen to the brain. Often, electrocardiography (ECG)■ is performed to rule out an abnormal heart rhythm as a possible cause of symptoms. Because an abnormal heart rhythm can reduce blood flow (and therefore the oxygen supply) to the brain, it can trigger seizures and cause loss of consciousness.

Computed tomography (CT) or magnetic resonance imaging (MRI) of the head is usually performed to check for structural damage to brain tissue (for example, by a stroke). Sometimes a spinal tap (lumbar puncture)★ is needed to determine whether the person has an infection of the layers of tissue covering the brain (meningitis) or of the brain (encephalitis).

▲ see page 445   ■ see page 122
★ see art on page 443

Treatment

If the cause can be identified and eliminated, no additional treatment is necessary. For example, if low sugar (glucose) levels in the blood (hypoglycemia)▲ caused the seizure, glucose is given to increase the levels and the disorder causing the low levels is treated. Other treatable causes include a tumor, an infection, and abnormal sodium levels.

Anticonvulsants may be needed to reduce the risk of having another seizure. Anticonvulsants are not usually prescribed for people who have had only one generalized seizure for which no cause can be found. But they are necessary for people who have had more than one, unless the cause has been identified and completely eliminated.

Anticonvulsants can completely prevent convulsive seizures in more than half of the people who have them and greatly reduce the frequency of seizures in another third. These drugs are only slightly less effective for absence seizures. Half of the people who respond to anticonvulsants can eventually discontinue them without having a relapse. However, for about 10 to 20% of people with a seizure disorder, anticonvulsants do not adequately prevent seizures.

No one drug can control all types of seizures. For most people, seizures can be controlled with a single drug. If seizures recur, different anticonvulsants are tried. Determining which anticonvulsant is effective may take several months. Some people have to take several drugs.

For women who have a seizure disorder and are pregnant, taking an anticonvulsant increases the risk of miscarrying or of having a baby with a birth defect.■ However, stopping the anticonvulsant may be more harmful to the woman and the baby.

Because status epilepticus is an emergency, large intravenous doses of one or more anticonvulsants are given as quickly as possible. Measures to prevent injuries are taken during the prolonged seizure.

Anticonvulsants, though very effective, may have side effects. Many cause drowsiness but, paradoxically, sometimes cause hyperactivity in children. Blood tests are performed periodically to determine whether an anticonvulsant is affecting the kidneys, liver, or blood cells. People taking anticonvulsants should be aware of possible side effects and should consult their doctor at the first sign of side effects.

The dose of an anticonvulsant is critical: The best dose of an anticonvulsant is the smallest dose that stops all seizures while causing the fewest side effects. Doctors ask the person about side effects, then adjust the dose if needed. Sometimes doctors also measure the level of anticonvulsant in the blood. Anticonvulsants should be taken just as prescribed. No other drugs should be taken at the same time without the doctor's or pharmacist's authorization because many drugs alter the level of anticonvulsant in the blood. People who take anticonvulsants should see a doctor regularly for dose adjustment and should always wear a Medic Alert bracelet inscribed with the type of seizure disorder and the drug being taken.

Exercise is recommended and social activities are encouraged. However, people who have a seizure disorder may have to make some adjustments. For example, they should not drink alcoholic beverages. They should not engage in activities where a sudden loss of consciousness could result in serious injury: They should not swim alone or operate power tools. In most states, laws prohibit people with a seizure disorder from driving until they have been free of seizures for at least 6 months to 1 year.

A family member or close friend should be trained to help if a seizure occurs. Attempting to put an object (such as a spoon) in the person's mouth to protect the person's tongue should not be tried, because such efforts can do more harm than good. The teeth may be damaged, or the person may bite the helper unintentionally as the jaw muscles contract. The important steps are protecting the person from falling, loosening clothing around the neck, and placing a pillow under the head. People who lose consciousness should be rolled onto one side to ease breathing. People who have had a seizure should not be left alone until they have awakened completely and can move about normally. Usually, their doctor should be notified.

If all drugs are ineffective in controlling seizures or if side effects of the drug cannot be tolerated, brain surgery is a possibility. If a defect in the brain (such as a scar) can be identified as the cause and is confined to a small area, surgically removing that area may eliminate the seizures or reduce their severity and frequency. Surgically cutting the nerve fibers that connect the two sides of the brain (corpus callosum) may help people who have seizures that originate in several areas of the brain or

▲ see page 970   ■ see table on page 1460

R_x DRUGS USED TO TREAT SEIZURES

DRUG	USE	POSSIBLE SIDE EFFECTS
Carbamazepine	Partial and generalized seizures	Low white blood cell count (granulocytopenia), low red blood cell count (anemia), digestive upset, and visual disturbances
Clonazepam	Absence, myoclonic, and atonic seizures and infantile spasms	Drowsiness, abnormal behavior, loss of muscle coordination, and tolerance of the drug after 1 to 6 months
Divalproex	Absence and complex partial seizures and, when the drug is given by injection, status epilepticus	Nausea, vomiting, abdominal pain, diarrhea, weakness, drowsiness, dizziness, tremor, weight gain, and liver damage
Ethosuximide	Absence seizures	Nausea, lethargy, dizziness, headache, low white blood cell count, and low red blood cell count
Felbamate	Complex partial seizures in conjunction with other anticonvulsants when all other drugs are ineffective	Headache, fatigue, liver failure, and, rarely, aplastic anemia (a fatal disorder)
Fosphenytoin	Status epilepticus	Loss of muscle coordination, drowsiness, dizziness, headache, rash, and tingling sensations
Gabapentin	Complex partial seizures in conjunction with other anticonvulsants	Drowsiness, dizziness, weight gain, and headache
Lamotrigine	Complex partial and generalized seizures in conjunction with other anticonvulsants	Rash, nausea, vomiting, indigestion, drowsiness, dizziness, runny nose, and abnormal menstrual periods in women
Levetiracetam	Complex partial seizures in conjunction with other anticonvulsants	Drowsiness, dizziness, and fatigue
Lorazepam	Status epilepticus	Drowsiness and slowing of heart and breathing rates

R DRUGS USED TO TREAT SEIZURES (Continued)

DRUG	USE	POSSIBLE SIDE EFFECTS
Midazolam	Status epilepticus	Drowsiness and slowing of heart and breathing rates
Oxcarbazepine	Complex partial seizures as the only anticonvulsant in adults or in conjunction with other anticonvulsants in children and adults	Headache, drowsiness, dizziness, fatigue, nausea, low sodium levels in the blood, and a low white blood cell count
Phenobarbital	Partial and generalized seizures and status epilepticus	Drowsiness, paradoxical hyperactivity in children, rapid movement of the eyes in one direction followed by a slower drift back to the original position (nystagmus), confusion, and loss of muscle coordination
Phenytoin	Partial and generalized seizures and, when the drug is given intravenously, status epilepticus	Swollen gums, low red blood cell count, loss of bone density, excessive hairiness (hirsutism), swollen glands, and, in children, impairment of cognitive development
Primidone	Partial and generalized seizures	Drowsiness, paradoxical hyperactivity in children, nystagmus, and loss of muscle coordination
Tiagabine	Complex partial seizures in conjunction with other anticonvulsants	Drowsiness, dizziness, confusion, weakness, nausea, abdominal pain, nervousness, muscle tremor, and knee buckling
Topiramate	Complex partial seizures in conjunction with other anticonvulsants in adults	Confusion, word-finding difficulties, depression, loss of appetite, and kidney stones
Valproate	Absence, myoclonic, generalized, and partial seizures and infantile spasms	Nausea, vomiting, weight gain, reversible hair loss, and temporary drowsiness
Vigabatrin	Complex partial seizures in conjunction with other anticonvulsants	Drowsiness, dizziness, headache, and fatigue
Zonisamide	Complex partial seizures in conjunction with other anticonvulsants	Drowsiness, loss of muscle coordination, kidney stones, loss of appetite, and nausea

that spread to all parts of the brain very quickly. This procedure usually has no appreciable side effects. After surgery, many people need to continue to take anticonvulsants.

Electrical stimulation of the vagus nerve (cranial nerve X) can reduce the number of partial seizures by one third. The vagus nerve is thought to have indirect connections to areas of the brain often involved in producing seizures. A device that looks like a heart pacemaker is implanted under the left collarbone and is connected to the vagus nerve in the neck with a wire that runs under the skin. The device causes a small bulge under the skin. The operation is performed on an outpatient basis and takes about 1 to 2 hours. When people who have such a device sense that a seizure is about to begin, they turn the device on with a magnet. Or, the device may be left on all the time. For some people, vagus nerve stimulation prevents seizures or reduces their frequency and severity. Vagus nerve stimulation is used in addition to anticonvulsants. Side effects include hoarseness, cough, and deepening of the voice.

Infantile Spasms and Febrile Seizures

Infantile spasms and febrile seizures occur almost exclusively in children.

In **infantile spasms** (salaam seizures), a child lying on his back suddenly raises and bends the arms, bends the neck and upper body forward, and straightens the legs. These spasms last for only a few seconds, but they may recur many times a day. They usually occur in children younger than 3 years. In many children, the spasms evolve into another type of seizure disorder later in life. In most children with infantile spasms, neurologic function develops slowly, and mental retardation is present. Usually, adrenocorticotropic hormone (ACTH) or another corticosteroid is used to treat these spasms. Usually, anticonvulsants are not effective in stopping the spasms; however, clonazepam and nitrazepam may have some benefit.

Febrile seizures (convulsive seizures) are seizures that are triggered by a fever. They occur in about 4% of children aged 6 months to 5 years but most often occur in children aged 9 to 20 months. Febrile seizures tend to run in families. Most children who have a febrile seizure have only one, and most seizures last for less than 15 minutes. Febrile seizures may be simple or complex. In simple febrile seizures, the entire body shakes (in a generalized seizure) for less than 15 minutes. In complex febrile seizures, the entire body shakes for more than 15 minutes, only one side of the body shakes—a partial seizure—for more than 15 minutes, or seizures occur at least twice within 24 hours. Children who have complex febrile seizures are slightly more likely to develop a seizure disorder later in life.

Children with febrile seizures should be taken to the emergency department for evaluation. Whether a child has meningitis or encephalitis may not be clear, and these disorders must be assessed and treated if present.▲ Usually, no treatment is given for a simple febrile seizure other than drugs to reduce the fever. For simple febrile seizures that recur or for complex febrile seizures, phenobarbital may be given to prevent seizures. However, phenobarbital can markedly interfere with the ability of the child to learn. Other anticonvulsants may be used instead.

CHAPTER 86

Stroke

A stroke is a disorder in which the arteries to the brain become blocked or rupture, resulting in death of brain tissue.

A stroke is a cerebrovascular disorder, so called because it affects the brain (cerebro-) and the blood vessels (vascular).

▲ see page 529

In Western countries, strokes are the third most common cause of death and the second most common cause of disabling neurologic damage after Alzheimer's disease. In the United States, over 600,000 people have a stroke and about 160,000 die of stroke each year. Strokes are much more common among older people than among younger adults, usually because the

Supplying the Brain With Blood

Blood is supplied to the brain through two pairs of large arteries: the internal carotid arteries and the vertebral arteries. The internal carotid arteries carry blood from the heart along the front of the neck, and the vertebral arteries carry blood from the heart along the back of the neck. In the skull, the vertebral arteries unite to form the basilar artery (at the back of the head). The internal carotid arteries and the basilar artery divide into several branches, including the cerebral arteries. These branches empty into a circle of other arteries (circle of Willis), which thus forms a connection between the vertebral and internal carotid arteries. Other small arteries branch off from the circle of Willis like roads from a traffic circle. The branches carry blood to all parts of the brain.

When the large arteries that supply the brain are blocked, some people have no symptoms or have only a small stroke. But others with the same blockage have a massive ischemic stroke. Why? Some people are born with arteries that can protect them from strokes. The circle of Willis is the key. If the diameter of this artery is large, the circle of Willis can redistribute blood to the whole brain when one or even two of the large arteries are blocked. If the diameter is small or if the circle is incomplete, redistribution of blood is more difficult. In addition, some people are born with a capability to grow new blood vessels (collateral vessels). When a carotid artery is blocked, these people can grow collateral vessels that bypass the blockage.

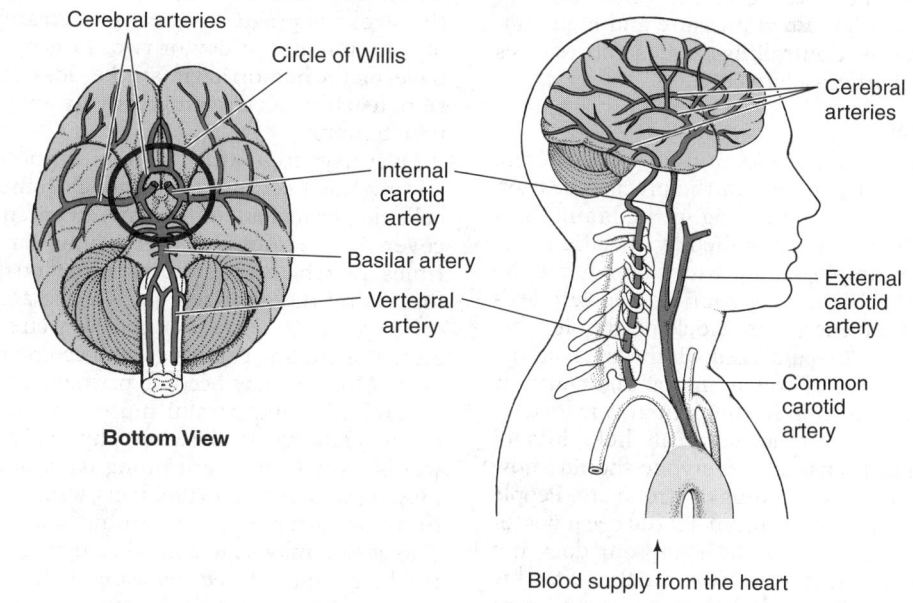

Cerebral arteries
Circle of Willis
Internal carotid artery
Basilar artery
Vertebral artery
Bottom View

Cerebral arteries
External carotid artery
Common carotid artery
Blood supply from the heart

disorders that lead to strokes progress over time. Over two thirds of all strokes occur in people older than 65. Slightly more than 50% of all strokes occur in men, but more than 60% of deaths due to stroke occur in women, possibly because women are on average older when the stroke occurs. Blacks are more likely than whites to have a stroke and to die of it.

There are two types of strokes: ischemic and hemorrhagic. About 80% of strokes are ischemic—due to a blocked artery. Brain cells, thus deprived of their blood supply, do not re-

ceive enough oxygen and glucose (a sugar), which are carried by blood. A transient ischemic attack (TIA), sometimes called a ministroke, is often an early warning sign of an impending ischemic stroke. TIAs are caused by an inadequate blood supply to part of the brain but only for a brief time. Because the blood supply is restored quickly, brain tissue does not die, as it does in a stroke.

The other 20% of strokes are hemorrhagic—due to bleeding in or around the brain. In this type of stroke, a blood vessel ruptures, interfering with normal blood flow and allowing blood to leak into brain tissue. Blood that comes into direct contact with brain tissue irritates the tissue and can cause scarring, leading to seizures.

The major risk factors for both types of stroke are atherosclerosis (the narrowing or blockage of arteries by patchy deposits of fatty material in the walls of arteries), high blood pressure, diabetes, and smoking. Atherosclerosis is a more important risk factor for ischemic stroke, and high blood pressure is a more important risk factor for hemorrhagic stroke. Other risk factors for hemorrhagic stroke include use of anticoagulants, cocaine, or amphetamines; aneurysms in arteries within the skull; blood vessel (arteriovenous) malformations; and vasculitis. The incidence of strokes has declined in recent decades, mainly because people are more aware of the importance of controlling high blood pressure and high cholesterol levels. Controlling these factors reduces the risk of atherosclerosis.

Symptoms

The effects of a stroke or transient ischemic attack vary depending on the precise location of the blockage or bleeding in the brain. Each area of the brain is supplied by specific arteries. For example, if an artery supplying the area of the brain that controls the left leg's muscle movements is blocked, the leg becomes weak or paralyzed. If the area of the brain that senses touch in the right arm is damaged, sensation in the right arm is lost.

Because early treatment can help loss of function and sensation, everyone should know what the early symptoms of stroke are. People who have such a symptom should see a doctor immediately, even if the symptom does not cause pain or if it goes away quickly. Starting treatment within 3 to 6 hours can help prevent the more severe consequences of a stroke.

The most common early symptoms of an ischemic stroke are sudden weakness or paralysis of the face and leg on one side of the body; slurred speech; sudden confusion with difficulty speaking or understanding speech; sudden dimness or loss of vision, particularly in one eye; loss of balance and coordination, leading to falls; sudden severe headache; and abnormal sensations or loss of sensation in an arm or a leg or on one side of the body. Symp-

toms of a transient ischemic attack are the same, but they usually disappear within minutes and rarely last more than 1 or 2 hours.

Symptoms of a hemorrhagic stroke are largely the same as those of an ischemic stroke but may also include sudden severe headache, nausea and vomiting, temporary or persistent loss of consciousness, and very high blood pressure.

In both types of stroke, an abnormal pattern of breathing can occur. Slow, irregular breathing may be caused by herniation of the brain.▲ Herniation may develop when very high pressure within the skull forces the brain downward in the skull and distorts the respiratory center in the lower part of the brain stem.

In most people who have had an ischemic stroke, the loss of function caused by a stroke is usually greatest immediately after the stroke occurs. However, in about 15 to 20%, the stroke is progressive, causing greatest loss of function after a day or two. In people who have had a hemorrhagic stroke, loss of function usually occurs progressively over minutes to hours.

Over days to months, some function is usually regained because even though some brain cells die, others are only damaged and may recover. Also, certain areas of the brain can sometimes switch to the functions previously performed by the damaged part—a characteristic called plasticity. However, the early effects of a stroke, including paralysis, can become permanent. Muscles may become permanently spastic and stiff, and painful muscle spasms may occur. Walking, swallowing, physically saying words clearly, and performing daily activities may remain difficult. Problems with memory, thinking, attention, or learning may persist. The person may be unable to recognize parts of the body and may be unaware of the stroke's effects. The person may continue to be unable to control emotions and to feel depressed. The peripheral field of vision may be reduced, and hearing may be partially lost. Dizziness and vertigo may be continuing problems. Control of bowel or bladder function may be permanently impaired.

Certain factors suggest that the outcome of a stroke is likely to be poor. Strokes that cause unconsciousness or that affect a large part of the left side of the brain (which is responsible for language) are particularly grave. In adults who have had an ischemic stroke, neurologic losses that remain after 6 months are likely to be permanent, although children continue to

▲ see art on page 515

improve slowly for many months. Older people fare less well than younger people. For people who already have other serious disorders (such as dementia), recovery is more limited.

If a hemorrhagic stroke is not massive and pressure within the brain is not very high, outcome is likely to be better after than that after an ischemic stroke. Blood (in a hemorrhagic stroke) does not damage brain tissue to the extent that an inadequate supply of oxygen (in an ischemic stroke) does. People who have had a hemorrhagic stroke may continue to improve for many months, even years.

Prevention

Preventing strokes is preferable to treating them. The main preventive strategy is managing the major risk factors. High blood pressure▲ and diabetes■ should be controlled; cholesterol levels should be measured and, if high, lowered to reduce the risk of atherosclerosis.★ Other recommendations include stopping smoking, not using amphetamines or cocaine, consuming alcohol only in moderation, exercising regularly, and, if overweight, losing weight.

Taking an antiplatelet drug, such as aspirin, reduces the risk of stroke (and heart attack). Antiplatelet drugs reduce the tendency of platelets to clump and to promote clot formation, a common cause of stroke. Aspirin, one of the most effective antiplatelet drugs, is usually prescribed as ½ of an adult's tablet or 1 children's tablet (which is ¼ of an adult's tablet) a day. Dipyridamole is sometimes prescribed, but for most people, it is not effective unless it is taken with aspirin. Taking aspirin with dipyridamole is more effective than taking aspirin alone. Ticlopidine or clopidogrel—other antiplatelet drugs—may be given to people who cannot tolerate or have not responded to aspirin. People who have had TIAs or strokes due to blood clots originating in the heart may be given warfarin, an anticoagulant.●

Rehabilitation

Intensive rehabilitation can help many people overcome disabilities after a stroke.◆ The exercises and training of rehabilitation help develop the plasticity of the brain (the ability of one area to shift to different functions) and teach the person new ways to use muscles unaffected by the stroke to compensate for losses in function.

The goals of rehabilitation are to regain as much normal function as possible, to main-

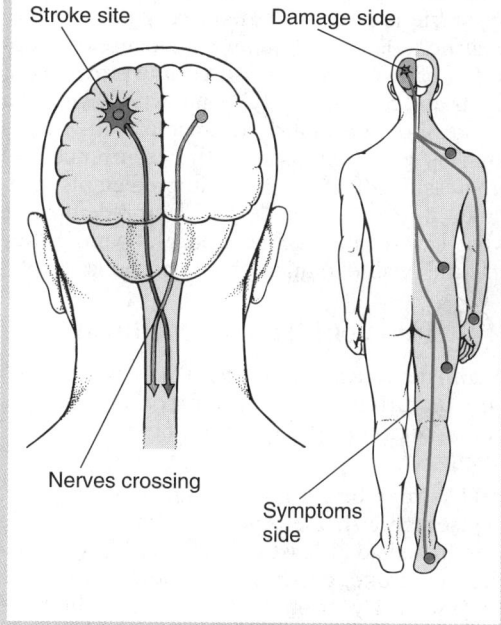

Why Strokes Affect Only One Side of the Body

Strokes usually damage only one side of the brain. Because nerves in the brain cross over to the other side of the body, symptoms appear on the side of the body opposite the damaged side of the brain.

Stroke site

Damage side

Nerves crossing

Symptoms side

tain and improve physical condition, and to help people relearn old skills and learn new ones as needed. Success depends on the area of the brain damaged and the person's general physical condition, functional and cognitive abilities before the stroke, social situation, learning ability, and attitude. Patience and perseverance are crucial.

Rehabilitation is started in the hospital as soon as the person is physically able—usually within 1 or 2 days of admission. After discharge from the hospital, rehabilitation can be continued on an outpatient basis, in a nursing home, in a rehabilitation center, or at home. Occupational and physical therapists can sug-

▲ see page 131   ■ see page 962
★ see page 922   ● see page 506
◆ see page 41

easier and the home
abilities.

ends can contribute
by keeping in mind
e, so that they can
t the person. Sup-
have had a stroke
care for them can help.

...-of-Life Issues

For some people who have had a stroke, quality of life is likely to remain very poor despite treatment. For such people, care focuses on control of pain, comfort measures, and provision of fluids and nourishment. People who have had a stroke should establish advance directives▲ as soon as possible, because the recurrence and progression of strokes are unpredictable. Advance directives can help a doctor determine what kind of medical care people want if they become unable to make these decisions.

Transient Ischemic Attacks

A transient ischemic attack (TIA) is a temporary disturbance in brain function resulting from a temporary blockage of the brain's blood supply.

TIAs may be a warning sign of an impending ischemic stroke. About one third of people who have had at least one TIA will have an ischemic stroke; about half of these strokes occur within 1 year of the TIA. People who have had a TIA are almost 10 times more likely to have a stroke than those who have not. Recognizing a TIA and having the cause identified can help prevent a stroke. Causes of TIAs and ischemic strokes are the same. Most TIAs occur when a piece of a blood clot (thrombus) or of fatty material (an atheroma) due to atherosclerosis breaks off from the heart or from the wall of an artery, travels through the bloodstream (becoming an embolus), and lodges in an artery that supplies the brain. Atherosclerosis causes recurring TIAs in about 5% of people.

Symptoms and Diagnosis

Symptoms of a TIA develop suddenly. They are identical to those of an ischemic stroke■ but are temporary and reversible. They usually last 2 to 30 minutes and rarely last more than 1 to 2 hours. By definition, they do not last longer than 24 hours. Apparently, no permanent damage results, because the blood supply to the affected area is restored relatively quickly. However, TIAs tend to recur. A person may have several in 1 day or only two or three in several years.

People who have a sudden, temporary symptom similar to any symptom of a stroke should report it to a doctor. Such a symptom suggests a TIA. However, other disorders, including seizures, brain tumors, migraine headaches, and abnormally low levels of sugar in the blood, have similar symptoms, so further evaluation is needed.

Doctors use several procedures to determine whether a an artery to the brain is blocked, which artery is blocked, and how complete the blockage is. These procedures include listening with a stethoscope for the sounds made by turbulent blood flow (bruits) in the internal carotid arteries (in the neck), color Doppler ultrasonography of the internal carotid and vertebral arteries, and sometimes magnetic resonance angiography★ and cerebral angiography.● Imaging procedures, such as computed tomography (CT) or magnetic resonance imaging (MRI), cannot be used to identify TIAs because TIAs, unlike strokes, usually do not cause brain damage. A specialized type of MRI, called diffusion MRI, can identify abnormal areas of brain tissue that are temporarily nonfunctional but that do not die (that is, that do not result in stroke).

Treatment

Treatment of TIAs is aimed at preventing a stroke. The first step in preventing a stroke is to control, if possible, the major risk factors for it: high blood pressure, high cholesterol levels, smoking, and diabetes. In addition, antiplatelet drugs, such as aspirin and dipyridamole, can be taken. When stronger drugs are needed (for example, for people who have atrial fibrillation, another abnormal heart rhythm, or a heart valve disorder), doctors may prescribe anticoagulants (drugs used to inhibit blood clotting), such as heparin or warfarin.

The degree of narrowing in the carotid arteries helps doctors determine the treatment. If the internal carotid artery is narrowed by more than 70% and the person has had stroke-like symptoms during the previous 6 months, an operation to widen the artery (called an endarterectomy) may be performed to reduce the risk of having a stroke. When the artery is less

▲ see page 54   ■ see page 507
★ see page 444   ● see page 445

narrowed, the operation is performed to prevent the blockage of the artery over time or to prevent additional TIAs or strokes if either are thought likely. An endarterectomy usually involves removing fatty deposits (atheromas) and clots in the internal carotid artery. The operation has a 2 to 6% risk of causing a stroke (because the operation may dislodge clots or other material that can then travel through the bloodstream and block an artery). For people who have minor narrowing and no symptoms, the risk of having a stroke is higher during the operation than it is with drug therapy. However, the risk is lower after the operation for several years than it is with drug therapy.

In other narrowed arteries, such as the vertebral arteries, endarterectomy may not be possible because the operation is more difficult to perform in these arteries than in the internal carotid arteries.

Alternatively, angioplasty▲ may be performed. In this procedure, a catheter with a balloon at its tip is threaded into the narrowed artery. The balloon is then inflated for several seconds to widen the artery. To keep the artery open, doctors insert a tube made of wire mesh (a stent) into the artery. This procedure is considered experimental but in the future is likely to replace endarterectomy.

Ischemic Stroke

An ischemic stroke is the death of brain tissue (cerebral infarction) resulting from an inadequate supply of blood and oxygen to the brain.

Causes

Ischemic strokes result from blockage of the arteries that supply the brain, most commonly in the branches of the internal carotid arteries. The blockage usually results when a piece of a blood clot (thrombus) or of a fatty deposit (atheroma) due to atherosclerosis breaks off (becoming an embolus), travels through the bloodstream, and lodges in an artery that supplies the brain.

Blood clots may form when a fatty deposit in the wall of an artery ruptures. The rupture of such a fatty deposit may also form when a large fatty deposit■ slows blood flow, reducing it to a trickle, like the flow of water through a clogged pipe. Blood that flows slowly is more likely to clot. Thus, the risk of a clot forming in and blocking a narrowed artery is high.

Blood clots may also form in other areas, such as in the heart or on a heart valve. Strokes due to such blood clots are most common among people who have recently had heart surgery and people who have a heart valve disorder or an abnormal heart rhythm (arrhythmia), especially atrial fibrillation. Also, in certain disorders such as an excess of red blood cells (polycythemia), the risk of blood clots is increased because the blood is thickened.

Rarely, a condition that resembles a stroke results when small pieces of fat from the marrow of a broken long bone, such as one in an arm or a leg, are released into the bloodstream. These pieces can clump together and block an artery. This condition is called fat embolism syndrome.

An ischemic stroke can result if the blood flow to the brain is reduced, as may occur when a person loses a lot of blood or has very low blood pressure. Occasionally, an ischemic stroke occurs when blood flow to the brain is normal but the blood does not contain enough oxygen. Disorders that reduce the oxygen content of blood include severe anemia (a deficiency of red blood cells), suffocation, and carbon monoxide poisoning. Usually, brain damage in such cases is widespread (diffuse), and coma results.

An ischemic stroke can occur if inflammation or infection narrows blood vessels that supply the brain. Drugs such as cocaine and amphetamines cause spasm of the arteries, which can narrow the arteries supplying the brain and cause a stroke.

Symptoms

Most ischemic strokes begin suddenly, develop rapidly, and cause death of brain tissue within minutes to hours. Then most strokes become stable, causing little or no further damage. (Strokes that remain stable for 2 to 3 days are called completed strokes.) Such strokes are more likely to be due to sudden blockage by an embolus. Less commonly, strokes may continue to worsen for several hours to a day or two, as a steadily enlarging area of brain tissue dies. (Such strokes are called evolving strokes.) The progression is usually interrupted by somewhat stable periods, during which the area temporarily stops enlarging or some improvement occurs. Such strokes are more likely to be due to formation of clots in a narrowed artery.

▲ see art on page 208   ■ see art on page 196

Recognizing an Ischemic Stroke

Because early treatment of stroke can help, everyone should know what the common early symptoms are:

- Sudden weakness or paralysis of an arm, a leg, or one side of the body
- Sudden dimness or loss of vision, particularly in one eye
- Sudden confusion, with difficulty speaking and understanding speech
- Loss of balance and coordination, leading to falls
- Sudden severe headache with no apparent cause
- Abnormal sensations or loss of sensation in an arm or a leg or on one side of the body

Many other symptoms may also occur. A transient ischemic attack causes the same symptoms. However, the symptoms usually disappear in 10 to 15 minutes and sometimes in 1 to 2 hours; they do not last longer than 24 hours. People who have a symptom that suggests an ischemic stroke should seek medical attention immediately.

Many different symptoms can occur, depending on which part of the brain is deprived of blood and oxygen. When the arteries that branch from the internal carotid artery are affected, blindness in one eye or abnormal sensations and weakness in one arm or leg or on one side of the body are most common. When the arteries that branch from the vertebral arteries in the back of the brain are affected, dizziness and vertigo, double vision, and generalized weakness of both sides of the body are more common. Many other symptoms, such as difficulty speaking (for example, slurred speech) and loss of coordination, can occur.

Large strokes may lead to stupor or coma. In addition, strokes, even small ones, can cause depression or an inability to control emotions (causing inappropriate crying or laughing).

Strokes can cause swelling in the brain due to accumulation of fluid (edema). Swelling in the brain is particularly dangerous because the skull does not expand. The resulting increase in pressure can cause the brain to shift and damage brain tissue further, making neurologic dysfunction worse, even if the area affected by the stroke itself does not enlarge. If the pressure becomes very high, the brain may be forced downward in the skull, resulting in herniation of the brain.▲

People who are immobilized by a stroke may develop certain complications. They may inhale vomit or other irritating materials into the lungs, resulting in aspiration pneumonia. Being in one position too long can result in bedsores (pressure sores). Not being able to move the legs can result in the formation of blood clots in the deep veins of the legs and groin (deep vein thrombosis).

Diagnosis

Doctors can usually diagnose an ischemic stroke based on the history of events and results of a physical examination. Doctors can usually identify which artery in the brain is blocked based on neurologic symptoms.■ For example, weakness or paralysis of the left leg suggests blockage of the artery supplying the area on the right side of the brain that controls the left leg's muscle movements. The sounds of turbulent blood flow (bruits) through the internal carotid arteries (heard using a stethoscope) may indicate narrowing.

Magnetic resonance imaging (MRI) or computed tomography (CT) is usually performed to confirm the diagnosis. Usually, MRI can detect ischemic strokes within minutes of their start. CT can detect ischemic strokes within 1 hour of their start. CT or MRI also helps distinguish an ischemic stroke from a hemorrhagic stroke, a brain tumor, an abscess, and other structural abnormalities. Cerebral angiography is performed when surgical removal of fatty deposits or clots (endarterectomy) is being considered or when inflammation of blood vessels (vasculitis) is suspected. Angiography provides detailed information about the blood supply to the brain.★ Magnetic resonance angiography or color Doppler ultrasonography, both less invasive procedures than cerebral angiography, are helpful. These imaging procedures can show which large artery is blocked, but they cannot show the medium and small arteries that may be affected by vasculitis.

Identifying the precise cause of the stroke, particularly whether the blockage is a blood clot or a fatty deposit, is important. If the blockage is a blood clot, another stroke is very likely unless the underlying disorder is corrected. For example, blood clots may form in the heart because it is beating irregularly. Treating the irregular heartbeat can prevent new clots from forming and causing another

▲ see art on page 515   ■ see art on page 476
★ see page 445

stroke. If doctors suspect an irregular heart-beat, electrocardiography (ECG) is usually performed to look for abnormal heart rhythms. Other procedures used to diagnose heart disorders may also be performed. They include continuous ambulatory ECG,▲ in which a Holter monitor records the heart rate and rhythms continuously for 24 hours, and echocardiography,■ which produces images of the chambers and valves of the heart.

Blood tests are performed to be sure that the stroke was not caused by a deficiency of red blood cells (anemia), polycythemia, cancer of the white blood cells (leukemia), or an infection. Rarely, a spinal tap (lumbar puncture) is performed—for example, after CT, when doctors still need to determine whether a stroke is due to an infection (such as herpes simplex) or whether a subarachnoid hemorrhage is present.★ This procedure can be performed only if doctors are sure that the brain is not under excess pressure (usually determined by CT or MRI).

Treatment

Symptoms that suggest an ischemic stroke require immediate medical attention; doctors can sometimes reduce the damage or prevent further damage by acting quickly.

When a person who has had a stroke arrives at the hospital, the first steps in treatment are to restore the person's breathing, heart rate, blood pressure, and temperature to normal. Fluids are given if blood pressure is low. Drugs (such as a beta-blocker) are given to stabilize the heart rate if it is too fast; a pacemaker may be inserted if the heart rate is too slow. If the person has a fever, it may be lowered using acetaminophen, ibuprofen, or a cooling blanket. An increase in body temperature by even a few degrees can dramatically worsen brain damage due to an ischemic stroke. Oxygen is usually administered through a face mask or nasal prongs, and an intravenous line to provide fluids and drugs is inserted. Generally, doctors do not immediately treat high blood pressure unless blood pressure is higher than 170/110 mm Hg, because if blood pressure becomes too low, brain tissue may not receive enough oxygen-rich blood.

A drug that breaks up clots (a thrombolytic drug), such as tissue plasminogen activator (tPA), can be given intravenously to help restore blood flow to the brain. Because thrombolytic drugs can cause bleeding in the brain and elsewhere, they should not be given to people who have had a hemorrhagic stroke. So before a thrombolytic drug is given, CT or MRI is performed to make sure that there is no bleeding in the brain. To be effective, a thrombolytic drug given intravenously must be started within 3 hours of the beginning of an ischemic stroke. However, most people who have had a stroke arrive at the hospital between 3 to 6 hours afterward—too late to be given a thrombolytic drug intravenously. Some of such people can be given a thrombolytic drug through an artery rather than through a vein (intravenously), so that a more concentrated dose of the drug can be applied directly to the clot. To give the drug through an artery, doctors make an incision in the skin and insert a thin, flexible tube (catheter) into an artery. The catheter is then threaded through other arteries to the clot.

For an evolving stroke, anticoagulants such as heparin may be given, but their effectiveness has not been proved. However, after the stroke is completed, anticoagulants are given to prevent subsequent strokes in people who have atrial fibrillation or a heart valve disorder. Because these drugs increase the risk of bleeding into the brain, doctors usually wait at least 24 hours after thrombolytic therapy is ended before anticoagulants are started. Anticoagulants are not given to people who have uncontrolled high blood pressure or who have had a hemorrhagic stroke.

Other new experimental measures that may improve the chances of a favorable outcome involve blocking the receptors of certain neurotransmitters in the brain. However, these measures are not yet available for routine use.

Once an ischemic stroke is completed, some brain tissue is dead, so reestablishing its blood supply by surgical removal of the blockage (endarterectomy) in an internal carotid artery cannot restore the lost function. Therefore, endarterectomy is not usually performed. However, removing blockages after a small stroke may reduce the risk of subsequent strokes.

If a stroke is very severe, drugs such as mannitol may be given to reduce swelling and the increased pressure on the brain. Some people need a ventilator to breathe adequately.

Measures to prevent aspiration pneumonia● and bedsore (pressure sores)◆ are started early.

▲ see art on page 124   ■ see page 125
★ see page 511   ● see page 271
◆ see page 1209

Heparin, injected under the skin, may be given to help prevent deep vein thrombosis.▲ The person is closely monitored to determine whether the bladder and intestines are functioning. Often, other disorders such as heart failure, abnormal heart rhythms, and lung infections must be treated. High blood pressure is often treated after the stroke has been stabilized. Because a stroke often causes mood changes, especially depression, family or friends should inform the doctor if the person seems depressed. Depression can be treated with drug therapy and psychotherapy.■

After a stroke, some people are given antiplatelet drugs or the anticoagulant warfarin to help prevent subsequent strokes.

Prognosis

About 10% of people who have an ischemic stroke recover almost all normal function, and about 25% recover most of it. About 40% of people have moderate to severe impairments requiring special care, and about 10% require care in a nursing home or other long-term care facility. Some people are physically and mentally devastated and unable to move, speak, or eat normally. About 15% of people who have a stroke die in the hospital. The proportion is higher among older people.

During the first few days after an ischemic stroke, doctors usually cannot predict whether a person will improve or worsen. About 50% of people with one-sided paralysis and most of those with less severe symptoms recover some function by the time they leave the hospital, and they can eventually take care of their basic needs. They can think clearly and walk adequately, although they may have limited use of the affected arm or leg. Use of an arm is more often limited than use of a leg.

Hemorrhagic Stroke

A hemorrhagic stroke is damage to brain tissue resulting from bleeding inside the skull.

There are two main types of hemorrhagic strokes: intracerebral hemorrhage and subarachnoid hemorrhage. Intracerebral hemorrhages occur within the brain. Subarachnoid hemorrhages occur between the inner layer (pia mater) and middle layer (arachnoid mater) of the tissue covering the brain (meninges).

Bleeding inside the skull can also result in epidural and subdural hematomas, which are usually caused by a head injury and cause different symptoms.★

INTRACEREBRAL HEMORRHAGE

An intracerebral hemorrhage is bleeding within the brain.

Intracerebral hemorrhage accounts for about 10% of all strokes but for a much higher percentage of deaths due to stroke. Among people older than 60, intracerebral hemorrhage is more common than subarachnoid hemorrhage. Causes of intracerebral hemorrhage include high blood pressure and, in older people, fragile blood vessels. Bleeding disorders and use of anticoagulants increase the risk of dying from an intracerebral hemorrhage.

Symptoms and Diagnosis

An intracerebral hemorrhage begins abruptly. In about half of the people, it begins with a severe headache. Neurologic symptoms develop and steadily worsen. They include weakness, paralysis, numbness, loss of speech or vision, and confusion. Symptoms worsen as the hemorrhage expands. Nausea, vomiting, seizures, and loss of consciousness are common and may occur within seconds to minutes.

Doctors can often diagnose intracerebral hemorrhages on the basis of symptoms and the results of a physical examination. However, computed tomography (CT) or magnetic resonance imaging (MRI) is usually performed when a stroke is suspected. Both procedures can help doctors distinguish a hemorrhagic stroke from an ischemic stroke. The procedures can also detect how much brain tissue has been damaged and whether pressure is increased in other areas of the brain.

A spinal tap (lumbar puncture) is not usually performed. A spinal tap can cause herniation of the brain,● a life-threatening disorder, when pressure within the skull is increased, as it is in people who have had a hemorrhagic stroke.

Treatment and Prognosis

Treatment of a hemorrhagic stroke differs from that of an ischemic stroke. Anticoagulants, thrombolytic drugs, and antiplatelet drugs (such as aspirin) are not given, and surgery may save the person's life. The goal of surgery is to remove blood that has accumulated in the brain and to relieve the resulting increased pressure.

Stroke due to intracerebral hemorrhage is more dangerous than ischemic stroke. The

---

▲ see page 232   ■ see page 617
★ see page 513   ● see art on page 515

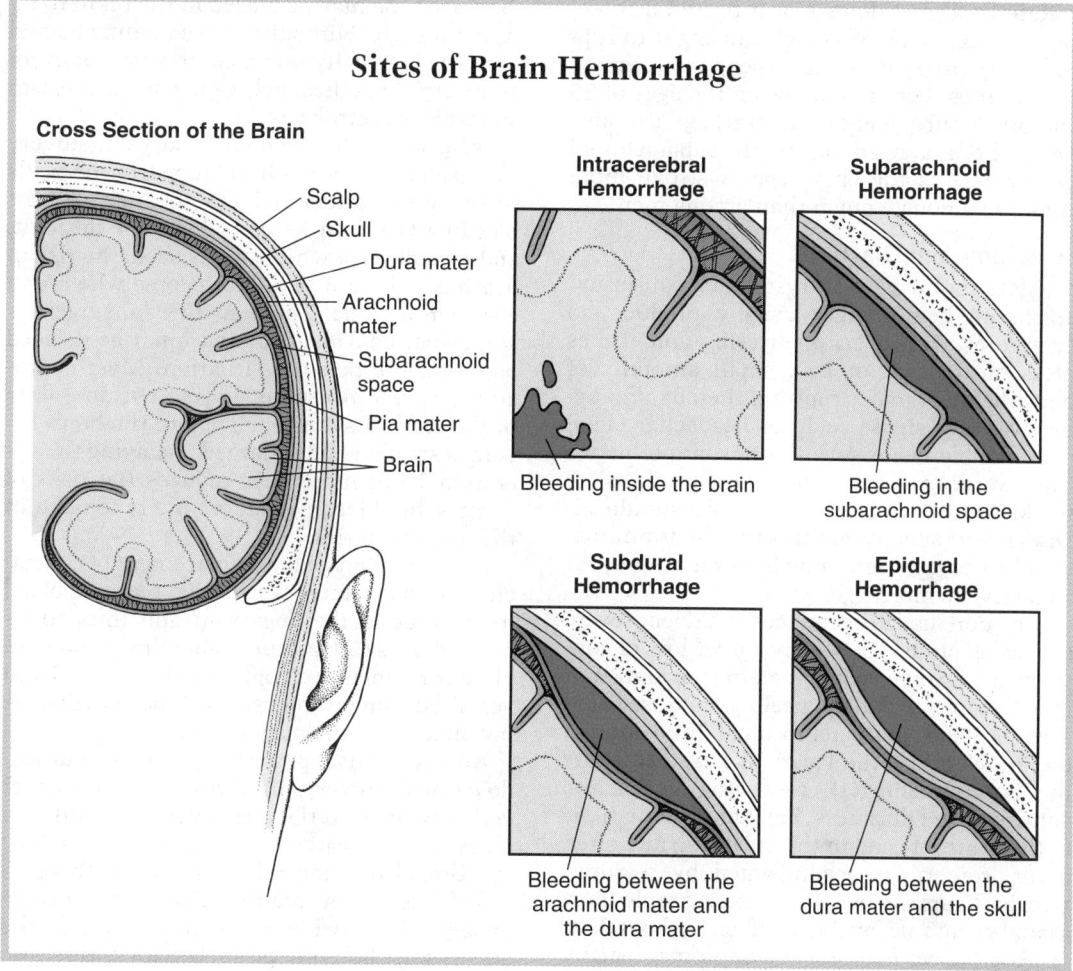

Sites of Brain Hemorrhage

Cross Section of the Brain

Scalp
Skull
Dura mater
Arachnoid mater
Subarachnoid space
Pia mater
Brain

Intracerebral Hemorrhage

Bleeding inside the brain

Subarachnoid Hemorrhage

Bleeding in the subarachnoid space

Subdural Hemorrhage

Bleeding between the arachnoid mater and the dura mater

Epidural Hemorrhage

Bleeding between the dura mater and the skull

stroke is usually large and catastrophic, especially in people who have chronic high blood pressure. More than half of the people who have large hemorrhages die within a few days. Those who survive usually recover consciousness and some brain function as the body absorbs the leaked blood. Even after surgery, many people continue to have some neurologic symptoms. Symptoms may include weakness, paralysis, loss of sensation on one side of the body, or difficulty understanding and using language (aphasia▲). However, people with small hemorrhages recover to a remarkable degree.

SUBARACHNOID HEMORRHAGE

A subarachnoid hemorrhage is sudden bleeding into the space (subarachnoid space) be-

tween the inner layer (pia mater) and middle layer (arachnoid mater) of the tissue covering the brain (meninges).

Usually, the cause is the sudden rupture of an aneurysm in a cerebral artery or a blood vessel (arteriovenous) malformation of the arteries or veins in or around the brain. An aneurysm may rupture because of the pressure of blood inside the artery; hemorrhage and stroke may result. An arteriovenous malformation may be present at birth, but it is identified only if symptoms develop. It may cause bleeding, usually during adolescence or young adulthood, and sudden collapse, stroke, and death may result.

▲ see page 477

Rarely, atherosclerosis or a bacterial infection damages a blood vessel, causing it to rupture. Ruptures can occur in people of any age but are most common between the ages of 25 and 50. A subarachnoid hemorrhage can also result from a head injury. A subarachnoid hemorrhage is the only type of stroke more common among women than among men.

Symptoms and Diagnosis

Before rupturing, aneurysms that cause subarachnoid hemorrhages usually produce no symptoms. However, aneurysms sometimes press on a nerve or leak small amounts of blood before a major rupture, thereby producing warning signs, such as headache, facial pain, double vision, or other visual problems. The warning signs can occur minutes to weeks before the rupture. People should always report such symptoms to a doctor immediately, because steps may be taken to prevent a massive hemorrhage.

A rupture usually produces a sudden, severe headache, often followed by a brief loss of consciousness. Some people remain in a coma, but more people wake up, feeling confused and sleepy. Blood and cerebrospinal fluid around the brain irritate the layers of tissue covering the brain (meninges), producing headaches, vomiting, and dizziness. Frequent fluctuations in the heart rate and in the breathing rate often occur, sometimes accompanied by seizures. Within hours or even minutes, people may again become sleepy and confused. About 25% of people have neurologic symptoms, usually paralysis on one side of the body.

A subarachnoid hemorrhage can usually be diagnosed using computed tomography (CT), which pinpoints the site of bleeding. Spinal tap (lumbar puncture), if necessary, can detect any blood in the cerebrospinal fluid. Cerebral angiography▲ is usually performed within 72 hours to confirm the diagnosis and to identify the site of the aneurysm or arteriovenous malformation causing the bleeding, so that surgery can be performed.

Treatment and Prognosis

People who may have had a subarachnoid hemorrhage are hospitalized immediately and instructed to avoid exertion. Analgesics such as opioids (but not aspirin or other nonsteroidal anti-inflammatory drugs) are given to control the severe headaches. Occasionally, a drainage tube may be placed in the brain to relieve pressure. Nimodipine, a calcium channel blocker, is usually given to prevent spasm of an artery. This drug helps prevent late spasm and ischemic stroke.

For people who have an aneurysm, surgery that isolates, blocks off, or supports the walls of the weak artery reduces the risk of fatal bleeding later. These procedures are difficult, and regardless of which one is used, the risk of death is high, especially for people who are in a stupor or coma. The best time for surgery is somewhat controversial and must be decided based on the person's situation. Most neurosurgeons recommend operating within 3 days of the start of symptoms, before the brain becomes swollen and inflamed. Delaying the operation 10 or more days reduces the risks of surgery, but bleeding is more likely to recur in the longer interim.

A common procedure is placement of a metal clip across the aneurysm, which prevents blood from entering the aneurysm and thus eliminates the risk of rupture. The clip remains in place permanently. People who had clips placed years ago cannot undergo MRI; newer clips are not affected by the magnetic forces.

An alternative procedure, called neuroendovascular surgery, involves the insertion of coiled wires into the aneurysm. The coils are placed using a catheter inserted into an artery and threaded to the aneurysm. Thus, this procedure does not require that the skull be opened. By slowing blood flow through the aneurysm, the coils promote clot formation, which seals off the aneurysm.

About 35% of people who have a subarachnoid hemorrhage due to an aneurysm die during the first episode because of extensive brain damage. Another 15% die within a few weeks because of subsequent bleeding. People who survive for 6 months but who do not have surgery for the aneurysm have a 3% chance of another rupture each year. The outlook is better when the cause is an arteriovenous malformation. Occasionally, the hemorrhage is caused by a small defect that is not detected by cerebral angiography because it has already sealed itself off. In such cases, the outlook is very good.

Many people recover most or all mental and physical function after a subarachnoid hemorrhage. However, neurologic symptoms, such as weakness, paralysis, loss of sensation on one side of the body, or difficulty understanding and using language (aphasia■), sometimes persist.

▲ see page 445   ■ see page 477

CHAPTER 87

Head Injuries

The thick, hard bones of the skull help protect the brain from injury. Also, the brain is surrounded by layers of tissue (meninges) containing cerebrospinal fluid, which cushions the brain. Consequently, most bumps and knocks on the head do not injure the brain, and most head injuries are minor.

Nonetheless, some head injuries are serious. Head injuries kill and disable more people younger than 50 than does any other type of neurologic damage. Head injuries occur in more than 70% of motor vehicle accidents, which are the leading cause of death in males younger than 35. Nearly 50% of people who have a severe head injury die.

About half of head injuries result from motor vehicle accidents. Other common causes are falls in the home, physical assaults, and accidents during sports, during recreational activities, or in the workplace (for example, while operating machinery).

Head injuries include external injury to the scalp, skull fractures, concussions, bruises (contusions) and tears (lacerations) of the brain, and accumulation of blood within the brain or between the brain and skull (intracranial hematoma). The brain can be damaged even if the skull is not fractured. Often, the severity of brain damage does not correlate with the severity of external injuries.

Symptoms

If the scalp is cut, bleeding may be profuse, because the scalp has many blood vessels close to the skin surface. Consequently, a scalp injury may appear to be more serious than it is.

After a concussion, consciousness may be lost, usually for less than 15 minutes. A bump may appear on the head, and headache, dizziness, nausea, and vomiting may occur. Usually, such symptoms resolve in days to weeks. Sometimes after a head injury, even a minor one, symptoms persist for a considerable time. Symptoms that persist are called the postconcussion syndrome. ▲

Certain symptoms indicate that the head injury is serious and that brain function is worsening. They include increasing sleepiness and confusion, vomiting that persists, severe headache, inability to feel or move an arm or leg, inability to recognize people or the surroundings, loss of balance, problems with speaking or seeing, lack of coordination, increasing blood pressure, slowing pulse, and drainage of clear fluid (cerebrospinal fluid) from the nose or mouth. These symptoms may develop hours or sometimes days after the original injury. Health care practitioners tell people who have a head injury what symptoms to watch for. Parents of small children are told how to monitor their children for these symptoms during the hours after an injury. If these symptoms occur, prompt medical attention is essential.

Symptoms of worsening brain function occur because pressure within the skull is increased. For example, pressure increases when blood vessels and tissues in or around the brain are torn, allowing blood and fluid to leak out. The result is accumulation of blood (hematoma) or of fluid (edema) and swelling. Pressure increases because the skull cannot expand to accommodate the increase in its contents. Increased pressure can damage or destroy brain tissue, causing loss of various functions, depending on which area of the brain is damaged.■ Increased pressure within the skull may force the brain downward, causing a herniation of the brain—an abnormal protrusion of brain tissue through a natural opening between the compartments of the brain. Herniation of the brain can be life threatening if pressure is put on the brain stem, the lower part of the brain, which controls such vital functions as heart rate and breathing. Unconsciousness, coma, and even death may result.

Posttraumatic epilepsy may occur months to years (usually not more than 4 years) after the brain is damaged by a severe head injury. Seizures ★ occur in about 70% of people who have had a severe head injury with penetration of the brain and in about 5 to 30% of those who have had a severe head injury without

---

▲ see page 517   ■ see page 476
★ see page 495

Recognizing a Serious Head Injury

Most head injuries are not serious. A serious head injury can be recognized based on certain symptoms. These symptoms indicate that brain functioning is worsening. If any of them occur in an adult or a child, medical attention should be sought immediately.

- Vomiting, paleness, irritability, or drowsiness without loss of consciousness that continues for more than 6 hours
- Loss of consciousness
- Inability to move or feel part of the body
- Inability to recognize people or the surroundings
- Inability to maintain balance
- Problems with speaking or seeing (for example, slurred speech or blurred vision)
- Drainage of clear fluid (cerebrospinal fluid) from the nose or mouth
- Severe headache

penetration of the brain. Symptoms often depend on where in the brain the seizure originates. For example, seizures originating in the frontal lobe cause twitches in specific muscles of the limbs on the opposite side of the body.

Prognosis

Most people who develop symptoms after a minor head injury recover completely within a few days.

For adults who have had a severe head injury, most recovery occurs within the first 6 months, although improvement may continue for up to 2 years. Children tend to recover more fully, regardless of the injury's severity, and they continue to improve for a much longer time.

The eventual consequences of a severe head injury range from complete recovery to permanent disability of varying degrees to death. The type and severity of disabilities depend on where and how badly the brain was damaged. Undamaged areas of the brain sometimes take over functions that were lost when another

area was damaged, resulting in partial recovery. However, as people age, the brain becomes less able to shift functions from one area to another. For example, language skills are handled by several parts of the brain in young children but are concentrated on one side of the brain in adults. If the left hemisphere's language areas are severely damaged before age 8, the right hemisphere can assume near-normal language function. However, damage to language areas during adulthood results in permanent disability.

Some functions, such as vision and control of arm and leg movements, are controlled by unique areas on one side of the brain. Damage to any of these areas usually causes permanent disability. Nonetheless, rehabilitation can help people minimize the effect of disabilities on function.▲

Recovery of memory after loss of consciousness due to a severe head injury depends on how quickly consciousness is regained. People who regain consciousness in the first week are most likely to recover their memory.

Diagnosis and Treatment

If a head injury is minor and causes no symptoms other than pain at the site of injury, acetaminophen■ (but not aspirin or any other nonsteroidal anti-inflammatory drug) may be taken. Applying cold compresses may also help relieve pain. Having another person check in with the injured person for a few hours to make sure that no symptoms develop is advisable. Children who have had a minor head injury may be allowed to sleep, but they should be awakened at regular intervals to make sure they can be aroused. The length of the interval (ranging from every 2 to 4 hours) depends on the relative severity of the injury and the appearance and behavior of the child.

If a head injury causes loss of consciousness, even briefly, or if symptoms of worsening brain function develop, immediate evaluation by a doctor is necessary.

If head injury is traumatic (for example, due to a motor vehicle accident) or the person is unconscious, an ambulance should be called. When emergency personnel are moving a person who has had a severe head injury, they take great care to avoid making the injuries worse. If the head injury was severe enough to cause loss of consciousness, the neck is assumed to be broken until proved otherwise. In such cases, the person's head, neck, and spine are stabilized. Usually, the person is strapped

▲ see page 41   ■ see page 454

Herniation: The Brain Under Pressure

Bleeding or swelling in the brain can cause pressure that forces the brain downward in the skull. The result may be a herniation, in which brain tissue is forced through a small natural opening in the relatively rigid sheets of tissue that separate the brain into right and left compartments and into upper and lower compartments. (These dividers are extensions of the outer layer of tissue covering the brain, the dura mater.) The most common type of herniation is a transtentorial herniation. Part of the temporal lobe is forced through the tentorial notch—the opening in the sheet of tissue between the temporal lobe and cerebellum. A transtentorial herniation can have catastrophic consequences, including paralysis, stupor, coma, abnormal heart rhythms, disturbances or cessation of breathing, cardiac arrest, and death.

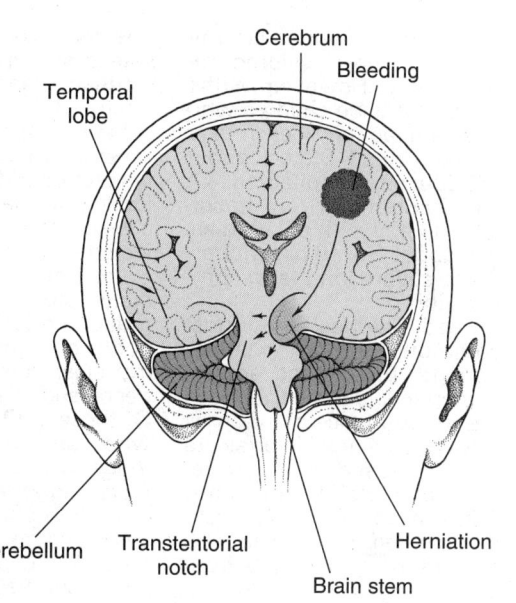

Cerebrum
Bleeding
Temporal lobe
Cerebellum
Transtentorial notch
Brain stem
Herniation

to a firm board and carefully padded to prevent movement.

When the person reaches the hospital, doctors and nurses perform a physical examination to determine whether the injury is serious. First, they check vital signs: heart rate, blood pressure, and breathing. A person who is not breathing adequately may need a ventilator. Level of consciousness, memory, and ability to use language are immediately assessed.▲ Basic brain function is evaluated by checking the size of the pupils and their reaction to light, by evaluating the response to sensations such as heat or pinpricks, and by testing the ability to move the arms and legs. Computed tomography (CT) or magnetic resonance imaging (MRI) is performed to check for possible brain damage. Standard x-rays can identify skull fractures but reveal very little about brain damage. These procedures are also used to determine whether the neck is broken.

If the head injury is severe and the person's condition is worsening, mannitol is usually given intravenously to reduce swelling (which can develop quickly) and thus reduce pressure within the skull. Mannitol draws fluid from the brain and promotes urine excretion. Sometimes corticosteroids are given intravenously to reduce swelling. A small pressure gauge

may be implanted inside the skull to measure pressure within the skull and to determine how well the treatments are working. Alternatively, a catheter may be inserted into one of the internal spaces (ventricles) within the brain. The ventricles contain cerebrospinal fluid, which flows over the surface of the brain between the meninges. The catheter can be used to monitor the pressure and to drain cerebrospinal fluid, reducing the pressure within the skull.

If a head injury is severe, most doctors recommend giving an anticonvulsant (such as phenytoin, carbamazepine, or valproate■) for up to 2 weeks to prevent seizures. If no seizures occur, the anticonvulsant is stopped. If a seizure occurs, the anticonvulsant is continued for several years or indefinitely.

Skull Fracture

A skull fracture is a break in a bone of the head.

Skull fractures can injure arteries and veins, which then bleed into the spaces around brain tissue. In people with a skull fracture, brain damage may be more severe than in people

▲ see table on page 441   ■ see table on page 500

Head Injuries in Children

Most head injuries are minor, and most children recover fully. However, of the nearly 1 million children who have a head injury each year in the United States, about 165,000 are hospitalized. Of the children who are hospitalized, about 1 of 20 dies, and about 1 of 10 has moderate to severe long-term complications.

Head injuries are most common among children younger than 1 and among teenagers older than 15. Boys are injured twice as often as girls. Severe head injuries are usually caused by motor vehicle and bicycle accidents. Minor head injuries are usually caused by falls in and around the home. Falls from heights is a common but preventable cause of death among children who live in high-rise apartment buildings. Almost two thirds of head injuries in infants are due to child abuse.

Headache is common after a head injury, even a minor one. Prompt evaluation by a doctor is required only if symptoms indicating worsening brain function occur.

In infants who have a skull fracture, the membranes surrounding the brain occasionally protrude through and become trapped by the fracture, forming a fluid-filled sac called a growing fracture.

The sac develops over 3 to 6 weeks and may be the first evidence that the skull was fractured.

Severe head injuries may severely damage the developing brain, interfering with physical, intellectual, and emotional development. Complications include memory loss for events that occurred immediately before the injury (retrograde amnesia), changes in behavior, emotional instability, sleep disturbances, and decreased intellectual ability. Of those with a severe injury who are unconscious for longer than 24 hours, 50% have long-term complications; 2 to 5% of these remain severely handicapped. Young children, especially infants, who have had a severe head injury are more likely to die than older children.

During the first week after a severe head injury, seizures occur in about 5% of children older than 5 years and in 10% of those younger than 5. Seizures that start soon after the injury are less likely to result in a long-term seizure disorder than those that start 7 or more days later.

Serious but relatively uncommon complications are intracranial hemorrhages and hematomas. Young children who have an epidural hematoma tend to gradually lose consciousness over a period

of minutes to hours, whereas in adults, symptoms may be delayed. In infants who have been shaken (a condition called shaken baby syndrome), bleeding often occurs in the back of the eyes, causing retinal hemorrhages.

Most children who have had minor head injuries are sent home, and their parents are instructed to observe them for persistent vomiting or increasing drowsiness. Children do not need to be kept awake during the night, but they do need to be awakened periodically (according to a doctor's instructions—for example, every 2 to 4 hours) to make sure they can be aroused. In some cases, children need to be observed in the hospital. They include children who are drowsy, who were unconscious even briefly, who have numbness or muscle weakness, who have pupils of unequal size, who have had a seizure, or who have had a particular type of skull fracture (such as a fracture at the back of the skull). Children who have a skull fracture without evidence of brain damage are not routinely hospitalized. In contrast, infants who have a skull fracture, especially if it is depressed, are almost always observed in the hospital. Children are also kept in the hospital if child abuse is suspected.

with a head injury but no fracture. Fractures, especially at the back and bottom (base) of the skull, can tear the meninges, the layers of tissue that cover the brain. Bacteria occasionally enter the skull through such fractures, causing infection and severe brain damage. However, a skull fracture often occurs without brain damage.

Certain symptoms suggest a fracture at the base of the skull: Cerebrospinal fluid—the clear fluid that flows over the surface of the brain between the meninges—may leak from the nose or ears. If the eardrum is ruptured, blood may collect behind the eardrum or

blood may drain from the ear. Bruises may develop behind the ear (Battle's sign) or around the eyes (raccoon's eyes). Blood may collect in the sinuses; it can be detected by x-rays, computed tomography (CT), or magnetic resonance imaging (MRI). Seizures may occur soon after the injury or later.

Many skull fractures do not require surgery. Depressed skull fractures are an exception. In this type of fracture, one or more fragments of bone may press inward on the brain, damaging the brain. The brain may be exposed to the outside. To prevent infection and the formation of abscesses, doctors remove foreign materials and dead tissue and repair as much of the damage as possible. They lift skull fragments back into position and stitch the wound closed.

Concussion

A concussion is a brief loss of consciousness after a head injury that does not cause visible physical damage.

Concussions result in a temporary malfunction of the brain but no visible physical damage. They may occur after even a minor head injury, depending on how the brain is jarred within the skull.

A person who has a concussion may temporarily feel dazed or mildly confused. Consciousness may be lost for a brief time. Memory for events just before or just after the injury may be lost. Most people recover completely within a few hours or days. Occasionally, symptoms of worsening brain function develop hours or sometimes days after the original injury, especially in older people. If these symptoms occur, prompt medical attention is essential.

Postconcussion syndrome is a group of symptoms that occur after a concussion. The syndrome lasts from a few days to several weeks but rarely longer. People may feel somewhat confused, headachy, and abnormally sleepy. Dizziness, difficulty concentrating, forgetfulness, depression, lack of feeling or emotion, and anxiety may develop. Meanwhile, people may have trouble working, studying, and socializing. Postconcussion syndrome is puzzling; why these problems commonly occur after a minor head injury is unknown. Experts disagree about whether the symptoms are caused by microscopic damage or psychologic factors.

Usually, once doctors have determined that severe damage has not occurred, no treatment is needed. As long as symptoms do not worsen, acetaminophen may be used for pain. Adults may take aspirin or another nonsteroidal anti-inflammatory drug (NSAID)▲ after the first 3 or 4 days if the injury is not severe and no bleeding is detected by computed tomography (CT). These drugs should not be taken any sooner, because they interfere with blood clotting and may prolong bleeding from damaged blood vessels.

People with postconcussion syndrome may be given drugs used to treat headache■ or dizziness.★ Psychiatric treatment helps some people.

Cerebral Contusions and Lacerations

Cerebral contusions are bruises on the brain, usually caused by a direct, strong blow to the head. Cerebral lacerations are tears in brain tissue, which often accompany visible head wounds and skull fractures.

Cerebral contusions and lacerations are usually more serious than concussions. Contusions may be caused by the sudden acceleration of the brain that follows a jolt—as may be delivered by a forceful blow to the head—or by the sudden deceleration that occurs when a moving head strikes an immovable object. The brain can be damaged at the point of impact and on the opposite side by striking the inside of the skull. Acceleration-deceleration injuries are sometimes called *coup contrecoup* (meaning hit-counterhit in French).

Contusions and lacerations may cause only minimal physical damage to the brain, with few symptoms. However, if swelling or bleeding is severe, these injuries can cause a severe headache, dizziness, and vomiting. One pupil may be larger than the other. Depending on which area of the brain is damaged, the ability to think, control emotions, move, feel, speak, see, hear, and remember may be impaired. The person may become irritable, restless, or agitated. One side of the body may become weak or feel numb. Confusion may develop. A more severe injury causes swelling within the brain, damaging brain tissue further. Herniation of the brain may result, sometimes leading to coma. Severe brain damage is often accompanied by other injuries, especially scalp injuries, skull fractures, and injuries of the chest and spine.

Magnetic resonance imaging (MRI), which can detect physical damage to the brain, is performed. If bleeding is minor, rest is the only treatment needed, but the person must be observed for a period of days up to 1 week. If bleeding is severe, the blood may have to be removed surgically. Other injuries, if present, must also be treated.

Intracranial Hematomas

Intracranial hematomas are accumulations of blood within the brain or between the brain and the skull.

▲ see page 452   ■ see page 456

★ see page 461

Intracranial hematomas include epidural hematomas, which form between the skull and the outer layer (dura mater) of tissue covering the brain (meninges); subdural hematomas, which form between the outer layer and the middle layer (arachnoid mater▲); and intracerebral hematomas, which form within the brain. Intracranial hematomas can result from an injury or a stroke. For people who are taking aspirin or anticoagulants (which increase the risk of bleeding), particularly in older people, the risk of developing a hematoma after even a minor head injury is increased.

Most hematomas develop rapidly and produce symptoms within minutes. Large hematomas press on the brain and may cause swelling and herniation of the brain. Hematomas may cause confusion and memory loss, especially in older people, as well as loss of consciousness, coma, paralysis on one or both sides of the body, breathing difficulties, slowing of the heart, and even death.

Recovery (after prompt treatment) is more likely to be rapid and complete if the hematoma is epidural or subdural than if it is intracerebral. The reason is that the blood in epidural and subdural hematomas, unlike that in intracerebral hematomas, does not touch brain tissue and therefore does not directly irritate the brain.

Epidural Hematomas: These hematomas are caused by bleeding from an artery or a large vein (venous sinus) located between the skull and the outer layer of tissue covering the brain. Bleeding occurs when a skull fracture tears the blood vessel. A severe headache may develop immediately or after several hours. The headache sometimes disappears but returns several hours later, worse than before. Deterioration in consciousness, including increasing confusion, sleepiness, paralysis, collapse, and a deep coma, can quickly follow. Some people lose consciousness after the injury, regain it, and have a period of unimpaired mental function (lucid interval) before consciousness begins to deteriorate again.

Early diagnosis is crucial and is usually based on results of magnetic resonance imaging (MRI) or computed tomography (CT). Epidural hematomas are treated as soon as they are diagnosed, because prompt treatment is necessary to prevent permanent damage. One or more

holes are drilled in the skull to drain the excess blood. The surgeon also seeks the source of the bleeding and stops the bleeding.

Subdural Hematomas: These hematomas are caused by bleeding from the bridging veins, located between the outer and middle layers of tissue covering the brain (meninges).

Subdural hematomas may be acute, subacute, or chronic. Rapid bleeding after a severe head injury can cause acute subdural hematomas, with immediate symptoms, or subacute subdural hematomas, with symptoms that develop over several hours. Chronic subdural hematomas result from a less severe head injury, in which bleeding starts more slowly, and symptoms develop after days, weeks, or even months. Symptoms are delayed because chronic subdural hematomas tend to enlarge very slowly.

Chronic subdural hematomas are more common among alcoholics and among older people. Alcoholics, who are relatively prone to falls and other injuries, may ignore minor to moderately severe head injuries. These injuries can lead to small subdural hematomas that may become chronic. In older people, the brain shrinks slightly, stretching the bridging veins and making them more likely to be torn if an injury, even a minor one, occurs. Also, bleeding tends to continue longer because older people heal more slowly. After the blood is resorbed from a hematoma, the brain may not re-expand as well in older people as in younger people. As a result, a fluid-filled space (hygroma) may be left. The hygroma may refill with blood or enlarge because small vessels tear, causing repeated bleeding.

Symptoms may include a persistent headache, fluctuating drowsiness, confusion, memory changes, paralysis on the opposite side of the body, and other symptoms depending on which area of the brain is damaged.■

In infants, a subdural hematoma can cause the head to enlarge (as in hydrocephalus), because the skull is soft and pliable. Therefore, pressure within the skull increases less in infants than it does in older children and adults.

Chronic subdural hematomas are more difficult to diagnose because of the length of time between the injury and the development of symptoms. However, MRI or CT can detect chronic as well as acute subdural hematomas.

Often, small subdural hematomas in adults do not require treatment because the blood is absorbed spontaneously. If a subdural hema-

---

▲ see art on page 435   ■ see page 476

toma is large and is causing symptoms such as persisting headache, fluctuating drowsiness, confusion, memory changes, and paralysis on the opposite side of the body, it is usually drained surgically by drilling a small hole in the skull. During surgery, a drain is usually inserted and left in place for several days, because subdural hematomas can recur. The person is monitored closely for recurrences. In infants, doctors usually drain the hematoma for cosmetic if for no other reasons.

Only about 50% of people who are treated for a large acute subdural hematoma survive.

People who are treated for a chronic subdural hematoma usually improve or do not worsen.

Intracerebral Hematomas: These hematomas are common after a severe head injury. They are due to a cerebral contusion. Fluid accumulation in the damaged brain (cerebral edema) is common and accounts for most deaths due to head injury. MRI or CT can detect intracerebral hematomas. Because these hematomas are caused by direct damage to the brain, surgery is less likely to restore function than when the brain is damaged primarily by bleeding, as occurs with epidural and subdural hematomas.

CHAPTER 88

Tumors of the Nervous System

A tumor is an abnormal growth, whether noncancerous (benign) or cancerous (malignant). In many parts of the body, a noncancerous tumor causes few or no problems. However, any abnormal growth or mass in the brain or spinal cord can cause considerable damage.

Cancers elsewhere in the body can cause symptoms of nervous system dysfunction even though there is no evidence that nerve tissue has been invaded. These disorders are called paraneoplastic syndromes.▲ Symptoms include dementia, mood swings, seizures, incoordination, dizziness, double vision, and abnormal eye movements. The most common effect, polyneuropathy, is a dysfunction of peripheral nerves,■ resulting in muscle weakness, numbness, and tingling.

Brain Tumors

A brain tumor is a noncancerous (benign) or cancerous (malignant) growth in the brain, whether it originates in the brain or has spread (metastasized) to the brain from another part of the body.

Brain tumors are equally common among men and women, but some types are more common among men and others are more common among women. Brain tumors are occurring with increasing frequency among older people.

Brain tumors may be primary or secondary. Primary brain tumors originate in the cells within or next to the brain. These tumors may be cancerous or noncancerous. Secondary brain tumors are metastases originating in another part of the body and thus are always cancerous.

Noncancerous tumors are named for the specific cells or tissues in which they originate. For example, hemangioblastomas originate in blood vessels ("hema" refers to blood vessels, and hemangioblasts are the cells that develop into blood vessel tissue). Some noncancerous tumors that originate in embryonic cells may be present at birth.

Most commonly, cancerous brain tumors are metastases from cancer that started in another part of the body. Metastases may grow in a single part of the brain or in several different parts. Many types of cancer—including breast cancer, lung cancer, cancer in the digestive tract, malignant melanoma, leukemia, and lymphoma—can spread to the brain. Lymphomas of the brain are common among people who have AIDS and, for unknown reasons, are becoming more common among people who have normal immune systems. The most common type of primary cancerous brain tumor is a glioma.

Symptoms

Symptoms occur whether a brain tumor is noncancerous or cancerous. A brain tumor can

---

▲ see box on page 1037   ■ see page 584

TUMORS THAT ORIGINATE IN OR NEAR THE BRAIN

TYPE OF TUMOR	ORIGIN	CANCER STATUS	PERCENTAGE OF ALL PRIMARY BRAIN TUMORS*	PEOPLE AFFECTED
Adenoma	Cells of the pituitary gland	Mostly non-cancerous	10%	Adults
Chordoma	Embryonic cells of the spinal column	Noncancerous but invasive	Less than 1%	Adults (may be present at birth)
Craniopharyn-gioma	Embryonic cells from the pituitary gland	Mostly non-cancerous	Less than 1%	Adults (may be present at birth)
Dermoid cysts and epidermoid tumors	Embryonic cells of the skin	Noncancerous	Less than 1%	Children and adults (dermoid cysts may be present at birth)
Ependymoma	Cells of the tissue that lines the spaces within the brain (ventricles)	Mostly non-cancerous	About 1% (and about 9% of childhood brain tumors)	Children
Germ cell tumors (including germi-nomas)	Embryonic cells near the pineal gland	Cancerous or noncancerous	1%	Children (germinomas may be present at birth)
Glioma			65%	
Astrocytoma	Cells of the tissue that supports nerve cells (glial cells)	Cancerous or noncancerous (some initially noncancerous astrocytomas become cancerous after 3–5 years, becoming anaplastic astrocytomas)		Children and adults
Oligoden-droglioma	Cells that form the myelin sheath around nerve fibers in the brain (oligo-dendrocytes)	Usually non-cancerous but sometimes becomes cancerous (becoming anaplastic oligoden-droglioma)		Children and adults
Glioblastoma-multiforme	Less differentiated forms of glial cells and oligodendro-cytes	Cancerous		Adults
Hemangioblas-toma	Embryonic cells that develop into blood vessels	Noncancerous	1–2%	Children and adults

TUMORS THAT ORIGINATE IN OR NEAR THE BRAIN (*Continued*)

TYPE OF TUMOR	ORIGIN	CANCER STATUS	PERCENTAGE OF ALL PRIMARY BRAIN TUMORS*	PEOPLE AFFECTED
Medulloblastoma	Embryonic cells of the cerebellum	Cancerous	(25% of childhood brain tumors)	Children (usually before puberty) and, rarely, adults
Meningioma	Cells of the layers of tissue covering the brain (meninges)	Noncancerous but may recur	20%	Adults
Osteoma	Bones of the skull	Noncancerous	2%	Children and adults
Osteosarcoma	Bones of the skull	Cancerous	Less than 1%	Children and adults
Pinealoma	Cells of the pineal gland	Noncancerous	Less than 1%	Children
Pituitary adenoma	Cells of the pituitary gland	Noncancerous	2%	Children and adults
Sarcoma	Connective tissue	Cancerous	1%	Children and adults

*Unless noted otherwise

cause many different symptoms, and symptoms may occur suddenly or develop gradually. Which symptoms develop first and how they develop depend on the tumor's size, growth rate, and location. In some parts of the brain, even a small tumor can have devastating effects. In other parts of the brain, tumors can grow relatively large before any symptoms appear. At first, the tumor pushes and stretches nerve tissue, which can compensate for these changes very well, so symptoms may not develop at first. Symptoms develop when brain tissue is destroyed or the pressure within the skull (intracranial pressure) increases, compressing the brain. Pressure may increase because the tumor is enlarging. Eventually, any brain tumor can increase pressure within the skull.

When the brain tumor is a metastasis from cancer in another part of the body, a person may also have symptoms related to that cancer. For example, a person with a metastasis from lung cancer may have a cough that brings up bloody mucus in addition to symptoms of a brain tumor.

A headache▲ is often the first symptom, although most headaches are not caused by brain tumors. A headache due to a brain tumor usually recurs more and more often as time passes. It eventually becomes constant without relief. It is often worse when the person lies down and may awaken the person from sleep. A gradually growing tumor causes a headache that typically is worse when the person first awakens. If headaches with these characteristics start in a person who has not had headaches before, a brain tumor may be the cause.

Brain tumors may produce a change in personality. For example, a person may become withdrawn, moody, and, often, inefficient at work. A person may feel drowsy, confused, and unable to think. Such symptoms are often more apparent to family members and co-workers than to the person. Depression and anxiety, especially if either develops suddenly, may be an early symptom of a brain tumor. Bizarre behavior is unusual. In older people, certain brain tumors cause symptoms that may be mistaken for those of dementia.■

Other common symptoms of a brain tumor include dizziness, loss of balance, and incoor-

▲ see page 456   ■ see page 484

Common Symptoms of Some Brain Tumors

Astrocytomas and Oligodendrogliomas

Some astrocytomas and oligodendrogliomas grow slowly and may initially cause only seizures. Others (anaplastic astrocytomas and anaplastic oligodendrogliomas) grow fast and are cancerous; they can produce various symptoms of brain dysfunction. Glioblastoma multiforme, a type of astrocytoma, grows so fast that it increases pressure in the brain, causing headaches and slowed thinking. If the pressure becomes high enough, drowsiness, then coma may result.

Symptoms vary depending on the tumor's location. Tumors in the frontal lobes (located behind the forehead) can cause weakness and personality changes. If they develop in the dominant frontal lobe (the left lobe in most people and the right lobe in some left-handers), they can cause speech disturbances. Tumors in the parietal lobes (located behind the frontal lobes) can cause loss of or changes in sensation; sometimes vision is lost in the eye on the side opposite the tumor. Tumors in the temporal lobes (located above the ears) can cause seizures and, if they develop on the dominant side, the inability to understand and use language. Tumors in the occipital lobes (toward the back of the head) can cause partial loss of vision in both eyes.

Tumors of or near the cerebellum (above the back of the neck), especially medulloblastomas in children, can cause alterations in eye movements, incoordination, unsteadiness in walking, and sometimes hearing loss and dizziness. They can block the drainage of cerebrospinal fluid, causing fluid to accumulate in the spaces within the brain (ventricles). As a result, the ventricles enlarge (a condition called hydrocephalus), and pressure within the skull increases. Symptoms include headaches, nausea, vomiting, difficulty turning the eyes upward, lethargy, and coma with herniation of the brain. In infants, the head enlarges.

Meningiomas

Meningiomas are usually noncancerous but may recur after they are removed. They occur more often in women and usually appear in people aged 40 to 60, but they can begin growing in childhood or later life. They may cause weakness or numbness, seizures, an impaired sense of smell, and changes in vision. If they become very large, they may cause mental deterioration, including memory loss, much like dementia.

Pineal Tumors

Pineal tumors usually develop during childhood and often cause early puberty. They can obstruct the drainage of cerebrospinal fluid around the brain, leading to

hydrocephalus. The most common type of pineal tumor is a germ cell tumor.

Pituitary Gland Tumors

The pituitary gland, located at the base of the skull, controls much of the body's endocrine system. Tumors of the pituitary gland (pituitary adenomas) are usually noncancerous. They secrete abnormally large amounts of pituitary hormones. Effects vary depending on which hormone is secreted in large amounts.

- For growth hormone, extreme height (gigantism) or disproportionate enlargement of the head, face, hands, feet, and chest (acromegaly)
- For corticotropin, Cushing's syndrome
- For thyroid-stimulating hormone (TSH), hyperthyroidism
- For prolactin, the cessation of menstrual periods (amenorrhea) in women, production of breast milk in women who are not breastfeeding (galactorrhea), and, in men, erectile dysfunction and enlargement of the breasts (gynecomastia)

Pituitary gland tumors can also destroy the tissues in the pituitary gland that secrete hormones, eventually resulting in insufficient levels of these hormones in the body. Headaches commonly occur. If the tumor enlarges, peripheral vision in both eyes is lost.

---

dination. Later, as the pressure within the skull increases, nausea, vomiting, lethargy, drowsiness, intermittent fever, and even coma may occur. Some brain tumors cause seizures.

Depending on which area of the brain is affected,▲ a tumor can cause an arm, a leg, or one side of the body to become weak or para-

lyzed or can impair the ability to feel heat, cold, pressure, a light touch, or sharp objects. The ability to express or understand language may be lost. Tumors can also affect hearing, smell, and sight (causing such symptoms as double vision and loss of vision). For example, a pituitary tumor may press on the nearby optic nerves (cranial nerve II), which are involved in vision, and thus impair peripheral vision. If

▲ see page 476

What Is Pseudotumor Cerebri?

In pseudotumor cerebri (also called benign intracranial hypertension), the pressure within the skull (intracranial pressure) increases without any evidence of a cause, such as a tumor, an infection, or a blockage that prevents the cerebrospinal fluid around the brain from draining. It is most common among women aged 20 to 50, especially those who are overweight.

In most people, neither the development nor the eventual disappearance of pseudotumor cerebri can be traced to a particular event. In about one third of people, the cause is blockage of the large veins (venous sinuses) that carry blood from the brain. In children, pseudotumor cerebri sometimes develops after corticosteroids are withdrawn or after a child has taken excessive amounts of vitamin A or the antibiotic tetracycline.

Pseudotumor cerebri usually begins with a headache, which is often mild at first but becomes severe. Late in the course of the disorder, about 5% of people lose their vision, partially or completely, in one or both eyes.

The increased pressure within the skull may cause the optic nerve to swell near the eyeball—a condition called papilledema. Doctors can observe the swelling by looking at the back of the eye through an ophthalmoscope.

When evaluating people with pseudotumor cerebri, doctors first rule out any possible treatable cause of the increased pressure within the skull. The results of computed tomography (CT) are usually normal, but spaces within the brain may appear slightly compressed. A spinal tap (lumbar puncture) is performed to measure pressure of the cerebrospinal fluid, which is usually increased, and to analyze the fluid, which is usually normal in content.

Pseudotumor cerebri often disappears without treatment within 6 months. Nonetheless, overweight people should lose weight. Aspirin or acetaminophen may relieve the headache. If the increased intracranial pressure is not relieved within a few weeks, doctors may prescribe the drug acetazolamide to help reduce the pressure.

Pseudotumor cerebri recurs in about 10% of people. It becomes chronic and progressively worse in some people, eventually causing blindness. Once vision is lost, it may never return, even if the pressure around the brain is relieved. However, vision need not be lost. People with the chronic form of the disorder should check their vision daily by reading small print and immediately report any changes in vision to their doctor or go to the emergency department. If vision is threatened, several procedures can reduce intracranial pressure.

Spinal taps can be performed daily or weekly to remove cerebrospinal fluid. Or, surgery on the optic nerve sheath (fenestration) may be performed. In this procedure, slits or patches are cut in the covering of the optic nerve behind the eyeball, allowing cerebrospinal fluid to escape into the tissues around the eye, where the fluid passes into veins. If the disorder persists, a permanent drain (shunt) can be surgically placed so that excess fluid can be removed.

---

the tumor compresses the brain stem, the pulse and breathing rate may become abnormally fast or slow. Any of these symptoms suggests a serious disorder and requires immediate medical attention.

If a tumor blocks the flow of cerebrospinal fluid through the spaces within the brain (ventricles), fluid may accumulate, causing the ventricles to enlarge (a condition called hydrocephalus). As a result, pressure within the skull increases. In addition to other symptoms of increased pressure, hydrocephalus causes difficulty turning the eyes upward. In infants, the head enlarges.

If the pressure within the skull is greatly increased, the brain may be pushed downward

because the skull cannot expand. Herniation of the brain▲ may result. There are two main types. In a transtentorial herniation, the upper part of the brain (cerebrum) is forced through the narrow opening (the tentorial notch) in the relatively rigid tissue that separates the cerebrum from the lower parts of the brain (cerebellum and brain stem). In people with this type of herniation, consciousness is reduced. The side of the body opposite the tumor may be paralyzed.

In a tonsillar herniation, a tumor that originates in the lower part of the brain pushes the lowest part of the cerebellum (the cerebellar tonsils) through the opening at the base of the skull (the foramen magnum). As a result, the brain stem, which controls breathing, heart rate, and blood pressure, is compressed and

---

▲ see art on page 515

malfunctions. If not diagnosed and treated immediately, a tonsillar herniation rapidly results in coma and death.

Diagnosis

Doctors consider the possibility of a brain tumor in people who have had a seizure for the first time or who have the characteristic symptoms. Although doctors can often detect brain dysfunction by performing a physical examination, other procedures are needed to diagnose a brain tumor.

Standard x-rays of the skull can detect tumors that erode bone (such as a meningioma or pituitary adenoma). However, magnetic resonance imaging (MRI) and computed tomography (CT) are more useful because they can detect all types of brain tumors. They can also show the tumor's size and exact position in great detail. When a brain tumor is detected, more diagnostic procedures are performed to determine the particular kind.

Sometimes a spinal tap (lumbar puncture)▲ is performed to obtain cerebrospinal fluid for examination under a microscope. This procedure is performed when doctors suspect that the tumor has invaded the meninges, is compressing the cranial nerves, and is blocking the flow of cerebrospinal fluid. The procedure may also help when the diagnosis or the type of tumor is unclear. Cerebrospinal fluid may contain cancer cells. However, a spinal tap cannot be performed in people who have a large tumor that is increasing pressure within the skull. The removal of cerebrospinal fluid during a spinal tap may cause the tumor to move, resulting in herniation of the brain.

A biopsy of the tumor (removal of a sample of the tumor for examination under a microscope) is usually needed to identify the type of tumor, including whether it is cancerous. A biopsy may be performed during surgery in which all or part of the tumor is removed. If a tumor is difficult to reach, a biopsy may be performed using three-dimensional needle placement (stereotactic biopsy) with CT.

Treatment and Prognosis

Treatment of a brain tumor depends on its location and type. When possible, the tumor is removed surgically. Some brain tumors can be removed with little or no damage to the brain. However, many grow in an area that makes removal difficult or impossible without destroy-

ing essential structures. Surgery sometimes causes brain damage that can lead to partial paralysis, changes in sensation, weakness, and impaired intellect. Nevertheless, removing a tumor—whether cancerous or noncancerous—is essential if its growth threatens important brain structures. Even when a cure is impossible, surgery may be useful to reduce the tumor's size, relieve symptoms, and help doctors determine whether other treatments, such as radiation therapy or chemotherapy, are warranted.

Removal of noncancerous tumors is often safe and cures the person. However, very small tumors and tumors in older people may be left in place as long as they are not causing symptoms. Sometimes radiation therapy is given after surgery to destroy any remaining tumor cells. Radiosurgery is used to treat tumors that are small and not readily accessible with traditional surgery. It is also used to treat meningiomas. Radiosurgery uses focused radiation to destroy a tumor rather than an incision to remove it. With radiosurgery, treatment is completed in 1 day.

Most cancerous brain tumors are treated with a combination of surgery, radiation therapy, and chemotherapy. As much of the tumor as can be removed safely is removed, and then radiation therapy is begun. Radiation therapy is given over a course of several weeks. It rarely cures but may shrink a tumor enough to keep it under control for many months or even years. Chemotherapy is used to treat some types of cancerous brain tumors. Chemotherapy appears to be particularly effective in treating anaplastic oligodendrogliomas. Radiosurgery is also used to treat cancerous brain tumors.

Increased pressure within the skull is extremely serious and requires immediate medical attention. Drugs such as mannitol and corticosteroids are usually given by injection to reduce the pressure and prevent herniation. Corticosteroids can often restore function within days, even if the tumor is large. If the tumor is blocking the flow of cerebrospinal fluid through the spaces within the brain, a device may be used to reduce the risk of herniation by draining the cerebrospinal fluid. The device consists of a small tube (catheter) connected to a gauge that measures the pressure within the skull. The tube is inserted through a tiny opening drilled in the skull. This procedure may be performed using a local anesthetic (usually plus a sedative) or a general anesthetic. The tube is removed or converted

---

▲ see art on page 443

Understanding Tumor Treatment

Craniotomy: After part of the scalp is shaved, an incision is made through the skin. A high-speed drill and a special saw are used to remove a small piece of bone above the tumor. The tumor is located and removed. Usually, the bone is then replaced and the incision stitched closed. A scalpel may be used to cut out the tumor; a laser (using heat) may be used to vaporize the tumor; or a device that emits ultrasound waves may be used to break the tumor apart, so that the pieces can be suctioned out (aspirated). Lasers and ultrasound devices are used to remove tumors that would be difficult to cut out.

Stereotactic techniques: Computers are used to produce a three-dimensional image of the tumor and thus to precisely locate a tumor and determine its relationship to other structures in the brain. The three-dimensional image can be obtained by attaching a metal imaging frame with a series of rods to the person's skull. The rods appear as dots on a CT scan, providing reference points, which help locate the tumor. Other devices, such as a viewing wand or compass system, do not involve attaching a frame and may be used instead. Stereotactic techniques can be used to biopsy or remove tumors or to insert implants containing a chemotherapy drug or radioactive pellets.

Radiosurgery: Radiosurgery is not really surgery because no incision is required. Focused radiation is used to destroy a tumor. Because the radiation is focused, a smaller dose can be used. Several machines, including a gamma knife and a linear accelerator, can produce this type of radiation.

When a **gamma knife** is used, an imaging frame is attached to the person's skull. The person lies on a sliding bed, and a large helmet with holes in it is placed over the frame. The head of the bed is then slid into a globe that contains radioactive cobalt. Radiation passes through the holes in the helmet and is aimed precisely at the tumor.

A **linear accelerator** circles the head of the person, who lies on a sliding bed. The linear accelerator aims radiation precisely at the tumor.

Implants: After a tumor is removed and before the skull and incision are closed, wafers soaked with a chemotherapy drug may be placed in the space where the tumor was. As the wafers gradually dissolve, they release the drug to destroy any remaining cancer cells.

A thin tube called a catheter may be inserted through an incision and used to place radioactive implants directly into the tumor. The implants may be removed after a few days or months or may be left in place. Unlike people who have externally applied radiation therapy, people who have radioactive implants are radioactive for a time and need to take precautions as advised by their doctor. After this procedure, surgery may be necessary to remove dead cancer cells.

Shunts: If a tumor causes pressure within the skull to increase, a shunt may be surgically placed. A shunt is a thin piece of tubing that is inserted into one of the spaces of the brain (ventricles) or sometimes into the space around the spine that contains cerebrospinal fluid (subarachnoid space). The other end of the tubing is threaded under the skin from the head usually to the abdominal cavity. Excess cerebrospinal fluid is drained from the brain and is absorbed in the abdominal cavity. The shunt contains a one-way valve that opens when there is too much fluid in the brain. Shunts may be temporary (until the tumor is removed) or permanent.

---

to a permanent drain (shunt) after a few days. During this time, doctors surgically remove all or part of the tumor or use radiosurgery or radiation therapy to reduce the size of the tumor and thus relieve the blockage.

Treatment of metastases to the brain depends largely on where the cancer originated. Radiation therapy directed at the metastases in the brain is often performed. Surgical removal may benefit people who have only a single metasta-

sis. In addition to traditional treatments, radiosurgery and some experimental treatments, involving chemotherapy and radioactive implants in the tumor, are being tried.

The prognosis for people who have a brain tumor ranges from complete recovery to death, depending on the type and location of the tumor.

End-of-Life Issues: Because people with cancerous brain tumors have a limited life expectancy, establishing advance directives is advisable.▲ Advance directives can help a

▲ see page 54

doctor determine what kind of care people want if they become unable to make decisions about medical care. Many cancer centers, especially those with hospice facilities, provide counseling and home health services.

Spinal Cord Tumors

A spinal cord tumor is a noncancerous (benign) or cancerous (malignant) growth in or around the spinal cord.

Spinal cord tumors are much less common than brain tumors. Spinal cord tumors may be primary or secondary. Primary spinal cord tumors originate in the cells within or next to the spinal cord. Only about 10% of primary spinal cord tumors originate in the cells within the spinal cord. The rest originate in cells next to the spinal cord. For example, some tumors develop on spinal nerve roots— the parts of spinal nerves that emerge from the spinal cord.▲ Primary spinal cord tumors may be cancerous or noncancerous.

Secondary spinal cord tumors, which are more common, are metastases of cancer originating in another part of the body and thus are always cancerous. Metastases most commonly spread to the vertebrae from cancers that originate in the lung, breast, prostate gland, kidney, or thyroid gland. Then they compress the spinal cord from the outside. Lymphomas also may spread to the spine and compress the spinal cord.

Symptoms

Symptoms of spine tumors are caused by pressure on the spinal cord and nerve roots. Pressure on the spinal cord may cause back pain, progressing paralysis, decreased sensation below the area compressed, impotence, and loss of bladder and bowel control. Pressure on the spinal cord may also block the blood supply to the cord, resulting in death of tissue, fluid accumulation, and swelling. Fluid accumulation may block more of the blood supply, leading to a vicious circle of damage. Pressure on spinal nerve roots can cause pain, numbness, tingling, and weakness of the muscles supplied by the compressed nerve root. Tumors originating in the spinal cord cause numbness, tingling, and weakness but may not cause pain.

Diagnosis

Compression of the spinal cord by a tumor must be diagnosed and treated immediately to prevent permanent damage to the spinal cord.

Doctors consider the possibility of a spinal cord tumor in people who have certain cancers in other parts of the body, who develop pain in a specific area of the spine, and who have weakness, tingling, or incoordination. Because the spinal cord is organized in a specific way, doctors can locate the tumor by determining which parts of the body are not functioning normally.■

Doctors must rule out other disorders that can affect the function of the spinal cord, such as sore back muscles, bone bruises, an inadequate blood supply to the spinal cord, fractured vertebrae, and a herniated disk, as well as syphilis, viral infections, multiple sclerosis, and disorders of the peripheral nerves such as amyotrophic lateral sclerosis.

Several procedures can help doctors diagnose a spinal cord tumor. Magnetic resonance imaging (MRI) is considered the best procedure for examining all the structures of the spinal cord and spine. When MRI is unavailable, myelography with computed tomography (CT) may be performed instead. X-rays of the spine can show only changes in the bones, and many tumors do not affect the bone when they are in an early stage.

A biopsy is usually needed to diagnose the precise type of tumor, especially primary spinal cord tumors. However, a biopsy is not needed for spinal cord tumors that result from metastases if cancer has been diagnosed elsewhere in the body. Often, a biopsy requires surgery, but sometimes it can be performed using a needle and computed tomography (CT) or MRI for guidance.

Prognosis and Treatment

Many tumors of the spinal cord and spine can be removed surgically. Others can be treated with radiation therapy or with surgery followed by radiation therapy. When a tumor is compressing the spinal cord, corticosteroids are given in high doses to reduce the swelling, and the tumor is surgically removed or treated with radiation therapy as soon as possible. Recovery generally depends on how long diagnosis and treatment were delayed and how much damage was done. Removal of meningiomas, neurofibromas, and some other primary spinal cord tumors may be curative.

▲ see art on page 436   ■ see art on page 562

TUMORS THAT ORIGINATE IN OR NEAR THE SPINAL CORD

TYPE OF TUMOR	ORIGIN	CANCER STATUS	PEOPLE AFFECTED
Astrocytoma	Cells of the tissue that supports nerve cells	Cancerous or noncancerous	Children and adults
Ependymoma	Cells lining the canal in the center of the spinal cord	Noncancerous	Children and adults
Meningioma	Cells of the layers of tissue covering the spinal cord (meninges)	Noncancerous but may recur	Children and adults
Neurofibroma	Cells that support peripheral nerves	Usually noncancerous	Children and adults (occurs in neurofibromatosis)
Sarcoma	Cells of connective tissue in the spine	Cancerous	Children and adults
Schwannoma	Cells that form the myelin sheath around peripheral nerve fibers (Schwann cells)	Usually noncancerous	Children and adults

Neurofibromatosis

Neurofibromatosis is a genetic disorder in which many soft, fleshy growths of nerve tissue (neurofibromas) grow under the skin and in other parts of the body.

Neurofibromas are growths of Schwann cells (which form a wrapping around peripheral nerve fibers) and other cells that support peripheral nerves. Neurofibromas, which can be felt under the skin as small lumps, usually start appearing after puberty. There are two types of neurofibromatosis: peripheral (type 1—also known as von Recklinghausen's disease) and central (type 2). Type 1 affects about 1 of 3,000 people, and type 2 affects about 1 of 40,000.

About half of the people with neurofibromatosis inherit it. Only one gene for neurofibromatosis—from one parent—is required for the disorder to develop, and each child of an affected parent has a 50% chance of inheriting the disorder. In the other half of the people with neurofibromatosis, it results from a spontaneous gene mutation. Thus, neurofibromatosis can occur in people who have no family history of the disorder.

Symptoms and Diagnosis

About one third of people with peripheral neurofibromatosis notice no symptoms, and the disorder is first diagnosed during a routine examination when doctors find lumps under the skin near nerves. Another third of the people seek help for a cosmetic problem caused by the disorder, leading to its diagnosis. In the remaining third, the disorder is diagnosed when people notice neurologic problems, such as weakness due to compression of the spinal cord or nerves.

Typically, medium-brown skin spots (café au lait spots) develop on the chest, back, pelvis, elbows, and knees. These spots may exist at birth or appear during infancy. Between ages 10 and 15, flesh-colored growths (neurofibromas) of varying sizes and shapes begin appearing on the skin. There may be fewer than 10 of these growths or thousands of them. In some people, neurofibromas under the skin or an overgrowth of the bone under the neurofibroma produces structural abnormalities, such as an abnormally curved spine (kyphoscoliosis), rib deformities, enlarged long bones in the arms and legs, and bone defects of the skull, including the part surrounding the eyeball (which results in bulging eyes).

Neurofibromas may affect any nerve in the body but frequently grow on spinal nerve roots. There, they often cause few or no problems. However, if they compress the spinal cord, they can become serious, causing paralysis or disturbances in sensation in different parts of the body, depending on what part of the spinal cord is compressed. If neurofibromas compress peripheral nerves, the nerves may not function normally, and pain or weakness may result. Neurofibromas that affect nerves in the head can cause blindness, dizziness, deafness, noise in the ears (tinnitus), and incoordination.

Neurofibromatosis usually progresses. As the number of neurofibromas increases, more neurologic problems develop.

People who have central neurofibromatosis develop tumors in the auditory nerves (auditory tumors, or acoustic neuromas) on both sides of the body. The tumors may cause hearing loss and sometimes dizziness, as early as age 20. People who have this disorder also may have gliomas or meningiomas,▲ and some develop cataracts prematurely. Because this disorder can be inherited, family members may also be affected.

Treatment

No known treatment can stop the progression of neurofibromatosis or cure it. Individual neurofibromas can usually be removed surgically or shrunk with radiation therapy. When they have grown close to a nerve, surgical removal often requires removing the nerve as well.

Because neurofibromatosis can be hereditary, genetic counseling is recommended when people with this disorder are considering having children. For people who have a child with the disorder but do not have the disorder themselves, the risk of having another child with the disorder is very small.

Radiation Damage to the Nervous System

Although doctors try to prevent radiation from damaging the nervous system during cancer treatments, such damage is sometimes unavoidable. Symptoms of injury due to radiation can appear suddenly or slowly, can remain the same or worsen, and can be temporary or permanent. Sometimes symptoms do not appear until months or years after radiation therapy is completed.

Exposing the brain to radiation can cause **acute encephalopathy,** with fluid accumulation in the brain (cerebral edema) and neurologic symptoms such as headaches, nausea, vomiting, drowsiness, and confusion. Acute encephalopathy usually begins shortly after the first or second dose of radiation is administered, but sometimes it begins 2 to 4 months after radiation therapy is completed. Usually, symptoms diminish during the radiation treatments, and corticosteroids such as dexamethasone may help prevent or reduce cerebral edema.

Symptoms of brain damage that appear many months or years after radiation therapy are called **late (delayed) radiation damage.** These effects may occur after treatment of brain tumors in adults or after preventive radiation therapy for leukemia in children. Such symptoms include progressively worsening dementia, memory loss, difficulty thinking, mistaken perceptions, personality changes, and unsteadiness in walking.

If radiation therapy to the neck or chest encompasses the spine, **radiation myelopathy** may result. This disorder sometimes causes a sensation like an electric shock. The sensation begins in the neck or back, usually when the neck is bent forward, and shoots down to the legs. People with this type of radiation myelopathy usually improve without treatment.

Radiation myelopathy that develops many months or years after radiation therapy is called **late (delayed) radiation myelopathy.** This disorder causes weakness, loss of sensation, and sometimes the Brown-Séquard syndrome. In this syndrome, one side of the spinal cord is damaged, resulting in weakness on one side of the body and loss of pain and temperature sensation on the other side. On the weak side of the body, people may lose the ability to know where the hands and feet are without looking at them (position sense). Late radiation myelopathy usually does not subside and often results in paralysis.

Nerves near the site of the radiation therapy may also become damaged. For example, radiation to the breast or lung may damage nerves in the arms, and radiation to the groin may damage nerves in the legs. Weakness or loss of sensation may result.

▲ see table on page 520

CHAPTER 89

Infections of the Brain and Spinal Cord

The brain and spinal cord are remarkably resistant to infection, but when they become infected, the consequences are usually very serious. Infections may be caused by bacteria, viruses, fungi, or, occasionally, protozoa or parasites. Another group of brain disorders that resemble infections, called spongiform encephalopathies, are caused by prions, which are abnormal tiny protein particles.▲

Infections usually cause inflammation. For example, meningitis, an inflammation of the layers of tissue covering the brain and spinal cord (meninges), is usually caused by a bacterial or viral infection. However, meningitis may be caused by other conditions, for example, by an allergic reaction to certain drugs or to a radiopaque dye injected into the spinal canal as part of a diagnostic procedure (myelography■). Encephalitis, an inflammation of the brain, is usually caused by a viral infection, but it may be caused by an autoimmune reaction, in which the body attacks its own tissues.★

Infections may affect a large area, or they may be localized as a collection of pus (abscess). An abscess, which resembles a boil, can form anywhere in the body, including the brain. Fungi (such as *Aspergillus*), protozoa (such as *Toxoplasma gondii*), and parasites (such as *Cysticercus*) may produce a localized brain infection similar to an abscess.

Bacteria and other infectious organisms can reach the meninges and other areas of the brain in several ways. They can be carried by the blood, enter the brain from the outside (for example, as the result of an injury or surgery), or spread from nearby infected structures, such as the sinuses or middle ear.

Acute Bacterial Meningitis

Acute bacterial meningitis is rapidly developing inflammation of the meninges caused by bacteria.

Acute bacterial meningitis is most common among children aged 1 month to 2 years.● It is much less common among adults. However, small epidemics of meningitis may occur among self-contained groups of people, such as those in military barracks or in college dormitories.

Causes

Two species of bacteria account for most cases of acute bacterial meningitis: *Neisseria meningitidis* and *Streptococcus pneumoniae*. Both are normally present in the external environment and may even reside in a person's nose and upper respiratory system without causing harm. Occasionally, these organisms infect the brain without an identifiable reason. In other cases, infection develops because the immune system is impaired—as it is in people who have an HIV (human immunodeficiency virus) infection. Or, infection may result from a head injury. For example, a skull fracture may create an opening between the nasal sinuses and the space around the meninges (which contains cerebrospinal fluid). Bacteria can travel from the sinuses through the opening and infect the meninges. People most at risk of developing meningitis due to *Neisseria meningitidis* and *Streptococcus pneumoniae* are those who abuse alcohol; those who have had a splenectomy (removal of the spleen); those who have chronic infections of the middle ear, nose, or sinuses; and those who have pneumococcal pneumonia or sickle cell disease.

Listeria monocytogenes causes about 10% of cases of bacterial meningitis. People who have kidney failure or who are taking corticosteroids (which suppress the immune system) have a higher-than-average risk of developing meningitis due to *Listeria* bacteria.

Other types of bacteria can also cause meningitis. Meningitis due to *Escherichia coli* (found normally in the colon and in feces) or *Klebsiella* bacteria usually develops after a head injury, brain or spinal cord surgery, a widespread infection of the blood (sepsis), or an infection acquired in a hospital. These infections are more common among people with

---

▲ see page 541　　■ see page 445
★ see page 1073　　● see also page 1562

an impaired immune system. Newborns, whose immune system is not completely formed, are at increased risk of developing infections due to *Escherichia coli* or group B streptococci.

Symptoms

Early symptoms of acute bacterial meningitis are a fever, headache, stiff neck, sore throat, and vomiting. These symptoms are sometimes preceded by a cough and other symptoms suggesting a respiratory illness. The stiff neck is more than just soreness: Trying to lower the chin to the chest causes pain and may be impossible. A skin rash (usually red and purple spots) may develop because of inflammation and bleeding in small blood vessels throughout the body, including those under the skin.

In children up to 2 years old, acute bacterial meningitis usually causes a fever, feeding problems, vomiting, irritability, seizures, and high-pitched crying. The skin over the fontanelles (soft spots between the skull bones) becomes taut, and the fontanelles may bulge. The flow of cerebrospinal fluid around the brain may become blocked, causing the fluid to accumulate and the skull to enlarge (a condition called hydrocephalus). Unlike older children or adults, infants younger than 1 year may not develop a stiff neck.▲

Adults may become desperately ill within 24 hours, and children even sooner. Older children and adults can become irritable, confused, then increasingly drowsy. Drowsiness can progress to stupor, coma, and death. The infection causes swelling of brain tissue, increasing pressure inside the skull, and hampers blood flow, causing stroke symptoms and paralysis. Some people have seizures.

Bacterial meningitis can spread from the meninges to the brain. In such cases, the disorder is technically called meningoencephalitis, but most doctors still refer to it as meningitis.

Infection with *Neisseria meningitidis* affects many organs. When it becomes very severe, it produces severe diarrhea, vomiting, internal bleeding, low blood pressure, shock, and death. These effects can develop rapidly and are called the Waterhouse-Friderichsen syndrome.

Diagnosis

If a child 2 years old or younger has an unexplained fever and the parent senses that the child is ill, the parent should call a doctor immediately. A child who becomes increasingly irritable or unusually sleepy, refuses to eat, vomits, has seizures, or develops a stiff neck requires immediate medical evaluation. In adults, fever, headache, skin rash, confusion, unresponsiveness (stupor), seizures, and a stiff neck also require immediate evaluation.

During the physical examination, doctors look for telltale signs of meningitis, such as a stiff neck and the characteristic skin rash. One way doctors test for meningitis is to bend the person's neck forward while the person is lying on the back. This maneuver causes a person with meningitis to involuntarily flex the knees. Doctors may then try to straighten the person's flexed knees; such straightening is difficult if the person has meningitis. The person with meningitis is thought to respond in these ways because the maneuvers stretch and therefore further irritate the inflamed meninges.

When doctors suspect meningitis, they must quickly decide whether to treat it immediately or to first perform procedures to determine the specific cause. If the person appears ill, one or more antibiotics are given immediately, before results of diagnostic procedures are known. If the person does not appear ill, treatment may be delayed until procedures are performed to determine whether meningitis is due to bacteria, a virus, another organism, or a noninfectious condition (such as an autoimmune reaction or use of certain drugs).

Usually, a spinal tap (lumbar puncture)■ is performed to diagnose meningitis and determine its cause. A thin needle is inserted between two vertebrae in the lower spine to withdraw a sample of cerebrospinal fluid. Sugar and protein levels and the number and type of white blood cells in the fluid are determined; this information helps doctors distinguish between bacterial and viral infections. Doctors examine the fluid under a microscope to check for and identify bacteria. If they do not see any bacteria, doctors perform other tests that can rapidly identify certain bacteria, such as *Neisseria meningitidis* and *Streptococcus pneumoniae*. These tests include analysis of the cerebrospinal fluid for evidence of antibodies against the bacteria and polymerase chain reaction (PCR) techniques, which cause DNA to make copies of itself.

A sample of the cerebrospinal fluid is sent to a laboratory, where the bacteria can be grown (cultured) and identified. The bacteria can be tested for susceptibility to treatment with dif-

---

▲ see page 1562   ■ see art on page 443

ferent antibiotics, so that the antibiotic therapy that was started immediately can be adjusted if necessary.

Doctors may also consider a different cause of the symptoms, such as infection by a virus or fungus. The cerebrospinal fluid may be analyzed further to identify viruses, such as herpes simplex, and other organisms that routine procedures do not identify.

Doctors may also culture samples of blood, urine, mucus from the nose and throat, and pus from skin infections to help make the diagnosis.

Treatment and Prognosis

Because acute bacterial meningitis, especially when caused by *Neisseria meningitidis*, can lead to death within hours or days, treatment is usually started immediately, without waiting for the results of diagnostic procedures. One or more antibiotics▲ are given intravenously. For people who are very ill, antibiotics are started even before a spinal tap is performed. Doctors base their choice of initial antibiotic therapy on the information available, including that from a quick examination of the cerebrospinal fluid. They choose antibiotics that are effective against the bacteria most likely to be causing the infection. Once the species of bacteria is identified (1 or 2 days later), the antibiotics may need to be changed to ones that are most effective against the species identified.

In children, corticosteroids, such as dexamethasone, are also given. After treatment with antibiotics, inflammation develops because the antibiotics break bacteria into fragments. Corticosteroids can suppress the inflammation and reduce the resulting swelling in the brain and increased pressure within the skull. Their use is beneficial in children, but their benefit is less clear in adults. Corticosteroids are not usually given to people who have a serious infection (because these drugs suppress the immune system), but bacterial meningitis is an exception. A corticosteroid is best started before or with the first dose of antibiotics and continued for only one or two days. Corticosteroids are especially dangerous when the cause of meningitis and thus the adequacy of antibiotic therapy are uncertain.

Treatment also includes replacing fluids lost because of fever, sweating, vomiting, and poor appetite.

Complications of acute bacterial meningitis may require specific treatment. If seizures occur, anticonvulsants are given.■ If shock★ develops (as can occur in the Waterhouse-Friderichsen syndrome), additional fluids and certain drugs (given intravenously) may be given to increase blood pressure.

If pressure within the skull is dangerously increased, the person is put on a ventilator to increase the breathing rate. Increasing the breathing rate reduces the carbon dioxide level in the blood, which controls the volume of blood in blood vessels within the skull. Thus, blood volume and pressure within the skull decrease. Mannitol may be given intravenously. It causes water in the brain to move into the bloodstream and thus reduces pressure within the skull. Corticosteroids are useful because they help the inflamed blood vessels repair themselves. The blood vessels can then actively move excess water in the brain into the bloodstream. Pressure within the skull may be monitored with a small tube (catheter) inserted through a tiny opening drilled through the skull. The tube is connected to a gauge, which registers the pressure.

If treated immediately, most people who have acute bacterial meningitis recover fully. But when diagnosis or treatment is delayed, permanent brain damage or death becomes more likely, especially in very young children and older people. Some people develop seizures that require lifelong treatment. Neurologic problems, such as permanent mental impairment and paralysis, may also result.

Prevention

A vaccine can help prevent meningitis caused by *Neisseria meningitidis.* The vaccine is used mainly when an epidemic occurs, when there is a threat of an epidemic in a self-contained group of people (such as those in military barracks), or when people may be repeatedly exposed to the bacteria. Family members, medical personnel, and others in close contact with people who have meningitis due to *Neisseria meningitidis* should be given an antibiotic (such as rifampin or minocycline) as a preventive measure. Children are now routinely immunized with *Haemophilus influenzae* type b vaccine, which has eliminated what once was the most common cause of meningitis in children.

▲ see page 1120   ■ see table on page 500

★ see page 148

Chronic Meningitis

Chronic meningitis is inflammation of the meninges that lasts a month or longer.

Chronic meningitis affects people whose immune system is impaired because of AIDS, cancer, use of chemotherapy, or long-term use of the corticosteroid prednisone. However, tuberculosis, Lyme disease, or another infection can cause chronic meningitis in people whose immune system is functioning competently.

The distinction between acute and chronic meningitis is not always clear, and sometimes the meningitis is described as subacute instead.

Causes

Some infectious organisms invade the brain or the meninges and multiply slowly over weeks, months, or even years. Such organisms include *Cryptococcus* fungus (in people with an impaired immune system, such as those with AIDS) and the bacteria that cause tuberculosis, syphilis, or Lyme disease. Acute bacterial meningitis that has been partially treated but not eliminated by antibiotics may evolve into chronic meningitis.

Some noninfectious disorders, such as sarcoidosis and some cancers (leukemia, lymphoma, brain tumors, and metastases to the brain), can invade and irritate the meninges, producing chronic meningitis. Chemotherapy drugs that are injected directly into the cerebrospinal fluid (such as methotrexate), drugs used in organ transplantation (such as cyclosporine and OKT3), and even nonsteroidal anti-inflammatory drugs (NSAIDs, such as ibuprofen)▲ can inflame the meninges, leading to chronic meningitis.

Symptoms and Diagnosis

The symptoms of chronic meningitis are similar to those of acute bacterial meningitis, but they develop more slowly and gradually, usually over weeks rather than days. Fever is often less severe than that in people with acute bacterial meningitis. Headache, confusion, and backache are common. Weakness, pins-and-needles sensations, numbness, and facial paralysis, which are also common, indicate that the cranial or peripheral nerves are affected.

Computed tomography (CT) or magnetic resonance imaging (MRI) of the head, followed by a spinal tap with examination of the cere-

brospinal fluid, can help with the diagnosis. In chronic meningitis due to bacterial infection, the number of white blood cells in the fluid is higher than normal but is usually lower than that in acute bacterial meningitis. Also, the type of white cells is different—lymphocytes rather than neutrophils.■ Some infectious organisms that cause chronic meningitis, such as *Cryptococcus* fungi, are readily visible under the microscope, but many, such as the bacteria that cause tuberculosis, are not.

The cerebrospinal fluid is always sent to be cultured, so that any organisms present can be identified. However, culturing may take weeks. The fluid may be analyzed for the bacteria that cause tuberculosis and syphilis and for certain fungi and viruses. For example, polymerase chain reaction (PCR) techniques, which cause DNA to make copies of itself, are used to detect the bacteria that cause tuberculosis. Results from these analyses may be available more quickly than those from culturing.

Treatment

Chronic meningitis due to sarcoidosis—which is thought to be a noninfectious disorder—is usually treated with corticosteroids (such as prednisone) for several weeks. Chronic meningitis due to cancer is treated with chemotherapy, radiation therapy, or both. The chemotherapy is injected directly into the cerebrospinal fluid through an Ommaya reservoir. This device is implanted under the scalp and delivers the drug slowly, over days or weeks, to the spaces around the brain through a small tube.

Treatment of chronic meningitis due to an infection depends on the organism. Chronic meningitis due to a fungus is usually treated with antifungal drugs given intravenously. Amphotericin B, flucytosine, and fluconazole are used most often. When the infection is particularly difficult to cure, amphotericin B is sometimes injected directly into the cerebrospinal fluid, either by repeated spinal taps or through an Ommaya reservoir. When chronic meningitis is due to the *Cryptococcus* fungus, amphotericin B is usually combined with flucytosine.

Viral Infections

Viral infections can produce inflammation of the meninges (causing viral meningitis), the brain (causing viral encephalitis), the spinal cord (causing myelitis), or spinal nerve roots (causing shingles). Viral encephalitis is often

---

▲ see page 452   ■ see page 1002

Some Infections That Can Cause Meningitis

Bacterial infections
- Brucellosis
- Cat-scratch disease
- Cerebral Whipple's disease
- Infection with *Escherichia coli*
- Infection with *Klebsiella* bacteria
- Infection with *Listeria monocyto-genes*
- Infection with *Neisseria meningitidis*
- Infection with *Streptococcus pneumonia*
- Leptospirosis
- Listerial infection
- Lyme disease
- Lymphogranuloma venereum
- Mycoplasmal pneumonia infection
- Tuberculosis
- Syphilis

Viral infections
- AIDS
- Chickenpox (varicella)
- Coxsackievirus infection
- Cytomegalovirus infection
- Eastern and western equine encephalitis

- Echovirus infection
- Herpes
- Infectious mononucleosis
- Lymphocytic choriomeningitis
- Mumps
- Polio
- St. Louis encephalitis

Viral infections that cause meningitis by an immune reaction
- Chickenpox
- Measles
- Rubella (German measles)

Other infections
- Amebiasis
- Coccidioidomycosis
- Coenurosis
- Cryptococcosis
- Cysticercosis
- Echinococcosis
- Malaria
- Rickettsiosis
- Schistosomiasis
- Toxoplasmosis
- Trichinosis

accompanied by viral meningitis. Viral encephalitis is more serious because it directly affects the brain rather than the meninges.

Some viruses can directly infect the brain and suddenly cause encephalitis. Infections due to some viruses, such as echovirus or coxsackievirus, can occur in epidemics. Other infections (such as herpes, mumps, and chickenpox) occur as isolated cases (sporadically). Rabies encephalitis, which is fatal, results from being bitten by an animal (such as a bat). Infections called arbovirus encephalitis are spread by mosquitoes, ticks, or other arthropods. Other viral infections, such as lymphocytic choriomeningitis, are spread by rodents. The human immunodeficiency virus (HIV) produces a chronic infection of the brain without the inflammation that occurs in acute encephalitis; this disorder is called HIV encephalopathy or AIDS dementia.

Some viruses do not directly infect the brain; instead, they trigger immune reactions that indirectly result in inflammation of the brain. This type of inflammation, which is called parainfectious or postinfectious en-

cephalitis, can follow measles, chickenpox, or rubella, typically developing 5 to 10 days later. It can cause severe damage. The spinal cord may also be affected, resulting in acute disseminated encephalomyelitis.▲

Very rarely, encephalitis develops weeks, months, or years after a viral infection. An example is subacute sclerosing panencephalitis, a brain inflammation that occasionally follows measles. This disorder most commonly occurs in children.■

Symptoms

Some viral infections are mild, causing fever and a general feeling of illness (malaise), often without specific symptoms. Usually, viral meningitis produces symptoms that are similar to those of bacterial meningitis (fever, headache, vomiting, weakness, and a stiff neck) but that are much less severe.

Viral encephalitis can cause personality changes, seizures, paralysis of the limbs, confusion, and sleepiness that can progress to coma

▲ see page 560   ■ see page 1582

Some Noninfectious Causes of Meningitis

Brain disorders
- Brain cancer
- Leukemia
- Lymphoma
- Multiple sclerosis
- Sarcoidosis
- Stroke

Drugs
- Azathioprine
- Carbamazepine
- Immunosuppressants, such as cyclosporine and OKT3
- Nonsteroidal anti-inflammatory drugs (NSAIDs), such as ibuprofen and naproxen
- Trimethoprim-sulfamethoxazole

Poisoning
- Lead poisoning

Reactions to substances injected into the spinal column
- Antibiotics
- Chemotherapy
- Dyes used in imaging procedures

Reactions to vaccines
- Pertussis vaccine
- Rabies vaccine

and death. In its early stages, encephalitis due to the herpes simplex virus (herpes encephalitis)—a treatable but potentially fatal infection—causes headache, fever, and flu-like symptoms. It also causes symptoms that indicate inflammation of the temporal lobes. They include seizures that usually involve strange smells, vivid flashbacks, or experience of a sudden, intense emotion. When this infection progresses, it causes severe brain damage resulting in confusion, repeated seizures, or coma.

When viral infections affect the spinal cord, the first symptom may be back pain at the site of the infection. Depending on which level of the spinal cord is affected,▲ the parts of the body supplied by the spinal cord below that level may feel numb and weak. Bladder and bowel function may be impaired. If the infec-

tion is severe, sensation may be lost, paralysis may occur, and bladder and bowel control may be lost.

Diagnosis

At first, doctors may have difficulty distinguishing viral meningitis and encephalitis from bacterial meningitis, abscesses in the brain, and other disorders that cause similar symptoms. At the first sign of any of these disorders, doctors try to pinpoint the cause. A spinal tap to examine the cerebrospinal fluid is almost always performed. In viral infections, the number of white blood cells is increased in the cerebrospinal fluid, and no bacteria are seen. Red blood cells are absent unless the inflammation is severe. Immunologic tests that detect antibodies against viruses in samples of cerebrospinal fluid may be performed, but these tests take days to complete. Even with these tests, a specific microorganism is identified less than half the time. Culturing most viruses from the fluid is difficult and takes many days; therefore, the fluid is rarely sent to be cultured. Polymerase chain reaction (PCR) techniques are used to identify organisms such as herpes viruses.

Doctors suspect herpes encephalitis when the case is not part of an epidemic and when symptoms indicate inflammation of the temporal lobes. Magnetic resonance imaging (MRI) can detect increased swelling in the temporal lobes and thus can help doctors make a quick diagnosis. Computed tomography (CT) is less helpful because it usually detects changes only after severe damage has occurred. When herpes encephalitis is severe (as it ultimately becomes), the cerebrospinal fluid contains many red blood cells. Occasionally, a biopsy of brain tissue (in which a tissue sample is removed for examination under a microscope) is needed to determine whether the herpes simplex virus is the cause.

CT or MRI is also performed to rule out a brain abscess, stroke, or another structural disorder, such as a hematoma, an aneurysm, or a tumor, which may cause similar symptoms.

Treatment and Prognosis

If a viral infection causes only headache and fever, the only treatment usually required is acetaminophen, given by mouth, and fluids, given by mouth or intravenous injection. Viral meningitis and many cases of mild viral encephalitis often resolve on their own and require no specific treatment.

▲ see art on page 562

8

For some severe viral infections, certain antiviral drugs are effective. For people with herpes encephalitis, prompt treatment with the antibiotic acyclovir is life-saving. If the diagnosis is in doubt, acyclovir is usually given because the herpes simplex virus is the cause in up to one third of people with encephalitis. Acyclovir is effective against herpes simplex and herpes zoster but not against most other viruses. Ganciclovir is effective against cytomegalovirus. For other infections, no specific treatment is available. Treatment involves relieving symptoms and, when necessary, providing life support.

For HIV infection, a combination of drugs▲ helps the immune system function better and delays the progression of the infection and its complications, including dementia.

Many people recover completely. The chances of survival and recovery depend largely on the type of virus and the promptness of treatment if available. For example, people who have encephalitis due to the herpes simplex virus must be treated with acyclovir before they lapse into a coma if they are to recover well. Infants are more likely to have permanent damage.

RABIES

Rabies is a viral infection of the brain that is transmitted by animals and causes inflammation of the brain and spinal cord.

Usually, rabies is eventually fatal once the rabies virus reaches the spinal cord and brain, but the virus takes at least 10 days—usually 30 to 50 days—to reach the brain (depending on where the bite is). During that interval, measures can be taken to eradicate the virus and help prevent death.

The rabies virus is present in many species of wild and domestic animals throughout most of the world. Animals with rabies may be sick for several weeks before they die. During that time, they often spread the disease.

The rabies virus, which is present in the saliva, is transmitted when a rabid animal bites or, very rarely, licks another animal or a person. The virus cannot pass through intact skin and can enter the body only through a puncture or another break in the skin. In the United States, almost all cases of rabies in people have been spread by bats but with no evidence of a bite, suggesting that the virus was probably inhaled.

From the point of entry, the virus travels along nerves to the spinal cord and then to the

What Is Aseptic Meningitis?

"Aseptic" is a term doctors may use to describe meningitis when no bacteria are identified during routine testing. Aseptic meningitis may be caused by noninfectious disorders, such as leukemia, lymphoma, or brain cancer, or by the use of certain drugs, such as chemotherapy drugs injected directly into the cerebrospinal fluid, drugs used to prevent rejection of transplanted organs (immunosuppressants), and even nonsteroidal anti-inflammatory drugs (NSAIDs). However, in most cases, a virus is the cause. Consequently, doctors often use aseptic meningitis and viral meningitis as synonyms.

Aseptic meningitis may be brief (acute) or prolonged (chronic). It is usually mild and does not require treatment. Rarely, it can be severe and life threatening.

brain, where it multiplies. From there, it travels along other nerves to the salivary glands and into the saliva.

Many different animals—such as cats, bats, raccoons, skunks, and foxes as well as dogs, the most common source—can transmit rabies to people. Rabies rarely affects rodents (such as mice, rats, hamsters, and squirrels), rabbits, or hares. In the United States, these animals have not been known to cause rabies among people. Birds and reptiles do not develop rabies. In the United States, vaccination has largely eliminated rabies in dogs. Worldwide, during the last 30 years, most people who have contracted rabies were bitten by rabid wild animals. However, rabies in dogs is still fairly common in most countries of Latin America, Africa, and Asia, where vaccination of dogs is not widespread.

Rabies has a furious and a dumb form. An animal with furious rabies is agitated and vicious, then becomes paralyzed and dies. An animal with dumb rabies is partially or generally paralyzed from the beginning. However, wild animals with furious rabies are less likely to appear vicious. Changes in their behavior are usually more subtle. For example, nocturnal animals (such as bats, skunks, raccoons, and foxes) may come out during the day and may not show normal fear of people.

▲ see table on page 1175

Who Should Receive a Rabies Vaccine?

> The decision to administer the rabies vaccine to a person who has been bitten by an animal depends on the type and status of the animal.
>
> **For people bitten by a pet dog, cat, or ferret:**
> If one of these animals appears healthy and can be observed for 10 days, the vaccine is not given unless the animal develops symptoms of rabies. If the animal develops any symptom suggesting rabies, the vaccine is given immediately. Animals that develop symptoms of rabies are put to sleep (euthanized), and their brain is examined for the rabies virus.
> If one of these animals has or appears to have rabies, the person who has been bitten is given the vaccine immediately.
> If the status of one of these animals cannot be determined—for example, because it escaped, public health officials are consulted to determine what the likelihood of rabies is and whether the vaccine should be given.
>
> **For people bitten by skunks, raccoons, foxes, most other carnivores, or bats:**
> Such an animal is considered rabid unless it can be tested and the results are negative. The person who has been bitten is usually given the vaccine immediately. Waiting to observe wild animals for 10 days is not recommended.
>
> **For people bitten by livestock, small rodents, large rodents (such as woodchucks and beavers), rabbits, or hares:**
> Each biting incident is considered individually, and public health officials are consulted. People who are bitten by squirrels, hamsters, guinea pigs, gerbils, chipmunks, rats, mice, other small rodents, rabbits, and hares almost never require rabies vaccination.

Symptoms

Symptoms appear when the rabies virus reaches the brain or spinal cord, usually 30 to 50 days after the person is bitten. However, this interval can vary from 10 days to more than a year. The closer the bite to the brain, the more quickly symptoms appear.

Rabies commonly begins with a short period of depression, restlessness, a general feeling of illness (malaise), and a fever. However, in 20% of people, rabies begins with paralysis in the lower legs that moves up through the body. Restlessness increases, leading to uncontrollable excitement, and saliva production greatly increases. Spasms of the muscles in the throat and voice box occur because rabies affects the area in the brain that controls swallowing and breathing. The spasms can be excruciatingly painful. A slight breeze or an attempt to drink water can trigger the spasms. Thus, a person with rabies cannot drink. For this reason, the disease is sometimes called hydrophobia (fear of water).

As the disease spreads through the brain, the person becomes more and more confused and very agitated. Eventually, coma and death result. The cause of death can be blockage of airways, seizures, exhaustion, or widespread paralysis.

Diagnosis

When a person is bitten by a pet that appears sick or by a wild animal, the biggest concern is rabies. No test can determine whether the rabies virus has been transmitted to the person immediately after the bite. So the animal is evaluated to determine whether the person requires treatment. A wild animal that has bitten a person is killed if possible, and a pet that appears sick is taken to the veterinarian to be put to sleep (euthanized), so that its brain can be examined for signs of rabies. Certain pets—dogs, cats, and ferrets—that do not appear sick may be confined and observed by a veterinarian for 10 to 14 days. If the pet remains healthy, it did not have rabies at the time of the bite. For other pets that appear healthy, the veterinarian or public health officials should be consulted.

If a person who has been bitten by an animal becomes increasingly confused and agitated or paralyzed, the diagnosis is probably rabies. At this point, tests can detect the rabies virus. A skin biopsy, in which a sample of skin is taken (usually from the neck) for examination under a microscope, can detect the virus.

Prevention and Treatment

The first step in prevention is to avoid being bitten by animals, especially wild animals. Pets that are not known and wild animals should not be approached. A wild animal that does not appear afraid of people is usually sick. An animal that appears sick should not be picked up to try to help it. A sick animal often bites.

People who are at high risk of exposure to the rabies virus should be given an injection of the rabies vaccine before exposure. High-risk people include veterinarians, laboratory workers who handle animals that may be rabid, people who live or stay more than 30 days in developing countries where rabies in dogs is widespread, and people who explore bat caves. Vaccination protects most people to some degree for the rest of their life. However, protection decreases with time, and people at high risk of continued exposure should receive a booster dose of vaccine every 2 years.

If a person is bitten by a rabid animal, the development of rabies can usually be prevented if appropriate measures are taken without delay.

The bite wound is treated immediately. It is cleaned thoroughly with soap and water. Deep puncture wounds are flushed out with soapy water. Sometimes doctors trim tissue from the edges of the wound.

People who have not been previously immunized with rabies vaccine may be given an injection of rabies immunoglobulin, depending on the status of the animal. Rabies immunoglobulin, which consists of antibodies against the virus, provides protection immediately but only for a short time. Several injections of rabies immunoglobulin are given initially (day 0), followed by injections of the rabies vaccine on days 3, 7, 14, and 28. Rabies vaccine stimulates the body to produce antibodies against the virus, providing protection that begins more gradually but that lasts for a much longer time than the protection provided by rabies immunoglobulin. Pain and swelling at the injection site are usually minor. Serious allergic reactions are rare.

If a person who is bitten has already been vaccinated, the risk of developing rabies is reduced. However, the wound must be cleaned promptly and an injection of rabies vaccine is given immediately and 2 days later (on day 3).

After a person develops symptoms, neither rabies vaccine nor rabies immunoglobulin is effective against the virus. Treatment is then directed at relieving symptoms and making the person as comfortable as possible. Death almost always results.

ARBOVIRUS ENCEPHALITIS

Arbovirus encephalitis is a severe inflammation of the brain caused by one of a group of viruses transmitted by certain arthropods, such as mosquitoes and ticks.

In the United States, the most common types of viral encephalitis are caused by arboviruses. Arboviruses are transmitted to people through the bite of mosquitoes, ticks or other arthro-

pods. (Arbovirus is short for *arthropod-borne virus.*) The viruses are transmitted to the arthropods when the arthropods bite infected animals. Many species of domestic animals and birds carry these viruses. Epidemics occur in people only periodically—when the population of mosquitoes or infected animals increases. Infection spreads from arthropod to person, not from person to person.

Many arboviruses can cause encephalitis. The different types of encephalitis that result are usually named for the place the virus was discovered or the animal species that typically carries it.

Several types of arbovirus encephalitis occur in the United States. All of the following are spread by mosquitoes. **Western equine encephalitis** occurs throughout the United States. It affects all age groups, but mainly children younger than 1 year. **Eastern equine encephalitis** occurs predominantly in the eastern United States. It affects mainly young children and people older than 55. The eastern type is more likely to be fatal than the western type. Both types tend to cause severe symptoms in children younger than 1 year, causing permanent nerve or brain damage. **St. Louis encephalitis** occurs throughout the United States, but particularly in Texas and some midwestern states. The risk of death is greatest in older people. Several related viruses cause **California encephalitis,** which affects mainly children. These viruses include the California virus (most common in the western United States), the La Crosse virus (most common in the midwestern United States), and the Jamestown Canyon virus (commonly in the area around the Great Lakes). **West Nile encephalitis,** once present only in Europe and Africa, first appeared in the New York City area in 1999. By 2000, cases were reported along the East Coast from Vermont to North Carolina. Several species of birds are the host for the virus. This encephalitis affects mainly older people. About 1 of 10 infected people die.

In other parts of the world, encephalitis is caused by different but related arboviruses. Examples are Venezuelan equine encephalitis and Japanese encephalitis, both spread by mosquitoes.

Symptoms and Diagnosis

The different types of arbovirus encephalitis produce similar symptoms. Usually, the first symptoms include headache, drowsiness, and fever. Vomiting and a stiff neck are less common. Muscles may tremble. Confusion, seizures, and coma may develop rapidly. Occasionally, the arms and legs become weak or paralyzed.

Arbovirus encephalitis is suspected on the basis of symptoms, especially if an epidemic is in progress. To confirm the diagnosis, doctors take a sample of blood or cerebrospinal fluid and test it for antibodies against the virus when the person is sick and later when the person is convalescing. If the test detects a marked increase in the level of antibodies, the diagnosis is confirmed. Alternatively, polymerase chain reaction (PCR) techniques, which cause DNA to make copies of itself, can be used to detect the genetic material of the virus.

Prevention and Treatment

The best way to prevent the encephalitis is to control the mosquitoes that spread it. Also, taking precautions against being bitten can help: using insect repellents, wearing a long-sleeve shirt and long pants, and avoiding standing water, where the mosquitoes can breed. No vaccines against arboviruses are available.

No specific treatment is available. Treatment usually involves relieving symptoms and, when necessary, providing life support until the infection subsides—in about 1 to 2 weeks.

LYMPHOCYTIC CHORIOMENINGITIS

Lymphocytic choriomeningitis is a flu-like disorder caused by an arenavirus and often followed by meningitis.

The arenavirus that causes lymphocytic choriomeningitis is commonly present in rodents, especially the gray house mouse and the hamster. These animals are usually infected by the virus for life and excrete it in urine, feces, semen, and nasal secretions. Most often, exposure to dust or food contaminated by these waste products causes the disorder in people. The disorder usually occurs in winter when wild rodents seek shelter indoors.

Symptoms

The disorder often occurs in two phases. In the first phase, flu-like symptoms develop 5 to 10 days after exposure to the virus. A fever of 101° to 104° F (38.3 to 40° C) typically occurs and may be accompanied by shaking. Other symptoms include a general feeling of illness (malaise), nausea, light-headedness, weakness, muscle pains, a headache behind the eyes worsened by bright light, and a poor appetite.

Sore throat may occur, and sensitivity to touch may be reduced.

After 5 days to 3 weeks, the flu-like symptoms may subside for 1 or 2 days. In the second phase of the disorder, these symptoms recur and other symptoms develop. Other symptoms may include painful and swollen finger joints, inflammation of the testes, loss of hair, and vomiting. Meningitis may develop, causing a headache and stiff neck. Most people who develop meningitis recover completely. Occasionally, encephalitis develops, causing a headache and drowsiness. Rarely, some symptoms persist because of brain damage due to encephalitis.

Diagnosis and Treatment

At first, the disorder cannot be distinguished from the flu, so usually no tests are performed. If symptoms suggest meningitis, a spinal tap is performed to obtain a sample of the cerebrospinal fluid. If lymphocytic choriomeningitis is present, the cerebrospinal fluid usually contains many white blood cells, mostly lymphocytes. The disorder is diagnosed by identifying the virus in the cerebrospinal fluid or by detecting increasing levels of the antibody against the virus in the blood.

No specific treatment is available. Doctors try to relieve the symptoms until the disorder subsides—in about 1 to 2 weeks.

PROGRESSIVE MULTIFOCAL LEUKOENCEPHALOPATHY

Progressive multifocal leukoencephalopathy is a rare infection of the brain and spinal cord that is caused by the JC virus.

Progressive multifocal leukoencephalopathy results from infection by the JC virus. The disorder affects mainly people whose immune system is impaired, such as people who have leukemia, lymphoma, or AIDS, or is suppressed by use of immunosuppressants, which may be used to prevent rejection of transplanted organs or to treat autoimmune disorders. About 4% of people with AIDS have this disorder.

Symptoms and Diagnosis

Many people who are infected with the JC virus have no apparent symptoms. The JC virus appears to remain inactive until something (such as an impaired immune system) allows it to be reactivated and start to multiply.

Symptoms vary depending on which part of the brain or spinal cord is infected. Symptoms may begin gradually, but they usually worsen rapidly. Paralysis commonly affects one side of the body. The hands rapidly become clumsy, making writing and grasping objects difficult. In about two of three people, mental function declines rapidly and progressively, causing dementia. Speaking becomes increasingly difficult, and partial blindness is characteristic. Rarely, headaches and seizures occur. Death is common within 1 to 6 months of when symptoms start, but a few people survive longer (about 2 years). Even fewer people improve for a few months and survive for up to 10 years.

Progressively worsening symptoms in a person with a severely impaired immune system suggest the diagnosis. Noninvasive procedures, such as computed tomography (CT) and magnetic resonance imaging (MRI), can help establish the diagnosis. However, the diagnosis is often not confirmed until after the person has died, when brain tissue can be examined. Polymerase chain reaction (PCR) techniques, which cause DNA to make copies of itself, can detect the JC virus in the cerebrospinal fluid of up to 90% of people.

Treatment

No treatment of progressive multifocal leukoencephalopathy has proved effective. However, longer survival results from treating the disorder that has impaired the immune system. Such treatment includes highly active antiretroviral therapy (antiviral drugs used to treat AIDS). Discontinuing immunosuppressants can cause progressive multifocal leukoencephalopathy to subside.

TROPICAL SPASTIC PARAPARESIS

Tropical spastic paraparesis is a slowly progressive viral infection of the spinal cord that causes weakness in the legs.

Tropical spastic paraparesis (also called HTLV-associated myelopathy) affects nerve bundles inside the spinal cord. The myelin sheath (which surrounds the part of the nerve that sends messages) is damaged or destroyed (demyelinated). This disorder results from infection by the human T-cell lymphotropic virus type I (HTLV-I). This virus, a retrovirus, can also cause a type of leukemia. Tropical spastic paraparesis may be transmitted through sexual contact or contaminated needles. It can also be transmitted from mother to child across the placenta or in breast milk.

Symptoms may begin years after exposure to the virus. Symptoms develop when the immune system damages nerve tissue in the process of responding to infection with HTLV-I. Muscles in both legs gradually become weak and stiff. These symptoms worsen over several years. Some sensation in the feet may be lost. Urinary problems, including frequent, strong urges to urinate and incontinence, are common. Bowel dysfunction may occur.

No cure is available. However, use of corticosteroids has produced marked improvement, and plasmapheresis has produced temporary improvement.

Brain Abscess

A brain abscess is a localized collection of pus in the brain.

Brain abscesses are fairly uncommon. They can result from the spread of an infection somewhere else in the head (such as in a tooth, in the nose, or in an ear), from a head wound that penetrates the brain, or from an infection in another part of the body that spreads through the bloodstream. Many types of bacteria, including *Staphylococcus aureus* and *Bacteroides fragilis,* can cause a brain abscess. *Toxoplasma gondii,*▲ a protozoan, is a common cause of brain abscess in people who have AIDS.

A brain abscess causes the surrounding brain tissue to swell and causes pressure to increase within the skull. The larger the abscess, the greater the swelling and the pressure.

Symptoms and Diagnosis

A brain abscess can cause many different symptoms, depending on its location, its size, and the extent of inflammation and swelling around the abscess. Symptoms include headache, nausea, vomiting, sleepiness, seizures, personality changes, and other signs of brain dysfunction. These symptoms can develop over days or weeks. A fever and chills may occur at first but then disappear as the body fights off the infection.

The best procedure for diagnosing a suspected brain abscess is computed tomography (CT) or magnetic resonance imaging (MRI). CT or MRI readily shows the abnormality. However, a brain tumor or damage from a stroke can resemble an abscess, and additional procedures may be needed to establish the diagnosis. A specialized form of MRI called MRI spectroscopy enables doctors to distinguish between the dead debris inside an abscess and the multiplying cells inside a tumor.

▲ see page 1144

Sometimes a biopsy of brain tissue (in which a tissue sample is removed for examination under a microscope) is necessary. The biopsy may be performed using CT to guide the placement of the needle. In this procedure (called a stereotactic biopsy), a metal imaging frame is attached to the person's skull. Attached to the frame are a series of rods that appear as dots on the CT scan. The frame and rods act as reference points for the placement of a biopsy needle. Also, a sample of the pus may be removed for examination under a microscope and for culture.

Treatment

A brain abscess may be fatal unless treated with antibiotics and possibly surgery. Those most commonly used are penicillin, metronidazole, nafcillin, and cephalosporins, such as ceftizoxime. An antibiotic is usually given for 4 to 6 weeks, and CT or MRI is repeated every 2 weeks to monitor the response to treatment. If the abscess does not shrink, a surgeon may have to drain the abscess with a needle (using stereotactic techniques to guide placement of the needle) or perform open surgery to remove the entire abscess. Recovery may be quick or slow depending on how successful surgery is, how many abscesses are present, and how well the person's immune system is functioning. People who have an abscess due to *Toxoplasma gondii* and an impaired immune system must take antibiotics for the rest of their life.

Doctors treat the swelling and increased pressure within the skull due to a brain abscess aggressively, because these effects can permanently damage the brain. Corticosteroids, such as dexamethasone, and other drugs that reduce swelling and pressure (such as mannitol) may be used.

Subdural Empyema

A subdural empyema is a collection of pus that develops between the brain and the layers of tissue covering it (meninges), rather than in the brain itself.

A subdural empyema may result from a sinus infection, a severe ear infection, a head injury, surgery, or a blood infection that develops after a lung infection. The same kinds of bacteria that cause brain abscesses can cause subdural empyemas.

Like a brain abscess, a subdural empyema can cause headache, sleepiness, seizures, and other signs of brain dysfunction. The symptoms can evolve over several days, and without treatment, they progress rapidly to coma and death.

Computed tomography (CT) and magnetic resonance imaging (MRI) are the best procedures for diagnosis. A spinal tap is of little help and may be dangerous. In infants, a needle can sometimes be inserted directly into the empyema through a fontanelle (a soft spot between the skull bones) to drain the pus, relieve pressure, and help doctors make the diagnosis.

Subdural empyemas must be drained surgically. If the infection occurred because of an abnormality in the sinuses, the surgeon usually repairs the abnormality at the same time. Antibiotics are given intravenously.

Parasitic Infections

In some parts of the world, brain infections due to worms or other parasites may occur.

Cysticercosis, an infection of pork tapeworm larvae, is the most common parasitic infection in the Western Hemisphere.▲ After a person eats food contaminated with *Cysticercus* eggs, secretions in the stomach cause the eggs to hatch into larvae. The larvae enter the bloodstream and are distributed to all parts of the body, including the brain. The larvae form cysts that can cause headaches and seizures. The cysts degenerate and the larvae die, triggering inflammation, swelling, and neurologic symptoms, such as headaches, seizures, and sometimes weakness in certain muscles or pins-and-needles sensations in certain areas. The infection is treated with albendazole or praziquantel. Corticosteroids are given to reduce the inflammation that occurs as the larvae die.

Echinococcosis (hydatid disease) and **coenurosis** are infections with other types of tapeworm larvae. Echinococcosis can produce large cysts in the brain. Coenurosis produces cysts, which can block the flow of fluid around the brain. **Schistosomiasis** is an infection with blood flukes.■ Echinococcosis, coenurosis, and schistosomiasis can cause neurologic symptoms similar to those of cysticercosis. These three infections can usually be controlled with drugs, such as albendazole, mebendazole, praziquantel, and pyrantel pamoate, but sometimes cysts must be removed surgically.

▲ see page 1143   ■ see page 1142

CHAPTER 90

Prion Diseases

Prion diseases (transmissible spongiform encephalopathies) are very rare degenerative diseases of the brain thought to be caused by a protein that converts to an abnormal form called a prion.

Before prions were identified, diseases such as Creutzfeldt-Jakob disease and other spongiform encephalopathies were thought to be caused by viruses. Prions are much smaller than viruses and differ from viruses, bacteria, and all living cells because they do not contain any genetic material. In prion diseases, a specific protein molecule called cellular prion protein (PrP^c) changes shape and becomes an abnormal protein molecule called scrapie prion protein (PrP^{sc})—a prion. (Scrapie refers to a prion disease first observed in sheep.) The newly formed prion then converts other nearby PrP^c into prions, and the process continues. When the prions reach a certain number, disease results. Prions never convert back into PrP^c.

PrP^c occurs in all cells of the body, with a high concentration in the brain. However, prion diseases affect the nervous system predominantly or exclusively. When these proteins are converted into prions, they usually cause tiny bubbles to develop in brain cells. Gradually, the affected cells die and the brain becomes filled with holes. When samples of brain tissue are viewed through a microscope, they somewhat resemble Swiss cheese or a sponge (hence the term "spongiform").

Prion disease may occur in families because of an inherited susceptibility that makes PrP^c molecules more likely to convert to prions. The susceptibility results from a mutation in the gene for PrP^c. Many different mutations exist. Each mutation generally causes different prion diseases, which, however, fit into three groups: fatal familial insomnia, familial Creutzfeldt-Jakob disease, and Gerstmann-Sträussler-Scheinker disease.

Prion disease may occur when prions are acquired from an external source, such as contaminated beef—as occurs in the so-called variant Creutzfeldt-Jakob disease. Or, prion disease may occur on its own (spontaneously).

There is no cure for prion diseases. All are fatal. The only available treatments are directed at keeping people comfortable and treating symptoms. A number of strategies can help caregivers of people with a prion disease cope with the dementia caused by the disease.▲ If possible, people who have a prion disease should establish advance directives■ about what kind of medical care they want at the end of life. Family members of people who develop the hereditary form of the disease may benefit from genetic counseling.

Creutzfeldt-Jakob Disease

Creutzfeldt-Jakob disease (subacute spongiform encephalopathy) is a prion disease characterized by progressive deterioration of mental function, muscle twitching, and staggering when walking.

Creutzfeldt-Jakob disease affects 1 of 1 million people each year throughout the world. It affects adults, mainly in their late 50s and 60s.

One form of Creutzfeldt-Jakob disease results from spontaneous conversion of the normal protein molecule PrP^c to a prion. Another form results from acquisition of the prion from an external source. However, doctors usually cannot determine which is the cause. In a few people, the prion has been transmitted through transplantation of contaminated corneas or possibly other tissues from affected donors. In some people, the prion has been transmitted during brain surgery using instruments previously used to operate on a person who had Creutzfeldt-Jakob disease. Routine cleansing and sterilization procedures do not destroy prions; however, bleach is effective.

The disease developed in some children who were treated with growth hormone derived from human pituitary glands. Other hormones derived from the pituitary gland have also caused Creutzfeldt-Jakob disease. These hormones are now genetically engineered rather than prepared from cadavers, so that there is no risk of Creutzfeldt-Jakob disease. There have been no reports of Creutzfeldt-Jakob disease being transmitted through blood transfusions nor through casual or even intimate contact with people who have the disease.

▲ see box on page 488   ■ see page 54

Of Sheep and Cows

Prion diseases occur in sheep, goats, cattle, and other animals, such as minks, elk, and goats. Like people with Creutzfeldt-Jakob disease, affected animals gradually become uncoordinated, then develop dementia. Scrapie, the disease in sheep, is so named because the sheep tend to scrape themselves against fence posts or other objects and tear their wool off. Mad cow disease is so named because the cattle become noticeably agitated. The disease can be transmitted from sheep to cattle by feeding cattle scrapie-infected sheep parts.

Eating contaminated beef or beef products is thought to be the cause of a new form of Creutzfeldt-Jakob disease in people. First described in 1996, this form is called variant Creutzfeldt-Jakob disease. The new form differs in many ways from the usual form: It causes different changes in brain tissue (seen under a microscope), and the first symptoms tend to be psychiatric symptoms, rather than the memory loss that occurs in people who have the usual form of Creutzfeldt-Jakob disease. By the year 2000, new variant Creutzfeldt-Jakob disease had been diagnosed in 90 people in the United Kingdom, 3 people in France, and 1 person in Ireland.

A new form of Creutzfeldt-Jakob disease, called variant Creutzfeldt-Jakob disease, has affected about 100 people to date. It is thought to be acquired from the consumption of contaminated beef or beef products. The variant form usually begins around age 30 in contrast to the spontaneous form of Creutzfeldt-Jakob disease, which usually begins around age 65.

Symptoms

In people who have acquired the prion from an external source, no symptoms appear for months or years after exposure. Then, symptoms of brain damage with dementia become apparent and usually progress gradually over months. Early symptoms—memory loss and confusion—may resemble those of other dementias, such as Alzheimer's disease. In people with variant Creutzfeldt-Jakob disease, the first symptoms tend to be psychiatric symp-

toms, rather than memory loss. Later symptoms are similar in both forms.

In about 10 to 20% of people, symptoms appear abruptly, starting with dizziness and double vision. Whether symptoms develop gradually or abruptly, mental decline progresses, often producing such symptoms as neglect of personal hygiene, apathy, and irritability. Some people tire easily and become sleepy; others cannot fall asleep.

Muscles usually begin to twitch in the first 6 months after symptoms begin. Trembling and clumsiness may also develop, and muscle coordination is lost. Walking becomes unsteady, resulting in staggering (similar to the walk of a person who is drunk). Movements may be slow. Impairment of muscle control may result in unusual postures, such as twisting of the trunk or limbs forward and sideways. Muscles may jerk when stretched. The muscles that control breathing and coughing are usually impaired, increasing the risk of pneumonia.

The person may be startled easily, and the resulting responses, such as jumping when a loud noise is heard, are exaggerated. Vision may become blurry or dim. The symptoms worsen, usually much more rapidly than in Alzheimer's disease, resulting in profound dementia.

Most people with Creutzfeldt-Jakob disease die after about 3 to 12 months of illness. About 10 to 20% of people survive for 2 years or more. Often, the cause of death is pneumonia.

Diagnosis and Treatment

Doctors consider Creutzfeldt-Jakob disease when mental function is deteriorating quickly, muscle twitching is present, walking is unsteady and staggering, and other dementias have been ruled out by routine testing. In about 70% of people with the disease, electroencephalography (EEG) detects specific abnormalities in the electrical activity of the brain.▲ In more than 80% of people, an unusual protein called 14-3-3 is detected in the cerebrospinal fluid. Abnormal EEG results plus the presence of the 14-3-3 protein in cerebrospinal fluid strongly support the diagnosis of Creutzfeldt-Jakob disease. The absence of the 14-3-3 protein does not rule out Creutzfeldt-Jakob disease. The definitive diagnosis of Creutzfeldt-Jakob disease is based on detecting prions in brain tissue by examination of a tissue sample under a microscope or by biochemical analysis.

▲ see page 445

Currently, Creutzfeldt-Jakob disease cannot be cured, and its progress cannot be slowed. However, certain drugs may be given to relieve symptoms. For example, the anticonvulsant valproate and the antianxiety drug clonazepam may reduce muscle jerking.

General support and care for the person and family members are important. Day care centers and respite and long-term care may be useful. Speech and occupational therapists can help with specific problems. Support groups are available.

Fatal Familial Insomnia

Fatal familial insomnia is a prion disease that interferes with sleep, leading to deterioration of mental function.

Fatal familial insomnia is a genetic disease, due to a specific mutation in the PrP^c gene. However, the disease can occur spontaneously, without a mutation. This form is called sporadic fatal insomnia. Fatal familial insomnia and sporadic fatal insomnia differ from other prion diseases because they affect predominantly one area of the brain, the thalamus, which influences sleep.

The disease usually begins between the ages of 40 and 60 but may begin in a person's late 30s. Most often, it runs in families. At first, people may have minor difficulties falling asleep and occasional problems with muscle movements. Eventually, they lose the ability to sleep. Other changes include muscle twitching, rapid heart rate, and dementia. Death usually occurs after about 7 to 36 months of illness. No treatment is available.

Gerstmann-Sträussler-Scheinker Disease

Gerstmann-Sträussler-Scheinker disease is a prion disease that causes muscle incoordination followed by slow deterioration of mental function.

Like Creutzfeldt-Jakob disease, Gerstmann-Sträussler-Scheinker disease may occur anywhere in the world. However, it is much less common than Creutzfeldt-Jakob disease, be-

gins earlier in life (affecting people in their 40s rather than in their late 50s and 60s), and progresses more slowly (with an average life expectancy of 5 years rather than 9 months). This disease usually runs in families.

Usually, the first symptoms are clumsiness and difficulty walking. Muscle twitching is much less common than in Creutzfeldt-Jakob disease. Eventually, speaking becomes difficult, and dementia develops. Nystagmus (rapid movement of the eyes in one direction followed by a slower drift back to the original position), blindness, and deafness may develop. Muscle coordination is lost. The muscles may tremble and become stiff. Usually, the muscles that control breathing and coughing are impaired, resulting in a high risk of pneumonia. Often, the cause of death is pneumonia. No treatment is available.

Kuru

Kuru is a prion disease that causes rapid deterioration of mental function and that used to occur in the Fore natives of the New Guinea highlands.

Until the early 1960s, kuru was fairly common in New Guinea. Prions were probably acquired during a cannibalistic ritual accompanying the care of the dead and involving eating tissues of a dead relative as a sign of respect. Kuru was more common among women and children because they were given the brain to eat. Many of these rituals have been abandoned, and kuru has been virtually eliminated.

Symptoms include loss of muscle coordination and difficulty walking. The limbs become stiff, and muscles twitch. Abnormal involuntary movements, such as repetitive, slow writhing or rapid jerking of the limbs and body, may develop. Emotions may switch suddenly from sadness to happiness with sudden outbursts of laughter. People with kuru become demented and eventually placid, unable to speak, and unresponsive to their surroundings. Most people die after about 3 to 24 months of illness, usually as a result of pneumonia or infection resulting from bedsores (pressure sores).

CHAPTER 91

Movement Disorders

Every body movement, from raising a hand to smiling, involves a complex interaction between the central nervous system (brain and spinal cord), nerves, and muscles. Damage to or malfunction of any of these components may result in a movement disorder.

Different types of movement disorders can develop, depending on the nature and location of the malfunction or damage. For example, damage to the connections between the brain and spinal cord can cause weakness or paralysis of the muscles involved in voluntary movements and can exaggerate reflexes. Damage to the basal ganglia (collections of nerve cells located at the base of the cerebrum, deep within the brain) can cause involuntary or decreased movements but not weakness or changes in reflexes. Damage to the cerebellum causes incoordination. Some movement disorders, such as hiccups, are temporary, usually causing little inconvenience. Others, such as Parkinson's disease, are serious and progressive, impairing the ability to walk, speak, use the hands, and stand.

Myoclonus

Myoclonus refers to quick, lightning-like jerks (contractions) of a muscle or a group of muscles.

Myoclonus is similar to sudden muscle cramps, but muscle contractions begin and end more rapidly, lasting only moments. Myoclonus may involve only one hand, a group of muscles in the upper arm or leg, or a group of facial muscles. Hiccups are a type of myoclonus that involves only the diaphragm, the muscle that separates the chest from the abdomen. Myoclonus may also involve many muscles at the same time.

Myoclonus may occur normally, often when a person is falling asleep. Or it may result from a disorder such as liver or kidney failure. Myoclonus may also occur after cardiac arrest—when the heart's pumping stops suddenly—or after taking high doses of certain drugs such as levodopa or bismuth. Other causes include certain types of seizure disorders (progressive myoclonic epilepsy), degenerative diseases that occur late in life (such as Alzheimer's disease), prion diseases (such as Creutzfeldt-Jakob disease), and head injuries.

If myoclonus is severe, anticonvulsants, such as clonazepam or valproate,▲ are sometimes helpful.

Tremor

A tremor is an involuntary, rhythmic, shaking movement produced when muscles repeatedly contract and relax.

Everyone has a tremor to some degree. For example, when held outstretched, the hands usually tremble slightly in most people. Such slight, rapid tremor is normal and reflects the precise moment-by-moment control of muscles by nerves. In most people, the tremor is too slight to be noticed.

Factors that can make the tremor more noticeable include stress, anxiety, fatigue, alcohol withdrawal, an overactive thyroid gland (hyperthyroidism), consumption of caffeine, and use of drugs that are stimulants (such as ephedrine).

There are several types of abnormal tremor. Tremors are classified according to how fast the shaking movements are (frequency); how wide (amplitude) they are, ranging from fine to coarse; how often the tremors occur; how severe they are; and whether they occur during rest, during movement, or at the end of a purposeful movement.

Essential Tremor: This tremor is rapid and fine. Essential tremor usually begins in early adulthood but can begin at any age. The tremor slowly becomes more obvious and becomes more noticeable among older age groups. It was once called senile tremor because it is more common among people older than 60. Some forms of essential tremor run in families and are sometimes called familial tremor. The cause is unknown.

Usually, essential tremor remains mild and does not indicate serious disease; however, it can be troublesome and embarrassing. It can affect handwriting and make using utensils difficult.

Essential tremor usually affects the arms and, rarely, the legs. The tremor usually stops when the arms or legs are at rest but becomes

---

▲ see table on page 500

Hiccups: Spasms of the Diaphragm

Almost everyone has had hiccups, so hiccups are hardly thought of as a movement disorder. But they are. They occur when there are spasms of the diaphragm, followed by quick, noisy closings of the glottis. (The diaphragm is the muscle that separates the chest from the abdomen and that is responsible for each breath; the glottis is the opening between the vocal cords that closes to stop the flow of air to the lungs.) Hiccups are more likely to occur when carbon dioxide levels in the blood decrease. Such a decrease can occur when people overbreathe (hyperventilate).

Most bouts of hiccups have no obvious cause. They usually start in a social situation, perhaps triggered by some combination of laughing, talking, eating, and drinking. Sometimes hot or irritating food or liquids are the cause. Less common but more serious causes of hiccups include irritation of the diaphragm, which may be due to pneumonia, chest or stomach surgery, or high levels of harmful substances in the blood, such as waste products that accumulate when the kidneys malfunction. Rarely, hiccups develop when a brain tumor or stroke interferes with the breathing center in the brain.

Hiccups usually begin suddenly and stop after several seconds or minutes, but occasionally, they persist for some time, even in healthy people. When due to a serious cause, hiccups tend to be prolonged and to persist until the cause is corrected. Hiccups due to a brain tumor or stroke may be very hard to stop and may become exhausting.

Many home remedies have been used to cure hiccups. Almost all involve ways to raise the level of carbon dioxide in the blood. Holding the breath is the simplest way. Breathing into a paper (not plastic) bag also raises the carbon dioxide level. Stimulating the vagus nerve, which runs from the brain to the stomach, may stop the hiccups. This nerve can be stimulated by drinking water quickly or by swallowing dry bread or crushed ice. Gently pulling on the tongue and gently rubbing the eyeballs are other ways to stimulate the vagus nerve. For most people with hiccups, any of these remedies work.

For persistent hiccups, treatment is needed, particularly when the cause cannot easily be corrected. Several drugs have been used with varying success. They include scopolamine, prochlorperazine, chlorpromazine, baclofen, metoclopramide, and valproate.

---

obvious when the limbs are outstretched and worsens when the limbs are held in uncomfortable positions. Essential tremor usually affects both sides of the body but may affect one side more than the other. Sometimes the tremor affects the head, causing it to tremble and bob, and the vocal cords, causing the voice to shake. In some people, the tremor gradually worsens over time, eventually resulting in disability.

Resting Tremor: This slow, coarse tremor occurs when the muscles are at rest, making an arm or a leg shake even when a person is completely relaxed. Resting tremor may develop when collections of nerve cells at the base of the cerebrum (including the basal ganglia) are disturbed. Such disturbances may result from Parkinson's disease, use of certain drugs (such as lithium and antipsychotic drugs), or heavy metal poisoning (such as occurs in Wilson's disease, in which copper accumulates in body tissues).

Resting tremor, although sometimes embarrassing, usually interferes little with voluntary movements, such as drinking a glass of water.

Intention (Cerebellar) Tremor: This relatively slow, broad tremor occurs at the end of a purposeful movement, such as trying to press a button. Intention tremor may result from a damage to the cerebellum or its connections. Multiple sclerosis and stroke are common causes. Wilson's disease, alcoholism, and overuse of sedatives or anticonvulsants can cause the cerebellum to malfunction, resulting in intention tremor.

Intention tremor may increase during an activity, such as touching an object with the hand. The tremor may cause a person to miss the targeted object.

Flapping Tremor (Asterixis): This tremor is a coarse, slow, nonrhythmic movement that occurs when a person stretches out the arms and extends the hands. This tremor commonly results from liver failure and so has been called liver flap. However, it may also result from kidney failure and brain damage (encephalopathy) due to a metabolic disorder.

Muscle tone lapses suddenly and temporarily. As a result, the hand flaps; that is, it quickly drops, then returns to its original position. This tremor may be accompanied by other tremors and by myoclonus.▲

Diagnosis and Treatment

The development of a noticeable tremor should be evaluated by doctors. Doctors can usually identify the type of tremor by its characteristics. The type of tremor determines which procedures are performed. For essential tremor, doctors ask what drugs are being used and whether the person is experiencing anxiety or stress. Often, a blood test to detect an overactive thyroid gland is performed. For a resting tremor, a complete neurologic evaluation and other procedures to check for Parkinson's disease are performed. For intention tremor, an imaging procedure, such as computed tomography (CT) or magnetic resonance imaging (MRI), is often performed to look for damage to the brain. For flapping tremor, blood tests to evaluate liver and kidney function are performed.

Usually, treatment for a tremor is not needed. Avoiding uncomfortable positions can help. Objects should be grasped firmly but comfortably and held close to the body.

For people with essential tremor, drinking alcohol in moderation may reduce the tremor. However, heavy drinking or alcohol withdrawal can make the tremor worse. If people with essential tremor have difficulty using utensils or do work that requires steady hands, drugs may help. A beta-blocker, such as propranolol, is most commonly prescribed. If it does not help, primidone, an anticonvulsant, is often tried.

A resting tremor due to Parkinson's disease is treated as part of that disease. Intention tremors are difficult to treat, but if the condition affecting the cerebellum can be corrected, the tremor may resolve. For flapping tremor, the underlying liver or kidney disorder is treated. The tremor may resolve as liver or kidney function improves.

Brain surgery is performed only when an essential or a resting tremor is severe and disabling and drugs are ineffective. There are two types of surgery. In thalamotomy, parts of the thalamus (located at the base of the cerebrum, deep within the brain) are destroyed, and thus

the pathways that produce the tremor are interrupted. In thalamic stimulation, an electrical probe is placed inside the thalamus. The probe delivers continuous high-frequency electrical stimulation to the thalamus, which generally reduces the tremor. Such procedures are available only at special centers.

Parkinson's Disease

Parkinson's disease is a slowly progressive degenerative disorder of the nervous system characterized by tremor when muscles are at rest (resting tremor), slowness of voluntary movements, and increased muscle tone (rigidity).

Parkinson's disease affects about 1 of 250 people older than 40 and about 1 of 100 people older than 65. It commonly begins between the ages of 50 and 79. It is twice as common among whites as among blacks.

When the brain initiates an impulse to move a muscle (for example, to lift an arm), the impulse passes through the basal ganglia (collections of nerve cells located at the base of the cerebrum, deep within the brain). The basal ganglia help smooth out muscle movements and coordinate changes in posture. Like all nerve cells, those in the basal ganglia release chemical messengers (neurotransmitters) that trigger the next nerve cell in the pathway to send an impulse. The main neurotransmitter in the basal ganglia is dopamine. Its overall effect is to increase nerve signals to muscles. In Parkinson's disease, nerve cells in part of the basal ganglia (called the substantia nigra) degenerate, reducing the production of dopamine and the number of connections between nerve cells in the basal ganglia. As a result, the basal ganglia cannot smooth out movements as they normally do, leading to tremor, incoordination, and slowed, reduced movement (bradykinesia).

The cause of nerve cell degeneration in Parkinson's disease is unknown. Genetics does not appear to play a large role, although the disease tends to occur in some families.

Parkinsonism is a disorder with many or all of the symptoms of Parkinson's disease. Various conditions can cause parkinsonism. It may be a complication of viral encephalitis, a rare disorder that follows a flu-like infection. Parkinsonism may also result when other degenerative diseases, drugs, or toxins interfere with or block the action of dopamine and other neurotransmitters. For example, anti-

▲ see page 544

psychotic drugs, used to treat paranoia and schizophrenia, block dopamine's action. Use of the substance MPTP (which was produced accidentally when illicit drugs users tried to synthesize the opioid meperidine) can cause sudden, severe, and irreversible parkinsonism in young people. Other causes include structural brain disorders (such as brain tumors and strokes) and head injury, particularly the repeated injury that occurs in boxing.

Corticobasal ganglionic degeneration is a rare cause of parkinsonism. It results from degeneration of brain tissue in the cerebral cortex and the basal ganglia. Corticobasal ganglionic degeneration is distinguished from other forms of parkinsonism by abnormalities in the cortex causing, for example, the inability to express or understand spoken or written language (aphasia), the inability to perform simple skilled tasks (apraxia), and the inability to associate objects with their usual role or function (agnosia). Symptoms begin after age 60, causing immobility after about 5 years and death after about 10 years.

Symptoms

Usually, Parkinson's disease begins subtly and progresses gradually. In many people, it begins with a coarse, rhythmic tremor in the hand while the hand is at rest. The tremor decreases when the hand is moving purposefully and disappears completely during sleep. Emotional stress or fatigue may increase the tremor. The tremor may eventually progress to the other hand, the arms, and the legs. A tremor may also affect the jaws, tongue, forehead, and eyelids. Tremor may become less obvious as the disease progresses. In about one third of people with Parkinson's disease, a tremor is not the first symptom. In some people, a tremor never develops. Other early symptoms may include a reduced sense of smell, a tendency to reduce body movements, difficulty walking, and lack of facial expression with infrequent blinking.

The sense of smell appears to be reduced partly because people with Parkinson's disease have difficulty sniffing—deliberately breathing in a large amount of air. (Degeneration of brain cells in the areas involved in smell may also contribute.) Although a reduced sense of smell may seem a minor problem, it can dampen the appetite, contributing to malnutrition.

Muscles become rigid, impairing movement. When the forearm is bent back or straightened out by another person, the movement may feel stiff and ratchet-like. Movements become slow and difficult to initiate, and mobility is decreased. Stiffness and decreased mobility can contribute to muscle ache and fatigue. Because the small muscles of the hands are often impaired, daily tasks, such as buttoning a shirt and tying shoelaces, become increasingly harder. Most people with Parkinson's disease have shaky, tiny handwriting (micrographia) because initiating and sustaining each stroke of the pen is difficult.

People with Parkinson's disease have difficulty walking, especially taking the first step. Once started, they often shuffle, taking short steps without swinging their arms as they walk. While walking, some people have difficulty stopping or turning. When the disease is advanced, some people suddenly stop walking because they feel as if their feet are glued to the ground. Other people unintentionally quicken their steps, breaking into a short stumbling run to avoid falling. Posture becomes stooped, and balance is difficult to maintain, leading to a tendency to fall forward. Because movements are slow, people often cannot move their hands quickly enough to break a fall.

The face becomes less expressive because the facial muscles that control expression do not move. This lack of expression may be mistaken for depression, or it may cause depression to be overlooked. (Depression is common among people with Parkinson's disease.) Eventually, the face can take on a blank stare with the mouth open, and the eyes may not blink often. Often, people drool or choke because muscle rigidity in the face and throat makes swallowing difficult. Malnutrition and dehydration can result. People with Parkinson's disease often speak softly in a monotone and may stutter because they have difficulty articulating words.

Constipation may develop. In many people with Parkinson's disease, intellect remains normal, but about half of the people develop dementia.

Diagnosis

Diagnosis is based on symptoms. Mild, early disease may be difficult for doctors to diagnose because it usually begins subtly. Diagnosis is especially difficult in older people, because aging can cause some of the same problems as Parkinson's disease, such as loss of balance, slow movements, muscle stiffness, and stooped posture. No tests or imaging procedures can directly confirm the diagnosis.

However, computed tomography (CT) and magnetic resonance imaging (MRI) may be performed to look for a structural disorder that may be the cause of the symptoms. The diagnosis of Parkinson's disease is likely if drug treatment for the disease results in improvement.

Treatment

The physical measures used to treat Parkinson's disease and parkinsonism are the same. However, the drugs used to treat Parkinson's disease are often not effective in people with parkinsonism. Treating the underlying disorder or discontinuing the drug causing parkinsonism is more effective and may result in a cure.

Physical Measures: Continuing to perform as many daily activities as possible and following a program of regular exercise can help people with Parkinson's disease maintain mobility. Physical and occupational therapy can help them maintain or regain muscle tone, maintain range of motion, and learn adaptive strategies.▲ Mechanical aids, such as wheeled walkers, can help them maintain independence.

A high-fiber diet can help counteract constipation, which may be worsened by the use of levodopa. Certain foods, such as prune juice and other juices, and stool softeners, such as senna concentrate, can help keep bowel movements regular. Difficulty swallowing can result in malnutrition, so doctors must ensure that the diet is nutritious. Learning to sniff more deeply may improve the ability to smell, enhancing the appetite.

Simple changes around the home can make the home safer for people with Parkinson's disease. For example, removing throw rugs can prevent tripping, and installing railings in bathrooms, hallways, and other locations reduces the risk of falling. Daily tasks can be simplified, for example by having buttons on clothing replaced with Velcro fasteners or buying shoes with such fasteners.

Drugs: No drug can cure Parkinson's disease or stop its progression, but many drugs can make movement easier and enable people to function effectively for many years. Two or more drugs may be needed.

Levodopa is most effective in reducing tremor and muscle rigidity and in improving movement. Treatment with levodopa can pro-

duce dramatic improvement in people with Parkinson's disease, but people with parkinsonism due to another disorder usually do not improve. Levodopa, taken by mouth, is converted to dopamine in the basal ganglia, thus compensating for the decrease in dopamine production. Taking levodopa enables many people with mild Parkinson's disease to return to a nearly normal level of activity and enables some people who are bedridden to walk again.

Levodopa is given with carbidopa. Carbidopa prevents levodopa from being converted to dopamine before it reaches the brain. When the two drugs are given together, a lower dose of levodopa can be used, and the side effects of levodopa (nausea and flushing) are reduced. Levodopa-carbidopa is the mainstay of treatment for Parkinson's disease.

To determine the best dose of levodopa for a particular person, doctors must balance control of the disease with the development of certain side effects, which may limit the amount of levodopa the person can tolerate. These side effects include involuntary movements of the mouth, face, and limbs; nightmares; hallucinations; and changes in blood pressure. Many experts believe that the development of involuntary movements can be delayed by using a drug that mimics the action of dopamine (a dopamine agonist) with or instead of levodopa during the early years of treatment.

After taking levodopa for 5 or more years, more than half of the people begin to alternate rapidly between a good response to the drug and no response—an effect called the on-off phenomenon. Within seconds, they may change from being fairly mobile to being severely impaired. The period of relief after each dose becomes shorter, and periods of immobility alternate with periods of improved mobility. However, improved mobility may be accompanied by writhing or hyperactivity—when the involuntary movements due to levodopa use are greatly increased. Taking lower, more frequent doses controls these effects at first, but after 15 to 20 years, these effects become hard to suppress. Surgery is then considered.

Other drugs are generally less effective than levodopa, but they may benefit some people, particularly if levodopa is not tolerated or is insufficient. Dopamine agonists (such as pramipexole and ropinirole), which mimic the action of dopamine, may be useful at any stage of the disease. Selegiline, a type of antidepressant called a monoamine oxidase inhibitor

▲ see pages 38 to 39

℞ DRUGS USED TO TREAT PARKINSON'S DISEASE

TYPE	DRUG	SELECTED SIDE EFFECTS	COMMENTS
Dopamine precursor (a substance that can be converted to dopamine)	Levodopa (given in combination with carbidopa)	For levodopa, involuntary movements of the mouth, face, and limbs; nightmares; changes in blood pressure; constipation; nausea; drowsiness; palpitations; and flushing	This combination is the mainstay of treatment of Parkinson's disease. Carbidopa helps increase the effectiveness of levodopa and reduce its side effects. After several years, the effectiveness of the combination may lessen
Dopamine agonists	Bromocriptine Pergolide Pramipexole Ropinirole	Drowsiness, nausea, changes in blood pressure, and hallucinations; with sudden withdrawal of the drugs, neuroleptic malignant syndrome (see box on page 644)	These drugs may be used alone in the early stages of the disease. Early use may delay the development of problems with levodopa's side effects
MAO-B inhibitor	Selegiline	Nausea, dizziness, confusion, dry mouth, and abdominal pain	Selegiline can be used alone but is often given as a supplement to levodopa. At best, selegiline is modestly effective
COMT inhibitors	Entacapone Tolcapone	Nausea, abnormal involuntary movements, diarrhea, back pain, and discoloration of the urine	Either of these drugs can be used to supplement levodopa late in the disease to extend the interval between doses of levodopa
Anticholinergic drugs	Benztropine Trihexyphenidyl Tricyclic antidepressants (such as amitriptyline—see table on page 618) Some antihistamines (such as diphen hydramine)	Drowsiness, dry mouth, blurred vision, dizziness, constipation, and difficulty urinating (see also box on page 79)	These drugs may be given alone in the early stages of the disease and with levodopa in the later stages. They can reduce the tremor but do not affect the slowed movements or muscle rigidity
Antiviral drug	Amantadine	Nausea, dizziness, insomnia, anxiety, and confusion; when the drug is withdrawn or the dose is reduced, life-threatening high fever with disturbances in blood pressure, breathing and heart rates, and other internal functions (similar to neuroleptic malignant syndrome)	Amantadine is used alone in the early stages for mild disease and in later stages to enhance levodopa's effects. If used alone, this drug may become ineffective after several months. Amantadine is thought to work by causing dopamine to be released
Beta-blockers	Propranolol	See table on page 138	Propranolol can be used to reduce the severity of tremor

MAO-B = monoamine oxidase, type B; COMT = catechol *O*-methyltransferase.

(MAOI),▲ prevents the breakdown of dopamine, thereby prolonging dopamine's action in the body. Tolcapone and entacapone also prevent the breakdown of dopamine and appear to be useful supplements to levodopa.

Anticholinergic drugs,■ such as benztropine and trihexyphenidyl, are effective in reducing the severity of a tremor and can be used in the early stages of Parkinson's disease. They can also be used in the later stages to supplement levodopa. Anticholinergic drugs may reduce tremor because they block the action of acetylcholine, and tremor is thought to be caused by an imbalance of acetylcholine (too much) and dopamine (too little). Other anticholinergic drugs, including some antihistamines and tricyclic antidepressants, are mildly effective and are used to supplement levodopa.

Amantadine, a drug sometimes used to treat influenza, may be used alone to treat mild disease or as a supplement to levodopa. Propranolol, a beta-blocker, may be prescribed to reduce the severity of a tremor.

Surgery: In a pallidotomy, a tiny area in one of the basal ganglia is surgically destroyed. This procedure can greatly reduce the "off" part—the difficulty initiating movements—of the on-off phenomenon and the involuntary movements that occur after years of levodopa therapy. Alternatively, tiny electrodes can be implanted in the same area. They provide high-frequency electrical stimulation to this area, often producing similar improvements.

Nerve cells that produce dopamine may be taken from human fetal tissue and implanted in the brain of a person with Parkinson's disease. These cells form connections with other nerve cells and produce dopamine, thus supplying the missing neurotransmitter. However, this procedure is still experimental and requires further study.

Caregiver and End-of-Life Issues: Because Parkinson's disease is progressive, people eventually need help performing normal daily activities, such as eating, bathing, dressing, and toileting. Caregivers can benefit from learning about the physical and psychologic effects of Parkinson's disease and about ways to enable people to function as well as possible. Because such care is tiring and stressful, caregivers may benefit from support groups.

Eventually, people with Parkinson's disease usually become severely disabled and immobile. They may be unable to eat, even with assistance. Dementia develops in about half of the people. Because swallowing becomes increasingly difficult, death due to aspiration pneumonia is a risk. For some people, depending on many factors, a nursing home may be the best place for care. Before people with this disease are incapacitated, they should establish advance directives, indicating what kind of medical care they want at the end of life.★

Progressive Supranuclear Palsy

Progressive supranuclear palsy is a disorder characterized by muscle stiffness (rigidity), an inability to move the eyes, and weakness of throat muscles.

Progressive supranuclear palsy, which is much rarer than Parkinson's disease, destroys parts of the basal ganglia and the brain stem. (The basal ganglia help smooth out muscle movements and coordinate changes in posture; the brain stem regulates critical body functions, such as breathing, heart rate, and swallowing, and helps adjust posture.) The cause of the damage to this part of the brain is unknown.

This disorder usually begins in late middle age with abnormalities in posture and an inability to roll the eyes downward. People with the disorder cannot fix their eyes on a stationary object or follow a moving object. They may have blurred or double vision. The upper eyelids may pull back, producing a look of astonishment. Walking is unsteady, with a tendency to fall backward. Speaking and swallowing are difficult, and movements are slow. Other symptoms include insomnia, agitation, irritability, apathy, and rapid changes in emotion.

In the late stages, depression and dementia are common. Like Parkinson's disease, progressive supranuclear palsy results in severe muscle rigidity and disability, usually within 3 to 5 years. Usually, death, often due to infection, occurs within 10 years after symptoms begin.

The diagnosis is based on symptoms. No effective treatment exists, but the drugs used to treat Parkinson's disease may provide some relief.

Shy-Drager Syndrome

Shy-Drager syndrome (idiopathic orthostatic hypotension) results in tremor when muscles

---

▲ see table on page 618

■ see box on page 79   ★ see page 54

are at rest (resting tremor) and in malfunction of the autonomic nervous system, including pronounced instability of blood pressure.

Shy-Drager syndrome usually develops between the ages of 37 and 75. It is 2 or 3 times more common among men than among women. It results from degeneration of the parts of the brain that control the autonomic nervous system,▲ including the motor nerve cells of the cerebellum, basal ganglia, and spinal cord. The cause of the degeneration is unknown. Shy-Drager syndrome is thought to be a form of multiple systems atrophy—a group of overlapping disorders that cause many symptoms and simultaneously affect several body systems.

Symptoms and Diagnosis

Shy-Drager syndrome is a progressive disorder. It is similar to Parkinson's disease, causing tremor, muscle rigidity, and problems with movements (such as difficulty walking and speaking). However, Shy-Drager syndrome also causes malfunction of the autonomic nervous system, which regulates internal body processes. This disorder therefore interferes with the regulation of blood pressure, heart rate, secretion of hormones, bladder and bowel function, body temperature, and focusing of the eyes. Blood pressure drops dramatically when a person stands up, causing dizziness, light-headedness, or fainting—a condition called orthostatic hypotension. Blood pressure may increase when a person lies down. The production of sweat, tears, and saliva decreases. Vision becomes poor. A person may have difficulty urinating or become constipated, and urinary or fecal incontinence may develop. In men, erectile dysfunction (impotence) may develop. Walking may become unsteady, and incoordination may develop. The disorder results in death 7 to 10 years after symptoms begin.

The diagnosis is based on symptoms.

Treatment

Generally, drugs used to treat Parkinson's disease are not effective in treating Shy-Drager syndrome, but response to them varies from person to person. Measures are taken to stabilize the sudden changes in blood pressure. The drug fludrocortisone can help increase blood pressure because it causes the body to retain salt and water. Adding salt to the diet and drinking a lot of water may increase the volume of blood and thus may also help increase blood pressure. Midodrine, which is used to treat orthostatic hypotension, may help prevent blood pressure from decreasing too much when a person stands, as may wearing fitted elastic stockings up to the waist. Raising the head of the bed can help prevent blood pressure from increasing too much when the person lies down. If blood pressure does increase, an antihypertensive drug may be given at night.

Avoiding extreme heat, abstaining from alcoholic beverages, eating small meals, getting up slowly, and not straining during a bowel movement may also help.

People with Shy-Drager syndrome should establish advance directives, indicating what kind of medical care they want at the end of life.■

Tics

Tics are brief, rapid, purposeless, simple or complex involuntary movements that are virtually identical to one another and are repetitive but not rhythmic.

Simple tics, such as excessive blinking, may begin as nervous mannerisms, often during childhood, and may disappear without any treatment. Complex tics, such as those that occur in Tourette's syndrome, often resemble fragments of normal behavior.

TOURETTE'S SYNDROME

Tourette's syndrome is a hereditary disorder in which muscle and vocal tics occur frequently throughout the day for at least one year.

Tourette's syndrome is 3 times more common among men than among women. It often begins in early childhood. The cause is unknown but is thought to be an abnormality in dopamine or another brain neurotransmitter (a chemical messenger that nerve cells use to communicate).

Symptoms and Diagnosis

Tourette's syndrome often begins with muscle tics. Many people who do not have this disorder have simple tics, such as repetitive eye blinks, which are nervous habits and may disappear with time. However, the tics in Tourette's syndrome consist of more than just a blink. For example, people with this disorder may repeatedly move the head from side to

▲ see page 437   ■ see page 54

side, blink the eyes, open the mouth, and stretch the neck. Before a tic occurs, the person may feel an urge to perform the movements of the tic. The tic can sometimes be postponed from seconds to hours but eventually becomes irresistible. Some people can suppress some of the tics, usually with difficulty. However, most people have trouble controlling the tics, especially during times of emotional stress.

The disorder progresses to bursts of complex tics, including vocal tics, hitting, kicking, and sudden, irregular, jerky breathing. Vocal tics may start as grunting, snorting, humming, or barking noises and progress to compulsive, involuntary bouts of cursing. For no apparent reason and often in the midst of conversation, some people with Tourette's syndrome may call out obscenities. Use of words related to feces (coprolalia) is common. These vocal outbursts are sometimes mistakenly thought to be intentional, especially in children. Repetition of words immediately after hearing them (echolalia) is also common.

People with Tourette's syndrome often have difficulty functioning and experience considerable anxiety in social situations. In the past, they were shunned, isolated, or even thought to be possessed by the devil. Many people with the disorder develop impulsive, aggressive, and self-destructive behaviors; about half of the people develop obsessive-compulsive behavior. Children with Tourette's syndrome often have difficulty learning. Whether the disorder itself or the extraordinary stresses of living with the disorder cause these behaviors is unclear.

Diagnosis is based on the symptoms. Early diagnosis can help parents understand that the tics their children have are not voluntary and that punishment cannot stop the tics.

Treatment

For simple tics, benzodiazepines (such as clonazepam and diazepam), which are mild sedatives, may help. Clonidine, a drug used to treat high blood pressure, occasionally helps because it blocks the action of norepinephrine, a neurotransmitter that is thought to contribute to the tics. Clonidine is more useful in controlling anxiety and obsessive-compulsive behavior; however, it may cause excessively low blood pressure.

▲ see page 643

When the disorder is severe, antipsychotic drugs may be used to help suppress the tics, even though psychosis is not the cause. Haloperidol, the most commonly used antipsychotic drug, is effective but can cause side effects such as repetitive involuntary movements of the mouth and tongue (tardive dyskinesia▲), stiffness, weight gain, blurred vision, sleepiness, and dulled, slowed thinking. Pimozide, fluphenazine, and risperidone—also antipsychotic drugs—can reduce the frequency and intensity of the tics. These drugs may have fewer side effects.

Injecting botulin into the muscles producing the tics may decrease the abnormal movements as well as the urge that precedes them. Botulin, the bacterial toxin that causes botulism, is used to paralyze muscles.

Chorea and Athetosis

Chorea consists of repetitive, brief, jerky, large-scale, dancelike, uncontrolled movements that start in one part of the body and move abruptly, unpredictably, and often continuously to another; *athetosis* is a continuous stream of slow, sinuous, writhing movements, generally of the hands and feet.

Chorea and athetosis, which may occur together as **choreoathetosis,** are not disorders. Rather they are symptoms that can result from several very different disorders. Chorea and athetosis result from abnormalities in the basal ganglia, the part of the brain that helps smooth out and coordinate movements initiated by nerve impulses from the brain. In most forms of chorea, an excess of dopamine, the main neurotransmitter used in the basal ganglia, prevents the basal ganglia from functioning normally. Drugs and disorders that increase dopamine levels or increase the sensitivity of nerve cells to dopamine tend to worsen chorea and athetosis.

Chorea and athetosis occur in Huntington's disease, a hereditary disease. Chorea may also be caused by Sydenham's disease (also called St. Vitus' dance or Sydenham's chorea), a complication of rheumatic fever (a childhood infection caused by certain streptococci). Sydenham's disease is characterized by jerky, uncontrollable movements and can last for several months.

Chorea sometimes develops in older people for no apparent reason, affecting particularly the muscles in and around the mouth. This disorder is called senile chorea. Chorea also can affect women in the first 3 months of pregnancy (a condition called chorea gravidarum), but it disappears without treatment shortly after they give birth. Rarely, a similar chorea develops in women taking oral contraceptives.

Hemiballismus, a type of chorea, consists of continuous violent flinging movements on one side of the body. It affects the arm more than the leg. It is usually caused by a stroke affecting a very small area just below the basal ganglia.

Treatment

If chorea is being caused by a drug, stopping the drug may help, but the chorea does not always disappear. Drugs that block dopamine's action may help control the abnormal movements. These drugs include antipsychotic drugs,▲ such as haloperidol and fluphenazine.

Antipsychotic drugs may also help people with hemiballismus. However, hemiballismus usually goes away on its own after several days, although it sometimes lasts for 6 to 8 weeks.

Huntington's Disease

Huntington's disease (Huntington's chorea) is a hereditary disease that begins with occasional jerks or spasms and gradual loss of brain cells and that progresses to more pronounced involuntary movements (chorea and athetosis) and mental deterioration.

Huntington's disease affects fewer than 1 of 10,000 people. Both sexes are affected equally. The gene for Huntington's disease is dominant; therefore, children of a person who has this disease have a 50% chance of developing it.■ Because Huntington's disease begins subtly, the exact age at which it begins is difficult to determine. Symptoms usually become obvious between the ages of 35 and 40.

Symptoms

During the early stages of Huntington's disease, people can blend the spontaneous abnormal movements into intentional ones so that the abnormal movements are barely noticeable. However, with time, the movements become more obvious. People grimace, flick the limbs, and blink more often. Muscles become uncoordinated, and movements slow. Eventually, the entire body is affected, making walking impossible and eating, speaking, dressing, and sitting still nearly impossible.

Mental changes are subtle at first. People with the disease may gradually become irritable and excitable; they may lose interest in

Genetic Testing for Huntington's Disease

The genetic mutation that causes Huntington's disease is located on chromosome 4. Because the gene for Huntington's disease is dominant, having only one copy of the abnormal gene, inherited from one parent, is sufficient to cause the disease. Most people who have the disease have only one copy of the abnormal gene. People with one copy of the abnormal gene may pass on either the abnormal gene or the normal gene to a child. Which gene is passed on is the crucial question—the odds are 50-50. A few people have two abnormal genes; their children always inherit the disease.

People who have a parent with Huntington's disease can find out whether they have inherited the gene for the disease by taking a genetic test. The test requires a blood sample. The test can detect the characteristic repetition of a particular section of the genetic code within the DNA. People who have a family history of Huntington's disease may or may not want to know whether they have inherited the gene. This issue should be discussed with an expert in genetic counseling before genetic testing.

their usual activities. They may be unable to control their impulses, losing their temper, having fits of despondency, or becoming promiscuous. As the disease progresses, people may behave irresponsibly and often wander aimlessly. Over years, they may lose their memory and the ability to think rationally. They may become severely depressed and attempt suicide. In advanced disease, almost all functions are impaired, and dementia is severe. Full-time assistance or nursing home care is needed. Death, often precipitated by pneumonia or by a fall, usually occurs 13 to 15 years after symptoms begin.

Diagnosis

Huntington's disease may be difficult to recognize in the early stages because symptoms are subtle. The disease may be suspected based on symptoms and a family history. Doctors should be told about relatives who have had mental problems or have been diagnosed as having a neurologic or psychiatric disorder

▲ see table on page 645　　■ see page 12

(such as Parkinson's disease or schizophrenia), because Huntington's disease may have been present but was not diagnosed. Computed tomography (CT) or magnetic resonance imaging (MRI) can detect wasting away (atrophy) of the basal ganglia, which is characteristic of the disease.

The disease can be easily diagnosed using genetic testing. However, whether people who have a family history of the disease but no symptoms should be tested is controversial. Such people should undergo genetic counseling before genetic testing.

Treatment

No cure exists for Huntington's disease. However, drugs, such as the sedative chlorpromazine, the antipsychotic haloperidol, and the antihypertensive reserpine, can help relieve symptoms and control behavior.

People with Huntington's disease should establish advance directives, indicating what kind of medical care they want at the end of life. ▲

Dystonia

Dystonia is involuntary, slow, repetitive, sustained muscle contractions that may cause freezing in the middle of an action, as well as twisting or turning of the trunk, the entire body, or part of the body.

Causes

Overactivity in several areas of the brain—the basal ganglia, thalamus, cerebellum, and cerebral cortex—seems to cause dystonia. Causes of dystonia include a severe lack of oxygen to the brain that occurs at birth or later in life, Parkinson's disease, multiple sclerosis, toxicity due to accumulation of certain metals (such as copper in Wilson's disease), and stroke. Antipsychotic drugs can cause various types of dystonia, including involuntary shutting of the eyelids (blepharospasm), involuntary twisting of the neck (spasmodic torticollis), grimacing, and repetitive involuntary movements of the mouth and tongue (tardive dyskinesia). Chronic dystonia usually has a genetic cause.

Types and Symptoms of Dystonia

Idiopathic torsion dystonia refers to dystonia that has no known cause. Episodes begin between the ages of 6 and 12. Early symptoms

can be mild or severe. Muscles contract slowly and abnormally, causing twisting and turning. The dystonia commonly starts in one foot or leg. It may remain limited to the trunk or a leg, but sometimes it affects the whole body, ultimately confining the child to a wheelchair. Another example of mild dystonia is persistent writer's cramp (however, not all writer's cramp is due to dystonia). When idiopathic torsion dystonia develops in adults, it usually begins in the face or arms and usually does not progress to other parts of the body.

Blepharospasm is a type of dystonia in which the eyelids are repeatedly and involuntarily forced shut. Occasionally, only one eye is affected at first, but ultimately, the other eye is also affected. It usually begins as excessive blinking, eye irritation, or extreme sensitivity to bright light. Many people with blepharospasm find ways to keep their eyes open, such as yawning, singing, or opening the mouth wide. These techniques become less effective as the disorder progresses. Blepharospasm can severely impair vision.

Spasmodic torticollis is dystonia involving the muscles of the neck.

Spasmodic dysphonia affects the muscles that control speech. People with this disorder usually have an essential tremor somewhere else as well. Spasms of the vocal cord muscles may block speech altogether or make speech sound strained, quavery, hoarse, whispery, jerky, creaky, staccato, or garbled and difficult to understand.

The **yips** are a type of dystonia experienced by some golfers who have muscle spasms. The muscles of the hands and wrists spontaneously contract, making putting nearly impossible. What is supposed to be a 3-foot putt can become a 15-foot putt when a golfer loses control because of the yips. Similarly, musicians who have bizarre spasms of the hands and arms that prevent them from performing may have dystonia.

Some dystonias are progressive; the movements may become more bizarre over time. Severe muscle contractions can force the neck and arms into odd, uncomfortable positions.

Treatment

Correcting or eliminating the cause of dystonia, if known, usually reduces the dystonia. For example, drugs used to treat Parkinson's disease may be effective for dystonia related to that disease. When dystonia is due to use of an antipsychotic drug, promptly taking diphenhydramine by injection or by mouth usually stops the episode quickly, and the antipsychotic is discontinued.

If the cause of dystonia is unknown, treatment is limited. Some people, especially children who have a hereditary form of dystonia (called dopa-responsive dystonia), improve dramatically when treated with levodopa. Benzodiazepines, a type of mild sedative, may be used. Baclofen, a muscle relaxant, may be given by mouth or by a pump implanted in the spinal canal. Anticholinergic drugs,▲ such as trihexyphenidyl and diphenhydramine, are sometimes helpful, but they also cause side effects, such as drowsiness, dry mouth, blurred vision, dizziness, constipation, difficulty urinating, and tremor, especially in older people. The antipsychotics clozapine and olanzapine may be useful.

Injections of botulin (a bacterial toxin used to paralyze muscles) into the overactive muscles have been the most successful treatment. These injections are particularly useful for blepharospasm, spasmodic torticollis, and spasmodic dysphonia.

If drug treatment is ineffective and symptoms are severe, surgery may be performed. Procedures include pallidotomy (surgical destruction of a tiny area in one basal ganglion) and implantation of electrodes to stimulate the same area of the brain.

Physical therapy helps some people, especially those who are treated with botulin.

SPASMODIC TORTICOLLIS

Spasmodic torticollis (cervical dystonia) is a disorder characterized by painful intermittent or continuous contractions or spasms of the neck muscles, forcing the head to rotate or tilt forward, backward, or sideways.

Spasmodic torticollis, a form of dystonia, is diagnosed in 3 of 10,000 people in the United States and is about 1½ times more common among women than among men. The disorder can occur at any age but usually develops between the ages of 25 and 55.

Usually, the cause is unknown. Dysfunction within the basal ganglia (collections of nerve cells located at the base of the cerebrum, deep within the brain) may be the cause. Sometimes spasmodic torticollis is caused by injury to the neck muscles during pregnancy or during a difficult delivery. This type of spasmodic torticollis is called congenital torticollis. Imbalanced eye muscles and bone or muscle deformities of the upper spine can cause torticollis in children.

Symptoms and Diagnosis

Initially, symptoms may be mild, but they may become severe. They include involuntary turning of the head, muscle pains, and slight tremor of the neck muscles. Usually, only one side of the neck is affected. The direction in which the head tilts and rotates depends on which neck muscles are affected. Sharp, painful neck muscle spasms may start suddenly and occur intermittently or continuously. The spasms occur without warning but rarely during sleep. One third of people who have this disorder also have spasms in other areas, usually in the eyelids, face, jaw, or hand.

To diagnose the disorder in children and adults, doctors ask detailed questions about past injuries and other neck problems. During a physical examination of a newborn, doctors can detect neck muscle damage that may cause congenital torticollis.

Imaging procedures, such as x-rays, computed tomography (CT), and magnetic resonance imaging (MRI), are sometimes used to look for specific causes of neck muscle spasms, although such causes are not commonly identified.

Treatment and Prognosis

When a cause, such as bone or muscle deformities, is identified, torticollis can usually be treated successfully. However, when the cause is unknown, treatment is less likely to control the spasms. Sometimes the spasm can be temporarily relieved by physical and occupational therapy, which may include biofeedback, electrical stimulation, massage, cold packs, heat, and deep heat with ultrasonography.

Certain drugs help reduce muscle spasms and involuntary movements in about one third of adults with spasmodic torticollis. Usually, these drugs also help control pain due to the spasms. Commonly used are anticholinergic drugs (such as trihexyphenidyl and benztropine), which block specific nerve impulses, and benzodiazepines (particularly clonazepam), which are mild sedatives. Less frequently, muscle relaxants (such as baclofen) and antidepressants (such as amitriptyline) are used.

For people with significant pain and an abnormal posture, several injections of botulin (a bacterial toxin used to paralyze muscles),

---

▲ see box on page 79

given in a low dose, is the best treatment. This toxin blocks muscle contractions. For most people, botulin injections reduce pain and spasms, so that the head can be held more normally. Improvement may last for a few months; then the treatment may be repeated as needed. Surgically removing the nerves to the dysfunctional neck muscles (called selective denervation) is sometimes successful and may be tried if other treatments do not provide relief. If emotional problems contribute to the spasms, psychiatric treatment may help.

For torticollis in newborns, intensive physical therapy to stretch the damaged muscle is begun within the first few months of life. If the physical therapy is unsuccessful or started too late, the muscle may have to be repaired surgically.

About 10 to 20% of people who have spasmodic torticollis—usually people younger than 40 with mild cases—recover without treatment within 5 years. However, in most adults, the disorder gradually worsens for 1 to 5 years, then stabilizes. Torticollis may persist for life, producing continued pain, restricted movement of the neck, and an abnormal posture.

Coordination Disorders

The cerebellum is the part of the brain most responsible for coordinating sequences of movements; it also controls balance and posture. Anything that damages the cerebellum can lead to incoordination (ataxia).

Prolonged alcohol abuse is the most common cause of damage to the cerebellum. Other causes include strokes, tumors, bleeding (hemorrhage) in the brain, repeated head injuries,

multiple sclerosis, birth defects of the brain, an underactive thyroid gland (hypothyroidism), a high fever, certain toxic substances (such as carbon monoxide and heavy metals), and undernutrition. Several rare hereditary disorders, such as Friedreich's ataxia and ataxia-telangiectasia, may also damage the cerebellum.

People with ataxia cannot control the position of their arms and legs or their posture, so they stagger and make broad, zigzag movements with their arms. There are several specific types of ataxia. People with dysmetria cannot control the accuracy of body movements. For example, in attempting to reach for an object, people with dysmetria may reach beyond the object. People with dysarthria have poor coordination of speech muscles, causing slurred speech and uncontrolled fluctuations in volume. Such people may also exaggerate movement of the muscles around the mouth. Damage to the cerebellum can cause intention tremor.

In Friedreich's ataxia, a progressive disorder, walking becomes unsteady between the ages of 5 and 15. Then arm movements become uncoordinated, and speech becomes slurred and hard to understand. Vibration sense, position sense (knowing where the arms and legs are), and reflexes are lost. Mental function may decrease. By their late 20s, people with this disorder may be confined to a wheelchair. Death, often due to an abnormal heart rhythm or heart failure, usually occurs by middle age.

For the hereditary disorders, such as Friedreich's ataxia and ataxia-telangiectasia, there is no treatment. Ataxia due to use of alcohol or a drug such as phenytoin can be treated by withdrawing that substance.

CHAPTER 92

Multiple Sclerosis and Related Disorders

Most nerve fibers inside and outside the brain are wrapped with many layers of tissue composed of a fat (lipoprotein) called myelin. These layers form the myelin sheath. Much like the insulation around an electrical wire, the myelin sheath enables electrical impulses to be con-

ducted along the nerve fiber with speed and accuracy. When the myelin sheath is damaged, nerves do not conduct impulses normally.

When babies are born, many of their nerves lack mature myelin sheaths. As a result, their movements are jerky, uncoordinated, and awkward. As myelin sheaths develop, movements become smoother, more purposeful, and more coordinated. Myelin sheaths do not develop normally in children with certain rare hereditary diseases, such as Tay-Sachs disease, Niemann-Pick disease, Gaucher's disease, and Hurler's syndrome. These children may have permanent, often extensive, neurologic problems.

In adults, the myelin sheath can be destroyed by stroke, inflammation, immune disorders, metabolic disorders, and nutritional deficiencies (for example, a lack of vitamin B_{12}). Such destruction is called demyelination. Poisons, drugs (such as the antibiotic ethambutol), and excessive use of alcohol can damage or destroy the myelin sheath. If the sheath is able to repair and regenerate itself, normal nerve function may return. However, if the sheath is severely damaged, the underlying nerve fiber can die, causing irreversible damage. Nerve fibers cannot regenerate themselves.

Disorders that cause demyelination in the central nervous system (the brain and spinal cord) and have no known cause are called primary demyelinating disorders. Multiple sclerosis is the most common of these disorders.

Multiple Sclerosis

Multiple sclerosis is a disorder in which patches of myelin and underlying nerve fibers in the eyes, brain, and spinal cord are damaged or destroyed.

The term "multiple sclerosis" refers to the many areas of scarring (sclerosis) that result from demyelination of nerves. In the United States, about 400,000 people, mostly young adults, have multiple sclerosis. Most commonly, it begins between the ages of 20 and 40. It is more common among women than among men. Most people with multiple sclerosis have periods of relatively good health (remissions) alternating with debilitating flare-ups (relapses). However, the disorder often worsens slowly over time.

Causes

The cause of multiple sclerosis is unknown, but a likely explanation is that a virus (possibly a herpesvirus or retrovirus) or some unknown antigen somehow triggers a reaction directed against the body's own tissues (autoimmune reaction▲), usually early in life. The autoimmune reaction results in inflammation, destruction of myelin, and damage to the myelin sheath and the underlying nerve fiber.

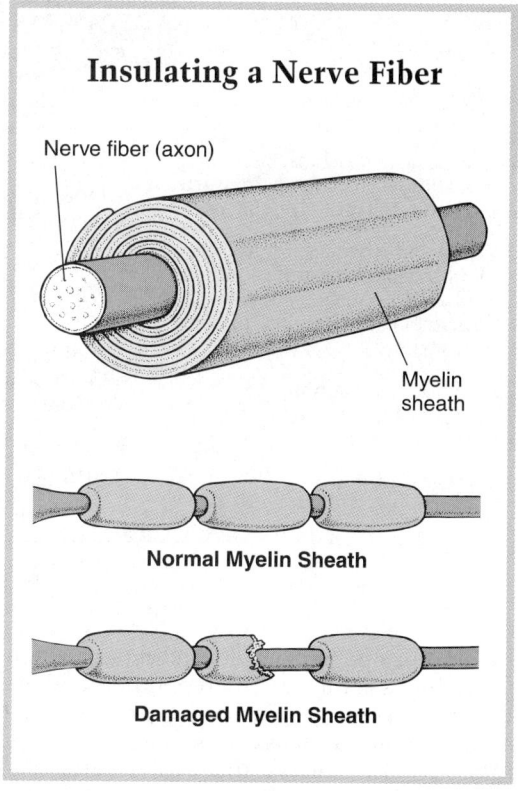

Insulating a Nerve Fiber

Nerve fiber (axon)

Myelin sheath

Normal Myelin Sheath

Damaged Myelin Sheath

Heredity seems to have a role in multiple sclerosis. About 5% of people with the disorder have a brother or sister who is affected, and about 15% have a close relative who is affected. Also, multiple sclerosis is more likely to develop in people with certain genetic markers for proteins (human leukocyte antigens■) that help the body to distinguish self from nonself.

Environment also has a role in multiple sclerosis. Where people spend the first 15 years of life affects their chance of developing multiple sclerosis. Multiple sclerosis occurs in 1 of 2,000 people who grow up in a temperate climate but in only 1 of 10,000 people who grow up in a tropical climate. Multiple sclerosis almost never occurs in people who grow up near the equator. The climate in which later years are spent does not change the chances of developing the disorder.

Symptoms

The symptoms of multiple sclerosis vary greatly, from person to person and from time

▲ see page 1073   ■ see page 1050

COMMON SYMPTOMS OF MULTIPLE SCLEROSIS

SENSORY SYMPTOMS	MOTOR SYMPTOMS	PSYCHOLOGIC OR NEUROLOGIC SYMPTOMS
Abnormal sensations, such as numbness, tingling, pain, burning, and itching	Weakness and clumsiness	Mood swings
	Difficulty walking or maintaining balance	Inappropriate elation or giddiness
Visual disturbances, including double vision, partial blindness and pain in one eye, dim or blurred vision, and loss of central vision	Tremor	Depression
	Uncoordinated eye movements	Inability to control emotions (for example, crying or laughing without reason)
Difficulty in reaching orgasm, lack of sensation in the vagina, and sexual impotence in men	Problems with control of urination and bowel movements	Subtle or obvious mental impairment
	Constipation	
Dizziness or vertigo	Stiffness, unsteadiness, and unusual fatigue	

to time in one person, depending on which nerve fibers are demyelinated. If nerve fibers that carry sensory information are demyelinated, abnormal sensations (sensory symptoms) result. If nerve fibers that carry signals to muscles are demyelinated, problems with movement (motor symptoms) result. Symptoms often come and go, affecting one or several parts of the body. The fluctuating symptoms result from damage to myelin sheaths, followed by repair, followed by more damage.

Multiple sclerosis may progress and regress unpredictably. However, there are several patterns of symptoms. In the relapsing-remitting pattern, flare-ups (relapses) alternate with remissions, in which symptoms are stable. Remissions may last months or years. Relapses can occur spontaneously or can be triggered by an infection such as influenza. High temperatures, such as very warm weather, a hot bath or shower, or a fever, can also trigger relapses or intensify symptoms. In the primary progressive pattern, the disease progresses gradually with no remissions, although there may be temporary plateaus during which the disease does not progress. The secondary progressive pattern begins with relapses alternating with remissions, followed by gradual progression of the disease. In the progressive relapsing pattern, the disease progresses gradually, but progression is interrupted by sudden relapses. This pattern is rare. About 20% of people with

multiple sclerosis have one episode, after which the disease progresses little if at all. Very rarely, multiple sclerosis progresses quickly, resulting in severe disability or death soon after the symptoms develop.

Common early symptoms include tingling, numbness, pain, burning, and itching in the arms, legs, trunk, or face and loss of strength or dexterity in a leg or hand. A person may feel unusually tired. Mild psychologic or neurologic symptoms (such as mood swings, inappropriate giddiness, euphoria, depression, and apathy) may occur. Cognitive problems include memory disturbances, decreased judgment, and inattention. These vague symptoms of demyelination in the brain sometimes begin long before the disorder is diagnosed.

Some people develop only eye symptoms, such as partial blindness and pain in one eye, dim or blurred vision, or loss of central vision; peripheral vision is not affected. Such symptoms are due to inflammation of the optic nerve (optic neuritis). Eye movements may be uncoordinated, sometimes resulting in double vision (a condition called internuclear ophthalmoplegia).

When the back part of the spinal cord in the neck is affected, bending the neck forward causes an electrical shock or a tingling sensation that shoots down the back, down both legs, down one arm, or down one side of the body (a response called Lhermitte's sign). Usually, the sensation lasts only a moment and disappears when the neck is straightened. Often, it is felt as long as the neck remains bent.

As the disorder progresses, movements may become shaky, irregular, and ineffective. Muscle weakness and spasticity may interfere with walking, sometimes eventually making it impossible. Multiple sclerosis can cause partial or complete paralysis. Speech may become slow, slurred, and hesitant. Late in the disorder, dementia and mania (excessive elation) may develop. The nerves that control urination or bowel movements can also be affected, leading to frequent and strong urges to urinate, retention of urine, constipation, and, occasionally, urinary and fecal incontinence.

If relapses become more frequent, people become increasingly disabled, sometimes permanently. Nonetheless, about 75% of people who have multiple sclerosis never need a wheelchair, and for about 40%, normal activities are not disrupted. Most people with multiple sclerosis have a normal life span.

Diagnosis

Because the symptoms vary widely, doctors may not recognize the disorder in its early stages. Doctors suspect multiple sclerosis in younger people who suddenly develop blurred vision, double vision, or movement problems and abnormal sensations in scattered parts of the body. Symptoms that fluctuate and a pattern of relapses and remissions support the diagnosis.

When doctors suspect multiple sclerosis, they thoroughly evaluate the nervous system during a physical examination.▲ The optic nerve may be inflamed or unusually pale, as detected by examination of the back of the eye (retina) with an ophthalmoscope.■

No single test is diagnostic, but laboratory tests can help doctors distinguish multiple sclerosis from other disorders that produce similar symptoms, such as AIDS, amyotrophic lateral sclerosis (Lou Gehrig's disease), arteritis, arthritis of the neck, Guillain-Barré syndrome, hereditary ataxias, lupus, Lyme disease, rupture of a spinal disk, syphilis, and a cyst in the spinal cord (syringomyelia).

Doctors may perform a spinal tap (lumbar puncture★) to obtain a sample of cerebrospinal fluid. The white blood cell count and protein content of the fluid may be higher than normal. The concentration of antibodies in the cerebrospinal fluid may be high, and a specific pattern of antibodies is detected in up to 90% of people with multiple sclerosis.

Magnetic resonance imaging (MRI) is the best imaging procedure for detecting multiple sclerosis and is used to confirm the diagnosis. It usually detects areas of demyelination in the brain and spinal cord. MRI with gadolinium, a paramagnetic contrast agent, helps distinguish areas of recent demyelination and active inflammation from areas of long-standing demyelination.

A procedure involving evoked responses● may be performed. Sensory stimuli, such as flashing lights, are used to activate certain areas of the brain, and the brain's electrical responses are recorded. In people with multiple sclerosis, the brain's response to stimuli may be slow because signal conduction along demyelinated nerve fibers is impaired. This procedure can also detect slight damage to the optic nerve.

Treatment

No treatment for multiple sclerosis is uniformly effective. Corticosteroids, the main form of therapy, are given for short periods to relieve immediate symptoms. For example, prednisone may be taken by mouth, or methylprednisolone may be given intravenously. Corticosteroids seem to work by suppressing the immune system. Although corticosteroids may shorten the duration of relapses, they do not stop disability from progressing over the long term.

Corticosteroids given intravenously are recommended for people who have inflammation of the optic nerve but do not have other symptoms of multiple sclerosis. For these people, taking corticosteroids by mouth may increase the risk of developing other symptoms of multiple sclerosis.

Corticosteroids are rarely used for a long time, because they can cause many side effects, such as increased susceptibility to infection, diabetes, weight gain, fatigue, decreased bone density (osteoporosis), and ulcers. Corticosteroids are started and stopped as needed.

Interferon-beta injections reduce the frequency of relapses and may help prevent or delay later disability. Glatiramer acetate injections may have similar benefits for people with early mild multiple sclerosis. The chemotherapy drug mitoxantrone can reduce the frequency of relapses and slow the progression

---

▲ see page 439   ■ see box on page 1284

★ see art on page 443   ● see page 446

of the disease. It can be given for only up to 3 years because it can eventually lead to heart damage. These drugs work by interfering with the immune system's attack on myelin sheaths.

Other promising treatments include other types of interferons and gamma globulins, which help keep the body from attacking its own myelin. The benefits of plasmapheresis (a procedure in which blood is withdrawn, the abnormal antibodies are removed from it, and the blood is returned to the person▲) have not been established. However, some experts continue to recommend it for severe relapses not controlled by corticosteroids.

Other drugs can be used to treat specific symptoms. For example, baclofen, tizanidine, or the sedative diazepam can relieve muscle spasms. Oxybutynin, bethanechol, or tamsulosin can help control urinary incontinence. The anticonvulsant gabapentin may be used to relieve the pain due to abnormalities in the nervous system. The beta-blocker propranolol may reduce the severity of tremors. Amantadine, a drug sometimes used to treat influenza, may help relieve fatigue. Antidepressants such as sertraline or amitriptyline may be given to treat depression.

People with multiple sclerosis can often maintain an active lifestyle, although they may tire easily and may not be able to keep up with a demanding schedule. Regular exercise such as riding a stationary bicycle, walking, swimming, or stretching reduces spasticity and helps maintain cardiovascular, muscular, and psychologic health. Physical therapy can help with maintaining balance, walking ability, and range of motion as well as reduce spasticity and weakness. Avoiding high temperatures—for example, by not taking hot baths or showers—can help prevent the aggravation of symptoms.

People with urine retention can learn to catheterize themselves to empty the bladder, and those with constipation can take stool softeners or laxatives regularly. People who become weak and unable to move easily may develop bedsores (pressure sores), so they and their caregivers must take extra care to prevent bedsores.■

▲ see box on page 986   ■ see page 1209
★ see also page 539

Other Primary Demyelinating Diseases

Acute disseminated encephalomyelitis (parainfectious or postinfectious encephalomyelitis) is a rare type of inflammation leading to demyelination of nerves in the brain and spinal cord. It usually develops after a viral infection (such as measles, chickenpox, or rubella) or vaccination. It is thought to be a misguided immune reaction triggered by the virus. Typically, the inflammation develops 5 to 10 days after the viral illness begins. It can be treated with corticosteroids given intravenously. Guillain-Barré syndrome seems to be a similar disorder of the peripheral nerves.

Adrenoleukodystrophy and **adrenomyeloneuropathy** are rare hereditary metabolic disorders. Adrenoleukodystrophy affects young boys, usually by the age of 7. A more slowly developing form of the disorder can begin in adults in their 20s. Adrenomyeloneuropathy affects adolescent boys. In these disorders, widespread demyelination is accompanied by adrenal gland dysfunction. Eventually, mental deterioration, spasticity, and blindness occur. No cure for either disorder is known. Dietary supplements with glycerol trioleate and glycerol trierucate (known as Lorenzo's oil) have not been shown to slow the progression of the disease. Bone marrow transplantation is an experimental treatment.

Leber's hereditary optic neuropathy causes demyelination leading to partial blindness. The disorder is more common among men. Usually, symptoms begin in the late teens or early 20s. This disorder is inherited through the mother, and the defective genes seem to be located in mitochondria, which are structures in cells that provide energy for the cell.

Tropical spastic paraparesis (HTLV-associated myelopathy★), a disorder that causes demyelination in the spinal cord, results from infection with the human T-cell lymphotropic virus (HTLV). The disorder worsens over several years, leading to gradual spasticity and weakness of the legs as well as frequent, strong urges to urinate, urinary incontinence, and bowel dysfunction. No cure is available, but use of corticosteroids has produced improvement, and plasmapheresis has produced temporary improvement.

CHAPTER 93

Spinal Cord Disorders

The spinal cord is the main pathway of communication between the brain and the rest of the body. It is a long, fragile, tubelike structure that extends downward from the base of the brain. The cord is protected by the back bones (vertebrae) of the spine (spinal column), which are separated and cushioned by disks made of cartilage.

Along the length of the spinal cord, 31 pairs of spinal nerves emerge through spaces between the vertebrae. The spinal nerves connect with nerves throughout the body. Each spinal nerve has two nerve roots (except the first, which has no sensory root). The root in the front, the motor root, transmits impulses from the spinal cord to the muscles. The root in the back, the sensory root, carries sensory information (about touch, position, pain, and temperature) from the body to the spinal cord.

The spinal cord is highly organized;▲ nerve pathways with similar functions are grouped together. The motor nerves, which transmit information to muscles and thus stimulate movement, are grouped together, as are the sensory nerves, which transmit sensory information to the brain. The motor and sensory nerves of the spinal cord connect with the motor and sensory roots of the spinal nerves, respectively.

Because of the function and organization of the spinal cord, damage to the cord can produce various patterns of symptoms, such as numbness, weakness, loss of sensation, loss of bowel and bladder function, and paralysis, as well as back pain. These patterns enable doctors to determine the location (level) of spinal cord damage.

Some spinal cord disorders originate outside the cord. They include injuries, infections, blockage of the blood supply, and compression. The spinal cord may be compressed by bone (as in cervical spondylosis or a fracture), an accumulation of blood (hematoma), a tumor, a localized collection of pus (abscess), or a ruptured or herniated disk. Other spinal cord disorders originate within the cord. They include fluid-filled cavities (syrinxes), acute transverse myelitis, tumors, abscesses, bleeding (hemorrhage), and multiple sclerosis.

Accident-Related Injuries

When the spinal cord is injured in an accident, it may be severed, jarred (by a blunt injury), or compressed (by broken bones, swelling, or bleeding).

Because of the way the cord is organized, injury to the spinal cord always results in loss of function below the site of the injury. For example, if the spinal cord is severely damaged in the middle of the back, the arms function normally but the legs may be paralyzed. Sensation in the affected area as well as muscle control is usually lost.

Reflex movements that are not controlled by the brain remain intact or may even be exaggerated below the site of the injury. An example is the knee jerk reflex, in which a tap with a small hammer just below the knee normally causes the lower leg to jerk upward. When the spinal cord is injured, a spastic type of paralysis with leg spasms may result: The muscles controlled by the knee jerk reflex tighten, feel hard, and twitch from time to time, causing the legs to jerk.

Paralysis and loss of sensation may be partial or total, temporary or permanent. An injury that severs the cord or destroys nerve pathways in the spinal cord causes permanent loss, but a blunt injury that jars the cord may cause temporary loss, which can last days, weeks, or months. Recovery is more likely if paralysis is incomplete and movement or sensation returns during the first week after the injury. If function is not regained within 6 months, loss is likely to be permanent.

People who are weak or paralyzed because of a spinal cord injury are at risk of developing bedsores, urinary tract infections, and pneumonia.

Treatment

The first goal is to prevent further damage. Emergency personnel take great care when moving a person with a possible spinal cord injury. Usually, the person is strapped to a firm board and carefully padded to prevent movement. When the spinal cord is damaged,

▲ see art on page 436

Which Area of the Spine Is Damaged?

The spine (spinal column) is divided into four areas: cervical (neck), thoracic (chest), lumbar (lower back), and sacral (pelvis). Each area is referred to by a letter (C, T, L, or S). The vertebrae in each area of the spine are numbered beginning at the top. For example, the first vertebra in the cervical spine is labeled C1, the second in the cervical spine is C2, the second in the thoracic spine is T2, the fourth in the lumbar spine is L4, and so forth.

Nerves run from the spine to specific areas of the body. By noting where a person has weakness, paralysis, or other loss of function (and thus nerve damage), a neurologist can trace back and pinpoint where the spine is damaged.

Effects of Spinal Injury

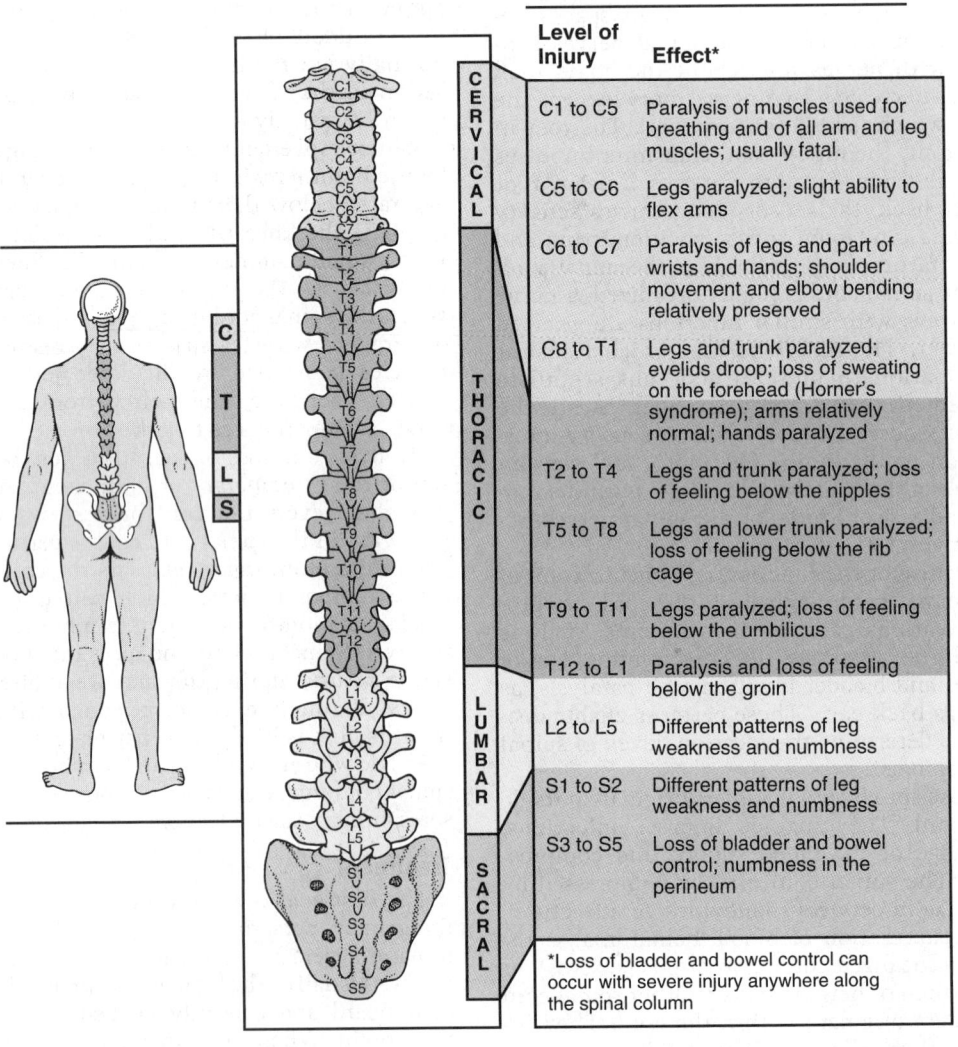

Level of Injury	Effect*
C1 to C5	Paralysis of muscles used for breathing and of all arm and leg muscles; usually fatal.
C5 to C6	Legs paralyzed; slight ability to flex arms
C6 to C7	Paralysis of legs and part of wrists and hands; shoulder movement and elbow bending relatively preserved
C8 to T1	Legs and trunk paralyzed; eyelids droop; loss of sweating on the forehead (Horner's syndrome); arms relatively normal; hands paralyzed
T2 to T4	Legs and trunk paralyzed; loss of feeling below the nipples
T5 to T8	Legs and lower trunk paralyzed; loss of feeling below the rib cage
T9 to T11	Legs paralyzed; loss of feeling below the umbilicus
T12 to L1	Paralysis and loss of feeling below the groin
L2 to L5	Different patterns of leg weakness and numbness
S1 to S2	Different patterns of leg weakness and numbness
S3 to S5	Loss of bladder and bowel control; numbness in the perineum

*Loss of bladder and bowel control can occur with severe injury anywhere along the spinal column

Dermatomes

The skin surface is divided into specific areas, called dermatomes, each of which is supplied by sensory nerve fibers of a single spinal nerve root. For the 7 cervical vertebrae, there are 8 pairs of sensory nerve roots—one of each pair on each side of the body. Each of the 12 thoracic, 5 lumbar, and 5 sacral vertebrae has one pair of spinal nerve roots—one root on each side of the body. In addition, there is a pair of coccygeal nerve roots, which supply a small area of the skin around the tailbone (coccyx). Sensory information from a specific dermatome is carried by sensory nerve fibers to the spinal nerve root of a specific vertebra. For example, sensory information from a strip of skin along the lower back, the outside of the thigh, the inside of the lower leg, and the heel is carried by sensory nerve fibers of the sciatic nerve to the fifth lumbar vertebra (L5).

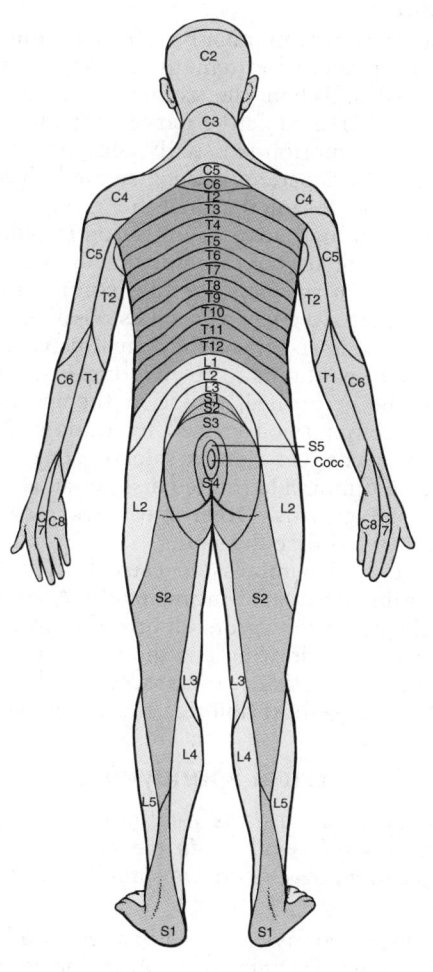

even slight shifting of the spine increases the possibility of permanent paralysis.

Usually, doctors immediately give corticosteroids (such as methylprednisolone) by injection to help prevent swelling around the injury. The drugs must be started within 8 hours of the injury to be effective and should be continued for about 24 hours. Muscle relaxants (such as cyclobenzaprine) and analgesics (such as ibuprofen) may be given to treat spasms. If the spine has been fractured or otherwise injured, a surgeon may implant steel rods to stabilize it because further movement may cause additional injury. A neurosurgeon removes any blood and bone fragments that have accumulated around the spinal cord.

While the spinal cord or spine is healing, skilled nursing care is needed to prevent complications. To help prevent bedsores (pressure sores)▲, nurses can inspect the person's skin daily, keep the skin dry and clean, and turn the person frequently. When necessary, a special bed called a Stryker frame is used. It can be turned to shift pressure on the body from front to back and from side to side. A urinary catheter may be needed if the person is immobile and cannot use a toilet. To help reduce the risk of a urinary tract infection, nurses can use sterile techniques when the catheter is inserted and apply antimicrobial ointments or solutions daily. To help reduce the risk of pneumonia, therapists and nurses can teach the person deep breathing exercises and use techniques such as placing the person at an angle to help drain secretions that accumulate in the lungs (postural drainage).

Extensive loss of body functions can be devastating, causing depression and loss of self-esteem. Learning exactly what has happened and what to expect in the near and distant future helps people cope with the loss. Physical and occupational therapy■ helps preserve muscle function. Therapists teach people special techniques to help them overcome lost functions. For most people, compassionate and skilled nursing care, psychologic counseling, and emotional support from family members and close friends help. Family members may also benefit from counseling.

Spinal Cord Compression

Normally the spinal cord is protected by the spine, but certain disorders may put pressure

▲ see page 1209   ■ see pages 38 and 39

on the spinal cord, disrupting its normal function. The spinal cord may be compressed suddenly, producing symptoms in minutes or over a few hours or days, or slowly, producing symptoms that progress over many weeks or months.

Sudden compression usually results from an injury, which can cause a fracture or dislocation of a vertebra. Sudden compression may also result from bleeding, an infection, an abscess, or a ruptured or herniated disk in the spine.▲

Slowly developing compression may be due to a tumor in the spinal cord or spine, an infection, a blood vessel (arteriovenous) malformation, or an abnormal bone growth. Spinal stenosis (narrowing of the spinal canal) can gradually compress the cord, causing back pain. An injury, cancer, or osteoporosis may cause vertebrae to collapse, compressing the spinal cord. Collapse of a vertebra is called a compression fracture.■

Symptoms

If compression of the spinal cord is minimal, only some nerve signals going up and down the spinal cord may be disrupted. Symptoms may include discomfort only in the back, minor weakness, tingling, other changes in sensation, or erectile dysfunction (impotence). If compression increases, symptoms may worsen. If compression is great, most nerve signals may be blocked, causing severe weakness, numbness, incontinence or retention of urine, and loss of bowel control. If all nerve signals are blocked, paralysis and complete loss of sensation result. A beltlike band of discomfort may be felt at the level of spinal cord compression. Once spinal cord compression begins to cause symptoms, the damage usually worsens from minimal to substantial unpredictably but rapidly in a few hours to a few days.

Diagnosis

Because the spinal cord is organized in a specific way, doctors can determine which part of the spinal cord is affected based on the symptoms and results of a physical examination. For example, if the legs (but not the arms) are weak and numb and bladder and bowel function are impaired, the midchest (thoracic) area of the spine may be damaged. The location of

pain or tenderness along the spine also helps doctors determine the site of the damage.

Magnetic resonance imaging (MRI) or myelography with computed tomography (CT) usually shows where the spinal cord is compressed and may indicate the cause. MRI or myelography with CT can detect a fracture or dislocation of a vertebra, a ruptured or herniated disk, an abnormal bone growth, an area of bleeding, an abscess, or a tumor.

The cause of the compression can be identified when surgery is performed immediately to relieve the pressure on the spinal cord. If surgery is not needed immediately or cannot be performed, a biopsy with a needle is performed to identify the cause. Placement of the needle is guided by CT. Occasionally, a biopsy is performed to determine whether an abnormal growth or a tumor is cancerous.

Treatment

The compression must be relieved immediately to prevent permanent damage to the spinal cord. When the compression is detected and treated before nerve pathways are destroyed, function is usually completely recovered. Corticosteroids (such as methylprednisolone or dexamethasone) are given intravenously in high doses by injection to reduce swelling in or around the spinal cord. Swelling may be contributing to the compression. These drugs are given as soon as possible, but if the cause is an injury, they must usually be given within 8 hours to be effective. If surgery cannot be performed, radiation therapy may relieve compression caused by tumors. Surgery is needed to remove blood, bone fragments, a tumor, a herniated disk, or an abnormal bone growth. Other measures may be needed to stabilize the spine.

Spinal cord compression caused by an abscess must be treated immediately. A doctor, usually a neurosurgeon, drains the abscess, sometimes by drawing out the pus through a syringe. Alternatively, the abscess can be surgically removed. Antibiotics are also given.

Cervical Spondylosis

Cervical spondylosis is a disorder in which the disks and vertebrae in the neck degenerate, putting pressure on the spinal cord in the neck.

Cervical spondylosis usually affects middle-aged and older people. With aging, the bone of the spine overgrows and narrows the spinal

---

▲ see art on page 570   ■ see page 357

canal in the neck. As a result, the spinal cord or the spinal nerve roots (the part of spinal nerves located next to the cord▲) are compressed, causing dysfunction.

Symptoms

Symptoms may reflect compression of the spinal cord, the spinal nerve roots, or both. If the spinal cord is compressed, a change in walking is usually the first sign. Leg movements may become jerky (spastic), and walking becomes unsteady. The neck may be painful. If the spinal nerve roots are compressed, weakness in one or both arms may develop, and the muscles may waste away. The neck is likely to be painful. Nerve root compression may be accompanied by or progress to spinal cord compression.

Diagnosis and Treatment

When doctors suspect cervical spondylosis, magnetic resonance imaging (MRI) or myelography with computed tomography (CT) is performed. MRI provides slightly more information, but myelography with CT may be more available. These procedures show where the spinal canal is narrowed, how compressed it is, and which spinal nerve roots may be affected. MRI has generally replaced x-rays of the neck.

Without treatment, spinal cord dysfunction due to cervical spondylosis sometimes lessens or stabilizes, but it may progress. Initially, a soft neck collar, neck traction, nonsteroidal anti-inflammatory drugs (NSAIDs) such as ibuprofen,■ and muscle relaxants such as cyclobenzaprine may provide relief. However, when the disorder progresses or when MRI shows severe compression or collapsed or displaced vertebrae, surgery is usually needed. As a rule, surgery does not reverse changes that have already occurred, because the pathways in the spinal cord become permanently damaged unless the disorder is treated very early.

Spinal Hematoma

A spinal hematoma is an accumulation of blood around the spinal cord.

A spinal hematoma may result from a back injury, a blood vessel (arteriovenous) malformation, a tumor, use of anticoagulants, or a bleeding disorder. A hematoma can compress the spinal cord. Hematomas within the spinal cord, often caused by injuries, are a common cause of compression. Hematomas outside the spinal cord are a relatively rare cause.

What Is the Cauda Equina Syndrome?

The bundle of nerves extending from the bottom of the spinal cord is called the cauda equina because it resembles a horse's tail. The cauda equina may be compressed by a ruptured or herniated disk, a tumor, an abscess, damage due to an injury, or swelling due to inflammation (as in ankylosing spondylitis). The symptoms that result are called the cauda equina syndrome. Pain is felt in the lower back, but sensation is reduced in the area of the body that would come in contact with a saddle (a condition called saddle anesthesia), including the buttocks, thighs, bladder, and rectum. Other symptoms include erectile dysfunction (impotence), urinary incontinence at night, and loss of reflexes in the ankle. If compression is great enough, bladder and bowel function may be lost. People who have this syndrome require immediate medical attention. The disorder causing the compression is treated, sometimes with surgery, and corticosteroids may be given to reduce swelling.

Symptoms

A spinal hematoma usually causes sudden pain and tenderness in the affected area, followed by weakness and loss of sensation below the level of the hematoma. Weakness may progress to complete paralysis in minutes or hours, although some people recover spontaneously. If an arteriovenous malformation near the spinal cord ruptures, blood flows upward into the brain, causing headaches and neck stiffness. A hematoma or an injury near the top of the spinal cord can interfere with breathing, because the nerves that supply the diaphragm originate there.

Diagnosis and Treatment

Doctors make a tentative diagnosis based on the symptoms and usually confirm it with magnetic resonance imaging (MRI). Myelography with computed tomography (CT)★ is sometimes used when MRI is not available.

Immediate removal of the accumulated blood by surgical drainage may prevent perma-

---

▲ see art on page 436   ■ see page 452
★ see page 445

nent injury to the spinal cord. Surgery using special techniques (microsurgery) can sometimes correct an arteriovenous malformation. People who are taking anticoagulants or who have a bleeding disorder are given injections of vitamin K and transfusions of plasma to eliminate or reduce the tendency to bleed. If the top of the spinal cord is damaged, a mechanical ventilator is often needed to assist breathing.

Syrinx

A syrinx is a fluid-filled cavity that develops in the spinal cord (called a syringomyelia), in the brain stem (called a syringobulbia), or in both.

Syrinxes are rare. In about half of the people who have a syrinx, it is present at birth, and then for poorly understood reasons, it enlarges during the teen or young adult years. Often, children who have a syrinx at birth also have other abnormalities. Usually, syrinxes that develop later in life are due to injury or tumors. About 30% of spinal cord tumors eventually result in a syrinx.

Symptoms

Syrinxes that grow in the spinal cord press on it from within. Although most common in the neck, a syrinx can occur anywhere along the length of the spinal cord and often extends to affect a long segment of the cord. Usually, the nerves that detect pain and temperature changes are most affected. Cuts and burns are common, because people with this type of nerve damage cannot feel pain or heat. As a syrinx extends further, it can cause spasms and weakness, usually beginning in the arms. Eventually, the muscles supplied by the affected nerves may begin to waste away.

Syrinxes in the brain stem can produce vertigo, nystagmus (rapid movement of the eyes in one direction followed by a slower drift back to the original position), unusual sensations (such as pins-and-needles) in the face, loss of taste, difficulty speaking, difficulty swallowing, and weakness and wasting away (atrophy) of the tongue.

Diagnosis and Treatment

Doctors may suspect a syrinx in a young child or teenager on the basis of symptoms. Magnetic resonance imaging (MRI) with a paramagnetic contrast agent, such as gadolinium, can outline the syrinx (and a tumor if present).

A neurosurgeon may make a hole in a syrinx to drain it and prevent it from expanding, but surgery does not always correct the problem. Even if the surgery successfully drains the syrinx, the nervous system may already be damaged irreversibly. Symptoms may not be relieved, or the syrinx may recur.

Hereditary Spastic Paraparesis

Hereditary spastic paraparesis is a rare hereditary disorder in which the legs gradually become spastic and weak.

Hereditary (familial) spastic paraparesis, also known as Strümpell-Lorrain disease, affects both sexes and may begin at any age. It affects about 3 of 100,000 people. Usually, the gene for this disorder is dominant;▲ therefore, children of a person who has the disorder have a 50% chance of developing it.

Symptoms and Diagnosis

Reflexes become exaggerated, and leg cramps, twitches, and spasms occur, making leg movements stiff and jerky. Walking becomes gradually more difficult. People may stumble or trip because they drag their toes. Babinski's sign, an abnormal reflex of the toes, may be present. Fatigue is common. In some people, muscles in the arms also become weak and stiff. Usually the symptoms continue to slowly worsen, but sometimes they level off after adolescence. Lifespan is not affected.

About 10% of people who have hereditary spastic paraparesis have other neurologic abnormalities, such as eye problems, lack of muscle control, hearing loss, mental retardation, dementia, and peripheral nerve disorders.

The disorder is diagnosed by excluding other disorders that produce similar symptoms (such as multiple sclerosis and spinal cord compression) and by determining whether other family members have hereditary spastic paraparesis. In the future, blood tests to detect the genes that cause the disorder may be available.

Treatment

Treatment is aimed at relieving symptoms. Physical therapy and exercise can help maintain mobility and muscle strength, improve range of motion and endurance, reduce fatigue, and prevent cramps and spasms.

▲ see page 12

Baclofen is the drug of choice to reduce spasticity. Alternatively, tizanadine, diazepam, clonazepam, or dantrolene may be used. Some people may benefit from using splints, a cane, or crutches. A few people require a wheelchair.

Acute Transverse Myelitis

Acute transverse myelitis is a localized inflammation of the spinal cord that blocks transmission of nerve impulses up and down the spinal cord.

The cause of acute transverse myelitis is unknown, but it may result from an autoimmune reaction (in which the immune system misinterprets the body's tissues as foreign and attacks them). About 30 to 40% of people with this disorder develop it after an otherwise minor viral infection. People who have multiple sclerosis or certain bacterial infections (such as Lyme disease, syphilis, or tuberculosis) and those who inject heroin or amphetamine intravenously are at increased risk of developing acute transverse myelitis.

Symptoms

Acute transverse myelitis usually begins with sudden back pain, followed by numbness and muscle weakness that start in the feet and move upward. Commonly, a beltlike tightness is felt around the chest or stomach at the level affected by the myelitis. People may have difficulty urinating. These effects may worsen over several hours or several days and may become severe, resulting in paralysis, loss of sensation, and loss of bladder and bowel control. The degree of disability depends on the location (level) of the inflammation in the spinal cord and the severity of the inflammation.

Diagnosis and Treatment

Acute transverse myelitis must be distinguished from other disorders that cause similar symptoms, such as Guillain-Barré syndrome, spinal cord compression, or blockage of the blood supply to the spinal cord. To exclude other possible diagnoses, doctors may perform a spinal tap (lumbar puncture).▲ In people with acute transverse myelitis, the number of certain types of white blood cells and the protein level in the spinal fluid are usually increased, but these findings are not conclusive. Magnetic resonance imaging (MRI) can detect swelling of the spinal cord. Blood tests are rarely helpful.

High doses of corticosteroids such as prednisone are often given to suppress the immune system, which is thought to be involved in acute transverse myelitis. However, the benefit of these drugs has been shown only in people who also have multiple sclerosis.

Most people with acute transverse myelitis recover at least partially, and many recover completely. However, many others continue to have weakness and numbness. Generally, the more quickly symptoms develop, the better the chance of recovery.

Blockage of the Blood Supply

Like all tissues in the body, the spinal cord requires a constant supply of oxygenated blood. Branches of the aorta supply most of the blood to the front part of the spinal cord. Blockage of any one of these arteries may be disastrous. Such a blockage occasionally results from severe atherosclerosis of the aorta, separation of the layers of the aorta's wall (aortic dissection), or a blood clot that breaks off from the wall of the heart and travels through the bloodstream (becoming an embolus). Occasionally, surgery to repair a bulge (aneurysm) in the abdominal aorta results in a blockage of an artery supplying the spinal cord.

Symptoms

The first symptoms are usually sudden back pain and pain in the areas supplied by the nerves branching from the affected area of the spinal cord. The pain is followed by weakness and an inability to feel heat, cold, or pain in areas below the level where the blood supply has been blocked. Symptoms are most noticeable during the first few days and may resolve, at least partially, over time. The blood supply to the front of the spinal cord is greatly reduced, but the back of the cord is unaffected because it receives blood from other sources. Therefore, the legs, which are controlled by the front part of the cord, are numb and paralyzed, but sensations transmitted in the back of the cord—including touch, the ability to feel vibration, and the ability to sense where the limbs are without looking at them (position sense)—remain intact.

Weakness and paralysis can lead to the development of bedsores and breathing difficulties. Bladder and bowel function may be impaired as may sexual function.

▲ see art on page 443

Diagnosis and Treatment

The diagnosis is usually based on symptoms. Magnetic resonance imaging (MRI) or myelography▲ can help doctors rule out other disorders that cause similar symptoms. A spinal tap■ may be performed to rule out transverse myelitis as the cause of the symptoms. Angiography can confirm that the artery to the front of the spinal cord is blocked, but it is usually unnecessary.

Treatment is aimed at relieving symptoms. Because some sensations are lost and paralysis may develop, preventing bedsores (pressure sores) from forming is important. Therapy to help fluids drain from the lungs (such as deep breathing exercises, postural drainage, and suctioning may be necessary. Physical and occupational therapy★ may be needed to help preserve muscle function. If bladder function is impaired, a catheter to drain urine from the bladder may be needed.

Subacute Combined Degeneration of the Spinal Cord

Subacute combined degeneration of the spinal cord is a progressive disorder that is due to vitamin B_{12} deficiency and produces weakness, clumsiness, tingling, and other abnormal sensations.

This disorder affects about 1 of 10,000 people, usually those who are older than 40. It is due to a deficiency of vitamin B_{12}, which typically also causes pernicious anemia. Usually,

the deficiency is not related to diet but to the body's inability to absorb vitamin B_{12} from the intestine. In this disorder, the columns of sensory nerve fibers in the spinal cord degenerate. The brain, nerves of the eyes, and peripheral nerves are sometimes damaged.

The disorder begins with a general feeling of weakness. Tingling, a pins-and-needles sensation, and numbness are felt in both hands and feet. These sensations tend to be constant and to gradually worsen. People who have this disorder may not be able to feel vibrations and may lose the sense of where their limbs are (position sense). The limbs feel stiff, movements become clumsy, and walking may become difficult. Reflexes may be decreased, increased, or absent. Vision may be reduced.

People who have this disorder may become irritable, apathetic, drowsy, suspicious, and confused. Their emotions may change rapidly and unpredictably. Rarely, dementia develops.

The diagnosis is made based on blood tests to measure levels of vitamin B_{12} and its breakdown products (metabolites).

Recovery is more likely if the disorder is treated early. When treated within a few weeks after symptoms appear, most people recover completely. If treatment is delayed, the progression of symptoms may be slowed or stopped, but recovery of lost function is unlikely. Injections of vitamin B_{12} should be given immediately and must be continued indefinitely to prevent symptoms from recurring. For some people, large doses of vitamin B_{12} taken by mouth are equally effective.

CHAPTER 94

Low Back Pain

Low back pain is very common. It affects 4 of 5 people at some time during their lives. It is the leading cause of disability for those aged 19 to 45 and is the second most common cause of missed work days (after the common cold) for adults younger than 45. Low back

pain becomes more common as people age. It affects half of the people older than 60 at any given time. Each year, the treatment of low back pain costs more than $80 billion, and insurance claims for disability due to low back pain exceed $8 billion. Thus, although low back pain rarely results from life-threatening disorders, it is a significant health problem. However, the number of back injuries in the workplace is decreasing, perhaps because

---

▲ see page 445   ■ see art on page 443
★ see pages 38 and 39

awareness of the problem has increased and preventive measures have improved.

The spine (spinal column) consists of the back bones (vertebrae), which are separated and cushioned by shock-absorbing disks made of cartilage. The vertebrae are also covered by a thin layer of cartilage. They are held in place by ligaments and muscles, which help stabilize the spine. These muscles include the two iliopsoas muscles (which run along both sides of the spine), the two erector spinae muscles (which run along the length of the spine behind it), and the many short paraspinal muscles (which run between the vertebrae). The abdominal muscles (which run from the bottom of the rib cage to the pelvis) also help stabilize the spine.

Enclosed in the spine is the spinal cord.▲ Along the length of the spinal cord, the spinal nerves emerge through spaces between the vertebrae to connect with nerves throughout the body. The part of the spinal nerve nearest the spinal cord is called the spinal nerve root. Because of their position, spinal nerve roots can be compressed when the spine is injured, resulting in pain.

The lower (lumbar) spine consists of five vertebrae. It connects the chest to the pelvis and legs, providing mobility—for turning, twisting, and bending. It also provides strength—for standing, walking, and lifting. Thus, the lower back is involved in almost all activities of daily living. Low back pain can limit many activities and reduce the quality of life.

Causes

Low back pain has many causes, although often no specific cause can be identified.

One of the most common causes is muscle and ligament strains and sprains. Strains and sprains may result from lifting, exercising, or moving in an unexpected way (such as when falling or when in a car accident). When due to exercise, injury to the lower back is sometimes called weight lifter's back (lumbar strain). Weight lifter's back may be caused not only by snatching a heavy weight from the ground in weight lifting but also by pushing against an opposing lineman in football, suddenly turning to dribble after a rebound in basketball, swinging a bat in baseball, or swinging a club in golf. The lower back is more likely to be injured when a person's physical conditioning is poor and the supporting muscles of the back are weak. Having poor posture, lifting improperly, being overweight, and being tired also contribute.

Osteoarthritis (degenerative arthritis) causes the cartilage that covers and protects the vertebrae to deteriorate. This disorder is thought to be due, at least in part, to the wear and tear of years of use. The disks between the vertebrae deteriorate, narrowing the spaces there and compressing spinal nerve roots. Irregular projections of bone (spurs) may develop on the vertebrae and also compress spinal nerve roots. All of these changes can cause low back pain as well as stiffness.

In osteoporosis, bone density decreases, making the bones more likely to fracture. The vertebrae are particularly susceptible to the effects of osteoporosis, often resulting in crush (compression) fractures (which may cause sudden, severe back pain) and compression of spinal nerve roots (which may cause chronic back pain). However, most fractures due to osteoporosis occur in the upper and middle back and cause upper and middle rather than low back pain.

A ruptured or herniated disk can cause low back pain. A disk has a tough covering and a soft, jelly-like interior. If a disk is suddenly squeezed by the vertebrae above and below it (as when lifting a heavy object), the covering may tear (rupture), causing pain. The interior of the disk can squeeze through the tear in the covering, so that part of the interior bulges out (herniates). This bulge can compress, irritate, and even damage the spinal nerve root next to it, causing more pain. A ruptured or herniated disk also commonly causes sciatica.

In older people, a common cause of low back pain is spinal stenosis (narrowing of the spinal canal, the passageway that runs through the center of the spine and contains the spinal cord). Spinal stenosis also develops in middle-aged people who were born with a narrow spinal canal. It is caused by such disorders as osteoarthritis and Paget's disease. Spinal stenosis may cause sciatica as well as low back pain.

In ankylosing spondylitis, the spine and large joints are inflamed, resulting in stiffness and back pain. This disorder is more common among men, usually starting between the ages of 20 and 40.

Sometimes low back pain is referred pain,■ which originates in another part of the body, such as the kidneys, bladder, uterus, or prostate, but is felt in the lower back. For example, pre-

---

▲ see pages 435 and 561   ■ see art on page 448

A Herniated Disk

The tough covering of a disk in the spine can tear (rupture), causing pain. The soft, jelly-like interior may bulge out (herniate) through the covering, causing more pain. Pain occurs because the bulge puts pressure on the spinal nerve root next to it. Sometimes the nerve is damaged.

More than 80% of herniated disks occur in the lower back. They are most common among people aged 30 to 50 years. Between these ages, the covering weakens. The interior, which is under high pressure, may squeeze through a tear or a weakened spot in the covering and bulge out. After age 50, the interior of the disk begins to harden, making a herniation less likely. A disk may herniate because of a sudden, traumatic injury or repeated minor injuries. Being overweight or lifting heavy objects, particularly lifting improperly, increases the risk.

Where the pain occurs depends on which disk is herniated and which spinal nerve root is affected. The pain is felt along the pathway of the nerve compressed by the herniated disk. For example, a herniated disk commonly causes sciatica. The pain varies from slight to debilitating, and movement intensifies the pain. Numbness and muscle weakness may also occur. If the pressure on the nerve root is great, the legs may be paralyzed. If the cauda equina (the bundle of nerves extending from the bottom of the cord) is affected, control of bladder and bowels can be lost. If these serious symptoms develop, medical attention is required immediately.

After about 2 weeks, many people recover without any treatment. Applying cold (such as ice packs) or heat (such as a heating pad) or using over-the-counter analgesics may help relieve the pain. Sometimes surgery to remove part or all the disk and part of a vertebra is necessary. In 10 to 20% of people who undergo surgery for sciatica due to a herniated disk, another disk ruptures.

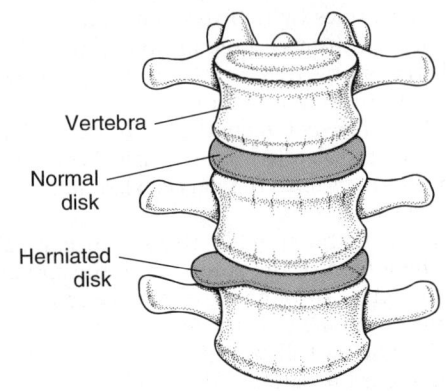

Front View

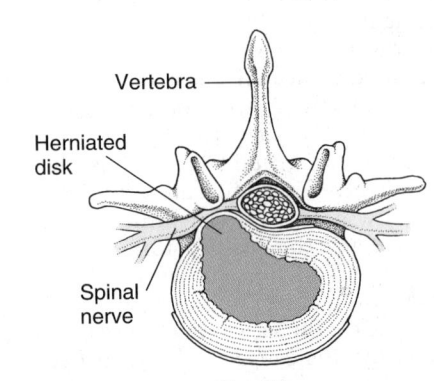

Top View

menstrual syndrome or a bladder infection can cause low back pain.

Other less common causes of low back pain include shingles; cancer that has spread to the spine from organs such as the breast, lung, prostate, or kidney; bone cancer (multiple myeloma); fibromyalgia; and birth defects such as scoliosis. Stress may contribute to low back pain, but how it does so is unclear. Heavy physical labor, obesity, smoking, and lack of exercise also contribute to low back pain.

Symptoms and Types of Low Back Pain

Low back pain may be intermittent or constant; superficial or deep; or dull and aching, throbbing, or sharp and stabbing, depending on the cause and type of pain. There are several types of low back pain.

Local pain occurs in a specific area of the lower back. It is usually due to sprains and strains. Sudden pain may be felt when the injury occurs. Local pain can often be relieved by changes in position or by light activity followed by stretching. Intense physical activity or inactivity tends to make it worse. Local pain may be constant and aching or, at times, can be intermittent and sharp. The lower back may be sore when touched. Muscle spasms may develop because the body moves in unusual ways as it tries to avoid the movements that trigger pain. Usually, local pain resolves gradually over days to weeks.

Pain due to compression of a spinal nerve root may be due to such disorders as a herniated disk, osteoarthritis, osteoporosis, spinal stenosis, or Paget's disease. The pain often occurs within minutes or hours of lifting a very heavy weight, but it may occur spontaneously. This type of pain tends to be a dull ache with a sharp, intense radiating pain sometimes su-perimposed on it. The pain can radiate to different parts of the body, depending on which nerve root is affected. Commonly, the pain extends from the lower back into the buttock and down the leg on the affected side, causing sciatica. Coughing, sneezing, straining, or bending over while keeping the legs straight can evoke the sharp, radiating pain. If a herniated disk is the cause, the pain is worsened by walking a distance. If spinal stenosis is the cause, the pain is typically increased by straightening the back (for example, when walking) and is relieved by bending the spine forward (for example, when leaning forward). If a compression fracture is the cause, the pain usually starts suddenly, stays in a particular area of the back, and worsens when a person

What Is Sciatica?

The two sciatic nerves are the largest and longest nerves in the body. Each is almost as large as a finger. On each side of the body, the sciatic nerve runs from the lower spine, behind the hip joint, down the buttock and back of the knee. There the sciatic nerve divides into several branches and continues to the foot. When the sciatic nerve is pinched, inflamed, or damaged, pain—sciatica—may radiate along the length of the sciatic nerve to the foot. Sciatica occurs in about 5% of people who have back pain.

In some people, no cause can be detected. In others, the cause may be a herniated disk, irregular projections of bone due to osteoarthritis, or swelling due to a sprained ligament. Rarely, spinal stenosis, Paget's disease, nerve damage due to diabetes (diabetic neuropathy), a tumor, or a blood clot causes sciatica. Some people seem to be prone to sciatica.

Sciatica usually affects only one side. It may cause a pins-and-needles sensation, a nagging ache, or a shooting pain. Numbness may be felt in the leg or foot. Walking, running, climbing stairs, and straightening the leg worsens the pain, which is relieved by bending the back or sitting.

Often, the pain goes away on its own. Resting, sleeping on a firm mattress, taking over-the-counter nonsteroidal anti-inflammatory drugs (NSAIDs), and applying heat and cold may be sufficient treatment. For many people, sleeping on their side with the knees bent and a pillow between the knees provides relief. Stretching the hamstring muscles gently after warming up may help.

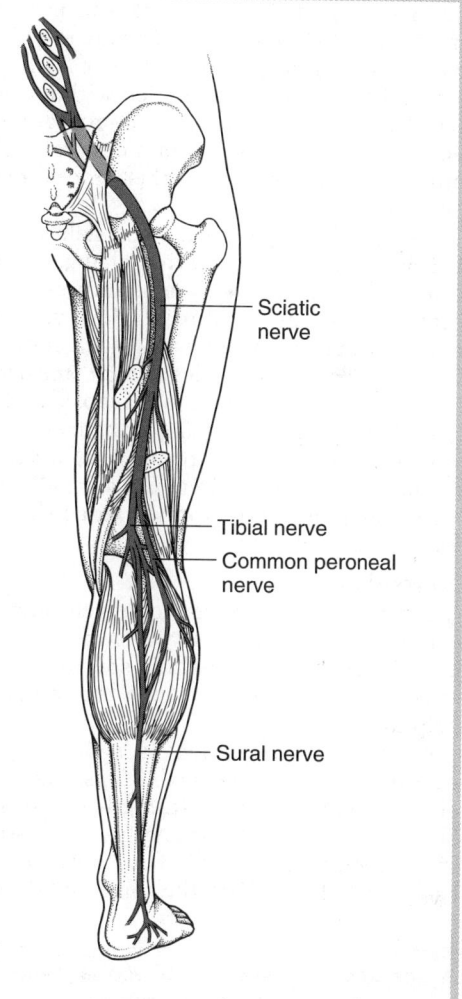

Sciatic nerve

Tibial nerve

Common peroneal nerve

Sural nerve

stands or walks. The area near the fracture may be tender.

Usually, the pain and tenderness disappear gradually after a few weeks or months. If pressure on the nerve root is great, the pain may be accompanied by muscle weakness in the leg, a pins-and-needles sensation, or even loss of sensation and of bladder and bowel control.

Referred pain (which originates in other organs)▲ tends to be deep, aching, constant, and relatively widespread (diffuse). Typically, movement does not affect it, and it worsens at night. For example, kidney infections can cause low back pain that is felt to the side rather than the center of the back.

Diagnosis

The symptoms, history, and results of a physical examination may suggest the cause of low back pain. As part of the physical examination, a doctor may ask the person to move in certain ways to determine the type of pain. For example, a doctor may ask the person to lie flat, then lift the leg without bending the knee. Usually, no other procedures are needed if the cause is a strain or sprain. If another cause is suspected, other procedures are often needed.

X-rays of the lower back can help detect a herniated disk, degenerative changes due to osteoarthritis, compression fractures due to osteoporosis, and scoliosis. However, magnetic resonance imaging (MRI) or computed tomography (CT) provides clearer images and can confirm or exclude the diagnosis of a herniated disk, spinal stenosis, or cancer. Rarely, when results of MRI are unclear, myelography■ with CT is required. Occasionally, electromyography★ is performed to confirm the location of nerve damage.

Prevention

The most effective way to prevent low back pain is to exercise regularly.● Two types of exercises—aerobic exercise and specific muscle-strengthening and stretching exercises—are helpful.

Aerobic exercise, such as swimming and walking, improves general fitness, decreases obesity, and generally strengthens muscles. Specific exercises to strengthen and stretch the muscles in the abdomen, buttocks, and back can help stabilize the spine and decrease

strain on the disks that cushion the spine and the ligaments that hold it in place.

Muscle-strengthening exercises include pelvic tilts and abdominal curls. Stretching exercises include the sitting leg stretch, knee-to-chest stretch, and hip and quadriceps stretch. Stretching exercises can increase back pain in some people and therefore should be performed carefully. As a general rule, any exercise that causes or increases back pain should be stopped. Exercises should be repeated until the muscles feel mildly but not completely fatigued. Breathing during each exercise is important. When lifting weights, wearing a weight-lifting belt may help prevent back injury. People who have back pain should consult a doctor before beginning to exercise.

Exercise can also help people maintain bone density and a desirable weight. Thus, exercise may reduce the risk of developing two conditions that can lead to low back pain—osteoporosis and obesity.

Maintaining good posture when standing and sitting reduces stress on the back; slouching should be avoided. Chair seats can be adjusted to a height that allows the feet to be flat on the floor, with the knees bent up slightly and the lower back flat against the back of the chair. If a chair does not support the lower back, a pillow can be used behind the lower back. Sitting with the feet on the floor rather than with the legs crossed is advised. People should avoid standing or sitting for long periods. If prolonged standing or sitting is unavoidable, changing positions frequently may reduce stress on the back.

Sleeping in a comfortable position on a firm mattress is recommended. Pillows under the waist and head can be used for support by people who sleep on their side, and a pillow under the knees can be used by those who sleep on their back. Pillows under the head should not force the neck to bend too much.

Learning to lift properly helps prevent back injury. The knees should be bent enough that the arms are level with the object to be lifted. The legs, not the back, should be used to lift. Lifting an object over the head increases the risk of back injury. Using a steady footstool makes such lifting unnecessary. Heavy objects should be carried close to the body. Stopping smoking is also recommended.

Treatment

For low back pain that has recently developed, treatment begins with avoiding activi-

---

▲ see art on page 448   ■ see page 445

★ see page 446   ● see page 31

Exercises to Prevent Low Back Pain

Pelvic Tilts

Lie on the back with the knees bent, the heels on the floor, and the weight on the heels. Press the small of the back against the floor, contract the buttocks (raising them about half an inch from the floor), and contract the abdominal muscles. Hold this position for a count of 10. Repeat 20 times.

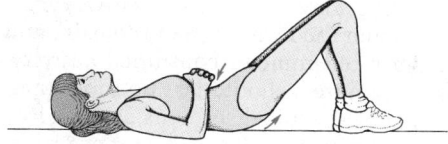

Abdominal Curls

Lie on the back with the knees bent and feet on the floor. Place the hands across the chest. Contract the abdominal muscles, slowly raising the shoulders 10 inches from the floor while keeping the head back (the chin should not touch the chest). Then release the abdominal muscles, slowly lowering the shoulders. Do 3 sets of 10.

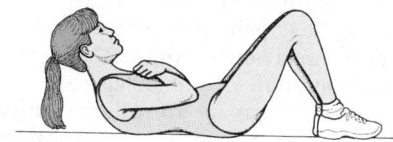

Knee-to-Chest Stretch

Lie on the back with the knees bent and both heels on the floor. While keeping the knees bent, place both hands behind one knee and bring it to the chest. Hold for a count of 10. Slowly lower that leg and repeat with the other leg. Do this exercise 10 times.

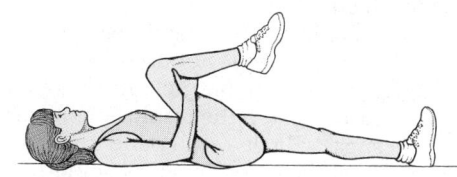

Sitting Leg Stretch

Sit on the floor with the knees straight but slightly flexed (not locked) and the legs as far apart as possible. Place both hands on the same knee. Slowly slide both hands toward the ankle. Stop if pain is felt and go no farther than a position that can be held comfortably for 10 seconds. Slowly return to a sitting position. Repeat with the other leg. Do this exercise 10 times for each leg.

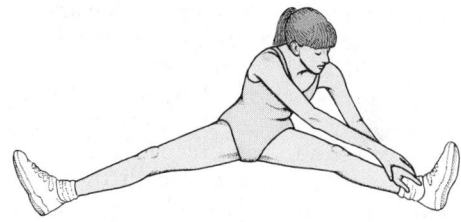

Hip and Quadriceps Stretch

Stand with one foot on the floor and the knee of the other leg bent at about a 90° angle. Grasp the front of the ankle of the bent leg with the hand on the same side. (The other hand may be placed on the back of a chair or on the wall for balance.) Keeping the knees together, press the foot against the hand and away from the body. Hold for a count of 10. Repeat with the other leg. Do this exercise 10 times.

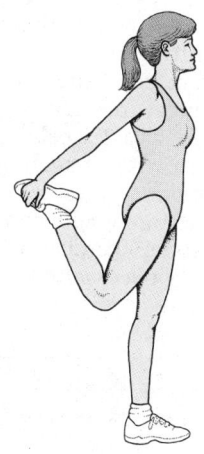

ties that stress the spine and cause pain—such as lifting heavy objects and bending. Bed rest for a few days may relieve pain. However, it does not hasten the resolution of the pain, and most experts recommend continued activity. Bed rest, if required, should last no more than 1 or 2 days. If a specific disorder is causing low back pain, treating that disorder—for example, giving antibiotics to treat a bladder infection—may relieve the low back pain.

Over-the-counter or prescription nonsteroidal anti-inflammatory drugs (NSAIDs)▲ can be taken to relieve pain and reduce inflammation. Muscle relaxants, such as methocarbamol, carisoprodol, cyclobenzaprine, or diazepam, may be given to relieve muscle spasms, although many experts question their usefulness. These drugs are not recommended for older people, who are more likely to experience side effects.

Application of heat or cold and massage may help.■ Usually, traction is not useful. Some reports suggest that acupuncture and chiropractic manipulation hasten the resolution of pain, but others suggest little or no benefit. During recovery, a back brace or corset is sometimes recommended for a short period or for use during back-stressing activities. However, these support garments can be uncomfortable and, if worn for a long time, may weaken the back muscles by doing their work for them.

After the pain has subsided, light activity, as recommended by a doctor or physical therapist, can speed healing and recovery. Specific exercises to strengthen and stretch the back are usually recommended to help prevent low back pain from becoming chronic or recurring. Other preventive measures (maintaining good posture, using a firm mattress with appropriately placed pillows, lifting properly, and stopping smoking) should be continued or started. In response to these measures, most episodes of back pain resolve in 1 to 2 weeks. Regardless of treatment, 80 to 90% of such episodes resolve within 6 weeks.

If low back pain is chronic, additional measures are needed. Aerobic exercise may help, and weight reduction, if necessary, is advised.

If the pain is severe, NSAIDs may not provide sufficient pain relief, and opioid analgesics★ may be required. If these analgesics are ineffective, some experts recommend that a corticosteroid, such as dexamethasone or methylprednisolone, plus a local anesthetic, such as lidocaine, be periodically injected around the spinal canal—as an epidural injection. However, these injections are effective usually only for several days to weeks.

Transcutaneous electrical nerve stimulation (TENS) is sometimes recommended.● A device that produces a gentle tingling sensation by generating a low oscillating current is used. A therapist applies the device to the painful area several times a day for 20 minutes to several hours at a time, depending on the severity of the pain. People are sometimes taught to use the device themselves.

If a disorder is causing severe and constant pain or serious symptoms, surgery may be necessary. If spinal nerve root compression due to a herniated disk is causing symptoms such as relentless sciatica, weakness, loss of sensation, or loss of bladder and bowel control, surgical removal of the disk (diskectomy) and part of the vertebra (laminectomy) may be necessary. A general anesthetic is usually required. The hospital stay after surgical removal of a disk is usually 1 or 2 days. Often, microsurgical techniques, with a small incision, can be used. A local anesthetic is used, and hospitalization is not required. However, when the incision is small, the surgeon may not be able to see and therefore may not remove all fragments of the herniated disk. After either procedure, most people can resume all of their activities after a few weeks. More than 90% of people recover fully.

For severe spinal stenosis, surgery to widen the spinal canal by removing a larger part of the vertebra may be performed. A general anesthetic is usually required. The hospital stay is usually 4 or 5 days. People may need 3 to 4 months before they can resume all of their activities. About two thirds of the people have a good or full recovery. For most of the rest, symptoms are prevented from worsening.

When the spine is unstable because of degeneration due to osteoarthritis, vertebrae may be fused together. However, fusion decreases mobility and may put additional stress on the rest of the spine.

▲ see pages 94 and 452   ■ see page 37

★ see table on page 451   ● see page 455

CHAPTER 95

Peripheral Nerve Disorders

The peripheral nervous system includes all the nerves outside the central nervous system, that is, all the nerves outside the brain and spinal cord. The nerves that connect the head, face, eyes, nose, muscles, and ears to the brain (cranial nerves)▲ and the nerves that connect the spinal cord to the rest of the body, including the 31 pairs of spinal nerves, are part of the peripheral nervous system.

Dysfunction of peripheral nerves may result from damage to any part of the nerve: the axon (the part that sends messages), to the body of the nerve cell, or to the myelin sheath (the membranes that surround the axon, enabling nerve impulses to travel quickly■). If motor nerves (which stimulate muscle action) are damaged, muscles may weaken or become paralyzed. If sensory nerves (which carry sensory information) are damaged, abnormal sensations may be felt or sensation may be lost.

Disorders of Muscle Stimulation

For normal muscle function, muscle tissue and nerve connections between the brain and muscle must be normal. If the motor nerves do not stimulate muscles normally, muscles weaken, waste away (atrophy), and can become completely paralyzed even though the muscles themselves are not the cause of the problem.

Muscle stimulation disorders (also called motor neuron disorders) include amyotrophic lateral sclerosis, primary lateral sclerosis, progressive pseudobulbar palsy, progressive muscular atrophy, progressive bulbar palsy, and postpolio syndrome. Motor neuron disorders are more common among men and usually develop in people who are in their 50s. In most people who have one of these disorders, the cause is unknown. About 10% of people who have a motor neuron disorder have a hereditary type and thus have family members who also have the disorder.

In all of these disorders, motor nerves in the spinal cord or brain progressively deteriorate, causing muscle weakness that can progress to paralysis. However, in each disorder, a different part of the nervous system is affected. Consequently, each disorder primarily affects different muscles and different parts of the body.

Symptoms

Amyotrophic Lateral Sclerosis (Lou Gehrig's Disease): This disorder is progressive. It begins with weakness, often in the hands and less frequently in the feet. Weakness may progress more on one side of the body than on the other and generally proceeds up the arm or leg. Cramps are also common and may precede the weakness, but no changes in sensation occur. Over time, weakness increases, and spasticity develops. Muscles twitch and become tight, followed by muscle spasms. Tremors may appear. Weakening of muscles in the throat may lead to difficulty speaking (dysarthria) and swallowing (dysphagia). Eventually, the muscles involved in breathing may weaken, leading to breathing problems; some people may need a ventilator to breathe.

How rapidly amyotrophic lateral sclerosis progresses varies. About 50% of people with the disorder die within 3 years of the first symptoms, 10% live 10 years or more, and a few people survive as long as 30 years.

Primary Lateral Sclerosis and Progressive Pseudobulbar Palsy: These disorders are rare, slowly progressive variants of amyotrophic lateral sclerosis. Primary lateral sclerosis affects mainly the arms and legs, and progressive pseudobulbar palsy affects mainly the muscles of the face, jaw, and throat. Emotions may be changeable: People with progressive pseudobulbar palsy may switch from happiness to sadness quickly and without reason. Inappropriate emotional outbursts are common. In both disorders, severe stiffness accompanies muscle weakness. The disorders usually progress for several years before total disability results.

Progressive Muscular Atrophy: This disorder is similar to amyotrophic lateral sclerosis, but it progresses more slowly, spasticity does not occur, and muscle weakness is less severe. Involuntary contractions or twitching of muscle fibers may be the earliest symptoms. Many people with this disorder survive 25 years or longer.

Progressive Bulbar Palsy: In this disorder, the nerves controlling the muscles of chewing, swallowing, and talking are affected, mak-

▲ see page 588   ■ see art on page 557

Using the Brain to Move a Muscle

Moving a muscle usually involves communication between the muscle and the brain through nerves. The impetus to move a muscle may originate with the senses. For example, the special nerve endings in the skin (sensory receptors) may sense pain when a person steps on a sharp rock or sense discomfort when a person picks up a very hot cup of coffee. This information is sent to the brain, and the brain sends a message to the muscle about how to respond. This type of exchange involves two complex nerve pathways: the sensory nerve pathway to the brain and the motor nerve pathway to the muscle. (A reflex may also be involved.▲)

1. If sensory receptors in the skin detect pain or a change in temperature, they transmit a signal, which ultimately reaches the brain.

2. The signal travels along a sensory nerve to the spinal cord.

3. The signal crosses a synapse (the junction between two nerve cells) between the sensory nerve and a spinal nerve in the spinal cord.

4. The spinal nerve carrying the signal crosses to the opposite side of the spinal cord.

5. The signal is sent up the spinal cord and through the brain stem to the thalamus.

6. The signal crosses a synapse in the thalamus to nerve fibers that carry the signal to the sensory cortex of the cerebrum.

7. The sensory cortex perceives the signal and triggers the motor cortex to generate a signal of movement.

8. The nerve carrying the signal crosses to the opposite side at the base of the brain.

9. The signal is sent down the spinal cord.

10. The signal crosses a synapse between the spinal cord nerve and a motor nerve.

11. The signal travels along the length of the motor nerve.

12. At the neuromuscular junction, the signal crosses from the motor nerve to the motor end plate on the muscle, where it stimulates muscle movement.

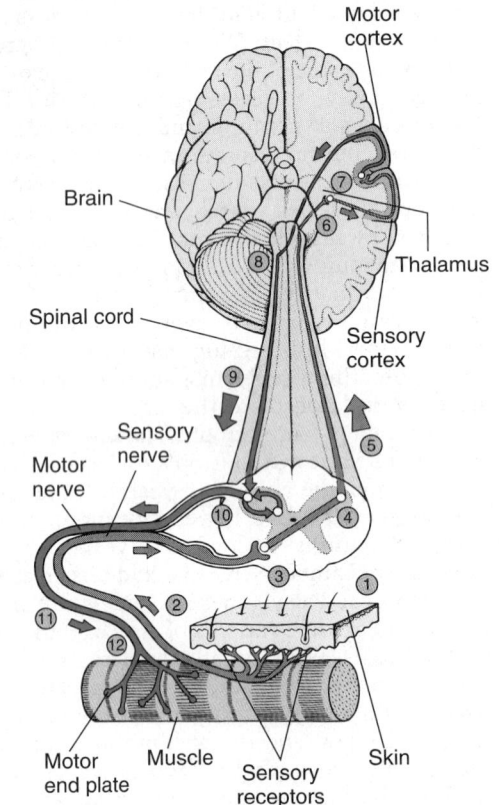

Motor cortex

Brain

Spinal cord

Thalamus

Sensory cortex

Sensory nerve

Motor nerve

Sensory receptors

Motor end plate

Muscle

Skin

ing these functions increasingly difficult. Because swallowing is difficult, food or saliva is often inhaled (aspirated) into the lungs, causing choking or gagging and increasing the risk of pneumonia. Death, which is often due to pneumonia, usually occurs 1 to 3 years after the disorder begins.

Postpolio Syndrome: Some people who have had polio may develop tired, painful, and weak muscles 15 years or more after their recovery from polio. Sometimes muscle tissue also wastes away, suggesting a reactivation of the polio infection. However, in most people who have had polio, such symptoms are not due to the postpolio syndrome but to the development of a new disorder, such as diabetes, a slipped (herniated) disk, or osteoarthritis.

Diagnosis

Doctors suspect one of these disorders in adults who have progressive muscle weakness without pain or loss of sensation. Muscle weakness can have many causes,■ so diagnostic procedures are performed to help narrow

▲ see art on page 442   ■ see table on page 340

the possibilities. For example, electromyography,▲ which records electrical activity in muscles, can help determine whether the problem is in the nerves or muscles. However, such procedures cannot determine which nerve disorder is causing the problem. The diagnosis is also based on which parts of the body are affected, when the disorder started, what symptoms appeared first, and how the symptoms changed over time.

Treatment

Motor neuron disorders have no specific treatment or cure. Physical therapy helps people maintain muscle strength and helps prevent tightening of the muscles (contractures). People with swallowing difficulties must be fed carefully to prevent choking; some must be fed through a tube inserted through the abdominal wall into the stomach (gastrostomy tube). Baclofen, phenytoin, or quinine may help decrease cramps. Amitriptyline, an antidepressant, may be given, not for its antidepressant effects, but for one of its anticholinergic effects—reduction of saliva formation.

Because amyotrophic lateral sclerosis and progressive bulbar palsy are progressive and incurable, people with one of these disorders are advised to establish advanced directives, specifying what kind of care they want at the end of life.■

Disorders of the Neuromuscular Junction

Nerves connect with muscles at the neuromuscular junction. There, the ends of nerve fibers connect to special sites on the muscle's membrane called motor end plates. These plates contain receptors that enable the muscle to respond to acetylcholine, the chemical messenger (neurotransmitter) released by the nerve to transmit a nerve signal across the neuromuscular junction. After a nerve stimulates a muscle at this junction, an electrical signal flows through the muscle, causing it to contract.

Disorders in which the neuromuscular junction malfunctions include myasthenia gravis, botulism, and Eaton-Lambert syndrome. In addition, many drugs (including very high doses of some antibiotics), certain insecticides (organophosphates), curare (an extract from plants used in hospitals to paralyze people in preparation for surgery), and the nerve gases used in chemical warfare can cause the neuromuscular junction

Overactive Nerves: Two Syndromes

Sometimes nerves repeatedly send electrical signals to muscles, resulting in overstimulation. This overactivity is thought to be a factor in stiff-person syndrome and Isaac's syndrome.

In **stiff-person syndrome,** the muscles of the trunk, abdomen, and legs gradually become stiffer. The muscles of the arms, head, and neck are affected to a lesser degree. The affected muscles enlarge. Stiff-person syndrome is more common among women. It may be due to an autoimmune reaction. Antibodies directed against an enzyme called glutamic acid decarboxylase are present, but whether they cause the symptoms is unknown. The sedative diazepam is effective; it consistently relieves the muscle stiffness. Plasmapheresis, in which toxic substances are filtered from the blood, is sometimes tried but often without success. Without treatment, the disorder progresses, leading to disability and stiffness throughout the body.

Isaac's syndrome is a rare disorder of unknown cause. The muscles, particularly those in the arms and legs, continually twitch, moving like a "bag of worms." This symptom is called myokymia. In addition, the hands and feet may intermittently have spasms and cramps. Muscle stiffness is common. Sweating may be increased. Symptoms can be relieved by carbamazepine or phenytoin, both of which are anticonvulsants.

to malfunction. For example, some of these substances prevent the normal breakdown of acetylcholine after the nerve impulse has been transmitted to the muscle.

MYASTHENIA GRAVIS

Myasthenia gravis is an autoimmune disorder in which communication between nerves and muscles is impaired, resulting in episodes of muscle weakness.

Myasthenia gravis is more common among women. It usually develops in women between the ages of 20 and 40. However, the disorder may affect men or women at any age.

▲ see page 446   ■ see page 54

In myasthenia gravis, the immune system produces antibodies that attack one type of receptor on the muscle side of the neuromuscular junction—the receptors that respond to the neurotransmitter acetylcholine. What causes the body to attack its own acetylcholine receptors—an autoimmune reaction—is unknown. According to one theory, a malfunction of the thymus gland may be involved. In the thymus gland, certain cells of the immune system learn how to differentiate between the body and foreign substances. The thymus gland also contains muscle cells (myocytes) with acetylcholine receptors. Myasthenia gravis may result because for unknown reasons, the thymus gland instructs the immune system cells to produce antibodies that attack the acetylcholine receptors. People may inherit a predisposition to this autoimmune abnormality. About 10% of people who have myasthenia gravis have a tumor of the thymus gland (thymoma). About half of thymomas are cancerous (malignant).

Antibodies against acetylcholine receptors, which circulate in the blood, may pass from a pregnant woman through the placenta to the fetus. In 12% of babies born to women who have this disorder, the transfer of antibodies produces **neonatal myasthenia,** in which the baby has muscle weakness that disappears several days to a few weeks after birth. The remaining 88% of babies are not affected.

Symptoms

Episodes during which symptoms worsen (exacerbations) are common. At other times, symptoms may be minimal or absent.

The most common symptoms are weak, drooping eyelids; weak eye muscles, which cause double vision; and excessive fatigue of specific muscles after exercise. In 40% of people with myasthenia gravis, the eye muscles are affected first, but 85% eventually have this problem. In 15% of people, only the eye muscles are affected, but in most people, the whole body is affected. Difficulty speaking and swallowing and weakness of the arms and legs are common. Hand grip may alternate between weak and normal; this fluctuating grip is called milkmaid's grip. The neck muscles may become weak. Sensation is not affected.

When a person with myasthenia gravis uses a muscle repetitively, the muscle usually becomes weak. For example, a person who once could use a hammer well becomes weak after hammering for several minutes. However, muscle weakness varies in intensity from hour to hour and from day to day, and the course of the disease varies widely.

About 15% of people have severe episodes (called myasthenia crisis). They may become extremely weak, but even then, they do not lose sensation. In about 10% of people who have a myasthenia crisis, the muscles needed for breathing weaken; this condition is life threatening.

Diagnosis

Doctors suspect myasthenia gravis in people with episodic weakness, especially when the muscles of the eyes or face are affected or when weakness increases with use of the affected muscles and disappears with rest. Because acetylcholine receptors are damaged, drugs that increase the levels of acetylcholine can be given as a test to help confirm the diagnosis. Edrophonium is most commonly used. When injected intravenously, it temporarily improves muscle strength in people with myasthenia gravis.

Other diagnostic procedures include electromyography to evaluate nerve and muscle function and blood tests to detect antibodies to acetylcholine. Computed tomography (CT) or magnetic resonance imaging (MRI) of the chest is performed to assess the thymus gland and to determine whether a thymoma is present.

Treatment

Drugs that increase the amount of acetylcholine, such as pyridostigmine (taken by mouth), may be given. Long-acting capsules are available for nighttime use to help people who experience severe weakness or difficulty swallowing when they awaken in the morning. Doctors must periodically adjust the dose, which may have to be increased during episodes of weakness. However, doses that are too high can cause weakness that is difficult to distinguish from that caused by the disorder. Also, the effectiveness of these drugs may decrease with long-term use. Increasing weakness, which may be due to a decrease in the drug's effectiveness, must be evaluated by a doctor with expertise in treating myasthenia gravis.

Common side effects of pyridostigmine include abdominal cramps and diarrhea. Drugs that slow the activity of the digestive tract, such as atropine or propantheline, may be needed to counteract these effects.

Doctors may also prescribe a corticosteroid, such as prednisone, or an immunosuppressant, such as azathioprine, to suppress the autoimmune reaction. These drugs may produce improvement within a few months.

When drugs do not provide relief or when a person has a myasthenic crisis, plasmapheresis▲ may be used. In plasmapheresis, toxic substances (in this case, the abnormal antibody) are extracted from the blood.

If a thymoma is present, the thymus gland must be surgically removed to prevent the thymoma from spreading. If no thymoma is present, the need to remove the thymus gland is uncertain.

BOTULISM

Botulism is an uncommon, life-threatening poisoning caused by toxins produced by the bacterium Clostridium botulinum.

The toxins that cause botulism, which are very potent poisons, can severely damage nerves. These toxins are called neurotoxins because they damage nerves. Botulism toxins paralyze muscles by inhibiting the release of the neurotransmitter acetylcholine from nerves. Botulism is usually a type of food poisoning. Another type of food poisoning may result from ingesting a neurotoxin sometimes present in shellfish.■

Causes

The bacterium *Clostridium botulinum* forms reproductive cells called spores. Like seeds, spores can exist in a dormant state for many years, and they are highly resistant to destruction. When moisture and nutrients are present and oxygen is absent (as in the intestine or sealed jars or cans), the spores start to grow and produce toxins. Some toxins produced by *Clostridium botulinum* are not destroyed by the intestine's protective enzymes. *Clostridium botulinum* is common in the environment, and spores can be transported by air. Many cases of botulism result from ingesting or inhaling small amounts of soil or dust.

Different forms of botulism are distinguished based on the cause.

Foodborne botulism occurs when food contaminated with the toxins is eaten. The most common sources of foodborne botulism are home-canned foods, particularly foods with a low acid content, such as asparagus, green beans, beets, and corn. Less common sources include chopped garlic in oil, chili peppers, tomatoes, foil-wrapped baked potatoes that have been left at room temperature too long, and home-canned or fermented fish. However, about 10% of outbreaks result from eating commercially prepared foods, most commonly, vegetables, fish, fruits, and condiments (such as salsa). Beef, milk products, pork, poultry, and other foods have also caused botulism.

Wound botulism occurs when a wound is contaminated with *Clostridium botulinum*. Inside the wound, the bacteria produce toxins that are absorbed into the bloodstream.

Infant botulism develops in infants who eat food containing spores of the bacteria rather than previously formed toxins. The spores then grow in the infant's intestine and produce toxins. The cause of most cases is unknown, but some cases have been linked to the ingestion of honey. Infant botulism occurs most commonly among infants aged 2 to 3 months.

Adult intestinal colonization botulism also results from eating food containing spores of the bacteria, but it occurs in older children and adults who have an intestinal disorder (such as colitis) or who have recently had surgery on the intestine. Only a few cases have been reported.

Symptoms

Symptoms of foodborne botulism develop suddenly, usually 18 to 36 hours after toxins enter the body, although symptoms can start as soon as 4 hours or as late as 8 days after ingesting the toxins. The more toxin ingested, the sooner the person becomes sick. Usually, people who become sick within 24 hours of eating contaminated food are the most severely affected.

The first symptoms of foodborne or wound botulism commonly include dry mouth, double vision, drooping eyelids, and an inability to focus on nearby objects. The pupils of the eyes do not constrict normally when exposed to light during an eye examination. However, in foodborne botulism, the first symptoms are often nausea, vomiting, stomach cramps, and diarrhea. People who have wound botulism do not have any digestive symptoms.

Nerve damage by the toxins affects muscle strength but not sensation. Speaking and swallowing become difficult. The muscles of the arms and legs and the muscles involved in breathing become progressively weaker as symptoms gradually move down the body. Breathing problems may be life threatening. The mind usually remains clear.

▲ see box on page 986   ■ see page 725

In about two thirds of infants with infant botulism, constipation is the first symptom. Then the muscles become paralyzed, beginning in the face and head and eventually reaching the arms, legs, and muscles involved in breathing. Problems range from mild lethargy and slowness in feeding to extensive loss of muscle tone and difficulty breathing.

Adult intestinal colonization botulism causes similar symptoms, but they are delayed. Symptoms develop up to 47 days after ingestion of the spores.

Diagnosis

Doctors may be able to diagnose foodborne botulism on the basis of symptoms. However, the symptoms are often mistakenly thought to result from more common causes of muscle weakness, such as stroke. A likely food source provides an additional clue. For example, when botulism occurs in two or more people who ate the same food prepared in the same place, the diagnosis is clearer. The diagnosis is confirmed when the toxins are detected in the person's blood or when the bacteria are detected in a culture of the person's stool. Toxins may also be identified in the suspected food.

The diagnosis of wound botulism is confirmed when the toxins are detected in the blood or when the bacteria are detected in a culture of tissue from the wound.

Detecting the bacteria or the toxins in a sample of an infant's stool confirms the diagnosis of infant botulism.

Electromyography (in which the electrical activity of muscles is recorded)▲ may be useful. It shows abnormal muscle responses after electrical stimulation in most cases of botulism.

Prevention and Treatment

The spores of *Clostridium botulinum* are highly resistant to heat and may survive boiling for several hours. However, the toxins are readily destroyed by heat. Therefore, cooking food at 176° F (79.9° C) for 30 minutes almost always destroys toxins and prevents foodborne botulism. Stored foods can cause botulism if they were inadequately cooked before they were stored. The bacteria can produce some toxins at temperatures as low as 37.4° F (3° C), a typical refrigerator temperature.

Proper home and commercial canning techniques and adequate heating of home-canned food before serving are essential. Boiling home-canned food for 10 minutes destroys the toxins. Canned foods that are discolored or smell spoiled should be discarded. Also, cans that are swollen or leaking should be discarded. Oils infused with garlic or herbs should be refrigerated. Potatoes that have been baked in aluminum foil should be kept hot until served. Children younger than 2 years should not be fed honey because *Clostridium botulinum* spores may be present.

Any food that may be contaminated should be disposed of carefully. Even tiny amounts of toxins ingested, inhaled, or absorbed through the eye or a break in the skin can cause serious illness. Skin contact should be avoided as much as possible, and the hands should be washed immediately after handling the food.

If a wound becomes infected, promptly seeking medical attention can reduce the risk of wound botulism.

A person who may have botulism should go to the hospital immediately. Laboratory procedures to confirm the diagnosis are performed, but treatment often cannot be delayed until the results are known. To rid the person's body of any unabsorbed toxin, doctors may induce vomiting, wash out the stomach (a procedure called gastric lavage), and give the person a laxative to speed the passage of intestinal contents.

Vital signs (pulse, breathing rate, blood pressure, and temperature) are measured often. If breathing problems begin, the person is transferred to an intensive care unit and may be temporarily placed on a ventilator. Such treatment has reduced the percentage of deaths due to botulism from about 70% in the early 1900s to less than 10%.

A substance that blocks the action of the toxins (antitoxin) is given as soon as possible after botulism has been diagnosed. It is most likely to help if given within 72 hours of when symptoms begin. The antitoxin may slow or stop further physical deterioration, so that the body can heal itself over a period of months. However, the antitoxin cannot undo damage already done. The antitoxin is not recommended for infant botulism, but its effectiveness for this type of botulism is being studied.

The person may need to be fed through an intravenous tube. Infants may need to be fed through a thin plastic feeding tube (a nasogastric tube) passed through the nose and down the throat.

Some people who recover from botulism feel tired and are short of breath for years

▲ see page 446

Nerve Junction Boxes: The Plexuses

Much like the electrical junction box in a house, a nerve plexus is a network of interwoven nerves. Nerve fibers from different spinal nerves are sorted and recombined in plexuses, so that all fibers going to a specific body part are put together in one nerve. Four nerve plexuses are located in the trunk of the body. The cervical plexus provides nerve connections to the head, neck, and shoulder. The brachial plexus provides connections to the chest, shoulders, upper arms, forearms, and hands. The lumbar plexus provides connections to the back, abdomen, groin, thighs, knees, and calves. The sacral plexus provides connections to the pelvis, buttocks, genitals, thighs, calves, and feet. Because the lumbar and sacral plexuses are interconnected, they are sometimes referred to as the lumbosacral plexus. The spinal nerves in the chest do not join a plexus; they are the intercostal nerves, which are located between the ribs.

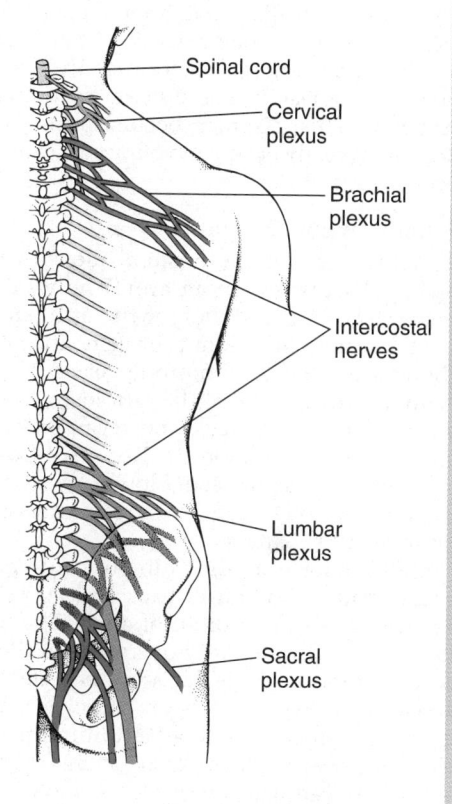

afterward. They may need long-term physical therapy.

EATON-LAMBERT SYNDROME

Eaton-Lambert syndrome is an autoimmune disease that causes weakness.

Eaton-Lambert syndrome is caused by antibodies that interfere with the release of acetylcholine rather than attack acetylcholine receptors (as in myasthenia gravis▲). Eaton-Lambert syndrome usually results from certain cancers, especially lung cancer.

Plexus Disorders

A plexus resembles an electrical junction box, which distributes wires to different parts of a house. In a plexus, nerve fibers from different spinal nerves are sorted and recombined so that all fibers going to a specific body part are put together in one nerve. Damage to nerves in the major plexuses causes problems in the arms or legs that these nerves supply. The major plexuses are the brachial plexus, which is located in the neck and distributes nerves throughout the arms, and the lumbosacral plexus, which is located in the lower back and distributes nerves to the pelvis and legs.

Causes

The most common causes of damage to a plexus are physical injury and cancer. An accident that pulls the arm or severely bends the arm at the shoulder may damage the brachial plexus (located near the shoulder). Similarly, a fall can injure the lumbosacral plexus (located near the hip). A cancer growing in the upper part of the lung can invade and destroy the brachial plexus. A cancer of the intestine, bladder, or prostate can invade the lumbosacral plexus. Other masses, such as a noncancerous (benign) tumor, an abscess, or a collection of blood (hematoma), may also cause plexus disorders by putting pressure on a plexus.

▲ see page 577

A plexus may be damaged when the body produces antibodies that attack its own tissues—an autoimmune reaction. **Acute brachial neuritis** (a sudden malfunction of the brachial plexus) is probably caused by an autoimmune reaction. This disorder occurs primarily in men. It typically occurs in young adults but can occur at any age.

Symptoms and Diagnosis

Malfunction of the brachial plexus causes pain and weakness in an arm. The weakness may affect only a portion of the arm, such as the forearm or biceps, or the entire arm. When the cause is an autoimmune reaction, as in acute brachial neuritis, the arm loses strength within a day to a week and regains strength slowly over a few months. Recovery from an injury also tends to occur slowly, over several months, although some severe injuries cause permanent weakness.

Malfunction of the lumbosacral plexus causes pain in the lower back and leg as well as weakness in part or all of a leg. The weakness may be limited to movements of the foot or calf, or the whole leg may become paralyzed. Recovery depends on the cause. Damage to the plexus due to an autoimmune reaction may resolve slowly over several months.

Doctors can determine that a plexus is involved based on the unpredictable, patchy pattern of sensory, muscle (motor), and reflex dysfunction. The location of the symptoms indicates which plexus is affected. Electromyography and nerve conduction studies can also help locate the damage.▲ Computed tomography (CT) or magnetic resonance imaging (MRI) can help determine whether a cancer, another mass, or an injury is causing the plexus disorder.

Treatment

Treatment depends on the cause of the plexus disorder. Cancer near the plexus may be treated with radiation therapy or chemotherapy. Occasionally, a cancer or another mass that is damaging the plexus must be removed surgically. Doctors sometimes prescribe corticosteroids for acute brachial neuritis and other plexus disorders thought to be caused by an autoimmune reaction, but these drugs have no proven benefit. When an injury is the cause, time for healing may be all that is needed.

Thoracic Outlet Syndromes

Thoracic outlet syndromes are an ill-defined group of disorders that cause pain and pins-and-needles sensations (paresthesias) in the hand, shoulder, and arm.

The thoracic outlet is the passageway between the neck and the chest, through which the esophagus, major blood vessels, trachea, and many nerves pass. Because this passageway is very crowded, problems can occur when blood vessels or nerves to the arm become compressed between a rib and the overlying muscle. However, the exact cause of these disorders is often unclear. Very rarely, the cause is a clear-cut anatomic abnormality, such as an extra little rib in the neck (cervical rib) that compresses an artery or a blockage of one of the subclavian arteries. (The subclavian arteries are located under the collarbone and supply blood to the arms.)

Symptoms and Diagnosis

Pain and pins-and-needles sensations are felt usually along the inner surface of the arm and sometimes down the side. If one of the subclavian arteries is compressed, the hands, arms, and shoulders may swell or the overlying skin may look bluish because the oxygen supply is inadequate (a condition called cyanosis). Sometimes the compression is severe enough to cause Raynaud's syndrome, in which the fingers turn white when exposed to cold. In severe cases, compression may cause gangrene in the fingers.

The diagnosis is suggested by a combination of information from the history, physical examination, and several diagnostic procedures. Nerve conduction studies and electromyography■ may detect abnormalities characteristic of thoracic outlet syndrome. Through a stethoscope placed on the collar bone or near the top of the armpit, doctors may hear sounds indicating abnormal blood flow (bruits) in a compressed artery. Angiography of the arteries in the arm (brachial arteries) may be performed to detect abnormal blood flow. In this procedure, x-rays are taken after a radiopaque dye is injected into the bloodstream. However, none of these procedures can definitively confirm or rule out the diagnosis of thoracic outlet syndrome.

Treatment

For most people with symptoms of thoracic outlet syndrome, physical therapy and exer-

▲ see page 446   ■ see page 446

cise result in improvement. Surgery may be needed if an anatomic abnormality or blockage of the subclavian artery is confirmed. However, because a definitive diagnosis is difficult to make and because symptoms often persist after surgery, most doctors try to avoid surgery.

Mononeuropathy

Mononeuropathy is damage to a single peripheral nerve.

Physical injury is the most common cause of a mononeuropathy. Often, the injury is caused by prolonged pressure on a nerve that runs close to the surface of the body near a bony prominence, such as a nerve in an elbow, a shoulder, a wrist, or a knee. Pressure on a nerve during a long, sound sleep (especially in alcoholics) may be prolonged enough to cause damage. Pressure may result from a misfitting cast, improper use of crutches, or staying in a cramped position for a long time, such as when gardening or when playing cards with the elbows resting on a table. Damage due to pressure may also occur in people who are under anesthesia for surgery, in those who are bedridden (particularly older people), and in those who are paralyzed.

Less commonly, strenuous activities, accidents, prolonged exposure to cold or heat, or radiation therapy for cancer may also damage a nerve. Repeated injuries, such as those due to tight gripping of small tools or to excessive vibration from an air hammer, can also damage nerves. Infections, such as leprosy and Lyme disease, may destroy a nerve, causing mononeuropathy. Cancer may cause mononeuropathy by directly invading a nerve. Some toxic substances and some drugs can cause mononeuropathy.

Certain peripheral nerves are more vulnerable to injury. Examples are the median nerve in the wrist (resulting in carpal tunnel syndrome▲), the ulnar nerve in the elbow, the radial nerve in the upper arm, and the peroneal nerve near the knee.

Ulnar Nerve Palsy: The ulnar nerve passes close to the surface of the skin at the elbow. This nerve is easily damaged by repeatedly leaning on the elbow or sometimes by an abnormal bone growth in the area. The result is ulnar nerve palsy, which consists of a pins-and-needles sensation and weakness in the hand. Severe, chronic ulnar nerve palsy can

When the Foot's Asleep

A sleeping foot can be considered a temporary neuropathy. The foot falls asleep when the nerve supplying it is compressed. Compression interferes with the blood supply to the nerve, making the nerve give off abnormal signals (a pins-and-needles sensation), called a paresthesia. Moving around relieves the compression and restores the blood supply. As a result, nerve function resumes, and the pins-and-needles sensation stops.

cause wasting away (atrophy) of muscles and a clawhand deformity (in which muscles tighten, causing the fingers to freeze in a bent position). Nerve conduction studies■ can help locate the damaged nerve. Because surgical repair is often unsuccessful, the disorder is usually treated with physical therapy, which helps prevent tightening of muscles. Avoiding pressure on the elbow is recommended.

Radial Nerve Palsy: The radial nerve passes along the underside of the bone in the upper arm. Prolonged compression of this nerve results in radial nerve palsy. This disorder is sometimes called Saturday night palsy because it occurs in people who drink heavily (often during weekends) and then sleep soundly with an arm draped over the back of a chair or under their partner's head. The nerve damage weakens the wrist and fingers so that the wrist may flop into a bent position with the fingers curved (a condition called wristdrop). Occasionally, the back of the hand may lose feeling. Usually, radial nerve palsy resolves once the pressure is relieved.

Peroneal Nerve Palsy: The peroneal nerve passes close to the surface of the skin on the outer part of the calf near the back of the knee. Compression of this nerve results in peroneal nerve palsy. This disorder weakens the muscles that lift the foot, so that the foot cannot be flexed upward (a condition called footdrop). It is most common among thin people who are bedridden, people who are improperly strapped into a wheelchair, and people who habitually cross their legs for long periods of time. Treatment involves avoiding pressure on the nerve—for example, by not crossing the legs.

▲ see page 398   ■ see page 446

Mononeuritis Multiplex

Mononeuritis multiplex is the simultaneous malfunction of two or several peripheral nerves in separate areas of the body.

Mononeuritis multiplex, which affects only a few nerves, is usually distinguished from polyneuropathy, which affects many nerves, usually in about the same areas on both sides of the body.

Several disorders can cause mononeuritis multiplex and each disorder produces characteristic symptoms. Diabetes is probably the most common cause of mononeuritis multiplex, although diabetes more commonly causes polyneuropathy. Other common causes of mononeuritis multiplex include polyarteritis nodosa, systemic lupus erythematosus, Sjögren's syndrome, rheumatoid arthritis, sarcoidosis, amyloidosis, and infections (for example, Lyme disease and HIV infection). Mononeuritis multiplex may result from direct invasion of the nerve by bacteria, as in leprosy. Treatment depends on the cause.

Polyneuropathy

Polyneuropathy is the simultaneous malfunction of many peripheral nerves throughout the body.

Polyneuropathy may be acute (beginning suddenly) or chronic (developing gradually, often over months or years).

Causes

Acute polyneuropathy has many causes. It may be caused by an infection involving a toxin produced by bacteria (as in diphtheria) or by an autoimmune reaction (as in Guillain-Barré syndrome). Toxic substances, including heavy metals such as lead and mercury, carbon monoxide, and some drugs can also cause acute polyneuropathy. The drugs include the anticonvulsant phenytoin, some antibiotics (such as chloramphenicol, nitrofurantoin, and sulfonamides), some chemotherapy drugs (such as vinblastine and vincristine), and some sedatives (such as barbital and hexobarbital). Cancer, such as multiple myeloma, may cause acute polyneuropathy by directly invading or compressing the nerves or by producing toxic substances.

The cause of chronic polyneuropathy is often unknown. The most common form of chronic polyneuropathy is most often due to diabetes but may be due to excessive use of alcohol. Nutritional deficiencies (such as vitamin B deficiency) are an uncommon cause of chronic polyneuropathy in the United States, except among alcoholics who are malnourished. Anemia due to vitamin B_{12} deficiency (pernicious anemia) may also cause chronic polyneuropathy. Other causes include an underactive thyroid gland (hypothyroidism), liver failure, and kidney failure. Rare causes include certain cancers, such as lung cancer, and taking excessive amounts of vitamin B_6 (pyridoxine).

Poor control of blood sugar levels in diabetes▲ causes several forms of polyneuropathy, collectively referred to as **diabetic neuropathy.** (Diabetes can also cause mononeuropathy or mononeuritis multiplex that leads to weakness, typically of the eye or thigh muscles.)

In some people, the cause is hereditary.

Symptoms

Acute polyneuropathy (for example, Guillain-Barré syndrome) begins suddenly in both legs and progresses upward to the arms. Symptoms include weakness and a pins-and-needles sensation or loss of sensation.

In the most common form of chronic polyneuropathy, only sensation is affected. Usually, the feet are affected first, but sometimes the hands are. A pins-and-needles sensation, numbness, burning pain, and loss of vibration sense and position sense (knowing where the arms and legs are) are prominent symptoms. Because position sense is lost, walking and even standing become unsteady. Consequently, muscles may not be used. Eventually, they may weaken and waste away.

Diabetic neuropathy commonly causes painful tingling or burning sensations in the hands and feet—a condition called distal polyneuropathy. Pain is often worse at night and may be aggravated by touch or by a change in temperature. People may lose the senses of temperature and pain, so they often burn themselves and develop open sores caused by prolonged pressure or other injuries. Without pain as a warning of too much stress, joints are susceptible to injuries; this type of injury is called Charcot's joints.

Polyneuropathy often affects the nerves of the autonomic nervous system, which controls involuntary functions in the body (such as blood pressure, heart rate, digestion, salivation, and urination). Typical symptoms are constipation, loss of bowel or bladder control (leading to fecal or urinary incontinence), sex-

▲ see page 962

No Pain: Charcot's Joints

When nerves that enable people to sense pain are damaged, people may become unable to sense pain. A variety of disorders, such as diabetes mellitus, spinal cord disorders, and syphilis, can damage these nerves. People with such nerve damage may injure a joint many times, or even fracture it, without noticing. Injuries may occur for years before the joint malfunctions. However, once it malfunctions, the joint may be permanently destroyed within a few months. This progressive malfunctioning is called Charcot's joints (neuropathic joint disease).

In its early stages, doctors may confuse Charcot's joints with osteoarthritis, because the joint is stiff, and fluid accumulates in it.

Usually, the joint is not painful or is less painful than would be expected considering the amount of joint damage. If the disorder progresses rapidly, the joint can become extremely painful. In these cases, the joint is usually swollen because of excess fluid and abnormal bone growth. It may look deformed because it has been fractured and ligaments have stretched, allowing the bones to slip out of place. Moving the joint may cause a coarse, grating sound because of bone fragments floating in the joint.

Any joint can be affected depending on where the nerve damage is—most commonly, the knee or, in people who have diabetes, the foot. Often, only one joint is

affected, and usually not more than two or three.

Doctors suspect Charcot's joints when people have a nerve disorder and joint problems. X-rays can detect joint damage, which often includes calcium deposits and abnormal bone growth. Sometimes Charcot's joints can be prevented by taking care of the feet and by avoiding injuries. Treatment of the underlying nerve disorder can slow or even reverse joint damage. Diagnosing and immobilizing painless fractures and splinting unstable joints can help stop or minimize the damage. Hips and knees may be surgically replaced if the nerve disorder is not progressing, but artificial joints often loosen prematurely.

---

ual dysfunction, and fluctuating blood pressure—most notably a sudden fall in blood pressure when a person stands up (orthostatic hypotension). The skin may become pale and dry, and sweating may be reduced.

People who have the hereditary form may have hammer toes, high arches, and a curved spine (scoliosis). Abnormalities in sensation and muscle weakness are mild. Affected people may not notice these symptoms or may consider them unimportant.

Diagnosis

Doctors easily recognize polyneuropathy by the symptoms. A physical examination and procedures such as electromyography and nerve conduction studies▲ can provide additional information about absent or reduced sensation in the feet. After polyneuropathy is diagnosed, causes that can be treated must be identified. Blood and urine tests may detect a disorder that is causing polyneuropathy—for example, diabetes, kidney failure, or a thyroid disorder. Infrequently, a nerve biopsy is necessary.

Treatment and Prognosis

Physical therapy sometimes reduces muscle weakness.

Specific treatment depends on the cause. When taking excessive amounts of vitamin B_6 is the cause, the disorder may resolve if the vitamin is discontinued. When neuropathy is related to diabetes, careful control of blood sugar levels may slow progression of the disorder and occasionally relieves symptoms. Transplantation of cells that produce insulin (islet cells ■), located in the pancreas, sometimes results in a cure. Treatment of multiple myeloma or liver or kidney failure may result in slow recovery. When polyneuropathy is due to cancer, the cancer may have to be surgically removed to relieve compression of the nerve. When polyneuropathy is due to an underactive thyroid gland, thyroid hormone is given.

The prognosis for people with acute or chronic polyneuropathy depends on the cause.

GUILLAIN-BARRÉ SYNDROME

Guillain-Barré syndrome (inflammatory demyelinating polyneuropathy) is a form of polyneuropathy that produces worsening muscle weakness, leading to paralysis.

The presumed cause is an autoimmune reaction: The body's immune system attacks

---

▲ see page 446   ■ see page 1081

the myelin sheath, which surrounds the axon of many nerves. In about 80% of people with this syndrome, symptoms begin about 5 days to 3 weeks after a mild infection, surgery, or an immunization.

There are two forms of Guillain-Barré syndrome. In the acute form, muscle weakness develops rapidly; in the chronic form, muscle weakness develops gradually.

Symptoms and Diagnosis

The acute form usually begins in both legs, then progresses upward to the arms. Occasionally, symptoms begin in the reverse order. Symptoms include weakness and a pins-and-needles sensation or loss of sensation. Weakness is more prominent than abnormal sensation. In 90% of people who have Guillain-Barré syndrome, weakness is most severe within 2 to 3 weeks. In 5 to 10%, the muscles that control breathing become so weak that a ventilator is needed. Because the facial and swallowing muscles become weak, about 10% of people need to be fed intravenously or through a tube placed directly through the abdominal wall into the stomach (gastrostomy tube). If the disorder is very severe, blood pressure may fluctuate, heart rhythm may become abnormal, or other functions controlled by the autonomic nervous system may be impaired.

In an unusual variant of the acute form called Miller-Fisher syndrome, only a few symptoms develop: Eye movements become paralyzed, walking becomes difficult, and normal reflexes disappear.

The chronic form produces symptoms similar to those of the acute form, but they develop more slowly, usually over a period of about 8 weeks. Symptoms also last longer and may become permanent.

The diagnosis is based on the pattern of symptoms and results of diagnostic procedures. Analysis of cerebrospinal fluid obtained by a spinal tap (lumbar puncture),▲ electromyography, nerve conduction studies, and blood tests can help doctors exclude other possible causes of severe weakness, such as transverse myelitis and spinal cord injuries. A combination of high protein levels and no inflammatory cells in the cerebrospinal fluid and specific results from electromyography strongly suggest Guillain-Barré syndrome.

Treatment and Prognosis

The acute form of Guillain-Barré syndrome, which can worsen rapidly, is a medical emergency. People who develop this syndrome should be hospitalized immediately. Establishing the diagnosis is crucial because the sooner appropriate treatment is started, the better the chance of a good outcome. In the hospital, the person is closely monitored so that breathing can be assisted with a ventilator if necessary. Nurses take precautions to prevent bedsores and injuries by providing soft mattresses and by turning the person every 2 hours. Physical therapy is started immediately to help preserve joint and muscle function.

Plasmapheresis, in which toxic substances are filtered from the blood,■ or infusion of immune globulin is the treatment of choice. Corticosteroids are no longer used because they have no proven benefit and may worsen the disorder.

People who have the chronic form may be given corticosteroids to help reduce weakness. These drugs may be needed for a long time. Immune globulins, plasmapheresis, and immunosuppressants (such as azathioprine) may also help.

Without treatment, most people improve slowly over several months. However, with early treatment, people can improve very quickly—in days or weeks. About 30% of adults and even more children with the disorder have residual weakness 3 years after the syndrome began. On average, less than 5% of people die during the early stage of the disease.

Hereditary Neuropathies

Hereditary neuropathies affect the peripheral nerves, causing subtle symptoms that worsen gradually.

Hereditary neuropathies may affect only motor nerves (motor neuropathies), only sensory nerves (sensory neuropathies), or both sensory and motor nerves (sensory-motor neuropathies). Some hereditary neuropathies are relatively common but often are not recognized. Hereditary sensory neuropathies are especially rare.

The genes responsible for many of these neuropathies have been identified. They include some forms of Charcot-Marie-Tooth disease, Refsum's disease,★ porphyria,● Fabry's disease,◆ and hereditary neuropathy with liability to pressure palsies.

▲ see art on page 443   ■ see box on page 986

★ see box on page 1621   ● see page 933

◆ see page 1620

CHARCOT-MARIE-TOOTH DISEASE

Charcot-Marie-Tooth disease (peroneal muscular atrophy) is a hereditary neuropathy in which the muscles of the lower legs become weak and waste away (atrophy).

Charcot-Marie-Tooth disease is the most common hereditary neuropathy, affecting 1 of 2,500 people. There are 3 types and several subtypes of the disease. In some types, axons (the part of the nerve that sends messages) die because the myelin sheath surrounding them is damaged or destroyed (demyelinated). In other types, axons die even though the sheath is not damaged. Most types of the disease are inherited as an autosomal (not sex-linked) dominant trait: only one gene from one parent is required for the disease to develop.

Symptoms vary by type of the disease. In type 1, symptoms begin in middle childhood, adolescence, or later. Weakness begins in the lower legs, which causes an inability to flex the foot (footdrop) and wasting away of the calf muscles (stork leg deformity). Later, hand muscles begin to waste away. There is little loss of sensation. In milder subtypes of type 1, high arches and hammer toes may be the only symptoms. In one subtype of type 1, males have severe symptoms, and females have mild symptoms or may be unaffected. The disease progresses slowly and does not affect life span.

People with type 2 disease, which progresses more slowly, develop somewhat similar symptoms, often beginning in their teens.

Type 3 disease starts in infancy. Walking and running are delayed, and the peripheral nerves become enlarged. Muscle weakness in the legs progresses at a faster rate than in type 1. Sensation in the legs is lost.

Diagnosis and Treatment

The distribution of weakness, the age at which the disease began, the family history, the presence of foot deformities (high arches and hammer toes), and the results of nerve conduction studies help doctors identify the different types of Charcot-Marie-Tooth disease and distinguish them from other causes of neuropathy. Genetic testing and counseling for Charcot-Marie-Tooth disease is available.

No treatment can stop the progression of the disease. Wearing braces helps correct footdrop, and sometimes orthopedic surgery is needed.

HEREDITARY NEUROPATHY WITH LIABILITY TO PRESSURE PALSIES

Hereditary neuropathy with liability to pressure palsies is malfunction or damage to one or more nerve resulting from slight pressure or injury.

People who have this neuropathy are susceptible to nerve damage resulting from relatively slight pressure or injury or from repetitive use. Usually, this neuropathy starts during adolescence or young adulthood, but it may start at any age. It affects both sexes equally. This neuropathy is inherited as an autosomal (not sex-linked) dominant trait.▲

Peroneal nerve palsy with footdrop, ulnar nerve palsy, and carpal tunnel syndrome commonly develop. Numbness or weakness occurs periodically in the affected area. Symptoms vary from unnoticeable and mild to severe and incapacitating. Episodes may last several minutes to months.

Doctors may have difficulty diagnosing this neuropathy because the symptoms come and go. Genetic testing for this neuropathy is available.

About half of the people who have this neuropathy recover completely within days to months. In people who do not recover completely, symptoms are rarely severe.

Spinal Muscular Atrophies

Spinal muscular atrophies are hereditary disorders in which nerve cells in the spinal cord and brain stem degenerate, causing progressive muscle weakness and wasting.

The disorders are usually inherited as a recessive autosomal (not sex-linked) trait: two genes are required, one from each parent.■ There are three main types of spinal muscular atrophy.

Symptoms

Symptoms first appear during infancy and childhood. In acute (type I) spinal muscular atrophy (Werdnig-Hoffmann disease), muscle weakness is apparent at or within a few days of birth. Death occurs in 95% of children by age 1½ years and in all by age 4 years, usually due to respiratory failure.

In children with intermediate (type II) spinal muscular atrophy, weakness develops by age 6

▲ see page 12   ■ see page 12

months. Most children are confined to a wheelchair by age 2 to 3 years. The disorder is often fatal in early life, usually because of respiratory problems, but some children survive with permanent weakness that does not continue to worsen.

Chronic (type III) spinal muscular atrophy (Wohlfart-Kugelberg-Welander disease) begins in children between the ages of 5 and 15 years and worsens slowly. Consequently, people with this disorder usually live longer than those with type I or II spinal muscular atrophy. Weakness and wasting of muscles begin in the legs and later spread to the arms.

Diagnosis and Treatment

Doctors test for these rare disorders when unexplained weakness and muscle wasting occur in young children. Because these disorders are inherited, a family history may help doctors make the diagnosis. Electromyography▲ also helps. The specific defective gene has been identified for some of the types and can be detected by blood tests. If there is a family history of one of the disorders, amniocentesis can be performed to help determine whether an unborn child has the defective gene.

No specific treatments are available. Physical therapy and wearing braces can sometimes help.

CHAPTER 96

Cranial Nerve Disorders

Twelve pairs of nerves—the cranial nerves—lead directly from the brain to various parts of the head and neck. A disorder may affect the connections between cranial nerves within the brain. An example is internuclear ophthalmoplegia. Or, a disorder may affect only one cranial nerve. Examples are trigeminal neuralgia, Bell's palsy, hemifacial spasms, and glossopharyngeal neuralgia. When doctors suspect a cranial nerve disorder, the function of a cranial nerve is tested by asking the person to perform simple tasks, such as to follow a moving target with the eyes.

Internuclear Ophthalmoplegia

Internuclear ophthalmoplegia is weakness or paralysis of eye movements caused by damage to the nerve fibers connecting collections of nerve cells (centers or nuclei) that give rise to cranial nerves III (oculomotor nerve) and VI (abducens nerve).

In internuclear ophthalmoplegia, nerve fibers necessary for the control of horizontal and vertical eye movements—looking from side to side and up and down—are damaged. The most

common causes are stroke in older people and multiple sclerosis in younger people.

Horizontal eye movements are impaired, but vertical ones are not. The eye on the affected side cannot turn inward when looking to the opposite side but can turn outward. Nystagmus occurs in the eye on the opposite side when it turns outward; that is, the eye moves rapidly in one direction, then drifts more slowly back to the original position.

A stroke may also damage the center for horizontal eye movements, resulting in the one-and-a-half syndrome. The eye on the affected side remains fixed in the middle. The other eye can turn outward but not inward. As in internuclear ophthalmoplegia, vertical eye movements are not affected.

Treatment of internuclear ophthalmoplegia depends on the cause. Whether internuclear ophthalmoplegia eventually resolves depends on the disorder that caused it.

Palsies of Cranial Nerves That Control Eye Movement

These disorders involve paralysis of cranial nerve III, IV, or VI, impairing the ability to move the eyes in certain directions depending on which nerve is affected.

▲ see page 446

The eye is moved by three pairs of muscles, controlled by cranial nerves III, IV, and VI. These muscles move the eye up and down, right and left, and diagonally.

Cranial Nerve III (Oculomotor Nerve): A palsy of this nerve can be caused by brain disorders (such as a head injury, an aneurysm in an artery supplying the brain, and a brain tumor) or by diabetes. The affected eye turns outward when the unaffected eye looks straight ahead, producing double vision. The affected eye can move only to the middle when looking inward and cannot look upward and downward. The eyelid droops, and the pupil may be dilated and sometimes fixed (that is, it does not change in size). Dilation and fixation of both pupils indicates deep coma and possibly brain death.▲ Development of a headache and a change in the level of consciousness (for example, if the person becomes drowsy) may indicate that the cause is a life-threatening disorder.

The diagnosis is based on results of a neurologic examination and computed tomography (CT) or magnetic resonance imaging (MRI). A spinal tap (lumbar puncture)■ is performed only if doctors suspect a hemorrhage and CT does not detect blood. Cerebral angiography is performed when a hemorrhage due to an aneurysm is suspected or when the pupil is affected but no head injury has occurred. Treatment depends on the cause of the palsy. Emergency treatment is required if a life-threatening disorder is the cause.

Cranial Nerve IV (Trochlear Nerve): In most cases, the cause of a palsy of this nerve is a head injury. Other causes, such as a tumor, are rare. The affected eye cannot turn inward and downward, resulting in vertical double vision. The person tends subconsciously to tilt the head, thereby using eye muscles that are unaffected by the palsy. This position can eliminate the double vision.

Usually, the diagnosis is suspected in a person who, after a head injury, has characteristic abnormal eye movements. CT or MRI may be performed. Treatment depends on the cause of the palsy. Eye exercises may help. Sometimes surgery is necessary to eliminate double vision.

Cranial Nerve VI (Abducens Nerve): The cause may be a head injury, a tumor, diabetes, multiple sclerosis, meningitis, blockage of an artery supplying the nerve, or increased pressure within the skull. The affected eye cannot fully turn outward and may be turned inward when the person looks straight ahead. Double

vision results when the person looks toward the side of the affected eye.

Usually, doctors can easily identify a palsy of cranial nerve VI, but the cause is less obvious. CT or MRI is performed to exclude tumors. A spinal tap (lumbar puncture) can determine whether pressure within the skull is increased and whether a tumor or swelling due to an infection is compressing the nerve. When no cause is identified, the cause is often thought to be blockage of an artery supplying the nerve or a transient ischemic attack that affects the nerve. These disorders are commonly the cause in people who have high blood pressure, diabetes, or atherosclerosis.

Treatment depends on the cause of the palsy. When the cause is treated, the palsy usually resolves. If the cause is a blockage of a blood vessel, the nerve regenerates, and the palsy usually resolves without treatment within 2 months.

Trigeminal Neuralgia

Trigeminal neuralgia (tic douloureux) is pain due to malfunction of cranial nerve V (trigeminal nerve), which carries sensory information from the face to the brain and controls the muscles involved in chewing.

Trigeminal neuralgia usually occurs in middle-aged and older people, although it can affect adults of all ages. It is more common among women.

In most cases, the cause is unknown. A common known cause is an abnormally positioned artery that compresses the trigeminal nerve near where it exits the brain. Occasionally in younger people, trigeminal neuralgia results from nerve damage due to multiple sclerosis. Rarely, trigeminal neuralgia results from damage due to herpes zoster (a viral infection) or compression by a tumor.

Symptoms

The pain can occur spontaneously but is often triggered by touching a particular spot (called a trigger point) on the face, lips, or tongue or by an activity such as brushing the teeth or chewing. Repeated short, lightning-like bursts of excruciating stabbing pain can be felt in any part of the lower portion of the face but are most often felt in the cheek next to the nose or in the jaw. Usually, only one side of the

▲ see page 490   ■ see art on page 443

TESTING THE CRANIAL NERVES

Cranial Nerve Number	Name	Function	Test
I	Olfactory	Smell	The ability to smell is tested by asking the person to identify items with very specific odors (such as soap, coffee, and cloves) placed under the nose. Each nostril is tested separately.
II	Optic	Vision and detection of light by the pupil	The ability to see is tested by asking the person to read an eye chart. Peripheral vision is tested by asking the person to detect objects or movement from the corners of the eyes.
III	Oculomotor	Eye movement upward, downward, and inward; narrowing (constriction) or widening (dilation) of the pupil in response to changes in light	The ability to move each eye upward, downward, and inward is tested by asking the person to follow a target moved by the examiner. The upper eyelid is checked for drooping (ptosis).
IV	Trochlear	Eye movement downward and inward	The ability to move each eye downward and inward is tested by asking the person to follow a target moved by the examiner.
V	Trigeminal	Facial sensation and chewing	Sensation in areas of the face is tested using a pin and a wisp of cotton. The blink reflex is tested by touching the cornea of the eye with a cotton wisp. Strength and movement of muscles that control the jaw are tested by asking the person to clench the teeth and open the jaw against resistance.
VI	Abducens	Side-to-side (lateral) eye movement	The ability to move each eye outward beyond the midline is tested.
VII	Facial	Facial expression and taste in the front two thirds of the tongue	The ability to move the face is tested by asking the person to smile, to open the mouth and show the teeth, and to close the eyes tightly. Taste is tested using substances that are sweet (sugar), sour (lemon juice), salty (salt), and bitter (aspirin, quinine, or aloes).
VIII	Acoustic	Hearing and balance	Hearing is tested with a tuning fork. Balance is tested by asking the person to walk a straight line.
IX	Glossopharyngeal	Swallowing, gag reflex, and speech	Because cranial nerves IX and X control similar functions, they are tested together. The person is asked to swallow. The person is asked to say "ah-h-h" to check the movement of the palate (roof of the mouth) and uvula (the small, soft projection that hangs down at the back of throat). The back of the throat is touched with a tongue blade, which evokes the gag reflex in most people. The person is asked to speak to check the voice for hoarseness.

TESTING THE CRANIAL NERVES (Continued)

CRANIAL NERVE NUMBER	NAME	FUNCTION	TEST
X	Vagus	Swallowing, gag reflex, and speech; control of muscle in internal organs (including the heart)	Same as for cranial nerve IX.
XI	Accessory	Neck turning and shoulder shrugging	The person is asked to turn the head and to shrug the shoulders against resistance provided by the examiner.
XII	Hypoglossal	Tongue movement	The person is asked to stick out the tongue, which is observed for deviation to one side or the other.

face is affected. The pain usually lasts seconds but may last up to 2 minutes. Recurring as often as 100 times a day, the pain can be incapacitating. Because the pain is intense, people tend to wince, and thus the disorder is sometimes called a tic. The disorder commonly resolves on its own, but bouts of the disorder often recur after a long pain-free interval.

Diagnosis and Treatment

Although no specific test exists for identifying trigeminal neuralgia, its characteristic pain makes it easy for doctors to diagnose. However, doctors must distinguish trigeminal neuralgia from other possible causes of facial pain, such as disorders of the jaw, teeth, or sinuses and trigeminal neuropathy (which is often due to compression of the trigeminal nerve by a tumor or an aneurysm). For example, trigeminal neuropathy causes loss of sensation in the face and trigeminal neuralgia does not.

Because the bouts of pain are brief and recurrent, typical analgesics are not usually helpful, but other drugs, especially certain anticonvulsants (which stabilize nerve membranes), may be helpful. The anticonvulsant carbamazepine is usually tried first. Phenytoin or valproate may be prescribed if carbamazepine is ineffective or produces intolerable side effects. Baclofen (a drug used to reduce muscle spasms) or a tricyclic antidepressant▲ may be used instead.

When trigeminal neuralgia results from an abnormally positioned artery, a surgeon separates the artery from the nerve and places a small sponge between them. This procedure usually relieves the pain for many years. If the cause is a tumor, the tumor can be surgically removed.

For people who have pain unrelieved by drugs and who may not be good candidates for surgery, a test can be performed to determine whether other procedures would be helpful. For the test, alcohol is injected into the nerve to temporarily block its function. If the pain is relieved by the alcohol, cutting the nerve surgically or with a radiofrequency probe (using heat) relieves the pain permanently. Alternatively, the nerve can be permanently destroyed by injecting a drug such as glycerol into it. However, these treatments are used as a last resort. They often provide only temporary relief—for months to a few years—and afterward, discomfort in the face recurs.

Bell's Palsy

Bell's palsy is sudden weakness or paralysis of the muscles on one side of the face due to malfunction of cranial nerve VII (facial nerve), which stimulates the facial muscles.

Bell's palsy affects about 23 of 100,000 people at some time. The cause of Bell's palsy is unknown, but it may involve swelling of the facial nerve as a reaction to an immune disorder or a viral infection. Swelling causes the nerve to be compressed and its blood supply to be reduced. Evidence suggests that herpes simplex, a viral infection, is usually the cause. Lyme disease is also a common cause of Bell's palsy, especially in the northeastern United States. In blacks, sarcoidosis is a common cause.

▲ see table on page 618

Horner's Syndrome: A Droopy Eye

Some of the nerve fibers that connect the eyes and the brain take a circuitous route. They travel down the spinal cord, emerge in the chest and then go back up the neck beside the carotid artery through the skull and into the eye. If these nerve fibers are disrupted anywhere along their pathway, Horner's syndrome results.

Horner's syndrome can develop in people of any age. The syndrome can be caused by disorders of the neck and spinal cord as well as by disorders of the head and brain. Causes include lung cancer; tumors in the brain or spinal cord; injuries to the neck, head, or spinal cord; thoracic aortic aneurysms; and dissection of the carotid artery or aorta. Horner's syndrome may be present at birth (congenital). In the congenital form, the affected eye remains blue-gray as at birth.

This syndrome affects the eye on the same side as the disrupted nerve fibers. The eyelid droops, the pupil decreases in size, and the eyeball sinks slightly into its orbit. In addition, the affected side of the face perspires less than normal.

The disorder is diagnosed on the basis of symptoms. Treatment depends on the cause, but often, no treatment is useful.

Symptoms

Pain behind the ear may be the first symptom, developing several hours or even a day or two before the facial muscles weaken. In Bell's palsy, facial weakness occurs suddenly and ranges from mild weakness to complete paralysis. The weakness reaches its maximum by 48 hours. Only one side of the face is affected. The weak side becomes flat and expressionless. However, people often feel as though the face is twisted because the muscles on the unaffected side tend to pull the face to that side every time a facial expression is made. Most people experience a numbness or heavy feeling in the face, even though sensation remains normal.

When the upper part of the face is affected, closing the eye on the affected side may be difficult and incomplete. Because the eye cannot close completely, it may become dry, resulting in pain, eye damage, and even blindness. The eye also tends to roll upward when it is closed.

Bell's palsy may interfere with the produc-

tion of saliva, the sensation of taste in the front part of the tongue, or the ability to produce tears. The ear on the affected side may perceive sounds as abnormally loud (a condition called hyperacusis) because the muscle that stretches the eardrum is paralyzed. This muscle is located in the inner ear.

Occasionally, as the facial nerve heals, it forms abnormal connections, resulting in unexpected movements of some facial muscles or in watering of the eyes ("crocodile tears") during salivation.

Diagnosis

Bell's palsy can usually be diagnosed based on symptoms. It can be distinguished from a stroke because stroke usually causes sudden weakness only in the lower part of the face rather than the entire face. Also, a stroke typically causes weakness of an arm and a leg.

Doctors can distinguish Bell's palsy from other disorders that are rare causes of facial nerve paralysis because the other disorders usually develop slowly. These disorders include brain tumors, other tumors that compress the facial nerve, infections in the middle ear or mastoid sinuses, and fractures of the bone at the base of the skull. Usually, doctors can exclude these disorders on the basis of the person's history and results of x-rays, computed tomography (CT), or magnetic resonance imaging (MRI). A blood test may be performed to check for Lyme disease or sarcoidosis. There is no specific test for Bell's palsy.

Treatment and Prognosis

Bell's palsy is treated as if the cause were herpes simplex. An antiviral drug called acyclovir is given to prevent the virus from replicating. Corticosteroids, such as prednisone, are given by mouth to reduce swelling of the nerve. For maximum benefit, treatment should start within 2 days of the development of symptoms and be continued for 1 to 2 weeks.

If paralyzed facial muscles prevent the eye from closing completely, the eye must be protected from dryness to reduce the risk of blindness. Eyedrops consisting of artificial tears or a salt (saline) solution are applied to the eye until it can close completely. An eye patch may also be needed.

Mild electrical stimulation of the nerve and massage of the facial muscles have no proven benefit. If no facial movement has returned after 6 to 12 months, an operation—called hypoglossal-facial anastomosis—may be performed to join cranial nerve XII (hypoglossal nerve) to the facial nerve. This operation may partially restore facial movement, but it also causes difficulties in eating and speaking and is therefore rarely performed.

When facial paralysis is partial, most people recover completely within 1 to 2 months whether they are treated or not. When the paralysis is total, the outcome varies. Many people do not recover completely; the facial muscles may remain weak, causing the face to droop.

Hemifacial Spasm

Hemifacial spasm is involuntary twitching of one side of the face.

Hemifacial spasm affects men and women but is more common among middle-aged and older women. The spasms are caused by an abnormally positioned artery or loop of an artery that compresses cranial nerve VII where it exits from the brain stem. Muscles on one side of the face twitch involuntarily, usually begin-ning with the eyelid and then spreading to the cheek and mouth. Twitching may be intermittent at first but may become almost continuous. The disorder is essentially painless but can be embarrassing.

The diagnosis is made by seeing the spasms. Magnetic resonance imaging (MRI) rarely detects the abnormal artery but should be performed to rule out a tumor.

Botulinum toxin is the drug of choice. It is injected into the affected muscles. If this treatment is unsuccessful, surgery may be performed to separate the abnormal artery from the nerve by placing a small sponge between them.

Glossopharyngeal Neuralgia

Glossopharyngeal neuralgia consists of recurring attacks of severe pain in the back of the throat near the tonsils and back of the tongue due to malfunction of cranial nerve IX (glossopharyngeal nerve), which supplies the throat, tonsils, and tongue.

Taking the Pressure Off a Nerve

When pain results from an abnormally positioned artery pressing on a cranial nerve, the pain can be relieved by a surgical procedure called vascular decompression. This procedure may be performed to treat trigeminal neuralgia, hemifacial spasms, or glossopharyngeal neuralgia.

If the trigeminal nerve is compressed, an area on the back of the head is shaved, and an incision is made. The surgeon cuts a small hole in the skull and lifts the edge of the brain to expose the nerve. Then the surgeon separates the artery from the nerve and places a small sponge between them. A general anesthetic is required, but the risk of side effects from the procedure is small. Side effects include facial numbness, facial weakness, double vision, infection, bleeding, alterations in hearing and balance, and paralysis. Usually, this procedure relieves the pain, but in about 15% of people, pain recurs.

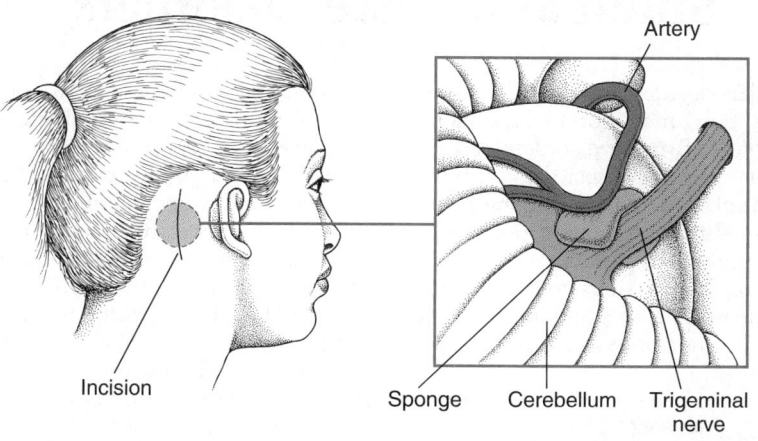

Incision   Sponge   Cerebellum   Artery   Trigeminal nerve

Glossopharyngeal neuralgia, a rare disorder, usually begins after age 40 and occurs more often in men. Its cause is unknown.

Symptoms

As in trigeminal neuralgia, attacks are brief, occur intermittently, but cause excruciating pain. Attacks may be triggered by a particular action, such as chewing, swallowing, coughing, or sneezing. The pain usually begins at the back of the tongue or back of the throat; sometimes pain spreads to the ear. The pain may last several seconds to a few minutes and usually affects only one side of the throat and tongue. The pain may radiate to the ear. In 1 to 2% of people, the heartbeat is affected: It slows so much that it stops temporarily, causing fainting.

Diagnosis and Treatment

Glossopharyngeal neuralgia is distinguished from trigeminal neuralgia based on the pain's location or results of a specific test. For the test, a doctor touches the back of the throat with a cotton-tipped applicator. If an attack results, the doctor applies a local anesthetic to the back of the throat and repeats the test. If the anesthetic prevents an attack, the diagnosis is glossopharyngeal neuralgia.

The same drugs used to treat trigeminal neuralgia—carbamazepine, phenytoin, baclofen, and tricyclic antidepressants▲—may be helpful. If these drugs are ineffective, applying a local anesthetic to the back of the throat may provide temporary relief. However, for permanent relief, surgery may be needed: The glossopharyngeal nerve is separated from the artery that is compressing it by placing a small sponge between them.

Hypoglossal Nerve Disorders

Disorders of cranial nerve XII (hypoglossal nerve) cause weakness or wasting (atrophy) of the tongue on the affected side.

Disorders of the hypoglossal nerve may result from a tumor at the base of the skull, a stroke, infections of the brain stem, or an injury to the neck, including that due to surgical removal of a blockage from an artery in the neck (endarterectomy■). Amyotrophic lateral sclerosis (Lou Gehrig's disease) can also damage the hypoglossal nerve.

The tongue becomes weak on the affected side and eventually wastes away (atrophies). As a result, people have difficulty speaking, chewing, and swallowing. Damage due to amyotrophic lateral sclerosis produces a distinctive wormlike movement of the tongue.

Magnetic resonance imaging (MRI) is usually performed to look for a tumor or evidence of a stroke. A spinal tap (lumbar puncture)★ may be necessary if cancer or infection is possible. Treatment depends on the cause.

CHAPTER 97

Smell and Taste Disorders

Because disorders of smell and taste are rarely life threatening, they may not receive close medical attention. Yet, these disorders can be frustrating because they can affect the ability to enjoy food and drink and to appreciate pleasant aromas. They can also interfere with the ability to notice potentially harmful chemicals and gases and thus may have serious consequences. Occasionally, impairment of smell and taste is due to a serious disorder, such as a tumor.

▲ see page 591   ■ see page 506
★ see art on page 443

Smell and taste are closely linked. The taste buds of the tongue identify taste; the nerves in the nose identify smell. Both sensations are communicated to the brain, which integrates the information so that flavors can be recognized and appreciated. Some tastes—such as salty, bitter, sweet, and sour—can be recognized without the sense of smell. However, more complex flavors (raspberry, for example) require both taste and smell sensations to be recognized.

Generally, when people are in their 50s, the ability to smell and to taste starts to diminish gradually. In about 40% of older people, the ability to smell is significantly reduced.

How People Sense Flavors

To distinguish most flavors, the brain needs information about both smell and taste. These sensations are communicated to the brain from the nose and mouth. Several areas of the brain integrate the information, enabling people to recognize and appreciate flavors.

A small area on the mucous membrane that lines the nose (the olfactory epithelium) contains specialized nerve cells called smell receptors. These receptors have hairlike projections (cilia) that detect odors. Airborne molecules entering the nasal passage stimulate the cilia, triggering a nerve impulse in nearby nerve fibers. The fibers extend upward through the bone that forms the roof of the nasal cavity (cribriform plate) and connect to enlargements of nerve cells (olfactory bulbs) that form the cranial nerves of smell (olfactory nerves). The impulse travels through the olfactory bulbs, along the olfactory nerves, to the brain. The brain interprets the impulse as a distinct odor. Also, the area of the brain where memories of odors are stored—the middle part of the temporal lobe—is stimulated. The memories enable a person to distinguish and identify many different odors experienced over a lifetime.

Thousands of tiny taste buds cover most of the tongue's surface. Food placed in the mouth stimulates taste receptors in the taste buds. Taste receptors have cilia that detect tastes. Food molecules stimulate the cilia, triggering a nerve impulse in nearby nerve fibers, which are connected to the cranial nerves of taste (the facial and glossopharyngeal nerves). The impulse travels along these cranial nerves to the brain, which interprets the impulse as a distinct taste. Taste buds can detect sweetness, saltiness, sourness, and bitterness. Combinations of the four basic tastes produce a wide spectrum of tastes.

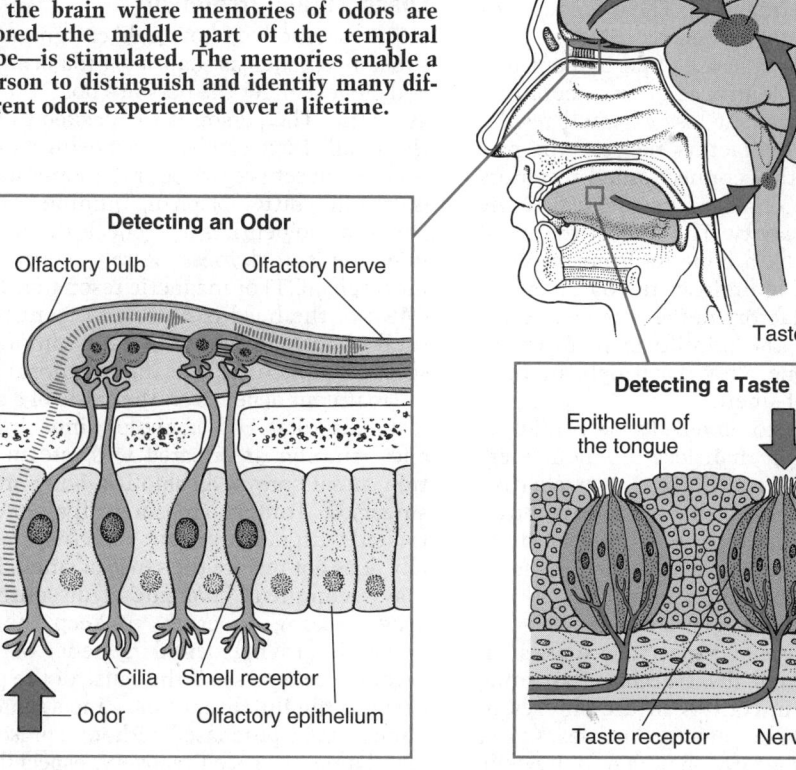

Smell signal

Smell and taste center

Taste signal

Detecting an Odor

Olfactory bulb   Olfactory nerve

Cilia   Smell receptor

Odor   Olfactory epithelium

Detecting a Taste

Epithelium of the tongue   Food   Cilia

Taste receptor   Nerve fiber

A reduced ability to smell (hyposmia) and loss of smell (anosmia) are the most common disorders of smell and taste. Because distinguishing one flavor from another is based largely on smell, people often first notice that their ability to smell is reduced when their food seems tasteless.

The ability to smell can be affected by changes in the nose, in the nerves leading from the nose to the brain, or in the brain. For example, if nasal passages are stuffed up from a common cold, the ability to smell may be reduced because odors are prevented from reaching the smell receptors (specialized nerve cells in the mucous membrane lining the nose). Because the ability to smell affects taste, food often does not taste right to people with colds. Smell receptors can be temporarily damaged by the influenza (flu) virus. Some people cannot smell or taste for several days or even weeks after a bout of the flu, and rarely, loss of smell or taste becomes permanent.

Occasionally, serious infections of the nasal sinuses or radiation therapy for cancer causes a loss of smell or taste that lasts for months or even becomes permanent. These conditions can damage or destroy smell receptors.

The most common cause of permanent loss of smell is a head injury, as often occurs in a car accident. Permanent loss of smell results when fibers of the olfactory nerves—the pair of cranial nerves that connect smell receptors to the brain—are damaged or sheared at the roof of the nasal cavity. The roof of the nasal cavity is formed by a bone (cribriform plate) that separates the brain from the nasal cavity. Damage to the olfactory nerves can also result from fractures of the cribriform plate or tumors near this bone. Very few people are born without a sense of smell.

Oversensitivity to smell (hyperosmia) is much less common than loss of smell. Pregnant women commonly become oversensitive to smell. Hyperosmia can also be psychosomatic. Psychosomatic hyperosmia is more likely to develop in people who have a histrionic personality (conspicuous seeking of attention with dramatic behavior▲).

A distorted sense of smell that makes innocuous odors smell disagreeable (dysosmia) may result from infections in the sinuses or partial damage to the olfactory nerves. Other causes of dysosmia are poor dental hygiene

and mouth infections. Dysosmia may be a symptom of depression. Seizures originating in the part of the brain where memories of smell are stored—the middle part of the temporal lobe—may produce brief, vivid, unpleasant smells (olfactory hallucinations). These smells are the part of the seizure called an aura, not a smell disorder.

A reduction in the ability to taste (hypogeusia) or loss of taste (ageusia) is usually caused by conditions that affect the tongue. Such conditions include a very dry mouth, heavy smoking (especially pipe smoking), radiation therapy to the head and neck, and side effects of drugs such as the chemotherapy drug vincristine and the antidepressant amitriptyline. In Bell's palsy, the sense of taste is often lost on the front two thirds of only one side of the tongue (the side affected by the palsy).

A distortion of taste (dysgeusia) may be caused by many of the same conditions that result in loss of taste, including depression and seizures. Burns to the tongue may temporarily destroy taste buds.

Diagnosis and Treatment

To test smell, doctors hold common fragrant substances (such as soap, a vanilla bean, coffee, and cloves) under the person's nose, one nostril at a time. The person is then asked to identify the smell. Taste can be tested using substances that are sweet (sugar), sour (lemon juice), salty (salt), and bitter (aspirin, quinine, or aloes). Doctors and dentists also check the mouth for infection and dryness. Rarely, computed tomography (CT) or magnetic resonance imaging (MRI) of the head is needed to identify structural abnormalities (such as a tumor, an abscess, or a fracture) near the cribriform plate.

Treatment depends on the cause of a smell or taste disorder. For example, sinus infections and irritation are treated with steam inhalation, nasal sprays, antibiotics, and sometimes surgery.■ Tumors are surgically removed or treated with radiation, but such treatment usually does not restore the sense of smell. Doctors may recommend changing or discontinuing a drug, sucking on candy to keep the mouth moist, improving dental hygiene, or waiting several weeks to see if the cause of the problem (such as the flu) disappears. Zinc supplements, which can be purchased without a prescription, are claimed to speed recovery, especially from taste disorders due to a bout of the flu. However, the claim has not been substantiated.

▲ see page 631   ■ see page 1267

MENTAL HEALTH DISORDERS

98   **Overview of Mental Health Care**..............................**598**

Mental Illness in Society ▪ Classification and Diagnosis of Mental Illness ▪ Treatment of Mental Illness

99   **Somatoform Disorders**..............................**601**

Somatization Disorder ▪ Conversion Disorder ▪ Hypochondriasis ▪ Body Dysmorphic Disorder

100   **Anxiety Disorders**..............................**605**

Generalized Anxiety Disorder ▪ Anxiety Induced by Drugs or Medical Problems ▪ Panic Attacks and Panic Disorder ▪ Phobic Disorders ▪ Obsessive-Compulsive Disorder ▪ Posttraumatic Stress Disorder ▪ Acute Stress Disorder

101   **Depression and Mania**..............................**613**

Depression ▪ Mania ▪ Manic-Depressive Illness

102   **Suicidal Behavior**..............................**622**

103   **Eating Disorders**..............................**624**

Anorexia Nervosa ▪ Bulimia Nervosa ▪ Binge Eating Disorder

104   **Sexuality**..............................**627**

Gender Identity ▪ Paraphilias

105   **Personality Disorders**..............................**631**

106   **Amnesia and Related Disorders**..............................**636**

Dissociative Amnesia ▪ Dissociative Fugue ▪ Dissociative Identity Disorder ▪ Depersonalization Disorder

107   **Schizophrenia and Delusional Disorder**..............................**640**

108   **Drug Use and Abuse**..............................**646**

Alcohol ▪ Opioids ▪ Antianxiety Drugs and Sedatives ▪ Nicotine ▪ Marijuana ▪ Amphetamines ▪ Cocaine ▪ Hallucinogens ▪ Phencyclidine ▪ Ketamine ▪ Gamma Hydroxybutyrate ▪ Solvent Inhalants

CHAPTER 98

Overview of Mental Health Care

Mental health (psychiatric) disorders involve disturbances in thinking, emotion, and behavior. These disorders are caused by complex interactions between physical, psychologic, social, cultural, and hereditary influences.

Mental Illness in Society

About 20% of adults will experience a mental illness at some point in their lives. In fact, 4 of the 10 leading causes of disability among people aged 5 and older are mental health disorders, with depression being the number one cause of all illnesses that cause disability. Unfortunately, despite this high prevalence of mental illness, only about half of people who have a mental illness seek professional help.

Although tremendous advances have been made in the understanding and treatment of mental illnesses, the stigma surrounding them persists. For example, people with mental illness may be blamed for their illness or viewed as lazy or irresponsible. Mental illness may be seen as less real or legitimate than physical illness, leading to reluctance on the part of policy makers and insurance companies to pay for treatment. Parents may be blamed for causing mental illness in their children. The public may shun people with mental illness and avoid living near them, working with them, and socializing with them.

Our current understanding of mental illness is that it is caused by a complex interaction of genetics and environment. Brain chemicals called neurotransmitters appear to be disordered in some mental illnesses. Research has shown that there is a hereditary component to many mental health disorders. Often, a genetic vulnerability interacts with certain stressors in a person's family life, social circle, or work situation to trigger an episode of mental illness.

Mental illness cannot always be clearly differentiated from normal behavior. Distinguishing normal bereavement from depression, for example, may be difficult in the face of a significant loss, such as the death of a spouse or child. Likewise, a diagnosis of anxiety disorder in relation to a person's worry and stress regarding his job is somewhat arbitrary, because most people experience these feelings at some time. The line between a person's

having certain personality traits and having a personality disorder can be blurry. Mental illness and mental health, therefore, are best thought of as residing on a continuum.

Deinstitutionalization

A movement in recent decades to bring mentally ill people out of institutions has been made possible by the development of effective drugs, along with some change in attitude about the mentally ill. With the deinstitutionalization movement, greater emphasis has been placed on viewing mentally ill people as members of families and communities.

Research has demonstrated that certain interactions between families and patients can improve or worsen mental illness. Therefore, family therapy techniques have been developed that dramatically prevent the chronically mentally ill from needing to be reinstitutionalized. Today, the family of a mentally ill person is more involved than ever as an ally in treatment. The family doctor also plays an important role in rehabilitating a mentally ill person into the community. In addition, mentally ill people who must be hospitalized are less likely to be isolated and restrained than in the past, and they are often discharged early into day treatment centers. These settings are less expensive because fewer staff members are needed, the emphasis is on group therapy rather than individual therapy, and people sleep at home or in halfway houses.

However, the deinstitutionalization movement has had its share of problems. Because mentally ill people who are not a danger to themselves or society can no longer be institutionalized or treated against their will, many have become homeless. Although these legal measures protect people's civil rights, they make it more difficult to provide needed treatment to many mentally ill people, some of whom may be extremely irrational. Homelessness also has an effect on society.

Social Support

Everyone requires a social network to satisfy the human need to be cared for, accepted, and emotionally supported, particularly in times of stress. Research has demonstrated that strong social support may significantly

TYPES OF MENTAL HEALTH CARE PROFESSIONALS

PROFESSIONAL	TRAINING AND EXPERTISE
Psychiatrist	Medical doctor with 4 years of psychiatric training after graduation from medical school. Can prescribe drugs and admit people to the hospital. Some practice psychotherapy, some only prescribe drugs, and many do both.
Psychologist	Professional who has a doctorate but not a medical degree. Many have post-doctoral training, and most are trained to administer psychologic tests that are helpful in diagnosis. May conduct psychotherapy but cannot perform physical examinations, prescribe drugs, or admit people to the hospital.
Psychiatric social worker	A professional with specialized training in certain aspects of psychotherapy, such as family/marital therapy or individual psychotherapy. Often trained to interface with the social service systems in the state. May have a master's degree, but some have doctorates as well. Cannot perform physical examinations or prescribe drugs.
Psychiatric nurse	Registered nurse who may practice psychotherapy independently in some states and may prescribe drugs under the supervision of a doctor.
Psychoanalyst	May be a psychiatrist, psychologist, or social worker who has many years of training in the practice of psychoanalysis, a type of intensive psychotherapy involving several sessions a week designed to explore unconscious patterns of thought, feeling, and behavior. Psychoanalysts who are also psychiatrists may prescribe drugs and admit people to hospitals in addition to conducting psychoanalysis.

improve recovery from both physical and mental illnesses. Changes in society have diminished the traditional support once offered by neighbors and families. As an alternative, self-help groups and mutual aid groups have sprung up throughout the country.

Some self-help groups, such as Alcoholics Anonymous and Narcotics Anonymous, focus on addictive behavior. Others act as advocates for certain segments of the population, such as the handicapped and older people. Still others, such as the National Alliance for the Mentally Ill, provide support for family members of people who have a severe mental illness.

Classification and Diagnosis of Mental Illness

In 1952, the American Psychiatric Association first published the *Diagnostic and Statistical Manual of Mental Disorders (DSM-I)*, marking the first attempt to approach the diagnosis of mental illness through standardized definitions and criteria. The latest edition, *DSM-IV*, published in 1994, provides a classification system that attempts to separate mental illnesses into diagnostic categories based on descriptions of symptoms (that is, what people say and do as a reflection of how they think and feel) and on the course of the illness.

The *International Classification of Disease, 10th Revision, Clinical Modification (ICD-10-CM)*, a book published by the World Health Organization, uses diagnostic categories similar to those in the *DSM-IV*. This similarity suggests that diagnoses of specific mental illnesses are becoming more standard and consistent throughout the world.

Advances have been made in diagnostic methods. Several brain imaging techniques are available, including computed tomography (CT), magnetic resonance imaging (MRI), and positron emission tomography (PET), a type of scan that measures blood flow to specific areas of the brain.▲ These imaging techniques are being used to map brain structure and function in people with normal and abnormal behavior, giving scientists greater understanding of how the brain functions in people with and without mental illness. Research that has differentiated one mental health disorder from another has led to greater precision in diagnosis.

Treatment of Mental Illness

Extraordinary advances have been made in the treatment of mental illness. An understanding of what causes some mental health

▲ see page 444

disorders has led to greater sophistication in tailoring treatment to the underlying basis of each disorder. As a result, many mental health disorders can now be treated nearly as successfully as physical disorders.

Most treatment methods for mental health disorders can be categorized as either somatic or psychotherapeutic. Somatic treatments include drug therapy and electroconvulsive therapy. Psychotherapeutic treatments include individual, group, or family and marital psychotherapy; behavior therapy techniques (such as relaxation training or exposure therapy); and hypnotherapy. Most studies suggest that for major mental health disorders, a treatment approach involving both drugs and psychotherapy is more effective than either treatment method used alone.

Psychiatrists are not the only mental health care professionals trained to treat mental illness. Others include clinical psychologists, social workers, nurses, and some pastoral counselors. However, psychiatrists are the only mental health care professionals licensed to prescribe drugs. Other mental health care professionals primarily practice psychotherapy.

Drug Therapy

Over the last 40 years, a number of psychoactive drugs have been developed that are highly effective and widely used by psychiatrists and other medical doctors. These drugs are often categorized according to the disorder for which they are primarily prescribed. For example, antidepressants are used to treat depression. Selective serotonin reuptake inhibitors are the newest and most widely used class of antidepressants. Other new classes of antidepressants are being developed. Antipsychotic drugs, such as chlorpromazine, haloperidol, and thiothixene, are helpful in treating psychotic disorders such as schizophrenia. Newer antipsychotic drugs, such as clozapine, risperidone, olanzapine, and quetiapine, are increasingly being used because they have fewer side effects. Antianxiety drugs, such as clonazepam and diazepam, as well as selective serotonin reuptake inhibitors (which are antidepressants), are used to treat anxiety disorders, such as panic disorder and phobias. Mood stabilizers, such as lithium, carbamazepine, and valproate, have been used with some success to treat manic-depressive illness (bipolar disorder).

Electroconvulsive Therapy

With electroconvulsive therapy, electrodes are attached to the head, and a series of electri-

cal shocks are delivered to the brain to induce seizures. This therapy has consistently been shown to be the most effective treatment for severe depression. Many people treated with electroconvulsive therapy experience temporary memory loss. However, contrary to its portrayal in the media, electroconvulsive therapy is safe and rarely causes any other complications. The modern use of anesthetics and muscle relaxants has greatly reduced any risk to the person.

Psychotherapeutic Treatments

In recent years, significant advances have been made in the field of psychotherapeutic treatments. Psychotherapy, sometimes referred to as "talk" therapy, works on the assumption that each person has within himself the cure for his own suffering and that this cure can be facilitated through a trusting, supportive relationship with a psychotherapist. By creating an empathetic and accepting atmosphere, the therapist often is able to help the person identify the source of his problems and consider alternatives for dealing with them. The emotional awareness and insight that the person gains through psychotherapy often results in a change in attitude and behavior that allows the person to live a fuller and more satisfying life.

Psychotherapy is appropriate in a wide range of conditions. Even people who do not have a mental health disorder may find psychotherapy helpful in coping with such problems as employment difficulties, bereavement, or chronic illness in the family. Group psychotherapy, couples' therapy, and family therapy are also widely used.

Most mental health professionals practice within one of five types of psychotherapy: psychoanalysis, psychodynamic psychotherapy, cognitive therapy, behavior therapy, or interpersonal therapy.

Psychoanalysis is the oldest form of psychotherapy and was developed by Sigmund Freud in the first part of the 20th century. The person typically lies on a couch in the therapist's office 4 or 5 times a week and attempts to say whatever comes into his mind, a practice called free association. Much of the focus is on understanding how past patterns of relationships repeat themselves in the present. The relationship between the person and the therapist is a key part of this focus. An understanding of how the past affects the present helps the person develop new and more adaptive ways of functioning in relationships and in work settings.

Psychodynamic psychotherapy, like psychoanalysis, emphasizes the identification of unconscious patterns in current thoughts, feelings, and behaviors. However, the person is usually sitting instead of lying on a couch and attends only 1 to 3 sessions per week. In addition, less emphasis is placed on the relationship between the person and therapist.

Cognitive therapy helps people identify distortions in thinking and understand how these distortions lead to problems in their lives. The underlying premise is that how people feel and behave are determined by how they interpret experiences. Through the identification of core beliefs and assumptions, people can begin to think in different ways about their experiences, resulting in improvement in symptoms, behavior, and feelings.

Behavior therapy is related to cognitive therapy. Sometimes, a combination of the two, known as cognitive-behavior therapy, is used. The theoretical basis of behavior therapy is learning theory, which holds that abnormal behaviors are due to faulty learning. Behavior therapy involves a number of interventions that are designed to help the person unlearn maladaptive behaviors while learning adaptive behaviors. Exposure therapy is one example of a behavior therapy.▲

Interpersonal therapy was initially conceived as a brief psychologic treatment for depression and is designed to improve the quality of a depressed person's relationships. It focuses on unresolved grief, conflicts that arise when people fill roles that differ from their expectations (such as when a woman enters a relationship expecting to be a stay-at-home mother and finds that she must also be the major provider for the family), social role transitions (such as going from being an active worker to being retired), and difficulty communicating with others. The therapist teaches the person to improve aspects of interpersonal relationships, such as overcoming social isolation and responding in a less habitual way to others.

Hypnosis and Hypnotherapy

Hypnosis and hypnotherapy are often used to manage pain and treat physical disorders that have a psychologic component. Hypnosis is simply the induction of a trance or altered state of consciousness, whereas hypnotherapy involves psychotherapeutic intervention in conjunction with the hypnotic state. These techniques may promote relaxation and thereby lower anxiety and reduce tension. For example, hypnosis and hypnotherapy can help people with cancer who have anxiety or depression in addition to pain.

CHAPTER 99

Somatoform Disorders

Somatoform disorders encompass several mental health disorders in which people report physical symptoms or concerns that suggest but are not explained by a physical disorder or report a perceived defect in appearance. These symptoms or concerns cause significant distress or interfere with daily functioning.

Somatoform disorder is a relatively new term for what many people used to refer to as psychosomatic disorder. In somatoform disorders, the physical symptoms cannot be explained by any underlying physical disease. In some cases of somatoform disorders, a physical disease is present that might explain the occurrence but not the severity or duration of

the physical symptoms. People with somatoform disorders are not faking illness; they sincerely believe that they have a serious physical problem.

The most commonly diagnosed somatoform disorders are somatization disorder, conversion disorder, hypochondriasis, body dysmorphic disorder, and pain disorder.■ The individual people who are diagnosed with a somatoform disorder vary greatly. Treatment approaches also vary according to which somatoform disorder a person has.

▲ see box on page 609   ■ see page 449

Münchausen Syndrome: Faking Illness for Attention

Münchausen syndrome is not a somatoform disorder, but its features are somewhat similar in that mental health problems underlie physical symptoms. The key difference is that people with Münchausen syndrome consciously *fake* the symptoms of a physical disorder. They repeatedly fabricate illnesses and often wander from hospital to hospital for treatment.

However, Münchausen syndrome is more complex than simple dishonest fabrication and simulation of symptoms. The disorder is associated with severe emotional problems. People with the disorder are usually quite intelligent and resourceful; they not only know how to mimic diseases but also are sophisticated with regard to medical practices. They can manipulate their care to be hospitalized and subjected to intense testing and treatment, including major operations. Their deceits are conscious, but their motivation and quest for attention are largely unconscious.

Münchausen by proxy is a bizarre variant of Münchausen syndrome in which a child is used as a surrogate patient, usually by a parent. The parent falsifies the child's medical history and may injure the child with drugs or add blood or bacterial contaminants to urine specimens, all in an effort to fake disease. The motivation underlying such bizarre behavior appears to be a pathologic need for attention and for an intense relationship with the child.

Somatization Disorder

Somatization disorder is a chronic, severe disorder characterized by many recurring physical symptoms, particularly some combination of pain and digestive, sexual, and neurologic symptoms, that cannot be explained by a physical disorder.

Somatization disorder often runs in families and occurs predominantly in women. Male relatives of women with the disorder tend to have a high incidence of socially disapproved behavior (antisocial personality▲) and substance-related disorders. People with somatization disorder tend to also have personality disorders

---

▲ see page 632   ■ see page 633

and exaggerated dependence on others (dependent personality■).

The physical symptoms that people with somatization disorder experience appear to be a way of communicating a plea for help and attention. The intensity and persistence of the symptoms reflect the person's intense desire to be cared for in every aspect of life. The symptoms may also serve other purposes, such as allowing the person to avoid the responsibilities of adulthood. The symptoms tend to be uncomfortable and prevent the person from engaging in many enjoyable pursuits, suggesting that the person also suffers feelings of worthlessness and guilt.

Symptoms

Symptoms appear first in adolescence or early adulthood. A person with somatization disorder has many vague physical complaints, often described as "unbearable," "beyond description," or "the worst imaginable." Any part of the body may be affected, and specific symptoms and their frequency vary among different cultures. Typical symptoms include headaches, nausea and vomiting, abdominal pain, diarrhea or constipation, painful menstrual periods, fatigue, fainting, pain during intercourse, and loss of sexual desire. Men frequently complain of erectile or other sexual dysfunction. Anxiety and depression also occur.

People with somatization disorder increasingly demand help and emotional support and may become enraged when they feel their needs are not being met. In an attempt to manipulate others, they may threaten or attempt suicide. Often dissatisfied with their medical care, they go from doctor to doctor.

Diagnosis

People with somatization disorder are not aware that their basic problem is psychologic, so they press their doctors for diagnostic tests and treatments. The doctor usually conducts many physical examinations and tests to determine whether the person has a physical disorder that adequately explains the symptoms. Referrals to specialists for consultations are common, even if the person has developed a reasonably satisfactory relationship with one doctor.

Once a doctor determines that the problem is psychologic, somatization disorder can be distinguished from similar mental health disorders by its many symptoms and their tendency to persist over a period of years. Adding to the diagnosis are the dramatic nature of the complaints and the person's dependent and sometimes suicidal behavior.

Prognosis and Treatment

Somatization disorder tends to fluctuate in severity but persists throughout life. Complete relief of symptoms for an extended period is rare. Some people become more depressed after many years. Suicide is a risk.

Treatment is extremely difficult. People with somatization disorder tend to be frustrated and angered by any suggestion that their symptoms are psychologic. Therefore, doctors cannot deal directly with the problem as a psychologic one, even when they recognize it. Drug therapy does not help much, and even if the person agrees to a mental health consultation, specific psychotherapeutic techniques are not likely to be beneficial. Usually, a person with this disorder is best helped by a trusting relationship with a doctor, who can offer symptomatic relief and protect the person from very costly and possibly dangerous diagnostic or therapeutic procedures. However, the doctor must remain alert to the possibility that the person may develop an actual physical disorder.

Conversion Disorder

In conversion disorder, physical symptoms that are caused by psychologic conflict are unconsciously converted to resemble those of a neurologic disorder.

Conversion disorder, once referred to as hysteria, is caused by psychologic stress and conflict, which people with this disorder unconsciously convert into physical symptoms. Although conversion disorder tends to occur during adolescence or early adulthood, it may first appear at any age. The disorder is generally believed to be somewhat more common in women than in men.

Symptoms and Diagnosis

The symptoms of conversion disorder are limited to those that suggest a nervous system dysfunction—usually paralysis of an arm or leg or loss of sensation in a part of the body. Other symptoms may include simulated seizures and the loss of one of the special senses, such as vision or hearing.

Generally, the onset of symptoms is linked to some distressing social or psychologic event. A person may have only a single episode in his lifetime or sporadic episodes, but usually the

episodes are brief. If people with conversion symptoms are hospitalized, they generally improve within 2 weeks. However, 20 to 25% of those people who are hospitalized have recurrences within a year, and for some people, symptoms become chronic.

The diagnosis tends to be initially difficult for a doctor to make because the person believes that the symptoms stem from a physical problem and does not want to be seen by a therapist. Also, doctors take great care to be certain no physical disorder is responsible for the symptoms. Thus, the diagnosis is usually considered only after extensive physical examinations and tests fail to reveal a physical disorder that can fully account for the symptoms.

Treatment

A trusting doctor-patient relationship is essential. As the doctor evaluates a possible physical disorder and reassures the person that the symptoms do not indicate a serious underlying disease, the person usually begins to feel better and the symptoms fade. When a psychologically distressing situation has preceded the onset of symptoms, psychotherapy can be particularly effective.

Various treatment methods have been tried. Although some may be helpful, none of them have been uniformly effective. In one method, hypnotherapy, the person is hypnotized, and psychologic issues that may be responsible for the symptoms are identified and discussed. Discussion continues after the hypnosis, when the person is fully alert. Another (rarely used) method is narcoanalysis, a procedure similar to hypnosis except that the person is given a sedative to induce a state of semisleep. Behavior therapy, including relaxation training, has also been effective for some people.

Hypochondriasis

Hypochondriasis is a disorder in which a person is preoccupied with the fear of having a serious disease.

Hypochondriasis occurs most commonly between the ages of 20 and 30 and appears to affect both sexes equally. Some people with hypochondriasis also have depression or anxiety.

In hypochondriasis, the person's concerns about having a serious disease are often based on a misinterpretation of normal bodily functions. Examination and reassurance by a doctor do not relieve their concerns; people with hypochondriasis tend to believe that the doc-

What Are Psychosomatic Disorders?

The term *psychosomatic disorder* usually is applied when a person has physical symptoms that appear to be caused or worsened by psychologic factors, rather than by some underlying physical disease. This does not imply, however, that physical symptoms are imaginary or are being faked (as in Munchausen syndrome); the symptoms are actually being experienced by the person. Thus, psychosomatic disorders require that the psychologic factors and the physical symptoms be consistently and closely connected in time.

Unlike somatoform disorders, psychosomatic disorders do not fit into specific diagnostic categories, and they manifest in a variety of ways. Social and psychologic stress can also aggravate a wide variety of physical diseases, including diabetes mellitus, coronary artery disease, and asthma.

Stress can cause physical symptoms even when no physical disease is present. For example, hives can be brought on entirely by a psychologic reaction. In some cases, physical symptoms result from the body's auto-matic response to emotional stress, as when heart rate and blood pressure increase in response to fear. In other cases, psychologic symptoms become physical symptoms in an unconscious attempt to divert attention away from a troublesome emotional issue.

Sometimes a physical symptom is a metaphor for the person's psychologic problem, as when a person with a "broken heart" experiences chest pain. Other times, a physical symptom reflects identification with another person's pain. For example, a person may have chest pain after a family member or friend has had a heart attack. Finally, a psychologic symptom may become a physical symptom as a way of reexperiencing a symptom of a previous physical disorder. For example, a person who once had a painful bone fracture may reexperience that sort of bone pain when a psychologic symptom becomes bone pain. Physical symptoms that evolve from psychologic symptoms tend to be mild and transient. The process of psychologic symptoms be-coming physical symptoms can affect people who do not have a serious underlying mental health disorder. Anyone can undergo this process. The resulting symptoms can be difficult for a doctor to diagnose, and a person is likely to undergo various diagnostic tests to eliminate the possibility of an underlying physical disorder.

Psychologic factors can also indirectly influence the course of a disease. For example, a person with high blood pressure may deny having it or deny its seriousness. Denial is a defense mechanism that helps reduce anxiety. However, denial may prevent a person from complying with treatment. In this case, the person with high blood pressure may fail to take his prescribed medication, thus worsening the condition. Conversely, physical disease can lead to a psychologic condition. For example, people with life-threatening, recurring, or chronic physical disorders commonly become depressed. The depression, in turn, may worsen the effects of the physical disease.

tor has somehow failed to find the underlying disease.

Symptoms and Diagnosis

Hypochondriasis is suspected when a healthy person with minor symptoms is preoccupied with the significance of those symptoms and does not respond to reassurance after thorough evaluation. Personal relationships and work performance often suffer as the person becomes increasingly concerned with health issues. The diagnosis of hypochondriasis is confirmed when the situation persists for at least 6 months and the person's symptoms cannot be attributed to depression or another mental health disorder.

Treatment

Treatment is difficult, because a person with hypochondriasis is convinced that some-thing inside the body is seriously wrong. Reassurance does not relieve these concerns. However, a trusting relationship with a caring doctor is beneficial, especially if regular visits are scheduled. If the person's symptoms are not adequately relieved, the person may benefit from referral to a therapist for further evaluation and treatment, along with continuation of the primary doctor's care. Treatment with serotonin reuptake inhibitors, a class of antidepressants, may be effective. Cognitive-behavior therapy may also relieve symptoms.

Body Dysmorphic Disorder

In body dysmorphic disorder, a preoccupation with a perceived defect in appearance results in significant distress or impaired functioning.

People with body dysmorphic disorder believe they have a defect in appearance that in reality is nonexistent or slight. The disorder usually begins in adolescence and is believed to occur in men and women equally.

Symptoms

Symptoms may develop gradually or abruptly, vary in intensity, and tend to persist without treatment. Concerns commonly involve the face or head but may involve any body part or several parts and may change from one body part to another. A person may be concerned about hair thinning, acne, wrinkles, scars, color of complexion, or excessive facial hair. Or a person may focus on the shape or size of a body part, such as the nose, eyes, ears, mouth, breasts, or buttocks. Some young men with athletic builds think that they are puny and obsessively try to gain weight and muscle.

Most people with body dysmorphic disorder have difficulty controlling their preoccupation and spend hours each day thinking about their perceived defect. Many people check themselves often in mirrors, others avoid mirrors, and still others alternate between the two behaviors. Most try to camouflage their imagined defect—for example, by growing a beard to hide "scars" or by wearing a hat to cover "thinning" hair. Many undergo medical, dental, or surgical treatment, sometimes repeatedly, to correct their perceived defect, which may intensify their preoccupation.

Because people with body dysmorphic disorder feel self-conscious, they may avoid appearing in public, including going to work and participating in social activities. Some leave their homes only at night; others not at all. This behavior can result in social isolation. Distress and dysfunction associated with the disorder can lead to repeated hospitalization and suicidal behavior.

Diagnosis and Treatment

Because people with body dysmorphic disorder are reluctant to reveal their symptoms, the disorder may go undiagnosed for years. It is distinguished from normal concerns about appearance because it is time-consuming and causes significant distress or impairs functioning.

Information regarding effective treatment is limited. Treatment with serotonin reuptake inhibitors, a class of antidepressants, is often effective. Cognitive-behavior therapy may also diminish symptoms.

CHAPTER 100

Anxiety Disorders

Anxiety disorders involve a state of distressing chronic but fluctuating nervousness that is inappropriately severe for the person's circumstances.

Anxiety is a normal response to a threat or to psychologic stress and is experienced occasionally by everyone. Normal anxiety has its root in fear and serves an important survival function. When someone is faced with a dangerous situation, anxiety induces the fight-or-flight response. With this response, a variety of physical changes, such as increased blood flow to the heart and muscles, provide the body with the necessary energy and strength to deal with life-threatening situations, such as running from an aggressive animal or fighting off an attacker. However, when anxiety occurs at inappropriate times, occurs frequently, or is so intense and long-lasting that it interferes with a person's normal activities, then it is considered a disorder.

Anxiety disorders are more common than any other category of mental health disorder and are believed to affect about 15% of adults in the United States. However, anxiety disorders often are not recognized by people who have them or by health care professionals and consequently are seldom treated.

Causes

The causes of anxiety disorders are not fully known, but both physical and psychologic factors are involved. Because anxiety disorders are prevalent in some families, heredity proba-

How Anxiety Affects Performance

The effects of anxiety on performance can be shown on a curve. As the level of anxiety increases, performance efficiency increases proportionately, but only up to a point. As anxiety increases further, performance efficiency decreases. Before the peak of the curve, anxiety is considered adaptive, because it helps people prepare for a crisis and improve their functioning. Beyond the peak of the curve, anxiety is considered maladaptive, because it produces distress and impairs their functioning.

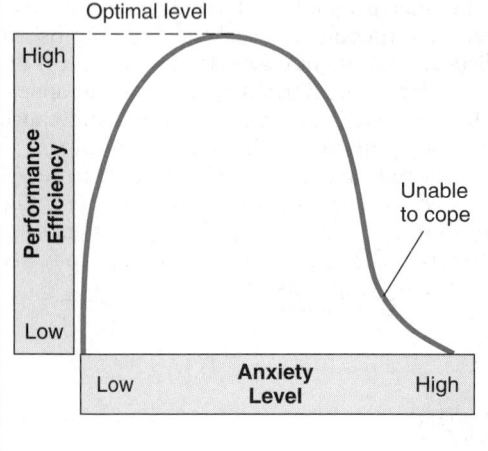

Symptoms and Diagnosis

Anxiety can arise suddenly, as in panic, or gradually over minutes, hours, or days. The anxiety itself can last for any length of time, from a few seconds to years. Anxiety ranges in intensity from barely noticeable qualms to full-blown panic attack,▲ during which a person may experience shortness of breath, dizziness, and increased heart rate.

Anxiety disorders can be so distressing and interfere so much with a person's life that they can lead to depression.■ Sometimes depression develops first and an anxiety disorder develops later.

The diagnosis of an anxiety disorder is based largely on its symptoms. The ability to tolerate anxiety varies, and determining what constitutes abnormal anxiety can be difficult. A family history of an anxiety disorder (except posttraumatic stress disorder) may help a doctor make the diagnosis.

Treatment

Accurate diagnosis is important, since treatment varies from one anxiety disorder to another. Additionally, anxiety disorders must be distinguished from anxiety that occurs in many other mental health disorders, for which different treatment approaches are used. Depending on the anxiety disorder, drug therapy or psychotherapy (such as behavior therapy), alone or in combination, can significantly relieve the distress and dysfunction for most people.

Generalized Anxiety Disorder

Generalized anxiety disorder consists of excessive, usually daily, nervousness and worry (lasting 6 months or longer) about a variety of activities or events.

Generalized anxiety disorder is common; about 3% of adults have it during any 12-month period. Women are twice as likely as men to have the disorder. It often begins in childhood or adolescence but may start at any age. For most people, the disorder fluctuates, worsening at times (especially during times of stress), and persists over many years.

People with generalized anxiety disorder constantly feel worried or distressed and find it difficult to control these feelings. The severity, frequency, or duration of the worries is disproportionately greater than the situation warrants. Worries are general in nature; common worries include work responsibilities, money, health, safety, car repairs, and chores.

bly plays a role. Anxiety is viewed at a psychologic level as a response to environmental stresses, such as the breakup of a significant relationship or exposure to a life-threatening disaster. When a person's response to stresses is improper or a person is overwhelmed by events, an anxiety disorder can arise. For example, some people find speaking before a group exhilarating, while others dread it, becoming anxious with symptoms such as sweating, fear, rapid heart rate, and tremor.

Anxiety disorders may also be caused by a physical disorder or the use of a drug. For example, an overactive thyroid gland, use of prescribed corticosteroids, or illicit use of cocaine may produce symptoms of an anxiety disorder.

▲ see page 608   ■ see page 614

℞ ANTIANXIETY DRUGS

DRUG	USES	SELECTED SIDE EFFECTS	COMMENTS
Benzodiazepines			
(alprazolam, chlordiazepoxide, clonazepam, clorazepate, diazepam, lorazepam, oxazepam)	Generalized anxiety disorder; panic disorder; phobic disorders	Sleepiness, impaired coordination, slowed reaction time. May lead to drug dependence; should not be used by people who have an alcohol dependency problem	Most commonly used type of antianxiety drug. Promote mental and physical relaxation by reducing nerve activity in the brain. Begin to work quickly, sometimes within an hour
Buspirone			
	Generalized anxiety disorder	Dizziness, headache	Does not cause sedation or interact with alcohol. Does not lead to drug dependence. Onset of antianxiety effects may take 2 weeks or longer
Antidepressants*			
(selective serotonin reuptake inhibitors, venlafaxine, monoamine oxidase inhibitors, tricyclic antidepressants)	Generalized anxiety disorder, panic disorder, phobic disorders, obsessive-compulsive disorder, posttraumatic stress disorder	See table on page 618	See table on page 618

*Not all of the antidepressants listed work for all of the uses that are listed.

The focus of worry may shift from one topic to another over time.

For a doctor to make a diagnosis of generalized anxiety disorder, a person must experience worry or anxiety and three or more of the following symptoms: restlessness, easy fatigue, difficulty concentrating, irritability, muscle tension, and disturbed sleep.

Treatment

Optimal management is best achieved with a combination of some form of counseling and drug therapy. Counseling can address the root causes of anxiety and ways to cope.

Antianxiety drugs such as benzodiazepines are usually prescribed. However, because long-term use of benzodiazepines can lead to drug dependence,▲ the drug, if discontinued, must be tapered off slowly rather than stopped abruptly. The relief that benzodiazepines bring usually outweighs any mild side effects and the possibility of drug dependence.

Buspirone is another antianxiety drug effective for some people with generalized anxiety disorder. Its use does not lead to drug dependence. However, buspirone may take 2 weeks or longer to start working, in contrast to benzodiazepines, which begin to work within an hour.

Some antidepressants, such as venlafaxine, paroxetine, and other selective serotonin reuptake inhibitors, are also effective for treatment of generalized anxiety disorder. These antidepressants start to relieve anxiety quickly, sometimes after a few days.

Herbal products such as kava and valerian■ appear to have antianxiety effects, although their effectiveness for treating anxiety disorders such as generalized anxiety disorder requires further study.

Cognitive-behavior therapy has been shown to be beneficial for generalized anxiety disorder. Relaxation, yoga, meditation, exercise, and biofeedback techniques may also be of some help.★

▲ see page 653   ■ see page 112
★ see page 1706

Anxiety Induced by Drugs or Medical Problems

Anxiety can be caused by a medical disorder or the use or discontinuation of a drug. Examples of medical disorders that may cause anxiety include neurologic disorders, such as a head injury, brain infection, or inner ear disorder; cardiovascular disorders, such as heart failure and abnormal heart rhythms (arrhythmias); endocrine disorders, such as an overactive adrenal or thyroid gland; and respiratory disorders, such as asthma and chronic obstructive pulmonary disease. Even fever can cause anxiety.

Drugs that can induce anxiety include alcohol, stimulants, caffeine, cocaine, and many prescription drugs, such as ephedrine (used, for example, in decongestants) and theophylline (used, for example, to treat asthma). Some over-the-counter weight-loss products contain both ephedrine and caffeine. Drugs that can induce anxiety when discontinued include benzodiazepines.

Anxiety may occur in dying people as a result of fear of death, pain, and difficulty breathing.▲

Treatment

A doctor aims to treat the primary causes rather than the secondary anxiety symptoms. Anxiety should subside after the medical disorder is treated or the drug has been discontinued long enough for any withdrawal symptoms to abate. A doctor can treat any remaining anxiety with appropriate antianxiety drugs or psychotherapy (such as behavior therapy). For people who are dying, strong analgesics with potent antianxiety effects, such as morphine, are often appropriate. No dying person should have to experience intense anxiety.

Panic Attacks and Panic Disorder

Panic is acute, short-lived, extreme anxiety with accompanying physical symptoms.

Panic *attacks* may occur in any anxiety disorder, usually in response to a specific situation tied to the main characteristic of the disorder. For example, a person with a phobia of snakes may panic when encountering a snake. However, these situational panic attacks differ from the spontaneous, unprovoked ones that define a person's problem as panic *disorder.*

Panic attacks are common, occurring in more than one third of adults each year. Women are 2 to 3 times more likely than men to have panic attacks and panic disorder. Most people recover from panic attacks without treatment; a few develop panic disorder. Panic disorder is present in 2% of the population during any 12-month period. Panic disorder usually begins in late adolescence or early adulthood.

A panic attack involves the sudden appearance of at least four of the following symptoms:
- Chest pain or discomfort
- Choking
- Dizziness, unsteadiness, or faintness
- Fear of dying
- Fear of "going crazy" or of losing control
- Feelings of unreality, strangeness, or detachment from the environment
- Flushes or chills
- Nausea, stomachache, or diarrhea
- Numbness or tingling sensations
- Palpitations or accelerated heart rate
- Shortness of breath or sense of being smothered
- Sweating
- Trembling or shaking.

Symptoms peak within 10 minutes and usually dissipate within minutes, leaving little for a doctor to observe except the person's fear of another terrifying attack. Since panic attacks sometimes are unexpected or occur for no apparent reason, especially when people experience them as part of panic disorder, people who have them frequently anticipate and worry about another attack—a condition called anticipatory anxiety—and try to avoid places where they have previously panicked.

Because symptoms of a panic attack involve many vital organs, people often worry that they have a dangerous medical problem involving the heart, lungs, or brain and seek help from a doctor or hospital emergency department. However, the correct diagnosis may not be made, leading to the additional worry that the medical problem is going untreated. Although panic attacks are uncomfortable—at times extremely so—they are not dangerous.

A diagnosis of panic disorder is made when a person experiences at least two unprovoked and unexpected panic attacks, which are followed by at least 1 month of fear that another attack will occur. The frequency of attacks can vary greatly; some people have weekly or even daily attacks that occur for months,

---

▲ see page 50

whereas others have several daily attacks followed by weeks or months of remission.

Treatment

People who experience panic attacks as part of an anxiety disorder other than panic disorder and some people with panic disorder who have recurring panic attacks, anticipatory anxiety, and avoidance recover without formal treatment. For others, panic disorder follows a waxing and waning course over years.

People with panic disorder are more receptive to treatment if they understand that the disorder involves both physical and psychologic processes and that treatment must address both. Drug therapy and behavior therapy can generally control the symptoms.

Drugs that are used to treat panic disorder include antidepressants and antianxiety drugs such as benzodiazepines. Most types of antidepressants—tricyclics, monoamine oxidase inhibitors (MAOIs), and selective serotonin reuptake inhibitors (SSRIs)—are effective.▲ Benzodiazepines work faster than antidepressants but can cause drug dependence■ and are probably more likely to cause sleepiness, impaired coordination, and slowed reaction time. SSRIs are preferred to other antidepressants and benzodiazepines because they are equally effective but have fewer side effects, especially considerably less sleepiness, and do not cause drug dependence.

When a drug is effective, it prevents or greatly reduces the number of panic attacks. A drug may have to be taken for a long time, because panic attacks often return once the drug is discontinued.

Exposure therapy, a type of behavior therapy in which the person is exposed repeatedly to whatever triggers a panic attack, often helps to diminish the fear. Exposure therapy is practiced until the person develops a high level of comfort with the anxiety-provoking situation. In addition, people who are afraid that they will faint during a panic attack can practice an exercise in which they spin in a chair or breathe quickly (hyperventilate) until they feel faint. This exercise teaches them that they will not actually faint during a panic attack. Practicing slow, shallow breathing (respiratory control) helps many people who tend to hyperventilate.

Supportive psychotherapy, which includes education and counseling, is beneficial because a therapist can provide general information about the disorder, its treatment, realistic hope

What Is Exposure Therapy?

Unlike systematic desensitization, which pairs relaxation with gradual exposure to the sources of anxiety (a process called reciprocal inhibition), exposure therapy purposefully generates anxiety. By being repeatedly exposed to the feared object or situation, either literally or using the imagination, the person experiences the anxiety over and over until the stimulating event eventually loses its effect. This process is called habituation

Two variants of exposure therapy are flooding and graduated exposure. Flooding exposes the person to the anxiety-producing stimulus for as long as 1 or 2 hours. Graduated exposure gives the person a greater degree of control over the length and frequency of exposures. Both types of exposure treatment may use the most fearful stimulus first, unlike systematic desensitization, which begins with the least fearful stimulus.

for improvement, and the support that comes from a trusting relationship with a doctor.

Phobic Disorders

Phobias involve persistent, unrealistic, intense anxiety and fear in response to specific external situations.

People who have a phobia avoid situations that trigger their anxiety and fear, or they endure them with great distress. However, they recognize that their anxiety is excessive and therefore are aware that they have a problem.

AGORAPHOBIA

Agoraphobia is characterized by anxiety about or avoidance of being trapped in situations or places with no way to escape easily if anxiety or panic develops.

Agoraphobia is diagnosed in about 4% of women and 2% of men during any 12-month period. Most people with this disorder develop it in their early 20s; agoraphobia rarely develops after age 40.

Although agoraphobia literally means "fear of the marketplace," the term more specifically describes the fear of being trapped, often

▲ see table on page 618   ■ see page 653

in a busy place filled with people, without a graceful and easy way to leave if anxiety becomes severe. Typical situations that are difficult for people with agoraphobia include standing in line at a bank or supermarket, sitting in the middle of a long row in a theater or classroom, and riding on a bus or airplane. Some people develop agoraphobia after experiencing a panic attack in one of these situations. Other people simply feel uncomfortable in these settings and may never, or only later, develop panic attacks. Agoraphobia often interferes with daily living, sometimes so drastically that it leaves the person housebound.

Treatment

If agoraphobia is not treated, it usually waxes and wanes in severity and may even disappear without formal treatment, possibly because the person has conducted some personal form of behavior therapy.

Exposure therapy, a type of behavior therapy in which the person is exposed repeatedly to the anxiety-provoking situation, is the best treatment for agoraphobia, helping more than 90% of people who practice this therapy faithfully.

People with agoraphobia who are deeply depressed may need to take an antidepressant. Substances that depress the central nervous system, such as alcohol or large doses of antianxiety drugs, may interfere with behavior therapy and are tapered off before therapy is begun.

SOCIAL PHOBIA

Social phobia (social anxiety disorder) is characterized by significant anxiety induced by exposure to certain social or performance situations, often resulting in avoidance.

Humans are social animals, and their ability to relate comfortably in social situations affects many important aspects of their lives, including family, education, work, leisure, dating, and mating.

Although some anxiety in social situations is normal, people with social phobia have so much anxiety that they either avoid social situations or endure them with distress. About 13% of people have social phobia sometime in their lives; the disorder affects about 9% of women and 7% of men during any 12-month period. Men are more likely than women to have the most severe form of social anxiety,

avoidant personality disorder.▲ Some people are shy by nature and show timidness early in life that later develops into social phobia. Others first experience anxiety in social situations around the time of puberty.

Some social phobias are tied to specific performance situations, producing anxiety only when the person must perform a particular activity in public. The same activity performed alone produces no anxiety. Situations that commonly trigger anxiety among people with social phobia include public speaking; performing publicly, such as reading in church or playing a musical instrument; eating with others; signing a document before witnesses; and using a public bathroom. People with social phobia are concerned that their performance or actions will seem inappropriate. Often they worry that their anxiety will be obvious—that they will sweat, blush, vomit, or tremble or that their voice will quaver; that they will lose their train of thought; or that they will not be able to find the words to express themselves.

A more general type of social phobia is characterized by anxiety in many social situations. In both types of social phobia, the person's anxiety comes from the belief that if his performance falls short of expectations, he will feel humiliated and embarrassed.

Treatment

Social phobia often persists if left untreated, causing many people to avoid activities in which they would otherwise like to participate.

Exposure therapy, a type of behavior therapy in which the person is exposed repeatedly to the anxiety-provoking situation, is effective, but arranging for exposure to last long enough to permit getting used to the anxiety-provoking situation and growing comfortable in that situation may not be easy. For example, a person who is afraid of speaking in front of his boss may not be able to arrange a series of speaking sessions in front of that boss. Substitute situations may help, such as joining Toastmasters (an organization for those who have anxiety about speaking in front of an audience) or reading a book to nursing home residents.

Antidepressants, such as selective serotonin reuptake inhibitors (SSRIs) and monoamine oxidase inhibitors (MAOIs), and antianxiety drugs can often help people with social phobia. Many people use alcohol as a social lubricant; for some people, however, alcohol abuse and dependence can result. Beta-blockers are commonly used to reduce the increased heart rate,

▲ see page 633

tremor, and sweating experienced by people who are distressed by performing in public.

SPECIFIC PHOBIAS

A specific phobia is an irrational fear of specific objects or situations.

Specific phobias, as a group, are among the most common anxiety disorders but are often less troubling than other anxiety disorders. During any 12-month period, about 13% of women and 4% of men have a specific phobia.

Some specific phobias cause little inconvenience, while others severely interfere with functioning. For example, a city dweller who is afraid of snakes may have no trouble avoiding them. However, a city dweller who fears small, closed places such as elevators will have a problem working on an upper floor in a skyscraper.

Some specific phobias, such as fear of large animals, the dark, or strangers, begin early in life. Many phobias stop as the person gets older. Other phobias, such as fear of rodents, insects, storms, water, heights, flying, or enclosed places, typically develop later in life.

At least 5% of people are to some degree phobic about blood, injections, or injury. These people can actually faint due to a decrease in heart rate and blood pressure, which does not happen with other phobias and anxiety disorders. In contrast, many people with other phobias and anxiety disorders hyperventilate, which can cause them to feel as though they might faint, although they virtually never faint.

Treatment

A person can often cope with a specific phobia by avoiding the feared object or situation. When treatment is needed, exposure therapy is the treatment of choice. A therapist can help ensure that the therapy is carried out properly, although it can be done without a therapist. Even people with a phobia of blood or needles respond well to exposure therapy. For example, a person who faints while blood is drawn can have a needle brought close to a vein and then removed when the heart rate begins to slow down. Repeating this process allows the heart rate to return to normal. Eventually, the person should be able to have blood drawn without fainting.

Drug therapy is not very useful in helping people overcome specific phobias. However, benzodiazepines (antianxiety drugs) may give a person short-term control over a phobia, such as the fear of flying.

SOME COMMON PHOBIAS

PHOBIA	DEFINITION
Acrophobia	Fear of heights
Amathophobia	Fear of dust
Astraphobia	Fear of lightning
Aviophobia	Fear of flying
Belonephobia	Fear of needles
Claustrophobia	Fear of confined spaces
Eurotophobia	Fear of female genitals
Gephyrophobia	Fear of crossing bridges
Hydrophobia	Fear of water
Odontiatophobia	Fear of dentists
Phasmophobia	Fear of ghosts
Spargarophobia	Fear of asparagus
Triskaidekaphobia	Fear of all things associated with the number thirteen
Zoophobia	Fear of animals (usually spiders, snakes, or mice)

Obsessive-Compulsive Disorder

Obsessive-compulsive disorder is characterized by the presence of recurring, unwanted, intrusive ideas, images, or impulses that may even seem silly, weird, nasty, or horrible (obsessions) to the person experiencing them, accompanied by urges to do something that will relieve the discomfort caused by the obsession (compulsions).

Obsessive-compulsive disorder occurs about equally in men and women and affects about 1.5% of the population during any 6-month period.

The obsessions are usually related to a sense of harm, risk, or danger. Common obsessions include concerns about contamination (for example, worrying that touching doorknobs will cause disease), doubts (for example, worrying that the front door was not locked), fear of loss, and fear of physically injuring someone.

More than 95% of people with obsessive-compulsive disorder feel compelled to perform rituals—repetitive, purposeful, intentional acts. Rituals used to control an obsession include washing or cleaning to be rid of contamination, checking to allay doubt, hoarding to prevent loss, and avoiding the people who might become objects of aggression. Most rituals, such as excessive hand washing or repeated checking to make sure a door has been locked, can be observed. Other rituals, such as repetitive counting or making statements intended to diminish danger, cannot be observed. Obsessions are not always accompanied by compulsions.

Most people with obsessive-compulsive disorder are aware that their obsessive thoughts do not reflect actual risks and that their compulsive behaviors are ineffective. Obsessive-compulsive disorder, therefore, differs from psychotic disorders, in which people lose contact with reality. Obsessive-compulsive disorder also differs from obsessive-compulsive personality disorder,▲ in which specific personality traits are defined (for example, being a perfectionist). Because people with obsessive-compulsive disorder are aware that their compulsive behaviors are excessive to the point of being bizarre and are afraid they will be embarrassed or stigmatized, they often perform their rituals secretly, even though the rituals may occupy several hours each day.

About one third of people with obsessive-compulsive disorder are depressed at the time the disorder is diagnosed. Altogether, two thirds become depressed at some point.

Treatment

Exposure therapy is effective in treating obsessive-compulsive disorder. Exposure therapy involves exposing the person to the situations or people that trigger obsessions, rituals, or discomfort. The person's discomfort or anxiety will gradually diminish if he prevents himself from performing the ritual during repeated exposure to the provocative stimulus. In this way, the person learns that rituals are unnecessary for decreasing discomfort. The improvement usually persists for years, probably because people who have mastered this self-help approach continue to practice it as a way of life without much effort after formal treatment has ended.

Selective serotonin reuptake inhibitors and clomipramine, a tricyclic antidepressant, are effective. Certain other antidepressant drugs are also used, but much less often. Many experts believe that a combination of behavior therapy and drug therapy is the best treatment for people with obsessive-compulsive disorder.

Psychodynamic psychotherapy and psychoanalysis have generally not been effective for people with obsessive-compulsive disorder.

▲ see page 633   ■ see box on page 1636

Posttraumatic Stress Disorder

Posttraumatic stress disorder is an anxiety disorder caused by exposure to an overwhelming traumatic event, in which the person later repeatedly reexperiences the event.

Experiences that threaten death or serious injury can affect people long after the experience is over. Intense fear, helplessness, or horror can haunt a person.

Traumatic events may involve having been threatened with death or serious injury or witnessing violence against another person. Examples include engaging in military combat, experiencing or witnessing sexual or physical assault, or being affected by a disaster, either natural (for example, a hurricane) or man-made (for example, a severe automobile accident). Sometimes symptoms do not begin until many months or even years after the traumatic event took place (delayed onset). If posttraumatic stress disorder has been present for 3 months or longer, it is considered chronic.

Posttraumatic stress disorder affects at least 8% of people sometime during their life, including childhood.■ Many people who undergo or witness traumatic events, such as combat veterans and victims of rape or other violent acts, experience posttraumatic stress disorder.

In posttraumatic stress disorder, the traumatic situation is reexperienced repeatedly, usually in nightmares or flashbacks. Intense distress often occurs when the person is exposed to an event or situation that reminds him of the original trauma. Examples of such reminders are anniversaries of the traumatic event; seeing a gun after being pistol-whipped during a robbery; and being in a small boat after a near-drowning accident.

The person persistently avoids things that are reminders of the trauma. He may also attempt to avoid thoughts, feelings, or conversations about the traumatic event and avoid activities, situations, or people who serve as reminders. Avoidance may also include memory loss (amnesia) for a particular aspect of the traumatic event. The person has a numbing or deadening of emotional responsiveness and symptoms of increased arousal (such as difficulty falling asleep or being easily startled). Symptoms of depression are common, and the person shows less interest in previously enjoyed activities. Feelings of guilt are also common.

Treatment

Treatment of posttraumatic stress disorder involves psychotherapy (including exposure therapy) and drug therapy. Because of the often intense anxiety associated with traumatic memories, supportive psychotherapy plays an especially important role in treatment. The therapist is openly empathic and sympathetic in recognizing the person's psychologic pain. The therapist reassures the person that his response is valid but encourages him to face his memories (as a form of exposure therapy). The person also is taught ways to control anxiety, which helps to modulate and integrate the painful memories into his personality.

Insight-oriented psychotherapy can help people with feelings of guilt understand why they are punishing themselves and help rid them of guilty feelings.

Antidepressants appear to provide some benefit, especially selective serotonin reuptake inhibitors (SSRIs), tricyclic antidepressants, and monoamine oxidase inhibitors (MAOIs).

Chronic posttraumatic stress disorder may not disappear but often becomes less intense over time even without treatment. Nevertheless, some people remain severely handicapped by the disorder.

Acute Stress Disorder

Acute stress disorder is similar to posttraumatic stress disorder, except that it begins within 4 weeks of the traumatic event and lasts only 2 days to 4 weeks.

A person with acute stress disorder has been exposed to a terrifying event. The person mentally reexperiences the traumatic event, avoids things that remind him of it, and has increased anxiety. The person also has three or more of the following symptoms:

• A sense of numbing, detachment, or lack of emotional responsiveness
• Reduced awareness of surroundings (for example, being dazed)
• A feeling that things are not real
• A feeling that he himself is not real
• An inability to remember an important part of the traumatic event.

The number of people with acute stress disorder is unknown. The likelihood of developing acute stress disorder is greater when traumatic events are severe.

Treatment

Many people recover from acute stress disorder once they are removed from the traumatic situation and given appropriate support in the form of understanding, empathy for their distress, and an opportunity to describe what happened and their reaction to it. Some people benefit from describing their experience several times.

Depression and Mania

Depression and mania represent the two extremes, or poles, of mood disorders. Mood disorders are mental health disorders in which emotional disturbances consist of prolonged periods of excessive sadness (depression) or excessive joyousness or elation (mania).

Mood disorders are sometimes called affective disorders. *Affect* (emphasis on the first syllable) means *emotional state* as revealed through facial expressions and gestures.

Sadness and joy are part of the normal experience of everyday life and differ from the depression and mania that characterize mood disorders. Sadness is a natural response to loss, defeat, disappointment, trauma, or catastrophe. Sadness may be psychologically beneficial because it permits a person to withdraw from offensive or unpleasant situations, which may aid recovery.

Grief or bereavement is the most common of the normal reactions to a loss or separation, such as the death of a loved one, divorce, or romantic disappointment. Bereavement and loss do not generally cause persistent, incapacitating depression except in people predisposed to mood disorders.

Joyousness or elation, usually linked to success and achievement, can sometimes be a defense against depression or a denial of the pain of loss. People who are dying sometimes have brief periods of elation and restless activity, and some recently bereaved people may even

What Is Seasonal Affective Disorder?

Many people report feeling sadder in late autumn and winter, blaming this tendency on the shortening of daylight hours and colder temperatures. However, some people develop a more intense sadness known as seasonal affective disorder, which is a type of depression. Seasonal affective disorder is characterized by recurring episodes of depression that usually begin in October or November and end by February or March (also called autumn-winter depression). The disorder is more common in extreme northern and southern latitudes, where the winter season is typically longer and harsher. It is believed that seasonal affective disorder may be caused by an increase in the duration of secretion of melatonin (a hormone produced by the pineal gland, which is located in the middle of the brain) that normally occurs at night.

Symptoms include lethargy, decreased interest in and withdrawal from usual activities, oversleeping, and overeating. In spring, the symptoms steadily resolve. However, in some people with seasonal affective disorder, with the coming of spring, there may be a rapid swing to symptoms that are almost the opposite of those experienced during the winter, such as increased energy and involvement in activities, decreased need for sleep, and decreased appetite (also called spring-summer hypomania).

Phototherapy is the most effective treatment for seasonal affective disorder. With phototherapy, the person is placed in a closed room that is bathed in artificial light. The light is controlled to mimic the season that the therapist is trying to create: longer days for summer and shorter days for winter.

become elated rather than grieve normally. In people predisposed to mood disorders, these reactions may be the prelude to mania.

Depression or mania is diagnosed when sadness or elation is overly intense and continues beyond what would be expected for a particular event. Unlike normal emotional reactions, depression and mania greatly impair a person's ability to function physically, socially, and at work.

▲ see page 1632

About 10% of the U.S. population experience depression severe enough to require medical attention. Of these people, one third have long-lasting (chronic) depression, and most of the remainder continue to have sporadic (recurring) episodes of depression separated by episodes of normal mood. Both chronic and recurring episodes of depression are termed unipolar. Nearly 2% of the U.S. population have a disorder called manic-depressive illness, or bipolar disorder, in which episodes of depression alternate with episodes of mania (or with episodes of less severe mania, known as hypomania). Mania without depression, also termed unipolar disorder, is very rare.

Depression

Depression is a feeling of intense sadness; it may follow a recent loss or other sad event but is out of proportion to that event and persists beyond an appropriate length of time.

After anxiety, depression is the most common mental health disorder. An estimated 10% of people who see their doctors for what they think is a physical problem are actually experiencing depression. People who become depressed typically do so in their 20s, 30s, or 40s, although depression can begin at almost any age. Depression affects a number of children and adolescents.▲ People born in the latter part of the 20th century seem to have higher rates of depression and suicide than those of previous generations, in part because of higher rates of substance abuse.

An episode of depression typically lasts about 6 months if untreated, but sometimes it lasts for 2 years or more. Episodes generally tend to recur several times over a lifetime.

Causes

A number of factors may make a person more likely to experience depression, such as a family tendency (heredity), side effects of certain drugs, and emotionally distressing events, particularly those involving a loss. Despite commonly held beliefs, however, depression does not necessarily reflect a personality disorder, childhood trauma, poor parenting, or weakness of character. Depression may arise or worsen without any apparent or significant life stresses.

Social class, race, and culture do not appear to affect the chance that a person will experience depression in his or her lifetime. However, a person's sex does appear to have an effect: Women are twice as likely as men to

Physical Disorders That Can Cause Depression

Side effects of drugs
- Amphetamines (withdrawal from)
- Antipsychotic drugs
- Beta-blockers
- Cimetidine
- Contraceptives (oral)
- Cycloserine
- Hormone (estrogen) replacement therapy
- Mercury
- Methyldopa
- Reserpine
- Thallium
- Vinblastine
- Vincristine

Infections
- AIDS
- Influenza
- Mononucleosis
- Syphilis (late stage)
- Tuberculosis
- Viral hepatitis
- Viral pneumonia

Hormonal disorders
- Addison's disease
- Cushing's syndrome

- High levels of parathyroid hormone
- Low and high levels of thyroid hormone
- Low levels of pituitary hormones (hypopituitarism)

Connective tissue diseases
- Rheumatoid arthritis
- Systemic lupus erythematosus

Neurologic disorders
- Brain tumors
- Dementia
- Head injury
- Multiple sclerosis
- Parkinson's disease
- Sleep apnea
- Stroke
- Temporal lobe epilepsy

Nutritional disorders
- Pellagra (vitamin B_6 deficiency)
- Pernicious anemia (vitamin B_{12} deficiency)

Cancers
- Abdominal cancers (ovary, colon)
- Cancer spreading in the entire body (metastatic)
- Cancer of the pancreas

experience depression, though the reasons are not entirely clear. Of physical factors, hormones are the ones most involved. Changes in hormone levels, which can create mood changes shortly before menstruation and after childbirth, might play some role in women. Similarly, the use of oral contraceptives or hormone (estrogen) replacement therapy may contribute to or cause mood changes. Abnormal thyroid function, which is fairly common in women, may also be a factor.

Transient depression is when someone becomes temporarily depressed in reaction to certain holidays (holiday blues) or meaningful anniversaries, such as the anniversary of a loved one's death; during the premenstrual phase (premenstrual dysphoric disorder); or during the first 2 weeks after giving birth (postpartum depression). Such reactions are normal, but people with an increased predisposition to depression may develop significant depression during such times. Depression without an apparent precipitating event is

called melancholia (formerly called endogenous depression). These distinctions, however, are not very important, since the effects and treatment of the depression are similar.

Depression may occur with, or be caused by, a number of physical disorders. Physical disorders may cause depression directly (such as when thyroid disease affects hormone levels, which can induce depression) or indirectly (such as when rheumatoid arthritis causes pain and disability, which can lead to depression). Often, depression that results from a physical disorder has both direct and indirect causes. For example, AIDS may cause depression directly if the human immunodeficiency virus (HIV), which causes AIDS, damages the brain; AIDS may cause depression indirectly by having an overall negative effect on the person's life.

The use of some prescription drugs can cause depression. For unknown reasons, corticosteroids often cause depression when they are produced in large amounts as part of a disease, as in Cushing's syndrome, but they tend to cause hypomania or, rarely, mania when they are given as medication.

A number of mental health disorders can predispose a person to depression, including certain anxiety disorders, alcoholism and other substance abuse disorders, and schizophrenia.

Symptoms

Symptoms typically develop gradually over days or weeks and can vary greatly depending on what type of depression the person is experiencing. For example, a person who is becoming depressed may appear sluggish and sad or irritable and anxious.

A person who is withdrawn, speaks little, stops eating, and sleeps little is experiencing what doctors call vegetative symptoms. In contrast, a person who appears anxious and fearful (especially in the evening), has an increased appetite resulting in weight gain, and, although initially unable to sleep, sleeps for increasingly longer periods is experiencing depression with atypical symptoms. A person who, in addition, is very restless—wringing the hands and talking continuously—is experiencing agitation.

Many people with depression cannot experience emotions—including grief, joy, and pleasure—in a normal way; in the extreme, the world appears to have become colorless and lifeless. Thinking, speech, and general activity may slow down so much that all voluntary activities stop. Depressed people may be preoccupied with intense feelings of guilt and self-denigration and may not be able to concentrate. They may experience feelings of despair, loneliness, and low self-esteem. They are often indecisive and withdrawn, feel progressively helpless and hopeless, and think about death and suicide.

Sleep problems are common. Most depressed people have difficulty falling asleep and awaken repeatedly, particularly early in the morning. A loss of sexual desire or pleasure is common. Poor appetite and weight loss sometimes lead to emaciation, and in women, menstrual periods may stop. However, overeating and weight gain are common in people with mild depression.

In some depressed people, the symptoms are mild but the disorder lasts for years, often decades. This type of depression, called dysthymia, often begins early in life and is associated with distinct changes in personality. People with dysthymia are gloomy, pessimistic, humorless, or incapable of having fun; passive

and lethargic; introverted; skeptical, hypercritical, or constantly complaining; and self-critical and full of self-reproach. They are preoccupied with inadequacy, failure, and negative events, sometimes to the point of morbid enjoyment of their own failures.

Some depressed people complain of having a physical illness, with various aches and pains or fears of calamity or of becoming insane. Others think they have illnesses they believe to be incurable or shameful, such as cancer or sexually transmitted diseases, and think they are infecting other people.

About 15% of depressed people, most commonly those with severe depression, have false beliefs (delusions), or they see or hear things that are not there (hallucinations). For example, they may believe that they have committed unpardonable sins or crimes or may hear voices accusing them of various misdeeds or condemning them to death. In rare cases, they may imagine that they see coffins or deceased relatives. Feelings of insecurity and worthlessness may lead people with severe depression to believe that they are being watched and persecuted. Depression with delusions or hallucinations is termed psychotic depression.

Thoughts of death are among the most serious symptoms of depression. Many depressed people want to die or feel they are so worthless that they should die. As many as 15% of untreated depressed people end their lives in suicide. A suicide threat represents an emergency situation.▲ When a person threatens to kill himself, a doctor may hospitalize the person so that he is kept under supervision until treatment reduces the risk of suicide. The risk is especially high when the person with depression continues to have feelings of excessive sadness even while returning to normal activities. The risk is also high around personally significant anniversaries and among people in a mixed bipolar state.■

Diagnosis

A doctor is usually able to diagnose depression from its signs and symptoms. A previous history of depression or a family history of depression helps to confirm the diagnosis. Excessive worrying, panic attacks, and obsession are common in depression and may lead the doctor to incorrectly think that the person has an anxiety disorder.

In older people, depression may be difficult to notice, especially among people who do not

▲ see also page 622   ■ see page 619

work or who have little social interaction. Depression may lead to slower thinking, decreased concentration, and memory impairment that simulates dementia. Indeed, the disorder can so resemble dementia that it is sometimes called pseudodementia.▲

Standardized questionnaires are used to help measure the degree of depression. Two such questionnaires are the Hamilton Depression Rating Scale, conducted verbally by an interviewer, and the Beck Depression Inventory, a self-administered questionnaire.

Laboratory tests may occasionally help a doctor determine if depression is caused by an endocrine or other physical disorder, but no simple laboratory test exists with which to diagnose depression.

In cases that are difficult to diagnose, doctors may perform other tests to confirm the diagnosis of depression. For example, because sleep problems are such a prominent sign of depression, doctors who specialize in diagnosing and treating mood disorders may use a sleep electroencephalogram to measure the time it takes for rapid eye movement sleep (the period during which dreaming occurs) to begin after the person falls asleep. Normally, progression to this stage of sleep takes about 90 minutes. In a person with depression, however, it usually takes less than 70 minutes.

Prognosis and Treatment

An untreated depression may last for about 6 months. Although mild symptoms persist in many people, functioning tends to return to normal. Nonetheless, most people with depression experience repeated episodes of depression, an average of 4 to 5 times over a lifetime. In older people, symptoms of pseudodementia (such as confusion), if present, clear up with treatment for depression.

Depression today is usually treated without hospitalization. However, sometimes a person should be hospitalized, especially if he is contemplating suicide or has attempted it, is too frail because of weight loss, or is at risk of heart problems because of severe agitation.

Drug therapy is the cornerstone of treatment for depression. Other treatments include psychotherapy and electroconvulsive therapy. Sometimes a combination of therapies is used. Depression can usually be treated successfully and does not represent a character flaw or weakness of mental abilities.

Drug Therapy: Several types of drugs—tricyclic antidepressants, selective serotonin reuptake inhibitors (SSRIs), monoamine oxidase inhibitors (MAOIs), psychostimulants, and other antidepressants—are available. Most must be taken regularly for at least several weeks before they begin to work. The chances that any given antidepressant will work for a particular person are about 65%. Side effects vary with each type of drug. Sometimes when treatment with one drug fails to relieve depression, a combination of antidepressant drugs is prescribed.

Tricyclic antidepressants, once the mainstay of treatment, are now used infrequently. They often cause sedation and lead to weight gain. They can also cause an increase in heart rate and a decrease in blood pressure when the person stands. Other side effects include blurred vision, dry mouth, confusion, constipation, and difficulty in starting to urinate. These other effects are called anticholinergic effects and are often more pronounced in older people.■

Selective serotonin reuptake inhibitors (SSRIs) are now the most commonly used class of antidepressants. SSRIs are effective in treating depression and dysthymia as well as other mental health disorders that often coexist with depression. Although SSRIs can cause nausea, diarrhea, tremor, weight loss, and headache, these side effects are usually mild or go away with continued use. Most people tolerate the side effects of SSRIs better than the side effects of tricyclics. SSRIs are safer than the tricyclics in their side effects on the heart. However, with long term use, SSRIs may cause additional side effects, such as weight gain. Abrupt discontinuation of some of the SSRIs may result in a withdrawal syndrome that includes dizziness, anxiety, irritability, and flu-like symptoms.

Monoamine oxidase inhibitors (MAOIs) represent another class of antidepressant drug. MAOIs may be effective when other antidepressants have failed but are rarely the first choice in treatment. People who use MAOIs must adhere to a number of dietary restrictions and follow special precautions. For example, they should not eat foods or beverages that contain tyramine, such as beer on tap, red wines (including sherry), liqueurs, overripe foods, salami, aged cheeses, fava or broad beans, yeast extracts (marmite), and soy sauce. They must avoid pseudoephedrine, found in

▲ see page 484   ■ see box on page 79

R_X DRUGS USED TO TREAT DEPRESSION

CLASS DRUG	SELECTED SIDE EFFECTS	COMMENTS
Tricyclics and related drugs		
Amitriptyline Amoxapine Clomipramine Desipramine Doxepin Imipramine Maprotiline Nortriptyline Protriptyline Trimipramine	Sedation, weight gain, increased heart rate, decreased blood pressure, dry mouth, confusion, blurred vision, constipation, difficulty in starting to urinate, delayed orgasm, seizures (clomipramine and maprotiline)	Side effects are usually more pronounced in older people. Serious, potentially life-threatening toxicity in overdosage.
Selective serotonin reuptake inhibitors		
Citalopram Fluoxetine Fluvoxamine Paroxetine Sertraline	Sexual dysfunction (primarily, delayed orgasm but also loss of desire in some people), nausea, diarrhea, headache, weight loss (short-term), weight gain (long-term), withdrawal syndrome, forgetfulness, blunting of emotions, easy bruising	Most commonly used class of antidepressants. Also effective for dysthymia, generalized anxiety disorder, obsessive-compulsive disorder, panic disorder, phobic disorder, posttraumatic stress disorder, premenstrual dysphoric disorder, and bulimia. Less serious risk of toxicity in overdosage.
Monoamine oxidase inhibitors		
Phenelzine Tranylcypromine	Insomnia, weight gain, sexual dysfunction (loss of desire and delayed orgasm), pins-and-needles sensation, lowered blood pressure, severe high blood pressure	Requires dietary restrictions and precautions when using certain drugs.
Psychostimulants		
Dextroamphet- amine Methylphenidate	Nervousness, tremor, insomnia, dry mouth	Generally not effective as antidepressants when used alone. Often used in combination with antidepressants.
Newer drugs		
Bupropion Mirtazapine Nefazodone Trazodone Venlafaxine	Headache and rarely seizures (bupropion); dry mouth (venlafaxine, mirtazapine); weight gain (mirtazapine); mild sedation and dizziness (nefazodone); prolonged sedation (trazodone)	Most of the side effects can be prevented or minimized when low doses are used and when changes in dosages are made slowly.

many over-the-counter cough and cold remedies. This drug, when combined with MAOIs, can cause a sudden and severe rise in blood pressure with a severe, throbbing headache (hypertensive crisis). People who take MAOIs should also avoid many other types of drugs, including tricyclic antidepressants, SSRIs, bupropion, mirtazapine, venlafaxine, nefa-

zodone, dextromethorphan (a cough suppressant), and meperidine (an analgesic).

People taking MAOIs usually are instructed to carry an antidote, such as chlorpromazine or nifedipine, at all times. If a severe, throbbing headache occurs, they should take the antidote at once and go to the nearest emergency room. Because of the risk of stroke and difficult dietary restrictions and necessary precautions, MAOIs are rarely prescribed except for depressed people whose condition has not improved with other antidepressants.

Psychostimulants, such as dextroamphetamine and methylphenidate, as well as other drugs, are sometimes used, often in combination with antidepressants.

Newer antidepressants have become available that are as effective and safe as SSRIs but may have fewer and less severe side effects for some people.

St. John's wort, an herbal dietary supplement, may help relieve mild depression. However, due to potentially harmful interactions between St. John's wort and many prescription drugs, people interested in taking this herbal supplement need to discuss possible drug interactions with their doctor.▲

Psychotherapy: Individual or group psychotherapy can help people with depression gradually resume former responsibilities and adapt to the normal pressures of life, building on the improvement made by antidepressant drug treatment. Interpersonal psychotherapy can provide the people with supportive guidance while adjusting to changes in life roles. Cognitive therapy can help change hopelessness and negative thinking. Psychotherapy alone may be just as effective as drug therapy for mild depression.

Electroconvulsive Therapy: Electroconvulsive therapy is sometimes used to treat people with severe depression, particularly when the person is psychotic, is threatening to commit suicide, or is refusing to eat. This type of therapy is usually very effective and can relieve depression quickly, unlike most antidepressants, which can take up to several weeks. The speed with which electroconvulsive therapy takes effect can save lives.

With electroconvulsive therapy, electrodes are placed on the head and an electrical current is applied to induce a seizure in the brain. For reasons that are not understood, the seizure relieves depression. Usually five to seven treatments, one treatment every other day, are given. Because the electrical current can cause muscle contractions and pain, the person undergoes general anesthesia during treatments. Electroconvulsive therapy may cause some temporary (rarely permanent) memory loss.

Mania

Mania is characterized by excessive physical activity and feelings of extreme elation that are grossly out of proportion to any positive event. Hypomania is a less severe form of mania.

Mania most commonly occurs as a part of manic-depressive illness (bipolar disorder■). The few people who appear to experience only mania (unipolar disorder) may actually have mild or brief episodes of depression. Mania and hypomania are less common than depression, and they are also less easily recognized. Whereas extreme and protracted sadness may prompt a visit to a doctor, elation much less commonly does, because people with mania are unaware that anything is wrong with their mental state or behavior. A doctor must rule out an underlying physical disorder in a person who is experiencing mania for the first time without a previous episode of depression.

Symptoms and Diagnosis

Manic symptoms typically develop rapidly over a few days. In the early (milder) stages of mania, the person feels better than normal, exuberant, and energetic.

A person who is manic may be irritable, cantankerous, or hostile. He typically believes he is quite well. A lack of insight into his condition, along with a huge capacity for activity, can make the person impatient, intrusive, meddlesome, and aggressively irritable when crossed. Mental activity speeds up (a condition called flight of ideas). The person is easily distracted and constantly shifts from one theme or endeavor to another. The person may have false convictions of personal wealth, power, inventiveness, and genius and may temporarily become delusional or assume a grandiose identity, sometimes believing that he is God.

The person may believe he is being assisted or persecuted by others or have hallucinations, hearing and seeing things that are not there. The need for sleep decreases. A manic person is inexhaustibly, excessively, and impulsively involved in various activities (such as risky business endeavors, gambling, or perilous sexual behavior) without recognizing the inherent social dangers. In extreme cases, mental and physical activity is so frenzied that any clear link between mood and behavior is lost in a kind of senseless agitation (delirious mania). Immediate treatment is then required, because the person may die of sheer physical exhaustion. In less severe mania, hospitalization may be needed during periods of overactivity to pro-

▲ see also page 111   ■ see page 620

Physical Disorders That Can Cause Mania

Side effects of drugs
- Amphetamines
- Antidepressants (most)
- Antidepressant withdrawal
- Bromocriptine
- Cocaine
- Corticosteroids
- Levodopa
- Methylphenidate

Infections
- AIDS
- Encephalitis
- Influenza
- Syphilis (late stage)

Hormonal disorders
- High levels of thyroid hormone

Connective tissue disease
- Systemic lupus erythematosus

Neurologic disorders
- Brain tumors
- Head injury
- Huntington's disease
- Multiple sclerosis
- Stroke
- Sydenham's disease
- Temporal lobe epilepsy

tect the person and his family from ruinous financial or sexual behavior.

Mania is diagnosed by its symptoms. However, because people with mania are notorious for denying that there is anything wrong with them, doctors usually have to obtain information from family members.

Treatment

Untreated episodes of mania end more abruptly than those of depression and are typically shorter, lasting from a few weeks to several months. Because mania is a medical and social emergency, a doctor makes all attempts to treat the person in a hospital.

The drug lithium can reduce the symptoms of mania. ▲ Because lithium takes 4 to 10 days to work, a drug that works rapidly, such as haloperidol, is often given at the same time to control excited thought and activity. How-

▲ see page 621

ever, haloperidol can cause muscle stiffness and unusual movements. Therefore, haloperidol is given in small doses, in combination with a benzodiazepine, such as lorazepam or clonazepam, which enhances the antimanic effects of haloperidol while reducing its unpleasant side effects. Haloperidol usually is stopped after about a week.

Manic-Depressive Illness

In manic-depressive illness, also called bipolar disorder, episodes of depression alternate with episodes of mania or lesser degrees of joyousness or elation.

Manic-depressive illness affects slightly less than 2% of the U.S. population to some degree. The disorder is believed to be hereditary, although the exact genetic defect is still unknown. Manic-depressive illness affects men and women equally. However, women are more likely to have symptoms of depression, whereas men are more likely to have symptoms of mania. Manic-depressive illness is more common among people in upper socioeconomic classes and usually begins in a person's teens, 20s, or 30s.

Symptoms and Diagnosis

Manic-depressive illness usually begins with depression and includes at least one episode of mania at some time during the disorder. Episodes of depression typically last for 3 to 6 months. In the most severe form of the disorder, called bipolar I disorder, depression alternates with intense mania. In the less severe form, called bipolar II disorder, short episodes of depression alternate with hypomania. The depressive and manic episodes often recur according to the season; for example, depression occurs in the fall and winter, and mania occurs in the spring or summer.

In an even less severe form of manic-depressive illness, called cyclothymic disorder, episodes of elation and sadness are less intense, typically last for only a few days, and recur fairly often at irregular intervals. Although cyclothymic disorder may ultimately evolve into a more severe form of manic-depressive illness, in many people cyclothymic disorder never progresses. Having cyclothymic disorder may contribute to a person's success in business, leadership, achievement, and artistic creativity. However, it may also cause uneven work and school records, frequent change of residence, repeated romantic breakups or marital failure, and alcohol and drug abuse. In about one third of people with cyclothymic disorder, these symptoms can lead to a mood disorder that requires treatment.

The diagnosis of manic-depressive illness is based on the distinctive pattern of symptoms. A doctor determines whether the person is experiencing an episode of mania or depression so that the correct treatment can be given. About one of three people with manic-depressive illness experiences symptoms of mania (or hypomania) and depression *simultaneously*. This condition is known as a mixed bipolar state.

Prognosis and Treatment

Manic-depressive illness recurs in nearly all cases. Episodes may sometimes switch from depression to mania, or vice versa, without any period of normal mood in between. Some people cycle more rapidly through episodes than do others. Up to 15% of people with manic-depressive illness, mostly women, have four or more episodes a year. People who cycle rapidly are more difficult to treat.

All antidepressants can cause swings from depression to hypomania or mania and sometimes cause rapid swings between them. Therefore, these drugs are used only for short periods, and their effect on mood is closely monitored. At the first sign of a swing to hypomania or mania, the antidepressant is discontinued. Optimally, most people with manic-depressive illness should be given mood-stabilizing drugs, such as lithium or an anticonvulsant, when they are treated with antidepressants.

Lithium has no effect on normal mood but reduces the tendency toward mood swings in about 70% of people with manic-depressive illness. A doctor monitors the level of lithium in the blood with blood tests. Possible side effects of lithium include tremor, fine muscle twitching, nausea, vomiting, diarrhea, thirst, excessive urination, and weight gain. However, these side effects are usually temporary, and the doctor can often lessen or relieve them by adjusting the dosage. Lithium can make acne or psoriasis worse and can cause the blood levels of thyroid hormone to fall, requiring the addition of thyroid hormone replacement. Reducing the dosage may lessen side effects, but sometimes lithium must be discontinued, in which case the undesirable side effects resolve. In rare cases, long-term use of lithium can affect kidney function. Therefore, kidney func-

tion must be monitored with blood and urine tests every 3 to 4 months.

A very high level of lithium in the blood can cause persistent headaches, mental confusion, drowsiness, seizures, and abnormal heart rhythms. Side effects are more likely to occur in older people. Women who are trying to become pregnant must stop taking lithium, because lithium can in rare cases cause heart defects in a developing fetus.

Newer drug treatments have evolved over the past several years. Sudden manic episodes are increasingly treated with risperidone, quetiapine, or olanzapine (drugs referred to as "atypical antipsychotics"), because they have a minimal risk of serious side effects. Other commonly used drugs for mania include the anticonvulsants carbamazepine and divalproex. However, carbamazepine can seriously reduce the number of red and white blood cells, and divalproex can cause liver damage (primarily in children) and in rare cases can cause severe damage to the pancreas. With close monitoring by a doctor, these problems can be caught in time, making carbamazepine and divalproex useful alternatives to lithium, especially for people who have not responded to other treatments.

Recently, the anticonvulsant lamotrigine has begun to be used to treat manic-depressive illness, especially in the depressed phase. Lamotrigine eliminates the need for antidepressants in some people. Like carbamazepine, lamotrigine can cause a serious rash. Oxcarbazepine and topiramate are other anticonvulsants being used as well.

Psychotherapy is often recommended for people taking mood-stabilizing drugs, mostly to help them stay with their treatment. Group therapy is often useful for helping people and their spouses or relatives understand the manic-depressive illness and better cope with it.

Phototherapy, which involves exposure to artificial light, is sometimes used to treat people with manic-depressive illness, especially those who have milder and more seasonal depression: autumn-winter depression and spring-summer hypomania (seasonal affective disorder). However, if the dose of light is excessive, the person may swing to hypomania or, in some cases, eye damage can occur. Therefore, phototherapy should be supervised by a doctor who specializes in the treatment of mood disorders.

CHAPTER 102

Suicidal Behavior

Suicidal behavior is characterized by a successful or unsuccessful attempt to kill oneself.

Suicidal behavior is an unmistakable signal that a person has feelings of desperation and hopelessness. Suicidal behavior includes attempted suicide, suicide gestures, and completed suicide. An attempted suicide is a suicidal action that is not fatal. If an attempted suicide involves a suicidal action unlikely to have any potential of being fatal, it is called a suicide gesture. A person taking such an action (for example, ingesting six acetaminophen tablets) may be making a plea for help or attention without having any intention of actually ending his life. A completed suicide is a suicidal action that results in death.

Information on the frequency of suicide comes mainly from death certificates and inquest reports and probably underestimates the true rate. Even so, suicidal behavior clearly is an all-too-common health problem. Although most suicidal behavior does not result in death, 10% of people who try to kill themselves using a potentially fatal means do die from their actions.

High-Risk Factors for Suicide

- Over age 55
- Male
- Painful or disabling illness
- Living alone
- Debt or poverty
- Bereavement
- Humiliation or disgrace
- Depression, especially associated with psychosis or anxiety
- Persistence of sadness even when other symptoms of depression are getting better
- History of drug or alcohol abuse
- History of prior suicide attempts
- Family history of suicide
- Family violence, including physical or sexual abuse
- Suicidal preoccupation and talk
- Well-defined plans for suicide

Suicidal behavior occurs in people of all ages and of both sexes. Suicide is the second leading cause of death among adolescents and is one of the top 10 causes of death among adults in the United States. The highest rate of completed suicide is among men older than 70. In contrast, suicide attempts are more common before middle age. Attempted suicide is particularly common among adolescent girls and single men in their 30s. Across all age groups, women attempt suicide 2 to 3 times more often than men, but men are more apt to die in their attempts.

Married people of either sex, particularly those in a secure relationship, have a much lower suicide rate than single people. People who live alone because of separation, divorce, or a spouse's death have higher rates of attempted and completed suicides. Having a family member who has attempted suicide may increase the risk as well.

Suicide among black women has increased 80% in the last 20 years, so that the overall rate for blacks now equals that for whites, especially in urban areas. Among Native Americans, the rate has also risen recently; in some tribes, it is 5 times the national average. Suicide rates are higher in urban areas than in rural areas worldwide. Many suicides take place in prisons.

Practicing members of most religious groups (particularly Roman Catholics and Jews) are less likely to commit suicide. Such people are generally supported by their beliefs and are provided with close social bonds protecting against acts of self-destruction. However, religious affiliation and strong religious beliefs do not necessarily prevent individual impetuous, unpremeditated suicidal acts during times of frustration, anger, and despair, especially when accompanied by delusions of guilt and unworthiness.

Suicide notes are left by about one of four people who complete suicide. The notes often refer to personal relationships and events that will follow the person's death. Notes left by older people often express concern for those left behind, whereas those of younger people may express anger or vindictiveness. The content of the note may indicate that the person had a mental health disorder that led to the suicidal act.

Causes

Suicidal behaviors usually result from the interaction of several factors, the most common of which is depression.▲ In fact, depression is involved in over 50% of attempted suicides. Marital problems, unhappy or ended love affairs, disputes with parents (among adolescents), or the recent loss of a loved one (particularly among older people) may precipitate the depression. Often, one factor, such as a disruption of an important relationship, is the last straw.

Depression associated with a medical disorder may lead to a suicide attempt. Most medical disorders associated with increased suicide rates either directly affect the nervous system and brain (such as AIDS, dementia, or temporal lobe epilepsy) or involve treatments that can cause depression (such as certain drugs used to treat high blood pressure). People whose depression includes anxiety or features of psychosis, such as false beliefs (delusions), may be at higher risk of suicide than those whose depression does not include these features.

People who have had traumatic childhood experiences, particularly the distresses of a broken home, parental deprivation, or abuse, are more likely to attempt suicide, perhaps because they are at higher risk of becoming depressed. Attempted suicide is also more likely among battered wives, many of whom were abused as children.

Depression may be intensified by the use of alcohol, which in turn makes suicidal behavior more likely. The use of alcohol diminishes self-control as well. About 30% of people who attempt suicide drink alcohol before the attempt. Because alcoholism, particularly binge drinking, often causes deep feelings of remorse during dry periods, alcoholics are suicide-prone even when sober.

In addition to depression, other mental health disorders put people at risk of suicide. People with schizophrenia■ and other psychotic disorders may hear voices (auditory hallucinations) commanding them to kill themselves. People with borderline personality disorder★ or antisocial personality disorder,● especially those with a history of violent behavior, may use suicide gestures or attempted suicide as a means of getting back at someone or of making a statement.

Suicide Intervention: Crisis Hot Lines

A person threatening suicide is in crisis, and suicide prevention centers, located around the country, provide 24-hour phone hot lines to those in distress. (E-mail hot lines on the Internet are available as well.) Suicide prevention centers are staffed by specially trained volunteers.

When a potentially suicidal person calls a hot line, a volunteer seeks to establish a relationship with the suicidal person, reminding him of his identity (for instance, by using his name repeatedly). The volunteer may offer constructive help for the problem that brought on the crisis and encourage the person to take positive action to resolve it. The volunteer may remind the person that he has family and friends who care and want to help. Finally, the volunteer may try to facilitate emergency face-to-face professional help for the suicidal person.

Sometimes a person may call a hot line to say that he has already committed a suicidal act (for example, taken a drug overdose or turned on the gas) or is in the process of doing so. In this case, the volunteer tries to obtain the person's address. If that is not possible, another volunteer contacts the police to trace the call and attempt a rescue. The person is kept talking on the telephone until the police arrive.

Methods

The choice of method often is influenced by cultural factors and availability and may or may not reflect the seriousness of intent. Some methods (for example, jumping from a tall building) make survival virtually impossible, whereas other methods (for example, overdosing on drugs) make rescue possible. However, even if a person uses a method that proves not to be fatal, the intent may have been just as serious as that of a person whose method was fatal.

Drug overdose and self-poisoning are two of the most common methods used in suicide attempts. Acetaminophen is now the most commonly used drug in attempted suicide, but antidepressants or a combination of drugs are also commonly used.

▲ see page 614   ■ see page 640
★ see page 633   ● see page 632

Violent methods, such as gunshots and hanging, are uncommon among attempted suicides because they usually result in death. Of completed suicides, a gunshot is the method most frequently used in the United States. It is a method predominantly used by males. Females are more likely to use nonviolent methods, such as poisoning, drug overdose, or drowning.

Prevention

Although some attempted or completed suicides come as a shock even to family and friends, clear warnings are given in most cases. Any suicide threat or suicide attempt is a plea for help and must be taken seriously. If the threat or attempt is ignored, a life may be lost.

If a person is threatening or has already attempted suicide, the police should be contacted immediately so that emergency services can arrive as soon as possible. Until help arrives, the person should be spoken to in a calm, supportive manner.

A doctor usually hospitalizes a person who has threatened or attempted suicide. Even if the person does not agree to hospitalization, most states allow a doctor to hospitalize a person against his wishes if the doctor believes that the person is at high risk of harming himself.

Impact of Suicide

Any suicidal act has a marked emotional effect on all involved. The person's family, friends, and doctor may feel guilt, shame, and remorse at not having prevented the suicide. They may also feel anger toward the person. Eventually, they may realize that they could not have prevented the suicide. Sometimes a grief counselor or a self-help group, such as Survivors of Suicide, can help family and friends deal with their feelings of guilt and sorrow. The primary care doctor or local mental health services (for example, at the county or state level) can often help locate these resources. In addition, national organizations, such as the American Foundation for Suicide Prevention, often maintain directories of local support groups. Resources are available on the Internet as well.

The effect of attempted suicide is similar. However, family members and friends have the opportunity to resolve their feelings by responding appropriately to the person's cry for help.

Assisted Suicide

Assisted suicide refers to the help given to a person who wishes to end his life by a doctor or other health care professional or even by a family member or friend. Assisted suicide is very controversial because it reverses the doctor's usual goal, which is to preserve life. Assisted suicide is illegal in all states except Oregon. In the rest of the United States, doctors can provide treatment intended to minimize physical and emotional suffering, but they cannot specifically intend to hasten death.

CHAPTER 103

Eating Disorders

Eating disorders are grouped into three categories: refusing to maintain a minimally normal body weight (anorexia nervosa), bingeing and purging (bulimia nervosa), and bingeing without purging (binge eating disorder). Bingeing is the rapid consumption of large amounts of food in a short period of time accompanied by a feeling of loss of control. Purging is self-induced vomiting or misuse of laxatives or enemas.

Eating disorders are far more common among women, especially younger women, than among men.

Anorexia Nervosa

Anorexia nervosa is characterized by a distorted body image, an extreme fear of obesity, refusal to maintain a minimally normal body weight, and in women, the absence of menstrual periods.

Hereditary factors have been shown to play a role in the development of anorexia nervosa. Social factors are also important. The desire to be thin pervades Western society, and obesity is considered unattractive, unhealthy, and undesirable. Even before adolescence, children are aware of these attitudes, and two thirds of all adolescent girls diet or take other measures to control their weight. Yet only a small percentage of these girls develop anorexia nervosa. Other factors, such as psychologic susceptibility, probably predispose certain people to developing anorexia nervosa. In areas with a genuine food shortage, anorexia nervosa is rare.

About 95% of people who have anorexia nervosa are female. The disorder usually begins in adolescence, occasionally earlier, and less commonly in adulthood. Anorexia nervosa primarily affects people in middle and upper socioeconomic classes. In Western society, the number of people who have this disorder seems to be increasing: it has been estimated to affect about 1% of girls aged 12 to 18.

Symptoms

Anorexia nervosa may be mild and transient or severe and persistent. Because many people who develop anorexia nervosa are meticulous, compulsive, and intelligent, with very high standards for achievement and success, an eating disorder may easily go undetected. The first indications of the impending disorder may be a subtle increased concern with diet and body weight. Such concerns seem out of place, because most people who have anorexia nervosa are already thin. Preoccupation and anxiety about weight intensify as the person becomes thinner. Even when emaciated, the person claims to feel fat, denies that anything is wrong, does not complain about weight loss, and usually resists treatment. The person usually does not see a doctor until brought to one by concerned family members.

Anorexia means "lack of appetite," but people who have anorexia nervosa are actually hungry and preoccupied with food. They study diets and count calories; they hoard, conceal, and deliberately waste food; they collect recipes; and they prepare elaborate meals for others. Half of the people who have anorexia nervosa binge and then purge by vomiting or taking laxatives. The other half simply restrict the amount of food they eat. They also frequently lie about how much they have eaten and conceal their vomiting and their peculiar dietary habits. Many also take diuretics to treat perceived bloating.

Women with anorexia nervosa stop having menstrual periods, sometimes before losing much weight. Women and men with the disorder may lose interest in sex. Typically, they have a low heart rate, low blood pressure, low body temperature, swelling of tissues caused by fluid accumulation (edema), and fine, soft hair or excessive body and facial hair. People with anorexia nervosa who become very thin tend to remain active, often exercising excessively to control their weight. Until they become emaciated, however, they have few symptoms of nutritional deficiencies. Depression is common.

Hormonal changes resulting from anorexia nervosa include markedly reduced levels of estrogen (in women) and thyroid hormone and increased levels of cortisol. If a person becomes seriously malnourished, every major organ system in the body is likely to be affected. When weight loss has been rapid or severe—for example, to more than 25% below the ideal body weight—restoring body weight quickly is crucial; such weight loss and the associated changes in electrolytes and fluid balance can be life threatening. Problems with the heart and with fluids and electrolytes (sodium, potassium, chloride) are the most dangerous. The heart gets weaker and pumps less blood through the body. The person may become dehydrated and prone to fainting. The blood may become alkaline (a condition called metabolic alkalosis▲), and potassium levels in the blood may decrease. Vomiting and taking laxatives and diuretics can worsen the situation. Sudden death, probably from abnormal heart rhythms, may occur.

Diagnosis and Treatment

Anorexia nervosa is usually diagnosed on the basis of severe weight loss and the characteristic psychologic symptoms. The typical person with anorexia nervosa is an adolescent girl who has lost at least 15% of her body weight, fears obesity, stops having menstrual periods, denies being sick, and otherwise appears healthy.

Treatment has two phases: short-term intervention to restore body weight and save the person's life and long-term therapy to improve psychologic functioning and prevent relapse.

The initial treatment of severe or rapid weight loss is best provided in a hospital where experienced staff members firmly but gently encourage the person to eat. Rarely, the person is fed intravenously or by a tube inserted through the nose and passed into the stomach. Sometimes doctors confine those with severe

▲ see page 932

disease in the hospital against their will after obtaining appropriate legal authorization from a parent, guardian, or the court.

When the person's nutritional status is acceptable and stabilized, long-term therapy is begun. Treatment is aimed at establishing a calm, concerned, stable environment while encouraging the consumption of an adequate amount of food. This treatment may include individual, group, and family psychotherapy as well as drug therapy. Combined treatment by the family doctor and a therapist often helps, and consultation with or referral to a specialist in eating disorders is wise.

When depression is diagnosed, antidepressants are prescribed. Certain antidepressants, particularly selective serotonin reuptake inhibitors, are useful for preventing relapse after weight has been restored.

As many as 10 to 20% of people diagnosed with anorexia nervosa die of it and its complications, which include fluid and electrolyte abnormalities, heart failure, and suicide resulting from depression. However, because mild cases may not be diagnosed, no one knows exactly how many people have anorexia nervosa or what percentage die of it.

Bulimia Nervosa

Bulimia nervosa is characterized by the repeated rapid consumption of large quantities of food (bingeing), followed by attempts to rid the body of the excess food consumed (purging).

As in anorexia nervosa, bulimia nervosa is influenced by hereditary and social factors. Also as in anorexia nervosa, most people who have bulimia nervosa are young women, are deeply concerned about body shape and weight, and belong to the middle or upper socioeconomic classes. About 2% of college women, the population believed to be at highest risk, are bulimics.

Symptoms

People with bulimia nervosa engage in repeated episodes of bingeing, which involves consuming large amounts of food within a relatively short period of time, often within 2 hours. Emotional stress often triggers the binge-purge cycle, which usually is done in secret. Bingeing, which is accompanied by a feeling of a loss of control, typically includes eating when not hungry and eating to the point of pain. In an attempt to counteract the effects of the binge, people with bulimia nervosa engage

in purging through such means as vomiting or taking laxatives; rigorously dieting; overexercising; or any combination of these. Many also take diuretics to treat perceived bloating. Unlike in anorexia nervosa, however, the body weight of people with bulimia nervosa tends to fluctuate around normal.

Self-induced vomiting can erode tooth enamel, enlarge the salivary glands in the cheeks (parotid glands), and inflame the esophagus. Vomiting and purging can lower potassium levels in the blood, causing abnormal heart rhythms. Sudden death from repeatedly taking large quantities of ipecac to induce vomiting can occur, the result of an abnormal heart rhythm. Rarely, people who have this disorder eat so much during a binge that their stomach ruptures or their esophagus tears, leading to life-threatening complications.

Compared with people who have anorexia nervosa, those who have bulimia nervosa tend to be more aware of their behavior and to feel remorseful or guilty about it. They are more likely to admit their concerns to a doctor or other confidant. Generally, people with bulimia nervosa are more outgoing. They also are more prone to impulsive behavior, drug or alcohol abuse, and depression.

Diagnosis and Treatment

A doctor suspects bulimia nervosa if a person, particularly a young woman, is overly concerned about weight gain and has wide fluctuations in weight, especially with evidence of excessive laxative use. Other clues include swollen salivary glands in the cheeks, scars on the knuckles from using the fingers to induce vomiting, erosion of tooth enamel from stomach acid, and a low level of potassium detected by a blood test. The diagnosis is not confirmed until the person describes binge-purge behavior and reports having two or more binge-eating episodes a week for at least 3 months.

The two most effective approaches to treatment are cognitive-behavior therapy and drug therapy.

In cognitive-behavior therapy, dysfunctional thoughts are identified and examined, and the person is helped to give them up. The person meets with the therapist once or twice a week over a period of 4 to 5 months, for a total of about 20 sessions. Cognitive-behavior therapy has been shown to reduce the frequency of bingeing in about two thirds of people with bulimia and to stop bingeing altogether in about one third. People who have undergone this type of therapy continue to reduce or refrain from bingeing for at least 1 year.

Drug therapy with selective serotonin reuptake inhibitors, a type of antidepressant, has been shown to work at least as well as cognitive-behavior therapy in the treatment of bulimia nervosa. However, when the drugs are stopped, bingeing recurs.

Binge Eating Disorder

Binge eating disorder is characterized by bingeing that is not followed by purging.

In this disorder, bingeing contributes to excessive caloric intake and consequent weight gain. Unlike bulimia nervosa, binge eating disorder occurs most commonly in people who are obese and becomes more prevalent with increasing body weight. People who have binge eating disorder tend to be older than those who have anorexia nervosa or bulimia nervosa, and more (nearly half) are men.

The foods that binge eaters typically choose (binge foods) are high in calories (for example, cake and ice cream), and binges usually occur in secrecy.

People who have binge eating disorder are distressed by it, and about 50% of obese binge eaters are depressed. Although this disorder does not cause the physical problems that can occur with bulimia nervosa, it may lead to complications of obesity.

Treatment

Behavior therapy, as it is used to treat obesity, may be the best treatment for binge eating disorder. Behavior therapy has been shown to reduce body weight and the frequency of bingeing, even when no special attention is given to binge eating. Cognitive-behavior therapy markedly reduces the frequency of bingeing as well, but without reducing body weight.

CHAPTER 104

Sexuality

Sexuality is a normal part of the human experience. However, the types of sexual behavior that are considered normal vary greatly within and among different cultures. In fact, it may be impossible to define "normal" sexuality. There are wide variations not only in "normal" sexual behavior but also in the frequency of or need for sexual release. Some people desire sexual activity several times a day, whereas others are satisfied with infrequent activity (for example, a few times a year).

Although younger people are often reluctant to view older people as sexually interested, most older people remain interested in sex and report quite satisfying sex lives well into old age. Problems with sexual function, such as erectile dysfunction in men▲ and dyspareunia, vaginismus, or anorgasmia in women,■ affect people of all ages, although such problems tend to be more common in older people.

Societal attitudes about sexuality change with time. Examples of such changes can be seen regarding masturbation, homosexuality, and frequent sexual activity with different sex partners.

Masturbation: Masturbation, which was once regarded as a perversion and even a cause of mental disease, is now recognized as a normal sexual activity throughout life. It is estimated that more than 97% of males and 80% of females have masturbated. In general, males masturbate more frequently than females, even if involved in a sexually gratifying relationship. Although masturbation is normal and is often recommended as a "safe sex" option, it may cause guilt and psychologic suffering that stems from the disapproving attitudes of others. This can result in considerable distress and can even affect sexual performance.

Homosexuality: As with masturbation, homosexuality, once considered abnormal by the medical profession, is no longer considered a disorder; it is widely recognized as a sexual ori-

---

▲ see page 1336   ■ see page 1382

entation that is present from childhood. An estimated 4 to 5% of adults are involved exclusively in homosexual relationships throughout their lives, with an additional 2 to 5% of people periodically engaging in sex with someone of the same sex (bisexuality). Adolescents may experiment with same-sex play, but this does not necessarily indicate an enduring interest in homosexual or bisexual activity as adults.▲

Homosexuals discover that they are attracted to people of the same sex, just as heterosexuals discover that they are attracted to people of the opposite sex. The attraction appears to be the end result of biologic and environmental influences and is not a matter of choice. Therefore, the popular term "sexual preference" makes little sense in matters of sexual orientation.

Most homosexuals adjust well to their sexual orientation, although they must overcome widespread societal disapproval and prejudice. This adjustment may take a long time and may be associated with substantial psychologic stress. Many homosexual men and women experience bigotry in social situations and in the workplace, adding to their stress. Discrimination based on sexual orientation (or perceived sexual orientation) remains widespread.

Frequent Sexual Activity With Different Partners: For some heterosexuals and homosexuals, frequent sexual activity with different partners is a common practice throughout life. This behavior may serve as a reason to seek professional counseling, because the transmission of certain diseases (for example, HIV infection, hepatitis, syphilis, gonorrhea, cervical cancer) is linked to having many sex partners and because having many sex partners may signify difficulty in forming meaningful, lasting relationships.

Gender Identity

Gender identity is how a person sees himself or herself, whether masculine, feminine, or somewhere in-between. Gender role is the objective, public presentation in our culture as masculine, feminine, or mixed. For most people, gender identity is consistent with gender role (as when a man has an inner sense of his masculinity and publicly acts in ways that support this feeling).

Gender identity is well established by early childhood (18 to 24 months of age). During

childhood, boys come to know they are boys, and girls come to know they are girls. Children sometimes prefer activities considered to be more appropriate for the other sex. However, this does not mean that a young girl who likes to play baseball and wrestle, for example, has a gender identity problem, as long as she sees herself as, and is content with being, female. Similarly, a boy who plays with dolls and prefers cooking to sports or to rough types of play does not have a gender identity problem as long as he identifies himself as, and is comfortable with being, male.

Children born with genitals that are not clearly male or female ■ usually do not have a gender identity problem if they are decisively reared as one sex or the other, even if they are raised in the gender role that is opposite their biologic sex pattern. There have been some highly publicized cases, however, in which this approach has failed.

Gender Identity Disorder and Transsexualism

People who experience a significant discrepancy between their anatomy and their inner sense of self as masculine, feminine, mixed, or neutral often have a gender identity disorder. The extreme form of gender identity disorder is called transsexualism.

People who are transsexuals believe that they are victims of a biologic accident and that they are cruelly imprisoned within a body incompatible with their gender identity. Most transsexuals are biologic males who identify themselves as females, usually early in childhood, and regard their genitals and masculine features with repugnance. Transsexualism appears to occur in about 1 of 30,000 males and 1 of 100,000 females.

Transsexuals may seek psychologic help, either to assist them in coping with the difficulties of living in a body that they do not feel comfortable with or to help them through a gender transition. Many transsexuals appear to be helped most by a combination of counseling, hormone therapy, electrolysis, and genital surgery.

Some transsexuals are satisfied with changing their gender role by working, living, and dressing in society as a member of the opposite sex, which may include obtaining identification (such as a driver's license) that reinforces their change in gender role. They may never seek to actually alter their anatomy in any way. Many of these people, who are some-

▲ see page 1554   ■ see page 1519

times referred to as "transgenderists," meet no criteria for a mental health disorder.

Other transsexuals, in addition to adopting the behavior, dress, and mannerisms of the opposite sex, also receive hormone treatments to change their secondary sex characteristics. In biologic males, use of the female hormone estrogen causes breast growth and other body changes, such as wasting of the genitals (genital atrophy) and the inability to maintain an erection. In biologic females, use of the male hormone testosterone causes such changes as the growth of facial hair, deepening of the voice, and changes in body odor.

Still other transsexuals seek to undergo sex reassignment surgery. For biologic males, this involves removal of the penis and testes and the creation of an artificial vagina. For biologic females, this involves removal of the breasts and the internal reproductive organs (uterus and ovaries), closure of the vagina, and creation of an artificial penis. For both sexes, surgery is preceded by use of the appropriate sex hormone (estrogen in male-to-female transformation, testosterone in female-to-male transformation).

Although transsexuals who undergo sex reassignment surgery are unable to have children, many are able to have quite satisfactory sexual relations. The ability to achieve orgasm is often retained after surgery, and some people report feeling comfortable sexually for the first time. However, few transsexuals endure the sex reassignment process for the sole purpose of being able to function sexually in the opposite sex. Confirmation of gender identity is the usual motivator.

Paraphilias

Paraphilias are attractions that in extreme forms are socially unacceptable deviations from the traditionally held norms of sexual relationships and attractions.

The key features of a paraphilia include repetitive, intense, sexually arousing fantasies or behaviors that usually involve objects (for example, shoes, underwear, leather or rubber products), the infliction of suffering or pain on oneself or one's partner, or having sex with nonconsenting people (for example, with children, with helpless people, or in rape situations). Once these arousal patterns are established, usually in late childhood or near puberty, they are often lifelong.

Some degree of variety is very common in healthy adult sexual relationships and fantasies. When people mutually agree to engage in them, noninjurious sexual behaviors of an unusual nature may be an intrinsic part of a loving and caring relationship. When taken to the extreme, however, such sexual behaviors are paraphilias, psychosexual disorders that seriously impair the capacity for affectionate, reciprocal sexual activity. Partners of people with a paraphilia may feel like an object or as if they are unimportant or unnecessary in the sexual relationship.

Paraphilias may take the form of fetishism, transvestic fetishism, pedophilia, exhibitionism, voyeurism, masochism, or sadism, among others. Most people with paraphilias are men, and many have more than one type of paraphilia.

Fetishism

In fetishism, sexual activity makes use of physical objects (the fetish), sometimes in preference to contact with humans. People with fetishes may become sexually stimulated and gratified by wearing another person's undergarments, wearing rubber or leather, or holding, rubbing, or smelling objects, such as high-heeled shoes. People with this disorder may not be able to function sexually without their fetish.

Transvestic Fetishism

In transvestic fetishism, a man prefers to wear women's clothing, or, far less commonly, a woman prefers to wear men's clothing (cross-dressing). In neither case, however, does the person wish to change his or her sex, as transsexuals do. Cross-dressing is not always considered a mental health disorder and may not adversely affect a couple's sexual relationship.

Transvestic fetishism is a disorder only if it causes distress, results in impairment of some type, or involves "daredevil" behavior likely to lead to injury, loss of a job, or imprisonment. Transvestites also cross-dress for reasons other than sexual stimulation, for example, to reduce anxiety, to relax, or, in the case of male transvestites, to experiment with the feminine side of their otherwise male personalities.

Pedophilia

Pedophilia is a preference for sexual activity with young children. In Western societies, pedophilia is defined as sexual fantasy about or sexual relations with a child younger than 13 by a person 16 or older. Some pedophiles are attracted only to children, often of a specific age range or developmental stage, whereas others are attracted to both children and adults.

Although state laws vary, the law generally considers a person older than 18 to be committing statutory rape if the victim is 16 or younger. Statutory rape cases often do not meet the definition of pedophilia, highlighting the somewhat arbitrary nature of selecting a specific age cutoff point in a medical or legal definition.

Pedophilia is much more common among men than among women. Both boys and girls can be victims, although more reported cases involve girls. Pedophiles may focus only on children within their families (incest), or they may prey on children in the community. Force or coercion may be used to engage children sexually, and threats may be invoked to prevent disclosure by the victim.

Pedophilia can be treated with psychotherapy and drugs that alter the sex drive, with varying results. Such treatment may be sought voluntarily or only after criminal apprehension and legal action. Incarceration, even long-term, does not change pedophilic desires or fantasies.

Exhibitionism

In exhibitionism, a person (usually male) exposes his genitals to unsuspecting strangers and becomes sexually excited when doing so. Further sexual contact is almost never sought, so exhibitionists rarely commit rape. Most exhibitionists are younger than 40 and may or may not be married. Exposure of genitals to unsuspecting strangers for sexual excitement is rare among women. Provocative dressing by women is increasingly accepted by society as normal. In addition, social venues in which women can expose themselves are not uncommon, and such behavior may not constitute a mental health disorder.

Voyeurism

In voyeurism, a person becomes sexually aroused by watching someone who is disrobing, naked, or engaged in sexual activity. It is the act of observing (peeping) that is arousing, not sexual activity with the observed person.

Some degree of voyeurism is particularly common, more among boys and men but increasingly among women. Society often regards mild forms of this behavior as normal. As a disorder, voyeurism is much more common among men; it may become the preferred method of sexual activity and consume countless hours of watching. The amount and variety of sexually explicit materials and shows available to men and women have increased significantly, but engaging in these activities lacks the element of secret observation that is the hallmark of voyeurism. The Internet has made voyeurism easier to engage in without the neighborhood prowling traditionally associated with this behavior.

Sexual Masochism and Sadism

Sexual masochism involves acts in which a person derives sexual excitement from being humiliated, beaten, bound, or otherwise abused. Sexual sadism involves acts in which a person derives sexual pleasure from inflicting physical or psychologic suffering on another person. Some people act out their sadistic urges with a consenting partner (who may have sexual masochism); rarely, some act them out on nonconsenting victims. Fantasies of total control and dominance are often important, and the sadist may bind and gag the partner in elaborate ways.

Some amount of sadism and masochism is commonly play-acted in healthy sexual relationships, and mutually compatible partners often seek one another out. For example, the use of silk handkerchiefs for simulated bondage and mild spanking during sexual activity are common practices between consenting partners and are not considered sadomasochistic.

In contrast, the disorder of sexual masochism or of sexual sadism takes these acts to an extreme and can result in severe bodily or psychologic harm and even death. For example, masochistic sexual activity may involve asphyxiophilia, whereby the person is partially choked or strangled (either by a partner or by the self-application of a noose around the neck). A temporary decrease in oxygen to the brain at the point of orgasm is sought as an enhancement to sexual release, but the practice may accidentally result in death.

CHAPTER 105

Personality Disorders

Personality disorders are characterized by patterns of perceiving, reacting, and relating that are relatively inflexible and socially maladaptive.

Everyone has characteristic patterns of perceiving and relating to other people and events (personality traits). Put another way, people tend to cope with stresses in an individual but repetitive style. For example, some people respond to a troubling situation by seeking someone else's help, whereas others prefer to deal with problems on their own. Some people minimize problems; others exaggerate them. Regardless of their usual style, however, mentally healthy people are likely to try an alternative approach if their first response is ineffective.

In contrast, people with personality disorders are rigid and tend to respond inappropriately to problems, to the point that relationships with family, friends, and coworkers are affected. These maladaptive responses usually begin in adolescence or early adulthood and do not change over time.

People with personality disorders are unaware that their thought or behavior patterns are inappropriate; thus they tend not to seek help on their own. Instead, they may be referred by their friends, their family, or a social agency because their behavior is causing difficulty for others. When they do seek help on their own, usually because of troubling symptoms (for example, anxiety, depression, or substance abuse), they tend to believe their problems are caused by other people or by circumstances beyond their control.

Personality disorders are grouped into three clusters. Cluster A personality disorders involve odd or eccentric behavior; cluster B, dramatic or erratic behavior; and cluster C, anxious or inhibited behavior.

Cluster A: Odd or Eccentric Behavior

Paranoid Personality: People with a paranoid personality are distrustful and suspicious of others. They suspect on the basis of little or no evidence that others are out to harm them, and they may retaliate at any time. This behavior often leads to rejection by others, which seems to justify their original feelings. They are generally cold and distant in their relationships.

People with a paranoid personality often take legal action against others, especially if they feel righteously indignant. They are unable to see their own role in a conflict. Although they usually work in relative isolation, they may be highly efficient and conscientious.

Sometimes people who already feel alienated because of a defect or handicap (such as deafness) are more likely to suspect that other people have negative ideas or attitudes toward them. Such heightened suspicion, however, is not evidence of a paranoid personality unless it involves wrongly attributing malevolence to others.

Schizoid Personality: People with a schizoid personality are introverted, withdrawn, and solitary. They are emotionally cold and socially distant. They are most often absorbed with their own thoughts and feelings and are fearful of closeness and intimacy with others. They talk little, are given to daydreaming, and prefer theoretical speculation to practical action. Fantasizing is a common coping mechanism (defense mechanism).

Schizotypal Personality: People with a schizotypal personality, like those with a schizoid personality, are socially and emotionally detached. In addition, they display oddities of thinking, perceiving, and communicating similar to those of people with schizophrenia.▲ Although schizotypal personality is sometimes found in people with schizophrenia before they become ill, most adults with a schizotypal personality do not develop schizophrenia.

Some people with a schizotypal personality show signs of magical thinking—that is, they believe that a particular thought or action can control something or someone. For example, a person may believe that he can cause harm to others by thinking angry thoughts. People with a schizotypal personality may also have paranoid ideas.

Cluster B: Dramatic or Erratic Behavior

Histrionic (Hysterical) Personality: People with a histrionic personality conspicuously seek attention, are dramatic and excessively

▲ see page 640

Consequences of Personality Disorders

- People with personality disorders are at high risk of behaviors that can lead to physical illness, such as alcohol or drug addiction; self-destructive behavior; reckless sexual behavior; hypochondriasis; and clashes with society's values.
- People with personality disorders may have inconsistent, detached, overemotional, abusive, or irresponsible styles of parenting, leading to medical and psychiatric problems in their children.
- People with personality disorders are vulnerable to mental breakdowns (a period of crisis when the person has difficulty performing even routine mental tasks) as a result of stress; the type of mental health disorder (for example, anxiety, depression, or psychosis) depends in part on the type of personality disorder.
- People with personality disorders are less likely to follow a prescribed treatment regimen; even when they follow the regimen, they are usually less responsive than most people to medications.
- People with personality disorders often have a poor relationship with their doctors because they refuse to take responsibility for their behavior or feel overly distrustful, deserving, or needy. The doctor may then become blaming, distrusting, and ultimately rejecting of the person.

emotional, and are overly concerned with appearance. Their lively, expressive manner results in easily established but often superficial and transient relationships. Their expression of emotions often seems exaggerated, childish, and contrived to evoke sympathy or attention (often erotic or sexual) from others.

People with a histrionic personality are prone to sexually provocative behavior or to sexualizing nonsexual relationships. However, they may not really want a sexual relationship; rather, their seductive behavior often masks their wish to be dependent and protected. Some people with a histrionic personality also are hypochondriacal and exaggerate their physical problems to get the attention they need.

Narcissistic Personality: People with a narcissistic personality have a sense of superiority, a need for admiration, and a lack of empathy. They have an exaggerated belief in their own value or importance, which is what therapists call "grandiosity." They may be extremely sensitive to failure, defeat, or criticism. When confronted by a failure to fulfill their high opinion of themselves, they can easily become enraged or severely depressed. Because they believe themselves to be superior in their relationships with other people, they expect to be admired and often suspect that others envy them. They believe they are entitled to having their needs met without waiting, so they exploit others, whose needs or beliefs they deem to be less important. Their behavior is usually offensive to others, who view them as being self-centered, arrogant, or selfish. This personality disorder typically occurs in high achievers, although it may also occur in people with few achievements.

Antisocial Personality: People with an antisocial personality (previously called psychopathic or sociopathic personality), most of whom are male, show callous disregard for the rights and feelings of others. Dishonesty and deceit permeate their relationships. They exploit others for material gain or personal gratification (unlike narcissistic people, who exploit others because they think their superiority justifies it).

Characteristically, people with an antisocial personality act out their conflicts impulsively and irresponsibly. They tolerate frustration poorly, and sometimes they are hostile or violent. Often they do not anticipate the negative consequences of their antisocial behaviors and, despite the problems or harm they cause others, do not feel remorse or guilt. Rather, they glibly rationalize their behavior or blame it on others. Frustration and punishment do not motivate people with an antisocial personality to modify their behaviors or improve their judgment and foresight but, rather, usually confirm their harshly unsentimental view of the world.

People with an antisocial personality are prone to alcoholism, drug addiction, sexual deviation, promiscuity, and imprisonment. They are likely to fail at their jobs and move from one area to another. They often have a family history of antisocial behavior, substance abuse, divorce, and physical abuse. As children, many were emotionally neglected and physically abused. People with an antisocial personality have shorter life expectancies than the general population. The disorder tends to diminish or stabilize with age.

Borderline Personality: People with a borderline personality, most of whom are women, are unstable in their self-image, moods, behavior, and interpersonal relationships. Their thought processes are more disturbed than those of people with an antisocial personality, and aggression is more often turned against the self. They are more angry, more impulsive, and more confused about their identity than are people with a histrionic personality. Borderline personality becomes evident in early adulthood, but prevalence decreases with age.

People with a borderline personality often were neglected or abused as children. Consequently, they feel empty, angry, and deserving of nurturing. They have far more dramatic and intense interpersonal relationships than people with cluster A personality disorders. When they feel cared for, they appear lonely and waiflike, often needing help for past mistreatment, depression, substance abuse, and eating disorders. However, when they fear being abandoned by a caring person, their mood shifts dramatically and is frequently expressed as inappropriate and intense anger. This shift in mood is accompanied by extreme changes in their view of the world, themselves, and others—things are black or white, good or evil, but never neutral.

People with a borderline personality who feel abandoned and alone may wonder whether they actually exist (that is, they do not feel real). They can become desperately impulsive, engaging in reckless promiscuity or substance abuse. At times they are so out of touch with reality that they have brief episodes of psychotic thinking, paranoia, and hallucinations.

People with a borderline personality are commonly seen by primary care doctors. Additionally, borderline personality is the most common personality disorder treated by therapists, because people with the disorder relentlessly seek someone to care for them. However, after repeated crises, vague unfounded complaints, and failures to comply with therapeutic recommendations, caretakers—including doctors—often become very frustrated with them and view them as help-rejecting complainers.

Cluster C: Anxious or Inhibited Behavior

Avoidant Personality: People with an avoidant personality are overly sensitive to rejection, and they fear starting relationships or anything new. They have a strong desire for affection and acceptance but avoid intimate relationships and social situations for fear of disappointment and criticism. Unlike those with a schizoid personality, they are openly distressed by their isolation and inability to relate comfortably to others. Unlike those with a borderline personality, they do not respond to rejection with anger; instead, they withdraw and appear shy and timid. Avoidant personality is similar to generalized social phobia.▲

Dependent Personality: People with a dependent personality routinely surrender major decisions and responsibilities to others and permit the needs of those they depend on to supersede their own. They lack self-confidence and feel intensely insecure about their ability to take care of themselves. They often protest that they cannot make decisions and do not know what to do or how to do it. This behavior is due partly to a belief that others are more capable and partly to a reluctance to express their views for fear of offending the people whom they need. People with other personality disorders often have aspects of a dependent personality, but these traits are usually hidden by the more dominant traits of the other disorder. Sometimes adults with prolonged illnesses develop a dependent personality.

Obsessive-Compulsive Personality: People with an obsessive-compulsive personality are preoccupied with orderliness, perfectionism, and control. They are reliable, dependable, orderly, and methodical, but their inflexibility makes them unable to adapt to change. Because they are cautious and weigh all aspects of a problem, they have difficulty making decisions. They take their responsibilities seriously, but because they cannot tolerate mistakes or imperfection, they often have trouble completing tasks. Unlike the mental health disorder called obsessive-compulsive disorder,■ obsessive-compulsive personality does not involve repeated, unwanted obsessions and ritualistic behavior.

People with an obsessive-compulsive personality are often high achievers, especially in the sciences and other intellectually demanding fields in which order and attention to detail are desirable. However, their responsibilities make them so anxious that they can rarely enjoy their successes. They are uncomfortable with their feelings, with relationships, and with situations in which they lack control or must rely on others or in which events are unpredictable.

▲ see page 610   ■ see page 611

COMMON COPING MECHANISMS

MECHANISM	DEFINITION	RESULT	PERSONALITY DISORDERS INVOLVED
Projection	Attributing one's own feelings or thoughts to others	Leads to prejudice, suspiciousness, and excessive worrying about external dangers	Typical of paranoid and schizotypal personalities; used by people with borderline, antisocial, or narcissistic personality when under acute stress
Splitting	Use of black-or-white, all-or-nothing thinking to divide people into groups of idealized all-good saviors and vilified all-bad evildoers	Allows a person to avoid the discomfort of having both loving and hateful feelings for the same person as well as feelings of uncertainty and helplessness	Typical of borderline personality
Acting out	A direct behavioral expression of an unconscious wish or impulse that enables a person to avoid thinking about a painful situation or experiencing a painful emotion	Leads to acts that are often irresponsible, reckless, and foolish. Includes many delinquent, promiscuous, and substance-abusing acts, which can become so habitual that the person remains unaware and dismissive of the feelings that initiated the acts	Very common in people with antisocial or borderline personality
Turning aggression against self	Expressing the angry feelings one has toward others by hurting one's self directly (for example, through self-mutilation) or indirectly (for example, body dysmorphic disorder); when indirect, it is called passive aggression	Includes failures and illnesses that affect others more than oneself and silly, provocative clowning	Dramatic in people with borderline personality
Fantasizing	Use of imaginary relationships and private belief systems to resolve conflict and to escape from painful realities, such as loneliness	Is associated with eccentricity, avoidance of interpersonal intimacy, and avoidance of involvement with the outside world	Used by people with avoidant or schizoid personality, who, in contrast to people with psychoses, do not believe and thus do not act on their fantasies
Hypochondriasis	Use of health complaints to gain attention	Provides one with nurturant attention from others; may be a passive expression of anger toward others	Used by people with dependent, histrionic, or borderline personality

Diagnosis

A doctor bases the diagnosis of a personality disorder on a person's history, specifically, repetitive displays of maladaptive thought or behavior patterns. These patterns tend to become apparent because the person stubbornly resists changing them despite their negative consequences. In addition, a doctor is likely to notice the person's inappropriate use of mental coping mechanisms (defense mechanisms). Although everyone unconsciously uses coping mechanisms, people with personality disorders use them in immature and maladaptive ways, such that it interferes with their daily functioning.

Treatment

Personality traits take many years to develop, thus the treatment of maladaptive traits takes many years as well. No short-term treatment can cure a personality disorder, although some changes may be accomplished faster than others. For example, drug therapy or reduction of environmental stresses can quickly relieve symptoms such as anxiety and depression. Behavioral changes can occur within a year; interpersonal changes take longer. For example, for a person with a dependent personality, a behavioral change might be to stop stating that he cannot make decisions; the interpersonal change might be to interact with others in a workplace or family setting in such a way that he actually seeks out or at least accepts some decision-making responsibilities.

Although treatments differ according to the type of personality disorder, some general principles apply to all treatments. Because the person with a personality disorder usually does not see a problem with his own behavior, he must be confronted with the harmful consequences of his maladaptive thoughts and behaviors. To do this, a therapist needs to repeatedly point out the undesirable consequences of the person's thought and behavior patterns. Sometimes the therapist finds it necessary to set limits on behavior (for example, the person might be told that he cannot raise his voice in anger but instead must use a regular speaking voice). The involvement of family members is helpful and often essential because they can act in ways that either reinforce or diminish the person's problematic behavior or thoughts. Group and family therapy, group living in designated residential settings, and participation in therapeutic social clubs or self-help groups can all be valuable in helping to change socially undesirable behaviors.

Psychotherapy (talk therapy) remains the cornerstone of most treatments and usually must continue for more than 1 year to effect change in a person's maladaptive behavior or interpersonal patterns. In the context of an intimate, cooperative, nonexploitative doctor-patient relationship, the person can begin to understand the sources of his distress and recognize his maladaptive behavior. Psychotherapy can help him more clearly recognize the attitudes and behaviors that lead to interpersonal problems, such as dependency, distrust, arrogance, and manipulativeness.

For some people with personality disorders, primarily those that involve maladaptive attitudes, expectations, and beliefs (such as narcissistic or obsessive-compulsive personality), psychoanalysis▲ is recommended and is usually continued for at least 3 years. Behavior therapy■ is helpful in changing behaviors such as recklessness, social isolation, lack of assertiveness, and temper outbursts. Behavioral change is most important for people with a borderline, antisocial, or avoidant personality. However, people with an antisocial or paranoid personality are rarely successfully treated by any therapy.

Drug therapy is sometimes appropriate for people with a personality disorder who have depression, phobia, or panic disorder. However, drugs usually provide only limited relief. In contrast, the feelings of anxiousness and sadness that result from a personality disorder are rarely satisfactorily relieved by drugs. Drug therapy for people with a borderline personality is frequently complicated by misuse of the drugs or by suicide attempts.

▲ see page 600   ■ see page 601

CHAPTER 106

Amnesia and Related Disorders

Amnesia and similar disorders are categorized by psychiatrists as dissociative disorders. They include dissociative amnesia, dissociative fugue, dissociative identity disorder, and depersonalization disorder. Dissociative disorders are usually triggered (precipitated) by overwhelming stress. The stress may be caused by experiencing or witnessing a traumatic event, accident, or disaster. Or a person may experience inner conflict so intolerable that his mind is forced to separate incompatible or unacceptable information and feelings from conscious thought.

Dissociative Amnesia

Dissociative amnesia is a type of amnesia caused by trauma or stress resulting in an inability to recall important personal information.

Dissociative amnesia is one type of amnesia. Amnesia is the total or partial inability to recall recent or remote experiences.▲ When amnesia is caused by a psychologic rather than a physical disturbance, it is called dissociative amnesia. Amnesia may also be a symptom of other disorders, such as acute stress disorder, posttraumatic stress disorder, or somatization disorder.

In dissociative amnesia, the lost memory usually involves information that is normally part of routine conscious awareness or "autobiographical" memory—who one is; what one did; where one went; to whom one spoke; what was said, thought, and felt; and so on. Sometimes the information, though forgotten, continues to influence the person's behavior.

People with dissociative amnesia usually have one or more memory gaps spanning a few minutes to a few hours or days. However, memory gaps spanning years or even a person's entire life may occur. Most people with dissociative amnesia are aware that they have "lost some time," but some become aware of time loss only when they realize or are confronted with evidence that they have done things that they do not recall. Some people with dissociative amnesia forget some but not all events over a period of time; others cannot recall their entire previous life or forget things as they occur.

The disorder is most common among young adults, more commonly among people who have been involved in wars, accidents, or natural disasters. It may also block memories of childhood sexual abuse, later recalled in adulthood. Dissociative amnesia can occur for some time after a traumatic event. Whether such recovered memories reflect real events in the person's past remains unknown, unless confirmed by another person.

Symptoms and Diagnosis

The most common symptom of dissociative amnesia is memory loss. Shortly after becoming amnesic, a person may seem confused. Many people with dissociative amnesia are somewhat depressed or very distressed by their amnesia.

To make the diagnosis, the doctor carefully reviews the person's symptoms and performs a physical examination to exclude physical causes of amnesia. Tests, including electroencephalography and blood testing for toxins and drugs, are sometimes needed to exclude physical causes. A psychologic examination is also performed. Special psychologic tests often help the doctor better characterize and understand the person's dissociative experiences to develop a treatment plan.

Treatment and Prognosis

A doctor begins treatment by helping the person to feel safe and secure. If the missing memories are not spontaneously recalled, or if the need to recall the memories is urgent, memory retrieval techniques are often successful. Using hypnosis or drug-facilitated interviews (interviews conducted after the person is calmed and sedated with an intravenous drug such as amobarbital or midazolam), the doctor questions the amnesic person about the past.

A doctor uses hypnosis and drug-facilitated interviews to reduce anxiety associated with the period for which there is amnesia, and to penetrate or bypass the defenses the amnesic person has created for protection from recalling painful experiences or conflicts. The doctor must be careful not to suggest what should be recalled or stimulate extreme anxiety.

▲ see page 479

Memories recalled through such techniques may not be accurate and may require external corroboration. Therefore, before hypnosis or a drug-facilitated interview is performed, the doctor informs the amnesic person that memories retrieved with these techniques may or may not be accurate and obtains the person's consent to proceed.

Filling in the memory gap to the greatest extent possible helps restore continuity to the person's identity and sense of self. Once the amnesia has disappeared, continued psychotherapy helps the person understand the trauma or conflicts that caused the disorder and find ways to resolve them.

Most people recover what appears to be their missing memories and resolve the conflicts that caused the amnesia. However, some people never break through the barriers that prevent them from reconstructing their missing past.

Dissociative Fugue

Dissociative fugue is a disorder in which one or more episodes of sudden, unexpected, and purposeful travel from home (fugue) occur, during which a person cannot remember some or all of his past life.

Dissociative fugue affects about 2 of 1,000 people in the United States. It is much more common in people who have been in wars, accidents, or natural disasters.

Causes

The causes of dissociative fugue are similar to those of dissociative amnesia. Dissociative fugue is often mistaken for malingering, because both conditions may occur under circumstances that a person might understandably wish to evade. However, dissociative fugue occurs spontaneously and is not faked. Malingering is a state in which a person feigns illness because it removes him from accountability for his actions, gives him an excuse to avoid responsibilities, or reduces his exposure to a known hazard, such as a dangerous job assignment. Many fugues seem to represent a disguised wish fulfillment (for example, an escape from overwhelming stresses, such as divorce or financial ruin). Other fugues are related to feelings of rejection or separation, or they may protect the person from suicidal or homicidal impulses.

When dissociative fugue recurs more than a few times, the person usually has an underlying dissociative identity disorder.

Symptoms and Diagnosis

A fugue may last from hours to weeks or months, or occasionally even longer. A person in a fugue state, having lost his customary identity, usually disappears from his usual haunts, leaving his family and job. If the fugue is brief, the person may appear simply to have missed some work or come home late or, if confused, may come to the attention of medical or legal authorities. If the fugue lasts several days or longer, the person may travel far from home and begin a new job with a new identity, unaware of any change in his life. During the fugue, the person may appear normal and attract no attention. However, at some point, the person may become aware of the memory loss (amnesia) or confused about his identity.

Often the person has no symptoms or is only mildly confused during the fugue. However, when the fugue ends, the person may experience depression, discomfort, grief, shame, intense conflict, and suicidal or aggressive impulses.

A doctor may suspect dissociative fugue when a person seems confused about his identity or is puzzled about his past, or when confrontations challenge the person's new identity or absence of one. The doctor makes the diagnosis by carefully reviewing the person's symptoms and performing a physical examination to exclude physical disorders that might be contributing to or causing memory loss. A psychologic examination is also performed.

Sometimes dissociative fugue cannot be diagnosed until the person abruptly returns to his pre-fugue identity and is distressed to find himself in unfamiliar circumstances. The diagnosis is usually made retroactively by a doctor reviewing the person's history and collecting information that documents the circumstances before the person left home, the travel itself, and the establishment of an alternate life.

Treatment and Prognosis

Most fugues last for hours or days and disappear on their own. Dissociative fugue is treated much the same as dissociative amnesia, and treatment may include the use of hypnosis or drug-facilitated interviews.▲ However, efforts to restore memories of the fugue period usually are unsuccessful. A therapist

▲ see page 636

may help the person to explore his patterns of handling the types of situations, conflicts, and moods that triggered (precipitated) the fugue episode to prevent subsequent fugue behavior.

Dissociative Identity Disorder

In dissociative identity disorder, formerly called multiple personality disorder, two or more identities or personalities alternate.

Dissociative identity disorder appears to be a rather common mental disorder. It can be found in 3 to 4% of people hospitalized for other mental health disorders and in a sizable minority of people in drug abuse treatment facilities. However, some authorities believe that many cases of this disorder reflect the influence of therapists on suggestible people.

Dissociative identity disorder appears to be caused by the interaction of several factors. These include overwhelming stress; an ability to separate one's memories, perceptions, or identity from conscious awareness; abnormal psychologic development, and insufficient protection and nurture during childhood.

Human development requires that children be able to integrate complicated and different types of information and experiences. As children learn to achieve a cohesive, complex identity, they go through phases in which different perceptions and emotions of themselves and others are kept segregated. These different perceptions and emotions become involved in the generation of different selves, but not every child who suffers abuse or a major loss or trauma has the capacity to develop multiple personalities. Those who do have the capacity also have normal ways of coping, and most of these vulnerable children are sufficiently protected and soothed by adults, so dissociative identity disorder does not develop.

Symptoms

People with dissociative identity disorder often describe an array of symptoms that can resemble those of other mental health disorders as well as many physical disorders. Some symptoms are an indication that another disorder is indeed present, but some symptoms may reflect the intrusions of past experiences into the present. For example, sadness may indicate coexisting depression, or it may be that one of the personalities is reliving emotions associated with past misfortunes.

Dissociative identity disorder is chronic and potentially disabling or fatal, although many with the disorder function very well and lead creative and productive lives. People with this disorder are prone to injuring themselves. They may engage in self-mutilation. Many attempt suicide.

In dissociative identity disorder, some of a person's personalities are aware of important personal information, whereas other personalities are unaware. Some personalities appear to know and interact with one another in an elaborate inner world. For example, personality A may be aware of personality B and know what B does, as if observing B's behavior; personality B may or may not be aware of personality A. Other personalities may or may not be aware of personality B, and personality B may or may not be aware of them.

The switching of personalities and the lack of awareness of one's behavior in the other personalities often make life chaotic for people with dissociative identity disorder. Because the personalities often interact with each other, people with dissociative personality disorder report hearing inner conversations and the voices of other personalities commenting on their behavior or addressing them. They experience distortion of time, with time lapses and amnesia. They have feelings of detachment from one's self (depersonalization) and feelings that one's surroundings are unreal (derealization). They often have concern with issues of control, both self-control and the control of others. In addition, people with dissociative identity disorder tend to develop severe headaches or other bodily pain and may experience sexual dysfunction. Different clusters of symptoms occur at different times.

People with dissociative identity disorder may not be able to recall things they have done or account for changes in their behavior. Often they refer to themselves as "we," "he," or "she." While most people cannot recall much about the first 3 to 5 years of life, people with dissociative identity disorder may have considerable amnesia for the period between the ages of 6 and 11 as well.

Diagnosis

To make the diagnosis of dissociative identity disorder, a doctor conducts a thorough psychologic interview. A medical examination may be needed to determine if a physical disorder is present that would explain certain symptoms. Special questionnaires have been developed to help doctors identify dissociative identity disorder.

Interviews may need to be prolonged and involve careful use of hypnosis or drug facilitation.▲ Hypnosis or drug-facilitated interviews may make the person more likely to allow the doctor to encounter other personalities or to reveal information about a period for which there is amnesia. However, some doctors feel that hypnosis and drug-facilitated interviews should not be performed because they believe the techniques can themselves generate symptoms of dissociative identity disorder.

Treatment and Prognosis

Some symptoms may come and go (fluctuate) spontaneously, but dissociative identity disorder does not clear up on its own. The goal of treatment is usually to integrate the personalities into a single personality. However, integration is not always possible. In these situations, the goal is to achieve a harmonious interaction among the personalities that allows more normal functioning.

Drug therapy can relieve some specific coexisting symptoms, such as anxiety or depression, but does not affect the disorder itself.

Psychotherapy is often arduous and emotionally painful. The person may experience many emotional crises from the actions of the personalities and from the despair that may occur when traumatic memories are recalled during therapy. Several periods of psychiatric hospitalization may be necessary to help the person through difficult times and to come to grips with particularly painful memories. Generally, two or more psychotherapy sessions a week for at least 3 to 6 years are necessary. Hypnosis may be helpful.

The prognosis of people with dissociative identity disorder depends on the symptoms and features they experience. For example, people who have additional serious mental health disorders, such as personality disorders, mood disorders, eating disorders, and substance abuse disorders, have a poorer prognosis.

Depersonalization Disorder

Depersonalization disorder is characterized by a persistent or recurring feeling of being detached from one's body or mental processes (depersonalization) and by a feeling of being an outside observer of one's life.

The symptom of depersonalization is the third most common psychologic symptom (after feelings of anxiety and feelings of depression) and often occurs after a person experi-

Dissociative Identity Disorder and Childhood Abuse

About 97 to 98% of adults with dissociative identity disorder report having been abused during childhood. Abuse can be documented for 85% of the adults and 95% of the children and adolescents with dissociative identity disorder.

Although childhood abuse is a major cause of dissociative identity disorder, that does not mean all the specific abuses alleged by people with this disorder really happened. Some aspects of some reported experiences clearly are not accurate. In addition, some people were not abused at all, but rather, suffered an important early loss, such as the death of a parent, a serious physical illness, or some other very stressful experience.

ences life-threatening danger, such as an accident, assault, or serious illness or injury. Depersonalization disorder has not been studied widely, and its cause and occurrence in the population are unknown.

Symptoms and Diagnosis

People with depersonalization disorder have a distorted perception of their identity, body, and life that makes them uncomfortable. Symptoms may be temporary or persist or recur for many years. People with the disorder often have a great deal of difficulty describing their symptoms and may fear or believe that they are going crazy.

Depersonalization disorder can be a minor, passing disturbance with little noticeable effect on behavior. Some people can adjust to it or even block its impact. Others are continually plagued with anxiety over their state of mind, worrying that they are going crazy or ruminating over the distorted perceptions of their body and their sense of estrangement from themselves and others. Mental anguish may disable them.

The diagnosis of depersonalization disorder is made on the basis of symptoms. A doctor evaluates the person to rule out physical disorders (such as a seizure disorder), drug abuse, and other mental health disorders. Psychologic tests and special interview procedures may help the doctor recognize the problem.

▲ see page 636

Treatment and Prognosis

Depersonalization disorder often disappears without treatment. Treatment is warranted only if the disorder persists, recurs, or causes distress. Psychodynamic psychotherapy, behavior therapy, and hypnosis have been effective for some people.▲ Sedatives and antidepressants help some people with the disorder. Depersonalization disorder is often associated with or triggered (precipitated) by other mental health disorders, which require treatment. Any stresses associated with the beginning (onset) of the depersonalization disorder must also be addressed.

Some degree of relief is usually achieved with treatment. Complete recovery is possible for many people, especially those whose symptoms occur in connection with stresses that can be addressed during treatment. Other people with depersonalization disorder do not respond well to treatment, although they may gradually improve on their own. A few remain unresponsive to all treatments.

▲ see page 601   ■ see page 1632

CHAPTER 107

Schizophrenia and Delusional Disorder

Schizophrenia and delusional disorder are distinct disorders that may share certain features, such as paranoia, suspiciousness, and unrealistic thinking. However, schizophrenia is associated with psychosis—a loss of contact with reality—and with a decline in general functioning. In contrast, in delusional disorder, contact with reality is preserved except for the very specific and focused unrealistic thinking that comprises the delusions; functioning is much less impaired. In addition, schizophrenia is relatively common, whereas delusional disorder is rare.

Schizophrenia

Schizophrenia is a mental disorder characterized by loss of contact with reality (psychosis), hallucinations (usually, hearing voices), delusions (false beliefs), abnormal thinking, flattened affect (restricted range of emotions), diminished motivation, and disturbed work and social functioning.

Schizophrenia is a major health problem throughout the world. The disorder typically strikes young people at the very time they are establishing their independence and can result in lifelong disability and stigma. In terms of personal and economic costs, schizophrenia has been described as among the worst disorders afflicting humankind.

Schizophrenia is listed by the World Health Organization as the ninth leading cause of disability worldwide and affects about 1% of the population, although pockets where schizophrenia is more or less common have been identified. Schizophrenia affects men and women equally. In the USA, schizophrenia accounts for about 1 of every 5 Social Security disability days and 2.5% of all health care expenditures. Schizophrenia is more common than Alzheimer's disease and multiple sclerosis.

Determining when onset occurs is often difficult because unfamiliarity with symptoms may delay medical care for several years. The average age for the onset of schizophrenia is 18 for men and 25 for women. Onset in childhood or early adolescence ■ is uncommon. Onset is also uncommon late in life.

Deterioration in social functioning can lead to substance abuse, poverty, and homelessness. People with untreated schizophrenia may lose contact with their families and friends and often find themselves living on the streets of large cities.

Causes

What precisely causes schizophrenia is not known, but current research suggests a combination of hereditary and environmental factors. Fundamentally, however, it is a biologic problem, not one caused by poor parenting or a mentally unhealthy environment. People who have a parent or sibling with schizophrenia have about a 10% risk of developing the disorder, compared with a 1% risk among the general population. An identical twin whose co-twin has schizophrenia has about a 50% risk of developing schizophrenia. These statistics suggest a hereditary risk.

Other causes may include problems that occurred before, during, or after birth, such as influenza infection during the 2nd trimester of pregnancy, oxygen deprivation at birth, low birth weight, and mother-infant blood type incompatibility.

Symptoms

The onset of schizophrenia may be sudden, over a period of days or weeks, or slow and insidious, over a period of years. Although the severity and types of symptoms vary among different people with schizophrenia, the symptoms are usually sufficiently severe as to interfere with the ability to work, interact with people, and care for oneself. In some people with schizophrenia, mental ability declines, leading to an impaired ability to pay attention, think in the abstract, and solve problems. The severity of mental impairment is a major determinant of overall disability in people with schizophrenia.

Symptoms may be triggered or worsened by environmental stresses, such as stressful life events. Drug use, including use of marijuana, may trigger or worsen symptoms as well. Overall, the symptoms of schizophrenia fall into three major groups: positive (nondeficit) symptoms, negative (deficit) symptoms, and cognitive impairment. A person may have symptoms from one, two, or all three groups.

Positive symptoms include delusions, hallucinations, thought disorder, and bizarre behavior. Delusions are false beliefs that usually involve a misinterpretation of perceptions or experiences. For example, people with schizophrenia may experience persecutory delusions, believing that they are being tormented, followed, tricked, or spied on. They may have delusions of reference, believing that passages from books, newspapers, or song lyrics are directed specifically at them. They may have delusions of thought withdrawal or thought insertion, believing that others can read their mind, that their thoughts are being transmitted to others, or that thoughts and impulses are being imposed on them by outside forces.

Hallucinations of sound, sight, smell, taste, or touch may occur, although hallucinations of sound (auditory hallucinations) are by far the most common. A person may "hear" voices commenting on his behavior, conversing with one another, or making critical and abusive comments.

Thought disorder refers to disorganized thinking, which becomes apparent when speech is rambling, shifts from one topic to another, and loses its goal-directed quality. Speech may be mildly disorganized or completely incoherent and incomprehensible. Bizarre behavior may take the form of childlike silliness, agitation, or inappropriate appearance, hygiene, or conduct. Catatonia is an extreme form of bizarre behavior in which a person maintains a rigid posture and resists efforts to be moved or, in contrast, displays purposeless and unstimulated motor activity.

Negative symptoms of schizophrenia include blunted affect, poverty of speech, anhedonia, and asociality. Blunted affect refers to a flattening of emotions. The person's face may appear immobile; he makes poor eye contact and lacks emotional expressiveness. Events that would normally make a person laugh or cry produce no response. Poverty of speech refers to a diminishment of thoughts reflected in a decreased amount of speech. Answers to questions may be terse, perhaps one or two words, creating the impression of an inner emptiness. Anhedonia refers to a diminished capacity to experience pleasure; the person may take little interest in previous activities and spend more time in purposeless ones. Asociality refers to a lack of interest in relationships with other people. These negative symptoms are often associated with a general loss of motivation, sense of purpose, and goals.

Cognitive impairment refers to difficulty in concentrating and remembering, organizing, planning, and problem solving. Some people are unable to concentrate sufficiently to read, follow the story line of a movie or television show, or follow directions. Others are unable to ignore distractions or remain focused on a task. Consequently, work that involves attention to detail, involvement in complicated procedures, and decision making may be impossible.

Types of Schizophrenia

Some researchers believe schizophrenia is a single disorder, whereas others believe it is a syndrome (a collection of symptoms) based on numerous underlying disorders. Subtypes of

Disorders That Resemble Schizophrenia

General medical and neurologic conditions such as thyroid disease, brain tumors, epilepsy, kidney failure, toxic reactions to drugs, and vitamin deficiencies can sometimes cause symptoms similar to those seen in schizophrenia. In addition, a number of mental disorders share features of schizophrenia.

- **Brief psychotic disorder:** Symptoms of this disorder resemble those of schizophrenia but last only for 1 day to 1 month. This time-limited disorder often occurs in people with a preexisting personality disorder or in people who have experienced a severe stress, such as the loss of a loved one.

- **Schizophreniform disorder:** The schizophrenia-like symptoms characteristic of this disorder last for 1 to 6 months. This disorder may resolve or may progress to manic-depressive illness or schizophrenia.

- **Schizoaffective disorder:** This disorder is characterized by the presence of mood symptoms, such as depression or mania, along with more typical symptoms of schizophrenia.

- **Schizotypal personality disorder:** This personality disorder▲ may share symptoms of schizophrenia, but they are generally not so severe as to meet the criteria for psychosis. People with this disorder tend to be shy and to isolate themselves and may show mild suspiciousness and other disturbances in thinking. Genetic studies indicate that schizotypal personality disorder may be a mild form of schizophrenia.

schizophrenia have been proposed in an effort to classify people into more distinct groups. However, among individuals, the subtype may change over time.

Paranoid schizophrenia is characterized by a preoccupation with delusions or auditory hallucinations; disorganized speech and inappropriate emotions are less prominent. Hebephrenic or disorganized schizophrenia is characterized by disorganized speech, disorganized behavior, and flat or inappropriate emotions. Catatonic schizophrenia is dominated by physical symptoms such as immobility, excessive motor activity, or the assumption of bizarre postures. Undifferentiated schizophrenia is characterized by a mixture of symptoms from the other subtypes: delusions and hallucinations, thought disorder and bizarre behavior, and negative symptoms.

Diagnosis

No definitive test exists to diagnose schizophrenia. A doctor makes the diagnosis on the basis of a comprehensive assessment of the person's history and symptoms. For a diagnosis of schizophrenia to be made, symptoms must persist for at least 6 months and be associated with significant deterioration of work, school, or social functioning. Information from family, friends, or teachers is often important in establishing when the disorder began.

Laboratory tests are often performed to rule out substance abuse or an underlying medical, neurologic, or hormonal disorder that can have features of psychosis. Examples of such disorders include brain tumors, temporal lobe epilepsy, thyroid disease, autoimmune disorders, Huntington's disease, liver disease, and side effects of drugs. Testing for drug abuse is sometimes warranted.

People with schizophrenia have brain abnormalities that may be seen on a computed tomography (CT) or magnetic resonance imaging (MRI) scan. However, the abnormalities are not specific enough to be of help in diagnosing schizophrenia.

Prognosis

Adherence to treatment is very important for people with schizophrenia. Without drug treatment, 70 to 80% of people with schizophrenia experience substantial recurrence of symptoms within the first year after diagnosis. Drugs taken continuously can reduce the relapse rate to about 20 to 30% and can lessen symptoms significantly in most people. After discharge from a hospital, a person with schizophrenia who does not take prescribed drugs is very likely to be readmitted within the year; taking drugs as directed dramatically reduces the likelihood of being readmitted.

Despite the proven benefit of drug therapy, half of people with schizophrenia do not take their prescribed drugs. Some do not recognize their illness and resist taking drugs. In other instances, unpleasant side effects lead people to decide to stop taking their drugs. Memory problems, disorganization, or simply a lack of money prevents others from taking their drugs.

Improving adherence to drug therapy is most successful when specific barriers to ad-

▲ see page 631

herence are addressed. If side effects of drugs are a major problem, a change to a different drug may help. A consistent, trusting relationship with a doctor or other therapist helps some people with schizophrenia to accept their illness more readily and recognize the need for adhering to prescribed treatment.

Over longer periods, the prognosis of schizophrenia varies. In general, one third of people achieve significant and lasting improvement, one third achieve some improvement with intermittent relapses and residual disabilities, and one third experience severe and permanent incapacity. Factors associated with a better prognosis include sudden onset of the disorder, late age at onset, a good level of skills and accomplishments before becoming ill, and having the positive (nondeficit) subtype of the disorder. Factors associated with a poor prognosis include early age of onset, poor social and vocational functioning before becoming ill, a family history of schizophrenia, and having the negative (deficit) subtype of the disorder.

About 10% of people with schizophrenia commit suicide.

Treatment

The general goals of treatment are to reduce the severity of psychotic symptoms, prevent the recurrence of symptomatic episodes and the associated deterioration in functioning, and provide support to allow functioning at the highest level possible. Antipsychotic drugs, rehabilitation and community support activities, and psychotherapy represent the three major components of treatment.

Antipsychotic Drugs: Drugs can be effective in reducing or eliminating symptoms, such as delusions, hallucinations, and disorganized thinking. After the immediate symptoms have cleared, the continued use of antipsychotic drugs substantially reduces the probability of future episodes.

Unfortunately, antipsychotic drugs have significant side effects that can include sedation, muscle stiffness, tremors, weight gain, and motor restlessness. Antipsychotic drugs may also cause tardive dyskinesia, an involuntary movement disorder most often characterized by puckering of the lips and tongue or writhing of the arms or legs. Tardive dyskinesia may not go away even after the drug is discontinued. For tardive dyskinesia that persists, there is no effective treatment. Another side effect of antipsychotic drugs, although rare but potentially fatal, is neuroleptic malig-

Antipsychotic Drugs: How Do They Work?

Antipsychotic drugs appear to be most effective in treating hallucinations, delusions, disorganized thinking, and aggression. Although antipsychotic drugs are most commonly prescribed for schizophrenia, they appear to be effective in treating these symptoms whether they arise from mania, schizophrenia, dementia, or acute intoxication with a substance such as amphetamines.

Antipsychotic drugs work by influencing how information is transmitted between individual brain cells. The adult brain is made up of more than 10 billion individual cells called neurons. Each neuron in the brain has a single long fiber called an axon, which transmits information to other neurons. Like wires connected in a vast telephone switchboard, each individual neuron makes contact with several thousand other neurons.

Information travels down a cell's axon as an electrical impulse. When the impulse reaches the end of the axon, a tiny amount of a specific chemical called a neurotransmitter is released to pass information on to the next cell down the line. A receptor on the receiving cell detects the neurotransmitter, which causes the receiving cell to generate a new signal.

Symptoms of psychosis appear to be caused by excessive activity of cells sensitive to the neurotransmitters dopamine and serotonin. Therefore, antipsychotic drugs work by blocking receptors so that communication between groups of cells is dampened.

Different antipsychotic drugs block different types of neurotransmitters. Every effective antipsychotic drug known blocks dopamine receptors. The new antipsychotic drugs (risperidone, olanzapine, quetiapine, ziprasidone, and clozapine) may be more effective because they also block serotonin receptors. They also appear to cause fewer side effects.

nant syndrome, which is characterized by muscle rigidity, fever, high blood pressure, and changes in mental function (for example, confusion and lethargy).

A number of new antipsychotic drugs that cause fewer side effects have become available. These drugs may relieve positive symptoms (such as hallucinations), negative symptoms (such as lack of emotion), and cognitive

What Is Neuroleptic Malignant Syndrome?

Neuroleptic malignant syndrome is a state of unresponsiveness caused by use of certain antipsychotic drugs. It develops in up to 3% of people who are treated with antipsychotic drugs, usually within the first few weeks of treatment. The syndrome is most common among men who, because they are agitated, are given rapidly increased doses of the drugs or high doses initially.

Symptoms include muscle rigidity, a high temperature, a fast heart rate, a fast breathing rate, high blood pressure, and coma. Damaged muscles release the protein myoglobin, which is excreted in the urine. Myoglobin turns the urine brown (myoglobinuria), and myoglobinuria can result in kidney damage or even kidney failure.

People with this syndrome are usually treated in an intensive care unit. The antipsychotic drug is discontinued, fever is controlled (usually with ice baths and wet towels or with special cooling blankets), and a muscle relaxant (such as bromocriptine or dantrolene) is given. Giving sodium bicarbonate intravenously helps prevent myoglobulinuria by making the urine alkaline. Most people recover completely; however, almost 30% of people with this syndrome die. After recovery, up to 30% of people develop the syndrome again if they are given the same antipsychotic drug.

impairment (such as reduced mental functioning and attention span) to a greater extent than the older antipsychotic drugs.

Clozapine has proven to be effective in up to half of the people for whom other drugs do not work. However, clozapine can cause serious side effects, such as seizures or potentially fatal bone marrow suppression; thus, it is generally used only for people who have not responded to other antipsychotic drugs. People who take clozapine must have their white blood cell count measured weekly, at least for the first 6 months, so that clozapine can be discontinued at the first indication that the number of white blood cells is dropping.

Rehabilitation and Community Support Activities: Community support activities, such as on-the-job coaching, are directed at teaching the skills needed to survive in the community. These skills enable a person with schizophrenia to work, shop, care for himself,

manage a household, and get along with others. Although hospitalization may be needed during severe relapses, and involuntary hospitalization may be needed if the person poses a danger to himself or others, the general goal is to have the person live in the community. To achieve this goal, some people may need to live in a supervised apartment or group home where someone can ensure that drugs are taken as prescribed.

A small number of people with schizophrenia are unable to live independently, either because they have severe and unresponsive symptoms or because they lack the skills necessary to live in the community. They usually require full-time care in a safe and supportive setting.

Psychotherapy: Generally, the goal of psychotherapy is to establish a collaborative relationship between the person, family, and doctor. That way the person might learn to understand and manage his disorder, to take antipsychotic drugs as prescribed, and to manage stresses that can aggravate the disorder. A good doctor-patient relationship is often a major determinant of successful treatment. Psychotherapy reduces symptoms in some cases and helps prevent relapse in others.

Delusional Disorder

Delusional disorder is characterized by one or more false beliefs that persist for at least 1 month.

Delusional disorder generally first affects people in middle or late adult life. Delusions tend to be nonbizarre and involve situations that could conceivably occur in real life, such as being followed, poisoned, infected, loved at a distance, or deceived by a spouse or lover. Several subtypes of delusional disorder are recognized.

In the erotomanic subtype, the central theme of the delusion is that another person is in love with the individual. Efforts to contact the object of the delusion through telephone calls, letters, or even surveillance and stalking may be common. Behavior related to the delusion may come in conflict with the law.

In the grandiose subtype, the person is convinced that he has some great talent or has made some important discovery.

In the jealous subtype, the person is convinced that a spouse or lover is unfaithful. This belief is based on incorrect inferences supported by dubious "evidence." Under such

℞ ANTIPSYCHOTIC DRUGS

TYPE	DRUG	SELECTED SIDE EFFECTS	COMMENTS
Older antipsychotics	Chlorpromazine Fluphenazine Haloperidol Loxapine Mesoridazine Molindone Perphenazine Pimozide Thioridazine Thiothixene Trifluoperazine	Dry mouth, blurred vision, seizures, increased heart rate, decreased blood pressure, constipation, sudden but often reversible tremor and muscle stiffness that may progress to rigidity, uncontrolled movements of the face and arms (tardive dyskinesia), fever and muscle damage (neuroleptic malignant syndrome)	Side effects are much more likely in older people and in people with impaired balance or serious medical disorders. Long-acting injectable forms of haloperidol and perphenazine are available Eye examination and electrocardiography (ECG) are recommended while taking thioridazine
Newer antipsychotics	Aripiprazole Clozapine Olanzapine Quetiapine Risperidone Ziprasidone	Drowsiness and weight gain, which can be substantial, are the most common side effects. May increase the risk of new-onset type II diabetes and high levels of triglycerides in the blood. Muscle tremor, uncontrolled movements of the face and arms (tardive dyskinesia), and muscle damage possible but occur less often compared to older antipsychotics.	Newer antipsychotics are less likely to cause tremor, muscle stiffness, uncontrolled movements, and fever and muscle damage Clozapine is used much less often because it can cause bone marrow suppression, reduced white blood cell count, and seizures. However, it is often effective in people who are not responsive to other drugs Clozapine and olanzapine are most likely to cause weight gain; aripiprazole is the least likely Ziprasidone does not cause weight gain but may lead to abnormalities on electrocardiogram

circumstances, physical assault may be a significant danger.

In the persecutory subtype, the person believes that he is being plotted against, spied on, maligned, or harassed. The person may repeatedly attempt to obtain justice by appealing to courts and other government agencies. Rarely, violence may be resorted to in retaliation for imagined persecution.

In the somatic subtype, the person is preoccupied with a bodily function or attribute, such as an imagined physical deformity or odor. The delusion can also take the form of an imagined general medical condition, such as a parasitic infection.

Symptoms and Diagnosis

A delusional disorder may arise from a pre-existing paranoid personality disorder.▲ Begin-ning in early adulthood, people with a paranoid personality disorder demonstrate a pervasive distrust and suspiciousness of others and their motives. Early symptoms may include feeling exploited, being preoccupied with the loyalty or trustworthiness of friends, reading threatening meanings into benign remarks or events, bearing grudges for a long time, and responding readily to perceived slights.

After ruling out other specific conditions that are associated with delusions, a doctor bases the diagnosis of delusional disorder largely on the person's history. It is particularly important for the doctor to assess the degree of dangerousness, particularly the extent to which the person is willing to act on his delusions.

▲ see page 631

Prognosis and Treatment

Delusional disorder does not generally lead to severe impairment. However, the person may become progressively involved with the delusion. Most people are able to remain employed.

A good doctor-patient relationship helps in the treatment of delusional disorder. Hospitalization may be needed if the doctor believes the person is dangerous. Antipsychotic drugs are not generally used but are sometimes effective in suppressing symptoms. A long-term treatment goal is to shift the person's focus away from the delusion to a more constructive and gratifying area, although this goal is frequently difficult to achieve.

CHAPTER 108

Drug Use and Abuse

Drugs are an integral part of everyday life for many people, and drug use among adolescents remains high.▲ The legality and social acceptance of a particular drug often depend on what it is used for, what its effects are, and who is using it. For example, use of marijuana for pleasure is illegal and considered socially unacceptable by many people, but use of marijuana to relieve nausea in a person with advanced cancer has been legalized by some governments and is viewed as acceptable by some people. The legality and social acceptance of a drug often vary among different societies or countries. Legality and acceptance may also change within a society or country over time, as has happened with alcohol in the United States.

Many drugs, some legal and some not, alter the mind. Some mind-altering drugs affect brain function each time they are used, regardless of how much is used. Other mind-altering drugs affect brain function only if a large amount is used or if it is used continually. Some drugs affect the brain in such a way that a person wants or feels a need to use the drug again and again (craving).

Doctors may suspect problems created by the use of mind-altering drugs when they notice changes in mood or behavior. Specific questions may then be asked about potential consequences of prolonged use of specific drugs. Blood and urine tests are sometimes used to confirm suspicions that a person has been taking certain mind-altering drugs.

The problems created by use of mind-altering drugs are given many different terms, for example, drug abuse, drug dependence, and drug addiction. Doctors and other experts, in treating these problems, often disagree about the exact meaning of these terms.

Drug Abuse: Drug abuse is the use of a mind-altering drug without medical need, in an amount large enough or over a period long enough to threaten the quality of life or health and safety of the user or others. Many people use drugs without medical need but keep that use under control so that it does not threaten their health or adversely affect their functioning.

Taking a drug that does not usually alter the mind is still considered abusive if the drug is taken without medical need and if the drug endangers the quality of life or health and safety of the user or others. Drug abuse occurs in all socioeconomic groups and involves highly educated and professional people as well as those who are uneducated and unemployed.

Overdose of a drug may occur as part of abuse. With some drugs, an overdose may be profoundly frightening or even fatal.

Drug Dependence: Drug dependence is a compelling need to continue taking a mind-altering drug to induce pleasure or to relieve anxiety and tension and avoid discomfort. Drug dependence is caused by a combination of biologic and psychologic factors. Drugs that cause dependence may produce euphoria, feelings of increased mental and physical ability, and altered sense perceptions.

Dependence can be very powerful and difficult to overcome. The body adapts to the continuous use of a drug that produces depen-

▲ see page 1559

dence, leading to tolerance and to withdrawal symptoms when use stops. Tolerance is the need to use progressively larger amounts of a drug to reproduce the effects originally achieved with the starting amount.

Withdrawal symptoms occur when drug use is stopped or when the drug's effects are blocked by another drug. A person undergoing withdrawal feels sick and may develop headaches, diarrhea, or shaking (tremors). Withdrawal can evoke a serious and even life-threatening illness.

Drug Addiction: Drug addiction is the disruptive behavior or activity associated with obtaining and using a drug that a person is dependent on. Addiction generally interferes with the ability to work, study, or interact normally with family and friends. A person can become dependent on illegal drugs or legal ones and can become dependent when a drug is used for a medical need or for less acceptable reasons. However, the behavior or activity associated with obtaining and using a drug is likely to vary tremendously based on the legality and acceptance of that drug. Obtaining a legal drug to meet a medical need is often as unremarkable as going to the doctor, getting a prescription, and then going to the pharmacy. However, for an illegal drug or a legal drug used without medical need and for unacceptable reasons, the behavior or activity may include lying and stealing.

When a person with advanced cancer becomes dependent on an opioid drug such as morphine, his behavior is not usually considered an addiction. However, when a person dependent on, for example, heroin steals to have money to buy heroin and lies to family and friends about his whereabouts or what he is doing, his behavior is considered an addiction.

At times, family members or friends may behave in ways that allow an addict to continue to use drugs or alcohol; these people are called enablers (also referred to as codependents when their own needs are intertwined with perpetuating the addict's use of his addictive substance). Enablers may call in sick for an addict or make excuses for the addict's behavior. The enabler may plead with the addict to stop using drugs or alcohol but rarely does anything else to help the addict change his behavior.

A pregnant addict exposes her fetus to the drugs she is using. Often, a pregnant addict does not admit to her doctor that she is using drugs or alcohol. The fetus may become dependent and may develop serious defects as a result of the mother's drug use.▲ Soon after delivery, the newborn can experience severe or even fatal withdrawal, particularly when the doctor has not been informed of the mother's addiction.

Alcohol

Nearly 8% of adults in the United States have some problem with alcohol use. Alcoholism is the most extreme alcohol use disorder. It is characterized by excessive drinking, unsuccessful attempts at stopping drinking, and continued drinking despite adverse social and occupational consequences. Men are 4 times more likely than women to become alcoholics.

Of the people who drink alcohol, about 10% become alcoholics. People who become alcoholics have been regularly using alcohol in excessive amounts over a prolonged period of time and are dependent on alcohol. The amount of drinking that takes place on an average day before a person becomes an alcoholic varies widely, but it may be as little as two drinks per day for women and three drinks for men (one drink is equivalent to 12 ounces of beer, 5 ounces of wine, or 1½ ounces of liquor, such as whiskey). Many alcoholics are also binge drinkers, meaning that they may drink five or more drinks on many days and little or none on a few days.

People of all ages are susceptible to alcoholism and other alcohol use disorders. Blood relatives of alcoholics have a higher rate of alcohol use disorders than do people at random, and alcohol use disorders are more likely to develop in biologic children of alcoholics than in adopted children. Increasingly, adolescents have alcohol problems, with especially disastrous consequences.■ Older adults develop higher alcohol levels in the blood per amount of alcohol consumed compared with younger adults. This tendency is primarily due to a decrease in muscle tissue and an increase in fat tissue that occurs in most people as they age.

Alcoholism leads to many destructive behaviors. Drunkenness may disrupt family and social relationships; married couples often divorce. Extreme absenteeism from work can lead to unemployment. Alcoholics often cannot control their behavior, tend to drive while drunk, and suffer physical injury from falls, fights, or motor vehicle accidents. Some alco-

Other Drugs of Abuse

Although mind-altering drugs typically are those that have potential for abuse, several other drugs that do not alter the mind (or do so only occasionally) are often taken without medical need, even when doing so endangers the quality of life or health and safety of the user. Using a drug this way is considered drug abuse.

People who stop abusing any of these drugs do not experience withdrawal symptoms, but they may experience medical problems when the drug is discontinued abruptly (problems that are usually preventable if discontinuation is supervised by a doctor).

Anabolic Steroids

Anabolic steroids are very similar to the hormone testosterone. Anabolic steroids have many physical effects on the body, including muscle growth and increased strength as well as increased energy level. Thus, anabolic steroids are often abused to gain a competitive edge in sports. Users are often athletes, typically football players, wrestlers, or weight lifters, and almost all users are male.

Many side effects are associated with the abuse of anabolic steroids. Very high doses of anabolic steroids may cause erratic mood swings, irrational behavior, and increased aggressiveness (often called steroid rage). Anabolic steroids can damage the liver and cause jaundice. Regular use of any amount also tends to increase body hair. Acne commonly gets worse with anabolic steroid use and is one of the few side effects for which an adolescent may visit a doctor. Laboratory tests can measure anabolic steroid breakdown products in the urine.

Growth Hormone

Growth hormone is produced by the brain to help the body control how protein, carbohydrates, and fats are used to stimulate growth. Growth hormone is also manufactured as a drug and is sometimes given to children of small stature because their body is unable to make enough growth hormone. Some athletes abuse growth hormone because they believe it will increase their muscle growth and strength while decreasing their body fat.

Use of growth hormone without medical need over a long period can cause an increase in fat levels in the blood, diabetes, and an increase in heart size that may result in heart failure. Laboratory tests to measure growth hormone not made by a person's body are not routinely available.

Erythropoietin and Darbepoietin

Erythropoietin is a hormone produced by the kidney that stimulates the bone marrow to produce red blood cells. Erythropoietin is also manufactured as a drug and is routinely given to many people with anemia resulting from kidney failure as well as to people with certain other types of anemia. Darbepoietin is a drug similar to erythropoietin that is also used for people with certain kinds of anemia. Some athletes abuse these drugs because they believe that with more red blood cells more oxygen will get to their muscles, enabling them to perform better.

Erythropoietin or darbepoietin use without medical need may change the body's regulation of red blood cell production, so that the number of red blood cells suddenly decreases when erythropoietin or darbepoietin use is discontinued. Laboratory tests to measure erythropoietin not made by a person's body are not routinely available.

Diuretics

Diuretics are drugs that speed elimination of salt and water by the kidneys. Diuretics are used to treat a variety of diseases, including heart failure and high blood pressure. However, some people, including athletes and people with eating disorders such as anorexia nervosa, abuse diuretics to help them lose weight quickly. Inappropriate use of diuretics may cause dehydration and severe deficiencies of electrolytes such as potassium.

Ipecac Syrup

Ipecac syrup is a drug that triggers vomiting. It is used to treat children who have swallowed chemicals or poisons. However, people with eating disorders such as anorexia nervosa often abuse ipecac syrup to help them lose weight. Inappropriate use of ipecac may cause diarrhea, severe deficiencies of electrolytes, weakness, irregular heart rhythms, and heart failure.

Laxatives

Laxatives are drugs that promote bowel movements and are used to treat constipation. However, people who falsely believe they must have frequent bowel movements as part of being healthy often abuse laxatives. In addition, people with eating disorders such as anorexia nervosa sometimes abuse laxatives because they believe doing so will help them lose weight.

Laxatives used often and without medical need may cause dehydration and severe deficiencies of electrolytes. Regular use of laxatives can also interfere with absorption of other drugs, causing them to stop working. Inappropriate use of laxatives over a long period can damage the muscle layers of the large intestine, which can lead to severe constipation.

holics become violent. Alcoholism in men is often associated with domestic violence against women.▲

Other alcohol use disorders may fall just short of the definition of alcoholism. A person can have a significant problem with alcohol use but be able to fulfill work and family responsibilities. However, the excessive alcohol use involved in these alcohol use disorders still exacts a terrible toll on the person's body, leading to many physical and mental health problems.

Causes

Alcohol use disorders involve heredity to some extent. Some research suggests that people at risk of alcoholism are less easily intoxicated than nonalcoholics; that is, their brains are less sensitive to the effects of alcohol.

Aside from a possible hereditary risk, certain background and personality traits may predispose a person to alcohol use disorders. Alcoholics frequently come from broken homes, and relationships with their parents are often disturbed. Alcoholics tend to feel isolated, lonely, shy, depressed, or hostile. They may exhibit self-destructive behavior and may be sexually immature. Whether such traits are the cause of alcoholism or the result is not certain.

Symptoms and Complications

Because alcohol is absorbed faster than it is processed (metabolized) and eliminated from the body, alcohol levels in the blood rise rapidly. Effects can occur within a few minutes of drinking.

Small amounts (for example, ½ to 1½ ounces of pure alcohol, or one to three drinks—resulting in a blood level of about 0.05 grams per deciliter, or 0.05%) can act as a stimulant, often making the person giddy and talkative, and perhaps even boisterous and violent. Larger amounts (usually resulting in blood levels above 0.08 grams per deciliter or 0.08%) depress brain function, resulting in slowed, impaired movements, unsteadiness, and sleepiness. As the alcohol is slowly metabolized, the process may reverse, such that a sedated person once again becomes agitated and violent. Very large amounts (resulting in blood levels above 0.30 grams per deciliter, or 0.3%) can lead to coma and death.

Prolonged use of excessive amounts of alcohol damages many organs of the body, particularly the liver, brain, and heart. Like many other drugs, alcohol tends to induce tolerance, so that people who regularly have more than two drinks a day can drink more alcohol than nondrinkers without becoming intoxicated. People who drink excessively over longer periods also can become tolerant to other drugs that depress brain function, such as barbiturates or benzodiazepines.

If an alcoholic who has been drinking continually for a period of time suddenly stops drinking, withdrawal symptoms are likely. Alcohol withdrawal usually begins 12 to 48 hours after drinking stops. Mild symptoms include tremor, weakness, sweating, and nausea. Some people develop seizures (called alcoholic epilepsy or rum fits). Heavy drinkers who stop drinking may develop alcoholic hallucinosis, in which they hear voices that seem accusatory and threatening, causing apprehension and terror. Alcoholic hallucinosis may last for days and can be controlled with antipsychotic drugs, such as chlorpromazine or thioridazine.

Delirium tremens (DTs), a very serious set of symptoms, may result if alcohol withdrawal is left untreated. Delirium tremens usually does not begin immediately; rather, it appears about 2 to 10 days after the drinking stops. In delirium tremens, the person is initially anxious and later develops increasing confusion, sleeplessness, nightmares, excessive sweating, and profound depression. The pulse rate tends to speed up. Fever typically develops. The episode may escalate to include fleeting hallucinations, illusions that arouse fear and restlessness, and disorientation with visual hallucinations that may incite terror. Objects seen in dim light may be particularly terrifying, and the person becomes extremely confused. The floor may seem to move, the walls fall, or the room rotates. As the delirium progresses, the hands develop a persistent tremor that sometimes extends to the head and body, and most people become severely uncoordinated. Delirium tremens can be fatal, particularly when untreated.

Other problems are directly related to the toxic effects of alcohol on the brain and liver. Prolonged use of excessive amounts of alcohol can lead to alcoholic liver disease.■ An alcohol-damaged liver is less able to rid the body of toxic substances, which can cause hepatic coma. A person developing hepatic coma becomes dull, sleepy, stuporous, and confused and usually develops an odd flapping tremor of

▲ see page 1410   ■ see box on page 799

EFFECTS OF PROLONGED ALCOHOL USE

Type of Deficit	Effects
Nutritional	
Low folic acid levels	Anemia (fatigue, weakness, light-headedness), birth defects
Low iron levels	Anemia
Low niacin levels	Pellagra (skin damage, diarrhea, depression)
Gastrointestinal	
Esophagus	Inflammation (esophagitis), cancer
Stomach	Inflammation (gastritis), ulcers
Liver	Inflammation (hepatitis), severe scarring (cirrhosis), fatty liver, cancer
Pancreas	Inflammation (pancreatitis), low blood sugar levels, cancer
Cardiovascular	
Heart	Abnormal heartbeat (arrhythmia), heart failure
Blood vessels	High blood pressure, atherosclerosis, stroke
Neurologic	
Brain	Confusion, reduced coordination, poor short-term memory (poor recall of recent events), psychosis (loss of contact with reality)
Nerves	Deterioration of nerves in arms and legs that control movements (reduced ability to walk)
Genitourinary	Decreased sex drive

the hands. Hepatic coma is life threatening and needs to be treated immediately.

Korsakoff's syndrome (Korsakoff's amnesic psychosis) usually occurs in people who regularly drink large amounts of alcohol, especially those who are malnourished and have a deficiency of B vitamins (particularly thiamin).▲ A person with Korsakoff's syndrome loses memory for recent events. Memory is so poor that a person often makes up stories to try to cover up the inability to remember (con-

fabulation). Korsakoff's syndrome sometimes follows a bout of delirium tremens. Korsakoff's syndrome can be fatal unless the thiamin deficiency is treated promptly. Some people with Korsakoff's syndrome also develop Wernicke's encephalopathy, which is due to a thiamin deficiency often resulting from prolonged heavy drinking. Symptoms occur suddenly and include abnormal eye movements, confusion, uncoordinated movements, and a decreased ability to sense pain.

Alcohol use disorders can lead to the development of a chronic tremor. Alcohol can damage the part of the brain that coordinates movement (cerebellum), leading to poorly controlled movement of the arms and legs (cerebellar degeneration). It can also damage the lining (myelin sheath) of nerves in the brain, resulting in a rare disorder called Marchiafava-Bignami disease. People with this disorder become agitated, confused, and demented. Some develop seizures and go into a coma before dying.

Drinking alcohol may worsen existing depression, and alcoholics have a higher likelihood of becoming depressed than do nonalcoholics. Because alcoholism, especially binge drinking, often causes deep feelings of remorse during dry periods, alcoholics are suicide-prone even when they are not drinking.

In a pregnant woman, alcohol use can cause severe birth defects in the developing fetus, including low birth weight, short body length, small head size, heart damage, muscle damage, and low intelligence or mental retardation.■ Avoidance of alcohol is therefore recommended during pregnancy.

Screening and Diagnosis

Doctors may suspect an alcohol use disorder in a person with an unexplained change in behavior, or when behavior becomes self-destructive. Doctors may also suspect an alcohol use disorder when medical problems, such as high blood pressure or stomach inflammation (gastritis), do not respond to usual treatment.

Some doctors periodically screen their patients for alcohol-related problems by asking about their use of alcohol. Questions that the doctor might ask include:

• On average, how many days per week do you drink alcohol?

• On a typical day when you drink, how many drinks do you have?

• What is the maximum number of drinks you had on any given occasion in the past month?

▲ see also page 479   ■ see page 1511

Doctors may ask more specific questions about consequences of drinking of people they suspect may be alcoholics. Questions may include:

- Have you ever felt you should cut down on your drinking?
- Does criticism of your drinking annoy you?
- Have you ever felt guilty about drinking?
- Have you ever had an "eye opener" (a drink first thing in the morning) to steady your nerves or to get rid of a hangover?

Two or more "yes" answers to these questions indicate a probable diagnosis of alcoholism.

Measuring the amount of alcohol in the blood may help the doctor confirm suspicions that a person has an alcohol use disorder, especially if the person's breath smells of alcohol. Alcohol levels can be measured in the blood or estimated by measuring the amount in a sample of exhaled breath.

Treatment

Emergency Treatment: Emergency treatment may occur when a person comes for medical care for intolerable withdrawal symptoms. Alternatively, a person may be brought in for care because of symptoms related to high alcohol levels. Alcoholics who develop withdrawal symptoms generally treat themselves by drinking. Some people seek medical attention because they do not want to continue drinking or because withdrawal symptoms are too severe. Because vitamin deficiency causes potentially life-threatening symptoms, doctors in emergency departments generally give large intravenous doses of vitamin C and B complex vitamins, especially thiamin. Intravenous fluids, magnesium, and glucose are often given to prevent some of the symptoms of alcohol withdrawal and to avoid dehydration.

Often, doctors prescribe a benzodiazepine drug for a few days to calm agitation and help prevent withdrawal symptoms. Antipsychotic drugs are sometimes given to people with alcoholic hallucinosis. Delirium tremens can be life threatening and is treated more aggressively to control the high fever and severe agitation. Intravenous fluids, drugs that lower fever (such as acetaminophen), sedatives, and close supervision usually are needed. With such treatment, delirium tremens generally begins to clear within 12 to 24 hours of onset.

Detoxification and Rehabilitation: After the urgent medical problems are resolved, a detox-

Alcoholics Anonymous: A Path to Recovery

No approach has benefited so many alcoholics as effectively as the help they can offer themselves by participating in Alcoholics Anonymous (AA). AA is an international fellowship of people who want to stop drinking. There are no dues or fees. The program operates on the basis of the "Twelve Steps," which offers the alcoholic a new way of living without alcohol. Members of the fellowship typically work with a sponsor—a fellow member who is abstaining from alcohol use—who offers guidance and support. AA operates within a spiritual context but is not affiliated with any ideology or religious doctrine; however, alternative organizations, such as LifeRing Recovery (Secular Organizations for Sobriety), exist for those seeking a more secular approach.

AA helps its members in other ways as well. It provides a place where the recovering alcoholic can socialize away from the tavern with nondrinking friends who are always available for support when the urge to start drinking again becomes strong. In meetings, the alcoholic hears other people relate—to the entire group—how they are struggling every day to avoid taking a drink. Finally, by providing a means to help others, AA builds self-esteem and confidence formerly found only in drinking alcohol.

Most metropolitan areas have many AA meetings available day and night, 7 days a week. An alcoholic is encouraged to try several different meetings and to attend those at which he feels most comfortable.

ification and rehabilitation program should be started. In the first phase of treatment, alcohol is completely withdrawn. Then an alcoholic has to modify his behavior. Without help, most alcoholics relapse within a few days or weeks. Treatment should be tailored to the individual. Enlisting the support of family members may be important as well.

Sometimes the prescription drug disulfiram can help an alcoholic avoid drinking alcohol. This drug interferes with alcohol metabolism for 3 to 7 days, causing acetaldehyde, a substance that results from the breakdown of alcohol, to build up in the bloodstream. Acetaldehyde produces facial flushing, a throbbing headache, a rapid heart rate, rapid breathing, and sweating within 5 to 15 minutes after the person drinks alcohol. Nausea and vomiting may follow 30 to 60 minutes later. These uncomfortable and potentially dangerous reactions last 1 to 3 hours. The discomfort from drinking alcohol after taking disulfiram is so intense that few people risk taking alcohol—even the small amount in some over-the-counter cough and cold preparations or some foods.

Disulfiram is given only as part of an ongoing intensive counseling regimen. Pregnant women, people who have a serious illness, and older people should not use disulfiram. Naltrexone can help people become less dependent on alcohol if it is used as part of a comprehensive treatment program that includes counseling. Naltrexone alters the effects of alcohol on certain chemicals made by the brain (endorphins), which may be associated with alcohol craving and consumption. A big advantage compared with disulfiram is that naltrexone does not make people sick. However, a person taking naltrexone can continue to drink. Naltrexone should not be taken by people who have hepatitis or certain other liver diseases.

Opioids

Opioids have a legitimate medical use as powerful pain relievers.▲ They include codeine (which has a low dependence potential), oxycodone (alone and in various combinations, such as oxycodone plus acetaminophen), meperidine, morphine, pentazocine, and hydromorphone. Heroin, which is illegal in the United States but is used in very limited treatment applications in other countries, is one of the strongest opioids. A person can become dependent on any opioid.

Some people become dependent on opioids after starting their use for appropriate medically prescribed control of pain. Although many people who use opioids for pain relief for more than several days feel some symptoms of withdrawal when they stop, serious dependence and addiction rarely occur when opioid use is medically supervised.

Tolerance can develop after 2 to 3 days of continued opioid use. People who have developed tolerance may show few signs of drug use and function normally in their usual activities as long as they have access to drugs.

Symptoms and Complications

Opioids have many effects. They are strong sedating drugs and cause people to become quiet and introspective. Opioids may also produce euphoria, sometimes simply because severe pain has finally been relieved. They dull pain and may enhance sexual pleasure. They also cause constipation; flushed or warm skin and lowered blood pressure; itching; constricted pupils; slow, shallow breathing; a slow heart rate; and low body temperature. Opioids may cause confusion, especially in older people.

Many complications can arise from opioid addiction, especially if the drugs are injected with shared unsterilized needles. For example, viral hepatitis, which causes liver damage, can be spread through shared needles. Infections can occur at the site of injection or be carried through the bloodstream (sepsis), causing infections in the brain and bones.

Drug abuser's elbow (myositis ossificans) is caused by repeated, inept needle punctures; the muscle around the elbow is replaced with scar tissue. Subcutaneous injections (skin popping) can cause skin sores. Intravenous injections lead to scarring of veins (tracks), which makes the veins more and more difficult to inject.

Opioid addicts can develop lung problems, such as lung irritations from aspiration (inhaling saliva or vomit), pneumonia, abscesses, pulmonary emboli, and scarring, which can develop from the talc in impure injections. Problems with the immune system can develop. Because the human immunodeficiency virus (HIV) can spread through shared needles, many people who inject opioids also develop AIDS. Needle sharing is now becoming the principal route of HIV infection in the United States.

Opioid addicts can develop neurologic problems, usually as the result of inadequate blood flow to the brain. Coma may result. Quinine, a common heroin contaminant, can cause double vision, paralysis, and other nerve injury symptoms, including Guillain-Barré syndrome.■ A contaminant sometimes present in homemade meperidine (MPTP) damages the brain and leads to severe parkinsonism.★

Drug overdose presents a serious threat to life. Opioids suppress breathing and can cause the lungs to fill with fluid.

Opioid use during pregnancy is especially serious. Heroin and methadone easily cross the placenta into the fetus. A baby born to an addicted mother may quickly develop withdrawal symptoms, including tremors, high-

▲ see page 450   ■ see page 585

★ see page 547

pitched crying, jitters, seizures, and rapid breathing.▲

Withdrawal symptoms can appear as early as 4 to 6 hours after the opioid use stops and generally peak within 36 to 72 hours. However, each opioid is eliminated from the body at a different rate, which alters the rate at which withdrawal occurs. The withdrawal symptoms are worse in people who have used large doses for longer times.

The first sign of withdrawal is generally rapid breathing, usually accompanied by yawning, perspiration, crying, and a runny nose. Other signs include hyperactivity, a sense of heightened alertness, rapid breathing, agitation, an increased heart rate, fever, dilated pupils, gooseflesh, tremors, muscle twitching, hot and cold flashes, aching muscles, loss of appetite, abdominal cramps, and diarrhea.

Treatment

Emergency Treatment: An opioid overdose is a medical emergency that must be treated quickly to prevent death. Breathing may require support, sometimes with a ventilator, if the overdose has suppressed breathing. A drug called naloxone is given intravenously as an antidote to the opioid.

Detoxification and Rehabilitation: Treatment is usually needed to lessen the symptoms of withdrawal. Symptoms of opioid withdrawal can also be relieved with a drug called clonidine. However, clonidine may cause some side effects, including low blood pressure, drowsiness, restlessness, insomnia, irritability, faster heartbeat, and headaches. Substituting methadone for the opioid provides another treatment for withdrawal. Methadone, itself an opioid, is taken by mouth and alters brain function less than do other opioids. Because methadone's effects last much longer than those of other opioids, it can be taken less frequently, usually once a day. The dose can then be decreased slowly.

Methadone may also be part of a long-term maintenance treatment program. Maintaining addicts with regular doses of methadone for months or years will enable them to be socially productive because their supply problems are met. For some, the treatment works. Others may not become socially rehabilitated. For many addicts, lifelong methadone maintenance is necessary. Opioid addicts must appear every day at a clinic, where methadone is dispensed in the smallest amount that prevents severe withdrawal symptoms from developing.

A few treatment centers may dispense l-alpha-acetylmethadol (LAAM), a longer-acting form of methadone. This eliminates the need to make daily clinic visits or to take drugs home. Buprenorphine, another maintenance drug, can be prescribed by doctors in their offices. This allows for treatment similar to methadone detoxification or maintenance without having to go to a methadone clinic.

Naltrexone is a drug that blocks the effects of opioids. Depending on the dose, naltrexone's effects last from 24 to 72 hours. Because of this, an addict who has a stable social background can take this drug daily (or possibly as few as 3 times a week) to avoid the temptation of using opioids.

The therapeutic community concept emerged nearly 25 years ago in response to the problems of heroin addiction. Daytop Village and Phoenix House pioneered this nondrug approach. Treatment involves a communal, relatively long-term (usually 15- to 18-month) stay in a residential setting to help addicts build new lives through training, education, and redirection. These programs have helped many people, but questions about precisely how well they have worked and how widely they should be applied remain unanswered.

The AIDS epidemic has motivated some people to suggest that sterile needles and syringes be provided to addicts who inject opioids intravenously. Such distribution has been shown to reduce HIV transmission.

Antianxiety Drugs and Sedatives

Prescription drugs used to treat anxiety (antianxiety drugs) and induce sleep (sedatives or sleep aids) can cause dependence. Such drugs include benzodiazepines, barbiturates, glutethimide, chloral hydrate, and meprobamate. Each works in a different way, and each has a different dependency and tolerance potential. Most people dependent on antianxiety drugs and sedatives started out taking them for a medical reason. Dependency can develop within as little as 2 weeks of continual use.

Symptoms and Complications

Antianxiety drugs and sedatives decrease alertness and can result in slurred speech, poor coordination, confusion, and slowed breathing. These drugs may make a person alternately depressed and anxious. Some people

▲ see page 1464

Classifying the Abuse Potential of Prescription Drugs

Prescription drugs that can cause dependency are subject to restrictions dictated by United States government regulations. All prescription drugs regulated under the Controlled Substances Act are assigned a schedule or class number that determines how they may be prescribed. Schedule I drugs are considered to have a high abuse potential, no accepted medical use, and no acceptable safety data. Schedule II drugs have a high abuse potential but have some appropriate medical uses. Schedule III drugs have less abuse potential; schedule IV and V drugs have the least abuse potential.

experience memory loss, faulty judgment, a shortened attention span, and frightening shifts in their emotions. Older people may appear demented, speaking slowly and have difficulty in thinking and in understanding others. Falls may occur that result in broken bones, especially hip fractures.

People who have used sedatives for more than a few days often feel that they cannot sleep without them. They may become anxious and nervous at bedtime without the drugs and may awaken irritable.

Abrupt withdrawal from antianxiety drugs and sedatives can produce a severe, frightening, and potentially life-threatening reaction, much like alcohol withdrawal (delirium tremens▲). The time course of withdrawal reactions varies from drug to drug. Within the first 12 to 24 hours, the person may become nervous, restless, tremulous, and weak. Seizures may occur in those taking high doses. Occasionally, a seizure may occur even 1 to 3 weeks after withdrawal.

Other effects that can occur during withdrawal include dehydration, delirium, insomnia, confusion, and visual and auditory hallucinations (seeing and hearing things that are not there). Serious withdrawal reactions are more common with barbiturates or glutethimide than with benzodiazepines. The person is usually hospitalized during the withdrawal process because of the possibility of a severe reaction.

▲ see page 649

Treatment

Emergency Treatment: A person who has overdosed on antianxiety drugs or sedatives requires hospitalization, usually in the intensive care unit. Benzodiazepines do have an antidote—flumazenil. Supportive care is given; which may include intravenous administration of fluids, drugs if blood pressure drops, and a ventilator.

Detoxification and Rehabilitation: People with mild withdrawal symptoms require social and psychologic support to help them overcome a strong urge to begin using the drug again to stop the feelings of anxiety. People with severe withdrawal symptoms usually need to begin taking the drug again at a lower dose and under close medical supervision, sometimes in the hospital. The dose is decreased gradually over days or weeks and then discontinued. Even with the best treatment, a person may not feel normal for a month or more.

Nicotine

Nicotine is the substance in cigarettes that smokers become dependent on. Thus, nicotine dependence is essentially dependence on cigarettes. About 70% of smokers have acknowledged that they desire to quit smoking but are unable to do so. Of people who quit, 90% do so on their own, but only about 3 to 4% successfully quit in any given year.

Symptoms and Complications

Nicotine, when obtained through smoking, generally produces few noticeable effects. Some people experience flushing. Nicotine withdrawal may result in many unpleasant symptoms, including craving for nicotine, irritability, anxiety, poor concentration, restlessness, headaches, drowsiness, and stomach upset. Many people gain weight while trying to stop smoking. Withdrawal is most troublesome in severely dependent people.

Treatment

Most smokers who quit do so for health or economic reasons. Behavior modification is a common method used in helping people to quit smoking. A behavior modification regimen may be established with the help of a professional, although other sources include the Internet and the package inserts in nicotine replacement products. Behavior modification deals with changing the habit patterns that are cues to smoking during the person's normal activities of daily living. These cues may be phone conversations, coffee breaks, meals, sexual activity, boredom, or traffic problems or other frustrations. People who recognize smoking cues may modify the cues (for example, taking a walk in place of a coffee break) or substitute oral activity (for example, sucking on candy or chewing on a toothpick or on chewing gum).

Quitting smoking abruptly (cold turkey) is generally preferable to tapering off. Selection of a quit date is very helpful. The quit date may be random or on a special occasion (for example, a holiday or anniversary). A stressful time, such as when a deadline (for example, tax deadline) needs to be met, is not a good time to try to quit.

Substituting a non-smoked version of nicotine for some period of time helps many people break the habit of smoking. Many over-the-counter and prescription nicotine-replacement products are available, including nicotine chewing gum, a nicotine patch, nicotine nasal spray, and a nicotine inhaler.

Bupropion can be combined with a nicotine-replacement product. Together, they have a higher success rate. The results of both drugs are best when used in conjunction with a behavior modification program.

Weight gain is a concern, particularly among women. Nicotine suppresses appetite and slightly increases the rate at which calories are burned. Exercise helps prevent weight gain and may also reduce the craving for nicotine.

A person with significant problems with depression who attempts to quit smoking should receive counseling. Bupropion is an antidepressant, making it particularly useful for people who are depressed or at risk of depression.

Many people dependent on nicotine relapse after the first attempt at quitting smoking. In fact, five to seven failures commonly precede success. The more often a person makes a serious attempt to quit smoking, the more likely the person ultimately will succeed.

Marijuana

Marijuana (cannabis) use is widespread. Surveys of high school students have periodically shown increases, decreases, and then increases in its use. In the United States, marijuana is commonly smoked in the form of cigarettes (joints) made from the stems, leaves, and flowering tops of the dried plant (*Cannabis sativa* or *Cannabis indica*). Marijuana is also used as hashish, the pressed resin (tarry substance) of the plant. The active in-

gredient of marijuana is tetrahydrocannabinol (THC), which occurs in many variations, the most active being delta-9-THC.

As with the use of alcohol, marijuana can be used intermittently by many people without causing noticeable social or psychologic dysfunction or dependence. However, some people become dependent on marijuana, and among those who become dependent, many will exhibit the characteristics of addiction.

Symptoms and Complications

Marijuana depresses brain activity, producing a dreamy state in which ideas seem disconnected and uncontrollable. It is mildly psychedelic, causing time, color, and spatial perceptions to distort and be enhanced. Colors may seem brighter, sounds may seem louder, and appetite may be increased. Marijuana generally relieves tension and provides a sense of well-being. The sense of exaltation, excitement, and inner joyousness (a high) seems to be related to the setting in which the drug is taken—such as whether the smoker is alone or in a group and the prevailing mood. Motor abilities decrease during marijuana use, so driving or operating heavy equipment is dangerous.

People who use large quantities of marijuana may become confused and disoriented. They may develop a toxic psychosis, not knowing who they are, where they are, or what time it is. Some people, particularly those with mental illness, are especially susceptible to these effects, and there is compelling evidence that schizophrenia may become worse with marijuana use. Occasionally, panic reactions occur, particularly in new users. Other effects include an increased heart rate, bloodshot eyes, and dry mouth.

Prolonged heavy use of marijuana among men may reduce testosterone levels, the size of the testes, and sperm count. Long-term use among women may lead to irregular menstrual cycles. However, these effects do not always occur, and the effects on fertility are uncertain. Pregnant women who use marijuana may have smaller babies than nonusers, and delta-9-THC passes into the breast milk and may intoxicate a breastfed infant.

Marijuana is eliminated from the body slowly over several weeks, so withdrawal reactions tend to be mild. Heavy users who stop abruptly may experience jerkiness and insomnia.

Diagnosis and Treatment

Urine test results for marijuana generally remain positive for several days or weeks after use, even for casual users. For regular users, test results may remain positive for several weeks or longer while the drug is slowly released from body fat. Urine testing is an effective means of identifying marijuana use, but a positive urine test result means only that the person has used marijuana; it does not prove that the user is currently impaired (intoxicated).

For those who want to stop using marijuana, counseling may be helpful. However, success relies heavily on the user's motivation to stop and for some willingness to disassociate from his social circle of regular users.

Amphetamines

Among the drugs classified as amphetamines are amphetamine, methamphetamine (speed, crystal), and methylenedioxymethamphetamine (MDMA, Ecstasy, or Adam). Methamphetamine is the most commonly used amphetamine in the United States. Use of MDMA is growing in popularity. Amphetamines are usually taken by mouth but can be snorted, smoked, or injected.

Amphetamines may be used almost continuously or used intermittently. Some amphetamines are not approved for medical use, and some are manufactured and used illegally.

Some amphetamine abusers are depressed and seek the mood-elevating effects of these stimulants to temporarily relieve the depression. Others tend to use them in high energy activities, such as at dance parties. Amphetamines cause the release of increased amounts of dopamine in the brain, which is the likely cause of mood elevation. MDMA differs from the other amphetamines, in that it interferes with the reuptake of serotonin (one of the body's neurotransmitters) in the brain. Amphetamine users frequently develop dependence.

Symptoms and Complications

Amphetamines increase alertness (reduce fatigue), heighten concentration, decrease appetite, and enhance physical performance. They may induce a feeling of well-being, euphoria, and disinhibition.

In addition to stimulating the brain, amphetamines increase blood pressure and heart rate. Heart attacks have occurred, even in healthy young athletes. Blood pressure may become so high that a blood vessel in the brain ruptures, causing a stroke. Complications are more likely when drugs such as MDMA are used in warm rooms with little ventilation,

when the user is very active physically (for example, dancing fast), or when the user sweats heavily and does not drink enough water to restore lost fluids.

People who habitually use amphetamines rapidly develop tolerance as part of their dependence. The amount used ultimately may exceed several *hundred* times the original dose. Most people using very high doses may become psychotic, because amphetamines can cause severe anxiety, paranoia, and a distorted sense of reality. Psychotic reactions include auditory and visual hallucinations (hearing and seeing things that are not there) and a feeling of having unlimited power (omnipotence). Although these effects can occur in any user, people with a mental health disorder, such as schizophrenia, are more vulnerable to them.

Symptoms opposite to the drug's effects occur when an amphetamine is suddenly discontinued. A person dependent on amphetamines becomes tired or sleepy—an effect that may last for 2 or 3 days after stopping the drug. Some people are severely anxious and restless, and some, especially those with a tendency toward depression, become depressed when they stop. They may become suicidal but may lack the energy to attempt suicide for several days.

Treatment

Emergency treatment is needed only rarely. A person experiencing delusions and hallucinations may be given an antipsychotic drug, such as chlorpromazine, which has a calming effect and relieves distress. However, an antipsychotic drug may sharply lower blood pressure. Usually, reassurance and a quiet, nonthreatening environment help a person to recover.

Treatment may be needed to correct dehydration and other complications of use. Long-term users may need to be hospitalized during drug withdrawal for observance of suicidal behavior. Otherwise, no treatment is generally needed for people experiencing withdrawal.

Cocaine

Cocaine produces effects similar to those of amphetamines but is a much more powerful stimulant. It may be taken by mouth, inhaled as a powder through the nose (snorted), or injected, usually directly into a vein (mainlining). When boiled with sodium bicarbonate, cocaine is converted into a freebase form called crack cocaine, which can then be smoked. Crack cocaine acts almost as fast as cocaine injected intravenously.

Symptoms and Complications

Cocaine produces a sense of extreme alertness, euphoria, and great power when injected intravenously or inhaled. Because cocaine's effects may last only about 30 minutes, the user takes repeated doses. Cocaine also increases blood pressure and heart rate and narrows (constricts) blood vessels. These effects can cause a heart attack, even in healthy young athletes. Other effects include constipation; intestinal damage; extreme nervousness; the feeling that something is moving under the skin (cocaine bugs), which is a sign of possible nerve damage; seizures; hallucinations; insomnia; paranoid delusions; and violent behavior. Long-term users may damage the tissue separating the two halves of the nose (septum), causing sores (ulcerations) that may require surgery.

Women who become pregnant while addicted to cocaine are more likely than nonaddicts to miscarry. If the woman does not miscarry, the fetus may be damaged by the cocaine, which easily travels into its bloodstream from the mother's blood. A baby born to an addicted mother may have abnormal sleep patterns and poor coordination.▲ Crawling, walking, and speech development may be delayed, although this may be the result of nutritional deficiencies, poor prenatal care, and maternal abuse of other drugs as well.

Withdrawal reactions include extreme fatigue and depression—the opposite of the drug's effects. Suicidal urges emerge when the addict stops taking the drug. After several days, when mental and physical strength have returned, the addict may attempt suicide.

Treatment

Emergency Treatment: Cocaine is a very short-acting drug, so treatment of uncomfortable reactions usually are not necessary. Emergency medical staff watch the person closely to see if the life-threatening effects subside. Drugs such as beta-blockers may be given to lower blood pressure or heart rate. Other drugs may be given to stop seizures. A very high fever may also need to be treated.

Detoxification and Rehabilitation: Withdrawing from long-term cocaine use may require close supervision because the person can become depressed and suicidal. Entering a hospital or a drug treatment center may be necessary. The most effective method of treating cocaine addiction is psychotherapy. Sometimes the mental health disorders common to cocaine addicts, such as depression, are treated with appropriate drugs.

Hallucinogens

Hallucinogens include LSD (lysergic acid diethylamide), psilocybin (magic mushroom), mescaline (peyote), and 2,5-dimethoxy-4-methylamphetamine (DOM, STP), an amphetamine derivative. Many new compounds are being synthesized, and the list of hallucinogens is growing.

Symptoms and Complications

Hallucinogens distort auditory and visual sensations. The actual effect can depend on the user's mood when the drug is taken and the setting in which the drug is taken. For example, users who were depressed before the drug was taken are likely to feel sadder when the drug takes effect. The chief dangers of using these drugs are the psychologic effects and impaired judgment they produce, which can lead to dangerous decision making or accidents. For example, a user might think he can fly and may even jump out a window to prove it.

The user's ability to cope with the visual and auditory distortions also affects the experience, often referred to as a "trip." An inexperienced, frightened user is less able to cope than someone who is more experienced and not afraid of the trip. A user under the influence of a hallucinogen, usually LSD, can develop extreme anxiety and begin to panic, resulting in a bad trip. The user may want to stop the trip, which is not possible.

Some users remain psychotic for many days (or longer) after the drug's effects have worn off. A prolonged psychosis is more likely in a user with a preexisting mental health disorder.

Some people—especially long-term or repeated users of hallucinogens, particularly LSD—may experience flashbacks after they have discontinued the drugs. Flashbacks are similar to but generally less intense than the original experience. Generally, flashbacks disappear over a 6- to 12-month period but can recur as long as 5 years after the last use of LSD, especially when the user still suffers from an anxiety or other mental health disorder.

Treatment

Most hallucinogen users never seek treatment. A quiet, dark room and calm, non-

▲ see page 1463

Common Substances That Contain Solvent Inhalants

Adhesives
Airplane glue
Rubber cement
Polyvinyl chloride cement

Aerosols
Spray paint
Hair spray

Solvents and gases
Nail polish remover
Paint remover
Paint thinner
Typing correction fluid and thinner
Fuel gas
Cigarette lighter fluid
Gasoline

Cleaning agents
Dry cleaning fluid
Spot remover
Degreaser

threatening talk can help a user who is having a bad trip. The user needs reassurance that the effects are caused by the drug and will end. A person who experiences a prolonged psychosis may need mental health treatment.

Phencyclidine

Phencyclidine (PCP, angel dust) is most often smoked after being sprinkled on plant material, such as parsley, mint leaves, tobacco, or marijuana. Occasionally PCP is taken by mouth or injected.

Symptoms and Complications

PCP depresses brain function, and users usually become confused and disoriented shortly after taking the drug. They may not know where they are, who they are, or what time or day it is. They may go into a trance as if hypnotized. PCP users can be combative, and because they do not feel pain, they may continue fighting even when hit hard. Salivation, sweating, blood pressure, and heart rate also increase. Muscle tremors (shaking) are common. High doses can cause hallucinations, seizures, a life-threatening high fever (hyperthermia), coma, and possibly death. Long-term PCP use may damage the brain, kidneys, and muscles.

Treatment

When PCP users become agitated (as most do when brought for treatment), they are put in a quiet room and allowed to relax, although their blood pressure, heart rate, and breathing are monitored frequently. Soothing talk does not help; in fact, the person may become even more agitated. If quiet surroundings do not calm an agitated person, the doctor may give a sedative such as diazepam. The treatment of an adverse reaction may require drugs to lower high blood pressure or to stop seizures. The stomach may be pumped and drugs given to hasten the excretion of PCP from the body.

Ketamine

Ketamine (Special K, Super K) induces a lack of awareness to pain and to one's general surroundings, leading to a scattered feeling or to a feeling of detachment. Ketamine is usually snorted but may be injected intravenously.

Ketamine reduces pain perception and causes sedation. Ketamine distorts the user's perceptions of his body, the environment, and time. At higher doses, hallucinations, paranoid delusions, and a complete sense of detachment from the world may occur (ketamine users often refer to these experiences as a k-hole). Ketamine also can disrupt memory for several hours.

Treatment

Usually, reassurance and a quiet, nonthreatening environment help a person to recover. The drug's effects generally abate in less than 2 hours.

Gamma Hydroxybutyrate

Gamma hydroxybutyrate (GHB) is taken by mouth. It is similar to ketamine in its effects.

GHB produces feelings of relaxation and tranquility. It may also cause fatigue and feelings of being uninhibited. At higher doses, GHB may produce dizziness and loss of coordination, nausea, and vomiting. Seizures and coma may also occur and can lead to respiratory failure and death. Combining GHB and any other sedative, especially alcohol, is extremely dangerous. Most deaths have occurred when GHB was taken with alcohol.

Withdrawal symptoms occur if GHB is not taken for several days after previous frequent use.

Treatment

Treatment is needed only for overdose. Use of a ventilator may be needed if breathing is affected. Most people recover rapidly.

Solvent Inhalants

Among teenagers, inhalants are used more frequently than cocaine or LSD but less frequently than marijuana or alcohol. Inhalant use is particularly a problem among children aged 12 and younger. Inhalants are found in many common household products.

The product may be sprayed into a plastic bag and inhaled (bagging, sniffing, or snorting), or a cloth soaked with the product may be placed next to the nose or in the mouth (huffing).

Symptoms and Complications

Users of solvent inhalants rapidly become intoxicated. Dizziness, drowsiness, confusion, slurred speech, and a reduced ability to stand and walk (unsteady gait) have been observed. These effects can last anywhere from a few minutes to more than an hour. The user may also become excited—not because the chemicals are stimulants. Death can occur, even the first time one of these products is directly inhaled, because of severely depressed breathing or an irregular heartbeat (cardiac arrhythmia).

Some people, usually teenagers or even young children, ignite the inhaled fumes with matches, producing a fire that travels right through the nose and mouth into the lungs. The severe burns to the skin and internal organs can be fatal. Others have died of oxygen deprivation (asphyxiation) because the inhaled spray coated the lungs, preventing oxygen from entering the bloodstream.

Chronic use or exposure to these chemicals (including exposure in the workplace) can severely damage the brain, heart, kidneys, liver, and lungs. In addition, the bone marrow may be damaged, affecting red blood cell production and causing anemia.

Abused Inhalants That Have Medical Uses

Amyl nitrite, an inhalant, has a legitimate medical use. By widening (dilating) the arteries of the heart, amyl nitrite allows more oxygen to reach the heart muscle, thus relieving chest pain caused by coronary artery disease. Two closely related drugs, butyl nitrite and isobutyl nitrite, are not used medically. Amyl nitrite can only be sold by prescription. Butyl nitrite and isobutyl nitrite can be sold legally for commercial purposes relating to their use as air-fresheners, but their noncommercial use is banned. All three of these nitrite drugs briefly lower blood pressure, produce dizziness, and cause flushing, followed by a rapid heartbeat; these effects combined may produce a sense of excitement and euphoria. People also use these drugs because they believe that they will enhance sexual pleasure. When used in conjunction with sildenafil (a drug used to treat erectile dysfunction), these nitrite drugs may severely lower blood pressure, which can cause fainting, heart attack, or stroke.

Nitrous oxide is a gas (laughing gas) that has legitimate medical use as an anesthetic. It is also used as a propellant in cans and dispensers of whipped cream. Nitrous oxide is sometimes abused because it produces a sense of euphoria and a pleasant dreamlike state. Prolonged exposure to nitrous oxide can cause numbness and weakness in the legs and arms, which can be permanent.

Treatment

Treating children and teenagers who use inhalants involves evaluating any organ damage. It also involves education and counseling to address mental health and sociologic problems. Recovery rates from inhalant use are among the poorest for any mood-altering substance.

MOUTH AND DENTAL DISORDERS

109   **Biology of the Mouth**..661

110   **Lip and Tongue Disorders**..664

111   **Salivary Gland Disorders**..666

112   **Mouth Sores**...667

Canker Sores ▪ Oral Herpes Simplex ▪ Other Mouth Sores

113   **Growths in the Mouth**...670

Noncancerous Growths ▪ Precancerous Lesions ▪ Cancerous Growths

114   **Tooth Disorders**..674

Cavities ▪ Pulpitis ▪ Periapical Abscess ▪ Impacted Teeth ▪ Malocclusion

115   **Periodontal Diseases**..681

Gingivitis ▪ Periodontitis ▪ Trench Mouth ▪ Gum Recession

116   **Temporomandibular Disorders**...685

117   **Urgent Dental Problems**...690

Toothaches ▪ Fractured, Loosened, and Knocked-Out Teeth ▪ Jaw Fracture ▪ Dislocated Jaw ▪ Problems After Dental Treatment

CHAPTER 109

Biology of the Mouth

The mouth is the entrance to both the digestive and the respiratory systems. The inside of the mouth is lined with mucous membranes. When healthy, the lining of the mouth (oral mucosa) is reddish pink; the gums are paler pink and fit snugly around the teeth.

The roof of the mouth (palate) is divided into two parts. The front part has ridges and is hard (hard palate); the back part is relatively smooth and soft (soft palate). The lips are distinctly divided by a wet-dry border (vermilion border); the inside surface is moist and the outside surface is skinlike.

On the floor of the mouth lies the tongue, which is used to taste and mix food. The tongue is not normally smooth; it is covered

A View of the Mouth

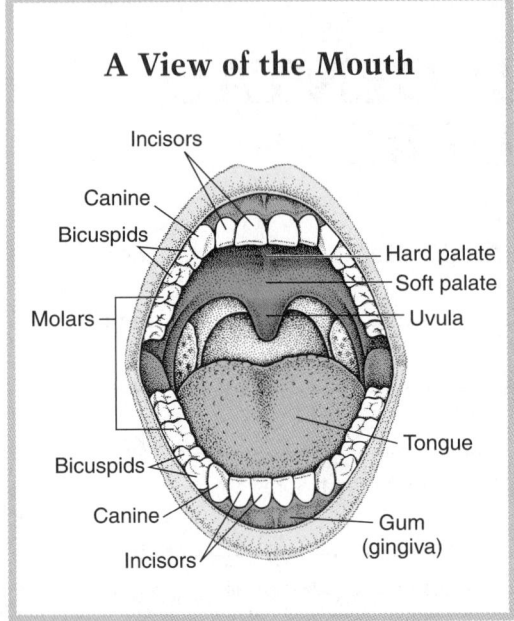

Incisors

Canine

Bicuspids

Hard palate

Soft palate

Molars

Uvula

Tongue

Bicuspids

Canine

Gum
(gingiva)

Incisors

with tiny projections (villi) that contain taste buds, which sense the taste of food. The sense of taste is relatively simple, distinguishing only sweet, sour, salty, and bitter. Smell is sensed by olfactory receptors high in the nose. The sense of smell is much more complex than that of taste, distinguishing many subtle variations. The senses of taste and smell work together to enable people to recognize and appreciate flavors.▲

The salivary glands produce saliva. There are three major pairs of salivary glands: parotid, submandibular, and sublingual. Besides the major salivary glands, many tiny salivary glands are distributed throughout the mouth. Saliva passes from the glands into the mouth through small tubes (ducts).

Saliva serves several purposes. It aids in chewing and eating by gathering food into lumps so that food can slide out of the mouth and down the esophagus, by beginning digestion, and by dissolving foods so that they can more easily be tasted. After food is eaten, saliva cleanses the mouth. Saliva helps keep the lining of the mouth healthy and prevents loss of minerals from teeth. It not only neutralizes acids produced by bacteria but also contains many substances such as antibodies

and enzymes that kill bacteria, yeasts, and viruses.

People have two sets of natural teeth: baby (deciduous) teeth and adult (permanent) teeth. There are 20 baby teeth: one pair each of upper and lower central (front) incisors, lateral incisors, canines (cuspids), first molars, and second molars. There are 32 permanent teeth: one pair each of upper and lower central incisors, lateral incisors, canines, bicuspids, second bicuspids, first molars, second molars, and third molars (wisdom teeth). Wisdom teeth, however, vary—not everyone gets all four wisdom teeth, and some people do not get any wisdom teeth. The wisdom teeth are the last permanent teeth to come in, typically between the ages of 17 and 21.

There is a broad range of normal times for teeth to push through the gum tissue (erupt) into the mouth. For baby teeth, the central incisors are the first teeth to erupt, occurring at about 6 months of age. These are followed by the lateral incisors, first baby molars, canines, and, finally, second baby molars. By about 2½ years of age, all the baby teeth can usually be seen in the child's mouth. Each of these baby teeth will be pushed out by a permanent tooth, starting at about age 6. The permanent 6-year molars come into the mouth just beyond the last baby molars and, therefore, do not replace any teeth. This lack of replacement is also true for the permanent second molars and third molars.

In rare cases, a child is born with a tooth (a natal tooth), or a baby tooth erupts in the mouth within a month of birth (a neonatal tooth). These teeth are usually baby lower incisors, but they may be extra (supernumerary) teeth. These teeth are removed only if they interfere with nursing or if they become exceedingly loose, which may pose a risk of choking.

In many children, the permanent lower incisors come in behind each other, resembling a cluster of grapes. Lack of space due to crowding or rotated permanent teeth may be the problem, and early orthodontic therapy (braces) may be necessary. Thumb or finger sucking may also affect the position of teeth, sometimes requiring early orthodontic therapy.

A tooth is divided into the crown, which is the part above the gum line, and the root, which is the part below the gum line. The crown is covered with shiny white enamel, which protects the tooth. Enamel is the hardest substance in the body, but if it is damaged,

▲ see art on page 595

Color Changes in the Mouth

White areas can appear anywhere in the mouth and often are simply food debris that can be wiped away. However, because white areas can be an early sign of mouth cancer, they should always be evaluated by a dentist or doctor. Other types of white areas include a white spongy patch (a hereditary condition called white sponge nevus); a white line running along the gum opposite the teeth (linea alba); and a grayish white area of the mucosa (leukoedema).

The mouth may have dark blue or black areas due to silver amalgam from a dental filling, graphite from falling with a pencil in the mouth, or a mole. Heavy cigarette smoking can lead to dark brown or black discoloration called smoker's melanosis. Ingestion of lead or of drugs containing silver can lead to gray discoloration of the gums. Minocycline, an antibiotic, discolors bone, which may show through near the teeth as gray or brown. Brown areas in the mouth can also be hereditary. For example, darkly pigmented areas are particularly common among dark-skinned and Mediterranean people.

Sometimes color changes in the mouth are a sign of a bodywide disease. Anemia may cause the lining of the mouth to be pale instead of the normal healthy reddish pink. Measles, a viral disease, can cause spots to form inside the cheeks. These spots, called Koplik's spots, resemble tiny grains of white sand surrounded by a red ring. Addison's disease and cancer (such as malignant melanoma) can cause color changes as well. In a person with AIDS, purplish patches caused by Kaposi's sarcoma may appear on the palate. Small red spots on the palate can be a sign of a blood disorder or infectious mononucleosis.

it has very little ability to repair itself. Under the enamel is dentin, which is similar to bone but is harder. Dentin surrounds the central (pulp) chamber, which contains blood vessels, nerves, and connective tissue.

The blood vessels and nerves enter the pulp chamber through the root canals, which are also surrounded by dentin. In the root, dentin is covered by cementum, a thin bonelike substance. Cementum is surrounded by a membrane (periodontal ligament) that cushions the tooth and attaches the cementum layer, and thereby the whole tooth, firmly to the jaw.

Cutting food with the front teeth and chewing with the back teeth break down food into more easily digestible particles. Saliva from the salivary glands coats food particles with digestive enzymes and begins digestion. Between meals, the flow of saliva washes away bacteria that can cause tooth decay (cavities) and other disorders.

At the back of the mouth hangs a narrow muscular structure called the uvula, which can be seen when a person says "Ahh." The uvula hangs from the back of the soft palate, which separates the back of the nose from the back of the mouth. Normally, the uvula hangs vertically. Its nerve supply comes from the vagus (10th cranial) nerve.

Effects of Aging

With age, taste sensation decreases. Older people are less able to identify food by taste, and many foods taste bitter. Older people may also have disorders or take drugs that affect their ability to taste.

Many older people retain their teeth, especially those people who do not develop cavities or periodontal disease, a destructive disease of the gums and supporting structures caused by the long-term accumulation of bacteria. Some older people lose some or all of their teeth and need partial or full dentures. Tooth loss is the major reason that older people cannot chew as well and thus may not consume enough calories.

Tooth enamel tends to wear away with age, making the teeth vulnerable to damage and decay. Periodontal disease, however, is the major cause of tooth loss. Periodontal disease is more likely to occur in people with poor oral hygiene, in people who smoke, and in people with certain disorders, such as diabetes mellitus, poor nutrition, leukemia, and AIDS.

A modest decrease in saliva production occurs with age. The significance of this change is uncertain; some experts believe that it may make the lining of the esophagus more susceptible to injury.

CHAPTER 110

Lip and Tongue Disorders

The lips and tongue may undergo changes in size, color, and surface. Some of these changes may indicate a medical problem. Other changes are harmless. For example, with age, the lips may grow thinner. Also, the side of the tongue may enlarge (bump out) where teeth are missing.

Lip Disorders

Swelling: An allergic reaction can make the lips swell. The reaction may be caused by sensitivity to certain foods or beverages, drugs, lipstick, or airborne irritants. When a cause can be identified and then eliminated, the lips usually return to normal. But at least half the time, the cause of the swelling remains a mystery. A condition called hereditary angioedema may cause recurring bouts of swelling. Nonhereditary conditions—such as erythema multiforme, sunburn, cold dry weather, or trauma—may also cause the lips to swell.

Treatment depends on the cause. A corticosteroid ointment is sometimes used to reduce swelling caused by an allergic reaction. Occasionally, excess lip tissue may be removed surgically to improve appearance.

Inflammation: With inflammation of the lips (cheilitis), the corners of the mouth may become painful, irritated, red, cracked, and scaly. Cheilitis may result from a deficiency of vitamin B_2 in the diet, but this deficiency is rare in the United States and can be treated by taking supplements of this vitamin.

Most commonly, vertical skinfolds and irritated skin (angular cheilitis) may develop in the corners of the mouth if a person has dentures that do not separate the jaws adequately. Treatment consists of replacing the dentures, which helps reduce the folds at the corners of the mouth.

Discoloration: Freckles and irregularly shaped brownish areas (melanotic macules) are common around the lips and may last for many years. These marks are not cause for

concern. Multiple, small, scattered brownish black spots may be a sign of a hereditary disease called Peutz-Jeghers syndrome, in which polyps form in the stomach and intestines.▲ Kawasaki syndrome, a disease of unknown cause that usually occurs in infants and children younger than 5 years of age, can cause dryness and cracking of the lips and reddening of the lining of the mouth.■

Sores: A raised area or a sore with hard edges on the lip may be a form of skin cancer.★ Other sores may develop as symptoms of other medical conditions, such as oral herpes simplex infection or syphilis.● Still others, such as keratoacanthoma, have no known cause.

Sun Damage: Sun damage may make the lips, especially the lower lip, hard and dry. Red speckles or a white filmy look signal damage that increases the chance of subsequent cancer. This type of damage can be reduced by covering the lips with a lip balm containing sunscreen or by shielding the face from the sun's harmful rays with a wide-brimmed hat.

Tongue Disorders

Injury: Traumatic injury is the most common cause of tongue discomfort. The tongue has many nerve endings for pain and touch and is more sensitive to pain than most other parts of the body. The tongue is frequently bitten accidentally but heals quickly. A sharp, broken filling or tooth can do considerable damage to this delicate tissue.

"Hairiness": An overgrowth of the normal projections on the top of the tongue (villi) can give it a hairy appearance. The tongue may also appear hairy after fever, after antibiotic treatment, or when peroxide mouthwash is used too often. These "hairs" on the top of the tongue should not be confused with hairy leukoplakia found on the side of the tongue, which is characteristic of AIDS.

Discoloration: The tongue's villi may become discolored if a person smokes or chews tobacco, eats certain foods, or has colored bacteria growing on the tongue.

The top of the tongue may look black if a person takes bismuth preparations for an

▲ see page 769   ■ see box on page 1581
★ see page 672   ● see page 668

Burning Mouth Syndrome

Burning mouth syndrome (also called stomatopyrosis, stomatodynia, and oral dysesthesia) occurs most commonly among women after menopause. The most commonly affected part of the mouth is the tongue (glossodynia). Burning mouth syndrome is not the same as the temporary discomfort that many people experience after eating irritating or acidic foods. Burning mouth syndrome is poorly understood. It probably represents a number of different conditions with different causes but a common symptom.

A common cause is use of antibiotics, which alters the balance of bacteria in the mouth, leading to an overgrowth of the fungus *Candida* (a condition called thrush). Ill-fitting dentures and allergies to dental materials may be causes as well. Overuse of mouth rinses and sprays may lead to burning tongue syndrome, as can anything that leads to a dry mouth. Sensitivities to certain foods and food additives, particularly to sorbic acid and benzoic acid (which are food preservatives), propylene glycol (found as a moisturizing agent in foods, drugs, and cosmetics), chicle (found in some chewing gums), and cinnamon, may play some role. Deficiencies of vitamins, including B_{12}, folic acid, and B-complex, can cause burning mouth syndrome. Iron deficiency has also been implicated.

A painful burning sensation may affect the entire mouth (particularly the tongue, lips, and roof of the mouth [palate]) or just the tongue. The sensation may be continuous or intermittent and may gradually increase throughout the day. Symptoms that commonly accompany the burning sensation include a dry mouth, thirst, and altered taste. Other possible symptoms include changes in eating habits, irritability, depression, and avoidance of other people.

The condition is easy for doctors to diagnose but difficult to treat. Frequent drinks of water or use of chewing gum may help keep the mouth moist. Antidepressants, such as nortriptyline, or antianxiety drugs, such as clonazepam, are sometimes helpful, although these drugs may make the symptoms worse by causing dry mouth. Sometimes symptoms disappear without treatment, although they may return later.

upset stomach. Brushing the tongue with a toothbrush or scraping it with a tongue scraper can remove such discoloration.

Redness of the tongue may be a sign of pernicious anemia or a vitamin deficiency. Iron deficiency anemia may make the tongue look pale and smooth. The first sign of scarlet fever may be a change from the tongue's normal color to a strawberry, and then raspberry, color. A strawberry-red tongue in a young child may also be a sign of Kawasaki syndrome. A smooth red tongue and painful mouth may indicate pellagra, a type of malnutrition caused by a deficiency of niacin (vitamin B_3) in the diet. A red tongue may also be inflamed (glossitis)—the tongue is red, painful, and swollen. A burning or painful sensation of the tongue may be due to burning mouth syndrome.

Whitish patches, similar to those sometimes found inside the cheeks, may accompany fever, dehydration, the second stage of syphilis, thrush, lichen planus, leukoplakia, or mouth breathing.

In geographic tongue, some areas of the tongue are white and rough, whereas others are red and smooth. The areas of discoloration move around over a period of weeks to years. The condition is usually painless, and no treatment is needed.

Sores and Bumps: Sores on the tongue can be caused by oral herpes simplex infection, canker sores, tuberculosis, bacterial infections, or early-stage syphilis. Sores can also be caused by allergies or other immune system disorders.

Although small bumps on both sides of the tongue are usually harmless, a bump on only one side may be cancerous. Unexplained red or white areas, sores, or lumps (particularly when hard) on the tongue—especially if painless—may be signs of cancer and should be examined by a doctor or dentist.▲ Most oral cancers grow on the sides of the tongue or on the floor of the mouth. Cancer almost never appears on the top of the tongue, except when the cancer has occurred as the result of syphilis.

Discomfort: Tongue discomfort can result from irritation by certain foods, especially acidic ones (for example, pineapple), or tooth-

▲ see page 672

pastes. Some drugs can cause tongue discomfort, as can injury and infection. A common infection causing tongue discomfort is thrush (candidiasis), in which an overgrowth of fungi forms a white film covering the tongue. Intense pain of the entire mouth can be caused by burning mouth syndrome.

Usually, it is a process of elimination to find out just what is causing the discomfort.

Tongue discomfort not caused by an infection is usually treated by eliminating the cause. For example, the person may try changing brands of toothpaste, discontinue irritating foods, or have a sharp or broken tooth repaired by a dentist. Warm salt-water rinses may help. Thrush can be treated with an antifungal drug, such as nystatin, in the form of a mouth rinse or lozenge.

CHAPTER 111

Salivary Gland Disorders

There are three major pairs of salivary glands in the mouth. The largest pair of salivary glands, called the parotid glands, lies just behind the angle of the jaw, below and in front of the ears. Two smaller pairs, the sublingual and submandibular glands, lie deep in the floor of the mouth. In addition to these major glands, many tiny salivary glands are distributed throughout the mouth. All of the glands produce saliva, which aids in breaking down food as part of the digestive process.

Other than cancer,▲ two major types of disorders affect the salivary glands: one that results in salivary gland malfunction, whereby not enough saliva is produced, and one that results in salivary gland swelling. When the flow of saliva is insufficient or almost nonexistent, the mouth feels dry. This condition is called dry mouth (xerostomia).

Salivary Gland Malfunction

Certain diseases and disorders can cause the salivary glands to malfunction and thus decrease saliva production, including Parkinson's disease, depression, chronic pain, HIV infection, and Sjögren's syndrome. Some drugs can decrease saliva production as well, including certain antidepressants, antihistamines, antipsychotics, sedatives, methyldopa, and diuretics.

The salivary glands often malfunction after a person has had chemotherapy or head and neck radiation for the treatment of cancer. Dry mouth due to radiation is usually permanent, especially if the radiation dose is high; that due to chemotherapy is usually temporary.

However, not all cases of dry mouth are caused by salivary gland malfunction. Drinking too little liquid and breathing through the mouth can dry the mouth. Anxiety or stress can also result in a dry mouth. The mouth may also dry somewhat as a person ages, although this is probably due to the greater likelihood of taking a drug that causes dry mouth than to the aging process itself.

Because saliva offers considerable natural protection against tooth decay, an inadequate amount of saliva leads to more cavities—especially on the roots of teeth. Dry mouth, if severe, can also lead to difficulty speaking and swallowing.

In rare cases, the salivary glands produce too much saliva. Increased saliva production is usually very brief and occurs in response to eating certain foods, such as sour foods. Sometimes even thinking about eating these foods can increase saliva production.

Salivary Gland Swelling

Salivary gland swelling can occur when one of the ducts that carry saliva from the salivary gland to the mouth is blocked. Pain may occur, especially during eating.

The most common cause of blockage is a stone. A stone can form from salts contained in the saliva. Blockage makes saliva back up inside the duct, causing the salivary gland to swell. A blocked duct and gland filled with stagnant saliva may become infected with bacteria. A typical symptom of a blocked salivary duct is swelling that worsens just before mealtime or particularly when a person eats a pickle (a sour pickle's taste stimulates saliva flow, but if the duct is blocked, the saliva has no place to go and the gland swells).

▲ see page 672

Mumps, certain bacterial infections, and other diseases (such as AIDS, Sjögren's syndrome, diabetes mellitus, and sarcoidosis) may be accompanied by swelling of the major salivary glands. Swelling also can result from cancerous or noncancerous tumors in the salivary glands. Swelling resulting from a tumor is usually firmer than that caused by an infection. If the tumor is cancerous, the gland may feel stone-hard and may be fixed firmly to surrounding tissues.▲

An injury to the lower lip—for instance, from accidental biting—may harm any of the minor salivary glands found there and block the flow of saliva. As a result, an affected gland may swell and form a small, soft lump (mucocele) that appears bluish. Over a few weeks, the lump usually disappears by itself.

Diagnosis and Treatment

There are no good quantitative tests to diagnose salivary gland malfunction. However, the salivary glands can be squeezed ("milked") and the ducts observed for saliva flow.

Swelling due to blockage of a salivary duct is diagnosed because of the relationship of pain to mealtimes. To diagnose other causes of swelling, a dentist or doctor may perform a biopsy to obtain a sample of salivary gland tissue and examine it under a microscope.

If a salivary duct is blocked by a stone, a dentist can sometimes push the stone out by pressing on both sides of the duct. If that fails, a fine-wire–like instrument can be used to pull the stone out. As a last resort, the stone can be removed surgically.

A mucocele that does not disappear on its own can be removed surgically if it becomes bothersome. Similarly, both noncancerous and cancerous salivary gland tumors can usually

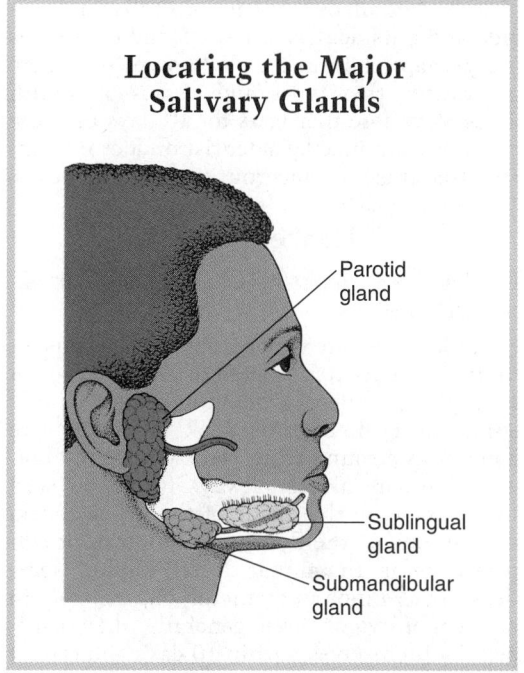

Locating the Major Salivary Glands

Parotid gland

Sublingual gland

Submandibular gland

be removed surgically. Treatment of other causes of salivary gland swelling varies with the cause.

Any person who has a disorder or who is taking a drug that dries the mouth must follow meticulous oral hygiene (brushing, flossing, and fluoride rinses), avoid sugars, and undergo dental examinations, cleanings, and fluoride treatments every 3 to 4 months.

When no specific treatment is available, saliva substitutes are marginally helpful. One drug that does help some people is pilocarpine, but the drug is often ineffective if the salivary glands have been damaged by radiation.

CHAPTER 112

Mouth Sores

Mouth sores vary in appearance and size. Some may be raised, usually filled with fluid (in which case it is called a vesicle or bulla); others may be ulcers. An ulcer is a hole that forms in the lining of the mouth when the top layer of cells breaks down and the underlying

tissue shows through. An ulcer appears white because of the dead cells and food debris inside the hole.

▲ see page 672

Sores can affect any part of the mouth, inside and outside. Canker sores and cold sores are perhaps the most well known, but there are many other types and causes of mouth sores. Any sore that lasts for 10 days or more must be examined by a dentist or doctor to ensure that it is not cancerous or precancerous.▲

Canker Sores

Canker sores (aphthous ulcers) are small, painful sores inside the mouth.

Canker sores are very common. The cause is unknown, but stress seems to play a role—for example, a college student may get canker sores during final exam week. A canker sore appears as a round white spot with a red border. The sore almost always forms on soft, loose tissue on the inside of the lip or cheek; on the tongue, the floor of the mouth, or soft palate; or in the throat. Small canker sores (less than $1/2$ inch in diameter) often appear in clusters of two or three; generally, they disappear by themselves within 10 days and do not leave scars. Larger canker sores are less common; they are irregularly shaped, can take many weeks to heal, and frequently leave scars. People with AIDS often have large canker sores that persist for weeks.

Many people who get canker sores get them repeatedly—often several times a year.

Symptoms and Diagnosis

The main symptom of a canker sore is pain—far more than would be expected from something so small. The pain, which lasts 4 to 7 days, worsens if the tongue or food rubs the sore or if hot or spicy foods are eaten. Severe canker sores can cause fever, swollen lymph nodes in the neck, and a generally run-down feeling.

A doctor or dentist identifies a canker sore by its appearance and the pain it causes.

Treatment

Treatment consists of relieving the pain until the sore heals by itself. An anesthetic such as dyclonine or lidocaine may be used as a mouth rinse. However, because these mouth rinses numb the mouth and throat and thus

---

▲ see page 670
■ see box on page 374
★ see page 1160

may make swallowing difficult, children using them should be watched to ensure that they do not choke on their food. Lidocaine in a thicker preparation (viscous lidocaine) can also be swabbed directly on the canker sore. A protective coating gel of carboxymethylcellulose, often combined with a corticosteroid (such as triamcinolone or betamethasone), may be applied to protect the sore and temporarily relieve pain by reducing inflammation.

If a person has many canker sores, a doctor or dentist may prescribe a tetracycline mouth rinse. People who have repeated outbreaks of canker sores may start using the tetracycline mouth rinse as soon as they feel a sore developing. Another treatment option, applying silver nitrate directly to the canker sore, destroys the nerves under the sore to relieve pain.

Finally, for the most severe cases, a corticosteroid may be prescribed as a dexamethasone mouth rinse or, rarely, as prednisone tablets taken by mouth. However, before prescribing a corticosteroid, a doctor ensures that the person does not also have oral herpes simplex infection, which can be further spread by corticosteroids. Corticosteroid rinses and tablets are absorbed into the body more than are corticosteroids given in gel form, so the side effects may be a concern.■

Oral Herpes Simplex

Infection of the mouth with herpes simplex virus causes recurring sores (often called cold sores), in which small fluid-filled sores develop on the skin, lips, or mouth in single or multiple clusters.

The first eruption of sores due to infection with oral herpes simplex virus is called primary herpes. It is usually contracted in childhood. Primary herpes may be mild or severe, but it often affects large areas of the mouth and always the gums. Any subsequent eruption of the sores is called secondary herpes. Secondary herpes is a reactivation of the virus rather than a new infection. There are at least two forms of herpes simplex virus. In the past, herpes simplex virus type 1 only caused sores above the waist, and type 2 only below the waist (genital herpes★). Now, however, either type can cause sores anywhere on the body. Herpes simplex virus type 2 tends to be more severe than type 1.

Typically, a previously uninfected child acquires the virus from contact with an adult who has a cold sore. In rare cases, a person first acquires herpes simplex virus in adulthood, also after contact with someone with a cold sore.

A person is capable of spreading the infection (contagious) from the time the tingling sensation that precedes the development of a sore (the prodrome) is experienced to the time at which the sore has completely crusted over. It is unknown whether herpes can be spread by sharing a glass or touching something that an infected person has touched.

Symptoms

When primary herpes is acquired in childhood, the infection causes gum inflammation and extensive mouth soreness. Fever, swollen lymph nodes in the neck, and general discomfort may develop. A child may be cranky and cry continually. However, many cases are mild and go unrecognized. Parents often mistake the problem for teething or another illness. In more severe cases, small blisters form in the child's mouth. These blisters may not be noticed because they rupture within a day or two, leaving many ulcers. The ulcers may occur anywhere in the mouth but always include the gums. Though the child gets better in a week to 10 days, the herpes simplex virus never leaves the body.

When primary herpes is acquired in adulthood, symptoms are usually more severe and include multiple rapidly developing painful sores on the gums and other parts of the mouth.

Unlike primary herpes, which causes widespread mouth soreness, the flare-ups of secondary herpes usually produce a single raw, weeping open sore on the outer lip that later crusts over before healing within 2 or 3 weeks. The sore is sometimes called a cold sore or fever blister. Less commonly, a cluster of blisters (vesicles) forms on the roof of the mouth. These small blisters run together and quickly break down into a sore. There is no crusting stage.

Flare-ups are commonly triggered by sunburn on the lips, certain foods, anxiety, a cold (hence the name "cold sore"), fever, or anything that lowers the body's resistance to infection. Certain dental procedures can cause a flare-up as well; if a cold sore already exists, dental visits should be postponed until the sore heals.

Although merely a painful annoyance for most people, flare-ups of oral herpes simplex infection can be life-threatening for a person with an impaired immune system. Impairment of the immune system can be caused by diseases (such as AIDS), chemotherapy, radiation therapy, or a bone marrow transplant. In such people, large, persistent sores in the mouth can interfere with eating; spread of the virus to the brain can be fatal.

Treatment

Treatment for primary herpes aims to relieve the pain so that the person can sleep, eat, and drink comfortably. Pain may keep a child from eating and drinking, which, combined with a fever, can quickly lead to dehydration. Thus, a child should drink as much fluids as possible. An adult or older child can use a prescribed anesthetic mouth rinse such as lidocaine to reduce pain. A mouth rinse containing baking soda may also be soothing.

Treatment for secondary herpes works best when started before the sore erupts—as soon as the person has the sensation (the prodrome) that an attack is starting. Taking vitamin C (1,000 to 2,000 milligrams per day) during the prodrome may make the attack less severe. A doctor may prescribe penciclovir cream or amlexanox paste, which is applied during the prodrome to shorten the duration and severity of the outbreak. The virus itself cannot be permanently eliminated.

Protecting the lips from direct sunlight by wearing a wide-brimmed hat or by using lip balm containing sunscreen can reduce the possibility of a flare-up. Also, a person should avoid activities and foods that are known to cause flare-ups. Anyone who suffers frequent, severe flare-ups may try taking lysine (available at health food stores) indefinitely. Levamisole, available by prescription, is another drug that seems to reduce recurrences.

For people with severe herpes simplex and for people with an impaired immune system, acyclovir or penciclovir capsules may be prescribed to prevent or limit the severity of the infection. Corticosteroids are not used for herpes simplex because they may allow the infection to spread.

Other Mouth Sores

Injury or irritation—for instance, when the inside of the cheek is accidentally bitten or scraped or when an irritating substance, such as an aspirin, is held against the gums—can cause blisters (vesicles, bullae) to form in the mouth. Typically, the surface of a blister breaks down quickly (ruptures), forming an ulcer. Noncancerous ulcers are invariably painful until healing is well under way. Red overgrown areas on the roof of the mouth can result from poorly fitting dentures or from dentures left in the mouth during sleep.

A rare condition called necrotizing sialo-metaplasia may follow injury to the mouth. In this condition, a large, gaping sore up to 1 inch in diameter forms on the roof of the mouth within 1 or 2 days of an injury. Despite its unsettling appearance, necrotizing sialo-metaplasia is relatively painless and heals without treatment in 2 months. A doctor may distinguish the condition from oral cancer on the basis of the symptoms (cancer would take a long time to reach the same size and by then would be painful) and sometimes by performing a biopsy (removing a tissue sample for examination under a microscope).

Bacterial infection can lead to sores and swelling in the mouth. Infections may be caused by an overgrowth of organisms normally present in the mouth or by newly introduced organisms. Bacterial infections from teeth or gums can spread to form a pus-filled pocket of infection (abscess) or cause widespread inflammation (cellulitis). Bacterial infections that spread from decayed lower teeth to the floor of the mouth can cause a very severe infection called Ludwig's angina. This swelling may force the tongue upward and block the airway. Infections from an upper tooth can spread to the brain.

Syphilis may produce a white, painless sore (chancre) that develops in the mouth or on the lips during the early stage of infection.▲ The sore usually heals after several weeks. About 1 to 4 months later, a white area (mucous patch) may form on the lip or inside the mouth if the syphilis has not been treated. Both the chancre and the mucous patch are highly contagious, and kissing may spread the disease during these stages. In late-stage syphilis, a hole (gumma) may appear in the palate or tongue; at this stage the disease is not contagious.

Herpes zoster, the virus responsible for chicken pox as well as the painful skin disorder called shingles,■ can cause multiple sores to form on one side of the mouth. These sores are the result of a flare-up of the virus, which, just like herpes simplex virus, never leaves the body. Herpes zoster is treated much like severe herpes simplex, but occasionally the mouth may remain painful for some time (weeks or months) after the sores are healed.

Behçet's syndrome, an inflammatory disease affecting many organs, including the eyes, genitals, skin, joints, blood vessels, brain, and digestive tract,★ can cause recurring, painful mouth sores. Lichen planus, a skin disease, can cause mouth sores as well, although most of the time these sores are not as uncomfortable as those on the skin.● Pemphigus and bullous pemphigoid, both skin diseases, can also cause blisters to form in the mouth.◆

CHAPTER 113

Growths in the Mouth

Noncancerous (benign) growths, precancerous (dysplastic) lesions, and cancerous (malignant) growths can originate in any type of tissue in and around the mouth, including bone, muscle, and nerve. Most commonly, growths form on the lips, the sides of the tongue, the floor of the mouth, and the back portion of the roof of the mouth (soft palate). Among people who use chewing tobacco and snuff, the insides of the cheeks and lips are common sites of cancer. Rarely, cancers found in the mouth region have spread there from other parts of the body, such as the lungs, breast, and prostate.

Noncancerous Growths

A variety of growths that are noncancerous may occur in and around the mouth. A lump or raised area on the gums (gingiva) is not a cause for alarm. Such a lump may be caused by a gum or tooth abscess or by irritation.

▲ see page 1176   ■ see page 1162
★ see page 390   ● see also page 1203
◆ see page 1216

Noncancerous growths due to irritation are relatively common and, if necessary, can be removed by surgery. In 10 to 40% of people, noncancerous growths on the gums recur because the irritant remains. Occasionally such irritation, particularly if it persists over a long period of time, can lead to cancer. Since any unusual growths in or around the mouth can be cancer, the growths should be checked by a doctor or dentist without delay.

Ordinary warts (verrucae) can infect the mouth if a person sucks one that is growing on a finger. A different type of wart—a genital wart▲—may be transmitted through oral sex. A doctor may remove an ordinary wart using one of several methods.■ Genital warts can be removed by several methods, but they tend to recur.

A slow-growing projection of bone (torus) may form in the middle of the roof of the mouth or on the lower jaw beneath the tongue. This hard growth is both common and harmless. It appears during puberty and persists throughout life. Even a large growth can be left alone unless it gets scraped during eating or the person needs a denture that will cover the area. However, multiple bony growths in the mouth may indicate Gardner's syndrome, a hereditary disorder of the digestive tract.★

Keratoacanthomas are noncancerous growths that form on the lips and other sun-exposed areas, such as the face and hands. A keratoacanthoma usually reaches its full size of ½ to 1 inch or more in diameter within 1 or 2 months, then begins to shrink after another few months and eventually disappears without treatment.

Many kinds of cysts (hollow, fluid-filled swellings) cause jaw pain and swelling. Often, they are next to an impacted wisdom tooth, and even though they are not cancerous, they can destroy considerable areas of the jawbone as they expand. Certain types of cysts are more likely to recur after surgical removal. Various types of cysts may also develop on the floor of the mouth. Often, these cysts are surgically removed because they make swallowing uncomfortable or because they are unattractive.

Odontomas are overgrowths of tooth-forming cells that look like small, misshapen extra teeth. In children, they may get in the way of normal teeth coming in. In adults, they may push teeth out of alignment. They are usually removed surgically.

Most tumors of the salivary glands (75 to 80%) are noncancerous, slow-growing, and painless. They usually occur as a single soft, movable lump beneath normal skin or under the lining (mucosa) of the inside of the cheek. Occasionally, when hollow and fluid-filled, they are firm. The most common type (called a mixed tumor or pleomorphic adenoma) occurs mainly in women older than 40. This type can become cancerous and is removed surgically. Unless completely removed, this type of tumor is likely to grow back. Other types of noncancerous tumors are also removed surgically but are much less likely to become cancerous or to grow back once removed.

Precancerous Lesions

White, red, or mixed white-red areas that are not easily wiped away, persist for more than 2 weeks, and are not definable as some other condition may be precancerous, that is, they tend to develop into cancer if left untreated. The same risk factors are involved in precancerous lesions as in cancerous growths, and precancerous lesions may become cancerous if not removed.

Leukoplakia is a flat white spot that may develop when the moist inner lining of the mouth (oral mucosa) is irritated for a long period. The injured spot appears white because it has a thickened layer of keratin—the same material that covers the outermost part of the skin and normally is less abundant in the lining of the mouth.

Erythroplakia is a reddened area that results when the lining of the mouth thins. The area appears red because the underlying capillaries are more visible. Erythroplakia is a much more ominous predictor of oral cancer than leukoplakia.

Cancerous Growths

Each year, cancerous growths of the mouth (oral cancer) develop in 30,000 people in the United States and cause 8,000 deaths, mostly in people older than 40. Oral cancer represents more than 2% of all cancers and 1.5% of all cancer-related deaths—a high rate considering the size of the mouth in relation to the rest of the body.

Because early detection vastly improves the likelihood of cure, screening for oral cancer should be an integral part of medical and den-

---

▲ see page 1183   ■ see page 1229
★ see page 768

tal examinations. Cancerous growths less than $1/2$ inch across usually can be cured. Unfortunately, most cancerous growths are not diagnosed until they are larger and have spread to the lymph nodes under the jaw and in the neck. Because of delayed detection, 25% of oral cancers are fatal.

Risk Factors

A hereditary factor, although not yet well understood, makes certain people more susceptible to developing oral cancer. The two greatest controllable risk factors for developing oral cancer are tobacco and alcohol use. Tobacco use— including smoking cigarettes (particularly more than 2 packs per day), cigars, or pipes; chewing tobacco; and dipping snuff—accounts for 80 to 90% of all oral cancers. Cigars and cigarettes are equally dangerous as risk factors in the development of oral cancer, followed in descending order by chewing tobacco and pipe smoking.

Chronic or heavy alcohol use (particularly more than 6 drinks per day) increases the risk of oral cancer. The combination of tobacco and alcohol is more likely to cause cancer than either one alone. There is some evidence that the alcohol contained in mouthwash can contribute to oral cancer. Therefore, people who smoke and drink alcohol should choose a mouthwash that contains the lowest concentration of alcohol (which is stated on the label).

People who have had oral cancer are at risk of recurrence. Hereditary predisposition may contribute to recurrence, as may the radiation used to treat the cancer. People who continue to use tobacco and alcohol after developing oral cancer have more than twice the chance as the rest of the population (30% vs. 12%) of developing a second oral cancer.

Other factors that add to the risk of oral cancer include repeated irritation from the sharp edges of broken teeth, fillings, or dental prostheses (dentures). Syphilis, if untreated for many years, may give rise to tongue cancer, the only cancer that forms on the top of the tongue. Sun damage can cause cancer of the lip.▲

About two thirds of oral cancers occur in men, but increased tobacco use among women over the past few decades is gradually closing the gender gap. As with most cancers, risk increases with age.

▲ see page 1230
■ see page 1240

Types of Oral Cancer

Squamous cell carcinoma is the most common type of oral cancer. Nearly 40% of squamous cell carcinomas affect the lower lip; many of the remainder affect the floor of the mouth or the tongue. These cancers form a hard lump or a firm-bordered sore (ulcer) that may bleed intermittently. Affected areas may appear white, red, or mixed white and red and can be smooth or raised. Another type of cancer is called verrucous (warty) carcinoma, which appears as a white grooved surface on the mucosa (lining of the mouth).

Other types of cancer are less common, such as malignant melanoma and Kaposi's sarcoma. Malignant melanoma is usually associated with a history of sunburns and occurs on the surface of the skin. However, it occasionally occurs in the mouth, most commonly on the roof of the mouth, usually as a result of spread from a skin site. A malignant melanoma often has uneven, irregularly shaped borders and ranges in color from dark blue or brown to black. Its color may be spotty, however, or even speckled. As with most cancers, it occasionally bleeds. Kaposi's sarcoma is a cancer of the blood vessels near the skin and in the lining of the mouth and throat.■ In people with AIDS, when Kaposi's sarcoma occurs in the mouth, it usually occurs on the roof of the mouth. The tumor is usually purple or brown and is slightly raised.

Cancers of the salivary glands are much less common than noncancerous growths. The most common cancer is mucoepidermoid carcinoma, which typically forms in a minor (small) salivary gland on the roof of the mouth. It may also occur as a lump in one of the major (large) salivary glands, either under or behind the lower jaw.

Cancers of the jawbone include osteosarcoma and metastatic tumors (those that have spread to the jaw from another part of the body).

Symptoms

Oral cancers are usually painless for a considerable length of time but eventually do cause pain. Pain usually starts when the cancer erodes into nearby nerves. When pain from cancer of the tongue or roof of the mouth begins, it usually occurs with swallowing, as with a sore throat.

The early growth of salivary gland tumors may or may not be painful. When these tumors do become painful, the pain may be worsened by food, which stimulates the secretion of saliva. Cancer of the jawbone often causes pain and a numb or pins-and-needles sensation (paresthesia), somewhat like the feeling of a dental anesthetic wearing off. Cancer of the lip or cheek may first become painful when the enlarged tissue is inadvertently bitten.

Squamous cell carcinomas often look like open sores (ulcers) and tend to grow into the underlying tissues. Cancers of the lip and other parts of the mouth often feel rock hard and are attached to the underlying tissues, whereas most noncancerous lumps in these areas are freely movable. A person who chews tobacco or uses snuff may develop white, ridged bumps on the insides of the cheeks that can develop into verrucous (warty) carcinoma. Cancerous tumors tend to grow fast and feel hard. Cancer beginning in the small salivary glands commonly appears as a small swelling.

Discolored areas on the gums, tongue, or lining of the mouth may be signs of cancer.▲ An area in the mouth that has recently become brown or darkly discolored may be a melanoma. Sometimes a brown, flat, freckle-like area (smoker's patch) develops at the site where a cigarette or pipe is habitually held in the lips.

Diagnosis

Oral cancers are suspected because of their appearance and symptoms. Doctors must distinguish a melanoma from normal pigmentation or from discoloration due to other causes. However, only a biopsy (removal of a tissue specimen for examination under a microscope) can determine whether a suspicious area is cancerous.

X-rays cannot always distinguish jaw cancers from cysts, noncancerous bone growths, or cancers that have spread from elsewhere in the body. However, x-rays may show irregular borders of jaw cancer and can show the loss of parts of neighboring teeth, which is characteristic of a rapidly growing cancer.

Prevention

Avoiding excessive alcohol and tobacco use can greatly reduce the risk of most oral cancers. Smoothing rough edges from broken teeth or fillings is another preventive measure. Some evidence indicates that antioxidant vitamins, such as vitamins C and E, may provide added protection, but further study is needed. Staying out of the sun reduces the risk of lip cancer. If sun damage covers a large area

of the lip, a lip shave in which all of the outer surface is removed, either by surgery or with a laser, may prevent a progression to cancer.

Prognosis and Treatment

Cancers originating in or around the mouth can spread to nearby lymph nodes, which become hard and swollen. Spread of cancers to more distant parts of the body is uncommon with squamous cell carcinoma but is more likely with osteosarcoma and is very likely with malignant melanoma, which can reach organs such as the brain.

The cure rate for squamous cell carcinoma is high if the entire cancer and the surrounding normal tissue is removed before the cancer has spread to the lymph nodes. On average, 68% of people survive at least 5 years after the diagnosis. However, if the cancer has spread to lymph nodes, the 5-year survival is only 25%. Regrettably, cure rates for squamous cell carcinoma have not improved much over the past several decades. However, verrucous carcinoma is rarely fatal because it develops late in life and grows slowly. The 5-year survival rate for malignant melanoma is only 5 to 10%.

For squamous cell carcinoma and most other types of oral cancer, the mainstays of treatment are surgery and radiation therapy. These two treatments are often used together, particularly for larger cancers. For malignant melanoma, surgery is the main approach because the cancer is generally not responsive to radiation therapy.

During surgery, the extent of the cancer can be determined. The lymph nodes under and behind the jaw and along the neck may be removed. Consequently, surgery for oral cancers can be disfiguring and psychologically traumatic. Newer methods are being used, however, to minimize disfigurement. In the case of the lips, the Mohs' technique—a method of determining the extent of disease during different phases of surgery by examining each slice of tissue under the microscope after its removal—minimizes disfigurement, as does the use of lasers to destroy cancer cells. Reconstructive surgery can improve function and restore normal appearance after the disease is controlled. Missing teeth and jaw parts can be replaced with prosthetic parts.

A person with oral cancer may receive radiation therapy after surgery or just radiation

▲ see page 671

therapy. Although radiation may not always be curative, especially if the cancer is extensive, it is sometimes used to shrink the cancer and thus relieve symptoms (palliation). Radiation therapy often destroys the salivary glands and leaves the person's mouth dry, which can lead to cavities and other dental problems. If the salivary glands have not been destroyed, saliva production usually recovers several weeks after the radiation treatment is completed. Because jawbones exposed to radiation do not heal well, dental problems should be completely treated before radiation is administered. Any teeth likely to become problematic are removed, and time is allowed for healing before radiation.

Good dental hygiene is critical for people who have had radiation therapy for oral cancer; the mouth heals poorly if dental surgery, such as tooth extractions, is ever needed. Such hygiene includes regular examinations and thorough home care, including daily home fluoride applications. If the person eventually has a tooth pulled, hyperbaric oxygen therapy may help the jaw heal without the death of bone and surrounding soft tissue in the area that receives the radiation (osteoradionecrosis).

Chemotherapy has been shown to have little value in the treatment of most oral cancers. For malignant melanoma, chemotherapy is used if surgery is not possible, but it generally only delays death and is usually not curative.

CHAPTER 114

Tooth Disorders

Tooth disorders include cavities (caused by tooth decay), pulpitis, periapical abscess, impacted teeth, and malocclusion. Fractured, loosened, and knocked-out teeth are considered urgent dental problems, as are some toothaches.▲ Tooth decay, which often leads to toothache and tooth loss, is largely preventable with good oral hygiene to remove plaque and prevent tartar buildup.

Plaque is a filmlike substance composed of a mixture of bacteria, saliva, and dead cells that is continually being deposited on teeth, day and night. It occurs in everyone. Because plaque can encourage growth of the kind of bacteria that leads to tooth decay, it needs to be removed by daily brushing and flossing.

Tartar (calculus) is hardened (calcified) plaque that forms a white covering at the base of the teeth, particularly the tongue side of the front lower teeth and the cheek side of the upper molars (the teeth at the back of the mouth). Because tartar is formed from plaque, daily brushing to remove plaque can significantly reduce the buildup of tartar. However, once tartar has formed, it can only be adequately removed by a dentist or dental hygienist.

Although a healthy mouth can be maintained with meticulous brushing and flossing, limiting sugar intake and using fluoridated water also help reduce the risk of tooth decay.

Symptoms of Tooth Disorders

Pain affecting an individual tooth (toothache) is probably the most recognized symptom of a tooth disorder. A tooth may be painful all the time or only under certain circumstances, such as when chewing or when tapped by a dental instrument. Pain in a tooth suggests tooth decay or gum disease. However, pain may also result when roots are exposed, when a person chews too forcefully or grinds his teeth (bruxism), or when a tooth is fractured. Sinus congestion can cause similar symptoms of pain in the area of the upper teeth.

Worn-down or loose teeth can be a symptom of bruxism, a disorder characterized by frequent clenching or grinding of the teeth. Bruxism occurs mostly during sleep, so that the person is unaware of it, but it may also occur during the day. People who have bruxism must concentrate on not clenching or grinding their teeth during the day. Attrition refers to the worn surfaces of the teeth where grinding of food occurs. Attrition may make chewing less effective.

▲ see page 690

Abnormally shaped teeth can be a symptom of genetic diseases, hormonal disorders, or infections acquired before birth. Teeth can be misshapen due to fractures or chipping from trauma to the mouth.

Abnormal tooth color is not the same as the darkening or yellowing of teeth that occurs as a person grows older or exposes his teeth to staining substances, such as coffee, tea, and cigarette smoke. Graying of a tooth may be a symptom of a previous infection within the tooth that has seriously damaged the pulp, which is the living center of the tooth. The same may occur when a permanent tooth replaces an infected baby tooth. Permanent discoloration of the teeth may be a result of having taken tetracycline as a child or of one's mother having taken tetracycline while pregnant. Excess fluoride ingestion during childhood can cause mottling of the enamel.

Abnormal tooth enamel (enamel is the hard outer surface of teeth) may be due to a diet containing insufficient vitamin D. Abnormal enamel may also be the result of a childhood infection (such as measles or chickenpox) occurring when the permanent teeth were forming. Abnormal enamel may also be due to repeated vomiting, as occurs in bulimia nervosa, because the stomach acid dissolves the surface of the teeth. Swimmers who spend a lot of time in chlorinated pools can lose tooth enamel, as can people who work with acids or chlorines. Damaged tooth enamel can allow bacteria to more easily invade the tooth and form a cavity.

Cavities

Cavities (dental caries) are decayed areas in the teeth, the result of a process that gradually dissolves a tooth's hard outer surface (enamel) and progresses toward the interior.

Along with the common cold and gum disease, cavities are among the most common human afflictions. If cavities are not properly treated by a dentist, they continue to enlarge. Ultimately, an untreated cavity can lead to tooth loss.

For tooth decay to develop, a tooth must be susceptible, acid-producing bacteria must be present, and food must be available for the bacteria to thrive. A susceptible tooth is one that has relatively little protective fluoride incorporated into the enamel or that has pronounced pits, grooves, or fissures that retain plaque. Poor oral hygiene that allows plaque

THE LANGUAGE OF DENTISTS

WHAT MOST PEOPLE CALL IT	WHAT DENTISTS CALL IT
Adult tooth	Permanent tooth
Baby tooth	Deciduous tooth
Back teeth	Molars
Bite	Occlusion
Braces	Orthodontic bands and wires, appliances
Cap	Crown
Cavities	Caries
Cleaning	Prophylaxis
Eye teeth	Canines or cuspids
Filling	Restoration
Front teeth	Incisors and canines
Gum	Gingiva
Gum disease	Periodontal disease, periodontitis
Harelip	Cleft lip
Laughing gas	Nitrous oxide
Lower jaw	Mandible
Plate	Complete or partial denture
Roof of the mouth	Palate
Side teeth	Bicuspids or premolars
Silver filling	Amalgam restoration
Tartar	Calculus
Uneven bite	Malocclusion
Upper jaw	Maxilla

and tartar to accumulate can accelerate this process. Although the mouth contains large numbers of bacteria, only certain types generate acid, which causes decay. The most common decay-causing bacterium is *Streptococcus mutans*.

Some people have especially active decay-causing bacteria in their mouth. A parent may pass these bacteria to a child through kissing or sharing eating utensils. The bacteria flourish in the child's mouth after the first teeth come in and can then cause cavities. So a tendency toward tooth decay that runs in families does not necessarily reflect poor oral hygiene or bad eating habits.

Progression of Tooth Decay: Decay in the enamel progresses slowly. After penetrating into the second layer of the tooth—the somewhat softer, less resistant dentin—decay spreads more rapidly and moves toward the pulp, the innermost part of the tooth, which contains the

Types of Cavities

The illustration on the left shows a tooth with no cavities; the illustration on the right shows a tooth with the three types of cavities.

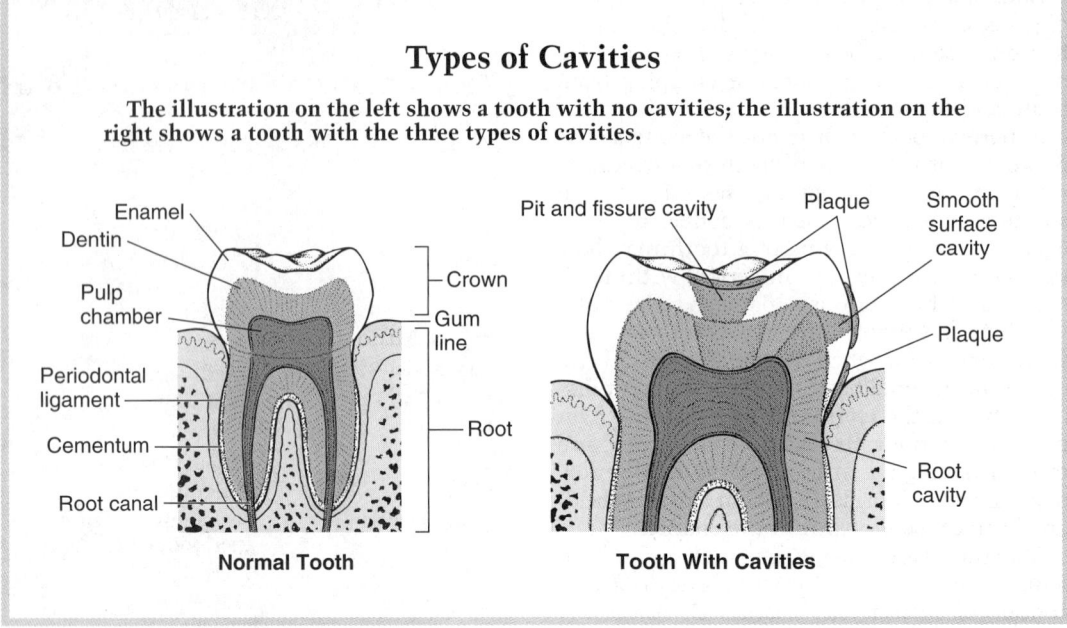

Normal Tooth   **Tooth With Cavities**

nerves and blood supply. Although a cavity may take 2 or 3 years to penetrate the enamel, it can travel from the dentin to the pulp—a much greater distance—in as little as a year. Thus, root decay that starts in the dentin can destroy a lot of tooth structure in a short time.

Smooth surface decay, the most preventable and reversible type, grows the slowest. In smooth surface decay, a cavity begins as a white spot where bacteria dissolve the calcium of the enamel. Smooth surface decay between the teeth usually begins between the ages of 20 and 30.

Pit and fissure decay, which usually starts during the teen years in the permanent teeth, forms in the narrow grooves on the chewing surface and on the cheek side of the back teeth; this decay progresses rapidly. Many people cannot adequately clean these cavity-prone areas because the grooves are narrower than the bristles of a toothbrush.

Root decay begins on the root surface covering (cementum) that has been exposed by receding gums, usually in people past middle age. This type of decay often results from difficulty cleaning the root areas, a lack of adequate saliva flow, a diet high in sugar, or a combination of these factors. Root decay can be the most difficult type of tooth decay to prevent.

Symptoms

Whether tooth decay causes pain depends on which part of the tooth is affected and how deeply the decay extends. A cavity in the enamel causes no pain; the pain starts when the decay reaches the dentin. A person may feel pain only when drinking something cold or eating candy. This indicates that the pulp is still healthy. If the cavity is treated at this stage, the dentist can restore the tooth, and most likely no further pain or chewing difficulties will develop.

A cavity that gets close to or actually reaches the pulp causes irreversible damage. Pain lingers even after a stimulus (cold water, for example) is removed. The tooth may even hurt without stimulation (spontaneous toothache).

If irreversible damage to the pulp occurs and the pulp subsequently dies, the pain may stop temporarily. The tooth then may become sensitive when the person bites or when the tongue or a finger presses on it, because the area at the end of the root has become inflamed or because infection has caused an abscess (a collection of pus). Pus accumulating around the tooth tends to push the tooth out of its socket. Biting pushes it back in place. This action causes extreme pain. Pus can continue to accumulate and cause swelling in the adjacent gum tissues or can spread more broadly through the jaw (cellulitis) and drain into the mouth or even through the skin near the jaw.

Diagnosis and Prevention

If a cavity is treated before it starts to hurt, the chance of damage to the pulp is reduced, and more of the tooth structure is saved. To detect cavities early, a dentist inquires about pain, examines the teeth, probes the teeth with dental instruments, and may take x-rays. A person should have a dental examination every 6 to 12 months, though not every examination will include x-rays. Depending on the dentist's assessment of a person's teeth, x-rays may be taken every 12 to 36 months.

Five general strategies are key to preventing cavities: good oral hygiene, proper diet, fluoride, sealants, and antibacterial therapy.

Oral Hygiene: Good oral hygiene, which involves brushing before or after breakfast and before bedtime and flossing daily to remove plaque, can effectively control smooth surface decay. Brushing helps prevent cavities from forming on the top and sides of the teeth, and flossing gets between the teeth where a brush cannot reach.

Electric and ultrasonic toothbrushes are excellent, but an ordinary toothbrush, used properly, is quite sufficient. Normally, proper brushing takes only about 3 minutes. Floss is gently moved back and forth between the teeth, then wrapped around the tooth and root surfaces in a "C" shape at the gum line. With the person using a vertical sliding motion, floss can remove plaque and food debris.

Initially, plaque is quite soft, and removing it with a soft-bristled toothbrush and dental floss at least once every 24 hours makes decay unlikely. Once plaque begins to harden, a process that begins after about 24 hours, removing it becomes more difficult.

Diet: Although all carbohydrates can cause tooth decay to some degree, the biggest culprits are sugars. All simple sugars, including table sugar (sucrose) and the sugars in honey (levulose and dextrose), fruit (fructose), and milk (lactose), have the same effect on the teeth. Whenever sugar comes in contact with plaque, *Streptococcus mutans* bacteria in the plaque produce acid. The amount of sugar eaten is of little consequence; the amount of time the sugar stays in contact with the teeth is the important issue. Thus, sipping a sugary soft drink over an hour is more damaging than eating a candy bar in 5 minutes, even though the candy bar may contain more sugar.

A person who tends to develop cavities should eat sweet snacks less often. Rinsing the mouth after eating a snack removes some of

A Brighter Smile Through Cosmetic Dentistry

Cosmetic dentistry can dramatically improve a person's appearance. The techniques used avoid the time involved with orthodontic therapy and the loss of tooth structure necessitated by crowns and bridges.

Bonding involves the attachment of tooth-colored fillings to natural teeth with minimal tooth preparation. Bonding is a conservative way to restore fractured or chipped teeth, to close spaces between the teeth, or to cover a portion of the tooth to change the shade, color, or shape. A mild acid solution is used to clean and mildly roughen the tooth surface so that a tooth-colored resin (generally made of a special type of plastic called a composite) can adhere to this surface. Bonding allows the dentist to improve the appearance of the teeth without removing large amounts of tooth structure.

Porcelain veneers are similar to bonding, but they use tooth-colored porcelain instead of composite to mask discoloration or change the shape of the teeth. The process requires two visits. An impression is made after the teeth are prepared. Porcelain veneers are then made in a dental prosthetic laboratory. The veneers are bonded to the teeth using a thin resin cement.

Bleaching, or tooth whitening, is a process used by dentists to lighten teeth. The effectiveness of bleaching varies according to the original color of the teeth. Products used for home bleaching usually contain a peroxide gel that is placed into a custom-made closely fitting mouthguard-like tray that holds the solution near the teeth. The bleaching agent is placed into the mouth for a few hours per day or even overnight for 2 to 4 weeks, depending on the concentration of the bleaching agent. Bleaching can also be done in a dentist's office, in which the process is much quicker. The most common side effect of bleaching is tooth sensitivity. Bleaching may not be effective for people whose teeth are darkened or discolored because of cavities, because of a side effect of some drugs or diseases, or because a tooth has died.

Root Canal Treatment for a Badly Damaged Tooth

1. The tooth is anesthetized.
2. A rubber dam is placed around the tooth to isolate it from bacteria in the rest of the mouth.
3. An opening is drilled through the chewing surface of a back tooth or the tongue side of a front tooth.
4. Fine instruments are passed through the opening, into the pulp canal space, and all the remaining pulp is removed.
5. The canal is smoothed and tapered from the opening to the end of the root.
6. The canal is sealed with a filling.

the sugar; brushing the teeth is more effective. Drinking artificially sweetened soft drinks also helps, although diet colas contain acid that can promote tooth decay. Drinking tea or coffee without sugar also can help people avoid cavities, particularly on exposed root surfaces.

Fluoride: Fluoride can make the teeth, particularly the enamel, more resistant to the acid that helps cause cavities. Fluoride taken internally is effective while the teeth are growing and hardening—until about age 11. Water fluoridation is the most efficient way to supply children with fluoride, and over half of the United States population now has drinking water with enough fluoride to reduce tooth decay. However, if a water supply has too much fluoride, the teeth can become spotted or discolored (fluorosis). If a child's water supply does not have enough fluoride, a doctor or dentist can prescribe sodium fluoride drops or tablets. A dentist may apply fluoride directly to the teeth of a person of any age who is prone to tooth decay. Fluoridated toothpaste and concentrated mouth rinses containing fluoride are beneficial for adults as well as children.

Sealants: Sealants protect hard-to-reach pits and fissures (grooves), particularly on the back teeth. After thoroughly cleaning the area to be sealed, a dentist roughens the enamel with an acid solution to help the sealant adhere to the teeth. The dentist then places a liquid plastic in and over the pits and fissures of the teeth. When the liquid hardens, it forms such an effective barrier that any bacteria inside a pit or fissure stop producing acid because food can

no longer reach them. About 90% of the sealant remains after 1 year and 60% after 10 years. The occasional need for repair or replacement of sealants can be assessed at periodic dental examinations.

Antibacterial Therapy: For people who are very prone to tooth decay, antibacterial therapy may be needed. The dentist first removes decayed areas and seals all pits and fissures in the teeth. Then the dentist prescribes a powerful mouth rinse (chlorhexidine) for several weeks to kill off the bacteria in any remaining plaque. The hope is that less harmful bacteria will replace the cavity-causing bacteria. To keep bacteria under control, the person may use daily home fluoride rinses and chew gum containing xylitol (a sweetener that inhibits the bacteria in plaque).

Treatment

If decay is halted before it reaches the dentin, the enamel can actually repair itself (remineralization) in conjunction with fluoride therapy. Fluoride treatment requires use of prescription-strength fluoride-containing mouthwash. Once decay reaches the dentin, the dentist drills out the decayed material inside the tooth and then fills the resulting space with a filling (restoration). Treating the decay at an early stage helps maintain the strength of the tooth and limits the chance of damage to the pulp.

Fillings: Fillings are made of various materials and may be put inside the tooth or around it. Silver amalgam (a combination of mercury, silver, copper, tin, and, occasionally, zinc, palladium, or indium) is most commonly used for fillings in back teeth, where strength is important and the silver color is relatively inconspicuous. Silver amalgam is relatively inexpensive and lasts an average of 14 years, but with good oral hygiene the amalgam can last for more than 40 years. The minute amount of mercury that escapes from silver amalgam is too small to affect health. Gold fillings (inlays and onlays) are more expensive, and at least two dental visits are required to permanently place them.

Composite resins and porcelain fillings are used in the front teeth, where silver would be conspicuous. Increasingly, these fillings are also being used in back teeth. Although they have the advantage of being the color of the teeth, they are more expensive than silver amalgam and may not last as long, particularly in the back teeth, which take the full force of chewing.

Glass ionomer, a tooth-colored filling, is formulated to release fluoride once in place, a benefit for people prone to tooth decay. Glass ionomer is also used to restore areas damaged by overzealous brushing.

Root Canal Treatment and Tooth Extraction: When tooth decay advances far enough to permanently harm the pulp, the only way to eliminate pain is to remove the pulp by root canal (endodontic) treatment or tooth extraction.

If a tooth is extracted, it should be evaluated for replacement as soon as possible. Otherwise, neighboring teeth may change position and alter the person's bite.

Bridges and Crowns: The replacement for an extracted tooth may be a bridge—a fixed partial denture in which teeth on either side of the missing tooth are covered with crowns—or a removable partial denture. Also, implants may be used to replace missing teeth.

A crown is a restoration that fits over a tooth. Getting a properly shaped crown usually takes two visits to the dentist, although sometimes several visits are needed. On the first visit, the dentist prepares the tooth by tapering it slightly, takes an impression of the prepared tooth, and puts a temporary crown on it. A permanent crown is then fashioned in a dental prosthetics laboratory, using the impression. On the next visit, the temporary crown is removed, and the final crown is permanently cemented onto the prepared tooth.

Usually, crowns are made of an alloy of gold or another metal. Porcelain can be used to mask the color of the metal. Crowns also may be made entirely of porcelain, although porcelain is harder and more abrasive than tooth enamel and may cause wear on the opposing tooth. Also, crowns made entirely of porcelain or similar material have a slightly greater tendency to break than those made of metal.

Pulpitis

Pulpitis is painful inflammation of the tooth pulp, the innermost part of the tooth that contains the nerves and blood supply.

Crowns, Bridges, and Implants

Damaged Tooth

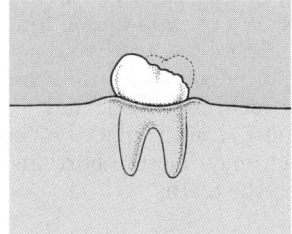

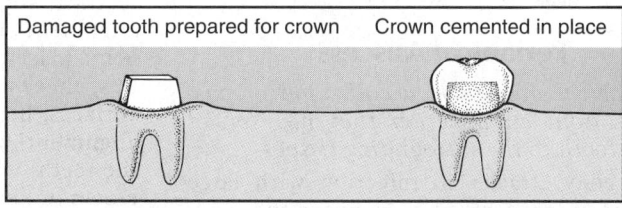

Damaged tooth prepared for crown   Crown cemented in place

To repair a damaged tooth, a dentist first prepares it by altering its shape. Then the dentist cements the crown onto the reshaped tooth.

Missing Tooth

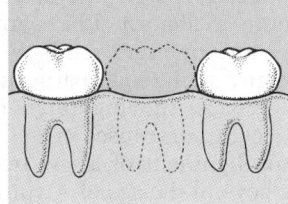

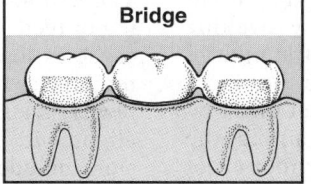

Bridge

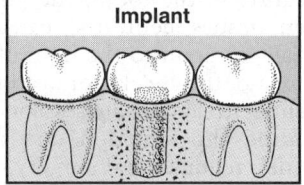

Implant

A dentist may replace a missing tooth using either a bridge or an implant.

The most common cause of pulpitis is tooth decay; the second most common cause is injury. Mild inflammation, if relieved, may not damage the tooth permanently. Severe inflammation may cause the pulp to die.

Symptoms and Diagnosis

Pulpitis can cause intense tooth pain. To determine if the pulp is healthy enough to save, a dentist can perform certain tests. For example, a dentist can apply a hot or cold stimulus. If pain persists after the stimulus is removed or if pain occurs spontaneously, the pulp may not be healthy enough to save.

A dentist may also use an electric pulp tester, which indicates whether the pulp is alive but not whether it is healthy. If the person feels the small electrical charge delivered to the tooth, the pulp is alive. Sensitivity to tapping on a tooth often means that inflammation has spread to the surrounding tissues.

Treatment

The inflammation stops when the cause is treated. When pulpitis is detected early, a temporary filling containing a sedative can eliminate the pain. This filling can be left in place for 6 to 8 weeks and then replaced with a permanent filling. Often a permanent filling can be put in immediately.

When pulp damage is extensive and cannot be reversed, the only way a dentist can stop the pain is by removing the pulp by root canal treatment or tooth extraction.

Periapical Abscess

A periapical abscess is a collection of pus, usually from an infection that has spread from a tooth to the surrounding tissues.

The body attacks an infection with large numbers of white blood cells; pus is the accumulation of these white blood cells, dead tissue, and bacteria. Usually, pus from a tooth infection drains into the gums first, so the gums swell near the root of the tooth. Depending on the location of the tooth, the pus may drain into soft tissues (cellulitis), causing swelling in the jaw, or drain to the floor of the mouth, in the area of the cheeks, or even to the skin.

A dentist treats an abscess or cellulitis by eliminating the infection and draining the pus, which requires oral surgery or root canal treatment. Dentists often prescribe antibiotics to help eliminate the infection, but removing the diseased pulp and draining the pus are more important.

Impacted Teeth

Impacted teeth are teeth that become stuck beneath the gum and are thus unable to emerge (erupt) properly.

Impaction is usually caused by the overcrowding of teeth, thus leaving insufficient room for a new tooth to emerge. Impaction can occur when a baby tooth is lost before the new tooth is ready to emerge, which allows the remaining teeth to drift into the space reserved for the new tooth. However, most teeth that become impacted are wisdom teeth because they are the last permanent teeth to come in and the jaw lacks enough room to accommodate them.

Impacted teeth are likely to become infected, thus they are usually removed. Often the removal can be done in the dentist's office with the person remaining awake, with use of a local anesthetic or with sedation to calm the person. Sometimes the surgery is performed in a hospital with the person asleep, with use of a general anesthetic.

Malocclusion

Malocclusion is an abnormal alignment of the upper and lower jaws that prevents the teeth from meeting properly.

Occlusion refers to the alignment of the teeth and the way in which the upper and lower teeth fit together. Ideally, the upper teeth fit slightly over the lower teeth. Proper alignment of teeth prevents undue force from being placed on just a few teeth and keeps the lips, cheeks, and tongue away from the biting surfaces. If the teeth are maloccluded (out of alignment), undue strain is placed on some of the teeth, which may fracture portions of the crown or loosen the teeth.

Causes

A common cause of malocclusion is disproportion between jaw size and tooth size or between the size of the upper and lower jaws. These differences can result in the overcrowding of teeth and in an abnormal bite. Another cause is loss of one or more teeth: When a tooth is lost, nearby teeth tend to drift into the newly available space, moving them out of alignment. Less common causes of malocclusion include misalignment of a jaw fracture, thumb sucking beyond the age of 4, tumors of the mouth or jaw, and improper fitting of crowns, fillings, retainers, or braces. Malocclusion may have a hereditary component.

Symptoms and Diagnosis

Malocclusion usually causes no symptoms at first. Eventually, though, it may result in a loosening or fracture of misaligned teeth because of the strain placed on them. Severe malocclusions may also cause difficulty or discomfort when biting or chewing, as well as speech difficulties. Malocclusions that prevent full access for proper oral hygiene may increase the risk of gum disease and cavities. Malocclusion can be diagnosed by the dentist during a dental examination.

Prevention and Treatment

After loss or removal of a tooth or teeth (for example, to make way for other permanent teeth), movement of remaining teeth can be prevented with braces or other orthodontic appliances. Once the teeth are properly aligned and the braces are removed, the person is usu-ally required to continue wearing a retainer at night for 2 to 3 years to maintain the position of the teeth.

Malocclusion can be corrected in a number of ways. Teeth can be realigned by applying a continuous mild force through the use of an orthodontic appliance, such as braces (wires and springs carried by brackets that are fixed to the teeth with dental adhesive) or a retainer (a removable brace combining wires and a plastic plate that snaps into the roof of the mouth). For some minor malocclusions, orthodontic therapy can be done with appliances that are barely visible. Occasionally, when an orthodontic appliance alone is not sufficient, jaw surgery may be necessary. Other methods of treating malocclusion include selective grinding of some teeth or building them up with the use of crowns or other dental restorations.

Periodontal Diseases

Periodontal diseases inflame and destroy the structures surrounding and supporting the teeth, primarily the gums, the jawbones, and the outer layer of the tooth root.

Periodontal diseases are caused mainly by accumulation of bacteria. They are more likely to occur in people with poor oral hygiene, in people who smoke, and in people with certain diseases and disorders, such as diabetes mellitus, poor nutrition, leukemia, and AIDS.

Gingivitis

Gingivitis is inflammation of the gums (gingiva).

Gingivitis is an extremely common disease in which the gums become red and swollen and bleed easily. Gingivitis causes little pain in its early stages and thus may not be noticed. However, gingivitis that is left untreated may progress to periodontitis, a more severe gum disease that can result in tooth loss.

Plaque-Induced Gingivitis

Inadequate brushing and flossing is by far the most common cause of gingivitis. Without proper brushing, plaque (a filmlike substance made up primarily of bacteria) remains along the gum line of the teeth. Plaque also accumulates in faulty fillings and around the teeth next to poorly cleaned partial dentures, bridges, and orthodontic appliances. When plaque stays on the teeth for more than 72 hours, it hardens into tartar (calculus), which cannot be completely removed by brushing and flossing.

The gums appear red rather than a healthy pink. They swell and become movable instead of being firm and tight against the teeth. The gums may bleed easily, especially while brushing or eating. In severe cases of plaque-induced gingivitis, the pillowcase may be bloodstained in the morning.

Plaque-induced gingivitis can be prevented with good oral hygiene—the daily use of a toothbrush and dental floss. Some mouthwashes also help control plaque. People who form a lot of tartar can use a tartar-control toothpaste that contains pyrophosphate. After tartar forms, it can only be removed by a dentist or dental hygienist. Depending on how fast tartar forms, a person may need professional cleanings every 3 to 12 months. People with poor oral hygiene, medical conditions that can lead to gingivitis, or a tendency to produce plaque may need professional cleanings more often. Because of their excellent blood supply, gums quickly become healthy again after tartar and plaque are removed, as long as the person brushes and flosses carefully.

Drug-Induced Gingivitis

Some drugs can cause an overgrowth of gum tissue, so that removing plaque becomes more difficult, and gingivitis often develops. Phenytoin (taken to control seizures), cyclosporine (taken by people who have had organ transplants), and calcium channel blockers such as nifedipine (taken to control blood pressure and heart rhythm abnormalities) can cause such an overgrowth. Also, oral or injectable contraceptives can aggravate gingivitis, as can exposure to lead or bismuth (which is used extensively in cosmetics) or to other heavy metals such as nickel (used in jewelry).

Medical conditions that might cause or worsen gingivitis should be treated or controlled. If a person must take a drug that causes gum tissue overgrowth, the excess gum tissue may need to be removed surgically. However, meticulous oral hygiene at home and frequent cleanings by a dentist or dental hygienist may slow the rate of tissue growth and eliminate the need for surgery.

Gingivitis due to Vitamin Deficiency

Vitamin deficiencies, in rare cases, can cause gingivitis. Vitamin C deficiency (scurvy) can lead to inflamed, bleeding gums. Niacin deficiency (pellagra) also causes inflamed, bleeding gums and a predisposition to certain mouth infections, such as thrush, or to inflammation of the tongue (glossitis).

Vitamin C and niacin supplements, together with a diet that includes more fresh fruits and vegetables, can be used to treat vitamin C and niacin deficiencies.

Gingivitis due to Infections

Viral infections can cause gingivitis. Acute herpetic gingivostomatitis is a painful viral infection of the gums and other parts of the mouth caused by the herpes virus.▲ The infection turns the gums bright red and causes many small white or yellow sores to form inside the mouth.

Acute herpetic gingivostomatitis usually gets better in 2 weeks without treatment. In-

tensive cleaning does not help, so a person should brush gently while the infection is still painful. A dentist may recommend an anesthetic mouth rinse to relieve discomfort while eating and drinking.

Fungal infections can cause gingivitis as well. Fungi commonly grow in the mouth in very small amounts. Use of antibiotics or a change in one's overall health can increase the number of fungi in the mouth. Thrush (candidiasis) is a fungal infection in which the overgrowth of fungi, particularly *Candida albicans*, forms a white film that irritates the gums. This film can also coat the tongue and corners of the mouth and leaves a bleeding surface if wiped away.■

Thrush can be treated with an antifungal drug, such as nystatin, in the form of a mouth rinse or a lozenge designed to dissolve slowly in the mouth. Good oral hygiene (proper brushing and flossing) and treatment of underlying dental problems, such as ill-fitting dentures, can also help. Dentures can be soaked overnight in nystatin solution as well.

Gingivitis due to Pregnancy

Pregnancy can worsen mild gingivitis, primarily because of hormonal changes. Some pregnant women may unknowingly contribute to the problem by neglecting oral hygiene because they feel nauseated in the morning (morning sickness). Also, during pregnancy, a minor irritation, often a buildup of tartar, may cause a lumplike overgrowth of gum tissue, called a pregnancy tumor. The bloated tissue bleeds easily if injured and may interfere with eating.

If a pregnant woman is neglecting oral hygiene because of morning sickness, a dentist can suggest ways to keep the teeth and gums clean without exacerbating the nausea. A bothersome pregnancy tumor can be surgically removed. However, such tumors tend to recur until, and even after, the pregnancy ends.

Gingivitis due to Menopause

Menopause can cause a condition called desquamative gingivitis, a poorly understood, painful condition that occurs most commonly in postmenopausal women. In this condition, the outer layers of the gums separate from the underlying tissue, exposing nerve endings. The gums become so loose that the outer layers can be rubbed away with a cotton swab or blown off with a dentist's air syringe.

If desquamative gingivitis develops during menopause, hormone replacement therapy

▲ see also page 668   ■ see also page 1150

may help. Otherwise, a dentist may prescribe corticosteroid tablets or a corticosteroid paste that is applied directly to the gums.

Gingivitis due to Leukemia

Leukemia can cause gingivitis. In fact, gingivitis is the first sign of disease in about 25% of children with leukemia. An infiltration of leukemia cells into the gums causes the gingivitis, and a reduced ability to fight infections worsens it. The gums appear red and bleed easily. Often, the bleeding continues for several minutes or more because blood does not clot normally in people with leukemia.

A person with gingivitis of leukemia can prevent bleeding by gently wiping the teeth and gums with a gauze pad or sponge instead of brushing and flossing. A dentist can prescribe chlorhexidine mouth rinse to control plaque and prevent mouth infections. When the leukemia is in remission (when evidence of the cancer disappears), good dental care can restore the gums to health.

Gingivitis due to an Impacted Tooth

Gingivitis can develop in the gums surrounding the crown of an impacted tooth (a tooth that has not fully emerged). In this condition, called pericoronitis, the gum swells over the tooth that has not fully emerged. The flap of gum over the partially emerged tooth can trap fluids, bits of food, and bacteria. Pericoronitis most commonly occurs with wisdom teeth, particularly the lower wisdom teeth. If the upper wisdom tooth emerges before the lower one, it may bite on this flap, increasing the irritation. Infections can develop and spread to the throat or cheek.

When a person has pericoronitis, a dentist may flush under the flap of gum to rinse out the debris and bacteria. If x-rays show that a lower tooth is not likely to emerge completely, a dentist may remove the upper tooth and prescribe antibiotics for a few days before removing the lower one. Sometimes a dentist removes the lower tooth immediately.

Periodontitis

Periodontitis (pyorrhea) is a severe form of gingivitis in which the inflammation of the gums extends to the supporting structures of the tooth.

Periodontitis is one of the main causes of tooth loss in adults and is the main cause in older people. Infection erodes the jawbone,

Periodontitis: From Plaque to Tooth Loss

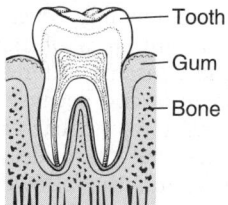

Healthy gums and bone hold the tooth firmly in place.

— Tooth
— Gum
— Bone

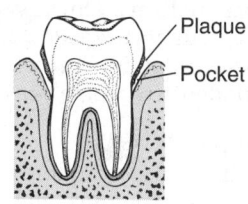

Plaque buildup irritates the gums, and they become inflamed. In time, the gums pull away from the tooth, creating a pocket that fills with more plaque.

— Plaque
— Pocket

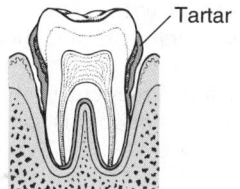

The pockets get deeper, and the plaque hardens into tartar. More plaque accumulates on top.

— Tartar

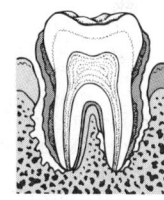

Tartar moves down to the root of the tooth and eventually destroys the bone supporting the tooth. Without this support, the tooth loosens and falls out.

which holds the teeth in place. The erosion weakens the attachments and loosens the teeth. An affected tooth may eventually fall out or need to be pulled out.

Causes

Most periodontitis results from a long-term accumulation of plaque and tartar between the teeth and the gums. Pockets form between the teeth and gums and extend downward between the root of the tooth and the underlying bone. These pockets collect plaque in an oxygen-free environment, which promotes the growth of aggressive forms of bacteria. If the disease continues, eventually so much jawbone near the pocket is destroyed that the tooth loosens and could fall out.

The rate at which periodontitis develops differs considerably, even among people with similar amounts of tartar. That is because plaque contains different types and numbers of bacteria and because people have different responses to the bacteria. Periodontitis may produce bursts of destructive activity that lasts for months followed by periods when the disease apparently causes no further damage.

Many diseases and disorders—including diabetes mellitus, Down syndrome, Crohn's disease, leukopenia, and AIDS—can predispose a person to periodontitis. In people with AIDS, periodontitis progresses quickly.

Symptoms

The early symptoms of periodontitis are bleeding, red gums, and bad breath (halitosis). Dentists measure the depth of the pockets in the gums with a thin probe, and x-rays show how much bone has been lost. As more and more bone is lost, the teeth loosen and shift position. Frequently, the front teeth tilt outward. Periodontitis usually does not cause pain until the teeth loosen enough to move while chewing or until an abscess (a collection of pus) forms.

Treatment

Unlike gingivitis, which usually disappears with good self-care, periodontitis requires repeat professional care. A person using good oral hygiene can clean only 2 to 3 millimeters ($\frac{1}{12}$ inch) below the gum line. A dentist can clean pockets up to 4 to 6 millimeters deep ($\frac{1}{5}$ inch) using scaling and root planing, which thoroughly remove tartar and the diseased root surface. For pockets of 5 millimeters ($\frac{1}{4}$ inch) or more, surgery is often required. A dentist or periodontist may access the tooth below the gum line surgically (periodontal flap surgery) to thoroughly clean the teeth and correct bone defects caused by the infection. A dentist or periodontist may also remove part of the infected and separated gum (a gingivectomy) so that the rest of the gum can reattach tightly to the teeth and the person can then remove the plaque at home.

A dentist may prescribe antibiotics (such as tetracyclines or metronidazole), especially if an abscess has developed. A dentist may also insert antibiotic-impregnated materials (filaments or gels) into deep gum pockets, so that

Understanding Halitosis

Halitosis (bad breath) can be real or imagined. When real, it is most often caused by a combination of food lodged between the teeth and poor oral hygiene that results in gum disease.

Odors from foods that contain volatile oils, such as onions and garlic, pass from the bloodstream into the lungs and are exhaled. Oral hygiene cannot remove these odors.

Certain diseases also produce bad breath. Liver failure gives the breath a mousy odor, kidney failure makes the breath smell like urine, and severe, uncontrolled diabetes makes the breath smell like nail polish remover (acetone). A lung abscess (a collection of pus) may cause very severe halitosis. Bad breath usually is not caused by problems in the intestine. However, a tumor in the esophagus or stomach may cause foul-smelling liquid or gas to be regurgitated into the mouth.

Halitosis that is imagined is called psychogenic halitosis, in which a person believes that his breath smells bad when it actually does not. This problem may occur in people who tend to exaggerate normal body sensations. Sometimes psychogenic halitosis is caused by a serious mental disorder, such as schizophrenia. A person with obsessional thoughts may have an overwhelming sense of feeling dirty. A person who is paranoid may have the delusion that his organs are rotting. Both may believe their breath smells bad.

Physical causes can be corrected or removed. For example, people can stop eating garlic, onions, and other spiced foods and can improve their oral hygiene. Daily use of a tongue scraper to clean the top and back of the tongue is effective. Many deodorant mouthwashes and sprays are available; one of the best active ingredients in these products is chlorophyll. The effects of most of these products, however, do not last more than a couple of hours.

Some people with psychogenic halitosis may be helped by having a doctor or dentist assure them that they do not have bad breath. If the problem continues, a person may benefit from seeing a psychotherapist.

high concentrations of the drug can reach the diseased area. Periodontal abscesses cause a burst of bone destruction, but immediate treatment with surgery and antibiotics may allow much of the damaged bone to grow back. If the mouth is sore after surgery, a chlorhexidine mouth rinse used for 1 minute twice a day may be temporarily substituted for brushing and flossing.

Trench Mouth

Trench mouth (Vincent's infection, acute necrotizing ulcerative gingivitis) is a painful, noncontagious infection of the gums, causing pain, fever, and sometimes fatigue.

The term trench mouth comes from World War I, when many soldiers in the trenches developed the infection. Trench mouth is now rare, although minor infection probably occurs relatively commonly. The severe form usually affects only people with an impaired immune system.

The infection is caused by an abnormal overgrowth of the bacteria that normally exist harmlessly in the mouth. Poor oral hygiene usually contributes to the development of trench mouth, as does physical or emotional stress, poor diet, and lack of sleep. The infection occurs most often in people who have gingivitis and experience a stressful event. Trench mouth is far more common among smokers than nonsmokers.

Usually, trench mouth begins abruptly with painful gums, an uneasy feeling, and fatigue. Foul breath also develops. The tips of the gums between the teeth erode and become covered with a gray layer of dead tissue. The gums bleed easily, and eating and swallowing cause pain. Often, the lymph nodes under the jaw swell, and a mild fever develops.

Treatment begins with a gentle, thorough cleaning. Rinsing several times a day with a hydrogen peroxide solution (3% hydrogen peroxide mixed half-and-half with water) may be recommended instead of brushing for the first few days because of the sensitivity of the gums. Antibiotics may be given for the first few days as well. The infection responds very well to good oral hygiene (daily brushing and flossing).

Gum Recession

Gum recession is the loss of gum tissue from the base of a tooth with exposure of the root surface.

Recession usually occurs in response to overaggressive brushing but can also result from injury or as the natural progression of thin, delicate gum tissue. Most people have some slight recession.

Recession may make the teeth very sensitive to cold, to sweet foods, or to touch. It may be accompanied by bone loss and may make the teeth more vulnerable to root cavities.

Treatment is needed when the gums or teeth are sensitive or when plaque accumulates and is difficult to remove. Treatment involves a grafting procedure, in which soft tissue is removed from the roof of the mouth or from donor tissues and stitched to the area.

CHAPTER 116

Temporomandibular Disorders

The temporomandibular joint is the connection between the temporal bone of the skull and the lower jawbone (mandible). There are two temporomandibular joints, one on each side of the face just in front of the ears. Ligaments, tendons, and muscles support the joints and are responsible for jaw movement.

The temporomandibular joint is one of the most complicated joints in the body: It opens and closes like a hinge and slides forward, backward, and from side to side. During chewing, it sustains an enormous amount of pressure. The temporomandibular joint contains a piece of special cartilage called a disk that

Locating the Temporomandibular Joint

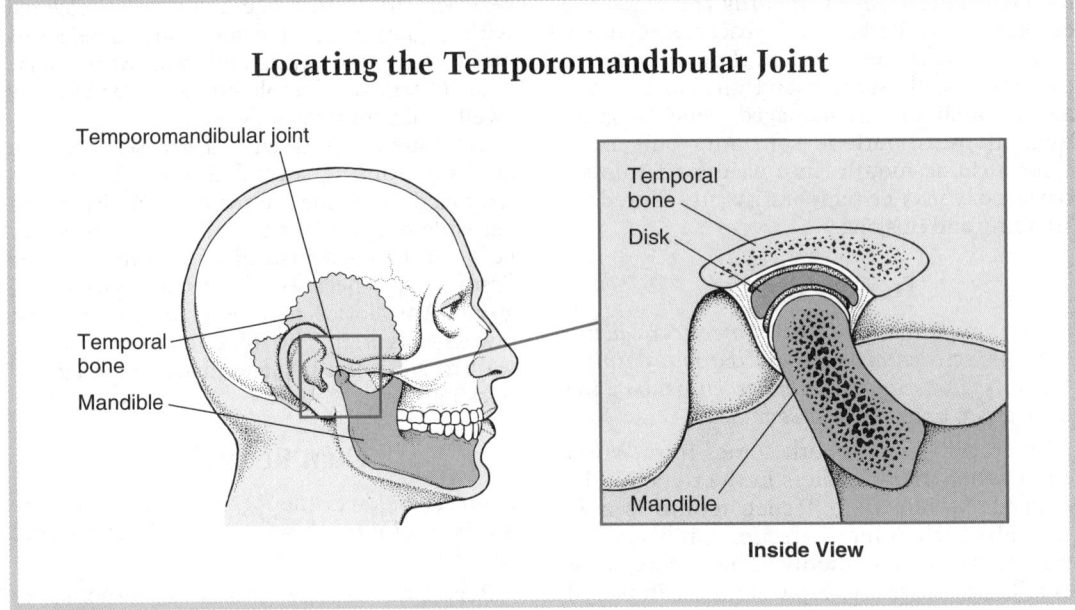

Inside View

keeps the skull and the lower jawbone from rubbing against each other.

Temporomandibular disorders, often called TMJ disorders (temporomandibular joint disorders), are most common in women in their early 20s and between the ages of 40 and 50 (in rare cases, babies are born with temporomandibular joint abnormalities). Temporomandibular disorders include problems with the joints, the muscles surrounding them, or both.

Causes

Most often, the cause of a temporomandibular disorder is a combination of muscle tension and anatomic problems within the joints. Sometimes, there is a psychologic component as well. Specific causes include muscle pain and tightness, internal joint derangement, arthritis, ankylosis, and hypermobility.

Muscle Pain and Tightness: Muscle pain and tightness around the jaw (myofascial pain syndrome) come mainly from muscle overuse, often brought on by problems of misalignment of the upper and lower sets of teeth, missing teeth, injury to the head or neck, or even toothache. Pain is also produced by trying to open the jaw too widely. Muscle pain and tightness can also result from clenching or

grinding the teeth (bruxism) at night due to psychologic or sleep-related stress. Clenching and grinding while asleep exert far more force than clenching and grinding while awake.

Internal Joint Derangement: In internal joint derangement, the disk inside the joint lies in front of its normal position. Internal joint derangement can occur with or without reduction. In internal joint derangement with reduction, which is the more common type (occurring in about one third of the adult population), the disk lies in front of its normal position only when the mouth is closed. As the mouth opens and the jaw slides forward, the disk slips back into its normal position. As the mouth closes, the disk slips forward again. In internal joint derangement without reduction, the disk never slips back into its normal position, and the degree to which the mouth can be opened is limited.

Arthritis: Arthritis in a temporomandibular joint may result from osteoarthritis, rheumatoid arthritis, infectious arthritis, or injury, particularly injury that causes bleeding into the joint. Such injuries are fairly common in children who are struck on the side of the chin.

Osteoarthritis, a type of arthritis in which the cartilage of the joints degenerates,▲ is most common in older people. The cartilage in the temporomandibular joints is not as

▲ see page 367

strong as the cartilage in other joints. Osteoarthritis occurs mainly when the disk is missing or has developed holes.

Rheumatoid arthritis, a disease in which the body attacks its own cells (an autoimmune disease), causing inflammation,▲ affects the temporomandibular joint in only about 17% of people with this type of arthritis. The temporomandibular joint generally is the last joint to be affected by rheumatoid arthritis.

Infectious arthritis is caused by an infection that has spread from an adjoining area of the head or neck or that has been carried by the bloodstream from another part of the body.■

Ankylosis: Ankylosis is loss of joint movement resulting from fusion of bones within the joint or calcification (the deposit of calcium into body tissues) of the ligaments around it.

Hypermobility: Hypermobility (looseness of the jaw) results when the ligaments that hold the joint together become stretched. In hypermobility, dislocation is usually caused by the shape of the joints, ligament looseness (laxity), and muscle tension. It may be caused by trying to open the mouth too wide or by being struck on the jaw.

Symptoms

Symptoms of temporomandibular disorders include headaches, tenderness of the chewing muscles, and clicking or locking of the joints. Sometimes the pain seems to occur near the joint rather than in it. Temporomandibular disorders may be the reason for recurring headaches that do not respond to usual medical treatment. Other symptoms include pain or stiffness in the neck radiating to the arms, dizziness, earaches or stuffiness in the ears, and disrupted sleep.

People with temporomandibular disorders have difficulty opening their mouth wide. For example, most people without temporomandibular disorders can place the tips of their index, middle, and ring fingers held vertically in the space between the upper and lower front teeth without forcing. For people with temporomandibular disorders (with the exception of hypermobility), this space usually is markedly smaller.

Muscle Pain and Tightness: People with muscle pain usually have very little pain in the joint itself. Rather, they feel pain and tightness on the sides of the face upon awakening or after stressful periods during the day. Nighttime clenching and grinding of the teeth may cause a person to awaken with a headache, which

may slowly diminish over the day. As the jaw opens, it may move slightly (deviate) to one side or the other. The chewing muscles are typically tender to the touch.

Internal Joint Derangement: Internal joint derangement with reduction usually causes a clicking or popping sound in the joint when the mouth opens wide or the jaw shifts from side to side. In many people, these joint sounds are the only symptoms. However, some people experience pain, particularly when chewing hard foods. In a small percentage of people who have missing teeth and who grind their teeth, these sounds progress to locking of the joints.

Internal joint derangement without reduction usually produces symptoms of pain and makes it difficult for people to open their mouth wide, as is typical of most temporomandibular disorders. After 6 to 12 months, the pain may decrease, but the limited degree to which the mouth can be opened generally persists.

Arthritis: With osteoarthritis, because it occurs mainly when the disk is missing or has developed holes, the person feels a grating sensation in the temporomandibular joints when opening and closing the mouth. When osteoarthritis is severe, the top of the jawbone flattens out, and the person cannot open the mouth wide. The jaw may also shift toward the affected side, and the person may be unable to move it back.

Rheumatoid arthritis usually affects both temporomandibular joints about equally, which is rarely the case in other types of temporomandibular disorders. When rheumatoid arthritis is severe, especially in young people, the top of the jawbone may degenerate and shorten. This damage can lead to sudden misalignment of many or all of the upper and lower teeth. If the damage is severe, the jawbone may eventually fuse to the skull (ankylosis).

Ankylosis: Typically, calcification (the deposit of calcium into body tissues) of the ligaments around the joint (extraarticular ankylosis) is not painful, but the mouth can open only about 1 inch or less. Fusion of bones within the joint (intraarticular ankylosis) causes pain and more severely limits jaw movement.

Hypermobility: In a person with hypermobility, the jaw may slip forward completely out of its socket (dislocate), causing pain and an inability to close the mouth. Dislocation may occur suddenly and repeatedly.

▲ see page 370   ■ see page 365

Diagnosis

A dentist or doctor almost always diagnoses a temporomandibular disorder based solely on a person's medical history and on a physical examination. Part of the examination involves gently pressing on the side of the face or placing the little finger in the person's ear and gently pressing forward while the person opens and closes the jaw. Also, the doctor gently presses on the chewing muscles to detect pain or tenderness and notes whether the jaw slides when the person bites.

When a doctor suspects internal joint derangement, further tests can be done. Magnetic resonance imaging (MRI) is now the gold standard with which doctors assess whether internal joint derangement has occurred or to find out why a person is not responding to treatment. Doctors occasionally use electromyography,▲ which analyzes muscle activity, to monitor treatment and, less commonly, to make a diagnosis. Laboratory tests are rarely useful.

A doctor suspects osteoarthritis when a creaking sound is heard when the person opens his mouth (crepitus). X-rays and a computed tomography (CT) scan can confirm the diagnosis. Infectious arthritis may be suspected when the area over and around the temporomandibular joint is inflamed and when movement of the joint is painful and limited. Infection in another part of the body serves as a clue as well. To confirm the diagnosis of infectious arthritis, the doctor may insert a needle into the temporomandibular joint and withdraw fluid (aspiration), which is then analyzed for bacteria.

If hypermobility is the cause, the person generally can open the mouth wider than the breadth of three fingers; the jaw may be chronically dislocated. If ankylosis is the cause, the jaw's range of motion tends to be markedly reduced.

Treatment

Treatment varies considerably according to the cause. Two common treatments are splint therapy and analgesics to relieve pain.

Muscle Pain and Tightness: Splint therapy usually is the main treatment for jaw muscle pain and tightness. For people who realize that they clench or grind their teeth, splint therapy can help them break the habit. A thin plastic splint is made to fit over either the upper or the lower set of teeth and is adjusted to give the

person an even bite. The splint, usually worn at night (a nightguard), reduces grinding, allowing the jaw muscles to rest and recover. For pain during the day, a splint allows the jaw muscles to remain relaxed and the bite to be stable, thereby reducing discomfort. The splint can also prevent damage to teeth that are under exceptional stress from the grinding. Day splints are worn only until symptoms subside, usually fewer than 8 weeks. Longer use may be warranted depending on the severity of symptoms.

Physical therapy may also be prescribed. Physical therapy may involve ultrasound treatment, electromyographic biofeedback (in which the person learns to relax the muscles), spray and stretch exercises (in which the jaw is stretched open with a passive jaw motion device after the skin over the painful area has been sprayed with a skin refrigerant or numbed with ice), or friction massage. Transcutaneous electrical nerve stimulation (TENS) also may help. Stress management, sometimes along with electromyographic biofeedback, often brings dramatic improvement.

Drug therapy may also be helpful. For instance, muscle-relaxing drugs, such as cyclobenzaprine, may be prescribed to ease tightness and pain, particularly while the person waits for a splint to be made. However, these drugs are not a cure, generally are not recommended for older people, and are prescribed for only a short time, usually for a month or less. Analgesics such as aspirin or other nonsteroidal anti-inflammatory drugs (NSAIDs) also relieve pain. A prescription for opioid analgesics is usually not given because treatment may be needed for some time and these drugs can be addictive. Sleep aids (sedatives) may be used occasionally and for a short time to help people who have trouble sleeping because of the pain.

Regardless of the type of treatment, most people experience significant relief within about 3 months. If the symptoms are not severe, many people recover without treatment within 2 to 3 years.

Internal Joint Derangement: In internal joint derangement with or without reduction, treatment is needed only if a person has jaw pain or trouble moving the jaw. If a person seeks treatment right after symptoms develop, a dentist or doctor may be able to manually move the disk back into its normal position. If a person has had the disorder for fewer than 3 months, a splint may be applied to hold the lower jaw forward. This splint keeps the disk in position, permitting the supporting liga-

▲ see page 446

ments to tighten. Over 2 to 4 months, the splint is adjusted to allow the jaw to return back to its normal position, with the expectation that the disk will remain in place.

A person with internal joint derangement with or without reduction should avoid opening the mouth wide—for instance, when yawning or biting into a thick sandwich—because injured joints are not as protected in these activities as would be a normal jaw. People with this disorder are advised to cut food into small pieces and to eat food that is easy to chew.

Sometimes the slipped disk becomes stuck in front of the temporomandibular joint, preventing the jaw from opening fully. The disk must then be manually moved out of position to allow the joint to move fully. Passive jaw motion devices, which stretch the jaw, have been used to slowly increase jaw motion. These devices are used several times a day. One such device is a threaded screw–type instrument that is placed between the front teeth and turned, much like a car jack, to gradually create a wider opening. If such a device is not available, then a doctor may use a stack of tongue depressors placed between the front teeth, with an additional tongue depressor being added to the middle of the stack.

If internal joint derangement cannot be treated by nonsurgical means, an oral-maxillofacial surgeon may need to reshape the disk and sew it back into place. However, the need for traditional surgery is relatively rare since the introduction of procedures such as arthroscopy.▲ All surgical procedures are used in combination with splint therapy.

Arthritis: A person with osteoarthritis in a temporomandibular joint needs to rest the jaw as much as possible, use a splint or other device to control muscle tightness, and take an analgesic (such as aspirin, acetaminophen, or another nonsteroidal anti-inflammatory drug) for pain. The pain usually goes away in 6 months with or without treatment. Even without treatment, most of the symptoms subside, probably because the band of tissue behind the disk becomes scarred and functions like the original disk. Usually, jaw movement is sufficient for normal activities, though the jaw may not open as wide as it used to.

Rheumatoid arthritis of the temporomandibular joint is treated with the drugs used for rheumatoid arthritis of any joint.■ Maintaining joint mobility and preventing fusion of the joint are particularly important. Usually, the best way to accomplish these goals is by exer-

Physical Therapy for Jaw Muscles

- Ultrasound is a method of delivering deep heat to painful areas. When warmed by the ultrasound, the blood vessels dilate, and the blood can more quickly carry away the accumulated lactic acid, a muscle waste product that may cause pain.

- Electromyographic biofeedback monitors muscle activity with a gauge. The person attempts to relax the entire body or a specific muscle while watching the gauge. In this way, the person learns to control or relax particular muscles.

- Spray and stretch exercises involve spraying a skin refrigerant over the cheek and temple, so the jaw muscles can be stretched.

- Friction massage consists of rubbing a rough towel over the cheek and temple to increase circulation and speed lactic acid removal.

- Transcutaneous electrical nerve stimulation (TENS) involves using a device that stimulates the nerve fibers that do not transmit pain. The resulting impulses are thought to block the painful impulses that the person has been feeling.

cising the jaw under a physical therapist's direction. To relieve symptoms, particularly muscle tightness, the person wears a splint at night that does not restrict jaw movement. If joint fusion freezes the jaw, the person may need surgery and, in rare cases, an artificial joint to restore jaw mobility.

Infectious arthritis is treated with antibiotics. Penicillin is usually the antibiotic used initially, until test results determine the type of bacteria present and thus the best antibiotic to use. Pus in the joint, if present, may be removed with a needle.

Ankylosis: Occasionally, stretching exercises help people with calcification, but people with calcification or bone fusion usually need surgery to restore jaw movement.

Hypermobility: Prevention and treatment of dislocation resulting from hypermobility are the same as those for other causes of a dislo-

▲ see page 343   ■ see table on page 372

cated jaw.▲ When dislocation occurs, a helper is sometimes needed to snap the jaw back into position. Many people who experience repeated dislocations, however, learn how to maneuver the joint back into place themselves by consciously relaxing the muscles and lightly shifting the lower jaw until it pops back into place. Surgery to tighten the ligaments of the temporomandibular joint is sometimes necessary to prevent recurrent dislocations.

CHAPTER 117

Urgent Dental Problems

Certain dental problems require prompt treatment to relieve discomfort and minimize damage to the structures of the mouth. Such urgent dental problems include toothaches; fractured, loosened, and knocked-out teeth; jaw fractures; a dislocated jaw; and certain complications that can develop after dental treatment.

Toothaches

Most toothaches result from cavities (caused by tooth decay). Some toothaches are caused by a tooth abscess or by inflammation of the gum around the crown of a tooth (pericoronitis). Much less commonly, toothaches result from inflammation of the nasal sinuses (sinusitis).

If several upper teeth hurt when a person is chewing or is bending down (for instance, to tie a shoe), the cause is probably sinusitis—especially if the toothache develops while the person has or recently has had a cold. Additional symptoms suggesting sinusitis are headache and tenderness and swelling of the skin above the affected sinus.

Fractured, Loosened, and Knocked-Out Teeth

A person who has brief, sharp pain while chewing or while eating something cold may have an incomplete (greenstick) fracture of a tooth. As long as the fracture is incomplete and part of the tooth has not split off, the dentist can correct the problem with a restoration.

The upper front teeth are prone to injury and fracture. If after an injury a tooth is not sensitive to air, most likely only the hard outer surface (enamel) has been harmed. Even if the enamel has sustained a small chip, immediate treatment is not required. Fractures of the intermediate layer of the tooth (dentin) are usually painful when exposed to air and food, so people with such fractures seek dental help quickly. If the fracture affects the innermost part of the tooth (pulp), a red spot and often some blood will appear in the fracture. Root canal treatment may be needed to remove the remaining pulp before it dies and causes severe pain.

If an injury loosens a tooth in the socket or if the surrounding gum tissue bleeds a great deal, a person should see a dentist immediately. Damaged baby (deciduous) teeth in the front of the mouth may be removed if the tooth is seriously loosened to prevent harm to the permanent teeth without losing space for those that are yet to come.

Knocked-out (avulsed) baby teeth should not be reimplanted for fear it will damage the permanent tooth bud. A knocked-out permanent tooth requires immediate treatment. The tooth should be rinsed off and placed back in its socket. If that is not possible, the tooth should be placed in a glass of milk (the milk provides a good medium for sustaining the tooth). In either case, the person and the tooth should be taken immediately to the nearest dentist.

If a tooth is reimplanted within 30 minutes, the likelihood that it will stay healthy is good. The longer the tooth is out of the socket, the worse the chance for long-term success. The dentist usually splints the tooth to the surrounding teeth for 7 to 10 days. Reimplanted teeth eventually need root canal treatment. If the bone around the tooth also has been fractured, the tooth may have to be splinted for 6 to 10 weeks.

▲ see page 691

Jaw Fracture

A fractured jaw causes pain and usually changes the way the teeth fit together. Often, the mouth cannot be opened wide, or it shifts to one side when opening or closing. Most jaw fractures occur in the lower jaw (mandible).

Fractures of the upper jaw (maxilla) may cause double vision (because the muscles of the eye attach nearby), numbness in the skin below the eye (because of injuries to nerves), or an irregularity in the cheekbone that can be felt when running a finger along it. Any injury forceful enough to fracture the jaw may also injure the spine in the neck. A blow powerful enough to fracture the jaw may also cause a concussion or bleeding within the skull.

If a person suspects a jaw fracture, the jaw should be held in place with the teeth together and immobile. The jaw may be held with a hand or preferably with a bandage wrapped under the jaw and over the top of the head several times (Barton's bandage). The person wrapping the bandage must be careful not to cut off breathing. Medical help should be sought as soon as possible because fractures can cause internal bleeding and airway obstruction.

At the hospital, before the jaw fracture is treated, neck x-rays are often taken to rule out spinal damage. The upper and lower jaws may be wired together; they remain wired for 6 weeks to allow the bone to heal. During this time, the person is able only to drink liquids through a straw. Many jaw fractures can be repaired surgically with a plate (a piece of metal that is screwed into the bone on each side of the fracture); the jaws are immobilized for only a few days, after which soft foods can be eaten for several weeks. In children, some jaw fractures are not immobilized. Instead, initial treatment allows restricted motion, and normal activity resumes in a few weeks. Antibiotics are usually given to a person with a compound fracture—one that extends through a tooth or its socket and opens to a contaminated area, such as the mouth.

Dislocated Jaw

A dislocated jaw (dislocated mandible) generally is very painful. The mouth usually cannot be closed, and the jaw may be twisted to one side. A dislocated jaw is typically caused by opening the mouth excessively wide or by an injury. Other causes include vomiting, yawning, looseness of the jaw (hypermobility), which

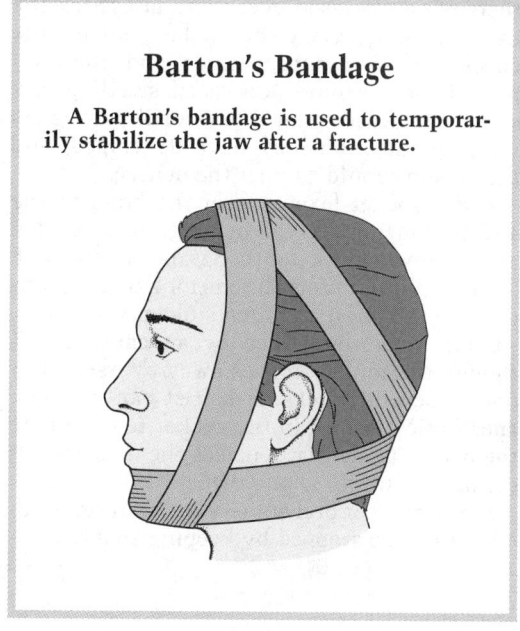

Barton's Bandage

A Barton's bandage is used to temporarily stabilize the jaw after a fracture.

often occurs due to a temporomandibular disorder,▲ and prolonged dental procedures.

The doctor typically maneuvers the jaw back into place (manual reduction). With his thumbs wrapped in gauze, the doctor places his thumbs on the gums next to the lower back teeth and presses downward and then slightly forward on the outer surface of the teeth. If necessary, he then exerts backward pressure.

Once the jaw is back in place, the person is told to avoid opening the mouth wide for at least 6 weeks. The person and his family usually can be taught how to repair the dislocation should it occur again. If the person has had more than one dislocation, surgery may be needed to reduce the risk of further dislocations. For instance, the ligaments connecting the jaw to the skull (at the temporomandibular joint) can be shortened, thereby tightening the joint.

Problems After Dental Treatment

Swelling is common after certain dental procedures, particularly tooth extractions and periodontal surgery. Holding an ice pack—or better yet, a plastic bag of frozen peas or corn (which adapts to facial contours)—to the cheek can prevent much of the swelling. Ice

▲ see page 685

therapy can be used every few hours for the first 18 hours. Cold should be held on the cheek for 25-minute periods and then removed for 5-minute periods. If swelling persists or increases after 3 days or if pain is severe, an infection may have developed, and the person should contact the dentist.

A dry socket (exposure of the bone in the socket, causing delayed healing) may develop after a lower back tooth has been removed. Typically, discomfort lessens for 2 or 3 days after the extraction and then suddenly worsens, sometimes accompanied by an earache. Although the condition goes away by itself after one to several weeks, a dentist can place an anesthetic dressing in the socket to eliminate the pain. The dentist replaces the dressing every day or two for about a week.

Bleeding after oral surgery is common. Usually, it can be stopped by keeping steady pressure on the surgical site for the first hour, normally by having the person bite down on a piece of gauze. Bleeding in the mouth can be deceptive because a small amount of blood may mix with saliva and appear worse than it is. If bleeding continues, the area can be wiped clean, and another piece of gauze or a moistened tea bag can be held against the area with steady biting pressure. If bleeding continues for more than a few hours, the dentist should be notified.

People who regularly take an anticoagulant (a drug that prevents clots) or aspirin (even if they only take one aspirin every few days) should mention it to the dentist a week before surgery, because these drugs increase the tendency to bleed. The dentist and the person's doctor may adjust the drug dosage or temporarily discontinue the drug.

DIGESTIVE DISORDERS

118 **Biology of the Digestive System** 694

Throat and Esophagus ▪ Stomach ▪ Small Intestine ▪
Pancreas ▪ Liver ▪ Gallbladder and Biliary Tract ▪ Large
Intestine ▪ Rectum and Anus ▪ Effects of Aging

119 **Symptoms and Diagnosis of Digestive Disorders** 699

Diarrhea ▪ Constipation ▪ Bleeding from the Digestive Tract ▪
Dyspepsia ▪ Regurgitation ▪ Difficulty Swallowing ▪ Globus
Sensation ▪ Abdominal Pain ▪ Chest or Back Pain ▪
Flatulence ▪ Loss of Appetite ▪ Nausea ▪ Vomiting ▪
Medical History and Physical Examination ▪ Psychologic
Evaluation ▪ Diagnostic Procedures

120 **Disorders of the Esophagus**...706

Obstruction of the Esophagus ▪ Abnormal Propulsion of Food ▪
Injury to the Esophagus

121 **Peptic Disorders** 711

Gastritis ▪ Peptic Ulcer ▪ Gastroesophageal Reflux

122 **Gastroenteritis**..719

Hemorrhagic Colitis ▪ Staphylococcal Food Poisoning ▪
Clostridium perfringens Food Poisoning ▪ Traveler's Diarrhea ▪
Chemical Food Poisoning

123 **Hiatus Hernia, Bezoars, and Foreign Bodies**..................................727

124 **Pancreatitis**...729

125 **Malabsorption** 734

Lactose Intolerance ▪ Celiac Disease ▪ Tropical Sprue ▪
Whipple's Disease ▪ Intestinal Lymphangiectasia

126 **Inflammatory Bowel Diseases** 738

Crohn's Disease ▪ Ulcerative Colitis ▪ Collagenous Colitis and
Lymphocytic Colitis ▪ Diversion Colitis

127 **Antibiotic-Associated Colitis** 745

128 **Diverticular Disease**...747

Diverticulosis ▪ Diverticulitis

129   **Bowel Movement Disorders**..750

Constipation ▪ Diarrhea ▪ Irritable Bowel Syndrome ▪ Fecal
Incontinence ▪ Flatulence

130   **Disorders of the Anus and Rectum**..759

Hemorrhoids ▪ Anal Fissure ▪ Anorectal Abscess ▪ Anorectal
Fistula ▪ Proctitis ▪ Pilonidal Disease ▪ Rectal Prolapse ▪
Anal Itching ▪ Foreign Objects

131   **Tumors of the Digestive System**..764

Noncancerous Tumors of the Esophagus ▪ Cancer of the
Esophagus ▪ Noncancerous Tumors of the Stomach ▪ Cancer
of the Stomach ▪ Noncancerous Tumors of the Small Intestine ▪
Cancer of the Small Intestine ▪ Polyps of the Large Intestine and
Rectum ▪ Colorectal Cancer ▪ Cancer of the Anus ▪ Cancer
of the Pancreas ▪ Other Tumors of the Pancreas

132   **Gastrointestinal Emergencies** 776

Gastrointestinal Bleeding ▪ Abdominal Abscesses ▪ Obstruction
of the Intestine ▪ Ileus ▪ Appendicitis ▪ Peritonitis ▪
Ischemic Colitis

CHAPTER 118

Biology of the Digestive System

The digestive system, which extends from the mouth to the anus, is responsible for receiving food, breaking it down into nutrients (a process called digestion), absorbing the nutrients into the bloodstream, and eliminating the undigestible parts of food from the body. The digestive tract consists of the mouth,▲ throat, esophagus, stomach, small intestine, large intestine, rectum, and anus. The digestive system also includes organs that lie outside the digestive tract: the pancreas, the liver, and the gallbladder.

The abdominal cavity is the space that holds the digestive organs. It is bordered by the abdominal wall (composed of layers of skin, fat, muscle, and connective tissue) in front, the spinal column in back, the diaphragm above, and the pelvic organs below. It is lined, as is the outer surface of the digestive organs, by a membrane called the peritoneum.

Experts have recognized a powerful connection between the digestive system and the brain. For example, psychologic factors greatly influence contractions of the intestine, secretion of digestive enzymes, and other functions of the digestive system. Even susceptibility to infection, which leads to various digestive system disorders, is strongly influenced by the brain. In turn, the digestive system influences the brain. For example, long-standing or recurring diseases such as irritable bowel syndrome, ulcerative colitis, and other painful diseases affect emotions, behaviors, and daily functioning. This two-way association has been called the brain-gut axis.

Throat and Esophagus

The throat (pharynx) lies behind and below the mouth. When food and fluids leave the mouth, they pass through the throat. Swallowing of food and fluids begins voluntarily and continues automatically. A small muscu-

▲ see page 661

Digestive System

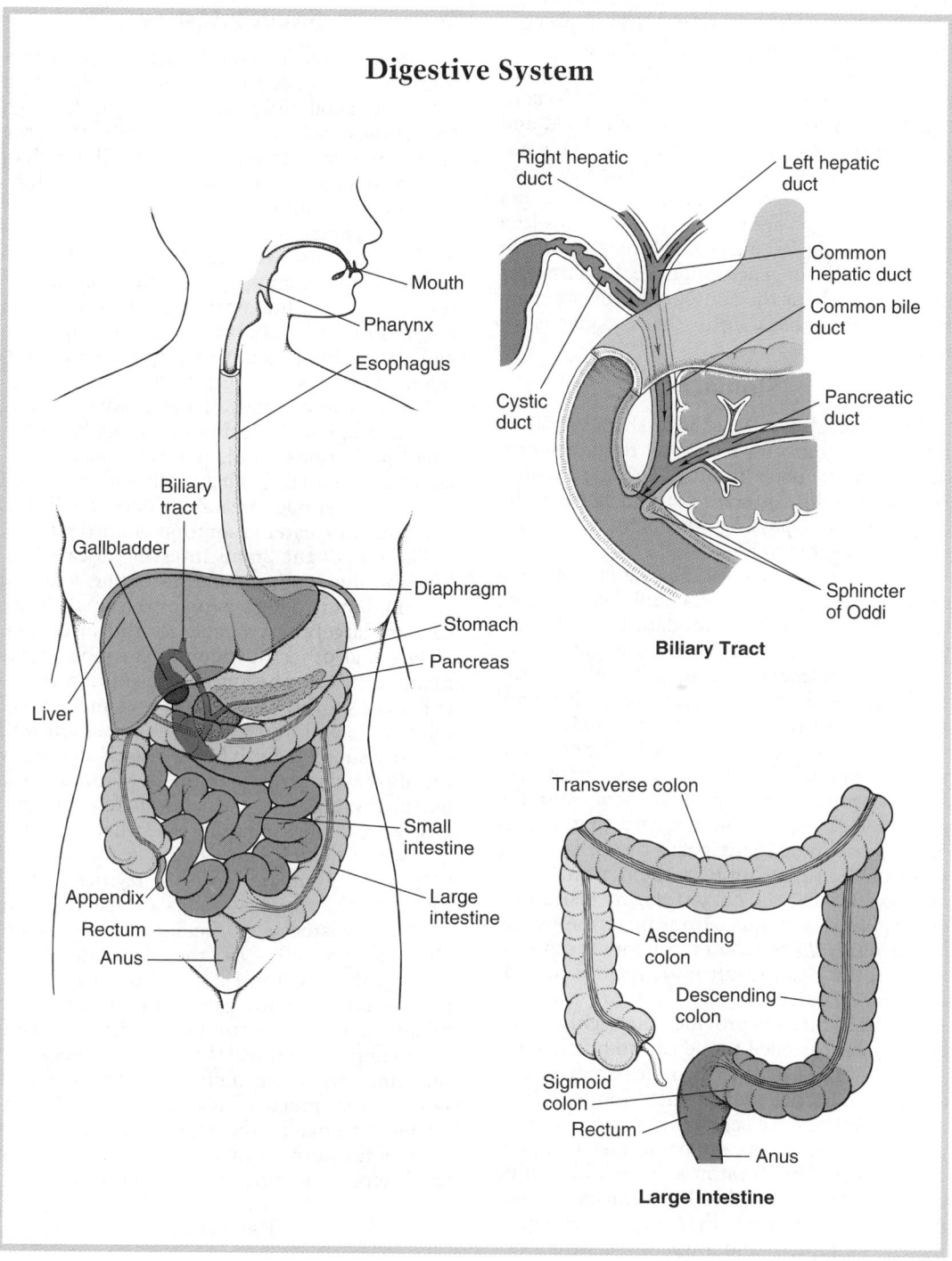

Mouth
Pharynx
Esophagus
Biliary tract
Gallbladder
Diaphragm
Stomach
Pancreas
Liver
Small intestine
Appendix
Large intestine
Rectum
Anus

Right hepatic duct
Left hepatic duct
Common hepatic duct
Common bile duct
Cystic duct
Pancreatic duct
Sphincter of Oddi

Biliary Tract

Transverse colon
Ascending colon
Descending colon
Sigmoid colon
Rectum
Anus

Large Intestine

lar flap (epiglottis) closes to prevent food and fluids from going down the windpipe (trachea) toward the lungs, and the back portion of the roof of the mouth (soft palate) lifts to prevent food and fluids from going up the nose.

The esophagus—a thin-walled, muscular channel lined with mucous membranes—connects the throat with the stomach. Food and fluids are propelled through the esophagus not by gravity but by waves of rhythmic muscular contractions, called peristalsis. At either end of the esophagus are ring-shaped muscles (the upper and lower esophageal sphincters), which open and close. The esophageal sphincters normally prevent the contents of the stomach from flowing back into the esophagus or throat.

Stomach

The stomach is a large, bean-shaped, hollow muscular organ consisting of three regions: the cardia, the body (fundus), and the antrum. Food and fluids enter the stomach from the esophagus by passing through the lower esophageal sphincter.

The upper stomach serves as a storage area for food. Here, the cardia and body of the stomach relax to accommodate food that enters the stomach. Then the antrum (lower stomach) contracts rhythmically, mixing the food with acid and enzymes (stomach juices) and grinding the food down into small pieces so that it is more easily digested. The cells lining the stomach secrete three important substances: mucus, hydrochloric acid, and the precursor of pepsin (an enzyme that breaks down proteins). Mucus coats the cells of the stomach lining to protect them from being damaged by acid and enzymes. Any disruption of this layer of mucus—from infection by the bacterium *Helicobacter pylori*, for example, or from aspirin—can result in damage that leads to a stomach ulcer.

Hydrochloric acid provides the highly acidic environment needed for pepsin to break down proteins. The stomach's high acidity also serves as a barrier against infection by killing most bacteria. Acid secretion is stimulated by nerve impulses to the stomach, gastrin (a hormone released by the stomach), and histamine (a substance released by the stomach). Pepsin is the only enzyme that digests collagen, which is a protein and a major constituent of meat.

Only a few substances, such as alcohol and aspirin, can be absorbed directly into the bloodstream from the stomach and only in small amounts.

Small Intestine

The stomach releases food into the duodenum, which is the first segment of the small intestine. Food enters the duodenum through the pyloric sphincter in amounts that the small intestine can digest. When full, the duodenum signals the stomach to stop emptying.

The duodenum receives pancreatic enzymes from the pancreas and bile from the liver and gallbladder. These fluids, which enter the duodenum through an opening called the sphincter of Oddi, are important in aiding digestion and absorption. Peristalsis also aids digestion and absorption by churning up food and mixing it with intestinal secretions.

The first few inches of the duodenal lining are smooth, but the rest of the lining has folds, small projections (villi), and even smaller projections (microvilli). These villi and microvilli increase the surface area of the duodenal lining, allowing for greater absorption of nutrients.

The rest of the small intestine, located below the duodenum, consists of the jejunum and the ileum. These parts of the small intestine are largely responsible for the absorption of fats and other nutrients. Churning movements facilitate absorption. Absorption is also enhanced by the vast surface area made up of folds, villi, and microvilli. The intestinal wall is richly supplied with blood vessels that carry the absorbed nutrients to the liver through the portal vein. The intestinal wall releases mucus, which lubricates the intestinal contents, and water, which helps dissolve the digested fragments. Small amounts of enzymes that digest proteins, sugars, and fats are also released.

The consistency of the intestinal contents changes gradually as the contents travel through the small intestine. In the duodenum, food is diluted with pancreatic enzymes and bile, which decrease stomach acidity. The contents continue to travel through the lower small intestine, becoming more liquid as they mix with water, mucus, bile, and pancreatic enzymes. Ultimately, the small intestine absorbs most of the nutrients and all but about 1 liter of fluid before emptying into the large intestine.

Pancreas

The pancreas is an organ that contains two basic types of tissue: the acini, which produce digestive enzymes, and the islets, which produce hormones. The pancreas secretes digestive enzymes into the duodenum and hormones into the bloodstream.

The digestive enzymes (such as amylase, lipase, and trypsin) are released from the cells of the acini and flow down various channels into the pancreatic duct. The pancreatic duct joins the common bile duct at the sphincter of Oddi, where both flow into the duodenum. The enzymes are secreted in an inactive form. They are activated only when they reach the digestive tract. Amylase digests carbohydrates; lipase digests fats; and trypsin digests proteins. The pancreas also secretes large amounts of sodium bicarbonate, which protects the duodenum by neutralizing the acid that comes from the stomach.

The three hormones produced by the pancreas are insulin, which lowers the level of sugar (glucose) in the blood by moving sugar into cells; glucagon, which raises the level of sugar in the blood by stimulating the liver to release its stores; and somatostatin, which prevents the other two hormones from being released.

Liver

The liver is a large organ with several functions,▲ only some of which are related to digestion.

The nutrients of food are absorbed into the intestinal wall, which is supplied with many tiny blood vessels (capillaries). These capillaries flow into veins that join larger veins and eventually enter the liver as the portal vein. This vein splits into tiny vessels inside the liver, where the incoming blood can be processed.

Blood in the liver is processed in two ways: Bacteria and other foreign particles absorbed from the intestine are removed, and many nutrients absorbed from the intestine are further broken down so they can be used by the body. The liver performs the necessary processing at high speed and passes the blood, laden with nutrients, into the general circulation.

The liver manufactures about half of the body's cholesterol; the rest comes from food. About 80% of the cholesterol made by the liver is used to make bile. The liver secretes bile, which is stored in the gallbladder until it is needed.

Gallbladder and Biliary Tract

Bile flows out of the liver through the right and left hepatic ducts,■ which come together to form the common hepatic duct. This duct then joins with a duct coming from the gallbladder, called the cystic duct, to form the common bile duct. The pancreatic duct joins the common bile duct just where it empties into the duodenum through the sphincter of Oddi.

Between meals, bile salts are stored in the gallbladder, and only a small amount of bile flows into the intestine. Food that enters the duodenum triggers a series of hormonal and nerve signals that cause the gallbladder to contract. As a result, bile flows into the duodenum and mixes with food contents.

Bile has two important functions: It assists in the digestion and absorption of fats, and it is responsible for the elimination of certain waste products from the body—particularly hemoglobin from destroyed red blood cells and excess cholesterol. Specifically, bile is responsible for these actions:

- Bile salts increase the solubility of cholesterol, fats, and fat-soluble vitamins to aid in their absorption.
- Bile salts stimulate the secretion of water by the large intestine to help move the contents along.
- Bilirubin (the main pigment in bile) is excreted in bile as a waste product of destroyed red blood cells, giving stool a green-brown color.
- Drugs and other waste products are excreted in bile and later eliminated from the body.
- Various proteins that play important roles in bile's absorptive function are secreted in bile.

Bile salts are reabsorbed by the last portion of the small intestine, extracted by the liver, and resecreted into bile. This recirculation of bile salts is known as the enterohepatic circulation. All the bile salts in the body circulate about 10 to 12 times a day. During each pass, small amounts of bile salts reach the large intestine, where bacteria break them down into various constituents. Some constituents are reabsorbed; the rest are excreted with the stool.

Large Intestine

The large intestine consists of the cecum and ascending (right) colon, the transverse colon, the descending (left) colon, and the sigmoid colon, which is connected to the rectum. The cecum, which is at the beginning of the

▲ see also page 786   ■ see also page 786

ascending colon, is the point at which the small intestine joins the large intestine. Projecting from the cecum is the appendix, which is a small finger-shaped tube that serves no known function. The large intestine secretes mucus and is largely responsible for the absorption of water from the stool.

Intestinal contents are liquid when they reach the large intestine but are normally solid by the time they reach the rectum as stool. The many bacteria that inhabit the large intestine can further digest some material, creating gas. Bacteria in the large intestine also make some important substances, such as vitamin K, which plays an important role in blood clotting. These bacteria are necessary for healthy intestinal function, and some diseases and antibiotics can upset the balance among the different types of bacteria in the large intestine. The result is irritation that leads to the secretion of mucus and water, causing diarrhea.

Rectum and Anus

The rectum is a chamber that begins at the end of the large intestine, immediately following the sigmoid colon, and ends at the anus. Ordinarily, the rectum is empty because stool is stored higher in the descending colon. Eventually, the descending colon becomes full, and stool passes into the rectum, causing an urge to move the bowels (defecate). Adults and older children can withstand this urge until they reach a bathroom. Infants and young children lack the muscle control necessary to delay bowel movement.

The anus is the opening at the far end of the digestive tract through which stool leaves the body. The anus is formed partly from the surface layers of the body, including the skin, and partly from the intestine. The anus is lined with a continuation of the external skin. A muscular ring (anal sphincter) keeps the anus closed until the person has a bowel movement.

Effects of Aging

Because the digestive system has a lot of reserve built into it, aging has relatively little effect on its function compared to its effects on other organ systems. Nonetheless, aging is a factor in several digestive system disorders. In

▲ see page 788

particular, older adults are more likely to develop diverticulosis and to experience digestive tract disorders (for example, constipation) as a side effect of taking certain drugs.

Esophagus: With age, the strength of esophageal contractions and the tension in the upper esophageal sphincter decrease, but the movement of food is not impaired by these changes. However, many older adults are likely to be affected by diseases that interfere with esophageal contractions.

Stomach: With age, the stomach lining's capacity to resist damage decreases, which in turn may increase the risk of peptic ulcer disease, especially in people who use aspirin and other nonsteroidal anti-inflammatory drugs (NSAIDs). Also with age, the stomach cannot accommodate as much food (because of decreased elasticity), and the rate at which the stomach empties food into the small intestine decreases, but these changes generally do not produce any noticeable symptoms. Aging has little effect on the secretion of stomach juices such as acid and pepsin, but conditions that decrease acid secretion, such as atrophic gastritis, become more common.

Small Intestine: Aging has only minor effects on the structure of the small intestine, so movement of contents through the small intestine and absorption of most nutrients do not change much. However, lactase levels decrease, leading to intolerance of dairy products by many older adults (lactose intolerance). Excessive growth of certain bacteria (bacterial overgrowth) becomes more common with age and can lead to weight loss. Bacterial overgrowth may lead to decreased absorption of certain nutrients, such as folic acid, iron, and calcium.

Pancreas, Liver, and Gallbladder: With age, the pancreas decreases in overall weight, and some tissue is replaced by scarring (fibrosis). However, these changes do not decrease the ability of the pancreas to produce digestive enzymes and sodium bicarbonate. As the liver and gallbladder age, a number of structural and microscopic changes occur.▲

Large Intestine and Rectum: The large intestine does not undergo much change with age. The rectum does enlarge somewhat. Constipation becomes more common. This may be due partly to a slight slowing in the movement of contents through the large intestine and a modest decrease in the contractions of the rectum when filled with stool.

CHAPTER 119

Symptoms and Diagnosis of Digestive Disorders

Disorders that affect the digestive (gastrointestinal) system are called digestive disorders. Some disorders simultaneously affect several parts of the digestive system, whereas others affect only one part or organ.

Symptoms

Some symptoms, such as diarrhea, constipation, bleeding from the digestive tract, regurgitation, and difficulty swallowing, usually suggest a digestive disorder. More general symptoms, such as abdominal pain, flatulence, loss of appetite, and nausea, may suggest a digestive disorder or another type of disorder.

Indigestion is an imprecise term that is used by different people to mean different things. The term covers a wide range of digestive tract problems, including dyspepsia, nausea and vomiting, regurgitation, and the sensation of having a lump in the throat (globus sensation).

Diarrhea

Diarrhea is the passing of frequent, loose stools. The consistency of the stool can be anything from soft and pasty to watery. The color can range from brown to clear. Black stools may indicate bleeding in the digestive tract. When a black color is caused by blood, the stools are usually tarry and foul-smelling (melena).

Cramping may occur before and with a bowel movement, and sometimes large amounts of gas are passed with the stool. Some people experience nausea, especially if the diarrhea is caused by an infectious organism or a toxic substance.

Constipation

Constipation is infrequent passage of bowel movements. A person with constipation often or always has hard stools that may be difficult to pass. The person also may feel as though the rectum has not been completely emptied.

Constipation can cause abdominal pain if the person strains during a bowel movement; in some people, the pain persists between movements. Constipation can cause nausea and curb appetite. Fecal impaction, in which the stool in the last part of the large intestine and the rectum hardens and blocks the flow from higher in the intestine, sometimes develops in people with severe constipation. Fecal impaction leads to cramps and rectal pain. Often, watery mucus oozes around the blockage, sometimes leading a person to conclude incorrectly that the problem is diarrhea and not constipation.

Constipation can result when the transit of stool through the large intestine is slowed by disease or certain drugs. Sometimes constipation is caused by dehydration or a low-fiber diet. Pain and psychologic conditions such as depression may also contribute to constipation. In many cases, however, the cause of constipation is unknown.

Bleeding from the Digestive Tract

Bleeding may occur anywhere along the digestive tract, from the mouth to the anus. Blood may be visible in vomit (hematemesis). When blood is vomited, it may be bright red if bleeding is brisk and ongoing. Alternatively, vomited blood may have the appearance of coffee grounds if bleeding has slowed or stopped, due to the partial digestion of the blood by acid in the stomach.

Blood may also be passed from the rectum, either as black tarry stools (melena) or as bright red blood (hematochezia). Melena is more likely when bleeding comes from the esophagus, stomach, or small intestine. The black color of melena results from blood that has been exposed for several hours to stomach acid and enzymes and to bacteria that normally reside in the large intestine. Hematochezia is more likely when bleeding comes from the large intestine, although it can result from very rapid bleeding from the upper portions of the digestive tract as well.

Bleeding from the digestive tract can have many causes, including peptic ulcers; abnormal connections between the arteries and veins of the intestines (arteriovenous malformations); dilated veins in the esophagus (esophageal varices); irritation from use of certain drugs, such as aspirin and other nonsteroidal anti-inflammatory drugs (NSAIDs); inflammatory bowel disease; and cancer of the digestive system.

Serious and sudden blood loss may be accompanied by a rapid pulse rate, low blood pressure, and reduced urine flow. A person may also have cold, clammy hands and feet. The decreased flow of blood to the brain that can occur with severe bleeding of the digestive tract may lead to confusion, disorientation, sleepiness, and even extremely low blood pressure (shock).

Dyspepsia

Dyspepsia is pain or discomfort in the middle of the upper abdomen often described as a gnawing or burning pain. Dyspepsia has many causes, including stomach ulcers, duodenal ulcers, and stomach cancer. Stomach inflammation (gastritis) may also cause dyspepsia. *Helicobacter pylori* bacteria may contribute to dyspepsia when they cause inflammation and ulcers of the stomach and duodenum (the first segment of the small intestine). Gallstones, when present in the tubes (ducts) that drain bile from the gallbladder, sometimes produce dyspepsia. Some drugs, especially aspirin and other nonsteroidal anti-inflammatory drugs (NSAIDs) cause symptoms. In many people, however, no abnormality can be found (functional dyspepsia), and symptoms are linked to increased sensitivity in the stomach or increased contractions (spasms).

Anxiety can cause or worsen dyspepsia—possibly because anxiety can increase a person's perception of unpleasant sensations, so that minor discomfort becomes very distressing. Sometimes, anxiety may worsen the abnormal stomach sensitivity and contractions or cause a person to sigh or gasp and swallow air (aerophagia).

The pain or discomfort in the upper abdomen varies in intensity and quality. Most people describe it as burning or gnawing. For some people, eating makes the pain worse; for others, eating relieves the pain. Other symptoms may include a poor appetite, nausea, constipation, diarrhea, flatulence, belching, and loud intestinal sounds (borborygmi).

Regurgitation

Regurgitation is the spitting up of food from the esophagus or stomach without nausea or forceful contractions of abdominal muscles. A ring-shaped muscle (sphincter) between the stomach and esophagus normally helps prevent regurgitation. Regurgitation of sour or bitter-tasting material can result from acid coming up from the stomach. Regurgitation of tasteless fluid containing mucus or undigested food can result from a narrowing (stricture) or a blockage of the esophagus. The blockage may result from acid damage to the esophagus, cancer of the esophagus, or abnormal nerve control that interferes with coordination between the esophagus and its sphincter at the opening to the stomach.

Regurgitation sometimes occurs with no apparent physical cause. Such regurgitation is called rumination. In rumination, small amounts of food are regurgitated from the stomach, usually 15 to 30 minutes after eating. The material often passes all the way to the mouth where a person may chew it again and reswallow it. Rumination occurs without pain or difficulty in swallowing. Rumination is common in infants. In adults, rumination most often occurs among people who have emotional disorders, especially during periods of stress.

Difficulty Swallowing

Difficulty swallowing (dysphagia) is the sensation that food is not moving normally from the throat to the stomach or that it has become stuck on the way down. A swallowing difficulty can result from impediments to the movement of liquids and solids by mechanical blockage of the throat, esophagus, and nearby organs, as is the case with esophageal cancer. A swallowing difficulty can also be caused by problems in the nervous system or muscles. Finally, a swallowing difficulty may be imagined (psychogenic).

Globus Sensation

Globus sensation (previously called globus hystericus) is the sensation of having a lump in the throat when there is no lump. Globus sensation may result from abnormal muscle activity or sensitivity of the esophagus. It sometimes occurs when stomach acid and enzymes flow backward from the stomach into the esophagus (gastroesophageal reflux). Globus sensation also may occur with frequent swallowing and drying of the throat brought on by anxiety or another strong emotion or by rapid breathing.

The feeling produced by globus sensation is similar to that experienced when feeling all choked up, such as during events that trigger grief, anxiety, anger, pride, or happiness.

Abdominal Pain

Abdominal pain can be an indication of problems in the digestive tract or elsewhere in the abdomen. Elderly people tend to have less abdominal pain than younger adults, and the pain develops more gradually. Abdominal pain also affects children.

Pain can arise from any of several causes, including infection, inflammation, formation of sores (ulcers), perforation or rupture of organs, muscle contractions that are uncoordinated or blocked by an obstruction, and lack of oxygen needed by digestive tract muscles.

Examples of disorders that result in abdominal pain include a perforated stomach ulcer, irritable bowel syndrome, infection and inflammation of the appendix (appendicitis) or pancreas (pancreatitis), and cancer. Some of these disorders are relatively minor; others may be life threatening.

Characteristics of abdominal pain vary depending on the cause of the pain. For example, pain that accompanies irritable bowel syndrome is often described as a dull aching or cramping, whereas pain produced by a peptic ulcer is often characterized as burning. The description of the pain's location may vary, from a vague sense of being present everywhere to being felt in one specific spot. For example, pain that accompanies diverticulitis is often limited to the lower left portion of the abdomen, whereas pain caused by inflammation of the lining of the abdominal cavity (peritonitis) is frequently felt throughout the abdomen.

Abdominal pain may be affected by a change in position or by functions such as eating or having a bowel movement. For example, inflammation of the pancreas (pancreatitis) often produces pain that is worsened by rolling over in bed and is relieved somewhat by sitting upright and leaning forward.

Chest or Back Pain

Chest or back pain that occurs as soon as a person swallows food or liquid may resemble the pain of heart disease; both are often perceived as a burning sensation or a tightness under the breastbone (sternum). Alternatively, the chest pain associated with esophageal disorders may be perceived as severe squeezing that occurs along with difficulty swallowing hot or cold beverages. This type of pain may result from esophageal muscle disorders, damage to the inner lining (mucosa) of the esophagus, infections (bacterial, viral, or fungal) of the throat, or tumors.

Flatulence

Flatulence is the presence of a large amount of gas in the digestive tract. Excess gas is expelled through the mouth (belching) or through the anus (flatulence), or it is absorbed through the walls of the digestive tract into the blood and then excreted by the lungs. Bacteria in the digestive system also break down (metabolize) some gases into a simpler, more easily excreted form.

Air is a gas that can be swallowed while eating (aerophagia). Swallowing small amounts of air is normal, but some people unconsciously swallow large amounts. Most swallowed air is later belched up, so only some of this air moves from the stomach into the rest of the digestive system. If large amounts of air are swallowed, the person may belch excessively or pass the air through the anus.

Other gases are produced in the digestive system by several means. Hydrogen, methane, and carbon dioxide are produced as bacteria break down and process food in the intestine (bacterial metabolism). People who have deficiencies of the enzymes that break down certain sugars, such as the sugar found in milk (lactose), also tend to produce large amounts of gas when they eat foods containing the sugars. Almost anyone who eats large amounts of proteins or fruits will develop some degree of flatulence.

Flatulence is often accompanied by abdominal pain and bloating. Some people are particularly sensitive to the effects of gas in the digestive system; others can tolerate large amounts without developing pain or bloating.

Loss of Appetite

Loss of appetite (anorexia) can result from many different digestive disorders. Anorexia implies that hunger is absent; a person with anorexia has no desire to eat. Anorexia can result from inflammation or infection of the digestive tract in disorders such as gastritis and gastroenteritis. Anorexia can occur when the digestive tract is obstructed. Cancer can also cause anorexia.

Diseases affecting other parts of the body can also cause or contribute to anorexia. Disorders that affect the part of the brain where appetite is regulated can cause anorexia as well.

Nausea

Nausea is an unpleasant feeling that may include dizziness, vague discomfort in the abdomen, an unwillingness to eat, and a feeling that the person will vomit. Nausea results when the vomiting center in the brain is activated. Nausea commonly occurs with any dysfunction of the digestive tract. Some people become nauseated from the movement of a boat, car, or airplane. Nausea may also occur during pregnancy, particularly in the early weeks and especially in the morning. Many drugs, including opioid analgesics, such as morphine, and chemotherapy drugs can cause nausea.

Vomiting

Vomiting is the forceful contraction of the stomach that propels its contents up the esophagus and out through the mouth. Vomiting usually occurs with nausea and can be caused by any of the conditions that cause nausea. Vomiting serves to empty the stomach of its contents and often makes a person with nausea feel considerably better, at least temporarily.

An obstruction of the intestine eventually causes vomiting, because food and fluids back up into the stomach from the blockage. Also, irritation or inflammation of the stomach, small intestine, or gallbladder can cause vomiting. Psychologic problems also can cause nausea and vomiting (functional, or psychogenic, vomiting). Such vomiting may be intentional—for instance, a person with bulimia vomits to lose weight. Or it may be unintentional—a conditioned response to address psychologic distress, such as to avoid going to school.

Vomitus—the material that is vomited up—can look like almost anything, usually reflecting what was recently eaten. Sometimes it contains chunks of food. When blood is vomited, the vomitus is usually bright red (hematemesis). When bile is present, the vomitus is green.

Even normal vomiting can be violent. A person who is vomiting typically doubles over and makes considerable noise during the process. Severe vomiting can project food many feet (projectile vomiting). Vomiting greatly increases pressure within the esophagus, and severe vomiting can tear the lining of the esophagus. People who are unconscious can inhale their vomitus. The acidic contents of the vomitus can severely irritate the lungs.

Diagnosis

Usually, a doctor can determine whether a person has a digestive disorder on the basis of

a medical history and a physical examination. The doctor can then select appropriate diagnostic procedures that help to confirm the diagnosis, determine the extent and severity of the disorder, and aid in planning treatment.

MEDICAL HISTORY AND PHYSICAL EXAMINATION

A doctor identifies symptoms by interviewing a person to obtain the medical history. The person is encouraged to describe symptoms in his own terms. The doctor can then ask specific questions to gain additional information. For example, in speaking with a person with abdominal pain, the doctor might first ask, "What is the pain like?". This question might be followed by questions like, "Does the pain get better after you eat?" or "Does the pain get worse when you bend over?".

During the physical examination, the doctor notes the person's weight and overall appearance, which may be indicators of digestive disorders. Although the doctor may examine the entire body, emphasis is placed on examining the abdomen, anus, and rectum.

First, the doctor observes the abdomen from different angles, looking for expansion (distension) of the abdominal wall that might accompany abnormal growth or enlargement of a particular part of the digestive tract. A stethoscope is placed on the abdomen, through which the doctor listens for sounds that normally accompany the movement of material through the intestines and for any abnormal sounds. The doctor feels for tenderness and any abnormal masses or enlarged organs. Pain that is caused by gentle pressure on the abdomen and that is relieved when the pressure is released (rebound tenderness) usually indicates inflammation and sometimes infection of the lining of the abdominal cavity (peritonitis).

The anus and rectum are examined with a gloved finger, and a small sample of stool is sometimes tested for hidden (occult) blood. In women, a pelvic examination often helps distinguish digestive problems from gynecologic ones.

PSYCHOLOGIC EVALUATION

Because the digestive system and the brain are so highly interactive,▲ psychologic evaluation is sometimes needed in the evaluation of digestive problems. In such cases, doctors are not implying that the digestive problems are imagined or made up. Rather, they may be the result of anxiety, depression, or other treatable mental

---

▲ see page 694

disorders, as appears to be true for as many as 50% of people with a digestive disorder.

DIAGNOSTIC PROCEDURES

On the basis of the findings of the medical history, physical examination, and, if applicable, psychologic evaluation, doctors choose the appropriate diagnostic tests. Tests performed on the digestive system make use of endoscopes (flexible tubes that doctors use to view internal structures and to obtain tissue samples from inside the body), x-rays, ultrasound scans, tiny amounts of radioactive materials, and chemical measurements. These tests can help a doctor locate, diagnose, and sometimes treat a problem. Some tests require the digestive system to be cleared of stool, some require 8 to 12 hours of fasting, and others do not require any preparation at all.

Although diagnostic tests can be very accurate, they can also be quite expensive and, in rare cases, can pierce (perforate) the digestive tract or cause bleeding or injury.

Endoscopy

Endoscopy is an examination of internal structures using a flexible viewing tube (endoscope). When passed through the mouth, an endoscope can be used to examine the esophagus (esophagoscopy), the stomach (gastroscopy), and most of the small intestine (upper gastrointestinal endoscopy). When passed through the anus, an endoscope can be used to examine the rectum (anoscopy); the lower portion of the large intestine, the rectum, and the anus (sigmoidoscopy); and the entire large intestine, the rectum, and the anus (colonoscopy). For procedures other than anoscopy and sigmoidoscopy, the person is given medication intravenously to prevent discomfort.

Endoscopes range in diameter from about $\frac{1}{4}$ inch to about $\frac{1}{2}$ inch and range in length from about 1 foot to about 5 feet. The choice of endoscope depends on which part of the digestive tract is to be examined. The endoscope is flexible and provides both a lighting source and a small camera, which allows doctors to get a good view of the lining of the digestive tract. The doctor can see areas of irritation, ulcers, inflammation, and abnormal tissue growth.

Many endoscopes are equipped with a small clipper with which tissue samples can be taken. These samples can then be evaluated for evidence of inflammation, infection, or cancer. Because the lining and the inner layers of the walls of the digestive tract do not have nerves

that sense pain (with the exception of the lower part of the anus), this procedure is painless.

Endoscopes can also be used for treatment. A doctor can pass different types of instruments through a small channel in the endoscope. An electric probe at the tip of the endoscope can be used to destroy abnormal tissue, to remove small growths, or to close off a blood vessel. A needle at the tip of the endoscope can be used to inject drugs into dilated veins in the esophagus and stop their bleeding.

Before having an endoscope passed through the mouth, a person usually must avoid food for several hours. Food in the stomach can obstruct the doctor's view and might be vomited up during the procedure. Before having an endoscope passed into the rectum and colon, a person usually takes laxatives and is sometimes given enemas to clear out any stool. In addition, the person must avoid food for several hours before the procedure because it might be vomited up and because it would reduce the effectiveness of the laxatives and enemas.

Complications from endoscopy are relatively rare. Although endoscopes can injure or even perforate the digestive tract, they more commonly cause only irritation of the digestive tract lining and a little bleeding.

Laparoscopy

Laparoscopy is an examination of the abdominal cavity using an endoscope. Laparoscopy is usually performed with the person under general anesthesia. After the appropriate area of the skin is washed with an antiseptic, a small incision is made, usually in the navel. Then an endoscope is passed into the abdominal cavity. A doctor can look for tumors or other abnormalities, examine virtually any organ in the abdominal cavity, obtain tissue samples, and even do reparative surgery. Complications include bleeding, infection, and perforation of the digestive tract.

X-ray Studies

X-rays often are used to evaluate digestive problems. Standard x-rays of the abdomen do not require any special preparation. These x-rays generally are used to show an obstruction or paralysis of the digestive tract or abnormal air patterns in the abdominal cavity. Standard x-rays can also show enlargement of the liver, kidneys, and spleen.

Barium studies often provide more information. X-rays are taken after a person swallows barium in a flavored liquid mixture or as bar-

Viewing the Digestive Tract With an Endoscope

A flexible tube called an endoscope is used to view different parts of the digestive tract. The tube contains several channels along its length. The different channels are used to transmit light to the area being examined, to view the area through a camera lens (with a camera at the tip of the tube), to pump fluids or air in or out, and to pass biopsy or surgical instruments through. When passed through the mouth, an endoscope can be used to examine the esophagus, the stomach, and some of the small intestine. When passed through the anus, an endoscope can be used to examine the rectum and the entire large intestine. The instrument used in the different procedures varies only in length and size of the tube.

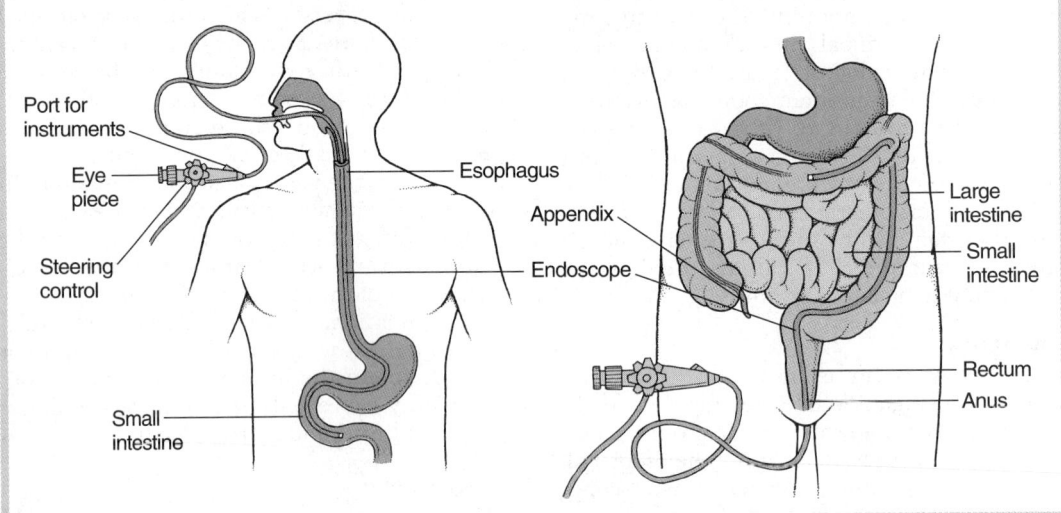

ium-coated food. The barium looks white on x-rays and outlines the digestive tract, showing the contours and lining of the esophagus, stomach, and small intestine. Barium collects in abnormal areas, showing ulcers, tumors, obstructions, erosions, and enlarged, dilated esophageal veins.

X-rays may be taken at intervals to determine where the barium is. Or, in a continuous x-ray technique called fluoroscopy, the barium is observed as it moves through the digestive tract. With this technique, doctors can see how the esophagus and stomach function, determine if their contractions are normal, and tell whether food is getting blocked in the digestive tract. The doctor may film this process for later review.

Barium also can be given in an enema to outline the lower part of the large intestine. Then, x-rays can show polyps, tumors, or other structural abnormalities. This procedure may cause crampy pain, producing slight to moderate discomfort.

Barium taken by mouth or given as an enema is eventually excreted in the stool, making the stool chalky white. Because barium can cause significant constipation, the doctor tries to make sure the barium is eliminated quickly after the studies. A gentle laxative can speed up the elimination of barium.

Ultrasound Scanning

Ultrasound scanning uses sound waves to produce pictures of internal organs. The examiner (a doctor or technician) usually performs an ultrasound scan by pressing a small probe against the person's abdominal wall. Sound waves are directed to various parts of the abdomen by moving the probe. The pictures are then displayed on a video screen and recorded on video film. An ultrasound scan can show the size and shape of many organs, such as the liver and pancreas, and can also show abnormal areas within them. It can show the presence of fluid as well. Ultrasound scanning with a probe on the abdominal wall is not a good method for examining the lining of the digestive tract, so it is less commonly used to look for tumors and causes of bleeding in the stomach, small intestine, or large intestine. Endoscopic ultrasound, a newer procedure, shows the lining of the digestive tract more clearly because the probe is placed on the tip of an endoscope.

An ultrasound scan is painless and poses no risk of complications. Endoscopic ultrasound poses the same risk of complications as endoscopy.

Computed Tomography and Magnetic Resonance Imaging

Computed tomography (CT) and magnetic resonance imaging (MRI) allow the doctor to view the abdomen at many different levels (cross-sections).

For either CT or MRI, the person is usually required to fast on the morning of the test. A radiopaque dye, which is visible on x-rays, is given intravenously before CT scanning; a paramagnetic contrast agent is given intravenously before an MRI. The person lies either on a table or in a tube-shaped device, and the machine slowly passes over the areas of interest.

In a CT scan, the machine gives off x-rays. In an MRI scan, the responses of the body's tissues to being in a magnetic field allow the machine to develop images of the underlying organs. Both of these tests require the person to lie still during the imaging process and may involve lying in a tube-like structure. People with fear of being in enclosed spaces (claustrophobia) may have difficulty with the test, although open scanners are becoming increasingly available. Also, some people may have a reaction to the dye used for the scan, including hives, shortness of breath, and rarely, dangerous lowering of the blood pressure.

CT and MRI scans are good for looking at the size and location of abdominal organs. Additionally, growths such as cancerous (malignant) or noncancerous (benign) tumors are often detected by these tests. Changes in the path or size of blood vessels can be detected as well. Inflammation, such as of the appendix (appendicitis) or diverticula (diverticulitis), is usually evident. Sometimes, these tests are used to help guide radiologic or surgical procedures.

Paracentesis

Paracentesis is the insertion of a needle into the abdominal cavity and the removal of fluid. Normally, the abdominal cavity outside of the digestive tract contains only a small amount of fluid. However, fluid can accumulate in certain circumstances, such as when a person has liver disease, heart failure, a ruptured stomach or intestine, cancer, or a ruptured spleen. A doctor may use paracentesis to aid in diagnosing a condition (for example, to obtain a fluid sample for analysis) or as part of treatment (for example, to remove excess fluid).

Before paracentesis, a physical examination, sometimes accompanied by an ultrasound scan, is performed to confirm that the abdominal cavity contains excess fluid. Next, an area of the skin, generally just below the navel, is washed with an antiseptic solution and numbed with a small amount of anesthetic. A doctor then pushes a needle attached to a syringe through the skin and muscles of the abdominal wall and into the area of fluid accumulation. A small amount of fluid may be removed for laboratory testing, or up to several quarts may be removed to relieve distention. Complications include perforation of the digestive tract and bleeding.

Occult Blood Tests

Bleeding in the digestive system can be caused by something as insignificant as a little irritation or as serious as cancer. When bleeding is profuse, a person can vomit blood (hematemesis), pass bright red blood in the stool (hematochezia), or pass black, tarry stool (melena). Amounts of blood too small to be seen or to change the appearance of stool can be detected chemically, and the detection of such small amounts may provide early clues to the presence of ulcers, cancers, and other abnormalities.

During a rectal examination, the doctor obtains a small amount of stool on a gloved finger. This sample is placed on a piece of filter paper impregnated with a chemical (guaiac). After another chemical is added, the color of the sample will change if blood is present. Alternatively, the person can take home a kit containing the impregnated filter papers. The person places samples of stool from about three different bowel movements on the filter papers, which are then mailed in special containers back to the doctor for testing. If blood is detected, further examinations are needed to determine the source.

Intubation of the Digestive Tract

Intubation of the digestive tract is the process of passing a small, flexible plastic tube through the nose or mouth into the stomach or small intestine. This procedure may be used for diagnostic or treatment purposes. Intubation may cause gagging and nausea in some people. The tube size varies according to the purpose.

Nasogastric intubation (passage of a tube through the nose into the stomach) can be used to obtain a sample of stomach fluid. The tube is passed through the nose rather than through the mouth, primarily because the tube can be more easily guided to the esophagus by this route. Also, passage of a tube through the nose is less irritating and is less likely to trigger coughing. By inserting a nasogastric tube, doctors can determine whether the stomach contains blood, or they can analyze the stomach's secretions for acidity, enzymes, and other characteristics. In poisoning victims, samples of the stomach fluid can be analyzed to identify the poison. In some cases, the tube is left in place, so that more samples can be obtained over several hours.

Nasogastric intubation may also be used to treat certain conditions. For example, poisons can be pumped out or neutralized with activated charcoal, or liquid food can be administered to people who cannot swallow.

Sometimes nasogastric intubation is used to continuously remove the contents of the stomach. The end of the tube is usually attached to a suction device, which removes gas and fluid from the stomach. This helps relieve pressure when the digestive system is blocked or otherwise not functioning properly. This type of tube is often used after abdominal surgery until the digestive system can resume its normal function.

In nasoenteric intubation, a longer tube is passed through the nose, through the stomach, and into the small intestine. This procedure can be used to remove a sample of intestinal contents, continuously remove fluids, or provide food.

Manometry

Manometry is a test in which a tube with pressure gauges along its surface is placed in the esophagus. Using this device (manometer), a doctor can determine whether contractions of the esophagus can propel food normally. Sometimes a doctor uses a similar device to measure pressure in the large intestine to determine the adequacy of muscle contractions, which are needed to move stool forward and to eventually result in a bowel movement.

An esophageal pH test (a test that measures acidity in the esophagus) can be performed during esophageal manometry. The test is used to determine if a person has backflow of stomach acid into the esophagus (gastroesophageal reflux). One or more measurements may be taken.

CHAPTER 120

Disorders of the Esophagus

The esophagus is the hollow tube that leads from the throat (pharynx) to the stomach. The walls of the esophagus propel food to the stomach not by gravity, but by rhythmic waves of muscular contractions called peristalsis.

Just below the junction of the throat and the esophagus is a band of muscle called the upper esophageal sphincter. Slightly above the junction of the esophagus and the stomach is another band of muscle called the lower esophageal sphincter. When the esophagus is not in use, these sphincters contract so that food and stomach acid do not flow up from the stomach to the mouth. During swallowing, the sphincters relax so food can pass to the stomach.

With age, the strength of esophageal contractions and the tension in the sphincters decrease. This condition, called presbyesophagus, makes older people more prone to backflow of acid from the stomach (gastroesophageal reflux), especially when lying down after eating.

Two of the most common symptoms of esophageal disorders are dysphagia (an awareness of difficulty in swallowing) and chest or back pain. Dysphagia and chest or back pain may occur in any esophageal disorder, the most serious of which is esophageal cancer.

The esophageal disorders discussed in this chapter are obstruction-related, propulsion-related, or injury-related. In another esophageal disorder, called esophageal varices, the veins at the lower end of the esophagus become dilated and twisted and bleed easily.▲

Obstruction of the Esophagus

The esophagus can be narrowed or completely blocked. In rare cases, the cause is hereditary (for example, congenital rings). In most cases, the cause is progression of an injury to the esophagus or tumor growth. Food and foreign bodies may obstruct the esophagus as well. Injuries that can progress to obstruction can result from damage caused by the repeated backflow of acid from the stomach (gastroesophageal reflux), usually over years. Injury can also result from damage caused by drugs taken in pill form or ingestion of corrosive substances.■ Narrowing may also be caused by compression against the outside of the esophagus. Compression can result from a number of causes, such as enlargement of the left atrium of the heart, an aortic aneurysm, an abnormally formed artery (dysphagia lusoria), an abnormal thyroid gland, a bony outgrowth from the spine, or cancer—most commonly lung cancer. Another serious cause of narrowing is noncancerous (benign) and cancerous (malignant) tumors of the esophagus.

Because all these conditions decrease the diameter of the esophagus, people with one of them usually have difficulty swallowing solid foods—particularly meat and bread. Difficulty in swallowing liquids develops much later, if at all.

A barium x-ray is usually taken to find the cause and location of the narrowing or obstruction. Treatment and outcome depend on the cause.

LOWER ESOPHAGEAL RING

A lower esophageal ring (Schatzki's ring), which results from chronic acid injury, narrows the lower esophagus.

Normally, the lower esophagus has a diameter of 1½ to 2 inches. However, it may be narrowed to ½ inch or less by a ring of tight tissue, which may cause difficulty in swallowing solids. This symptom can begin at any age but usually does not begin until after age 25, because it takes time for acid injury to cause a ring to form. The swallowing difficulty comes and goes and is especially aggravated by meat and dry bread. Often, barium x-rays are taken to detect the problem.

How the Esophagus Works

As a person swallows, food moves from the mouth to the throat, also called the pharynx (1). The upper esophageal sphincter opens (2) so that food can enter the esophagus, where waves of muscular contractions, called peristalsis, propel the food downward (3). The food then passes through the lower esophageal sphincter (4) and moves into the stomach (5).

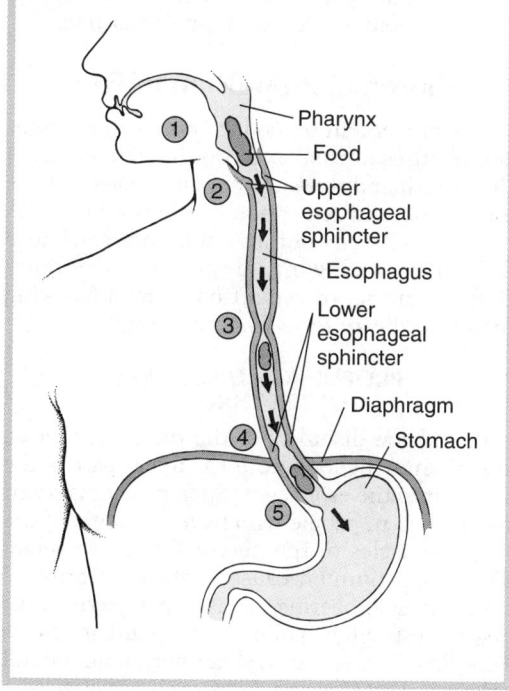

Chewing food thoroughly followed by sips of water usually prevents symptoms. A doctor may fix the narrowing by passing an endoscope (a flexible viewing tube with attachments) through the mouth and throat and into the esophagus or may use a dilator (called a bougie) to widen the passageway. In rare cases, the constricting ring is opened surgically.

ESOPHAGEAL WEBS

Esophageal webs (Plummer-Vinson syndrome, sideropenic dysphagia) are thin mem-

▲ see pages 776 and 794   ■ see page 710

branes that grow across the inside of the upper one third of the esophagus from its surface lining (mucosa).

Although rare, esophageal webs occur most often in people who have untreated severe iron deficiency anemia. The means by which anemia leads to the development of webs is unknown. Webs in the upper esophagus usually make swallowing solids difficult. A cineradiograph (an x-ray that produces a moving image as a person swallows barium) is usually the best procedure with which to diagnose the problem.

Once the iron deficiency has been treated, the web usually disappears. If not, a doctor can rupture it using a dilator or an endoscope.

Abnormal Propulsion of Food

The movement of food from mouth to stomach requires normal and coordinated action of the mouth and throat, propulsive waves of the esophagus, and relaxation of the sphincters. A problem with any of these functions can cause difficulty swallowing (dysphagia), regurgitation, vomiting, or aspiration of food (sucking food into the airways when inhaling).

PROPULSION DISORDERS OF THE THROAT

Propulsion disorders of the throat can cause trouble moving food from the upper part of the throat into the esophagus. Such problems occur most often in people who have disorders of the throat muscles or the nerves that serve them. The most common cause is stroke. Dermatomyositis, scleroderma, myasthenia gravis, muscular dystrophy, polio, pseudobulbar palsy, Parkinson's disease, and amyotrophic lateral sclerosis (Lou Gehrig's disease) all can affect the throat muscles or nerves. Difficulty swallowing may also result from the use of a phenothiazine (a class of antipsychotic drug), because these drugs can impair the normal function of the throat muscles. A person with a propulsion disorder of the throat often regurgitates food through the back of the nose or inhales it into the windpipe (trachea) and then coughs.

In cricopharyngeal incoordination, the upper esophageal sphincter (cricopharyngeal muscle) remains closed, or it opens in an uncoordinated way. An abnormally functioning sphincter may allow food to repeatedly enter the windpipe and lungs, which may lead to recurring lung infections and eventually to chronic lung disease. A surgeon can cut the sphincter so that it is permanently relaxed. If left untreated, the condition may lead to the formation of a diverticulum, a sac formed when the lining of the esophagus pushes outward and backward through the cricopharyngeal muscle.

ESOPHAGEAL SPASM

Esophageal spasm (rosary bead or corkscrew esophagus) is a disorder of the propulsive movements (peristalsis) of the esophagus caused by malfunctioning nerves.

In this disorder, the normal propulsive contractions that move food through the esophagus are replaced periodically by nonpropulsive contractions. In addition, in 30% of people with this disorder, the lower esophageal sphincter opens and closes abnormally.

Symptoms

Muscle spasms throughout the esophagus typically are felt as chest pain under the breastbone coinciding with difficulty in swallowing liquids (especially those that are very hot or cold) or solids. Pain also occurs at night and may be severe enough to awaken a person. Esophageal spasm also may produce severe pain without swallowing difficulty. This pain, often described as a squeezing pain under the breastbone, may accompany exercise or exertion, making it difficult for a doctor to distinguish it from angina (chest pain stemming from heart disease). Over many years, this disorder may evolve into achalasia, a disorder in which the rhythmic contractions of the esophagus are greatly decreased.

Diagnosis

X-rays taken while the person swallows a barium drink may show that food does not move normally down the esophagus and that contractions of the esophageal wall are uncoordinated and do not propel the food. Esophageal scintigraphy (an imaging test that shows the movement of food that has been labeled or tagged with a tiny amount of radioactive tracer) is used to detect abnormal movements of food through the esophagus. Pressure measurements by manometry (a test in which a tube placed in the esophagus measures the pressure of contractions)▲ provide the most sensitive and detailed analysis of the spasms. If these studies are inconclusive, a doctor may conduct manometry after the person eats a

▲ see page 706

meal or takes a drug called edrophonium to provoke the painful spasms.

Treatment

Esophageal spasm is often difficult to treat. Nitroglycerin, long-acting nitrates, anticholinergics such as dicyclomine, or calcium channel blockers such as nifedipine may relieve the symptoms by relaxing the muscles of the esophagus. Sometimes, strong analgesics are needed. In many cases, a narrowing is treated by inflating a balloon inside the esophagus or by inserting bougies (progressively larger dilators) to dilate the esophagus. In rare cases, a surgeon must cut the muscle layer along the full length of the esophagus if other less radical forms of treatment are not effective.

ACHALASIA

Achalasia (cardiospasm, esophageal aperistalsis, megaesophagus) is a disorder in which the rhythmic contractions of the esophagus are greatly decreased and the lower esophageal sphincter fails to relax normally.

Achalasia results from a malfunction of the nerves controlling the rhythmic contractions of the esophagus. The cause of the nerve malfunction is not known.

Symptoms

Achalasia may occur at any age but usually begins, almost unnoticed, between the ages of 20 and 60 and then progresses gradually over many months or years. The tight lower esophageal sphincter causes the part of the esophagus above it to enlarge greatly. This enlargement contributes to many of the symptoms. Difficulty swallowing both solids and liquids is the main symptom. Other symptoms may include chest pain, regurgitation of the bland, nonacidic contents of the enlarged esophagus, and coughing at night. Although uncommon, chest pain may occur during swallowing or for no apparent reason. About one third of people who have achalasia regurgitate undigested food while sleeping. They may inhale food into their lungs, which can cause coughing, a lung abscess, infection of the airways, bronchiectasis, or aspiration pneumonia.

Diagnosis

X-rays of the esophagus taken while the person is swallowing barium show an absence of peristalsis. The esophagus is widened, usually only moderately but occasionally to enormous proportions, but is narrow at the lower esophageal sphincter.

Esophagoscopy (an examination of the esophagus through a flexible viewing tube)▲ shows widening of the esophagus but no obvious obstruction. A doctor performs a biopsy (removal of tissue samples for examination under a microscope) to make sure the symptoms are not caused by cancer at the lower end of the esophagus.

Treatment

The aim of treatment is to relieve symptoms by getting the lower esophageal sphincter to open more easily. Nitrates (for example, nitroglycerin placed under the tongue before meals) or calcium channel blockers (for example, nifedipine) may delay the need for dilation by helping to relax the sphincter.

Dilation widens the sphincter mechanically—for example, by inflating a large balloon inside it. This procedure helps about 70% of the time, but repeated dilations may be needed. In fewer than 5% of people with achalasia, the esophagus ruptures during the dilation procedure. Esophageal rupture leads to inflammation of the surrounding tissue (mediastinitis) and in rare cases is fatal if not treated appropriately. Immediate surgery is needed to close the rupture in the wall of the esophagus.

As an alternative to mechanical dilation, a doctor may inject botulinum toxin into the lower esophageal sphincter. This newer therapy is as effective as mechanical dilation with balloons. Thus far, this method appears to be more successful in providing sustained symptom relief to older people than to younger people, but the long-term effects are not fully known.

If dilation or botulinum toxin therapy does not work, surgery to cut the muscular fibers in the lower esophageal sphincter (myotomy) is usually performed. Surgery can be done laparoscopically.■ This surgery is successful about 85% of the time. A procedure to prevent backflow of acid from the stomach (gastroesophageal reflux) is usually performed during the same surgery, but about 15% of people still experience episodic backflow of acid after surgery.

ESOPHAGEAL POUCHES

Esophageal pouches (diverticula) are abnormal protrusions from the esophagus that in rare cases cause swallowing difficulties.

▲ see page 703   ■ see page 703

There are three types of esophageal pouches: pharyngeal pouch or Zenker's diverticulum, midesophageal pouch or traction diverticulum, and epiphrenic pouch. Each has a different cause, but probably all are related to uncoordinated swallowing and muscle relaxation, as may occur in disorders such as esophageal spasm and achalasia.

A large pouch can fill with food that may be regurgitated later, when the person bends over or lies down. This may cause food to be inhaled into the lungs during sleep, resulting in aspiration pneumonia. Rarely, the pouch enlarges and causes swallowing difficulty.

A video x-ray or cineradiograph (an x-ray that produces a moving image as a person swallows barium) is used to diagnose a pouch.

Treatment is not usually needed. If symptoms are severe, however, the pouch can be removed surgically. When esophageal spasm or achalasia is present, treatment of sphincter tightness may be needed.

Injury to the Esophagus

The esophagus is relatively impervious to injury but can be harmed gradually by backflow of acid from the stomach (gastroesophageal reflux) or, more suddenly, by caustic or acidic chemicals, some irritating drugs, a sharp object, or extreme pressure. Extreme pressure can occur during violent vomiting.

The more sudden types of injuries can cause pain, often experienced as sharp pain under the breastbone, and bleeding, which may be vomited up or present in the stool. Fainting may occur, especially if the esophagus ruptures, allowing blood and food contents to spill into the mediastinum (the area of the chest bordered by the sternum in front, the spinal column in back, the entrance to the chest cavity above, and the diaphragm below).

EROSIVE ESOPHAGITIS

Erosive esophagitis is a condition in which areas of the esophageal lining are inflamed and worn away.

The most common cause of erosive esophagitis is chronic acid reflux. Corrosive substances, such as cleaning solutions, can erode the esophagus if they are swallowed accidentally or deliberately, as in a suicide attempt. Some pills (for example, aspirin or other nonsteroidal anti-inflammatory drugs [NSAIDs], alendronate, doxycycline, and certain large iron and potassium tablets) can cause painful erosions if they lodge temporarily in the esophagus.

Diagnosis of erosive esophagitis is made by esophagoscopy. If an erosion results from a pill, the pill usually can be washed down with large quantities of water; the pain often resolves within hours. Rarely, erosions caused by corrosive substances or pills persist, leading to narrowing of the esophagus.

ESOPHAGEAL LACERATION

An esophageal laceration is a tear that does not penetrate the wall of the esophagus.

A laceration of the lower esophagus and the upper part of the stomach during forceful vomiting, retching, or hiccups is called Mallory-Weiss syndrome. The first symptom is usually bleeding from a ruptured blood vessel in the esophagus. Mallory-Weiss syndrome is the cause of about 5% of bleeding episodes in the upper digestive tract.

Diagnosis is made by esophagoscopy or angiography. The laceration cannot be detected on routine x-rays.

Most bleeding episodes stop by themselves, but sometimes a surgeon must tie off the bleeding vessel. Bleeding may also be controlled by injecting vasopressin or epinephrine during arteriography to reduce blood flow into the bleeding vessel.

ESOPHAGEAL RUPTURES AND PERFORATIONS

Esophageal ruptures and perforations are tears that penetrate the wall of the esophagus; a perforation has defined borders, whereas a rupture does not.

Ruptures of the esophagus are usually caused by violent vomiting. Perforations can occur during endoscopy (examination of the esophagus with a flexible viewing tube)▲ or other procedures in which instruments are inserted through the mouth and throat. An esophageal rupture or perforation leads to tissue inflammation in the chest outside the esophagus and allows fluid to enter the space between the membrane layers (pleura) covering the lungs, a condition called pleural effusion.■ The risk of death is very high, especially with esophageal ruptures. Surgical repair of the esophagus and drainage of the area surrounding it are performed immediately.

▲ see page 703   ■ see page 314

CHAPTER 121

Peptic Disorders

Peptic disorders include gastritis, peptic ulcer, and gastroesophageal reflux. They involve damage to the lining of the esophagus, stomach, or duodenum (the first segment of the small intestine). These disorders are usually caused by stomach acids (especially hydrochloric acid), digestive enzymes (especially pepsin), infection with the bacterium *Helicobacter pylori*, and use of certain drugs, such as nonsteroidal anti-inflammatory drugs (NSAIDs).

Gastritis

Gastritis is inflammation of the stomach lining.

The stomach lining resists irritation and can usually withstand very strong acid. Nevertheless, in gastritis, the stomach lining becomes irritated and inflamed.

Causes

Gastritis can be caused by many factors, including infection, injury, and disorders of the immune system.

Gastritis may be caused by infections with bacteria, viruses, or fungi. Worldwide, the most common cause of gastritis is infection with *Helicobacter pylori* bacteria. Viral or fungal gastritis may develop in people with a prolonged illness or an impaired immune system, such as those with AIDS or cancer or those taking immunosuppressant drugs.

Erosive gastritis involves both inflammation and wearing away of the stomach lining. Erosive gastritis results from irritants such as drugs, especially aspirin and other NSAIDs; Crohn's disease; bacterial and viral infections; and the ingestion of corrosive substances. In some people, even a daily baby aspirin can injure the stomach lining. Erosive gastritis can develop suddenly but more commonly develops slowly, usually in people who are otherwise healthy.

Acute stress gastritis, actually a form of erosive gastritis, is caused by a sudden illness or injury. The injury may not even be to the stomach. For example, extensive skin burns and injuries involving major bleeding are typical causes. Exactly why serious illness can lead to gastritis is not known but may be related to decreased blood flow to the stomach or to impairment of the stomach lining's ability to protect and renew itself.

Radiation gastritis can occur if radiation is delivered to the lower left side of the chest or upper abdomen, where it can irritate the stomach lining.

Postgastrectomy gastritis occurs in people who have had part of their stomach surgically removed (a procedure called partial gastrectomy). The inflammation usually occurs where tissue has been sewn back together. Postgastrectomy gastritis is thought to result when surgery impairs blood flow to the stomach lining or exposes the stomach lining to an excessive amount of bile (the greenish yellow digestive fluid produced by the liver).

Atrophic gastritis occurs when antibodies▲ attack the stomach lining, causing it to become very thin and to lose many or all of the cells that produce acid and enzymes. This condition usually affects older people, particularly those who are chronically infected with *Helicobacter pylori* bacteria. It also tends to occur in those who have had part of their stomach removed.

Eosinophilic gastritis may result from an allergic reaction to an infestation with roundworms. In other cases, the cause is unknown. In this type of gastritis, eosinophils (a type of white blood cell) accumulate in the stomach wall.

Ménétrier's disease, whose cause is unknown, is a type of gastritis in which the stomach wall develops thick, large folds; enlarged glands; and fluid-filled cysts. The disease may be due to an abnormal immune reaction and has also been associated with *H. pylori* infection.

In plasma cell gastritis, plasma cells (a type of white blood cell) accumulate in the stomach wall and other organs. Why this happens is not known.

Symptoms and Complications

Gastritis usually causes no symptoms. When symptoms do occur, they vary depending on the cause and may include pain or dis-

▲ see page 1055

When the Stomach Is Infected

Infection with *Helicobacter pylori,* a type of bacteria, is the most common cause of gastritis worldwide. Infection with *H. pylori* is also one of the most common causes of peptic ulcer.

H. pylori bacteria grow in the protective mucus layer of the stomach lining, where they are less exposed to the highly acidic juices produced by the stomach. Virtually all people with *H. pylori* infection have gastritis, which may affect the entire stomach or only the lower part (antrum). Infection can sometimes lead to erosive gastritis. *H. pylori* contributes to ulcer formation by interfering with the normal defenses against stomach acid and by producing toxins. A small number of people develop other diseases that have been linked to long-standing *H. pylori* infection, such as stomach cancer.

Most people with gastritis from *H. pylori* infection do not develop symptoms, but people who do develop symptoms experience those typical of gastritis, such as indigestion and pain or discomfort of the upper abdomen. Ulcers from *H. pylori* infection cause symptoms similar to ulcers from other causes, including pain in the upper abdomen.

H. pylori can be detected with tests that use breath or stool samples. These tests identify only people with active *H. pylori* infection. A blood test to measure the level of antibodies to *H. pylori* is also available. However, antibody levels can remain detectable for years after the *H. pylori* infection has been eliminated.

H. pylori infection must be treated with antibiotics. The most popular treatment for *H. pylori* infection includes a proton pump inhibitor to reduce acid production along with two antibiotics, such as amoxicillin and clarithromycin given twice daily for 7 to 14 days. The combination of bismuth subsalicylate (a drug similar to sucralfate), tetracycline (an antibiotic), and metronidazole (an antibiotic) with a proton pump inhibitor is another popular option. However, this treatment entails taking four drugs up to 4 times a day for 7 to 14 days. The likelihood that a peptic ulcer will recur over 1 year goes from 60 to 80% in people not treated with antibiotics to less than 20% in people treated with antibiotics. In addition, treatment of *H. pylori* infection may heal ulcers that have resisted previous treatment.

comfort or nausea or vomiting, problems that are often simply referred to as indigestion. Gastritis can lead to ulcers, at which time the symptoms may get worse.

Nausea and intermittent vomiting can result from erosive gastritis, radiation gastritis, Ménétrier's disease, and plasma cell gastritis. Pain or discomfort (dyspepsia) can occur, especially with erosive gastritis, radiation gastritis, postgastrectomy gastritis, and atrophic gastritis. Very mild pain or discomfort also occurs with acute stress gastritis.

Ulcers can develop with several types of gastritis, especially acute stress gastritis, erosive gastritis, and radiation gastritis. Ulcers may bleed, causing a person to vomit blood (hematemesis) or pass tarry black stools (melena). Acute stress gastritis may lead to bleeding from ulcers within a few days after an illness or injury, whereas bleeding tends to develop more slowly in the case of erosive gastritis or radiation gastritis. Persistent bleeding can lead to symptoms of anemia, including fatigue, weakness, and light-headedness. If an ulcer perforates (pierces) the stomach wall, stomach contents may spill into the abdominal cavity, resulting in peritonitis (inflammation and usually infection of the lining of the abdominal cavity) and sudden worsening of pain.

Some complications of gastritis are slow to develop. The scarring and narrowing of the stomach outlet that can result from gastritis, especially from radiation gastritis and eosinophilic gastritis, can cause severe nausea and frequent vomiting. In Ménétrier's disease, fluid retention and swelling of the tissues (edema) may occur because of loss of protein from the inflamed stomach lining. About 10% of people with Ménétrier's disease develop stomach cancer some years later. Postgastrectomy gastritis and atrophic gastritis may cause symptoms of anemia, such as fatigue and weakness, because of decreased production of intrinsic factor (a protein that binds vitamin B_{12}, allowing the B_{12} to be absorbed and used in the production of red blood cells). A small percentage of people with atrophic gastritis develop a condition called metaplasia, in which cells lining the stomach change and become precancerous. In an even smaller percentage of people, metaplasia leads to stomach cancer.

Diagnosis

A doctor suspects gastritis when a person has upper abdominal discomfort or pain or nausea. Tests usually are not needed. However, if the doctor is uncertain of the diagnosis, or if symptoms do not resolve with treatment, an examination of the stomach using an endoscope (a flexible viewing tube)▲ may be needed. If necessary, the doctor can perform a biopsy (removal of a tissue sample for examination under a microscope) of the stomach lining.

Treatment

Regardless of the cause of gastritis, symptoms can be relieved with drugs that neutralize or reduce the production of stomach acid.■ For mild symptoms, taking antacids, which neutralize acid that has already been produced and released in the stomach, is often sufficient. However, antacids have to be taken several times a day and often produce diarrhea or constipation. Drugs that reduce acid production include histamine-2 (H_2) blockers and proton pump inhibitors. H_2 blockers are usually more effective than antacids in relieving symptoms, and many people find them far more convenient. Proton pump inhibitors are prescribed when the strongest treatment is needed. When infection is a part of gastritis, antibiotics are also prescribed. Doctors may prescribe sucralfate, which helps to prevent irritation. When gastritis leads to ulceration that perforates the stomach wall, immediate surgery is usually needed.

People with erosive gastritis must avoid taking drugs, such as NSAIDs, that irritate the stomach lining. Some doctors prescribe proton pump inhibitors or misoprostol to help protect the stomach lining. However, the coxibs (COX-2 inhibitors such as celecoxib and rofecoxib) are less likely to irritate the stomach lining than the older NSAIDs.

Most people with acute stress gastritis recover fully when the underlying illness, injury, or bleeding is controlled. However, 2% of people in intensive care units have heavy bleeding from acute stress gastritis, which is often fatal. Therefore, doctors try to prevent acute stress gastritis after a major illness, major injury, or severe burn. Drugs that reduce acid production are commonly given after surgery and in most intensive care units to prevent acute stress gastritis. These drugs are also used to treat any ulcers that form. For people with heavy bleeding from acute stress gastritis, a wide variety of treatments have

been used. Few of these treatments, however, improve the outcome. Blood transfusions may actually make bleeding worse. Bleeding points can be temporarily heat-sealed (cauterized) during an endoscopy, but bleeding often starts again if the underlying illness persists. If bleeding continues, the entire stomach may have to be removed as a lifesaving measure.

There is no cure for postgastrectomy gastritis or atrophic gastritis. People with anemia resulting from decreased absorption of vitamin B_{12} that occurs with atrophic gastritis must take supplemental injections of the vitamin for the rest of their lives.

Corticosteroids or surgery may be needed to relieve a blocked stomach outlet in eosinophilic gastritis. Removing part or all of the stomach may cure Ménétrier's disease. No drug treatment is effective.

Peptic Ulcer

A peptic ulcer is a round or oval sore where the lining of the stomach or duodenum has been eaten away by stomach acid and digestive juices.

Ulcers penetrate into the lining of the stomach or duodenum (the first part of the small intestine). Gastritis may develop into ulcers.

The names given to specific ulcers identify their anatomic locations or the circumstances under which they developed. Duodenal ulcers, the most common type of peptic ulcer, occur in the duodenum, the first few inches of the small intestine just below the stomach. Gastric ulcers, which are less common, usually occur along the upper curve of the stomach. Marginal ulcers can develop when part of the stomach has been removed surgically, at the point where the remaining stomach has been reconnected to the intestine. As with acute stress gastritis, stress ulcers can occur under the stress of severe illness, skin burns, or trauma. Stress ulcers occur in the stomach and the duodenum.

Causes

Ulcers develop when the lining of the stomach or duodenum is chronically inflamed or exposed to irritants, such as excess stomach acid, and digestive enzymes, such as pepsin.

Almost everyone produces stomach acid, but only 1 of 10 people develops ulcers at some

▲ see page 703   ■ see page 716

point during his or her lifetime. Different people generate different amounts of stomach acid, and a person's pattern of acid secretion tends to persist throughout life. People who normally secrete more acid (high secretors) have a greater tendency to develop peptic ulcers than those who secrete less acid (low secretors). However, other factors besides acid secretion are involved, because most people who are high secretors never develop ulcers, and some people who are low secretors do develop them. In addition, ulcers are common among older people, even though less acid is produced with age.

By far, the two most common causes of peptic ulcer are infection with *Helicobacter pylori* bacteria and use of certain drugs. Many drugs, especially aspirin, other nonsteroidal anti-inflammatory drugs (NSAIDs), and corticosteroids, irritate the stomach lining and can cause ulcers. However, most people who take NSAIDs or corticosteroids do not develop peptic ulcers. Regardless, some experts suggest that people at high risk of developing peptic ulcers should use a new type of NSAID called a coxib (COX-2 inhibitor) rather than one of the older types of NSAIDs, because coxibs are less likely to irritate the stomach.▲

People who smoke are more likely to develop a peptic ulcer than people who do not smoke, and their ulcers heal more slowly. Although psychologic stress can increase acid production, no link has been found between psychologic stress and peptic ulcers.

A rare cause of ulcers is cancer. The symptoms of cancerous ulcers are very similar to those of noncancerous ulcers. However, cancerous ulcers usually do not respond to the treatments used for noncancerous ulcers.

Symptoms

The typical ulcer tends to heal and recur; thus, pain may occur for days or weeks and then wane or disappear. Symptoms can vary with the location of the ulcer and the person's age. For example, children and older people may not have the usual symptoms or may have no symptoms at all. In these instances, ulcers are discovered only when complications develop.

Only about half of the people with duodenal ulcers have the typical symptoms of gnawing, burning, aching, soreness, an empty feeling, and hunger. The pain is steady and mild or moderately severe, and it is usually located just below the breastbone. For many people with a duodenal ulcer, pain is usually absent on awakening but appears by midmorning. Drinking milk or eating (which buffers stomach acid) or taking antacids generally relieves the pain, but it usually returns 2 or 3 hours later. Pain that awakens the person during the night is common. Frequently, the pain erupts once or more a day over a period of one to several weeks and then may disappear without treatment. However, pain usually recurs, often within the first 2 years and occasionally after several years. People generally develop patterns and often learn by experience when a recurrence is likely (commonly in spring and fall and during periods of stress).

The symptoms of gastric, marginal, and stress ulcers, unlike those of duodenal ulcers, do not follow any pattern. Eating may relieve pain temporarily or may cause pain rather than relieve it. Gastric ulcers sometimes cause swelling of the tissues (edema) that lead into the small intestine, which may prevent food from easily passing out of the stomach. This blockage may cause bloating, nausea, or vomiting after eating.

Complications of peptic ulcers, such as bleeding or rupture, are accompanied by symptoms of low blood pressure, such as dizziness and fainting.

Diagnosis

A doctor suspects an ulcer when a person has characteristic stomach pain. Sometimes the doctor simply treats the person for an ulcer to see if the symptoms resolve, which suggests that the person had an ulcer that has healed.

Tests may be needed to confirm the diagnosis, especially when symptoms do not resolve after a few weeks of treatment, because stomach cancer can cause similar symptoms. Also, when severe ulcers resist treatment, particularly if a person has several ulcers or the ulcers are in unusual places, a doctor may suspect an underlying condition that causes the stomach to overproduce acid.

To help diagnose ulcers and determine their cause, the doctor may use endoscopy (a procedure performed using a flexible viewing tube) or barium contrast x-rays (x-rays taken after a substance that outlines the digestive tract has been swallowed).

Endoscopy is usually the first diagnostic procedure ordered by a doctor. Endoscopy is more reliable than barium contrast x-rays for

▲ see page 454

What Are the Complications of Peptic Ulcers?

Most ulcers can be cured without complications. However, in some cases, peptic ulcers can develop potentially life-threatening complications, such as penetration, perforation, bleeding (hemorrhage), and obstruction.

Penetration

An ulcer can go through the muscular wall of the stomach or duodenum (the first segment of the small intestine) and continue into an adjacent organ, such as the liver or pancreas. This causes intense, piercing, persistent pain, which may be felt outside of the area involved—for example, the back may hurt when a duodenal ulcer penetrates the pancreas. The pain may intensify when the person changes position. If drugs do not heal the ulcer, surgery may be needed.

Perforation

Ulcers on the front surface of the duodenum, or less commonly the stomach, can go through the wall, creating an opening to the free space in the abdominal cavity. The resulting pain is sudden, intense, and steady. It rapidly spreads throughout the abdomen. The person may feel pain in one or both shoulders, which may intensify with deep breathing. Changing position worsens the pain, so the person often tries to lie very still. The abdomen is tender when touched, and the tenderness worsens if a doctor presses deeply and then suddenly releases the pressure. (Doctors call this rebound tenderness.) Symptoms may be less intense in older people, in people taking corticosteroids, or in very ill people. A fever indicates an infection in the abdominal cavity. If the condition is not treated, shock may develop. This emergency situation requires immediate surgery and intravenous antibiotics.

Bleeding

Bleeding is a common complication of ulcers even when they are not painful. Vomiting bright red blood or reddish brown clumps of partially digested blood that look like coffee grounds and passing black or obviously bloody stools can be symptoms of a bleeding ulcer. Such bleeding may result from other digestive conditions as well, but doctors begin their investigation by looking for the source of bleeding in the stomach and duodenum. Unless bleeding is massive, a doctor performs an endoscopy (an examination using a flexible viewing tube). If a bleeding ulcer is seen, the endoscope can be used to cauterize it (that is, destroy it with heat). A doctor may also use the endoscope to inject a material that causes clotting of a bleeding ulcer. If the source cannot be found and the bleeding is not severe, treatments include taking ulcer drugs, such as histamine-2 (H_2) blockers or proton pump inhibitors. The person also receives intravenous fluids and takes nothing by mouth, so the digestive tract can rest. If these measures fail, surgery is needed.

Obstruction

Swelling of inflamed tissues around an ulcer or scarring from previous ulcer flare-ups can narrow the outlet from the stomach or narrow the duodenum. A person with this type of obstruction may vomit repeatedly—often regurgitating large volumes of food eaten hours before. A feeling of being unusually full after eating, bloating, and a lack of appetite are symptoms of obstruction. Over time, vomiting can cause weight loss, dehydration, and an imbalance in body chemicals (electrolytes). Treating the ulcers relieves the obstruction in most cases, but severe obstructions may require endoscopy or surgery.

detecting ulcers in the duodenum and on the back wall of the stomach; endoscopy is also more reliable if the person has had stomach surgery. However, even a highly skilled endoscopist may miss a small number of gastric and duodenal ulcers. With an endoscope, a doctor can perform a biopsy (removal of a tissue sample for examination under a microscope) to determine if a gastric ulcer is cancerous and to help identify the presence of *Helicobacter pylori* bacteria. An endoscope also can be used to stop active bleeding and decrease the likelihood of recurring bleeding from an ulcer.

Barium contrast x-rays of the stomach and duodenum (also called a barium swallow or an upper gastrointestinal series) can help determine the severity and size of an ulcer, which sometimes cannot be completely seen on endoscopy.

Treatment

Because infection with *H. pylori* bacteria is a major cause of ulcers, antibiotics are often used. Sometimes bismuth subsalicylate is used in combination with antibiotics. Neutralizing or reducing stomach acid by using drugs that directly inhibit the stomach's production of acid promotes healing of peptic ulcers regardless of the cause. In most people, treatment is continued for 4 to 8 weeks. Although bland diets may help reduce acid, no evidence supports the belief that such diets speed healing or keep ulcers from recurring. Nevertheless, it makes sense for people to avoid foods that seem to make pain and bloating worse. Eliminating possible stomach irritants, such as NSAIDs, alcohol, and nicotine, is also important.

Antacids: Antacids relieve symptoms of ulcers by neutralizing stomach acid. Their effectiveness varies with the amount of antacid taken and the amount of acid a person produces. Almost all antacids can be purchased without a doctor's prescription and are available in tablet or liquid form. Generally, antacids are not effective in healing ulcers.

Sodium bicarbonate and calcium carbonate, the strongest antacids, may be taken occasionally for short-term relief. However, because they are absorbed by the bloodstream, continual use of these drugs may make the blood too alkaline (alkalosis▲), resulting in nausea, headache, and weakness. Therefore, these antacids generally should not be used in large amounts for more than a few days. These products also contain a lot of salt and should not be used by people who need to follow a low-sodium diet.

Aluminum hydroxide is a relatively safe, commonly used antacid. However, aluminum may bind with phosphate in the digestive tract, reducing phosphate levels in the blood and causing weakness and a loss of appetite. The risk of these side effects is greater in alcoholics and in people with kidney disease, including those receiving dialysis. Aluminum hydroxide may also cause constipation.

Magnesium hydroxide is a more effective antacid than aluminum hydroxide. Bowel movements usually remain regular if only four doses of 1 to 2 tablespoons a day are taken; more than four doses a day may cause diarrhea. Because small amounts of magnesium are absorbed into the bloodstream, people with kidney damage should take magnesium hydroxide only in small doses. Many antacids contain both magnesium hydroxide and aluminum hydroxide.

Acid-reducing Drugs: Histamine-2 (H2) blockers, such as cimetidine, famotidine, nizatidine, and ranitidine, relieve symptoms and promote ulcer healing by reducing the production of stomach acid. These highly effective drugs are taken once or twice a day. H2 blockers usually do not cause serious side effects. However, cimetidine is more likely to cause side effects, particularly in older people, in whom the drug may cause confusion. In addition, cimetidine may interfere with the body's elimination of certain drugs—such as theophylline for asthma, warfarin for excessive blood clotting, and phenytoin for seizures.

Proton pump inhibitors are the most potent of the drugs that reduce acid production. Proton pump inhibitors promote healing of ulcers in a greater percentage of people in a shorter period of time than do H2 blockers. They are also very useful in treating conditions that cause excessive stomach acid secretion, such as Zollinger-Ellison syndrome.

Miscellaneous Drugs: Sucralfate may work by forming a protective coating in the base of an ulcer to promote healing. It works well on peptic ulcers and is a reasonable alternative to antacids. Sucralfate is taken 2 to 4 times a day and is not absorbed into the bloodstream, so it causes few side effects. It may, however, cause constipation, and in some cases it reduces the effectiveness of other drugs.

Misoprostol may be used to reduce the likelihood of developing stomach and duodenal ulcers caused by NSAIDs. Misoprostol may work by reducing production of stomach acid and by making the stomach lining more resistant to acid. People who are at higher risk of developing an ulcer caused by NSAIDs for other reasons, including older people, people taking corticosteroids, and people who have a history of ulcers, may also be potential candidates for misoprostol. However, misoprostol causes diarrhea and other digestive problems in more than 30% of people who take it. In addition, this drug can cause spontaneous abortions in pregnant women. Alternatives to misoprostol are available for people taking aspirin, NSAIDs, or corticosteroids. These alternatives, such as proton pump inhibitors, are just as effective for reducing the likelihood of developing an ulcer and cause fewer side effects.

Surgery: Surgery for ulcers is now seldom needed because drugs so effectively heal peptic ulcers and endoscopy so effectively stops active bleeding. Surgery is used primarily to deal with complications of a peptic ulcer, such as a perforation, an obstruction that fails to respond to drug therapy or that recurs, two or more major episodes of bleeding ulcers, a gastric ulcer suspected of being cancerous, or se-

▲ see page 932

vere and frequent recurrences of peptic ulcers. A number of different operations may be performed to treat these problems. However, ulcers may recur after surgery, and each procedure may cause problems of its own, such as weight loss, poor digestion, and anemia.

Gastroesophageal Reflux

In gastroesophageal reflux (gastroesophageal reflux disease [GERD]), stomach acid and enzymes flow backward from the stomach into the esophagus, causing inflammation and pain in the esophagus.

The stomach lining protects the stomach from the effects of its own acid. Because the esophagus lacks a similar protective lining, stomach acid and enzymes that flow backward (reflux) into the esophagus routinely cause symptoms and in some cases damage.

Acid and enzymes reflux when the lower esophageal sphincter, the ring-shaped muscle that normally prevents the contents of the stomach from flowing back into the esophagus, is not functioning properly. When a person is standing or sitting, gravity helps to prevent the reflux of stomach contents into the esophagus. This explains why reflux can worsen when a person is lying down. Smoking and certain foods, such as chocolate, interfere with the sphincter muscle, making reflux more likely. Reflux is also more likely to occur soon after meals, when the volume and acidity of contents in the stomach are higher. Alcohol and coffee also stimulate acid production. Delayed emptying of the stomach (for example, due to diabetes or use of opioids) can also worsen reflux.

Symptoms and Complications

Heartburn (a burning pain behind the breastbone) is the most obvious symptom of gastroesophageal reflux. Sometimes the pain even extends to the neck, throat, and face. Heartburn may be accompanied by regurgitation, in which the stomach contents reach the mouth.

Inflammation of the esophagus (esophagitis) may cause bleeding that is usually slight but can be massive. The blood may be vomited up or may pass through the digestive tract, resulting in the passage of dark, tarry stools (melena) or bright red blood, if the bleeding is brisk enough.

Esophageal ulcers, which are open sores on the lining of the esophagus, can result from re-

Zollinger-Ellison Syndrome: An Acid-Generating Cancer

Zollinger-Ellison syndrome causes the stomach to produce too much acid. In this syndrome, a cancerous (malignant) tumor, usually in the duodenum, pancreas, or bile ducts, produces gastrin. Gastrin is a hormone that stimulates the stomach to produce large amounts of acid. People with Zollinger-Ellison syndrome almost always develop many ulcers that recur despite treatment to control ulcer disease.

People with this disease typically have an elevated level of gastrin in their blood. Testing involves administration of a hormone called secretin. In people with Zollinger-Ellison syndrome, gastrin levels in the bloodstream greatly increase when secretin is injected into a vein. In addition, testing can reveal increased production of stomach acid. A number of tests can be used in an attempt to localize the tumor, including computed tomography (CT) scanning, endoscopic ultrasound, and radionuclide scanning.

Proton pump inhibitors help control the excess production of stomach acid. Surgery to remove the tumor can be curative. Even when not curative, surgery can shrink the tumor, which in turn reduces the amount of acid produced by the stomach and prevents local complications, such as blockage of the intestine. Radiation and chemotherapy are not helpful.

peated reflux. They can cause pain that is usually located behind the breastbone or just below it, similar to the location of heartburn.

Narrowing (stricture) of the esophagus from reflux makes swallowing solid foods increasingly more difficult. Narrowing of the airways can cause shortness of breath and wheezing. Other symptoms of gastroesophageal reflux include chest pain, sore throat, hoarseness, excessive salivation (water brash), a sensation of a lump in the throat (globus sensation), and inflammation of the sinuses (sinusitis).

With prolonged irritation of the lower part of the esophagus from repeated reflux, the cells lining the esophagus may change (resulting in a condition called Barrett's esophagus). Changes may occur even in the absence of symptoms. These abnormal cells are precancerous and progress to cancer rarely.

℞   DRUGS USED TO TREAT PEPTIC DISORDERS

TYPE DRUG	SELECTED SIDE EFFECTS	COMMENTS
Antacids		
Aluminum hydroxide Calcium carbonate Magnesium hydroxide Sodium bicarbonate	Nausea, headache, weakness, loss of appetite, constipation (aluminum hydroxide) or diarrhea (magnesium hydroxide)	Used mainly to relieve symptoms, not as a cure
Histamine-2 blockers		
Cimetidine Famotidine Nizatidine Ranitidine	Rash, fever, muscle pains; may cause breast enlargement and erectile dysfunction in men; may interfere with elimination of certain drugs (cimetidine); confusion (cimetidine, ranitidine)	The once-daily dose is taken in the evening or at bedtime; doses taken in the morning are less effective
Proton pump inhibitors		
Lansoprazole Omeprazole Pantoprazole Rabeprazole Esomeprazole	Diarrhea, constipation, headache	Usually well tolerated; most effective means of reducing stomach acid
Antibiotics		
Amoxicillin Clarithromycin Metronidazole Tetracycline	Diarrhea (amoxicillin, clarithromycin, tetracycline), altered taste, nausea	Effective for treating peptic ulcers caused by *Helicobacter pylori* infection
Miscellaneous		
Bismuth subsalicylate Misoprostol Sucralfate	Diarrhea (bismuth subsalicylate, misoprostol); darkening of the tongue and stool (bismuth subsalicylate); spontaneous abortion (misoprostol); constipation (bismuth subsalicylate); may reduce effectiveness of other drugs (sucralfate)	Bismuth subsalicylate is used in combination with antibiotics to cure *H. pylori* infection

Diagnosis

The symptoms point to the diagnosis, and treatment can be started without detailed diagnostic testing. Specific testing is usually reserved for situations in which the diagnosis is not clear or treatment has failed to control symptoms. Examination of the esophagus using an endoscope (a flexible viewing tube), x-ray studies, pressure measurements (manometry) of the lower esophageal sphincter, and esophageal pH (acidity) tests are sometimes needed to help confirm the diagnosis and check for complications.

Endoscopy may confirm the diagnosis if the doctor finds that the person has esophagitis or Barrett's esophagus. Endoscopy also helps to exclude the presence of esophageal cancer. X-rays taken after a person drinks a barium solution and then lies on an incline with the head lower than the feet may show reflux of the barium from the stomach into the esophagus. A doctor may press on the abdomen to increase the likelihood of reflux. The x-rays taken after the barium is swallowed also can reveal esophageal ulcers or a narrowed esophagus.

Pressure measurements at the lower esophageal sphincter indicate the strength of the sphincter and can distinguish a normal sphincter from a poorly functioning one. The information gained from this test helps the doctor decide whether surgery is an appropriate treatment.

Some doctors believe that the best test for gastroesophageal reflux is esophageal pH testing. In this test, a thin, flexible tube with a sensor probe on the tip is placed through the nose and into the lower esophagus. The other end of this tube is attached to a monitor that the person wears on his belt. The monitor records the acid levels in the esophagus, usually for 24 hours. Besides determining how much reflux is occurring, this test identifies the relationship between symptoms and reflux and is particularly helpful for people with symptoms that are not typical of reflux. The esophageal pH test is needed for all people being considered for surgery for gastroesophageal reflux.

Prevention and Treatment

Several measures may be taken to relieve gastroesophageal reflux. Raising the head of the bed about 6 inches can prevent acid from flowing into the esophagus as a person sleeps. Specific foods (for example, fats and chocolate) should be avoided, as should smoking and certain drugs (for example, anticholinergics, certain antidepressants, calcium channel blockers, and nitrates), all of which increase the tendency of the lower esophageal sphincter to leak. A doctor may prescribe a cholinergic drug (for example, bethanechol or metoclopramide) to make the lower sphincter close more tightly. Coffee, alcohol, and other substances that strongly stimulate the stomach to produce acid or that delay stomach emptying should be avoided as well.

Many of the drugs used to treat gastritis and peptic ulcers also help prevent and treat gastroesophageal reflux.▲ Antacids taken at bedtime, for example, are often helpful. Antacids can usually relieve the pain of esophageal ulcers by reducing the amount of acid that reaches the esophagus. However, proton pump inhibitors, the most powerful drugs for reducing acid production, are usually the most effective treatment for gastroesophageal reflux, because even a small amount of acid can cause significant symptoms. Healing requires drugs that reduce stomach acid over a 4- to 12-week period. The ulcers heal slowly, tend to recur, and, when chronic and severe, can leave a narrowed esophagus after healing.

Esophageal narrowing is treated with drug therapy and repeated dilation, which may be performed using balloons or progressively larger dilators (bougies). If dilation is successful, narrowing does not seriously limit what a person can eat.

Barrett's esophagus may or may not disappear when treatment relieves symptoms. Therefore, people with Barrett's esophagus are asked to undergo an endoscopic examination every 2 to 3 years to ensure that it is not progressing to cancer.

Surgery is an option for people whose symptoms are unresponsive to drug therapy or for people with esophagitis that persists even after symptoms are relieved. In addition, surgery may be the preferred treatment for people who do not like the prospect of having to take drugs for many years. A minimally invasive procedure performed through a laparoscope is available. However, 20 to 30% of people who undergo this procedure experience side effects, most commonly difficulty swallowing and a sensation of bloating or abdominal discomfort after eating.

CHAPTER 122

Gastroenteritis

Gastroenteritis describes a group of conditions usually caused by infection with a microorganism or ingestion of chemical toxins.

Gastroenteritis usually consists of mild to severe diarrhea that may be accompanied by loss of appetite, nausea, vomiting, cramps, and discomfort in the abdomen. Although gastroenteritis usually is not serious in a healthy adult, causing only discomfort and inconvenience, it can cause life-threatening dehydra-

▲ see page 716

MICROORGANISMS THAT CAUSE GASTROENTERITIS

MICROORGANISM	COMMON SOURCES	SYMPTOMS	ANTIMICROBIAL USE
Campylobacter	Eating contaminated meat (especially under-cooked poultry); drinking contaminated water or unpasteurized milk	Often bloody, some-times watery diarrhea lasting 1 day to a week or more	Antibiotics given in the early stages of ill-ness may shorten the duration of symp-toms (for example, erythromycin, ciprofloxacin)
Salmonella	Eating contaminated food; contact with rep-tiles (iguanas, snakes, turtles)	High fever, abdominal cramps, nausea, vomit-ing, diarrhea that may or may not be bloody. Symptoms usually last 3 to 7 days	Antibiotics usually not given
Shigella	Person-to-person con-tact, especially in day-care centers	May be mild or severe. In mild cases, watery, loose stools. In severe cases, high fever, severe abdominal cramps, painful passage of stool containing blood and mucus. Symptoms usu-ally last about a week without treatment	Antibiotics shorten the duration of the illness and decrease chance of spread to another person (for example, ciprofloxacin, trimethoprim-sulfamethoxazole)
Escherichia coli O157:H7	Eating undercooked ground beef or drinking unpasteurized milk or juice; swimming in con-taminated pools; person-to-person contact; touching infected ani-mals and then putting fingers in one's mouth	Sudden abdominal cramps, watery diarrhea that usually becomes bloody within 24 hours, hemolytic-uremic syndrome	Antibiotics not given
Clostridium difficile	Usually due to bacterial overgrowth in people who have been taking antibiotics	Diarrhea	Antibiotic use is stopped. In some cases, however, metronidazole is given by mouth
Entamoeba histolytica	Eating or drinking con-taminated food or water	Bloody diarrhea, abdom-inal pain, weight loss lasting 1 to 3 weeks. Can cause infection in liver and other organs	Antiparasitic drugs given (for example, metronidazole, iodoquinol, paro-momycin)
Enterotoxigenic *E. coli*	Eating or drinking con-taminated food or water	Frequent watery diar-rhea. Usually lasts 3 to 5 days	Antibiotics (for ex-ample, ciprofloxacin, azithromycin) may help shorten duration of illness
Vibrio cholerae	Eating or drinking con-taminated food or water	Painless, watery diarrhea; vomiting. Can lead to massive fluid loss, shock	Antibiotics given (for example, ciproflox-acin, doxycycline)
Other types of *Vibrio*	Shellfish	Watery diarrhea, often with little nausea or vomiting	Antibiotics given (for example, ciproflox-acin, doxycycline)

MICROORGANISMS THAT CAUSE GASTROENTERITIS (Continued)

MICROORGANISM	COMMON SOURCES	SYMPTOMS	ANTIMICROBIAL USE
Staphylococcus aureus	Eating food contaminated by toxins produced by bacteria	Severe nausea and vomiting beginning about 2 to 8 hours after eating contaminated food	Antibiotics not given
Clostridium perfringens	Eating food contaminated by toxins produced by bacteria	Usually mild. When severe, abdominal pain, abdominal expansion, severe diarrhea, dehydration, shock. Symptoms usually begin 8 to 16 hours after eating contaminated food	---
Viral infections (rotaviruses, Norwalk virus, astroviruses, enteric adenoviruses)	Epidemic and often seasonal	Frequent watery diarrhea; vomiting and fever (milder in astroviruses). Usually last 2 to 7 days (10 days or more for enteric adenoviruses)	Antibiotics and antiviral drugs not given
Giardia	Drinking contaminated stream water; person-to-person contact, particularly in day-care centers	Diarrhea, nausea, loss of appetite. More long-term illness (lasting several days to several weeks) may occur, with greasy stools, abdominal bloating, gas, and weight loss	Antiparasitic drugs given (for example, metronidazole, furazolidone)
Cryptosporidium	Drinking contaminated water; person-to-person contact. People with AIDS are particularly susceptible	Watery diarrhea, crampy abdominal pain, nausea, vomiting	Antibiotics and antiparasitic drugs not given

tion▲ and electrolyte imbalance■ in the very ill, the very young, and the very old.

Causes

Infections that produce gastroenteritis can be transmitted from person to person, especially if someone with diarrhea does not thoroughly wash his hands after a bowel movement. A person, and sometimes large numbers of people (in which case an outbreak of illness is called an epidemic), can also become infected by eating food or drinking water that has been contaminated by infected stool. Most foods can be contaminated with bacteria and cause gastroenteritis if not cooked thoroughly or pasteurized. Contaminated water is sometimes ingested in unexpected ways, such as when swimming in a pond contaminated by

stool from an animal or in a swimming pool contaminated by stool from another person. In some cases, gastroenteritis is acquired through contact with animals that carry the infectious microorganism.

Certain bacteria produce toxins that cause the cells in the intestinal wall to secrete electrolytes and water. One such toxin, produced by the bacterium *Vibrio cholerae*, is responsible for the watery diarrhea that is the main symptom of cholera; other *Vibrio* species, often present in raw shellfish, produce a similar but less severe gastroenteritis. A toxin produced by the common bacterium *Escherichia coli (E. coli)* may cause traveler's diarrhea and some outbreaks of diarrhea in hospital nurseries.

▲ see page 928   ■ see page 901

Some bacteria (such as certain strains of *E. coli, Campylobacter, Shigella,* and *Salmonella*) invade the lining of the intestine. There, they damage cells, causing tiny sores (ulcerations) that bleed and allow a considerable leakage of fluid containing proteins, electrolytes, and water.

Besides bacteria, several types of viruses, such as rotaviruses and the Norwalk virus, cause gastroenteritis. During the winter in temperate climates, rotaviruses cause most cases of diarrhea that are serious enough to send infants and toddlers to the hospital.

Certain intestinal parasites, particularly *Giardia lamblia,* stick to or invade the lining of the intestine and cause nausea, vomiting, diarrhea, and a general sick feeling. The resulting infection, called giardiasis, is more common in cold climates but occurs in every region of the United States and throughout the world. If the disease becomes persistent (chronic), it can keep the body from absorbing nutrients, a condition known as a malabsorption syndrome. Another intestinal parasite, called *Cryptosporidium,* causes watery diarrhea that is sometimes accompanied by abdominal cramps, nausea, and vomiting. The resulting infection, called cryptosporidiosis, is usually mild in otherwise healthy people, but it may be severe or even fatal in people with a weakened immune system. Both *Giardia* and *Cryptosporidium* are most commonly acquired by drinking contaminated water.

Gastroenteritis may result from eating chemical toxins. These toxins are usually produced by a plant, such as poisonous mushrooms, or by certain kinds of exotic seafood and thus are not the product of an infection. Gastroenteritis due to chemical toxicity can also occur after ingesting water or food contaminated by chemicals such as arsenic, lead, mercury, or cadmium. Eating large amounts of acidic foods, such as citrus fruits and tomatoes, gives some people a chemical-induced gastroenteritis.

Symptoms

The type and severity of the symptoms depend on the type and quantity of microorganism or toxin ingested. Symptoms also vary according to the person's resistance. Symptoms often begin suddenly—sometimes dramatically—with a loss of appetite, nausea, or vomiting. Audible rumbling of the intestine and

abdominal cramping may occur. Diarrhea is the most common symptom and may be accompanied by visible blood and mucus. Loops of intestine may be painfully swollen (distended) with gas. The person may have a fever, feel generally sick, and experience aching muscles and extreme exhaustion.

Severe vomiting and diarrhea can lead to marked dehydration.▲ Symptoms of dehydration include weakness, decreased frequency of urination, dry mouth, and, in infants, lack of tears when crying. Excessive vomiting or diarrhea can result in low levels of potassium in the blood (hypokalemia). Low levels of sodium in the blood (hyponatremia) also may develop, particularly if the person replaces lost fluids by drinking fluids that contain little or no salt, such as water and tea. Water and electrolyte imbalances are potentially serious, especially in the young, the old, and people with chronic diseases.

Diagnosis

The diagnosis of gastroenteritis is usually obvious from the symptoms alone, but the cause often is not. Sometimes other family members or coworkers have recently been ill with similar symptoms. Other times, gastroenteritis can be traced to inadequately cooked, spoiled, or contaminated food, such as raw seafood or mayonnaise left out of the refrigerator too long. Recent travel, especially to certain foreign countries, may give clues as well.

If the symptoms are severe or last for more than 48 hours, stool samples may be examined in a laboratory for white blood cells and bacteria, viruses, or parasites. In rare cases, laboratory analysis of vomit, food, or blood may help identify the cause.

If the symptoms persist beyond a few days, a doctor may need to examine the large intestine with a colonoscope (a flexible viewing tube) to determine whether the person has a disease such as ulcerative colitis.

Prevention and Treatment

Because most infections that cause gastroenteritis are transmitted by person-to-person contact, particularly through direct or indirect contact with infected stool, good hand washing with soap and water after a bowel movement is the most effective means of prevention. To prevent food-borne infections, meat and eggs should be cooked thoroughly, and leftovers should be refrigerated promptly after cooking. Only pasteurized dairy products

▲ see page 928

and pasteurized apple juice should be used. For infants, a simple and effective way to prevent gastroenteritis is breastfeeding.

Usually the only treatment needed for gastroenteritis is to drink an adequate amount of fluids. Even a person who is vomiting should drink as much as can be tolerated, taking small frequent sips. If vomiting or diarrhea is prolonged or the person becomes severely dehydrated, intravenous fluids and electrolytes may be needed. Because children can become dehydrated more quickly, they should be given fluids with the appropriate mix of salts and sugars. Any of the commercially available solutions designed to replace lost fluids and electrolytes (rehydration solutions) are satisfactory. Carbonated beverages, teas, sports drinks, beverages containing caffeine, and fruit juices are not appropriate. For adults, a doctor may give a drug, either as an injection or as a suppository, to control severe vomiting. These drugs usually are not given to young children.

As the symptoms subside, the person may gradually add bland foods—such as cooked cereals, bananas, rice, applesauce, and toast—to the diet. If the diarrhea continues after following the bland diet for 12 to 24 hours and there is no blood in the stool to indicate a more serious bacterial infection, the doctor may prescribe a drug such as diphenoxylate or instruct the person to use an over-the-counter drug such as loperamide or bismuth subsalicylate. Again, these drugs usually are not given to young children.

Because antibiotics can cause diarrhea and may encourage the growth of organisms resistant to antibiotics, they are rarely appropriate, even when a known bacterium is causing gastroenteritis. Antibiotics may be used, however, when certain bacteria, such as *Campylobacter*, *Shigella*, and *Vibrio*, are the cause.

Hemorrhagic Colitis

Hemorrhagic colitis is a type of gastroenteritis in which certain strains of the bacterium Escherichia coli (E. coli) *infect the large intestine and produce a toxin that causes bloody diarrhea and other serious complications.*

Hemorrhagic colitis can occur in people of all ages but is most common in children and older people. In North America, the most common strain of *E. coli* that causes hemorrhagic colitis is found in the intestines of healthy cattle. Outbreaks can be caused by eating undercooked beef, especially ground beef, or by drink-

Gastroenteritis as a Side Effect of Drugs

Nausea, vomiting, and diarrhea are common side effects of many drugs. Common culprits include antacids containing magnesium as a major ingredient, antibiotics, chemotherapy drugs, colchicine (for gout), digoxin (usually used for heart failure or certain irregular heart rhythms), and laxatives. Laxative abuse can lead to weakness, vomiting, diarrhea, electrolyte loss, and other disturbances.

Recognizing that a drug is causing gastroenteritis can be difficult. In mild cases, a doctor can have a person stop taking the drug, then later start taking it again. If the symptoms subside when the person stops taking the drug and resume when the person starts taking the drug again, then the drug may be the cause of the gastrointestinal symptoms. In severe cases of gastroenteritis, a doctor may instruct the person to stop taking the drug permanently.

ing unpasteurized milk. Unpasteurized juice can also be contaminated. The disease can be transmitted from person to person, particularly among children in diapers.

E. coli toxins damage the lining of the large intestine. If they are absorbed into the bloodstream, they can also affect other organs, such as the kidney.

Symptoms

Severe abdominal cramps begin suddenly along with watery diarrhea, which typically becomes bloody within 24 hours. The diarrhea usually lasts 1 to 8 days. Fever is usually absent or mild but occasionally can exceed 102° F (38.9° C).

About 5% of people with hemorrhagic colitis develop a severe complication called hemolytic-uremic syndrome.▲ Symptoms include anemia (characterized by fatigue, weakness, and light-headedness) caused by the destruction of red blood cells (hemolytic anemia), a low platelet count (thrombocytopenia), and sudden kidney failure. Some people with hemolytic-uremic syndrome also develop complications of nerve or brain damage,

▲ see page 998

such as seizures or strokes. These complications typically develop in the second week of illness and may be preceded by increasing fever. Hemolytic-uremic syndrome is more likely to occur in children younger than 5 years and in older people. Even without hemolytic-uremic syndrome and its complications, hemorrhagic colitis may cause death in older people.

Diagnosis and Treatment

A doctor usually suspects hemorrhagic colitis when a person reports bloody diarrhea. To make the diagnosis, a doctor has stool specimens tested for strains of *E. coli*. Other tests, such as colonoscopy, may be performed if a doctor suspects that other diseases may be causing the bloody diarrhea.

The most important aspect of treatment is drinking enough fluids. Sometimes so much fluid is lost, however, that a doctor has to replace them intravenously. The diet is kept bland, with cooked cereals, bananas, rice, applesauce, and toast. Antibiotics are not given because they increase the risk of developing hemolytic-uremic syndrome. People who develop complications are likely to require intensive care in the hospital and may need kidney dialysis.▲

Staphylococcal Food Poisoning

Staphylococcal food poisoning results from eating food contaminated with toxins produced by certain types of staphylococci, resulting in diarrhea and vomiting.

The staphylococci bacteria grow in food, in which they produce their toxins. Thus, staphylococcal food poisoning does not result from ingesting the bacteria but rather from ingesting the toxins that are already present in the contaminated food. Typical contaminated foods include custard, cream-filled pastry, milk, processed meats, and fish. The risk of an outbreak is high when food handlers with skin infections contaminate foods left at room temperature.

Symptoms and Diagnosis

Symptoms usually begin abruptly with severe nausea and vomiting starting about 2 to 8 hours after the contaminated food is eaten. Other symptoms may include abdominal cramping, diarrhea, and sometimes headache and fever. Severe fluid and electrolyte loss may cause weakness and very low blood pressure (shock). Symptoms usually last less than 12 hours, and recovery is usually complete. Occasionally, staphylococcal food poisoning is fatal, especially in the very young, the very old, and people weakened by long-term illness.

The symptoms are usually all a doctor needs to make the diagnosis of gastroenteritis. A more specific diagnosis of staphylococcal food poisoning may be suspected when other people who ate the same food are similarly affected and when the disorder can be traced to a single source of contamination. To confirm the diagnosis, a laboratory analysis must identify staphylococci in the suspected food, but this analysis is not usually performed. Microscopic specimens of vomit may also show staphylococci.

Prevention and Treatment

Careful food preparation can prevent staphylococcal food poisoning. Anyone who has a skin infection should not prepare food for others until the infection heals.

Treatment usually consists of only drinking an adequate amount of fluids. A doctor may give a drug, either as an injection or as a suppository, to help control severe nausea and vomiting. Sometimes so much fluid is lost that fluids have to be given intravenously.

Clostridium perfringens Food Poisoning

Clostridium perfringens *food poisoning results from eating food contaminated by the bacterium* Clostridium perfringens; *once in the small intestine, the bacterium releases a toxin that often causes diarrhea.*

Some strains cause a mild to moderate disease that gets better without treatment; other strains cause severe gastroenteritis that can damage the small intestine and sometimes lead to death. Contaminated meat is usually responsible for outbreaks of *Clostridium perfringens* food poisoning. Some strains cannot be destroyed by cooking the food thoroughly; others can.

Symptoms, Diagnosis, and Treatment

The gastroenteritis is usually mild, although it can cause abdominal pain, abdominal expansion (distention) from gas, severe diarrhea, de-

▲ see page 833

hydration, and a severe decrease in blood pressure (shock). A doctor usually suspects the diagnosis when a local outbreak of the disease has occurred. The diagnosis is confirmed by testing contaminated food for *Clostridium perfringens*. The person is given fluids and is encouraged to rest.

Traveler's Diarrhea

Traveler's diarrhea (turista) is characterized by diarrhea, nausea, and vomiting that commonly occur in travelers to areas of the world with poor water purification.

Traveler's diarrhea occurs when people are exposed to bacteria in food and water to which they have had little exposure and thus no immunity. It occurs mostly in developing countries where the water supply is inadequately treated. The organisms most likely to cause traveler's diarrhea are the types of *Escherichia coli (E. coli)* that produce certain toxins and some viruses such as the Norwalk virus.

Symptoms and Diagnosis

Nausea, vomiting, intestinal rumbling, abdominal cramping, and diarrhea can occur in any combination and with any degree of severity. Vomiting, headache, and muscle pain are particularly common in infections caused by the Norwalk virus. Most cases are mild and disappear without treatment within 3 to 5 days. Diagnostic tests are rarely needed.

Prevention and Treatment

Travelers should patronize only those restaurants with a reputation for safety and should not purchase any food or beverages from street vendors. Cooked foods that are still hot when served are generally safe. Salads containing uncooked vegetables should be avoided, and all fruit should be peeled by the traveler. Travelers should drink only bottled carbonated beverages or beverages made with water that has been boiled. Even ice cubes should be made with water that has been boiled.

Preventive antibiotics are recommended only for people who are particularly susceptible to the consequences of traveler's diarrhea, such as those whose immune system is impaired. The antibiotic most commonly recommended is ciprofloxacin. Bismuth subsalicylate, a nonprescription drug, can help.

When symptoms occur, treatment includes drinking plenty of fluids and eating a bland diet (for example, cooked cereals, bananas, rice, applesauce, and toast). In addition, antibiotics (such as ciprofloxacin) and antidiarrheal drugs (such as loperamide or bismuth) are usually recommended. Travelers are encouraged to seek medical care if they develop fever or blood in the stool.

Chemical Food Poisoning

Chemical food poisoning results from eating a plant or animal that contains a toxin.

Mushroom (Toadstool) Poisoning: Mushroom poisoning can result from ingesting any of several species of mushroom. The potential for poisoning may vary within the same species, at different times of the growing season, and with cooking. In poisoning caused by many species of *Inocybe* and some species of *Clitocybe,* the dangerous substance is muscarine. Symptoms, which begin a few minutes to 2 hours after eating, may include increased tearing and salivation, narrowing (constriction) of the pupils, sweating, vomiting, stomach cramps, diarrhea, dizziness, confusion, coma, and occasionally, seizures. With appropriate treatment, the person usually recovers in 24 hours. Without treatment, death can occur in a few hours.

In phalloidine poisoning, caused by eating *Amanita phalloides* and related species of mushroom, symptoms start in 6 to 24 hours. People develop intestinal symptoms similar to those of muscarine poisoning, and kidney damage may reduce or stop urination. Jaundice from liver damage is common and develops in 2 or 3 days. Sometimes the symptoms disappear on their own, but about half of the people who have phalloidine poisoning die in 5 to 8 days.

Plant and Shrub Poisoning: This type of poisoning can result from ingesting the leaves and fruits of many wild and domestic plants and shrubs. Green or sprouting underground roots that contain solanine may produce mild nausea, vomiting, diarrhea, and weakness. Fruit of the Koenig tree causes the vomiting sickness of Jamaica.

Seafood Poisoning: Gastroenteritis may be caused by eating bony fish or shellfish. Usually, poisoning caused by eating bony fish results from one of three toxins—ciguatera, tetraodon, or histamine.

Ciguatera poisoning can occur after eating any of more than 400 species of fish from the tropical reefs of Florida, the West Indies, or the

Chinese Restaurant Syndrome

What is popularly called the Chinese restaurant syndrome is not a type of chemical food poisoning. Rather, it is a sensitivity to monosodium glutamate (MSG), a flavor enhancer often used in Chinese cooking. In susceptible people, MSG can produce facial pressure, chest pain, and burning sensations throughout the body. Many people feel anxious as well. The amount of MSG that can cause these symptoms varies considerably from person to person.

Pacific. The toxin is produced by certain dinoflagellates, microscopic sea organisms that the fish eat and that accumulate in their flesh. Larger, older fish are more toxic than smaller, younger ones. The flavor of the fish is not affected. Current processing procedures cannot destroy the toxin. The initial symptoms—abdominal cramps, nausea, vomiting, and diarrhea—may begin 2 to 8 hours after the person eats the fish and last 6 to 17 hours. Later symptoms may include itchiness, a pins-and-needles sensation, headache, muscle aches, a reversal of sensations of hot and cold, and facial pain. For months afterward, the sensations may be disabling.

Tetraodon poisoning from the puffer fish, which is found most commonly in the seas surrounding Japan, is similar to ciguatera poisoning. Death may result from paralysis of the muscles that regulate breathing.

Histamine poisoning from fish such as mackerel, tuna, and blue dolphin (mahimahi) occurs when the tissues of the fish break down after it has been caught, producing high levels of histamine. When ingested, histamine causes immediate facial flushing. It can also cause nausea, vomiting, stomach pain, and hives (urticaria) a few minutes after a person eats the fish. Symptoms usually last less than 24 hours.

Neurotoxin poisoning can occur from June to October, especially on the Pacific and New England coasts. Shellfish such as mussels,

clams, oysters, and scallops may ingest certain poisonous dinoflagellates at certain times when the water has a red cast, called the red tide. They produce a toxin that attacks nerves (such toxins are called neurotoxins▲). The toxin, which produces paralytic shellfish poisoning, persists even after the food has been cooked. The first symptom, a pins-and-needles sensation around the mouth, begins 5 to 30 minutes after eating. Nausea, vomiting, and abdominal cramps develop next. About 25% of people develop muscle weakness over the next few hours; occasionally, the weakness progresses to paralysis of the arms and legs. Weakness of the muscles needed for breathing may even be severe enough to cause death.

Contaminant Poisoning: Gastroenteritis may affect people who have ingested unwashed fruits and vegetables sprayed with arsenic, lead, or organic insecticides; acidic fluids served in lead-glazed pottery; or food stored in cadmium-lined containers.

Treatment

Most people with chemical food poisoning recover fully and rapidly with nothing more than replacement of fluids and electrolytes. As soon as symptoms begin, a person should try to consume large amounts of fluids. If fluids cannot be tolerated, the person needs to go to an emergency room for intravenous fluid replacement.

If possible, it is often a good idea to rid the stomach of the toxic substance as quickly as possible. For most people, vomiting accomplishes this. Saving a small amount of the first vomitus may be useful if tests are needed later. If a person cannot vomit adequately and symptoms are severe, a doctor may empty the stomach by placing a small tube through the nose or mouth into the stomach. A laxative helps to pass the toxins from the intestines more quickly.

Specific treatments are sometimes given when the toxin is known. For example, atropine is given for certain types of mushroom poisoning. Phalloidine poisoning is treated with a diet high in carbohydrates and sugar given intravenously. Ciguatera poisoning is sometimes treated with mannitol given intravenously. Antihistamines help block the symptoms of histamine poisoning.

▲ see page 579

CHAPTER 123

Hiatus Hernia, Bezoars, and Foreign Bodies

The stomach is a large, bean-shaped organ that receives food and fluids after they are eaten. The stomach normally resides below the diaphragm in the abdomen. The stomach may move upward through the diaphragm or become clogged with undigested material.

Hiatus Hernia

Hiatus hernia is a protrusion of a portion of the stomach from its normal position in the abdomen through the diaphragm.

The cause of hiatus hernia is usually unknown. Sometimes it exists from birth. The stomach sometimes protrudes upward through the diaphragm from its normal position in the upper abdomen. This condition sometimes occurs as a birth defect, in which case it is called a diaphragmatic hernia;▲ in adults, the condition is called hiatus (hiatal) hernia.

In a sliding hiatus hernia, the junction between the esophagus and the stomach as well as a portion of the stomach itself, all of which are normally below the diaphragm, protrude above it.

In a paraesophageal hiatus hernia, the junction between the esophagus and stomach is in its normal place below the diaphragm, but a portion of the stomach is pushed above the diaphragm and lies beside the esophagus.

Symptoms

More than 40% of the people in the United States have a sliding hiatus hernia. The frequency increases with age, so that the rate climbs to 60% of people older than 60 years of age. Most sliding hiatus hernias are very small, and most people with sliding hiatus hernias have no symptoms. Symptoms that do occur are usually minor. They are usually related to gastroesophageal reflux■ leading to indigestion, typically when a person lies down after eating.

A paraesophageal hiatus hernia may get trapped or pinched by the diaphragm and lose its blood supply. Such a trapping is a serious and painful condition, called strangulation, that re-

quires immediate surgery. Rarely, microscopic or massive bleeding from the lining of the hernia occurs with either type of hiatus hernia.

Diagnosis and Treatment

Usually, x-rays clearly reveal a hiatus hernia, although a doctor may have to press on the abdomen during the procedure.

Often, elevating the head of the bed while sleeping prevents symptoms. Antacids and drugs that prevent acid production also relieve symptoms.★ A paraesophageal hiatus hernia may be corrected surgically to prevent strangulation, but such surgery is rarely needed.

Bezoars and Foreign Bodies

Bezoars are tightly packed collections of partially digested or undigested material stuck in the stomach or other parts of the digestive tract. **Foreign bodies** *are small ingested objects that can also get stuck in the digestive tract and sometimes perforate (pierce) it.*

The stomach is a common collection site for hardened masses of food materials or other objects. This is due in part to the shape of the stomach and to the narrow opening (pyloric sphincter) through which the stomach's contents must empty in order to enter the first segment of the small intestine (duodenum). Undigestible masses (bezoars) or foreign objects (bodies) larger than 2 centimeters (about $3/4$ of an inch) in diameter are rarely able to pass out of the stomach.

Bezoars consist of partially digested hair or fiber from fruits or vegetables that accumulate most often in the stomach but sometimes elsewhere in the digestive tract. These hairballs or foodballs cannot pass through narrow openings or spaces and thus get stuck in the digestive tract. Even hardened blocks of drugs, such as antacids, can accumulate and become stuck.

▲ see page 1522   ■ see page 717
★ see table on page 718

Understanding Hiatus Hernia

A hiatus hernia is an abnormal bulging of a portion of the stomach through the diaphragm.

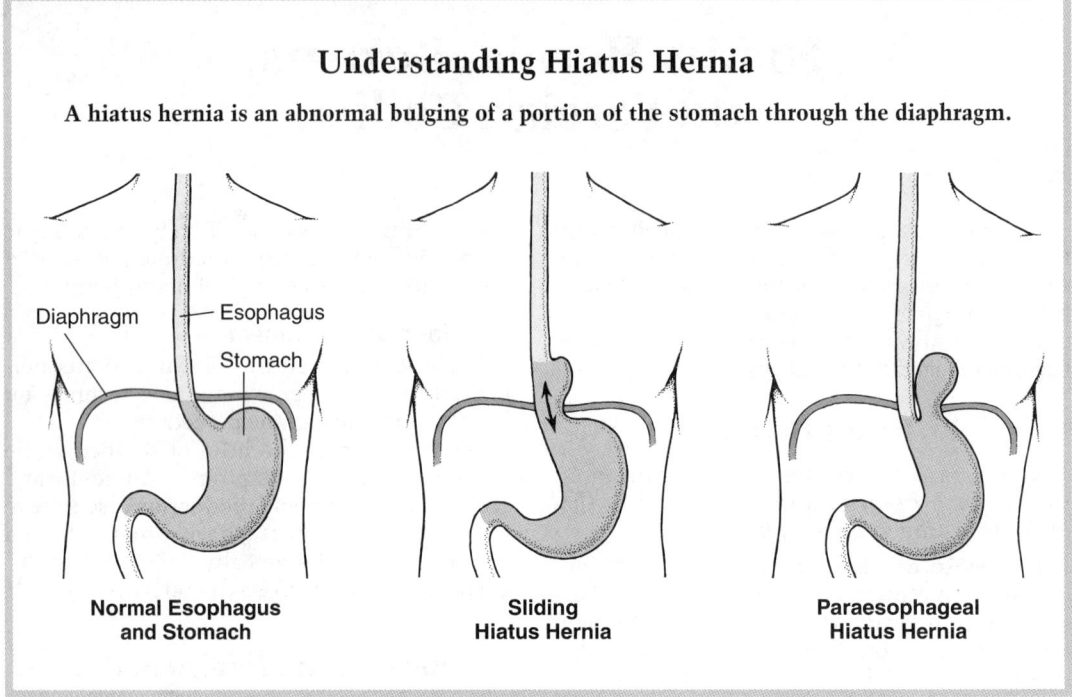

| Normal Esophagus and Stomach | Sliding Hiatus Hernia | Paraesophageal Hiatus Hernia |

Foreign bodies are sometimes swallowed by children and even adults, especially intoxicated adults. If these undigestible objects are small, they pass through the digestive system until they are excreted with stool. However, larger objects or sharp ones, such as fish bones, may get stuck in the esophagus or stomach or, less often, in other parts of the digestive tract. Sometimes foreign bodies are swallowed purposely, such as when smugglers swallow balloons filled with illegal drugs to get through customs; the foreign bodies may become stuck in the stomach.

Food or other materials can collect in anyone but do so more often under certain circumstances. People who have undergone surgery to their digestive tract, particularly if they have had part of their stomach or intestines removed, are particularly prone to bezoars and foreign bodies becoming stuck. People with diabetes sometimes develop a condition in which the stomach does not empty properly, resulting in problematic collections of food.

Symptoms and Diagnosis

Most bezoars and foreign bodies cause no symptoms.

A small blunt object that is swallowed may produce the sensation of something being stuck in the esophagus. This feeling may persist for a short time even after the object has passed into the stomach. A small sharp object that is swallowed may become lodged in the esophagus and cause pain, even though the person is able to swallow normally. When the esophagus is completely blocked, the person is unable to swallow anything, even saliva, and drools and spits constantly. The person may try to vomit, but nothing comes up.

Sometimes bezoars or foreign bodies lead to blood in the stool. If they are partially or completely obstructing the stomach, the small intestine, or, rarely, the large intestine, they cause cramps, bloating, loss of appetite, vomiting, and sometimes fever. If a sharp object has pierced the stomach or intestines, stool spills into the area around the intestines, causing severe abdominal pain, fever, fainting, and sometimes shock. Such a leakage is a medical emergency because it can cause peritonitis.▲ If a person has swallowed a drug-filled balloon,

▲ see page 782

the balloon may rupture, which can then lead to an overdose of the drug.

Often an obstructing object can be seen on x-rays of the abdomen. Sometimes endoscopy (a visual examination of the digestive tract using a flexible tube)▲ is performed to determine the nature of the obstructing object and to exclude a tumor as the cause. Rarely, computed tomography (CT) and ultrasound scans are used to identify the problem.

Treatment

Most bezoars and foreign bodies require no treatment. Even a small coin is likely to pass without problem. A doctor advises the person to check the stool to see when the object is excreted. Sometimes a doctor recommends that the person consume a liquid diet to help excrete the object.

To help break down a bezoar, a doctor may prescribe a regimen of dissolved cellulase, which is taken by mouth for several days.

When a doctor suspects that a blunt foreign body is stuck in the esophagus, the drug glucagon may be given intravenously to relax the esophagus and allow the object to pass through the digestive tract. Other drugs such as metoclopramide taken by mouth can help bezoars or blunt foreign objects pass through the digestive tract by causing muscles to contract.

Doctors can remove some objects that are stuck in the esophagus by passing a small tube (catheter) with a balloon on the end of it through the mouth and below the object. The balloon is inflated and the catheter is pulled out, removing the object.

Sharp objects may pierce the wall of the esophagus, with serious consequences. Therefore, they must be removed, either by endoscopy or surgery. Batteries are also removed because they can cause internal burns. When an object suspected of being a drug-filled balloon is detected, it is removed to prevent the drug overdose that can occur if the object ruptures.

CHAPTER 124

Pancreatitis

Pancreatitis is inflammation of the pancreas.

The pancreas is a leaf-shaped organ about 5 inches long. It is surrounded by the lower edge of the stomach and the wall of the duodenum (the first portion of the small intestine leading out of the stomach). The pancreas has three major functions: to secrete fluid containing digestive enzymes into the duodenum; to secrete the hormones insulin and glucagon, which help regulate sugar levels in the bloodstream; and to secrete into the duodenum the large quantities of sodium bicarbonate (the chemical in baking soda) needed to neutralize the acid coming from the stomach.

Inflammation of the pancreas can be caused by gallstones, alcohol, various drugs, some viral infections, and digestive enzymes. Pancreatitis usually develops quickly and subsides quickly (acute pancreatitis). In some cases, however, inflammation persists and gradually destroys pancreatic function (chronic pancreatitis).

Acute Pancreatitis

Acute pancreatitis is sudden inflammation of the pancreas that may be mild or life threatening but that usually subsides.

Gallstones and alcohol abuse account for almost 80% of the hospital admissions for acute pancreatitis. About $1\frac{1}{2}$ times as many women as men experience acute pancreatitis caused by gallstones. Normally, the pancreas secretes pancreatic fluid through the pancreatic duct to the duodenum. This pancreatic fluid contains digestive enzymes in an inactive form and inhibitors that inactivate any enzymes that become activated on the way to the duodenum. Blockage of the pancreatic duct by a gallstone stuck in the sphincter of Oddi stops the flow of pancreatic fluid. Usually, the blockage is temporary and causes limited damage, which

---

▲ see page 703

Locating the Pancreas

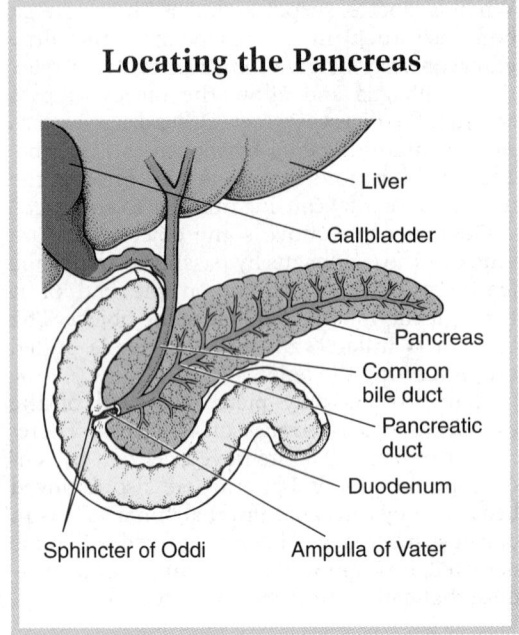

is soon repaired. But if the blockage continues, activated enzymes accumulate in the pancreas, overwhelm the inhibitors, and begin to digest the cells of the pancreas, causing severe inflammation.

Drinking as little as 2 ounces of alcohol a day (half a bottle of wine, four bottles of beer, or 5 ounces of liquor) for several years may cause the small ductules in the pancreas that drain into the pancreatic duct to clog, eventually causing acute pancreatitis. An attack of pancreatitis may be precipitated by an alcoholic binge or by an excessively large meal. Many other conditions can also cause acute pancreatitis.

Many drugs can irritate the pancreas. Usually, the inflammation resolves when the drugs are stopped. Viruses can cause pancreatitis, which is usually short-lived.

Symptoms

Almost everyone with acute pancreatitis suffers severe abdominal pain in the upper midabdomen, below the breastbone (sternum). The pain often penetrates to the back. Rarely, the pain is first felt in the lower abdomen.

▲ see page 292   ■ see page 314
★ see page 1054   ● see page 781

When acute pancreatitis is caused by gallstones, the pain usually starts suddenly and reaches its maximum intensity in minutes. The pain then remains steady and severe, has a penetrating quality, and persists for days.

Coughing, vigorous movement, and deep breathing may worsen the pain; sitting upright and leaning forward may provide some relief. Most people feel nauseated and have to vomit, sometimes to the point of dry heaves—retching without producing any vomit. Often, even large doses of an injected opioid analgesic do not relieve pain completely.

Some people, especially those who develop acute pancreatitis because of alcohol abuse, may never develop any symptoms other than moderate pain. Others feel terrible. They look sick and sweaty and have a fast pulse (100 to 140 beats a minute) and shallow, rapid breathing. Rapid breathing may occur secondary to inflammation of the lungs, areas of collapsed lung tissue (atelectasis▲), and accumulation of fluid in the chest cavity (pleural effusion■). These conditions decrease the amount of lung tissue available to transfer oxygen from the air to the blood.

At first, body temperature may be normal, but it increases in a few hours to between 100° F and 101° F (37.7° C and 38.3° C). Blood pressure may be high or low, but it tends to fall when the person stands, causing faintness. As acute pancreatitis progresses, people tend to be less and less aware of their surroundings: Some are nearly unconscious. Occasionally, the whites of the eyes (sclera) become yellowish.

Complications

Damage to the pancreas may permit activated enzymes and toxins such as cytokines★ to ooze out and enter the abdominal cavity, where they cause irritation and inflammation of the lining of the cavity (peritonitis) or of other organs. Activated enzymes and cytokines may be absorbed from the abdominal cavity into lymph vessels and eventually the bloodstream, which can lead to low blood pressure and damage to organs outside of the abdominal cavity, such as the lungs. The part of the pancreas that produces hormones, especially insulin, tends not to be damaged or affected. One of five people with acute pancreatitis develops some swelling in the upper abdomen. This swelling may occur because the movement of stomach and intestinal contents stops (a condition called ileus●) or because the inflamed pancreas enlarges and pushes the stomach forward.

Fluid also may accumulate in the abdominal cavity (a condition called ascites▲).

In severe acute pancreatitis (necrotizing pancreatitis), blood and pancreatic fluid may escape into the abdominal cavity, diminishing blood volume and resulting in a large drop in blood pressure, possibly causing shock.■ Severe acute pancreatitis can be life threatening.

Infection of an inflamed pancreas is a risk, particularly after the first week of illness. Sometimes, a doctor suspects an infection because the person's condition worsens and because a fever and high white blood cell count develop after other symptoms had initially started to subside. The diagnosis is made by culturing blood samples (growing large numbers of bacteria) to identify bacteria that are causing the infection and performing a computed tomography (CT) scan. A doctor may be able to withdraw a sample of infected material from the pancreas by inserting a needle through the skin and into the pancreas. An infection is treated with antibiotics, and surgical removal of infected and dead tissue usually is necessary.

Sometimes, a collection of pancreatic enzymes, fluid, and tissue debris resembling a cyst (a pseudocyst) but without the usual lining found in other types of cysts forms in the pancreas and expands like a balloon. If a pseudocyst grows larger and causes pain or other symptoms, a doctor drains it quickly because death can result if the pseudocyst expands further, becomes infected, bleeds, or ruptures. Depending on its location, the pseudocyst is drained either by performing a surgical procedure or by inserting a catheter through the skin or through an endoscope (a flexible viewing tube) that is passed through the mouth and into the stomach or intestine and allowing the pseudocyst to drain for several weeks.

Diagnosis

Characteristic abdominal pain leads a doctor to suspect acute pancreatitis, especially in a person who has gallbladder disease or who is an alcoholic. On examination, a doctor often notes that the abdominal wall muscles are rigid. When listening to the abdomen with a stethoscope, a doctor may hear few or no bowel (intestinal) sounds.

No single blood test proves the diagnosis of acute pancreatitis, but certain tests corroborate it. Blood levels of two enzymes produced by the pancreas, amylase and lipase, usually increase on the first day of the illness but return to normal in 3 to 7 days. If the person has

Causes of Acute Pancreatitis

- Gallstones
- Alcohol abuse
- Drugs such as furosemide and azathioprine
- Estrogen use associated with high lipid levels
- Hyperparathyroidism and high levels of calcium in the blood
- Mumps
- High levels of lipids (especially triglycerides) in the blood
- Damage to the pancreas from surgery or endoscopy
- Damage to the pancreas from blunt or penetrating injuries
- Cancer of the pancreas
- Reduced blood supply to the pancreas, for example, from severely low blood pressure
- Hereditary pancreatitis
- Kidney transplantation

had other flare-ups (bouts or attacks) of pancreatitis, however, the levels of these enzymes may not increase, because so much of the pancreas may have been destroyed that few cells are left to release the enzymes. The white blood cell count is usually increased.

Standard x-rays of the abdomen may show dilated loops of intestine or, rarely, one or more gallstones. Chest x-rays may reveal areas of collapsed lung tissue or accumulation of fluid in the chest cavity. Ultrasound scans may show gallstones in the gallbladder or sometimes in the common bile duct and also may detect swelling of the pancreas.

A CT scan is particularly useful in detecting changes in the size of the pancreas and is used in people with severe acute pancreatitis and in people with complications, such as extremely low blood pressure. Because the images are so clear, a CT scan helps a doctor make a precise diagnosis.

Prognosis

In severe acute pancreatitis, a CT scan helps determine the prognosis. If the scan indicates that the pancreas is only mildly swollen, the prognosis is excellent. If the scan shows large

▲ see page 794   ■ see page 148

areas of destroyed pancreas, the prognosis is poor.

When acute pancreatitis is mild, the death rate is about 5%. However, in pancreatitis with severe damage and bleeding, or when the inflammation is not confined to the pancreas, the death rate can be as high as 10 to 50%. Death during the first several days of acute pancreatitis is usually caused by failure of the heart, lungs, or kidneys. Death after the first week is usually caused by pancreatic infection or by a pseudocyst that bleeds or ruptures.

Treatment

Treatment of mild pancreatitis, particularly when flare-ups are recurrent, usually involves taking analgesics for pain relief and ingesting only clear liquids. Usually, normal eating can resume after 2 to 3 days without further treatment.

Moderate to severe pancreatitis usually requires hospitalization. All people with moderate to severe acute pancreatitis must initially avoid food and liquids, because eating and drinking stimulate the pancreas to produce more enzymes. If symptoms such as pain and nausea subside quickly and complications such as ileus do not develop, food and liquids can be resumed through a tube (tube feeding). However, if symptoms do not subside quickly or if complications do develop, fluids are given intravenously to prevent or treat dehydration and low blood pressure, which could worsen the pancreatitis.

People with severe acute pancreatitis generally are admitted to an intensive care unit, where vital signs (pulse, blood pressure, and rate of breathing) and urine production can be monitored continuously. Blood samples are repeatedly drawn to monitor various components of the blood, including hematocrit, sugar (glucose) levels, electrolyte levels, white blood cell count, and amylase and lipase levels. A tube may be inserted through the nose and into the stomach to remove fluid and air, particularly if nausea and vomiting persist and gastrointestinal ileus is present.

For people with a drop in blood pressure or who are in shock, blood volume is carefully maintained with intravenous fluids, and heart function is closely monitored. Some people need supplemental oxygen and the most seriously ill require a ventilator. Severe pain usually is treated with opioids.

▲ see page 789 and art on page 790

Occasionally, surgery is needed during the first few days of severe acute pancreatitis. For instance, surgery may be undertaken to clarify an uncertain diagnosis (exploratory surgery) or to relieve pancreatitis that stems from an injury. Sometimes, if a person's condition deteriorates after the first week of the illness, surgery is performed to remove infected or dead pancreatic tissue.

When acute pancreatitis results from gallstones, treatment depends on the severity. If the pancreatitis is mild, removal of the gallbladder can usually be delayed until symptoms subside. Severe pancreatitis caused by gallstones can be treated with endoscopic retrograde cholangiopancreatography (ERCP)▲ or surgery. Although more than 80% of people with gallstone pancreatitis pass the stone spontaneously, ERCP with stone removal is usually needed for people who do not improve over the initial 24 hours of hospitalization. The surgical procedure consists of removing the gallbladder and clearing out the ducts. In an older person with a coinciding illness, such as heart disease, endoscopy often is used first, but if this treatment fails, surgery is necessary.

Chronic Pancreatitis

Chronic pancreatitis is long-standing inflammation of the pancreas that results in irreversible deterioration of pancreatic structure and function.

In the United States, the most common cause of chronic pancreatitis is alcohol abuse. Other causes include a hereditary predisposition and an obstruction of the pancreatic duct resulting from narrowing of the duct or pancreatic cancer. Rarely, an attack of severe acute pancreatitis makes the pancreatic duct so narrow that chronic pancreatitis results. In many cases, the cause of chronic pancreatitis is not known. In tropical countries (for example, India, Indonesia, and Nigeria), chronic pancreatitis of unknown cause occurs commonly in children and young adults.

Symptoms

Symptoms of chronic pancreatitis may be identical to those of acute pancreatitis and generally fall into two patterns. In one, a person has persistent midabdominal pain that varies in intensity. In this pattern, a complication of chronic pancreatitis, such as an inflammatory mass, a cyst, or even pancreatic cancer, is more likely. In the other, a person has intermittent flare-ups of pancreatitis with symptoms similar to those of mild to moderate acute pancreatitis; the pain sometimes is severe and lasts for many hours or several days. With either pattern, as chronic pancreatitis progresses, cells that secrete the digestive enzymes are slowly destroyed, so eventually the pain stops.

As the number of digestive enzymes decreases, food is inadequately absorbed (resulting in a condition called malabsorption), and the person may produce bulky, unusually foul-smelling stools. The stool is light-colored and greasy and may even contain oil droplets. The inadequate absorption of food also leads to weight loss. Eventually, the insulin-secreting cells of the pancreas may be destroyed, gradually leading to diabetes.

Diagnosis

A doctor suspects chronic pancreatitis because of a person's symptoms or history of acute pancreatitis flare-ups. Blood tests are less useful in diagnosing chronic pancreatitis than in diagnosing acute pancreatitis, but they may indicate elevated levels of amylase and lipase. Also, blood tests can be used to check the level of sugar (glucose) in the blood, which may be elevated.

Tests such as x-rays, ultrasound scans, and computed tomography (CT) scans are not routinely done for people with chronic pancreatitis. However, abdominal x-rays and ultrasound scans can be used to show stones in the pancreas. Endoscopic retrograde cholangiopancreatography (ERCP)▲ may reveal a dilated duct, narrowing of the duct, or stones in the duct. A CT scan may show these abnormalities as well as the size, shape, and texture of the pancreas. And unlike ERCP, a CT scan does not require the use of an endoscope.

People with chronic pancreatitis are at increased risk of pancreatic cancer. Worsening of symptoms, especially narrowing of the pancreatic duct, makes doctors suspect cancer. In such cases, a doctor is likely to order an ultrasound scan, CT scan, or endoscopic study.

Treatment

Treatment of repeated flare-ups of chronic pancreatitis is similar to that of acute pancreatitis. During a flare-up, avoiding alcohol is essential. Avoiding all food and receiving only intravenous fluids can rest the pancreas and intestine and may relieve a painful flare-up. In addition, opioid analgesics are sometimes needed to relieve the pain.

Later, eating four or five meals a day consisting of food low in fat and protein and high in carbohydrate may help reduce the frequency and intensity of the flare-ups. The person also must continue to avoid alcohol. If pain continues, a doctor searches for complications, such as an inflammatory mass in the head of the pancreas or a pseudocyst (a collection of pancreatic enzymes, fluid, and tissue debris resembling a cyst but without the usual lining found in other types of cysts). An inflammatory mass may require surgery; a pancreatic pseudocyst that causes pain as it expands may have to be drained (decompressed).

If the person has continuing pain and no complications, usually a doctor injects a combination of lidocaine and corticosteroids into the nerves from the pancreas to block pain impulses from reaching the brain. If this procedure fails, surgery may be performed. For instance, when the pancreatic duct is dilated, creating a bypass from the pancreas to the small intestine relieves the pain in about 60 to 80% of people. When the duct is not dilated, part of the pancreas may have to be removed. Removing part of the pancreas means that cells that produce insulin will be removed as well, and diabetes may develop.

For people who no longer produce adequate digestive enzymes, taking tablets or capsules of pancreatic enzyme extracts with meals can make the stool less greasy and improve food absorption, but these problems are rarely eliminated. If necessary, a liquid antacid, a histamine-2 (H_2) blocker, or a proton pump inhibitor (drugs that reduce or prevent the production of stomach acid) may be taken with the pancreatic enzymes. With such treatment, the person usually gains some weight, has fewer daily bowel movements, has no more oil droplets in the stool, and generally feels better. If these measures are ineffective, the person can try decreasing fat intake. Supplements of the fat-soluble vitamins (A, D, E, and K) also may be needed.

Oral hypoglycemic drugs rarely can be used in the treatment of diabetes caused by chronic pancreatitis. Insulin is generally needed but can cause a problem, because these people also have decreased levels of glucagon, which is a hormone that acts to balance the effects of insulin. An excess of insulin in the bloodstream causes low sugar levels in the blood, which can result in a hypoglycemic coma.■

▲ see page 789 and art on page 790
■ see page 971

CHAPTER 125

Malabsorption

Malabsorption refers to a number of disorders in which nutrients from food are not absorbed properly in the small intestine.

Normally, foods are digested and nutrients are absorbed into the bloodstream mainly in the small intestine. Malabsorption may occur if a disorder interferes with the digestion of food or if a disorder interferes directly with the absorption of nutrients.

Digestion can be affected by disorders that prevent adequate mixing of food with digestive enzymes and acid from the stomach. Inadequate mixing may occur in a person who has had part of the stomach surgically removed. In some disorders, the body produces inadequate amounts or types of digestive enzymes, which are necessary for the breakdown of food. For example, a common cause of malabsorption is insufficient production of digestive enzymes by the pancreas, as occurs with some pancreatic diseases, or by the small intestine, as occurs in lactase deficiency. Decreased production of bile, too much acid in the stomach, or too many of the wrong kinds of bacteria growing in the small intestine may also interfere with digestion.

Absorption of nutrients into the bloodstream can be affected by disorders that injure the lining of the small intestine. The normal lining consists of small projections called villi and even smaller projections called microvilli, which create an enormous surface area for absorption. Surgical removal of a large section of the small intestine substantially reduces the surface area for absorption (short bowel syndrome). Infections (bacterial, viral, or parasitic), drugs such as neomycin and alcohol, celiac disease, and Crohn's disease all may injure the intestinal lining. Disorders that affect the remaining layers of the intestinal wall, such as blockage of the lymph vessels by lymphoma (cancer of the lymphatic system) or poor blood supply to the small intestine, also reduce absorption.

Symptoms

Symptoms of malabsorption are caused by the increased passage of unabsorbed nutrients through the digestive tract or by the nutritional deficiencies that result from inadequate absorption.

The inadequate absorption of fats in the digestive tract results in stool that is light-colored, soft, bulky, and unusually foul smelling (such stool is called steatorrhea). The stool may float or stick to the side of the toilet bowl and be difficult to flush away. The inadequate absorption of certain sugars can cause explosive diarrhea, abdominal bloating, and flatulence.

Malabsorption can cause deficiencies of all nutrients or selective deficiencies of proteins, fats, sugars, vitamins, or minerals. People with malabsorption usually lose weight. The symptoms vary depending on the specific deficiencies. For example, a protein deficiency can cause swelling (edema) anywhere throughout the body, dry skin, and hair loss.

Diagnosis

A doctor suspects malabsorption when a person has chronic diarrhea, nutritional deficiencies, and substantial weight loss despite a healthy diet. Malabsorption is less obvious and often more difficult to recognize in older people than in younger people.

Laboratory tests can help confirm the diagnosis. Tests that directly measure fat in stool samples collected over 2 or 3 days are the most reliable ones for diagnosing malabsorption of fat, which is present in almost all malabsorption disorders. A finding of more than 6 grams of fat in the stool daily is the hallmark of malabsorption. Other laboratory tests can detect malabsorption of other specific substances, such as lactose or vitamin B_{12}.

Stool samples are examined with the unaided eye as well as under the microscope. Undigested food fragments may mean that food passes through the intestine too rapidly. In a person with jaundice, stool with excess fat indicates decreased production or secretion of bile. Sometimes parasites or their eggs are seen under the microscope, suggesting that malabsorption is caused by a parasitic infection.

A biopsy (removal of a tissue specimen for examination under a microscope) may be needed to detect abnormalities in the lining of the small intestine. The tissue is removed through an endoscope (a flexible viewing tube equipped with a light source and a small clipper) passed through the mouth and into the small intestine.

Pancreatic function tests are performed if the doctor thinks that the cause of malabsorption may be the insufficient production of digestive enzymes by the pancreas. However, some of these tests are complex, time-consuming, and invasive. In one test, a tube is passed through the mouth and guided to the small intestine, so that intestinal fluids containing pancreatic secretions can be collected and measured. In another test, the person swallows a substance that requires pancreatic enzymes for its digestion. The products of digestion are then measured in the urine.

Lactose Intolerance

Lactose intolerance is the inability to digest the sugar lactose (which is present in all dairy products) because of a deficiency of the digestive enzyme lactase, leading to diarrhea and abdominal cramping.

Between 30 million and 50 million people in the United States are lactose intolerant. Lactose, the predominant sugar found in milk and other dairy products, is broken down by the enzyme lactase, which is produced by the cells in the inner lining of the small intestine. Normally, the enzyme lactase breaks down lactose, a complex sugar, into its two components, glucose and galactose. These simple sugars are then absorbed into the bloodstream through the intestinal wall. If lactase is lacking, lactose cannot be digested and absorbed. The resulting high concentration of lactose draws fluid into the small intestine, causing diarrhea. The unabsorbed lactose then passes into the large intestine, where it is fermented by bacteria, resulting in flatulence and acidic stool.

Intolerances to other sugars can also occur but are relatively rare. For example, a lack of the enzyme sucrase prevents the sugar sucrose from being absorbed into the bloodstream, and a lack of the enzymes maltase and isomaltase prevents the sugar maltose from being absorbed into the bloodstream.

Symptoms

People with lactose intolerance usually cannot tolerate milk and other dairy products, all of which contain lactose. Some people recognize this early in life and consciously or unconsciously avoid dairy products.

A child who is lactose intolerant has diarrhea and may not gain weight when milk is part of the diet. An adult may have abdominal bloating, cramps, diarrhea, flatulence, nausea,

SYMPTOMS OF NUTRIENT DEFICIENCIES

NUTRIENT	SYMPTOMS
Calcium	Bone pain and deformities; greater likelihood of fractures (due to bone thinning or osteoporosis); muscle spasms; tooth discoloration and greater susceptibility to painful tooth decay
Folic acid	Fatigue and weakness (due to anemia)
Iron	Fatigue and weakness (due to anemia)
Magnesium	Muscle spasms
Niacin	Diarrhea; skin disorders; confusion (pellagra), sore tongue
Protein	Tissue swelling (edema), usually in legs; dry skin; hair loss
Vitamin A	Night blindness
Vitamin B_1	Pins-and-needles sensation, especially in the feet; heart failure
Vitamin B_2	Sore tongue; cracks at edge of mouth
Vitamin B_{12}	Fatigue and weakness (due to anemia); pins-and-needles sensation; confusion
Vitamin C	Weakness; bleeding gums
Vitamin D	Bone thinning; bone pain
Vitamin K	Tendency to bruise and bleed

audible bowel sounds (borborygmi), and an urgent need to have a bowel movement between 30 minutes and 2 hours after eating a meal containing lactose. For some people, severe diarrhea may prevent proper absorption of nutrients because they are expelled from the body too quickly. However, the symptoms that result from lactose intolerance are usually mild. In contrast, symptoms that result from malabsorption in such conditions as celiac disease, tropical sprue, and infections of the intestine are more severe.

Diagnosis and Treatment

A doctor suspects lactose intolerance when a person has symptoms after consuming dairy products. If a 3- to 4-week trial period of a diet free of dairy products eliminates the symptoms, the diagnosis is confirmed. Specific tests are rarely necessary.

Lactose intolerance can be controlled through diet by avoiding foods containing lactose, primarily dairy products. Lactase enzymes are available in liquid and tablet forms without a prescription and can be added to milk. Lactose-reduced milk and other products are available at many supermarkets. People who must avoid dairy products should take calcium supplements to prevent calcium deficiency.

Celiac Disease

Celiac disease (nontropical sprue, gluten enteropathy, celiac sprue) is a hereditary intolerance to gluten, a protein found in wheats, barley, and oats, which causes characteristic changes in the lining of the small intestine, resulting in malabsorption.

Celiac disease affects as many as 1 of 300 people in Italy and southwestern Ireland, yet it is extremely rare in Africa, Japan, and China. There is a genetic component; about 10% of people with celiac disease have a close relative with the disease. In this disease, gluten, a protein found in wheat and, to a lesser extent, barley, rye, and oats, is believed to stimulate the production of certain antibodies. These antibodies damage the inner lining of the small intestine, resulting in flattening of the villi. The resulting smooth surface leads to malabsorption of nutrients. However, the small intestine's normal brushlike surface and function are restored when the person stops eating foods containing gluten.

Symptoms

Some people develop symptoms as children, others not until adulthood. The severity of symptoms depends on how much of the small intestine is affected.

Adults with the more classic or typical form of the disease experience diarrhea, malnutrition, and weight loss. However, some people have no digestive symptoms at all. About 10% of people with celiac disease develop a painful, itchy skin rash with small blisters—a disease called dermatitis herpetiformis.▲

In children, symptoms do not appear until foods containing gluten are introduced. Some children experience only mild upset stomach, whereas others develop painful abdominal bloating and have light-colored, unusually foul-smelling, bulky stools (steatorrhea).

The nutritional deficiencies resulting from malabsorption in celiac disease can cause additional symptoms, which tend to be more prominent in children. Some children develop growth abnormalities, such as short stature. Anemia, causing fatigue and weakness, develops as a result of iron deficiency. Low protein levels in the blood can lead to fluid retention and tissue swelling (edema). Malabsorption of vitamin B_{12} can lead to nerve damage, causing a pins-and-needles sensation in the arms and legs. Poor calcium absorption results in abnormal bone growth, a higher risk of broken bones, and painful bones and joints. Lack of calcium can also cause tooth discoloration and greater susceptibility to painful tooth decay. Girls with celiac disease may not have menstrual periods because of a low production of hormones, such as estrogen.

Diagnosis

The diagnosis is suspected when a person has the above-mentioned symptoms. Measurement of the level of specific antibodies produced when a person with celiac disease consumes gluten is a new and helpful test. The diagnosis is confirmed by an initial microscopic examination of a biopsy specimen revealing flattened villi of the small intestine and by a subsequent improvement in the lining after the person stops eating foods containing gluten.

Treatment and Prognosis

People with celiac disease must exclude all gluten from their diet, since eating even small amounts may cause symptoms. The response to a gluten-free diet is usually rapid. Once gluten is avoided, the brushlike surface of the small intestine and its absorptive function return to normal. Gluten is so widely used in food products that people with celiac disease need detailed lists of foods to be avoided and expert advice from a dietitian. Gluten is found, for example, in commercial soups, sauces, ice cream, and hot dogs.

Some people continue to have symptoms even when gluten is avoided. In such cases, either the diagnosis is incorrect or the disease has progressed to a condition called refractory celiac disease. In refractory celiac disease, treatment with corticosteroids, such as prednisone, may

▲ see page 1217

help. In rare cases, if there is no response to either gluten withdrawal or drug treatment, intravenous feeding is needed. Sometimes children are seriously ill when first diagnosed and need a period of intravenous feeding before a gluten-free diet is begun.

Although most people do well if they avoid gluten, long-standing celiac disease can be fatal in a small percentage of people who develop intestinal lymphoma. Whether strictly adhering to a gluten-free diet decreases the risk of long-term complications such as intestinal cancers or lymphoma is not known.

Tropical Sprue

Tropical sprue is a disorder of unknown cause affecting people living in tropical and subtropical areas who develop abnormalities of the lining of the small intestine, leading to malabsorption and deficiencies of many nutrients.

Tropical sprue occurs chiefly in the Caribbean, southern India, and Southeast Asia. Both natives and visitors may be affected, but children are rarely affected. The cause is unknown, but available evidence suggests an infectious cause.

Symptoms and Diagnosis

Light-colored stools, chronic diarrhea, and weight loss are typical symptoms of tropical sprue. Other symptoms of malabsorption of specific nutrients may also develop. A sore tongue develops from vitamin B_2 deficiency. A deficiency of prothrombin, which is important in blood clotting, leads to easy bruising and prolonged bleeding after an injury. Anemia usually develops as a result of iron, vitamin B_{12}, or folic acid deficiency, causing fatigue and weakness.

A doctor considers the diagnosis of tropical sprue in a person with anemia and symptoms of malabsorption who lives in or has recently visited one of the areas in which the disorder commonly occurs. X-rays of the small intestine may or may not be abnormal. An endoscopic biopsy (in which a tissue sample is obtained through a flexible tube and examined microscopically) of the small intestine can show some characteristic but not specific abnormalities. A stool sample may be analyzed to exclude parasites or bacteria as a cause.

Treatment

A person suspected of having tropical sprue is treated with an antibiotic. Either tetracycline or oxytetracycline is given over several months. Nutritional supplements, especially folic acid and vitamin B_{12}, are given as needed. Treatment usually results in a full recovery.

Whipple's Disease

Whipple's disease (intestinal lipodystrophy) is the result of a rare bacterial infection that damages the lining of the small intestine and may involve other organs of the body.

Whipple's disease affects mainly men aged 30 to 60. It is caused by an infection with the organism *Tropheryma whippelii*. The infection usually involves the small intestine but can affect other organs, such as the heart, lung, brain, joints, and eye.

Symptoms

Symptoms of Whipple's disease include diarrhea, inflamed and painful joints, fever, and skin darkening. Severe malabsorption results in weight loss along with fatigue and weakness caused by anemia. Other common symptoms are abdominal pain, cough, and pain when breathing caused by inflammation of the membrane layers covering the lungs (pleura). Fluid may collect in the space between the pleural layers (a condition called pleural effusion▲). The lymph nodes may become enlarged. People with Whipple's disease may develop heart murmurs. Confusion, memory loss, or uncontrolled eye movements indicate that the infection has spread to the brain. If left untreated, the disease is progressive and fatal.

Diagnosis and Treatment

A doctor can make the diagnosis of Whipple's disease when a biopsy (a microscopic examination of tissue) of the small intestine or of an enlarged lymph node demonstrates the bacteria.

Whipple's disease can be cured with antibiotics such as tetracycline, ampicillin, trimethoprim/sulfamethoxazole, or penicillin taken for 6 to 12 months. Symptoms subside rapidly. Despite initial response to antibiotics, however, the disease can recur.

Intestinal Lymphangiectasia

Intestinal lymphangiectasia (idiopathic hypoproteinemia) is a disorder in which the lymph vessels supplying the lining of the small intestine become enlarged and obstructed.

▲ see page 314

The lymph vessels from the digestive tract, which carry white blood cells called lymphocytes, may be enlarged at birth. Less commonly, these lymph vessels may enlarge later in life as a result of such conditions as inflammation of the pancreas (pancreatitis) or stiffening of the sac that envelops the heart (constrictive pericarditis). Lymphatic fluid leaks from the swollen lymph vessels in the wall of the intestine, preventing fat and proteins from being absorbed into the bloodstream.

Symptoms and Diagnosis

A person with intestinal lymphangiectasia has diarrhea. Nausea, vomiting, fatty stools, and abdominal pain may also develop. The person may also have swelling (edema) if lymph vessels elsewhere in the body are blocked.

Levels of protein in the blood are low. The low protein levels result in tissue swelling. The number of lymphocytes in the blood is decreased, and cholesterol levels in the blood may be normal or low.

The diagnosis is established by a biopsy of the small intestine showing enlargement of the lymph vessels. Measurement of a certain protein, called alpha$_1$-antitrypsin, in the stool can indicate the severity of protein loss into the intestines.

Treatment

When intestinal lymphangiectasia is caused by a specific condition, the underlying condition is treated. Symptoms can be relieved by eating a low-fat diet and taking supplements of certain triglycerides, which are absorbed directly into the blood and not through the lymph vessels.

CHAPTER 126

Inflammatory Bowel Diseases

In inflammatory bowel diseases, the intestine (bowel) becomes inflamed, often causing recurring abdominal cramps and diarrhea.

The two primary types of inflammatory bowel disease are Crohn's disease and ulcerative colitis. These two diseases have many similarities and sometimes are difficult to distinguish from each other. However, there are several differences. For example, Crohn's disease can affect almost any part of the digestive tract, whereas ulcerative colitis almost always affects only the large intestine. The cause of these diseases is not known. More recently recognized inflammatory bowel diseases include collagenous colitis, lymphocytic colitis, and diversion colitis.

To make a diagnosis of inflammatory bowel disease, a doctor must first exclude other possible causes of inflammation. For example, infection with parasites or bacteria may cause inflammation. Therefore, the doctor performs several tests. Stool samples obtained during a sigmoidoscopy▲ are analyzed for evidence of a bacterial or parasitic infection (acquired during travel, for example). Blood samples can determine the presence of a parasitic infection as well, or of a second infection resulting from antibiotic use.■ A doctor also checks for sexually transmitted diseases of the rectum, such as gonorrhea, herpesvirus infection, and chlamydial infection. Tissue samples may be taken from the lining of the rectum and examined microscopically for evidence of colorectal cancer and other diseases that sometimes cause bloody diarrhea. Other possible causes of inflammation that a doctor tries to exclude are ischemic colitis, which occurs more often in people older than 50; pelvic inflammatory disease, ectopic pregnancy, and ovarian cysts and tumors in women; celiac disease; and tropical sprue.

Crohn's Disease

Crohn's disease (regional enteritis, granulomatous ileitis, ileocolitis) is a chronic inflammation of the intestinal wall that may affect any part of the digestive tract.

▲ see page 703   ■ see page 745

The cause of Crohn's disease is not known. Researchers believe that a dysfunction of the immune system results in the intestine overreacting to an environmental, dietary, or infectious agent. Certain people may have a hereditary predisposition to this immune system dysfunction. Cigarette smoking appears to contribute to both the development and the periodic flare-ups (bouts or attacks) of Crohn's disease.

In the past few decades, Crohn's disease has become more common worldwide. It occurs about equally in both sexes, is more common among Jews, and tends to run in families. Most people develop Crohn's disease before age 35, usually between the ages of 15 and 25.

Most commonly, Crohn's disease occurs in the last portion of the small intestine (ileum) and in the large intestine, but it can occur in any part of the digestive tract, from the mouth to the anus and even in the skin around the anus. Crohn's disease affects the small intestine alone (35% of people), the large intestine alone (20% of people), or both the last portion of the small intestine and the large intestine (45% of people). The disease may affect some segments of the intestinal tract while leaving normal segments (skip areas) between the affected areas. Where Crohn's disease is active, the full thickness of the bowel is involved.

Symptoms and Complications

The most common early symptoms of Crohn's disease are chronic diarrhea (which sometimes is bloody), crampy abdominal pain, fever, loss of appetite, and weight loss. Symptoms may continue for days or weeks and may resolve without treatment. Complete and permanent recovery after a single attack is extremely rare. Crohn's disease almost invariably flares up at irregular intervals throughout a person's life. Flare-ups can be mild or severe, brief or prolonged. Severe flare-ups can lead to intense pain, dehydration, and blood loss. Why the symptoms come and go and what triggers new flare-ups or determines their severity are not known. The inflammation tends to recur in the same area of the intestine, but it may spread to other areas after a diseased area has been removed surgically.

Common complications of inflammation include the development of an intestinal obstruction, pus-filled pockets of infection (abscesses), and abnormal connecting channels (fistulas). Fistulas may connect two different parts of the intestine. Fistulas also may connect the intestine and bladder or the intestine and the skin surface, especially around the anus. Although fistulas from the small intestine are common, wide-open perforations are rare.

When the large intestine is affected extensively by Crohn's disease, rectal bleeding commonly occurs; after many years, the risk of colon cancer (cancer of the large intestine) is greatly increased. About one third of people who develop Crohn's disease have problems around the anus, especially fistulas and cracks (fissures) in the lining of the mucus membrane of the anus. Crohn's disease may be complicated by certain disorders affecting other parts of the body—such as gallstones, inadequate absorption of nutrients, urinary tract infections, kidney stones, and deposits of the protein amyloid in several organs (amyloidosis).

When Crohn's disease causes a flare-up of gastrointestinal symptoms, the person may also experience inflammation of the joints (arthritis), inflammation of the whites of the eyes (episcleritis), mouth sores (aphthous stomatitis), inflamed skin nodules on the arms and legs (erythema nodosum), and blue-red skin sores containing pus (pyoderma gangrenosum). When Crohn's disease is not causing a flare-up of gastrointestinal symptoms, the person still may experience inflammation of the spine (ankylosing spondylitis), inflammation of the pelvic joints (sacroiliitis), inflammation inside the eye (uveitis), and inflammation of the bile ducts (primary sclerosing cholangitis).

In children, gastrointestinal symptoms such as abdominal pain and diarrhea often are not the main symptoms and may not appear at all. Instead, the main symptom may be slow growth, joint inflammation, fever, or weakness and fatigue resulting from anemia.

Diagnosis

A doctor may suspect Crohn's disease in a person with recurring crampy abdominal pain and diarrhea, particularly if the person has a family history of Crohn's disease or a history of problems around the anus. Other clues to the diagnosis may include inflammation in the joints, eyes, or skin. The doctor may feel a lump or fullness in the lower part of the abdomen, most often on the right side.

No laboratory test specifically identifies Crohn's disease, but blood tests may show anemia, abnormally high numbers of white blood cells, low levels of the protein albumin, and other indications of inflammation.

A colonoscopy (an examination of the large intestine with a flexible viewing tube) and a biopsy (removal of a tissue specimen for microscopic examination) are usually the first tests performed after a physical examination and blood tests have been completed.

If Crohn's disease is limited to the small intestine, a colonoscopy will not detect the disease. However, Crohn's disease can almost always be detected on x-rays after barium is swallowed. X-rays taken after barium is given by enema can reveal the characteristic appearance of Crohn's disease in the large intestine. Computed tomography (CT) can show changes that are helpful in distinguishing between Crohn's disease and ulcerative colitis and is the best way to identify complications that occur outside the walls of the intestinal tract, such as abscesses or fistulas.

Treatment and Prognosis

Although Crohn's disease has no known cure, many treatments help reduce inflammation and relieve symptoms.

Antidiarrheal Drugs: These drugs may relieve cramps and diarrhea.▲ These drugs, which include anticholinergic drugs (drugs that block the normal action of part of the nervous system),■ diphenoxylate, loperamide, deodorized opium tincture, and codeine, are taken by mouth—preferably before meals. Taking methylcellulose or psyllium preparations sometimes helps prevent anal irritation by making the stool firmer.

Anti-inflammatory Drugs: Sulfasalazine and mesalamine, olsalazine, and balsalazide (drugs chemically related to sulfasalazine) reduce inflammation. These drugs can suppress symptoms when they occur and reduce inflammation, especially in the large intestine. Mesalamine is marginally effective in preventing recurrences. However, all of these drugs work less well for relieving severe flare-ups.

Corticosteroids such as prednisone, which is given by mouth, may dramatically reduce fever and diarrhea, relieve abdominal pain and tenderness, and improve appetite and sense of well-being. However, long-term corticosteroid therapy invariably results in side effects.★ Generally, high doses are taken to relieve major inflammation and symptoms; then the dose is reduced, and the drug is discontinued

as soon as possible. A new corticosteroid called budesonide has fewer side effects than prednisone, although it is not as effective and generally does not prevent relapses beyond 6 to 9 months.

If the disease becomes severe, the person is hospitalized, and corticosteroids are given intravenously. Initially, the person is given nothing by mouth, and intravenous fluids are given to restore and maintain body fluids (hydration). People with heavy rectal bleeding may require blood transfusions; those people with mild anemia require iron supplements by mouth.

Immunomodulating Drugs: Drugs such as azathioprine and mercaptopurine, which modify the actions of the immune system, are effective for people with Crohn's disease who do not respond to other drugs and are especially effective for maintaining long periods of remission. They significantly improve the person's overall condition, decrease the need for corticosteroids, and often heal fistulas. However, these drugs often do not produce benefits for 2 to 4 months and may have potentially serious side effects. Therefore, a doctor closely monitors the person for allergy, inflammation of the pancreas (pancreatitis), and a low white blood cell count. Newly available blood tests may help the doctor ensure safe and effective drug dosages.

Methotrexate, given by injection once a week, benefits some people who do not respond to or who cannot tolerate corticosteroids, azathioprine, or mercaptopurine. High-dose cyclosporine may help reduce inflammation and heal fistulas, but it cannot safely be used long-term.

Infliximab, derived from monoclonal antibodies, is another modifier of the immune system's actions. Infliximab can be given intravenously for moderate to severe Crohn's disease that has not responded to other drugs. However, because the benefits of each infusion are short-lived, other treatments are needed between infusions of infliximab. Because infliximab is a relatively new drug, its long-term benefit and all of its side effects are not yet known. Many other drugs that focus on regulating the immune system are being developed.

Broad-spectrum Antibiotics: Antibiotics that are effective against many types of bacteria are often prescribed to treat infectious complications. The antibiotic metronidazole is the most common choice for the treatment of abscesses and fistulas around the anus. Metronidazole may also help relieve the noninfectious symp-

▲ see table on page 756
■ see box on page 79   ★ see box on page 374

℞ DRUGS THAT REDUCE BOWEL INFLAMMATION

TYPE DRUG	SELECTED SIDE EFFECTS	COMMENTS
Aminosalicylates		
Balsalazide Mesalamine Olsalazine Sulfasalazine	Nausea, headache, dizziness, fatigue; rarely, inflammation of the liver (hepatitis) and pancreas (pancreatitis)	Abdominal pain, dizziness, and fatigue are related to dose; hepatitis and pancreatitis are unrelated to dose. Side effects are more common with sulfasalazine than with any of the other aminosalicylates
Corticosteroids		
Prednisone	Diabetes mellitus, high blood pressure, cataracts, osteoporosis; thinning of skin, mental problems (see also box on page 374)	Diabetes and high blood pressure more likely to occur in people with other risk factors
Budesonide	Diabetes mellitus, high blood pressure, cataracts, osteoporosis (decreased bone density)—see also box on page 374	Lower rate of side effects than many other corticosteroids
Immunomodulators		
Azathioprine Mercaptopurine	Allergic reactions, pancreatitis, low white blood cell count	
Cyclosporine	High blood pressure, kidney failure, development of lymphomas (cancers of the lymphatic system)	Side effects become more likely with long-term use
Methotrexate	Scarring of the liver (cirrhosis), low white blood cell count	
Infliximab	Abdominal pain, bronchitis (inflammation of the major airways of the lungs), infection	Numerous potential immediate side effects during infusion, such as fever, hives, decreased blood pressure, difficulty breathing

toms of Crohn's disease, such as diarrhea and abdominal cramps. However, when used for a long time, metronidazole can damage nerves, resulting in a pins-and-needles sensation in the arms and legs. This side effect usually disappears when the drug is stopped, but relapses of Crohn's disease after discontinuing metronidazole are common. Some other antibiotics, such as ciprofloxacin or levofloxacin, may be used in place of or in combination with metronidazole.

Dietary Regimens: Defined-formula diets, in which each nutritional component is precisely measured, may improve the condition of an intestinal obstruction or fistula at least for a short time and also may help children grow more than they might otherwise. These diets may be tried before or in addition to surgery. Occasionally, concentrated nutrients are given intravenously to compensate for the poor absorption of nutrients that is typical of Crohn's disease.

Surgery: Surgery may be needed when the intestine is obstructed or when abscesses or fistulas do not heal. An operation to remove diseased sections of the intestine may relieve symptoms indefinitely, but it does not cure the disease. Crohn's disease tends to recur where the remaining intestine is rejoined, although several drug therapies initiated after surgery reduce this tendency. A second operation is ultimately needed in nearly half of the people. Consequently, surgery is performed only if specific complications or the failure of drug therapy makes it necessary. Still, most people who have undergone surgery consider their quality of life to be better than it was before the operation.

Crohn's disease usually does not shorten a person's life. However, some people die of cancer of the digestive tract, which may develop in long-standing Crohn's disease.

Ulcerative Colitis

Ulcerative colitis is a chronic disease in which the large intestine becomes inflamed and ulcerated (pitted or eroded), leading to flare-ups (bouts or attacks) of bloody diarrhea, abdominal cramps, and fever.

Ulcerative colitis may start at any age but usually begins between the ages of 15 and 30. A small group of people have their first attack between the ages of 50 and 70.

Ulcerative colitis usually does not affect the full thickness of the wall of the large intestine and rarely affects the small intestine. The disease usually begins in the rectum or the sigmoid colon (the lower end of the large intestine) and eventually spreads along the partial or entire length of the large intestine. In some people, most of the large intestine is affected early on.

Ulcerative proctitis, which is confined to the rectum, is a very common and more benign form of ulcerative colitis.

The cause of ulcerative colitis is not known, but heredity and an overactive immune response in the intestine may be contributing factors. Cigarette smoking, which is detrimental in Crohn's disease, appears to actually decrease the risk of ulcerative colitis. However, smoking in order to reduce the risk of ulcerative colitis is ill-advised in light of the many health problems that smoking can cause.

Symptoms

The symptoms of ulcerative colitis occur in flare-ups. A flare-up may be sudden and severe, producing violent diarrhea, high fever, abdominal pain, and peritonitis (inflammation of the lining of the abdominal cavity). During such flare-ups, the person is profoundly ill. More often, a flare-up begins gradually, and the person has an urgency to have a bowel movement (defecate), mild cramps in the lower abdomen, and visible blood and mucus in the stool. A flare-up can last days or weeks and can recur at any time.

When the disease is limited to the rectum and the sigmoid colon, the stool may be normal or hard and dry; however, mucus containing large numbers of red and white blood cells is discharged from the rectum during or between bowel movements. General symptoms of illness, such as fever, are mild or absent.

If the disease extends farther up the large intestine, the stool is looser, and the person may have 10 to 20 bowel movements a day. Often, the person has severe abdominal cramps and distressing, painful rectal spasms that accompany the urge to defecate. There is no relief at night. The stool may be watery and contain pus, blood, and mucus. Frequently, the stool consists almost entirely of blood and pus. The person also may have a fever and a poor appetite and may lose weight.

Complications

Bleeding, the most common complication, often causes iron deficiency anemia. In nearly 10% of people with ulcerative colitis, a rapidly progressive first attack becomes very severe, with massive bleeding, perforation, or widespread infection.

Toxic colitis, a particularly severe complication, involves damage to the entire thickness of the intestinal wall. The damage causes ileus—a condition in which the normal contractile movements of the intestinal wall temporarily stop—so that the intestinal contents are not propelled along their way. Abdominal expansion (distention) develops. As toxic colitis worsens, the large intestine loses muscle tone, and within days—or even hours—it starts to expand. X-rays of the abdomen show gas inside the paralyzed sections of intestine.

Toxic megacolon occurs when the large intestine greatly expands (distends). The person is severely ill and may have a high fever. The person also has pain and tenderness in the abdomen and a high white blood cell count. If the intestine ruptures, the risk of death is great. However, of the people who receive prompt treatment before rupture occurs, fewer than 4% die.

Colon cancer occurs in as many as 1 of 100 people with ulcerative colitis each year in the later stages of their illness; 10 of 100 people with extensive ulcerative colitis develop colon cancer over their lifetime. The risk of colon cancer is highest when the entire large intestine is affected and the person has had ulcerative colitis for more than 8 years, regardless of how active the disease is. Colonoscopy (examination of the large intestine using a flexible viewing tube) every 1 to 2 years is advised for people who have had ulcerative colitis for at least 8 years. During colonoscopy, tissue samples are obtained throughout the large intestine for microscopic examination. Most people survive if the diagnosis of cancer is made during the cancer's early stages.

Other complications can occur, as in Crohn's disease. When ulcerative colitis causes a flare-up of gastrointestinal symptoms, the person also may experience inflammation of the joints (arthritis), inflammation of the whites of the eyes (episcleritis), inflamed skin nodules (erythema nodosum), and blue-red skin sores containing pus (pyoderma gangrenosum). When ulcerative colitis is not causing a flare-up of gastrointestinal symptoms, the person still may experience inflammation of the spine (ankylosing spondylitis), inflammation of the pelvic joints (sacroiliitis), and inflammation of the inside of the eye (uveitis).

Although people with ulcerative colitis commonly have minor liver dysfunction, only about 1 to 3% have symptoms of mild to severe liver disease. Severe liver disease can include inflammation of the liver (chronic active hepatitis); inflammation of the bile ducts (primary sclerosing cholangitis), which narrow and eventually close; and replacement of functional liver tissue with scar tissue (cirrhosis). Inflammation of the bile ducts may appear many years before any intestinal symptoms of ulcerative colitis; bile duct inflammation greatly increases the risk of cancer of the bile ducts and may even increase the risk of colon cancer.

Diagnosis

The person's symptoms and a stool examination help the doctor establish the diagnosis. Blood tests reveal anemia, increased numbers of white blood cells, a low level of the protein albumin, and an elevated erythrocyte sedimentation rate (ESR), which indicates active inflammation. A sigmoidoscopy (an examination of the sigmoid colon using a flexible viewing tube) confirms the diagnosis and permits a doctor to directly observe the severity of the inflammation. Even during symptom-free intervals, the intestine rarely appears entirely normal, and tissue samples removed for microscopic examination usually show chronic inflammation.

X-rays of the abdomen may indicate the severity and extent of the disease. Barium enema x-ray studies and colonoscopy are not usually done before treatment begins because they pose a risk of perforation when done during the active stages of the disease. At some point, however, the entire large intestine is usually evaluated by colonoscopy to determine the extent of the disease.

Prognosis and Treatment

Usually, ulcerative colitis is chronic, with repeated flare-ups and remissions. A rapidly progressive initial attack results in serious complications in about 10% of people. Complete recovery after a single attack may occur in another 10%. However, some people who have only a single attack may actually have ulcerations from an undetected infection rather than true ulcerative colitis.

People who have ulcerative proctitis (inflammation and ulceration that are confined to the rectum) have the best prognosis. Severe complications are unlikely; however, in about 10 to 30% of people, the disease eventually spreads to the large intestine (thus evolving into ulcerative colitis).

Treatment aims to control the inflammation, reduce symptoms, and replace any lost fluids and nutrients.

Dietary Restrictions: Iron supplements may offset anemia caused by ongoing blood loss in the stool. Raw fruits and vegetables should be avoided to reduce injury to the inflamed lining of the large intestine. A diet free of dairy products may decrease symptoms and is worth trying but need not be continued if no benefit is noted.

Antidiarrheal Drugs: Anticholinergic drugs or small doses of loperamide or diphenoxylate are taken for relatively mild diarrhea. For more intense diarrhea, higher doses of diphenoxylate or deodorized opium tincture, loperamide, or codeine may be needed. In severe cases, a doctor closely monitors the person taking these antidiarrheal drugs to avoid precipitating toxic megacolon.

Anti-inflammatory Drugs: Drugs such as sulfasalazine, olsalazine, mesalamine, and, most recently, balsalazide, are used to reduce the inflammation of ulcerative colitis and to prevent flare-ups of symptoms. These drugs usually are taken by mouth, but mesalamine can also be given as an enema or a suppository. Whether given by mouth or rectally, these drugs are at best moderately effective for treating mild or moderately active disease and for maintaining remission.

People with moderately severe disease who are not confined to bed usually take oral corticosteroids such as prednisone. Prednisone in fairly high doses frequently induces a dramatic remission. After prednisone controls the inflammation of ulcerative colitis, sulfasalazine, olsalazine, or mesalamine often is given to maintain the improvement. Gradually, the prednisone dosage is decreased, and ultimately, the prednisone is discontinued. Prolonged corticosteroid treatment almost invariably produces side effects. The new corticosteroid budesonide has fewer side effects than prednisone but may not be as effective. When mild or moderate ulcerative colitis is limited to the left side of the large intestine (descending colon) and the rectum, enemas with a corticosteroid or mesalamine may be given.

If the disease becomes severe, the person is hospitalized, and corticosteroids and fluids are given intravenously. People with heavy rectal bleeding may require blood transfusions.

Immunomodulating Drugs: Drugs such as azathioprine and mercaptopurine have been used to maintain remissions in people with ulcerative colitis who would otherwise need long-term corticosteroid therapy. These drugs inhibit the function of T cells, which are an important component of the immune system. However, these drugs are slow to act, and a benefit may not be seen for 2 to 4 months. They also have potentially serious side effects that require close monitoring by the doctor. Cyclosporine has been given to some people who are suffering severe flare-ups and have not responded to corticosteroid therapy. Many of these people respond initially to the cyclosporine, but some may still ultimately require surgery.

Surgery: Surgery may be necessary for unremitting chronic disease that would otherwise make the person an invalid or chronically dependent on high doses of corticosteroids. In rare cases, severe colitis-related problems outside the intestine, such as blue-red skin sores containing pus (pyoderma gangrenosum) or severe blood clotting in deep veins of the legs or arms, may make surgery necessary.

Surgery is performed on a nonemergency basis when cancer is diagnosed or precancerous changes (dysplasia) are identified in the large intestine. Surgery also may be performed because of a narrowing of the large intestine or growth retardation in children. Complete removal of the large intestine and rectum permanently cures ulcerative colitis. Living with a permanent ileostomy (a surgically created connection between the lowest portion of the

small intestine and an opening in the abdominal wall) and an ileostomy bag has been the traditional price of this cure. However, various alternative procedures are available, the most common one being a procedure called ileo-anal anastomosis. In this procedure, the large intestine and most of the rectum are removed, and a small reservoir is created out of the small intestine and attached to the remaining rectum just above the anus. This procedure maintains continence, although some complications, such as inflammation of the reservoir, may occur.

For people with ulcerative proctitis, surgery is rarely needed, and life expectancy is normal. In some people, though, the symptoms may prove exceptionally resistant to treatment.

Toxic colitis is an emergency that may require surgery. As soon as a doctor detects it or suspects impending toxic megacolon, all antidiarrheal drugs are discontinued, the person is given nothing to eat, a tube is inserted through the nose and into the stomach or small intestine and attached to intermittent suction, and all fluids, nutrition, and drugs are given intravenously. The person is monitored closely for signs of peritonitis or a perforation. If these measures fail to improve the person's condition in 24 to 48 hours, emergency surgery is needed: All or most of the large intestine is removed.

Collagenous Colitis and Lymphocytic Colitis

Collagenous colitis and lymphocytic colitis are chronic diseases in which certain kinds of white blood cells infiltrate the lining of the large intestine, leading to watery diarrhea.

These chronic diseases can affect the entire length of the large intestine, including the sigmoid colon and the rectum, but often in a patchy distribution. The lining of the intestine develops a thicker layer of a type of connective tissue (collagen) or an accumulation of lymphocytes (a certain type of white blood cell).

The cause is unknown, although an overactive immune response to some unidentified triggering factor seems possible. Many people who develop collagenous colitis or lymphocytic colitis have been regular users of nonsteroidal anti-inflammatory drugs (NSAIDs), but these drugs have not been proven to be a cause of the diseases. Unlike Crohn's disease and ulcerative colitis, collagenous colitis and lymphocytic colitis do not increase the risk of colon cancer.

Collagenous colitis develops primarily in middle-aged or older women; lymphocytic colitis may develop in younger people and occurs in both sexes equally.

Symptoms and Diagnosis

In addition to nonbloody, watery diarrhea, people with collagenous colitis or lymphocytic colitis often experience crampy abdominal pain, nausea, abdominal expansion (distention), and weight loss. Fasting for a few days often leads to a decrease in the frequency and amount of diarrhea. Diarrhea and other symptoms often fluctuate, with periods of worsening symptoms and periods of improvement or complete resolution.

A doctor considers the diagnosis of collagenous colitis or lymphocytic colitis when a person has persistent watery diarrhea and when tests do not reveal another cause. The diseases are diagnosed by microscopic examination of several samples of tissue taken from the lining of the large intestine obtained during colonoscopy (examination of the large intestine with a flexible viewing tube).

Treatment

Antidiarrheal drugs, such as anticholinergic drugs or small doses of loperamide or diphenoxylate, are effective for many people with these diseases. Anti-inflammatory drugs, such as salicylates (for example, bismuth subsalicylate), sulfasalazine, and mesalamine, are effective as well. Antibiotics such as metronidazole and erythromycin also seem to help, although infection has not been found to be a cause of the diseases. Corticosteroids (such as prednisone) also work well but are usually reserved for people who do not respond to other drug treatment.

Diversion Colitis

Diversion colitis is inflammation that develops in a lower part of the large intestine after the passage of stool above this part has been surgically diverted.

Some people undergo an ileostomy (a surgically created connection between the lowest portion of the small intestine and an opening in the abdominal wall) or a colostomy (the surgical creation of an opening between the large intestine and the abdominal wall). Ileostomies and colostomies may be performed for treatment of diseases such as cancer, ulcerative colitis, and diverticulitis or for treatment of damage to the intestine due to an injury. In many people, especially when the doctor expects the need for the bypass of the large intestine to be temporary, either the entire large intestine or a portion of the large intestine is left in place below the point where the flow of stool is diverted.

In about one third of people who have all or a portion of their large intestine left in place after an ileostomy or colostomy, symptoms of diversion colitis, ranging from passage of mucus from the rectum to rectal bleeding and pain, may develop within 1 year after surgery. Most people do not require treatment because the symptoms remain mild. Surgery to reattach the two separated portions of the intestine and restore the normal flow of stool usually leads to resolution of the inflammation and symptoms.

CHAPTER 127

Antibiotic-Associated Colitis

Antibiotic-associated colitis is inflammation of the large intestine caused by the growth of unusual bacteria that results from the use of antibiotics.

Many antibiotics alter the balance among the types and quantity of bacteria in the intestine, thus allowing certain disease-causing bacteria to multiply and replace other bacteria. The type of bacteria that most commonly overgrows and causes infection is *Clostridium difficile*. *Clostridium difficile* infection releases two toxins that can damage the protective lining of the large intestine.

Almost any antibiotic can cause this disorder, but clindamycin, penicillins such as ampi-

When *Clostridium difficile* Colitis Is Not Caused by Antibiotics

Colitis with evidence of *Clostridium difficile* infection sometimes occurs when there has not been any recent use of antibiotics. Physically stressful events, such as surgery, can likely lead to the same kind of imbalance among the types and quantity of bacteria in the intestine, which in turn allows *Clostridium difficile* infection and colitis to develop. People who are hospitalized or who live in a nursing home may become infected and develop colitis when *Clostridium difficile* is spread from other infected people. The bacteria can be inadvertently carried on a person's hands; spread among people can be prevented by meticulous hand-washing. Some otherwise healthy people may be carriers of *Clostridium difficile* bacteria without having symptoms of colitis themselves.

cillin, and cephalosporins such as cephalexin are implicated most often. Other commonly involved antibiotics include erythromycin, sulfonamides such as sulfamethoxazole, chloramphenicol, tetracycline, and quinolones such as norfloxacin.

Clostridium difficile infection is most common when an antibiotic is taken by mouth, but it also occurs when antibiotics are injected or administered intravenously. The risk of developing antibiotic-associated colitis increases with age.

Symptoms

Symptoms usually begin while the person is taking antibiotics. However, in one third of people who have this disorder, symptoms do not appear until 1 to 10 days after treatment has stopped, and in some people, symptoms do not appear for as long as 6 weeks afterward.

Symptoms vary according to the degree of inflammation caused by the bacteria, ranging from slightly loose stools to bloody diarrhea, abdominal pain, and fever. The most severe cases may involve life-threatening dehydration, low blood pressure, toxic megacolon,▲ and perforation of the large intestine.

Diagnosis

The diagnosis of antibiotic-associated colitis is confirmed when one of the toxins produced by *Clostridium difficile* is identified in

▲ see page 742

a stool sample. A toxin is found in about 20% of people with mild antibiotic-associated colitis and in more than 90% of those with severe antibiotic-associated colitis. Sometimes two or three stool samples must be obtained before the toxin is detected.

A doctor can also diagnose antibiotic-associated colitis by inspecting the lower part of the inflamed large intestine (the sigmoid colon), usually through a sigmoidoscope (a rigid or flexible viewing tube). A colonoscope (a longer flexible viewing tube) is used to examine the entire large intestine if the diseased section of intestine is higher than the reach of the sigmoidoscope. These procedures, however, usually are not required.

Treatment

If a person with antibiotic-associated colitis has diarrhea while taking antibiotics, the drugs are discontinued immediately unless they are essential. Drugs that slow the movement of the intestine, such as diphenoxylate, generally are avoided because they may prolong the disorder by keeping the disease-causing toxin in contact with the large intestine. Antibiotic-induced diarrhea without complications usually subsides on its own within 10 to 12 days after the antibiotic has been stopped. When it does, no other therapy is required. However, if mild symptoms persist, cholestyramine may be effective, probably because it binds itself to the toxin.

For most cases of more severe antibiotic-associated colitis, the antibiotic metronidazole is effective against *Clostridium difficile*. The antibiotic vancomycin is reserved for the most severe or resistant cases. Symptoms return in up to 20% of people with this disorder, and treatment with antibiotics is repeated. If diarrhea returns repeatedly, prolonged antibiotic therapy may be needed. Some people are treated with preparations of lactobacillus given by mouth or bacteroides given rectally to restock the intestine with normal bacteria; however, these treatments are not used routinely.

Rarely, antibiotic-associated colitis is so severe that the person must be hospitalized to receive intravenous fluids, electrolytes (such as sodium, magnesium, calcium, and potassium), and blood transfusions. A temporary ileostomy (a surgically created connection between the small intestine and an opening in the abdominal wall that diverts stool from the large intestine and rectum) or surgical removal of the large intestine occasionally is needed in these severe cases as a lifesaving measure.

CHAPTER 128

Diverticular Disease

Diverticular disease is characterized by small, balloon-like sacs (diverticula) protruding through the muscular layer of the gastrointestinal (digestive) tract.

By far, the most common site for diverticula to develop is in the large intestine. Rarely, diverticula develop in the stomach and small intestine. Meckel's diverticulum is the most common diverticular disease of the small intestine; it is present at birth in about 3% of people.▲ The presence of diverticula is called diverticulosis—a condition that tends to develop during middle age. If diverticula become inflamed, the condition is called diverticulitis.

Diverticulosis

Diverticulosis is the presence of multiple diverticula, usually in the large intestine.

Diverticula may develop anywhere in the large intestine, but they are more common in the sigmoid colon, which is the last part of the large intestine just before the rectum. Diverticula vary in diameter from one tenth of an inch to 1 inch. They are uncommon before age 40 but become more common rapidly thereafter; just about everyone who reaches age 90 has many diverticula. Giant diverticula, which are rare, range from 1 to 6 inches in diameter. A person may have only a single giant diverticulum.

Cause

The development of diverticula is thought to be caused by spasms of the muscular layer of the intestine. The cause of these intestinal spasms is unknown but may be related to a low-fiber diet or to inadequate fluid intake. The resulting pressure that these spasms exert on the intestinal wall causes a part of the wall to bulge at a point of weakness, usually near to where an artery penetrates the muscular layer of the large intestine. An increase in the thickness of the muscular layer is a common finding in the sigmoid colon of people with diverticulosis. The cause of a giant diverticulum is unclear.

Symptoms

Diverticula themselves are not dangerous. In fact, most people with diverticulosis do not have symptoms. However, diverticulosis can sometimes cause unexplained painful cramps, diarrhea or other bowel movement disturbances, and blood in the stool. The narrow opening of a diverticulum can bleed, sometimes heavily, into the intestine and out through the rectum. Bleeding may also result when stool gets wedged in the diverticulum and damages a blood vessel (usually the artery beside the diverticulum). Stool that is trapped in a diverticulum may cause not only bleeding but also inflammation and infection, resulting in diverticulitis.

Diagnosis

Diverticulosis is suspected when symptoms such as unexplained painful cramps, diarrhea or other bowel movement disturbances, or rectal bleeding are present. The diagnosis is confirmed by barium enema x-ray study or by colonoscopy. However, if the person has severe abdominal pain, computed tomography (CT) is performed instead, so as not to rupture the inflamed intestine.

If blood is present in the stool, colonoscopy is usually the best method with which to identify the source. However, angiography or radionuclide scans taken after an intravenous injection of radioactive red blood cells may be required to determine the source of bleeding.

Treatment

The goal of treatment is usually to reduce intestinal spasms, which is best achieved by maintaining a high-fiber diet (which consists of vegetables, fruits, and whole grains) and drinking plenty of fluids. An increased bulk in the large intestine reduces spasms, which in turn decreases the pressure on the walls of the large intestine. If a high-fiber diet alone is not effective, a diet supplemented daily with bran or a bulking agent, such as psyllium or methylcellulose, may help.

Uncomplicated diverticulosis, in which a person has no evidence of inflammation, infection, or complications, does not require surgery. If bleeding recurs often or if the source of the

---

▲ see page 1590

What Is Diverticulosis?

In diverticulosis, many balloon-like sacs (diverticula) develop in the large intestine, most commonly in the last part of it (sigmoid colon). Most diverticula vary in diameter from $\frac{1}{10}$ inch to more than 1 inch. For unclear reasons, some diverticula become very large—up to 6 inches in diameter.

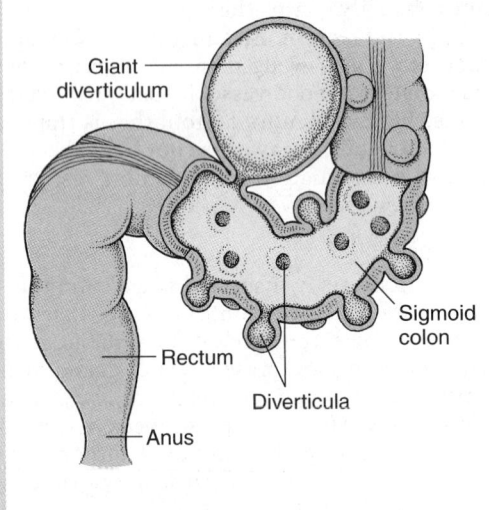

bleeding cannot be determined, surgery to remove most of the large intestine may be needed, but such surgery is not commonly done.

A giant diverticulum usually requires surgery, because it is likely to become infected and to rupture.

Diverticulitis

Diverticulitis is inflammation or infection of one or more diverticula.

Diverticulitis occurs in people with diverticulosis. It most commonly affects the sigmoid colon, which is the last part of the large intestine just before the rectum. Diverticulitis is more common in people older than 40. It can be severe in people of any age, although it is most serious in the elderly, especially those taking corticosteroids or other drugs that suppress the immune system and thus increase the hazards of infection. Among people younger than 50 who must undergo surgery for diverticulitis, men outnumber women three to one;

among those older than 70, women outnumber men three to one.

Symptoms and Diagnosis

Diverticulitis typically produces pain, tenderness (usually in the left lower part of the abdomen), and fever. Unlike diverticulosis, diverticulitis generally does not cause gastrointestinal bleeding.

If a doctor knows that the person already has diverticulosis, a diagnosis of diverticulitis may be made almost entirely on the basis of the symptoms. However, many other conditions involving the large intestine and other organs in the abdomen and pelvis can produce symptoms similar to diverticulitis, including appendicitis, colon or ovarian cancer, a pus-filled pocket of infection (abscess), and noncancerous growths on the wall of the uterus (uterine fibroids).

A CT or ultrasound scan may be helpful for determining that the problem is diverticulitis and not appendicitis or an abscess.

Once inflammation has subsided or infection has been treated, a doctor may perform a colonoscopy (an examination of the large intestine using a flexible viewing tube) or a barium enema x-ray study. These tests are performed to either confirm the presence or assess the severity of diverticula. Colonoscopy or barium enema x-rays usually need to be delayed for several weeks after treatment, because they could damage or rupture an inflamed intestine. Exploratory surgery may be needed to confirm the diagnosis.

Complications

The inflammation of the intestinal wall can lead to the development of fistulas (abnormal channels) that connect the large intestine with other organs. Fistulas usually form when a diverticulum in the large intestine is touching another organ (such as the bladder), and the diverticulum ruptures. The resulting inflammation along with the bacterial contents of the large intestine slowly penetrates the adjacent organ, resulting in a fistula. Most fistulas form between the sigmoid colon and the bladder. These fistulas are more common in men than in women, although women who have had a hysterectomy (removal of the uterus) are at increased risk, because the large intestine and bladder are no longer separated by the uterus. When fistulas form between the large intestine and bladder, intestinal contents, including normal bacteria, enter the

Complications of Diverticular Disease

In diverticular disease, a diverticulum may bleed into the intestine. If a diverticulum ruptures, the contents of the intestine, including bacteria and blood, spill into the abdominal cavity, often causing infection. An abnormal channel (fistula) may form between the large intestine and another organ, usually when a diverticulum that touches another organ ruptures.

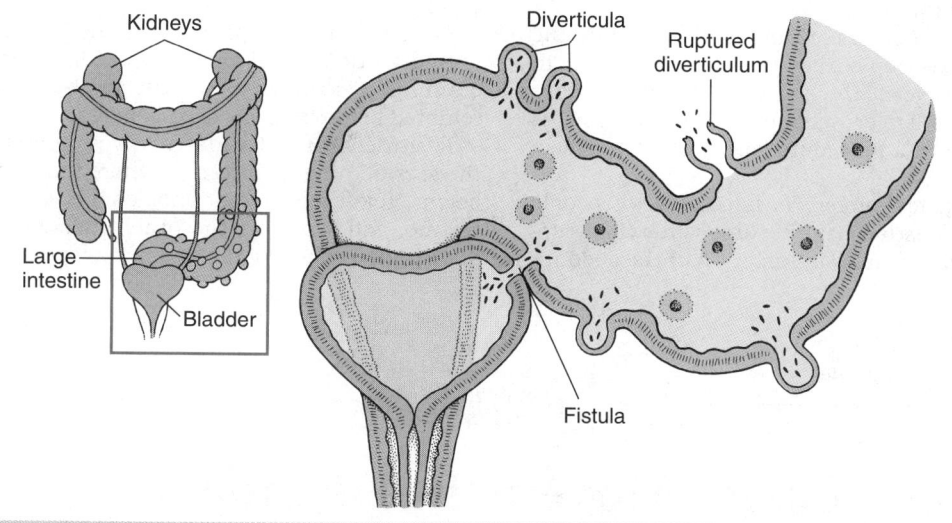

bladder and cause urinary tract infections. Less commonly, a fistula can develop between the large intestine and the small intestine, uterus, vagina, abdominal wall, or even the thigh or chest.

Other possible complications of diverticulitis include inflammation of nearby organs (such as the uterus, bladder, or other areas of the digestive tract), rupture of the wall of a diverticulum, abscess (a pus-filled pocket of infection), infection of the lining of the abdominal cavity (peritonitis), and bleeding. Repeated bouts of diverticulitis can lead to intestinal obstruction, because the resulting scarring and muscle thickening can narrow the inside of the large intestine and prevent solid stool from passing through.

Treatment

Mild diverticulitis can be treated with rest, a liquid diet, and oral antibiotics. Symptoms usually disappear rapidly. After a few days, the person can begin a soft, low-fiber diet and take a daily psyllium seed preparation. After 1 month, a high-fiber diet can be started.

People with more severe symptoms—such as abdominal pain, body temperature above 101° F (38.3° C), poor response to oral antibi-

DIVERTICULITIS: REASONS FOR ELECTIVE SURGERY

Condition	Reason
Two or more severe attacks of diverticulitis (or one severe attack in someone younger than 50)	High risk of serious complications
Narrowing of the sigmoid colon (lower part of the large intestine) due to scarring	High risk of serious complications
Persistent tender mass in the abdomen	May be cancer
X-ray showing suspicious changes in the sigmoid colon	May be cancer
Pain when urinating	May be a warning of impending fistula formation between the large intestine and the bladder
Sudden abdominal pain in people taking corticosteroids	Large intestine may have ruptured into the abdominal cavity

otics, and other evidence of serious infection or complications—are generally admitted to the hospital. There they are given intravenous fluids and antibiotics, kept on bedrest, and given nothing by mouth until the symptoms subside. About 20% of people who have diverticulitis require surgery because the condition does not improve.

If the source of bleeding is known, only the affected section of the intestine is removed, in most people. If the source of bleeding is not known, a larger section of the intestine is removed in a procedure called subtotal colectomy.

Emergency surgery is necessary for people whose intestine has ruptured; intestinal rupture always results in infection of the abdominal cavity. The surgeon generally removes the ruptured section and creates an opening between the large intestine and the skin surface. This opening is called a colostomy.▲ About 10 to 12 weeks later (or sometimes longer), the cut ends of the intestine are rejoined during a follow-up operation, and the colostomy is closed.

Surgery may be optional for some people with diverticulitis. If an abscess is discovered, draining it through the skin might be attempted before surgery is considered.

Treatment of a fistula involves removing the section of large intestine where the fistula begins, rejoining the cut ends of the large intestine, and repairing the other affected area (for example, the bladder or small intestine).

CHAPTER 129

Bowel Movement Disorders

Bowel (intestinal) function varies greatly not only from one person to another but also for any one person at different times. Most people find it easiest to move their bowels in the morning. The urge tends to be strongest about 30 to 60 minutes after first eating in the morning. Bowel function can be affected by diet, stress, drugs, disease, and even social and cultural patterns. In most Western societies, the normal number of bowel movements ranges from 2 or 3 a week to as many as 2 or 3 a day. Changes in the frequency, consistency, or volume of bowel movements or the presence of blood, mucus, pus, or excess fatty material (oil or grease) in the stool may indicate a bowel disorder.

Constipation

Constipation is a condition in which a person has uncomfortable or infrequent bowel movements.

Constipation may be acute or chronic. Acute constipation begins suddenly and conspicuously. Chronic constipation may begin insidiously and persist for months or years.

A person with constipation often or always produces hard stools that may be difficult to pass. The person also may feel as though the rectum has not been completely emptied. Bowel movements are likely to be infrequent as well. Many people believe they are constipated if they do not have a bowel movement (defecate) every day. However, daily bowel movements are not normal for everyone, and having less frequent bowel movements does not necessarily indicate a problem unless there has been a substantial change from previous patterns. The same is true of the color and consistency of stool; unless there is a substantial change, the person probably does not have constipation.

Causes

Slowed Transit of Stool: Constipation tends to occur when the transit (passage) of stool along the large intestine slows. Under normal circumstances, water is pulled from the stool as it passes through the large intestine. Slowed transit of stool allows the large intestine to pull more water from the stool, resulting in the hard, dry stools and associated difficult passage of stools that characterize constipation.

▲ see box on page 772

Drugs that slow transit, including aluminum hydroxide (common in over-the-counter antacids), bismuth subsalicylate, iron salts, anticholinergic drugs, certain antihypertensives, opioids, and many sedatives, frequently cause constipation. Because physical activity helps the intestines move stool along, lack of activity tends to slow transit and lead to constipation. For this reason, people who are confined to bed because of illness often are constipated.

Disorders and diseases that can slow transit time of stool include an underactive thyroid gland (hypothyroidism), high blood calcium levels (hypercalcemia), and Parkinson's disease. People with diabetes often develop a condition in which parts of the digestive system slow down. Other conditions, including poor blood supply to the large intestine and nerve or spinal cord injury, can also cause constipation by slowing transit.

In an extreme case of slowed transit, called colonic inertia (inactive colon), the large intestine stops responding to the stimuli that usually cause bowel movements: eating, a full stomach, a full large intestine, and stool in the rectum. A decrease in contractions in the large intestine or an insensitivity of the rectum to the presence of stool results in severe, chronic constipation. Colonic inertia often occurs in people who are older, debilitated, or bedridden, but it can occasionally occur in otherwise healthy younger women (and, much less commonly, in healthy younger men). Colonic inertia sometimes occurs in people who habitually delay moving their bowels or who have used laxatives or enemas for a long time.

Dehydration and Low-Fiber Diet: Dehydration causes constipation because the body tries to conserve water in the blood by removing additional water from the stool. Lack of fiber (the indigestible part of food) in the diet can lead to constipation because fiber helps hold water in the stool and increases its bulk, making it easier to pass.

Obstruction: Constipation is sometimes caused by obstruction of the large intestine. Obstruction can be caused by cancer, especially in the last portion of the large intestine, if it blocks the movement of stool. Bezoars (tightly packed collections of partially digested or undigested material) and foreign bodies can also block the intestinal tract.▲ People who previously had abdominal surgery may develop obstruction, usually of the small intestine, because of formation of bands of fibrous tissues (adhesions).

Dyschezia: Dyschezia is difficulty in defecating caused by an inability to control the pelvic and anal muscles. Having a normal bowel movement requires relaxing the pelvic floor muscles (the muscles that support the bladder, uterus, and rectum) and the circular muscles (sphincters) that keep the anus closed. Otherwise, efforts to defecate are futile, even with severe straining. People with dyschezia sense the need to have a bowel movement but cannot. Even stool that is not hard may be difficult to pass.

Conditions that can cause dyschezia include pelvic floor dyssynergia (a disturbance of muscle coordination), anismus (a failure of the sphincter muscles to relax during defecation), rectocele (hernia of the rectum into the vagina), enterocele (hernia of the small intestine into the rectum), rectal ulcer, and rectal prolapse.

Aging: Constipation is particularly common among older people. Age-related changes in the large intestine■ along with increased use of medications and reduced physical activity tend to slow the transit of stool through the large intestine. Slowed transit is particularly common during periods of illness. The rectum enlarges with age, and increased storage of stool in the rectum allows hard stool to become impacted.

Pain and Psychogenic Factors: Chronic pain and psychologic conditions, especially depression, are common causes of acute and chronic constipation. Constipation may result from changes in the levels of certain substances in the brain, such as serotonin, that can affect the intestinal tract.

Symptoms and Complications

Constipation can cause abdominal pain. The pain may occur only when straining during a bowel movement, although in some people the pain persists between bowel movements. Constipation can cause nausea and impair appetite.

Straining during a bowel movement increases pressure on the veins around the anus and can lead to hemorrhoids. Straining also increases blood pressure, which, although only temporary, may be extreme.

Constipation is one of the major risk factors for the development of diverticular disease. The walls of the large intestine are damaged by the increased pressure required to move small hard stools. Damage to the walls of the large intestine leads to the formation

▲ see page 727   ■ see page 698

of balloon-like sacs (diverticula), which can become clogged and inflamed.

Fecal impaction, in which the stool in the last part of the large intestine and rectum hardens and blocks the transit of other stool, sometimes develops in people with constipation. This condition is particularly common among older people, pregnant women, and people with colonic inertia. Fecal impaction leads to cramps, rectal pain, and strong but futile efforts to defecate. Often, watery mucus or liquid stool oozes around the blockage, sometimes giving the false impression of diarrhea. Fecal impaction can aggravate or further worsen constipation.

Diagnosis

When constipation develops in someone who has not had it before and there is not an easy explanation, such as a change in diet or physical activity or new use of one of the many drugs known to cause constipation, a doctor may perform blood tests to check for an underactive thyroid gland (hypothyroidism) or high calcium levels in the blood (hypercalcemia), both of which can cause constipation. If there is any question about cancer as a cause, a barium enema x-ray study or colonoscopy is performed.

Prevention and Treatment

Constipation is best prevented and treated with a combination of adequate exercise, a high-fiber diet, an adequate intake of fluids, and the occasional use of laxatives. When a potentially constipating drug has been prescribed, a laxative along with increased intake of dietary fiber and fluids helps to prevent constipation.

Vegetables, fruits, and bran are excellent sources of fiber. Many people find it convenient to sprinkle 2 or 3 teaspoons of unrefined miller's bran on high-fiber cereal or fruit 2 or 3 times a day. To work well, fiber must be consumed with plenty of fluids.

When an underlying disease is causing constipation, the disease must be treated.

Dyschezia is not easily treated with laxatives. Relaxation exercises and biofeedback are used for pelvic floor dyssynergia and are effective for some people. Surgery may be needed to repair an enterocele or a large rectocele.

Fecal impaction cannot be treated with diet or easily with laxatives. The hard stool usually has to be removed by a doctor or nurse using a gloved finger. Sometimes, the impaction can be resolved with an enema.

Overzealous treatment, especially the long-term use of stimulant laxatives, irritant suppositories, and enemas, can lead to diarrhea, dehydration, cramps, or dependence on laxatives.

Laxatives: Many people use laxatives to relieve constipation. Some laxatives are safe for long-term use; others should be used only occasionally. Some are good for preventing constipation; others can be used to treat it.

Bulking agents, such as bran and psyllium (also available in the fiber of many vegetables), add bulk to the stool. The increased bulk stimulates the natural contractions of the intestine, and bulkier stools are softer and easier to pass. Bulking agents act slowly and gently and are among the safest ways to promote regular bowel movements. These agents generally are taken in small amounts at first. The dose is increased gradually until regularity is achieved. People who use bulking agents should always drink plenty of fluids.

Stool softeners, such as docusate, increase the amount of water that the stool can hold. Actually, these laxatives are detergents that decrease the surface tension of the stool, allowing water to penetrate the stool more easily and soften it. In addition, the slightly increased bulk that results from these drugs stimulates the natural contractions of the large intestine and thus promotes easier elimination. Some people, however, find the softened nature of the stool unpleasant. These softeners are best reserved for people who must avoid straining, for example, people with hemorrhoids or people who recently underwent surgery.

Osmotic agents pull large amounts of water into the large intestine, making the stool soft and loose. The excess fluid also stretches the walls of the large intestine, stimulating contractions. These laxatives consist of salts or sugars that are poorly absorbed. They may cause fluid retention in people with kidney disease or heart failure, especially when given in large or frequent doses. Osmotic agents containing magnesium and phosphate are partially absorbed into the bloodstream and can be harmful in people with kidney failure. These laxatives generally work within 3 hours. They are also used to clear stool from the intestine before x-rays of the digestive tract are taken or before colonoscopy is performed.

Stimulant laxatives contain irritating substances, such as senna and cascara, that directly stimulate the walls of the large intestine, causing them to contract and move the stool. Taken by mouth, stimulant laxatives generally cause a semisolid bowel movement in 6 to 8 hours but often cause cramping as

℞ DRUGS USED TO PREVENT OR TREAT CONSTIPATION

TYPE	DRUG	SELECTED SIDE EFFECTS	COMMENTS
Bulking agents			
	Bran Polycarbophil Methylcellulose Psyllium	Flatulence, bloating	Bulking agents generally are used to prevent or control chronic constipation
Stool softeners			
	Docusate	Nausea (especially with syrup/liquid formulation)	Stool softeners may be used to treat constipation and are often used to help prevent it
Osmotic agents			

	Lactulose
	Magnesium salts
	  (magnesium hydroxide,
	  magnesium citrate)
	Sodium phosphate
	Sorbitol
		Cramps, flatulence (lactulose, sorbitol)	Osmotic agents are better for treating constipation than for preventing it

Stimulant laxatives			
	Bisacodyl Cascara Castor oil Senna	Abdominal pain (cramps); prolonged use can damage large intestine	Stimulant laxatives are not used if there is a possibility of an intestinal obstruction

well. In suppositories, these laxatives often work in 15 to 60 minutes.

Prolonged use of stimulant laxatives can create abnormal changes in the lining of the large intestine caused by deposits of a pigment (a condition called melanosis coli). Also, stimulant laxatives can become addictive, leading to the development of lazy bowel syndrome, which in turn causes the large intestine to become dependent on the laxatives. For all these reasons, stimulant laxatives should be used only for brief periods of time to treat constipation. They are useful for preventing constipation in people who are taking drugs that will almost certainly cause constipation, such as opioids. Stimulant laxatives are often used to empty the large intestine before diagnostic procedures are performed.

Enemas: Enemas mechanically flush stool from the rectum and lower part of the large intestine. Small-volume enemas can be purchased in squeeze bottles at a pharmacy. They can also be administered with a reusable squeeze-ball device. However, small-volume enemas are often inadequate, especially in older people, whose rectal capacity increases as advancing age makes the rectum more easily stretched. Larger-volume enemas are administered with an enema bag.

Plain water is often the best fluid to be used as an enema. The water should be room temperature to slightly warm, but not hot or cold. Water (in volumes of about 5 to 10 fluid ounces [150 to 300 milliliters]) is gently directed into the rectum; adding additional force is dangerous. The water is then expelled, washing stool out with it.

Prepackaged enemas often contain small amounts of salts, often phosphates. Appropriate salts can also be added to homemade enemas. They offer little advantage, however, to plain water.

The addition of small amounts of soap to the water (soap-suds enema) adds the stimulant laxative effects of soap. Soap-suds enemas are sometimes useful when plain water enemas fail, but they can cause cramping.

Many other substances, including mineral oil, are sometimes added to water-based enemas. However, they offer little advantage.

Very large volume enemas, called colonic enemas, are rarely used in medical practice. Doctors use colonic enemas only in people with very severe constipation (obstipation).

Some practitioners of alternative medicine use colonic enemas in the belief that cleansing the large intestine is beneficial. Tea, coffee, and other substances are often added to colonic enemas but have no proven health value and may be dangerous.

Diarrhea

Diarrhea is an increase in the volume, wateriness, or frequency of bowel movements.

The frequency of bowel movements alone is not the defining feature of diarrhea. Some people normally move their bowels 3 to 5 times a day. People who eat large amounts of vegetable fiber may produce more than a pound of stool a day, but the stool in such cases is well formed and not watery. Diarrhea occurs when not enough water is removed from the stool, making the stool loose and poorly formed. Diarrhea is often associated with gas, cramping, an urgency to move the bowels (defecate), nausea, and vomiting.

Causes

Normally, stool is 60 to 90% water; diarrhea mainly results when the percentage exceeds 90%. Stool may contain too much water if it travels too quickly through the digestive tract, if certain components of the stool prevent the large intestine from absorbing water, or if water is being secreted by the large intestine into the stool. Many different causes, including drugs; infection with viruses, bacteria, or parasites; components of food; stress; chemicals; tumors; chronic disorders such as irritable bowel syndrome and inflammatory bowel disease; and stress can lead to diarrhea. Malabsorption syndromes, in which food cannot be digested normally, can lead to diarrhea as well.

Rapid Transit of Stool: Rapid transit of stool is one of the most common causes of diarrhea. For stool to have normal consistency, it must remain in the large intestine for a certain amount of time. Stool that leaves the large intestine too quickly is watery. Many medical conditions and treatments can decrease the amount of time that stool stays in the large intestine, including an overactive thyroid (hyperthyroidism) or Zollinger-Ellison syndrome; surgical removal of part of the stomach, small intestine, or large intestine; treatment of ulcers in which the vagus nerve is cut; surgical bypass of part of the intestine; and drugs such as antacids containing magnesium, laxatives, prostaglandins, serotonin, and even caffeine. Many foods, especially those that are acidic,

can increase transit. Some people are intolerant of specific foods and always develop diarrhea after eating them. Stress and anxiety are also common causes.

Retention of Water in the Stool: Osmotic diarrhea occurs when certain substances that cannot be absorbed into the bloodstream remain in the intestine. These substances cause excessive amounts of water to remain in the stool, leading to diarrhea. Certain foods (such as some fruits and beans) and hexitols, sorbitol, and mannitol (used as sugar substitutes in dietetic foods, candy, and chewing gum) can cause osmotic diarrhea. Also, lactase deficiency can lead to osmotic diarrhea. (Lactase is an enzyme normally found in the small intestine that converts lactose [milk sugar] to glucose and galactose, so that it can be absorbed into the bloodstream.) When people with lactase deficiency drink milk or eat dairy products, lactose is not digested. As lactose accumulates in the intestine, it causes osmotic diarrhea. The severity of osmotic diarrhea depends on how much of the osmotic substance is consumed. Diarrhea stops soon after the person stops eating or drinking the substance.

Blood in the digestive tract also acts as an osmotic agent and results in black, tarry stools (melena). Another cause of osmotic diarrhea is an overgrowth of normal intestinal bacteria or the growth of bacteria normally not found in the intestines. Infection by certain parasites (for example, amebas) can also cause osmotic diarrhea. Antibiotics can cause osmotic diarrhea by destroying the normal intestinal bacteria.

Secretion of Water Into the Stool: Secretory diarrhea occurs when the small and large intestines secrete salts (especially sodium chloride) and water into the stool. Certain toxins—such as the toxin produced during a cholera infection or during some viral infections—can cause these secretions. Infections by certain bacteria (for example, *Campylobacter*) and parasites (for example, *Cryptosporidium*) can also stimulate secretions. The diarrhea can be massive—more than a quart of stool an hour in cholera. Other substances that cause salt and water secretion include certain laxatives, such as castor oil, and bile acids (which may build up after surgery to remove part of the small intestine). Certain rare tumors—such as carcinoid, gastrinoma, and vipoma—also can cause secretory diarrhea, as can some polyps.

Exudative diarrhea occurs when the lining of the large intestine becomes inflamed, ulcerated, or engorged, and it releases proteins, blood, mucus, and other fluids, which increase the bulk and fluid content of the stool. This type of diarrhea can be caused by many diseases, including ulcerative colitis, Crohn's disease (regional enteritis), tuberculosis, and cancers such as lymphoma and adenocarcinoma. When the lining of the rectum is affected, the person often feels an urgent need to move his bowels and has frequent bowel movements because the inflamed rectum is more sensitive to expansion (distention) by stool.

Symptoms and Complications

Diarrhea is characterized by frequent loose stools. The consistency of the stool can be anything from soft and pasty to completely watery. The color can range from brown to clear. Black stools may indicate bleeding in the digestive tract, although some drugs used to treat diarrhea (those containing bismuth subsalicylate) turn the stools black as well. When a black color is caused by blood (melena), the stools are usually tarry and foul-smelling.

Cramping may occur before and with a bowel movement, and sometimes large amounts of gas are passed with the stool. Some people experience nausea, especially if the diarrhea is caused by an infectious organism or a toxic substance.

Diarrhea can lead to dehydration and a loss of electrically charged particles (electrolytes), such as sodium, potassium, magnesium, and chloride, from the blood. If large amounts of fluid and electrolytes are lost, blood pressure can drop enough to cause fainting (syncope), heart rhythm abnormalities (arrhythmias), and other serious disorders. At particular risk are the very young, older people, the debilitated, and people with very severe diarrhea. Bicarbonate may be lost in the stool as well, leading to metabolic acidosis.▲

Diagnosis

A doctor first tries to establish whether the diarrhea appeared suddenly and has been present for a short time (acute) or whether it is persistent (chronic). If acute diarrhea persists for more than 72 hours (or sooner if blood is present), it should be evaluated by a doctor. A doctor tries to determine whether changes in diet may be the cause; whether the person has other symptoms, such as a fever, pain, and rash; and whether the person has been exposed to people with a similar condition. When diarrhea is not severe and has lasted for less than a

FOODS AND DRUGS THAT CAN CAUSE DIARRHEA	
FOODS AND DRUGS	**INGREDIENT CAUSING DIARRHEA**
Apple juice, pear juice, sugar-free gum, mints	Hexitols, sorbitol, mannitol
Apple juice, pear juice, grapes, honey, dates, nuts, figs, soft drinks (especially fruit flavors)	Fructose
Table sugar	Sucrose
Milk, ice cream, yogurt, frozen yogurt, soft cheese, chocolate	Lactose
Antacids containing magnesium	Magnesium
Coffee, tea, cola drinks, some over-the-counter headache remedies	Caffeine
Fat-free potato chips, fat-free ice cream	Olestra

week, the symptoms and physical examination alone are usually enough to determine the cause and necessary treatment. If needed, stool samples can be examined. This examination determines if the stool is formed or watery, if it has an unusual odor, and if it contains fat, blood, or undigested materials. The volume of stool over a 24-hour period is also determined.

When diarrhea persists, often a sample of the stool must be examined microscopically for cells, mucus, fat, and other substances. The stool also can be tested for blood and substances that might cause osmotic diarrhea. Samples can be tested for infectious organisms that stimulate secretion, including certain bacteria (for example, *Campylobacter* and *Yersinia*) and parasites (for example, amebas, *Giardia*, and *Cryptosporidium*). If the person is surreptitiously taking a laxative, it also can be identified in the stool sample. A sigmoidoscopy may be performed, so that a doctor can examine the lining of the anus and rectum. Sometimes a biopsy (removal of a tissue specimen for examination under a microscope) of the rectal lining is performed.

▲ see page 931

℞ DRUGS USED TO TREAT DIARRHEA

TYPE	DRUG	SELECTED SIDE EFFECTS	COMMENTS
Adsorbents			
	Bismuth subsalicylate Kaolin Pectin	Well tolerated	Adsorbents are less potent than intestinal muscle relaxants
Intestinal muscle relaxants			
	Codeine Diphenoxylate Loperamide* Paregoric (tincture of opium)	Obstruction of the large intestine	Used carefully if infectious cause of diarrhea is suspected

*Some formulations of loperamide are available over-the-counter.

Treatment

Diarrhea is a symptom, and its treatment depends on the cause. Most people with diarrhea only have to remove the cause and suppress the diarrhea until the body heals itself. For example, sometimes chronic diarrhea is cured when a person stops drinking coffee or cola drinks containing caffeine. A viral cause generally resolves by itself in 24 to 48 hours.

Many prescription and over-the-counter drugs are available for the treatment of diarrhea. Over-the-counter drugs include adsorbents (for example, kaolin-pectin), which adhere to chemicals, toxins, and infectious organisms. Some adsorbents can also help firm up the stool. Bismuth subsalicylate helps many people with diarrhea. It has a normal side effect of turning the stool black. Other drugs used are loperamide, codeine, and diphenoxylate.

Prescription drugs used to treat diarrhea include opioids and other drugs that relax the muscles of the intestines. Bulking agents used for chronic constipation, such as psyllium or methylcellulose, can sometimes help relieve chronic diarrhea as well.

When severe diarrhea causes dehydration, hospitalization and treatment with intravenous water and salts may be necessary. As long as the person is not vomiting and does not feel nauseated, drinking liquids containing a balance of water, sugars, and salts can be very effective.

Irritable Bowel Syndrome

Irritable bowel syndrome is a disorder of motility of the entire digestive tract that causes abdominal pain, constipation, or diarrhea.

In this disorder, the digestive tract is especially sensitive to many stimuli. Stress, diet, drugs, hormones, or minor irritants may cause the digestive tract to contract abnormally, usually leading to diarrhea. Periods of constipation may occur between bouts of diarrhea. Irritable bowel syndrome affects women 3 times more often than men.

The brain has enormous control over the digestive system. Stress, anxiety, depression, fear, and virtually any strong emotion can lead to diarrhea, constipation, and other changes in bowel function and can further worsen a flare-up (bout or attack) of irritable bowel syndrome.

During a flare-up, the contractions of the digestive tract become stronger and more frequent, and the resulting rapid transit of food and stool through the large intestine often leads to diarrhea. Crampy pain seems to result from the strong contractions of the large intestine and increased sensitivity of the receptors in the large intestine that sense stretching and pressure. Flare-ups almost always occur when a person is awake; they rarely wake a person from sleep.

For some people, high-calorie meals or a high-fat diet may be to blame. For other people, wheat, dairy products, coffee, tea, or citrus fruits appear to aggravate the symptoms, but it is not clear whether these foods are actually the cause. Others find that eating too quickly or eating after too long a period without food stimulates a flare-up of irritable bowel syndrome.

Symptoms

Symptoms are commonly triggered by eating, often by eating too quickly or too much. A few minutes later, diarrhea with pain occurs. The diarrhea may begin very suddenly and with extreme urgency. Sometimes the urgency is so strong that the person loses control and cannot reach a bathroom in time. Diarrhea during the night is rare. Sometimes constipation and diarrhea alternate. Mucus often appears in the stool. The pain may come in bouts of continuous dull aching or cramps, usually over the lower abdomen. The person may experience bloating, gas, nausea, headaches, fatigue, depression, anxiety, and difficulty concentrating. Having a bowel movement often relieves the pain. Periods of stress may worsen symptoms.

Diagnosis

Most people with irritable bowel syndrome appear healthy. A physical examination generally does not reveal anything unusual except sometimes tenderness over the large intestine. Doctors generally perform some tests—for example, blood tests, a stool examination, and a sigmoidoscopy—to differentiate irritable bowel syndrome from Crohn's disease, ulcerative colitis, collagenous and lymphocytic colitis, and the many other diseases that can cause abdominal pain and changes in bowel habits. These test results are usually normal, although the stool may be watery. The results of a sigmoidoscopy, which may cause spasms and pain, are normal. Sometimes other tests—such as abdominal ultrasound, x-rays of the intestines, or a colonoscopy—are used.

Treatment

The treatment for irritable bowel syndrome differs from person to person. People who can identify particular foods or types of stress that bring on the problem should avoid them if possible. For most people, especially those who tend to be constipated, regular physical activity helps keep the digestive tract functioning normally.

In general, a normal diet is best. Many people do better eating frequent, smaller meals rather than less frequent, larger meals (for example, five or six small meals rather than three large meals a day). People with abdominal expansion (distention) and increased gas (flatulence) should avoid beans, cabbage, and other foods that are difficult to digest. Sorbitol, an artificial sweetener used in dietetic foods and in some drugs and chewing gums, should not be consumed in large amounts. Fructose, a common constituent of fruits, berries, and some plants, should be eaten only in small amounts. A low-fat diet helps some people. People who have both irritable bowel syndrome and lactase deficiency should not eat dairy products.

Some people with irritable bowel syndrome can improve their condition by eating more fiber. They can take a tablespoon of raw bran with plenty of water and other fluids at each meal, or they can take psyllium mucilloid supplements with two glasses of water. However, increasing the dietary fiber may aggravate some symptoms, such as flatulence and bloating.

Antispasmodic drugs, which slow the function of the digestive tract, are frequently prescribed but have not been proved effective in all people with irritable bowel syndrome. Antidiarrheal drugs help people with diarrhea. Aromatic oils, such as oil of peppermint, often help symptoms of flatulence and cramping.

If an emotional disorder is identified as the cause, treatment of the disorder may relieve irritable bowel syndrome symptoms. Such treatment may include the use of antidepressants, mild tranquilizers, psychotherapy, hypnosis, and behavior modification techniques.

Fecal Incontinence

Fecal incontinence is the loss of control over bowel movements.

Fecal incontinence can occur briefly during bouts of diarrhea or when hard stool becomes lodged in the rectum (fecal impaction). People with injuries to the anus or spinal cord, rectal prolapse (protrusion of the rectal lining through the anus), dementia, neurologic injury from diabetes, tumors of the anus, or injuries to the pelvis during childbirth can develop persistent fecal incontinence.

A doctor examines the person for any structural or neurologic abnormality that may be causing fecal incontinence. This involves examining the anus and rectum, checking the extent of sensation around the anus, and usually performing a sigmoidoscopy. Other tests, including an examination of the function of nerves and muscles lining the pelvis, may be needed.

The first step in correcting fecal incontinence is to try to establish a regular pattern of bowel movements that produces well-formed stool. Dietary changes, including the addition of a small amount of fiber, often help. If such changes do not help, a drug that slows bowel movements, such as loperamide, may succeed.

Exercising the anal muscles (sphincters) by squeezing and releasing them increases their tone and strength and helps prevent fecal incontinence from recurring. Using biofeedback, a person can retrain the sphincters and increase the sensitivity of the rectum to the presence of stool. About 70% of well-motivated people benefit from biofeedback.

If fecal incontinence persists, surgery may help in a small number of cases—for instance, when the cause is an injury to the anus or an anatomic defect in the anus. As a last resort, a colostomy (the surgical creation of an opening between the large intestine and the abdominal wall)▲ may be performed. The anus is sewn shut, and stool is diverted into a removable plastic bag attached to the opening in the abdominal wall. A colostomy does not always have to be permanent.

Flatulence

Flatulence is the sensation of an increased amount of gas in the digestive tract.

Increased amounts of gas can gather in the stomach or farther along the digestive tract. Excess gas is expelled through the mouth (belching) or through the anus (known colloquially as farting and called flatus by doctors), or it is absorbed through the walls of the digestive tract into the blood and then excreted by the lungs. Bacteria in the digestive system also break down (metabolize) some gases.

Air is a gas, which can be swallowed with food. Swallowing small amounts of air is normal, but some people unconsciously swallow large amounts (aerophagia), especially when they feel anxious. Most swallowed air is later belched up, so only some air passes from the stomach into the rest of the digestive system. Swallowing large amounts of air may make a person feel full, and the person may belch excessively or pass the air through the anus.

Other gases are produced in the digestive system by several means. Hydrogen, methane, and carbon dioxide are produced by bacterial metabolism of food in the intestine, especially after a person eats certain foods such as beans and cabbage. People who have deficiencies of the enzymes that break down certain sugars also tend to produce large amounts of gas when they eat foods containing these sugars. Lactase deficiency, tropical sprue, and pancreatic insufficiency all may lead to the produc-

tion of large amounts of gas. People with irritable bowel syndrome do not produce large amounts of gas, although the passage of normal volumes of gas through the bowel may be changed. Almost anyone who eats large amounts of proteins or fruits will develop some degree of flatulence.

Symptoms

Flatulence is often associated with abdominal pain and bloating; however, the exact relationship between flatulence and any of these symptoms is not really known. Some people appear to be particularly sensitive to the effects of gas in the digestive system; others can tolerate large amounts without developing any symptoms.

Belching is more likely to occur shortly after eating or during periods of stress. Drinking carbonated beverages sometimes leads to belching. Some people feel a tightness in their chest or stomach just before belching that is relieved as the gas is expelled.

People normally pass gas through the anus more than 10 times a day, but flatulence may cause a person to pass gas more often. Gas passed through the anus may or may not have an odor. On occasion, fecal incontinence occurs as a person tries to pass gas, only to be surprised by the expulsion of stool as well.

Infants with crampy abdominal pain sometimes pass excessive amounts of gas. Whether these children actually produce more gas than others or are simply more sensitive to gas is not clear.

Treatment

Bloating and belching are difficult to relieve. If belching is the main problem, reducing the amount of air being swallowed can help, which is difficult because people generally are not aware of swallowing air. Avoiding chewing gum and eating more slowly in a relaxed atmosphere may help.

People who belch or pass gas excessively may need to change their diet by avoiding foods that are difficult to digest. Discovering which foods are causing the problem may require eliminating one food or one group of foods at a time. A person can start by eliminating milk and dairy products, then fresh fruits, and then certain vegetables and other foods. Avoiding carbonated beverages helps some people.

Although drugs generally are not very effective, simethicone, which is present in some antacids and is also available sepa-

▲ see box on page 772

rately, can provide a little relief. Sometimes other drugs—including other types of antacids (including those that contain baking soda), metoclopramide, and bethanechol—may help. Aromatic oils, such as peppermint oil, help some people, especially those who experience cramps with flatulence. Eating more fiber helps some people but worsens the symptoms in others. Chlorophyll, an ingredient in many over-the-counter products, and charcoal tablets do not decrease flatulence but help reduce its offensive odor.

Disorders of the Anus and Rectum

The anus is the opening at the end of the digestive tract where stool leaves the body; the rectum is the section of the digestive tract above the anus where stool is held before it passes out of the body through the anus.

The anus is formed partly from the surface layers of the body, including the skin, and partly from the intestine. The rectal lining consists of glistening orange-tan tissue containing mucus glands—much like the rest of the intestinal lining. The lining of the rectum is relatively insensitive to pain, but the nerves from the anus and nearby external skin are very sensitive to pain.

The veins from the rectum and anus drain into the portal vein, which leads to the liver, and then into the general circulation. The lymph vessels of the rectum drain into lymph nodes in the lower abdomen; those of the anus drain into the lymph nodes in the groin.

A muscular ring (anal sphincter) keeps the anus closed. This sphincter is controlled subconsciously by the autonomic nervous system;▲ however, the lower part of the sphincter can be relaxed or tightened at will.

To diagnose disorders of the anus and rectum, a doctor inspects the skin around the anus for any abnormality. With a gloved finger, the doctor probes the rectum. For women, this is often done along with a manual examination of the vagina.

Next, a doctor looks into the anus and rectum with a 3- to 10-inch rigid viewing tube (anoscope or proctoscope). A longer, flexible tube (sigmoidoscope)■ may then be inserted so that the doctor can observe as much as 2 or more feet of the large intestine. An anoscopy or sigmoidoscopy is generally uncomfortable but not painful; however, if the area in or around the anus proves to be painful because of an abnormal condition, a local, regional, or even general anesthetic may be given before examination proceeds. Sometimes a cleansing enema to rid the lower part of the large intestine of stool is given before sigmoidoscopy. Tissue and stool samples for microscopic examination and cultures may be obtained during sigmoidoscopy. A barium enema x-ray may also be performed.

Hemorrhoids

Hemorrhoids are dilated, twisted (varicose) veins located in the wall of the rectum and anus.

Hemorrhoids occur when the veins in the rectum or anus become enlarged; they may eventually bleed. Hemorrhoids may also become inflamed or may develop a blood clot (thrombus). Hemorrhoids that form above the boundary between the rectum and anus (anorectal junction) are called internal hemorrhoids; those that form below the anorectal junction are called external hemorrhoids. Both internal and external hemorrhoids may remain in the anus or protrude outside the anus.

Increased pressure in the veins of the anorectal area leads to hemorrhoids. This pressure may result from pregnancy, from frequent heavy lifting, or from repeated straining during bowel movements (defecation). Constipation may contribute to straining. In a few people, hemorrhoids develop from increased blood pressure in the portal vein. A doctor can distinguish the dilated, twisted veins that occur in this condition from common hemorrhoids.

▲ see page 437   ■ see page 703

Symptoms and Diagnosis

Hemorrhoids can bleed, typically after a bowel movement, producing blood-streaked stool or toilet paper. The blood may turn water in the toilet bowl red. However, the amount of blood is usually small, and hemorrhoids rarely lead to severe blood loss or anemia.

Hemorrhoids that protrude from the anus may need to be pushed back gently with a finger, or they may go back by themselves. A hemorrhoid may swell further and become painful if its surface is rubbed raw or if a blood clot forms in it. Less commonly, hemorrhoids may discharge mucus and create a feeling that the rectum is not completely emptied after a bowel movement. Itching in the anal region (pruritus ani) is usually not a symptom of hemorrhoids, but itching may develop if hemorrhoids make proper cleaning of the anal region difficult.

A doctor can readily diagnose swollen, painful hemorrhoids by inspecting the anus and rectum. An examination with an anoscope or sigmoidoscope helps a doctor determine if the person has a more serious condition, such as a tumor.

Treatment

Usually, hemorrhoids do not require treatment unless they cause symptoms. Taking stool softeners or a bulking type of laxative such as psyllium may relieve straining with bowel movements. Symptoms can sometimes be relieved by soaking the anus in warm water in what is known as a sitz bath. The soaking is accomplished by squatting in a partially filled tub or using a container filled with warm water placed on the toilet bowl or commode.

Bleeding hemorrhoids can be treated with an injection of a substance that causes the hemorrhoids to become obliterated with scar tissue; this procedure is called injection sclerotherapy.

Large internal hemorrhoids and those that do not respond to injection sclerotherapy can be tied off with rubber bands (a procedure called rubber band ligation). The band causes the hemorrhoid to wither and drop off painlessly. The treatment is usually applied to one hemorrhoid at a time at intervals of 2 weeks or longer. Internal hemorrhoids may also be destroyed with a laser (laser destruction), an infrared light (infrared photocoagulation), or an electrical current (electrocoagulation).

Surgery to remove the hemorrhoids may be used if other treatments fail. However, hemorrhoid surgery may result in severe pain. New, less painful techniques are being investigated, including Doppler-guided hemorrhoid artery ligation, in which hemorrhoid arteries are identified and tied off, thus reducing the blood supply to the hemorrhoids; and circumferential stapled hemorrhoidectomy.

When a hemorrhoid with a blood clot causes pain, it is treated with warm sitz baths, local anesthetic ointments, or witch-hazel compresses. Pain and swelling usually diminish after a short while, and clots disappear over 4 to 6 weeks. Alternatively, especially when the pain is severe, a doctor may cut the vein and remove the clot, which sometimes relieves the pain rapidly.

Anal Fissure

An anal fissure is a tear or ulcer in the lining of the anus.

Anal fissures may be caused by an injury from a hard or large bowel movement. Uncommonly, they may also be caused by penetration of the anus during anal sex. Fissures cause the anal sphincter to go into spasm, which prevents healing.

Fissures cause pain and bleeding, usually during or shortly after a bowel movement. The pain lasts for several minutes to several hours and then subsides until the next bowel movement. A doctor diagnoses a fissure by inspecting the anus.

Treatment

A stool softener or psyllium may reduce the possibility of reinjury by hard bowel movements, while lubricating and soothing the lower rectum. Lubricant suppositories also can be helpful. A warm sitz bath for 10 to 15 minutes after each bowel movement eases discomfort and helps increase blood flow, which promotes healing.

Promising experimental treatments have been developed to reduce sphincter spasm and promote healing of fissures, including injection of the sphincter with toxins from *Clostridium botulinum* bacteria and application of nitroglycerin ointment or calcium channel blockers to the area of the fissure.

When these measures fail, surgery may be needed. Sphincter spasm can be relieved either by stretching (dilating) the anus or by cutting the internal sphincter (internal anal sphincterotomy).

Banding a Hemorrhoid

Some internal hemorrhoids are removed by tying them off with rubber bands in an outpatient procedure called rubber band ligation. The instrument used (ligator) consists of forceps surrounded by a cylinder with ¼-inch rubber bands placed on one end. The ligator is inserted into the anus through an anoscope (a short, rigid viewing tube), and the hemorrhoid is grasped with the forceps. The cylinder is slid upward over the forceps and the hemorrhoid, pushing the rubber bands off the cylinder and around the base of the hemorrhoid. The rubber bands cut off the hemorrhoid's blood supply, causing it to wither and drop off painlessly in a few days.

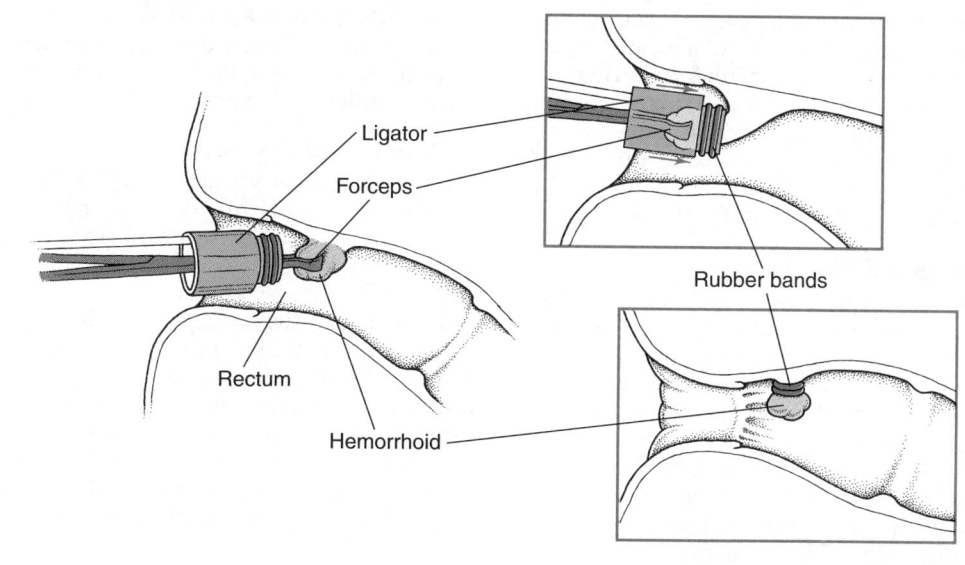

Ligator
Forceps
Rubber bands
Rectum
Hemorrhoid

Anorectal Abscess

An anorectal abscess is a pus-filled cavity caused by bacteria invading a mucus-secreting gland in the anus and rectum.

An abscess may be deep in the rectum or close to the opening of the anus. An abscess develops when bacteria invade a mucus-secreting gland in the anus or rectum, where they multiply. Although the anus is an area that is rich in bacteria, infection generally does not occur because the internal sphincter acts as a barrier and blood flow to the area is rich. When infection does occur, it usually is caused by a combination of different types of bacteria. An abscess can cause substantial damage to nearby tissues and may lead to incontinence of stool.

Symptoms and Diagnosis

Abscesses just under the skin can be swollen, red, tender, and very painful. Abscesses higher in the rectum often cause fewer symptoms but may produce fever and pain in the lower abdomen. A doctor can usually see an abscess if it is in the skin around the anus. When no external swelling or redness is seen, however, a doctor can make the diagnosis by examining the rectum with a gloved finger. A tender swelling in the rectum indicates an abscess.

Treatment

Antibiotics have limited value except for people who have a fever, diabetes, or an infection elsewhere in the body. Usually, treatment consists of cutting into the abscess and draining the pus after a local anesthetic has been given. Occasionally, a person is hospitalized and undergoes general anesthesia before a doctor cuts and drains an abscess. Even with proper treatment, in about two thirds of people, an abscess leads to the formation of an abnormal channel from the anus or rectum to the skin (anorectal fistula).

Anorectal Fistula

An anorectal fistula is an abnormal channel from the anus or rectum usually to the skin near the anus but occasionally to another organ, such as the vagina.

Most fistulas begin in a deep gland in the wall of the anus or rectum. Sometimes fistulas occur after drainage of an anorectal abscess, but often the cause cannot be identified. Fistulas are more common among people with Crohn's disease or tuberculosis. They also occur in people with diverticulitis, cancer, or an anal or rectal injury. A fistula in an infant is usually a birth defect; such fistulas are more common among boys than girls. Fistulas that connect the rectum and vagina may result from radiation therapy, cancer, Crohn's disease, or an injury to a mother during childbirth.

Symptoms and Diagnosis

A fistula may be painful and may discharge pus. A doctor can usually see one or more openings of a fistula or can feel the fistula beneath the surface. A probe may be inserted to determine its depth and direction. Looking through an anoscope inserted into the rectum and exploring with the probe, a doctor may locate the internal opening. Inspection with a sigmoidoscope, which is a much longer viewing scope, helps a doctor determine whether the problem is being caused by cancer, Crohn's disease, or another disorder.

Treatment

The only effective treatment is surgery to remove the fistula (fistulotomy). During surgery, sometimes the sphincter is inadvertently partially cut. If too much of the sphincter is cut, the person may have difficulty controlling bowel movements. If the person has diarrhea or Crohn's disease, which may delay wound healing, the operation usually is not performed.

Proctitis

Proctitis is inflammation of the lining of the rectum (rectal mucosa).

Proctitis, which is becoming increasingly common, has several causes. It may result from Crohn's disease or ulcerative colitis. It can also result from a sexually transmitted disease (such as gonorrhea, syphilis, *Chlamy-*

dia trachomatis infection, herpes simplex virus infection, or cytomegalovirus infection), especially in homosexual men.

A person whose immune system is impaired is also at increased risk of developing proctitis, particularly from infections by the herpes simplex virus or cytomegalovirus. Proctitis may also be caused by some bacteria not transmitted sexually, such as *Salmonella,* or by the use of an antibiotic that destroys normal intestinal bacteria, thus allowing other bacteria to grow in their place.▲ Another cause of proctitis is radiation therapy directed at or near the rectum, which is commonly used to treat prostate and rectal cancer.

Symptoms and Diagnosis

Proctitis typically causes painless bleeding or the passage of mucus from the rectum. When the cause is gonorrhea, herpes simplex virus, or cytomegalovirus, the anus and rectum may be intensely painful.

To make the diagnosis, a doctor looks inside the rectum with an anoscope or sigmoidoscope and takes a tissue sample of the rectal lining for examination. The laboratory then can identify the bacterium, fungus, or virus that may be causing the proctitis. A doctor may also examine other areas of the intestine using colonoscopy or barium enema x-rays.

Treatment

Antibiotics are the best treatment for proctitis caused by a specific bacterial infection. When proctitis is caused by use of an antibiotic that destroys normal intestinal bacteria, a doctor may prescribe metronidazole or vancomycin, which should destroy the harmful bacteria that have displaced the normal ones.

When the cause is radiation therapy or is unknown, anti-inflammatory drugs such as hydrocortisone (a corticosteroid) or mesalamine may provide relief. Both hydrocortisone and mesalamine can be administered as either an enema or a suppository. Some corticosteroids are available in a foam preparation that can be inserted with a cartridge and plunger. Mesalamine and other anti-inflammatory drugs, such as sulfasalazine and olsalazine, may be taken by mouth at the same time that drugs are administered rectally, for added benefit. If these forms of treatment do not relieve the inflammation, formalin can be applied directly to the area or oral corticosteroids may be used. Laser or Argon plasma coagulation has also been used.

▲ see page 745

Pilonidal Disease

Pilonidal disease is an infection caused by a hair that injures the skin at the top of the cleft between the buttocks.

A pilonidal abscess is a collection of pus at the infection site; a pilonidal sinus is a chronic draining wound at the site.

Pilonidal disease usually occurs in young, hairy white men but can also occur in women. A pilonidal sinus can cause pain and swelling. To distinguish pilonidal disease from other infections, a doctor looks for pits—tiny holes in or next to the infected area.

Generally, a pilonidal abscess must be cut and drained by a doctor. Usually, a pilonidal sinus must be removed surgically.

Rectal Prolapse

Rectal prolapse is protrusion of the rectum through the anus.

Rectal prolapse causes the rectum to turn inside out, so that the rectal lining is visible as a dark red, moist fingerlike projection from the anus. Less commonly, the rectum protrudes into the vagina (rectocele▲).

A temporary prolapse of only the rectal lining (mucosa) often occurs in otherwise healthy infants, probably when the infant strains during a bowel movement, and is rarely serious. In adults, prolapse of the rectal lining tends to persist and may worsen, so that more of the rectum protrudes. A complete prolapse of the rectum is called procidentia; this occurs most often in women older than age 60.

To determine the extent of a prolapse, a doctor examines the area after the person strains. By feeling the anal sphincter with a gloved finger, a doctor often detects diminished muscle tone. A sigmoidoscopy and barium enema x-rays■ of the large intestine may reveal an underlying disease.

Treatment

In infants and children, a stool softener eliminates the urge to strain. Strapping the buttocks together between bowel movements usually helps the prolapse heal on its own.

In adults, surgery is usually needed to correct the problem. Surgery often cures procidentia. During one kind of abdominal operation, the entire rectum is lifted, pulled back, and attached to the sacral bone in the pelvis. In another, a segment of the rectum is removed, and the remainder of the rectum is stitched to the sacral bone.

For people who are too weak to undergo surgery because of extreme old age or poor health, surgery to the rectum is preferred to surgery to the abdomen. One type of surgery to the rectum is performed by inserting a wire or plastic loop to encircle the sphincter in a technique called the Thiersch procedure. Alternatively, a segment of the rectum or the excess lining of the rectum may be cut out (excised).

Anal Itching

Itchy skin around the anus (pruritus ani) can have many causes, including skin disorders such as psoriasis and atopic dermatitis, diseases such as diabetes or liver disease, anal disorders such as skin tags or draining fistulas, and cancers such as Bowen's disease. Allergic reactions such as contact dermatitis caused by anesthetic preparations applied to the skin, various ointments, or chemicals used in soap are another cause. Infections with fungi, bacteria, or parasites (such as pinworms and, less commonly, scabies or lice) can produce anal itching. Or itching can be a side effect of antibiotics, especially tetracycline.

Spices, citrus fruits, coffee, beer, and cola as well as vitamin C tablets can cause irritation of the anus when they are expelled in feces, causing itching. Poor hygiene that leaves stool residue (especially in people with large external hemorrhoids) or overly meticulous hygiene with excessive rubbing and use of soap can also lead to irritation and itching. Excessive sweating because of pantyhose, tight underwear (especially non-cotton underwear), obesity, or hot weather may be a factor. Or the itching may be rooted in anxiety, leading to the anxiety-itch-anxiety cycle (in which an anxious person develops an urge to scratch, scratching causes irritation possibly followed by infection, irritation/infection leads to itching, and itching leads to more anxiety).

Treatment

After bowel movements, the anal area should be cleaned with absorbent cotton or soft, plain toilet or facial tissue, which may be moistened with warm water. Dusting with cornstarch or a small amount of talc may combat moisture. Corticosteroid creams, antifungal creams such as miconazole, or soothing suppositories may be used. Foods that can cause anal itching are avoided for a while to see if the condition

▲ see page 1379   ■ see page 703

improves. Clothing should be loose and bed clothing lightweight. If the condition does not improve and a doctor suspects cancer, a skin specimen may be obtained for examination.

Foreign Objects

Swallowed objects, such as toothpicks, chicken bones, or fish bones, may become lodged at the junction between the rectum and anus.▲ Also, enema tips, thermometers, and objects used for sexual stimulation may become lodged unintentionally in the rectum after being passed through the anus.

Sudden, excruciating pain during bowel movements suggests that a foreign object, usually at the anorectal junction, is penetrating the lining of the anus or rectum. Other symptoms depend on the size and shape of the object, how long it has been there, and whether it has perforated (pierced) the anus or rectum or caused an infection.

A doctor can feel the object by probing with a gloved finger during an examination. An abdominal examination, sigmoidoscopy, and x-rays may be needed to make sure the wall of the large intestine has not been perforated.

Treatment

If a doctor can feel the object, a local anesthetic is usually injected under the skin and lining of the anus to numb the area. The anus can then be spread wider with an instrument called a rectal retractor, and the object can be grasped and removed. Natural movements of the wall of the large intestine (peristalsis) generally bring higher foreign objects down, making removal possible.

Occasionally, if a doctor cannot feel the object or if the object cannot be removed through the anus, exploratory surgery is needed. The person is given a regional or general anesthetic so that the object can be gently moved toward the anus or so that the rectum can be cut open to remove the object. After the object is removed, the doctor performs a sigmoidoscopy to determine whether the rectum has been perforated or otherwise injured.

CHAPTER 131

Tumors of the Digestive System

A variety of abnormal growths (tumors) can develop throughout the digestive system, from the esophagus to the anus, as well as in the liver,■ gallbladder,★ and pancreas. Some of these tumors are noncancerous (benign); others are cancerous (malignant).

Noncancerous Tumors of the Esophagus

Noncancerous tumors of the esophagus are rare and are usually more bothersome than harmful.

The most common type of noncancerous tumor is a leiomyoma, a tumor of the smooth muscle. It occurs most frequently in people between the ages of 30 and 60. Most leiomyomas are small and do not require treatment. A small number of leiomyomas grow large enough to cause partial obstruction of the esophagus, which may lead to difficulty swallowing (dysphagia) and pain or discomfort. Analgesic drugs may provide temporary relief, but surgical removal is needed for permanent relief.

Other types of noncancerous tumors, including those consisting of connective tissue (fibrovascular polyps) and tissues related to nerves (schwannomas), are rare.

Cancer of the Esophagus

The most common types of esophageal cancer are squamous cell carcinoma and adenocarcinoma, which develop in the cells that line the wall of the esophagus. These cancers may develop anywhere in the esophagus and may appear as a narrowing (stricture) of the esophagus, a lump, an abnormal flat area (plaque), or an abnormal connection (fistula) between the esophagus and the airways that supply the lungs.

▲ see also page 727   ■ see page 810
★ see page 817

Cancer of the esophagus affects about 3 of 100,000 people each year in the United States. Both squamous cell carcinoma and adenocarcinoma are more common among men than women. Squamous cell carcinoma is more common among blacks, whereas adenocarcinoma is more common among whites. The frequency of adenocarcinoma has been increasing rapidly in the United States since the 1970s, especially among white men.

Risk Factors

Smoking and alcohol are the most important risk factors for developing esophageal cancer, although more so for squamous cell carcinoma than for adenocarcinoma. People who have had certain human papillomavirus infections, who have had head and neck cancer, or who have undergone radiation therapy to the esophagus for treatment of other nearby cancers are at greater risk of developing esophageal cancer.

People with an existing disorder of the esophagus, such as achalasia, esophageal webs, or narrowing due to having once swallowed a corrosive substance, are at greater risk of developing esophageal cancer. Prolonged irritation of the esophagus from the repeated backflow of stomach acid (gastroesophageal reflux) can cause a precancerous condition called Barrett's esophagus. Although esophageal cancer from Barrett's esophagus remains relatively rare in most industrialized countries, its frequency is increasing faster than all other esophageal cancers.

Symptoms

Early-stage esophageal cancer may go unnoticed. The first symptom is usually difficulty in swallowing solid foods, which develops as the growing cancer narrows the esophagus. Several weeks later, swallowing soft foods and then liquids becomes difficult. Weight loss is common, even when the person continues to eat well.

As the cancer progresses, it commonly invades various nerves and other tissues and organs. The tumor may compress the nerve that controls the vocal cords, which can lead to hoarseness. Compression of surrounding nerves may produce Horner's syndrome,▲ pain, and hiccups. The cancer usually spreads to the lungs, where it may cause shortness of breath, and to the liver, where it may cause fever and abdominal swelling. Spread to bones may cause pain. Spread to the brain may produce headache, confusion, and seizures. Spread to the intestines may produce vomiting, blood in the

Rare Types of Esophageal Cancer

Types of esophageal cancer that are much less common include lymphomas (cancers of the lymphatic system), leiomyosarcomas (cancers of the smooth muscle of the esophagus), and metastatic cancer (cancer that has spread from elsewhere in the body). All of these types are more common among men than women.

The risk factors for developing lymphoma may include infection, possibly with the bacterium *Helicobacter pylori* (which plays a role in producing ulcers); impairment of the immune system; and exposure to radiation (either unintentionally or as the result of receiving radiation therapy for cancer of sites near the esophagus). The risk of developing metastatic cancer of the esophagus depends on where the cancer originated; liver cancer, breast cancer, and melanoma (a type of skin cancer) are more likely than other cancers to spread (metastasize) to the esophagus. The risk factors for developing leiomyosarcoma are unknown.

Lymphomas are treated with chemotherapy and radiation therapy, which may lengthen survival time and possibly cure the cancer. Leiomyosarcomas are treated with surgery, which may relieve symptoms temporarily but is unlikely to cure the cancer. Chemotherapy after surgery may slightly lengthen survival time. Metastatic cancer often leads to obstruction of the esophagus, which requires the use of a tube (stent) or laser therapy. Use of chemotherapy or radiation therapy for metastatic cancer depends on the type of cancer that has spread to the esophagus.

stool, and iron-deficiency anemia. Spread to the kidneys often produces no symptoms.

In late stages, the cancer may completely block the esophagus. Swallowing becomes impossible so that secretions build up in the mouth, which can be very distressing.

Diagnosis

Endoscopy, in which a flexible viewing tube (endoscope) is passed through the mouth to view the esophagus, is the best diagnostic procedure if esophageal cancer is suspected. Endoscopy also allows the doctor to remove a tissue sample (biopsy) and loose cells (brush cytology) for examination under a microscope.

▲ see box on page 592

An x-ray procedure called a barium swallow (in which the person swallows a solution of barium, which shows up on x-rays) can also show the obstruction, but does not supply a sample of tissue. Computed tomography (CT) and ultrasound scans as well as a newer imaging study called endoscopic ultrasound may be used to further assess the extent of the cancer.

Prognosis and Treatment

Because esophageal cancer usually is not diagnosed until the disease has spread, the death rate is high. Fewer than 5% of people survive more than 5 years. Many die within a year of noticing the first symptoms. Because nearly all cases of esophageal cancer are fatal, the doctor's main objective is to control symptoms, especially pain and the inability to swallow, which can be very frightening to the person and loved ones.▲

Surgery to remove a tumor offers the most prolonged relief but seldom cures, because the cancer usually has spread by the time of surgery. Chemotherapy, alone or with radiation therapy, may relieve symptoms and lengthen survival time by a few months. Sometimes preoperative radiation therapy combined with chemotherapy can increase the surgical cure rate. Other measures that aim only to relieve symptoms include widening (dilating) the narrowed area of the esophagus and then inserting a tube (a stent) to keep the esophagus open; bypassing the tumor using a loop of intestine; and performing laser phototherapy, in which a high-energy beam of light is directed at the growth to destroy the cancer tissue obstructing the esophagus.

A more recent technique for symptom relief is photodynamic therapy, in which a light-sensitive dye (contrast agent) is administered intravenously 48 hours before treatment. The dye is absorbed by cancer cells to a much greater degree than by the cells of normal surrounding esophageal tissue. When activated by light from a laser passed into the esophagus through an endoscope, the dye destroys cancer tissue, thus opening the esophagus. Photodynamic therapy destroys obstructing lesions more rapidly than radiation or chemotherapy in people who cannot tolerate surgery because of poor health.

Adequate nutrition makes any type of treatment more feasible and tolerable. If the person can swallow, he may receive concentrated liquid nutritional supplements. If the person cannot swallow, temporary tube feeding or intravenous feeding may be necessary.

Because death is likely, a person with esophageal cancer should make all necessary plans. The person should have frank discussions with the doctor about wishes for medical care (advance directives)■ and the need for end-of-life care.

Noncancerous Tumors of the Stomach

Noncancerous tumors of the stomach are unlikely to cause symptoms or medical problems, so they often remain undiagnosed and untreated. Occasionally, however, some bleed and are then removed during endoscopy or surgery.

Stomach polyps, uncommon noncancerous round growths that project into the stomach cavity, may become cancerous (that is, they may be precancerous). Therefore, polyps are usually removed using endoscopy. Through the endoscope, an electrical current (electrocautery) or heat (thermal obliteration) is applied directly to the growth, or a high-energy beam of light is directed at the growth (laser phototherapy).

Cancer of the Stomach

About 95% of stomach cancers are adenocarcinomas. Adenocarcinomas of the stomach originate from the glandular cells of the stomach lining.

In the United States, adenocarcinoma of the stomach occurs in about 8 of 100,000 people each year and is the seventh most common cause of cancer death. It is more common among certain populations: people aged 50 and older, poor people, blacks, and people who live in northern climates. For unknown reasons, adenocarcinoma of the stomach is becoming less common in the United States. It is far more common in Japan, China, Chile, and Iceland; in these nations, screening programs are an important means of early detection.

Causes and Risk Factors

The cause of adenocarcinoma of the stomach is unknown. It often begins at a site where the stomach lining is inflamed. However, many experts now believe that inflammation is the result of adenocarcinoma rather than the cause of it. Certain foods, especially smoked foods, are suspected as contributing to stomach cancer.

· ▲ see page 49   ■ see page 54

Some experts suggest that peptic ulcers in the stomach can lead to adenocarcinoma, but most people with ulcers and adenocarcinoma probably had an undetected cancer before the ulcers developed. The bacterium *Helicobacter pylori*, which plays a role in producing ulcers, likely plays a role in the development of adenocarcinoma.

Stomach polyps may become cancerous and are thus removed. Adenocarcinoma of the stomach is particularly likely to develop if the polyps consist of glandular cells, if the polyps are larger than $3/4$ inch, or if several polyps exist.

Certain dietary factors were once thought to play a role in the development of adenocarcinoma of the stomach. These factors included a high intake of salt, a high intake of carbohydrates, a high intake of preservatives called nitrates (often present in smoked foods), and a low intake of fruit and green leafy vegetables. However, none of these factors has been proven to be a cause.

Symptoms

In the early stages, symptoms are vague and easily ignored. Early symptoms may mimic peptic ulcer disease, with burning abdominal pain. Therefore, peptic ulcer symptoms that do not resolve with treatment may indicate stomach cancer. The person may notice a feeling of fullness after a small meal (early satiety).

Weight loss or weakness usually results from difficulty in eating or from an inability to absorb some vitamins and minerals. Anemia, characterized by fatigue, weakness, and lightheadedness, may result from very gradual bleeding that causes no other symptoms, from malabsorption of vitamin B_{12} (a vitamin needed for red blood cell formation), or from malabsorption of iron (a mineral needed for red blood cell formation) due to a lack of stomach acid. Uncommonly, a person may vomit large amounts of blood (hematemesis) or pass black tarry stools (melena). When adenocarcinoma is advanced, a doctor may be able to feel a mass when pressing on the abdomen.

Even in the early stages, a small adenocarcinoma may spread (metastasize) to distant sites. The spread of the tumor may cause liver enlargement, jaundice (a yellowish discoloration of the skin and the whites of the eyes), ascites (fluid accumulation and swelling in the abdominal cavity), and cancerous skin nodules. The spreading cancer also may weaken bones, leading to bone fractures.

Rare Types of Stomach Cancer

Lymphoma is cancer of the lymphatic system. Lymphoma can develop within the stomach. The bacterium *Helicobacter pylori* is believed to play a role in the development of some lymphomas of the stomach. Surgery is often the initial treatment. Chemotherapy and radiation therapy are more successful in treating lymphoma than adenocarcinoma. Longer survival and even cure are possible.

Leiomyosarcoma (also called stromal cell tumor or spindle cell tumor) is cancer of the smooth muscle of the stomach. It is best treated with surgery. If cancer has already spread (metastasized) to other parts of the body at the time a leiomyosarcoma is found, then chemotherapy may lead to slightly longer survival. A newer drug, imatinib, has been found to be effective for treating leiomyosarcoma that cannot be treated with surgery.

Diagnosis

Endoscopy (an examination in which a flexible tube is used to visualize the inside of the digestive tract) is the best diagnostic procedure. It allows a doctor to view the stomach directly, to check for *Helicobacter pylori*, and to remove tissue samples for examination under a microscope (biopsy). Barium x-rays are used less often because they rarely reveal small early-stage cancers and do not allow for biopsy.

Prognosis and Treatment

Fewer than 20% of people with adenocarcinoma of the stomach survive longer than 5 years. The cancer tends to spread early to other sites. If the cancer is confined to the stomach, surgery is usually performed to try to cure it. Removal of the entire tumor before it has spread offers the only hope of cure. Most or all of the stomach and nearby lymph nodes are removed. The prognosis is good if the cancer has not penetrated the stomach wall too deeply. In the United States, the results of surgery are often poor, because most people have extensive cancer by the time a diagnosis is made. In Japan, where stomach cancer is very common, mass public health screening programs help to detect it early so that a cure is more likely. Chemotherapy and radiation therapy do not usually improve survival time after surgery.

If the cancer has spread beyond the stomach, surgery cannot cure the condition, but it is sometimes used to relieve symptoms. For example, if the passage of food is obstructed at the far end of the stomach, a bypass operation, in which an alternate connection is made between the stomach and the small intestine, allows food to pass. This connection relieves the symptoms of obstruction—pain and vomiting—at least for a while. Chemotherapy and radiation therapy may relieve symptoms as well, but their effectiveness is limited.

Noncancerous Tumors of the Small Intestine

Most tumors of the small intestine are noncancerous. These include tumors of fat cells (lipomas), nerve cells (neurofibromas), connective tissue cells (fibromas), and muscle cells (leiomyomas).

Most noncancerous tumors of the small intestine do not cause symptoms. However, larger ones may cause blood in the stool, a partial or complete intestinal obstruction, or intestinal strangulation if one part of the intestine telescopes into an adjacent part (a condition called intussusception).

Small noncancerous growths may be destroyed through an endoscope by applying an electrical current (electrocautery) or heat (thermal obliteration) directly to the growth, or by directing a high-energy beam of light at the growth (laser phototherapy). For large growths, surgery may be needed.

Cancer of the Small Intestine

Cancerous tumors in the small intestine are very uncommon, occurring in fewer than 2 of 100,000 people in the United States each year. Adenocarcinoma is the most common type of cancer of the small intestine. Adenocarcinomas develop in the glandular cells of the lining of the small intestine. People with Crohn's disease of the small intestine are more likely than others to develop adenocarcinoma.

Symptoms and Diagnosis

Adenocarcinoma may produce bleeding into the intestine, which shows up as blood in the stool, and obstruction, which in turn may lead to crampy abdominal pain, expansion (distention) of the abdomen, and vomiting.

A doctor may use an endoscope (a flexible viewing tube) passed through the mouth and down to the duodenum and part of the jejunum (the upper section of the small intes-

tine) to locate the tumor and perform a biopsy (remove a tissue sample for examination under a microscope). A doctor can sometimes see tumors of the ileum (the lower section of the small intestine) by passing a colonoscope (an endoscope used to view the lower part of the digestive tract) through the anus, through the entire large intestine, and up into the ileum. A barium x-ray can show the entire small intestine and may be used to outline the tumor. Arteriography (an x-ray taken after a radiopaque dye is injected into an artery) of intestinal arteries may be performed, especially if the tumor is bleeding. Similarly, radioactive technetium can be injected into the artery and observed on x-rays as it leaks into the intestine; this procedure helps locate sites where the tumor is bleeding. The bleeding can then be corrected surgically. Sometimes exploratory surgery is needed to identify a tumor in the small intestine.

Treatment

The best treatment for all types of cancerous growths is surgical removal of the tumor. Chemotherapy and radiation therapy after surgery do not lengthen survival time.

Polyps of the Large Intestine and Rectum

A polyp is a growth of tissue from the intestinal or rectal wall that protrudes into the intestine or rectum and may be noncancerous or cancerous. Polyps vary considerably in size; the bigger the polyp, the greater the risk that it is cancerous or precancerous. Polyps may grow with or without a stalk; those without a stalk are more likely to be cancerous than those with a stalk. Adenomatous polyps, which consist primarily of glandular cells that line the inside of the large intestine, are likely to become cancerous (that is, they are precancerous).

Some polyps are the result of hereditary conditions, such as familial polyposis, Gardner's syndrome, and Peutz-Jeghers syndrome. In familial polyposis, 100 or more precancerous polyps develop throughout the large intestine and rectum during childhood or adolescence. In nearly all untreated people, the polyps develop into cancer of the large intestine or rectum (colorectal cancer) before age 40. In Gardner's syndrome, various types of noncancerous tumors develop elsewhere in the body (for example, on the skin, skull, or jaw) in addition to the precancerous polyps that develop in the large intestine and rectum. In Peutz-Jeghers syndrome, small lumps called juvenile polyps develop in the stomach, small intestine, large intestine, and rectum. These polyps develop before birth (in utero) or during early childhood. Although polyps in Peutz-Jeghers syndrome do not increase the risk of developing cancer of the intestinal tract, people with Peutz-Jeghers syndrome do have an increased risk of developing cancer of the pancreas, breast, lung, ovary, and uterus.

Symptoms and Diagnosis

Most polyps do not cause symptoms. When they do, the most common symptom is bleeding from the rectum. A large polyp may cause cramps, abdominal pain, or obstruction. Large polyps with fingerlike projections (villous adenomas) may excrete water and salts, causing profuse watery diarrhea that may result in low levels of potassium in the blood (hypokalemia). Rarely, a rectal polyp on a long stalk drops down and dangles through the anus. People with Peutz-Jeghers syndrome have brown skin and brown mucous membranes, especially of the lips and gums.

A doctor may be able to feel polyps by inserting a gloved finger into the rectum, but usually polyps are discovered during flexible sigmoidoscopy (examination of the lower portion of the large intestine with a viewing tube). If flexible sigmoidoscopy reveals a polyp, colonoscopy is performed to examine the entire large intestine. This more complete and reliable examination is performed because more than one polyp is usually present and may be cancerous. Colonoscopy also allows a doctor to perform a biopsy (removal of a tissue sample for examination under a microscope) of any area that appears cancerous.

Treatment

Doctors generally recommend removing all polyps from the large intestine and rectum because of their potential to become cancerous. Polyps are removed during a colonoscopy procedure using a cutting instrument or an electrified wire loop. If a polyp has no stalk or cannot be removed during colonoscopy, abdominal surgery may be needed.

If a polyp that has been removed is found to be cancerous, treatment depends on whether the cancer is likely to have spread. If the risk is low, no further treatment is necessary. If the risk is high, particularly if the cancer has invaded the polyp's stalk, the affected segment

Rare Types of Small-Intestinal Cancer

Carcinoid tumors can develop in the glandular cells that line the small intestine. Carcinoid tumors often secrete hormones that cause diarrhea and flushing of the skin. Chemotherapy and other types of drugs sometimes help control the symptoms produced by carcinoid tumors.

Lymphoma (cancer of the lymphatic system) may develop in the middle section (jejunum) or the lower section (ileum) of the small intestine. Lymphoma may cause a segment of intestine to become rigid or elongated. This cancer is more common in people with celiac disease. Chemotherapy and radiation therapy can help control symptoms and sometimes lengthen survival time.

Leiomyosarcomas develop in the muscle cells in the wall of the small intestine. Chemotherapy may slightly lengthen survival time after surgery to remove leiomyosarcomas.

of the large intestine is removed surgically, and the cut ends of the intestine are rejoined.

When a person has a polyp removed, the entire large intestine and rectum are examined by colonoscopy a year later and then at intervals determined by the doctor. If such an examination is impossible because of a narrowing of the large intestine, a barium enema may be used to view the large intestine on x-ray.

For people with familial polyposis, complete removal of the large intestine and rectum eliminates the risk of cancer. Alternatively, the large intestine is removed and the rectum is joined to the small intestine; this procedure sometimes eliminates the rectal polyps and thus is preferred by many experts. The remaining part of the rectum is inspected by sigmoidoscopy every 3 to 6 months, so that new polyps can be removed. If new polyps appear too rapidly, however, the rectum must also be removed. If the rectum is removed, a surgical opening is created through the abdominal wall from the small intestine; this procedure is called an ileostomy. Bodily wastes are eliminated through the ileostomy into a disposable bag.

Some nonsteroidal anti-inflammatory drugs (NSAIDs) are being studied for their ability to reverse the growth of polyps in people with familial polyposis. Their effects are temporary, however, and once these drugs are discontinued, the polyps begin to grow again.

Colorectal Cancer

Almost all colorectal cancers are adenocarcinomas, which develop from the lining of the large intestine (colon) and rectum. Colorectal cancer usually begins as a buttonlike swelling on the surface of the intestinal or rectal lining or on a polyp. As the cancer grows, it begins to invade the wall of the intestine or rectum. Nearby lymph nodes also may be invaded. Because blood from the wall of the intestine and much of the rectum is carried to the liver, colorectal cancer usually spreads (metastasizes) to the liver soon after spreading to nearby lymph nodes.

In Western countries, cancer of the large intestine and rectum is the second most common type of cancer and the second leading cause of cancer death. The incidence of colorectal cancer begins to rise at age 40 and peaks between the ages of 60 and 75. The rate for the entire U.S. population is about 50 new instances of colorectal cancer for every 100,000 people each year. Colon cancer is more common among women; rectal cancer is more common among men. About 5% of the people with colon or rectal cancer have cancer in two or more sites in the colon and rectum that do not appear to simply be spread from one site to another.

Risk Factors

People with a family history of colorectal cancer have a higher risk of developing the cancer themselves. A family history of polyps▲ also increases the risk of colorectal cancer. People with ulcerative colitis or Crohn's disease are at greater risk as well; this risk is related to the person's age when the disease developed and the length of time the person has had the disease.

People at highest risk tend to consume a high-fat, low-fiber diet. Greater exposure to air and water pollution, particularly to industrial cancer-causing substances (carcinogens), may play a role.

Symptoms

Colorectal cancer grows slowly and does not cause symptoms for a long time. Symptoms depend on the type, location, and extent of the cancer.

Fatigue and weakness resulting from occult bleeding (bleeding not visible to the naked eye) may be the person's only symptoms. A tumor in the left (descending) colon is likely to cause obstruction at an earlier stage, because the left colon has a smaller diameter and the stool is semisolid. Cancer tends to encircle this part of the colon, causing alternating constipation and frequent bowel movements before obstruction. The person may seek medical treatment because of crampy abdominal pain or severe abdominal pain and constipation. A tumor in the right (ascending) colon does not cause obstruction until late in the course of the cancer, because the ascending colon has a large diameter and the contents flowing through it are liquid. By the time the tumor is discovered, therefore, it may be so large that a doctor can feel it through the abdominal wall.

Most colon cancers bleed, usually slowly. The stool may be streaked or mixed with blood, but often the blood cannot be seen; a test of the stool for occult blood is needed to detect it.■ The most common first symptom of rectal cancer is bleeding during a bowel movement. Whenever the rectum bleeds, even if the person is known to have hemorrhoids or diverticular disease, doctors must consider cancer as part of their differential diagnosis. Painful bowel movements and a feeling that the rectum has not been completely emptied are other symptoms of rectal cancer. Sitting may be painful, but otherwise the person usually feels no pain from the cancer itself unless it spreads to tissue outside the rectum.

Diagnosis

Early diagnosis depends on routine screening. The stool can be tested for occult blood. To help ensure accurate test results, the person eats a high-fiber diet that is free of red meat for 3 days before providing a stool sample. Alternatively, a doctor can test stool obtained during a digital rectal examination, in which he places a gloved finger in the person's rectum. If blood is detected, further testing is needed.

Sigmoidoscopy (examination of the lower portion of the large intestine with a viewing tube) is another diagnostic procedure performed for screening. People at high risk may undergo colonoscopy, in which the entire large intestine is evaluated. Some growths that appear cancerous are removed using surgical instruments passed through the scope; other growths must be removed during regular surgery.

Blood tests are not used to diagnose colorectal cancer, but they can help the doctor monitor the effectiveness of treatment after a tumor has been removed. For example, if levels

▲ see page 768   ■ see page 705

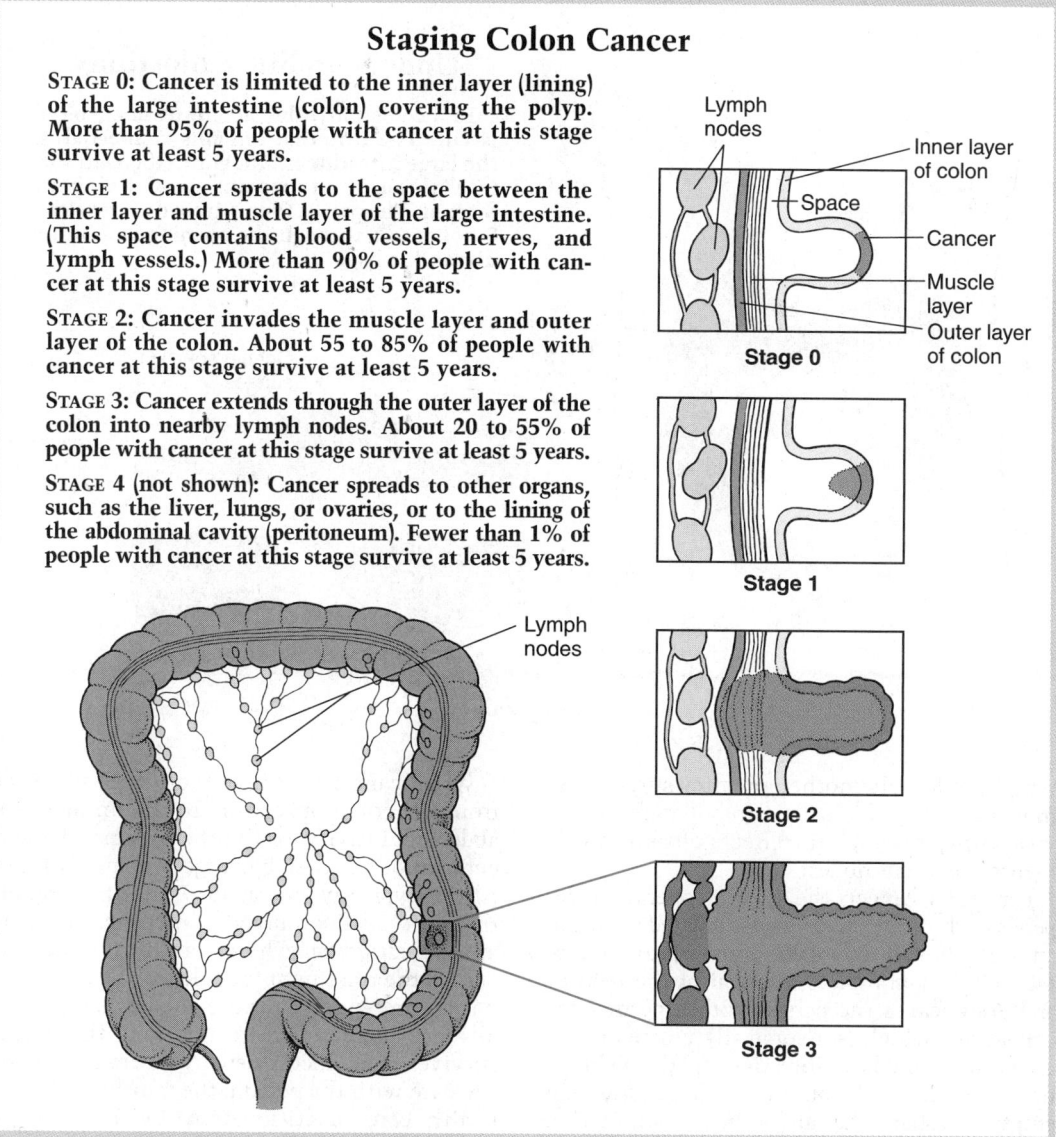

Staging Colon Cancer

STAGE 0: Cancer is limited to the inner layer (lining) of the large intestine (colon) covering the polyp. More than 95% of people with cancer at this stage survive at least 5 years.

STAGE 1: Cancer spreads to the space between the inner layer and muscle layer of the large intestine. (This space contains blood vessels, nerves, and lymph vessels.) More than 90% of people with cancer at this stage survive at least 5 years.

STAGE 2: Cancer invades the muscle layer and outer layer of the colon. About 55 to 85% of people with cancer at this stage survive at least 5 years.

STAGE 3: Cancer extends through the outer layer of the colon into nearby lymph nodes. About 20 to 55% of people with cancer at this stage survive at least 5 years.

STAGE 4 (not shown): Cancer spreads to other organs, such as the liver, lungs, or ovaries, or to the lining of the abdominal cavity (peritoneum). Fewer than 1% of people with cancer at this stage survive at least 5 years.

Lymph nodes

Inner layer of colon

Space

Cancer

Muscle layer

Outer layer of colon

Stage 0

Stage 1

Stage 2

Stage 3

Lymph nodes

of carcinoembryonic antigen (CEA) are high before surgery to remove a known cancer and low after surgery, monitoring for another increase in the CEA level may help detect an early recurrence of the cancer. Two other cancer markers, CA 19-9 and CA 125, are similar to CEA and are sometimes elevated in colorectal cancer.

Prognosis and Treatment

Colon cancer is most likely to be cured if it is removed early, before it has spread. Cancers that have grown deeply or through the wall of the colon have often spread, even if metastases (spread) cannot be detected. Surgery, the main treatment for colorectal cancer, is curative in about 70% of cases.

In most cases of colon cancer, the cancerous segment of the intestine and any nearby lymph nodes are removed surgically, and the remaining ends of the intestine are joined. When people have colon cancer that has penetrated the wall of the large intestine and spread to a very limited number of nearby

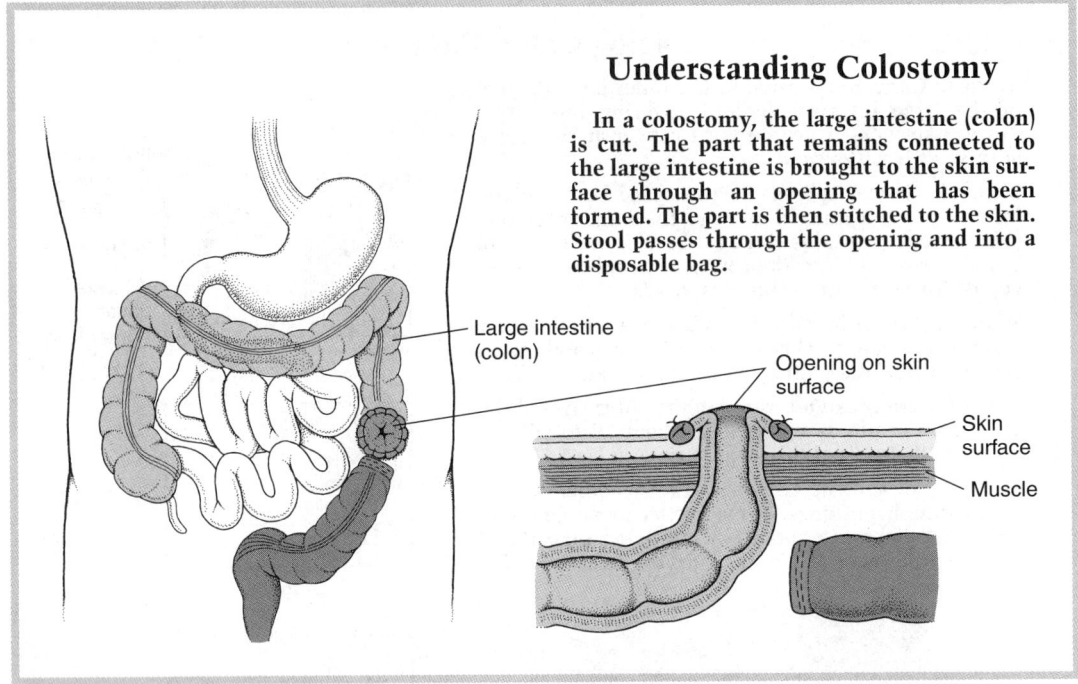

Understanding Colostomy

In a colostomy, the large intestine (colon) is cut. The part that remains connected to the large intestine is brought to the skin surface through an opening that has been formed. The part is then stitched to the skin. Stool passes through the opening and into a disposable bag.

Large intestine (colon)

Opening on skin surface

Skin surface

Muscle

lymph nodes, chemotherapy after surgical removal of all visible cancer may lengthen survival time, although the effects of these treatments are often modest.

For rectal cancer, the type of operation depends on how far the cancer is located from the anus and how deeply it has grown into the rectal wall. The complete removal of the rectum and anus leaves the person with a permanent colostomy, which is a surgically created opening between the large intestine and the abdominal wall. The contents of the large intestine empty through the abdominal wall into a colostomy bag. If possible, however, only part of the rectum is removed, leaving a rectal stump and the anus intact. Then the rectal stump is rejoined to the end of the large intestine.

When rectal cancer has penetrated the rectal wall and spread to a very limited number of nearby lymph nodes, chemotherapy after surgical removal of all visible cancer may lengthen survival time. Also, radiation therapy after surgical removal of visible rectal cancer may help control the growth of any residual tumors, delay a recurrence, and lengthen survival time.

When cancer has spread to lymph nodes far from the colon or rectum, to the lining of the abdominal cavity, or to other organs, the cancer cannot be cured by surgery alone. Survival time is typically only about 7 months. Chemotherapy with fluorouracil (sometimes also with another drug) may be given after surgery as part of the treatment for colorectal cancer that has spread widely, but the chemotherapy usually has little effect on how long the person survives. The doctor usually discusses end-of-life care with the person, the family, and other health care practitioners.▲ Even when the cancer has spread widely, surgery is sometimes performed to relieve the intestinal obstruction and ease symptoms.

When the cancer has spread only to the liver, chemotherapy drugs can be injected directly into the artery supplying the liver. A small pump inserted surgically beneath the skin or an external pump worn on a belt allows the person to be mobile during the treatment. This treatment may provide more benefit than ordinary chemotherapy, but more research is needed. When cancer has spread beyond the liver, this approach has no advantage.

For people who cannot tolerate surgery because of poor health, treatment may involve

▲ see page 45

drying out and shrinking the tumor in a procedure called desiccation. Desiccation is performed either with a probe that applies an electrical charge to the surface of the tumor (cautery device) or with a device that dries the tumor with electrified Argon gas (Argon plasma coagulator); both devices can be passed through a colonoscope. Desiccation may relieve symptoms and lengthen survival time modestly by reducing tumor mass but rarely cures the cancer.

Cancer of the Anus

Anal cancer develops in the skin cells of the immediate area around the anus or in the lining of the transitional zone between the anus and the rectum (the anal canal). Unlike the rectum and the large intestine, in which cancers are almost always adenocarcinomas, cancers of the anus are primarily squamous cell carcinomas.

Cancer of the anus occurs in about 1 of 100,000 people in the United States each year. Anal cancer is almost twice as common in women as in men. The cause of anal cancer is unknown. Receptive anal intercourse has been linked to anal cancer, and infection with a specific type of sexually transmitted human papillomavirus (HPV type 16) has been identified as a likely cause.

Symptoms and Diagnosis

People with anal cancer often experience bleeding with bowel movements, pain, and sometimes itching around the anus. About 25% of people with anal cancer have no symptoms; in these instances, the cancer is found only during a routine examination.

To diagnose anal cancer, a doctor first inspects the skin around the anus for any abnormalities. With a gloved hand, the doctor probes the anus and lower rectum, checking for any portions of the lining that feel different from surrounding areas. The doctor then removes a sample of tissue from an abnormal area and examines it under a microscope (performs a biopsy).

Treatment

Radiation therapy combined with chemotherapy may be used instead of or in addition to surgery. Surgery alone is avoided so as not to interfere with the functioning of the muscular ring that keeps the anus closed until the person has a bowel movement (the anal sphincter), which could lead to loss of control over bowel movements (fecal incontinence). A combination of radiation with chemotherapy, or radiation with surgery, cures many anal cancers, with 70% or more of people surviving longer than 5 years. More extensive surgery is sometimes needed if the results of follow-up biopsies performed after initial treatment show recurrence of the cancer.

Cancer of the Pancreas

About 95% of cancerous tumors of the pancreas are adenocarcinomas. Adenocarcinomas usually originate in the glandular cells lining the pancreatic duct. Most adenocarcinomas occur in the head of the pancreas, the part nearest the first segment of the small intestine (duodenum).

Adenocarcinoma of the pancreas has become increasingly common in the United States, occurring in about 10 of 100,000 people each year. Adenocarcinoma usually does not develop before age 50; the average age at diagnosis is 55. These tumors are nearly twice as common in men as in women and are slightly more common in blacks than in whites. Adenocarcinoma of the pancreas is 2 to 3 times more common in heavy smokers than in nonsmokers. People with chronic pancreatitis are at greater risk as well.

Symptoms and Complications

Tumors in the head of the pancreas can interfere with the drainage of bile (the digestive fluid produced by the liver) into the small intestine.▲ Therefore, jaundice (a yellowish discoloration of the skin and the whites of the eyes) caused by obstruction of bile flow is typically an early symptom. The jaundice is accompanied by itchiness all over the body resulting from the deposit of bile salt crystals under the skin. Vomiting may result from instances when cancer in the head of the pancreas obstructs the flow of stomach contents into the small intestine (gastric outlet obstruction) or obstructs the small intestine itself.

Adenocarcinoma of the body or tail of the pancreas (the middle part of the pancreas and the part farthest from the duodenum) typically causes no symptoms until the tumor has grown large. Thus, at the time of diagnosis, the tumor has already spread (metastasized) beyond the

▲ see art on page 730 and page 817

Rare Types of Pancreatic Cancer

Cystadenocarcinoma of the pancreas is a rare type of pancreatic cancer that develops from a fluid-filled noncancerous tumor called a cystadenoma. It often causes upper abdominal pain and may grow large enough for a doctor to feel it through the abdominal wall. Diagnosis is usually made by ultrasound or computed tomography (CT) scan of the pancreas. Only 20% of these cancers have spread by the time surgery is performed. Therefore, cystadenocarcinoma has a much better prognosis than adenocarcinoma. If the cancer has not spread and the whole pancreas is removed surgically, the person has a 65% chance of surviving for at least 5 years.

Intraductal tumor is a newly recognized type of pancreatic tumor characterized by enlargement (dilation) of the main pancreatic duct, mucus overproduction, and occasional pain. More than 30% of these tumors are cancerous, but it is not yet known how intraductal tumors develop and progress. Because diagnostic tests cannot distinguish between noncancerous and cancerous forms of this tumor, surgery is the best diagnostic and treatment option for all people suspected of having an intraductal tumor.

pancreas in 90% of the cases. It usually spreads to the neighboring lymph nodes, the liver, or the lung. Typically, the first symptoms are pain and weight loss. At the time of diagnosis, 90% of people have abdominal pain—usually severe pain in the upper abdomen that penetrates to the back—and significant weight loss.

Adenocarcinoma of the body or tail of the pancreas may obstruct the vein draining the spleen (the organ that produces, monitors, stores, and destroys blood cells), resulting in enlargement of the spleen (splenomegaly). Obstruction can also cause the veins to become swollen and twisted (varicose) around the esophagus (esophageal varices) and stomach. Severe bleeding may result, particularly from the esophagus, if these varicose veins rupture.

Diagnosis

Early diagnosis of tumors in the body or tail of the pancreas is difficult because symptoms occur late and physical examination and blood test results are often normal. When adenocar-

▲ see page 789 and art on page 790

cinoma of the pancreas is suspected, the most accurate diagnostic test is computed tomography (CT). Other commonly used tests are ultrasound scans, endoscopic retrograde cholangiopancreatography,▲ and magnetic resonance imaging (MRI).

To confirm the diagnosis, a doctor may obtain a sample of the pancreas for examination under a microscope (biopsy) by inserting a needle through the skin using a CT or ultrasound scan as a guide. However, this approach often misses the tumor and may spread cancer cells out of the local area along the track of the needle. The same approach may be used to obtain a biopsy sample from the liver to look for cancer that has spread to the pancreas. If the results of these tests are normal but the doctor still strongly suspects adenocarcinoma, the pancreas may be evaluated surgically.

Prognosis and Treatment

Because adenocarcinoma of the pancreas has usually spread to other parts of the body before it is discovered, the prognosis is very poor. Fewer than 2% of people with adenocarcinoma of the pancreas survive for 5 years after the diagnosis. The only hope of a cure is surgery, which is performed on about 10% of people in whom it is believed that the cancer has not spread. Either the pancreas alone or the pancreas and the duodenum are removed. After such surgery, only 15 to 20% of people live for 5 years. Additional chemotherapy and radiation therapy are not likely to improve survival time or rates substantially.

Mild pain may be relieved by aspirin or acetaminophen. Most often, stronger painkillers, such as oral codeine or morphine, are needed. For 70 to 80% of people with severe pain, injections into nerves to block pain sensations may provide relief. The lack of pancreatic digestive enzymes can be treated with oral enzyme preparations. If diabetes develops, insulin treatment may be needed.

Obstruction of bile flow may be temporarily relieved by placement of a tube (stent) in the lower portion of the duct that drains bile from the liver and gallbladder. In most cases, however, the tumor eventually obstructs the duct above and below the stent. An alternative treatment method is the surgical creation of a channel that bypasses the obstruction. For example, an obstruction of the small intestine can be bypassed by a channel that connects the stomach with a portion of the small intestine that is beyond the obstruction.

Because adenocarcinoma of the pancreas is fatal in most cases, a doctor usually discusses end-of-life care with the person, family members, and other health care practitioners.▲

Other Tumors of the Pancreas

INSULINOMA

An insulinoma is a rare type of pancreatic tumor that secretes insulin, a hormone that lowers the levels of sugar (glucose) in the blood.

Only 10% of insulinomas are cancerous.

Symptoms

Symptoms result from low levels of sugar in the blood, which occur when the person does not eat for several hours (most often in the morning after an all-night fast). The symptoms include faintness, weakness, trembling, awareness of the heartbeat (palpitations), sweating, nervousness, and profound hunger. Other symptoms include headache, confusion, vision abnormalities, unsteadiness, and marked changes in personality. The low levels of sugar in the blood may even lead to a loss of consciousness, seizures, and coma.

Diagnosis and Treatment

Diagnosing an insulinoma can be difficult. The person fasts for at least 24 hours, sometimes up to 72 hours, and is closely monitored, often in the hospital. During that time, the symptoms usually appear, and blood tests are performed to measure the levels of sugar and insulin. Very low levels of sugar and high levels of insulin in the blood indicate the presence of an insulinoma. The location must then be pinpointed. Imaging tests—such as computed tomography (CT), ultrasound scans, and arteriography (an x-ray taken after a radiopaque dye is injected into an artery) of the intestinal arteries—can be used to locate the tumor, but sometimes exploratory surgery is needed.

The primary treatment for an insulinoma is surgical removal, which has a cure rate of about 90%. When the insulinoma cannot be completely removed and symptoms continue, several drugs (for example, streptozocin and octreotide) can be helpful.

GASTRINOMA

A gastrinoma is a tumor usually in the pancreas or duodenum (the first segment of the small intestine) that produces excessive levels of the hormone gastrin, which stimulates

the stomach to secrete acid and enzymes, causing peptic ulcers.

Most people with gastrinomas have several tumors clustered in or near the pancreas. About half of the tumors are cancerous. Sometimes a gastrinoma occurs as part of multiple endocrine neoplasia, a hereditary disorder in which tumors arise from the cells of various endocrine glands, such as the insulin-producing cells of the pancreas.

Symptoms and Diagnosis

The excess gastrin secreted by the gastrinoma causes Zollinger-Ellison syndrome,■ in which a person suffers the symptoms of aggressive peptic ulcers in the stomach, duodenum, and elsewhere in the intestine. However, as many as 25% of people with Zollinger-Ellison syndrome may not have an ulcer when the diagnosis is made. Rupture, bleeding, and obstruction of the intestine can occur and are life threatening. For more than half of the people with a gastrinoma, symptoms are no worse than those experienced by people with ordinary peptic ulcer disease. In 25 to 40% of people, diarrhea is the first symptom.

A doctor suspects a gastrinoma when a person has frequent peptic ulcers or several peptic ulcers that do not respond to the usual ulcer treatments. Blood tests to detect abnormally high levels of gastrin are the most reliable diagnostic tests. Also, samples of gastric juice—obtained by inserting a slender tube through the nose and into the stomach—show very high levels of acid. Doctors use several imaging techniques, such as computed tomography (CT), ultrasound scans, and arteriography, to locate tumors. These tumors may be difficult to find, however, because usually they are small.

Treatment

High doses of proton pump inhibitors★ may be effective for reducing acid levels and relieving symptoms temporarily. About 20% of people who do not have multiple endocrine neoplasia can be cured with surgical removal of the gastrinoma. If these treatments fail, an operation to remove the stomach completely (total gastrectomy) may be necessary. This operation does not remove the tumor, but the gastrin can no longer create ulcers after the acid-producing stomach is removed. If the stomach is removed, daily oral iron and cal-

---

▲ see page 45   ■ see also box on page 717

★ see page 716 and table on page 718

cium supplements and monthly injections of vitamin B_{12} are needed, because absorption of these nutrients is impaired when stomach juices that prepare these nutrients for absorption are no longer available.

If cancerous tumors have spread to other parts of the body, chemotherapy may help reduce the number of tumor cells and the levels of gastrin in the blood. However, such therapy does not cure the cancer, which is ultimately fatal.

GLUCAGONOMA

A glucagonoma is a tumor of the pancreas that produces the hormone glucagon, which raises the level of sugar (glucose) in the blood and produces a distinctive rash.

About 80% of glucagonomas are cancerous. However, they grow slowly, and many people survive for 15 years or more after the diagnosis. The average age at which symptoms begin is 50. About 80% of people with glucagonomas are women.

Symptoms and Diagnosis

High levels of glucagon in the blood cause the symptoms of diabetes mellitus. Often, the person loses weight. In 90% of people, the most distinctive features are a chronic reddish brown skin rash (necrolytic migratory erythema) and a smooth, shiny, bright red-orange tongue. The mouth also may have cracks at the corners. The rash, which causes scaling, starts in the groin and moves to the buttocks, forearms, and legs.

The diagnosis is made by identifying high levels of glucagon in the blood and then locating the tumor by arteriography▲ and abdominal surgery.

Treatment

Ideally, the tumor is surgically removed, which eliminates all symptoms. However, if removal is not possible or if the tumor has spread, chemotherapy may reduce the levels of glucagon and lessen the symptoms. However, chemotherapy does not improve survival. The drug octreotide also reduces glucagon levels, may clear up the rash, and may restore appetite, facilitating weight gain. But octreotide may elevate the levels of sugar in the blood even more. Zinc ointment may be used to treat the skin rash. Sometimes the rash is treated with intravenous amino acids or fatty acids.

CHAPTER 132

Gastrointestinal Emergencies

Certain gastrointestinal disorders can be life threatening and require emergency treatment—surgery, in many cases. Abdominal pain, often severe, usually accompanies these gastrointestinal emergencies. If a person is experiencing abdominal pain, a doctor must decide if there is a need for immediate surgery to both identify and treat the problem or whether surgery can wait until diagnostic test results are available. Emergency surgery of the abdomen is often performed when the abdominal pain seems to result from an intestinal obstruction; a ruptured organ, such as the gallbladder, appendix, or intestine; or an abscess (a pus-filled pocket of infection).

Gastrointestinal Bleeding

Bleeding may occur anywhere along the digestive tract, from the mouth to the anus, for a variety of reasons. Blood may be visible in the stool or in vomit or may be hidden (occult) and detectable only by diagnostic tests.

Abnormal connections between the arteries and veins (arteriovenous malformations) sometimes form in the stomach and in the small and large intestines. These abnormal blood vessels are fragile and are likely to rupture and bleed intermittently, sometimes heavily, especially in older people. Veins in the esophagus can become dilated and twisted, a condition called esophageal varices (varicose veins in the esophagus), making them fragile and prone to bleeding.■

▲ see page 789   ■ see also page 794

Certain drugs, such as aspirin and many other nonsteroidal anti-inflammatory drugs (NSAIDs), can irritate the digestive tract and cause bleeding. Drugs that reduce the blood's tendency to clot (anticoagulants) or that dissolve clots once they have formed (thrombolytics such as streptokinase or tissue plasminogen activator) can cause gastrointestinal bleeding as well.

Symptoms

Symptoms of gastrointestinal bleeding include vomiting blood (hematemesis), passing black tarry stools (melena), and passing visible blood from the rectum (hematochezia). Black tarry stools usually result from bleeding that occurs high up in the digestive tract—for example, in the stomach or first segment of the small intestine (duodenum); blood in the stomach turns black when exposed to stomach acid and enzymes. A single severe bleeding episode can produce tarry stools for as long as a week, so continuing tarry stools do not necessarily indicate persistent bleeding.

People with long-term bleeding that tends to occur in small amounts or intermittently may develop symptoms of anemia, such as tiring easily and looking unnaturally pale. In the absence of such symptoms, a doctor may be able to detect an abnormal drop in blood pressure when a person sits or stands up after lying down.

Symptoms indicating a serious and sudden blood loss include a rapid pulse rate, low blood pressure, and reduced urine flow. A person may also have cold, clammy hands and feet. The reduced supply of blood to the brain caused by the bleeding may lead to confusion, disorientation, sleepiness, and even shock.▲

Symptoms of serious blood loss may differ, depending on whether the person has certain other diseases. For instance, a person with coronary artery disease may suddenly develop chest pain (angina) or symptoms of a heart attack. The symptoms of other diseases—such as heart failure, lung disease, and kidney failure—may worsen. In people with liver disease, bleeding into the intestine can cause a buildup of toxins that, in turn, may cause a condition called liver encephalopathy, characterized by changes in personality, awareness, and mental ability.■

Diagnosis

A doctor may suspect gastrointestinal bleeding after reviewing symptoms and examining a stool sample. If blood is not visible in the stool,

CAUSES OF BLEEDING

Location	Causes
Esophagus	Torn tissue Irritation (esophagitis) Esophageal varices Cancer
Stomach	Ulcer Cancer or noncancerous (benign) tumor Irritation (gastritis) Rupture of abnormal blood vessels connecting veins and arteries (arteriovenous malformation)
Small intestine	Duodenal ulcer Cancer or noncancerous tumor Arteriovenous malformation
Large intestine	Cancer Noncancerous polyp Inflammatory bowel disease (Crohn's disease or ulcerative colitis) Diverticular disease Arteriovenous malformation Impaired blood flow (ischemic colitis)
Rectum	Cancer Noncancerous tumor
Anus	Hemorrhoids Torn tissue
Throughout digestive tract	Foreign objects

a chemical (guaiac) can be added to the stool sample to reveal hidden blood.★ It may be necessary to obtain a sample from the stomach; if vomit is not available to test for blood, a doctor may have to pass a tube through the mouth into the stomach to obtain the sample.

Once it has been established that bleeding has occurred or is continuing to occur, a doctor performs a rectal examination to determine the source of the bleeding. For example, a doctor feels for hemorrhoids, rectal tears

▲ see page 148   ■ see page 795
★ see page 705

(fissures), and tumors. Then, tests that may include different types of x-rays and endoscopy (examination with a flexible viewing tube) are chosen according to whether the doctor suspects that the bleeding is coming from the upper digestive tract (esophagus, stomach, and first segment of the small intestine) or lower digestive tract (lower small intestine, large intestine, rectum, and anus).

Knowing about the symptoms that led up to a bleeding episode may help a doctor determine its cause. Pain in the abdomen that is relieved by food or antacids suggests a peptic ulcer; however, bleeding ulcers often are not painful. A doctor will ask about use of aspirin or other nonsteroidal anti-inflammatory drugs, which can damage the lining of the stomach.

Cancer is suspected when bleeding is accompanied by loss of appetite and weight that occurs for no obvious reason. A person who has difficulty swallowing is examined for a narrowing of the esophagus, which could be caused by cancer. Very forceful vomiting and retching immediately before bleeding occurs suggests a torn esophagus, but about half of people with such a tear do not vomit beforehand. New or worsening constipation or diarrhea, along with bleeding or hidden blood in the stool, may be caused by cancer or a polyp in the lower intestine, particularly in someone older than 45. Fresh blood on the surface of the stool may result from rectal cancer or from another problem with the rectum, such as hemorrhoids.

Knowing that a person has certain other diseases may also help a doctor determine the cause of bleeding. For example, people with liver disease are more likely to develop arteriovenous malformations in the stomach or intestines and varicose veins in the esophagus (esophageal varices).

Treatment

In more than 80% of people with gastrointestinal bleeding, the body is able to stop the bleeding on its own. People who continue to bleed or who have symptoms of a sudden loss of a large amount of blood usually are hospitalized and often are admitted to an intensive care unit.

If a large amount of blood has been lost, fluids are given intravenously, and a blood transfusion may be needed. After a blood transfusion, the person is observed closely for evidence of continued bleeding, such as an in-

creased pulse rate, a drop in blood pressure, or a loss of blood from the mouth or anus.

Bleeding from esophageal varices can be treated in several ways. In one method, an irritating chemical is injected into the bleeding vessels through an endoscope, causing inflammation and scarring of the veins, which stops the bleeding (sclerotherapy). In a second, more frequently used method, the varices are tied off with rubber bands during endoscopy (rubber band ligation). In a third method, now rarely used, a catheter with a deflated balloon at its tip is inserted through the mouth into the esophagus, and the balloon is then inflated to apply pressure on the bleeding area (esophageal tamponade).

Bleeding in the stomach often can be stopped with one of several procedures performed with an endoscope; these involve using an electrical current to destroy the portion of a vessel that is bleeding (cauterization) or injecting a material that causes clotting within the bleeding vessel. If these procedures fail, surgery may be needed.

Bleeding of the lower intestine usually does not require emergency treatment unless the person loses a large amount of blood quickly. Tests to locate the bleeding precisely, such as endoscopy or radionuclide scans, may be needed. Surgery can be performed if bleeding does not stop.

Abdominal Abscesses

An abscess is a pocket of pus, usually caused by a bacterial infection.

Abdominal abscesses may form below the diaphragm, in the middle of the abdomen, in the pelvis, or behind the abdominal cavity. Abscesses also may form in or around any abdominal organ, such as the kidneys, spleen, pancreas, or liver, or in the prostate gland. Often, abdominal abscesses are caused by injury, infection or rupture of the intestine, or infection of another abdominal organ.

Causes and Symptoms

An abscess below the diaphragm may form when infected fluid, for example, from a ruptured appendix, is moved upward by the pressure of abdominal organs and by the suction created when the diaphragm moves during breathing. Symptoms may include a cough, painful breathing, and pain in one shoulder—an example of referred pain that occurs because the shoulder and the diaphragm share the same nerves, and the brain incorrectly interprets the source of the pain.▲

▲ see box on page 448

Abscesses in the midabdomen may result from a ruptured appendix, a ruptured intestine, inflammatory bowel disease, diverticular disease, or an abdominal wound. The abdomen is usually painful in the area of the abscess.

Pelvic abscesses can result from the same disorders that cause abscesses in the midabdomen or from gynecologic infections. Symptoms may include abdominal pain, diarrhea from intestinal irritation, and an urgent or frequent need to urinate caused by bladder irritation.

Abscesses behind the abdominal cavity (called retroperitoneal abscesses) lie behind the peritoneum, the membrane that lines the abdominal cavity and organs. The causes, which are similar to those of abscesses in the abdomen, include inflammation and infection of the appendix (appendicitis) and of the pancreas (pancreatitis). Pain, usually in the lower back, worsens when the person moves the leg at the hip.

Abscesses inside the pancreas typically form after an attack of acute pancreatitis. Symptoms such as fever, abdominal pain, nausea, and vomiting often begin a week or more after a person recovers from pancreatitis.

Liver abscesses may be caused by bacteria or by amebas (single-celled parasites). Bacteria can reach the liver from an infected gallbladder; a penetrating or blunt wound; an infection in the abdomen, such as a nearby abscess; or an infection carried by the bloodstream from elsewhere in the body. Amebas from an intestinal infection reach the liver through the lymph vessels. Symptoms of liver abscesses include loss of appetite, nausea, and a fever. A person may or may not have abdominal pain.

Abscesses in the spleen are caused by an infection traveling through the bloodstream to the spleen, by an injury to the spleen, or by the spread of an infection from a nearby abscess, such as one below the diaphragm. Pain may occur in the left side of the abdomen, the back, or the left shoulder.

Diagnosis and Treatment

Doctors can easily misdiagnose an abscess, because the symptoms are commonly caused by less serious problems. When a person has an abscess, blood tests often reveal an abnormally large number of white blood cells. X-rays, ultrasound scanning, computed tomography (CT), or magnetic resonance imaging (MRI) can be used to distinguish an abscess from other problems (for example, tumors or cysts), as well as to determine the size and

position of an abscess once it has been diagnosed. Because abscesses and tumors often cause the same symptoms and produce similar results on imaging tests, a definitive diagnosis sometimes requires that a doctor obtain a sample of the pus or surgically remove the abscess for examination under a microscope.

In nearly all people with an abdominal abscess, the pus must be drained, either by surgery or by a needle inserted through the skin. To guide the placement of the needle, a doctor uses CT or ultrasound scanning. Antibiotics are usually used in conjunction with drainage to prevent the infection from spreading and to help completely eliminate the infection. Laboratory analysis of the pus identifies the infecting organism so that the most effective antibiotic can be selected. It is uncommon for antibiotics to cure an abscess without drainage.

Obstruction of the Intestine

An obstruction of the intestine is a blockage that completely stops or seriously impairs the passage of intestinal contents.

An obstruction may occur anywhere along the small or large intestine. The part of the intestine above the obstruction continues to function. The intestine enlarges as it fills with food, fluid, digestive secretions, and gas. The intestinal lining becomes swollen and inflamed. If the condition is not treated, the intestine can rupture, leaking its contents and causing inflammation and infection of the abdominal cavity.

In newborns and infants, intestinal obstruction is commonly caused by a birth defect, a hard mass of intestinal contents (meconium), or a twisting of a loop of intestine (volvulus).

In adults, an obstruction of the first segment of the small intestine (duodenum) may be caused by cancer of the pancreas; scarring from an ulcer, a previous operation, or Crohn's disease; or adhesions, in which a fibrous band of connective tissue traps the intestine. An obstruction also can occur when part of the intestine bulges through an abnormal opening (hernia), such as a weakness in the muscles of the abdomen, and becomes trapped. Rarely, a gallstone, a mass of undigested food, or a collection of parasitic worms may block the intestine.

An obstruction of the large intestine is commonly caused by cancer. Obstruction also tends to occur (as a result of scarring and connective bands of scar tissue [adhesions]) in

What Causes Intestinal Strangulation?

Intestinal strangulation (cutting off of the blood supply to the intestine) usually results from one of three causes.

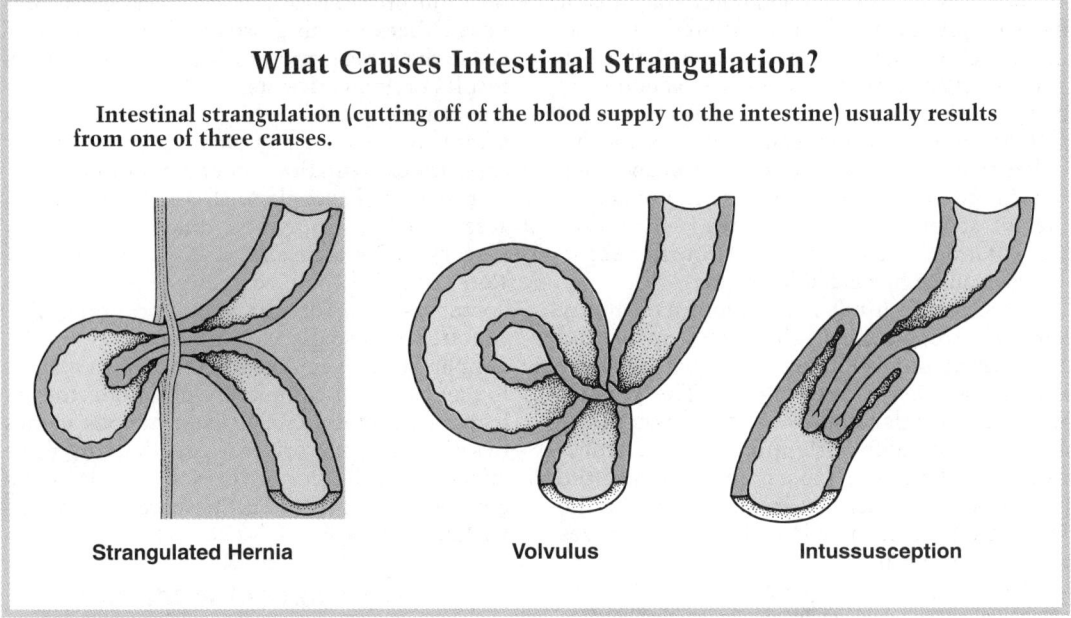

| Strangulated Hernia | Volvulus | Intussusception |

people who have previously undergone abdominal surgery. A hard lump of stool (fecal impaction) also may cause a blockage.

If an obstruction cuts off the blood supply to the intestine, the condition is called strangulation. Strangulation occurs in nearly 25% of people with small-intestinal obstruction. Usually, strangulation results from the trapping of part of the intestine in an abnormal opening (strangulated hernia); the twisting of a loop of intestine (volvulus); or the telescoping of a loop of intestine into another loop (intussusception). Gangrene can develop in as few as 6 hours. With gangrene, the intestinal wall dies, usually causing rupture, which leads to inflammation of the lining of the abdominal cavity (peritonitis) and infection. Without treatment, the person may die.

Symptoms and Diagnosis

Intestinal obstruction usually causes cramping pain in the abdomen, accompanied by bloating and disinterest in eating (anorexia). The pain may become severe and steady. Vomiting, which is common, begins later with large-intestinal obstruction than it does with small-intestinal obstruction. Complete obstruction causes severe constipation, while partial obstruction may cause diarrhea. A fever

is common and is particularly likely if the intestinal wall ruptures. Rupture can rapidly lead to severe inflammation and infection, causing shock.▲

A doctor examines the abdomen for tenderness, swelling, or masses. When an obstruction occurs, the sounds normally made by a functioning intestine (bowel sounds), which can be heard through a stethoscope, may be much louder and higher pitched, or they may be absent. If rupture has caused peritonitis, the person will feel pain when the doctor presses on the abdomen; often the pain increases when the doctor suddenly releases the pressure (rebound tenderness).

X-rays may show dilated loops of intestine that indicate the location of the obstruction. The x-rays also may reveal air around the intestine or under the layer of muscle that separates the abdomen and the chest (diaphragm). Air normally is not found in those places and thus is a sign of rupture.

Treatment

Anyone suspected of having an intestinal obstruction is hospitalized. Usually, a long, thin tube is passed through the nose and placed in the stomach or intestine. Suction is applied to the tube to remove the material that has accumulated above the blockage. Fluid and electrolytes (sodium, chloride, and potassium) are

▲ see page 148

given intravenously to replace water and salts lost from vomiting or diarrhea.

Sometimes an obstruction resolves without further treatment, especially if caused by scarring or bands of connective tissue (adhesions). Occasionally, an endoscope (a flexible viewing tube), which is advanced through the anus, or a barium enema, which inflates the large intestine, may be used to treat some disorders, such as a twisted intestinal segment in the lower part of the large intestine. Most often, however, surgery is performed as soon as possible. The cause of the obstruction determines whether the surgeon can relieve the blockage without removing a segment of the intestines. Sometimes fibrous bands can be released, although they tend to recur.

Ileus

Ileus (paralytic ileus, adynamic ileus) is temporary absence of the normal contractile movements of the intestinal wall.

Like an obstruction of the intestines, ileus prevents the passage of intestinal contents. Unlike a mechanical obstruction, though, ileus rarely leads to rupture.

Ileus commonly occurs for 24 to 72 hours after abdominal surgery. It may also be caused by an infection or a blood clot inside the abdomen, atherosclerosis that reduces the blood supply to the intestine, or an injury to an intestinal artery or vein. Disorders outside the intestine may cause ileus, such as kidney failure or abnormal levels of blood electrolytes—low potassium or high calcium levels, for example. Other causes of ileus are use of certain drugs (especially opioid analgesics and anticholinergic drugs▲) and an underactive thyroid gland.

Symptoms and Diagnosis

The symptoms of ileus are abdominal bloating, vomiting, severe constipation, loss of appetite, and cramps.

A doctor hears few bowel sounds or none at all through a stethoscope. An x-ray of the abdomen shows bulging loops of intestine. Occasionally, doctors evaluate the situation using colonoscopy (examination of the large intestine with a flexible viewing tube).

Treatment

The buildup of gas and liquid caused by ileus must be relieved. Sometimes a tube is passed through the anus into the large intestine to relieve the pressure. In addition, a tube is passed through the nose into the stomach or small intestine, and suction is applied to relieve pressure and expansion (distention). The person is not allowed to eat or drink anything until intestinal function normalizes (or returns). Fluids and electrolytes (such as sodium, chloride, and potassium) are given intravenously.

Appendicitis

Appendicitis is inflammation and infection of the appendix.

The appendix is a small finger-shaped tube projecting from the large intestine near the point where it joins the small intestine. The appendix may have some immune function, but it is not an essential organ.

Except for trapped hernias, appendicitis is the most common cause of sudden, severe abdominal pain and abdominal surgery in the United States. Appendicitis is most likely to occur between the ages of 10 and 30.

The cause of appendicitis is not fully understood. In most cases, a blockage inside the appendix probably starts a process in which the appendix becomes inflamed and infected. If inflammation continues without treatment, the appendix can rupture. A ruptured appendix spills bacteria-laden intestinal contents into the abdominal cavity, causing peritonitis,■ which may result in a life-threatening infection. A rupture also may cause an abscess (a pus-filled pocket of infection) to form. In a woman, the ovaries and fallopian tubes may become infected, and the resulting blockage of the fallopian tubes may cause infertility. A ruptured appendix also may allow bacteria to infect the bloodstream—a life-threatening condition called sepsis.★

Symptoms

Fewer than 50% of people with appendicitis have the traditionally described symptoms of nausea, vomiting, and severe pain in the lower right abdomen. Pain may begin suddenly in the upper abdomen or around the navel; then nausea and vomiting develop. After a few hours, the nausea passes, and the pain shifts to the right lower portion of the abdomen. When a doctor presses on this area, it is tender, and when the pressure is released, the pain may

▲ see box on page 79   ■ see page 782
★ see page 1118

increase sharply (rebound tenderness). A fever of 100 to 101° F (37.7 to 38.3° C) is common.

Pain, particularly in infants and children, may be widespread rather than confined to the right lower portion of the abdomen. In older people and in pregnant women, the pain is usually less severe, and the area is less tender.

If the appendix is ruptured, pain and fever may become severe. Worsening infection can lead to shock.▲

Diagnosis

A doctor may suspect appendicitis after reviewing the person's symptoms and examining the abdomen. A blood test shows a moderate increase in the white blood cell count in response to the infection. Usually, in the early stages of appendicitis, most tests—including x-rays, ultrasound scanning, and computed tomography (CT)—are useless. Typically, exploratory surgery is performed immediately if the suspicion of appendicitis is strong.

Treatment

Surgery is the main treatment. In nearly 15% of operations for appendicitis, the appendix is found to be normal. However, delaying surgery until the cause of the abdominal pain is certain can be fatal: An infected appendix can rupture less than 24 hours after symptoms begin. If appendicitis is found, the appendix is removed (appendectomy). Even when appendicitis is not found to be the cause, the appendix is usually removed.

With an early operation, the chance of death from appendicitis is very low. The person can usually leave the hospital in 2 or 3 days, and convalescence is normally quick and complete.

For a ruptured appendix, the prognosis is more serious. Fifty years ago, a rupture often was fatal. Surgery and antibiotics have lowered the death rate to nearly zero, but repeated operations and a long convalescence may be necessary.

Peritonitis

Peritonitis is inflammation and usually infection of the abdominal cavity and its lining.

Peritonitis is usually caused by an infection spreading from an infected organ in the abdominal cavity. Common sources are perforations of the stomach, intestine, gallbladder, or appendix. Infection can also spread to the peritoneum

from other parts of the body through the blood. The peritoneum (the membrane that lines the abdominal cavity and organs) is remarkably resistant to infection. Unless contamination continues, peritonitis does not progress, and the peritoneum tends to heal with treatment.

Pelvic inflammatory disease■ in sexually active women is a common cause of peritonitis. An infection of the uterus and fallopian tubes—which may be caused by several types of bacteria, including the ones that cause gonorrhea and chlamydial infection—spreads into the abdominal cavity.

Peritonitis can develop after surgery for several reasons. An injury to the gallbladder, ureter, bladder, or intestine during an operation can spill bacteria into the abdominal cavity. Leakage also can occur during operations in which intestinal segments are joined.

Peritoneal dialysis (a treatment for kidney failure) frequently results in peritonitis. The usual cause is an infection gaining access through the drains placed in the abdominal cavity. In liver or heart failure, fluid may accumulate in the abdominal cavity (ascites) and become infected.

Peritonitis can also result from irritation of abdominal organs without any infection. For example, inflammation of the pancreas (acute pancreatitis) can produce peritonitis. Also, talc or starch on a surgeon's gloves can cause inflammation of the peritoneum without infection.

Spontaneous peritonitis occurs in people with an accumulation of fluid in their abdomen (ascites). Many such people have liver disease, often from alcohol abuse. Infection of the fluid occurs without an obvious source.

Symptoms

Usually, vomiting, a fever (100.5° F [38.0° C] or higher), and abdominal tenderness occur. Other symptoms depend on whether infection follows inflammation and on the type and extent of the infection. Pain may be limited to a small area of the abdomen or may be present throughout the abdomen. Abdominal pain is usually severe.

Unless peritonitis is treated promptly, complications develop rapidly. One or more pus-filled pockets (abscesses) may form, and the infection can leave scar tissue that eventually may obstruct the intestine. The normal propulsion of stool through the intestines (peristalsis) stops (ileus). Fluid leaks from the bloodstream into the abdominal cavity. Severe dehydration

▲ see page 148   ■ see page 1377

develops, and the bloodstream loses electrolytes (such as sodium and potassium). Major complications—such as lung, kidney, or liver failure and widespread clotting—can follow.

Diagnosis

Rapid diagnosis is crucial. X-rays are taken with the person lying down and standing. Free gas in the abdominal cavity can be seen on x-rays and indicates a rupture. Occasionally, a needle is used to withdraw fluid from the abdominal cavity so that laboratory personnel can detect and identify any infectious organism and test its sensitivity to various antibiotics. This procedure is relatively simple and is done while the person sits up or lies in bed. The most reliable means of diagnosis, however, is exploratory surgery.

Treatment

Usually, the first step is emergency exploratory surgery, particularly when appendicitis, a pierced (perforated) peptic ulcer, or diverticulitis seems likely. When the cause is thought to be inflammation of the pancreas (acute pancreatitis), pelvic inflammatory disease in women, or spontaneous peritonitis, emergency surgery usually is not performed.

Antibiotics, often several at once, are given promptly. Also, a tube may be inserted through the nose and into the stomach or intestine to drain fluid and gas. Fluids and electrolytes may also be given intravenously to replace those that have been lost.

Ischemic Colitis

Ischemic colitis is injury of the large intestine that results from an interruption of its blood supply.

Ischemic colitis may result from sudden (acute) or, more commonly, long-term (chronic) blockage of blood flow through arteries that supply the large intestine. Blood clots can produce acute blockage; deposits of fatty material (atherosclerosis) can lead to chronic blockage. Damage of the inside lining and inner layers of the wall of the large intestine results; the degree of damage depends on the duration and severity of the blockage. The damage produces ulcers (sores) in the lining of the large intestine. Ischemic colitis affects primarily people who are 50 or older.

Symptoms and Diagnosis

Usually, the person experiences abdominal pain. The pain is felt more often on the left side, but it can occur anywhere in the abdomen. The person frequently passes loose stools that are often accompanied by dark red clots. Sometimes bright red blood is passed without stool. Low-grade fevers (usually below 100° F [37.7° C]) are common.

A doctor may suspect ischemic colitis on the basis of the symptoms, especially in a person older than 50. An abdomen that is tender when pressed gently is further evidence of ischemic colitis. A colonoscopy or barium enema is needed to distinguish ischemic colitis from other forms of inflammation, such as infection or inflammatory bowel disease.

Prognosis and Treatment

People with ischemic colitis are hospitalized. Initially, the person is given neither fluids nor food by mouth so that the intestine can rest. Instead, intravenous fluids, electrolytes, and nutrients are given. Antibiotics are often given to prevent infection that might follow the inflammation. Within a few days, antibiotics are usually stopped and eating is resumed. More than 50% of people with ischemic colitis improve and recover over a period of 1 to 2 weeks. However, when the interruption to the blood supply is more severe or more prolonged, the affected portion of the large intestine may have to be surgically removed.

LIVER AND GALLBLADDER DISORDERS

133   **Biology of the Liver and Gallbladder** 786

Liver ▪ Gallbladder and Biliary Tract ▪ Effects of Aging

134   **Diagnostic Tests for Liver and Gallbladder Disorders** 788

Imaging Tests ▪ Liver Biopsy

135   **Clinical Manifestations of Liver Disease** 791

Jaundice ▪ Cholestasis ▪ Liver Enlargement ▪ Portal
Hypertension ▪ Ascites ▪ Liver Encephalopathy ▪ Liver
Failure

136   **Fatty Liver, Cirrhosis, and Related Disorders** 797

Fatty Liver ▪ Cirrhosis ▪ Primary Biliary Cirrhosis ▪ Primary
Sclerosing Cholangitis ▪ Alpha$_1$-Antitrypsin Deficiency

137   **Hepatitis** 802

Acute Viral Hepatitis ▪ Chronic Hepatitis

138   **Blood Vessel Disorders of the Liver** 806

Abnormalities of the Hepatic Artery ▪ Veno-occlusive Disease ▪
Budd-Chiari Syndrome ▪ Portal Vein Thrombosis ▪ Blood Vessel
Disorders Resulting From Other Diseases

139   **Liver Tumors** 810

Hemangioma ▪ Hepatocellular Adenoma ▪ Hepatoma ▪
Other Primary Liver Cancers ▪ Metastatic Liver Cancer

140   **Gallbladder Disorders** 813

Gallstones ▪ Cholecystitis ▪ Bile Duct Tumors

CHAPTER 133

Biology of the Liver and Gallbladder

Located in the upper right portion of the abdomen, the liver and gallbladder are interconnected by ducts known as the biliary tract, which drains into the first segment of the small intestine (the duodenum). Although the liver and gallbladder participate in some of the same functions, they are very different.

Liver

The wedge-shaped liver is the largest—and in some ways the most complex—organ in the body. It serves as the body's chemical factory, performing many vital functions, from regulating the levels of chemicals in the body to producing substances that make the blood clot during bleeding.

Functions of the Liver

The liver manufactures about half of the body's cholesterol; the rest comes from food. Most of the cholesterol made by the liver is used to make bile, a greenish yellow, viscid fluid that aids in digestion. Cholesterol is also needed to make certain hormones, including estrogen, testosterone, and the adrenal hormones, and is a vital component of every cell membrane. The liver manufactures other substances as well, especially proteins, which the body uses to carry out its functions. Clotting factors, for example, are proteins needed to stop bleeding. Albumin is a protein needed to maintain fluid pressure in the bloodstream.

Sugars are stored in the liver as glycogen and then broken down and released into the bloodstream as glucose when needed—for example, when sugar levels in the blood become too low, such as during sleep when a person spends many hours without eating.

Another one of the liver's main functions is to break down harmful or toxic substances absorbed from the intestine or manufactured elsewhere in the body and then to excrete them as harmless by-products into the bile or the blood. By-products excreted into the bile enter the intestine, then leave the body in the stool. By-products excreted into the blood are filtered out by the kidneys, then leave the body in the urine. The liver also chemically alters (metabolizes) drugs,▲ rendering them inactive or allowing them to be more easily excreted from the body.

Disorders of liver function can be divided broadly into two groups: those caused by a malfunction of the cells in the liver itself (such as cirrhosis and hepatitis) and those caused by an obstruction of bile flow from the liver through the biliary tract (such as bile stones and cancer).

Blood Supply of the Liver

The liver receives blood from the intestines and directly from the heart. Tiny capillaries in the intestinal wall drain into the portal vein, which enters the liver. The blood then flows through a latticework of tiny channels inside the liver, where digested nutrients and any harmful substances are processed. The hepatic artery brings blood to the liver from the heart. This blood carries oxygen for the liver tissue itself as well as cholesterol and other substances for processing. Blood from the intestines and heart then mix together in the tissues of the liver and flow back to the heart through the hepatic vein.

Gallbladder and Biliary Tract

The gallbladder is a small, pear-shaped, muscular storage sac that holds bile. Bile flows out of the liver through the left and right hepatic ducts, which come together to form the common hepatic duct. This duct then joins with a duct connected to the gallbladder, called the cystic duct, to create the common bile duct. The common bile duct enters the small intestine at the sphincter of Oddi (a ring-shaped muscle), a few inches below the stomach.

About half the bile secreted between meals is diverted through the cystic duct and into the gallbladder, where bile is stored. In the gallbladder, up to 90% of the water in the bile is absorbed into the bloodstream, making the remaining bile very concentrated. The rest of

▲ see page 68

View of the Liver and Gallbladder

Liver cells produce bile, which flows into channels called bile ductules. These channels join to form the left and right hepatic ducts, which join to form the common hepatic duct. The common hepatic duct joins with a duct connected to the gallbladder, called the cystic duct, to form the common bile duct. The common bile duct is joined by the pancreatic duct just before it enters the small intestine at the sphincter of Oddi.

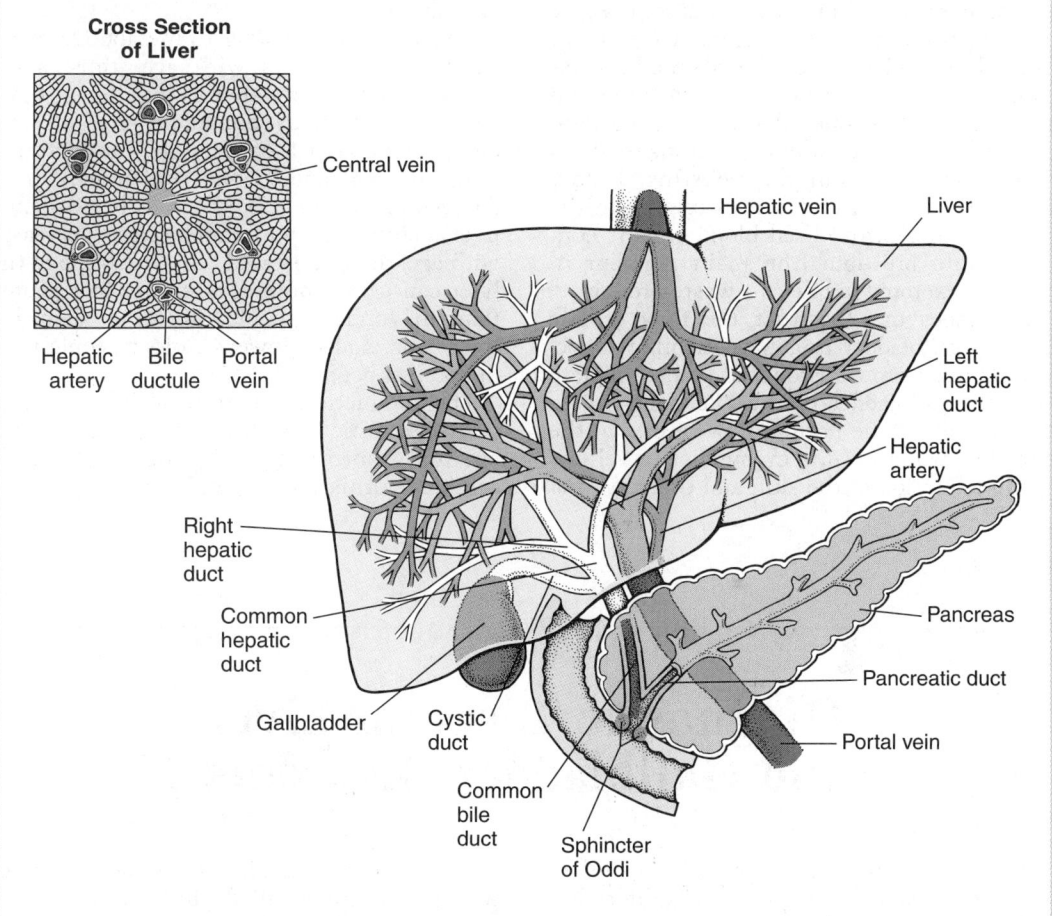

the bile produced by the liver flows directly through the common bile duct into the small intestine. When food enters the small intestine, a series of hormonal and nerve signals trigger the gallbladder to contract and the sphincter of Oddi to relax and thus open. Bile then flows from the gallbladder into the small intestine to mix with food contents and perform its digestive functions.

After bile enters and passes down the small intestine, about 95% of the bile salts are reabsorbed into the bloodstream through the wall of the lower small intestine. The liver then extracts these bile salts from the blood and resecretes them back into the bile. The bile salts in the body go through this cycle about 10 to 12 times a day. Each time, small amounts of bile salts escape absorption and reach the large intestine, where they are broken down by bacteria. Some bile salts are reabsorbed in the large intestine; the rest are excreted in the stool.

Although the gallbladder is useful, it is not necessary. Thus, if the gallbladder is removed (for example, in someone with cholecystitis), bile is able to move directly from the liver to the small intestine.

Bile consists of bile salts; electrolytes (dissolved charged particles, such as sodium and bicarbonate); bile pigments, such as bilirubin; cholesterol; and other fats (lipids). Bile is responsible for the elimination of certain waste products from the body—particularly pigment from destroyed red blood cells and excess cholesterol—and assists in the digestion and absorption of fats. Bile salts increase the solubility of fats and fat-soluble vitamins to aid in their absorption from the intestine. Hemoglobin (the protein that carries oxygen in the blood) from destroyed red blood cells is converted into bilirubin (the main pigment in bile) and excreted in bile as a waste product.

Gallstones may obstruct the flow of bile from the gallbladder, causing pain (biliary colic) or inflammation. Gallstones may also migrate from the gallbladder to the bile duct, where they can block the normal flow of bile to the intestine, which results in jaundice, a yellowish discoloration of the skin and the whites of the eyes. The flow of bile can also be blocked by tumors and by other less common causes.

Effects of Aging

A number of structural and microscopic changes occur as the liver ages. With age, the color of the liver changes from lighter to darker brown. Its size and blood flow decrease. However, liver function test results generally remain normal.

The ability of the liver to metabolize many substances decreases with age; thus, some drugs are not inactivated as quickly in older people as they are in younger people. This puts older people at risk of receiving too high of a drug dosage▲ and is one reason why their dosages must be checked carefully. Also, the liver's ability to withstand stress decreases with age; thus, substances that are toxic to the liver can cause more damage in older people than in younger people. Repair of damaged liver cells is also slower in older people than in younger people.

The production and flow of bile decrease with age. This probably has no significance but may contribute to the increased risk of gallstone formation as people age.

CHAPTER 134

Diagnostic Tests for Liver and Gallbladder Disorders

A variety of diagnostic tests can help doctors assess disorders of the liver, gallbladder, and biliary tract. Among the most important are a group of blood tests known as liver function tests. The term is misleading, however, since liver function tests do not really test the function of the liver. Rather, liver function tests indicate inflammation of or damage to the liver.

Depending on the suspected problem, a doctor may also order certain imaging tests, such as ultrasound scanning, computed tomography (CT), or magnetic resonance imaging (MRI). Also, a doctor may take a sample of liver tissue for examination under a microscope, a procedure called a liver biopsy.

Imaging Tests

Ultrasound scanning uses sound waves to provide images of the liver, gallbladder, and biliary tract. The test is better for detecting structural abnormalities, such as tumors, than diffuse abnormalities, such as cirrhosis (severe scarring of the liver) or fatty liver (excess fat in the liver). It is the least expensive and safest technique for creating images of the gallbladder and biliary tract.

Using ultrasound, a doctor can readily detect gallstones in the gallbladder. Ultrasound

▲ see also page 79

of the abdomen easily distinguishes jaundice (a yellowish discoloration of the skin and the whites of the eyes) caused by bile duct obstruction from jaundice caused by liver cell malfunction; ultrasound shows that the ducts are dilated (widened) in obstruction. A type of ultrasound, called vascular Doppler ultrasound, can show the flow of blood in the blood vessels of the liver. A doctor also may use ultrasound scanning as a guide when inserting a needle to obtain a tissue sample for biopsy.

Radionuclide (radioisotope) imaging uses a substance containing a radioactive tracer that is injected into the body and taken up by a particular organ. The radioactivity is detected by a gamma-ray camera (positioned over the upper abdomen) attached to a computer that generates an image. Liver scanning is a type of radionuclide imaging that uses a radioactive substance taken up by liver cells. Cholescintigraphy (hepatobiliary scintigraphy), another type of radionuclide imaging, follows the movement of a radioactive substance through the biliary tract after it has been excreted by the liver. This technique can detect blockage of the cystic duct, which leads to acute inflammation of the gallbladder (cholecystitis).▲

Computed tomography (CT) provides excellent images of the liver. Doctors find it particularly useful for detecting tumors. It can also be used to detect diffuse disorders, such as fatty liver (excess fat in the liver), collections of pus (abscesses), and abnormally dense liver tissue caused by iron overload (hemochromatosis). Because CT involves exposure to x-rays (which are potentially harmful) and is more expensive than ultrasound, it is not as widely used, even though it often provides more information about the liver.

Magnetic resonance imaging (MRI) provides images similar to those obtained with CT. An advantage over CT is that it does not involve exposure to x-rays. Its drawbacks include being more expensive than CT and taking longer to perform than other imaging methods do. Its major use is in providing images of the biliary tract, termed magnetic resonance cholangiopancreatography (MRCP). The quality of the image produced can reduce the need for more invasive tests, in which dye is directly injected into the biliary and pancreatic ducts.

Hepatic arteriography uses a radiopaque dye (a dye that can be seen on x-rays) that is injected into the hepatic artery. X-rays then display the hepatic artery and its branches. Hepatic arteriography is particularly useful in investigating

Liver Function Tests

Liver function tests are performed on blood samples. Most tests measure the levels of enzymes or other substances in the blood as a way of diagnosing liver problems. One test measures the time needed for blood to clot. Values that are higher than normal may indicate inflammation of or damage to the liver.

- Alanine transaminase (ALT)
- Albumin
- Alkaline phosphatase
- Alpha-fetoprotein
- Aspartate transaminase (AST)
- Bilirubin
- Gamma-glutamyl transpeptidase
- Lactic dehydrogenase
- Mitochondrial antibodies
- 5'-nucleotidase
- Prothrombin time

and sometimes treating a type of liver cancer called hepatoma (a cancer that begins in the liver cells).■

Endoscopic retrograde cholangiopancreatography (ERCP) is a test in which an endoscope (a flexible viewing tube) is passed through the mouth, esophagus, and stomach and into the duodenum (the first segment of the small intestine). A fine tube is inserted through the endoscope and into the biliary tract. A radiopaque dye is then injected into the bile ducts, and x-rays are taken of the biliary tract and pancreatic duct and its tributaries. This test causes inflammation of the pancreas (pancreatitis) in 3 to 5% of the people who undergo it.

Percutaneous transhepatic cholangiography involves inserting a long needle through the skin into the liver and then injecting a radiopaque dye into one of the liver's bile ducts. A doctor uses ultrasound for guidance when inserting the needle. The x-rays clearly reveal the biliary tract, particularly any blockage within the bile ducts.

Operative cholangiography involves the injection of a radiopaque dye directly into the ducts of the biliary tract at the time of gallbladder surgery. X-rays then reveal clear images of the biliary tract.

▲ see page 815   ■ see page 811

Diagnostic Imaging Techniques for Assessing the Biliary Tract

Computed tomography (CT) and ultrasound scanning are used most commonly to view the biliary tract. If additional imaging is needed, the following diagnostic procedures may be used. In these procedures, a radiopaque dye (a dye visible on x-rays) is injected in the biliary tract, then x-rays are taken. These procedures can detect blockages and other abnormalities in the biliary tract.

Endoscopic Retrograde Cholangiopancreatography	Percutaneous Transhepatic Cholangiography	Operative Cholangiography
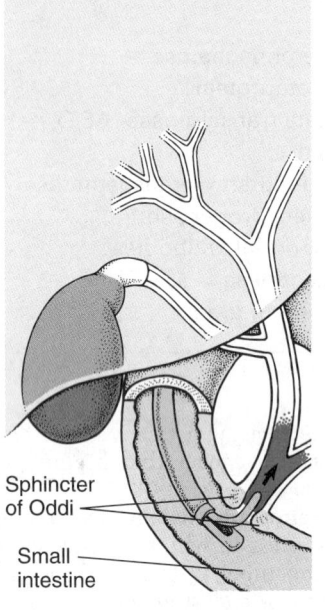	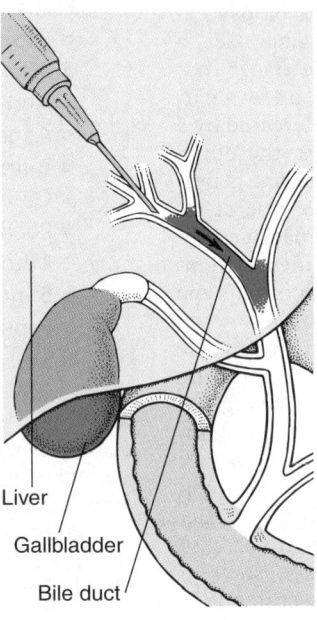	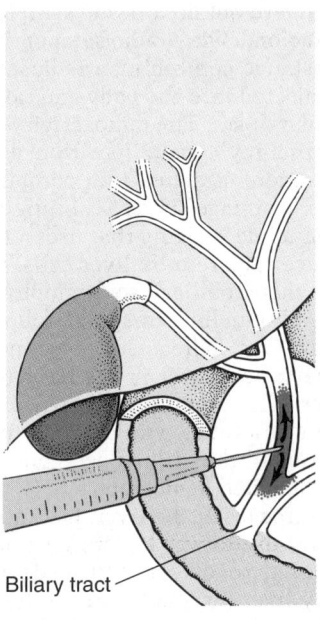

In endoscopic retrograde cholangiopancreatography (ERCP), a radiopaque dye (a dye visible on x-rays) is introduced through an endoscope (a flexible viewing tube), which is inserted into the mouth and through the stomach into the duodenum (the upper portion of the small intestine). The radiopaque dye is introduced past the sphincter of Oddi and then flows back up the biliary tract.

In percutaneous transhepatic cholangiography, a radiopaque dye is injected through the skin directly into a small bile duct in the liver. The radiopaque dye then flows through the biliary tract.

In operative cholangiography, a radiopaque dye is injected directly into the biliary tract during gallbladder surgery.

Simple x-rays of the abdomen can often reveal a gallstone that contains calcium. Gallstones that are not calcified are not generally seen.

Liver Biopsy

A liver specimen can be obtained during exploratory surgery but is more often obtained by inserting a needle through the skin and into the liver. Before this procedure, called percutaneous liver biopsy, is performed, the person receives a local anesthetic. Ultrasound or CT scans may be used to locate the abnormal area from which the specimen is to be taken. In most medical centers, a liver biopsy is performed as an outpatient procedure.

After the specimen is obtained, the person remains in the outpatient department for 3 to 4 hours because of a small risk of complications, such as laceration of the liver. If the liver is lacerated, bleeding into the abdomen may occur, which can lead to shock. In addition, bile may leak into the abdomen, causing inflammation of the abdominal lining (peritonitis). Because bleeding can start up to 15 days after the biopsy, the person is instructed to stay within an hour's drive of the hospital during that period. These complications can cause serious problems; 1 of 10,000 people die as a result of the procedure. Mild pain in the upper right abdomen, sometimes extending to the right shoulder, is common after a liver biopsy and is usually relieved by analgesics.

In transvenous liver biopsy, a catheter is inserted into a neck vein, threaded through the heart, and placed into one of the hepatic veins that drain the liver. The needle of the catheter is then inserted through the wall of the vein into the liver. This procedure is less likely to injure the liver than is percutaneous liver biopsy. It is especially useful in people who bleed easily, which is a complication of severe liver disease.

CHAPTER 135

Clinical Manifestations of Liver Disease

Liver disease can manifest itself in many different ways. Manifestations of liver disease that are particularly important include jaundice (a yellowish discoloration of the skin and the whites of the eyes), cholestasis (reduction or stoppage of bile flow), liver enlargement, portal hypertension (abnormally high blood pressure in the veins that bring blood from the intestines to the liver), ascites (accumulation of fluid in the abdominal cavity), liver (hepatic) encephalopathy (a liver disorder in which toxins build up in the blood, leading to brain dysfunction), and liver failure.

Sometimes the manifestations of liver disease are not obvious. For example, symptoms may include fatigue, a feeling of unwellness, loss of appetite, and mild weight loss, yet these symptoms are also typical of many other diseases. Thus, liver disease can easily be overlooked, particularly in its early stages.

Jaundice

Jaundice is a yellowish discoloration of the skin and of the whites of the eyes caused by abnormally high levels of the pigment bilirubin in the bloodstream.

Old or damaged red blood cells are constantly being removed from the circulation, mainly by the spleen. During this process, hemoglobin, the part of red blood cells that carries oxygen in the blood, is broken down into a dark greenish yellow pigment called bilirubin. Bilirubin is then carried in the bloodstream to the liver and is excreted into the intestine as a component of bile (the digestive fluid produced by the liver). If bilirubin cannot be excreted into the bile quickly enough, it builds up in the blood. The excess bilirubin gets deposited in the skin, resulting in the yellowish discoloration called jaundice.

High levels of bilirubin in the blood may result from problems originating either within the liver or outside the liver. Damage to the liver, such as from inflammation or scarring, can hinder its ability to excrete bilirubin into bile. Alternatively, the bile ducts, which carry the bile from the liver to the small intestine, may be blocked, for example, by a gallstone or a tumor. Less commonly, an overproduction of bilirubin, due to excessive breakdown of red blood cells, can overwhelm the liver with more than the liver is capable of processing. This is most common in newborns with jaundice.▲

In Gilbert's syndrome, bilirubin levels are slightly increased but usually not enough to cause jaundice. This disorder, which is sometimes hereditary, is most often detected in young adults during routine screening tests. It has no other symptoms and causes no problems.

▲ see page 1505

Major Clinical Features of Liver Disease

Jaundice

Enlarged liver

Fluid in the abdomen (ascites)

Confusion from deterioration of brain function due to buildup of toxins in the blood (encephalopathy)

Gastrointestinal bleeding from varices (large, tortuous veins)

Portal hypertension (unusually high blood pressure in the portal vein)

Skin
- Spiderlike blood vessels
- Red palms
- Bright red complexion
- Itching

Blood
- Decreased number of red blood cells (anemia)
- Decreased number of white blood cells (leukopenia)
- Decreased number of platelets (thrombocytopenia)
- A tendency to bleed (coagulopathy)

Hormones
- High levels of insulin but poor response to it, leading to high blood sugar levels
- Cessation of menstrual periods and decreased fertility (in women)
- Impotence and feminization (in men)

Heart and blood vessels
- Increased heart rate and amount of blood pumped
- Low blood pressure (hypotension)

General
- Fatigue
- Weakness
- Weight loss
- Poor appetite
- Nausea
- Fever

People who eat large amounts of carrots may develop a mild yellow tint to the skin, but their eyes do not turn yellow. This is not jaundice and is unrelated to liver disease.

▲ see page 703   ■ see page 799

★ see page 1453

Symptoms

In jaundice, the skin and the whites of the eyes appear yellow. The urine is often dark because excess bilirubin is excreted through the kidneys. Other symptoms, such as itching and light-colored stools, may appear, depending on the underlying cause of the jaundice. For example, acute inflammation of the liver (acute hepatitis) may cause loss of appetite, nausea, vomiting, and fever. Blockage of bile may produce the symptoms of cholestasis.

Diagnosis and Treatment

A doctor uses laboratory tests and imaging studies to determine the cause of the jaundice. If the problem is a disease of the liver itself, such as acute viral hepatitis, the jaundice usually gradually disappears as the condition of the liver improves. If the problem is blockage of a bile duct, then surgery or endoscopy (a procedure involving use of a flexible viewing tube with surgical attachments)▲ is usually performed as soon as possible to reopen the affected bile duct.

Cholestasis

Cholestasis is a reduction or stoppage of bile flow.

With cholestasis, the flow of bile, the digestive fluid produced by the liver, is impaired at some point between the liver cells and the duodenum (the first segment of the small intestine). Even when bile flow is stopped, the liver continues to process the pigment bilirubin, which escapes into the bloodstream.

The causes of cholestasis are divided into two groups: those originating within the liver and those originating outside the liver. Causes within the liver include acute hepatitis, alcoholic liver disease, primary biliary cirrhosis (inflammation and scarring of the bile ducts),■ the effects of drugs, and the effects of hormonal changes during pregnancy (a condition called cholestasis of pregnancy).★ Causes outside the liver include a stone in a bile duct, a narrowing (stricture) of a bile duct, cancer of a bile duct, cancer of the pancreas, and inflammation of the pancreas (pancreatitis).

Symptoms

Jaundice, dark urine, pale stools, and generalized itchiness are characteristic symptoms of cholestasis. Jaundice results from excess bilirubin deposited in the skin, and dark urine results from excess bilirubin excreted by the kidney. Retention of bile products in the skin may cause itching, with subsequent scratching and skin damage. Stool may become pale because of a lack of bilirubin in the intestine. The stool may also contain too much fat (a condition called steatorrhea), because bile is not available in the intestine to help digest dietary fat. The lack of bile in the intestine also means that calcium and vitamin D are not properly absorbed. If the cholestasis persists, a lack of these nutrients can cause bone loss. Vitamin K, which is needed for blood clotting, is also poorly absorbed from the intestine, creating a tendency to bleed easily.

Prolonged jaundice from cholestasis produces a muddy skin color and fatty yellow deposits in the skin. The underlying cause of cholestasis determines whether the person has other symptoms, such as abdominal pain, loss of appetite, vomiting, or fever.

Diagnosis

A doctor tries to determine whether the cause is within or outside the liver on the basis of symptoms and the results of a physical examination.

Symptoms that suggest a cause within the liver include loss of appetite, nausea, and vomiting (all of which are symptoms of hepatitis). Heavy alcohol intake or recent use of drugs that can cause cholestasis also suggests a cause within the liver. Small, spiderlike blood vessels visible in the skin, an enlarged spleen, and fluid in the abdominal cavity (ascites) are signs of chronic liver disease.

Features that suggest a cause outside the liver include intermittent pain in the upper right side of the abdomen and sometimes also in the right shoulder or an enlarged gallbladder (which a doctor can feel or imaging studies can detect).

Typically, the blood levels of an enzyme called alkaline phosphatase are very high in people with cholestasis. A blood test that measures the level of bilirubin indicates the severity of the cholestasis but not its cause. An ultrasound or computed tomography (CT) scan or both are almost always done if blood test results are abnormal. If the cause appears to be within the liver, a liver biopsy▲ may be performed and usually establishes the diagnosis. If the cause appears to be blockage of the bile ducts, endoscopy (a procedure involving use of a flexible viewing tube with surgical attachments)■ is often performed to determine the nature of the blockage.

Treatment

A blockage of the bile ducts can usually be treated with surgery or therapeutic endoscopy. A blockage within the liver may be treated in various ways depending on the cause. If a particular drug is the suspected cause, then the doctor discontinues its use. If acute hepatitis is responsible for the blockage, then the cholestasis and jaundice usually disappear when the hepatitis has run its course. The person is advised to avoid or discontinue using any substance that is toxic to the liver, such as alcohol and certain drugs.

Cholestyramine, taken by mouth, can be used to treat the itchiness. This drug binds with certain bile products in the intestine, so they cannot be reabsorbed to irritate the skin. Unless the liver is severely damaged, taking vitamin K can improve blood clotting. Supplements of calcium and vitamin D are often taken if the cholestasis persists, but they are not very effective in preventing bone loss.

Liver Enlargement

An enlarged liver (hepatomegaly) usually indicates liver disease. However, many people with liver disease have a normal-sized or even a shrunken liver. An enlarged liver usually causes no symptoms. However, if the enlargement is extreme, it may cause abdominal discomfort or a feeling of fullness. If the enlargement occurs quickly, the liver may be tender to the touch. When performing a physical examination, a doctor can usually estimate the size of the liver by feeling whether it extends below the level of the ribs.

When feeling an enlarged liver, a doctor also notes its texture. The liver usually feels soft if it is enlarged because of acute hepatitis, fatty infiltration, congestion with blood, or early obstruction of the bile ducts. The liver feels firm and irregular if it is enlarged because of cirrhosis (severe scarring of the liver). Distinct lumps usually suggest cancer. Treatment depends on the underlying cause.

Portal Hypertension

Portal hypertension is abnormally high blood pressure in branches of the portal vein, the large vein that brings blood from the intestines to the liver.

▲ see page 790   ■ see page 703

The portal vein receives blood drained from the entire intestine and from the spleen, pancreas, and gallbladder. After entering the liver, the vein divides into right and left branches and then into tiny channels that run through the liver. When blood leaves the liver, it drains back into the general circulation through the hepatic vein.▲

Two factors can increase blood pressure in the portal blood vessels: increased volume of blood flowing through the vessels and increased resistance to the blood flow through the liver. In Western countries, the most common cause of portal hypertension is increased resistance to blood flow caused by cirrhosis (most often due to excessive alcohol intake).

Portal hypertension leads to the development of veins (called collateral vessels) that directly connect the portal blood vessels to the general circulation, thus bypassing the liver. Because of this bypass, substances that are normally removed from the blood by the liver are able to pass into the general circulation. Collateral vessels develop at specific places, the most important of which is at the lower end of the esophagus. Here the vessels become engorged and tortuous—that is, they become esophageal varices (varicose veins in the esophagus). These engorged vessels are fragile and prone to bleeding, sometimes seriously. Other collateral vessels may develop around the navel and at the rectum.

Symptoms and Diagnosis

Portal hypertension often enlarges the spleen (which drains its blood supply into the portal vessels via the splenic vein). Protein-containing fluid (ascitic fluid) may leak from the surface of the liver and intestines and expand (distend) the abdominal cavity, a condition called ascites. Varicose veins in the esophagus (esophageal varices) and in the upper part of the stomach bleed easily and sometimes massively. Varicose veins in the rectum may also bleed, though this is much less common.

Doctors can usually feel an enlarged spleen through the abdominal wall. They can detect fluid in the abdomen by noting abdominal swelling and by listening for a dull sound when tapping (percussing) the abdomen. An ultrasound scan may be used to examine the blood flow in the portal blood vessels and to detect the presence of fluid in the abdomen. A computed tomography (CT) scan can also be used to look for and examine any collateral vessels. In rare cases, a needle can be inserted through the abdominal wall and into the liver or spleen to directly measure pressure in the portal system (manometry).

Treatment

To reduce the risk of bleeding from esophageal varices, a doctor may try to reduce the pressure in the portal vein. One way is to give propranolol.

Bleeding from esophageal varices is a medical emergency.■ Drugs such as vasopressin or octreotide may be given intravenously to constrict the bleeding veins, and blood transfusions are given to replace lost blood. An endoscopic examination is usually done to confirm that the bleeding is from varices. The veins can then be blocked off with rubber bands or with injections of a chemical given through the endoscope.

If the bleeding continues or recurs repeatedly, a surgical procedure may be done to create a bypass (called a shunt) between the portal venous system and the general (systemic) venous system. This lowers the pressure in the portal vein, because the pressure is much lower in the general venous system.

There are various types of portal-systemic shunt operations. In one type, called transjugular intrahepatic portal-systemic shunting (TIPS), an x-ray–guided needle is passed through the liver to create a shunt connecting the portal vein directly with one of the hepatic veins. Shunt operations are usually successful in stopping the bleeding but pose certain risks, such as liver (hepatic) encephalopathy.★ The TIPS procedure, although less dangerous than other surgical procedures involving portal-systemic shunts, may need to be repeated periodically because of narrowing of the shunt in some people.

Ascites

Ascites is the accumulation of protein-containing (ascitic) fluid in the abdominal cavity.

Ascites tends to occur in long-standing (chronic) rather than in short-lived (acute) disorders. It occurs most commonly in cirrhosis (severe scarring of the liver), especially in cirrhosis caused by alcoholism. Other liver disorders in which ascites may occur include alcoholic hepatitis without cirrhosis, chronic hepatitis, and

▲ see art on page 807   ■ see also page 776

★ see page 795

obstruction of the hepatic vein. Ascites can also occur in nonliver diseases, such as cancer, heart failure, kidney failure, inflammation of the pancreas (pancreatitis), and tuberculosis affecting the lining of the abdominal cavity.

In people with liver disease, ascitic fluid leaks from the surface of the liver and intestine. A combination of factors is responsible, including portal hypertension, decreased ability of the blood vessels to retain fluid, fluid retention by the kidneys, and alterations in various hormones and chemicals that regulate bodily fluids.

Symptoms and Diagnosis

Small amounts of fluid in the abdomen usually produce no symptoms, but massive amounts may cause abdominal expansion (distention) and discomfort. Pressure on the stomach from the swollen abdomen may lead to loss of appetite, and pressure on the lungs may lead to shortness of breath. When a doctor taps (percusses) the abdomen, the fluid makes a dull sound. When the abdomen contains large amounts of fluid, the abdomen is taut, and the navel is flat or even pushed out. In some people with ascites, the ankles swell with excess fluid (edema).

If the presence of ascites or its cause is not clear, the doctor may use ultrasound scanning. In addition, a small sample of ascitic fluid can be withdrawn by inserting a needle through the abdominal wall—a procedure called diagnostic paracentesis.▲ Laboratory analysis of the fluid can help determine the cause.

Treatment

The basic treatment for ascites is bed rest and a salt-restricted diet, usually combined with drugs called diuretics, which make the kidneys excrete more water into the urine. If ascites makes breathing or eating difficult, the fluid may be removed through a needle—a procedure called therapeutic paracentesis. The fluid tends to reaccumulate unless the person also takes a diuretic. Because a large amount of albumin (the major protein in plasma) is usually lost from the blood into the abdominal fluid, albumin may be administered intravenously.

An infection called spontaneous bacterial peritonitis occasionally develops in ascitic fluid for no apparent reason, especially in people with alcoholic cirrhosis. Untreated, this infection can be fatal. Survival depends on early vigorous treatment with antibiotics.

Liver Encephalopathy

Liver encephalopathy (portal-systemic encephalopathy, hepatic encephalopathy, hepatic coma) is a disorder in which brain function deteriorates because toxic substances normally removed by the liver build up in the blood.

Substances absorbed into the bloodstream from the intestines pass through the liver, where toxins are normally removed. Many of these toxins are normal breakdown products of the digestion of protein. In liver encephalopathy, toxins are not removed because liver function is impaired. Also, some toxins may bypass the liver altogether through connections formed between the portal venous system (which supplies blood to the liver) and the general (systemic) venous system as a result of liver disease. A surgical bypass (portal-systemic shunt) to correct portal hypertension may have the same effect. Whatever the cause, the outcome is the same: Toxins can pass to the brain and affect its function. Exactly which substances are toxic to the brain is not known; however, high levels of protein breakdown products in the blood, such as ammonia, appear to play a role.

In a person with long-standing (chronic) liver disease, encephalopathy is usually triggered by an event such as an acute infection or an alcoholic binge, which increases liver damage. Or encephalopathy may be triggered by eating too much protein, which increases the levels of protein breakdown products in the blood. Bleeding in the digestive tract, such as from dilated, twisted veins in the esophagus (esophageal varices), can also lead to a buildup of protein breakdown products, which may directly affect the brain. Certain drugs—especially some sedatives, analgesics, and diuretics—may also trigger encephalopathy. When such a precipitating cause is removed, the encephalopathy may disappear.

Symptoms and Diagnosis

The symptoms of liver encephalopathy are those of decreased brain function, especially impaired consciousness. In the earliest stages, subtle changes appear in logical thinking, personality, and behavior. The person's mood may change, and judgment may be impaired. Normal sleep patterns may be disturbed. The person's breath may have a musty sweet odor. When the person stretches out the arms, the

▲ see page 705

hands cannot be held steady and the person displays a crude flapping motion of the hands (asterixis). As the disorder progresses, the person usually becomes drowsy and confused, and movements and speech become sluggish. Disorientation is common. A person with encephalopathy may be agitated and excited, but this is uncommon. Seizures are also uncommon. Eventually, the person may lose consciousness and lapse into a coma.

An electroencephalogram (EEG)▲ may help in diagnosing early encephalopathy. Even in mild cases, an EEG shows abnormal brain waves. Blood tests usually show abnormally high levels of ammonia.

In an older person, liver encephalopathy may be more difficult to recognize in its early stages, because its initial symptoms (such as disturbed sleep patterns and mild confusion) may be attributed to dementia or are erroneously labeled as delirium.■

Treatment

A doctor looks for and tries to remove any precipitating cause of the deterioration in brain function, such as an infection or a drug that the person is taking. A doctor also tries to eliminate toxic substances from the intestines, usually by restricting the person's diet. Protein is reduced or eliminated from the diet, and oral or intravenous carbohydrates serve as the main source of calories. Later, a doctor may increase the amount of vegetable protein (such as soy protein) rather than animal protein, thereby improving the protein balance without worsening the encephalopathy. The higher fiber content of a vegetable diet tends to speed up the passage of food through the intestines and alter the acidity in the intestines, thereby helping reduce absorption of ammonia. A synthetic sugar (lactulose), taken by mouth, has similar beneficial effects: It alters the acidity of the intestines, and it acts as a laxative, which tends to speed up the passage of food through the intestines, helping to decrease the absorption of ammonia. Cleansing enemas also may be given. Occasionally, a person may take neomycin, an antibiotic. Neomycin reduces the quantity of intestinal bacteria that normally help digest protein; however, prolonged use of neomycin can impair kidney function and cause deafness.

With treatment, liver encephalopathy is frequently reversible. In fact, complete recovery is possible, especially if the encephalopathy was precipitated by a reversible cause. However, for a person in a severe coma as a result of acute liver inflammation, the disorder is fatal up to 80% of the time despite intensive treatment.

Liver Failure

Liver failure is a severe deterioration in liver function.

Liver failure can result from any type of liver disorder, including viral hepatitis, cirrhosis, and liver damage from alcohol or drugs such as acetaminophen. A large portion of the liver must be damaged before liver failure occurs. Liver failure may develop rapidly over days or weeks (acute liver failure) or gradually over months or years (chronic liver failure).

Symptoms and Diagnosis

A person with liver failure usually has jaundice, a tendency to bruise or bleed, ascites, liver encephalopathy, and generally failing health. Other common symptoms include fatigue, weakness, nausea, and a loss of appetite. In acute liver failure, a person may go from being healthy to near death within a few days. In chronic liver failure, the deterioration in health may be very gradual until a dramatic event, such as bleeding varices (large, tortuous veins), occurs.

The clinical manifestations alone provide strong evidence of liver failure. Blood tests usually show severely deteriorated liver function.

Prognosis and Treatment

Treatment depends on the cause and on the specific clinical manifestations. The urgency of treatment depends on whether the liver failure is acute or chronic, but the principles of treatment are the same. The person is usually placed on a restricted diet. Protein consumption is carefully controlled: Too much protein can cause brain dysfunction; too little can cause weight loss. Sodium consumption is kept low to help keep ascitic fluid from accumulating in the abdomen. Alcohol is completely avoided because it can worsen the liver damage.

Ultimately, liver failure is fatal if it is not treated or if the liver disease is progressive. Even after treatment, liver failure may be irreversible. In terminal cases, the person may die of kidney failure (hepatorenal syndrome), because liver failure can eventually lead to kidney failure. Liver transplantation,★ if performed soon enough, can restore a person to normal health, but it is suitable for only a small number of people with liver failure.

▲ see page 445   ■ see page 480
★ see page 1077

CHAPTER 136

Fatty Liver, Cirrhosis, and Related Disorders

Fatty liver, cirrhosis, primary biliary cirrhosis, primary sclerosing cholangitis, and alpha$_1$-antitrypsin deficiency are all disorders that result from an injury to the liver. Injury can be caused by toxins, including alcohol, some drugs, impurities in foods, and the abnormal buildup of normal substances in the blood. Injury to the liver can also be caused by infection or by a disease in which the body attacks its own tissues (an autoimmune reaction▲). Sometimes the exact cause of the injury is not known.

Fatty Liver

Fatty liver is an excessive accumulation of a type of fat (triglyceride) inside the liver cells.

In the United States and other Western countries, the most common causes of fatty liver are alcoholism, obesity, diabetes, and elevated serum triglyceride levels. Other causes include malnutrition, hereditary disorders of metabolism (such as the glycogen storage diseases■), and drugs (such as corticosteroids, tetracycline, and aspirin). The mechanism by which these diseases or factors cause fat to accumulate within liver cells is not known. Simply eating a high-fat diet, for example, does not produce a fatty liver. One possible explanation is that these diseases or factors slow the rate at which fat is processed (metabolized) and excreted by the body. The resulting buildup of fat within the body, according to this theory, is then stored inside the liver cells.

Sometimes the cause of fatty liver is not clear, especially when it occurs in newborns; however, it is likely to be a defect in the mitochondria of the liver cells.

In some people, a fatty liver not due to alcohol abuse or drugs and toxins but associated with obesity, diabetes mellitus, and raised serum triglycerides will progress to scarring (fibrosis) and cirrhosis, possibly because of underlying inflammation. This type of fatty liver is sometimes referred to as nonalcoholic steatohepatitis.

Symptoms and Diagnosis

Fatty liver usually produces no symptoms. In rare cases, however, it results in jaundice (a yellowish discoloration of the skin and the whites of the eyes), nausea, vomiting, pain, and abdominal tenderness.

A physical examination that reveals an enlarged liver without any other symptoms suggests fatty liver. Liver function tests are also performed to determine if there is a liver abnormality, such as inflammation,★ which sometimes accompanies the extra fat in the liver cells and can be associated with the development of cirrhosis in nonalcoholic steatohepatitis. Excess fat in the liver can be detected on abdominal ultrasound. The diagnosis may be confirmed by a liver biopsy, in which a doctor inserts a long hollow needle through the skin to obtain a small piece of liver tissue for examination under a microscope.●

Prognosis and Treatment

Although excessive fat in the liver may not in itself be a serious problem (the fat can disappear, for example, if the person stops drinking), its underlying cause might be. For example, repeated liver injury from toxic substances such as alcohol may eventually progress from fatty liver to cirrhosis (severe scarring of the liver). Therefore, treatment of fatty liver aims at minimizing or eliminating the underlying cause of the disorder.

Cirrhosis

Cirrhosis is the destruction of normal liver tissue that leaves nonfunctioning scar tissue surrounding areas of functioning liver tissue.

Most of the common causes of liver injury, when repeated or sustained over a long time, can result in cirrhosis. In the United States, the most common cause of cirrhosis is alcohol abuse—continued excessive intake of alcohol over a prolonged period. In many parts of Asia and Africa, chronic hepatitis is a major cause of cirrhosis.

Cirrhosis is the third most common cause of death after heart disease and cancer among people aged 45 to 65. The scar tissue that

---

▲ see page 1073　　■ see pages 412 and 1616
★ see box on page 789　　● see page 790

Known Causes of Fatty Liver _____

- Obesity
- Diabetes
- Chemicals and drugs (such as alcohol, corticosteroids, tetracyclines, valproate, methotrexate, carbon tetrachloride, and yellow phosphorus)
- Malnutrition and a low-protein diet
- Pregnancy
- Vitamin A toxicity
- Bypass surgery of the small intestine
- Cystic fibrosis (most likely accompanied by malnutrition)
- Hereditary defects in glycogen, galactose, tyrosine, or homocystine metabolism
- Medium-chain aryl dehydrogenase deficiency
- Cholesterol esterase deficiency
- Phytanic acid storage disease (Refsum's disease)
- Abetalipoproteinemia
- Reye's syndrome

forms impairs the liver's ability to function and obstructs the flow of blood through the portal vein (the vein that carries blood from the intestines to the liver). As a result of this obstruction, high blood pressure (portal hypertension▲) occurs.

Symptoms and Complications

Many people with mild cirrhosis have no symptoms and appear to be well for years. Others are weak, have a poor appetite, feel sick, and lose weight. If the flow of bile (the greenish yellow digestive fluid produced by the liver) is chronically obstructed, the person develops jaundice,■ overall itchiness, and small yellow skin nodules, especially around the eyelids. The reduced production of bile salts by the damaged liver means that the absorption of fats and fat-soluble vitamins is impaired. Malnutrition commonly results from the impaired absorption of vitamins and from the loss of appetite.

Other effects of cirrhosis (which are also found in other causes of severe liver failure) include the wasting away of muscle (atrophy),

▲ see page 793   ■ see page 791
★ see page 794   ● see page 794
◆ see page 828   ▼ see page 795

redness of the palms (palmar erythema), a curling up of the fingers (Dupuytren's contracture), small spiderlike veins in the skin, salivary gland enlargement in the cheeks, axillary hair loss, abnormal nerve function (peripheral neuropathy), and, in men, breast enlargement (gynecomastia) and shrinking of the testes (testicular atrophy) due to a failure of the damaged liver to break down estrogens.

Some complications of cirrhosis result from the high blood pressure. High blood pressure can cause dilated, twisted veins to form at the lower end of the esophagus (esophageal varices★). A person may vomit large amounts of blood because of bleeding from esophageal varices. High blood pressure in the portal vein along with poor liver function may also lead to fluid accumulation in the abdomen (ascites●). Other complications of cirrhosis include kidney failure◆ and a deterioration of brain function due to liver failure (liver encephalopathy▼).

Liver cancer (hepatoma) is another complication of cirrhosis, particularly when the cirrhosis is due to chronic hepatitis B or hepatitis C infection, iron overload (hemochromatosis), or glycogen storage diseases. Liver cancer may result from cirrhosis due to alcohol abuse.

Diagnosis

The diagnosis of cirrhosis is generally made on the basis of the symptoms and physical examination, together with a history of risk factors such as alcohol abuse. On physical examination, a doctor may feel a small, firm liver; occasionally, small lumps (nodules) on the surface of the liver are felt as well.

Liver function tests often are normal because of the tremendous reserve of the liver and the relative insensitivity of these biochemical tests. The liver can carry out essential functions even when its total activity is 85% below normal. An ultrasound or computed tomography scan (CT) may show that the liver is shrunken or abnormally patterned, suggesting cirrhosis. A liver scan using a radioactive isotope creates an image showing which areas of the liver are functioning and which are scarred. The diagnosis can be confirmed by a liver biopsy (removal of a tissue sample for examination under a microscope).

Prognosis and Treatment

Cirrhosis is usually progressive. If someone with early-stage cirrhosis stops drinking alcohol, the process of further liver scarring may stop, but scar tissue, once formed, remains

Alcohol's Toll on the Liver

In alcoholic liver disease, damage to the liver results from excessive alcohol use. In general, the amount of alcohol consumed (how much and how often) determines the risk and the degree of liver damage. Women are more vulnerable to liver damage than men. Among people who drink over a period of years, the equivalent of as little as $2/3$ ounce of pure alcohol a day in women (6$1/2$ ounces of wine, 13 ounces of beer, or 2 ounces of whiskey) or 2 ounces a day in men (20 ounces of wine, 40 ounces of beer, or 6 ounces of whiskey) can cause liver damage. However, the amount of alcohol that causes liver damage varies from person to person. Heavy drinkers usually first develop symptoms during

their 30s and tend to develop severe problems by their 40s.

Alcohol may cause three types of liver damage: fat accumulation (fatty liver), inflammation (alcoholic hepatitis), and severe scarring (cirrhosis). People with fatty liver usually have no symptoms. In one third of these people, the liver is enlarged and occasionally tender. People with alcoholic hepatitis may have a fever, jaundice, an increased white blood cell count, and a tender, painful, enlarged liver. The skin may develop spiderlike veins. People with cirrhosis may have few symptoms or the same symptoms as those of a person with alcoholic hepatitis. Such people may also have complications such as high blood pressure in the portal

vein (the vein that carries blood from the intestines to the liver), spleen enlargement, fluid accumulation in the abdominal cavity (ascites), kidney failure from liver failure, confusion, and liver cancer.

If the person with alcoholic liver disease continues to drink alcohol, liver damage progresses and usually is fatal. If the person stops drinking, some of the liver damage may repair itself, although the scarring remains. The chances are good that the person will live longer.

The only effective treatment is to stop drinking alcohol. Doing so can be extremely difficult, and most people need to participate in a formal program, such as Alcoholics Anonymous (AA), to help them stop drinking.

indefinitely. In general, the prognosis is poorer if serious complications—such as vomiting of blood, accumulation of fluid in the abdominal cavity, or deterioration in brain function—have occurred.

No cure exists for cirrhosis. Thus, it is a disorder that should be prevented or arrested at its earliest stages. Treatment includes withdrawing toxic agents such as alcohol and treating complications as they arise. If the person needs to take drugs that are processed (metabolized) by the liver, much smaller doses must be given to avoid overdosage. Attention is given to proper nutrition, which usually involves carefully controlling protein and sodium intake and taking supplemental vitamins.

Liver transplantation can be lifesaving for a person with advanced cirrhosis. If the person continues to abuse alcohol, or if another underlying cause cannot be altered, a transplanted liver will also eventually develop cirrhosis, and liver transplantation is not usually done.

Primary Biliary Cirrhosis

Primary biliary cirrhosis is inflammation and eventual scarring and obstruction of the bile ducts inside the liver.

Primary biliary cirrhosis is most common among women aged 35 to 60, though it can oc-

cur in men and women of any age. The cause, though not clear, is probably autoimmune; the person's immune system attacks the body's own tissues.▲ Primary biliary cirrhosis occurs in association with rheumatoid arthritis, scleroderma, or autoimmune thyroiditis. Unlike primary sclerosing cholangitis, primary biliary cirrhosis affects only the bile ducts inside the liver.

Primary biliary cirrhosis begins with inflammation of the bile ducts inside the liver. The inflammation blocks the flow of bile (the greenish yellow digestive fluid) out of the liver; thus, bile remains in the liver cells or spills over into the bloodstream. As inflammation spreads from the bile ducts to the rest of the liver, a latticework of scar tissue develops throughout the liver.

Symptoms and Diagnosis

Usually, primary biliary cirrhosis starts gradually. Itchiness and sometimes fatigue are often the first symptoms. Other features, which may not occur until months or years later, include enlargement of the tips of the fingers (clubbing) and abnormalities of the bone, nerves, and kidney. The stool may be pale and greasy and have an unusually offensive odor (steatorrhea). Later, any of the symp-

▲ see page 1073

toms and complications of cirrhosis can develop.▲ Metabolic bone disease (osteoporosis) develops in most people.

On physical examination, a doctor feels an enlarged, firm liver in about 50% of people and an enlarged spleen in about 25%. In the late stages, the scarred liver shrinks in size. About 15% of people have small yellow deposits in the skin (xanthoma) or eyelids (xanthelasma). About 10% have increased skin pigmentation. Fewer than 10% have only jaundice (a yellowish discoloration of the skin and the whites of the eyes) early on; jaundice tends to develop in others later.

In about 50% of people with primary biliary cirrhosis, the disorder is discovered before symptoms even develop because of abnormalities detected during routine blood testing. Antibodies against mitochondria (tiny structures contained within cells) are found in the blood of more than 90% of people with the disorder.

When jaundice is evident or results of liver function tests indicate abnormalities, an ultrasound scan, or occasionally an MRI of the bile duct system (magnetic resonance cholangiogram) can be used to show any abnormalities or obstruction of the bile ducts outside the liver. The diagnosis of primary biliary cirrhosis is supported by finding that the bile ducts outside the liver are unobstructed, thus identifying the liver as the site of the problem. Finding antibodies against mitochondria clinches the diagnosis. A liver biopsy (removal of a tissue sample for examination under a microscope)■ confirms the diagnosis and stages the disease (such as early or late with cirrhosis established).

Prognosis and Treatment

The progression of primary biliary cirrhosis varies greatly. People who initially have no symptoms often develop symptoms after 2 to 7 years. Others have virtually no symptoms for 10 to 15 years. Still others become very ill in 3 to 5 years. The disorder eventually culminates in severe cirrhosis. The outcome is poor for people who develop jaundice.

No cure is known. The drug cholestyramine may control itchiness. Supplements of calcium and vitamins A, D, and K in a water-soluble form may be needed, because the natural

forms of these nutrients are fat-soluble and are therefore not properly absorbed from the intestine when there is insufficient bile. The drug ursodeoxycholic acid appears to somewhat lessen the progression of the disorder and is generally well tolerated. Liver transplantation★ is the best treatment for people entering the final stages of the disorder.

Primary Sclerosing Cholangitis

Primary sclerosing cholangitis is inflammation and eventual scarring and obstruction of the bile ducts inside and outside the liver.

In primary sclerosing cholangitis, scarring narrows and eventually blocks the bile ducts, leading to cirrhosis. It differs from primary biliary cirrhosis because the bile ducts both inside and outside the liver are affected. The cause is not known but is likely autoimmune, in which the person's immune system attacks the body's own tissues.● The disorder most often affects young men. It commonly occurs in people with inflammatory bowel disease, especially ulcerative colitis.

Symptoms and Complications

Symptoms usually begin gradually with worsening fatigue, itchiness, and jaundice (yellowish discoloration of the skin and the whites of the eyes). Attacks of upper abdominal pain and fever caused by inflammation and recurring infection of the bile ducts (bacterial cholangitis) may occur. However, bacterial cholangitis is uncommon unless the duct system has been manipulated. Sometimes stents, which keep the bile ducts open, are placed endoscopically, and this procedure can result in bacterial cholangitis. An affected person may have an enlarged liver and spleen or symptoms of cirrhosis.◆ The person also may develop increased blood pressure in the vein that carries blood from the intestines to the liver (portal hypertension), accumulation of fluid in the abdominal cavity (ascites), and liver failure, which can be fatal.

Cancer of the bile ducts (cholangiocarcinoma) develops in 10 to 15% of people with primary sclerosing cholangitis.

Diagnosis

Because some people have no symptoms for as long as 10 years, the disorder may be detected by abnormal results of liver function tests performed as part of an annual physical examination or for some unrelated medical

▲ see page 797　■ see page 790
★ see page 1077　● see page 1073
◆ see page 797

reason. The diagnosis is usually confirmed by endoscopic retrograde cholangiopancreatography (ERCP) or percutaneous cholangiography.▲ In ERCP, x-rays are taken after a radiopaque dye, which is visible on x-rays, is injected into the bile ducts through an endoscope (a flexible viewing tube). In percutaneous cholangiography, x-rays are taken after a radiopaque dye is injected directly into the bile ducts. Increasingly, abdominal ultrasound and especially magnetic resonance imaging (MRI) scans of the bile ducts (magnetic resonance cholangiography) can be used to make the diagnosis. A liver biopsy (removal of a tissue sample for examination under a microscope)■ may be necessary to help confirm the diagnosis.

Prognosis and Treatment

Usually, primary sclerosing cholangitis worsens gradually. Drugs such as corticosteroids, azathioprine, penicillamine, and methotrexate have been used in an attempt to slow the progression of the disorder but have not proved very effective and can cause severe side effects. The value of the drug ursodeoxycholic acid remains unclear. Primary sclerosing cholangitis may require liver transplantation,★ which is the only known cure for this otherwise fatal disorder.

Recurring infection of the bile ducts (bacterial cholangitis) requires treatment with antibiotics and, when possible, drainage of obstructed parts of the bile ducts using ERCP.

If cancer of the bile ducts (cholangiocarcinoma) develops and removal of the cancer is not possible by surgery, an endoscope may be used to place tubes (stents) into major bile ducts obstructed by the cancer, to open them up.

Alpha₁-Antitrypsin Deficiency

Alpha₁-antitrypsin deficiency is a hereditary disorder in which a lack of the enzyme alpha₁-antitrypsin may cause lung and liver disease.

Alpha₁-antitrypsin is an enzyme that the liver produces and secretes into the bloodstream. Certain tissues then take up this enzyme and, in turn, secrete it into fluids that they produce. Thus alpha₁-antitrypsin is normally present in saliva, duodenal fluid (the fluid present in the first segment of the small

intestine), lung secretions, tears, nasal secretions, and cerebrospinal fluid.

Alpha₁-antitrypsin inhibits the action of enzymes that break down proteins (proteases). A lack or reduced level of alpha₁-antitrypsin allows proteases to damage tissue, particularly in the lungs and liver. In alpha₁-antitrypsin deficiency, the liver is unable to secrete (export) this enzyme, which then accumulates inside the liver cells, leading to their destruction. The disorder is usually identified in children, many of whom die before they reach adulthood. Therefore, this disorder is uncommon in adults.

Symptoms and Prognosis

About 25% of children with alpha₁-antitrypsin deficiency develop cirrhosis and excessive pressure in the portal vein (the vein that carries blood from the intestines to the liver) and die before age 12. About 25% die by age 20. Another 25% have only minor liver abnormalities and survive into adulthood. The remaining 25% do not develop liver abnormalities and have no evidence of progressive disease.

Adults with alpha₁-antitrypsin deficiency commonly develop emphysema, a lung disease that results in increasing shortness of breath. Less commonly, adults with this disorder develop cirrhosis, which may eventually lead to liver cancer.

Treatment

Replacement of the missing enzyme using synthetic alpha₁-antitrypsin has shown some promise in the treatment of children, but liver transplantation● remains the only fully successful treatment. Liver damage does not usually recur in the transplanted liver, which is able to produce and secrete alpha₁-antitrypsin normally.

Treatment in adults is usually directed at the lung disease.◆ Measures include preventing lung infection and getting a person who smokes to stop smoking. Liver transplantation is also successful in adults.

▲ see art on page 790   ■ see page 790

★ see page 1077   ● see page 1077

◆ see also page 285

CHAPTER 137

Hepatitis

Hepatitis is inflammation of the liver from any cause.

Hepatitis commonly results from a virus, particularly one of the five hepatitis viruses—A, B, C, D, or E (a sixth category called hepatitis virus G had been created but has since been retracted). Less commonly, hepatitis results from other viral infections, such as infectious mononucleosis, yellow fever, or cytomegalovirus infection. The major nonviral causes of hepatitis are excessive alcohol intake and use of certain drugs, such as isoniazid (used to treat tuberculosis).

Hepatitis can be acute (short-lived) or chronic (lasting at least 6 months). It is common throughout the world.

Acute Viral Hepatitis

Acute viral hepatitis is inflammation of the liver caused by infection with one of the five hepatitis viruses; for most people, the inflammation begins suddenly and lasts only a few weeks.

Symptoms

Acute viral hepatitis can produce anything from a minor flu-like illness to fatal liver failure. The severity of symptoms and speed of recovery vary considerably, depending on the particular virus and on the person's response to the infection. Hepatitis A and C often produce very mild symptoms, or none at all, and may go unnoticed, whereas B and E are more likely to produce severe symptoms. Co-infection of hepatitis B with hepatitis D may make the symptoms even more severe.

Symptoms of acute viral hepatitis usually begin suddenly. They include a poor appetite, nausea, vomiting, and often a fever. In people who smoke, a distaste for cigarettes is a typical symptom. Occasionally, especially with hepatitis B infection, an affected person develops joint pains and itchy red hives on the skin (wheals).

After a few days, the urine becomes dark, and jaundice (a yellowish discoloration of the skin and the whites of the eyes) may develop. Both of these symptoms occur because bilirubin (the main pigment in bile, the greenish yellow digestive fluid produced by the liver) builds up in the blood. Most symptoms typically disappear at this point, and the person feels better even though the jaundice gets worse. The jaundice usually peaks in 1 to 2 weeks, then fades over 2 to 4 weeks. Symptoms of cholestasis (a reduction or stoppage of bile flow)—such as pale stools and overall itchiness—may develop.

Rarely, particularly with hepatitis B, symptoms may become extremely severe (fulminant), with liver failure, which may be fatal, especially in adults.

Diagnosis

Doctors suspect acute viral hepatitis on the basis of the person's symptoms. On physical examination, a doctor finds the liver to be tender and somewhat enlarged in about half of the people with acute viral hepatitis. Results of liver function tests indicate that the liver is inflamed and can help doctors distinguish hepatitis due to alcohol abuse from that due to a virus. Usually the specific virus causing the hepatitis or the specific antibodies produced by the body to fight it can be identified as well.

Prevention

Vaccines are available to prevent hepatitis A and B infections. As with most vaccines, however, protection requires allowing a number of weeks for the vaccine to reach its full effect as the person's immune system gradually creates antibodies against the particular virus. People who have not been vaccinated and who are exposed to hepatitis A or B virus can obtain immediate protection with an injection of an antibody preparation called immune globulin. The amount of protection varies, however, and is only temporary. No vaccines are available against hepatitis C, D, or E virus. However, vaccination against hepatitis B virus also eliminates the risk of infection with hepatitis D virus.

A number of other preventive measures against infection with the hepatitis viruses can be taken, such as washing the hands thoroughly before handling food, refraining from high-risk behavior such as sharing needles to inject illicit drugs and having unprotected sex, and avoiding blood transfusions except when absolutely essential.

Treatment and Prognosis

In most people, special treatment is not necessary, although people with unusually severe acute hepatitis may require hospitalization. After the first several days, appetite usually returns and the person does not need to stay in bed. Severe restrictions of diet or activity are unnecessary, and vitamin supplements are not required. Most people can safely return to work after the jaundice clears, even if their liver function test results are not quite normal.

People with hepatitis should avoid alcohol until they fully recover.▲ A doctor may need to discontinue or reduce the dosage of certain drugs that could build to harmful levels in the body (for example warfarin or theophylline) because of the liver's inability to process (metabolize) them. Thus the person should disclose to the doctor all drugs being taken (both prescription and over-the-counter, including any herbal medicines), so that dosage adjustments can be made if necessary.

A person with acute viral hepatitis usually recovers in 4 to 8 weeks, even without treatment. However, those people infected with hepatitis C and to a lesser extent with hepatitis B may become chronic carriers of the virus. In the carrier state, the person has no symptoms but is still infected, may develop chronic hepatitis even though the disease is not apparent, and is able to transmit the virus to others. A chronic carrier may eventually develop cirrhosis (severe scarring of the liver)■ or liver cancer.★

Chronic Hepatitis

Chronic hepatitis is inflammation of the liver that lasts at least 6 months.

Chronic hepatitis, though much less common than acute hepatitis, can persist for years, even decades. In most people, it is quite mild and does not cause significant liver damage. In some people, though, continued inflammation slowly damages the liver, eventually producing cirrhosis (severe scarring of the liver), liver failure, and sometimes liver cancer.

Causes

About one third of people with chronic hepatitis develop it after a bout of acute viral hepatitis. The remaining two thirds of people develop the disease gradually without any obvious symptoms, although most cases of chronic hepatitis are still caused by one of the hepatitis viruses.

Hepatitis C virus is the most common cause of chronic hepatitis; at least 75% of acute hepatitis C cases become chronic. Hepatitis B virus, sometimes together with hepatitis D virus, causes a smaller percentage of chronic infections. Hepatitis A and E viruses do not cause chronic hepatitis.

Drugs such as methyldopa, isoniazid, nitrofurantoin, and possibly acetaminophen can cause chronic hepatitis, particularly when they are taken for prolonged periods. Wilson's disease, a rare hereditary disease involving abnormal retention of copper in the liver,● may cause chronic hepatitis in children and young adults.

No one knows exactly why a particular virus or drug causes chronic hepatitis in some people but not in others, or why the degree of severity varies. In many people with chronic hepatitis, no obvious cause can be found. In some of these people, there appears to be an overactive immune system response that is responsible for the chronic inflammation. This response may occur because the body is attacking its own tissues (an autoimmune reaction◆), although this has not been proven. This disease, called autoimmune hepatitis, is more common among women than men.

Symptoms and Diagnosis

Many people with chronic hepatitis have no symptoms at all. For those who do, the symptoms often include a feeling of illness, poor appetite, and fatigue. Sometimes an affected person also has a low-grade fever and some upper abdominal discomfort. Jaundice may or may not develop. Features of chronic liver disease may eventually develop. These can include an enlarged spleen, spiderlike blood vessels in the skin, and fluid retention. Other features may occur, especially in young women with autoimmune hepatitis. Such features can involve virtually any body system and include acne, cessation of menstrual periods, joint pain, lung scarring, inflammation of the thyroid gland and kidneys, and anemia.

Many people have chronic hepatitis for years without developing progressive liver damage.

▲ see box on page 799   ■ see page 797
★ see page 810   ● see box on page 905
◆ see page 1073

THE HEPATITIS VIRUSES

Virus	Transmission	Symptoms and Prognosis	Prevention
Hepatitis A	Hepatitis A is spread primarily from the stool of one person to the mouth of another, usually as the result of poor hygiene, such as when food is prepared by the unwashed hands of an infected person. It is sometimes spread in day care centers, where caregivers can come in contact with infected stool in diapers. Raw shellfish are sometimes contaminated when taken from waters where raw sewage drains. Waterborne and food-borne epidemics are common, especially in developing countries. Hepatitis A also can be transmitted through sexual contact.	Most hepatitis A infections cause no symptoms and go unrecognized, though typical symptoms of acute hepatitis can occur. Except for rare full-blown (fulminant) cases (rarer than with hepatitis B), recovery from the acute infection is complete, and the virus does not cause a carrier state or chronic hepatitis.	Good hygiene in handling food and avoiding contamination of water supplies is important. Vaccination against hepatitis A is given to people at high risk of acquiring the infection, such as travelers to parts of the world where the disease is widespread. Standard immune globulin is useful immediate protection for people exposed to hepatitis A. It can be given in addition to vaccination.
Hepatitis B	Hepatitis B is less easily transmitted than hepatitis A. One mode of transmission, now rare in the United States, is through contaminated blood. Transmission commonly occurs among people who share needles to inject illicit drugs. Hepatitis B is also spread through contact with saliva, tears, breast milk, urine, vaginal fluid, and semen. Transmission commonly occurs between sex partners, both heterosexual and male homosexual. Also at increased risk are people in closed environments (such as prisons and institutions for the mentally retarded), because body fluid contact is more likely. A pregnant woman infected with hepatitis B can transmit the virus to her baby during birth. Hepatitis B can be transmitted by healthy people who are chronic carriers of the virus. Whether insect bites can transmit this virus is not clear. Many cases of hepatitis B have no known source.	In general, hepatitis B is more serious than hepatitis A and is occasionally fatal, especially in older people or after a blood transfusion, and can be mild or full-blown (fulminant). When a person with hepatitis B has hepatitis D as well, symptoms are more severe. Joint pains and itchy red hives on the skin (wheals) are more likely in a person with hepatitis B than with the other viruses. Hepatitis B becomes chronic in 5 to 10% of infected people. In the Far East and parts of Africa, hepatitis B virus is responsible for many cases of chronic hepatitis, cirrhosis, and liver cancer.	High-risk behavior such as sharing needles and sexual promiscuity should be avoided, as should unnecessary blood transfusions. Vaccination against hepatitis B stimulates the body's immune defenses and protects most people. However, people undergoing dialysis, people with cirrhosis, and people with an impaired immune system may derive less protection from vaccination. Vaccination is especially important for people at risk of contracting hepatitis B. Universal vaccination of all people against hepatitis B is being increasingly recommended. Standard immune globulin provides immediate but weak protection for people exposed to hepatitis B. Hepatitis B immune globulin provides better protection. Infants born to mothers with hepatitis B are given hepatitis B immune globulin and are vaccinated; this combination prevents chronic hepatitis B in about 70%.

Virus	Transmission	Symptoms and Prognosis	Prevention
Hepatitis C	Hepatitis C until 1992 was responsible for at least 80% of hepatitis cases arising from blood transfusions. Now it is rarely transmitted that way. It is most commonly transmitted among people who share needles to inject illicit drugs. Sexual transmission is uncommon. Transmission from a pregnant woman infected with hepatitis C to her baby is also uncommon. For unknown reasons, people with alcoholic liver disease often also have hepatitis C. A small proportion of healthy people appear to be chronic carriers.	Hepatitis C is somewhat unpredictable: The acute illness is usually mild and often without symptoms. However, liver function may improve and then fluctuate repeatedly for several months or years. Hepatitis C has at least a 75% chance of becoming chronic. About 20% of affected people develop cirrhosis, and liver cancer may occur once cirrhosis has developed.	Illicit drug use and related high-risk behavior such as tattoos and body piercing should be avoided, as should unnecessary blood transfusions. No vaccine is currently available. Standard immune globulin is not useful.
Hepatitis D	Hepatitis D occurs most often among people who share needles to inject illicit drugs.	Hepatitis D occurs only as a co-infection with hepatitis B virus and usually makes the hepatitis B infection more severe.	Vaccination against hepatitis B virus eliminates the risk of hepatitis D virus as well. Hepatitis B immune globulin also protects against hepatitis D infection.
Hepatitis E	Hepatitis E is spread primarily from the stool of one person to the mouth of another. It causes occasional epidemics, which are often waterborne, similar to those caused by hepatitis A virus. So far, these epidemics have occurred only in underdeveloped countries.	Hepatitis E may produce severe symptoms of acute viral hepatitis, especially in pregnant women. Chronic hepatitis or a chronic carrier state does not occur.	No vaccine is currently available. The usefulness of standard immune globulin is not known.

Standard immune globulin: a formulation of antibodies that fight a variety of diseases.

For others, the disease gradually worsens. Over a period of years, about 20% of people with chronic hepatitis C and about 50% of people with autoimmune hepatitis develop cirrhosis, with or without liver failure.

Although the person's symptoms and liver function test results provide helpful diagnostic information, a liver biopsy▲ is essential for a definite diagnosis. The liver biopsy allows a doctor to determine the severity of the inflammation and whether any scarring or cirrhosis has developed. The biopsy may also reveal the underlying cause of the hepatitis. Occasionally, a biopsy needs to be performed more than once.

Treatment

In people with progressive chronic hepatitis C infection, a combination of the antiviral agent interferon-alpha plus ribavirin is most commonly used. This combination may stop the inflammation. However, hepatitis tends to recur once treatment is stopped, and the overall success rate is only about 30 to 40%. Side effects are common. In people with chronic hepatitis B, treatment with interferon-alpha or lamivudine is sometimes effective.

▲ see page 790

If use of a particular drug is suspected of causing the hepatitis, then discontinuing the drug may effectively treat the disease.

Autoimmune hepatitis is usually treated with corticosteroids, sometimes in combination with azathioprine. These drugs suppress the inflammation, resolve the symptoms, and improve long-term survival. Nevertheless, scarring in the liver may gradually worsen. Discontinuing therapy usually leads to a recurrence of the inflammation, so most people have to take the drugs indefinitely.

Regardless of the cause or type of chronic hepatitis, any complications—such as fluid in the abdominal cavity (ascites▲) or abnormal brain function (liver encephalopathy■)—require treatment.

Liver transplantation★ may be considered for a person with severe liver failure. However, liver transplantation is not generally suitable for a person with hepatitis B infection, because recurrence of the infection tends to occur early and severely in the transplanted liver. For people with hepatitis C, the infection virtually always recurs in the transplanted liver, but the disease is usually so mild that the person is likely to survive for many years.

CHAPTER 138

Blood Vessel Disorders of the Liver

The liver receives three quarters of its blood supply from the portal vein, which carries nutrient-rich blood from the intestines. This blood carries digested food substances to the liver for processing. The liver receives the remaining quarter of its blood supply from the hepatic artery, which carries oxygen-rich blood from the heart.

Blood leaves the liver through the hepatic veins. This blood is a mixture of blood from the hepatic artery and blood from the portal vein. The hepatic veins drain into the inferior vena cava—the largest vein in the body—which then empties into the heart.

With age, the overall flow of blood through the liver decreases. The decreased blood flow reduces the liver's ability to inactivate some drugs and to remove toxins from the blood.

Abnormalities of the Hepatic Artery

The hepatic artery carries oxygen-rich blood to the liver from the heart or its branches. It is the main supply of blood and oxygen to the liver. The portal artery also supplies blood to the liver, helping ensure that this vital organ always receives enough blood.

Narrowing or Blockage: A narrowing or blockage can reduce the flow of blood through the hepatic artery. If this happens, blood flow to the liver is reduced. Narrowing or blockage of the hepatic artery can have various causes, including injuries, such as a gunshot wound or surgical trauma, or blood clots. Blood clots generally are caused by inflammation of the arterial wall (arteritis) or by an infusion of chemotherapy drugs or other toxic or irritating substances into the artery. Blockage of the hepatic artery can be detected using x-rays enhanced with the injection of radiopaque dye (arteriography) or through magnetic resonance angiography (MRA).

Reduced blood flow through the hepatic artery can be due to other causes as well, including shock (for example, due to heart failure, severe blood or body fluid loss, or infection) and sickle cell disease.

Because the liver has a dual blood supply, reduced blood flow through the hepatic artery usually does not damage the liver or causes only minor problems. However, severe damage to the liver resulting from reduced blood flow, called ischemic hepatitis, can occur in a person who has had a liver transplant or a previous blood clot of the portal vein. Ischemic hepatitis is often of less immediate concern than are the problems resulting from the cause of the reduced blood flow, such as shock resulting from severe heart failure. Symptoms of

---

▲ see page 794   ■ see page 795
★ see page 1077

Blood Supply of the Liver

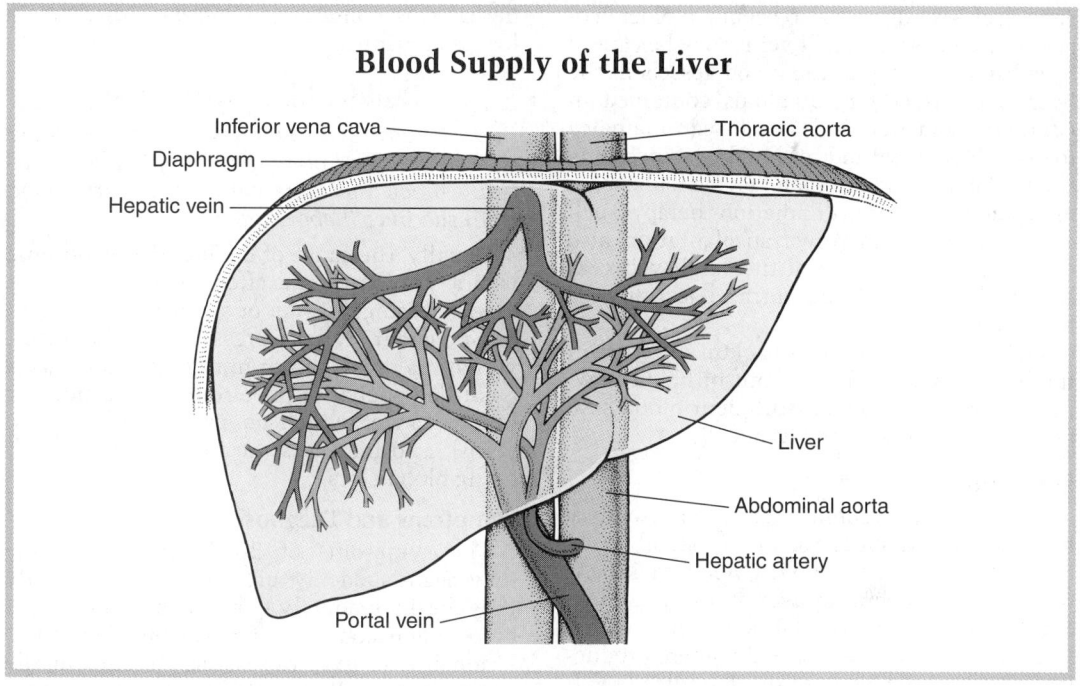

Inferior vena cava
Diaphragm
Hepatic vein
Thoracic aorta
Liver
Abdominal aorta
Hepatic artery
Portal vein

ischemic hepatitis include nausea, vomiting, and liver enlargement and tenderness. Abnormal results of liver function tests help confirm the diagnosis. Treatment of ischemic hepatitis is concentrated on treating the underlying cause and thereby restoring blood flow to the liver. There is no specific treatment for the liver itself.

Unlike the liver, the large bile ducts outside the liver, such as the left and right hepatic ducts and the common bile duct, do not have a dual blood supply. They receive their blood exclusively from the hepatic artery. Thus, any obstruction of blood flow through the hepatic artery to the ducts can result in damage (ischemia), causing death of some of the cells forming the ducts. Death of some of the cells can result in a narrowing (stricture) of the affected bile duct, which leads to obstruction and may result in jaundice (a yellowish discoloration of the skin and the whites of the eyes). The obstruction is treated with endoscopic retrograde cholangiopancreatography▲ and the insertion of a stent (stenting).

Aneurysms: An aneurysm is a bulge at a weak spot in an artery;■ an aneurysm in the hepatic artery is usually caused by infection, atherosclerosis, injury, or polyarteritis nodosa.★ An aneurysm that presses on a nearby bile duct may narrow or even block it, which

then blocks bile flow from the liver. This blockage results in jaundice. An aneurysm may also bleed into a nearby bile duct. Unless treated, up to 75% of aneurysms of the hepatic artery rupture, often causing massive bleeding and possible death.

Imaging tests, such as x-rays enhanced by injection of a radiopaque dye (a dye visible on x-rays) in a technique called arteriography or computed tomography (CT) scanning enhanced by injection of a radiopaque dye, may be used to diagnose an aneurysm.

An aneurysm may be treated by inserting a catheter into the hepatic artery and injecting an irritating substance that causes a clot to form, thereby blocking the artery. If this procedure (called embolization) fails, surgery is performed to tie off (ligate) the artery directly.

Veno-occlusive Disease

Veno-occlusive disease is a blockage of the small veins in the liver.

Veno-occlusive disease may occur at any age. Children aged 1 to 3 are particularly vulnerable because they have smaller blood vessels, but

▲ see art on page 790   ■ see page 226
★ see page 387

veno-occlusive disease also occurs in older people. Blockage of the small veins may be caused by substances toxic to the blood vessels in the liver, such as certain alkaloids contained in *Crotalaria* and *Senecio* leaves (used in Jamaica to make herbal tea) and certain drugs, including chemotherapy drugs, such as cyclophosphamide and azathioprine. Radiation therapy (such as is used in bone marrow transplantation) also can produce a blockage of the small veins, as can antibodies produced during rejection of a transplanted liver.

Such blockage causes a backup of blood in the liver, reducing the amount of blood flowing into the liver. The insufficient blood supply, in turn, damages the liver cells.

Symptoms

Symptoms of veno-occlusive disease may begin suddenly. Blockage of the small veins causes the liver to swell with blood, making it tender when a doctor presses on the abdomen. Fluid may leak from the surface of the swollen liver and accumulate in the abdomen, producing a condition called ascites. Jaundice (a yellowish discoloration of the skin and the whites of the eyes) may occur. The backup of blood in the liver also raises the pressure in the portal vein (a condition called portal hypertension) and in the veins that empty into it. This higher pressure may cause dilated, twisted (varicose) veins in the esophagus (esophageal varices), which may rupture and bleed, sometimes massively. The bleeding results in vomiting of blood and the passage of blood through the digestive tract, resulting in black stools (melena) and even shock if the bleeding is severe.

Prognosis and Treatment

The prognosis depends on the extent of damage and whether the injury (exposure to a toxin) recurs. Typically, a blockage disappears quickly, and the person recovers regardless of any treatment. However, 25% of people with veno-occlusive disease die of liver failure within about 3 months. In most affected people, the pressure in the portal vein remains high and the injury leads to cirrhosis (severe scarring of the liver).

There is no specific treatment for the blocked veins. In cases caused by the ingestion of a toxic substance, the only treatment is to stop taking that substance. Recurrences are common, particularly if consumption of

herbal teas containing *Crotalaria* or *Senecio* leaves continues.

Budd-Chiari Syndrome

Budd-Chiari syndrome is a rare disorder caused by blood clots that completely or partially block the large veins that carry blood from the liver (hepatic veins).

Usually, the cause of Budd-Chiari syndrome is not known. Some affected people have a blood clotting disorder or sickle cell disease or are pregnant. Direct pressure on the veins, which may result from injury, liver abscess (a pus-filled pocket of infection), liver cancer, or kidney cancer (which can press on the hepatic veins), also increases the likelihood of developing blood clots.

Symptoms and Diagnosis

The symptoms of Budd-Chiari syndrome may begin suddenly and severely, but usually they begin gradually. The liver swells with blood and becomes tender. The blood accumulation in the liver raises the pressure in the portal vein, although the consequences may not develop for months. One such consequence of this raised pressure is the formation of dilated, twisted (varicose) veins in the esophagus (esophageal varices), which may rupture and bleed, sometimes massively, often with vomiting of blood. In addition, fluid leaks from the surface of the swollen liver into the abdominal cavity (ascites), and abdominal pain and mild jaundice (a yellowish discoloration of the skin and the whites of the eyes) occur.

Within a few days to several months, other symptoms of liver failure may occur.▲ The blood clots occasionally extend to block the inferior vena cava—the largest vein entering the heart. This blockage causes considerable swelling in the legs and abdomen.

The characteristic symptoms are the main clues used by the doctor to make the diagnosis. X-rays of the veins taken after injection of a radiopaque dye (a dye visible on x-rays) may reveal the precise location of the blockage. Ultrasound or magnetic resonance imaging (MRI) scanning or a liver biopsy (in which a sample of liver tissue is removed by needle for examination under a microscope) may be used to confirm the diagnosis.■

Prognosis and Treatment

Fewer than one third of people with Budd-Chiari syndrome survive for 1 year without prompt and effective treatment.

▲ see page 796   ■ see page 790

If the vein is narrowed rather than blocked, anticoagulants (drugs that prevent clots) or thrombolytics (drugs that dissolve clots) may be used. If esophageal varices develop and bleed, surgery may be performed to reduce the pressure in the portal vein. During surgery, the portal vein is connected to the inferior vena cava, causing blood flow to bypass the liver. However, this newly created connection (shunt) can increase the risk of liver encephalopathy (brain damage from liver disease). Liver transplantation▲ can be an effective treatment, particularly for people with severe liver failure.

Portal Vein Thrombosis

Portal vein thrombosis is a blockage (by a blood clot) of the portal vein, which brings blood to the liver.

Portal vein thrombosis can be caused by any blood clotting disorder or by any condition that backs up blood in the portal vein, such as Budd-Chiari syndrome, chronic heart failure,■ or chronic constrictive pericarditis.★ It may also be caused by cirrhosis (severe scarring of the liver) or by cancer of the liver, pancreas, or stomach. Or it may be caused by inflammation of the bile ducts (cholangitis), inflammation of the pancreas (pancreatitis), or a liver abscess (a pus-filled pocket of infection). In newborns, portal vein thrombosis may result from an infection of the navel. Portal vein thrombosis can occur in pregnant women, especially in those with eclampsia.● However, in more than half of the people with portal vein thrombosis, the cause cannot be found.

Symptoms and Diagnosis

Blockage of the portal vein raises the pressure in the portal vein and in the other veins that drain into it (portal hypertension). This higher pressure may cause dilated, twisted (varicose) veins in the esophagus (esophageal varices) to form, which may rupture and bleed, sometimes massively. The bleeding results in vomiting of blood. Such bleeding is often the first symptom of portal vein thrombosis. The spleen typically enlarges, especially in children. A doctor can feel an enlarged spleen, which may be tender.

In about one third of people with portal vein thrombosis, blockage of the portal vein develops slowly, allowing other blood channels (collateral channels) to become established around the block. Rarely, the portal vein re-

opens. Even with such reopening, high pressure in the portal vein may persist.

A doctor suspects portal vein thrombosis based on the findings during a physical examination: primarily, sudden bleeding in the upper digestive tract and an enlarged spleen. Ultrasound, CT, or MRI can be helpful. To confirm the diagnosis, a doctor may perform a liver biopsy,◆ in which a small piece of liver tissue is removed with a needle and examined under a microscope. If the person has high pressure in the portal vein and the biopsy reveals that the cells are normal, portal vein thrombosis is a possible culprit. Ultrasound or computed tomography (CT) scans may show the blockage. The diagnosis is confirmed by angiography—an x-ray technique that creates images of the veins after a radiopaque dye (a dye visible on x-rays) is injected into the portal vein—or by magnetic resonance imaging (MRI).

Treatment

Treatment is aimed at reducing the pressure in the portal vein and preventing bleeding of esophageal varices.

Surgery may be performed to create a connection (shunt) between the portal vein and the inferior vena cava, causing blood flow to bypass the liver, thereby reducing the pressure in the portal vein. If cirrhosis is present or liver function is impaired, bypass surgery increases the risk of liver encephalopathy (brain damage from liver disease).▼ Sometimes, instead of surgery, a radiologist can connect the hepatic venous system to the portal vein by passing a needle through the skin and directly into the liver; guide wires and catheters are then inserted through the needle and used to create a shunt.

In some people, liver transplantation may be the most effective treatment, depending on the underlying cause and on the condition of the person.▶

A doctor may try to close the esophageal varices by applying rubber bands to them (ligation) or by injecting them with irritating chemicals (sclerotherapy) given through an endoscope (a flexible viewing tube with surgical attachments).

▲ see page 1077	■ see page 150
★ see page 190	● see page 1452
◆ see page 790	▼ see page 795
▶ see page 1077	

Blood Vessel Disorders Resulting From Other Diseases

Severe heart failure can cause increased pressure in the hepatic veins (the veins through which blood leaves the liver). This increased pressure can eventually cause liver damage. Treating the heart failure often allows normal liver function to resume.

Sickle cell disease is an inherited disorder that affects red blood cells.▲ In this disorder, abnormally shaped red blood cells may block blood vessels inside the liver, causing liver damage.

Hereditary hemorrhagic telangiectasia (Rendu-Osler-Weber disease)■ is an inherited disorder that can affect the liver. When the liver is affected, small areas of abnormally wide blood vessels (telangiectasia) develop in the liver. These abnormal blood vessels create short connections (shunts) between arteries and veins. The shunts can cause severe heart failure, which can further damage and enlarge the liver. The shunted blood flow also produces a continuous roaring noise (bruit) that can be heard through a stethoscope. Also typical in hereditary hemorrhagic telangiectasia are scars affecting parts of the liver (cirrhosis and fibrosis) and noncancerous (benign) tumors composed of blood vessels (hemangiomas).

CHAPTER 139

Liver Tumors

Liver tumors may be noncancerous (benign) or cancerous (malignant). Cancerous liver tumors are classified as primary (originating in the liver) or metastatic (spreading from elsewhere in the body). Most liver cancers are metastatic; the liver is particularly vulnerable to metastatic cancer because of the large volume of blood that it filters from the heart and the digestive tract.

Noncancerous liver tumors are relatively common and usually cause no symptoms. Most are detected only when people happen to undergo a scanning test—such as an ultrasound, computed tomography (CT), or magnetic resonance imaging (MRI)—for an unrelated reason. However, in rare cases, some noncancerous tumors cause the liver to enlarge or to bleed into the abdominal cavity. The liver usually functions normally even when a noncancerous tumor is present, and results of liver function tests are usually within normal limits.

Hemangioma

A hemangioma is a noncancerous liver tumor composed of a mass of abnormal blood vessels.

In the United States, an estimated 1 to 5% of adults have small hemangiomas that cause no symptoms. These tumors are usually detected only if a person with them happens to undergo an ultrasound or computed tomography (CT) scan. Such tumors do not require treatment. Hemangiomas that do cause symptoms are very rare. In infants, large hemangiomas occasionally produce symptoms that lead to their detection, such as widespread blood clotting and heart failure. Surgery may be required to remove these large hemangiomas.

Hepatocellular Adenoma

A hepatocellular adenoma is a common noncancerous liver tumor that may be mistaken for a cancerous tumor and that in rare cases may rupture and bleed.

Hepatocellular adenomas occur mainly in women of childbearing age, particularly among those who use oral contraceptives.

These tumors usually cause no symptoms, so most remain undetected. Rarely, a hepatocellular adenoma suddenly ruptures and bleeds into the abdominal cavity, requiring emergency surgery. Hepatocellular adenomas caused by oral contraceptive use often disappear when the woman stops taking the drug. In extremely rare cases, a hepatocellular adenoma becomes cancerous, in which case treatment is the same as that for a hepatoma.

▲ see page 992   ■ see page 996

Hepatoma

A hepatoma (hepatocellular carcinoma) is a cancer that begins in the liver cells (a primary liver cancer).

Hepatomas are the most common type of cancer originating in the liver. In certain areas of Africa and Southeast Asia, hepatomas are even more common than metastatic liver cancer, and they are a prominent cause of death. These areas have a high prevalence of chronic infection with the hepatitis B virus, which increases the risk of hepatomas more than 100-fold. Chronic infection with hepatitis C also increases the risk of hepatomas. Finally, certain cancer-causing substances (carcinogens) produce hepatomas. In subtropical regions where hepatomas are common, food is often contaminated by carcinogens called aflatoxins, substances that are produced by certain types of fungi.

In North America, Europe, and other geographic areas where hepatomas are less common, most people with hepatomas are alcoholics with long-standing cirrhosis (severe scarring of the liver). Additional types of cirrhosis may lead to hepatomas, although the risk is lower with primary biliary cirrhosis than with other types.

Fibrolamellar carcinoma is a rare type of hepatoma that usually affects relatively young adults. It is not caused by preexisting cirrhosis, hepatitis B or C virus infection, or other known risk factors.

Symptoms

Usually, the first symptoms of a hepatoma are abdominal pain, weight loss, and a large mass that can be felt in the upper right abdomen. Alternatively, a person who has had cirrhosis for a long time may unexpectedly become much more ill. A fever may occur. Occasionally, the first symptoms are sudden abdominal pain and shock (extremely low blood pressure) caused by a rupture or bleeding of the tumor.

Diagnosis

In people with a hepatoma, levels of alpha-fetoprotein in the blood typically are high. Rarely, blood tests reveal low levels of blood sugar (glucose) or high levels of calcium, fats (lipids), or red blood cells.

At first, the symptoms do not provide many clues to the diagnosis. However, once the liver enlarges enough to be felt, a doctor may suspect a hepatoma, especially if the person has long-standing cirrhosis. Occasionally, a doctor can hear rushing sounds (hepatic bruits—due to the blood rushing through blood vessels inside the cancer) and scratchy sounds (friction rubs—due to irritation caused by the cancer rubbing against the liver surface and surrounding structures) when a stethoscope is placed over the liver.

Cancers that have not yet caused symptoms can sometimes be detected by abdominal ultrasound, computed tomography (CT) scans, or magnetic resonance imaging (MRI). In some countries where the hepatitis B virus is common, such as Japan, ultrasound scans are used to screen people with hepatitis B infection for liver cancer. X-rays taken after a radiopaque dye (a dye visible on x-rays) is injected into the main artery in the liver (hepatic artery) may reveal a hepatoma. This is particularly useful before surgical removal of the hepatoma because it shows the doctor the precise location of the liver's blood vessels.

A liver biopsy, in which a small sample of liver tissue is removed with a needle for examination under a microscope, can confirm the diagnosis.▲ The risk of bleeding or other injury during a liver biopsy generally is low.

Prognosis and Treatment

Usually, the survival rate for people in the United States with a hepatoma is poor because the tumor is detected at a late stage. In some other countries, such as Japan, the survival rate is higher because of routine screening and thus earlier detection. Occasionally, a person with a small tumor may do very well after the tumor is surgically removed. Chemotherapy drugs can be injected into a vein or into the hepatic artery, which then delivers a high concentration of the drugs directly to the cancer cells in the liver. Although chemotherapy drugs can temporarily slow the growth of the tumor, they do not cure the cancer.

Other Primary Liver Cancers

A **cholangiocarcinoma** is a relatively slow-growing cancer that originates in the lining of the bile channels in the liver or bile ducts outside the liver. In China, infestation with liver flukes (a type of parasite) may be partly responsible for this cancer. People with long-standing ulcerative colitis and sclerosing cholan-

▲ see page 790

gitis occasionally develop cholangiocarcinoma. Symptoms of the cancer are often vague but may include sudden deterioration of the person's general health, with jaundice (a yellowish discoloration of the skin and the whites of the eyes), weight loss, and abdominal discomfort.

A **hepatoblastoma** is one of the more common cancers in infants, boys being affected twice as often as girls are. Occasionally, it occurs in older children and may produce hormones called gonadotropins that result in early (precocious) puberty.▲ No underlying cause is known.

An **angiosarcoma** is a rare cancer originating in the blood vessels of the liver. An angiosarcoma may be caused by exposure to vinyl chloride in the workplace, such as in the manufacture of polyvinyl chloride (PVC), or by exposure to arsenic. However, in most people, there is no discernible cause.

Diagnosis and Treatment

A hepatoblastoma is usually suspected when a doctor feels a large mass in an infant's upper right abdomen and the infant is in overall failing health. Cholangiocarcinoma within the liver, hepatoblastoma, and angiosarcoma are diagnosed by liver biopsy, in which a sample of liver tissue is removed with a needle for examination under a microscope.■ Cholangiocarcinoma of the bile ducts outside the liver is usually diagnosed by special x-ray techniques (endoscopic retrograde cholangiopancreatography [ERCP] or percutaneous transhepatic cholangiography★) or at surgery. In two thirds of people with this type of cancer, the cancer has already spread to nearby lymph nodes by the time it is detected.

Usually, treatment of these cancers has little value, and most people die within a few months of when the tumor was detected. If the cancer is detected relatively early, however, the tumor may be surgically removed, offering the hope of long-term survival.

Metastatic Liver Cancer

Metastatic liver cancer is a cancer that has spread to the liver from elsewhere in the body.

Metastatic liver cancer most commonly originates in the lung, breast, large intestine, pan-

creas, or stomach. Leukemia (a cancer of white blood cells) and lymphoma (a cancer of the lymph system) may involve the liver. Sometimes the discovery of a metastatic liver cancer is the first indication that a person has cancer.

Symptoms

Often, the first symptoms include weight loss and poor appetite. Fever may be present. Typically, the liver is enlarged and hard and may be tender; often the liver feels lumpy as well. Occasionally the spleen is enlarged, especially if the cancer originated in the pancreas. At first, the person has mild or no jaundice (a yellowish discoloration of the skin and the whites of the eyes) unless the cancer is blocking the bile ducts. Later, the abdominal cavity may become swollen (distended) with fluid, a condition called ascites.● In the weeks before the person dies, jaundice progressively worsens. Also, the person may become confused and drowsy as toxins accumulate in the brain, a condition called liver encephalopathy.◆

Diagnosis

The diagnosis is often difficult in the early stages of the disease but becomes fairly easy in the late stages. The tumors often damage the liver, causing it to malfunction and resulting in abnormal liver function test results. Ultrasound, computed tomography (CT), and magnetic resonance imaging (MRI) of the liver may reveal the cancer, but these scans cannot always detect small tumors or distinguish a tumor from cirrhosis or other abnormalities.

A liver biopsy, in which a sample of liver tissue is removed with a needle for examination under a microscope,▼ confirms the diagnosis in only about 75% of cases. To improve the chances of obtaining cancerous tissue, a doctor sometimes uses ultrasound to guide the insertion of the biopsy needle. Alternatively, a biopsy specimen may be obtained while a doctor looks at the liver through a laparoscope (a flexible viewing tube that is inserted through the abdominal wall).

Treatment

Depending on the type of cancer, chemotherapy drugs may be used to temporarily shrink the tumor and prolong life, but they do not cure the cancer. Chemotherapy drugs may be injected into the liver's main artery (the hepatic artery), which then delivers a high concentration of the drugs directly to the can-

---

▲ see box on page 1557   ■ see page 790

★ see art on page 790   ● see page 794

◆ see page 795   ▼ see page 790

cer cells in the liver. Radiation therapy to the liver can sometimes reduce severe pain, but it has little other benefit.

If only a single tumor is found in the liver, it may be surgically removed, especially if it originated in the intestines. However, not all experts consider this surgery worthwhile. For most people with extensive cancer, all a doctor can do is relieve the symptoms.▲ A person may develop an advance directive ■ to specify the type of care desired if he becomes unable to make decisions about care.

CHAPTER 140

Gallbladder Disorders

The gallbladder is a small, pear-shaped organ located beneath the liver. The gallbladder stores bile, the greenish yellow digestive fluid produced by the liver. When bile is needed, the gallbladder contracts, pushing the bile through the lower portion of the bile duct into the small intestine.

Disorders such as gallstones and tumors can obstruct the flow of bile through the bile ducts. Occasionally, an injury during gallbladder surgery may cause an obstruction, or the duct may be narrowed as it passes through a chronically diseased pancreas. Rarer causes of bile duct obstruction include infection by the parasite *Ascaris lumbricoides* or *Clonorchis sinensis*. Cancer of the gallbladder itself is extremely rare.

Gallstones

Gallstones are collections of solid crystals (predominantly cholesterol) in the gallbladder or in the bile ducts (biliary tract). When stones are in the gallbladder, the condition is called **cholelithiasis;** *when stones are in the bile ducts, the condition is called* **choledocholithiasis.**

Gallstones are more common among women and among certain groups of people, such as Native Americans. The risk factors for gallstone formation include increased age, obesity, a typical Western diet, and a family history of gallstones. In the United States, about 20% of people older than age 65 have gallstones. Generally, gallstones do not cause symptoms; about 80% of affected people never experience any problems. Each year, more than half a million people in the United States have their gallbladder surgically removed.

In the Western world, the major component of most gallstones is cholesterol, which is insoluble in water yet can dissolve in bile. Bile contains large amounts of cholesterol that usually remains dissolved in the bile. When bile becomes oversaturated with cholesterol, however, the cholesterol becomes insoluble and crystallizes. The microscopic crystals accumulate. Some gallstones are made up of calcium salts and bilirubin, the main pigment in bile (these are called pigmented stones).

Most gallstones form in the gallbladder, which retains the small crystals and allows them to grow. Stones in the bile ducts have usually traveled there from the gallbladder. Stones that form in a bile duct are usually associated with infection or inflammation and consist of pigment material. Any stone in the bile duct system, however, can cause obstruction with inflammation and bacterial infection. A stricture (narrowing) can result, leading to further obstruction of bile flow even after the stone passes.

Symptoms

Most gallstones do not cause any symptoms for many years, if ever, particularly if they remain in the gallbladder.

Typically, gallstones pass from the gallbladder into the bile ducts. If tiny, they may pass through these ducts and into the small intestine without incident, or they may remain in the ducts without obstructing the flow of bile or causing symptoms. Stones that obstruct a bile duct, however, may cause pain as well as nausea and vomiting. Obstruction can allow bacteria to flourish and quickly establish in-

---

▲ see page 48   ■ see page 54

What Are Gallstones?

Gallstones are usually composed mainly of cholesterol that has crystallized from bile. Gallstones usually form in the gallbladder and may lodge in the cystic duct, the common bile duct, or the pancreatic duct.

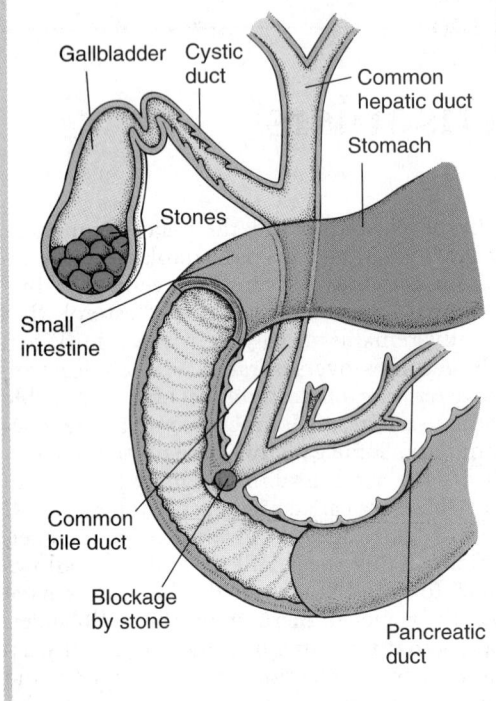

abdomen, usually on the right side under the ribs. This pain comes on gradually, can last from 30 minutes to 12 hours, and resolves. Continued obstruction causes the gallbladder to become inflamed (a condition called acute cholecystitis▲). The pain persists and may extend to the right shoulder blade. The person may have a fever as well.

Stones also can obstruct the pancreatic duct (which joins the pancreas with the common bile duct), causing inflammation of the pancreas (pancreatitis) as well as pain.

Rarely, large gallstones gradually erode the gallbladder wall and enter the small intestine. A gallstone in the small intestine can cause an intestinal obstruction, called a gallstone ileus. This condition occurs more commonly in older people.

Diagnosis

With simple biliary colic, blood test results usually are normal. In acute cholecystitis, the white blood cell count is elevated. With stones obstructing the bile ducts, liver function tests are abnormal, exhibiting a pattern of impaired bile secretion (cholestasis), often with a rise in the amount of the pigment bilirubin. Ultrasound scanning is essential. This method is 95% accurate in detecting gallstones in the gallbladder. Although less accurate in detecting stones in the bile ducts, ultrasound may show that the obstruction has caused the ducts to dilate. Other diagnostic techniques may be necessary, such as endoscopic retrograde cholangiopancreatography (ERCP),■ computed tomography (CT), or magnetic resonance imaging (MRI) of the biliary and pancreatic system.

Treatment

Most people with gallstones that do not cause any symptoms ("silent" gallstones) do not require treatment. People with intermittent episodes of pain can try avoiding or reducing their intake of fatty foods, but dietary restriction rarely prevents pain or changes the progression of symptoms.

Gallstones in the Gallbladder: If gallstones in the gallbladder cause disruptive recurring attacks of pain, a doctor may recommend surgical removal of the gallbladder (cholecystectomy). Removal of the gallbladder causes no change in digestion. No special dietary restrictions are required after surgery. During cholecystectomy, the doctor may investigate the possibility of stones in the bile ducts.

fection in the ducts and occasionally to cause abscesses (pus-filled pockets of infection) in the liver. If an infection develops, it may be accompanied by fever, chills, and jaundice (a yellowish discoloration of the skin and the whites of the eyes). Occasionally, a life-threatening infection called bacterial cholangitis develops. In bacterial cholangitis, the bacteria may spread to the bloodstream and cause infections elsewhere in the body, increasing the risk of death.

Stones that obstruct the outlet of the gallbladder or the cystic duct (the duct that joins the gallbladder with the common bile duct) result in steady pain (biliary colic) in the upper

▲ see page 815

■ see art on page 790 and page 815

About 90% of cholecystectomies are performed laparoscopically. In this method, the gallbladder is removed through tubes inserted through small incisions in the abdominal wall. Laparoscopic cholecystectomy has lessened the discomfort after surgery, shortened the length of hospital stays, and reduced sick leave time.

An alternative method of treating gallstone disease without removing the gallbladder involves dissolving gallstones with drugs. Ingestion of bile acids (ursodeoxycholic acid), for example, can dissolve some gallstones. Daily therapy can dissolve tiny stones in 6 months; larger stones may take up to 1 to 2 years. The success rate varies from about 80% for very small stones to less than 40% for large stones, which are the most common. However, even if the stones are successfully dissolved, half of the people so treated develop gallstones again within 5 years.

Gallstones in the Bile Ducts: Stones in the bile ducts can cause serious problems; therefore, they should be removed surgically or by endoscopic retrograde cholangiopancreatography (ERCP). With ERCP, an endoscope (a flexible viewing tube with surgical attachments) is passed through the mouth, down the esophagus, through the stomach, and into the small intestine.▲ A thin catheter is passed through the endoscope, into the sphincter of Oddi, and up into the common bile duct. Radiopaque dye (a dye that is visible on x-rays) is then injected through the catheter into the bile ducts, and x-rays are taken to detect any abnormalities.

Most stones can be removed from the bile duct during the ERCP procedure. An instrument passed through the endoscope is used to cut the lower bile duct where it joins the duodenum (endoscopic sphincterotomy). Sometimes the stones spill out spontaneously into the duodenum once the cut is made. If not, a basket is passed up into the bile ducts, where it encircles and traps the stone. The basket is then pulled out through the endoscope. When the cut is made, the sphincter of Oddi (between the bile ducts and the duodenum) is opened wide enough to let any future stones that might obstruct the bile duct pass spontaneously into the small intestine and eventually exit in the stool.

ERCP in combination with endoscopic sphincterotomy is successful in 90% of people. Gallstones located only in the gallbladder cannot be removed by this technique. Fewer than 1% of people who undergo this procedure

die, and 3 to 7% experience complications, making this procedure a safer option than open abdominal surgery and exploration of the common duct. Immediate complications include bleeding, inflammation of the pancreas (pancreatitis), and perforation or infection of the bile ducts. In 2 to 6% of the people who undergo this procedure, the inflamed ducts narrow (stricture), and stones may develop here in the future.

Most people who have undergone ERCP and endoscopic sphincterotomy later have their gallbladder removed. Otherwise, they are at risk of developing acute gallbladder problems in later years or passing stones into the duct system, causing recurrent obstruction.

Cholecystitis

Cholecystitis is inflammation of the gallbladder wall, usually resulting from a gallstone obstructing the cystic duct.

Acute cholecystitis is the sudden onset of inflammation of the gallbladder, resulting in severe, steady upper abdominal pain (biliary colic), which may occur repeatedly. Chronic cholecystitis is long-standing inflammation of the gallbladder characterized by repeated attacks of pain (gallbladder attacks) over a prolonged period.

At least 95% of people with acute cholecystitis have gallstones. The inflammation almost always begins without infection, although infection may follow later. Rarely, acute cholecystitis occurs in a person without gallstones (acalculous cholecystitis). Acalculous cholecystitis is a serious disease. It tends to occur after major injuries, operations, burns, bodywide infections (sepsis), and critical illnesses—particularly in people receiving prolonged intravenous feedings. It can occur in young children as well, perhaps originating as an infection (viral or other).

In chronic cholecystitis, the gallbladder is damaged by repeated attacks of acute inflammation, usually from gallstones, and may become thick-walled, scarred, and small. The gallbladder generally contains sludge or gallstones that often obstruct its outlet or the cystic duct.

Symptoms

A gallbladder attack, whether in acute or chronic cholecystitis, begins as severe, steady

▲ see art on page 790

pain (biliary colic), usually in the right upper part of the abdomen. The person typically feels a sharp pain when a doctor presses on the upper right part of the abdomen. The pain may worsen when the person breathes deeply and often extends to the lower part of the right shoulder blade. The pain may become excruciating; nausea and vomiting are usual. The pain usually lasts more than 12 hours.

Within a few hours, the abdominal muscles on the right side become rigid. Fever occurs in about one third of people but is less likely in older people. The fever tends to be slight at first, then rises gradually to above 100° F (38° C).

Typically, an attack of cholecystitis subsides in 2 to 3 days and completely disappears in a week. If the attack persists, it may signal a serious complication. A high fever, chills, a marked increase in the white blood cell count, and a cessation of the normal propulsive movements of the intestine (ileus▲) suggest formation of an abscess (a pus-filled pocket of infection), gangrene (death of tissue), or a perforated (pierced) gallbladder.

Other complications may occur. A gallbladder attack accompanied by jaundice■ and other evidence of a backup of bile into the liver (cholestasis), such as passing light-colored stools, indicates that the common bile duct is obstructed (usually partially) by a stone. If blood test results reveal an increased level of a pancreatic enzyme (amylase or lipase), the person may have inflammation of the pancreas (pancreatitis) caused by a stone obstructing the pancreatic duct.

In acalculous cholecystitis, typically the person has no previous symptoms or other evidence of gallbladder disease and experiences sudden, excruciating pain in the upper abdomen. Usually, the disease is very severe and can lead to gangrene or rupture of the gallbladder. If the person has other severe problems (for example, the person is in the intensive care unit), acalculous cholecystitis at first may be overlooked.

Diagnosis

Doctors diagnose cholecystitis, both acute and chronic, based on the person's symptoms and the results of tests that suggest gallbladder inflammation. Increased levels of white blood cells suggest inflammation or infection or both. Ultrasound scans often confirm the presence of gallstones in the gallbladder, which may be responsible for the attacks. Ultrasound scans can also show thickening of the gallbladder wall, which is typical of chronic cholecystitis.

Cholescintigraphy is an imaging technique that is useful when acute cholecystitis is difficult to diagnose. In this test, a radioactive tracer is injected intravenously and its movement from the liver through the biliary tract is followed. Images are taken of the liver, bile ducts, gallbladder, and upper part of the small intestine. If the tracer does not fill the gallbladder, it is presumed that the cystic duct is obstructed by a gallstone.

Treatment

A person with acute or chronic cholecystitis who experiences a gallbladder attack usually is hospitalized, is given fluids and electrolytes intravenously, and is not allowed to eat or drink. A doctor may pass a tube through the nose and into the stomach, so that suctioning can be used to keep the stomach empty and reduce fluid accumulating in the intestines, which do not work properly because of the inflammation of the abdominal cavity. Antibiotics usually are given.

In acute cholecystitis, if the diagnosis is certain and the risk of surgery is small, the gallbladder usually is removed during the first day or two of the illness. If necessary, gallbladder removal may be delayed; if the attack subsides, removal may wait 6 weeks or more. If a complication such as an abscess, gangrene, or perforation of the gallbladder is suspected, immediate surgery is necessary.

In chronic cholecystitis, treatment generally involves surgical removal of the gallbladder, usually by laparoscopic cholecystectomy, once the acute episode subsides.

In acalculous cholecystitis, immediate surgery is necessary to remove the diseased gallbladder.

After gallbladder removal for cholecystitis with gallstones, a small percentage of people develop new or recurring episodes of pain that feel like gallbladder attacks even though they no longer have a gallbladder. The cause of these episodes is not known, but episodes may result from an abnormal function of the sphincter of Oddi, the opening at the base of the bile duct that controls the release of bile into the small intestine. Pain is believed to result from increased pressure in the ducts caused by resistance to the flow of bile or pan-

▲ see page 781   ■ see page 791

creatic secretions. In some people, small gallstones remaining after surgery may cause pain. A doctor can use endoscopic retrograde cholangiopancreatography to widen (by cutting) the sphincter of Oddi. This procedure usually relieves symptoms in people who have a recognizable abnormality of the sphincter. In many others, the pain is caused by another problem, such as the irritable bowel syndrome or even peptic ulcer disease.

Bile Duct Tumors

Cancer is a far less common cause of bile duct obstruction than stones. Most cancers originate in the head of the pancreas, through which the common bile duct runs.▲ Less commonly, cancers originate in the biliary tract itself at the junction of the common bile duct and the pancreatic duct, in the gallbladder, or in the liver. Much less commonly, the bile ducts are obstructed by cancer that has spread (metastasized) from elsewhere in the body, or the bile ducts are compressed by lymph nodes affected with lymphoma.■ Noncancerous (benign) tumors in bile ducts also cause obstruction.

Symptoms and Diagnosis

The symptoms of bile duct obstruction are progressive jaundice, abdominal discomfort, loss of appetite, weight loss, and itchiness, usually without fever and chills. Symptoms gradually worsen. When the obstruction is due to cancer, the person may experience fatigue, discomfort, and itchiness that may be particularly distressing.

A tumor in the bile ducts may be detected using ultrasound scanning or computed tomography (CT). A tissue sample can usually be obtained by inserting a thin needle through the skin under ultrasound or CT guidance. Endoscopic retrograde cholangiopancreatography (ERCP) may also be used to provide a tissue sample.★

Treatment

ERCP allows bypass tubes (stents) to be inserted to ensure that bile can flow around the obstruction, which also helps control pain and relieve itchiness. A cancerous tumor usually cannot be completely removed surgically. Most cancerous tumors do not respond well to radiation therapy. Chemotherapy for tumors that have spread from other parts of the body (metastatic tumors) may provide some relief from the symptoms but ultimately does not dramatically improve survival.

▲ see page 773   ■ see page 1016

★ see art on page 790

KIDNEY AND URINARY TRACT DISORDERS

141   Biology of the Kidneys and Urinary Tract.................................820

Kidneys ▪ Ureters ▪ Bladder ▪ Urethra ▪ Effects of Aging

142   Symptoms and Diagnosis of Kidney and Urinary Tract Disorders 823

Fever ▪ Pain ▪ Fatigue, Nausea, Vomiting, and Itching ▪ Swelling ▪ Problems with Urination ▪ Urinalysis ▪ Kidney Function Tests ▪ Imaging Tests ▪ Cystoscopy ▪ Tissue and Cell Sampling

143   Kidney Failure..828

Acute Kidney Failure ▪ Chronic Kidney Failure ▪ Dialysis

144   Nephritis 837

Nephritic Syndrome ▪ Nephrotic Syndrome ▪ Asymptomatic Proteinuria and Hematuria Syndrome ▪ Tubulointerstitial Nephritis

145   Blood Vessel Disorders of the Kidneys 844

Blockage of the Renal Arteries ▪ Atheroembolic Kidney Disease ▪ Cortical Necrosis ▪ Malignant Nephrosclerosis ▪ Renal Vein Thrombosis

146   Tubular and Cystic Kidney Disorders 849

Renal Tubular Acidosis ▪ Renal Glucosuria ▪ Nephrogenic Diabetes Insipidus ▪ Cystinuria ▪ Fanconi's Syndrome ▪ Hypophosphatemic Rickets ▪ Hartnup Disease ▪ Bartter's Syndrome ▪ Liddle's Syndrome ▪ Polycystic Kidney Disease ▪ Medullary Cystic Disease ▪ Medullary Sponge Kidney ▪ Alport's Syndrome ▪ Nail-Patella Syndrome

147   Urinary Incontinence 857

148   Urinary Tract Obstruction 862

Hydronephrosis ▪ Stones in the Urinary Tract

149   Urinary Tract Infections 866

Urethritis ▪ Cystitis ▪ Ureteritis ▪ Pyelonephritis

150   Injury to the Urinary Tract 872

Kidney Injuries   ▪   Ureteral Injuries   ▪   Bladder Injuries   ▪
Urethral Injuries

151   Cancers of the Kidney and Urinary Tract 875

Kidney Cancer   ▪   Cancers of the Renal Pelvis and Ureters   ▪
Bladder Cancer   ▪   Cancer of the Urethra

CHAPTER 141

Biology of the Kidneys and Urinary Tract

Normally, a person has two kidneys. The remainder of the urinary tract consists of two ureters (the tubes attached to the kidneys and to the bladder), the bladder, and the urethra (a tube attached to the bladder that leads to the outside of the body). Each kidney continuously produces urine, which then drains through the ureter into the bladder at a low pressure. From the bladder, urine drains through the urethra and exits the body through the penis in males and the vulva in females. Under normal circumstances, urine is free of bacteria and other infectious organisms.

Kidneys

The kidneys are bean-shaped organs, each about 4 to 5 inches long. One lies on each side of the spinal column, just behind the space that contains the digestive organs (abdominal cavity). Each kidney receives blood through a branch of the aorta, called the renal artery. Blood flows from the renal artery into progressively smaller arteries, the smallest being the arterioles. From the arterioles, blood flows into glomeruli, which are tufts of microscopic vessels that are called capillaries. Blood exits each glomerulus through another arteriole, which connects to a small vein. The small veins join to form a single large renal vein, which carries blood away from each kidney.

Nephrons are microscopic units that filter the blood and produce urine. Each kidney contains about one million nephrons. Each nephron consists of a glomerulus surrounded

by a thin-walled, bowl-shaped structure (Bowman's capsule), a tiny tube (tubule) that drains fluid from a space in Bowman's capsule, and a collecting duct that drains urine (the fluid becomes urine by the time it reaches the collecting ducts) from the tubule. Each tubule has three interconnected parts: the proximal convoluted tubule, the loop of Henle, and the distal convoluted tubule. The kidneys consist of an outer part (cortex) and an inner part (medulla). All of the glomeruli are located in the cortex, while the tubules reside in both the cortex and the medulla. The urine drains from the collecting ducts of many thousands of nephrons into a cuplike structure (calix). Each kidney has several calices, all of which drain into a single central chamber (renal pelvis). Urine drains from the renal pelvis of each kidney into a ureter.

The Kidney's Functions

All of the functions normally performed by two kidneys can be carried out adequately by one healthy kidney. Some people are born with only one kidney and others choose to donate one kidney. In other cases, one kidney may be severely damaged by disease or injury.

Filtration and Excretion of Waste Products: The primary functions of the kidneys are to filter the blood and eliminate (excrete) metabolic waste products and excess water and electrolytes (for example, sodium, potassium, chloride, glucose, and bicarbonate). In addition, many drugs are excreted by the kidneys.

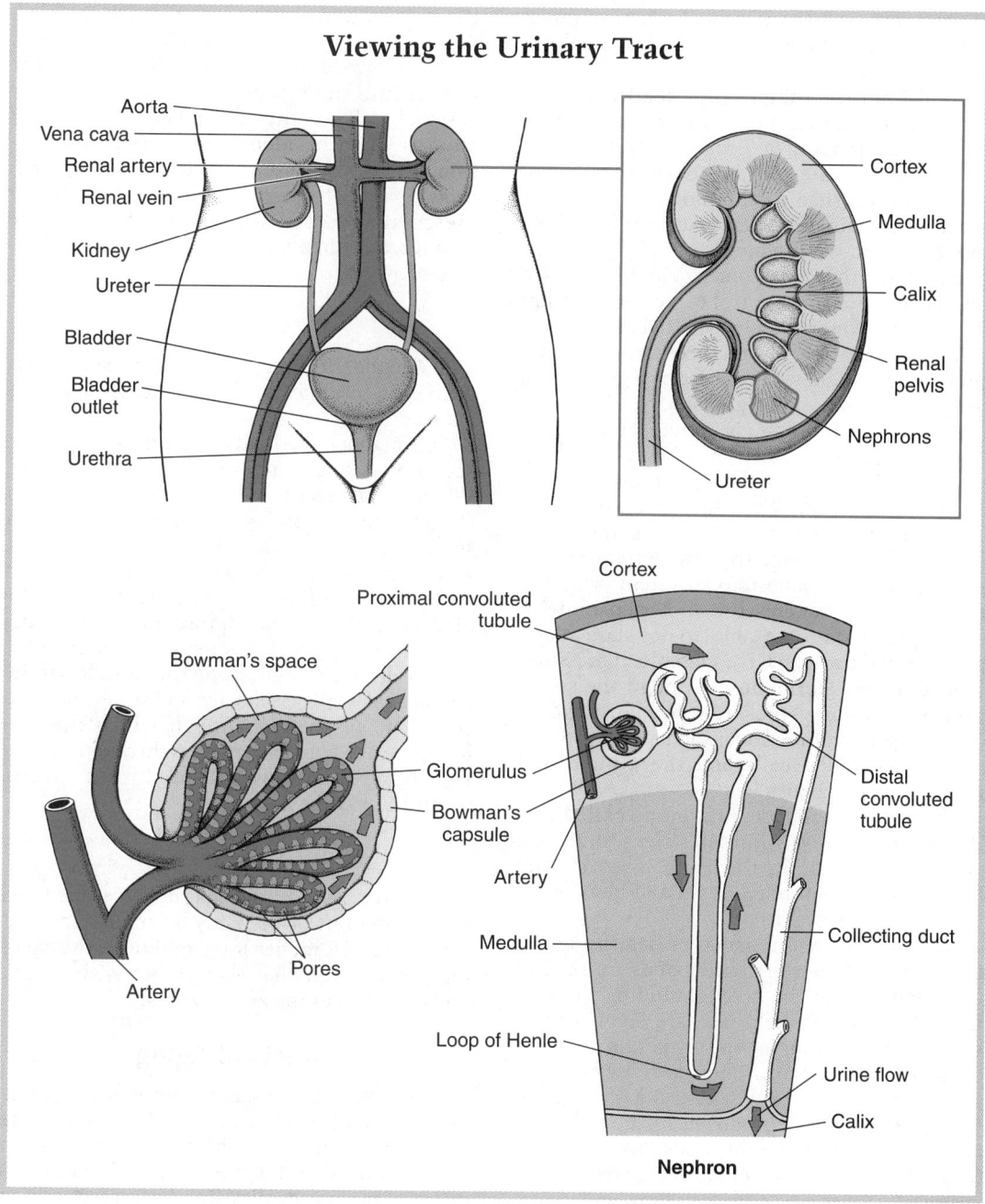

Viewing the Urinary Tract

Nephron

Blood enters a glomerulus at high pressure. Much of the fluid part of blood is filtered through small pores in the glomerulus, leaving behind blood cells and most large molecules, such as proteins. The clear, filtered fluid enters Bowman's space and passes into the tubule leading from Bowman's capsule. In the first part of the tubule, most of the sodium, water, glucose, and other filtered substances are reabsorbed and ultimately returned to the blood. In the next part of the tubule, sodium, potassium, and chloride are pumped out, and the remaining fluid becomes increasingly dilute. The dilute fluid passes through the next part of the tubule, where more sodium is pumped out in exchange for potassium and acid, which are pumped in.

Fluid from the tubules of several nephrons enters a collecting duct. In the collecting ducts, fluid (now urine) may continue as dilute urine, or water can be absorbed from the urine and returned to the blood, making the urine more concentrated. Antidiuretic hormone, which is produced by the pituitary gland, and other hormones help to regulate kidney function and control urine composition to maintain water and electrolyte balance.

Regulation of Blood Pressure: Another function of the kidneys is to help regulate the body's blood pressure by excreting excess sodium. If too little sodium is excreted, blood pressure is likely to increase. The kidneys also help regulate blood pressure by producing an enzyme called renin. When blood pressure falls below normal levels, the kidneys secrete renin into the bloodstream, thereby activating the renin-angiotensin-aldosterone system, which in turn raises blood pressure.▲ A person with kidney failure is less able to regulate blood pressure and tends to have high blood pressure.

Secretion of Hormones: Through the secretion of hormones, the kidneys help regulate other important functions, such as the production of red blood cells and the growth and maintenance of bones.

The kidneys produce a hormone called erythropoietin, which stimulates the production of red blood cells in the bone marrow. The bone marrow then releases the red blood cells into the bloodstream.

Growth and maintenance of healthy bones is a complex process that depends on several organ systems of the body, including the kidneys. The kidneys help regulate levels of calcium and phosphorus, the minerals that are critical to bone health. They do so by converting an inactive form of vitamin D (a type of hormone), which is produced in the skin and is also present in many foods, to an active form of vitamin D (calcitriol). Calcitriol then stimulates absorption of calcium and phosphorus from the small intestine.

Ureters

The ureters are muscular tubes—about 16 inches long—that attach at their upper end to the kidneys and at their lower end to the bladder.

Urine formed in the kidneys flows down the ureters into the bladder, but it does not flow passively. The ureters push each small amount of urine along in waves of contraction, at low pressure. At the bladder, each ureter passes through a sphincter, a circular muscular structure that opens to let the urine through and then closes tightly like the aperture of a camera.

Bladder

The bladder is an expandable, muscular sac. Urine accumulates in the bladder as it arrives from the ureters.

The bladder gradually increases in size to accommodate an increasing volume of urine. When the bladder is full, nerve signals are sent to the brain to convey the need to urinate. A sphincter located at the bladder's outlet, where the bladder and urethra meet, opens to allow urine to flow out. Simultaneously, the bladder wall contracts automatically, creating pressure that forces the urine down the urethra. Voluntarily tightening the muscles of the abdominal wall assists by adding extra pressure. The sphincters through which the ureters enter the bladder remain tightly shut to prevent urine from flowing back up the ureters toward the kidneys.

Urethra

The urethra is a tube that drains urine from the bladder out of the body. In males, the urethra is about 8 inches long, ending at the tip of the penis. In females, the urethra is about $1\frac{1}{2}$ inches long, ending at the vulva.

Effects of Aging

As people age, there is a slow, steady decline in the weight of the kidneys. After about age 30 to 40, about two thirds of people (even those who do not have kidney disease) undergo a gradual decline in the rate at which their kidneys filter blood. However, the rate does not change in the remaining one third of older people, which suggests that factors other than age may affect kidney function.

As people age, many glomeruli are lost because of thickening of the walls, or even blockage, of some of the small arteries that flow into the glomeruli. Accompanying the loss of glomeruli is a decline in the ability of the nephrons to concentrate or dilute urine and to excrete acid. Despite age-related changes, however, sufficient kidney function is preserved to meet the needs of the body. Changes that occur with age do not in and of themselves cause disease, but the changes do reduce the amount of reserve kidney function that is available.

The ureters do not change much with age, but the bladder and the urethra do undergo some changes. The maximum volume of urine that the bladder can hold decreases. A person's ability to delay urination after first sensing a need to urinate also declines. The rate of urine flow out of the bladder and into the urethra

slows. Throughout life, sporadic contractions of bladder wall muscles occur separate from any need or appropriate opportunity to urinate. In younger people, most of these contractions are blocked by spinal cord and brain controls, but the number of sporadic contractions that are not blocked rises with age. There is an increase in the amount of urine that remains in the bladder after urination is completed. In women, the urethra shortens and its lining becomes thinner; these changes in the urethra decrease the ability of the urinary sphincter to close tightly. The trigger for these changes in a woman's urethra seems to be a declining level of estrogen during menopause.

CHAPTER 142

Symptoms and Diagnosis of Kidney and Urinary Tract Disorders

Kidney and urinary tract disorders can affect one or both kidneys, one or both ureters, the bladder, or the urethra.

Symptoms

Symptoms of urinary tract disorders often provide important clues to doctors. However, some urinary tract disorders, including infection, stones, urinary tract obstruction, and tumors, may be present even when the person does not have symptoms. Chronic kidney failure, in particular, produces no symptoms until the disease has progressed to an advanced stage. The first symptom is often a general feeling of illness (malaise), or loss of appetite, which may lead to weight loss. In older people, mental confusion may be the first recognized symptom.

Fever

Fever can be a symptom of kidney inflammation (nephritis) or kidney stones due to infection. A bacterial infection of the kidney (pyelonephritis) almost always causes a high fever. Kidney cancer sometimes causes fever. A bladder infection (cystitis) rarely causes a fever unless complicated by stones or obstruction.

Pain

Pain caused by kidney disorders usually is felt in the side (flank) or small of the back. Occasionally, the pain radiates to the center of the abdomen. Usually pain occurs because the kidney's outer covering (renal capsule) is stretched because of a disorder that produces swelling of the kidney tissue.

A kidney stone causes excruciating pain when it enters a ureter. The ureter contracts in response to the stone, causing severe, crampy pain (renal colic) in the lower back, often radiating to the groin. The pain stops when the ureter relaxes or once the stone passes into the bladder.

Pain in the bladder is most often caused by a bacterial infection. The discomfort is usually felt above the pubic bone and at the outer end of the urethra while the person is urinating. Blocked urine outflow causes pain above the pubic bone. However, a blockage that develops slowly may enlarge the bladder painlessly.

Fatigue, Nausea, Vomiting, and Itching

Fatigue, nausea, vomiting, and overall itching of the skin commonly develop in people who have kidney failure. These symptoms result from the accumulation of metabolic waste, including acids, which the diseased kidneys are unable to excrete. Fatigue may also result from decreased production of red blood cells, a frequent problem in chronic kidney failure.

Swelling

Swelling results from accumulation of fluid in the tissues (edema). The swelling may cause weight gain. Swelling is usually most noticeable in the ankles and feet, but it may also involve the abdomen, lower back, hands, and face.

Swelling may occur if the kidneys are unable to excrete excess water and sodium from the body. Swelling may also develop from a kidney disorder that causes the loss of large amounts of protein (especially albumin) in the urine (nephrotic syndrome). When the albumin level in the blood drops sufficiently, swelling occurs as fluid leaks from the circulation into the tissues.

Problems with Urination

Most people urinate about 4 to 6 times a day, mostly in the daytime. Normally, adults pass about 3 cups to 2 quarts of urine a day. Infants may pass as little as 1 cup per day.

Frequency: Anything that increases urine production, such as diuretics and a high level of sugar in the blood, can cause frequency. A frequent need to urinate without an increase in the total daily output of urine is a symptom of a urinary tract infection (UTI) or of something irritating the bladder, such as a stone or tumor. A tumor or other mass pressing on the outside of the bladder can also cause a frequent urge to urinate because the mass reduces the capacity of the bladder. An inability to fully empty the bladder because of partial obstruction, often from an enlarged prostate, can produce frequency.

Changes in Output: A kidney disorder can impair the kidney's ability to concentrate urine, increasing the daily output of urine. Very large amounts of urine are often a response to a high level of glucose (sugar) in the blood (as in diabetes mellitus), decreased production of antidiuretic hormone by the pituitary gland (diabetes insipidus), or the kidneys' lack of response to antidiuretic hormone (nephrogenic diabetes insipidus).

Certain kidney disorders (such as kidney failure) and urinary tract disorders (such as obstruction of both ureters, an obstruction of the outlet of the bladder, or an obstruction of the urethra) may cause the daily output of urine to suddenly decrease to less than 2 cups a day. A persistently reduced output of less than about 1 cup of urine a day leads to the buildup of metabolic wastes in the blood (azotemia).

Urinating at Night: In the early stages of many kidney disorders, a person may need to urinate frequently during the night (nocturia). Nocturia is also common in people with heart failure, liver failure, poorly controlled diabetes mellitus, or diabetes insipidus. A person may have nocturia if the kidneys cannot concentrate urine normally. Frequent urination of very small amounts at night may result when the flow of urine into and through the urethra is obstructed and urine backs up in the bladder; an enlarged prostate is the most common cause of obstruction in older men.▲ Sometimes, however, the cause of nocturia may simply be drinking a large amount of fluids, especially alcohol, coffee, or tea, in the late evening.

Bed-wetting (enuresis) is normal in young children. After about age 5 or 6, it may indicate a delay in the maturation of the muscles and nerves of the lower urinary tract, which most often resolves without treatment. If bed-wetting persists, other causes are considered, such as an infection or narrowing (stricture) of the urethra, inadequate control of the nerves of the bladder, or psychologic causes.

Hesitating, Straining, and Dribbling: A hesitating start when urinating, a need to strain, a weak and trickling stream of urine, and dribbling at the end of urination are common symptoms of a partially obstructed urethra. In men, these symptoms are caused most commonly by an enlarged prostate that compresses the urethra and less often by a narrowing (stricture) of the urethra. Similar symptoms in a boy may mean that he was born with an abnormally narrow urethra or has a urethra with an abnormally narrow external opening. The opening may also be abnormally narrow in women.

Urgency: A compelling need to urinate (urgency), which may feel like almost constant painful straining (tenesmus), can be caused by bladder irritation. Incontinence may occur if a person does not urinate immediately.

Incontinence: An uncontrollable loss of urine (incontinence) can have a variety of causes.■

▲ see page 1329   ■ see page 857

Blood or Gas in the Urine: Blood in the urine (hematuria) can make the urine appear red or brown, depending on the amount of blood, how long it has been in the urine, and how acidic the urine is. An amount of blood too small to turn the urine red may be detected by chemical tests or microscopic examination. Blood in the urine without pain may be caused by problems in the bladder, urethra, ureters, or kidneys. Causes of blood in the urine that may or may not be accompanied by pain include kidney stones, kidney cysts, sickle cell disease, hydronephrosis, and cancer. Blood in the urine with pain is often the result of a kidney or bladder infection, or of a stone, or a blood clot moving through one of the ureters or the urethra.

Passing gas (air) in the urine, a rare symptom, usually indicates an abnormal connection (fistula) between the urinary tract and the intestine. A fistula may be a complication of diverticulitis, other types of intestinal inflammation, an abscess, or cancer. A fistula between the bladder and the vagina may also cause gas to escape into the urine. Rarely, bacteria in the urine may produce gas.

Changes in the Urine's Color: Normally, dilute urine is nearly colorless. Concentrated urine is deep yellow. Colors other than yellow are abnormal. Food pigments can make the urine red, and drugs can produce a variety of colors: brown, black, blue, green, or red. Brown urine may contain broken-down hemoglobin (the protein that carries oxygen in red blood cells), which is present if blood leaks into the urine from kidney, ureter, or bladder disease. Less commonly, broken-down hemoglobin may be present because of certain disorders, such as hemolytic anemia. Brown urine may contain muscle proteins excreted into the urine after severe muscle injury. Urine may be red because of pigments caused by porphyria, or black because of pigments produced by melanoma. Cloudy urine suggests the presence of pus from a urinary tract infection or the presence of crystals of salts from uric acid or from phosphoric acid. Doctors usually can identify the cause of an abnormal color with chemical tests or by examining the urine under a microscope.

Changes in the Urine's Odor: The odor of urine may provide clues about certain diseases and conditions. The odor is usually stronger if the urine is more concentrated, as occurs in dehydration. The urine may smell foul in a person who has a bacterial infection of the kidneys or the urinary tract. The urine may smell sweet in a person with uncontrolled diabetes mellitus. The urine may smell musty in a child with phenylketonuria.▲

Diagnosis

During a physical examination, a doctor attempts to feel the kidneys. Except for newborn infants, normal kidneys cannot usually be felt in children or adults. Enlarged kidneys or a kidney tumor may be detectable. Often, a distended bladder also can be felt. The doctor performs a rectal examination in a man to determine whether the prostate gland is enlarged, although the size of the prostate as ascertained by rectal examination does not always correlate with the degree of urethral obstruction. A vaginal examination in a woman may provide information about the bladder and urethra.

Additional procedures may need to be performed to diagnose a kidney or urinary tract disorder.

Urinalysis

Urinalysis can be used to detect and measure the level of a variety of substances in the urine, including protein, glucose (sugar), ketones, blood, and other substances. These tests use a thin strip of plastic (dipstick) impregnated with chemicals that react with substances in the urine and change color. Sometimes, the test results are confirmed with more sophisticated and accurate laboratory analysis of the urine. The urine is examined under a microscope to check for the presence of red and white blood cells, crystals, and casts.

Protein: Protein in the urine (proteinuria) can usually be detected quickly by dipstick. Protein may appear constantly or only intermittently in the urine, depending on the cause. Proteinuria is usually a sign of kidney disorders, but it may occur normally after strenuous exercise such as marathon running.

Glucose: Glucose in the urine (glucosuria) can be accurately detected by dipstick. The most common cause of glucose in the urine is diabetes mellitus. If glucose continues to appear in the urine while glucose levels in the blood are normal, impaired reabsorption of glucose by the kidney tubules (renal glucosuria) is the cause of the glucosuria.

▲ see page 1618

Obtaining a Clean-Catch Urine Sample

1. The head of a man's penis or opening of a woman's urethra is cleansed, usually with a small pad that contains an antiseptic substance.

2. The first few drops of urine are allowed to flow into the toilet, washing out the urethra.

3. Urination is resumed, and a sample is collected from the stream into a sterile cup.

Ketones: Ketones in the urine (ketonuria) can be detected by dipstick. Ketones are formed when the body breaks down fat. Starvation, uncontrolled diabetes mellitus, and occasionally alcohol intoxication can produce ketones in the urine.

Blood: Blood in the urine (hematuria) is detectable by dipstick and confirmed by viewing the urine with a microscope and other tests. Sometimes the urine contains enough blood to be visible, making the urine appear red or brown.

Nitrites: Nitrites in the urine (nitrituria) are also detectable by dipstick. High nitrite levels indicate an infection.

Leukocyte Esterase: Leukocyte esterase (an enzyme found in certain white blood cells) in the urine can be detected by dipstick. Leukocyte esterase is a sign of inflammation, which is most commonly caused by a urinary tract infection.

Acidity: The acidity of urine is measured by dipstick. Certain foods and metabolic disorders may change the acidity of urine.

Concentration: The concentration of urine (also called the osmolality or specific gravity) may be important in diagnosing abnormal kidney function. The kidneys lose their capacity to concentrate urine at an early stage of a disorder that leads to kidney failure. In one special test, a person drinks no water or other fluids for 12 to 14 hours; in another, a person receives an injection of antidiuretic hormone. Afterward, urine concentration is measured. Normally, either test should make the urine highly concentrated. However, in certain kidney disorders (such as nephrogenic diabetes insipidus), the urine cannot be concentrated even though other kidney functions are normal.

Sediment: Sediment in urine can be examined under a microscope to provide information about a possible kidney or urinary tract disorder. Normally, urine contains a small number of cells and other debris shed from the inside of the urinary tract. A person who has a kidney or urinary tract disorder usually sheds more cells, which form a sediment if urine is centrifuged or allowed to settle.

Urine Cultures: Urine cultures, in which bacteria are grown in a urine sample in a laboratory, are performed to diagnose a urinary tract infection. The sample of urine must be obtained by the clean-catch method. Other methods to obtain an uncontaminated urine sample include passing a catheter through the urethra into the bladder or inserting a needle through the abdominal wall into the bladder (suprapubic needle aspiration).

Kidney Function Tests

Doctors can assess kidney function by performing tests on blood and urine samples. The kidney filtration rate can be estimated by measuring creatinine, a waste product, in the serum. Creatinine clearance—a more accurate test—can be approximated from a blood sample using a formula that relates the serum creatinine level to a person's age, weight, and sex. Determining creatinine clearance more precisely requires an accurately timed urine collection in conjunction with the serum creatinine determination. The level of blood urea nitrogen (BUN) can also indicate how well the kidneys are functioning, although many other factors can alter the BUN level.

Imaging Tests

X-rays: An x-ray of the abdomen can confirm that a person has two kidneys, helps assess kidney size and position, and shows stones that contain calcium in the urinary tract. However, x-rays are rarely used as the initial imaging technique in evaluating urinary tract disorders.

Ultrasonography: Ultrasonography uses reflected sound waves to produce an image of the kidney, ureters, and bladder. It is often the initial imaging technique because it can be performed safely even when kidney function is impaired. It is noninvasive, painless, and requires no radiopaque dye. Ultrasound scans provide some indirect information about kidney function, are an excellent way to estimate kidney size and position, readily detect obstruction, and help diagnose structural abnormalities. Although less accurate than computed tomography (CT) in initially detecting kidney tumors, ultrasonography is particularly useful in distinguishing a simple benign (noncancerous) cyst from a more complex cyst, or a solid mass that may be cancerous. Doctors also use ultrasonography to locate the best place for a kidney biopsy.

All types of urinary tract stones, including those that do not contain calcium, may be detected by ultrasonography, although stones smaller than 5 mm (about ¼ inch) may be missed. When doctors suspect that the flow of urine from the bladder is obstructed, they sometimes use ultrasonography to measure the amount of urine that remains in the bladder after a person makes every effort possible to urinate. Although doctors may be able to identify a bladder tumor using ultrasonography, CT is more reliable.

Computed Tomography: Computed tomography (CT) is used to evaluate kidney masses. Spiral CT, performed by continuous movement of a person through the CT scanner, permits special images of certain structures and more rapid completion of the scanning process. Spiral CT is often used in the initial evaluation of people suspected of having kidney stones because all stones can be seen with this technique. Spiral CT without the use of a radiopaque dye is useful for the investigation of stones or bleeding into the kidney or surrounding tissues. A radiopaque dye is often used to enhance images with spiral CT to evaluate obstruction of the kidney arteries.

Magnetic Resonance Imaging: Magnetic resonance imaging (MRI) can provide three-dimensional images of the kidneys, blood vessels, and structures surrounding the kidneys. MRI helps distinguish tumors from cysts. When used with a paramagnetic contrast agent to enhance images, MRI can identify disorders of kidney blood vessels.

Intravenous Urography: Intravenous urography uses a radiopaque dye to provide an image of the kidneys, ureters, and bladder. Intravenous urography is sometimes used to locate the site and identify the underlying problem when the flow of urine is obstructed. Intravenous urography can also show abnormal connections (fistulas) between the urinary tract and the skin or other organs. Intravenous urography does not work well in people with poorly functioning kidneys because the kidneys cannot excrete and concentrate the radiopaque dye normally.

Problems With Using Radiopaque Dye

Radiopaque dyes are commonly used in kidney and urinary tract imaging procedures. There are a number of such compounds that may cause two types of problems. Some people react to a radiopaque dye in a way that is very similar to an allergic reaction. Some people develop kidney problems because of the toxic effects of the dye.

About 5% of people who receive an intravenous injection of a radiopaque dye have an allergic-like reaction, which can include a rash of red, itchy welts (hives), difficulty breathing, and a drop in blood pressure. Very rarely, the reaction may be fatal. Although it is not possible for a doctor to determine with certainty whether someone will have a reaction, certain drugs (such as prednisone or diphenhydramine) can be given to someone with a history of a previous reaction to a radiopaque dye before the dye is injected. This measure reduces the chances of a reaction and the severity of reactions that do occur.

Kidney problems that develop because of the toxic effects of the dye vary. A mild decrease in kidney function is common. More severe, sometimes irreversible, kidney failure may occur in people who already have some impairment of kidney function and in people who have other medical disorders that reduce blood flow to the kidneys, such as dehydration, heart failure, or diabetes mellitus. When a radiopaque dye must be used in a person at high risk of kidney problems, the person may be given acetylcysteine by mouth in combination with fluids intravenously beforehand. The lowest dose of the dye is used. Sometimes an alternative test can be performed without the use of a dye, such as computed tomography (CT) or magnetic resonance imaging (MRI).

A **cystogram,** an x-ray image of the bladder, is obtained as part of intravenous urography. When films of the bladder and urethra are taken during and immediately after urination, the study is called a voiding cystourethrogram, which is especially useful in evaluating recurring urinary tract infections.

Retrograde Urography: In retrograde urography, a radiopaque dye similar to that used in intravenous urography is injected directly through a scope or catheter passed through the bladder and into the ureter. This technique provides good images of the bladder, ureters, and renal pelvis when intravenous urography has been unsuccessful. Retrograde urography is also useful in investigating an obstruction of a ureter. Disadvantages include the risk of infections and the need for anesthesia.

Radionuclide Scanning: A radionuclide scan of the kidneys is an imaging technique that relies on the detection of small amounts of radiation by a special gamma camera after the injection of a radioactive chemical. One type of radionuclide scan assesses kidney blood flow (renogram). Other types of scans are useful in evaluating other kidney problems.

Angiography: Angiography involves injecting a radiopaque dye into an artery. Because it has higher risks than all other kidney imaging procedures, angiography is reserved for special situations, such as the assessment of the blood supply to the kidneys. Complications of angiography may include injury to the injected arteries and neighboring organs, bleeding, an allergic-like reaction to the radiopaque dye, and acute kidney failure triggered by the radiopaque dye.

Cystoscopy

A doctor can diagnose some disorders of the bladder and urethra by looking through a flexible viewing tube (cystoscope, a type of endoscope). A cystoscope, which has a diameter about the size of a pencil, may be between 1 and 5 feet in length. Most contain a light source and a small camera, which allows the doctor to view the inside of the bladder and urethra. Many cystoscopes also contain a small clipping device on the tip, allowing the doctor to obtain a biopsy of the bladder lining.

Tissue and Cell Sampling

Kidney Biopsy: A kidney biopsy (in which a sample of kidney tissue is removed and examined under a microscope) is primarily used to help a doctor diagnose disorders that affect the specialized blood vessels of the kidney (glomeruli) or unusual causes of acute kidney failure. A biopsy is often performed on a transplanted kidney to look for signs of rejection.

When undergoing a kidney biopsy, the person lies face down, and a local anesthetic is injected into the skin and muscles of the back over the kidney. Ultrasonography or CT is used to locate the part of the kidney where the glomeruli are located and to avoid large blood vessels. The biopsy needle is inserted through the skin and into the kidney.

This procedure is not recommended for anyone with uncontrolled high blood pressure, bleeding disorders, active urinary tract infection, or only one kidney (except for a transplanted kidney). Complications include bleeding around the kidney and formation of small arteriovenous fistulas (abnormal connections between very small arteries and veins within the kidney).

Urine Cytology: Urine cytology, which is a microscopic examination of the urine to look for cancer cells, is sometimes useful in diagnosing cancers of the kidneys and urinary tract. For people at high risk—for example, smokers, petrochemical workers, and people with painless bleeding—urine cytology may be used to screen for cancer of the bladder and kidneys. For people who have had a bladder or kidney tumor removed, the technique may be used for follow-up evaluation. However, the results can sometimes indicate cancer when none is present, or they can fail to indicate cancer when it is present, especially if the cancer is very new or very slow growing.

CHAPTER 143

Kidney Failure

Kidney (renal) failure is the inability of the kidneys to adequately filter metabolic waste products from the blood.

Kidney failure has many possible causes. Some lead to a rapid decline in kidney function (acute kidney failure); others lead to a gradual decline in kidney function (chronic kidney failure). In addition to the kidneys being unable to filter metabolic waste products (such as creatinine and blood urea nitrogen) from the blood, the kidneys are less able to control the amount and distribution of body water (fluid balance) and the levels of electrolytes (sodium, potassium, calcium, phosphate) in the blood.

When kidney failure becomes chronic, blood pressure often rises. The kidneys lose their ability to produce sufficient amounts of a hormone (erythropoietin) that stimulates the formation of new red blood cells, resulting in a low red blood cell count (anemia). In children, kidney failure affects the growth of bones. In both children and adults, kidney failure can lead to weaker, abnormal bones.

Although kidney failure can affect people of all ages, both acute and chronic kidney failure are more common in older than in younger people. Many causes of kidney failure can be treated, and kidney function may recover. The availability of dialysis has transformed kidney failure from a fatal disease to a chronic one.

Acute Kidney Failure

Acute kidney failure is a rapid decline (days to weeks) in the kidneys' ability to filter metabolic waste products from the blood.

Acute kidney failure can result from any condition that decreases the blood supply to the kidneys or that obstructs urine flow anywhere along the urinary tract. Kidney failure may also result from disease affecting the kidneys themselves. In many people, no cause of acute kidney failure can be identified.

Symptoms

Symptoms depend on the severity of kidney failure, its rate of progression, and its underlying cause.

In some people, the first symptom of acute kidney failure is fluid retention, with swelling of the feet and ankles or puffiness of the face and hands. The person may notice the passage of cola-colored urine, which may indicate a number of kidney diseases. The amount of urine (which for most healthy adults is between 3 cups and 2 quarts per day) often decreases to less than 1 pint per day or stops completely. Very little urine production is called oliguria, and no urine production is called anuria. However, some people with acute kidney failure continue to produce normal amounts of urine.

As acute kidney failure persists and metabolic waste products accumulate in the body, a person may experience fatigue, a de-creased ability to concentrate on mental tasks, loss of appetite, nausea, and overall itchiness (pruritus). A person with acute kidney failure may experience a rapid heart rate (tachycardia) and lightheadedness.

If the cause is an obstruction, the backup of urine within the kidneys causes the drainage system to stretch (a condition called hydronephrosis). Urinary obstruction may produce crampy pain—ranging from mild to excruciating—usually along the sides (flanks) of the body. Some people with hydronephrosis have blood in their urine. If the obstruction is located below the bladder, the bladder will enlarge. If the bladder enlarges rapidly, the person is likely to feel severe pain. If the bladder enlarges slowly, pain may be minimal, but the lower part of the abdomen may swell from the markedly distended bladder.

If acute kidney failure develops during hospitalization, the condition often relates to some recent injury, surgical event, drug, or medical illness such as infection. The symptoms of the underlying cause of the acute kidney failure may predominate. For example, high fever, life-threatening low blood pressure (shock), and symptoms of heart failure or liver failure may occur before symptoms of kidney failure and be more obvious and urgent.

Some of the conditions that cause acute kidney failure also affect other parts of the body. For example, Wegener's granulomatosis,▲ which damages blood vessels in the kidneys, may also damage blood vessels in the lungs, causing a person to cough up blood. Skin rashes are typical of some causes of acute kidney failure, including polyarteritis nodosa, systemic lupus erythematosus, and some toxic drugs.

Diagnosis

Blood tests that measure levels of creatinine and blood urea nitrogen in the blood are needed to confirm the diagnosis. A progressive daily rise in creatinine indicates acute kidney failure. The level of creatinine is also the best indicator of the degree or severity of kidney failure; the higher the level, the more severe the failure is likely to be. Other blood tests detect metabolic imbalances that occur as kidney failure persists, such as a high acid level (acidosis), a high potassium level (hyperkalemia), a low sodium level (hyponatremia), and a high phosphorus level (hyperphosphatemia).

▲ see page 389

MAJOR CAUSES OF ACUTE KIDNEY FAILURE

CAUSE	UNDERLYING PROBLEM
Insufficient blood supply to the kidneys	Not enough blood because of blood loss, severe sodium and water loss, or physical injury that blocks blood vessels
	Heart pumping too weakly (heart failure)
	Extremely low blood pressure (shock)
	Liver failure (hepatorenal syndrome)
Obstructed urine flow	Enlarged prostate
	Tumor pressing on the urinary tract or within urinary tract
	Stones
Injuries within the kidneys	Allergic reactions (for example, to radiopaque dyes used for x-ray imaging)
	Toxic substances (drugs, poisons)
	Conditions affecting the filtering units (nephrons) of the kidneys (acute glomerulonephritis or vascular injury, such as occurs with hemolytic-uremic syndrome, systemic lupus erythematosus, atheroembolic renal disease, Wegener's granulomatosis, polyarteritis nodosa)
	Blocked arteries or veins within the kidneys
	Obstruction within the kidneys (for example, crystals such as oxalate, uric acid)
	Surgery, which can injure the kidneys
	Injury to the kidney itself, such as from an abdominal wound

The physical examination may help the doctor identify the cause of the acute kidney failure. Enlarged or tender kidneys give clues to the cause, such as obstruction with hydronephrosis. Urine tests, such as a urinalysis and a measurement of certain electrolytes, may enable the doctor to categorize the cause of kidney failure.

Imaging of the kidneys using ultrasound or computed tomography (CT) is helpful, sometimes by providing such basic information as the size of the kidneys. For example, an ultrasound can be used to identify hydronephrosis or to detect an enlarged bladder. X-rays of the renal arteries or veins (angiography) may be performed if obstruction of blood vessels is the suspected cause. Alternatively, magnetic resonance imaging (MRI) can be used. If these studies do not reveal the cause of kidney failure, a biopsy may be necessary to determine the diagnosis and the prognosis.

Prognosis and Treatment

Acute kidney failure and its immediate complications, such as fluid retention, high acid and potassium levels in the blood, and increased urea in the blood, can often be treated successfully. The overall survival rate is about 60%. Survival is less than 50% for people who have several organs failing at the same time. Yet, survival is about 90% for people whose kidney failure is due to decreased blood flow because body fluids have been lost through bleeding, vomiting, or diarrhea—conditions that are reversible with treatment.

Any treatable cause of kidney failure is addressed as soon as possible. For example, if obstruction is the cause, endoscopy or surgery may be needed to relieve the obstruction.

Often, simple but meticulous supportive care is all that is needed for the kidneys to heal themselves, especially if the kidney failure has existed for less than 5 days and has been uncomplicated by other problems such as infection.

The doctor strictly limits the person's intake of all substances that are eliminated through the kidneys, including many drugs, such as digoxin, and many antibiotics. Water intake is restricted to replacing the amount lost from the body, unless hydration is needed. A person's weight is measured every day to monitor fluid intake because measured intake may be inaccurate. A weight gain from one day to the next indicates that the person is receiving excessive fluid.

In addition to receiving nutrients such as glucose, a person with acute kidney failure receives certain amino acids (the building blocks of protein) by mouth or intravenously to maintain adequate protein levels. Salt (sodium) and potassium intake is usually restricted.

Sodium polystyrene sulfonate is sometimes given by mouth or rectally to treat a high level of potassium in the blood. Calcium salts (calcium carbonate or calcium acetate) may be given to prevent or treat a high level of phosphorus in the blood.

Fluids are not restricted in a person who is recovering from acute kidney failure caused by obstruction. During this time, the kidneys are unable to reabsorb sodium and water normally, and a large amount of urine is produced for a period of time after the obstruction is relieved. Such a person may also need replacement of fluids and electrolytes, such as sodium, potassium, and magnesium.

Acute kidney failure may be prolonged, necessitating that waste products and excess water be removed through dialysis, usually hemodialysis.▲ In these cases, dialysis is started as soon as possible after diagnosis. Dialysis may be needed only temporarily, until the kidneys recover their function, usually in several days to several weeks. If the kidneys are too badly damaged to recover, then the acute kidney failure will become chronic.

Chronic Kidney Failure

Chronic kidney failure is a slowly progressive decline (months to years) in the kidneys' ability to filter metabolic waste from the blood.

Many diseases can irreversibly damage or injure the kidneys. Acute kidney failure can become chronic if kidney function does not recover after treatment. Therefore, anything that can cause acute kidney failure can cause chronic kidney failure. However, the most common cause of chronic kidney failure is diabetes mellitus, followed by high blood pressure (hypertension). Both of these conditions directly harm the kidneys' small blood vessels. Other causes of chronic kidney failure include urinary tract obstruction; kidney abnormalities (such as polycystic kidney disease and glomerulonephritis); and autoimmune disorders (such as systemic lupus erythematosus), in which antibodies damage the tiny blood vessels (glomeruli) and the tiny tubes (tubules) of the kidneys.

Symptoms

Symptoms may develop slowly or evolve from acute kidney failure. A person with mild to moderate kidney failure may have only mild symptoms despite the increase in the levels of urea and other metabolic waste products in the blood. At this stage, the person may need to urinate several times during the night (nocturia), because the kidneys cannot absorb water from the urine to reduce the volume and concentrate it as normally occurs during the night.

As kidney failure progresses and metabolic wastes build up in the blood, the person may feel fatigued and generally weak and may become less mentally alert. These symptoms progress as the blood becomes more acidic, a condition called acidosis. A loss of appetite and shortness of breath can result. Fatigue and generalized weakness may also be attributed in part to a decline in red blood cell production and the resulting anemia. People with chronic kidney failure tend to bruise easily or bleed for an unusually long time after cuts or other injuries. Chronic kidney failure also diminishes the body's ability to fight infections.

As metabolic wastes build up in the blood, damage to muscles and nerves can cause muscle twitches, muscle weakness, cramps, and pain. The person may also feel a pins-and-needles sensation in the arms and legs and may lose sensation in certain areas of the body. Encephalopathy, a condition in which the brain malfunctions, may ensue from the buildup of metabolic waste products in the blood. This condition may lead to confusion, lethargy, and seizures.

High blood pressure often develops in people who have kidney failure, because the diseased kidneys produce hormones that raise blood pressure. In addition, diseased kidneys cannot excrete excess salt and water. Salt and fluid retention can lead to heart failure, which may cause shortness of breath. The sac that surrounds the heart (pericardium) may be-

▲ see page 834

come inflamed (pericarditis) as metabolic waste products accumulate. This complication may cause chest pain and low blood pressure. The level of triglycerides in the blood is often elevated, which, along with hypertension, increases the risk for atherosclerosis. The buildup of metabolic waste in the blood also causes nausea, vomiting, and an unpleasant taste in the mouth, which may lead to malnutrition and weight loss. People who have advanced chronic kidney failure commonly develop gastrointestinal ulcers and bleeding. The skin may turn yellow-brown, and occasionally, the concentration of urea is so high that it crystallizes from sweat, forming a white powder on the skin. Some people with chronic kidney failure itch all over their body.

The formation and maintenance of bone tissue may be impaired (renal osteodystrophy) if certain conditions that accompany chronic kidney failure are present for a long time. These conditions include a high level of parathyroid hormone, low concentration of calcitriol (the active form of vitamin D) in the blood, impaired absorption of calcium, and a high concentration of phosphate in the blood. Renal osteodystrophy may lead to bone pain and an increased risk of fractures.

Diagnosis

Blood tests are essential and show increased levels of urea and creatinine, metabolic waste products that are normally filtered out by the kidneys. Typically, the blood becomes moderately acidic. The level of potassium in the blood is normal or only slightly increased but can become dangerously high when kidney failure reaches an advanced stage or if a person ingests large amounts of potassium. Usually, the person has some decline in red blood cell count (anemia). The level of triglycerides in the blood is likely to be elevated. The calcium and calcitriol levels decrease, and the phosphate and parathyroid hormone levels increase.

Urine volume often stays about the same, regardless of the amount of fluid consumed. Analysis of the urine may detect many abnormalities, including protein and abnormal cells.

Determining a precise cause becomes increasingly difficult as the kidney failure reaches an advanced stage. A kidney biopsy may be the most accurate test, but it is not recommended if results of an ultrasound show that the kidneys are small and scarred.

Prognosis and Treatment

Ultimately, chronic kidney failure progresses in most people regardless of treatment. It is fatal if not treated. Survival when kidney failure is severe (sometimes called end-stage kidney failure) is usually limited to several months in people who are not treated, but those who are treated with dialysis can live many years. The doctor must pay attention to conditions that can cause or worsen kidney failure and consequences of the kidney failure that might adversely affect overall health. For example, infections are treated promptly with antibiotics, and any obstructions in the urinary tract are removed or relieved.

The rate of decline in kidney function depends somewhat on the underlying disorder causing the kidney failure. For example, controlling the level of sugar in the blood as well as hypertension in people with diabetes substantially slows deterioration in kidney function. Drugs called angiotensin-converting enzyme (ACE) inhibitors and also angiotensin receptor blockers may decrease the rate of decline in kidney function in some people with chronic kidney failure.

Meticulous attention to diet helps control a number of potential problems. Sometimes mild acidosis can be controlled by increasing the intake of carbohydrates and reducing proteins. However, moderate or severe acidosis may require treatment with sodium bicarbonate. The decline in kidney function can be slowed slightly by restricting the amount of protein consumed daily. The person needs to consume sufficient carbohydrates to offset the reduction in protein. The triglyceride level may be lowered somewhat by limiting fat in the diet. Drugs such as gemfibrozil may be required to reduce the triglyceride level.

The intake of salt (sodium) usually does not have to be restricted unless fluid accumulates and is retained in the tissues or high blood pressure develops. A person with heart failure needs to restrict the intake of sodium. Diuretics may also relieve symptoms of heart failure, even when kidney function is poor, but dialysis may be needed to remove the excess fluid.

During chronic kidney failure, changes in thirst usually determine how much water is consumed. Occasionally, water intake needs to be restricted to prevent the sodium concentration in the blood from becoming too low. Foods that are extremely high in potassium, such as salt substitutes, must be avoided, and foods that are somewhat high in potassium, such as dates and figs, should not be consumed in excess. A high potassium level in the blood increases the risk of abnormal heart rhythms and cardiac arrest. If the potassium level becomes too high, drugs may help, but emergency dialysis may be required.

The elevated phosphorus level in the blood can cause deposits of calcium and phosphorus to form in tissues, including the blood vessels. Restricting the intake of foods high in phosphorus, such as dairy products, liver, legumes, nuts, and most soft drinks, lowers the phosphate concentration in the blood. Drugs that bind phosphate, such as calcium carbonate and calcium acetate, taken by mouth, may also lower the phosphorus level in the blood.

The anemia caused by kidney failure responds to the drugs erythropoietin or darbepoietin. Blood transfusions are given only if the anemia is severe, is causing symptoms, and does not respond to erythropoietin or darbepoietin. Doctors also look for and treat other causes of anemia, particularly dietary deficiencies of iron, folic acid (folate), and vitamin B_{12} or excesses of aluminum in the body. Most people receiving erythropoietin or darbepoietin regularly need to be given iron intravenously to prevent iron deficiency, which impairs the body's response to these drugs. Anemia often requires more aggressive treatment in older people, because they are more likely to have heart disease, which can be aggravated by the anemia. The tendency to bleed can be temporarily suppressed by transfusions of platelets or fresh frozen plasma or by such drugs as desmopressin or estrogens. Such treatment may be needed after an injury or before a surgical procedure or a tooth extraction.

A moderate or severe increase in blood pressure is treated with blood pressure drugs to prevent further impairment of heart and kidney function.

When the treatments for chronic kidney failure are no longer effective, the only option is long-term dialysis or kidney transplantation.▲ Despite the advent of dialysis, most people with advanced kidney failure die within 5 to 10 years. End-of-life care is important.■

Dialysis

Dialysis is the process of removing waste products and excess fluids from the body.

There are a number of reasons why a person may need dialysis. Making the decision to be-

Reasons for Dialysis

Doctors decide to place a person on dialysis when the person's kidney failure is causing certain conditions:

- Abnormal brain function (uremic encephalopathy)
- Inflammation of the sac around the heart (pericarditis)
- High level of acid in the blood (acidosis) that does not respond to other treatments
- Heart failure
- Total body fluid overload
- Fluid overload in the lungs (pulmonary edema) that does not respond to other treatments
- A very high level of potassium in the blood (hyperkalemia)

gin dialysis is not easy because it entails a major change in lifestyle, including a dependency on machines to maintain life. However, for most people, a successful dialysis program results in a reasonably normal life. Most people undergoing dialysis are able to eat a tolerable diet, have normal blood pressure, do not have anemia, and avoid progression of nerve damage and other complications.

For acute kidney failure, many doctors recommend dialysis when urine output is low, and they continue the dialysis until the person's blood tests indicate that adequate kidney function has been restored. Short-term or urgent dialysis can also be used to remove certain drugs or poisons from the body.

For chronic kidney failure, doctors may recommend dialysis when tests indicate that the kidneys are not removing metabolic waste products adequately or when a person can no longer perform normal daily activities. Dialysis may be used as long-term therapy for chronic kidney failure or as an interim measure before kidney transplantation.

Dialysis usually requires the effort of a team of people. A doctor completes a dialysis prescription, manages complications, and monitors the process. A nurse monitors the person's general well-being and mental health and educates the person about such issues as exercise. A social worker arranges transportation and home assistance. A dietitian recom-

▲ see page 1077   ■ see page 45

mends an appropriate diet and monitors the person's response to dietary changes.

Types of Dialysis

There are two types of dialysis: hemodialysis and peritoneal dialysis.

Hemodialysis: In hemodialysis, blood is removed from the body and pumped by a machine outside the body into a dialyzer (artificial kidney). The dialyzer filters metabolic waste products from the blood and then returns the purified blood to the person. The total amount of fluid returned can be adjusted. A person typically undergoes hemodialysis at a dialysis center, usually outside of a hospital but sometimes located in a hospital.

Hemodialysis requires repeated access to the bloodstream. A doctor can achieve temporary access by inserting a large intravenous catheter in a big vein, usually one near the neck. An artificial connection between an artery and a vein (an arteriovenous fistula) is surgically created to make long-term access easier. In this procedure, typically the radial artery in the forearm is joined with the cephalic vein. As a result, the cephalic vein subsequently enlarges and becomes suitable for repeated puncture with a needle. When a fistula cannot be created, a synthetic graft may be surgically connected to an artery and vein. In this situation, the synthetic graft is punctured by the needle for hemodialysis.

Heparin, a drug that prevents clotting, is administered during hemodialysis to prevent blood from clotting in the dialyzer. Inside the dialyzer, a porous artificial membrane separates the blood from a fluid (the dialysate). Fluid, waste products, and electrolytes in the blood filter through the membrane into the dialysate. Blood cells and large proteins are unable to filter through the small pores of the membrane and so remain in the blood. The dialyzed (purified) blood is then returned to the person's body.

Dialyzers have different sizes and degrees of efficiency. Dialysis treatment time is usually about 3 to 4 hours. Most people who have chronic kidney failure need hemodialysis 3 times a week.

Peritoneal Dialysis: In peritoneal dialysis, the peritoneum—a membrane that lines the abdomen and covers the abdominal organs—acts as a filter. This membrane has a large surface area and a rich network of blood vessels. Substances from the blood can easily pass through the peritoneum into the abdominal cavity. A fluid (dialysate) is infused through a catheter inserted through the abdominal wall into the peritoneal space within the abdomen. The dialysate must be left in the abdomen for a sufficient time to allow metabolic waste products from the bloodstream to pass slowly into it. Then the dialysate is drained out, discarded, and replaced with fresh dialysate.

A soft silicone rubber or porous polyurethane catheter allows the dialysate to flow smoothly and is unlikely to cause damage. A catheter can be put in place temporarily at the person's bedside, or it may be surgically put in place permanently. One type of permanent catheter eventually forms a seal with the skin and can be capped when not in use.

Various techniques are used for peritoneal dialysis. In the simplest technique, manual intermittent peritoneal dialysis, bags containing dialysate are warmed to body temperature and infused into the peritoneal (abdominal) cavity for 10 minutes. The dialysate is allowed to remain there (dwell time) for 60 to 90 minutes and then drained out in about 10 to 20 minutes. The entire treatment can take 12 hours.

POSSIBLE COMPLICATIONS OF HEMODIALYSIS

COMPLICATION	CAUSE
Fever	Bacteria or fever-causing substances (pyrogens) in the bloodstream
	Overheated dialysate
Life-threatening allergic reaction (anaphylaxis)	Allergy to a substance in the dialyzer or blood tubing
Low blood pressure	Removal of too much fluid
Abnormal heart rhythms	Abnormal levels of potassium and other substances in the blood
Air embolus	Air entering blood in the machine
Bleeding in the intestine, brain, eyes, or abdomen	Heparin being used to prevent clotting in the machine
Infection	Insertion of a needle into veins for hemodialysis access

Another technique is automated cycler intermittent peritoneal dialysis, which can reduce the need for nursing attention.

In continuous ambulatory peritoneal dialysis, the dialysate is kept in the abdomen for much longer intervals. Typically, the dialysate is drained and replenished 4 or 5 times a day. Generally three of these dialysate exchanges are performed during the day, at intervals of 4 hours or longer. Each exchange takes 30 to 45 minutes. An exchange is performed at night with a long dwell time of 8 to 12 hours during sleep.

Another technique, continuous cycler-assisted peritoneal dialysis, uses an automated cycler to perform short exchanges at night during sleep, whereas longer exchanges are performed manually—without the cycler—during the day. This technique minimizes the number of exchanges during the day but prevents mobility at night because of cumbersome equipment.

Choosing a Type of Dialysis

Many factors, including lifestyle, must be considered in determining which type of dialysis is best for a person. Peritoneal dialysis can be performed at home, eliminating the need for travel to a hemodialysis center.

Doctors recommend hemodialysis for people with recent abdominal wounds or abdominal surgery. Peritoneal dialysis is better tolerated in people whose blood pressure fluctuates frequently between periods of high or normal pressure and periods of low blood pressure. With hemodialysis, blood pressure may be controlled simply by removing a sufficient amount of fluid during dialysis. Otherwise, drugs to lower blood pressure may be needed.

Special Considerations

People undergoing dialysis need a special diet. In people undergoing peritoneal dialysis, appetite is generally poor, and protein is lost during dialysis. The diet should be relatively high in protein, roughly ½ gram of protein per pound of ideal body weight a day. Salt, both the usual salt containing sodium and the salt containing potassium, is restricted.

For those undergoing hemodialysis, daily consumption of sodium and potassium is even more restricted. Foods high in phosphorus also may have to be limited. Daily fluid intake is limited for people who have a persistently low or a decreasing sodium concentration in the blood. Daily weighing is important to monitor

POSSIBLE COMPLICATIONS OF PERITONEAL DIALYSIS

COMPLICATION	CAUSE
Bleeding	A doctor may unintentionally perforate an internal organ during placement of the catheter, or bleeding may occur where the catheter leaves the body or within the abdomen
Leakage of fluid	The catheter did not seal to abdominal wall
Infection	May occur if the dialysis procedure is not sterile
Low level of albumin (a protein) in the blood	Albumin loss in fluid removed during peritoneal dialysis
Scarring of the peritoneum	Inflammation and infection, the electrolyte content of dialysis fluid, or the use of certain drugs
High sugar (glucose) level in the blood	Use of a peritoneal dialysate that has a high concentration of glucose to remove water and sodium during dialysis
Hernias of the abdomen and groin	Continuous fluid expansion of peritoneal (abdominal) cavity weakens barriers that normally prevent excessive movement of organs and other structures
Constipation	Poor dietary fiber intake or calcium salts used for treatment of high phosphate levels in the blood; may interfere with dialysate flow into and out of the abdomen

weight gain. Excessive weight gain between hemodialysis treatments indicates that the person is consuming excessive fluid.

Multivitamin supplements are needed to replace the nutrients lost through hemodialysis

Comparing Hemodialysis With Peritoneal Dialysis

When the kidneys fail, waste products and excess water can be removed from the blood by hemodialysis or peritoneal dialysis.

In hemodialysis, blood is removed from the body into a dialyzer (called an artificial kidney), which filters the blood. An artificial connection between an artery and a vein (arteriovenous fistula) is made to facilitate the removal of blood.

In peritoneal dialysis, the peritoneum is used as a filter. The peritoneum is a membrane that lines the abdomen and covers the abdominal organs, creating a space within the abdomen called the peritoneal space or abdominal cavity.

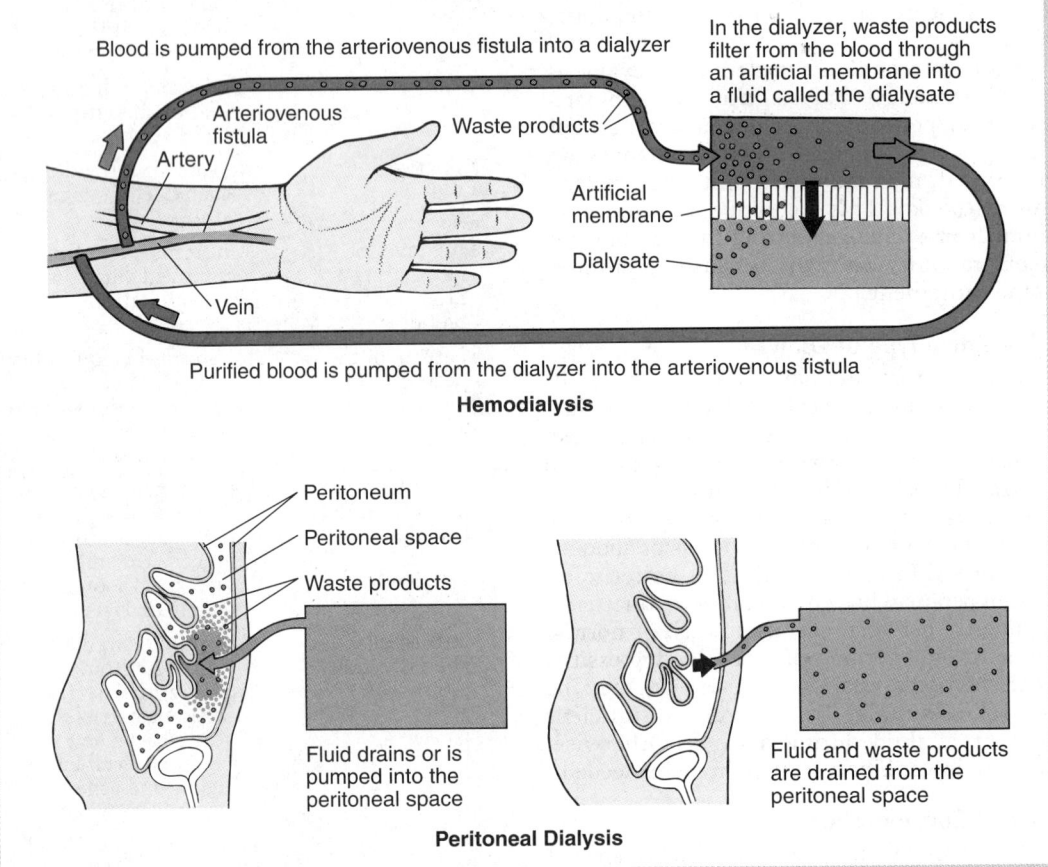

Blood is pumped from the arteriovenous fistula into a dialyzer

In the dialyzer, waste products filter from the blood through an artificial membrane into a fluid called the dialysate

Arteriovenous fistula

Artery

Waste products

Artificial membrane

Dialysate

Vein

Purified blood is pumped from the dialyzer into the arteriovenous fistula

Hemodialysis

Peritoneum

Peritoneal space

Waste products

Fluid drains or is pumped into the peritoneal space

Fluid and waste products are drained from the peritoneal space

Peritoneal Dialysis

or peritoneal dialysis. Erythropoietin or darbepoietin may be given to stimulate the production of red blood cells. Phosphate binders, such as calcium carbonate or calcium acetate, are used to remove excess dietary phosphate.

A low calcium level in the blood and severe renal osteodystrophy may be treated with calcitriol (the active form of vitamin D) and supplemental calcium.

People undergoing dialysis may experience losses in every aspect of their lives. The poten-

tial loss of independence can be especially distressing; coping with disruptions in lifestyles can be difficult. Many people undergoing dialysis become depressed and anxious. Psychologic and social counseling is often helpful to families as well as to those undergoing dialysis. Many dialysis centers provide psychologic and social support. Dealing with a loss of independence is helped when people are encouraged to pursue their previous interests. People undergoing hemodialysis need to arrange for transportation to and from dialysis centers on a regular basis. Dialysis sessions may interfere with work, school, or leisure activities.

More than half of the people on long-term dialysis are 60 years of age or older. Older people often are better able to adapt to long-term dialysis than are younger people. However, older people undergoing dialysis may become more dependent on their grown children or may not be able to continue living alone. Older people are more likely to experience fatigue from treatments. Often, family roles and responsibilities must be modified to fit the dialysis routine, creating stress and feelings of guilt and inadequacy.

Children whose growth has been stunted may feel isolated and different from their peers.▲ Young adults and adolescents coping with identity, independence, and body image issues may find these issues further complicated by dialysis. Diet is an important issue for children undergoing dialysis because children must receive enough nutrients to support their growth.

CHAPTER 144

Nephritis

Nephritis is inflammation of the kidneys. It may be caused by a bacterial infection of the kidneys (pyelonephritis)■ or exposure to a toxin. However, it more commonly develops from an abnormal immune reaction, which can occur in two ways: (1) an antibody can attack either the kidney itself or a substance that stimulates an immune reaction (antigen) attached to kidney cells, or (2) an antigen and antibody can combine somewhere else in the body, forming an immune complex, and then attach to cells in the kidney.

Some types of nephritis involve infiltration of kidney tissues by white blood cells and deposits of antibodies. In other types of nephritis, inflammation may consist of tissue swelling or scarring without white blood cells or antibodies. Nephritis can occur anywhere in the kidneys.

Nephritis most often affects the tufts of microscopic blood vessels (glomeruli) with small pores through which blood is filtered. Such inflammation is called glomerulonephritis.

When a glomerulus is damaged, substances not normally filtered out of the bloodstream— such as proteins, red blood cells, and white blood cells—can pass through the glomerulus and enter the fluid that becomes urine. Progressive damage to glomeruli causes urine production to fall and metabolic waste products to build up in the blood. When damage is severe, inflammatory cells and injured glomerular cells accumulate, compressing the capillar-

ies within the glomerulus and interfering with filtration. Scarring may develop, impairing kidney function and reducing urine production. In some cases, tiny blood clots (microthrombi) may form in the small blood vessels, further decreasing kidney function.

There are three major types of glomerulonephritis: nephritic syndrome, nephrotic syndrome, and asymptomatic proteinuria and hematuria syndrome. The three types are not exclusive; a person may have two types simultaneously, or have one type that later develops into another type.

Less commonly, nephritis involves the tubules and the tissues that surround them (tubulointerstitial tissues). Such inflammation is called tubulointerstitial nephritis. A kidney tubule is a microscopic tube that carries fluid and substances filtered from the blood in the glomerulus to the duct that drains urine into the pelvis of the kidney. Tubulointerstitial tissues surround each of the tubules and separate one tubule from another. When inflammation damages the tubules and the tubulointerstitial tissues, the kidneys may become unable to concentrate urine, eliminate (excrete) metabolic waste products from the body, or balance the excretion of sodium and other electrolytes, such as potassium. When the tubules and tubulointerstitial

---

▲ see page 1639   ■ see page 871

tissues are damaged, kidney failure often develops.

Nephritis may also involve the blood vessels within the kidneys. Inflammation of the blood vessels is called vasculitis.

Nephritic Syndrome

Nephritic syndrome is a disorder of glomeruli characterized by tissue swelling (edema), high blood pressure, and the presence of red blood cells in the urine.

Nephritic syndrome can develop suddenly or over a short time period (acute nephritic syndrome) or develop and progress slowly (chronic nephritic syndrome). In 1% of children and 10% of adults, the acute nephritic syndrome evolves into rapidly progressive glomerulonephritis, in which most of the glomeruli are destroyed, resulting in kidney failure.

Causes

Acute nephritic syndrome most often results from infection by streptococcus, a type of bacteria. Acute nephritic syndrome after a streptococcal infection (post-streptococcal glomerulonephritis) typically develops following a throat or skin infection in children between the ages of 2 and 14. Infections by other types of bacteria, such as staphylococcus and pneumococcus, viral infections such as chickenpox, and parasitic infections such as malaria can also result in acute nephritic syndrome. Membranoproliferative glomerulonephritis, IgA nephropathy, Henoch-Schönlein purpura, systemic lupus erythematosus, mixed cryoglobulinemia, Goodpasture's syndrome, and Wegener's granulomatosis are all noninfectious causes of acute nephritic syndrome. Acute nephritic syndrome that develops into rapidly progressive glomerulonephritis most often results from conditions that involve an abnormal immune reaction.

The cause of chronic nephritic syndrome cannot be identified in many people. Often, chronic nephritic syndrome seems to result from one of the same conditions that causes acute nephritic syndrome.

Symptoms

About half of the people with acute nephritic syndrome have no symptoms. If symptoms do occur, the first to appear are fluid retention and tissue swelling (edema), low urine volume, and dark urine that contains blood. Edema may first appear as puffiness of the face and eyelids but later is prominent in the legs. Blood pressure increases as kidney function becomes impaired. In turn, high blood pressure and swelling of the brain may produce headaches, visual disturbances, and more serious disturbances of brain function. In older people, nonspecific symptoms, such as nausea and a general feeling of illness (malaise), are more common.

When rapidly progressive glomerulonephritis develops, weakness, fatigue, and fever are the most obvious early symptoms. Loss of appetite, nausea, vomiting, abdominal pain, and joint pain are also common. About 50% of people had a flu-like illness in the month before kidney failure started to develop. These people have edema and usually produce very little urine. High blood pressure is uncommon and rarely severe when it does occur.

Because chronic nephritic syndrome usually causes only very mild or subtle symptoms for years, it goes undetected in most people. Fluid retention (edema) may occur. High blood pressure is common. The disease may progress to kidney failure, which can cause itchiness, fatigue, decreased appetite, nausea, vomiting, and difficulty breathing.

Diagnosis

Doctors investigate the possibility of acute nephritic syndrome in people who develop symptoms of the disorder after having had strep throat or another infection and whose laboratory test results indicate kidney dysfunction. Laboratory tests show variable amounts of protein and blood cells in the urine and a high concentration of urea and creatinine (metabolic waste products) in the blood.

In people with rapidly progressive glomerulonephritis, protein clumps (casts) of red blood cells or white blood cells are almost always visible under a microscope, and blood tests detect anemia and often an abnormally high number of white blood cells. When doctors suspect nephritic syndrome, a biopsy is usually performed to confirm the diagnosis, help determine the cause, and determine the amount of scarring and potential for reversibility.

Additional tests are sometimes helpful for identifying the cause of nephritic syndrome. For example, a throat culture may provide evidence of streptococcal infection. Blood levels of antibodies against streptococci may be higher than normal or progressively increase over several weeks. Acute nephritic syndrome that follows an infection other than strep throat is usually easier to diagnose, because its symptoms often begin while the infection is still obvious. Cultures and blood tests that help identify the organisms that cause these other types of infections are sometimes needed to confirm the diagnosis.

Chronic nephritic syndrome develops gradually, and therefore, a doctor may not be able to tell exactly when it began. It may be discovered when a urine test performed as part of a medical examination reveals the presence of protein and blood cells in a person who is feeling well, has normal kidney function, and has no symptoms. A kidney biopsy is the most reliable way to distinguish chronic nephritic syndrome from other kidney diseases. A biopsy, however, is rarely performed in advanced stages, when the kidneys are shrunken and scarred, because the chance of obtaining specific information about the cause is small.

Prognosis

Acute nephritic syndrome resolves completely in about 80 to 90% of children and about 60% of adults.

The prognosis for people with rapidly progressive glomerulonephritis depends on the severity of glomerular scarring and whether the underlying cause, such as infection, can be cured. In about half of the people who are treated early (within weeks to a few months), kidney function is preserved and dialysis is not needed. However, because the early symptoms can be subtle and vague, many people who have rapidly progressive glomerulonephritis are not aware of the underlying disease and do not seek medical care until kidney failure develops. People with advanced kidney failure die within a few weeks unless they undergo dialysis. The prognosis also depends on the cause, the person's age, and any other diseases the person might have. When the cause is unknown or the person is older, the prognosis is worse.

In some children and adults who do not recover completely from acute nephritic syndrome, other types of kidney disorders develop, such as asymptomatic proteinuria and hematuria syndrome or nephrotic syndrome. Other people with acute nephritic syndrome, especially older adults, develop chronic nephritic syndrome.

Treatment

No specific treatment is available in most cases of acute nephritic syndrome. Following a diet that is low in protein and sodium may be necessary until kidney function recovers. Diuretics may be prescribed to help the kidneys excrete excess sodium and water. High blood pressure needs to be treated.

When a bacterial infection is suspected as the cause of acute nephritic syndrome, antibiotics are usually ineffective because the nephritis begins 1 to 6 weeks (average, 2 weeks) after the infection. However, if a bacterial infection is still present when acute nephritic syndrome is discovered, antibiotic therapy is started. Antimalarial drugs may be beneficial if the cause of the syndrome is malaria.

For rapidly progressive glomerulonephritis, drugs to suppress the immune system are started promptly. High doses of corticosteroids are usually given intravenously for about a week, followed by a variable period of time when they are taken by mouth. Cyclophosphamide, an immunosuppressant, may also be given. In addition, plasmapheresis is sometimes used to remove antibodies from the blood. If treatment is delayed, there is an increased likelihood of kidney failure and the need for dialysis. Kidney transplantation is sometimes considered for people who have chronic kidney failure, but rapidly progressive glomerulonephritis may recur in the transplanted kidney.

Angiotensin-converting enzyme (ACE) inhibitors often slow progression of chronic nephritic syndrome. Taking drugs to reduce high blood pressure and reducing sodium intake are considered beneficial. Restricting the amount of protein in the diet is modestly helpful in reducing the rate of kidney deterioration. Kidney failure must be treated with dialysis or a kidney transplant.

Nephrotic Syndrome

Nephrotic syndrome is a glomerular disorder characterized by severe loss of protein in the urine, typically leading to accumulation of fluid (edema) and low levels of the protein albumin in the blood.

Nephrotic syndrome can develop from gradual progression of a mild loss of protein in the urine (sometimes called microalbuminuria), or it can develop suddenly. Nephrotic syndrome can occur at any age. In children, it is most common between the ages of 18 months and 4 years, and more boys than girls are af-

What Causes Nephrotic Syndrome?

Diseases
- Amyloidosis
- Cancer (lymphoma, leukemia, various solid tumors)
- Diabetes mellitus*
- Pregnancy-associated (toxemia)
- Nephritic syndrome
- Systemic lupus erythematosus*
- Vasculitic-immunologic disorders (Henoch-Schönlein purpura, polyarteritis, rapidly progressive glomerulonephritis)
- Viral infections (hepatitis B,* hepatitis C,* HIV*)

Drugs
- Gold
- Nonsteroidal anti-inflammatory drugs (NSAIDs)*
- Penicillamine
- Heroin taken intravenously

Allergies
- Insect bites
- Pollens
- Poison ivy and poison oak

* Asterisks indicate the most common causes.

fected. In older people, both sexes are more equally affected.

Protein loss in the urine (proteinuria) is accompanied by low levels of important proteins, such as albumin, in the blood, increased levels of fats (lipids) in the blood, a tendency for increased blood clotting, and a greater susceptibility to infection. The decreased level of albumin in the blood leads to edema in spaces where normally there is no fluid and the retention of excess sodium.

Causes

Nephrotic syndrome can be due to a vast array of diseases that affect other parts of the body, most commonly diabetes mellitus, systemic lupus erythematosus, and certain viral infections. Nephrotic syndrome can also result from nephritic syndrome. A number of drugs that are toxic to the kidneys can also cause nephrotic syndrome, especially nonsteroidal anti-inflammatory drugs (NSAIDs). The syndrome may be caused by certain allergies, including allergies to insects and poison

ivy. Some types of the syndrome are hereditary.

Symptoms

Early symptoms include loss of appetite, a general feeling of illness (malaise), puffy eyelids and tissue swelling from excess sodium and water retention, abdominal pain, wasting of muscles (atrophy), and frothy urine. The abdomen may be swollen because of a large accumulation of fluid in the abdominal cavity (ascites), and shortness of breath may develop because fluid accumulates in the space surrounding the lungs (pleural effusion). Other symptoms may include swelling of the knees and, in men, the scrotum. Most often, the fluid that causes tissue swelling is affected by gravity and therefore moves around. During the night, fluid accumulates in the upper parts of the body, such as the eyelids. During the day, fluid accumulates in the lower parts of the body, such as the ankles, when the person is sitting or standing. Swelling that worsens may hide the muscle wasting that is progressing at the same time.

In children, blood pressure is generally low, and blood pressure may fall when the child stands up (orthostatic hypotension). Shock may also develop. Adults may have low, normal, or high blood pressure. Urine production may decrease and kidney failure may develop if the leakage of fluid from blood vessels into tissues depletes the liquid component of blood and blood supply to the kidney is diminished. Occasionally, kidney failure with low urine output occurs suddenly.

Nutritional deficiencies may result from the loss of nutrients in the urine. In children, growth may be stunted. Calcium may be lost from bones. The hair and nails may become brittle, and some hair may fall out. Horizontal white lines may develop in fingernail beds for unknown reasons.

The membrane that lines the abdominal cavity and abdominal organs (peritoneum) may become inflamed and infected. Opportunistic infections—infections caused by normally harmless bacteria—are common. The higher likelihood of infection is thought to occur because the antibodies that normally combat infections are lost in the urine or not produced in normal amounts. The tendency for blood clotting (thrombosis) increases, particularly inside the main vein from the kidney. Less commonly, the blood may not clot when clotting is needed, generally leading to excessive bleeding. High blood pressure accompanied by complications affecting the heart and brain is most likely to occur in people who have diabetes and in those who have systemic lupus erythematosus.

Diagnosis

A doctor bases the diagnosis of nephrotic syndrome on the symptoms, physical examination findings, and laboratory findings. A laboratory test of urine collected over a 24-hour period is useful for measuring the degree of protein loss, but collection of urine over such a long period is difficult for many people to accomplish. Alternatively, a randomly collected urine specimen can be tested to measure the ratio of the level of urine protein to that of urine creatinine. Blood tests and other urine tests detect additional characteristics of the syndrome. The level of albumin in the blood is low because this vital protein is lost in the urine and its production is impaired. The urine often contains clumps (casts) of cells that may be combined with protein and fat. The urine contains low levels of sodium and high levels of potassium.

Blood fat (lipid) concentrations are high, sometimes exceeding 10 times that of a normal concentration. Levels of lipid in the urine are also high. Anemia may be present. Blood clotting proteins may be increased or decreased.

The doctor investigates possible causes of nephrotic syndrome, including drugs. Analysis of the urine and blood may reveal an underlying disorder. If the person has lost weight or is older, a search for cancer is undertaken. A kidney biopsy is especially useful in determining the cause and extent of kidney tissue damage.

Prognosis

The prognosis varies depending on the cause of the nephrotic syndrome, the person's age, and the type and degree of kidney damage. Symptoms may disappear completely if the nephrotic syndrome is caused by a treatable disorder, such as an infection, cancer, or drugs. This situation occurs in about half the cases in children but less often in adults. If the underlying disorder responds to corticosteroids, sometimes progression of the disease is halted, and less often the condition partially, or rarely, completely reverses. When the syndrome is caused by HIV infection, it usually progresses relentlessly, often resulting in complete kid-

ney failure in 3 or 4 months. Children born with the nephrotic syndrome rarely live beyond their first birthday, although a few have survived by means of dialysis treatments or a kidney transplant.

When the cause is systemic lupus erythematosus or diabetes mellitus, treatment with an angiotensin-converting enzyme (ACE) inhibitor often stabilizes or decreases the amount of protein in the urine. However, some people do not respond to treatment with an ACE inhibitor and develop progressive kidney failure within a few years.

In cases of nephrotic syndrome resulting from conditions such as an infection, allergy, or intravenous heroin use, the prognosis varies, depending on how early and effectively the underlying condition is treated.

Prevention and Treatment

Use of an angiotensin-converting enzyme (ACE) inhibitor, such as enalapril, quinapril, and lisinopril, is the mainstay of both prevention and treatment. When a person with a disease such as systemic lupus erythematosus or diabetes mellitus has mild or moderate proteinuria, an ACE inhibitor is used as soon as possible because it may prevent proteinuria from worsening and becoming nephrotic syndrome.

When a person who already has nephrotic syndrome is treated with an ACE inhibitor, symptoms may improve, the amount of protein excreted in the urine usually decreases, and lipid concentrations in the blood are likely to decline. However, these drugs can increase the potassium levels in the blood in people who have moderate to severe kidney failure.

General therapy for nephrotic syndrome includes a diet that contains normal amounts of protein and potassium but that is low in saturated fat and sodium. Eating too much protein increases protein levels in the urine.

If fluid accumulates in the abdomen, the person may need to eat frequent, small meals because of the reduced capacity of the stomach. High blood pressure is usually treated with diuretics. Diuretics can also reduce fluid retention and tissue swelling but may increase the risk of blood clots. Anticoagulants may help control clot formation if it occurs. Infections can be life threatening and must be treated promptly.

Whenever possible, specific treatment is aimed at the cause. Treating an infection that

PROGNOSIS OF CERTAIN GLOMERULAR DISORDERS THAT CAN CAUSE NEPHROTIC SYNDROME

GLOMERULAR DISORDER	DESCRIPTION	PROGNOSIS
Minimal change disease	A mild type of glomerulonephritis	Good prognosis: 90% of children and nearly as many adults respond to treatment, but 30 to 50% of adults relapse; rarely progresses to kidney failure; likely to recur unless the person has been free of the disease for 1 year
Focal segmental glomerulosclerosis	A disease that damages glomeruli; affects mainly adolescents but also young and middle-aged adults	The prognosis is poor because treatment is not very effective. Most adults and children progress to end-stage kidney failure 5 to 20 years after being diagnosed
Membranous glomerulonephritis	A more serious type of glomerulonephritis; affects mainly adults	Spontaneous remission of proteinuria occurs in 5 to 20% of people. Partial remission occurs in 25 to 40%. The likelihood of end-stage kidney failure rises steadily over time to about 40% at 15 years
Congenital and infantile nephrotic syndrome	A rare inherited disease; congenital nephrotic syndrome (Finnish type) and diffuse mesangial sclerosis are the two main causes; they closely resemble focal segmental glomerulosclerosis; symptoms are present at birth in the Finnish type and develop during childhood in the infantile variety	The disorder does not respond to corticosteroids. Because of severe hypoalbuminemia, removal of both kidneys is often considered. Supportive therapy, including dialysis, is given until the child is eligible for a kidney transplant
Membranoproliferative glomerulonephritis	An uncommon type of glomerulonephritis; primarily occurs between the ages of 8 and 30; sometimes the cause is unknown, or it may be caused by immune complex disease	If caused by immune complex disease, a partial remission may occur; the outcome is not as good in people in whom the cause remains unknown. About half of untreated people will progress to end-stage kidney failure within 10 to 15 years, while in most others the kidney function stabilizes or improves
Mesangial proliferative glomerulonephritis	Accounts for about 3 to 5% of people with idiopathic nephrotic syndrome; affects all ages; may be a severe form of minimal change disease	About 50% initially respond to corticosteroids; 10 to 30% develop progressive kidney failure; relapses may respond to cyclophosphamide

causes nephrotic syndrome may cure the syndrome. If a treatable disease, such as certain cancers, causes the syndrome, treating that disease can eliminate the syndrome. If a heroin user with the nephrotic syndrome stops using heroin in the early stages of the disease, the syndrome may resolve. If other drugs are responsible for the syndrome, discontinuing the drugs may be curative. People who are sensitive or allergic to poison oak, poison ivy, or insect bites should avoid these irritants. Allergy shots (desensitization) may reverse the nephrotic syndrome caused by poison oak, poison ivy, or insect bites.

If no reversible cause can be found, the person may be given corticosteroids and other drugs that suppress the immune system, such as cyclophosphamide. However, corticosteroids cause problems for children because they can stunt growth and suppress sexual development.▲

Asymptomatic Proteinuria and Hematuria Syndrome

Asymptomatic proteinuria and hematuria syndrome is a disorder of glomeruli characterized by steady or intermittent loss of small amounts of protein and blood in the urine.

Mild proteinuria and hematuria are sometimes discovered in people without symptoms, when urine tests are performed for routine purposes. The presence of clumps of red blood cells (casts) or abnormally shaped red blood cells is a clue for doctors that the blood in the urine came from glomeruli. A kidney biopsy may show that glomeruli contain deposits of antibodies or slight changes in the cells that filter the blood. However, a kidney biopsy is rarely performed because the likelihood of finding a treatable disease is very low.

Doctors usually recommend that people with this syndrome have a physical examination and undergo urine testing once or twice a year. Additional tests are performed if the amount of protein or blood increases much, or if symptoms occur that suggest the development of a specific disease. Most people with asymptomatic proteinuria and hematuria syndrome do not worsen, and the condition may persist indefinitely.

Tubulointerstitial Nephritis

Tubulointerstitial nephritis is inflammation that affects the tubules of the kidneys and the tissues that surround them (tubulointerstitial tissue).

Tubulointerstitial nephritis may be acute or chronic, and it often results in kidney failure. It may be caused by various diseases, drugs, or toxins that damage the kidneys.

Causes

The most common cause of acute tubulointerstitial nephritis is an allergic reaction to a drug. Antibiotics such as penicillin and the sulfonamides, diuretics, and nonsteroidal anti-inflammatory drugs (NSAIDs)—including as-

pirin—may trigger an allergic reaction. The interval between the exposure to the allergen that caused the reaction and the development of acute tubulointerstitial nephritis varies from 5 days to 5 weeks.

Bacterial infection of the kidneys (pyelonephritis) can also cause acute or chronic tubulointerstitial nephritis.

Symptoms and Diagnosis

Some people have few or no symptoms. When symptoms develop, they are highly variable, and they may develop suddenly or gradually.

When tubulointerstitial nephritis develops suddenly, the amount of urine produced may be normal or less than normal. Some people develop the symptoms of a urinary tract infection: fever, painful urination, pus in the urine, and pain in the lower back or side (flank). If the cause is an allergic reaction, symptoms may include a fever and a rash.

When tubulointerstitial nephritis develops gradually, the first symptoms to appear are those of kidney failure, such as itchiness, fatigue, decreased appetite, nausea, vomiting, and difficulty breathing. Blood pressure is normal or only slightly above normal in the early stages of the disease.

Laboratory tests usually detect signs of kidney failure, such as an increase in the level of waste products in the blood. A kidney biopsy is the only conclusive means of diagnosing this disorder, although a biopsy is rarely performed except when the cause cannot be found or treatment with corticosteroids is being considered.

When tubulointerstitial nephritis develops suddenly, the urine may be almost normal, with only a trace of protein or pus, but often the abnormalities are striking. The urine may show large numbers of white blood cells, including eosinophils. Eosinophils rarely appear in the urine, but when they do, a person almost certainly has acute tubulointerstitial nephritis caused by an allergic reaction. Also, the number of eosinophils in the blood may be increased.

When an allergic reaction is the cause, the kidneys usually are large because of inflammation caused by the allergic reaction. This enlargement can be seen with x-rays or ultrasound scanning.

▲ see box on page 374

Prognosis and Treatment

Kidney function usually improves when an offending drug is discontinued or treatment of the underlying disease is effective, although some kidney scarring is common. Treatment with a corticosteroid may speed the recovery of kidney function when the disorder is caused by an allergic reaction. If kidney function worsens and kidney failure develops, dialysis is usually needed. In some cases, the damage is irreversible, and kidney failure becomes chronic.

When the inflammation occurs gradually, kidney damage may develop at different rates in different portions of the kidney. When the proximal tubule is damaged, the normal reabsorption of sodium, potassium, bicarbonate, uric acid, and phosphate may be altered, resulting in low bicarbonate (metabolic acidosis), low potassium (hypokalemia), low uric acid (hypouricemia), and low phosphate (hypophosphatemia). Injuries to the distal tubule are usually associated with a loss of urine concentrating ability and an increase in daily urine volume (polyuria). Kidney damage usually progresses to involve most or all of the kidney, resulting in the need for dialysis or kidney transplantation.

CHAPTER 145

Blood Vessel Disorders of the Kidneys

The blood flow to the kidneys needs to be intact for the kidneys to function properly. Any interruption or reduction in the blood flow can cause kidney damage, dysfunction, and increased blood pressure. When blood flow in the arteries supplying the kidneys is completely blocked, the entire kidney or a portion of the kidney supplied by that artery dies (kidney infarction); this condition can lead to kidney failure.

Blood vessel disorders of the kidneys have a number of causes, including blockages in the renal (kidney) arteries or veins, inflammation of blood vessels (vasculitis), and injury to the kidneys or blood vessels.

Blockage of the Renal Arteries

There are two renal arteries—one supplies blood to the right kidney, the other to the left kidney. These arteries branch into many smaller arteries. Blockage of the renal artery or one of its large or medium-sized branches is rare. Most often a blockage occurs when a clot moves from elsewhere in the body and lodges in the renal artery (embolus). Typically, such clots originate as fragments from a larger clot in the heart or from the breakup of a fatty deposit (atheroma) in the aorta.

Alternatively, a blockage may result when a blood clot forms in the renal artery itself, usually where the artery has been injured. A sudden injury may be caused by a medical procedure, such as surgery, angiography, or angioplasty. A clot may also develop where the renal artery has been gradually injured or damaged by atherosclerosis, arteritis (inflammation of arteries), or an aneurysm (a slow-forming bulge in the wall of the artery).

A tear in the lining of the aorta or the renal artery can cause a sudden obstruction of blood flow; a tear may also cause the artery to rupture. Diseases that cause the walls of arteries to become thicker and less elastic because of deposits of fatty material (atherosclerosis) or the development of fibrous material (fibrodysplasia) may predispose vessels to tears. These disorders can lead to significant narrowing and partial blockage of the renal arteries even when there is no blood clot; when this occurs, the condition is called renal artery stenosis.

Symptoms

A partial blockage of the renal arteries usually does not cause any symptoms. However, as the blockage worsens, a person may have a steady aching pain in the lower back or occasionally in the lower abdomen. A partial blockage may gradually lead to high blood pressure, or a sudden worsening of previous high blood pressure may occur when a person has gradual and progressive narrowing of one or both renal arteries. If the person is given an angiotensin-converting enzyme (ACE) inhibitor or an angiotensin II blocker to treat high blood pressure, kidney function may decline rapidly. The effect is reversible if the drug is discontinued promptly.

If a blockage is the result of a clot that has moved to and lodged in one of the renal artery segments, the person may have clots elsewhere in the body, such as in the intestines, brain, and the skin of the fingers and toes. These clots may cause pain in these areas as well as small ulcers or gangrene, or a small stroke.

A complete blockage of one of the renal arteries may cause fever, nausea, vomiting, and back pain. Rarely, a blockage causes bleeding that turns the urine red or dark brown. Complete blockage of both renal arteries—or of one renal artery in people who have only one kidney—completely stops urine production and shuts down the kidneys (acute kidney failure).

Diagnosis

A doctor may suspect a blockage based on the person's symptoms. Laboratory tests, such as a complete blood count and urinalysis (microscopic examination of the urine), may add further clues. The amount of lactate dehydrogenase in the blood is often increased; lactate dehydrogenase is an enzyme that is often released when organ damage has occurred.

Because none of the symptoms or laboratory tests can specifically identify a blockage, a doctor needs to perform imaging tests of the kidneys to demonstrate that they are not functioning properly. Intravenous urography or radionuclide scanning can show absent or diminished blood flow to the affected kidney. However, neither of these procedures can distinguish between kidney infarction and other conditions that result in poor kidney function. Retrograde urography or ultrasound may be needed to make this distinction.

Angiography is one of the best procedures a doctor can use to confirm the diagnosis. However, angiography is performed only if the doctor is considering surgery to relieve the blockage. An alternative is a special type of computed tomography (spiral CT), which can accurately show a blockage. Doctors may monitor how well kidney function recovers by

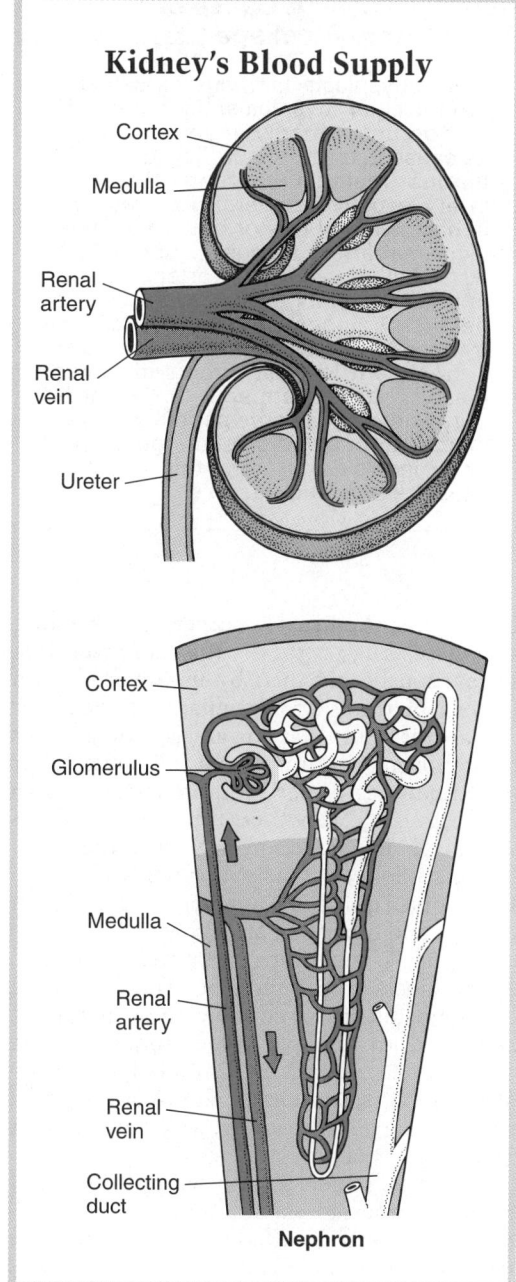

Kidney's Blood Supply

Cortex

Medulla

Renal artery

Renal vein

Ureter

Cortex

Glomerulus

Medulla

Renal artery

Renal vein

Collecting duct

Nephron

repeating ultrasound or radionuclide scanning at frequent intervals.

Treatment

Treatment is aimed at preventing further deterioration of blood flow and restoring blood flow that has been blocked. In the case of

Fibrodysplasia: A Cause of Renal Artery Blockage

Fibrodysplasia (sometimes called fibromuscular dysplasia) is a disorder that occurs primarily in young women. Its cause is unknown. In fibrodysplasia, fibrous material narrows the renal artery, usually in several sites, resulting in narrowing of one or both renal arteries (renal artery stenosis). About 10 to 30% of all cases of renal artery stenosis in adults are due to fibrodysplasia. Renal artery stenosis from fibrodysplasia frequently causes high blood pressure.

Treatment is most often with angioplasty. After treatment, the disorder may not recur in some people, and usually the high blood pressure goes away or is improved. Rarely, this condition causes kidney failure.

blood clots, the usual treatment is with anticoagulant drugs;▲ these drugs are given first intravenously and then by mouth for longer periods of time. Anticoagulants prevent the initial clot from enlarging and additional clots from forming. Drugs that dissolve clots (thrombolytics)■ may be more effective than anticoagulants. However, thrombolytic drugs improve kidney function only when the artery is not completely blocked or when clots can be dissolved quickly. After 3 hours, permanent damage and infarction are likely.

Surgery is sometimes performed to open an artery blocked by a clot, but this treatment has a greater risk of complications and death and does not improve kidney function more than anticoagulant or thrombolytic drugs alone. Drug treatment is almost always preferred to surgery. However, when the cause is injury, the artery must be repaired.

To relieve a blockage caused by atherosclerosis or fibrodysplasia of a renal artery, a doctor may thread a balloon catheter from the femoral artery in the groin to the renal artery. The balloon is then inflated to force open the obstructed area. This procedure is called percutaneous transluminal angioplasty. When doctors perform this procedure, they may place a short hollow tube (stent) in the artery to prevent the blockage from occurring again. Anti-

coagulant drugs are also often used after this procedure. When angioplasty is unsuccessful, surgery is needed to remove or bypass a blockage caused by atherosclerosis or fibrodysplasia.

Although kidney function may improve with treatment, it usually is not restored completely. The person's outlook is poor when clot fragments from other parts of the body are involved because similar clots often cause problems in the brain, liver, intestines, and feet at the same time.

Atheroembolic Kidney Disease

In atheroembolic kidney disease, numerous small pieces of fatty material (atheroemboli) travel from arteries above the kidneys to clog the smallest branches of the renal arteries, causing the kidneys to fail.

Tiny pieces of hard fatty material adhering to a blood vessel wall, usually the aorta, break off and travel to the smallest renal arteries, blocking the blood supply. Usually, this process affects both kidneys equally and at the same time.

The fatty material may break off spontaneously when there is severe atherosclerosis of the aorta. It may also occur as a complication of surgery or angioplasty, or imaging procedures that involve the aorta, such as angiography, when pieces of fatty material adhering to the walls of the aorta are unintentionally broken off. Atheroembolic kidney disease is much more common in older people.

Symptoms and Diagnosis

Atheroembolic kidney disease usually produces slowly progressive failure of the kidneys that causes no symptoms until the failure is advanced. If the blockage of arteries results from a surgical or imaging procedure involving the aorta, the kidneys often fail suddenly. Urine production is often decreased.

As the duration and severity of kidney failure increase, a wide variety of symptoms may appear, beginning with fatigue, nausea, loss of appetite, itching, and difficulty concentrating. The symptoms reflect disturbances in the muscles, brain and nerves, heart, digestive tract, and skin that result from kidney failure.

Atheroemboli may cause symptoms in other organs. If atheroemboli travel to the arms or legs, particularly the toes, such symptoms as a lacy purplish discoloration of the skin and even gangrene may result. Pieces of

▲ see box on page 997

■ see box on page 997

atheroemboli that travel to an eye may cause sudden blindness.

A kidney biopsy is the best way for a doctor to make the diagnosis; microscopic examination of a tissue sample shows characteristic evidence of fatty material in the smallest arteries. If the skin is discolored, a skin biopsy may be helpful.

Prognosis and Treatment

If the emboli travel to the brain, they may cause small strokes. Prognosis depends on how soon the body reacts to prevent additional pieces of fatty material from breaking off as fatty emboli. If the body reacts quickly, minimal damage may result. If pieces continue to break off, parts of the body may fail and death can follow.

The only treatments for advanced kidney failure are kidney dialysis and, in some cases, transplantation.

Cortical Necrosis

Cortical necrosis is tissue death that results from blockage of the small arteries that supply blood to the outer part of kidney (cortex) and causes acute kidney failure.

Cortical necrosis can occur at any age. About 10% of the cases occur in infants and children. More than half of the newborns with this condition had deliveries complicated by premature detachment of the placenta; the next most common cause is a bacterial infection of the bloodstream (sepsis). In children, cortical necrosis may follow an infection, dehydration, shock, or the hemolytic-uremic syndrome.▲

In adults, sepsis causes one third of all cases of cortical necrosis. About half of the reported cases in women follow complications of pregnancy, such as premature detachment of or abnormal position of the placenta, bleeding from the uterus, infections immediately after childbirth, blockage of arteries by amniotic fluid, death of the fetus within the uterus, and preeclampsia.

Other causes of cortical necrosis in adults include rejection of a transplanted kidney, burns, inflammation of the pancreas, injury, snakebite, and poisoning from certain chemicals.

Symptoms and Diagnosis

The urine often becomes red or dark brown because of the presence of blood. Pain along both sides of the lower back may occur. A fever is often present. Changes in blood pressure, including mildly high pressure or even low pressure, are common.

Doctors may have difficulty making a diagnosis of cortical necrosis because it may resemble other types of acute kidney failure. A doctor may suspect cortical necrosis when the flow of urine suddenly greatly decreases or stops completely in a person who has a predisposing condition.

Blood tests may reveal an increase in the number of white blood cells and abnormally shaped red blood cells circulating in the blood. Blood tests may also reveal an increase in the levels of substances typically released when kidney tissue is damaged, such as the enzyme lactic dehydrogenase. The small amount of urine that is produced contains protein and many white and red blood cells, along with kidney cells and other debris.

Initially the kidneys may appear enlarged on ultrasound and then shrink to about half of the normal size after 6 to 8 weeks. Calcium deposits seen on x-rays suggest cortical necrosis, but these deposits are found in only 20 to 50% of people. A doctor can usually confirm the diagnosis by performing a computed tomography (CT) scan. Kidney biopsy and arteriography give important information but are invasive and are not used in most people.

Treatment

Treatment is often complicated, because the underlying condition must be treated. Kidney failure requires dialysis, although 20 to 40% of people recover partially and regain enough kidney function to discontinue dialysis after several months. For most people with cortical necrosis, however, kidney transplantation or lifelong dialysis is the only solution.

Malignant Nephrosclerosis

In malignant nephrosclerosis, severe high blood pressure (malignant hypertension) damages the smallest arteries in the kidneys, and kidney failure progresses rapidly.

Malignant nephrosclerosis occurs in about 1% of people with high blood pressure and is more common among blacks than whites. It is most common in men during their 40s and 50s and women during their 30s.

▲ see page 997

Malignant hypertension most commonly results from poorly controlled high blood pressure. It may also result from other conditions, such as glomerulonephritis, chronic kidney failure, narrowing of the renal artery (renal vascular hypertension), inflammation of renal blood vessels (vasculitis), or, rarely, hormonal disorders such as pheochromocytoma, Conn's syndrome, or Cushing's syndrome.

Symptoms and Diagnosis

Symptoms initially are caused by the effects of the severe high blood pressure on the brain and heart. Symptoms, which may include restlessness, blurred vision, headache, nausea, vomiting, sleepiness, and confusion, result from swelling of brain tissue. Seizures and coma may also occur if swelling is severe or if there is bleeding within the brain.

By viewing the back of the eye with an ophthalmoscope, a doctor can see areas of bleeding, collections of fluid, and swelling of the optic nerve. The doctor may also detect heart enlargement and heart failure.

Damage to the kidneys eventually produces the symptoms of kidney failure, such as fatigue and weakness. Protein leaking from the kidneys can be detected in the urine, along with blood cells. Anemia often results from the breakdown and impaired production of red blood cells. Widespread clotting within the blood vessels is also common (disseminated intravascular coagulation▲). Blood levels of substances produced by the kidneys that help regulate blood pressure (renin and aldosterone) are extremely high.

Prognosis and Treatment

If malignant nephrosclerosis is not treated, about 50% of people who have it die within 6 months, and most of the remainder die within a year. About 60% of the deaths result from kidney failure, 20% from heart failure, 19% from strokes, and 1% from heart attacks. Aggressive lowering of blood pressure with diet and drugs and treating the kidney failure significantly reduce the death rate.

People who have less severe kidney failure improve the most with treatment. Those who have progressive kidney failure can be maintained by dialysis and occasionally improve enough that dialysis can be discontinued.

▲ see page 1001
■ see page 285

Renal Vein Thrombosis

Renal vein thrombosis is blockage of the renal vein, which carries blood away from the kidney.

In adults, renal vein thrombosis usually occurs with other kidney disorders that cause the nephrotic syndrome, in which large amounts of protein are lost in the urine. Renal vein thrombosis may also be caused by kidney cancer or conditions that put pressure on the renal vein (for example, a tumor) or on the inferior vena cava, which the renal vein drains into. Other possible causes are oral contraceptive use, injury, or, rarely, thrombophlebitis migrans—a condition in which clotting occurs sequentially in different veins all over the body.

Symptoms and Diagnosis

Blockage of the renal vein is usually gradual (chronic) but may be sudden (acute). Depending on whether the onset is gradual or sudden, the disorder follows one of two patterns.

In adults, onset and progression are usually gradual and without symptoms, and the disorder goes undetected. An occasional clue to doctors is when a piece of clot breaks off and travels from the renal vein to the lungs (pulmonary embolism■). This event causes sudden pain in the chest made worse by breathing, along with shortness of breath. In other people, urine production diminishes.

In most children and a limited number of adults, onset and progression are usually sudden and with symptoms, and the disorder is detected. Pain, often the first symptom, typically occurs in the back behind the lower ribs and in the hips. The person may have fever, less than a normal amount of urine, protein and blood in the urine, and retention of fluid and salt (sodium) causing tissue swelling (edema). Blood tests may indicate an abnormally high number of white blood cells and evidence of kidney failure.

An ultrasound shows an enlarged kidney if the blockage developed suddenly; it shows a shrunken kidney if the blockage developed gradually. Imaging tests, such as intravenous urography and radionuclide scanning, show poor kidney function. X-rays of the inferior vena cava or the renal vein (venography) may reveal the outline of the blockage, and Doppler ultrasound studies, which use sound waves, are often helpful. When additional information is needed, computed tomography

(CT) or angiography of the renal arteries may be performed.

Prognosis and Treatment

The outcome depends on the cause of the thrombosis, complications, and the degree of kidney damage. Death from renal vein thrombosis is rare and usually results from a fatal underlying cause or from complications, such as a pulmonary embolism. The effects on kidney function depend on whether one or both kidneys are affected, whether blood flow is restored, and what the state of kidney function was before the blockage occurred.

The primary treatment is with anticoagulant drugs, which usually improve kidney function by preventing additional clot formation and can reduce the risk of pulmonary embolism. Using drugs that dissolve clots (thrombolytics) is a newer treatment that is still not routine. Rarely, surgery is performed to remove clots in the renal vein. A kidney is rarely removed and then only if other complications develop, such as high blood pressure.

CHAPTER 146

Tubular and Cystic Kidney Disorders

The primary function of the kidneys is to filter and cleanse the blood. They also maintain the body's balance of water, dissolved salts (electrolytes), and nutrients in the blood. The kidneys begin these tasks by filtering the blood as it flows through tiny blood vessels (glomeruli). This process moves a large amount of water and electrolytes and other substances into small tubules. The cells lining these tubules reabsorb and return needed water, electrolytes (sodium, potassium, calcium), and nutrients (glucose, amino acids) to the blood. The cells also move waste products and drugs from the blood into the fluid (which becomes urine) as it flows through the tubules.

Disorders that interfere with the function of the cells lining the tubules are called tubular disorders. Some conditions, called cystic disorders, interfere with these tubular cell functions by causing fluid-filled sacs (cysts) to form and in doing so compress normal tubules. Many of these tubular and cystic disorders are hereditary; of these hereditary disorders, some are present at birth. The effects of other hereditary disorders are not obvious until years later.

Renal Tubular Acidosis

In renal tubular acidosis, the kidney tubules cannot adequately remove acids from the blood to excrete them in the urine.

Normally, the breakdown of food produces acids that circulate in the blood. The kidneys remove acids from the blood and excrete them in the urine. This function is predominantly performed by the kidney tubules. In renal tubular acidosis, one of several causes of metabolic acidosis, the ability of the kidneys to excrete acids is partially impaired, and acid levels build up in the blood. The balance of electrolytes is also affected. Renal tubular acidosis may lead to the following problems:

- Low or high potassium levels in the blood
- Calcium deposits in the kidneys
- Dehydration
- Painful softening and bending of the bones (osteomalacia or rickets)

Renal tubular acidosis may be hereditary or may be caused by drugs, such as acetazolamide and amphotericin B; poisoning by some heavy metals; or an autoimmune disease, such as systemic lupus erythematosus or Sjögren's syndrome.

Symptoms and Diagnosis

Three types of renal tubular acidosis exist: type 1, type 2, and type 4. Each type produces slightly different symptoms. When potassium levels in the blood are low, as occurs in types 1 and 2, neurologic problems may develop, including muscle weakness, diminished reflexes, and even paralysis. In type 4, potassium levels typically increase, although it is un-

TYPES OF RENAL TUBULAR ACIDOSIS

TYPE	CAUSE	UNDERLYING ABNORMALITY	RESULTING SYMPTOMS AND METABOLIC ABNORMALITIES
1	May be hereditary; may be triggered by an autoimmune disease or certain drugs; cause usually not known, especially in women	Inability to excrete acid into the urine	High blood acidity; mild dehydration; low potassium levels in the blood, leading to muscle weakness and paralysis; fragile bones; bone pain; kidney stones (calcium deposits); kidney failure
2	Usually caused by a hereditary disease such as Fanconi's syndrome, hereditary fructose intolerance, Wilson's disease, or Lowe's syndrome; may also be caused by heavy metal poisoning or certain drugs	Inability to reabsorb bicarbonate from the urine, so bicarbonate is lost	High blood acidity, mild dehydration, and low potassium levels in the blood
4	Not hereditary; caused by diabetes, an autoimmune disease, sickle cell disease, or an obstruction in the urinary tract	Deficiency of or inability to respond to aldosterone, a hormone that helps regulate potassium and sodium excretion in the kidneys	High blood acidity and high potassium levels in the blood that rarely cause symptoms, unless the potassium level is so high that irregular heartbeats and muscle paralysis develop

Note: There is no type 3.

common for the level to rise high enough to cause symptoms. If the level becomes too high, irregular heartbeats and muscle paralysis may develop. In type 1, kidney stones may develop, causing damage to kidney cells and, in some cases, chronic kidney failure.

A doctor considers the diagnosis of type 1 or type 2 renal tubular acidosis when a person has certain characteristic symptoms (muscle weakness, diminished reflexes) and when tests reveal high levels of acid and low levels of bicarbonate and potassium in the blood. Type 4 renal tubular acidosis is usually suspected when high potassium levels accompany high acid levels and low bicarbonate levels in the blood. Special tests help to determine the type of renal tubular acidosis.

Treatment

Treatment depends on the type. Types 1 and 2 are treated by drinking a solution of sodium bicarbonate (baking soda) every day to neutralize the acid that is produced from food. This treatment relieves the symptoms and prevents kidney failure and bone disease or keeps these problems from becoming worse. Other specially prepared solutions are available, and potassium supplements may also be required. In type 4, the acidosis is so mild that bicarbonate may not be needed. High potassium levels in the blood can usually be kept in check by restricting the potassium intake and, if necessary, taking diuretics.

Renal Glucosuria

In renal glucosuria (glycosuria), glucose (sugar) is excreted in the urine, despite normal or low glucose levels in the blood.

Normally, the body excretes glucose in the urine only when glucose levels in the blood are very high. In most healthy people, glucose that is filtered from the blood by the kidneys is completely reabsorbed back into the blood. In people with renal glucosuria, glucose may be excreted in the urine despite normal or low levels of glucose in the blood. This happens because of a defect in the tubular cells that decreases the reabsorption of glucose. Renal glucosuria may be a hereditary condition.

Renal glucosuria has no symptoms or serious consequences. A doctor makes the diagnosis when a routine urine test detects glucose in the urine even though glucose levels in the blood are normal. In a small number of people, renal glucosuria may be an early sign of diabetes mellitus. No treatment is needed.

Nephrogenic Diabetes Insipidus

In nephrogenic diabetes insipidus, the kidneys produce a large volume of dilute urine because they fail to respond to antidiuretic hormone and are unable to concentrate urine.

Both diabetes insipidus and the better-known type of diabetes, diabetes mellitus, result in the excretion of large volumes of urine. Otherwise, the two types of diabetes are very different.

Two types of diabetes insipidus exist. In nephrogenic diabetes insipidus, the kidneys do not respond to antidiuretic hormone, so they continue to excrete a large amount of dilute urine. In the other, more common type (central diabetes insipidus), the pituitary gland fails to secrete antidiuretic hormone.▲

Causes

Normally, the kidneys adjust the concentration of urine according to the body's needs. The kidneys make this adjustment in response to the level of antidiuretic hormone in the blood. Antidiuretic hormone, which is secreted by the pituitary gland, signals the kidneys to conserve water and concentrate the urine. In nephrogenic diabetes insipidus, the kidneys fail to respond to the signal.

Nephrogenic diabetes insipidus may be hereditary. The gene that causes the disorder is recessive and carried on the X chromosome, so usually only males develop symptoms. However, females who carry the gene can transmit the disease to their sons. In other people, nephrogenic diabetes insipidus may be caused by certain drugs that block the action of antidiuretic hormone, such as lithium. Also, high levels of calcium or low levels of potassium in the blood partially block the action of antidiuretic hormone.

Symptoms and Diagnosis

The symptoms of nephrogenic diabetes insipidus are excessive thirst (polydipsia) and the excretion of large volumes of dilute urine (polyuria). When nephrogenic diabetes insipidus is hereditary, symptoms usually start soon after birth. Because infants cannot communicate thirst, they may become very dehydrated. They may develop a high fever accompanied by vomiting and seizures.

If nephrogenic diabetes insipidus is not quickly diagnosed and treated, the brain may be damaged, leaving the infant with permanent mental retardation. Frequent episodes of dehydration can also retard physical development. With treatment, however, an infant who has this disorder is likely to develop normally.

Laboratory tests reveal high sodium levels in the blood and very dilute urine. A doctor may use a water deprivation test to help make the diagnosis.■

Prognosis and Treatment

The prognosis is good if nephrogenic diabetes insipidus is diagnosed before the person suffers severe episodes of dehydration. In adults, correction of the underlying cause usually helps kidney function return to normal.

To prevent dehydration, people with nephrogenic diabetes insipidus must always drink adequate amounts of water as soon as they feel thirsty. Infants and young children must be given water often. People who drink enough water are not likely to become dehydrated, but several hours without water can lead to serious dehydration. A diet low in salt may help. Nonsteroidal anti-inflammatory drugs (NSAIDs) and thiazide diuretics are sometimes used to treat this disorder. NSAIDs and thiazide diuretics act by different mechanisms to increase the amount of sodium and water that is reabsorbed by the kidney; these changes decrease excretion of urine. Because most people with nephrogenic diabetes insipidus respond slightly to antidiuretic hormone, desmopressin (a drug very similar to antidiuretic hormone) may reduce urine volume.

Cystinuria

Cystinuria is a rare disorder that results in excretion of the amino acid cystine into the urine, often causing cystine stones to form in the urinary tract.

Cystinuria is caused by an inherited defect of the kidney tubules. The gene that causes cystinuria is recessive, so people with the dis-

▲ see page 944   ■ see page 944

order must have inherited two abnormal genes, one from each parent.▲ People who carry the gene but do not have the disorder have one normal and one abnormal gene. These people may excrete larger than normal amounts of cystine into the urine, but seldom enough to form cystine stones.

Symptoms and Diagnosis

Cystine stones form in the bladder, renal pelvis (the area where urine collects and flows out of the kidney), or ureters (the long narrow tubes that carry urine from the kidneys to the bladder). Symptoms usually start between the ages of 10 and 30. Often, the first symptom is intense pain caused by a spasm of the ureter where a stone becomes lodged. Blockage of the urinary tract by stones reduces the ability of one or both kidneys to excrete waste products and excess fluid and salts. The stone may also become a site where bacteria can cause infection.

A doctor tests for cystinuria when a person has recurring kidney stones. Cystine crystals may be seen during a microscopic examination of the urine (urinalysis), and cystine levels are measured in the urine.

Treatment

Treatment consists of preventing cystine stones from forming by keeping the concentration of cystine in the urine low. To keep the cystine concentration low, a person must drink enough fluids to produce at least 8 pints of urine each day. During the night, however, when the person is not drinking, less urine is produced and stone formation is more likely. This risk is reduced by drinking fluids before going to bed. Another treatment approach involves taking potassium citrate or sodium bicarbonate to make the urine more alkaline, because cystine dissolves more easily in alkaline urine than in acidic urine. Efforts to increase intake of water and make the urine more alkaline can lead to abdominal bloating, making the treatment difficult for some people to tolerate.

If stones continue to form despite these measures, drugs such as penicillamine, tiopronin, or captopril may be tried. These drugs react with cystine to keep it dissolved. Captopril is slightly less effective than the other drugs, but has fewer serious side effects. Although the treatments are usually effective, there is a fairly high risk that stones will continue to form.

Fanconi's Syndrome

Fanconi's syndrome is a rare disorder of tubule function that results in excess amounts of glucose, bicarbonate, phosphates, uric acid, potassium, sodium, and certain amino acids being excreted in the urine.

Fanconi's syndrome may be hereditary or may be caused by exposure to heavy metals or other chemical agents, vitamin D deficiency, kidney transplantation, multiple myeloma, or amyloidosis.

Symptoms and Diagnosis

In hereditary Fanconi's syndrome, symptoms usually begin during infancy. A child with Fanconi's syndrome may excrete a large amount of urine. Other symptoms include weakness and bone pain.

The symptoms and a test that shows a high level of acid in the blood may lead a doctor to suspect Fanconi's syndrome. The diagnosis is confirmed when high levels of glucose, bicarbonate, phosphate, uric acid, potassium, and sodium are detected in the urine. Most often, some damage to bones or kidney tissue has occurred before the diagnosis is made.

Treatment

Fanconi's syndrome cannot be cured, but it can be controlled with proper treatment. Effective treatment can keep the damage to bones or kidney tissue from getting worse and in some cases correct it. The high acid level of the blood (acidosis) may be neutralized by drinking sodium bicarbonate. People with low potassium levels in the blood may need to take potassium supplements by mouth. Bone disease requires treatment with phosphates and vitamin D supplements given by mouth. Kidney transplantation may be lifesaving if a child with the disorder develops kidney failure.

Hypophosphatemic Rickets

Hypophosphatemic rickets (previously called vitamin D–resistant rickets) is a disorder in which the bones become painfully soft and bend easily because the blood contains low levels of phosphate and has inadequate amounts of the active form of vitamin D.

▲ see art on page 12

This very rare disorder is nearly always hereditary, passed as a dominant gene that is carried on the X chromosome. The genetic defect causes a kidney abnormality that allows an inappropriately high amount of phosphate to be excreted into the urine, resulting in low levels of phosphate in the blood. Because bones need phosphate to grow, this deficiency causes defective bones. Females with hypophosphatemic rickets have less severe bone disease than males. In rare cases, the disorder develops as a result of certain cancers, such as giant cell tumors of bone, sarcomas, prostate cancer, and breast cancer. Hypophosphatemic rickets is not the same as rickets caused by vitamin D deficiency.▲

Symptoms and Treatment

Hypophosphatemic rickets usually begins in the first year of life. It ranges from so mild that it produces no noticeable symptoms to so severe that it produces bowing of the legs and other bone deformities, bone pain, and a short stature. Bony outgrowth where muscles attach to bones may limit movement at those joints. A baby's skull bones may close too soon, leading to seizures. Laboratory tests show that calcium levels in the blood are normal, but phosphate levels are low.

The aim of treatment is to raise phosphate levels in the blood, which will promote normal bone formation. Phosphate can be taken by mouth and should be combined with calcitriol, the activated form of vitamin D. Taking vitamin D alone is not helpful. However, treatment often leads to high levels of calcium in the blood, the accumulation of calcium in kidney tissue, or kidney stones. These effects can harm the kidneys and other tissues. In some adults, hypophosphatemic rickets resulting from cancer improves dramatically after the cancer is removed.

Hartnup Disease

Hartnup disease is a rare hereditary disorder that results in a skin rash and brain abnormalities because tryptophan and certain other amino acids are not well absorbed from the intestine and not well reabsorbed by the kidneys.

Hartnup disease occurs when a person inherits two copies of the abnormal gene for the disorder, one from each parent. The defective gene controls the absorption of certain amino acids from the intestine and the reabsorption

of those amino acids in the kidneys. Consequently, a person with Hartnup disease cannot absorb amino acids properly from the intestine and cannot reabsorb them properly from tubules in the kidneys. Excessive amounts of amino acids, such as tryptophan, are excreted in the urine. The body is thus left with inadequate amounts of amino acids, which are the building blocks of protein. With too little tryptophan in the blood, the body is unable to make a sufficient amount of the B-complex vitamin niacinamide, particularly under stress when more vitamins are needed.

Symptoms

Symptoms may begin in infancy or early childhood, but sometimes as late as early adulthood. Symptoms may be triggered by sunlight, fever, drugs, or emotional or physical stress. A period of poor nutrition nearly always precedes an attack. The attacks usually become progressively less frequent with age. Most symptoms occur sporadically and are caused by a deficiency of niacinamide. A rash develops on parts of the body exposed to the sun. Mental retardation, short stature, headaches, an unsteady gait, and collapsing or fainting are common. Psychologic problems (such as anxiety, rapid mood changes, delusions, and hallucinations) may also result.

Diagnosis and Treatment

Laboratory tests performed on urine samples reveal abnormally high excretion of amino acids and their breakdown products.

People with Hartnup disease can prevent attacks by maintaining good nutrition and supplementing their diet with niacinamide or niacin, a B-complex vitamin very similar to niacinamide. A diet that is adequate in protein can overcome the deficiency caused by poor gastrointestinal absorption and excess excretion of amino acids into the urine.

Bartter's Syndrome

In Bartter's syndrome, the kidneys excrete excessive amounts of electrolytes (potassium, sodium, and chloride), resulting in electrolyte abnormalities.

Bartter's syndrome is usually hereditary and is caused by a recessive gene; thus, a person with the disorder has inherited two recessive genes for the disorder, one from each parent.

▲ see page 894

The abnormal gene causes the kidney to excrete excessive amounts of sodium, chloride, and potassium. The loss of sodium and chloride leads to mild dehydration, which causes the body to produce more renin and aldosterone. The increase in aldosterone increases potassium and acid secretion in the kidneys, leading to hypokalemia and metabolic alkalosis.▲

Symptoms and Diagnosis

Children with Bartter's syndrome grow slowly and appear malnourished. They may have muscle weakness and excessive thirst, may produce large amounts of urine, and may be mentally retarded. The loss of sodium and chloride leads to chronic mild dehydration.

The diagnosis of Bartter's syndrome in young children is based on a physical examination and low levels of potassium, sodium, and chloride in the blood. However, similar findings occur when children with certain eating disorders, such as bulimia nervosa, self-induce vomiting and misuse diuretics.

Treatment

Many of the consequences of Bartter's syndrome can be prevented by taking potassium supplements and a drug that reduces excretion of potassium into the urine, such as spironolactone (which also blocks the action of aldosterone), triamterene, amiloride, captopril, propranolol, or nonsteroidal anti-inflammatory drugs (NSAIDs), such as indomethacin. Drinking adequate amounts of fluids is necessary to compensate for the excessive fluid losses.

Liddle's Syndrome

Liddle's syndrome is a rare hereditary disorder in which the kidneys excrete potassium but retain too much sodium and water, leading to high blood pressure.

The gene that causes Liddle's syndrome is dominant, meaning that children of a person with the disorder have a 50% chance of inheriting the defective gene. The disorder does not always cause symptoms. When it does, symptoms such as high blood pressure often begin during childhood.

The condition is effectively treated by drugs that increase sodium excretion and lessen potassium excretion, such as triamterene or

amiloride. These drugs effectively lower the blood pressure. The prognosis is very good.

Polycystic Kidney Disease

Polycystic kidney disease is a hereditary disorder in which many fluid-filled sacs (cysts) form in both kidneys; the kidneys grow larger but have less functioning kidney tissue.

The genetic defect that causes polycystic kidney disease may be dominant or recessive. That is, a person with the disease has inherited either one copy of a dominant gene from one parent or two copies of a recessive gene, one from each parent. Those with dominant gene inheritance usually have no symptoms until adulthood; those with recessive gene inheritance develop severe illness in childhood.

The genetic defect leads to the widespread formation of cysts in the kidneys. Gradual enlargement of the cysts with increasing age is accompanied by a reduction of blood flow and scarring within the kidneys. Kidney stones may develop. Kidney failure can occur eventually. The genetic defect may also cause cysts to develop in other parts of the body, such as the liver and pancreas.

Symptoms and Complications

In the recessive form of this disease that begins during childhood, the cysts become very large and cause the abdomen to protrude. A severely affected newborn may die shortly after birth, because kidney failure can develop in the fetus, leading to poor development of the lungs. The liver is also affected, and at 5 to 10 years of age, a child with this disorder tends to develop high pressure in the blood vessels that connects the intestine and the liver (portal system). Eventually, liver failure and kidney failure occur.

In the dominant form of polycystic kidney disease, the cysts develop slowly in number and size. Typically, symptoms begin in early or middle adulthood, although occasionally the disease is not discovered until after death at autopsy. Symptoms usually include discomfort or pain in the abdomen or side (flank), blood in the urine, frequent urination, and intense crampy (colicky) pain from kidney stones. In other cases, fatigue, nausea, and other consequences of kidney failure may result because the person has less functioning kidney tissue. Chronic urinary tract infections can worsen the kidney failure. At least half of the people with polycystic kidney disease

▲ see page 932

have high blood pressure at the time of diagnosis.

About one third of people who have polycystic kidney disease also have cysts in their liver, but these cysts do not affect liver function. As many as 10% of people have dilated blood vessels (aneurysms) in their brain. Usually, the dilated blood vessels cause headaches when they expand. Many of these brain aneurysms bleed and cause strokes.

Diagnosis, Prognosis, and Treatment

A doctor suspects this disease on the basis of family history and laboratory tests of kidney function. When the disease is advanced and the kidneys are very large, the diagnosis is obvious. Ultrasonography and computed tomography (CT) reveal the characteristic moth-eaten appearance of the kidneys and liver caused by the cysts.

Treating urinary tract infections and high blood pressure may prolong life. However, more than half of the people who have this disease develop kidney failure at some time in their life. Without dialysis or kidney transplantation, kidney failure is fatal.

Genetic testing is available to help people with polycystic kidney disease understand the probability that their children will inherit the condition.

Medullary Cystic Disease

Medullary cystic disease is a rare disorder in which fluid-filled sacs (cysts) develop deep within the kidneys, leading to kidney failure.

Medullary cystic disease either is hereditary or is caused by a non-genetic abnormality that occurs during development of the fetus. The disorder damages microscopic tubules within the kidneys. The damaged tubules are less able to concentrate urine and reabsorb sodium. Dehydration, a low level of sodium in the blood, and an elevated concentration of urea and creatinine in the blood may occur if sodium intake is not adequate.

Symptoms and Diagnosis

Symptoms usually begin before age 20, but symptoms vary greatly, and a few people do not have any symptoms until much later. A person starts to produce excessive amounts of urine as the kidneys' responsiveness to antidiuretic hormone diminishes. Retarded growth and evidence of bone disease are common in children. In many people, these problems de-

Polycystic Kidney Disease

In polycystic kidney disease, many cysts form in both kidneys. The cysts gradually enlarge, destroying some or most of the normal tissue in the kidneys.

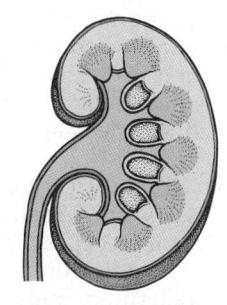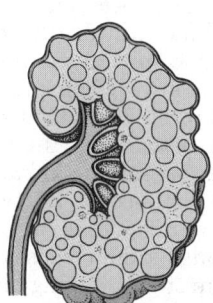

Normal Kidney   **Polycystic Kidney**

velop slowly over several years, and the body compensates so well that the problems are not recognized until kidney failure is advanced.

Laboratory tests reveal poor kidney function. The level of sodium in the blood is often low. X-rays show that the kidneys are small. Ultrasonography may detect cysts deep within the kidneys, although the cysts may be too small to be detected. Computed tomography (CT) is the test that is most likely to detect cysts.

Prognosis and Treatment

The disease progresses slowly but relentlessly. A large daily intake of fluids and salt (sodium) is needed to compensate for the excessive excretion of sodium and the production of large volumes of dilute urine. When kidney failure occurs, dialysis or kidney transplantation is needed.

Medullary Sponge Kidney

Medullary sponge kidney is an uncommon disorder in which the urine-containing tubules of the kidneys are dilated.

Medullary sponge kidney is usually caused by a non-genetic abnormality that occurs during development of the fetus. Much less often, the abnormality is hereditary. Medullary sponge kidney causes no symptoms most of the time, but a person with the disorder is prone to developing painful kidney stones, blood in the urine, and kidney infections. Calcium deposits in the kidneys occur in more than half of the people with the disorder.

A doctor may suspect medullary sponge kidney based on the symptoms. X-rays of the kidneys reveal calcium deposits if there are any. The diagnosis can be confirmed by an imaging technique in which a radiopaque dye, which is visible on x-rays, is injected intravenously and then observed on x-rays as it is excreted by the kidneys. Ultrasound scans may help but may not detect tiny fluid-filled sacs (cysts) lying deep within the kidneys.

Most people do well without treatment. Treatment may be necessary if medullary sponge kidney causes calcium to deposit and form stones. Taking thiazide diuretics, drinking a lot of fluids, and eating a diet that is low in calcium may prevent stones from forming and obstructing the urinary tract. Surgery may be needed if the urinary tract becomes obstructed. Infections are treated with antibiotics.

Alport's Syndrome

Alport's syndrome (hereditary nephritis) is a hereditary disorder in which kidney function is poor, blood is present in the urine, and deafness and eye abnormalities sometimes occur.

Alport's syndrome is usually caused by a defective gene on the X chromosome, but it sometimes results from an abnormal gene on a nonsex (autosomal) chromosome. Other factors influence how severe the disorder is in a person who has the gene. Females with the defective gene on one of their two X chromosomes usually do not have symptoms, although their kidneys may perform somewhat less efficiently than normal; most of these females have some blood in the urine. Males with the defective gene (males do not have a second X chromosome to compensate for the defect) usually develop kidney failure between the ages of 20 and 30. Many people with the defective gene on only one autosomal chromosome have no symptoms other than blood in the urine, but the urine may also contain varying amounts of protein, white blood cells, and casts (small clumps of material) visible under a microscope. Kidney function in people who have the defective gene on two autosomal chromosomes slowly worsens, and kidney failure usually occurs.

Alport's syndrome can affect organs other than the kidneys. Hearing problems, usually an inability to hear sounds in the higher frequencies, are common. Cataracts can also occur, although less often than hearing loss. Abnormalities of the cornea, lens, or retina sometimes cause blindness. Other problems include a low number of platelets in the blood (thrombocytopenia) and abnormalities that affect several nerves (polyneuropathy).

People who develop kidney failure need to undergo dialysis or receive a kidney transplant. Genetic testing is usually offered to people with Alport's syndrome who want to have children.

Nail-Patella Syndrome

The nail-patella syndrome is a rare hereditary disorder that results in abnormalities of the kidneys, bones, joints, and fingernails.

The gene that causes nail-patella syndrome is dominant. Commonly, people who have this syndrome have one or both kneecaps (patellas) missing, one of the arm bones (the radius) dislocated at the elbow, and the pelvic bone abnormally shaped. They have either no fingernails or poorly developed ones, with pitting and ridges. The irises of the eyes may be variably colored.

High blood pressure may develop. The urine may contain proteins, usually in small amounts, and rarely blood, which may prompt the doctor to order kidney function tests. Kidney failure eventually develops in about 30% of the people with affected kidneys. The diagnosis is confirmed by bone x-rays and a biopsy of kidney tissue.

There is no effective treatment for this syndrome. Controlling blood pressure may slow the rate of deterioration of kidney function. Those who develop kidney failure need dialysis or a kidney transplant. Genetic testing is usually offered to people who want to have children.

CHAPTER 147

Urinary Incontinence

Urinary incontinence is the uncontrollable loss of urine.

Urinary incontinence mostly affects older people but can occur at any age. It may affect as many as 1 of 5 younger adults to some extent; the rate rises to about 1 of 3 older people. In most age groups, urinary incontinence is more common in women than in men.

Urinary incontinence differs somewhat among age groups. Incontinence experienced by younger adults tends to begin suddenly, and it often resolves quickly with little or no treatment. Also, when younger adults experience incontinence, they usually maintain control without leakage for most of their episodes of urination. Older adults are often more frequently and severely affected. In addition, incontinence is less likely to resolve quickly or without treatment in older adults.

Although urinary incontinence is common, highly treatable, and very often curable, it is often not diagnosed or treated. People often live with incontinence without seeking professional help because they are afraid, embarrassed, or mistakenly believe it is a normal part of aging. A person with incontinence often feels isolated or depressed. In addition, urinary incontinence is often a reason for institutionalization because of the substantial burden it places on caregivers. More than 50% of nursing home residents are incontinent.

Urinary incontinence can lead to many complications. For example, incontinence that is not properly managed can contribute to the development of bladder and kidney infections. Particularly among older adults, incontinence can also increase the risk for skin rashes and pressure sores (because urine can irritate the skin), and falls (because an incontinent person may fall when rushing to use the toilet).

Control of Urination

The kidneys constantly produce urine, which flows through two tubes (the ureters) to the bladder, where urine is stored. The lowest part of the bladder (the neck) is encircled by a muscle (the urinary sphincter) that remains contracted to close off the channel that carries urine out of the body (the urethra), so that urine is retained in the bladder until it is full.

When the bladder is full, messages travel along nerves from the bladder to the spinal cord; they are then relayed to the brain and the person becomes aware of the urge to urinate. A person who has control of urination can then consciously and voluntarily decide whether to release the urine from the bladder or to hold it for a while. When the decision is made to urinate, the sphincter muscle relaxes, allowing urine to flow out through the urethra, and the bladder wall muscles contract to push the urine out. Muscles in the abdominal wall and floor of the pelvis can be contracted to increase the pressure on the bladder.

Several changes occur with age that affect the person's ability to control urination. The maximum amount of urine that the bladder can hold (bladder capacity) declines. A person's ability to postpone urination after feeling a need to urinate also decreases with age. The rate of urine flow out of the bladder and through the urethra slows. At any age, sporadic contractions of bladder wall muscles occur regardless of need or appropriate opportunity to urinate; most contractions are blocked by normal spinal cord and brain controls at younger ages, but the number that are not blocked increases with age. The amount of urine remaining in the bladder after urination is finished (residual urine) also increases with age. In women, the urethra shortens and its lining becomes thinner as the level of estrogen declines during menopause; these changes decrease the ability of the urinary sphincter to close tightly. In men, the prostate gland enlarges, sometimes impeding the flow of urine through the urethra. Although all of these age-related changes increase the odds that incontinence will occur, it usually only occurs when another factor is in place, for example, when the person has a medical disorder. Many disorders can impair or disrupt the ability to control urination.

Types and Causes

Incontinence can be categorized according to whether it started recently and suddenly (acute urinary incontinence) or slowly and gradually (chronic or persistent urinary incontinence). A bladder infection is the most common cause of acute urinary incontinence. Several reversible factors can contribute to incontinence. Examples include conditions that result in confusion (a severe infection such as pneumonia) or impaired mobility (a leg or hip fracture). Other causes include excess intake of alcohol or beverages that contain caffeine and conditions that can result in irritation of the bladder or urethra, such as atrophic vaginitis or severe constipation. Persistent urinary incontinence may be caused by brain disorders such as stroke, diseases that affect the nerves leading to and from the bladder, conditions in the lower urinary tract, and conditions that impair mental function or mobility.

Urinary incontinence can also be categorized into five basic types based on the pattern of symptoms: urge, stress, overflow, functional, and mixed.

Urge Incontinence: Urge incontinence is an abrupt and intense urge to urinate that cannot be suppressed, followed by an uncontrollable loss of urine. Some people experience the abrupt and intense urge to urinate but are still able to remain continent. People with urge incontinence usually have little time to get to the bathroom before they have an "accident." An illness or injury that interferes with mobility makes it even harder for a person to get to the bathroom quickly.

Urge incontinence is the most common type of persistent incontinence in older people and often has no clear cause. Urge incontinence in older people may be caused by a combination of overactivity of the muscles in the bladder along with poor squeezing ability of those muscles. Part of the cause of persistent urge incontinence relates to changes in the part of the brain in the frontal lobe that inhibits urination. These changes may accompany brain disorders, especially stroke and dementia, which disrupt the nervous system's ability to inhibit the bladder. Chronic overactivity of the bladder—overactive bladder—is common in older people and causes the abrupt and intense urge to urinate as well as frequent urination during the day and night.

Stress Incontinence: Stress incontinence is the uncontrollable loss of small amounts of urine when coughing, straining, sneezing, lifting heavy objects, or performing any maneuver that suddenly increases pressure within the abdomen. Stress incontinence is the most common type of incontinence among young and middle-aged women. It can be caused by weakness of the urinary sphincter, which sometimes results from childbirth, pelvic surgery, or an abnormal position of the urethra or uterus. In postmenopausal women, a lack of estrogen reduces the urethra's resistance to urine flow. In men, stress incontinence may follow prostate surgery if the upper part of the urethra or the bladder neck is injured. In both men and women, obesity can cause or worsen stress incontinence because extra weight stresses the bladder.

Some people with severe stress incontinence have nearly constant urine loss (sometimes referred to as total incontinence). In adults, this usually occurs because the urinary sphincter does not close adequately. Some children have total incontinence because a birth defect prevents the urethra from developing completely.

Overflow Incontinence: Overflow incontinence is the uncontrollable leakage of small amounts of urine, usually caused by some type of blockage or by weak contractions of the bladder muscles. When urine flow is blocked or the bladder muscles can no longer contract, the bladder becomes overfilled and enlarged. Pressure in the bladder increases until small amounts of urine dribble out.

In children, blockage of urine flow may be caused by narrowing of the end of the urethra or the bladder neck because of a birth defect. In men, an enlarged prostate can block the opening into the urethra from the bladder. Less commonly, blockage is caused by narrowing of the bladder neck or the urethra (urethral stricture), which may occur after prostate surgery. In men and women, constipation can cause overflow incontinence if stool fills the rectum to the point of putting pressure on the bladder neck and urethra. A number of drugs that affect the brain or spinal cord or that interfere with nerve messages, such as anticholinergic drugs and opioids, may impair bladder contractions and cause overflow incontinence. Nerve damage that paralyzes the bladder (neurogenic bladder) can also cause overflow incontinence. Diabetes mellitus can also cause a form of neurogenic bladder and overflow incontinence.

Functional Incontinence: Functional incontinence refers to urine loss resulting from the inability (or sometimes unwillingness) to get to a toilet. The most common causes are con-

DRUGS THAT MAY CAUSE OR WORSEN URINARY INCONTINENCE

Type of Drug	Examples	Effects
Alcohol	Wine, beer, liquor	Increases urine production
Alpha-adrenergic agonists	Nasal decongestants (containing pseudoephedrine)	Tighten the urinary sphincter; can cause urinary retention and overflow incontinence
Alpha-adrenergic blockers	Prazosin, terazosin, doxazosin, tamsulosin	Relax the bladder outlet and urethra; can cause stress incontinence
Angiotensin-converting enzyme (ACE) inhibitors	Captopril, benazepril, others	Can cause cough and worsen stress incontinence
Anticholinergics	Antihistamines, benztropine, antidepressants	Interfere with bladder contraction and worsen constipation; can cause urinary retention and overflow incontinence
Antidepressants	Amitriptyline, desipramine, nortriptyline	Interfere with bladder contraction and worsen constipation; can cause urinary retention and overflow incontinence
Antipsychotics	Haloperidol, thioridazine, thiothixene, risperidone, others	Can cause slow mobility and worsen urge incontinence
Calcium channel blockers	Diltiazem, verapamil	Interfere with bladder contraction and worsen constipation; can cause urinary retention and overflow incontinence
Diuretics	Caffeine, thiazides, furosemide, others	Increase urine production
Opioids	Morphine, codeine, oxycodone, others	Interfere with bladder contraction and worsen constipation; can cause urinary retention and overflow incontinence
Sedatives and hypnotics	Diazepam, flurazepam, lorazepam, others	Can cause slow mobility and worsen urge incontinence

ditions that cause immobility, such as stroke or severe arthritis, and conditions that interfere with mental function, such as dementia due to Alzheimer's disease. In rare situations, people may become so depressed or otherwise emotionally disturbed that they do not go to the toilet. This is sometimes referred to as psychogenic incontinence.

Mixed Incontinence: Mixed incontinence involves more than one type of incontinence. For example, a child may have incontinence resulting from both nerve damage and psycho-

logic factors. A man may have overflow incontinence from prostate enlargement and urge incontinence from a stroke. The most common type of mixed incontinence occurs in older women, who often have a mixture of urge and stress incontinence.

Diagnosis

As a first step, a doctor asks specific questions about the history of the problem. The doctor also asks how much the incontinence is affecting the person's quality of life and abil-

Neurogenic Bladder: One Cause of Overflow Incontinence

A neurogenic bladder functions abnormally because of damage to the nerve connections between the brain, spinal cord, and bladder. Diseases such as diabetes mellitus, stroke, and multiple sclerosis can cause neurogenic bladder. The bladder can be underactive and unable to contract well (hypotonic) or overactive (spastic), emptying too often and when it should not. Spinal cord injuries are a common cause of an overactive bladder. An underactive bladder in children is commonly caused by spina bifida (myelomeningocele).

An underactive bladder usually stretches and enlarges painlessly. In some cases, the enlarged bladder constantly leaks small amounts of urine (overflow incontinence). Bladder infections are common, and stones tend to form.

An overactive bladder may fill and empty without control and with varying degrees of warning. Pressure can increase in an overactive bladder when it contracts while the sphincter is closed, causing a damaging backward flow (reflux) of urine toward the kidneys.

Although total recovery is uncommon with any type of neurogenic bladder, symptoms and complications may be reduced with vigorous and appropriate therapy.

When an underactive bladder develops suddenly after an injury, a catheter is promptly inserted to prevent stretching and infection. If the bladder underactivity persists, some people can be trained to insert the catheter periodically—3 to 6 times a day—and remove it after the bladder is empty (intermittent self-catheterization). Drugs offer very limited benefit for an underactive bladder. Electrical stimulation may be applied to the bladder, the nerves that control the bladder, or the spinal cord to induce the bladder to contract, but this treatment is experimental.

People with an overactive bladder may also need to have a catheter inserted if the bladder does not empty completely. Anticholinergic drugs can usually relax an overactive bladder, but these drugs commonly cause dry mouth and constipation, and they may impair normal contractions that are needed for bladder emptying. Sometimes sympathetic blocking drugs improve coordination between the bladder and the sphincter, which must open for the bladder to empty. Electrical stimulation may reduce bladder overactivity in many people who do not respond to drug treatment. Surgery to enlarge the bladder with a segment of the intestine (augmentation cystoplasty) can help some people with an overactive bladder. After the procedure, catheterization through the urethra is necessary to drain urine.

If kidney function is deteriorating or if drainage of urine through a permanent catheter is not feasible, surgery may be needed to divert the urine to an external opening (ostomy) made in the abdominal wall.

Extensive efforts are made to reduce the risk of stones forming in the urine. Kidney function is closely monitored. A kidney or urinary tract infection is treated promptly. Drinking at least eight glasses of fluids a day helps by diluting the urine. Finally, because immobility increases the risk of complications in people with a neurogenic bladder, those who can walk are encouraged to do so as soon as possible. In a person who is paralyzed, changing positioning often helps to prevent complications.

ity to function. These questions can help the doctor determine the cause of the problem and guide an appropriate treatment plan.

A person with urinary incontinence may be asked to record the pattern of urination for at least 3 days (a "bladder diary"). This diary can help the doctor evaluate the cause of the incontinence. Useful information for the doctor might include how often and when the person urinates, whether or not control was lost, and estimates of how much urine leaked when incontinence did occur.

A physical examination can provide valuable information. A rectal examination can confirm whether the person is severely constipated. A pelvic examination in women can help identify problems that may contribute to or cause incontinence, such as atrophy of the lining of urethra and prolapse of the bladder (cystocele). Stress incontinence is sometimes diagnosed simply by observing the loss of urine while the person is coughing or straining. The amount of urine left in the bladder after urination (residual urine) can be measured using ultrasound or urinary catheterization (placing a small tube called a catheter into the bladder). A large amount of residual urine indicates an obstruction or a problem with nerves or the bladder muscle, which may indicate overflow incontinence. Urinalysis is performed to determine whether an infection is present.

For some people, special tests during urination (urodynamic evaluation) may be helpful. These tests measure the pressure in the bladder at rest and when filling. A catheter is inserted through the urethra into the bladder and water is passed through the catheter while the pressure within the bladder is recorded. Normally, the pressure increases slowly. In some people, pressure builds in sudden spasms or rises too sharply before the bladder is completely filled. The pattern of pressure change helps the doctor determine the type of incontinence and the best treatment. The rate of urine flow can also be measured; this measurement can help determine whether urine flow is obstructed and whether the bladder muscles can contract strongly enough to expel the urine.

Treatment

Treatment varies according to the type and cause of incontinence. Most people can be either cured or helped considerably.

The person should receive education about bladder functioning, the effects of medications and fluid intake, and bladder and bowel habits. Treatment often requires taking only some simple steps to change behavior, such as deliberately urinating at regular intervals—every 2 to 3 hours—to keep the bladder relatively empty. Avoiding fluids that may irritate the bladder, such as beverages that contain caffeine, may help. The person should drink adequate amounts of fluids (six to eight 8-ounce glasses a day) to prevent the urine from becoming too concentrated—which can irritate the bladder. Drugs that adversely affect bladder function can often be discontinued. For people taking diuretics, the timing of the dose can be adjusted so that the person can be close to a bathroom when the drug takes effect.

Specially designed incontinence pads and undergarments can protect the skin and enable people to remain dry, comfortable, and socially active. These items are unobtrusive and readily available.

Episodes of **urge incontinence** often can be prevented by urinating at regular intervals before the urge occurs (scheduled voiding). Bladder training techniques, which include pelvic

muscle (Kegel) exercises, can be very helpful. Learning how to contract these muscles is not easily self-taught, so biofeedback is often used to help with training. Nurses or physical therapists can help teach these exercises. The exercises involve repeatedly contracting the muscles many times a day to build up strength and learning to use the muscles properly in situations that cause incontinence, such as coughing.

Drugs that relax the bladder may help. The two most commonly used drugs of this class are oxybutynin and tolterodine. Both can be taken once a day. Although these drugs can help by reducing bladder irritability and the strong urge to urinate, they have potential side effects, such as dryness of the mouth, constipation, gastroesophageal reflux, or even retention of urine.

For people with **stress incontinence,** urinating frequently to avoid a full bladder and pelvic muscle (Kegel) exercises are usually helpful. In women with stress incontinence, applying estrogen cream to the vagina or taking estrogen tablets may be helpful. Other drugs that help tighten the sphincter, such as pseudoephedrine, should be used with estrogen. Incontinence pads may be used to absorb the small amount of urine that usually leaks during stress.

More severe cases of stress incontinence that do not respond to treatment can be corrected surgically using any of several procedures that lift up the bladder and strengthen the bladder outlet (the portion of the bladder that empties into the outflow passage or urethra). Injections of collagen around the urethra are effective in some cases. A urinary sphincter that does not close adequately may be replaced with an artificial one.

For **overflow incontinence** caused by an enlarged prostate or other blockage, surgery is usually necessary. A variety of procedures are available to remove part or all of the prostate. The drug finasteride, when taken over a period of months, can reduce the size of the prostate or stop its growth, so that surgery can be avoided or deferred. Drugs that relax the sphincter, such as terazosin and tamsulosin, can be quite effective.

When the cause of overflow incontinence is weak contraction of the bladder muscles, drugs are usually not helpful. Gentle pressure applied by squeezing the lower abdomen with the hands just over the bladder may help, especially for people who can empty the bladder but have difficulty emptying it completely. In some cases, a catheter may need to be inserted into the bladder to drain the bladder and prevent complications, such as recurring infections and kidney damage. The catheter may be placed permanently, or it may be inserted and removed several times a day.

Treatment for **functional incontinence** involves regular toileting assistance. For example, another person can remind the incontinent person to urinate on a schedule, usually every 3 to 4 hours, so that the bladder is emptied before episodes of incontinence can occur (prompted scheduled voiding). If depression is a contributing factor, it should be treated. The use of garments and pads is also helpful; however, a person should not become unnecessarily dependent on them.

CHAPTER 148

Urinary Tract Obstruction

An obstruction anywhere along the urinary tract—from the kidneys, where urine is produced, to the urethra, through which urine leaves the body—can increase pressure inside the urinary tract and slow the flow of urine. An obstruction may occur suddenly or develop slowly over days, weeks, or even months. An obstruction may completely or only partially block part of the urinary tract.

Urinary tract obstruction can make the kidneys distend (dilate). Distention damages the kidneys. Although the kidneys can usually recover if the obstruction is relieved quickly, permanent damage may occur. Severe damage can result in loss of kidney function (kidney failure). Obstruction can also lead to stone formation and urinary tract infections. An infection may develop because bacteria that enter the urinary tract are not flushed out when the flow of urine is obstructed.

Hydronephrosis

Hydronephrosis is distention (dilation) of the kidney with urine, caused by backward pressure on the kidney when the flow of urine is obstructed.

Normally, urine flows out of the kidneys at extremely low pressure. If the flow of urine is obstructed, urine backs up in the small tubes of the kidney and its collecting area (renal pelvis), distending the kidney and increasing the pressure on its internal structures. The elevated pressure from obstruction may ultimately damage the kidney and can result in loss of kidney function.

Long-standing distention of the renal pelvis and ureter can also inhibit the rhythmic muscular contractions that normally move urine down the ureter from the kidney to the bladder. Scar tissue may then replace the normal muscular tissue in the walls of the ureter, resulting in permanent damage.

Causes

Hydronephrosis commonly results from an obstruction located at the junction of the ureter and renal pelvis. Causes of this type of obstruction include the following:
• Structural abnormalities—for example, when the insertion of the ureter into the renal pelvis is too high
• Kinking at this junction resulting from a kidney shifting downward
• Stones (calculi) in the renal pelvis
• Compression of the ureter by bands of fibrous tissue, an abnormally located artery or vein, or a tumor

Hydronephrosis can also result from an obstruction below the junction of the ureter and renal pelvis or from backflow (reflux) of urine from the bladder. Causes of this type of obstruction include the following:
• Stones in the ureter
• Tumors in or near the ureter
• Narrowing of the ureter resulting from a birth defect, an injury, an infection, radiation therapy, or surgery
• Disorders of the muscles or nerves in the ureter or bladder
• Formation of fibrous tissue in or around the ureter resulting from surgery, x-rays, or drugs (especially methysergide)

• Bulging of the lower end of the ureter into the bladder (ureterocele)

• Cancers of the bladder, cervix, uterus, prostate, or other pelvic organs

• Obstruction that prevents urine flow from the bladder to the urethra, resulting from prostate enlargement (most often caused by a condition called benign prostatic hyperplasia▲), or rectal impaction with feces

• Abnormal contractions of the bladder resulting from a birth defect or an injury

Hydronephrosis of both kidneys can occur during pregnancy as the enlarging uterus compresses the ureters. Hormonal changes during pregnancy may aggravate the problem by reducing the muscular contractions that normally move urine down the ureters. The hydronephrosis usually ends when the pregnancy ends, although the renal pelvis and ureters may remain somewhat distended afterward.

Symptoms

Symptoms depend on the cause, location, and duration of the obstruction. When the obstruction begins quickly (acute hydronephrosis), it usually produces renal colic—an excruciating, intermittent pain in the flank (the area between the ribs and hip) on the affected side. Partial obstruction may reduce the rate of urine flow. A total stoppage of the flow of urine most often occurs with complete blockage of the ureters from both kidneys or complete blockage of the urethra.

People who have slowly progressive (chronic) hydronephrosis may have no symptoms, or they may have attacks of dull, aching discomfort in the flank on the affected side. Sometimes a kidney shifts downward, causing temporary overfilling of the renal pelvis or temporary blockage of the ureter and producing painful hydronephrosis that occurs intermittently.

Hydronephrosis may cause vague intestinal symptoms, such as nausea, vomiting, and abdominal pain. These symptoms sometimes occur in children when hydronephrosis results from a birth defect in which the junction of the ureter and renal pelvis is too narrow. Urinary tract infections—with pus in the urine, fever, and discomfort in the area of the bladder or kidneys—are fairly common. When the flow of urine is obstructed, stones may form. If both kidneys are obstructed, kidney failure may result.

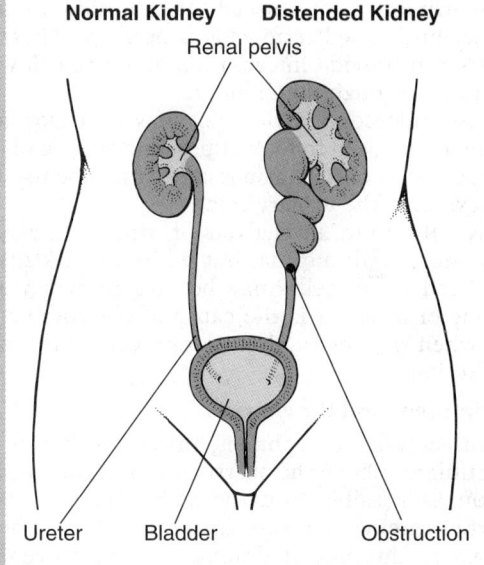

Hydronephrosis: A Distended Kidney

In hydronephrosis, the kidney is distended because the flow of urine is obstructed and urine backs up in the kidney's small tubes and central collecting area (renal pelvis).

Normal Kidney   **Distended Kidney**
Renal pelvis

Ureter   Bladder   Obstruction

Diagnosis

Early diagnosis is important, because most cases of obstruction can be corrected and a delay in treatment can lead to irreversible kidney damage. The doctor may suspect hydronephrosis during a physical examination. A distended kidney can sometimes be felt in the flank, particularly if the kidney is greatly enlarged in an infant or a child or a thin adult.

The doctor depends on testing to make the diagnosis. Bladder catheterization (insertion of a hollow, flexible tube through the urethra) is often performed as the first diagnostic test. If the catheter drains a large amount of urine from the bladder, then either the bladder outlet or the urethra is the site of the obstruction.

Ultrasound is a very useful test in most people (particularly children and pregnant

▲ see page 1329

women) because it has fewer complications than x-ray studies that use radiocontrast chemicals. Usually it can detect the cause of the obstruction.

Sometimes intravenous urography is used. In this procedure, the kidneys are x-rayed after a radiopaque dye, which can be seen on x-rays, is injected into the bloodstream. X-ray images of the bladder and urethra can be produced after the injected radiopaque dye passes through the kidneys or after this dye is introduced into the urinary tract through the urethra in a procedure called retrograde urography. These tests can provide information about the flow of urine through the kidneys.

An endoscope (a flexible viewing tube) is sometimes used to look at possible sites of obstruction as closely as possible; it can be used to examine the urinary tract.

Results from an analysis of urine (urinalysis) are usually normal but white blood cells and red blood cells may be present when a stone or a cancer is the cause of obstruction, or when the obstruction is complicated by an infection.

Treatment and Prognosis

In acute hydronephrosis, urine that has accumulated above the obstruction is drained as soon as possible, usually with a needle inserted through the skin into the kidney. The goals of this urgent drainage are to prevent loss of kidney function or prevent further loss if function is already impaired. The obstruction must also be relieved quickly. The method used depends on the cause, but most obstructions require surgery of some kind. For example, surgery may be needed to remove a stone from the renal pelvis or the ureter.

Complications of acute hydronephrosis, such as urinary tract infections and kidney failure, if present, are treated promptly. The cause of the obstruction that led to acute hydronephrosis is corrected whenever possible.

Urgent treatment of chronic hydronephrosis is usually not required. Chronic hydronephrosis is corrected by draining urine above the obstruction. For example, soft tubes (ureteral stents) may be inserted into the ureter to bypass an obstruction. Complications of ureteral stents can include movement of the tube, infection, irritation, and discomfort.

The cause of the obstruction that led to chronic hydronephrosis is also treated when-

ever possible. A narrow or abnormal section of a ureter may be surgically removed and the cut ends joined together. Sometimes surgery is needed to remove fibrous tissue from the ureter. If the junction of the ureter and bladder is obstructed, the ureter can be surgically detached, then attached to a different part of the bladder.

If the urethra is obstructed because of an enlarged or cancerous prostate, treatment can include drugs, such as hormone therapy for prostate cancer,▲ surgery, or enlargement of the urethra with dilators. Other treatments may be needed for stones that block the flow of urine.

Treatment to correct acute hydronephrosis in one or both kidneys is usually successful when the obstruction can be relieved and the kidneys are functioning adequately. The prognosis is less certain for chronic hydronephrosis.

Stones in the Urinary Tract

Stones (calculi) are hard masses that form anywhere in the urinary tract and may cause pain, bleeding, obstruction of the flow of urine, or an infection.

Depending on where a stone forms, it may be called a kidney stone, ureteral stone, or bladder stone. The process of stone formation is called urolithiasis, renal lithiasis, or nephrolithiasis.

Every year, about 1 of 1,000 adults in the United States is hospitalized because of stones in the urinary tract. Stones are more common in older adults and men. Stones may form because the urine becomes too saturated with salts that can form stones or because the urine lacks the normal inhibitors of stone formation. Citrate is such an inhibitor, because it normally binds with calcium that is often involved in forming stones. About 80% of the stones are composed of calcium; the remainder are composed of various substances, including uric acid, cystine, and struvite. Stones are more common in people with certain diseases (for example, hypertension and short bowel syndrome) and in people whose diet is very high in protein or who do not consume enough water. Struvite stones—a mixture of magnesium, ammonium, and phosphate—are also called infection stones, because they form only in infected urine.

Stones vary in size from too small to be seen with the naked eye to 1 inch or more in diam-

▲ see page 1331

eter. A large so-called staghorn stone may fill almost the entire renal pelvis and the tubes that drain into it (calices).

A urinary tract infection may result when bacteria become trapped in urine that pools above a blockage. When stones block the urinary tract for a long time, urine backs up in the tubes inside the kidney, producing excessive pressure that can distend the kidney (hydronephrosis) and eventually damage it.

Symptoms

Stones, especially tiny ones, may not cause any symptoms. Stones in the bladder may cause pain in the lower abdomen. Stones that obstruct the ureter or renal pelvis or any of its drainage tubes may cause back pain or renal colic. Renal colic is characterized by an excruciating intermittent pain, usually in the flank (the area between the ribs and hip), that spreads across the abdomen, often to the genital area and inner thigh.

Other symptoms include nausea and vomiting, abdominal distention, chills, fever, and blood in the urine. A person may have an urge to urinate frequently, particularly as a stone passes down the ureter.

Diagnosis

Stones that cause pain are generally diagnosed on the basis of the symptoms of renal colic, together with tenderness over the back and groin or pain in the genital area without an obvious cause. Usually, no additional tests are needed, unless the pain persists for more than a few hours or the diagnosis is uncertain. Urinalysis may show blood or pus in the urine whether or not symptoms are present.

X-rays or an ultrasound of the abdomen can show stones made of calcium, cystine, and struvite, but usually not of uric acid. If needed, other diagnostic procedures can be performed. In intravenous urography, a radiopaque dye, which is visible on x-rays, is injected into a vein and travels to the kidneys where it outlines uric acid stones so they can be seen on x-rays. In retrograde urography, the radiopaque dye is introduced into the urinary tract through the urethra. Computed tomography (CT) is usually reserved for situations in which the diagnosis has not been made with other procedures.

Treatment

Small stones that are not causing symptoms, obstruction, or an infection usually do

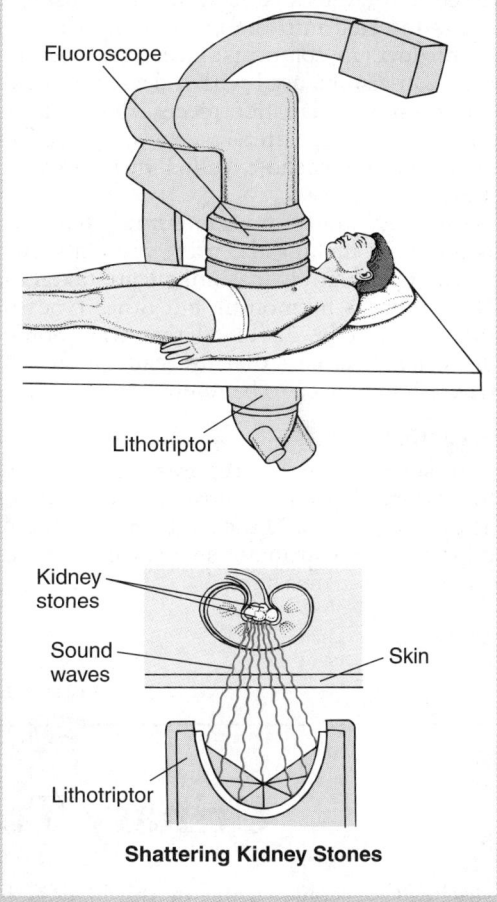

Removing a Stone With Sound Waves

Kidney stones can sometimes be broken up by sound waves produced by a lithotriptor in a procedure called extracorporeal shock wave lithotripsy. After an ultrasound device or fluoroscope is used to locate the stone, the lithotriptor is placed against the back, and the sound waves are focused on the stone, shattering it. Then the person drinks fluids to flush the stone fragments out of the kidney, to be eliminated in the urine. Sometimes blood appears in the urine or the abdomen is bruised after the procedure, but serious problems are rare.

Fluoroscope

Lithotriptor

Kidney stones

Sound waves

Skin

Lithotriptor

Shattering Kidney Stones

not need to be treated. Drinking plenty of fluids or receiving large amounts of fluids intravenously if oral intake is not feasible increases urine production and helps wash out some stones; once a stone is passed, no other immediate treatment is needed. The pain of renal colic may be relieved with nonsteroidal anti-inflammatory drugs (NSAIDs) or opioids.

Often, a stone in the renal pelvis or uppermost part of the ureter that is ½ inch or less in diameter can be broken up by ultrasound waves directed at the body by a sound wave generator (a procedure called extracorporeal shock wave lithotripsy). The pieces of stone are then passed in the urine. Sometimes, a stone is removed with grasping forceps through a small incision in the skin (percutaneous nephrostolithotomy), or the stone can be fragmented using a lithotripsy probe.

Small stones in the lower part of the ureter may be removed with a small, flexible scope (called a ureteroscope, a kind of endoscope) that is inserted into the urethra and through the bladder. In some instances, the ureteroscope can also be used with a device to break stones up into smaller pieces that can be removed with the ureteroscope or passed in the urine (a procedure called intracorporeal lithotripsy).

Uric acid stones are sometimes dissolved gradually by making the urine more alkaline (for example, with potassium citrate taken for 4 to 6 months by mouth), but other types of stones cannot be dissolved this way. Sometimes, larger stones that are causing an obstruction may need to be removed surgically.

Prevention

Measures to prevent the formation of new stones vary, depending on the composition of the existing stones. These stones are analyzed, and levels in the urine of substances that can form stones are measured.

Drinking large amounts of fluids—8 to 10 ten-ounce glasses a day—is recommended. Following a diet moderately low in calcium and taking sodium cellulose phosphate, a resin, may help, but such measures can cause levels of calcium to become too low. Many people with calcium stones have a condition called hypercalciuria, in which excess calcium is excreted in the urine. Thiazide diuretics, such as hydrochlorothiazide, reduce the concentration of calcium in the urine and help prevent the formation of new stones in such people. Potassium citrate may be given to increase a low urine level of citrate, a substance that inhibits calcium stone formation.

A high level of oxalate in the urine, which contributes to calcium stone formation, may result from excess consumption of foods high in oxalate, such as rhubarb, spinach, cocoa, nuts, pepper, and tea, or from certain intestinal disorders. A change in diet may help, and the underlying disorder can be treated.

In rare cases when calcium stones result from hyperparathyroidism, sarcoidosis, vitamin D toxicity, renal tubular acidosis, or cancer, the underlying disorder must be treated.

For stones that contain uric acid, a diet low in meat, fish, and poultry is recommended, because these foods increase the level of uric acid in the urine. Allopurinol may be given to reduce the production of uric acid. Potassium citrate should be given to all people who have uric acid stones to make the urine alkaline, because uric acid stones form when urine acidity increases.

Struvite stones usually need to be removed by extracorporeal shock wave lithotripsy or surgery. Antibiotics are not helpful for urinary tract infections until the stones are removed.

CHAPTER 149

Urinary Tract Infections

In healthy people, urine in the bladder is sterile—no bacteria or other infectious organisms are present. The channel that carries urine from the bladder out of the body (urethra) contains no bacteria or too few to cause an infection. However, any part of the urinary tract can become infected; an infection any-

where along the urinary tract is called a urinary tract infection (UTI).

UTIs are usually classified as upper or lower according to where they occur along the urinary tract. Lower UTIs are infections of the urethra (urethritis) or bladder (cystitis); upper UTIs are infections of the kidneys (pyelonephritis) or ureters (ureteritis). UTIs can occur in children▲ as well as in adults.

Causes

The organisms that cause infection usually enter the urinary tract by one of two routes. The most common route by far is through the lower end of the urinary tract—the opening of a man's urethra at the tip of the penis or the opening of a woman's urethra at the vulva. The result is an ascending infection that spreads up the urethra. The other possible route is through the bloodstream, usually directly to the kidneys.

UTIs are almost always caused by bacteria, although some viruses, fungi, and parasites can infect the urinary tract as well. More than 85% of UTIs are caused by bacteria from the intestine or vagina. Ordinarily, however, bacteria that enter the urinary tract are washed out by the flushing action of the bladder as it empties.

Bacteria: Bacterial infections of the lower urinary tract—the bladder and urethra—are very common, especially in adolescent girls. *Escherichia coli* is the most common bacteria. When the person has a kidney stone, *Proteus* bacteria may be able to grow. Among people between the ages of 20 and 50, UTIs caused by bacteria are about 50 times more common in women than in men. In men, the urethra is longer, so it is more difficult for bacteria to ascend far enough to cause an infection. In people older than 50, UTIs become more common in both men and women, with less difference between the sexes.

Viruses: The herpes simplex virus type 2 (HSV-2) may infect the urethra to cause a UTI, making urination painful and emptying of the bladder difficult.

Fungi: Certain fungi or yeasts can infect the urinary tract to cause a UTI. The most common type is *Candida*, which causes candidiasis. *Candida* frequently infects people who have an impaired immune system or a bladder catheter in place. Rarely, other types of fungi, including those that cause blastomycosis (*Blastomyces*) or coccidiomycosis (*Coccidioides*), infect the urinary tract. Fungi and bacteria often infect the kidneys at the same time.

Parasites: A number of parasites, including certain types of worms, can infect the urinary tract.

Trichomoniasis, caused by a type of microscopic parasite, is a sexually transmitted dis-

Factors Contributing to Bacterial Urinary Tract Infections

Ascending Infections

- Blockage (for example, by stones) anywhere in the urinary tract
- Abnormal bladder function that prevents proper emptying, such as occurs in neurologic diseases
- Leaking of the valve between the ureter and the bladder, allowing urine and bacteria to flow backward from the bladder up the ureters, possibly reaching the kidneys
- Insertion of a urinary catheter or an instrument by a doctor
- Sexual intercourse
- Use of a diaphragm with spermicide
- Presence of fistulas between the vagina and the bladder or the intestine and the bladder
- Prostatitis

Blood-borne Infections

- Infection in the bloodstream (septicemia)
- Infection of the heart valves (infective endocarditis)

ease that can produce a copious greenish yellow, frothy discharge from the vagina in women. Rarely, the bladder or urethra becomes infected. Trichomoniasis in men usually produces no symptoms, although it can cause inflammation of the prostate gland (prostatitis).

Schistosomiasis, an infection caused by a type of worm called a fluke, can affect the kidneys, ureters, and bladder. This infection is a common cause of severe kidney failure among people who live in Africa, South America, and Asia. Persistent bladder infections with schistosomiasis may eventually result in bladder cancer.

Malaria, a disease caused by a type of microscopic parasite carried by mosquitoes, can destroy the small blood vessels (glomeruli) of the kidneys or can rapidly damage red blood cells, causing acute kidney failure.

Filariasis, a threadworm infection, obstructs lymphatic vessels, causing lymph fluid to en-

▲ see page 1567

ter the urine (chyluria). Filariasis can cause enormous swelling of tissues (elephantiasis), which, in men, may involve the scrotum.

Urethritis

Urethritis is infection of the urethra, the channel that carries urine from the bladder out of the body.

Urethritis may be caused by bacteria, fungi, or viruses. In women, the organisms generally travel to the urethra from the vagina. In most women, the bacteria come from the lower intestine and reach the vagina from the anus. Men are much less likely to develop urethritis because the opening of the male urethra is far removed from the anus and is not as easily injured during sexual intercourse.

Sexually transmitted organisms—such as *Neisseria gonorrhoeae*, which causes gonorrhea—can spread to the urethra during sexual intercourse with an infected partner.▲ *Chlamydia* and the herpes simplex virus are also commonly transmitted sexually and can cause urethritis.■ When men develop urethritis, the gonorrheal organism is a very common cause. Although this organism may infect the urethra in women, the vagina, cervix, uterus, ovaries, and fallopian tubes are more likely to be infected. Trichomonas, a type of microscopic parasite, also causes urethritis in men.

Symptoms

In women, urethritis may gradually cause pain during urination and urination may also cause pain if vaginitis is present. The urine, which is acidic, may cause a burning pain as it passes over the inflamed labia. In men, urethritis usually begins with a discharge from the urethra. The discharge contains pus (which is yellowish green) when the gonococcal organism is involved or mucus (which is clear) when other organisms are involved. Other symptoms of urethritis in men include pain during urination and a frequent, urgent need to urinate.

A gonorrheal infection of the urethra that is not treated or is inadequately treated eventually can cause a narrowing (stricture) of the urethra. A stricture increases the risk that infections will develop in the bladder (cystitis) or the kidneys (pyelonephritis). Untreated gonorrhea occasionally leads to an accumula-

tion of pus (abscess) around the urethra. An abscess can produce outpouchings from the urethral wall (urethral diverticula), which can also become infected. If the abscess perforates the skin, urine may flow through a newly created abnormal connection (urethral fistula).

Diagnosis, Prevention, and Treatment

A doctor can usually make a diagnosis of urethritis based on the symptoms alone. A sample of the discharge, if present, is collected by inserting a soft-tipped swab into the end of the urethra. The urethral swab is then sent to a laboratory for analysis so that the infecting organism can be identified.

Sexually transmitted diseases that cause urethritis can be prevented by using a condom. Treatment depends on the cause of the infection. Antibiotics are given for a bacterial infection. Antifungal drugs are used to treat fungal infections. An antiviral drug, such as acyclovir, may be needed for a herpes simplex infection.

Cystitis

Cystitis is infection of the bladder.

Cystitis is common in women, particularly during the reproductive years. Some women have recurring episodes of cystitis. There are a number of reasons for this—the short length of the urethra and the closeness of the urethra to the vagina and anus, where bacteria are commonly found. Sexual intercourse can contribute, too, because the motion can cause slight injuries to the urethra and a tendency for bacteria to ascend to the bladder. Pregnant women are especially likely to develop cystitis because the pregnancy itself can interfere with emptying of the bladder.

Use of a diaphragm increases the risk of developing cystitis, possibly because spermicide used with the diaphragm suppresses the normal vaginal bacteria and allows bacteria that cause cystitis to flourish in the vagina. Rarely, cystitis recurs because of an abnormal connection between the bladder and the vagina (vesicovaginal fistula).

Cystitis is less common in men. In men, cystitis generally starts with an infection in the urethra that moves into the prostate, then into the bladder. The most common cause of recurring cystitis in men is a persistent bacterial infection of the prostate. Although antibiotics quickly clear bacteria from the urine in the bladder, most of these drugs cannot pene-

▲ see page 1179   ■ see page 1180

trate well enough into the prostate to cure an infection there. Consequently, when drug therapy is discontinued, bacteria that remain in the prostate tend to reinfect the bladder. Cystitis can also be caused by a catheter or an instrument used during surgery that introduces bacteria into the bladder.

If the flow of urine becomes partly obstructed because of a kidney stone or an enlarged prostate, infected urine cannot pass and the number of bacteria increases so that bacteria have a greater opportunity to cause an infection above the point of obstruction.

In men and women, an abnormal connection between the bladder and the intestine (vesicoenteric fistula) can develop, allowing air to enter the bladder and sometimes enabling bacteria that produce gas to enter and grow in the bladder. Air bubbles can appear in the urine (pneumaturia). A structural abnormality (such as a drooping uterus and bladder) may cause poor emptying of the bladder and predispose a person to cystitis.

Sometimes the bladder can become inflamed without an infection being present (interstitial cystitis).

Symptoms

Cystitis usually produces a frequent, urgent need to urinate and a burning or painful sensation while urinating. The urgent need to urinate may cause an uncontrollable loss of urine (incontinence), especially in older people. Fever is rarely present. Pain is usually felt above the pubic bone and often in the lower back as well. Frequent urination during the night (nocturia) is another symptom. The urine is often cloudy and contains visible blood in about 30% of people. Symptoms may disappear without treatment.

Sometimes cystitis produces no symptoms, particularly in older people, and is discovered when urine tests are performed for other reasons. A person whose bladder is malfunctioning because of nerve damage (neurogenic bladder▲) or a person who has a permanently placed catheter may have cystitis with no symptoms until a kidney infection or an unexplained fever develops.

Diagnosis

A doctor can diagnose cystitis based on its typical symptoms. A midstream (clean-catch) urine specimen■ is collected so that the urine is not contaminated with bacteria from the vagina or the tip of the penis. A strip of test pa-

Interstitial Cystitis: Bladder Inflammation, Not Infection

Interstitial cystitis is painful inflammation of the bladder without evidence of infection. The cause is unknown. No infectious organisms are found in the urine. Typically, middle-aged women are affected; it is very unusual for men to be affected.

Symptoms include very frequent, painful urination, and the urine often contains pus and blood detected by microscopic examination. Occasionally, blood is visible in the urine. Over time, the chronic inflammation may cause the bladder to shrink. An examination of the bladder by cystoscopy may detect small superficial areas of bleeding and ulcers.

A number of treatments have been tried, but none is routinely satisfactory. Drugs to relieve pain, anticholinergic drugs, or antidepressants sometimes help. Pentosan polysulfate is a newer drug taken by mouth that may provide pain relief for some people. Dimethyl sulfoxide, a drug injected directly into the bladder, benefits some people. When the person has intolerable symptoms that do not respond to treatment, the bladder may need to be surgically removed. This situation is rare, but when it does occur, a doctor may create a new bladder from a segment of the small intestine (ileum) or insert a tube directly into the kidney; the tube allows urine to drain externally into a bag.

per is sometimes dipped into the urine to perform two quick and simple tests for substances that are normally not found in the urine. The testing strip can detect nitrites that are released by bacteria. The testing strip can also detect the presence of leukocyte esterase (an enzyme found in certain white blood cells), which may indicate that the body is trying to clear the urine of bacteria.

The urine specimen is examined under a microscope to see whether it contains red or white blood cells or other substances. Bacteria are counted, and the sample is cultured to identify the type of bacteria. If the person has an infection, one type of bacteria is usually present in large numbers.

▲ see box on page 860   ■ see box on page 826

In men, a midstream urine specimen is usually sufficient for the diagnosis. In women, a specimen is more likely to be contaminated with bacteria from the vagina or vulva. When the urine contains only small numbers of bacteria, or several different types of bacteria simultaneously, the urine has likely been contaminated during the collection process. To ensure that the urine is not contaminated, a doctor sometimes must obtain a specimen directly from the bladder with a catheter.

It is important for the doctor to find the cause of urinary tract infections in several different groups. The cause should be found in children younger than 5, in men at any age, and in women with frequently recurring infections (3 or more per year), especially when accompanied by symptoms of obstruction, an upper urinary tract infection, or infection with the *Proteus* bacteria. In these types of people, there is a greater likelihood of finding a cause that requires specific treatment other than giving drugs to treat the infection (for example, a large kidney stone). Doctors may perform an x-ray study in which a radiopaque dye, visible on x-rays, is injected into a vein, then excreted into the urine by the kidneys. The x-ray films then provide images of the kidneys, ureters, and bladder. Performing

Preventing Bladder Infections in Women

In women who experience three or more bladder infections in a year, these measures may help:

- Drinking cranberry juice, because the juice contains a substance that directly inhibits bacterial growth and because it acidifies the urine (making it a less hospitable environment for bacterial growth)
- Increasing the intake of fluids
- Urinating often
- Urinating within a short time after sexual intercourse
- Avoiding the use of spermicides in conjunction with a diaphragm for birth control
- Taking antibiotics continually in low doses; the yearly cost is only one fourth the cost of treating three or four infections a year. Typically, the antibiotic is taken daily, 3 times a week, or immediately after sexual intercourse

voiding cystourethrography, which involves injecting a radiopaque dye into the bladder and filming its exit, is a good way to investigate the backflow (reflux) of urine from the bladder, up the ureters, particularly in children, and may also identify any narrowing (stricture) of the urethra. Retrograde urethrography, in which the radiopaque dye is injected directly into the urethra, is useful for detecting stricture, outpouching, or an abnormal connection (fistula) of the urethra in both men and women. Looking directly into the bladder with a flexible viewing tube (cystoscopy) may help diagnose the problem when cystitis does not improve with treatment.

Treatment

People who have frequent bladder infections may continuously take low doses of antibiotics. The antibiotic can be taken daily, 3 times a week, or immediately after sexual intercourse.

Drinking plenty of fluids may help to prevent cystitis. The flushing action of the urine washes many bacteria out of the bladder; the body's natural defenses eliminate the remainder.

Cystitis is usually treated with antibiotics. Treating cystitis that has no symptoms may be harmful, because bacteria that are resistant to many antibiotics may flourish. However, cystitis is treated during pregnancy even when the woman has no symptoms, because of a higher risk that organisms might reach and infect the kidneys. Before prescribing antibiotics, the doctor determines whether the person has a condition that would make cystitis more severe, such as a structural abnormality, diabetes, or a weakened immune system (which reduces the person's ability to fight infection). Such conditions may require more potent antibiotics taken for a longer period of time, particularly because the infection is likely to return as soon as the person stops taking antibiotics.

For women, taking an antibiotic by mouth for 3 days is usually effective if the infection has not led to any complications, although some doctors prefer to use a single dose. For more stubborn infections, an antibiotic is usually taken for 7 to 10 days. For men, an antibiotic is usually taken for 10 to 14 days because a shorter duration of treatment is associated with frequent recurrences.

A variety of drugs are used to relieve symptoms, especially the frequent, insistent urge to urinate and painful urination. Certain drugs, such as atropine, may relieve bladder spasms that cause the sense of urgency. Other drugs, such as phenazopyridine, reduce the pain by soothing the inflamed tissues.

Surgery may be necessary to relieve any physical obstruction to the flow of urine or to correct a structural abnormality that makes infection more likely, such as a drooping uterus and bladder. Draining urine from an obstructed area through a catheter helps control the infection. Usually, an antibiotic is given before surgery to reduce the risk of the infection spreading throughout the body.

Ureteritis

Ureteritis is infection of one or both ureters, the tubes that connect the kidneys to the bladder.

The spread of an infection from the kidneys or bladder is the most common cause of ureteritis. Another cause is a slowing of the flow of urine because of a defective nerve supply to part of the ureter. An underlying kidney or bladder infection is treated with an antibiotic. The sections of the ureter in which nerves are defective may need to be removed surgically.

Pyelonephritis

Pyelonephritis is a bacterial infection of one or both kidneys.

Pyelonephritis is more common in women than in men. *Escherichia coli*, a type of bacteria that is normally found in the large intestine, causes about 90% of cases of pyelonephritis among people who live in the community. Infections usually ascend from the genital area through the urethra to the bladder, up the ureters, into the kidneys. In a person with a healthy urinary tract, an infection is usually prevented from moving up the ureters into the kidneys by the flow of urine washing organisms out and by closure of the ureters at their entrance to the bladder. However, any physical obstruction to the flow of urine, such as a structural abnormality, kidney stone, or an enlarged prostate, or the backflow (reflux) of urine from the bladder into the ureters increases the likelihood of pyelonephritis.

Infections can also be carried to the kidneys from another part of the body through the

bloodstream. For instance, a staphylococcal skin infection can spread to the kidneys through the bloodstream.

The risk of pyelonephritis is increased in people with obstruction of the ureters, diabetes, in people with a weakened immune system (which reduces the body's ability to fight infection), and in pregnant women. During pregnancy, the enlarging uterus puts pressure on the ureters, which partially obstructs the normal downward flow of urine. Pregnancy also increases the risk of reflux of urine up the ureters by causing the ureters to dilate and reducing the muscle contractions that propel urine down the ureters into the bladder.

Symptoms and Complications

Symptoms of pyelonephritis often begin suddenly with chills, fever, pain in the lower part of the back on either side, nausea, and vomiting.

About one third of people with pyelonephritis also have symptoms of cystitis, including frequent, painful urination. One or both kidneys may be enlarged and tender, with tenderness felt in the small of the back on the affected side. Sometimes the muscles of the abdomen are tightly contracted. Irritation from the infection or the passing of a kidney stone can cause spasms of the ureters. If the ureters go into spasms, the person may experience episodes of intense pain (renal colic). In children, symptoms of a kidney infection often are slight and more difficult to recognize.▲

In a long-standing infection (chronic pyelonephritis), the pain may be vague, and fever may come and go or not occur at all. Chronic pyelonephritis occurs only in people who have major underlying abnormalities, such as a urinary tract obstruction, large kidney stones that persist or, most commonly, reflux of urine from the bladder into the ureters (which occurs mostly in young children). Tuberculosis and fungal infections rarely cause pyelonephritis. Rarely, chronic pyelonephritis can eventually severely damage the kidneys.

Diagnosis

The typical symptoms of pyelonephritis lead a doctor to perform two common laboratory tests to determine whether the kidneys are infected: examining a urine specimen under a microscope and culturing bacteria in a urine specimen to determine which bacteria

▲ see page 1567

are present. Blood tests are also performed to check for elevated white blood cells or bacteria in the blood.

Additional tests are performed in people who have intense back pain from renal colic, in those who do not respond to antibiotic treatment within 48 hours, in those whose symptoms return shortly after antibiotic treatment is finished, and in men (because they so rarely develop pyelonephritis). Ultrasound or x-ray studies performed in these situations may reveal kidney stones, structural abnormalities, or other causes of urinary obstruction.

Treatment

Antibiotics are started as soon as the doctor suspects pyelonephritis and urine and blood samples have been taken for laboratory tests. The choice of drug or its dosage may be modified based on the laboratory test results, how sick the person is, and whether the infection started in the hospital, where bacteria tend to be resistant to antibiotics.

Treatment with antibiotics given by mouth for 14 days is sometimes successful if the person has no nausea or vomiting, no signs of dehydration, pain that is controlled with drugs taken by mouth, and no high fever or chills. Otherwise, the person is usually treated initially in the hospital. If hospitalization is needed, after 1 or 2 days of injected or intravenous antibiotics, treatment can usually be switched to antibiotics given by mouth.

Antibiotic treatment to prevent recurrence of the infection usually continues for 2 weeks but may last as long as 6 weeks for men, in whom the infection is commonly more difficult to eradicate. A final urine sample is usually taken 4 to 6 weeks after the antibiotic treatment is finished to make sure the infection has been eradicated.

Surgery may be needed if tests reveal a predisposing condition, such as an obstruction, a structural abnormality, or a stone.

People who have frequent episodes of pyelonephritis or whose infection returns after antibiotic treatment is finished may be advised to take a small dose of antibiotic every day as preventive therapy. The ideal duration of such therapy is unknown, but it is often discontinued after a year. If the infection returns, therapy may be continued indefinitely.

CHAPTER 150

Injury to the Urinary Tract

The kidneys and the rest of the urinary tract may become injured in a number of ways. Examples include injuries from a blunt or penetrating force (most commonly motor vehicle accidents, falls, and gunshot or stab wounds), surgery, or radiation therapy for cancer treatment. Injuries to the urinary tract often occur with injuries to other organs, especially abdominal organs.

Because the function of the kidneys is to continuously filter out metabolic wastes from the blood and remove them from the body through the urinary tract, injuries to the kidneys or urinary tract can lead to kidney failure. Other complications of injury include bleeding, leakage of urine from the urinary tract into surrounding tissues, and infection. Preventing permanent damage to the urinary tract and even death may depend on prompt diagnosis and treatment.

Kidney Injuries

The kidney is injured more often than any of the organs along the urinary tract. Blunt force due to motor vehicle accidents, falls, or sports injuries is the usual cause of injury. Penetrating kidney injuries can result from gunshot or stab wounds. Less commonly, injuries can occur during diagnostic tests, such as a kidney biopsy. Injuries may also occur occasionally during various treatments, such as

Kidney Injuries: Minor to Severe

The severity of kidney injuries varies widely. When an injury is minor, the kidney may be only bruised. When an injury is more severe, the kidney may be lacerated, and urine may leak into the surrounding tissue. If the kidney is torn from its attachment to blood vessels, bleeding may be profuse, resulting in shock or death. Most kidney injuries result in blood in the urine.

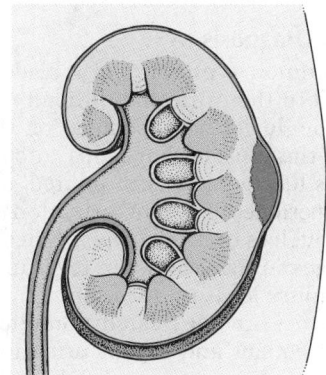 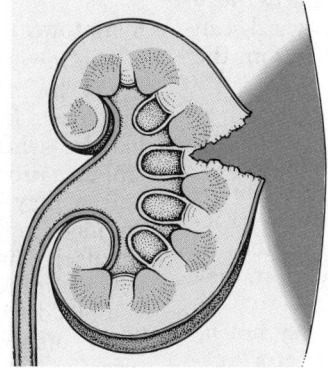 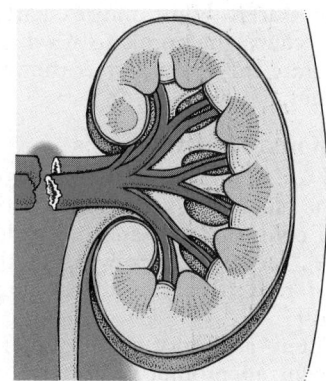

| Bruise | Laceration | Torn Attachment |

those for kidney stones, including extracorporeal shock wave lithotripsy or percutaneous procedures.

Symptoms and Diagnosis

If kidney injuries are not treated or are very serious, complications, such as kidney failure, high blood pressure, delayed bleeding, and infection may result.

The history of events, the person's complaints, and a physical examination help a doctor diagnose a kidney injury. Blood in the urine (visible or microscopic) is the strongest indicator of a kidney injury. With major kidney injuries, low blood pressure and anemia may occur if the person loses a significant amount of blood. Other indicators of a kidney injury include bruising of the flank (the area between the ribs and hip), marks made from a seat belt, fractures of the lower ribs, or pain in the upper abdomen. Most blunt kidney injuries are minor and may result in nothing more than a microscopic amount of blood in the urine. With penetrating injuries, the location of the wound (whether in the upper or mid abdomen, back, or flank) may help a doctor determine if the kidney is involved.

A suspicion of an injury can be evaluated by imaging the kidneys and urinary tract. This is best accomplished using computed tomography (CT) or intravenous urography to accurately determine the location and extent of the injury. Occasionally, additional imaging tests may be needed to confirm the diagnosis.

Treatment

In general, most people recover from their kidney injuries, provided they are diagnosed and treated promptly. Treatment begins with steps to control blood loss and to prevent shock. Fluids are given intravenously to help keep blood pressure within a normal range and stimulate urine production. For minor kidney injuries, careful control of fluid intake and bed rest are often the only treatment needed, because these measures allow the kidney to heal itself. Major injuries usually require surgical repair. Blood transfusions may be needed; rarely, the injured kidney needs to be removed.

Kidney failure may require lifelong treatment. Other complications of kidney injuries that require treatment include high blood pressure, delayed bleeding, and infection.

Ureteral Injuries

Most injuries to the ureter occur during pelvic or abdominal operations, such as removal of the uterus (hysterectomy) or the colon, or during ureteroscopy (an examination of the ureter with a flexible viewing tube). Another cause of ureteral injury is penetration by either a gunshot or stab wound. A ureteral injury from a direct blow to the body is uncommon. Rarely, blunt injuries, particularly those that cause the trunk to bend backward, can separate the upper part of the ureter from the kidney.

Symptoms and Diagnosis

If ureteral injuries are untreated, complications, such as formation of a fistula (abnormal connection to another abdominal structure), stricture (narrowing of the ureter), or persistent urinary leakage and infection, may result.

Often, an injury to the ureters may not be recognized promptly. Usually a doctor suspects an injury when the person has had a recent operation or notices a wound that has penetrated the abdomen. People may complain simply of pain in the abdomen or flank, or they may notice urine leaking from their wound. Fever may accompany an infection caused by persistent urinary leakage. Blood may appear in the urine.

When a ureteral injury is suspected, imaging tests are needed. The initial test is often intravenous urography or computed tomography (CT), but if both are inconclusive, retrograde urography may be performed. Sometimes surgery may be needed to identify an injury.

Treatment

If a ureter is injured, surgery is often needed to repair it. Some minor ureteral injuries can be treated by placing a flexible tube either directly in the ureter or through the kidney via a small incision in the side (percutaneous nephrostomy). The purpose of these procedures is to divert urine from flowing through the ureter, usually for 2 to 6 weeks, allowing the ureter to heal. If the ureteral injury does not resolve using this procedure, additional surgery may be needed.

Treatment helps to prevent complications of ureteral injuries. If complications occur despite efforts to prevent them, they must be treated.

Bladder Injuries

A bladder injury often occurs when the pelvis is injured, as may occur in a high-speed motor vehicle accident or a fall. Penetrating wounds, usually from gunshots, also can injure the bladder. In addition, a bladder injury may occur unintentionally during diagnostic tests or surgery involving the pelvis or lower abdomen.

Symptoms and Diagnosis

The most common symptoms of a bladder injury are blood in the urine and difficulty in urinating. If the lowermost portion of the bladder (where the muscle that helps to control urination is located) has been injured, the person may experience frequent urination or an uncontrollable loss of urine (urinary incontinence). Changes in urination and fever may develop if the injury leads to infection.

If bladder injuries are not treated, complications, such as frequent and urgent urination, infection, and incontinence, may develop.

The diagnosis of a bladder injury is best established by cystography, a procedure in which a radiopaque dye, which is visible on x-rays, is injected into the bladder and x-rays are taken to look for leakage.

Treatment

Minor bladder injuries, either bruises or tears (lacerations), may be treated by inserting a catheter into the urethra for 5 to 10 days while the bladder heals. For more extensive bladder injuries or any injury resulting in leakage of urine into the abdominal cavity, surgery should be performed to determine the extent of the injury and to repair all tears. The urine can then be more effectively drained from the bladder using two catheters, one inserted through the urethra (a transurethral catheter) and one inserted directly into the bladder through the skin over the lower abdomen (a suprapubic catheter). These catheters are removed in 7 to 10 days or once the bladder has healed satisfactorily. If complications develop, they must be treated.

Urethral Injuries

Common causes of injury to the urethra include pelvic fractures in men and women and straddle injuries (between the legs) in men. The urethra can also be injured unintentionally during surgical procedures performed directly on the urethra or during procedures in which instruments are passed into the urethra, such as bladder catheterization or cystoscopy (passing a flexible viewing tube through the urethra into the bladder). Rarely, urethral injuries can be self-inflicted when a person inserts a foreign object directly into the urethra.

Some injuries to the urethra are limited to bruising. Injury to the urethra can also tear the lining, resulting in leakage of urine into the tissues of the penis, scrotum, abdominal wall, or perineum (the area between the anus and vulva or scrotum).

Symptoms and Diagnosis

The most common symptoms occurring with a urethral injury include blood at the tip of the penis in men or the urethral opening in women, blood in the urine, and an inability to urinate. Other symptoms may arise when complications develop. If urine leaks into surrounding tissues, infection may result, causing fever and other symptoms. Over time, the injury may cause the urethra to narrow (constrict) near or at the site of injury. When an injury occurs during a surgical procedure, uncontrollable loss of urine (urinary incontinence) may also develop. Men may also experience impairment in the ability to have an erection (erectile dysfunction), caused by damage to the nerves or blood supply to the penis.

If urethral injuries are not treated, complications, such as narrowing of the urethra, persistent infection, urinary incontinence, and erectile dysfunction, may develop.

The diagnosis of a urethral injury is usually confirmed by retrograde urography, an x-ray taken after a radiopaque dye is injected directly into the urethra.

Treatment

For urethral bruises (contusions) that do not result in any leakage of urine, a doctor can place a catheter through the urethra into the bladder for several days to drain the urine while the urethra heals itself. For urethral tears, the urine must be diverted from the urethra using a catheter placed directly into the bladder through the skin over the lower abdomen. The urethra is not repaired surgically until all other injuries have healed or for at least 8 to 12 weeks (when inflammation has resolved).

Treatment helps to prevent complications of urethral injuries. Complications must be treated if efforts to prevent them are unsuccessful.

CHAPTER 151

Cancers of the Kidney and Urinary Tract

Tumors of the kidney and urinary tract affect men and women alike and may occur in people of any age. Most of these tumors are cancerous (malignant).

Kidney Cancer

Kidney cancer accounts for about 2 to 3% of cancers in adults, affecting twice as many men as women. Smokers are about twice as likely to develop kidney cancer as nonsmokers. Other risk factors include exposure to toxic chemicals and obesity. For unknown reasons, between 1975 and 1995, the rate of new kidney cancers rose 2 to 4% per year. People affected are usually between 50 and 70 years of age.

Most solid kidney tumors are cancerous, but fluid-filled tumors (cysts) generally are not. Almost all kidney cancer is renal cell carcinoma. Another kind of kidney cancer, Wilms' tumor, occurs in children.▲

Symptoms and Diagnosis

Blood in the urine is the most common first symptom, but the amount of blood may be so small that it can be detected only under a microscope. On the other hand, the urine may be

---

▲ see page 1622

visibly red. The next most common symptoms are pain in the flank (the area between the ribs and hip), fever, and weight loss. Sometimes kidney cancer is first detected when a doctor feels an enlargement or lump in the abdomen, or a cancer may be discovered by chance during evaluation of another problem, such as high blood pressure. If the cancer interferes with the blood supply to part or all of the kidney, an enzyme called renin is released, which leads to an increase in blood pressure.

The red blood cell count may become abnormally high, resulting in secondary polycythemia, because high levels of the hormone erythropoietin (which is produced by the diseased kidney or by the tumor itself) stimulate the bone marrow to increase the production of red blood cells. Conversely, kidney cancer may lead to a drop in the red blood cell count because of bleeding into the urine. Some people develop high levels of calcium in the blood (hypercalcemia).

If doctors suspect kidney cancer, they may use intravenous urography, ultrasound, or computed tomography (CT) to confirm the diagnosis. Magnetic resonance imaging (MRI) may be used to provide more information about whether the cancer has spread into nearby structures, including veins. If a fluid-filled tumor (cyst) is found, fluid may be withdrawn with a needle to determine if the tumor is cancerous.

Treatment

When the cancer has not spread (metastasized) beyond the kidney, surgically removing the affected kidney and lymph nodes provides a reasonable chance of cure. A doctor may remove only the tumor plus a rim of adjacent normal tissue, which spares the remainder of the kidney. Sometimes the entire kidney needs to be removed.

If the cancer has spread into the renal vein or even the large vein that carries blood to the heart (vena cava) but has not spread to distant sites, surgery may still provide a chance for cure. However, kidney cancer has a tendency to spread early, especially to the lungs. Treating the cancer by enhancing the immune system's ability to destroy it causes some cancers to shrink and may prolong survival.▲ One such treatment, interleukin-2, is used for kidney cancer. Various combinations of interleukin-2, interferon, and other biologic agents and even vaccines developed from cells removed from the kidney cancer are being investigated. Rarely (in less than 1% of people), removing the affected kidney causes tumors elsewhere in the body to shrink. However, the slim possibility that this will occur is not considered sufficient reason to remove a cancerous kidney when the cancer has already spread, unless removal is part of an overall plan that includes traditional anticancer drugs (chemotherapy) or biologic agents.

Distant spread of kidney cancer cannot always be detected when kidney cancer is diagnosed. Therefore, spread of the kidney cancer sometimes becomes apparent after the doctor has surgically removed all of the kidney cancer that could be found; cancer that has spread to new areas is usually unresponsive to traditional chemotherapy. However, treatment with interleukin-2 or interferon may be beneficial, although their effects are modest.

Prognosis

Many factors affect prognosis, but the 5-year survival rate for people with cancer confined to the kidney is 85% or better. If the cancer has spread into the renal vein and the vena cava but has not spread to distant sites, the 5-year survival rate is 35 to 60%. When cancer has spread to distant sites, the 5-year survival rate is no higher than 10%. In some instances, the goal is to focus on pain relief and other means to improve the person's comfort.■ As with all terminal illnesses, planning for end-of-life issues, including creating advance directives, is essential.★

Cancers of the Renal Pelvis and Ureter

Cancer can occur in the cells lining the central collecting area of the kidney (the renal pelvis—called transitional cell carcinoma of the renal pelvis) and in the slender tubes that carry urine from the kidney to the bladder (ureters). Cancers of the renal pelvis and ureter are much less common than cancers of the rest of the kidney or bladder; they probably occur in fewer than 6,000 people in the United States each year.

Symptoms and Diagnosis

Blood in the urine is usually the first symptom. Crampy pain in the flank (the space be-

---

▲ see page 1044   ■ see page 48

★ see pages 51 and 54

tween the ribs and hip) or lower abdomen may occur if the flow of urine is obstructed.

The diagnosis is made by intravenous urography or retrograde urography. Computed tomography (CT) can help a doctor distinguish a kidney stone from a cancer or blood clot and may help show how much the cancer has grown. Microscopic examination of a urine sample may show cancer cells. A flexible viewing tube—a ureteroscope or nephroscope—threaded up through the bladder or passed through the abdominal wall may be used to view, and occasionally even treat, small cancers.

Treatment and Prognosis

If the cancer has not spread beyond the area of the renal pelvis and ureter, the usual treatment is surgical removal of the entire kidney and ureter (nephroureterectomy) along with a small part of the bladder. However, in some situations—for example, when the kidneys are not functioning well or a person has only one kidney—the kidney is usually not removed, because the person would then become dependent on dialysis. Some cancers in the renal pelvis and ureter may be treated with a laser to destroy the cancer cells or with surgery that removes only the cancer itself while leaving the kidney, the noncancerous portion of the ureter, and the bladder in place. If the cancer has spread, chemotherapy is used.

A person may be cured if the cancer has not spread and if it can be completely removed surgically. A cystoscopy (insertion of a flexible viewing tube to examine the inside of the bladder) is performed periodically after surgery, because people who have had this type of cancer are at risk of developing bladder cancer.

Bladder Cancer

An estimated 54,300 new cases of bladder cancer are diagnosed every year in the United States. About 2½ times as many men as women develop bladder cancer. Smoking is the strongest single risk factor and appears to be one of the underlying causes in at least half of all new cases. Certain chemicals that are used in industry can become concentrated in the urine and cause cancer, although exposure to these chemicals is decreasing. The chronic irritation that occurs with a parasitic infection called schistosomiasis or with bladder stones also predisposes people to bladder cancer, al-

though irritation accounts for only a small proportion of all cases.

Most cases of bladder cancer are of transitional cells (called transitional cell carcinoma of the bladder), the same type of cells that line the renal pelvis and ureters.

Symptoms and Diagnosis

Bladder cancer is often first suspected when blood is found in the urine. Blood may be detected when a routine microscopic examination of a urine specimen detects red blood cells. However, the urine may be visibly red. Later symptoms may include pain and burning during urination and an urgent, frequent need to urinate. The symptoms of bladder cancer may be identical to those of a bladder infection (cystitis),▲ and the two problems may occur together. Bladder cancer may be suspected if the symptoms do not disappear with treatment for the cystitis. Special microscopic evaluation of urine (cytology)■ frequently detects cancer cells.

Cystography or intravenous urography—x-ray films taken after a radiopaque dye is injected intravenously—may show an irregularity in the bladder wall, suggesting a possible cancer. Ultrasound, computed tomography (CT), or magnetic resonance imaging (MRI) may also show an abnormality in the bladder, usually by chance during evaluation of another problem. If any of these tests detect a growth, the doctor looks inside the bladder with a cystoscope passed through the urethra and removes samples of any suspicious areas for examination under a microscope (biopsy).

Prognosis

For superficial tumors that grow and divide slowly, the risk of death from bladder cancer is less than 5%, but the risk may rise to about 15 to 20% for tumors that grow and divide rapidly or that have invaded almost as far as the muscle layer of the bladder. The 5-year survival rate for tumors that invaded the superficial layer of muscle is a little worse, with the risk of death probably rising to 20 to 35%; some of these people may benefit from chemotherapy. For tumors extending into or through the deep muscle layer, the 5-year survival rate is 45 to 60%. If the cancer has spread to the lymph nodes or beyond, the 5-year survival rate is 20 to 45%.

▲ see page 868   ■ see page 828

Treatment

Cancers that remain on the bladder's inner surface or invade only the most superficial part of the muscle layer under the surface may be removed completely during cystoscopy. However, people commonly develop new cancers later, sometimes in the same place or, more commonly, elsewhere in the bladder. Doctors may be able to prevent the recurrence of cancers that are limited to the inner surface of the bladder by repeatedly instilling anticancer drugs or BCG (a substance that stimulates the body's immune system) into the bladder after all of the cancer has been removed during cystoscopy. These instillations may serve as treatment for people with cancers that cannot be removed during cystoscopy.

Cancers that have grown deep into or through the bladder wall cannot be completely removed through a cystoscope. They are usually treated by total or partial removal of the bladder (cystectomy). Radiation therapy alone or in combination with chemotherapy may also be used in an attempt to cure the cancer.

If the entire bladder needs to be removed, the doctor must devise a method for the person to be able to drain urine. Usually, urine is routed to an opening (stoma) made in the abdominal wall through a passageway made of intestine, called an ileal loop. The urine is then collected in a bag worn on the outside of the body.

Several alternative methods of diverting urine are becoming increasingly common and are appropriate for some people. These methods can be grouped into two categories: an orthotopic neobladder and a continent urinary diversion. In both, an internal reservoir for urine is constructed from the intestine.

For an orthotopic neobladder, the reservoir is connected to the urethra. The person learns to empty this reservoir by relaxing the pelvic floor muscles and increasing pressure within the abdomen, so that urine passes through the urethra very much as it would naturally. Most people are dry during the day, but some incontinence may occur at night.

For a continent urinary diversion, the reservoir is connected to a stoma in the abdominal wall. A collecting bag is not needed, because the urine remains in the reservoir until the person empties it by inserting a catheter through the stoma into the reservoir, which is emptied at regular intervals throughout the day.

Cancer that has spread beyond the bladder to the lymph nodes or other organs is treated with chemotherapy. Several different combinations of drugs are active against this type of cancer, particularly when the spread is confined to the lymph nodes. Cystectomy or radiation may be offered to people who respond well to chemotherapy. However, a relatively small number of people are cured. For people who are not cured, efforts are directed at pain relief and end-of-life issues.▲

Cancer of the Urethra

Cancer of the urethra (the channel that carries urine from the bladder out of the body) is rare, occurring most commonly after age 50. It can occur in men and women. Certain types of human papillomavirus are suspected as the cause of cancer of the urethra in some people. Otherwise, the cause is unknown.

The first symptom is usually blood in the urine. The amount of blood may be so small that it can be detected only under a microscope. On the other hand, the urine may be visibly red. The flow of urine may become obstructed, making urination difficult or the stream of urine slow and thin. Fragile, bleeding growths at the external opening of a woman's urethra may be cancerous. A biopsy must be performed to positively identify a cancer.

Radiation therapy, surgical removal, or a combination of both has been used to treat cancer of the urethra with variable results. The prognosis of cancer of the urethra depends on the precise location and extent of the cancer.

▲ see page 48

DISORDERS OF NUTRITION AND METABOLISM

152   Overview of Nutrition 880

Carbohydrates, Proteins, and Fats • Vitamins and Minerals •
Fiber • Calories • Nutritional Requirements • Diets •
Weight Loss Diets

153   Undernutrition 887

154   Vitamins 890

Vitamin A • Vitamin D • Vitamin E • Vitamin K • Vitamin
B_1 • Vitamin B_2 • Niacin • Vitamin B_6 • Vitamin B_{12} •
Folic Acid • Vitamin C

155   Minerals and Electrolytes...900

Calcium • Copper • Fluoride • Iodine • Iron •
Magnesium • Phosphate • Potassium • Selenium •
Sodium • Zinc

156   Obesity 914

157   Disorders of Cholesterol..920

Hyperlipoproteinemia • Hereditary Hyperlipoproteinemias •
Hypolipoproteinemia

158   Water Balance 927

Dehydration • Overhydration • Effects of Aging

159   Acid-Base Balance...930

Acidosis • Alkalosis

160   Porphyrias 933

Porphyria Cutanea Tarda • Acute Intermittent Porphyria •
Erythropoietic Protoporphyria

CHAPTER 152

Overview of Nutrition

Nutrition is the process of consuming, absorbing, and using nutrients needed by the body for growth, development, and maintenance of life.

To receive adequate, appropriate nutrition, people need to consume a healthy diet, which consists of a variety of nutrients (the chemical substances in foods that nourish the body). A healthy diet enables people to maintain a desirable body weight and composition (the percentage of fat and muscle in the body) and to perform their daily physical and mental activities.

If a person does not consume sufficient amounts of nutrients, a nutritional deficiency disorder may result. To determine whether a person is consuming enough nutrients, a doctor asks about eating habits and diet and performs a physical examination to assess the composition and functioning of the body. Body composition, including the proportion of body fat, can be determined accurately by weighing the person under water (hydrostatic weighing) and can be approximated by measuring skinfold thickness or performing bioelectrical impedance analysis. Laboratory tests to measure the levels of nutrients in blood and tissues can be performed. For example, the level of albumin, the main protein in blood, can be measured. Nutrient levels decrease when nutrition is inadequate.

Generally, nutrients are divided into two classes: macronutrients and micronutrients. Macronutrients are required daily in large quantities. They include proteins, fats, carbohydrates, some minerals, and water. Water is required in amounts of 1 milliliter for each calorie of energy expended or about 2.6 quarts (2,500 milliliters) a day. Micronutrients are required daily in small quantities—in milligrams (one thousandth of a gram) to micrograms (one millionth of a gram). They include vitamins and trace minerals that enable the body to use macronutrients.

Foods consumed in the daily diet contain as many as 100,000 substances. But only 300 are classified as nutrients, and only 45 are classified as essential nutrients. However, food contains many other useful components, including some fibers, such as cellulose, pectins, and gums. Food contains additives (such as preservatives, emulsifiers, antioxidants, and stabilizers), which improve the production, processing, storage, and packaging of foods. Spices, flavors, substances that add odor or color, phytochemicals (substances in plants that have biologic activity in animals), and many other natural products improve the appearance, taste, and stability of food.

Carbohydrates, Proteins, and Fats

Carbohydrates, proteins, and fats supply 90% of the dry weight of the diet and 100% of its energy. As sources of energy, carbohydrates, proteins, and fats are interchangeable in proportion to their energy content. The energy content is 4 calories in a gram of carbohydrate or protein and 9 calories in a gram of fat

HEIGHT-WEIGHT REFERENCE CHART FOR ADULTS*

| Height | WEIGHT (POUNDS) | |
	Women	Men
4' 10"	92–121	—
4' 11"	95–124	—
5' 0"	98–127	—
5' 1"	101–130	105–134
5' 2"	104–134	108–137
5' 3"	107–138	111–141
5' 4"	110–142	114–145
5' 5"	114–146	117–149
5' 6"	119–150	121–154
5' 7"	122–154	125–159
5' 8"	126–159	129–163
5' 9"	130–164	133–167
5' 10"	134–169	137–172
5' 11"	—	141–177
6' 0"	—	145–182
6' 1"	—	149–187
6' 2"	—	153–192
6' 3"	—	157–197

*Height is without shoes; weight is without clothes.

(1 gram equals ¹⁄₂₈ ounce). However, these nutrients differ in how quickly they supply energy; carbohydrates are the quickest, and fats are the slowest.

Carbohydrates, proteins, and fats are digested in the intestine, where they are broken down into their basic units: carbohydrates into sugars, proteins into amino acids, and fats into fatty acids and glycerol. The body uses these basic units to build substances it needs for growth, maintenance, and activity (including other carbohydrates, proteins, and fats).

Carbohydrates: Depending on the size of the molecule, carbohydrates may be simple or complex. Simple carbohydrates are various forms of sugar, such as glucose and fructose. Because they are small molecules, they can be broken down by the body quickly and are the quickest source of energy. Fruits, dairy products, honey, and maple syrup contain large amounts of simple carbohydrates, which provide the sweet taste in most candies and cakes.

Complex carbohydrates are composed of long strings of simple carbohydrates. Because complex carbohydrates are larger molecules than simple carbohydrates, they are slower sources of energy. However, energy can be generated from them relatively quickly. Complex carbohydrates occur in wheat products (such as breads and pastas), other grains (such as rye and corn), beans, and root vegetables (such as potatoes).

The body stores very small amounts of excess energy as carbohydrates. The liver stores some as glycogen, a complex carbohydrate that the body can easily and rapidly convert to energy. Muscles also store glycogen, which they use during periods of intense exercise. The amount of carbohydrates stored as glycogen provides almost a day's worth of calories. A few other body tissues store carbohydrates as complex carbohydrates that cannot be used to provide energy.

Most authorities recommend that about 50 to 55% of the total daily calories should consist of carbohydrates.

Proteins: Proteins consist of units called amino acids, strung together in complex formations. Because proteins are complex molecules, the body takes longer to break them down. As a result, they are a much slower and longer-lasting source of energy than carbohydrates. There are 20 amino acids. The body synthesizes some of them from components within the body, but it cannot

Fat Versus Lean: Body Composition

Maintaining an appropriate weight is important for physical and psychologic health. A standardized height-weight table can be used as a guide. But body mass index is more reliable. It is calculated by dividing the weight (in kilograms) by the height (in meters squared).▲ A body mass index between 18 and 25 is usually considered normal for men and women. A less obvious but important consideration is how much of the body is fat and how much is muscle (body composition). There are several ways to determine body composition.

Underwater (hydrostatic) weighing in an immersion pool can determine body composition. Bone and muscle are denser than water, so a person with a high percentage of lean tissue weighs more in water and a person with a high percentage of fat weighs less. Although this method is considered the most accurate, it requires special equipment, considerable time, and expertise to perform.

Body composition can be estimated by measuring the amount of fat under the skin (skinfold thickness) or by bioelectric impedance analysis. For skinfold thickness, a fold of skin on the back of the left upper arm (triceps skinfold) is pulled away from the arm and measured with a caliper. A skinfold measurement of about ¹⁄₂ inch in men and about 1 inch in women is considered normal. This measurement plus the circumference of the left upper arm can be used to estimate the amount of skeletal muscle in the body (lean body mass).

Bioelectric impedance analysis measures the resistance of body tissues to the flow of an undetectable low-voltage electrical current. Typically, a person stands barefoot on metal footplates, and the electrical current is sent up one foot and down the other. Body fat and bone resist the flow much more than does muscle tissue. By measuring the resistance to the current, doctors can estimate the percentage of body fat. This test takes only about 1 minute.

Dual-energy x-ray absorptiometry (DEXA) accurately determines the amount and distribution of body fat. This imaging procedure uses a very low dose of radiation and is safe. However, it is too expensive to use routinely.

▲ see table on page 916

synthesize nine of the amino acids—called essential amino acids. They must be consumed in the diet. They include histidine, isoleucine, leucine, lysine, methionine, phenylalanine, threonine, tryptophan, and valine.

The body contains large amounts of protein. Protein, the main building block in the body, is the primary component of most cells. For example, muscle, connective tissues, and skin are all built of protein.

Adults need to eat about 60 grams of protein per day (0.8 grams per kilogram of weight or 10 to 15% of total calories). Adults who are trying to build muscle need slightly more. Children also need more. If more protein is consumed than is needed, the body does not build more protein (or muscle). Instead, the body breaks the protein down and stores its components as fat, which can be broken down and used for energy later as needed.

Fats: These complex molecules are composed of fatty acids and glycerol. Fats are the slowest source of energy but the most energy-efficient form of food. Each gram of fat supplies the body with about 9 calories, more than twice that supplied by proteins or carbohydrates. Because fats are such an efficient form of energy, the body stores any excess energy as fat. The body deposits excess fat in the abdomen (omental fat) and under the skin (subcutaneous fat) to use when it needs more energy. The body also stores excess fat in blood vessels and within organs, where it blocks blood flow and damages the organs, often with devastating results.

The body cannot synthesize some fatty acids—called essential fatty acids. They must be consumed in the diet. The essential fatty acids make up about 7% of the fat consumed in a normal diet and about 3% of total calories (about 8 grams). They include linoleic acid, linolenic acid, arachidonic acid, eicosapentaenoic acid, and docosahexaenoic acid. Linoleic acid and linolenic acid are found in vegetable oils. Eicosapentaenoic acid and docosahexaenoic acid, which are essential for brain development, are found in fish oils. In the body, arachidonic acid can be formed from linoleic acid, and eicosapentaenoic and docosahexaenoic acid can be formed from linolenic acid, although fish oil is a more efficient source.

There are different kinds of fat: monounsaturated, polyunsaturated, and saturated.▲ In general, saturated fats are more likely to increase cholesterol levels and increase the risk of atherosclerosis. Some evidence suggests that consuming trans fatty acids, a different category of fat, may increase cholesterol levels in the body and thus may contribute to the risk of atherosclerosis.■

Authorities generally recommend that fat be limited to less than 30% of daily total calories, or fewer than 90 grams per day, and that the amount of saturated fat, trans fatty acids, and cholesterol in the diet be reduced. However, people with high cholesterol levels may need to reduce their fat intake even more. When fat intake is reduced to 10% or less of daily total calories, cholesterol levels tend to decrease dramatically.

Vitamins and Minerals

Most vitamins and all minerals are essential nutrients. That is, they cannot be synthesized by the body and so must be consumed in the diet.

Vitamins are classified as water soluble—vitamin C and the eight members of the vitamin B complex—or fat soluble—vitamins A, D, E, and K.

Some minerals are required in fairly large quantities (about 1 or 2 grams a day) and are considered macronutrients. They include calcium, chloride, magnesium, phosphorus (occurring mainly as phosphate in the body), potassium, and sodium. Minerals required in small amounts are considered micronutrients and are called trace minerals. They include copper, fluoride, iodine, iron, selenium, and zinc. Except for fluoride, all of these minerals activate enzymes required in metabolism. Fluoride forms a stable compound with calcium, helping stabilize the mineral content of bones and teeth and helping prevent tooth decay. Trace minerals such as arsenic, chromium, cobalt, nickel, silicon, and vanadium, which may be essential in animal nutrition, have not been established as requirements in human nutrition. All trace minerals are toxic at high levels, and some (arsenic, nickel, and chromium) have been identified as causes of cancer.

Some vitamins and minerals (such as vitamins C and E and selenium) act as antioxidants, as do other substances in fruits and vegetables (such as beta-carotene). Antioxidants protect cells against damage by free radicals,

---

▲ see page 200

■ see box on page 201

which are reactive by-products of the normal activity of cells. Free radicals are thought to contribute to such disorders as heart disease and cancer. People who eat adequate amounts of fruits and vegetables, which are rich in antioxidants, are less likely to develop heart disease and certain cancers. However, whether these benefits are due to antioxidants, other substances in the fruits and vegetables, or other factors is not known.

Fiber

Some foods contain fiber, a tough complex carbohydrate that is only partially digested by the body. The digestible part provides some calories; the indigestible part provides bulk to the feces. This bulk helps the intestine move feces along, thereby preventing constipation, and it reduces pressure in the intestine, helping prevent diverticular disease. Eating fiber also helps increase the elimination of cancer-causing substances produced by the bacteria in the large intestine and helps moderate the changes in sugar and cholesterol levels in the blood that occur after eating a meal. Authorities generally recommend that about 30 grams of fiber be consumed daily. In the United States, the average amount of fiber consumed daily is about 25 grams. An average serving of fruit, a vegetable, or cereal contains 2 to 4 grams of fiber.

Calories

A calorie is a measure of energy. Foods have calories; that is, foods supply the body with energy, which is released when foods are broken down during digestion. Energy enables cells to perform all of their functions, including building proteins and other substances needed by the body. The energy can be used immediately or stored to be used later.

When the supply of energy—that is, the number of calories consumed in foods—exceeds the body's immediate needs, the body stores the excess energy. Most excess energy is stored as fat. Some is stored as carbohydrates, usually in the liver and muscles. As a result, weight is gained. An excess of only 200 calories per day for 10 days is likely to result in a weight gain of nearly ½ pound, mostly as fat.

When the intake of energy is insufficient for the body's needs, the body begins to use carbohydrates stored in the liver and muscle. Because the body mobilizes stored carbohydrates quickly and because water is usually excreted

How Are Calories in Foods Measured?

Food labels always contain the number of calories per serving. But how is this number determined? The answer is surprisingly simple: The food is burned. A sample of the food is placed in an insulated, oxygen-filled chamber that is surrounded by water; this chamber is called a bomb calorimeter. The sample is burned completely. The heat from the burning increases the temperature of the water, which is measured and which indicates the number of calories in the food. For example, if water temperature increases by 20 degrees, the food contains 20 calories. This method of measuring calories is called direct calorimetry.

as carbohydrates are mobilized, weight loss tends to be fast initially. However, the small amount of stored carbohydrates provides energy for only a short time. Next, the body uses stored fat. Converting fat to energy is a slower process, so weight loss is slower as the body uses fat for energy. However, the amount of fat stored is much larger and can, in most people, provide energy for a long time. Only during prolonged, severe shortages of energy, does the body break down protein. For normally nourished people who experience total starvation (who do not consume any food to supply energy), death occurs in 8 to 12 weeks.

Energy requirements vary markedly from about 1,000 to more than 4,000 calories a day depending on age, sex, and physical activity. Typically, to maintain body weight, sedentary women, young children, and older adults need about 1,600 calories a day; older children, active adult women, and sedentary men need about 2,000 calories; and active adolescent boys and young men need about 2,400 calories. However, division of caloric intake by a 24-hour period (daily intake) is arbitrary. Furthermore, the needs of the body vary depending on its activity at any particular time. Vigorous activity, especially aerobic exercise, increases needs substantially, and a lack of activity decreases needs.

Nutritional Requirements

Although daily nutritional requirements, including those for essential nutrients, depend on a person's age, sex, height, weight, and metabolic and physical activity, general guidelines for a healthy diet have been developed. The Food and Nutrition Board of the National Academy of Sciences—National Research Council and the U.S. Department of Agriculture periodically publish recommended dietary allowances for protein, vitamins,▲ and minerals.■ These allowances are intended to meet the needs of healthy people.

The U.S. Department of Agriculture has also proposed the food guide pyramid as a guide to a balanced diet. This guide is intended to help people choose a diet that provides a balance of different types of food, supplies essential nutrients, and helps reduce the risk of such disorders as cancer, high blood pressure, coronary artery disease, and stroke. In this guide, the number of servings a day for each food group varies, depending on energy needs that range from 1,600 to more than 2,400 calories a day. For example, a person who consumes 1,600 calories a day could eat 6 servings from the bread group and 3 from the vegetable group, whereas a person who consumes 2,400 calories a day could eat 10 servings from the bread group and 5 from the vegetable group. In general, authorities recommend that fat intake be reduced to about 30% of calories and the intake of fruits, vegetables, and cereals be increased.

Diets

A diet is whatever a person eats, regardless of the goal—whether it is losing weight, gaining weight, reducing fat intake, avoiding carbohydrates, or having no particular goal. However, the term is often used to imply a goal of losing weight, which is an obsession for many people.

Standard healthy diets for children and adults are based on the needs of average people who do not need to lose or gain weight; who do not need to restrict any component of the diet because of disorders, risk, or advanced age; and who expend average amounts of energy through exercise or other vigorous activities. Thus, for a particular person, a healthy diet may vary substantially from what is recommended in standard diets. For example, special diets are required by people who have diabetes, certain kidney disorders, certain

---

▲ see table on pages 892 and 893

■ see table on pages 902 and 903

---

liver disorders, coronary artery disease, high cholesterol levels, osteoporosis, diverticular disease, chronic constipation, or food sensitivities. There are special dietary recommendations for young children, but little guidance is available for other specific age groups, such as older people.

WEIGHT LOSS DIETS

Weight loss requires consuming fewer calories than the body uses. Losing 1/2 pound of fat by dieting requires 10 days of consuming 200 fewer calories per day than the body uses. If 400 fewer calories are consumed than needed, a dieter can hope to lose 1/2 pound every 5 to 7 days. One pound of body fat stores about 3,500 calories.

In most conservative weight loss diets, the number of calories consumed is usually reduced to 1,200 to 1,500 a day. Diets containing fewer than 1,200 calories often lack essential nutrients, such as protein, iron, and calcium. To be healthy, weight loss diets should provide about the same volume of food (by including more fiber and fluids) as the normal diet. They should also be low in saturated fat and sugar and include essential nutrients, including antioxidants. Reading food labels makes people aware of the composition and calorie (energy) content of food, including beverages. Counting calories helps people control calorie intake. Using sugar and fat substitutes and eating foods that contain them help some people reduce calorie intake.

Combining increased exercise with dieting greatly enhances weight loss because exercise increases the number of calories the body uses. For example, vigorous walking burns about 4 calories per minute, so that 1 hour of brisk walking per day burns about 240 calories. Running is even better, burning about 6 to 8 calories per minute.

Eating small meals frequently can help with weight loss for several reasons. Insulin levels usually increase after eating, and more insulin is produced when many calories are consumed, especially when the meal is rich in carbohydrates. High insulin levels promote the deposition of fat and increase appetite. Eating small, frequent meals prevents insulin levels from increasing, thus discouraging fat deposition and helping suppress appetite. Eating certain types of foods at certain times of the day may also promote weight loss. For example, fast-energy foods, such as carbohydrates, are best eaten when the body needs a

Food Guide Pyramid

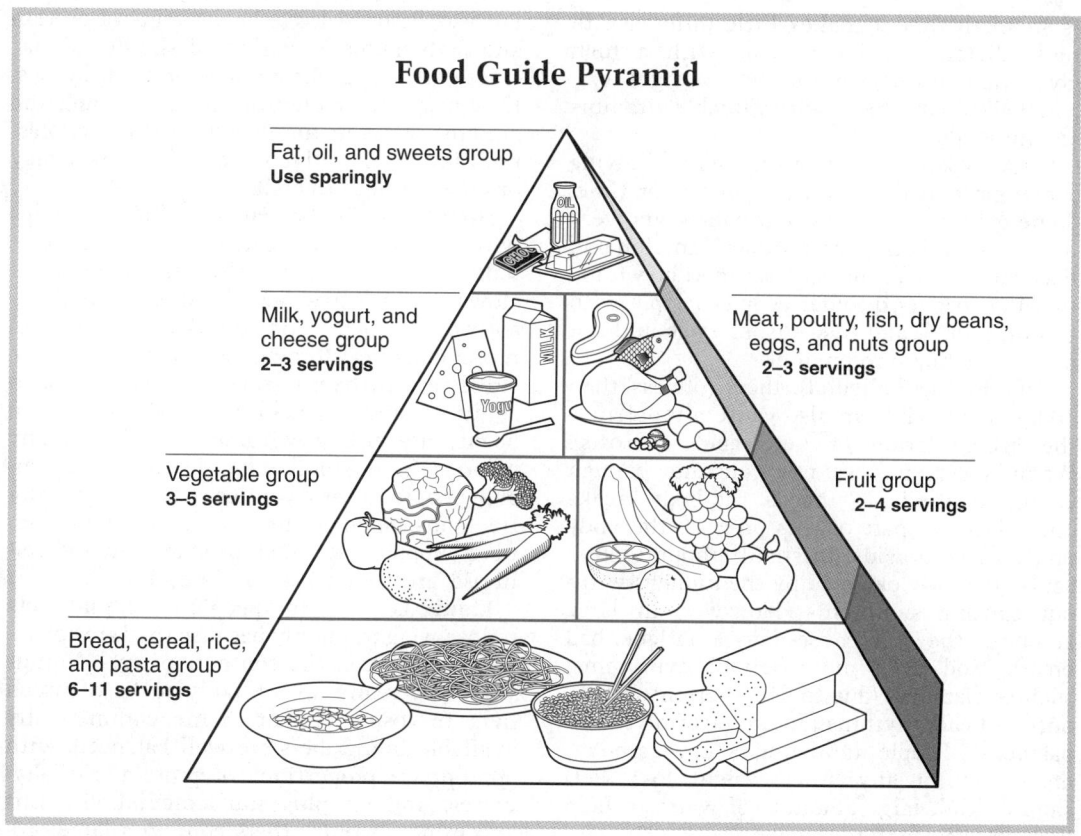

Fat, oil, and sweets group
Use sparingly

Milk, yogurt, and cheese group
2–3 servings

Meat, poultry, fish, dry beans, eggs, and nuts group
2–3 servings

Vegetable group
3–5 servings

Fruit group
2–4 servings

Bread, cereal, rice, and pasta group
6–11 servings

large supply of energy—that is, in the morning and during vigorous exercise. The body's need for energy is lowest at night, so avoiding carbohydrates in the evening may help.

High Protein–Low Carbohydrate Diets: Diets high in protein and low in simple carbohydrates have become popular as a way to lose weight. Such diets usually also restrict fat, because each gram supplies so many calories. However, some high protein–low carbohydrate diets, such as the Atkins diet, do not restrict fat.

The theory behind these diets is that slower-burning energy sources—protein and fat—provide a steady supply of energy and thus are less likely to lead to weight gain. In addition, people tend to feel full longer after eating protein than after eating carbohydrates, because carbohydrates empty from the stomach quickly and are digested quickly. Carbohydrates also strongly stimulate insulin production, which promotes fat deposition and increases appetite.

Some of these diets recommend avoiding foods with a high glycemic index. Foods that contain carbohydrates are given a glycemic index, which indicates how quickly the carbohydrates are digested and thus how a food affects the level of sugar in the blood. Foods that contain large amounts of sugar (such as maple syrup, honey, and candy) and starchy foods (such as carrots, potatoes, and some cereals) have a high glycemic index because they are quickly digested and quickly increase blood sugar levels. Foods that are high in fiber (such as whole-grain rye bread and all-bran cereals) have a low glycemic index because they are digested more slowly and do not quickly increase blood sugar levels. This index is useful for diabetics who need to control their blood sugar levels and for athletes who need to restore their blood sugar levels after an athletic performance. However, the glycemic index is not useful for dieters. The difference between the speed of carbohydrate digestion for foods with the highest and lowest glycemic indexes is so small that it makes little difference to most dieters. Avoiding foods with a high glycemic index does not promote weight loss, and it eliminates foods with valuable vitamins and minerals.

Some experts do not recommend following a high-protein diet for long periods of time. Some evidence suggests that over years, very high protein diets impair kidney function and may contribute to the decrease in kidney function that occurs in older people. People with certain kidney and liver disorders should not consume a high-protein diet.

Very low carbohydrate diets (of less than 100 grams a day) can also cause a problem— the accumulation of keto acids (ketosis). When a person does not consume enough energy for the body's needs, the body breaks down fats. As part of this process, the body produces keto acids. In small amounts, keto acids are easily excreted by the kidneys without causing symptoms. However, in large amounts, they can cause nausea, fatigue, bad breath, and even more serious symptoms, such as dizziness (due to dehydration) and abnormal heart rhythms (due to electrolyte imbalances). People following a low-carbohydrate diet (or any other weight loss diet) should drink large amounts of water to help flush keto acids from the body.

Low-carbohydrate diets tend to cause large amounts of weight to be lost during the first week or so, as the body converts stored carbohydrates (glycogen) to energy. As glycogen is broken down, the body also excretes large amounts of water, adding to the weight loss. However, once the body begins to use stored fat for energy, weight loss slows. Low carbohydrate diets may be high in fat and thus the total caloric intake may exceed what the body uses; in such cases, weight loss may stop after glycogen is used up.

Low-Fat Diets: This type of diet is the most effective for losing weight and maintaining weight loss. Fat supplies a large number of calories per gram and is more readily deposited as body fat than are proteins and carbohydrates. Reducing the amount of fat rather than the amount of protein or carbohydrate may be an easier way to reduce total caloric intake because a small reduction in fat saves so many calories. A reduction of only 10 grams of fat per day saves about 900 calories.

For weight to be lost, the amounts of protein and carbohydrates consumed should not increase greatly as the amount of fat decreases. However, the main reason for reducing the amount of fat in the diet is to lower cholesterol levels in the blood—which a dieter may or may not need to do.▲

High-Fiber Diets: Fiber indirectly helps with weight loss in several ways. It provides bulk, which makes people feel full faster. It slows the rate at which the stomach empties so people feel full longer. Fiber also requires more chewing, forcing people to eat more slowly and perhaps less. High-fiber foods, such as fruits and vegetables, wheat bread, and beans, are filling without providing many calories. Eating more high-fiber foods may enable people to eat fewer less filling, high-calorie foods, such as high-fat foods. However, fiber supplements, such as guar gum and cellulose, are not effective for weight loss.

Liquid Diets: Many people use liquid diets to lose weight, mainly because they are convenient. However, the contents of such liquids vary, and many are unlikely to be of much help in losing weight. Some commercially available liquid diets are well balanced, with appropriate proportions of protein, carbohydrates, and fat plus supplemental vitamins and minerals. But others contain a large proportion of carbohydrates, producing a sweet and tasty drink, and are not necessarily low in calories. Such liquid diets are more useful as a supplement to other foods for people who are trying to gain weight.

Very low calorie commercial liquid diets contain all needed nutrients. Usually, a drink that contains 220 calories is consumed 4 times a day instead of meals. Such diets are effective for short-term weight loss. For long-term weight loss, two or three meals are replaced with a liquid-diet drink. The remaining one or two meals should be low-fat, low-calorie, and nutritious.

An alternative to commercial diets is the all milk diet. This diet is simple and inexpensive and may be useful for short-term weight loss.

Grapefruit Diet: One popular fad diet involves consuming large amounts of grapefruit and grapefruit juice. The theory behind this diet is that grapefruit contains an enzyme that helps burn fat, but this theory has never been proved.

Although grapefruits are a healthful food—containing no fat, little sodium, and large amounts of vitamin C, beta-carotene (at least

▲ see pages 200 and 923

in pink grapefruits), and fiber—a diet based primarily on one fruit is nutritionally unsound. A grapefruit diet may help some people reduce total caloric intake, but it does not supply a balance of nutrients, which is needed for good health. Furthermore, eating grapefruit alters the levels of several drugs in the blood,▲ and eating large amounts of grapefruit often causes diarrhea.

Food-Combining and Food-Cycling Diets: Other fad diets are based on a theory that eating certain kinds of foods at different times promotes weight loss. An example is the Beverly Hills Diet, which recommends cycling different foods, usually over a 6-week period. For part of the time, a person eats nothing but fruits. Later, the person eats only breads, then only protein, then only fats. No scientific evidence supports this approach to weight loss, and the diet is intrinsically unhealthful.

Other Fad Diets: There are many fad diets. Some require extreme reductions in the number of calories consumed; others rely on supplements alleged to help burn fat; and still others are based on eating a single type of food. The Richard Simmons diet (900 calories a day) and the Atkins Diet (2,000 calories a day) are both low in carbohydrates and may result in dehydration if not enough fluids are consumed. Following the Richard Simmons diet for a long time may lead to deficiencies of iron, calcium, and protein as well as vitamins A, B_1 (thiamin), B_2 (riboflavin), and B_3 (niacin). The Atkins diet is particularly high in fat and cholesterol. The Beverly Hills, Rice, and Pritikin diets are low in fat and protein and high in carbohydrates. The Beverly Hills and Rice diets are deficient in protein, iron, calcium, zinc, and vitamin B_{12}. The Pritikin diet is relatively adequate in nutrition, but its low-fat content makes it unpalatable and less likely to be followed. These diets have not been shown to lead to sustained weight loss, and many are dangerous, supplying inadequate amounts of essential nutrients and leading to serious metabolic disturbances, such as loss of bone density and strength (including osteoporosis), problems with menstruation, abnormal heart rhythms, high cholesterol levels, kidney stones, and worsening of gout.

CHAPTER 153

Undernutrition

Undernutrition is a deficiency of calories or of one or more essential nutrients.

Undernutrition is usually thought of as a deficiency primarily of calories (that is, overall food consumption) or protein. Deficiencies of vitamins and minerals are usually considered as separate disorders. However, when calories are deficient, vitamins and minerals are likely to be also.

In developed countries, undernutrition is usually far less common than overnutrition (in which too many calories or too much of any specific nutrient—protein, fat, vitamin, mineral, or other dietary supplement—is consumed). However, undernutrition does occur, especially in people who are very poor, most notably the homeless, and in those who have psychiatric disorders. Also, people who become very ill may be unable to eat enough food because appetite is lost or their body's need for nutrients is greatly increased.

Undernutrition also occurs in older people. About 1 of 7 older people who live in the community consume less than 1,000 calories a day—not enough for adequate nutrition. As many as half of older people in hospitals and long-term care institutions do not consume enough calories. A deficiency of calories is the leading cause of death in children who live in developing countries.

A severe deficiency of calories causes a disorder called marasmus. Marasmus is common in many developing countries. It tends to develop in infants and very young children, who typically become thin and dehydrated. Breast-

▲ see table on page 77

feeding usually protects against marasmus. A severe deficiency primarily of proteins causes a disorder called kwashiorkor. Kwashiorkor is less common than marasmus. The term is derived from an African word meaning "first child–second child," because a first-born child often develops kwashiorkor when the second child is born and replaces the first-born child at the mother's breast. Because children tend to develop kwashiorkor after they are weaned, they are usually older than those who have marasmus. Kwashiorkor tends to be confined to certain areas of the world where staple foods and foods used to wean babies are deficient in protein even though they provide enough calories as carbohydrates. Examples of such foods are yams, cassava, rice, sweet potatoes, and green bananas. However, anyone can develop kwashiorkor if their diet consists mainly of carbohydrates. People with kwashiorkor retain fluid, making them appear puffy and swollen.

If both calories and proteins are deficient, the resulting disorder is called marasmic kwashiorkor.

Starvation is the most extreme form of undernutrition. It results from a partial or total lack of essential nutrients for a long time.

Causes

Undernutrition may result from lack of access to food; disorders that interfere with the intake, metabolism or absorption of nutrients; or a greatly increased need for calories.

The use of certain drugs may contribute to undernutrition. Many drugs decrease appetite. Some drugs cause nausea, which decreases appetite. Others (such as thyroxine and theophylline) increase metabolism, and still others (such as cholestyramine) interfere with the absorption of nutrients in the intestine, causing malabsorption. Also, withdrawal from certain drugs (such as antianxiety drugs and antipsychotics) or from alcohol may lead to weight loss.

Many factors work together to cause undernutrition in older people. Older people tend to consume less food. Those who eat alone may be less inclined to prepare and eat meals. Physical impairments or reduced mobility may make shopping for or preparing food difficult. Older people seem to require less food to feel full, possibly because age-related chemical changes decrease their drive to eat and increase their sense of satiety. A diminished sense of smell and taste may decrease the pleasure of eating. Also, as people age, the ability to absorb some nutrients is reduced.

Many disorders that are more common among older people can contribute to undernutrition. A stroke or tremors may make chewing, swallowing, or preparing food difficult. If tremors are continuous, as they are in Parkinson's disease, they cause weight loss by increasing the rate at which the body uses calories (metabolic rate). Dental problems, such as ill-fitting dentures or gum disease, may make eating painful or difficult. Malabsorption disorders, cancer (which can reduce appetite and increase the body's need for calories), and depression (which can decrease appetite) are common among older people. People with dementia may forget to eat and so lose weight. When dementia is advanced, people cannot feed themselves and may resist at-

Causes of Undernutrition

Lack of access to food
- Poverty
- Famine
- Inability to obtain food (for example, due to lack of transportation or physical disability)
- Voluntary restriction of calories (as for a strict reducing diet or a fast)

Disorders that interfere with the intake, metabolism, or absorption of nutrients
- Malabsorption disorders
- Inflammatory bowel disorders
- Liver disorders
- Anorexia nervosa
- Depression
- Alcoholism
- Drug abuse

Greatly increased need for calories
- Cancer
- Injury, such as burns
- Surgery
- An overactive thyroid gland (hyperthyroidism)
- Infections
- Kidney disorders
- High fever
- Demanding exercise, such as rehabilitation or training for athletic competition
- Pregnancy and breastfeeding
- Growth and development in infants, children, and adolescents

tempts to feed them. Older people also take many drugs that can result in weight loss.

Symptoms

The most obvious sign of a deficiency of calories is loss of body fat (adipose tissue). When not enough calories are consumed, the body breaks down its own tissues and uses them for calories—much like burning the furniture to keep a house warm. The loss of fat is often first noticeable in the face: The cheeks are hollow, and the eyes seem sunken.

If the deficiency of calories is severe, adults can lose up to half of their body weight, and children can lose even more. Bones protrude, and the skin becomes thin, dry, inelastic, pale, and cold. The hair becomes dry and sparse, falling out easily. When this wasting away is due to a disorder, it is called cachexia.

Other symptoms include fatigue, an inability to stay warm, diarrhea, loss of appetite, irritability, and apathy, sometimes leading to unresponsiveness (stupor). In children who are severely undernourished, behavioral development may be markedly slow, and mental retardation may occur. The number of some types of white blood cells decreases, resembling what happens in people who have AIDS. As a result, the immune system is weakened, increasing the risk of infections. If the deficiency of calories continues for a long time, heart and respiratory failure may develop. Total starvation (when no food is consumed) is fatal in 8 to 12 weeks.

Diagnosis and Treatment

Doctors can usually diagnose undernutrition based on the person's appearance. Blood tests may be performed to measure the level of albumin, which decreases when people do not consume enough protein. A physical examination, x-rays, and blood tests may be performed to determine the effects of undernutrition.

For most people, treatment involves gradually increasing the number of calories consumed. Eating several small, nutritious meals each day is the best way. For people who have been starving, foods are reintroduced carefully.

Feeding Methods: Sometimes nutrients cannot be given by mouth. In such cases, nutrients may be given through a tube inserted into the digestive tract or into a vein (intravenously).

Tube feeding may be used to feed people whose digestive tract is functioning normally

HOW STARVATION AFFECTS THE BODY

AREA	EFFECTS
Digestive system	Decreased production of acid by the stomach Reduced size of the interior of the digestive tract Frequent, often fatal diarrhea
Cardiovascular system (heart and blood vessels)	Reduced heart size, reduced amount of blood pumped, slow heart rate, and low blood pressure Ultimately, heart failure
Respiratory system	Slow breathing and reduced lung capacity Ultimately, respiratory failure
Reproductive system	Reduced size of ovaries in women and testes in men Loss of sex drive (libido) Cessation of menstrual periods in women
Nervous system	Apathy and irritability In children, mental retardation (sometimes) In older people, mental dysfunction
Muscles	Reduced muscle size and strength, reducing the ability to exercise or work
Blood	Anemia
Metabolism (chemical alteration of substances by the body to produce energy and to synthesize needed substances)	Low body temperature (hypothermia) Fluid accumulation in the arms, legs, and abdomen Disappearance of fat under the skin
Skin and hair	Thin, dry, inelastic skin and dry, sparse hair that falls out easily
Immune system	Impaired ability to fight infections and repair wounds

but who cannot eat enough to meet their nutritional needs (such as people with severe burns) or who cannot swallow (such as some people who have had a stroke). For tube feeding, a thin plastic tube (a nasogastric tube) is passed through the nose and down the throat until it reaches the stomach or small intestine. If tube feeding is needed for a long time, the tube can be inserted directly into the stomach or small intestine through a small incision in the abdomen.

Food given through a tube (enteral nutrition) should contain all the nutrients a person needs. Special solutions are available, but solid foods may be processed and given through a nasogastric tube. Food solutions may be slowly and continuously given or given in a more concentrated amount every few hours.

Tube feeding causes many problems, and the problems may be life threatening. The most common problem among older people is the inhalation (aspiration) of food into the lungs, causing pneumonia. Aspiration of food can be lessened by elevating the head of the bed to reduce the risk of spitting food up (regurgitation) and by giving the solution slowly. Some people have diarrhea and abdominal discomfort. The risks of administering too much water and of nutritional imbalances can be reduced by calculating the amount of water required and measuring the levels of dissolved minerals (electrolytes) and urea in the blood.

Intravenous feeding is used when the digestive tract cannot adequately absorb nutrients (for example, in people with a malabsorption disorder) or must be temporarily kept free of food (for example, in people with ulcerative colitis or severe pancreatitis). Food given intravenously (parenteral nutrition) can supply part of a person's nutritional requirements (partial parenteral nutrition) or all of them (total parenteral nutrition). Because total parenteral nutrition requires a large intravenous tube (catheter), it is inserted into a large vein, such as the subclavian vein, located under the collarbone.

With intravenous feeding, infection is a constant risk because the catheter is usually left in place for a long time and the solutions that pass through it contain a lot of glucose—a sugar—which promotes the growth of bacteria. People receiving total parenteral nutrition are closely monitored for signs of infection as well as for changes in weight and urine output.

People who are very undernourished are sometimes given drugs such as recombinant growth hormone, medroxyprogesterone (a progestin used as a contraceptive), or dronabinol (used to treat nausea) to promote weight gain.

CHAPTER 154

Vitamins

Vitamins are a vital part of a healthy diet. The recommended dietary allowance (RDA)—the amount most healthy people need each day to remain healthy—has been determined for most vitamins. A safe upper limit has been determined for some vitamins. Intake above this level increases the risk of a harmful effect (toxicity).

Consuming too little or too much of certain vitamins can cause a nutritional disorder. People who eat a variety of foods are unlikely to develop a vitamin deficiency. However, people who follow restrictive diets may not consume enough of a particular vitamin. For example, strict vegetarians, who consume no animal products, may become deficient in vitamin B_{12}, which is available only in animal products. On the other hand, consuming large amounts (megadoses) of vitamin supplements, without medical supervision, may have harmful effects.

Vitamins are called essential micronutrients because they are required by the body in small amounts. Some vitamins—A, D, E, and K—are fat soluble. Other vitamins—B vitamins and vitamin C—are water soluble. B vitamins include vitamins B_1 (thiamin), B_2 (riboflavin), niacin, pantothenic acid, B_6 (pyridoxine), biotin, B_{12} (cobalamin), and folic acid (folate).

The body does not store most vitamins. Therefore, a person must consume them regularly. Vitamins A, D, and B_{12} are stored in significant amounts, mainly in the liver.

Disorders that impair the intestine's absorption of fats can reduce the absorption of fat-soluble vitamins—A, D, E, and K—and increase the risk of a deficiency. Such disorders include Crohn's disease, cystic fibrosis, obstruction of the bile ducts, and malabsorption disorders.

Vitamin A

There are several forms of vitamin A. One form is a component of nerve cells that are sensitive to light (photoreceptors) in the eye's retina. Another form keeps the skin and the lining of the lungs, intestine, and urinary tract healthy. Carotenoids, such as beta-carotene, are slowly converted to vitamin A in the body. Drugs related to vitamin A (retinoids) are used to treat severe acne and psoriasis and are being investigated for the treatment of certain types of cancer.

VITAMIN A DEFICIENCY

Vitamin A deficiency is common in areas of the world where the intake of animal and fish liver, yellow and green leafy vegetables, eggs, and whole milk products is inadequate. Disorders that impair the intestine's absorption of fats can reduce the absorption of vitamin A and increase the risk of vitamin A deficiency. Surgery on the intestine or pancreas can have the same effect. Liver disorders can interfere with the storage of vitamin A.

Symptoms, Diagnosis, and Treatment

An early symptom of vitamin A deficiency is night blindness, which is caused by a disorder of the retina. The whites (sclera) and corneas of the eyes may become dry—a condition called xerophthalmia. Xerophthalmia is particularly common among children who have a severe deficiency of calories (energy) or protein,▲ which includes an inadequate intake of vitamin A. Foamy deposits (Bitot's spots) may appear in the whites of the eyes. The dry cornea may soften and ulcerate, and blindness may result. Vitamin A deficiency is a common cause of blindness in developing countries.

The diagnosis is based on symptoms and a low level of vitamin A in the blood. People who are at high risk of developing this deficiency and people who have it should take vitamin A supplements. If symptoms persist after 2 months, doctors usually evaluate the person for a disorder that causes malabsorption.

VITAMIN A EXCESS

Too much vitamin A can cause toxicity. Taking daily doses 10 times the RDA or greater for a period of months can cause toxicity due to excess vitamin A. A smaller dose can cause toxicity in infants, sometimes within a few weeks.

Carotenoids can be consumed in foods without causing toxicity. However, when large amounts are consumed, the skin turns a deep yellow (carotenosis), especially on the palms and soles. High-dose supplements of beta-carotene may increase the risk of cancer.

Symptoms, Diagnosis, and Treatment

Very large amounts of vitamin A consumed all at once can cause drowsiness, irritability, headache, and vomiting within hours, followed by peeling of the skin. In children, pressure within the brain (intracranial pressure) is increased and vomiting occurs. Coma and death may occur unless vitamin A is discontinued.

When too much vitamin A is consumed over a period of time, symptoms include coarse hair, partial loss of hair (including the eyebrows), cracked lips, and dry, rough skin, which may peel. Later symptoms include severe headaches, increased pressure within the brain, and general weakness. Bone and joint pain are common, especially among children. The liver and spleen may enlarge.

Taking isotretinoin (a vitamin A derivative used to treat severe acne) during pregnancy may cause birth defects. Women who are or who may become pregnant should not consume vitamin A in amounts above the safe upper limit (3,000 micrograms) because birth defects are a risk.

The diagnosis of vitamin A excess is based on symptoms and a high level of vitamin A in the blood. Treatment involves discontinuing vitamin A supplements.

▲ see page 887

VITAMINS

VITAMIN	GOOD SOURCES	MAIN FUNCTIONS	RECOMMENDED DIETARY ALLOWANCE FOR ADULTS	SAFE UPPER LIMIT
Fat-soluble vitamins				
Vitamin A (retinol)	As vitamin A: Fish liver oils, beef liver, egg yolk, butter, and cream As carotenoids such as beta-carotene: Dark green leafy vegetables, yellow vegetables and fruits, and red palm oil	Used to form light-sensitive nerve cells (photoreceptors) in the retina, helping maintain normal vision Helps maintain the health of the skin and the lining of the lungs, intestine, and urinary tract Helps protect against infections Used as the basis for drugs called retinoids that are used to treat severe acne and possibly some cancers	700–900 micrograms 1,300 micrograms for pregnant and breastfeeding women	3,000 micrograms
Vitamin D	As vitamin D_2 (ergocalciferol) or D_3 (cholecalciferol): Fortified milk and cereals, fatty fish, fish liver oils, and egg yolk; also formed in the skin when it is exposed to direct sunlight	Promotes the absorption of calcium and phosphorus from the intestine Required for bone mineralization, growth, and repair	200 IU for people aged 50 and younger 400 IU for people aged 51 to 70 600 IU for people older than 70	2,000 IU
Vitamin E	Vegetable oil, wheat germ, leafy vegetables, egg yolk, margarine, and legumes	Acts as an antioxidant, protecting cells against damage by free radicals	15 milligrams (22 IU of natural; 33 IU of synthetic)	1,500 IU
Vitamin K	As phylloquinone: Green leafy vegetables (such as collards, spinach, salad greens), soybeans, and vegetable oils (such as canola oil) As menaquinone: Produced by bacteria in the intestine	Helps in the formation of blood clotting factors and thus is necessary for normal blood clotting	65 micrograms for women 80 micrograms for men	—
Water-soluble vitamins				
Vitamin B_1 (thiamin)	Dried yeast, whole grains, meat (especially pork and liver), enriched cereals, nuts, legumes, and potatoes	Required for the metabolism of carbohydrates and for normal nerve and heart function	1.1 milligrams for women 1.2 milligrams for men	—
Vitamin B_2 (riboflavin)	Milk, cheese, liver, meat, fish, eggs, and enriched cereals	Required for the metabolism of carbohydrates and amino acids and for healthy mucous membranes, such as those lining the mouth	1.1 milligrams for women 1.3 milligrams for men	—

Vitamin	Good Sources	Main Functions	Recommended Dietary Allowance for Adults	Safe Upper Limit
Niacin (nicotinamide or nicotinic acid)	Dried yeast, liver, meat, fish, legumes, and whole-grain or enriched cereal products	Required for the metabolism of carbohydrates, fats, and many other substances	14 milligrams for women 16 milligrams for men	35 milligrams
Pantothenic acid	Liver, meats, egg yolk, yeast, and vegetables	Required for the metabolism of carbohydrates and fats	5 milligrams (but no RDA has been established)	—
Vitamin B$_6$ (pyridoxine)	Dried yeast, liver, organ meats, whole-grain cereals, fish, and legumes	Required for the metabolism of amino acids and fatty acids, for nerve function, for the formation of red blood cells, and for healthy skin	1.5 milligrams for women 1.7 milligrams for men	100 milligrams
Biotin	Liver, kidneys, egg yolk, milk, fish, yeast, cauliflower, nuts, and legumes	Required for the metabolism of carbohydrates and fatty acids	30 micrograms (but no RDA has been established)	—
Vitamin B$_{12}$ (cobalamin)	Liver, meats (especially beef, pork, and organ meats), eggs, milk, and milk products	Required for the maturation of red blood cells, for nerve function, and for DNA synthesis	2.4 micrograms	—
Folic acid	Fresh leafy green vegetables, asparagus, broccoli, tomatoes, fruits (especially citrus), liver and other organ meats, dried yeast, and enriched breads, pastas, and cereals (but extensive cooking destroys 50–95% of the folic content of food)	Required for the maturation of red blood cells and for DNA and RNA synthesis	400 micrograms	1,000 micrograms
Vitamin C (ascorbic acid)	Citrus fruits, tomatoes, potatoes, cabbage, and green peppers	Required for the formation and growth of bone and connective tissue, for healing of wounds and burns, and for normal function of blood vessels

Acts as an antioxidant, protecting cells against damage by free radicals

Helps the body absorb iron | 75 milligrams for women 90 milligrams for men 35 milligrams more for smokers | 2,000 milligrams |

IU = international unit; DNA = deoxyribonucleic acid; RNA = ribonucleic acid.

Vitamin D

Vitamin D exists in two forms that are important for nutrition. Vitamin D_2 (ergocalciferol), which is produced by plants, is consumed in the diet. The most common food source of vitamin D_2 is fortified foods, such as cereals and dairy products. Vitamin D_2 is present in fish liver oils and fatty fish. Vitamin D_3 (cholecalciferol) is formed in the skin when the skin is exposed to sunlight. Vitamin D is stored mainly in the liver. Vitamin D must be processed (metabolized) by the liver and kidneys before it is converted to the active form. The active form promotes the absorption of calcium and phosphorus from the intestine and thus is necessary for the formation and maintenance of bones.

VITAMIN D DEFICIENCY

In vitamin D deficiency, calcium and phosphate levels in the blood decrease because vitamin D is necessary for absorption of these minerals. The level of parathyroid hormone, which increases the calcium level in the blood, may increase as the body tries to compensate for the vitamin D deficiency. Because not enough calcium and phosphate are available to maintain healthy bones, vitamin D deficiency may result in a bone disorder called rickets in children or osteomalacia in adults.

Vitamin D deficiency can be caused by a lack of vitamin D in the diet or by inadequate exposure to sunlight. A pregnant woman with vitamin D deficiency may develop osteomalacia, and the newborn has a high risk of developing rickets. Because breast milk does not contain large amounts of vitamin D, breastfed infants who are not exposed to enough sunlight may develop rickets and usually require supplements. Vitamin D deficiency may occur in older people because their skin, when exposed to sunlight, produces less vitamin D. Also, older people tend to spend less time outdoors, and their diet may be deficient in vitamin D (because they tend to consume fewer fortified dairy products). Because people with kidney or liver disorders may be unable to convert vitamin D into a usable form, they are at risk of osteomalacia. Malabsorption disorders and the use of certain anticonvulsants increase the risk of vitamin D deficiency. Several rare hereditary forms of rickets develop

because the body cannot process (metabolize) vitamin D normally.

Symptoms, Diagnosis, and Treatment

Muscle spasms caused by a low calcium level may be the first sign of rickets in infants. (However, spasms may occur at any age.) Older infants may be slow to sit and crawl, and the spaces between the skull bones (fontanelles) may be slow to close. In children aged 1 to 4 years, bone growth may be abnormal, causing an abnormal curve in the spine and bowlegs or knock-knees. These children may be slow to walk. For older children and adolescents, walking is painful. The pelvic bones may flatten, narrowing the birth canal in adolescent girls. In adults, the bones, particularly the spine, pelvis, and legs, weaken. Affected areas may be painful to touch, and fractures may occur.

The diagnosis of rickets or osteomalacia is based on symptoms, the appearance of bones on x-rays, and a low level of vitamin D byproducts in the blood.

Treatment involves taking daily vitamin D and calcium supplements by mouth. People with a chronic liver or kidney disorder may require special formulations of vitamin D supplements.

VITAMIN D EXCESS

Taking very high daily doses of vitamin D over several months can cause toxicity and a high calcium level in the blood (hypercalcemia). ▲

Early symptoms are loss of appetite, nausea, and vomiting, followed by excessive thirst, weakness, nervousness, and high blood pressure. Because the calcium level is high, calcium may be deposited throughout the body, particularly in the kidneys, blood vessels, lungs, and heart. The kidneys may be permanently damaged and malfunction. As a result, urination increases, protein passes into the urine, and the level of urea (a waste product) increases in the blood. Kidney failure may result.

Vitamin D excess is usually diagnosed when blood tests detect a high calcium level in a person who takes high doses of vitamin D. The diagnosis is confirmed by measuring the level of vitamin D in the blood. Treatment consists of discontinuing vitamin D supplements, following a low-calcium diet for a while to offset the effects of a high calcium level in the body, and taking drugs to suppress the release of calcium from the bones.

▲ see page 904

Vitamin E

Vitamin E is an antioxidant: It protects cells against damage by free radicals, which are reactive by-products of normal cell activity.

VITAMIN E DEFICIENCY

Consuming a low-fat diet may reduce consumption of vitamin E, because vegetable oils are the main source of this vitamin. Disorders that impair fat absorption can also reduce the absorption of vitamin E and increase the risk of vitamin E deficiency. Newborns have a relatively low reserve of vitamin E, because only small amounts of vitamin E cross the placenta. Thus, newborns are at increased risk of a vitamin E deficiency.

Vitamin E deficiency is rare among older children and adults. Symptoms may include reduced reflexes, difficulty walking, loss of coordination, loss of position sense (knowing where the limbs are without looking at them), and muscle weakness.

Premature infants who have a vitamin E deficiency are at risk of several serious disorders. They may develop a form of anemia in which red blood cells rupture (hemolytic anemia). Other disorders include bleeding (hemorrhage) within the brain and retinopathy of prematurity, in which blood vessels in the eyes grow abnormally.▲

Blood tests to detect vitamin E deficiency are not routinely available. Treatment involves taking vitamin E supplements by mouth.

VITAMIN E EXCESS

High doses of vitamin E may increase the risk of bleeding (including hemorrhagic stroke in adults), particularly for people who are also taking an anticoagulant (especially warfarin). Premature infants may be given high doses to reduce the risk of retinopathy. Occasionally, adults who take very high doses develop muscle weakness, fatigue, nausea, and diarrhea.

The diagnosis is based on the person's circumstances and symptoms. Treatment involves discontinuing vitamin E supplements. If necessary, vitamin K is given to stop bleeding.

Vitamin K

Vitamin K has two forms. The most important form nutritionally (phylloquinone) occurs in plants and is consumed in the diet. The other form (menaquinone) is produced by bacteria in the intestine, but only limited amounts of this form can be absorbed. Vitamin K is necessary for the synthesis of the proteins that help control bleeding (clotting factors) and thus for the normal clotting of blood. It is also needed for healthy bones.

VITAMIN K DEFICIENCY

Disorders that interfere with fat absorption can reduce the absorption of vitamin K and cause vitamin K deficiency. Taking large amounts of mineral oil may reduce the absorption of vitamin K. Vitamin K deficiency can develop in people who take certain drugs, including anticoagulants, anticonvulsants, and certain antibiotics.

One form of vitamin K deficiency is hemorrhagic disease of the newborn, characterized by a tendency to bleed. A vitamin K injection is usually given to newborns to protect them from this disease. Breastfed infants who have not received this injection at birth are especially susceptible to vitamin K deficiency.

Symptoms, Diagnosis, and Treatment

The main symptom is bleeding (hemorrhage)—into the skin (causing bruises), from the nose, from a wound, in the stomach (sometimes with vomiting of blood), or in the intestine. Blood may be seen in the urine or stool. In newborns, life-threatening bleeding within or around the brain may occur. Vitamin K deficiency may also weaken bones.

When vitamin K deficiency is suspected, a blood test to measure clotting function is performed. An abnormal test result can also be caused by use of anticoagulants or by liver damage.

Treatment consists of vitamin K injections or adjusting the dose of the anticoagulant. People who have vitamin K deficiency and a severe liver disorder may also need blood transfusions to replenish the clotting factors. The damaged liver may be unable to synthesize prothrombin and other clotting factors even after vitamin K injections.

Vitamin B$_1$

Vitamin B$_1$ (thiamin) is essential for the metabolism of carbohydrates (to produce energy) and for normal nerve and heart function.

▲ see page 1504

VITAMIN B₁ DEFICIENCY

Vitamin B₁ (thiamin) deficiency may result from a deficiency in the diet. People whose diet consists mainly of polished (refined) white rice are at risk of vitamin B₁ deficiency, because polishing removes almost all of the vitamins. Alcoholics, who often substitute alcohol for food, are at high risk of developing this deficiency.

Symptoms

Early symptoms are vague. They include fatigue, irritability, memory impairment, loss of appetite, sleep disturbances, abdominal discomfort, and weight loss. Eventually, a severe vitamin B₁ deficiency (beriberi) may develop, characterized by nerve, heart, and brain abnormalities.

Beriberi causes different symptoms in different people. One form, called dry beriberi, causes nerve and muscle abnormalities. Symptoms include a prickling (pins-and-needles) sensation in the toes, a burning sensation in the feet that is particularly severe at night, and pain, weakness, and wasting (atrophy) of muscles in the legs.

Wet beriberi causes heart abnormalities. Symptoms include a high output of blood from the heart, a fast heart rate, and dilation of blood vessels, causing the skin to be warm and moist. Because the heart cannot maintain the high output, heart failure eventually develops, causing fluid accumulation in the legs (edema) and in the lungs (congestion). As a result, blood pressure may fall, leading to shock and death.

Brain abnormalities due to vitamin B₁ deficiency occur primarily in alcoholics. Brain abnormalities may develop when a chronic vitamin B₁ deficiency is suddenly worsened by a rapid, substantial decrease in the vitamin B₁ level (which can be caused by an alcoholic binge) or by a sudden increase in vitamin B₁ requirements (which may occur when an undernourished alcoholic is fed intravenously).

Brain abnormalities may develop in two stages: an early stage called Korsakoff's syndrome and a later stage called Wernicke's encephalopathy. Together, these stages are called the Wernicke-Korsakoff syndrome.▲ Korsakoff's syndrome causes memory loss, and Wernicke's encephalopathy causes mental confusion, difficulty walking, and eye problems (including nystagmus and paralysis of the eyes). If Wernicke's encephalopathy is not promptly treated, symptoms may worsen, resulting in coma and even death.

Diagnosis and Treatment

The diagnosis is based on symptoms. Tests to confirm the diagnosis are not readily available. All forms of the deficiency are treated with vitamin B₁ supplements.

Wernicke's encephalopathy, a medical emergency, is treated with high doses of vitamin B₁ for several days. When people who may be alcoholics must be fed intravenously, they are often given vitamin B₁ supplements as a preventive measure. For people who have the Wernicke-Korsakoff syndrome, recovery is often incomplete because some brain damage may be permanent. Symptoms of beriberi may recur years after apparent recovery.

Vitamin B₂

Vitamin B₂ (riboflavin) is essential for the metabolism of carbohydrates (to produce energy) and amino acids. It also helps keep mucous membranes (such as those lining the mouth) healthy.

VITAMIN B₂ DEFICIENCY

Vitamin B₂ deficiency by itself is uncommon. It usually occurs with deficiencies of other B vitamins in people who have a protein and calorie deficiency. Chronic disorders, such as heart disease, cancer, and diabetes mellitus, and malabsorption disorders increase the risk of vitamin B₂ deficiency, as can hemodialysis and peritoneal dialysis—procedures that filter the blood.■

Symptoms are vague. They include painful cracks in the corners of the mouth and on the lips and a sore mouth and tongue. The tongue may turn magenta, and greasy (seborrheic) patches may appear around the nose and in the area between the nose and the lips.

The diagnosis is based on the symptoms and evidence of general undernutrition.★ Tests to confirm the diagnosis are not readily available. High doses of vitamin B₂ are taken by mouth until symptoms resolve. Supplements of other B vitamins are also taken. People who are undergoing hemodialysis or peritoneal dialysis or who have a malabsorption disorder should take vitamin B₂ supplements.

▲ see page 479   ■ see art on page 836

★ see page 889

Niacin

Niacin is essential for the metabolism of carbohydrates, fats, and many other substances in the body.

NIACIN DEFICIENCY

Niacin (nicotinamide or nicotinic acid) deficiency causes pellagra only if tryptophan, an amino acid, is also deficient. Tryptophan can be converted to niacin in the body. People who live in areas where maize (Indian corn) is the main food source are at risk of developing pellagra because maize is low in niacin and tryptophan. Furthermore, the niacin in maize cannot be absorbed in the intestine unless the maize is treated with alkali (as it is when tortillas are prepared). Pellagra may be a seasonal disorder, appearing each spring and lasting through the summer, when the diet consists mainly of maize products.

Alcoholics and other undernourished people are at risk of developing pellagra. Inadequate intake of iron and vitamins B_2 and B_6 increase the risk of niacin deficiency. Pellagra develops in people who have Hartnup disease, a rare hereditary disorder in which tryptophan absorption is impaired.▲

Symptoms, Diagnosis, and Treatment

Pellagra affects the skin, digestive tract, and brain. A symmetric, reddened rash that resembles a sunburn and becomes worse when exposed to sunlight (a condition called photosensitivity) may occur. Skin abnormalities are persistent, and the affected areas may become brown and scaly.

The whole digestive tract is affected. The tongue and mouth may become inflamed and red. The tongue may swell, the mouth may burn, and sores may develop on both. The throat and esophagus may also burn. Other symptoms include nausea, vomiting, constipation, and diarrhea.

Later, fatigue, insomnia, and apathy develop. Malfunction of the brain (encephalopathy) usually follows. It is characterized by confusion, disorientation, hallucinations, and memory loss.

The diagnosis is based on the diet history, symptoms, and circumstances of the person. Tests to confirm the diagnosis are not readily available.

Pellagra is treated with high daily doses of nicotinamide, a form of niacin, taken by mouth. Supplements of other B vitamins are also taken.

NIACIN EXCESS

Niacin (but not nicotinamide) in high doses may be prescribed to lower high fat (lipid) levels in the blood. Such doses can cause flushing, itching, gout, liver damage, and an increase in the levels of sugar (glucose) in the blood. Most side effects can be minimized by starting with a relatively low dose and gradually increasing the dose. Taking aspirin before taking niacin also helps. If the side effects of niacin are intolerable, the dose may be decreased, other (especially slow-release) formulations may be tried, or niacin may be discontinued and another lipid-lowering drug substituted.■

Vitamin B₆

Vitamin B_6 (pyridoxine) is essential for the metabolism of amino acids and fatty acids, for normal nerve function, and for the formation of red blood cells. It also helps keep the skin healthy.

VITAMIN B₆ DEFICIENCY

Vitamin B_6 deficiency may result from inadequate intake or from use of drugs that deplete vitamin B_6 reserves in the body. These drugs include the antibiotic isoniazid, the antihypertensive hydralazine, and penicillamine (used to treat such disorders as rheumatoid arthritis and Wilson's disease).

Vitamin B_6 deficiency can cause seizures in infants. In adults, it can cause anemia and inflammation of the skin (dermatitis) with redness and greasy scaling. The hands and feet may feel numb and prickling—a pins-and-needles sensation. The tongue may become sore and red, and cracks may form in the corners of the mouth. The person may become confused, irritable, and depressed.

The diagnosis is based on the person's circumstances, symptoms, and response to vitamin B_6 supplements. Blood tests to confirm the diagnosis are not readily available. People who have the deficiency or who are taking a drug that depletes vitamin B_6 reserves should take vitamin B_6 supplements.

VITAMIN B₆ EXCESS

Vitamin B_6 in very high doses may be prescribed for such disorders as carpal tunnel syndrome, premenstrual syndrome, and nerve

▲ see page 853　　■ see table on page 925

damage (neuropathy), although there is little evidence of benefit. Taking such high doses may cause pain and numbness in the feet and legs.

The diagnosis is based on symptoms and a history of taking high doses of vitamin B_6. Treatment involves discontinuing vitamin B_6 supplements. Recovery from this disorder may be slow, and some difficulty walking may persist.

Vitamin B_{12}

Vitamin B_{12} (cobalamin), with folic acid, is necessary for the maturation of red blood cells and the synthesis of DNA (deoxyribonucleic acid), the genetic material of cells. Vitamin B_{12} is also necessary for normal nerve function. Unlike most other vitamins, B_{12} is stored in substantial amounts, mainly in the liver. The body's stores of this vitamin would take about 3 to 5 years to exhaust.

VITAMIN B_{12} DEFICIENCY

Usually, vitamin B_{12} deficiency is due to inadequate absorption. The cause may be lack of intrinsic factor, a protein produced in the stomach. Normally, vitamin B_{12} is readily absorbed in the last part of the small intestine (ileum), which leads to the large intestine. However, to be absorbed, the vitamin must combine with intrinsic factor. Without intrinsic factor, vitamin B_{12} remains in the intestine and is excreted in the stool. Intrinsic factor may be lacking because, for example, abnormal antibodies, produced by an overactive immune system, attack and destroy the stomach cells that produce intrinsic factor—an autoimmune reaction.

Older people may have a vitamin B_{12} deficiency because stomach acidity is low, reducing the body's ability to remove vitamin B_{12} from the protein in meat. Abnormal growth of bacteria in the small intestine may reduce the absorption of vitamin B_{12}. Disorders that impair the absorption of nutrients in the intestine can reduce the absorption of vitamin B_{12}. Fish tapeworm infection may also reduce the absorption of vitamin B_{12} in the intestine. Liver disorders may interfere with the storage of vitamin B_{12}. Surgery that removes the stomach (where intrinsic factor is produced) or the part of the small intestine where vitamin B_{12} is absorbed can result in a deficiency. A strict vegetarian diet may also cause vitamin B_{12} deficiency because vitamin B_{12} is available only in animal products. Infants who are breastfed by a mother who is a strict vegetarian are at risk of vitamin B_{12} deficiency.

Symptoms

Because vitamin B_{12} is necessary for the production of mature blood cells, deficiency of this vitamin can result in anemia, characterized by abnormally large red blood cells (macrocytes) and white blood cells with abnormal nuclei. The type of anemia that results when an autoimmune reaction destroys the stomach cells that produce intrinsic factor is called pernicious anemia. Because the liver stores a large amount of vitamin B_{12}, pernicious anemia may not develop until 3 to 5 years after the body stops absorbing vitamin B_{12}.

Vitamin B_{12} deficiency anemia develops gradually, allowing the body to adapt somewhat. Consequently, the anemia may be more severe than the symptoms indicate. Anemia causes paleness, weakness, and fatigue. Severe anemia causes shortness of breath, dizziness, and a rapid heart rate.

Vitamin B_{12} deficiency can also cause nerve damage (neuropathy) even when no anemia develops, particularly in people older than 60. The legs are affected earlier and more often than the arms. Tingling is felt in the feet and hands, and sensation in the legs, feet, and hands is lost. Vibration and position senses are also lost. Mild to moderate muscle weakness develops, and reflexes may be lost. Walking becomes difficult. Some people become confused, irritable, and mildly depressed. Advanced vitamin B_{12} deficiency may lead to delirium, paranoia, and impaired mental function, including dementia.

Diagnosis

Usually, vitamin B_{12} deficiency is suspected when routine blood tests detect large red blood cells. If this deficiency is suspected, the level of vitamin B_{12} in the blood is measured. If a deficiency is confirmed in an older person, no other tests are performed, because the cause, such as low stomach acidity, is usually not serious. In a younger person, tests to determine the cause may be performed, usually focusing on intrinsic factor.

If the cause of vitamin B_{12} deficiency is still unclear, a Schilling test may be performed. A tiny amount of radioactive vitamin B_{12} is given by mouth, and the amount absorbed is measured. Then vitamin B_{12} is given with intrinsic factor, and the amount absorbed is measured. If vitamin B_{12} is absorbed only when given with intrinsic factor, the diagnosis of pernicious anemia is confirmed.

Treatment

Treatment of vitamin B_{12} deficiency or pernicious anemia consists of replacing vitamin B_{12}. People who have symptoms due to nerve damage are usually given vitamin B_{12} by injection. Injections, which may be self-administered, are given daily or weekly for several weeks until the level of vitamin B_{12} returns to normal. Then injections are given once a month indefinitely, unless the disorder causing it can be corrected. For people who have the deficiency but no symptoms, the vitamin may be taken by mouth or as a nasal gel, but blood tests are performed periodically to make sure the vitamin B_{12} level returns to and remains normal. Severe symptoms—for example, dementia in an older person—may not resolve.

Folic Acid

Folic acid (folate), with vitamin B_{12}, is necessary for the formation of normal red blood cells and the synthesis of DNA, the genetic material of cells.

FOLIC ACID DEFICIENCY

Because the body stores only a small amount of folic acid (folate), a diet lacking in folic acid leads to a deficiency within a few months. Folic acid deficiency is common because many people do not eat enough raw leafy vegetables or citrus fruits. Undernutrition associated with alcoholism is a common cause. Also, alcohol consumed in large amounts interferes with the absorption and processing (metabolism) of folic acid. Certain anticonvulsants (such as phenytoin and phenobarbital) and drugs used to treat ulcerative colitis (such as sulfasalazine) decrease the absorption of this vitamin. Methotrexate (used to treat cancer and rheumatoid arthritis) and trimethoprim-sulfamethoxazole (an antibiotic) interfere with the metabolism of folic acid.

Women who are pregnant or breastfeeding and people undergoing dialysis may develop this deficiency, because their need for folic acid is increased.

Symptoms, Diagnosis, and Treatment

People who have folic acid deficiency develop anemia similar to that due to vitamin B_{12} deficiency.

Homocysteine: A Diet–Heart Disease Connection?

Homocysteine is an amino acid in the blood. A high level of homocysteine is associated with an increased risk of atherosclerosis, which can result in a heart attack (due to coronary artery disease) and stroke.

The homocysteine level may be increased by a genetic disorder. The homocysteine level may also increase in some people when they do not consume enough folic acid and vitamins B_6 and B_{12} in their diet. These vitamins help break down homocysteine in the body. People who have high levels of these vitamins often have a relatively low level of homocysteine. However, folic acid supplements have not yet been shown to reduce the risk of atherosclerosis, and there are no guidelines for how much of a vitamin B supplement should be taken to decrease the homocysteine level. Consequently, taking supplements is not routinely recommended. Rather, people are advised to eat foods that are rich in these vitamins.

Fatigue may be the first symptom. In addition to the general symptoms of anemia (such as paleness, irritability, shortness of breath, and dizziness), folic acid deficiency may cause a red and sore tongue, a reduced sense of taste, weight loss, and diarrhea. If a pregnant woman has folic acid deficiency, the baby may have a birth defect of the spinal cord (neural tube defect).

If a blood test detects large red blood cells in a person who has anemia or who is undernourished, doctors measure the folic acid level in a blood sample. A low level indicates this deficiency.

Treatment consists of taking daily doses of a folic acid supplement. People who are taking drugs that interfere with the absorption or metabolism of folic acid should take a folic acid supplement as a preventive measure. Women who are pregnant or who are planning to become pregnant should take higher doses to reduce the risk of having a baby with a birth defect.

FOLIC ACID EXCESS

Folic acid is generally not toxic. Very high doses may worsen nerve damage in people who have vitamin B_{12} deficiency.

Vitamin C

Vitamin C (ascorbic acid) is essential for the formation of bone and connective tissue (which binds other tissues and organs together). Vitamin C helps the body absorb iron, and it helps burns and wounds heal. Like vitamin E, vitamin C is an antioxidant: It protects cells against damage by free radicals, which are reactive by-products of normal cell activity.

VITAMIN C DEFICIENCY

Vitamin C deficiency causes scurvy. In adults, the deficiency usually results from a diet low in vitamin C. For example, vitamin C deficiency may develop in people who eat only such foods as dried meat, tea, toast, and canned vegetables. Pregnancy, breastfeeding, surgery, and burns can significantly increase the body's requirements for vitamin C and the risk of vitamin C deficiency. Smoking increases the vitamin C requirement by 30 to 50%.

Scurvy in infants is rare because breast milk usually supplies enough vitamin C and infant formulas are fortified with the vitamin.

In adults, a few months of a diet low in vitamin C can cause bleeding under the skin (particularly around hair follicles or as bruises), around the gums, and into the joints. Symptoms may include irritability, depression, weight loss, fatigue, and general weakness. The gums become swollen, purple, and spongy. The teeth eventually loosen. Infections may develop, and wounds do not heal.

In infants, symptoms include irritability, pain during movement, and loss of appetite. Infants do not gain weight as they normally do. Bone growth is impaired, and bleeding and anemia may occur.

The diagnosis of scurvy is based on symptoms. Blood tests detect a very low level of vitamin C. Scurvy is treated with daily vitamin C supplements. Such treatment plus iron supplements can cure the anemia.

VITAMIN C EXCESS

Some people take high doses of vitamin C because it is an antioxidant, which protects cells against damage by free radicals. Free radicals, which are reactive by-products of normal cell activity, are thought to contribute to many disorders, such as atherosclerosis, cancer, lung disorders, the common cold, eye cataracts, and memory loss. Whether taking high doses of vitamin C protects against these disorders is unclear. Evidence of a protective effect against cataracts is strongest. In any case, high doses (up to the safe upper limit) of vitamin C are usually not toxic, although they occasionally cause nausea or diarrhea and interfere with the interpretation of some blood test results.

CHAPTER 155

Minerals and Electrolytes

Minerals are necessary for the normal functioning of the body's cells. The body needs large quantities of sodium, potassium, calcium, magnesium, chloride, and phosphate. These minerals are called macrominerals. The body needs small quantities of copper, fluoride, iodine, iron, selenium, and zinc. These minerals are called trace minerals.

Minerals are an essential part of a healthy diet. The recommended dietary allowance (RDA)—the amount most healthy people need each day to remain healthy—has been determined for most minerals. People who have a disorder may need more or less than this amount.

Consuming too little or too much of certain minerals can cause a nutritional disorder. People who eat a balanced diet containing a variety of foods are unlikely to develop a nutritional disorder or a major mineral deficiency, except iron or iodine deficiency. However, people who follow restrictive diets may not consume enough of a particular mineral. For example, vegetarians, including those who eat eggs and dairy products, are at risk of iron deficiency. Consuming large amounts (megadoses) of mineral supplements without medical supervision may have harmful (toxic) effects.

Some minerals—especially the macrominerals—are important as electrolytes. The body uses electrolytes to help regulate nerve and muscle function and acid-base balance.▲ Also, electrolytes help the body maintain normal volume in its different fluid-containing areas (compartments). Electrolytes are dissolved in three main compartments: the fluid within the cells, the fluid in the space surrounding the cells, and the blood.

To function normally, the body must keep the concentration of electrolytes in its compartments within very narrow limits. The body maintains the concentration of electrolytes in each compartment by moving electrolytes into or out of the cells. The kidneys filter the electrolytes in the blood and excrete any excess in the urine to maintain a balance between daily intake and output.

If the balance of electrolytes is disturbed, disorders can develop. An electrolyte imbalance can occur when a person becomes dehydrated; uses certain drugs; has certain heart, kidney, or liver disorders; or is given intravenous fluids or feedings in inappropriate amounts.

To detect nutritional disorders or an electrolyte imbalance, doctors measure the levels of minerals in a sample of blood or urine.

Calcium

Most of the body's calcium is stored in the bones, but calcium is also found in cells (particularly muscle cells) and in the blood. Calcium is essential to muscle contraction and to the normal functioning of many enzymes. It is necessary for the formation of bone and teeth, for blood clotting, and for normal heart rhythm.

The body precisely controls the amount of calcium in the cells and the blood. Maintaining a normal level of calcium in the blood depends on consuming at least 1,000 to 1,500 milligrams of calcium a day and excreting excess calcium in urine. Calcium moves out of the bones into the bloodstream as needed to

maintain a steady level of calcium in the blood. However, mobilizing too much calcium from the bones weakens them and can lead to osteoporosis.

The level of calcium in the blood is regulated primarily by two hormones: parathyroid hormone and calcitonin. Parathyroid hormone is produced by the four parathyroid glands, located around the thyroid gland in the neck. When the calcium level in the blood falls, the parathyroid glands produce more parathyroid hormone. When the calcium level in the blood rises, the parathyroid glands produce less hormone. Parathyroid hormone stimulates the digestive tract to absorb more calcium and causes the kidneys to activate vitamin D. Vitamin D further enhances the ability of the digestive tract to absorb calcium. Parathyroid hormone also stimulates the bones to release calcium into the blood and causes the kidneys to excrete less calcium in urine. Calcitonin, a hormone produced by cells of the thyroid gland, lowers the calcium level in the blood by slowing the breakdown of bone.

HYPOCALCEMIA

In hypocalcemia, the level of calcium in the blood is too low. Most of the calcium in the blood is carried by (bound to) the protein albumin. Albumin-bound calcium acts as a reserve but has no active function in the body. By contrast, unbound (ionized) calcium affects the body's functions. Thus, a low level of albumin in the blood usually causes no problems as long as the amount of unbound calcium remains normal. The total calcium level in the blood usually parallels the level of unbound calcium.

Hypocalcemia is most commonly caused by excessive calcium loss in the urine or a failure to move calcium out of the bones into the bloodstream. Hypocalcemia may result when the level of parathyroid hormone is low (for example, if the parathyroid glands are damaged during thyroid gland surgery), when a person is born without parathyroid glands, or when the body responds poorly to a normal level of parathyroid hormone (pseudohypoparathyroidism). A low level of magnesium may cause hypocalcemia by reducing the activity of parathyroid hormone. Other causes of hypocalcemia include vitamin D deficiency (due to poor nutri-

▲ see page 930

MINERALS

Mineral	Good Sources	Main Functions	Recommended Dietary Allowance for Adults	Safe Upper Limit
Calcium	Milk and milk products, meat, fish, eggs, cereal products, beans, fruits, and vegetables	Required for the formation of bone and teeth, for blood clotting, for normal muscle function, and for normal heart rhythm	1,000 milligrams 1,200 milligrams for people older than 50	2,500 milligrams
Chloride	Salt, beef, pork, sardines, cheese, green olives, corn bread, potato chips, sauerkraut, and processed or canned foods	Involved in electrolyte balance	1,000 milligrams	—
Copper	Organ meats, shellfish (especially oysters), chocolate, mushrooms, nuts, dried legumes, and whole-grain cereals	Used to form enzymes that are necessary for energy production, for antioxidation (protection against cell damage due to reactive by-products of normal cell activity called free radicals), and for formation of the hormone epinephrine, red blood cells, bone, and connective tissue	900 micrograms	10,000 micrograms
Fluoride	Saltwater fish, tea, coffee, and fluoridated water	Required for the formation of bone and teeth	3 milligrams for women 4 milligrams for men	10 milligrams
Iodine	Seafood, iodized salt, dairy products, and drinking water (in amounts that vary by the iodine content of local soil)	Required for the formation of thyroid hormones	150 micrograms	1,100 micrograms
Iron	As heme iron: Meats, poultry, fish, kidneys, and liver As nonheme iron: Soybean flour, beans, molasses, spinach, clams, dried fruit, and fortified cereals	Required for the formation of many enzymes in the body Is an important component of muscle cells and of hemoglobin (which enables red blood cells to carry oxygen and deliver it to the body's tissues)	8 milligrams 18 milligrams for women younger than 50 (premenopause) 27 milligrams for pregnant women 9 milligrams for breastfeeding women	45 milligrams
Magnesium	Leafy green vegetables, nuts, cereal grains, and seafood	Required for the formation of bone and teeth, for normal nerve and muscle function, and for the activation of enzymes	320 milligrams for women 420 milligrams for men	—

MINERALS (*Continued*)

MINERAL	GOOD SOURCES	MAIN FUNCTIONS	RECOMMENDED DIETARY ALLOWANCE FOR ADULTS	SAFE UPPER LIMIT
Phosphorus	Milk, cheese, meat, poultry, fish, cereals, nuts, and legumes	Required for the formation of bone and teeth and for energy production Used to form nucleic acids, including DNA (deoxyribonucleic acid)	700 milligrams	4,000 milligrams
Potassium	Whole and skim milk, bananas, tomatoes, oranges, melons, potatoes, sweet potatoes, prunes, raisins, spinach, turnip greens, collard greens, kale, other green leafy vegetables, most peas and beans, and salt substitutes (potassium chloride)	Required for normal nerve and muscle function Involved in electrolyte balance	3.5 grams	—
Selenium	Meats, seafood, and cereals (depending on the selenium content of soil where grains were grown)	Acts as an antioxidant, with vitamin E, protecting cells against damage by free radicals, which are reactive by-products of normal cell activity Required for thyroid gland function	55 micrograms	400 micrograms
Sodium	Salt, beef, pork, sardines, cheese, green olives, corn bread, potato chips, sauerkraut, and processed or canned foods	Required for normal nerve and muscle function Involved in electrolyte balance	1,000 milligrams	2,400 milligrams
Zinc	Organ meats such as liver, eggs, and seafood	Used to form many enzymes and insulin Required for healthy skin, healing of wounds, and growth	15 milligrams	—

tion or inadequate exposure to sunlight), kidney damage (which increases loss of calcium in urine and reduces the kidneys' ability to activate vitamin D), inadequate intake of calcium in the diet, disorders that affect calcium absorption, and pancreatitis.

The calcium level in the blood can be moderately low without producing any symptoms.

Over time, hypocalcemia can affect the brain and cause neurologic or psychologic symptoms, such as confusion, memory loss, delirium, depression, and hallucinations. These symptoms are reversible if the calcium level is restored. An extremely low calcium level may cause tingling (often in the lips, tongue, fingers, and feet), muscle aches, spasms of the

What Is Hyperparathyroidism?

The parathyroid glands release parathyroid hormone, which increases the absorption of calcium from the digestive tract and causes the bones to release stored calcium. If the parathyroid glands release too much parathyroid hormone, hyperparathyroidism results. People with hyperparathyroidism have too much calcium and a normal or low level of phosphate in their blood. Parathyroid hormone causes the kidneys to excrete more phosphate, but it also causes the bones to release phosphate into the blood. The balance between these two effects determines whether the phosphate level remains normal or falls.

Primary hyperparathyroidism occurs when an abnormality causes the release of too much parathyroid hormone. In about 90% of people with primary hyperparathyroidism, the abnormality is a noncancerous tumor (adenoma) in one of the parathyroid glands. In the remaining 10%, the glands simply enlarge and produce too much hormone. Rarely, cancers of the parathyroid glands cause hyperparathyroidism.

Primary hyperparathyroidism is more common among women than among men. It is more likely to develop in older people and in people who have received radiation therapy to the neck. Sometimes it occurs as part of syndrome of multiple endocrine neoplasia, a rare hereditary disorder▲.

Secondary hyperparathyroidism occurs when excess parathyroid hormone is released in response to a severe decrease in the calcium level in the blood. For example, chronic kidney disease and vitamin D deficiency cause a severe decrease in the calcium level and thus are causes of secondary hyperparathyroidism. Continuous stimulation of the parathyroid glands, as occurs in hypocalcemia, can cause secondary hyperparathyroidism.

Primary hyperparathyroidism is usually treated by surgically removing one or more of the parathyroid glands. The surgery aims for the removal of all parathyroid tissue that is producing excess hormone. Surgery is successful in almost 90% of cases. Treatment of secondary hyperparathyroidism depends on the cause.

▲ see page 972   ■ see box on page 1037

muscles in the throat (leading to difficulty breathing), stiffening and spasms of muscles (tetany), and abnormal heart rhythms.

Hypocalcemia is often detected by routine blood tests before symptoms become obvious.

Oral calcium supplements are often all that is needed to treat hypocalcemia. Once symptoms appear, intravenous administration of calcium is usually warranted. Taking vitamin D supplements helps increase the absorption of calcium from the digestive tract.

HYPERCALCEMIA

In hypercalcemia, the level of calcium in the blood is too high. Hypercalcemia is commonly caused by hyperparathyroidism (the excessive secretion of parathyroid hormone by one or more of the four parathyroid glands).

Another cause of hypercalcemia is the ingestion of large amounts of calcium. Occasionally, hypercalcemia develops in people with peptic ulcers if they drink a lot of milk and take calcium-containing antacids for relief. The resulting disorder is called the milk-alkali syndrome. An overdose of vitamin D can also affect the calcium level in the blood by greatly increasing the absorption of calcium from the digestive tract.

Hypercalcemia often occurs in people who have cancer. Cancers of the kidneys, lungs, and ovaries may secrete large amounts of a protein that has effects similar to those of parathyroid hormone. These effects are considered a paraneoplastic syndrome.■ Calcium can also be released into the blood when cancer spreads (metastasizes) to bone and destroys bone cells. Such bone destruction occurs most commonly with cancers of the prostate, breast, and lung. Multiple myeloma (a cancer involving bone marrow) can also lead to the destruction of bone and result in hypercalcemia. Other cancers can raise the calcium level in the blood by means not yet fully understood.

Disorders in which bone is broken down (resorbed) or destroyed, causing calcium to be released, may also cause hypercalcemia. In Paget's disease, bone is broken down, but the calcium level in the blood is usually normal. However, the calcium level can become too high if people with the disease become dehydrated or spend too much time sitting or lying down—when the bones are not bearing weight. Rarely, other people who are immobilized, such as paraplegics, quadriplegics, or people who require prolonged bed rest, develop hypercalcemia because calcium in bone is released into the blood when the bones do not bear weight for long periods of time.

Hypercalcemia often produces no symptoms. The earliest symptoms are usually constipation, nausea, vomiting, abdominal pain, loss of appetite, and abnormally large amounts of urine. Very severe hypercalcemia often causes brain dysfunction with confusion, emotional disturbances, delirium, hallucinations, and coma. Muscle weakness may occur, and abnormal heart rhythms and death can follow. Kidney stones containing calcium may form in people with chronic hypercalcemia.

Hypercalcemia is usually discovered during routine blood tests.

If the hypercalcemia is not severe, correcting the cause is often sufficient. People who have normal kidney function and a tendency to develop hypercalcemia are usually advised to drink plenty of fluids, which stimulates the kidneys to excrete calcium and helps prevent dehydration.

If the calcium level is very high or if symptoms of brain dysfunction or muscle weakness appear, fluids and diuretics are given intravenously as long as kidney function is normal. Dialysis is a highly effective, safe, reliable treatment, but it is usually reserved for people with severe hypercalcemia that cannot be treated by other methods.

Several other drugs (including plicamycin, gallium nitrate, calcitonin, bisphosphonates, and corticosteroids) can be used to treat hypercalcemia. These drugs work primarily by slowing the release of calcium from bone.

Hypercalcemia caused by cancer is particularly difficult to treat. If the cancer cannot be controlled, hypercalcemia usually returns despite the best treatment.

Copper

Most of the copper in the body is located in the liver, bones, and muscle, but traces of copper occur in all tissues of the body. The liver excretes excess copper into the bile for elimination from the body. Copper is a component of many enzymes. Some of these enzymes are necessary for energy production or for the formation of the hormone epinephrine, red blood cells, bone, or connective tissue (which binds other tissues and organs together). Other enzymes act as antioxidants. They help protect cells against damage by free radicals, which are reactive by-products of normal cell activity.

Wilson's Disease: When Copper Accumulates

In Wilson's disease, a rare hereditary disorder, the liver does not excrete excess copper into the bile as it normally does. As a result, copper accumulates in and damages the liver. The damaged liver releases copper directly into the bloodstream, and copper is carried to other organs, such as the brain and eyes, where it also accumulates.

Symptoms usually begin after age 5. In almost half of affected people, the first symptoms result from brain damage. They include tremors, difficulty speaking and swallowing, incoordination, involuntary jerky movements (chorea), personality changes, and even psychosis (such as schizophrenia or manic-depressive illness). In most of the other people, the first symptoms result from liver damage, which causes hepatitis and eventually cirrhosis. In the cornea of the eyes, the accumulated copper produces gold or greenish gold rings.

Doctors suspect Wilson's disease on the basis of symptoms, such as unexplained hepatitis, tremors, and personality changes. The diagnosis is confirmed by blood tests and a liver biopsy. For children who have a family history of the disease, tests are performed at about age 2 years.

Treatment consists of drugs that bind with copper, such as penicillamine, taken by mouth. Taking zinc supplements may help decrease absorption of copper. Without lifelong treatment, Wilson's disease is fatal. People who do not take the drugs as directed, especially younger people, may develop liver failure. Liver transplantation can cure the disease.

COPPER DEFICIENCY

Copper deficiency is rare among healthy people. It occurs most commonly among infants who are premature, who are recovering from severe undernutrition, or who have persistent diarrhea. A severe disorder that impairs absorption of nutrients (such as celiac disease, Crohn's disease, cystic fibrosis, or tropical sprue) may cause this deficiency. A high intake of zinc or iron can decrease the absorption of copper.

Symptoms of copper deficiency include fatigue, bleeding under the skin, damage to blood vessels, and an enlarged heart. Anemia is common, and the number of white blood cells is decreased.

The diagnosis of copper deficiency is based on symptoms and on blood tests that detect low levels of copper and ceruloplasmin (a protein that contains copper). Copper deficiency is treated with a copper supplement.

COPPER EXCESS

Excess consumption of copper is rare. Any copper not bound to a protein is toxic. Acidic food or beverages in prolonged contact with copper vessels, tubing, or valves can be contaminated with small amounts of unbound copper. Consuming even relatively small amounts of unbound copper may cause nausea, vomiting, and diarrhea. Large amounts can damage the kidneys, inhibit urine production, and cause anemia due to the rupture of red blood cells (hemolysis) and even death.

The diagnosis is made by measuring copper and ceruloplasmin levels in the blood or urine. Treatment involves use of drugs that bind with copper.

Fluoride

In the body, most fluoride occurs in bones and teeth. Fluoride is necessary for the formation and health of bones and teeth.

FLUORIDE DEFICIENCY

Fluoride deficiency can lead to tooth decay and possibly osteoporosis. Consuming enough fluoride can prevent tooth decay and may strengthen bones. The addition of fluoride (fluoridation) to drinking water that is low in fluoride or the use of fluoride supplements significantly reduces the risk of tooth decay.

FLUORIDE EXCESS

People who live in areas where the drinking water has a naturally high fluoride level may consume too much fluoride—a condition called fluorosis. Fluoride accumulates in the teeth, particularly permanent teeth. Chalky white, irregular patches appear on the surface of the tooth enamel, causing the enamel to appear mottled. The teeth may also become pitted. These defects appear to affect appearance only and may even make the enamel more resistant to cavities. Fluoride also accumulates

in bones. Rarely, consuming too much fluoride for a long time results in dense but weak bones, abnormal bone growths (spurs) on the spine, and crippling due to calcium accumulation (calcification) in ligaments.

The diagnosis is based on symptoms. Treatment involves reducing fluoride consumption. For example, people who live in areas with fluoridated water should not drink fluoridated water or take fluoride supplements. Children should always be instructed not to swallow fluoridated toothpaste.

Iodine

Most of the iodine in the body occurs in the thyroid gland. Iodine in the thyroid gland is necessary for the formation of thyroid hormones.

IODINE DEFICIENCY

Iodine deficiency is rare, because in most countries, iodine (as iodide) is added to commercial table salt.

When iodine is deficient, the thyroid gland enlarges, forming a goiter, as it attempts to capture more iodine for the production of thyroid hormones. Iodine deficiency causes the same symptoms as an underactive thyroid gland (hypothyroidism).▲ In adults, such symptoms include puffy skin, a hoarse voice, impaired mental function, dry and scaly skin, sparse and coarse hair, and weight gain. If a pregnant woman has this deficiency, the growth and brain development of the fetus may be abnormal. Unless the baby is treated soon after birth, mental retardation with short stature (cretinism) develops. If a nuclear radiation accident occurs, iodine deficiency increases the risk of thyroid cancer in children because the deficient thyroid gland collects the radioactive iodine.

The diagnosis of iodine deficiency is based on blood tests indicating low levels of iodine and thyroid hormones or a high level of thyroid-stimulating hormone (TSH) or on the presence of a goiter (only in adults). Treatment consists of iodine supplements. Infants may also require supplements of thyroid hormone, sometimes throughout life.

IODINE EXCESS

Excess consumption of iodine is uncommon. It usually results from taking iodine supplements to treat a prolonged iodine defi-

▲ see page 952

ciency. Sometimes people who live near the sea consume too much iodine because they eat a lot of seafood and drink water that is high in iodine. Iodine excess may cause the thyroid gland to become overactive and produce excess thyroid hormones (a disorder called hyperthyroidism).▲ As a result, the thyroid gland enlarges, forming a goiter.

The diagnosis is based on symptoms and on high levels of iodine and thyroid hormones and a low level of thyroid-stimulating hormone (TSH) in the blood. Treatment involves using salt that is not fortified with iodine and reducing consumption of foods that contain iodine.

Iron

Much of the iron in the body occurs in hemoglobin. Hemoglobin is the component of red blood cells that enables them to carry oxygen and deliver it to the body's tissues. Iron is an important component of hemoglobin and muscle cells. Iron is also necessary for the formation of many enzymes in the body.

The body recycles iron: When red blood cells die, the iron in them is returned to the bone marrow to be used again in new red blood cells. A small amount of iron is lost each day, mainly in cells shed from the lining of the intestine. This amount is usually replaced by the 1 to 2 milligrams of iron absorbed from food each day.

Food contains two types of iron: heme iron (found in animal products) and nonheme iron (found in most foods and in iron supplements). Nonheme iron accounts for more than 85% of iron in the average diet. However, less than 20% of nonheme iron that is consumed is absorbed into the body. Nonheme iron is absorbed better when it is consumed with animal protein and with vitamin C. Heme iron is absorbed much better than nonheme iron.

IRON DEFICIENCY

Iron deficiency is the most common mineral deficiency in the world, causing anemia in men, women, and children.

In adults, iron deficiency is most commonly caused by loss of blood. In premenopausal women, monthly menstrual bleeding may cause the deficiency. In men and post-menopausal women, iron deficiency usually indicates bleeding in the digestive tract—for example, from a bleeding ulcer or a polyp in the colon. The deficiency may also result from bleeding in other areas of the body, such as the kidneys.

Iron deficiency may result from an inadequate diet, primarily in infants and small children, who need more iron because they are growing. Adolescent girls who do not eat meat are at risk of developing iron deficiency because they are growing and starting to menstruate. Pregnant women are also at risk of this deficiency, because the growing fetus requires large amounts of iron.

Symptoms

When iron reserves in the body are exhausted, anemia develops.■ Anemia causes paleness, weakness, irritability, drowsiness, and fatigue. Concentration and learning ability may be impaired. When severe, anemia may cause headache, ringing in the ears (tinnitus), spots before the eyes, digestive upset, shortness of breath, dizziness, and a rapid heart rate. Occasionally, severe anemia causes chest pain and heart failure. Menstrual periods may stop.

In addition to anemia, iron deficiency may produce such symptoms as pica (a craving for nonfoods such as ice, dirt, or pure starch), spoon nails (a deformity in which the fingernails are thin and concave), and leg cramps at night. Rarely, iron deficiency may cause a thin membrane to grow across part of the esophagus, resulting in difficulty swallowing.

Diagnosis

The diagnosis of iron deficiency is based on symptoms and on blood test results. Results include a low level of hemoglobin (which contains iron), a low hematocrit (the proportion of red blood cells to the total volume of blood), and a low number of red blood cells, which are abnormally small. The amount of iron in transferrin—the protein that carries iron in blood when iron is not inside red blood cells—is determined. If the amount is less than 10%, iron deficiency is likely. Iron deficiency is confirmed if the level of ferritin (a protein that stores iron) in the blood is low. However, inflammation, infection, cancer, or liver damage can result in a normal or high ferritin level even when iron deficiency is present.

Occasionally, a bone marrow examination is needed to make the diagnosis. A sample of bone marrow cells is removed, usually from

---

▲ see page 949   ■ see also page 989

the hipbone, through a needle and examined under a microscope to determine the iron content.

Treatment

Because the most common cause of iron deficiency in adults is excessive bleeding, doctors first look for a source of bleeding. Drugs, such as oral contraceptives (birth control pills), may be needed to control excessive menstrual bleeding. Surgery may be needed to repair a bleeding ulcer or remove a polyp in the colon. A blood transfusion may be necessary if the anemia is severe.

General treatment includes daily doses of an iron supplement taken by mouth. Normal dietary intake of iron may not be sufficient to replace lost iron (because less than 20% of iron in a typical diet is absorbed into the body). Iron is absorbed best when the supplement is taken on an empty stomach, 30 minutes before meals or 2 hours after meals, particularly if the meals include foods that reduce the absorption of iron (such as vegetable fibers, phytates, bran, coffee, and tea). However, taking iron supplements on an empty stomach can cause indigestion and constipation. So some people must take the supplements with meals. Antacids and calcium supplements can also reduce iron absorption. Consuming vitamin C in juices or taking it as a supplement enhances iron absorption. Eating small amounts of meat, which contains the easily absorbed form of iron (heme iron), enhances the absorption of the poorly absorbed form of iron (nonheme iron). Iron supplements almost always turn stools black—a harmless side effect.

Rarely, iron is given by injection. Injections are necessary for people who cannot tolerate tablets or for a few people who cannot absorb enough iron from the digestive tract.

Correcting iron deficiency anemia usually takes 3 to 6 weeks, even after the bleeding has stopped. After the anemia is corrected, an iron supplement should be taken for 6 months to replenish the body's reserves. Blood tests are usually performed periodically to determine whether the person is receiving enough iron and to check for continued bleeding.

Women who are not menstruating and men should not take iron supplements or multiple vitamins with iron unless specifically instructed to do so by a doctor. Taking such supplements can make diagnosing bleeding from the intestine difficult. Such bleeding may be due to serious disorders including colon cancer.

Because a developing fetus requires iron, iron supplements are recommended for most pregnant women. Most babies, particularly those who are premature or who have a low birth weight, need an iron supplement. It is given as an iron-fortified formula or, to breast-fed babies, as a separate liquid supplement.

IRON EXCESS

Excess iron can accumulate in the body. Causes include many blood transfusions and iron therapy given in excessive amounts or for too long. Another cause is hemochromatosis, a hereditary disorder. Excess iron consumed all at once causes vomiting, diarrhea, and damage to the intestine. Excess iron consumed over a period of time may damage coronary arteries. Treatment often consists of the drug deferoxamine, which binds with iron and carries it out of the body in urine. Treatment of hemachromatosis consists of bloodletting (phlebotomy).

Magnesium

Most of the body's magnesium occurs in bone; very little is present in the blood. Magnesium is necessary for the formation of bone and teeth and for normal nerve and muscle function. Many enzymes in the body depend on magnesium to function normally. The body takes in magnesium from the diet and excretes it in urine and stool.

HYPOMAGNESEMIA

In hypomagnesemia, the level of magnesium in the blood is too low. The most common causes of hypomagnesemia are decreased dietary intake (due to starvation) and decreased intestinal absorption (malabsorption). Hypomagnesemia occurs frequently in people who consume large amounts of alcohol and in people who have protracted diarrhea. Hypomagnesemia can also be caused by increased excretion of magnesium by the kidneys. High levels of aldosterone, antidiuretic hormone, or thyroid hormones can cause hypomagnesemia by increasing the excretion of magnesium by the kidneys. Diuretics, the antifungal drug amphotericin B, or the chemotherapy drug cisplatin can also cause hypomagnesemia.

Symptoms of hypomagnesemia include nausea, vomiting, sleepiness, weakness, personality changes, muscle spasms, tremors, and loss of appetite. The diagnosis is made by determining that the magnesium level in the blood is low.

Magnesium is replaced when the deficiency causes symptoms or when the magnesium level is very low. Magnesium can be taken by mouth (usually as small amounts of magnesium hydroxide) or by injection into a muscle or vein.

HYPERMAGNESEMIA

In hypermagnesemia, the level of magnesium in the blood is too high. Hypermagnesemia usually develops only in people with kidney failure who are given magnesium salts or who take drugs that contain magnesium (such as some antacids or laxatives).

Symptoms of hypermagnesemia include weakness, low blood pressure, and impaired breathing. When hypermagnesemia is severe, the heart can stop beating. The diagnosis is made by determining that the magnesium level in the blood is high.

People with severe hypermagnesemia are given intravenous calcium gluconate. Intravenous diuretics can increase the kidneys' excretion of magnesium, but if the kidneys are not functioning well, dialysis is usually needed.

Phosphate

Phosphorus is present in the body almost exclusively in the form of phosphate. Most of the body's phosphate is contained in bone. The rest is located primarily inside the cells, where it is involved in energy metabolism. Phosphate is necessary for the formation of bone and teeth. Phosphate is also used as a building block for several important substances, including those used by the cell for energy and DNA (deoxyribonucleic acid). Phosphate is taken in from the diet and excreted in urine and stool.

HYPOPHOSPHATEMIA

In hypophosphatemia, the level of phosphate in the blood is too low. Chronic hypophosphatemia occurs in people who have hyperparathyroidism, hypothyroidism (an underactive thyroid gland), or impaired kidney function or who use diuretics for a long time. Taking large amounts of aluminum-containing antacids for a long time or large amounts of the drug theophylline can also deplete the

Hemochromatosis: When Iron Accumulates

In hemochromatosis, a hereditary disorder, too much iron is absorbed, resulting in the accumulation of iron in the body. Hemochromatosis is potentially fatal but usually treatable. The gene associated with hemochromatosis has been identified.

Usually, symptoms develop gradually, often not appearing until middle age or later. In women, symptoms usually start after menopause, because menstrual bleeding and pregnancy provide some protection.

Symptoms vary because iron accumulation can damage any part of the body, including the brain, liver, pancreas, lungs, or heart. The liver and pancreas may be damaged first, causing symptoms of cirrhosis or diabetes. Or, the first symptoms may be vague and affect the whole body. Fatigue is an example. Later, the skin may become bronze-colored.

Diabetes develops in 50 to 60% of people. Heart disorders (such as heart failure and abnormal heart rhythms) develop in some people. Liver cancer may eventually develop. In many men, levels of male hormones decrease. Other symptoms may include arthritis, erectile dysfunction (impotence), infertility, an underactive thyroid gland (hypothyroidism), and chronic fatigue. Hemochromatosis can worsen neurologic disorders that are already present.

Identifying hemochromatosis based on symptoms may be difficult. However, blood tests to measure the levels of two substances can identify people who should be further evaluated. These substances are ferritin, a protein that stores iron, and the iron in transferrin, the protein that carries iron when it is not inside red blood cells. If these levels are high, genetic testing is usually performed to confirm the diagnosis. A liver biopsy may be necessary to determine whether the liver has been damaged. All relatives of an affected person should undergo genetic testing.

Usually, bloodletting (phlebotomy) is the best treatment. It prevents additional organ damage but does not reverse existing damage. Bloodletting is performed once or sometimes twice a week. Each time, about 500 milliliters (1 pint) of blood is removed until the level of ferritin is normal.

With early diagnosis and treatment of hemochromatosis, a long, healthy life is possible.

body's stores of phosphate. Phosphate stores are depleted in people with severe undernutrition, diabetic ketoacidosis, severe alcohol intoxication, or severe burns. The level of phosphate in the blood can fall dangerously low very quickly in people recovering from these conditions, because the body uses large amounts of phosphate during recovery.

Symptoms occur only when the phosphate level in the blood falls very low. Muscle weakness progresses to stupor, coma, and death. With prolonged mild hypophosphatemia, the bones can weaken, resulting in bone pain and fractures. The diagnosis is made by determining that the phosphate level in the blood is low.

Drinking one quart of low-fat or skim milk, which provides a large amount of phosphate, may help. A person with mild hypophosphatemia and no symptoms can take phosphate by mouth, but doing so usually causes diarrhea. If hypophosphatemia is very severe or if phosphate cannot be taken by mouth, intravenous phosphate may be given.

HYPERPHOSPHATEMIA

In hyperphosphatemia, the level of phosphate in the blood is too high. Hyperphosphatemia rarely occurs except in people with severe kidney dysfunction. Dialysis is not very effective at removing phosphate.

Hyperphosphatemia rarely causes symptoms. Progressive bone weakness can occur, resulting in pain and increased susceptibility to fractures. Calcium and phosphate can crystallize in the walls of the blood vessels and heart, causing severe arteriosclerosis (hardening of the arteries) and leading to strokes, heart attacks, and poor circulation. Crystals can also form in the skin, where they cause severe itching. The diagnosis is made by determining that the phosphate level in the blood is high.

Hyperphosphatemia in people with kidney damage is treated by decreasing phosphate intake and reducing the absorption of phosphate from the digestive tract. Foods that are high in phosphate should be avoided. Phosphate-binding antacids should be taken with meals as prescribed by a doctor. These antacids bind to the phosphate and prevent it from being absorbed.

Potassium

Most of the body's potassium is located inside the cells. Potassium is necessary for the normal functioning of cells, nerves, and muscles.

The level of potassium in the blood must be maintained within a narrow range. A potassium level that is too high or too low can have serious consequences, such as an abnormal heart rhythm or even cardiac arrest. The potassium stored within the cells can be used by the body to help maintain a constant level of potassium in the blood.

Potassium balance is achieved by matching the amount of potassium taken in with the amount lost. Potassium is taken in through food and electrolyte-containing drinks and lost primarily in urine, although some potassium is also lost through the digestive tract and in sweat. Healthy kidneys are able to adjust the excretion of potassium to match changes in dietary intake. Some drugs and certain conditions affect the movement of potassium into and out of cells, which greatly influences the potassium level in the blood.

HYPOKALEMIA

In hypokalemia, the level of potassium in the blood is too low. Excessive potassium loss usually results from vomiting, diarrhea, chronic laxative use, or colon polyps. Very occasionally, excessive loss results from excessive sweating in conditions of extreme heat and humidity. Many foods contain potassium, so hypokalemia is rarely caused by too little intake in people who eat a balanced diet.

There are several reasons why potassium may be lost in the urine. By far the most common is the use of diuretics that cause the kidneys to excrete excess sodium, water, and potassium. In Cushing's syndrome, the adrenal glands produce excess amounts of aldosterone, a hormone that causes the kidneys to excrete large amounts of potassium.▲ Excessive potassium is also excreted by people who eat large amounts of licorice or chew certain types of tobacco. People with Liddle's syndrome,■ Bartter's syndrome,★ and Fanconi's syndrome● have rare defects that interfere with the kidneys' ability to conserve potassium.

Certain drugs (such as insulin and the antiasthmatic drugs albuterol, terbutaline, and theophylline) increase the movement of potassium into the cells and can result in hy-

▲ see page 958   ■ see page 854
★ see page 853   ● see page 852

pokalemia. However, use of these drugs is rarely the sole cause of hypokalemia.

A mild decrease in the potassium level in the blood usually causes no symptoms. A more severe decrease can cause muscle weakness, twitches, and even paralysis. Abnormal heart rhythms may develop, especially in people with heart disease. Even mild hypokalemia is dangerous in people taking the heart drug digoxin. The diagnosis is made by determining that the potassium level in the blood is low.

Potassium usually can be replaced by eating potassium-rich foods or by taking potassium supplements by mouth. Because potassium can irritate the digestive tract, supplements should be taken in small doses with food several times a day rather than in a single large dose. Special types of potassium supplements, such as wax-impregnated or microencapsulated potassium chloride, are much less likely to irritate the digestive tract.

Most people who take diuretics do not need to take potassium supplements. Nevertheless, doctors periodically check the potassium level in the blood so that the drug regimen can be altered if necessary. Alternatively, potassium-conserving diuretics (such as triamterene, amiloride, or spironolactone) can be added to the diuretic therapy, but only in people whose kidneys are functioning normally.

HYPERKALEMIA

In hyperkalemia, the level of potassium in the blood is too high. Hyperkalemia usually results when the kidneys do not excrete enough potassium. Probably the most common cause of mild hyperkalemia is the use of drugs that decrease blood flow to the kidneys or prevent the kidneys from excreting normal amounts of potassium. Such drugs include triamterene, spironolactone, and angiotensin-converting enzyme (ACE) inhibitors. Hyperkalemia can also be caused by Addison's disease, in which the adrenal glands do not produce sufficient amounts of the hormone aldosterone, which stimulates the kidneys to excrete potassium.▲ Kidney failure can result in severe hyperkalemia.

Hyperkalemia can also result when a large amount of potassium is suddenly released from the cells. A sudden release of potassium from the cells can result from crush injuries (involving the destruction of large amounts of muscle tissue), severe burns, or overdoses of crack cocaine. The rapid movement of potas-

sium from the cells into the bloodstream can overwhelm the kidneys and result in life-threatening hyperkalemia.

Mild hyperkalemia causes few, if any, symptoms. Usually, hyperkalemia is first detected when routine blood tests are performed or when a doctor notices changes on an electrocardiogram. A high level of potassium in the blood is dangerous. It can cause the heart rhythm to become abnormal. If the level is very high, the heart can stop beating.

For mild hyperkalemia, reducing the potassium intake or discontinuing drugs that prevent the kidneys from excreting potassium may be the only treatment that is needed. If the kidneys are functioning, a diuretic may be given to increase potassium excretion.

For severe hyperkalemia, immediate treatment is essential. A resin that absorbs potassium from the digestive tract and passes out of the body in the stool can be given by mouth or enema. When this treatment is given, doctors also induce diarrhea so that the resin, with potassium absorbed into it, is quickly expelled.

When more rapid treatment is needed, the person may be given an intravenous solution containing calcium, glucose, or insulin. Calcium helps protect the heart from the effects of a high potassium level but does not actually affect the potassium level. This protective effect lasts only a few minutes. Glucose and insulin drive potassium from the blood into the cells, thus lowering the potassium level in the blood. If these measures do not work or if a person has kidney failure, dialysis may be necessary to remove the excess potassium.

Selenium

Selenium occurs in all tissues. Selenium works with vitamin E as an antioxidant. It helps protect cells against damage by free radicals, which are reactive by-products of normal cell activity. Selenium is also necessary for the thyroid gland to function normally.

SELENIUM DEFICIENCY

Selenium deficiency is rare, even in New Zealand and Finland, where selenium intake is much lower than in the United States and Canada. In China, where selenium intake is even lower, selenium deficiency occurs in association with Keshan disease, a viral disease

---

▲ see page 956

that affects mainly children and young women. Keshan disease damages the heart, resulting in cardiomyopathy.

In selenium deficiency, antioxidants are lacking in the heart and muscles. As a result, cardiomyopathy and muscle weakness may occur.

Doctors suspect selenium deficiency on the basis of the person's circumstances and symptoms. Treatment with a selenium supplement may result in a complete recovery.

SELENIUM EXCESS

Taking more than 1 milligram of a nonprescription selenium supplement each day can have harmful effects. Symptoms include nausea and vomiting, loss of hair and nails, a skin rash, and nerve damage. The diagnosis is based on symptoms, particularly rapid hair loss. Treatment involves reducing selenium consumption.

Sodium

Most of the body's sodium is located in the blood and in the fluid in the space surrounding the cells. Sodium is required by all cells in the body to maintain a normal fluid balance.▲ Sodium plays a key role in normal nerve and muscle function. Sodium is taken in through food and drink and lost primarily in sweat and urine. Healthy kidneys maintain a consistent level of sodium in the body by adjusting the amount excreted in the urine.

When sodium intake and loss are not in balance, the total amount of sodium in the body is affected. Changes in the total amount of sodium are closely linked to changes in the volume of water in the blood. A loss of sodium from the body does not necessarily cause the level of sodium in the blood to decrease but does cause blood volume to decrease. When blood volume decreases, blood pressure also decreases, heart rate increases, and light-headedness and sometimes shock occur.

Conversely, the blood volume increases when there is too much sodium in the body. When excess sodium accumulates in the body, extra fluid accumulates in the space surrounding the cells. As a result, the tissues, especially in the feet and ankles, swell (a condition called edema).

The body continually monitors blood volume. Sensors in the heart, blood vessels, and kidneys detect when blood volume becomes too high and stimulate the kidneys to increase sodium excretion, thus returning blood volume to normal. Sensors in the blood vessels and kidneys detect when blood volume is becoming low and trigger one of several mechanisms that result in an increase in blood volume. One such mechanism involves the adrenal glands, which secrete the hormone aldosterone. Aldosterone causes the kidneys to retain sodium and to excrete potassium.■ Another mechanism involves the pituitary gland, which secretes antidiuretic hormone. Antidiuretic hormone causes the kidneys to conserve water. The retained sodium and water lead to decreased urine production, which eventually leads to an increase in blood volume.

Blood volume most closely parallels the total amount of sodium in the body, which cannot be directly measured with a laboratory test and requires assessment by a doctor. The sodium level in the blood, on the other hand, can be easily measured. Changes in the sodium level in the blood do not necessarily parallel changes in the total amount of sodium in the body or changes in blood volume and have a different set of causes.

HYPONATREMIA

In hyponatremia, the level of sodium in the blood is too low. Hyponatremia occurs when sodium has been overdiluted in the body. Sodium can be overdiluted when people drink enormous amounts of water—as people with certain psychiatric disorders occasionally do— or when people who are hospitalized receive large amounts of water intravenously. In either case, the amount of fluid taken in exceeds the kidneys' capacity to eliminate the excess. Intake of smaller amounts of water—sometimes as little as 1 quart a day—can lead to hyponatremia in people whose kidneys are not functioning normally, such as people with kidney failure. Hyponatremia also often occurs in people with heart failure or cirrhosis. Excessive chronic loss of fluids, as occurs with chronic diarrhea, can also result in hyponatremia.

Another cause of hyponatremia is the syndrome of inappropriate secretion of antidiuretic hormone (SIADH). People who have SIADH have a low sodium level because the pituitary gland secretes too much antidiuretic hormone. Hyponatremia also occurs in people who have underactive adrenal glands (Addi-

---

▲ see page 927   ■ see page 956

When the Body Has Too Much Antidiuretic Hormone

Antidiuretic hormone (vasopressin) regulates the amount of water in the body and the level of sodium in the blood. The pituitary produces and releases antidiuretic hormone when a person becomes dehydrated or when electrolyte levels become too high. Pain, stress, exercise, and a low level of sugar in the blood can also stimulate the release of antidiuretic hormone from the pituitary gland, as can the following drugs:

- Chlorpropamide (a drug that lowers the sugar level in the blood)
- Carbamazepine (an anticonvulsant)
- Vincristine (a chemotherapy drug)
- Clofibrate (a drug that lowers cholesterol levels)
- Antipsychotic drugs

- Aspirin, ibuprofen, and many other nonprescription analgesics
- Vasopressin and oxytocin (synthetic antidiuretic hormones)

When too much antidiuretic hormone is released, the sodium level in the blood falls and the body retains water. This condition is called syndrome of inappropriate secretion of antidiuretic hormone (SIADH). Symptoms of SIADH tend to be those of the hyponatremia (low sodium level in the blood) that accompanies it.

SIADH is most common among older people. This syndrome occurs in people with heart failure and, rarely, in people with disorders of the hypothalamus (a part of the brain), including brain tumors in this area. SIADH is also associated with several other disorders, including meningitis, encephalitis, psychosis, and some lung disorders (including pneumonia and acute respiratory failure).

Antidiuretic hormone is sometimes produced outside the pituitary gland, especially by some lung cancers. Thus, when doctors discover SIADH, they check the function of the pituitary but also search for cancer.

For people with SIADH, doctors restrict fluid intake and identify and treat the cause of the disorder if possible. Drugs that decrease the effect of antidiuretic hormone on the kidneys (for example, demeclocycline or thiazide diuretics) may be given if the sodium level in the blood falls even more or does not rise despite restriction of fluid intake.

son's disease)▲ and who thus excrete too much sodium in the urine.

When the sodium level in the blood falls quickly, symptoms tend to develop rapidly and be more severe. The brain is particularly sensitive to changes in the sodium level in the blood. Therefore, symptoms such as lethargy and confusion occur first. As hyponatremia becomes more severe, muscle twitching and seizures may occur; stupor, coma, and death may follow. The diagnosis of hyponatremia is made by measuring the sodium level in the blood. Determining the cause of hyponatremia is more difficult and requires a full assessment by a doctor.

Mild hyponatremia can be treated by restricting fluid intake to less than 1 quart per day. Severe hyponatremia is an emergency. To treat it, doctors slowly increase the level of sodium in the blood with drugs, intravenous fluids, or sometimes both. Increasing the level too rapidly can result in severe and often permanent brain damage.

HYPERNATREMIA

In hypernatremia, the level of sodium in the blood is too high. The body contains too little

water relative to the amount of sodium. The sodium level in the blood becomes abnormally high when water loss exceeds sodium loss, as occurs with dehydration. In most people, hypernatremia results from dehydration.■

Hypernatremia occurs in people who drink too little water and in those who have diarrhea, vomiting, fever, excessive sweating (particularly during hot weather), or abnormal kidney function. For example, hypernatremia may occur in diabetes insipidus, in which the kidneys excrete too much water.★ Other causes of hypernatremia include head trauma or neurosurgery involving the pituitary gland, disorders of other electrolytes (a high calcium level or low potassium level), sickle cell disease, and use of drugs (such as lithium, demeclocycline, or diuretics).

Hypernatremia is most common among older people, who tend to sense thirst more gradually and less intensely than younger people do. Older people who are bedridden or demented may be unable to obtain water even if they feel thirsty. In addition, the kidneys' abil-

▲ see page 956   ■ see page 928
★ see page 944

ity to concentrate urine declines in advanced age, so older people are less able to conserve water. Older people who take diuretics, which force the kidneys to excrete more water, are at particular risk of hypernatremia—especially when the weather is hot or they become ill and do not drink enough water.

The most important symptoms of hyperna-tremia result from brain dysfunction. Severe hypernatremia can lead to confusion, muscle twitching, seizures, coma, and death. The di-agnosis is made by determining that the sodium level in the blood is high.

Hypernatremia is treated by replacing wa-ter. In all but the mildest cases, dilute fluids (containing water and a small amount of sodium in carefully adjusted concentrations) are given intravenously. The sodium level in the blood is reduced very slowly, because cor-recting the condition too rapidly can cause permanent brain damage.

Zinc

Zinc is widely distributed in the body. It is a component of more than 100 enzymes, includ-ing those involved in the formation of RNA (ribonucleic acid) and DNA (deoxyribonucleic acid). The level of zinc in the body depends on the amount of zinc consumed in the diet. Zinc is necessary for healthy skin, healing of wounds, and growth. Much of the zinc con-sumed in the diet is not absorbed.

ZINC DEFICIENCY

Zinc deficiency is most likely to develop in people who eat little meat, liver, eggs, or seafood. Consuming phytic acid (found in grains) and large amounts of iron and calcium may reduce the absorption of zinc. Liver and

pancreatic disorders, alcoholism, diabetes mellitus, and disorders that impair absorption can cause zinc deficiency. Taking diuretics can also cause zinc deficiency. People who must be fed intravenously for a long time may develop this deficiency. Acrodermatitis en-teropathica, a rare hereditary disorder in which zinc cannot be absorbed, may result in zinc deficiency as well as diarrhea and rashes.

Early symptoms include a loss of appetite and slowed growth in infants and children. Other symptoms include patchy hair loss, im-paired taste and smell, inflammation of the skin (dermatitis), and night blindness. In men, sperm production may be reduced. The body's immune system and ability to heal wounds may be impaired. In acrodermatitis entero-pathica, symptoms usually appear when an af-fected infant is weaned.

Doctors suspect zinc deficiency on the basis of the person's circumstances, symptoms, and response to zinc supplements.

ZINC EXCESS

Consumption of excess zinc is rare. It usu-ally results from consuming acidic foods or beverages packaged in a zinc-coated (galva-nized) container. Symptoms include a metallic taste in the mouth, nausea, vomiting, and di-arrhea. Consumption of 1 gram or more (about 70 times the RDA) may be fatal. In certain in-dustries, inhaling zinc oxide fumes can cause rapid breathing, sweating, and weakness—a disorder called metal fume fever. Consuming too much zinc for a long time can reduce the absorption of copper and impair the immune system.

Doctors suspect the diagnosis based on the person's circumstances and symptoms. Treat-ment involves reducing zinc consumption.

CHAPTER 156

Obesity

Obesity is the accumulation of excessive body fat.

For most people, the condition of being overweight is easy to recognize. But medi-cally, a distinction is made between being

overweight and being obese. The body mass index (BMI) is used to define these conditions. BMI is weight (in kilograms) divided by height (in meters squared). Overweight is defined as a BMI of 25 to 29.9, and obesity is defined as a BMI of 30 or more.

Body composition—the percentage of fat and muscle in the body—is also considered when obesity is defined. Women who have more than 30% body fat or men who have more than 25% body fat are considered obese.▲ Thus, people who are very muscular and have low body fat (such as body builders) may have a high BMI without being obese and without increasing health risks.

Obesity is becoming increasingly common throughout the world. In the United States, this increase has been dramatic: Between 1980 and 1999, the percentage of overweight people increased from 47 to 61%, and the percentage of obese people increased from 15 to 26%.

Obesity is more common among women than among men. How common it is (prevalence) varies by age and race. For example, prevalence increases from about 14% at age 25 to 32% at age 55, then decreases to 22% at age 75. Obesity is equally common among black and white men and is slightly more common among Hispanic men. However, obesity is much more common among black and Hispanic women than among white women. About 67% of middle-aged black women are overweight or obese compared with 45% of middle-aged white women.

Causes

Obesity results from consuming more calories than the body uses. The number of calories needed varies from person to person, depending on age, sex, physical activity, and the person's metabolic rate—the rate at which the body burns calories.

Genetic and environmental factors influence body weight, but precisely how they interact is unclear. One proposed explanation is that body weight is regulated around a set point, similar to a thermostat setting. Some people may have a higher-than-normal set point, which may explain why they are obese and why losing weight and maintaining weight loss are difficult for them.

Obesity tends to run in families. However, families share not only genes but also environment, and separating the two influences is difficult. Genetic factors explain about one third to two thirds of the variability in body weight.

Several genes influence weight. One gene that has been identified—the *ob* gene—controls the production of leptin. Leptin is a protein made by fat cells. Leptin travels to the brain and acts on receptors in the hypothalamus (the part of the brain that helps regulate appetite). The message carried by leptin is to decrease food intake and increase the amount of calories (energy) burned. Researchers discovered that mutations in the *ob* gene prevent leptin production and result in severe obesity in mice and in a very small number of children. In these cases, administration of leptin effectively reduces weight to a normal amount. However, most experts think that in most people, many genes influence weight, and each has a very small effect. These genes have not been identified. Thus, genetic treatment of obesity is unlikely in the near future.

Physical inactivity is one of the main reasons for the increase in obesity among people in affluent societies. It is also a common cause of obesity as people age. Sedentary people need fewer calories. When physical activity increases, food intake usually increases. However, when physical activity decreases, food intake does not always decrease accordingly, and for some people, it even increases.

In affluent societies, the diet has become higher in fats. One problem with a high-fat diet is that fats do not appear to trigger the stop-eating (satiety) response as quickly as carbohydrates or proteins. Thus, when a diet is high in fat, more food tends to be eaten. Furthermore, fats have twice as many calories per gram as carbohydrates and proteins.

Drinking alcohol can contribute to obesity. Alcohol tends to increase the number of calories taken in because it is usually consumed in addition to food. A single shot (1 ounce) of liquor has 80 to 90 calories. A 12-ounce regular beer (which is about 8% alcohol) has 150 calories. As soon as alcohol is consumed, it is used as energy, causing the calories from food to be stored as fat. Furthermore, alcohol tends to stimulate the appetite and reduce self-control.

Socioeconomic factors strongly influence obesity, especially among women. In the United States and other developed countries, obesity is more than twice as common among women of lower socioeconomic class as it is among women of higher ones.

People who were obese as children■ are more likely to be obese as adults, largely because when weight is gained during infancy and early childhood, new fat cells form. People who become obese during childhood may have up to 5 times more fat cells than people who maintained a normal weight. Because the number of cells cannot be decreased, weight

---

▲ see box on page 881   ■ see page 1557

DETERMINING BODY MASS INDEX

HEIGHT	WEIGHT (POUNDS)					
	100	110	120	130	140	150
4' 10"	21	23	25	27	29	31
4' 11"	20	22	24	26	28	30
5' 0"	20	21	23	25	27	29
5' 1"	19	21	23	25	26	28
5' 2"	18	20	22	24	26	27
5' 3"	18	19	21	23	25	27
5' 4"	17	19	21	22	24	26
5' 5"	17	18	20	22	23	25
5' 6"	16	18	19	21	23	24
5' 7"	16	17	19	20	22	23
5' 8"	15	17	18	20	21	23
5' 9"	15	16	18	19	21	22
5' 10"	14	16	17	19	20	22
5' 11"	14	15	17	18	20	21
6' 0"	13	15	16	18	19	20
6' 1"	13	15	16	17	18	20
6' 2"	12	14	15	17	18	19
6' 3"	12	14	15	16	17	19
6' 4"	12	13	15	16	17	18
6' 5"	12	13	14	15	17	18
6' 6"	12	13	14	15	16	17

Underweight: Less than 17.9
Normal: 18 to 25
Overweight: 25.1 to 29.9
Obese:
  Moderate 30 to 40
  Severe More than 40

can be lost only by markedly decreasing the amount of fat in each cell. This fact may limit how much weight can be lost and make maintaining a normal body weight more difficult.

Gaining weight during pregnancy is normal and necessary. However, for a few women, pregnancy is the beginning of weight problems: They gain a large amount of weight and do not lose it afterward. Having several children close together may compound the problem.

After menopause, many women gain weight. At this time, hormonal changes cause fat to be redistributed in the body and to tend to accumulate around the waist rather than the hips and thighs (This redistribution increases health risks.▲) Becoming less active, which may occur gradually and unconsciously at this age, also contributes to weight gain.

Psychologic factors, such as emotional disturbances, are no longer considered an important cause of obesity. However, stress can af-

fect weight. When under stress, some people eat more, and some people eat less.

Hormonal disorders rarely cause obesity. Excess production of cortisol by the adrenal glands (Cushing's syndrome) causes an unusual type of obesity in which fat accumulates only in the trunk while the arms and legs remain thin. Polycystic ovary syndrome■ may be associated with obesity. Occasionally, an increased level of insulin in the blood (hyperinsulinemia) causes obesity.

Many drugs used for common disorders promote weight gain. Examples are drugs used to treat psychologic and neurologic disorders (including many antidepressants and antipsychotics), some antihypertensives (such as beta-blockers), corticosteroids, and some drugs used to treat diabetes (such as insulin).

Stopping smoking usually results in weight gain. Nicotine decreases appetite and increases the metabolic rate. Thus, when nicotine is stopped, food intake increases and the metabolic rate decreases, so that fewer calories are burned. As a result, body weight may increase by 5 to 10%.

▲ see page 918   ■ see page 1367

DETERMINING BODY MASS INDEX *(Continued)*

WEIGHT (POUNDS)

160	170	180	190	200	210	220	230	240	250	260
33	36	38	40	42	44	46	48	50	52	54
32	34	36	38	40	42	45	47	49	51	53
31	33	35	37	39	41	43	45	47	49	51
30	32	34	36	38	40	42	43	45	47	49
29	31	33	35	37	38	40	43	44	46	48
28	30	32	34	35	37	39	41	43	44	46
27	29	31	33	34	36	38	39	41	43	45
27	28	30	32	33	35	37	38	40	42	43
26	27	29	31	32	34	36	37	39	40	42
25	27	28	30	31	33	31	36	38	39	41
24	26	27	29	30	32	33	35	36	38	40
24	25	27	28	30	31	32	34	35	37	38
23	24	26	27	29	30	32	33	34	36	37
22	24	25	26	28	29	31	32	33	35	36
22	23	24	26	27	28	30	31	33	34	35
21	22	24	25	26	28	29	30	32	33	34
21	22	23	24	26	27	28	30	31	32	33
20	21	22	24	25	26	27	29	30	31	33
19	21	22	23	24	26	27	28	29	30	32
19	20	21	23	24	25	26	27	29	30	31
19	20	21	22	23	24	25	27	28	29	30

Symptoms

Accumulation of excess body fat changes overall appearance. Severely obese people often walk abnormally to accommodate their weight. They widen their stance, making walking less steady and stressing the joints. As a result, osteoarthritis may develop or worsen, particularly in the hips, knees, and ankles, and walking may become even more difficult. Low back pain may also result. Fatigue is common. Physical and social activities may be decreased because of fatigue, lack of mobility, or other complications. The feet and ankles often swell because fluid accumulates (a condition called edema).

Because obese people have relatively little body surface for their weight, they cannot eliminate body heat efficiently and they sweat more than thinner people. Skin disorders are particularly common because moisture is trapped in skin folds.

Obese people may have difficulty breathing and may become short of breath, even when exertion is minimal. These problems occur when the lungs are compressed by accumulation of excess fat below the diaphragm (the muscle that divides the chest from the abdomen) and in the chest wall. Furthermore, airflow may be reduced if excess fat accumulates in the tissues that line the throat, narrowing the airway. Sleeping on the back makes breathing even more difficult (regardless of weight). Breathing problems may disturb sleep, and breathing may stop momentarily but repeatedly (a condition called sleep apnea).▲ Sleep apnea can lead to daytime sleepiness and other problems, such as high blood pressure and strokes.

Obesity increases the risk of developing many disorders. For example, because the heart has to work harder, heart failure is more common among obese people. Certain cancers—of the breast, uterus, and ovaries in women and of the colon, rectum, and prostate in men—are more common among people who are obese than among those who are not. Menstrual disorders, osteoarthritis, gout, and gallbladder disease are also more common.

▲ see page 472

The risk of developing some disorders is affected by the location of excess fat. In men and in women after menopause, fat tends to accumulate in the abdomen (abdominal obesity), producing a so-called apple shape. In women, fat tends to accumulate in the thighs and buttocks (described as lower-body obesity), producing a so-called pear shape. Abdominal obesity has been linked with a high risk of coronary artery disease, stroke, high blood pressure, type 2 diabetes, and high levels of fats (lipids) in the blood. For people with abdominal obesity, losing as little as 5 to 10% of their weight dramatically reduces these risks. Blood pressure decreases in most people who have high blood pressure, and more than half of the people with type 2 diabetes can discontinue insulin or other drugs that lower blood sugar. Losing weight and changing to a low-fat diet can reduce levels of fats in the blood.

Obesity doubles or triples the risk of premature death. The more severe the obesity, the higher the risk. In the United States, 300,000 deaths a year are attributed to obesity.

In a culture that values thinness, being obese can cause psychologic or emotional problems. Many young obese women have a poor body image, which leads to self-consciousness and discomfort in social situations. People who are obese may experience prejudice and job discrimination, causing feelings of rejection and low self-esteem. However, depression does not appear to be more common among obese people than among other people.

Diagnosis and Treatment

Obesity is readily diagnosed, and its severity is determined by the BMI. Other tests, such as those used to determine body composition, are rarely needed.▲

Untreated obesity tends to worsen. Even though progress has been made in helping people lose weight and maintain weight loss, most people who lose weight regain it, usually within 3 years. The concern that losing and regaining weight (weight cycling) causes health problems is unfounded and should not prevent obese people from trying to lose weight.

To lose weight, people must consume fewer calories than they burn. They can reduce their intake of calories or exercise more (to burn more calories). Usually, both should be done.

Different approaches help different people. Some people work on their own or join a group of like-minded people. These groups include Overeaters Anonymous (OA), Take Off Pounds Sensibly (TOPS), and community-based and work-site programs. Books and magazine articles, special diet plans, and weight loss products such as meal replacement formulas may be used. There is little information about the success of these approaches.

Other people choose organized programs. Typically, weekly meetings are conducted by counselors and supplemented by instructional and guidance materials. Counselors may be licensed health care practitioners or not. Such programs tend to be limited in duration, and many people drop out of them. Costs vary from about $15 per week to $3,000 per 6 months of treatment. There is little information about their effectiveness. Nevertheless, their ready availability and the desire for treatment have made them popular.

Most weight management programs focus on diet with nutritional counseling and exercise. Most programs include behavior modification techniques to facilitate diet and exercise. These techniques help people identify and change the behaviors that trigger overeating (such as shopping for food when they are hungry or keeping high-calorie snacks at home). Doctors may prescribe drugs that help reduce body weight as part of a weight management program.

Diet and Nutritional Counseling: Dieting is useful only when it includes permanent changes in eating habits. Reputable programs teach people how to make safe, sensible, gradual changes in eating habits to increase the consumption of complex carbohydrates (fruits, vegetables, breads, and pasta) and decrease the consumption of fat. Fad diets may be dangerous and are best avoided.■ For mildly obese people, only a modest restriction of calories and dietary fat is recommended. Usually, the number of calories consumed is reduced to 1,200 to 1,500 a day. Very low calorie diets of 800 calories per day, or even fewer, have been used in the past but have been largely abandoned. After these diets, body weight is usually rapidly regained.

Exercise: Regular moderate exercise can help with weight loss. One commonly suggested goal is 30 minutes or more 5 to 7 days a week.★ Exercise increases the number of calories the body uses. Yet, exercise cannot substitute for controlling caloric intake. It takes

▲ see box on page 881   ■ see page 884
★ see page 32

about 1 hour of walking to burn the calories in one alcoholic drink and about 1 hour of running to burn those in one piece of cheesecake.

Aerobic exercise, such as jogging, walking briskly (3 to 4 miles an hour), biking, singles tennis, skating, and cross-country skiing, burn more calories than less active exercises.▲ For example, vigorous walking burns about 4 calories per minute, so that 1 hour of brisk walking per day burns about 240 calories. Running is more effective. It burns about 6 to 8 calories per minute.

Drugs: The combination of fenfluramine and phentermine (often called fen-phen) was the most effective treatment used so far. However, fenfluramine was removed from the market because of heart valve problems in people who took this combination. Seven weight loss drugs are currently available by prescription: orlistat, sibutramine, phentermine, benzphetamine, diethylpropion, mazindol, and phendimetrazine. Orlistat limits the breakdown and absorption of fats in the intestine, producing, in effect, a low-fat diet. Sibutramine, phentermine, benzphetamine, diethylpropion, mazindol, and phendimetrazine are all believed to reduce appetite by affecting chemical messengers in the part of the brain that controls appetite. Weight loss with these drugs is rarely more than 10%. Some nonprescription diet aids, including medicinal herbs, claim to enhance weight loss by increasing metabolism or by increasing a feeling of fullness. Although usually harmless, they are ineffective and, if they contain stimulants (such as ephedra), should be avoided. New drugs for the treatment of obesity are being developed.

Surgery: For severe obesity (BMI of more than 40), surgery is the treatment of choice. There are two major types of surgery. In vertical banded gastroplasty, rows of staples and a band that limits the entrance of food into the stomach are used to form a 1-ounce stomach pouch, which drastically reduces the amount of food that can be eaten at one time. In gastric bypass surgery (which is somewhat more effective), some of the small intestine is bypassed, thus reducing the absorption of food. These operations were originally performed by opening the abdomen. More and more commonly, they are being performed through a laparoscope, a viewing tube that is inserted into the abdominal cavity through a small incision just below the navel.

▲ see table on page 34

Bypassing Part of the Digestive Tract

In gastric bypass surgery, rows of staples are used to divide the stomach into two parts. Food can enter only the smaller upper part, called a stomach pouch. The small intestine is cut, and the section of the small intestine below the cut is attached to the stomach pouch. Thus, the lower part of the stomach and the upper part of the small intestine are bypassed. As a result, the amount of food that can be eaten at one time is drastically reduced and less food is absorbed. The section of the small intestine above the cut is then attached to the small intestine further down. Thus, digestive juices produced in the bypassed part of the stomach can reach the rest of the small intestine and can be mixed with food.

Usually, surgery is performed using a laparoscope inserted through a small incision in the abdomen. Laparoscopic surgery requires an anesthetic, usually a general anesthetic. A person may go home the same day or stay overnight in the hospital. Afterward, for many people, eating foods high in fat and refined sugar can cause indigestion, nausea, diarrhea, sweating, weakness, or palpitations. But these symptoms usually last only a short time. Sometimes the reduced absorption of food results in anemia due to iron deficiency and in nutritional deficiencies. Taking the appropriate supplements can almost always prevent these deficiencies.

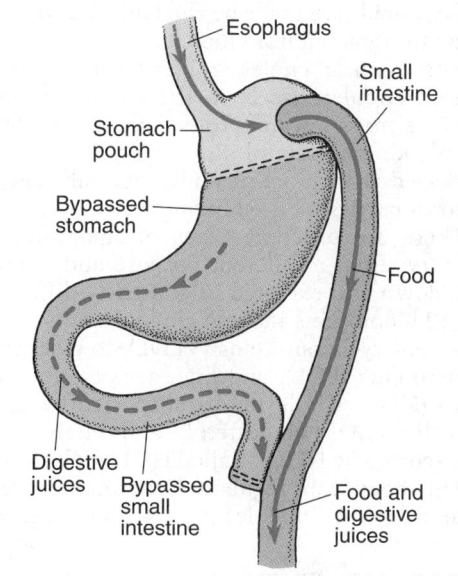

Surgery using a laparoscope is much less traumatic and recovery after surgery is much more rapid.

These operations result in a large weight loss—half or even more of the person's excess weight and as much as 80 to 160 pounds. Weight loss is rapid at first, then slows gradually over a period of about 2 years. The loss is often maintained for years. The loss greatly reduces obesity-related complications (such as high blood pressure and diabetes) and improves the person's mood, self-esteem, body image, activity level, and ability to work and interact with other people.

When conducted at specialized centers, surgery is well tolerated. Fewer than 10% of people develop complications from surgery, and fewer than 1% die.

CHAPTER 157

Disorders of Cholesterol

Cholesterol and triglycerides are important fats (lipids) in the blood. Cholesterol is an essential component of cell membranes, brain and nerve cells, and bile, which helps the body absorb fats and fat-soluble vitamins. The body uses cholesterol to make vitamin D and various hormones, such as estrogen, testosterone, and cortisol. The body can produce all the cholesterol that it needs, but it also obtains cholesterol from food. Triglycerides, which are contained in fat cells, can be broken down, then used to provide energy for the body's metabolic processes, including growth. Triglycerides are produced in the intestine and liver from smaller fats called fatty acids. Some types of fatty acids are made by the body, but others must be obtained from food.▲

Fats, such as cholesterol and triglycerides, cannot circulate freely in the blood, because blood is mostly water. To be able to circulate in blood, cholesterol and triglycerides are packaged with proteins and other substances to form particles called lipoproteins.

There are different types of lipoproteins. Each type has a different purpose and is broken down and excreted in a slightly different way. Lipoproteins include chylomicrons, very low density lipoproteins (VLDL), low-density lipoproteins (LDL), and high-density lipoproteins (HDL). Cholesterol transported by LDL is called LDL cholesterol, and cholesterol transported by HDL is called HDL cholesterol.

The body can regulate lipoprotein levels (and therefore lipid levels) by increasing or decreasing the production rate of lipoproteins. The body can also regulate how quickly lipoproteins enter and are removed from the bloodstream.

Levels of cholesterol and triglycerides vary considerably from day to day. From one measurement to the next, cholesterol levels can vary by about 10%, and triglyceride levels can vary by up to 25%.

Lipid levels may become abnormal because of changes that occur with aging, various disorders (including some hereditary ones), use of certain drugs, or lifestyle (consuming a high-fat diet, being physically inactive, or being overweight).

Abnormal levels of lipids (especially cholesterol) can lead to long-term problems, such as atherosclerosis. Generally, a high total cholesterol level (which includes LDL, HDL, and VLDL cholesterol) or a high level of LDL (the "bad") cholesterol increases the risk of atherosclerosis and thus the risk of heart attack and stroke. However, not all types of cholesterol increase this risk. A high level of HDL (the "good") cholesterol may decrease risk, and conversely, a low level of HDL cholesterol increases risk. The effect of triglyceride levels on the risk of heart attack is less clear-cut. But very high levels of triglycerides (higher than 500 milligrams per deciliter of blood, or mg/dL) can increase the risk of pancreatitis. For people older than 20, levels of total cholesterol, triglycerides, LDL cholesterol, and HDL cholesterol after fasting should be measured at least once every 5 years. Collectively, these measurements are called the fasting lipoprotein profile.

▲ see page 882

LIPOPROTEINS: LIPID CARRIERS

Type	Formation	Lipid Content	Function
Chylomicrons	Formed from fats in food processed by the intestine	Mostly triglycerides	To transport digested fats (as triglycerides) to muscle and fat cells
Very low density lipoprotein	Formed in the liver	More than $1/2$ triglycerides About $1/4$ cholesterol	To transport triglycerides from the liver to fat cells
Low-density lipoprotein	Formed from VLDL after it delivers triglycerides to fat cells	More than $1/2$ cholesterol Less than $1/10$ triglycerides	To transport cholesterol to various cells
High-density lipoprotein	Formed in the liver and small intestine	About $1/4$ cholesterol About $1/20$ triglycerides	To remove cholesterol from tissues in the body and transport it to the liver

Hyperlipoproteinemia

Hyperlipoproteinemia (hyperlipidemia) is abnormally high levels of lipids (cholesterol, triglycerides, or both) carried by lipoproteins in the blood.

Levels of lipoproteins (and therefore lipids, particularly LDL cholesterol) increase slightly as people age. Levels are normally slightly higher in men than in women, but levels increase in women after menopause. The increase in levels of lipoproteins that occurs with age can result in hyperlipoproteinemia and increase the risk of atherosclerosis. (A high level of HDL—the good—cholesterol is beneficial and is not considered a disorder.)

Factors that increase the risk of hyperlipoproteinemia include having close relatives who have had hyperlipoproteinemia (having a family history of the disorder), being overweight, consuming a diet high in saturated fats and cholesterol, being physically inactive, and consuming a moderate to excessive amount of alcohol.

Some people are more sensitive to the effects of diet than others, but most people are affected to some degree. One person can eat large amounts of animal fat, and the total cholesterol level does not rise above 200 mg/dL. Another person can follow a strict low-fat diet, and the total cholesterol does not fall below 260 mg/dL. This difference seems to be mostly genetically determined. A person's genetic makeup influences the rate at which the body makes, uses, and disposes of these fats. Eating excess calories can result in high triglyceride levels, as can excessive consumption of alcohol.

Some disorders, including some hereditary disorders,▲ cause lipid levels to increase. Diabetes that is poorly controlled or kidney failure can cause total cholesterol levels or triglyceride levels to increase. Obstructive liver disease and an underactive thyroid gland (hypothyroidism) can cause the total cholesterol level to increase.

Use of drugs such as estrogens (taken by mouth), oral contraceptives, corticosteroids, and thiazide diuretics (to some extent) can cause triglyceride levels to increase.

Symptoms

High lipid levels in the blood usually cause no symptoms. Occasionally, when levels are particularly high, fat is deposited in the skin and tendons and forms bumps called xanthomas. Very high triglyceride levels can cause the liver or spleen to enlarge and may increase the risk of developing pancreatitis. Pancreatitis can cause severe abdominal pain and is occasionally fatal.

The risk of developing atherosclerosis increases as the total cholesterol level increases. Atherosclerosis can affect the arteries that supply blood to the heart (causing coronary

▲ see page 925

Metabolic Syndrome: A Cluster of Problems

> The metabolic syndrome, also called the syndrome of insulin resistance, includes high triglyceride levels, a low HDL cholesterol level, high blood pressure, resistance to the effects of insulin, a high level of sugar (glucose) in the blood, and an increased tendency to form blood clots. It also includes being overweight (particularly if fat accumulates in the abdomen). All of these problems work together to increase the risk of coronary artery disease. One fourth of the people in the United States may have this disorder.
>
> Treatment consists of weight loss, increased physical activity, use of antihypertensive drugs (to lower blood pressure), and use of aspirin (to reduce the risk of blood clotting). Many people with metabolic syndrome need to take lipid-lowering drugs.

artery disease), those that supply blood to the brain (causing cerebrovascular disease), and those that supply the rest of the body (causing peripheral arterial disease). Therefore, having a high total cholesterol level also increases the risk of having a heart attack or stroke. Having a low total cholesterol level is generally considered better than having a high one. However, having a very low cholesterol level may not be healthy either.▲ For adults, a total cholesterol level of less than 200 mg/dL is desirable. In parts of the world (such as China and Japan) where the average cholesterol level is 150 mg/dL, coronary artery disease is less common than it is in countries such as the United States. The risk of a heart attack more than doubles when the total cholesterol level approaches 300 mg/dL.

The total cholesterol level is only a general guide to the risk of atherosclerosis. Levels of the components of total cholesterol—particularly LDL and HDL cholesterol—are more important. A high level of LDL (bad) cholesterol increases the risk. A high level of HDL (good) cholesterol decreases the risk, and a low level of HDL cholesterol (defined as less than 40 mg/dL) increases the risk. Experts consider an LDL cholesterol level of less than 100 mg/dL optimal.

Whether high triglyceride levels increase the risk of a heart attack or stroke is uncertain. Triglyceride levels higher than 150 mg/dL are considered abnormal, but high levels do not appear to increase risk for everyone. For people with high triglyceride levels, the risk of heart attack or stroke is increased if they also have a low HDL cholesterol level, diabetes, kidney disease, or many close relatives who have had atherosclerosis (family history).

Diagnosis

Levels of total cholesterol, LDL cholesterol, HDL cholesterol, and triglycerides—the lipid profile—are measured in a blood sample. Because consuming food or beverages may cause triglyceride levels to increase temporarily, a person must fast at least 12 hours before the blood sample is taken.

When lipid levels in the blood are very high, special blood tests are performed to identify the specific underlying disorder. Specific disorders include several hereditary disorders (hereditary hyperlipoproteinemias), which produce different lipid abnormalities and have different risks, as well as other disorders such as hypothyroidism.

Treatment

Usually, the best treatment for people who have high cholesterol or triglyceride levels is to lose weight if they are overweight, stop smoking if they smoke, decrease the total amount of fat and cholesterol in their diet, increase physical activity, and, if necessary, take a lipid-lowering drug.

A diet low in fats and cholesterol can lower the LDL cholesterol level. Experts recommend

DESIRABLE LIPID LEVELS IN ADULTS

LIPID	GOAL (MG/DL)*
Total cholesterol	Less than 200 mg/dL
Low-density lipoprotein (LDL) cholesterol	Less than 100 mg/dL
High-density lipoprotein (HDL) cholesterol	More than 40 mg/dL
Triglycerides	Less than 150 mg/dL

▲ see page 926

*mg/dL = milligrams per deciliter of blood.

LIMITING FAT AND CHOLESTEROL IN THE DIET

TYPE OF FAT	RECOMMENDED AMOUNTS	FOOD SOURCES
Saturated	7–10% of total calories Less than 7% for people who have high lipid levels or coronary artery disease	Meats Nonskim dairy products, such as whole milk, cheese, and butter Artificially hydrogenated vegetable oils
Polyunsaturated Omega-3 fats	Up to 10% of total calories	Fatty fish, such as mackerel, salmon, and tuna
Omega-6 fats		Vegetable oils, such as corn oil and safflower oil
Monounsaturated	Up to 20% of total calories	Canola oil Olive oil Nuts Avocado
Cholesterol	Less than 300 mg a day (less than 200 mg a day for people with high lipid levels or heart disease)	Egg yolks Organ meats, such as liver Meat Poultry Fish and other seafood Nonskim dairy products

limiting calories from fat to no more than 25 to 35% of the total calories consumed over several days.

The type of fat consumed is also important.▲ Fats may be saturated, polyunsaturated, or monounsaturated. Saturated fats increase cholesterol levels more than other forms of fat. Saturated fats should provide no more than 7 to 10% of total calories consumed each day. Polyunsaturated fats (which include omega-3 fats and omega-6 fats) and monounsaturated fats may help decrease levels of triglycerides and LDL cholesterol in the blood. The fat content of most foods is included on the label of the container.

Large amounts of saturated fats occur in meats, egg yolks, full-fat dairy products, some nuts (such as macadamia nuts), and coconut. Vegetable oils contain smaller amounts of saturated fat, but only some vegetable oils are truly low in saturated fats.

Margarine, which is produced from polyunsaturated vegetable oils, was once thought to be a healthier substitute for butter, which is high in saturated fat (about 60%). However, some margarines (and some processed foods) contain trans fatty acids, which may increase LDL (bad) cholesterol levels and lower HDL (good) cholesterol levels.■ Margarines made primarily from liquid oil (squeeze or tub margarines) contain less saturated fat than butter, contain no cholesterol, and contain fewer trans fatty acids. Margarines that contain plant stanols or sterols can lower total and LDL cholesterol levels.

Eating lots of fruits, vegetables, and grains, which are naturally low in fat and contain no cholesterol, is recommended. Also recommended are foods rich in soluble fiber, which binds fats in the intestine and helps lower the cholesterol level. Such foods include oat bran, oatmeal, beans, peas, rice bran, barley, citrus fruits, strawberries, and apple pulp.

Regular physical activity can help lower the LDL cholesterol level and increase the HDL cholesterol level. An example is walking briskly for 30 to 45 minutes 3 to 4 times a week.

Treatment with lipid-lowering drugs depends not only on what the person's lipid levels are but also on whether the person has coronary artery disease, diabetes, or other major risk factors for coronary artery disease.★ For people who have coronary artery disease or diabetes, the goal for the LDL cholesterol

▲ see page 200   ■ see box on page 201
★ see page 199

level is 100 mg/dL or less. Consequently, such people usually require lipid-lowering drugs. For people who do not have coronary artery disease or diabetes but have two or more other risk factors for coronary artery disease, the goal is 130 mg/dL or less. For those with one or no risk factors, the goal is 160 mg/dL or less.

There are different types of lipid-lowering drugs: bile acid binders, fibric acid derivatives, niacin (a lipoprotein synthesis inhibitor), and

A PRACTICAL APPROACH TO A LOW-CHOLESTEROL, LOW–SATURATED FAT DIET

Food Category	Foods to Reduce	Foods to Choose
Meats and meat products	Fatty cuts of beef, lamb, and pork; spareribs; organ meats; regular cold cuts; sausage; and hot dogs	Fish; chicken and turkey (without the skin); and lean cuts of beef, lamb, pork, and veal
Dairy products	Whole milk, evaporated or condensed whole milk, cream, half-and-half, most nondairy creamers, and whipped toppings	Skim milk, $\frac{1}{2}$% fat milk, 1% fat milk, and buttermilk
	Whole-milk yogurt, whole-milk cottage cheese, cheeses (such as blue, Roquefort, Camembert, cheddar, and Swiss), cream cheese, sour cream, and ice cream	Nonfat or low-fat yogurt, low-fat cottage cheese, low-fat cheeses, sherbet, sorbet, and frozen low-fat yogurt
	Butter and butter-margarine mixtures	Less solid forms of margarines made from liquid vegetable oils (packaged in a tub or squeeze bottle), olive oil, canola oil, and margarine products containing a plant sterol or stanol
	Egg yolks (to less than 3 a week)	Cholesterol-free egg substitutes and egg whites (2 whole egg whites can be substituted for 1 egg in recipes)
Commercial baked goods	Pies, cakes, doughnuts, croissants, pastries, muffins, biscuits, high-fat crackers, high-fat cookies, egg noodles, and breads made with several eggs	Homemade baked goods made with unsaturated oils; angel food cake; low-fat cookies and crackers; rice; pasta; and whole-grain* (oatmeal, bran, rye, and multigrain) breads and cereals
Saturated fats and oils	Chocolate	Cocoa powder, carob, and nonfat chocolate syrup
	Coconut oil, palm oil, lard, and bacon	Unsaturated vegetable oils: canola, olive, corn, safflower, sesame, soybean, and sunflower
Dressings	Dressings made with egg yolk	Low-fat mayonnaise and salad dressings made with liquid oils
Fruits and vegetables	Fruits and vegetables prepared in butter, saturated fats, cream, or sauces made with saturated fat	Fresh, frozen, canned, and dried fruits or vegetables*
	Coconut	Seeds and nuts*

*Fruits, vegetables, grains, seeds, and nuts contain no cholesterol, and most contain no saturated fat.

℞ LIPID-LOWERING DRUGS

TYPE	MECHANISM OF ACTION	INDICATIONS	SIDE EFFECTS
Bile acid binders			
Cholestyramine Colesevelam Colestipol	Binds bile acids in the intestine, causing the acids to be excreted rather than used to make bile and causing the liver to remove more LDL cholesterol from the bloodstream to make bile	High LDL cholesterol	Constipation, abdominal pain, nausea, bloating, binding of other drugs (reducing their effectiveness), and an increased triglyceride level
Fibric acid derivatives			
Fenofibrate Gemfibrozil	Increases the breakdown of lipids and speeds the removal of VLDL from the bloodstream and may decrease VLDL production by the liver	High VLDL cholesterol Low HDL cholesterol Dysbetalipoproteinemia	Diarrhea, nausea, bloating, abdominal pain, rash, abnormal levels of liver enzymes, muscle inflammation, and gallstones
Lipoprotein synthesis inhibitors			
Niacin	Decreases the production rate of VLDL, which is used to synthesize LDL	High LDL and VLDL cholesterol and low HDL cholesterol Dysbetalipoproteinemia	Flushing, itching, digestive upset, ulcers, increased levels of liver enzymes, gout, and a high blood sugar level (hyperglycemia)
Statins (HMG-CoA reductase inhibitors)			
Atorvastatin Fluvastatin Lovastatin Pravastatin Simvastatin	Blocks the synthesis of cholesterol, increasing the removal of LDL from the bloodstream	High LDL cholesterol Combined hyperlipidemia	Mild constipation, loose stools, bloating, headaches, rashes, fatigue, and, rarely, increased levels of liver enzymes, muscle aches due to inflammation (myositis) and muscle degeneration (rhabdomyolysis)

HMG-CoA = 3-hydroxy-3-methylglutaryl coenzyme A.

statins. Each type lowers lipid levels by a different mechanism. Consequently, the different types of drugs have different side effects and may affect lipid levels differently. Following a low-fat diet when drugs are used is recommended.

Lipid-lowering drugs do more than lower lipid levels—they can also prevent coronary artery disease. In addition, niacin and statins have been shown to reduce the risk of early death.

HEREDITARY HYPERLIPOPROTEINEMIAS

Cholesterol and triglyceride levels are highest in people with hereditary hyperlipoproteinemias, which interfere with the body's metabolism and elimination of lipids.

In **familial hyperchylomicronemia**, a rare disorder, the body cannot remove chylomicrons from the bloodstream, resulting in very high triglyceride levels. Without treatment, levels are often considerably higher than 1,000 mg/dL. Symptoms appear during childhood and young adulthood. They include recurring bouts of abdominal pain, an enlarged liver and spleen, and pinkish yellow bumps in the skin on the elbows, knees, buttocks, back, front of the legs, and back of the arms. These bumps, called eruptive xanthomas, are deposits of fat.

Eating fats worsens symptoms. Although this disorder does not lead to atherosclerosis, it can cause pancreatitis, which is occasionally fatal. People who have this disorder must avoid eating fats of all types—saturated, unsaturated, and polyunsaturated.

In **familial hypercholesterolemia,** the total cholesterol level is high. This severe disorder affects about 1 of 500 people. Affected people may have fatty deposits (xanthomas) in the tendons at the heels, knees, elbows, and fingers. Rarely, xanthomas appear by age 10. Familial hypercholesterolemia can result in rapidly progressive atherosclerosis and early death due to coronary artery disease. One sixth of men with this disorder have a heart attack by age 40, and two thirds have a heart attack by age 60. Women with this disorder are also at increased risk, but the risk starts later. About two fifths of women with the disorder have a heart attack by age 60.

Treatment begins with following a diet that is low in saturated fats and cholesterol. When applicable, losing weight, stopping smoking, and increasing physical activity are advised. One or more lipid-lowering drugs are usually needed.

In **familial combined hyperlipidemia,** the levels of cholesterol, triglycerides, or both may be high. This disorder affects about 1 to 2% of people. The lipid levels typically become abnormal after age 30 but sometimes at a younger age, especially in people who are overweight, who have a diet that is very high in fat, or who have metabolic syndrome.

Treatment involves limiting intake of fat, cholesterol, and sugar as well as exercising and, when applicable, losing weight. Many people with this disorder need to take lipid-lowering drugs.

In **familial dysbetalipoproteinemia (type III hyperlipoproteinemia),** levels of VLDL and total cholesterol and triglycerides are high. These levels are high because an unusual form of VLDL accumulates in the blood. Fatty deposits (xanthomas) may form in the skin over the elbows and knees. This uncommon disorder results in the early development of severe atherosclerosis. By middle age, atherosclerosis often produces blockages in the coronary and peripheral arteries. Decreased blood flow to the legs may cause pain during walking (claudication).▲

Treatment involves achieving and maintaining recommended body weight and limiting intake of cholesterol, saturated fats, and carbohydrates. A lipid-lowering drug is usually needed. With treatment, lipid levels can be improved, the progression of atherosclerosis may be slowed, and the fatty deposits in the skin may become smaller or disappear.

In **familial hypertriglyceridemia,** triglyceride levels are high. This disorder affects about 1% of people. In some families affected by this disorder, atherosclerosis tends to develop at a young age, but in others, it does not. When applicable, losing weight and limiting alcohol often lower triglyceride levels to normal. If these measures are ineffective, use of a lipid-lowering drug can help. For people who also have diabetes, good control of the diabetes is important.

In **severe mixed hyperlipoproteinemia,** the triglyceride level is very high. In the severe form of this disorder (which is rare), the body cannot adequately metabolize and eliminate excess triglycerides. In people who have a milder form of the disorder, the triglyceride level can become very high if other conditions (such as excessive alcohol intake, poorly controlled diabetes, or kidney failure) are also present. Symptoms can include many fatty deposits (eruptive xanthomas) in the skin on the front of the legs and back of the arms, an enlarged spleen and liver, abdominal pain, and a decreased sensitivity to touch due to nerve damage. Eating fats or drinking alcohol makes symptoms worse. This disorder can cause pancreatitis, which is occasionally fatal. Eating fats can also cause recurring bouts of pancreatitis and increases the risk of death. Limiting fat intake (to less than 50 grams a day) can prevent nerve damage and pancreatitis. Losing weight and not drinking alcohol can also help. Lipid-lowering drugs may be effective.

Hypolipoproteinemia

Hypolipoproteinemia is abnormally low levels of lipids in the blood.

Having low lipid levels rarely causes a problem, but it may indicate the presence of another disorder. For example, a low cholesterol level may indicate an overactive thyroid gland (hyperthyroidism), anemia, undernutrition, cancer, or impaired absorption of foods from the digestive tract (malabsorption). Therefore, doctors may suggest further evaluation when the total cholesterol is less than 120 mg/dL. A

▲ see page 217

few rare hereditary disorders, such as abeta-lipoproteinemia and hypoalphalipoproteine-mia, result in lipid levels low enough to have serious consequences.

In **abetalipoproteinemia,** a rare disorder, no LDL cholesterol is present, and the body cannot make chylomicrons. As a result, the absorption of fat and fat-soluble vitamins is greatly impaired. Bowel movements contain excess fat (a condition called steatorrhea). Red blood cells are misshapen. The retina of the eye degenerates, causing blindness (this condition is similar to retinitis pigmentosa). The central nervous system may be damaged, resulting in loss of coordination (ataxia). Although abetalipoproteinemia cannot be cured, taking massive doses of vitamin E may delay or slow the damage to the central nervous system.

In **hypobetalipoproteinemia,** the LDL cholesterol level is very low. Usually, there are no symptoms and no treatment is required. In the most severe form of hypobetalipoproteinemia, almost no LDL cholesterol is present. The symptoms are similar to those of abetalipoproteinemia.

In **hypoalphalipoproteinemia,** the HDL cholesterol level is low. A low HDL cholesterol level is often inherited. Obesity, physical inactivity, cigarette smoking, diabetes, or kidney disorders (such as nephrotic syndrome) may contribute to a low HDL cholesterol level. Drugs such as beta-blockers and anabolic steroids can lower the HDL cholesterol level. Having a low HDL cholesterol level increases the risk of atherosclerosis.▲ Therefore, lifestyle changes to eliminate conditions that lower the HDL cholesterol level are advised when applicable: losing weight, increasing physical activity, and stopping smoking. Some lipid-lowering drugs increase the HDL cholesterol level and may be used in people who also have high LDL cholesterol or triglyceride levels.

CHAPTER 158

Water Balance

Water accounts for about one half to two thirds of an average person's weight. Fat tissue has a lower percentage of water and women tend to have more fat, so the percentage of water in the average woman is lower (52 to 55%) than it is in the average man (60%). The percentage of water is also lower in older people and in obese people. A 150-pound man has about 10 gallons of water in his body: 6 to 7 gallons inside the cells, 2 gallons in the space around the cells, and slightly less than 1 gallon (or about 8% of the total amount of water) in the bloodstream. The body regulates the amount of water in each of these areas. Water is moved as needed to keep the amount in each area relatively constant, thus enabling the body to function normally.

Water intake must balance water loss. To maintain water balance—and to protect against dehydration, the development of kidney stones, and other medical problems—healthy adults should drink at least 1½ to 2 quarts of fluids a day. Drinking too much is better than drinking too little, because excret-ing excess water is much easier for the body than conserving water. However, when the kidneys are functioning normally, the body can handle wide variations in fluid intake.

The body obtains water primarily by absorbing it from the digestive tract. Additionally, a small amount of water is produced when the body processes (metabolizes) certain nutrients.

The body loses water primarily by excreting it in urine from the kidneys. Depending on the body's needs, the kidneys may excrete less than a pint or up to several gallons of urine a day. About 1½ pints of water are lost daily when water evaporates from the skin and is breathed out by the lungs. Profuse sweating—which may be caused by vigorous exercise, hot weather, or a fever—can dramatically increase the amount of water lost through evaporation. Normally, little water is lost from the digestive tract. However, prolonged vomiting or se-

---

▲ see page 194

A Careful Balancing Act

In the body, several mechanisms work together to maintain water balance. One of the most important is thirst. When the body needs water, nerve centers deep within the brain are stimulated, resulting in the sensation of thirst. The sensation becomes stronger as the body's need for water increases, motivating a person to drink the needed fluids. When the body has excess water, thirst is suppressed.

Another mechanism for maintaining water balance involves the pituitary gland (located at the base of the brain) and the kidneys. When the body is low in water, the pituitary gland secretes antidiuretic hormone (vasopressin) into the bloodstream. Antidiuretic hormone stimulates the kidneys to conserve water and excrete less urine. When the body has excess water, the pituitary gland secretes little antidiuretic hormone, enabling the kidneys to excrete excess water in the urine.

The body can move water from one area to another as needed. When water loss is severe, the amount of water in the bloodstream decreases, so the body moves water from inside the cells to the bloodstream until it can be replaced through increased intake of fluids. When the body has excess water, the amount of water in the bloodstream increases, so the body moves water from the bloodstream into and around the cells. In this way, blood volume and blood pressure can be kept relatively constant.

vere diarrhea can result in the loss of a gallon or more a day.

Usually, a person can drink enough fluids to compensate for excess water loss. However, a person may be unable to drink enough fluids to compensate for water loss caused by prolonged vomiting or severe diarrhea, and dehydration may result. Also, confusion, restricted mobility, or loss of consciousness can prevent a person from being able to drink enough fluids.

Mineral salts (electrolytes), such as sodium and potassium, are dissolved in the water in the body. Water balance and electrolyte bal-

ance▲ are closely linked. The body works to keep the total amount of water and the levels of electrolytes in the bloodstream constant. For example, when the sodium level becomes too high, thirst develops, leading to an increased intake of fluids. In addition, a hormone secreted by the brain in response to thirst causes the kidneys to excrete less urine. The combined effect is an increased amount of water in the bloodstream. As a result, sodium is diluted and the balance of sodium and water is restored. When the sodium level becomes too low, the kidneys excrete more urine, which decreases the amount of water in the bloodstream, again restoring the balance.

Dehydration

Dehydration is a deficiency of water in the body.

Dehydration occurs when the body loses more water than it takes in. Vomiting, diarrhea, the use of diuretics (drugs that increase excretion of water and salt by the kidneys), profuse sweating (for example, because of excessive heat), and decreased water intake can lead to dehydration.

Dehydration is particularly common in older people, because their thirst center does not function as well as a younger person's. Therefore, an older person may not recognize that he is becoming dehydrated. Certain disorders such as diabetes mellitus,■ diabetes insipidus,★ and Addison's disease● can increase the excretion of urine and thereby lead to dehydration.

At first, dehydration stimulates the thirst center of the brain, causing a person to drink more fluids. If water intake cannot keep up with water loss, dehydration becomes more severe. Sweating decreases, and less urine is excreted. Water moves from inside the cells to the bloodstream to maintain the needed amount of blood (blood volume) and blood pressure. If dehydration continues, tissues of the body begin to dry out, and cells begin to shrivel and malfunction. Symptoms of mild to moderate dehydration include thirst, reduced sweating, reduced skin elasticity, reduced urine production, and dry mouth. Brain cells are particularly susceptible to more severe levels of dehydration. Consequently, confusion is one of the best indicators that dehydration has become severe. Very severe dehydration can lead to coma.

▲ see page 901   ■ see page 962
★ see page 944   ● see page 956

Dehydration causes the sodium level in the bloodstream to increase.▲ However, the common causes of dehydration (such as profuse sweating, vomiting, and diarrhea) usually result in a loss of electrolytes (especially sodium and potassium). Thus, dehydration is often accompanied by a deficiency of electrolytes—sodium is lost, but because even more water is lost, the level of sodium rises. When electrolytes in the bloodstream are also deficient, water moves less readily from inside the cells to the bloodstream. As a result, the amount of water in the bloodstream is not replenished as it would normally be. Blood pressure can fall, causing light-headedness or faintness, particularly upon standing (a condition called orthostatic hypotension). If water and electrolytes continue to be lost, blood pressure can fall dangerously low, resulting in shock and severe damage to many internal organs, such as the kidneys, liver, and brain.

Treatment

Prevention is better than cure. Adults should drink at least 6 glasses of fluids daily. Fluid intake should be increased on hot days. Exercise, fever, and hot weather increase the body's need for water. For mild dehydration, drinking plenty of water may be all that is needed. If electrolytes (especially sodium and potassium) are also lost, they must be replaced. Flavored sports drinks have been formulated to replace electrolytes lost during vigorous exercise. These drinks can be used to prevent dehydration or treat mild dehydration. Drinking plenty of fluids and consuming a small amount of salt (for example, by taking salt tablets or drinking a sports drink) during or after exercise works as well. Before exercising, people with heart or kidney disorders should consult their doctor about how to safely replace fluids.

More severe dehydration requires treatment by a doctor. If blood pressure becomes very low, a solution containing sodium chloride is usually given intravenously. The intravenous solution is given rapidly at first and then more slowly as the person's physical condition improves.

Treatment is also directed at the cause of dehydration. For example, if the person has diarrhea, drugs to control or stop the diarrhea may be necessary in addition to replacement of fluids.

After treatment, people who are recovering from dehydration are monitored to make sure that they are drinking enough fluids to prevent dehydration.

Overhydration

Overhydration is an excess of water in the body.

Overhydration occurs when the body takes in more water than it loses. The result is too much water and not enough sodium. Thus, overhydration generally results in low sodium levels in the blood (hyponatremia).■ Usually, drinking large amounts of water does not cause overhydration if the pituitary gland, kidneys, liver, and heart are functioning normally. To exceed the body's ability to excrete water, an adult with normal kidney function would have to drink more than 2 gallons of water a day on a regular basis.

Overhydration is much more common among people whose kidneys do not excrete urine normally—for example, among people with a disorder of the heart, kidneys, or liver. Overhydration may also result from syndrome of inappropriate secretion of antidiuretic hormone (SIADH). In this syndrome, the pituitary gland secretes too much antidiuretic hormone, stimulating the kidneys to conserve water.★

Brain cells are particularly susceptible to overhydration (as well as dehydration). When overhydration occurs slowly, brain cells have time to adapt, so few symptoms occur. When overhydration occurs quickly, confusion, seizures, or coma may develop.

Doctors try to distinguish between overhydration and excess blood volume. With overhydration and normal blood volume, the excess water usually moves into the cells, and tissue swelling (edema) does not occur. With overhydration and excess blood volume, an excess amount of sodium prevents the excess water from moving into the cells; instead, the excess water accumulates around the cells, resulting in edema in the chest, abdomen, and lower legs.

Treatment

Regardless of the cause of overhydration, fluid intake usually must be restricted (but only as advised by a doctor). Drinking less than a quart of fluids a day usually results in

▲ see page 913   ■ see page 912

★ see box on page 913

improvement over several days. If overhydration occurs because of heart, liver, or kidney disease, restricting the intake of sodium (sodium causes the body to retain water) is also helpful.

Sometimes, doctors prescribe a diuretic to increase urine excretion. In general, diuretics are more useful when overhydration is accompanied by excess blood volume.

Effects of Aging

The very young (especially premature infants) and the very old are more susceptible to disturbances in water balance. In both groups, the kidneys may function less well than during the rest of life. Thus, premature infants can very easily become dehydrated, usually due to diarrhea. They may become overhydrated if they receive too large an amount of intravenous fluids.

Older people are particularly susceptible to dehydration. In older people, common causes of dehydration include confusion and disorders that make obtaining fluids difficult (usually because of restricted mobility). Additionally, older people sense thirst more slowly and less intensely than younger people do, so those who are otherwise well may not drink enough fluids. Also, older people have a higher percentage of body fat. Because fat tissue contains less water than lean tissue, the total amount of water in the body tends to decrease with age.

CHAPTER 159

Acid-Base Balance

An important property of blood is its degree of acidity or alkalinity. Body acidity increases when the level of acidic compounds in the body rises (through increased intake or production, or decreased elimination) or when the level of basic (alkaline) compounds in the body falls (through decreased intake or production, or increased elimination). Body alkalinity increases with the reverse of these processes. The body's balance between acidity and alkalinity is referred to as acid-base balance.

The blood's acid-base balance is precisely controlled, because even a minor deviation

What Is the Blood pH?

Acidity and alkalinity are expressed on the pH scale, which ranges from 0 (strongly acidic) to 14 (strongly basic, or alkaline). A pH of 7.0, in the middle of this scale, is neutral. Blood is normally slightly basic, with a pH range of 7.35 to 7.45. To function properly, the body maintains the pH of blood close to 7.4.

from the normal range can severely affect many organs. The body uses different mechanisms to control the blood's acid-base balance.

One mechanism the body uses to control blood pH involves the release of carbon dioxide from the lungs. Carbon dioxide, which is mildly acidic, is a waste product of the metabolism of oxygen (which all cells need) and, as such, is constantly produced by cells. As with all waste products, carbon dioxide gets excreted into the blood. The blood carries carbon dioxide to the lungs, where it is exhaled. As carbon dioxide accumulates in the blood, the pH of the blood decreases. The brain regulates the amount of carbon dioxide that is exhaled by controlling the speed and depth of breathing. The amount of carbon dioxide exhaled, and consequently the pH of the blood, increases as breathing becomes faster and deeper. By adjusting the speed and depth of breathing, the brain and lungs are able to regulate the blood pH minute by minute.

The kidneys are also able to affect blood pH by excreting excess acids or bases. The kidneys have some ability to alter the amount of acid or base that is excreted, but because the kidneys make these adjustments more slowly than the lungs do, this compensation generally takes several days.

Yet another mechanism for controlling blood pH involves the use of buffer systems, which guard against sudden shifts in acidity and alkalinity. The pH buffer systems are combinations of a weak acid and weak base that exist in balance under normal pH conditions. The pH buffer systems work chemically to minimize changes in the pH of a solution by adjusting the proportion of acid and base. The most important pH buffer system in the blood involves carbonic acid (a weak acid formed from the carbon dioxide dissolved in blood) and bicarbonate ions (the corresponding weak base).

Acidosis and alkalosis are the two abnormalities of acid-base balance. In acidosis, the blood has too much acid (or too little base), resulting in a decrease in blood pH. In alkalosis, the blood has too much base (or too little acid), resulting in an increase in blood pH. Acidosis and alkalosis are not diseases, but rather are the result of a wide variety of disorders. The presence of acidosis or alkalosis provides an important clue to doctors that a serious problem exists.

Acidosis and alkalosis are categorized as metabolic or respiratory, depending on their primary cause. Metabolic acidosis and metabolic alkalosis are caused by an imbalance in the production of acids or bases and their excretion by the kidneys. Respiratory acidosis and respiratory alkalosis are caused primarily by lung or breathing disorders.

Acidosis

Acidosis is excessive blood acidity caused by an overabundance of acid in the blood or a loss of bicarbonate from the blood (metabolic acidosis), or by a buildup of carbon dioxide in the blood that results from poor lung function or slow breathing (respiratory alkalosis).

If an increase in acid overwhelms the body's pH buffering systems, the blood will become acidic. As the blood pH drops, the parts of the brain that regulate breathing are stimulated to produce faster and deeper breathing, which increases the amount of carbon dioxide exhaled.

The kidneys also try to compensate by excreting more acid in the urine. However, both mechanisms can be overwhelmed if the body continues to produce too much acid, leading to severe acidosis and eventually coma.

Causes

Metabolic acidosis develops when the amount of acid in the body is increased through ingestion of a substance that is, or can be metabolized to, an acid—such as wood alcohol (methanol), antifreeze (ethylene glycol), or large doses of aspirin (acetylsalicylic acid). Metabolic acidosis can also occur as a result of abnormal metabolism. The body produces excess acid in the advanced stages of shock and in poorly controlled type 1 diabetes mellitus. Even the production of normal amounts of acid may lead to acidosis when the kidneys are not functioning normally and are therefore not able to excrete sufficient amounts of acid in the urine.

Respiratory acidosis develops when the lungs do not expel carbon dioxide adequately, a problem that can occur in diseases that severely affect the lungs (such as emphysema, chronic bronchitis, severe pneumonia, pulmonary edema, and asthma). Respiratory acidosis can also develop when diseases of the nerves or muscles of the chest impair breathing. In addition, a person can develop respiratory acidosis if overly sedated from opioids (narcotics) and strong sleeping medications that slow respiration.

Symptoms

A person with mild metabolic acidosis may have no symptoms but usually experiences nausea, vomiting, and fatigue. Breathing becomes deeper and slightly faster (as the body tries to correct the acidosis by expelling more carbon dioxide). As the acidosis worsens, the person begins to feel extremely weak and drowsy and may feel confused and increasingly nauseated. Eventually, blood pressure can fall, leading to shock, coma, and death.

The first symptoms of respiratory acidosis may be headache and drowsiness. Drowsiness may progress to stupor and coma. Stupor and coma can develop within moments if breathing stops or is severely impaired, or over hours if breathing is less dramatically impaired.

Diagnosis

The diagnosis of acidosis generally requires the measurement of blood pH in a sample of arterial blood, usually taken from the radial artery in the wrist. Arterial blood is used because venous blood contains high levels of bi-

Major Causes of Metabolic Acidosis and Metabolic Alkalosis

Metabolic acidosis

- Kidney failure
- Renal tubular acidosis (a form of kidney malfunction)
- Diabetic ketoacidosis (buildup of ketones)
- Lactic acidosis (buildup of lactic acid)
- Poisons such as ethylene glycol, methanol, paraldehyde, acetazolamide, ammonia chloride, or aspirin overdose
- Loss of bases, such as bicarbonate, through the digestive tract from diarrhea, an ileostomy, or a colostomy

Metabolic alkalosis

- Use of diuretics (thiazides, furosemide, ethacrynic acid)
- Loss of acid from vomiting or drainage of the stomach
- Overactive adrenal gland (Cushing's syndrome or use of corticosteroids)

carbonate and thus is not an accurate measure of blood pH.

To learn more about the cause of the acidosis, doctors also measure the levels of carbon dioxide and bicarbonate in the blood. Additional blood tests may be performed to help determine the cause.

Treatment

The treatment of metabolic acidosis depends primarily on the cause. For instance, treatment may be needed to control diabetes with insulin or to remove the toxic substance from the blood in cases of poisoning.

The treatment of respiratory acidosis aims at improving the function of the lungs. Drugs to improve breathing may help people who have lung diseases such as asthma and emphysema. People who have severely impaired lung function, for whatever reason, may need mechanical ventilation to aid breathing.▲

Acidosis may also be treated directly. If the acidosis is mild, the administration of intra-venous fluids may be all that is needed. When acidosis is severe, bicarbonate may be given intravenously; however, bicarbonate provides only temporary relief and may cause harm—for instance, by overloading the body with sodium and water.

Alkalosis

Alkalosis is excessive blood alkalinity caused by an overabundance of bicarbonate in the blood or a loss of acid from the blood (metabolic alkalosis), or by a low level of carbon dioxide in the blood that results from rapid or deep breathing (respiratory alkalosis).

Metabolic alkalosis develops when the body loses too much acid or gains too much base. For example, stomach acid is lost during periods of prolonged vomiting or when stomach acids are suctioned with a stomach tube (as is sometimes done in hospitals). In rare cases, metabolic alkalosis develops in a person who has ingested too much base from substances such as baking soda (bicarbonate of soda). In addition, metabolic alkalosis can develop when excessive loss of sodium or potassium affects the kidneys' ability to control the blood's acid-base balance. For instance, loss of potassium sufficient to cause metabolic alkalosis may result from the use of diuretics or corticosteroids.

Respiratory alkalosis develops when rapid, deep breathing (hyperventilation) causes too much carbon dioxide to be expelled from the bloodstream. The most common cause of hyperventilation, and thus respiratory alkalosis, is anxiety. Other causes of hyperventilation and consequent respiratory alkalosis include pain, cirrhosis, low levels of oxygen in the blood, fever, and aspirin overdose (which can also cause metabolic acidosis).■

Symptoms and Diagnosis

Alkalosis may cause irritability, muscle twitching, muscle cramps, or no symptoms at all. If the alkalosis is severe, prolonged contraction and spasms of muscles (tetany) can develop.

A sample of blood taken from an artery shows that the blood is alkaline.

Treatment

Doctors usually treat metabolic alkalosis by replacing water and electrolytes (sodium and potassium) while treating the underlying

▲ see page 316   ■ see page 931

cause. Occasionally, when metabolic alkalosis is very severe, dilute acid in the form of ammonium chloride is given intravenously.

With respiratory alkalosis, usually the only treatment needed is slowing down the rate of breathing. When respiratory alkalosis is caused by anxiety, a conscious effort to slow breathing may make the condition disappear. If pain is causing the person to breathe rapidly, relieving the pain usually suffices. Breathing into a paper (not a plastic) bag may help raise the carbon dioxide level in the blood as the person breathes carbon dioxide back in after breathing it out.

CHAPTER 160

Porphyrias

Porphyrias are a group of disorders caused by deficiencies of enzymes involved in the production of heme.

Heme, a chemical compound that contains iron and gives blood its red color, is the key component of several important proteins in the body. The essential functions of heme depend on its ability to bind oxygen. Heme is incorporated into hemoglobin, a protein that enables red blood cells to carry oxygen from the lungs to all parts of the body. Heme is also a component of cytochromes (a type of protein). Some cytochromes in the liver process (metabolize) chemicals—including drugs and hormones—so that they are more easily removed from the body.

Heme is produced in the bone marrow and liver through a complex process regulated by eight different enzymes. As this production process progresses, several different intermediate compounds (heme precursors) are created and modified. If there is a deficiency in one of the enzymes that are essential for heme production, certain heme precursors may accumulate in tissues (especially in the bone marrow or liver), appear in excess in the blood, and get excreted in the urine or stool. The specific precursors that accumulate depend on which enzyme is deficient. One group of heme precursors is called the porphyrins.

Porphyrias are a number of different diseases, each caused by a specific abnormality in the heme production process. Most porphyrias are hereditary. All people with a particular porphyria have a deficiency of the same enzyme. The result is a deficiency or inactivity of a specific enzyme in the heme production process, with resulting accumulation of heme precursors.

Some porphyrias result in photosensitivity (extreme sensitivity to sunlight) because certain porphyrins are deposited in the skin. When exposed to light and oxygen, these porphyrins can generate a charged, unstable form of oxygen capable of damaging the skin. Nerve damage, leading to pain and even paralysis, can also occur in some porphyrias. Some porphyrias result in abdominal pain and liver damage.

The three most common porphyrias are porphyria cutanea tarda, acute intermittent porphyria, and erythropoietic protoporphyria. These disorders are very distinct: their symptoms differ considerably, different tests are required for their diagnosis, and different treatments are involved. Some features of these porphyrias are shared with the other, less common forms (which include delta-aminolevulinic acid dehydratase deficiency, congenital erythropoietic porphyria, hepatoerythropoietic porphyria, hereditary coproporphyria, and variegate porphyria).

Porphyria Cutanea Tarda

Porphyria cutanea tarda is the most common porphyria and causes blistering of skin exposed to sunlight.

Porphyria cutanea tarda occurs throughout the world. As far as is known, this porphyria is the only one that can occur in someone without an inherited deficiency of an enzyme involved in heme production.

Porphyria cutanea tarda results from under-activity of the enzyme uroporphyrinogen de-

Classifying Porphyrias

Porphyrias can be classified in several ways. Classification according to the specific enzyme deficiency is the most accurate. Another classification system distinguishes porphyrias that cause neurologic symptoms (acute porphyrias) from those that cause photosensitivity (cutaneous porphyrias). A third classification system is based on whether the excess precursors originate primarily in the liver (hepatic porphyrias) or primarily in the bone marrow (erythropoietic porphyrias). Some porphyrias are classified into more than one of these categories.

carboxylase, which leads to accumulation of porphyrins in the liver. Skin damage occurs because porphyrins produced in the liver are transported by the blood plasma to the skin.

Several common factors (precipitating factors) are associated with porphyria cutanea tarda; these include excess iron in body tissues, moderate or heavy alcohol use, taking estrogens, infection with hepatitis C virus, and possibly smoking. Infection with the human immunodeficiency virus (HIV) is a less common precipitating factor. These factors are thought to interact with iron and oxygen in the liver and thereby inhibit or damage the enzyme uroporphyrinogen decarboxylase.

In about 80% of people with porphyria cutanea tarda, the disorder does not appear to be hereditary and is called sporadic. In the remaining 20%, the disorder is hereditary and is called familial.

Symptoms and Diagnosis

People with porphyria cutanea tarda experience chronic, recurring blisters of various sizes on sun-exposed areas such as the arms, face, and especially the backs of the hands. Crusting and scarring follow the blisters and take a long time to heal. The skin, especially on the hands, is also sensitive to minor injury. Hair growth on the face and other sun-exposed area may increase. Liver damage usually occurs; cirrhosis and even liver cancer may eventually develop.

To diagnose porphyria cutanea tarda, a doctor tests the blood plasma, urine, and stool for increased levels of porphyrins. The specific porphyrins that are increased provide a pattern that distinguishes porphyria cutanea tarda from other porphyrias.

Treatment

Porphyria cutanea tarda is the most readily treated porphyria. Avoiding alcohol and other precipitating factors is beneficial.

A procedure called phlebotomy, in which a pint of blood is removed, is the most widely recommended treatment. With phlebotomy, the excess iron is gradually removed, the activity of uroporphyrinogen decarboxylase in the liver returns toward normal, and porphyrin levels in the liver and blood plasma fall gradually. The skin symptoms improve, and the skin eventually returns to normal. Phlebotomy is discontinued when the person becomes slightly iron deficient. Anemia develops if too many phlebotomy sessions are performed.

Very low doses of chloroquine or hydroxychloroquine are also effective in treating porphyria cutanea tarda. These drugs remove excess porphyrins from the liver. However, doses that are too high cause porphyrins to be removed too rapidly, resulting in a temporary worsening of the disorder and damage to the liver.

For women taking estrogen, doctors discontinue the estrogen therapy (because it is a precipitating factor of the porphyria) until phlebotomy has been completed and porphyrin levels are normal. The estrogen is then restarted and seldom causes a recurrence of the porphyria.

Acute Intermittent Porphyria

Acute intermittent porphyria, which causes neurologic symptoms, is the most common acute porphyria.

Acute intermittent porphyria occurs in people of all races but may be more common in those from Northern Europe. In most countries, it is the most common of the acute porphyrias. People first experience acute intermittent porphyria with acute onset of neurologic symptoms. Attacks are more common in women than in men.

Acute intermittent porphyria is due to a deficiency of the enzyme porphobilinogen deaminase (also known as hydroxymethylbilane synthase) that leads to accumulation of the heme precursors delta-aminolevulinic acid and porphobilinogen initially in the liver. The disorder is inherited due to a single abnormal gene from one parent. The normal gene from the other parent keeps the deficient enzyme at half-normal levels, which is sufficient to produce normal amounts of heme. Very rarely, the disease is inherited from both parents (and therefore two abnormal genes are present); symptoms may then appear in childhood and include developmental abnormalities.

Most people with a deficiency of porphobilinogen deaminase never develop symptoms. In some people, however, certain factors—drugs, hormones, or diet—can precipitate symptoms, producing an attack. Many drugs (including barbiturates, anticonvulsants, and sulfonamide antibiotics) can bring on an attack. Hormones, such as progesterone and related steroids, can precipitate symptoms, as can low-calorie and low-carbohydrate diets, large amounts of alcohol, or smoking. Stress resulting from an infection, another illness, surgery, or a psychologic upset is also sometimes implicated. Usually a combination of factors is involved. Sometimes the factors that cause an attack cannot be identified.

Symptoms

Symptoms occur as attacks lasting several days or weeks, and sometimes even longer. Such attacks usually first appear after puberty. In some women, attacks develop during the second half of the menstrual cycle.

Abdominal pain is the most common symptom. The pain can be so severe that the doctor may mistakenly think that abdominal surgery is needed. Gastrointestinal symptoms include nausea, vomiting, constipation or diarrhea, and abdominal bloating. The bladder may be affected, making urination difficult and sometimes resulting in an overfull bladder. A rapid heart rate, high blood pressure, sweating, and restlessness are also common during attacks; interference with sleep is typical. High blood pressure can continue after the attack.

All of these symptoms, including the gastrointestinal ones, result from effects on the nervous system. Nerves that control muscles can be damaged, leading to weakness, usually beginning in the shoulders and arms. The weakness can progress to virtually all the muscles, including those involved in breathing. Tremors and seizures may develop.

Recovery from symptoms may occur within a few days, although complete recovery from severe muscle weakness may take several

months or years. Attacks are rarely fatal; however, in a few people, attacks are disabling.

Diagnosis and Prognosis

The severe gastrointestinal and neurologic symptoms resemble those of many more common disorders. Laboratory tests performed on samples of urine show increased levels of two heme precursors (delta-aminolevulinic acid and porphobilinogen). Levels of these precursors are very high during attacks and remain high in people who have repeated attacks. The precursors can form porphyrins, which are reddish in color, and other substances that are brownish. These turn the urine dark, especially after exposure to light.

Relatives without symptoms can be identified as carriers of the disorder by measuring porphobilinogen deaminase in red blood cells or sometimes by DNA testing. Diagnosis before birth is also possible but usually is not needed because most affected people never get symptoms.

Prevention and Treatment

Attacks of acute intermittent porphyria can be prevented by maintaining good nutrition and avoiding the drugs that can provoke them. Crash diets to lose weight rapidly should be avoided. Heme can be given to prevent attacks. Premenstrual attacks in women can be prevented with one of the gonadotropin-releasing hormone agonists used to treat endometriosis,▲ although this treatment is still investigational.

People who have attacks of acute intermittent porphyria are often hospitalized for treatment of severe symptoms. People with severe attacks are treated with heme given intravenously. Blood and urine levels of delta-aminolevulinic acid and porphobilinogen are promptly lowered and symptoms improve, usually within several days. If treatment is delayed, recovery takes longer, and some nerve damage may be permanent.

Glucose given intravenously or a diet high in carbohydrates can also be beneficial, particularly in people whose attacks are brought on by a low-calorie or low-carbohydrate diet, but these measures are less effective than heme. Pain can be controlled with drugs (such as opioids) until the person responds to heme or glucose.

▲ see page 1369

Nausea, vomiting, anxiety, and restlessness are treated with a phenothiazine for a short time. Insomnia may be treated with chloral hydrate or low doses of a benzodiazepine but not a barbiturate. An overfull bladder may be treated by draining the urine with a catheter.

The doctor ensures that the person does not take any of the drugs known to precipitate an attack, and—if possible—addresses other factors that may have contributed to the attack. Treatment of seizures is problematic, because almost any anticonvulsant would worsen an attack. Beta-blockers may be used to treat rapid heart rate and high blood pressure but are not used in people who are dehydrated, in whom a rapid heart rate is needed to maintain the blood circulation.

Erythropoietic Protoporphyria

Erythropoietic protoporphyria is a condition characterized by photosensitivity.

Erythropoietic protoporphyria is the third most common porphyria. It occurs most often in whites but can also occur in people of any origin. Erythropoietic protoporphyria occurs equally in men and women.

In erythropoietic protoporphyria, a deficiency of the enzyme ferrochelatase leads to accumulation of the heme precursor protoporphyrin in the bone marrow, red blood cells,

blood plasma, skin, and liver. The enzyme deficiency is usually inherited from one parent.

Accumulation of protoporphyrin in the skin results in extreme sensitivity to sunlight. The sunlight activates the protoporphyrin molecules, which damage the surrounding tissue. Accumulation of protoporphyrins in the liver can cause liver damage. Protoporphyrins in the bile can lead to bile stones.

Symptoms and Diagnosis

Symptoms usually start in childhood. Pain and swelling develop soon after the skin is exposed to sunlight. Because blistering and scarring seldom occur, doctors do not always recognize the disorder. Gallstones cause characteristic abdominal pain.▲ Liver damage may lead to increasing liver failure, with jaundice and enlargement of the spleen.

Porphyrin levels in urine are not increased. The diagnosis is therefore made when increased levels of protoporphyrin are detected in the plasma and red blood cells.

Prevention and Treatment

Extreme care should be taken to avoid exposure to sunlight. Accidental sun exposure is given the same treatment as is sunburn.■ Beta-carotene, when taken in sufficient amounts to cause slight yellowing of the skin, makes many people more tolerant of sunlight; however, sunlight should still be avoided. People who develop gallstones that contain protoporphyrin may need to have them surgically removed. Liver damage, if severe, may necessitate liver transplantation.

▲ see page 813   ■ see page 1230

HORMONAL DISORDERS

161 Biology of the Endocrine System..937

Endocrine Glands ▪ Endocrine Function ▪ Endocrine Controls

162 Pituitary Gland Disorders...940

Enlargement of the Pituitary Gland ▪ Hypopituitarism ▪
Central Diabetes Insipidus ▪ Acromegaly and Gigantism ▪
Galactorrhea ▪ Empty Sella Syndrome

163 Thyroid Gland Disorders..948

Hyperthyroidism ▪ Hypothyroidism ▪ Thyroiditis ▪ Thyroid
Cancer

164 Adrenal Gland Disorders..956

Addison's Disease ▪ Cushing's Syndrome ▪ Virilization ▪
Hyperaldosteronism ▪ Pheochromocytoma

165 Diabetes Mellitus...962

166 Hypoglycemia..970

167 Multiple Endocrine Neoplasia Syndromes...............................972

168 Carcinoid Tumors..974

CHAPTER 161

Biology of the Endocrine System

The endocrine system consists of a group of glands and organs that regulate and control various body functions by producing and secreting hormones. The glands of the endocrine system do not have ducts but rather release their hormones directly into the bloodstream.

Endocrine Glands

The major glands of the endocrine system, each of which produces one or more specific hormones, are the hypothalamus, the pituitary gland, the thyroid gland, the parathyroid glands, the islets of the pancreas, the adrenal glands, the testes in men, and the ovaries in women. During pregnancy, the placenta also acts as an endocrine gland in addition to its other functions.

Not all organs that secrete hormones or hormonelike substances are considered part of the endocrine system. For example, the kidneys produce the hormones renin and angio-

Major Endocrine Glands

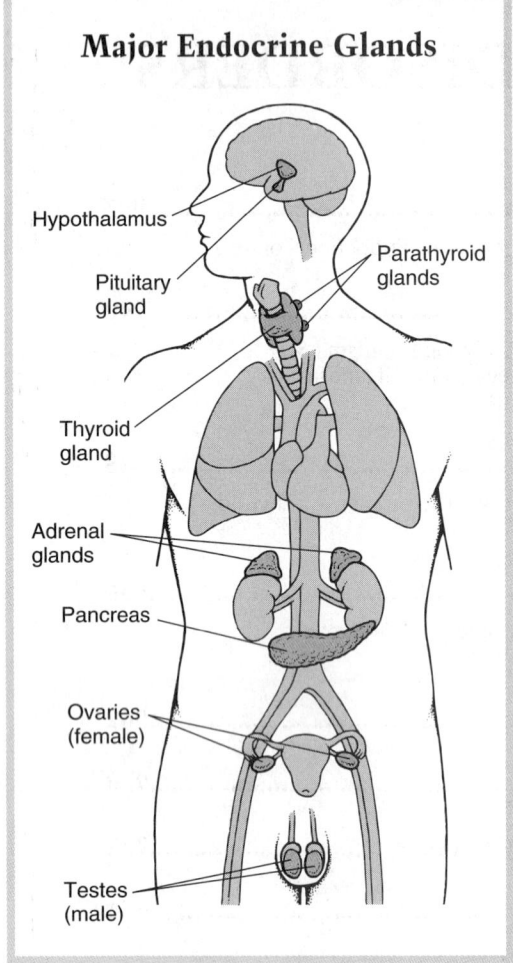

Hypothalamus

Pituitary
gland

Parathyroid
glands

Thyroid
gland

Adrenal
glands

Pancreas

Ovaries
(female)

Testes
(male)

stream. Hormones are chemical substances that affect the activity of another part of the body (target site). In essence, hormones serve as messengers, controlling and coordinating activities throughout the body.

Upon reaching a target site, hormones bind to receptors, much like a key fits into a lock. Once the hormone locks into its receptor, it transmits a message that causes the target site to take a specific action. Hormone receptors may be within the nucleus or on the surface of the cell.

Ultimately, hormones control the function of entire organs, affecting such diverse processes as growth and development, reproduction, and sexual characteristics. Hormones also influence the way the body uses and stores energy and control the volume of fluid and the levels of salts and sugar in the blood. Very small amounts of hormones can trigger very large responses in the body.

Although hormones circulate throughout the body, each type of hormone influences only certain organs and tissues. Some hormones affect only one or two organs, whereas others have influence throughout the body. For example, thyroid-stimulating hormone, produced in the pituitary gland, affects only the thyroid gland. In contrast, thyroid hormone, produced in the thyroid gland, affects cells throughout the body and is involved in such important functions as regulating growth of cells, controlling the heart rate, and affecting the speed at which calories are burned. Insulin, secreted by the islet cells of the pancreas, affects the metabolism of glucose, protein, and fat throughout the body.

Most hormones are proteins. Others are steroids, which are fatty substances derived from cholesterol.

Endocrine Controls

To control endocrine functions, the secretion of each hormone must be regulated within precise limits. The body is able to sense whether more or less of a given hormone is needed.

Many endocrine glands are controlled by the interplay of hormonal signals between the hypothalamus, located in the brain, and the pituitary gland, which sits at the base of the brain. This interplay is referred to as the hypothalamic-pituitary axis. The hypothalamus secretes several hormones that control the pituitary gland. The pituitary, sometimes called the master gland, in turn controls the func-

tensin to help control blood pressure and the hormone erythropoietin to stimulate the bone marrow to produce red blood cells. In addition, the digestive system produces a variety of hormones that control digestion, affect insulin secretion from the pancreas, and alter behaviors, such as those associated with hunger. Fat tissue also produces hormones that regulate metabolism and appetite. Additionally, the term "gland" does not mean that the organ is part of the endocrine system. For example, sweat glands, glands in mucus membranes, and mammary glands secrete substances other than hormones.

Endocrine Function

The main function of endocrine glands is to secrete hormones directly into the blood-

MAJOR HORMONES

Where Hormone Is Produced	Hormone	Function
Pituitary gland	Antidiuretic hormone (vasopressin)	Causes kidneys to retain water and, along with aldosterone, helps control blood pressure
	Corticotropin (ACTH)	Controls the production and secretion of hormones by the adrenal cortex
	Growth hormone	Controls growth and development; promotes protein production
	Luteinizing hormone and follicle-stimulating hormone	Control reproductive functions, including the production of sperm and semen, egg maturation, and menstrual cycles; control male and female sexual characteristics (including hair distribution, muscle formation, skin texture and thickness, voice, and perhaps even personality traits)
	Oxytocin	Causes muscles of the uterus and milk ducts in the breast to contract
	Prolactin	Starts and maintains milk production in the ductal glands of the breast (mammary glands)
	Thyroid-stimulating hormone	Stimulates the production and secretion of hormones by the thyroid gland
Parathyroid glands	Parathyroid hormone	Controls bone formation and the excretion of calcium and phosphorus
Thyroid gland	Thyroid hormone	Regulates the rate at which the body functions (metabolic rate)
Adrenal glands	Aldosterone	Helps regulate salt and water balance by retaining salt and water and excreting potassium
	Cortisol	Has widespread effects throughout the body; especially has anti-inflammatory action; maintains blood sugar level, blood pressure, and muscle strength; helps control salt and water balance
	Dehydroepiandrosterone (DHEA)	Has effects on bone, mood, and the immune system
	Epinephrine and norepinephrine	Stimulate the heart, lungs, blood vessels, and nervous system
Pancreas	Glucagon	Raises the blood sugar level
	Insulin	Lowers the blood sugar level; affects the processing (metabolism) of sugar, protein, and fat throughout the body
Kidneys	Erythropoietin	Stimulates red blood cell production
	Renin	Controls blood pressure
	Angiotensin	Controls blood pressure
Ovaries	Estrogen	Controls the development of female sex characteristics and the reproductive system
	Progesterone	Prepares the lining of the uterus for implantation of a fertilized egg and readies the mammary glands to secrete milk
Testes	Testosterone	Controls the development of male sex characteristics and the reproductive system
Digestive tract	Cholecystokinin	Controls muscle contractions that move food through the intestine and gallbladder contractions
	Glucagon-like peptide	Increases insulin release from pancreas
	Ghrelin	Controls growth hormone release from the pituitary gland
Adipose (fat) tissue	Resistin	Blocks the effects of insulin on muscle
	Leptin	Controls appetite

tions of many other endocrine glands.▲ The pituitary controls the rate at which it secretes hormones through a feedback loop in which the blood levels of other endocrine hormones signal the pituitary to slow down or speed up.

Many other factors can control endocrine function as well. For example, a baby sucking on its mother's nipple stimulates the pituitary gland to secrete prolactin and oxytocin, hormones that stimulate breast milk production and flow. Rising blood sugar levels stimulate the islet cells of the pancreas to produce insulin. Part of the nervous system stimulates the adrenal gland to produce epinephrine.

CHAPTER 162

Pituitary Gland Disorders

The pituitary is a pea-sized gland that is housed within a bony structure (sella turcica) at the base of the brain. The sella turcica protects the pituitary but allows very little room for expansion.

The pituitary controls the function of most other endocrine glands and is therefore sometimes called the master gland. In turn, the pituitary is controlled in large part by the hypothalamus, a region of the brain that lies just above the pituitary. By detecting the levels of hormones produced by glands under the pituitary's control (target glands), the hypothalamus or the pituitary can determine how much stimulation the target glands need.

The pituitary has two distinct parts: the anterior (front) lobe, which accounts for 80% of the pituitary gland's weight, and the posterior (back) lobe. The lobes are connected to the hypothalamus by a stalk that contains blood vessels and nerve cell projections (nerve fibers, or axons). The hypothalamus controls the anterior lobe by releasing hormones through the connecting blood vessels; it controls the posterior lobe through nerve impulses.

The **anterior lobe** of the pituitary produces and releases (secretes) six main hormones: growth hormone, which regulates growth and physical development and has important effects on body shape by stimulating muscle formation and reducing fat tissue; thyroid-stimulating hormone, which stimulates the thyroid gland to produce thyroid hormones; corticotropin (also called adrenocorticotropic hormone or ACTH), which stimulates the adrenal glands to produce cortisol and other hormones; follicle-stimulating hormone and luteinizing hormone (the gonadotropins), which stimulate the testes to produce sperm, the ovaries to produce eggs, and the sex organs to produce sex hormones (testosterone and estrogen); and prolactin, which stimulates the mammary glands of the breast to produce milk.

The anterior lobe also produces hormones that cause the skin to darken (melanocyte-stimulating hormone) and that inhibit pain sensations and help control the immune system (endorphins).

The **posterior lobe** of the pituitary produces only two hormones: antidiuretic hormone and oxytocin. Antidiuretic hormone (also called vasopressin) regulates the amount of water excreted by the kidneys and is therefore important in maintaining water balance in the body.■ Oxytocin causes the uterus to contract during childbirth and immediately after delivery to prevent excessive bleeding. Oxytocin also stimulates contractions of the milk ducts in the breast, which moves milk to the nipple (the let-down) in lactating women.

The hormones produced by the pituitary are not all produced continuously. Most are released in bursts every 1 to 3 hours, with alternating periods of activity and inactivity. Some of the hormones, such as corticotropin, which controls the adrenal glands; growth hormone, which controls growth; and prolactin, which controls milk production, follow a circadian rhythm: The levels rise and fall predictably during the day, usually peaking just before awakening and dropping to their lowest levels just before sleep. The levels of other hormones

---

▲ see box on page 941   ■ see also page 927

vary according to other factors. For example, in women, the levels of luteinizing hormone and follicle-stimulating hormone, which control reproductive functions, vary during the menstrual cycle.

The pituitary gland can malfunction in several ways, usually as a result of developing a noncancerous tumor (adenoma). The tumor may overproduce one or more pituitary hormones; it may press on the normal pituitary cells, causing underproduction of one or more pituitary hormones; or it may cause enlargement of the pituitary gland, with or without disturbing hormone production. Sometimes there is overproduction of one hormone by a pituitary tumor and underproduction of another at the same time due to pressure. Too little or too much of a pituitary hormone results in a wide variety of symptoms.

Doctors can diagnose pituitary gland malfunction using several tests. Imaging tests, such as a computed tomography (CT) or magnetic resonance imaging (MRI) scan, can show whether the pituitary has enlarged or shrunk and can usually determine whether a tumor exists in the gland.

Doctors can measure the levels of pituitary hormones, usually by a simple blood test. Doctors select which pituitary hormone levels they want to measure depending on the person's symptoms. Some pituitary hormones are not easy to measure because their levels vary greatly during the day and according to the body's needs; measuring a random blood sample does not provide useful information.

For some of those hormones, doctors give a substance that would normally affect hormone production; then they measure the level of the hormone. For example, if a doctor injects insulin, the levels of corticotropin, growth hormone, and prolactin should increase. Rather than measuring growth hormone levels directly, doctors often measure another hormone, insulin-like growth factor I (IGF-I). Growth hormone is produced in bursts and its levels quickly fall, but IGF-I levels reflect the overall daily production of growth hormone. For all of these reasons, interpreting the results of blood tests for pituitary hormones is complex.

Enlargement of the Pituitary Gland

Enlargement of the pituitary gland is usually due to a tumor but may be due to bleeding into the gland or involvement by some other

Pituitary: The Master Gland

The pituitary, a pea-sized gland at the base of the brain, produces a number of hormones, each of which affects a specific part of the body (a target organ). Because the pituitary controls the function of most other endocrine glands, it is often called the master gland.

HORMONE	TARGET ORGAN
Antidiuretic hormone	Kidney
Beta-melanocyte–stimulating hormone	Skin
Corticotropin	Adrenal glands
Endorphins	Brain
Enkephalins	Brain
Follicle-stimulating hormone	Ovaries or testes
Growth hormone	Muscles and bones
Luteinizing hormone	Ovaries or testes
Oxytocin	Uterus and mammary glands
Prolactin	Mammary glands
Thyroid-stimulating hormone	Thyroid gland

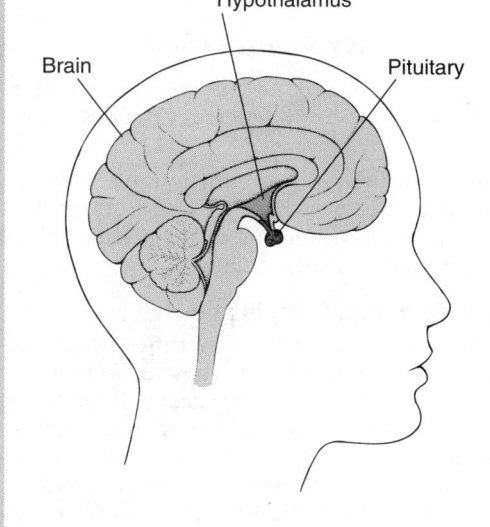

disease, such as tuberculosis or sarcoidosis. An enlarged pituitary gland may produce symptoms such as headaches and, because the growing gland often presses on the optic nerve above the pituitary gland, a loss of vision. Vision loss often initially affects only the upper,

What Causes an Underactive Pituitary?

Causes affecting primarily the pituitary gland
- Pituitary tumors
- Inadequate blood supply to the pituitary (from severe bleeding, blood clots, anemia, or other causes)
- Infections and inflammatory diseases
- Sarcoidosis or amyloidosis (unusual diseases)
- Irradiation
- Surgical removal of pituitary tissue
- Autoimmune disease

Causes affecting primarily the hypothalamus, which then affects the pituitary
- Tumors of the hypothalamus
- Inflammatory diseases
- Head injuries
- Surgical damage to the pituitary or to the blood vessels or nerves leading to it

outermost fields of vision in both eyes. Underproduction or overproduction of pituitary hormones may also occur.

Hypopituitarism

Hypopituitarism is an underactive pituitary gland that results in deficiency of one or more pituitary hormones.

Hypopituitarism, an uncommon disorder, can be caused by a number of factors, including a pituitary tumor or an insufficient blood supply to the pituitary gland.

Symptoms and Complications

Although symptoms sometimes begin suddenly and dramatically, they usually begin gradually and may go unrecognized for a long time. Symptoms depend on which pituitary hormones are deficient. In some cases, the pituitary gland's production of a single hormone decreases; more typically, the levels of several hormones decrease at the same time (panhypopituitarism). Production of growth hormone, luteinizing hormone, and follicle-stimulating hormone often decreases before that

of thyroid-stimulating hormone and corticotropin.

Growth Hormone Deficiency: A lack of growth hormone typically leads to poor overall growth and short height (dwarfism) if it occurs in childhood. In adults, growth hormone deficiency does not affect height, because the bones have finished growing, but it can cause increased fat and reduced muscle tissue, thinning of bones, and reduced energy and quality of life.

Deficiency of Gonadotropins (follicle-stimulating hormone and luteinizing hormone): In premenopausal women, deficiencies of these hormones cause menstrual periods to stop (amenorrhea), infertility, vaginal dryness, and loss of some female sexual characteristics. In men, deficiencies of these hormones result in wasting away (atrophy) of the testes, decreased sperm production and consequent infertility, and loss of some male sexual characteristics. Deficiencies of luteinizing hormone and follicle-stimulating hormone can also occur in Kallmann's syndrome, in which people may also have a cleft lip or palate,▲ are color-blind, and are unable to sense smells.

Thyroid-stimulating Hormone Deficiency: Thyroid-stimulating hormone deficiency leads to an underactive thyroid gland (hypothyroidism), which results in such symptoms as confusion, intolerance to cold, weight gain, constipation, and dry skin.■ Most cases of hypothyroidism, however, are due to a problem originating in the thyroid gland itself, not to low levels of pituitary hormones.

Corticotropin Deficiency: Corticotropin deficiency leads to an underactive adrenal gland (Addison's disease),★ which results in fatigue, low blood pressure, low levels of sugar in the blood, and low tolerance for stress. This is the most serious pituitary hormone deficiency; if the body is unable to make any corticotropin, it can be fatal.

Prolactin Deficiency: Prolactin deficiency reduces or eliminates a woman's ability to produce breast milk after childbirth. One cause of low prolactin levels and deficiency of other pituitary hormones is Sheehan's syndrome, a rare complication of childbirth. Sheehan's syndrome typically develops because of excessive blood loss and shock during childbirth, which results in partial destruction of the pituitary gland. Symptoms include fatigue, loss of pubic and underarm hair, and inability to produce breast milk. Prolactin deficiency has no known ill effects in men.

▲ see page 1523   ■ see page 952
★ see page 956

Diagnosis

Because the pituitary gland stimulates other glands, a deficiency in pituitary hormones often reduces the amount of hormones the other glands produce. Therefore, a doctor considers the possibility of pituitary malfunction when investigating a deficiency in another gland, such as the thyroid or adrenal gland. When symptoms suggest that several glands are underactive, a doctor may suspect hypopituitarism or a polyglandular deficiency syndrome.

An evaluation usually begins by measuring levels of the hormones that the pituitary gland produces and at the same time measuring levels of the hormone produced by the target organ. For example, a person with hypothyroidism due to failure of the pituitary gland has low levels of thyroid hormone and low or inappropriately normal levels of thyroid-stimulating hormone, which is produced by the pituitary gland. In contrast, a person with hypothyroidism due to failure of the thyroid gland itself has low levels of thyroid hormone and high levels of thyroid-stimulating hormone.

Growth hormone production by the pituitary is difficult to evaluate because no test accurately measures it. The body produces growth hormone in several bursts each day, and the hormone is quickly used. Thus, the blood level at any given moment does not indicate whether production is normal over the course of a day. Instead, doctors measure the levels of insulin-like growth factor I (IGF-I) in the blood. Production of IGF-I is controlled by growth hormone, and the level of IGF-I tends to change slowly in proportion to the overall amount of growth hormone produced by the pituitary.

Because the levels of luteinizing hormone and follicle-stimulating hormone fluctuate with the menstrual cycle, their measurement in women may be difficult to interpret. However, in postmenopausal women who are not taking estrogen, luteinizing hormone and follicle-stimulating hormone levels normally are high.

Production of corticotropin is usually measured by assessing the response of its target hormone (cortisol) to stimuli, such as a low level of sugar in the blood after an insulin injection. If the level of cortisol does not change and the level of corticotropin in the blood is normal or low, a deficiency of corticotropin production is confirmed.

Polyglandular Deficiency Syndromes

Polyglandular deficiency syndromes are hereditary disorders in which several endocrine glands malfunction simultaneously. The actual cause of the malfunction may be related to an autoimmune reaction in which the body's immune defenses mistakenly attack the body's own cells. Polyglandular deficiency syndromes are classified into three types:

Type 1: In this type, which develops in children, the parathyroid and adrenal glands are underactive, which can lead to diabetes, hepatitis, gallstones, hair loss, and malabsorption. These children are prone to chronic yeast infections as well.

Type 2: In this type, which develops in adults, the adrenal and thyroid glands are underactive, although the thyroid gland sometimes becomes overactive. People with type 2 polyglandular deficiency also develop diabetes.

Type 3: This type is very similar to type 2, except that the adrenal glands remain normal.

Once hypopituitarism is established by blood tests, the pituitary gland is usually evaluated with a computed tomography (CT) or magnetic resonance imaging (MRI) scan to identify structural problems. CT or MRI scans help reveal individual (localized) areas of abnormal tissue growth as well as general enlargement or shrinkage of the pituitary gland. The blood vessels that supply the pituitary can be examined with cerebral angiography. ▲

Treatment

When possible, treatment is aimed at removing the cause of the pituitary hormone deficiency, such as a tumor. Surgical removal of a tumor is often the most appropriate first treatment, and removal also usually reduces any pressure symptoms and vision problems caused by the tumor. For all but the largest tumors, surgery can usually be done through the nose (transphenoidal).

Supervoltage or proton beam irradiation of the pituitary gland can be used to destroy a tu-

▲ see page 445

mor. Large tumors and those that have extended beyond the sella turcica may be impossible to remove with surgery alone. If so, doctors use supervoltage irradiation after surgery to kill the remaining tumor cells. Irradiation of the pituitary gland tends to cause a slow loss of pituitary function. The loss may be partial or complete. Therefore, the function of the target glands is generally evaluated every 3 to 6 months for the first year and yearly thereafter. Tumors that produce prolactin can be treated with dopamine agonist drugs, such as bromocriptine or cabergoline. These drugs shrink the tumor while also lowering prolactin levels.

When it is not possible to remove the cause of the hormone deficiency, such as an insufficient blood supply to the pituitary gland, treatment focuses on replacing the deficient hormones, usually by replacing the target hormones. For example, people deficient in thyroid-stimulating hormone are given thyroid hormone, those deficient in corticotropin are given adrenocortical hormones such as hydrocortisone, and those deficient in luteinizing hormone and follicle-stimulating hormone are given estrogen, progesterone, or testosterone.

Growth hormone is the one pituitary hormone that is replaced. Growth hormone treatment must be given by injection. When given to children who have growth hormone deficiency before the growth plates in their bones close, replacement growth hormone prevents them from being exceptionally short. Growth hormone is now also being used to treat some adults with growth hormone deficiency to improve body composition, increase bone density, and enhance quality of life.

Central Diabetes Insipidus

Central diabetes insipidus is a lack of antidiuretic hormone that causes excessive production of very dilute urine (polyuria).

Causes

Central diabetes insipidus usually results from the decreased production of antidiuretic hormone (vasopressin), the hormone that helps regulate the amount of water in the body.▲ Antidiuretic hormone is unique in that it is produced in the hypothalamus but is

then stored and released into the bloodstream by the pituitary gland.

Central diabetes insipidus may be caused by insufficient production of antidiuretic hormone by the hypothalamus. Alternatively, the disorder may be caused by failure of the pituitary gland to release antidiuretic hormone into the bloodstream. Other causes of central diabetes insipidus include damage done during surgery on the hypothalamus or pituitary gland; a brain injury, particularly a fracture of the base of the skull; a tumor; sarcoidosis or tuberculosis; an aneurysm (a bulge in the wall of an artery) or blockage in the arteries leading to the brain; some forms of encephalitis or meningitis; and the rare disease Langerhan's cell granulomatosis (histiocytosis X). Another type of diabetes insipidus, nephrogenic diabetes insipidus, may be caused by abnormalities in the kidneys.■

Symptoms and Diagnosis

Symptoms may begin gradually or suddenly at any age. Often the only symptoms are excessive thirst and excessive urine production. A person may drink huge amounts of fluid—4 to 40 quarts a day—to compensate for the fluid lost in urine. Ice-cold water is often the preferred drink. When compensation is not possible, dehydration can quickly follow, resulting in low blood pressure and shock. The person continues to urinate large quantities of dilute urine, and this is particularly noticeable during the night.

Doctors suspect diabetes insipidus in people who produce large amounts of urine. They first test the urine for sugar to rule out diabetes mellitus. Blood tests show abnormal levels of many electrolytes, including a high level of sodium. The best test is a water deprivation test, in which urine production, blood electrolyte (sodium) levels, and weight are measured regularly for a period of about 12 hours, during which the person is not allowed to drink. A doctor monitors the person's condition throughout the course of the test. At the end of the 12 hours—or sooner if the person's blood pressure falls or heart rate increases or if he loses more than 5% of his body weight—the doctor stops the test and injects antidiuretic hormone. The diagnosis of central diabetes insipidus is confirmed if, in response to antidiuretic hormone, the person's excessive urination stops, the urine becomes more concentrated, the blood pressure rises, and the heart beats more normally. The diagnosis of

▲ see box on page 928

■ see page 851

nephrogenic diabetes insipidus is made if, after the injection, the excessive urination continues, the urine remains dilute, and blood pressure and heart rate do not change.

Treatment

Vasopressin or desmopressin, which are modified forms of antidiuretic hormone, may be taken as a nasal spray several times a day. The dose is adjusted to maintain the body's water balance and a normal urine output. Taking too much of these drugs can lead to fluid retention, swelling, and other problems. People with central diabetes insipidus who are undergoing surgery or are unconscious are generally given injections of antidiuretic hormone.

Sometimes central diabetes insipidus can be controlled with drugs that stimulate production of antidiuretic hormone, such as chlorpropamide, carbamazepine, clofibrate, and various diuretics (thiazides). These drugs are unlikely to relieve symptoms completely in people whose diabetes insipidus is severe.

Acromegaly and Gigantism

Overproduction of growth hormone causes excessive growth. In children, the condition is called gigantism; in adults, it is called acromegaly.

Growth hormone stimulates the growth of bones, muscles, and many internal organs. Excessive growth hormone, therefore, leads to abnormally robust growth of all of these tissues. Overproduction of growth hormone is almost always caused by a noncancerous (benign) pituitary tumor (adenoma). Certain rare tumors of the pancreas and lungs also can produce hormones that stimulate the pituitary to produce excessive amounts of growth hormone, with similar consequences.

Symptoms

If excessive growth hormone production starts before the growth plates have closed (that is, in children), the condition produces gigantism. The long bones grow enormously. A person grows to unusually great stature, and the arms and legs lengthen. Puberty may be delayed, and the genitals may not develop fully.

In most cases, excessive production of growth hormone begins between the ages of 30 and 50, long after the growth plates of the bones have closed. Increased growth hormone

in adults produces acromegaly, in which the bones become deformed rather than elongated. Because changes occur slowly, they are usually not recognized for years.

The person's facial features become coarse, and the hands and feet swell. Larger rings, gloves, shoes, and hats are needed. Overgrowth of the jawbone (mandible) can cause the jaw to protrude (prognathism). Cartilage in the voice box (larynx) may thicken, making the voice deep and husky. The ribs may thicken, creating a barrel chest. Joint pain is common; after many years, crippling degenerative arthritis may occur.

In both gigantism and acromegaly, the tongue may enlarge and become more furrowed. Coarse body hair, which typically darkens, increases as the skin thickens. The sebaceous and sweat glands in the skin enlarge, producing excessive perspiration and often an offensive body odor. The heart usually enlarges, and its function may be so severely impaired that heart failure occurs. Sometimes a person feels disturbing sensations and weakness in the arms and legs as enlarging tissues compress the nerves. Nerves that carry messages from the eyes to the brain may also be compressed, causing loss of vision, particularly in the outer visual fields. The pressure on the brain may also cause severe headaches.

Nearly all women with acromegaly have irregular menstrual cycles. Some women produce breast milk even though they are not breastfeeding (galactorrhea) because of either too much growth hormone or a related increase in prolactin. About one third of men who have acromegaly develop erectile dysfunction (impotence). There is also an increased likelihood of developing diabetes mellitus, high blood pressure (hypertension), heart failure, sleep apnea, and certain tumors, particularly affecting the large intestine, which may become cancerous. Life expectancy is reduced in people with untreated acromegaly.

Diagnosis

In children, rapid growth may not seem abnormal at first. Eventually, however, the abnormality of the extreme growth becomes clear.

In adults, because the changes induced by high levels of growth hormone occur slowly, acromegaly often is not diagnosed until many years after the first symptoms appear. Serial photographs (those taken over many years) may help a doctor establish the diagnosis. An x-ray of the skull may show thickening of the bones and enlargement of the nasal sinuses. X-rays of the hands show thickening of the bones under the fingertips and swelling of the tissue around the bones. Blood sugar levels and blood pressure may be high.

The diagnosis is confirmed by blood tests, which usually show high levels of both growth hormone and insulin-like growth factor I (IGF-I). Because growth hormone is released in short bursts and the levels of growth hormone often fluctuate dramatically even in people without acromegaly, a single high level of growth hormone in the blood is insufficient to make the diagnosis. Doctors must give something that would normally suppress growth hormone levels, most commonly a glucose drink (the oral glucose tolerance test), and show that normal suppression does not occur. This test is not necessary when the clinical features of acromegaly are obvious, the IGF-I level is high, or a tumor is seen in the pituitary on scanning.

A computed tomography (CT) or magnetic resonance imaging (MRI) scan is usually performed to look for abnormal growths in the pituitary gland. Because acromegaly is usually present for some years before being diagnosed, a tumor is seen on these scans in most people.

Treatment

Stopping or reducing the overproduction of growth hormone is not easy; thus, doctors may need to use a combination of surgery, radiation, and drug therapy.

Surgery by an experienced surgeon is currently regarded as the best first treatment for most people with acromegaly caused by a tumor. It results in an immediate reduction in tumor size and growth hormone production, most often without causing deficiency of other pituitary hormones. Unfortunately, tumors are often large by the time they are found, and surgery alone does not usually produce a cure. Radiation therapy is often used as a follow-up treatment, particularly if a substantial amount of the tumor remains after surgery and acromegaly persists.

Radiation therapy involves the use of supervoltage irradiation, which is less traumatic than surgery. This treatment may take several years to have its full effect, however, and often results in later deficiencies of other pituitary hormones, as normal tissue is often also affected. More directed radiation therapy, such as stereotactic radiosurgery, is being tried to speed results and spare the normal pituitary tissue.

Drug therapy can also be used to lower growth hormone levels. Occasionally, bromocriptine and other dopamine agonists are of some benefit. The most effective drugs, however, are those that are forms of somatostatin, the hormone that normally blocks growth hormone production and secretion. These drugs include octreotide and its new long-acting analogs, which only have to be given about once a month. These drugs are effective in controlling acromegaly in many people as long as they continue to be taken (they do not provide a cure). Their use has been limited by the need to inject them and by their high cost. This may change as such drugs become longer acting and more readily available. Several new growth hormone blocker drugs are being investigated.

Galactorrhea

Galactorrhea is the production of breast milk in men or in women who are not breastfeeding.

In both sexes, the most common cause of galactorrhea is a prolactin-secreting tumor (prolactinoma) in the pituitary gland. Prolactinomas usually are very small when first diagnosed; however, they tend to be larger in men than in women, probably because they come to attention later. Overproduction of prolactin and the development of galactorrhea may also be induced by drugs, including phenothiazines, certain drugs given for high blood pressure (especially methyldopa), opioids, and even licorice. There are other causes of galactorrhea that do not involve high levels of prolactin, such as an underactive thyroid gland (hypothyroidism).

Symptoms

Although breast milk production may be the only symptom of a prolactinoma, many women also stop menstruating (amenorrhea) or have less frequent menstrual periods. Women with prolactinomas often develop hot flashes and vaginal dryness, which causes discomfort with sexual intercourse, because of low estrogen levels. About two thirds of men with prolactinomas lose interest in sex (reduced libido) and have erectile dysfunction (impotence). A high prolactin level can cause infertility in both men and women.

speeds the release of TSH, depending on whether the levels of thyroid hormones circulating in the blood are getting too high or too low.

The thyroid gland also produces the hormone calcitonin, which may contribute to bone strength by helping calcium to be incorporated into bone.

Diagnostic Tests

To determine how well the thyroid gland is functioning, doctors use several tests. Usually the first and best test of thyroid function is measurement of the level of TSH in the blood. Because this hormone stimulates the thyroid gland, blood levels of TSH are high when the thyroid gland is underactive (and thus needs more stimulation) and low when the thyroid gland is overactive (and thus needs less stimulation). However, in rare cases in which the pituitary gland is not functioning normally, the level of TSH does not accurately reflect thyroid gland function.

Doctors can also measure the level of thyroid hormones in the blood. In some cases, the level of a protein called thyroxine-binding globulin is measured as well because it binds the thyroid hormones in the blood. Abnormal levels of this protein can lead to misinterpretation of a person's total thyroid hormone levels but will not affect the levels of unbound or free hormones in the blood, which are the effective forms. The level of thyroxine-binding globulin is lower in people who have kidney disease or who take anabolic steroids. The level is higher in women who are pregnant or taking oral contraceptives or other forms of estrogen and in people in the early stages of hepatitis.

If a doctor feels one or more growths (nodules) in the thyroid gland, he may order a scanning procedure. An ultrasound scan uses sound waves to measure the size of the gland and to determine whether the growth is solid or filled with fluid (cystic). A thyroid scan uses radioactive iodine or technetium and a device to produce a picture of the thyroid gland that will show any physical abnormalities. Thyroid scanning can also help determine whether the functioning of a specific area of the thyroid is normal, overactive, or underactive compared with the rest of the gland.

Additional testing may be necessary in rare cases in which a doctor cannot determine whether the problem lies in the thyroid or in the pituitary gland. One of these tests involves

Euthyroid Sick Syndrome

In euthyroid sick syndrome, thyroid test results are abnormal even though the thyroid gland is functioning normally.

Euthyroid sick syndrome commonly occurs in people who have a severe illness other than thyroid disease. When people are sick or malnourished or have had surgery, the thyroid hormone T_4 is not converted normally to the active T_3 hormone. Large amounts of reverse T_3, an inactive thyroid hormone, accumulate. Despite this abnormal conversion, the thyroid gland continues to function and to control the body's metabolic rate normally. Because no problem exists with the thyroid gland, no treatment is needed. Laboratory tests show normal results once the underlying illness resolves.

injecting thyrotropin-releasing hormone intravenously and then measuring the level of TSH in the blood to determine the pituitary gland's response. If cancer of the thyroid gland is suspected, a biopsy is performed. When medullary thyroid cancer is suspected, blood levels of calcitonin are checked, because these cancers always secrete calcitonin.

Hyperthyroidism

Hyperthyroidism is overactivity of the thyroid gland that leads to high levels of thyroid hormones and speeding up of vital body functions.

Hyperthyroidism affects about 1% of the U.S. population and can occur at any age but is more common in women during menopause and after childbirth.

Causes

Hyperthyroidism has several causes, including Graves' disease, thyroiditis, inflammation from toxic substances or radiation exposure, toxic thyroid nodules, and overstimulation due to an overactive pituitary gland.

Graves' disease, the most common cause of hyperthyroidism, is an autoimmune disorder caused by an abnormal protein (antibody) in the blood that stimulates the thyroid to produce and secrete excess thyroid hormones into the blood. This cause of hyperthyroidism is often hereditary, especially in women, and almost always leads to a diffusely enlarged thyroid. Graves' disease may go into spontaneous remission, and therapy is required only during the hyperthyroid phase.

Thyroiditis is inflammation of the thyroid gland. In subacute painful thyroiditis, subacute painless thyroiditis, and, much less often, Hashimoto's thyroiditis, as stored hormone is released from the inflamed gland, hyperthyroidism occurs. Hypothyroidism usually follows because the levels of stored hormones are depleted. Finally, the gland usually returns to normal function.

Inflammation from toxic substances or radiation exposure, like the three main types of thyroiditis, can also cause hyperthyroidism.

A **toxic thyroid nodule** (adenoma) is an area of abnormal local tissue growth within the thyroid gland. This abnormal tissue produces thyroid hormone even without stimulation by thyroid-stimulating hormone. Thus, a nodule escapes the mechanisms that normally control the thyroid gland and produces thyroid hormone in large quantities. Toxic multinodular goiter (Plummer's disease), in which there are many nodules, is uncommon in adolescents and young adults and tends to become more common with age.

An **overactive pituitary gland** can produce too much thyroid-stimulating hormone, which in turn leads to overproduction of thyroid hormone. However, this is an extremely rare cause of hyperthyroidism.

Symptoms

Most people with hyperthyroidism have an enlarged thyroid gland (goiter). The entire gland may be enlarged, or nodules may develop within certain areas. The gland may be tender and painful.

Symptoms of hyperthyroidism, regardless of the cause, reflect the speeding up of body functions: increased heart rate and blood pressure, abnormal heart rhythms (arrhythmias), excessive sweating, hand tremors (shakiness), nervousness and anxiety, difficulty sleeping (insomnia), weight loss despite increased appetite, increased activity level despite fatigue and weakness, and frequent bowel movements, occasionally with diarrhea. Older people with hyperthyroidism may not develop these characteristic symptoms but have what is sometimes called apathetic or masked hyperthyroidism, in which they become weak, sleepy,

confused, withdrawn, and depressed. Hyperthyroidism can cause changes in the eyes. A person with hyperthyroidism may appear to be staring.

If the cause of hyperthyroidism is Graves' disease, eye symptoms include puffiness around the eyes, increased tear formation, irritation, and unusual sensitivity to light. Two distinctive additional symptoms may occur: bulging eyes (exophthalmos)▲ and double vision (diplopia). The eyes bulge outward because of a substance that builds up in the orbits behind the eyes. The muscles that move the eyes become inflamed and unable to function properly, making it difficult or impossible to move the eyes normally or to coordinate eye movements, resulting in double vision. The eyelids may not close completely, exposing the eyes to injury from foreign particles and dryness. These eye changes may begin before any other symptoms of hyperthyroidism, providing an early clue to Graves' disease, but most often occur when other symptoms of hyperthyroidism are noticed. Eye symptoms may even appear or worsen after the excessive thyroid hormone secretion has been treated and controlled.

When Graves' disease affects the eyes, a substance similar to the one deposited behind the eyes is also occasionally deposited in the skin, usually over the shins. The thickened area may be itchy and red and feels hard when pressed with a finger. As with deposits behind the eyes, this problem may begin before or after other symptoms of hyperthyroidism are noticed.

Diagnosis

A doctor usually suspects hyperthyroidism on the basis of the symptoms. Blood tests are used to confirm the diagnosis. Often, testing begins with measurement of thyroid-stimulating hormone (TSH). If the thyroid gland is overactive, the level of TSH is low. However, in rare cases in which the pituitary gland is overactive, the level of TSH is normal or high. If the level of TSH in the serum is low, doctors measure the levels of the thyroid hormones in the blood. If there is a question of whether Graves' disease is the cause, doctors check a sample of blood for the presence of antithyroid antibodies. More specific antibodies can be measured, but such a test is rarely needed.

If a toxic thyroid nodule is suspected as the cause, a thyroid scan will show whether the nodule is overactive, that is, whether it is pro-

▲ see page 1319

Rx DRUGS USED TO TREAT HYPERTHYROIDISM

TYPE	DRUG	SELECTED SIDE EFFECTS	COMMENTS
Thionamides			
	Carbimazole Methimazole Propylthiouracil	Allergic reactions (usually skin rashes); nausea; loss of taste; infection (rare) due to a low white blood cell count; liver dysfunction	Decrease the production of thyroid hormone
Nonmetallic elements			
	Iodine	Skin rash	Decreases the production and release of thyroid hormone
Radioactive isotope			
	Radioactive iodine	Causes hypothyroidism	Destroys the thyroid gland
Beta-blockers			
	Atenolol Metoprolol Propranolol	In people with respiratory disease, may cause wheezing; can cause worsening of peripheral vascular disease and depression; may reduce blood pressure (hypotension)	Block many of the stimulating effects of excess thyroid hormone on other organs

ducing excess hormone. Such a scan may also help doctors in their evaluation of Graves' disease: In a person with Graves' disease, the scan shows the entire gland to be overactive, not just one area. In thyroiditis, the scan shows low activity.

Prognosis and Treatment

Treatment of hyperthyroidism depends on the cause. In most cases, the problem causing hyperthyroidism can be cured, or the symptoms can be eliminated or greatly reduced. If left untreated, however, hyperthyroidism places undue stress on the heart and many other organs.

Beta-blockers such as propranolol help control many of the symptoms of hyperthyroidism. These drugs can slow a fast heart rate, reduce tremors, and control anxiety. Doctors therefore find beta-blockers particularly useful for people with extreme hyperthyroidism and for people with bothersome or dangerous symptoms that have not responded to other treatments. However, beta-blockers do not control abnormal thyroid function. Therefore, they are given until other treat-

ments bring hormone production to normal levels.

Propylthiouracil or methimazole are the drugs most commonly used to treat hyperthyroidism; they work by decreasing the gland's production of thyroid hormone. Each drug is taken by mouth, beginning with high doses that are later adjusted according to blood test results. These drugs can usually control thyroid function in 6 to 12 weeks. Larger doses of these drugs may work more quickly but increase the risk of side effects. Pregnant women who take propylthiouracil or methimazole are closely monitored, because these drugs cross the placenta and can induce goiter or hypothyroidism in the fetus. Carbimazole, a drug that is widely used in Europe, is converted into methimazole in the body.

Iodine, given by mouth, is sometimes used to treat hyperthyroidism. It is reserved for those in whom rapid treatment is needed. It may also be used to control hyperthyroidism until the person can have surgery to remove the thyroid. It is not used long-term.

Radioactive iodine may be given by mouth to destroy part of the thyroid gland. Very little

Thyroid Storm

> Thyroid storm, which is sudden extreme overactivity of the thyroid gland, is a life-threatening emergency. All of the body functions are accelerated to dangerously high levels. Severe strain on the heart can lead to a life-threatening irregular heartbeat (arrhythmia), extremely fast pulse, and shock. Thyroid storm may also cause fever, extreme weakness and loss of muscle, restlessness, mood swings, confusion, altered consciousness (even coma), and an enlarged liver with mild jaundice (a yellowish discoloration of the skin and the whites of the eyes).
>
> Thyroid storm is generally caused by untreated or inadequately treated hyperthyroidism and can be triggered by infection, injury, surgery, poorly controlled diabetes, pregnancy or labor, discontinuance of thyroid drugs, or other stresses. It is rare in children.

radioactivity is introduced to the body as a whole but a great deal is delivered to the thyroid gland because the thyroid gland takes up the iodine and concentrates it. Hospitalization is rarely necessary. After treatment, the person should probably not be near infants and young children for 2 to 4 days. No special precautions are needed in the workplace. There are no precautions needed for sleeping with a partner. Pregnancy should be avoided for about 6 months.

Some doctors try to adjust the dose of radioactive iodine to destroy only enough of the thyroid gland to bring its hormone production back to normal, without reducing thyroid function too much; others use a larger dose to completely destroy the thyroid. Most of the time, people who undergo this treatment must take thyroid hormone replacement therapy for the rest of their lives.▲ Concern that radioactive iodine may cause cancer has never been confirmed. Radioactive iodine is not given to pregnant or nursing women, because it crosses the placenta and enters the milk and may destroy the fetus's or breastfed infant's thyroid gland.

Surgical removal of the thyroid gland, called thyroidectomy, is a treatment option for young people with hyperthyroidism. Surgery is also an option for people who have a very large goiter as well as for those who are allergic to or who develop severe side effects from the drugs used to treat hyperthyroidism. Hyperthyroidism is permanently controlled in more than 90% of those who choose this option. Hypothyroidism often occurs after surgery, and people then have to take replacement thyroid hormone for the rest of their lives. Rare complications of surgery include paralysis of the vocal cords and damage to the parathyroid glands (the tiny glands behind the thyroid gland that control calcium levels in the blood).

In Graves' disease, additional treatment may be needed for the eye and skin symptoms. Eye symptoms may be helped by elevating the head of the bed, by applying eye drops, by sleeping with the eyelids taped shut, and, occasionally, by taking diuretics (drugs that hasten fluid excretion). Double vision may be helped by using eyeglass prisms. Finally, corticosteroids taken by mouth, x-ray treatment to the orbits, or eye surgery may be needed if the eyes are severely affected. Corticosteroid creams or ointments can help relieve the itching and hardness of the abnormal skin. Often the problem disappears without treatment months or years later.

Hypothyroidism

Hypothyroidism is underactivity of the thyroid gland that leads to inadequate production of thyroid hormone and a slowing of vital body functions.

Hypothyroidism is common, especially among older people, particularly women; it affects about 10% of older women. It can, however, occur at any age. Very severe hypothyroidism is called myxedema.

Causes

Hypothyroidism has several causes. The most common cause is Hashimoto's thyroiditis.■ As the thyroid is gradually destroyed, hypothyroidism develops.

Subacute painless thyroiditis and subacute painful thyroiditis can both cause transient hypothyroidism. The hypothyroidism is transient because the thyroid is not destroyed.

Hypothyroidism can develop from complete lack of thyroid hormone production because of radioactive iodine or surgical removal of the thyroid gland, both of which are used to treat hyperthyroidism and thyroid cancer.

▲ see page 953   ■ see page 953

A chronic lack of iodine in the diet is the most common cause of hypothyroidism in many developing countries. However, this is rare in the United States because iodine is added to table salt; iodine is also used to sterilize the udders of dairy cattle and thus is present in dairy products. Rarer causes of hypothyroidism include some inherited disorders in which an abnormality of the enzymes in thyroid cells prevents the gland from making or secreting enough thyroid hormones. In other rare disorders, either the hypothalamus or the pituitary gland fails to secrete enough thyroid-stimulating hormone, which is necessary for normal stimulation of the thyroid.

Symptoms

Insufficient thyroid hormone causes body functions to slow. Symptoms are subtle and develop gradually. They may be mistaken for depression, especially among older people. Facial expressions become dull, the voice is hoarse and speech is slow, eyelids droop, and the eyes and face become puffy. Many people with hypothyroidism gain weight, become constipated, and are unable to tolerate cold. The hair becomes sparse, coarse, and dry, and the skin becomes coarse, dry, scaly, and thick. Some people develop carpal tunnel syndrome, which makes the hands tingle or hurt.▲ The pulse may slow, the palms and soles may appear slightly orange (carotenemia), and the side parts of the eyebrows slowly fall out. Some people, especially older people, may appear confused, forgetful, or demented—signs that can easily be mistaken for Alzheimer's disease or other forms of dementia.

If untreated, hypothyroidism can eventually cause anemia, a low body temperature, and heart failure. This situation may progress to confusion, stupor, or coma (myxedema coma), a life-threatening complication in which breathing slows, seizures occur, and blood flow to the brain decreases. Myxedema coma can be triggered in a person with hypothyroidism by physical stresses, such as exposure to the cold, as well as by an infection, injury, surgery, and drugs such as sedatives that depress brain function.

Diagnosis

Usually hypothyroidism can be diagnosed with one simple blood test: the measurement of thyroid-stimulating hormone. Many experts suggest that the test be performed at least every other year in people older than 55,

because hypothyroidism is so common among older people yet so difficult, in its mild stages, for doctors to distinguish from other disorders that affect people in this age group.

In those rare cases of hypothyroidism caused by inadequate secretion of thyroid-stimulating hormone, a second blood test is needed to measure the level of the thyroid hormone T_4 that is not bound by protein (free). A low level confirms the diagnosis of hypothyroidism.

Treatment

Treatment involves replacing thyroid hormone using one of several oral preparations. The preferred form of hormone replacement is synthetic T_4. Another form, desiccated (dried) thyroid, is obtained from the thyroid glands of animals. In general, desiccated thyroid is less satisfactory than synthetic T_4 because the content of thyroid hormones in the tablets may vary. In emergencies, such as myxedema coma, doctors may give synthetic T_4, T_3, or both intravenously.

Treatment begins with small doses of thyroid hormone, because too large a dose can cause serious side effects, although large doses may be necessary. The starting dose and the rate of increase are especially small in older people, who are often most at risk of side effects. The dose is gradually increased until the levels of thyroid-stimulating hormone in the person's blood return to normal. During pregnancy, doses may need to be adjusted.

Thyroiditis

Thyroiditis is inflammation of the thyroid gland.

The three types of thyroiditis are Hashimoto's thyroiditis (autoimmune thyroiditis), subacute painful thyroiditis (granulomatous thyroiditis), and subacute painless thyroiditis (silent lymphocytic thyroiditis, postpartum thyroiditis).

Hashimoto's Thyroiditis: Hashimoto's thyroiditis is the most common type of thyroiditis and the most common cause of hypothyroidism. For unknown reasons, the body turns against itself (an autoimmune reaction);■ the thyroid is invaded by white blood cells, and antibodies are created that attack the thyroid gland. Many people with Hashimoto's thyroiditis have other endocrine disorders, such

▲ see page 398   ■ see page 1073

as diabetes, an underactive adrenal gland, or underactive parathyroid glands, and other autoimmune diseases, such as pernicious anemia, rheumatoid arthritis, Sjögren's syndrome, or systemic lupus erythematosus (lupus).

Hashimoto's thyroiditis is most common among women, particularly older women, and tends to run in families. The condition occurs more frequently among people with certain chromosomal abnormalities, including Down, Turner's, and Klinefelter's syndromes.

Hashimoto's thyroiditis often begins with a painless, firm enlargement of the thyroid gland or a feeling of fullness in the neck. The gland usually has a rubbery texture and sometimes feels lumpy. In about 50% of people with Hashimoto's thyroiditis, the thyroid becomes underactive. In most of the rest, the thyroid remains normal. In a small number of people, the gland initially becomes overactive, after which it usually becomes underactive.

Doctors perform thyroid function tests on blood samples to determine whether the gland is functioning normally; however, the diagnosis is based on a physical examination and the results of a blood test to determine whether the person has antithyroid antibodies, which attack the thyroid gland. The level of thyroid-stimulating hormone (TSH) is measured to be sure that hypothyroidism is not present.

No specific treatment is available for Hashimoto's thyroiditis.

Most people eventually develop hypothyroidism and then must take thyroid hormone replacement therapy for the rest of their lives. Thyroid hormone may also be useful in reducing the size of the enlarged thyroid gland. People with Hashimoto's thyroiditis should avoid excess iodine (which can cause hypothyroidism) from natural sources, such as kelp tablets and seaweed.

Subacute Painful Thyroiditis: Subacute painful thyroiditis, which is probably caused by a virus, usually begins suddenly. In this disorder, inflammation causes the thyroid gland to release excessive amounts of thyroid hormones, resulting in hyperthyroidism, almost always followed by transient hypothyroidism and finally normal thyroid function.

Subacute painful thyroiditis often follows a viral illness and begins with what many people call a sore throat but actually proves to be neck pain localized to the thyroid. Many people with subacute painful thyroiditis feel extremely tired. The thyroid gland becomes increasingly tender, and the person usually develops a low-grade fever (99 to 101° F). The pain may shift from one side of the neck to the other, spread to the jaw and ears, and hurt more when the head is turned or when the person swallows. Subacute painful thyroiditis is often mistaken at first for a dental problem or a throat or ear infection.

Most people recover completely from this type of thyroiditis. Generally the thyroiditis resolves by itself within a few months, but sometimes it comes back or, more rarely, damages enough of the thyroid gland to cause permanent hypothyroidism.

Aspirin or other nonsteroidal anti-inflammatory drugs (NSAIDs) can relieve the pain and inflammation. In severe cases, a doctor may recommend corticosteroids, such as prednisone, which are tapered off over 6 to 8 weeks. When corticosteroids are discontinued abruptly or too early, symptoms often return in full force. When symptoms of hyperthyroidism are severe, a beta-blocker may be recommended.

Subacute Painless Thyroiditis: Subacute painless thyroiditis occurs most often among women, typically just after childbirth, and causes the thyroid to become enlarged without becoming tender. The disorder recurs with each subsequent pregnancy. For several weeks to several months, a person with subacute painless thyroiditis has hyperthyroidism followed by hypothyroidism before eventually recovering normal thyroid function.

Hyperthyroidism may require treatment for a few weeks, often with a beta-blocker, such as propranolol. During the period of hypothyroidism, the person may need to take thyroid hormone, usually for no longer than a few months. However, hypothyroidism becomes permanent in about 10% of people with subacute painless thyroiditis, and these people must take thyroid hormone for the rest of their lives.

Thyroid Cancer

The cause of thyroid cancer is not known, but the thyroid gland is very sensitive to radiation. Thyroid cancer is more common among people who were treated with radiation to the head, neck, or chest, most often for noncancerous (benign) conditions, when they were children (although radiation treatment for noncancerous conditions is no longer used).

Rather than causing the whole thyroid gland to enlarge, a cancer usually causes small growths (nodules) to develop within the thyroid. However, most thyroid nodules are not cancerous (malignant). Nodules are more likely to be cancerous if only one nodule is found rather than several, if the nodule is solid rather than filled with fluid (cystic), if the nodule is not producing much thyroid hormone, if the nodule is hard, if the nodule is growing quickly, or if the nodule occurs in a man.

A painless lump in the neck is usually the first sign of thyroid cancer. When doctors find a nodule in the thyroid gland, they request several tests. The first test is generally a measurement of the level of thyroid-stimulating hormone (TSH) in the blood to determine if hyperthyroidism is present. A thyroid scan determines whether the nodule is producing thyroid hormone and is done when the level of TSH is low. An ultrasound scan is less helpful but may be performed to determine whether the nodule is solid or filled with fluid or whether other nodules are present.

A fine-needle biopsy, in which a sample of the nodule is removed through a small needle and then examined under a microscope, is usually performed. This procedure is almost always painless, is carried out in the doctor's office, and may involve the use of a local anesthetic as well as ultrasound to guide needle placement.

Cancer can develop in any of several types of cells within the thyroid gland.

Papillary cancer is the most common type, accounting for 60 to 70% of all thyroid cancers. About 2 to 3 times as many women as men have papillary cancer. Papillary cancer is more common in young people but grows and spreads more quickly in older people. People who have received radiation treatment to the neck, usually for a noncancerous condition in infancy or childhood or for some other cancer in adulthood, are at greater risk of developing papillary cancer.

Papillary cancer grows within the thyroid gland but sometimes spreads (metastasizes) to nearby lymph nodes. If left untreated, papillary cancer may spread to more distant sites.

Papillary cancer is almost always curable. Nodules smaller than $3/4$ inch are removed along with the thyroid tissue immediately surrounding them, although some experts recommend removing the entire thyroid gland. For larger nodules, most or all of the thyroid gland is usually removed. Radioactive iodine is often given to destroy any remaining thyroid tissue or cancer. Thyroid hormone is also given in large doses to suppress the growth of any remaining thyroid tissue.

Follicular cancer accounts for about 15% of all thyroid cancers and is more common among older people. Follicular cancer is also more common in women than in men.

Much more aggressive than papillary cancer, follicular cancer tends to spread (metastasize) through the bloodstream, spreading cancerous cells to various parts of the body. Treatment for follicular cancer requires surgically removing as much of the thyroid gland as possible and destroying any remaining thyroid tissue, including the metastases, if present, with radioactive iodine. It is often curable, but less so than papillary cancer.

Anaplastic cancer accounts for less than 5% of thyroid cancers and is most common among older women. This cancer grows very quickly and usually causes a large growth in the neck. It also tends to spread throughout the body.

About 80% of people with anaplastic cancer die within 1 year, even with treatment. However, treatment with chemotherapy and radiation therapy before and after surgery has resulted in some cures. Radioactive iodine is not helpful in the treatment of this type of cancer.

Medullary cancer begins in the thyroid gland but in a different type of cell than that which produces thyroid hormone. The origin of this cancer is the C-cell, which is normally dispersed throughout the thyroid and secretes the hormone calcitonin. The cancer produces excessive amounts of calcitonin. Because medullary thyroid cancer can also produce other hormones, it can cause unusual symptoms.

This cancer tends to spread (metastasize) through the lymphatic vessels to the lymph nodes and through the blood to the liver, lungs, and bones. Medullary cancer can develop along with other types of endocrine cancers in what is called multiple endocrine neoplasia syndrome.▲

Treatment requires surgically removing the thyroid gland. Additional surgery may be needed to determine whether the cancer has spread to the lymph nodes. More than two thirds of people whose medullary thyroid cancer is part of multiple endocrine neoplasia syndrome are cured. When medullary thyroid cancer occurs alone, the chances of survival are not as good.

▲ see page 972

CHAPTER 164

Adrenal Gland Disorders

The body has two adrenal glands, one near the top of each kidney. The inner part (medulla) of the adrenal glands secretes hormones, such as adrenaline (epinephrine), that help control blood pressure, heart rate, sweating, and other activities also regulated by the sympathetic nervous system. The outer part (cortex) secretes different hormones, including corticosteroids (cortisone-like hormones, such as cortisol) and mineralocorticoids (particularly aldosterone, which controls blood pressure and the levels of salt and potassium in the body). The adrenal glands also play a role in stimulating the production of androgens (testosterone and similar hormones).

The adrenal glands are controlled in part by the brain. The hypothalamus, a small gland in the brain involved in hormonal regulation, produces corticotropin-releasing hormone and vasopressin. These two hormones trigger the pituitary gland to secrete corticotropin (also known as adrenocorticotropic hormone or ACTH), which stimulates the adrenal glands to produce corticosteroids. The renin-angiotensin-aldosterone system, regulated mostly by the kidneys, causes the adrenal glands to produce more or less aldosterone.

The body controls the levels of corticosteroids according to need. The levels tend to be much higher in the early morning than later in the day. When the body is stressed, from illness or otherwise, the levels of corticosteroids increase dramatically.

Addison's Disease

In Addison's disease, the adrenal glands are underactive, resulting in a deficiency of all adrenal hormones.

Addison's disease can start at any age and affects males and females about equally. In 70% of people with Addison's disease, the cause is not precisely known, but the adrenal glands are affected by an autoimmune reaction▲ in which the body's immune system attacks and destroys the adrenal cortex. In the other 30%, the adrenal glands are destroyed by cancer, an infection such as tuberculosis, or another identifiable disease. In infants and children, Addison's disease may be due to a genetic abnormality of the adrenal glands.

Secondary adrenal insufficiency is a term given to a disorder that resembles Addison's disease. In this disorder, the adrenal glands are underactive because the pituitary gland is not stimulating them, not because the adrenal glands have been destroyed or have otherwise directly failed.

When the adrenal glands become underactive, they tend to produce inadequate amounts of all of the adrenal hormones. Thus, Addison's disease affects the balance of water, sodium, and potassium in the body, as well as the body's ability to control blood pressure and react to stress. In addition, loss of androgens, such as dehydroepiandrosterone (DHEA), may cause a loss of body hair in women. In men, testosterone from the testes more than makes up for this loss. DHEA has additional effects that do not relate to androgens.

When the adrenal glands are destroyed by infection or cancer, the adrenal medulla and thus the source of epinephrine is lost. However, this loss does not cause symptoms.

A deficiency of aldosterone in particular causes the body to excrete large amounts of sodium and retain potassium, leading to low levels of sodium and high levels of potassium in the blood. The kidneys are not able to concentrate urine, so when a person with Addison's disease drinks too much water or loses too much sodium, the level of sodium in the blood falls. Inability to concentrate urine ultimately causes the person to urinate excessively and become dehydrated. Severe dehydration and a low sodium level reduce blood volume and can culminate in shock.

Corticosteroid deficiency leads to an extreme sensitivity to insulin so that the level of sugar in the blood may fall dangerously low. The deficiency prevents the body from manufacturing carbohydrates from protein, fighting infections, and healing wounds very well. Muscles weaken, and even the heart can become weak and unable to pump blood adequately. In addition, the blood pressure may become dangerously low.

▲ see page 1073

People with Addison's disease are not able to produce additional corticosteroids when they are stressed. They therefore are susceptible to serious symptoms and complications when confronted with illness, extreme fatigue, severe injury, surgery, or, possibly, severe psychologic stress.

In Addison's disease, the pituitary gland produces more corticotropin in an attempt to stimulate the adrenal glands. Corticotropin also stimulates melanin production, so dark pigmentation of the skin and the lining of the mouth often develop.

Symptoms

Soon after developing Addison's disease, a person feels weak, tired, and dizzy when standing up after sitting or lying down. These problems may develop gradually and insidiously. People with Addison's disease develop patches of dark skin; this darkness may seem like tanning, but it appears on areas not even exposed to the sun. Even people with dark skin can develop excessive pigmentation, although the change may be harder to recognize. Black freckles may develop over the forehead, face, and shoulders; a bluish black discoloration may develop around the nipples, lips, mouth, rectum, scrotum, or vagina.

Most people lose weight, become dehydrated, have no appetite, and develop muscle aches, nausea, vomiting, and diarrhea. Many become unable to tolerate cold. Unless the disease is severe, symptoms tend to become apparent only during times of stress. Periods of hypoglycemia, with nervousness and extreme hunger, can occur, particularly in children.

If Addison's disease is not treated, severe abdominal pains, profound weakness, extremely low blood pressure, kidney failure, and shock may occur (adrenal crisis). An adrenal crisis often occurs if the body is subjected to stress, such as an accident, injury, surgery, or severe infection. Death may quickly follow.

Diagnosis

Because the symptoms may start slowly and subtly, and because no single laboratory test is definitive in the early stages, doctors often do not suspect Addison's disease at the outset. Sometimes a major stress makes the symptoms more obvious and precipitates a crisis.

Blood tests may show low sodium and high potassium levels and usually indicate that the kidneys are not working well. A doctor who

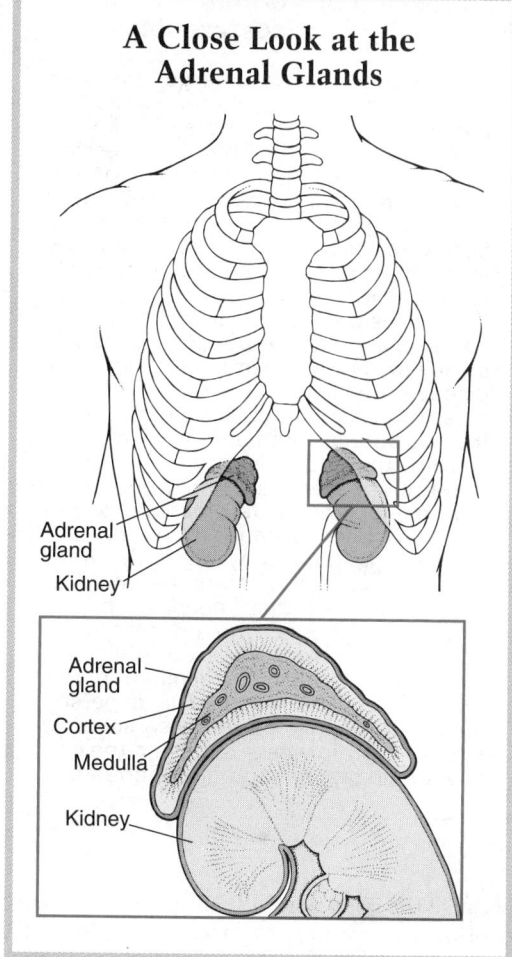

A Close Look at the Adrenal Glands

Adrenal gland

Kidney

Adrenal gland

Cortex

Medulla

Kidney

suspects Addison's disease measures cortisol levels, which may be low, and corticotropin levels, which may be high. However, a doctor usually confirms the diagnosis by measuring cortisol levels after they have been stimulated with corticotropin. If cortisol levels are low, further tests are needed to determine if the problem is Addison's disease or secondary adrenal insufficiency.

Treatment

Regardless of the cause, Addison's disease can be life threatening and must be treated with corticosteroids. Usually treatment can be started with hydrocortisone or prednisone (a synthetic corticosteroid) taken by mouth. However, people who are severely ill may be given cortisol intravenously or intramuscularly at first and then hydrocortisone tablets.

Suppression of Adrenal Function by Corticosteroids

In people who take large doses of corticosteroids, such as prednisone, the function of the adrenal glands can become suppressed. This suppression occurs because large doses of corticosteroids prevent the hypothalamus and pituitary glands from producing the hormones that normally stimulate adrenal function. If the person abruptly stops taking corticosteroids, the body cannot restore adrenal function quickly enough, and temporary adrenal insufficiency (a condition similar to Addison's disease) results. Also, when stress occurs, the body is not able to stimulate the additional production of corticosteroids that are needed.

Therefore, doctors never discontinue the use of corticosteroids abruptly if they have been taken for more than 2 or 3 weeks. Instead, they taper the dose over weeks and sometimes months. Also, the dose may need to be increased in people who become ill or otherwise severely stressed while taking corticosteroids. Corticosteroid use may need to be resumed in a person who becomes ill or otherwise severely stressed within weeks of having the corticosteroid tapered and discontinued.

Because the body normally produces most cortisol in the morning, replacement hydrocortisone should also be taken in divided doses, with the largest dose in the morning. Hydrocortisone will need to be taken every day for the rest of the person's life. Larger doses of hydrocortisone may be needed when the body is stressed, especially from an illness, and may need to be given by injection if the person has severe diarrhea or vomiting.

Most people also need to take fludrocortisone tablets every day to help restore the body's normal excretion of sodium and potassium. Supplemental testosterone is not usually needed, although there is some evidence that replacement with DHEA improves the quality of life. Although treatment must be continued for life, the outlook is excellent.

Cushing's Syndrome

In Cushing's syndrome, the level of corticosteroids is excessive, usually from overproduction by the adrenal glands.

The adrenal glands may overproduce corticosteroids because of a problem in the adrenal glands or because of too much stimulation from the pituitary gland. An abnormality in the pituitary gland, such as a tumor, can cause the pituitary to produce large amounts of corticotropin, the hormone that controls the production of corticosteroids from the adrenal glands. Tumors outside the pituitary gland, such as small-cell lung cancer, can produce corticotropin as well (a condition called ectopic corticotropin syndrome). Corticotropin may also be produced by a tumor called a carcinoid, which may occur almost anywhere in the body.

Sometimes a noncancerous tumor (adenoma) develops in the adrenal glands, which causes them to overproduce corticosteroids. Adrenal adenomas are extremely common; half of all people have them by the age of 70. Only a small fraction of adenomas produce excess hormone, however. Cancerous tumors of the adrenal glands are very rare.

Cushing's syndrome can also develop in people who must take large doses of corticosteroids because of a serious medical condition. Those who must take large doses have the same symptoms as those who produce too much of the hormone. The symptoms can occasionally occur even if the corticosteroids are inhaled, as for asthma, or are used topically for a skin condition.

Symptoms

Corticosteroids alter the amount and distribution of body fat. Excessive fat develops throughout the torso and may be particularly noticeable at the top of the back. A person with Cushing's syndrome usually has a large, round face (moon face). The arms and legs are usually slender in proportion to the thickened trunk. Muscles lose their bulk, leading to weakness. The skin becomes thin, bruises easily, and heals poorly when bruised or cut. Purple streaks that look like stretch marks may develop over the abdomen. People with Cushing's syndrome tend to tire easily.

High corticosteroid levels over time raise the blood pressure, weaken bones (osteoporosis), and diminish resistance to infections. The risk of developing kidney stones and diabetes is increased, and mental disturbances, including depression and hallucinations, may occur. Women usually have an irregular menstrual cycle. Children with Cushing's syndrome grow slowly and remain short. In some people, the adrenal glands also produce large amounts of androgens (testosterone and similar hormones), leading to increased facial and body hair in women, balding, and an increased sex drive.

Diagnosis

When doctors suspect Cushing's syndrome, they measure the level of cortisol, the main corticosteroid hormone, in the blood. Normally, cortisol levels are high in the morning and lower late in the day. In people who have Cushing's syndrome, cortisol levels are very high throughout the day.

If the cortisol levels are high, the doctor may recommend a dexamethasone suppression test. Dexamethasone suppresses the pituitary gland and should lead to suppression of cortisol secretion by the adrenal glands. If Cushing's syndrome is caused by too much pituitary stimulation, the level of cortisol will fall to some extent, although not as much as in people who do not have Cushing's syndrome. If Cushing's syndrome has another cause, the level of cortisol will remain high. A high corticotropin level further suggests overstimulation of the adrenal gland.

Other laboratory tests may be needed to determine the exact cause, including a computed tomography (CT) or magnetic resonance imaging (MRI) scan of the pituitary or adrenal glands and a chest x-ray or CT scan of the lungs; however, these tests often fail to find the tumor.

When overproduction of corticotropin is thought to be the cause, blood samples are taken from different parts of the body to determine the source.

Treatment

Treatment depends on whether the problem is in the adrenal glands, the pituitary gland, or elsewhere. Surgery or radiation therapy may be needed to remove or destroy a pituitary tumor. Tumors of the adrenal gland (usually adenomas) can often be removed surgically. Both adrenal glands may have to be removed if these treatments are not effective or if no tumor is present. People who have both adrenal glands removed, and many people who have part of their adrenal glands removed, must take corticosteroids for life. Tumors outside the pituitary and adrenal glands that secrete excess hormones are usually surgically removed. Certain drugs can lower cortisol levels and can be used while awaiting more definitive treatment such as surgery.

What Is Nelson's Syndrome?

People who have both their adrenal glands removed for Cushing's disease may develop Nelson's syndrome. In this disorder, a pituitary tumor develops, producing large amounts of corticotropin and other hormones that stimulate melanocytes, leading to darkening of the skin. The enlarging pituitary tumor may compress nearby structures in the brain, producing headaches and defects in vision. Some experts believe that this may be prevented, at least in some people, by radiation therapy to the pituitary gland. If necessary, Nelson's syndrome can be treated with radiation or surgical removal of the pituitary gland.

Virilization

Virilization is the development of exaggerated masculine characteristics, usually in women, often as a result of the adrenal glands overproducing androgens (testosterone and similar hormones).

The most common cause of virilization is an enlargement of the hormone-producing portions of the adrenal cortex (adrenal hyperplasia). Sometimes the cause is a small hormone-producing tumor (adenoma or cancer) in the gland. Occasionally, virilization occurs when a cancer outside the adrenal gland produces androgens. Athletes who take large amounts of androgens (anabolic steroids) to increase their muscle bulk may develop symptoms of virilization.▲ Cystic enlargement of the ovaries may cause virilization, but such cases are almost always mild. Sometimes an abnormality in an enzyme (a protein) in the adrenal glands can also produce virilization.

Symptoms and Diagnosis

Symptoms of virilization include excess facial and body hair (hirsutism), baldness, acne, deepening of the voice, increased muscularity, and an increased sex drive. In women, the uterus shrinks, the clitoris enlarges, the breasts become smaller, and normal menstruation stops.

The combination of body changes makes virilization relatively easy for a doctor to rec-

▲ see box on page 648

ognize. A test can determine the level of androgens in the blood. If the level is very high, a dexamethasone suppression test can help determine if the problem is coming from the adrenal glands and whether the problem is an adenoma or adrenal hyperplasia. If the problem is adrenal hyperplasia, dexamethasone prevents the adrenal glands from producing androgens. If the problem is an adenoma or cancer, dexamethasone reduces androgen production only partially or not at all. The doctor may also order a computed tomography (CT) or magnetic resonance imaging (MRI) scan to obtain a view of the adrenal glands. In women with cystic ovaries, the testosterone level may appear to be normal, but its binding protein is low so that the free (unbound) fraction is relatively high.

Treatment

Androgen-producing adenomas and adrenal cancers are usually treated by surgically removing the adrenal gland that contains the tumor. For adrenal hyperplasia, small amounts of corticosteroids, such as dexamethasone, generally reduce the production of androgens. The mild virilization caused by cystic ovaries may need no treatment. It can be treated with drugs that lower the free testosterone levels, such as oral contraceptives, or that block the effects of testosterone.

Hyperaldosteronism

In hyperaldosteronism, overproduction of aldosterone leads to fluid retention and increased blood pressure, weakness, and, rarely, periods of paralysis.

Aldosterone, a hormone produced and secreted by the adrenal glands, signals the kidneys to excrete less sodium and more potassium. Aldosterone production is regulated partly by corticotropin (secreted by the pituitary gland) and partly through the renin-angiotensin-aldosterone system.▲ Renin, an enzyme produced in the kidneys, controls the activation of the hormone angiotensin, which stimulates the adrenal glands to produce aldosterone.

Hyperaldosteronism can be caused by a tumor (usually a noncancerous adenoma) in the adrenal gland (a condition called Conn's syndrome), although sometimes both glands are involved and are overactive. Sometimes hyperaldosteronism is a response to certain diseases, such as very high blood pressure (hypertension) or narrowing of one of the arteries to the kidneys.

Symptoms and Diagnosis

High aldosterone levels can lead to low potassium levels. Low potassium levels often produce no symptoms but may lead to weakness, tingling, muscle spasms, and periods of temporary paralysis. Some people become extremely thirsty and urinate frequently.

A doctor who suspects hyperaldosteronism first tests the levels of sodium and potassium in the blood. The doctor may also measure aldosterone levels. If they are high, spironolactone, a drug that blocks the action of aldosterone, may be given to see if the levels of sodium and potassium return to normal. In Conn's syndrome, the levels of renin are also very low.

When too much aldosterone is being produced, doctors examine the adrenal glands for a noncancerous tumor (adenoma). Computed tomography (CT) or magnetic resonance imaging (MRI) can be helpful, but sometimes blood samples from different parts of the body must be tested to localize the source of the hormone.

Treatment

If a tumor is found, it can usually be surgically removed. When the tumor is removed, blood pressure returns to normal, and other symptoms disappear about 70% of the time. If no tumor is found and both glands are overactive, partial removal of the adrenal glands may not control high blood pressure, and complete removal will produce Addison's disease, requiring treatment for life. However, spironolactone can usually control the symptoms, and drugs for high blood pressure are readily available. Rarely do both adrenal glands have to be removed.

Pheochromocytoma

A pheochromocytoma is a tumor that usually originates from the adrenal glands' chromaffin cells, causing overproduction of catecholamines, powerful hormones that induce high blood pressure and other symptoms.

Pheochromocytomas may grow within the adrenal glands or in chromaffin cells outside the adrenal glands. Only 5% of pheochromo-

---

▲ see art on page 133

cytomas that grow within the adrenal glands are cancerous, but this percentage is higher for those outside the adrenal glands. Pheochromocytomas may occur in men or women at any age, but they are most common in people between the ages of 30 and 60.

Some people who develop pheochromocytomas have a rare inherited condition, called multiple endocrine neoplasia, that makes them prone to tumors in the thyroid, parathyroid, and adrenal glands.▲ Pheochromocytomas may also develop in people who have von Hippel-Lindau disease and in those who have neurofibromatosis (von Recklinghausen's disease).

Symptoms

Pheochromocytomas are usually very small. However, even a small pheochromocytoma can produce large amounts of potent catecholamines. Catecholamines are hormones such as adrenaline (epinephrine), norepinephrine, and dopamine, which tend to greatly increase blood pressure, heart rate, and other symptoms usually associated with life-threatening situations.

The most prominent symptom of a pheochromocytoma is high blood pressure, which may be very severe. Other symptoms include a fast and pounding heart rate, excessive sweating, light-headedness when standing, rapid breathing, cold and clammy skin, severe headaches, chest and stomach pain, nausea, vomiting, visual disturbances, tingling fingers, constipation, and an odd sense of impending doom. When these symptoms appear suddenly and forcefully, they can feel like a panic attack. In half of the people, symptoms come and go, sometimes triggered by pressure on the tumor, massage, drugs (especially anesthesia and beta-blocking drugs), emotional trauma, and, on rare occasions, the simple act of urination. However, many people may have these symptoms as manifestations of an anxiety state, not a glandular disorder.

Diagnosis

A doctor may not suspect a pheochromocytoma, because almost half of the people have no symptoms other than persistent high blood pressure. However, when high blood pressure occurs in a young person, comes and goes, or accompanies other symptoms of pheochromocytoma, the doctor may request certain labo-

Eating Real Licorice

Eating large amounts of real licorice can produce all the symptoms of hyperaldosteronism. Real licorice contains a chemical that can act like aldosterone; however, most candy sold as licorice contains little or no real licorice.

ratory tests. For example, the level of certain catecholamines may be measured in blood or urine samples. Because of high blood pressure and other symptoms, a doctor may prescribe a beta-blocker before knowing that the cause is a pheochromocytoma. Beta-blockers can make high blood pressure worse in people with pheochromocytoma. This paradoxical reaction often makes the diagnosis of pheochromocytoma clear.

If the level of catecholamines is high, a computed tomography (CT) or magnetic resonance imaging (MRI) scan can help locate the pheochromocytoma. A test using injected radioactive chemicals that tend to accumulate in pheochromocytomas is also useful. A scan is then performed to see where the radioactive chemicals are.

Treatment

Usually the best treatment is to remove the pheochromocytoma. Surgery is often delayed, however, until a doctor can bring the tumor's secretion of catecholamines under control with drugs, because having high levels of catecholamines can be dangerous during surgery. Phenoxybenzamine is generally given to stop hormone secretion. Once this step is accomplished, a beta-blocker can safely be given to further control symptoms.

If the pheochromocytoma is cancerous and has spread, chemotherapy with cyclophosphamide, vincristine, and dacarbazine may help slow the tumor's growth. Treatment with a radioisotope known as MIBG that targets the tumor tissue can also be highly effective. The dangerous effects of the excess catecholamines secreted by the tumor can almost always be blocked by continuing to take phenoxybenzamine or a similar drug and beta-blockers.

▲ see page 972

CHAPTER 165

Diabetes Mellitus

Diabetes mellitus is a disorder in which blood sugar (glucose) levels are abnormally high because the body does not produce enough insulin.

Insulin, a hormone released from the pancreas, controls the amount of sugar in the blood. When a person eats or drinks, food is broken down into materials, including sugar, that the body needs to function. Sugar is absorbed into the bloodstream and stimulates the pancreas to produce insulin. Insulin allows sugar to move from the blood into the cells. Once inside the cells, sugar is converted to energy, which is either used immediately or stored until it is needed.

The levels of sugar in the blood vary normally throughout the day. They rise after a meal and return to normal within about 2 hours after eating. Once the levels of sugar in the blood return to normal, insulin production decreases. The variation in blood sugar levels is usually within a narrow range, about 70 to 110 milligrams per deciliter (mg/dL) of blood. If a person has eaten a large amount of carbohydrates, the levels may increase more. People older than 65 years tend to have slightly higher levels, especially after eating.

If the body does not produce enough insulin to move the sugar into the cells, the resulting high levels of sugar in the blood and the inadequate amount of sugar in the cells together produce the symptoms and complications of diabetes.

Doctors often use the full name diabetes mellitus, rather than diabetes alone, to distinguish this disorder from diabetes insipidus, a relatively rare disease that does not affect blood sugar levels.▲

Types

Type 1: In type 1 diabetes (formerly called insulin-dependent diabetes or juvenile-onset diabetes), more than 90% of the insulin-producing cells of the pancreas are permanently destroyed. The pancreas, therefore, produces little or no insulin. Only about 10% of all people with diabetes have type 1 disease. Most people who have type 1 diabetes develop the disease before age 30.

Scientists believe that an environmental factor—possibly a viral infection or a nutritional factor in childhood or early adulthood—causes the immune system to destroy the insulin-producing cells of the pancreas. A genetic predisposition may make some people more susceptible to the environmental factor.

Type 2: In type 2 diabetes (formerly called non–insulin-dependent diabetes or adult-onset diabetes), the pancreas continues to produce insulin, sometimes even at higher-than-normal levels. However, the body develops resistance to the effects of insulin, so there is not enough insulin to meet the body's needs.

Type 2 diabetes may occur in children and adolescents, but usually begins in people older than 30 and becomes progressively more common with age. About 15% of people older than 70 have type 2 diabetes. Certain racial and cultural groups are at increased risk of developing type 2 diabetes: blacks and Hispanics who live in the United States have a twofold to threefold increased risk. Type 2 diabetes also tends to run in families.

Obesity is the chief risk factor for developing type 2 diabetes, and 80 to 90% of people with this disease are obese. Because obesity causes insulin resistance, obese people need very large amounts of insulin to maintain normal blood sugar levels.

Certain diseases and drugs can affect the way the body uses insulin and can lead to type 2 diabetes. High levels of corticosteroids (from Cushing's disease or from taking corticosteroid drugs) and pregnancy (gestational diabetes)■ are the most common causes of altered insulin use. Diabetes also may occur in people with excess production of growth hormone (acromegaly) and in people with certain hormone-secreting tumors. Severe or recurring pancreatitis and other diseases that directly damage the pancreas can lead to diabetes.

Symptoms

The two types of diabetes have very similar symptoms. The first symptoms are related to the direct effects of high blood sugar levels.

▲ see page 944   ■ see page 1452

LONG-TERM COMPLICATIONS OF DIABETES

TISSUE OR ORGAN AFFECTED	WHAT HAPPENS	COMPLICATIONS
Blood vessels	Atherosclerotic plaque builds up and blocks large or medium-sized arteries in the heart, brain, legs, and penis. The walls of small blood vessels are damaged so that the vessels do not transfer oxygen normally and may leak	Poor circulation causes wounds to heal poorly and can lead to heart disease, stroke, gangrene of the feet and hands, erectile dysfunction (impotence), and infections
Eyes	The small blood vessels of the retina become damaged	Decreased vision and, ultimately, blindness
Kidney	Blood vessels in the kidney thicken; protein leaks into the urine; the blood is not filtered normally	Poor kidney function; kidney failure
Nerves	Nerves are damaged because glucose is not metabolized normally and because the blood supply is inadequate	Sudden or gradual weakness of a leg; reduced sensations, tingling, and pain in the hands and feet; chronic damage to nerves
Autonomic nervous system	The nerves that control blood pressure and digestive processes become damaged	Swings in blood pressure; swallowing difficulties and altered digestive function, with bouts of diarrhea
Skin	Poor blood flow to the skin and loss of feeling result in repeated injury	Sores, deep infections (diabetic ulcers); poor healing
Blood	White blood cell function is impaired	Increased susceptibility to infection, especially of the urinary tract and skin
Connective tissue	Glucose is not metabolized normally, causing tissues to thicken or contract	Carpal tunnel syndrome; Dupuytren's contracture

When the blood sugar level rises above 160 to 180 mg/dL, sugar spills into the urine. When the level of sugar in the urine rises even higher, the kidneys excrete additional water to dilute the large amount of sugar. Because the kidneys produce excessive urine, a person with diabetes urinates large volumes frequently (polyuria). The excessive urination creates abnormal thirst (polydipsia). Because excessive calories are lost in the urine, the person loses weight. To compensate, the person often feels excessively hungry. Other symptoms include blurred vision, drowsiness, nausea, and decreased endurance during exercise.

Type 1: In people with type 1 diabetes, the symptoms often begin abruptly and dramatically. A condition called **diabetic ketoacidosis** may quickly develop. Without insulin, most cells cannot use the sugar that is in the blood. Cells still need energy to survive, and they switch to a back-up mechanism to obtain energy. Fat cells begin to break down, producing compounds called ketones. Ketones provide some energy to cells but also make the blood too acidic (ketoacidosis). The initial symptoms of diabetic ketoacidosis include excessive thirst and urination, weight loss, nausea, vomiting, fatigue, and—particularly in children—abdominal pain. Breathing tends to become deep and rapid as the body attempts to correct the blood's acidity.▲ The person's breath smells like nail polish remover, the smell of the ketones escaping into the breath. Without treatment, diabetic ketoacidosis can progress to coma and death, sometimes within a few hours.

Type 2: People with type 2 diabetes may not have any symptoms for years or decades before

▲ see page 931

they are diagnosed. Symptoms may be subtle. Increased urination and thirst are mild at first and gradually worsen over weeks or months. Eventually, the person feels extremely fatigued, is likely to develop blurred vision, and may become dehydrated.

Sometimes during the early stages of diabetes, the blood sugar level is abnormally low, a condition called hypoglycemia.▲

Because people with type 2 diabetes produce some insulin, ketoacidosis does not usually develop. However, the blood sugar levels can become extremely high (often exceeding 1,000 mg/dL). Such high levels often happen as the result of some superimposed stress, such as an infection or drug use. When the blood sugar levels get very high, the person may develop severe dehydration, which may lead to mental confusion, drowsiness, and seizures, a condition called nonketotic hyperglycemic-hyperosmolar coma.

Complications

People with diabetes may experience many serious, long-term complications. Some of these complications begin within months of the onset of diabetes, although most tend to develop after a few years. Most of the complications are progressive. The more tightly a person with diabetes is able to control the levels of sugar in the blood, the less likely it is that these complications will develop or become worse.

High sugar levels cause narrowing of both the small and large blood vessels. Complex sugar-based substances build up in the walls of small blood vessels, causing them to thicken and leak. As they thicken, they supply less blood, especially to the skin and nerves. Poor control of blood sugar levels also tends to cause the levels of fatty substances in the blood to rise, resulting in atherosclerosis■ and decreased blood flow in the larger blood vessels. Atherosclerosis is between 2 and 6 times more common in people with diabetes than in people who do not have the disease and tends to occur at younger ages.

Over time, elevated levels of sugar in the blood and poor circulation can harm the heart, brain, legs, eyes, kidneys, nerves, and skin, resulting in angina, heart failure, strokes, leg cramps on walking (claudication), poor vision,

renal failure, damage to nerves (neuropathy), and skin breakdown. Heart attacks and strokes are more common among people with diabetes.

Poor circulation to the skin can lead to ulcers and infections, and all wounds heal slowly. People with diabetes are particularly likely to have ulcers and infections of the feet and legs. Too often, these wounds heal slowly or not at all, and amputation of the foot or part of the leg may be needed.

People with diabetes often develop bacterial and fungal infections, typically of the skin. When the levels of sugar in the blood are high, white blood cells cannot effectively fight infections. Any infection that develops tends to be more severe.

Damage to the blood vessels of the eye can cause loss of vision (diabetic retinopathy).★ Laser surgery can seal the leaking blood vessels of the eye and prevent permanent damage to the retina. Therefore, people with diabetes should have yearly eye examinations to check for damage.

The kidneys can malfunction, resulting in kidney failure that may require dialysis or kidney transplantation. Doctors usually check the urine of people with diabetes for abnormally high levels of protein (albumin), which is an early sign of kidney damage. At the earliest sign of kidney complications, the person is often given angiotensin-converting enzyme (ACE) inhibitors, drugs that slow the progression of kidney disease.

Damage to nerves can manifest in several ways. If a single nerve malfunctions, an arm or leg may suddenly become weak. If the nerves to the hands, legs, and feet become damaged (diabetic polyneuropathy), sensation may become abnormal, and tingling or burning pain and weakness in the arms and legs may develop.● Damage to the nerves of the skin makes repeated injuries more likely because the person cannot sense changes in pressure or temperature.

Diagnosis

The diagnosis of diabetes is made when a person has abnormally high levels of sugar in the blood. Blood sugar levels are often checked during a routine physical examination. Checking the levels of sugar in the blood annually is particularly important in older people, because diabetes is so common in later life. A person may have diabetes, particularly type 2 diabetes, and not know it. A doctor may also

---

▲ see page 970 ■ see page 194
★ see page 1313 ● see page 584

check blood sugar levels if a person has increased thirst, urination, or hunger; frequent infections; or signs of any of the complications associated with diabetes.

To measure the blood sugar levels, a blood sample is usually taken after the person has fasted overnight. However, it is possible to take the blood sample after the person has eaten. Some elevation of blood sugar levels after eating is normal, but even after a meal the levels should not be very high. Fasting blood sugar levels should never be higher than 126 mg/dL. Even after eating, blood sugar levels should not be higher than 200 mg/dL.

Doctors can also measure the level of a protein in the blood, hemoglobin A_{1C} (also called glycolated or glycosylated hemoglobin). This test is most useful in confirming the diagnosis in adults in whom the levels of sugar in the blood are only mildly elevated.▲

Another kind of blood test, an oral glucose tolerance test, may be performed in certain situations, such as when a doctor suspects that a pregnant woman has gestational diabetes■ or in older people who have symptoms of diabetes but normal glucose levels when fasting. However, it is not routinely used for testing for diabetes. In this test, a person fasts, has a blood sample taken to determine the fasting blood sugar level, and then drinks a special solution containing a large, standard amount of glucose. More blood samples are then obtained over the next 2 to 3 hours and are tested to determine whether the level of sugar in the blood rises abnormally high.

Treatment

Treatment of diabetes involves diet, exercise, education, and, for most people, drugs. If a person with diabetes keeps blood sugar levels tightly controlled, complications are less likely to develop. The goal of diabetes treatment, therefore, is to keep blood sugar levels within the normal range as much as possible. Treatment of high blood pressure and cholesterol levels can prevent some of the complications of diabetes as well. A low dose of aspirin taken daily is also helpful.

People with diabetes benefit greatly from learning about the disease, understanding how diet and exercise affect their blood sugar levels, and knowing how to avoid complications. A nurse trained in diabetes education can provide information.

People with diabetes should always carry or wear a medical identification bracelet or tag to

The Foot in Diabetes

Diabetes causes many changes in the body. The following changes in the feet are common and difficult to treat.

- Neuropathy (damage to the nerves) affects sensation to the feet, so that pain is not felt. Irritation and other forms of injury may go unnoticed; an injury may wear through the skin before any pain is felt.

- Other changes in sensation alter the way people with diabetes carry weight on their feet, concentrating weight in certain areas so that calluses form. Calluses (along with dry skin) increase the risk of skin breakdown.

- Diabetes can cause poor circulation in the feet, making it more likely that ulcers will form when the skin is damaged and making the ulcers slower to heal.

In addition to the changes in the foot, diabetes can affect the body's ability to fight infections. Therefore, once an ulcer forms, it easily becomes infected; the infection may become serious and difficult to treat, leading to gangrene. People with diabetes are more than 30 times more likely to require an amputation of a foot or leg than are people without diabetes.

Foot care is critical.★ The feet should be protected from injury, and the skin should be kept moist with a good skin moisturizer. Shoes should fit properly and not cause areas of irritation. Shoes should have appropriate cushioning to spread out the pressure caused by standing. Going barefoot is ill advised. Regular care from a podiatrist, such as having toenails cut and calluses removed, may also be helpful. Also, sensation and blood flow to the feet should be regularly evaluated by a doctor.

alert health care professionals to the presence of diabetes. This information allows health care professionals to start life-saving treatment quickly, especially in the case of injury or altered mental status.

Diet management is very important in people with both types of diabetes. Doctors rec-

▲ see page 969   ■ see page 1452

★ see also box on page 222

ommend a healthy, balanced diet and efforts to maintain a healthy weight. Some people benefit from meeting with a dietitian to develop an optimal eating plan.

People with type 1 diabetes who are able to maintain a healthy weight may be able to avoid the need for large doses of insulin. People with type 2 diabetes may be able to avoid the need for all drugs by achieving and maintaining a healthy weight. In general, people with diabetes should not eat much sweet food. They should also try to eat meals on a regular schedule; long periods between eating should be avoided. People with diabetes also tend to have high levels of cholesterol in the blood, so limiting the amount of saturated fat in the diet is important. Drugs may also be needed to help control the level of cholesterol in the blood.

Appropriate amounts of exercise can also help people control their weight and maintain blood sugar levels within the normal range.

Keeping blood sugar levels from getting too high is difficult. The main difficulty with trying to tightly control the levels of sugar in the blood is that low blood sugar levels (hypoglycemia) may occur.▲ Treatment of hypoglycemia is an emergency. Sugar must get into the body within minutes to prevent permanent harm and relieve symptoms. Most of the time, the diabetic person can eat sugar. Almost any form of sugar will do, although glucose works more quickly than table sugar (typical table sugar is sucrose). Many people with diabetes carry glucose tablets or foil packets of a glucose-containing liquid. Other options are to drink a glass of milk (which contains lactose, a type of sugar), sugar water, or fruit juice or to eat a piece of cake, some fruit, or another sweet food. In more serious situations, it may be necessary for an emergency medical professional to inject glucose into a vein.

Another treatment for hypoglycemia involves the use of glucagon. Glucagon can be injected into the muscle and causes the liver to release large amounts of glucose within minutes. Small transportable kits containing a syringe filled with glucagon are available for people with diabetes to use in emergency situations.

Diabetic ketoacidosis is also a medical emergency, because it can cause coma and death. Hospitalization, usually in an intensive care unit, is necessary. Large amounts of fluids are given intravenously along with electrolytes, such as sodium, potassium, chloride, and phosphate, to replace those lost through excessive urination. Insulin is generally given intravenously so that it works quickly and the dose can be adjusted frequently. Levels of sugar, ketones, and electrolytes are measured every few hours. Doctors also measure the blood's acid level. Sometimes, additional treatments are needed to correct a high acid level. However, controlling the levels of sugar in the blood and replacing electrolytes usually allow the body to restore the normal acid-base balance.

The treatment of nonketotic hyperglycemic-hyperosmolar coma is similar to that of diabetic ketoacidosis. Fluids and electrolytes must be replaced. The levels of sugar in the blood must be restored to normal levels gradually to avoid sudden shifts of fluid into the brain. The blood sugar levels tend to be more easily controlled than in diabetic ketoacidosis, and blood acidity problems are not severe.

Insulin Replacement Therapy

People with type 1 diabetes almost always require insulin therapy, and many people with type 2 diabetes require it as well. Insulin is usually injected; it currently cannot be taken by mouth because insulin is destroyed in the stomach. New forms of insulin, such as a nasal spray and a form that can be taken by mouth, are being tested.

Insulin is injected under the skin into the fat layer, usually in the arm, thigh, or abdominal wall. Small syringes with very thin needles make the injections nearly painless. An air pump device that blows the insulin under the skin can be used for people who cannot tolerate needles. An insulin pen, which contains a cartridge that holds the insulin, is a convenient way for many people to carry insulin, especially for those who take several injections a day outside the home. Another device is an insulin pump, which pumps insulin continuously from a reservoir through a small needle left in the skin. Additional doses of insulin can be released at programmed times, or release can be triggered as needed; the pump more closely mimics the way the body normally produces insulin. For some people, the pump offers an added degree of control, whereas others find wearing the pump annoying or develop sores at the needle site.

▲ see page 970

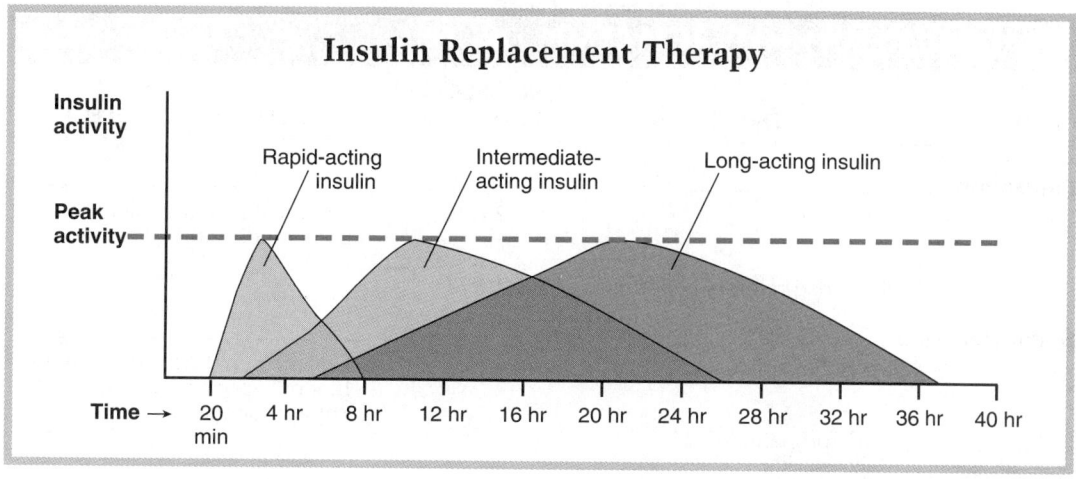

The easiest regimen to follow is a single
daily injection of an intermediate-acting insulin. However, such a regimen provides the
least control over blood sugar levels and is,
therefore, rarely the best approach. Tighter
control may be achieved by combining two
insulins—a rapid-acting and an intermediate-
acting insulin—in one morning dose. This
combination requires more skill, but it offers
the person greater opportunity to adjust the
blood sugar levels. A second injection of one
insulin or both may be taken at dinner or at
bedtime. Tightest control is usually achieved
by injecting a rapid-acting and an intermediate-acting insulin in the morning and evening
along with several additional injections of
rapid-acting insulin during the day. Adjustments can be made as the person's insulin
needs change. Although this regimen requires
the most knowledge of the disease and attention to the details of treatment, it is considered the best option for most people who are
treated with insulin.

Some people, especially older people, take
the same amount of insulin every day; others
adjust the insulin dose daily depending on
their diet, exercise, and blood sugar patterns.
In addition, insulin needs may change if a
person experiences weight changes, emotional
stress, or illness, especially infection.

Over time, some people develop resistance
to insulin. Because the injected insulin is not
exactly like the insulin the body manufactures, the body can produce antibodies to the
insulin. These antibodies interfere with the

Insulin is available in three basic forms,
each with a different speed of onset and duration of action. Rapid-acting insulin, such as
regular insulin, is the fastest and shortest acting. Lispro insulin, a type of regular insulin, is
the fastest of all. Rapid-acting insulin is often
used by people who take several daily injections and is injected 15 to 20 minutes before
meals or just after eating. It reaches its maximum activity in 2 to 4 hours and works for 6
to 8 hours.

Intermediate-acting insulin (such as insulin
zinc suspension, lente, or isophane insulin
suspension) starts to work in 1 to 3 hours,
reaches its maximum activity in 6 to 10 hours,
and works for 18 to 26 hours. This type of insulin may be used in the morning to provide
coverage for the first part of the day or in the
evening to provide coverage during the night.
Long-acting insulin (such as extended insulin
zinc suspension, ultra-lente, or glargine) has
very little effect for about 6 hours but provides
coverage for 28 to 36 hours.

Insulin preparations are stable at room temperature for months, allowing them to be carried, brought to work, or taken on a trip. Insulin should not, however, be exposed to
extreme temperatures.

The choice of insulin is complex. The following factors are considered before deciding
which insulin is best:

• How willing and able the person is to
monitor the blood sugar levels and adjust the
insulin dosage

• How varied the person's daily activity is

• How adept the person is at learning about
and understanding the disease

• How stable the person's blood sugar levels
are during the day and from day to day

Ｒ ORAL ANTIHYPERGLYCEMIC DRUGS

CLASS	DRUG	NUMBER OF DAILY DOSES	SELECTED SIDE EFFECTS
Biguanides			
	Metformin	2 to 3	Diarrhea; increased acidity of body fluids (rare); liver failure (rare)
	Extended-release metformin	1 to 2	
Sulfonylureas			
	Acetohexamide	1 to 2	Weight gain; low sodium in blood (hyponatremia) with chlorpropamide
	Chlorpropamide	1	
	Glimepiride	1	
	Glipizide	1 to 2	
	Glyburide	1 to 2	
	Micronized glyburide	1 to 2	
	Tolazamide	1 to 2	
	Tolbutamide	1 to 2	
Meglitinides			
	Nateglinide	3	Weight gain
	Repaglinide	3	
Thiazolidinediones			
	Pioglitazone	1	Weight gain; fluid retention (edema)
	Rosiglitazone	1 to 2	
Glucosidase inhibitors			
	Acarbose	3	Diarrhea; abdominal pain; bloating
	Miglitol	3	

insulin's activity, so a person with insulin resistance must take very large doses.

Insulin injections can affect the skin and underlying tissues. An allergic reaction, which occurs rarely, produces pain and burning, followed by redness, itchiness, and swelling around the injection site for several hours. More commonly, the injections either cause fat deposits, making the skin look lumpy, or destroy fat, causing indentation of the skin. Many people rotate the injection sites, for example, using the thigh one day, the stomach another, and an arm the next, to avoid these problems.

Oral Antihyperglycemic Drugs

Oral antihyperglycemic drugs can often lower blood sugar levels adequately in people with type 2 diabetes. However, they are not effective in type 1 diabetes. There are several types. Sulfonylureas (for example, glyburide) and meglitinides (for example, repaglinide) stimulate the pancreas to produce more insulin (insulin secretagogues). Biguanides (for example, metformin) and thiazolidinediones (for example, rosiglitazone) do not affect the release of insulin but increase the body's response to it (insulin sensitizers). A doctor may prescribe one of these drugs alone or with a sulfonylurea drug. Another class of drug is the glucosidase inhibitors, such as acarbose, which work by delaying absorption of glucose in the intestine.

Oral antihyperglycemic drugs are usually prescribed for people with type 2 diabetes if diet and exercise fail to lower the levels of sugar in the blood adequately. The drugs are sometimes taken only once a day, in the morning, although some people need two or three doses. More than one type of oral drug may be used if one is not adequate. If oral anti-hyperglycemic drugs cannot control blood sugar levels well enough, insulin injections alone or in combination with the oral drugs may be needed.

Monitoring Treatment

Monitoring blood sugar levels is an essential part of diabetes care. People with diabetes must adjust their diet, exercise, and drugs to control blood sugar levels. Monitoring blood sugar levels provides the information needed to make those adjustments. Waiting until symptoms of low or high blood sugar levels develop is a recipe for disaster.

Many things cause blood sugar levels to change: diet, exercise, stress, illness, drugs, and even the time of day. The blood sugar levels may jump after a person eats foods he did not realize were high in carbohydrates. Exercise may cause the levels of sugar in the blood to fall low, requiring that additional sugar be eaten. Emotional stress, an infection, and many drugs tend to increase blood sugar levels. Blood sugar levels increase in many people in the early morning hours because of the normal release of hormones (growth hormone and corticosteroids), a reaction called the dawn phenomenon. And blood sugar may shoot too high if the body releases sugar in response to low blood sugar levels (Somogyi effect).

Blood sugar levels can be measured easily at home or anywhere. Most blood sugar monitoring devices use a drop of blood obtained by pricking the tip of the finger with a small lancet. The lancet holds a tiny needle that can be jabbed into the finger or placed in a spring-loaded device that easily and quickly pierces the skin. Most people find the pricking nearly painless. Then, a drop of blood is placed on a reagent strip. In response to sugar, the reagent strip undergoes some chemical changes. A machine reads the changes in the test strip and reports the result on a digital display. Most of these machines time the reaction and read the result automatically. The machines are smaller than a deck of cards.

A new device reads blood sugar through the skin without needing a sample of blood. The device is worn like a wristwatch and can measure the level of sugar in the blood every 15 minutes. Alarms on the device can be set to sound when blood sugar levels drop too low or climb too high. Disadvantages of this device are that it must be calibrated periodically with a blood test, it may irritate the skin, and it is somewhat large.

Most people with diabetes should keep a record of their blood sugar levels and report them to their doctor or nurse for advice in adjusting the dose of insulin or the oral anti-hyperglycemic drug. Many people can learn to adjust the insulin dose on their own as necessary.

Although urine can also be tested for the presence of sugar, checking urine is not a good way to monitor treatment or adjust therapy. Urine testing can be misleading because the amount of sugar in the urine may not reflect the current level of sugar in the blood. Blood sugar levels can get very low or reasonably high without any change in the sugar levels in the urine.

Doctors can monitor treatment using a blood test called hemoglobin A_{1C}. When the blood sugar levels are high, changes occur in hemoglobin, the protein that carries oxygen in the blood. These changes are in direct proportion to the blood sugar levels over an extended period. Thus, unlike the blood sugar measurement, which reveals the level at a particular moment, the hemoglobin A_{1C} measurement demonstrates whether the blood sugar levels have been controlled over the previous few weeks. The normal level for hemoglobin A_{1C} is less than 7%. People with diabetes rarely achieve such levels, but tight control aims to come close. Levels above 9% show poor control, and levels above 12% show very poor control. Most doctors who specialize in diabetes care recommend that hemoglobin A_{1C} be measured every 3 to 6 months. Fructosamine, a glycolated amino acid, is also useful for measuring glucose control over a period of a few weeks.

Experimental Treatments

Experimental treatments are also showing promise for the treatment of type 1 diabetes. In one such treatment, insulin-producing cells are transplanted into body organs. This procedure is not yet routinely performed, however, because immunosuppressant drugs must be given to prevent the body from rejecting the transplanted cells. Newer techniques may make suppression of the immune system unnecessary.

Hypoglycemia

Hypoglycemia is abnormally low levels of sugar (glucose) in the blood.

Normally, the body maintains the levels of sugar in the blood within a range of about 70 to 110 milligrams per deciliter (mg/dL) of blood. In hypoglycemia, the sugar levels in the blood become too low. In diabetes mellitus, the sugar levels in the blood become too high, a condition called hyperglycemia. Although diabetes is characterized by high levels of sugar in the blood, many people with diabetes periodically experience hypoglycemia. Hypoglycemia is uncommon among people without diabetes.

Low levels of sugar in the blood interfere with the function of many organ systems. The brain is particularly sensitive to low sugar levels, because sugar is the brain's major energy source. If the sugar levels in the blood fall far below their usual range, the brain responds by stimulating the adrenal glands to release epinephrine (adrenaline), the pancreas to release glucagon, and the pituitary gland to release growth hormone, all of which cause the liver to release sugar into the blood.

Causes

Drugs: Most cases of hypoglycemia occur in people with diabetes and are caused by the insulin or other drugs (for example, sulfonylureas) they take to lower the levels of sugar in their blood. People with diabetes sometimes call the hypoglycemia that can occur after taking insulin an "insulin reaction" or "being shaky." Insulin reactions are more common when intense efforts are made to keep the sugar levels in the blood as close to normal as possible. People who are losing weight or who develop kidney failure are more likely to have hypoglycemia. Older people are more susceptible than younger people to hypoglycemia resulting from sulfonylurea drugs.

If, after taking a dose of a drug for diabetes, a person eats less than usual or is more physically active than normal, the drug may lower the level of sugar in the blood too much. People with long-standing severe diabetes are par-

ticularly prone to hypoglycemia in these situations because they do not produce enough glucagon or epinephrine. The amounts of glucagon and epinephrine that are released are often too low to counteract a low level of sugar in the blood.

Many drugs other than those for diabetes, most notably pentamidine, used to treat a form of pneumonia that occurs most often as part of AIDS, and quinine, used to treat muscle cramps, can cause hypoglycemia.

An uncommon type of drug-related hypoglycemia sometimes occurs in people with Münchausen syndrome, who secretly take insulin or other drugs as part of their attention-seeking behavior.▲

Fasting: In fasting hypoglycemia, the body is not able to maintain adequate levels of sugar in the blood after a period without food. Prolonged fasting and prolonged strenuous exercise, even after a period of fasting, are unlikely to cause hypoglycemia in otherwise healthy people, but they can do so occasionally.

There are several diseases or conditions that can cause fasting hypoglycemia. In people who drink heavily without eating, alcohol can block the release of stored sugar from the liver. In people with liver disease, such as viral hepatitis, cirrhosis, or cancer, the liver may not store sufficient sugar. Infants and children who have an abnormality of the enzyme systems that control sugar use also may have fasting hypoglycemia.

Reaction to Eating: Hypoglycemia can occur as a reaction to eating, usually carbohydrates. The body's response to food is excessive, so the body produces more insulin than is needed.

After certain types of stomach surgery, such as removal of part of the stomach, sugars are absorbed very quickly, stimulating excess insulin production. Problems with digestion of some sugars (fructose and galactose) and amino acids (leucine) may also cause reactive hypoglycemia. An uncommon form of reactive hypoglycemia can occur after drinking alcohol in combination with sugar (for example, a gin and tonic).

Other Causes: Some causes of hypoglycemia seem to have no specific relation to

▲ see box on page 602

Chapter 166   HYPOGLYCEMIA   **971**

food, but fasting or vigorous exercise can trigger or worsen an episode of hypoglycemia. Rarely, a tumor in the pancreas can produce large amounts of insulin, leading to hypoglycemia. In some people, an autoimmune disorder lowers sugar levels in the blood by changing insulin secretion or by some other means. Disorders that lower hormone production by the pituitary and adrenal glands (most notably Addison's disease) can cause hypoglycemia. Certain severe diseases, such as kidney or heart failure, cancer, and shock, may also cause hypoglycemia, particularly in a person who is also being treated for diabetes.

Symptoms

The symptoms of hypoglycemia rarely develop until the level of sugar in the blood falls below 60 milligrams per deciliter of blood. Some people develop symptoms at slightly higher levels, especially when blood sugar levels fall quickly, and some do not develop symptoms until the sugar levels in their blood are much lower.

The body first responds to a fall in the level of sugar in the blood by releasing epinephrine (adrenaline) from the adrenal glands. Epinephrine stimulates the release of sugar from body stores but also causes symptoms similar to those of an anxiety attack: sweating, nervousness, shaking, faintness, palpitations, and hunger. More severe hypoglycemia reduces the sugar supply to the brain, causing dizziness, fatigue, weakness, headaches, inability to concentrate, confusion, inappropriate behavior that can be mistaken for drunkenness, slurred speech, blurred vision, seizures, and coma. Prolonged hypoglycemia may permanently damage the brain. Symptoms can begin slowly or suddenly, progressing from mild discomfort to severe confusion or panic within minutes. On the infrequent occasions when people who have well-controlled diabetes develop hypoglycemia, awareness of the symptoms of hypoglycemia may be lost, and faintness or even coma may develop without any other warning.

In a person with an insulin-producing pancreatic tumor, symptoms are likely to occur early in the morning after an overnight fast, especially if the sugar stores in the blood are further depleted by exercise before breakfast. At first, people with a tumor usually have only occasional episodes of hypoglycemia, but over months or years, episodes become more frequent and severe.

Diagnosis

In someone who is known to have diabetes, a doctor may suspect hypoglycemia when symptoms of hypoglycemia are described. The diagnosis may be confirmed when low sugar levels in the blood are measured while the person is experiencing symptoms.

In an otherwise healthy person who does not have diabetes, a doctor is usually able to recognize hypoglycemia based on the symptoms, medical history, a physical examination, and simple tests.

Doctors first measure the level of sugar in the blood. A low sugar level in the blood found at the time a person is experiencing typical symptoms of hypoglycemia confirms the diagnosis in a person without diabetes, especially if the relationship between a low sugar level in the blood and symptoms is demonstrated more than once. If symptoms are relieved as the sugar levels in the blood rise within a few minutes of ingesting sugar, the diagnosis is supported.

When the relationship between a nondiabetic person's symptoms and the level of sugar in the blood remains unclear, additional tests may be needed. Often, the next step is measurement of the sugar level in the blood after a night of fasting in a hospital or other closely supervised setting. More extensive tests may also be needed.

If the use of a drug such as pentamidine or quinine is thought to be the cause of hypoglycemia, the drug is stopped and blood sugar levels are measured to determine if they increase. If the cause remains unclear, other laboratory tests may be needed.

If an insulin-producing tumor is suspected, measurements of insulin levels in the blood during fasting (sometimes up to 72 hours) may be needed. If the insulin measurements reveal a tumor, the doctor will try to locate it before treatment.

Treatment

The symptoms of hypoglycemia are relieved within minutes of consuming sugar in any form, such as candy or glucose tablets, or of drinking a sweet drink, such as a glass of fruit juice. People with recurring episodes of hypoglycemia, especially those with diabetes, often prefer to carry glucose tablets because the tablets take effect quickly and provide a consistent amount of sugar. Both diabetic and nondiabetic people with hypoglycemia may benefit from consuming sugar followed by a food that provides longer-lasting carbohydrates (such as bread or crackers). When hypoglycemia is severe or prolonged and taking sugar by mouth is not possible, doctors quickly give sugar intravenously to prevent brain damage.

People who are known to be at risk of severe episodes of hypoglycemia may keep glucagon on hand for emergencies. Glucagon administration stimulates the liver to release large amounts of sugar. It is given by injection and generally restores blood sugar to an adequate level within 5 to 15 minutes.

Insulin-producing tumors should be removed surgically. However, because these tumors are small and difficult to locate, a specialist should perform the surgery. Before surgery, the person may be given a drug such as diazoxide to inhibit the tumor's insulin production. Sometimes more than one tumor is present, and if the surgeon does not find them all, a second operation may be necessary.

Nondiabetic people who are prone to hypoglycemia often can avoid episodes by eating frequent small meals rather than the usual three meals a day. People prone to hypoglycemia should carry or wear a medical identification bracelet or tag to inform health care professionals of their condition.

CHAPTER 167

Multiple Endocrine Neoplasia Syndromes

Multiple endocrine neoplasia syndromes are rare conditions in which several endocrine glands develop noncancerous (benign) or cancerous (malignant) tumors or grow excessively without forming tumors.

Multiple endocrine neoplasia syndromes can appear in infants or in those as old as age 70. Almost all the multiple endocrine neoplasia syndromes are inherited.

Multiple endocrine neoplasia syndromes occur in three patterns, called types 1, 2A, and 2B, although the types occasionally overlap. The tumors and the abnormally large glands often produce excess hormones. Although tumors or abnormal growth may occur in more than one gland at the same time, changes often take place over time.

Types

Type 1 Disease: People with multiple endocrine neoplasia type 1 develop tumors, or excessive growth and activity, of two or more of the following glands: the parathyroid glands (the small glands located next to the thyroid gland), the pancreas, the pituitary gland, and,

less often, the thyroid gland and the adrenal glands.

Almost all people with type 1 disease have tumors of the parathyroid glands; most of the tumors are noncancerous, but they cause the glands to produce too much parathyroid hormone (hyperparathyroidism).▲ The excess parathyroid hormone usually raises the levels of calcium in the blood, sometimes leading to kidney stones.

Most people with type 1 disease also develop tumors of the hormone-producing cells (islet cells) of the pancreas. Some of these tumors produce high levels of insulin and, consequently, low levels of sugar in the blood (hypoglycemia), especially if the person has not eaten for several hours. More than half of islet cell tumors produce excessive gastrin, which stimulates the stomach to overproduce acid. People with tumors that produce gastrin generally develop peptic ulcers that often bleed, perforate and leak stomach contents into the abdomen, or obstruct the stomach. The high acid levels commonly interfere with the activity of enzymes from the pancreas, resulting in diarrhea and fatty, smelly stools (steatorrhea). The remaining islet cell tumors may produce other hormones, such as vasoactive intestinal

---

▲ see box on page 904

polypeptide, which can cause severe diarrhea and lead to dehydration.

Some of the islet cell tumors are cancerous and able to spread (metastasize) to other areas of the body. Cancerous islet cell tumors tend to grow more slowly than other types of cancer that develop in the pancreas.

Most people with type 1 disease develop pituitary gland tumors. Some of these tumors produce the hormone prolactin, leading to menstrual abnormalities in women and erectile dysfunction (impotence) in men. Others produce growth hormone, leading to acromegaly.▲ A small percentage of pituitary tumors produce corticotropin, which overstimulates the adrenal glands, leading to high levels of corticosteroid hormones and Cushing's syndrome.■ A few pituitary tumors produce no hormones at all. Some pituitary tumors cause headaches, impaired vision, and decreased pituitary gland function by pressing against nearby parts of the brain.

In some people with type 1 disease, tumors or excessive growth and activity of the thyroid and adrenal glands develop. A small percentage of people develop a different type of tumor, known as carcinoid tumors.★ Some people also develop soft, noncancerous fatty growths just below the skin (lipomas).

Type 2A Disease: People with multiple endocrine neoplasia type 2A develop tumors or excessive growth and activity in two or three of the following glands: the thyroid gland, the adrenal glands, and the parathyroid glands.

Almost everyone with type 2A disease develops medullary thyroid cancer.● About 50% develop pheochromocytomas, tumors of the adrenal glands,◆ which usually raise blood pressure because of the epinephrine and other substances they produce. The high blood pressure may be intermittent or constant and is often very severe.

Some people with type 2A disease have overactive parathyroid glands and therefore have increased levels of calcium in the blood, which may lead to kidney stones. In others, the parathyroid glands increase in size without producing large amounts of parathyroid hormone, so the people do not have problems related to high calcium levels.

Type 2B Disease: Multiple endocrine neoplasia type 2B can consist of medullary thyroid cancer, pheochromocytomas, and neuromas (growths around the nerves). Some people with type 2B disease have no family history of it.

The medullary thyroid cancer that occurs in type 2B disease tends to develop at an early age and has been found in infants as young as 3 months of age. The medullary thyroid tumors in type 2B grow faster and spread more rapidly than those in type 2A disease.

Most people with type 2B disease develop neuromas in their mucous membranes. The neuromas appear as glistening bumps around the lips, tongue, and lining of the mouth. Neuromas may also occur on the eyelids and glistening surfaces of the eyes, including the conjunctiva and cornea. The eyelids and lips may thicken.

Digestive tract abnormalities cause constipation and diarrhea. Occasionally, the colon develops large, dilated loops (megacolon). These abnormalities probably result from neuromas growing on the intestinal nerves.

People with type 2B disease often develop spinal abnormalities, especially curvature of the spine. They may also have abnormalities of the bones of the feet and thighs. Many people have long limbs and loose joints.

Screening

Because about half of the children of people with a multiple endocrine neoplasia syndrome inherit the disease, screening is important for early diagnosis and treatment. Tests for identification of each type of tumor are available. A single gene responsible for type 1 disease has been identified, and a test for abnormalities in this gene is available. Abnormalities in a different gene have been identified in people with types 2A and 2B disease, and tests for mutations in this gene are also available. These genetic tests permit earlier and more effective diagnosis and treatment in people who have a family history of multiple endocrine neoplasia syndromes.

Treatment

No cure is known for any of the multiple endocrine neoplasia syndromes. Doctors treat the changes in each gland individually. A tumor is treated either by removing it or by correcting the hormone imbalance, using drugs that counteract the effects of gland overactivity. An excessively large and overactive gland

▲ see page 945   ■ see page 958

★ see page 974   ● see page 955

◆ see page 960

without a tumor is treated with drugs to counteract the effects of gland overactivity.

Because medullary thyroid cancer is ultimately fatal if untreated, a doctor will most likely recommend surgical removal of the thyroid gland if a person has evidence of type 2A or type 2B disease, even if the diagnosis of medullary thyroid cancer cannot be established before the surgery. Unlike other types of thyroid cancer, this aggressive type of thyroid cancer cannot be treated with radioactive iodine. Once the thyroid is removed, a person must take thyroid hormone for the rest of his life.

CHAPTER 168

Carcinoid Tumors

Carcinoid tumors are noncancerous (benign) or cancerous (malignant) growths that produce excessive amounts of hormonelike substances.

Carcinoid tumors usually originate in hormone-producing cells that line the small intestine or other cells of the digestive tract. They can also occur in the pancreas, testes, ovaries, or lungs. Carcinoid tumors can produce an excess of hormonelike substances, such as serotonin, bradykinin, histamine, and prostaglandins. Excess levels of these substances can sometimes result in a diverse set of symptoms called carcinoid syndrome.

When carcinoid tumors occur in the digestive tract or pancreas, the substances they produce are released into a blood vessel that flows directly to the liver (portal vein), where enzymes destroy them. Therefore, carcinoid tumors that originate in the digestive tract generally do not produce symptoms unless the tumors have spread to the liver.

If the tumors have spread to the liver, the liver is unable to process the substances before they begin circulating throughout the body. Depending on which substances are being released by the tumors, the person will have the various symptoms of carcinoid syndrome. Carcinoid tumors of the lungs, testes, and ovaries also cause symptoms because the substances they produce bypass the liver and circulate widely in the bloodstream.

Symptoms

Most people with carcinoid tumors have symptoms similar to those of other intestinal tumors, mainly cramping pain and changes in bowel movements as a result of obstruction.

Fewer than 10% of people with carcinoid tumors develop symptoms of carcinoid syndrome. Uncomfortable flushing, typically of the head and neck, is the most common and often the earliest symptom of carcinoid syndrome. Flushing, the result of blood vessel dilation, is often triggered by emotions, by eating, or by drinking alcohol or hot liquids. The flushing may be followed by periods when the skin is bluish (cyanosis). Excessive contraction of the intestines may result in abdominal cramping and diarrhea. The intestine may not be able to absorb nutrients properly, resulting in malnutrition and fatty, foul-smelling stools.

Heart damage may occur, resulting in swelling of the feet and legs (edema). Wheezing and shortness of breath may result from obstructed airflow in the lungs. Some people with carcinoid syndrome lose interest in sex, and some men have erectile dysfunction (impotence).

Diagnosis

When symptoms lead a doctor to suspect a carcinoid tumor, the diagnosis can often be confirmed by measuring the amount of 5-hydroxyindoleacetic acid (5-HIAA)—one of the chemical by-products of serotonin—in the person's urine, which is collected over a 24-hour period. For at least 3 days before undergoing this test, the person refrains from eating foods that are rich in serotonin—bananas, tomatoes, plums, avocados, pineapples, eggplants, and walnuts. Certain drugs, including guaifenesin (found in many cough syrups), methocarbamol (a muscle relaxant), and phenothiazines (antipsychotics), also interfere with test results.

Different tests are used to locate carcinoid tumors. These tests include computed tomography (CT), magnetic resonance imaging (MRI), and arteriography. Sometimes exploratory surgery is needed to locate the tumor.

Radionuclide scanning is another useful test. Most carcinoid tumors have receptors for the hormone somatostatin. Doctors can therefore inject a radioactive form of somatostatin into the blood and use radionuclide scanning to locate a carcinoid tumor and determine if it has spread. About 90% of tumors can be located using this technique. MRI or CT can be helpful in confirming whether the tumor has spread to the liver.

Treatment

When a carcinoid tumor is restricted to a specific area, such as the appendix, small intestine, rectum, or lungs, surgical removal may cure the disease. If the tumor has spread to the liver, surgery rarely cures the disease but may help relieve symptoms. The tumors grow so slowly that even people whose tumors have spread often survive for 10 to 15 years.

Neither radiation therapy nor chemotherapy is effective in curing carcinoid tumors. However, combinations of certain chemotherapy drugs (streptozocin with fluorouracil and sometimes doxorubicin) may relieve symptoms. A drug called octreotide can also relieve symptoms, and tamoxifen, interferon alfa, and eflornithine may reduce the tumor's growth. Phenothiazines, cimetidine, and phentolamine are used to control flushing in people with carcinoid syndrome. Prednisone is sometimes given to people with carcinoid tumors of the lung who have episodes of severe flushing. Diarrhea may be controlled with codeine, tincture of opium, diphenoxylate, or cyproheptadine.

BLOOD DISORDERS

169 **Biology of Blood** 978
Blood Components ▪ Blood Cell Formation ▪ Effects of Aging

170 **Symptoms and Diagnosis of Blood Disorders** 979

171 **Blood Transfusion**..982
The Donation Process ▪ Types of Transfusions ▪ Special
Donation Procedures ▪ Precautions and Adverse Reactions

172 **Anemia** 987
Anemia From Excessive Bleeding ▪ Iron Deficiency Anemia ▪
Vitamin Deficiency Anemia ▪ Anemia of Chronic Disease ▪
Autoimmune Hemolytic Anemia ▪ Sickle Cell Disease ▪
Hemoglobin C, S-C, and E Diseases ▪ Thalassemias

173 **Bleeding and Clotting Disorders** 995
Hereditary Hemorrhagic Telangiectasia ▪ Allergic Purpura ▪
Thrombocytopenia ▪ Von Willebrand's Disease ▪ Hemophilia ▪
Thrombophilia ▪ Disseminated Intravascular Coagulation

174 **White Blood Cell Disorders** 1001
Neutropenia ▪ Neutrophilic Leukocytosis ▪ Lymphocytopenia ▪
Lymphocytic Leukocytosis ▪ Monocyte Disorders ▪ Eosinophilic
Disorders ▪ Basophilic Disorders

175 **Plasma Cell Disorders** 1006
Monoclonal Gammopathies of Undetermined Significance ▪
Multiple Myeloma ▪ Macroglobulinemia ▪ Heavy Chain Diseases

176 **Leukemias** 1010
Acute Lymphocytic Leukemia ▪ Acute Myelocytic Leukemia ▪
Chronic Lymphocytic Leukemia ▪ Chronic Myelocytic Leukemia

177 **Lymphomas**..1016
Hodgkin's Disease ▪ Non-Hodgkin's Lymphomas

178 **Myeloproliferative Disorders** 1023
Polycythemia Vera ▪ Myelofibrosis ▪ Thrombocythemia

179 **Spleen Disorders** 1027
Enlarged Spleen ▪ Ruptured Spleen

CHAPTER 169

Biology of Blood

Blood is a complex mixture of plasma (the liquid component), white blood cells, red blood cells, and platelets. The body contains about 5 to 6 quarts of blood. Once blood is pumped out of the heart, it takes 20 to 30 seconds to make a complete trip through the circulation and return to the heart.

Blood performs a variety of essential functions as it circulates through the body. It delivers oxygen and essential nutrients (such as fats, sugars, minerals, and vitamins) to the body's tissues. It carries carbon dioxide to the lungs and other waste products to the kidneys for elimination from the body. It transports hormones (chemical messengers) to allow various parts of the body to communicate with each other. Also, it carries components that fight infection and stop bleeding.

Blood Components

Plasma

Plasma is the liquid component of blood, in which the red blood cells, white blood cells, and platelets are suspended. It constitutes more than half of the blood's volume and consists mostly of water containing dissolved salts (electrolytes) and proteins. The major protein in plasma is albumin. Albumin helps keep fluid from leaking out of blood vessels and into tissues, and albumin binds to and carries substances such as hormones and certain drugs. Other proteins in plasma include antibodies (immunoglobulins), which actively defend the body against viruses, bacteria, fungi, and cancer cells, and clotting factors, which control bleeding.

Plasma has other functions. It acts as a reservoir that can either replenish insufficient water or absorb excess water from tissues. When tissues of the body are in need of additional liquid, water from plasma is the first resource to meet that need. Plasma also prevents blood vessels from collapsing and clogging and helps maintain blood pressure and circulation throughout the body simply by filling blood vessels and flowing through them continuously. Plasma also plays a role in warming and cooling the body as needed, by carrying heat from body tissues to where it is needed and by passing through areas that lose heat more readily, such as the arms, legs, and head.

Red Blood Cells

Red blood cells (also called erythrocytes) make up about 40% of the blood's volume. Red blood cells contain hemoglobin, a protein that gives blood its red color and enables it to carry oxygen from the lungs and deliver it to all body tissues. Oxygen is used by cells to produce energy that the body needs, leaving carbon dioxide as a waste product. Red blood cells carry carbon dioxide away from the tissues and back to the lungs. When the number of red blood cells is too low (anemia), blood carries less oxygen, and fatigue and weakness develop. When the number of red blood cells is too high (polycythemia), blood can become too thick, which may cause the blood to clot more easily and increase the risk of heart attacks and strokes.

White Blood Cells

White blood cells (also called leukocytes) are fewer in number than red blood cells, with a ratio of about 1 white blood cell to every 660 red blood cells. White blood cells are responsible primarily for defending the body against infection. There are five main types of white blood cells. **Neutrophils,** the most numerous type, help protect the body against infections by killing and ingesting bacteria and fungi and by ingesting foreign debris. **Lymphocytes** consist of three main types: T lymphocytes and natural killer cells, which both help protect against viral infections and can detect and destroy some cancer cells, and B lymphocytes, which develop into cells that produce antibodies. **Monocytes** ingest dead or damaged cells and help defend against many infectious organisms. **Eosinophils** kill parasites, destroy cancer cells, and are involved in allergic responses. **Basophils** also participate in allergic responses.

Some white blood cells flow smoothly through the bloodstream, but many adhere to blood vessel walls or even penetrate the vessel walls to enter other tissues. When white blood cells reach the site of an infection or other problem, they release substances that attract more white blood cells. The white blood cells function like an army, dispersed throughout the body but ready at a moment's notice to gather and fight off an invading organism. White blood cells accomplish this by engulfing and digesting organisms and by producing antibodies that attach to organisms so that they can be more easily destroyed.▲

When the number of white blood cells is too low (leukopenia), infections are more likely to occur. A higher than normal number of white blood cells (leukocytosis) may not directly cause symptoms, but the high number of cells can be an indication of a disease such as an infection or leukemia.

Platelets

Platelets (also called thrombocytes) are cell-like particles smaller than red or white blood cells. Platelets are fewer in number than red blood cells, with a ratio of about 1 platelet to every 20 red blood cells. Platelets help in the clotting process by gathering at a bleeding site and clumping together to form a plug that helps seal the blood vessel. At the same time, they release substances that help promote further clotting. When the number of platelets is too low (thrombocytopenia), bruising and abnormal bleeding become more likely. When the number of platelets is too high (thrombocythemia), blood may clot excessively, producing a stroke or heart attack.

Blood Cell Formation

Red blood cells, most white blood cells, and platelets are produced in the bone marrow, the soft fatty tissue inside bone cavities. Two types of white blood cells, T and B lymphocytes, are also produced in the lymph nodes and spleen, and T lymphocytes are produced and mature in the thymus gland.

Within the bone marrow, all blood cells originate from a single type of unspecialized cell called a stem cell. When a stem cell divides, it first becomes an immature red blood cell, white blood cell, or platelet-producing cell. The immature cell then divides, matures further, and ultimately becomes a mature red blood cell, white blood cell, or platelet.

The speed of blood cell production is controlled by the body's needs. Normal blood cells last for a limited time (ranging from a few hours to a few days for white blood cells, to about 10 days for platelets, to about 120 days for red blood cells) and must be replaced constantly. Certain conditions may trigger additional production of blood cells. When the oxygen content of body tissues or the number of red blood cells decreases, the kidneys produce and release erythropoietin, a hormone that stimulates the bone marrow to produce more red blood cells. The bone marrow produces and releases more white blood cells in response to infections. It produces and releases more platelets in response to bleeding.

Effects of Aging

Aging has some effect on bone marrow and blood cells. The amount of fat in the marrow increases so that the amount of cell-producing marrow decreases. While this decrease generally does not cause problems, it may when the body experiences an increased demand for blood cells: the marrow of an older person may be less able to meet those increased demands. Anemia is the most common result.

CHAPTER 170

Symptoms and Diagnosis of Blood Disorders

Disorders that affect the cells in the blood (blood cells) or proteins in the blood clotting system are called blood disorders or hematologic disorders. Depending on the person's symptoms, a doctor usually recommends a variety of tests to help determine the person's exact blood disorder.

Symptoms

Symptoms of blood disorders are often vague and nonspecific, that is, they could indicate a disorder of almost any part of the body.

▲ see also page 1050

Such symptoms include fatigue, weakness, shortness of breath, fever, weight loss, pain, dizziness, fainting, excessive bleeding, easy bruising, and very small red or purple spots on the skin.

Although no single symptom unmistakably indicates a blood disorder, certain groups of symptoms suggest the possibility. Such groups of symptoms most commonly relate to decreases in blood cells, such as a reduced number of red blood cells (anemia), a reduced number of white blood cells (leukopenia), or a reduced number of platelets (thrombocytopenia). For example, a person who has weakness and shortness of breath may have anemia. A person who has fever and infection may have too few white blood cells. A person who bleeds or bruises easily may have too few platelets.

Occasionally, symptoms may relate to increased numbers of blood cells. For example, people with thickened (more viscous) blood due to increased numbers of red blood cells or white blood cells may experience symptoms such as shortness of breath, headaches, dizziness, and confusion.

Finally, disorders of factors responsible for normal blood clotting may result in insufficient blood clotting (manifesting as bruising or bleeding) or formation of abnormal blood clots (producing warm, painful areas in the legs or sudden shortness of breath or chest pain).

Diagnosis

Laboratory Blood Tests

Doctors depend on many different laboratory tests of blood samples to diagnose and monitor diseases. Because the liquid portion of the blood (plasma) carries so many substances essential to the body's functioning, blood tests can be used to find out what is happening in many parts of the body.

Testing blood is easier than obtaining a tissue sample from a specific organ. For example, thyroid function can be evaluated more easily by measuring the level of thyroid hormones in the blood than by directly sampling the thyroid. Likewise, measuring liver enzymes and proteins in the blood▲ is easier than sampling the liver. However, certain blood tests are used to measure the components and function of the blood itself. These

are the tests that are mostly used to diagnose blood disorders.

Complete Blood Count: The most commonly performed blood test is the complete blood count (CBC), which is a basic evaluation of the cellular components of blood (red blood cells, white blood cells, and platelets). Automated machines perform this test in less than 1 minute on a small drop of blood. The CBC is supplemented in most instances by examination of blood cells under a microscope.

The CBC determines the number of red blood cells and the amount of hemoglobin (the protein that enables the cells to carry oxygen) in the blood. In addition, the size of red blood cells is usually assessed and can alert laboratory workers to the presence of abnormally shaped red blood cells (which may then be further characterized by microscopic examination). Abnormal red blood cells may be fragmented or shaped like teardrops, crescents, needles, or a variety of other forms. Knowing the specific shape or size of red blood cells can help a doctor diagnose a particular cause of anemia. For example, sickle-shaped cells are characteristic of sickle cell disease, small cells containing insufficient amounts of hemoglobin may signal iron deficiency anemia, and large oval cells suggest anemia due to folic acid or vitamin B_{12} deficiency (pernicious anemia).

After putting together information about the number, size, and shape of the red blood cells, a doctor might order additional tests to evaluate the cause of an anemia. These include tests for increased red blood cell fragility, abnormal types of hemoglobin, and the quantities of certain other substances contained within red blood cells.

The CBC also determines the number of white blood cells. The specific types of white blood cells can be counted (differential white blood cell count) when a doctor needs more detailed information on a person's condition. If the total number of white blood cells or the number of one of the specific types of white blood cells is above or below normal, the doctor can examine these cells under a microscope. The microscopic examination can identify features that are characteristic of certain diseases. For example, large numbers of white blood cells that have a very immature appearance (blasts) may suggest leukemia (cancer of the white blood cells).

Platelets are usually also counted as part of a CBC. The number of platelets is an important measure of the blood's protective mecha-

▲ see page 788

COMPLETE BLOOD COUNT (CBC)

TEST	WHAT IT MEASURES	NORMAL VALUES
Hemoglobin	Amount of this oxygen-carrying protein within red blood cells	Men: 14 to 17 grams per deciliter Women: 12.5 to 15 grams per deciliter
Hematocrit	Proportion of total blood volume made up of red blood cells	Men: 42 to 50% Women: 36 to 45%
Mean corpuscular volume	Average volume of individual red blood cells	86 to 98 femtoliters
White blood cell count	Number of white blood cells in a specified volume of blood	4,500 to 10,500 per microliter
Differential white blood cell count	Percentages of the different types of white blood cells	Segmented neutrophils: 34 to 75% Band neutrophils: 0 to 8% Lymphocytes: 12 to 50% Monocytes: 2 to 9% Eosinophils: 0 to 5% Basophils: 0 to 3%
Platelet count	Number of platelets in a specified volume of blood	140,000 to 450,000 per microliter
Mean platelet volume	Average volume of platelets	7 to 10 femtoliters

nisms for stopping bleeding (clotting). A high number of platelets (thrombocytosis or thrombocythemia) can lead to blood clots in small blood vessels, especially those in the heart or brain.

Reticulocyte Count: The reticulocyte count measures the number of newly formed (young) red blood cells (reticulocytes) in a specified volume of blood. Reticulocytes normally make up about 1% of the total number of red blood cells. When the body needs more red blood cells, as in anemia, the bone marrow normally responds by producing more reticulocytes. Thus, the reticulocyte count is a measure of bone marrow function.

Blood Typing: Blood type, which is determined by the presence of proteins on the surface of red blood cells, can be identified by measuring the reaction of a small sample of a person's blood to certain antibodies. Blood typing must be done before blood can be transfused.▲

Bleeding Time and Other Clotting Tests: The body's ability to stop bleeding may be determined by the bleeding time (in addition to a count of the number of platelets). In this test, a small cut is made on the person's forearm, and the examiner measures the amount of time that elapses before bleeding stops. This

test is largely a measure of platelet function; most tests of platelet function are done by automated methods. Other tests can be performed to measure the overall function of the many proteins needed for normal blood clotting (clotting factors). The most common of these tests are the prothrombin time (PT) and the partial thromboplastin time (PTT). The levels of individual clotting factors can also be determined.

Other Blood Tests: Specialized blood tests can be used to determine other blood disorders. For example, on rare occasions, doctors must measure the total volume of blood or the total number of certain blood cells in the body. These measurements can be done using radioactive isotopes that mix in the blood or attach to blood cells.

Bone Marrow Examination

Sometimes a sample of bone marrow must be examined to determine why blood cells are abnormal. A doctor can take two different types of bone marrow samples: a bone marrow aspirate and a bone marrow core biopsy. Both types are usually taken from the hipbone (iliac

▲ see art on page 984

Taking a Bone Marrow Sample

Bone marrow samples are usually taken from the hipbone (iliac crest). The person may lie on one side, facing away from the doctor, with the knee of the top leg bent. After numbing the skin and tissue over the bone with a local anesthetic, the doctor inserts a needle into the bone and withdraws the marrow.

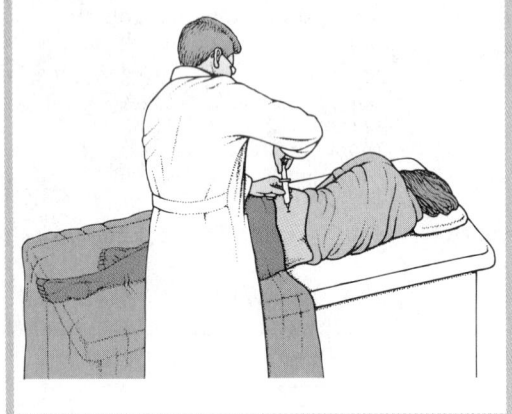

children, bone marrow samples are occasionally taken from a leg bone (tibia).

When both types of samples are needed, they are taken at the same time. After the skin and tissue over the bone are numbed with a local anesthetic, the sharp needle of a syringe is inserted into the bone. For a bone marrow aspirate, the doctor pulls back on the plunger of the syringe and draws out a small amount of the soft bone marrow, which can be spread on a slide and examined under a microscope. Special tests, such as cultures for bacteria, fungi, or viruses, chromosomal analysis, and analysis of cell surface proteins (flow cytometry), can be performed on the sample. Although the aspirate often provides enough information for a diagnosis to be made, the process of drawing the marrow into the syringe breaks up the fragile bone marrow. As a result, determining the original arrangement of the cells is difficult.

When the exact anatomic relationships of cells must be determined and the structure of the tissues evaluated, the doctor also performs a core biopsy. A small core of intact bone marrow is removed with an internal coring device. This core is preserved and sliced into thin sections that are examined under a microscope.

A bone marrow sampling generally involves a slight jolt of pain, followed by minimal discomfort. The procedure takes a few minutes.

crest), although aspirates are sometimes taken from the breastbone (sternum). In very young

---

CHAPTER 171

Blood Transfusion

A blood transfusion is the transfer of blood or a blood component from one person (a donor) to another (a recipient).

In the United States, about 27 million blood transfusions are performed every year. Transfusions are given to increase the blood's ability to carry oxygen, restore the body's blood volume, improve immunity, and correct clotting problems. Accident victims, people undergoing surgery, and people receiving treatment for cancers (such as leukemia) or other diseases (such as the blood diseases sickle cell anemia and thalassemia) are typical recipients.

The Food and Drug Administration (FDA) strictly regulates the collection, storage, and transportation of blood and its components. These regulations were developed to protect both the donor and the recipient. Additional standards are upheld by many state and local health authorities, as well as by organizations such as the American Red Cross and the American Association of Blood Banks. Because of these regulations, giving and receiving blood has become very safe. However, transfusions still pose risks for the recipient, such as allergic reactions, fever and chills, blood volume overload, and bacterial and viral infections. Even though the chance of contracting AIDS or hepatitis from transfusions is remote, doctors are well aware of these risks and order transfusions only when there seems to be no alternative.

The Donation Process

The entire process of donating whole blood takes about 1 hour. Blood donors must be at least 17 years old and weigh at least 110 pounds. In addition, they must be in good health: their pulse, blood pressure, and temperature are measured, and a blood sample is tested to check for anemia. They are asked a series of questions about their health, factors that might affect their health, and countries they have visited.

Conditions that permanently disqualify a person from donating blood include hepatitis B or C, heart disease, certain types of cancer (leukemia, lymphoma, and any type of cancer that has recurred after treatment or that has ever been treated with chemotherapy drugs), severe asthma, bleeding disorders, possible exposure to prion diseases (such as variant Creutzfeldt-Jakob disease),▲ AIDS, and possible exposure to the human immunodeficiency virus (HIV, the virus that causes AIDS) due to high-risk behaviors.■ Conditions that temporarily disqualify a person include malaria (if less than 3 years since last experiencing symptoms), cancer that has been treated with surgery or radiation (if less than 5 years since last receiving treatment), pregnancy, recent major surgery, poorly controlled high blood pressure, low blood pressure, anemia, the use of certain drugs, exposure to some forms of hepatitis, and a recent blood transfusion.

Generally, donors are not allowed to give blood more than once every 56 days. The practice of paying donors for blood has almost disappeared; it encouraged needy people to present themselves as donors and then sometimes to deny having any conditions that would disqualify them.

After a person is deemed eligible to donate blood, he sits in a reclining chair or lies on a cot. A health care worker examines the inside surface of the person's elbow and determines which vein to use. After the area immediately surrounding the vein is cleaned, a needle is inserted into the vein and temporarily secured with a sterile covering. A stinging sensation is usually felt when the needle is first inserted, but otherwise the procedure is painless. Blood

Testing Donated Blood for Infections

Blood transfusions can transmit infectious organisms carried in the donor's blood. That is why health officials have further restricted blood donor eligibility and made blood testing more thorough. Today, all blood donations are tested for infection with the organisms that cause viral hepatitis, AIDS, selected other viral disorders, and syphilis.

Viral Hepatitis

Donated blood is tested for infection with the viruses that cause the types of viral hepatitis (types B and C) that are transmitted by blood transfusions. These tests cannot identify all cases of infected blood, but with recent improvements in testing and donor screening, a transfusion poses almost no risk of transmitting hepatitis B. Hepatitis C remains the most common potentially serious disorder transmitted by blood transfusions, with a current risk of about 1 infection for every 100,000 units of blood transfused.

AIDS

In the United States, donated blood is tested for the human immunodeficiency virus (HIV), the cause of AIDS. The test is not 100% accurate, but potential donors are interviewed as part of the screening process. Interviewers ask about risk factors for AIDS—for instance, whether the potential donors or their sex partners have injected drugs or had sex with a male homosexual. Because of the blood test and the screening interview, the risk of contracting HIV infection through a blood transfusion is extremely low—1 in 825,000, according to recent estimates.

Syphilis

Blood transfusions rarely transmit syphilis. Not only are blood donors screened and donations tested for the organism that causes syphilis, but the donated blood is also refrigerated at low temperatures, which kills the infectious organisms.

moves through the needle and into a collecting bag. The actual collection of blood takes only about 10 minutes.

The standard unit of donated blood is about 1 pint. Freshly collected blood is sealed in

▲ see page 541   ■ see page 1168

Blood Typing

Because transfusing blood that does not match the recipient's can be dangerous, donated blood is classified by type. A person's blood type is determined by testing for the presence or absence of certain proteins (Rh factor and blood group antigens A and B) on the surface of red blood cells.

The four main blood types are A, B, AB, and O, and for each type the blood is either Rh-positive or Rh-negative. For example, a person with O-negative blood has red blood cells that lack both A and B antigens and the Rh factor. A person with AB-positive blood has red blood cells that have A and B antigens and the Rh factor. Some blood types are far more common than others. The most common blood types in the United States are O-positive and A-positive, followed by B-positive, O-negative, A-negative, AB-positive, B-negative, and AB-negative.

In an emergency, anyone can receive type O red blood cells; thus people with type O blood are known as universal donors. People with type AB blood can receive red blood cells from any blood type and are thus known as universal recipients. Recipients whose blood is Rh-negative must receive blood from Rh-negative donors, but recipients whose blood is Rh-positive may receive Rh-positive or Rh-negative blood.

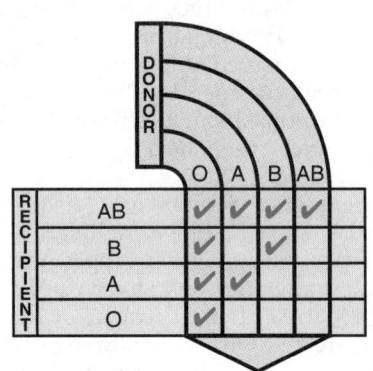

plastic bags containing preservatives and an anticlotting compound. A small sample from each donation is tested for the infectious organisms that cause AIDS, viral hepatitis, and syphilis.

Types of Transfusions

Most blood donations are divided (fractionated) into their components: red blood cells, platelets, plasma, clotting factors, antibodies (immunoglobulins), and white blood cells. Depending on the situation, people may receive only the cells from blood, only the clotting factors from blood, or some other blood component. Transfusing only selected blood components allows the treatment to be specific, reduces the risks of side effects, and can efficiently use the different components from a single unit of blood to treat several people.

Red Blood Cells: Packed red blood cells, the most commonly transfused blood component, can restore the blood's oxygen-carrying capacity. This component may be given to a person who is bleeding or who has severe anemia. The red blood cells are separated from the fluid component of the blood (plasma) and from the other cellular and cell-like components. After this step, the red blood cells are concentrated so that they occupy less space, thus the term "packed." Red blood cells can be refrigerated for up to 42 days. In special circumstances—for instance, to preserve a rare type of blood—red blood cells can be frozen for up to 10 years.

Platelets: Platelets can help restore the blood's clotting ability. They are usually given to people with too few platelets (thrombocytopenia), which may result in severe and spontaneous bleeding. Platelets can be stored for only 5 days.

Blood Clotting Factors: Blood clotting factors are plasma proteins that normally work with platelets to help the blood clot. Clotting factors may be produced from plasma products or manufactured artificially using a special technological procedure; manufactured proteins are called recombinant factor concentrates. Without clotting factors, bleeding would not stop after an injury. Individual concentrated blood clotting factors can be given to people who have an inherited bleeding disorder, such as hemophilia or von Willebrand's disease, and to those who are unable to produce enough clotting factors (usually because of severe infection or liver disease).

Plasma: Plasma is a source of blood clotting factors. Plasma is used for bleeding disorders in which the missing clotting factor is unknown or when the specific clotting factor is not available. Plasma also is used when bleeding is caused by insufficient production of all or many of the different clotting factors, as a result of liver failure or severe infection. Plasma that is frozen right after it is separated from the cells of donor blood (fresh frozen plasma) can be stored for up to 1 year.

Antibodies: Antibodies (immunoglobulins), the disease-fighting components of blood, are sometimes given to build up immunity in people who have been exposed to an infectious disease, such as chickenpox or hepatitis, or who have low antibody levels. Antibodies are produced from treated plasma donations.

White Blood Cells: White blood cells are transfused to treat life-threatening infections in people who have a greatly reduced number of white blood cells or whose white blood cells are functioning abnormally. White blood cell transfusions are rare, because improved antibiotics and the use of cytokine growth factors have greatly reduced the need for such transfusions. White blood cells are obtained by hemapheresis and can be stored for up to 24 hours.

Special Donation Procedures

Plateletpheresis

In plateletpheresis, a donor gives only platelets rather than whole blood. Whole blood is drawn from the donor, and a machine that separates the blood into its components selectively removes the platelets and returns the rest of the blood to the donor. Because donors get most of their blood back, they can safely give 8 to 10 times as many platelets during one of these procedures as they would give in a single donation of whole blood. Collecting platelets from a donor takes about 1 to 2 hours, compared with collecting whole blood, which takes about 10 minutes.

Autologous Transfusion

In an autologous transfusion, the donor is the recipient of his own blood. For example, in the weeks before undergoing surgery, a person may donate several units of blood to be transfused if needed during or after the operation. Or, during surgery, if a person is bleeding, the

blood can be collected and given back. An autologous transfusion is the safest type of blood transfusion, because it eliminates the risk of incompatibility and blood-borne disease.

Directed or Designated Donation

Family members or friends can donate blood specifically for one another if the recipient's and donor's blood types and Rh factors are compatible. For some recipients, knowing who donated the blood is comforting, although a donation from a family member or friend is not necessarily safer than one from an unrelated person. Blood from a family member is treated with radiation to prevent graft-versus-host disease, which, although rare, occurs more often when the recipient and donor are related.

Stem Cell Pheresis

In stem cell pheresis, a donor gives only stem cells rather than whole blood. Prior to the donation procedure, the donor receives an injection of a special type of protein (growth factor) that stimulates the bone marrow to release stem cells into the bloodstream. Whole blood is drawn from the donor, and a machine that separates the blood into its components selectively removes the stem cells and returns the rest of the blood to the donor.

Precautions and Adverse Reactions

To minimize the chance of an adverse reaction during a transfusion, health care practitioners take several precautions. Before starting the transfusion, usually a few hours or even a few days beforehand, a technician mixes a drop of the donor's blood with the recipient's to make sure they are compatible; this is called cross-matching. When a person's blood has been adequately tested and antibodies are not present, this process may be performed electronically by the blood bank computer system.

After double-checking labels on the bags of blood that are about to be given to ensure the units are intended for that recipient, the health care practitioner gives the blood to the recipient slowly, generally over 1 to 2 hours for each unit of blood. Because most adverse reactions occur during the first 15 minutes of the transfusion, the recipient is closely observed at first. After that, a nurse checks on the recipient periodically and must stop the transfusion if an adverse reaction occurs.

Controlling Diseases by Purifying the Blood

In hemapheresis, blood is removed from a person and then returned after fluids, substances in the fluid, blood cells, or platelets are removed or reduced in quantity. Sometimes this process is used to obtain needed blood cells or platelets from a donor (for example, stem cell pheresis or plateletpheresis). This process is also used to purify blood by removing harmful substances or excessive numbers of blood cells or platelets in people with serious illnesses who have not responded to conventional treatment. To be helpful for purifying blood, hemapheresis must remove the undesirable substance or blood cell faster than the body produces it.

The two most common types of hemapheresis that are used to purify blood are plasmapheresis and cytapheresis. In plasmapheresis, harmful substances are removed from the plasma. Plasmapheresis is used to treat such disorders as myasthenia gravis and Guillain-Barré syndrome (neurologic disorders that cause muscle weakness), Goodpasture's syndrome (an allergic disorder involving bleeding in the lungs and kidney failure), pemphigus vulgaris (severe, sometimes fatal, blistering of the skin), cryoglobulinemia (a type of abnormal antibody formation), and thrombotic thrombocytopenic purpura (a rare clotting disorder). In cytapheresis, excess numbers of certain blood cells are removed. Cytapheresis can be used to treat polycythemia (an excess of red blood cells), certain types of leukemia (an excess of white blood cells), and thrombocythemia (an excess of platelets).

Hemapheresis is repeated only as often as necessary, because the large fluid shifts between blood vessels and tissues that occur as blood is removed and returned may cause complications in people who are already ill. Hemapheresis can help control some diseases but generally does not cure them.

Most transfusions are safe and successful; however, mild reactions occur occasionally, and severe and even fatal reactions, rarely. The most common reactions are fever and allergic reactions (hypersensitivity), which occur in about 1 to 2% of transfusions. Symptoms of an allergic reaction include itching, a widespread rash, swelling, dizziness, and headache. Less common symptoms are breathing difficulties, wheezing, and muscle spasms. Rarely, an allergic reaction is severe enough to cause low blood pressure and shock.

Treatments are available that allow transfusions to be given to people who previously had allergic reactions to them. People who have allergic reactions to donated blood may have to be given washed red blood cells. Washing the red blood cells removes components of the donor blood that may cause allergic reactions. More commonly, the transfused blood is filtered to reduce the number of white blood cells (a process called leukocyte reduction). Leukocyte reduction is usually done by placing a special filter in the line through which the transfusion is flowing. Alternatively, the blood may be filtered before it is stored.

Despite careful typing and cross-matching of blood, mismatches can still occur that cause the transfused red blood cells to be destroyed shortly after the transfusion (a hemolytic reaction). Usually, this reaction starts as a general discomfort or anxiety during or immediately after the transfusion. Sometimes breathing difficulty, chest pressure, flushing, and severe back pain develop. Very rarely, the reactions become more severe and even fatal. A doctor can confirm that a hemolytic reaction is destroying red blood cells by checking to see whether hemoglobin released from these cells is in the person's blood and urine.

Transfusion recipients can become overloaded with fluid. Recipients who have heart disease are most vulnerable, so their transfusions are given more slowly and they are monitored closely.

Graft-versus-host disease is an unusual complication that affects primarily people whose immune system is impaired by drugs or disease. In this disease, the recipient's (host's) tissues are attacked by the donated white blood cells (the graft). The symptoms include fever, rash, low blood pressure, low blood counts, tissue destruction, and shock. These reactions can be fatal but are eliminated by treating with radiation those blood products that are intended for people with a weakened immune system.

CHAPTER 172

Anemia

Anemia is a condition in which the number of red blood cells or the amount of hemoglobin (the protein that carries oxygen in them) is low.

Red blood cells contain hemoglobin, a protein that enables them to carry oxygen from the lungs and deliver it to all parts of the body. When the number of red blood cells is reduced or the amount of hemoglobin in them is low, the blood cannot carry an adequate supply of oxygen. An inadequate supply of oxygen in the tissues produces the symptoms of anemia.

Causes

The individual causes of anemia are numerous, but most can be grouped within three major mechanisms that produce anemia: blood loss (excessive bleeding), inadequate production of red blood cells, or excessive destruction of red blood cells.

Anemia may be caused by excessive bleeding. Bleeding may be sudden, as may occur in an accident or during surgery. Often, bleeding is gradual and repetitive, typically from abnormalities in the digestive or urinary tract. Chronic bleeding typically leads to low levels of iron, which leads to worsening anemia.

Anemia may also result when the body does not produce enough red blood cells. Many nutrients are needed for red blood cell production. The most critical are iron, vitamin B_{12}, and folic acid, but the body also needs trace amounts of vitamin C, riboflavin, and copper, as well as a proper balance of hormones, especially erythropoietin (a hormone that stimulates red blood cell production). Without these nutrients and hormones, production of red blood cells is slow and inadequate, or the red blood cells may be deformed and unable to carry oxygen adequately. Chronic disease also may affect red blood cell production. In some circumstances, the bone marrow space may be invaded and replaced (for example, by leukemia, lymphoma, or metastatic cancer), and this results in decreased production of red blood cells.

Anemia may also result when too many red blood cells are destroyed. Normally, red blood cells live about 120 days; scavenger cells in the bone marrow, spleen, and liver detect and destroy red blood cells that are near or beyond their usual life span. If red blood cells are destroyed prematurely (hemolysis), the bone marrow tries to compensate by producing new cells faster. When destruction of red blood cells exceeds their production, hemolytic anemia results. Hemolytic anemia is relatively uncommon compared with the anemia caused by excessive bleeding and decreased red blood cell production.

Symptoms and Diagnosis

Symptoms vary depending on the severity of the anemia and how rapidly it develops. Some people with mild anemia, particularly when it develops slowly, have no symptoms at all; others may experience symptoms only with physical exertion. More severe anemia may produce symptoms even when a person is resting. Symptoms are more severe when mild or severe anemia develops rapidly, such as with bleeding that occurs when a blood vessel ruptures.

Mild anemia often causes fatigue, weakness, and paleness. In addition to these symptoms, more severe anemia may produce faintness, dizziness, increased thirst, sweating, a weak and rapid pulse, and rapid breathing. Severe anemia may produce painful lower leg cramps during exercise, shortness of breath, and chest pain, especially if a person already has impaired blood circulation in the legs or certain types of lung or heart disease.

Sometimes anemia is detected before a person notices symptoms, when routine blood tests are performed.

Low levels of hemoglobin and a low hematocrit (the percentage of red blood cells in the total blood volume) confirm the anemia. Other tests help determine the cause of the anemia.

Anemia From Excessive Bleeding

Anemia from excessive bleeding results when loss of red blood cells through bleeding exceeds production of new red blood cells.

Excessive bleeding is the most common cause of anemia. When blood is lost, the body quickly pulls water from tissues outside the

THE MAJOR CAUSES OF ANEMIA

EXCESSIVE BLEEDING	DECREASED RED BLOOD CELL PRODUCTION	INCREASED RED BLOOD CELL DESTRUCTION
Sudden	Iron deficiency	Enlarged spleen
Accidents	Vitamin B_{12} deficiency	Mechanical damage to red blood
Surgery	Folic acid deficiency	cells
Childbirth	Vitamin C deficiency	Autoimmune reactions against
Ruptured blood vessel	Chronic disease	red blood cells
	Aplastic anemia	Paroxysmal nocturnal
Chronic	Myelofibrosis	hemoglobinuria
Nosebleeds	Myelodysplasia	Hereditary spherocytosis
Hemorrhoids	Multiple myeloma	Hereditary elliptocytosis
Ulcers in the stomach or small	Leukemia	G6PD deficiency
intestine	Lymphoma	Sickle cell disease
Cancer or polyps in the digestive	Metastatic cancer	Hemoglobin C disease
tract		Hemoglobin S-C disease
Kidney or bladder tumors		Hemoglobin E disease
Heavy menstrual bleeding		Thalassemia

bloodstream in an attempt to keep the blood vessels filled. As a result, the blood is diluted, and the hematocrit (the percentage of red blood cells in the total blood volume) is reduced. Eventually, increased production of red blood cells may correct the anemia. Over time, bleeding can reduce the amount of iron in the body, so that the bone marrow is not able to increase production of new red blood cells to replace those lost.

The symptoms may be severe initially, especially if anemia develops rapidly from a sudden loss of blood, such as from an accident, surgery, childbirth, or a ruptured blood vessel. Losing large amounts of blood suddenly can create two problems: Blood pressure falls because the amount of fluid left in the blood vessels is insufficient, and the body's oxygen supply is drastically reduced because the number of oxygen-carrying red blood cells has diminished so quickly. Either problem may lead to a heart attack, stroke, or death.

Far more common than a sudden loss of blood is chronic (continuous or repeated) bleeding, which may occur in various parts of the body. Bleeding from nosebleeds and hemorrhoids is obvious. Bleeding from other common sources—such as ulcers in the stomach or small intestine and polyps or cancers in the large intestine—may not be obvious. The amount of blood is small and may not be visible in the stool. This type of blood loss is described as occult. Other sources of chronic bleeding include kidney or bladder tumors,

which may cause blood to be lost in the urine, and heavy menstrual bleeding.

Symptoms and Diagnosis

Symptoms are similar to those of other types of anemia and vary from mild to severe, depending on how much blood is lost.

How rapidly the blood is lost also determines whether symptoms are mild or severe. When the blood loss is rapid—over several hours or less—loss of just one third of the blood volume can be fatal. Dizziness upon sitting or standing after a period of lying down (orthostatic hypotension) is common when blood loss is rapid. When the blood loss is slower—over several days, weeks, or longer—loss of up to two thirds of the blood volume may cause only fatigue and weakness or no symptoms at all, if the person drinks enough fluids.

A doctor may suspect blood loss is causing anemia when a person describes symptoms of anemia and has noticed bleeding. Stool and urine are tested for blood in an effort to identify the source of bleeding. Imaging tests or endoscopy may be needed to identify the source of bleeding.

Treatment

For large or rapid blood loss, transfusion of red blood cells is the only reliable treatment. Also, the source of bleeding must be found and stopped. With slow or small blood loss, the body may produce enough red blood cells to correct the anemia without the need for blood transfusions. Because iron, which is required to produce red blood cells, is lost during bleeding, most people who have anemia from bleeding need to take iron supplements, usually tablets, for several months.

Iron Deficiency Anemia

Iron deficiency anemia results from low or depleted stores of iron, which is needed to produce red blood cells.

Iron deficiency anemia usually develops slowly, because it may take several months for the body's iron reserves to be used up. As the iron reserves are decreasing, the bone marrow gradually produces fewer red blood cells. When the reserves are depleted, the red blood cells are not only fewer in number but also abnormally small.

Iron deficiency is one of the most common causes of anemia, and blood loss is the most common cause of iron deficiency in adults. In

OTHER CAUSES OF ANEMIA

Cause	Mechanism	Treatment	Comments
Enlarged spleen	An enlarged spleen traps and destroys too many red blood cells	Treatment is aimed at the disorder that has caused the spleen to enlarge. Sometimes the spleen must be removed surgically	Symptoms tend to be mild; often an enlarged spleen reduces the number of platelets and white blood cells
Damage to red blood cells	Abnormalities in the blood vessels (such as an aneurysm), an artificial heart valve, or extremely high blood pressure can break apart normal red blood cells	The cause of the damage is identified and corrected	The kidneys eventually filter the broken-apart red blood cell components out of the blood but may also be damaged by them
Paroxysmal nocturnal hemoglobinuria	The immune system destroys red blood cells in a sudden (paroxysmal) way, not just at night	Corticosteroids relieve symptoms, but no cure is available. People with blood clots may need to take an anticoagulant. Bone marrow transplantation may be needed	Can cause severe stomach cramps and clotting in the large veins of the abdomen and legs
Hereditary spherocytosis	Red blood cells become misshapen and rigid, getting trapped and destroyed in the spleen	Treatment is usually not needed, but severe anemia may require removal of the spleen	An inherited disorder that can also cause bone abnormalities, such as a tower-shaped skull and extra fingers and toes
Hereditary elliptocytosis	Red blood cells are oval or elliptical in shape rather than the normal disk shape	Severe anemia may require removal of the spleen	The anemia is usually mild and requires no treatment
G6PD deficiency	The G6PD enzyme is missing from red blood cell membranes. Without the enzyme, red blood cells are more likely to break apart	Anemia can be prevented by avoiding the situations or substances (fever, diabetic crisis, aspirin, vitamin K, fava beans) that trigger it	An inherited disorder that almost always affects only males. About 10% of black males and a smaller percentage of white people of Mediterranean origin have the disorder

men and postmenopausal women, iron deficiency usually indicates bleeding in the digestive tract. Monthly menstrual bleeding may cause iron deficiency in premenopausal women. Iron deficiency may also result from too little iron in the diet,▲ especially in infants, young children, adolescent girls, and pregnant women.

Symptoms and Diagnosis

Symptoms of iron deficiency anemia tend to develop gradually and are similar to symptoms produced by other types of anemia.

Once a doctor diagnoses anemia, tests for iron deficiency are often performed. With iron deficiency, the red blood cells tend to be small and pale. Blood levels of iron and transferrin (the protein that carries iron when it is not inside red blood cells) are measured and compared. The most accurate test for iron deficiency is a measurement of the blood level of ferritin (a protein that stores iron). A low level of ferritin indicates iron deficiency. However, sometimes ferritin levels are misleading because they can be falsely elevated by liver damage, inflammation, infection, or cancer. In this case, the doctor may measure the level of a protein on the surface of cells that binds to transferrin (transferrin receptor).

Occasionally, the diagnosis requires a bone marrow biopsy to determine the iron content of blood cells in the bone marrow.

Treatment

Because excessive bleeding is the most common cause of iron deficiency, the first step is to locate its source.

Normal dietary iron intake usually cannot compensate for iron loss from chronic bleeding, and the body has a very small iron reserve. Consequently, lost iron must be replaced by taking iron supplements.

Correcting iron deficiency anemia with iron supplements usually takes 3 to 6 weeks, even after the bleeding has stopped. Iron supplements are usually taken by mouth. An iron supplement is absorbed best when taken 30 minutes before breakfast with a source of vitamin C (either orange juice or a vitamin C supplement). Iron supplements are typically continued for 6 months after the blood counts return to normal to fully replenish the body's reserves. Blood tests are performed periodically to ensure that the person's iron supply is sufficient.

Vitamin Deficiency Anemia

Vitamin deficiency anemia results from low or depleted levels of vitamin B_{12} or folic acid (folate).

Vitamin B_{12} deficiency and folic acid deficiency cause megaloblastic anemia. In megaloblastic anemia, the bone marrow produces red cells that are large and abnormal (megaloblasts).

Deficiency of vitamin B_{12}■ or folic acid★ most often develops due to a lack of these vitamins in the diet or an inability to absorb these vitamins from the digestive tract. Deficiency of these vitamins is sometimes caused by drugs used to treat cancer, such as methotrexate, hydroxyurea, fluorouracil, and cytarabine.

Symptoms and Diagnosis

Symptoms of anemia due to vitamin B_{12} or folic acid deficiency develop slowly and are similar to symptoms produced by other types of anemia. Vitamin B_{12} deficiency can also cause nerves to malfunction.●

Once anemia has been diagnosed, tests are performed to determine if a deficiency of vitamin B_{12} or folic acid is the cause. Anemia due to vitamin B_{12} or folic acid deficiency is suspected when large abnormal cells (megaloblasts) are seen in a blood sample that is examined under a microscope. Changes in white blood cells and platelets also can be detected, especially when a person has had megaloblastic anemia for a long time.

The blood levels of vitamin B_{12} and folic acid are measured, and other tests may be performed to determine the cause of the vitamin deficiency.

Treatment

The treatment of anemia due to vitamin B_{12} or folic acid deficiency consists of replacing the deficient vitamin.

Commonly, vitamin B_{12} is administered by injection. At first, injections are given daily or weekly for several weeks until the blood levels of vitamin B_{12} return to normal; then injections are given once a month. Vitamin B_{12} can also be taken daily as a nose spray, a tablet placed under the tongue, or a tablet that is swallowed. People who have anemia due to vitamin B_{12} deficiency usually must take vitamin B_{12} supplements for life.

▲ see page 907   ■ see page 898
★ see page 899   ● see page 898

Folic acid can be taken as one tablet daily. People who have trouble absorbing folic acid take supplements for life.

Anemia of Chronic Disease

In anemia of chronic disease, some chronic disorder slows the production of red blood cells, the result of production of proteins called cytokines that interfere with the production of red blood cells.

Chronic disease often leads to anemia, especially in older adults. Conditions such as infections, inflammation, and cancer particularly suppress production of red blood cells in the bone marrow. Since the suppression is usually not severe, anemia develops slowly and is evident only after time. Because the bone marrow is unable to use stored iron in the developing red blood cells, this type of anemia is often called iron-reutilization anemia.

Because this type of anemia develops slowly and is generally mild, it usually produces few or no symptoms. When symptoms do occur, they usually result from the disease causing the anemia rather than from the anemia itself. There are no specific laboratory tests, so the diagnosis is typically made by excluding other causes.

Because no specific treatment exists for this type of anemia, doctors treat the disease causing it. Taking additional iron or vitamins does not help. On the rare occasion that the anemia becomes severe, transfusions may help. Alternatively, erythropoietin or darbepoietin, drugs that stimulate the bone marrow to produce red blood cells, may be given.

Autoimmune Hemolytic Anemia

Autoimmune hemolytic anemia is a group of disorders characterized by a malfunction of the immune system that produces autoantibodies, which attack red blood cells as if they were substances foreign to the body.

Autoimmune hemolytic anemia is an uncommon group of disorders that can occur at any age. These disorders affect women more often than men. About half of the time, the cause of autoimmune hemolytic anemia cannot be determined (idiopathic autoimmune hemolytic anemia). Autoimmune hemolytic anemia can also be caused by or occur with another disease, such as systemic lupus ery-

Aplastic Anemia: When the Bone Marrow Shuts Down

When the bone marrow cells that develop into mature blood cells and platelets (stem cells) are damaged or suppressed, the bone marrow can shut down. This bone marrow failure is called aplastic anemia. The most common cause of aplastic anemia may be an autoimmune disorder, in which the immune system suppresses bone marrow stem cells. Other causes include infection with parvovirus, radiation exposure, toxins (such as benzene), chemotherapy drugs, and other drugs (such as chloramphenicol).

The bone marrow failure leads to too few red blood cells (anemia), too few white blood cells (leukopenia), and too few platelets (thrombocytopenia). The anemia causes fatigue, weakness, and paleness; the leukopenia causes increased susceptibility to infection; the thrombocytopenia causes easy bruising and bleeding. In some people, only red blood cell production is affected (resulting in a condition called pure red blood cell aphasia); this is particularly true when parvovirus infection is the cause. Aplastic anemia is diagnosed when microscopic examination of a sample of bone marrow (bone marrow biopsy) reveals a sharp decrease in the number of stem cells and in the maturation of blood cells.

People with aplastic anemia quickly die unless immediately treated. Transfusions of red blood cells, platelets, and substances called growth factors may temporarily increase the numbers of red blood cells, white blood cells, and platelets. Stem cell or bone marrow transplantation can cure aplastic anemia in younger and middle-aged people. Older adults and people without a suitable bone marrow donor often respond to treatment with corticosteroids and drugs that suppress the immune system.

thematosus, and rarely it follows the use of certain drugs, such as penicillin.

Destruction of red blood cells by autoantibodies may occur suddenly, or it may develop gradually. In some people, the destruction may stop after a period of time; whereas in other people, it persists and becomes chronic. There are two main types of autoimmune hemolytic anemia: warm antibody hemolytic anemia and cold antibody hemolytic anemia. In the warm antibody type, the autoantibodies attach to and destroy red blood cells at temperatures equal to or in excess of normal body temperature. In the cold antibody type, the autoantibodies become most active and attack red blood cells only at temperatures well below normal body temperature.

Symptoms

Some people with autoimmune hemolytic anemia may have no symptoms, especially when the destruction of red blood cells is mild and develops gradually. Others have symptoms similar to those that occur with other types of anemia, especially when the destruction is more severe or rapid. When severe or rapid destruction of red blood cells occurs, mild jaundice may also develop. When destruction persists for a few months or longer, the spleen may enlarge, resulting in a sense of abdominal fullness and, occasionally, discomfort.

When the cause of autoimmune hemolytic anemia is another disease, symptoms of the underlying disease, such as swollen and tender lymph nodes and fever, may dominate.

Diagnosis

Once a doctor diagnoses anemia, increased destruction of red blood cells is suspected when a blood test shows an increase in the number of red blood cells that are immature (reticulocytes). Alternatively, a blood test may show an increased amount of a substance called bilirubin and a decreased amount of a protein called haptoglobin.

Autoimmune hemolytic anemia as the cause is confirmed when blood tests detect increased amounts of certain antibodies, either attached to red blood cells (direct antiglobulin or Coombs test) or in the liquid portion of the blood (indirect antiglobulin or Coombs test). Other tests sometimes help determine the cause of the autoimmune reaction that is destroying red blood cells.

Treatment

If symptoms are mild or if destruction of red blood cells seems to be slowing on its own, no treatment is needed. If red blood cell destruction is worsening, a corticosteroid drug such

as prednisone is usually the first choice for treatment. High doses are used at first, followed by a gradual tapering of the dose over many weeks or months. When people do not respond to corticosteroids or when the corticosteroid causes intolerable side effects, surgery to remove the spleen (splenectomy) is often the next treatment. When destruction of red blood cells persists after removal of the spleen or when surgery cannot be performed, immunosuppressive drugs, such as cyclophosphamide or azathioprine, are used.

Plasmapheresis, which involves filtering blood to remove antibodies, is occasionally helpful when other treatments fail.▲ When red blood cell destruction is severe, blood transfusions are sometimes needed, but they do not treat the cause of the anemia and provide only temporary relief.

Sickle Cell Disease

Sickle cell disease is an inherited condition characterized by sickle (crescent)-shaped red blood cells and chronic anemia caused by excessive destruction of red blood cells.

Sickle cell disease affects blacks almost exclusively. About 10% of blacks in the United States have one copy of the gene for sickle cell disease (that is, they have sickle cell trait); they do not develop sickle cell disease, although rarely they may notice blood in their urine. About 0.3% of blacks have two copies of the gene; they develop the disease.

In sickle cell disease, the red blood cells contain an abnormal form of hemoglobin (the protein that carries oxygen) that reduces the amount of oxygen in the cells. The reduced oxygen causes some of the red blood cells to become sickle-shaped. Because these deformed cells are fragile, they break apart as they travel through the smallest blood vessels, causing severe anemia, blocked blood flow, and reduced oxygen supply. The deformed cells also damage the spleen, kidneys, brain, bones, and other organs.

Symptoms and Complications

People who have sickle cell disease always have some degree of anemia and mild jaundice, but they may have few other symptoms. Anything that reduces the amount of oxygen in their blood, such as vigorous exercise, mountain climbing, flying at high altitudes without sufficient oxygen, or an illness, may

▲ see box on page 986

bring on a sickle cell "crisis." A crisis may consist of a sudden worsening of anemia, pain (often in the abdomen or long bones of the arms and legs), fever, and sometimes shortness of breath. Abdominal pain may be severe, and vomiting may occur.

In children, sickle cell crisis may take the form of a chest syndrome, characterized by severe chest pain and difficulty breathing. The exact cause of the chest syndrome is unknown but may be related to or produced by an infection or a blocked blood vessel resulting from a blood clot or an embolus (a piece of a blood clot that has broken off and lodged in a blood vessel).

Most people who have sickle cell disease develop an enlarged spleen during childhood. By the time the person reaches adolescence, the spleen is often so badly injured that it shrinks and no longer functions. Because the spleen helps fight infection, people with sickle cell disease are more likely to develop pneumococcal pneumonia and other infections. Viral infections, in particular, can decrease blood cell production, so anemia becomes more severe. The liver becomes progressively larger throughout life, and gallstones often form from the pigment of broken-apart red blood cells. The heart usually enlarges, and heart murmurs are common.

Children who have sickle cell disease often have a relatively short torso but long arms, legs, fingers, and toes. Changes in the bones and bone marrow may cause bone pain, especially in the hands and feet. Episodes of joint pain with fever may occur, and the hip joint may become so damaged that it eventually needs to be replaced.

Poor circulation to the skin may cause sores on the legs, especially at the ankles. Young men may develop persistent, often painful erections (priapism). Blocked blood vessels may cause strokes that damage the nervous system. In older people, lung and kidney function may deteriorate.

Diagnosis

Doctors recognize anemia, stomach and bone pain, and nausea in a young black person as signs of a sickle cell crisis. Sickle-shaped red blood cells and fragments of destroyed red blood cells can be seen in a blood sample examined under a microscope.

A blood test called electrophoresis can detect abnormal hemoglobin and indicate whether a person has sickle cell trait or sickle

Red Blood Cell Shapes

Normal red blood cells are flexible and disk-shaped, thicker at the edges than in the middle. In several hereditary disorders, red blood cells become spherical (in hereditary spherocytosis), oval (in hereditary elliptocytosis), or sickle-shaped (in sickle cell disease).

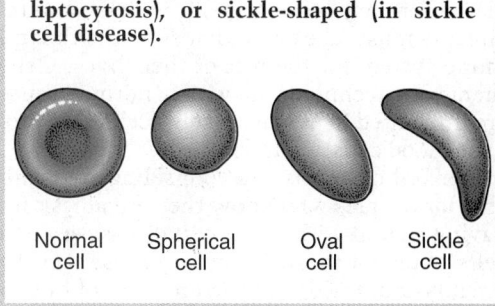

| Normal cell | Spherical cell | Oval cell | Sickle cell |

cell disease. Discovering the trait may be important for family planning, to determine the risk of having a child with sickle cell disease.

Treatment and Prevention

Sickle cell disease can be a relatively mild disease that requires little treatment or a severe, recurring disease that causes enormous disability and early death. Rarely, a person who has sickle cell trait dies suddenly while undergoing very strenuous exercise that has caused severe dehydration, such as during military or athletic training.

Sickle cell disease cannot be cured, so treatment is aimed at preventing crises, controlling the anemia, and relieving symptoms. People who have this disease should try to avoid activities that reduce the amount of oxygen in their blood and should seek prompt medical attention for even minor illnesses, such as viral infections. Because they are at increased risk of infection, they should be immunized with pneumococcal and *Haemophilus influenzae* vaccines.

Sickle cell crisis may require hospitalization. The person is given large amounts of fluid intravenously and drugs to relieve pain. Blood transfusions and oxygen may be given if a doctor suspects that anemia is severe enough to pose a risk of stroke, heart attack, or lung damage. Conditions that may have caused the crisis, such as an infection, are treated.

Drugs can help control sickle cell disease. Hydroxyurea increases the production of a form of hemoglobin found predominantly in fetuses, which decreases the number of red blood cells becoming sickle-shaped. Therefore, it reduces the frequency of sickle cell crises. Bone marrow or stem cells from a family member or other donor who does not have the sickle cell gene may be transplanted in a person with the disease. Although such transplantation may be curative, it is risky, and recipients must take drugs that suppress the immune system for the rest of their lives. Gene therapy, a technique in which normal genes are implanted in precursor cells (cells that produce blood cells), is under study.

Prenatal diagnosis and counseling are available for couples who know they are at risk for having a child with sickle cell disease.▲ Fetal cells obtained through amniocentesis can be directly examined, and the presence of one or two copies of the sickle cell gene can be accurately determined.

Hemoglobin C, S-C, and E Diseases

Hemoglobin C, S-C, and E diseases are inherited conditions characterized by abnormally shaped red blood cells and chronic anemia that is caused by excessive destruction of red blood cells.

Hemoglobin C disease occurs mostly in blacks, affecting 2 to 3% of blacks in the United States. A person must inherit two copies of the abnormal gene that causes the disease in order to develop it. In general, symptoms are few. Anemia varies in severity. People who have this disease, particularly children, may have episodes of abdominal and joint pain, an enlarged spleen, and mild jaundice, but they do not have severe crises, as occur in sickle cell disease.

Hemoglobin S-C disease occurs in people who have one copy of the gene for sickle cell disease and one copy of the gene for hemoglobin C disease. Hemoglobin S-C disease is much more common than hemoglobin C disease, and its symptoms are similar to those of sickle cell disease but much milder.

Hemoglobin E disease affects primarily blacks and people from Southeast Asia. This disease produces anemia but none of the other symptoms that occur in sickle cell disease and hemoglobin C disease.

Thalassemias

Thalassemias are a group of inherited disorders resulting from an imbalance in the production of one of the four chains of amino acids that make up hemoglobin (the oxygen-carrying protein found in red blood cells).

Thalassemias are categorized according to the amino acid chain affected. The two main types are alpha-thalassemia (the alpha chain is affected) and beta-thalassemia (the beta chain is affected). Alpha-thalassemia is most common in blacks (25% carry at least one copy of the defective gene), and beta-thalassemia is most common in people from the Mediterranean area and Southeast Asia. Thalassemias are also categorized according to whether a person has one copy of the defective gene (thalassemia minor) or two copies of the defective gene (thalassemia major).

All thalassemias have similar symptoms, but they vary in severity. In alpha-thalassemia minor and beta-thalassemia minor, people have mild anemia with no symptoms. In alpha-thalassemia major, people have moderate or severe symptoms of anemia and an enlarged spleen.

In beta-thalassemia major, people have severe symptoms of anemia, and they may also have jaundice, skin ulcers, gallstones, and an enlarged spleen. Overactive bone marrow may cause some bones, especially those in the head and face, to thicken and enlarge. The long bones in the arms and legs may weaken and fracture easily.

Children who have beta-thalassemia major may grow more slowly and reach puberty later than they normally would. Because iron absorption may be increased and frequent blood transfusions (providing even more iron) are needed, excessive iron may accumulate and be deposited in the heart muscle, eventually causing iron overload disease and heart failure.

Thalassemias are more difficult to diagnose than other hemoglobin disorders. Testing a drop of blood by electrophoresis is helpful but may be inconclusive, especially for alpha-thalassemia. Therefore, the diagnosis is usually based on special hemoglobin tests and determination of hereditary patterns.

Most people who have a thalassemia do not need treatment, but people who have a severe form may need bone marrow transplantation. Gene therapy, in which normal genes are inserted in the person, is being studied but to date has been unsuccessful.

▲ see page 1429

CHAPTER 173

Bleeding and Clotting Disorders

An abnormality in any part of the system that controls bleeding (hemostasis) can lead to excessive bleeding or excessive clotting, both of which can be dangerous. When clotting is poor, even a slight injury to a blood vessel may lead to major blood loss. When clotting is uncontrolled, small blood vessels in critical places can become clogged with clots. Clogged vessels in the brain can cause strokes; clogged vessels leading to the heart can cause heart attacks; and pieces of clots from veins in the legs, pelvis, or abdomen can travel through the bloodstream to the lungs and block major arteries there (pulmonary embolism).

Hemostasis is the body's way of stopping injured blood vessels from bleeding. It involves three major processes: narrowing (constriction) of blood vessels, activity of platelets, and activity of blood clotting factors.

An injured blood vessel constricts so that blood flows out more slowly and clotting can start. At the same time, the accumulating pool of blood outside the blood vessel (a hematoma) presses against the vessel, helping prevent further bleeding.

As soon as a blood vessel wall is damaged, a series of reactions activates platelets so that they stick to the injured area. The "glue" that holds platelets to the blood vessel wall is von Willebrand factor, a protein produced by the cells of the vessel wall. The proteins collagen and thrombin act at the site of the injury to induce platelets to stick together. As platelets accumulate at the site, they form a mesh that plugs the injury. The platelets change shape from round to spiny, and they release proteins and other substances that entrap more platelets and clotting proteins in the enlarging plug that becomes a blood clot.

Thrombin converts fibrinogen, a blood clotting factor that is normally dissolved in blood, into long strands of fibrin that radiate from the clumped platelets and form a net that entraps more platelets and blood cells. The fibrin strands add bulk to the developing clot and help hold it in place to keep the vessel wall plugged. Formation of a clot also involves activation of a sequence of blood clotting factors that generate thrombin.

The reactions that result in the formation of a blood clot are balanced by other reactions that stop the clotting process and dissolve clots after the blood vessel has healed. Without this control system, minor blood vessel injuries could trigger widespread clotting

Blood Clots: Plugging the Breaks

When an injury causes a blood vessel wall to break, platelets are activated. They change shape from round to spiny, stick to the broken vessel wall and each other, and begin to plug the break. They also interact with other blood proteins to form fibrin. Fibrin strands form a net that entraps more platelets and blood cells, producing a clot that plugs the break.

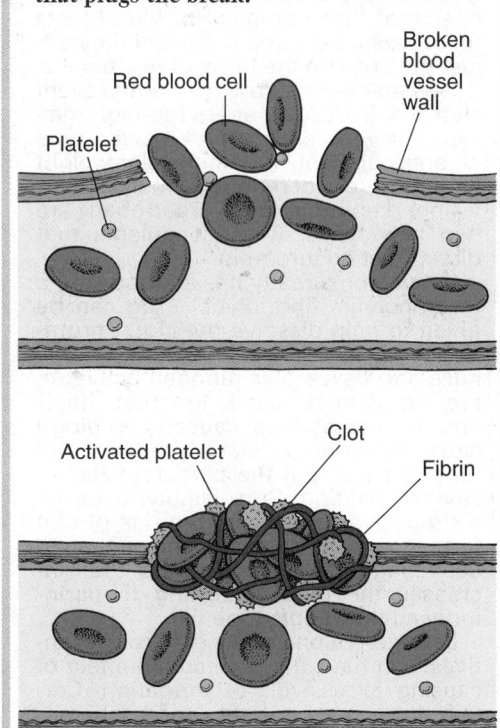

Drugs and Blood Clots:
A Complicated Relationship

The relationship between drugs and the body's ability to control bleeding (hemostasis) is complicated. The body's ability to form blood clots is vital to hemostasis, but too much clotting increases the risk of a heart attack, stroke, or pulmonary embolism. Many drugs, either intentionally or unintentionally, affect the body's ability to form blood clots.

Some people are at high risk of forming blood clots and are intentionally given drugs to decrease the risk. Drugs may be given that reduce the stickiness of platelets, so that they will not clump together to block a blood vessel. Aspirin, ticlopidine, clopidogrel, abciximab, and tirofiban are examples of drugs that interfere with the activity of platelets.

Other people at risk of forming blood clots may be given an anticoagulant, a drug that inhibits the action of blood proteins called clotting factors. Although often called "blood thinners," anticoagulants do not really thin the blood. Commonly used anticoagulants are warfarin, given by mouth, and heparin, given by injection. People who take these drugs must be under close medical supervision. Doctors monitor the effects of these drugs with blood tests that measure clotting time, and they adjust the dose on the basis of test results. Doses that are too low may not prevent clots, while doses that are too high may cause severe bleeding. A newer type of anticoagulant, low-molecular-weight heparin, does not require as much supervision. Lepirudin and argatroban are two new types of anticoagulants that directly act on thrombin.

If a person already has a blood clot, a thrombolytic (fibrinolytic) drug can be given to help dissolve the clot. Thrombolytic drugs, which include streptokinase and tissue plasminogen activator, are sometimes used to treat heart attacks and strokes caused by blood clots. These drugs may save lives, but they can also put the person at risk of severe bleeding. Surprisingly, heparin, a drug given to reduce the risk of clot formation, sometimes has an unintended activating effect on platelets that increases the risk of clotting (heparin-induced thrombocytopenia).

Estrogen, alone or in oral contraceptives, can have the unintended effect of causing excessive clot formation. Certain drugs used to treat cancer (chemotherapy drugs), such as asparaginase, can also increase the risk of clotting.

throughout the body—which actually happens in some diseases.

Hereditary Hemorrhagic Telangiectasia

Hereditary hemorrhagic telangiectasia (Rendu-Osler-Weber disease) is a hereditary disorder in which blood vessels are malformed, making them fragile and prone to bleeding.

Blood vessels under the skin may break and bleed, causing small, red-to-violet discolorations, especially on the face, lips, lining of the mouth and nose, and tips of the fingers and toes. Severe nosebleeds may also occur. Small blood vessels in the digestive and urinary tracts, as well as in the brain and spinal cord, may also be affected, causing bleeding in these sites.

Treatment is aimed at stopping an occurrence of bleeding. Treatment may involve applying pressure, using a topical drug that narrows blood vessels (astringent), or using a laser beam to destroy the leaking blood vessel. Severe bleeding may require more invasive techniques. Bleeding almost always recurs, resulting in iron deficiency anemia; consequently, people with hereditary hemorrhagic telangiectasia need to take iron supplements.

Allergic Purpura

Allergic purpura (Henoch-Schönlein purpura) is a disease in which blood vessels in the skin, joints, digestive tract, or kidneys may become inflamed and leak.

Allergic purpura, an uncommon disease, affects mainly young children but can affect older children and adults. The disease is believed to be the result of an autoimmune reaction, in which the body attacks its own tissues. Usually, allergic purpura develops after a respiratory tract infection, but it can be caused by an allergic reaction to drugs. The rate at which the disease develops and its duration vary.

Symptoms and Diagnosis

The disease may begin with the appearance of small, bluish purple bruises (purpura)—most often on the feet, legs, arms, and buttocks—as blood leaks from vessels in the skin. Over several days, the purpura may become raised and hard; crops of new purpura may break out for several weeks after the first one appears. Swollen, achy joints are common, usually accompanied by fever. Bleeding in the digestive tract may cause abdominal cramps and pain. Blood in the urine (hematuria) may develop. Most people recover completely within a month, but symptoms may recur several times. Bleeding in the kidneys may cause kidney damage.

The diagnosis is based on the symptoms.

Treatment

A drug that may be causing an allergic reaction is discontinued immediately. Corticosteroids (for example, prednisone) may help relieve swelling, joint pain, and abdominal pain, but they do not prevent or reverse kidney damage. Drugs that reduce the activity of the immune system (immunosuppressive drugs), including azathioprine or cyclophosphamide, are sometimes used if kidney damage develops, but it is not known if they are helpful.

Thrombocytopenia

Thrombocytopenia is a deficiency of platelets (thrombocytes).

The blood usually contains about 150,000 to 350,000 platelets per microliter. Bleeding can occur with relatively minor trauma when the platelet count falls below 20,000 to 30,000 platelets per microliter of blood. The most serious risk of bleeding, however, generally does not occur until the platelet count falls below 10,000 platelets per microliter. At these very low levels, bleeding may occur without any injury.

Causes

Many diseases can cause thrombocytopenia. Thrombocytopenia can occur when the bone marrow does not produce enough platelets, as happens in leukemia and some anemias. Infection with HIV, the virus that causes AIDS, often results in thrombocytopenia. Platelets can become entrapped in an enlarged spleen, as happens in myelofibrosis and Gaucher's disease, reducing the number of platelets in the bloodstream. Massive blood transfusions can dilute the concentration of platelets in the blood. Finally, the body may use or destroy too many platelets, as occurs in many disorders, three of the most notable being idiopathic thrombocytopenic purpura, thrombotic thrombocytopenic purpura, and hemolytic-uremic syndrome.

Idiopathic thrombocytopenic purpura is a disease in which antibodies form and destroy the body's platelets. Why the antibodies form is

Causes of Thrombocytopenia

Bone marrow does not produce enough platelets

- Leukemia
- Lymphoma
- Aplastic anemia
- Heavy alcohol consumption
- Megaloblastic anemias, including vitamin B_{12} and folic acid deficiency anemias
- Some bone marrow disorders

Platelets become entrapped in an enlarged spleen

- Cirrhosis with congestive splenomegaly
- Myelofibrosis
- Gaucher's disease

Platelets become diluted

- Massive blood replacement or exchange transfusion with stored blood containing too few platelets
- Cardiopulmonary bypass surgery

Use or destruction of platelets increases

- Idiopathic thrombocytopenic purpura
- HIV infection
- Drugs such as heparin, quinidine, quinine, sulfa-containing antibiotics, some oral diabetes drugs, gold salts, and rifampin
- Conditions involving disseminated intravascular coagulation within blood vessels, such as can occur with obstetric complications, cancer, blood poisoning (septicemia) from gram-negative bacteria, and traumatic brain damage
- Thrombotic thrombocytopenic purpura
- Hemolytic-uremic syndrome
- Paroxysmal nocturnal hemoglobinuria

not known. Although the bone marrow increases platelet production to compensate for the destruction, the supply cannot keep up with the demand.

Thrombotic thrombocytopenic purpura is a rare disease in which small blood clots form suddenly throughout the body. The blood clots mean that an abnormally high number of platelets are being used, which leads to a sharp decrease in the number of platelets in the bloodstream.

Hemolytic-uremic syndrome is a disorder in which the number of platelets suddenly decreases, red blood cells are destroyed, and the kidneys stop functioning. Hemolytic-uremic syndrome is rare but can occur with certain bacterial infections and with the use of certain chemotherapy drugs, including mitomycin. It is most common in infants, small children, and women who are pregnant or have just given birth, although it can occur in older children, adults, and women who are not pregnant.

Symptoms and Complications

Bleeding in the skin may be the first sign of a low platelet count. Many tiny red dots often appear in the skin on the lower legs, and minor injuries may cause small scattered bruises. The gums may bleed, and blood may appear in the stool or urine. Menstrual periods may be unusually heavy. Bleeding may be hard to stop.

Bleeding worsens as the number of platelets decreases. People who have very few platelets may lose large amounts of blood into the digestive tract or may develop life-threatening bleeding in the brain even though they have not been injured.

The rate at which symptoms develop can vary depending on the cause of thrombocytopenia. For example, in thrombotic thrombocytopenic purpura and hemolytic-uremic syndrome, symptoms develop suddenly. In idiopathic thrombocytopenic purpura, symptoms may develop suddenly or gradually and subtly.

Symptoms in thrombotic thrombocytopenic purpura and hemolytic-uremic syndrome are quite distinct. In thrombotic thrombocytopenic purpura, the small blood clots that develop (using up platelets) cause a wide range of symptoms and complications, some of which can be life threatening. Symptoms that result from clots in the brain may include headache, confusion, seizures, and coma. Symptoms that result from clots elsewhere in the body include abnormal heart rhythms, blood in the urine that accompanies kidney damage, and abdominal pain. The predominant symptoms and complications of hemolytic-uremic syndrome are related to kidney damage, which is usually severe and may progress to kidney failure.

Diagnosis

Doctors suspect thrombocytopenia in people who have abnormal bruising and bleeding.

They often check the number of platelets routinely in people who have disorders that cause thrombocytopenia. Sometimes they discover thrombocytopenia when blood tests are performed for other reasons in people who have no bruising or bleeding.

Determining the cause of thrombocytopenia is critical to treating the condition. Certain symptoms may help determine the cause. For example, people usually have a fever when thrombocytopenia results from an infection. In contrast, they usually do not have a fever when the cause is idiopathic thrombocytopenia, thrombotic thrombocytopenic purpura, or hemolytic-uremic syndrome. An enlarged spleen, which a doctor may be able to feel during a physical examination, suggests that the spleen is trapping platelets and that thrombocytopenia results from a disorder that causes the spleen to enlarge. Hemolytic-uremic syndrome is diagnosed when poor kidney function is identified by blood tests that show high levels of urea nitrogen and creatinine.

A sample of blood may be examined under a microscope, or the platelet count may be measured with an electronic counter to determine the severity of thrombocytopenia and provide clues to its cause. A sample of bone marrow removed and examined under a microscope (bone marrow aspiration and biopsy)▲ may be needed to provide information about platelet production.

Treatment

People who have a very low platelet count are often treated in a hospital or advised to stay in bed to avoid accidental injury. When bleeding is severe, platelets may be transfused.

Addressing the underlying cause can often treat the thrombocytopenia. Thrombocytopenia caused by a drug usually is corrected by discontinuing the drug. The effects produced by antibodies that destroy platelets in idiopathic thrombocytopenic purpura can be blocked temporarily with a corticosteroid (for example, prednisone), allowing the number of platelets to increase. Danazol may have similar effects as prednisone. Drugs that suppress the immune system, including cyclophosphamide and sometimes azathioprine, may reduce the formation of antibodies. Most people with idiopathic thrombocytopenic purpura eventually require surgical removal of the spleen (splenectomy) to increase the number of platelets. People with thrombotic thrombocytopenic purpura are often treated with

▲ see page 981

plasma transfusions along with plasmapheresis.▲ The two procedures together are called plasma exchange.

Complications that require long-term treatment can result from some causes of thrombocytopenia. For example, the number of platelets usually increases as people recover from the hemolytic-uremic syndrome; however, lifelong dialysis or kidney transplantation may be needed if the kidney failure persists.

Von Willebrand's Disease

Von Willebrand's disease is a hereditary deficiency or abnormality of the von Willebrand factor in the blood, a protein that affects platelet function.

The von Willebrand factor is found in plasma, platelets, and the walls of blood vessels. When the factor is missing or defective, platelets cannot adhere to the vessel wall at the site of an injury. As a result, bleeding does not stop as quickly as it should.

Symptoms and Diagnosis

Often, a person with von Willebrand's disease has a parent who has a history of bleeding problems. Typically, a child bruises easily or bleeds excessively after a cut, tooth extraction, or surgery. A young woman may have increased menstrual bleeding. Bleeding may worsen at times. On the other hand, hormonal changes, stress, pregnancy, inflammation, and infections may stimulate the body to increase production of the von Willebrand factor and temporarily improve the capacity of platelets to stick to the blood vessel wall and stop bleeding.

Laboratory tests typically show that the bleeding time is abnormally long. Bleeding time is the amount of time that elapses before bleeding stops after a small cut is made on the forearm. Doctors may order tests that measure the amount of von Willebrand factor in the blood. Because the von Willebrand factor is the protein that carries an important clotting factor (factor VIII) in the blood, the level of factor VIII in the blood may also be decreased.

Treatment

Many people with von Willebrand's disease never need treatment. If excessive bleeding occurs, a transfusion of concentrated blood clotting factors containing von Willebrand factor may be given. For some mild forms of the disease, drug treatment with desmopressin may be given to increase the amount of the von Willebrand factor long enough for surgery or dental procedures to be performed without transfusions.

Hemophilia

Hemophilia is a bleeding disorder caused by a deficiency in one of two blood clotting factors: factor VIII or factor IX.

There are two forms of hemophilia. Hemophilia A, which accounts for about 80% of all cases, is a deficiency in clotting factor VIII. Hemophilia B is a deficiency in clotting factor IX. The bleeding patterns and consequences of these two types of hemophilia are similar.

Hemophilia is caused by several different gene abnormalities. They are sex-linked, which means that the gene abnormalities are inherited through the mother and that nearly everyone with hemophilia is male.

Symptoms and Complications

The severity of the symptoms depends on how a particular gene abnormality affects the blood clotting activity of factor VIII or IX. People whose clotting activity is 5 to 25% of normal have very mild hemophilia that may go undiagnosed; however, these people may bleed more than expected after surgery, dental extractions, or a major injury. People whose blood clotting activity is 1 to 5% of normal may have only mild hemophilia. They have few unprovoked bleeding episodes, but surgery or injury may cause uncontrolled and fatal bleeding. When the clotting activity is less than 1% of normal, hemophilia is severe. Serious episodes of bleeding occur and recur for no apparent reason.

In severe hemophilia, the first bleeding episode generally occurs before 18 months of age and may follow a minor injury. A child who has hemophilia bruises easily. Even an injection into a muscle can cause bleeding that results in a large bruise and hematoma. Recurring bleeding into the joints and muscles can lead to crippling deformities. Bleeding can swell the base of the tongue until it blocks the airway, making breathing difficult. A slight bump on the head can trigger substantial bleeding in the skull, causing brain damage and death.

▲ see box on page 986

Diagnosis and Treatment

A doctor may suspect hemophilia in a child (especially a boy) who bleeds without an apparent cause or bleeds more than expected after injury. A laboratory analysis of blood samples can determine whether the boy's clotting is abnormally slow. If it is, the doctor can confirm the diagnosis of hemophilia and can determine the type and severity by testing the activity of the clotting factors.

People who have hemophilia should avoid situations that might provoke bleeding and should avoid drugs (for example, aspirin) that interfere with the function of platelets. They should be conscientious about dental care so that they will not need to have teeth extracted. If people who have milder forms of hemophilia need to have dental or other surgery, the drugs aminocaproic acid or desmopressin may be given to improve temporarily the body's ability to control bleeding so that transfusions can be avoided.

Often, treatment involves transfusions to replace the deficient clotting factor. These factors are found in normal plasma. Clotting factors may be concentrated or produced in purified form from plasma products, or they may be produced using special technological procedures as highly purified recombinant factor concentrates. Recombinant forms of both factor VIII and IX are available; the dose, frequency, and duration of therapy are determined by the site and severity of the bleeding problem. They may also be used to prevent bleeding before surgery or at the first sign of bleeding.

Some people with hemophilia develop antibodies to transfused clotting factors, which destroy the factors. As a result, factor replacement therapy becomes less effective. If antibodies are detected in the blood of a person with hemophilia, the dosage of the recombinant factor or plasma concentrates may be increased, or different types of clotting factors or drugs to reduce the antibody levels may be needed.

Thrombophilia

Thrombophilia is a disorder in which the blood clots easily or excessively.

Most disorders that cause thrombophilia increase the risk of blood clot formation in veins; a few increase the risk of clot formation in both arteries and veins.

Causes

Some of the disorders that cause thrombophilia are inherited. Many of these result from changes in the amount or function of certain proteins in the blood that control clotting. For example, activated protein C resistance (Factor V Leiden mutation), a specific mutation in the prothrombin gene, and a deficiency of protein C, protein S, or antithrombin all cause an increase in the production of fibrin, an important protein involved in clot formation. Hyperhomocysteinemia, an increase in the amount of homocysteine (a type of amino acid) in the blood, results in an increased risk of clotting in veins and arteries.

Other disorders that cause thrombophilia are acquired after birth. These disorders include disseminated intravascular coagulation (often associated with cancer), the presence of the lupus "anticoagulant," and antiphospholipid (anticardiolipin) syndrome, which increase the risk of clotting because of overactivation of blood clotting factors.

Other factors may increase the risk of clotting along with thrombophilia. Many involve conditions that result in a person not moving around sufficiently, causing blood to pool in the veins. Examples include paralysis, prolonged sitting (especially in confined spaces as in a car or airplane), prolonged bed rest, recent surgery, or heart attack. Heart failure, a condition in which the blood is not pumped sufficiently through the bloodstream, is a risk factor. Conditions that result in increased pressure on veins, including obesity or pregnancy, also increase risk.

Symptoms and Complications

Most of the inherited disorders do not begin to cause an increased risk of clotting until young adulthood, although clots can form at any age. Many people with inherited disorders develop a deep vein clot (deep vein thrombosis) in the legs, which can result in leg swelling. Formation of a deep leg clot may be followed by pulmonary embolism. After experiencing several deep vein clots, more serious swelling and skin discoloration may develop (chronic deep vein insufficiency). Sometimes, clots form in superficial leg veins, causing pain and redness (superficial thrombophlebitis). Less commonly, clots may form in arm veins, abdominal veins, and veins inside the skull. Hyperhomocysteinemia, the presence of the lupus "anticoagulant," and the antiphospholipid syndrome may result in venous or arterial clots. Arterial clots can damage and cause death of tissues that lose their supply of blood when clots form and obstruct blood flow.

Diagnosis and Treatment

A person who has had at least two separate instances of a blood clot may have an inherited thrombophilia disorder. An inherited disorder may also be suspected if a person with an initial blood clot has a family history of blood clots. A young healthy person who develops an initial clot for no apparent reason may have an inherited disorder.

Blood tests that measure the amount or activity of different proteins that control clotting are used to identify specific inherited disorders of thrombophilia. These tests are usually more accurate when performed after a blood clot has been treated.

The inherited disorders that cause thrombophilia are incurable. People who have had two or more clots are especially likely to be advised to take the anticoagulant warfarin for the rest of their lives. When a person has had only one clot, warfarin or heparin to prevent future clots may be used only when the person is at higher risk for clot formation, including during a period of prolonged bed rest.

People with hyperhomocysteinemia may be advised to take vitamin supplements with folic acid, vitamin B_6 (pyridoxine), and vitamin B_{12} (cobalamin), which can reduce homocysteine levels.

Disseminated Intravascular Coagulation

Disseminated intravascular coagulation is a condition in which small blood clots develop throughout the bloodstream, blocking small blood vessels and depleting the platelets and clotting factors needed to control bleeding.

Disseminated intravascular coagulation (DIC) begins with excessive clotting. The excessive clotting is usually stimulated by a substance that enters the blood as part of a disease (such as an infection or certain cancers) or as a complication of childbirth, retention of a dead fetus, or surgery. People who have a severe head injury or who have been bitten by a poisonous snake are also at risk. As the clotting factors and platelets are depleted, excessive bleeding occurs.

Symptoms and Diagnosis

DIC may appear suddenly and be very severe. If the condition follows surgery or childbirth, bleeding may be uncontrollable. Bleeding may occur at the site of an intravenous injection or in the brain, digestive tract, skin, muscles, and cavities of the body. If DIC develops more slowly, as in people with cancer, then clots in veins are more common than bleeding.

Blood tests may show that the number of platelets in a blood sample has dropped and that the blood is taking a long time to clot. The diagnosis of DIC is confirmed if test results show diminished amounts of clotting factors and large quantities of proteins that are produced when clots are broken up by the body (fibrin degradation products).

Treatment

The underlying cause must be identified and corrected, whether it is an obstetric problem, an infection, or a cancer. The clotting problems subside when the cause is corrected.

DIC that develops suddenly is life threatening and is treated as an emergency. Platelets and clotting factors are transfused to replace those depleted and to stop bleeding. Heparin may be used to slow the clotting in people who have more chronic, milder DIC in which clotting is more of a problem than bleeding.

CHAPTER 174

White Blood Cell Disorders

White blood cells (leukocytes) are an important part of the body's defense against infective organisms and foreign substances. To defend the body adequately, a sufficient number of white blood cells must receive a message that an infective organism or foreign substance has invaded the body, get to where they are needed, and then kill and digest the harmful organism or substance. ▲

Like all blood cells, white blood cells are produced in the bone marrow. They develop from stem (precursor) cells that mature over time into one of the five major types of white blood cells—neutrophils, lymphocytes, monocytes, eosinophils, and basophils.

Normally, a person produces about 100 billion white blood cells a day. The number of white blood cells in a given volume of blood is expressed as cells per microliter of blood. The total white blood cell count normally ranges between 4,000 and 11,000 cells per microliter. The proportion of each of the five major types of white blood cells and the total number of cells of each type can also be determined in a given volume of blood.

Too few or too many white blood cells indicates a disorder. Leukopenia, a decrease in the number of white blood cells to fewer than 4,000 cells per microliter of blood, makes a person more susceptible to infections. Leukocytosis, an increase in the number of white blood cells to more than 11,000 cells per microliter of blood, may result from the normal response of the body to help fight an infection. However, an increase in the number of white blood cells can also result when the regulation of white blood cell development is disrupted and immature or abnormal cells are released into the blood.

Some white blood cell disorders involve only one of the five types of white blood cells; other disorders may involve a few types together or all five types. Disorders of neutrophils and disorders of lymphocytes are the most common. Disorders that involve monocytes and eosinophils are less common, and disorders involving basophils are rare.

Neutropenia

Neutropenia is an abnormally low number of neutrophils in the blood.

Neutrophils serve as the major defense of the body against acute bacterial and certain fungal infections. Neutrophils usually constitute about 45 to 75% of all white blood cells in the bloodstream. When the neutrophil count falls below 1,000 cells per microliter of blood,

the risk of infection increases somewhat; when it falls below 500 cells per microliter, the risk of infection increases greatly. Without the key defense provided by neutrophils, a person has problems controlling infections and is at risk of dying from an infection.

Causes

Neutropenia can develop if neutrophils are used up or destroyed in the bloodstream faster than the bone marrow can make new ones. With some bacterial infections, some allergic disorders, and some drug treatments, neutrophils are destroyed faster than they are produced. People with an autoimmune disease can make antibodies that destroy neutrophils and result in neutropenia. People with an enlarged spleen■ may have a low neutrophil count because the enlarged spleen traps and destroys neutrophils.

Neutropenia can also develop if the production of neutrophils in the bone marrow is reduced, as can occur in some people with cancer, viral infections such as influenza, bacterial infections such as tuberculosis, myelofibrosis, or deficiencies of vitamin B_{12} or folic acid. People who have received radiation therapy that involves the bone marrow may also develop neutropenia. Many drugs, including phenytoin, chloramphenicol, sulfa drugs, and many drugs used in cancer treatment (chemotherapy), as well as certain toxins (benzene and insecticides) can also impair the bone marrow's ability to produce neutrophils.

Production of neutrophils in the bone marrow is also affected by a severe disorder called aplastic anemia (in which the bone marrow may shut down production of all blood cells). ★ Certain rare hereditary diseases also cause the number of neutrophils to decrease.

Symptoms and Diagnosis

Neutropenia can develop suddenly over a few hours or days (acute neutropenia), or it can develop gradually and last for months or years (chronic neutropenia). Because neutropenia itself has no specific symptoms, it is usually diagnosed when an infection occurs. In acute neutropenia, a person can develop fever and painful sores (ulcers) around the mouth and anus. Bacterial pneumonia and other severe infections can follow. In chronic neutropenia, the course may be less severe if the number of neutrophils is not extremely low, and the course can occasionally be intermittent (cyclic neutropenia).

▲ see page 1050 and art on page 1053
■ see page 1028   ★ see box on page 991

When a person has frequent or unusual infections, a doctor suspects neutropenia and orders a complete blood cell count to make the diagnosis. A low neutrophil count indicates neutropenia. In many cases, the neutropenia is expected and the cause is known, as in those receiving chemotherapy or radiation therapy. When the cause is not known, it must be determined.

A doctor usually takes a sample of bone marrow through a needle.▲ The bone marrow sample is examined under a microscope to determine whether it looks normal, has a normal number of neutrophil stem cells, and shows normal development of neutrophils. By determining whether the number of stem cells is decreased and whether these cells are maturing normally, the doctor may be able to determine whether the problem lies in faulty production of the cells or whether too many cells are being used or destroyed in the bloodstream. Sometimes, the bone marrow examination indicates that other diseases, such as leukemia or other cancers, or infections, such as tuberculosis, are affecting the bone marrow.

Treatment

The treatment of neutropenia depends on its cause and severity. Drugs that may cause neutropenia are discontinued whenever possible, and exposures to suspected toxins are avoided. Sometimes the bone marrow recovers by itself without treatment. The neutropenia accompanying viral infections (such as influenza) may be transient and resolve after the infection has cleared. People who have mild neutropenia generally have no symptoms and may not need treatment.

People who have severe neutropenia can rapidly succumb to infection because their bodies lack the means to fight invading organisms. When these people develop infections, they are generally hospitalized and immediately given strong antibiotics, even before the cause and exact location of the infection are identified. Fever, the symptom that usually indicates infection in a person who has neutropenia, is an important sign that immediate medical attention is needed.

Growth factors called colony-stimulating factors, which stimulate the production of white blood cells, are sometimes helpful. Corticosteroids may help if the neutropenia is caused by an autoimmune reaction. Antithymocyte globulin or other types of therapy that suppresses the activity of the immune system may be used when a disease such as aplastic anemia is present. Removing an enlarged spleen may cure the neutropenia involved with hypersplenism.

When neutropenia is caused by another disease (such as tuberculosis or leukemia or other cancers), treatment of the underlying disease may resolve the neutropenia. Bone marrow (or stem cell) transplantation is not used to treat neutropenia per se, but it may be recommended to treat certain serious causes of neutropenia, such as aplastic anemia or leukemia.

Neutrophilic Leukocytosis

Neutrophilic leukocytosis is an abnormally high number of neutrophils in the blood.

Neutrophils help the body to fight infections and to heal injuries. Neutrophils may increase in response to a number of conditions or diseases. In many instances, the increased number of neutrophils is a necessary reaction by the body, as it tries to heal or to ward off an invading microorganism or foreign substance. Infections by bacteria, viruses, fungi, and parasites may all increase the number of neutrophils in the blood. The number may rise in a person who has an injury, such as a hip fracture or burn. Inflammatory disorders, including autoimmune diseases such as rheumatoid arthritis, can cause an increase in the number and activity of neutrophils. Some drugs, such as corticosteroids, also lead to an increased number of neutrophils in the blood. Myelocytic leukemias can lead to an increased number of immature or mature neutrophils in the blood.

When a doctor discovers an increased number of neutrophils, a blood sample is viewed under a microscope to determine if immature neutrophils (myeloblasts) are leaving the bone marrow and entering the bloodstream. Immature neutrophils in the bloodstream may indicate the presence of a disease in the bone marrow, such as leukemia. When immature neutrophils are found in the bloodstream, a doctor usually takes a sample of bone marrow (bone marrow biopsy).■

An increased number of mature neutrophils in the blood is not usually a problem in itself. Therefore, doctors focus on treating the condition or disease that caused the number of neutrophils to increase.

▲ see page 981   ■ see page 981

Causes of Lymphocytopenia

AIDS

Cancer (leukemias, lymphomas, Hodgkin's disease)

Chronic infections (such as miliary tuberculosis)

Hereditary disorders (certain agammaglobulinemias, DiGeorge anomaly, Wiskott-Aldrich syndrome, severe combined immunodeficiency syndrome, and ataxia-telangiectasia)

Rheumatoid arthritis

Some viral infections

Systemic lupus erythematosus

Lymphocytopenia

Lymphocytopenia is an abnormally low number of lymphocytes in the blood.

Lymphocytes usually constitute 20 to 40% of all white blood cells in the bloodstream. The lymphocyte count is normally above 1,500 cells per microliter of blood in adults and above 3,000 cells per microliter of blood in children. A reduction in the number of lymphocytes may not cause a significant decrease in the total number of white blood cells.

A variety of diseases and conditions, including infection with human immunodeficiency virus (HIV)—the virus that causes AIDS, can decrease the number of lymphocytes in the blood. Also, the number of lymphocytes can decrease briefly during times of severe stress and during use of corticosteroids (such as prednisone), chemotherapy for cancer, and radiation therapy. Severe reduction in lymphocytes can occur in certain hereditary disorders (the hereditary immunodeficiency diseases).▲

There are three types of lymphocytes: B lymphocytes, T lymphocytes, and natural killer cells, all of which have very important functions in the immune system. Too few B lymphocytes can lead to a decrease in the number of plasma cells and reduced antibody production. People who have too few T lymphocytes or too few natural killer cells have problems controlling certain infections, especially viral, fungal, and parasitic infections.

▲ see page 1057

Severe lymphocyte deficiencies can result in uncontrolled infections that can be fatal.

Symptoms and Diagnosis

Mild lymphocytopenia may cause no symptoms and is usually detected by chance when a complete blood cell count is conducted for other reasons. Drastically reduced numbers of lymphocytes lead to infections with bacteria, viruses, fungi, and parasites.

When the numbers of lymphocytes are drastically reduced, a doctor usually takes a sample of bone marrow to examine under a microscope (bone marrow biopsy). The number of specific types of lymphocytes (T lymphocytes, B lymphocytes, and natural killer cells) can also be determined in the blood. A decrease in certain types of lymphocytes may help a doctor diagnose some diseases, such as AIDS or certain hereditary immunodeficiency disorders.

Treatment

Treatment depends mainly on the cause. Lymphocytopenia caused by a drug usually begins to resolve within days after a person stops taking the drug. If the lymphocytopenia is the result of AIDS, combination therapy with at least three antiviral agents of different classes can increase the number of T lymphocytes and improve survival.

Gamma globulin (a substance rich in antibodies) may be given to help prevent infections in people with too few B lymphocytes (who therefore have a deficiency of antibody production). People with a hereditary immunodeficiency may benefit from bone marrow (stem cell) transplantation. If an infection develops, a specific antibiotic, antifungal, antiviral, or antiparasitic drug directed against the infective organism is given.

Lymphocytic Leukocytosis

Lymphocytic leukocytosis is an abnormally high number of lymphocytes in the blood.

The number of lymphocytes can increase in response to infections, especially by viruses. Some bacterial infections, such as tuberculosis, may also increase the number. Certain types of cancer, such as lymphoma and acute or chronic lymphocytic leukemia, may produce an increase in the number of lymphocytes, in part by releasing immature lymphocytes (lymphoblasts) or the lymphoma cells into the bloodstream. Graves' disease and

Crohn's disease may also result in an increase in the number of lymphocytes in the bloodstream.

When the number of lymphocytes increases, symptoms usually result from the infection or other disease that has caused the number of lymphocytes to increase, rather than from the increase in lymphocytes per se. When a doctor discovers an increased number of lymphocytes, a blood sample is examined under a microscope to determine if the lymphocytes in the bloodstream appear activated (as occurs in response to viral infections) or if they appear immature or abnormal (as occurs in certain leukemias or lymphomas).

Treatment for lymphocytic leukocytosis depends on the cause.

Monocyte Disorders

Monocytes help other white blood cells to remove dead or damaged tissues, destroy cancer cells, and regulate immunity against foreign substances. Monocytes are produced in the bone marrow and then enter the bloodstream, where they account for about 1 to 10% of the circulating leukocytes (200 to 600 monocytes per microliter of blood). After a few hours in the bloodstream, they migrate to tissues (such as spleen, liver, lung, and bone marrow tissue), where they mature into macrophages, the main scavenger cells of the immune system. Genetic abnormalities that affect the function of monocytes and macrophages and cause buildup of debris within the cells result in the lipid storage diseases (such as Gaucher's disease and Niemann-Pick disease).▲

An increased number of monocytes in the blood (monocytosis) occurs in response to chronic infections, in autoimmune disorders, in blood disorders, and in cancers. A proliferation of macrophages in tissues can occur in response to infections, sarcoidosis,■ and Langerhans' cell granulomatosis.★

A low number of monocytes in the blood (monocytopenia) can occur in response to the release of toxins into the blood by certain types of bacteria (endotoxemia), as well as in people receiving chemotherapy or corticosteroids.

Eosinophilic Disorders

Eosinophils usually account for less than 7% of the circulating leukocytes (100 to 500 eosinophils per microliter of blood). These cells have a role in the protective immunity against certain parasites but also contribute to the inflammation that occurs in allergic disorders.

An increased number of eosinophils in the blood (eosinophilia) usually indicates the response of the body to abnormal cells, parasites, or substances that cause an allergic reaction (allergens). A low number of eosinophils in the blood (eosinopenia) can occur with Cushing's syndrome and stress reactions but does not usually cause problems because other parts of the immune system compensate adequately.

Idiopathic hypereosinophilic syndrome is a disorder in which the number of eosinophils increases to more than 1,500 cells per microliter of blood for more than 6 months without an obvious cause.

People of any age can develop idiopathic hypereosinophilic syndrome, but it is more common in men older than 50. The increased number of eosinophils can damage the heart, lungs, liver, skin, and nervous system. For example, the heart can become inflamed in a condition called Löffler's endocarditis, leading to formation of blood clots, heart failure, heart attacks, or malfunctioning heart valves.

Symptoms may include weight loss, fevers, night sweats, fatigue, cough, chest pain, swelling, stomachache, skin rashes, pain, weakness, confusion, and coma. Additional symptoms of this syndrome depend on which organs are damaged. The syndrome is suspected when the number of eosinophils is persistently increased in people who have these symptoms. The diagnosis is confirmed when a doctor determines that the eosinophilia is not caused by a parasitic infection, an allergic reaction, or another diagnosable disorder.

Without treatment, generally more than 80% of the people who have this syndrome die within 2 years; with treatment, more than 80% survive. Heart damage is the principal cause of death. Some people need no treatment other than close observation for 3 to 6 months, but most need drug treatment with prednisone or hydroxyurea. If these drugs fail, a variety of other drugs may be used, and they can be combined with a procedure to remove eosinophils from the blood (leukapheresis).

▲ see page 1620   ■ see page 304
★ see page 303

Basophilic Disorders

Basophils account for less than 3% of the circulating leukocytes (0 to 300 basophils per microliter of blood). These cells have some role in immune surveillance and wound repair. Basophils can release histamine and other mediators and play a role in the initiation of allergic reactions. A decrease in the number of basophils (basopenia) can occur as a response to thyrotoxicosis, acute hypersensitivity reactions, and infections. An increase in the number of basophils (basophilia) can be seen in people with hypothyroidism. In the myeloproliferative disorders (for example, polycythemia vera and myelofibrosis), a marked increase in the number of basophils can occur.

CHAPTER 175

Plasma Cell Disorders

Plasma cell disorders (plasma cell dyscrasias) are uncommon. They begin when a single group (clone) of plasma cells multiplies excessively and produces a large quantity of abnormal antibodies. Plasma cells develop from B lymphocytes, a type of white blood cell, and normally produce antibodies (immunoglobulins), which help the body fight infection. Plasma cells are found mainly in bone marrow and lymph nodes. Every plasma cell divides repeatedly to form a clone, composed of many identical cells. The cells of a clone produce only one specific type of antibody. Thousands of different clones exist; thus, the body can produce a vast number of different antibodies▲ to fight the body's frequent exposure to infectious microorganisms.

In plasma cell disorders, one clone of plasma cells multiplies uncontrollably; as a result, this clone produces vast amounts of a single antibody (monoclonal antibody) known as the M-protein. In some cases (such as with monoclonal gammopathies), the antibody produced is incomplete, consisting of only light chains or heavy chains (functional antibodies normally consist of two pairs of two different chains called a light chain and heavy chain). These abnormal plasma cells and the antibodies they produce are limited to one type, and levels of other types of antibodies that help fight infections fall. Thus, people with plasma cell disorders are often at higher risk of infections. The ever-increasing number of abnormal plasma cells also invades and damages various tissues and organs, and the antibody produced by the clone of plasma cells can sometimes damage vital organs, especially the kidneys.

Plasma cell disorders include monoclonal gammopathies of undetermined significance, multiple myeloma, macroglobulinemia, and heavy chain diseases. These disorders are more common among older people.

Monoclonal Gammopathies of Undetermined Significance

A monoclonal gammopathy of undetermined significance is a buildup of monoclonal antibodies produced by abnormal but noncancerous plasma cells.

In general, monoclonal gammopathies of undetermined significance do not cause significant health problems. These disorders do not usually cause symptoms, so they are almost always discovered by chance when laboratory tests are performed for other purposes, such as to measure protein in the blood. However, the monoclonal antibody can bind to nerves and lead to numbness, tingling, and weakness.

The M-protein levels in people with a monoclonal gammopathy of undetermined significance often remain stable for years—25 years in some people—and do not require treatment.

For unknown reasons, in about one quarter of people with these disorders, there is a progression to a cancerous disorder, such as multiple myeloma, macroglobulinemia, or B-cell lymphoma, often after many years. This progression cannot be prevented. People with a monoclonal gammopathy of undetermined sig-

▲ see page 1055

nificance are usually monitored with a physical examination and blood and sometimes urine tests about twice a year, to determine if a progression to cancer is beginning to occur. If progression is detected early, symptoms and complications of the cancerous disorder may be prevented or treated sooner.

Multiple Myeloma

Multiple myeloma is a cancer of plasma cells in which abnormal plasma cells multiply uncontrollably in the bone marrow and occasionally in other parts of the body.

Typically, multiple myeloma occurs in people at least 60 years of age. Although its cause is not certain, the increased occurrence of multiple myeloma among close relatives indicates that heredity plays a role. Exposure to radiation is thought to be a possible cause, as is exposure to benzene and other solvents. A herpesvirus, HHV-8, may play some role in the disease.

Normally, plasma cells make up less than 1% of the cells in the bone marrow; in multiple myeloma, typically the vast majority of bone marrow elements are cancerous plasma cells. The overabundance of these cancerous plasma cells in the bone marrow leads to the increased production of proteins that suppress the development of other normal bone marrow elements, including white blood cells, red blood cells, and platelets (cell-like particles that help the body form blood clots). In addition, the abnormal plasma cells almost always produce a large amount of a single type of antibody accompanied by a markedly reduced amount of all other types of normal antibodies.

Often, collections of cancerous plasma cells develop into tumors that lead to loss of bone, most commonly in the pelvic bones, spine, ribs, and skull. Infrequently, these tumors develop in areas other than bone, particularly in the lungs, liver, and kidneys.

Symptoms and Complications

Because plasma cell tumors often invade bone, bone pain, often in the back, ribs, and hips, may occur. Loss of bone density (osteoporosis) resulting from plasma cell tumors weakens bones, which can lead to fractures. In addition, calcium released from the bones may result in abnormally high levels of calcium in the blood, possibly causing constipation, increased frequency of urination, weakness, and confusion.

The reduced production of red blood cells often leads to anemia, which causes fatigue, weakness, and pallor, and may lead to heart problems. Decreased production of white blood cells leads to repeated infections, which may cause fever and chills. Decreased platelet production impairs the blood's ability to clot and results in easy bruising or bleeding.

Pieces of monoclonal antibodies, known as light chains, frequently end up in the collecting system of the kidneys, sometimes permanently damaging them by interfering with their filtering function and leading to kidney failure. The light chain pieces of the antibody in the urine (or blood) are called Bence Jones proteins. The increased number of growing cancerous cells can lead to the overproduction and excretion of uric acid in the urine, which can lead to kidney stones. Calcium levels may become high, affecting the heart, kidneys, and brain. Deposits of certain types of antibody pieces in the kidneys or other organs can lead to amyloidosis,▲ another serious disorder found in a small number of people with multiple myeloma.

In rare instances, multiple myeloma interferes with blood flow to the skin, fingers, toes, nose, kidneys, and brain because the blood thickens (hyperviscosity syndrome).■

Diagnosis

Multiple myeloma may be discovered even before a person has symptoms, when an x-ray performed for another reason shows a loss of bone density. Bone loss may be widespread or limited to scattered punched-out areas of a few bones.

Multiple myeloma is sometimes suspected because of symptoms, such as back pain or other sites of bone pain, fatigue, fevers, and bruising. Blood tests performed to investigate such symptoms may reveal that a person has anemia, a decreased white blood cell count, a decreased platelet count, or kidney failure.

The two most useful blood tests are serum protein electrophoresis and immunoelectrophoresis. They detect and identify an overabundance of a single type of antibody found in most people who have multiple myeloma. Doctors also measure the different types of antibodies, especially IgG, IgA, and IgM.

Calcium levels are usually measured as well. A 24-hour collection of urine is analyzed for the amount and types of protein in it. Bence

▲ see page 1715   ■ see page 1009

Jones proteins are found in the urine of half of the people who have multiple myeloma.

A bone marrow biopsy▲ is almost always performed to confirm the diagnosis. When a person has multiple myeloma, the biopsy shows a large number of plasma cells abnormally arranged in sheets and clusters; the individual cells also may appear abnormal.

In addition, other blood tests are useful in determining the overall outlook for the person. Higher levels of beta$_2$-microglobulin and C-reactive protein in the person's blood when the disease is diagnosed usually indicate the likelihood of a shortened survival and are likely to affect treatment decisions.

Treatment and Prognosis

Multiple myeloma remains incurable despite recent advances in therapy. Treatment is aimed at preventing or relieving symptoms and complications, destroying abnormal plasma cells, and slowing progression of the disorder.

The most consistently helpful group of drugs for multiple myeloma is corticosteroids, such as prednisone or dexamethasone. In addition, chemotherapy slows the progression of multiple myeloma by killing the abnormal plasma cells. Because chemotherapy kills normal cells as well as abnormal ones, the blood cells are monitored and the dose is adjusted if the number of normal white blood cells and platelets decreases too much. Melphalan, and less often cyclophosphamide, are the chemotherapy drugs most often added to corticosteroids. Vincristine and doxorubicin are also effective and may have less severe side effects, particularly on the bone marrow, than melphalan and cyclophosphamide. Thalidomide may help nearly one third of people whose multiple myeloma is worsening with other treatments. For people who have a good response to chemotherapy, the drug interferon may prolong the response somewhat but has little impact on survival.

Many new combinations of treatment are being used. One involves several months of conventional chemotherapy followed by high-dose chemotherapy. Because this high-dose treatment is also toxic to normal blood cells made in the bone marrow, stem cells (unspecialized cells that transform into immature blood cells, which eventually mature to become red blood cells, white blood cells, and

platelets) are collected from the person's blood before the high-dose chemotherapy is administered. These stem cells are then returned (transplanted) to the person after the high-dose treatment.■ Generally, this procedure is reserved for people who are younger than 70.

Strong analgesics and radiation therapy directed at the affected bones can help relieve bone pain, which can be severe. Radiation therapy may also prevent the development of fractures. Monthly intravenous administration of pamidronate (a bisphosphonate) and the more potent drug zoledronic acid can reduce the development of bony complications, and most people with multiple myeloma receive these drugs as part of their treatment forever. Staying active is also important; prolonged bed rest tends to accelerate bone loss and makes the bones more vulnerable to fractures. Most people can enjoy a normal lifestyle that includes most activities. Drinking plenty of fluids dilutes the urine and helps prevent dehydration, which can make kidney failure more likely.

People who have signs of infection—fever, chills, cough productive of sputum, or reddened areas of the skin—should seek attention from a doctor promptly because they may need antibiotics. Those who have severe anemia may need transfusions of red blood cells. Erythropoietin or darbepoietin, drugs that stimulate red blood cell formation, may adequately treat the anemia in some people. High levels of calcium in the blood can be treated with intravenous fluids and often require intravenous bisphosphonates. People who have high levels of uric acid in the blood may benefit from allopurinol, a drug that blocks the body's production of uric acid.

Currently, no cure is available for multiple myeloma. However, treatment slows disease progression in more than 60% of people. The average survival is more than 3 years after the disorder is diagnosed, but survival time varies widely depending on the features at the time of diagnosis and the response to treatment. Importantly, bisphosphonates to reduce bony complications, substances that stimulate the production of blood cells (growth factors) to increase the number of red and white blood cells, and better pain relievers have greatly improved the quality of life of these people. Occasionally, people who survive for many years after successful treatment of multiple myeloma develop leukemia or irreversible loss of bone marrow function. These late complica-

---

▲ see page 981   ■ see page 1081

tions may result from chemotherapy and often lead to severe anemia and an increased susceptibility to infections and bleeding.

Because multiple myeloma is ultimately fatal, people with multiple myeloma are likely to benefit from discussions of end-of-life care that involve their doctors and appropriate family and friends. Points for discussion may include advance directives,▲ the use of feeding tubes, and pain relief.■

Macroglobulinemia

Macroglobulinemia (Waldenström's macroglobulinemia) is a plasma cell cancer in which a single clone of plasma cells produces excessive amounts of a certain type of large antibody (IgM) called macroglobulins.

Men are affected by macroglobulinemia more often than women, and the average age at which the disorder appears is 65 years. Its cause is unknown.

Symptoms and Complications

Many people who have macroglobulinemia have no symptoms, and the disorder is discovered by chance when an elevated level of blood proteins is found during routine blood tests. Others have symptoms resulting from interference with blood flow to the skin, fingers, toes, nose, and brain that occurs when the large quantity of macroglobulins thickens the blood (hyperviscosity syndrome). These symptoms include bleeding from the skin and mucous membranes (such as the lining of the mouth, nose, and digestive tract), fatigue, weakness, headache, confusion, dizziness, and even coma. The thickened blood also may aggravate heart conditions and cause increased pressure in the brain. Tiny blood vessels in the back of the eyes can become filled with blood and may bleed, resulting in damage to the retina and impaired eyesight.

People who have macroglobulinemia may also have swollen lymph nodes and an enlarged liver and spleen due to infiltration by cancerous plasma cells. Recurring bacterial infections resulting from inadequate production of normal antibodies may cause fever and chills. Anemia, which may result in weakness and fatigue, occurs when cancerous plasma cells prevent normal blood-forming cells in the bone marrow from being produced. Infiltration of bones by cancerous plasma cells may cause loss of bone density (osteoporosis), which can weaken bones and increase the risk of fractures.

What Is Cryoglobulinemia?

Cryoglobulins are abnormal antibodies produced by plasma cells and dissolved in the blood. When cooled below normal body temperature, cryoglobulins form large collections of solid particles (precipitates). When warmed to normal body temperature, they redissolve.

The formation of cryoglobulins (cryoglobulinemia) is uncommon. In most instances, people who form cryoglobulins have an underlying disorder as the cause. These disorders include cancers such as macroglobulinemia and chronic lymphocytic leukemia, autoimmune disorders such as systemic lupus erythematosus, and infections by such organisms as hepatitis C virus. Rarely, a cause for the formation of cryoglobulins cannot be found.

Precipitates of cryoglobulins can trigger inflammation of blood vessels (vasculitis), which causes a wide variety of symptoms, such as bruises, joint aches, and weakness. People with cryoglobulinemia may also be very sensitive to cold or develop Raynaud's phenomenon, in which the hands and feet become very painful and turn white when chilled. The vasculitis may damage the liver and kidneys. Damage may progress to liver failure and kidney failure in some people and can be fatal.

Avoiding cold temperatures helps prevent vasculitis. Treating the underlying disorder may reduce the formation of cryoglobulins; for example, using interferon to treat hepatitis C virus infection helps to reduce formation of cryoglobulins. Plasmapheresis may help, especially when combined with interferon.

Many people develop a condition called cryoglobulinemia. Cryoglobulinemia involves the development of antibodies that clog up the blood vessels in cold temperatures.

Diagnosis

Blood tests are performed when macroglobulinemia is suspected; the three most useful are serum protein electrophoresis, measurement of immunoglobulins, and immunoelectrophoresis.

A doctor may perform other laboratory tests as well. For example, the doctor may check a

▲ see page 54   ■ see page 48

blood sample to determine if the numbers of red and white blood cells and platelets are normal. In addition, serum viscosity, which is a test to check the thickness of the blood, is often performed. Blood clotting test results may be abnormal, and other tests may detect cryoglobulins. An examination of a urine sample may show Bence Jones proteins (pieces of abnormal antibodies). A bone marrow biopsy may reveal an increased number of lymphocytes and plasma cells, which helps confirm the diagnosis of macroglobulinemia, and the appearance of these cells helps differentiate this disease from multiple myeloma.

X-rays may show a loss of bone density (osteoporosis). Computed tomography (CT) scans may reveal an enlarged spleen, liver, or lymph nodes.

Treatment and Prognosis

Chemotherapy, usually with chlorambucil or fludarabine, can slow the growth of abnormal plasma cells but does not cure macroglobulinemia. Other drugs, such as melphalan or cyclophosphamide, are sometimes used, alone or in combination. Recent results show that the monoclonal antibody rituximab may also be effective at slowing the growth of the abnormal plasma cells.

A person whose blood is thickened must be treated promptly with plasmapheresis, a procedure in which blood is withdrawn, the abnormal antibodies are removed from it, and the red blood cells are returned to the person.▲ However, only a small number of people with macroglobulinemia require this procedure.

The course of the disorder varies from person to person. Even without treatment, many people survive for 5 years or more.

Heavy Chain Diseases

Heavy chain diseases are plasma cell cancers in which a clone of plasma cells produces a large quantity of pieces of abnormal antibodies called heavy chains.

Heavy chain diseases are categorized according to the type of heavy chain produced: alpha, gamma, or mu.

Alpha heavy chain disease affects mainly younger adults of Middle Eastern or Mediterranean ancestry. Infiltration of the intestinal tract wall by cancerous plasma cells often prevents proper absorption of nutrients from food (malabsorption), resulting in severe diarrhea and weight loss. Alpha heavy chain disease progresses rapidly, and half of the affected people die within 1 year. Treatment with cyclophosphamide, prednisone (a corticosteroid), and antibiotics may slow the progression of the disease.

Gamma heavy chain disease affects mainly older adults. Some people with gamma heavy chain disease have no symptoms. Infiltration of the bone marrow by cancerous plasma cells causes other people to have symptoms of recurring infections, such as repeated episodes of fever and chills associated with a decreased number of white blood cells, and fatigue and weakness associated with severe anemia. Cancerous plasma cells may also enlarge the liver and spleen. People with symptoms may respond to therapy with cyclophosphamide and prednisone.

Mu heavy chain disease, the rarest of the three heavy chain diseases, may cause enlargement of the liver and spleen as well as enlargement of the lymph nodes in the abdomen. Length of survival and response to chemotherapy drugs vary widely.

CHAPTER 176

Leukemias

Leukemias are cancers of white blood cells or of cells that develop into white blood cells.

White blood cells develop from stem cells in the bone marrow. Sometimes the develop-

▲ see box on page 986

ment goes awry, and pieces of chromosomes get rearranged. The resulting abnormal chromosomes interfere with normal control of cell division, so that affected cells multiply uncontrollably and become cancerous (malignant), resulting in leukemia. Leukemia cells ultimately occupy the bone marrow, replacing or suppressing the function of cells that develop into normal blood cells. Leukemia cells may also invade other organs, including the liver, spleen, lymph nodes, testes, and brain.

Leukemias are grouped into four main types—acute lymphocytic leukemia, acute myelocytic leukemia, chronic lymphocytic leukemia, and chronic myelocytic leukemia—according to how quickly they progress and the type of cell that becomes cancerous. Acute leukemias progress rapidly; chronic leukemias progress slowly. Lymphocytic leukemias develop from cancerous changes in lymphocytes or in cells that normally produce lymphocytes; myelocytic (myeloid) leukemias develop from cancerous changes in cells that normally produce neutrophils, basophils, eosinophils, and monocytes.

The cause of most types of leukemia is not known. Exposure to radiation or to some types of chemotherapy increases the risk of developing some types of leukemia, although leukemia develops in a very small number of people receiving such treatments. Certain hereditary disorders, such as Down syndrome and Fanconi's syndrome, increase the risk as well. A virus known as HTLV-I (human T-cell lymphotropic virus type I), which is similar to the virus that causes AIDS, is strongly suspected of causing a rare type of lymphocytic leukemia called adult T-cell leukemia. Infection with the Epstein-Barr virus has been associated with an aggressive form of lymphocytic leukemia called Burkitt's leukemia.

Many leukemias can be effectively treated; some can be cured. When a leukemia is under control, the person is said to be in remission. If leukemia cells appear again, the person is said to have a relapse. For some people in relapse, quality of life may eventually deteriorate, and the potential benefit for further treatment may be extremely limited. Keeping the person comfortable may become more important than trying to modestly prolong his or her life. The person and family members must be involved in these decisions. Much can be done to provide compassionate care, relieve symptoms,▲ and maintain the person's dignity.

Acute Lymphocytic Leukemia

Acute lymphocytic (lymphoblastic) leukemia is a life-threatening disease in which the cells that normally develop into lymphocytes become cancerous and rapidly replace normal cells in the bone marrow.

Acute lymphocytic leukemia (ALL) occurs in people of all ages but is the most common cancer in children, accounting for 25% of all cancers in children younger than 15 years. ALL most often affects young children between the ages of 2 and 5 years. Among adults, it is somewhat more common in those older than 65.

In ALL, very immature leukemia cells accumulate in the bone marrow, destroying and replacing cells that produce normal blood cells. The leukemia cells are also carried in the bloodstream to the liver, spleen, lymph nodes, brain, and testes, where they may continue to grow and divide. They can irritate the layers of tissue covering the brain and spinal cord, causing inflammation (meningitis), and can cause anemia, liver and kidney failure, and other organ damage.

Symptoms and Diagnosis

Early symptoms result from the inability of the bone marrow to produce enough normal blood cells. Fever and excessive sweating, which may indicate infection, result from too few normal white blood cells. Weakness, fatigue, and paleness, which indicate anemia, result from too few red blood cells. Easy bruising and bleeding, sometimes in the form of nosebleeds or bleeding gums, result from too few platelets. Leukemia cells in the brain may cause headaches, vomiting, and irritability, and those in the bone marrow may cause bone and joint pain. A sense of fullness in the abdomen and sometimes pain can result when leukemia cells enlarge the liver and spleen.

Blood tests, such as a complete blood count,■ can provide the first evidence that a person has ALL. The total number of white blood cells may be decreased, normal, or increased, but the number of red blood cells and platelets is almost always decreased. In addition, very immature white blood cells (blasts) are seen in blood samples examined under a microscope. A bone marrow biopsy★ is almost always performed to confirm the diagnosis and to distinguish ALL from other types of leukemia.

Prognosis and Treatment

Before treatment was available, most people who had ALL died within 4 months of the di-

---

▲ see page 48   ■ see page 980
★ see page 981

agnosis. Now, nearly 80% of children and 30 to 40% of adults with ALL are cured. For most people, the first course of chemotherapy brings the disease under control (complete remission). Children between the ages of 3 and 7 have the best prognosis; children younger than 2 and older adults fare the least well. The white blood cell count and particular chromosome abnormalities in the leukemia cells also influence outcome.

Chemotherapy is highly effective and is administered in phases. The goal of initial treatment (induction chemotherapy) is to achieve remission by destroying leukemia cells so that normal cells can once again grow in the bone marrow. The person may need to stay in the hospital for a few days or weeks, depending on how quickly the bone marrow recovers. Blood and platelet transfusions may be necessary to treat anemia and to prevent bleeding, and antibiotics may be needed to treat infections. Intravenous fluids and therapy with a drug called allopurinol may also be used to help rid the body of harmful substances, such as uric acid, that are released when leukemia cells are destroyed.

One of several combinations of chemotherapy drugs is used, and doses are repeated for several days or weeks. One combination consists of prednisone taken by mouth and weekly doses of vincristine given with an anthracycline drug (usually daunorubicin), asparaginase, and sometimes cyclophosphamide, given intravenously. Other drugs are being investigated.

For treatment of leukemia cells in the meninges (the layers of tissue covering the brain and spinal cord), methotrexate, cytosine arabinoside, or both is usually injected directly into the cerebrospinal fluid. This chemotherapy may be given in combination with radiation therapy to the brain. Even when there is little evidence that the leukemia has spread to the brain, a similar type of treatment is usually given as a preventive measure because of the high likelihood of spread to the meninges.

A few weeks after the initial, intensive treatment, additional treatment (consolidation chemotherapy) is given to destroy any remaining leukemia cells. Additional chemotherapy drugs, or the same drugs as were used during the induction phase, may be used a few times over a period of several weeks. Further treat-

ment (maintenance chemotherapy), which usually consists of fewer drugs, sometimes at lower doses, may continue for 2 to 3 years. For some people who are at high risk of relapse because of particular chromosomal changes found in their cells, stem cell transplantation▲ during the first remission is often recommended.

Leukemia cells may begin to appear again (a condition termed relapse), often in the blood, bone marrow, brain, or testes. Reappearance in the bone marrow is particularly serious. Chemotherapy is given again, and although most people respond to treatment, the disease has a strong tendency to come back, especially in children younger than 2 and in adults. When leukemia cells reappear in the brain, chemotherapy drugs are injected into the cerebrospinal fluid 1 or 2 times a week. When leukemia cells reappear in the testes, radiation therapy is given along with chemotherapy.

For people who have relapsed, high-dose chemotherapy along with allogeneic stem cell transplantation offers the best chance of cure, but this procedure can be performed only if stem cells can be obtained from a person who has a compatible tissue type (HLA-matched). The donor is usually a sibling, but cells from matched, unrelated donors (or occasionally partially matched cells from family members or unrelated donors, as well as umbilical stem cells) are sometimes used. Stem cell transplantation is rarely used for people older than 65, because it is much less likely to be successful and side effects are much more likely to be fatal.

After relapse, additional treatment for a person who is unable to undergo stem cell transplantation is often poorly tolerated and ineffective, frequently causing the person to feel much sicker. However, remissions can occur. End-of-life care should be considered for people who do not respond to treatment.■

Acute Myelocytic Leukemia

Acute myelocytic (myeloid, myelogenous, myeloblastic, myelomonocytic) leukemia is a life-threatening disease in which the cells that normally develop into neutrophils, basophils, eosinophils, and monocytes become cancerous and rapidly replace normal cells in the bone marrow.

Acute myelocytic leukemia (AML) is the most common type of leukemia among adults, although it affects people of all ages.

▲ see page 1081   ■ see page 45

In AML, immature leukemia cells rapidly accumulate in the bone marrow, destroying and replacing cells that produce normal blood cells. The leukemia cells are released into the bloodstream and are transported to other organs, where they continue to grow and divide. They can form small masses (chloromas) in or just under the skin or gums or in the eyes.

Acute promyelocytic leukemia is a subtype of AML. In this subtype, chromosomal changes in promyelocytes—cells that are at an early stage in the development into mature neutrophils—prevent binding and activity of vitamin A. Without vitamin A activity, normal cell maturation is disrupted, and abnormal promyelocytes accumulate.

Symptoms and Diagnosis

The first symptoms of AML are very similar to those of acute lymphocytic leukemia.▲ Although meningitis occurs less often than in acute lymphocytic leukemia, AML cells can cause inflammation of the layers of tissue covering the brain and spinal cord (meninges).

The diagnosis of AML is also similar to that of acute lymphocytic leukemia. A bone marrow biopsy■ is almost always performed to confirm the diagnosis and to distinguish AML from other types of leukemia.

Prognosis and Treatment

Without treatment, most people with AML die within a few weeks to months of the diagnosis. With therapy, between 20% and 40% of people survive at least 5 years, without any relapse. Because relapses almost always occur within the first 5 years after initial treatment, most people who remain leukemia-free after 5 years are considered cured. People who have the poorest prognosis are those older than 60, those who develop AML after undergoing chemotherapy and radiation therapy for other cancers, and those whose leukemia evolved slowly after a period of months to years of abnormal blood counts.

Treatment is aimed at bringing about prompt remission—the destruction of all leukemia cells. However, AML responds to fewer drugs than does acute lymphocytic leukemia. In addition, treatment often makes people sicker before they get better, because the treatment suppresses bone marrow activity, resulting in fewer white blood cells, particularly neutrophils. Having too few neutrophils makes infection likely. Meticulous care is taken to prevent infections, and any

Myelodysplastic Syndromes

In myelodysplastic syndromes, a line of identical cells (clone) develops and occupies the bone marrow. These abnormal cells do not grow and mature normally, resulting in deficits of red blood cells, white blood cells, and platelets. In some people, red blood cell production is predominantly affected. Myelodysplastic syndromes occur most often in people older than 50 years. Men are more than twice as likely as women to be affected.

The cause is usually not known. However, in some people, exposure of bone marrow to radiation therapy or certain types of chemotherapy drugs may play a role.

Symptoms develop very slowly. Fatigue, weakness, and other symptoms of anemia are common. Fever due to infections may develop if the number of white blood cells decreases. Easy bruising and abnormal bleeding can result if the number of platelets drops. A myelodysplastic syndrome may be suspected when someone has unexplained persistent anemia, but diagnosis requires a bone marrow biopsy.

People with myelodysplastic syndromes often need transfusions of red blood cells. Platelets are transfused only if a person has uncontrolled bleeding, or if surgery is needed and the number of platelets is low. People who have very low numbers of neutrophils—the white blood cells that fight infection—may benefit from intermittent injections of a special type of protein called a colony-stimulating factor.

Although these syndromes are thought to be a type of leukemia, they progress gradually, over a period of several months to years. In 10 to 30% of people, a myelodysplastic syndrome transforms into acute myelocytic leukemia (AML). Treatment with chemotherapy during the early stages of a myelodysplastic syndrome does not help prevent transformation to AML. If transformation to AML occurs, chemotherapy may be helpful, but the AML is unlikely to be curable.

that occur are promptly treated with antibiotics. Red blood cell and platelet transfusions are invariably also needed.

▲ see page 1011   ■ see page 981

The first course of drug treatment (induction chemotherapy) generally includes cytarabine for 7 days by a continuous infusion and daunorubicin (or idarubicin or mitoxantrone) for 3 days.

Once AML is in remission, the person usually receives a few courses of additional chemotherapy (consolidation chemotherapy) a few weeks or months after the initial treatment to help ensure that as many leukemia cells as possible are destroyed. A preventive treatment to the brain usually is not needed, and long-term lower-dose chemotherapy (as is used in acute lymphocytic leukemia) has not been shown to improve survival.

People who have not responded to treatment and younger people who are in remission but who are likely to have a high rate of relapse (generally identified by certain chromosomal abnormalities) may be given high-dose chemotherapy with stem cell transplantation.▲

When relapse occurs, additional chemotherapy for people unable to undergo stem cell transplantation is less effective and often poorly tolerated. Another course of chemotherapy is most effective in younger people and in people whose initial remission lasted more than 1 year. Doctors take many factors into consideration when determining the advisability of additional intensive chemotherapy for people with AML in relapse. A new drug, gemtuzumab ozogamicin, which combines an antibody with a chemotherapy drug as an attempt to specifically "target" the leukemia cells, is effective in some people after relapse has occurred. The long-term benefits of the drug have not been determined.

People with acute promyelocytic leukemia can be treated with a type of vitamin A called all-*trans*-retinoic acid. Results are best when chemotherapy is used also; currently more than 70% of people with acute promyelocytic leukemia can be cured. Arsenic chemical compounds are also uniquely effective in this subtype of AML.

Chronic Lymphocytic Leukemia

Chronic lymphocytic leukemia is a disease in which mature lymphocytes become cancerous and gradually replace normal cells in lymph nodes.

More than three fourths of the people who have chronic lymphocytic leukemia (CLL) are older than 60, and the disease does not occur in children. This type of leukemia affects men 2 to 3 times more often than women. CLL is the most common type of leukemia in North America and Europe. It is rare in Japan and Southeast Asia, which indicates that heredity plays some role in its development.

The number of cancerous mature lymphocytes increases first in the blood and lymph nodes. They then spread to the liver and spleen, both of which begin to enlarge. Cancerous lymphocytes also invade the bone marrow, where they crowd out normal cells, resulting in a decreased number of red blood cells and a decreased number of normal white blood cells and platelets in the blood. The level of antibodies, proteins that help fight infections, also decreases. The immune system, which ordinarily defends the body against foreign organisms and substances, sometimes becomes misguided, reacting to and destroying normal body tissues. This misguided activity can sometimes result in the destruction of red blood cells and platelets.

In 95% of cases, CLL is a disorder of B lymphocytes (B cells).■ There are other types of CLL other than B-cell CLL. Hairy cell leukemia, a slow-growing uncommon type of B-cell leukemia, produces a large number of abnormal white blood cells with distinctive hairlike projections that are visible under a microscope. T-cell leukemia (leukemia of T lymphocytes) is much less common than B-cell leukemia. Sézary syndrome is a rare type of T-cell leukemia in which cancerous T lymphocytes that start as a skin cancer called mycosis fungoides★ grow and divide more rapidly and enter the bloodstream, becoming leukemia cells.

Symptoms and Diagnosis

In early stages of CLL, most people have no symptoms, and the disease is diagnosed only because of an increased white blood cell count. Later symptoms may include enlarged lymph nodes, fatigue, loss of appetite, weight loss, shortness of breath when exercising, and a sense of abdominal fullness resulting from an enlarged spleen.

As CLL progresses, the person may appear pale and bruise easily. Bacterial, viral, and fungal infections generally do not occur until late in the course of the disease.

Sometimes the disease is discovered accidentally when blood counts ordered for some

▲ see page 1081   ■ see page 1054

★ see box on page 1020

other reason show an increased number of lymphocytes. A bone marrow biopsy is usually not needed to confirm the diagnosis because specialized tests to characterize the lymphocytes can be performed on the cells in the blood. Blood tests also may show that the person has a decreased number of red blood cells, platelets, and antibodies.

Prognosis

Most types of CLL progress slowly. A doctor determines how far the disease has progressed (staging) to predict the person's survival time. Staging is based on factors such as the number of lymphocytes in the blood and bone marrow, size of the spleen and liver, presence or absence of anemia, and platelet count.

People who have B-cell leukemia often survive 10 to 20 years or longer after the diagnosis is made and usually do not need treatment in the early stages. People who are anemic or who have a low number of platelets need more immediate treatment and have a less favorable prognosis. Usually, death occurs because the bone marrow can no longer produce a sufficient number of normal cells to carry oxygen, fight infections, and prevent bleeding. The prognosis for people who have T-cell leukemia is usually worse.

For reasons probably related to changes in the immune system, people who have CLL are more likely to develop other cancers, such as skin or lung cancers. CLL can also transform into a more aggressive type of lymphoma.

Treatment

Because CLL progresses slowly, many people do not need treatment for years—until the number of lymphocytes begins to increase, the lymph nodes begin to enlarge, or the number of red blood cells or platelets decreases.

Drugs used to treat the leukemia itself help relieve symptoms and eliminate enlarged lymph nodes and spleen but do not cure the disease. For B-cell CLL, initial drug treatment includes alkylating drugs such as chlorambucil, which kill cancer cells by interacting with their DNA, or a drug called fludarabine, which is given intravenously. Either treatment can control CLL for months to many years and can be used again with success when the leukemia regrows. Eventually CLL becomes resistant to these drugs, and sometimes experimental treatments with other drugs or monoclonal antibodies (such as alemtuzumab) are considered. For hairy cell leukemia, 2-chlorodeoxyadeno-

sine and pentostatin are highly effective and can control the disease for more than 15 years.

Anemia due to a decreased number of red blood cells is treated with blood transfusions and occasionally with injections of erythropoietin or darbepoietin (drugs that stimulate red blood cell formation). Low platelet counts are treated with platelet transfusions, and infections are treated with antibiotics. Radiation therapy is used to shrink enlarged lymph nodes or an enlarged liver or spleen if the enlargement is causing discomfort and chemotherapy is ineffective.

Chronic Myelocytic Leukemia

Chronic myelocytic (myeloid, myelogenous, granulocytic) leukemia is a disease in which cells that normally would develop into neutrophils, basophils, eosinophils, and monocytes become cancerous.

Chronic myelocytic leukemia (CML) may affect people of any age and of either sex but is uncommon in children younger than 10 years. The disease most commonly develops in adults between the ages of 40 and 60.

In CML, most of the leukemia cells are produced in the bone marrow, but some are produced in the spleen and liver. In contrast to the acute leukemias, in which large numbers of immature blasts are seen, the chronic stage of CML is characterized by marked increases in the numbers of normal-appearing white blood cells and sometimes platelets. During the course of the disease, more and more leukemia cells fill the bone marrow and others enter the bloodstream.

Eventually the leukemia cells undergo more changes, and the disease progresses to an accelerated phase and then inevitably to blast crisis. In blast crisis, only immature leukemia cells are produced, a sign that the disease has become much worse. Massive enlargement of the spleen is common in blast crisis, as well as fever and weight loss.

Symptoms and Diagnosis

Early on, in its chronic stage, CML may produce no symptoms. However, some people become fatigued and weak, lose their appetite, lose weight, develop a fever or night sweats, and notice a sensation of being full—which is usually caused by an enlarged spleen. As the disease progresses to blast crisis, people become sicker because the number of red blood cells and platelets decreases, leading to paleness, bruising, and bleeding.

The diagnosis of CML is suspected based on the results of a simple blood test. The test may show an abnormally high white blood cell count. In blood samples examined under a microscope, less mature white blood cells, normally found only in bone marrow, are seen.

Tests that analyze chromosomes (cytogenetics or molecular genetics) are needed to confirm the diagnosis. Chromosomal analysis of the leukemia cells always shows a rearrangement of two particular chromosomes into what is called the Philadelphia chromosome. The Philadelphia chromosome produces an abnormal enzyme (tyrosine kinase), which is responsible for the abnormal growth pattern of the white blood cells in CML.

Prognosis and Treatment

Although most treatments do not cure the disease, they do slow its progress. About 20% of people who have CML die within 2 years of the diagnosis, and about 15 to 20% die each year after that. However, more than 50% of people with CML survive 4 to 5 years or more after the diagnosis, ultimately dying during the accelerated phase or a blast crisis. Treatment of a blast crisis is similar to treatment of acute leukemia. The average survival time after a blast crisis is only 2 months, but chemotherapy can sometimes extend survival to 8 to 12 months.

Treatment in the chronic phase is considered successful if the white blood cell count is reduced to no more than what would be considered a moderately high level. Even the best treatment cannot destroy all of the leukemia cells. The only chance for cure is high-dose chemotherapy with stem cell transplantation.▲ The transplantation of stem cells—which must come from a donor who has a compatible tissue type, usually a sibling—is most effective during the early stages of the disease and is considerably less effective during the accelerated phase or blast crisis.

Hydroxyurea, which can be taken by mouth, is the most widely used chemotherapy drug for CML. The drug interferon-alpha helps return the bone marrow to normal function. Interferon-alpha can sometimes reduce the percentage of cells with the Philadelphia chromosome, and some people in whom the chromosome is eliminated enjoy prolonged survival.

A new drug, imatinib, has been found to control blood counts and reduce the Philadelphia chromosome more effectively than interferon-alpha, with many fewer side effects. The drug works by inhibiting the abnormal enzyme produced by the Philadelphia chromosome. Because imatinib is so new, its long-term benefits in terms of prevention or delay of blast crisis remain to be determined. It is also effective initial treatment for blast crisis, although most people eventually relapse.

In addition to chemotherapy, radiation therapy to the spleen is sometimes given to help reduce the number of leukemia cells. Occasionally, the spleen must be surgically removed (splenectomy) to relieve abdominal discomfort, increase the number of platelets, and decrease the need for blood transfusions.

In people for whom stem cell transplantation is not an option, or in people whose transplant fails to cure CML, chemotherapy sometimes provides temporary benefit. When no options are left and the person is clearly at the end of life, then palliative care that focuses on relief of pain and other symptoms is appropriate.■

CHAPTER 177

Lymphomas

Lymphomas are cancers of lymphocytes, which reside in the lymphatic system and in blood-forming organs.

▲ see page 1081   ■ see page 48

Lymphomas are cancers of a specific type of white blood cells known as lymphocytes. These cells help fight infections. Lymphomas can develop from either B or T lymphocytes. T lymphocytes are important in regulating the immune system and in fighting viral infections. B lymphocytes produce antibodies.

Lymphocytes move about to all parts of the body through the bloodstream and through a network of tubular channels (lymphatic vessels).▲ Scattered throughout the network of lymphatic vessels are lymph nodes, which house collections of lymphocytes. Lymphocytes that become cancerous (lymphoma cells) may remain confined to a single lymph node or may spread to the bone marrow, the spleen, or virtually any other organ.

The two major types of lymphoma are Hodgkin's lymphoma, more commonly known as Hodgkin's disease, and non-Hodgkin's lymphoma. Non-Hodgkin's lymphoma is a much more common disease than Hodgkin's disease. Burkitt's lymphoma and mycosis fungoides are subtypes of non-Hodgkin's lymphoma.

Hodgkin's Disease

Hodgkin's disease is a type of lymphoma distinguished by the presence of a particular kind of cancer cell called a Reed-Sternberg cell.

In the United States, about 8,000 new cases of Hodgkin's disease occur every year. The disease is more common in males than in females—about three men are affected for every two women. Hodgkin's disease rarely occurs before age 10. It is most common in people between the ages of 15 and 34 and in those older than 60.

The cause of Hodgkin's disease is unknown. There is strong evidence that, in some people, Epstein-Barr virus infection causes B lymphocytes to become cancerous and transform into Reed-Sternberg cells. Although there are some families in which more than one person has Hodgkin's disease, the disease does not appear to be contagious.

Symptoms

A person with Hodgkin's disease usually becomes aware of one or more enlarged lymph nodes, most often in the neck but sometimes in the armpit or groin. Although usually painless, sometimes the enlarged lymph nodes may be painful for a few hours after a person drinks large amounts of alcohol.

People with Hodgkin's disease sometimes experience fever, night sweats, and weight loss. They can also have itching and fatigue. Some people have Pel-Ebstein fever, an unusual pattern of high temperature for several

SYMPTOMS OF HODGKIN'S DISEASE

SYMPTOMS*	CAUSE
Weakness and shortness of breath, resulting from too few red blood cells (anemia); infection and fever, resulting from too few white blood cells; and bleeding, resulting from too few platelets; possibly bone pain	Lymphoma is invading bone marrow
Loss of muscle strength; hoarseness	Enlarged lymph nodes are compressing nerves in the spinal cord or nerves to the vocal cords
Jaundice	Lymphoma is blocking flow of bile from the liver
Swelling of the face, neck, and upper extremities (superior vena cava syndrome)	Enlarged lymph nodes are blocking flow of blood returning from the head to the heart
Swelling of legs and feet (edema)	Lymphoma is blocking lymphatic flow from the legs
Cough and shortness of breath	Lymphoma is invading the lungs
Decreased ability to fight infection and increased susceptibility to fungal and viral infections	Disease is continuing to spread

*Some of these symptoms may occur for more than one reason.

days alternating with normal or below-normal temperature for days or weeks. Other symptoms may develop, depending on where the cancerous cells are growing. For example, enlargement of lymph nodes in the chest may partially narrow and irritate airways, resulting in a cough, chest discomfort, or shortness of breath. Enlargement of the spleen or lymph

▲ see art on page 1053

nodes in the abdomen may cause discomfort in the abdomen.

Diagnosis

A doctor suspects Hodgkin's disease when a person with no apparent infection develops persistent and painless enlargement of lymph nodes that lasts for several weeks. The suspicion is stronger when lymph node enlargement is accompanied by fever, night sweats, and weight loss. Rapid and painful enlargement of lymph nodes—which may occur when a person has a cold or infection—is not typical of Hodgkin's disease. Sometimes enlarged lymph nodes deep within the chest or abdomen are found unexpectedly on a chest x-ray or computed tomography (CT) scan performed for another reason.

Abnormalities in blood cell counts and other blood tests may provide supportive evidence. However, to make the diagnosis, a doctor must perform a biopsy of an affected lymph node to see if it is abnormal and if Reed-Sternberg cells are present. Reed-Sternberg cells are large cancerous cells that have more than one nucleus. Their distinctive appearance can be seen when a biopsy specimen of lymph node tissue is examined under a microscope.

The type of biopsy depends on which node is enlarged and how much tissue is needed. A doctor must remove enough tissue to be able to distinguish Hodgkin's disease from other diseases that can cause lymph node enlargement, including non-Hodgkin's lymphoma, infections, or other cancers.

The best way to obtain enough tissue is with an excisional biopsy. A small incision is made to remove a piece of the lymph node. Occasionally, when an enlarged lymph node is close to the body's surface, a sufficient amount of tissue can be obtained by inserting a hollow needle through the skin and into the lymph node (needle biopsy). When an enlarged lymph node is deep inside the abdomen or chest, surgery may be needed to obtain a piece of tissue.

Staging

Before treatment is started, doctors must determine how extensively the lymphoma has spread—the stage of the disease. The choice of treatment and the prognosis are based on the stage. An initial examination may detect only a single enlarged lymph node, but procedures to find if and where the lymphoma has spread (staging) may detect considerably more disease.

The disease is classified into four stages based on the extent of its spread (I, II, III, IV; the higher the number, the more the lymphoma has spread). The four stages are subdivided, based on the absence (A) or presence (B) of one or more of the following symptoms: unexplained fever (more than 100° F for 3 consecutive days), night sweats, and unexplained loss of more than 10% of body weight in the preceding 6 months. For example, a person with a stage II lymphoma who has experienced night sweats is said to have stage IIB Hodgkin's disease.

Several procedures are used to stage or assess Hodgkin's disease. Basic blood tests, including tests of liver and kidney function, along with computed tomography (CT) scans of the chest, abdomen, and pelvis are standard. CT scans are quite accurate in detecting enlarged lymph nodes or spread of the lymphoma to the liver and other organs.

Positron emission tomography (PET) scanning is the most sensitive technique for determining the stage of Hodgkin's disease and for evaluating the person's response to treatment. Because living tissue can be identified on a PET scan, doctors can use this imaging technique to distinguish scar tissue from active Hodgkin's disease after the person has undergone treatment. Gallium scanning is another procedure that is used for staging and for following the effects of treatment. A small dose of radioactive gallium is injected into the bloodstream, and 3 to 4 days later, the person is scanned with a device that detects the radioactivity and then produces an image of the internal organs.

Uncommonly, a person with Hodgkin's disease needs surgery to determine whether the disease has spread to the abdomen. During this surgery, the spleen is often removed and a liver biopsy is performed to determine whether the disease has spread to these organs. Abdominal surgery is performed only when its results are likely to affect the choice of treatment—for example, when a doctor needs to know whether to use radiation therapy alone.

Treatment and Prognosis

With radiation therapy, chemotherapy, or both, most people who have Hodgkin's disease can be cured.

Radiation therapy alone cures about 80% of people who have stage IA or IIA disease. Treatments are usually given on an outpatient basis over about 4 or 5 weeks. Radiation is beamed at the affected areas and at the surrounding lymph nodes. Alternatively, chemotherapy is used, followed by radiation therapy for those with stage IB or IIB disease or for those whose chest lymph nodes are greatly enlarged. With this dual approach, about 85% of people are cured.

In stage III and IV disease, a combination of chemotherapy drugs is used. The most common combination for Hodgkin's disease is ABVD (doxorubicin [Adriamycin], bleomycin, vinblastine, and dacarbazine). Each cycle of chemotherapy lasts for 1 month, with a total treatment time of 6 or more months. Other combinations of chemotherapy drugs are sometimes used, but whether these are better than ABVD remains unknown.

It is uncertain whether people with stage III disease receive added benefit when radiation therapy is given along with chemotherapy. For people with very large lymph nodes in the chest, adding radiation therapy to chemotherapy is often recommended. The cure rate of people with stage III disease ranges from 70 to 80%. Cure rates for people with stage IV disease, while not as high, are above 50%.

Although chemotherapy greatly improves the chances for a cure, side effects can be serious. The drugs may cause temporary or permanent sterility, an increased risk of infection, potential damage to other organs, such as the heart or lungs, and reversible hair loss. Sometimes leukemia can develop 5 to 10 years after chemotherapy for Hodgkin's disease. There is also an increased risk of non-Hodgkin's lymphoma or other cancers such as lung, breast, or stomach cancers 10 or more years after treatment with chemotherapy drugs; the risk may increase further when a person is also treated with radiation therapy.

A person who has a remission (with the disease under control) after initial treatment, but then relapses (lymphoma cells reappear), has less of a chance for long-term survival. The cure rate for people who relapse ranges from 10 to 50%. Among those who relapse in the first 12 months after initial treatment, cure rates are somewhat lower, whereas the rates for those who relapse later tend to be somewhat higher. People who relapse after initial treatment generally are treated with additional chemotherapy at usual doses followed by high doses. This is likely to be followed by autologous stem cell transplantation, which

STAGES OF HODGKIN'S DISEASE

STAGE	EXTENT OF SPREAD	LIKELIHOOD OF CURE*
I	Limited to one lymph node	More than 95%
II	Involves two or more lymph nodes on the same side of the diaphragm, either above or below it (for example, some enlarged nodes in the neck and some in the armpit)	90%
III	Involves lymph nodes both above and below the diaphragm (for example, some enlarged nodes in the neck and some in the groin)	80%
IV	Involves lymph nodes and other parts of the body (such as the bone marrow, lungs, or liver)	60 to 70%

*Survival for 15 years with no further disease.

involves using the person's own stem cells.▲ People who relapse more than a year after initial treatment do not always require stem cell transplantation. High-dose chemotherapy with stem cell transplantation is generally a safe procedure, with less than a 5% risk of death related to the treatment.

Non-Hodgkin's Lymphomas

Non-Hodgkin's lymphomas are a diverse group of cancers that develop in B or T lymphocytes.

This group of cancers is actually more than 20 different diseases, which have distinct appearances under the microscope, different cell patterns, and different clinical courses. Most non-Hodgkin's lymphomas (85%) are from B cells; less than 15% develop from T cells. Non-Hodgkin's lymphoma is more common than Hodgkin's disease. In the United States, about 65,000 new cases are diagnosed every

▲ see page 1081

Unusual Non-Hodgkin's Lymphomas

Mycosis fungoides is a rare, persistent, very slow-growing non-Hodgkin's lymphoma. Most people who develop it are older than 50. It originates from mature T lymphocytes and first affects the skin. Mycosis fungoides starts so subtly and grows so slowly that it may not be noticed initially. It causes a long-lasting, itchy rash—sometimes a small area of thickened, itchy skin that later develops nodules and slowly spreads. In some people, it develops into a form of leukemia (Sézary syndrome). In other people, it progresses to the lymph nodes and internal organs. Even with a biopsy, doctors have trouble diagnosing this disease in its early stages. However, later in the course of the disease, a biopsy shows lymphoma cells in the skin.

The thickened areas of skin are treated with a form of radiation called beta rays or with sunlight and corticosteroid drugs. Nitrogen mustard applied directly to the skin can help reduce the itching and size of the affected areas. Interferon drugs can also reduce symptoms. If the disease spreads to lymph nodes and other organs, chemotherapy may be needed. Without treatment, most people can expect to live 7 to 10 years after the diagnosis is made. Treatment does not cure the disease, but it slows it down even further.

Burkitt's lymphoma is a very fast-growing non-Hodgkin's lymphoma that originates from B lymphocytes. Burkitt's lymphoma can develop at any age, but it is most common in children and young adults, particularly males. Unlike other lymphomas, Burkitt's lymphoma has a specific geographic distribution: It is most common in central Africa and rare in the United States. The Epstein-Barr virus causes it, but it does not appear to be contagious. It is more common in people who have AIDS.

Burkitt's lymphoma grows and spreads quickly, often to the bone marrow, blood, and central nervous system. When it spreads, weakness and fatigue often develop. Large numbers of lymphoma cells may accumulate in the lymph nodes and organs of the abdomen, causing swelling. Lymphoma cells may invade the small intestine, resulting in blockage or bleeding. The neck and jaw may swell, sometimes painfully. To make the diagnosis, a doctor performs a biopsy of the abnormal tissue and orders procedures to stage the disease.

Without treatment, Burkitt's lymphoma is fatal. Surgery may be needed to remove affected parts of the intestine, which otherwise may bleed, become blocked, or rupture. Intensive chemotherapy can cure 70 to 80% of people if the disease has not spread widely. If the lymphoma has spread to the bone marrow, blood, or central nervous system at the time of diagnosis, the prognosis is much worse.

---

year, and the number of new cases is increasing, especially among older people and people whose immune system is not functioning normally. Those at risk include people who have had organ transplants and some people who have been infected with the human immunodeficiency virus (HIV).

Although the cause of non-Hodgkin's lymphoma is not known, evidence strongly supports a role for viruses in some of the less common types of non-Hodgkin's lymphomas. A rare type of rapidly progressive non-Hodgkin's lymphoma, which occurs in southern Japan and the Caribbean, may result from infection with human T-cell lymphotropic virus type I (HTLV-I), a retrovirus similar to HIV. The Epstein-Barr virus is the cause of many cases of Burkitt's lymphoma, another type of non-Hodgkin's lymphoma.

Symptoms

The first symptom is often painless enlargement of lymph nodes in the neck, under the arms, or in the groin. Enlarged lymph nodes within the chest may press against airways, causing cough and difficulty in breathing. Deep lymph nodes within the abdomen may press against various organs, causing loss of appetite, constipation, abdominal pain, or progressive swelling of the legs.

Since some lymphomas can appear in the bloodstream and bone marrow, people can develop symptoms related to too few red blood cells, white blood cells, or platelets. Too few red blood cells can cause anemia; and the person may have fatigue, shortness of breath, and pale skin. Too few white blood cells can lead to infections. Too few platelets may lead to increased bruising or bleeding. Non-Hodgkin's lymphomas also commonly invade the bone marrow, digestive tract, skin, and occasionally the nervous system, causing a variety of symptoms. Some people have persistent fever without an evident cause, the so-called fever of unknown origin. This commonly reflects an advanced stage of disease.

In children, the first symptoms—anemia, rashes, and neurologic symptoms, such as weakness and abnormal sensation—are likely to be caused by infiltration of lymphoma cells into the bone marrow, blood, skin, intestine, brain, and spinal cord. Lymph nodes that become enlarged are usually deep ones, leading to accumulation of fluid around the lungs, which causes difficulty in breathing; pressure on the intestine, which causes loss of appetite or vomiting; and blocked lymph vessels, which causes fluid retention, most noticeably in the arms and legs.

Diagnosis and Classification

Doctors perform a biopsy of an enlarged lymph node to diagnose non-Hodgkin's lymphoma and to distinguish it from Hodgkin's disease and other problems that cause enlarged lymph nodes.

Although more than 20 different diseases can be called non-Hodgkin's lymphoma, doctors sometimes group them into three broad categories. Indolent lymphomas are characterized by a survival of many years even when a person does not undergo treatment. Aggressive lymphomas are characterized by survival limited to several months in someone who goes untreated. Highly aggressive lymphomas are characterized by survival of only weeks when a person does not undergo treatment. Although non-Hodgkin's lymphomas are usually diseases of middle-aged and older people, children and young adults may develop lymphomas, and these lymphomas are commonly more aggressive.

Staging

Many people with a non-Hodgkin's lymphoma have disease that has spread at the time of diagnosis. In only 10 to 30% of people, the disease is limited to one specific area. People with the disease undergo similar staging procedures as those with Hodgkin's disease.▲ In addition, a bone marrow biopsy is almost always performed.

Treatment and Prognosis

Almost everyone benefits from treatment. For some people, complete cure is possible; for others, treatment extends life and relieves symptoms for many years. The likelihood of cure or long-term survival depends on the type of non-Hodgkin's lymphoma and the stage when treatment starts. It is somewhat of a paradox that indolent lymphomas usually re-

SYMPTOMS OF NON-HODGKIN'S LYMPHOMA

SYMPTOMS	CAUSE
Difficulty in breathing, swelling of the face	Enlarged lymph nodes in the chest
Loss of appetite, severe constipation, abdominal pain or distention	Enlarged lymph nodes in the abdomen
Progressive swelling of the legs	Blocked lymph vessels in the groin or abdomen
Weight loss, diarrhea, malabsorption (interference with digestion and passage of nutrients into the blood)	Invasion of the small intestine
Fluid accumulation around the lungs (pleural effusion)	Blocked lymph vessels in the chest
Thickened, dark, itchy areas of skin	Infiltration of the skin
Weight loss, fever, night sweats	Spread of the disease throughout the body
Anemia (an insufficient number of red blood cells)	Bleeding into the digestive tract, destruction of red blood cells by an enlarged spleen or by abnormal antibodies, destruction of bone marrow because of invasion by the lymphoma, inability of the bone marrow to produce sufficient numbers of red blood cells because of drugs or radiation therapy
Susceptibility to severe bacterial infections	Invasion of the bone marrow and lymph nodes, causing decreased antibody production

spond readily to treatment by going into remission (in which the disease is under control), often followed by long-term survival, but

▲ see page 1018

the disease usually is not cured. In contrast, aggressive and highly aggressive non-Hodgkin's lymphomas, which usually require very intensive treatment to achieve remission, have a good chance of being cured.

Stage I and II Non-Hodgkin's Lymphomas: People with indolent lymphomas who have very limited disease (stages I and II) are often treated with radiation limited to the site of the lymphoma and adjacent areas. With this approach, 20 to 30% of people may have long-term remission and are probably cured. People with aggressive or highly aggressive lymphomas at a very early stage need to be treated with combinations of chemotherapy, often with the addition of localized radiation therapy. With this approach, 70 to 90% of people are cured.

Stage III and IV Non-Hodgkin's Lymphomas: Almost all people with indolent lymphomas have stage III or IV disease. They do not always require treatment, but they are closely monitored for evidence of complications that could signal more rapid progression of the disease. There is no evidence that early treatment in people with indolent lymphomas at more advanced stages extends survival. If the disease begins to progress more rapidly, there are many treatment choices.

Treatment may include chemotherapy with a single drug or as a combination of several different drugs. No treatment is clearly superior, so the choice of treatment is influenced by the extent of disease and the symptoms a person is having. Treatment usually produces a remission, but the average length of remission ranges from 2 to 4 years. A decision about treatment after a relapse (in which lymphoma cells reappear) again depends on the extent of the disease and the symptoms. After an initial relapse, remissions tend to become shorter.

Many new treatments are now available for indolent lymphomas. These include monoclonal antibodies, which bind to lymphoma cells and kill them. These antibodies (immunoglobulins), such as rituximab, are given intravenously. Sometimes, the monoclonal antibodies are modified so that they can carry radioactive particles or toxic chemicals directly to the cancer cells in different parts of the body. It remains uncertain whether these mon-

oclonal antibodies can cure non-Hodgkin's lymphomas, or if they can achieve better results when combined with chemotherapy.

Another new approach to treating indolent lymphomas involves vaccinating the person with proteins taken from his own lymphoma. The person's immune system recognizes the proteins as "foreign" and then fights the lymphoma in much the same way that it fights an infection.

For people with aggressive or highly aggressive stage III or IV non-Hodgkin's lymphomas, combinations of chemotherapy drugs are given promptly. Many potentially effective combinations of chemotherapy drugs are available. Combinations of chemotherapy drugs are often given names created by using single letters from each of the drugs that are included. For example, one of the oldest and still most commonly used combinations is known as CHOP (cyclophosphamide, [hydroxy]doxorubicin, vincristine [Oncovin], and prednisone). About 50% of people with aggressive or highly aggressive non-Hodgkin's lymphomas at an advanced stage are cured with CHOP chemotherapy. Newer combinations of drugs have not produced much improvement in cure rates. However, chemotherapy, which often causes different types of blood cells to decrease in number, is sometimes better tolerated if special proteins (called growth factors) are given to stimulate growth and development of blood cells. Chemotherapy for some people with aggressive or highly aggressive lymphomas is now combined with monoclonal antibodies. For example, results from the combination of CHOP with rituximab may be better than from CHOP alone, but studies are still ongoing.

Chemotherapy at usual doses is of very limited value when relapse occurs. Many people who have a relapse of an aggressive or highly aggressive lymphoma at an advanced stage receive high-dose chemotherapy combined with autologous stem cell transplantation, involving the person's own stem cells.▲ With this type of treatment, up to 40% of people may be cured. Some stem cell transplants for people with an aggressive or highly aggressive lymphoma use stem cells from a matched or unrelated donor (allogeneic transplant), but this type of transplantation has a greater risk of complications.

▲ see page 1081

CHAPTER 178

Myeloproliferative Disorders

In myeloproliferative disorders (myelo = bone marrow, proliferative = rapid multiplication), the blood-producing cells in the bone marrow (precursor cells) develop and reproduce abnormally or are crowded out by an overgrowth of fibrous tissue.

Three major myeloproliferative disorders are polycythemia vera, myelofibrosis, and thrombocythemia. The proliferation of blood-producing cells is always clinically noncancerous (benign) when it begins. However, in a small number of people, a myeloproliferative disorder progresses or transforms to a cancerous (malignant) condition (leukemia).

Polycythemia Vera

Polycythemia vera (primary polycythemia) is a disorder of the blood-producing cells of the bone marrow that results in overproduction of red blood cells.

In polycythemia vera, the excess of red blood cells increases the volume of blood and makes it thicker, so that it flows less easily through small blood vessels.

Polycythemia vera is rare, occurring in about 5 of every 1 million people. The average age at which the disorder is diagnosed is 60, and it rarely occurs before age 20. More men than women develop polycythemia vera. The cause is not known.

Symptoms and Complications

Often, people with polycythemia vera have no symptoms for years. The earliest symptoms usually are weakness, fatigue, headache, light-headedness, shortness of breath, and night sweats. Vision may be distorted, and a person may have blind spots or may see flashes of light. Bleeding from the gums and more bleeding than would be expected from small cuts are common. The skin, especially the face, may look red. A person may itch all over, particularly after bathing or showering. Burning sensations in the hands and feet or, more rarely, bone pain may be felt.

In some people, the number of platelets (cell-like particles that help the body form blood clots) in the bloodstream increases. The liver and spleen may enlarge, as both organs begin to produce blood cells and as the spleen removes more red blood cells from the circulation. As the liver and spleen enlarge, a sense of fullness in the abdomen may develop. Pain can suddenly become intense should a blood clot develop in blood vessels of the liver or spleen.

The excess of red blood cells may be associated with other complications, including

MAJOR MYELOPROLIFERATIVE DISORDERS

Disorder	Bone Marrow Characteristics	Blood Characteristics
Polycythemia vera	Increased number of the cells that produce the circulating blood cells	Increased number of red blood cells, often accompanied by an increased number of platelets and white blood cells
Myelofibrosis	Excess fibrous tissue	Increased number of immature red and white blood cells and misshapen red blood cells; decrease in the overall number of red blood cells (anemia); eventually, the number of white blood cells and platelets decreases
Thrombocythemia	Increased number of megakaryocytes (cells that produce platelets)	Increased number of platelets

What Are Secondary and Relative Polycythemia?

Secondary and relative polycythemia differ from polycythemia vera (which literally translates as "true polycythemia") in that their causes are known.

Secondary polycythemia is caused by oxygen deprivation, which can result, for example, from smoking, severe lung disease, or heart disease. In secondary polycythemia, a high concentration of red blood cells results from an actual increase in the erythropoietin level in the blood. People who spend long periods of time in circumstances low in oxygen, such as fighter pilots and those who live at high altitude, sometimes develop polycythemia but do not have polycythemia vera.▲

Secondary polycythemia may be treated with oxygen. Smokers are advised to quit and are offered specific treatment to assist quitting. Any underlying disease that is causing the oxygen deprivation and secondary polycythemia is treated as effectively as possible. Phlebotomy is used to lower the number of red blood cells.

In relative polycythemia, a high concentration of red blood cells results from abnormally low levels of fluid (plasma). The low plasma level can occur as the result of burns, vomiting, diarrhea, drinking an inadequate amount of fluids, and the use of diuretics (drugs that speed elimination of salt and water by the kidneys). Relative polycythemia is treated by giving fluids by mouth or intravenously and by treating any underlying conditions that are contributing to the low plasma level.

stomach ulcers, gout, and kidney stones. The increase in the thickness (viscosity) of the blood can cause heart attacks and strokes and can block blood flow to the arms and legs, lungs, and eyes. Rarely, polycythemia vera progresses to leukemia.

Diagnosis

Polycythemia vera may be discovered through routine blood tests performed for another reason, even before a person has any symptoms. Levels of hemoglobin (the protein that carries oxygen in red blood cells) and the

▲ see box on page 1673   ■ see page 981

hematocrit (the percentage of red blood cells in the total blood volume) are abnormally high. The number of platelets and white blood cells may also be increased.

Most doctors consider a high hematocrit result to be an indication of polycythemia. However, the diagnosis cannot be based solely on the hematocrit result. Therefore, to help make the diagnosis, a test that uses radioactively labeled red blood cells to determine the total number of red blood cells in the body (red blood cell mass) is sometimes performed.

Once polycythemia is discovered, the doctor must determine if it is polycythemia vera or polycythemia due to another cause (secondary polycythemia). The person's medical history may help differentiate the two, but sometimes the doctor must investigate further.

Blood levels of erythropoietin, a hormone that stimulates the bone marrow to produce red blood cells, also may be measured. Levels of erythropoietin are extremely low in polycythemia vera but are normal or high in secondary polycythemia. Rarely, cysts in the liver or kidneys and tumors in the kidneys or brain produce erythropoietin; people with these conditions have high levels of erythropoietin and may develop secondary polycythemia.

Removal of a sample of bone marrow for examination under a microscope (bone marrow biopsy)■ can also be helpful to diagnose polycythemia vera.

Prognosis and Treatment

Without treatment, about half of the people who have polycythemia vera with symptoms die in less than 2 years. With treatment, they live an average of 15 to 20 years.

Treatment does not cure polycythemia vera, but it does control it and can decrease the likelihood of complications, such as the formation of blood clots. The aim of treatment is to decrease the number of red blood cells. Usually, blood is removed from the body in a procedure called phlebotomy, similar to the way blood is removed when donating blood. A pint of blood is removed every other day until the hematocrit reaches a normal level, which is then maintained by removing blood every few months, as needed.

Because phlebotomy may increase the number of platelets and does not reduce the size of an enlarged liver or spleen, people who undergo phlebotomy may need drugs to suppress production of red blood cells and platelets. Hydroxyurea, a chemotherapy drug, is frequently given, but when used for many years there is concern that it may increase the risk of transformation to leukemia. Alternative drugs for lowering the number of platelets, such as interferon-alpha and anagrelide, are sometimes used in younger people who may need treatment for long periods. Some people are given radioactive phosphorus intravenously, but doctors restrict this type of treatment to people older than 70 because of the potential for transformation to leukemia.

Other drugs can help control some of the symptoms. For example, antihistamines can help relieve itching, and aspirin can relieve burning sensations in the hands and feet as well as bone pain.

Myelofibrosis

Myelofibrosis is a disorder in which fibrous tissue replaces the blood-producing cells in the bone marrow, resulting in abnormally shaped red blood cells, anemia, and an enlarged spleen.

In normal bone marrow, cells called fibroblasts produce fibrous (connective) tissue that supports the blood-producing cells. In myelofibrosis, the fibroblasts produce too much fibrous tissue, which crowds out the blood-producing cells. Consequently, red blood cell production decreases, fewer red blood cells are released into the bloodstream, and anemia develops, becoming progressively more severe. In addition, many of these red blood cells are immature or misshapen. Variable numbers of immature white blood cells and platelets also may be seen in the blood. As myelofibrosis progresses, the number of white blood cells may increase or decrease, and the number of platelets typically decreases.

Myelofibrosis is rare, affecting less than 2 of 100,000 people in the United States. It occurs most commonly among people between the ages of 50 and 70.

Myelofibrosis may develop on its own (in which case it is also called idiopathic myelofibrosis or agnogenic myeloid metaplasia) or may accompany other blood disorders, such as chronic myelocytic leukemia, polycythemia vera, thrombocythemia, multiple myeloma, lymphoma, and myelodysplasia; tuberculosis; or bone infections. People who have been exposed to certain toxic substances, such as benzene and radiation, are at increased risk of developing myelofibrosis.

Symptoms, Complications, and Diagnosis

Often, myelofibrosis produces no symptoms for years. Eventually, anemia becomes severe enough to cause weakness, fatigue, weight loss, and a general feeling of illness (malaise). Fever and night sweats may occur. With the reduced number of white blood cells, the body is at risk for infections. With the reduced number of platelets, the body is at risk for bleeding.

The liver and spleen often enlarge as they try to take over some of the job of making blood cells. Enlargement of these organs may cause pain in the abdomen and may lead to abnormally high blood pressure in certain veins (portal hypertension)▲ and bleeding from varicose veins in the esophagus (esophageal varices).■

Anemia and the misshapen, immature red blood cells, seen in blood samples viewed under a microscope, suggest myelofibrosis. However, a bone marrow biopsy★ is needed to confirm the diagnosis.

Prognosis and Treatment

Because myelofibrosis generally progresses slowly, people who have it usually live for 10 years or longer, but outcomes are determined by how well the bone marrow functions. Occasionally, however, the disorder worsens rapidly. This rapidly progressive form, called malignant myelofibrosis or acute myelofibrosis, is a type of cancer involving uncontrolled growth of cells that would normally develop into platelets.

No available treatment can effectively reverse or permanently slow the progression of myelofibrosis. Treatment aims to delay and relieve complications.

The combination of androgen (a male sex hormone) and prednisone temporarily lessens the severity of the anemia in about one third of people with myelofibrosis. In a few people, red blood cell production can be stimulated with erythropoietin or darbepoietin, drugs that stimulate the bone marrow to produce red blood cells. In others, blood transfusions are needed to treat the anemia. Infections are treated with antibiotics.

▲ see page 793

■ see pages 776 and 794

★ see page 981

Other Causes of a High Platelet Count

When the cause of thrombocythemia is known, the disorder is called secondary thrombocythemia. Bleeding, removal of the spleen, infections, rheumatoid arthritis, certain cancers, and sarcoidosis can cause secondary thrombocythemia.

People with secondary thrombocythemia may have no symptoms related to a high number of platelets; symptoms of the underlying condition usually dominate. When symptoms from a high number of platelets do occur, they are similar to those of primary thrombocythemia. Secondary thrombocythemia is diagnosed—and distinguished from primary thrombocythemia—when a person with a high platelet count has a condition that readily accounts for the high platelet count.

Treatment is aimed at the cause. If the treatment is successful, the platelet count usually returns to normal.

Hydroxyurea, a chemotherapy drug, or interferon-alpha, a drug that affects the immune system, may decrease the size of the liver or spleen, but either drug may worsen the anemia. Rarely, the spleen becomes extremely large and painful and may have to be removed.

Bone marrow or stem cell transplantation is sometimes offered to people who are in otherwise good health and who have an appropriate matched donor.▲ A transplant is the only treatment available that may cure myelofibrosis, but it also has significant risks associated with it.

Thrombocythemia

Thrombocythemia (primary thrombocythemia) is a disorder in which excess platelets are produced, leading to abnormal blood clotting or bleeding.

Platelets (thrombocytes) are normally produced in the bone marrow by cells called megakaryocytes. In thrombocythemia, megakaryocytes increase in number and produce too many platelets.

▲ see page 1081
■ see page 981

Thrombocythemia is rare, affecting about 2 to 3 of 100,000 people. It usually occurs in people older than 50 and more frequently in women. The cause of thrombocythemia is unknown.

Symptoms

Often, thrombocythemia does not produce symptoms. However, an excess of platelets can cause blood clots to form spontaneously, blocking the flow of blood through blood vessels, especially smaller ones. Older people with thrombocythemia are much more likely to form clots than are younger people.

Symptoms are due to the blockage of blood vessels and may include tingling and other abnormal sensations in the hands and feet (paresthesias), cold fingertips, headaches, weakness, and dizziness. Bleeding, usually mild, may occur, often consisting of nosebleeds, easy bruising, slight oozing from the gums, or bleeding in the digestive tract. The spleen and liver may enlarge.

Diagnosis

A doctor makes a diagnosis of thrombocythemia on the basis of the person's symptoms or after finding increased platelets during routine screening of the blood. Blood tests may be used to confirm the diagnosis. In thrombocythemia, the platelet count is usually 2 to 4 times higher than normal. In addition, a microscopic examination of the blood reveals abnormally large platelets, clumps of platelets, and fragments of megakaryocytes.

To distinguish primary thrombocythemia, whose cause is unknown, from secondary thrombocythemia, which has a known cause, a doctor looks for signs of other conditions that could increase the platelet count. Removal of a sample of bone marrow for examination under a microscope (bone marrow biopsy)■ is sometimes helpful and can exclude chronic myelocytic leukemia as a cause of an increased platelet count.

Treatment

Thrombocythemia may require treatment with a drug that decreases platelet production. Such drugs include hydroxyurea, anagrelide, and interferon-alpha. Treatment with one of these drugs is typically started when the platelet count becomes exceedingly high or when bleeding or clotting complications develop. The age of the person, the other risks present, and previous history of thrombosis determine the need for such treatment. The drug is continued until the platelet count falls into a safe range. The dose must be adjusted to maintain an adequate number of platelets and other circulating cells. Small doses of aspirin, which makes platelets less sticky and impairs clotting, may also be used.

If drug treatment does not slow platelet production quickly enough, it may be combined with or replaced by plateletpheresis, a procedure reserved for emergency situations. In this procedure, blood is withdrawn, platelets are removed from it, and the platelet-depleted blood is returned to the person.

Spleen Disorders

The spleen, a spongy, soft organ about as big as a person's fist, is located in the upper left part of the abdomen, just under the rib cage. The splenic artery brings blood to the spleen from the heart. Blood leaves the spleen through the splenic vein, which drains into a larger vein (the portal vein) that carries the blood to the liver. The spleen has a covering of fibrous tissue (the splenic capsule) that supports its blood vessels and lymphatic vessels.

The spleen is made up of two basic types of tissue: the white pulp and the red pulp, each with different functions. The white pulp is part of the infection-fighting (immune) system. It produces white blood cells called lymphocytes, which in turn produce antibodies (specialized proteins that protect against invasion by a foreign substance). The red pulp filters the blood, removing unwanted material. The red pulp contains other white blood cells called phagocytes that ingest microorganisms, such as bacteria, fungi, and viruses. It also monitors red blood cells, destroying those that are abnormal or too old or damaged to function properly. In addition, the red pulp serves as a reservoir for different elements of the blood, especially white blood cells and platelets (cell-like particles involved in clotting). However, releasing these elements is a minor function of the red pulp.

A person can live without a spleen. Sometimes the spleen must be removed surgically (splenectomy) because of irreparable damage (for example, due to an injury sustained in a car accident). When the spleen is removed, the body loses some of its ability to produce protective antibodies and to remove unwanted microorganisms from the blood. As a result,

the body's ability to fight infections is impaired. People who do not have a spleen are at particularly high risk of pneumococcal infec-

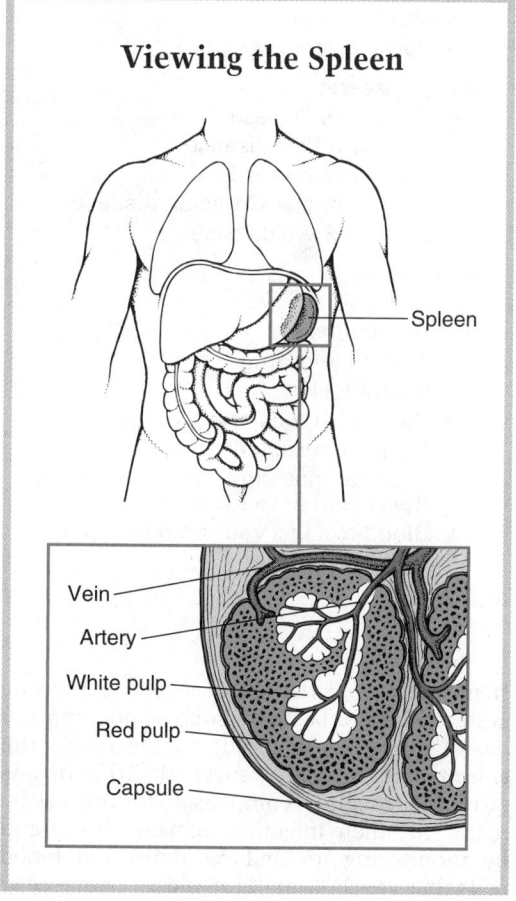

Viewing the Spleen

Spleen

Vein

Artery

White pulp

Red pulp

Capsule

Causes of an Enlarged Spleen

Infections
- Hepatitis
- Infectious mononucleosis
- Psittacosis
- Subacute bacterial endocarditis
- Brucellosis
- Kala-azar
- Malaria
- Syphilis
- Tuberculosis

Anemias
- Hereditary elliptocytosis
- Hereditary spherocytosis
- Sickle cell disease (mainly in children)
- Thalassemia

Blood cancers and myeloproliferative disorders
- Hodgkin's disease and other lymphomas
- Leukemia
- Myelofibrosis
- Polycythemia vera

Storage diseases
- Gaucher's disease
- Niemann-Pick disease
- Wolman's disease
- Hand-Schüller-Christian disease
- Letterer-Siwe disease

Other causes
- Cirrhosis
- Amyloidosis
- Felty's syndrome
- Sarcoidosis
- Systemic lupus erythematosus
- Cysts in the spleen
- External pressure on veins from the spleen or to the liver
- Blood clot in a vein from the spleen or to the liver

tions because of the spleen's role in fighting certain kinds of bacteria, such as pneumococcus. Despite these problems, however, the spleen is not critical to survival: Other organs (primarily the liver) compensate for the loss by increasing their infection-fighting ability and by monitoring for and removing red blood cells that are abnormal, too old, or damaged.

Enlarged Spleen

An enlarged spleen (splenomegaly) is not a disease in itself but the result of an underlying disorder. Many disorders can make the spleen enlarge. To pinpoint the cause, a doctor must consider disorders ranging from chronic infections to blood cancers.

When the spleen enlarges, it traps and stores an excessive number of blood cells and platelets (hypersplenism), thereby reducing the number of blood cells and platelets in the bloodstream. This process creates a vicious circle: the more cells and platelets the spleen traps, the larger it grows; the larger it grows, the more cells and platelets it traps. Eventually, the greatly enlarged spleen also traps normal red blood cells, destroying them along with the abnormal ones. In addition, excessive numbers of blood cells and platelets can clog the spleen, interfering with its functioning.

An enlarged spleen may outgrow its own blood supply. When parts of the spleen do not get enough blood, they may become damaged, causing them to bleed or die.

Symptoms

An enlarged spleen does not cause many symptoms, and the symptoms that it does cause may be mistaken for many other medical conditions. Because the enlarged spleen lies next to the stomach and sometimes presses against it, a person may feel full after eating a small snack or even without eating. A person may also have abdominal or back pain in the area of the spleen; the pain may spread to the left shoulder, especially if parts of the spleen do not get enough blood and start to die.

When the spleen removes too many blood cells and platelets from the bloodstream, a variety of problems may develop. These problems include anemia as a result of too few red blood cells, frequent infections as a result of too few white blood cells, and the tendency to bleed as a result of too few platelets.

Diagnosis

A doctor may suspect that the spleen is enlarged when the person complains of fullness or pain in the upper left portion of the abdomen or back. Usually, the doctor can feel an enlarged spleen during a physical examination. An x-ray of the abdomen may also show that the spleen is enlarged. In some cases, an ultrasound or computed tomography (CT) scan is needed to determine how large the spleen is and whether it is pressing on other organs. A magnetic resonance imaging (MRI) scan provides similar information and also traces blood flow through the spleen. Other specialized scanning devices use mildly radioactive particles to assess the spleen's size and function and to determine whether it is accumulating or destroying large numbers of blood cells.

Blood tests show decreased numbers of red blood cells, white blood cells, and platelets. When blood cells are examined under a microscope, their shape and size may provide clues to the cause of the spleen enlargement. An examination of bone marrow▲ may show cancer of the blood cells (such as leukemia or lymphoma) or an accumulation of unwanted substances (such as occurs in storage diseases).■ Blood protein measurement can determine whether other conditions are present that can cause the spleen to enlarge, such as amyloidosis, sarcoidosis, malaria, kala-azar, brucellosis, and tuberculosis. Liver function tests help determine whether the liver is also diseased.

Doctors cannot easily remove a sample of the spleen for examination because inserting a needle or cutting spleen tissue may cause uncontrollable bleeding. If a person's enlarged spleen is removed during surgery to diagnose or treat certain diseases, the spleen is sent to a laboratory, where the cause of enlargement can usually be determined.

Treatment

When possible, a doctor treats the underlying disease that caused the enlarged spleen. Surgical removal of the spleen (splenectomy) may be necessary but can cause problems, including an increased susceptibility to infections. However, the risks are worth taking in certain critical situations: when the spleen destroys red blood cells so rapidly that severe anemia develops; when it so depletes stores of white blood cells and platelets that infection and bleeding are likely; when it is so large that it causes pain or puts pressure on other organs; or when it is so large that parts of it bleed or die. As an alternative to surgery, radiation therapy can sometimes be used to shrink the spleen.

Ruptured Spleen

Because of the spleen's position in the abdomen, a severe blow to the stomach area can rupture the spleen, tearing its covering and the tissue inside. A ruptured spleen is the most common serious complication of abdominal injury resulting from car accidents, athletic mishaps, and beatings.

When the spleen ruptures, a large volume of blood may pour out into the abdomen. The spleen's tough outer covering may contain the bleeding temporarily, but surgery is needed immediately to prevent life-threatening blood loss.

Symptoms

A ruptured spleen makes the abdomen painful and tender. Blood in the abdomen acts as an irritant and causes pain; the abdominal muscles contract reflexively and feel rigid. If the blood leaks out gradually, no symptoms may occur until the body's blood supply is so depleted that blood pressure falls and not enough oxygen can reach the brain and heart. Symptoms of low blood pressure and lack of oxygen include light-headedness, blurred vision, confusion, and loss of consciousness (fainting). Such a situation is an emergency requiring immediate blood transfusions to maintain adequate circulation and surgery to stop the leak; without these actions, the person could go into shock and die.

Diagnosis and Treatment

X-rays of the abdomen are taken to determine if the symptoms may be caused by something other than a ruptured spleen. Scanning procedures using radioactive material to trace blood flow and find leaks may be performed, or fluid in the abdomen may be withdrawn by a needle and tested to see if it contains blood. When doctors strongly suspect that the spleen has ruptured, the person is rushed to surgery to stop the potentially fatal loss of blood. Usually the entire spleen is removed (splenectomy), but sometimes surgeons are able to repair a small rupture.

Before and after a splenectomy, certain precautions are needed to prevent infections. For example, vaccinations against pneumococcus are given before a splenectomy whenever possible, and yearly vaccinations against influenza are recommended after a splenectomy. Under some circumstances, antibiotics are recommended to prevent infections, particularly when the person has another condition (such as a sickle-cell disease or cancer) that increases the risk of developing life-threatening infections.

▲ see page 981   ■ see page 1616

CANCER

180 Overview of Cancer 1031

How Cancer Develops and Spreads ▪ Types of Cancer ▪ Risk Factors ▪ Bodily Defenses Against Cancer

181 Symptoms and Diagnosis of Cancer 1035

Pain ▪ Bleeding ▪ Weight Loss and Fatigue ▪ Swollen Lymph Nodes ▪ Depression ▪ Neurologic and Muscular Symptoms ▪ Respiratory Symptoms ▪ Screening ▪ Diagnostic Tests and Staging

182 Prevention and Treatment of Cancer 1042

Surgery ▪ Radiation Therapy ▪ Chemotherapy ▪ Immunotherapy ▪ Combination Therapy ▪ Alternative Medicine ▪ Side Effects of Treatments

CHAPTER 180

Overview of Cancer

A cancer is a group of cells (usually derived from a single cell) that has lost its normal control mechanisms and thus has unregulated growth. Cancerous (malignant) cells can develop from any tissue within any organ. As cancerous cells grow and multiply, they form a mass of cancerous tissue—called a tumor—that invades and destroys normal adjacent tissues. The term "tumor" refers to an abnormal growth or mass; tumors can be cancerous or noncancerous. Cancerous cells from the primary (initial) site can spread (metastasize) throughout the body.

How Cancer Develops and Spreads

Cancerous cells develop from healthy cells in a complex process called transformation. The first step in the process is **initiation,** in which a change in the cell's genetic material (in the DNA and sometimes in the chromosome structure) primes the cell to become cancerous. The change in the cell's genetic material may occur spontaneously or be brought on by an agent that causes cancer (a carcinogen). Carcinogens include many chemicals, tobacco, viruses, radiation, and sunlight. However, not all cells are equally susceptible to carcinogens. A genetic flaw in a cell may make it more susceptible. Even chronic physical irritation may make a cell more susceptible to carcinogens.

The second and final step in the development of cancer is called **promotion.** Agents that cause promotion are called promoters. Promoters may be substances in the environment or even some drugs (such as barbiturates). Unlike carcinogens, promoters do not cause cancer by themselves. Instead, promoters allow a cell that has undergone initiation to become cancerous. Promotion has no effect on noninitiated cells. Thus, several factors, often the combination of a susceptible cell and a carcinogen, are needed to cause cancer.

Talking About Cancer

Aggressiveness: The degree to which (or speed at which) a tumor grows and spreads.

Anaplasia: A lack of differentiation. Thus, an anaplastic cancer is highly undifferentiated and usually very aggressive.

Benign: Noncancerous.

Carcinogen: An agent that causes cancer.

Carcinoma-in-situ: Cancerous cells that are still contained within the tissue where they have started to grow and that have not yet become invasive or spread to other parts of the body.

Cure: Complete elimination of the cancer with the result that the specific cancer will not grow back.

Differentiation: The extent to which the cancerous cells resemble normal cells— less resemblance means the cancer is less differentiated and more aggressive.

Invasion: The capacity of a cancer to infiltrate and destroy surrounding tissue.

Malignant: Cancerous.

Metastasis: Cancerous cells that have spread to a completely new location.

Neoplasm: General term for a tumor, whether cancerous or noncancerous.

Recurrence (relapse): Cancerous cells return after treatment, either in the primary location or as metastases (spread).

Remission: Absence of all evidence of a cancer after treatment.

Survival rate: The percentage of people who survive for a given time period after treatment (for example, the 5-year survival rate is the percentage of people who survive 5 years).

Tumor: Abnormal growth or mass.

Some carcinogens are sufficiently powerful to be able to cause cancer without the need for promotion. For example, ionizing radiation (which is used in x-rays and is produced in nuclear power plants and atomic bomb explosions) can cause a variety of cancers, particularly sarcomas, leukemia, thyroid cancer, and breast cancer.

Cancer can grow directly into surrounding tissue or spread to tissues or organs, nearby or distant. Cancer can spread through the lymphatic system. This type of spread is typical of carcinomas. For example, breast cancer usually spreads first to the nearby lymph nodes; only later does it spread more extensively throughout the body. Cancer can also spread via the bloodstream. This type of spread is typical of sarcomas.

Types of Cancer

Cancerous tissues (malignancies) can be divided into those of the blood and blood-forming tissues (leukemias and lymphomas) and "solid" tumors, often termed cancer. Cancers can be carcinomas or sarcomas.

Leukemias and **lymphomas** are cancers of the blood and blood-forming tissues. Rather than forming a lump, they may remain as separate cancerous cells. Thus, they often harm the body by crowding out normal blood cells in the bone marrow and bloodstream, so that normal functioning cells are gradually replaced by cancerous blood cells.

Carcinomas are cancers of epithelial cells, which are cells that cover the surface of the body, produce hormones, and make up glands. Examples of carcinomas are cancer of the skin, lung, colon, stomach, breast, prostate, and thyroid gland. Typically, carcinomas occur more often in older than in younger people.

Sarcomas are cancers of mesodermal cells, which are the cells that form muscles and connective tissue. Examples of sarcomas are leiomyosarcoma (cancer of smooth muscle that is found in the wall of digestive organs) and osteosarcoma (bone cancer). Typically, sarcomas occur more often in younger than in older people.

Risk Factors

Many genetic and environmental factors increase the risk of developing cancer.

Family History and Genetic Factors: Some families have a significantly higher risk of developing certain cancers. Sometimes the increased risk is due to a single gene and sometimes it is due to several genes interacting together. Environmental factors—common to the family—may alter this genetic interaction and produce cancer.

An extra or abnormal chromosome may increase the risk of cancer. For example, people with Down syndrome, who have three instead of the usual two copies of chromosome 21, have a 12 to 20 times higher risk of developing acute leukemia.

Age: Some cancers, such as Wilms' tumor, retinoblastoma, and neuroblastoma, occur almost exclusively in children. Why these cancers occur in the young is not well understood, but genetics is one factor. However, most cancers are more common in older people. In the United States, more than 60% of cancers occur in people older than 65; the risk of developing cancer doubles every 5 years after age 25. The increased cancer rate is probably due to a combination of increased and prolonged exposure to carcinogens and weakening of the body's immune system.

Environmental Factors: Numerous environmental factors increase the risk of developing cancer.

Pollution in the air, whether from industrial waste or cigarette smoke, can increase the cancer risk. Many chemicals are known to cause cancer and many others are suspected of doing so. For example, asbestos exposure may cause lung cancer and mesothelioma (cancer of the pleura), especially in smokers. The time between exposure to the chemicals and development of the cancer may be many years.

Smoking cigarettes produces carcinogens that substantially increase the risk of developing cancers of the lung, mouth, larynx, kidney, and bladder.

Exposure to radiation is a risk factor in the development of cancer. Extended exposure to ultraviolet radiation, primarily from sunlight, causes skin cancer. Ionizing radiation is particularly carcinogenic. Exposure to the radioactive gas radon, which is released from soil, increases the risk of lung cancer. Normally, radon disperses rapidly into the atmosphere and produces no harm. However, when a building is placed on soil with a high radon content, radon can accumulate within the building, sometimes producing sufficiently high levels in the air to cause harm. Radon is breathed into the lungs, where it may eventually cause lung cancer. If an exposed person also smokes, the risk of lung cancer is further increased.

Geography: The risk of cancer varies according to where people live, although the reasons for the geographic differences are often complex and poorly understood. This geographic variation in cancer risk is probably multifactorial: a combination of genetics, diet, and environment.

For example, the risk of colon and breast cancers is low in Japan, yet in Japanese people who immigrate to the United States, the risk increases and eventually equals that of the rest of the American population. In contrast, the Japanese have extremely high rates of stomach cancer. When these people immigrate to the United States and eat a Western diet, the risk declines to that of the United States, although the decline may not be evident until the next generation.

Diet: Substances consumed in the diet can increase the risk of cancer. For instance, a diet high in fat has been linked to an increased risk of colon, breast, and possibly prostate cancer. People who drink large amounts of alcohol are at much higher risk of developing esophageal cancer. A diet high in smoked and pickled foods or in barbecued meats increases the risk of developing stomach cancer.

SOME CARCINOGENS

CARCINOGEN	TYPE OF CANCER
Environmental and industrial	
Arsenic	Lung
Asbestos	Lung, pleura
Aromatic amines	Bladder
Benzene	Leukemia
Chromates	Lung
Nickel	Lung, nasal sinuses
Vinyl chloride	Liver
Soot and mineral oil	Skin
Diesel exhaust	Lung
Associated with lifestyle	
Alcohol	Esophagus, mouth, throat
Betel nuts	Mouth, throat
Tobacco	Mouth, throat, lung, esophagus, bladder, kidney
Used in medicine	
Alkylating agents	Leukemia, bladder
Chemotherapy drugs (such as topoisomerase inhibitors)	Leukemia
Diethylstilbestrol	Liver, vagina (if exposed before birth)
Oxymetholone	Liver
Radiation therapy	Sarcomas
Thorotrast	Blood vessels

MOST COMMON CANCERS IN MEN AND WOMEN*

MEN	WOMEN
Prostate	Breast
Lung	Lung
Colon and rectum	Colon and rectum
Bladder	Uterus
Non-Hodgkin's lymphoma	Non-Hodgkin's lymphoma

*Based on statistics from the American Cancer Society. Skin cancer is probably the most common cancer in both sexes, but only one type of skin cancer—melanoma—is required to be reported. Thus, reports of other types of skin cancer are incomplete and therefore generally excluded from statistics.

Viral Infections: Several viruses are known to cause cancer in humans, and several others are suspected of causing cancer. The papillomavirus (which causes genital warts) is one cause of cervical cancer in women. Hepatitis B virus can cause liver cancer. Some human retroviruses cause lymphomas and other cancers of the blood system.

Some viruses produce cancer in certain countries but not in others. For instance, the Epstein-Barr virus causes Burkitt's lymphoma (a type of cancer) in Africa and cancers of the nose and pharynx in China.

Inflammatory Diseases: Inflammatory diseases often produce an increased risk of cancer. Such diseases include ulcerative colitis (which can result in colon cancer). Infection with certain parasites can produce inflammation that may result in cancer. For example, infection with the parasite *Schistosoma (Bilharzia)* may cause bladder cancer by chronically irritating the bladder.

Bodily Defenses Against Cancer

Even when a cell becomes cancerous, the immune system is thought to be able to recognize it as abnormal and destroy it before it

▲ see page 1049   ■ see table on page 1039

replicates or spreads. Cancer is more likely to progress in people whose immune system is altered or impaired, as in people with AIDS, those receiving immunosuppressive drugs, those with certain autoimmune diseases, and older people, in whom the immune system works less well than in younger people. However, even when a person's immune system is functioning normally, cancer can escape the immune system's protective surveillance.

Tumor Antigens: An antigen is a foreign substance recognized and targeted for destruction by the body's immune system.▲ Antigens are found on the surface of all cells, but normally a person's immune system does not react to his own cells. When a cell becomes cancerous, new antigens—unfamiliar to the immune system—appear on the cell's surface. The immune system may regard these new antigens, called tumor antigens, as foreign and may be able to contain or destroy the cancerous cells. This is the mechanism by which the body destroys abnormal cells and is often able to destroy cancerous cells before they can become established. However, even a fully functioning immune system cannot always destroy all cancerous cells. And, once cancerous cells reproduce and form a mass of cancerous cells (a cancerous tumor), the body's immune system is highly unlikely to be able to destroy it.

Tumor antigens have been identified in several types of cancer, including malignant melanoma, bone cancer (osteosarcoma), and some cancers of the digestive tract. People with these cancers may have antibodies against the tumor antigens. However, the antibodies are usually not powerful enough to control the cancer. In other cancers, such as choriocarcinoma (a cancerous tumor developing in the uterus from parts of a developing embryo), the immune system is much more likely to be able to destroy cancerous cells early.

Certain tumor antigens can be detected with blood tests. These antigens are sometimes called **tumor markers.** Measurements of some of these tumor markers can be used as screening tests in people who have no symptoms of cancer. Sometimes these markers are used for diagnosis and sometimes to evaluate the person's response to treatment.■

CHAPTER 181

Symptoms and Diagnosis of Cancer

Cancer can produce many different symptoms, some subtle and some not at all subtle. Some symptoms develop early in the course of cancer and are therefore important warning signs that should be evaluated by a doctor. Other symptoms develop only after the cancer progresses and are therefore not helpful in the early detection of cancer. Still other symptoms, such as nausea, loss of appetite, fatigue, and vomiting, may be the result of treatment or may be warning signs. Some symptoms occur with many or almost all cancers, and others are specific to the type of cancer and where it is growing.

Screening programs allow early detection and diagnosis of cancer. The earlier cancer is diagnosed, the more effective treatment is likely to be.

Symptoms

At first, cancer, as a tiny mass of cells, produces no symptoms whatsoever. When cancer grows in an area with a lot of space, such as in the wall of the large intestine, it may not cause any symptoms until it becomes quite large. In contrast, a cancer growing in a more restricted space, such as on a vocal cord, may cause symptoms (such as hoarseness) when it is relatively small.

Cancers produce symptoms by growing into and thus irritating or destroying other tissues, putting pressure on other tissues, producing toxic substances, and using energy and nutrients normally available for other bodily functions. Cancer may cause one set of symptoms as it grows in its initial site and cause different symptoms as it spreads (metastasizes) to other parts of the body.

As a cancer grows and spreads throughout the body, a number of complications can result. Some of these complications can be serious and require emergency treatment. Certain complications, called paraneoplastic syndromes, result when substances produced by cancers spread throughout the body.

Pain

Cancers are typically painless at first. However, as they grow, the first symptom is often a mild discomfort, which may steadily worsen into increasingly severe pain as the cancer enlarges. The pain may result from the cancer compressing or eroding into nerves or other structures.

Bleeding

At first, a cancer may bleed slightly because its cells are not well attached to each other

Warning Signs of Cancer

Because cancer is more likely to be cured if treated early, it is critical that cancer be discovered early. Some symptoms may give early warning of cancer and should, therefore, trigger a person to seek medical care. Fortunately, most of these symptoms are usually caused by far less serious conditions. Nonetheless, the development of any of the warning signs of cancer should not be ignored.

Some of the warning signs are general; that is, they are vague changes that do not help pinpoint any particular cancer. Still, their presence can help direct doctors to perform the physical examinations and laboratory tests necessary to exclude or confirm a diagnosis. Other symptoms are much more specific and steer doctors to a particular kind of cancer or location. Some warning signs of cancer are:

- Weight loss
- Fatigue
- Night sweats
- Loss of appetite
- New, persistent pain
- Recurrent nausea or vomiting
- Blood in urine
- Blood in stool (either visible or detectable by special tests)
- Sudden depression
- A recent change in bowel habits (constipation or diarrhea)
- Recurrent fever
- Chronic cough
- Changes in the size or color of a mole or changes in a skin ulcer that does not heal
- Enlarged lymph nodes

SOME COMPLICATIONS OF CANCER

Type	Description
Cardiac tamponade	Occurs when fluid accumulates in the baglike structure surrounding the heart (pericardium, or pericardial sac). This fluid puts pressure on the heart and interferes with its ability to pump blood. Fluid can accumulate when a cancer invades the pericardium and irritates it. The cancers most likely to invade the pericardium are lung cancer, breast cancer, and lymphoma.
Pleural effusion	Occurs when fluid accumulates in the baglike structure around the lungs (pleural sac), causing shortness of breath.
Superior vena cava syndrome	Occurs when cancer partially or completely blocks the vein (superior vena cava) that drains blood from the upper part of the body into the heart. Blockage of the superior vena cava causes the veins in the upper part of the chest and neck to swell, resulting in swelling of the face, neck, and upper part of the chest.
Spinal cord compression	Occurs when cancer compresses the spinal cord or the spinal cord nerves, resulting in pain and loss of function. The longer the compression of the spinal cord or spinal cord nerves persists, the less likely normal nerve function will return when the compression is relieved.
Brain dysfunction	Occurs when the brain functions abnormally as a result of a cancer growing within it, either as a brain cancer or more commonly as a metastasis from a cancer elsewhere in the body. Many different symptoms can occur, including confusion, sedation, agitation, headaches, abnormal vision, abnormal sensations, weakness, nausea, vomiting, and seizures.

and its blood vessels are fragile. Later, as the cancer enlarges and invades surrounding tissues, it may grow into a nearby blood vessel, causing bleeding. The bleeding may be slight and undetectable or detectable only with testing. Such is often the case in early-stage colon cancer. Or, particularly with advanced cancer, the bleeding may be massive and even life threatening.

The site of the cancer determines the site of the bleeding. Cancer anywhere along the digestive tract can cause bleeding in the stool. Cancer anywhere along the urinary tract can cause bleeding in the urine. Other cancers can bleed into internal areas of the body. Bleeding into the lungs can cause the person to cough up blood.

Weight Loss and Fatigue

Typically, a person with cancer experiences weight loss and fatigue, which increase as the cancer progresses. Some people notice weight loss despite a good appetite. Others lose their appetite and may even become nauseated by food. They may become very thin; the loss of underlying fat is particularly noticeable in the face. People with advanced stage cancer are often very tired and sleep many hours a day. If anemia develops, these people may find that they feel tired or become short of breath when exerting themselves.

Swollen Lymph Nodes

As a cancer begins to spread around the body, it may first spread to nearby lymph nodes, which become swollen and may feel hard or rubbery. The swollen lymph nodes may be painless or tender. They may be freely moveable or, if the cancer is more advanced, they may be stuck to the skin above, the deeper layers of tissue below, or to each other.

Depression

Cancer often results in depression. Depression can be related to the symptoms of the illness, a fear of dying, and a loss of independence. Additionally, some cancers may produce substances that directly cause depression by affecting the brain.

Neurologic and Muscular Symptoms

Cancer can grow into or compress nerves, causing any of several neurologic and muscular symptoms, including a change in sensations (such as tingling sensations) or muscle weakness. When a cancer grows in the brain, symptoms may be hard to pinpoint but can include confusion, dizziness, headaches, nausea, changes in vision, and seizures. Neurologic symptoms may also be part of a paraneoplastic syndrome.

Respiratory Symptoms

Cancer can compress or block structures, such as the airways in the lungs, causing shortness of breath or pneumonia and the inability to cough up secretions. Shortness of breath can also occur when the cancer causes bleeding into the lungs or anemia.

Diagnosis

Diagnosis encompasses screening, testing, and a physical examination. After cancer is diagnosed, it is staged. Staging is a way of noting how advanced the cancer has become, including such criteria as how big it is and whether it has spread to other organs.

Screening

Screening tests serve to detect the *possibility* that a cancer is present before symptoms occur. Screening tests usually are not defini-

What Are Paraneoplastic Syndromes?

Paraneoplastic syndromes occur when a cancer produces one or more substances that circulate in the bloodstream, such as hormones, cytokines (a type of protein), or other proteins. These substances can affect the function of other tissues and organs, resulting in a variety of symptoms termed paraneoplastic syndromes. Some substances damage organs or tissues by causing an autoimmune reaction. Others directly interfere with the function of different organs or actually destroy tissues. Symptoms such as low blood sugar, diarrhea, and high blood pressure can result.

Polyneuropathy occurs as a dysfunction of peripheral nerves, resulting in weakness, loss of sensation, and reduced reflexes. Subacute sensory neuropathy occurs as a rare form of polyneuropathy that sometimes develops before the cancer is diagnosed. It causes a disabling loss of sensation and incoordination but little weakness. Subacute cerebellar degeneration occurs in women with breast or ovarian cancer. This disorder may be caused by an autoantibody (an antibody that attacks the body's own tissues) that destroys the cerebellum. Symptoms— unsteadiness in walking, in-

coordination of the arms and legs, difficulty speaking, dizziness, and double vision—may appear weeks, months, or even years before the cancer is detected. Subacute cerebellar degeneration usually worsens over weeks or months, often resulting in severe disability.

Spasms of the eye and muscles and lack of coordination of movements can occur in some children with neuroblastoma. Uncontrollable eye movements (opsoclonus) and quick lightning-like muscle contractions (myoclonus) occur in the muscles of the trunk, arms, and legs.

Subacute motor neuropathy occurs in some people with Hodgkin's disease. The nerve cells of the spinal cord are indirectly affected, weakening the arms and legs in a pattern similar to that due to polyneuropathy. Polymyositis occurs as muscle weakness and soreness resulting from muscle inflammation. When polymyositis is accompanied by skin inflammation, the condition is called dermatomyositis.

Eaton-Lambert syndrome occurs in some people with lung cancer. This syndrome is characterized by extreme muscle weakness caused by lack of proper activation of the muscle by the nerve.

Hypertrophic osteoarthropathy can also occur in people with lung cancer. This syndrome alters the shape of the fingers and toes and causes changes at the ends of long bones that can be seen on x-rays.

Other paraneoplastic syndromes linked to lung cancer include the following: small cell carcinoma may secrete corticotropin, causing Cushing's syndrome, or antidiuretic hormone, causing water retention and low sodium levels in the blood (hyponatremia). Excessive hormone production can also cause the carcinoid syndrome— flushing, wheezing, diarrhea, and heart valve problems. Squamous cell carcinoma may secrete a hormonelike substance that leads to very high calcium levels in the blood (hypercalcemic syndrome). High calcium levels may also result if the cancer directly invades bone, thereby releasing calcium into the bloodstream. As a result of the high calcium levels in the blood, the person develops confusion, which can progress to coma and even death. Other problems include breast enlargement in men (gynecomastia), an excess of thyroid hormone (hyperthyroidism), and skin changes, including darkening of the skin in the armpits.

CANCER SCREENING RECOMMENDATIONS

PROCEDURE	FREQUENCY
Skin cancer	
Physical examination	Should be part of a routine checkup; more frequent examinations may be needed for people at high risk for the development of skin cancer
Whole-body photography	Not routinely needed; may be helpful for people with multiple moles or in whom examination of the skin is difficult
Lung cancer	
Chest x-ray	Not recommended on a routine basis
Sputum cytology	Not recommended on a routine basis
Low-dose spiral computed tomography	Not recommended on a routine basis, but is under investigation
Rectal and colon cancer	
Stool examination for occult blood	Yearly after age 50
Rectal examination	Yearly after age 40
Sigmoidoscopic or colonoscopic examination	Every 3 to 5 years after age 50
Prostate cancer	
Rectal examination	Yearly after age 50
Blood test for prostate-specific antigen	Yearly after age 50
Testicular cancer	
Testicle self-examination	Monthly after age 14
Cervical, uterine, and ovarian cancers	
Pelvic examination	Every 1 to 3 years between ages 18 and 40, then yearly
Cervical cancer	
Papanicolaou (Pap) test	Yearly between ages 18 and 65. After 3 or more consecutive normal examinations, a Pap test may be performed less often at the doctor's discretion. Most women older than 65 need Pap tests less often
Breast cancer	
Breast self-examination	Monthly after age 18
Breast physical examination	Every 3 years between ages 18 and 40, then yearly
Mammography	Initial baseline exam between ages 35 and 40, every 1 to 2 years from age 40 to 49, and yearly after age 50

tive; results are confirmed or disproved with further examinations and tests. Diagnostic tests are performed once a doctor suspects that a person has cancer.

Although screening tests can help save lives, they can be costly and sometimes have psychologic or physical repercussions. Screening tests can produce false-positive results—results that suggest a cancer may be present when it actually is not. False-positive results can create undue psychologic stress and can lead to other tests that are expensive and risky. Screening tests can also produce false-negative results—results that show no hint of a cancer that is actually present. False-negative results can lull people into a false sense of security. For these reasons, health care practitioners carefully consider whether or not to perform such tests. Doctors try to determine whether a particular person is at special risk

SELECTED TUMOR MARKERS

Tumor Marker	Description	Comment about Testing
Carcinoembryonic antigen (CEA)	Levels are raised in the blood of people with cancer of the colon, breast, pancreas, bladder, ovary, or cervix. Levels may also be raised in people who are heavy cigarette smokers and in those who have cirrhosis of the liver or ulcerative colitis	Testing can be useful in screening for cancer and in monitoring treatment and detecting recurrence
Alpha-fetoprotein (AFP)	Normally produced by fetal liver cells, AFP is found in the blood of people with liver cancer (hepatoma). In addition, AFP is often found in people with certain cancers of the ovary or testis and in children and young adults with pineal gland tumors	Testing can be useful in diagnosing cancer and in monitoring its treatment
Beta–human chorionic gonadotropin (β–HCG)	This hormone is produced during pregnancy but also occurs in women who have a cancer originating in the placenta and in men with various types of testicular cancer	Testing can be useful in diagnosing cancer and in monitoring its treatment
Prostate-specific antigen (PSA)	Levels are raised in men with non-cancerous (benign) enlargement of the prostate and are considerably higher in men with prostate cancer. What constitutes a meaningfully abnormal level is somewhat uncertain, but men with an elevated PSA level should be evaluated further by a doctor	Testing can be useful in screening for cancer and in monitoring its treatment
Carbohydrate antigen 125 (CA-125)	Levels are raised in women with a variety of ovarian diseases, including cancer	Because ovarian cancer is often difficult to diagnose, some cancer experts recommend using this test in women older than 40. However, it is not routinely used
Carbohydrate antigen 15-3 (CA 15-3)	Levels are raised in people with breast cancer	This test cannot be recommended for cancer screening. However, it can be useful in monitoring treatment
Carbohydrate antigen 19-9 (CA 19-9)	Levels are raised in people with cancers of the digestive tract, particularly pancreatic cancer	This test cannot be recommended for cancer screening. However, it can be useful in monitoring treatment
Beta$_2$ (β$_2$)-microglobulin	Levels are raised in people with multiple myeloma, chronic lymphocytic leukemia, and in many forms of lymphoma	This test cannot be recommended for cancer screening. However, it can be useful in monitoring treatment
Lactate dehydrogenase	Levels can be raised for a variety of reasons	This test cannot be recommended for cancer screening. However, it is useful in assessing prognosis and monitoring treatment, particularly for people with testicular cancer, melanomas, and lymphomas

for cancer—because of age, sex, family history, previous history, and lifestyle—before they choose which screening tests to perform.

In women, two of the most widely used screening tests are the Papanicolaou (Pap) test to detect cervical cancer and mammography to detect breast cancer. Both screening tests have been successful in reducing the death rates from these cancers in certain age groups.

In men, a common screening test involves measuring the level of prostate-specific antigen (PSA) in the blood. PSA levels are high in men with prostate cancer, but levels are also elevated in men with noncancerous (benign) enlargement of the prostate. Whether the PSA test should be used routinely to screen for prostate cancer is unresolved. The main drawback to its use as a screening test is the large

TESTS FOR DIAGNOSING AND STAGING CANCERS

CANCER SITE	TYPE OF BIOPSY PERFORMED	OTHER TESTS PERFORMED
Breast	Needle or lump biopsy	Mammogram Bone scans Computed tomography (CT) scan Estrogen-, progesterone-receptor testing on the biopsy sample; testing for other receptors
Digestive tract	Tissue for biopsy taken with endoscopy or with a needle (usually guided by a CT scan) through the skin for liver, pancreas, or other organs	Chest x-ray Barium x-ray Ultrasound CT scan Blood tests for liver enzymes
Lung	Tissue for biopsy usually taken by bronchoscopy	Chest x-ray CT scan Sputum cytology Mediastinoscopy Positron emission tomography (PET) scan
Lymphatic system	Lymph node biopsy Bone marrow biopsy	Chest x-ray Blood cell counts CT scan Radioisotope scan Exploratory surgery Splenectomy
Prostate	Needle biopsy	Blood tests for acid phosphatase and prostate-specific antigen (PSA) Ultrasound Bone scan CT scan
Testes	Testis removed for biopsy	Chest x-ray CT scan Blood tests for alpha-fetoprotein (AFP), beta–human chorionic gonadotropin (β–HCG), lactate dehydrogenase
Uterus, cervix, ovaries	Tissue for biopsy of uterus or fractional dilation and curettage with hysteroscopy; colposcopy for biopsy of cervix; sample taken during exploratory surgery for biopsy of ovaries	Pelvic examination under anesthesia Ultrasound CT scan Barium enema examination

number of false-positive results, which generally lead to more invasive tests.

In both men and women older than 40, a common screening test involves checking the stool for blood that cannot be seen by the naked eye (occult blood). Finding occult blood in the stool is an indication that something is wrong in the colon. The problem may be cancer, although many other disorders can also cause small amounts of blood to leak into the stool. In addition, taking an aspirin or another nonsteroidal anti-inflammatory drug (NSAID) or even eating red meat can temporarily produce a positive result. Positive results can occasionally be caused by consuming poultry, fish, certain raw fruits and vegetables (turnips, cauliflower, red radishes, broccoli, cantaloupe, horseradish, and parsnips), and vitamin C.

Some screening tests can be done at home. For example, monthly breast self-examinations are valuable in helping women detect breast cancer. Periodically examining the testes can help men detect testicular cancer, one of the most curable forms of cancer, especially when diagnosed early. Periodically checking the mouth for sores can help detect mouth cancer in an early stage.

Diagnostic Tests and Staging

Tumor markers are substances secreted into the bloodstream by certain tumors. However, tumor markers sometimes are present in the blood of people who do not have cancer. Thus, finding a tumor marker does not necessarily mean a person has cancer. However, in people who do have cancer, tumor markers can be used to monitor the effectiveness of treatment and to detect possible recurrence of the cancer. The level of a tumor marker increases if the cancer recurs.

When cancer is diagnosed, staging tests help determine how advanced the cancer is in terms of its location, size, growth into nearby structures, and spread to other parts of the body. People with cancer sometimes become impatient and anxious during staging tests, wishing for a prompt start of treatment. However, staging allows doctors to determine the most appropriate treatment as well as helping to determine prognosis.

Staging may use scans, such as bone scans, or other imaging tests, such as computed tomography (CT) or magnetic resonance imaging (MRI), to determine whether the cancer has spread.

Ultrasound scanning is a painless, noninvasive procedure that uses sound waves to show the structure of internal organs. It is helpful for identifying and determining the size of certain cancers, particularly of the kidneys, liver, pelvis, and prostate. It can also be used in staging a cancer. Doctors often use ultrasound to guide the removal of tissue samples during a needle biopsy.

Computed tomography (CT) scanning is used to detect cancer in many parts of the body, including the brain and lungs and parts of the abdomen, including the adrenal glands, lymph nodes, liver, and spleen. Such detection is useful in diagnosing and staging a cancer. Magnetic resonance imaging (MRI) is an alternative to CT. With this procedure, a very powerful magnetic field generates exquisitely detailed anatomic images. MRI is of particular value in detecting cancers of the brain, bone, and spinal cord. No x-rays are involved, and MRI is extremely safe. An MRI can often be used for people who have allergic or other reactions to the radiopaque dye that is commonly injected during CT. CT and MRI scans have largely replaced the use of liver scans for evaluation of the liver and the use of lymphangiograms for the evaluation of abdominal and pelvic lymph nodes.

Positron emission tomography (PET) can also be used to help diagnose and stage cancer. A PET scan images a cancer by measuring biochemical processes within it. The test is not routinely used as a part of screening for cancer.

Biopsies are often needed to be sure that an abnormality discovered on an imaging test is cancer; biopsies are important in both diagnosis and staging. Many kinds of biopsies can be performed with a needle and do not require surgery. Sometimes, however, surgery is needed to obtain a sample of tissue. For example, a laparotomy (an abdominal operation) allows the surgeon to sample internal lymph nodes while at the same time removing a colon cancer. During the operation, the surgeon can inspect the area, including the liver, to check for spread of the cancer. During surgery for breast cancer, the surgeon performs a biopsy of lymph nodes in the armpit to determine how far breast cancer has spread and whether further treatment is needed after surgery. An operation to remove the spleen (splenectomy) for examination helps in staging Hodgkin's disease.

CHAPTER 182

Prevention and Treatment of Cancer

Reducing the risk of certain cancers may be possible through dietary and other lifestyle changes. How risk can be reduced depends on the specific cancer. For example, not smoking and avoiding exposure to tobacco smoke can greatly reduce the risk of lung, kidney, bladder, and head and neck cancer. Avoiding the use of smokeless tobacco (snuff, chew) decreases the risk of cancer of the mouth and tongue. Avoiding sun exposure (especially during the middle of the day) can reduce the risk of skin cancer. Covering exposed skin and using sunblock lotion with a high sun protection factor (SPF) against ultraviolet light also helps reduce the risk of skin cancer.

Other lifestyle changes reduce the risk of several types of cancer. A reduced intake of fat in the diet appears to decrease the risk of breast and colon cancer. Use of aspirin and other nonsteroidal anti-inflammatory drugs (NSAIDs) reduces the risk of colon cancer.

Treating cancer is one of the most complex aspects of medical care. It involves a team that encompasses many types of doctors working together (for example, primary care doctors, gynecologists, oncologists, surgeons, radiotherapists, and pathologists) and many other types of health care workers (for example, nurses, physiotherapists, social workers, and pharmacists). Treatment decisions take into account many factors, including the likelihood of cure or of prolonging life when cure is not possible, the effect of treatment on symptoms, the side effects of treatment, and the person's wishes regarding all of these issues. People undergoing cancer treatment hope for the best outcome and the longest survival with the highest quality of life. However, people who are candidates for radiation therapy or anti-cancer drugs must understand the risks involved with treatment. People with cancer should discuss their wishes regarding medical care with all of their doctors, including the level of treatment desired when no cure is possible.▲

When the diagnosis of cancer is first made, the main goals of treatment are to remove the cancer if possible (through a single treatment or a combination of surgery, radiation therapy, or chemotherapy) and reduce the chance of spread (metastases). Chemotherapy is usually the only way to treat the cancer cells that have spread beyond the original (primary) site. Using combinations of chemotherapy drugs may help eradicate the original cancer and kill cancer cells elsewhere in the body.

Even when a cure is impossible, symptoms resulting from the cancer can often be relieved with treatment that improves the quality and length of life (palliative therapy). For example, if a tumor cannot be removed surgically, radiation of the tumor may shrink it, temporarily reducing pain and symptoms in the immediate vicinity of the tumor (local symptoms).

As treatments become more complex, specific approaches to care, called treatment protocols, have been developed for many types of cancer to ensure that people receive the most effective care with the fewest side effects. Thus, the use of treatment protocols assures that people with the same type and stage of cancer are treated with some standard sequence and dose of therapies. Such protocols are derived from careful scientific experiments. Protocols are constantly being refined to improve their effectiveness.

Surgery

Surgery is one of the oldest forms of cancer treatment and often is the most effective. Surgery is usually the sole or primary means of treating tumors that have not spread beyond their original site of growth. However, surgery cannot be used for all early-stage cancers. Some tumors occur in inaccessible sites. In other instances, removing the tumor might require removing a necessary function or organ. In some instances, surgery must be combined with other treatments. In some cases, surgery is intended to remove part of the cancer in a process doctors call debulking. Debulking may reduce

▲ see page 54

symptoms and improve the likelihood that radiation therapy or chemotherapy will be effective.

Radiation Therapy

Radiation is a beam or field of intense energy focused on a certain area or organ of the body. It can be generated by a radioactive substance (such as cobalt) or with an atomic particle (linear) accelerator. In other strategies, a radioactive substance may be injected into a vein to travel to the cancer (for example, radioactive iodine, which is used in treatment of thyroid cancer, or radioactive implants, which may be placed directly into the cancer). A linear accelerator directs the radiation to the tumor, while normal tissue is shielded as much as possible. To reduce exposure of normal tissue to the beam, multiple beam paths are used.

Radiation preferentially kills cells that divide rapidly. Cancer cells divide more often than normal cells and therefore are more likely than most normal cells to be killed by radiation. Nonetheless, cancer cells differ in how easily they are killed by radiation; some are very resistant and thus cannot be effectively treated with radiation therapy. Unfortunately, radiation can damage normal tissues adjacent to the tumor, especially tissues in which cells normally divide rapidly, such as skin, the bone marrow, hair follicles, and the lining of the mouth, esophagus, and intestines. Radiation can also damage the ovaries or testes. A doctor tries to accurately target the radiation therapy to protect normal cells.

Radiation therapy is divided into a series of doses over a prolonged period of time. This method increases the lethal effects of the radiation on tumor cells, while decreasing the toxic effects of the radiation on normal cells. The latter effect occurs because normal cells have the capacity to repair themselves quickly after being exposed to radiation.

Radiation therapy plays a key role in curing many cancers, including Hodgkin's disease, early-stage non-Hodgkin's lymphoma, squamous cell cancer of the head and neck, seminoma (a testicular cancer), prostate cancer, early-stage breast cancer, early-stage nonsmall cell lung cancer, and medulloblastoma (a brain or spinal cord tumor). For early-stage cancers of the larynx and prostate, the rate of cure is essentially the same with radiation therapy as with surgery.

Preventing Cancer

According to the American Cancer Society, the risk of developing certain cancers may be reduced by making lifestyle changes.

Measures known to reduce the risk of cancer:
- Avoiding smoking or exposure to tobacco smoke
- Avoiding occupational carcinogens (for example, asbestos)
- Avoiding prolonged exposure to sunlight without sunscreen protection

Measures that possibly reduce the risk of cancer:
- Limiting intake of high-fat foods, particularly from animal sources (for example, high-fat meats, whole-fat dairy products)
- Increasing intake of fruits and vegetables
- Being physically active
- Achieving and maintaining a healthy weight

Radiation therapy can reduce symptoms when a cure is not possible, as in multiple myeloma and advanced lung, esophageal, head and neck, and stomach cancers. By temporarily shrinking the tumors, radiation therapy can be given as palliative therapy to relieve symptoms caused by spread of cancer to bone or brain.

New techniques of intense and highly focused radiation therapy, such as proton radiation, can effectively treat certain tumors in areas where damage to normal tissue is a worry, such as the eye, brain, or spinal cord. Radioactive seed implants (small pellets of a radioactive substance) are often used to treat prostate cancer. These seed implants provide intense radiation to the cancer and little to surrounding tissues.

Chemotherapy

Chemotherapy involves the use of drugs to destroy cancer cells. Although an ideal chemotherapy drug would destroy cancer cells without harming normal cells, few such drugs exist. Instead, in chemotherapy, drugs are designed to inflict greater damage on cancer cells than on normal cells. Nonetheless, all chemotherapy drugs affect normal cells and cause side effects.

Response to Treatment

While being treated for cancer, the person is assessed to see how the cancer is responding to therapy. When a cancer disappears for any length of time after treatment, a person is said to have had a **complete response (remission).** The most successful treatment produces a **cure.** A cure means that all evidence of cancer disappears and never recurs. Doctors sometimes consider cures in terms of the 5-year or 10-year disease-free survival rates, in which the cancer completely disappears and does not recur within these (or some other usually long) time periods. With a **partial response,** the size of one or more tumors is reduced by more than half; this response can reduce symptoms and may prolong life, although the cancer eventually grows back. The least successful treatment produces **no response.**

Sometimes a cancer completely disappears but returns later **(relapse);** the interval between these two events is called the **disease-free interval.** The interval from diagnosis of cancer to the time of death is the **total survival time.** In people who have a partial response, the duration of response is measured from the time of the partial response to the time when the cancer begins to enlarge or spread again.

Some cancers respond well to chemotherapy or radiation therapy and are termed **responsive.** Some cancers respond poorly to chemotherapy or radiation therapy and are termed **resistant.** Other cancers may have excellent initial responses but may develop resistance after repeated treatment.

Some cancers produce substances that are termed **tumor markers.** Most of these tumor markers are not specific enough to be useful in screening—a number of disorders other than cancer can cause many of these substances to appear in the blood. However, they can often be useful to assess response to treatment. If the tumor marker was present before treatment but no longer appears in a blood sample after treatment, the treatment has probably been successful. If the tumor marker disappears after treatment then later reappears, the cancer has probably returned.

Not all cancers respond to chemotherapy. The type of cancer determines which drugs are used, in what combination, and at what dose. Chemotherapy may be used as the sole treatment or combined with radiation therapy and surgery.

One approach is to use a variety of "molecularly targeted" drugs that can enter cancerous (malignant) cells and interrupt important pathways of information flow in the cell. These molecules render the cells defective, and they die. Imatinib, the first such drug, alters the energy site in the malignant cell and is highly effective in chronic myelocytic leukemia and certain tumors of the digestive tract. Other such drugs target cell surface receptors in nonsmall cell lung cancer and colon cancer, but are not yet available for general use.

Dose-intensity chemotherapy is a new but risky approach in which especially high doses of drugs are used. This therapy is used for a few types of cancer (including some types of myeloma, lymphoma, and leukemia) that have recurred even though the person had a good response when first treated with drugs. Because such tumors have already demonstrated sensitivity to the drug, the strategy is to markedly increase the drug dose to kill more cancer cells and thus prolong the person's survival.

However, dose-intensity chemotherapy can cause life-threatening injury to the bone marrow. Therefore, dose-intensity chemotherapy is commonly combined with bone marrow rescue strategies, in which marrow cells are harvested before the chemotherapy is administered and returned to the person after chemotherapy. In some cases, stem cells can be isolated from a blood sample and used instead of bone marrow to restore the bone marrow.

Immunotherapy

The purpose of immunotherapy is to stimulate the body's immune system against cancer. Some forms of immunotherapy use vaccines composed of antigens derived from tumor cells to boost the body's production of antibodies or immune cells (T lymphocytes). Substances such as extracts of weakened tuberculosis bacteria, which are known to boost the immune response, have been successful when applied locally to bladder cancers. To date, other vaccines have not proven useful in the treatment of cancer.

Monoclonal antibody therapy involves the use of experimentally produced antibodies to specific proteins on the cell surface.

℞ CHEMOTHERAPY DRUGS

CLASS	EXAMPLES	HOW THE DRUG WORKS	SIDE EFFECTS
Alkylating agents	Cyclophosphamide Chlorambucil Melphalan	Form chemical bond with DNA, causing breaks in DNA and errors in replication of DNA	Suppress bone marrow, injure lining of stomach, cause hair loss; may decrease fertility
Antimetabolites	Methotrexate Cytarabine Fludarabine 6-Mercaptopurine 5-Fluorouracil	Block synthesis of DNA	Same as for alkylating agents
Antimitotics	Vincristine Paclitaxel Vinorelbine	Block division of cancer cells	Same as for alkylating agents; also can cause nerve damage
Topoisomerase inhibitors	Doxorubicin Irinotecan	Prevent DNA synthesis and repair through blockage of enzymes called topoisomerases	Same as for alkylating agents; doxorubicin can cause heart damage
Platinum derivatives	Cisplatin Carboplatin	Form bonds with DNA causing breaks	Same as for alkylating agents; also can cause nerve and kidney damage, hearing loss
Hormonal therapies	Tamoxifen	Blocks estrogen action (in breast cancer)	Can cause endometrial cancer, blood clots, hot flashes
	Bicalutamide	Blocks androgen action (in prostate cancer)	Can cause erectile dysfunction (impotence)
Signaling inhibitors	Imatinib	Blocks signal for cell division in chronic myelocytic leukemia	Can cause abnormal liver function test results; can also cause fluid retention
Monoclonal antibodies	Rituximab	Induces cell death through binding to cell surface receptor on lymphocyte-derived tumors	Can cause allergic reaction
	Trastuzumab	Blocks growth factor receptor on breast cancer cells	
	Gemtuzumab ozogamicin	Contains a specific antibody that attaches to a receptor found on leukemic cells and then delivers a toxic dose of its chemotherapeutic component to the leukemic cells	
Biologic response modifiers	Interferon-alpha	Unknown	Can cause fever, chills, bone marrow suppression
Differentiating agents	Tretinoin	Induces differentiation and death of leukemic cells	Can cause severe difficulty with breathing (respiratory distress)

Trastuzumab is one such antibody. It helps women with advanced breast cancer when given alone or in combination with a variety of chemotherapy drugs. Rituximab may be helpful for lymphomas and chronic lymphocytic leukemia. Gemtuzumab ozogamicin, a combined antibody and drug, is effective in some people with acute myelocytic leukemia. Antibodies linked to a radioactive isotope can be used to deliver radiation directly to the cancer cells.

Biologic response modifiers are used to improve the immune system's ability to find and destroy cancer cells, such as by stimulating normal cells to produce chemical messengers (mediators). Interferon (of which there are several types) is the best-known and most widely used biologic response modifier. Almost all human cells produce interferon naturally, but it can also be made artificially using recombinant technology. Although its precise mechanisms of action are not totally clear, interferon has a role in the treatment of several cancers. Measurable responses have occurred in about 30% of people with Kaposi's sarcoma, the majority of people with chronic myelocytic leukemia, and in 10 to 15% of people with renal cell carcinoma and malignant melanoma.

Combination Therapy

Commonly, several chemotherapy drugs are combined (combination chemotherapy). The rationale for combination chemotherapy is to use drugs that work on different parts of the cancer cell's life cycle, thereby increasing the likelihood that more cancer cells will be killed. When drugs with different toxicities are combined, each drug can be used at its optimal dose, helping avoid intolerable side effects. Finally, drugs with very different properties are sometimes combined. For example, drugs that kill tumor cells may be combined with antibodies or with drugs that stimulate the body's immune system against cancer (biologic response modifiers).

For some cancers, the best approach is a combination of surgery, radiation, and chemotherapy. Surgery or radiation therapy treats cancer that is confined locally, while chemotherapy also kills cancer cells that may have spread.

Sometimes radiation or chemotherapy is given before surgery to shrink a tumor, thereby making the complete removal of the tumor using surgery more likely, or after surgery to destroy any remaining cancer cells. The stage of the cancer often determines whether single therapy or a combination is needed. For example, early-stage breast cancer may be treated with surgery alone or surgery combined with radiation therapy, chemotherapy, or with all three treatments, depending on the size of the tumor and the risk of recurrence. Locally advanced breast cancer is usually treated with chemotherapy, radiation therapy, and surgery.

Sometimes combination chemotherapy is used not to cure but to reduce symptoms and prolong life. Combination chemotherapy can be useful for people with advanced cancers that are not suitable for irradiation or surgical treatment (for example, those with nonsmall cell lung cancer, esophageal cancer, or bladder cancer).

Alternative Medicine

Some people turn to alternative medicine, including certain medicinal herbs,▲ to treat their cancer, instead of or in addition to standard treatment. However, most types of alternative medicine have not been subjected to careful scientific studies. Thus, very little is known about the effectiveness of alternative medicine in treating cancer.

Although benefits of alternative medicine for cancer have not been scientifically proven, there is significant potential for harm because:
• The use of alternative medicine may be toxic
• The use of alternative medicine may interact with standard treatment, thus reducing the effectiveness of chemotherapy
• The use of alternative medicine may be costly, reducing the person's ability to afford standard treatment
• If alternative medicine is used instead of standard treatment, the person will not obtain the proven benefits of standard treatment

A person using alternative medicine should inform his doctor. Hiding the use of alternative medicine could be harmful.

Side Effects of Treatment

Almost everyone who receives cancer treatment experiences side effects. Relieving side effects is an important part of treatment.

▲ see page 103

Chemotherapy commonly causes nausea, vomiting, loss of appetite, weight loss, fatigue, and low blood cell counts that lead to anemia and risk of infections. With chemotherapy, people often lose their hair, but side effects vary according to the type of drug.

Side effects from radiation therapy depend on how large an area is being treated, the dose given, and the tumor's proximity to sensitive tissues. For example, radiation to head and neck tumors often causes damage to the overlying skin. Radiation to the stomach or abdomen often causes irritation of the stomach (gastritis) and of the intestine (enteritis), resulting in nausea, lack of appetite, and diarrhea.

Nausea and vomiting can usually be prevented or relieved with drugs (antiemetics). Nausea may be reduced without using drugs by eating small meals and by avoiding foods that are high in fiber, that produce gas, or that are very hot or very cold.

Low blood cell counts (cytopenia, a deficiency of one or more types of blood cell) can develop during cancer treatment because of the toxic effect of drugs on bone marrow. For example, a person may develop abnormally low numbers of red blood cells (anemia), white blood cells (neutropenia or leukopenia), or platelets (thrombocytopenia). If anemia is severe, erythropoietin or darbepoietin can be given to increase red blood cell formation, or packed red blood cells can be transfused. Similarly, if thrombocytopenia is severe, platelets can be transfused to lower the risk of bleeding.

A person with neutropenia is at increased risk of developing an infection. A fever higher than 100.4° F in a person with neutropenia is treated as an emergency. Such a person must be evaluated for infection and may require antibiotics and even hospitalization. White blood cells are rarely transfused because, when transfused, they survive only a few hours and produce many side effects. Instead, certain substances (such as granulocyte-colony stimulating factor) can be administered to stimulate white blood cell production.

Other common side effects include inflammation or even ulcers of the mucous membranes, such as the lining of the mouth. Mouth ulcers are painful and can make eating difficult. A variety of oral solutions (usually containing an antacid, an antihistamine, and a local anesthetic) can reduce the discomfort. On rare occasions, nutritional support must be given by a feeding tube that is placed directly into the stomach or small intestine or even by vein. A variety of drugs can reduce the diarrhea caused by radiation therapy to the abdomen.

IMMUNE DISORDERS

183 Biology of the Immune System **1049**

Nonspecific Immunity ▪ Specific Immunity ▪ Effects of Aging

184 Immunodeficiency Disorders...**1057**

X-Linked Agammaglobulinemia ▪ Selective Antibody Deficiency ▪ Common Variable Immunodeficiency ▪ Transient Hypogammaglobulinemia of Infancy ▪ Chronic Mucocutaneous Candidiasis ▪ DiGeorge Anomaly ▪ Ataxia-Telangiectasia ▪ Severe Combined Immunodeficiency Disease ▪ Wiskott-Aldrich Syndrome ▪ Hyperimmunoglobulinemia E Syndrome ▪ Chronic Granulomatous Disease ▪ Immunodeficiency due to Spleen Disorders

185 Allergic Reactions..**1063**

Seasonal Allergies ▪ Year-Round Allergies ▪ Food Allergy ▪ Mastocytosis ▪ Physical Allergy ▪ Exercise-Induced Allergic Reactions ▪ Hives and Angioedema ▪ Anaphylactic Reactions

186 Autoimmune Disorders **1073**

187 Transplantation...**1075**

Principles of Organ Transplantation ▪ Kidney Transplantation ▪ Liver Transplantation ▪ Heart Transplantation ▪ Lung and Heart-Lung Transplantation ▪ Pancreas Transplantation ▪ Stem Cell Transplantation ▪ Transplantation of Other Organs

CHAPTER 183

Biology of the Immune System

The immune system is designed to defend the body against foreign or dangerous substances that invade it. Such substances include microorganisms (commonly called germs, such as bacteria, viruses, and fungi), parasites (such as worms), cancer cells, and even transplanted organs and tissues.▲ Substances that stimulate an immune response in the body are called antigens. Antigens may be contained within or on bacteria, viruses, other microorganisms, or cancer cells. Antigens may also exist on their own—for example, as pollen or food molecules. A normal immune response consists of recognizing a foreign antigen, mobilizing forces to defend against it, and attacking it.

▲ see page 1075

Disorders of the immune system occur
• when the body generates an immune response against itself (an autoimmune disorder)▲
• when the body cannot generate appropriate immune responses against invading microorganisms (an immunodeficiency disorder)■
• when a normal immune response to foreign antigens damages normal tissues (an allergic reaction).★

The first line of defense against invaders is mechanical or physical barriers: the skin; the cornea of the eye; and the membranes lining the respiratory, digestive, urinary, and reproductive tracts. As long as these barriers remain unbroken, many invaders cannot penetrate them. If a barrier is broken—for example, if extensive burns damage much of the skin—the risk of infection is increased. In addition, the barriers are defended by secretions containing enzymes that can destroy bacteria. Examples are tears in the eyes and secretions in the digestive tract and vagina.

The next line of defense involves white blood cells that travel through the bloodstream and into tissues, searching for and attacking microorganisms and other invaders. This defense has two parts. The first part, called nonspecific (innate) immunity, involves several types of white blood cells that usually act on their own to destroy invaders. The second part, called specific (adaptive) immunity, involves white blood cells that work together to destroy invaders. Some of these cells do not directly destroy invaders but enable other white blood cells to recognize and destroy invaders.

Nonspecific immunity and specific immunity interact, influencing each other directly or through substances that attract or activate other cells of the immune system—part of the mobilization step in defense. These substances include cytokines (which are the messengers of the immune system), antibodies, and complement proteins (which form the complement system). These substances are not contained in cells but are dissolved in a body fluid, such as plasma, the liquid part of blood.

To be able to destroy invaders, the immune system must first recognize them. That is, the immune system must be able to distinguish what is nonself (foreign) from what is self. The immune system can make this distinction because all cells have identification molecules on their surface. Microorganisms are recognized because they have unique, foreign identification molecules on their surface. In people, identification molecules are called human leukocyte antigens (HLA), or the major histocompatibility complex (MHC). HLA molecules are called antigens because they can provoke an immune response in another person (normally, they do not provoke an immune response in the person who has them). Each person has unique human leukocyte antigens. A cell with molecules on its surface that are not identical to those on the body's own cells is identified as being foreign. The immune system then attacks that cell. Such a cell may be a microorganism, a cell from transplanted tissue, or one of the body's cells that has been infected by an invading microorganism.

Some white blood cells—B lymphocytes—recognize invaders directly. But others—T lymphocytes—need help from other cells of the immune system—called antigen-presenting cells. These cells ingest an invader and break it into fragments. Antigen fragments from the invader are then "presented" in a way that T lymphocytes can recognize.

The immune system includes several organs in addition to cells dispersed throughout the body. These organs are classified as primary or secondary lymphoid organs. The primary lymphoid organs—the thymus gland and bone marrow—are the sites where white blood cells are produced. In the thymus gland, T lymphocytes—a type of white blood cell—are produced and trained to recognize foreign antigens and ignore the body's own antigens. (T lymphocytes are critical for specific immunity.) The bone marrow produces several types of white blood cells, including neutrophils, monocytes, and B lymphocytes. When needed to defend the body, the white blood cells are mobilized, mainly from the bone marrow. They then move into the bloodstream and travel to wherever they are needed.

The secondary lymphoid organs include the spleen, lymph nodes, tonsils, liver, appendix, and Peyer's patches in the small intestine. These organs trap microorganisms and other foreign substances and provide a place for mature cells of the immune system to collect, interact with each other and with the foreign

---

▲ see page 1073   ■ see page 1057

★ see page 1063

How T Lymphocytes Recognize Antigens

T lymphocytes are part of the immune surveillance system. They travel through the bloodstream and lymphatic system, looking for foreign substances (antigens) in the body. However, a T lymphocyte cannot recognize an antigen unless it has been processed and "presented" to the T lymphocyte by another white blood cell, called an antigen-presenting cell. Antigen-presenting cells consist of dendritic cells (which are the most effective), macrophages, and B lymphocytes.

1. By itself, a T lymphocyte cannot recognize an antigen circulating in the body.

2. A cell that can process antigens, such as a dendritic cell, ingests the antigen.

3. Enzymes in the antigen-processing cell break the antigen into fragments.

4. Some antigen fragments are picked up by human leukocyte antigen (HLA) molecules as they are assembled inside the antigen-processing cell. Then the molecules with the antigen fragments are transported to the cell's surface.

5. A special molecule called a T-cell receptor, which is located on the surface of a T lymphocyte, can recognize the antigen fragment when it is attached to and presented by an HLA molecule. The T-cell receptor then attaches to the part of the HLA molecule presenting the antigen fragment, fitting in it as a key fits in a lock.

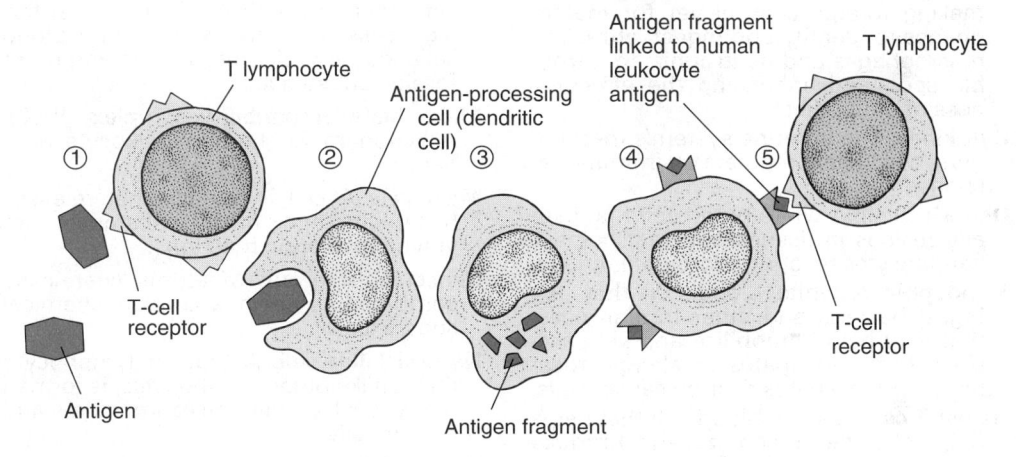

substances, and generate a specific immune response.

The lymph nodes are strategically placed in the body and are connected by an extensive network of lymphatic vessels, which act as the immune system's circulatory system. The lymphatic system transports microorganisms, other foreign substances, cancer cells, and dead or damaged cells from the tissues to the lymph nodes and then to the bloodstream. Lymph nodes are one of the first places that cancer cells can spread. Thus, doctors often evaluate lymph nodes to determine whether a cancer has spread. Cancer cells in a lymph node can cause the node to swell. Lymph nodes can also swell after an infection, because immune responses to infections are generated in lymph nodes.

Nonspecific Immunity

Nonspecific (innate) immunity is present at birth. Nonspecific immunity is so named because its components treat all foreign substances in much the same way.

The white blood cells involved in nonspecific immunity are monocytes (which develop into macrophages), neutrophils, eosinophils, basophils, and natural killer cells. Each type has a slightly different function. The complement system and cytokines also participate in nonspecific immunity.

Macrophages

Macrophages develop from a type of white blood cell called monocytes after monocytes move from the bloodstream to the tissues.

Understanding the Immune System

Antibody (immunoglobulin): A protein that is produced by B lymphocytes and that interacts with a specific antigen.

Antigen: Any substance that can stimulate an immune response.

Basophil: A white blood cell that releases histamine (a substance involved in allergic reactions) and that produces substances to attract neutrophils and eosinophils to a trouble spot.

Cell: The smallest unit of a living organism, composed of a nucleus and cytoplasm surrounded by a membrane.

Chemotaxis: The process of attracting cells by means of a chemical substance.

Complement system: A group of proteins with various immune functions, such as killing bacteria and other foreign cells, making foreign cells easier for macrophages to identify and ingest, attracting macrophages and neutrophils to a trouble spot, and enhancing the effectiveness of antibodies.

Cytokines: The immune system's messengers, which help regulate an immune response.

Dendritic cell: A white blood cell that usually resides in tissues and that helps T lymphocytes recognize foreign antigens.

Eosinophil: A white blood cell that can ingest bacteria and other foreign cells, that may help immobilize and kill parasites, that participates in allergic reactions, and that helps destroy cancer cells.

Helper T cell: A white blood cell that helps B lymphocytes recognize and produce antibodies against foreign antigens.

Histocompatibility: Literally, compatibility of tissue; determined by human leukocyte antigens (the major histocompatibility complex) and used to determine whether a transplanted tissue or organ will be accepted by the recipient.

Human leukocyte antigens (HLA): A group of molecules that are located on the surface of cells and that are unique in each organism, enabling the body to distinguish self from nonself; also called the major histocompatibility complex.

Immune response: The reaction of the immune system to an antigen.

Immunoglobulin: A synonym for antibody.

Interleukin: A type of cytokine secreted by some white blood cells to affect other white blood cells.

Killer (cytotoxic) T cell: A lymphocyte that attaches to foreign or abnormal cells and kills them.

Leukocyte: A white blood cell, such as a monocyte, a neutrophil, an eosinophil, a basophil, or a lymphocyte.

Lymphocyte: The white blood cell responsible for specific immunity, including producing antibodies (by B lymphocytes) and distinguishing self from nonself (by T lymphocytes).

Macrophage: A large cell that is derived from a white blood cell called a monocyte, that ingests bacteria and other foreign cells, and that helps white blood cells identify microorganisms and other foreign substances.

Major histocompatibility complex (MHC): A synonym for human leukocyte antigens.

Mast cell: A cell in tissues that releases histamine and other substances involved in allergic reactions.

Molecule: A group of atoms chemically combined to form a unique chemical substance.

Natural killer cell: A type of lymphocyte that, unlike other lymphocytes, is formed ready to kill certain microorganisms and cancer cells.

Neutrophil: A white blood cell that ingests and kills bacteria and other foreign cells.

Phagocyte: A cell that ingests and kills invading microorganisms, other cells, and cell fragments.

Phagocytosis: The process of a cell ingesting an invading microorganism, another cell, or a cell fragment.

Receptor: A molecule on a cell's surface or inside the cell that allows only molecules that fit precisely to it—as a key fits in its lock—to attach to it.

Suppressor T cell: A white blood cell that helps end an immune response.

When infection occurs, monocytes leave the bloodstream and move into the tissues. There, over a period of about 8 hours, monocytes enlarge greatly and produce granules within themselves. The granules are filled with en-zymes and other substances that help digest bacteria and other foreign cells. Monocytes that have enlarged and contain granules are macrophages. Macrophages stay in the tissues. They ingest bacteria, foreign cells, and damaged and dead cells. (The process of a cell ingesting a microorganism, another cell, or cell fragments is called phagocytosis, and cells that ingest are called phagocytes.)

Neutrophils

Neutrophils ingest bacteria and other foreign cells. Neutrophils contain granules that release enzymes to help kill and digest these cells. Neutrophils circulate in the bloodstream and must be signaled to leave the bloodstream and enter tissues. The signal of-

ten comes from the bacteria themselves, from complement proteins, or from macrophages, all of which produce substances that attract neutrophils to a trouble spot. (The process of attracting cells is called chemotaxis.)

Eosinophils

Eosinophils can ingest bacteria and other foreign cells, contain granules filled with enzymes to digest the ingested bacteria and cells, and circulate in the bloodstream. However, they are less active against bacteria than are

Lymphatic System: Helping Defend Against Infection

The lymphatic system is a vital part of the immune system, along with the thymus gland, bone marrow, spleen, tonsils, liver, appendix, and Peyer's patches in the small intestine.

The lymphatic system is a network of lymph nodes connected by lymphatic vessels. This system transports lymph. Fluids that contain oxygen, proteins, and other nutrients seep through the thin walls of capillaries into the body's tissues to nourish them. Some of these fluids enter the lymphatic vessels to be returned eventually to the bloodstream. The fluids also transport foreign substances (such as bacteria), cancer cells, and dead or damaged cells that may be present in tissues into the lymphatic vessels. Lymph also contains many white blood cells.

All substances transported by the lymph pass through at least one lymph node, where foreign substances can be filtered out and destroyed before fluids are returned to the bloodstream. In the lymph nodes, white blood cells can collect, interact with each other and antigens, and generate immune responses to foreign substances. Lymph nodes contain a mesh of tissue in which lymphocytes are tightly packed. Harmful microorganisms are filtered through the mesh, then attacked by lymphocytes and macrophages (which are also present in the lymph nodes). Lymph nodes are often clustered in areas where the lymphatic vessels branch off, such as the neck, armpits, and groin.

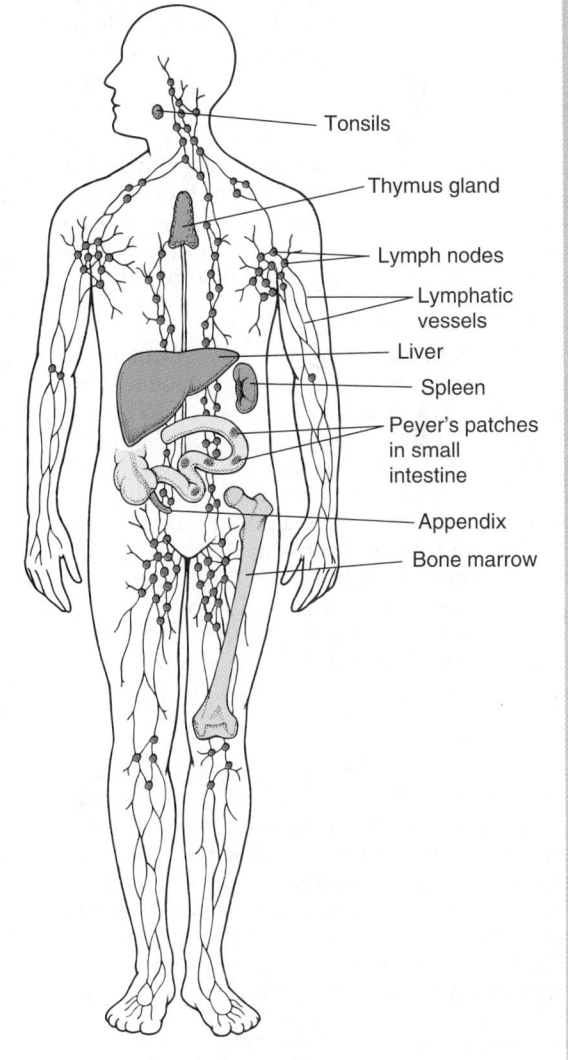

Tonsils

Thymus gland

Lymph nodes

Lymphatic vessels

Liver

Spleen

Peyer's patches in small intestine

Appendix

Bone marrow

neutrophils and macrophages. Their main function may be to attach to and thus help immobilize and kill parasites. Eosinophils also participate in allergic reactions (such as asthma).▲

Basophils

Basophils do not ingest foreign cells. They contain granules that release histamine, a substance involved in allergic reactions. Basophils also produce substances that attract neutrophils and eosinophils to a trouble spot.

Natural Killer Cells

Natural killer cells are lymphocytes, a type of white blood cell. Natural killer cells are called "natural" killers because they are ready to kill as soon as they are formed. Natural killer cells attach to foreign cells and release enzymes and other substances that damage the outer membranes of the foreign cells. Natural killer cells kill certain microorganisms, cancer cells, and cells infected by viruses. Thus, natural killer cells are often the body's first line of defense against viral infections. Also, natural killer cells produce cytokines that regulate some of the functions of T lymphocytes, B lymphocytes, and macrophages.

Complement System

The complement system consists of more than 30 proteins that act in a sequence: One protein activates another and so on. This sequence is called the complement cascade. Complement proteins can kill bacteria directly or help destroy bacteria by attaching to them, thus making the bacteria easier for neutrophils and macrophages to identify and ingest. Other functions include attracting macrophages and neutrophils to a trouble spot, causing bacteria to clump together, and neutralizing viruses. The complement system also participates in specific immunity.

Cytokines

Cytokines are the messengers of the immune system. White blood cells and certain other cells of the immune system produce cytokines when an antigen is detected. There are many different cytokines, which affect different parts of the immune system. Some stimulate activity. They stimulate certain white blood cells to become more effective killers and to attract other white blood cells to a trou-

ble spot. Other cytokines inhibit activity, helping end an immune response. Some cytokines, called interferons, interfere with the reproduction (replication) of viruses. Cytokines also participate in specific immunity.

Specific Immunity

Specific (adaptive) immunity is not present at birth; it is acquired. As a person's immune system encounters antigens, it learns the best way to attack each antigen and begins to develop a memory for that antigen. Specific immunity is so named because it tailors its attack to a specific antigen previously encountered. The hallmarks of specific immunity are its ability to learn, adapt, and remember. Specific immunity takes time to develop after initial exposure to a new antigen. However, because a memory is formed, subsequent responses to a previously encountered antigen are more effective and more rapid than those generated by nonspecific immunity.

Lymphocytes are the most important type of white blood cell involved in specific immunity. Dendritic cells, antibodies, cytokines, and the complement system (which enhances the effectiveness of antibodies) are also involved.

Lymphocytes

Lymphocytes enable the body to remember antigens and to distinguish self from nonself (foreign). Lymphocytes circulate in the bloodstream and lymphatic system and move into tissues as needed.

The immune system can remember every antigen encountered because lymphocytes live a long time—for years or even decades. When lymphocytes encounter an antigen for the second time, they respond quickly, vigorously, and specifically to that particular antigen. This specific immune response is the reason that people do not contract chickenpox or measles more than once and that vaccination can prevent certain disorders.

Lymphocytes include B lymphocytes, T lymphocytes, and natural killer cells (which are involved in nonspecific immunity).

B Lymphocytes: B lymphocytes (B cells) are formed in the bone marrow. B lymphocytes have particular sites (receptors) on their surface where specific antigens can attach. When a B lymphocyte encounters an antigen, the antigen attaches to the receptor, stimulating the B lymphocyte to change into a plasma cell.

▲ see page 1063

Plasma cells produce antibodies. These antibodies are specific to the antigen that stimulated their production.

T Lymphocytes: T lymphocytes (T cells) are produced in the thymus gland. There, they learn how to distinguish self from nonself. Only the T lymphocytes that tolerate the self-identification molecules are allowed to mature and leave the thymus. Without this training process, T lymphocytes could attack the body's cells and tissues.

Mature T lymphocytes are formed and stored in secondary lymphoid organs (such as the spleen), bone marrow, and lymph nodes. They circulate in the bloodstream and the lymphatic system, where they search for particular foreign or abnormal cells, such as particular bacteria or cells infected by particular viruses. T lymphocytes can attack particular foreign or abnormal cells.

There are different types of T lymphocytes:

• **Killer (cytotoxic) T cells** attach to foreign or abnormal cells (because they recognize the antigens on these cells). Killer T cells kill foreign or abnormal cells by making holes in the cell membrane and injecting enzymes into the cells.

• **Helper T cells** help B lymphocytes recognize and produce antibodies against foreign antigens. Helper T cells also help killer T cells kill foreign or abnormal cells.

• **Suppressor T cells** produce substances that help end the immune response.

Sometimes T lymphocytes—for reasons that are not completely understood—develop without or lose the ability to distinguish self from nonself. The result is an autoimmune disorder, in which the body attacks its own tissues.▲

Dendritic Cells

Dendritic cells develop from monocytes and reside mainly in tissues. Newly developed dendritic cells ingest and break antigens into fragments so that other immune cells can recognize them—an activity called antigen processing. A dendritic cell matures after it is stimulated by cytokines at a site of infection or inflammation. Then, it moves from tissues to the lymph nodes where it shows (presents) the antigen fragments to T lymphocytes, which generate a specific immune response.

Antibodies

When a B lymphocyte encounters an antigen, it is stimulated to mature into a plasma

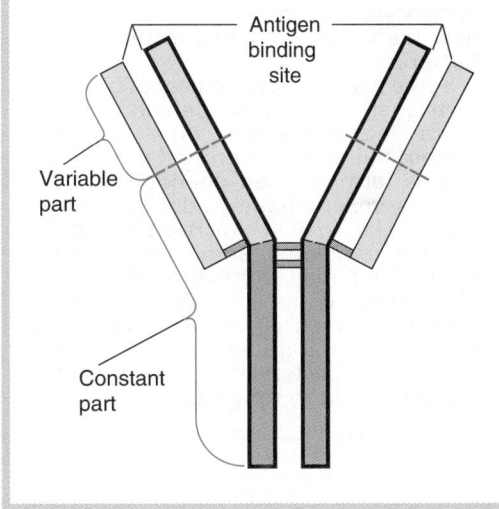

Basic Y Structure of Antibodies

An antibody molecule is basically shaped like a Y. The molecule has two parts. One part varies from antibody to antibody, depending on which antigen the antibody targets. The antigen attaches to the variable part. The other part (constant part) is one of five structures, which determines the antibody's class—IgG, IgM, IgD, IgE, or IgA. This part is the same within each class.

Antigen binding site

Variable part

Constant part

cell, which then produces antibodies (also called immunoglobulins, or Ig). Antibodies protect the body by helping other immune cells ingest antigens, by inactivating toxic substances produced by bacteria, and by attacking bacteria and viruses directly. Antibodies also activate the complement system. Antibodies are essential for fighting off certain types of bacterial infections.

Each antibody molecule has two parts. One part varies; it is specialized to attach to a specific antigen. The other part is one of five structures, which determines the antibody's class—IgG, IgM, IgD, IgE, or IgA. This part is the same within each class.

IgM: This class of antibody is produced when a particular antigen is encountered for the first time. The response triggered by the

▲ see page 1073

Strategies for Attack

Different types of invading microorganisms are attacked and destroyed in different ways. Some microorganisms are directly recognized, ingested, and destroyed by phagocytes, such as neutrophils and macrophages. However, phagocytes cannot recognize certain bacteria, because the bacteria are enclosed in a capsule. In these cases, B lymphocytes have to help phagocytes with recognition. B lymphocytes produce antibodies against the antigens contained in the bacteria's capsule. The antibodies attach to the capsules. The phagocyte can then recognize and ingest the whole complex, including the bacteria.

Some microorganisms cannot be completely eliminated. To defend against these microorganisms, the immune system builds a wall around them. The wall is formed when phagocytes, particularly macrophages, adhere to each other. The walled microorganism is called a granuloma. Some bacteria thus imprisoned may survive in the body indefinitely. If the immune system is weakened (even 50 or 60 years later), the walls of the granuloma may crumble, and the bacteria may start to multiply, producing symptoms.

first encounter with an antigen is called the primary antibody response. Normally, IgM is present in the bloodstream but not in the tissues.

IgG: The most prevalent class of antibody, IgG is produced when a particular antigen is encountered again. This response is called the secondary antibody response. It is faster and results in more antibodies than the primary antibody response. IgG is present in the bloodstream and tissues. It is the only class of antibody that crosses the placenta from mother to fetus. The mother's IgG protects the fetus and infant until the infant's immune system can produce its own antibodies.

IgA: These antibodies help defend against the invasion of microorganisms through body surfaces lined with a mucous membrane, including those of the nose, eyes, lungs, and digestive tract. IgA is present in the bloodstream, in secretions produced by mucous membranes, and in breast milk.

▲ see page 1063

IgE: These antibodies trigger immediate allergic reactions.▲ IgE binds to basophils (a type of white blood cell) in the bloodstream and mast cells in tissues. When basophils or mast cells with IgE bound to them encounter allergens (antigens that cause allergic reactions), they release substances that cause inflammation and damage surrounding tissues. Thus, IgE is the only class of antibody that often seems to do more harm than good. However, IgE may help defend against certain parasitic infections that are common in some developing countries.

IgD: Small amounts of these antibodies are present in the bloodstream. The function of IgD is not well understood.

Effects of Aging

The immune system changes throughout life. At birth, specific immunity is not fully developed. However, newborns have some antibodies, which crossed the placenta from the mother during pregnancy. These antibodies protect newborns against infections until their own immune system fully develops. Breastfed newborns also receive antibodies from the mother in the breast milk.

As people age, the immune system becomes less effective. It becomes less able to distinguish self from nonself. As a result, autoimmune disorders become more common. Macrophages destroy bacteria, cancer cells, and other antigens more slowly. This slowdown may be one reason that cancer is more common among older people. T lymphocytes respond less quickly to antigens, and there are fewer lymphocytes capable of responding to new antigens. Thus, when older people encounter a new antigen, the body is less able to recognize and defend against it.

Older people have smaller amounts of complement proteins than younger people, especially during bacterial infections. The amount of antibody produced in response to an antigen and the antibody's ability to attach to the antigen are reduced. These changes may partly explain why pneumonia, influenza, infectious endocarditis, and tetanus are more common among older people and result in death more often. Also, vaccines are less likely to produce immunity in older people.

These changes in immune function may contribute to the greater susceptibility of older people to some infections and cancers.

CHAPTER 184

Immunodeficiency Disorders

Immunodeficiency disorders involve malfunction of the immune system, resulting in infections that develop and recur more frequently, are more severe, and last longer than usual.

Immunodeficiency disorders impair the immune system's ability to defend the body against foreign or abnormal cells that invade or attack it (such as bacteria, viruses, fungi, and cancer cells). As a result, unusual bacterial, viral, or fungal infections and rare cancers may develop.

An immunodeficiency disorder may be present at birth (congenital, or primary) or may develop later in life, often as a result of another disorder (acquired, or secondary). Congenital immunodeficiency disorders are usually hereditary. They typically become evident during infancy or childhood. There are more than 70 congenital immunodeficiency disorders; all are relatively rare. Acquired immunodeficiency disorders are much more common. Some immunodeficiency disorders shorten lifespan, others persist throughout life but do not affect lifespan, and a few resolve with or without treatment.

Immunodeficiency disorders are grouped by which part of the immune system▲ is affected. They may involve problems with antibodies (due to abnormalities in B lymphocytes, a type of white blood cell), T lymphocytes (a type of white blood cell that helps identify and destroy foreign or abnormal cells), both B and T lymphocytes, phagocytes (cells that ingest and kill microorganisms), or complement proteins. The affected component of the immune system may be missing, reduced in number, or abnormal and malfunctioning.

Causes

Congenital immunodeficiency disorders are caused by a genetic abnormality, which is often X-linked.■ That is, boys are more likely to be affected than girls. As a result, about 60% of affected people are male.

Acquired immunodeficiency disorders may result from almost any prolonged serious disorder. Examples are cancer, blood disorders (such as aplastic anemia, leukemia, and myelofibrosis), kidney failure, diabetes, liver disorders, and spleen disorders. Diabetes can result in an immunodeficiency disorder because white blood cells do not function well when the blood sugar level is high. Infections can also cause immunodeficiency disorders. Human immunodeficiency virus (HIV) infection results in acquired immunodeficiency syndrome (AIDS), the most common severe acquired immunodeficiency disorder.

Undernutrition—whether of all nutrients or only one—can impair the immune system. When undernutrition causes weight to decrease to less than 80% of recommended weight, the immune system is usually impaired. A decrease to less than 70% usually results in severe impairment.

Use of certain drugs called immunosuppressants may result in an acquired immunodeficiency disorder. These drugs are intentionally used to suppress the immune system. For example, immunosuppressants are used to prevent rejection of a transplanted organ or tissue,★ and corticosteroids, a type of immunosuppressant, are used to suppress inflammation due to various disorders. However, immunosuppressants also suppress the body's ability to fight infections and perhaps to destroy cancer cells. Chemotherapy and radiation therapy can also result in immunodeficiency disorders.

Symptoms

People with an immunodeficiency disorder tend to have one infection after another. Usually, respiratory infections develop first and recur often. Most people eventually develop severe bacterial infections that persist, recur, or lead to complications. For example, sore throats and head colds may progress to pneumonia. However, having many colds does not suggest an immunodeficiency disorder.

Infections of the skin and the membranes lining the mouth, eyes, and digestive tract are common. Thrush, a fungal infection of the mouth, may be an early sign of an immunodeficiency disorder. Skin infections by bacteria

---

▲ see page 1049   ■ see page 12

★ see table on page 1078

SOME CONGENITAL IMMUNODEFICIENCY DISORDERS

CLASSIFICATION	DISORDER
Problems with antibodies (due to abnormalities in B lymphocytes)	Common variable immunodeficiency Selective antibody deficiency (such as IgA deficiency) Transient hypogamma-globulinemia of infancy X-linked agammaglobulinemia
Problems with T lymphocytes	Chronic mucocutaneous candidiasis DiGeorge anomaly
Problems with B and T lymphocytes	Ataxia-telangiectasia Severe combined immunodeficiency disease Wiskott-Aldrich syndrome X-linked lymphoproliferative syndrome
Problems with the movement or killing activity of phagocytes	Chédiak-Higashi syndrome Chronic granulomatous disease Hyperimmunoglobulinemia E syndrome Leukocyte adhesion defects Leukocyte glucose-6-phosphate dehydrogenase deficiency Myeloperoxidase deficiency
Problems with complement proteins	Complement component 1 (C1) inhibitor deficiency (hereditary angioedema) C3 deficiency C6 deficiency C7 deficiency C8 deficiency

or viruses are also common. Bacterial infections (with staphylococci, for example) may cause pyoderma, in which the skin is covered with pus-filled sores. Warts (caused by viruses) may occur.

▲ see page 1168

Many people lose weight. Children tend to develop slowly. Other symptoms vary depending on the severity and duration of the infections.

Diagnosis

Doctors first establish that an immunodeficiency exists. Then they identify the abnormality in the immune system.

Doctors suspect immunodeficiency when a severe or an unusual infection recurs often or when an organism that normally does not cause infection (such as pneumocystis or cytomegalovirus) causes infection. The results of a physical examination may also suggest immunodeficiency. Evidence of recurring infections—such as rashes, hair loss, many skin infections, chronic cough, weight loss, and an enlarged liver and spleen—is often present.

To help identify the type of immunodeficiency disorder, doctors ask at what age the person began to have recurring or unusual infections. Infections in infants younger than 6 months usually indicate an abnormality in T lymphocytes. Infections in older children usually indicate an abnormality in B lymphocytes and antibody production. The type of infection may also help doctors identify the type of immunodeficiency disorder.

Doctors ask the person about risk factors, such as diabetes, use of certain drugs, exposure to toxic substances, and the possibility of having close relatives with immunodeficiency disorders (family history). The person is asked about past and current sexual activity and use of intravenous drugs to determine whether HIV infection could be the cause. ▲

Laboratory tests are needed to confirm the diagnosis of immunodeficiency and identify the type of immunodeficiency disorder. A blood sample is taken and analyzed to determine the total number of white blood cells and the percentages of each main type of white blood cell. The white blood cells are examined under a microscope for abnormalities. Antibody levels, the number of red blood cells and platelets, and the levels of complement proteins are determined. If any results are abnormal, additional tests are usually performed.

A laboratory test using a chemical to stimulate lymphocytes or skin tests may be performed if the immunodeficiency is thought to be due to a T-lymphocyte abnormality. The skin test resembles the tuberculin skin test, which is used to screen for tuberculosis: Small amounts of proteins from common infectious organisms such as yeast are injected under the skin. If a reaction (redness, warmth, and swelling) occurs within 48 hours, the T lymphocytes are functioning normally. No reaction suggests a T-lymphocyte abnormality. These skin tests are not useful in children younger than 2 years.

People whose families are known to carry a gene for a hereditary immunodeficiency disorder may wish to have genetic testing to learn whether they carry the gene for the disorder and what the chances are of having an affected child. Genetic counseling before testing is helpful. Several immunodeficiency disorders, such as X-linked agammaglobulinemia, Wiskott-Aldrich syndrome, severe combined immunodeficiency disease, and chronic granulomatous disease, can be detected in a fetus by testing a sample of the fluid around the fetus (amniotic fluid) or the fetus's blood.

Prevention and Treatment

Some of the disorders that can cause immunodeficiency disorders can be prevented or treated. For example, the spread of HIV infection can be reduced by following safe sex guidelines and by not sharing needles to inject drugs. Successful treatment of cancer usually restores the function of the immune system. Treatment with antiviral drugs can help improve white blood cell function, thus preventing additional infections due to immunodeficiency. Good control of diabetes can help white blood cells function better and thus prevent infections.

Strategies for reducing the risk of and for treating infections depend on the type of immunodeficiency disorder. For example, people who have an immunodeficiency disorder due to a deficiency of antibodies are at risk of bacterial infections. Periodic treatment with immune globulin given intravenously and good personal hygiene (including conscientious dental care) reduce this risk, as does not eating undercooked food, drinking bottled water and avoiding contact with people who have infections. Antibiotics are given as soon as a fever or another sign of an infection develops and before surgical and dental procedures, which may introduce bacteria into the bloodstream.

For people who have an immunodeficiency disorder that increases the risk of viral infections (particularly immunodeficiency due to a T-lymphocyte abnormality, such as AIDS), antiviral drugs, such as amantadine for influenza

or acyclovir for herpes, are promptly given at the first sign of infection.

People who can produce antibodies are vaccinated. However, people who have a B- or T-lymphocyte abnormality are given only killed viral and bacterial vaccines rather than live vaccines. Live viruses may cause an infection in such people. Live vaccines include oral poliovirus vaccine, measles-mumps-rubella vaccine, chicken pox (varicella) vaccine, and bacille Calmette-Guérin (BCG) vaccine. An influenza vaccine given once a year is recommended for people who can produce antibodies and for their immediate family members.

Stem cell transplantation▲ can correct some immunodeficiency disorders, particularly severe combined immunodeficiency disease. Stem cells are usually obtained from bone marrow but occasionally from blood (including umbilical cord blood). Stem cell transplantation, which is available at some major medical centers, is usually reserved for severe disorders.

Transplantation of thymus tissue is sometimes helpful. Gene therapy for a few congenital immunodeficiency disorders is being studied.

X-Linked Agammaglobulinemia

X-Linked agammaglobulinemia (Bruton's agammaglobulinemia) is a hereditary immunodeficiency disorder due to an abnormality in the X chromosome and resulting in few or no B lymphocytes and very low levels of antibodies.

X-Linked agammaglobulinemia affects only boys. For about the first 6 months after birth, antibodies from the mother protect against infection. At about age 6 months, affected infants start having recurring infections of the ears, sinuses, lungs, and bones, usually due to bacteria such as pneumococcus, haemophilus, and streptococcus. Some unusual viral infections of the brain may develop. The risk of cancer is increased.

Infusions of immune globulin are given throughout life to help prevent infections. Antibiotics are promptly given to treat bacterial infections and may be given continuously. Despite these measures, chronic sinus and lung infections often develop. With treatment, lifespan may be unaffected.

▲ see page 1081

Selective Antibody Deficiency

Selective antibody deficiency is a usually acquired but sometimes hereditary immunodeficiency disorder resulting in a low level of a specific class of antibody, even though the total level of antibodies is normal.

There are several classes of antibodies (immunoglobulins). Each helps protect the body from infection in a different way.▲ The level of any class of antibody may be low, but the most commonly affected class is immunoglobulin A (IgA). Selective IgA deficiency usually persists throughout life. The disorder sometimes results from a chromosomal abnormality or from taking phenytoin, an anticonvulsant.

Most people with selective IgA deficiency have few or no symptoms. Others develop chronic respiratory infections, allergies, chronic diarrhea, or autoimmune disorders. If given blood transfusions or immune globulin that contains IgA, some people with selective IgA deficiency produce antibodies against IgA. Such people may have a severe allergic (anaphylactic) reaction■ the next time they are given a blood transfusion or immune globulin. They should wear a medical identification bracelet or tag to alert doctors to take precautions against such reactions.

Usually, no treatment of selective IgA deficiency is needed. Antibiotics are given to people who have recurring infections. Lifespan is usually unaffected. Selective IgA deficiency that results from taking phenytoin may resolve if the drug is discontinued.

Common Variable Immunodeficiency

Common variable immunodeficiency is an acquired immunodeficiency disorder resulting in very low antibody levels despite a normal number of B lymphocytes.

Common variable immunodeficiency usually develops between the ages of 10 and 20. In some people with this disorder, T lymphocytes malfunction. Recurring lung infections, particularly pneumonia, are common. Autoimmune disorders, including Addison's disease, thyroiditis, and rheumatoid arthritis,

often develop. Diarrhea may occur, and food may not be absorbed well from the digestive tract.

Infusions of immune globulin are given throughout life, and antibiotics are promptly given to treat infections. Lifespan may be shortened.

Transient Hypogammaglobulinemia of Infancy

Transient hypogammaglobulinemia of infancy is an immunodeficiency disorder in which antibody production by an infant is delayed.

At birth, the immune system is not fully developed. Most of the antibodies in infants are those produced by the mother and transferred via the placenta before birth. Antibodies from the mother protect infants against infection until infants start to produce their own antibodies, usually by age 6 months. Infants who have transient hypogammaglobulinemia of infancy do not start producing antibodies until later. As a result, antibody levels become low starting at age 3 to 6 months and return to normal at about age 12 to 36 months. This disorder is more common among premature infants, because they receive fewer antibodies from the mother. Although the disorder is present at birth, it is not hereditary.

Most infants with the disorder have some antibodies. Therefore, they do not have a problem with infections and need no treatment. However, some infants, particularly those born prematurely, develop infections frequently. Immune globulin can prevent and help treat infections. It is usually given for about 6 to 12 months. Antibiotics are given when needed. Lifespan is unaffected.

Chronic Mucocutaneous Candidiasis

Chronic mucocutaneous candidiasis is a hereditary immunodeficiency disorder in which T lymphocytes malfunction.

Because the T lymphocytes malfunction, the body is less able to fight fungal infections, including yeast infections. The ability to fight other infections is not reduced. Infections with the *Candida* fungus (candidiasis)★ develop and persist, usually beginning during infancy but sometimes during early adulthood. The fungus may cause mouth infections (thrush) as well as infections of the scalp, skin;

▲ see page 1055   ■ see page 1072
★ see page 1150

nails; and membranes lining the mouth, eyes, digestive tract, and reproductive tract. Severity varies: The disorder may affect one nail or cause a disfiguring rash that covers the face and scalp. Hair may fall out. Hepatitis and chronic lung disorders sometimes develop. Many people also have endocrine disorders, such as underactive parathyroid glands (hypoparathyroidism).

Usually, the infections can be treated with an antifungal drug—nystatin or clotrimazole—applied to the skin. Severe infections, which are rare, require a stronger antifungal drug, such as itraconazole given by mouth. Usually, this disorder is chronic but does not affect lifespan.

DiGeorge Anomaly

DiGeorge anomaly is a congenital immunodeficiency disorder in which the thymus gland is absent or underdeveloped at birth.

Usually, DiGeorge anomaly is due to a chromosomal abnormality but is not usually hereditary. The fetus does not develop normally, and abnormalities of the heart, parathyroid gland, face, and thymus gland often result. The thymus gland is necessary for the normal development of T lymphocytes. Consequently, people with this disorder have a low number of T lymphocytes, limiting their ability to fight many infections. Infections begin soon after birth and recur often. However, the degree to which the immune system is affected varies considerably.

Typically, children with DiGeorge anomaly also have symptoms that are unrelated to immunodeficiency, such as congenital heart disease and unusual facial features, with low-set ears, a small jawbone that recedes, and wide-set eyes. They also are born without parathyroid glands, which help regulate the calcium levels in the blood. The resulting low calcium levels lead to muscle spasms (tetany).

For children who have some T lymphocytes, the immune system may function adequately without treatment. Infections that develop are treated promptly. For children who have very few or no T lymphocytes, transplantation of stem cells or thymus tissue can cure the immunodeficiency.

A low calcium level is treated with calcium supplements to prevent muscle spasms. Sometimes the heart disease is worse than the immunodeficiency, and surgery to prevent se-

vere heart failure or death may be needed. The prognosis usually depends on the severity of the heart disease.

Ataxia-Telangiectasia

Ataxia-telangiectasia is a hereditary disorder characterized by incoordination, dilated capillaries, and increased susceptibility to infections.

The increased susceptibility to infections in people with ataxia-telangiectasia results from malfunction of B and T lymphocytes. Often, levels of the antibody classes IgA and IgE are also deficient. Sinus and respiratory infections recur, often leading to pneumonia and chronic lung disorders such as bronchitis. The risk of cancer, especially leukemia, brain tumors, and stomach cancer, is increased.

Abnormalities in the cerebellum (which are unrelated to the immunodeficiency disorder) lead to incoordination (ataxia). Incoordination usually develops when the child begins to walk but may be delayed until age 4. Speech becomes slurred, and muscles progressively weaken, leading to severe disability. Mental retardation may develop and progress. Between the ages of 1 and 6, capillaries in the skin and eyes become dilated and visible. The dilated capillaries (telangiectasia), called spider veins, are usually most obvious on the eyeballs and ears. The endocrine system may be affected, resulting in small testes (in boys), infertility, and diabetes.

Antibiotics and immune globulin help prevent infections but do not relieve the problems with the nervous system. Ataxia-telangiectasia usually progresses to paralysis, dementia, and death, usually by age 30.

Severe Combined Immunodeficiency Disease

Severe combined immunodeficiency disease is a congenital immunodeficiency disorder resulting in low levels of antibodies and a low number and malfunction of T lymphocytes.

Severe combined immunodeficiency disease is the most serious immunodeficiency disorder. It can be caused by several different genetic defects, most of which are hereditary. One form of the disorder is due to a deficiency of the enzyme adenosine deaminase. In the past, children with this disorder were kept in strict isolation, sometimes in a plastic tent, leading to the disorder being called "bubble boy syndrome."

Most infants with severe combined immunodeficiency disease develop pneumonia, thrush, and diarrhea, usually by age 3 months. More serious infections, including pneumocystis pneumonia, can also develop. If not treated, these children usually die before age 2.

Treatment with antibiotics and immune globulin is helpful. The best treatment is transplantation of stem cells from bone marrow or umbilical cord blood. For a deficiency of adenosine deaminase, replacement of that enzyme can be effective. Gene therapy seems to be effective in some infants who have one form of severe combined immunodeficiency disease. Gene therapy consists of removing some white blood cells from the infant, inserting a normal gene into the cells, and returning the cells to the infant.

Wiskott-Aldrich Syndrome

Wiskott-Aldrich syndrome is a hereditary immunodeficiency disorder characterized by abnormal antibodies and T lymphocytes, a low platelet count, and eczema.

Wiskott-Aldrich syndrome affects only boys. The number of platelets is low. Consequently, bleeding problems, usually bloody diarrhea, may be the first symptom. Eczema also develops at an early age. Susceptibility to infections, particularly of the respiratory tract, is increased because the antibody levels are low and T lymphocytes malfunction. The risk of developing cancers such as lymphoma and leukemia is increased.

Stem cell transplantation is necessary to preserve life. Without it, most boys with this disorder die by age 15. Surgical removal of the spleen may relieve the bleeding problems. Antibiotics are given continuously to prevent infections, and immune globulin may help.

Hyperimmunoglobulinemia E Syndrome

Hyperimmunoglobulinemia E syndrome (hyper-IgE syndrome, or Job-Buckley syndrome) is a hereditary immunodeficiency disorder with very high levels of IgE and normal levels of other antibody classes, resulting in recurring infections.

In most people with hyperimmunoglobulinemia E syndrome, neutrophils—a type of white blood cell that is also a phagocyte—are abnormal. (Phagocytes are cells that ingest and kill bacteria.) The cause is unknown. The skin, joints, lungs, or other organs may be infected, usually with *Staphylococcus* bacteria. Many people with this disorder have weak bones and therefore many fractures. Some people have symptoms of allergy, such as eczema, nasal stuffiness, and asthma. Facial features may be coarse.

Antibiotics, often trimethoprim-sulfamethoxazole, are given continuously or intermittently for the staphylococcal infections. Lifespan depends on the severity of the lung infections.

Chronic Granulomatous Disease

Chronic granulomatous disease is a hereditary immunodeficiency disorder in which phagocytes (neutrophils, eosinophils, monocytes, and macrophages) malfunction.

In this disorder, neutrophils, eosinophils, monocytes, and macrophages do not produce hydrogen peroxide, superoxide, and other substances that kill certain bacteria and fungi. Chronic granulomatous disease usually affects boys.

Symptoms usually first appear during early childhood but sometimes not until adolescence. Chronic infections occur in the skin, lungs, lymph nodes, mouth, nose, and intestines. Pockets of pus (abscesses) can develop around the anus and in the lungs, bones, and liver. The lymph nodes tend to fill with bacteria and enlarge. The skin over the lymph nodes may break down. As a result, the abscess drains. The liver and spleen enlarge. Children may grow slowly.

Antibiotics are given continuously or intermittently. Interferon-gamma, injected 3 times a week, can reduce the number and severity of infections. Stem cell transplantation has been successful in some people but because of the risks is not usually recommended.

Immunodeficiency due to Spleen Disorders

The spleen is crucial to the function of the immune system: The spleen traps and destroys bacteria and other infectious organisms in the bloodstream and produces antibodies. For people whose spleen is absent at birth, damaged, or removed because of disease, the risk of developing severe bacterial infections is increased.

People who do not have a spleen are given pneumococcal and meningococcal vaccines in addition to the usual childhood vaccines. People who have a spleen disorder or no spleen are given antibiotics at the first sign of infection.

Children who do not have a spleen should take antibiotics continuously until at least age 5. An antibiotic, usually penicillin or ampicillin, is often given to prevent an infection in the bloodstream.

Allergic Reactions

Allergic reactions (hypersensitivity reactions) are inappropriate immune responses to a normally harmless substance.

Normally, the immune system—which includes antibodies, white blood cells, mast cells, complement proteins, and other substances—defends the body against foreign substances (called antigens). However, in susceptible people, the immune system can overreact to certain antigens (called allergens), which are harmless in most people. The result is an allergic reaction. Some people are allergic to only one substance; others are allergic to many. About one third of the people in the United States have an allergy.

Allergens may cause an allergic reaction when they land on the skin or in the eye, are inhaled, are eaten, or are injected. An allergic reaction can occur as part of a seasonal allergy (such as hay fever), caused by exposure to such substances as grass or ragweed pollen. Or an allergic reaction can be triggered by taking a drug, eating certain foods, or breathing in dust or animal dander.

In most allergic reactions, the immune system, when first exposed to an allergen, produces a type of antibody called immunoglobulin E (IgE). IgE binds to a type of white blood cell called basophils in the bloodstream and to a similar type of cell called mast cells in the tissues. The first exposure may make a person sensitive to the allergen but does not cause symptoms. When the sensitized person subsequently encounters the allergen, the cells that have IgE on their surface release substances (such as histamine, prostaglandins, and leukotrienes) that cause swelling or inflammation in the surrounding tissues. Such substances begin a cascade of reactions that con-

tinue to irritate and harm tissues. These reactions range from mild to severe.

Symptoms and Diagnosis

Most allergic reactions are mild, consisting of watery, itchy eyes, a runny nose, itchy skin, and some sneezing. Rashes (including hives) are common and often itch. Swelling may occur in small areas of the skin (with hives) or in larger areas under the skin (as angioedema).▲ Swelling is caused by fluids leaking from blood vessels. Depending on which areas of the body are affected, angioedema may be serious. Allergies may trigger attacks of asthma. Certain allergic reactions, called anaphylactic reactions,■ can be life threatening. The airways can constrict (causing wheezing), and blood vessels can dilate (causing a fall in blood pressure).

Doctors first determine whether a reaction is allergic. They may ask whether the person has close relatives with allergies, because a reaction is more likely to be allergic in such cases. Blood tests are usually performed to detect a type of white blood cell called eosinophils. Eosinophils are produced in large numbers as a result of an allergic reaction.

Because each allergic reaction is triggered by a specific allergen, the main goal of diagnosis is to identify that allergen. Often, the person and doctor can identify the allergen based on when the allergy started and when and how often the reaction occurs (for example, during certain seasons or after eating certain foods).

Skin tests are the most useful way to identify specific allergens. Usually, a skin prick test is performed first. Dilute solutions are

▲ see page 1071   ■ see page 1072

made from extracts of pollens (from trees, grasses, weeds, or fungal spores), dust, animal dander, insect venom, foods, and some drugs. A drop of each solution is placed on the person's skin, which is then pricked with a needle. If the person is allergic to one or more of these substances, the person has a wheal and flare reaction: A pale, slightly elevated swelling—the wheal—appears at the pinprick site within 15 to 20 minutes. The wheal is surrounded by a well-defined area of redness—the flare. The resulting area is about $1/2$ inch in diameter. The skin prick test can identify most allergens. If no allergen is identified, a tiny amount of each solution can be injected into the person's skin. This type of skin test is more likely than the skin prick test to detect a reaction to an allergen. Antihistamines should not be taken before skin tests, because they may suppress a reaction to the tests.

The radioallergosorbent test (RAST) is used when skin tests cannot be used—for example, when a skin rash is widespread. This test measures blood levels of different types of IgE that are specific to particular allergens and thus helps doctors identify the allergen.

Prevention

Avoiding an allergen, if possible, is the best approach. Avoiding an allergen may involve discontinuing a drug, keeping a pet out of the house, installing high-efficiency air filters, or not eating a particular food. A person with severe seasonal allergies may consider moving to an area that does not have the allergen. A person with an allergy to house dust should remove items that collect dust.

Allergen Immunotherapy: Because some allergens, especially airborne allergens, cannot be avoided, allergen immunotherapy, commonly called allergy shots or injections, can be given to desensitize a person to the allergen. With allergen immunotherapy, allergic reactions can be prevented or reduced in number or severity. However, allergen immunotherapy is not always effective. Some people and some allergies tend to respond better than others. Immunotherapy is used most often for allergies to pollens, house dust mites, insect venoms, and animal dander. Immunotherapy for food allergies is usually not advised because it can cause severe reactions and is less effective. Also, foods can usually be avoided.

In immunotherapy, tiny amounts of the allergen are injected under the skin. The dose is gradually increased until a dose adequate to control symptoms (maintenance dose) is reached. A gradual increase is necessary because exposure to a high dose of the allergen too soon can produce an allergic reaction. Injections are usually given once or twice a week until the maintenance dose is reached. Then injections are usually given every 2 to 6 weeks. The procedure is most effective when maintenance injections are continued throughout the year, even for seasonal rhinitis. Allergen immunotherapy may take 3 to 4 years to complete.

Because immunotherapy injections occasionally cause dangerous allergic reactions, the person remains in the doctor's office for at least 20 minutes afterward. If the person has mild reactions to immunotherapy (such as sneezing, coughing, flushing, tingling sensations, itching, chest tightness, wheezing, and hives), a drug—usually an antihistamine, such as diphenhydramine or loratadine—may help. For more severe reactions, epinephrine (adrenaline) is injected.

Allergen immunotherapy may be used to prevent anaphylactic reactions▲ in people who are allergic to unavoidable allergens, such as insect stings. Immunotherapy is not used when the allergen, such as penicillin and other drugs, can be avoided. However, for people who need to take a drug they are allergic to, immunotherapy, closely monitored by a doctor, can be rapidly performed to desensitize them.

Treatment

Antihistamines: The drugs most commonly used to relieve the symptoms of allergies are antihistamines. Some antihistamines are available without a prescription, and some require a prescription. Nonprescription (over-the-counter) antihistamines are a particular problem for older people.■ Often, prescription antihistamines have fewer side effects (such as sleepiness, dry mouth, blurred vision, constipation, and difficulty with urination). Antihistamines block the effects of histamine rather than stop its production. Taking antihistamines partially relieves the itching and reduces the swelling due to hives or mild angioedema.

Cromolyn: Cromolyn may help control allergic symptoms. It is available by prescription for use with an inhaler or nebulizer

Rx   SOME ANTIHISTAMINES

DRUG	DEGREE OF ANTICHOLINERGIC EFFECTS*	DEGREE OF DROWSINESS†
Nonprescription		
Brompheniramine	Moderate	Some
Chlorpheniramine	Moderate	Some
Clemastine	Strong	Moderate
Diphenhydramine	Strong	Extreme
Loratadine	Few to none	Little to none
Triprolidine	Moderate	Some
Prescription**		
Azatadine	Moderate	Moderate
Cetirizine	Few to none	Moderate in some people
Cyproheptadine	Moderate	Some
Dexchlorpheniramine	Moderate	Some
Fexofenadine	Few to none	Little to none
Hydroxyzine	Moderate	Extreme
Promethazine	Strong	Extreme

*Anticholinergic effects include confusion, dry mouth, blurred vision, constipation, difficulty with urination, and light-headedness (particularly after a person stands up). Older people are particularly susceptible to these effects.

† The degree of drowsiness varies, depending on the other active ingredients in the formulation (as in decongestants) and on the person.

**Some prescription antihistamines may also be available in nonprescription form.

(which delivers the drug to the lungs) or as eye drops. It is available without a prescription as a nasal spray. Cromolyn usually affects only the areas where it is applied, such as the back of the throat, lungs, eyes, or nose. When taken by mouth, cromolyn is not absorbed into the bloodstream, but it can relieve the digestive symptoms of mastocytosis. Cromolyn inhibits mast cells from releasing substances that damage nearby tissues.

Corticosteroids: When antihistamines and cromolyn cannot control allergy symptoms, a corticosteroid may help. Corticosteroids can be taken as a nasal spray to treat nasal symptoms or through an inhaler, usually to treat asthma. If symptoms are very severe or widespread, taking a corticosteroid (such as prednisone) by mouth may be necessary. If taken by mouth for more than 3 to 4 weeks, corticosteroids have many, sometimes serious side effects.▲ Therefore, corticosteroids taken by mouth are prescribed only for severe symptoms when all other treatments are ineffective, and they are given for as short a time as possible.

Emergency Treatment: Severe allergic reactions, such as an anaphylactic reaction, re-

quire prompt emergency treatment. People who have severe allergic reactions should always carry a self-injecting syringe of epinephrine. Such people often also carry antihistamine tablets, which are also taken as quickly as possible. Usually, the combination of epinephrine and an antihistamine stops the reaction. Nonetheless, people who have had a severe allergic reaction should go to the hospital emergency department where they can be closely monitored and treatment can be repeated or adjusted as needed.

Seasonal Allergies

Seasonal allergies result from exposure to airborne substances (such as pollens) that appear only during certain times of the year.

Seasonal allergies are common. Seasonal allergies (commonly called hay fever) occur only during certain times of the year—particularly the spring, summer, or fall—depending on what a person is allergic to. Symptoms involve primarily the membrane lining the nose, caus-

▲ see box on page 374

ing allergic rhinitis, or the membrane lining the eyelids and covering the whites of the eyes (conjunctiva), causing allergic conjunctivitis. (Rhinitis and conjunctivitis may be caused by other disorders.▲)

The term hay fever is somewhat misleading, because symptoms do not occur only in the summer when hay is traditionally gathered and never include fever. Hay fever is usually a reaction to pollens and grasses. Different parts of the country have very different pollen seasons. In the eastern, southern, and midwestern United States, the pollens that cause hay fever in the spring usually come from trees, such as oak, elm, maple, alder, birch, juniper, and olive. In the early summer, pollens come from grasses, such as bluegrasses, timothy, redtop, and orchard grass; in the late summer, pollens come from ragweed. In the western United States, mountain cedar (a juniper) is one of the main sources of tree pollen from December to March. In the arid Southwest, grasses pollinate for much longer, and in the fall, pollen from other weeds, such as sagebrush and Russian thistle, can cause hay fever. People may react to one or more pollens, so a person's pollen allergy season may be from early spring to late fall. Seasonal allergy is also caused by mold spores, which can be airborne for long periods of time during the spring, summer, and fall.

Allergic conjunctivitis may result when airborne substances, such as pollens, contact the eyes directly.

Symptoms and Diagnosis

Hay fever can cause itching of the nose, roof of the mouth, back of the throat, and eyes. Itching may start gradually or abruptly. The nose runs, producing a clear watery discharge, and may become stuffed up. Sneezing is common.

Hay fever causes the eyes to water, sometimes profusely, and itch. The whites of the eyes and the eyelids may become red and swollen. Wearing contact lenses can irritate the eyes further. The lining of the nose may become swollen and bluish red. Other symptoms include headache, coughing, wheezing, and irritability. More rarely, depression, loss of appetite, and insomnia develop.

Many people who have a seasonal allergy also have asthma (which results in wheezing), caused by the same allergens that contribute to allergic rhinitis and conjunctivitis.

The diagnosis is based on symptoms plus the circumstances under which they occur— that is, during certain seasons. This information can also help doctors identify the allergen. The nasal discharge may be examined to see if it contains eosinophils (a type of white blood cell produced in large numbers as a result of an allergic reaction). Skin tests can help confirm the diagnosis and the identity of the allergen.■

Treatment

For allergic rhinitis, antihistamines are usually used first. Sometimes a decongestant, such as pseudoephedrine, is taken by mouth with the antihistamine to help relieve a stuffy nose. Many antihistamine-decongestant combinations are available as a single tablet. However, people with high blood pressure should not take a decongestant unless a doctor recommends it and monitors its use. Nonprescription decongestant nose drops or sprays should not be used for more than a few days at a time, because using them continually for a week or more may worsen or prolong nasal congestion. This reaction is called a rebound effect, which may eventually result in chronic congestion.

Cromolyn, which is available as a nonprescription nasal spray, may be useful. To be effective, it must be used regularly. Its effects are usually limited to the areas where it is applied.

When antihistamines and cromolyn cannot control allergy symptoms, doctors may prescribe a corticosteroid nasal spray. Corticosteroid nasal sprays are very effective, and most have minimal side effects. However, these sprays can cause nosebleeds and a sore nose. Azelastine, an antihistamine taken as a nasal spray, may be effective. But it can cause side effects similar to those of antihistamines taken by mouth, especially drowsiness.

When these treatments are ineffective, a corticosteroid may be taken by mouth or by injection for a short time (usually for fewer than 10 days). If taken by mouth or injection for a long time, corticosteroids can produce serious side effects.

Certain people can benefit from allergen immunotherapy.★ They include people who have severe side effects from taking drugs usu-

---

▲ see pages 1264 and 1298

■ see page 1063

★ see page 1064

ally used to treat allergic rhinitis, who need to take corticosteroids by mouth to control allergic rhinitis, or who also develop asthma. Allergen immunotherapy for hay fever should be started after the pollen season to prepare for the next season. Immunotherapy is most effective when continued year-round.

For allergic conjunctivitis, bathing the eyes with plain eyewashes (such as artificial tears) can help reduce irritation. Any substance that may be causing the allergic reaction should be avoided. Contact lenses should not be worn during episodes of conjunctivitis.

For allergic conjunctivitis, antihistamines are usually taken as eye drops, although they can be effective when taken by mouth. Usually, nonprescription antihistamine eye drops also contain a drug that causes blood vessels to narrow (a vasoconstrictor) and thus reduces the redness. However, something in the eye drops—the antihistamine or another component—sometimes makes the allergic reaction worse. Also, long-term use of a vasoconstrictor may worsen or prolong the inflammation. Prescription eye drops may be more effective.

Eye drops containing cromolyn, available by prescription, are used to prevent rather than relieve allergic conjunctivitis. They can be used when exposure to the allergen is anticipated. Eye drops containing olopatadine, available by prescription, can be very effective. This drug is an antihistamine and, like cromolyn, inhibits mast cells from releasing damaging substances.

If symptoms are very severe, eye drops containing corticosteroids, available by prescription, may be used as a last resort. During treatment with corticosteroid eye drops, eye pressure should be checked regularly, because use of these eye drops can lead to glaucoma. Eyes should also be checked for infection, because corticosteroids suppress the immune system and thus increase the risk of infection. Use of these eye drops is best supervised by an ophthalmologist. If other treatments are ineffective, allergen immunotherapy may be beneficial.

Year-Round Allergies

Year-round (perennial) allergies result from exposure to airborne substances, such as house dust.

Perennial allergies may occur at any time of year—unrelated to the season—or may last year-round. Perennial allergies are often a re-

action to house dust. House dust may contain mold and fungal spores, fibers of fabric, animal dander, dust mites, and bits of insects. Substances in and on cockroaches are often the cause of allergic symptoms. These substances are present in houses year-round but may cause more severe symptoms during the cold months when more time is spent indoors.

Usually, perennial allergies cause nasal symptoms (allergic rhinitis) but not eye symptoms (allergic conjunctivitis). However, allergic conjunctivitis can result when certain substances are purposely or inadvertently placed in the eyes. These substances include drugs used to treat eye disorders, cosmetics such as eyeliner and face powder, and hair dye. The cleaning solutions for contact lenses can cause a chemical allergic reaction.

Symptoms and Diagnosis

Perennial allergies can cause itching of the nose, roof of the mouth, back of the throat, and eyes. Itching may start gradually or abruptly. The nose runs, producing a clear watery discharge, and may become stuffed up. Sneezing is common. The nose may become chronically stuffy. The eustachian tube, which connects the middle ear and the back of the nose, may become swollen. As a result, hearing can be impaired, especially in children. Some people also have recurring sinus infections (chronic sinusitis) and growths inside the nose (nasal polyps).

When affected, the eyes water and itch. The whites of the eyes and the eyelids may become red and swollen.

Many people who have a perennial allergy also have asthma, caused by the same allergens that contribute to the allergic rhinitis and allergic conjunctivitis.

Diagnosis is based on symptoms plus the circumstances under which they occur—that is, in response to certain activities—for example, when petting a cat.

Prevention and Treatment

Avoiding the allergen, if possible, is recommended, thus preventing the development of symptoms. If a person is allergic to house dust, removing items that collect dust, such as knickknacks, magazines, and books, may help. Upholstered furniture can be replaced or vacuumed frequently. Draperies and shades can be replaced with blinds, and carpets can be removed or replaced with throw rugs. Mattresses and pillows can be covered with finely woven fabrics that cannot be penetrated by dust mites and allergen particles. Frequently dusting and wet-mopping rooms may help. Air conditioners can reduce the high indoor humidity that encourages the breeding of dust mites, and high-efficiency air filters can be installed. If a person is allergic to animal dander, the family pet may be limited to certain rooms of the house or, if possible, kept out of the house. Washing the pet weekly can also help.

Drug treatment is similar to that for seasonal allergies.

For people with chronic sinusitis and nasal polyps, surgery is sometimes needed to improve sinus drainage and remove infected material or to remove the polyps. Before and after surgery, regularly flushing out the sinuses with a warm water and salt (saline) solution may be helpful. This technique is called sinus irrigation.

Food Allergy

A food allergy is an allergic reaction to a particular food.

Many different foods can cause allergic reactions. However, food allergies are most commonly triggered by certain nuts, peanuts, shellfish, fish, milk, eggs, wheat, and soybeans. Allergic reactions to foods may be severe and sometimes include an anaphylactic reaction.▲

Food allergies may start during infancy. They are most common among children whose parents have food allergies, allergic rhinitis, or allergic asthma. Children with food allergies tend to be allergic to the most common allergens, such as those in eggs, milk, peanuts, and soybeans.

Food allergies are sometimes blamed for such disorders as hyperactivity in children, chronic fatigue, arthritis, poor athletic performance, and depression. However, these associations have not been substantiated.

Some reactions to food are not an allergic reaction. For example, food intolerance differs from a food allergy because it does not involve the immune system. Instead it involves a reaction in the digestive tract that results in digestive upset. For example, some people lack an enzyme necessary for digesting the sugar in milk (lactose).■ Other reactions to a food may result from contamination or deterioration of the food.

In some people, food additives can cause a reaction that resembles but is not an allergic reaction. For example, monosodium glutamate (MSG),★ some preservatives (such as metabisulfite), and dyes (such as tartrazine, a yellow dye used in candies, soft drinks, and other foods) can cause symptoms such as asthma and hives. Similarly, eating certain foods, such as cheese, wine, and chocolate, triggers migraine headaches in some people.

Symptoms

In infants, the first symptom of a food allergy may be a rash such as eczema (atopic dermatitis) or a rash that resembles hives. The rash may be accompanied by nausea, vomiting, and diarrhea. By about age 1 year, the rash often lessens. By about age 10, food allergies—most commonly to milk and less commonly to eggs and peanuts—tend to subside. Allergies to airborne substances, such as allergic asthma and hay fever, may develop as food allergies subside.

In adults, food allergies cause itching of the mouth, hives, eczema, and, occasionally, a runny nose and asthma. For some adults with a food allergy, eating a tiny amount of the food may trigger a severe reaction. A rash may cover the entire body, the throat may swell, and the airways may narrow, making breathing difficult. Occasionally, this reaction is a life-threatening anaphylactic reaction. For some people, allergic reactions to food occur only if they exercise immediately after eating the food.

Diagnosis

Doctors suspect a food allergy primarily on the basis of the person's history. Then skin tests with extracts from various foods may be performed. A reaction to a food tested does not necessarily mean that a person is allergic to that food, but no skin reaction means that an allergy to that food is unlikely. If the person reacts to the food tested, an oral challenge test may be performed to confirm the diagnosis. In this test, the suspected food is given in a carrier food such as milk or applesauce, and the doctor observes as the person eats the food. If no symptoms develop, the person is not allergic to the food.

Another way to identify the food allergy is an elimination diet. The person stops eating all foods that may be causing the symptoms

---

▲ see box on page 1069   ■ see page 735

★ see box on page 726

for about 1 week. The doctor provides the diet the person is to follow. Only the foods or fluids specified in the diet may be eaten, and only pure products should be used. Following such a diet is not easy, because many food products have ingredients that are not obvious or expected. For example, many rye breads contain some wheat flour. Eating in restaurants is not advisable, because the person and the doctor need to know the ingredients of every meal eaten. If no symptoms occur, foods are added back one at a time. Each added food is given for several days or until symptoms appear, and thus the allergen is identified.

Treatment

People with food allergies must eliminate the foods that trigger their allergies from their diet. Desensitization by first eliminating the food, then eating small amounts of the food or placing drops of food extracts under the tongue is not effective. Antihistamines are useful only for relieving hives and swelling. People with severe food allergies often carry antihistamines to take immediately if a reaction starts. They should also carry a self-injecting syringe of epinephrine to use when needed for severe reactions.

Mastocytosis

Mastocytosis is an abnormal accumulation of mast cells in the skin and sometimes in various other parts of the body.

Mastocytosis is rare. It differs from typical allergic reactions because it is chronic rather than episodic. Mastocytosis develops when mast cells increase in number and accumulate in tissues over a period of years. Mast cells, a component of the immune system, produce histamine, a substance involved in allergic reactions and the production of stomach acid. Because the number of mast cells increases, levels of histamine increase.

There are three main forms of mastocytosis. In a rare form, mast cells accumulate as a single mass in the skin (mastocytoma). Typically, a mastocytoma develops before age 6 months. In a form called urticaria pigmentosa, mast cells accumulate in many areas of the skin, forming small reddish brown spots or bumps. Rarely, urticaria pigmentosa progresses to systemic mastocytosis during adulthood. In systemic mastocytosis, mast cells accumulate in the skin, stomach, intestines, liver, spleen, lymph nodes, and bones.

Symptoms and Diagnosis

A single mastocytoma does not cause symptoms. Rubbing or scratching the spots of urticaria pigmentosa may make the spots itch. Itching may be worsened by changes in temperature, contact with clothing or other materials, or use of some drugs. Consuming hot beverages, spicy foods, or alcohol may also make itching worse. Rubbing or scratching the spots may result in hives and make the skin turn red. Flushing and widespread reactions, including anaphylactic reactions, may occur.

Systemic mastocytosis causes itching and flushing. It can cause widespread reactions, which tend to be severe and include anaphylactoid reactions. Anaphylactoid reactions resemble anaphylactic reactions, but no allergen triggers them. Bone pain and abdominal pain are common. Peptic ulcers and chronic diarrhea may develop because the stomach produces too much histamine, which stimulates the production of stomach acid.

Urticaria pigmentosa may be diagnosed based on the presence of the typical spots that,

Anaphylactoid Versus Anaphylactic

Anaphylactoid reactions resemble anaphylactic reactions. However, anaphylactoid reactions may occur after the first exposure to a substance—for example, after the first injection of certain drugs, such as polymyxin, pentamidine, opioids, or the radiopaque dyes sometimes used with x-ray procedures. Anaphylactoid reactions are not allergic reactions because IgE, the class of antibodies involved in allergic reactions, does not cause them. Rather, the reaction is caused by the substance itself. Aspirin and other nonsteroidal anti-inflammatory drugs (NSAIDs) can cause anaphylactoid reactions in some people, particularly those with year-round allergic rhinitis and nasal polyps.

If possible, doctors avoid using dyes with x-ray procedures in people who have anaphylactoid reactions to such dyes. However, some disorders cannot be diagnosed without dyes. In such cases, special dyes that reduce the risk of reactions are used. In addition, drugs that block anaphylactoid reactions, such as prednisone, diphenhydramine, or ephedrine, are usually given before the dye is injected.

when scratched, result in hives and redness. A biopsy may also be performed. If mastocytosis affecting the skin is suspected, a sample of skin tissue is removed and examined under a microscope for mast cells. If systemic mastocytosis is suspected, a sample is taken from the bone marrow or other tissues.

Treatment

In children, a mastocytoma usually disappears spontaneously. Itching due to urticaria pigmentosa may be treated with antihistamines. Systemic mastocytosis is treated with antihistamines and histamine-2 (H₂) blockers (which reduce acid production in the stomach).▲ Cromolyn given by mouth can relieve digestive problems. A self-injecting syringe of epinephrine should always be carried for prompt emergency treatment of anaphylactic reactions. Ultraviolet light and corticosteroid creams applied to the skin may be used to treat the skin symptoms of mastocytosis.

Physical Allergy

A physical allergy is an allergic reaction triggered by a physical stimulus.

A physical allergy differs from other allergic reactions because the trigger is a physical stimulus. The physical stimulus can be cold, sunlight, heat, other stimuli that cause sweating (such as emotional stress or exercise), vibration, a minor injury (such as that due to scratching), or physical pressure. For some people, symptoms occur only in response to a physical stimulus. For some people who have other allergies, a physical stimulus makes symptoms worse.

What causes this type of allergic reaction is not understood. One theory suggests that the physical stimulus changes a protein in the skin. The immune system mistakes this protein for a foreign substance and attacks it. Sensitivity to sunlight (photosensitivity) is sometimes triggered by the use of drugs, such as antibiotics, or other substances, including some cosmetics such as skin creams, lotions, and oils. A few people who are sensitive to cold have abnormal proteins (called cryoglobulins or cryofibrinogen) in the blood. Sometimes the presence of these proteins indicates a serious disorder such as cancer, a connective tissue disorder, or chronic infection.

▲ see table on page 718

Itching, skin blotches, hives, and angioedema are the most common symptoms. The symptoms tend to develop within minutes of exposure to the physical stimulus.

When people who are sensitive to heat are exposed to heat or engage in any activity that causes sweating, they may develop small, intensely itchy hives that are surrounded by a ring of redness—a condition called cholinergic urticaria.

When people who are sensitive to cold are exposed to cold, they may develop hives, asthma, a runny nose, nasal stuffiness, or swelling of tissues under the skin (angioedema). Rarely, a widespread anaphylactic reaction occurs.

Diagnosis and Treatment

The diagnosis is based on symptoms and the circumstances under which they occur. To diagnose reactions caused by cold, doctors place an ice cube on the skin for 4 minutes, remove the ice cube, then watch for the development of a hive.

The best treatment is to avoid the stimulus that causes the physical allergy. Not using cosmetics and skin creams, lotions, and oils for a while enables the person to determine whether one of these substances may be worsening the allergy.

An antihistamine can usually relieve itching. Cyproheptadine tends to work best for hives caused by cold, and hydroxyzine for hives caused by heat or emotional stress. People who are very sensitive to sunlight should use a sunscreen and avoid exposure to the sun as much as possible.

Exercise-Induced Allergic Reactions

Exercise-induced allergic reactions occur during or after exercise.

Exercise often triggers an asthma attack in people who have asthma, but some people have asthma only when they exercise. Exercise may trigger or worsen asthma because breathing fast cools and dries the airways, and as the airways warm again, they narrow. Exercise-induced asthma is more likely to occur when the air is cold and dry. The chest feels tight. The person may wheeze and have difficulty breathing.

Rarely, vigorous exercise triggers an anaphylactic reaction. In some people, this reaction occurs only if they eat a specific food before exercising. Breathing becomes difficult or blood pressure falls, leading to dizziness and collapse. An anaphylactic reaction can be life threatening.

Typically, symptoms triggered by exercise—asthma or an anaphylactic reaction—occur after 5 to 10 minutes of vigorous exercise. Often, symptoms begin after exercise has stopped.

The diagnosis is based on the symptoms and their relationship to exercise. An exercise challenge test can also help doctors make the diagnosis. For this test, measurements of lung function are made before and after exercise on a treadmill or stationary bicycle.▲

Treatment

For people with exercise-induced asthma, the goal of treatment is to be able to exercise without symptoms. Becoming more physically fit may make the development of symptoms during exercise less likely. Inhaling a beta-adrenergic drug (such as those used to treat asthma)■ about 15 minutes before starting to exercise often helps prevent reactions. Cromolyn, usually taken through an inhaler, may be helpful.

For people who have asthma, taking the drugs usually used to control asthma often prevents symptoms from developing during exercise. For some people with asthma, taking drugs to treat asthma and gradually increasing the intensity and duration of exercise enables them to tolerate exercise.

People who have had an exercise-induced anaphylactic reaction should avoid the form of exercise that triggered the attack. If eating a specific food before exercise triggers symptoms, they should not eat the food before exercise. A self-injecting syringe of epinephrine should always be carried for prompt emergency treatment. Exercising with other people is recommended.

Hives and Angioedema

*Hives, also called urticaria, is a skin reaction characterized by pale, slightly elevated swellings (wheals) surrounded by an area of redness with clearly defined borders. **Angioedema** is swelling of larger areas of tissue under the skin, sometimes affecting the face and throat.*

Hives and angioedema, which may occur together, can be severe. Common triggers are drugs, insect stings or bites, allergy injections (allergen immunotherapy), and certain foods—particularly eggs, shellfish, nuts, and fruits.

Eating even a tiny amount of some foods can suddenly result in hives or angioedema. But with other foods (such as strawberries), these reactions occur only after a large amount is eaten. Also, hives sometimes follow viral infections such as hepatitis, infectious mononucleosis, and German measles.

Hives or angioedema can be chronic, recurring over weeks or months. In most cases, no specific cause is identified. The cause may be habitual, unintentional intake of a substance—for example, a food additive, such as a preservative or food dye. In some people, antibodies to thyroid hormone may be the cause. Use of certain drugs, such as aspirin or other nonsteroidal anti-inflammatory drugs (NSAIDs),★ can also cause chronic hives or angioedema. In many cases, no specific cause can be identified. Chronic angioedema that occurs without hives may be hereditary angioedema.

Symptoms and Diagnosis

Hives usually begin with itching. Then wheals quickly develop. The wheals usually remain small (less than $1/2$ inch across). Wheals that are larger (up to 4 inches across) may look like rings of redness with a pale center. Typically, crops of hives come and go. One spot may remain for several hours, then disappear, and later, another may appear elsewhere. After the hive disappears, the skin usually looks completely normal.

Angioedema may affect part or all of the hands, feet, eyelids, lips, or genitals. Sometimes the membranes lining the mouth, throat, and airways swell, making breathing difficult.

In children, when hives appear suddenly, disappear quickly, and do not recur, an examination by a doctor is usually unnecessary, because the cause is usually a viral infection. If the cause is a bee sting, seeing a doctor is important. A person can obtain advice about treatment if another bee sting occurs. When angioedema or hives recur without an obvious cause, an examination by a doctor is recommended.

Treatment

Usually, if hives appear suddenly, they subside without any treatment within days and sometimes within minutes. If the cause is not

---

▲ see page 276   ■ see table on page 278

★ see page 452

Hereditary Angioedema: Not an Allergy

Hereditary angioedema looks much like the angioedema of an allergic reaction. However, the cause is different. Hereditary angioedema is a genetic disorder due to a deficiency or malfunction of C1 inhibitor. C1 inhibitor is part of the complement system, which is part of the immune system. In this disorder, an injury, a viral infection, or stress (such as that due to anticipating a dental or surgical procedure) may trigger attacks of swelling (angioedema).

Areas of the skin, the tissue under the skin, or the membranes lining the mouth, throat, windpipe, and digestive tract may swell. Typically, the swollen areas are painful, not itchy. Hives do not appear. Nausea, vomiting, and cramps are common. Swelling of the windpipe can interfere with breathing. Doctors diagnose the disorder by measuring C1 inhibitor levels or activity in a sample of blood.

The drug aminocaproic acid can sometimes relieve the swelling. Epinephrine, antihistamines, and corticosteroids are often given, although there is no proof that these drugs are effective. If a sudden attack interferes with breathing, the airway must be opened—for example, by inserting a breathing tube in the windpipe.

Certain treatments may help prevent subsequent attacks. For example, before a dental or surgical procedure, people with hereditary angioedema may be given a transfusion of fresh plasma to increase levels of C1 inhibitor in the blood. For long-term prevention, anabolic steroids (androgens) taken by mouth, such as stanozolol or danazol, can stimulate the body to produce more C1 inhibitor. Because these drugs can have masculinizing side effects, the dose is reduced as soon and as much as possible when these drugs are given to women.

obvious, the person should stop taking all nonessential drugs until the hives subside.

For hives and mild angioedema, taking antihistamines partially relieves the itching and reduces the swelling. Corticosteroids are prescribed only for severe symptoms when all other treatments are ineffective, and they are

▲ see box on page 374

given for as short a time as possible. When taken by mouth for more than 3 to 4 weeks, they cause many, sometimes serious side effects.▲

In about half of the people with chronic hives, the hives disappear without treatment within 2 years. For some adults, the antidepressant doxepin, which is also a potent antihistamine, helps relieve chronic hives.

If severe angioedema results in difficulty swallowing or breathing or in collapse, prompt emergency treatment is necessary. Affected people should always carry a self-injecting syringe of epinephrine and antihistamine tablets to be used immediately if a reaction occurs. After a severe allergic reaction, such people should go to the hospital emergency department, where they can be checked and treated as needed.

Anaphylactic Reactions

Anaphylactic reactions (anaphylaxis) are sudden, widespread, potentially severe and life-threatening allergic reactions.

Anaphylactic reactions are most commonly caused by drugs (such as penicillin), insect stings, certain foods, and allergy injections (allergen immunotherapy). But they can be caused by any allergen. Like other allergic reactions, an anaphylactic reaction does not usually occur after the first exposure to an allergen but may occur after a subsequent exposure. However, many people do not recall a first exposure. Any allergen that causes an anaphylactic reaction in a person is likely to cause that reaction with subsequent exposures, unless measures are taken to prevent it.

Symptoms

Anaphylactic reactions begin within 1 to 15 minutes of exposure to the allergen. Rarely, reactions begin after 1 hour. The heart beats quickly. The person may feel uneasy and become agitated. Blood pressure may fall, causing fainting. Other symptoms include tingling (pins-and-needles) sensations, itchy and flushed skin, throbbing in the ears, coughing, sneezing, hives, and swelling (angioedema). Breathing may become difficult and wheezing may occur because the windpipe (upper airway) constricts or becomes swollen.

An anaphylactic reaction may progress so rapidly that it leads to collapse, cessation of breathing, seizures, and loss of consciousness within 1 to 2 minutes. The reaction may be fatal unless emergency treatment is given immediately.

Prevention and Treatment

People who are allergic to unavoidable allergens (such as insect stings) may benefit from long-term allergen immunotherapy.▲

If an anaphylactic reaction occurs, an epinephrine injection should be given imme-diately. People who have these reactions should always carry a self-injecting syringe of epinephrine and antihistamine tablets for prompt treatment. Usually, this treatment stops the reaction. Nonetheless, after a severe allergic reaction, such people should go to the hospital emergency department, where they can be closely monitored and treatment can be adjusted as needed.

CHAPTER 186

Autoimmune Disorders

An autoimmune disorder is a malfunction of the body's immune system, causing the body to attack its own tissues.

Normally, the immune system can distinguish what is self from what is not self (or foreign)■ and reacts against foreign substances called antigens. Antigens may be contained within or on bacteria, viruses, other microorganisms, or cancer cells. Or antigens may exist on their own—for example, as pollen or food molecules. Sometimes the immune system malfunctions, interpreting the body's own tissues as foreign and producing abnormal antibodies (called autoantibodies) or immune cells that target and attack particular cells or tissues of the body. This response is called an autoimmune reaction. It results in inflammation and tissue damage. Different cells or tissues are targeted in different autoimmune disorders.

Causes

Autoimmune reactions can be triggered in several ways:

• A substance in the body that is normally confined to a specific area (and thus is hidden from the immune system) is released into the bloodstream. For example, a blow to the eye can cause the fluid in the eyeball to be released into the bloodstream. The fluid stimulates the immune system to attack.

• A normal body substance is altered, for example, by a virus, a drug, sunlight, or radiation. The altered substance may appear foreign to the immune system. For example, a virus can infect and thus alter cells in the body. The virus-infected cells stimulate the immune system to attack.

• A foreign substance that resembles a natural body substance may enter the body. The immune system may inadvertently target the similar body substance as well as the foreign substance.

• The cells that control antibody production—for example, B lymphocytes (a type of white blood cell)—may malfunction and produce abnormal antibodies that attack some of the body's cells.

Heredity may be involved in some autoimmune disorders. Susceptibility, rather than the disorder itself, may be inherited. In susceptible people, a trigger, such as a viral infection or tissue damage, may cause the disorder to develop. Hormonal factors may also be involved, because many autoimmune disorders are more common among women.

Symptoms and Diagnosis

Autoimmune disorders commonly cause a fever. However, symptoms vary depending on the disorder and the part of the body affected. Some autoimmune disorders affect certain types of tissue throughout the body—for example, blood vessels, cartilage, or skin. Other autoimmune disorders affect a particular organ. Virtually any organ, including the kidneys, lungs, heart, and brain, can be affected. The resulting inflammation and tissue damage can cause pain, deformed joints, weakness,

---

▲ see page 1064   ■ see page 1050

SOME AUTOIMMUNE DISORDERS

DISORDER	MAIN TISSUES AFFECTED	CONSEQUENCES
Autoimmune hemolytic anemia	Red blood cells	Anemia with fatigue, weakness, and light-headedness develops, and the spleen enlarges. The anemia can be severe and even fatal.
Bullous pemphigoid	Skin	Large blisters, surrounded by red, swollen areas, form on the skin. Itching is common. With treatment, the prognosis is good.
Graves' disease	Thyroid gland	The thyroid gland is inflamed, stimulated, and enlarged, resulting in high levels of thyroid hormones (hyperthyroidism). With treatment, the prognosis is good.
Hashimoto's thyroiditis	Thyroid gland	The thyroid gland is inflamed and damaged, resulting in low levels of thyroid hormones (hypothyroidism). Lifelong treatment with thyroid hormone is necessary.
Type 1 diabetes	Beta cells of pancreas (which produce insulin)	The beta cells are destroyed, so the body lacks insulin. Treatment with insulin is needed lifelong even if the reaction terminates because the cells in the pancreas have been destroyed.
Lupus (systemic lupus erythematosus)	Joints, kidneys, skin, lungs, heart, and brain	The affected tissues are inflamed and often damaged, but the joints, although inflamed, do not become deformed. The prognosis varies widely, but most people can lead an active life despite occasional flare-ups of the disorder.
Myasthenia gravis	The connection between nerves and muscles (neuromuscular junction)	Muscles, particularly those of the eyes, weaken and tire easily, but the weakness varies in intensity. The pattern of progression varies widely, but drugs can usually control the symptoms. Rarely, the disorder is fatal.
Pemphigus	Skin	Large blisters form on the skin. The disorder can be life threatening.
Pernicious anemia	Cells in the stomach's lining and red and white blood cells	Because the stomach's lining is damaged, it is less able to absorb vitamin B_{12} (which is necessary for the production of mature blood cells). Anemia results, and nerves are damaged. Without treatment, the spinal cord may be damaged. The risk of stomach cancer is increased. Otherwise, with treatment, the prognosis is good.

jaundice, itching, difficulty breathing, accumulation of fluid (edema), delirium, and even death.

Blood tests may detect an autoimmune disorder. For example, the erythrocyte sedimentation rate (ESR) is often increased, because proteins, produced in response to inflammation, interfere with the ability of red blood cells (erythrocytes) to remain suspended in blood. Typically, the number of red blood cells is decreased, resulting in anemia. Blood tests can also detect different antibodies, some of which typically occur in people who have an autoimmune disorder. Examples of these antibodies are antinuclear antibodies (which attack the nuclei of cells) and rheumatoid factor.

Treatment

Treatment involves control of the autoimmune reaction by suppressing the immune system. However, many of the drugs used to control the autoimmune reaction interfere with the body's ability to fight disease, especially infections. Treatment to relieve symptoms may also be needed.

Drugs that suppress the immune system (immunosuppressants), such as azathioprine, chlorambucil, cyclophosphamide, cyclosporine, or methotrexate, are often given, usually by mouth and often for a long time.▲ However, these drugs suppress not only the autoimmune reaction but also the body's ability to defend itself against foreign substances, including microorganisms that cause infection and cancer cells. Consequently, the risk of infection and of certain cancers increases.

Often, corticosteroids, such as prednisone, are given, usually by mouth. These drugs relieve inflammation as well as suppress the immune system. Corticosteroids given for a long time have many side effects.■ When possible, corticosteroids are used for a short time—when the disorder begins or when symptoms

worsen. However, corticosteroids must sometimes be used indefinitely.

Etanercept and infliximab block the action of tumor necrosis factor (TNF), a substance that can cause inflammation in the body. These drugs are very effective in treating rheumatoid arthritis and inflammatory bowel disease, but they may be harmful if used to treat certain other autoimmune disorders, such as multiple sclerosis.

Plasmapheresis is used to treat a few autoimmune disorders. Blood is withdrawn and filtered to remove the abnormal antibodies. Then the filtered blood is returned to the person.

Some autoimmune disorders resolve as inexplicably as they began. However, most autoimmune disorders are chronic. Drugs are often required throughout life to control symptoms. The prognosis varies depending on the disorder.

CHAPTER 187

Transplantation

Transplantation is the transfer of living cells, tissues, or organs from one person to another or from one part of the body to another.

The most common type of transplantation is a blood transfusion,★ which is used to treat millions of people each year. Some organs or tissues can also be transplanted.

Tissues or organs come from a donor. A donor can be a living person or a person who has recently died. Tissues and organs from a living donor are preferable because transplantation is more likely to be successful. However, some organs, such as the heart, obviously cannot be taken from a living donor.

Stem cells (from bone marrow or blood) and kidneys are the tissues most often donated by a living donor. Usually, a kidney can be safely donated because the body has two kidneys and can function well with only one. Living donors can also donate a part of the liver or a lung. An organ from a living donor is transplanted within minutes of being removed.

After a person dies, organs deteriorate quickly. Consequently, organs from a donor who has died usually come from a person who was expected to die and who had previously agreed to donate organs. Permission for donation may be given by the person's closest family member. Often, such donors are otherwise healthy people who have been in a major accident, rather than those who die of a disorder. Sometimes one donor can provide several people with transplants. For example, one donor could provide two people with corneas, two with kidneys, one with a liver, two with lungs, and another with a heart. Some organs last only a few hours outside the body. Other organs, if kept cold, last up to several days.

In the United States, a national organization (United Network for Organ Sharing) matches

---

▲ see table on page 1078   ■ see box on page 374
★ see page 982

donors and recipients for transplantation through the use of a computer database. The database includes all people who are on a waiting list for a transplant, along with their tissue type. When organs become available, that information is entered and a match is made. Thus, transplantation can be performed without delay. In many states, people can indicate the wish to donate organs when they register with the Department of Motor Vehicles. This wish is recorded on their driver's license. In the United States, being paid to donate an organ is illegal.

Principles of Organ Transplantation

Organ transplantation, unlike a blood transfusion, involves major surgery, the use of drugs to suppress the immune system (immunosuppressants), and the possibility of transplant rejection and serious complications, including death. However, for people whose vital organs malfunction irreversibly, organ transplantation may offer the only chance of a normal life or of survival.

Tissue Matching

Matching the tissues of an organ donor and those of the recipient is desirable because the immune system normally attacks foreign tissue,▲ including transplants. This reaction is called rejection. However, tissue matching may have to be balanced with other factors that affect the quality of the transplant, such as the time involved in reaching the recipient. Some people are too ill to wait for a highly compatible donor. For organs (such as the heart) that cannot be donated by a living family member, a highly compatible donor is rarely available. With the use of immunosuppressants, the success of transplantation is less affected by the compatibility of the donor. Consequently, transplants, even of organs (such as a kidney) that may be donated by a living family member who is highly compatible, may come from less compatible donors. Nonetheless, doctors try to find a donor whose tissue type matches the recipient's tissue type as closely as possible. A close match reduces the severity of rejection and improves the long-term outcome for the recipient.

Tissue type is determined by molecules on the surface of every cell in the body. These

molecules are called human leukocyte antigens (HLA) or the major histocompatibility complex. Each person has unique HLAs. When a person receives a transplant, the HLAs on the cells of the transplant signal the body that the tissue is foreign, stimulating an immune response.

For blood transfusions, matching is relatively simple, because red blood cells have only three main antigens on their surface—A, B, and Rh. For organ transplantation, many antigens are involved.

The recipient's blood is screened for antibodies against the tissues of the specific potential donor. The body may produce such antibodies in response to a blood transfusion, a previous transplantation, or a pregnancy. If these antibodies are present, transplantation is usually not performed, because immediate, severe rejection often results.

Suppression of the Immune System

Even if tissue types are closely matched, transplanted organs, unlike transfused blood, are usually rejected unless measures are taken to prevent rejection. Rejection results not only in destruction of the transplanted organ but also in fever, chills, nausea, fatigue, and sudden changes in blood pressure. Rejection, if it occurs, usually begins soon after transplantation but can occur after weeks, months, or even years. Rejection can be mild and easily controlled or severe, worsening despite treatment.

Rejection can usually be controlled by using drugs called immunosuppressants, which suppress the immune system and the body's ability to recognize and destroy foreign substances. With the use of these drugs, transplantation is more likely to be successful. However, while immunosuppressants suppress the immune system's reaction to the transplanted organ, they also reduce the ability of the immune system to fight infections and perhaps to destroy cancer cells. Thus, transplant recipients are at increased risk of developing infections and certain cancers.

Many different types of immunosuppressants can be used to prevent or control rejection. Most of them, including corticosteroids, suppress the immune system as a whole. Antilymphocyte globulin, antithymocyte globulin, and monoclonal antibodies suppress only specific parts of the immune system.

Immunosuppressants must be taken indefinitely. However, high doses are usually neces-

▲ see page 1050

sary only during the first few weeks after transplantation or during an episode of rejection. After that, smaller doses can usually prevent rejection. At the first sign of rejection, doctors increase the dose of the immunosuppressant, change the type of immunosuppressant, or use more than one immunosuppressant.

Sometimes radiation is directed at the transplant and surrounding tissue to suppress the immune system. Before bone marrow transplantation in people with leukemia, radiation of the whole body is necessary to destroy the bone marrow, which is producing cancer cells. Radiation of all lymph nodes (total lymphatic irradiation) appears to be a safe, effective way to suppress the immune system, but this treatment is still being studied.

Kidney Transplantation

For people of all ages whose kidneys do not function despite other treatments (irreversible kidney failure), kidney transplantation is a lifesaving alternative to dialysis. In the United States, about 11,000 kidneys are transplanted each year. About 90% of kidneys obtained from living donors are functioning 1 year after transplantation; 3 to 5% of these kidneys stop functioning during each year that follows. About 70 to 90% of kidneys from someone who has just died are functioning after 1 year; 5 to 8% stop functioning during each year that follows. Transplanted kidneys sometimes function for more than 30 years. People with successful kidney transplants can usually lead normal, active lives.

More than two thirds of transplanted kidneys come from people who have died, usually in an accident. The kidneys are removed, cooled, and transported quickly to a medical center for transplantation to a person who has a compatible tissue type and whose blood does not contain antibodies to the tissues of the donor.

Kidney transplantation is a major operation. The donated kidney is placed in the pelvis through an incision and is attached to the recipient's blood vessels and bladder. Usually, the nonfunctioning kidneys are left in place. Occasionally, they are removed because they are causing uncontrollable high blood pressure or are infected.

Despite the use of immunosuppressants, one or more episodes of rejection often occur shortly after transplantation. Rejection of a kidney may cause fever as well as weight gain due to fluid retention (because the kidneys are not removing enough fluids from the bloodstream). The area over the transplanted kidney may be tender and swollen, less urine may be produced, and blood pressure may increase. Blood tests can detect deteriorating kidney function. If doctors are not sure whether the kidney is being rejected, they can perform a biopsy using a needle.

Rejection can usually be stopped by increasing the dose of the immunosuppressant, changing the type, or using more than one immunosuppressant. If rejection cannot be stopped, the transplantation is unsuccessful. The rejected kidney may be left in place unless fever, tenderness, blood in the urine, or high blood pressure persists. When transplantation is unsuccessful, dialysis must be started again. Often, another kidney can be transplanted after the person has recovered from the first attempt. The chance of success with second transplants is almost as good as that with first transplants.

Rejection and other complications usually occur within 3 to 4 months of transplantation. After that, the recipient continues to take immunosuppressants indefinitely, unless they cause side effects or a severe infection develops. If immunosuppressants are discontinued even briefly, the body could reject the new kidney. Rejection that develops over many weeks or months is relatively common and may cause kidney function to gradually deteriorate.

Compared with the general population, kidney transplant recipients are 10 to 15 times more likely to develop cancer, probably because the drugs needed to prevent rejection of the transplanted kidney also suppress the immune system, which helps defend the body against cancer. Kidney transplant recipients are about 30 times more likely to develop cancer of the lymphatic system (lymphoma) than the general population. However, even among kidney transplant recipients, this cancer is still relatively uncommon.

Liver Transplantation

Liver transplantation is the only option for people whose liver can no longer function. A complete liver can be obtained only from a person who has died, but a living donor can provide a part of the liver. A donated liver can be stored for 8 to 15 hours, sometimes up to 24

℞   DRUGS USED TO PREVENT TRANSPLANT REJECTION

TYPE	DRUG	POSSIBLE SIDE EFFECTS	COMMENTS

Corticosteroids
(potent anti-inflammatory drugs that suppress the immune system as a whole)

	Dexamethasone Prednisolone Prednisone	High blood sugar levels (as occur in diabetes mellitus), muscle weakness, osteoporosis, water retention, stomach ulcers, a puffy face, fragile skin, and excess hair on the face	Given by vein in a high dose at the time of transplantation; then gradually reduced to a maintenance dose given by mouth, usually indefinitely

Globulins
(natural substances produced by the body that suppress specific parts of the immune system)

	Antilymphocyte globulin Antithymocyte globulin	Severe allergic (anaphylactic) reactions with fever and chills, usually occurring only after the first or second dose	Given by vein; used with other immunosuppressants so that the other immunosuppressant can be started later or its dose can be reduced (to reduce side effects)

Macrolide immunosuppressants
(drugs that suppress specific parts of the immune system)

	Sirolimus	Increased cholesterol levels, high blood pressure, rash, anemia, joint pain, diarrhea, low potassium levels, and increased risk of lymphoma	Taken by mouth and used with corticosteroids or cyclosporine in people who have received a kidney transplant
	Tacrolimus	Tremor, headache, diarrhea, high blood pressure, nausea, liver and kidney damage, insomnia, an enlarged heart, and increased risk of lymphoma	Given by vein or by mouth at the time of transplantation or later; used as an alternative to cyclosporine in people who have received a liver transplant

Mitotic inhibitors
(drugs that suppress cell division and thus the production of white blood cells)

	Azathioprine	Fatigue, increased risk of infection, a tendency to bleed, nausea, vomiting, hepatitis (rarely), and a low white blood cell count	Given by vein or by mouth at the time of transplantation and often continued indefinitely sometimes at a reduced dose; may be used with cyclosporine
	Cyclophospha-mide	Fatigue, increased risk of infection, a tendency to bleed, nausea, vomiting, hair loss, bladder inflammation (cystitis) with bleeding, and infertility	Given by vein or by mouth; used for people who cannot tolerate azathioprine; used in high doses in people who have received a bone marrow transplant
	Methotrexate	Fatigue, increased risk of infection, a tendency to bleed, nausea, vomiting, mouth sores, digestive upset, general feeling of illness, chills, fever, and dizziness	Given by mouth or injected in muscle

℞ DRUGS USED TO PREVENT TRANSPLANT REJECTION (Cont'd)

TYPE	DRUG	POSSIBLE SIDE EFFECTS	COMMENTS
Monoclonal antibodies (substances that target and suppress specific parts of the immune system)			
	Basiliximab Daclizumab Infliximab Muromonab (OKT3)	Severe allergic (anaphylactic) reactions, fever, shaking (rigors), muscle and joint pain, irritation of the digestive tract, seizures, and drug tolerance (the drug becomes less effective for subsequent rejection episodes); severe side effects usually only occur after the first few doses	Given by vein at the time of a rejection episode or transplantation
Fungal metabolite (a substance that is produced by a fungus and that inhibits the activity of T lymphocytes)			
	Cyclosporine	Liver and kidney damage, high blood pressure, tremor, enlarged gums, excessive hairiness (hirsutism), and increased risk of cancer	Given by vein at first, then by mouth; usually given with azathioprine or prednisone
Others			
	Glatiramer acetate	Inflammation at the site of injection, chest pain, weakness, infection, pain, nausea, and joint pain	Injected under the skin; used in people who have received liver transplants
	Mycophenolate mofetil	Diarrhea, a blood infection (sepsis), nausea, vomiting, and increased risk of lymphoma	Given by vein at first, then by mouth; used with corticosteroids or cyclosporine

hours. Some people die while waiting for a compatible liver to become available.

About 80% of liver transplant recipients survive for at least 1 year. Most recipients are people whose liver was destroyed by primary biliary cirrhosis, hepatitis, or use of a drug toxic to the liver (such as high doses of acetaminophen). People whose liver has been destroyed by alcoholism can receive a transplant if they stop drinking. In people who have primary biliary cirrhosis, liver transplantation is often lifesaving. In people who have liver cancer, liver transplantation is rarely successful. The cancer usually returns in the transplanted liver or elsewhere. Fewer than 20% of recipients who have liver cancer survive for even 1 year. In people who have viral hepatitis, the virus tends to infect the transplanted liver.

The damaged liver is removed through an incision in the abdomen. Then the donated liver is put in place and connected to the recipient's blood vessels and bile ducts. Usually, blood transfusions are required. Typically, the operation lasts $4\frac{1}{2}$ hours or more, and the hospital stay is 7 to 12 days.

Liver transplants are rejected somewhat less vigorously than transplants of other organs, such as the kidney and heart. Nonetheless, immunosuppressants must be taken after transplantation. If the recipient develops an enlarged liver, nausea, pain, fever, jaundice, or abnormal liver function (detected by blood tests), doctors may perform a biopsy using a needle. Biopsy results help doctors determine whether the liver is being rejected and whether immunosuppressant therapy should be adjusted.

Heart Transplantation

Heart transplantation is reserved for people who have severe heart failure and who cannot be treated effectively with drugs or other forms of surgery. In some medical centers, heart machines can keep people alive for weeks or months until a compatible heart can be found. Also, newly developed, implantable artifical hearts are being used to tide people over until a heart is available or, in some experimental situations, to be used as a long-term replacement. Nonetheless, many people die while waiting.

About 95% of people who have had a heart transplant are substantially better able to exercise and perform daily activities than they were before the transplantation. About 85% of heart transplant recipients survive for at least 1 year.

Through an incision in the chest, most of the damaged heart is removed, but the back walls of the upper heart chambers (atria) are left. The donated heart is then attached to what remains of the recipient's heart. The procedure takes about 3 to 5 hours. The hospital stay after this operation is usually 7 to 14 days.

Immunosuppressants must be taken to prevent rejection of a transplanted heart. Rejection, if it occurs, usually causes fever, weakness, and a rapid or other abnormal heart rhythm. Because the transplanted heart is not functioning well, blood pressure falls, and fluid accumulates in the limbs, especially the legs, and sometimes the abdomen, causing swelling—a condition called edema. Fluid may also accumulate in the lungs. If rejection is mild, no symptoms may occur, but electrocardiography (ECG) may detect changes in the heart's electrical activity. If doctors suspect rejection, they usually perform a biopsy. A catheter is inserted through an incision in the neck into a vein and is threaded to the heart. A device at the end of the catheter is used to remove a small piece of heart tissue, which is examined under a microscope. If doctors find evidence of rejection, they increase the dose of the immunosuppressant, change the type, or use more than one immunosuppressant.

Nearly half of all deaths that occur after heart transplantation are due to infections. About one fourth of people who have a heart transplant develop atherosclerosis in the coronary arteries.

Lung and Heart-Lung Transplantation

Usually, one lung is transplanted, but two lungs can be transplanted. When a lung disor-

der has also damaged the heart, one or both lungs and a heart may be transplanted at the same time. Because preserving a lung for transplantation is difficult, lung transplantation must be performed as soon as possible after a lung has been obtained.

Lung transplants can come from a living donor or from someone who has recently died. A living donor cannot donate more than one entire lung and usually donates only one lobe. A person who has died can provide both lungs or the heart and lungs.

Through an incision in the chest, the recipient's lung or lungs are removed and replaced with those of the donor. The blood vessels to and from the lung (pulmonary artery and pulmonary vein) and the main airway (bronchus) are connected to the transplanted lung or lungs. The operation takes 4 to 8 hours for one lung and 6 to 12 hours for two lungs. A heart and lung may be transplanted at the same time. The hospital stay after these operations is usually 7 to 14 days.

About 70% of people who receive a lung transplant survive for at least 1 year. The risk of infection is high because the lungs are continually exposed to air, which contains bacteria and other microorganisms that can cause disease. The site at which the airway is attached sometimes heals poorly. Scar tissue may form, narrowing the airway, reducing air flow, and causing shortness of breath. Treatment of this complication consists of widening (dilating) the airway—for example, by placing a stent (a wire-mesh tube) in the airway.

Rejection of a lung transplant can be difficult to detect, evaluate, and treat. More than 80% of people who receive a lung transplant develop some symptoms of rejection within a month of transplantation. Symptoms include fever, shortness of breath, and weakness. Weakness develops because the transplanted lung cannot provide enough oxygen to supply the body. Later, scar tissue may form in the small airways and gradually block them, possibly indicating gradual rejection. Rejection of a lung transplant may be controlled by increasing the dose of an immunosuppressant, changing the type, or using more than one immunosuppressant.

Pancreas Transplantation

The entire pancreas or only the cells that produce insulin (islet cells) may be transplanted. Islet cell transplants may consist of the person's own cells (a procedure called islet cell autotransplantation) or cells from another person (a procedure called islet cell allotransplantation). A person's own islet cells can sometimes be used to prevent diabetes from developing when the pancreas must be removed—for example, in people who have chronic pancreatitis causing pain that is difficult to control. Transplantation of another person's islet cells or sometimes the entire pancreas is used to treat people who have diabetes that is difficult to control and has not yet caused serious complications. However, this procedure may have other uses in the future.

Transplantation of an entire pancreas is a major operation, requiring an incision into the abdomen and a general anesthetic. The recipient's pancreas is not removed. Typically, the operation takes about 3 hours and the hospital stay is about 1 to 3 weeks.

In contrast, transplantation of islet cells is not a major operation and requires only a local anesthetic and no hospital stay or only a brief one. Islet cells may be injected through a thin needle into the recipient's umbilical vein in the abdomen or through a tube inserted into a vein to the liver.

More than 80% of people with diabetes who receive a pancreas transplant and about 75% of those who receive an islet cell transplant have normal blood sugar levels afterward and do not need to use insulin. However, people who receive a pancreas or islet cell transplant from another person must take immunosuppressants—a major disadvantage because these drugs increase the risk of infection and have other side effects. Thus, the risk of taking insulin (which can cause abnormally low blood sugar levels) and having less control of diabetes is traded for the risk of taking immunosuppressants (which increases the risk of infection) and having better control of diabetes. Because of the risk of taking immunosuppressants, these transplantations have usually been reserved for people who are already taking immunosuppressants for another reason—for example, those who have received a kidney transplant because of kidney failure. The pancreas and kidney are often transplanted at the same time.

Stem Cell Transplantation

Stem cells are unspecialized cells from which all specialized cells are derived. Adults,

What Are Stem Cells?

Stem cells are undifferentiated cells. That means that they have the potential to become one of many different kinds of specialized cells. Some stem cells can be triggered to become any kind of cell in the body. Others are already partially differentiated; these stem cells can become, for example, any kind of nerve or glandular cell. Stem cells divide, producing more stem cells, until they are triggered to specialize. Then as they continue to divide, they become more and more specialized until they lose the ability to be anything but one kind of cell. Stem cells produce all the cells in the body—over 200 types of cells, including blood, nerve, muscle, heart, glandular, and skin cells.

Researchers think that stem cells can be directed to repair or replace cells or tissues damaged or destroyed by such disorders as Alzheimer's disease, Parkinson's disease, diabetes, and spinal injuries. Stem cells can be directed by stimulating the genetic code that causes them to specialize. Stem cells can be obtained from four sources (but other sources may soon be discovered):

Embryos: Stem cells are taken from embryos produced in fertility clinics by test tube (in vitro) fertilization. Sperm from the man and several eggs from the woman are placed in a culture dish. The sperm fertilizes the egg and the resulting cell divides, forming an embryo. Several of the healthiest-looking embryos are placed in the woman's uterus. The rest are discarded or frozen to be used later if needed. Stem cells can be obtained from the embryos that are not used. In the process, the embryos are destroyed. For this reason, the use of stem cells from embryos is controversial. Researchers think that these stem cells have the most potential for producing different kinds of cells and for surviving after being transplanted.

Fetuses: After 8 weeks of development, the embryo is called a fetus. Stem cells can be obtained from fetuses that have been miscarried or aborted.

Umbilical Cord: Stem cells can be obtained from the blood in the umbilical cord or placenta after a baby is born. These stem cells can produce only blood cells.

Children and Adults: The bone marrow and blood of children and adults contain stem cells. These stem cells can produce only blood cells. Currently, the only stem cells used for transplantation are these cells.

Corneal Transplants and Why They Usually Work

Corneal transplantation is a common and highly successful type of transplantation. A scarred or cloudy cornea can be replaced with a clear, healthy one using a microscopic surgical procedure that takes about 1 hour. Donated corneas come from people who have recently died. A general or local anesthetic is used. The donated cornea is cut to the right size, the damaged cornea is removed, and the donated cornea is sewn in place. The recipient usually stays in the hospital 1 or 2 nights but may go home the same day.

A cornea is rarely rejected because it does not have its own blood supply. It receives oxygen and other nutrients from nearby tissues and fluid. The components of the immune system that initiate rejection in response to a foreign substance—certain white blood cells and antibodies—are carried in the bloodstream. Thus, these cells and antibodies do not reach the transplanted cornea, do not encounter the foreign tissue there, and do not initiate rejection. Tissues with a rich blood supply are much more likely to be rejected.

as well as embryos, have stem cells. Stem cells for different kinds of blood cells can be obtained from the bone marrow or, in small numbers, from the blood. Stem cells obtained from fetuses are thought to be best because they are more likely to survive transplantation than those obtained from children or adults. **Bone marrow transplantation** is one type of stem cell transplantation, because bone marrow contains stem cells that produce more blood cells.

Stem cell transplantation can be used as part of the treatment of leukemia, certain types of lymphoma (including Hodgkin's disease), and aplastic anemia. It can also be used to treat children with certain genetic disorders, including thalassemia, sickle cell anemia, and some congenital metabolic or immunodeficiency disorders (such as chronic granulomatous disease). Certain types of stem cells can also be used as transplants for people whose bone marrow is destroyed by high doses

of chemotherapy or radiation therapy used to treat cancers such as breast cancer. Stem cell transplantation may become useful for treating other disorders, such as Parkinson's disease and Alzheimer's disease, in which the transplanted stem cells can become brain cells.

Stem cells may be the person's own cells (a procedure called autologous transplantation) or those of a donor (a procedure called allogeneic transplantation). When the person's own stem cells are used, they are collected before chemotherapy or radiation therapy because these treatments can damage stem cells. They are injected back into the body after the treatment.

For bone marrow transplantation, the donor is usually given a general anesthetic. Then a doctor removes marrow from the donor's hip bone with a syringe. Removal of bone marrow takes about 1 hour.

Sometimes stem cells from adults are obtained from blood in an outpatient procedure. First, the donor is given a drug that causes the bone marrow to release more stem cells into the bloodstream. Then blood is removed through a catheter inserted in one arm and is circulated through a machine that removes stem cells. The rest of the blood is returned to the person through a catheter inserted in the other arm. Usually, about six 2- to 4-hour sessions during a period of 1 to 2 weeks are required to obtain enough stem cells. Stem cells can be preserved for later use by freezing them.

The doctor injects the stem cells into the recipient's vein. The injected stem cells migrate to and begin to multiply in the recipient's bones and produce blood cells.

Stem cell transplantation is risky because the recipient's white blood cells have been destroyed or reduced in number by chemotherapy or radiation therapy. As a result, the risk of infection is very high for about 2 to 3 weeks—until the donated stem cells can produce enough white blood cells to protect against infections.

Another problem is that the new bone marrow obtained from another person may produce cells that attack the recipient's cells, causing graft-versus-host disease.▲ Furthermore, the original disorder may recur.

The risk of infection can be reduced by keeping the recipient in isolation for a period of time (until the transplanted cells begin to produce blood cells). During this time, staff

▲ see page 986

members and visitors must wear masks and gowns and wash their hands thoroughly before entering the room. Antibodies isolated from the donor's blood may be given intravenously to the recipient to help protect against infection. Growth factors, which stimulate the production of blood cells, can help reduce the risk of infection and graft-versus-host disease.

Recipients of a stem cell transplant usually remain in the hospital for 1 to 2 months. After discharge from the hospital, follow-up visits are necessary at regular intervals. Most people need at least 1 year to recover.

Transplantation of Other Organs

Skin grafts can be used in people who have lost large areas of skin—for example, because of extensive burns. Skin grafting is most successful when healthy skin is removed from one part of the body and grafted to another part. When such grafting is not possible, skin from a donor or even from animals (such as pigs) can be used as a temporary measure. Such grafts last only a short time, but they can provide temporary protection until normal skin grows to replace them. The amount of skin available for grafting may be increased by growing small pieces of the person's skin in a tissue culture or by making many tiny cuts in the grafted skin, so that it can be stretched to cover a much larger area.

Cartilage may be transplanted successfully without the use of immunosuppressants. The body's immune system attacks transplanted cartilage much less vigorously than other tissues. In children, cartilage is usually used to repair defects in the ears or nose. In adults, it can be used to repair joints damaged by arthritis.

Corneas, the transparent domes on the surface of the eyes, can usually be transplanted successfully without the use of immunosuppressants.

Bone from one part of the body can be used to replace bone in another part. Bone transplanted from one person to another survives only a short time. However, it stimulates

Reattaching a Body Part

If fingers, hands, and arms are relatively undamaged after being severed from the body, they can sometimes be reattached successfully. Reattachment of legs is less successful. The severed part is kept clean and is packed in ice until it can be used. Prompt reattachment is crucial so that the blood supply to the severed part can be restored. Rarely, transplantation of such parts from one person to another has been attempted, but this technique is experimental.

growth of new bone, stabilizes the area until new bone can form, and provides a framework for new bone to fill in.

Transplantation of the small intestine is experimental. It may be used as a last resort when the intestine has been destroyed by a disorder or does not function well enough to sustain life. Because the small intestine contains a large amount of lymphatic tissue, the new intestinal tissue may produce cells that attack the recipient's cells, causing graft-versus-host disease.

Parkinson's disease can be treated by transplanting tissue from a person's adrenal glands to that person's brain. Alternatively, brain tissue from aborted fetuses can be used. Both procedures can relieve symptoms. However, whether using tissue from aborted fetuses is ethically acceptable is controversial.

Thymus glands from aborted or miscarried fetuses can be transplanted into children who are born without a thymus gland (a disorder called DiGeorge anomaly). When the thymus gland is missing, the immune system is impaired, because white blood cells, which are a vital part of the immune system's defense against foreign substances, mature in the thymus gland. Transplantation of a thymus gland restores the impaired immune system in these children. However, the new thymus may produce cells that attack the recipient's cells, causing graft-versus-host-disease.

SECTION 17

INFECTIONS

188 Biology of Infectious Disease.................................**1086**

Resident Flora ▪ How Infection Develops ▪ The Body's
Defenses Against Infection ▪ Prevention of Infection ▪
Infections in People With Impaired Defenses

189 Immunization.................................**1092**

Common Vaccinations ▪ Vaccination Before Foreign Travel

190 Bacterial Infections.................................**1095**

Actinomycosis ▪ Anthrax ▪ Bejel, Yaws, and Pinta ▪
Campylobacter Infections ▪ Cholera ▪ Gas Gangrene ▪
Enterobacteriaceae Infections ▪ *Haemophilus* Infections ▪
Leptospirosis ▪ Listeriosis ▪ Lyme Disease ▪ Plague ▪
Pneumococcal Infections ▪ *Pseudomonas* Infections ▪
Salmonella Infections ▪ Shigellosis ▪ Staphylococcal
Infections ▪ Streptococcal Infections ▪ Tetanus ▪ Toxic
Shock Syndrome ▪ Tularemia ▪ Typhoid Fever

191 Bacteremia, Sepsis, and Septic Shock.................................**1118**

192 Antibiotics.................................**1120**

193 Tuberculosis.................................**1125**

194 Leprosy.................................**1130**

195 Rickettsial and Ehrlichial Infections.................................**1132**

Rocky Mountain Spotted Fever ▪ Ehrlichioses

196 Parasitic Infections.................................**1135**

Amebiasis ▪ Ascariasis ▪ Babesiosis ▪ Cryptosporidiosis ▪
Giardiasis ▪ Hookworm Infection ▪ Malaria ▪ Pinworm
Infection ▪ Schistosomiasis ▪ Tapeworm Infection ▪
Toxocariasis ▪ Toxoplasmosis ▪ Trichinosis ▪ Whipworm
Infection

197 Fungal Infections.................................**1148**

Aspergillosis ▪ Blastomycosis ▪ Candidiasis ▪
Coccidioidomycosis ▪ Cryptococcosis ▪ Histoplasmosis ▪
Mucormycosis ▪ Paracoccidioidomycosis ▪ Sporotrichosis

198   Viral Infections **1154**

Common Cold ▪ Influenza ▪ Herpes Simplex Virus
Infections ▪ Shingles ▪ Epstein-Barr Virus Infection ▪
Cytomegalovirus Infection ▪ Hemorrhagic Fevers ▪
Hantavirus Infection ▪ Yellow Fever ▪ Dengue Fever

199   Human Immunodeficiency Virus Infection **1168**

200   Sexually Transmitted Diseases **1176**

Syphilis ▪ Gonorrhea ▪ Nongonococcal Urethritis and
Chlamydial Cervicitis ▪ Lymphogranuloma Venereum ▪
Chancroid ▪ Granuloma Inguinale ▪ Trichomoniasis ▪
Genital Warts ▪ Other Sexually Transmitted Diseases

CHAPTER 188

Biology of Infectious Disease

Microorganisms are tiny living creatures, such as bacteria and viruses. Microorganisms are present everywhere. Despite their overwhelming abundance, relatively few of the thousands of species of microorganisms invade, multiply, and produce illness in people.

Many microorganisms live on the skin and in the mouth, upper airways, intestine, and genitals (particularly the vagina) without causing disease. Whether a microorganism lives as a harmless companion to a person or invades and causes disease depends on the nature of the microorganism and on the state of the person's natural defenses.

Resident Flora

A healthy person lives in harmony with most microorganisms that establish themselves on (colonize) the body. The microorganisms that usually occupy a particular body site are called the resident flora. The resident flora at each site includes several different types of microorganisms; some sites are normally colonized by several hundred different types of microorganisms. Rather than causing disease, the resident flora often protects the body against disease-causing organisms. If disturbed, the resident flora promptly reestablishes itself. Microorganisms that colonize the host for hours to weeks but do not establish themselves permanently are called transient flora.

Environmental factors—such as diet, sanitary conditions, air pollution, and hygienic habits—influence what species make up a person's resident flora. Under certain conditions, microorganisms that are part of a person's resident flora may cause disease. Such conditions include the use of antibiotics and a weakening of the immune system (as occurs in people with AIDS and cancer, people taking corticosteroids, and those receiving chemotherapy). When antibiotics used to treat an infection kill a large proportion of the resident flora of the skin, vagina, or intestine, other resident bacteria or fungi can grow without being held in check. An example is a vaginal yeast infection occurring in a woman taking antibiotics for a bladder infection.

How Infection Develops

Infectious diseases are usually caused by microorganisms that invade the body and multiply. Invasion by most microorganisms begins when they adhere to a person's cells.

Adherence is a very specific process, involving "lock-and-key" connections between the microorganism and cells in the person's body. Whether the microorganism remains near the invasion site or spreads to other sites depends on such factors as whether it produces toxins, enzymes, or other substances.

Some microorganisms that invade the body produce toxins. For example, *Clostridium tetani* in an infected wound produces a toxin that causes tetanus. Some illnesses are caused by toxins produced by microorganisms outside the body. Food poisoning caused by staphylococci is one example. Most toxins contain components that bind specifically with molecules on certain cells (target cells). Toxins play a central role in such diseases as tetanus, toxic shock syndrome, botulism, anthrax, and cholera.

After invading the body, microorganisms must multiply to produce infection. After multiplication begins, one of three things can happen: the microorganisms can continue to multiply and overwhelm the body's defenses; a state of balance can be achieved, producing a chronic infection; or the body—with or without medical treatment—can destroy and eliminate the invading microorganism.

Many disease-causing microorganisms have properties that increase the severity of the diseases they cause (virulence) and help them resist the body's defense mechanisms. For example, some bacteria produce enzymes that break down tissue, allowing the infection to spread faster.

Some microorganisms have ways of blocking the body's defense mechanisms. For example, a microorganism may be able to interfere with the body's production of antibodies or T cells (a type of white blood cell) specifically armed to attack them. Others have outer coats (capsules) that resist being ingested by white blood cells. The fungus *Cryptococcus* actually develops a thicker capsule after it enters the lungs for the specific purpose of resisting the invaded body's defenses. Some bacteria resist being split open (lysed) by substances circulating in the bloodstream. Some even produce substances that counter the effects of antibiotics.

The Body's Defenses Against Infection

Physical barriers and the immune system defend the body against organisms that can

Types of Infectious Organisms

Bacteria: Bacteria are microscopic, single-celled organisms. Examples: *Streptococcus pyogenes* (strep throat); *Escherichia coli* (urinary tract infection).

Viruses: A virus is a small infectious organism—much smaller than a fungus or bacterium—that cannot reproduce on its own; it must invade a living cell and use that cell's machinery to reproduce. Examples: *Varicella zoster* (chickenpox, shingles); *Rhinovirus* (common cold).

Fungi: Fungi are actually a type of plant. Yeasts, molds, and mushrooms are all types of fungi. Examples: *Candida albicans* (vaginal yeast infection); *Tinea pedis* (athlete's foot).

Parasites: A parasite is an organism, such as a worm or single-celled animal (protozoan) that survives by living inside another, usually much larger, organism (the host). Examples: *Enterobius vermicularis* (pinworm); *Plasmodium falciparum* (malaria).

cause infection. Physical barriers include the skin, mucous membranes, tears, earwax, mucus, and stomach acid. Also, the normal flow of urine washes out microorganisms that enter the urinary tract. The immune system uses white blood cells and antibodies to identify and eliminate organisms that get through the body's physical barriers.▲

Physical Barriers

Usually, the skin prevents invasion by microorganisms unless it is damaged—for example, from an injury, insect bite, or burn. Other effective physical barriers are the mucous membranes, such as the linings of the mouth, nose, and eyelids. Typically, mucous membranes are coated with secretions that fight microorganisms. For example, the mucous membranes of the eyes are bathed in tears, which contain an enzyme called lysozyme that attacks bacteria and helps protect the eyes from infection.

The airways filter out particles that are present in the air that is breathed in. The walls of the passages in the nose and airways are coated with mucus. Microorganisms in the air

▲ see page 1049

Identifying an Infectious Organism

It is usually important to know what specific microorganism is causing an illness. Many different microorganisms can cause a given condition (for example, pneumonia can be caused by viruses, bacteria, or fungi), and the treatment is different for each organism.

There are many ways to identify microorganisms. Despite the development of rapid identification systems, direct microscopic examination of samples taken from the site of infection is often the most rapid method of identifying microorganisms capable of causing disease. But the microorganisms must be of sufficient size and number to be seen with a regular microscope. Sometimes microorganisms can be seen with a microscope and recognized by characteristic shapes and colors. Usually, however, the microorganisms are too few or too small to see, so they may be grown in the laboratory until there are enough to be recognized with chemical tests. The process of growing the organism is called a culture. Many microorganisms can be grown this way; such as the bacteria that cause gonorrhea and strep throat. Cultures can also be used to test the sensitivity of microorganisms to various antibiotics, which can help a doctor determine what drug to use in treating an infected person. This strategy is particularly important because microorganisms are constantly developing resistance to antibiotics that were previously effective.

Some microorganisms, such as the bacterium that causes syphilis and the virus that causes AIDS, are very difficult to culture. These infections, and many others, can be identified by finding antibodies to the microorganisms in the infected person's blood or body fluids (for example, cerebrospinal fluid). Antibody-based tests are used to identify many infections, but they are not always reliable. Antibodies often stay in the body for many years after an infection has gone away. New tests, such as the polymerase chain reaction (PCR), identify pieces of the microorganism's genetic material (DNA), which are only present when the organism is present.

These tests are performed only when a doctor already suspects a particular disease. Therefore, a doctor's understanding of all the features of a person's illness, including symptoms, physical examination, and risk factors, is essential for diagnosing an infection.

become stuck to the mucus, which is coughed up or blown out of the nose. Mucus removal is aided by the coordinated beating of tiny hairlike projections (cilia) that line the air passages. The cilia sweep the mucus up the airways, away from the lungs.

The digestive tract has a series of effective barriers, including stomach acid, pancreatic enzymes, bile, and intestinal secretions. The contractions of the intestine (peristalsis) and the normal shedding of cells lining the intestine help remove harmful microorganisms.

The bladder is protected by the urethra, the tube through which urine passes as it leaves the body. In males older than 6 months of age, the urethra is long enough that bacteria are seldom able to pass through it to reach the bladder, unless the bacteria are unintentionally placed there by catheters or surgical instruments. In females, the urethra is shorter, occasionally allowing for passage of external bacteria into the bladder. The flushing effect as the bladder empties is another defense mechanism in both sexes. The vagina is protected by its normal acidic environment.

The Blood

One way the body defends against infection is by increasing the number of certain types of white blood cells (neutrophils and monocytes), which engulf and destroy invading microorganisms. The increase can occur within several hours, largely because of the release of white blood cells from the bone marrow. The number of neutrophils increases first. If an infection persists, the number of monocytes increases. The number of eosinophils, another type of white blood cell, increases in allergic reactions and many parasitic infections, but usually not with bacterial infections.

Certain infections, such as typhoid fever, actually lead to a decrease in the white blood cell count, but how these infections do this is not known.

Inflammation

Any injury, including an invasion by microorganisms, causes a complex reaction called inflammation in the affected area. Inflammation occurs as a result of many different conditions. Through the release of different substances from the damaged tissue, inflammation directs the body's defenses to wall off the area, attack and kill any invaders, dispose of dead and damaged tissue, and begin

Biological Warfare and Terrorism

Biological warfare is the use of microbiological agents for hostile purposes. Such use is contrary to international law and in fact has rarely taken place during formal warfare in modern history, despite the extensive preparations and stockpiling of biological agents carried out in the 20th century by most major powers. Currently, the NATO nations have taken biological weapons out of service. Some other nations (including Iraq, Iran, and North Korea) are thought to maintain biological warfare capability. For a variety of reasons—including uncertain military efficacy and the threat of massive retaliation—experts consider the use of biological agents in formal warfare unlikely. However, biological agents are thought by some people to be an ideal weapon for terrorists. These agents may be delivered clandestinely, and they have delayed effects—allowing the user to remain undetected.

Potential biological agents include anthrax, botulism toxin, brucellosis, encephalitis viruses, hemorrhagic fever viruses (Ebola and Mar-

burg), plague, tularemia, and smallpox. Each of these is potentially fatal and, except for anthrax and botulism toxin, can be passed from person to person. Anthrax spores are relatively easy to prepare and, unlike most other agents, can be spread through the air, creating the potential for distribution by airplane. Theoretically, 1 kilogram of anthrax could kill 10,000 people, although technical difficulties with preparing the spores in a sufficiently fine powder would probably limit actual deaths to a fraction of this.

Despite these theoretical concerns, the only successful terrorist use of anthrax—multiple pieces of contaminated mail delivered to a variety of locations in the United States in 2001—resulted in only a handful of deaths and serious infections. A larger number of people were contaminated with anthrax spores without developing illness, possibly because of extensive use of the antibiotic ciprofloxacin. However, there was extreme public anxiety related to these incidents, which may have been a major goal of

the terror group responsible.

In addition to these actual infections, an even greater number of false threats of anthrax have been reported. In 1999, the FBI received an average of one false report per day of alleged anthrax use. False reports, both hoaxes and alarmed citizens misperceiving harmless material for anthrax, increased even more following the 2001 anthrax attack.

The only other successful use of a biological agent by a terror group in the United States occurred in 1984. In this event, 751 people were stricken with diarrhea resulting from the intentional contamination with *Salmonella* of a salad bar in Oregon. The bacteria were introduced by a religious cult trying to influence the results of a local election. No one died.

Defense against bioterrorism involves several factors: intelligence to disrupt the terrorists before they can use the weapons; early detection; availability of protective antibiotics; and immunization of selected populations (such as the military).

the process of repair. However, inflammation may not be able to overcome large numbers of microorganisms.

During inflammation, the blood supply increases. An infected area near the surface of the body becomes red and warm. The walls of blood vessels become more porous, allowing fluid and white blood cells to pass into the affected tissue. The increase in fluid causes the inflamed tissue to swell. The white blood cells attack the invading microorganisms and release substances that continue the process of inflammation. Other substances trigger clotting in the tiny vessels (capillaries) in the inflamed area, which delays the spread of the infecting microorganisms and their toxins. Many of the substances produced during in-

flammation stimulate the nerves, producing pain. Reactions to the substances released during inflammation include the chills, fever, and muscle aches that commonly accompany infection.

Immune Response

When an infection develops, the immune system responds by producing several substances and agents that are designed to attack the specific invading microorganisms.▲ For example, the immune system may create killer T cells (a type of white blood cell) that can recognize and kill the invading microor-

▲ see page 1049

ganism. Also, the immune system produces antibodies that are specific to the invading microorganism. Antibodies attach to and immobilize microorganisms—killing them outright or helping the neutrophils target and kill them.

Fever

Body temperature increases (fever) as a protective response to infection and injury. The elevated body temperature enhances the body's defense mechanisms, although it can cause discomfort for the person. Temperature is considered elevated when it is higher than 100° F as measured by an oral thermometer. Although 98.6° F is considered "normal" temperature, body temperature varies throughout the day, being lowest in the early morning and highest in the late afternoon—sometimes reaching 99.9° F.

A part of the brain called the hypothalamus controls body temperature. Fever results from an actual resetting of the hypothalamus's thermostat. The body raises its temperature to a higher level by moving (shunting) blood from the skin surface to the interior of the body, thus reducing heat loss. Shivering (chills) may occur to increase heat production through muscle contraction. The body's efforts to conserve and produce heat continue until blood reaches the hypothalamus at the new, higher temperature. The new, higher temperature is then maintained. Later, when the thermostat

is reset to its normal level, the body eliminates excess heat through sweating and shunting of blood to the skin.

Fever may follow a pattern: sometimes temperature peaks every day and then returns to normal. Alternatively, fever may be remittent, in which the temperature varies but does not return to normal. Certain people (for example, alcoholics, the very old, and the very young) may experience a *drop* in temperature as a response to severe infection.

Substances that cause fever are called pyrogens. Pyrogens can come from inside or outside the body. Microorganisms and the substances they produce (such as toxins) are examples of pyrogens formed outside the body. Pyrogens formed inside the body are usually produced by monocytes. Pyrogens from outside the body cause fever by stimulating the body to release its own pyrogens. However, infection is not the sole cause of fever; fever also may result from inflammation, cancer, or an allergic reaction.

Usually, fever has an obvious cause, which is often—but not always—an infection (such as influenza, pneumonia, a urinary tract infection, or some other infection) that a doctor can easily diagnose with a brief history, physical examination, and occasionally a few simple tests, such as a chest x-ray and urine tests. Sometimes, however, the cause is not readily discernible.

If fever continues for several days and has no obvious cause, a more detailed investigation is required. There are many potential causes of such a fever; common causes in adults include infections, diseases caused by antibodies against the person's own tissues (autoimmune diseases), and an undetected cancer (especially leukemia or lymphoma).

To determine the cause of a fever, a doctor begins by asking a person about present and previous symptoms and diseases, drugs currently being taken, exposure to infections, and recent travel. The pattern of the fever usually does not help with the diagnosis. There are, however, some exceptions: a fever that recurs every other day or every third day is typical of malaria.

Recent travel (especially overseas) may give clues to the cause of a fever, because some infections occur only in certain areas. For example, coccidioidomycosis (a fungal infection) occurs almost exclusively in the southwestern United States. A history of exposure to certain materials or animals also is important. For ex-

Some Causes of Fever

- Infection
- Cancer
- An allergic reaction
- Hormone disorders, such as pheochromocytoma or hyperthyroidism
- Autoimmune diseases, such as rheumatoid arthritis
- Excessive exercise, especially in hot weather
- Excessive exposure to the sun, especially in hot weather
- Certain drugs, including anesthetics, antipsychotics, and anticholinergics; also, overdoses of aspirin
- Damage to the hypothalamus (the part of the brain that controls temperature), such as from a brain injury or tumor

ample, a person who works in a meatpacking plant is more likely to develop brucellosis.

After asking questions, the doctor performs a thorough physical examination to find a source of infection or evidence of disease. Blood and other body fluids may be sent to the laboratory to try to grow the microorganism in a culture. Other blood tests can be used to detect antibodies against specific microorganisms. Increases in the white blood cell count usually indicate infection. The differential count (the proportion of different types of white blood cells) gives further clues. An increase in neutrophils, for example, suggests an acute bacterial infection. An increase in eosinophils suggests the presence of parasites—for example, tapeworms or roundworms.

When a person has a fever of at least 101° F for several weeks and extensive investigation fails to reveal a cause, a doctor may refer to it as a **fever of unknown origin.** In such cases, the cause may be an unusual chronic infection or something other than infection, such as a connective tissue disease, cancer, or some other disease. Ultrasonography, computed tomography (CT), or magnetic resonance imaging (MRI) may help a doctor diagnose the cause. Injection of white blood cells labeled with a radioactive marker can be used to identify areas of infection or inflammation. If these test results are negative, the doctor may need to obtain a biopsy specimen from the liver, bone marrow, or another suspected site. The specimen is then examined under a microscope and cultured.

Because fever helps the body defend against infection, there is some debate as to whether it should be routinely treated. However, a person with a high fever generally feels much better when the fever is treated.

Drugs used to lower body temperature are called antipyretics. The most effective and widely used antipyretics are acetaminophen and the nonsteroidal anti-inflammatory drugs (NSAIDs), such as aspirin and ibuprofen. However, aspirin should not be given to children and teenagers to treat a fever because it increases the risk of Reye's syndrome,▲ which can be fatal.

Prevention of Infection

Several steps help protect people against infection. Hand washing is an effective way of preventing the transmission of infectious microorganisms from one person to another.

Infection From Medical Devices

Usually, people think of infection as occurring when microorganisms invade the body and adhere to specific cells. But microorganisms can also adhere to medical devices placed in the body—such as catheters, artificial joints, and artificial heart valves—and begin to grow. The microorganisms may be present on the device when inserted if the device was accidentally contaminated. Or infecting organisms from another site may spread through the bloodstream and lodge on an already implanted device. Because implanted material has no natural defenses, it is easy for the microorganisms to grow and spread, causing illness.

Hand washing is particularly important for people who handle food or who have frequent physical contact with other people. People visiting hospital patients who are seriously ill may be asked to wash their hands and put on a gown, mask, and gloves before entering the person's room.

Sometimes, to prevent an infection, antibiotics are given to people who do not yet have an infection. This preventive measure is called prophylaxis. Antibiotics are given prophylactically before dental procedures to people with abnormal heart valves.■ Many healthy people who undergo certain types of surgery—particularly abdominal surgery and organ transplantation—also require prophylactic antibiotics.

Vaccination also can prevent infections.★ People who are at increased risk of developing infections (especially infants, children, older people, and people with AIDS) should receive all the vaccinations necessary to reduce this risk.

Infections in People With Impaired Defenses

Many diseases, drugs, and other treatments can cause a breakdown in the body's natural defenses. Such a breakdown can lead to infections, which can even be caused by microorganisms that normally live harmlessly on or in the body.

▲ see box on page 1572   ■ see table on page 187
★ see page 1092

People with extensive burns have an increased risk of infection because damaged skin cannot prevent invasion by harmful microorganisms. People undergoing medical procedures that introduce foreign material into the body have an increased risk of infection. Such procedures include the insertion of a catheter into the urinary tract or a blood vessel, or the insertion of a tube into the windpipe. Many drugs can suppress the immune system, including anticancer drugs (chemotherapy), drugs used to prevent organ rejection after a transplant (such as azathioprine, methotrexate, and cyclosporine), and corticosteroids (such as prednisone). Radiation treatments may suppress the immune system, particularly when the bone marrow receives radiation.

The ability to fight certain infections decreases dramatically in people with AIDS, especially late in the disease.▲ People with AIDS are at particular risk for opportunistic infections (infections by microorganisms that generally do not cause infection in people with a healthy immune system). They also become more severely ill from many common infections.

Infections are more likely and usually more severe in older people than in younger people, probably because aging reduces the immune system's effectiveness.■ Many long-term (chronic) disorders that are common in older people—such as chronic obstructive pulmonary disease, cancer, and diabetes mellitus—also increase the risk of infection. In addition, older people are more likely to be in a hospital or a nursing home, where the risk of acquiring a serious infection is greater. In hospitals, the widespread use of antibiotics allows antibiotic-resistant organisms to thrive, and infections with these microorganisms are often more difficult to treat than infections acquired at home.

CHAPTER 189

Immunization

In immunization, the body's ability to fight off certain disease-causing bacteria or viruses is stimulated or enhanced. There are two types of immunization, active and passive. Immunization is a method doctors use to protect people against certain diseases caused by bacteria and viruses.

In **active immunization,** vaccines are used to help prevent infection by stimulating the body's natural defense mechanisms. Vaccines are preparations that contain either noninfectious fragments of bacteria or viruses or whole forms of these organisms that have been weakened such that they do not cause infection. The body's immune system responds to a vaccine by producing substances (such as antibodies and white blood cells) that recognize and attack the specific bacterium or virus contained in the vaccine. These antibodies and other substances are then automatically produced whenever the person is exposed to that specific bacterium or virus. The process of giving a vaccine is called vaccination, although many doctors use the more general term immunization.

In **passive immunization,** antibodies against a specific infectious organism are given directly to a person. Passive immunization is used for people whose immune system does not respond adequately to an infection or for people who acquire an infection before they can be vaccinated (for example, after exposure to the rabies virus). Passive immunization can also be used to prevent disease when exposure is likely and the person does not have time to get or complete a vaccination series. An example of this is the use of gamma globulin (an antibody preparation) to help prevent hepatitis in people who travel to certain parts of the world. Passive immunization lasts for only a

▲ see page 1168
■ see page 1056

few days or weeks, until the body eliminates the injected antibodies.

Vaccines available today are highly reliable and most people tolerate them well. They do not work in everyone, however, and rarely they have side effects.

Some vaccines are given routinely—for example, the tetanus toxoid is given to adults preferably every 10 years. Several different vaccines are routinely given to children. Other vaccines are given mainly to specific groups of people—for instance, the yellow fever vaccine is given only to people traveling to certain parts of Africa and South America. Still other vaccines are given after possible exposure to a specific disease—for instance, the rabies vaccine may be given to a person who has been bitten by a dog.

Common Vaccinations

Children typically receive a number of vaccines according to a standard schedule.▲ Depending on their circumstances, adults may also be advised to receive certain vaccines. Factors that a doctor considers when advising adults about vaccination include the person's age, health history, childhood vaccinations, occupation, geographic location, and travel plans.

Measles, Mumps, and Rubella

Measles, mumps, and rubella (German measles) are all viral infections. Anyone born after 1956 who has never had one of these infections and who has not received two doses of the vaccine—but who is likely to be exposed to these diseases—should be vaccinated. People likely to be exposed to these diseases include those beginning college, joining the military, or working in schools or child care centers. Pregnant women and people who are allergic to eggs or the antibiotic neomycin should *not* be vaccinated.

A person can receive individual vaccines for measles, mumps, or rubella. However, a combination vaccine that helps protect against all three of these diseases is more often administered. This vaccine is recommended because anyone who needs protection against one of these infections usually also needs protection against the other two.

Tetanus

Tetanus vaccination protects the body against the toxin produced by the tetanus bacterium, not the bacterium itself. Because

tetanus is often fatal, vaccination is particularly important. A primary series of three injections over a 6-month period should be administered to any adult who was not vaccinated in childhood. A booster dose of the vaccine is recommended every 10 years. Adults receive the tetanus vaccine alone or in combination with a diphtheria vaccine administered in a single injection. Children receive a combination vaccine against tetanus, diphtheria, and pertussis (whooping cough). Pertussis vaccination is not necessary for adults.

Hepatitis A

Vaccination against the hepatitis A virus is recommended for adults and children older than age 2 traveling outside of the United States (except to Canada, Northern/Western Europe, Australia, New Zealand, and Japan) and for injecting drug users, male homosexuals, and people with chronic liver disease or blood clotting disorders. Two doses, 6 to 12 months apart, are given. In communities with high rates of hepatitis A, children should routinely be given the vaccine.

Hepatitis B

Hepatitis B vaccination is recommended for all children and for any adult who is at high risk of exposure to the hepatitis B virus. People at high risk include health care workers, mortuary workers, people receiving frequent blood transfusions or dialysis, injecting drug users, people who have multiple sex partners, and sex partners and household contacts of people known to be carriers of hepatitis B.

The vaccine is given in a series of three or four injections. However, if a person who has been vaccinated is exposed to the virus, a doctor measures that person's antibody levels against hepatitis B. If the antibody levels are low, the person may need another injection of hepatitis B vaccine. People with a history of severe allergic reaction to baker's yeast, which is used in the production of the vaccine, should not receive the vaccine.

Haemophilus influenzae type b

All children should be vaccinated against the bacterium *Haemophilus influenzae* type b. Protection is not required by adults, in whom the infection is very uncommon.

▲ see box on page 1493

PROTECTING AGAINST DISEASE

In the United States, vaccines are available for the following diseases:

DISEASE	WHO SHOULD RECEIVE VACCINE
Adenovirus	Selected people (available only to the United States Armed Forces)
Anthrax	Selected people
Cholera	Selected people
Diphtheria	All children and adults
Haemophilus influenzae type b infections (meningitis)	All children, selected adults
Hepatitis A	All children, selected adults
Hepatitis B	All children, selected adults
Influenza	Selected people
Japanese encephalitis	Selected people
Measles	All children and adults
Meningococcal meningitis	Selected people
Mumps	All children and adults
Pertussis (whooping cough)	All children and adults
Plague	Selected people
Pneumococcal infection (meningitis, pneumonia)	All children, selected adults
Polio	All children and adults
Rabies	Selected people
Rubella (German measles)	All children and adults
Smallpox	Not currently recommended
Tetanus	All children and adults
Tuberculosis	Selected people
Typhoid	Selected people
Varicella (chickenpox)	All children, selected adults
Yellow fever	Selected people

Influenza

Vaccination against the influenza virus is recommended for people at high risk of developing influenza or its complications. People at risk include residents of nursing homes, those older than 50, and health care workers. Others at risk include people with chronic heart or lung disease, diabetes, kidney failure, sickle cell disease, a weakened immune system, or human immunodeficiency virus (HIV) infection.

Influenza epidemics usually begin in late December or midwinter. Therefore, the best time to receive the vaccine is in September or October. Influenza vaccination must be repeated every year because the virus changes from year to year.

Pneumococcal Infection

Vaccination against pneumococcal infection is recommended for all children; a newly developed vaccine for children is highly effective. Adults who are at high risk of developing pneumonia should receive the adult vaccine. People at high risk of pneumonia include those with chronic disease (especially lung and heart disease), those who do not have a functioning spleen, those with cancer of the blood cells, those with spinal fluid leakage, and alcoholics.

The adult vaccine is effective in about two of three adults, although it is less effective in debilitated older people. It is more effective in preventing some of the serious complications of pneumococcal pneumonia than in preventing the pneumonia itself. Although one injection of the vaccine may provide lifetime protection, people at high risk are advised to receive the vaccine every 6 years.

Polio

All children should be vaccinated against polio. Until recently, the vaccine most often used contained live, weakened virus and was given by mouth. However, about 1 in every 2.4 million people who receives this oral polio vaccine develops a case of polio (the chance of getting polio from the oral vaccine is higher in people with a weakened immune system). Because of this, doctors in the United States now use an injectable polio vaccine that contains killed virus that cannot cause the disease.

Because polio is now so rare in the United States, unvaccinated people older than 18 do not receive the polio vaccine unless they are traveling to an area where polio is common.

Varicella

Vaccination against varicella (the virus that causes chickenpox) is part of the routine vaccination schedule recommended for children. The vaccine is relatively new, however, so older children and adults who have never had chickenpox may want to consider vaccination, especially because the infection tends to be more serious when acquired in adulthood. The vaccine does not completely prevent chickenpox, but vaccinated people who do get the disease usually have milder symptoms. It is likely that the varicella vaccine helps prevent shingles,▲ a complication of chickenpox that can produce painful skin sores years later.

The vaccine is administered in two doses 4 to 8 weeks apart. The vaccine is not given to pregnant women, people with a weakened immune system, or people with cancer affecting the bone marrow or lymphatic system.

Smallpox

Vaccination against smallpox was once routine for everyone in the United States. Smallpox vaccination was discontinued over 20 years ago because of the elimination of the disease. Because the vaccine's protective effects wear off after about 10 years, most people are now susceptible to smallpox. Recent fears about the possible use of smallpox by terrorists have led to the suggestion that smallpox vaccination resume. The vaccine is generally safe, although serious adverse reactions develop in about 100 of every million previously unvaccinated people, and death occurs in 1 per million. The risk of serious adverse effects and death is lower in previously vaccinated people. If smallpox vaccination is resumed, it is likely to be recommended only for people in the area of a smallpox outbreak. The vaccine is most effective when given very early after exposure, but may also benefit people who have contracted smallpox if given in the first days after symptoms appear.

Vaccination Before Foreign Travel

Residents of the United States may be required to receive specific vaccines before traveling to areas that have infectious diseases not normally found in the United States.■ Recommendations change frequently in response to disease outbreaks. The Centers for Disease Control and Prevention (CDC) provide the most up-to-date information on vaccination requirements in their Travelers' Health Section.★

CHAPTER 190

Bacterial Infections

Bacteria are microscopic, single-celled organisms. Thousands of different kinds of bacteria live throughout the world. Some live in the environment, and others live on the skin, in the airways, in the mouth, and in the digestive and genitourinary tracts of people and animals. Only a few kinds of bacteria cause disease.

Bacteria are classified in several ways. One way is by their distinctive shapes. Spherical bacteria are cocci, rod-like bacteria are bacilli, and spiral or helical bacteria are spirochetes.

Another way bacteria are classified is by their color after a particular chemical stain (Gram stain) is applied. Some bacteria stain blue and are called gram-positive, whereas others stain pink and are called gram-negative. Gram-positive and gram-negative bacteria differ in the kinds of infections they produce and in the kinds of antibiotics that are likely to kill them.

Gram-negative bacteria have a unique outer membrane that prevents many drugs from penetrating them, making gram-negative bacteria generally more resistant to antibiotics than are gram-positive bacteria. The outer

---

▲ see page 1162   ■ see table on page 1709

★ see page 1768

Shapes of Bacteria

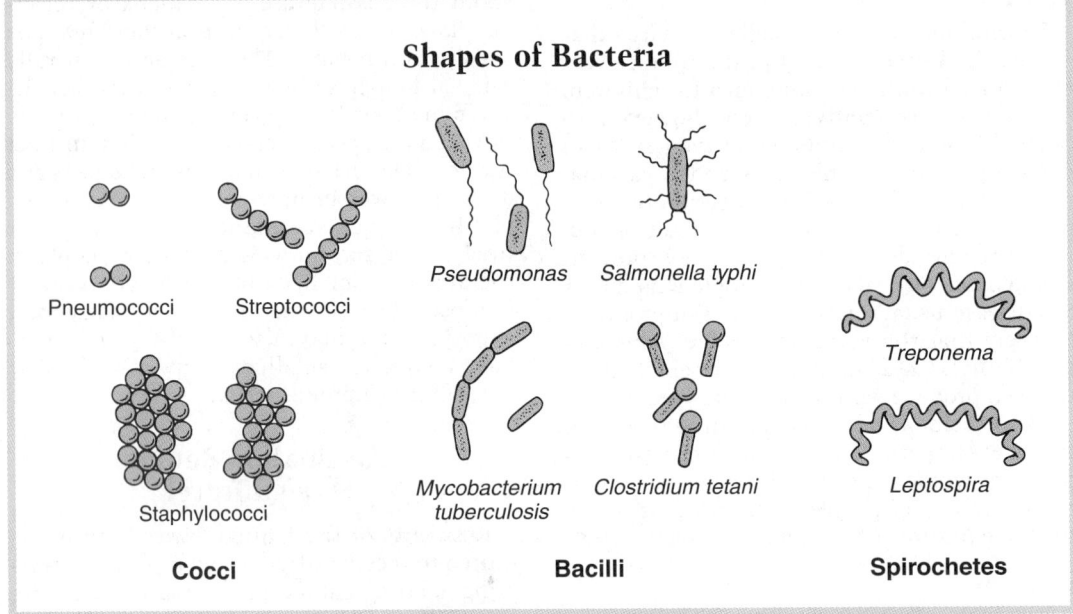

Pneumococci Streptococci

Pseudomonas *Salmonella typhi*

Treponema

Staphylococci

Mycobacterium tuberculosis *Clostridium tetani*

Leptospira

Cocci **Bacilli** **Spirochetes**

membrane of gram-negative bacteria is also rich in molecules called lipopolysaccharides. If gram-negative bacteria enter the bloodstream, their lipopolysaccharides can trigger high fever and a life-threatening drop in blood pressure.▲ For this reason, bacterial lipopolysaccharides are referred to as endotoxins.

Gram-negative bacteria have a great facility for exchanging genetic material (DNA) with other strains of the same species and even with different species. Thus, if gram-negative bacteria undergo a genetic change (mutation) that produces resistance to an antibiotic and then share DNA with another strain of bacteria, the second (recipient) strain becomes resistant as well.

Gram-positive bacteria are usually slow to develop resistance to antibiotics. Some gram-positive bacteria (for example, *Bacillus anthracis* and *Clostridium botulinum*) produce potent poisons (toxins) that cause serious illness.

A third way of classifying bacteria is by their use of oxygen. Most bacteria can live and grow in the presence of oxygen; these bacteria are called aerobes. Bacteria that can tolerate only low levels of oxygen, or are poisoned by oxygen, are called anaerobes. Anaerobes thrive in areas of the body that have low levels of

oxygen—such as the intestine, decaying tissue, and wounds that are particularly deep and dirty.

Hundreds of species of anaerobes normally live harmlessly on the skin and mucous membranes (such as the lining of the mouth, intestine, and vagina); several hundred billion bacteria may exist in a cubic inch of stool. Most anaerobic infections arise from the body's own pool of bacteria.

Anaerobes tend to invade skin and muscle tissue that has been damaged by injury or surgery—particularly if the tissue has a poor blood supply. Spontaneous infections sometimes develop in people who have certain cancers or a weakened immune system. Also common are infections in the mouth. Anaerobes sometimes cause chronic (but not acute) infections of the sinuses and middle ear. Anaerobic infections tend to form collections of pus (abscesses). Severe anaerobic infections often release gas into the surrounding tissue.

Disease-causing anaerobes include clostridia (which live in the intestinal tract of humans and animals, as well as in dust, soil, and decaying vegetation) and *Peptococci* and *Peptostreptococci*—which are part of the normal bacterial population (flora) of the mouth, upper respiratory tract, and large intestine. Other anaerobes include *Bacteroides*, which is part of the normal flora of the large intestine, and

▲ see page 1118

Actinomyces, Prevotella, and *Fusobacterium,* which are part of the normal flora of the mouth.

Actinomycosis

Actinomycosis is a chronic infection caused mainly by Actinomyces israelii, *an anaerobic bacterium present on the gums, teeth, and tonsils.*

Actinomycosis occurs in four forms, all of which cause abscesses (collections of pus). Adult men are affected most often, but the infection occasionally develops in women who use an intrauterine device (IUD).

The **abdominal form** is caused by swallowing saliva contaminated with the bacteria. The infection affects the intestines and the lining of the abdominal cavity (peritoneum). Pain, fever, vomiting, diarrhea or constipation, and severe weight loss are common symptoms. If an abscess develops in the abdomen, pus may drain through the skin by way of channels connecting the abscess to the abdominal wall.

The **cervicofacial form** (lumpy jaw) usually begins as small, flat, hard, sometimes painful swellings in the mouth, on the skin of the neck, or below the jaw. These swellings may soften and discharge pus that contains small, round, yellowish granules. Because of their resemblance to sulfur, these granules are sometimes called sulfur granules: they do not, however, contain sulfur. The infection may extend to the cheek, tongue, throat, salivary glands, skull, facial bones, brain, or the tissues covering the brain (meninges).

The **thoracic form** causes chest pain, fever, and a cough that brings up sputum. These symptoms, however, may not appear until the lungs are severely infected. If an abscess develops in the chest, pus may drain through the skin by way of channels connecting the abscess to the chest wall.

The **generalized form** of actinomycosis results when the bacteria are carried in the blood to the skin, vertebrae, brain, liver, kidneys, ureters, and, in women, the uterus and ovaries.

Diagnosis, Prognosis, and Treatment

The symptoms, x-ray findings, and isolation of *Actinomyces israelii* in samples of pus, sputum, or tissue help the doctor make the diagnosis. With some intestinal infections, a sample cannot be obtained, and surgery is needed to make the diagnosis.

What Are Clostridia?

Clostridia are toxin-producing anaerobic bacteria that cause a number of serious diseases, including tetanus, botulism, and tissue infections.

Clostridia normally inhabit the human intestinal tract, soil, and decaying vegetation. All species of clostridia produce toxins. Some clostridial diseases, such as botulism and the various diarrheal illnesses, result solely from the toxin without any bacterial invasion of tissue. In other clostridial diseases, such as tetanus and clostridial wound infections, there is both tissue invasion and toxin production.

The most common toxin-only clostridial diseases are short-lived and relatively mild food poisonings caused by *Clostridium perfringens.* Sometimes, clostridial food poisoning is more severe, resulting in necrotizing enteritis, an inflammation that destroys the walls of the intestines, producing severe, bloody diarrhea. This infection can occur as an isolated case or in outbreaks caused by eating contaminated meat. People who have taken antibiotics for a long time may have colitis produced by an overgrowth of toxin-producing *Clostridium difficile.*▲ Botulism, a disease causing muscle paralysis and sometimes death, occurs from eating food contaminated with a toxin produced by *Clostridium botulinum.*■

Clostridia, particularly *Clostridium perfringens,* also infect wounds. Clostridial wound infections, including skin gangrene, muscle gangrene (clostridial myonecrosis), and tetanus, are relatively rare but may be lethal. These infections are more likely in contaminated wounds, deep puncture wounds, and wounds in which much tissue is crushed. Injecting drug users are more susceptible. The risk of death is high, especially in older people and people with cancer.

Lumpy jaw is the most easily treated form of actinomycosis and has the best prognosis. The thoracic, abdominal, and generalized forms are harder to treat and have a worse prognosis. More than 50% of people with actinomycosis of the brain and spinal cord have persisting neurologic damage, and more than 25% die.

▲ see page 745   ■ see page 579

To treat actinomycosis, doctors drain abscesses and give high doses of antibiotics such as penicillin or tetracycline. To prevent relapse, antibiotics are taken for as long as 6 to 12 months.

Anthrax

Anthrax is infection with the gram-positive bacterium Bacillus anthracis *that typically involves the skin, lungs, or digestive tract.*

Anthrax is a potentially fatal disease that usually spreads to people from animals, especially cows, goats, and sheep. Dormant bacteria (spores) can live in soil and in animal products (such as wool) for decades and are not easily killed by cold or heat. Even minimal contact is likely to result in infection. Although infection in people usually occurs through the skin, it can also result from inhaling spores or from eating contaminated, poorly cooked meat. Infection cannot spread from person to person.

Because anthrax is highly lethal when inhaled, it has been considered and used by some countries and terrorists as an agent of biological warfare.▲ Anthrax bacilli produce several toxins, which are responsible for many of the symptoms.

Symptoms and Diagnosis

Anthrax skin infection begins as a painless, red-brown bump that appears 1 to 5 days after infection. The bump forms a blister, which hardens and eventually breaks open to form a black scab (eschar). Lymph nodes in the affected area may swell, and the person may feel ill—sometimes experiencing muscle aches, headache, fever, nausea, and vomiting. One in five untreated people dies.

Pulmonary anthrax (woolsorter's disease) results from inhaling the spores of the anthrax bacterium. The spores multiply in the lymph nodes near the lungs. Toxins produced by the bacteria cause the lymph nodes to swell, break down, and bleed, spreading the infection to nearby structures in the chest. Infected fluid builds up in the lungs and in the space between the lungs and the chest wall. Symptoms develop in two stages. For the first 2 to 3 days, the symptoms are vague and similar to those of influenza, with mild aches, fever, and dry cough. The person then suddenly develops severe difficulty breathing, high fever, and

sweating, rapidly followed by shock and coma. This second stage is probably the result of a massive release of toxins. Infection of the brain and meninges (meningoencephalitis) may also occur. Many people die 24 to 36 hours after severe symptoms start, even with early treatment.

Anthrax of the digestive tract (gastrointestinal anthrax) is rare. When a person eats contaminated meat, the bacteria grow in the mouth, throat, or intestines and release toxins that cause extensive bleeding and tissue death. Sore throat, neck swelling, abdominal pain, vomiting, and bloody diarrhea also develop. At least half of the untreated people die.

Anthrax skin sores are diagnosed by their typical appearance. Knowing that a person had contact with animals or was in an area where other people developed anthrax also helps a doctor make the diagnosis. Anthrax bacteria are easily recognized under a microscope in samples from skin or body fluids. Also, the bacteria may be grown in culture. Blood tests can be used to detect fragments of bacterial DNA or antibodies to one of the bacterial toxins. In a person with pulmonary anthrax, the bacteria are sometimes, but not always, present in the sputum. In serious infections, the person may die before any test results are complete, so treatment is usually started when anthrax is first suspected.

Prevention and Treatment

People at high risk of contracting anthrax—such as veterinarians, laboratory technicians, and employees of textile mills that process animal hair—can be vaccinated. Because of anthrax's potential as a biological weapon, most members of the armed forces are also vaccinated. Despite widely publicized anxiety, well over 1.25 million people have received anthrax vaccine without serious adverse reactions. People exposed to anthrax may be given preventive treatment using either oral ciprofloxacin or doxycycline if the bacteria's susceptibility to penicillin is unknown. If susceptibility to penicillin is documented, children should be given preventive treatment with oral amoxicillin.

Anthrax infection is treated with a combination of antibiotics, including intravenous ciprofloxacin or doxycycline, plus clindamycin, rifampin, or penicillin. Corticosteroids may also be used to reduce any swelling in the throat. The longer treatment is delayed, the greater the risk of death.

▲ see box on page 1089

Bejel, Yaws, and Pinta

Bejel (previously called endemic syphilis), yaws (frambesia), and pinta are nonsexually transmitted infections caused by treponemal spirochetes closely related to Treponema pallidum, *the bacterium that causes the sexually transmitted disease syphilis.*

Bejel, yaws, and pinta (collectively referred to as treponematoses) are diseases closely related to syphilis▲ that mainly occur in the tropics and subtropics. Unlike syphilis, they are transmitted by nonsexual skin contact—chiefly between children living in conditions of poor hygiene.

Like syphilis, these diseases begin with skin sores and have a latent period that is followed by more destructive disease. Bejel occurs mainly in the arid countries of the eastern Mediterranean region and West Africa. Yaws occurs in humid equatorial countries. Pinta is common among the Indians of Mexico, Central America, and South America.

Symptoms

Bejel affects the skin, bones, and mucous membranes of the mouth. Symptoms begin with a slimy patch on the inside of the mouth followed by blisters on the trunk, arms, and legs. Bone infection develops later, mainly in the legs. Also in later stages, soft, gummy lumps may appear in the nose and on the roof of the mouth (soft palate).

Yaws affects the skin and bones. It begins several weeks after exposure to *Treponema* as a slightly raised sore at the site of infection, usually on a leg. The sore heals, but soft nodules of tissue (granulomas) erupt on the face, arms, legs, and buttocks. These granulomas heal slowly and may recur. Painful open sores may develop on the soles of the feet (crab yaws). Later, areas of the shinbones may be destroyed, and many other disfiguring growths, especially around the nose (gangosa), may develop.

Pinta involves only the skin. It begins as flat, reddened areas on the hands, feet, legs, arms, face, or neck. After several months, slate blue patches develop in the same areas on both sides of the body and over bony places, such as the elbow. Later, the patches lose their pigmentation. Thickened skin may develop in the patches on the palms and soles.

Diagnosis and Treatment

A doctor makes the diagnosis when typical symptoms appear in a person who lives in or has visited an area where such diseases are common. Because the bacteria causing the treponematoses and syphilis are so similar, a person with one of these infections tests positive for syphilis. Standard tests cannot distinguish between treponematoses and syphilis.

The lesions are destructive and leave scars. However, a single injection of penicillin kills the bacteria, so the skin can heal. Tetracycline and chloramphenicol given by mouth are also effective. Because the diseases are very contagious, public health measures seek out and treat infected people and their close contacts.

Campylobacter Infections

Several species of the gram-negative bacilli Campylobacter *can infect the digestive tract and rarely other organs.*

Campylobacter normally inhabits the digestive tract of many domestic animals and fowl. Water may become contaminated from the feces of infected animals. The most common form of *Campylobacter* infection is gastroenteritis,■ which may be acquired by drinking contaminated water, eating undercooked poultry or meat, or having contact with infected animals.

Campylobacter is also a common cause of diarrhea among people who travel to developing countries. Very rarely, *Campylobacter* causes a bloodstream infection (bacteremia), most often in people with an existing disease such as diabetes or cancer. Bacteria in the bloodstream may lead to infections in many different organs.

Symptoms

The symptoms of *Campylobacter* gastroenteritis include diarrhea, abdominal pain, and cramps, which may be severe. The diarrhea may be bloody, and a fever ranging from 100 to 104° F may develop.

A fever that comes and goes may be the only symptom of a *Campylobacter* infection outside the digestive tract. Additional symptoms of a bodywide (systemic) *Campylobacter* infection may include a joint that becomes painful, red, and swollen; abdominal pain; and enlargement of the liver or spleen. Rarely, the infection involves the heart valves (endocarditis) or the tissues covering the brain and spinal cord (meningitis).

▲ see page 1176   ■ see table on page 720

Diagnosis and Treatment

The diagnosis of *Campylobacter* gastroenteritis can be made by finding the organism in a culture of stool. This is not always done, however, because infectious diarrhea is usually effectively treated without knowing which bacteria caused it. Doctors perform a blood culture if they suspect a bloodstream infection.

Many people get better in a week or so without specific treatment, although some people require extra fluids intravenously or by mouth. Some people, especially those with bloodstream infections, require antibiotics such as ciprofloxacin or azithromycin.

Cholera

Cholera is a serious infection of the intestine caused by the gram-negative bacterium Vibrio cholerae *that produces severe diarrhea.*

Several species of *Vibrio* bacteria cause diarrhea,▲ but the type that produces the most serious illness is *Vibrio cholerae*, the bacterium that causes cholera. Cholera may occur in large outbreaks of diarrheal illness. The disease is fatal in one third to one half of the people who do not receive proper medical care. Once common throughout the world, cholera is now largely confined to developing countries in the tropics and subtropics.

Vibrio cholerae normally lives in aquatic environments, attached to particular types of algae and plankton. People acquire the infection by ingesting water, seafood, or other foods contaminated with the bacteria. Once infected, people return the bacteria to the environment in their stool (particularly in regions where human waste is untreated), allowing explosive spread of the infection. The most recent cholera outbreak is still ongoing in Africa, where more than 400,000 people contracted the disease from 1998 to 1999.

Vibrio cholerae produces a toxin that causes the small intestine to secrete enormous amounts of fluid (in the form of watery diarrhea) that is rich in salts and minerals. It is the loss of fluid and minerals that causes death. The bacteria remain within the small intestine and do not invade tissues. Because the bacteria are sensitive to stomach acid, people with lower amounts of acid (such as young children and older people) are more susceptible to the disease. People living in areas where

cholera is common (endemic) gradually acquire some immunity.

Symptoms and Diagnosis

Symptoms begin 1 to 3 days after infection and range from mild, uncomplicated diarrhea to severe, potentially fatal disease. Some infected people have no symptoms.

The disease starts with sudden, painless, watery diarrhea and vomiting. The amount of fluid lost through diarrhea and vomiting is proportional to the severity of the infection. In severe infections, the diarrhea causes a loss of more than 1 quart per hour. Within hours, the resulting depletion of fluid and salts leads to severe dehydration, with intense thirst, muscle cramps, weakness, and minimal urine production. Severe loss of fluid from tissues causes the eyes to become sunken and the skin on the fingers to become severely wrinkled. If the dehydration is not treated, the loss of fluid and salts can lead to kidney failure, shock, coma, and death.

Symptoms usually subside in 3 to 6 days. Most people are free of the bacteria in 2 weeks, but a few become long-term carriers.

A doctor confirms a diagnosis of cholera by recovering the bacteria from rectal swabs or from fresh stool samples.

Prevention and Treatment

Purification of water supplies and proper disposal of human waste are essential for controlling cholera. Other precautions include using boiled water and avoiding uncooked vegetables or inadequately cooked fish or shellfish. Shellfish tend to carry other forms of *Vibrio* as well.

Several vaccines for cholera are available outside the United States. These vaccines provide only partial protection and only for a limited time, and therefore are not generally recommended; new vaccines are currently being tested. Prompt treatment with the antibiotic tetracycline may help prevent the disease in household contacts of a person infected with cholera.

Rapid replacement of lost body fluids and salts is lifesaving, because people die from dehydration, not bacterial invasion. Most people with cholera can be treated effectively with fluids and salts given by mouth. Premixed packets of salts are available for use in areas prone to cholera epidemics, allowing people to make their own rehydration solution for home treatment when health care facilities are over-

---

▲ see table on page 720

whelmed. The solution contains 20 grams of glucose, 3.5 grams of sodium chloride, 2.9 grams of sodium citrate, and 1.5 grams of potassium chloride per liter of boiled water. For severely dehydrated people who cannot drink, a salt solution is given intravenously. In epidemics, people sometimes receive fluids through a tube inserted through the nose into the stomach, because sufficient supplies for intravenous therapy are not available. Once dehydration is corrected, the goal of treatment is replacement of the exact amount of fluid lost through diarrhea and vomiting. Solid foods can be eaten after vomiting stops and appetite returns.

Early treatment with tetracycline or another antibiotic kills the bacteria and usually stops the diarrhea in 48 hours.

More than 50% of untreated people with severe cholera die. Less than 1% of people who receive prompt, adequate fluid replacement die.

Gas Gangrene

Gas gangrene (clostridial myonecrosis) is a life-threatening infection of muscle tissue caused mainly by the anaerobic bacterium Clostridium perfringens *and several other* Clostridium *species.*

Gas gangrene is a fast-spreading clostridial infection of muscle tissue that quickly leads to death if untreated. The bacteria produce gas that becomes trapped in the infected tissue. Several thousand cases occur in the United States every year. Gas gangrene usually develops after trauma or surgery, although spontaneous infections can occur—usually in people with colon cancer or leukemia. Surgery on the colon and gallbladder are the procedures most likely to be complicated by gas gangrene. High-risk injuries are those that become contaminated with dirt and vegetable matter or that contain crushed and dead tissue. People with open fractures and frostbite are also particularly susceptible to gas gangrene.

Symptoms and Diagnosis

Gas gangrene produces severe pain in the infected area. Initially, the area is swollen and pale, but eventually turns red, then bronze, and finally blackish green. Large blisters often form. Gas bubbles may be visible in the blister fluid or may be felt under the skin. The odor of any wound drainage is described as sweet or mousy, unlike the putrid odor typical of other anaerobic infections.

As the infection progresses, the person becomes sweaty and very anxious; vomiting may also occur. Rapid heart rate and rapid breathing are common. These effects are caused by toxins produced by the bacteria. Typically, the person remains very alert until late in the illness, when very low blood pressure (shock) and coma develop, followed rapidly by death.

The initial diagnosis of gas gangrene is based on the person's symptoms and a physical examination. Finding gas bubbles in the muscle tissue on x-ray increases a doctor's suspicion of a clostridial infection, but gas bubbles may also occur with non-clostridial anaerobic infections. Examination of secretions from the wound under a microscope may reveal the clostridia, and cultures can confirm their presence—but because gas gangrene is so rapidly fatal, treatment is always begun before the culture results are available.

Prevention, Prognosis, and Treatment

Cleaning wounds thoroughly and removing foreign objects and dead tissue is the best way to prevent clostridia from infecting a wound. Intravenous antibiotics are used before, during, and after abdominal surgery to prevent postoperative infection. There are no vaccines to prevent clostridial infection.

Without treatment, gas gangrene is fatal within 48 hours. Even with treatment, death occurs in about one of eight people with infection of a limb and in about two of three people with infection on the trunk.

If gas gangrene is suspected, treatment must begin immediately. High doses of antibiotics, typically penicillin and clindamycin, are given, and all dead and infected material is removed surgically. About one of five people with gas gangrene in a limb requires amputation of the infected limb. Treatment in a high-pressure oxygen (hyperbaric oxygen) chamber is of uncertain value; moreover, such chambers are not readily available.

Enterobacteriaceae Infections

Enterobacteriaceae is a group of gram-negative bacteria that can cause infections of the digestive tract or other organs of the body.

The group Enterobacteriaceae includes the bacteria *Enterobacter, Escherichia, Klebsiella, Morganella, Proteus, Providencia, Salmonella, Serratia, Shigella,* and *Yersinia*. Although *Escherichia coli* (*E. coli*) normally inhabits the intestines, certain strains of *E. coli* can cause

OTHER BACTERIAL INFECTIONS

Infection	Cause and Source of Infection	Symptoms and Treatment	Comments
Brucellosis	**Cause:** Brucella **Source:** Domestic animals; buffalo; unpasteurized milk; contaminated dairy products	**Symptoms:** Fever that may return repeatedly for months to years; abdominal pain; vomiting; diarrhea; bone and joint pain **Treatment:** Oral doxycycline combined with daily injections of streptomycin	Meat packers, veterinarians, farmers, and livestock producers are at increased risk
Cat-scratch disease	**Cause:** Bartonella henselae **Source:** Domestic cats	**Symptoms:** Red, crusted blisters at site of a cat scratch; swollen lymph nodes that fill with pus and may drain through the skin **Treatment:** Heat application; pain relievers; azithromycin may be given	Most domestic cats throughout the world are infected (most show no signs of illness)
Erysipelothricosis	**Cause:** Erysipelothrix rhusiopathiae **Source:** Puncture wound that occurs while handling animal matter	**Symptoms:** Purplish red, hard area on skin at site of injury; itching; burning; swelling **Treatment:** Single penicillin injection or a 1-week course of oral erythromycin; infection usually resolves without treatment	Rarely infects joints or heart valves
Neisserial infections	**Cause:** Neisseria meningitidis **Source:** Neisseria meningitidis is part of the resident flora of people **Cause:** Neisseria gonorrhoeae **Source:** Neisseria gonorrhoeae is sexually transmitted	**Symptoms:** Symptoms of meningitis (headache, confusion, lethargy, coma, and death) **Treatment:** Ceftriaxone **Symptoms:** Urethral or vaginal discharge **Treatment:** Single dose of ceftriaxone or azithromycin	Vaccine is available for most types
Nocardiosis	**Cause:** Nocardia (usually Nocardia asteroides) **Source:** Nocardia inhabits decaying matter in soil; lung infection can result from inhalation of contaminated dust; skin infection can result from puncture wounds	**Symptoms:** Cough; general weakness; chills; chest pain; shortness of breath; fever; lung abscesses; skin sores **Treatment:** Trimethoprim-sulfamethoxazole or imipenem plus amikacin for many months to a year	People who are chronically ill or who are receiving drugs that suppress the immune system are at increased risk; infection spreads to the brain in one third of people and causes abscesses; infection is potentially fatal

OTHER BACTERIAL INFECTIONS (Continued)

Infection	Cause and Source of Infection	Symptoms and Treatment	Comments
Rat-bite fever	**Cause:** *Streptobacillus moniliformis* **Source:** Wild rats or mice; occasionally, dogs, cats, ferrets, weasels, or other carnivores that have fed on infected rodents; food contaminated by rodents	**Symptoms:** Chills; fever that may recur for months; vomiting; headache; back and joint pain; rash on hands and feet; joint swelling **Treatment:** Penicillin or erythromycin	Doctors often give antibiotics to people with rat bites to prevent disease; rat-bite fever caused by *Streptobacillus moniliformis* is common in the United States. A type of rat-bite fever caused by *Spirillum minus* is common in Asia. The symptoms are similar, except that the person also has inflammation at the site of the bite, swollen lymph nodes, fatigue, and a rash. Treatment for that type of rat-bite fever is with penicillin or erythromycin
Relapsing fever	**Cause:** *Borrelia* **Source:** Body lice; soft-bodied ticks	**Symptoms:** Sudden chills followed by high fever (fevers come and go at 1 to 2 week intervals); severe headache; vomiting; muscle and joint pain; reddish rash over trunk, arms, and legs; jaundice; enlargement of liver and spleen; heart inflammation; heart failure **Treatment:** Tetracycline, erythromycin, or doxycycline	In the United States, infection is generally confined to western states; complications can include eye inflammation, eruption of red rash all over the body (erythema multiforme), and miscarriage in pregnant women

intestinal infections that produce bloody, watery, or inflammatory diarrhea (traveler's diarrhea). In children, diarrhea caused by certain strains of E. coli may lead to destruction of red blood cells and kidney failure (hemolytic-uremic syndrome). E. coli can also cause urinary tract infections (particularly in women) and bacteremia and meningitis in newborns (particularly premature newborns). Infections caused by E. coli are diagnosed by finding the bacteria in cultures of blood or body fluids. The infection is treated with antibiotics, such as trimethoprim-sulfamethoxazole or, for more serious infections, ceftriaxone.

Klebsiella, Enterobacter, and Serratia infections are usually acquired in the hospital, mainly by people who have a reduced ability to fight infections. These bacteria typically infect the urinary or respiratory tract, although burns and wounds are sometimes infected. Pneumonia caused by Klebsiella is an uncommon, but severe, lung infection that is most common in alcoholics, older people, and people with diabetes. Typically, people with this infection cough up sticky sputum that is dark brown or dark red. The pneumonia may lead to the formation of abscesses (collections of pus) in the lung or in the lining of the lungs (empyema). If treated early enough, this pneumonia can be cured with intravenous antibiotics, usually cephalosporins or quinolones.

Proteus is normally present in soil, water, and stool. It can also cause deep infections, particularly in the urinary tract and the abdominal cavity. Doctors treat Proteus infections with intravenous antibiotics such as quinolones.

Haemophilus Infections

Haemophilus *are gram-negative bacilli that can cause infections almost anywhere in the body.*

Many species of *Haemophilus* grow in the upper airways of children and adults. Most of these rarely cause disease, but *Haemophilus influenzae* is a common cause of infection in children and sometimes in adults with chronic lung disease. In children, *Haemophilus influenzae* can cause infection of the bloodstream, joints, lungs, ears, eyes, sinuses, epiglottis (the area just above the voice box), and the tissues covering the brain and spinal cord (meninges). The symptoms vary depending on the part of the body affected.

Some of the other *Haemophilus* bacteria cause respiratory tract infections, infections of the heart (endocarditis), and brain abscesses (collections of pus). *Haemophilus ducreyi* causes chancroid, a sexually transmitted disease.▲

Haemophilus infections are diagnosed by finding the bacteria in cultures of blood, pus, or other body fluids.

Children are routinely vaccinated against *Haemophilus influenzae* type b; the vaccine is very effective, especially in preventing meningitis.

Treatment of *Haemophilus influenzae* meningitis requires intravenous ceftriaxone or cefotaxime. Corticosteroids may help prevent brain damage. Other *Haemophilus influenzae* infections are treated with a variety of antibiotics, including amoxicillin-clavulanate and trimethoprim-sulfamethoxazole. If the household of a person with a serious *Haemophilus influenzae* infection has someone younger than 4 years who is not fully immunized against *Haemophilus influenzae*, all members of the household are given a preventive antibiotic such as rifampin.

Leptospirosis

Leptospirosis is a potentially serious illness caused by species of the spirochete Leptospira.

Leptospirosis occurs in many wild and domestic animals. Some animals act as carriers and pass the bacteria in their urine; others become ill and die. People acquire these infections through contact with infected animals, their urine, or soil and water contaminated by infected urine.

Although leptospirosis is an occupational disease of farmers and sewer and slaughterhouse workers, most people become infected while engaging in outdoor activities such as swimming or wading in contaminated water. The 40 to 100 infections reported every year in the United States occur mainly in the late summer and early fall. Because mild leptospirosis typically causes vague, flu-like symptoms, many infections probably go unreported.

Symptoms and Diagnosis

Leptospirosis causes mild disease in about 90% of infected people, whereas 10% have severe, potentially fatal, disease that affects many organs. The first phase starts 2 to 20 days after infection with *Leptospira*. Symptoms begin abruptly with a fever, headache, severe muscle aches, and chills. The eyes usually become very red on the third or fourth day. Nausea and vomiting are common. Symptoms involving the lungs (including the coughing up of blood) occur in 10 to 15% of infected people. Episodes of chills and fever, which often reaches 102° F, continue for 4 to 9 days.

The fever clears for a few days, marking the beginning of the second phase. During this phase, the body's immune reaction against the bacteria causes inflammation, producing many symptoms. The fever returns, and there is often inflammation of the tissues covering the brain (meningitis), causing a stiff neck, headache, and sometimes stupor and coma. In the severe form of the infection, people may also have inflammation of the liver, kidneys, and lungs, resulting in jaundice, kidney failure, and bloody cough. Sometimes the heart is inflamed, causing palpitations and dangerously low blood pressure (shock). A pregnant woman who develops leptospirosis may miscarry.

Weil's syndrome is a severe form of leptospirosis that causes a continuous fever, stupor, and a reduction in the blood's ability to clot, which leads to bleeding within tissues. Blood tests reveal anemia. By the third to sixth day, signs of kidney damage and liver injury appear. Kidney abnormalities may cause blood in the urine and painful urination. Liver injury tends to be mild and usually heals completely.

A doctor can confirm the diagnosis of leptospirosis by identifying *Leptospira* in cul-

▲ see page 1181

tures of blood, urine, or cerebrospinal fluid samples or, more commonly, by detecting antibodies against the bacteria in the blood.

Prognosis and Treatment

Infected people who do not develop jaundice usually recover. Jaundice indicates liver damage and increases the death rate to 10% or higher in people older than 60.

The antibiotic doxycycline can prevent the disease and is given to people who were exposed to the same source as an infected person. Penicillin, ampicillin, or similar antibiotics are given to treat the disease. In severe infections, antibiotics may be given intravenously. People with the disease do not have to be isolated, but care must be taken when handling and disposing of their urine.

Listeriosis

Listeriosis is infection with the gram-positive bacillus Listeria monocytogenes *that can cause many problems, including meningitis, eye infections, miscarriage, vomiting, and diarrhea.*

Listeria monocytogenes occurs worldwide in the environment and in the intestines of many animals. Most cases of listeriosis occur in July and August and result from consumption of contaminated food—typically meat, dairy products, and raw vegetables. Surveys of common fresh foods have found the bacteria in 15 to 70% of samples. Despite the high prevalence of the bacteria, listeriosis is rare, with about 1,000 cases each year in the United States. Newborns, people older than 70, and those with a weakened immune system are most susceptible.

Symptoms and Diagnosis

Listeriosis can affect almost any organ in the body, but in adults and newborns the most common site of infection is the meninges (the tissues covering the brain and spinal cord), causing meningitis. Meningitis produces fever and a stiff neck; without treatment, confusion, coma, and death can result. Brain abscesses (collections of pus) may form in up to 20% of people with meningitis.

The bacteria may sometimes infect the eyes, making them red and painful. The infection can spread to the lymph nodes, blood, and meninges. In rare instances, infection of the heart valves (endocarditis) can produce heart failure and lead to death.

While listeriosis during pregnancy may not be recognized in the mother, the fetus may die in the womb, leading to miscarriage, or the infant may die shortly after delivery. Sometimes well-appearing infants that are born to infected mothers develop meningitis a week or two after birth.

Diagnosis usually requires culture of a sample of tissue or body fluid. Antibodies against the bacteria can also be detected in blood samples.

Treatment

Treatment with the antibiotic ampicillin generally cures listeriosis. If the heart valves are infected, a second antibiotic (such as tobramycin) may be given at the same time. Eye infections can be treated with oral erythromycin.

Lyme Disease

Lyme disease is caused by the spirochete Borrelia burgdorferi, *which is usually transmitted to people by deer ticks.*

Lyme disease was recognized and named in 1975 when a cluster of cases occurred in Lyme, Connecticut. It is now the most common insect-borne infection in the United States, occurring in 47 states. About 80% of the cases in the United States occur along the northeastern coast from Massachusetts to Maryland. Most of the remaining reported cases are from Wisconsin, Minnesota, and the coastal regions of northern California and Oregon. Lyme disease also occurs in Europe and has been reported in China, Japan, Australia, and the former Soviet Union.

Usually, Lyme disease occurs in the summer and early fall. Children and young adults who live in wooded areas are most often infected.

The bacteria that cause Lyme disease are transmitted by the deer tick (*Ixodes*), so named because the adult ticks often feed on the blood of deer. The young forms of these ticks (nymphs) feed on the blood of rodents, particularly the white-footed mouse, which is a carrier of Lyme disease bacteria. Deer do not carry or transmit Lyme disease bacteria—they are simply another food source for the adult ticks.

The bacteria that cause Lyme disease are transmitted to people when an infected tick bites and stays attached for one or two days. Brief periods of attachment rarely transmit disease. At first, the bacteria multiply at the site of the tick bite. After 3 to 32 days, the bacteria migrate from the site of the bite into the surrounding skin and also spread through the blood to other organs or sites in the skin.

Symptoms

Lyme disease has three stages: early-localized, early-disseminated (widespread), and late. The early and late stages are usually separated by a period without symptoms.

The early-localized stage typically begins with a large, red spot at the site of the bite, usually on the thigh, buttock, trunk, or armpit. The spot (erythema migrans) typically expands to a diameter of 6 inches (15 centimeters), often with a central clearing (bull's eye). Although erythema migrans does not itch or hurt, it may be warm to the touch. About 25% of infected people never develop—or at least never notice—any red spot.

The symptoms of early-disseminated Lyme disease begin when the bacteria spread through the body from the initial bite area. In this stage, many people feel ill with fatigue, chills and fever, headaches, stiff neck, and aches in muscles and joints. Nearly half develop more, usually smaller, erythema migrans spots on other parts of the body. Less common symptoms include backache, nausea and vomiting, sore throat, swollen lymph nodes, and an enlarged spleen. Although most symptoms may come and go, feelings of illness and fatigue may persist for weeks. These symptoms are often mistaken for influenza or common viral infections, especially if erythema migrans is not present.

Sometimes symptoms that are more serious develop in the early-disseminated stage. Overall, abnormalities of nerve function develop in about 15% of people. The most common problems are headache, stiff neck, involvement of the tissues covering the brain and spinal cord (aseptic meningitis), and weakness on one side of the face (Bell's palsy); these may persist months before disappearing. Nerve pain and weakness may develop in other areas and persist longer. Irregular heartbeats (arrhythmias) and inflammation of the sac around the heart (pericarditis) that causes chest pain develop in 8% of infected people.

In untreated Lyme disease, the late stage begins months to years after the initial infection. Arthritis develops in about half of the people with late-stage Lyme disease. Episodes of swelling and pain in a few large joints, especially the knee, typically recur for several years. The knees are commonly more swollen than painful, often hot to the touch, and, in rare instances, red. Cysts may develop and rupture behind the knee, suddenly increasing the pain. About 10% of people with Lyme arthritis develop persistent knee problems. A smaller number of people develop neurologic abnormalities, including problems with mood, speech, memory, and sleep. Sometimes people who develop neurologic abnormalities have numbness or shooting pains in the back, legs, and arms.

Diagnosis

Cultures are not helpful because *Borrelia burgdorferi* is very difficult to grow in the laboratory. The most commonly used tests measure antibodies to the bacterium in the blood. However, antibody tests alone are not adequate because they are often negative in the early stages of Lyme disease and are sometimes positive in people who do not have the disease. Accordingly, the diagnosis depends on both test results and the presence of typical symptoms in a person who lives in (or has visited) an area where Lyme disease is common.

The lack of a definitive test for Lyme disease causes some difficulties. In areas where Lyme disease is common, many people who have painful joints, have trouble concentrating, or are always tired (chronic fatigue) often become concerned that they have late-stage Lyme disease, even though they never had a rash or any other symptoms of early-stage Lyme disease. Few of these people actually have Lyme disease; most of the time their symptoms are caused by other conditions. In people who never had symptoms of early-stage Lyme disease, the tests for Lyme antibodies are not reliable enough to make an accurate diagnosis. If a doctor makes the diagnosis based solely on the results of antibody tests, many people who do not have Lyme disease will be diagnosed with it. This typically leads to long and fruitless courses of antibiotic therapy.

Treatment

Most doctors do not give antibiotics to people who were simply bitten by ticks but have no rash or other symptoms. Sometimes an exception is made if the person lives in an area endemic for Lyme disease and the tick was engorged (indicating long attachment).

Although all stages of Lyme disease respond to antibiotics, early treatment is the most effective in helping to prevent complications.

Preventing Tick Bites

People can reduce their chances of picking up a tick by staying on paths and trails when walking in wooded areas and by not sitting on the ground or on stone walls. Wearing light-colored clothing makes ticks crawling on clothing easier to see. Applying an insecticide containing diethyltoluamide (DEET) to the skin and one containing permethrin to clothing may help protect against tick bites. People who may have been exposed to ticks should inspect their whole body for ticks daily. Deer ticks, which transmit Lyme disease, are very small, much smaller than dog ticks. So people should check the whole body very carefully, especially hairy areas. Inspection is effective because ticks must be attached for more than a day to transmit Lyme disease.

To remove a tick, a person should use fine-pointed tweezers to grasp the tick by the head or mouthparts right where they enter the skin and should pull the tick straight off. The tick's body should not be grasped or squeezed. Petroleum jelly, alcohol, lit matches, or any other irritants should not be used.

Actual size

| Deer tick (nymph) | Deer tick (adult) | Dog tick (adult) |

Antibiotics such as doxycycline, amoxicillin, penicillin, or erythromycin may be taken by mouth and are effective in the early stages of the disease. Antibiotics are given intravenously for severe neurologic disease. Treatment is given for 3 to 4 weeks.

Antibiotics eradicate the bacteria in late-stage disease, and in most people this relieves the arthritis. However, a few people have persistent arthritis even after all the bacteria are gone because of continued inflammation. Nonsteroidal anti-inflammatory drugs (NSAIDs), such as aspirin or ibuprofen, may relieve the pain of swollen joints. Fluid that collects in affected joints may be drained. The use of crutches may be helpful.

A vaccine against Lyme disease was available but was removed from the market.

Plague

Plague is a severe infection caused by the gram-negative bacterium Yersinia pestis.

The bacterium that causes plague primarily infects wild rodents, such as rats, mice, squirrels, and prairie dogs. In the past, massive plague epidemics, such as the Black Death of the Middle Ages, killed large numbers of people. Large numbers of rodents and poor sanitation were the major factors contributing to these epidemics. More recent outbreaks have been limited to one person or small clusters of people. More than 90% of the plague infections in the United States occur in the southwestern states, particularly Arizona, California, Colorado, and New Mexico.

The bacteria that cause plague are usually transmitted from infected animals to people by fleas. Coughing or sneezing, which disperse bacteria in droplets, can spread the infection from one person to another. Transmission from household pets, especially cats, can also occur through fleabites or the inhalation of infected droplets.

Symptoms and Diagnosis

Plague takes one of several forms—bubonic, pneumonic, septicemic, or pestis minor. The symptoms vary depending on the form of plague.

Bubonic plague symptoms usually appear 2 to 5 days after exposure to the bacterium, but they can appear any time from a few hours to 12 days later. Symptoms start suddenly with chills and a fever of up to 106° F. The heartbeat becomes rapid and weak, and the blood pressure may drop. Swollen lymph nodes (buboes) appear in the groin, armpit, or neck shortly before or along with the fever. Typically, the swollen lymph nodes are firm and extremely tender. The overlying skin is smooth and red but not warm. The person is likely to become restless, delirious, confused, and uncoordinated. The liver and spleen may enlarge and can be felt easily during examination. Lymph nodes may fill with pus and drain spontaneously during the second week. More than 60% of untreated people die. Most deaths occur between the third and fifth day.

Pneumonic plague is infection of the lungs with plague bacteria that have spread through the blood from another site of infection or that have been inhaled during exposure to a source of the bacteria—such as a person with pneumonic plague who is coughing. This form of plague is highly contagious; experts believe that the pneumonic form could result if plague were disseminated by terrorists. Symptoms, which begin abruptly 2 or 3 days after exposure to the bacteria, include a high fever, chills, rapid heartbeat, and often a severe headache. A cough develops within 24 hours. The sputum is clear at first, but rapidly becomes flecked with blood, and then becomes uniformly pink or bright red (resembling raspberry syrup) and foamy. Rapid and labored breathing is common. Most untreated people die within 48 hours of the start of symptoms.

Septicemic plague is infection that spreads into the blood. Death may occur even before other symptoms of bubonic or pneumonic plague appear.

Pestis minor is a mild form of plague that usually occurs only in a geographic area where the disease is common (endemic). Its symptoms—swollen lymph nodes, fever, headache, and exhaustion—subside within a week.

Plague is diagnosed by analyzing laboratory cultures of bacteria grown from samples of blood, sputum, or lymph nodes.

Prevention and Treatment

Prevention strategies are based on controlling rodents and using repellents to avoid fleabites. Vaccination is no longer available. People who live in, or are traveling to, locations with a plague outbreak may take preventive doses of the antibiotic tetracycline.

When a person is thought to have plague, a doctor begins treatment immediately. Treatment of septicemic or pneumonic plague must start within 24 hours. Prompt treatment reduces the chance of death to less than 5%. Streptomycin injections are given for 10 days; many other antibiotics are effective also.

People with pneumonic plague—unlike those with bubonic plague—must be isolated. Anyone who has had contact with a person with pneumonic plague must be treated or observed closely by a doctor for signs of infection.

Pneumococcal Infections

Pneumococcal infections are caused by Streptococcus pneumoniae *(pneumococcus), a gram-positive coccus that usually infects the lungs.*

Pneumococci commonly inhabit the upper respiratory tract of people, their natural host, particularly during the winter and early spring. Despite their presence, pneumococci only occasionally cause illness. The most common serious pneumococcal disease is pneumonia, an infection of the tissues of the lungs.▲

Pneumococci may also cause infections in the ear (otitis media), paranasal sinuses (sinusitis), the tissues covering the brain and spinal cord (meningitis), and, less often, the heart valves, joints, and abdominal cavity. Sometimes these areas become infected because the pneumococci have spread through the bloodstream from another site of infection.

People at particular risk of developing pneumococcal infection include those with chronic illnesses and a weakened immune system—for example, people with Hodgkin's disease, lymphoma, multiple myeloma, malnutrition, and sickle cell disease. Older people also often develop pneumococcal infections. Because antibodies produced in the spleen normally help prevent pneumococcal infection, people who have had their spleen removed or who have a nonfunctioning spleen are also at risk. Pneumococcal pneumonia also may develop after chronic bronchitis or if a common respiratory virus, notably the influenza virus, damages the lining of the respiratory tract.

Symptoms and Diagnosis

Symptoms begin suddenly with sharp chest pains and shaking chills. Sometimes, these symptoms follow the symptoms of a viral upper respiratory tract infection (sore throat,

▲ see page 267

stuffed nasal passages, runny nose, and non-productive cough). Fever and cough develop, and the cough produces sputum, which may have a rusty color. The person feels generally sick and is often short of breath.

Sometimes, doctors can recognize pneumococci when examining a sample of sputum under a microscope. Usually, however, a sample of sputum, pus, or blood is sent for culture. Chest x-rays are taken to look for pneumonia.

People with pneumococcal meningitis have fever, headache, and a general feeling of illness (malaise). The neck becomes stiff and painful to move, although this is not always obvious early in the disease. As soon as doctors suspect meningitis, they perform a spinal tap (lumbar puncture)▲ to look for signs of infection, such as white blood cells and bacteria, in the cerebrospinal fluid.

Pneumococcal ear infections are common in children. These infections cause ear pain and a red, bulging eardrum. Cultures and other diagnostic tests are usually not done. The use of a vaccine against pneumococci in children very significantly lowers the rate of serious infection.

Prevention and Treatment

Two types of pneumococcal vaccines are available. One (conjugate vaccine) can be given to children as young as 2 months of age.■ The other (nonconjugate vaccine) is for older children and adults; this vaccine protects against the most common strains of pneumococci, substantially reducing the chance of developing pneumococcal pneumonia and bacteremia. Pneumococcal vaccine is recommended for people 55 and older, infants, and some older children, and should also be given to people with chronic heart and lung diseases, diabetes, sickle cell disease, Hodgkin's disease, HIV infection, and metabolic disorders. People who have had their spleen removed or who have a nonfunctioning spleen also should be given pneumococcal vaccine.

Penicillin is the preferred antibiotic for most pneumococcal infections. It is taken by mouth for ear and sinus infections and given intravenously for more severe infections. Pneumococci that are resistant to penicillin are becoming increasingly common, so newer quinolone antibiotics are often used.

Pseudomonas Infections

Pseudomonas *infections are caused by any of several types of the gram-negative bacteria* Pseudomonas, *especially* Pseudomonas aeruginosa.

Pseudomonas is present throughout the world in soil, water, and on the skin of animals and people. *Pseudomonas* favors moist areas, such as sinks, toilets, pools, and hot tubs, and usually can withstand standard levels of pool chlorination. The bacteria have even been known to live in antiseptic solutions.

Pseudomonas can cause minor skin infection or serious, life-threatening illness. The most serious infections from *Pseudomonas* develop in debilitated and hospitalized people, particularly those with a weakened immune system. People with diabetes are particularly prone to *Pseudomonas* infections. *Pseudomonas* can infect the blood, skin, bones, ears, eyes, urinary tract, heart valves, and lungs.

Symptoms and Diagnosis

Two minor *Pseudomonas* infections that can affect otherwise healthy people are **swimmer's ear** and **hot-tub folliculitis.** Swimmer's ear (otitis externa) is infection of the external ear canal that produces pain and drainage.★ Hot-tub folliculitis is an itchy skin rash consisting of tiny pimples, some of which may contain a drop of pus in their center.●

Malignant external otitis, a deeply penetrating *Pseudomonas* ear infection, can cause severe ear pain and nerve damage and is most common in people with diabetes.

Pseudomonas can cause ulcers in the eye after gaining entry through an eye injury, a contaminated contact lens, or contaminated contact lens fluid. The ulcers are painful and may lead to a loss of vision. *Pseudomonas* can cause infection in deep puncture wounds, especially those occurring in the feet of children. When *Pseudomonas* infects a wound, growth in the soiled dressings often gives off a characteristic fruity odor.

Pseudomonas can cause severe pneumonia in hospitalized people, especially those in intensive care. *Pseudomonas* can also cause urinary tract infections, usually in people who have had urologic procedures or those who have an obstruction of the urinary tract.

These bacteria often invade the blood of people with burns and those who have cancer. Without treatment, an overwhelming infection can lead to dangerously low blood pres-

▲ see page 442   ■ see box on page 1493

★ see also page 1254   ● see page 1223

sure (shock) and death. The infection usually causes purple-black spots to appear on the skin. These spots are about ³⁄₈ inch in diameter with a sore at the center surrounded by redness and swelling. The spots often occur in the underarm and groin.

Rarely, *Pseudomonas* infects heart valves. People who have received an artificial heart valve are more vulnerable; however, natural heart valves can be infected, especially in injecting drug users.

Doctors diagnose *Pseudomonas* infections by growing the bacteria in cultures of blood or other body fluids.

Prevention and Treatment

Swimmer's ear can usually be prevented by irrigating the ears with a mixture of alcohol and acetic acid before and after swimming. If infection is treated with acetic acid drops and locally applied antibiotics, it usually improves quickly. Hot-tub folliculitis usually goes away without treatment.

Pseudomonas eye infections are treated with highly concentrated antibiotic drops. Sometimes, antibiotics must be injected directly into the eye.

Serious *Pseudomonas* infections are difficult to treat. Malignant external otitis, internal infections, and blood infections require weeks of intravenous antibiotic therapy, usually with a combination of antibiotics. Sometimes an infected heart valve can be cured with antibiotics, but often open-heart surgery to replace the valve is needed.▲

Salmonella Infections

Infection with any of several species of the gram-negative bacilli Salmonella *results in gastroenteritis and sometimes local tissue infections.*

About 2,200 types of *Salmonella* are known, including the one that causes typhoid fever.■ Each type can produce gastrointestinal upset, enteric fever, and specific localized infections. With the exception of the type that causes typhoid fever, *Salmonella* infects the digestive tracts of many domestic and wild animals, birds, and reptiles. Contaminated foods—particularly meat, poultry, eggs, egg products, and raw milk—are common sources of *Salmonella*. Another source is infected pet reptiles

(snakes, lizards, turtles). Up to 90% of pet reptiles in the United States are infected with *Salmonella*. *Salmonella* infections are a significant public health problem in the United States.

Symptoms and Diagnosis

Symptoms of *Salmonella* infection are usually confined to the digestive tract and start 12 to 48 hours after ingesting *Salmonella*. The first symptoms are nausea and cramping abdominal pain, soon followed by watery diarrhea, fever, and sometimes vomiting. The infection is often gone within 1 to 4 days, but it may last much longer. Some people become carriers and continue to pass the bacteria in their stool well after symptoms are gone.

Very rarely, *Salmonella* leaves the intestines and travels through the bloodstream to infect other sites, such as the bones (particularly in people with sickle cell disease), joints, or heart valves. Occasionally, a tumor may become infected and develop an abscess that provides a source for continued blood infection.

Diagnosis is confirmed in a laboratory by culturing a rectal swab or sample of stool or blood taken from an infected person.

Treatment

Salmonella gastroenteritis is treated with fluids and a bland diet. Antibiotics do not shorten recovery time but do prolong the excretion of bacteria in the stool and are therefore usually not given. However, infants, people in nursing homes, and those with a weakened immune system are given antibiotics because they are at higher risk for complications. In carriers who do not have symptoms, the infection usually resolves on its own; antibiotic treatment is rarely needed and may not be effective.

People with *Salmonella* in their blood must take antibiotics for 4 to 6 weeks. Abscesses (collections of pus) are treated by surgical drainage and 4 weeks of antibiotic therapy. People with infection in blood vessels, heart valves, or other sites generally require surgery and prolonged antibiotic therapy.

Shigellosis

Shigellosis is infection with species of the gram-negative bacillus Shigella, *which results in dysentery that is characterized by frequent watery stools, often with mucus and blood, pain, fever, and dehydration.*

▲ see art on page 179   ■ see page 1117

Shigella is a major cause of dysentery throughout the world and is responsible for 5 to 10% of diarrheal illnesses in many areas. About half a million people in the United States develop shigellosis every year. The bacteria appear in the stool of infected people and are usually spread by person-to-person contact. Sometimes, contaminated food serves as a common source of infection. Epidemics are most frequent in overcrowded populations with inadequate sanitation. High-risk sites include child-care centers, long-term care facilities, and military camps. Children are especially likely to become infected and usually develop more severe symptoms.

The bacteria cause disease by penetrating the lining of the intestine—primarily, the large intestine—resulting in swelling and sometimes shallow sores.

Symptoms

The first symptoms are abdominal pain and watery diarrhea that start 1 to 4 days after infection. Fever is frequently present and may reach 106° F. Vomiting is not common but may occur. After 1 or 2 days, many people have pain on passing stool, which contains blood and mucus. The number of bowel movements generally increases rapidly, possibly exceeding 20 per day. Weight loss and dehydration become severe. Severe dehydration that leads to shock and death occurs mainly in chronically ill adults and children younger than 2 years of age.

Some children develop seizures. It is not known if these seizures occur simply from the high fever or as a specific complication of shigellosis. Some adults develop eye inflammation and reactive arthritis (Reiter's syndrome).▲ Rarely, intestinal perforation occurs. Severe straining during bowel movements may cause part of the rectum to be pushed out of the body (rectal prolapse). Permanent loss of bowel control can result.

Diagnosis and Treatment

A doctor suspects shigellosis from the typical symptoms of pain, fever, and bloody diarrhea in a person who lives in an area where *Shigella* is common. The diagnosis is confirmed by culturing freshly passed stool.

Treatment consists mainly of replacing fluids and salts lost because of diarrhea. Oral replacement is satisfactory for most people, but some may need to receive fluids intravenously. In most cases, the disease resolves

within 4 to 8 days without antibiotics. Severe infections may last 3 to 6 weeks. Antibiotics such as trimethoprim-sulfamethoxazole, norfloxacin, ciprofloxacin, or furazolidone may be given when the person is very young or very old, when the disease is severe, or when there is a high risk of the infection spreading to other people. The severity of the symptoms and the length of time the stool contains *Shigella* are reduced with antibiotics. Antidiarrheal drugs (such as diphenoxylate or loperamide) may prolong the infection and should not be used.

Staphylococcal Infections

Staphylococcal infections are caused by the common gram-positive cocci Staphylococcus *(staphylococci).*

Staphylococci normally grow in the nose and on the skin of 20 to 30% of healthy adults (and less commonly in the mouth; mammary glands; and urinary, intestinal, and upper respiratory tracts). These bacteria do no harm most of the time; however, a break in the skin, burn, or other injury may allow the bacteria to penetrate the body's defenses and cause infection. Commonly, staphylococcal infections produce collections of pus (abscesses), which can appear not only on the skin but also in internal organs. Staphylococcal infections range from mild to life threatening.

People prone to staphylococcal infections include newborns; injecting drug users; breast-feeding women; and people with skin disorders, surgical incisions, a weakened immune system, or chronic diseases (especially diabetes, lung disease, disease of the veins and arteries, and cancer). Intravenous catheters, particularly those that remain in the body for more than 1 or 2 days, often become contaminated with staphylococci, allowing the bacteria to enter the bloodstream (bacteremia). Postoperative staphylococcal infections usually appear a few days to several weeks after surgery but may develop more slowly if the person received antibiotics at the time of surgery.

Staphylococci tend to infect the skin,■ but they can travel through the bloodstream and involve almost any site in the body, particularly the heart (endocarditis)★ and the bones

▲ see page 376   ■ see page 1220
★ see page 184

(osteomyelitis).▲ Staphylococcal endocarditis is common in injecting drug users. Staphylococcal osteomyelitis predominantly affects children, although it also develops in older people—especially those with deep skin ulcers (bedsores or pressure sores).

Staphylococcal pneumonia is a severe infection■ that develops mainly in people with chronic lung diseases (such as chronic bronchitis and emphysema) or influenza.

Some strains of staphylococci produce toxins. These toxins cause staphylococcal food poisoning,★ toxic shock syndrome, and scalded skin syndrome.●

Symptoms

There are many kinds of staphylococcal skin infections. The least serious is folliculitis, an infection of a hair root (follicle) that produces a slightly painful, tiny white pimple at the base of a hair. Impetigo consists of shallow, fluid-filled blisters surrounded by yellow crusts. Impetigo may itch or hurt. Staphylococcal skin abscesses (boils, furuncles) are warm, painful, collections of pus below the skin surface. Staphylococcal cellulitis is a spreading infection that develops under the skin, producing pain and redness. Two particularly serious staphylococcal skin infections are toxic epidermal necrolysis and, in newborns, scalded skin syndrome, both of which lead to large-scale peeling of skin. All staphylococcal skin infections are very contagious.

Staphylococcal breast infections (mastitis) and abscesses typically develop 1 to 4 weeks after delivery. The infected area is red and painful. Breast abscesses often release large numbers of bacteria into the mother's milk, and these milk-borne bacteria may infect the nursing infant.

Staphylococcal pneumonia often causes a high fever, shortness of breath, rapid breathing, and a cough that produces sputum that may be tinged with blood. In both newborns and adults, staphylococcal pneumonia can cause lung abscesses. These abscesses may extend to involve the membranes surrounding the lungs (empyema), which adds to the breathing difficulties caused by the pneumonia.

Staphylococcal bacteremia is a common cause of death in people with severe burns.

Typically, the bacteremia causes a persistent, high fever, and sometimes shock.

Staphylococcal endocarditis can quickly damage the heart valves, leading to heart failure (with weakness and difficulty breathing) and death.

Staphylococcal osteomyelitis causes chills, fever, and bone pain. Redness and swelling appear over the infected bone, and fluid may build up in joints near the areas invaded by the bacteria.

Diagnosis and Treatment

Staphylococcal skin infections are usually diagnosed by their appearance without laboratory testing. Other more serious staphylococcal infections require samples of blood or infected fluids for culture. The laboratory establishes the diagnosis and determines which antibiotics can kill the staphylococci. Sometimes x-rays and other imaging scans can identify an area of infection, but they generally do not help the doctor make an early diagnosis.

Minor skin infections—such as folliculitis and tiny patches of impetigo—are usually treated with an ointment such as nonprescription triple-antibiotic mixture (bacitracin, neomycin, polymyxin B) or prescription mupirocin. For most other skin infections, oral antibiotics (such as cloxacillin, dicloxacillin, and cephalexin) are adequate. More severe infections, especially blood infections, require intravenous antibiotic therapy, often for up to 6 weeks.

The choice of antibiotic depends on the site of infection, the severity of the illness, and the susceptibility of the particular staphylococcal strain. Some strains are resistant to many antibiotics. Methicillin-resistant *Staphylococcus aureus* (MRSA) is resistant to nearly all antibiotics and is increasingly common in big city and university hospitals. Among the few antibiotics that are still effective against MRSA are vancomycin and trimethoprim-sulfamethoxazole.

Antibiotics alone do not cure abscesses; they must also be drained. Abscesses deeper in the body may require surgery.

Streptococcal Infections

Streptococcal infections are caused by species of the gram-positive cocci Streptococcus (streptococci).

The various disease-causing forms of streptococci are divided into groups based on their

---

▲ see page 364   ■ see page 269
★ see page 724   ● see page 1223

behavior, chemistry, and appearance. Each group tends to produce specific kinds of infections and symptoms. Many forms of streptococci live harmlessly in and on the body. Sometimes, even disease-causing streptococci can be found in healthy people (carrier state). When the laboratory finds these bacteria in sick people, it can be difficult to tell whether they are the cause of illness or not.

Infections with certain types of streptococci can cause an autoimmune reaction in which the body attacks its own tissues.▲ Autoimmune reactions can develop after an infection such as strep throat and may lead to rheumatic fever and kidney damage (glomerulonephritis).

Symptoms

Streptococci typically infect the throat and skin, although many other parts of the body can become infected, particularly the heart (endocarditis). Skin infections include cellulitis, erysipelas, impetigo, and necrotizing fasciitis.■

Strep throat is the most common streptococcal infection. Symptoms appear suddenly and include sore throat, sometimes with chills, fever, headache, nausea, vomiting, a rapid heartbeat, and a general feeling of illness (malaise). The throat is beefy red, the tonsils are swollen, and the lymph nodes in the neck may be enlarged and tender. Cough, inflammation of the larynx (laryngitis), and a stuffy nose are uncommon in streptococcal infections; these symptoms suggest another cause, such as a cold or allergy. However, in children younger than 4 years, the only symptom may be a runny nose.

Scarlet fever results when streptococci infecting a person—usually in the throat—release a toxin. This toxin leads to a widespread, pink-red rash that is most obvious on the abdomen, on the sides of the chest, and in the skinfolds. The rash does not itch or hurt. Other symptoms include a pale area around the mouth, a flushed face, and dark red lines in the skinfolds. Also, the tongue develops a white coating with red spots (white-strawberry tongue). After several days, the coating disappears and the tongue turns beefy red. The outer layer of reddened skin often peels after the fever subsides.

Diagnosis

Because of their characteristic symptoms, some streptococcal infections (such as cellulitis and impetigo) can usually be diagnosed without any tests. Other streptococcal infections, strep throat in particular, resemble illnesses caused by other bacteria and viruses. For these conditions, doctors try to confirm the diagnosis by obtaining a sample from the infected area for culture. Unfortunately, many infections (especially skin infections) are difficult to culture. Many bacteria live on or in the skin, so finding them in culture does not mean that they are the cause of the infection. Also, cultures must be allowed to grow overnight, so results are not immediately available. Certain rapid tests for streptococci produce results within a few hours. If the result of a rapid test is positive, a culture is not needed. However, if the rapid test is negative, most doctors recommend doing the overnight culture as well. These tests are important because most sore throats, even ones that look very bad, are caused by viruses and should not be treated with antibiotics.

Treatment

People with strep throat and scarlet fever usually get better in 2 weeks, even without treatment. Nevertheless, antibiotics can shorten the duration of symptoms and help prevent serious complications (such as rheumatic fever). Antibiotics also help prevent the spread of the infection to the middle ear, sinuses, and mastoid bone as well as to other people. An antibiotic, usually oral penicillin V, is started promptly after the appearance of symptoms and continued for 10 days.

Other streptococcal infections (such as cellulitis, necrotizing fasciitis, and endocarditis) are very serious and require intravenous penicillin, sometimes together with other antibiotics. In necrotizing fasciitis, surgical removal of dead, infected tissue is essential. Penicillin is effective against most streptococci, but some are resistant to penicillin and many other antibiotics.

Fever, headache, and sore throat can be treated with drugs (such as acetaminophen or nonsteroidal anti-inflammatory drugs [NSAIDs]) that reduce pain and fever. Neither bed rest nor isolation is necessary. However, family members or friends who have similar symptoms or who have had complications from earlier streptococcal infections may be given preventive therapy.

▲ see page 1073   ■ see page 1220

Tetanus

Tetanus (lockjaw) is a disease in which a toxin produced by the anaerobic bacterium Clostridium tetani *causes severe muscle spasms.*

Although rare in the United States, tetanus occurs in many parts of the world, especially in developing countries. Worldwide, as many as 50,000 people die each year from tetanus.

Spores of *Clostridium tetani* can live for years in animal feces and soil. Once tetanus spores gain entry into a person's body—typically through a wound—they begin to grow (germinate). Only growing tetanus bacilli produce toxin; it is the toxin—not the bacteria themselves—that causes disease.

Tetanus sometimes develops after cuts with dirty, rusty objects or deep punctures from stepping on a nail; the infection can also result from clean, superficial wounds. In the United States, injecting drug users and people with burns or surgical wounds are at particular risk of developing tetanus. After childbirth, tetanus infection of the woman's uterus and the umbilical stump of the newborn (tctanus neonatorum) can occur—a hazard in developing countries.

Symptoms

Symptoms usually appear 5 to 10 days after infection, but they can start as soon as 2 days or as late as 50 days after infection. The most common symptom is stiffness of the jaw, which accounts for the name "lockjaw." Other symptoms include restlessness, difficulty in swallowing, irritability, headache, fever, sore throat, chills, and muscle spasms and stiffness in the neck, arms, and legs. As the disease progresses, a person may have difficulty opening the jaw (trismus). Spasm of the facial muscles produces a facial expression of a fixed smile and raised eyebrows (risus sardonicus). Rigidity or spasm of abdominal, neck, and back muscles can cause a distinctive posture with the head and heels pulled back and the body arched forward (opisthotonos). Spasms of sphincter muscles in the lower abdomen can lead to constipation and retention of urine.

Minor disturbances—such as noise, a draft, or the bed being jarred—can trigger painful muscle spasms and profuse sweating. During full-body spasms, a person cannot cry out or speak because of rigid chest muscles or throat spasm. This condition also prevents normal breathing, causing oxygen deprivation or fatal suffocation.

Tetanal spasms may be limited to muscle groups near the wound. Such local tetanus may persist for weeks.

Diagnosis and Prognosis

A doctor suspects tetanus when muscle stiffness or a spasm occurs after a person has suffered a wound. Although *Clostridium tetani* can sometimes be cultured from a swab sample taken from the wound, negative culture results do not always mean tetanus is not present.

Tetanus has a worldwide mortality rate of 50%. Death is most likely in injecting drug users, the very young, and the very old. The prognosis is grave if symptoms worsen rapidly or treatment is delayed.

Prevention

Preventing tetanus is far better than treating tetanus once it develops. Tetanus rarely develops in a person who has completed a primary series of tetanus vaccinations (three or more injections). The tetanus vaccine stimulates the body to neutralize the toxin rather than the bacteria themselves. In young children, the tetanus vaccine is given as part of a series that includes the diphtheria and pertussis (whooping cough) vaccines. Adults who have completed the primary series of tetanus vaccination should also receive tetanus boosters every 10 years.

The guidelines for vaccination of injured people are complex: in general, people who have completed a primary series do not need a booster if they had one in the previous 5 years. People who have not completed a primary series or who have gone more than 10 years without a booster require a booster and may also require tetanus immune globulin.

The other preventive measure is prompt, thorough cleaning of wounds (especially deep puncture wounds), because dirt and dead tissue promote the growth of *Clostridium tetani*. Surgical removal of foreign material and damaged tissue may be necessary.

Treatment

Once symptoms of tetanus appear, the person is hospitalized and kept in a quiet room. Antibiotics (for example, metronidazole, penicillin, or tetracycline) are given to kill the bacteria and prevent further production of toxin; however, antibiotics have no effect on toxin

WHO NEEDS A TETANUS BOOSTER?

| Number of previous vaccinations | CLEAN, MINOR WOUNDS | | DEEP OR DIRTY WOUNDS[1] | |
	Td[2]	Tetanus immune globulin	Td	Tetanus immune globulin
Uncertain or less than 3	Yes	No	Yes	Yes
3 or more[3]	Yes, if it is more than 10 years since last dose	No	Yes, if it is more than 5 years since last dose	No

1 Such as, but not limited to, wounds contaminated with dirt, stool, or saliva; puncture wounds; wounds involving loss of tissue; and wounds resulting from foreign bodies, crushing, burns, and frostbite.
2 Td = Tetanus and diphtheria toxoids, adsorbed (for adult use); for children younger than 7, DTP.
3 If only three injections of tetanus vaccine have been received, a fourth dose should be given.

that has already been produced. Tetanus immune globulin is given to neutralize the toxin. Other drugs may be given to provide sedation; relax the muscles; relieve pain; and control seizures, heart rate, and blood pressure.

For people with moderate to severe infections, a ventilator may be required to assist breathing. Because people with tetanus have trouble swallowing, nourishment is given intravenously or through a tube inserted through the nose and into the stomach.

Although many other diseases (for example, chickenpox) leave a person immune to further episodes of the disease, people who survive a tetanus infection are not immune to tetanus. Thus, the full series of vaccinations must be given after the person recovers.

Toxic Shock Syndrome

Toxic shock syndrome is a group of severe symptoms, including dangerously low blood pressure, usually caused by toxins produced by staphylococci (and sometimes streptococci).

Toxic shock syndrome is the result of toxins produced by bacteria, usually staphylococci. The toxins may come from bacteria infecting the body or from bacteria simply growing on the body—for example, in a tampon (especially the high-absorbant type) held in the vagina. Certain types of super-absorbant tampons, particularly those containing polyacrylate, have been removed from the market because of this.

The toxin may enter the blood through small cuts in the vaginal lining or through the uterus into the abdominal cavity. However, toxic shock syndrome also occurs in women who do not use tampons and in men. Although the strain of *Staphylococcus* that causes most cases of toxic shock syndrome is known, the event that triggers the syndrome is not. A person who has had toxic shock syndrome is at increased risk of developing it again.

Symptoms and Diagnosis

Symptoms start suddenly with a fever of 102 to 105° F. A severe headache, sore throat, red eyes, extreme tiredness, confusion, vomiting, profuse watery diarrhea, and a sunburn-like rash all over the body quickly develop. Within 48 hours, the person may also faint and develop dangerously low blood pressure (shock). Between the third and seventh day, the skin peels, particularly on the palms and soles.

Toxic shock syndrome affects many parts of the body. Damage to the kidneys, liver, and muscles is very common, especially during the first week. Heart and lung problems, as well as anemia, may also develop. Most organs recover fully after the symptoms disappear.

The diagnosis is usually based on the person's symptoms. Although there is no laboratory test available that specifically identifies toxic shock syndrome, blood tests usually are performed to look for other possible causes of the symptoms.

Prevention, Treatment, and Prognosis

There are no recommendations for preventing toxic shock syndrome in women who do not wear tampons or in men. Tampon-related disease is less likely in women who avoid constant tampon use during menstruation. Because of their association with toxic shock syndrome, super-absorbent tampons should not be used when the menstrual flow is mild or moderate.

Ideally, a person suspected of having toxic shock syndrome is hospitalized immediately. Tampons, diaphragms, and other foreign objects are removed from the vagina, and antibiotic therapy is started.

About 8 to 15% of people with severe toxic shock syndrome die. Recurrences are common in women who continue to use tampons in the 4 months after an episode of toxic shock syndrome, unless antibiotic treatment has eliminated the staphylococci.

Tularemia

Tularemia (rabbit fever, deer fly fever) is infection caused by the gram-negative bacterium Francisella tularensis *that is contracted from wildlife, usually rabbits.*

People become infected with *Francisella tularensis* mainly by eating or touching infected animals. Hunters, butchers, farmers, fur handlers, and laboratory workers are most commonly infected. In the winter, most infections result from contact with wild rabbits (especially while skinning them). In the summer, infection usually results from being bitten by infected ticks or deer flies. Rarely, tularemia may be caused by eating undercooked meat or drinking contaminated water, or by inhaling bacteria that have become airborne (as occurs during butchering, or may occur while mowing if an infected animal is run over). The bacterium can penetrate unbroken skin. Person-to-person transmission has not been reported.

Symptoms

The symptoms start suddenly 1 to 10 days—usually 2 to 4 days—after contact with the bacterium. Initial symptoms include headaches, chills, nausea, vomiting, a fever of up to 104° F, and severe exhaustion. Extreme weakness, recurring chills, and profuse drenching sweats develop. In 24 to 48 hours, an inflamed blister appears at the infection site—usually the finger, arm, eye, or roof of the mouth—except in the glandular and typhoidal types of tularemia. The blister rapidly fills with pus and opens to form a sore. Single sores commonly appear on the arms or legs, but many sores usually appear in the mouth or eye. Lymph nodes around the sore enlarge and may produce pus, which later drains. A rash may appear at any time during the course of the disease.

Pneumonia sometimes develops, although the pneumonia may cause only mild symptoms, such as a dry cough that causes a burning sensation in the middle of the chest. Other people with pneumonia become delirious.

Diagnosis and Treatment

A doctor suspects tularemia in a person who develops sudden fever, swollen lymph nodes, and characteristic sores after having been exposed to ticks or deer flies or after having had even slight contact with a wild mammal (especially a rabbit). Infections acquired by laboratory workers frequently affect only the lymph nodes or lungs and are difficult to diagnose. The bacteria may be grown on special laboratory cultures.

Tularemia is treated with injections of streptomycin for 7 to 14 days. Moist bandages are placed on the sores and changed frequently. These bandages help prevent the spread of infection. Rarely, large abscesses (collections of pus) need to be drained by surgical incision. Applying warm compresses to an affected eye and wearing dark glasses may give some relief. People with intense headaches are usually treated with opioid pain relievers, such as codeine.

About one third of untreated people die, but people who are treated almost always survive.

Types of Tularemia

There are four types of tularemia. In the most common type (**ulceroglandular type**), sores develop on the hands and fingers, and the lymph nodes swell on the same side as the infection. The second type (**oculoglandular type**) involves the eye, causing redness and swelling along with swollen lymph nodes; this type probably results from touching the eye with a contaminated or infected finger, or from having infected fluid splashed into the eye. In the third type (**glandular type**), lymph nodes swell but no sores develop, suggesting that the source is ingested bacteria. The fourth type (**typhoidal type**) leads to a high fever, abdominal pain, and exhaustion. If the bacteria that cause tularemia are inhaled, pneumonia can result.

Death usually results from overwhelming infection, pneumonia, infection of the tissues covering the brain and spinal cord (meningitis), or infection of the lining of the abdominal cavity (peritonitis). Relapses are uncommon but can occur if treatment is inadequate. A person who has had tularemia develops immunity to reinfection.

Typhoid Fever

Typhoid fever (enteric fever) is caused by the gram-negative bacilli Salmonella typhi *and is characterized by prolonged fever, abdominal pain, and a rash.*

Salmonella typhi is passed in the stool and urine of infected people. Inadequate hand washing after defecation or urination may spread the bacteria to food or drink; inadequate treatment of sewage may lead to contamination of water supplies. Flies may spread the bacteria directly from stool to food. Rarely, hospital workers who have not taken adequate precautions develop typhoid fever after handling soiled bed linens or contaminated bandages from infected people.

About 3% of the infected people who do not receive treatment continue to pass bacteria in their stool for more than a year. Some of these carriers never have symptoms. Most of the estimated 2,000 carriers in the United States are older women with chronic gallbladder disease. In the past, one such woman (a cook named Mary Mallon) was responsible for spreading typhoid fever to numerous people and became known as Typhoid Mary.

Typhoid bacteria enter the digestive tract and gain access to the bloodstream. Inflammation of the small and large intestine follows. In severe infections, which can be life threatening, sores may develop in the small intestine. These sores bleed and sometimes perforate the intestinal wall.

Symptoms and Diagnosis

Usually, symptoms begin gradually 8 to 14 days after infection. The first symptoms include loss of appetite, fever, headache, joint pain, sore throat, constipation (or, less commonly, diarrhea), and abdominal pain and tenderness. A brassy, nonproductive cough is common. Nosebleed may occur.

As the illness progresses, fever remains high, and the person may become delirious. This sustained fever is often accompanied by a slow heartbeat and extreme exhaustion. Diarrhea may continue, although some people become constipated. In about 10% of infected people, clusters of small, pink spots appear on the chest and abdomen during the second week and last 2 to 5 days. After 2 weeks, intestinal bleeding or perforation occurs in 3 to 5% of infected people.

Pneumonia may develop during the second or third week and usually results from a pneumococcal infection, although typhoid bacteria can also cause pneumonia. Infection of the gallbladder and liver also may occur. A blood infection (bacteremia) occasionally leads to infection of bones (osteomyelitis), heart valves (endocarditis), kidneys (glomerulitis), the genitourinary tract, or the tissues covering the brain and spinal cord (meningitis). Infection of muscles may lead to abscesses (collections of pus).

Although the history and symptoms of illness may suggest typhoid fever, the diagnosis must be confirmed by identifying the bacteria in cultures of blood, stool, urine, or other body fluids or tissues.

Prevention and Treatment

People who travel to areas where typhoid fever is common should avoid eating raw vegetables and other foods served or stored at room temperature. Foods served very hot, bottled carbonated beverages, and raw foods that can be peeled are generally safe. Unless water is known to be safe, it should be boiled or chlorinated before being used for drinking or brushing teeth.

Both oral and injectable vaccines against typhoid fever are available, but they provide only partial protection. The vaccine is given only to people who have been exposed to the bacterium and to those who are at high risk of exposure, including laboratory workers studying the organism and people traveling to areas where the disease is common.

With prompt antibiotic therapy, more than 99% of the people with typhoid fever are cured, although convalescence may last several months. The antibiotic chloramphenicol is used worldwide, but increasing resistance to it has prompted the use of other antibiotics (such as trimethoprim-sulfamethoxazole or ciprofloxacin). If the person is delirious, comatose, or in shock, corticosteroids may be given to reduce brain inflammation. Typically, people who die are malnourished, very young, or very old. Stupor, coma, and shock are signs of severe infection and a poor prognosis.

People who recover do so in 3 to 4 weeks. Between 10 and 30% of untreated people with typhoid fever die. In about 10% of untreated people, symptoms of the initial infection recur 2 weeks later. For unknown reasons, antibiotics taken during the initial illness increase the recurrence rate to 15 to 20%. If antibiotics are given for the relapse, the fever goes away much more quickly than in the original illness, but occasionally another relapse occurs.

Relapses are treated the same way as the initial illness, but antibiotics are usually needed for only 5 days. Carriers (people who do not have symptoms but who pass the bacteria in their stool) must report to the local health department and are prohibited from working with food. The bacteria may be eradicated in many carriers after 4 to 6 weeks of antibiotic therapy.

CHAPTER 191

Bacteremia, Sepsis, and Septic Shock

Bacteria commonly enter the bloodstream (a condition called bacteremia or blood poisoning), but usually only a small number of bacteria do so at a time, and no symptoms develop. Most bacteria that enter the bloodstream are rapidly removed by white blood cells.▲ Sometimes, however, there are too many bacteria to be removed easily, and an infection develops. An infection that is widespread throughout the bloodstream is called sepsis (or septicemia) and causes severe symptoms. Sepsis can lead to a life-threatening condition called septic shock.

Bacteremia and Sepsis

Bacteremia is the presence of bacteria in the bloodstream; sepsis is a bacterial infection in the bloodstream.

Temporary bacteremia may occur during dental procedures or toothbrushing, because bacteria living on the gums around the teeth are forced into the bloodstream. Bacteria may also enter the bloodstream from the intestine, but they are rapidly removed when the blood passes through the liver. These conditions are usually not serious.

Sepsis is less common. It most often occurs when there is another infection somewhere within the body, such as in the lungs, abdo-men, urinary tract, or skin. Although bacteria typically stay at the original site of infection, they sometimes spread into the bloodstream. Sepsis can also result when surgery is performed on an infected area or on a part of the body where bacteria normally grow, such as the intestine. The presence of a foreign object—such as an intravenous line, urinary catheter, drainage tube, prosthetic joint, or artificial heart valve—may increase the risk of sepsis. The likelihood of sepsis increases the longer the object is left in place. Sepsis is more common in injecting drug users, who rarely use sterile drugs and needles. It is also more likely to occur in a person whose immune system is not functioning properly—for example, a person receiving chemotherapy. Rarely, nonbacterial infections can cause sepsis.

The circulating bacteria may settle in sites throughout the body if treatment is not given quickly. An infection can develop in the tissues surrounding the brain (meningitis), the sac around the heart (pericarditis), the inside lining of the heart (endocarditis), the bones (osteomyelitis), the joints (infectious arthritis), and other areas. Certain types of bacteria, such as staphylococci, may produce abscesses (collections of pus) in the organs they infect.

Symptoms and Diagnosis

Because the body is usually able to clear small numbers of bacteria quickly, temporary bacteremia rarely causes symptoms. Symp-

▲ see page 1050

toms such as shaking, chills, fever, weakness, confusion, nausea, vomiting, and diarrhea indicate sepsis. Depending on the type and location of the initial infection (if any), other symptoms may also be present.

A doctor usually suspects sepsis when a person who has an infection suddenly develops a high fever. Bacteria in the bloodstream are usually difficult to detect directly. To make the diagnosis, a doctor takes several blood samples to try to grow the bacteria in the laboratory (blood culture)—a process that takes 1 to 3 days. However, bacteria may not always grow in a blood culture, particularly if the person is taking antibiotics. Cultures from other fluids and substances—for example, urine, cerebrospinal fluid, tissue from wounds, and material coughed up from the lungs (sputum)—may also be analyzed for the presence of bacteria. Sometimes catheters are removed from the body and the tips are cut off and sent for culture.

Treatment and Prognosis

Bacteremia caused by surgery or dental procedures usually requires no treatment. Bacteremia caused by insertion of a catheter (catheterization) into the urinary tract may not require treatment, as long as the catheter is removed quickly. However, to prevent bacteremia and sepsis, people at risk of developing serious infections (such as those with heart valve disease or a weakened immune system) generally are given antibiotics before undergoing such procedures.

Sepsis is very serious, and the risk of death is high. Sepsis requires immediate treatment with antibiotics—even if test results confirming the diagnosis are not yet available. A delay in starting antibiotic treatment greatly decreases the person's chances of survival. Initially, a doctor bases the choice of antibiotic on which bacteria are most likely to be present, which depends on where the infection started. Often, two or three antibiotics are given together to increase the chances of killing the bacteria, particularly when the source of the bacteria is unknown. Later, when the test results are available, the doctor can substitute the antibiotic that is most effective against the specific bacteria causing the infection. Surgery may sometimes be needed to eliminate the source of the infection.

The drug drotrecogin alfa (activated), an artificially produced human protein that prevents inflammation and blood clotting, may improve survival in people with severe sepsis.

Septic Shock

Septic shock is a condition caused by an infection in the bloodstream (sepsis) in which blood pressure falls dangerously low and many organs malfunction because of inadequate blood flow.

There are several causes of shock,▲ one of which is sepsis. Septic shock occurs most often in newborns,■ people older than age 50, and people with a weakened immune system. People whose white blood cell counts are low (such as those who have AIDS or cancer or are receiving chemotherapy) and people who have a chronic disease (for example, diabetes or cirrhosis) are at greater risk of developing septic shock.

Septic shock is caused by cytokines (substances made by the immune system to fight an infection)★ and by the toxins produced by some bacteria. These substances cause the blood vessels to widen (dilate), which results in a drop in blood pressure. Consequently, blood flow to vital organs—particularly the kidneys and brain—is reduced. This reduction in blood flow occurs despite the body's attempts to compensate by increasing both the heart rate and the volume of blood pumped. Eventually, the toxins and the increased work of pumping weaken the heart, resulting in a decreased output of blood and even poorer blood flow to vital organs. The walls of the blood vessels may leak, allowing fluid to escape from the bloodstream into tissues and causing swelling. Leakage and swelling can develop in the lungs, causing difficulty breathing (respiratory distress).

Symptoms and Diagnosis

Often, the first indications of septic shock are confusion and reduced mental alertness; these symptoms may be evident 24 or more hours before blood pressure drops. Other early symptoms may include a shaking chill; a rapid rise in temperature; warm, flushed skin; a rapid, pounding pulse; excessively rapid breathing; and blood pressure that rises and falls. Urinary output decreases. Tissues with

---

▲ see page 148   ■ see page 1510
★ see page 1054

poor blood flow release excess lactic acid into the bloodstream, causing the blood to become more acidic, which results in malfunction of many different organs. In later stages, the body temperature often falls below normal.

As septic shock worsens, several organs may fail. For example, the kidneys may fail, resulting in very low or no urine output and the accumulation of metabolic waste products (such as urea nitrogen) in the blood. The lungs may fail, resulting in breathing difficulties and a reduction in the level of oxygen in the blood. The heart may fail, resulting in fluid retention and swelling of tissues. Additionally, blood clots may form inside blood vessels.

To confirm the diagnosis of septic shock, a doctor may take and analyze blood samples. High or low levels of white blood cells, a decrease in the level of oxygen, a reduction in the number of platelets, excess lactic acid, and increased levels of metabolic waste products are all signs that a person may be in septic shock. A doctor may also use a fingertip sensor to monitor the level of oxygen in the blood. An electrocardiogram (ECG) may show irregularities in heart rhythm, indicating inadequate blood supply to the heart. Blood cul-

tures are performed to identify the infecting organisms. Because there are other causes of shock besides sepsis, additional tests may be needed.

Treatment and Prognosis

As soon as symptoms of septic shock are apparent, the person must be admitted to an intensive care unit for treatment. Large amounts of fluid are given intravenously to increase the blood pressure. Drugs are given to increase blood flow to the brain, heart, and other organs. Extra oxygen is given. If the lungs fail, the person may need a mechanical ventilator to help breathing.

High doses of intravenous antibiotics are given as soon as blood samples have been taken for laboratory cultures. Until the laboratory identifies the infecting bacteria, two or more antibiotics are usually given together to increase the chances of killing the bacteria.

Any abscesses are drained, and any catheters that may have started the infection are removed. Surgery may be performed to remove any dead tissue, such as gangrenous tissue of the intestine. Despite all efforts, more than 25% of people with septic shock die.

CHAPTER 192

Antibiotics

Antibiotics are drugs derived wholly or partially from certain microorganisms and are used to treat bacterial or fungal infections. They are ineffective against viruses. Antibiotics either kill microorganisms or stop them from reproducing, allowing the body's natural defenses to eliminate them. Antifungal and antiviral drugs are discussed elsewhere.▲

Selecting an Antibiotic

Each antibiotic is effective only against certain bacteria. In selecting an antibiotic to treat a person with an infection, a doctor makes a

---

▲ see tables on pages 1152 and 1156

■ see box on page 1088

best guess as to which bacterium is responsible. For some infections, doctors know that only certain types of bacteria may be responsible. If there is one antibiotic that is predictably effective against all of these bacteria, further testing is not needed. For infections that may be caused by many different types of bacteria or by bacteria whose susceptibility to antibiotics is not predictable, a laboratory will be asked to identify the infecting bacterium from samples of blood, urine, or tissue taken from the person.■ The infecting bacterium is then tested for susceptibility to a variety of antibiotics. These tests generally take a day or two to yield results and thus cannot guide the initial choice of which antibiotic is given.

Antibiotics that are effective in the laboratory do not necessarily work in an infected person, however. The effectiveness of the treatment depends on how well the drug is absorbed into the bloodstream, how much of the drug reaches the sites of infection in the body, and how quickly the body eliminates the drug. In selecting which antibiotic to use, a doctor also considers the nature and seriousness of the infection, the drug's possible side effects, the possibility of allergies or other serious reactions to the drug, and the cost of the drug.

Combinations of antibiotics are sometimes needed to treat severe infections, particularly in the first days when the bacterium's sensitivity to antibiotics is not known. Combinations are also important for certain infections in which the bacterium rapidly develops resistance to a single antibiotic. Infections caused by more than one bacterium, in which each bacterium is susceptible to a different antibiotic, are also treated with a combination of antibiotics.

Antibiotic Resistance

Bacteria, like all living organisms, change over time in response to environmental challenges. Because of the widespread use and misuse of antibiotics in modern society, bacteria are constantly exposed to these agents. Although many bacteria die when exposed to antibiotics, some develop resistance to the drugs' effects. For example, 50 years ago the bacterium *Staphylococcus aureus* (a common cause of skin infections) was very sensitive to penicillin. Over time, strains of *Staphylococcus aureus* developed an enzyme able to break down penicillin, making the drug ineffective. Researchers responded by developing a form of penicillin that the enzyme could not split, but after a few years the bacteria adapted and became resistant to even this modified penicillin. Other bacteria have developed resistance to antibiotics using different mechanisms.

Medical researchers continually work to ensure that there are effective drugs to combat bacteria. Taking antibiotics only when necessary (not for viral infections such as a cold or the flu) and for the full prescribed course helps limit the development of antibiotic-resistant bacteria.

Taking Antibiotics

For severe bacterial infections, antibiotics are usually first given by injection. When the infection is under control, antibiotics can then be taken by mouth. Less severe infections can be treated from the start with oral antibiotics. Antibiotics need to be taken until the infecting organism is eliminated from the body, which may be days after the symptoms disappear. Antibiotics are rarely given for fewer than 5 days (an exception is certain uncomplicated urinary tract infections). Discontinuing treatment too soon can result in a relapse of infection or the development of antibiotic-resistant bacteria.

A doctor, nurse, or pharmacist can explain how the prescribed antibiotic should be taken. Some antibiotics must be taken on an empty stomach, whereas others may be taken with food. Metronidazole, a common antibiotic, causes an unpleasant reaction with alcohol. Also, some antibiotics can interact with other drugs a person may be taking, possibly reducing the effectiveness or increasing the side effects of the antibiotic or the other drugs. Some antibiotics make the skin sensitive to sunlight.

In addition to treating existing infections, antibiotics are sometimes used to prevent infections (prophylaxis). Antibiotics may be used to prevent meningitis in people who have been exposed to someone with meningitis. Some people with abnormal or artificial heart valves take antibiotics before dental and surgical procedures to prevent bacteria from infecting the damaged valves. Prophylactic antibiotics may also be given to people who have a weakened immune system, such as people with leukemia, people receiving chemotherapy for cancer, or people with AIDS. People undergoing surgery that has a high risk of introducing infection (such as major orthopedic or intestinal surgery) may also be given antibiotics. To be effective, and to avoid the development of resistance in bacteria, prophylactic antibiotic therapy is used for only a short time.

Home Antibiotic Therapy

Usually, antibiotics are given by mouth and the duration of treatment does not cause hardship. However, the treatment of some infections—such as those involving bone (osteomyelitis) or the heart (endocarditis)—requires antibiotics to be given intravenously for a long time, often 4 to 6 weeks. If the person has no other conditions that need treatment in the hospital and is feeling relatively well, intravenous antibiotics may be administered at home. Short intravenous (IV) cathe-

℞ ANTIBIOTICS

TYPE	DRUG	COMMON USES	SIDE EFFECTS
Aminoglycosides	Amikacin Gentamicin Kanamycin Neomycin Netilmicin Streptomycin Tobramycin	Infections caused by gram-negative bacteria, such as *Escherichia coli* and *Klebsiella*	Hearing loss Dizziness Kidney damage
Carbecephem	Loracarbef		
Carbapenems	Ertapenem Imipenem/ cilastatin Meropenem	Gangrene, sepsis, pneumonia, abdominal and urinary infections, and (except for ertapenem) *Pseudomonas* infections	Seizures Confusion
Cephalosporins, 1st generation	Cefadroxil Cefazolin Cephalexin	Skin and soft tissue infections	Gastrointestinal upset and diarrhea Nausea Allergic reactions
Cephalosporins, 2nd generation	Cefaclor Cefamandole Cefotetan Cefoxitin Cefprozil Cefuroxime	Some respiratory and abdominal infections	Gastrointestinal upset and diarrhea Nausea Allergic reactions
Cephalosporins, 3rd generation	Cefixime Cefdinir Cefditoren Cefoperazone Cefotaxime Cefpodoxime Ceftazidime Ceftibuten Ceftizoxime Ceftriaxone	Broad coverage of many bacteria for people with mild-to-moderate infections (oral) and serious illness (by injection)	Gastrointestinal upset and diarrhea Nausea Allergic reactions
Cephalosporins, 4th generation	Cefepime	Serious infections, particularly in people with a weakened immune system	Gastrointestinal upset and diarrhea Nausea Allergic reactions
Macrolides	Azithromycin Clarithromycin Dirithromycin Erythromycin Troleandomycin	Streptococcal infections, syphilis, respiratory infections, mycoplasmal infections, Lyme disease	Nausea, vomiting, and diarrhea (especially at higher doses) Jaundice

R_x   ANTIBIOTICS (Continued)

TYPE	DRUG	COMMON USES	SIDE EFFECTS
Monobactam			
	Aztreonam	Infections caused by gram-negative bacteria	Allergic reactions
Penicillins			
	Amoxicillin Ampicillin Carbenicillin Cloxacillin Dicloxacillin Nafcillin Oxacillin Penicillin G Penicillin V Piperacillin Ticarcillin	Wide range of infections; penicillin used for streptococcal infections, syphilis, and Lyme disease	Nausea, vomiting, and diarrhea Allergy with serious anaphylactic reactions Brain and kidney damage (rare)
Polypeptides			
	Bacitracin Colistin Polymyxin B	Ear, eye, skin, or bladder infections; usually applied directly to the skin or eye; rarely given by injection	Kidney and nerve damage (when given by injection)
Quinolones			
	Ciprofloxacin Enoxacin Gatifloxacin Levofloxacin Lomefloxacin Moxifloxacin Norfloxacin Ofloxacin Trovafloxacin	Urinary tract infections, bacterial prostatitis, bacterial diarrhea, gonorrhea	Nausea (rare) Nervousness, tremors, seizures Inflammation or rupture of tendons
Sulfonamides			
	Mafenide Sulfacetamide Sulfamethizole Sulfasalazine Sulfisoxazole Trimethoprim-sulfamethoxazole	Urinary tract infections (except sulfasalazine, sulfacetamide, and mafenide); mafenide is used topically for burns	Nausea, vomiting, and diarrhea Allergy (including skin rashes) Crystals in urine (rare) Decrease in white blood cell count Sensitivity to sunlight
Tetracyclines			
	Demeclocycline Doxycycline Minocycline Oxytetracycline Tetracycline	Syphilis, chlamydial infections, Lyme disease, mycoplasmal infections, rickettsial infections	Gastrointestinal upset Sensitivity to sunlight Staining of teeth Potential toxicity to mother and fetus during pregnancy

Table continues on the following page.

Rx   ANTIBIOTICS (Continued)

TYPE	DRUG	COMMON USES	SIDE EFFECTS
Miscellaneous antibiotics			
	Chloramphenicol	Typhoid and other *Salmonella* infections, meningitis	Severe decrease in white blood cell count (rare)
	Clindamycin	Streptococcal and staphylococcal infections, respiratory infections, lung abscess	Severe diarrhea
	Ethambutol	Tuberculosis	Vision disturbances
	Fosfomycin	Bladder infections	Diarrhea
	Isoniazid	Tuberculosis	Nausea and vomiting Jaundice
	Linezolid	Serious infections caused by gram-positive bacteria that are resistant to other antibiotics	Nausea Headache Diarrhea Low platelet count
	Metronidazole	Vaginitis caused by *Trichomonas* or *Gardnerella*; pelvic and abdominal infections	Nausea Headache (especially if taken with alcohol) Metallic taste Dark urine
	Nitrofurantoin	Urinary tract infections	Nausea and vomiting Allergy
	Pyrazinamide	Tuberculosis	Liver dysfunction Gout (occasional)
	Quinupristin/ dalfopristin	Serious infections caused by gram-positive bacteria that are resistant to other antibiotics	Aching muscles and joints
	Rifampin	Tuberculosis and leprosy	Rash Liver dysfunction Red-orange saliva, sweat, tears, and urine
	Spectinomycin	Gonorrhea	Allergy Fever
	Vancomycin	Serious infections resistant to other antibiotics	Flushing, itching

ters inserted into small veins in the arm or hand (such as are used in most routine hospital procedures) do not last more than 3 days, so a special type of IV catheter inserted into a large central vein may be needed. Some devices for infusing antibiotics are simple enough that people and their families can learn to operate them on their own. In other cases, a visiting nurse must come to the home to administer each dose. In either situation, careful supervision is required to assist the person and watch for possible complications and side effects.

People who receive antibiotics at home through an IV catheter are at increased risk of developing an infection at the site where the catheter is inserted and in the bloodstream. Pain, redness, and pus at the catheter insertion site, or chills and fever (even in the absence of problems at the insertion site) are signs that a catheter-related infection may have developed.

Side Effects and Allergies

Common side effects of antibiotics include upset stomach, diarrhea, and, in women, vaginal yeast infections. Some side effects are more severe and, depending on the antibiotic, may disrupt the function of the kidneys, liver, bone marrow, or other organs. Blood tests are used to monitor such adverse reactions.

Some people who receive antibiotics develop colitis, an inflammation of the large intestine. The colitis results from a toxin produced by the bacterium *Clostridium difficile*, which grows unchecked when other antibacteria are killed by the antibiotics.

Antibiotics can also cause allergic reactions. Mild allergic reactions consist of an itchy rash or slight wheezing. Severe allergic reactions (anaphylaxis) can be life threatening and usually include swelling of the throat, inability to breathe, and low blood pressure.

Many people tell their doctor that they are allergic to an antibiotic when in fact they have only experienced side effects from it that are not allergy-related. The distinction is important because people who are allergic to an antibiotic should not be given that drug or one closely related to it. However, people who have experienced minor side effects can usually take related drugs or even continue taking the same one. The doctor can determine the significance of any unpleasant reaction a person has to an antibiotic.

CHAPTER 193

Tuberculosis

Tuberculosis is a contagious infection caused by an airborne bacterium, Mycobacterium tuberculosis.

Tuberculosis usually affects the lungs, although it can attack almost any organ in the body. Other mycobacteria (such as *Mycobacterium bovis* or *Mycobacterium africanum*) occasionally can cause a similar disease.

Tuberculosis has been a serious public health problem for a long time. In the 1800s, the disease was responsible for more than 30% of all deaths in Europe. With the advent of antituberculosis antibiotics in the 1940s, the battle against tuberculosis seemed to be won. Unfortunately—because of factors such as inadequate public health resources, reduced immune response due to AIDS, the development of drug resistance, and extreme poverty in many parts of the world—tuberculosis continues to be a deadly disease. Worldwide, there are 8 million new cases of symptomatic tuberculosis and 3 million deaths from the disease every year. It is believed that one third of all the people in the world have a dormant (latent) tuberculosis infection, although only about 5 to 10% progress to active tuberculosis disease.

In the United States and other developed countries, tuberculosis has been more common among older people, whereas it is a disease of young adults in poorer countries. Of the cases reported in the United States in 2000, 22% involved people older than age 65. There were more cases among older people because they were more likely to have acquired the infection in an era when tuberculosis was more common. As the body's immune system weakens with age, dormant bacteria become reactivated. Fortunately, the incidence of tuberculosis among older people is declining because each generation entering old age has a lower rate of latent infection.

Because tuberculosis has existed in Europe longer than anywhere else, people of European descent are somewhat more resistant to the disease than people whose ancestors lived in parts of the world where tuberculosis was introduced more recently. Thus, in the United States, tuberculosis is more common among blacks, Native Americans, certain other minorities, and immigrants from non-European countries. Additionally, people in these groups tend to be poorer, live in crowded conditions, and have less access to medical care—all conditions that are conducive to the spread of tuberculosis.

How Infection Develops

With most infectious diseases (such as strep throat or pneumonia), a person becomes sick right after the microorganism enters the body and is noticeably ill within 1 or 2 weeks. Tuberculosis does not follow this pattern.

Diseases Resembling Tuberculosis

Many types of mycobacteria exist; many can cause infections that produce symptoms similar to tuberculosis.

The most common are a group known as *Mycobacterium avium* complex (MAC). Although these mycobacteria are common, they generally cause infection only in people with a weakened immune system or with lungs that have been damaged by prolonged smoking, an old tuberculosis infection, bronchitis, emphysema, or other diseases. Similar to tuberculosis, a MAC infection primarily affects the lungs but may also attack the lymph nodes, bones, skin, and other tissues. Unlike tuberculosis, a MAC infection cannot be passed from one person to another.

The infection usually develops slowly. The first symptoms include coughing and spitting up mucus. As the infection progresses, the person may regularly spit up blood and have trouble breathing. A chest x-ray may or may not reveal an infection. A laboratory analysis of sputum taken from an infected person is needed to distinguish the infection from tuberculosis.

In people with AIDS or other diseases that weaken the immune system, MAC infection can spread throughout the body. Symptoms include a fever, anemia, blood disorders, diarrhea, and stomach pain.

MAC infection of the lymph nodes may develop in children, generally those between the ages of 1 and 5 years. The infection is usually caused by eating soil or drinking water that is contaminated with the mycobacteria. Antibiotics do not usually cure the infection, but the infected lymph nodes can be removed by surgery.

MAC infections were very difficult to treat until recently, because the bacteria were resistant to most of the antibiotics effective against tuberculosis. Newer antibiotics, such as clarithromycin and azithromycin—which do not work in tuberculosis—have been found to be effective against MAC when used in combination with ethambutol and rifabutin.

Other mycobacteria grow in swimming pools and even in home aquariums and can cause skin disorders. These infections may clear up without treatment. However, people with chronic infections usually need treatment with tetracycline, clarithromycin, or another antibiotic for 3 to 6 months. Another type of mycobacteria, *Mycobacterium fortuitum*, can infect wounds and artificial body parts, such as a mechanical heart valve or breast implant. Antibiotics and surgical removal of the infected areas usually cure the infection.

Stages of Infection: Except for very young children, few people become sick immediately after tuberculosis bacteria enter their body (primary infection). Many tuberculosis bacteria that enter the lungs are immediately killed by the body's defenses. Those that survive are captured inside white blood cells called macrophages. The captured bacteria can remain alive inside these cells in a dormant state for many years, walled off inside tiny scars (latent infection). In 90 to 95% of cases, the bacteria never cause any further problem, but in about 5 to 10% of infected people they start to multiply (active disease). It is in this active phase that an infected person actually becomes sick and can spread the disease.

More than half the time, activation of dormant bacteria happens within the first 2 years, but it may not occur for a very long time. Doctors do not always know why the dormant bacteria become active, but it often occurs when the person's immune system becomes impaired—for example, from very advanced age, the use of corticosteroids, or AIDS. Like many infectious diseases, tuberculosis spreads more quickly and is much more dangerous in people who have a weakened immune system. For such people (including the very young, the very old, and those who are also infected with HIV), tuberculosis can be life threatening.

Transmission of Infection: *Mycobacterium tuberculosis* can live only in people; it cannot be carried by animals, insects, soil, or other nonliving objects. A person can be infected with tuberculosis only from another person who has active disease. Touching someone who has the disease does not spread it, because the bacteria are transmitted only through the air. *Mycobacterium bovis*, a bacterium that can live in animals, is an exception. In developing countries, children become infected with it by drinking unpasteurized milk from infected cattle.

People with active tuberculosis in their lungs contaminate the air with bacteria when they cough, sneeze, or even speak. These bacteria can stay in the air for several hours. If another person breathes them in, that person may become infected. People who have latent disease or tuberculosis that is not in their lungs do not spread bacteria into the air and cannot transmit the infection.

Progression and Spread of Infection: The progression of tuberculosis from latent infection to active disease varies greatly. For example, tuberculosis often progresses more rapidly in blacks and Native Americans than in whites because of inherited differences in resistance. Impaired immunity also plays a role. Progression to an active disease is far more likely and much faster in people with AIDS. A person with AIDS who becomes infected with *Mycobacterium tuberculosis* has a 50% chance of developing active tuberculosis within 2 months and a 5 to 10% chance of developing active disease each year thereafter.

In people with a fully functioning immune system, active tuberculosis is usually limited to the lungs (pulmonary tuberculosis). Tuberculosis that affects other parts of the body (extrapulmonary tuberculosis) comes from pulmonary tuberculosis that has spread through the blood. As in the lungs, the infection may not cause disease, but the bacteria may remain dormant in a very small scar. Latent organisms in these scars can reactivate later in life, leading to symptoms in the organs involved. In pregnant women, the tuberculosis bacteria may spread to the fetus and cause disease; however, such congenital tuberculosis is uncommon.

Symptoms and Complications

Cough is the most common symptom of tuberculosis. Because the disease comes on slowly, an infected person at first may blame the cough on smoking, a recent episode of flu, or asthma. The cough may produce a small amount of green or yellow sputum in the morning. Eventually, the sputum may be streaked with blood, although large amounts of blood are rare.

Another symptom is awakening in the night drenched with a cold sweat. Sometimes there is so much sweat that the person has to change nightclothes or even the bed sheets. However, these night sweats are not specific to tuberculosis. Along with the cough and night sweats, the person feels generally unwell, with decreased energy and appetite. Weight loss often occurs after the illness has been present for a while.

Rapidly developing shortness of breath along with chest pain may signal the presence

TUBERCULOSIS: A DISEASE OF MANY ORGANS

SITE OF INFECTION	SYMPTOMS OR COMPLICATIONS
Abdominal cavity	Fatigue, swelling, slight tenderness, appendicitis-like pain
Bladder	Painful urination, blood in urine
Bones (mainly children)	Swelling, minimal pain
Brain	Fever, headache, nausea, drowsiness; coma and brain damage if untreated
Pericardium (the membrane around the heart)	Fever, enlarged neck veins, shortness of breath
Joints	Arthritis-like symptoms
Kidneys	Kidney damage, infection around the kidneys
Lymph nodes	Painless, red swelling; may drain pus
Reproductive organs	
Men	Lump in scrotum
Women	Sterility
Spine	Pain, leading to collapsed vertebrae and leg paralysis

of air (pneumothorax)▲ or fluid (pleural effusion) in the space between the lungs and the chest wall.■ About one third of tuberculosis infections first show up as a pleural effusion. Eventually, many people with untreated tuberculosis develop shortness of breath as the infection spreads in the lungs.

In a new tuberculosis infection, the bacteria may travel from the lungs to the lymph nodes that drain the lungs. If the body's natural defenses can control the infection, it goes no further, and the bacteria become dormant. However, very young children have weaker defenses and these lymph nodes may become large enough to compress the bronchial tubes, causing a brassy cough and possibly a collapsed lung. Occasionally, bacteria spread up the lymph channels to the lymph nodes in the neck. An infection in these lymph nodes may break through the skin and discharge pus.

▲ see page 316   ■ see page 314

The Tuberculin Skin Test

A tuberculin skin test is performed by injecting a small amount of protein derived from tuberculosis bacteria between the layers of the skin, usually on the forearm. About 2 days later, the injection site is checked and measured: swelling that feels firm to the touch and is larger than a certain size indicates a positive result. Redness around the site without swelling is not positive. Some people who are very ill or who have a weakened immune system may not respond to the skin test even if they are infected with tuberculosis.

The kidneys and lymph nodes are probably the most common sites for tuberculosis that develops outside the lungs (extrapulmonary tuberculosis). It can also affect the bones, brain, abdominal cavity, membrane around the heart (pericardium), joints (especially weight-bearing joints, such as the hips and knees), and reproductive organs. Tuberculosis in these areas can be difficult to diagnose.

The symptoms of extrapulmonary tuberculosis are vague, usually with fatigue, poor appetite, intermittent fevers, sweats, and possibly weight loss. Sometimes the infection causes pain or discomfort, depending on the area involved, but not always.

Tuberculosis that infects the tissues covering the brain (tuberculous meningitis) is life threatening. In the United States and other developed countries, tuberculous meningitis most commonly occurs among older people. In developing countries, tuberculous meningitis is most common among children from birth to age 5. Symptoms include fever, constant headache, neck stiffness, nausea, and drowsiness that can lead to coma. Tuberculosis also may infect the brain itself, forming a mass called a tuberculoma. The tuberculoma may cause symptoms such as headaches, seizures, or muscle weakness.

Tuberculous pericarditis is tuberculosis affecting the pericardium. This infection causes the pericardium to thicken and sometimes leak fluid into the space between the pericardium and the heart. This limits the heart's ability to pump and causes swollen neck veins and difficulty breathing.

▲ see box on page 1126

Intestinal tuberculosis occurs mainly in developing countries. This infection may not produce any symptoms but can produce abnormal growth of tissue, which may be mistaken for cancer, at the infected area.

Diagnosis

Sometimes the first indication of tuberculosis is an abnormal chest x-ray or positive tuberculin skin test (also known as a Mantoux test or PPD for purified protein derivative), because these tests are often done as routine screening tests. When a person has symptoms that suggest tuberculosis, a chest x-ray is taken, a tuberculin skin test is performed, and a sputum sample is sent to the laboratory. The sputum sample is examined under a microscope to look for tuberculosis bacteria and used to grow the bacteria in a culture. The microscopic examination is much faster than a culture but is less accurate. Cultures do not provide results for many weeks because tuberculosis bacteria grow slowly.

Chest x-ray findings in tuberculosis often resemble those from other diseases, so the diagnosis may depend on the results of the tuberculin skin test and examination of sputum for *Mycobacterium tuberculosis.* Although a tuberculin skin test is one of the most useful tests for diagnosing tuberculosis, it indicates only that an infection by the bacteria has occurred some time in the past. It does not reveal whether the infection is currently active. False-positive results can occur because of an infection with one of the close, generally harmless, relatives of tuberculosis▲ or by recent vaccination against tuberculosis.

Sputum usually provides an adequate sample from the lung, but occasionally a doctor may use an instrument called a bronchoscope to inspect the bronchial tubes and obtain samples of mucus or lung tissue. This procedure is most often performed when other diseases, such as lung cancer, are suspected.

When symptoms indicate the possibility of tuberculous meningitis, a doctor may need to perform a spinal tap to obtain a sample of spinal fluid for analysis. Because tuberculosis bacteria are hard to find in spinal fluid, and cultures usually take weeks, the sample is often sent for a test called polymerase chain reaction (PCR), which can detect tiny amounts of the bacteria's DNA. Although test results are available quickly, a doctor generally begins antibiotic therapy on the mere suspicion of tuberculous meningitis to prevent death and minimize brain damage.

Treatment

A number of antibiotics are effective against tuberculosis. But because tuberculosis bacteria are very slow-growing, the antibiotics must be taken for a long time—usually for 6 months or longer. Treatment must be continued long after the person feels completely well; otherwise, the disease tends to relapse because it was not fully eliminated.

Most people find it difficult to remember to take their drugs every day for such a long time. Other people, for various reasons, discontinue treatment as soon as they feel better. Because of these problems, many experts recommend that people with tuberculosis receive their drugs from a health care worker. This is called Directly Observed Therapy (DOT). Because DOT ensures that the person takes every dose, DOT treatments are often shorter, and the drugs are usually given just 2 or 3 times per week.

To treat tuberculosis, two or more antibiotics with different mechanisms of action are always given, because treatment with only one drug can leave behind a few bacteria resistant to that drug. With most other bacteria, this would not be enough to cause a relapse, but people treated with only one drug develop tuberculosis resistant to that drug. A third and fourth drug are usually used during the initial, intensive phase of treatment to shorten the duration of treatment and to ensure success even if drug resistance exists at the outset.

The most commonly used antibiotics are isoniazid, rifampin, pyrazinamide, streptomycin, and ethambutol. Isoniazid causes liver injury in 1 person in 10,000, resulting in nausea, vomiting, and jaundice. Rifampin also may injure the liver, particularly when combined with isoniazid. These effects go away when the person discontinues the drug. Pyrazinamide also causes liver injury and sometimes gout. Streptomycin can damage the nerves of the inner ear, producing dizziness and slight hearing loss. Ethambutol sometimes affects the optic nerve, causing blurred vision and decreased color perception. However, 95% of the people with tuberculosis successfully complete therapy and are cured with these drugs and do not experience any serious side effects.

There are many different combinations and dose schedules for these drugs. Isoniazid, ri-

What Is Miliary Tuberculosis?

A potentially life-threatening type of tuberculosis may result when a large number of the bacteria spread throughout the body by way of the bloodstream. This infection is called miliary tuberculosis because the millions of tiny lesions formed are the size of millet, the small round seeds in bird food.

Symptoms of miliary tuberculosis can be vague and difficult to identify; they include weight loss, fever, chills, weakness, general discomfort, and difficulty in breathing. Involvement of the bone marrow may cause severe anemia and other blood abnormalities, suggesting leukemia. An intermittent release of bacteria into the bloodstream from a hidden lesion may cause a fever that comes and goes, with gradual wasting of the body.

fampin, and pyrazinamide may be contained in the same capsule, reducing the number of pills a person has to take each day and reducing the chance of developing drug resistance.

Surgery to remove a portion of the lung is seldom needed if the person faithfully follows the drug treatment plan. However, surgery is sometimes needed for very drug-resistant infections and to drain pus from wherever it has accumulated. When tuberculous pericarditis causes significant restriction of the motion of the heart, the pericardium may need to be removed surgically. A tuberculoma in the brain may need to be surgically removed.

Prevention

There are two aspects of prevention: stopping the spread of disease and treating early infection before it becomes active disease.

Because tuberculosis bacteria are airborne, good ventilation with fresh air lowers the concentration of bacteria and limits their spread. Also, a germicidal ultraviolet light can be used to kill airborne tuberculosis bacteria in places where people at risk are gathered, such as homeless shelters, jails, and hospital and emergency department waiting areas.

Since tuberculosis is transmitted only by people with active disease, early recognition and treatment of active disease is one of the best ways to stop it from spreading. People with active tuberculosis should cough into a tissue to reduce the spread of bacteria, and they should remain in isolation until they are no longer coughing. After only a few days of treatment with the correct antibiotics, a person is less likely to spread the disease and usually does not need to be isolated for longer than a week or two. However, if a person works with people who are at high risk (such as young children or people with AIDS), repeated analyses of sputum samples may be needed to determine when there is no danger of transmission of the infection. Also, people who continue to cough during treatment, fail to take their drugs properly, or have drug-resistant tuberculosis may need to be isolated longer so that they do not spread the disease.

The second aspect of prevention consists of treating people with a positive tuberculin skin test who are not yet ill. The drug isoniazid is very effective at stopping the infection before it becomes active disease. It is given daily for 6 to 9 months. Newer, shorter treatments use rifampin plus pyrazinamide daily for 2 months or rifampin alone daily for 4 months. Preventive therapy definitely benefits younger people who have a positive tuberculin skin test. It also is likely to help older people at high risk for tuberculosis (for example, people whose tuberculin skin test result recently changed from negative to positive, people who have been recently exposed, or those with a weakened immune system). The risk of toxicity from the antibiotics in older adults with long-standing dormant (latent) disease may be greater than the risk of developing tuberculosis.

A person with a positive tuberculin skin test who becomes infected with HIV is at very high risk of developing active infection; similarly, a person who takes corticosteroids has a greatly increased risk of activation of latent tuberculosis. Thus, such people usually need treatment of latent tuberculosis infection.

In much of the developing world, a vaccine called BCG is used to prevent development of serious complications, such as meningitis, in people who are at high risk of becoming infected with *Mycobacterium tuberculosis*. The value of BCG is the subject of debate, and the vaccine continues to be used only in countries where the likelihood of contracting tuberculosis is very high. Research is under way to develop a more effective vaccine. About 10% of people who have received BCG at birth have a positive reaction to the tuberculin skin test 15 years later, even if they are not infected with tuberculosis bacteria. However, it is common for people vaccinated at birth to incorrectly attribute a positive PPD reaction later in life to having received BCG. In most countries, tuberculosis is stigmatized and many people are reluctant to believe they have even latent infection, much less active disease.

CHAPTER 194

Leprosy

Leprosy (Hansen's disease) is a chronic infection caused by the bacterium Mycobacterium leprae *that results in damage primarily to the peripheral nerves (the nerves outside the brain and spinal cord), skin, testes, eyes, and mucous membrane of the nose.*

Because of the visible disfigurement in untreated people, people with leprosy have long been feared and shunned by others. Although leprosy is not highly contagious, does not cause death, and can be effectively treated with antibiotics, the disease still causes widespread anxiety. As a result, people with leprosy often suffer psychologic and social problems.

More than 1 million people worldwide have leprosy. Leprosy is most common in Asia (especially India and Nepal), Africa, Latin America, and the islands of the Pacific Ocean. About 4,000 people in the United States are infected, most of them in California, Hawaii, and Texas. Almost all cases of leprosy in the United States involve people who emigrated from developing countries. The infection can start at any age but most commonly begins in the 20s and 30s.

It is not clear how leprosy is spread. However, one way the disease is likely passed from person to person is through droplets expelled from the nose and mouth of an infected person and breathed in or touched by an uninfected person. But even with the bacteria in the air, most people do not contract leprosy. About half of the people with leprosy probably contracted it through close, long-term contact with an infected person. Casual and short-term contact do not seem to spread the disease. Leprosy cannot be contracted by simply touching someone with the disease, as is commonly believed. Health care workers often work for many years with people who have leprosy without contracting the disease. Other potential sources of *Mycobacterium leprae* are soil, armadillos, and possibly bedbugs and mosquitoes.

About 95% of people who are exposed to *Mycobacterium leprae* do not develop leprosy because their immune system fights off the infection. In people who do develop the disease, the infection can range from mild (tuberculoid leprosy) to severe (lepromatous leprosy). The tuberculoid form of leprosy is not contagious.

Symptoms

Because the bacteria that cause leprosy multiply very slowly, symptoms usually do not begin until at least 1 year after a person has been infected; on average, symptoms appear 5 to 7 years after infection. Once symptoms do begin, they progress slowly.

Leprosy mainly affects the skin and peripheral nerves. The skin develops characteristic rashes and bumps. Infection of the nerves makes the skin numb or the muscles weak in areas controlled by those nerves.

Leprosy is categorized as tuberculoid, lepromatous, or borderline according to the type and number of skin spots. The type of leprosy dictates the long-term prognosis, likely complications, and how long antibiotic treatment is needed.

In tuberculoid leprosy, a rash appears, consisting of one or a few flat, whitish areas. Areas affected by this rash are numb because the bacteria damage the underlying nerves.

In lepromatous leprosy, many small bumps or larger raised rashes of variable size and shape appear on the skin. There are more areas of numbness than in tuberculoid leprosy, and certain muscle groups may be weak.

Borderline leprosy shares features of both tuberculoid and lepromatous leprosy. If not treated, borderline leprosy may improve to resemble the tuberculoid form or worsen to become more like the lepromatous form.

The most severe symptoms of leprosy result from infection of the peripheral nerves, which causes a deterioration of a person's sense of touch and a corresponding inability to feel pain and temperature. People with peripheral nerve damage may unknowingly burn, cut, or otherwise harm themselves. Repeated damage may eventually lead to loss of fingers and toes. Also, damage to peripheral nerves may cause muscle weakness, at times resulting in clawing of the fingers and a "drop foot" deformity. Skin infection can lead to areas of swelling and lumps, which can be particularly disfiguring on the face.

People with leprosy also may develop sores on the soles of the feet. Damage to the nasal passages can result in a chronically stuffy nose and, if untreated, complete erosion of the nose. Eye damage may lead to blindness. Men with lepromatous leprosy may experience erectile dysfunction (impotence) and become infertile, because the infection can reduce the amount of testosterone and sperm produced by the testes.

During the course of untreated or even treated leprosy, the body's immune response may produce inflammatory reactions. These reactions can produce fever and inflammation of the skin, peripheral nerves, and less commonly the lymph nodes, joints, testes, kidneys, liver, and eyes.

Diagnosis

The symptoms (such as distinctive skin rashes that do not disappear, loss of the sense of touch, and deformities that result from muscle weakness) provide strong clues to the diagnosis of leprosy. Microscopic examination of a sample of infected skin tissue confirms the diagnosis. Because leprosy bacteria will not grow in the laboratory, tissue cultures and blood tests are not useful.

Prevention and Treatment

In the past, the deformities caused by leprosy led to ostracism, and people with the disease often were isolated in institutions or colonies. In some countries, this practice is still common. Isolation, however, is unnecessary. Leprosy is contagious only in the untreated lepromatous form, and even then the disease is not easily transmitted to others. Once treatment has begun, the disease cannot be passed to others. Furthermore, most people are naturally immune to leprosy, and only those who have close, long-term contact with an infected person are at risk of developing an infection. People at risk should be monitored by a doctor, but preventive antibiotics are not used. The BCG vaccine, which is used to prevent tuberculosis, offers some protection against leprosy—but is not often used.

Antibiotic treatment can stop the progression of leprosy but does not reverse any nerve damage or deformity. Thus, early detection and treatment are vitally important. Because some leprosy bacteria may be resistant to certain antibiotics, doctors prescribe more than one drug. The standard combination is dapsone and rifampin. Dapsone is relatively inexpensive and generally safe to use; it only occasionally causes allergic skin rashes and anemia. Rifampin, which is more expensive, is even stronger than dapsone; its most serious side effects are damage to the liver and flu-like symptoms. Clofazimine is often added to the treatment regimen for severe cases. Other antibiotics that may be given to people with leprosy include ethionamide, minocycline, clarithromycin, and ofloxacin.

Antibiotic therapy must be continued for a long time, because the bacteria are difficult to eradicate. Depending on the severity of the infection and the doctor's judgment, treatment continues from 6 months to many years. Some doctors recommend lifelong treatment for people with lepromatous leprosy.

CHAPTER 195

Rickettsial and Ehrlichial Infections

Rickettsiae are an unusual type of bacteria that cause several diseases, including Rocky Mountain spotted fever and epidemic typhus. Rickettsiae differ from most other bacteria in that they can live and multiply only inside the cells of another organism (host) and cannot survive on their own in the environment. Ehrlichiae are similar to rickettsiae and cause similar diseases.

People are the main host for some rickettsiae and ehrlichiae. For most species, however, animals are the usual host. This population of animals is called the reservoir of infection. Animals in the reservoir may or may not be ill from the infection. Rickettsiae are usually spread to people through the bites of ticks, mites, fleas, and lice (vectors) that previously fed on an infected animal. Q fever can be spread through the air or in food. Each of the rickettsiae and ehrlichiae has its own hosts and vectors.

In people, rickettsiae infect the cells lining small blood vessels, causing the blood vessels to become inflamed or blocked or to bleed into the surrounding tissue. The part of the body where this occurs determines what symptoms develop.

Symptoms and Diagnosis

The different rickettsial infections tend to produce similar symptoms. Fever, severe headache, a characteristic skin rash, and a general feeling of illness (malaise) typically develop. Because the rash often does not appear for several days, early rickettsial infection is often mistaken for a common viral infection, such as influenza.

As rickettsial disease progresses, a person typically experiences confusion and severe weakness—often with cough, difficulty breathing, and sometimes vomiting and diarrhea. In some people, the liver or spleen enlarges, the kidneys fail, and blood pressure falls dangerously low. Death can occur.

Because rickettsiae are transmitted by ticks, mites, fleas, and lice, a history of a bite from one or more of these vectors is a helpful clue—particularly in geographic areas where rickettsial infection is common. However, many people do not recall such a bite.

The diagnosis of a rickettsial infection is difficult for a doctor to confirm quickly, because rickettsiae cannot be identified using commonly available laboratory tests. Special cultures and blood tests for rickettsiae are not

SOME OTHER RICKETTSIAL INFECTIONS

DISEASE	INFECTING ORGANISM	WHERE THE INFECTION IS FOUND	FEATURES OF THE INFECTION
Epidemic typhus	*Rickettsia prowazekii*, transmitted by lice **Host:** People	Throughout the world	After an incubation of 7 to 14 days, onset is sudden, with fever, headache, and extreme fatigue (prostration). A rash appears on the 4th to 6th day. Untreated, the infection may be fatal, especially in people older than age 50
Murine typhus	*Rickettsia typhi*, transmitted by fleas **Host:** Rodents, opossums	Throughout the world	Very similar to epidemic typhus, but symptoms are less severe
Scrub typhus	*Rickettsia tsutsugamushi*, transmitted by mites **Host:** Rodents	Asiatic-Pacific area, bounded by Japan, India, Australia, and Thailand	After an incubation of 6 to 21 days, onset is sudden, with fever, chills, and headache. A rash appears on the 5th to 8th day
Rickettsial-pox	*Rickettsia akari*, transmitted by mites **Host:** Rodents	First observed in New York City, has also occurred in other areas in the United States and in Russia, Korea, and Africa	About 1 week before the onset of fever, a small buttonlike ulcer (sore) with a black center appears on the skin; fever comes and goes, lasts about a week, and is accompanied by chills, profuse sweating, headache, sensitivity to the sun, and muscle pains
Q fever	*Coxiella burnetii* (*Rickettsia burnetii*), transmitted by inhaling infected droplets containing the rickettsiae or by consuming contaminated raw milk **Host:** Sheep, cattle, and goats	Throughout the world	After an incubation of 9 to 28 days, onset is sudden, with fever, severe headache, chills, extreme weakness, muscle aches, chest pain, and pneumonitis, but no rash

routinely available and take so long to process that the person usually needs to be treated before the test results are available. The doctor's suspicion of rickettsial infection remains the most important factor in diagnosis.

Treatment

Rickettsial infections respond promptly to early treatment with the antibiotics tetracycline, doxycycline, or chloramphenicol. These antibiotics are given by mouth unless the person is very sick, in which case they are given intravenously. Noticeable improvement usually takes place in 1 or 2 days, and fever usually disappears in 2 to 3 days. The person continues to take antibiotics for a minimum of 1 week—longer if the fever persists. When treatment begins late, improvement is slower and the fever lasts longer. Death can occur if the infection is untreated, or if treatment is begun too late.

Rocky Mountain Spotted Fever

Rocky Mountain spotted fever (spotted fever, tick fever, tick typhus) is a rickettsial disease that is transmitted by dog ticks and wood ticks and causes a rash, headache, and high fever.

Rocky Mountain spotted fever (RMSF) is caused by the bacterium *Rickettsia rickettsii* and is probably the most common rickettsial infection in the United States. Despite its name, this disease is found throughout most of the continental United States. It is most common in the Midwest and on the southern Atlantic seaboard. The disease occurs mainly from March to September, when adult ticks are active and people are likely to be in tick-infested areas. In the southern states, the disease may occur throughout the year. People who spend a lot of time in tick-infested areas—such as children younger than age 15—have an increased risk of infection.

Ticks acquire rickettsiae by feeding on infected mammals. Infected female ticks can also transmit rickettsiae to their offspring. Rickettsial disease is not transmitted directly from person to person.

Rickettsiae live and multiply in the cells lining blood vessels. Blood vessels in and under the skin and in the brain, lungs, heart, kidneys, liver, and spleen are commonly infected. Small blood vessels that develop the infection may become blocked by blood clots.

Symptoms

Typically, symptoms include a severe headache, chills, extreme exhaustion (prostration), and muscle pains. Symptoms begin suddenly 3 to 12 days after a tick bite. A high fever develops within several days and, in severe infections, persists for 1 to 2 weeks. A hacking, dry cough may also develop.

On about the fourth day of the fever, a rash appears on the wrists and ankles and rapidly extends to the palms, soles, forearms, neck, face, armpits, buttocks, and trunk. At first, the rash is flat and pink, but later darkens and becomes slightly raised. It does not itch. Warm water—for example, from a bath—makes the rash more evident. In about 4 days, small purplish areas (petechiae) develop because of bleeding in the skin. An ulcer may form where these areas merge.

If the blood vessels in the brain are affected, the person may have a headache, restlessness, insomnia, or delirium. Coma may develop. Nausea and vomiting and abdominal pain may also occur. Inflammation of the airways (pneumonitis) and pneumonia can develop. Also, heart damage and anemia may occur. Although uncommon, low blood pressure and death occur in severe cases.

Prevention and Treatment

There is no vaccine against RMSF, so avoiding tick bites is the best prevention. Tucking trousers into boots or socks and applying permethrin-containing insecticide to clothing limits tick access to skin. Tick repellents such as DEET (diethyltoluamide) may be applied to the skin. These repellents are effective but rarely cause toxic reactions, such as seizures, in small children. Conducting frequent searches for ticks is an important strategy for preventing infection, because the tick must be attached for 24 hours on average to transmit infection. Attached ticks should be removed carefully with tweezers; the head of the tick should be grasped as close to the skin as possible. Rickettsiae may be transmitted if an infected tick that is engorged with blood is crushed while being removed.

Because RMSF can cause serious illness or death, a doctor immediately prescribes antibiotics if he suspects RMSF based on a person's symptoms and potential for exposure to the disease—even if laboratory test results are not yet available. Tetracycline, doxycycline, and chloramphenicol are effective antibiotics for RMSF. They are given by mouth for mild disease and intravenously for more serious infections. Antibiotic therapy has significantly reduced the death rate from about 20% to 5%. Death is more likely when treatment is delayed. However, because most tick bites do not result in RMSF, a doctor usually does not prescribe antibiotics for a person who has simply had a tick bite. Instead, the doctor may ask the person to immediately report symptoms.

Ehrlichioses

Ehrlichioses are tick-borne infections that cause an abrupt onset of fever, chills, headache, and a general feeling of illness (malaise).

Ehrlichiae are very similar to rickettsiae: they are bacteria that can live only inside the cells of an animal or person. Unlike rickettsiae, however, ehrlichiae inhabit white blood cells (such as granulocytes and monocytes). Different species of ehrlichiae inhabit different types of white blood cells. In general, however, ehrlichioses are very similar in the symptoms they produce and in the way they are diagnosed and treated.

Ehrlichioses occur in the United States and Europe, but are most common in the midwestern, southeastern, and south-central United States. Ehrlichioses are most likely to develop between spring and late fall, when ticks are most active.

Symptoms, Diagnosis, and Treatment

Ehrlichioses begin 1 to 2 weeks after a tick bite. The first symptoms are fever, severe headache, body aches, and malaise. As the illness progresses, vomiting and diarrhea may develop, along with confusion and even coma. Sometimes cough and difficulty breathing develop. Skin rash is much less common than in rickettsial disease. Death is uncommon, but can occur in people with a poorly functioning immune system or in those who are not treated soon enough.

A person with an ehrlichial infection may have a low white blood cell count, a low blood count (anemia), and abnormal blood clotting, but these findings occur in many other illnesses. Blood tests for antibodies to ehrlichiae may be helpful, but usually do not give positive results until several weeks after the beginning of the illness. Polymerase chain reaction (PCR), a test that identifies the organism's DNA in the person's blood, may be more useful. Sometimes the person's white blood cells contain characteristic spots (morulae) that can be seen under a microscope. The presence of morulae confirms the diagnosis of ehrlichiosis, but they are often not visible.

Treatment is usually started based on the person's symptoms. Tetracycline, doxycycline, and chloramphenicol are all effective against ehrlichioses.

CHAPTER 196

Parasitic Infections

A parasite is an organism that lives on or inside another organism (the host) and causes harm to the host.

Parasitic infections are common in rural parts of Africa, Asia, and Latin America and less prevalent in industrialized countries. A person who visits a developing country can unknowingly acquire a parasitic infection; a doctor may not readily diagnose the infection when the person returns home.

Parasites generally enter the body through the mouth or skin. Parasites that enter through the mouth are swallowed and can remain in the intestine or burrow through the intestinal wall and invade other organs. Parasites that enter through the skin bore directly through the skin or are introduced through the bites of infected insects (the vector). Some parasites enter through the soles of the feet when a person walks barefoot or through the skin when a person swims or bathes in water where the parasites are present.

A doctor who suspects that a person may have a parasitic infection may take samples of blood, stool, or urine for laboratory analysis. The doctor may also take a sample of tissue that may contain the parasite. Repeated sample collections and examinations may be necessary to find the parasite.

Some parasites, particularly those that are single-celled, reproduce inside the host. Other parasites have complex life cycles, producing eggs or larvae that spend time in the environment or in an insect vector before becoming infective. If egg-laying parasites live in the digestive tract, their eggs may be found in the person's stool when a sample is examined under a microscope. Antibiotics, laxatives, and antacids can reduce the number of parasites enough to make their detection in a stool sample more difficult.

Food, drink, and water are often contaminated with parasites in regions of the world with poor sanitation and unhygienic practices. Thus, wise advice for travelers is to "cook it, boil it, peel it, or forget it" when eating in developing areas. Because some organisms survive freezing, ice cubes sometimes transmit disease unless made from purified water.

Amebiasis

Amebiasis is an infection of the large intestine or other organs caused by the single-celled parasite Entamoeba histolytica.

Amebiasis is relatively common in areas where sanitation is poor and fecal contamination of food and water occurs. It can also be acquired through certain sexual practices. *Entamoeba histolytica* initially infects the intestine, although it sometimes reaches other organs, such as the liver. Amebic infections are common in Latin America, Africa, and the Indian subcontinent.

Entamoeba histolytica exists in two forms: as an active parasite (trophozoite) and as a dormant parasite (cyst). Infection begins when cysts are swallowed. The cysts hatch, releasing trophozoites that multiply, cause ulcers on the lining of the intestine, and produce diarrhea. Some of the trophozoites form cysts, which are excreted in the feces along with trophozoites. Outside the body, the fragile trophozoites die, but the cysts are hardy. Cysts can be spread directly from person to person or indirectly through food or water.

In places with poor sanitation, transmission of amebiasis occurs through ingestion of fecally contaminated food or water. Fruits and vegetables may be contaminated when grown in soil fertilized by human stool, washed in polluted water, or prepared by someone who is infected. Amebiasis also may occur and spread in places with proper sanitation if incontinence and poor hygiene are present (for example, day care centers, or mental institutions). Amebiasis can be spread by sexual contact.

Symptoms

Only a few people infected with *Entamoeba* species develop symptoms. In the United States, most cases of symptomatic amebiasis occur among immigrants and, less commonly, people who have traveled to developing countries.

Infected people who develop symptoms typically have intermittent diarrhea, increased gas (flatulence), and cramping abdominal pain. In more severe cases, the abdomen is tender when touched, and the stool contains mucus and blood. The person may also have a fever. Wasting of the body (emaciation) and anemia can occur in people with chronic infection. Sometimes a large lump (ameboma) forms and blocks the intestine. Occasionally, the trophozoites perforate the intestinal wall and enter the abdominal cavity, causing severe abdominal pain and an abdominal infection (peritonitis) that requires immediate medical attention.

In some people, *Entamoeba histolytica* forms an abscess in the liver. Symptoms include fever, sweats, chills, weakness, weight loss, and pain or discomfort in the area over the liver.

Occasionally, *Entamoeba histolytica* spreads to other organs (including the lungs or brain). The skin may also become infected, especially around the buttocks, genitals, or wounds caused by abdominal surgery or injury.

Diagnosis

To diagnose amebiasis, a doctor collects stool samples for analysis. Three samples may be needed to make the diagnosis. A flexible tube (colonoscope) may be used to look inside the large intestine and to obtain a tissue sample if any ulcers are found there.

It can be difficult for a doctor to diagnose amebiasis when the disease spreads to sites outside the intestine (such as the liver), because the parasites may no longer be present in the stool. Ultrasound or computed tomography (CT) scans can be performed to confirm an abscess in the liver, but these tests do not indicate the cause. Blood tests for antibodies to the amebas may be helpful. Sometimes, doctors who suspect that a person has an amebic liver abscess simply try antiamebic drugs to see if they work. A positive response confirms the diagnosis.

Treatment

A person with symptomatic amebiasis involving the intestinal tract, or amebiasis that occurs in the liver or elsewhere outside the intestine, is given the antiamebic drug metronidazole. Nausea and vomiting develop if people taking metronidazole drink alcohol.

Metronidazole does not always kill cysts that are in the stool. Several drugs (such as iodoquinol, paromomycin, and diloxanide) can be used to kill the cysts in the stool.

Ascariasis

Ascariasis is infection caused by Ascaris lumbricoides, *an intestinal roundworm.*

Ascariasis is the most common roundworm infection in people, occurring in over 1 billion people worldwide. The infection is most common in areas with poor sanitation, where it persists largely because of indiscriminate defecation and other unsanitary practices. In the United States, infections are most often encountered in people who have traveled to areas with poor sanitation.

Infection begins when a person swallows food contaminated with *Ascaris* eggs. Food usually becomes contaminated through contact with soil or other objects. *Ascaris* eggs are hardy and can survive in the soil for years.

Once swallowed, *Ascaris* eggs hatch and release larvae into the intestine. Each larva migrates through the wall of the small intestine and is carried through the lymphatic vessels and bloodstream to the lungs. Once inside the lungs, the larva passes into the air sacs (alveoli), moves up the respiratory tract, and is swallowed. The larva matures in the small intestine, where it remains as an adult worm. Adult worms range from 6 to 20 inches in length and from $^1/_{10}$ to $^2/_{10}$ inch in diameter.

Symptoms and Diagnosis

Many people who have ascariasis do not develop symptoms, although the migration of larvae through the lungs can cause fever, coughing, and wheezing. A large number of worms in the intestine can cause abdominal cramps and, occasionally, a blockage of the intestine, most commonly in children. Sometimes adult worms are vomited up or passed in the stool, a situation that can be psychologically distressing. Adult worms occasionally block the appendix, biliary tract, or pancreatic duct, producing severe abdominal pain.

Diagnosis of ascariasis is made by identifying eggs or adult worms in a stool sample, or rarely by seeing adult worms that have migrated to the throat or nose. Rarely, the effects of larvae migrating through the lungs can be seen on an x-ray of the chest.

Prevention and Treatment

The best strategies for preventing ascariasis include using adequate sanitation and avoiding uncooked foods.

To treat a person with ascariasis, a doctor prescribes mebendazole, albendazole, or pyrantel pamoate. However, these drugs cannot be taken by pregnant women, because they may harm the fetus.

Babesiosis

Babesiosis is infection of red blood cells caused by the one-celled parasite Babesia.

Babesiosis is transmitted by the same deer tick that transmits Lyme disease. Although infection in animals is common, people are rarely infected. In the United States, babesiosis usually affects people on the offshore islands or coastal regions of New York and Massachusetts. It also occurs in Europe.

Babesia lives inside red blood cells and eventually destroys them, producing fever, headache, and muscle aches. Anemia may result from the breakdown of red blood cells.

In people whose spleen has been removed, the risk of severe disease and death is high. In these people, babesiosis resembles malaria (causing a high fever, anemia, dark urine, jaundice, and kidney failure). A person with a functioning spleen usually has a mild illness that disappears on its own without treatment.

To diagnose babesiosis, a doctor examines a blood sample under a microscope. Treatment consists of taking quinine and clindamycin; an alternative combination is atovaquone plus azithromycin.

Cryptosporidiosis

Cryptosporidiosis is a diarrhea-producing intestinal infection caused by the one-celled parasite Cryptosporidium parvum.

Cryptosporidium infects people and many species of animals throughout the world. The infection is acquired by ingesting fecally contaminated water or food or by touching the mouth after having contact with soil, a person, or an item that has been contaminated with the organism. Cryptosporidiosis is a common cause of diarrhea among children living in developing areas where sanitation is poor. It also occasionally occurs among people who travel to these areas. People with a weakened immune system, particularly those with AIDS, are prone to infection with *Cryptosporidium* and are more likely to have severe disease.

The egg cysts (oocysts) of *Cryptosporidium* are very hardy and are frequently present in surface water in the United States. Many farm animals also harbor the organism. *Cryptosporidium* is not killed by freezing or by the usual levels of chlorine in swimming pools or drinking water.

Symptoms and Diagnosis

Symptoms begin 7 to 10 days after infection and consist mainly of cramps and watery diarrhea. Vomiting, fever, and weakness also may occur. The severity of the diarrhea varies from mild to severe (as much as 3 to 4 gallons of watery stool per day in people with AIDS).

To diagnose cryptosporidiosis, a doctor takes a stool sample for examination.

Prevention and Treatment

Prevention of cryptosporidiosis involves proper sanitation and hand washing, particularly in health care facilities and day care centers and after contact with soil, animals, or infected people. When public health departments discover a municipal outbreak of the disease, they typically advise people to boil drinking water (including water for toothbrushing and food washing), to eat only cooked foods, and to avoid unpasteurized milk and juice. Bottled water cannot be presumed to be safe. Tap water filters that use reverse osmosis or have the words "absolute 1 micron" or "tested and certified by NSF Standard 53 for cyst removal/reduction" are effective. Other types of filters may not be.

People with a healthy immune system typically recover on their own. A person with severe diarrhea may require treatment with oral or intravenous fluids and antidiarrheal drugs such as loperamide. No drugs have been found that kill *Cryptosporidium* in people with diarrhea. In people with AIDS, treatment with antiretroviral therapy can improve immune function and relieve diarrhea caused by *Cryptosporidium*; however, they may remain permanently infected.

Giardiasis

Giardiasis is a diarrhea-producing infection of the small intestine caused by the single-celled parasite Giardia lamblia.

Giardiasis occurs worldwide and is the most common parasitic infection of the intestine in the United States. *Giardia* is a common contaminant of fresh water, including many lakes and streams—even ones that appear clean. Most people acquire the infection from drinking contaminated water, but direct person-to-person transmission of cysts passed in the stool also occurs—typically between children or sex partners. Giardiasis is more common among homosexual men with multiple partners, children in day care centers, and people who have traveled to developing countries. Backpackers and hikers who drink untreated water from streams and lakes are also at risk.

Symptoms and Diagnosis

Some infected people have no symptoms. When symptoms occur, they typically consist of cramps, increased gas (flatulence), and foul-smelling diarrhea. If untreated, the diarrhea may persist for weeks, and the person may not absorb enough nutrients from food, resulting in weight loss.

The symptoms often suggest the diagnosis. Microscopic examination of stool samples or secretions taken from the small intestine may reveal the parasite. Because people who have been infected for a long time tend to excrete the parasites at unpredictable intervals, repeated stool examinations may be needed. A stool antigen test can also confirm infection.

Treatment

Metronidazole taken by mouth is effective against *Giardia*. Nausea and vomiting develop if people drink alcohol while taking it. Furazolidone is available in liquid form and is given to children. People who live with or have had close contact with an infected person and develop symptoms of giardiasis should consult their doctor to see whether they need to be tested or treated for the disease.

Hookworm Infection

Hookworm infection (ancylostomiasis) is a disease of the intestines, resulting in anemia and occasionally skin rash, respiratory problems, or abdominal pain.

About 1 billion people are infected with hookworms, which are intestinal roundworms. The infection is most common in warm, moist places where sanitation is poor. Two species of hookworm cause infection in people: *Ancylostoma duodenale*, which is present in India, China, Japan, and the Mediterranean area; and *Necator americanus*, which is present in the tropical areas of Africa, Asia, and the Americas. *Necator americanus* also occasionally causes infection in the southern part of the United States.

Eggs are passed in stool and hatch in the soil after incubating for 1 to 2 days. Larvae emerge to live in the soil. When fully developed, the larvae can penetrate the skin. A person can become infected by walking barefoot or sitting in contaminated soil. Once they enter the body, the larvae move through the lymphatic vessels and the bloodstream to the lungs. The larvae pass into the air spaces, climb the respiratory tract into the throat, and are swallowed. About a week after penetrating the skin, they reach the intestine. Once inside the intestine, the larvae develop to adults, attach themselves by their mouths to the lining of the upper small intestine, produce substances that keep blood from clotting, and live on blood from the wall of the host's intestine.

Life Cycle of the Hookworm

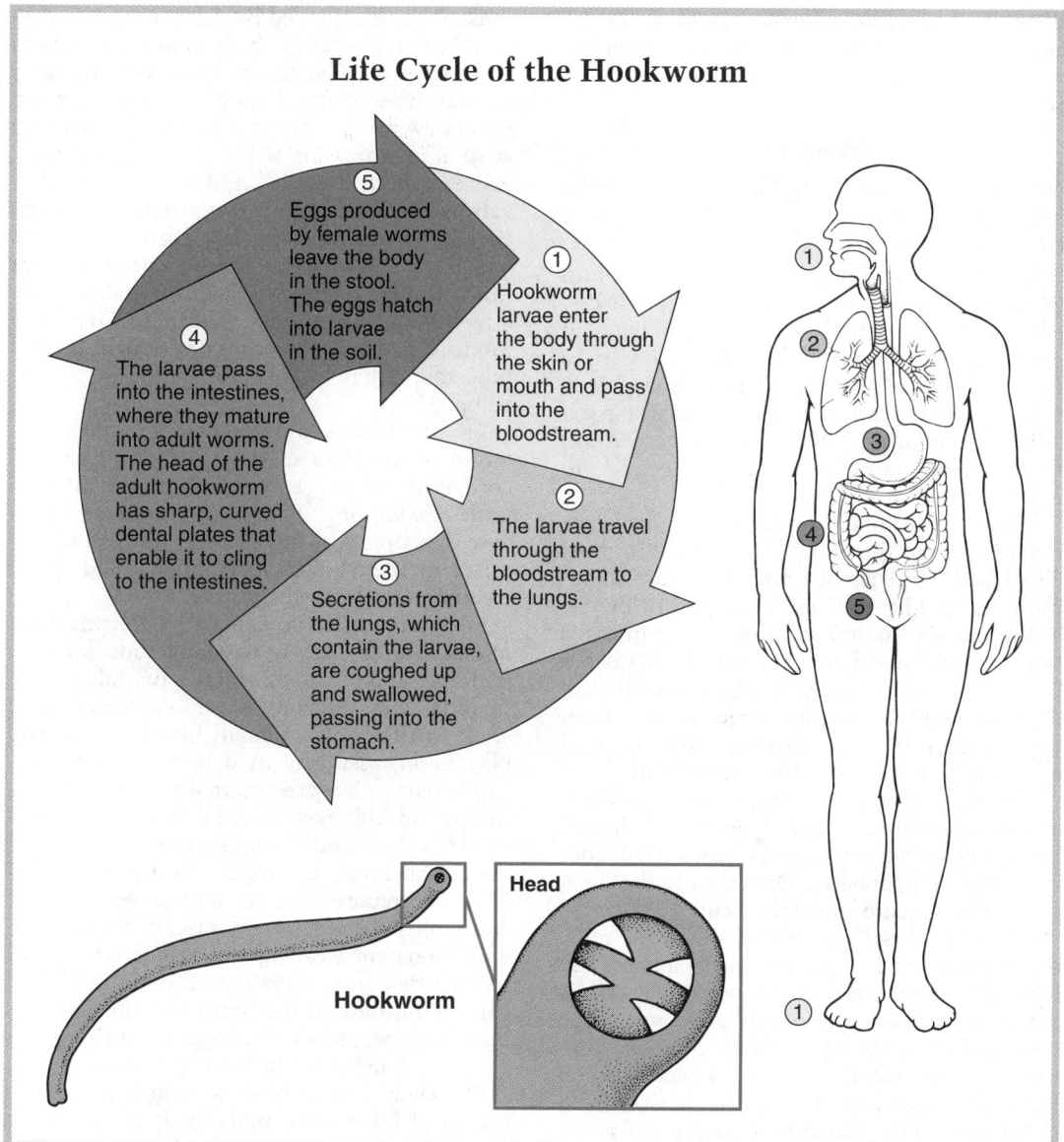

⑤ Eggs produced by female worms leave the body in the stool. The eggs hatch into larvae in the soil.

④ The larvae pass into the intestines, where they mature into adult worms. The head of the adult hookworm has sharp, curved dental plates that enable it to cling to the intestines.

③ Secretions from the lungs, which contain the larvae, are coughed up and swallowed, passing into the stomach.

① Hookworm larvae enter the body through the skin or mouth and pass into the bloodstream.

② The larvae travel through the bloodstream to the lungs.

Head

Hookworm

Symptoms and Diagnosis

An itchy, red, raised rash (ground itch) may develop where the larvae penetrated the skin. The migration of the larvae through the lungs can cause fever, coughing, and wheezing. Adult worms can cause pain in the upper abdomen when they first attach in the intestine. Over time, anemia develops as blood is lost and the person becomes iron deficient. In children, slow growth, heart failure, and widespread tissue swelling may develop when the resulting anemia is severe.

The diagnosis is made by identifying hookworm eggs in a sample of stool. If the stool is not examined for several hours, the eggs may hatch and release larvae.

Treatment

A doctor prescribes an oral drug, such as albendazole, mebendazole, or pyrantel pamoate.

Because of possible adverse effects to the fetus, these drugs cannot be taken by pregnant women. Iron supplements are given to people with anemia.

Malaria

Malaria is infection of red blood cells with the single-celled parasite Plasmodium, *which causes fever, an enlarged spleen, and anemia.*

Malaria is usually spread by the bite of an infected female mosquito. Very rarely, the disease is transmitted through a transfusion of contaminated blood or an injection with a needle that was previously used by a person with malaria. Four species of malaria parasites—*Plasmodium falciparum, Plasmodium vivax, Plasmodium ovale,* and *Plasmodium malariae*—can infect people.

Although drugs and insecticides have made malaria rare in the United States and in most developed countries, the disease remains common and deadly in tropical areas worldwide. There are 300 to 500 million people infected with malaria, and 1 to 2 million deaths occur each year. Most of these deaths occur in children younger than 5 years of age. Visitors from the tropics or travelers returning from tropical areas can bring the infection with them.

The cycle of malarial infection begins when a female mosquito bites a person with malaria. The mosquito ingests blood that contains malarial parasites. Once inside the mosquito, the parasite multiplies and migrates to the mosquito's salivary gland. When the mosquito bites another person, the parasites are injected along with the mosquito's saliva. Inside the person, the parasites move to the liver and multiply again. They typically mature over an average of 1 to 3 weeks, then leave the liver and invade the person's red blood cells. The parasites multiply yet again inside the red blood cells, eventually causing the infected cells to rupture.

Plasmodium vivax and *Plasmodium ovale* can remain in the liver in a dormant form that periodically releases mature parasites into the bloodstream, causing recurring attacks of symptoms. *Plasmodium falciparum* and *Plasmodium malariae* do not persist in the liver. However, mature forms of *Plasmodium malariae* can persist in the bloodstream for months or even years before causing an attack of symptoms.

Symptoms and Complications

As the infected red blood cells rupture and release parasites, a person suddenly develops a shaking chill followed by a fever that can exceed 104° F. Headache, body aches, and nausea are common. The fever typically falls after several hours, and heavy sweating occurs. Fevers eventually become periodic, occurring at 48-hour intervals with *Plasmodium vivax* and *Plasmodium ovale* and at 72-hour intervals with *Plasmodium malariae*. The fevers caused by *Plasmodium falciparum* are often not periodic, but sometimes occur at 48-hour intervals. Travelers who acquire malaria usually develop symptoms within the first few months after their return, although it may take more than a year for symptoms to develop.

As the illness progresses, the spleen enlarges. A decrease in the level of sugar (glucose) in the blood can occur in people infected with *Plasmodium falciparum* and may be severe in people who have a large number of parasites in their blood—particularly if they are treated with the drug quinine.

Falciparum malaria, caused by *Plasmodium falciparum,* is the most dangerous form of malaria and can be fatal. In falciparum malaria, the infected red blood cells often stick to the walls of small blood vessels and clog them, resulting in damage to many organs—particularly the brain (cerebral malaria), lungs, and kidneys. Cerebral malaria is a particularly dangerous complication that can produce high fever, headache, drowsiness, delirium, confusion, seizure, and coma. It most commonly occurs in infants or young children, pregnant women, and people who travel to high-risk areas. In falciparum malaria, fluid can accumulate in the lungs and cause severe breathing problems. Damage to multiple organs can cause a fall in blood pressure.

Blackwater fever is an uncommon complication of falciparum malaria. It is caused by the rupture of large numbers of red blood cells, which releases blood pigment (hemoglobin) into the bloodstream. The released hemoglobin is excreted in the urine, which turns the urine dark. Kidney damage may be severe enough to require dialysis. Blackwater fever is more likely to develop in people who have taken quinine for treatment.

Malaria caused by *Plasmodium vivax, Plasmodium ovale,* and *Plasmodium malariae* tends to be less severe, although these parasites can remain in the blood for long periods, producing fever, chills, headache, poor appetite, fatigue, and a general feeling of illness (malaise).

Diagnosis

A doctor suspects malaria when a person develops fever and accompanying symptoms during or after traveling to an area where malaria is present. Periodic fever develops in less than half of American travelers with malaria, but when present, suggests the diagnosis. Identification of parasites in a blood sample confirms the diagnosis. More than one sample may be needed. The laboratory identifies the species of *Plasmodium* found in the sample, because the treatment, complications, and prognosis vary depending on the species involved. *Plasmodium falciparum* infection is an emergency and requires immediate evaluation and treatment.

Prevention and Treatment

Mosquito control measures, which include eliminating breeding areas and killing larvae in the standing water where they live, are very important. People who live in or travel to malaria-infested areas can also take precautions to limit mosquito exposure, such as using insecticide sprays in homes and outbuildings, placing screens on doors and windows, using permethrin-impregnated mosquito netting over beds, and applying mosquito repellents containing DEET on exposed areas of the skin. People can wear long pants and long-sleeved shirts, particularly between dusk and dawn, to protect against mosquito bites. People subject to intense mosquito exposure can spray permethrin on their clothing before it is worn.

Vaccines for preventing malaria are still in the experimental stage.

Drugs should be taken to prevent malaria during travel in areas where malaria is prevalent. The preventive drug is started before travel begins, continued throughout the stay, and extended for a period of time that varies for each drug but is usually 4 weeks after the person leaves the high-risk area.

Many drugs are used to prevent and treat malaria. Drug resistance is a serious problem, particularly with the dangerous *Plasmodium falciparum* species. The prevalence of drug-resistant strains varies in different parts of the world. Thus, the choice of drug for prevention varies by geographic location. Information about specific sites is available from the Centers for Disease Control and Prevention. The choice of drug for treatment is based on the infecting species of *Plasmodium* and its known or suspected sensitivities.

Chloroquine is the preferred drug for prevention of malaria caused by *Plasmodium falciparum* in Mexico, areas of Central America west of the Panama Canal, Haiti, the Dominican Republic, and some areas of the Middle East. Strains of *Plasmodium falciparum* that are resistant to chloroquine are present in most other areas of the world where malaria occurs. In those areas, the recommended preventive drugs include mefloquine, doxycycline, or the combination atovaquone-proguanil.

Chloroquine is the drug of choice for treatment in a person who has malaria caused by *Plasmodium vivax*, *Plasmodium ovale*, or *Plasmodium malariae*—except in a very few areas where resistance to chloroquine in people with *Plasmodium vivax* has been reported. Chloroquine also is acceptable for *Plasmodium falciparum* infections acquired in areas without known drug resistance. Primaquine is added to kill persistent parasites in the liver of a person infected with *Plasmodium vivax* or *Plasmodium ovale*. Before primaquine is given, a blood test is done to look for a relatively common enzyme deficiency (G6PD deficiency). People with G6PD deficiency who are given primaquine may have a breakdown of their red blood cells.

Falciparum malaria in areas with known chloroquine resistance is treated with quinine plus doxycycline or, if uncomplicated, atovaquone-proguanil. Atovaquone-proguanil has fewer side effects than quinine. Mefloquine can be used but side effects are common. If the person cannot take drugs by mouth, quinidine may be given intravenously under careful observation in the hospital.

Travelers who develop a fever while in areas where malaria is prevalent should be examined by a doctor immediately. If medical care is not available, self-treatment for presumed malaria is sometimes recommended with pyrimethamine-sulfadoxine or atovaquone-proguanil until medical evaluation is possible. This approach should be discussed with a doctor before traveling.

Chloroquine is relatively safe and is approved for use in children and pregnant women. Mefloquine sometimes causes nausea, dizziness, and trouble sleeping. It may rarely produce seizures or psychiatric problems. It should also be avoided in people with certain heart conditions. Quinine is often associated with headache, nausea, vomiting, visual disturbances, and ringing in the ears—a condition known as cinchonism. Quinine may also cause low blood sugar in people infected with *Plasmodium falciparum*. Atovaquone-proguanil may cause nausea, vomiting, or abdominal pain and is not used in people with poor kidney function, pregnant women, or infants.

Pinworm Infection

Pinworm infection (enterobiasis) is a disease caused by intestinal roundworms.

Pinworms are the most common parasite in children in the United States.

Infection follows ingestion of pinworm eggs (ova). Eggs can be transferred from the area around the anus of an infected child to clothing, bedding, or toys. Eggs can survive outside the body for as long as 3 weeks at normal room temperature. These eggs can be transferred, often by the fingers, to the mouth of another child, who swallows them. Eggs sometimes are ingested in contaminated food. Children may reinfect themselves by transferring eggs from the area around the anus to their mouth. Children who suck their thumbs are at increased risk of infection.

After ingestion, the eggs hatch in the intestinal tract, and young worms migrate to the rectum and lower intestine. Pinworms mature in the lower intestine within 2 to 6 weeks. The female worm then moves to the area around the anus, usually at night, to deposit her eggs. The eggs are deposited in a sticky, gelatinous substance that adheres to the skin. The eggs and gelatinous material cause itching.

Symptoms and Diagnosis

Most children who carry pinworms have no symptoms. Some, however, feel an itching sensation around the anus and scratch the area. The skin can become raw and superficially infected with bacteria. In girls, pinworms may cause vaginal itching and irritation.

The diagnosis of pinworm infection is made by finding the worms or eggs. The search for adult pinworms is best conducted by examining the child's anus about 1 to 2 hours after the child has been put to bed for the night. The worms are white and hair-thin, but they wiggle and are visible to the naked eye. Eggs can be obtained by patting the skin folds around the anus with the sticky side of a strip of transparent tape in the early morning before the child wakes up. The tape can be taken to the doctor for microscopic examination.

Treatment

A single dose of mebendazole, albendazole, or pyrantel pamoate, repeated after 2 weeks, effectively cures pinworm infection. Many doctors recommend treating the entire family. Despite drug therapy, reintroduction of the disease is common after treatment. Clothing, bedding, and toys should be washed and the environment vacuumed to try to eliminate any eggs. Anti-itching creams or ointments applied directly to the area around the anus may provide relief from itching.

Schistosomiasis

Schistosomiasis (bilharziasis) is infection caused by blood flatworms (flukes) that often produces symptoms in the intestine, liver, or urinary tract.

Schistosomiasis affects over 200 million people in tropical and subtropical regions of South America, Africa, and Asia. Three species cause most of the cases of schistosomiasis in people: *Schistosoma hematobium* infects the urinary tract and bladder, and *Schistosoma mansoni* and *Schistosoma japonicum* infect the intestine. The infection is acquired by swimming or bathing in fresh water that is contaminated with the parasites. Schistosomes multiply inside specific types of water-dwelling snails, from which they are released to swim free in the water. If they encounter a person's skin, they burrow in and migrate through the bloodstream to the lungs, where the schistosomes mature into adult flukes. The adults pass through the bloodstream to their final home in small veins in the bladder or intestines, where they may remain for years. The adult flukes lay large numbers of eggs in the walls of the intestines or bladder, some of which flow through the bloodstream to the liver. These eggs elicit an inflammatory response that blocks veins in the intestines, bladder, and liver—resulting in ulcers, local bleeding, and scar tissue formation. Eggs produce enzymes that allow them to pass into the stool and urine. When people with the disease urinate or defecate in fresh water, these eggs are passed, and the cycle begins again.

The eggs of *Schistosoma mansoni* and *Schistosoma japonicum* typically lodge in the intestine and liver, whereas those of *Schistosoma hematobium* typically lodge in the bladder. The resulting inflammation can lead to scarring, and increased pressure in the veins that carry blood between the digestive tract and the liver (portal vessels). This high portal pressure can cause enlargement of the spleen and bleeding from veins in the esophagus. Other organs (such as the lungs, spinal cord, and brain▲) can also be involved.

Symptoms and Diagnosis

When schistosomes first penetrate the skin, an itchy rash (swimmer's itch) may develop. Fever, chills, body aches, headache, and cough may develop when the adult flukes begin laying eggs (4 to 8 weeks after entering the body). The liver, spleen, and lymph nodes may temporarily enlarge and then return to normal. A person may develop abdominal cramps and pass blood in the stool or urine. Blood loss may result in anemia. Chronic infection of the urinary tract can produce obstruction and is associated with later development of cancer of the bladder.

A doctor diagnoses schistosomiasis by examining samples of stool or urine for the presence of eggs. Blood tests are also available. Ultrasound scans can be used to assess the severity of infections in the urinary tract or liver.

Prevention and Treatment

Prevention of schistosomiasis is best achieved by avoiding swimming, bathing, or wading in fresh water in areas known to contain schistosomes. To treat the disease, a doctor prescribes praziquantel to be taken by mouth in 2 or 3 doses over 1 day.

Tapeworm Infection

Tapeworm infection is an intestinal disease caused by one of several species of tapeworms, including Taenia saginata *(beef tapeworm),* Taenia solium *(pork tapeworm), and* Diphyllobothrium latum *(fish tapeworm).*

Tapeworms are large, flat worms that live in the intestine and can grow 15 to 30 feet in length. Egg-bearing sections of the worm (proglottids) are passed in the stool. If untreated human waste is released into the environment, the eggs may be ingested by intermediate hosts, such as pigs, cattle, or (in the case of fish tapeworms) small crustaceans, which are in turn ingested by fish. The eggs hatch in the intermediate host, then the larvae invade the intestinal wall and are carried through the bloodstream to skeletal muscle and other tissues, where they form cysts. People acquire the parasite by eating the cysts in raw or undercooked meat or fish. The cysts

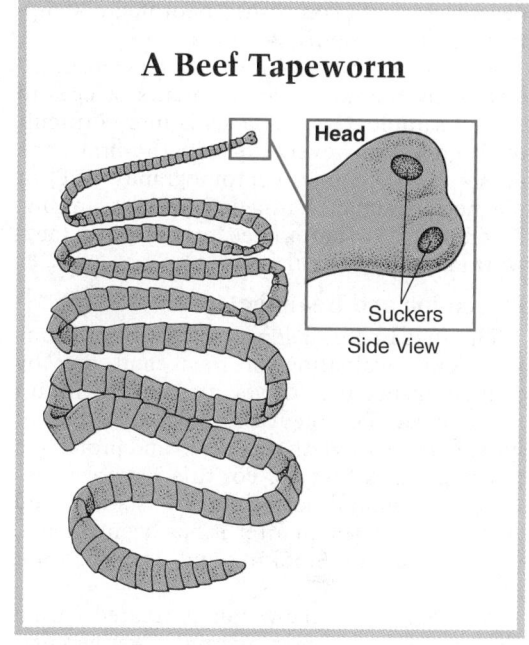

A Beef Tapeworm

Head

Suckers

Side View

hatch and develop into adult worms, which latch onto the person's intestinal wall. The worms then grow in length.

People may also act as an intermediate host for the pork tapeworm, *Taenia solium.* Pork tapeworm eggs reach the stomach when a person swallows them in food or water contaminated with human feces or from contact with the unclean hands of a person infected with adult worms. The eggs may also reach the stomach when proglottids are regurgitated from the intestine. Once the larvae are released, they penetrate the intestinal wall and travel to muscles, internal organs, the brain,■ or tissue under the skin, where they form cysts (cysticerci). This form of the disease is called cysticercosis.

Symptoms and Diagnosis

Although tapeworms in the intestine usually cause no symptoms, some people experience upper abdominal discomfort, diarrhea, and loss of appetite. Occasionally, a person with tapeworms may feel a piece of the worm move out through the anus. Rarely, tapeworms acquired from fish cause anemia.

Cysts in the brain and meninges (the tissues covering the brain) in people with cysticercosis may cause inflammation, resulting in

▲ see page 540   ■ see page 540

headache, confusion, other neurologic symptoms, and commonly, seizures.

A doctor diagnoses intestinal tapeworm infection by finding worm segments or eggs in a stool sample. Cysticercosis is more difficult to diagnose; however, cysts in the brain can be seen with computed tomography (CT) or magnetic resonance imaging (MRI) scanning. Blood tests for antibodies to the pork tapeworm also are helpful.

Prevention and Treatment

The first line of defense against tapeworms is careful evaluation of meat and fish by trained inspectors. Cysts are visible in infected meat. Thorough cooking (such that all meat reaches more than 135° F) and prolonged freezing will kill cysts. For this reason, freshwater fish should not be served as sushi, and should only be eaten after it has been cooked, frozen, or cured. Smoking and drying do not kill cysts.

A person with tapeworms is treated with a single oral dose of praziquantel. Cysticercosis is usually not treated unless it involves the brain, in which case antiparasitic drugs (such as albendazole or praziquantel) may be given along with corticosteroids, which help reduce inflammation.

Toxocariasis

Toxocariasis (visceral larva migrans) is infection caused by larvae of the parasitic roundworms Toxocara canis *or* Toxocara cati.

Toxocariasis occurs mainly in young children, who acquire *Toxocara* eggs through contact with soil contaminated by the feces of dogs and cats that carry the parasite. Children's sandboxes, where dogs and cats often defecate, pose a particular hazard for exposure to the eggs. Children frequently transfer the eggs from their hands to their mouth and may eat the contaminated sand. Occasionally, adults who eat clay become infected. After the eggs are swallowed, larvae hatch in the intestine. The larvae penetrate the intestinal wall and are spread through the bloodstream. Almost any tissue of the body may be involved, but the liver and lung are most commonly affected. The larvae can remain alive for many months, causing damage by migrating through tissues and stimulating inflammation.

Symptoms and Diagnosis

Symptoms may start within several weeks of ingestion of the eggs; fever, cough or wheezing, and liver enlargement are the most common. Some people have a skin rash, spleen enlargement, and recurring pneumonia. When larvae infect the eye, inflammation and decreased vision may result.

A doctor may suspect toxocariasis in a person who has an enlarged liver, inflammation of the lungs, a fever, and high levels of eosinophils (a type of white blood cell). The diagnosis is confirmed by identifying *Toxocara* antibodies in the blood. Rarely, a sample of liver tissue is obtained and examined (biopsy) for evidence of larvae or inflammation resulting from their presence.

Prevention and Treatment

To prevent toxocariasis, dogs and cats should be dewormed regularly, starting before they are 4 weeks old. Covering sandboxes when not in use prevents animals from defecating in them.

The effectiveness of treatment is uncertain. In people, toxocariasis usually goes away without treatment. For people with severe symptoms, diethylcarbamazine or mebendazole may be helpful. Corticosteroids are sometimes prescribed to control the symptoms of inflammation.

Toxoplasmosis

Toxoplasmosis is infection caused by Toxoplasma gondii, *a single-celled parasite.*

Toxoplasma is present worldwide and infects people and a large number of animals and birds. Many people in the United States have been infected with *Toxoplasma*, although few ever develop symptoms. Severe illness generally develops only in fetuses and people with a weakened immune system.

Although the parasite can grow in the tissues of many animals, it produces eggs (oocysts) only in cells lining the intestine of cats. Eggs are shed in a cat's stool and can survive for up to 18 months in the soil.

People who touch soil contaminated with *Toxoplasma* eggs may acquire the infection from direct hand-to-mouth contact or by contaminated food, which is then eaten. Occasionally animals such as pigs acquire toxoplasmosis from contaminated soil. People can become infected by eating raw or undercooked meat from infected animals. Both freezing and thoroughly cooking meat destroy *Toxoplasma*.

A woman who acquires the infection while pregnant can transfer *Toxoplasma* to her fetus through the placenta. The result may be a miscarriage, stillbirth, or a baby born with congenital toxoplasmosis.▲ A woman who was infected before the pregnancy will not pass the parasite on to the fetus.

People with a weakened immune system, primarily those with AIDS or cancer, or those who have received an organ transplant and drugs to suppress rejection, are especially at risk of toxoplasmosis. Symptoms usually develop in these people because of reactivation of a previously acquired *Toxoplasma* infection. The infection usually occurs in the brain, but it may affect the eye or be spread (disseminated) throughout the body. In these people, toxoplasmosis is very serious and nearly always fatal when untreated.

Symptoms and Diagnosis

Children born with congenital toxoplasmosis may be severely ill and die shortly after birth, or they may have no symptoms until months or years later. Some never develop illness. Typical symptoms in newborns can include inflammation of the eyes (chorioretinitis), which can result in blindness, enlargement of the liver and spleen, jaundice, easy bruising, seizures, a large or small head, and mental retardation.

Toxoplasmosis acquired after birth in otherwise healthy people seldom causes symptoms. When symptoms occur, they are usually mild and include painless, swollen lymph nodes; intermittent low fevers; and a vague ill feeling. Sometimes people develop only chorioretinitis, with blurred vision, eye pain, and sensitivity to light.

Symptoms of toxoplasmosis in people with a weakened immune system depend on the site of infection. Toxoplasmosis of the brain (encephalitis) produces symptoms such as weakness on one side of the body, trouble speaking, headache, confusion, and seizures. Acute disseminated toxoplasmosis can cause a rash, high fever, chills, trouble breathing, and fatigue. In some people, infection causes inflammation of the brain and its lining (meningoencephalitis), liver (hepatitis), lungs (pneumonitis), or heart (myocarditis).

The diagnosis of toxoplasmosis is usually based on a blood test that reveals antibodies against the parasite. However, if the person's immune system is impaired by AIDS, the blood test may be falsely negative. A doctor may instead depend on computed tomography (CT) and magnetic resonance imaging (MRI) of the brain. Less commonly, a piece of infected tissue is removed and examined under a microscope (biopsy) to make the diagnosis.

Treatment and Prognosis

Infected adults without symptoms and with a healthy immune system do not require treatment. Those with symptoms are treated with sulfadiazine plus pyrimethamine, with the addition of leucovorin to protect the bone marrow from the toxic effects of pyrimethamine. Alternatively, people with chorioretinitis can be given clindamycin, along with prednisone or another corticosteroid to reduce inflammation.

Toxoplasmosis in people with AIDS tends to recur, so drugs are often given indefinitely. To prevent toxoplasmosis, some people with AIDS are placed on preventive treatment with trimethoprim-sulfamethoxazole, which also helps prevent *Pneumocystis carinii* infection.

Women who are known to have acquired toxoplasmosis during pregnancy may be treated with spiramycin to prevent transmission to the fetus. Pregnant women should avoid cleaning cat litter boxes or should wear gloves when doing so. Meat should be cooked thoroughly before ingestion.

Trichinosis

Trichinosis is infection caused by the roundworm Trichinella spiralis.

Trichinella larvae live in the muscle tissue of animals, typically pigs, wild bears, horses, and many carnivores. People develop trichinosis if they eat uncooked or poorly cooked meat from an animal that carries the parasite. Most human infections result from pork, particularly in regions where pigs are fed uncooked meat scraps and garbage. Trichinosis is now rare in the United States.

When a person eats meat containing live *Trichinella* cysts, the cyst wall is digested, releasing larvae that quickly mature to adulthood and mate in the intestine. The male worms play no further role in illness. The females burrow into the intestinal wall and, by the seventh day, begin to produce larvae.

Production of larvae continues for about 4 to 6 weeks, after which the female worm dies. The tiny larvae are carried through the body by the lymphatic vessels and bloodstream.

▲ see table on page 1508

OTHER PARASITES

PARASITE	SOURCE AND SITE OF ENTRY	COMMON SYMPTOMS	DIAGNOSTIC CLUES	TREATMENT
Roundworms				
Strongyloides (threadworm); occurs in moist tropics, also in the southeastern United States	**Source:** Fecal contamination of soil (larvae) **Entry site:** Skin, usually feet	Pain in pit of stomach; diarrhea, hives or rash in a linear pattern, wheezing and asthma	Larvae in stool or duodenum Disseminated hyperinfection; larvae in sputum; polymicrobial bacterial sepsis or meningitis	Ivermectin
Tapeworms				
Hymenolepis nana (dwarf tapeworm); occurs worldwide	**Source:** Eggs that contaminate the environment **Entry site:** Mouth	Diarrhea, abdominal discomfort in children with a heavy infection	Eggs in stool	Praziquantel Niclosamide
Echinococcus; occurs in sheep- or cattle-raising areas of the world; can also occur in wild animals	**Source:** Animal feces **Entry site:** Mouth	Liver or lung mass, abdominal pain, biliary tract disease, chest pain, coughing up blood or cyst contents	Living in area where the infection is present; liver or lung cyst; antibodies to tapeworm in a blood sample; abnormal chest x-ray	Albendazole Surgical removal Percutaneous drainage, injection of a concentrated salt into the cyst, and aspiration
Flukes				
Intestinal flukes; most common in the Far East	**Source:** Vegetation or freshwater fish **Entry site:** Mouth	Usually no symptoms; sometimes, abdominal pain, diarrhea	Eggs in stool	Praziquantel
Sheep liver fluke (*Fasciola hepatica*); occurs worldwide in sheep-raising countries	**Source:** Watercress or other water plants that contain cysts **Entry site:** Mouth	Acute abdominal pain, inflammation of the liver or gallbladder	Eggs in stool or bile	Bithionol
Liver flukes (clonorchiasis); occurs in the Far East	**Source:** Freshwater fish **Entry site:** Mouth	Abdominal pain, jaundice, diarrhea; cancer of the biliary tract years later	Eggs in stool and intestinal contents	Praziquantel
Lung flukes; most common in the Far East	**Source:** Freshwater crabs and crayfish containing cysts **Entry site:** Mouth	Difficulty breathing, coughing up blood	Eggs in stool or sputum; positive blood test; multiple small, grapelike cavities on chest x-ray	Praziquantel
Trypanosomes				
Trypanosoma cruzi (Chagas' disease); occurs in North, Central, and South America	**Source:** Triatomine bugs ("kissing bugs") **Entry site:** Skin (site of bug bite) or area around eyes; sometimes acquired in blood transfusions	Acute: Fever, generalized weakness, potentially fatal heart or brain infection Chronic: Survivors often have long-term heart and digestive tract symptoms	Trypanosomes in blood	Nifurtimox Benzimidazole (often ineffective and toxic)

	OTHER PARASITES *(Continued)*			
PARASITE	**SOURCE AND SITE OF ENTRY**	**COMMON SYMPTOMS**	**DIAGNOSTIC CLUES**	**TREATMENT**
Trypanosoma brucei (sleeping sickness); occurs in parts of equatorial Africa	**Source:** Tsetse flies **Entry site:** Skin (site of fly bite)	Painful bump at bite site, followed later by fever, headache, rash, and eventually sleepiness, difficulty walking, coma, and death	Trypanosomes in blood or the cerebrospinal fluid	Suramin Pentamidine Eflornithine (for *T. brucei gambiense* only) Melarsoprol (for brain infection)

The larvae penetrate muscles, causing inflammation. By the end of the third month, they form cysts.

Certain muscles, such as those in the tongue and around the eyes, and between the ribs, are most often infected. Larvae that reach the heart muscle are usually killed by the intense inflammatory reaction they provoke.

Symptoms

The symptoms of trichinosis vary, depending on the number of invading larvae, the tissues invaded, and the general physical condition of the person. Many people have no symptoms at all. Sometimes, diarrhea, abdominal cramps, and a slight fever begin 1 to 2 days after eating contaminated meat. However, symptoms from the larval invasion usually do not start for 7 to 15 days.

The main symptoms of trichinosis are muscle pain, weakness, fever, muscle soreness, and swelling of the upper eyelids. The soreness is often most pronounced in the muscles used to breathe, speak, chew, and swallow. A non-itchy skin rash may occur, and some people develop diarrhea. Some people develop redness in the whites of the eyes, pain in the eyes, and sensitivity to bright light. Death can occur but is rare.

Without treatment, most symptoms disappear by the third month of infection, although vague muscle pain and fatigue can persist longer.

Diagnosis

Unlike most other worm infections, trichinosis cannot be diagnosed by microscopic examination of the stool. Blood tests for antibodies to *Trichinella* are fairly reliable but only when performed 2 to 3 weeks after the start of the disease. A doctor bases an initial diagnosis of trichinosis on the symptoms and the presence of elevated levels of eosinophils (a type of white blood cell) in a blood sample. A biopsy of muscle tissue (in which a sample of tissue is removed and examined under a microscope), performed after the fourth week of infection, may reveal larvae or cysts, but it is seldom necessary.

Prevention and Treatment

Trichinosis is prevented by thoroughly cooking (to a temperature of more than 140° F) meats, especially pork and pork products. Alternatively, larvae can usually be killed by freezing meat at 5° F for 3 weeks or at −4° F for 1 day. Larvae of worms that infect arctic mammals are able to survive these temperatures.

Oral doses of mebendazole or albendazole are effective against the parasite. Bed rest and analgesics help relieve muscle pain. Corticosteroids (such as prednisone) may be prescribed to reduce inflammation of the heart or brain. Most people with trichinosis recover fully.

Whipworm Infection

Whipworm infection (trichuriasis) is an intestinal infection caused by the roundworm Trichuris trichiura.

Trichuriasis is a very common disorder, occurring mainly in the subtropics and tropics, where poor sanitation and a warm, moist climate provide the conditions needed for *Trichuris* eggs to incubate in the soil.

People acquire the parasite by swallowing food that contains eggs that have incubated in the soil. The larvae hatch in the small intestine, migrate to the large intestine, and embed their heads in the intestinal lining. Each larva grows into a worm that is about 4½ inches long. Eggs are passed in the stool.

Symptoms and Diagnosis

Symptoms such as abdominal pain and diarrhea occur when a large number of worms are present in the colon. People with an extremely large number of worms may have chronic diarrhea, weight loss, bleeding from the intestine, and anemia. Occasionally, the rectum may protrude through the anus (rectal prolapse), especially in heavily infected children.

A doctor bases a diagnosis of trichuriasis on seeing the typical barrel-shaped eggs in stool samples examined under a microscope or occasionally by observing adult worms during a colonoscopy.

Prevention and Treatment

Prevention depends on using sanitary toilet facilities, maintaining good personal hygiene, and avoiding unwashed vegetables. Albendazole or mebendazole are effective but cannot be used in pregnant women because of harmful effects on the fetus.

CHAPTER 197

Fungal Infections

Fungi are a type of plant that can infect people. Yeasts, molds, and mushrooms are all examples of fungi.

Some fungi reproduce by spreading microscopic spores. These spores are often present in the air, where they can be inhaled or come into contact with the surfaces of a person's body. Consequently, fungal infections usually begin in the lungs or on the skin. Of the wide variety of spores that land on the skin or are inhaled into the lungs, most do not cause infection. Except for some superficial skin conditions, fungal infections are rarely passed from one person to another.

Certain types of fungi (such as *Candida*) are normally present on body surfaces or in the intestines. Although normally harmless, these fungi sometimes cause local infections of the skin and nails,▲ vagina,■ or mouth,★ or sinuses.● They seldom cause serious harm, except in people with a weakened immune system or with foreign material (such as an intravenous catheter) in their body.

Sometimes, the normal balances that keep fungi in check are upset and infections occur. For example, the bacteria normally present in the digestive tract and vagina limit the growth of certain fungi in those areas. When a person

takes antibiotics, those helpful bacteria can be killed—allowing the fungi to grow unchecked. The resulting overgrowth of fungi can cause symptoms, which are usually mild. As the bacteria grow back, the balance is restored, and the problem usually resolves.

Some fungal infections (for example, histoplasmosis, blastomycosis, and coccidioidomycosis) can be serious in otherwise healthy people.

Some fungal infections are more common in certain geographic areas. For example, in the United States coccidioidomycosis occurs almost exclusively in the Southwest, whereas histoplasmosis is especially common in the Ohio and Mississippi River valleys. Blastomycosis is particularly common in the eastern and central United States and in Africa.

Because many fungal infections develop slowly, months or years may pass before a person seeks medical attention. In people with a weakened immune system (for example, people who have received an organ transplant, are being treated for cancer with immunosuppressive drugs, or who have AIDS), fungal infections can be very aggressive—spreading quickly to other organs and often leading to death.

Several drugs effective against fungal infections are available, but the structure and chemical makeup of fungi make them difficult to kill. Antifungal drugs may be applied directly to a fungal infection of the skin or other surface, such as the vagina or the inside

---

▲ see page 1225   ■ see page 1374

★ see pages 666 and 682   ● see box on page 1266

of the mouth. Antifungal drugs may also be taken by mouth or injected when needed to treat more serious infections. Several months of treatment are often needed.

Aspergillosis

Aspergillosis is infection caused by the fungus Aspergillus *that usually affects the lungs.*

Aspergillus is very common and is frequently found in compost heaps, air vents, and airborne dust. Inhalation of *Aspergillus* spores is the primary cause of aspergillosis.

Aspergillosis usually affects open spaces in the body, such as cavities that have formed in the lungs from preexisting lung diseases. The infection may also occur in the ear canals and sinuses. In the sinuses and lungs, aspergillosis shows up as a ball (aspergilloma) composed of a tangled mass of fungus fibers, blood clots, and white blood cells. The fungus ball gradually enlarges, destroying lung tissue in the process, but usually does not spread to other areas.

Less often, aspergillosis can become very aggressive and rapidly spread throughout the lungs and often through the bloodstream to the brain and kidneys. This rapid spread occurs mainly in people with a weakened immune system.

In addition to causing infection, *Aspergillus* sometimes produces an allergic reaction when it is present on a person's skin or mucous membranes.▲

Symptoms and Diagnosis

A fungus ball in the lungs may cause no symptoms and may be discovered only with a chest x-ray. Or it may cause repeated coughing up of blood and—rarely—severe, even fatal, bleeding. A rapidly invasive *Aspergillus* infection in the lungs often causes cough, fever, chest pain, and difficulty breathing.

Aspergillosis affecting the deeper tissues makes a person very ill. Symptoms include fever, chills, shock, delirium, and blood clots. The person may develop kidney failure, liver failure (causing jaundice), and breathing difficulties. Death can occur quickly.

Aspergillosis of the ear canal causes itching and occasionally pain. Fluid draining overnight from the ear may leave a stain on the pillow. Aspergillosis of the sinuses causes a feeling of congestion and sometimes pain or discharge.

In addition to the symptoms, an x-ray or computed tomography (CT) scan of the in-

Risk Factors for Developing Fungal Infections

Use of drugs that suppress the immune system
- Anticancer drugs (chemotherapy)
- Corticosteroids and other immunosuppressant drugs

Diseases and conditions
- AIDS
- Kidney failure
- Diabetes
- Lung disease, such as emphysema
- Hodgkin's disease or other lymphomas
- Leukemia
- Extensive burns
- Organ transplantation

fected area provides clues for making the diagnosis. Whenever possible, a doctor sends a sample of infected material to a laboratory to confirm identification of the fungus.

Prognosis and Treatment

Aspergillosis that is present only in a sinus or a single spot in the lung progresses slowly. The infection requires treatment but does not pose an immediate danger. However, if the infection is widespread or the person appears seriously ill, treatment is started immediately. Aspergillosis is treated with antifungal drugs, such as amphotericin B, itraconazole, or voriconazole. Some forms of *Aspergillus* are resistant to these drugs, however, and may need to be treated with a caspofungin, a newer antifungal drug.

Doctors treat aspergillosis in the ear canal by scraping out the fungus and applying drops of antifungal drugs. Fungus collections in the sinuses must usually be removed surgically. If fungus balls in the lungs grow near large blood vessels, they may also need to be removed surgically because they may invade the blood vessel and cause bleeding.

Blastomycosis

Blastomycosis (North American blastomycosis, Gilchrist's disease) is infection caused by the fungus Blastomyces dermatitidis.

▲ see page 311

Spores of *Blastomyces* probably enter the body through the airways when they are inhaled. Thus, blastomycosis primarily affects the lungs▲ but occasionally spreads through the bloodstream to other areas of the body, including the skin. Most infections occur in the United States, chiefly in the Southeast and the Mississippi River valley. Infections have also occurred in widely scattered areas of Africa. Men between the ages of 20 and 40 years are most commonly infected. Unlike most other fungal infections, blastomycosis is not more common in people with AIDS.

Symptoms and Diagnosis

Blastomycosis of the lungs begins gradually with a fever, chills, and drenching sweats. Chest pain, difficulty breathing, and a cough that may or may not bring up sputum may also develop. The lung infection usually progresses slowly, although it sometimes gets better without treatment.

When blastomycosis spreads, it can affect many areas of the body, but the skin, bones, and genitourinary tract are the most common sites. A skin infection begins as very small, raised bumps (papules), which may contain pus. Raised, warty patches then develop, surrounded by tiny, painless abscesses (collections of pus). Painful swelling in the bones may occur. Also, men may experience painful swelling of the epididymis (a cordlike structure attached to the testes) or discomfort from an infection of the prostate gland (prostatitis).

A doctor diagnoses blastomycosis by sending a sample of sputum or infected tissue to a laboratory to be examined under a microscope and cultured.

Prognosis and Treatment

Blastomycosis may be treated with intravenous amphotericin B or oral itraconazole. With treatment, the person begins to feel better fairly quickly, but the drug must be continued for months. Without treatment, the infection slowly worsens and leads to death.

Candidiasis

Candidiasis (candidosis, moniliasis, "yeast infection") is infection caused by species of Candida, *especially* Candida albicans.

▲ see also page 271   ■ see page 1226

★ see pages 666 and 682

● see page 1374

Candida is normally present on the skin, in the intestinal tract, and—in women—in the genital region. Usually, *Candida* in these areas does not cause problems. Sometimes, however, the fungus can cause infection of the skin ■ or the mucous membranes of the mouth★ or vagina.● Such infections can develop in people with a healthy immune system, but they are more common or persistent in people with diabetes, cancer, or AIDS and in pregnant women. Candidiasis is also common in people who are given antibiotics, because the bacteria that normally compete with *Candida* are killed and the fungus is able to grow unchecked.

Some people, mainly those with a weakened immune system, develop candidiasis that spreads through the bloodstream to other parts of the body.

Symptoms and Diagnosis

Infection of the mouth (thrush or trench mouth) causes creamy, white, painful patches to form inside the mouth. Skin infections can cause a burning rash. Patches in the esophagus cause pain with swallowing.

More serious infections, such as those in the heart valves, can cause fever, heart murmur, and enlargement of the spleen. An infection of the retina and inner parts of the eye can cause blindness. An infection of the blood (candidemia) or kidney can cause fever, very low blood pressure (shock), and a decrease in urine production.

Many candidal infections are apparent from the symptoms alone. To confirm the diagnosis, however, a doctor must identify the fungi in a skin sample under a microscope. Samples of blood or spinal fluid that have been cultured may also reveal the presence of the fungus.

Prognosis and Treatment

Candidiasis that occurs only on the skin or in the mouth or vagina can be treated with antifungal drugs that are applied directly to the affected area (for example, clotrimazole and nystatin). A doctor may prescribe the antifungal drug fluconazole to be taken by mouth.

Candidiasis that has spread throughout the body is a severe, progressive, and potentially fatal infection that is usually treated with intravenous amphotericin B, although fluconazole is effective for some people. Caspofungin and voriconazole, drugs that are still being studied, may be useful as well.

Certain medical conditions, such as diabetes, can worsen candidiasis. In people with diabetes, control of the blood sugar levels facilitates cure of the infection.

Coccidioidomycosis

Coccidioidomycosis (San Joaquin fever, valley fever) is infection caused by the fungus Coccidioides immitis *that usually affects the lungs).*▲

The spores of *Coccidioides* can be found in soil in the southwestern United States, Central America, and South America. Farmers and others who work with soil are most likely to inhale the spores and become infected. People who become infected while traveling may not develop symptoms of the disease until after they leave the area.

Coccidioidomycosis occurs either as a mild lung infection that disappears without treatment (acute primary coccidioidomycosis) or as a severe, progressive infection that spreads throughout the body and is often fatal (progressive coccidioidomycosis). The progressive form is often a sign that the person has a weakened immune system, usually because of AIDS.

Symptoms and Diagnosis

Most people with acute primary coccidioidomycosis have no symptoms. If symptoms develop, they appear 1 to 3 weeks after the person becomes infected. The symptoms are usually mild and include a cough, fever, chills, chest pain, and sometimes shortness of breath. The cough may produce sputum and even occasionally blood. Some people develop "desert rheumatism"—inflammation of the surface of the eye (conjunctivitis) and joints (arthritis) and the formation of skin nodules (erythema nodosum).

The progressive form of the disease is unusual and may develop weeks, months, or even years after the acute primary infection. Symptoms include mild fever and losses of appetite, weight, and strength. The lung infection may worsen, causing increased shortness of breath. The infection also may spread from the lungs to the bones, joints, liver, spleen, and kidneys. Infection of the brain and the tissues covering the brain (meninges) is often chronic.

A doctor may suspect coccidioidomycosis if a person develops symptoms after living in or recently traveling through an area where the disease is common. Chest x-rays usually reveal abnormalities, but further testing (of blood, sputum, or pus samples) may be needed to confirm the diagnosis.

Prognosis and Treatment

Acute primary coccidioidomycosis typically goes away without treatment, and recovery usually is complete. However, some doctors prefer to treat the person if coccidioidomycosis affects the lungs. Oral fluconazole or intravenous amphotericin B is given to people with the progressive form of the disease. Alternatively, the doctor may treat the infection with itraconazole or ketoconazole. If a person develops meningitis (infection of the tissues covering the brain and spinal cord), intravenous fluconazole is given. Alternatively, amphotericin B may be injected into the spinal fluid. Untreated meningitis is always fatal. Although drug treatment can be effective in localized infections—for example, in the skin, bones, or joints—relapses often occur after treatment is discontinued. Treatment must therefore be continued for years, often for life.

Cryptococcosis

Cryptococcosis is infection caused by the fungus Cryptococcus neoformans.

Cryptococcus is present around the world, but infection was relatively rare until the AIDS epidemic began. The fungus sometimes infects people with Hodgkin's disease or sarcoidosis and those who are on long-term corticosteroid treatment.

Cryptococcosis mainly occurs in the tissues covering the brain and spinal cord (meninges), resulting in meningitis; in the lungs; and on the skin. Other organs are sometimes involved.

Symptoms and Diagnosis

Cryptococcosis usually produces mild and vague symptoms. People with meningitis develop headache and confusion. People with lung infection may not have any symptoms, although some have cough or an aching chest. A severe lung infection causes difficulty breathing.

To diagnose the infection a doctor takes and analyzes samples of tissue and body fluids. Blood and spinal fluid may be tested for antibodies to *Cryptococcus*.

Prognosis and Treatment

People with a functioning immune system who have *Cryptococcus* in only a small part of

---

▲ see also page 270

℞ DRUGS FOR SERIOUS FUNGAL INFECTIONS

DRUG	COMMON USES	SIDE EFFECTS
Amphotericin B	Wide variety of fungal infections	Chills, fever, headache, vomiting; lowered blood potassium levels, kidney damage, anemia
Caspofungin	*Aspergillus* and possibly *Candida*	Fever, nausea, inflammation of veins
Fluconazole	*Candida* and other fungal infections, including cryptococcus	Liver toxicity but less than that with ketoconazole
Flucytosine	*Candida* and *Cryptococcus* infections	Bone marrow and kidney damage
Itraconazole	*Candida* and other fungal infections	Nausea, diarrhea, liver toxicity but less than that with ketoconazole
Ketoconazole	*Candida* and other fungal infections	Nausea and vomiting, blocked production of testosterone and cortisol, liver toxicity
Voriconazole	*Aspergillus* and *Candida*	Visual disturbance

their lungs usually do not require any treatment. Drugs used to treat people with a weakened immune system include fluconazole, amphotericin B, and sometimes flucytosine.

Histoplasmosis

Histoplasmosis is infection caused by the fungus Histoplasma capsulatum *that occurs mainly in the lungs▲ but can sometimes spread throughout the body.*

The spores of *Histoplasma* are present in the soil and are particularly common in the eastern and midwestern United States. Farmers and others who work with soil are most likely to inhale the spores; severe disease can result when large numbers of spores are inhaled. People with human immunodeficiency virus (HIV) infection are more likely to develop histoplasmosis, especially the form that spreads throughout the body.

Symptoms and Diagnosis

Most people with histoplasmosis do not have any symptoms. However, three forms of histoplasmosis do cause symptoms: acute, progressive disseminated, and chronic cavitary.

In **acute histoplasmosis,** symptoms usually appear 3 to 21 days after a person inhales the spores. The person may feel sick and have a fever and a cough. Symptoms usually disappear without treatment in 2 weeks and rarely last longer than 6 weeks. This form of histoplasmosis is very rarely fatal.

Progressive disseminated histoplasmosis does not normally affect healthy adults. This infection usually occurs in infants and in people with a weakened immune system (such as those with AIDS). Symptoms are vague at first. People may experience fatigue, weakness, and a general feeling of illness (malaise). Symptoms may worsen very slowly or extremely rapidly. The liver, spleen, and lymph nodes may enlarge. Less commonly, the infection causes ulcers to form in the mouth and intestines. In rare cases, the adrenal glands may be damaged, causing Addison's disease.■ Without treatment, this form of histoplasmosis is fatal in 90% of people. Even with treatment, death may occur rapidly in people with AIDS.

Chronic cavitary histoplasmosis is a lung infection that develops gradually over several

▲ see also page 270
■ see page 956

weeks, producing a cough and increased difficulty in breathing. Symptoms include weight loss, a mild fever, and a general feeling of illness (malaise). Most people recover without treatment within 2 to 6 months. However, breathing difficulties may gradually worsen, and some people may cough up blood, sometimes in large amounts. Lung damage or bacterial invasion of the lungs eventually may cause death.

To make the diagnosis, a doctor obtains samples of an infected person's sputum, bone marrow, urine, or blood. Samples may also be taken from the liver, lymph nodes, or any mouth ulcers that are present. These samples are sent to a laboratory for culture and analysis.

Prognosis and Treatment

People with the acute form of histoplasmosis rarely require drug treatment. Those with the progressive disseminated form do need treatment and often respond well to amphotericin B given intravenously or to itraconazole given by mouth. In the chronic cavitary form, itraconazole or amphotericin B may eliminate the fungus, although the destruction caused by the infection leaves behind scar tissue. Breathing problems similar to those caused by chronic obstructive pulmonary disease usually remain. Therefore, treatment should begin as soon as possible to limit lung damage.

Mucormycosis

Mucormycosis (phycomycosis) is infection caused by a fungus of the group Mucorales.

Mucormycosis is caused by inhalation of spores. It most commonly affects the nose and brain (rhinocerebral mucormycosis) and is a severe and potentially fatal infection. This form of mucormycosis typically affects people whose immune system is weakened by disease, such as uncontrolled diabetes. The other common site of infection is the lung. Rarely, the skin and digestive system are involved.

Symptoms and Diagnosis

The symptoms of rhinocerebral mucormycosis include pain, fever, and an infection of the eye socket (orbital cellulitis) with a bulging of the affected eye (proptosis). Pus is discharged from the nose. The roof of the mouth (palate), the facial bones surrounding the eye socket or sinuses, or the divider be-

tween the nostrils (septum) may be destroyed by the infection. Infection in the brain may cause seizures, partial paralysis, and coma.

Mucormycosis in the lungs causes fever, cough, and sometimes breathing difficulty.

Because the symptoms of mucormycosis can resemble those of other infections, a doctor may not be able to diagnose it immediately. Usually the diagnosis is made when a doctor sees the organism in tissue samples and grows it in culture.

Prognosis and Treatment

A person with mucormycosis generally is treated with amphotericin B given intravenously or injected directly into the spinal fluid. Infected tissue may be removed by surgery. In people with diabetes, blood sugar levels are brought down to within the normal range. The disease is very serious, and many people die.

Paracoccidioidomycosis

Paracoccidioidomycosis (South American blastomycosis) is infection caused by the fungus Paracoccidioides brasiliensis.

Paracoccidioidomycosis is a fungal infection that usually involves the skin, mouth, throat, and lymph nodes, although it sometimes appears in the lungs, liver, or spleen. It is very common in South America but rare in the United States.

Symptoms and Diagnosis

Lymph nodes become swollen when they are infected by *Paracoccidioides*, and they may drain pus, but there is little pain. The lymph nodes most commonly infected are those in the neck and under the arms. Painful ulcers may form in the mouth. If the lungs are affected, the person may have a cough and difficulty breathing.

To diagnose the infection, a doctor takes tissue samples for analysis under a microscope.

Prognosis and Treatment

Symptoms are long lasting but rarely fatal. The drug itraconazole is the treatment of choice. Amphotericin B is also effective, but because of its side effects it is reserved for very severe cases.

Sporotrichosis

Sporotrichosis is infection caused by the fungus Sporothrix schenckii.

Sporothrix typically grows on rosebushes, barberry bushes, sphagnum moss, and other mulches. Most often, farmers, gardeners, and horticulturists are infected, usually from a small puncture wound.

Sporotrichosis mainly affects the skin and nearby lymphatic vessels. Very rarely, the bones, joints, lungs, or other tissues are infected.

Symptoms and Diagnosis

An infection of the skin typically starts on a finger as a small, nontender bump (nodule) that slowly enlarges and forms a sore. Over the next several days or weeks, the infection spreads through the lymphatic vessels of the finger, hand, and arm to the lymph nodes, forming nodules and sores along the way. Even at this stage, there is little or no pain. Usually, the person has no other symptoms.

An infection in the lungs may cause pneumonia, with a slight chest pain and cough.

Lung infection usually occurs in people who have another lung disease, such as emphysema. Joint infection produces swelling and makes movement painful. Rarely, an infection develops in other areas.

The characteristic nodules and sores may lead a doctor to suspect sporotrichosis. The diagnosis is confirmed by culturing and identifying *Sporothrix* in samples of infected tissue.

Prognosis and Treatment

Sporotrichosis that affects the skin usually spreads very slowly and is seldom fatal. The skin infection is treated with oral itraconazole. Oral potassium iodide may be prescribed instead, but it is not as effective and causes side effects (such as a rash; runny nose; and inflammation of the eyes, mouth, and throat) in most people. Lung and bone infection may also be treated with itraconazole. For life-threatening, bodywide infection, amphotericin B is given intravenously.

CHAPTER 198

Viral Infections

A virus is a small infectious organism— much smaller than a fungus or bacterium— that must invade a living cell to reproduce (replicate). The virus attaches to a cell, enters it, and releases its DNA or RNA inside the cell. The virus's DNA or RNA is the genetic code containing the information needed to replicate the virus. The viral genetic material takes control of the cell and forces it to replicate the virus. The infected cell usually dies because the virus keeps it from performing its normal functions. Before it dies, however, the cell releases new viruses, which go on to infect other cells.

Some viruses do not kill the cells they infect, but instead alter the cells' functions. Sometimes the infected cell loses control over normal cell division and becomes cancerous. Some viruses that do not kill the cells they infect leave their genetic material in the host cell where it remains dormant for an extended time (latent infection). When the cell is disturbed, the virus may be able to begin growing again and cause disease.

Viruses usually infect one particular type of cell. For example, cold viruses infect only cells of the upper respiratory tract. Additionally, most viruses infect only a few species of plants or animals; some infect only people.

Viruses are transmitted in a variety of ways. Some are swallowed, some are inhaled, and some are transmitted by the bites of insects and other parasites (for example, mosquitoes and ticks).

The body has a number of defenses against viruses. Physical barriers, such as the skin, discourage easy entry. Infected cells also make interferons, substances that can make non-infected cells more resistant to infection by many viruses.

Upon entering the body, a virus triggers the body's immune defenses. These defenses begin with white blood cells, such as lymphocytes, which learn to attack and destroy the virus or the cells it has infected.▲ If the body survives the virus attack, the lymphocytes "remember" the invader and are able to respond more quickly and effectively to a subsequent infection by the same virus. This is called immunity. Immunity can also be produced by receiving a vaccine.

Drugs that combat viral infections are called antiviral drugs. Antiviral drugs work by interfering with viral replication. Because viruses are tiny and replicate inside cells using the cells' own metabolic pathways, there are only a limited number of metabolic functions that antiviral drugs can target. In contrast, bacteria are relatively large organisms, commonly reproduce by themselves outside of cells, and have many metabolic functions against which antibiotics can be directed. Therefore, antiviral drugs are much more difficult to develop. Antiviral drugs can be toxic to human cells. Viruses can develop resistance to antiviral drugs.

Antibiotics are not effective against viral infections, but if a person has a bacterial infection in addition to a viral infection, an antibiotic is often necessary.

Probably the most common viral infections are those of the nose, throat, and airways. These infections include sore throat, sinusitis, the common cold, and influenza. Doctors often refer to these as upper respiratory infections (URIs). In small children, viruses also commonly cause croup and inflammation of the windpipe (laryngitis) or other airways deeper inside the lungs (bronchiolitis, bronchitis■).

Some viruses (for example, rabies, West Nile virus, and several different encephalitis viruses) infect the nervous sytem.★ Viral infections also develop in the skin, sometimes resulting in warts or other blemishes.● Additionally, many viruses commonly infect infants and children.◆

Other common viral infections are caused by the herpesviruses. Eight different herpesviruses infect people. Three of these—herpes simplex virus type 1, herpes simplex virus type 2, and varicella-zoster virus—cause infections that produce blisters on the skin. Another herpesvirus, Epstein-Barr virus, causes infectious mononucleosis. Cytomegalovirus is a cause of serious infections in newborns and in people with a weakened immune system. It can also produce an illness similar to infectious mononucleosis in people with a healthy immune system. Human herpesviruses 6 and

VIRUSES AND CANCER: A LINK

Some viruses affect the DNA of their host cells in such a way as to help cancer develop. Only a few viruses are known to cause cancer, but there may be others.

VIRUS	CANCER
Epstein-Barr virus	Burkitt's lymphoma
Certain nose and throat cancers
Other lymphomas (in people with AIDS)
Hepatitis B and C viruses	Liver cancer
Herpesvirus 8	Kaposi's sarcoma (in people with AIDS)
B cell lymphomas (in people with AIDS)
Human papillomavirus	Cervical cancer

7 cause a childhood illness known as roseola infantum.▼ Human herpesvirus 8 has been implicated as a cause of cancer (Kaposi's sarcoma) in people with AIDS.

All of the herpesviruses cause lifelong infection because the virus remains within its host cell in a dormant (latent) state. Sometimes, the virus reactivates and produces further episodes of disease. Reactivation may occur rapidly or many years after the initial infection.

Common Cold

The common cold is a viral infection of the lining of the nose, sinuses, throat, and large airways.

Common colds are among the most common illnesses. Many different viruses cause colds, but the rhinoviruses (of which there are 100 subtypes) are implicated more often than others. Colds caused by rhinoviruses occur more commonly in the spring and fall; different viruses cause colds during other times of the year.

▲ see page 1050   ■ see page 1585
★ see page 532   ● see page 1228
◆ see page 1568   ▼ see page 1580

℞ ANTIVIRAL DRUGS

DRUG	COMMON USES	SIDE EFFECTS
Acyclovir	Genital herpes, herpes zoster, and chickenpox	Side effects are few
Amantadine	Influenza A	Nausea or loss of appetite Nervousness Light-headedness Slurred speech Unsteadiness Sleeplessness
Cidofovir	Cytomegalovirus infections	Kidney damage Low white blood cell count
Famciclovir	Genital herpes, herpes zoster, and chickenpox	Side effects are few
Fomivirsen	Cytomegalovirus retinitis	Mild eye inflammation
Foscarnet	Cytomegalovirus and herpes simplex virus infections	Kidney damage Seizures
Ganciclovir	Cytomegalovirus infections	Low white blood cell count
Interferon-alpha	Hepatitis B and C	Flu-like symptoms Bone marrow suppression Depression or anxiety
Oseltamivir	Influenza A and B	Nausea and vomiting
Penciclovir	Cold sores (topical application)	Side effects are few
Ribavirin	Respiratory syncytial virus Hepatitis C	Breakdown of red blood cells, causing anemia
Rimantadine	Influenza A	Similar to amantadine, but milder nervous system problems
Trifluridine	Herpes simplex keratitis	Stinging of eyes Swelling of eyelids
Valacyclovir	Genital herpes, herpes zoster, and chickenpox	Side effects are few
Valganciclovir	Cytomegalovirus infections	Low white blood cell count
Vidarabine	Herpes simplex keratitis	Side effects are few
Zanamivir	Influenza A and B (inhaled powder)	Irritation of the airways

Colds mainly spread when a person's hands come in contact with nasal secretions from an infected person. These secretions contain cold viruses. When the person touches his mouth, nose, or eyes, the viruses gain entry to the body and produce a new cold. Less often, colds are spread when a person breathes air that contains droplets that were coughed or sneezed out by an infected person. A cold is most contagious in the first 1 or 2 days after symptoms develop. Becoming chilled does not cause colds, nor does it increase a person's susceptibility to infection. A person's general health and eating habits also do not seem to affect susceptibility to infection, nor does having an abnormality of the nose or throat (such as enlarged tonsils or adenoids).

Symptoms and Diagnosis

Symptoms of the cold start 1 to 3 days after infection. Usually, the first symptom is discomfort in the nose or throat. Later, the person starts sneezing, has a runny nose, and feels mildly ill. Fever is not common, but a mild fever may develop at the beginning of the illness. At first, the secretions from the nose are watery and clear and can be annoyingly plentiful; eventually they become thicker, opaque, yellow-green, and less abundant. Many people also develop a cough. Symptoms usually disappear in 4 to 10 days, although a cough often lasts into the second week.

Complications may prolong the illness. Rhinovirus infection often triggers asthma attacks in people with asthma. Some people develop bacterial infections of the middle ear (otitis media) or sinuses because of a cold. These infections develop because congestion in the nose blocks the normal drainage of those areas, allowing bacteria to grow in collections of blocked secretions. Other people develop bacterial infections of the lower airways (secondary bronchitis or pneumonia).

Doctors are usually able to diagnose a cold from the typical symptoms. A high fever, severe headache, rash, difficulty breathing, or chest pain suggests that the infection is not a simple cold. Laboratory tests usually are not needed to diagnose a cold. If complications are suspected, doctors may order blood tests and x-rays.

Prevention

Because so many different viruses cause colds and because each virus changes slightly over time, an effective vaccine has not yet been developed. The best preventive measure is practicing good hygiene. Because many cold viruses are spread through contact with the secretions of an infected person, both the sick person and the people in his household and office should wash their hands frequently. Sneezing and coughing should be done into tissues, which should then be carefully disposed of. When possible, the sick person should sleep in a separate room. People who are coughing or sneezing from a cold should not go to work or school where they might infect others. Cleaning shared objects and surfaces can also help to reduce the spread of common cold viruses.

Despite their popularity, echinacea and high-dose vitamin C (up to 2,000 milligrams per day) have not been shown to prevent colds. When sprayed into the nose, the substance interferon reduces the chance of acquiring a rhinovirus cold. However, interferon causes irritation and bleeding of the nose and does not work against other cold viruses. Interferon nasal spray is not commercially available in the United States.

Treatment

A person with a cold should stay warm and comfortable and try to avoid spreading the infection to others. Anyone with a fever or severe symptoms should rest at home. Drinking fluids and inhaling steam or mist from a vaporizer may help to keep secretions loose and easier to expel.

Currently available antiviral drugs are not effective against colds. An experimental antiviral drug called pleconaril reduces the duration and severity of cold symptoms and may become available in the near future. Antibiotics do not help people with colds, even when the nose or cough produces colored mucus.

Echinacea,▲ zinc preparations, and vitamin C have been suggested as therapy for colds. Small studies have shown them to be effective, but the effectiveness has not been confirmed in rigorous, large clinical studies.

Several popular nonprescription remedies that help the symptoms of a cold are available.■ Because they do not cure the infection, which usually resolves after a week anyway, doctors feel that their use is optional, depending on how bad the person feels. Several different types of drugs are used to relieve cold

▲ see page 108   ■ see page 95

R̲ₓ   NONPRESCRIPTION COLD REMEDIES

TYPE	DRUG	SIDE EFFECTS
Analgesics/Antipyretics		
(relieve aches and pains, reduce fever)		
	Acetaminophen	Minimal
	Aspirin	Reye's syndrome possible in children with influenza, stomach irritation
	Nonsteroidal anti-inflammatory drugs such as ibuprofen and naproxen	Stomach irritation
Antihistamines		
(open nasal passages, help relieve sneezing)		
	Brompheniramine Chlorpheniramine Clemastine Diphenhydramine	All can cause drowsiness, dry mouth, blurred vision, difficulty urinating, constipation, and, in older people, light-headedness on standing and confusion
Cough suppressants		
(reduce cough)		
	Benzonatate	Confusion, stomach upset
	Codeine	Constipation, drowsiness, difficulty urinating, stomach upset
	Dextromethorphan	Minimal; confusion, nervousness and irritability at high doses
Decongestants (nasal spray)		
(open clogged nasal passages)		
	Naphazoline Oxymetazoline Phenylephrine Xylometazoline	Rebound congestion (worse congestion when drug wears off)
Decongestant (oral)		
(dries runny nose)		
	Pseudoephedrine	Palpitations, high blood pressure, nervousness, insomnia
Expectorant		
(loosens mucus)		
	Guaifenesin	Minimal, headache and stomach upset at high doses
Other		
	Zinc (lozenges or nasal gel)	Metallic taste

symptoms: decongestants help open clogged nasal passages, antihistamines help dry a runny nose, and cough syrups make coughing easier by thinning secretions or suppressing cough. These drugs are most often sold as combinations but can also be obtained individually. Antihistamines can cause drowsiness and are particularly problematic in older people.

Aspirin is generally not recommended for children because in that age group it is associated with an increased risk of Reye's syndrome.

Cough suppressants are not routinely recommended because coughing is a good way to clear secretions and debris from the airways during a viral infection. However, a severe cough that interferes with sleep or causes great discomfort can be treated with a cough suppressant.

Influenza

Influenza (flu) is infection of the lungs and airways with one of the influenza viruses, causing a fever, runny nose, sore throat, cough, headache, muscle aches (myalgias), and a general feeling of illness (malaise).

Every year, throughout the world, widespread outbreaks of influenza occur during late fall or early winter. Influenza occurs in epidemics, in which many people get sick all at once. In each epidemic, usually only one strain of influenza virus is responsible for the disease. Strains are often named after the first location (for example, Hong Kong flu) or animal (for example, swine flu) in which it was found.

There are two types of influenza virus, type A and type B, and many different strains within each type. The illnesses produced by the different types and strains are similar. The strain of influenza virus causing outbreaks is always changing, so every year the influenza virus is a little different from the previous year's. It often changes enough that previously effective vaccines no longer work.

Influenza is distinctly different from the common cold. It is caused by a different virus and produces symptoms that are more severe. Also, influenza affects cells much deeper down in the respiratory tract.

Influenza virus is spread by inhaling droplets that have been coughed or sneezed out by an infected person or by having direct contact with an infected person's secretions. Handling household articles that have been in contact with an infected person or an infected person's secretions may sometimes spread the disease.

Symptoms and Diagnosis

Symptoms start 24 to 48 hours after infection and can begin suddenly. Chills or a chilly sensation are often the first indication of influenza. Fever is common during the first few days, and the temperature may rise to 102 to 103° F. Many people feel sufficiently ill to remain in bed for days; they have aches and pains throughout the body, most pronounced in the back and legs. Headache is often severe, with aching around and behind the eyes. Bright light may make the headache worse.

At first, the respiratory symptoms may be relatively mild, with a scratchy sore throat, a burning sensation in the chest, a dry cough, and a runny nose. Later, the cough can become severe and bring up sputum. The skin may be warm and flushed, especially on the face. The mouth and throat may redden, the eyes may water, and the whites of the eyes may become bloodshot. The ill person, especially a child, may have nausea and vomiting. A small percentage of people with influenza lose their sense of smell for a few days or weeks; rarely, the loss is permanent.

Most symptoms subside after 2 or 3 days. However, fever sometimes lasts up to 5 days, cough may persist for 10 days or longer, and airway irritation may take 6 to 8 weeks to completely resolve. Weakness and fatigue may persist for several days or occasionally for weeks.

The most common complication of influenza is pneumonia. This can be viral pneumonia, in which the influenza virus itself spreads into the lungs, or bacterial pneumonia, in which unrelated bacteria (such as pneumococci) attack the person's weakened defenses. In both cases, the person may have a worsened cough, difficulty breathing, persistent or recurring fever, and sometimes bloody sputum. Pneumonia is more common in older people and in people with heart or lung disease. As many as 7% of older people in long-term care facilities who develop influenza have to be hospitalized, and 1 to 4% die. Younger people with chronic illnesses are also at risk of developing severe complications.

Because most people are familiar with the symptoms of influenza, and because influenza occurs in epidemics, the illness is often correctly diagnosed by the person who has it or by family members. The severity of the illness and the presence of a high fever and body aches help distinguish influenza from a cold. Tests on samples of blood or respiratory secretions can identify the influenza virus but are useful only in special circumstances.

Prevention

Vaccination is the best way to avoid contracting influenza. Influenza vaccines contain inactivated (killed) influenza virus or pieces of the virus. Modern vaccines protect against three different strains of influenza virus. Different vaccines may be given every year to

Preventing Influenza With a Vaccine

Who should get the flu vaccine

- Anyone 50 years of age or older
- Residents of nursing homes
- Adults and children 6 months of age or older with diabetes, heart disease, chronic lung disease, or immune system problems
- Family members and caregivers of people in the above groups
- Doctors and health care workers
- Women who will be in the second or third trimester of pregnancy during the influenza season (women who have medical conditions that increase their risk for complications from influenza should be vaccinated before the influenza season, regardless of the stage of pregnancy)
- Children younger than 18 years of age on chronic aspirin therapy (who are at risk for Reye's syndrome if they develop influenza)

Who should not get the flu vaccine

- People with severe allergy to eggs
- People who have had Guillain-Barré syndrome
- People who currently have a febrile illness (other than a mild cold)

keep up with changes in the virus. Doctors try to predict the strain of virus that will attack each year based on the strain of virus that predominated during the previous flu season and the strain causing disease in other parts of the world.

Vaccination is particularly important for people who are likely to become very ill if infected. People in this group include the young, those older than 50, and anyone with a chronic illness such as diabetes, lung disease, or heart disease. Other than occasional soreness at the injection site, vaccine side effects are rare.

In the United States, vaccination takes place during the fall so that levels of antibodies are highest during the peak influenza months: November through March. For most people, about 2 weeks is needed for the vaccination to provide protection.

Several antiviral drugs can be used to prevent infection with influenza virus. Doctors may prescribe these drugs when a person has a clear, recent exposure to someone with influenza. In addition, these drugs are used during epidemics of influenza to protect unvaccinated people who are at high risk of complications of influenza: older people and people with chronic illnesses.

Amantadine and rimantadine are older antiviral drugs that offer protection against influenza type A but not influenza type B. These drugs can cause stomach upset, nervousness, sleeplessness, and other side effects, especially in older people and in those with brain or kidney disease. Rimantadine tends to cause fewer side effects than amantadine. Another drawback of both amantadine and rimantadine is that the influenza virus rapidly develops resistance to them.

Two new drugs, oseltamivir and zanamivir, can prevent infection with either influenza virus type A or type B. These drugs produce minimal side effects.

Treatment

The main treatment for influenza is to rest adequately, drink plenty of fluids, and avoid exertion. Normal activities may resume 24 to 48 hours after the body temperature returns to normal, but most people take several days to recover. People may treat fever and aches with acetaminophen or nonsteroidal anti-inflammatory drugs (NSAIDs, such as aspirin or ibuprofen). Because of the risk of Reye's syndrome, children should not be given aspirin. Acetaminophen and ibuprofen can be used in children if needed. Other measures as listed for the common cold, such as nasal decongestants and steam inhalation, may help relieve symptoms.

The same antiviral drugs that prevent infection (amantadine, rimantadine, oseltamivir, and zanamivir) are also helpful in treating people who have influenza. However, these drugs work only if taken in the first day or two of illness, and they shorten fever and respiratory symptoms only by a day or so. Nevertheless, these drugs are very effective in some people. Most doctors recommend zanamivir and oseltamivir, which work against both influenza type A and type B. If a secondary bacterial infection develops, antibiotics are added.

Herpes Simplex Virus Infections

Herpes simplex virus (HSV) infection produces recurring episodes of small, painful, fluid-filled blisters on the skin or mucous membranes.

There are two types of herpes simplex virus, HSV-1 and HSV-2. HSV-1 is the usual cause of cold sores on the lips (herpes labialis▲) and sores on the cornea of the eye (herpes simplex keratitis■). HSV-2 causes genital herpes. This distinction is not absolute: genital infections are sometimes caused by HSV-1. These infections can be transmitted by direct contact with sores and sometimes by contact with the oral and genital areas of chronically infected people in between episodes of sores.

HSV infections produce an eruption of tiny blisters on the skin or mucous membranes. After the eruption of blisters subsides, the virus remains in a dormant (latent) state inside the group of nerve cells (ganglia) that supply the nerve fibers to the infected area. Periodically, the virus reactivates, begins growing again, and travels through the nerve fibers back to the skin—causing eruptions of blisters in the same area of skin as the earlier infection. Sometimes the virus may be present on the skin or mucous membranes even when there is no obvious blister.

Reactivation of latent oral or genital HSV infection may be triggered by a fever, menstruation, emotional stress, or suppression of the immune system. An episode of cold sores can develop following physical trauma, such as a dental procedure or overexposure of the lips to sunlight. Often the trigger is unknown.

Symptoms and Complications

The first oral infection with HSV usually causes sores inside the mouth (herpetic gingivostomatitis). In addition, the person generally feels sick and has fever, headache, and body aches. The mouth sores last 10 to 14 days and are often very severe, making eating and drinking extremely uncomfortable. In some first oral infections, swollen gums are the only symptom; occasionally, no symptoms develop. Herpetic gingivostomatitis most commonly develops in children.

Recurrences of oral HSV infection produce what are called "cold sores" (so named because they are often triggered by colds). These sores typically develop on the lips. An episode of cold sores begins with tingling at the site, lasting from minutes to a few hours, followed by redness and swelling. Usually, fluid-filled blisters form and break open, leaving sores. The sores quickly form into a scab. After a week, the scab falls off and the episode ends. Less frequently, tingling and redness occur without blister formation. Sometimes small clusters of herpes sores develop on the gums or the roof of the mouth; these sores also last about a week and then go away.

The first genital HSV infection can be severe and prolonged, with multiple painful blisters in the genital area. Fever and a general feeling of illness (malaise) are common, and some people have burning during urination. Occasionally, an infected person may have no symptoms. A recurring attack of genital herpes begins with symptoms (including local tingling, discomfort, itching, or aching in the groin) that precede the blisters by several hours to 2 to 3 days. Painful blisters surrounded by a reddish rim appear on the skin or mucous membranes of the genitals. The blisters quickly break open, leaving sores. Blisters also may appear on the thighs, buttocks, or around the anus. In women, genital blisters may develop on the vulva, in which case they are usually obvious and very painful. Internal blisters may develop in the vagina or on the cervix; they are less painful and are not visible. A typical episode of recurring genital herpes lasts a week.

In people with a weakened immune system, recurring outbreaks of genital or oral herpes can result in progressive, gradually enlarging sores that take weeks to heal. The infection may progress inside the body, moving down into the esophagus and lungs. Ulcers in the esophagus cause pain during swallowing, and infection of lungs produces pneumonia with cough and shortness of breath.

Sometimes HSV-1 or HSV-2 enters through a break in the skin of a finger, causing a swollen, painful, red fingertip (herpetic whitlow).

HSV-1 sometimes infects the cornea of the eye (herpes simplex keratitis★). This produces a painful sore and blurred vision. Over time, the cornea can become cloudy, causing a significant loss of vision and requiring corneal transplantation.

Infants or adults with a skin condition called atopic eczema can develop a potentially fatal HSV infection in the area of skin that has the eczema (eczema herpeticum●). Therefore, people with atopic eczema should avoid being near anyone with an active herpes infection.

Although it usually infects only the skin and outer surfaces of the body, HSV may

---

▲ see page 668   ■ see page 1301

★ see page 1301   ● see page 1195

rarely infect internal organs, such as the brain (herpes encephalitis). Herpes encephalitis begins with confusion, fever, and seizures and can be fatal.

Although an infrequent event, a pregnant woman can transmit HSV infection to her baby (neonatal herpes). Transmission usually occurs at birth, when the baby comes into contact with infected secretions in the birth canal. Infection of the baby is most likely when the woman has visible herpes sores in the vaginal area, although many babies become infected from mothers who have no apparent sores. Rarely, HSV can be transmitted to the fetus during pregnancy. Newborns with HSV infection become very ill. They may have widespread disease, brain infection, or skin infection. Without treatment, two thirds die, and even with treatment, many suffer brain damage.

Diagnosis

HSV infection is usually easy for a doctor to recognize. If the doctor is unsure, he may swab the sore and send the swab to the laboratory to grow and identify the virus. Sometimes doctors examine material scraped from the blisters under a microscope. Although the virus itself cannot be seen, scrapings sometimes contain enlarged infected cells (giant cells) that are characteristic of a viral infection. Blood tests to identify antibodies to HSV and biopsy of the sores can also be helpful. A new kind of blood test can distinguish between HSV-1 infection and HSV-2 infection.

Treatment

No current antiviral treatments can eradicate HSV infection, and treatment of the first oral or genital infection does not prevent chronic infection of nerves. However, treatment may relieve the discomfort of a recurring outbreak slightly and shorten its duration by a day or two. Treatment is most effective if started early, usually within a few hours of the start of symptoms—preferably at the first sign of tingling or discomfort, before blisters appear. In people who have frequent, painful attacks, the number of outbreaks can be reduced by continuous therapy (suppression) with antiviral drugs.

Penciclovir cream can shorten the healing time and duration of symptoms of a cold sore by about a day. Nonprescription creams containing docosanol or tetracaine may have a modest effect. Acyclovir, valacyclovir, or famciclovir taken by mouth for a few days may be the most effective treatment. Severe HSV infections are treated with intravenous acyclovir. People with herpes simplex keratitis are usually given trifluridine eye drops.

For people who have minimal discomfort, the only treatment needed for recurring herpes of the lips or genitals is to keep the infected area clean by gentle washing with soap and water. Application of ice may be soothing and reduce swelling.

Because herpes simplex is contagious, people with infection of the lips should avoid kissing during eruptions. People with genital herpes should use condoms at all times. Even when there are no visible blisters, the virus may be present on the genital surfaces and potentially transmissible to sex partners.

Shingles

Shingles (herpes zoster) is infection with the varicella-zoster virus that produces a severely painful skin eruption of fluid-filled blisters.

Chickenpox and shingles are caused by the varicella-zoster virus. Chickenpox is the initial infection with varicella-zoster virus,▲ and shingles is a reemergence of the virus, usually years later. During the chickenpox infection, the virus spreads in the bloodstream and infects many nerve cells (ganglia) of the spinal or cranial nerves, remaining there in a dormant (latent) state. The virus may never cause symptoms again, or it may reactivate many years later. When it reactivates, the virus travels back down the nerve fibers to the skin, where it creates painful sores resembling those of chickenpox. This outbreak of sores (shingles) is almost always limited to a strip of the skin on one side of the body that contains a group of infected nerve fibers. This area is called a dermatome.■ Unlike HSV infections, there is usually only one outbreak of shingles in a person's lifetime.

Shingles may develop at any age but is most common after age 50. Most often, the reason for reactivation is unknown, although reactivation sometimes occurs when the body's immunity is reduced by another disorder, such as AIDS or Hodgkin's disease, or by use of drugs that impair the immune system. However, the occurrence of shingles does not usually mean that the person has another serious disease.

▲ see page 1571   ■ see art on page 563

Symptoms and Complications

Some people with shingles feel unwell and have chills, a fever, nausea, diarrhea, or difficulties with urination in the 3 or 4 days before shingles develops. Others experience pain, a tingling sensation, or itching in an area of skin. Clusters of small, fluid-filled blisters surrounded by a small red area then develop. The blisters occupy only the limited area of skin served by the infected nerves. Most often, blisters appear on the trunk, usually on only one side. However, a few blisters may appear elsewhere as well. The involved area of the body is usually sensitive to any stimulus, including light touch, and may be severely painful. Children with shingles usually have less severe symptoms than adults.

The blisters begin to dry and scab about 5 days after they appear. Until scabbing occurs, the blisters contain varicella-zoster virus, which can cause chickenpox if transmitted to susceptible people. Blisters that cover large areas of skin or persist for more than 2 weeks usually indicate that the immune system is not functioning properly.

One attack of shingles usually gives a person lifelong immunity from further attacks; fewer than 5% of people have further attacks. Scarring of the skin, which can be extensive, may occur, but most people recover without any lasting effects.

A few people, more commonly older people, continue to have chronic pain in the area (postherpetic neuralgia). Involvement of the part of the facial nerve leading to the eye can be quite serious, and if it is not treated properly, vision may be affected.

Diagnosis

A doctor may have trouble diagnosing shingles before the blisters appear, but the location of the initial pain in a vague band on one side of the body can be a useful clue. Depending on the nerves involved, the pain may resemble that caused by appendicitis, a kidney stone or gallstone, or inflammation of the large intestine. However, once the blisters appear in the typical pattern following a nerve root, the diagnosis is usually clear. Laboratory tests are seldom performed but may be used to confirm the diagnosis.

Treatment

There are several effective antiviral drugs for shingles. Oral antiviral drugs such as famciclovir, valacyclovir, and acyclovir are often

What Is Postherpetic Neuralgia?

Chronic pain in areas of skin supplied by nerves infected with herpes zoster is called postherpetic neuralgia. This pain may persist for months or years after an episode of shingles. It does not indicate that the virus continues to be actively replicating. Exactly why the pain occurs is not well understood. The pain of postherpetic neuralgia may be constant or intermittent, and it may worsen at night or in response to heat or cold. Sometimes the pain is incapacitating.

Postherpetic neuralgia occurs most often in older people: 25 to 50% of people older than 50 years who have shingles also have some postherpetic neuralgia. However, only about 10% of all people with shingles develop postherpetic neuralgia. Few have severe pain.

In most instances, the pain subsides within 1 to 3 months, but in 10 to 20% of cases, the pain may persist for more than 1 year, but rarely more than 10 years.

Although a number of treatments for postherpetic neuralgia have been tried, no treatment has been found routinely successful. Direct injection of a corticosteroid into the cerebrospinal fluid may be helpful. In most instances, pain is mild and requires no specific treatment, but some people require strong pain drugs.

given, particularly to older people and to those with an impaired immune system. These drugs do not cure the disease, but they can help relieve the symptoms and shorten the duration of illness. There is also evidence that taking corticosteroids along with these drugs may help. To prevent secondary bacterial infections, the skin should be kept clean and dry.

Pain-relieving drugs are often required. Nonsteroidal anti-inflammatory drugs (NSAIDs) or acetaminophen may be tried, but oral opioids are often necessary.▲

Epstein-Barr Virus Infection

Epstein-Barr virus (EBV) causes a number of diseases, including infectious mononucleosis.

Infection with EBV is very common. In the United States, about 50% of all children 5 years of age and nearly 95% of adults have had an EBV infection. Most of these infections pro-

▲ see page 450

duce symptoms similar to those of a cold or other mild viral illness. Sometimes, however, teenagers and young adults develop different and more severe symptoms from EBV infection. This illness is called infectious mononucleosis. Infectious mononucleosis is named for the presence of large numbers of white blood cells (mononuclear cells) in the bloodstream. Teenagers and young adults usually catch infectious mononucleosis by kissing or having other intimate contact with someone infected with EBV.

Rarely, EBV contributes to the development of several uncommon types of cancer, such as Burkitt's lymphoma and certain cancers of the nose and throat. It is thought that specific viral genes alter the growth cycle of infected cells and cause them to become cancerous. EBV has been implicated in chronic fatigue syndrome,▲ although evidence for it as a cause is scanty and controversial.

Symptoms and Complications

EBV can produce a number of different symptoms, depending on the strain of the virus and several other, poorly understood factors. In most children younger than 5, the infection produces no symptoms. In adolescents and adults, it may or may not produce symptoms. The usual time between infection and the appearance of symptoms (incubation period) is thought to be 30 to 50 days.

The four major symptoms of infectious mononucleosis are extreme fatigue, fever, sore throat, and swelling of the lymph nodes. Not everyone has all four symptoms. Usually, the infection begins with a general feeling of illness (malaise) that lasts several days to a week. This vague discomfort is followed by a fever, sore throat, and enlarged lymph nodes. The fever usually peaks at around 103° F in the afternoon or early evening. The throat is often very sore, and puslike material may be present at the back of the throat. Any lymph node may be enlarged; most commonly, the nodes of the neck are affected. Fatigue is usually most pronounced in the first 2 to 3 weeks but may last 6 weeks or more.

The spleen is enlarged in more than 50% of the people with infectious mononucleosis. In most infected people, this enlargement causes few if any symptoms, but an enlarged spleen may rupture if injured. The liver may also enlarge slightly. Less commonly, jaundice and swelling around the eyes occur. Skin rashes develop infrequently; however, people with EBV infection who receive the antibiotic ampicillin usually develop a rash. Other very rare complications include seizures, various nerve abnormalities, behavioral abnormalities, and inflammation of the brain (encephalitis) or tissues covering the brain (meningitis).

The duration of the illness varies. The acute phase lasts about 2 weeks, after which most people are able to resume their usual activities. However, fatigue may persist for several more weeks and, occasionally, for months or longer.

Diagnosis

The symptoms of infectious mononucleosis also occur in many other viral and bacterial infections. Therefore, to confirm the diagnosis, doctors perform a blood test to detect antibodies to EBV. Sometimes, the first sign of infectious mononucleosis is large numbers of characteristic mononuclear white blood cells (atypical lymphocytes) in a blood sample.

Treatment

People with infectious mononucleosis should rest until the fever, sore throat, and feeling of illness disappear. Because of the risk of rupturing the spleen, heavy lifting and contact sports should be avoided for 6 to 8 weeks, even if the spleen is not noticeably enlarged.

Acetaminophen or NSAIDs (such as aspirin or ibuprofen) can relieve fever and pain. However, aspirin should be avoided in children because of the risk of Reye's syndrome, which can be fatal. Some complications, such as severe swelling of the airway, may be treated with corticosteroids. Currently available antiviral drugs have little effect on the symptoms of infectious mononucleosis and should not be used.

Cytomegalovirus Infection

Cytomegalovirus is a common herpesvirus that generally causes disease only in infants infected before birth and in people who have a weakened immune system.

Infection with cytomegalovirus (CMV), a type of herpesvirus, is very common. Blood tests show that 60 to 90% of adults have had a CMV infection at some time. Usually this infection produces no symptoms. Serious infections generally develop only in babies infected before birth■ and in people with an impaired

---

▲ see page 1717   ■ see table on page 1508

immune system—for example, people with AIDS or those who have received an organ transplant. People who have received an organ transplant are particularly susceptible to CMV infection because of the immunosuppressant drugs they receive as part of the transplantation process.

CMV spreads very easily. Infected people may shed the virus in their urine or saliva for months. The virus is also excreted in cervical mucus, semen, stool, and breast milk. Thus, both sexual and nonsexual transmission of the virus takes place. CMV infection may develop in people who receive infected blood.

CMV may cause symptoms soon after infection. It also has the ability to remain dormant in various tissues for the person's lifetime. Various stimuli can cause the dormant CMV to become active and cause disease.

Symptoms

The vast majority of people infected with CMV have no symptoms. Occasionally, a healthy person who is infected may feel ill and have a fever. CMV infection in adolescents and young adults can produce an illness with symptoms of fever and fatigue that resembles infectious mononucleosis. If a person receives a transfusion of blood containing CMV, fever and sometimes liver inflammation may develop 2 to 4 weeks later.

A person with a weakened immune system who becomes infected with CMV is particularly likely to develop a severe infection; serious illness and death may result. In people with AIDS, CMV infection is the most common viral complication. The virus tends to infect the retina of the eye (CMV retinitis), which can cause blindness. Infection of the brain (encephalitis) or ulcers of the intestine or esophagus may also develop.

In a pregnant woman, CMV infection can cause miscarriage, stillbirth, or death of the newborn. Death is caused by bleeding, anemia, or extensive damage to the liver or brain. Other disorders that may occur in the newborn include hearing loss and mental retardation.

Diagnosis and Treatment

CMV infection may develop gradually and not be recognized immediately. However, doctors always consider the possibility of CMV infection in a person with an impaired immune system. Once CMV infection is suspected, a doctor conducts tests to detect the virus in body fluids or tissues. In newborns, the diagnosis is usually made by culturing the urine. In other people, doctors may be able to grow the virus from blood or lung specimens. In a person with CMV retinitis, an eye doctor can see characteristic abnormalities using an ophthalmoscope (an instrument that allows viewing of the internal eye structures).

Mild CMV infection usually is not treated but subsides by itself. When the infection threatens a person's life or eyesight, the antiviral drugs ganciclovir, valganciclovir, cidofovir, or foscarnet may be given. For people with CMV retinitis, a small device containing sustained-release ganciclovir can be implanted in the eye, or fomivirsen may be injected directly into the eye. These drugs have serious side effects and they may not cure the infection; however, treatment slows the disease's progression. CMV infections usually subside without treatment when the body's immune system recovers or immunosuppressant drugs are discontinued.

Hemorrhagic Fevers

Hemorrhagic fevers are a group of serious infections caused by certain viruses and characterized by bleeding.

Ebola and **Marburg virus** are two dangerous African viruses classified as filoviruses. The natural hosts (reservoir or species that maintains the virus in nature) of these viruses are not known. To date, no infections of people have occurred in the United States.

Both viruses can be transmitted from person to person by exposure to blood or infected body tissues. Person-to-person transmission occurs when family members and health care workers come into contact with blood and secretions from infected people.

Symptoms include fever, vomiting, diarrhea, bleeding, and loss of consciousness. Both infections are often fatal, with mortality varying from 25% for Marburg virus to 80 to 90% for some strains of Ebola virus.

There is no specific treatment for these infections except for general support of the person. Strict isolation precautions are necessary to prevent further spread. There is always fear that these viruses will spread from within local outbreaks to large regions, although this has not yet happened.

Lassa fever and the **South American hemorrhagic fevers** are infections caused by arenaviruses. These infections are transmitted from

Smallpox: New Risks From an Old Disease

Smallpox (variola) is a highly contagious and very deadly disease caused by the smallpox virus. The virus can exist only in people—not in animals.

Over 200 years ago, a vaccine against smallpox (the first vaccine ever) was invented. The vaccine proved very effective and was given to people throughout the world. The number of smallpox cases declined steadily until the last case was reported in 1977. In 1980, the World Health Organization (WHO) declared the disease eliminated and recommended discontinuing vaccination.

Because the vaccine's protective effects gradually wear off, nearly all people—even those previously vaccinated—are now susceptible to smallpox. This lack of protection would not be of concern, except that samples of the virus remain in storage at two research facilities, one in the United States and one in Russia. Also, there are reports that the Russian military has a large stockpile of smallpox virus that was created for use as a biological weapon. If the smallpox virus from one of these sources was somehow reintroduced into the population, the resultant epidemic would be devastating.

The smallpox virus spreads from person to person and is acquired by breathing air contaminated with drop-lets of moisture breathed or coughed out by an infected person. Contact with clothing or bed linens used by an infected person also can spread the disease. Smallpox usually spreads to close personal contacts of an infected person. A large outbreak in a school or workplace would be uncommon. The virus survives no more than 2 days in the environment—less, if temperature and humidity are high.

Symptoms of smallpox begin 12 to 14 days after infection. An infected person develops fever, headache, and backache and feels extremely ill. The person may have severe abdominal pain and become delirious. After 2 to 4 days, a rash of flat, red spots develops on the face and arms and inside the mouth, spreading shortly thereafter to the trunk and legs. A person is contagious only after the rash has started. After 1 or 2 days, the spots turn into blisters and then pustules. After 8 or 9 days, the pustules become crusted. About 30% of people with smallpox die, usually in the second week of illness. Some people who survive would be left with large, disfiguring scars.

A doctor would suspect smallpox when a person has the disease's characteristic spots—particularly when there is an outbreak of the disease. The diagnosis can be confirmed by identifying the smallpox virus in a culture or under a microscope in a sample taken from the blisters or pustules.

Prevention is the best response to the threat of smallpox. Vaccination within the first few days of exposure can prevent or limit the severity of illness. People with symptoms suggestive of smallpox would need to be isolated to prevent spread of the disease. Contacts of these people would not need to be isolated because they could not spread the infection unless they became sick and developed a rash. These contacts would need to be watched closely, however, and isolated at the first sign of illness.

Vaccination is dangerous for some people, especially those with a weak immune system. Even some healthy people have adverse reactions to smallpox vaccination, although these are rare. Adverse reactions are less common in previously vaccinated people than in those who have never received the vaccine. About 1 in every million previously unvaccinated people and 1 in every 4 million previously vaccinated people die from the vaccine.

There is no specific treatment for smallpox, although certain antiviral drugs are being studied. Doctors support the person's breathing and blood pressure. Any bacterial infections that develop are treated.

rodents to people or from person to person. Lassa fever occurs mainly in West Africa. The South American fevers are mostly confined to Bolivia and Argentina.

The infections cause fever, chest pain, diffuse body aches, and vomiting. Bleeding from the mouth, nose, stomach, and intestinal tract is common in the South American hemorrhagic fevers. Overt bleeding is less common in Lassa fever, but small spots of blood are often present under the skin. When death occurs, it is usually as a result of shock caused by diffuse leakage of fluid from blood vessels. These infections are often fatal and require strict isolation of cases to prevent transmission to health care workers and family members. There is an experimental vaccine effective against some of the South American hemorrhagic fevers. The antiviral drug rib-avirin does not cure the infection but reduces the death rate.

Hantavirus Infection

Hantavirus infection is a viral disease that is spread from rodents to people and causes severe infections of the lungs and kidneys.

Hantaviruses are present throughout the world in the urine, feces, and saliva of various rodents. People acquire the infection by having contact with rodents or their droppings, or possibly by inhaling virus particles in places with large amounts of rodent droppings. No evidence of person-to-person spread has been found.

There are five different strains of hantavirus, some of which affect different parts of the body. Recent outbreaks of infection with a hantavirus strain affecting the lungs have occurred in the southwestern United States.

Symptoms of hantavirus infection begin with fever and muscle pain. Abdominal pain, diarrhea, or vomiting also may develop. Other symptoms depend on which virus strain is involved. After 4 to 5 days, a person with infection involving the lungs develops a cough and shortness of breath, which may become severe within hours. Lung infection can be fatal. Other virus strains mainly affect the kidney. People with kidney infection have fever, headache, backache, abdominal pain, rash, and very low blood pressure (shock). Urine output may cease (anuria). In some people, symptoms of kidney infection are mild and complete recovery occurs. In others, symptoms become severe, with death occurring in 5% of cases.

Treatment mostly involves supportive care. Providing oxygen and treatment to stabilize the blood pressure appear to be most crucial to recovery from illness. For kidney damage, dialysis may be needed and can be lifesaving.

Yellow Fever

Yellow fever is a mosquito-borne viral disease that can cause bleeding from the digestive tract and inflammation of the liver that results in jaundice.

Yellow fever is caused by an arbovirus (*ar*thropod-[insect]-*bo*rne *virus*). Mosquitoes are the particular arthropod responsible for transmitting yellow fever. Yellow fever is one of the most recognized and historically important viral infections. In the past, major epidemics of yellow fever have been responsible for tens of thousands of deaths. Once common in tropical and temperate zones around the world, the disease now occurs only in Central Africa and Central and South America.

The first symptoms of yellow fever are headache, muscle aches, and mild fever, all of which subside after a few days. Some people then recover, but others develop high fevers, nausea and vomiting, and severe generalized pain. The skin turns yellow because of infection of the liver. Often there is bleeding from the nose, mouth, and digestive tract. Some people develop very low blood pressure (shock) and coma. Up to 50% of people with these more severe symptoms die.

Doctors diagnose yellow fever by growing the virus and detecting antibodies to the virus in the blood. A vaccine that is 95% effective at preventing yellow fever is available, but there is no specific treatment for the infection.

Dengue Fever

Dengue fever is a mosquito-borne viral infection that causes fever and generalized pain.

Dengue fever is common worldwide in the tropics and subtropics. Recently, some cases have occurred in Southern Texas. The infection is caused by an arbovirus and is transmitted by mosquitoes.

Dengue fever varies in severity. Children typically have a mild illness with low fever, fatigue, runny nose, and cough. The disease is more severe in adults, with fever, headache, and severe generalized body aches. These aches are often so painful that the disease has been called "breakbone fever." Some people develop bleeding from the nose, mouth, and digestive tract—usually after a second infection. Sometimes the blood vessels leak fluid into the lungs, causing difficulty breathing. Dengue fever is occasionally fatal.

Doctors diagnose dengue fever by growing the virus from blood specimens and by tests for antibodies to the virus. There is no specific treatment, but an experimental vaccine to prevent dengue fever is currently undergoing tests.

CHAPTER 199

Human Immunodeficiency Virus Infection

Human immunodeficiency virus (HIV) infection is an infection by one of two viruses, HIV-1 and HIV-2. The HIV viruses progressively destroy some types of white blood cells called lymphocytes. Lymphocytes are an important part of the body's immune defenses.▲ When lymphocytes are destroyed, the body becomes susceptible to attack by many other infectious organisms. Many of the complications of HIV infection, including death, are usually the result of these other infections and not of the HIV infection itself.

Acquired immunodeficiency syndrome (AIDS) is the most severe form of HIV infection. A person with HIV infection is considered to have AIDS when at least one complicating illness develops or his ability to defend against infection significantly declines as measured by a low CD4+ lymphocyte count.

HIV infection and AIDS have reached epidemic proportions. Through December 2000, more than 770,000 cases of AIDS and 448,000 deaths were reported in the United States. At the end of 2000, 36 million people worldwide were infected with HIV. More than 800,000 people in the United States are thought to be infected with HIV, and 40,000 new infections occur in this country each year. In parts of Africa, more than 30% of the adult population (between the ages of 15 and 45) is infected, threatening to nearly eliminate a whole generation.

Infections with HIV-1 and HIV-2 are serious and tend to occur in different regions. HIV-1 is most common in the Western Hemisphere; Europe; Asia; and Central, South, and East Africa. HIV-2 is common in West Africa, although many people there are infected with HIV-1.

Transmission of Infection

The transmission of HIV requires contact with a body fluid that contains the virus or infected cells. HIV can appear in nearly any body fluid, but transmission mainly comes from blood, semen, vaginal secretions, and breast milk. Although low concentrations of HIV are also present in tears, urine, and saliva, transmission from these fluids is extremely rare.

HIV is transmitted in the following ways:
• Sexual contact with an infected person, during which the mucous membrane lining the mouth, vagina, penis, or rectum is exposed to contaminated body fluids (unprotected sex)
• Injection or infusion of contaminated blood, as occurs with blood transfusions, the sharing of needles, or an accidental prick from an HIV-contaminated needle
• Transfer of the virus from an infected mother to a child before birth, during birth, or after birth through the mother's milk

Susceptibility to HIV infection increases when the skin or a mucous membrane is torn or damaged—even minimally—as can happen during vigorous vaginal or anal intercourse. Sexual transmission of HIV is more likely if either partner has herpes, syphilis, or another sexually transmitted disease (STD) that produces breaks in the skin or inflammation of the genitals. However, HIV can be transmitted even if neither partner has other STDs or obvious breaks in the skin. HIV transmission also can occur during oral sex, although it is far less common than during vaginal or anal intercourse.

In the United States, Europe, and Australia, HIV has mainly been transmitted through male homosexual contact and the sharing of needles among injecting drug users, but transmission through heterosexual contact has been rapidly increasing. In 2000, 42% of new HIV infections in the United States developed in homosexual men, 33% in heterosexual men and women, and 25% in injecting drug users. HIV transmission in Africa, the Caribbean, and Asia occurs primarily between heterosexuals, and HIV infection occurs equally among men and women. Through December 2000, more than 17% of the adults in the United States reported to have AIDS were women. HIV infection is increasing at a faster rate among women than among men. In areas of the United States where HIV infection is reported, 31% of new HIV infections occur in women. Before 1992, most American women

---

▲ see page 1054

with HIV were infected by injecting drugs with contaminated needles. In 2000, however, 75% of women were infected by sexual contact.

A health care worker who is accidentally pricked with an HIV-contaminated needle has about a 1 in 300 chance of contracting HIV. The risk increases if the needle penetrates deeply or if contaminated blood is injected. Infected fluid splashing into the mouth or eyes has less than a 1 in 1,000 chance of causing infection. Taking a combination of antiretroviral drugs soon after exposure appears to reduce, but not eliminate, the risk of becoming infected and is recommended.

People with hemophilia require frequent infusions of whole blood or other blood products. Before 1985, many people with hemophilia in the United States became infected with HIV because the blood products they received were contaminated with HIV. AIDS became the leading cause of death among these people. Since 1985, all blood collected for transfusion has been tested for HIV, and when possible, some blood products are treated with heat to eliminate the risk of HIV infection. The current risk of HIV infection from a single blood transfusion is estimated to be less than 1 in 500,000.

HIV infection in a large number of women of childbearing age has led to HIV infection in children.▲ In about 25 to 35% of the pregnancies involving women infected with HIV, the virus is transmitted to the fetus through the placenta or, more commonly, at birth during passage through the birth canal. Infants who are breastfed can contract HIV infection through breast milk. A few children contract HIV infection through sexual abuse.

HIV is not transmitted by casual contact or even by close, nonsexual contact at work, school, or home. No case of HIV transmission has been traced to the coughing or sneezing of an infected person or to a mosquito bite. Transmission from an infected doctor or dentist to a patient is extremely rare.

Mechanism of Infection

Once in the body, HIV attaches to several types of white blood cells, the most important being the helper T lymphocyte. Helper T lymphocytes activate and coordinate other cells of the immune system. These lymphocytes have a receptor protein called CD4 in their outer membrane (and are therefore designated as CD4+). HIV has its genetic material encoded in RNA. Once inside a CD4+ lymphocyte, the

What Is a Retrovirus?

The human immunodeficiency virus (HIV) is a retrovirus, which like many other viruses stores its genetic information as RNA rather than as DNA. When the virus enters a targeted host cell, it releases its RNA and an enzyme (reverse transcriptase), and then makes DNA using the viral RNA as a pattern. The viral DNA is then incorporated into the host cell DNA. This reverses the pattern of human cells, which copy RNA from the pattern of human DNA (thus, the term "retro" for "backward"). Other RNA viruses, such as polio or measles, do not make DNA copies but simply copy their own RNA.

Each time a host cell divides, it makes a new copy of the integrated viral DNA along with its own genes. The viral DNA can either lie latent (hidden) and do no damage or activate to take over the functions of the cell, causing the cell to produce new viruses. These new viruses are released from the infected cell to invade other cells.

virus turns its RNA into DNA by means of an enzyme called reverse transcriptase. The viral DNA is incorporated into the DNA of the infected lymphocyte. The lymphocyte's own machinery then reproduces (replicates) the virus inside the cell, eventually destroying the cell. The thousands of new viruses produced by each infected cell infect other lymphocytes and can destroy them as well. Within a few days or weeks, enough HIV may be produced to reduce numbers of lymphocytes substantially and enable the person to spread the HIV infection to others.

Because HIV infection destroys CD4+ lymphocytes, it weakens the body's system for protecting itself against certain infections and cancers. This weakening of the immune system is part of the reason that the body is unable to eliminate HIV infection once it has started. However, the immune system is able to mount some response. Within a month or two of infection, the body produces lymphocytes and antibodies that help to lower the amount of HIV in the blood and keep the infection under control. For this reason, HIV infection can continue for a long time in some people before it causes serious problems.

▲ see page 1573

The HIV Transmission Risk of Several Sexual Activities

No risk (unless sores are present)
- Dry kissing
- Body-to-body rubbing and massage
- Using unshared inserted sexual devices
- Being masturbated by a partner, without semen or vaginal fluids
- Bathing and showering together
- Contact of intact skin with feces or urine

Theoretical risk (extremely low risk unless sores are present)
- Wet kissing
- Oral sex performed on male (no ejaculation, with or without a condom)
- Oral sex performed on female (with barrier)
- Oral-anal contact
- Digital vaginal or anal penetration, with or without a glove
- Using shared but disinfected inserted sexual devices

Low risk
- Oral sex performed on male (with ejaculation, with or without ingestion of semen)
- Oral sex performed on female (no barrier)
- Vaginal or anal intercourse (with proper use of a condom)
- Using shared but not disinfected inserted sexual devices

High risk
- Vaginal or anal intercourse (with or without ejaculation, condom not used or used improperly)

Because the number of CD4+ lymphocytes in the blood helps determine the ability of the immune system to protect the body from infections, it is a good measure of the severity of the damage done by HIV infection. A healthy person has a CD4+ lymphocyte count of roughly 800 to 1,300 cells per microliter of blood. Typically, 40 to 60% of CD4+ lymphocytes are destroyed in the first few months of infection. After about 6 months, the CD4+ count stops falling so quickly, but it continues to decline.

If the CD4+ count falls below about 200 cells per microliter of blood, the immune system becomes less able to fight certain infections (for example, the fungal infection that causes *Pneumocystis carinii* pneumonia [PCP]). These infections do not usually appear in people with a healthy immune system and are called opportunistic infections. A count below about 50 cells per microliter of blood is particularly dangerous, because additional opportunistic infections that can rapidly cause severe weight loss, blindness, or death commonly occur.

The amount of virus in the blood is called the **viral load.** In the first few months after infection, a large number of virus particles circulate in the blood. The infection is very contagious at this stage. Later, the viral load drops to a lower level that remains constant for some time. This level is an important indicator of how contagious a person's infection is and how fast the disease is likely to progress. Doctors measure the viral load during treatment, because a decreasing or very low level indicates that treatment is working. The goal of treatment is to lower the viral load to the point where it is undetectable (suppressed) in the blood, although some virus is probably still present. A rise in the viral load may indicate the development of drug resistance or failure to take the drugs.

Symptoms

Most people experience no noticeable symptoms upon initial infection. However, fever, rashes, swollen lymph nodes, fatigue, and a variety of less common symptoms may develop within a few weeks of HIV infection and last a few weeks. The symptoms disappear, although the lymph nodes may stay enlarged. An infected person is able to spread the virus soon after becoming infected; this is true even if there are no symptoms.

A person can have HIV infection for years—even a decade or longer—before developing AIDS. Before AIDS develops, many people feel well, although some develop a variety of nonspecific symptoms. These symptoms include swollen lymph nodes, weight loss, fatigue, recurring fever or diarrhea, anemia, and thrush (a fungal infection of the mouth).

The main symptoms of AIDS are those of the specific opportunistic infections and cancers that develop. HIV can also directly infect the brain, causing memory loss, weakness, difficulty walking, and difficulty in thinking and

Simplified Life Cycle of the Human Immunodeficiency Virus

Like all viruses, human immunodeficiency virus (HIV) reproduces (replicates) using the genetic machinery of its host cell, usually a CD4+ lymphocyte. Currently licensed drugs inhibit two critical enzymes (reverse transcriptase and protease) that the virus uses to replicate. Drugs targeted at a third enzyme, integrase, are being developed.

1. HIV first attaches to and penetrates its target cell.

2. HIV releases RNA, the genetic code of the virus, into the cell. For the virus to replicate, its RNA must be converted into DNA; the enzyme that performs the conversion is called reverse transcriptase. HIV mutates easily at this point, because reverse transcriptase is prone to errors during the conversion of viral RNA to DNA.

3. The viral DNA enters the cell's nucleus.

4. With the help of an enzyme called integrase, the viral DNA becomes integrated with the cell's DNA.

5. The DNA now replicates and reproduces RNA and proteins. The proteins are in the form of a long chain that must be cut into pieces after the virus leaves the cell.

6. A new virus is assembled from RNA and short pieces of protein.

7. The virus buds through the membrane of the cell, wrapping itself in a fragment of the cell membrane (envelope).

8. To be able to infect other cells, the budded virus must mature. It becomes mature when another viral enzyme (HIV protease) cuts structural proteins within the virus, causing them to rearrange.

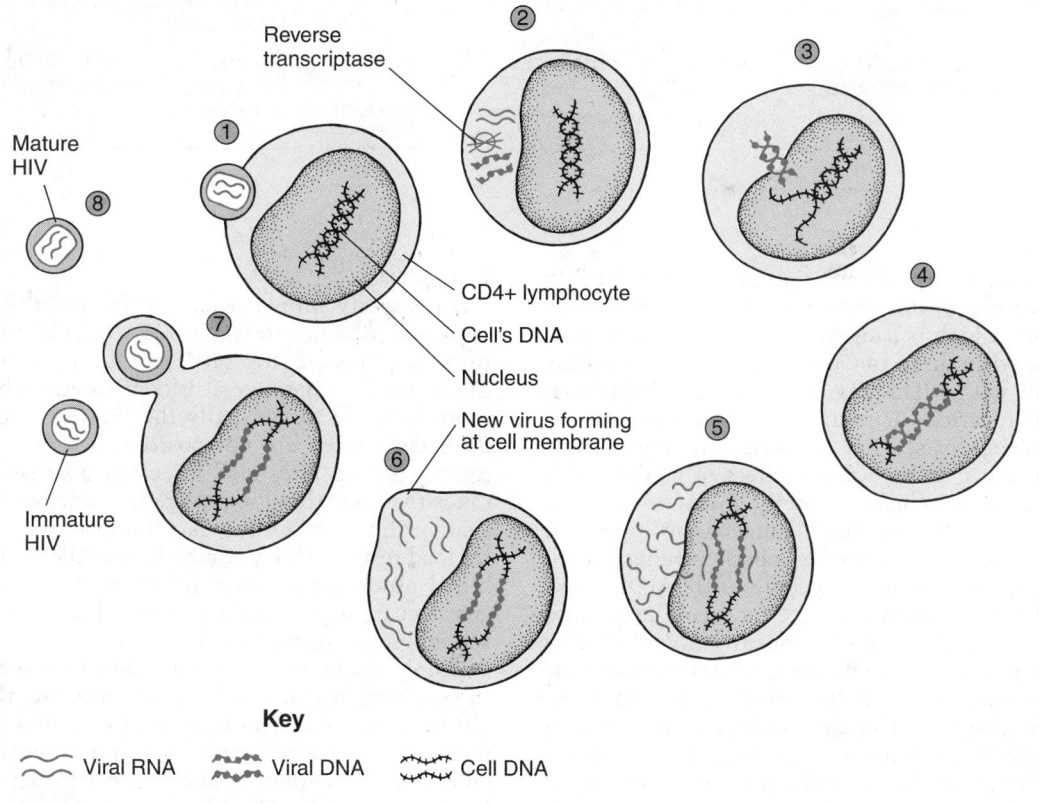

Reverse transcriptase

Mature HIV

CD4+ lymphocyte

Cell's DNA

Nucleus

New virus forming at cell membrane

Immature HIV

Key

〜 Viral RNA   ⌇⌇ Viral DNA   ⌇⌇ Cell DNA

COMMON OPPORTUNISTIC INFECTIONS ASSOCIATED WITH AIDS

INFECTION	DESCRIPTION	SYMPTOMS
Candida esophagitis	A yeast infection of the esophagus	Painful swallowing, burning in chest
Pneumocystis carinii pneumonia	An infection of the lungs with *Pneumocystis* fungus	Difficulty breathing, cough, fever
Toxoplasmosis	Infection with the parasite *Toxoplasma*, which usually affects the brain	Headache, confusion, lethargy, seizures
Tuberculosis	Infection of the lungs and sometimes other organs with tuberculosis bacteria	Cough, fevers, night sweats, weight loss, chest pain
Mycobacterium avium complex	Infection of the intestines or lungs with a type of bacteria that resembles tuberculosis bacteria	Fever, weight loss, diarrhea, cough
Cryptosporidiosis	Infection of the intestines with the parasite *Cryptosporidium*	Diarrhea, abdominal pain, weight loss
Cryptococcal meningitis	Infection of the lining of the brain with the yeast *Cryptococcus*	Headache, fever, confusion
Cytomegalovirus infection	Infection of the eyes or intestinal tract with cytomegalovirus	Eye: blindness Intestinal tract: diarrhea, weight loss
Progressive multifocal leukoencephalopathy	Infection of the brain with a polyomavirus	Weakness on one side of the body, loss of coordination or balance

concentrating (dementia). In some people, HIV is probably directly responsible for AIDS wasting, which is a significant loss of weight with or without an obvious cause. Wasting in people with AIDS may also be caused by a series of infections or an untreated infection (such as tuberculosis) that persists. Kidney failure, which may be a direct effect of HIV, is more common in blacks than in whites.

Kaposi's sarcoma, a cancer that appears as painless, red to purple, raised patches on the skin, affects many people with AIDS, especially homosexual men. Cancers of the immune system (lymphomas, typically non-Hodgkin's lymphoma) may develop, sometimes first appearing in the brain, where they can cause confusion, personality changes, and memory loss. Women are prone to developing cancer of the cervix. Homosexual men are prone to developing cancer of the rectum.

Usually, death is caused by the cumulative effects of wasting, dementia, opportunistic infections, or cancers.

Diagnosis

A relatively simple, accurate blood test that detects antibodies to HIV (ELISA test) is used to screen people for HIV infection. If the ELISA result is positive, it is confirmed with a more accurate test, usually the Western Blot. Both tests often are not positive in the first month or two after HIV infection because it takes the body that long to produce antibodies against the virus. Other tests (for example, viral load tests or P24 antigen) detect HIV in the blood much sooner after infection. P24 antigen is currently used along with other tests to screen blood donated for transfusions.

People diagnosed with HIV infection have their blood tested regularly to measure the CD4+ count and viral load. CD4+ counts indicate the health of a person's immune system and, when low, their chances of becoming ill from an infection. Viral load is a predictor of how fast the CD4+ count is likely to drop over the next year. Doctors use these two measurements to decide when to start drugs for both the treatment of HIV and the prevention of the complicating infections. Doctors also use these tests to monitor the effects of treatment. With successful treatment, the viral load falls to low levels within weeks and the CD4+ count begins a long, slow recovery toward normal levels. AIDS is diagnosed when the CD4+ count falls below 200 cells per microliter of blood, there is extreme wasting, or certain opportunistic infections and cancers develop.

Prevention

Because HIV is nearly always transmitted by sexual contact or the sharing of needles, infection is almost completely preventable. Unfortunately, the measures required for prevention—sexual abstinence or condom use▲ and access to clean needles—are sometimes personally or socially unpopular. Many people have difficulty changing their addictive or sexual behaviors, so they continue to engage in behavior that puts them at risk for HIV infection. Additionally, safe sex practices are not foolproof: condoms can leak or break.

Vaccines for preventing HIV infection or slowing the progression of AIDS in people who are already infected have so far proved elusive. Research continues, and several promising vaccines are being tested.

Because HIV is not transmitted through the air or by casual contact (such as touching, holding, or dry kissing), hospitals and clinics do not isolate HIV-infected people unless they have another contagious infection. HIV-contaminated surfaces can easily be cleaned and disinfected because HIV is inactivated by heat and by common disinfectants such as hydrogen peroxide and alcohol. People who are likely to come into contact with blood or other body fluids at their job should wear protective gear, including latex gloves, masks, and eye shields. These universal precautions apply to body fluids from all people, not just those from someone with HIV, for two reasons: people with HIV may not know that they are infected, and other viruses can be transmitted by body fluids.

People who have been exposed to HIV from a blood splash, needlestick, or sexual contact may reduce the chance of infection by taking a brief course of anti-HIV drugs. These drugs must be started as soon as possible after the exposure. Four weeks of preventive treatment with two or three drugs is currently recommended. Because the risk of infection varies, doctors and infected people make treatment

Strategies for Preventing the Transmission of HIV

- Abstain from sexual activity
- Use a latex condom for each act of intercourse with an infected partner or a partner whose HIV status is unknown (vaginal spermicides and sponges do not protect against HIV infection)
- If engaging in oral sex, withdraw before ejaculation; avoid brushing teeth for several hours before and after oral sex
- Newly monogamous couples should get tested for HIV and other sexually transmitted diseases (STDs) before engaging in unprotected sexual intercourse
- Never share needles or syringes
- Wear rubber gloves (preferably latex) when touching body fluids of a person who might be infected with HIV
- If exposed to HIV by needlestick, seek treatment to prevent infection

decisions individually based on the type of exposure.

Treatment

Three classes of drugs are available to treat HIV infection: nucleoside reverse transcriptase inhibitors, non-nucleoside reverse transcriptase inhibitors, and protease inhibitors. Both types of reverse transcriptase inhibitors work by interfering with the HIV enzyme reverse transcriptase, which converts viral RNA into DNA. Protease inhibitors interfere with the HIV enzyme protease, which is needed to activate certain proteins inside newly produced viruses. Failure to activate these proteins results in immature, defective HIV that does not infect new cells. None of these drugs kill HIV; they prevent the virus from replicating. If replication is sufficiently slowed, the destruction of CD4 cells by HIV is decreased dramatically and CD4+ counts begin to rise. The result can be reversal of much of the damage to the immune system caused by HIV.

HIV usually develops resistance to any of these drugs when they are used alone. Resistance can develop after a few days to several months of use, depending on the drug and the person. Therefore, treatment is most effective

▲ see box on page 1178

when at least two or three of the drugs are given in combination—usually one or two reverse transcriptase inhibitors plus a protease inhibitor. This combination of drugs is sometimes referred to as a "drug cocktail." Combinations of drugs are used for three reasons. First, combinations are more powerful than single drugs in reducing levels of HIV in the blood. Second, combinations help prevent the development of drug resistance. Third, some HIV drugs (like ritonavir) boost the blood levels of other HIV drugs (including most protease inhibitors) by slowing their removal from the body. Drug combinations have delayed the onset of AIDS in HIV-infected people, thus extending their lives.

Combinations of HIV drugs have both unpleasant and serious side effects. Disturbances in the metabolism of fats appear to be caused primarily by the protease inhibitors. Symptoms are the slow migration of body fat from the face, arms, and legs to the abdomen ("protease paunch") and sometimes to the breasts of women. Blood levels of cholesterol and triglycerides, two forms of fat in the blood, are increased—probably increasing the risk of future heart attacks and strokes.

Nucleoside reverse transcriptase inhibitors damage mitochondria, a critical site of energy generation in human cells. Their side effects include anemia, painful feet caused by nerve damage, and liver damage that rarely progresses to liver failure. Individual drugs differ in their tendency to cause these problems. Careful monitoring and changes of drugs can usually prevent serious problems.

Drug treatment is beneficial only when the drugs are taken on schedule. Missed doses allow the virus to replicate and develop resistance. The goal of combination therapy is to reduce the viral load so it is below detectable levels. No treatments have proven able to eliminate the virus from the body, although levels often fall below what can be measured; if treatment is stopped, viral load increases and CD4+ counts begin to fall.

It is not yet clear for which infected people drug treatment should be started, but people with low CD4+ counts or high viral loads require treatment, even if they have no symptoms. Because of the many significant and unpleasant side effects and because the drugs are very expensive, it is not easy for people with HIV infection to take the drugs for many years without fail. Because taking HIV drugs irregularly often leads to drug resistance, doctors try

to ensure that anyone prescribed these drugs is both willing and able to adhere to the treatment schedule.

People with low CD4+ counts are routinely prescribed drugs to prevent opportunistic infections. To prevent *Pneumocystis* pneumonia, the combination of sulfamethoxazole and trimethoprim is given when the CD4+ count drops below 200 cells per microliter of blood. This combination of drugs also prevents toxoplasmosis, which can damage the brain of a person with AIDS. For people with CD4+ counts below 50 cells per microliter of blood, azithromycin taken weekly or clarithromycin or rifabutin taken daily may prevent *Mycobacterium avium* infections. People recovering from cryptococcal meningitis or those experiencing repeated infections of the mouth, esophagus, or vagina with the fungus *Candida* may be given the antifungal drug fluconazole for prolonged periods. People with recurring episodes of herpes simplex infections of the mouth, lips, genitals, or rectum may require prolonged treatment with an antiviral drug (such as acyclovir) to prevent relapses.

Other drugs may help with the weakness and weight loss associated with AIDS. Megestrol and dronabinol (a marijuana derivative) stimulate appetite. Many people with AIDS claim that natural marijuana is even more effective, and use of marijuana for this purpose has been legalized in a few states. Anabolic steroids (such as testosterone) can also significantly reverse the loss of muscle tissue. Testosterone levels are reduced in some men and can be replaced by use of injections or patches on the skin.

Prognosis

Exposure to HIV does not always lead to infection, and some people who have had repeated exposures over many years remain uninfected. Moreover, many infected people have remained well for more than a decade. Doctors do not fully understand why some people become ill so much sooner than others, but a number of genetic factors appear to influence both susceptibility to infection and progression to AIDS after infection.

Of the people infected with HIV who do not receive drug treatment, each year 1 to 2% develop AIDS for the first several years after infection. Every year thereafter, about 5% of the people with untreated HIV infection develop AIDS. Within 10 to 11 years of contracting HIV infection, half of the people who have not

℞ DRUGS FOR HIV INFECTION

TYPE	DRUG	SIDE EFFECTS

Non-nucleoside reverse transcriptase inhibitors

	Delavirdine	Rash, headaches
	Efavirenz	Dizziness, sleepiness, nightmares, confusion, agitation, forgetfulness, euphoria, rash
	Nevirapine	Rash (occasionally severe or life threatening), liver dysfunction

Nucleoside and nucleotide reverse transcriptase inhibitors

		All may cause lactic acidosis and liver damage
	Abacavir	Fever, rash (occasionally severe or life threatening), nausea and vomiting, low white blood count
	Didanosine (ddI)	Peripheral nerve damage, pancreas inflammation, nausea, diarrhea
	Lamivudine (3TC)	Headache, fatigue
	Stavudine (d4T)	Peripheral nerve damage, loss of facial fat
	Tenofovir	Mild to moderate diarrhea, nausea and vomiting, flatulence
	Zalcitabine (ddC)	Peripheral nerve damage, pancreas inflammation, mouth sores
	Zidovudine (AZT)	Anemia and susceptibility to infection (resulting from bone marrow toxicity), headache, insomnia, weakness, muscle aches

Protease inhibitors

		All produce nausea, vomiting, diarrhea, and abdominal discomfort; high blood sugar and cholesterol are common; increased abdominal fat ("protease paunch") may occur; bleeding in hemophilia; liver dysfunction
	Amprenavir	
	Indinavir	Kidney stones
	Lopinavir	Mouth tingling, altered taste
	Nelfinavir	
	Ritonavir	Mouth tingling, altered taste
	Saquinavir	

received treatment develop AIDS. Eventually, more than 95% of untreated infected people develop AIDS, and it is possible that they all will if they live long enough, although a few people have remained well for more than 15 years.

Early in the AIDS epidemic, many people with AIDS experienced a rapid decline in their quality of life after first being hospitalized for the infection—often spending much of their remaining time in the hospital. Most people died within 2 years of developing AIDS. However, current therapy has changed AIDS into a more stable, manageable disease. Many people have lived for years with AIDS, continuing to lead productive and active lives. Nevertheless, illness from infections and the expense and side effects of drugs may reduce quality of life. For people unable to tolerate or take drugs consistently, the natural progression of the disease resumes. Cure is not yet possible, although intensive research on a cure continues.

CHAPTER 200

Sexually Transmitted Diseases

Sexually transmitted (venereal) diseases are infections that are passed from person to person through sexual contact.

Because sexual activity includes intimate contact, it provides an easy opportunity for organisms to spread from one person to another. A variety of infectious microorganisms can be spread by sexual contact. Bacterial sexually transmitted diseases (STDs) include syphilis, gonorrhea, nongonococcal urethritis and chlamydial cervicitis, lymphogranuloma venereum, chancroid, granuloma inguinale, and trichomoniasis. Viral STDs include genital warts, genital herpes,▲ molluscum contagiosum,■ and HIV infection or AIDS.★

STDs are among the most common infectious diseases. It is estimated that over 3 million people contract gonorrhea and chlamydia every year in the United States—making these the two most common STDs in the country.

Although STDs usually result from having vaginal, oral, or anal sex with an infected partner, genital penetration is not necessary to spread an infection. Some diseases may also be transmitted by kissing or by close body contact. Also, the organisms responsible for some STDs (for example, HIV and hepatitis viruses) can be transmitted through nonsexual means, such as from mother to child at birth or through breastfeeding or exposure to contaminated food, water, blood, medical instruments, or needles.

Effective drugs are available for most STDs caused by bacteria, although a number of new antibiotic-resistant strains of bacteria have become widespread. Viral STDs, especially herpes and HIV, persist for life and have effective treatment but no known cure.

Preventing or controlling STDs depends on practicing safe sex and getting prompt diagnosis and treatment. Knowing how to prevent the spread of STDs—in particular, knowing the proper method for using a condom—is crucial.

One strategy health care workers use to help control the spread of some STDs is contact tracing. Health care workers try to trace and treat (if treatment is available) all of an infected person's sexual contacts. People who have been treated are reexamined to make sure they are cured.

Syphilis

Syphilis is a sexually transmitted disease caused by the bacterium Treponema pallidum.

Syphilis is highly contagious during the primary and secondary stages: a single sexual encounter with a person who has syphilis results in infection about one third of the time. The bacterium enters the body through mucous membranes, such as those in the vagina or mouth, or through the skin. Within hours, the bacterium reaches nearby lymph nodes, then spreads throughout the body by way of the bloodstream. Syphilis can infect a fetus during pregnancy,● causing birth defects and other problems.

The annual number of people with newly diagnosed symptomatic syphilis last peaked in 1990, with 50,000 cases in the United States. Since then—largely because of focused public health measures—numbers have been dropping; 35,600 total and slightly more than 6,000 symptomatic cases were reported in 1999. Thus, most cases are detected in people without symptoms.

Symptoms

Symptoms of syphilis usually begin 3 to 4 weeks after infection, although they may start as early as 1 week or as late as 13 weeks after infection. Syphilis progresses through several stages (primary, secondary, latent, and tertiary) if not treated. Infection can persist for many years and may cause heart damage, brain damage, and death.

In the **primary stage,** a painless sore or ulcer (chancre) appears at the infection site—typically the penis, vulva, or vagina. The chancre may also appear on the anus, rectum, lips, tongue, throat, cervix, fingers, or, rarely, other parts of the body. Usually, a person has only one chancre, but occasionally several develop.

The chancre begins as a small red raised area, which soon turns into a painless open sore. The chancre does not bleed and is hard to

---

▲ see page 1160   ■ see page 1229
★ see page 1168   ● see table on page 1509

the touch. Nearby lymph nodes usually swell and are also painless. About half of infected women and one third of infected men are unaware of it. Others ignore the chancre because it causes few symptoms. The chancre usually heals in 3 to 12 weeks, after which the person appears to be completely healthy.

The **secondary stage** usually begins with a skin rash, which typically appears 6 to 12 weeks after infection. About 25% of infected people still have a healing chancre at this time. The rash usually does not itch or hurt and can have many different appearances. Unlike rashes from most other diseases, the rash of secondary syphilis commonly appears on the palms or soles. The skin rash may be short-lived or may last for months. Even if a person is not treated, the rash eventually clears up. New rashes, however, may appear weeks or months later.

Secondary-stage syphilis is a generalized disease that can cause fever, fatigue, loss of appetite, and weight loss. Mouth sores develop in more than 80% of people. About 50% have enlarged lymph nodes throughout the body, and about 10% develop inflammation of the eyes. The eye inflammation usually causes no symptoms, although occasionally the optic nerve swells, which may cause some blurring of vision. About 10% of people have inflamed bones and joints that ache. Jaundice may result from inflammation of the liver. A small number of people develop acute syphilitic meningitis, which causes headaches, neck stiffness, and sometimes deafness.

Raised areas (condylomata lata) may develop where the skin adjoins mucous membrane (for example, at the inner edges of the lips and vulva) and in moist areas of the skin. These extremely infectious areas may flatten and turn a dull pink or gray. The hair often falls out in patches, leaving a moth-eaten appearance.

After the person has recovered from the secondary stage, the disease enters a **latent stage,** in which the infection persists but no symptoms occur. This stage may last for years to decades—or for the rest of the person's life. Syphilis is generally not contagious in the latent stage.

During the **tertiary (third) stage,** syphilis is also not contagious but produces symptoms that range from mild to devastating. Three main types of tertiary syphilis may occur: benign tertiary syphilis, cardiovascular syphilis, and neurosyphilis.

Diseases That May Be Sexually Transmitted

- Amebiasis
- Campylobacteriosis
- Pediculosis pubis (crabs, lice)
- Cytomegalovirus infection
- Giardiasis
- Hepatitis A, B, and C
- Salmonellosis
- Scabies
- Shigellosis

Benign tertiary syphilis is rare today. Lumps called gummas appear on the skin or in various organs. These lumps grow slowly, heal gradually, and leave scars. The lumps can develop almost anywhere in the body but are most common on the scalp, face, upper trunk, and leg (just below the knee). The bones may be affected, resulting in a deep, penetrating pain that is usually worse at night.

Cardiovascular syphilis usually appears 10 to 25 years after the initial infection. A person may develop an aneurysm (weakening and dilation) of the aorta (the main artery leaving the heart) or leakage of the aortic valve. These changes may lead to chest pain, heart failure, or death.

Neurosyphilis (syphilis of the nervous system) affects about 5% of all people with untreated syphilis, although it is rare in developed countries. It can cause many serious problems in the brain and spinal cord, interfering with thinking, walking, talking, and many other activities of daily life.

Neurosyphilis occurs in three forms: meningovascular, paretic (also called general paralysis of the insane), and tabetic (tabes dorsalis). Meningovascular neurosyphilis is a chronic form of meningitis that affects the brain and spinal cord. Paretic neurosyphilis usually does not start until the person is 40 or 50. It begins with gradual behavioral changes, such as deterioration in personal hygiene, mood swings, and progressive confusion. Tabetic neurosyphilis is a progressive disease of the spinal cord that begins gradually, typically with an intense, stabbing pain in the legs that comes and goes irregularly. Later, the person becomes unsteady while walking.

Diagnosis

A chancre or a typical rash on the palms and soles usually leads a doctor to suspect

Proper Condom Use

- Use a new condom for each act of sexual intercourse.
- Use the correct size condom.
- Carefully handle the condom to avoid damaging it with fingernails, teeth, or other sharp objects.
- Put the condom on after the penis is erect and before any genital contact with the partner.
- Place the rolled condom over the tip of the erect penis.
- Leave 1/2 inch at the tip of the condom to collect semen.
- With one hand, squeeze trapped air out of the tip of the condom.
- If uncircumcised, pull the foreskin back before rolling the condom down.
- With the other hand, roll the condom over the penis to its base and smooth out any air bubbles.
- Make sure that lubrication is adequate during intercourse.
- With latex condoms, use only water-based lubricants. Oil-based lubricants (such as petroleum jelly, shortening, mineral oil, massage oils, body lotions, and cooking oil) can weaken latex and cause the condom to break.
- Hold the condom firmly against the base of the penis during withdrawal, and withdraw the penis while it is still erect to prevent slippage.

syphilis. A definitive diagnosis is based on the results of laboratory tests.

Two types of blood test are used. The first is a screening test, such as the Venereal Disease Research Laboratory (VDRL) or the rapid plasma reagin (RPR) test. Screening tests are inexpensive and easy to perform, but they may need to be repeated because the results can be falsely negative in the first few weeks of primary syphilis. Screening tests sometimes come back falsely positive because of diseases other than syphilis. Therefore, a positive screening test result usually must be confirmed with a second, specialized blood test that measures antibodies to syphilis bacteria. Screening test results become negative after successful treatment, but the second, confirmatory test stays positive indefinitely.

In the primary or secondary stages, syphilis may also be diagnosed by obtaining fluid from a skin or mouth sore and identifying the bacteria under a microscope. For neurosyphilis, a spinal tap (lumbar puncture) is needed to obtain spinal fluid for antibody testing. In the latent stage, syphilis is diagnosed only by antibody tests of the blood and spinal fluid. In the tertiary stage, syphilis is diagnosed from the symptoms and an antibody test.

Treatment and Prognosis

Because people with primary and secondary syphilis can pass the disease to others, they must avoid sexual contact or take careful precautions until they and their sex partners have completed treatment. With primary-stage syphilis, all sex partners for the previous 3 months are at risk of being infected. With secondary-stage syphilis, all sex partners for the previous year are at risk. Sex partners in these categories need to be screened with an antibody test performed on a blood sample. If the test is positive, they need to be treated. Some doctors simply treat all sex partners without waiting for test results.

Penicillin given by injection is the best antibiotic for all stages of syphilis. For primary-stage syphilis, a one-time treatment with penicillin is adequate, although some doctors repeat the dose in one week. For secondary-stage syphilis, the second dose is always given. Penicillin is also given for latent-stage syphilis and for all forms of tertiary-stage syphilis, although more frequent or longer treatment given intravenously may be needed. People who are allergic to penicillin may receive azithromycin once by mouth, ceftriaxone by injection daily for 10 days, or doxycycline by mouth for 14 days.

More than half of the people with syphilis in its early stages, especially those with secondary-stage syphilis, develop a reaction 2 to 12 hours after the first treatment. This reaction is called the Jarisch-Herxheimer reaction and is believed to result from the sudden death of millions of bacteria. Symptoms of the reaction include a feeling of overall illness, fever, headache, sweating, shaking chills, and temporary worsening of the syphilitic sores. Rarely, people with neurosyphilis may experience seizures or paralysis. The symptoms of this reaction are temporary and rarely cause permanent harm.

After treatment, the prognosis for primary-, secondary-, and latent-stage syphilis is excellent. The prognosis is poor for tertiary-stage syphilis of the brain or heart, because existing damage usually cannot be reversed. A person who has been cured of syphilis does not become immune to it and can acquire the infection again.

Gonorrhea

Gonorrhea is a sexually transmitted disease caused by the bacterium Neisseria gonorrhoeae *that infects the inner lining of the urethra, cervix, rectum, and throat, or the membranes (conjunctivae) of the eyes.*

While the rate of gonorrhea has declined by 75% since 1975, there were still 360,000 reported cases in the United States in 1999. Gonorrhea usually causes problems only at the site of infection, although the disease can spread through the bloodstream to other parts of the body, especially the skin and joints. In women, the disease may ascend the genital tract and infect the membranes inside the pelvis, causing pelvic pain and reproductive problems.

Symptoms

In men, the first symptoms usually appear 2 to 7 days after infection. Symptoms start with mild discomfort in the urethra, followed a few hours later by mild to severe pain during urination, discharge of pus from the penis, and a frequent and urgent need to urinate, which worsens as the disease spreads to the upper part of the urethra. The penile opening may become red and swollen.

Infected women often have no symptoms for weeks or months, and the disease may only be discovered after the woman's male partner is diagnosed and she is examined as a contact. If symptoms do occur, they usually appear 7 to 21 days after infection and are usually mild. However, some women have severe symptoms, such as a frequent need to urinate, pain while urinating, a discharge from the vagina, and fever. The cervix, uterus, fallopian tubes, ovaries, urethra, and rectum may be infected, causing tenderness or severe deep pelvic pain, especially during intercourse. Pus, which appears to come from the vagina, may be coming from the cervix, urethra, or glands near the vaginal opening.

Anal sex with an infected partner may result in gonorrhea of the rectum. The disease may cause discomfort around the anus and a discharge from the rectum. The area around the anus may become red and raw, and the stool may be coated with mucus and pus. When a doctor examines the rectum with a viewing tube (anoscope), mucus and pus may be visible on the wall of the rectum.

Oral sex with an infected partner may result in gonorrhea of the throat (gonococcal pharyngitis). Usually, the infection produces no symptoms, but sometimes it causes a sore throat and discomfort during swallowing.

If infected fluids come into contact with the eyes, gonococcal conjunctivitis may develop,▲ causing swelling of the eyelids and a discharge of pus from the eyes. A pregnant woman with gonorrhea can infect the eyes of her baby during birth. In adults, often only one eye is affected. Newborns usually have infection in both eyes. Blindness may result if the infection is not treated early.

Gonorrhea in infant and young girls is usually the result of sexual abuse by adults or teens. Symptoms may include irritation, redness, and swelling of the vulva, with a discharge of pus from the vagina. The girl may be sore in the vaginal area or have pain during urination. The rectum also may be inflamed. The underpants may be stained with discharge.

In some people, gonorrhea spreads through the bloodstream to one or more joints, causing them to become swollen, tender, and extremely painful and limiting movement. A bloodstream infection may also cause fever, a general feeling of illness, pain that moves from joint to joint, and the formation of red pus-filled spots on the skin (arthritis-dermatitis syndrome).

The interior of the heart may become infected (endocarditis). Infection of the covering of the liver (perihepatitis) causes pain in the upper right part of the abdomen similar to that of gallbladder disease. These infections are treatable and rarely fatal, but recovery from arthritis or endocarditis may be slow.

Diagnosis

A doctor can make a diagnosis almost immediately by identifying the bacterium (gonococcus) under a microscope. In more than 90% of infected men, this diagnosis can be made using a sample of discharge from the penis. The sample is usually obtained by passing a

▲ see page 1296

small swab a few centimeters into the urethra. Microscopic examination of a sample of the discharge from the cervix is less reliable; gonococci can be seen in only about 60% of infected women. The sample of discharge is also sent to the laboratory for culture, which is very reliable in both sexes but takes longer than a microscopic examination. If a doctor suspects an infection of the throat or rectum, samples from these areas are sent for culture.

Recently developed, highly sensitive methods for finding the DNA of the bacteria that cause gonorrhea and chlamydia allow laboratories to test for both infections in a single specimen. Because these tests can be performed on urine samples from both sexes, they are convenient for screening people who have no symptoms or who are unwilling to have urethral, rectal, or cervical specimens taken.

Because a person may have more than one STD, a doctor may take a sample of blood to determine whether the person also has syphilis or human immunodeficiency virus (HIV) infection.

Treatment

People with gonorrhea are usually given antibiotics to kill both *Chlamydia* and gonococci, because people with gonorrhea are often infected with *Chlamydia* at the same time. A single injection of ceftriaxone into a muscle or a single dose of cefixime, levofloxacin, ciprofloxacin, or ofloxacin by mouth is usually adequate to cure gonorrhea but a week-long course of another oral antibiotic (doxycycline or levofloxacin) is routinely given to cure chlamydia. Alternatively, a single large dose of azithromycin can be used to cure both infections. If gonorrhea has spread through the bloodstream, the person usually is treated in the hospital with intravenous antibiotics.

If symptoms recur or persist at the end of treatment, the doctor may obtain specimens for culture to make sure the person is cured. Symptoms of urethritis may recur in men (postgonococcal urethritis) and are most commonly caused by *Chlamydia* and other organisms that do not respond to treatment with ceftriaxone.

Nongonococcal Urethritis and Chlamydial Cervicitis

Nongonococcal urethritis and chlamydial cervicitis are sexually transmitted diseases caused by the bacterium Chlamydia tra-

chomatis *and various other microorganisms that produce inflammation of the urethra and cervix.*

Several different microorganisms cause diseases that resemble gonorrhea. These microorganisms include *Chlamydia trachomatis, Trichomonas vaginalis,* and several different types of *Mycoplasma.* In the past, these microorganisms were hard for laboratories to identify, so the infections they caused were simply called "nongonococcal" to indicate that they were not caused by *Neisseria gonorrhoeae,* the bacterium that causes gonorrhea.

Chlamydia trachomatis infection (chlamydia) is very common, with 659,000 reported cases in the United States in 1999. Because the infection sometimes produces no symptoms, even more people may be affected. In men, chlamydia causes about half of the urethral infections not caused by gonorrhea. Most of the remaining male urethral infections are caused by *Ureaplasma urealyticum.* In women, chlamydia accounts for virtually all of the pus-forming cervical infections not caused by gonorrhea. Both sexes may acquire gonorrhea and chlamydia at the same time.

Symptoms and Diagnosis

Between 4 and 28 days after intercourse with an infected person, an infected man typically has a mild burning sensation in his urethra while urinating. A clear or cloudy discharge from the penis may be evident. The discharge is usually less thick than the discharge that occurs in gonorrhea. Early in the morning, the opening of the penis is often red and stuck together with dried secretions. Occasionally, the disease begins more dramatically. The man needs to urinate frequently, finds urinating painful, and has discharge of pus from the urethra.

Although most women infected with *Chlamydia* have few or no symptoms, some experience frequent urges to urinate and pain while urinating, pain in the lower abdomen, pain during sexual intercourse, and secretions of yellow mucus and pus from the vagina.

Anal infections may cause pain and a yellow discharge of pus and mucus.

In most cases, a doctor can diagnose chlamydia by examining discharge from the penis or cervix in a laboratory. Newer tests that amplify DNA or RNA, such as the polymerase chain reaction (PCR), enable a doctor to diagnose chlamydia or gonorrhea from a urine sample. These tests are recommended for screening of sexually active women between the ages of 15 and 25. Genital infections with *Ureaplasma* and *Mycoplasma* are not diagnosed specifically in routine medical settings, because culturing of these microorganisms is difficult and other techniques for diagnosis are expensive. The diagnosis of nongonococcal infections is often presumed if the person has characteristic symptoms and no evidence of gonorrhea.

If chlamydia is not treated, symptoms usually disappear in 4 weeks. However, an untreated infection can cause a number of complications. Untreated chlamydial cervicitis often ascends to the fallopian tubes (tubes that connect the ovaries to the uterus), where inflammation may cause pain and scarring. The scarring can cause infertility and ectopic pregnancy.▲ These complications can occur in women without symptoms and result in considerable suffering and medical costs. In men, chlamydia may cause epididymitis, which produces painful swelling of the scrotum on one or both sides.■ Whether *Ureaplasma* has a role in these complications is unclear.

Treatment

Chlamydial and ureaplasmal infections are usually treated with tetracycline, doxycycline, or levofloxacin taken by mouth for at least 7 days or with a single dose of azithromycin taken by mouth. Because the symptoms are so similar to those of gonorrhea, doctors usually give an antibiotic such as ceftriaxone to treat gonorrhea at the same time. Pregnant women are given erythromycin instead of tetracycline or doxycycline. If symptoms persist or return, treatment is then repeated for a longer period.

Infected people who have sexual intercourse before completing treatment may infect their partners. Also, partners who are infected may re-infect the treated person. Thus, sex partners are treated simultaneously if possible. The risk of a repeat infection of chlamydia or another STD within 3 to 4 months is high enough that screening may be repeated at that time.

Lymphogranuloma Venereum

Lymphogranuloma venereum is a sexually transmitted disease caused by Chlamydia trachomatis *that produces painful swellings in the groin.*

Lymphogranuloma venereum is caused by types of *Chlamydia trachomatis* other than

Complications of Chlamydial and Ureaplasmal Infections

In men
- Infection of the epididymis
- Narrowing (stricture) of the urethra

In women
- Infection of the fallopian tubes and linings of the pelvic cavity
- Infection of the surface of the liver

In men and women
- Infection of the membranes of the eyes (conjunctivitis)

In newborns
- Conjunctivitis
- Pneumonia

those that cause nongonococcal urethritis and chlamydial cervicitis. The disease occurs mostly in tropical and subtropical areas and is uncommon in the United States, afflicting about 100 people each year.

Symptoms begin 3 or more days after infection. A small, painless, fluid-filled blister develops usually on the penis or in the vagina. Typically, the blister becomes a sore that quickly heals—often going unnoticed. Next, lymph nodes in the groin on one or both sides may swell and become tender. With prolonged or repeated episodes of infection, the lymphatic vessels may become obstructed, causing tissue to swell. Rectal infection may cause scarring, which can result in a narrowing of the rectum.

A doctor suspects lymphogranuloma venereum based on its characteristic symptoms. The diagnosis can be confirmed by a blood test that identifies antibodies against *Chlamydia trachomatis*. If given early in the disease, treatment with oral doxycycline, erythromycin, or tetracycline for 3 weeks results in rapid healing.

Chancroid

Chancroid is a sexually transmitted disease caused by the bacterium Haemophilus ducreyi *that produces painful genital sores.*

While quite common in other parts of the world, chancroid is rare in the United States,

▲ see art on page 1455   ■ see page 1328

with only 143 cases reported in 1999—three quarters of which occurred in local outbreaks in New York, South Carolina, and Texas.

Symptoms begin 3 to 7 days after infection. Small, painful blisters form on the genitals or around the anus and rapidly rupture to form shallow sores. These sores may enlarge and connect. The lymph nodes in the groin may become tender, enlarged, and matted together, forming an abscess (a collection of pus). The skin over the abscess may become red and shiny and may break down and discharge pus onto the skin.

Several antibiotics are effective for chancroid. A single injection of ceftriaxone is effective, as is a single oral dose of azithromycin, 3 days of oral ciprofloxacin, or 7 days of oral erythromycin.

Granuloma Inguinale

Granuloma inguinale is a rare sexually transmitted disease caused by the bacterium Calymmatobacterium granulomatis *that leads to chronic inflammation of the genitals.*

Granuloma inguinale is rare in developed countries, with only eight cases reported in the United States in 1999. It is more common in people living under primitive conditions in Papua New Guinea, Australia, and South Africa.

Symptoms usually begin 1 to 12 weeks after infection. The first symptom is a painless, red nodule that slowly grows into one or more round, raised lumps that then break down to form a sore. Sites of infection include the penis, scrotum, groin, and thighs in men and the vulva, vagina, and surrounding skin areas in women. Either trimethoprim-sulfamethoxazole or doxycycline taken by mouth for at least 3 weeks is effective.

Trichomoniasis

Trichomoniasis is a sexually transmitted disease of the vagina or urethra caused by Trichomonas vaginalis, *a single-celled organism.*

Trichomonas vaginalis commonly infects the genitals and urinary tract of men and women. However, women are more likely to develop symptoms. About 20% of women develop trichomoniasis of the vagina during their reproductive years.

In men, urethral infection with no or minimal symptoms is common, although rarely the epididymis and prostate are infected. In some populations, *Trichomonas* may account for 5 to 10% of all cases of nongonococcal urethritis.

Symptoms and Diagnosis

In women, the disease usually starts with a greenish yellow, frothy vaginal discharge. In some women the discharge is slight. The vulva may be irritated and sore, and sexual intercourse may be painful. In severe cases, the vulva and surrounding skin may be inflamed and the labia swollen. Pain on urination or frequency of urination, such as occurs in a bladder infection, may occur alone or with the other symptoms.

Men with trichomoniasis may have no symptoms but still infect their sex partners. Many men have nongonococcal urethritis with symptoms of discharge from the urethra, pain during urination, and a need to urinate frequently. The role of *Trichomonas* in prostate infections is unclear.

The organism is more difficult to detect in men than in women. In women, the diagnosis can usually be made quickly by seeing the organism in a sample of vaginal secretions under a microscope or after several days by culture. Tests for other STDs are usually performed as well, because *Trichomonas* is common in people with gonorrhea or chlamydia. In men, secretions from the end of the penis (obtained in the morning, before urination) may be examined under a microscope and sent to the laboratory for culture. Microscopic examination of the urine may also detect *Trichomonas*.

Treatment

A single dose of metronidazole taken by mouth cures up to 95% of infected women; however, they may become reinfected unless their sex partners are treated simultaneously. It is not known whether a single-dose treatment is effective in men, but men are usually cured after 7 days of treatment.

If taken with alcohol, metronidazole may cause nausea and flushing of the skin. The drug also may cause a metallic taste in the mouth, nausea, or a decrease in the number of white blood cells and, in women, an increased susceptibility to vaginal yeast infections (genital candidiasis). Metronidazole is best avoided during pregnancy, at least during the first 3 months. Infected people who have sexual intercourse before the infection is cured are likely to infect their partners.

Genital Warts

Genital warts (condylomata acuminata) are growths in or around the vagina, penis, or rectum caused by sexually transmitted papillomaviruses.

Genital warts are common; in the United States an estimated 500,000 people per year develop genital warts. As many as 20 to 46% of sexually active young women have been infected with one of the viruses that causes these warts. Because of the location of these warts, condoms may not protect against infection.

Genital warts are caused by certain types of papillomavirus, other types of which cause the common warts that appear on other parts of the body. Several types of papillomavirus infect the genitals, but not all of them cause plainly visible external genital warts. Some types cause tiny raised areas on the cervix that may only be visible with a magnifying instrument called a culposcope. Although these less-visible spots generally do not cause symptoms, the papillomaviruses causing them increase the risk of developing cervical cancer and therefore should be treated.▲

Symptoms and Diagnosis

Genital warts occur most often on warm, moist surfaces. In men, the usual areas are on the penis, especially below the foreskin (if the penis is uncircumcised). In women, genital warts occur on the vulva, vaginal wall, cervix, and skin surrounding the vaginal area. Genital warts may develop in the area around the anus and in the rectum, especially in people who engage in anal sex. Many people have no symptoms from the warts, but some feel occasional burning pain.

The warts usually appear 1 to 6 months after infection with papillomavirus, beginning as tiny, soft, moist, pink or red swellings. They grow rapidly and appear as rough, irregular bumps, which sometimes grow out from the skin on narrow stalks. Groups of warts often grow in the same area, and their rough surfaces give them the appearance of a small cauliflower. The warts may grow very rapidly in pregnant women, in people with an impaired immune system (for example, people with AIDS or those who are taking immunosuppressive drugs), and in people who have inflammation of the skin.

Genital warts usually can be diagnosed from their appearance. Unusual-looking or persistent warts may be removed surgically and examined under a microscope to make sure that they are not cancerous. Regular Papanicolaou (Pap) tests to detect the early stages of cancer are very important in women who have warts on the cervix.

Treatment

In many people, the immune system eventually controls the papillomavirus. Half the time, the infection is gone after 8 months; less than 10% of people are infected longer than 2 years.

No treatment is completely satisfactory, and some treatments are uncomfortable and leave scars. External genital warts may be removed by laser, freezing (cryotherapy), or surgery using local anesthetics. Podophyllin toxin, imiquimod, or trichloroacetic acid can be applied directly to the warts. This approach, however, requires many applications over weeks to months, may burn the surrounding skin, and frequently fails. Imiquimod cream produces less burning but may be less effective. The warts may return after apparently successful treatment.

Warts in the urethra may be removed by endoscopic surgery (a procedure in which a flexible viewing tube with surgical attachments is used). This is sometimes followed by injection of the wart with a chemotherapy drug, 5-fluorouracil. Interferon-alpha injections into the wart are somewhat effective, but they must be administered several times a week for many weeks and are very expensive.

In uncircumcised men, circumcision may help prevent recurrence. All sex partners should be examined for warts and other STDs and treated, if necessary.

Other Sexually Transmitted Diseases

Some bacteria (*Shigella, Campylobacter,* and *Salmonella*), viruses (hepatitis A, B, and C), and parasites (*Giardia* and other amebas) that are usually transmitted nonsexually can sometimes be transmitted during sex. Infection by these organisms, with the exception of hepatitis B and C, is usually acquired by mouth. Thus, activities in which the mouth comes into contact with the anus of an in-

▲ see page 1406

fected person can transmit these infections. Symptoms are typically those of the specific organism transmitted and may involve diarrhea, fever, abdominal pain or bloating, nausea and vomiting, and jaundice. Infections recur frequently, especially in homosexual men with many sex partners. Some infections cause no symptoms, but may lead to serious long-term complications, such as chronic hepatitis B or C.

SKIN DISORDERS

201   Biology of the Skin **1186**

Structure and Function ▪ Effects of Aging

202   Diagnosis and Treatment of Skin Disorders **1188**

203   Itching and Noninfectious Rashes..**1191**

Itching ▪ Dermatitis ▪ Drug Rashes ▪ Stevens-Johnson Syndrome and Toxic Epidermal Necrolysis ▪ Erythema Multiforme ▪ Erythema Nodosum ▪ Granuloma Annulare ▪ Psoriasis ▪ Pityriasis Rosea ▪ Rosacea ▪ Lichen Planus ▪ Keratosis Pilaris

204   Acne...**1204**

205   Pressure Sores **1208**

206   Sweating Disorders **1210**

Prickly Heat ▪ Excessive Sweating

207   Hair Disorders..**1211**

Excessive Hairiness ▪ Hair Loss ▪ Ingrown Beard Hairs

208   Pigment Disorders **1214**

Albinism ▪ Vitiligo ▪ Melasma

209   Blistering Diseases **1216**

Pemphigus ▪ Bullous Pemphigoid ▪ Dermatitis Herpetiformis

210   Parasitic Skin Infections **1218**

Scabies ▪ Lice Infestation ▪ Creeping Eruption

211   Bacterial Skin Infections **1220**

Cellulitis ▪ Necrotizing Skin Infections ▪ Erythrasma ▪ Impetigo ▪ Staphylococcal Scalded Skin Syndrome ▪ Folliculitis, Skin Abscesses, and Carbuncles ▪ Hidradenitis Suppurativa

212   Fungal Skin Infections **1225**

Ringworm ▪ Candidiasis ▪ Tinea Versicolor

213   **Viral Skin Infections**...**1228**

Warts   ▪   Molluscum Contagiosum

214   **Sunlight and Skin Damage**..**1230**

Sunburn   ▪   Skin Photosensitivity Reactions

215   **Noncancerous Skin Growths** **1233**

Moles   ▪   Skin Tags   ▪   Lipomas   ▪   Dermatofibromas   ▪
Hemangiomas   ▪   Port-wine Stains   ▪   Lymphangiomas   ▪
Pyogenic Granulomas   ▪   Spider Angiomas   ▪   Seborrheic
Keratoses   ▪   Keratoacanthomas   ▪   Keloids   ▪   Epidermal Cysts

216   **Skin Cancers** **1238**

Basal Cell Carcinoma   ▪   Squamous Cell Carcinoma   ▪
Melanoma   ▪   Kaposi's Sarcoma   ▪   Paget's Disease

CHAPTER 201

Biology of the Skin

The skin is the largest organ of the body. It serves many important functions, including regulating body temperature, maintaining water and electrolyte balance, and sensing painful and pleasant stimuli. The skin keeps dangerous substances from entering the body and provides a shield from the sun's harmful effects. In addition, skin color, texture, and folds help mark people as individuals. Anything that goes wrong with skin function or appearance can have important consequences for physical and mental health.

Structure and Function

The skin has three layers—the epidermis, dermis, and fat layer (also called the subcutaneous layer). Each layer of skin performs specific tasks.

Epidermis: The epidermis is the thin, tough, top layer of skin. The outer portion of the epidermis, the stratum corneum, is waterproof and, when undamaged, prevents most bacteria, viruses, and other foreign substances from entering the body. The epidermis also protects the internal organs, muscles, nerves, and blood vessels against trauma. The dead flat cells on the surface of the epidermis are composed of a tough, fibrous protein called keratin, which is also found in the hair and fingernails. As these dead cells at the surface are worn away, they are continuously replaced by newer cells that are pushed up from below. The outer keratin layer of the epidermis is thicker on skin surfaces that require greater protection, such as the palms of the hands and the soles of the feet.

At the bottom of the epidermis are the melanocytes, the cells that produce melanin—the dark pigment of skin. Melanin filters out ultraviolet radiation from sunlight▲ and provides color to the skin.

The epidermis also contains Langerhans' cells, which are part of the skin's immune system. These cells help detect foreign substances and play a role in the development of skin allergies.

▲ see page 1230

Dermis: The dermis, the next layer of skin, is a thick layer of fibrous and elastic tissue (made mostly of the proteins collagen and fibrillin) that gives the skin its flexibility and strength. The dermis contains nerve endings, glands, hair follicles, and blood vessels.

The nerve endings sense pain, touch, pressure, and temperature. Some areas of the skin contain more nerve endings than others. For example, the fingertips and toes contain many nerves and are extremely sensitive to touch.

The sweat glands produce sweat in response to heat. Sweat is composed of water, salt, and other chemicals. As sweat evaporates off the skin, it helps cool the body. Specialized sweat glands of the armpit and genital region (apocrine sweat glands) secrete a thick, oily sweat that produces a characteristic body odor when the sweat is digested by the skin bacteria in those areas. Sebaceous glands produce oil, which keeps the skin moist and soft and acts as a barrier against foreign substances.

The blood vessels of the dermis provide nutrients to the skin and help regulate body temperature. Heat makes the blood vessels widen (dilate), allowing large amounts of blood to circulate near the skin surface, where the heat can be released. Cold makes the blood vessels narrow (constrict), retaining the body's heat.

Over different parts of the body, the number of nerves, sweat glands, sebaceous glands, hair follicles, and blood vessels varies. The top of the head, for example, has many hair follicles; the soles of the feet have none.

Fat Layer: Below the dermis lies a layer of fat that helps insulate the body from heat and cold, provides protective padding, and serves as an energy storage area. The fat is contained in living cells, called fat cells, held together by fibrous tissue. The fat layer varies in thickness, from a fraction of an inch on the eyelids up to several inches on the abdomen and buttocks in some people.

Effects of Aging

The skin tends to change throughout a person's lifetime. A baby's skin is very soft and smooth and provides a less effective barrier against harmful substances. A baby's skin has a much thicker fat layer and a much thinner layer of protective keratin. A young adult's skin is strong and supple. With age, the skin becomes thinner and finely wrinkled, with less underlying fat.

Getting Under the Skin

The skin consists of three layers. Beneath the surface of the skin are nerves, nerve endings, glands, hair follicles, and blood vessels.

Aging itself results in thinning of the dermis and epidermis. Much of the underlying fat is lost as well, except on the thighs and abdomen, resulting in less insulation from cold. The skin loses some of its elasticity and becomes drier. The number of nerve endings in the skin decreases, so sensation is diminished. The number of sweat glands and blood vessels decreases as well, reducing the ability to respond to heat exposure. The number of melanocytes tends to decrease with age, so the skin has less protection against ultraviolet radiation. All of these changes make the skin both more susceptible to damage and slower to heal.

Sun damage produces many of the skin changes that people commonly associate with aging.▲ Long-term exposure to the ultraviolet radiation in sunlight is responsible for wrinkles, both fine and coarse; irregular pigmentation; brown and red spots; and the rough texture of sun-exposed skin.

CHAPTER 202

Diagnosis and Treatment of Skin Disorders

Many problems that appear on the skin are limited to the skin. Sometimes, however, the skin reveals a disorder that affects the entire body. Consequently, doctors often must consider many possible diseases when evaluating skin problems. They may need to order blood tests or other laboratory tests to look for an internal disease in people who come to them with a skin problem.

Diagnosis

Doctors can identify many skin disorders simply by looking at the skin. Revealing characteristics include size, shape, color, and location of the abnormality as well as the presence or absence of other signs or symptoms. To check the distribution of a skin problem, the doctor usually asks the person to undress completely, even though the person may have noticed an abnormality on only a small area of skin.

Sometimes, a biopsy must be performed, in which a small piece of skin is removed for examination under a microscope. For this simple procedure, the doctor generally numbs a small area of skin with a local anesthetic and, using a small knife (scalpel), scissors, or round cutter (punch biopsy), removes a piece of skin about ⅛ inch in diameter.

When an infection is suspected, a doctor may scrape off some material from the skin and examine it under a microscope. The material can also be sent to a laboratory, where the specimen is placed in a culture medium (a substance that allows microorganisms to grow). If the specimen contains any bacteria, fungi, or viruses, they grow in the culture and can be identified.

In a Wood's light examination, also used when certain skin infections are suspected, the skin is illuminated with an ultraviolet light in a dark room. The ultraviolet light makes some fungi or bacteria glow brightly and may make some pigmentation abnormalities, such as vitiligo, more visible.

Skin tests, including a patch test, a prick test, and an intradermal test, may be performed if a doctor suspects an allergic reaction as the cause of a rash. In the patch test, small samples of possible causative agents are held against the skin for 1 to 2 days. If the substance produces a rash, the person is allergic to it. In the prick test and intradermal test,■ tiny amounts of a substance are injected under the skin. The area is then watched for redness and swelling, which indicate an allergic reaction.

Treatment

Topical drugs are a mainstay of treating skin disorders. They are applied directly to the affected area of the skin. Systemic drugs are usually taken by mouth and are distributed throughout the body. Rarely, when a high concentration of a drug is needed at the affected area, a doctor injects the drug just under the skin (intradermal injection).

Topical Preparations

The active ingredient, or drug, in a topical preparation is mixed with an inactive ingredient (vehicle). The vehicle determines the consistency of the product (for example, thick and

---

▲ see page 1230   ■ see page 1063

Medical Names for Marks and Growths on the Skin

Atrophic skin: Paper-thin, wrinkled skin.

Crust (scab): Dried blood, pus, or skin fluids on the surface of the skin. A crust can form wherever the skin has been damaged.

Erosion: Loss of part or all of the top surface of the skin. Erosions occur when infection, pressure, irritation, or temperature has damaged the skin.

Excoriation: A hollowed-out or linear crusted area caused by scratching, rubbing, or picking at the skin.

Lichenification: Thickened skin that has accentuated skinfolds or creases that appear as deep grooves and wrinkles. Lichenification is produced by prolonged scratching.

Macule: A flat, discolored spot of any shape less than 3/8 inch in diameter. Freckles, flat moles, port-wine stains, and many rashes are macular. A patch is like a macule, but larger.

Nodule: A solid bump, deeper and easier to feel than a papule, that may be raised. A nodule sometimes appears to form below the surface of the skin and press upward.

Papule: A solid bump less than 3/8 inch in diameter. Warts, insect bites, skin tags, and some skin cancers are papules.

Plaque: A flat, raised bump or group of bumps typically more than 3/8 inch in diameter.

Pustule: A blister containing pus.

Scales: Areas of heaped-up, dead epidermal cells, producing a flaky, dry patch. Scales occur with psoriasis, seborrheic dermatitis, and many other disorders.

Scar: An area where normal skin has been replaced by fibrous (scar-forming) tissue. Scars form after destruction of some part of the dermis.

Telangiectasia: Dilated blood vessels within the skin that have a twisted appearance and that whiten (blanch) on pressure.

Ulcer: Like an erosion, only deeper, penetrating at least part of the dermis. The causes are the same as for erosions.

Vesicle: A small, fluid-filled spot less than 1/5 inch in diameter. A blister (bulla) is a larger vesicle. Insect bites, herpes zoster (shingles), chickenpox, burns, and irritations form vesicles and blisters.

Wheal (hive): Swelling in the skin that produces an elevated, soft, spongy area that appears relatively suddenly and then disappears. Wheals are common allergic reactions to drugs, insect bites, or something that touches the skin.

---

greasy or light and watery) and whether the active ingredient remains on the surface or penetrates the skin. Depending on the vehicle used, the same drug can be placed in an ointment, cream, lotion, solution, powder, or gel. In addition, many preparations are available in different strengths (concentrations).

Creams, the most commonly used preparations, are emulsions of oil in water. They are easy to apply and appear to vanish when rubbed into the skin.

Ointments are oily and contain very little water. They are messy, greasy, and difficult to wash off. Ointments are most appropriate when the skin needs lubrication or moisture. Ointments are usually better than creams at delivering active ingredients into the skin. The same concentration of drug in an ointment may have more effect than in a cream.

Lotions are similar to creams but contain more water. They are actually suspensions of finely dispersed powdered material in a base of water or oil and water. Lotions are easy to apply and are particularly useful for cooling or drying the skin.

Solutions are liquids in which a drug is dissolved. Solutions tend to dry rather than moisturize the skin. The most commonly used liquids are alcohol, propylene glycol, polyethylene glycol, and plain water.

Powders are dried forms of substances that are used to protect areas where skin rubs against skin—for instance, between the toes or buttocks, in the armpits or groin, or under the breasts. Powders are used on skin that has been softened and damaged by moisture (macerated).

Gels are water-based substances thickened without oil or fat. The skin does not absorb gels as well as it absorbs preparations containing oil or fat.

Types of Topical Drugs

Topical drugs can be divided into several overlapping categories: cleansing agents, protective agents, moisturizing agents, drying agents, symptom-relieving agents, anti-inflammatory agents, and anti-infective agents.

Cleansing Agents: The principal cleansing agents are soaps, detergents, and solvents (a liquid substance capable of dissolving other substances). Soap is the most popular cleanser, but detergents are used as well. Certain soaps dry the skin; others have a creamy base that is nondrying.

Because baby shampoos are excellent cleansing agents and are usually gentle to the skin, they are good for cleansing wounds, cuts, and abrasions. Also, people with psoriasis, eczema, and other scaling diseases can use baby shampoos to wash away dead scaly skin. Oozing (weeping) lesions, however, should generally be cleaned only with water and gentle soaps; detergents and harsher soaps can irritate the area.

Many chemicals are added to cleansing agents. For example, some soaps have antibacterial substances added to them. Antibacterial soap does not improve hygiene or prevent disease, and routine use may disrupt the normal balance of bacteria on the skin. Antidandruff shampoos and lotions may contain zinc dipyrithione, selenium sulfide, or tar extracts to help treat flaking skin, eczema, and psoriasis of the scalp.

Solvents include petroleum jelly, which can cleanse the skin of material that cannot be dissolved with soap and water, such as tar. Small amounts of alcohol, which dissolves fats and oils, can safely be used to cleanse the skin before injections or blood drawing. Alcohol is not needed for routine skin hygiene. Other solvents, such as acetone (nail polish remover), gasoline, and paint thinner, are rarely used for skin cleansing. These solvents dissolve the skin's natural oils, causing significant drying, and may also be absorbed through the skin, resulting in poisoning. Gasoline and paint thinner are also irritating to the skin.

Protective Agents: Many different kinds of preparations help protect the skin. Oils and ointments supply an oil-based barrier that can help protect scraped or irritated skin and retain moisture. Powders may protect skin that rubs against skin or clothing. Synthetic hydrocolloid dressings protect pressure sores (bedsores, decubitus ulcers) and other areas of raw skin. Sunscreens and sunblocks reflect or filter out harmful ultraviolet light.

Moisturizing Agents: Moisturizers (emollients) restore water and oils to the skin. The best time to apply a moisturizer is when the skin is already moistened—immediately after a bath or shower, for instance. Moisturizers typically contain glycerin, mineral oil, or petrolatum and are available as lotions, creams, ointments, and bath oils. Some stronger moisturizers contain compounds such as urea, lactic acid, and glycolic acid.

Drying Agents: Excessive moisture in areas where skin rubs against skin can cause irritation and skin breakdown (maceration), particularly under hot, humid conditions. The areas most commonly affected are between the toes or buttocks, in the armpits or groin, and under the breasts. These moist areas also provide fertile breeding grounds for infections, especially with fungi and bacteria.

Talcum powder is the most commonly used drying agent. Talc absorbs moisture from the skin surface. Most of the many talc preparations vary only in their scents and packaging. Cornstarch, another good drying agent, has the disadvantage of encouraging the growth of fungi. For this reason, talc is generally preferred, except for babies, because babies sometimes accidentally inhale the powder, and cornstarch is less dangerous to breathe than talc. Solutions containing aluminum salts are drying agents.

Symptom-relieving Agents: Skin disease is often accompanied by itching. Itching and mild pain can sometimes be controlled with soothing agents such as chamomile, eucalyptus, camphor, menthol, zinc oxide, talc, glycerin, and calamine. Antihistamines, such as diphenhydramine, are sometimes included in topical preparations to relieve the itching associated with allergic reactions. Although antihistamines block certain types of allergic reactions, they sometimes actually trigger an allergic reaction when applied to the skin. Taking antihistamines by mouth does not seem to produce this type of reaction, so oral rather than topical antihistamines are preferred to relieve itching.

Anti-inflammatory Agents: Corticosteroids are the main topical drugs used to relieve inflammation (swelling, itching, and redness) of the skin. Corticosteroids are most effective for rashes caused by allergic or inflammatory reactions to poison ivy, metals, cloth, or other substances. Because they lower resistance to bacterial and fungal infections, corticosteroids usually should not be used on infected areas or wounds. However, corticosteroids are sometimes mixed with antifungal drugs to help reduce itching caused by a fungus.

Topical corticosteroids are sold as lotions, creams, ointments, and gels. Creams are most effective if rubbed in gently until they vanish. In general, the ointments are the most potent. The type and concentration of corticosteroid in the preparation determines the overall strength. Hydrocortisone is available in concentrations of up to 1% without a prescription; concentrations of 0.5% or less offer little benefit. Stronger corticosteroid preparations require a prescription. Doctors usually prescribe potent corticosteroids first, then less potent corticosteroids as the disorder improves. Generally, topical corticosteroids are applied 2 to 3 times a day in a thin layer. Where the skin is already thin, such as on the face, corticosteroids should be used sparingly and not for more than a few days.▲

When a stronger dose is needed, a doctor may inject a corticosteroid just under the skin. Another way to deliver a strong dose is to apply a thin plastic film, such as household plastic wrap, over the topical corticosteroid (oc-

clusive dressing). The plastic film increases the drug's absorption and effectiveness and is usually left on overnight. Occlusive dressings increase the penetration of corticosteroids and thereby increase their effects. Such dressings are generally reserved for disorders such as psoriasis and severe eczema.

Anti-infective Agents: Viruses, bacteria, fungi, and parasites can all infect the skin. By far, the best way to prevent such infections is by carefully washing the skin with soap and water. Stronger disinfecting agents are only used on healthy skin by nurses and doctors to disinfect their own skin and the person's skin before surgery. Once infection has occurred, it may be treated with topical or systemic drugs. The type of infection dictates which drug is given.

CHAPTER 203

Itching and Noninfectious Rashes

Itching and rashes may develop as the result of infection or irritation or from a reaction of the immune system. Some rashes occur mostly in children,■ whereas others almost always occur in adults. Sometimes an immune reaction is triggered by substances a person touches or eats, but many times doctors do not know why the immune system reacts to produce a skin rash.

The diagnosis of most noninfectious skin rashes is based on the appearance of the rash. The cause of a rash cannot be determined by blood tests, and tests of any kind are rarely performed. However, persistent rashes, particularly those that do not respond to treatment, may lead the doctor to perform a skin biopsy, in which a small piece of skin is surgically removed for examination under a microscope. Also, if the doctor suspects a contact allergy as the cause, skin tests may be performed.★

Itching

Itching (pruritus) is a sensation that instinctively demands scratching.

Itching may be caused by a skin disorder or by a disease that affects the whole body (sys-

temic disease). Skin disorders that cause severe itching include infestations with parasites (scabies, mites, or lice), insect bites, hives, atopic dermatitis, and allergic and contact dermatitis. These disorders usually also produce a rash. Systemic diseases that can cause itching include liver disease, kidney failure, lymphomas, leukemias and other blood disorders, and, occasionally, thyroid disease, diabetes, and cancer. However, itching from these diseases usually does not result in a rash.

Many drugs can cause itching, including barbiturates and aspirin as well as any drug to which a person has an allergy.

Itching is also common during the later months of pregnancy. Usually, pregnancy-related itching does not indicate any abnormality, but it can result from mild liver problems.

Often, contact with wool clothing or irritants, such as solvents or cosmetics, causes itching. Dry skin (xerosis), which is especially common in older people, can cause severe, widespread itching. Dry skin also can result

---

▲ see box on page 374   ■ see page 1534

★ see page 1188

When the Skin Is Dry

> Normal skin owes its soft, pliable texture to its water content. To help protect against water loss, the outer layer of skin contains oil, which slows evaporation and holds moisture in the deeper layers of skin. If the oil is depleted, the skin becomes dry.
>
> Dry skin (xerosis) is common, especially in people past middle age. Common causes are cold weather and frequent bathing. Bathing washes away surface oils, allowing the skin to dry out. Dry skin may become irritated and often itches—sometimes it sloughs off in small flakes and scales. Scaling most often affects the lower legs. Rubbing or scratching dry skin can lead to infection and scarring.
>
> A form of severe dry skin is called ichthyosis. Ichthyosis can be an inherited disorder or can result from a number of other medical problems, such as an underactive thyroid gland, lymphoma, AIDS, and sarcoidosis.
>
> The key to treating simple dry skin is keeping the skin moist. Taking fewer baths allows protective oils to remain on the skin. Moisturizing ointments or creams containing petroleum jelly, mineral oil, or glycerin also can hold water in the skin. Harsh soaps, detergents, and the perfumes in some moisturizers irritate the skin and may further dry it.
>
> When scaling is a problem, solutions or creams containing salicylic or lactic acid or urea may help remove the scales. For some forms of severe ichthyosis, creams containing substances related to vitamin A, such as tretinoin, help the skin shed excessive scales.

from cold weather or prolonged exposure to water. Hot baths typically worsen itching.

The act of scratching can itself irritate the skin and lead to more itching, creating an itching-scratching-itching cycle. Vigorous scratching may cause redness and deep scrapes in the skin. In some people, even gentle scratching causes raised, red streaks that can itch intensely. Prolonged scratching and rubbing can thicken and scar the skin.

Diagnosis

Doctors try to determine the cause of itching to eliminate it. Often, the cause is obvi-

---

▲ see pages 1063 and 1188

■ see page 1188   ★ see box on page 374

ous, such as an insect bite or poison ivy. Itching that lasts longer than a few days or that comes and goes frequently without an obvious cause usually requires testing. If an allergy is suspected, skin tests may be performed.▲ If a systemic disease is suspected, blood tests are usually performed to check liver function, kidney function, and blood sugar levels. The number of eosinophils, a type of white blood cell, may be checked as well, because a high number may indicate an allergic reaction. Sometimes, the doctor may have a person discontinue one or more drugs to see if the itching is relieved. A biopsy or skin scraping■ may help identify the cause, including an infectious one.

Treatment

For itching of any cause, bathing should be kept brief and preferably in cool or lukewarm water with very little or no soap. The skin should be patted dry gently rather than rubbed vigorously. Many people with itching benefit from an over-the-counter moisturizing cream applied right after bathing. The moisturizer should be odorless and colorless, because additives that provide color or scent may irritate the skin and even cause itching. Fingernails, especially children's, should be kept short to minimize abrasions from scratching. Coating the affected area with soothing compounds, such as menthol, camphor, chamomile, eucalyptus, or calamine, also can help.

Taking antihistamines by mouth may decrease itching. Some antihistamines, such as hydroxyzine and diphenhydramine, usually cause sleepiness and dry mouth and are mainly used at bedtime. Other antihistamines, such as loratadine and cetirizine, usually do not cause sleepiness. Generally, creams containing antihistamines (such as diphenhydramine) should not be used, because they can themselves cause an allergic reaction.

Corticosteroid creams decrease inflammation and control itching and may be used when itching is limited to a small area. Itching from some conditions, such as poison ivy, may require high-strength corticosteroid creams. However, only mild corticosteroids, such as 1% hydrocortisone, should be applied to the face and genitals, because stronger corticosteroids may thin the sensitive skin in these areas. Also, powerful corticosteroid creams applied over large areas or for a long time can cause serious medical problems,★ especially in infants, because these drugs are absorbed into the bloodstream. Oral corticosteroids are sometimes used when large areas of the body are involved.

Specific treatments may be needed. For example, when fungal, parasitic, or bacterial infections cause itching, topical or systemic drugs may be required. Topical drugs are applied directly to the affected area of the skin. Systemic drugs are taken by mouth or injected and are distributed throughout the body.

Dermatitis

Dermatitis (eczema) is inflammation of the upper layers of the skin, causing itching, blisters, redness, swelling, and often oozing, scabbing, and scaling.

Dermatitis is a broad term covering many different disorders that all result in a red, itchy rash. The term eczema is sometimes used for dermatitis. Some types of dermatitis affect only specific parts of the body, whereas others can occur anywhere. Some types of dermatitis have a known cause; others do not. However, dermatitis is always the skin's way of reacting to severe dryness, scratching, a substance that is causing irritation, or an allergen. Typically, that substance comes in direct contact with the skin, but sometimes the substance is swallowed. In all cases, continuous scratching and rubbing may eventually lead to thickening and hardening of the skin.

Dermatitis may be a brief reaction to a substance. In such cases it may produce symptoms, such as itching and redness, for just a few hours or a day or two. Chronic dermatitis persists over a period of time. The hands and feet are particularly vulnerable to chronic dermatitis, because the hands are in frequent contact with many foreign substances and the feet are in the warm, moist conditions created by socks and shoes that favor fungal growth.

Chronic dermatitis may represent a contact, fungal, or other dermatitis that has been inadequately diagnosed or treated, or it may be one of several chronic skin disorders of unknown origin, such as pompholyx▲ or hyperkeratotic palmar eczema. Because chronic dermatitis produces cracks and blisters in the skin, any type of chronic dermatitis may lead to bacterial infection.

CONTACT DERMATITIS

Contact dermatitis is skin inflammation caused by direct contact with a particular substance; the rash is very itchy, is confined

Common Causes of Allergic Contact Dermatitis

Cosmetics: Hair-removing chemicals, nail polish, nail polish remover, deodorants, moisturizers, aftershave lotions, perfumes, sunscreens

Metal compound (in jewelry): Nickel

Plants: Poison ivy, poison oak, poison sumac, ragweed, primrose, thistle

Drugs in skin creams: Antibiotics (sulfonamides, neomycin), antihistamines (diphenhydramine, promethazine), anesthetics (benzocaine), antiseptics (thimerosal), stabilizers

Chemicals used in clothing manufacturing: Tanning agents in shoes; rubber accelerators and antioxidants in gloves, shoes, undergarments, other apparel

to a specific area, and often has clearly defined boundaries.

Substances can cause skin inflammation by one of two mechanisms—irritation (irritant contact dermatitis) or allergic reaction (allergic contact dermatitis).

Irritant contact dermatitis occurs when a chemical substance causes direct damage to the skin. Typical irritating substances are acids, alkalis (such as drain cleaners), solvents (such as acetone in nail polish remover), and strong soaps. Some of these chemicals cause skin changes within a few minutes, whereas others require longer exposure. People vary in the sensitivity of their skin to irritants. Even very mild soaps and detergents may irritate the skin of some people after frequent or prolonged contact.

Allergic contact dermatitis is a reaction by the body's immune system to a substance contacting the skin. Sometimes a person can be sensitized by only one exposure, and other times sensitization occurs only after many exposures to a substance. After a person is sensitized, the next exposure causes itching and dermatitis within 4 to 24 hours, although some people, particularly older people, do not develop a reaction for 3 to 4 days.

Thousands of substances can result in allergic contact dermatitis. The most common include substances found in plants such as poison ivy, rubber (latex), antibiotics, fragrances,

▲ see page 1198

preservatives, and some metals (nickel, cobalt). About 10% of women are allergic to nickel, a common component of jewelry. People may use (or be exposed to) substances for years without a problem, then suddenly develop an allergic reaction. Even ointments, creams, and lotions used to treat dermatitis can cause such a reaction. People may also develop dermatitis from many of the materials they touch while at work (occupational dermatitis).

Sometimes contact dermatitis results only after a person touches certain substances and then exposes the skin to sunlight (photoallergic or phototoxic contact dermatitis). Such substances include sunscreens, aftershave lotions, certain perfumes, antibiotics, coal tar, and oils.

Symptoms and Diagnosis

Regardless of cause or type, contact dermatitis results in itching and a rash. The itching is usually severe, but the rash varies from a mild, short-lived redness to severe swelling and large blisters. Most commonly, the rash contains tiny blisters. The rash develops only in areas contacted by the substance. However, the rash appears earlier in thin, sensitive areas of skin, and later in areas of thicker skin or on skin that had less contact with the substance, giving the impression that the rash has spread. Touching the rash or blister fluid cannot spread contact dermatitis to other people or to other parts of the body that did not make contact with the substance.

Determining the cause of contact dermatitis is not always easy. Most people are unaware of all the substances that touch their skin. Often, the location of the initial rash is an important clue, particularly if it occurs under an item of clothing or jewelry or only in areas exposed to sunlight. However, many substances that people touch with their hands are unknowingly transferred to the face, where the more sensitive facial skin may react even if the hands do not.

If a doctor suspects contact dermatitis and a process of elimination does not pinpoint the cause, patch testing can be performed. For this test, small patches containing substances that commonly cause dermatitis are placed on the skin for 1 to 2 days to see if a rash develops beneath one of them. Although useful, patch

testing is complicated. People may be sensitive to many substances, and the substance they react to on a patch may not be the cause of their dermatitis. A doctor must decide which substances to test based on what a person might have been exposed to.

Prevention and Treatment

Contact dermatitis can be prevented by avoiding contact with the causative substance. If contact does occur, the material should be washed off immediately with soap and water. If circumstances risk ongoing exposure, gloves and protective clothing may be helpful. Barrier creams are also available that can block certain substances, such as poison ivy and epoxy resins, from contacting the skin. Desensitization with injections or tablets of the causative substance is not effective in preventing contact dermatitis.

Treatment is not effective until there is no further contact with the substance causing the problem. Once the substance is removed, the redness usually disappears after a week. Blisters may continue to ooze and form crusts, but they soon dry. Residual scaling, itching, and temporary thickening of the skin may last for days or weeks.

Itching can be relieved with a number of topical or oral drugs.▲ In addition, small areas of dermatitis can be soothed by applying pieces of gauze or thin cloth dipped in cool water or aluminum acetate (Burow's solution) several times a day for an hour. Larger areas may be treated with short, cool tub baths with or without colloidal oatmeal. The doctor may drain fluid from large blisters, but the blister is not removed.

ATOPIC DERMATITIS

Atopic dermatitis is chronic, itchy inflammation of the upper layers of the skin that often develops in people who have hay fever or asthma and in people who have family members with these conditions.

Atopic dermatitis is one of the most common skin diseases, affecting 15 million people in the United States. Almost 66% of people with the disorder develop it before age 1, and 90% by age 5. In half of these people, the disorder will be gone by the teenage years; in others, it is lifelong.

Doctors do not know what causes atopic dermatitis, but people with it usually have many allergic disorders, particularly asthma,

---

▲ see page 1192

Poison Ivy Dermatitis

About 50 to 70% of people are sensitive to the plant oil *urushiol* contained in poison ivy, poison oak, and poison sumac. Similar oils are also present in the shells of cashew nuts; the leaves, sap, and fruit skin of the mango; and Japanese lacquer. Once a person has been sensitized by contact with these oils, subsequent exposure produces a contact dermatitis.

The oils are quickly absorbed into the skin but may remain active on clothing, tools, and pet fur for long periods of time. Smoke from burning plants also contains the oil and may cause a reaction in certain people. Sensitivity to poison ivy tends to run in families.

Symptoms begin from 8 to 48 hours after contact and consist of intense itching, a red rash, and multiple blisters, which may be tiny or very large. Typically, the blisters occur in a straight line following the track where the plant brushed along the skin. The rash may appear at different times in different locations either because of repeat contact with contaminated clothing and other objects or because some parts of the skin are more sensitive than others. The blister fluid itself is not contagious. The itching and rash last for 2 to 3 weeks.

Recognition and avoidance of contact with the plants is the best prevention. A number of commercial barrier creams and lotions can be applied before exposure to minimize, but not completely prevent, absorption of oil by the skin. The oil can soak through latex rubber gloves. Washing of the skin with soap and water prevents absorption of the oil if done immediately. Stronger solvents, such as acetone, alcohol, and various commercial products, are probably no more effective. Desensitization with various shots or pills or by eating poison ivy leaves is not effective.

Treatment helps relieve symptoms but does not shorten the duration of the rash. The most effective treatment is with corticosteroids. Small areas of rash are treated with strong topical corticosteroids, such as triamcinolone, clobetasol, or diflorasone—except on the face and genitals, where only mild corticosteroids, such as 1% hydrocortisone, should be applied. People with large areas of rash or significant facial swelling are given high-dose corticosteroids taken by mouth. Cool compresses wet with water or aluminum acetate may be used on large blistered areas. Antihistamines given by mouth may help with itching. Lotions and creams containing antihistamines are seldom used.

hay fever, and food allergies. The relationship between the dermatitis and these disorders is not clear; atopic dermatitis is not an allergy to a particular substance. Atopic dermatitis is not contagious.

Many conditions can make atopic dermatitis worse, including emotional stress, changes in temperature or humidity, bacterial skin infections, and contact with irritating clothing (especially wool). In some infants, food allergies may provoke atopic dermatitis.

Symptoms

Infants may develop red, oozing, crusted rashes on the face, scalp, diaper area, hands, arms, feet, or legs. Large areas of the body may be affected. In older children and adults, the rash often occurs (and recurs) in only one or a few spots, especially on the hands, upper arms, in front of the elbows, or behind the knees.

Although the color, intensity, and location of the rash vary, the rash always itches. The itching often leads to uncontrollable scratching, triggering a cycle of itching-scratching-itching that makes the problem worse. Scratching and rubbing can also tear the skin, leaving an opening for bacteria to enter and cause infections.

In people with atopic dermatitis, infection with the herpes simplex virus, which usually affects a small area with tiny, slightly painful blisters,▲ may produce a serious illness with widespread dermatitis, blistering, and high fever (eczema herpeticum).

Diagnosis and Treatment

A doctor makes the diagnosis based on the typical pattern of the rash and often on whether other family members have allergies.

No cure exists, but itching can be relieved with topical or oral drugs.■ Certain other measures can help. Avoiding contact with substances known to irritate the skin or foods that the person is sensitive to can prevent a

▲ see page 1160

■ see page 1192

rash. The skin should be kept moist, either with commercial moisturizers or with petroleum jelly or vegetable oil. Moisturizers are best applied after bathing, while the skin is damp. To limit the use of corticosteroids in people being treated for long periods, doctors sometimes replace the corticosteroids with petroleum jelly for a week or more at a time. Corticosteroid tablets are a last resort for people with stubborn cases.

Phototherapy (exposure to ultraviolet light) often helps adults.▲ This treatment is rarely recommended for children because of its potential long-term side effects, including skin cancer and cataracts.

For severe cases, the immune system can be suppressed with cyclosporine taken by mouth or tacrolimus used as an ointment. Zafirlukast, a new oral drug used to prevent asthma attacks, may also be helpful in treating atopic dermatitis.

SEBORRHEIC DERMATITIS

Seborrheic dermatitis is chronic inflammation of unknown cause that causes scales on the scalp and face and occasionally on other areas.

Seborrheic dermatitis occurs most often in infants, usually within the first 3 months of life, and between the ages of 30 and 70. The disorder is more common in men, often runs in families, and is worse in cold weather. A form of seborrheic dermatitis also occurs in as many as 85% of people with AIDS.

Symptoms

Seborrheic dermatitis usually begins gradually, causing dry or greasy scaling of the scalp (dandruff), sometimes with itching but without hair loss. In more severe cases, yellowish to reddish scaly pimples appear along the hairline, behind the ears, in the ear canal, on the eyebrows, on the bridge of the nose, around the nose, on the chest, and on the upper back. In infants younger than 1 month of age, seborrheic dermatitis may produce a thick, yellow, crusted scalp rash (cradle cap) and sometimes yellow scaling behind the ears and red pimples on the face. Frequently, a stubborn diaper rash accompanies the scalp rash. Older children and adults may develop a thick, tenacious, scaly rash with large flakes of skin.

Treatment

The scalp can be treated with a shampoo containing pyrithione zinc, selenium sulfide, an antifungal drug, salicylic acid and sulfur, or tar. The person usually uses the medicated shampoo every other day until the dermatitis is controlled and then twice weekly. Ketoconazole cream is often effective as well. In adults, thick crusts and scales, if present, can be loosened with overnight application of corticosteroids or salicylic acid under a shower cap.

Often, treatment must be continued for many weeks; if the dermatitis returns after the treatment is discontinued, treatment can be restarted. Topical corticosteroids are also used on the head and other affected areas. On the face, only mild corticosteroids, such as 1% hydrocortisone, should be used. Even mild corticosteroids must be used cautiously, because long-term use can thin the skin and cause other problems.

In infants and young children who have a thick scaly rash on the scalp, salicylic acid in mineral oil can be rubbed gently into the rash with a soft toothbrush at bedtime. The scalp can also be shampooed daily with mild baby shampoo, and 1% hydrocortisone cream can be rubbed into the scalp.

NUMMULAR DERMATITIS

Nummular dermatitis is a persistent, usually itchy, rash and inflammation characterized by coin-shaped spots with tiny blisters, scabs, and scales.

The cause is unknown. Nummular dermatitis usually affects middle-aged people, occurs along with dry skin, and is most common in winter. However, the rash may come and go without any apparent reason.

The round spots start as itchy patches of pimples and blisters that later ooze and form crusts. The rash may be widespread. Often, spots are more obvious on the backs of the arms or legs and on the buttocks, but they also appear on the torso.

Most people benefit from skin moisturizers. Other treatments include antibiotics taken by mouth, corticosteroid creams and injections, and phototherapy (exposure to ultraviolet light). All treatments, however, are often unsatisfactory.

GENERALIZED EXFOLIATIVE DERMATITIS

Generalized exfoliative dermatitis (erythroderma) is severe inflammation that causes

▲ see box on page 1202

the entire skin surface to become red, cracked, and covered with scales.

Certain drugs (especially penicillins, sulfonamides, isoniazid, phenytoin, and barbiturates) may cause this disorder. In some cases, it is a complication of other skin diseases, such as atopic dermatitis, psoriasis, and contact dermatitis. Certain lymphomas (cancers of the lymph nodes)▲ may also cause generalized exfoliative dermatitis. In many cases, the cause is unknown.

Symptoms and Diagnosis

Exfoliative dermatitis may start rapidly or slowly. At first the entire skin surface becomes red and shiny. Then the skin becomes scaly, thickened, and sometimes crusted. Sometimes the hair and nails fall out. Some people have itching and swollen lymph nodes. Although many people have a fever, they may feel cold because so much heat is lost through the damaged skin. Large amounts of fluid and protein may seep out, and the damaged skin is a poor barrier against infection.

Because symptoms of exfoliative dermatitis are similar to those of skin infection, doctors send samples of skin and blood to the laboratory to exclude infection as a cause.

Treatment

Early diagnosis and treatment are important in preventing infection from developing in the affected skin and in keeping fluid and protein loss from becoming life threatening.

People with severe exfoliative dermatitis often need to be hospitalized and given antibiotics (for infection), intravenous fluids (to replace the fluids lost through the skin), and nutritional supplements. Care may include the use of drugs and heated blankets to control body temperature. Cool baths followed by applications of petroleum jelly and gauze may help protect the skin. Corticosteroids (such as prednisone) given by mouth or intravenously are used only when other measures are unsuccessful or the disease worsens. Any drug or chemical that could be causing the dermatitis should be eliminated. If lymphoma is causing the dermatitis, treatment of the lymphoma is helpful.

STASIS DERMATITIS

Stasis dermatitis is inflammation on the lower legs from pooling of blood and fluid.

Stasis dermatitis tends to occur in people who have varicose (dilated, twisted) veins■

and swelling (edema). It usually occurs on the ankles but may spread upward to the knees. At first, the skin becomes reddened and mildly scaly. Over several weeks or months, the skin turns dark brown. Eventually, areas of the skin may break down and form an open sore (ulcer), typically near the ankle. Ulcers sometimes become infected with bacteria. Stasis dermatitis makes the legs feel itchy and swollen, but not painful. Ulcers are usually painful.

Treatment

Long-term treatment is aimed at keeping blood from pooling in the veins around the ankles. When sitting, the person should elevate the legs above the level of the heart. Properly fitted prescription support hose (compression stockings) also prevent pooling of blood and decrease swelling. Department store "support" stockings are not adequate.

For dermatitis of recent onset, soothing compresses, such as gauze pads soaked in tap water or aluminum acetate (Burow's solution), may make the skin feel better and can help prevent infection by keeping the skin clean. If the disorder worsens, as evidenced by increased warmth, redness, small ulcers, or pus, a more absorbent dressing can be used. Corticosteroid creams are also helpful and are often combined with zinc oxide paste and applied in a thin layer. Corticosteroids should not be applied directly to an ulcer because this will interfere with healing.

When a person has large or extensive ulcers, special moisture-containing hydrocolloid or hydrogel dressings may be used. Antibiotics are used only when the skin is already infected. Sometimes, skin from elsewhere on the body may be grafted to cover very large ulcers.

Some people may need an Unna's boot, which is a woven stretch wrap filled with a gelatin paste that contains zinc. The wrap is applied to the ankle and lower leg where it hardens, similar to but softer than a cast. The boot limits swelling and helps protect the skin from irritation, and the paste helps heal the skin. At first the boot is changed every 2 or 3 days, but later it is left on for a week at a time.

In stasis dermatitis, the skin is easily irritated; antibiotic creams, first-aid (anesthetic)

▲ see page 1016

■ see page 236

creams, alcohol, witch hazel, lanolin, or other chemicals should not be used because they can make the disorder worse.

LOCALIZED SCRATCH DERMATITIS

Localized scratch dermatitis (lichen simplex chronicus, neurodermatitis) is chronic, itchy inflammation of the top layer of the skin.

Localized scratch dermatitis is caused by chronic scratching of an area of skin. The act of scratching triggers more itching, beginning a vicious circle of itching-scratching-itching. Sometimes the scratching begins for no apparent reason. Other times scratching starts because of a contact dermatitis, parasitic infestation, or other condition, but the person continues to scratch long after the inciting cause is gone. Doctors do not know why this happens, but psychologic factors may play a role. The disorder does not seem to be allergic. More women than men have localized scratch dermatitis, and it is common among Asians and Native Americans. It usually develops between the ages of 20 and 50.

Symptoms and Diagnosis

Localized scratch dermatitis can occur anywhere on the body, including the anus (pruritus ani)▲ and the vagina (pruritus vulvae),■ but is most common on the head, arms, and legs. In the early stages, the skin looks normal, but it itches. Later, dryness, scaling, and dark patches develop as a result of the scratching and rubbing.

Doctors try to discover any possible underlying allergies or diseases that may be causing the initial itching. When the disorder occurs around the anus or vagina, the doctor may investigate the possibility of pinworms, trichomoniasis, hemorrhoids, local discharges, fungal infections, warts, contact dermatitis, or psoriasis as the cause.

Treatment

For the disorder to clear up, the person must stop all scratching and rubbing of the area. Standard treatments for itching should be followed.★ Using surgical tape saturated with a corticosteroid helps relieve itching and inflammation and protects the skin from scratching. The doctor may inject longer-acting cor-

ticosteroids under the skin to control the itching.

When this disorder develops around the anus or vagina, the best treatment is a corticosteroid cream. Zinc oxide paste may be applied over the cream to protect the area; the paste can be removed with mineral oil.

PERIORAL DERMATITIS

Perioral dermatitis is a red, bumpy rash around the mouth and on the chin.

The disorder, whose cause is unknown, mainly affects women between the ages of 20 and 60.

Treatment is with tetracyclines or other antibiotics taken by mouth. If these antibiotics do not clear up the rash and the disorder is particularly severe, isotretinoin, an acne drug, may help. Corticosteroids and some oily cosmetics, especially moisturizers, tend to worsen the disorder.

POMPHOLYX

Pompholyx is a chronic dermatitis characterized by itchy blisters on the palms and sides of the fingers and sometimes on the soles of the feet.

Pompholyx is sometimes called dyshidrosis, which means "abnormal sweating," but the disorder has nothing to do with sweating. Doctors do not know what causes pompholyx, but stress may be a factor as well as some ingested substances such as nickel, chromium, and cobalt. It is more common in adolescents and young adults.

The blisters are often scaly, red, and oozing. Pompholyx comes and goes in attacks that last 2 to 3 weeks. Pompholyx takes weeks to go away on its own. Wet compresses with potassium permanganate or aluminum acetate (Burow's solution) may help the blisters resolve. Strong topical corticosteroids may help itching and inflammation.

Drug Rashes

Drug rashes are a side effect of a drug that manifests as a skin reaction.

Most drug rashes result from an allergic reaction to the drug.● The drug does not have to be applied to the skin to cause a drug rash. Sometimes a person can be sensitized to a drug by one exposure, and other times sensitization occurs only after many exposures to a

---

▲ see page 763   ■ see page 1349
★ see page 1192   ● see page 85

substance. Later exposure to the drug may trigger an allergic reaction, such as a rash.

Sometimes a rash develops directly without involving an allergic reaction. For example, corticosteroids and lithium produce a rash that looks like acne, and anticoagulants (blood thinners) may cause bruising when blood leaks under the skin. Other important nonallergic rashes that may result from drugs are those that occur in Stevens-Johnson syndrome, toxic epidermal necrolysis, and erythema nodosum.

Certain drugs make the skin particularly sensitive to the effects of sunlight (photosensitivity). These drugs include certain antipsychotics, tetracycline, sulfa antibiotics, chlorothiazide, and some artificial sweeteners. No rash appears when the drug is taken, but later exposure to the sun produces a reddened area of skin that is sometimes itchy or that appears grayish blue.

Symptoms

Drug rashes vary in severity from mild redness with tiny bumps over a small area to peeling of the entire skin. Rashes may appear suddenly within minutes after a person takes a drug, or they may be delayed for hours or days. People with an allergic rash often have other allergic symptoms—runny nose, watery eyes, wheezing, and even collapse from dangerously low blood pressure. Hives are very itchy,▲ whereas other drug rashes itch little, if at all.

Diagnosis and Treatment

Figuring out whether a drug is responsible may be difficult because a rash can result from only a minute amount of a drug, it can erupt long after a person has taken a drug, and it can persist for weeks or months after a person has discontinued a drug. Every drug a person has taken is suspect, including those bought without a prescription; even eye drops, nose drops, and suppositories are possible causes. Sometimes the only way to determine which drug is causing a rash is to have the person discontinue all but life-sustaining drugs. Whenever possible, chemically unrelated drugs are substituted. If there are no such substitutes, the person starts taking the drugs again one at a time to see which one causes the reaction. However, this method can be hazardous if the person had a severe allergic reaction to the drug. Skin testing is not helpful, except when penicillin is the suspect drug.

Most drug reactions disappear when the responsible drug is discontinued. Standard itching treatments are used as needed.■ Serious allergic eruptions, particularly those accompanied by significant symptoms such as wheezing or difficulty breathing, are treated with injections of epinephrine, diphenhydramine, and a corticosteroid.

Stevens-Johnson Syndrome and Toxic Epidermal Necrolysis

Stevens-Johnson syndrome and toxic epidermal necrolysis are two forms of the same life-threatening skin disease that cause rash, skin peeling, and sores on the mucous membranes.

In Stevens-Johnson syndrome, a person has blistering of mucous membranes, typically in the mouth, eyes, and vagina, and patchy areas of rash. In toxic epidermal necrolysis, there is a similar blistering of mucous membranes, but in addition the entire top layer of the skin (the epidermis) peels off in sheets from large areas of the body. Both disorders can be life threatening.

Nearly all cases are caused by a reaction to a drug, most often sulfa antibiotics; barbiturates; anticonvulsants, such as phenytoin and carbamazepine; certain nonsteroidal anti-inflammatory drugs (NSAIDs); or allopurinol. A very few cases are caused by a bacterial infection. In some cases, a cause cannot be identified. The disorder occurs in all age groups but is more common in older people, probably because older people tend to use more drugs. The disorder is also more likely to occur in people with AIDS.

Symptoms

Stevens-Johnson syndrome and toxic epidermal necrolysis usually begin with fever, headache, cough, and body aches, which may last from 1 to 14 days. Then a flat red rash breaks out on the face and trunk, often spreading later to the rest of the body in an irregular pattern. The areas of rash enlarge and spread, often forming blisters in their center. The skin of the blisters is very loose and easy to rub off. In toxic epidermal necrolysis, large areas of skin peel off, often with just a gentle touch or pull. In many people, 30% or more of the body surface peels away. The affected areas of skin are painful, and the person feels very ill with

---

▲ see page 1071   ■ see page 1192

chills and fever. In some people, the hair and nails fall out.

In both disorders, blisters break out on the mucous membranes lining the mouth, throat, anus, genitals, and eyes. The damage to the lining of the mouth makes eating difficult, and closing the mouth may be painful, so the person may drool. The eyes may become very painful, swell, and become so filled with pus that they seal shut. The corneas can become scarred. The opening through which urine passes (urethra) may also be affected, making urination difficult and painful. Sometimes the mucous membranes of the digestive and respiratory tracts are involved, resulting in diarrhea and difficulty breathing.

The skin loss in toxic epidermal necrolysis is similar to a severe burn and is equally life threatening. Huge amounts of fluids and salts can seep from the large, raw, damaged areas. A person who has this disorder is very susceptible to infection at the sites of damaged, exposed tissues; such infections are the most common cause of death in people with this disorder.

Treatment

People with Stevens-Johnson syndrome or toxic epidermal necrolysis are hospitalized. Any drugs suspected of causing the disorder are immediately discontinued. When possible, these people are treated in a burn unit and given scrupulous care to avoid infection. If the person survives, the skin grows back on its own, and unlike burns, skin grafts are not needed. Fluids and salts, which are lost through the damaged skin, are replaced intravenously.

Use of corticosteroids to treat the disorder is controversial: Some doctors believe that giving large doses within the first few days is beneficial; others believe that corticosteroids should not be used. These drugs suppress the immune system, which increases the potential for serious infection. If infection develops, doctors give antibiotics immediately.

Erythema Multiforme

Erythema multiforme is a recurring disorder characterized by patches of red, raised skin that often look like targets and usually are distributed symmetrically over the body.

▲ see page 1160

Most cases are caused by a reaction to infection with the herpes simplex virus.▲ This viral infection is apparent as visible cold sores in about two thirds of people before the erythema multiforme appears. Doctors are not sure if other infectious diseases also cause erythema multiforme. Doctors are unsure exactly how herpes simplex causes this disorder, but a type of immune reaction is suspected.

Symptoms

Usually, erythema multiforme appears suddenly, with reddened patches erupting on the arms, legs, and face. Sometimes the rash is also present on the palms or soles. The red patches are distributed equally on both sides of the body; these red areas often develop red concentric rings with purple-gray centers (target or iris lesions) and small blisters. The reddened areas usually are symptomless, although they sometimes itch mildly. Painful blisters often form on the lips and lining of the mouth but do not involve the eyes.

Attacks of erythema multiforme may last 2 to 4 weeks. Some people have only one attack, but some have recurrences an average of 6 times a year for almost 10 years. Recurrences are more common in the spring and can probably be triggered by sunlight. The frequency of recurrence usually decreases with time.

Treatment

Erythema multiforme may resolve on its own. If itching is bothersome, standard treatments may be used. Corticosteroids given by mouth may be helpful. If painful mouth blisters make eating difficult, a topical anesthetic, such as lidocaine, may be applied. If oral intake is still poor, nutrition and fluids are given intravenously. People with frequent recurrences may benefit from an antiviral drug, such as acyclovir, given at the first sign of an outbreak.

Erythema Nodosum

Erythema nodosum is an inflammatory disorder that produces tender red bumps (nodules) under the skin, most often over the shins but occasionally on the arms and other areas.

Quite often, erythema nodosum is a symptom of some other disease or of sensitivity to a drug. Young adults, particularly women, are most prone to the disorder, which may recur for months or years. Bacterial, fungal, or viral infections may also cause erythema nodosum.

Streptococcal infection is one of the most common causes of erythema nodosum, particularly in children. Sarcoidosis, ulcerative colitis, and various drugs, such as sulfa antibiotics and oral contraceptives, are other common causes. Numerous other infections and several types of cancer are also thought to cause the eruption.

Erythema nodosum nodules usually appear on the shins and resemble raised bumps and bruises that gradually change from pink to bluish brown. Fever and joint pain are common; lymph nodes in the chest occasionally become enlarged and are detected with a chest x-ray. The painful nodules are usually the telltale sign for the doctor. Evaluation includes chest x-ray, blood tests, and skin biopsy.

Treatment

Drugs that might be causing erythema nodosum are discontinued, and any underlying infections are treated. If the disorder is caused by a streptococcal infection, a person may have to take antibiotics, such as penicillin, or a cephalosporin.

The nodules may go away in 3 to 6 weeks without treatment. Bed rest and nonsteroidal anti-inflammatory drugs (NSAIDs) may help relieve the pain caused by the nodules. Individual nodules may also be treated by injecting them with a corticosteroid; when a person has many nodules, corticosteroid or potassium iodide tablets sometimes are prescribed to speed relief of pain.

Granuloma Annulare

Granuloma annulare is a chronic, harmless skin disorder of unknown cause in which small, firm, raised bumps form a ring with normal or slightly sunken skin in the center.

The bumps are red, violet, or flesh-colored; a person may have one ring or several. The bumps usually cause no pain or itching; they most often form on the feet, legs, hands, or fingers of children and adults. In a few people, clusters of granuloma annulare bumps erupt when the skin is exposed to the sun.

Most often, granuloma annulare heals without any treatment. Corticosteroid creams under waterproof bandages, surgical tape saturated with a corticosteroid, or injected corticosteroids may help clear up the rash. People with large affected areas often benefit from treatment that combines phototherapy (exposure to ultraviolet light) with the use of psoralens (drugs that make the skin more sensitive to the effects of ultraviolet light). This treatment is called PUVA (psoralens plus ultraviolet A).

Psoriasis

Psoriasis is a chronic, recurring disease that causes one or more raised, red patches that have silvery scales and a distinct border between the patch and normal skin.

The patches of psoriasis occur because of an abnormally high rate of growth of skin cells. The reason for the rapid cell growth is unknown, but a problem with the immune system is thought to play a role. The disorder often runs in families. Psoriasis is common, affecting 2 to 4% of whites; blacks are less likely to get the disease.

Symptoms

Psoriasis begins most often in people aged 10 to 40, although people in all age groups are susceptible.

It usually starts as one or more small patches on the scalp, elbows, knees, back, or buttocks. The first patches may clear up after a few months or remain, sometimes growing together to form larger patches. Some people never have more than one or two small patches, and others have patches covering large areas of the body. Thick patches or patches on the palms of the hands, soles of the feet, or skinfolds of the genitals are more likely to itch or hurt, but many times the person has no symptoms. Although the patches do not cause extreme physical discomfort, they are very obvious and often embarrassing to the person. The psychologic distress caused by psoriasis can be severe. Many people with psoriasis also have deformed, thickened, pitted nails.

Psoriasis persists throughout life but may come and go. Symptoms are often diminished during the summer when the skin is exposed to bright sunlight. Some people may go for years between occurrences. Psoriasis may flare up for no apparent reason or as a result of a variety of circumstances. Flare-ups often result from conditions that irritate the skin, such as minor injuries and severe sunburn. Sometimes flare-ups follow infections, such as colds and strep throat. Flare-ups are more common in the winter and after stressful situations. Many drugs, such as antimalarial drugs, lithium, and beta-blockers, can also cause psoriasis to flare up.

Phototherapy: Using Ultraviolet Light to Treat Skin Disorders

For many years, people have known that exposure to sunlight is helpful for certain skin disorders. Doctors now know that one component of sunlight—ultraviolet (UV) light—is responsible for this effect. UV light has many different effects on skin cells, including altering the amounts and kinds of chemicals they make and causing the death of certain cells that can be involved in skin diseases. The use of UV light to treat disease is called phototherapy. Psoriasis and atopic dermatitis are the disorders most commonly treated with phototherapy.

Because natural sunlight exposure varies in intensity and is not practical for a large part of the year in certain climates, phototherapy is nearly always performed with artificial UV light. Treatments are given in a doctor's office or in a specialized treatment center. Ultraviolet light, which is invisible to the human eye, is classified as A, B, or C, depending on its wavelength. Ultraviolet A (UVA) penetrates deeper into the skin than ultraviolet B (UVB). UVA or UVB is chosen based on the type and severity of the person's disorder. Ultraviolet C is not used in phototherapy. Some lights produce only certain specific wavelengths of UVA or UVB (narrow-band therapy), which are used to treat specific disorders. Narrow-band therapy helps limit the sunburning associated with phototherapy.

Phototherapy is sometimes combined with the use of psoralens. Psoralens are drugs that may be taken by mouth before treatment with ultraviolet light. Psoralens sensitize the skin to the effects of UV light, allowing shorter, less intense exposure. The combination of psoralens plus UVA is known as PUVA therapy.

Side effects of phototherapy include pain and reddening similar to sunburn with prolonged exposure to UV light. UV light exposure also increases the long-term risk of skin cancer, although the risk is small for brief courses of treatment. Psoralens often cause nausea. In addition, because psoralens enter the lens of the eye, UV-resistant sunglasses must be worn for at least 12 hours after undergoing PUVA therapy.

Some uncommon types of psoriasis can have more serious effects. Psoriatic arthritis produces joint pain and swelling.▲ Erythrodermic psoriasis causes all of the skin on the body to become red and scaly. This form of psoriasis is serious because, like a burn, it keeps the skin from serving as a protective barrier against injury and infection. In another uncommon form of psoriasis, pustular psoriasis, large and small pus-filled blisters (pustules) form on the palms of the hands and soles of the feet. Sometimes, these pustules are scattered on the body.

Treatment

Many drugs are available to treat psoriasis. Most often, a combination of drugs is used, depending on the severity and extent of the person's symptoms.

Topical drugs (drugs applied to the skin) are used most commonly. Nearly everyone with psoriasis benefits from skin moisturizers (emollients). Other topical agents include corticosteroids, often used together with calcipotriene, a vitamin D derivative, or coal or pine tar. Tazarotene or anthralin may also be used. Very thick patches can be thinned with ointments containing salicylic acid, which make the other drugs more effective. Many of these drugs are irritating to the skin, and doctors must find which ones work best for each person.

Phototherapy (exposure to ultraviolet light) also can help clear up psoriasis for several months at a time. Phototherapy is often used in combination with various topical drugs, particularly when large areas of skin are involved. Traditionally, treatment has been with phototherapy combined with the use of psoralens (drugs that make the skin more sensitive to the effects of ultraviolet light). This treatment is called PUVA (psoralens plus ultraviolet A). Some doctors are now using narrow-band ultraviolet B (UVB) treatments, which are equally effective but avoid the need to use psoralens and the side effects they cause, such as extreme sensitivity to sunshine.

For serious forms of psoriasis and psoriatic arthritis, drugs taken by mouth are used. These drugs include cyclosporine, methotrexate, and acitretin. Cyclosporine is an immunosuppressant drug. Cyclosporine may cause high blood pressure and damage the kidneys. Methotrexate interferes with the growth and multiplication of skin cells. Doctors use methotrexate for people whose psoriasis does not respond to other forms of therapy. Liver

▲ see page 375

damage and impaired immunity are possible side effects. Acitretin is similar to the acne drug isotretinoin▲ and is particularly effective in pustular psoriasis but often raises fat (lipid) levels in the blood and might cause problems with the liver and bones. It can also cause birth defects and should not be taken by a woman who might get pregnant.

Pityriasis Rosea

Pityriasis rosea is a mild disease that causes many small patches of scaly, rose-colored, inflamed skin.

The cause of pityriasis rosea is not certain but may be an infectious agent; however, the disorder is not thought to be contagious. It can develop at any age but is most common in young adults. It usually appears during spring and autumn.

Symptoms

Pityriasis rosea causes a rose-red or light-tan patch of skin about 1 to 4 inches in diameter that doctors call a herald or mother patch. This round or oval area usually develops on the torso. Sometimes the patch appears without any previous symptoms, but some people have a vague feeling of illness, loss of appetite, fever, and joint pain a few days before. In 5 to 10 days, many similar but smaller patches appear on other parts of the body. These secondary patches are most common on the torso, especially along and radiating from the spine. Most people with pityriasis rosea have some itching, and in some people the itching can be severe.

Diagnosis and Treatment

A doctor usually makes the diagnosis based on the appearance of the rash, particularly the herald patch. Usually the rash goes away in 4 to 5 weeks without treatment, although sometimes it lasts for 2 months or more. Both artificial and natural sunlight may speed clearing and relieve the itching. Other standard treatments for itching may be used as needed.■ Corticosteroids taken by mouth are necessary only for very severe itching.

Rosacea

Rosacea is a persistent skin disorder that produces redness, tiny pimples, and noticeable blood vessels, usually on the central area of the face.

The cause of rosacea is not known. The disorder usually appears during or after middle age and is most common in people of Celtic or Northern European descent who have fair complexions. Alcoholics tend to develop rosacea. Although usually easy for doctors to recognize, rosacea sometimes looks like acne and certain other skin disorders. It is often called "adult acne."

The skin over the cheeks and nose becomes red, often with small pimples. The skin may appear thin and frail, with small blood vessels visible just below the surface. The skin around the nose may thicken, making it look red and bulbous (rhinophyma), which is particularly common in alcoholics. Occasionally, rosacea appears on the torso, arms, and legs rather than on the face.

Treatment

People with rosacea should avoid foods that cause the blood vessels in the skin to dilate—for example, spicy foods, alcohol, coffee, and other caffeinated beverages.

Certain antibiotics taken by mouth relieve rosacea; tetracyclines are usually most effective and produce the fewest side effects. Antibiotics that are applied to the skin, such as metronidazole, clindamycin, and erythromycin, are also effective. In rare cases, antifungal creams, such as ketoconazole or terbinafine cream, are used.

Isotretinoin is effective when taken by mouth or when applied to the skin. Corticosteroids applied to the skin tend to make rosacea worse. Severe rhinophyma is unlikely to improve completely with drugs; a person with this disorder may need surgery or laser treatment.★

Lichen Planus

Lichen planus, a recurring itchy disease, starts as a rash of small, discrete red or purple bumps that then combine and become rough, scaly patches.

The cause of lichen planus is not known, but it may be a reaction by the immune system to a variety of drugs (especially gold, bismuth, arsenic, quinine, quinidine, and quinacrine), chemicals (especially certain chemicals used to develop color photographs), and infectious organisms. The disorder itself is not infectious.

▲ see page 1206

■ see page 1192

★ see box on page 1235

Symptoms

The rash of lichen planus almost always itches, sometimes severely. The bumps are usually violet and have angular borders; when light is directed at them from the side, the bumps display a distinctive sheen. New bumps may form wherever scratching or a mild skin injury occurs. Sometimes a dark discoloration remains after the rash heals.

Usually, the rash is evenly distributed on both sides of the body—most commonly on the torso, on the inner surfaces of the wrists, on the legs, on the head of the penis, and in the vagina. About half of those who get lichen planus also develop mouth sores. The face is less often affected. On the legs, the rash may become especially large, thick, and scaly. The rash sometimes results in patchy baldness on the scalp.

Lichen planus in the mouth usually results in a bluish white patch that forms in lines. This type of mouth patch often does not hurt, and the person may not know it is there. Sometimes painful sores form in the mouth, which often interfere with eating and drinking.

Prognosis and Treatment

Lichen planus usually clears up by itself after 1 or 2 years, although it sometimes lasts longer, especially when the mouth is involved. Symptoms recur in about 20% of people. Prolonged treatment may be needed during outbreaks of the rash; between outbreaks, no treatment is needed. People with mouth sores have a slightly increased risk of oral cancer, but the rash on the skin does not turn cancerous.

Drugs or chemicals that may be causing lichen planus should be avoided, and standard treatments can be used to relieve itching.▲

Corticosteroids may be injected into the bumps, applied to the skin, or taken by mouth, sometimes with other drugs, such as acitretin or cyclosporin. Phototherapy (exposure to ultraviolet light) combined with the use of psoralens (drugs that make the skin more sensitive to the effects of ultraviolet light) may also be helpful. This treatment is called PUVA (psoralens plus ultraviolet A). For painful mouth sores, a mouthwash containing lidocaine, an anesthetic, may be used before meals to form a pain-killing coating.

Keratosis Pilaris

Keratosis pilaris is a common disorder in which dead cells shed from the upper layer of skin plug the openings of hair follicles.

The cause is not known, although heredity probably plays a role. Also, people with atopic dermatitis are more likely to have keratosis pilaris.

The plugs or bumps that occur in keratosis pilaris make the skin feel rough (like chicken skin) and dry. Sometimes the plugs resemble small pimples. Generally, these plugs do not itch or hurt and cause only cosmetic problems. The upper arms, thighs, and buttocks are most commonly affected. The face may break out as well, particularly in children. Plugs are more likely to develop in cold weather and to clear up in the summer.

Treatment is not needed unless the person is bothered by the appearance of the disorder. Skin moisturizers are the main treatment. Creams with salicylic acid, lactic acid, or tretinoin can also be used. Keratosis pilaris is likely to come back when treatment is stopped.

CHAPTER 204

Acne

Acne is a common skin condition producing pimples on the face and upper torso.

Acne is caused by an interaction between hormones, skin oils, and bacteria that results in inflammation of hair follicles. Acne occurs mostly on the face, upper chest, shoulders, and back and is characterized by pimples, cysts, and sometimes abscesses. Both cysts and abscesses are pus-filled pockets, but abscesses are somewhat larger and deeper.

▲ see page 1192

Comparing Mild Acne and Severe Acne

Epidermis | Hair follicle | Hair | Oil (sebum) | Sebaceous gland | Dermis

Dead skin cells | Trapped sebum | Blackhead

Pus | Inflamed tissue | Rupture

Cross Section of Normal Skin

Mild Acne

Severe Acne

Sebaceous glands, which secrete an oily substance (sebum), lie in the dermis, the middle layer of skin. These glands are attached to the hair follicles. The sebum, along with dead skin cells, passes up from the sebaceous gland and hair follicle and out to the surface of the skin through the pores.

Acne results when a collection of dried sebum, dead skin cells, and bacteria clog the hair follicles, blocking the sebum from leaving through the pores. If the blockage is incomplete, a blackhead (open comedone) develops; if the blockage is complete, a whitehead (closed comedone) develops. The blocked sebum-filled hair follicle promotes overgrowth of the bacteria *Propionibacterium acnes*, which are normally present in the hair follicle. These bacteria break down the sebum into substances that irritate the skin. The resulting inflammation and infection produce the skin eruptions that are commonly known as acne pimples. If the infection worsens, an abscess may form, which may rupture into the skin, creating even more inflammation.

Acne occurs mainly during puberty, when the sebaceous glands are stimulated by increased hormone levels, especially the androgens (such as testosterone), resulting in excessive sebum production. By a person's early to mid 20s, hormone production stabilizes and acne usually disappears. Other conditions that involve hormonal changes can affect the occurrence of acne as well. For example, acne may occur with each menstrual period in young women and may clear up or substantially worsen during pregnancy. The use of certain drugs, particularly corticosteroids and anabolic steroids, can cause acne by stimulating the sebaceous glands. Certain cosmetics may worsen acne by clogging the pores.

Because acne naturally varies in severity for most people—sometimes worsening, sometimes improving—pinpointing the factors that may produce an outbreak is difficult. Acne is often worse in the winter and better in the summer, for unknown reasons. There is no relationship, however, between acne and specific foods or sexual activity.

Symptoms

Acne ranges from mild to very severe. Yet, even mild acne can be vexing, especially to teenagers, who see each pimple as a major cosmetic challenge.

People with mild (superficial) acne develop only a few noninflamed blackheads or a moderate number of small, mildly irritated pimples. Most acne occurs on the face but is also common on the shoulders, back, and upper chest. Anabolic steroid use typically causes acne on the shoulders and upper back. Blackheads appear as tiny, dark dots at the center of a small swelling of normal-colored skin. Pimples are mildly uncomfortable and have a white center surrounded by a small area of reddened skin. People with severe (deep, or cystic) acne have numerous large, red, painful pus-filled lumps (nodules) that sometimes even join together under the skin into giant, oozing abscesses.

Mild acne usually does not leave scars. However, squeezing pimples or trying to open them in other ways increases inflammation and the depth of injury to the skin, making scarring more likely. The nodules and abscesses of severe acne often rupture and, after healing, typically leave scars. Scars may be tiny, deep holes (ice pick scars); wider pits of varying depth; or large, irregular indentations. Acne scars last a lifetime and, for some people, are cosmetically significant and a source of psychologic stress.

Treatment

General care of acne is very simple. Affected areas should be gently washed once or twice a day with a mild soap. Antibacterial or abrasive soaps, alcohol pads, and heavy frequent scrubbing provide no added benefit and may further irritate the skin. Cosmetics should be water-based; very greasy products can worsen acne. Although there are no restrictions on specific foods (for example, pizza or chocolate), a healthy, balanced diet should be followed.▲

Beyond these routine measures, acne treatment depends on the severity of the condition. Mild acne requires the simplest treatment, which poses the fewest risks of side effects. More severe acne or acne that does not respond to preliminary treatment requires additional treatment.

Mild Acne: Drugs used to treat mild acne are applied to the skin (topical drugs). They work by either killing bacteria (antibacterials) or drying up or unclogging the pores.

The two most commonly prescribed antibacterials are the antibiotics clindamycin and erythromycin. Benzoyl peroxide, another effective antibacterial, is available with or without a prescription.

Older nonprescription creams that contain salicylic acid, resorcinol, or sulfur work by drying out the pimples and causing slight scaling. These drugs, however, are less effective than antibiotics or benzoyl peroxide.

If topical antibacterials fail, doctors use other topical prescription drugs that help unclog the pores. The most common such drug is tretinoin. Tretinoin is very effective but is irritating to the skin and makes it more sensitive to sunlight. Doctors therefore use this drug cautiously, starting with low concentrations and infrequent applications, which can be gradually increased. Benzoyl peroxide inactivates tretinoin, so the two must not be applied together. Newer drugs with effects similar to tretinoin include adapalene, azelaic acid, and tazarotene.

Blackheads and whiteheads can be removed by a doctor. A large pimple may be opened with a sterile needle. Other instruments, such as a loop extractor, can also be used to drain plugged pores and pimples.

Severe Acne: Antibiotics given by mouth, including tetracycline, doxycycline, minocycline, and erythromycin, are reserved for the treatment of severe acne. People may need to take one of these drugs for weeks, months, or even years to prevent a recurrence. Some of these drugs have potentially serious side effects, so close monitoring by a doctor is necessary. Women who take antibiotics for a long time sometimes develop vaginal yeast infections that may require treatment with other drugs. If controlling the yeast infection proves difficult, oral antibiotic therapy for acne may not be practical.

For the most severe acne, when antibiotics do not work, oral isotretinoin is the best treatment. Isotretinoin, which is related to the topical drug tretinoin, is the only drug that can potentially cure acne. However, isotretinoin can have very serious side effects. *Isotretinoin can harm a developing fetus, and women taking it must use strict contraceptive measures so they do not become pregnant.* Other, less serious side effects may occur as well. Therapy generally continues for 20 weeks. If more therapy is needed, it should not be restarted for at least 4 months.

Other acne treatments are useful for specific people. For example, a woman with severe acne that worsens with her menstrual period may be helped by taking oral contraceptives. This treatment takes 2 to 4 months to produce results.

Doctors sometimes treat large, inflamed nodules or abscesses by injecting cortico-

▲ see page 884

℞ DRUGS USED TO TREAT ACNE

ACTION	DRUG	SELECTED SIDE EFFECTS	COMMENTS
Kills bacteria			
(applied topically)	Clindamycin	Diarrhea (rarely)	—
	Erythromycin	—	Well tolerated
	Benzoyl peroxide	Dries the skin; may discolor clothing and hair	Especially effective when combined with erythromycin
Unclogs pores			
(applied topically)	Tretinoin	Irritates skin; sensitizes skin to sunlight	Acne appears to worsen when tretinoin is started; may take 3 to 4 weeks to notice any improvement; protective clothing and sunscreen should be worn during sun exposure
	Tazarotene	Irritates skin; sensitizes skin to sunlight	Acne appears to worsen when tazarotene is started; may take 3 to 4 weeks to notice any improvement; protective clothing and sunscreen should be worn during sun exposure
	Adapalene	Some redness, burning, and increased sun sensitivity	As effective as tretinoin but less irritating; protective clothing and sunscreen should be worn during sun exposure
	Azelaic acid	May lighten skin	Minimally irritating; may be used by itself or with tretinoin; should be used cautiously in people with darker skin because of skin-lightening effects
Kills bacteria			
(taken by mouth)	Tetracycline	Sensitizes skin to sunlight	Inexpensive and safe, but must be taken on an empty stomach; protective clothing and sunscreen should be worn during sun exposure
	Doxycycline	Sensitizes skin to sunlight	Protective clothing and sunscreen should be worn during sun exposure
	Minocycline	Headache, dizziness, skin discoloration	Most effective antibiotic
	Erythromycin	Stomach upset	Bacteria frequently become resistant to erythromycin
Unclogs pores			
(taken by mouth)	Isotretinoin	Can harm a developing fetus; can affect blood cells, liver, and fat levels; dry eyes, chapped lips, drying of the mucous membranes; pain or stiffness of large joints and lower back with high dosages; has been associated with depression, suicidal thoughts, attempted suicide, and (in rare cases) completed suicide	A sexually active woman should have a pregnancy test before she starts taking isotretinoin and at monthly intervals while she is taking it; contraception or sexual abstinence should begin 1 month before she starts taking the drug and should continue while she takes it and for 1 month after she discontinues it. Blood tests are necessary to make sure the drug is not affecting blood cells, the liver, or fat (triglyceride and cholesterol) levels

steroids into them. Occasionally, a doctor cuts open a nodule or abscess to drain it.

Treatment of severe acne scars depends on their shape, depth, and location. Individual scars of any depth may be cut out and the skin sewn back together. Wide indented scars can be improved cosmetically in a procedure called subcision, in which small cuts are made under the skin to release the scar tissue. This procedure often allows the skin to resume its nor-mal contours. Multiple shallow scars may be treated with chemical peels or laser resurfac-ing.▲ Dermabrasion, a procedure in which the skin surface is rubbed with an abrasive metal instrument to remove the top layer, also may help remove small scars. Sometimes scars are injected with various substances such as colla-gen, fat, or a variety of synthetic materials. These substances may raise the scarred area to make it level with the rest of the skin.

CHAPTER 205

Pressure Sores

Pressure sores (bedsores, decubitus ulcers) are areas of skin damage resulting from a lack of blood flow due to pressure.

Pressure sores can occur in people of any age who are bedridden, chairbound, or unable to reposition themselves. However, they fre-quently affect older people. Pressure sores usually develop below the waist, although they can occur anywhere on the body. They tend to occur over bony projections where pressure is concentrated, such as the lower back, heels, elbows, and hips. They may occur where pressure from a bed, wheelchair, cast, splint, or other hard object contacts and presses on the skin. Pressure sores may be painful and can be life threatening. They lengthen the time spent in hospitals or nurs-ing homes and increase the cost of care.

Causes

The skin has a rich blood supply that deliv-ers oxygen to all its layers. If that blood supply is cut off for more than 2 or 3 hours, the skin dies, beginning at its outer layer (the epider-mis). The dead skin breaks down and forms an open sore or ulcer. Once the skin is broken, bacteria may enter the opening and cause an infection.

Pressure reduces blood flow to the skin. The intense pressure created by sitting in a chair or lying on a mattress cuts off blood flow over bony areas. Most people do not normally de-velop pressure sores because they constantly shift position without thinking, even when asleep. However, some people are incapable of normal movement and are therefore at high risk of developing pressure sores. This group includes people who are paralyzed, comatose, very weak, or restrained. Paralyzed and coma-tose people are at particular risk because they may be unable to sense discomfort or pain, signals that normally motivate people to move or to ask to be moved.

Traction also reduces blood flow to the skin and can lead to pressure sores. Traction occurs when the skin sticks to something, often bed linens. When the skin is pulled, the effect is much like pressure.

Friction can lead to pressure sores as well. Repeated irritation may wear away the top layers of skin. Such irritation may occur if a person scrapes the heels, elbows, or knees or wears poorly fitted shoes.

Skin moisture can lead to the development of pressure sores. Prolonged exposure to mois-ture—often perspiration, urine, or feces—weakens and damages the skin surface, mak-ing pressure sores more likely.

Inadequate nutrition increases the risk of developing pressure sores and slows the heal-ing process of sores that do develop. Malnour-ished people lack the protective layer of fat that helps pad the skin and that keeps the blood vessels from being squeezed shut. Peo-ple whose diets are deficient in protein, vita-min C, or zinc, which are essential for normal skin repair, are at increased risk as well.

▲ see box on page 1235

Symptoms

For most people, pressure sores cause some pain and itching. However, in people whose senses are dulled, even severe, deep sores may be painless.

Pressure sores are categorized into four stages according to the severity of damage, from redness and inflammation (stage 1) to destruction of muscle, fat, and bone (stage 4).

Infection delays healing of shallow sores and can be life threatening in deeper sores. Infection can even penetrate the bone (osteomyelitis), requiring weeks of treatment with antibiotics. In the most severe cases, infection can spread into the bloodstream (sepsis).

Prevention

Prevention is the best strategy for dealing with pressure sores. In most cases, pressure sores can be prevented by meticulous attention from all caregivers, including nurses, nurses' aides, and family members. Close daily inspection of a bedridden or chairbound person's skin can detect early redness or discoloration. Any sign of redness or discoloration is a signal that the person needs to be repositioned and kept from lying or sitting on the discolored area until it returns to normal.

Because shifting position is necessary to keep the blood flowing to the skin, oversedation should be avoided and activity encouraged. People who cannot move themselves should be repositioned every 2 hours—more often if possible. The skin must be kept clean and dry, because moisture increases the risk of developing pressure sores. Dry skin is less likely to stick to fabrics and cause traction.

Bony projections (such as heels and elbows) can be protected with soft materials, such as cotton or fluffy wool. Special beds, mattresses, and seat cushions can be used to reduce pressure in people who are wheelchair-bound or bedridden. These products can reduce pressure and offer extra relief. A doctor or nurse can recommend the most appropriate mattress surface or seat cushion. It is important to remember that none of these devices eliminate pressure completely or are a substitute for frequent repositioning.

Treatment

Treating a pressure sore is much more difficult than preventing one. Adequate nutrition is important in helping pressure sores heal and in preventing new sores from forming. A well-

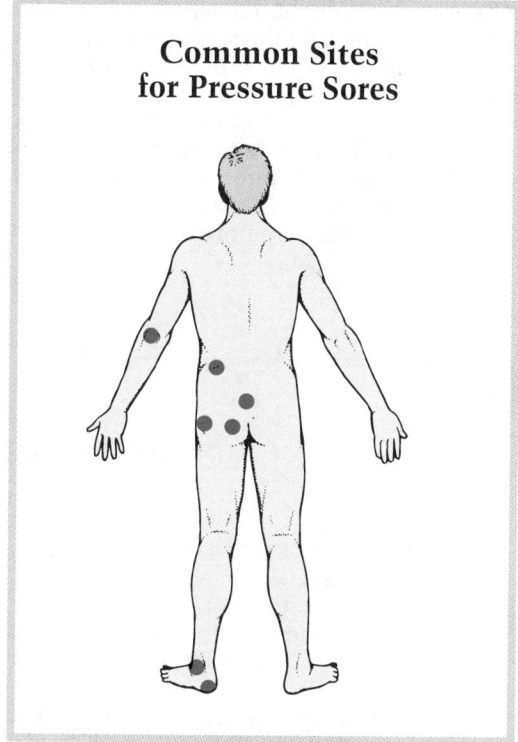

Common Sites for Pressure Sores

balanced, high-protein diet is recommended as well as a daily high-potency vitamin and mineral supplement. Supplemental vitamin C and zinc may help with healing as well.

In the early stages, pressure sores usually heal by themselves once pressure is removed. When the skin is broken, a doctor or nurse will consider the location and condition of the pressure sore when recommending a dressing. Film (see-through) dressings help protect early-stage pressure sores and allow them to heal more quickly. Hydrocolloid (oxygen- and moisture-retaining) patches protect, keep the skin appropriately moist, and provide a healthy environment for deep sores. Other types of dressings may be used for deeper sores, those that ooze a lot of fluids, and those that are infected.

If the sore appears infected or oozes, rinsing with saline and wiping gently with a gauze pad is helpful. Sometimes stronger cleansing agents are used. A doctor may need to remove (debride) the dead material with a scalpel or with chemical agents.

Newer treatments for wound care include vacuum-assisted closure devices, which apply suction to a wound; growth factors, which are substances (usually proteins) that stimulate cells to grow; hyperbaric oxygen treatment, in which a person is placed in a chamber with oxygen at increased pressure;▲ and synthetic skin grafts.

Deep pressure sores are difficult to treat. Sometimes they require skin grafting, in which healthy skin is transplanted to the damaged area. This type of surgery is not al-ways successful, however, especially for frail older people who are malnourished. Often, when infections develop deep within a sore, antibiotics are given. When bones beneath a sore become infected, the bone infection (osteomyelitis) is extremely difficult to cure and may spread through the bloodstream, requiring many weeks of treatment with an antibiotic.■

CHAPTER 206

Sweating Disorders

Sweat is made by sweat glands in the skin and carried to the skin's surface by ducts. Sweating helps keep the body cool. Thus, people sweat more when it is warm. They also sweat when they are nervous, under stress, or exercising.

Sweat is composed mostly of water, but it also contains salt (mostly sodium chloride) and other chemicals. When a person sweats a lot, the lost salt and water must be replaced.

Prickly Heat

Prickly heat (miliaria) is an itchy skin rash caused by trapped sweat.

Prickly heat develops when the narrow ducts carrying sweat to the skin surface get clogged. The trapped sweat causes inflammation, which produces irritation (prickling), itching, and a rash of very tiny blisters. Prickly heat also can appear as large, reddened areas of skin.

Prickly heat is most common in warm, humid climates. It tends to occur on areas of the body where skin touches skin, such as under the breasts, on the inner thighs, and under the arms.

The condition is controlled by keeping the skin cool and dry. Use of powders and antiperspirants often helps. Conditions that increase sweating should be avoided; an air-conditioned environment is ideal.

Once the rash develops, corticosteroid creams or lotions are used, sometimes with a bit of menthol added; however, these topical treatments are not as effective as keeping the skin cool and dry.

Excessive Sweating

People with excessive sweating (hyperhidrosis) sweat profusely, and some sweat almost constantly. Although people with a fever or those exposed to very warm environments sweat, people with excessive sweating tend to sweat even without these circumstances. Excessive sweating may affect the entire surface of the skin, but often it is limited to the palms of the hands, soles of the feet, armpits, or genital area.

Usually, no specific cause is found. However, medical disorders that can cause excessive sweating include hyperthyroidism, a low level of sugar in the blood, and, rarely, pheochromocytoma. An abnormality in the part of the nervous system that controls sweating can cause excessive sweating as well. Also, people with a spinal cord injury or disease may have episodes of excessive sweating. People with excessive sweating are frequently anxious about their condition. This anxiety often makes the sweating worse.

Severe, chronic wetness can make the affected area white, wrinkled, and cracked. Sometimes the area becomes red and inflamed. The area may emit a foul odor (bromhidrosis) due to the breakdown of sweat by bacteria and yeasts that normally live on the skin.

▲ see page 1671

■ see page 364

Treatment

Excessive sweating can be controlled to some degree with commercial antiperspirants. However, stronger treatment is often needed, especially for the palms of the hands, soles of the feet, armpits, or genital area. Nighttime application of aluminum chloride solution may help; prescription and nonprescription strengths of this drug are available. A person first dries the sweaty area and then applies the solution. If the response is inadequate, a plastic film can be applied over the solution to enhance the effectiveness of the treatment. In the morning, the person removes the film and washes the area. Some people need two applications daily; this regimen usually gives relief in a week. If the solution irritates the skin, the plastic film should be left off.

A solution of methenamine also may help. Tap water iontophoresis, a process in which a weak electrical current is applied to the sweaty area, is sometimes used. Drugs taken by mouth, such as phenoxybenzamine and propantheline, sometimes control sweating, and injections of botulinum toxin into the affected area diminish sweating. If drugs are not effective, a more drastic measure to control severe sweating is surgical cutting of the nerves leading to the sweat glands. Excessive sweating limited to the armpits is sometimes treated by liposuction to remove the sweat glands. Psychologic counseling or antianxiety drugs may relieve sweating caused by anxiety.

For the few people in whom odor is a problem, cleansing twice daily with soap and water usually removes the bacteria and yeast that

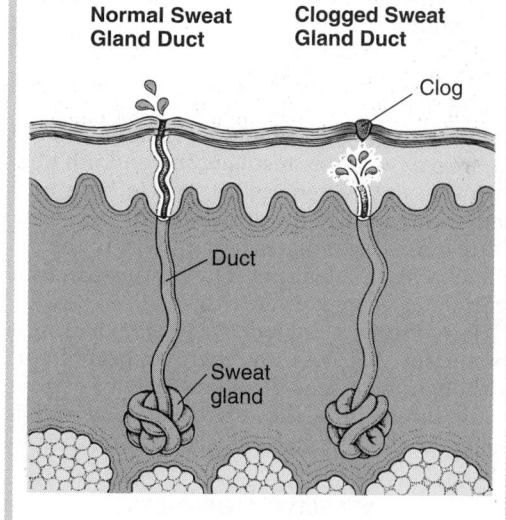

What Causes Prickly Heat?

Prickly heat results when sweat glands are blocked and ruptured, and sweat is trapped below the skin.

Normal Sweat Gland Duct

Clogged Sweat Gland Duct

Clog

Duct

Sweat gland

cause odor. In some people, a few days of washing with an antiseptic soap, which may be combined with use of antibacterial creams containing clindamycin or erythromycin, may be necessary. Shaving the hair in the armpits may also help control odor.

CHAPTER 207

Hair Disorders

Hair originates in the hair follicles, which are located in the dermis, the skin layer just below the surface layer. Hair follicles are present everywhere on the surface of the body except the lips, palms of the hands, and soles of the feet. New hair is made in the hair bulb at the base of the hair follicle. Living cells in the hair bulb multiply and push upward. These cells rapidly dehydrate, die, and compact into a dense, hard mass that forms the hair shaft. The hair shaft, which is made up of dead protein, is covered by a delicate covering (cuticle) composed of platelike scales.

Hair is colored by the pigment melanin, which is also responsible for skin color. Human hair colors come from two types of melanin: eumelanin in black or brown hair and pheomelanin in auburn or blond hair.

Hair grows in cycles. Each cycle consists of a long growing phase followed by a short resting phase. At the end of the resting phase, the hair falls out and a new hair starts growing in the follicle, beginning the cycle again. Eyebrows and eyelashes have a growing phase of 1 to 6 months. Scalp hairs have a growing phase of 2 to 6 years. Normally, about 100 scalp hairs reach the end of the resting phase each day and fall out.

Hair growth is regulated by male hormones (androgens, such as testosterone and dihydrotestosterone), which are present in both men and women, although in different amounts. Testosterone stimulates hair growth in the pubic area and underarms. Dihydrotestosterone stimulates beard hair growth.

Hair disorders include excessive hairiness (hirsutism), hair loss, and ingrown beard hairs. Although most hair disorders are not serious or life threatening, they are often perceived as major cosmetic issues that require treatment.

Excessive Hairiness

Different people have widely varying amounts of body hair. A person's age, sex, racial and ethnic origin, and hereditary factors determine the amount of body hair. The definition of "excessive" hair is subjective. In some cultures, hairy men are considered masculine; in others, hairiness is eschewed. Some women detest having any body hair, whereas others are not concerned by it. Rarely, excessive hairiness is present at birth (because of a hereditary disorder) but usually develops later in life. In women and children, excessive hairiness can be caused by disorders of the pituitary gland, adrenal glands, or ovaries that result in overproduction of male hormones. The condition may also result from the use of certain drugs, such as minoxidil, phenytoin, cyclosporine, and anabolic steroids. Porphyria cutanea tarda, an enzyme deficiency disorder,▲ also may cause excessive hair growth.

Diagnosis and Treatment

Because some medical disorders stimulate excessive hair growth, doctors must distinguish excessive hairiness that is the result of

an underlying medical problem from hair growth that is simply a cosmetic concern.

A doctor first looks for other symptoms of excess androgens, such as irregular menstrual cycles, deepening voice, baldness, or features of Cushing's syndrome,■ such as a large round face and a pad of fat between the shoulders. If any of these symptoms are present, doctors perform various blood tests to measure levels of certain hormones.

Drugs possibly causing excessive hairiness are discontinued unless this would cause a health problem. If high testosterone levels are determined to be the cause, drugs that block the effects of testosterone, such as spironolactone, flutamide, or finasteride, can be helpful but are rarely used.

Temporary hair removal methods include shaving or clipping the hair. Although shaving does not make hair grow faster, as is sometimes thought, it does make the hair appear thicker. Other common temporary measures include plucking and waxing, which pull the hairs out at the roots, and using a depilatory (a liquid or cream preparation), which chemically removes the hair at the surface. Eflornithine cream substantially slows hair growth in many people and may decrease the need to manually remove hair. Hair bleach may mask excessive hairiness if the hair texture is fine.

Permanent hair removal requires that the hair follicles be destroyed. Electrolysis, in which an electric needle is inserted into each hair follicle, destroys the hair follicles by heat and electrical current. Multiple treatments are often necessary, and many follicles often survive the procedure, allowing hair regrowth. Laser treatments also may reduce unwanted hair.★ Although multiple laser treatments may permanently destroy some hair follicles, much hair eventually grows back.

Hair Loss

Hair loss (alopecia), most common on the head, may affect any part of the body.

Hair loss may develop gradually or suddenly. It results from hereditary factors, aging, local skin conditions, and diseases that affect the body generally (systemic diseases). Many different drugs can also cause hair loss. When it occurs on the head, hair loss is generally referred to as baldness.

Androgenetic alopecia is the most common type of hair loss, eventually affecting about half of all men (male-pattern baldness) and 10

▲ see page 933   ■ see page 958

★ see box on page 1235

to 20% of women (female-pattern baldness). A slightly elevated level of the male hormone dihydrotestosterone probably plays a major role, along with genetic factors. The hair loss can begin at any age, even during the teenage years.

In men, hair loss usually begins at the forehead or on the top of the head toward the back. Some men lose only some hair and have only a receding hairline or a small bald spot in the back. Others, especially men whose hair loss began at a young age, lose all of the hair on the top of the head but retain hair on the sides and back of the scalp.

In women, hair loss begins on the top of the head and is usually a thinning of the hair rather than a complete loss of hair. The hairline typically stays intact. This pattern is referred to as female-pattern baldness.

Toxic alopecia is hair loss resulting from physical or psychologic stress. Sudden weight loss, many severe illnesses (particularly those that involve a high fever), or surgery may cause hair loss. Some drugs—including chemotherapy drugs, blood pressure drugs, lithium, valproate, oral contraceptives, vitamin A, and retinoids—can also cause the condition. Toxic alopecia may also result from an underactive thyroid gland or pituitary gland and commonly occurs after pregnancy.

The hair may fall out soon after the disease or condition that is causing the hair loss occurs or as long as 3 or 4 months later. Usually, the hair loss is temporary, and the hair grows back.

Alopecia areata is a common skin disorder in which round, irregular patches of hair are suddenly lost. The cause is believed to be an autoimmune reaction, in which the body's immune defenses mistakenly attack the hair follicles. The site of hair loss is usually the scalp or beard. Rarely, all body hair is lost, a condition called alopecia universalis. Alopecia areata occurs in both sexes and at all ages but is most common in children and young adults. Alopecia areata is not the result of another disease, although some people also have a thyroid disorder. The hair usually grows back in several months. In people with widespread hair loss, regrowth is unlikely.

Hair pulling (trichotillomania) is the habitual pulling out of normal hair. The habit is most common in children but may occur in adults. The hair pulling may not be noticed for a long time, making doctors and parents think that an illness such as alopecia areata or a fungal infection is causing the hair loss.

Scarring alopecia is hair loss that occurs at scarred or damaged areas. The skin may be damaged from burns and other physical injuries or from x-ray therapy. Diseases that cause scarring include lupus erythematosus, lichen planus, and persistent bacterial or fungal infections. Skin cancers also may scar the skin.

Diagnosis and Treatment

A doctor diagnoses male-pattern or female-pattern baldness based on its typical appearance. Determining the cause of other types of hair loss simply by observation is sometimes difficult. A doctor usually examines the hair shafts under a microscope and may perform a biopsy of the skin.▲ A biopsy helps determine if the hair follicles are normal; if they are not, the biopsy may indicate possible causes. If the doctor's examination finds signs of hormonal irregularities or other serious illness, blood tests to identify those disorders may be needed.

Male-pattern and female-pattern baldness can sometimes be treated effectively with drugs. Minoxidil may stimulate and support hair growth when applied directly to the scalp daily. Finasteride works by blocking the effects of male hormones on the hair follicles and is taken by mouth daily. Improvement may occur with either of these drugs when taken for several months. The most important effect of these drugs may be to prevent further hair loss. The effects last only as long as the drugs are taken.

A more permanent solution is hair transplantation, in which hair follicles are removed from one part of the scalp and transplanted to the bald area. In a newer hair transplantation technique, only one or two hairs are transplanted at a time. Although this technique is more time consuming, it does not require removal of large plugs of skin and allows the implants to be oriented in the same direction as the natural hair.

Toxic alopecia generally resolves after the toxic substance is discontinued. Because the hair loss is usually temporary, wigs often offer the best treatment. A person undergoing chemotherapy should consult a wig maker even before therapy begins so that an appropriate wig can be ready when needed.

Alopecia areata can be treated with corticosteroids. For small bald patches, corticosteroids

▲ see page 1188

are typically injected under the skin of the bald patch, and minoxidil may be applied topically as well. For larger patches, corticosteroids are sometimes taken by mouth, but hair often falls out again when treatment is discontinued. Another treatment for alopecia areata involves applying irritating chemicals, such as anthralin, to the scalp to induce a mild allergic reaction or irritation. The irritation sometimes promotes hair growth.

Scarring alopecia is particularly difficult to treat. When possible, the cause of the scarring is treated, but after an area is fully scarred, hair growth is unlikely.

Ingrown Beard Hairs

A hair that curls so that the tip punctures the skin can cause inflammation (pseudofolliculitis barbae). This most often happens with the curly hairs of the beard, especially in black men. Each ingrown hair results in a tiny, mildly painful pimple with a barely visible hair curling into the center.

Doctors diagnose the condition by its typical appearance. Treatment involves teasing the tips of any ingrown hairs out of the skin with the point of a needle or sharp scalpel. The best preventive treatment is to grow the beard: When the hairs are longer, they do not curl back and puncture the skin. A man who does not want a beard can use a depilatory (a liquid or cream preparation that removes unwanted hair) made of thioglycolate, although it often irritates the skin. People who must shave should shave in the same direction in which the hair grows. Shaving closely with multiple razor strokes should be avoided. People who continue to have problems may undergo laser therapy.▲

CHAPTER 208

Pigment Disorders

Various shades and colors of human skin are created by the brown pigment, melanin. Without melanin, the skin would be pale white with varying shades of pink caused by the blood flowing through it. Fair-skinned people produce very little melanin; darker-skinned people produce moderate amounts; and very dark skinned people produce a great deal. People with albinism have no melanin.

Melanin is produced by special cells (melanocytes) that are interspersed among the other cells in the top layer of the skin, the epidermis. After melanin is produced, it spreads into other nearby skin cells.

When exposed to sunlight, melanocytes produce increased amounts of melanin, causing the skin to darken, or tan. In some fair-skinned people, certain melanocytes produce more melanin than others in response to sunlight. This uneven melanin production results in spots of pigmentation known as freckles.

A tendency to freckles runs in families. Increased amounts of melanin can also occur in response to hormonal changes, such as those that may take place in Addison's disease, in pregnancy, or with oral contraceptive use. Some cases of skin darkening, however, are not related to increased melanin at all, but rather to abnormal pigments that make their way into the skin. Diseases such as hemochromatosis or hemosiderosis or some drugs that are applied to the skin, swallowed, or injected can cause skin darkening. A buildup of bilirubin (the main pigment in bile) causes the skin to turn yellow (jaundice).

An abnormally low amount of melanin (hypopigmentation) may affect large areas of the body or small patches. Decreased melanin usually results from a previous injury to the skin such as a blister, ulcer, burn, or skin infection. Sometimes pigment loss results from an inflammatory condition of the skin or, in rare instances, is hereditary. A common skin infection, tinea versicolor,■ can also cause pigment loss in patches of skin.

▲ see box on page 1235   ■ see page 1227

Albinism

Albinism is a rare hereditary disorder in which little or no melanin is formed.

Albinism occurs in people throughout the world and in all races.

Albinism is easily recognized by its typical appearance. People with albinism (albinos) have white hair, pale skin, and pink or pale blue eyes. The genetic disorder causing albinism also results in abnormal vision and involuntary eye movements (nystagmus).

Because melanin protects the skin from the sun, people with albinism are very prone to sunburn and, therefore, to skin cancer. Even a few minutes of bright sunlight can cause serious burns.

There is no cure for albinism. People with the disorder can minimize problems by staying out of direct sunlight, wearing sunglasses, and applying sunscreen with the highest sun protection factor (SPF) rating.▲ Even while wearing sunscreen, people with albinism should not expose their skin to bright sunlight for any prolonged period.

Vitiligo

Vitiligo is a disorder in which a localized loss of melanocytes results in smooth white patches of skin.

The cause of vitiligo is unknown, but it may involve an attack by the person's immune system on melanocytes. Vitiligo tends to run in families and may occur with certain other diseases. Thyroid disease is present in almost one third of people with vitiligo, but the relationship between the disorders is unclear. People with diabetes, Addison's disease, and pernicious anemia also are somewhat more likely to develop vitiligo. The disorder may occur after physical trauma or a sunburn.

Although vitiligo does not pose a medical problem, it may cause considerable psychologic distress.

Symptoms and Diagnosis

In some people, one or two sharply demarcated patches of vitiligo appear; in others, patches appear over a large part of the body. The changes are most striking in dark-skinned people. Commonly affected areas are the face, elbows and knees, hands and feet, and genitals. The unpigmented skin is extremely prone to sunburn. The areas of skin affected

by vitiligo also produce white hair, because the melanocytes are lost from the hair follicles. Premature graying of scalp hair may occur even when the underlying skin is unaffected by vitiligo.

Vitiligo is recognized by its typical appearance. A Wood's light examination is often performed to help distinguish vitiligo from other causes of lightened skin.■ Other tests and biopsies are rarely necessary.

Treatment

No cure is known for vitiligo, although some people regain their color spontaneously. Treatment may be helpful. Small patches sometimes darken when treated with corticosteroid creams. Some people use bronzers, skin stains, or makeup to darken the area. Because many people still have a few melanocytes in the patches of vitiligo, phototherapy restimulates pigment production in more than half of them.★ In particular, psoralens (light-sensitive drugs) combined with ultraviolet A light (PUVA) and narrow-band ultraviolet B light treatments are most beneficial. However, phototherapy takes months to be effective and must be continued indefinitely.

Areas that do not respond to phototherapy may be treated with various skin-grafting techniques and even transplantation of melanocytes grown from unaffected areas of the person's skin. All affected areas of skin must be protected from the sun with sunscreen and clothing.

Some people who have very large areas of vitiligo sometimes prefer to bleach the pigment out of the unaffected skin to achieve an even color. Bleaching is done with repeated applications of hydroquinone cream to the skin for weeks to years. The effects of bleaching are irreversible.

Melasma

Melasma produces dark brown patches of pigmentation on sun-exposed areas, usually the face.

Melasma tends to appear during pregnancy (mask of pregnancy) and in women who take oral contraceptives, although it can occur in

---

▲ see also page 1231

■ see page 1188

★ see box on page 1202

anyone. The disorder is most common in sunny climates and in people of Latin or Asian origin.

Melasma produces irregular, patchy areas of dark color that are the same on both sides of the face. The pigmentation most often occurs in the center of the face and on the cheeks, forehead, upper lip, and nose. Sometimes people have the patches only on the sides of the face. Rarely, melasma appears on the forearms.

The patches do not itch or hurt and are only of cosmetic significance.

Melasma usually fades after pregnancy or when an oral contraceptive is discontinued. People with melasma can use sunscreens on the dark patches and avoid sun exposure to prevent the condition from getting worse. Skin-bleaching creams containing hydroquinone and retinoic acid can help lighten the dark patches.

CHAPTER 209

Blistering Diseases

A blister (bulla) is a bubble of fluid that forms beneath a thin layer of dead skin. The fluid is a mixture of water and proteins that oozes from injured tissue. Blisters most commonly form in response to a specific injury, such as a burn or irritation, and usually involve only the topmost layers of skin. These blisters heal quickly, usually without leaving a scar. Blisters that develop as part of a systemic (bodywide) disease may start in the deeper layers of the skin and cover widespread areas. These blisters heal more slowly and may leave scars.

Many diseases and injuries can cause blistering, but three autoimmune diseases—pemphigus, bullous pemphigoid, and dermatitis herpetiformis—are among the most serious. In an autoimmune disease, the body's immune system, which normally protects the body against foreign invaders, mistakenly attacks the body's own cells▲—in this case, the skin.

Pemphigus

Pemphigus (pemphigus vulgaris) is a rare, severe autoimmune disease in which blisters of varying sizes break out on the skin, the lining of the mouth, the genitals, and other mucous membranes.

Pemphigus develops most often in middle-aged or older people. It rarely develops in children. In this disease, the immune system produces antibodies that attack specific proteins that connect the epidermal cells (the cells in the top layer of skin) to each other. When these connections are disrupted, the cells separate from the lower layers of the skin, and blisters form. A similar-appearing but less dangerous disease, bullous pemphigoid, results in shallower blisters.

Symptoms

The major symptom of pemphigus is the development of clear, soft, painful blisters of various sizes. In addition, the top layer of skin may detach from the lower layers in response to slight pinching or rubbing, causing it to peel off in sheets.

The blisters that develop often first appear in the mouth and soon rupture, forming painful ulcers (sores). More blisters and ulcers may follow until the entire lining of the mouth is affected, causing difficulty swallowing. Blisters form on the skin as well. These blisters then rupture, leaving raw, painful, crusted wounds. The person feels generally ill. Blisters may be widespread, and once ruptured, they may become infected. When severe, pemphigus is as harmful as a serious burn. Similar to a burn, the damaged skin oozes large amounts of fluid and is prone to infection by many types of bacteria.

Diagnosis and Treatment

Doctors usually recognize pemphigus by its characteristic blisters, but the disorder is diagnosed with certainty by examining a sample of

---

▲ see page 1073

skin under a microscope (skin biopsy). Sometimes doctors use special chemical stains that allow antibody deposits to be seen under the microscope. Doctors differentiate pemphigus from bullous pemphigoid by noting the layers of skin involved and the particular appearance of the antibody deposits.

Without treatment, pemphigus is usually fatal. With treatment, 90% of people with pemphigus survive. High doses of corticosteroids are the mainstay of treatment. If the disease is controlled, the dose of corticosteroids is tapered. If the person does not respond to treatment or the disease flares up as the dose is tapered, an immunosuppressant, such as azathioprine or cyclophosphamide, is also given. People with severe pemphigus may also undergo plasmapheresis, a process in which antibodies are filtered from the blood.▲ Injections of gold salts are sometimes used. Immune globulin given intravenously is a new, safe and effective treatment for severe pemphigus. Some people respond well enough to discontinue drug therapy, whereas others must continue taking low doses of the drugs for long periods.

In a hospital, the raw skin surfaces require extraordinary care, similar to the care given to people with severe burns. Antibiotics may be needed to treat infections in ruptured blisters. Dressings, sometimes filled with petroleum jelly, can protect raw, oozing areas.

Bullous Pemphigoid

Bullous pemphigoid is an autoimmune disease that causes blistering of the skin.

Bullous pemphigoid tends to occur mainly in older people. It is a less serious disease than pemphigus, is rarely fatal, and does not result in widespread peeling of skin. It can involve a large portion of the skin, however, and can be very uncomfortable.

In bullous pemphigoid, the immune system forms antibodies directed against the skin, resulting in large, tense, very itchy blisters surrounded by areas of red, inflamed skin. Blisters in the mouth are uncommon and are not severe. The areas of skin that are not blistered appear normal.

Diagnosis and Treatment

Doctors usually recognize bullous pemphigoid by its characteristic blisters. However, it is not always easy to distinguish from pemphigus and other blistering conditions, such as

severe poison ivy; it is diagnosed with certainty by examining a sample of skin under a microscope (skin biopsy). Doctors differentiate bullous pemphigoid from pemphigus by noting the layers of skin involved and the particular appearance of the antibody deposits.

Mild bullous pemphigoid sometimes resolves without treatment, but resolution usually takes months or years. Therefore, most people receive drug therapy. Nearly everyone responds quickly to high-dose corticosteroids, which are tapered after several weeks. Sometimes azathioprine or cyclophosphamide is given as well. Immune globulin given intravenously is a safe, promising new treatment, especially for people who do not respond to conventional drug therapy. Although some local skin care may be needed, most people do not require hospitalization or intensive skin care treatment.

Dermatitis Herpetiformis

Dermatitis herpetiformis is an autoimmune disease causing clusters of intensely itchy small blisters and hivelike swellings.

Despite its name, dermatitis herpetiformis has nothing to do with the herpes virus. In people with dermatitis herpetiformis, glutens (proteins) in wheat, rye, and barley products somehow activate the immune system, which attacks parts of the skin and causes the rash and itching. People with dermatitis herpetiformis may develop celiac disease,■ which is caused by the gluten sensitivity. These people have a higher incidence of other autoimmune diseases, such as thyroiditis, systemic lupus erythematosus, sarcoidosis, and diabetes. People with dermatitis herpetiformis occasionally develop lymphoma in the intestines.

Small blisters usually develop gradually, mostly on the elbows, knees, buttocks, lower back, and back of the head. Sometimes blisters break out on the face and neck. Itching and burning are likely to be severe. Anti-inflammatory drugs, such as ibuprofen, may worsen the rash.

Diagnosis and Treatment

The diagnosis is based on a skin biopsy, in which doctors find particular kinds and patterns of antibodies in the skin samples.

▲ see box on page 986

■ see page 736

The blisters do not go away without treatment. The drug dapsone, taken by mouth, almost always provides relief in 1 to 2 days, but requires that blood counts be checked regularly. Once the disease has been brought under control with drugs and the person has followed a strict gluten-free diet (a diet that is free of wheat, rye, and barley) for 6 months or longer, drug treatment usually can be discontinued. However, some people can never discontinue the drug. In most people, any reexposure to gluten, however small, will trigger another outbreak. A gluten-free diet may prevent the development of intestinal lymphoma.

CHAPTER 210

Parasitic Skin Infections

Most skin parasites are tiny insects or worms that burrow into the skin and make their home there. Some parasites live in the skin for part of their life cycle; others would be permanent residents.

Scabies

Scabies is a mite infestation that produces tiny reddish bumps and severe itching.

Scabies is caused by the itch mite *Sarcoptes scabiei.* The infestation spreads easily from person to person on physical contact, often spreading through an entire household. In rare cases, mites can be spread on clothing, bedding, and other shared objects, but their survival is brief, and normal laundering destroys them.

The female itch mite tunnels in the topmost layer of the skin and deposits her eggs in burrows. Young mites (larvae) then hatch in a few days. The infestation causes intense itching, probably from an allergic reaction to the mites.

Symptoms and Diagnosis

The hallmark of scabies is intense itching, which is usually worse at night. The burrows of the mites are often visible as very thin lines up to ½ inch long, sometimes with a tiny bump at one end. Sometimes, only tiny bumps are seen, many of which are scratched open because of the itching. The burrows can be anywhere on the body except the face. Common sites are the webs between the fingers and toes, the wrists, ankles, buttocks, and, in males, the genitals. Over time, the burrows may become difficult to see because they are obscured by inflammation induced by scratching. People with a weakened immune system may develop severe infestations, which produce large areas of thickened, crusted skin.

Usually, itching and the appearance of burrows are all that are needed to make a diagnosis of scabies. However, a doctor can confirm the diagnosis by taking a scraping from the bumps or burrows and looking at it under a microscope to confirm the presence of mites, eggs, or mite feces.

Treatment

Scabies can be cured by applying a cream containing 5% permethrin, which is left on the skin overnight and then washed off. Although only one treatment is usually needed, some people require a second treatment a week later. Ivermectin taken by mouth in two doses given a week apart also is effective and is especially helpful for severe infestations in people with a weakened immune system.

Even after successful treatment, itching may persist for up to 2 weeks because of a continued allergic reaction to the mite bodies, which remain in the skin for a while. The itching can be treated with mild corticosteroid cream and antihistamines taken by mouth.▲ Occasionally, the skin irritation and deep scratches lead to a bacterial infection, which may require antibiotics given by mouth.

Family members and people who have had close physical contact, such as sexual contact,

---

▲ see page 1192

with a person with scabies should be treated as well. Clothing and bedding used during the preceding few days should be washed in hot water and dried in a hot dryer or can be dry cleaned.

Lice Infestation

Lice infestation (pediculosis) is a skin infestation by tiny wingless insects.

Lice are barely visible wingless insects that spread easily from person to person by body contact and shared clothing and other personal items. Three species of lice inhabit different parts of the body.

Head lice infest the scalp hair. The infestation is spread by personal contact and possibly by shared combs, brushes, hats, and other personal items. Head lice are a common scourge of school children of all social strata. Head lice are less common among blacks.

Body lice usually infest people who have poor hygiene and those living in close quarters or crowded institutions. They live in the seams of garments that are in contact with the skin.

Pubic lice ("crabs"), which infest the genital area, are typically spread during sexual contact. These lice may infest the chest hair, underarm hair, beard hair, eyebrows, and eyelashes as well.

Symptoms and Diagnosis

Lice infestation causes severe itching in the infested area. Intense scratching often breaks the skin, which can lead to bacterial infections. Children may hardly notice head lice or may have only a vague scalp irritation.

Lice themselves are sometimes hard to find, but their eggs are readily apparent. Female lice lay shiny grayish white eggs (nits) that can be seen as tiny globules firmly stuck to hairs near their base. With chronic scalp infestations, the nits grow out with the hair and therefore can be found some distance from the scalp, depending on the duration of the infestation.

Nits are distinguished from other foreign material present on hair shafts by the fact that they are so strongly attached. Adult body lice and their eggs also may be found in the seams of clothing worn close to the skin.

Treatment

Several effective prescription and nonprescription drugs are available to treat lice. Non-

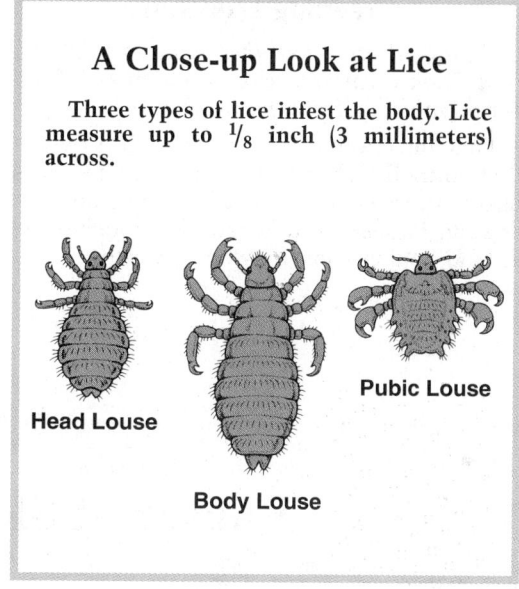

A Close-up Look at Lice

Three types of lice infest the body. Lice measure up to 1/8 inch (3 millimeters) across.

Head Louse

Body Louse

Pubic Louse

prescription shampoos and creams containing pyrethrins plus piperonyl butoxide are applied for 10 minutes and are then rinsed out. Prescription permethrin, applied as a liquid or as a cream, is also effective. Lindane—a prescription drug that can be applied as a cream, lotion, or shampoo—also cures lice infestation but is not as effective as the other preparations and is not recommended for children because of possible neurologic side effects. Prescription malathion, although highly effective at killing both adult lice and eggs, is not considered a first line of treatment because it is flammable, has an objectionable odor, and must remain on the skin for 8 to 12 hours. All louse treatments are repeated in 7 to 10 days to kill newly hatched lice.

After a drug application, nits must be removed manually, because drugs do not kill all nits and because it is not possible to distinguish between living and dead nits. Removal requires a fine-tooth comb—which is often packaged with the medication—and careful searching (hence the term "nit-picking"). Because the nits are so strongly stuck to the hair, several nonprescription preparations are available to loosen them. The nits of body lice are destroyed simply by throwing away infested clothing.

Sources of infestation (combs, hats, clothing, and bedding) should be decontaminated by laundering or dry cleaning.

Creeping Eruption

Creeping eruption (cutaneous larva migrans) is a hookworm infection transmitted from warm, moist soil to exposed skin.

This infection is caused by a hookworm that normally inhabits dogs and cats. The eggs of the parasite are deposited on the ground in dog and cat feces. When bare skin touches the ground, which happens when a person walks barefoot or sunbathes, the hookworm gets into the skin. Starting from the site of infection—usually the feet, legs, buttocks, or back—the hookworm burrows along a haphazard tract, leaving a winding, threadlike, raised, red rash. The eruption itches intensely.

A liquid preparation of thiabendazole applied to the area effectively treats the infection. Thiabendazole or ivermectin given by mouth also is effective.

CHAPTER 211

Bacterial Skin Infections

The skin provides a remarkably good barrier against bacterial infections. Although many bacteria come in contact with or reside on the skin, they are normally unable to establish an infection. When bacterial skin infections do occur, they can range in size from a tiny spot to the entire body surface. They can range in seriousness as well, from harmless to life threatening.

Many types of bacteria can infect the skin. The most common are *Staphylococcus* and *Streptococcus*. Skin infections caused by less common bacteria may develop in hospitals or nursing homes or while gardening or swimming in a pond, lake, or ocean.

Some people are at particular risk of contracting skin infections—for example, people with diabetes because they are likely to have poor blood flow, especially to the hands and feet, and because high levels of sugar in the blood decrease the ability of white blood cells to fight infections. People with AIDS or other immune disorders and those undergoing chemotherapy are at higher risk as well, because they have a weakened immune system. Skin that is inflamed or damaged by sunburn, scratching, or other trauma is more likely to be infected. In fact, any break in the skin predisposes a person to infection.

Prevention involves keeping the skin undamaged and clean. When the skin is cut or scraped, the injury should be washed with soap and water and covered with a sterile bandage. Antibiotic creams and ointments may be applied to open areas to keep the tissue moist and to try to prevent bacterial invasion. If an infection develops, small areas may be treated with antibiotic creams. Larger areas require antibiotics taken by mouth or given by injection. Abscesses (pus-filled pockets) should be cut open by the doctor and allowed to drain, and any dead tissue must be surgically removed.

Cellulitis

Cellulitis is a spreading bacterial infection of the skin and the tissues immediately beneath the skin.

Cellulitis may be caused by many different bacteria; the most common are those of the *Streptococcus* species. Streptococci spread rapidly in the skin because they produce enzymes that hinder the ability of the tissue to confine the infection. *Staphylococcus* bacteria can also cause cellulitis, as can many other bacteria, especially after bites by humans or animals or after injuries in water or dirt.

Bacteria usually enter through small breaks in the epidermis that result from scrapes, punctures, burns, and skin disorders such as dermatitis.▲ Areas of the skin that become swollen with fluid (edema) are especially vulnerable. However, cellulitis can also occur in skin that is not overtly injured.

▲ see page 1193

Symptoms and Complications

Cellulitis most commonly develops on the legs but can occur anywhere. The first symptoms are redness, pain, and tenderness over an area of skin. These symptoms are caused both by the bacteria themselves and by the body's attempts to halt the infection. The infected skin becomes hot and slightly swollen and may look slightly pitted, like an orange peel. Fluid-filled blisters, which may be small (vesicles) or large (bullae), sometimes appear on the infected skin. **Erysipelas** is one form of streptococcal cellulitis in which the skin is bright red and noticeably swollen and the edges of the infected area are raised. The swelling occurs because the infection blocks the lymphatic vessels in the skin.

Most people with cellulitis feel only mildly ill, but some may have a fever, chills, rapid heart rate, headache, low blood pressure, and confusion.

As the infection spreads, nearby lymph nodes may become enlarged and tender (lymphadenitis). Other complications—lymphangitis,▲ skin abscesses,■ and spread through the blood (sepsis★)—are also possible.

When cellulitis affects the same site repeatedly, especially the leg, lymphatic vessels may be damaged, causing permanent swelling of the affected tissue.

Diagnosis and Treatment

A doctor usually diagnoses cellulitis based on its appearance and symptoms. Laboratory identification of the bacteria from blood, pus, or tissue specimens usually is not necessary unless a person is seriously ill. Sometimes, doctors need to perform tests to differentiate cellulitis from a blood clot in the deep veins of the leg (deep vein thrombosis,● because the symptoms of these disorders are similar.

Prompt treatment with antibiotics can prevent the infection from spreading rapidly and reaching the blood and organs. Antibiotics, such as dicloxacillin or cephalexin, that are effective against both streptococci and staphylococci are used. People with mild cellulitis may take antibiotics by mouth; those with rapidly spreading cellulitis, high fever, or other evidence of serious infection often receive intravenous antibiotics. Also, the affected part of the body, when possible, is kept immobile and elevated to help reduce swelling. Cool, wet dressings applied to the infected area may relieve discomfort.

Symptoms of cellulitis usually disappear after a few days of antibiotic therapy. However, symptoms often get worse before they get better, probably because with the death of the bacteria, substances that cause tissue damage are released. When this occurs, the body continues to react even though the bacteria are dead. Antibiotics are continued for 10 days or longer even though the symptoms may disappear earlier.

Necrotizing Skin Infections

Necrotizing skin infections, including necrotizing cellulitis and necrotizing fasciitis, are severe forms of cellulitis characterized by death of infected tissue (necrosis).

Most skin infections do not result in death of skin and nearby tissues. Sometimes, however, bacterial infection can cause small blood vessels in the infected area to clot. This clotting causes the tissue fed by these vessels to die from lack of blood. Because the body's immune defenses that travel through the bloodstream (such as white blood cells and antibodies) can no longer reach this area, the infection spreads rapidly and may be difficult to control. Death is not uncommon, even with appropriate treatment.

Some necrotizing skin infections spread deep in the skin along the surface of the muscle (fascia) and are termed necrotizing fasciitis. Other necrotizing skin infections spread on the outer layers of skin and are termed necrotizing cellulitis. Several different bacteria, such as *Streptococcus* and *Clostridia*, may cause necrotizing skin infections, although in many people the infection is caused by a combination of bacteria. The streptococcal infection in particular has been termed "flesh-eating disease" by the lay press, although it differs little from the others.

Some necrotizing skin infections begin at puncture wounds or lacerations, particularly wounds contaminated with dirt and debris. Other infections begin in surgical incisions or even healthy skin. Sometimes people with diverticulitis, intestinal perforation, or tumors of the intestine develop necrotizing infections of the abdominal wall, genital area, or thighs.

▲ see page 241   ■ see page 1224
★ see page 1118
● see page 232

These infections occur when certain bacteria escape from the intestine and spread to the skin. The bacteria may initially create an abscess in the abdominal cavity and spread directly outward to the skin, or they may spread through the bloodstream to the skin and other organs.

Symptoms and Diagnosis

Symptoms often begin just as for cellulitis.▲ The skin may look pale at first, but quickly becomes red or bronze and warm to the touch, and sometimes becomes swollen. Later, the skin turns violet, often with the development of large fluid-filled blisters (bullae). The fluid from these blisters is brown, watery, and sometimes foul smelling. Areas of dead skin (gangrene) turn black. Some types of infection, including those produced by *Clostridia* and mixed bacteria, produce gas.■ The gas creates bubbles under the skin and sometimes in the blisters themselves, causing the skin to feel crackly when pressed. Initially the infected area is painful, but as the skin dies, the nerves stop working and the area loses sensation.

The person usually feels very ill and has a fever, a rapid heart rate, and mental deterioration ranging from confusion to unconsciousness. Blood pressure may fall because of toxins secreted by the bacteria and the body's response to the infection (septic shock★).

A doctor makes a diagnosis of necrotizing skin infection based on its appearance, particularly the presence of gas bubbles under the skin. X-rays may show gas under the skin as well. The specific bacteria involved are identified by laboratory analysis of infected fluid and tissue samples. However, treatment must begin before a doctor can be certain which bacteria are causing the infection.

Treatment and Prognosis

The treatment for necrotizing fasciitis is intravenous antibiotic therapy and surgical removal of the dead tissue. Large amounts of skin, tissue, and muscle must often be removed, and in some cases, an affected arm or leg may have to be amputated. People with necrotizing infections caused by anaerobic bacteria (for example, *Clostridium perfrin-*

▲ see page 1220

■ see page 1101

★ see page 1119

● see box on page 1097

gens)● may benefit from treatment in a high-pressure (hyperbaric) oxygen chamber.

The overall death rate is about 30%. Older people, those who have other medical disorders, and those in whom the disease has reached an advanced stage have a poorer outcome.

Erythrasma

Erythrasma is infection of the top layers of the skin caused by the bacterium Corynebacterium minutissimum.

Erythrasma affects mostly adults, especially those with diabetes; it is most common in the tropics. Erythrasma often appears in areas where skin touches skin, such as under the breasts and in the armpits, webs of the toes, and genital area—especially in men, where the thighs touch the scrotum. The infection can produce irregularly shaped pink patches that may later turn into fine brown scales. In some people, the infection spreads to the torso and anal area.

Although erythrasma may be confused with a fungal infection, doctors can easily diagnose erythrasma because skin infected with *Corynebacterium* glows coral red under an ultraviolet light.

An antibiotic given by mouth, such as erythromycin or tetracycline, can eliminate the infection. Antibacterial soaps, such as chlorhexidine, may also help. Topical drugs such as clindamycin and miconazole cream are also effective. Erythrasma may recur in 6 to 12 months, necessitating a second treatment.

Impetigo

Impetigo is a skin infection, caused by Staphylococcus aureus, Streptococcus pyogenes, *or both, that leads to the formation of scabby, yellow-crusted sores and, sometimes, small blisters filled with yellow fluid.*

Impetigo is common. It affects mostly children. Impetigo can occur anywhere on the body but most commonly occurs on the face, arms, and legs. The blisters that may form (bullous impetigo) can vary from pea-sized to large rings and can last for days to weeks. Impetigo often affects normal skin but may follow an injury or a condition that causes a break in the skin, such as a fungal infection, sunburn, or an insect bite.

Impetigo is itchy and slightly painful. The itching often leads to extensive scratching, particularly in children, which serves to spread the infection. Impetigo is very contagious—both to other areas of the person's own skin and to other people.

The infected area should be washed gently with soap and water several times a day to remove any crusts. Small areas are treated with bacitracin ointment or mupirocin cream or ointment. If large areas are involved, an antibiotic taken by mouth, such as a cephalosporin, may be needed.

Staphylococcal Scalded Skin Syndrome

Staphylococcal scalded skin syndrome is a reaction to a staphylococcal skin infection in which the skin peels off as though burned.

Certain types of staphylococci bacteria secrete toxic substances that cause the top layer of the epidermis to split from the rest of the skin. Because the toxin spreads throughout the body, staphylococcal infection of a small area of skin may result in peeling over the entire body. Staphylococcal scalded skin syndrome occurs almost exclusively in infants, young children, and people with a weakened immune system. Like other staphylococcal infections, staphylococcal scalded skin syndrome is contagious.

Symptoms

Symptoms begin with an isolated, crusted infection that may look like impetigo. In newborns, the infection may appear in the diaper area or around the stump of the umbilical cord. In adults, the infection may begin anywhere. In all people with this disorder, scarlet-colored areas appear around the crusted area within a day of the beginning of infection. These areas may be painful. Then, other large areas of skin distant from the initial infection redden and develop blisters that break easily.

The top layer of the skin then begins peeling off, often in large sheets, with even slight touching or gentle pushing. Within another 1 to 2 days, the entire skin surface may be involved, and the person becomes very ill with a fever, chills, and weakness. With the loss of the protective skin barrier, other bacteria and infective organisms can easily penetrate the body, causing what doctors call superinfections. Also, critical amounts of fluid can be lost because of oozing and evaporation, resulting in dehydration.

Diagnosis and Treatment

A diagnosis is made by the appearance of skin peeling after an apparent staphylococcal infection. If no signs of staphylococcal infection are observed, doctors often perform a biopsy, in which a small piece of skin is removed, examined under a microscope, and sent to the laboratory to be cultured for bacteria.▲

Antibiotics given intravenously, such as nafcillin or cefazolin, are started quickly. Treatment continues for at least 10 days. With early treatment, healing takes 5 to 7 days.

The skin must be protected to help prevent further peeling; it should be treated as if it were burned.

Folliculitis, Skin Abscesses, and Carbuncles

Folliculitis, skin abscesses, and carbuncles are pus-filled pockets in the skin resulting from bacterial infection.

Most skin infections involving pus-filled pockets are caused by *Staphylococcus aureus* bacteria.■ Sometimes the bacteria enter the skin through a hair follicle, small scrape, or puncture, although often there is no obvious point of entry. People who have poor hygiene or chronic skin diseases or whose nasal passages contain *Staphylococcus* are more likely to have episodes of these skin infections. Some people may have recurring episodes of infection for unknown reasons.

Doctors may try to eliminate *Staphylococcus* from people prone to recurring infections by instructing them to wash the entire body with antibacterial soap, apply antibiotic ointment inside the nose, and take antibiotics by mouth.

Folliculitis, skin abscesses, and carbuncles differ in the size and depth of the pus-filled pockets.

Folliculitis: Folliculitis is an infection of a hair follicle. It looks like a tiny white pimple at the base of a hair. There may be only one infected follicle or many. Each infected follicle is slightly painful, but the person otherwise does not feel sick.

Some people develop folliculitis after exposure to a poorly chlorinated hot tub or whirl-

---

▲ see page 1188

■ see also page 1111

pool. This condition, sometimes called "hot-tub folliculitis" or "hot-tub dermatitis," is caused by the bacterium *Pseudomonas aeruginosa*. It begins anytime from 6 hours to 5 days after the exposure. Areas of skin covered by a bathing suit, such as the torso and buttocks, are the most common sites.

Sometimes stiff hairs in the beard area curl and reenter the skin (ingrown hair) after shaving, producing irritation without substantial infection. This type of folliculitis (pseudofolliculitis barbae) is particularly common in black men.

Folliculitis is treated with warm compresses. Sometimes, topical antibiotics with mupirocin or clindamycin are applied 2 to 3 times per day. Large areas of folliculitis may require antibiotics, such as dicloxacillin or cephalexin, taken by mouth. Hot-tub folliculitis goes away in a week without any treatment. Folliculitis caused by ingrown hairs is treated by a number of methods with varying success. For severe, recurring problems, shaving may need to be discontinued.

Skin Abscesses: Skin abscesses, also called boils or furuncles, are warm, painful pus-filled pockets of infection below the skin surface. Abscesses may be from one to several inches in diameter. If not treated, they often come to a point and rupture. Bacteria may spread from the abscess to infect the surrounding tissue and lymph nodes. The person may have a fever and feel generally sick.

A doctor treats an abscess by cutting it open and draining the pus. After draining the abscess, a doctor makes sure all of the pus has been removed by washing out the pocket with a sterile salt solution. Sometimes the drained abscess is packed with gauze, which is removed 24 to 48 hours later.

If the abscess is completely drained, antibiotics usually are not needed. However, if the infection has spread or if the abscess is on the middle or upper part of the face, antibiotics that kill staphylococci, such as dicloxacillin and cephalexin, may be used because of the high risk that the infection will spread to the brain.

Carbuncles: Carbuncles are clusters of small, shallow abscesses that connect with each other under the skin. Multiple areas may

open and drain pus spontaneously. The person often has a fever and feels fatigued and sick. Carbuncles are more common in men and usually occur on the back of the neck. They often result in extensive peeling of skin and scar formation. Older people, people with diabetes, and people with serious medical disorders are more prone to carbuncles.

Treatment is with antibiotics taken by mouth. Any large abscesses are cut open to allow pus to drain. Carbuncles are hard to eliminate because many small pus-filled pockets are difficult to find and drain. Therefore, antibiotics must sometimes be continued for several months.

Hidradenitis Suppurativa

Hidradenitis suppurativa is inflammation of the apocrine sweat glands resulting in painful accumulations of pus under the skin.

Hidradenitis suppurativa develops in some people after puberty because of chronic blockage of the apocrine sweat glands (the specialized sweat glands under the arms, in the genital area, around the anus, and under the breasts). Doctors do not know why the blockage occurs, but it is not related to the use of deodorants or powders or to underarm shaving. The blockage causes the glands to swell and rupture, frequently leading to infection by various bacteria. The abscesses (pus-filled pockets) that result are painful and foul smelling and tend to recur. After several recurrences, the skin in the area becomes thick and scarred.

Hidradenitis suppurativa resembles common skin abscesses. A doctor makes the diagnosis based on the location of the abscesses and on the fact that they recur often.

For people with mild cases, a doctor injects corticosteroids into the area and prescribes antibiotics, such as tetracycline or erythromycin, to be taken by mouth. Clindamycin applied topically is also effective. In some cases, a doctor cuts open the abscesses to drain the pus. For severe cases, isotretinoin, an anti-inflammatory drug, may be given by mouth. Laser treatment has also been used. In severe cases, cutting out the involved area followed by skin grafting may be necessary.

CHAPTER 212

Fungal Skin Infections

Fungi usually make their homes in moist areas of the body where skin surfaces meet: between the toes, in the genital area, and under the breasts. Many fungi that infect the skin (dermatophytes) live only in the topmost layer of the epidermis (stratum corneum) and do not penetrate deeper. Obese people are more likely to get these infections because they have excessive skinfolds. People with diabetes tend to be more susceptible to fungal infections as well.

Strangely, fungal infections on one part of the body can cause rashes on other parts of the body that are not infected. For example, a fungal infection on the foot may cause an itchy, bumpy rash on the fingers. These eruptions (dermatophytids, or id reactions) are allergic reactions to the fungus. They do not result from touching the infected area.

A doctor may suspect a fungal infection upon seeing a red, irritated, or scaly rash in one of the commonly affected areas. The doctor can usually confirm the diagnosis by scraping off a small amount of skin and having it examined under a microscope or placed in a culture medium that will grow the specific fungus so that it can be identified.▲

Ringworm

Ringworm (tinea) is a fungal skin infection caused by several different fungi and generally classified by its location on the body.

Despite its name, ringworm infection does not involve worms. The name arose because of the ring-shaped skin patches created by the infection.

Athlete's foot (tinea pedis) is a common fungal infection that usually appears during warm weather. The infection may spread from person to person in communal showers and bathrooms or in other moist areas where infected people walk barefoot. It is usually caused by either *Trichophyton* or *Epidermophyton*. These fungi most commonly grow in the warm, moist areas between the toes. The fungus can produce mild scaling with or without redness and itching. The scaling may involve a small area or the entire sole of the foot; sometimes even the toenails are involved. Sometimes scaling is severe, with breakdown and painful cracking (fissuring) of the skin. Fluid-filled blisters can also form. Because the fungus may cause the skin to crack, athlete's foot can lead to bacterial infection,■ especially in older people and in people with inadequate blood flow to the feet.

Nail ringworm (tinea unguium, onychomycosis★) is an infection of the nail most often caused by *Trichophyton*. The fungus may get into the nail, producing a thickened, lusterless, and deformed nail. Infection is much more common on the toenails than on the fingernails. An infected toenail may separate from the toenail bed, crumble, or flake off.

Jock itch (tinea cruris) is much more common in men than in women and develops most frequently in warm weather. The infection begins in the skinfolds of the genital area and can spread to the upper inner thighs. Usually the scrotum is not involved (unlike in yeast infection). The rash has a scaly, pink border. Jock itch can be quite itchy and may be painful. A susceptible person may have repeated infections.

Scalp ringworm (tinea capitis) is primarily caused by *Trichophyton*. Scalp ringworm is highly contagious and is common among children,● especially black children. It may produce a pink scaly rash that may be somewhat itchy, or it may produce a patch of hair loss without a rash. Less commonly it can cause a painful, inflamed, swollen patch on the scalp that sometimes oozes pus (a kerion). A kerion is caused by an allergic reaction to the fungus.

Body ringworm (tinea corporis) may be caused by *Trichophyton*, *Microsporum*, or *Epidermophyton*. The infection generally produces round patches with pink scaly borders and clear areas in the center. Sometimes the rash is itchy. Body ringworm can develop anywhere on the skin and can spread rapidly to other parts of the body or to other people with whom there is close bodily contact.

▲ see page 1188
■ see page 1220
★ see also page 409
● see also page 1535

Topical Antifungal Drugs

Amorolfine	Oxiconazole
Butenafine	Selenium sulfide
Ciclopirox	(shampoo for
Clotrimazole	tinea versicolor)
Econazole	Sulconazole
Haloprogin	Terbinafine
Ketoconazole	Terconazole
Miconazole	Tioconazole
Naftifine	Tolnaftate
Nystatin (*Candida*	Undecylenate
only)	

Beard ringworm (tinea barbae) is rare. Most skin infections in the beard area are caused by bacteria, not fungi.

Treatment

Most ringworm infections, except those of the scalp and nails, are mild. Antifungal creams usually cure them. Many effective antifungal creams can be purchased without a prescription; antifungal powders are generally not as good. The active ingredients in topical antifungal drugs include miconazole, clotrimazole, econazole, oxiconazole, ciclopirox, ketoconazole, terbinafine, and butenafine.

Usually, creams are applied once or twice a day, and treatment should continue for 7 to 10 days after the rash completely disappears. If the cream is discontinued too soon, the infection may not be eradicated, and the rash will return. Ciclopirox in the form of a nail lacquer may be painted on fungal nail infections. This treatment may take up to 1 year, however, and still may not be effective.

Several days may pass before antifungal creams reduce symptoms. Corticosteroid creams are often used to help relieve itching and pain for the first few days. Low-dose hydrocortisone is available over the counter; more potent corticosteroids require a prescription and may be added to the antifungal cream.

For more serious or stubborn skin infections and for scalp and nail infections, a doctor may prescribe an antifungal drug to be taken by mouth. Itraconazole, terbinafine, and griseofulvin are all effective. These drugs are taken daily. Some doctors prescribe fluconazole, which may be given once a week for 3 or 4 weeks for body ringworm. Nail ringworm re-

quires longer treatment with itraconazole or terbinafine: 6 weeks for fingernails and 12 weeks or longer for toenails. Up to 1 year is required for new toenails to grow out. Terbinafine is the most effective drug available for treating nail ringworm. Griseofulvin requires more prolonged treatment. However, nail ringworm does not always respond to drugs taken by mouth and may recur even after apparently successful treatment. Scalp ringworm may need to be treated with drugs taken by mouth for 4 to 6 weeks—or even longer if griseofulvin is used. Some doctors give corticosteroids by mouth to children with a kerion of the scalp.

If the ringworm infection oozes, a bacterial infection also may have developed. Such an infection may require treatment with antibiotics, either applied to the skin or taken by mouth.▲

Candidiasis

Candidiasis (yeast infection, moniliasis) is infection by the yeast Candida, *formerly called* Monilia.

Candida is a normal resident of the mouth, digestive tract, and vagina that usually causes no harm. Under certain conditions, however, *Candida* can infect mucous membranes and moist areas of the skin. Typical areas of infection are the lining of the mouth and vagina, the genital area and anus, the armpits, the skin under the breasts in women, and the skinfolds of the stomach. Conditions that enable *Candida* to infect the skin include hot, humid weather; tight, synthetic underclothing; poor hygiene; and inflammatory diseases, such as psoriasis, occurring in the skinfolds.

People taking antibiotics may develop candidiasis because the antibiotics kill the bacteria that normally reside on the body, allowing *Candida* to grow unchecked. Corticosteroids or immunosuppressive therapy after organ transplantation can also lower the body's defenses against candidiasis. Inhaled corticosteroids, often used by people with asthma, sometimes produce candidiasis of the mouth. Pregnant women, obese people, and people with diabetes also are more likely to be infected by *Candida*.

In some people (usually people with a weakened immune system), *Candida* invades deeper tissues as well as the blood, causing life-threatening systemic candidiasis.■

▲ see page 1220   ■ see page 1150

Symptoms

Symptoms vary, depending on the location of the infection.

Infections in skinfolds (intertriginous infections) or in the navel usually cause a bright red rash, sometimes with softening and breakdown of skin. Small pustules may appear, especially at the edges of the rash, and the rash may itch intensely or burn. A *Candida* rash around the anus may be raw, white or red, and itchy. Babies may develop a *Candida* rash in the diaper area.▲

Vaginal candidiasis (vulvovaginitis, yeast infection■) is common, especially in women who are pregnant, have diabetes, or are taking antibiotics. Symptoms of these infections include a white or yellow cheeselike discharge from the vagina and burning, itching, and redness along the walls and external area of the vagina.

Penile candidiasis most often affects men with diabetes, uncircumcised men, or men whose female sex partners have vaginal candidiasis. Usually the infection produces a red, raw, sometimes painful rash on the head of the penis and sometimes the scrotum. Sometimes the rash may not cause any symptoms.

Thrush is candidiasis inside the mouth.★ The creamy white patches typical of thrush cling to the tongue and sides of the mouth and may be painful. The patches cannot be scraped off easily with a finger or blunt object. Thrush in otherwise healthy children is not unusual, but in adults it may signal a weakened immune system, possibly caused by diabetes or AIDS. The use of antibiotics that kill off competing bacteria increases the chances of getting thrush.

Perlèche is candidiasis at the corners of the mouth, creating cracks and tiny cuts. It may stem from chronic lip licking, thumb sucking, ill-fitting dentures, or any other condition that leaves the corners of the mouth moist enough so that yeast can grow.

Candidal paronychia is candidiasis in the nail beds, producing painful redness and swelling.● Nails infected with *Candida* may turn white or yellow and separate from the nail bed. This disorder typically occurs in people with diabetes or a weakened immune system or in otherwise healthy people whose hands are subjected to frequent wetting or washing.

Diagnosis and Treatment

Usually, a doctor can identify candidiasis by observing its distinctive rash or the thick, white, pasty residue it generates. To confirm the diagnosis, a doctor may scrape off some of the skin or residue with a scalpel or tongue depressor. The sample is then examined under a microscope or placed in a culture medium (a substance that allows microorganisms to grow) to identify the specific fungus.◆

Generally, candidiasis of the skin is easily cured with creams containing miconazole, clotrimazole, oxiconazole, ketoconazole, econazole, ciclopirox, or nystatin. The cream is usually applied twice daily for 7 to 10 days. Corticosteroid creams are sometimes used along with antifungal creams because they quickly reduce itching and pain (although they do not help cure the infection itself). Candidiasis that does not respond to antifungal creams and liquids may be treated with gentian violet, a purple dye that is painted on the infected area to kill the yeast.

Keeping the skin dry helps clear up the infection and prevents it from returning. Talcum powder helps keep the surface area dry, and talcum powder with nystatin may further help prevent a recurrence.

Different treatments are prescribed for vaginal yeast infections, thrush, and nail infections.

Tinea Versicolor

Tinea versicolor (pityriasis versicolor) is a fungal infection of the topmost layer of the skin causing scaly, discolored patches.

The infection, caused by the yeast *Malassezia furfur*, is quite common, especially in young adults. It rarely causes pain or itching, but it prevents areas of the skin from tanning, producing patches that are lighter in color than surrounding skin. People with naturally dark skin may notice lighter patches; people with naturally fair skin may get dark or lighter patches. The color depends on how the yeast affect the melanocytes, the cells that make the pigment.▼ The patches are often on the chest or back and may scale slightly. Over

---

▲ see page 1534

■ see page 1374

★ see also page 682

● see also page 409

◆ see page 1188

▼ see page 1214

time, small areas can join to form large patches.

Diagnosis and Treatment

Doctors can diagnose tinea versicolor by its appearance. A doctor may use an ultraviolet light to show the infection more clearly or may examine scrapings from the infected area under a microscope to confirm the diagnosis.

Topical antifungal cream such as ketoconazole may be used, as well as terbinafine solution spray. Prescription selenium sulfide shampoo is effective if applied full-strength to the affected areas (including the scalp) at bedtime, left on overnight, and washed off in the morning. Treatment is usually continued for 3 or 4 nights. Alternatively, the shampoo can be applied for 10 minutes a day for 10 days. Prescription ketoconazole shampoo is also effec-

tive; it is applied and washed off in 5 minutes. It is used as a single application or daily for 3 days.

Antifungal drugs taken by mouth, such as itraconazole, ketoconazole, or fluconazole, are sometimes used to treat widespread, resistant infection.▲ However, because these drugs may cause unwanted side effects, topical drugs are usually preferred.

The skin may not regain its normal pigmentation for many months after the infection is gone. Tinea versicolor commonly comes back after successful treatment because the fungus that causes it normally lives on the skin. Therefore, many doctors recommend use of 2.5% selenium sulfide shampoo or ketoconazole shampoo monthly or every other month to prevent recurrences.

CHAPTER 213

Viral Skin Infections

Many viral infections—such as measles, chickenpox, and rubella—result in rashes, spots, or sores on the skin. Herpesviruses often produce rashes and sores.■ However, in two common infections, warts and molluscum contagiosum, the virus remains solely within the skin.

Warts

Warts (verrucae) are small skin growths caused by any of 80 or more related human papillomaviruses.

Warts can develop at any age but are most common in children and least common in older people. People may have one or two warts or hundreds. Because prolonged or repeated contact is necessary for the virus to spread, warts are most often spread from one area of the body to another rather than from one person to another. Sexual contact, however, is often sufficient to spread genital warts.★

Most warts are harmless, although they may be quite bothersome. The exceptions are certain types of genital warts that sometimes cause cervical cancer in women.

Classification

Some warts grow in clusters (mosaic warts); others appear as isolated, single growths. Warts are classified by their location and shape.

Common warts (verrucae vulgaris), which almost everyone gets, are firm growths that usually have a rough surface. They are round or irregularly shaped; are gray, yellow, or brown; and are usually less than ½ inch across. Generally, they appear on areas that are frequently injured, such as the knees, face, fingers, and around the nails (periungual warts). Common warts may spread to surrounding skin.

Plantar warts develop on the sole of the foot, where they are usually flattened by the pressure of walking and are surrounded by thickened skin. They tend to be hard and flat, with a rough surface and well-defined boundaries. Warts may appear on the top of the foot or on the toes, where they are usually raised and fleshier. Warts are often gray or brown and

---

▲ see table on page 1152   ■ see page 1160

★ see page 1183

have a small black center. Unlike corns and calluses, plantar warts tend to bleed from many tiny spots, like pinpoints, when a doctor shaves or cuts the surface away with a knife.

Filiform warts are long, narrow, small growths that usually appear on the eyelids, face, neck, or lips.

Flat warts, which are more common in children and young adults, usually appear in groups as smooth yellow-brown, pink, or flesh-colored spots, most frequently on the face and tops of the hands. The beard area in men and the legs in women are also common locations for flat warts, where they may be spread by shaving.

Genital warts (venereal warts, condylomata acuminata) occur on the penis, anus, vulva, vagina, and cervix. They are irregular, bumpy growths often with the texture of a small cauliflower.▲

Symptoms and Diagnosis

Warts are painless, except for plantar warts. Plantar warts can be very painful when pressure is placed on them in the course of weight bearing.

Doctors recognize warts by their typical appearance. Growths on the skin that cannot be definitely identified may need to be removed for examination under a microscope (biopsy).

Treatment

Many warts, particularly common warts, disappear on their own within a year or two. Because warts rarely leave a scar when they heal spontaneously, they do not need to be treated unless they cause pain or psychologic distress. Genital warts are more likely to persist and are more contagious, so doctors often remove them or treat them with drugs. All types of warts may recur after removal. Plantar warts are the most difficult to cure.

In general, warts can be removed with chemicals, cut off, frozen off, or burned off with a laser or electrical current.

Typical chemicals used for removal include salicylic acid, formaldehyde, glutaraldehyde, trichloroacetic acid, cantharidin, and podophyllin. Flat warts are often treated with peeling agents such as retinoic or salicylic acid. 5-Fluorouracil cream or solution may also be used. Some chemicals can be applied by the person, whereas others must be applied by a doctor. Most of these chemicals can burn normal skin, so when they are applied at home, it is essential to follow directions carefully. Chemicals usually require multiple applications over several weeks to months. The wart is scraped to remove dead tissue before each treatment.

Freezing (cryotherapy) is safe and does not usually require any numbing of the area but may be too painful for children to tolerate. Warts may be frozen with various commercial freezing probes or with liquid nitrogen sprayed on or applied with a cotton swab. Cryotherapy is often used for plantar warts and warts under the fingernails. Multiple treatments at monthly intervals are often required, especially for large warts.

Burning and cutting warts off is effective but is more painful and usually leaves a scar. A pulsed dye laser is also effective but, like freezing, usually requires multiple treatments.■

Imiquimod is a new cream for the treatment of genital warts, which some doctors are using on other kinds of warts as well.

Molluscum Contagiosum

Molluscum contagiosum is infection of the skin by a poxvirus that causes flesh-colored or white smooth, waxy bumps.

The bumps are usually less than ¼ inch in diameter and have a tiny dimple in the center. The virus that causes molluscum is contagious; it spreads by direct skin contact and is common in children.★ Genital lesions are often transmitted sexually in adults.

Molluscum can infect any part of the skin. The bumps usually are not itchy or painful and may be discovered only coincidentally during a physical examination. However, the bumps can become very inflamed (resembling a boil) and itchy as the body fights off the virus. This inflammatory response may herald the disappearance of the lesions.

Most growths disappear spontaneously in 1 to 2 years; no treatment is needed unless they are disfiguring or otherwise bothersome. The growths can be treated by freezing or removing their core with a needle or sharp scraping instrument (curette). Sometimes doctors give high doses of cimetidine by mouth or apply trichloroacetic acid or cantharidin to molluscum. Others prescribe retinoic acid or imiquimod cream, which is applied for weeks or months.

▲ see page 1183   ■ see box on page 1235
★ see page 1535

CHAPTER 214

Sunlight and Skin Damage

The skin shields the rest of the body from the sun's rays. Ultraviolet (UV) light, although invisible to the human eye, is the component of sunlight that has the most effect on skin. UV light is classified into three types, ultraviolet A (UVA), ultraviolet B (UVB), and ultraviolet C (UVC), depending on its wavelength.

UV light in small amounts is beneficial, because it helps the body produce vitamin D. However, larger amounts of UV light damage DNA (the body's genetic material) and alter the amounts and kinds of chemicals that the skin cells make. UV light also may break down folic acid, sometimes resulting in deficiency of that vitamin in fair-skinned people. Although UVA penetrates deeper into the skin, UVB is responsible for at least three quarters of the damaging effects of UV light, including tanning, burning, premature skin aging, wrinkling, and skin cancer.

The amount of UV light reaching the earth's surface is increasing, especially in the northern latitudes. This increase is attributable to chemical reactions between ozone and chlorofluorocarbons (chemicals in refrigerants and spray can propellants) that are depleting the protective ozone layer, creating a thinner atmosphere with some holes. UV light is more intense between 10 A.M. and 3 P.M., in the summer, and at higher altitudes.

The skin undergoes certain changes when exposed to UV light to protect against damage. The epidermis (the skin's uppermost layer) thickens, blocking UV light. The melanocytes (the pigment-producing skin cells) make increased amounts of melanin, which darkens the skin, resulting in a tan. Melanin absorbs the energy of UV light and prevents the light from penetrating deeper into the tissues.

Sensitivity to sunlight varies according to the amount of melanin in the skin. Darker-skinned people have more melanin and therefore greater protection against the sun's harmful effects, although they are still vulnerable to some extent. The amount of melanin present in a person's skin depends on heredity as well as on the amount of recent sun exposure.

Some naturally pale people are able to produce large amounts of melanin in response to UV light, whereas others produce very little. People with albinism▲ have little or no melanin at all.

Exposure to sunlight prematurely ages the skin. Exposure to ultraviolet light is responsible for the wrinkles, both fine and coarse; irregular pigmentation; brown and red spots; and leathery, rough texture of sun-exposed skin. Although fair-skinned people are most vulnerable, with enough exposure, anyone's skin will change.

The more sun exposure a person has, the higher the risk of skin cancers, including squamous cell carcinoma, basal cell carcinoma, and, to some degree, malignant melanoma.■

The key to minimizing the damaging effects of the sun is avoiding further sun exposure; damage that is already done is difficult to reverse. Moisturizing creams and makeup help hide wrinkles. Chemical peels, alpha-hydroxy acids, tretinoin creams, and laser skin resurfacing may improve the appearance of thin wrinkles and irregular pigmentation. Deep wrinkles and significant skin damage, however, are unlikely to be reversed.

Sunburn

Sunburn results from a brief (acute) overexposure to ultraviolet (UV) light. The amount of sun exposure required to produce a burn varies with each person's pigmentation and ability to produce more melanin.

Sunburn results in painful reddened skin. Severe sunburn may produce swelling and blisters. Symptoms may begin as soon as 1 hour after exposure and typically reach their peak after 1 day. Some severely sunburned people develop a fever, chills, and weakness and on rare occasions even may go into shock (characterized by very low blood pressure, fainting, and profound weakness). Several days after a sunburn, people with naturally fair skin may have peeling in the burned area, usually accompanied by itching. These peeled areas are even more sensitive to sunburn for several weeks. People who have had severe sunburns when young are at greater risk of

---

▲ see page 1215   ■ see page 1239

skin cancer in later years even if they have not had long-term sun exposure.

Prevention

The best—and most obvious—way to prevent sun damage is to stay out of strong, direct sunlight. If sun exposure is necessary, the person should get out of the sun quickly at the first sign of tingling or redness. Clothing and ordinary window glass filter out most of the damaging rays. Water is not a good filter: UVA and UVB light can penetrate a foot of clear water. Clouds and fog are also not good filters of UV light; a person can get sunburned on a cloudy or foggy day. Snow, water, and sand reflect sunlight, magnifying the amount of UV light that reaches the skin. People also burn more quickly at high altitudes, where the thin air allows more burning UV light to reach the skin.

Before exposure to strong direct sunlight, a person should apply a sunscreen, an ointment or cream containing chemicals that protect the skin by filtering out UV light. Most sunscreens tend to filter only UVB light, although some newer sunscreens are somewhat effective at filtering UVA light as well.

Sunscreens contain substances, such as para-aminobenzoic acid (PABA) and benzophenone, that absorb UV light. Because PABA does not immediately bind strongly to the skin, sunscreens containing PABA must be applied 30 to 45 minutes before going out in the sun or into the water. PABA may irritate the skin or cause an allergic reaction in some peo-

Are Tans Healthy?

In a word—no. Although a suntan is often considered an emblem of good health and of an active, athletic life, tanning for its own sake has no health benefit and is actually a health hazard. Any exposure to ultraviolet A or ultraviolet B light can alter or damage the skin. Long-term exposure to natural sunlight causes skin damage and increases the risk of skin cancer. Exposure to the artificial sunlight used in tanning salons is harmful as well, even though the UVA lights used in these establishments are somewhat less likely to produce skin cancer. Quite simply, there is no "safe tan."

Self-tanning, or sunless, lotions do not really tan the skin but, rather, stain it. They therefore provide a safe way to achieve a tanned look without risking dangerous exposure to UV rays. However, because they do not increase melanin production, self-tanning lotions do not offer protection from the sun. Therefore, sunscreens should still be used during exposure to sunlight. Results with the use of self-tanning lotions may vary, depending on a person's skin type, the formulation used, and the manner in which the lotion is applied.

Actinic Keratoses: Precancerous Growths

Actinic keratoses (solar keratoses) are precancerous growths caused by long-term sun exposure. These growths appear as flaky, scaly areas that do not heal; they may also be darkened or gray and feel hard. The surrounding skin often appears thin.

Actinic keratoses usually can be removed by freezing them with liquid nitrogen; however, if a person has too many growths, a liquid or cream containing fluorouracil may be applied. Often, during such treatment, the skin temporarily looks worse because fluorouracil causes redness, scaling, and burning of the keratoses and of the surrounding sun-damaged skin.

ple. Many sunscreens contain both PABA and benzophenone or other chemicals; these combinations provide protection from a broader range of UV light. Many sunscreens claim to be either waterproof or water-resistant, but most of these nonetheless require more frequent application in people who are swimming or sweating.

Other sunscreens, called sunblocks, contain physical barriers such as zinc oxide or titanium dioxide; these thick, white ointments block almost all sunlight from the skin and can be used on small, sensitive areas, such as the nose and lips. Some cosmetics contain zinc oxide or titanium dioxide.

In the United States, sunscreens are rated by their sun protection factor (SPF) number—the higher the SPF number, the greater the protection. Sunscreens rated between 0 and 12 provide minimum protection; those rated between 13 and 29 provide moderate protection; those rated 30 and above provide maximum protection.

Some Substances That Sensitize the Skin to Sunlight

Antianxiety drugs
Alprazolam
Chlordiazepoxide

Antibiotics
Quinolones
Sulfonamides
Tetracyclines
Trimethoprim

Antidepressants
Tricyclic anti-
depressants

**Antifungal drugs
(taken by mouth)**
Griseofulvin

Antihyperglycemics
Sulfonylureas

Antimalarial drugs
Chloroquine
Quinine

Antipsychotics
Phenothiazines

Diuretics
Furosemide
Thiazides

Chemotherapy drugs
Dacarbazine
Fluorouracil
Methotrexate
Vinblastine

**Drugs used to treat
acne (taken by
mouth)**
Isotretinoin

Heart drugs
Amiodarone
Quinidine

Skin preparations
Antibacterials
(chlorhexidine,
hexachloro-
phene)
Antifungal drugs
Coal tar
Fragrances
Sunscreens

Treatment

Cold tap water compresses can soothe raw, hot areas, as can skin moisturizers without anesthetics or perfumes that might irritate or sensitize the skin. Nonsteroidal anti-inflammatory drugs (NSAIDs)▲ help relieve pain and inflammation. Corticosteroid tablets also may help relieve the inflammation but are used only for the most serious burns. Specific antibiotic burn creams are required only for severe blistering. Most sunburn blisters break on their own: they do not need to be popped and drained unless they are still intact after 3 or 4 days. Sunburned skin rarely becomes infected, but if an infection develops, healing may be delayed. A doctor can determine the severity of an infection and prescribe antibiotics if necessary.

Sunburned skin begins healing by itself within several days, but complete healing may take weeks. After burned skin peels, the newly exposed layers are thin and initially very sensitive to sunlight and must be protected for several weeks.

Skin Photosensitivity Reactions

Photosensitivity, sometimes referred to as a sun allergy, is an immune system reaction that is triggered by sunlight. Photosensitivity reactions include solar urticaria, chemical photosensitization, and polymorphous light eruption and are usually characterized by an itchy eruption on patches of sun-exposed skin. People may inherit a tendency to these reactions. Certain diseases, such as systemic lupus erythematosus and some porphyrias, also may cause the skin to break out in response to sunlight.

Solar urticaria are hives (large, itchy red bumps) that develop after only a few minutes of exposure to sunlight. The hives appear within 10 minutes of sun exposure and go away within an hour or two after leaving the sunlight. People with large affected areas often have headaches and feel weak and nauseated.

Chemical photosensitivity is a condition in which people develop redness, inflammation, and sometimes brown or blue discoloration in areas of skin that have been exposed to sunlight for a brief period. This reaction differs from sunburn in that it occurs only after the person has swallowed certain drugs or chemicals or has applied them to the skin. These substances make some people's skin more sensitive to the effects of ultraviolet light. Some people develop hives with itching, which indicates a type of drug allergy that is triggered by sunlight.

Polymorphous light eruption is an unusual reaction to sunlight, the cause of which is not understood. It is one of the most common sun-related skin problems and is more common in women and in people who are not regularly exposed to the sun. The eruption appears as multiple red bumps and irregular red patches appearing on sun-exposed skin. These patches, which are itchy, generally appear between 30 minutes and several hours after sun exposure; however, new patches may develop many hours or several days later. The bumps and patches usually go away within a week. Typically, people with this condition who continue to go out in the sun gradually become less sensitive to the effects of sunlight.

▲ see page 452

Diagnosis, Prevention, and Treatment

There are no specific tests for photosensitivity reactions. A doctor suspects a photosensitivity reaction when a rash appears only in areas exposed to sunlight. A close review of any diseases, drugs taken by mouth, or substances applied to the skin (such as drugs or cosmetics) may help a doctor pinpoint the cause of the photosensitivity reaction. Doctors may perform tests to rule out diseases, such as systemic lupus erythematosus, that are known to make someone susceptible to such reactions.

A person with sensitivity to sunlight from any cause should wear protective clothes, avoid sunlight as much as possible, and use sunscreens. If possible, any drugs or chemicals that could cause photosensitivity should be discontinued.

People with polymorphous light eruption or lupus photosensitivity sometimes benefit from treatment with hydroxychloroquine or corticosteroids taken by mouth. For certain types of photosensitivity, treatment can consist of phototherapy (exposure to ultraviolet light) with the use of psoralens (drugs that sensitize the skin to the effects of ultraviolet light). This treatment is called PUVA (psoralens plus ultraviolet A).▲ However, people with systemic lupus erythematosus cannot tolerate PUVA therapy.

CHAPTER 215

Noncancerous Skin Growths

Skin growths are accumulations of various types of cells that look different than the surrounding skin. They may be raised or flat and range in color from dark brown or black to flesh-colored to red. Skin growths may be present at birth or develop later.

When the growth is controlled and the cells do not spread to other parts of the body, the skin growth (tumor) is noncancerous (benign). When the growth is uncontrolled, the tumor is cancerous (malignant), and the cells invade normal tissue and even spread (metastasize) to other parts of the body. Noncancerous skin growths are often more of a cosmetic problem than anything else.

Doctors do not know what causes most noncancerous skin growths. Some growths, however, are known to be caused by viruses (for example, warts), systemic (bodywide) disease (for example, xanthelasmas or xanthomas caused by excess fats in the blood), and environmental factors (for example, moles and epidermal cysts stimulated by sunlight).

Moles

Moles (nevi) are small, usually dark, skin growths that develop from pigment-producing cells in the skin (melanocytes).

Moles vary in size from small dots to more than 1 inch in diameter. They may be flat or raised, smooth or rough (wartlike), and may have hairs growing from them. Although they are usually dark brown or black, some moles are flesh-colored or yellow-brown. They may be red at first but often darken.

Almost everyone has a few moles, and many people have large numbers of moles. Moles commonly develop in childhood or adolescence, although in some people they continue to develop throughout life. Moles respond to changes in hormone levels in women and may appear, enlarge, or darken during pregnancy. Once formed, moles remain for a lifetime. In fair-skinned people, moles occur more commonly on sun-exposed areas of the skin.

Moles usually are easily recognized by their typical appearance. They do not itch or hurt, and they are not a form of cancer. However, moles sometimes develop into or resemble malignant melanoma, a cancerous growth of melanocytes.■ In fact, many malignant melanomas begin in moles, so a mole that looks sus-

---

▲ see box on page 1202
■ see page 1239

picious should be removed and examined under a microscope. *Changes in a mole—such as enlargement (especially with an irregular border), darkening, inflammation, spotty color changes, bleeding, broken skin, itching, or pain—are warnings of malignant melanoma.* People with more than 10 or 20 moles have a somewhat increased risk of melanoma and should be checked every year by a doctor. If a mole proves to be cancerous, additional surgery may be needed to remove the skin surrounding it.

Most moles, however, are harmless and do not require removal. Depending on their appearance and location, some moles may even be considered beauty marks. Normal moles that are unattractive or located where clothing can irritate them can be removed by a doctor using a scalpel and a local anesthetic.

Atypical moles (dysplastic nevi) tend to be larger than normal moles. Like cancerous skin growths, they tend to be multicolored and have irregular shapes and borders. People with even a few atypical moles have a slightly increased risk of developing malignant melanoma. This risk increases greatly if the person has close family members with malignant melanoma. The tendency to grow atypical moles is hereditary.

People with atypical moles—particularly those with a family history of melanoma—must look for any changes that might indicate malignant melanoma. They should have their skin checked at least yearly by a dermatologist to look for changes in the color or size of a mole. To help monitor such changes, dermatologists often use full-body color photographs. Atypical moles that change should be removed.

Sunlight accelerates the development of and changes in atypical moles. Even moderate sun exposure during childhood may be harmful and increase the risk of developing melanoma decades later. Therefore, fair-skinned people or those with atypical moles should avoid sun exposure. When in the sun, they should always use a sunblock with a high sun protection factor (SPF) rating to help shield against cancer-producing ultraviolet (UV) rays.▲

Skin Tags

Skin tags are soft, small, flesh-colored or slightly darker skin growths that develop mostly on the neck, in the armpits, or in the genital area.

Usually, skin tags cause no trouble, but they may be unattractive, and clothing or nearby skin may rub and irritate them so that they bleed or hurt. A doctor can easily remove a skin tag by burning it off with an electric needle or by cutting it off with a scalpel or scissors.

Lipomas

Lipomas are soft deposits of fatty material that grow under the skin, causing round or oval lumps.

A lipoma appears as a smooth, soft bump under the skin. Lipomas range in firmness, some feeling rather hard. The skin over the lipoma has a normal appearance. Lipomas rarely grow more than 2 or 3 inches across. They can develop anywhere on the body but are particularly common on the forearms, torso, and back of the neck. Some people have only one, whereas others develop many lipomas. Lipomas rarely cause problems, although they may occasionally be painful if they grow against a nerve. Lipomas are more common in women than in men.

Usually, a doctor can easily recognize lipomas, and no tests are required for diagnosis. Lipomas are not a form of cancer, and they rarely become cancerous. If a lipoma begins to change in any way, a doctor may perform a biopsy (removal of a tissue sample for examination under a microscope). Treatment usually is not required, but bothersome lipomas may be removed by surgery or by liposuction (removal of fat with a suction device).

Dermatofibromas

Dermatofibromas are small red-to-brown bumps (nodules) that result from an accumulation of collagen, which is a protein made by the cells (fibroblasts) that populate the soft tissue under the skin.

Dermatofibromas are common and usually appear as single firm bumps, often on the legs, particularly in women. Some people develop many dermatofibromas. Causes include trauma, insect bites, and cuts caused by shaving. Dermatofibromas are harmless and usually do not cause any symptoms, except for occasional itching. Usually, dermatofibromas are

▲ see page 1230

not treated unless they become bothersome or enlarge. A doctor can remove them with a scalpel.

Growths and Malformations of the Vessels

Growths and malformations of the vessels (angiomas) are collections of abnormally dense blood or lymph vessels, usually located in and below the skin, that cause red or purple discolorations.

Growths and malformations of the vessels often appear at birth or soon afterward, and some may be referred to as birthmarks. Examples include hemangiomas, port-wine stains, lymphangiomas, pyogenic granulomas, and spider angiomas. These different growths and malformations are usually recognized by their appearances, thus biopsies are rarely necessary. About one third of all newborns have some type of growth or malformation of the vessels, many of which disappear by themselves.

HEMANGIOMAS

Hemangiomas are abnormal overgrowths of blood vessels that can appear as red or purple lumps in the skin and on other parts of the body.

Hemangiomas develop soon after birth and tend to enlarge rapidly during the first 6 to 18 months of life. After this, they begin to shrink. About three quarters of hemangiomas disappear by age 7, although the skin that remains is often slightly discolored or scarred.

Superficial hemangiomas (strawberry hemangiomas, cherry angiomas), the most common type of blood vessel growth, occur on or near the surface of the skin. They appear as raised, red, irregular growths or patches that range from tiny bumps to large, deforming swellings 3 or 4 inches across. They usually occur on the torso and can number from a few to dozens. Superficial hemangiomas are harmless; if they are bothersome, a doctor can remove them with an electric needle or laser.

Deep hemangiomas (cavernous hemangiomas) grow within the skin and deep beneath it. They cause the skin to bulge and may be purple or, if they are very deep, flesh-colored. Most deep hemangiomas grow between ¼ inch and 2 inches across, although sometimes they grow much larger. More than half occur on the head and neck. Sometimes,

Using Lasers to Treat Skin Problems

A laser is a device that produces a thin, very intense beam of light that has one particular color (wavelength). Laser beams can be very powerful, containing thousands of watts of energy. But because this energy is in the form of light, it does not affect human tissue until it is absorbed. Whether tissue absorbs laser light depends on the color of the tissue and the color of the light. For example, red blood vessels absorb yellow, blue, and green light best, so lasers of these colors are used to selectively target blood vessels in the treatment of hemangiomas. Other colors are used to target different conditions. Laser beams may be continuous, like a flashlight, or briefly pulsed in individual flashes. The pulse duration helps determine the depth and amount of effect of the laser beam.

Laser treatments are sometimes combined with photodynamic therapy, in which certain light-absorbing chemicals are applied to skin tumors or given intravenously. When these chemicals are struck by laser light, they break apart into substances that help destroy the tumor.

Blood vessel growths, such as hemangiomas, and malformations, such as port-wine stains, are commonly treated with laser therapy. Laser therapy is also used to remove unwanted hair, tattoos, skin discoloration, scars from acne or sun damage, and cancerous tumors.

hemangiomas develop in organs, such as the liver.▲

Superficial and deep hemangiomas do not cause pain but occasionally break open (ulcerate) and bleed, which can be difficult to stop. Hemangiomas around the eye may grow large enough to block vision, which can lead to permanent vision loss if uncorrected. Hemangiomas may also block the nose or throat, which can obstruct breathing.

Because hemangiomas often go away on their own, doctors do not treat them when they first appear unless they grow rapidly, obstruct vision or breathing, ulcerate, or are cos-

▲ see page 810

metically distressing. Doctors usually treat any facial hemangiomas that have not gone away by age 5 or 6.

When treatment is required, doctors inject small superficial hemangiomas with corticosteroids or surgically remove them if the injections do not work. People with rapidly growing or large, ulcerating hemangiomas take corticosteroids by mouth. For older children in whom the hemangioma has shrunken, laser therapy or surgery may improve the appearance of the skin.

PORT-WINE STAINS

Port-wine stains (capillary malformations, nevi flammeus) are flat pink, red, or purplish discolorations present at birth due to malformed blood vessels.

Port-wine stains are harmless, permanent discolorations. However, their cosmetic appearance may be psychologically bothersome or even devastating. The stains appear as smooth, flat pink, red, or purple patches of skin. Port-wine stains may be small or may cover large areas of the body. Stains that appear on the nape of the neck of newborns have been referred to as stork bites. Very rarely, port-wine stains appear in conjunction with Sturge-Weber syndrome, a rare hereditary disorder that leads to mental retardation and growth deformities.

Small port-wine stains can be covered with cosmetic cover-up cream. If a stain is bothersome, its appearance can be greatly improved with laser therapy.▲

LYMPHANGIOMAS

Lymphangiomas (lymphatic malformations) are skin bumps caused by a collection of enlarged lymph vessels—the channels that carry lymph (a clear fluid related to blood) throughout the body.

Lymphangiomas are uncommon, but usually appear between birth and age 2. They may be tiny bumps or large, deforming growths. Lymphangiomas do not itch or hurt and are not a form of cancer. Most lymphangiomas are yellowish tan, but a few are reddish. When injured or punctured, they release a colorless fluid. Although treatment is not usually needed, lymphangiomas can be removed surgically. However, such surgery requires the re-

moval of many layers of skin and underlying tissue, because lymphangiomas grow deep beneath the surface.

PYOGENIC GRANULOMAS

Pyogenic granulomas are scarlet, brown, or blue-black slightly raised areas caused by increased growth of capillaries (the smallest blood vessels) and swelling of the surrounding tissue.

The condition develops rapidly, usually after injury to the skin. For unknown reasons, large pyogenic granulomas may develop during pregnancy, appearing even on the gums (pregnancy tumors). Pyogenic granulomas appear as $1/4$- to $1/2$-inch growths that rise from the surface of the skin. They do not hurt, but they bleed easily when bumped or scratched because they consist almost entirely of capillaries.

Pyogenic granulomas sometimes disappear by themselves, but if they persist, a doctor usually removes them surgically, with laser therapy, or with an electric needle (electrocoagulation). A sample of tissue may be sent to a laboratory to ensure that the growth is not a type of melanoma or other skin cancer. Sometimes pyogenic granulomas recur after treatment.

SPIDER ANGIOMAS

Spider angiomas are small, bright red spots consisting of a central dilated blood vessel surrounded by slender dilated capillaries that resemble spider legs.

Many people have a few spider angiomas, which are often referred to as "broken" blood vessels. Spider angiomas on the face are commonly seen in fair-skinned people and are thought to be due to sun exposure. In most people, there is no known cause, but people with cirrhosis often develop many spider angiomas, as do many women who are pregnant or who are using oral contraceptives. Spider angiomas are not present at birth.

Spider angiomas appear as tiny, hard-to-see red spots less than $1/4$ inch across. They are harmless and generally cause no symptoms; they are only of cosmetic significance. Spider angiomas that develop during pregnancy or oral contraceptive use usually disappear on their own 6 to 9 months after childbirth or after discontinuing oral contraceptive use. If treatment is desired for cosmetic reasons, a doctor can destroy the central blood vessel with laser therapy or with an electric needle.

▲ see box on page 1235

Seborrheic Keratoses

Seborrheic keratoses (seborrheic warts) are flesh-colored, brown, or black growths that can appear anywhere on the skin.

These harmless growths are very common in middle-aged and older people. Some people have a hundred or more. Although these growths can appear anywhere, they most often appear on the torso and the temples.

Seborrheic keratoses are round or oval and vary in size from less than ¼ inch to several inches. They appear to be stuck on the skin and often have a waxy or scaly surface. These growths develop slowly. They are not cancerous and do not become so. Dark brown keratoses may sometimes be mistaken for atypical moles or melanomas.

Treatment is not needed unless the keratoses become irritated or itchy or are cosmetically undesirable. They are best removed by freezing them with liquid nitrogen. Laser removal is also effective.▲ Alternatively, a doctor can cut them out with a scissors, scalpel, or other sharp instrument.

Keratoacanthomas

Keratoacanthomas are round, firm, usually flesh-colored growths that have a central crater that is scaly or crusted.

Keratoacanthomas appear most commonly on the face, forearm, and back of the hand and grow quickly. In 1 or 2 months, they can grow into lumps up to 1 inch wide, after which they begin to shrink. They usually disappear within 6 months, often leaving a scar. They may be caused by a virus, but doctors are not sure.

Keratoacanthomas closely resemble squamous cell carcinoma, a type of skin cancer,■ and some doctors believe that they may actually be an unusual form of squamous cell carcinoma. Therefore, doctors often perform a biopsy, in which a piece of skin is removed and examined under a microscope. Keratoacanthomas can be cut out or scraped (curetted). Alternatively, they can be treated with injections of corticosteroids or fluorouracil.

Keloids

Keloids are smooth, shiny, flesh-colored, raised growths of fibrous tissue that form over areas of injury or surgical wounds.

Keloids are an extreme overgrowth of scar tissue over healed wounds. They may form in the months after an injury. They may be raised as much as ¼ inch above the surface of the skin. Keloids may form in any scar, even those resulting from severe acne. They are much more common in blacks than in whites and typically develop on the chest, shoulders, back, and, sometimes, face and earlobes. Keloids do not hurt, but they may itch or be sensitive to touch.

Keloids respond poorly to therapy, but monthly injections of corticosteroids may flatten them somewhat. A doctor may try surgical or laser removal followed by corticosteroid injections, but new keloids often form in the scar resulting from the treatment. Some doctors have applied silicone patches to keloids and have had some success in flattening them.

Epidermal Cysts

An epidermal cyst is a common slow-growing bump consisting of a thin sac of skinlike material containing a cheesy substance composed of skin secretions.

Epidermal cysts, often incorrectly referred to as sebaceous cysts, are flesh-colored and range from ½ to 2 inches across. They can appear anywhere but are most common on the scalp, back, and face. They tend to be firm and easy to move within the skin. Epidermal cysts are not painful unless they become infected or inflamed.

Large epidermal cysts are removed surgically after an anesthetic is injected to numb the area. The thin sac wall must be removed completely or the cyst will grow back. Small cysts may be injected with corticosteroids if they become inflamed. Infected cysts are treated with an antibiotic and cut open to drain. Tiny cysts that are bothersome can be burned out with an electric needle.

Because sunlight may stimulate growth of epidermal cysts, fair-skinned people are advised to stay out of the sun and to use protective clothing and sunscreen.★

▲ see box on page 1235

■ see page 1238

★ see page 1230

CHAPTER 216

Skin Cancers

Skin cancer is the most common form of cancer in the United States. The three main types of skin cancer—basal cell carcinoma, squamous cell carcinoma, and melanoma—are caused, at least in part, by long-term sun exposure. Lymphoma can also develop in the skin.▲ Fair-skinned people are particularly susceptible to developing most forms of skin cancer because they produce less melanin, the protective pigment in the epidermis that filters out ultraviolet (UV) light. However, skin cancer also can develop in dark-skinned people and in people whose skin has not had significant sun exposure. Most skin cancers are curable, especially when treated at an early stage. Therefore, any unusual skin growth that persists for more than a few weeks is best examined by a doctor.

Doctors treat most skin cancers by removing them surgically. Usually, the defect that is left in the skin is small. Larger or more invasive cancer may require removal of a significant amount of skin, which may have to be replaced with a skin graft.■

Basal Cell Carcinoma

Basal cell carcinoma is a cancer that originates in cells of the epidermis.

Basal cells are found in the lowest layer of the epidermis. Although basal cell carcinoma may not originate in the basal cells, the disease is so named because the cancer cells resemble basal cells. Basal cell carcinoma is the most common human cancer. More than 1 million people develop this type of cancer in the United States each year. Basal cell carcinoma usually develops on skin surfaces that are exposed to sunlight, commonly on the head or neck. The tumors usually begin as small, shiny, firm raised growths (papules) that enlarge very slowly, sometimes so slowly that they go unnoticed as new growths. However, the growth rate varies greatly from tumor to tumor, with some growing as much as ½ inch in a year.

Basal cell carcinomas can vary greatly in their appearance. Some are raised bumps that may break open and form scabs in the center. Some are flat pale or red patches that look somewhat like scars. The border of the cancer is sometimes thickened and pearly white. The cancer may alternately bleed and form a scab and heal, leading a person to falsely think that it is a sore rather than a cancer.

Basal cell carcinomas rarely spread (metastasize) to distant parts of the body. Instead, they invade and slowly destroy surrounding tissues. When basal cell carcinomas grow near the eye, mouth, bone, or brain, the consequences of invasion can be serious. Yet, for most people, the tumors simply grow slowly into the skin.

Diagnosis, Treatment, and Prevention

A doctor often can recognize a basal cell carcinoma simply by looking at it, but a biopsy is the standard procedure for confirming the diagnosis.★

A doctor removes the cancer in the office by scraping and burning it with an electric needle (curettage and electrodesiccation) or by cutting it out. A technique called Mohs' microscopically controlled surgery may be required for some basal cell carcinomas that regrow or occur in certain areas, such as around the nose and eyes. Rarely, radiation treatment is used.

Treatment is nearly always successful, and basal cell carcinoma is rarely fatal. However, in almost 25% of people who have been treated successfully, another basal cell carcinoma develops within 5 years. Thus, anyone with one basal cell carcinoma should have yearly skin examinations.

Because basal cell carcinoma is often caused by sun exposure, people can help prevent this cancer by staying out of the sun and using protective clothing and sunscreen. In addition, any skin change that persists for more than a few weeks should be evaluated by a doctor.

Squamous Cell Carcinoma

Squamous cell carcinoma is cancer that originates in the squamous cells (keratinocytes).

▲ see page 1016   ■ see page 1083
★ see page 1188

Squamous cells (keratinocytes) are the main structural cells of the epidermis. Squamous cell carcinoma usually develops on sun-exposed areas but may grow anywhere on the skin or in the mouth, where sun exposure is minimal. It may develop on normal skin but is more likely to develop in precancerous skin growths caused by previous sun exposure (actinic keratosis▲). Squamous cell carcinoma is characterized by its thick, scaly, irregular appearance. Fair-skinned people are much more susceptible to squamous cell carcinoma than darker-skinned people. This type of cancer is also more likely to develop in chronic sores—such as chronic skin ulcers—or in skin that has been scarred, particularly by burns.

Squamous cell carcinoma begins as a red area with a scaly, crusted surface that does not heal. As it grows, the tumor may become somewhat raised and firm, sometimes with a wartlike surface.■ Eventually, the cancer becomes an open sore and grows into the underlying tissue.

Most squamous cell carcinomas affect only the area around them, penetrating into nearby tissues. But some spread (metastasize) to distant parts of the body and can be fatal. Those that occur near the ears and lower lip are more likely to spread. Squamous cell carcinoma in the mouth often spreads.

Bowen's disease is an early form of squamous cell carcinoma that is confined to the epidermis and has not yet invaded the deeper layers of the skin. The affected skin is red-brown and scaly or crusted and flat, sometimes looking like a patch of psoriasis or dermatitis or a fungal infection (ringworm).

Diagnosis, Treatment, and Prevention

When doctors suspect squamous cell carcinoma, they perform a biopsy to differentiate this skin cancer from similar-looking diseases.

Doctors treat squamous cell carcinoma and Bowen's disease by scraping and burning the tumor with an electric needle (curettage and electrodesiccation) or by cutting the tumor out. A technique called Mohs' microscopically controlled surgery may be used. Sometimes radiation treatments are used. These treatments are usually effective, and most people survive.

Squamous cell carcinoma that has spread to other parts of the body can be fatal. It is treated with radiation or chemotherapy, but treatment may not be effective.

Because squamous cell carcinoma is often caused by sun exposure, people can help pre-

Mohs' Microscopically Controlled Surgery

Because skin cancer cells often have spread beyond the edges of the visible patch on the skin, doctors sometimes use a special surgical technique to make sure they remove all of the cancer. In this technique, called Mohs' microscopically controlled surgery or Mohs' micrographic surgery, doctors first remove the visible tumor and then begin cutting away the edges of the wound bit by bit. While they are still performing surgery, doctors examine pieces of tissue immediately to look for cancer cells. Tissue removal from the area continues until the samples no longer contain cancer cells. Mohs' surgery is useful for basal cell and squamous cell cancer. The procedure limits the amount of tissue removed, which is especially important for cancer near important sites such as the eye. Mohs' surgery also reduces recurrence rates for skin cancers. It is rarely used for melanoma.

After removing all of the cancer, the surgeon decides how best to replace the skin that has been cut away. The surgeon may decide to use a skin graft,★ to bring the edges of the remaining skin together with sutures, or to let the skin heal on its own with dressings placed on top of the wound.

vent this cancer by staying out of the sun and using protective clothing and sunscreen.

Melanoma

Melanoma is a cancer that originates in the pigment-producing cells of the skin (melanocytes).

Melanocytes are the pigmented cells in the skin that give skin its distinctive color. Sunlight stimulates melanocytes to produce more melanin (the pigment that darkens the skin) and increases the risk of melanoma.

Melanoma can begin as a new, small, pigmented skin growth on normal skin, most often on sun-exposed areas, or it may develop from preexisting pigmented moles.● Some-

▲ see box on page 1231
■ see page 673
★ see page 1083   ● see page 1233

Warning Signs of Melanoma

- Enlarging pigmented (especially black or deep blue) spot or mole
- Changes in color of an existing mole, especially the spread of red, white, brown, or blue pigmentation to surrounding skin
- Changes in characteristics of skin over the pigmented spot, such as changes in size or shape
- Bleeding or breaking open (ulceration) of an existing mole

times melanoma runs in families. Melanoma readily spreads (metastasizes) to distant parts of the body, where it continues to grow and destroy tissue.

Melanomas can vary in appearance. Some are flat, irregular brown patches containing small black spots. Others are raised brown patches with red, white, black, or blue spots. Sometimes melanoma appears as a firm black or gray lump.

Diagnosis, Treatment, and Prevention

A new mole or changes in a mole—such as enlargement (especially with an irregular border), darkening, inflammation, spotty color changes, bleeding, broken skin, itching, and pain—are warnings of possible melanoma. If these or other findings lead a doctor to suspect melanoma, he performs a biopsy. Growths are usually removed entirely. The tissue is then examined under a microscope to determine whether the growth is a melanoma and, if so, whether all the cancer has been removed.

Most darkly pigmented growths that are sent for biopsy are not melanoma but, rather, simple moles. Nonetheless, it is preferable to remove a harmless mole than to allow a cancer to grow. Some growths are neither simple moles nor melanomas but something in between. These tumors, called **dysplastic nevi,** or atypical moles, sometimes later turn into melanoma.

The less a melanoma has grown into the skin, the greater the chance that surgery will cure it. Almost 100% of the earliest, most shallow melanomas are cured by surgery. Thus, doctors treat melanomas by cutting them out, taking at least a ½-inch border of skin around the tumor. However, melanomas that have grown deeper than 1/32 inch into the

skin are very likely to have spread (metastasized) through the lymphatic and blood vessels. Melanomas that have spread are often fatal.

Chemotherapy is used to treat melanomas that have spread, but few are cured. Some of the people treated live less than 9 months. However, the course of the disease varies greatly and depends in part on the strength of the body's immune defenses. Some people survive in apparent good health for several years despite the spread of the melanoma. New experimental treatments with interleukin-2 and vaccines that stimulate the body to attack the melanoma cells have yielded promising results.

Because melanoma is often caused by long-term sun exposure, people can help prevent this cancer by staying out of the sun and using protective clothing and sunscreen, starting in early childhood. Anyone who has had a melanoma is at risk of developing other melanomas. Therefore, such people need yearly skin examinations. People with a lot of moles should have total body skin examinations at least once a year.

Kaposi's Sarcoma

Kaposi's sarcoma is a cancer that produces multiple flat pink, brown, or purple patches or bumps on the skin; it is caused by herpesvirus type 8.

Kaposi's sarcoma occurs in several distinct groups of people and acts differently in each group. It occurs in older men, usually of Mediterranean or Jewish heritage; in children and young men from certain parts of Africa; in people receiving immunosuppressants after organ transplantation; and in people with AIDS (which accounts for most of the cases in the United States).

Symptoms

In older men, Kaposi's sarcoma usually appears as a single purple or dark brown spot on the toes or leg. The cancer may grow to several inches or more as a deeply colored, flat or slightly raised area that tends to bleed and break open. Several additional spots may appear on the leg, but the cancer rarely spreads to other parts of the body and is almost never fatal.

In the other groups, Kaposi's sarcoma is more aggressive. Similar appearing spots develop, but they are often multiple and may occur anywhere on the body. Within several months, the spots spread to other parts of the body, often including the mouth, where they cause pain with eating. They may also develop in lymph nodes and internal organs, especially the digestive tract, where they can cause diarrhea and internal bleeding that leads to blood in the stool.

Diagnosis and Treatment

Doctors usually recognize Kaposi's sarcoma by its appearance. A biopsy is usually performed to confirm the diagnosis.

Older men with slow-growing Kaposi's sarcoma in one or two spots may have the tumors removed surgically or by freezing. People with multiple spots usually receive radiation therapy. Some people with very few spots and no other symptoms may choose to receive no treatment unless the condition spreads.

People who have the more aggressive form, but whose immune system is normal, often respond to interferon-alpha or chemotherapy drugs.

In people taking immunosuppressants, the tumors sometimes disappear when immunosuppressants are discontinued. If these drugs must be continued because of the person's underlying condition, however, chemotherapy and radiation therapy are used. However, these treatment methods are less successful than in people with a healthy immune system.

In people with AIDS, treatment with chemotherapy and radiation has not been very successful. The best results are achieved in people whose immune system improves as a result of intensive treatment with AIDS drugs. In general, treating Kaposi's sarcoma does not appear to prolong the lives of people with AIDS.

Paget's Disease

Paget's disease is a rare type of skin cancer that originates in glands in or under the skin.

The term Paget's disease also refers to an unrelated metabolic bone disease;▲ these distinct diseases should not be confused with each other.

Paget's disease occurs mainly on the nipple and is the result of a cancer of the breast milk ducts that has spread to the skin of the nipple. Men and women are both affected. The underlying cancer may or may not be felt by the person or the doctor. Sometimes, Paget's disease develops in the genital area or around the anus as the result of a cancer originating in underlying sweat glands or even in nearby structures such as the genitals, intestines, or urinary tract.

The skin in Paget's disease appears red, oozing, and crusting. It looks like an inflamed, reddened patch of skin (dermatitis). Itching and pain are common. Because Paget's disease looks very much like common dermatitis, a biopsy is necessary to make the diagnosis.

Paget's disease of the nipple is managed like other types of breast cancer.■ Paget's disease outside the breast area is treated by surgically removing the entire growth.

▲ see page 346   ■ see page 1400

Epithelium: Surfaces of the Body

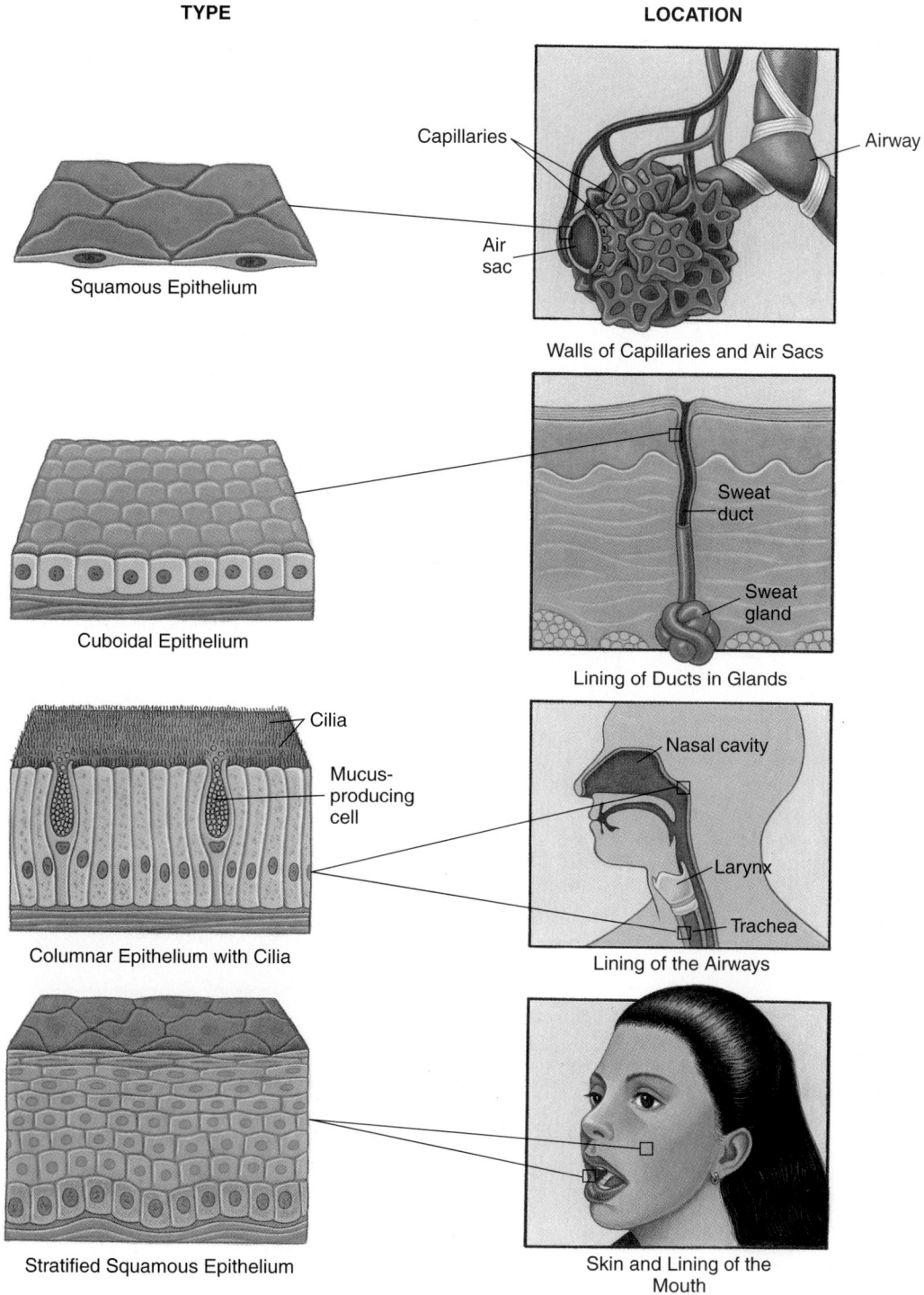

TYPE

LOCATION

Squamous Epithelium

Capillaries

Airway

Air sac

Walls of Capillaries and Air Sacs

Cuboidal Epithelium

Sweat duct

Sweat gland

Lining of Ducts in Glands

Cilia

Mucus-producing cell

Columnar Epithelium with Cilia

Nasal cavity

Larynx

Trachea

Lining of the Airways

Stratified Squamous Epithelium

Skin and Lining of the Mouth

Blood Vessels and Lymph Nodes

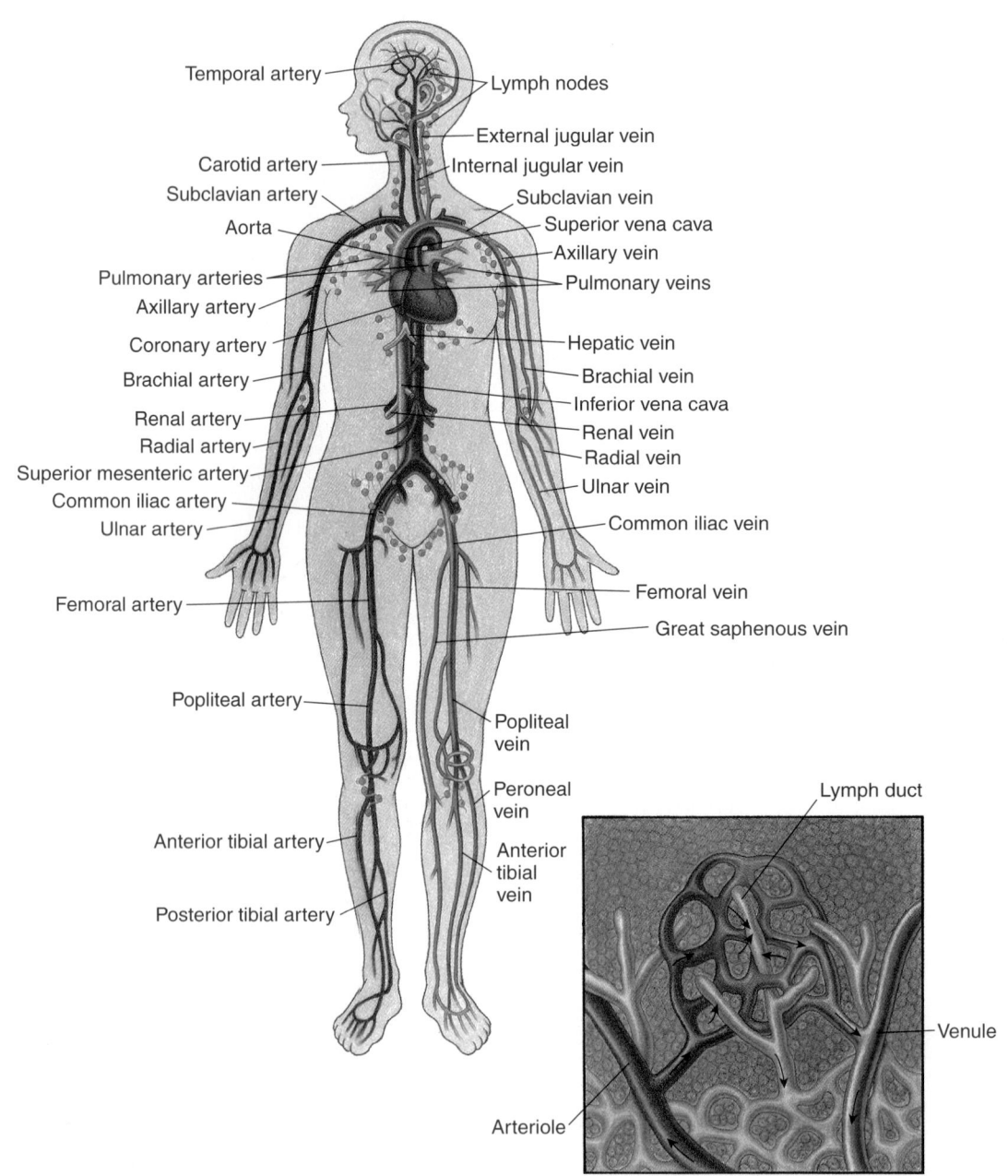

Temporal artery

Lymph nodes

External jugular vein

Carotid artery

Internal jugular vein

Subclavian artery

Subclavian vein

Aorta

Superior vena cava

Pulmonary arteries

Axillary vein

Axillary artery

Pulmonary veins

Coronary artery

Hepatic vein

Brachial artery

Brachial vein

Renal artery

Inferior vena cava

Radial artery

Renal vein

Superior mesenteric artery

Radial vein

Common iliac artery

Ulnar vein

Ulnar artery

Common iliac vein

Femoral artery

Femoral vein

Great saphenous vein

Popliteal artery

Popliteal vein

Peroneal vein

Anterior tibial artery

Anterior tibial vein

Posterior tibial artery

Lymph duct

Venule

Arteriole

Capillary Bed

Heart-Lung Connections

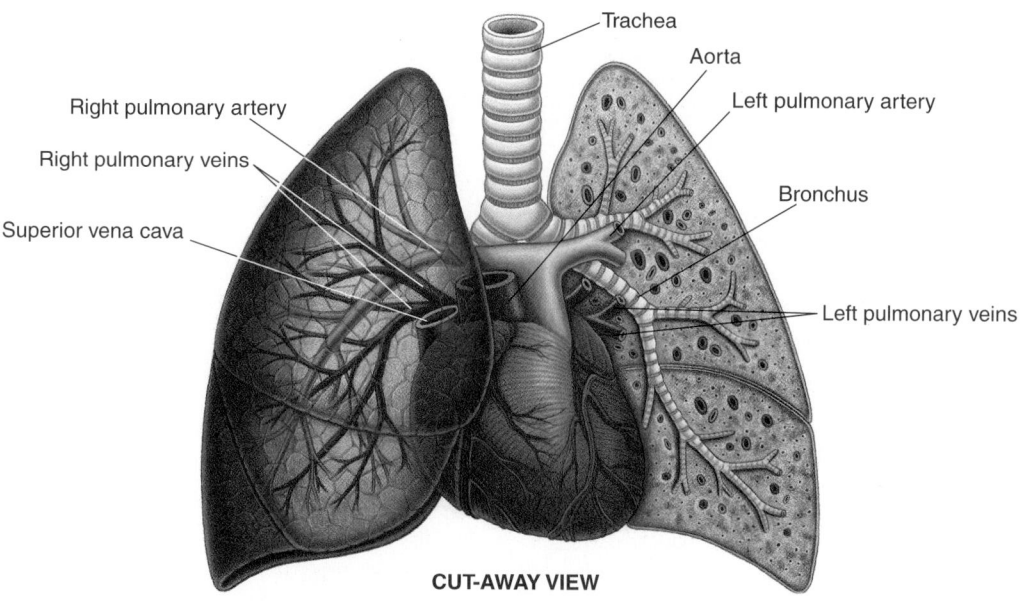

Trachea

Aorta

Right pulmonary artery

Left pulmonary artery

Right pulmonary veins

Bronchus

Superior vena cava

Left pulmonary veins

CUT-AWAY VIEW

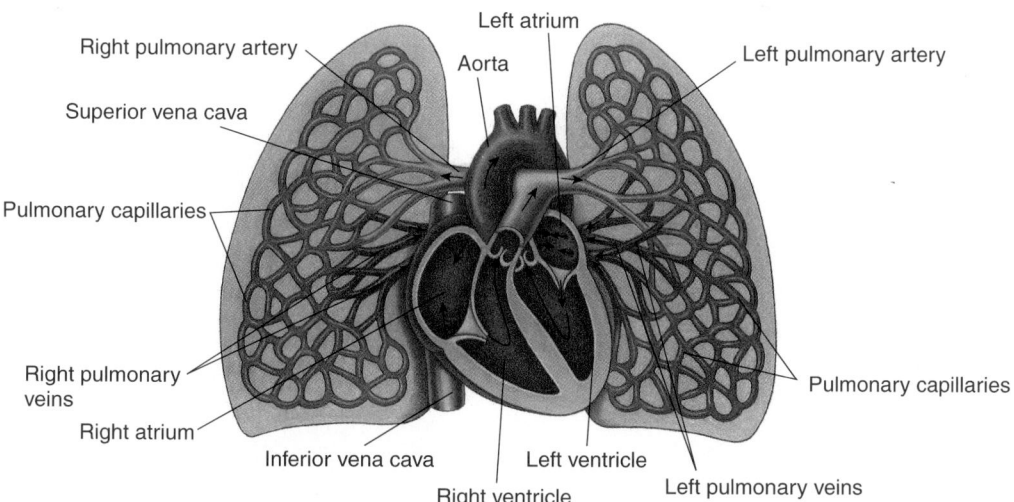

Left atrium

Right pulmonary artery

Left pulmonary artery

Aorta

Superior vena cava

Pulmonary capillaries

Pulmonary capillaries

Right pulmonary veins

Right atrium

Inferior vena cava

Left ventricle

Left pulmonary veins

Right ventricle

SCHEMATIC VIEW OF BLOOD FLOW

Brain and Spinal Cord

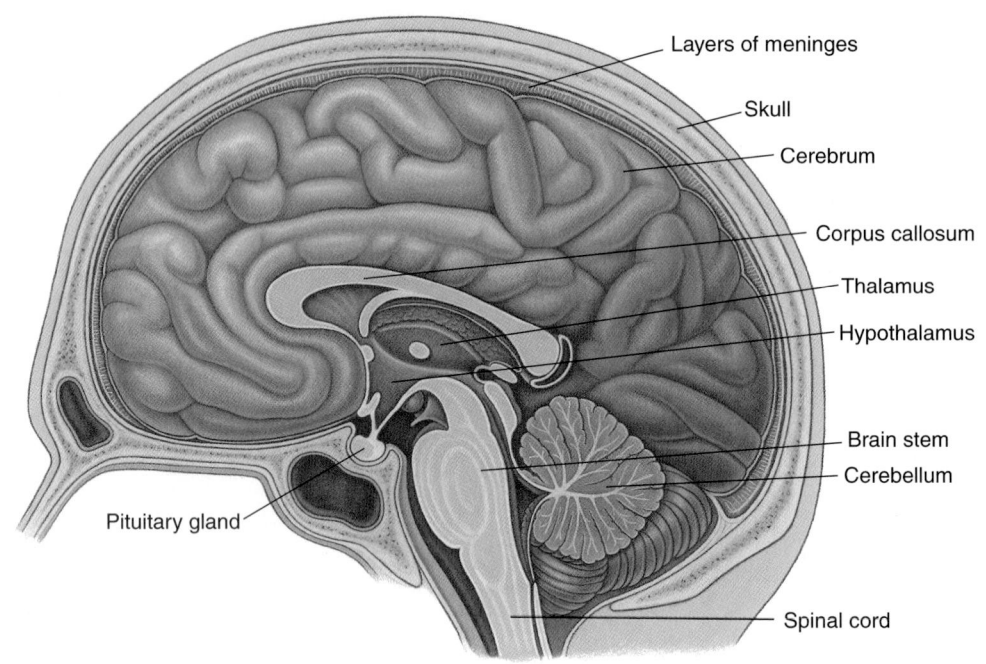

Layers of meninges

Skull

Cerebrum

Corpus callosum

Thalamus

Hypothalamus

Brain stem

Cerebellum

Pituitary gland

Spinal cord

SIDE VIEW

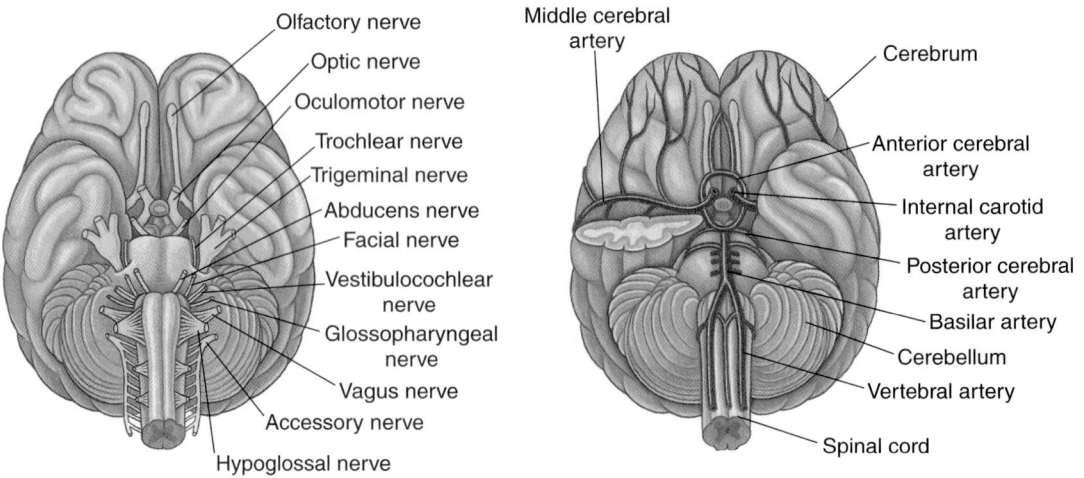

Olfactory nerve
Optic nerve
Oculomotor nerve
Trochlear nerve
Trigeminal nerve
Abducens nerve
Facial nerve
Vestibulocochlear nerve
Glossopharyngeal nerve
Vagus nerve
Accessory nerve
Hypoglossal nerve

**CRANIAL NERVES
BOTTOM VIEW**

Middle cerebral artery
Cerebrum
Anterior cerebral artery
Internal carotid artery
Posterior cerebral artery
Basilar artery
Cerebellum
Vertebral artery
Spinal cord

**ARTERIES OF THE BRAIN
BOTTOM VIEW**

Head and Neck

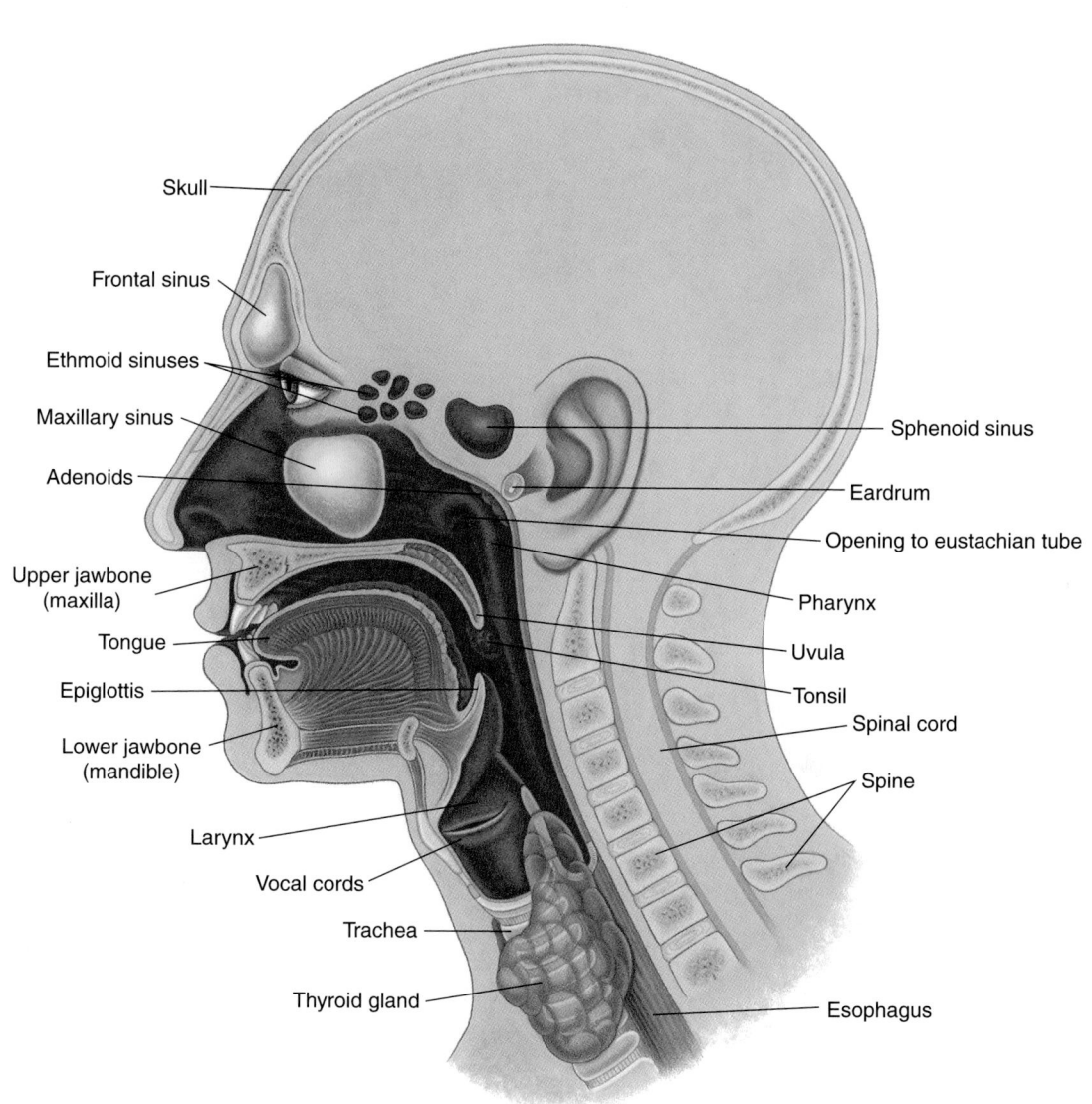

Skull

Frontal sinus

Ethmoid sinuses

Maxillary sinus

Adenoids

Upper jawbone (maxilla)

Tongue

Epiglottis

Lower jawbone (mandible)

Larynx

Vocal cords

Trachea

Thyroid gland

Sphenoid sinus

Eardrum

Opening to eustachian tube

Pharynx

Uvula

Tonsil

Spinal cord

Spine

Esophagus

Muscle-Bone Connections

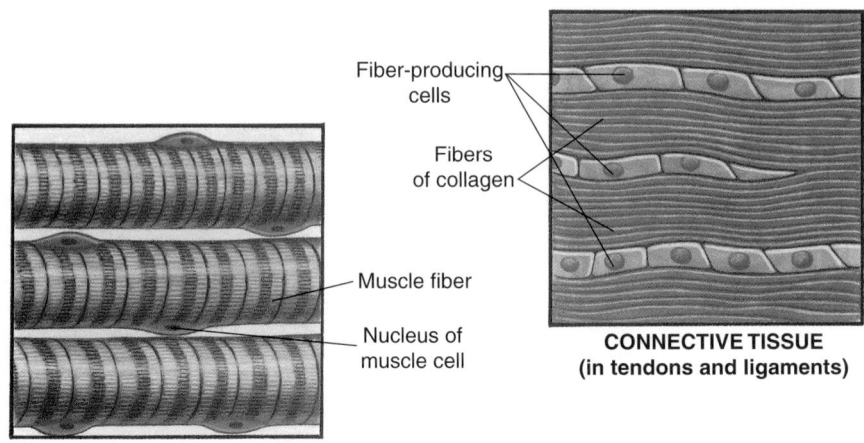

Fiber-producing cells

Fibers of collagen

Muscle fiber

Nucleus of muscle cell

**CONNECTIVE TISSUE
(in tendons and ligaments)**

SKELETAL MUSCLE TISSUE

Skeletal muscle

Bundle of bundles

Muscle fiber

Bundle of muscle fibers

Bone

Tendon

Ligament

Bone

Bone cells

BONE TISSUE

Digestive System

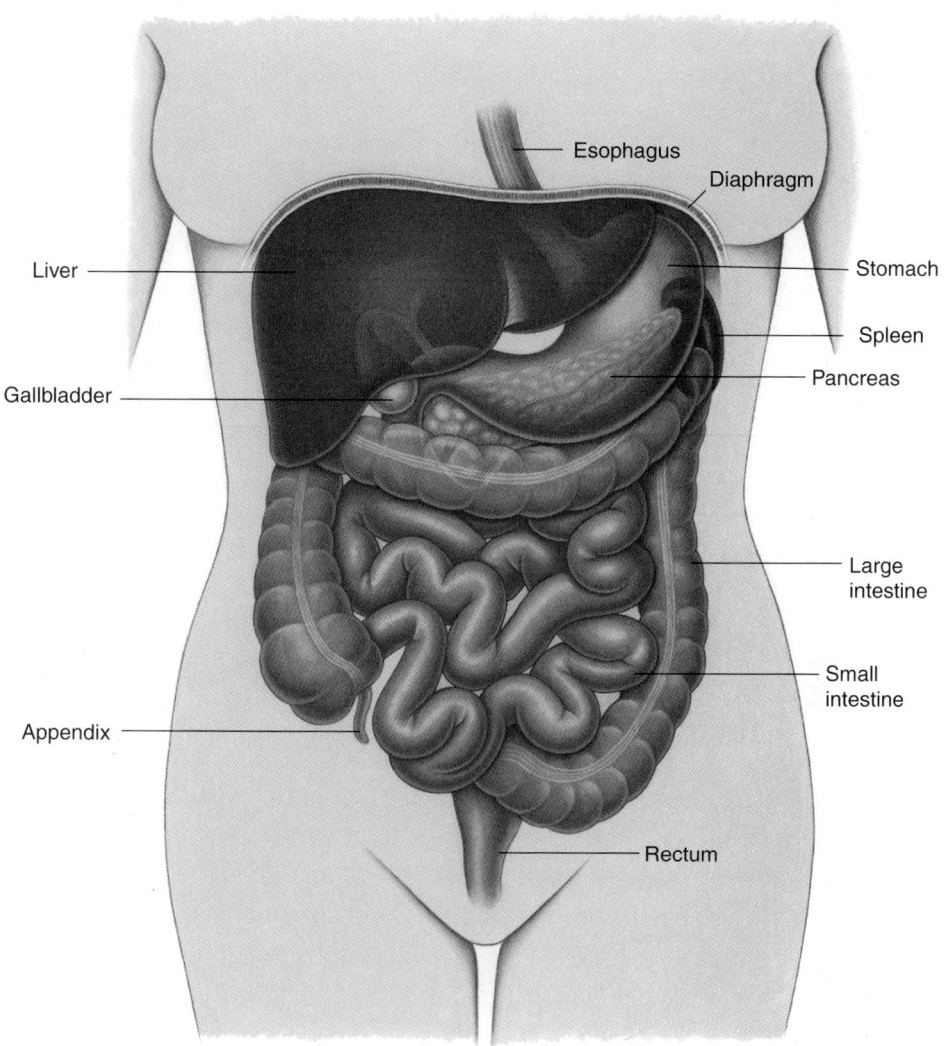

Esophagus

Diaphragm

Liver

Stomach

Spleen

Pancreas

Gallbladder

Large intestine

Small intestine

Appendix

Rectum

Urinary System

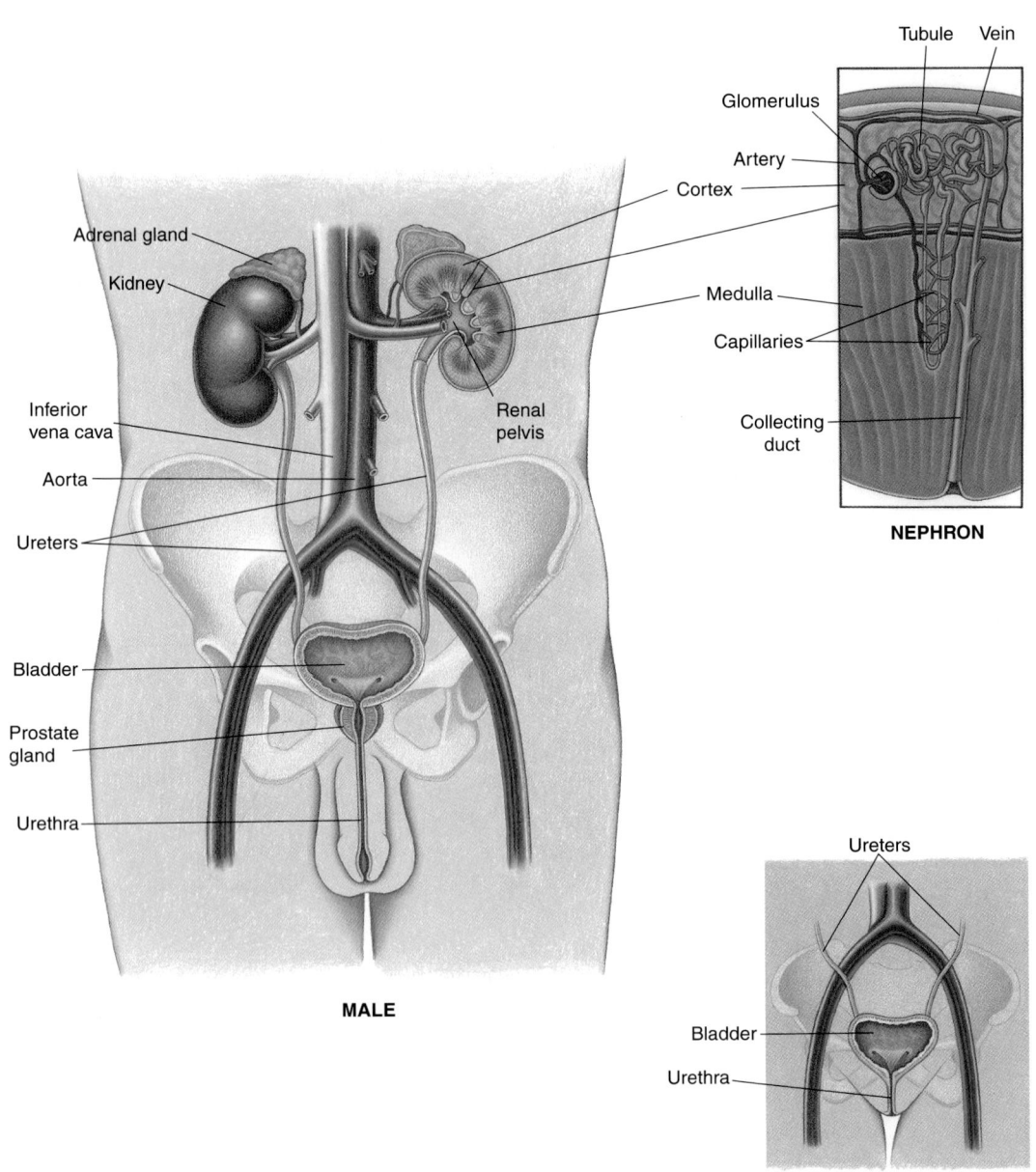

Tubule

Vein

Glomerulus

Artery

Cortex

Medulla

Capillaries

Collecting duct

NEPHRON

Adrenal gland

Kidney

Inferior vena cava

Aorta

Ureters

Bladder

Prostate gland

Urethra

Renal pelvis

MALE

Ureters

Bladder

Urethra

FEMALE

EAR, NOSE, AND THROAT DISORDERS

217   Biology of the Ears, Nose, and Throat 1244

Ears ▪ Nose and Sinuses ▪ Throat ▪ Effects of Aging

218   Hearing Loss and Deafness..1247

219   Outer Ear Disorders 1253

Blockages ▪ External Otitis ▪ Perichondritis ▪ Tumors ▪ Injury

220   Middle and Inner Ear Disorders 1255

Perforation of the Eardrum ▪ Barotrauma ▪ Infectious Myringitis ▪ Acute Otitis Media ▪ Serous Otitis Media ▪ Chronic Otitis Media ▪ Mastoiditis ▪ Meniere's Disease ▪ Vestibular Neuronitis ▪ Temporal Bone Fracture ▪ Auditory Nerve Tumors ▪ Tinnitus

221   Disorders of the Nose and Sinuses..1262

Fractures of the Nose ▪ Deviated Septum ▪ Perforations of the Septum ▪ Nosebleeds ▪ Nasal Vestibulitis ▪ Rhinitis ▪ Nasal Polyps ▪ Sinusitis

222   Throat Disorders 1267

Tonsillar Cellulitis and Abscess ▪ Epiglottitis ▪ Laryngitis ▪ Vocal Cord Nodules and Polyps ▪ Contact Ulcers of the Vocal Cords ▪ Vocal Cord Paralysis ▪ Laryngoceles

223   Nose and Throat Cancers 1271

Cancer of the Larynx ▪ Cancer of the Paranasal Sinuses ▪ Cancer of the Nasopharynx ▪ Cancer of the Tonsils

CHAPTER 217

Biology of the Ears, Nose, and Throat

The ears, nose, and throat have two things in common: they are located near each other and have separate but related functions. The ears and nose are sensory organs—necessary for the senses of hearing, balance, and smell. The throat mainly functions as a pathway through which food and fluids travel to the esophagus and air passes to the lungs. Primary care doctors often diagnose and treat disorders involving these organs, but doctors called otolaryngologists specialize in them.

Ears

The ear, which is the organ of hearing and balance, consists of the outer, middle, and inner ear. The outer, middle, and inner ear function together to convert sound waves into nerve impulses that travel to the brain, where they are perceived as sound. The inner ear also helps to maintain balance.

Outer Ear

The outer ear consists of the external part of the ear (pinna or auricle) and the ear canal (external auditory meatus). The pinna consists of cartilage covered by skin and is shaped to capture sound waves and funnel them through the ear canal to the eardrum (tympanic membrane), a thin membrane that separates the outer ear from the middle ear.

Middle Ear

The middle ear consists of the eardrum and a small air-filled chamber containing a chain of three tiny bones (ossicles) that connect the eardrum to the inner ear. The ossicles are named for their shapes. The hammer (malleus) is attached to the eardrum. The anvil (incus) is the middle bone between the hammer and the stirrup (stapes), which is attached to the oval window, a thin membrane at the entrance to the inner ear. Vibrations of the eardrum are amplified mechanically by the ossicles and transmitted to the oval window.

The middle ear also contains two tiny muscles. The tensor tympani muscle is attached to the hammer; it helps to tune and protect the ear. The stapedius muscle is attached to the stirrup and oval window; it contracts in response to a loud noise, making the chain of ossicles more rigid so that less sound is transmitted. This response, called the acoustic reflex, helps protect the delicate inner ear from sound damage.

The eustachian tube, a small tube that connects the middle ear with the back of the nose, allows outside air to enter the middle ear. This tube, which opens when a person swallows, helps maintain equal air pressure on both sides of the eardrum and prevents fluid from accumulating in the middle ear. If air pressure is not equal, the eardrum may bulge or retract, which can be uncomfortable and distort hearing. Swallowing or voluntary "popping" of the ears can relieve pressure on the eardrum caused by sudden changes in air pressure, as often occurs when flying in an airplane. The eustachian tube's connection with the middle ear explains why upper respiratory infections (such as the common cold), which inflame and block the eustachian tube, can lead to middle ear infections or changes in middle ear pressure, resulting in pain.

Inner Ear

The inner ear (labyrinth) is a complex structure consisting of two major parts: the cochlea, the organ of hearing; and the vestibular system, the organ of balance. The vestibular system consists of the saccule and the utricle, which determine position sense, and the semicircular canals, which help maintain balance.

The cochlea, a hollow tube coiled in the shape of a snail's shell, is filled with fluid. Within the cochlea is the organ of Corti, which consists, in part, of about 20,000 specialized cells, called hair cells. These cells have small hairlike projections (cilia) that extend into the fluid. Sound vibrations transmitted from the ossicles in the middle ear to the oval window in the inner ear cause the fluid and cilia to vibrate. Hair cells in different parts of the cochlea vibrate in response to different sound frequencies and convert the vibrations into nerve impulses. The nerve impulses are transmitted along fibers of the cochlear nerve to the brain.

Despite the protective effect of the acoustic reflex, loud noise can damage and destroy hair cells. Once a hair cell is destroyed, it does not appear to regrow. Continued exposure to loud noise causes progressive damage, eventually resulting in hearing loss and sometimes noise or ringing in the ears (tinnitus).

The semicircular canals are three fluid-filled tubes at right angles to one another. Movement of the head causes the fluid in the canals to move. Depending on the direction the head moves, the fluid movement will be greater in one of the canals than in the others. The canals contain hair cells that respond to this movement of fluid. The hair cells initiate nerve impulses that tell the brain which way the head is moving, so that appropriate action can be taken to maintain balance.

If the semicircular canals malfunction, as may occur in an upper respiratory infection and other conditions both temporary and permanent, a person's sense of balance may be lost or a whirling sensation (vertigo) may develop.

Nose and Sinuses

The nose is the organ of smell and a main passageway for air into and out of the lungs. The nose warms, moistens, and cleans air before it enters the lungs. The bones of the face around the nose contain hollow spaces called paranasal sinuses. There are four groups of paranasal sinuses: the maxillary, ethmoid, frontal, and sphenoid sinuses. Sinuses reduce the weight of the facial bones while maintaining bone strength and shape. The air-filled spaces of the nose and sinuses also add resonance to the voice.

The supporting structure of the upper part of the external nose consists of bone, while the lower part consists of cartilage. Inside the nose is the nasal cavity, which is divided into two passages by the nasal septum. The nasal septum is composed of both bone and cartilage and extends from the nostrils to the back of the throat. Bones called nasal conchae project into the nasal cavity, forming a series of folds (turbinates). These folds greatly increase the surface area of the nasal cavity.

Lining the nasal cavity is a mucous membrane rich with blood vessels. The increased surface area and the many blood vessels enable the nose to warm and humidify incoming air quickly. Cells in the mucous membrane

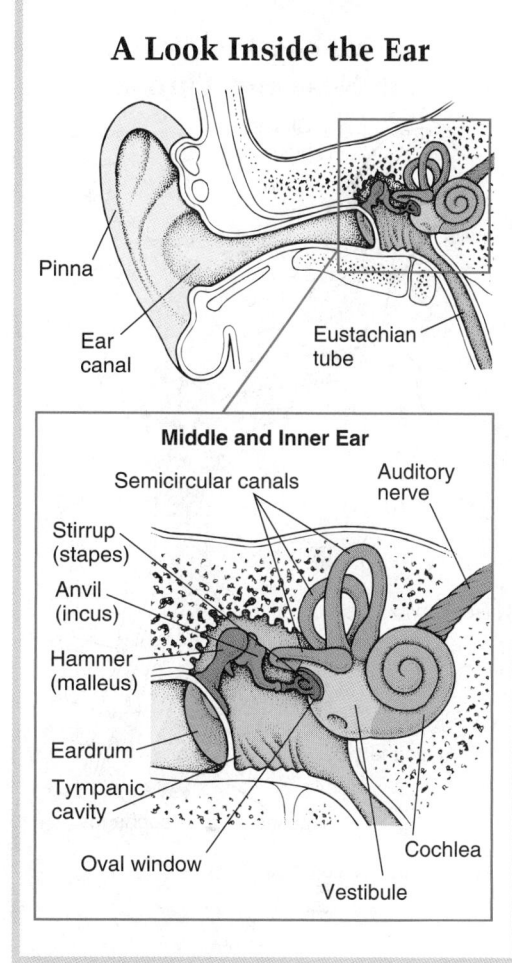

A Look Inside the Ear

Pinna

Ear canal

Eustachian tube

Middle and Inner Ear

Semicircular canals

Auditory nerve

Stirrup (stapes)

Anvil (incus)

Hammer (malleus)

Eardrum

Tympanic cavity

Oval window

Cochlea

Vestibule

produce mucus and have tiny hairlike projections (cilia). Usually, the mucus traps incoming dirt particles, which are then moved by the cilia toward the front of the nose or down the throat to be removed from the airway. This action helps clean the air before it goes to the lungs. Sneezing automatically clears the nasal passages in response to irritation, just as coughing clears the lungs.

Like the nasal cavity, the sinuses are lined with a mucous membrane composed of cells that produce mucus and have cilia. Incoming dirt particles are trapped by the mucus, then moved by the cilia into the nasal cavity, through small sinus openings (ostia). Because these openings are so small, the drainage can easily be blocked by conditions such as colds or allergies, which produce swelling of the mucous membranes. Blockage of normal sinus

A Look Inside the Nose and Throat

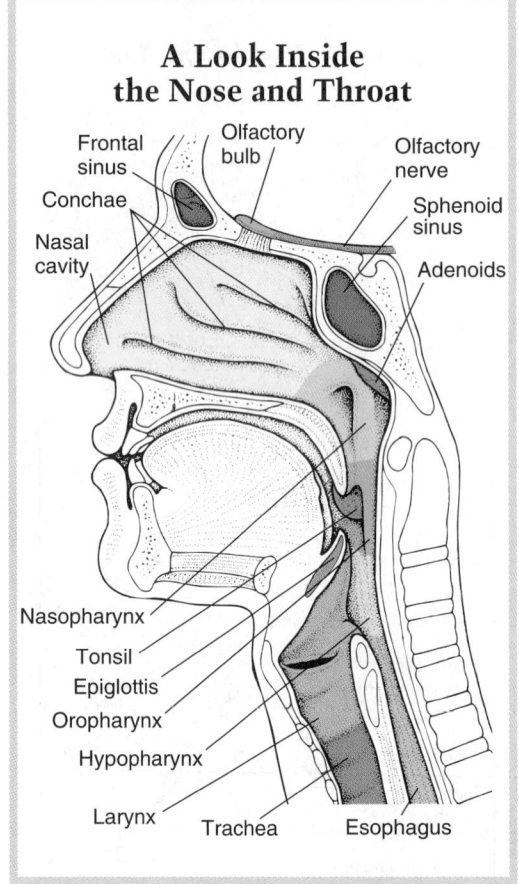

Frontal sinus
Olfactory bulb
Olfactory nerve
Conchae
Sphenoid sinus
Nasal cavity
Adenoids
Nasopharynx
Tonsil
Epiglottis
Oropharynx
Hypopharynx
Larynx
Trachea
Esophagus

smell▲ as well as texture and temperature. This is why food seems somewhat tasteless when a person has a decreased sense of smell, as may occur when the person has a cold. Because the smell receptors are located in the upper part of the nose, normal breathing does not draw much air over them. Sniffing, however, increases the flow of air over the smell receptor cells, greatly increasing their exposure to odors.

Throat

The throat (pharynx) is located behind the mouth, below the nasal cavity, and above the esophagus and windpipe (trachea). It consists of an upper part (nasopharynx), a middle part (oropharynx), and a lower part (hypopharynx). The throat is a muscular passageway through which food is carried to the esophagus and air to the lungs. Like the nose and mouth, the throat is lined with a mucous membrane composed of cells that produce mucus and have hairlike projections (cilia). Dirt particles caught in the mucus are carried by the cilia toward the esophagus and are swallowed.

The tonsils are located on both sides of the back of the mouth, and the adenoids at the back of the nasal cavity. The tonsils and adenoids consist of lymphoid tissue and help fight off infections. They are largest during childhood and gradually shrink throughout life. The uvula is a small flap of tissue visible in the back of the throat between the tonsils. It helps prevent food and fluids from entering the nasal cavity during swallowing.

At the top of the trachea is the voice box (larynx), which contains the vocal cords and is primarily responsible for producing the sound of the voice. When relaxed, the vocal cords form a V-shaped opening that air can pass through freely. When contracted, they vibrate as air from the lungs passes over them, generating sounds that can be modified by the tongue, nose, and mouth to produce speech.

The epiglottis is a stiff flap of cartilage located above and in front of the larynx. During swallowing, the epiglottis covers the opening to the larynx to prevent food and fluids from entering the trachea. Thus, the epiglottis protects the lungs.

Effects of Aging

Aging greatly affects the function of the ears, nose, and throat. The effects of aging result from many factors such as wear and tear,

drainage leads to sinus inflammation and infection (sinusitis).

One of the most important functions of the nose is its role in the sense of smell. Smell receptor cells are located in the upper part of the nasal cavity. These cells are special nerve cells that have cilia. The cilia of each cell are sensitive to different chemicals and, when stimulated, create a nerve impulse that is sent to the nerve cells of the olfactory bulb, which lies inside the skull just above the nose. The olfactory nerves carry the nerve impulse from the olfactory bulb directly to the brain, where it is perceived as a smell.

The sense of smell, which is not fully understood, is much more sophisticated than the sense of taste. Distinct smells are far more numerous than tastes. The subjective sense of taste while eating (flavor) involves taste and

▲ see art on page 595

noise, and the cumulative effect of infections, as well as the effect of substances such as alcohol and tobacco.

A progressive loss of hearing, especially for higher-pitched sounds, is common (presbycusis). This change can alter a person's ability to understand speech. Vestibular imbalance and ringing in the ears (tinnitus) are also more common in older people but are not normal.

The sense of smell may decline with age, making tastes less distinct. Changes in the voice also occur with age. The tissues in the larynx may stiffen, affecting the pitch and quality of the voice and causing hoarseness. Changes in the tissues of the pharynx may lead to the leakage of food or fluids into the trachea during swallowing (aspiration). If persistent or severe, aspiration may cause pneumonia.

CHAPTER 218

Hearing Loss and Deafness

*Hearing loss is deterioration in hearing; **deafness** is profound hearing loss.*

More than 28 million people in the United States are deaf or have hearing loss. Older people are the most affected: 30 to 40% of people aged 65 and older have significant hearing loss. Children also develop hearing loss,▲ which can be detrimental to language and social development. Every year, about 1 of 5,000 people develops sudden deafness. Sudden deafness is severe hearing loss, usually in only one ear, that develops over a period of a few hours or less.

Causes

Hearing loss has many causes. It may be caused by a mechanical problem in the external ear canal or middle ear that blocks the conduction of sound (conductive hearing loss). Blockage of the external ear canal can be due to something as mundane as an accumulation of wax or something as uncommon as a tumor. The most common cause of conductive hearing loss in the middle ear, especially in children, is an accumulation of fluid. Fluid can accumulate in the middle ear as a result of ear infections or conditions, such as allergies or tumors, that block the eustachian tube, which drains the middle ear.

Hearing loss also may be due to damage to the sensory structures (hair cells) of the inner ear, auditory nerve, or auditory nerve pathways in the brain (sensorineural hearing loss). These sensory structures may be damaged by drugs, infections, tumors, and skull injuries. Hearing loss is often a mixture of a conductive and sensorineural loss.

Age: Age-related hearing loss is called presbycusis. As some people age, structures of the ear become less elastic and undergo other changes that make them less able to respond to sound waves, contributing to hearing loss. In many people, exposure to noise over many years worsens the changes caused by aging. Age-related hearing loss begins early, starting some time after age 20. However, it progresses very slowly, and most people do not notice any changes until well after age 50.

Age-related hearing loss first affects the highest pitches (frequencies) and only later affects lower pitches. Loss of the ability to hear high-pitched sounds often makes it more difficult to understand speech. Although the loudness of speech appears normal to the person, certain consonant sounds—such as the sound of letters C, D, K, P, S, and T—become hard to hear, so that many people with hearing loss think the speaker is mumbling. Indeed, some people complain more that others are not speaking clearly than that they cannot hear well. Women and children, whose voices tend to be higher in pitch than those of men, are particularly difficult to understand. Many people also notice a change in the vibrancy of certain musical sounds, such as those of violins and flutes.

Otosclerosis: In otosclerosis, a hereditary disorder, the bone surrounding the middle and inner ear grows excessively. This exuberant growth immobilizes the stirrup (the ear bone attached to the inner ear) so that it cannot transmit sounds properly. Sometimes the

---

▲ see page 1597

Causes of Hearing Loss

Conductive hearing loss
- Cholesteatoma (noncancerous tumor caused by an ear infection)
- Chronic middle ear fluid (otitis media with effusion)
- Middle ear infection (otitis media)
- Obstruction of external ear canal (with wax, a tumor, or pus from an infection)
- Otosclerosis (bony overgrowth of the ossicles)
- Perforated eardrum

Sensorineural hearing loss
- Aging
- Brain tumors
- Certain drugs
- Childhood infections (mumps, meningitis)
- Congenital infection (toxoplasmosis, rubella, cytomegalovirus, herpes, syphilis)
- Congenital abnormality
- Demyelinating diseases (diseases that destroy the myelin sheath covering nerves)
- Genetic
- Loud noise
- Meniere's disease
- Sudden pressure changes from flying, diving, and strenuous exercise
- Viral infection of the inner ear (labyrinthitis)

bone's growth also pinches and damages the nerves connecting the inner ear with the brain. Otosclerosis tends to run in families and may develop in someone who had a childhood measles infection. Hearing loss first becomes evident in late adolescence or early adulthood. About 10% of adults have some evidence of otosclerosis, but only about 1% develop hearing loss as a result.

Noise: About 30 million people in the United States are exposed to levels of noise that can cause hearing loss. Noise destroys the hair cells in the inner ear. Although people vary greatly in their sensitivity to loud noise, everyone loses some hearing if exposed to sufficiently loud noise long enough.

▲ see page 1261

Both the loudness and duration of exposure are important—the louder the noise, the less time it takes to produce hearing loss. Extremely loud noise can cause hearing loss with even a single, brief exposure. Although brief exposure to loud noise usually produces only temporary hearing loss lasting a few hours to a day or so (called a temporary threshold shift), loss can be permanent, especially when the person is exposed many times. The person may have high-pitched ringing in the ears (tinnitus)▲ and problems comprehending speech. When a person experiences these symptoms, it is a warning that a sound is too loud and must be avoided.

Common sources of potentially damaging noise include highly amplified music, power tools, heavy machinery, and many types of powered vehicles, such as snowmobiles. Many people are exposed to injurious levels of noise during the course of their jobs, and hearing loss is a significant occupational hazard for many people. Explosions and gunfire also damage hearing.

Ear Infections: Young children commonly have some degree of conductive hearing loss after an ear infection (otitis media), because infection may lead to accumulation of fluid (effusion) in the middle ear. Most children regain normal hearing in 3 to 4 weeks after the infection resolves, but a few have persistent hearing loss. Chronic, long-standing infections of the middle ear often result in both conductive and sensorineural losses. Hearing loss is more likely in children who have recurring ear infections.

Autoimmune Disorders: Autoimmune disorders are sometimes a cause of hearing loss. The hearing loss may occur in people who have rheumatoid arthritis, systemic lupus erythematosus, Paget's disease, and polyarteritis nodosa. A fluctuating hearing loss, which may be progressive, occurs in both ears. The cause is an attack by the immune system on the cells of the cochlea.

Drugs: Drugs sometimes cause hearing loss. The aminoglycoside family of intravenous antibiotics are the drugs most commonly implicated, particularly when given in high doses. Some people have a rare hereditary disorder that makes them extremely susceptible to hearing loss due to aminoglycosides. Other drugs include vancomycin, quinine, and the cancer chemotherapy drugs cisplatin and nitrogen mustard. Hearing loss can be caused by aspirin (salicylate), but the hearing can come back when the drug is discontinued.

Diagnosis

All hearing loss needs to be evaluated by an otolaryngologist—a doctor who specializes in the care of the ear. An audiologist is a trained professional who tests hearing and performs hearing evaluation tests that measure the degree of hearing loss and the particular sound frequencies that are impaired. If hearing loss is present, other tests help determine how much the hearing loss affects the person's ability to understand speech and whether the hearing loss is sensorineural, conductive, or mixed. Some hearing tests also help identify possible causes of hearing loss. Although many hearing tests require the person's active participation, some do not.

Audiometry is the first step in hearing testing. In this test, a person wears headphones that play tones of different frequency (pitch) and loudness into one ear or the other. The person signals when he hears a tone, usually by raising his hand on the side the tone was heard. For each pitch, the test identifies the quietest tone the person can hear in each ear. The results are presented in comparison to what is considered normal hearing. Because loud tones presented to one ear may also be heard by the other ear, a sound other than the test tone (usually noise) is presented to the ear not being tested.

Speech threshold audiometry measures how loudly words have to be spoken to be understood. A person listens to a series of two-syllable, equally accented words (spondees), such as "railroad," "stairway," and "baseball"; presented at different volumes. The volume at which the person can correctly repeat half of the words (spondee threshold) is recorded.

Discrimination, the ability to hear differences between words that sound similar, is tested by presenting pairs of similar one-syllable words. The percentage of words correctly repeated is the discrimination score. People with a conductive hearing loss usually have a normal discrimination score, although at a higher volume. People with sensorineural loss often have abnormal discrimination at all volumes.

Tympanometry tests how well sound can pass through the eardrum and middle ear. This procedure does not require the active participation of the person being tested and is commonly used in children. A device containing a microphone and a sound source is placed snugly in the ear canal, and sound waves are bounced off the eardrum as the device varies the pressure in the ear canal. Abnormal tympanometry results suggest a conductive type of hearing loss.

The **Rinne tuning fork test** is a screening test that helps distinguish between conductive and sensorineural hearing loss. This test compares how well a person hears sounds conducted by air with how well the person hears sounds conducted by the skull bones. To test hearing by air conduction, the tuning fork is placed near the ear. To test hearing by bone conduction, the base of a vibrating tuning fork is placed against the head so the sound bypasses the middle ear and goes directly to the nerve cells of the inner ear. If hearing by air conduction is reduced but hearing by bone

Measurement of Loudness

Loudness is measured on a logarithmic scale. This means that an increase of 10 decibels (dB) represents a 10-fold increase in sound intensity, and a doubling of the perceived loudness. Thus, 20 dB is 100 times the intensity of 0 dB and appears 4 times as loud; 30 dB is 1000 times the intensity of 0 dB and appears 8 times as loud.

Decibels	Example
0	Faintest sound heard by human ear
30	Whisper, quiet library
60	Normal conversation, sewing machine, typewriter
90	Lawnmower, shop tools, truck traffic (8 hours per day is the maximum exposure without protection*)
100	Chainsaw, pneumatic drill, snowmobile (2 hours per day is the maximum exposure without protection)
115	Sandblasting, loud rock concert, automobile horn (15 minutes per day is the maximum exposure without protection)
140	Gun muzzle blast, jet engine (Noise causes pain and even brief exposure injures unprotected ears; injury may occur even with hearing protectors)
180	Rocket launching pad

*Mandatory federal standard, but protection is recommended for sound levels above 85 decibels.

conduction is normal, the hearing loss is conductive. If both air and bone conduction hearing are reduced, the hearing loss is sensorineural or mixed. People with sensorineural hearing loss may need further evaluation to look for other conditions, such as Meniere's disease or brain tumors.

Auditory brain stem response is a test that measures nerve impulses in the brain stem resulting from sound signals in the ears. The information helps determine what kind of signals the brain is receiving from the ears. Test results are abnormal in people with some sensorineural types of hearing loss and in people with many types of brain tumors. Auditory brain stem response is used to test infants and also can be used to monitor certain brain functions in people who are comatose or undergoing brain surgery.

Electrocochleography measures the activity of the cochlea and the auditory nerve by means of an electrode placed on, or through, the eardrum. This test and the auditory brain stem response can be used to measure hearing in people who cannot or will not respond voluntarily to sound. For example, these tests are used to find out whether infants and very young children have profound hearing loss (deafness) and whether a person is faking or exaggerating hearing loss (psychogenic hypacusis).

Otoacoustic emissions testing uses sound to stimulate the inner ear (cochlea). The ear itself then generates a very low intensity sound that matches the stimulus. These cochlear emissions are recorded using sophisticated electronics and are used routinely in many newborn nurseries to screen newborns for congenital hearing loss. This test is also used in adults to help determine the reason for a hearing loss.

Other tests can measure the ability to interpret and understand distorted speech, understand a message presented to one ear when a competing message is presented to the other ear, fuse incomplete messages to each ear into a meaningful message, and determine where a sound is coming from when it is presented to both ears at the same time. Depending on the person's symptoms and the results of the hearing tests, some people need computed tomography (CT) or magnetic resonance imaging (MRI) to look for tumors invading structures of the ear or blocking the eustachian tube.

▲ see art on page 1595

Prevention and Treatment

Age-related hearing loss and most other causes of hearing loss are not preventable. However, many measures can be taken to help prevent noise-induced hearing loss, such as limiting exposure to loud noise, reducing noise levels whenever possible, and staying away from the source of the noise. The volume of music played through headphones should always be kept at a reasonable level. The louder the noise, the less time a person should spend near it. For occupational or firearm exposure, the use of hearing protectors, such as plastic or foam rubber plugs in the ear canals or glycerin-filled muffs over the ears, is essential. Plastic plugs can also be used in other loud environments.

Treatment of hearing loss depends on the cause. When the cause is fluid in the middle ear, children and adults may need to have a small tube placed in the eardrum (tympanostomy).▲ The tube helps prevent fluid from accumulating. Some children also need to have their adenoids removed (adenoidectomy), which helps keep the eustachian tube open. Tumors blocking the eustachian tube are removed. Hearing loss caused by autoimmune disorders is treated with corticosteroids, such as prednisone.

Damage to the eardrums or the bones in the middle ear may require reconstructive surgery. For some people with otosclerosis, hearing may be restored by removing the stirrup surgically and replacing it with an artificial one. Brain tumors causing hearing loss may, in some cases, be removed and the hearing preserved.

Most other causes of hearing loss have no cure. In these cases, treatment involves compensating for the hearing loss as much as possible. Most people with moderate to severe loss use hearing aids. Those with severe to profound loss are greatly helped by a cochlear implant.

Hearing Aids: Sound amplification with a hearing aid helps people who have either conductive or sensorineural hearing loss. Unfortunately, a hearing aid does not restore hearing to normal. A hearing aid should, however, significantly improve a person's ability to communicate and enjoy sounds.

All hearing aids have a microphone to pick up sounds, a battery-powered amplifier to increase their volume, and a means of transmitting the sound to the person. Most hearing aids transmit the sounds through a small

Hearing Aids: Amplifying the Sound

The behind-the-ear hearing aid is the most powerful but least attractive hearing aid. The in-the-ear hearing aid is the best choice for severe hearing loss. It is easy to adjust but is difficult to use with telephones. The in-the-canal hearing aid is used for mild to moderate hearing loss. This aid is relatively inconspicuous but is difficult to use with telephones. The completely-in-the-canal hearing aid is used for mild to moderate hearing loss. This aid has good sound, is nearly invisible, and can be easily used with telephones. It is removed by pulling on a small string. However, it is the most expensive and hard to adjust.

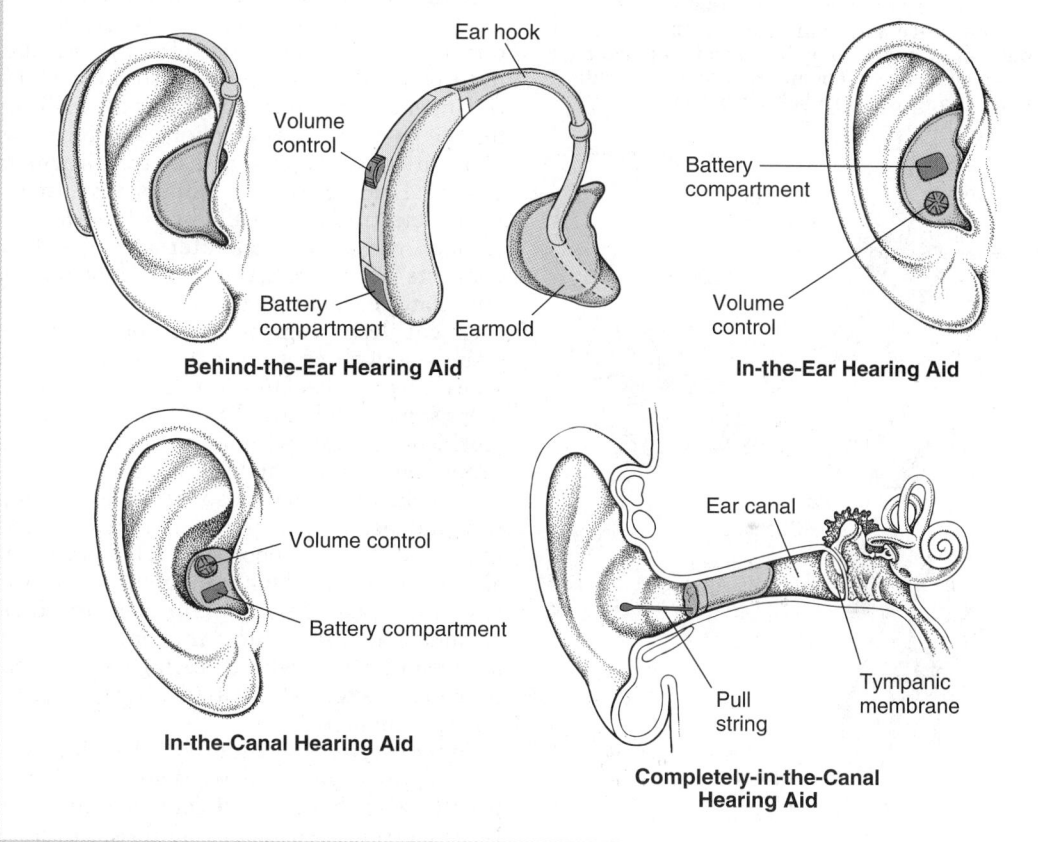

Behind-the-Ear Hearing Aid

In-the-Ear Hearing Aid

In-the-Canal Hearing Aid

Completely-in-the-Canal Hearing Aid

speaker placed in the ear canal. Other hearing aids, which require surgical implantation, transmit sounds directly to the bones of the middle ear (ossicles) or the skull instead of through a speaker. Hearing aids differ in how big the components are and where they are located. As a general rule, larger hearing aids are more noticeable and less attractive but are easier to adjust. Larger aids can often accommodate features that are not available in small ones.

Hearing aids have different electronic characteristics that are chosen to suit the person's particular type of hearing loss. For example, people whose hearing loss affects mainly higher frequencies do not benefit from simple amplification, which merely makes the mumbled speech they hear sound louder. Hearing aids that selectively amplify the high frequencies markedly improve speech recognition. Other hearing aids contain vents in the ear mold, which facilitate the passage of high-

Cochlear Implant: Aid for the Profoundly Deaf

A cochlear implant, a type of hearing aid for profoundly deaf people, consists of an internal coil, electrodes, an external coil, a speech processor, and a microphone. The internal coil is surgically implanted in the skull behind and above the ear, and the electrodes are implanted in the cochlea. The external coil is held in place by magnets on the skin over the internal coil. The speech processor, connected to the external coil by a wire, may be worn in a pocket or special holster. The microphone is placed in a hearing aid worn behind the ear.

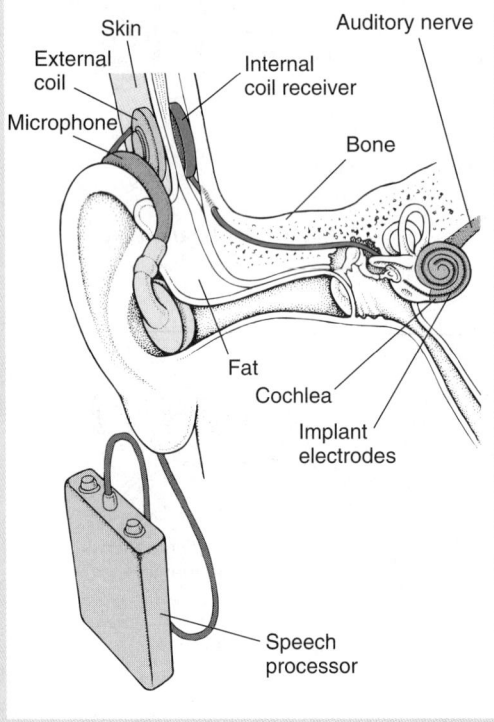

phone coil: With the flip of a switch the microphone is turned off, and the phone coil links electromagnetically to the magnet in the phone handle. As long as the hearing aid has the proper features, this setup can be arranged by the phone company with simple changes to the phone. Hearing aids with complex features tend to be the most expensive but are often essential to meet hearing needs.

Cochlear Implants: Most profoundly deaf people who cannot hear sounds even with a hearing aid benefit from a cochlear implant. Cochlear implants provide electrical signals directly into the auditory nerve by means of multiple electrodes inserted into the cochlea, the inner ear structure containing the auditory nerve. An external microphone and processor pick up sound signals and convert them to electrical impulses. The impulses are transmitted electromagnetically by an external coil through the skin to an internal coil, which connects to the electrodes. The electrodes stimulate the auditory nerve.

A cochlear implant does not transmit sounds as well as a normal cochlea but provides different benefits to different people. It helps some people read lips. Others can distinguish some words without reading lips. Some people can hear on the telephone.

A cochlear implant also helps deaf people hear and distinguish environmental and warning signals, such as doorbells, telephones, and alarms. It helps them modulate their own voices to make their speech easier for others to understand. A cochlear implant is more effective in a person whose hearing loss is recent or who had successfully used a hearing aid before the implant.

Other Means of Coping With Hearing Loss: Several other types of devices are available for people who have significant hearing loss. Light alerting systems enable these people to know when the doorbell is ringing or a baby is crying. Special sound systems help people hear in theaters, churches, or other places where there is competing noise. Many television programs carry closed captioning, with the dialog shown as visible text. Telephone communication devices are also available.

Lip reading (speech reading) is an important skill for people who have decreased hearing. It is particularly important for people who can hear but have trouble discriminating sounds, typically those with age-related hearing loss. Observing the position of a speaker's lips allows people to recognize which consonant is

frequency sound waves into the ear. Many hearing aids use digital sound processing with multiple frequency channels so that the amplification can even more precisely match the person's hearing loss. People who cannot tolerate loud sounds may need hearing aids with special electronic circuitry, which keeps the maximum volume of sound at a tolerable level.

Telephone use can be difficult for people with hearing aids. With typical hearing aids, placing the ear next to the phone handle causes squealing. Some hearing aids have a being spoken. Because people whose hearing loss affects high frequencies are unable to understand consonant sounds, lip reading can significantly improve the comprehension of speech.

Lip reading and other strategies for coping with hearing loss are sometimes taught by hearing professionals in a program called aural rehabilitation.▲ In addition to training in lip reading, people are taught to gain control over their listening environment by learning to anticipate difficult communication situations and modifying or avoiding them. For example, people can visit a restaurant during off-peak hours, when it is quieter. They can ask for a booth, which blocks out some extraneous sounds. They can request that "specials of the day" be written rather than spoken. In direct conversations, people may ask the speaker to face them. At the beginning of a telephone conversation, people can identify themselves as being hearing-impaired.

People with profound hearing loss often communicate using sign language. American Sign Language (ASL) is the version most widely used in the United States. Other forms include Signed English, Signing Exact English, and Cued Speech.

CHAPTER 219

Outer Ear Disorders

The outer ear consists of the external part of the ear (pinna or auricle) and the ear canal (external auditory meatus).■ Disorders of the outer ear include blockages, infections (external otitis and perichondritis), eczema, and tumors. The outer ear is also prone to certain types of injury.

Blockages

Earwax (cerumen) may block the ear canal. Even large amounts of wax often produce no symptoms. Symptoms can range from itching to a loss of hearing. A doctor may remove the earwax by gently flushing out the ear canal with warm water (irrigation). However, if a person has had a perforated eardrum, irrigation is not used because water can enter the middle ear if the perforation is still present. Similarly, irrigation is not used if there is any discharge from the ear, because the discharge may be coming from a perforated eardrum. In these situations, a doctor may remove earwax with a blunt instrument, an instrument with a loop at the end, or a vacuum device.

Earwax solvents help soften wax, but they usually must be followed by irrigation, because the solvent rarely dissolves all of the wax. People should not attempt earwax removal at home with cotton swabs, bobby pins, pencils, or any other implements. Such attempts usually just pack the wax in more and can damage the eardrum. Soap and water on a washcloth provide adequate external ear hygiene.

Other blockages can occur when people, particularly children, put foreign objects, such as beads, erasers, and beans, into the ear canal. Usually, a doctor removes such objects with a blunt hook or small vacuum device. Sometimes metal and glass beads can be flushed out by irrigation, but water causes some objects, such as beans, to swell, complicating removal. Objects that are deep in the canal are more difficult to remove because of the risk of injury to the eardrum. A general anesthetic is used when a child does not cooperate or when removal is particularly difficult.

Insects, particularly cockroaches, may also block the ear canal. To kill the insect, a doctor fills the canal with mineral oil or lidocaine, a numbing agent. This measure also provides immediate pain relief and enables the doctor to remove the insect.

External Otitis

External otitis is infection of the ear canal.

External otitis may affect the entire canal, as in generalized external otitis, or just one small area, as in a boil (furuncle) or pimple.

Causes

A variety of bacteria or, rarely, fungi can cause generalized external otitis. Certain peo-

---

▲ see page 45   ■ see art on page 1245

Irrigating the Ear Canal

The tip of a water-filled syringe is placed just inside the ear canal, and a stream of warm water is gently directed into the canal to remove earwax. This procedure should be performed by a doctor or a nurse.

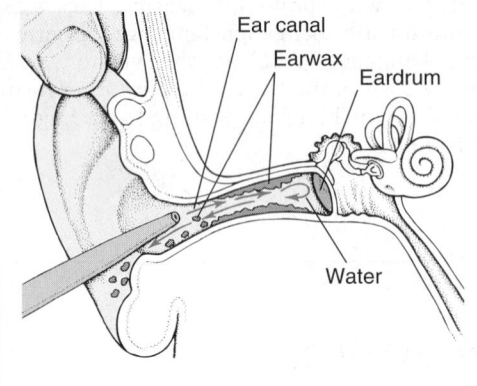

ple, including those who have allergies, psoriasis, eczema, or scalp dermatitis, are particularly prone to external otitis. Injuring the ear canal while cleaning it or getting water or irritants such as hair spray or hair dye in the canal often leads to external otitis. External otitis is particularly common after swimming in fresh water pools, in which case it is sometimes called **swimmer's ear.** Earplugs and hearing aids make external otitis more likely, particularly if these devices are not properly cleaned.

Symptoms and Diagnosis

Symptoms of generalized external otitis are itching and pain. Sometimes an unpleasant-smelling white or yellow discharge drains from the ear. The ear canal may have no swelling, slight swelling, or in severe cases be swollen completely closed. If the ear canal swells or fills with pus and debris, hearing is impaired. Usually, the canal is tender and hurts if the external ear (pinna) is pulled or if pressure is placed on the fold of skin in front of the ear canal. To a doctor looking into the ear canal through an otoscope (a device for viewing the canal and eardrum), the skin of the canal appears red and swollen and may be littered with pus and debris.

▲ see page 1220

Boils cause severe pain. When they rupture, a small amount of blood and pus may leak from the ear.

Prevention and Treatment

Swimmer's ear may be prevented by putting drops of a solution containing half rubbing alcohol and half vinegar in the ear before and after swimming. The person should avoid swimming in polluted water, using hair spray, and spending much time in warm, humid climates.

Attempting to clean the canal with cotton swabs interrupts the normal, self-cleaning mechanism and can push debris toward the eardrum, where it accumulates. Also, these actions may cause minor damage that predisposes to external otitis.

To treat generalized external otitis from any cause, a doctor first removes the infected debris from the canal with suction or dry cotton wipes. After the ear canal is cleared, hearing often returns to normal. Usually, a person is given antibiotic ear drops to use several times a day for up to a week. Some ear drops also contain a corticosteroid to reduce swelling and analgesics to reduce pain. Often, external otitis is successfully treated with ear drops containing vinegar. Bacteria do not grow as well once the normal acidity of the ear canal is restored. If the ear canal is very swollen, a doctor inserts a small wick in the canal to allow the drops to penetrate.

Analgesics such as acetaminophen or codeine may help reduce pain for the first 24 to 48 hours, until the inflammation begins to subside. An infection that has spread beyond the ear canal (cellulitis▲) may be treated with an antibiotic given by mouth.

Treatment of boils depends on how advanced the infection is. In an early stage of infection, a heating pad can be applied for a short time and analgesics can be given to help relieve pain; the heat may also help speed healing. A boil that has come to a head is cut open to drain the pus. An antibiotic is then applied directly to the area or given by mouth.

Perichondritis

Perichondritis is infection of the cartilage of the external ear.

Injury, burns, insect bites, ear piercing, or a boil on the ear may cause perichondritis. The infection also tends to occur in people whose immune system is weakened and in people who have diabetes. The first symptoms are redness, pain, and swelling of the ear. The person may have a fever. Pus accumulates between the cartilage and the layer of connective tissue around it (perichondrium). Sometimes the pus cuts off the blood supply to the cartilage, destroying it and leading eventually to a deformed ear. Although destructive and long-lasting, perichondritis tends to produce only mild discomfort.

A doctor makes an incision to drain the pus, allowing blood to reach the cartilage again. Antibiotics are given by mouth for milder infections and intravenously for severe infections. The choice of antibiotic depends on how severe the infection is and which bacteria are causing it.

Tumors

Tumors of the ear may be noncancerous (benign) or cancerous (malignant). Most ear tumors are found when a person sees them, or when a doctor looks in the ear because the person notices his hearing seems decreased.

Noncancerous tumors may develop in the ear canal, blocking it and causing hearing loss and a buildup of earwax. Such tumors include small sacs filled with skin secretions (sebaceous cysts), osteomas (bone tumors), and growths of excess scar tissue after an injury (keloids). The most effective treatment is surgical removal of the tumor. After treatment, hearing usually returns to normal.

Basal cell and squamous cell cancers▲ are common skin cancers that often develop on the external ear after repeated and prolonged exposure to the sun. When these cancers first appear, they can be successfully treated by removing them surgically or by applying radiation therapy. More advanced cancers may re-

quire surgical removal of a larger area of the external ear.

Ceruminoma (cancer of the cells that produce earwax) develops in the outer third of the ear canal and can spread. Ceruminomas have nothing to do with earwax buildup. Treatment consists of removing the cancer and the surrounding tissue surgically.

Injury

A number of different injuries can affect the outer ear. A blunt blow to the external ear can cause bruising between the cartilage and the layer of connective tissue around it (perichondrium). When blood collects in this area, the external ear becomes swollen and purple. The collected blood (hematoma) can cut off the blood supply to the cartilage, allowing that portion of the cartilage to die, leading in time to a deformed ear. This deformity, called a cauliflower ear, is common among wrestlers, boxers, and rugby players.

A doctor cuts open the hematoma and removes the blood with suction. After the hematoma is empty, the doctor applies a compression dressing, which is left on for 3 to 7 days to keep the hematoma from coming back. The dressing keeps the skin and perichondrium in their normal positions, allowing blood to reach the cartilage again.

If a cut (laceration) goes all the way through the ear, the area is cleansed thoroughly and the skin is sewn back together and a dressing is applied to protect the area and allow the cartilage to heal. The cartilage is not sewn.

A forceful blow to the jaw may fracture the bones surrounding the ear canal and distort the canal's shape, often narrowing it. The shape can be corrected surgically.

CHAPTER 220

Middle and Inner Ear Disorders

The middle ear consists of the eardrum (tympanic membrane) and an air-filled chamber containing a chain of three bones (ossicles) that connect the eardrum to the inner ear.■ The fluid-filled inner ear (labyrinth) consists of two major parts: the organ of hearing (cochlea) and the organ of balance (vestibular

system, which consists of the semicircular canals, the saccule, and the utricle). The middle ear acts as an amplifier of sound, while the inner ear is a transducer, changing mechanical

▲ see also page 1238   ■ see page 1244

sound waves into an electrical signal that is sent to the brain via the nerve of hearing (statoacoustic nerve). Middle and inner ear disorders produce many of the same symptoms, and a disorder of the middle ear may affect the inner ear and vice versa.

Perforation of the Eardrum

A perforation is a hole in the eardrum.

A middle ear infection (otitis media) is the most common cause of eardrum perforation. The eardrum can also be perforated by a sudden change in pressure—either an increase, such as that caused by an explosion, a slap, or diving underwater; or a decrease, such as occurs while flying in an airplane. Another cause is burns from heat or chemicals. The eardrum may also be perforated (punctured) by objects placed in the ear, such as a cotton-tipped swab, or by objects entering the ear accidentally, such as a low-hanging twig or a thrown pencil. An object that penetrates the eardrum can dislocate or fracture the chain of small bones (ossicles) that connect the eardrum to the inner ear. Pieces of the broken ossicles or the object itself may even penetrate the inner ear. A blocked eustachian tube may lead to the perforation because of severe imbalance of pressure (barotrauma).

Symptoms and Diagnosis

Perforation of the eardrum causes sudden severe pain, sometimes followed by bleeding from the ear, hearing loss, and noise in the ear (tinnitus).▲ The hearing loss is more severe if the chain of ossicles has been disrupted or the inner ear has been injured. Injury to the inner ear may also cause vertigo (a whirling sensation). Pus may begin to drain from the ear in 24 to 48 hours, particularly if water or other foreign material enters the middle ear. A doctor diagnoses eardrum perforation by looking in the ear with a special instrument called an otoscope.

Treatment

The ear is kept dry. Ear drops containing an antibiotic may be used if the ear becomes infected. Usually, the eardrum heals without further treatment, but if it does not heal within 2 months, surgery to repair the eardrum (tympanoplasty) may be needed. If a perforation is not repaired, the person may develop a smoldering infection—chronic otitis media—in the middle ear.

A persistent conductive hearing loss ■ following perforation of the eardrum suggests a disruption or fixation of the ossicles, which may be repaired surgically. A sensorineural hearing loss or vertigo that persists for more than a few hours after the injury suggests that something has injured or penetrated the inner ear.

Barotrauma

Barotrauma is damage to the middle ear caused by unequal air pressure on the two sides of the eardrum.

The eardrum separates the ear canal and the middle ear. If air pressure in the ear canal from outside air and air pressure in the middle ear are unequal, the eardrum can be damaged. Normally, the eustachian tube, which connects the middle ear and the back of the nose, helps maintain equal pressure on both sides of the eardrum by allowing outside air to enter the middle ear. When outside air pressure changes suddenly—for example, during the ascent or descent of an airplane or a deep-sea dive★—air must move through the eustachian tube to equalize the pressure in the middle ear.

If the eustachian tube is partly or completely blocked because of scarring, a tumor, an infection, the common cold, or an allergy, air cannot move in and out of the middle ear. The resulting pressure difference may bruise the eardrum or even cause it to rupture and bleed. If the pressure difference is very great, the oval window (the entrance into the inner ear from the middle ear) may rupture, allowing fluid from the inner ear to leak into the middle ear. Hearing loss or vertigo occurring during descent in a deep-sea dive suggests that such leakage is taking place. The same symptoms occurring during ascent suggest that an air bubble has formed in the inner ear.

When sudden changes in pressure cause a sense of fullness or pain in the ear, often the pressure in the middle ear can be equalized and the discomfort relieved by several maneuvers. If outside pressure is decreasing, as in a plane climbing upward, the person should try breathing with the mouth open, chewing gum, or swallowing. Any of these measures may open the eustachian tube and allow air out of the middle ear. If outside pressure is increas-

---

▲ see page 1261   ■ see page 1247
★ see page 1667

The Eustachian Tube: Keeping Air Pressure Equal

The eustachian tube helps maintain equal air pressure on both sides of the eardrum by allowing outside air to enter the middle ear. If the eustachian tube is blocked, air cannot reach the middle ear, so the pressure there decreases. When air pressure is lower in the middle ear than in the ear canal, the eardrum bulges inward. The pressure difference can cause pain and can bruise or rupture the eardrum.

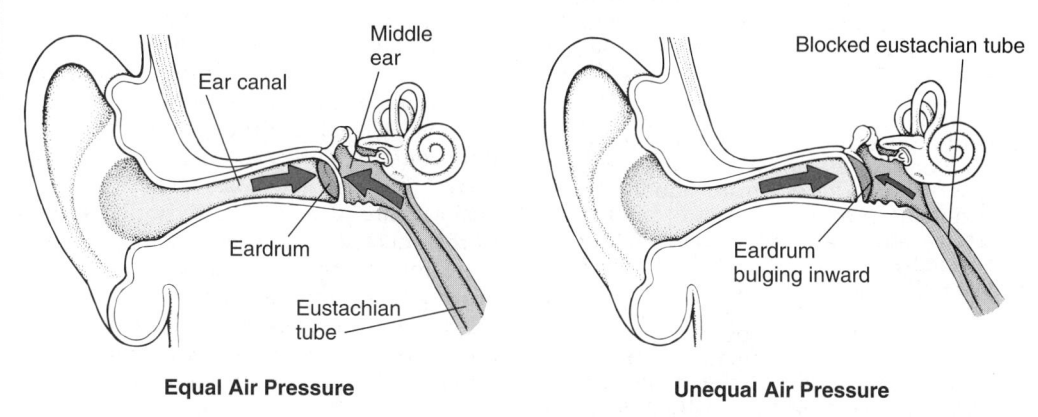

Equal Air Pressure   **Unequal Air Pressure**

ing, as in a plane descending or a diver going deeper underwater, the person should pinch his nose shut, hold the mouth closed, and try to blow gently out through the nose. This will force air through the blocked eustachian tube. People who have an infection or an allergy affecting the nose and throat may experience discomfort when they fly in a plane or dive. However, if flying is necessary, a decongestant, such as phenylephrine nose drops or nasal spray, relieves congestion and helps open the eustachian tubes, equalizing pressure on the eardrums. Diving should be avoided until the infection or allergy is controlled.

Infectious Myringitis

Infectious myringitis is infection of the eardrum by a virus or bacteria.

Myringitis is caused by a variety of viruses and bacteria; the bacteria *Mycoplasma* is a common cause. The eardrum becomes inflamed, and small, fluid-filled blisters (vesicles) form on its surface. Blisters may also be present in otitis media; however, in myringitis, there is no pus or fluid in the middle ear.

Pain begins suddenly and lasts for 24 to 48 hours. There may be some hearing loss.

Doctors diagnose myringitis by looking at the eardrum with an otoscope. Because it is

difficult to tell if the infection is viral or bacterial, most people are treated with antibiotics and analgesics. A doctor may need to rupture the vesicles with a small blade to relieve the pain.

Acute Otitis Media

Acute otitis media is a bacterial or viral infection of the middle ear.

Acute otitis media results from infection by viruses or bacteria, often as a complication of the common cold or of allergies. Acute otitis media is more common in children than in adults. Symptoms and treatment are similar in adults and older children.▲

The infected ear is painful, with a red, bulging eardrum. Most people with acute otitis media get better on their own. However, because it is hard to predict who will not improve, most doctors treat all people with antibiotics, such as amoxicillin. Acetaminophen or nonsteroidal anti-inflammatory drugs (NSAIDs) can relieve pain. Decongestants containing phenylephrine may help, and antihistamines are useful for people who have allergies but not for those with colds.

▲ see page 1594

When the Ear Aches

An earache is a pain that appears to originate in the ear. The actual source of pain may be within the ear or in nearby structures that share the same nerves to the brain; this type of pain is called referred pain.

Pain originating in the ear is most likely the result of infection. Infection of the middle ear (otitis media) is the most common cause of earaches in children. Infection of the ear canal (otitis externa) is also very painful and occurs in both children and adults. Ear pain also occurs when blockage of the eustachian tube (the tube that connects the middle ear and back of the nose) prevents pressure in the middle ear from equalizing with outside pressure. Pressure mainly causes symptoms during airplane flights and undersea diving. Swallowing or blowing the nose sometimes relieves the pressure and pain.

Ear pain that originates outside the ear may come from infections or tumors of many areas of the nose and throat. If a person with earache has no apparent ear disorder, doctors look for problems with the nose, sinuses, teeth, gums, jaw joint (temporomandibular joint), tongue, tonsils, throat (pharynx), voice box (larynx), windpipe (trachea), esophagus, and salivary glands in the cheek (parotid glands). Sometimes, the first symptom of cancer in any of these structures is pain that feels like an earache.

If a person has severe or persistent pain and fever, and the eardrum is bulging, a doctor may perform a myringotomy, in which an opening is made through the eardrum to allow fluid to drain from the middle ear. The opening, which does not affect hearing, usually heals on its own. People who have repeated bouts of otitis media may need to have drainage tubes (tympanostomy tubes) placed in their eardrums.▲

Serous Otitis Media

Serous otitis media is an accumulation of fluid in the middle ear.

Serous (secretory) otitis media can develop from acute otitis media that has not com-

---

▲ see art on page 1595   ■ see page 1594
★ see page 1249   ● see art on page 1595

pletely cleared or from a blocked eustachian tube. Allergies are a common cause of eustachian tube blockage. Serous otitis media can occur at any age but is particularly common in children.■

Normally, pressure in the middle ear is equalized 3 or 4 times a minute as the eustachian tube opens during swallowing. If the eustachian tube is blocked, pressure in the middle ear tends to decrease as oxygen is absorbed into the bloodstream from the middle ear. As the pressure decreases, fluid accumulates in the middle ear, reducing the eardrum's ability to move. Usually, although not always, the fluid contains some bacteria, but symptoms of active infection (such as redness, pain, and pus) are rare. People usually notice a fullness in the affected ear and may hear a popping or crackling sound when they swallow. Some hearing loss commonly develops.

A doctor examines the ear to make the diagnosis. Tympanometry★ helps diagnose the presence of fluid in the middle ear.

Treatment

Decongestants, such as phenylephrine and ephedrine, and, in people with allergies, antihistamines, can be taken to reduce congestion and help open the eustachian tube. Although most people are treated with antibiotics in the United States, they usually are not necessary. Low pressure in the middle ear can be temporarily increased by forcing air past the blockage in the eustachian tube. To do this, the person breathes out with the mouth closed and the nostrils pinched shut.

If symptoms become chronic (lasting more than 3 months), a doctor may perform a myringotomy, in which an opening is made through the eardrum to allow fluid to drain from the middle ear. A tiny drainage tube (tympanostomy tube)● can be inserted into the opening in the eardrum to help fluid drain and allow air to enter the middle ear.

Chronic Otitis Media

Chronic otitis media is a long-standing infection of the middle ear.

Chronic otitis media is caused by a permanent hole (perforation) in the eardrum or a noncancerous growth of white skinlike material (cholesteatoma). People may have a perforation without ever getting any symptoms, but sometimes a chronic bacterial infection develops.

Chronic otitis media may flare up after an infection of the nose and throat, such as the common cold, or after water enters the middle ear while bathing or swimming. Usually, flare-ups result in a painless discharge of pus, which may be malodorous, from the ear. Persistent flare-ups may result in the formation of protruding growths called polyps, which extend from the middle ear through the perforation and into the ear canal. Persistent infection can destroy parts of the ossicles—the small bones in the middle ear that connect the eardrum to the inner ear and conduct sounds from the outer ear to the inner ear—causing conductive hearing loss.▲ Other serious complications include inflammation of the inner ear, facial paralysis, and brain infections. Some people with chronic otitis media develop cholesteatomas in the middle ear. Cholesteatomas, which destroy bone, greatly increase the likelihood of other serious complications. A doctor diagnoses chronic otitis media when seeing pus or skinlike material accumulating in a hole or in a pocket in the eardrum that often drains.

Treatment

When chronic otitis media flares up, a doctor thoroughly cleans the ear canal and middle ear with suction and dry cotton wipes, then prescribes a solution of acetic acid with hydrocortisone or antibiotic ear drops. Water must be kept out of the ear when a perforation is present.

Usually, the eardrum can be repaired in a procedure called tympanoplasty. If the ossicle chain has been disrupted, it may be repaired at the same time. Cholesteatomas must be removed surgically. If a cholesteatoma is not removed, serious complications can develop.

Mastoiditis

Mastoiditis is a bacterial infection in the mastoid process, the prominent bone behind the ear.

This disorder usually occurs when untreated or inadequately treated acute otitis media spreads from the middle ear into the surrounding bone—the mastoid process.

Usually, symptoms appear 2 or more weeks after acute otitis media develops, as the spreading infection destroys the inner part of the mastoid process. A collection of pus (abscess) may form in the bone. The skin covering the mastoid process may become red, swollen, and tender, and the external ear is pushed sideways and down. Other symptoms are fever, pain around and within the ear, and a creamy, profuse discharge from the ear. The pain tends to be persistent and throbbing. Hearing loss is progressive.

Computed tomography (CT) shows that the air cells (spaces in bone that normally contain air) in the mastoid process are filled with fluid. As mastoiditis progresses, the spaces enlarge. Inadequately treated mastoiditis can result in deafness, blood poisoning (sepsis), infection of the tissues covering the brain (meningitis), brain abscess, or death.

Treatment is with intravenous antibiotics. A sample of ear discharge is examined to identify the organism causing the infection and to determine the antibiotics most likely to eliminate the bacteria. Antibiotics may be given by mouth once the person starts to recover and are continued for at least 2 weeks. If an abscess has formed in the bone, surgical drainage (mastoidectomy) is required.

Meniere's Disease

Meniere's disease is a disorder characterized by recurring attacks of disabling vertigo (a whirling sensation), hearing loss, and tinnitus.

Meniere's disease is thought to be caused by an imbalance in the fluid that is normally present in the inner ear. This fluid is continually being secreted and reabsorbed, maintaining a constant amount. Either an increase in production of inner ear fluid or a decrease in its reabsorption results in an imbalance of fluid. Why either happens is not known.

Symptoms include sudden, unprovoked attacks of severe, disabling vertigo, nausea, and vomiting; these symptoms usually last for 2 to 3 hours but can rarely last up to 24 hours. Periodically, a person may feel a fullness or pressure in the affected ear. Hearing tends to fluctuate but progressively worsens over the years. Tinnitus, which may be constant or intermittent, may be worse before, during, or after an attack of vertigo. Both hearing loss and tinnitus usually affect only one ear.

In one form of Meniere's disease, hearing loss and tinnitus precede the first attack of vertigo by months or years. After the attacks of vertigo begin, hearing may improve.

Diagnosis and Treatment

A doctor suspects Meniere's disease because of the typical symptoms of vertigo with tinni-

▲ see page 1247

tus and hearing loss in one ear. Doctors usually perform hearing tests and sometimes magnetic resonance imaging (MRI) to look for other causes. A low-salt diet and a diuretic lower the frequency of attacks in some people. When attacks do occur, vertigo may be relieved temporarily with drugs given by mouth, such as meclizine, lorazepam, or scopolamine. Scopolamine is also available in skin patches. Nausea and vomiting may be relieved by suppositories containing the drug prochlorperazine.

Several procedures are available for people who are disabled by frequent attacks of vertigo despite drug treatment. The procedures aim either to reduce fluid pressure in the inner ear or to destroy inner ear balance function. The endolymphatic shunt procedure, in which a thin sheet of flexible plastic material is placed in the inner ear, is the least destructive of these procedures. To destroy inner ear balance function, a solution of gentamicin can be injected through the eardrum into the middle ear. Several injections over time provide the best result. However, severe hearing loss or chronic imbalance can result from this treatment. Cutting the vestibular nerve permanently destroys inner ear balance, while preserving hearing, and is successful 99% of the time in controlling vertigo. This procedure is usually performed on people who do not improve after an endolymphatic shunt or those who never want to experience another spell of vertigo. Finally, when vertigo is disabling and hearing has deteriorated in the involved ear, the entire semicircular canals can be drilled away in a procedure called a labyrinthectomy. The hearing loss that often accompanies Meniere's disease does not improve with any of the procedures to treat the severe vertigo.

Vestibular Neuronitis

Vestibular neuronitis is a disorder characterized by a sudden severe attack of vertigo (a whirling sensation), caused by inflammation of the nerve to the semicircular canals.

Vestibular neuronitis is probably caused by a virus. It may occur as a single, isolated attack of vertigo lasting several days, although many people have additional attacks of milder vertigo for several weeks thereafter. The first attack of vertigo is usually the most severe. The attack, which is accompanied by nausea

and vomiting, lasts for 3 to 7 days. The eyes flicker involuntarily away from the affected side (a sign called nystagmus). Each subsequent attack is shorter and less severe than the previous one, and typically occurs only when the head is in certain positions. Hearing is usually not affected.

Diagnosis involves hearing tests and tests for nystagmus.▲ Magnetic resonance imaging (MRI) of the head may be performed to make sure the symptoms are not caused by another disorder, such as a tumor.

Treatment of vertigo is the same as in Meniere's disease and consists of drugs such as meclizine, lorazepam, or scopolamine. Nausea and vomiting may be relieved by suppositories containing the drug prochlorperazine. If vomiting continues for a long time, a person may need to be given fluids and electrolytes intravenously. The disorder eventually goes away on its own.

Temporal Bone Fracture

The temporal bone (the skull bone containing part of the ear canal, the middle ear, and the inner ear) can be fractured by a blow to the head.

Temporal bone fractures frequently rupture the eardrum and may also damage the ossicles and the cochlea.

Symptoms include facial paralysis on the side of the fracture and profound hearing loss, which may be conductive, sensorineural, or both. People may have bleeding from the ear, blood behind the eardrum, or patchy bruising of the skin behind the ear. Sometimes, cerebrospinal fluid leaks from the brain through the fracture and appears as clear fluid draining from the ear or nose. Leakage of this fluid indicates that the brain is exposed to infection.

Diagnosis is made with computed tomography (CT). Treatment usually requires an antibiotic given intravenously to prevent infection of the tissues covering the brain (meningitis). Sometimes, persistent facial paralysis caused by pressure on the facial nerve can be relieved by surgery. Damage to the eardrum and structures of the middle ear is repaired surgically weeks or months later if necessary.

Auditory Nerve Tumors

An auditory nerve tumor (acoustic neuroma, acoustic neurinoma, vestibular schwannoma, eighth nerve tumor) is a noncancerous (be-

▲ see page 464

nign) tumor that originates in the cells that wrap around the auditory nerve (Schwann cells).

Auditory nerve tumors usually grow from the vestibular (balance) nerve. Hearing loss, tinnitus, dizziness, and unsteadiness are early symptoms. If the tumor grows larger and compresses other parts of the brain, such as the facial nerve or the trigeminal nerve, weakness and numbness of the face may result. Early symptoms include ringing in one ear (tinnitus), hearing loss, and imbalance or unsteadiness when the person turns quickly.

Early diagnosis is based on a magnetic resonance imaging (MRI) scan and hearing tests.

Tumors are removed by surgery, which may be performed with a microscope (microsurgery) to avoid damaging the facial nerve.

Tinnitus

Tinnitus is noise originating in the ear rather than in the environment.

Tinnitus is a symptom and not a specific disease. It is very common—10 to 15% of people experience some degree of tinnitus.

More than 75% of ear-related problems include tinnitus as a symptom, including injury from loud noises or explosions, ear infections, a blocked ear canal or eustachian tube, otosclerosis (a type of hearing loss), tumors of the middle ear, and Meniere's disease. Certain drugs (such as aminoglycoside antibiotics and high doses of aspirin) also may cause tinnitus.

Tinnitus may also occur with disorders outside the ears, including anemia, heart and blood vessel disorders such as hypertension and arteriosclerosis, an underactive thyroid gland (hypothyroidism), and head injury. Tinnitus that is only in one ear or that pulsates is a more serious sign. A pulsating sound may result from certain tumors, a blocked artery, an aneurysm, or other blood vessel disorders.

The noise heard by people with tinnitus may be a buzzing, ringing, roaring, whistling, or hissing sound. Some people hear more complex sounds that vary over time. These sounds are more noticeable in a quiet environment and when the person is not concentrating on something else. Thus, tinnitus tends to be most disturbing to people when they are trying to sleep. However, the experience of tinnitus is highly individual; some people are very disturbed by their symptoms, and others find them quite bearable.

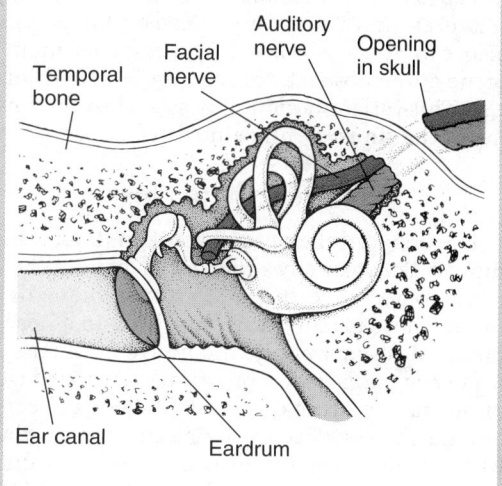

How Ear Disorders Affect the Facial Nerve

Because the facial nerve winds through the ear, disorders of the middle and inner ear can affect it. For example, herpes zoster of the ear may affect the facial nerve as well as the auditory nerve. The facial nerve then swells and presses against the opening in the skull that it passes through. The pressure on this nerve can cause temporary or permanent facial paralysis. Treatment depends on the disorder causing the problem.

Diagnosis and Treatment

Because a person who has tinnitus usually has some hearing loss, thorough hearing tests are performed as well as magnetic resonance imaging (MRI) of the head and computed tomography (CT) of the temporal bone (the skull bone that contains part of the ear canal, the middle ear, and the inner ear).

Attempts to identify and treat the disorder causing tinnitus are often unsuccessful. Various techniques can help make tinnitus tolerable, although the ability to tolerate it varies from person to person. Often a hearing aid helps suppress tinnitus. Many people find relief by playing background music to mask the tinnitus. Some people use a tinnitus masker, a device worn like a hearing aid that produces a constant level of neutral sounds. For the profoundly deaf, a cochlear implant may reduce tinnitus.

CHAPTER 221

Disorders of the Nose and Sinuses

The upper part of the nose consists mostly of bone; the lower part gains its support from cartilage. Inside the nose is a hollow cavity (nasal cavity), which is divided into two passages by a thin sheet of cartilage and bone called the nasal septum. The bones of the face contain the paranasal sinuses, which are hollow cavities that open into the nasal cavity.▲

Because of its prominent position, the nose is especially vulnerable to injury, including fractures. Infections, nosebleeds, and polyps also can affect the nose. The mucous membrane of the nose may become inflamed (rhinitis). This inflammation may spread to the lining of the sinuses (rhinosinusitis).

Fractures of the Nose

The bones of the nose are broken (fractured) more often than any other facial bone. When nasal bones break, the mucous membrane lining the nose usually tears, resulting in a nosebleed. Most commonly, the bridge of the nose is pushed to one side. Sometimes, the cartilage of the nasal septum can break. If blood collects around the cartilage of the nasal septum, the cartilage may die. The dead cartilage may disintegrate, resulting in a saddle nose deformity, in which the bridge of the nose sags in the middle.

Diagnosis and Treatment

A person whose nose bleeds, hurts, and is swollen after a blunt injury may have a broken nose. Applying ice packs every 2 hours for 15 minutes at a time and sleeping with the head elevated help limit pain and swelling; however, medical attention is needed.

The mucous membrane and other soft tissues swell quickly, making the break difficult for a doctor to find, so the evaluation needs to be done very quickly (within the first few hours) or after the swelling has started to subside but before the bones become fixed in their new position. Ordinarily, a doctor diagnoses a broken nose by gently feeling the bridge of the nose for irregularities in shape and alignment, unusual movement of bones, the rough sensation of broken bones moving against one another, and tenderness. X-rays of the nose may not be as accurate as the doctor's eyes and fingers for determining proper bone alignment.

Doctors usually wait 3 to 5 days after an injury for the swelling to go down before they push the broken pieces of bone back into place (reduce them). Waiting makes it easier for the doctor to see and feel when the pieces are perfectly aligned. Many nasal fractures are in a good position and do not have to be reduced. Before reducing a fracture, a doctor usually gives an adult a local anesthetic and a child a general anesthetic. Blood that has collected in the septum is drained; the doctor places a small incision in the mucous membrane of the septum to prevent the destruction of the cartilage. By pressing with his fingers, the doctor manipulates the bones into their normal position. The nose is then stabilized with an external splint. Internal packing (stenting) may also be used. Nasal bone fractures heal in about 6 weeks. Fractures of the septum are difficult to set and often require surgery later.

Deviated Septum

Usually, the nasal septum is straight, lying about in the middle of the two nostrils. Occasionally, it may be bent (deviated) because of a birth defect or injury and positioned so that one nostril is much smaller than the other. Most people have some minor deviation of the septum so that one nostril is tighter than the other. A minor deviation usually causes no symptoms and requires no treatment. However, if severe, a deviation may block one side of the nose, making a person prone to inflammation of the sinuses (sinusitis), particularly if the deviated septum blocks drainage from a sinus into the nasal cavity. Also, a deviated septum may make a person prone to nosebleeds because of the drying effect of airflow over the deviation. A deviated septum that causes breathing problems can be surgically repaired.

Perforations of the Septum

Ulcers and holes (perforations) in the nasal septum may occur as a result of nasal surgery, repeated injury such as that resulting from

▲ see also page 1245

picking the nose, or diseases such as Wegener's granulomatosis and syphilis. Frequent use of cocaine snorted through the nose causes ulcerations and perforations because it decreases blood flow.

Symptoms may include crusting around the nostrils and repeated nosebleeds. People who have small perforations in the septum may make a whistling sound when they breathe.

Bacitracin ointment reduces the crusting. Doctors can sometimes surgically repair perforations using a person's own tissue from another part of the nose or with an artificial membrane made of a soft, pliable plastic. Most perforations do not need to be repaired unless bleeding or crusting is a major problem.

Nosebleeds

Nosebleeds (epistaxis) have a variety of causes, the most common of which are nose picking and injury. The cold, dry air of winter also makes nosebleeds more likely. People who take aspirin or other drugs that interfere with the blood's ability to clot (anticoagulants) commonly develop nosebleeds. Some people get them rather often, and others rarely get them.

Bleeding usually comes from the front part of the nasal septum, which contains many blood vessels. There may be just a trickle of blood or a strong stream. Most nosebleeds are more frightening than serious. However, bleeding from the back part of the nose—which is uncommon—is more dangerous and difficult to treat.

Prevention and Treatment

Important steps to prevent nosebleeds include avoiding picking the nose, humidifying the air during the winter, and, for some people, moistening the front of the nasal septum with petroleum jelly.

Bleeding usually can be controlled at home by pinching the sides of the nose together for 5 to 10 minutes. It is important to hold the nose with a firm pinch and not let go even once until the 10 minutes is up. Other home techniques, such as ice packs to the nose, wads of tissue paper in the nostrils, and placing the head in various positions, are not as effective.

If the pinch technique does not stop the bleeding, the person should see a doctor. The doctor packs the bleeding nostril with a piece of cotton saturated with a drug that causes blood vessels in the nose to narrow (constrict),

such as phenylephrine. A local anesthetic, such as lidocaine, numbs the nose so the doctor can look in the nose and find the bleeding site. For minor bleeds, often nothing more is done. For more severe or recurring bleeding, sometimes the doctor seals (cauterizes) the bleeding source with a chemical, silver nitrate, or electrocautery (cauterization using an electrical current to produce heat). Another treatment is to place a long absorbent sponge in the nostril. The sponge swells in contact with moisture and compresses the bleeding site. The sponge is removed after 2 to 4 days. Rarely, the doctor may need to pack the entire nasal cavity on one side with a long strip of gauze. Nasal packing is usually removed after 3 or 4 days.

In some people, particularly those who are older and have narrowing of the arteries (arteriosclerosis), the bleeding source is sometimes further back in the nose (posterior nosebleed). Bleeding in this area is very difficult to stop and can be life threatening. For a posterior nosebleed, doctors may place a specially shaped balloon in the nose and inflate it to compress the bleeding site. However, this and other types of nasal packing are very uncomfortable and interfere with the person's breathing. Therefore, people who have had this type of packing are admitted to the hospital and given oxygen and antibiotics to prevent an infection of the sinuses. Because of the discomfort and breathing risks associated with nasal packing, doctors sometimes cauterize or clip the bleeding vessel while looking in the nose through a small visualizing device (endoscope). Occasionally, doctors, guided by x-ray techniques, can pass a small catheter through the person's blood vessels to the bleeding site and inject material to block the bleeding vessel.

Nasal Vestibulitis

Nasal vestibulitis is infection of the area just inside the opening of each nostril (the nasal vestibule).

Minor infections at the opening of the nose may result in pimples at the base of nasal hairs (folliculitis) and sometimes crusts around the nostrils. The cause is usually the bacteria, *Staphylococcus*. Bacitracin ointment usually cures these infections.

More serious infections result in boils (furuncles) in the nasal vestibule. Boils may develop into a spreading infection under the skin (cel-

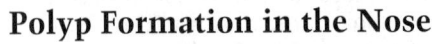

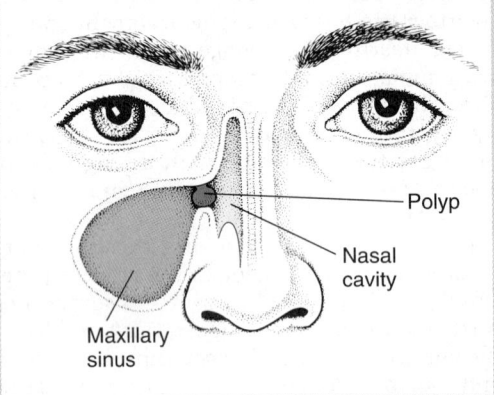

Polyp Formation in the Nose

Polyps usually develop in the area where the sinuses open into the nasal cavity. Polyps may block drainage from the sinuses. Fluid may accumulate in the blocked sinuses, causing a sinus infection.

Polyp

Nasal cavity

Maxillary sinus

lulitis) at the tip of the nose. A doctor becomes concerned about infections in this part of the face because veins lead from there to the brain. A life-threatening condition called cavernous sinus thrombosis can develop if the bacteria spread to the brain through these veins.▲

A person with nasal vestibulitis usually takes an antibiotic by mouth and applies moist hot cloths 3 times a day for about 15 to 20 minutes at a time. A doctor may need to surgically drain large boils or those that fail to respond to antibiotic therapy.

Rhinitis

Rhinitis is inflammation and swelling of the mucous membrane of the nose, characterized by a runny nose and stuffiness and usually caused by the common cold■ or an allergy.★

The nose is the most commonly infected part of the upper airways. Rhinitis may be acute (short-lived) or chronic (long-standing). Acute rhinitis commonly results from viral infections but may also be a result of allergies or other causes. Chronic rhinitis usually occurs with chronic sinusitis (chronic rhinosinusitis).

▲ see box on page 1318   ■ see page 1155
★ see page 1065   ● see table on page 80

Viral Rhinitis: Acute viral rhinitis (the common cold) can be caused by a variety of viruses. Symptoms consist of runny nose, congestion, post-nasal drip, cough, and a low-grade fever. Stuffiness can be relieved by taking phenylephrine as a nasal spray or pseudoephedrine by mouth. These drugs, available over the counter, cause the blood vessels of the nasal mucous membrane to narrow (constrict). Nasal sprays should be used for only 3 or 4 days because after that period of time, when the effects of the drugs wear off, the mucous membrane often swells even more than before. This phenomenon is called rebound congestion. Antihistamines help control runny nose but cause drowsiness and other problems, especially in older people.● Antibiotics are not effective for acute viral rhinitis.

Allergic Rhinitis: Allergic rhinitis is caused by a reaction of the body's immune system to an environmental trigger. The most common environmental triggers include dust, molds, pollens, grasses, trees, and animals. Symptoms include sneezing, runny nose, stuffiness, and itchy, watery eyes. A doctor may diagnose allergic rhinitis based on a person's history of symptoms. Often, the person has a family history of allergies. More detailed information may be obtained using blood tests or skin testing.

Avoiding the substance that triggers the allergy prevents symptoms but is often not possible. Nasal corticosteroid sprays decrease nasal inflammation caused by many sources and are relatively safe for long-term use. Antihistamines help prevent the allergic reaction and thus symptoms. Antihistamines dry the mucous membrane of the nose but many of them also cause sleepiness and other problems, especially in older people. Newer ones require a prescription but do not have these side effects. Allergy shots (desensitization) help to build long-term tolerance to specific environmental triggers, but they may take months or years to become fully effective. Antibiotics do not relieve the symptoms of allergic rhinitis.

Atrophic Rhinitis: Atrophic rhinitis is a form of chronic rhinitis in which the mucous membrane thins (atrophies) and hardens, causing the nasal passages to widen (dilate) and dry out. The cells normally found in the mucous membrane of the nose—cells that secrete mucus and have hairlike projections to move dirt particles out—are replaced by cells like those normally found in the skin. The disorder can develop in someone who had sinus surgery in which a significant amount of intranasal structures and mucous membranes were removed. A prolonged bacterial infection of the lining of the nose is also a factor.

Crusts form inside the nose, and an offensive odor develops. A person may have recurring severe nosebleeds and can lose his sense of smell (anosmia).

Treatment is aimed at reducing the crusting, eliminating the odor, and reducing infections. Topical antibiotics, such as bacitracin applied inside the nose, kill bacteria. Estrogens and vitamins A and D sprayed into the nose or taken by mouth may reduce crusting by promoting mucosal secretions. Other antibiotics, given by mouth or intravenously, may also be helpful. Surgery to narrow the nasal passages may reduce crusting because the decreased airflow prevents drying of the thinned mucous membrane.

Vasomotor Rhinitis: Vasomotor rhinitis is a form of chronic rhinitis. Nasal stuffiness, sneezing, and a runny nose—common allergic symptoms—occur when allergies do not appear to be present. In some people, the nose reacts strongly to irritants (such as dust and pollen), perfumes, and pollution. The disorder comes and goes but is worsened by dry air. The swollen mucous membrane varies from bright red to purple. Sometimes, people also have slight inflammation of the sinuses. When persistent, endoscopy of the nose or computed tomography (CT) of the sinuses may be needed. If inflammation of the sinus is not significant, treatment is aimed at relieving symptoms. Avoiding smoke and irritants and using a humidified central heating system or vaporizer to increase humidity may be beneficial.

Nasal Polyps

Nasal polyps are fleshy outgrowths of the mucous membrane of the nose.

Polyps are common teardrop-shaped growths that form around the openings to the sinus cavities. A polyp resembles a peeled, seedless grape. Unlike polyps in the colon or bladder, polyps in the nose are not tumors and do not suggest an increased risk of cancer. They are merely a reflection of inflammation, although there may be a family history of the problem. The doctor may perform a biopsy of the polyp to ensure that it is not a cancer.

Polyps may develop during infections and may disappear after the infection subsides, or they may begin slowly and persist. Many people are not aware that they have nasal polyps,

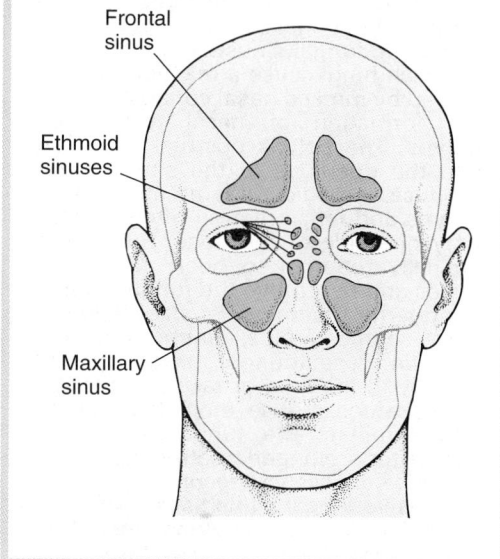

Locating the Sinuses

The sinuses are hollow cavities in the bones around the nose. The two frontal sinuses are located just above the eyebrows; the two maxillary sinuses, in the cheekbones; and the two groups of ethmoid sinuses, on either side of the nasal cavity. The two sphenoid sinuses (not shown) are located behind the ethmoid sinuses.

Frontal sinus

Ethmoid sinuses

Maxillary sinus

although they may have nasal congestion, obstruction, drainage, and chronic infections.

People with nasal polyps may be seriously allergic to aspirin and other nonsteroidal anti-inflammatory drugs (NSAIDs).▲ People with nasal polyps often develop asthma as well.

Corticosteroids in the form of nasal sprays or oral tablets may shrink or eliminate polyps. Endoscopic surgery or oral corticosteroids are needed if polyps block the airways or cause frequent sinus infections by blocking drainage from the sinuses. Polyps tend to grow back unless the underlying irritation, allergy, or infection is controlled. Using an aerosol corticosteroid spray may slow or prevent recurrences. However, a doctor may need to examine the person periodically with endoscopy to evaluate and treat persistent or recurring problems.

▲ see page 452

Fungal Sinus Infections

A variety of fungi that are normally found throughout the environment can be present in the nose and sinuses of most healthy people. In certain situations, however, fungi can cause significant nasal and sinus inflammation.

Fungus balls are an overgrowth of fungi in otherwise healthy people. Symptoms include sinus pain, pressure, nasal congestion, drainage of fluids, and chronic infections. Surgery is needed to open the affected sinus and remove the fungal debris.

Allergic fungal sinusitis is a disorder in which fungi cause a reaction characterized by marked nasal congestion and the formation of nasal and sinus polyps. The polyps obstruct the nose and the openings to the sinuses and produce chronic inflammation. The polyps and inflammation often involve only one side of the nose. Surgery is typically required to open up the sinuses and to remove the fungal debris. Long-term treatment is also required with corticosteroids, antibiotics, and sometimes, antifungal drugs applied directly to the area or taken by mouth. These drugs reduce the inflammation and eliminate the fungus. However, even after prolonged treatment, the disorder is very likely to recur.

Invasive fungal sinusitis is a very serious disorder that develops most often in people whose immune system is impaired by chemotherapy or by diseases such as poorly controlled diabetes, leukemia, lymphoma, multiple myeloma, or AIDS. It may spread rapidly. Symptoms include pain, fever, and discharge of pus from the nose. The fungus may spread to the eye socket, causing a bulging of the affected eye (proptosis) and blindness. A doctor makes the diagnosis by biopsy. Treatment is with surgery and antifungal drugs given intravenously. Doctors also must control the underlying disease and stimulate a weakened immune system.

Sinusitis

Sinusitis is inflammation of the sinuses, most commonly caused by an allergy or infection.

Sinusitis is one of the most common medical conditions. About 10 to 15 million people each year develop symptoms of sinusitis. Sinusitis may occur in any of the four groups of sinuses: maxillary, ethmoid, frontal, or sphe-

noid. Sinusitis nearly always occurs in conjunction with inflammation of the nasal passages (rhinitis), and some doctors refer to the disorder as rhinosinusitis. It may be acute (short-lived) or chronic (long-standing).

Acute Sinusitis: Acute sinusitis may be caused by a variety of bacteria and often develops after something blocks the openings to the sinuses. Such blockage commonly results from a viral infection of the upper airways, such as the common cold. During a cold, the swollen mucous membranes of the nasal cavity tend to block the openings of the sinuses. Air in the sinuses is absorbed into the bloodstream, and the pressure inside the sinuses decreases, causing pain and drawing fluid into the sinuses. This fluid is a breeding ground for bacteria. White blood cells and more fluid enter the sinuses to fight the bacteria; this influx increases the pressure and causes more pain.

Allergies also cause mucous membrane swelling, which blocks the openings to the sinuses. Additionally, people with a deviated septum are more prone to obstructed sinuses.

Chronic Sinusitis: Sinusitis is defined as chronic if it has been ongoing for more than 8 to 12 weeks. Doctors do not understand exactly what causes chronic sinusitis but it may follow a viral infection, a severe allergy, or exposure to an environmental pollutant. Often the person has a family history; a genetic predisposition appears to be a factor. If the person has a bacterial or fungal infection, the inflammation is much worse. Occasionally, chronic sinusitis of the maxillary sinus results when an upper tooth abscess spreads into the sinus above.

Symptoms and Diagnosis

Acute sinusitis usually results in pain, tenderness, and swelling over the affected sinus. Maxillary sinusitis produces pain over the cheeks just below the eyes, toothache, and headache. Frontal sinusitis produces headache over the forehead. Ethmoid sinusitis produces pain behind and between the eyes and headache, often described as splitting, over the forehead. The pain produced by sphenoid sinusitis does not occur in well-defined areas and may be felt in the front or back of the head.

In acute sinusitis, yellow or green pus may be discharged from the nose. Fever and chills also can occur, but their presence may suggest that the infection has spread beyond the sinuses. Any change in vision or swelling around the eye is a very serious condition that can quickly—within minutes to hours—result in blindness. Such a change should be evaluated by a doctor as soon as possible.

The symptoms of chronic sinusitis are usually much more subtle, and pain occurs less often. The most common symptoms of chronic sinusitis are nasal obstruction, nasal congestion, and post-nasal drip. People with sinusitis may have colored discharge and a decreased sense of smell. A person also may feel generally ill (malaise).

A doctor makes the diagnosis based on the typical symptoms and, sometimes, on x-ray studies. X-rays may show fluid in the sinuses, but computed tomography (CT) is better able to determine the extent and severity of sinusitis. If a person has maxillary sinusitis, the teeth may be x-rayed to check for tooth abscesses. Sometimes a doctor passes a thin viewing scope (endoscope) into the nose to inspect the sinus openings and to obtain samples of fluid for culture. This procedure, which requires a local anesthetic, can be done in the doctor's office.

Treatment

Treatment of acute sinusitis is aimed at improving sinus drainage and curing the infection. Nasal sprays, such as phenylephrine, which cause blood vessels to narrow (constrict), can be used for a limited time. Similar drugs, such as pseudoephedrine, taken by mouth are not as effective. For both acute and chronic sinusitis, antibiotics such as amoxicillin or trimethoprim-sulfamethoxazole are given, but people who have chronic sinusitis take antibiotics for a longer period of time. Nasal corticosteroid sprays and corticosteroid tablets are helpful in reducing the inflammation in the mucous membranes. If significant allergy symptoms are present, antihistamines may be useful. Nasal irrigations with salt water can help to cleanse the sinuses and keep them moist. When antibiotics are not effective, surgery may be performed either to wash out the sinus and obtain material for culture or to improve sinus drainage, which allows the inflammation to resolve.

CHAPTER 222

Throat Disorders

Disorders of the throat (pharynx) and voice box (larynx) include inflammation and infections, vocal cord polyps and nodules, cancer,▲ contact ulcers, vocal cord paralysis, and laryngoceles. Laryngeal papillomas usually affect children.■

Throat infections (pharyngitis) are particularly common in children, although adults get them as well. Causes, symptoms, and treatment are similar in both groups,★ except that in adults, gonorrhea, a sexually transmitted disease, sometimes infects the throat.

Tonsillar Cellulitis and Abscess

*Tonsillar cellulitis is a bacterial infection of the tissues around the tonsils; a **tonsillar abscess** is a collection of pus in the area of the tonsils.*

Sometimes, bacteria, usually streptococci, that infect the throat can spread deeper into the surrounding tissues. This condition is called cellulitis. If the bacteria grow unchecked, a collection of pus (abscess) may form. Abscesses may form next to the tonsils (peritonsillar) or in the side of the throat (parapharyngeal). Abscesses occur in children but are more common in young adults.

Symptoms

With tonsillar cellulitis or an abscess, swallowing causes severe pain. A person feels ill, has a fever, and may tilt his head toward the side of the abscess to help relieve pain. Spasms of the chewing muscles make opening the mouth difficult (trismus). Cellulitis produces general redness and swelling above the tonsil and on the soft palate. An abscess pushes the tonsil forward, and the uvula (the small, soft projection that hangs down at the back of the throat) is swollen and can be pushed to the side opposite the abscess.

▲ see page 1271   ■ see page 1600
★ see page 1595

Diagnosis and Treatment

A doctor makes the diagnosis by viewing the throat. Tests are not usually performed, but if the doctor is not sure whether an abscess is present, computed tomography (CT) can be used to identify one. Sometimes if the doctor suspects an abscess, he inserts a needle into the area and tries to draw out pus.

Antibiotics, such as penicillin or clindamycin, are given intravenously. If no abscess is present, the antibiotic usually starts to clear the infection in 24 to 48 hours. If an abscess is present, a doctor must insert a needle in it or cut into it to drain the pus. The area is first numbed with an anesthetic spray or injection. Treatment with antibiotics is continued by mouth.

Peritonsillar abscesses tend to recur; recurrences can be prevented by removing the tonsils (tonsillectomy),▲ which is usually performed 4 to 6 weeks after the infection has subsided or earlier if the infection is not controlled with antibiotics.

Epiglottitis

Epiglottitis is a bacterial infection of the epiglottis.

The epiglottis is a small flap of stiff tissue that closes the entrance to the voice box (larynx) and windpipe (trachea) during swallowing. Sometimes, the epiglottis becomes infected with bacteria, usually *Haemophilus influenzae.* The infection is most common in children, but routine vaccination against *Haemophilus* has recently made this organism less common. The swelling produced by this infection may block the airway and lead to difficulty breathing and death. Because children have a smaller airway than adults, epiglottitis is more dangerous in children.■

Symptoms are severe throat pain, fever, and a muffled voice. Because the infection is in the epiglottis, the back of the throat often does not appear infected. As swelling of the epiglottis starts to narrow the airway, the person first begins to make a squeaking noise when breathing in (stridor) and then has progressively worse trouble breathing. The condition progresses rapidly.

A doctor suspects the diagnosis based on the person's symptoms. If the person is not having trouble breathing, the doctor may look down the throat with a mirror or take x-rays, which often show the swollen epiglottis. Sometimes the doctor looks down the throat with a thin, flexible viewing tube inserted through the nose (nasopharyngeal laryngoscopy).

A person without difficulty breathing is given antibiotics and is closely observed in an intensive care unit. If the person has difficulty breathing, doctors insert a plastic breathing tube through the mouth or nose into the trachea (endotracheal intubation). The tube keeps the airway from swelling shut. Sometimes the airway is so swollen that the doctor cannot insert a tube this way and must cut open the front of the neck and insert the tube directly into the trachea (tracheotomy or cricothyroidotomy).

Laryngitis

Laryngitis is inflammation of the voice box (larynx).

The most common cause of laryngitis is a viral infection of the upper airways, such as the common cold. Laryngitis also may accompany bronchitis or any other inflammation or infection of the upper airways. Excessive use of the voice, an allergic reaction, and inhalation of irritants such as cigarette smoke can cause short-lived (acute) or persistent (chronic) laryngitis. Bacterial infections of the larynx are extremely rare.

Symptoms are an unnatural change of voice, such as hoarseness, or even loss of voice that develops within hours to a day or so. The throat may tickle or feel raw, and a person may have a constant urge to clear the throat. Symptoms vary with the severity of the inflammation. Fever, a general feeling of illness (malaise), difficulty in swallowing, and a sore throat may occur in severe infections.

A diagnosis is based on the typical symptoms and voice changes. Sometimes a doctor looks down the throat with a mirror or a thin, flexible viewing tube, which shows some reddening and sometimes some swelling of the lining of the larynx. Because cancer of the larynx may cause hoarseness, a person whose symptoms persist more than a few weeks should be evaluated for cancer.★

Treatment of viral laryngitis depends on the symptoms. Resting the voice (by not speaking), drinking extra fluids, and inhaling steam relieve symptoms and help healing. Whispering, however, may irritate the larynx even

---

▲ see page 1597   ■ see page 1564

★ see page 1271

Vocal Cord Problems

When relaxed, the vocal coards normally form a **V**-shaped opening that allows air to pass freely through to the trachea. The cords open during speech and close during swallowing.

Holding a mirror in the back of a person's mouth, a specially trained doctor can often see the vocal cords and check for problems, such as contact ulcers, polyps, nodules, paralysis, and cancer, all of which affect the voice. Paralysis may affect one (one-sided) or both vocal cords (two-sided—not shown).

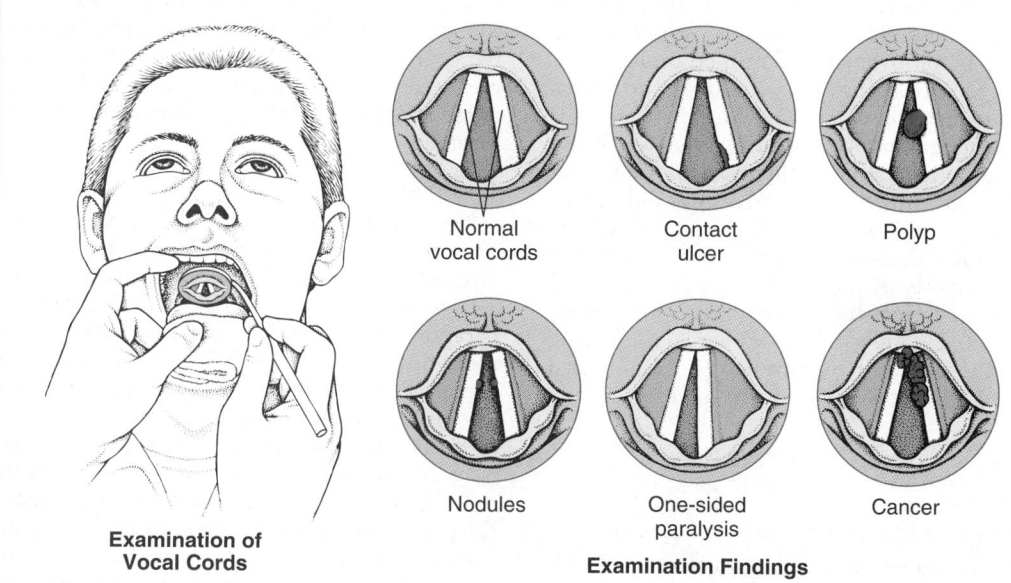

Normal vocal cords

Contact ulcer

Polyp

Nodules

One-sided paralysis

Cancer

Examination of Vocal Cords

Examination Findings

more. Treating bronchitis, if present, may improve the laryngitis. An antibiotic is given only for infection caused by bacteria.

Vocal Cord Nodules and Polyps

Vocal cord nodules and polyps are noncancerous growths that produce hoarseness.

Vocal cord nodules and polyps are similar conditions that develop mainly from abuse of the voice (prolonged singing or shouting). Chronic irritation of the larynx, such as occurs with inhalation of cigarette smoke or industrial fumes, or backflow (reflux) of stomach acid at night may also cause a nodule or polyp to form. The growths are similar, but polyps tend to be larger and protrude somewhat more than nodules.

Symptoms include chronic hoarseness and a breathy voice, which tend to develop over days to weeks. A doctor makes the diagnosis by examining the vocal cords with a thin, flexible viewing tube. Sometimes the doctor removes a small piece of tissue for examination under a microscope (biopsy) to make sure the growth is not cancerous.

Treatment is to avoid whatever is irritating the larynx and rest the voice. If abuse of the voice is the cause, voice therapy conducted by a speech therapist may be needed to teach the person how to speak or sing without straining the vocal cords. Most nodules go away with this treatment, but most polyps must be surgically removed to restore the person's normal voice.

Contact Ulcers of the Vocal Cords

Contact ulcers are raw sores on the mucous membrane covering the cartilage to which the vocal cords are attached.

Contact ulcers are usually caused by abusing the voice with forceful speech, particularly as a person starts to speak. These ulcers typically occur in teachers, preachers, sales representatives, lawyers, and other people whose occupation requires them to talk a lot. Smoking, persistent coughing, and backflow (reflux) of stomach acid also may cause contact ulcers.

Symptoms include mild pain while speaking or swallowing and varying degrees of hoarseness. A doctor makes the diagnosis by examining the vocal cords with a thin, flexible viewing tube. Occasionally, a small tissue sample is removed and examined under a microscope (biopsy) to make sure that the ulcers are not cancerous.

Treatment involves resting the voice by talking as little as possible for at least 6 weeks so that the ulcers can heal. To avoid recurrences, people who develop contact ulcers need voice therapy to learn how to use the voice properly. A speech therapist can provide such instruction. If the person has acid reflux, treatment includes taking antacids, not eating within 2 hours of retiring for the night, and keeping the head elevated while sleeping.

Vocal Cord Paralysis

Vocal cord paralysis is the inability to move the muscles that control the vocal cords.

Vocal cord paralysis may affect one or both vocal cords. Paralysis can result from brain disorders, such as brain tumors, strokes, and demyelinating diseases,▲ or damage to the nerves that lead to the larynx. Nerve damage may be caused by noncancerous and cancerous tumors; injury; a viral infection of the nerves; or neurotoxins (substances that poison or destroy nerve tissue), such as lead or the toxins produced in diphtheria.

Symptoms and Diagnosis

Vocal cord paralysis may affect speaking, breathing, and swallowing. Paralysis may allow food and fluids to be inhaled into the windpipe (trachea) and lungs. If only one vocal cord is paralyzed, the voice is hoarse and breathy. Usually, the airway is not obstructed because the normal cord on the other side

▲ see page 556

opens sufficiently. When both vocal cords are paralyzed, the voice is reduced in strength but otherwise sounds normal. However, the space between the paralyzed cords is very small, and the airway is inadequate so that even moderate exercise causes difficulty in breathing and a harsh, high-pitched sound with each breath.

A doctor tries to find the cause of the paralysis. Examination of the larynx, bronchial tubes, or esophagus with a thin, flexible viewing tube may be performed. Magnetic resonance imaging (MRI) or computed tomography (CT) of the head, neck, chest, and thyroid gland and x-rays of the esophagus also may be needed.

Treatment

The first goal of treatment is to prevent closure of the airway from the paralyzed cord. If only one side is paralyzed, an operation called a thyroplasty can be performed to move the paralyzed vocal cord to the best position for more normal speech. When both sides are paralyzed, keeping the airway open adequately is difficult. A tracheostomy (surgery to create an opening into the trachea through the neck) may be needed. The tracheostomy opening may be permanent or may be used only when the person has an upper respiratory tract infection. In another procedure, called an arytenoidectomy, the vocal cords are permanently separated, thus widening the airway. However, this procedure may worsen voice quality.

Laryngoceles

Laryngoceles are outpouchings of the mucous membrane of a part of the voice box (larynx).

Laryngoceles may bulge inward, resulting in hoarseness and airway obstruction, or outward, producing a visible lump in the neck. Laryngoceles are filled with air and can be expanded when a person breathes out forcefully with the mouth closed and the nostrils pinched shut. Laryngoceles tend to occur in musicians who play wind instruments.

On a computed tomography (CT) scan, laryngoceles appear smooth and egg-shaped. They may become infected or filled with mucuslike fluid and are usually removed surgically.

CHAPTER 223

Nose and Throat Cancers

Often, cancers of the nose and throat are considered together by doctors because of certain similarities. Nose and throat cancers occur in the voice box (larynx), the hollow spaces located in the bones around the nose (paranasal sinuses), the nasal passages and upper throat (nasopharynx), and the tonsils. Cancer of the mouth is very similar to nose and throat cancers in a number of ways.▲ Because these cancers can cause death, a person with nose and throat cancer that has not responded to treatment should make all necessary plans; the person should have frank discussions with the doctor about wishes for medical care and the need for end-of-life care.■

Cancer of the Larynx

Cancer of the voice box (larynx), a common area of cancer within the head and neck, occurs more often in men than in women. It is linked to cigarette smoking and alcohol consumption.

Symptoms and Diagnosis

This cancer commonly originates on the vocal cords or the surrounding structures and often causes hoarseness. A person who has been hoarse for more than 2 weeks should seek medical attention. Cancer in other parts of the larynx causes pain and difficulty in swallowing or breathing. Sometimes, however, a lump in the neck resulting from the cancer's spread to a lymph node (metastasis) may be noticed before any other symptoms.

To make the diagnosis, a doctor looks at the larynx through a laryngoscope (a thin viewing tube used for direct viewing of the larynx) and performs a biopsy (removal of a tissue sample for examination under a microscope). A biopsy is most often performed in the operating room, while the person is under general anesthesia. Occasionally, it may be performed in the doctor's office, after a topical anesthetic has been applied.

Staging and Prognosis

Staging is a way for doctors to describe how advanced the cancer has become, taking into account both the size and spread of the can-

cer.★ Staging helps the doctor guide therapy and assess prognosis. Cancer of the larynx is staged according to the size and location of the original tumor, the number and size of metastases to the lymph nodes in the neck, and evidence of metastases in distant parts of the body. Stage I cancer is the least advanced, and stage IV is the most advanced.

The larger the cancer and the more it has spread, the worse the prognosis. If the tumor has also invaded muscle, bone, or cartilage, cure is less likely. Almost 90% of people with small cancers that have not spread anywhere survive for 5 years, compared with fewer than 50% of those who have cancer that has spread to the local lymph nodes. For people who have metastases beyond the local lymph nodes, the chance of surviving longer than 2 years is poor.

Treatment

Treatment depends on the stage and the precise location of the cancer within the larynx. For cancer in an early stage, doctors may use either surgery or radiation therapy. Usually, radiation is aimed not only at the cancer but also at the lymph nodes on both sides of the neck, because many of these cancers spread to those lymph nodes. When the vocal cords are affected, radiation therapy may be preferred over surgery because it may preserve a more normal voice. However, for very early cancers of the larynx, microsurgery, sometimes performed with a laser, provides identical cure rates with equal preservation of the voice and can be completed in a single treatment.

Tumors larger than $3/4$ inch and those that have invaded bone or cartilage are usually treated with combination therapy. One combination consists of radiation therapy plus surgery to remove part or all of the larynx and vocal cords (partial or total laryngectomy). Radiation therapy also may be combined with chemotherapy. This treatment provides equivalent cure rates to the radiation and surgery

▲ see page 671   ■ see page 51
★ see page 1041

Speech Without Vocal Cords

Speech requires a source of sound waves (vibrations) and a means of shaping those vibrations into words. The vocal cords normally provide the vibrations, which are then shaped into words by the tongue, palate, and lips. People whose vocal cords have been removed can regain their voice if a new source of sound vibrations can be provided, because their tongue, palate, and lips remain able to shape these new vibrations into words. There are three ways that people with no larynx can produce sound vibrations: esophageal speech, an electrolarynx, or a tracheoesophageal puncture (TEP).

For esophageal speech, a person is taught to swallow air into the esophagus and gradually expel the air, as in a belch, to produce a sound. Esophageal speech is difficult for the person to learn and may be hard for other people to understand, but it requires no surgery or mechanical accessories.

The electrolarynx is a vibrating device that acts as a sound source when it is held against the neck; it produces an artificial, mechanical sound. An electrolarynx is easier to use and understand than esophageal speech, but it requires batteries and must be carried with the person.

A TEP is a one-way valve surgically inserted between the windpipe (trachea) and the esophagus. The valve diverts air into the esophagus while the person exhales, producing a sound. TEP requires significant practice but can eventually produce easy and fluent speech in many people. The valve may stay in place for many months, but it requires daily cleaning. If the valve malfunctions, fluids and food may accidentally enter the windpipe. Some types of valves require the person to block the opening in the windpipe with a finger to operate the valve, while others can be operated hands-free.

combination, and the voice is preserved in a significant number of people. However, surgery may still be required to remove any cancer that remains after this treatment. If the cancer is too advanced for surgery or radiation

therapy, chemotherapy can help reduce the pain and the size of the tumor but is unlikely to provide a cure.

Treatment almost always has significant side effects. Surgery often affects swallowing and speaking; in such cases, rehabilitation is necessary. A number of methods have been developed that allow people without vocal cords to speak, often with excellent results. Depending on the specific tissue removed, reconstructive surgery may be performed. Radiation may cause skin changes (such as inflammation, itching, and loss of hair), scarring, loss of taste, and dry mouth, and occasionally, destruction of normal tissues. People whose teeth will be exposed to the radiation treatments must have dental problems corrected and any unhealthy teeth removed, because radiation will make any subsequent dental work more likely to fail, and severe infections of the jawbone may occur. Chemotherapy typically produces a variety of side effects, depending on the drug used; these effects may include nausea, vomiting, hearing loss, and infections.

Cancer of the Paranasal Sinuses

Cancer of the paranasal sinuses occurs mainly in the maxillary and ethmoid sinuses.▲ Although rare in the United States, these cancers are more common in Japan and among the Bantu people of South Africa. Doctors are not sure what causes these cancers, but they are more common in people who regularly inhale certain types of wood and metal dust. Doctors do not think chronic sinusitis causes these cancers.

Because the sinuses provide room for the cancer to grow, most people do not develop symptoms until the cancer is far advanced. Symptoms, including pain, a sensation of nasal obstruction, double vision, nosebleeds, and loosened teeth in the jawbone underneath the affected sinus, result from the pressure of the cancer on nearby structures.

Doctors treat cancer of the sinuses with a combination of surgery and radiation therapy. Recent advances in surgical techniques have allowed doctors to remove the tumors completely, spare uninvolved parts of the face, such as the eye, and reconstruct the area with much better appearance. The earlier the cancer is treated, the better the prognosis. However, survival is generally poor; only about 10 to 20% of people live more than 5 years.

▲ see art on page 1265

Cancer of the Nasopharynx

Cancer of the nasal passages and upper throat (nasopharynx) may occur in children and young adults. Although rare in North America, cancer of the nasopharynx is one of the most common cancers in Asia. This cancer is also more common among Chinese people who immigrated to North America than other Americans. It is slightly less common among American-born Chinese than their immigrant parents.

The Epstein-Barr virus, which causes infectious mononucleosis, plays a role in the development of nasopharyngeal cancer. In addition, children and young adults who eat large amounts of salted fish (especially people with a poor intake of vitamins) are more likely to develop nasopharyngeal cancer.

Often, the first symptom is persistent blockage of the nose or eustachian tubes, which causes a sensation of fullness or pain in the ears and may cause hearing loss, particularly in one ear. If an eustachian tube is blocked, fluid may accumulate in the middle ear. A person may have a discharge of pus and blood from the nose. Rarely, part of the face or an eye becomes paralyzed. Often, the cancer spreads to lymph nodes in the neck.

A doctor diagnoses the cancer by performing a biopsy of the tumor, in which a sample of tissue is removed and examined under a microscope. Computed tomography (CT) or magnetic resonance imaging (MRI) of the head and neck is performed to evaluate the extent of the cancer. The tumor is treated with radiation therapy and chemotherapy. If the tumor is large or persists, surgery may be needed. Overall, 35% of the people survive for at least 5 years after diagnosis; early treatment improves prognosis significantly.

Cancer of the Tonsils

Cancer of the tonsils occurs predominantly in men. It is strongly linked to smoking and alcohol consumption. This cancer often spreads to the lymph nodes in the neck. Cancer of the tonsils occurs most often in people between the ages of 50 and 70.

A sore throat is often the first symptom. Pain usually radiates to the ear on the same side as the affected tonsil. Sometimes, however, a lump in the neck resulting from the cancer's spread to a lymph node (metastasis) may be noticed before any other symptoms. A doctor di-

Finding a Lump in the Neck

A doctor may discover an abnormal lump in the neck of a person who has no other symptoms. Most lumps are enlarged lymph nodes, which may enlarge because of a nearby infection, such as of the throat. However, an enlarged lymph node may also be caused by cancer, either a cancer of the lymph node (lymphoma) or a cancer that has spread to the lymph node from elsewhere in the body (metastasis). Lymph nodes in the neck are a common site for the spread of cancer from many parts of the body. Painless lumps are somewhat more worrisome than painful ones. Any lump that stays more than a few days should be evaluated by a doctor.

A doctor first examines the ears, nose, pharynx, larynx, tonsils, base of the tongue, and thyroid and salivary glands. This examination often includes looking down the throat with a mirror or a thin flexible viewing tube. If there is no obvious source of infection or a visible cancerous spot, further tests are needed. The initial test is often a needle biopsy of the enlarged lymph node but may be computed tomography (CT) or magnetic resonance imaging (MRI) of the head and neck. Children, in whom lumps are caused most often by infection, are usually first given a trial of antibiotics. To look for cancer originating in other parts of the body, doctors usually obtain x-rays of the upper digestive tract, a thyroid scan, and a CT scan of the chest. Direct examination of the larynx (laryngoscopy), lungs (bronchoscopy), and esophagus (esophagoscopy) may be needed.

When cancer cells are found in an enlarged lymph node in the neck and there are no signs of cancer anywhere else, the entire lymph node containing the cancer cells is removed along with additional lymph nodes and fatty tissue within the neck. If the tumor is large enough, doctors may also remove the internal jugular vein, along with nearby muscles and nerves. Radiation therapy is often given as well.

agnoses the cancer by performing a biopsy of the tonsil, in which a sample of tissue is removed for examination under a microscope. Evaluation usually includes laryngoscopy (examination of the larynx), bronchoscopy (examination of the lungs), and esophagoscopy (examination of the esophagus). These areas are evaluated because of the high risk of additional cancers being present (up to 10%).

Treatment typically includes radiation therapy and surgery. Certain types of chemotherapy are effective as well, when combined with radiation therapy. Surgery may involve removal of the tumor, lymph nodes in the neck, and part of the jaw. There have been notable advances in the reconstruction used after surgery to remove the cancer, resulting in significant improvements in function and appearance. About 50% of the people survive for at least 5 years after diagnosis, although the exact number depends on the stage of the cancer at the time of treatment.

EYE DISORDERS

224 Biology of the Eyes 1276

Structure and Function ▪ Muscles, Nerves, and Blood Vessels ▪ Protective Features ▪ Effects of Aging

225 Symptoms and Diagnosis of Eye Disorders............................1278

226 Refractive Disorders 1286

227 Eye Injuries 1290

Blunt Injuries ▪ Foreign Objects ▪ Burns

228 Eyelid and Tear Gland Disorders 1292

Dacryostenosis ▪ Dacryocystitis ▪ Eyelid Swelling ▪ Blepharitis ▪ Stye ▪ Chalazion ▪ Entropion and Ectropion ▪ Eyelid Tumors

229 Disorders of the Conjunctiva and Sclera...............................1296

Infectious Conjunctivitis ▪ Trachoma ▪ Allergic Conjunctivitis ▪ Episcleritis ▪ Scleritis ▪ Noncancerous Growths

230 Corneal Disorders..1299

Superficial Punctate Keratitis ▪ Corneal Ulcer ▪ Keratoconjunctivitis Sicca ▪ Keratomalacia ▪ Herpes Simplex Keratitis ▪ Herpes Zoster Ophthalmicus ▪ Peripheral Ulcerative Keratitis ▪ Keratoconus ▪ Bullous Keratopathy

231 Cataract 1303

232 Uveitis 1305

233 Glaucoma 1306

234 Retinal Disorders 1309

Age-related Macular Degeneration ▪ Macular Pucker ▪ Retinal Detachment ▪ Retinitis Pigmentosa ▪ Blockage of Central Retinal Arteries and Veins ▪ Hypertensive Retinopathy ▪ Diabetic Retinopathy ▪ Endophthalmitis ▪ Cancers Affecting the Retina

235 Optic Nerve Disorders 1315

Papilledema ▪ Optic Neuritis ▪ Optic Neuropathy

236 Eye Socket Disorders 1317

Fractures ▪ Infections ▪ Inflammation ▪ Tumors ▪ Exophthalmos

CHAPTER 224

Biology of the Eyes

The structures and functions of the eyes are complex. Each eye constantly adjusts the amount of light it lets in, focuses on objects near and far, and produces continuous images that are instantly transmitted to the brain.

Structure and Function

The orbit is the bony cavity that contains the eyeball, muscles, nerves, and blood vessels, as well as the structures that produce and drain tears. Each orbit is a pear-shaped structure that is formed by several bones.

The eye has a relatively tough white outer layer (sclera or white of the eye). Near the front of the eye, the sclera is covered by a thin membrane (conjunctiva), which runs to the edge of the cornea and also covers the insides of the eyelids.

Light enters the eye through the cornea, a transparent dome on the front surface of the eye. The cornea serves as a protective covering for the front of the eye and also helps focus light on the retina at the back of the eye. After passing through the cornea, light travels through the pupil, the black area in the middle of the iris. The iris, the circular, colored area of the eye, controls the amount of light that enters the eye so that the pupil dilates and constricts like the aperture of a camera lens. The iris allows more light into the eye when the environment is dark and allows less light into the eye when the environment is bright. The size of the pupil is controlled by the pupillary sphincter muscle.

Behind the iris sits the lens. By changing its shape, the lens focuses light onto the retina. For the eye to focus on nearby objects, small muscles (called the ciliary muscles) contract, allowing the lens to become thicker. For the eye to focus on distant objects, the same muscles relax, allowing the lens to become thinner.

The retina contains the cells that sense light (photoreceptors) and the blood vessels that nourish them. The most sensitive part of the retina is a small area called the macula, which has millions of tightly packed photoreceptors. The high density of photoreceptors in the macula makes the visual image sharp, just as high-resolution film has more tightly packed grains. Each photoreceptor is linked to a nerve fiber. The nerve fibers from the photoreceptors are bundled together to form the optic nerve. The optic disk, the first part of the optic nerve, is at the back of the eye. The photoreceptors in the retina convert the image into electrical impulses, which are carried to the brain by the optic nerve.

There are two main types of photoreceptor, cones and rods. Cones are responsible for sharp vision and color vision and are clustered mainly in the macula. The rods are responsible for night and peripheral vision; they are more numerous than cones and much more sensitive to light, but they do not register color. Rods are grouped mainly in the peripheral areas of the retina and do not contribute to visual clarity as the cones do.

The optic nerve connects the retina to the brain in a split pathway. Half the fibers of this nerve cross over to the other side at the optic chiasm, an area immediately in front of the pituitary gland just below the front portion of the brain. The bundles of nerve fibers then come together again just before they reach the back portion of the brain, where vision is sensed and interpreted. In this arrangement, impulses from each side of the eye's visual field are sent to the other side of the brain. Because of this

An Inside Look at the Eye

Posterior chamber
Anterior chamber
Lens
Cornea
Pupil
Iris
Conjunctiva
Optic nerve
Macula
Retina
Sclera

structure, damage to the optic chiasm can lead to specific patterns of vision loss.▲

The eyeball is divided into two sections, each of which is filled with fluid. The front section (anterior segment) extends from the inside of the cornea to the front surface of the lens. It is filled with a fluid called the aqueous humor that nourishes the internal structures. The back section (posterior segment) extends from the back surface of the lens to the retina. It contains a jellylike fluid called the vitreous humor. These fluids fill out the eyeball and help maintain its shape.

The anterior segment itself is divided into two chambers. The front (anterior) chamber extends from the cornea to the iris; the back (posterior) chamber extends from the iris to the lens. Normally, the aqueous humor is produced in the posterior chamber, flows slowly through the pupil into the anterior chamber, and then drains out of the eyeball through outflow channels at the edge of the iris.

Muscles, Nerves, and Blood Vessels

Several muscles working together move the eye. Each muscle is stimulated by a specific cranial nerve.■ The optic nerve (a cranial nerve), which carries impulses from the retina to the brain, the lacrimal nerve, which stimulates the tear glands to produce tears, and other nerves, which transmit sensation to the brain from the various parts of the eye, travel through the orbit.

An ophthalmic artery and a retinal artery provide blood to each eye, and an ophthalmic vein and a retinal vein drain blood from the eye. These blood vessels enter and leave through the back of the eye.

Protective Features

The bony cavity of the orbit protects the eye, while allowing it to move freely in a wide arc.

The eyelashes are short hairs that grow from the edge of the eyelid. The upper lashes are longer than the lower lashes and turn upward. The lower lashes turn downward. Eyelashes act as a barrier by sweeping foreign particles away from the eye.

The upper and lower eyelids are thin folds of skin that can cover the eye. They reflexively close quickly (blink) to form a mechanical barrier that protects the eye from foreign objects, wind, dust, and very bright light. The reflex is triggered by the sight of an approaching object,

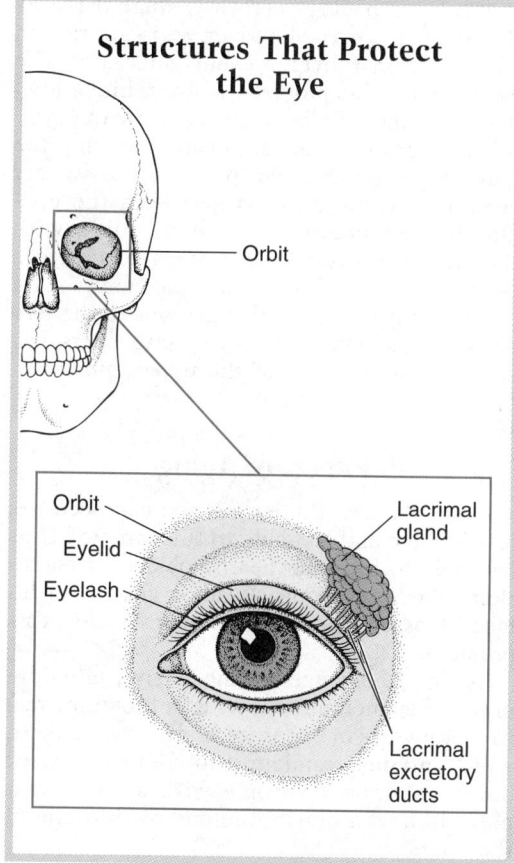

Structures That Protect the Eye

Orbit

Orbit

Eyelid

Eyelash

Lacrimal gland

Lacrimal excretory ducts

the touch of an object on the surface of the eye, or the eyelashes being exposed to wind or small particles such as dust or sand. On the inner surface of the eyelid, the conjunctiva loops back to cover the front surface of the eye, right up to the edge of the cornea. The conjunctiva protects the sensitive tissues underneath it.

When blinked, the eyelids help spread tears over the surface of the eye. Tears consist of a salty fluid that continuously bathes the surface of the eye to keep it moist. When closed, the eyelids help trap the moisture against the surface of the eye. Small glands at the edge of the upper and lower eyelids secrete an oily substance that contributes to the tear film and keeps tears from evaporating. Tears keep the surface of the eye moist. Without such moisture, the normally transparent cornea can become dried, injured, infected, and opaque.

▲ see art on page 1316   ■ see page 588

Tears also trap and sweep away small particles that enter the eye. Moreover, tears are rich in antibodies that help prevent infection. The eyelids and tears protect the eye while allowing clear access to light rays entering the eye.

The lacrimal glands, located at the top outer edge of each eye, produce the watery portion of tears. Mucous glands in the conjunctiva produce mucus, which mixes with the watery portion of the tears to create a more protective tear film. Tears drain from each eye into the nose through one of the two nasolacrimal ducts; each of these ducts has openings at the edge of the upper and lower eyelids near the nose.

Effects of Aging

In middle age, the lens of the eye becomes less flexible and less able to thicken, and thus less able to focus on nearby objects, a condition called presbyopia. Reading glasses, or bifocal lenses, can help compensate for this problem.

In old age, changes to the sclera (the white of the eyes) include yellowing or browning due to many years of exposure to ultraviolet light, wind, and dust; random splotches of pigment (more common in people with a dark complexion); and a bluish hue due to thinning of the sclera.

The number of mucous cells in the conjunctiva may decrease with age. Tear production may also decrease with age, so that fewer tears are available to keep the surface of the eye moist. Both of these changes explain why older people are more likely to have dry eyes.

Arcus senilis (a deposit of calcium and cholesterol salts) appears as a gray-white ring at the edge of the cornea. It is common in people older than 60. Arcus senilis does not affect vision.

Some diseases of the retina▲ are more likely to occur in old age, including macular degeneration, diabetic retinopathy, and retinal detachment. Other eye diseases, such as cataracts and dry eye, become common.

The muscles that squeeze the eyelids shut decrease in strength with age; this, combined with age-related looseness of the eyelids, sometimes results in the lower eyelid falling away from the eyeball, a condition called ectropion. In some older people the fat around the orbit shrinks, causing the eyeball to sink into the orbit.

The muscles that work to regulate the size of the pupils weaken with age. The pupils become smaller, react more sluggishly to light, and dilate more slowly in the dark. Therefore, people older than 60 may find that objects are not as bright, that they are dazzled initially when going outdoors (or when facing oncoming cars during night driving), and that they have difficulty going from a brightly lit environment to a darker one. These changes may be particularly bothersome when combined with the effects of a cataract.

Other changes in eye function also occur as people age. The sharpness of vision (acuity) is reduced despite the use of the best glasses. The amount of light that reaches the back of the retina is reduced, increasing the need for brighter illumination and for greater contrast between objects and the background. Color perception and depth perception are reduced. Older people may also see increased numbers of floating black spots (floaters). Floaters do not significantly interfere with vision.

CHAPTER 225

Symptoms and Diagnosis of Eye Disorders

Eye symptoms may involve changes in vision, changes in appearance of the eye, or changes in sensation of the eye. Eye symptoms typically develop because of a problem in the eye but occasionally may indicate a problem elsewhere, particularly in the brain. Sometimes eye symptoms develop as part of an illness that affects several organ systems.

A person who experiences eye symptoms should be checked by his doctor. However,

▲ see page 1309

many eye diseases cause few or no symptoms in their early stages, so the eyes should be checked regularly (every 1 to 2 years or more frequently if there is an eye condition) by an ophthalmologist (a physician who specializes in the diagnosis and medical and surgical treatment of eye diseases) or by an optometrist (a nonphysician who specializes in refraction problems).

A person with eye or vision problems describes the location and duration of the symptoms, and then the doctor examines the eye, the area around it, and possibly other parts of the body, depending on the suspected cause.

Symptoms

Changes in Vision

Changes in vision may involve loss of vision or distortion of vision.

Loss of Vision: Loss of vision is a complete or nearly complete absence of sight. A person with loss of vision may see nothing whatsoever or he may be able to distinguish light from dark and may even be able to detect vague shapes. Loss of vision may involve part or all of the visual field of one or both eyes and may be temporary or permanent. Depending on the particular type of vision loss and how rapidly it develops, the person may immediately notice the problem, or it may not be discovered for some time—perhaps not until a car accident or other event prompts a thorough vision examination.

Complete loss of vision may occur in one or both eyes. Common causes include blockage of the blood supply to the retina, diabetes, optic nerve disease, glaucoma, and, in tropical areas, infections such as trachoma.

There are many types of loss of vision that involve only part of the visual field. People who have had certain kinds of strokes may not be able to see anything on one side but see normally on the other. People with a tumor of the pituitary gland (which lies just below the brain, behind a cross-over of the optic nerve fibers) may not be able to see things on either side but see normally in the middle (tunnel vision). Before a migraine headache, some people are temporarily (usually about 20 minutes) unable to see things above or below or to the right or left of their line of sight. People with macular degeneration lose the ability to see things they directly look at, but they retain their side or peripheral vision (the things seen out of the "corner of the eye"). Smaller, irregu-

lar patches of vision may be lost as a result of many disorders that damage the retina, such as diabetic retinopathy and hypertensive retinopathy. Glaucoma, if left untreated, can cause loss of part of the peripheral visual field, tunnel vision, and eventually total blindness.

Distortion of Vision: Distortion of vision is an inability to see clearly and correctly. This distortion may involve a refractive error, lack of depth perception, double vision, glare or halos, flashes of light, or floaters. It may also involve color blindness.

Refractive error causes objects to appear blurred and out of focus. Refractive error usually results from a mismatch between the shape of the cornea or lens and the length of the eye. If only distant objects are blurred, the person is nearsighted or myopic. If only nearby objects are blurred, the person is farsighted or hyperopic. Upon reaching middle age, most people—even those with previously excellent vision—develop difficulty focusing on nearby objects (presbyopia). Astigmatism, another type of refractive error, is caused by an irregularity in the curvature of the cornea or lens and results in slight blurring of vision. Astigmatism may occur on its own or together with any of the other types of refraction error.

Depth perception is the ability to determine the relative position of objects in space. People with impaired depth perception may have difficulty distinguishing which of two objects is closer. Depth perception is reduced when one eye is blind or has an uncorrected refractive error. It also may be impaired by a failure of the brain to integrate the two images—one from each eye—into a single three-dimensional image (fusion), resulting in double vision. However, many depth perception clues come from only one eye; therefore, if a person closes one eye and looks at two objects, he can usually tell which object is closer, even with only one eye.

Double vision (diplopia) is seeing two images of one object. Double vision may result from weakness in one or more of the muscles that control eye movements, resulting in cross-eye (strabismus).▲ Other causes include fatigue, alcohol intoxication, multiple sclerosis, trauma, or cataract. The sudden appearance of double vision may indicate a serious disorder of the brain or nervous system, such as a tumor, aneurysm, or blood clot.

▲ see page 1601

How and Why Blindness Develops

Anything that disrupts the passage of light from the environment to the back of the eye, or the nerve impulses from the back of the eye to the brain, will interfere with vision. Legally, blindness is defined as visual acuity worse than 20/200 even after correction with eyeglasses or contact lenses. Many people who are considered legally blind can distinguish shapes and shadows but not normal detail.

Blindness can occur under the following circumstances:

- **Light cannot reach the retina**

  Damage to the cornea from infections such as trachoma, leprosy, or onchocerciasis, which results in an opaque corneal scar

  Damage to the cornea from vitamin A deficiency, which causes dry eyes (keratomalacia) and results in an opaque corneal scar

  Cataracts

- **Light rays do not focus on the retina properly**

  Severe focusing (refraction) errors that are not fully correctible by eyeglasses or contact lenses

- **The retina cannot sense light rays normally**

  Detached retina

  Diabetes mellitus

  Glaucoma

  Macular degeneration

  Retinitis pigmentosa

- **Nerve impulses from the retina are not transmitted to the brain normally**

  Brain tumors that push on the optic nerve or on its pathways inside the brain

  Disorders of the nervous system, such as multiple sclerosis

  Inadequate blood supply to the retina (usually due to a blood clot in the retinal artery or vein or due to temporal arteritis)

  Inflammation of the optic nerve (optic neuritis)

- **The brain cannot interpret information sent by the eye**

  Strokes or brain tumors that affect the areas of the brain that interpret visual impulses (visual cortex)

Some people experience glare or halos around bright lights, especially when driving at night. Such symptoms are more common in older people and in those who have had certain types of refractive surgery or who have certain types of cataracts. Glare and halos can also occur in people whose pupils are widely dilated (for example those who have been given eye drops for an examination or who have large pupils). When the pupil is widely dilated, light is able to pass through the peripheral part of the lens, where it is bent differently from that passing through the more central parts of the lens and therefore causes glare.

Older people frequently have difficulty seeing in low light. Such symptoms are sometimes referred to as night blindness. Most commonly this results from a cataract, although certain forms of retinal degeneration, such as retinitis pigmentosa, have night blindness as a feature.

Some people experience bright flashing or flickering lights. This sensation most commonly results from shifting of the jellylike substance that fills the back of the eye (vitreous humor) or less commonly from a detached retina or a migraine headache. Flashes of light can also result from a blow to the back of the head ("seeing stars"), probably because of stimulation of the part of the brain where vision is interpreted.

Floating spots (floaters) are dark specks that appear to move in front of the eye. They are fast-moving or slow-moving clumps of the microscopic fibers that make up the vitreous humor. Floaters become increasingly common with aging. Floaters rarely affect vision and are generally considered normal; however, a sudden increase in the number of floaters (especially in association with flashing lights) may indicate a serious problem, such as a detached retina. A person with these symptoms should be evaluated by an ophthalmologist.

People with color blindness are unable to perceive certain colors, or they may perceive certain colors with different intensity than do people with normal color vision. For instance, in the most common form of color blindness (red-green color blindness), people may have a reduced ability to distinguish dark or pastel green or red or both. Often, the changes are subtle, and many people are unaware they have color blindness until they are tested.

Changes in the Appearance of the Eyes

The most common change in appearance is a red eye. Many conditions dilate the blood vessels in the conjunctiva, causing the white of the eye to appear red. Such conditions include fatigue, allergies, infections, abrasions or ulcers of the cornea, and foreign bodies in the eye. Sometimes, a forceful cough or a direct blow causes a blood vessel in the conjunctiva to burst, resulting in a bright red patch in the white of the eye. Sometimes the bleeding turns the whole white of the eye bright red. With a chalazion,▲ allergy, or a bacterial infection of the eyelids or sinuses, typically the eyelids and other tissue around the eye may become red.

In jaundice, the whites of the eyes (the sclera) become yellow, as does the skin.■

Sometimes dark spots appear on the iris or conjunctiva. Some are present at birth, and others may appear as a person ages. Often they are of no significance; however, any dark spot that grows should be evaluated by an ophthalmologist to ensure that it is not cancer.

The pupils normally are the same size; they become large (dilate) in the dark and become small (constrict) in bright light. Certain drugs used to treat eye diseases dilate or constrict the pupils. Opioid drugs, such as morphine, constrict the pupils. Amphetamines, antihistamines, cocaine, and marijuana may dilate the pupils.

Unequal pupils (one large and one small) may be caused by injury or inflammation of the eye, injury of the nerves that control the pupil, head injury, or brain tumors or by using eye drops in only one eye. People with syphilis may have small, irregularly shaped pupils (Argyll Robertson pupils). A few people are born with pupils of different sizes.

Changes may also be visible in the structures around the eye, such as the eyelids. For instance, the eyelids may droop (ptosis). This may occur in myasthenia gravis.★ Sometimes the eyes are unusually wide open and prominent, usually because they are being pushed forward (exophthalmos), which can occur in Graves' disease.●

The eyelids may become swollen, due to allergy, infection, or inflammation (as in a chalazion or stye). The roots of the eyelashes may become infected, sometimes resulting in the eyelashes falling out. Allergies or infections may also lead to abnormal secretions from the eyes, which may harden (crusting) and cause difficulty in opening the eyes.

Changes in Eye Sensation

Pain may occur around the eye, in the eye, or behind the eye. Pain from the cornea tends

What Causes Color Blindness?

Color blindness (dyschromatopsia) affects how people perceive certain colors. It is usually present from birth and is nearly always due to an X-linked recessive gene, which means that it nearly always occurs in men who have the gene. Women, who are not usually affected themselves, can pass the gene for color blindness on to their children.

Although color blindness is sometimes due to a problem with how the brain interprets color (rather than a problem with the eyes), usually people with color blindness lack certain photoreceptors at the back of the eye.

Most cases of color blindness are due to a relative deficiency or abnormality of one of the photoreceptor types. Red-green color blindness is the most common form. Blue-yellow color blindness is usually due to acquired rather than inherited disease and may be caused by optic nerve disease.

A person may be tested for color blindness if it is known that a family member has the abnormality. Some people may be tested because they have difficulty in matching colors. Other people, such as airline pilots, may be unaware of any problem but are tested because their jobs require that they be able to distinguish colors.

to be sharp and is usually worsened by blinking; it may give a sensation of "something in the eye." Corneal pain may be caused by an abrasion, foreign body, dry eye, ulcer, or infection. Acute closed-angle glaucoma produces a deep, aching pain in the eye. However, most chronic glaucoma is not painful. Pain originating within the eye may occur together with tenderness of the eyeball (when gently pressed, it hurts). A deep, boring pain in the eye can be a symptom of scleritis, a potentially serious inflammation of the thick fibrous coat of the eye, or uveitis, an inflammation of the inner structures of the eye.

Sensitivity to bright light (photophobia) occurs normally during extremely sunny conditions or when coming out of a dark environment into bright sunlight. However, unusual

▲ see page 1295   ■ see page 791

★ see page 577   ● see page 949

What Is Astigmatism?

Astigmatism is an irregularity in the curvature (curved differently in different directions) of the cornea or lens that causes light traveling in different planes to be focused differently. For example, vertical lines may be in focus when horizontal lines are not (or vice versa). The irregularity can be in any plane, however, and is often different in each eye. A person with astigmatism (each eye should be tested separately) tends to see certain lines more boldly (that is, in better focus) than the others. Astigmatism is correctible with prescription eyeglasses or contact lenses. It often occurs together with nearsightedness or farsightedness.

The following diagram is of a standard chart used to test for astigmatism in one eye at a time:

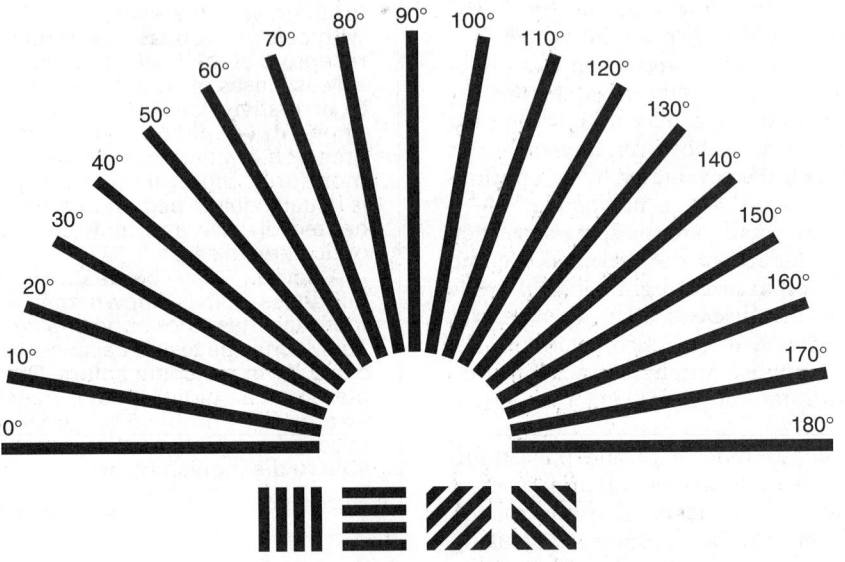

sensitivity to light can also be a symptom of a migraine headache or a number of eye disorders, for example, due to inflammation or infection within the front part of the eye (keratitis and uveitis) or an eye injury. It may also be due to meningitis (which also results in a severe headache with neck stiffness▲). Photophobia can also be caused by the use of drugs to dilate the pupils (mydriatics).

Itching may result from allergy and is usually accompanied by watering of the eyes (tearing). Inflammation of the eyelids (blepharitis) may also cause itching. Itching may also result from infection or infestation with lice or other parasites.

The sensation of dryness of the eyes can be caused by a variety of conditions, including inadequate tear production, accelerated tear evaporation, or less commonly, vitamin A deficiency and Sjögren's syndrome.■

Diagnosis

Diagnosis of eye disorders is initially based on the appearance of the eyes and on the symptoms that the person is experiencing. A variety of tests can be carried out to confirm a problem or to determine the extent or severity of the disorder.

Refraction

Refraction is the procedure by which focusing error is assessed. Problems with visual acuity (sharpness of vision) that result from refractive errors, such as nearsightedness, far-

---

▲ see page 529

■ see page 1292

sightedness, astigmatism, and presbyopia, are diagnosed by refraction. Acuity is usually measured on a scale that compares a person's vision at 20 feet with that of someone who has perfect vision. Thus, a person who has 20/20 vision sees objects that are 20 feet away with the same clarity as a person with normal vision, but a person who has 20/200 vision sees at 20 feet what a person with perfect vision sees at 200 feet. One important visual acuity test uses the **Snellen chart** (eye chart), which is a large card or lighted box that displays rows of letters in smaller and smaller sizes. The card is read from a standard distance. The degree of visual acuity is determined by the size of the row of letters that the person can read. For those who are unable to read, a modified chart can be used in which the letters are represented by an upper case "E," which is rotated randomly. The person is asked to describe the way the letter is facing.

Automated refraction is performed with machines that determine the refractive error of the eye by measuring how light is changed when it enters a person's eye. A person sits in front of the autorefractor, a beam of light is emitted from the device, and the eye's response is measured. The machine uses this information to calculate the lens prescription needed to correct the person's refractive error. This measurement takes only a few seconds.

A **phoropter** is the device commonly used, in conjunction with a Snellen chart, to allow determination of the best corrective lenses for a person being assessed for eyeglasses or contact lenses. The phoropter contains a complete range of corrective lenses, allowing the person to compare different levels of correction while viewing the chart. Typically, the eye doctor will use the phoropter to refine the information obtained from the autorefractor before prescribing lenses.

Visual Field Testing

The visual field is the entire area of vision that one sees out of each eye, including the corners (peripheral vision). The visual field is often tested as a regular part of an eye examination. It may also be tested if a person notices specific changes in vision, for example, if he keeps bumping into objects on one side. The simplest way to test peripheral vision is for a doctor to face the person and gradually move a finger from the left and the right at face level in toward the center of vision. The person tells the doctor when the moving fin-

ger is first detected. The person must fix his vision on the doctor's face (and not look for the finger) in order for the result of the test to be valid. Each eye is tested separately.

The visual field may be measured more precisely with a "tangent screen" or a Goldmann perimeter. With these tests, the person stares at the center of a black screen or a hollow, white, spherical device (which resembles a small satellite dish). An object or a light is moved slowly from the periphery toward the center of vision from many different directions. The person indicates when he first sees the light out of the corner of his eye. The doctor places a mark on the screen or perimeter indicating where the person can see, thus allowing recognition of blind spots. Visual fields can be measured using computerized automated perimetry. Here, the person stares at the center of a large shallow bowl and presses a button whenever he sees a flash of light.

The Amsler grid is used to test the central area of vision. The grid consists of a black card covered with a white grid and with a white dot in its center. Looking through one eye, the person notes any distortion in the lines of the grid, while staring at the white dot. Each eye is tested separately at a normal reading distance and while using reading glasses if the person normally uses them. If a person cannot see an area of the grid, an abnormal blind spot may exist. (There is a normal but very small blind spot in the area where the optic nerve leaves the eye; however, people are not aware of it.) Wavy lines suggest a possible problem with the macula. The test is simple enough to be used by people at home and is useful for monitoring macular degeneration.

Color Vision Testing

A variety of tests can be used to detect a reduced ability to perceive certain colors (color blindness). The Ishihara plates, which are most commonly used, are patterns of small, colored circles crowded together on a white background to form a large circle. The small circles are usually arranged so that people with normal color vision see a particular number. Those who have color blindness see another number or no number, depending on the type of color blindness.

Ophthalmoscopy

A direct ophthalmoscope is a handheld device like a small flashlight with magnifying lenses that shines a light into the eye to en-

What Is an Ophthalmoscope?

An ophthalmoscope is an instrument that enables a doctor to examine the inside of a person's eye. The instrument has an angled mirror, various lenses, and a light source. With it, a doctor can see the vitreous humor (the jellylike substance in the eye), the retina, the optic nerve, and the retinal veins and arteries.

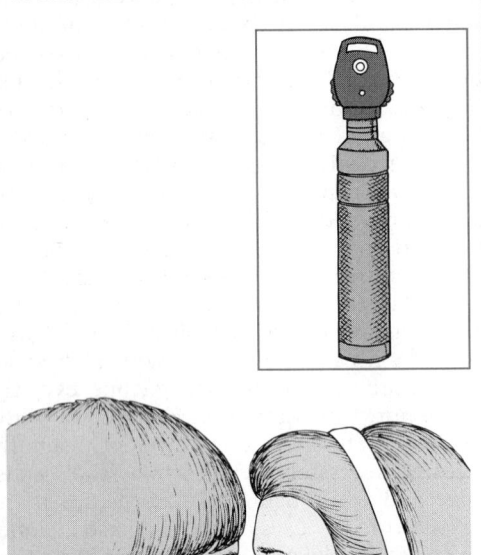

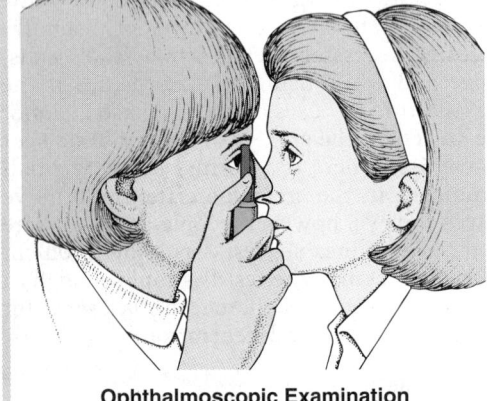

Ophthalmoscopic Examination

able a doctor to examine the cornea, lens, and retina. The person looks straight ahead as the beam of light is shone into the eye. Often, eye drops are given to dilate the pupil, which allows the doctor to have a better view. Ophthalmoscopy is painless, but if eye drops are used to dilate the pupils, vision may be blurred and the person will be more sensitive to light for a few hours afterward.

▲ see page 1306

Ophthalmoscopy is a standard part of every regular eye examination. Ophthalmoscopy is useful to detect not only changes in the retina due to eye disease but also changes due to certain diseases affecting other parts of the body. For instance, it is useful to detect the changes that occur in the retinal blood vessels in people with high blood pressure, arteriosclerosis, and diabetes mellitus. Ophthalmoscopy can also be used to diagnose elevated pressure within the brain, which results in a swelling (pushing-out) of the normally cupped optic disk (papilledema). Tumors on the retina can be seen with ophthalmoscopy. Macular degeneration can be diagnosed with ophthalmoscopy as well.

Sometimes the doctor uses an instrument called an indirect ophthalmoscope, in which a binocular device is placed on the doctor's head and a handheld lens is used in front of the person's eye to focus the image inside the eye. This method gives a three-dimensional view, allowing a better view of objects that have depth, including a detached retina or a swollen optic disk. It also allows a brighter light source to be used, which is important if the interior of the eye is cloudy, for instance due to infection or cataract. The indirect ophthalmoscope also allows a much wider field of view than a regular ophthalmoscope, so that the doctor can examine more of the retina at once.

Slit Lamp Examination

The slit lamp is a table-mounted binocular microscope that shines a light into the eye to allow the doctor to examine the entire eye under high magnification. The slit lamp has better optics than the ophthalmoscope, providing magnification and a three-dimensional view, which allows measurement of depth. Often, eye drops are used to dilate the pupils so that the doctor can view even more of the eye, including the lens, vitreous humor, retina, and optic nerve. Sometimes, in people with suspected or known glaucoma,▲ an additional lens is placed on or held in front of the eye to allow examination of the "angle" between the iris and the front part of the eye (inside surface of the cornea). This examination is called gonioscopy.

Tonometry

With tonometry, the pressure of the aqueous humor within the eye can be measured. The aqueous humor is the fluid in the front part of the eye. Normal pressure within the eye is 8 to 21 millimeters of mercury (mm

Hg). Pressure in the eye is measured to detect certain types of glaucoma and monitor its treatment.

The noncontact ("air-puff") tonometer is used to screen for elevated pressure in the eye. This device is not highly accurate, but it is useful in screening. A small puff of air is blown against the cornea, which causes the person to blink but is not uncomfortable. The puff of air flattens the cornea, and the device measures the time (in thousandths of a second) it takes to flatten the cornea. It takes less time for the puff of air to flatten the cornea in an eye with normal pressure than it does an eye in which pressure is elevated.

Portable, handheld instruments are also used for tonometry. Eye drops that contain a drug to numb the eye are given, then the instrument is gently placed on the cornea, and a reading is obtained. Portable tonometers can be used in the emergency department or a doctor's office to quickly detect increased pressure in the eye.

Applanation tonometry is a more accurate method. The applanation tonometer is usually attached to a slit lamp. After numbing the eye with drops, the instrument is gently moved until it rests upon the cornea, while the doctor observes the cornea through a slit lamp. The amount of pressure it takes to indent the cornea is related to the pressure within the eye.

Fluorescein Angiography

Fluorescein angiography allows a doctor to clearly see the blood vessels at the back of the eye. A fluorescent dye, which is visible in blue light, is injected into a vein in the person's arm. The dye circulates throughout the person's bloodstream, including the blood vessels in the retina. Shortly after the dye is injected, a rapid sequence of photographs is taken of the retina. The dye inside the blood vessels fluoresces, making the vessels stand out. Fluorescein angiography is particularly useful in the diagnosis of macular degeneration, blocked retinal blood vessels, and diabetic retinopathy.

Electroretinography

Electroretinography allows a doctor to examine the function of the photoreceptors in the retina by measuring the response of the retina to flashes of light. Eye drops numb the eye and dilate the pupil. A recording electrode in the form of a contact lens is then placed on the cornea and another electrode is placed on the skin of the face nearby. The eyes are then

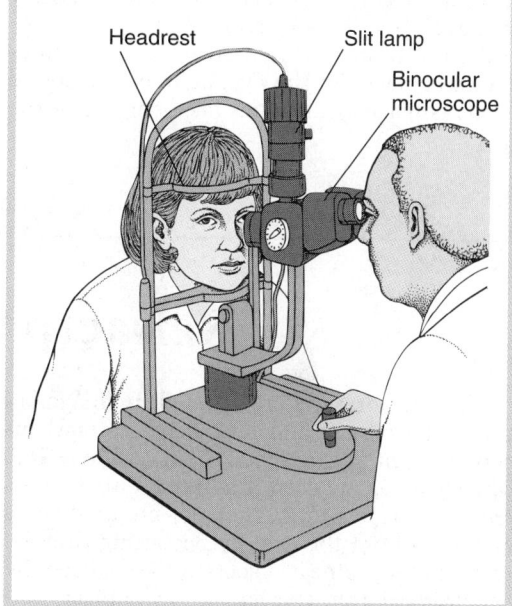

What Is a Slit Lamp?

A slit lamp is an instrument that enables a doctor to examine the entire eye under high magnification. The slit lamp focuses a bright light into the eye.

Headrest   Slit lamp

Binocular microscope

propped open. The room is darkened and the person stares at a light source that emits flashes of light. The electrical activity generated by the retina in response to the flashes of light is recorded by the electrodes. Electroretinography is particularly useful for evaluating diseases, such as retinitis pigmentosa, in which the retina or photoreceptors are affected.

Ultrasound

The eye can be examined by ultrasound. A probe is placed gently against the closed eyelid and painlessly bounces sound waves off the eyeball. The reflected sound waves produce a two-dimensional image of the inside of the eye. Ultrasound is useful when an ophthalmoscope or slit lamp cannot show the retina because the inside of the eye is cloudy or something is blocking the line of sight. Ultrasound can also be used to determine the nature of abnormal structures, such as a tumor, inside the eye. Ultrasound also can be used to examine blood vessels supplying the eye (Doppler ultrasound) and to determine the thickness of the cornea in pachymetry.

Pachymetry

Pachymetry (measuring the thickness of the cornea) is usually carried out using ultrasound. Accurate measurement of the thickness of the cornea is very important in refractive eye surgery, such as LASIK.▲

For ultrasound pachymetry, a drop of anesthetic is placed in the eye, and an ultrasound probe is placed gently onto the surface of the cornea. Optical pachymetry methods do not require anesthetic eye drops because the instruments do not touch the eye.

Computed Tomography and Magnetic Resonance Imaging

These imaging techniques can be used to provide detailed information about the structures inside the eye and the bony structure that surrounds the eye (the orbit). Computed tomography (CT) is particularly useful to locate foreign bodies inside the eye.

CHAPTER 226

Refractive Disorders

The eye normally creates a clear image because the cornea and lens bend (refract) incoming light rays to focus them on the retina. The shape of the cornea is fixed, but the lens changes shape to focus on objects at various distances from the eye. By becoming thicker, the lens allows near objects to be focused; by becoming flatter, the lens allows objects farther away to be focused. A refractive error occurs when the cornea and lens cannot focus the image of an object sharply on the retina.

Causes

The lens and cornea may not bend light correctly for several reasons. The eyeball may be too large for the optical power of the focusing system. Because of this, light is focused in front of (rather than directly on) the retina, and the person has trouble clearly seeing distant objects. This is called nearsightedness (myopia). In some people, the eyeball is too small for the optical power of the focusing system, so light is focused behind the retina. This is called farsightedness (hyperopia). People who are farsighted have trouble clearly seeing anything close. Some people have an imperfectly shaped cornea, which may cause objects to appear blurred from any distance. This condition is called astigmatism.■

As people reach their early 40s, the lens becomes increasingly stiff; it does not change shape easily, so it cannot focus on nearby objects, a condition called presbyopia. If a person has had a lens removed to treat cataracts but has not had a lens implant, objects look blurred from any distance.★ The absence of a lens (as a result of birth defect, eye injury, or eye surgery for cataract) is called aphakia.

Symptoms and Diagnosis

A person who has a refractive error may notice that vision is blurred. For example, a child who becomes nearsighted may have difficulty with schoolwork.

Everyone should have regular eye examinations by a family doctor, internist, ophthalmologist (a physician who specializes in diagnosing and treating eye diseases and performing eye surgery), or optometrist (a nonphysician specialist in eye defects and refractive errors). A Snellen eye chart is used to determine visual acuity. Visual acuity (sharpness of vision) is measured in relation to what a person with normal vision sees. For example, a person with 20/60 vision sees at 20 feet what a person with normal vision sees at 60 feet. Although refractive errors usually occur in otherwise healthy eyes, testing generally also includes assessments unrelated to refractive error, such as a test of the visual fields● and eye movements. The eyes are tested together and individually.

Treatment

The usual treatment for refractive errors is to wear corrective lenses. However, certain surgical procedures and laser treatments that

---

▲ see page 1288   ■ see box on page 1282
★ see page 1303   ● see page 1283

change the shape of the cornea also can correct refractive errors.

Corrective Lenses

Refractive errors can be corrected with glass or plastic lenses mounted in a frame (eyeglasses) or with small pieces of plastic placed directly over the cornea (contact lenses). Good vision correction is possible with both eyeglasses and contact lenses; for most people, the choice is a matter of appearance, convenience, and comfort.

Plastic lenses for eyeglasses are lighter but tend to scratch; glass lenses are more durable but are more likely to break. Plastic lenses are more commonly used because they are thinner; they can also be coated with a chemical that helps them resist scratches. Both glass and plastic lenses can be tinted or treated with a chemical that darkens them automatically on exposure to light. Lenses can also be coated to reduce the amount of potentially damaging ultraviolet light that reaches the eye.

Bifocals contain two lenses—an upper lens that corrects the view of distant objects and a lower lens that corrects the view of nearby objects, as in reading. However, people also need to focus at middle distances, such as when viewing a computer screen. Trifocals meet this need by adding a lens for middle distance. Continuously variable lenses (progressive add lenses) also permit focusing at middle distances and have a cosmetic advantage in that there is no line or sharp division between the lenses.

Many people think contact lenses are more attractive than eyeglasses, and some think that vision is more natural with contact lenses. However, contact lenses require more care than eyeglasses, and, rarely, they can damage the eye. For some people, contact lenses cannot correct vision as well as eyeglasses can. However, newer types of contact lenses have been developed to allow correction of a wider range of refractive errors. For example, soft toric lenses allow correction of astigmatism. Some people, particularly older people and people with arthritis, may have trouble handling contact lenses and placing them in their eyes.

Rigid contact lenses, which include hard and gas-permeable contact lenses, are thin disks made of hard plastic. Oxygen, which the cornea needs to survive, does not pass easily through the plastic of the older style hard contact lenses. Gas-permeable contact lenses, which are made of plastics such as newer sili-

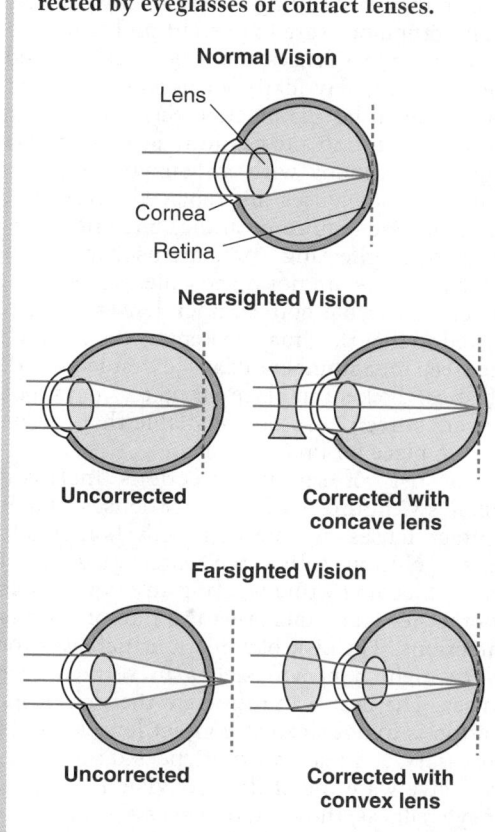

Understanding Refraction

Normally, the cornea and lens bend (refract) incoming light rays to focus them on the retina. When there is a refractive error, the cornea and lens cannot focus light rays on the retina. Refractive errors can be corrected by eyeglasses or contact lenses.

Normal Vision

Lens

Cornea

Retina

Nearsighted Vision

Uncorrected

Corrected with concave lens

Farsighted Vision

Uncorrected

Corrected with convex lens

cone compounds, permit more oxygen to reach the cornea. Rigid contact lenses can be used to correct irregularities in the cornea (astigmatism).

Rigid contact lenses usually need to be worn for up to a week before they feel comfortable for a prolonged period. The contact lenses are worn for a gradually increasing number of hours each day. Although rigid contact lenses may be uncomfortable at first, they should not be painful. Pain indicates an improper fit.

Soft hydrophilic (water-absorbing) contact lenses are made of flexible plastic. They are larger than rigid contact lenses and cover the entire cornea. Soft contact lenses allow oxygen to reach the cornea easily.

Soft contact lenses are easier to handle than are rigid contact lenses, because they are larger. They are also less likely than rigid contact lenses to fall out or to allow dust and other particles to get trapped underneath. In addition, soft contact lenses are usually comfortable on the first wearing. They do, however, require scrupulous care to prevent problems.

Most contact lenses must be removed and cleaned every day (daily wear). Most contact lenses must be disinfected each night and cleaned of protein and calcium deposits. Some require treatment with an enzyme weekly. Some contact lenses are replaced every day. They do not require cleaning, enzyme treatment, or disinfecting. Some are used for 1 to 4 weeks. Others are not disposable. Some regular or disposable soft contact lenses are designed so that they may be kept in the eye during sleep for a number of days (extended wear). Most can be kept in place for up to 7 days, but newer contact lenses are available that can be kept in place for up to 30 days.

The risk of serious infections increases when swimming with contact lenses and if contact lenses are cleaned with homemade saline solution, saliva, tap water, or distilled water. Sleeping while wearing any type of soft contact lens also increases the risk of serious infections. The risk of infection increases for every night a person sleeps in soft contact lenses. The best way to reduce the risk of infection is to not sleep in contact lenses unless necessary. If a person experiences discomfort, excessive watering of the eye, vision changes, or eye redness, the contact lenses should be removed immediately. If the symptoms do not resolve quickly, the person should contact an eye doctor.

Wearing contact lenses poses a risk of serious, vision-threatening, painful complications, including the formation of ulcers on the cornea. Ulcers can be caused by an infection, which can lead to a loss of vision.▲ The risks can be greatly reduced by following the instructions of the eye doctor and the manufacturer and by using common sense.

Surgery for Refractive Errors

Surgical and laser procedures (refractive surgery) can be used to correct nearsighted-

ness, farsightedness, and astigmatism. These procedures are used to reshape the cornea so that it is better able to focus light on the retina. These procedures usually correct vision about as well as eyeglasses and soft contact lenses do. Before deciding on such a procedure, a person should have a thorough discussion with an ophthalmologist and should carefully consider his own needs and expectations, along with the risks and benefits.

The best candidates for refractive surgery are people who cannot tolerate contact lenses and those who enjoy activities, such as swimming or skiing, that are difficult to do with eyeglasses or contact lenses. Many people undergo this surgery for convenience and cosmetic purposes. However, refractive surgery is not recommended for all people with refractive errors. For example, people whose eyeglass or contact lens prescription has changed in the past year and those with autoimmune or connective tissue diseases, with signs of keratoconus, who are taking certain drugs (for example, isotretinoin or amiodarone), and with a few exceptions, people younger than 21 years of age, usually should not have laser refractive surgery.

The doctor determines the exact refractive error (eyeglass prescription) before surgery. The eyes are thoroughly examined, and special attention is paid to the surface cells of the cornea (including whether the cornea has loose or well anchored surface skin), the cornea's shape and thickness (using pachymetry■), the pupil size in light and dark, the intraocular pressure, the optic nerve, and the retina. Refractive surgical procedures are generally brief and cause little discomfort. Eye drops are used to numb the eye. The eye is held still, but the person must also not move the eye during the procedure. Usually, a person can go home soon after the procedure.

After refractive surgery, most people have distance vision that is good enough to do most things well (for example, driving or going to the movies), although not everyone has perfect 20/20 vision without eyeglasses after the procedure. If a person has a weak eyeglass prescription before refractive surgery, he is most likely to have 20/20 distance vision after surgery. Even if they do not wear eyeglasses for distance vision, most people older than 40 still need to wear eyeglasses for reading after refractive surgery.

Complications include overcorrection, undercorrection, excessive inflammation, infection, double vision, sensitivity to bright light,

▲ see page 1300   ■ see page 1286

glare and halos around lights, difficulty with seeing or driving at night, wrinkling of the cornea, and deposition of cells or other material in the cornea. Rarely, even with eyeglasses, a person may have worse vision after refractive surgery. Because treating undercorrection is usually easier than treating overcorrection, surgeons prefer not to overcorrect. If undercorrection or overcorrection occurs, further correction can usually be done.

LASIK (Laser in situ Keratomileusis): LASIK, the most common refractive surgical procedure, is used to correct nearsightedness, farsightedness, and astigmatism. In LASIK, a very thin flap is cut in the central part of the cornea with a knife called a microkeratome. Pulses from an excimer laser vaporize tiny amounts of corneal tissue under the flap to reshape the cornea. The flap is then laid back in place and heals over several days. LASIK causes little discomfort during and after surgery. Vision improvement is rapid; many people are able to go back to work within 1 to 3 days. People who have any conditions that preclude refractive surgery, as well as those who have thin corneas, loose corneal surface skin, and large pupils, may not be good candidates for LASIK.

Photorefractive Keratectomy (PRK): This procedure uses an excimer laser to reshape the cornea. It is used primarily to correct moderate nearsightedness, mild astigmatism, and farsightedness. Computer-controlled pulses of highly focused ultraviolet light remove small amounts of the cornea and thus change its shape to better focus light onto the retina and improve vision without eyeglasses. This procedure usually takes less than 1 minute per eye. Although there is more discomfort and longer healing time than with LASIK, PRK can be performed on people who cannot have LASIK, such as those with loose corneal surface cells or thin corneas.

Radial and Astigmatic Keratotomy: These are surgical procedures used to treat nearsightedness and astigmatism by making very deep cuts in the cornea with a small blade.

In radial keratotomy, the surgeon makes small radial (or wheel spoke) cuts in the cornea. Usually, four to eight cuts are made. Because the cornea is only $\frac{1}{2}$ millimeter thick, the depth of the cuts must be determined precisely. The surgeon determines where to make each cut after analyzing the shape of the cornea and the person's visual acuity.

The surgery flattens the central part of the cornea, so it can better focus incoming light on the retina. This change improves vision without eyeglasses, and about 90% of those who have the surgery can function well and drive without eyeglasses or contact lenses. Sometimes, a second or third procedure (enhancement) is needed to sufficiently improve vision without eyeglasses. For some people who have radial keratotomy, the vision without eyeglasses fluctuates slightly throughout the day, and for some, the effect of the surgery may increase over years. Since the development of laser refractive procedures with lower risks and better results, radial keratotomy is rarely performed now.

Astigmatic keratotomy is used to correct naturally occurring astigmatism and astigmatism that occurs after cataract surgery or corneal transplantation. In this procedure, the surgeon makes one or two curved or straight deep cuts in the peripheral part of the cornea parallel to the edge of the cornea.

No surgical procedure is risk free, but the risks from radial and astigmatic keratotomy are small. The major risks are overcorrection and undercorrection of the vision problem. Because overcorrection usually cannot be treated effectively, a surgeon tries to avoid doing too much correction at one time. Undercorrection can be treated by a second or third procedure. Vision can fluctuate with changes in atmospheric oxygen, such as at high altitudes. The most serious complication is infection, which is rare. When it does develop, it must be treated with antibiotics.

Other Refractive Surgery: Other techniques are available that may have advantages over or different risks than LASIK. For people who are very nearsighted, surgical procedures in which a plastic lens is placed inside the eye, in front of the iris (phakic intraocular lens implantation), between the iris and the natural lens (implantable contact lens), or behind the iris after the natural lens has been removed (clear lensectomy with intraocular lens implantation) may be best. Because these techniques make an opening into the eye, there is a very small risk (but significantly higher than for LASIK) of severe infection inside the eye.

Intracorneal ring segments are used for people with mild nearsightedness without astigmatism. Small plastic arcs are implanted into the middle layer of the cornea. Because no tissue is removed during the procedure, the intracorneal ring segment procedure can be reversed by removing the small plastic arcs.

Laser thermal keratoplasty (LTK) is used for people with mild farsightedness without astigmatism. It is a quick surgical procedure that does not involve any cutting; several small laser burns are made in the cornea. There are few risks, but some people lose some or most of the effect over time.

Laser epithelial keratomileusis (LASEK), a modification of the LASIK technique, may be used for nearsightedness, farsightedness, or astigmatism. Like PRK, LASEK is better than LASIK for people with thin corneas.

CHAPTER 227

Eye Injuries

The structure of the face and eyes is well suited for protecting the eyes from injury. The eyeball is set into a socket surrounded by a strong, bony ridge. The eyelids can close quickly to form a barrier to foreign objects,▲ and the eye can tolerate a minor impact without damage.

Even so, injury may damage the eye, sometimes so severely that vision is lost and, in rare instances, the eye must be removed. Most eye injuries are minor, but because of extensive bruising to surrounding structures, they may look worse than they are. Any injury to the eye should be examined by a doctor to determine the extent of injury and the treatment that is needed.

Blunt Injuries

A blunt impact may damage the structures near the surface of the eye (the eyelid, conjunctiva, sclera, cornea, iris, and lens) and those at the back of the eye (retina and optic nerve). Such an impact may also break the bones that surround the eye. Even blunt trauma may result in cuts (lacerations) to the tissues of the eye.

Symptoms

In the first 24 hours after a blunt eye injury, blood may leak into the skin of the eyelid and surrounding areas, producing a bruise (contusion), commonly called a black eye. If a blood vessel on the surface of the eye breaks, the conjunctiva will become red. The superficial bleeding may look alarming but is usually minor. It resolves without treatment. The red area may become slightly green and then yel-

low within a few days; all traces of the bleeding typically disappear within 1 to 2 weeks. Lacerations, small or large, commonly occur as well and lead to bleeding from the skin.

Damage to the inside of the eye is more serious than damage to the surface. Bleeding into the front chamber of the eye (hyphema or anterior chamber hemorrhage) is serious and requires examination by an ophthalmologist (a medical doctor trained in the medical and surgical treatment of eye disease). Symptoms of bleeding into the front chamber of the eye include reduced vision and light sensitivity. Blood within the front chamber of the eye may cause pressure within the eye to increase (glaucoma). Further bleeding within the eye may occur days after the original injury.

Bleeding can also occur in the back section (posterior segment) of the eye (vitreous hemorrhage), the iris (the colored part of the eye) can be torn, or the lens can be dislocated. Bleeding may also occur in the retina (retinal hemorrhage). The retina can also be torn by injury and may become detached from its underlying surface at the back of the eye (retinal detachment). Initially, retinal detachment may create images of irregular floating shapes or flashes of light and may blur vision, but then vision greatly decreases.■ In severe injuries, the thick, fibrous coat of the eyeball (the sclera) can be ruptured.

Treatment

If there is uncertainty about the seriousness of a blunt injury to the eye or if vision is affected, the person should seek immediate medical advice. Generally, an ophthalmologist should evaluate the injury.

During the first 24 to 48 hours, ice packs may help reduce swelling and ease the pain of a black eye. If the skin around the eye or on

▲ see page 1277   ■ see page 1311

the eyelid has been cut, stitches may be needed. When possible, stitches near the edge of the eyelids should be placed by an ophthalmologist to ensure that no deformities develop that will affect the way the eyelids close. An injury that affects the tear ducts should be repaired by an ophthalmologist.

A laceration of the eye needs to be evaluated by an ophthalmologist who can determine how deep the cut is and whether surgery is needed to repair the injury. Many injuries involve only the conjunctiva and may not require surgical repair. Cuts involving the deeper layers of the eye (the sclera) or the cornea typically require stitches. Drugs are usually given to ease pain until the cut has healed.

Treatment for bleeding into the anterior chamber of the eye usually involves bed rest with the head of the bed elevated to encourage the blood to settle and eye drops to dilate the pupil and reduce inflammation within the eye. Aspirin and other nonsteroidal anti-inflammatory drugs (NSAIDs), which can predispose to bleeding, should be avoided for several weeks.

If there has been a cut that penetrates into the interior of the eye, antibiotics are usually given intravenously first and then occasionally by mouth to prevent infection within the eyeball (endophthalmitis). Eye drops that dilate the pupil can prevent bleeding from the iris and may reduce the sensitivity to light that often accompanies eye injuries. Corticosteroid eye drops are often given to reduce inflammation. A metal shield is often used to protect the eye from further injury. Serious damage may result in a partial or a total loss of vision, even after surgical treatment. Very rarely, after a severe laceration of one eye, the uninjured eye becomes inflamed (sympathetic ophthalmia), which may result in partial loss of vision or even blindness.

Foreign Objects

The most common eye injuries are those to the cornea and outer surface of the eye (conjunctiva) caused by foreign objects. Although most of these injuries are minor, some—such as penetration of the cornea or development of an infection from a cut or scratch on the cornea—can be serious.

Perhaps the most common source of surface injuries is contact lenses. Poorly fitting lenses, lenses left in the eyes too long, lenses left in inappropriately during sleep, inadequately

sterilized lenses, and forceful or inept removal of lenses can scratch the surface of the eye.

Other causes of surface injuries include glass particles, wind-borne particles, tree branches, and falling debris. People with certain occupations or hobbies are particularly likely to have small particles fly in their faces. For example, hammering a nail or other metal object with a steel hammer produces white-hot particles of steel that resemble sparks. Any of these white-hot particles can enter the unprotected eye and embed themselves deep within it. Protective eyewear (safety glasses) can help prevent injuries.

Symptoms

Injury to the surface of the eye usually causes pain and a feeling that there is something in the eye. It may also produce an increased sensitivity to light, redness, bleeding from blood vessels on the surface of the eye, or swelling of the eye and eyelid. Vision may become blurred.

Foreign bodies that penetrate the inside of the eye or injuries that are contaminated with soil or vegetable matter (for example, an injury caused by a tree branch) are particularly likely to become infected. Prompt diagnosis and appropriate treatment can help prevent infection.

Diagnosis and Treatment

Diagnosis of eye injury is based on the person's symptoms and the circumstances of the injury. Examination of the eye is carried out simultaneously with the procedure to remove the foreign object. Sometimes, additional tests, such as computed tomography (CT), may be needed.

Eye drops containing a dye that glows under special lighting make the object more visible and reveal surface abrasions. The surface of the eye is usually numbed with anesthetic drops. Using a special lighting and magnifying instrument, such as a binocular lens or slit lamp, to view the surface of the eye in detail, the doctor then removes the foreign object. Often the foreign object can be lifted out with a moist sterile cotton swab or flushed out with sterile water. Foreign objects that cannot be dislodged easily can often be removed painlessly with a needle or a special instrument. When metal foreign bodies are removed, they can leave a ring of rust, which may need to be removed with a special burr (a small surgical tool with a tiny, rotating, grinding and drilling surface).

An antibiotic ointment is usually applied for several days. Large abrasions of the cornea may require additional treatment: The pupil is kept dilated with eye drops, and an antibiotic ointment is applied; a patch may be placed over the eye to keep it closed. An abrasion that results from a contact lens or an object that may be contaminated with soil or vegetation is not patched, because patching can worsen the risk of a serious infection of the cornea (corneal ulcer). Fortunately, the surface cells of the eye regenerate rapidly. Even large abrasions tend to heal in 1 to 3 days. Follow-up examination by an ophthalmologist 1 or 2 days after injury is wise. Corneal abrasions are uncomfortable, so drugs to relieve pain are often given by mouth.

When a foreign object has pierced the deeper layers of the eye, an ophthalmologist should be consulted immediately for emergency surgical treatment to remove the object. Prompt removal reduces the risk of infection.

Burns

Exposure to extreme heat or chemicals makes the eyelids close quickly in a reflex reaction to protect the eyes from burns. Thus, only the eyelids may be burned; however, extreme heat can also burn the eye itself. The severity of the injury, the amount of pain, and the appearance of the eyelids depend on the depth of the burn.

Chemical burns can occur when an irritating substance gets into the eye. Even mildly irritating substances can cause substantial pain and damage the eye. Because the pain is so great, there is a tendency to keep the eyelids closed. This keeps the substance against the eye for a prolonged period, which may worsen the damage.

Treatment

To treat heat burns on the eyelids, a doctor or other health care practitioner washes the area with a sterile solution and then applies an antibiotic ointment or a strip of gauze saturated with petroleum jelly. The treated area is covered with sterile dressings held in place with a plastic bandage or stockinette to allow the burn to heal.

A chemical burn of the eye is treated by immediately flooding the open eye with water. This treatment must be started even before medical personnel arrive. Although a person may have difficulty keeping the injured eye open because of pain, quick removal of the chemical is essential. The injured person or a colleague may have to hold the eyelids open while flushing the eye with large amounts of room-temperature water.

A doctor may begin treatment by placing anesthetic drops and a drug to keep the pupil dilated in the eye. An antibiotic ointment is applied. Corticosteroid eye drops may be used to help reduce inflammation. Drugs to relieve pain may also be needed.

Severe burns need to be treated by an ophthalmologist to preserve vision and prevent major complications, such as damage to the cornea and iris, perforation of the eye, and deformities of the eyelids. However, even with the best treatment, severe chemical burns of the cornea, especially alkali injuries (such as from lye [caustic soda], which is often found in drain cleaners), can lead to scarring, perforation of the eye, and blindness. Using safety glasses when handling potentially hazardous chemicals is essential to help prevent these injuries.

CHAPTER 228

Eyelid and Tear Gland Disorders

The eyelids play a key role in protecting the eyes. They sweep away debris when the eyes close and help spread moisture (tears) over the surface of the eyes when they open. The eyelids provide a mechanical barrier against injury by closing rapidly when needed.

An abnormality of the tear (lacrimal) glands can lead to insufficient tear production or to a deficiency in the composition of the tears themselves. Without adequate or normal tear production, the eyes can dry and may be unable to normally fight infections from airborne particles, fingertips, or surrounding skin. Abnormal tear production may be due to a problem within the tear glands (lacrimal glands) and ducts (lacrimal excretory ducts, which carry tears into the eye) or due to a systemic disease that affects the tear glands, such as Sjögren's syndrome.▲

Dacryostenosis

Dacryostenosis is blockage of the drainage of tears from the eye, usually due to narrowing of the nasolacrimal ducts.

The nasolacrimal ducts are responsible for draining tears from the eye. Dacryostenosis can result from inadequate development of any part of the nasolacrimal ducts, chronic nasal infection, severe or recurring eye infections, or fractures of the nasal or facial bones.

Inadequate development of the nasolacrimal ducts at birth usually results in an overflow of tears that run down the cheek (epiphora). One eye or, rarely, both eyes are affected. The problem is usually first noticed in 3- to 12-week-old infants. This type of blockage usually disappears without treatment by the age of 6 months, as the nasolacrimal system develops. Sometimes the blockage resolves faster when parents are taught to gently massage the area above the duct with a fingertip.

Dacryostenosis may not resolve spontaneously and can lead to infection of the lacrimal sac (dacryocystitis).

If the blockage does not clear up, an ear, nose, and throat specialist (otorhinolaryngologist) or an eye specialist (ophthalmologist) may have to open the nasolacrimal duct with a small probe, which is usually inserted through the duct opening at the corner of the eyelid. Children are given general anesthesia for this procedure, but adults need only local anesthesia. If the nasolacrimal duct or gland is completely blocked, more extensive surgery may be needed.

Dacryocystitis

Dacryocystitis is infection of the lacrimal sac.

The lacrimal sac is a small chamber into which tears drain. Usually, dacryocystitis results from a blockage of the nasolacrimal duct, which leads from the lacrimal sac into the nose. Dacryocystitis may occur suddenly (acute) or be longstanding (chronic). In acute infection, the area around the lacrimal sac is painful, red, and swollen. The eye becomes red and watery and oozes pus. Slight pressure applied to the lacrimal sac may push pus through the opening at the inner corner of the eye, near the nose. Fever is common.

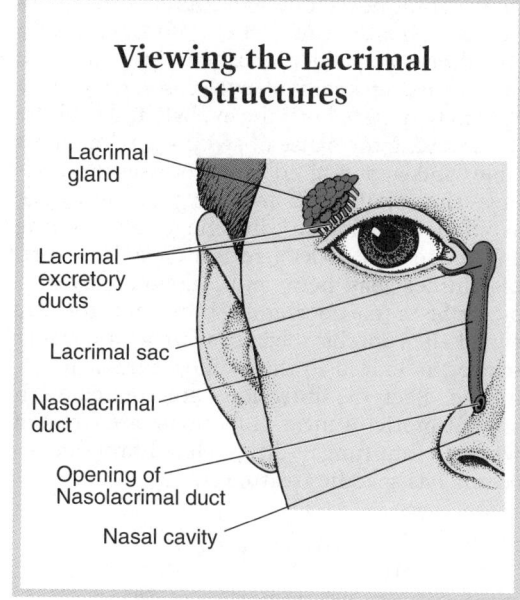

Viewing the Lacrimal Structures

Lacrimal gland

Lacrimal excretory ducts

Lacrimal sac

Nasolacrimal duct

Opening of Nasolacrimal duct

Nasal cavity

Often the infection is mild, and most symptoms disappear. Sometimes, an infection causes fluid to be retained in the lacrimal sac; a large fluid-filled lacrimal sac is called a mucocele. An abscess may form and rupture through the skin, creating a passage for drainage.

An acute infection is treated with oral or intravenous antibiotics. Applying warm compresses to the area several times a day also helps. If an abscess develops, surgery is performed to open and drain it. For chronic infections, the blocked nasolacrimal duct may be opened with a probe or by surgery. In rare instances, surgical removal of the entire lacrimal sac may be necessary.

Eyelid Swelling

Anything that irritates the eyes can also irritate the eyelids and cause swelling (eyelid edema). The most common cause of irritation is an allergy, which can make one or both lids crinkled or swollen. Allergic reactions may be caused by cosmetics, pollen or other particles in the air, metals such as nickel, or drugs placed into the eye as eye drops. Stings or bites from insects or infections from bacteria, viruses, or fungi can also cause the eyelids to

▲ see page 382

swell. Trichinosis, due to a roundworm infection,▲ can also cause the eyelids to swell. Hereditary angioedema, a genetic disorder,■ may cause episodes of eyelid swelling. Dry eyes may irritate both the eyeball and eyelids.

Removing the cause of swelling, where possible, and applying cold compresses may relieve the swelling. If an allergy is the cause, avoiding the allergen can relieve the swelling and reduce the risk of future episodes. Antihistamines may help, and a doctor may also prescribe a corticosteroid ointment for the eyelid. If a foreign object, such as an insect stinger, is lodged in the eyelid, it must be removed. Bacterial infections are treated with an antibiotic; fungal infections are treated with an antifungal drug. Hereditary angioedema has specific treatment.

Blepharitis

Blepharitis is inflammation of the edges of the eyelids, possibly with thickening scales, crusts, shallow ulcers, or inflamed oil glands at the edges of the eyelids.

Disorders that may cause blepharitis include staphylococcal infection of the eyelids or the ducts of the deeper glands that open at the edges of the eyelids, seborrheic dermatitis of the face and scalp, and acne rosacea.

Blepharitis may produce the feeling that something is in the eye. The eyes and eyelids may itch and burn, and the edges of the eyelids may become red. The eyes may become watery and sensitive to bright light. The eyelid may swell, and some of the eyelashes may fall out. Sometimes, small abscesses containing pus (pustules) develop in the sacs at the base of the eyelashes and eventually form shallow ulcers (ulcerative blepharitis). A crust may form and stick tenaciously to the edges of the eyelid; when the crust is removed, it may leave a bleeding surface. During sleep, secretions dry and make the eyelids sticky.

Blepharitis tends to recur and stubbornly resist treatment. It is inconvenient and unattractive but usually does not damage the cornea or result in loss of vision. Occasionally, ulcerative blepharitis can result in a loss of the eyelashes, scarring of the eyelid margins, and even damage to the cornea.

Diagnosis is usually based on the symptoms and the appearance of the eyelids. A doctor may use a slit lamp to examine the eyelids more closely. Occasionally, a sample of pus is taken from the edges of the eyelids and is cultured to identify the type of bacteria responsible and the antibiotics to which they are susceptible.

For blepharitis caused by seborrheic dermatitis, treatment usually consists of keeping the eyelids clean by gently scrubbing the edges of the eyelids each day with a wash cloth or cotton swab dipped in a dilute solution of baby shampoo (two to three drops in $1/2$ cup of warm water). For inflamed oil glands at the edge of the eyelids, warm compresses may ease the itching and burning. Occasionally, a doctor may prescribe an antibiotic ointment, such as bacitracin plus polymyxin B or sulfacetamide, or an oral antibiotic, such as doxycycline. When seborrheic dermatitis is the cause, the face and scalp must be treated as well.★ If acne rosacea is the cause, it can be treated.

Stye

A stye (hordeolum) is an acute infection of one or more of the glands at the edge of the eyelid or under it.

A stye is usually caused by a staphylococcal infection. An abscess forms and tends to rupture, releasing a small amount of pus. A stye usually lasts 2 to 4 days. Styes sometimes form simultaneously with or as a result of blepharitis. A person may have one or two styes in a lifetime, but some people develop them repeatedly.

A stye usually begins with redness, tenderness, and pain at the edge of the eyelid. Then a small, round, tender, swollen area forms. The eye may water, become sensitive to bright light, and feel as though something is in it. Usually, only a small area of the eyelid is swollen, but sometimes the entire eyelid swells. Often a tiny, yellowish spot develops at the center of the swollen area.

Rarely, a stye forms in one of the deeper glands of the eyelid, a condition called an internal stye. The pain and other symptoms are usually more severe with an internal stye. Pain, redness, and swelling tend to occur in just a very small area, usually at the edge of the eyelid.

Although antibiotics are sometimes used to treat styes, they do not really help much. The

---

▲ see page 1145   ■ see box on page 1072
★ see page 1196

best treatment is to apply hot compresses for 10 minutes several times a day followed by a gentle eyelid massage. The warmth helps the stye come to a head, rupture, and drain. Because an internal stye rarely ruptures by itself, a doctor may have to open it to drain the pus. Internal styes tend to recur.

Chalazion

A chalazion is an enlargement of a deeper oil gland in the eyelid that results from an obstruction of the gland opening at the edge of the eyelid.

At first, a chalazion looks and feels like a stye: swollen eyelid, mild pain, and irritation. However, these symptoms disappear after a few days, leaving a round, painless swelling in the eyelid that grows slowly for the first week. Occasionally, the swelling continues to grow and may press on the eyeball and cause vision changes. A red or gray area may develop on the underside of the eyelid.

Most chalazions disappear without treatment after 1 to 3 months. If hot compresses are applied several times a day, chalazions may disappear sooner. If they remain after 2 weeks or longer or if they cause vision changes, a doctor can drain them or inject a corticosteroid.

Entropion and Ectropion

Entropion is a condition in which the eyelid is turned in against the eyeball. Ectropion is a condition in which the eyelid is turned outward and does not come in contact with the eyeball.

Normally, the upper and lower eyelids close tightly, protecting the eye from damage and preventing tear evaporation. If the edge of one eyelid turns in (entropion), the eyelashes rub against the eye, which can lead to ulcer formation and scarring of the cornea. If the edge of one eyelid turns outward (ectropion), the two eyelids cannot meet properly, and tears are not spread over the eyeball. These conditions are more common in older people (generally the result of tissue relaxation with aging) and in those who have had an eyelid injury that caused scar formation.

Both entropion and ectropion can irritate the eyes, causing watering and redness. Eye drops and ointments can be used to keep the eye moist and soothe the irritation. Occasionally, entropion can lead to corneal ulcer.▲ En-

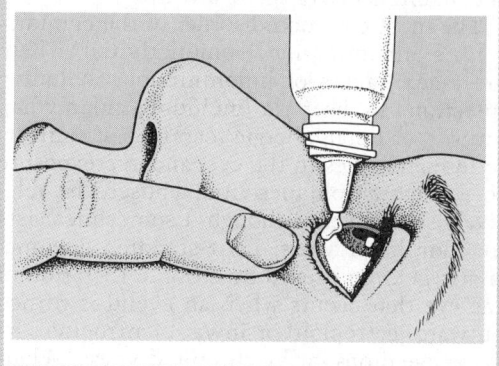

Using Eye Drops and Eye Ointments

The person receiving the drug should lean back and look up. With a clean forefinger, the lower eyelid is gently pulled down to create a pocket. Eye drops are then dropped into the pocket, not directly onto the eye. When using eye ointments, a small strip of ointment is placed in the pocket. Blinking distributes the drug over the eye.

tropion and ectropion can be treated by surgery—for instance, to preserve sight if damage to the eyes (such as corneal ulcer with entropion) is likely or has occurred, for comfort, or for cosmetic reasons.

Eyelid Tumors

Noncancerous (benign) and cancerous (malignant) growths can form on the eyelids. One of the most common types of benign tumor is xanthelasma, a yellow-white, flat growth that consists of fatty material. Xanthelasmas need not be removed unless their appearance becomes bothersome. Because xanthelasmas may indicate elevated cholesterol levels (especially in young people), a doctor checks the person's cholesterol level by taking a blood sample.

Squamous cell and basal cell carcinoma,■ both malignant growths, can develop on the eyelid. If a growth on the eyelid does not disappear after several weeks, a doctor may perform a biopsy (removal of a tissue sample for examination under a microscope). The growth is treated, usually with surgery.

▲ see page 1300   ■ see page 1238

CHAPTER 229

Disorders of the Conjunctiva and Sclera

The conjunctiva is the thin, transparent lining that covers the back of the eyelid and loops back to cover the sclera (the white of the eye), right up to the edge of the cornea.▲ The conjunctiva helps protect the eye by keeping small foreign objects and infection-causing microorganisms out and by contributing to the maintenance of the tear film.

The most common disorder of the conjunctiva is inflammation (conjunctivitis). There are many causes of inflammation, including infections by bacteria (including chlamydia), viruses, or fungi; allergic reactions; chemicals or foreign bodies in the eye; and overexposure to sunlight. Conjunctivitis tends to be relatively short-lived, although it sometimes lasts for months or years. Long-standing conjunctivitis is often caused by chronic irritation of the eye that occurs when an eyelid is turned outward (ectropion) or inward (entropion), by some eye drops, or by chronic dryness. Whatever the cause, people with conjunctivitis typically have similar symptoms, such as redness, itching or pain, discharge, and, sometimes, blurred vision.

The sclera is the tough, white, outer coat of the eyeball. The sclera provides the eyeball with structural strength and protects against penetration and rupture. Rarely, the sclera becomes inflamed (scleritis).

Infectious Conjunctivitis

Infectious conjunctivitis is inflammation of the conjunctiva caused by viruses, bacteria, or fungi.

A variety of microorganisms may infect the conjunctiva. The most common organisms are viral, particularly those from the group known as adenoviruses. Bacterial infections are less frequent. Both viral and bacterial conjunctivitis are quite contagious, easily passing from one person to another, or from a person's infected eye to his uninfected eye. Fungal infections are rare and occur mainly in people who use corticosteroid eye drops for a long time and in eye injuries involving vegetable matter. Newborns are particularly susceptible to eye

infections, which they acquire from organisms in the mother's birth canal (neonatal conjunctivitis■).

Inclusion conjunctivitis is a particularly long-lasting form of conjunctivitis caused by certain strains of the bacterium *Chlamydia trachomatis*. Inclusion conjunctivitis spreads by contact with genital secretions from a person who has a genital chlamydial infection. Another type of conjunctivitis is caused by *Neisseria gonorrhea* (gonorrhea), a sexually transmitted disease that also may spread to the eye.

Severe infections may scar the conjunctiva, causing abnormalities in the tear film. Sometimes, severe conjunctival infections spread to the cornea, the transparent part of the eye.

Symptoms and Diagnosis

When infected, the eye sometimes feels irritated, and bright light may cause discomfort. The conjunctiva becomes pink from dilated blood vessels, and a discharge appears in the eye. The discharge tends to be watery in viral conjunctivitis and thicker white or yellow in bacterial infection, but this distinction is not absolute. Often the discharge causes the person's eyes to stick shut, particularly overnight. This discharge may also cause the vision to blur; vision improves when the discharge is washed away. If the cornea is infected, vision also blurs but does not improve with washing. Very rarely, severe infections that have scarred the conjunctiva lead to long-term vision difficulties.

People with inclusion conjunctivitis or with conjunctivitis from gonorrhea often have symptoms of a genital infection, such as penile or vaginal discharge and burning during urination.

Doctors diagnose infectious conjunctivitis by its symptoms and appearance. The eye is closely examined with a slit lamp, an instrument that magnifies the surface of the eye. The slit lamp allows the doctor to see inflammation of the conjunctiva or infection of the cornea and front part of the eye (anterior chamber).

It is difficult to distinguish viral from bacterial conjunctivitis by appearance, although the presence of an upper respiratory infection increases the likelihood of a viral cause. Upper respiratory infections often accompany con-

▲ see also page 1276   ■ see table on page 1509

junctivitis caused by viruses, but they are rare in bacterial conjunctivitis. Samples of infected secretions may be sent to a laboratory to identify the infecting organism by a culture. However, doctors usually do this when the symptoms are severe or recurrent or when *Chlamydia* or *N. gonorrhea* is thought to be the cause.

Prognosis and Treatment

Most people with infectious conjunctivitis eventually get better on their own. However, some infections, particularly those caused by some bacteria, may last a long time if not treated. Inclusion conjunctivitis persists for months.

People with conjunctivitis should gently wash the eyelid with tap water and a clean washcloth to keep it clean and free of discharge. Cool compresses sometimes soothe the feeling of irritation. Because infective (bacterial or viral) conjunctivitis is highly contagious, a person should wash his hands before and after cleaning the eye or applying drugs. Also, a person should be careful not to touch the infected eye and then touch the other eye. Towels and washcloths used to clean the eye should be kept separate from other towels and washcloths. People with infectious conjunctivitis generally stay home from work or school for a few days, just as they would with a cold.

Antibiotics are helpful only in bacterial conjunctivitis. However, because it is difficult to distinguish between bacterial and viral infection, doctors often prescribe antibiotics for everyone with conjunctivitis. Antibiotic eye drops or ointments, such as sulfacetamide or trimethoprim-polymyxin, that are effective against many types of bacteria are used for 7 to 10 days. Eye drops must be applied every 2 to 3 hours, because the drug is washed away by tears. Ointments last longer and are applied every 6 hours but blur vision.

Inclusion conjunctivitis requires antibiotics, such as erythromycin, azithromycin, or doxycycline, which are taken by mouth. Gonococcal conjunctivitis may be treated with an injection of ceftriaxone. Corticosteroid eye drops may be needed in some people with severe adenoviral conjunctivitis, particularly in those in whom inflammation of the eye is interfering with important daily activities. In a person with viral conjunctivitis caused by herpes, antiviral drugs may be applied to the eyes (trifluridine or idoxuridine eye drops or vidarabine ointment) or given by

What Is Pinkeye?

Although most eye inflammations result in a pink discoloration of the eye (because of dilated blood vessels in the conjunctiva), doctors usually use the term pinkeye for conjunctivitis caused by infection with a bacteria or virus. One of the most severe forms of pinkeye is the result of infection with several particular strains of adenovirus. This infection, epidemic keratoconjunctivitis, is extremely contagious and often results in large outbreaks within a community or school. The infection is spread through contact with infected secretions. Such contact may take place person-to-person or through contaminated objects, including doctors' instruments.

The symptoms of this infection are similar to other types of viral conjunctivitis—redness, irritation, light sensitivity, and thin, watery discharge. Many people develop a swollen lymph node in front of the ear on the affected side. These symptoms typically last from 1 to 3 weeks. Some people have blurred vision, which may last for weeks or months before resolving.

Epidemic keratoconjunctivitis resolves completely without specific treatment. Doctors sometimes give corticosteroid drops to people with blurred vision or severe light sensitivity. Good hygiene, particularly hand washing, is needed to minimize the spread of the infection. People generally stay home from work or school for several days.

mouth (acyclovir). Antiviral drugs are not useful for infections caused by other viruses.

Trachoma

Trachoma (granular conjunctivitis, Egyptian ophthalmia) is a prolonged infection of the conjunctiva caused by the bacterium Chlamydia trachomatis.

Trachoma is the leading preventable cause of blindness in the world; it results from chronic or repeated infections with certain nonsexually transmitted strains of *C. trachomatis*. Trachoma is common in poverty-stricken parts of dry, hot countries in North Africa, the Middle East, the Indian Subcontinent, and Southeast Asia. In the United States, trachoma is rare, occurring occasionally among Native Americans and among immigrants from areas where trachoma is common. The disease occurs mainly in children, particularly those between the ages of 3 and 6. Older children and adults are much less likely to have the disease because of increased immunity and better personal hygiene. Trachoma is contagious in its early stages and may be transmitted by eye-hand contact, by certain flies, or by sharing contaminated articles, such as towels, handkerchiefs, and eye makeup.

Symptoms

Trachoma usually affects both eyes. The conjunctivae become inflamed, red, and irritated, and the eyes water excessively. Sensitivity to bright light occurs.

In the later stages, blood vessels gradually grow across the cornea (neovascularization), obstructing vision. In some people, the eyelid is scarred in such a way that the eyelashes turn inward (trichiasis). As the person blinks, the eyelashes rub against the cornea, causing infection and permanent damage; impaired vision or blindness occurs in about 5% of people with trachoma.

Diagnosis and Treatment

Doctors suspect trachoma because of the appearance of the eyes and the duration of symptoms. The diagnosis can be confirmed by sending a sample from the eye to a laboratory, where the infecting organism is identified.

Treatment consists of the antibiotic erythromycin or a tetracycline, which is taken by mouth for 3 to 5 weeks. The newer antibiotic, azithromycin, can be used once per week for 1 to 3 weeks. Tetracycline or erythromycin eye ointments are effective, but they must be applied for 4 to 6 weeks. If the condition damages the eyelid, conjunctiva, or cornea, surgery may be needed.

Because the disease is contagious, reinfection commonly occurs. Regular hand and face washing helps prevent the spread of infection. Doctors often give antibiotics to entire neighborhoods where there are many people with trachoma.

Allergic Conjunctivitis

Allergic conjunctivitis is inflammation of the conjunctiva caused by an allergic reaction.

The conjunctiva contains a large number of cells from the immune system (mast cells) that release chemical substances (mediators) in response to a variety of stimuli (such as pollens or dust mites). These mediators produce inflammation in the eyes, which may be brief or long-lasting. About 20% of people have some degree of allergic conjunctivitis.

Seasonal allergic conjunctivitis and **perennial allergic conjunctivitis** are the most common types of allergic reaction in the eyes. Seasonal allergic conjunctivitis is often caused by trees or grass pollens, leading to its typical appearance in the spring and early summer. Weed pollens are responsible for symptoms of allergic conjunctivitis in the summer and early fall. Perennial allergic conjunctivitis occurs year-round; it is most often caused by dust mites, animal dander, and feathers.

Vernal conjunctivitis is a more serious form of allergic conjunctivitis in which the stimulant is not known. The condition is most common in boys, particularly those younger than 10 who also have eczema, asthma, or seasonal allergies. Vernal conjunctivitis typically reappears each spring and subsides in the fall and winter. Many children outgrow the condition by early adulthood.

Symptoms

People with all forms of allergic conjunctivitis develop intense itching and burning in both eyes. Although usually equal, occasionally, one eye may be more affected than the other. The conjunctiva becomes red, and sometimes the conjunctiva swells, giving the surface of the eyeball a puffy appearance that many people find disturbing. With seasonal and perennial conjunctivitis, there is a large amount of thin, watery discharge. Vision is seldom affected.

With vernal conjunctivitis, the eye discharge is thick and mucuslike. Unlike other types of allergic conjunctivitis, vernal conjunctivitis often affects the cornea, and painful ulcers develop. These ulcers cause extreme sensitivity to bright light and sometimes lead to a permanent decrease in vision.

Diagnosis and Treatment

Doctors recognize allergic conjunctivitis by its typical appearance and symptoms. The condition is treated with allergy eye drops. Such drugs include cromolyn, lodoxamide, olopatadine, and antihistamine eye drops, such as emedastine and levocabastine. Ketorolac eye drops have anti-inflammatory properties and help relieve symptoms. Corticosteroid eye drops have more potent anti-inflammatory effects; however, they should not be used for more than a few weeks without close monitoring because they may produce increased pressure in the eyes (glaucoma), cataracts, and an increased risk of eye infections. Recently, eye drops that block both the release and the effects of the inflammatory mediators, such as azelastine, nedocromil, and pemirolast, have been used successfully.

Episcleritis

Episcleritis is inflammation of the tissue lying between the sclera and the conjunctiva.

Episcleritis occurs in young adults and affects women more often than men. Usually, the inflammation affects only a small patch of the eyeball and causes a red, and sometimes slightly yellow, raised area. Symptoms include eye tenderness and irritation, with increased watering of the eye and mildly increased sensitivity to bright light. The condition is not usually a sign of any other disease and tends to disappear and recur. The diagnosis is based on the symptoms and on the appearance of the eye.

Treatment is often unnecessary. Eye drops that constrict blood vessels in the eye, such as tetrahydrozoline, can improve the appearance of the eyes. To shorten an attack, corticosteroid eye drops or an oral nonsteroidal antiinflammatory drug (NSAID) can be used.

Scleritis

Scleritis is a deep, extremely painful inflammation and purple discoloration of the sclera that may severely damage vision.

Scleritis is most common among people in their 30s through 50s and affects women more often than men. In one third of cases, it affects both eyes. Scleritis may accompany rheumatoid arthritis, systemic lupus erythematosus, or another autoimmune disorder. About half of the cases of scleritis have no known cause.

Symptoms include pain in the eye (typically a deep, boring ache) that often interferes with sleep and reduces appetite. Other symptoms include eye tenderness, increased watering of the eye, and sensitivity to bright light. In some people, inflammation is severe enough to cause perforation of the eyeball and loss of the eye.

Doctors diagnose scleritis by its symptoms and appearance on slit lamp examination. Sometimes signs of scleritis can be seen on an ultrasound or computed tomography (CT) scan.

Doctors treat scleritis with nonsteroidal antiinflammatory drugs (NSAIDs) or a corticosteroid, such as prednisone, which is given by mouth. Eye drops and ointments rarely help scleritis. If the person has rheumatoid arthritis or does not respond to corticosteroids, drugs that suppress the immune system, such as cyclophosphamide or azathioprine, may be needed.

Noncancerous Growths

Two kinds of noncancerous (benign) growths can develop on the conjunctiva— pinguecula and pterygium. They both are more common in older people and probably occur as a result of long-term ultraviolet light exposure. Doctors easily recognize these growths by their typical appearance. A **pinguecula** is a raised yellowish white growth next to, but not overlapping, the cornea. This growth is unsightly, but it generally does not cause any serious problem and need not be removed. A **pterygium** is a similar fleshy growth of the conjunctiva next to the cornea that spreads across the cornea. Most pterygia do not produce symptoms, but sometimes they cause irritation or distort the shape of the cornea, possibly causing a change in vision. Sometimes removal is appropriate to reduce irritation and to prevent changes in vision.

CHAPTER 230

Corneal Disorders

The cornea is the domed covering in the front of the eye that protects the iris and lens and helps focus light on the retina. It is composed of cells, protein, and fluid. The cornea is normally as stiff as a fingernail, transparent, and very sensitive to touch. Corneal disease or damage can cause pain and loss of vision.

Superficial Punctate Keratitis

Superficial punctate keratitis is death of cells on the surface of the cornea.

The cause of this disorder may be a viral infection, a bacterial infection (including trachoma▲), dry eyes, strong chemicals splashed in the eye, exposure to ultraviolet light (sunlight, sunlamps, or welding arcs), irritation from prolonged use of contact lenses, or irritation from or an allergy to eye drops. The disorder can also be a side effect of certain drugs taken by mouth or intravenously.

In superficial punctate keratitis, the eyes are generally painful, watery, sensitive to bright light, and bloodshot, and vision may be slightly blurred. Often there will be a burning, gritty feeling or a feeling as if a foreign object is trapped in the eye. When ultraviolet light causes the disorder, symptoms usually do not occur until several hours after exposure; they last for 1 to 2 days. When a virus causes the disorder, a lymph node in front of the ear on the affected side may be swollen and tender.

The diagnosis is based on the symptoms, on whether the person has been exposed to any of the known causes, and on an examination of the cornea with a slit lamp.■

Almost everyone who has this disorder recovers completely. When the cause is a virus, (other than herpes simplex or herpes zoster [shingles]), no treatment is needed, and recovery usually occurs within 3 weeks. When the cause is a bacterial infection or contact lens irritation, antibiotics are used. When the cause is dry eyes, ointments and artificial tears (eye drops prepared with substances that simulate real tears) are effective. When the cause is exposure to ultraviolet light, an antibiotic ointment, an eye drop that dilates the pupil,★ and an eye patch may provide relief. And when the cause is a drug reaction or irritation from allergy to eye drops, the drug or eye drops must be discontinued.

Corneal Ulcer

A corneal ulcer is an open sore on the cornea.

Corneal ulcers may begin with a corneal injury, which then becomes infected with bacteria, fungi, or the protozoan *Acanthamoeba* (which lives in contaminated water). Viral ulcers (often due to a herpes virus) can be triggered to recur by physical stress or may recur spontaneously. Ulcers can also occur if a foreign object lodges in the eye or the eye is irritated by a contact lens, especially when contact lenses are worn during sleep or are not

adequately disinfected. A deficiency of vitamin A and protein may lead to the formation of a corneal ulcer; however, such ulcers are rare in the United States.

When the eyelids do not close properly, the cornea may become dry and irritated; such irritation can lead to injury and the development of a corneal ulcer. These ulcers usually become infected. Corneal injury may result from in-growing eyelashes (trichiasis) or an inturned eyelid (entropion).

Symptoms

Corneal ulcers cause pain, usually a feeling like a foreign object is in the eye, with aching and sensitivity to bright light and increased tear production. A white spot of pus may appear in the cornea. Sometimes, ulcers develop over the entire cornea and may penetrate deeply. Additional pus may accumulate behind the cornea. The deeper the ulcer, the more severe the symptoms and complications. The conjunctiva usually is bloodshot.

Corneal ulcers may heal with treatment, but they may leave a cloudy scar that impairs vision. Other complications may include deep-seated infection, perforation of the cornea, displacement of the iris, and destruction of the eye.

Diagnosis and Treatment

A corneal ulcer is an emergency that should be treated immediately. To see an ulcer clearly, a doctor may apply eye drops that contain a dye called fluorescein, which temporarily stains the ulcer and allows it to be examined more clearly. Treatment depends on the underlying cause. For instance, antibiotic, antiviral, or antifungal drugs may be needed. Corneal transplantation (keratoplasty) is sometimes needed also.●

Keratoconjunctivitis Sicca

Keratoconjunctivitis sicca (dry eye) is dryness of the conjunctiva and cornea.

Dry eyes may be due to inadequate tear production (aqueous tear deficient dry eyes). With this type of dry eyes, the tear gland (lacrimal gland) does not produce enough tears to keep the entire conjunctiva and cornea covered by a complete layer of tears. This is the most common type found in postmenopausal women.

Dry eyes may also be due to an abnormality of tear composition that results in rapid evaporation of the tears (evaporative dry eyes). Al-

---

▲ see page 1297   ■ see art on page 1285

★ see art on page 1295   ● see box on page 1082

though the tear gland produces a sufficient amount of tears, the rate of evaporation is so rapid that the entire conjunctiva and cornea cannot be kept covered with a complete layer of tears during certain activities or in certain environments.

Rarely, aqueous tear deficient dry eyes may be a symptom of diseases such as rheumatoid arthritis, systemic lupus erythematosus, or Sjögren's syndrome.

Symptoms

Symptoms of dry eyes include irritation, burning, itching, a pulling sensation, pressure behind the eye, and a feeling like something is in the eye. Damage to the surface of the eye increases discomfort and sensitivity to bright light. Symptoms are worsened by activities in which the rate of blinking is reduced, specifically those that involve prolonged use of the eyes, such as reading, working on a computer, driving, or watching television. Symptoms are also worse in dusty or smoky areas and dry environments, such as in airplanes or in shopping malls; on days with low humidity; and in areas where air conditioners (especially in the car), fans, or heaters are being used. Certain drugs can worsen symptoms, including isotretinoin, tranquilizers, diuretics, antihypertensives, oral contraceptives, and antihistamines. Symptoms improve during cool, rainy, or foggy weather and in humid places, such as in the shower.

Even with the most severe dry eyes, it is rare that vision is lost; however, people sometimes feel that their vision blurs with use, or the irritation is so severe that it is difficult to use the eyes. In some people with severe dryness, the surface of the cornea can thicken or ulcers and scars can develop. Occasionally blood vessels can grow across the cornea. Scarring and blood vessel growth can impair vision.

Diagnosis and Treatment

Although a doctor can usually diagnose dry eyes by the symptoms alone, a Schirmer test—in which a strip of filter paper is placed at the edge of the eyelid—can measure the amount of moisture bathing the eye. Doctors examine the eyes with a slit lamp▲ to determine if the eye has been damaged.

Artificial tears (eye drops prepared with substances that simulate real tears) applied every few hours can generally control the problem. Avoiding dry, drafty environments and using

humidifiers can help also. Minor surgery can be done to block the flow of tears into the nose, so that more tears are available to bathe the eyes. In people with very dry eyes, the eyelids may be partially sewn together to decrease tear evaporation.

Keratomalacia

Keratomalacia (xerophthalmia, xerotic keratitis) is drying and clouding of the cornea due to vitamin A deficiency and insufficient protein and calories in the diet.

The surface of the conjunctiva and cornea dries, then corneal ulcers and bacterial infections may occur. The tear glands are also affected, resulting in an inadequate tear film and dry eyes. Night blindness (poor vision in the dark) may develop because of vitamin A deficiency. The diagnosis is based on the presence of a dry or ulcerated cornea in a malnourished person.

Antibiotic eye drops or ointments can help cure an infection, but correcting the vitamin A deficiency and malnutrition with an improved diet or supplements is also important.

Herpes Simplex Keratitis

Herpes simplex keratitis is infection of the cornea caused by herpes simplex virus.

When herpes simplex keratitis (herpes simplex keratoconjunctivitis)■ begins, the symptoms may resemble a mild bacterial infection: the eyes are slightly painful, watery, red, and sensitive to bright light. Rarely, the infection worsens and the cornea swells, making vision hazy.

Most often, the initial infection produces only mild changes in the cornea and goes away without treatment. However, sometimes the infection returns and symptoms worsen. If the infection recurs, further damage to the surface of the cornea may result. Several recurrences may result in the formation of deep ulcers, permanent scarring, and a loss of feeling when the eye is touched. The herpes simplex virus can also cause blood vessels to grow onto the cornea and, occasionally, can lead to significant visual impairment. To diagnose a herpes simplex infection, a doctor examines the eye with a slit lamp.★ Sometimes, the doctor may

---

▲ see art on page 1285   ■ see also page 1160
★ see art on page 1285

take a sample from the infected area to identify the virus (viral culture).

The doctor may prescribe an antiviral drug, such as trifluridine eye drops or vidarabine ointment. Acyclovir, an antiviral drug, can be taken by mouth. Treatment should be started as soon as possible. Occasionally, to help speed healing, after numbing the eye, an ophthalmologist may have to gently swab the cornea with a soft cotton-tipped applicator to remove infected and damaged cells.

Herpes Zoster Ophthalmicus

Herpes zoster ophthalmicus is infection of the eye caused by varicella-zoster virus.

Herpes zoster is a virus that grows in nerves and may spread to the skin, causing shingles.▲ If the forehead or nose becomes infected, the eye is also likely to become infected, on the same side as the skin involvement.

Infection of the eye produces pain, redness, and eyelid swelling. An infected cornea can become swollen, severely damaged, and scarred. The structures behind the cornea can become inflamed (uveitis), the pressure in the eye can increase (glaucoma), and the cornea can become numb, which can lead to injuries. The appearance of active shingles, a history of the typical rash, or old scars from a shingles rash help a doctor make the diagnosis.

When herpes zoster infects the face and threatens the eye, early treatment with acyclovir, valacyclovir or famciclovir, which are taken by mouth, reduces the risk of eye complications. Corticosteroids, usually in eye drops, may also help. Eye drops, such as atropine, are used to keep the pupil dilated, to help prevent a severe form of glaucoma, and to relieve pain.

Peripheral Ulcerative Keratitis

Peripheral ulcerative keratitis is inflammation and ulceration of the cornea that often occurs in people who have connective tissue diseases such as rheumatoid arthritis.

Peripheral ulcerative keratitis is probably caused by an autoimmune reaction.■ Blurred vision, increased sensitivity to bright light,

and a sensation of a foreign object trapped in the eye develop. The ulcer is located in the periphery of the cornea and is usually oval in shape.

Of the people who have rheumatoid arthritis and peripheral ulcerative keratitis, about 40% die (mostly due to a heart attack) within 10 years of developing peripheral ulcerative keratitis unless they are treated. Treatment with drugs that suppress the immune system, such as cyclophosphamide, reduces the death rate to about 8% in 10 years.

Keratoconus

Keratoconus is a gradual change in the shape of the cornea that causes it to become cone shaped.

The condition usually begins between the ages of 15 and 25. Both eyes are usually affected, producing major changes in vision and requiring frequent changes in the prescription for eyeglasses or contact lenses. Contact lenses often correct the vision problems better than eyeglasses, but sometimes the change in corneal shape is so severe that contact lenses either cannot be worn or cannot correct vision. In severe cases, corneal transplantation★ may be needed.

Bullous Keratopathy

Bullous keratopathy is a swelling of the cornea.

Bullous keratopathy is most common in older people. Occasionally, bullous keratopathy occurs after eye surgery, such as cataract removal. The swelling leads to the formation of fluid-filled blisters on the surface of the cornea. The blisters can rupture, causing pain, often with the sensation of a foreign object trapped in the eye, and impairing vision. The diagnosis is based on the typical appearance of a swollen, cloudy cornea with blisters on the surface. Pachymetry (an ultrasound measurement of the cornea's thickness) is useful to confirm the diagnosis.

Bullous keratopathy is treated by reducing the amount of fluid in the cornea. Salty eye drops can be used to draw the fluid out. Occasionally, soft contact lenses can be used to decrease discomfort. If vision is insufficient for daily activities or discomfort is significant, corneal transplantation● is needed.

▲ see page 1162   ■ see page 1073

★ see box on page 1082   ● see box on page 1082

CHAPTER 231

Cataract

A cataract is a clouding (opacity) of the lens of the eye that causes a progressive, painless loss of vision.

Cataracts are the leading cause of blindness worldwide. Cataracts are common in the United States, where they affect mostly older adults. Almost one in five people between the ages of 65 and 74 develop cataracts severe enough to reduce vision, and almost one in two people older than 75 have them. Fortunately, people in the United States can often get their cataracts treated before they cause blindness.

Cataracts usually develop without any apparent cause; however, they can result from injury to the eye, prolonged exposure to certain drugs (such as corticosteroids) or to x-rays (such as with radiation therapy to the eye), inflammatory and infectious eye diseases, and as a complication of diseases such as diabetes. Cataracts also seem to be more common in people with dark eyes, those who have had prolonged exposure to direct sunlight, those with poor nutrition, and smokers. People who have had a cataract in one eye are more likely to develop one later in the other eye. Sometimes cataracts can develop in both eyes at the same time. Babies can be born with them (congenital cataracts▲), and children can also develop cataracts, usually as a result of injury or illness.

Symptoms and Diagnosis

Because all light entering the eye passes through the lens, any clouding of the lens that blocks, distorts, or diffuses light can cause poor vision. The first symptom of a cataract is usually blurred vision. Glare and halos and, less commonly, double vision can also be early symptoms of cataracts. A person may also notice that colors seem more yellow and less vibrant. Reading may become more difficult because of a worsening ability to distinguish between the light and dark of printed letters on a page.

How much vision is changed by a cataract depends on the intensity of light entering the eye and on the location of the cataract. In bright light, the pupil constricts and narrows the pathway through which light enters the eye, and light cannot easily pass around a cataract that is centrally located (nuclear cataract). In dim light, the pupil dilates; bright lights, such as oncoming headlights, are scattered by the edge of the cataract, causing halos and glare, which may be especially disturbing during night driving. People with cataracts who take drugs that constrict their pupils (certain glaucoma eye drops, for example) may also have greater vision loss.

In normal light, however, a nuclear cataract may at first improve vision without eyeglasses for farsighted people. The cataract acts as a stronger lens, thus refocusing light, improving vision for objects close to the eye (near vision). Older people, who generally have trouble seeing things that are close without eyeglasses, may discover that they can read again without eyeglasses, a phenomenon often described as gaining second sight. Unfortunately, a nuclear cataract eventually blocks and blurs light entering the eye and impairs vision.

A cataract at the back of the lens (posterior subcapsular cataract) affects vision more than a cataract in another location because the clouding is at the point where light rays are focused in a narrow beam. This type of cataract impairs vision more in bright light and is more likely to cause glare and halos.

Although cataracts almost never cause pain, rarely they can swell and increase the pressure in the eye (glaucoma), which can be painful.

A doctor can usually detect a cataract while examining the eye with an ophthalmoscope (a handheld instrument used to view the inside of the eye). Using an instrument called a slit lamp that allows examination of the eye in more detail, a doctor can identify the exact location of the cataract and the extent to which it blocks light.

Prevention

There are several things people can do to try to prevent cataracts. Consistent use of sunglasses with a coating to filter ultraviolet (UV) light will protect the eyes from bright sunlight and may help. Not smoking is useful and has other health advantages. People with diabetes should work with their doctor to be sure the

---

▲ see table on page 1512

How Cataracts Affect Vision

On the left, a normal lens receives light and focuses it on the retina. On the right, a cataract blocks some light from reaching the lens and distorts the light being focused on the retina.

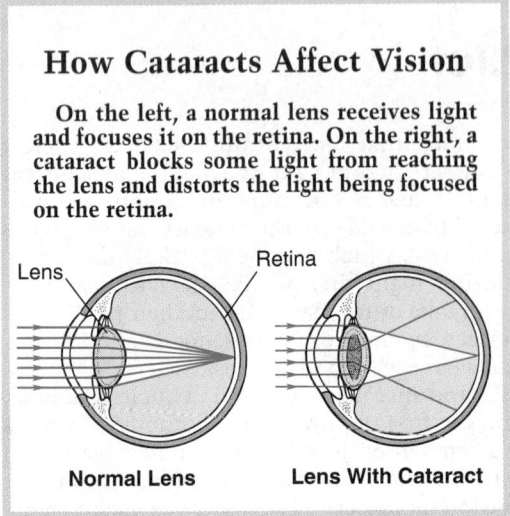

Normal Lens   Lens With Cataract

level of sugar in their blood is well controlled. A diet high in vitamin C, vitamin A, and substances known as carotenoids (contained in vegetables such as spinach and kale) may protect against cataracts. Estrogen use by women after menopause may also be protective, but estrogen should not be used solely for this purpose. Finally, people who are taking corticosteroids for extended periods might discuss with their doctor the possibility of using a different drug.

Treatment

Until vision is significantly impaired, eyeglasses and contact lenses may improve a person's vision. Wearing sunglasses in bright light and using lamps that provide over-the-shoulder lighting may decrease glare and aid vision. Rarely, drugs that keep the pupil dilated may be used to help vision if the cataract is located in the center of the lens.

The only treatment that provides a cure for cataracts is surgery; there are no eye drops or drugs that will make cataracts go away. Occasionally, cataracts will cause changes (such as swelling of the cataract or glaucoma) that lead doctors to recommend the cataract be removed quickly. However, most times people should have surgery only when their vision is so impaired by cataracts that they feel unsafe, uncomfortable, or unable to perform daily tasks. There is no advantage to having cataracts removed before then.

Cataract surgery can be performed on a person of any age and is generally safe even for people with illnesses such as heart disease and diabetes. Usually, the doctor makes a small incision in the eye and removes the cataract by breaking it up with ultrasound and taking out the pieces (phacoemulsification). When all the cataract pieces have been removed, the surgeon replaces the cataract with an artificial lens (intraocular lens). The intraocular lens cannot always be safely placed, however; when this is the case, people must wear thick eyeglasses or contact lenses after the cataract has been removed.

Surgery to remove cataracts is almost always performed under local anesthesia, in which the eye surface is numbed with an injection or eye drops. Rarely, children or adults who cannot hold still during surgery require general anesthesia. The procedure normally takes about 30 minutes, and the person can go home the same day. No sutures are usually needed, because the incision into the eye is small and can seal itself.

People should make arrangements in advance to get extra help at home for a few days after surgery because activity may be restricted (for example, bending over and heavy lifting may be prohibited) and vision changes, such as blurred vision and discomfort with bright light, may occur for a short time after surgery. For a few weeks after surgery, eye drops or ointments are used to prevent infection, reduce inflammation, and promote healing. A person is given eyeglasses or a metal shield to wear to protect the eye from injury until healing is complete, usually a few weeks. The person visits the doctor the day after surgery and then typically one week and one month later. If a person has cataracts in both eyes, many doctors wait several months after the first eye has healed to remove a cataract from the other eye.

Many people notice improved distance vision within a few weeks after cataract surgery. Almost everyone will need eyeglasses for reading, and some people will need eyeglasses to obtain the best possible distance vision as well. The doctor makes calculations before the surgery to decide how powerful the artificial lens should be. Thus, it is possible to go from wearing very thick eyeglasses before the surgery to wearing much thinner eyeglasses after it.

Complications after cataract surgery are rare. A person may develop an infection or serious bleeding in the eye, which can lead to a loss of vision. Eye pressure may become too high, which if left untreated, leads to glaucoma, or the implant can become displaced. The back of the eye (retina) can become swollen or detached.▲ Rarely, people with retinal disorders, such as diabetic retinopathy, may notice their vision worsen after the operation. Proper follow-up with the doctor can lead to early detection and treatment of these unusual complications.

Sometimes people develop a haziness of the tissue (capsule) left behind in the eye when the original lens was removed (secondary cataract). This occurs in about one in four people who have had cataract surgery, months or even years after an artificial lens is implanted. Typically, it is treated by using a laser to make a small opening in the hazy capsule to let light through.

CHAPTER 232

Uveitis

Uveitis is inflammation anywhere in the uvea.

The pigmented inside lining of the eye, called the uvea or the uveal tract, consists of three structures: the iris, the ciliary body, and the choroid. The iris, the colored ring around the black pupil, opens and closes like the aperture of a camera lens to let light into the eye. The ciliary body is the set of muscles that, by contracting, allows the lens to become thicker so the eye can focus on nearby objects and, by relaxing, allows the lens to become thinner so the eye can focus on distant objects. The choroid, the inner lining of the eyeball, extends from the edge of the ciliary muscles to the optic nerve at the back of the eye. The choroid lies between the retina on the inside and the sclera on the outside. The choroid contains layers of blood vessels that nourish the inside parts of the eye, particularly the retina.

Part or all of the uvea may become inflamed. Inflammation limited to part of the uvea is named, according to its location, as anterior uveitis, intermediate uveitis, or posterior uveitis. Inflammation that affects the entire uvea is called diffuse uveitis or panuveitis. Sometimes, uveitis is referred to by the name of the specific part that is inflamed—for example, iritis (inflammation of the iris), choroiditis (inflammation of the choroid), or chorioretinitis (inflammation that involves both the choroid and the overlying retina). Inflammation of the uvea is limited to one eye in many people with uveitis but may involve both eyes.

The inflammation has many possible causes—some that are limited to the eye itself and others that affect the entire body. In most people, no cause is identified, and they are said to have idiopathic uveitis. About 40% of people with uveitis have a disease that also affects organs elsewhere in the body. These include inflammatory diseases such as ankylosing spondylitis and juvenile rheumatoid arthritis, sarcoidosis, and widespread infections.

Symptoms

The early symptoms of uveitis may be mild or severe, depending on which part of the uvea is affected and the amount of inflammation. Anterior uveitis has the most dramatic symptoms. Severe pain in the eye, redness of the conjunctiva, sensitivity to bright light, and a decrease in vision are typical. A doctor may be able to see a small pupil with prominent blood vessels on the conjunctiva near the edge of the iris, white blood cells floating in the fluid that fills the front part of the eye (aqueous humor), and deposits of white blood cells (keratic precipitates) on the inside surface of the cornea. Intermediate uveitis is typically painless. Vision may be decreased, and the person may see irregular floating black spots (floaters). Posterior uveitis typically produces decreased vision. Floaters are also common. There may also be retinal detachment (early symptoms may include blurred vision) and inflammation of the optic nerve (symptoms include loss of vision, which may vary from a small blind spot to total blindness).■ Diffuse uveitis may produce any or all of these symptoms.

Uveitis can rapidly damage the eye; it can produce long-term, vision-threatening complications, such as swelling of the macula, glaucoma, and cataracts. Many people have only

---

▲ see page 1311   ■ see page 1315

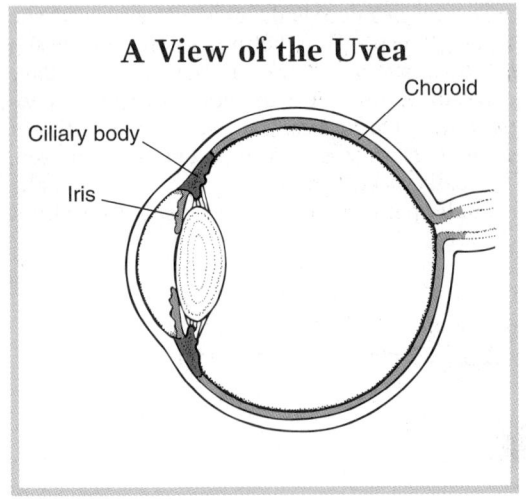

A View of the Uvea

Choroid

Ciliary body

Iris

one episode of uveitis. Others have periodic recurrences over months to years.

Diagnosis and Treatment

A doctor makes the diagnosis based on the symptoms and the findings from a physical examination. If the doctor suspects a disease that also affects other organs, appropriate tests are carried out.

Treatment must start early to prevent permanent damage. Treatment almost always includes using corticosteroids, usually given as eye drops. Drugs to dilate the pupils, such as scopolamine, cyclopentolate, or atropine eye drops, are also used. Other drugs may be used to treat specific causes of uveitis; for example, if infection is the cause, drugs may be given to eliminate bacteria or parasites.

CHAPTER 233

Glaucoma

Glaucoma is optic nerve damage, often associated with increased eye pressure, that leads to progressive, irreversible loss of vision.

Almost 3 million people in the United States and 14 million people worldwide have glaucoma. People older than age 40; African-Americans; people whose family members have (or had) the disease; and people who are farsighted or nearsighted, have diabetes, have used corticosteroid drugs for a long time, or who have previously injured their eye are at highest risk. Glaucoma is the third leading cause of blindness worldwide.

Glaucoma occurs when an imbalance in production and drainage of fluid in the eye (aqueous humor) increases eye pressure to unhealthy levels. Normally the aqueous fluid, which nourishes the eye, is produced by the ciliary body behind the iris (in the posterior chamber) and flows to the front of the eye (anterior chamber), where it drains into drainage canals between the iris and cornea (the "angle"). When functioning properly, the system works like a faucet (ciliary body) and sink (drainage canals). Balance between fluid production and drainage—between an open faucet and a properly draining sink—keeps the

fluid flowing freely and prevents pressure in the eye from building up.

In glaucoma, the canals through which the fluid drains become clogged, blocked, or covered. Fluid cannot leave the eye even though new fluid is being produced in the posterior chamber. In other words, the sink "backs up" while the faucet is still running. Because there is nowhere in the eye for the fluid to go, pressure in the eye increases. When the pressure becomes higher than the optic nerve can tolerate, glaucoma results. Sometimes eye pressure increases within the range of normal but is nonetheless too high for the optic nerve to tolerate.

Most glaucoma falls into two categories: open-angle or closed-angle glaucoma.

Open-angle glaucoma is most common. In open-angle glaucoma, the drainage canals in the eyes become clogged gradually over months or years. Pressure in the eye rises slowly because fluid is produced at a normal rate but drains sluggishly.

Closed-angle glaucoma is far less common than open-angle glaucoma. In closed-angle glaucoma, the drainage canals in the eyes suddenly become blocked or covered. Pressure in the eye rises rapidly, because fluid drainage is abruptly blocked while production continues.

In most people, the underlying cause of glaucoma is not known, although both open-angle and closed-angle glaucoma tend to run in families. In others, damage to the eye caused by infection, inflammation, tumor, large cataracts or surgery for cataracts, or other conditions keeps the fluid from draining freely and leads to increased eye pressure and optic nerve damage (secondary glaucoma).

Symptoms

Open-Angle Glaucoma: Open-angle glaucoma is painless and causes no early symptoms. The most important symptom of open-angle glaucoma is the development of blind spots, or patches of vision loss, over months to years. The blind spots slowly grow larger and coalesce. Peripheral (side) vision is usually lost first; vision loss occurs so gradually that it is often not noticed until much of it is lost. Because central vision is generally lost last, many people develop tunnel vision; they see straight ahead perfectly but become blind in all other directions. If glaucoma is left untreated, eventually even tunnel vision is lost, and a person becomes totally blind.

Closed-Angle Glaucoma: Eye pressure rises rapidly in closed-angle glaucoma, so people with this form of the disease typically notice an abrupt onset of severe eye pain and headache, redness, blurred vision, rainbow-colored halos around lights, and sudden loss of vision. They may also have nausea and vomiting as a response to the increase in eye pressure.

Closed-angle glaucoma is considered a medical emergency, because people can lose their vision as quickly as 2 to 3 hours after the appearance of symptoms if the condition is not treated.

People who have had open-angle or closed-angle glaucoma in one eye are likely to develop it in the other.

Screening and Diagnosis

Because the most common types of glaucoma can cause slow and silent loss of vision over years, early detection of the disease is extremely important. All people at high risk for glaucoma—people older than 40; African-Americans; relatives of people with glaucoma; and people who are very nearsighted or farsighted, have diabetes, have used corticosteroid drugs for a long time, or have had a previous eye injury—should have a comprehensive eye examination every 1 to 2 years.

There are four parts to a comprehensive eye examination for glaucoma. First, pressure in

Normal Fluid Drainage

Fluid is produced in the ciliary body behind the iris (posterior chamber), passes into the front of the eye (anterior chamber), and then drains through the drainage canals.

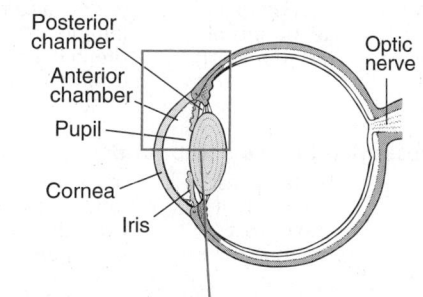

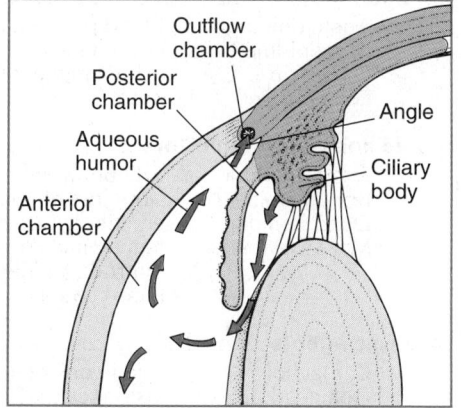

the eye is measured. This is done painlessly with an instrument called a tonometer.▲ In general, eye pressure readings of greater than 20 to 22 millimeters of mercury (mm Hg) are considered higher than normal.

But measuring eye pressure is not enough, because a third or more of people with glaucoma have normal eye pressure. So doctors also use an ophthalmoscope and a slit lamp to look for changes in the optic nerve that indicate damage from glaucoma.■

In addition, visual field (peripheral or side vision) testing allows a doctor to detect blind spots. Most often, visual field testing is done with a machine that determines the person's

▲ see page 1284

■ see art on pages 1284 and 1285

℞   DRUGS USED TO TREAT GLAUCOMA

TYPE	DRUG	SELECTED SIDE EFFECTS	COMMENTS
Beta blockers	Betaxolol Carteolol Levobetaxalol Levobunolol Metipranolol Timolol	Shortness of breath, slow heart beat, lightheadedness, cold fingers and toes, insomnia, fatigue, depression, vivid dreams, hallucinations, sexual dysfunction; hair loss; see also table on page 138	**How they work:** Decrease aqueous humor production **Given as:** Eye drops **Other comments:** Some side effects are worse in people with heart, lung, and blood vessel disease
Prostaglandin-like compounds	Bimatoprost Latanoprost Travoprost Unoprostone	Increased eye and skin pigmentation; elongated and thickened eyelashes; muscle, joint, and back pain; skin rash	**How they work:** Increase aqueous humor outflow **Given as:** Eye drops
Alpha-agonists	Apraclonidine Brimonidine Dipivefrin Epinephrine	Blood pressure changes, abnormal heart rhythm, headache, fatigue, dry mouth, dry nose	**How they work:** Decrease aqueous humor production and increase aqueous humor outflow **Given as:** Eye drops
Carbonic anhydrase inhibitors	Acetazolamide Brinzolamide Dorzolamide Methazolamide	Fatigue, weight loss, depression, loss of appetite, nausea, erectile dysfunction (impotence), metallic or bitter taste, diarrhea, kidney stones, low blood counts	**How they work:** Decrease aqueous humor production **Given as:** Brinzolamide and dorzolamide are given as eye drops; acetazolamide and methazolamide are given by mouth
Cholinergic agents	Carbachol Demecarium Echothiophate Physostigmine Pilocarpine	Pupil constriction, blurred vision, cataract formation, sweating, headache, tremor, excess saliva production, diarrhea, abdominal cramps, nausea	**How they work:** Increase aqueous humor outflow and may widen "angle" of eye **Given as:** Eye drops; physostigmine given as ointment **Other comments:** Demecarium, echothiophate, and physostigmine are more potent and are more likely to cause cataracts and systemic side effects than are carbachol and pilocarpine

ability to see small dots of light in all areas of the visual field.▲

Finally, doctors may also use a special lens to examine the drainage channels in the eye, a procedure known as gonioscopy. The gonioscope allows the doctor to determine if the glaucoma is of the open-angle or closed-angle type.

▲ see page 1283

Treatment

Once a person loses vision because of glaucoma, the loss cannot be reversed. But if glaucoma is detected, proper treatment can prevent further vision loss. So the goal of glaucoma treatment is to prevent the onset of vision loss or stop its progression.

Treatment of glaucoma is lifelong. It involves decreasing eye pressure by reducing the amount of fluid produced by the eye or by increasing fluid drainage. Some people with high eye pressure who do not have signs of optic nerve damage (known as glaucoma "suspects") can be monitored closely without treatment.

Eye drops and surgery are the main treatments for open-angle and closed-angle glaucoma.

Eye drops containing beta-blockers, prostaglandin analogs, alpha-agonists, carbonic anhydrase inhibitors, or cholinergic agents are commonly used to treat glaucoma. Most people with open-angle glaucoma respond well to these drugs. These drugs are also used for people with closed-angle glaucoma, although surgery, not eye drops, is the main treatment. Glaucoma eye drops are generally safe, but they may cause a variety of side effects. People need to use them for the rest of their lives, and regular check-ups are necessary to monitor eye pressure, optic nerves, and visual fields.

Surgery may be needed if eye drops cannot effectively control eye pressure, if a person cannot take eye drops, or if a person develops side effects while using the eye drops. Laser surgery can be used to open clogged drainage canals in people with open-angle glaucoma (laser trabeculoplasty) or to make an opening in the iris (laser peripheral iridectomy or iridotomy) in people with closed-angle glaucoma. Both techniques improve fluid drainage. Laser surgery is done in the doctor's office or in a hospital or clinic. Anesthetic eye drops are used to prevent pain. People are usually able to go home the same day.

Glaucoma filtration surgery is the other form of surgery doctors use to treat glaucoma. With glaucoma filtration surgery, doctors manually create a new drainage system (trabeculectomy) to allow fluid to bypass the clogged or blocked canals and filter out of the eye. Glaucoma filtration surgery is generally performed in a hospital. People are usually able to return home the same day.

The most common complication of glaucoma laser surgery is a temporary increase in eye pressure, which is treated with glaucoma eye drops. Rarely, the laser used in laser surgery may burn the cornea, but these burns usually heal quickly. With laser and glaucoma filtration surgery, inflammation and bleeding within the eye may occur but are usually short-lived. Glaucoma filtration surgery may occasionally lead to double vision, cataracts, or infection.

After glaucoma surgery, doctors prescribe eye drops and examine the eye after the procedure to monitor eye pressure and to make sure the procedure was effective.

Because severe closed-angle glaucoma is a medical emergency, doctors may use treatments that have larger and more immediate effects than those of eye drops or surgery. Doctors may use glycerin or acetazolamide pills or intravenous drugs such as mannitol if they think the eye is vulnerable to high pressure. Eye drops are also given as soon as possible. Emergency surgery is performed if necessary.

The treatment of glaucoma caused by other disorders depends on the cause. For infection or inflammation, antibiotic, antiviral, or corticosteroid eye drops may provide a cure. A tumor obstructing fluid drainage should be treated, as should a cataract that is so large it causes eye pressure to rise. High eye pressure that results from cataract surgery is treated with glaucoma eye drops that reduce eye pressure. If eye drops do not work, glaucoma filtration surgery can be performed to create a new pathway for fluid to leave the eye.

CHAPTER 234

Retinal Disorders

The cornea and lens focus light onto the retina, the transparent, light-sensitive membrane on the inner surface of the back of the eye. The central area of the retina, called the macula, primarily contains a high density of color-sensitive photoreceptor cells. These cells, called cones, produce the sharpest visual images and are responsible for central vision. The peripheral area of the retina, which surrounds the macula, contains photoreceptor cells called rods, which respond to lower lighting levels but are not color sensitive. The rods are responsible for peripheral vision and night vision.

The optic nerve carries signals generated by the photoreceptors (cones and rods). Each photoreceptor sends a tiny branch to join the optic

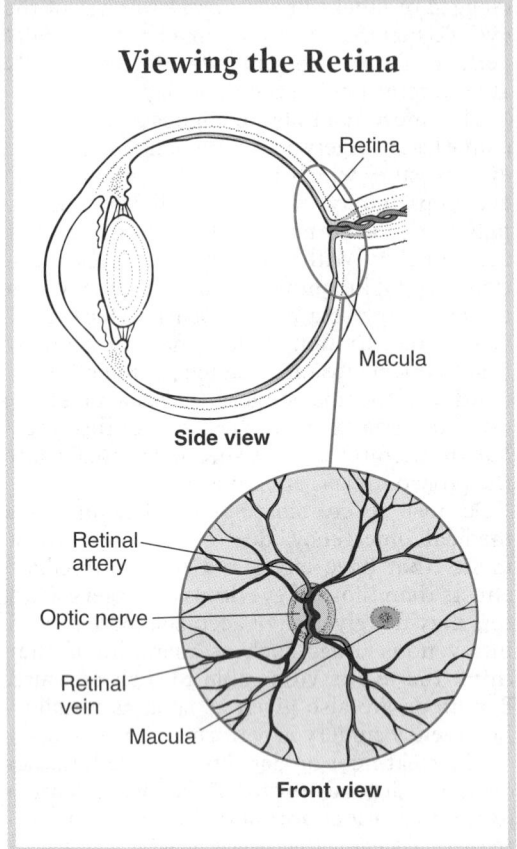

Viewing the Retina

Retina

Macula

Side view

Retinal artery

Optic nerve

Retinal vein

Macula

Front view

nerve. The optic nerve extends into the brain and connects to neurons that carry signals to the vision center of the brain, where they are interpreted as visual images.

The optic nerve and the retina have a rich supply of blood vessels that carry blood and oxygen. Part of this supply of blood vessels comes from the choroid, which is the layer of blood vessels that lies between the retina and the outer white coat of the eye (the sclera). The central retinal artery (the other major source of blood to the retina) reaches the retina near the optic nerve and then branches out within the retina.

Age-related Macular Degeneration

Age-related macular degeneration (age-related maculopathy) causes progressive damage to the macula, the central and most vital area of the retina, resulting in gradual loss of vision.

Age-related macular degeneration affects older people and is equally common in men and women; it is more common in fair-skinned people and in those who smoke. The cause is unknown, but the condition tends to run in families.

There are two forms of age-related macular degeneration, dry (atrophic) and wet (neovascular or exudative) macular degeneration. In dry macular degeneration, the tissues of the macula thin as cells disappear. There is no evidence of scarring or of bleeding or other fluid leakage in the retina. In wet macular degeneration, abnormal blood vessels develop in the layer of tissue under the macula. These vessels may leak fluid and blood under the retina in that area. Eventually a mound of scar tissue develops under the retina. Macular degeneration is a slow process. Both eyes may be affected simultaneously in the dry form. The wet form develops in one eye first but eventually affects both eyes.

Symptoms and Diagnosis

In dry macular degeneration, central vision slowly and painlessly worsens. Objects may appear washed out, or fine detail may be lost. Sometimes a doctor can see early physical changes near the macula, even before symptoms develop. In wet macular degeneration, loss of vision tends to progress quickly and may be particularly sudden if one of the abnormal blood vessels bleeds. The first symptom may be distortion of vision in one eye, so that fine, straight lines appear wavy. Often, difficulty with reading or watching television results.

Macular degeneration can severely damage vision, but it rarely leads to complete blindness. Vision at the outer edges of the visual field (peripheral vision) and the ability to see color are generally not affected. The dry type tends to result in less sudden or severe vision loss and generally develops more slowly than the wet type.

A doctor can usually diagnose macular degeneration by examining the eyes with an ophthalmoscope or a slit lamp. Sometimes fluorescein angiography—a procedure in which a doctor injects dye into a vein and photographs the retina—is used to determine the diagnosis.

Treatment

No treatment is currently available for the dry type. No treatment is currently recommended for mild or severe disease. People with moderate disease may benefit from high doses of antioxidants (vitamin C, vitamin E, and beta-carotene) and zinc and copper. Transplantation of retinal tissue is being studied and may eventually be available.

In the wet type, when new blood vessels grow in or around the macula, a laser can be used to destroy them before they do further harm. If the laser is used to destroy retinal and choroidal tissue as well, this treatment is called thermal laser. Another promising treatment is photodynamic therapy. In this treatment, a substance that sensitizes the blood vessels in the eye to laser light is given intravenously, and then a beam of laser light is used to destroy these abnormal blood vessels. Transpupillary thermotherapy is an alternative treatment, in which an infrared laser is used. Both photodynamic therapy and transpupillary thermotherapy are used to damage the new blood vessels without damaging the retina or choroid.

Magnifiers, reading glasses, telescopes, and closed-circuit television magnifying devices may help people with poor vision. There are also a variety of low-vision aids for computer users. For instance, one device projects an enhanced image from the computer onto an undamaged part of the retina. Software is available that displays computer data in large print or reads the data aloud in a synthetic voice. Counseling regarding the types of services that are available for people with poor vision is advisable and is typically given by a low-vision specialist (an ophthalmologist or optometrist who specializes in treating those with very poor vision).

Macular Pucker

Macular pucker (cellophane maculopathy, premacular fibrosis, or epiretinal membrane) is formation of a thin membrane over the retina, which interferes with vision.

Macular pucker typically occurs after age 50 and is most common in people older than 75. A macular pucker is a thin membrane of scar tissue that forms over the retina and contracts, wrinkling the retina underneath.

With aging, the vitreous humor (the jelly-like substance inside the back part of the eye; also called the vitreous) shrinks. Various conditions that can cause wrinkling of the retina include diabetic retinopathy, uveitis, retinal detachment, or injury to the eye.

Symptoms may include blurred vision or distorted vision (straight lines may appear wavy). A doctor confirms the diagnosis by looking at the back of the eye with an ophthalmoscope. Fluorescein angiography may also be helpful.

Most people need no treatment. If problems with vision are significant, the membrane can be removed surgically, using a procedure called a membrane peel. This procedure can be done under local anesthesia in an operating room and usually takes about 30 minutes.

Retinal Detachment

Retinal detachment is separation of the retina from the underlying layer of blood vessels.

When the retina detaches, it separates from part of its blood supply, preventing it from working properly. Unless the retina is reattached, it may be permanently damaged.

Detachment may begin in a small area, usually as the result of a retinal tear. If the small area is not reattached, the entire retina can detach. Retinal tears that can lead to retinal detachment are more likely to occur in people who are highly nearsighted (myopic) or who have had cataract surgery. Tears are also more likely to occur after an eye injury. Fluid or blood from a damaged blood vessel may collect between the retina and the underlying tissue, further worsening vision.

Symptoms

A retinal detachment is painless. People usually see small, floating objects (floaters) or flashes of bright light that last less than a second. Loss of peripheral vision typically begins first, and vision loss spreads as the detachment progresses. The loss of vision resembles a curtain or veil falling across the line of sight. If the macula becomes detached, vision rapidly deteriorates, and everything becomes blurred.

A doctor examines the retina through an ophthalmoscope and can usually see a detachment. If the detachment is not visible, an ultrasound scan of the eye can reveal it.

Treatment and Prognosis

Anyone who experiences a sudden loss of vision should see an ophthalmologist immediately. Depending on the cause of the detachment, laser surgery or freezing therapy (cryopexy) may be used to repair the retina. Laser surgery seals holes in the retina. Freezing therapy causes a scar to form, which holds the retina in place.

If the retina is reattached within 2 to 7 days, the likelihood that sight will improve is usually good. If the retina has been detached for a longer time or if bleeding or scarring has occurred, the likelihood that sight will improve is decreased.

Retinitis Pigmentosa

Retinitis pigmentosa is a rare, progressive degeneration of the retina that eventually causes blindness.

Retinitis pigmentosa is often inherited. One form has a dominant pattern of inheritance, requiring only one abnormal gene from either parent. Other forms are recessive and require an abnormal gene from both parents. An X-linked recessive form is exhibited mainly in males who inherit one abnormal gene from their mother. In some people, mostly males, an inherited form of hearing loss may be associated (Usher's syndrome).

The photoreceptors of the retina that are responsible for vision when light is low (rods) gradually degenerate, so that vision becomes poor in the dark. The first symptoms often begin in early childhood. Over time, peripheral vision progressively deteriorates. In the late stages of the disease, the person typically has a small area of central vision and possibly some peripheral vision remaining (tunnel vision).

When examining the retina with an ophthalmoscope, a doctor sees specific changes that suggest the diagnosis. Several tests, such as the electroretinogram, which is a test of the electrical response of the retina to light, may help make the diagnosis. No conventional treatment can slow the progression of retinal damage. High doses of vitamin A are recommended by some doctors, but the value of this treatment is unknown. However, an experimental treatment in which fetal retinal tissue is transplanted into people with retinitis pigmentosa has been reported to improve vision.

Blockage of Central Retinal Arteries and Veins

The central retinal artery, the main vessel that supplies blood to the retina, can become completely blocked because of atherosclerosis or particles, such as blood clots, that float in the bloodstream and block a vessel (emboli). Inflammation of the blood vessels is also a possible cause of retinal artery blockage. In people with glaucoma, diabetes, or high blood pressure, various processes may occur, which can lead to blockage of the veins.

If the central retinal artery is blocked, the affected eye has a sudden but painless loss of vision. Blockage of the central retinal vein causes engorged veins and swelling of the front of the optic nerve. Vision loss ranges from mild to severe as in central retinal artery blockage. Recurrences are common.

In addition to severe vision loss, complications of blockage of the central retinal artery or vein include hemorrhage into the eye and glaucoma caused by growth of abnormal blood vessels on the iris and angle, where fluid drains from the eye.

Diagnosis and Treatment

Using an ophthalmoscope, a doctor can see changes in blood vessels and other indications of decreased blood supply to the retina, such as paleness of the retina in the case of arterial blockage or engorged veins and swelling of the front of the optic nerve in the case of venous blockage. Fluorescein angiography—a procedure in which a doctor injects dye into a vein and then photographs the retina—helps determine the extent of damage to the retina and helps the doctor plan treatment. Doppler ultrasound scanning may sometimes be used to observe blood flow in the vessels.

Immediate treatment is often given in an attempt to unblock the retinal artery. However, treatments are rarely effective. Pressure inside the eye can be lowered by intermittently massaging the closed eyelids with the fingers. Alternatively, a procedure called anterior chamber paracentesis may help lower pressure inside the eye. In this procedure, drops are placed in the eye to numb the eye, and then a needle is inserted into the anterior chamber of the eye to withdraw a small amount of fluid, thereby rapidly lowering the pressure in the eye. Lowering the pressure inside the eye by massage or by anterior chamber paracentesis may dislodge a blood clot or other embolus and allow it to enter a smaller branch of the vessel, thereby reducing the area of damage to the retina. There is no generally accepted drug therapy. Laser treatment may be used to destroy abnormal blood vessels if they develop on the iris or angle.

Hypertensive Retinopathy

Hypertensive retinopathy is damage to the retina as a result of high blood pressure.

When blood pressure becomes high, as it does in hypertension, the retina may become damaged. Even mild hypertension may damage the retinal blood vessels if it goes untreated for years. Hypertension damages the small blood vessels in the retina, causing their walls to thicken and thereby narrowing the blood vessels' openings and reducing the blood supply to the retina. Patches of the retina may become damaged because the blood supply is inadequate. As hypertensive retinopathy progresses, blood may leak into the retina. These changes lead to a gradual loss of vision, particularly if they affect the macula, the central part of the retina.

A doctor makes the diagnosis using an ophthalmoscope to see the typical appearance of the retina in a person with high blood pressure. When blood pressure is extremely high, doctors may be able to see other changes in the eye, such as swelling of the front of the optic nerve.

The goal of treatment is to lower the blood pressure. When high blood pressure is severe and life threatening, treatment may be needed immediately to save vision and avoid other complications, including stroke, heart failure, kidney failure, and heart attack.

Diabetic Retinopathy

Diabetic retinopathy is damage to the retina as a result of diabetes.

Diabetes mellitus can produce two types of changes in the eye. These changes, nonproliferative and proliferative retinopathy, are among the leading causes of blindness in the United States and other developed countries. Some retinal change occurs in virtually all people with diabetes, whether or not they use insulin therapy. People with diabetes who also have high blood pressure are at higher risk of developing diabetic retinopathy because both conditions tend to damage the retina.

High levels of sugar (glucose) in the blood make the walls of small blood vessels, including those in the retina, weaker and, therefore, more prone to damage. Damaged retinal blood vessels leak blood and plasma into the retina.

The extent of retinopathy and vision loss is related to how poorly blood sugar levels are controlled and how long a person has had diabetes. In general, retinopathy develops after a person has had diabetes for at least 10 years.

Symptoms and Diagnosis

In **nonproliferative retinopathy,** small blood vessels in the retina leak. The area around the leak may swell, causing damage to parts of the field of vision. If the leakage is near the macula, central vision may blur. At first, the effects on vision may be minimal, but gradually vision may become impaired. A blue-yellow color vision abnormality may develop, interfering with color perception. Blind spots may occur, although these may not be noticed by the person and are usually discovered only if testing is carried out. Swelling of the macula (macular edema), due to leakage of fluid from blood vessels, can eventually lead to significant loss of vision.

In **proliferative retinopathy,** damage to the retina stimulates the growth of new blood vessels. The new blood vessels grow abnormally, sometimes leading to hemorrhage or development of scars. Extensive scarring may lead to retinal detachment. Proliferative retinopathy tends to result in greater loss of vision than does nonproliferative retinopathy. It can result in total or near-total blindness due to massive hemorrhage into the vitreous humor (the jelly-like substance inside the back part of the eye) or to retinal detachment.

A doctor diagnoses nonproliferative and proliferative retinopathy by examining the retina with an ophthalmoscope or a slit lamp. Fluorescein angiography helps to determine the location of the leaks.▲

Prevention and Treatment

The best way to prevent diabetic retinopathy is to control the diabetes and keep blood pressure at normal levels. People with diabetes should have annual eye examinations, so that retinopathy can be detected and any necessary treatment can be started early.

Treatment consists of laser photocoagulation, in which a laser beam is aimed into the eye at the retina to slow the growth of abnormal new retinal blood vessels and decrease leakage. Laser photocoagulation may need to be repeated. If bleeding from damaged vessels has been extensive, a procedure called vitrectomy may be needed. In this procedure, blood is removed from the cavity in which the vitreous humor lies. Vision often improves after vitrectomy for vitreous hemorrhage, and vision may improve after vitrectomy for retinal

▲ see page 1285

detachment. Laser treatment only rarely improves vision, but it commonly prevents further deterioration.

Endophthalmitis

Endophthalmitis is infection inside the eye.

Endophthalmitis is caused by organisms that have traveled through the bloodstream into the eye or have entered the eye through a surgical incision or an injury. Infection in the blood comes from intravenous drug administration, an abscess (a collection of pus), or surgery anywhere in the body. Infection is usually due to bacteria, but fungi or protozoa may also be responsible. Viruses can also cause extensive eye infections, but these are generally not called endophthalmitis.

Symptoms may be severe and include pain, redness in the white of the eye, extreme sensitivity to bright light, and partial or complete loss of vision. The diagnosis is based on the symptoms, an examination of the eye, cultures, and sometimes antibody or DNA testing. Cultures may be taken from the aqueous humor (fluid inside the front of the eye; also called the aqueous) and the vitreous humor (the jellylike substance inside the back part of the eye) to determine which organisms are responsible and which drugs are most active against them.

Endophthalmitis is a medical emergency. Rapid treatment is generally needed if vision is to be preserved. Treatment usually begins immediately; a delay of even a few hours can result in vision loss in extreme cases. Antibiotics are given; the choice of antibiotic may be adjusted depending on which organism is found to be causing the endophthalmitis. Corticosteroids may also be given. Surgery may be needed to remove infected tissue from inside the eye, which may improve the chances of stopping the infection.

Cancers Affecting the Retina

Cancers affecting the retina generally begin in the choroid, a dense layer of blood vessels that supplies the retina. The choroid is sandwiched between the retina and the sclera (the outer white part of the eye). Because the retina depends on the choroid for its blood supply and support, damage to the choroid by a cancer is likely to affect vision.

Choroidal Melanoma: Choroidal melanoma is a cancer that originates in the pigment-producing cells (melanocytes) of the choroid. Choroidal melanoma is the most common cancer originating in the eye. It is most common in people with fair complexions and blue eyes. In its early stages, the cancer usually does not interfere with vision. Later, it may cause blurred vision or complete loss of vision due to retinal detachment. Metastases to other parts of the body may occur.

Early diagnosis is important, because the likelihood of curing choroid melanoma is related to the size of the tumor. Diagnosis is made using an ophthalmoscope, ultrasound scanning, and serial photographs.

If the melanoma is small, treatment with a laser, radiation, or an implant of radioactive materials may preserve vision and save the eye. If the cancer is large, the eye must be removed. If a large cancer is not removed, it can spread directly into the eye socket (orbit) or through the bloodstream (metastasize) to other organs, causing death.

Choroidal Metastases: Choroidal metastases are cancers that have spread to the eye from other parts of the body. Because of its excellent blood supply, the choroid is often a place to which cancers from other parts of the body may spread. In women, breast cancer is the most common cause. In men, cancers of the lung or prostate are the most common causes.

Often, these cancers produce no symptoms and may be discovered during a routine eye examination. In those with symptoms, initial symptoms are decreasing vision and flashes of light. Retinal detachment and severe vision loss may occur.

The diagnosis is sometimes made during a routine eye examination with an ophthalmoscope. Diagnosis is aided by ultrasound scanning. Confirmation of the diagnosis may involve using a fine needle to remove a sample of tissue for examination under a microscope (biopsy). Treatment is usually with chemotherapy and radiation therapy.

CHAPTER 235

Optic Nerve Disorders

The small photoreceptors of the retina (the inner surface at the back of the eye) sense light and transmit impulses to the optic nerve. The optic nerve carries impulses to the brain. A problem anywhere along the optic nerve or damage to the areas at the back of the brain that sense visual information can result in loss of vision. A common cause of damage to the optic nerve is a tumor of the pituitary gland that presses on the nerve.

The two optic nerves carry signals from the eyes to the back of the brain. At a structure in the brain called the optic chiasm, each nerve splits, and half of its fibers cross over to the other side. Because of this anatomic arrangement, damage along the optic nerve pathway causes specific patterns of vision loss. By understanding the pattern of vision loss, a doctor can often determine where in the pathway the problem is.

Papilledema

Papilledema is a condition in which increased pressure in or around the brain causes the optic nerve to swell where it enters the eye.

The condition is usually caused by a brain tumor or abscess, head injury, bleeding in the brain, infection of the brain or its tissue coverings (meninges), pseudotumor cerebri (which is not a tumor and is also called benign intracranial hypertension,▲ or severe high blood pressure. Severe lung disease can also increase pressure in the brain, leading to papilledema. These conditions typically result in papilledema in both eyes.

At first, papilledema may be present without affecting vision. Fleeting visual changes—blurred vision or complete loss of vision—typically lasting seconds are characteristic of papilledema. They may occur when arising from sitting or lying down. Other symptoms may occur due to the elevated pressure in the brain rather than the effects on the eye. Headache may occur.

An ophthalmologist uses an ophthalmoscope to diagnose papilledema. Computed tomography (CT) and magnetic resonance imaging (MRI) may be used to monitor papilledema

and help determine its cause. A spinal tap is performed to measure the pressure of the cerebrospinal fluid. A sample of the cerebrospinal fluid may be examined for evidence of a brain tumor or infection.

If the high pressure of the cerebrospinal fluid is due to a brain tumor, corticosteroids are usually given, but surgery to remove the tumor may be needed. Papilledema that occurs as a result of pseudotumor cerebri can be treated with weight loss and a diuretic. Other treatments of papilledema depend on the cause. For example, a brain abscess is drained and antibiotics are given, high blood pressure is lowered with drug therapy,■ and an infection, if bacterial, can be treated with antibiotics. If headaches persist, surgery may be needed.

Optic Neuritis

Optic neuritis is inflammation of the optic nerve anywhere along its course.

Optic neuritis may be caused by a viral infection (especially in children), vaccination, meningitis, syphilis, certain autoimmune diseases such as multiple sclerosis, and intraocular inflammation (uveitis★). However, the cause of optic neuritis is often unknown.

Optic neuritis causes vision loss, which may be mild or severe and may occur in one or both eyes. Loss of vision may occur over days. Vision in the involved eye or eyes can range from almost normal to complete blindness. There may be pain with eye movement. Depending on the cause, vision may recover only to deteriorate later in repeat episodes of worsening vision.

Diagnosis involves examination of the reactions of the pupils and observing the back of the eyes with an ophthalmoscope; the optic disk (the head of the optic nerve at the back of the eye) may appear swollen. Testing peripheral vision may reveal loss of vision at the periphery (side) of the visual field. Magnetic resonance imaging (MRI) may show evidence of multiple sclerosis or, rarely, a tumor pressing on the optic nerve.

▲ see box on page 523

■ see table on page 138　　★ see page 1305

Tracing the Visual Pathways

Nerve signals travel along the optic nerve from each eye. The two optic nerves meet at the optic chiasm. There, the optic nerve from each eye divides, and half of the nerve fibers from each side cross to the other side. Because of this arrangement, the brain receives information via both optic nerves for the left visual field and for the right visual field.

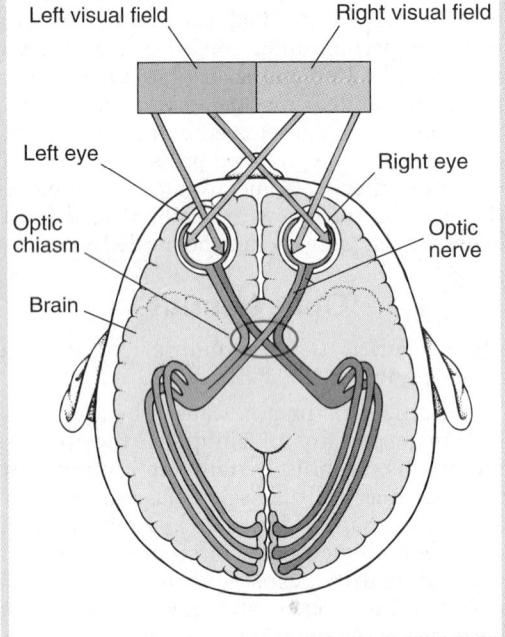

Left visual field

Right visual field

Left eye

Right eye

Optic chiasm

Optic nerve

Brain

Most cases of optic neuritis will improve over a few months without treatment. However, in some instances, treatment with intravenous corticosteroids and other drugs may hasten recovery and reduce the chance of a recurrence. If a tumor is pressing on the optic nerve, vision usually improves once the pressure caused by the tumor is relieved.

Optic Neuropathy

Optic neuropathy is damage of the optic nerve due to a blockage of its blood supply, to nutritional deficiencies, or to toxins.

▲ see page 388

Blockage of the blood supply to the part of the optic nerve within the eye can lead to death or dysfunction of optic nerve cells and is called ischemic optic neuropathy. Two types can occur: nonarteritic and arteritic.

Nonarteritic ischemic optic neuropathy usually occurs in people older than 50. Risk factors include high blood pressure, diabetes, and atherosclerosis. Rarely, it occurs in younger people with severe migraines. Arteritic ischemic optic neuropathy usually occurs in people older than 70. The blood supply to the optic nerve is blocked due to inflammation of the arteries (arteritis), most notably the temporal artery, which causes temporal arteritis (giant cell arteritis).▲

Damage to the optic nerve can also be caused by exposure to a substance that is harmful to the optic nerve, such as lead, methanol, ethylene glycol (antifreeze), tobacco, or arsenic. This type is sometimes called toxic amblyopia. Optic neuropathy may be caused by a nutritional deficiency (sometimes called nutritional amblyopia), especially of vitamin B_{12}. Alcoholics are particularly susceptible, although the cause may be malnutrition, not alcohol. Rarely, optic neuropathy may be caused by drugs such as chloramphenicol, isoniazid, ethambutol, and digoxin.

Loss of vision may be rapid (over minutes or hours), but it can develop gradually over 2 to 7 days. Depending on the cause, vision may be impaired in one or both eyes. Vision in the involved eye or eyes can range from almost normal to complete blindness. In people with optic neuropathy caused by exposure to a toxin or to a nutritional deficiency, both eyes are usually affected. A small area of vision loss at the center of the visual field slowly enlarges and can progress to complete blindness. People with temporal arteritis tend to be older, and their loss of vision tends to be more severe.

About 40% of people with nonarteritic ischemic optic neuropathy experience spontaneous improvement over time. In this condition, repeat episodes in the same eye are extremely rare. Involvement of the other eye is estimated to occur in 10 to 34% of affected people over a 5-year period.

Diagnosis involves examination of the back of the eyes with an ophthalmoscope. Determining the cause involves obtaining a careful history of possible exposures to toxic substances and determining whether the person is suffering from any of the disorders known to be a risk factor. If temporal arteritis is suspected as a cause, blood tests and a biopsy of the temporal artery may be done to confirm the diagnosis.

In people with nonarteritic ischemic optic neuropathy, treatment involves controlling blood pressure, diabetes, cholesterol levels, and other factors that affect the blood supply to the optic nerve. In people with arteritic ischemic optic neuropathy due to temporal arteritis, high doses of corticosteroids are given to prevent loss of vision in the second eye, which occurs in 25 to 50% of people within days to weeks if treatment is not started. The role of aspirin in preventing involvement of the second eye is being investigated, although at this time there is no evidence to support its use.

People with optic neuropathy caused by exposure to chemicals or drugs should avoid tobacco, alcohol, or other responsible toxic chemical or drug if it is known. If alcohol use is a contributing cause, the person should eat a well-balanced diet and take vitamin supplements. If lead is the cause, chelating drugs (such as succimer or dimercaprol) help remove it from the body.

In people with optic neuropathy caused by a nutritional deficiency, treatment usually involves correction of the deficiency with di-

Some Patterns of Vision Loss

Depending on where the damage to the visual pathway occurs, the type of vision loss varies.

For instance, if the optic nerve is damaged somewhere between an eyeball and the optic chiasm, the person may become blind in only that eye. If the optic chiasm is damaged, both eyes lose some vision—the right eye loses vision in the right portion of its visual field, and the left eye loses vision in the left portion of its visual field.

In hemianopia, damage farther back in the optic nerve pathway (which is often the result of a stroke or a tumor) produces yet another pattern of vision loss. Half of the visual field in both eyes is affected. For example, with damage to the left portion of the brain, both eyes lose the right half of their visual field.

etary supplements. However, if the cause is vitamin B_{12} deficiency, treatment with dietary supplements alone is not enough. Vitamin B_{12} deficiency is typically treated with injections of supplemental vitamin B_{12}. Unless the optic nerve shows evidence of wasting (atrophy), recovery of some of the lost vision is expected.

CHAPTER 236

Eye Socket Disorders

The eye sockets (orbits) are bony cavities that contain and protect the eyes. Disorders affecting the orbits include fractures, infections, inflammation, and tumors. Thyroid disease can also affect the orbit.

Fractures

An injury to the face can fracture any of several bones that form each orbit.

Vision may be impaired when blood that accumulates after a fracture, typically from torn blood vessels, puts pressure on the eye or on the nerves and blood vessels going to and from it (retrobulbar hematoma). Pressure on the nerves may impair vision by interfering with

nerve impulses going from the eye to the brain. The fracture (or a bone fragment) may also impair the function of the muscles that move the eye (possibly by damaging the muscles themselves or the nerves that move the muscles). Damage to these muscles may inhibit eye movement up, down, or to the right or left and thereby produce double vision. The eyeball may become sunken (enophthalmos) if the fracture is large. The eyeball itself also may be damaged in these injuries.

Diagnosis and Treatment

Diagnosis is suspected based on the symptoms. X-rays of the skull and computed tomography (CT) or magnetic resonance imag-

Cavernous Sinus Thrombosis

Cavernous sinus thrombosis is the blockage of a large vein at the base of the brain (the cavernous sinus). It is usually caused by the spread of bacteria from a sinus infection or from an infection in the eye or around the nose. Thus, infections in the area around the nose to the rim of the eyes are always considered serious.

Cavernous sinus thrombosis causes bulging eyes, severe headache, drowsiness or coma, seizures, a high fever, and abnormal sensations or muscle weakness in certain areas. To identify the bacteria, a blood sample and samples of fluid, mucus, or pus from the throat and nose are sent to a laboratory to be cultured. Computed tomography (CT) of the sinuses, eyes, and brain is usually performed.

High doses of intravenous antibiotics are given immediately. If the condition does not improve after 24 hours of antibiotic treatment, the sinus may be drained surgically.

ing (MRI) confirm the diagnosis. When a fracture traps muscles or soft tissues of the orbit and produces double vision or makes the eyeball sunken, surgical repair of the facial bones is usually necessary. After ensuring that the fracture has not damaged a vital structure, the surgeon restores the bones to their proper positions, sometimes using small metal plates and screws or wires to hold them in place. The surgeon may use a thin plastic sheet or a bone graft to connect the broken parts and assist healing.

Infections

An infection may spread from the sinuses, teeth, or bloodstream to the orbit. Infection of the orbit is called orbital cellulitis. Eye infections may develop after an injury. Symptoms include pain, a bulging eye, reduced eye movement, swollen eyelids, and fever. The eyeball has a swollen, indistinct appearance. Vision may be impaired.

Without adequate treatment, orbital cellulitis can lead to blindness. Infection can spread to the brain and spinal cord, or blood clots can

▲ see art on page 1293

form and spread from the veins around the eye to involve a large vein at the base of the brain (the cavernous sinus) and result in cavernous sinus thrombosis.

Diagnosis and Treatment

Doctors can usually recognize orbital cellulitis without using diagnostic tests. However, determining the cause may require further assessment, including examination of the teeth and mouth and x-rays or computed tomography (CT) of the sinuses. Often, doctors obtain samples from the lining of the eye and from the skin, throat, or sinuses as well as blood samples and send them to a laboratory for testing. The samples are cultured (to grow organisms) to determine where the infection that gave rise to the orbital cellulitis is located, which type of organism is causing the infection, and which treatment should be used.

Antibiotics are started before the results of the laboratory testing are known. Oral antibiotics are given for mild cases; intravenous antibiotics are given for severe cases. The antibiotic used at first may be changed if the culture results suggest that another drug would be more effective. Sometimes surgery is needed to drain a collection of pus (abscess) or an infected sinus.

Inflammation

Any or all of the structures within the orbit may become inflamed. The inflammation can be part of another disease process, such as Wegener's granulomatosis, in which inflammation affecting blood vessels (called vasculitis) occurs, or inflammation may occur for no apparent reason. Inflammation affecting the white coat (sclera) of the eye is called scleritis. Inflammation affecting the lacrimal gland, located at the upper outer edge of the orbit,▲ is called inflammatory dacryoadenitis. If inflammation affects one of the muscles that move the eye, it is called myositis. Inflammation affecting the entire orbit and its contents is called inflammatory orbital pseudotumor (which is not really a tumor and is not a cancer) or nonspecific orbital inflammation.

Symptoms vary depending on which structures are actually inflamed. In general, symptoms start rather suddenly, typically over a few days. Pain and redness of the eyeball or eyelid occur. Pain can be severe and incapacitating at times. A doctor may take a sample from the inflamed area for examination under a microscope (biopsy) to determine the cause.

Inflammation is usually treated with a corticosteroid drug, which can be given by mouth. Corticosteroids can be given intravenously if the inflammation is severe.

Tumors

Rarely, tumors, either cancerous or noncancerous, can form in the tissues behind the eye. Tumors can form within the tissues behind the eye, or cancerous tumors from elsewhere in the body can spread (metastasize) to the tissues behind the eye.

These tumors can push the eye forward (exophthalmos). Usually a biopsy is needed to determine what type of tumor is present, and treatment depends on these results. Treatment may include surgical removal, radiation therapy, chemotherapy, or a combination of these treatments.

Exophthalmos

Exophthalmos is an abnormal bulging of one or both eyes.

Many conditions can cause exophthalmos. In some types of thyroid disease, especially Graves' disease,▲ the tissues in the orbit swell and accumulate certain types of cells (such as lymphocytes), which push the eyeball forward. Exophthalmos can develop rapidly from bleeding behind the eye or from inflammation in the orbit. Tumors, either cancerous or noncancerous, can form in the orbit behind the eyeball and push it forward. An unusual noncancerous accumulation of inflammatory and fibrous tissue (pseudotumor) may produce exophthalmos with pain and swelling. Cavernous sinus thrombosis causes swelling because blood in the veins cannot exit the eye. Abnormal connections between the arteries and veins (arteriovenous malformations) behind the eye may produce a pulsating exophthalmos, in which the eye bulges forward and pulses along with the heartbeat.

The protruding eye is less protected by the eyelids, and the cornea may become too dry. As a result, corneal ulcers may form, which can become infected. Prolonged exophthalmos can impair vision because the optic nerve is stretched. The increased pressure within the orbit may also result in compression of the optic nerve, which can also impair vision.

Diagnosis and Treatment

All people with protruding eyes do not necessarily have exophthalmos. Some people simply have prominent eyes with more white showing than normal. The extent of the protrusion can be measured with an ordinary ruler or with an instrument called an exophthalmometer. Further diagnostic tests may include computed tomography (CT) and thyroid function tests.

The treatment depends on the cause. If the problem is an abnormal connection between arteries and veins, surgery may be needed to close off certain blood vessels. Thyroid disease that is severe enough to cause exophthalmos may need to be treated. But it is unclear if treating the thyroid condition actually improves bulging of the eyes. Treatment of exophthalmos includes eyeshades and eye drops if symptoms are mild, or corticosteroids, radiation therapy, or surgery if the condition is more severe. Treatment of bleeding or inflammation involves treating the underlying disorder.■ Tumors (depending on type) are treated with chemotherapy, radiation therapy, or surgery. Corticosteroids may help the inflammation caused by a pseudotumor.

▲ see page 949   ■ see page 1318

MEN'S HEALTH ISSUES

237 Male Reproductive System 1321

Structure ▪ Function ▪ Puberty ▪ Effects of Aging

238 Disorders of the Penis and Testes 1324

Penile Inflammation ▪ Urethral Stricture ▪ Penile Growths ▪
Priapism ▪ Peyronie's Disease ▪ Penile and Testicular Injury ▪
Testicular Cancer ▪ Testicular Torsion ▪ Inguinal Hernia ▪
Epididymitis and Epididymo-orchitis ▪ Hydrocele ▪
Varicocele ▪ Testicular Swelling

239 Prostate Disorders..1329

Benign Prostatic Hyperplasia ▪ Prostate Cancer ▪ Prostatitis

240 Sexual Dysfunction 1335

Erectile Dysfunction ▪ Decreased Libido ▪ Premature
Ejaculation ▪ Retrograde Ejaculation

CHAPTER 237

Male Reproductive System

The external structures of the male reproductive system include the penis and scrotum. The internal structures include the vas deferens, testes (testicles), urethra, prostate gland, and seminal vesicles.

The sperm, which carries the man's genes, is made in the testes and stored in the seminal vesicles. During ejaculation, the sperm is transported along with a fluid called semen through the vas deferens and the erect penis.

Structure

The penis consists of the root (which is attached to the abdominal wall), the body (the middle portion), and the glans penis (the cone-shaped end). The opening of the urethra (the channel that transports semen and urine) is lo-

cated at the tip of the glans penis. The base of the glans penis is called the corona. In uncircumcised males, the foreskin (prepuce) extends from the corona to cover the glans penis.

The body of the penis primarily consists of three cylindrical spaces (sinuses) of erectile tissue. The two larger ones, the corpora cavernosa, occur side by side. The third sinus, the corpus spongiosum, surrounds the urethra. When these spaces fill with blood, the penis becomes large and rigid (erect).

The scrotum is the thin-skinned sac that surrounds and protects the testes. The scrotum also acts as a climate-control system for the testes, because they need to be slightly cooler than body temperature for normal sperm development. The cremaster muscles in the scrotal wall relax or contract to allow

Male Reproductive Organs

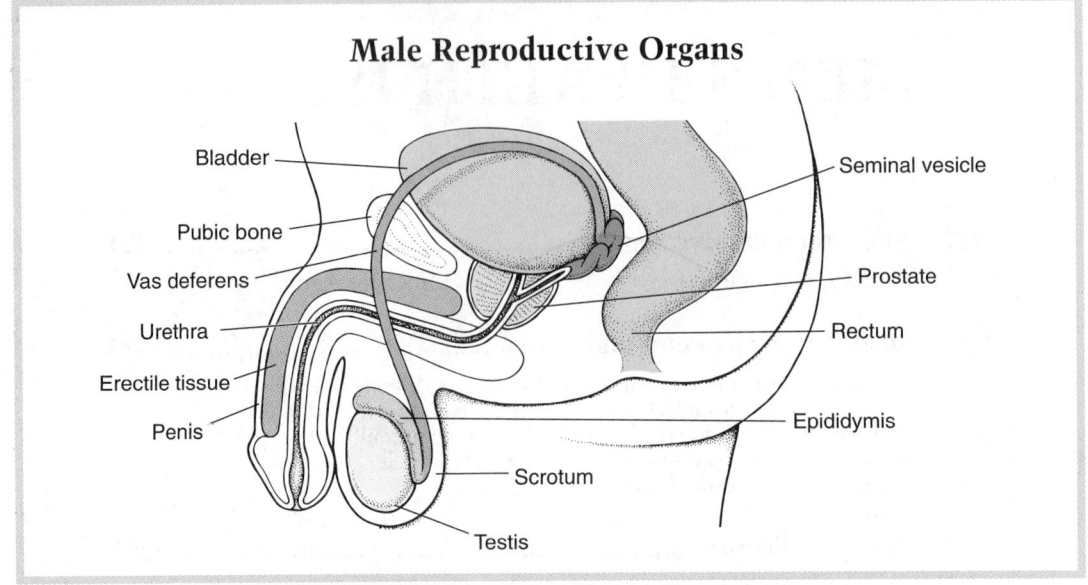

Bladder
Pubic bone
Vas deferens
Urethra
Erectile tissue
Penis

Seminal vesicle
Prostate
Rectum
Epididymis

Scrotum
Testis

the testes to hang farther from the body to cool or to be pulled closer to the body for warmth or protection.

The testes are oval bodies the size of large olives that lie in the scrotum; usually the left testis hangs slightly lower than the right one. The testes have two functions: producing sperm and testosterone (the primary male sex hormone). The epididymis is a coiled tube almost 20 feet long. It collects sperm from the testis and provides the space and environment for sperm to mature. One epididymis lies against each testis.

The vas deferens is a firm duct that transports sperm from the epididymis. One such duct travels from each epididymis to the back

Testosterone Replacement Therapy

Beginning at about age 30, the production of testosterone (the main male sex hormone) in men usually decreases an average of 1 to 2% per year. This decline differs from the usually rapid and nearly universal hormonal changes of menopause in women, but the decline in testosterone is sometimes referred to as male menopause or andropause. The rate of testosterone decline also varies greatly among men; many men in their 70s have testosterone levels that match those of the average man in his 30s.

All men with low testosterone levels develop certain characteristics associated with aging, including decreased libido, decreased muscle mass, increased abdominal fat, thin bones that easily fracture, decreased energy level, slow mathematical and spatial thinking, and a low blood count. Many men are interested in taking testosterone to slow or reverse development of these characteristics, but this is only helpful for men with abnormally low levels of testosterone.

The most worrisome side effect of testosterone replacement therapy is worsening of prostate disease. Without knowing it, many men have small prostate cancers that would likely never

produce symptoms. Testosterone can make prostate cancers grow, so testosterone replacement therapy could cause an unnoticed prostate cancer to produce symptoms or become lethal. Testosterone also worsens benign prostatic hyperplasia, a noncancerous enlargement of the prostate.

Testosterone replacement therapy is recommended only for men whose blood tests show low testosterone levels and who have no prostate disease. Men taking testosterone need to be checked frequently for prostate cancer. Such testing may detect cancers early, when they are more often curable.

of the prostate and enters the urethra. Other structures, such as blood vessels and nerves, also travel along with each vas deferens and together form an intertwined structure, the spermatic cord.

The urethra serves a dual function in males. This channel is the part of the urinary tract that transports urine from the bladder and the part of the reproductive system through which semen is ejaculated.

The prostate gland lies just under the bladder and surrounds the urethra. Walnut-sized in young men, the prostate gland enlarges with age. When the prostate enlarges too much, it can block urine flow through the urethra. The seminal vesicles, located above the prostate, join with the vas deferens to form the ejaculatory ducts. The prostate and the seminal vesicles produce fluid that nourishes the sperm. This fluid provides most of the volume of semen, the secretion in which the sperm is expelled during ejaculation. Other fluid that makes up the semen comes from the vas deferens and from mucous glands in the head of the penis.

Function

During sexual activity, the penis becomes erect, enabling penetration during sexual intercourse. An erection results from a complex interaction of neurologic, vascular, hormonal, and psychologic actions. Pleasurable stimuli cause the brain to send nerve signals through the spinal cord to the penis. The arteries supplying blood to the corpora cavernosa and corpus spongiosum respond by dilating. The widened arteries dramatically increase blood flow to these erectile areas, which become engorged with blood and expand. Muscles tighten around the veins that normally drain blood from the penis, slowing the outflow of blood and elevating blood pressure in the penis. This elevated blood pressure causes the penis to increase in length and diameter.

At the climax of sexual excitement (orgasm), ejaculation usually occurs, caused when friction on the glans penis and other stimuli send signals to the brain and spinal cord. Nerves stimulate muscle contractions along the seminal vesicles, prostate, and the ducts of the epididymis and vas deferens. These contractions force semen into the urethra. Contraction of the muscles around the urethra further propels the semen through and out of the penis. The neck of the bladder also

Breast Disorders in Men

Breast disorders, which include breast enlargement and breast cancer, occur infrequently in men.

Breast Enlargement

Breast enlargement in males (gynecomastia) sometimes occurs during puberty. The enlargement is usually normal and transient, lasting a few months to a few years. Breast enlargement commonly takes place after age 50.

Male breast enlargement may be caused by certain diseases (particularly liver disease), certain drug therapies (including the use of female sex hormones and anabolic steroids), or heavy use of marijuana, beer, or heroin. Less commonly, male breast enlargement results from a hormonal imbalance, which can be caused by rare estrogen-producing tumors in the testes or adrenal glands.

One or both breasts may become enlarged. The enlarged breast may be tender. If tenderness is present, cancer is probably not the cause. Breast pain in men, as in women, is not usually a sign of cancer.

Generally, no specific treatment is needed. Breast enlargement often disappears on its own or after its cause is identified and treated. Surgical removal of excess breast tissue is effective but rarely necessary. Liposuction, a surgical technique that removes tissue through a suction tube inserted through a small incision, is becoming increasingly popular and sometimes is followed by additional cosmetic surgery.

Breast Cancer

Men can develop breast cancer, although 99% of all breast cancers develop in women. Because male breast cancer is uncommon, it may not be suspected as a cause of symptoms. As a result, male breast cancer often progresses to an advanced stage before it is diagnosed. The prognosis is the same as that for a woman whose cancer is at the same stage.

Treatment options are generally the same as those used for women (surgery, radiation therapy, and chemotherapy), except that breast-conserving surgery is rarely used. If an examination of tissue samples shows that sex hormones are making the cancer grow, those hormones are suppressed with the drug tamoxifen.

constricts to keep semen from flowing backward into the bladder.

Once ejaculation takes place—or the stimulation stops—the arteries constrict and the veins relax. This reduces blood inflow and increases blood outflow, causing the penis to become limp (detumescence). After detumescence, erection cannot be obtained for a period of time (refractory period), commonly about 20 minutes in young men.

Puberty

Puberty is the stage during which a person reaches full reproductive ability and develops the adult features of their gender. In boys, puberty usually occurs between the ages of 10 and 14 years. However, it is not unusual for puberty to begin as early as age 9 or to continue until age 16.

The pituitary gland, which is located in the brain, initiates puberty. The pituitary gland secretes luteinizing hormone and follicle-stimulating hormone, which stimulate the testes to produce testosterone. Testosterone is responsible for the development of secondary

sex characteristics, such as facial hair growth and voice change.

Testosterone also produces many changes in the male reproductive organs, including elongation and thickening of the penis; enlargement of the scrotum, testes, epididymis, and prostate; darkening of the skin of the scrotum; and growth of pubic hair. Sperm usually develops by age 14. Ejaculation first occurs during late puberty.

Effects of Aging

It is not clear whether aging itself or the diseases associated with aging cause the gradual changes that occur in men's sexual functioning. The frequency, length, and rigidity of erections gradually decline throughout adulthood. Levels of the male sex hormone (testosterone) decrease also, reducing sex drive (libido). Blood flow to the penis decreases. Other changes include decreases in penile sensitivity and ejaculatory volume, reduced forewarning of ejaculation, orgasm without ejaculation, more rapid detumescence, and a longer refractory period.

CHAPTER 238

Disorders of the Penis and Testes

The penis and testes (testicles) can be affected by inflammation, scar tissue, infection (including sexually transmitted diseases), or injury. Skin cancer can also develop on the penis. Birth defects can cause difficulty in urinating and in engaging in sexual intercourse. Disorders of the penis and testes can be psychologically disturbing as well as physically damaging.

Penile Inflammation

Balanitis is inflammation of the glans penis (the cone-shaped end of the penis). **Posthitis** is inflammation of the foreskin. Commonly, a yeast or bacterial infection beneath the foreskin causes posthitis. Inflammation of both the glans penis and the foreskin (**balanoposthi-**

tis) can also develop. The inflammation causes pain, itching, redness, and swelling and can ultimately lead to a narrowing (stricture) of the urethra. Men who develop balanoposthitis have an increased chance of later developing balanitis xerotica obliterans, phimosis, paraphimosis, and cancer.

In **balanitis xerotica obliterans,** chronic inflammation causes the skin near the tip of the penis to harden and turn white. The opening of the urethra is often surrounded by this hard white skin, which eventually blocks the flow of urine and semen. Antibacterial or anti-inflammatory creams may relieve the inflammation, but often the urethra must be reopened surgically.

In **phimosis,** the foreskin is tight and cannot be retracted over the glans penis. This condition is normal in a newborn or young child and usually resolves without treatment by puberty. In older men, phimosis may result from prolonged irritation or recurring balanoposthitis. The tightened foreskin can interfere with urination and sexual activity and may increase the risk of urinary tract infections. The usual treatment is circumcision.

In **paraphimosis,** the retracted foreskin cannot be pulled forward to cover the glans penis. The condition most commonly develops after a medical professional retracts the foreskin as part of a medical procedure or if someone pulls back the foreskin to clean the penis of a child and forgets to pull it back forward. The glans penis swells, increasing pressure around the trapped foreskin. The increasing pressure eventually prevents blood from reaching the penis, which could result in the destruction of penile tissue if the foreskin is not pulled back forward. Circumcision or slitting the foreskin relieves paraphimosis.

Erythroplasia of Queyrat usually occurs in uncircumcised men. It produces a discrete, reddish, velvety area on the penis, usually on or at the base of the glans penis. The cause may be long-standing irritation of the penis under the foreskin. While not cancer itself, erythroplasia of Queyrat can become cancerous if left untreated. Removal of a tissue sample for examination under a microscope (biopsy) confirms the diagnosis. Erythroplasia of Queyrat is treated with a cream containing the drug fluorouracil.

Urethral Stricture

A urethral stricture is scarring that narrows the urethra.

A urethral stricture most commonly results from previous infection or injury. A less forceful urinary stream or a double stream usually occurs with mild strictures. Severe strictures may completely block the stream of urine. The buildup of pressure behind the stricture may cause the formation of passages from the urethra into the surrounding tissues (diverticula). By decreasing the frequency or completeness of urination, strictures often lead to urinary tract infections.

A urologist diagnoses a stricture by looking directly into the urethra through a flexible viewing tube (cystoscope) after administering a lubricant containing a local anesthetic. To widen the urethra, a urologist may dilate or cut (urethrotomy) the stricture. Urethral stric-

tures can recur and may require excision of the scar and surgical reconstruction of the urethra, sometimes with a skin graft.

Penile Growths

Growths on the penis are sometimes caused by infections. One example is syphilis,▲ which may cause flat pink or gray growths (condylomata lata). Also, certain viral infections can produce one or more small, firm, raised skin growths (genital warts, or condylomata acuminata) or small, firm, dimpled growths (molluscum contagiosum).

Skin cancer can occur anywhere on the penis, most commonly at the glans penis, especially its base. Cancers affecting the skin of the penis, uncommon in the United States, are even rarer in men who have been circumcised. The cause of cancer of the penis may be long-standing irritation, usually under the foreskin. Squamous cell carcinoma■ occurs most commonly; less common cancers include Bowen's disease★ and Paget's disease.● Cancer usually first appears as a painless, reddened area with sores that do not heal for weeks.

To diagnose cancer of the penis, a doctor removes a tissue sample for examination under a microscope (biopsy). To treat the cancer, a surgeon removes it and some normal surrounding tissue, sparing as much of the penis as possible. If a lot of tissue is removed, the penis can often be rebuilt surgically.

Most men with small cancers that have not spread survive for many years after treatment. Most men with cancer that has spread die within 5 years.

Priapism

Priapism is a painful, persistent erection unaccompanied by sexual desire or excitement.

Priapism probably results from abnormalities of the blood vessels and nerves that cause blood to become trapped in the erectile tissue (corpora cavernosa) of the penis. In most cases, priapism is caused by drugs taken by mouth or injected into the penis to cause erection. Other known causes of priapism include blood clots, leukemia, sickle cell disease, a tumor in the pelvis, and an injury to the spinal cord. Sometimes, however, no cause can be found.

▲ see page 1176   ■ see page 1238
★ see page 1239   ● see page 1241

Several symptoms help differentiate priapism from normal erections. Priapism lasts longer, usually several hours. Sexual excitement does not accompany priapism, and the erection is painful. Also, in priapism, the glans penis may be soft.

The treatment of priapism depends on the cause. Any drug that appears to cause the priapism is discontinued immediately. Injection into the penis of a drug that decreases erection (for example, epinephrine, phenylephrine, terbutaline, or ephedrine) can relieve priapism caused by penile drug injection. Spinal anesthesia may relieve priapism caused by a spinal cord injury. If a blood clot is the probable cause, surgery to remove the clot or restore normal circulation in the penis is necessary. Usually, if other treatments are ineffective, priapism can be treated by draining excess blood from the penis with a needle and syringe and using fluid to wash out any blood clots or other blockages from the blood vessels. One or more of many possible drugs may also be used, depending on the underlying cause. Prolonged priapism usually impairs erectile function permanently.

Peyronie's Disease

Peyronie's disease is a fibrous thickening that contracts and deforms the penis, distorting the shape of an erection.

Many men have a small degree of curvature of their erect penis. Peyronie's disease produces a more severe deformity. Inflammation in the penis results in the formation of fibrous scar tissue that causes curvature in the erect penis, making penetration difficult or impossible. However, what causes the inflammation is not known.

The condition can make an erection painful. The scar tissue can extend into the erectile tissue (corpora cavernosa), preventing erection from occurring.

Minor curvature or disease that does not impair sexual function does not require treatment. Peyronie's disease may resolve over several months without treatment. No treatment has proven clearly successful.

Vitamin E, which can aid wound healing and decrease scarring, may be taken by mouth. Corticosteroids or verapamil can be injected into the scar tissue to decrease inflammation and reduce scarring. Ultrasound treatments can stimulate blood flow, which may prevent

further scarring. Radiation therapy may decrease pain; however, radiation often worsens tissue damage. Surgery is not recommended unless the disease has progressed and the curvature has become too severe for successful intercourse. Surgery to excise the scar may worsen the disease or result in erectile dysfunction (impotence).

Penile and Testicular Injury

Several types of injuries can affect the penis. Catching the penis in a pants zipper is common, but the resulting cut usually heals quickly. Cuts and irritations heal quickly without treatment but may need antibiotics if they become infected. Injuries to the urethra (the opening at the end of the penis) may require other specific treatment, usually provided by a urologist (a doctor who specializes in the diagnosis and treatment of genitourinary disorders).

Fracture of the penis can occur from excessive bending of an erect penis. Pain and swelling from damage to the structures that control the erection and difficulty with intercourse or urination follow. Fractures of the penis usually occur during vigorous sexual intercourse. Emergency surgery is usually necessary to repair such a fracture to prevent abnormal curvature of the penis or permanent erectile dysfunction (impotence). The penis can also be partially or fully severed. Reattachment of a severed penis is sometimes possible, but full sensation and function are rarely recovered.

The location of the scrotum makes it susceptible to injury. Blunt forces (for example, a kick or crushing blow) cause most injuries. However, occasionally gunshot or stab wounds penetrate the scrotum or testes. Rarely, the scrotum is torn off the testes. Testicular injury causes sudden, severe pain, usually with nausea and vomiting. Ultrasound may show whether the testes have ruptured. Ice packs, a jockstrap, and drugs for pain and nausea usually effectively treat internal bleeding in or around the testes. Ruptured testes require surgical repair. When the scrotum is torn off, the testes can die or lose their capacity for hormone or sperm production. Surgery to bury them under the skin of the thigh or abdomen may save the testes.

Testicular Cancer

Most testicular cancers develop in men younger than age 40. Among the types of cancer that develop in the testes are seminoma, teratoma, embryonal carcinoma, and choriocarcinoma.

The cause of testicular cancer is not known, but men whose testes did not descend into the scrotum (cryptorchidism▲) by age 3 have a greater chance of developing the disease than do men whose testes descended by that age. Cryptorchidism is best corrected surgically in childhood. Sometimes, removal of a single undescended testis in adults is recommended to reduce the risk of cancer.

Symptoms and Diagnosis

Testicular cancer may cause an enlarged testis or a lump elsewhere in the scrotum. Most lumps elsewhere in the scrotum are not caused by testicular cancer, but most lumps in the testes are. A testis normally feels like a smooth oval, with the epididymis attached behind and on top. Testicular cancer produces a firm, growing lump in or attached to the testis. With cancer, the testis loses its normal shape, becoming large, irregular, or bumpy. Although testicular cancer is often painless, the testis or lump may hurt when lightly touched and may even hurt without being touched. A firm lump on the testis requires prompt medical attention. Occasionally, blood vessels rupture within the tumor, yielding a suddenly enlarged, severely painful swelling.

Physical examination and ultrasound scanning may indicate whether a lump is part of the testis and whether it is solid (and thus more likely to be cancer) or filled with fluid (cystic). Determining the blood levels of two proteins, alpha-fetoprotein and human chorionic gonadotropin, may help in diagnosis. The levels of these proteins often increase in men with testicular cancer. If cancer is suspected, surgery to examine the testis is performed.

Treatment

The initial treatment for testicular cancer is surgical removal of the entire affected testis (radical orchiectomy). The other testis is not removed, so the man retains adequate levels of male hormones and remains fertile. Infertility sometimes occurs with testicular cancer but may subside after treatment.

With certain types of cancers, lymph nodes in the abdomen are also removed (retroperito-

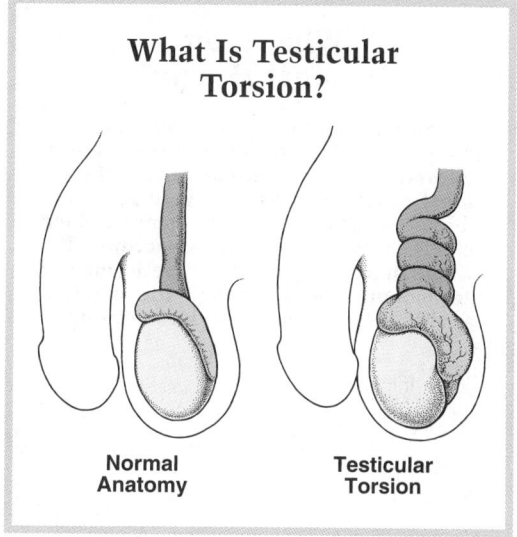

What Is Testicular Torsion?

Normal Anatomy	Testicular Torsion

neal lymph node dissection) because the cancer often spreads there first. Radiation therapy may also help, especially for a seminoma.

A combination of surgery and chemotherapy often cures testicular cancer that has spread. Blood levels of alpha-fetoprotein and human chorionic gonadotropin that were elevated at diagnosis decline after successful treatment. If levels rise after treatment, the cancer may have recurred. After surgery and any other necessary treatments are completed, a surgeon can replace the removed testis with an artificial one.

The prognosis for a man with testicular cancer depends on the type and extent of the cancer. Almost all men with seminomas, teratomas, or embryonal carcinomas that are not widespread survive 5 years or more. Most men with cancer that has spread survive 5 years or more. However, very few men with choriocarcinomas, which spread rapidly, survive even 5 years.

Testicular Torsion

Testicular torsion is the twisting of a testis on its spermatic cord so that the testis's blood supply is blocked.

Testicular torsion usually occurs in men between puberty and about age 25; however, it can occur at any age. Abnormal development of the spermatic cord or the membrane covering the testis makes testicular torsion possible

---

▲ see page 1535

What Is an Inguinal Hernia?

In an inguinal hernia, a loop of intestine pushes through an opening in the abdominal wall into the inguinal canal. The inguinal canal contains the spermatic cord, which consists of the vas deferens, blood vessels, nerves, and other structures. Before birth, the testes, which are formed in the abdomen, pass through the inguinal canal as they descend into the scrotum.

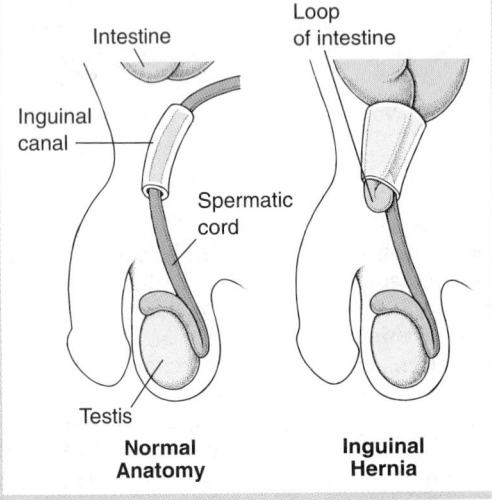

Intestine

Loop of intestine

Inguinal canal

Spermatic cord

Testis

Normal Anatomy

Inguinal Hernia

in later life. With torsion, the testis usually dies within 6 to 12 hours after the blood supply is cut off unless it is treated.

Severe pain and swelling develop suddenly in the testis. The pain may seem to come from the abdomen, and nausea and vomiting may develop. A doctor may diagnose the condition based on the man's description of his symptoms and the physical examination findings. Alternatively, the doctor may use a scan, usually an ultrasound scan, for diagnosis. Because the testis may die rapidly, emergency surgery to untwist the spermatic cord is required. Urologists usually secure both testes during surgery to prevent future episodes of torsion.

Inguinal Hernia

An inguinal hernia is a protrusion of a piece of the intestine through an opening in the abdominal wall.

An inguinal hernia extends into the groin, and can extend into the scrotum. The opening

in the abdominal wall can be present from birth or develop later in life.

Inguinal hernias usually produce a painless bulge in the groin or scrotum. The bulge may enlarge when the man stands and shrink when he lies down because the intestine slides back and forth with gravity. Sometimes a portion of the intestine is trapped in the scrotum (incarceration); this can cut off the intestine's blood supply (strangulation). Strangulated intestines may die (become gangrenous) within hours.

Surgical repair may relieve the symptoms of a hernia, depending on its size and the amount of discomfort it causes. For strangulated hernias, emergency surgery is needed to pull the intestine out of the inguinal canal and tighten the opening so the hernia cannot recur.

Epididymitis and Epididymo-orchitis

Epididymitis is inflammation of the epididymis; epididymo-orchitis is inflammation of the epididymis and testes.

Epididymitis and epididymo-orchitis are usually caused by a bacterial infection. Infection can result from surgery, the insertion of a catheter into the bladder, or the spread of infections from elsewhere in the urinary tract.

Symptoms of epididymitis and epididymo-orchitis include swelling and tenderness of the infected area, pain that may become constant and severe, fluid around the testes (hydrocele), and sometimes a fever. Rarely, an abscess (collection of pus) that feels like a soft lump develops in the scrotum.

Epididymitis and epididymo-orchitis are usually treated with antibiotics taken by mouth, bed rest, pain relievers, and ice packs applied to the scrotum. Immobilizing the scrotum with a jockstrap decreases pain from repetitive, minor bumps. Abscesses tend to drain on their own, but occasionally surgical drainage is necessary.

Hydrocele

A hydrocele is a collection of fluid in the membrane that covers the testis or testes.

A hydrocele may be present at birth or develop later in life. It is most common after age 40. Usually the cause is unknown. However, the condition occasionally results from a testicular disorder (for example, injury, epididymitis, or cancer).

Usually, a hydrocele does not cause symptoms; it is found as a painless swelling surrounding the testis. A doctor may shine a bright light on the swelling (transillumination) to confirm the diagnosis. Ultrasound examination of the testis is performed in unusual instances—for example, in a young man with no apparent cause for the hydrocele. The ultrasound may reveal an infection or tumor.

Most hydroceles need no treatment. However, surgical removal is sometimes performed for unusually large hydroceles.

Varicocele

Varicocele is a condition in which the blood supply of the testis develops varicose veins.

Veins contain valves that prevent blood from flowing backward. Faulty valves can result in a varicocele. Varicoceles usually develop on the left side of the scrotum and may produce no symptoms. Alternatively, varicoceles may cause pain and a sense of fullness that becomes bothersome. The varicocele feels like a bag of worms when the man is standing. However, the swelling usually disappears when he reclines because blood flow to the enlarged veins decreases. Rarely, a varicocele impairs fertility.

If symptoms are severe, a doctor may treat it by surgically tying off the affected veins.

Testicular Swelling

The testes can swell for many reasons. Possible causes include cancer, testicular torsion, inguinal hernia, epididymitis, hydrocele, and varicocele. Other causes are far less common in adults.

Lymphedema causes painless swelling of the entire scrotum. Lymphedema results most often from blockage of genital blood or lymph fluid returning to the body. Cirrhosis and heart failure are common causes. Lymphedema can also result from compression of the abdominal or pelvic veins or lymph glands (for example, by a tumor). A doctor makes a diagnosis of lymphedema based on findings from a physical examination. Treating the underlying cause usually gives better results than surgery.

Mumps, a viral infection, usually affects children. If an adult contracts mumps, the testes can become painful and swollen and may sometimes shrink and stop working (atrophy). Mumps can permanently damage the ability of the testes to produce sperm but does not usually cause complete infertility unless it affects both testes.

A **spermatocele** is a collection of sperm in a sac that develops next to the epididymis. Most are painless. While most spermatoceles need no treatment, one that becomes large or bothersome can be removed surgically.

CHAPTER 239

Prostate Disorders

The prostate gland lies just under the bladder and surrounds the urethra. It produces the fluid in the semen that nourishes sperm. Walnut-sized in young men, the prostate gland enlarges with age. Three common disorders affect the prostate: benign prostatic hyperplasia, prostate cancer, and prostatitis.

Benign Prostatic Hyperplasia

Benign prostatic hyperplasia is a noncancerous (benign) enlargement of the prostate gland that can make urination difficult.

Benign prostatic hyperplasia (BPH) becomes increasingly common as men age, especially after age 50. The precise cause is not known but probably involves changes induced by hormones, especially testosterone.

As the prostate enlarges, it gradually compresses the urethra and blocks the flow of urine (urinary obstruction). When a man with BPH urinates, the bladder may not empty completely. Consequently, urine stagnates in the bladder, making the man susceptible to kidney stones and urinary tract infections. Prolonged obstruction can damage the kidneys.

Drugs such as over-the-counter antihistamines and nasal decongestants can increase resistance to the flow of urine or reduce the bladder's ability to contract, causing temporary urinary retention in a man with BPH.

Symptoms

BPH first causes symptoms when the enlarged prostate begins to block the flow of urine. At first, a man may have difficulty starting urination. Urination may also feel incomplete. Because the bladder does not empty completely, he has to urinate more frequently, often at night (nocturia). Also, the need to urinate becomes more urgent. The volume and force of the urinary flow may diminish noticeably, and urine may dribble at the end of urination.

Other problems can develop, but these problems affect only a small number of men with BPH. Obstruction of urine flow with urinary retention may increase the pressure in the bladder and slow the flow of urine from the kidneys, putting increased stress on the kidneys. This increased pressure may impede kidney function, although the effect is usually temporary if the obstruction is relieved early. If obstruction is prolonged, the bladder may overstretch, causing overflow incontinence.▲ As the bladder stretches, small veins in the bladder and urethra also stretch. These veins sometimes burst when the man strains to urinate, causing blood to enter the urine. Urinary retention can develop, making urination impossible and leading to a full feeling and severe pain in the lower abdomen.

Diagnosis

By feeling the prostate during a rectal examination, a doctor can usually determine if it is enlarged. The doctor inserts his gloved and lubricated finger into the man's rectum. The prostate can be felt just in front of the rectum. A prostate affected by BPH feels enlarged and smooth but is not painful to the touch.

A doctor may take a blood sample, which can be used to assess kidney function. A test to measure the level of prostate-specific antigen in the blood (PSA test) may also be performed in men with BPH in whom prostate cancer is suspected. A urine sample can be examined to make sure there is no infection.

Further tests are not usually needed. However, if the diagnosis is unclear or the severity of BPH is not known, other tests can be useful. An ultrasound scan can measure the size of the prostate or the amount of urine remaining in the bladder after urination. Alternatively, to check for urinary retention, a doctor can insert a catheter through the urethra after the man has tried to empty his bladder.

▲ see page 858

Treatment

Treatment is not necessary unless BPH causes especially bothersome symptoms or complications (such as urinary tract infections, impaired kidney function, blood in the urine, kidney stones, or urinary retention).

When BPH is treated, drugs are usually tried first. Alpha-adrenergic blockers (such as terazosin, doxazosin, or tamsulosin) relax certain muscles of the prostate and bladder and may ease the flow of urine. Some drugs (such as finasteride) may reverse the effects of the male hormones responsible for the prostate's growth, shrinking the prostate and helping delay the need for surgery or other treatments. However, finasteride may need to be taken for 3 months or more before symptoms are relieved. Also, many men who take finasteride never experience relief of their symptoms.

If drugs are ineffective, surgery can be performed. Surgery offers the greatest relief of symptoms but may cause complications. The most common surgical procedure is transurethral resection of the prostate (TURP), in which a doctor passes an endoscope (a flexible viewing tube) up the urethra. Attached to the endoscope is a surgical instrument that is used to remove part of the prostate. TURP is usually performed using spinal anesthesia. The procedure spares the man from a surgical incision.

TURP requires overnight hospital admission and can lead to such complications as infection and bleeding. Also, about 5% of the men who undergo the procedure have urinary incontinence afterward, which is usually temporary; permanent incontinence develops in about 1% of men. The procedure causes permanent erectile dysfunction (impotence) in about 5 to 10% of men. About 10% of men undergoing TURP need the procedure repeated within 5 years. Various alternative surgical treatments offer less symptom relief than TURP; however, the risk of complications is lower. Most of these procedures are done with instruments inserted through the urethra. These treatments destroy prostate tissue with microwave heat (transurethral thermotherapy or hyperthermia), a needle (transurethral needle ablation), ultrasound (high intensity focused ultrasound), electric vaporization (transurethral electrovaporization), or lasers (laser therapy). Inflating a balloon inserted through the urethra can also forcibly widen the prostate (transurethral balloon dilation).

Problems resulting from urine obstruction may need treatment prior to definitive treatment of BPH. Urinary retention can be treated by draining the bladder with a catheter inserted through the urethra. Infections can be treated with antibiotics.

Prostate Cancer

Among men in the United States, prostate cancer is the most common cancer and the second most common cause of cancer death. The chance of developing prostate cancer increases with age and is greater for African-Americans and Hispanics, men whose close relatives had the disease, and men receiving testosterone treatment. Prostate cancer usually grows very slowly and may take decades to produce symptoms. Thus, far more men have prostate cancer than die from it. Many men with prostate cancer die without ever knowing that the cancer was present.

Prostate cancer begins as a small bump in the gland. Most prostate cancers grow very slowly and never cause symptoms. Some, however, grow rapidly or spread outside the prostate. The cause of prostate cancer is not known.

Symptoms

Prostate cancer usually causes no symptoms until it reaches an advanced stage. Sometimes, symptoms similar to those of benign prostatic hyperplasia (BPH) develop, including difficulty urinating and a need to urinate frequently or urgently. However, these symptoms do not develop until after the cancer grows large enough to compress the urethra and partially block the flow of urine. Later, prostate cancer may cause bloody urine or a sudden inability to urinate.

In some men, symptoms of prostate cancer develop after it spreads (metastasizes). The areas most often affected by cancer spread are bone (typically the pelvis, ribs, or vertebrae) and the kidneys. Bone cancer tends to be painful and may weaken the bone enough for it to easily fracture. Prostate cancer can also spread to the brain, which eventually causes seizures, confusion, headaches, weakness, or other neurologic symptoms. Spread to the spinal cord, which is also common, can cause pain, numbness, weakness, or incontinence. After the cancer spreads, anemia is common.

Screening

Because prostate cancer is common, many doctors check for it in men with no symptoms (screening). However, experts disagree about whether screening is helpful. In theory, screening offers the advantage of finding more prostate cancers early—when the disease is most easily cured. However, because prostate cancer grows so slowly and often never causes symptoms or death, determining the advantages of screening (and thus early treatment) is difficult. Screening may find cancers that would probably not hurt or kill a man even if they were never detected. Treating such a cancer can prove more damaging than leaving the cancer untreated. It is not clear whether the benefits of screening outweigh the harm from unnecessary treatment and testing. Additionally, screening often indicates the possibility of prostate cancer in men without the disease. When screening indicates the possibility of disease, more tests are done to find the cancer. These further tests are expensive, sometimes harmful, and often stressful.

To screen for prostate cancer, a doctor performs a blood test and a digital rectal examination. If the man has prostate cancer, a doctor sometimes feels a lump in the prostate gland. The lump is often hard. A blood test is performed to measure the level of prostate-specific antigen (PSA), a substance that is usually elevated in men with prostate cancer. PSA levels can be misleading: they can be normal when prostate cancer is present or elevated when prostate cancer is absent. PSA levels normally increase with age, but cancer increases the age-related change. Also, PSA levels can be slightly elevated in men with disorders other than prostate cancer (such as BPH or prostatitis) and in men who have undergone procedures involving the urinary tract within the previous 2 days.

Diagnosis

A doctor may suspect prostate cancer based on the man's symptoms or the results of screening tests. The first steps in diagnosing suspected cancer are digital rectal examination and measurement of PSA levels. If results of these tests suggest cancer, ultrasound scanning is usually performed. In men with prostate cancer, ultrasound scans may or may not reveal the cancer.

If the results of a digital rectal examination or PSA test suggest prostate cancer, tissue samples from the prostate are taken and analyzed (biopsy). When performing a biopsy, a doctor usually first obtains images of the prostate by inserting an ultrasound transducer, or probe, into the rectum (transrectal ultrasound). The doctor then obtains tissue samples with a needle inserted through the probe. This procedure takes only a few minutes and may be done with or without local anesthesia.

Two features help a doctor determine the likely course and the best treatment of the cancer: how distorted (malignant) the cells look under a microscope (grading) and how far the cancer has spread (staging).

Grading: Prostate cancer cells that are distorted tend to grow and spread quickly. The Gleason scoring system is the most common way to grade prostate cancer. Based on the microscopic examination and biochemical tests of tissues obtained from the biopsy, a number between 2 and 10 is assigned to the cancer. Scores between 4 and 6 are most common. The higher the number (high grade), the more likely it is that the cancer will spread. Cancers that are confined to a small area within the prostate and have Gleason scores of 5 or lower (low grade) rarely kill a man within 15 years of diagnosis. This is true regardless of the man's age. In contrast, up to 80% of men die within 15 years if the Gleason score is higher than 7. Large, low-grade cancers are more aggressive and may require treatment.

Staging: Testing to stage the cancer often proceeds when cancer is diagnosed. However, such testing may not be necessary when the likelihood of spread beyond the prostate is extremely low.

Prostate cancers are staged according to three criteria: how far the cancer has spread within the prostate, whether the cancer has spread to lymph nodes in areas near the prostate, and whether the cancer has spread to organs far from the prostate. Results of the digital rectal examination, ultrasound scan, and biopsy reveal how far the cancer has spread within the prostate. Computed tomography (CT) or radiolabeled antibody nuclear medicine scans of the pelvis may be performed to detect spread to the lymph nodes, and bone scanning is performed to reveal spread of the cancer to bone. If spread to the brain or spinal cord is suspected, CT or magnetic resonance imaging (MRI) of those organs is performed.

Treatment

Choosing among treatment options can be complicated and often depends on the man's lifestyle preferences. For many men, doctors are uncertain about which treatments are most effective and how likely it is that a particular treatment will prolong a man's life. Some treatments can impair quality of life. For example, major surgery, radiation therapy, and hormonal therapy often cause incontinence and erectile dysfunction (impotence). When choosing among treatment options, men need to weigh the advantages and disadvantages. For these reasons, a man's preferences are a bigger consideration in choosing treatment for prostate cancer than they might be in choosing treatment for many other diseases.

Treatment for prostate cancer usually involves one of three strategies: watchful waiting, curative treatment, and palliative therapy.

Watchful waiting foregoes all treatment until symptoms develop, if they develop at all. This strategy is best for men whose cancers are unlikely to spread or cause symptoms. For example, most cancers that are confined to a small area within the prostate and have low Gleason scores grow very slowly. These cancers usually do not spread for many years. Older men are far more likely to die before such cancers kill them or cause symptoms. Watchful waiting avoids the incontinence and erectile dysfunction associated with many treatments. During watchful waiting, symptoms can be treated if necessary. Periodic testing may also be done to see if the cancer is growing rapidly or spreading. The man may later decide to pursue a cure for the cancer if testing shows growth or spread.

Curative treatment is a common strategy for men with cancers confined to the prostate that are likely to cause troublesome symptoms or death. Such cancers include any that are growing rapidly. Curative (also called definitive) therapy may also help men with small, slowly growing cancers if the man expects to otherwise live many years. Symptoms from such cancers are unlikely to develop in less than a decade and may not do so for 15 or more years. Curative therapy can also benefit men with cancers that have spread outside the prostate and thus are likely to cause symptoms in a relatively short period. However, curative therapy is likely to be successful only with cancers that are still confined to the area near the prostate. Curative therapy can prolong life and reduce or eliminate severe symptoms resulting from some cancers. However, side effects of curative therapy, most significantly permanent erectile dysfunction and incontinence, can impair quality of life.

COMMON METHODS AND STRATEGIES FOR TREATING PROSTATE CANCER

CHARACTERISTICS OF THE CANCER	TREATMENT STRATEGY	METHOD OF TREATMENT
Small, slow-growing cancer, confined to prostate; man expected to live many years	Definitive therapy	Surgery or radiation therapy
Small, slow-growing cancer, confined to prostate; man not expected to live many years	Watchful waiting	No treatment
Large or fast-growing cancer, confined to prostate	Definitive therapy	Surgery or radiation therapy
Cancer spread to areas around the prostate, but not to distant areas	Definitive therapy	Radiation therapy
Widespread cancer	Palliative therapy	Hormonal therapy

Palliative therapy aims at treating the symptoms rather than the cancer itself. This strategy is best suited to men with widespread prostate cancer that is not curable. The growth or spread of such cancers can usually be slowed or temporarily reversed, relieving symptoms. Since these treatments cannot cure the cancer, symptoms eventually worsen. Death from the disease eventually follows.

Three forms of treatment can be used to treat prostate cancer: surgery, radiation therapy, and hormonal therapy. Chemotherapy is not usually used.

Surgery: Surgically removing the prostate (prostatectomy) is useful for cancer that is confined to the prostate. Prostatectomy is less effective in curing fast-growing cancers because they are more likely to have spread at the time of diagnosis. Prostatectomy requires general anesthesia, an overnight hospital stay, and a surgical incision, but treatment is accomplished with one procedure. Prostatectomy may lead to permanent erectile dysfunction and urinary incontinence.

There are three forms of prostatectomy: radical prostatectomy, nerve-sparing radical prostatectomy, and laparoscopic radical prostatectomy.

In radical prostatectomy, the entire prostate, the seminal vesicles, and part of the vas deferens are removed. This is the surgery most likely to cure prostate cancer. However, the procedure causes complete incontinence in about 3% of men and partial or stress incontinence in up to 20%. Temporary incontinence develops in most men and may last for several months. Incontinence is less likely in younger men. Erectile dysfunction commonly develops

after radical prostatectomy. More than 90% of men with cancer confined to the prostate live at least 10 years after radical prostatectomy. Younger men who can otherwise expect to live at least 10 to 15 more years are most likely to benefit from radical prostatectomy.

Sometimes, depending on the estimated size and location of the cancer, surgery can be performed in such a way that some of the nerves needed to achieve erection are spared—this procedure is called nerve-sparing radical prostatectomy. This procedure cannot be used to treat cancer that has invaded the nerves and blood vessels of the prostate. Nerve-sparing radical prostatectomy is less likely than non-nerve–sparing radical prostatectomy to cause erectile dysfunction.

Another form of prostatectomy is laparoscopic radical prostatectomy. The advantages of this procedure are that it requires a smaller incision and produces less postoperative pain. Disadvantages include increased expense and longer operative time. Because this procedure is technically demanding, it is offered only at certain centers.

Radiation Therapy: The goal of radiation therapy is to kill the cancer and preserve healthy tissue. Radiation may cure cancers that are confined to the prostate, as well as cancers that have invaded tissues around the prostate (but not cancer that has spread to distant organs). Radiation therapy can also relieve the pain resulting from the spread of prostate cancer to bone but cannot cure the cancer itself.

For many stages of prostate cancer, 10-year survival rates with radiation therapy are nearly as high as those achieved with surgery: more than 90% of men with cancer confined to the prostate live at least 10 years after undergoing radiation therapy. Whereas surgery is accomplished in one procedure, radiation therapy usually requires many separate treatment sessions over the course of several weeks.

During traditional radiation therapy, a machine sends beams of radiation to the prostate and surrounding tissues (traditional external beam radiation). A CT scanner is used to identify the prostate and surrounding tissues that are affected by the cancer. Treatments are usually given 5 days per week for 5 to 7 weeks. Although erectile dysfunction can occur in 30% of men, it is less likely to develop after radiation therapy than after prostatectomy. Traditional external beam radiation therapy causes incontinence in fewer than 5% of men. Urethral strictures—scars that narrow the urethra and impede the flow of urine—develop in about 7% of men. Other troublesome but usually temporary side effects of traditional external radiation therapy include burning during urination, having to urinate frequently, blood in the urine, diarrhea that is sometimes bloody, irritation of the rectum and diarrhea (radiation proctitis), and sudden urges to defecate.

With recent technical advances, doctors can more precisely focus the radiation beam on the cancer (a procedure called three-dimensional conformal radiotherapy). Cure rates for traditional external beam radiation and three-dimensional conformal radiotherapy have not yet been compared. However, conformal radiotherapy causes fewer temporary side effects.

Radiation can also be delivered by inserting radioactive implants into the prostate (brachytherapy). The implants are placed using images obtained from ultrasound or CT scans. Brachytherapy offers many advantages: it can deliver high doses of radiation to the prostate while sparing healthy surrounding tissues and producing fewer side effects. Brachytherapy can be performed in a few hours, does not require repeated treatment sessions, and uses only spinal anesthesia. However, brachytherapy may cause urethral strictures in up to 20% of men. Cure rates for brachytherapy have not yet been compared to those from other treatments. Combined treatment with brachytherapy and external beam radiation is sometimes recommended.

Prostate cancer can be resistant to radiation therapy or can recur after treatment.

Hormonal Therapy: Because most prostate cancers require testosterone to grow or spread, treatments that block the effects of this hormone (hormonal therapy) can slow progression of the tumors. Hormonal therapy is commonly used to delay the spread of the cancer or to treat widespread (metastatic) prostate cancer and is sometimes combined with other treatments. Growth and spread of metastatic prostate cancer can be slowed or temporarily reversed with hormonal therapy. Hormonal therapy can prolong life as well as improve symptoms. Eventually, however, hormonal therapy becomes ineffective, and the disease progresses.

Drugs used to treat prostate cancer in the United States include leuprolide and goserelin, which prevent the pituitary gland from stimulating the testes to make testosterone. These drugs are administered by injection in a doctor's office every 1, 3, 4, or 12 months, usually for the rest of the man's life.

Drugs that block testosterone's effects (such as flutamide, bicalutamide, and nilutamide) may also be used. These drugs are taken daily by mouth. However, drugs that block testosterone produce changes associated with low testosterone levels, such as hot flashes, osteoporosis, loss of energy, reduced muscle mass, fluid weight gain, reduced libido, reduced body hair, and often erectile dysfunction and breast enlargement (gynecomastia).

The oldest form of hormonal therapy involves the removal of both testes (bilateral orchiectomy). The effects of bilateral orchiectomy on testosterone level are equivalent to those produced by leuprolide and goserelin. Bilateral orchiectomy greatly slows the growth of the prostate cancer but produces the side effects of low testosterone levels. The physical and psychologic effects of bilateral orchiectomy make the procedure difficult for some men to accept.

Hormonal therapy usually becomes ineffective within 3 to 5 years in men with widespread prostate cancer. When cancer eventually progresses despite hormonal therapy, most men die within 1 or 2 years. When hormonal therapy fails (hormone resistance), alternative hormone drugs or chemotherapy may be tried.

After all forms of treatment, PSA levels are measured at regular intervals depending on the risk for recurrence and the time from treatment completion (usually every 3 to 4 months for the first year, every 6 months for the next year, and then every year for the rest of the man's life). Increases in the PSA levels may indicate that the cancer has recurred.

Prostatitis

Prostatitis is pain and swelling of the prostate gland.

Prostatitis usually develops for unknown reasons. Prostatitis can result from a bacterial infection that spreads to the prostate from the urinary tract or from bacteria in the bloodstream. Bacterial infections may develop slowly and tend to recur (chronic bacterial prostatitis) or develop rapidly (acute bacterial prostatitis). Rarely, fungal, viral, or protozoal infections can cause prostatitis.

Symptoms

Spasm of the muscles in the bladder and pelvis, especially in the perineum (the area between the scrotum and the anus), causes many of the symptoms of prostatitis. Prostatitis causes pain in the perineum, the lower back, and often the penis and testes. The man also may need to urinate frequently and urgently, and urinating may cause pain or burning. Pain may make obtaining an erection or ejaculating difficult or even painful. Constipation can develop, making defecation painful. Some symptoms tend to occur more often with acute bacterial prostatitis, such as fever, difficulty urinating, and blood in the urine. Bacterial prostatitis can result in a collection of pus (abscess) in the prostate or in epididymitis (inflammation of the epididymis). Chronic prostatitis can impair fertility.

Diagnosis and Treatment

The diagnosis of prostatitis is usually based on the symptoms and a physical examination. The prostate, examined through the rectum by a doctor, may be swollen and tender to the touch. Cultures are taken of urine and, sometimes, of fluids expressed from the penis after massaging the prostate during the examina-

tion. Urine cultures reveal bacterial infections located anywhere in the urinary tract. In contrast, when infection is found by culturing fluid from the prostate, the prostate is clearly the cause of the infection.

When cultures reveal no bacterial infection, prostatitis is usually difficult to cure. Most treatments for this kind of prostatitis relieve symptoms but may not cure the prostatitis. These treatments for symptoms can also help in chronic bacterial prostatitis.

Non-drug treatments include periodic prostate massage (done by a doctor by placing a finger in the rectum), frequent ejaculation, and sitting in a warm bath. Relaxation techniques (biofeedback) may relieve spasm and pain of the pelvic muscles. Among drug therapies, stool softeners can relieve painful defecation resulting from constipation. Analgesics and anti-inflammatory drugs may relieve pain and swelling regardless of its source. Alpha-adrenergic blockers that are used to treat prostate enlargement (such as doxazosin, terazosin, and tamsulosin) may help relieve symptoms by relaxing the muscles within the prostate. For reasons that are not understood, antibiotics sometimes relieve symptoms. If symptoms are severe despite other treatments, surgery, such as partial or complete removal of the prostate, may be considered as a last resort. Destruction of the prostate by microwave or laser treatments is another alternative.

When prostatitis results from a bacterial infection, an oral antibiotic that can penetrate prostate tissue (such as ofloxacin, levofloxacin, ciprofloxacin, or trimethoprim-sulfamethoxazole) is taken for 30 to 90 days. Taking antibiotics for less time may lead to a chronic infection. Chronic bacterial prostatitis can be difficult to cure. If a prostate abscess occurs, surgical drainage is usually necessary.

CHAPTER 240

Sexual Dysfunction

In men, sexual dysfunction refers to difficulties engaging in sexual intercourse. Sexual dysfunction encompasses a variety of disorders that affect sex drive (libido), the ability to achieve or maintain an erection (erectile dys-

function, or impotence), ejaculation, and the ability to achieve orgasm.

Sexual dysfunction may result from either physical or psychologic factors; many sexual problems result from a combination of both. A

Psychologic Causes of Sexual Dysfunction

- Anger toward a partner
- Anxiety
- Depression
- Discord or boredom with a partner
- Fear of pregnancy, dependence on another person, or losing control
- Feelings of detachment from sexual activities or one's partner
- Guilt
- Inhibitions or ignorance about sexual behavior
- Performance anxiety (worrying about performance during intercourse)
- Previous traumatic sexual experiences (for example, rape, incest, sexual abuse, or previous sexual dysfunction)

physical problem may lead to psychologic problems (such as anxiety, fear, or stress), which can in turn aggravate the physical problem. Men sometimes pressure themselves or feel pressured by a partner to perform well sexually and become distressed when they cannot (performance anxiety). Performance anxiety can be troublesome and further worsen a man's ability to enjoy sexual relations.

Erectile dysfunction is the most common sexual dysfunction in men. Decreased libido also affects some men. Problems with ejaculation include uncontrolled ejaculation before or shortly after penetrating the vagina (premature ejaculation), ejaculation into the bladder (retrograde ejaculation), and blockage (obstruction) of the ejaculatory ducts.

Normal Sexual Function

Normal sexual function is a complex interaction involving both the mind (thoughts, memories, and emotions) and the body. The nervous, circulatory, and endocrine (hormonal) systems all interact with the mind to produce a sexual response. A delicate and balanced interplay among all parts of the nervous system controls the sexual response in men.

Desire (also called sex drive or libido) is the wish to engage in sexual activity. It may be triggered by thoughts, words, sights, smell, or touch. Desire leads to the first stage of the sex-

ual response cycle, excitement. Excitement is sexual arousal. During excitement, blood flow to the penis increases, leading to an erection. Also, muscle tension increases throughout the body. In the plateau stage, excitement and muscle tension are maintained or intensified. Orgasm is the peak or climax of sexual excitement. At orgasm, muscle tension throughout the body further increases. The man experiences contractions of the pelvic muscles followed by a release of muscle tension. Semen is usually, but not always, ejaculated from the penis. Although ejaculation and orgasm often occur nearly simultaneously, they are separate events. Ejaculation can occur without orgasm. Also, orgasm can occur in the absence of ejaculation, especially before puberty, or with the use of certain drugs (such as some antidepressants). Most men find orgasm highly pleasurable. In resolution, a man returns to an unaroused state. After orgasm, men cannot have another erection for some time (refractory period), often as short as 20 minutes or less in young men but much longer in older men. The time between erections generally increases as men age.

Erectile Dysfunction

Erectile dysfunction (impotence) is the inability to achieve or maintain an erection.

Every man is occasionally unable to achieve an erection; this is normal. Erectile dysfunction occurs when the problem is frequent or continuous.

Erectile dysfunction can range from mild to severe. A man with mild erectile dysfunction may occasionally achieve a full erection, but more often he achieves an erection that is inadequate for penetration. He may frequently be unable to achieve an erection at all. A man with severe erectile dysfunction is rarely able to achieve an erection.

Erectile dysfunction becomes more common with age but is not part of the normal aging process. About half of men 65 years of age and three fourths of men 80 years of age have erectile dysfunction.

Causes

To achieve an erection, the penis needs both an adequate inflow of blood and a slowing of blood outflow.▲ Disorders that narrow arteries and decrease blood inflow (such as atherosclerosis, diabetes, or a blood clot) or surgery

---

▲ see page 1322

on the blood vessels can cause erectile dysfunction. Also, abnormalities in the veins of the penis can sometimes drain blood back to the body so rapidly that erections cannot be sustained despite adequate blood inflow.

Neurologic damage is another possible cause of erectile dysfunction. Damage to the nerves leading to or from the penis produces erectile dysfunction. Such damage could result from surgery (most commonly prostate surgery), spinal disease, diabetes, multiple sclerosis, peripheral nerve disorders, stroke, alcohol, and drugs.

Occasionally, hormonal disturbances (such as abnormally low levels of testosterone) cause erectile dysfunction. Also, factors that decrease a man's energy level (such as illness, fatigue, and stress) can make erections difficult.

Many drugs can interfere with the ability to achieve an erection, especially among older men. Drugs that commonly cause erectile dysfunction include antihypertensives, antidepressants, some sedatives, cimetidine, digoxin, lithium, and antipsychotics.

Psychologic issues (such as depression, performance anxiety, guilt, fear of intimacy, and ambivalence about sexual orientation) can impair the ability to achieve erections. Psychologic causes are more common in younger men. Any new stressful situation, such as a change of sex partners or problems with relationships or at work, can also contribute.

Symptoms

Sex drive (libido) often decreases in men with erectile dysfunction, although some men do maintain a normal libido. Regardless of whether libido changes, men with erectile dysfunction have difficulty engaging in intercourse either because the erect penis is not sufficiently hard, long, or elevated for penetration or because the erection cannot be sustained. Some men stop having erections during sleep or upon awakening. Others may attain strong erections sometimes but be unable to attain or maintain erections other times.

When testosterone levels are low, the result is more likely to be a drop in libido than erectile dysfunction. Low testosterone levels can cause gradual development of many symptoms, including enlargement of the breasts (gynecomastia▲), raised pitch of the voice, shrinking of the testes (testicles), and loss of pubic hair. Low testosterone may also cause thinning of the bones, loss of energy, and loss of muscle mass.

Sexual Activity and Heart Disease

Sexual activity is generally less taxing than moderate to heavy physical activity and is therefore usually safe for men with heart disease. Although the risk of a heart attack is higher during sexual activity than it is during rest, the risk is still very low during sexual activity.

Still, sexually active men with diseases of the heart and cardiovascular system (which include angina, high blood pressure, heart failure, abnormal rhythms of the heart, and blockage of the aortic valve [aortic stenosis]) need to take reasonable precautions. Usually, sexual activity is safe if the disease is mild, if it causes few symptoms, and if blood pressure is normal. If the disease is moderate in severity or if the man has other conditions that make a heart attack likely, testing may be necessary to determine how safe sexual activity is. If the disease is severe or if the man has an enlarged heart that blocks the flow of blood leaving the left ventricle (obstructive cardiomyopathy), sexual activity should be deferred until after treatment reduces the severity of the symptoms. Use of sildenafil may be dangerous; men taking nitroglycerine should not use sildenafil. Sexual activity should also be deferred until at least 2 to 6 weeks after a heart attack.

Most often, testing to determine the safety of sexual activity involves monitoring the heart for signs of poor blood supply while exercising on a treadmill. If the blood supply is adequate during exercise, a heart attack during sexual activity is very unlikely.

Diagnosis

To diagnose erectile dysfunction, a doctor performs a general physical examination and examines the man's genitals. The doctor may also assess the function of the nerves and blood vessels that supply the genitals. Measurement of blood pressure in the legs may reveal a problem with the arteries in the pelvis and groin that supply blood to the penis. Examination of the man's rectum may reveal a problem with the nerve supply of the penis.

A blood sample is taken to measure the level of testosterone. Certain blood tests can help identify diseases that may lead to temporary or permanent erectile dysfunction. For

▲ see box on page 1323

example, blood tests can reveal evidence of diabetes (which can lead to permanent erectile dysfunction) or infection (which can lead to temporary erectile dysfunction).

If a problem with the arteries or veins is suspected, specialized tests may be performed. Ultrasound examination can reveal narrowing or blockage within the arteries of the penis.

Treatment

Some men and their partners may choose not to pursue treatment for erectile dysfunction. Physical contact without an erection may satisfy their needs for intimacy and fulfillment.

Sometimes, discontinuing use of a particular drug can improve erections.

For men who choose to pursue treatment, there are many choices.

Drug Treatment: Many drugs are used to treat erectile dysfunction. Most drugs given to treat erectile dysfunction increase blood flow to the penis. Most of these drugs are given by mouth, but some drugs can be applied locally—by injection or insertion into the penis.

Sildenafil is the drug most frequently used to treat erectile dysfunction. Sildenafil, which is taken by mouth, increases the frequency and rigidity of erections within 30 to 60 minutes; erections last about 10 to 30 minutes. The drug is effective only when the man is sexually aroused. Side effects of sildenafil include headache, flushing, runny nose, upset stomach, and vision problems. More serious side effects, including dangerously low blood pressure, can occur when sildenafil is taken with certain other drugs (such as nitroglycerin or amyl nitrite). Because of this, a man should not take sildenafil while taking drugs such as nitroglycerin. Drugs similar to sildenafil are likely to become available in the future.

Other oral drugs that have been used in the treatment of erectile dysfunction are phentolamine, yohimbine, and testosterone. Phentolamine is sometimes prescribed for erectile dysfunction but is less effective than sildenafil. Yohimbine is occasionally used to treat men whose erectile dysfunction is caused by psychologic factors, but the drug can cause side effects (including anxiety, shaking, rapid heart rate, and increased blood pressure) and is only minimally effective.

Drugs injected or inserted into the penis widen the arteries that supply blood to the penis. Men who cannot tolerate drugs taken by mouth can often be treated with these drugs.

Alprostadil, in the form of a pellet (suppository), can be inserted into the penis through the urethra. When used alone, alprostadil may result in an erection, but it is more effective when combined with another treatment, such as a binding device. Alprostadil may cause lightheadedness, a burning sensation of the penis, or, occasionally, a prolonged, painful erection (priapism▲). Because these serious side effects occasionally occur, a man usually takes his first dose under observation in a doctor's office.

A man can also induce an erection by injecting drugs (such as alprostadil alone or a combination of alprostadil, papaverine, and phentolamine) into the shaft of his penis. Injection is one of the most effective ways to obtain an erection. However, many men are unwilling to inject their penis. Also, the injection can cause priapism, and repeated injections may eventually produce scar tissue.

Testosterone replacement therapy may help men whose erectile dysfunction is caused by abnormally low testosterone levels. Unlike other drugs, which work by increasing blood flow to the penis, testosterone works by correcting a hormonal deficiency. Testosterone can be taken in many forms, including pills, patches, topical creams, and injections. Side effects can include liver dysfunction, increased red blood cell counts, increased risk of stroke, and enlargement of the prostate.■

Constriction (binding) and Vacuum Devices: Most men with erectile dysfunction can achieve erections by using a constriction device with or without a vacuum device. These devices are among the least expensive treatments for erectile dysfunction, and they enable a man to avoid the side effects that can occur with drug treatment. However, the devices can cause excessive bruising in men who are taking blood-thinning (anticoagulant) drugs and in those with diseases that interfere with blood clotting. Constriction devices should not be left on for longer than 30 minutes.

Constriction devices (such as bands and rings made of metal, rubber, or leather) are placed at the base of the penis to slow the outflow of blood. These medically engineered devices can be purchased with a doctor's prescription in a pharmacy, but inexpensive versions (often called "cock rings") can be purchased in stores that sell sexual paraphernalia.

A constriction device used alone may produce an erection in a man with mild erectile

---

▲ see page 1325   ■ see box on page 1322

dysfunction, especially when the problem is maintenance of the erection. A constriction device can also be used in combination with a vacuum device. A binding device occasionally causes pain or interferes with ejaculation.

Vacuum devices (which consist of a hollow chamber attached to a source of suction) fit over the penis, creating a seal. Suction applied to the chamber draws blood into the penis, producing an erection. Once an erection is achieved, a binding device is applied to prevent the blood from flowing out of the penis.

Surgery: When erectile dysfunction does not respond to other treatments, a device that simulates an erection (prosthesis) can be surgically implanted in the penis.

A variety of prostheses are available. One type consists of firm rods that are inserted into the penis to create a permanently hard penis. Another prosthesis is an inflatable balloon that is inserted into the penis; before having intercourse, the man inflates the balloon with a small pump (which may be part of the prosthesis). Surgical implantation of a penile prosthesis requires at least a 3-day hospitalization and a 6-week recovery before intercourse is attempted.

Psychologic Therapy: Some types of psychologic therapy (which include behavior-modification techniques, such as the sensate focus technique▲) can improve the mental and emotional factors that contribute to erectile dysfunction. Psychologic therapy can even help when the erectile dysfunction has a physical cause, because psychologic factors often compound the problem.

Specific therapies are selected based on the particular psychologic cause of the man's erectile dysfunction. For example, if the man is suffering from depression, psychotherapy or antidepressants may help with erectile dysfunction. Sometimes psychotherapy can reduce anxiety about sexual performance in men with erectile dysfunction from any cause. Improvement may take a long time, and many sessions are usually required. A man, and often his partner, must be highly motivated for psychotherapy to work.

Several folk remedies for erectile dysfunction exist, but none have proven to be effective.

Decreased Libido

Decreased libido is a reduction in sex drive.

Sex drive (libido) varies greatly among men. Different men find different degrees of libido

The Stop-and-Start Technique

One technique used to treat premature ejaculation is the stop-and-start technique, which trains the man to experience high levels of excitement without ejaculating. The technique involves stimulation of the penis until the man feels that he will soon ejaculate unless the stimulation stops. He signals his partner to stop stimulation, which is resumed after 20 to 30 seconds. The partners rehearse this technique at first with hand stimulation and later during intercourse. With practice, more than 95% of the men learn to delay ejaculation for 5 to 10 minutes or even longer. The technique also helps reduce the anxiety that often aggravates the problem.

satisfactory. Libido may be decreased temporarily by conditions such as fatigue or anxiety. Libido also tends to gradually decrease as a man ages. Persistent low libido may cause a man and his sex partner distress.

Occasionally, libido can be low throughout a man's life. Lifelong low libido can result from traumatic childhood sexual experiences or from learned suppression of sexual thoughts. Most often, however, low libido develops after years of normal sexual desire. Psychologic factors, such as depression, anxiety, and relationship problems, are often the cause. Some drugs (such as those used to treat high blood pressure, depression, or anxiety) and decreased levels of testosterone can also lower libido.

A man with decreased libido thinks less about sex. He loses interest in sexual fantasy and masturbation, and also in sexual activity. Even sexual stimulation, by sights, words, or touch, may fail to provoke interest. The man often retains the capacity for sexual function. Some men continue to engage in sexual activity to satisfy their partner.

A blood test can measure the level of testosterone in the blood. However, the diagnosis is usually based on the man's description of his symptoms.

If the cause is psychologic, various psychologic therapies—including behavioral therapies, such as the sensate focus technique■—can help. If the testosterone level is low, testosterone can be given, usually as a patch or

---

▲ see box on page 1385

■ see box on page 1385

gel applied to the skin or as an injection. If a drug appears to be the cause, a doctor can often try treating the man with a different drug.

Premature Ejaculation

Premature ejaculation is ejaculation that occurs too early, usually before, upon, or shortly after penetration.

Many males, especially adolescents, ejaculate sooner than they or their partners would like. Premature ejaculation is not just ejaculation that occurs before a man wants it to but rather ejaculation that occurs very soon—often within a minute or two—after penetration.

Many experts believe that premature ejaculation almost always results from anxiety or other psychologic causes. Others think that unusually sensitive penile skin may be a cause. Premature ejaculation is rarely caused by a disease, although inflammation of the prostate gland or a nervous system disorder can cause the condition.

Premature ejaculation can distress a man and his partner. If the man ejaculates too early, the partner may be left unsatisfied sexually and may become resentful.

Behavior modification therapy can help most men overcome premature ejaculation. A therapist provides reassurance, explains why premature ejaculation occurs, and teaches the man strategies for delaying ejaculation.

Other methods that can help a man delay ejaculation include drug treatment (with a selective serotonin reuptake inhibitor such as fluoxetine, paroxetine, or sertraline), application of an anesthetic to the penis, and use of condoms, which tend to decrease sensation. Sometimes a combination of drug treatment and behavioral therapy enables a man to delay

ejaculation even longer than he might be able to with only one of these treatments. When premature ejaculation is caused by more serious psychologic problems, psychologic therapy may help.

Retrograde Ejaculation

Retrograde ejaculation is a condition in which semen is ejaculated backward into the bladder rather than out through the penis.

In retrograde ejaculation, the part of the bladder that normally closes during ejaculation (the bladder neck) remains open, causing the ejaculatory fluid to travel backward into the bladder. Common causes of retrograde ejaculation include diabetes, spinal cord injuries, certain drugs, and some surgical operations (including major abdominal or pelvic surgery—one of the most common causes is transurethral resection of the prostate).

Men with retrograde ejaculation can still have orgasms. However, retrograde ejaculation decreases the amount of fluid ejaculated out of the penis; sometimes, no fluid comes out. The condition can cause infertility but is otherwise not harmful.

A doctor makes the diagnosis of retrograde ejaculation by finding a large amount of sperm in a urine sample. Most men need no treatment. About one third of men with retrograde ejaculation improve after treatment with drugs that close the bladder neck (such as pseudoephedrine, phenylephrine, chlorpheniramine, brompheniramine, or imipramine). However, most of these drugs can increase heart rate and blood pressure, which can be dangerous in men with high blood pressure or heart disease.

If infertility requires treatment and drugs do not help, doctors can sometimes collect a man's sperm for insemination.▲

▲ see page 1416

WOMEN'S HEALTH ISSUES

241 Biology of the Female Reproductive System..........................1343

External Genital Organs ▪ Internal Genital Organs ▪ Puberty ▪
Menstrual Cycle ▪ Effects of Aging

242 Symptoms and Diagnosis of Gynecologic Disorders 1349

Vaginal Itching ▪ Abnormal Vaginal Discharge ▪ Abnormal
Vaginal Bleeding ▪ Excessive Hairiness ▪ Pelvic Pain ▪
Breast Symptoms ▪ Gynecologic History ▪ Gynecologic
Examination ▪ Diagnostic Procedures

243 Menopause 1356

Premature Menopause

244 Menstrual Disorders and Abnormal Vaginal Bleeding............1361

Premenstrual Syndrome ▪ Dysmenorrhea ▪ Amenorrhea ▪
Abnormal Vaginal Bleeding ▪ Dysfunctional Uterine Bleeding ▪
Polycystic Ovary Syndrome

245 Endometriosis 1369

246 Fibroids 1372

247 Vaginal Infections..1374

248 Pelvic Inflammatory Disease...1377

249 Pelvic Floor Disorders 1379

250 Sexual Dysfunction 1382

Dyspareunia ▪ Vaginismus ▪ Vulvodynia ▪ Decreased
Libido ▪ Sexual Arousal Disorder ▪ Orgasmic Disorder

251 Breast Disorders 1387

Breast Cysts ▪ Fibroadenomas ▪ Fibrocystic Breast Disease ▪
Breast Infection and Abscess ▪ Breast Cancer

252 Cancers of the Female Reproductive System 1401

Cancer of the Uterus ▪ Cancer of the Ovaries ▪ Cancer of the
Cervix ▪ Cancer of the Vulva ▪ Cancer of the Vagina ▪
Cancer of the Fallopian Tubes ▪ Hydatidiform Mole

253   **Violence Against Women**..**1410**

Domestic Violence ▪ Rape

254   **Infertility**..**1414**

Problems With Sperm ▪ Problems With Ovulation ▪ Problems
With the Fallopian Tubes ▪ Problems With Mucus in the Cervix ▪
Fertilization Techniques

255   **Family Planning** **1419**

Contraception ▪ Abortion ▪ Sterilization

256   **Detection of Genetic Disorders** **1429**

Genetic Screening ▪ Prenatal Diagnostic Testing

257   **Normal Pregnancy** **1434**

Detecting and Dating a Pregnancy ▪ Stages of Development ▪
Physical Changes in a Pregnant Woman ▪ Medical Care During
Pregnancy ▪ Self-Care During Pregnancy

258   **High-Risk Pregnancy** **1444**

Risk Factors Present Before Pregnancy ▪ Risk Factors That Develop
During Pregnancy ▪ Miscarriage

259   **Drug Use During Pregnancy** **1458**

Social Drugs ▪ Illicit Drugs ▪ Drugs Used During Labor and
Delivery

260   **Normal Labor and Delivery** **1464**

261   **Complications of Labor and Delivery** **1470**

Problems With the Timing of Labor ▪ Problems Affecting the Fetus
or Newborn ▪ Problems Affecting the Woman ▪ Procedures
Used During Labor

262   **Postdelivery Period**...**1476**

What to Expect in the Hospital ▪ What to Expect at Home ▪
Postpartum Infections ▪ Blood Clots ▪ Thyroid Disorders ▪
Postpartum Depression

CHAPTER 241

Biology of the Female Reproductive System

The female reproductive system consists of the external and internal genital organs. (The breasts are sometimes considered part of the reproductive system.▲) However, other parts of the body also affect the development and functioning of the reproductive system. They include the hypothalamus (an area of the brain), the pituitary gland (located directly below the hypothalamus), and the adrenal glands (located on top of the kidneys). The hypothalamus orchestrates the interactions among the genital organs, pituitary gland, and adrenal glands. These parts of the body interact with each other by releasing hormones. Hormones are chemical messengers that control and coordinate activities in the body. The hypothalamus produces gonadotropin-releasing hormone, which stimulates the pituitary gland to produce luteinizing hormone and follicle-stimulating hormone. These hormones stimulate the ovaries to produce the female sex hormones, estrogen and progesterone, and some male sex hormones (androgens). (Male sex hormones stimulate the growth of pubic and underarm hair at puberty and maintain muscle mass in girls as well as boys.) After childbirth, the hypothalamus signals the pituitary gland to produce prolactin, a hormone that stimulates milk production. The adrenal glands produce small amounts of female and male sex hormones.

External Genital Organs

The external genital organs consist of the mons pubis, labia majora, labia minora, Bartholin's glands, and clitoris. The area containing these organs is called the vulva. The external genital organs have three main functions: enabling sperm to enter the body, protecting the internal genital organs from infectious organisms, and providing sexual pleasure.

The mons pubis is a rounded mound of fatty tissue that covers the pubic bone. During puberty, it becomes covered with hair. The mons pubis contains oil-secreting (sebaceous) glands that release pheromones, which are involved in sexual attraction. The labia majora (liter-ally, large lips) are relatively large, fleshy folds of tissue that enclose and protect the other external genital organs. They are comparable to the scrotum in males. The labia majora contain sweat and sebaceous glands, which produce lubricating secretions. After puberty, hair appears on the labia majora.

The labia minora (literally, small lips) can be very small or up to 2 inches wide. The labia minora lie just inside the labia majora and surround the openings to the vagina and urethra. A rich supply of blood vessels gives the labia minora a pink color. During sexual stimulation, these blood vessels become engorged with blood, causing the labia minora to swell and become more sensitive to stimulation.

The area between the vaginal opening and the anus, at the back of the labia majora, is called the perineum. It varies in length from almost 1 to more than 2 inches (2 to 5 centimeters). A long perineum is less likely to tear during childbirth.

The labia majora and the perineum are covered with skin similar to that on the rest of the body. The skin is thick, dry, and sometimes scaly. In contrast, the labia minora are lined with a mucous membrane, whose surface is kept moist by fluid secreted by specialized cells.

The opening to the vagina is called the introitus. The vaginal opening is the entryway for the penis during sexual intercourse and the exit for menstrual blood and vaginal discharge as well as a baby. When stimulated, Bartholin's glands (located beside the vaginal opening) secrete a thick fluid that supplies lubrication for intercourse. The opening to the urethra, which carries urine from the bladder to the outside, is located above and in front of the vaginal opening.

The clitoris, located between the labia minora, is a small protrusion that corresponds to the penis in the male. The clitoris, like the penis, is very sensitive to sexual stimulation and can become erect. Stimulating the clitoris can result in an orgasm.

▲ see page 1387

External Female Genital Organs

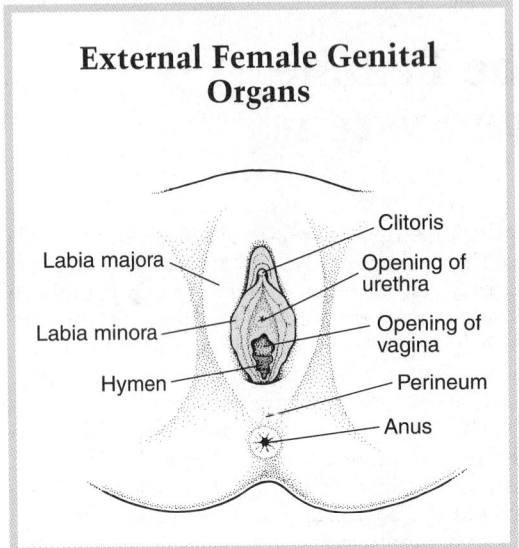

- Labia majora
- Labia minora
- Hymen
- Clitoris
- Opening of urethra
- Opening of vagina
- Perineum
- Anus

Internal Genital Organs

The internal genital organs form a pathway (the genital tract). This pathway consists of the following:

- the vagina (part of the birth canal), where sperm are deposited and from which a baby can emerge
- the uterus, where an embryo can develop into a fetus
- the fallopian tubes (oviducts), where a sperm can fertilize an egg
- the ovaries, which produce and release eggs.

Sperm can travel up the tract, and eggs down the tract.

At the beginning of the tract, just inside the vaginal opening is the hymen, a mucous membrane. In virgins, the hymen usually encircles the opening like a tight ring, but it may completely cover the opening. The hymen helps protect the genital tract but is not necessary for health. It may tear at the first attempt at sexual intercourse, or it may be so soft and pliable that no tearing occurs. The hymen may also be torn during exercise or insertion of a tampon or diaphragm. Tearing usually causes slight bleeding. In women who have had intercourse, the hymen may be unnoticeable or may form small tags of tissue around the vaginal opening.

▲ see page 1176

The vagina is a narrow, muscular but elastic organ about 4 to 5 inches long in an adult woman. It connects the external genital organs with the uterus. The vagina is the main female organ of sexual intercourse, into which the penis is inserted. It is the passageway for sperm to the egg and for menstrual bleeding or a baby to the outside.

Usually, there is no space inside the vagina unless it is stretched open—for example, during an examination or sexual intercourse. The lower third of the vagina is surrounded by elastic muscles that control the diameter of its opening. These muscles contract rhythmically during sexual intercourse and can be toned by Kegel exercises.

The vagina is lined with a mucous membrane, kept moist by fluids oozing from cells on its surface and by secretions from glands in the cervix (the lower part of the uterus). These fluids may pass to the outside as a vaginal discharge, which is normal. During a woman's reproductive years, the lining of the vagina has folds and wrinkles. Before puberty and after menopause (if the woman is not taking estrogen), the lining is smooth.

The uterus is a thick-walled, muscular, pear-shaped organ located in the middle of the pelvis, behind the bladder, and in front of the rectum. The uterus is anchored in position by several ligaments. The main function of the uterus is to sustain a developing fetus. The uterus consists of the cervix and the main body (the corpus).

The cervix, the lower part of the uterus, protrudes into the upper end of the vagina and can be seen during a pelvic examination. Like the vagina, the cervix is lined with a mucous membrane, but the mucous membrane of the cervix is smooth.

Sperm can enter and menstrual blood can exit the uterus through a channel in the cervix. The channel is narrow. During labor, the channel widens to let the baby through. The cervix is usually a good barrier against bacteria, except during the menstrual period, around the time an egg is released by the ovaries (ovulation), or during labor. Bacteria can enter the uterus through the cervix during sexual intercourse. Unlike the bacteria that cause sexually transmitted diseases,▲ bacteria normally found in the vagina rarely cause problems.

The channel through the cervix is lined with glands that secrete mucus. This mucus is thick and impenetrable to sperm until just be-

Internal Female Genital Organs

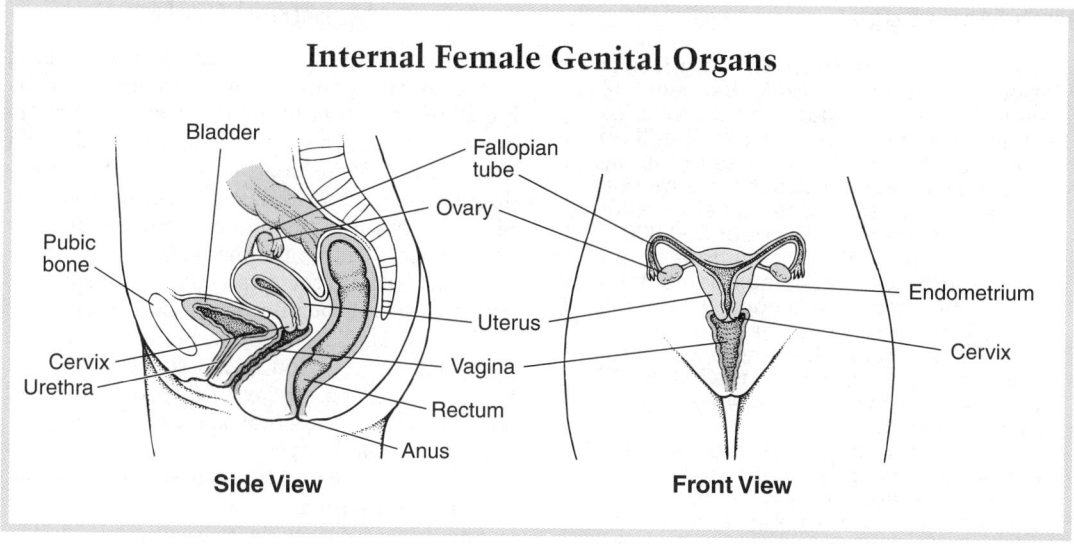

Side View · Front View

Bladder, Fallopian tube, Ovary, Pubic bone, Endometrium, Cervix, Uterus, Cervix, Urethra, Vagina, Rectum, Anus

fore ovulation. At ovulation, the consistency of the mucus changes so that sperm can swim through it and fertilization can occur. At this time, the mucus-secreting glands of the cervix can store live sperm for 2 or 3 days. These sperm can later move up through the corpus and into the fallopian tubes to fertilize an egg. Thus, intercourse 1 or 2 days before ovulation can lead to pregnancy. For some women, the time between a menstrual period and ovulation varies from month to month. Consequently, pregnancy can occur at different times during a menstrual cycle.

The corpus of the uterus, which is highly muscular, can stretch to accommodate a growing fetus. Its muscular walls contract during labor to push the baby out through the cervix and the vagina. During the reproductive years, the corpus is twice as long as the cervix. After menopause, the reverse is true.

As part of a woman's reproductive cycle (which usually lasts about a month), the lining of the corpus (endometrium) thickens. If the woman does not become pregnant during that cycle, most of the endometrium is shed and bleeding occurs, resulting in the menstrual period.

The two fallopian tubes, which are about 2 to 3 inches long, extend from the upper edges of the uterus toward the ovaries. The tubes do not connect with the ovaries. Instead, the end of each tube flares into a funnel shape with fingerlike extensions (fimbriae). When an egg is released from an ovary, the fimbriae guide the egg into the relatively large opening of a fallopian tube.

The fallopian tubes are lined with tiny hairlike projections (cilia). The cilia and the muscles in the tube's wall propel an egg downward through the tube to the uterus. The egg may be fertilized by a sperm in the fallopian tube.▲

The ovaries are usually pearl-colored, oblong, and somewhat smaller than a chicken egg. They are attached to the uterus by ligaments. In addition to producing female sex hormones (estrogen and progesterone) and male sex hormones, the ovaries produce and release eggs. The developing egg cells (oocytes) are contained in fluid-filled cavities (follicles) in the wall of the ovaries. Each follicle contains one oocyte.

Puberty

The physical changes that occur at puberty are regulated by changes in levels of hormones that are produced by the pituitary gland—luteinizing hormone and follicle-stimulating hormone. At birth, the levels of these hormones are high, but they decrease within a few months and remain low until puberty. Early in puberty, levels of luteinizing hormone and follicle-stimulating hormone increase, stimulating the production of sex hormones. The increased levels of sex hormones

▲ see page 1435

How Many Eggs?

A baby girl is born with egg cells (oocytes) in her ovaries. Between 16 and 20 weeks of pregnancy, the ovaries of a female fetus contain 6 to 7 million oocytes. Most of the oocytes gradually waste away, leaving about 1 to 2 million present at birth. None develop after birth. At puberty, only about 300,000— more than enough for a lifetime of fertility—remain. Only a small percentage of oocytes mature into eggs. The many thousands of oocytes that do not mature degenerate. Degeneration progresses more rapidly in the 10 to 15 years before menopause. All are gone by menopause.

Only about 400 eggs are released during a woman's reproductive life, usually one during each menstrual cycle. Until released, an egg remains dormant in its follicle—suspended in the middle of a cell division. Thus, the egg is one of the longest-lived cells in the body. Because a dormant egg cannot perform the usual cellular repair processes, the opportunity for damage increases as a woman ages. A chromosomal or genetic abnormality is thus more likely when a woman conceives a baby later in life.

result in physical changes, including maturation of the breasts, ovaries, uterus, and vagina. Normally, these changes occur sequentially during puberty, resulting in sexual maturity.▲

The first change of puberty is usually the start of breast development (breast budding). In girls who live in the United States, this change usually occurs around age 9 to 11. Shortly afterward, pubic and underarm hair begin to grow. The interval from breast budding to the first menstrual period is usually about $2\frac{1}{2}$ years. In the United States, girls, on average, have their first period when they are almost 13. The girl's body shape changes, and the percentage of body fat increases. The growth spurt accompanying puberty typically begins even before the breasts start to develop. Growth is fastest relatively early in puberty (before menstrual periods begin) and peaks at about age 12. Then growth slows considerably, usually stopping between the ages of 14 and 16.

Menstrual Cycle

Menstruation is the shedding of the lining of the uterus (endometrium) accompanied by bleeding. It occurs in approximately monthly cycles except during pregnancy and after menopause. Menstruation marks the reproductive years of a woman's life, from the start of menstruation (menarche) during puberty until its cessation (menopause■).

By definition, the first day of bleeding is counted as the beginning of each menstrual cycle (day 1). The cycle ends just before the next menstrual period. Menstrual cycles range from about 21 to 40 days. Only 10 to 15% of women have cycles that are exactly 28 days. The intervals between periods are usually longest in the years immediately after menarche and before menopause.

The menstrual cycle is regulated by hormones: luteinizing hormone and follicle-stimulating hormone, which are produced by the pituitary gland, and estrogen and progesterone, which are produced by the ovaries. The cycle has three phases: follicular, ovulatory, and luteal.

The **follicular phase** lasts from the first day of bleeding to immediately before a surge in the level of luteinizing hormone. The surge results in release of the egg (ovulation). During this phase, the follicles in the ovaries develop. The follicular phase varies in length, averaging about 13 days of the cycle. This phase tends to become shorter at the end of the reproductive years, near menopause.

At the beginning of the follicular phase, the lining of the uterus (endometrium) thickens with fluids and nutrients designed to nourish an embryo. If no egg has been fertilized, estrogen and progesterone levels decrease, the endometrium is shed, and menstrual bleeding occurs. Menstrual bleeding lasts 3 to 7 days, averaging 5 days. Blood loss during a cycle ranges from $\frac{1}{2}$ to 10 ounces, averaging $4\frac{1}{2}$ ounces. A sanitary pad or tampon, depending on the type, can hold up to an ounce of blood. Menstrual blood, unlike blood resulting from an injury, usually does not clot unless the bleeding is very heavy.

During the first part of the follicular phase, the pituitary gland increases slightly its production of follicle-stimulating hormone. This hormone then stimulates the growth of 3 to 30 follicles, each containing an egg. Later in the phase, as the level of this hormone decreases, only one of these follicles—the dominant follicle—continues to grow. It soon be-

▲ see box on page 1553   ■ see page 1356

Changes During the Menstrual Cycle

A menstrual cycle is regulated by the complex interaction of hormones: luteinizing hormone and follicle-stimulating hormone, which are produced by the pituitary gland, and the female sex hormones estrogen and progesterone, which are produced by the ovaries.

The menstrual cycle begins with menstrual bleeding (menstruation), which marks the first day of the follicular phase. Bleeding occurs when levels of estrogen and progesterone decrease, causing the thickened lining of the uterus (endometrium) to degenerate and be shed. During the first half of this phase, the follicle-stimulating hormone level increases slightly, stimulating the development of several follicles. Each follicle contains an egg. Later, as the follicle-stimulating hormone level decreases, only one follicle continues to develop. This follicle produces estrogen.

The ovulatory phase begins with a surge in luteinizing hormone and follicle-stimulating hormone levels. Luteinizing hormone stimulates egg release (ovulation), which usually occurs 16 to 32 hours after the surge begins. The estrogen level peaks during the surge, and the progesterone level starts to increase.

During the luteal phase, levels of luteinizing hormone and follicle-stimulating hormone decrease. The ruptured follicle closes after releasing the egg and forms a corpus luteum, which produces progesterone. Later in this phase, the level of estrogen increases. Progesterone and estrogen cause the lining of the uterus to thicken more. If the egg is not fertilized, the corpus luteum degenerates and no longer produces progesterone, the estrogen level decreases, the lining degenerates and is shed, and a new menstrual cycle begins.

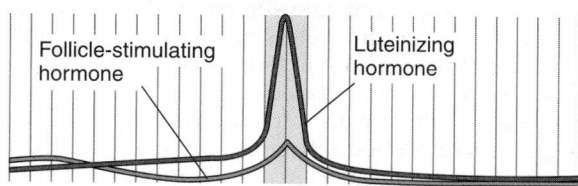

Pituitary Hormone Cycle

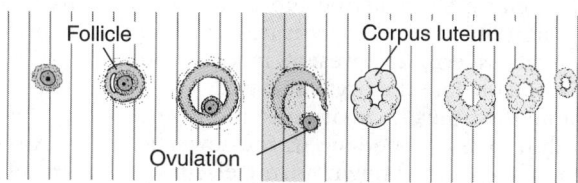

Ovarian Cycle

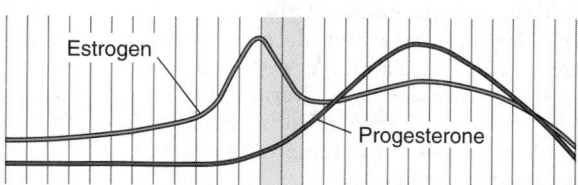

Sex Hormone Cycle

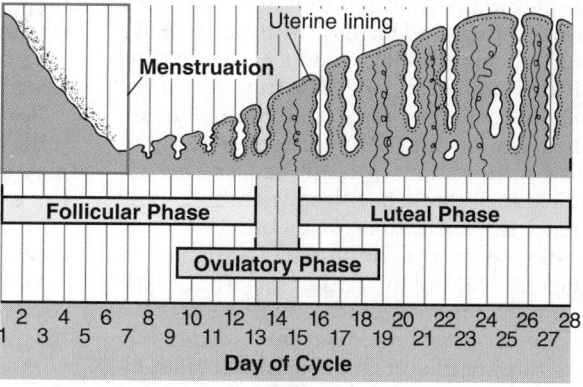

Endometrial Cycle

gins to produce estrogen, and the other stimulated follicles begin to degenerate.

The **ovulatory phase** starts with a surge in the levels of luteinizing hormone and, to a lesser degree, follicle-stimulating hormone. Luteinizing hormone stimulates the dominant follicle to bulge from the surface of the ovary and finally rupture, releasing the egg. (The function of the increase in follicle-stimulating hormone is not understood.)

The ovulatory phase ends with the release of the egg, usually 36 hours after the surge in luteinizing hormone begins. About 12 to 24 hours after the egg is released, this surge can be detected by measuring the luteinizing hormone level in the urine. The egg can be fertilized for only a short period (up to about 12 hours) after its release. Fertilization is more likely when sperm are present in the reproductive tract before the egg is released.

Around the time of ovulation, some women feel a dull pain on one side of the lower abdomen. This pain is known as mittelschmerz (literally, middle pain). The pain may last for a few minutes to a few hours. The pain is felt on the same side as the ovary that released the egg, but the precise cause of the pain is unknown. The pain may precede or follow the rupture of the follicle and may not occur in all cycles. Egg release does not alternate between the two ovaries and appears to be random. If one ovary is removed, the remaining ovary releases an egg every month.

The **luteal phase** follows ovulation. It lasts about 14 days, unless fertilization occurs, and ends just before a menstrual period. In the luteal phase, the ruptured follicle closes after releasing the egg and forms a structure called a corpus luteum, which produces increasing quantities of progesterone. The function of the corpus luteum is to prepare the uterus in case fertilization occurs. The progesterone produced by the corpus luteum causes the endometrium to thicken, filling with fluids and nutrients in preparation for a potential fetus. Progesterone causes the mucus in the cervix to thicken, making the entry of sperm or bacteria into the uterus less likely. Progesterone also causes body temperature to increase slightly during the luteal phase and remain elevated until a menstrual period begins. This increase in temperature can be used to estimate whether ovulation has occurred.▲ In the

second part of the luteal phase, the estrogen level increases, also stimulating the endometrium to thicken.

In response to the increase in estrogen and progesterone levels, the milk ducts in the breasts increase. As a result, the breasts may swell and become tender.

If the egg is not fertilized, the corpus luteum degenerates after 14 days, and a new menstrual cycle begins. If the egg is fertilized, the cells around the developing embryo begin to produce a hormone called human chorionic gonadotropin. This hormone maintains the corpus luteum, which continues to produce progesterone, until the growing fetus can produce its own hormones. Pregnancy tests are based on detecting an increase in the human chorionic gonadotropin level.

Effects of Aging

Around menopause,■ changes in the genital organs occur rapidly. Menstrual cycles stop, and the ovaries stop producing estrogen. After menopause, the tissues of the labia minora, clitoris, vagina, and urethra thin (atrophy). This thinning can result in chronic irritation, dryness, and a discharge from the vagina. Vaginal infections are more likely to develop. Also after menopause, the uterus, fallopian tubes, and ovaries become smaller.

With aging, there is a decrease in the amount of muscle and connective tissue, including that in muscles, ligaments, and other tissues that support the bladder, uterus, vagina, and rectum. As a result, these organs may sag or drop down (prolapse), sometimes causing difficulty urinating, loss of control over urination or bowel movements (incontinence), or pain during sexual intercourse.

Because there is less estrogen to stimulate milk ducts, the breasts decrease in size and may sag. The connective tissue that supports the breast also decreases, contributing to sagging. Fibrous tissue in the breasts is replaced with fat, making the breasts less firm.

Despite these changes, many women enjoy sexual activity more after menopause, possibly because they are no longer able to become pregnant. In addition, after menopause, the ovaries continue to produce male sex hormones. Male sex hormones help maintain the sex drive, slow the loss of muscle tissue, and contribute to an overall sense of well-being.

▲ see page 1416   ■ see page 1356

CHAPTER 242

Symptoms and Diagnosis of Gynecologic Disorders

Disorders that affect the female reproductive system, including the breasts, are called gynecologic disorders. Various diagnostic procedures are performed when a woman has specific symptoms (to determine the cause) or when a woman has a routine physical examination (to check for certain disorders). These procedures help prevent problems and maintain a woman's health.

Symptoms

The most common symptoms due to gynecologic disorders include vaginal itching, a vaginal discharge, abnormal bleeding from the vagina, pain in the pelvic area, and breast pain. The significance of gynecologic symptoms often depends on the age of the woman, because hormonal changes that occur with age may be involved.

Vaginal Itching

Vaginal itching may involve the area containing the external genital organs (vulva) as well as the vagina. Many women have occasional vaginal itching that resolves without treatment. Itching is considered a problem only when it is persistent, is severe, or recurs.

Vaginal itching may result from irritation by chemicals, such as those in laundry detergents, bleaches, fabric softeners, synthetic fibers, bubble baths, soaps, feminine hygiene sprays, perfumes, menstrual pads, fabric dyes, toilet tissue, vaginal creams, douches, and contraceptive foams. Vaginal itching may result from an infection,▲ such as bacterial vaginosis, candidiasis (a yeast infection), or trichomoniasis (a protozoan infection). Vaginal itching may also result from vaginal dryness due to hormonal changes at menopause. Other causes include skin disorders such as psoriasis or lichen sclerosus. Lichen sclerosus is characterized by thin white patches that develop around the opening of the vagina. If untreated, lichen sclerosus can cause scarring and may increase the risk of cancer. Treatment consists of a cream or an ointment containing a high dose of a corticosteroid (such as clobetasol).

Itching may be accompanied by a discharge. If itching persists or is accompanied by a vaginal discharge that looks or smells abnormal, a woman should see her doctor.

Abnormal Vaginal Discharge

A small amount of vaginal discharge is usually normal. The discharge consists of secretions (mucus) produced mainly by the cervix but also in the vagina. The discharge is usually thin and clear, milky white, or yellowish. Its amount and appearance vary with age. Typically, the discharge has no odor. It is not accompanied by itching or burning.

Newborn girls normally have a vaginal discharge of mucus, often mixed with a small amount of blood. This discharge is due to estrogen absorbed from the mother before birth. It usually stops within 2 weeks, as the level of estrogen in the blood decreases. Normally, older infants and girls, except those near puberty, do not have any significant vaginal discharge.

During a woman's reproductive years, the amount and appearance of the normal vaginal discharge vary with the menstrual cycle. For example, at the middle of the cycle (at ovulation), more mucus is usually produced and the mucus is thinner. Pregnancy, use of oral contraceptives, and sexual arousal also affect the amount and appearance of the discharge. After menopause, the estrogen level decreases, often reducing the amount of normal discharge.

A vaginal discharge is considered abnormal if it is

- heavier than usual
- thicker than usual
- puslike
- white and clumpy (like cottage cheese)
- grayish, greenish, yellowish, or blood-tinged
- foul-smelling (fishy)
- accompanied by itching, burning, a rash, or soreness.

A discharge may indicate inflammation of the vagina (vaginitis), which may be due to a

▲ see page 1374

chemical irritant (as for vaginal itching) or to an infection.▲ In some women, spermicides, vaginal lubricants or creams, or diaphragms can irritate the vagina or vulva, causing inflammation. For women who are allergic to latex, contact with latex condoms can irritate the area. In young girls, a foreign object in the vagina can cause inflammation of the vagina, with a vaginal discharge that may contain blood. Most commonly, the foreign object is a piece of toilet paper that has worked its way into the vagina. Sometimes it is a toy.

A white, gray, or yellowish cloudy discharge with a foul or fishy odor is typically caused by bacterial vaginosis. A thick, white, and clumpy discharge (which looks like cottage cheese) is typically caused by candidiasis, a yeast infection. A heavy, greenish yellow, frothy discharge that may have a bad odor is typically caused by trichomoniasis, a protozoan infection.

A watery, blood-tinged discharge may be caused by cancer of the vagina, cervix, or lining of the uterus (endometrium). Radiation therapy to the pelvis may also cause an abnormal discharge.

Doctors may identify the cause of the abnormal discharge based on the appearance of the discharge, the woman's age, and other symptoms. A sample of the discharge is examined under a microscope to check for an infection and to identify it. Treatment depends on the cause. If a product (such as a cream, powder, soap, feminine hygiene spray, or brand of condom) causes persistent irritation, it should not be used.

Abnormal Vaginal Bleeding

Bleeding from the vagina may originate in the vagina or another reproductive organ, particularly the uterus. Abnormal vaginal bleeding includes menstrual bleeding that is excessively heavy or light, occurs too frequently, or is irregular. Any vaginal bleeding that is not associated with a menstrual period or that occurs before puberty or after menopause is also considered abnormal.■

Abnormal vaginal bleeding may result from a disorder (such as an injury, infection, or cancer) or from changes in the normal hormonal control of menstruation. Such hormonal changes are more likely to occur when menstrual periods are just starting (in teenagers) or nearing an end (in women in their 40s★).

Excessive Hairiness

Excessive body hair, particularly on the face and trunk (in a male pattern) and on the limbs, is called hirsutism. Excessive hairiness may not seem like a gynecologic disorder, but it is considered one. It usually results from abnormal levels of female and male hormones.

Hirsutism is more common among postmenopausal women, because levels of female hormones have decreased. Hirsutism may be due to a disorder of the pituitary gland or adrenal glands that results in overproduction of male hormones (such as testosterone). Sometimes exaggerated masculine characteristics (virilization) result. Hirsutism may also be due to polycystic ovary syndrome.● Rare causes include tumors in the ovaries, porphyria cutanea tarda (a form of porphyria that affects the skin), and use of drugs such as anabolic steroids, corticosteroids, and minoxidil.

Blood tests may be performed to measure male and female hormone levels. Drugs that may be the cause are discontinued. Temporary solutions include shaving, plucking, waxing, and using depilatories. Eflornithine, a topical cream available by prescription, may be used. It can slow the growth of hair, causing a gradual reduction of unwanted facial hair. This drug may temporarily irritate the skin, causing redness, burning, stinging, or a rash. Bleaching may be effective if the hair is fine. Laser phototherapy is temporarily effective. The only safe permanent treatment is electrolysis, which destroys the hair follicles. The disorder causing hirsutism is treated when possible.

Pelvic Pain

Many women experience pelvic pain—pain that occurs in the lowest part of the trunk, below the abdomen and between the hipbones. Pelvic pain may be caused by problems related to any of the organs in the pelvis: the reproductive organs (the uterus, fallopian tubes, ovaries, and vagina), bladder, rectum, or appendix. However, pelvic pain sometimes originates in organs outside the pelvis, such as the intestine, ureters, and gallbladder. Psychologic factors, especially stress and depression, may contribute to pelvic pain.

The pain may be sharp, intermittent, or crampy (like menstrual cramps). It may be sudden and excruciating, or it may be dull and constant. The pain may gradually increase in

▲ see page 1374   ■ see page 1361
★ see page 1361   ● see page 1367

intensity. The area may feel tender to the touch. The pain may be accompanied by fever, nausea, and vomiting.

When a woman suddenly develops very severe pain in the lower abdomen or pelvis, doctors must quickly decide whether the cause requires emergency surgery. Examples of emergencies are appendicitis, a perforated ulcer, an aortic aneurysm, a twisted ovarian cyst, pelvic infections due to sexually transmitted diseases, and a pregnancy that develops outside of the uterus (ectopic pregnancy), usually in a fallopian tube.

To identify the cause, doctors may ask the woman to describe the pain, including its duration and location, and other symptoms. Doctors also ask about previous episodes of similar pain. Information about the timing of the pain in relation to eating, sleeping, sexual intercourse, activity, urination, and defecation may also be useful, as is information about any other factors that worsen or ease the pain.

Doctors gently feel the entire abdomen, checking for tenderness and abnormal growths. A pelvic examination helps doctors determine which organs are affected and whether an infection is present. Other procedures may include a complete blood cell count, urine tests, a pregnancy test, ultrasonography, computed tomography (CT), magnetic resonance imaging (MRI), and cultures to check for infections. Sometimes surgery or laparoscopy (use of a viewing tube to examine the abdominal and pelvic cavities) is needed to identify the cause of the pain.

Treating the disorder causing the pain, if identified, may relieve the pain. If a psychologic disorder is contributing to the pain, counseling or other therapy may help.

Breast Symptoms

Symptoms related to the breast are common. They include breast pain, lumps (including solid masses and cysts), pitting or dimpling in the skin of the breast, and a discharge from the nipple.▲ Breast symptoms may or may not indicate a serious disorder. For example, diffuse breast pain that is related to hormonal changes before a menstrual period does not indicate a serious disorder. However, because breast cancer is a concern and because early detection is essential to the successful treatment of breast cancer, any change in the breast should be evaluated by a doctor. In addition, women should examine their breasts themselves once a month.■

What Causes Pelvic Pain?

Disorders related to the reproductive organs

- Ectopic pregnancy
- Endometriosis
- Fibroids
- Mittelschmerz (pain that occurs in the middle of the menstrual cycle and is caused by ovulation)
- Engorgement of blood vessels in the pelvis with blood about a week before the menstrual period (pelvic congestion syndrome)
- Ovarian cysts that are large, that rupture, or that twist
- Pelvic inflammatory disease

Disorders not related to the reproductive organs

- Appendicitis
- Urinary tract infections, such as cystitis
- Diverticulitis
- Gastroenteritis
- Ulcer disease
- Inflammatory bowel disease
- Inflammation of the lymph nodes in the abdomen (mesenteric lymphadenitis)
- Stones in the urinary tract, such as kidney stones

Gynecologic Evaluation

A healthy lifestyle includes having regular gynecologic examinations and screening tests for disorders that can be prevented or treated effectively if detected early.★ The main tests specific to women are the Papanicolaou (Pap) test or other similar tests to detect cancer of the cervix and mammography to detect breast cancer.

For gynecologic care, a woman should choose a health care practitioner with whom she can comfortably discuss sensitive topics, such as sex, birth control, pregnancy, and problems related to menopause. The practitioner may be a gynecologist, an internist, a nurse-midwife, or a general, family, or nurse practitioner. During the gynecologic visit, a

---

▲ see page 1387

■ see art on page 1395

★ see table on page 29

woman can ask this practitioner any questions she has about reproductive and sexual function and anatomy, including safe sex practices.

GYNECOLOGIC HISTORY

A gynecologic evaluation starts with a series of questions related to reproductive function, which usually focus on the reason for the visit to the doctor's office. The answers form the gynecologic history. A complete gynecologic history includes information about the age at which menstrual bleeding began (menarche); the frequency, regularity, and duration of menstrual periods; the amount of flow; and the dates of the last two menstrual periods. Questions about abnormal bleeding—too much, too little, or between menstrual periods—are included.

A doctor may ask about sexual activity to assess the possibility of gynecologic infections, injuries, and pregnancy. A woman is asked whether she uses or wants to use birth control and whether she is interested in counseling or other information. The number of pregnancies, dates that they occurred, outcomes, and complications are recorded.

The doctor asks the woman whether she has pain during menstrual periods, during intercourse, or under other circumstances. If the woman has pain, she is asked how severe it is and what provides relief. Questions are also asked about breast problems, such as pain, lumps, areas of tenderness or redness, and discharge from the nipples. The woman is asked whether she is examining her breasts, how often, and whether she needs any instruction on technique.

The doctor reviews the woman's history of past gynecologic disorders and usually obtains a medical and surgical history that includes all previous health problems. The doctor reviews all the drugs a woman is taking, including prescription and nonprescription drugs, illicit drugs, tobacco, and alcohol, because many of them affect gynecologic function. The woman is asked about mental, physical, or sexual abuse in the present and the past. Some questions about urination are asked to find out whether the woman has a urinary tract infection or has problems with leakage of urine (incontinence).

GYNECOLOGIC EXAMINATION

If a woman has any questions or fears about the gynecologic examination, she should talk with the doctor beforehand about her concerns. If any part of the examination causes pain, the woman should let the doctor know. A woman is usually asked to empty her bladder before the physical examination and may be asked to collect a urine sample for analysis.

A breast examination may be performed before or after the pelvic examination. With the woman sitting, the doctor inspects the breasts for irregularities, dimpling, tightened skin, lumps, and a discharge. The woman then sits or lies down, with her arms above her head, while the doctor feels (palpates) each breast with a flat hand and examines each armpit for enlarged lymph nodes. The doctor also feels the neck and the thyroid gland for lumps and abnormalities. While performing the examination, the doctor can review the technique for breast self-examination with the woman.▲

The doctor gently feels the entire abdomen, looking for abnormal growths or enlarged organs, especially the liver and spleen. Although the woman may experience some discomfort when the doctor presses deeply, the examination should not be painful. To estimate the size of the liver and spleen, the doctor may tap with the fingers (percuss) and listen for differences in sound between hollow-sounding and dull-sounding areas. A stethoscope may be used to listen for the activity of the intestines and for any abnormal noises made by blood flowing through narrowed blood vessels.

During the pelvic examination, the woman lies on her back with her hips and knees bent and her buttocks moved to the edge of the examining table. Most examining tables have heel stirrups that help a woman maintain this position. If a woman wants to observe the pelvic examination, she should let the doctor know ahead of time. The doctor can provide a mirror as well as explanations or a diagram. First, the doctor inspects the external genital area and notes the distribution of hair and any abnormalities, discoloration, discharge, or inflammation. This examination may indicate that all is well or give clues to hormonal problems, cancer, infections, injury, or physical abuse.

The doctor spreads the tissues around the opening of the vagina (labia) and examines the opening. Using a speculum (a metal or plastic instrument that spreads the walls of the vagina apart), the doctor examines the deeper

▲ see art on page 1395

areas of the vagina and the cervix. The cervix is examined closely for signs of irritation or cancer. The doctor checks for a protrusion of the bladder, rectum, or intestine into the vagina.▲

For a Papanicolaou (Pap) test or another similar test, the doctor collects cells from the surface of the cervix with a plastic spatula similar to a tongue depressor. Then, a small bristle brush is used to obtain cells from the cervix. Usually, these tests feel scratchy or crampy, but they are not painful and take only a few seconds. The cells removed with the spatula or brush are placed on a glass slide and sprayed with a preservative or rinsed into a vial of liquid. The sample is sent to a laboratory, where it is examined under a microscope for abnormal cells, which may indicate cervical cancer. Such tests identify 80 to 85% of cervical cancers, even in their earliest stages. They can also detect changes in cells of the cervix that can lead to cancer. The changes can be treated, thus helping prevent cancer.

Pap and similar tests are most accurate if the woman is not having her period and does not douche or use vaginal creams for at least 24 hours before the examination. Most women should have such a test once a year. The first test is usually performed when a woman becomes sexually active or reaches age 18. If test results are normal for 3 consecutive years, the woman can discuss with her health care practitioner whether scheduling tests every 1, 2, or 3 years is appropriate.

If an infection is suspected, the doctor uses a swab to obtain a small amount of vaginal discharge from the vagina and cervix. The sample is sent to a laboratory for culture and evaluation. Tests for sexually transmitted diseases are not part of a routine examination. If a woman thinks she may have one of these diseases, she can request testing.

After removing the speculum, the doctor feels the vaginal wall to determine its strength and support. The doctor inserts the index and middle fingers of one gloved hand into the vagina and places the fingers of the other hand on the lower abdomen above the pubic bone. Between the two hands, the uterus can usually be felt as a pear-shaped, smooth, firm structure, and its position, size, consistency, and degree of tenderness (if any) can be determined. Then the doctor attempts to feel the ovaries by moving the hand on the abdomen more to the side and exerting slightly more pressure. More pressure is required because

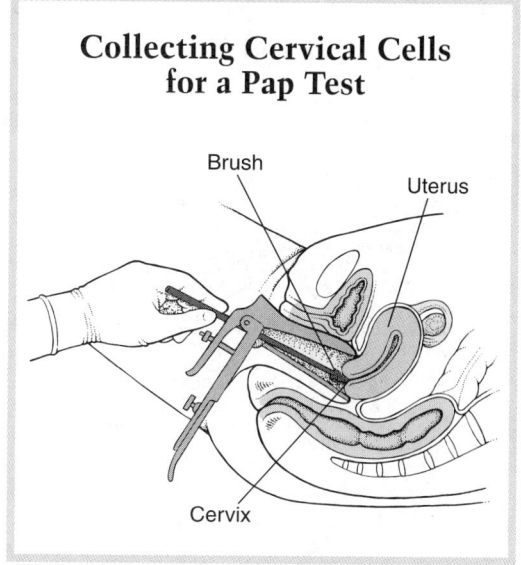

Collecting Cervical Cells for a Pap Test

Brush

Uterus

Cervix

the ovaries are small and much more difficult to feel than the uterus. The woman may find this part of the examination to be slightly uncomfortable, but it should not be painful. The doctor determines how large the ovaries are and whether they are tender. The doctor also feels for growths or tender areas within the vagina.

Finally, the doctor performs a rectovaginal examination by inserting the index finger into the vagina and the middle finger into the rectum. In this way, the back wall of the vagina can be examined for abnormal growths or thickness. In addition, the doctor can examine the rectum for hemorrhoids, fissures, polyps, and lumps. A small sample of stool can be obtained with a gloved finger and tested for unseen (occult) blood. A woman may be given a take-home kit to test for occult blood in the stool.

DIAGNOSTIC PROCEDURES

Occasionally, more extensive diagnostic procedures are needed.

Colposcopy

For colposcopy, a binocular magnifying lens (similar to that of a microscope) can be used to inspect the cervix for signs of cancer. The procedure is often performed after an abnormal

▲ see page 1379

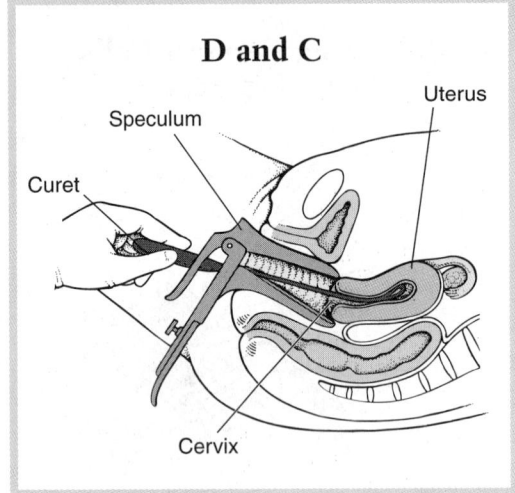

D and C

Speculum

Uterus

Curet

Cervix

Pap test result. A speculum is used to spread the walls of the vagina so that the cervix can be seen. Colposcopy is painless and requires no anesthetic. It takes 15 to 30 minutes to perform.

Biopsy

A biopsy consists of removing a small sample of tissue for examination under a microscope. This procedure is performed when a precancerous condition (a condition that is likely to eventually lead to cancer) or cancer is suspected. A biopsy of the vulva can usually be performed in the doctor's office with use of a local anesthetic. A biopsy of the cervix and vagina is usually performed during colposcopy. Colposcopy enables doctors to take tissue samples from the area that looks most abnormal. Usually, biopsy of the cervix or vagina does not require an anesthetic. Typically, this procedure feels like a pinch or a cramp.

For biopsy of the lining of the uterus (endometrial biopsy), a small metal or plastic tube is inserted through the cervix into the uterus. The tube is moved back and forth and around to dislodge and suction out tissue from the uterine lining. This procedure is usually performed to determine the cause of abnormal vaginal bleeding. Also, infertility specialists use this procedure to determine whether ovulation is occurring normally or whether the uterus is ready for implantation of embryos. An endometrial biopsy can be performed in a doctor's office and usually does not require an anesthetic. Typically, it feels like strong menstrual cramps.

Endocervical Curettage

Endocervical curettage consists of inserting a small, sharp instrument (curet) inside the cervix to obtain tissue. This tissue is examined under a microscope by a pathologist. It is performed when endometrial or cervical cancer is suspected or needs to be ruled out. This procedure is usually performed during colposcopy and usually does not require an anesthetic.

Loop Electrical Excision Procedure

In a loop electrical excision procedure (LEEP), a thin wire loop through which an electrical current can pass is used to remove a piece of tissue. This procedure may be performed after an abnormal Pap test result to evaluate the abnormality more accurately and to remove the abnormal tissue. LEEP requires an anesthetic (often a local one), takes about 5 to 10 minutes, and can be performed in a doctor's office. Afterward, a woman may feel mild discomfort and have a small amount of bleeding.

Dilation and Curettage

For dilation and curettage (D and C), the cervix is stretched open (dilated) with metal rods so that a small, sharp instrument (curet) can be inserted to remove tissue lining the uterus. This procedure may be used to identify abnormalities of the uterine lining if biopsy results are inconclusive or to treat women who have had an incomplete miscarriage. D and C is often performed in a hospital, and a general anesthetic may be used. However, most women do not have to stay overnight in the hospital.

Hysteroscopy

To view the interior of the uterus, doctors can insert a thin viewing tube (hysteroscope) through the vagina and cervix into the uterus. The tube is about $1/4$ inch in diameter and contains cables that transmit light. A biopsy, an electrocautery (heat), or a surgical instrument may be threaded through the tube. The site of abnormal bleeding or other abnormalities can usually be seen and can be sampled for a biopsy, sealed off using heat, or removed. This procedure may be performed in a doctor's office or in a hospital at the same time as a dilation and curettage.

Ultrasonography

Ultrasonography uses ultrasound waves, produced at a frequency too high to be heard.

The ultrasound waves are emitted by a hand-held device that is placed on the abdomen or inside the vagina. The waves reflect off internal structures, and the pattern of this reflection can be displayed on a monitor. In pregnant women, ultrasonography can help determine the condition and size of a fetus and can detect the presence of more than one fetus. It can often identify the sex of the fetus. Ultrasonography can also be used to monitor the fetus and to detect fetal abnormalities. It can be used to guide the placement of instruments during amniocentesis and chorionic villus sampling, which are used to detect genetic disorders in the fetus. Ultrasonography can detect an ectopic pregnancy, tumors, cysts, and other abnormalities in the pelvic organs. Ultrasonography is painless and has no known risks.

Sonohysterography

For sonohysterography, fluid is placed in the uterus through a thin tube (catheter) inserted through the vagina. Then ultrasonography is performed. The fluid fills and stretches (distends) the uterus so that abnormalities inside the uterus, such as polyps or fibroids, can be more easily detected. The procedure is performed in a doctor's office and may require a local anesthetic. A nonsteroidal anti-inflammatory drug (NSAID), such as ibuprofen, may be taken 20 minutes before the procedure to help relieve the cramping that may occur.

Laparoscopy

To directly examine the uterus, fallopian tubes, or ovaries, doctors use a viewing tube called a laparoscope. The laparoscope is attached to a thin cable containing flexible plastic or glass rods that transmit light. The laparoscope is inserted into the abdominal cavity through a small incision just below the navel. A probe is inserted through the vagina and into the uterus. The probe enables doctors to manipulate the organs for better viewing. Carbon dioxide is pumped through the laparoscope to inflate the abdomen, so that organs in the abdomen and pelvis can be seen clearly. Laparoscopy is performed in a hospital and requires an anesthetic, usually a general anesthetic. An overnight stay in the hospital is usually not required. Laparoscopy may cause mild abdominal discomfort, but normal activities can usually be resumed in 1 or 2 days.

Often, laparoscopy is used to determine the cause of pelvic pain, infertility, and other gynecologic disorders. Instruments can be threaded

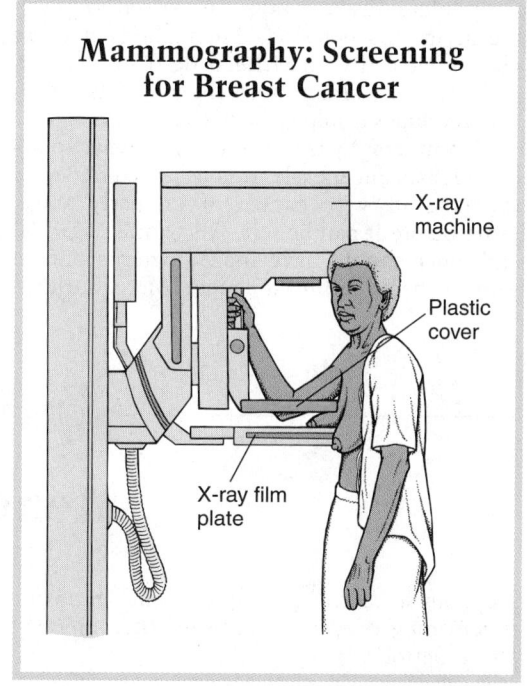

Mammography: Screening for Breast Cancer

- X-ray machine
- Plastic cover
- X-ray film plate

through the laparoscope to perform some surgical procedures, such as biopsies, sterilization procedures, and removal of an ectopic pregnancy in a fallopian tube or an ovary.

Hysterosalpingography

For hysterosalpingography, x-rays are taken after a radiopaque dye, which can be seen on x-rays, is injected through the cervix to outline the interior of the uterus and fallopian tubes. The procedure is often used to help determine the cause of infertility. The procedure is performed in a place where x-rays can be taken, such as a hospital or the radiology suite of a doctor's office. Hysterosalpingography usually causes discomfort, such as cramps.

Mammography

For mammography, x-rays of the breasts are taken to detect abnormal areas.▲ A technician positions the woman's breast on top of an x-ray plate. An adjustable plastic cover is lowered on top of the breast, firmly compressing the breast. Thus, the breast is flattened so that the maximum amount of tissue can be imaged and examined. X-rays are aimed downward through the breast, producing an image on the

▲ see page 1392

x-ray plate. Two x-rays are taken of each breast in this position. Then plates may be placed vertically on either side of the breast, and x-rays are aimed from the side. This position produces a side view of the breast.

Mammography is one of the best ways to detect breast cancer early. It is designed to detect the possibility of cancer at an early stage, years before it can be felt. All women aged 50 and older should have mammograms once a year to check for breast cancer. Many authori-

ties recommend that women aged 40 to 49 have mammograms every 1 to 2 years.

The dose of radiation used is very low and is considered safe. This procedure may cause some discomfort, but the discomfort lasts only a few seconds. Mammography should be scheduled at a time during the menstrual period when the breasts are less likely to be tender. Deodorants should not be used on the day of the procedure, because they can affect it. The entire procedure takes about 15 minutes.

CHAPTER 243

Menopause

Menopause is the permanent end of cyclic functioning of the ovaries and thus of menstrual periods.

Menopause occurs because as women age, the ovaries produce smaller and smaller amounts of estrogen and progesterone. Estrogen and progesterone are the hormones that control the monthly cycle of egg release (ovulation▲). Thus, as women approach menopause, an egg is released in fewer and fewer cycles, and eventually, egg release stops. As a result, menstrual periods end and pregnancy is no longer possible. A woman's last period can be identified only later, after she has had no periods for at least 6 months. (Women who do not wish to become pregnant should use birth control until 1 year has passed since their last menstrual period.)

A distinctive transitional period called perimenopause occurs before and just after menopause. During perimenopause, estrogen and progesterone levels fluctuate widely. Estrogen levels may be high at the beginning of this transitional period, but for short intervals, no estrogen may be produced. These fluctuations explain why many women in their 40s report bouts of menopausal symptoms, which may subside without treatment.

In the United States, the average age at which menopause occurs is about 51 to 52. However, menopause may occur normally in

women as young as 40. Premature menopause is menopause occurring before age 40.■

Artificial menopause results from a medical treatment that reduces or stops hormone production by the ovaries. Examples are surgery to remove the ovaries, surgery that unintentionally reduces the blood supply to the ovaries, and chemotherapy or radiation therapy to the pelvis, including the ovaries, to treat cancer. Surgery to remove the uterus (hysterectomy) ends menstrual periods but does not cause menopause as long as the ovaries are functioning.

Symptoms

During perimenopause, symptoms may be nonexistent, mild, moderate, or severe. Perimenopausal symptoms are thought to be caused by the fluctuations in hormone levels that occur as women approach menopause.

Irregular menstrual periods, which occur more or less often, may be the first symptom of perimenopause. Periods may be shorter or longer, lighter or heavier. They may not occur for months, then become regular again. However, periods may occur regularly until menopause.

Hot flashes affect three fourths of women. Most women have hot flashes for more than 1 year, and up to one half of women have them for more than 5 years. What causes hot flashes in unknown, but they may be related to fluctuations in hormone levels. Hot flashes seem to result in the widening (dilating) of blood vessels near the skin's surface. As a result,

---

▲ see page 1346   ■ see page 1361

blood flow increases, causing the skin, especially on the head and neck, to become red and warm (flushed). Perspiration may be profuse. Hot flashes are sometimes called hot flushes because of this warming effect. A hot flash lasts from 30 seconds to 5 minutes and may be followed by chills.

Other symptoms that may occur around the time of menopause include mood changes, depression, irritability, anxiety, nervousness, insomnia, loss of concentration, headache, and fatigue. These symptoms may be related to the decreases in estrogen levels occurring at the same time. But the precise relationship between estrogen levels and symptoms is unclear. Night sweats, which are related to hot flashes, may disturb sleep, contributing to fatigue and irritability. However, sleep disorders are common even among women who do not have hot flashes.

Women may feel dizzy occasionally or have tingling (pins-and-needles) sensations. They may feel the heart beating very forcefully or rapidly (have palpitations). Weight gain may occur during perimenopause and continue after menopause. But this weight gain is unrelated to the changes in hormone levels and may just be part of normal aging.

Many of the symptoms of perimenopause, although disturbing, become less frequent and less intense after menopause. In contrast, the complications of menopause, which result from the decrease in estrogen, are progressive, unless measures to prevent them are taken.

After menopause, the decrease in estrogen causes changes in the reproductive tract over a period of months or years. The lining of the vagina becomes thinner, drier, and less elastic (a condition called vaginal atrophy). These changes may make sexual intercourse painful and may increase the risk of inflammation (vaginitis). Other genital organs—the labia minora, clitoris, uterus, and ovaries—decrease in size. Sex drive (libido) commonly decreases. The effect of menopause on the ability to have an orgasm varies from woman to woman. In many women, the ability is unaffected. It improves in some women but is lost in others.

The lining of the urethra becomes thinner, and the muscles that control the outflow of urine (around the bladder outlet) become weaker. As a result, a burning sensation may occur when urinating, and urinary tract infections may develop more easily. Many postmenopausal women have stress incontinence, in which small amounts of urine escape from the bladder during laughing, coughing, or other activities that put pressure on the bladder.▲ Some women develop urge incontinence, which is an abrupt, intense urge to urinate that cannot be suppressed.

As estrogen decreases, the amount of collagen, a protein that makes skin strong, and elastin, a protein that makes skin elastic, also decrease. Thus, the skin may become thinner, dryer, less elastic, and more vulnerable to injury.

The decrease in estrogen often leads to a decrease in bone density and sometimes to osteoporosis,■ because estrogen helps maintain bone. Bone becomes less dense and weaker, making fractures more likely. During the first 2 years after menopause, bone density decreases by about 3 to 5% each year. After that, it decreases by about 1 to 2% each year.

After menopause, levels of lipids, particularly LDL cholesterol, increase in women. The increase in lipid levels may partly explain why coronary artery disease becomes more common among women after menopause. Also, until menopause, the high estrogen levels seems to protect against the disease.

Diagnosis

In about three fourths of women, menopause is obvious. If menopause needs to be confirmed (particularly in younger women), blood tests are performed to measure levels of estrogen and follicle-stimulating hormone (which stimulates the ovaries to produce estrogen and progesterone).

Before any treatment is started, doctors ask women about their medical and family history and perform a physical examination, including breast and pelvic examinations and measurement of blood pressure. Mammography is also performed. Blood tests may be performed, and bone density may be measured. The information thus obtained helps doctors determine the woman's risk of developing disorders after menopause. For women with a history of abnormal bleeding from the vagina, an endometrial biopsy★ may be performed to check for signs of cancer. A small sample of tissue is removed from the lining of the uterus (endometrium) and is examined under a microscope.

▲ see page 858

■ see page 343

★ see page 1354

Treatment

Not consuming spicy foods, hot beverages, caffeine, and alcohol may help prevent hot flashes, because these substances can trigger hot flashes. Eating foods rich in B vitamins or vitamin E or foods rich in plant estrogens (phytoestrogens), such as tofu, soy milk, tempeh, and miso, may also help. Not smoking, avoiding stress, and exercising regularly may help improve sleep as well as relieve hot flashes. Wearing layers of clothing, which can be taken off when a woman feels hot and put on when she feels cold, can help her cope with hot flashes. Wearing clothing that breathes, such as cotton underwear and sleepwear, may enhance comfort.

Aerobic exercise, relaxation techniques, meditation, massage, and yoga may help relieve depression, irritability, and fatigue, as well as reduce hot flashes. Reducing the number of calories consumed and exercising more can help prevent weight gain. Weight-bearing exercise (such as walking, jogging, and weight lifting) and taking calcium and vitamin D supplements slow the loss of bone density.

Many of these measures—losing weight if needed, stopping smoking, and exercising regularly—plus decreasing the total amount of fat and cholesterol in the diet may be recommended to help lower cholesterol levels and thus reduce the risk of atherosclerosis.

If vaginal dryness makes sexual intercourse painful, an over-the-counter vaginal lubricant may help. Staying sexually active also helps by stimulating blood flow to the vagina and surrounding tissues and by keeping tissues flexible. Kegel exercises may help with bladder control.▲ For these exercises, a woman tightens the pelvic muscles as if stopping urine flow.

Hormone Therapy: For women who have a uterus, hormone therapy usually includes a progestin, such as medroxyprogesterone, as well as estrogen. A progestin, a drug similar to the hormone progesterone, is given with estrogen to reduce the risk of cancer of the uterine lining (endometrial cancer). A progestin without estrogen may be prescribed for women who have endometrial cancer or breast cancer. Progestins are available in synthetic and natural forms. The natural forms are identical to a woman's own progesterone.

Benefits and risks: Hormone therapy (estrogen plus a progestin) can relieve many symptoms of menopause and may be appropriate if the benefits seem to outweigh the risks. Whether to take hormone therapy is a difficult decision that must be made by a woman and her doctor based on the woman's individual situation. The decision is complicated because interpreting and applying the information about estrogen's benefits and risks is difficult. Recent evidence suggests that hormone therapy is not appropriate for all women. Recent evidence has also raised questions about the long-term use of hormone therapy. For this reason, taking hormone therapy for more than 5 years is no longer recommended.

Estrogen is the most effective treatment for hot flashes. It can prevent the drying and thinning of vaginal and urinary tract tissues, thus improving sexual function and helping prevent infections. Estrogen may help prevent the skin from becoming dry and inelastic.

Estrogen helps prevent or slow the progression of osteoporosis. During the first year estrogen is taken, bone density may increase by 3% and remain at that level as long as estrogen is taken. Women who are taking hormone therapy to relieve symptoms experience this benefit. However, for most women, taking hormone therapy with the sole purpose of preventing osteoporosis is no longer recommended.

The effect of estrogen on the development of atherosclerosis, including the risk of heart attack and stroke, is not as clear-cut. Estrogen decreases the level of low-density lipoprotein (LDL) cholesterol, the bad cholesterol, and increases the level of high-density lipoprotein (HDL) cholesterol, the good cholesterol. However, estrogen does not appear to improve outcome after a heart attack, increases the risk of blood clots, and may increase the risk of heart attack and stroke. Therefore, taking hormone therapy (estrogen plus a progestin) to prevent coronary artery disease or its consequences (such as heart attack or stroke) is no longer recommended regardless of whether or not a woman has had a heart attack, a stroke, or blood clots.

Estrogen used alone increases the risk of endometrial cancer from about 1 to 4 in 1,000 women each year. The risk is higher with higher doses and longer use of estrogen. Taking a progestin with estrogen almost eliminates the risk of endometrial cancer and reduces the risk below that for women who do

---

▲ see box on page 1384

not take hormone therapy. A woman whose uterus has been removed has no risk of developing this cancer and thus does not need to take a progestin. Usually, estrogen, with or without a progestin, is not prescribed for women who have or have had advanced endometrial cancer or who have vaginal bleeding of unknown cause.

Taking hormone therapy for more than 4 years appears to increase the risk of breast cancer. The longer women take hormone therapy and the higher the dose, the higher the risk of developing breast cancer.

During the first year of estrogen therapy, the risk of developing gallstones is modestly increased.

Estrogen therapy may worsen liver disorders and acute intermittent porphyria. Therefore, this therapy is usually not prescribed for women who have or have had these disorders.

Estrogen, especially at high doses, may have side effects, including nausea, breast tenderness, headache, fluid retention, and mood changes.

A progestin taken alone may relieve hot flashes and may help prevent osteoporosis but does not affect vaginal dryness. Synthetic progestins increase the LDL (the bad) cholesterol level and decrease the HDL (the good) cholesterol level and may increase the risk of atherosclerosis. Side effects of progestins include abdominal bloating, breast discomfort, headache, mood changes, and acne. However, a type of progestin called micronized progesterone appears to have fewer side effects and may not adversely affect cholesterol levels.

Dosage forms: Estrogen and a progestin can be taken in several ways. They may be taken as two tablets or a combination tablet. Commonly, estrogen and a progestin are taken every day. This schedule typically causes irregular vaginal bleeding for the first year or more of therapy. Alternatively, a cyclic monthly schedule may be followed: Estrogen is taken daily, and a progestin is taken for 12 to 14 days each month. With this schedule, most women have monthly vaginal bleeding.

Other forms include progestin injections, an estrogen skin patch (transdermal estrogen), a combination estrogen-progestin patch, and estrogen creams.

An estrogen cream may be applied to the vagina, or a ring may be inserted into the vagina (similar to a diaphragm). Or an estrogen tablet may be inserted into the vagina. Applied in these ways, estrogen may help prevent thin-

ning and drying of the vaginal lining. Such treatment helps prevent intercourse from being painful. Some of the estrogen cream is absorbed into the bloodstream, particularly as the vaginal lining becomes healthier. Theoretically, the cream form of estrogen can increase the risk of endometrial cancer. Therefore, if women use this form, they should also take a progestin. The vaginal tablet and ring forms (which do not enter the bloodstream in substantial amounts) may be suggested for women who have breast cancer or a high risk of developing it.

Selective Estrogen Receptor Modulators (SERMs): These drugs function like estrogen in some parts of the body. The only SERM currently used to prevent problems related to menopause is raloxifene. Like estrogen, raloxifene helps prevent bone density from decreasing in postmenopausal women and increases the chance of developing blood clots (from 1 to 2 or 3 in 10,000 women). Raloxifene also prevents fractures of the bones in the spine (vertebrae). However, raloxifene may have effects opposite to those of estrogen in other parts of the body. For example, hot flashes worsen in about 1 in 10 women. It also does not appear to increase the risk of endometrial cancer, and it inhibits the growth of breast tissue.

Tamoxifen, another SERM, is used to treat breast cancer and prevent its recurrence and to prevent breast cancer in women who have a high risk of developing it. Because raloxifene is similar to tamoxifen, raloxifene is being studied for the prevention of breast cancer.

Other Drugs: Several other types of drugs can help reduce the severity of some of the symptoms associated with menopause. Clonidine, which is used to treat high blood pressure, can reduce the intensity of hot flashes. An antidepressant, such as paroxetine, sertraline, or venlafaxine, may relieve hot flashes. Antidepressants may also help relieve depression, anxiety, and irritability.▲ Sleep aids may help relieve insomnia.■

Lipid-lowering drugs★ may be taken to lower cholesterol levels, reducing the risk of atherosclerosis. Bisphosphonates, used alone or taken with estrogen, can be taken to reduce the risk of osteoporosis.● They increase bone density and are the only drugs proved to reduce the risk of spine and hip fractures.

▲ see page 617   ■ see page 469

★ see table on page 925   ● see page 345

TYPE	DRUG	ADVANTAGES	DISADVANTAGES
Female hormones			
	Estrogen	Relieves hot flashes, night sweats, and vaginal dryness Helps prevent osteoporosis Has positive effects on cholesterol levels	Increases the risk of endometrial cancer if not taken with a progestin Increases the risk of blood clots Appears to increase the risk of breast cancer May increase the risk of athero-sclerosis, heart attack, and stroke Increases triglyceride levels Modestly and temporarily increases the risk of developing gallstones
	A progestin, such as medroxy-progesterone	Reduces the risk of endometrial cancer associated with taking estrogen alone May help relieve hot flashes May help prevent osteoporosis	Does not relieve vaginal dryness May increase the risk of atherosclerosis In synthetic forms, may have nega-tive effects on cholesterol levels
Selective estrogen receptor modulators (SERMs)			
	Raloxifene	Prevents and treats osteoporosis Does not appear to increase the risk of endometrial cancer Inhibits the growth of breast tissue	Increases the risk of blood clots May mildly worsen hot flashes
Bisphosphonates			
	Alendronate Risedronate	Prevent and treat osteoporosis	Can irritate the lining of the esophagus if taken improperly Must be taken with a glass of water after awakening, followed by 30 minutes without consuming any food, liquid, or drug and without lying down
Antidepressants			
	See table on page 618	Relieve depression, anxiety, irritability, and insomnia May relieve hot flashes	See table on page 618
Lipid-lowering drugs			
	See table on page 925	Prevent atherosclerosis (including coronary artery disease)	See table on page 925
One type of antihypertensive drug			
	Clonidine	Lessens hot flashes	Can cause side effects, such as drowsiness, dry mouth, fatigue, an abnormally slow heart rate, rebound high blood pressure when the drug is withdrawn, and sexual dysfunction
Male hormone			
	Testosterone (used in combin-ation with estrogen)	May increase sex drive and energy Prevents osteoporosis Improves mood	Decreases the HDL (good) cholesterol level In high doses, may have some masculinizing effects, such as facial hair growth Has not been studied extensively, so risks are unknown

Testosterone, the main male sex hormone, taken with estrogen is an option for relief of some symptoms of menopause. Taking testosterone may help increase sex drive, increase bone density, improve mood, and increase energy. Synthetic testosterone is available as a tablet (combined with estrogen). Natural testosterone is available as an injection or a cream. Side effects include decreasing the HDL (the good) cholesterol level. When taken in usual doses, testosterone may have some masculinizing effects.

Alternative Medicine: Some women take medicinal herbs and other supplements to relieve hot flashes, irritability, mood changes, and memory loss. Examples are black cohash, DHEA (dehydroepiandrosterone), dong quai, evening primrose, ginseng, and St. John's wort. However, such remedies are not regulated. That is, they have not been shown to be safe or effective for this use, and what their ingredients are and how much of each ingredient a product contains are not standardized.▲ Furthermore, some supplements can interact with other drugs and can worsen some disorders. Women who are considering taking such supplements are advised to discuss them with a doctor.

Premature Menopause

Premature menopause (premature ovarian failure) is the permanent end of the cyclic functioning of the ovaries and thus of menstrual periods before age 40.

Hormonally, premature menopause resembles natural menopause. Estrogen levels are low.

Premature menopause may result from genetic abnormalities, including chromosomal abnormalities, or from an autoimmune disorder, in which the body produces abnormal antibodies that attack the body's tissues (including the ovaries). Other possible causes of premature menopause include metabolic disorders and chemotherapy for cancer. Premature menopause has the same symptoms as natural menopause, such as hot flashes and mood swings.

Diagnosis and Treatment

Identifying the cause of premature menopause can help doctors evaluate a woman's health risks and recommend treatment.

For women younger than 30, a chromosome analysis may be performed. If a chromosomal abnormality is detected, additional procedures and treatment may be required.

Estrogen therapy can prevent or reverse the symptoms of menopause. However, a woman with premature menopause has less than a 10% chance of becoming pregnant. She has up to a 50% chance of becoming pregnant by having another woman's eggs (donor eggs) implanted in her uterus after they have been fertilized in the laboratory.■

CHAPTER 244

Menstrual Disorders and Abnormal Vaginal Bleeding

Complex interactions among hormones control the start of menstruation during puberty, the rhythms and duration of menstrual cycles during the reproductive years, and the end of menstruation at menopause. Hormonal control of menstruation begins in the hypothalamus (the part of the brain that coordinates and controls hormonal activity). The hypothalamus releases gonadotropin-releasing hormone in pulses. This hormone stimulates the pituitary gland to produce two hormones called gonadotropins: luteinizing hormone and follicle-stimulating hormone. These hormones stimulate the ovaries. The ovaries produce the female hormones estrogen and progesterone,★ which ultimately control

---

▲ see page 106   ■ see page 1419
★ see page 1346

DECIPHERING MEDICAL TERMS FOR MENSTRUAL DISORDERS

TERM	DESCRIPTION
Amenorrhea	Absence of periods
Dysmenorrhea	Painful periods
Hypomenorrhea	Unusually light periods
Menometror- rhagia	Prolonged bleeding that occurs at irregular intervals
Menorrhagia	Unusually long and heavy periods
Metrorrhagia	Bleeding that occurs at frequent, irregular intervals
Oligomenorrhea	Unusually infrequent periods
Polymenorrhea	Unusually frequent periods
Postmenopausal bleeding	Bleeding that occurs after menopause
Premenstrual syndrome (PMS)	Physical and psycho- logic symptoms that occur before the start of a period
Primary amenorrhea	No periods ever starting at puberty
Secondary amenorrhea	Periods that have stopped

menstruation. Hormones produced by other glands, such as the adrenal glands and the thyroid gland, can also affect the functioning of the ovaries and menstruation.

Menstrual disorders include premenstrual syndrome, dysmenorrhea, and amenorrhea. Vaginal bleeding may be abnormal during the reproductive years when menstrual periods are too heavy or too light, last too long, occur too often, or are irregular. Any vaginal bleeding that occurs before puberty or after menopause is abnormal until proven otherwise.

Premenstrual Syndrome

Premenstrual syndrome (PMS) is a group of physical and psychologic symptoms that occur before a menstrual period begins.

Because so many monthly symptoms, such as bad mood, irritability, bloating, and breast tenderness, have been ascribed to PMS, defining and identifying PMS can be difficult. PMS affects 20 to 50% of women. About 5% of women of reproductive age have a severe form of PMS called premenstrual dysphoric disorder.

PMS may occur partly because estrogen and progesterone levels fluctuate during the menstrual cycle. Also, in some women with PMS, progesterone may be broken down differently. Progesterone is usually broken down into two components that have opposite effects on mood. Women with PMS may produce less of the component that tends to reduce anxiety and more of the component that tends to increase anxiety.

Symptoms and Diagnosis

The type and intensity of symptoms vary from woman to woman and from month to month in the same woman. The various physical and psychologic symptoms of PMS can temporarily upset a woman's life.

Symptoms may begin a few hours up to about 14 days before a menstrual period, and they usually disappear completely after the period begins. Women who are approaching menopause may have symptoms that persist through and after the menstrual period. The symptoms of PMS are often followed each month by a painful period (dysmenorrhea), particularly in teenagers.

Other disorders may worsen while PMS symptoms are occurring. Women who have a seizure disorder may have more seizures than usual. Women who have a connective tissue disease, such as lupus or rheumatoid arthritis, may have flare-ups. Respiratory disorders (such as allergies and congestion of the nose and airways) and eye disorders (such as conjunctivitis) may worsen.

In premenstrual dysphoric disorder, premenstrual symptoms are so severe that they interfere with work, social activities, and relationships.

The diagnosis is based on symptoms. To identify it, doctors ask a woman to keep a daily record of her symptoms. This record helps the woman be aware of changes in her body and moods and helps doctors determine what treatment is best. Premenstrual dysphoric disorder cannot be diagnosed until a woman has recorded her symptoms for at least two menstrual cycles. Doctors can distinguish premenstrual syndrome and premenstrual dysphoric disorder from mood disorders, such as depression, because the symptoms disappear soon after the menstrual period begins.

Treatment

Treatment involves relieving symptoms. Reducing the intake of salt often reduces fluid retention and relieves bloating. Diuretics (which help the kidneys eliminate salt and water from the body) may be prescribed to help reduce the buildup of fluid. For most women who have mild to moderate symptoms, exercise and stress reduction techniques (meditation or relaxation exercises) help relieve nervousness and agitation. Reducing the consumption of beverages and foods containing caffeine (including chocolate) may also help. Taking calcium supplements (1,000 milligrams a day) lessens the physical and emotional symptoms of PMS. There are claims that other supplements such as magnesium and the B vitamins, especially B_6 (pyridoxine), taken daily, lessen symptoms. However, the usefulness of these supplements has not been confirmed. Taking vitamin B_6 in high doses may be harmful. Nerve damage has been reported with as little as 200 milligrams a day.

Taking nonsteroidal anti-inflammatory drugs (NSAIDs)▲ may help relieve headaches, pain due to abdominal cramps, and joint pain. Taking combination oral contraceptives (birth control pills that contain estrogen and a progestin) reduces pain, breast tenderness, and changes in appetite in some women but worsens these symptoms in a few. Taking oral contraceptives that contain only a progestin does not help.

Women who have more severe symptoms may benefit from taking fluoxetine, paroxetine, or sertraline, which are antidepressants.■ They are most effective for reducing irritability, depression, and some of the other psychologic and physical symptoms of PMS. Buspirone or alprazolam (both antianxiety drugs) may reduce irritability and nervousness and help reduce stress. However, taking alprazolam can result in drug dependency. Doctors may ask a woman to continue keeping a record of her symptoms so that they can judge the effectiveness of treatment.

Women who have premenstrual dysphoric disorder may benefit from taking antidepressants. Taking a gonadotropin-releasing hormone (GnRH) agonist (such as leuprolide or goserelin★), given by injection, plus estrogen, given in a low dose by mouth or patch, may control symptoms. GnRH agonists cause the body to produce less estrogen and progesterone.

Symptoms of Premenstrual Syndrome

Physical
- Awareness of heartbeats (palpitations)
- Backache
- Bloating
- Breast fullness and pain
- Changes in appetite and cravings for certain foods
- Constipation
- Cramps, heaviness, or pressure in the lower abdomen
- Dizziness
- Easy bruising
- Fainting
- Fatigue
- Headaches
- Hot flashes
- Insomnia, including difficulty falling or staying asleep at night
- Joint and muscle pain
- Lack of energy
- Nausea and vomiting
- Pins-and-needles sensations in the hands and feet
- Skin problems, such as acne and localized scratch dermatitis
- Swelling of hands and feet
- Weight gain

Psychologic
- Agitation
- Confusion
- Crying spells
- Depression
- Difficulty concentrating
- Emotional hypersensitivity
- Forgetfulness or memory loss
- Irritability
- Mood swings
- Nervousness
- Short temper
- Social withdrawal

▲ see page 452

■ see table on page 618

★ see table on page 1371

Dysmenorrhea

Dysmenorrhea is pelvic pain during a menstrual period.

About three fourths of women with dysmenorrhea have primary dysmenorrhea, for which no cause can be identified. The rest have secondary dysmenorrhea, for which a cause is identified.

Primary dysmenorrhea may affect more than 50% of women, usually starting during adolescence. In about 5 to 15%, primary dysmenorrhea is sometimes severe, interfering with daily activities and resulting in absence from school or work. Primary dysmenorrhea may become less severe with age and after pregnancy.

In primary dysmenorrhea, the pain occurs only during menstrual cycles in which an egg is released. The pain is thought to result from prostaglandins released during menstruation. Prostaglandins are hormonelike substances that cause the uterus to contract, reduce the blood supply to the uterus, and increase the sensitivity of nerve endings in the uterus to pain. Women who have primary dysmenorrhea have higher levels of prostaglandins.

Common causes of secondary dysmenorrhea include endometriosis, fibroids, adenomyosis, pelvic congestion syndrome, and pelvic infection. In a few women, the pain results from passage of menstrual blood through a narrow cervix (cervical stenosis). A narrow cervix may be present at birth or result from removal of polyps or treatment of a precancerous condition (dysplasia) or cancer of the cervix. Abdominal pain due to other disorders, such as inflammation of the fallopian tubes or abnormal bands of fibrous tissue (adhesions) between structures in the abdomen, may be worse during a menstrual period.

Symptoms and Diagnosis

Pain occurs in the lower abdomen and may extend to the lower back or legs. The pain is usually crampy and comes and goes, but it may be a dull, constant ache. Usually, the pain starts shortly before or during the menstrual period, peaks after 24 hours, and subsides after 2 days. Other common symptoms include headache, nausea, constipation, diarrhea, and an urge to urinate frequently. Occasionally, vomiting occurs. Premenstrual irritability,

nervousness, depression, and abdominal bloating may persist during part or all of the menstrual period.

Diagnosis is based on symptoms and the results of a physical examination. To identify possible causes (such as fibroids), doctors may examine the abdominal cavity using a viewing tube (laparoscope) inserted through a small incision just below the navel. They may examine the interior of the uterus using a similar tube (hysteroscope) inserted through the vagina and cervix. Other procedures may include dilation and curettage (D and C) and hysterosalpingography.▲

Treatment

Nonsteroidal anti-inflammatory drugs (NSAIDs) usually relieve pain effectively. NSAIDs may be more effective if started 1 or 2 days before a menstrual period begins and continued for 1 or 2 days after it begins. An antiemetic drug may relieve nausea and vomiting, but these symptoms usually disappear without treatment as the pain subsides. Getting enough rest and sleep and exercising regularly may also help relieve symptoms.

If the pain continues to interfere with daily activities, oral contraceptives that contain estrogen in a low dose plus a progestin may be prescribed to suppress the release of eggs from the ovaries (ovulation). If these treatments are ineffective, procedures to identify the cause of the pain may be performed.

When dysmenorrhea results from another disorder, that disorder is treated if possible. A narrow cervical canal can be widened surgically. However, this operation usually relieves the pain only temporarily. If needed, fibroids or misplaced endometrial tissue (due to endometriosis) is surgically removed.

When other treatments are ineffective and the pain is severe, the nerves to the uterus may be cut surgically. However, this operation occasionally injures other pelvic organs, such as the ureters. Alternatively, hypnosis or acupuncture may be tried.

Amenorrhea

Amenorrhea is the absence of menstrual periods.

Some women never go through puberty, so periods never start. This disorder is called primary amenorrhea. In other women, periods start at puberty, then stop. This disorder is called secondary amenorrhea. Amenorrhea is

---

▲ see pages 1354 and 1355

normal only before puberty, during pregnancy, while breastfeeding, and after menopause.

Causes

Primary amenorrhea may be caused by a birth defect in which the uterus or fallopian tubes do not develop normally or by a chromosomal disorder, such as Turner syndrome (in which the cells contain one X chromosome instead of the usual two). Primary amenorrhea can also result from malfunction of the hypothalamus (a part of the brain), pituitary gland, or ovaries. Sometimes it results from malfunction of the thyroid gland (hyperthyroidism or hypothyroidism). Young women who are very thin, particularly those who have anorexia nervosa, may never menstruate.

Secondary amenorrhea can result from malfunction of the hypothalamus, pituitary gland, ovaries, thyroid gland, adrenal glands, or almost any part of the reproductive tract. Malfunction of these organs may result from a tumor, an autoimmune disorder, or use of certain drugs (including hallucinogenic drugs, chemotherapy drugs, antipsychotic drugs, and antidepressants). Cushing's syndrome and polycystic ovary syndrome (both of which involve hormonal abnormalities) may cause periods to stop or to be irregular. Other causes of secondary amenorrhea include a hydatidiform mole (a tumor that develops from an abnormal fertilized egg or the placenta) and Asherman's syndrome (scarring of the lining of the uterus resulting from an infection or surgery).

Stress due to internal or situational concerns can cause secondary amenorrhea, because stress interferes with the brain's control (through hormones) of the ovaries. Exercising too much or eating too little (as in anorexia nervosa) also affects the brain's control of the ovaries. Either behavior can cause the brain to signal the pituitary gland to decrease its production of the hormones that stimulate the ovaries. As a result, the ovaries produce less estrogen and periods stop.

Symptoms and Diagnosis

Amenorrhea may or may not be accompanied by other symptoms, depending on the cause.

Primary amenorrhea is diagnosed when periods have not started by age 16. Girls who have no signs of puberty by age 13 or who have not started having periods within 5 years of starting puberty are evaluated for possible problems.

Adenomyosis: Noncancerous Growth of the Uterus

In adenomyosis, glandular tissue from the lining of the uterus (endometrium) grows into the muscular wall of the uterus. The uterus becomes enlarged, sometimes doubling or tripling in size. This common disorder causes symptoms in only a small percentage of women, usually between the ages of 35 and 50. It is more common among women who have had children. The cause is unknown.

Symptoms include heavy and painful periods, bleeding between periods, vague pain in the pelvic area, and a feeling of pressure on the bladder and rectum. Sometimes sexual intercourse is painful.

Doctors suspect adenomyosis when they perform a pelvic examination and discover that the uterus is enlarged, round, and softer than normal. Pelvic ultrasound or magnetic resonance imaging (MRI) helps confirm the diagnosis. Sometimes when adenomyosis causes abnormal bleeding, a biopsy is performed. Usually, no treatment is effective, although oral contraceptives and gonadotropin-releasing hormone agonists (such as leuprolide or goserelin) may be tried. Analgesics may be taken for pain. In some cases, a hysterectomy may be performed.

Secondary amenorrhea is diagnosed when a woman of reproductive age (who is not pregnant or breastfeeding) has had no menstrual periods for at least 3 months. A physical examination can help doctors determine whether puberty occurred normally and may provide evidence of the cause of amenorrhea. But other procedures may be needed to confirm or identify the cause. Hormone levels in the blood may be measured. X-rays of the skull may be taken to look for a pituitary tumor. Computed tomography (CT), magnetic resonance imaging (MRI), or ultrasonography may be used to look for a tumor in the ovaries or adrenal glands.

Treatment

The underlying disorder is treated if possible. For example, a tumor is removed. Some disorders, such as Turner syndrome and other genetic disorders, cannot be cured.

If a girl's periods have never started and all test results are normal, she is examined every 3 to 6 months to monitor the progression of

What Is Pelvic Congestion Syndrome?

Sometimes pain that occurs before or during menstrual periods results from a problem with veins in the pelvis. The veins may widen and become convoluted and blood accumulates in them. The result is varicose veins in the pelvis— a disorder called pelvic congestion syndrome. Pain, sometimes debilitating, can result. Estrogen may contribute because it causes some veins supplying the ovaries and uterus to widen. Up to 15% of women of reproductive age have varicose veins in their pelvis, but not all of them have symptoms.

Typically, the pain is dull and aching, but it may be sharp or throbbing. It is worse at the end of the day (after a woman has been sitting or standing a long time) and is relieved when she lies down. The pain is also worse during or after sexual intercourse. It is often accompanied by low back pain, aches in the legs, abnormal menstrual bleeding, and a vaginal discharge. Occasionally, fatigue, mood swings, headache, and abdominal bloating occur.

Doctors may suspect pelvic congestion syndrome when a woman has pelvic pain but a pelvic examination does not detect inflammation or another abnormality. Ultrasonography can help doctors confirm the diagnosis. Alternatively, the veins can be viewed with a viewing tube inserted through a small incision just below the navel in a procedure called laparoscopy. Nonsteroidal anti-inflammatory drugs (NSAIDs) usually relieve the pain.

puberty. A progestin and sometimes estrogen may be given to start her periods and to stimulate the development of secondary sexual characteristics, such as breasts.

Abnormal Vaginal Bleeding

During the reproductive years, bleeding from the vagina may be abnormal when menstrual periods are too heavy or too light, last too long, occur too frequently, or are irregular. Any vaginal bleeding that occurs before puberty or after menopause is abnormal. Bleeding from the vagina may originate in the vagina or other reproductive organs, particularly the uterus.

▲ see box on page 1557

Many disorders, including inflammation, infection, and cancer, can cause bleeding from the vagina. Injuries, including that due to sexual abuse, can also cause bleeding. The cause may be hormonal changes, resulting in a type of bleeding called dysfunctional uterine bleeding. Some causes are more common among certain age groups.

In children, vaginal bleeding is rare and should be evaluated by a doctor. The most common cause is injury to the vulva or vagina (sometimes due to insertion of an object, such as a toy). Vaginal bleeding may also result from prolapse of the urethra (in which the urethra bulges outside of the body) or tumors of the reproductive tract. Tumors of the ovaries usually cause bleeding only if they produce hormones. Bleeding may also be caused by vaginal adenosis (overgrowth of glandular tissue in the vagina). Having vaginal adenosis increases the risk of developing clear cell adenocarcinoma (a cancer of the cervix and vagina) later in life.

Bleeding in children may also result from puberty that starts very early (precocious puberty▲). This cause can be easily recognized because pubic hair and breasts also develop.

In women of reproductive age, abnormal bleeding may be caused by birth control methods, such as oral contraceptives (a combination of a progestin and estrogen or a progestin alone) or an intrauterine device (IUD). Abnormal bleeding may also be caused by complications of pregnancy, such as an ectopic pregnancy, or by infections of the uterus, usually after delivery of a baby or an abortion.

Other causes of bleeding include blood disorders involving abnormal clotting (such as leukemia or a low platelet count), a hydatidiform mole, endometriosis, and noncancerous growths (such as adenomyosis, fibroids, cysts, and polyps). Cancer may cause bleeding in women of reproductive age, but not commonly. Bleeding from the vulva is usually due to injury. Thyroid disorders can cause menstrual periods to be irregular, to be heavy and occur more frequently, or to occur less frequently (as well as to stop).

In postmenopausal women, bleeding from the vagina may be due to thinning of the lining of the vagina (atrophic vaginitis), thinning or thickening (hyperplasia) of the lining of the uterus, or polyps in the uterus. Cancer, such as cancer of the cervix, vagina, or lining of the uterus (endometrial cancer) can also cause bleeding.

Diagnosis and Treatment

The cause of abnormal bleeding may be suggested by symptoms and the results of a physical examination (including a pelvic examination). But additional procedures may be needed. If doctors suspect vaginal adenosis, a biopsy of the vagina is performed. Usually, women who have abnormal bleeding from the vagina, particularly after menopause, are evaluated to determine whether they have cancer of the vagina, cervix, or lining of the uterus.▲ Procedures may include a Papanicolaou (Pap) test, a biopsy of the cervix, and dilation and curettage (D and C). Ultrasonography using an ultrasound device inserted through the vagina into the uterus (transvaginal ultrasonography) can determine whether the uterine lining is thickened. A biopsy of cells obtained during dilation and curettage can determine if the thickening is due to cancer.

Treatment varies, depending on the cause. Usually, a girl who has vaginal adenosis does not need to be treated unless cancer is detected. However, she is reexamined at regular intervals for signs of cancer. Uterine polyps, fibroids, and cancers may be surgically removed.

Dysfunctional Uterine Bleeding

Dysfunctional uterine bleeding is abnormal bleeding resulting from changes in the normal hormonal control of menstruation.

Dysfunctional uterine bleeding occurs most commonly at the beginning and end of the reproductive years: 20% of cases occur in adolescent girls, and more than 50% occur in women older than 45.

Dysfunctional uterine bleeding commonly results when the level of estrogen remains high. The high level of estrogen is not balanced by an appropriate level of progesterone, and release of an egg (ovulation) does not occur. As a result, the lining of the uterus (endometrium) thickens. This condition is called endometrial hyperplasia. The lining is then shed incompletely and irregularly, causing bleeding. Bleeding is irregular, prolonged, and sometimes heavy. This type of bleeding is common among women who have polycystic ovary syndrome.

Diagnosis and Treatment

Dysfunctional uterine bleeding is diagnosed when all other possible causes of vaginal bleeding have been excluded. The results of a blood test can help doctors estimate the extent of the blood loss. Transvaginal ultrasonography may be used to determine whether the uterine lining is thickened. If the risk of cancer of the uterine lining (endometrial cancer) is high, an endometrial biopsy is performed before drug treatment is started. Women at risk include those who are 35 or older, those who are substantially overweight, and those who have polycystic ovary syndrome, high blood pressure, or diabetes.

Treatment depends on how old the woman is, how heavy the bleeding is, whether the uterine lining is thickened, and whether the woman wishes to become pregnant.

When the uterine lining is thickened but its cells are normal, hormones may be used. Women who have heavy bleeding may be treated with an oral contraceptive containing estrogen and a progestin. When bleeding is very heavy, estrogen may be given intravenously until the bleeding stops. Sometimes a progestin is given by mouth at the same time or started 2 or 3 days later. Bleeding usually stops in 12 to 24 hours. Low doses of the oral contraceptive may then be prescribed for at least 3 months.

Treatment with an oral contraceptive or estrogen given intravenously is inappropriate for some women (such as postmenopausal women and women with significant risk factors for heart or blood vessel disease). These women may be given a progestin alone by mouth for 10 to 14 days each month. For women who wish to become pregnant, clomiphene may be given by mouth instead. It stimulates ovulation.

If the uterine lining remains thickened or the bleeding persists despite treatment with hormones, dilation and curettage (D and C) is usually needed. In this procedure, tissue from the uterine lining is removed by scraping. When the uterine lining is thickened and contains abnormal cells (particularly in women who are older than 35 and do not want to become pregnant), treatment begins with a high dose of a progestin. If the cells continue to be abnormal after treatment, a hysterectomy is performed, because the abnormal cells may become cancerous.

Polycystic Ovary Syndrome

Polycystic ovary syndrome (Stein-Leventhal syndrome) involves enlarged ovaries, which contain many fluid-filled sacs (cysts), and a

▲ see page 1401

tendency to have high levels of male hormones (androgens).

Polycystic ovary syndrome affects about 7 to 10% of women. A common cause is excess production of luteinizing hormone by the pituitary gland. The excess luteinizing hormone increases the production of male hormones (androgens). If the disorder is not treated, some of the male hormones may be converted to estrogen. Not enough progesterone is produced to balance the estrogen's effects. If this situation continues a long time, the lining of the uterus (endometrium) may become extremely thickened (a condition called endometrial hyperplasia). Also, the risk of cancer of the lining of the uterus (endometrial cancer) may be increased.

Symptoms and Diagnosis

Symptoms typically develop during puberty. In some women, menstrual periods do not start at puberty. Thus, these women do not release an egg from the ovaries (ovulate). These women also develop symptoms related to the high levels of male hormones—a process called masculinization or virilization. Symptoms include acne, a deepened voice, a decrease in breast size, and an increase in muscle size and in body hair (hirsutism) growing in a male pattern, such as on the chest and face. Many women with polycystic ovary syndrome produce too much insulin, or the insulin they produce does not function normally. Consequently, these women tend to gain weight or have a hard time losing weight. Most women are obese. Other women have irregular vaginal bleeding, with no increase in weight or body hair. Women with polycystic ovary syndrome also have an increased risk of heart disease, diabetes, and high blood pressure.

Often, the diagnosis is based on symptoms. Blood tests to measure levels of luteinizing hormone and male hormones are performed, and ultrasonography of the ovaries may be performed. Ultrasonography or computed tomography (CT) may be used to determine whether the male hormones are being produced by a tumor in an ovary or adrenal gland.

Treatment

No ideal treatment is available. The choice of treatment depends on the type and severity of symptoms, the woman's age, and her plans regarding pregnancy. Often, a biopsy of the uterine lining is performed to make sure no cancer is present.

If insulin levels are high, lowering them may help. Exercising (at least 30 minutes a day) and reducing consumption of carbohydrates (found in breads, pasta, potatoes, and sweets) can help lower insulin levels. In some women, weight loss lowers insulin levels enough that ovulation can begin. Weight loss may help reduce hair growth and the risk of thickening of the uterine lining.

Women who do not wish to become pregnant may take a progestin by mouth or a combination oral contraceptive (which contains estrogen and a progestin). Either treatment may reduce the risk of cancer of the uterine lining due to the high estrogen level and help lower the levels of male hormones. However, oral contraceptives are not given to women who have reached menopause or who have other significant risk factors for heart or blood vessel disorders.

Women who wish to become pregnant may take clomiphene. This drug stimulates ovulation. If clomiphene is not effective, other hormones may be tried. They include follicle-stimulating hormone (to stimulate the ovaries), a gonadotropin-releasing hormone agonist (to stimulate the release of follicle-stimulating hormone), and human chorionic gonadotropin (to trigger ovulation).

Increased body hair can be bleached or removed by electrolysis, plucking, waxing, hair-removing liquids or creams (depilatories), or laser. No drug treatment for removing excess hair is ideal or completely effective. Oral contraceptives may help, but they must be taken for several months before any effect, which is often slight, can be seen. Spironolactone, a drug that blocks the production and action of male hormones, can reduce unwanted body hair. Side effects include increased urine production and low blood pressure (sometimes causing fainting). Spironolactone may not be safe for a developing fetus, so sexually active women taking the drug are advised to use effective birth control methods. Cyproterone, a strong progestin that blocks the action of male hormones, reduces unwanted body hair in 50 to 75% of affected women. It is used in many countries but is not approved in the United States. Gonadotropin-releasing hormone agonists and antagonists are being studied as treatment for unwanted body hair. Both types of drugs inhibit the production of sex hormones by the ovaries. But both can cause bone loss and lead to osteoporosis.

CHAPTER 245

Endometriosis

Endometriosis is a noncancerous disorder in which pieces of endometrial tissue—normally occurring only in the lining of the uterus (endometrium)—grow outside the uterus.

Endometriosis is a chronic disorder that may be painful. Exactly how many women have endometriosis is unknown because it can usually be diagnosed only by directly viewing the endometrial tissue (which requires a surgical procedure). Endometriosis probably affects about 10 to 15% of menstruating women aged 25 to 44. It can also affect teenagers.

Endometriosis sometimes runs in families. It is more likely to occur in women who have their first baby after age 30, who have never had a baby, who are of Asian descent, or who have structural abnormalities of the uterus.

The cause of endometriosis is unclear, but there are several theories: Small pieces of the uterine lining that are shed during menstruation may flow backward through the fallopian tubes toward the ovaries into the abdominal cavity, rather than flow through the vagina and out of the body with the menstrual period. Cells from the uterine lining (endometrial cells) may be transported through the blood or lymphatic vessels to another location. Or cells located outside the uterus may change into endometrial cells.

Common locations of misplaced endometrial tissue are the ovaries and the ligaments that support the uterus. Less common locations are the outer surface of the small and large intestines, the ureters (tubes leading from the kidneys to the bladder), the bladder, the vagina, and surgical scars in the abdomen. Rarely, endometrial tissue grows on the membranes covering the lungs (pleura), the sac that envelops the heart (pericardium), the vulva, or the cervix.

As the disorder progresses, the misplaced endometrial tissue tends to gradually increase in size. It may also spread to new locations.

Symptoms

The main symptom associated with endometriosis is pain in the lower abdomen and pelvic area. The pain usually varies during the menstrual cycle. Menstrual irregularities, such as heavy menstrual bleeding and spotting before menstrual periods, may occur. Misplaced endometrial tissue responds to the same hormones—estrogen and progesterone (produced by the ovaries)—as normal endometrial tissue in the uterus. Consequently, the misplaced tissue may also bleed during menstruation, often causing cramps and pain.

Some women with severe endometriosis have no symptoms. Others, even some with minimal disease, have incapacitating pain. In many women, endometriosis does not cause pain until it has been present for several years. For such women, sexual intercourse tends to be painful before or during menstruation.

Endometrial tissue attached to the large intestine or bladder may cause abdominal bloating, pain during bowel movements, rectal bleeding during menstruation, or pain above the pubic bone during urination. Endometrial tissue attached to an ovary or a nearby structure can form a blood-filled mass (endometrioma). Occasionally, an endometrioma ruptures or leaks, causing sudden, sharp abdominal pain.

The misplaced endometrial tissue may irritate nearby tissues. As a result, scar tissue may form, sometimes as bands of fibrous tissue (adhesions) between structures in the abdomen. The misplaced endometrial tissue and adhesions can interfere with the functioning of organs. Rarely, adhesions block the intestine.

Severe endometriosis may block the egg's passage from the ovary into the uterus, causing infertility. Mild endometriosis may also cause infertility, but how it does so is less clear. Endometriosis affects as many as 25 to 50% of infertile women.

Diagnosis

A doctor may suspect endometriosis in a woman who has certain symptoms or unexplained infertility. Occasionally, during a pelvic examination, a woman may feel pain or tenderness or a doctor may feel a mass of tissue behind the uterus or near the ovaries.

However, the diagnosis can usually be confirmed only if a doctor examines the abdominal cavity and sees pieces of endometrial tissue. For this examination, a viewing tube

Endometriosis: Misplaced Tissue

In endometriosis, small or large patches of tissue that usually occurs only in the lining of the uterus (endometrium) appear in other parts of the body. How and why the tissue appears in other locations is unclear. The misplaced endometrial tissue may adhere to the ovaries, the ligaments supporting the uterus, the small and large intestines, the ureters, the bladder, the vagina, surgical scars, or the lining of the chest cavity. The misplaced endometrial tissue can irritate nearby tissues, causing large bands of scar tissue (adhesions) to form between structures in the abdomen.

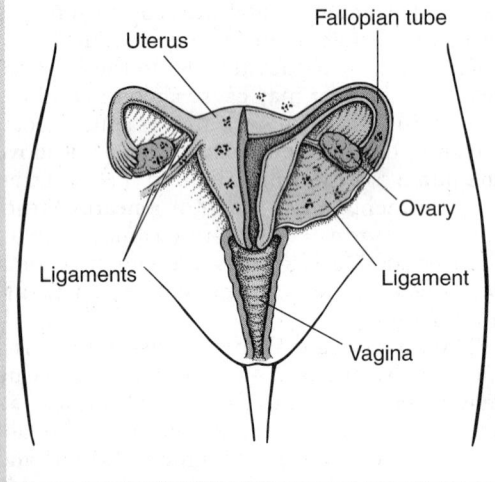

(laparoscope) is usually used. It is inserted into the abdominal cavity through a small incision just below the navel. Carbon dioxide gas is injected into the abdominal cavity to distend it so that organs can be viewed more easily. Laparoscopy usually requires a general anesthetic, so that the entire abdominal cavity can be examined. An overnight stay in the hospital is not required. Laparoscopy may cause mild abdominal discomfort, but normal activities can usually be resumed in 1 or 2 days.

Sometimes a biopsy is necessary. A small sample of tissue is removed, usually through the laparoscope, and examined under a microscope.

▲ see page 1418   ■ see page 452

Other procedures, such as ultrasonography, barium enemas with x-ray, computed tomography (CT), and magnetic resonance imaging (MRI), may be used to determine the extent of endometriosis and follow its course, but their usefulness for diagnosis is limited. Blood tests may be performed to measure levels of substances (called markers) that increase when endometriosis is present. Markers include cancer antigen 125 and antibodies to endometrial tissue. Such measurements may help a doctor follow the course of endometriosis. However, because these markers may be increased in several other disorders, they are not useful in establishing the diagnosis. Tests may also be performed to determine whether the endometriosis is affecting the woman's fertility.▲

Treatment

Treatment depends on a woman's symptoms, pregnancy plans, and age, as well as the extent of endometriosis.

Drugs can be given to suppress the activity of the ovaries and thus slow the growth of the misplaced endometrial tissue and reduce bleeding and pain. However, these drugs do not eliminate endometriosis. They include combination oral contraceptives (estrogen plus a progestin), progestins (such as medroxyprogesterone), danazol (a synthetic hormone related to testosterone), and gonadotropin-releasing hormone agonists (GnRH agonists—such as buserelin, goserelin, leuprolide, and nafarelin). GnRH agonists turn off the brain's signal to the ovaries to produce estrogen and progesterone. As a result, production of these hormones decreases. Continued use of GnRH agonists causes a decrease in bone density and may lead to osteoporosis unless small doses of estrogen plus a progestin or of a progestin alone are also taken. Even when taken this way, GnRH agonists are not usually given for longer than 1 year. New types of drugs, such as GnRH antagonists, antiprogestins, and aromatase inhibitors, are being studied for the treatment of endometriosis.

Nonsteroidal anti-inflammatory drugs (NSAIDs)■ may be given to relieve pain. For persistent pain, options include surgery to remove the misplaced endometrial tissue, surgery to interrupt the nerve pathways that conduct pain sensation from the pelvic area to the brain, and surgery to do both.

Often, misplaced endometrial tissue can be removed during laparoscopy when the diagno-

℞ DRUGS COMMONLY USED TO TREAT ENDOMETRIOSIS

DRUG	SOME SIDE EFFECTS AND COMPLICATIONS	COMMENTS
Combination estrogen-progestin oral contraceptives		
	Abdominal bloating, breast tenderness, increased appetite, ankle swelling, nausea, bleeding between periods, and deep vein thrombosis	Oral contraceptives may be useful for women who wish to delay childbearing. They may be taken cyclically or continuously
Progestins		
	Bleeding between periods, mood swings, depression, and atrophic vaginitis	Progestins are drugs similar to the hormone progesterone. They can be given by mouth or by injection into a muscle
Danazol		
	Weight gain, acne, a lowered voice, an increase in body hair, hot flashes, vaginal dryness, ankle swelling, muscle cramps, bleeding between periods, decreased breast size, mood swings, liver malfunction, carpal tunnel syndrome, and adverse effects on cholesterol levels in the blood	Danazol, a synthetic hormone related to testosterone, inhibits the activity of estrogen and progesterone. It is given by mouth. The usefulness of danazol may be limited by its side effects
GnRH agonists		
	Hot flashes, vaginal dryness, a decrease in bone density, and mood swings	GnRH agonists may be injected into a muscle once a month, used as a nasal spray, or implanted as a pellet under the skin. These drugs are often given with estrogen, a progestin, or both to reduce the side effects of a decrease in estrogen levels, including decreased bone density. (This use of estrogen and a progestin or of a progestin alone is called add-back therapy.)

GnRH = gonadotropin-releasing hormone.

sis is made. However, if endometriosis is moderate to severe, more extensive surgery requiring an incision into the abdomen (abdominal surgery) may be necessary. This type of surgery is usually necessary when pieces of endometrial tissue are larger than 1½ to 2 inches in diameter, when adhesions in the lower abdomen or pelvis cause significant symptoms, when endometrial tissue blocks one or both fallopian tubes, or when drugs cannot relieve severe lower abdominal or pelvic pain.

Sometimes electrocautery (a device that uses an electrical current to produce heat), an ultrasound device, or a laser (which concentrates light into an intense beam to produce heat) is used to destroy or remove endometrial tissue during laparoscopic or abdominal surgery. Doctors remove as much misplaced endometrial tissue as possible without damaging the ovaries. Thus, the woman's ability to have children may be preserved. Depending on the extent of the endometriosis, 40 to 70% of women who have surgery may become pregnant.

Surgical removal of misplaced endometrial tissue is only a temporary measure. After treatment, endometriosis recurs in most women, although the use of oral contraceptives or other drugs may slow its progression.

The drugs used to suppress endometriosis may be started immediately after surgery.

Some women who have endometriosis can become pregnant through the use of assisted reproductive techniques, such as in vitro fertilization.▲

Both ovaries and the uterus are removed only when drugs do not relieve abdominal or pelvic pain and the woman does not plan to become pregnant. Because removal of the ovaries and uterus has the same effects as menopause (effects that result from the decrease in estrogen levels),■ estrogen therapy may be started. Some experts recommend the use of estrogen plus a progestin (because a progestin can suppress the growth of endometriosis). When estrogen is given alone, it may be started after a delay of 4 to 6 months after surgery, because estrogen may stimulate any remaining pieces of endometrial tissue. The delay gives the endometrial tissue time to disappear.

CHAPTER 246

Fibroids

A fibroid is a noncancerous tumor composed of muscle and fibrous tissue.

Fibroids are also known as fibromyomas, fibromas, myofibromas, leiomyomas, and myomas. Fibroids in the uterus are the most common noncancerous tumor of the female reproductive tract. They occur in one fourth of white women and one half of black women.

What causes fibroids to grow in the uterus is unknown. High estrogen levels seem to stimulate their growth. Thus, fibroids often grow larger during pregnancy and shrink after menopause. If fibroids grow too large, they may not be able to get enough blood. As a result, they begin to degenerate.

Fibroids may be microscopic or as large as a basketball. They may grow in the wall of the uterus, from the wall into the interior of the uterus (sometimes from a stalk), under the lining of the uterus, or on the outside of the uterus. Usually, more than one fibroid is present. Large fibroids that grow in the wall or under the lining of the uterus can distort the shape or interior of the uterus.

Symptoms

Symptoms depend on the number of fibroids present, their size, and their location in the uterus. Many fibroids, even large ones, do not cause symptoms. However, large fibroids, particularly those that grow in the wall of the uterus, may cause pain, pressure, or a feeling of heaviness in the pelvic area during or between menstrual periods. Fibroids may press on the bladder, making a woman need to urinate more frequently or more urgently. They may press on the rectum, causing discomfort and constipation. Large fibroids may cause the abdomen to enlarge. A fibroid growing from a stalk inside the uterus may twist and cause severe pain. Fibroids that are growing or degenerating usually cause pressure or pain. Pain due to degenerating fibroids can last as long as they continue to degenerate.

Fibroids, particularly those just under the lining of the uterus, commonly cause menstrual bleeding to be heavier or to last longer than usual. Anemia may result from the loss of blood. Less often, fibroids cause bleeding between menstrual periods, after sexual intercourse, or after menopause. Rarely, fibroids cause infertility by blocking the fallopian tubes or distorting the shape of the uterus, making implantation of a fertilized egg difficult or impossible.

Fibroids that cause no symptoms before pregnancy may cause problems during pregnancy. Problems include miscarriage, early (preterm) labor, abnormal positioning (presentation) of the baby before delivery, and excessive blood loss after delivery (postpartum hemorrhage).

Rarely, cancerous tumors that resemble fibroids (sarcomas) develop in the uterus.★

▲ see page 1419   ■ see page 1356
★ see page 1403

Diagnosis

Doctors can often detect fibroids during a pelvic examination. Several procedures that enable doctors to examine the uterus can confirm the diagnosis. For transvaginal ultrasonography, an ultrasound device is inserted into the vagina. For saline infusion sonohysterography, ultrasonography is performed after a small amount of fluid is infused into the uterus to outline its interior. For hysteroscopy, a flexible viewing tube is inserted through the vagina and cervix into the uterus. A local, regional, or general anesthetic is used. Sometimes magnetic resonance imaging (MRI) or computed tomography (CT) is also performed. Additional tests are usually unnecessary.

If bleeding (other than menstrual) has occurred, doctors may want to exclude cancer of the uterus. So they may perform a Papanicolaou (Pap) test, biopsy of the uterine lining (endometrial biopsy), ultrasonography, sonohysterography, or hysteroscopy.

Treatment

For most women who have fibroids but no symptoms, treatment is not required. They are reexamined every 6 to 12 months to determine whether the fibroid is growing.

Several treatment options, including drugs and surgery, are available if bleeding or other symptoms worsen or if fibroids enlarge substantially.

Drugs: Drugs may be used to relieve symptoms or to shrink fibroids, but only temporarily. No drug can permanently shrink a fibroid. Nonsteroidal anti-inflammatory drugs (NSAIDs), alone or given with a progestin (a drug similar to the hormone progesterone), can reduce bleeding caused by fibroids. Both are usually taken by mouth, but the progestin may be injected into muscle. Danazol (a synthetic hormone related to testosterone) can suppress the growth of a fibroid, but it is rarely used because of its side effects.▲ Hormonal contraceptives■ can control bleeding in some women. However, when women discontinue contraceptives, abnormal bleeding and pain tend to recur. Also, when some women are treated with contraceptives, the fibroids grow.

Synthetic forms of gonadotropin-releasing hormone (GnRH agonists) can shrink fibroids and reduce bleeding by causing the body to produce less estrogen (and progesterone). GnRH agonists may be given before surgery to make removal of fibroids easier. They are injected once a month, used as a nasal spray, or

implanted as a pellet under the skin. They can be given only for a few months, because if taken for a long time, they may cause a decrease in bone density and increase the risk of osteoporosis.★ Estrogen may be given in low doses with GnRH agonists to help prevent side effects. Fibroids often regrow within 6 months after the GnRH agonist is discontinued.

Surgery: Surgery may involve removal of the fibroids (myomectomy) or removal of the entire uterus (hysterectomy). In contrast with hysterectomy, myomectomy usually preserves the ability to have children and avoids the psychologic effects of removing the uterus. However, fibroids regrow in up to 50% of women.

For myomectomy, an incision may be made in the abdomen. Or a viewing tube with surgical attachments may be inserted through a small incision just below the navel (laparoscopy) or through the vagina into the uterus (hysteroscopy). Which method is used depends on the size, number, and location of fibroids. Laparoscopy and hysteroscopy are outpatient procedures, and recovery is faster than recovery after an abdominal incision. However, laparoscopy often cannot be used to remove large fibroids, and the risk of complications after laparoscopy can be higher.

Hysterectomy is usually considered when symptoms, such as pain and bleeding, are severe enough to interfere with daily activities and other treatments have been ineffective. If a woman is bothered by large fibroids that she can feel, she may choose to have a hysterectomy. Hysterectomy is performed only in women who do not wish to become pregnant. It is the only permanent solution to fibroids. For treatment of fibroids, only the uterus is removed, not the ovaries.

Other Treatments: New procedures that destroy rather than remove fibroids appear to shrink fibroids. In myolysis, a needle that transmits an electrical current is inserted into the fibroid during laparoscopy. The current is used to destroy the core of the fibroid, causing the fibroid to shrink. In cryomyolysis, a similar procedure, a cold probe (containing liquid nitrogen) is used to destroy the core of the fibroid. Whether these procedures affect the ability to become pregnant is unknown. Also,

---

▲ see table on page 1371   ■ see page 1419

★ see table on page 1371

fibroids tend to grow back after these procedures.

In uterine artery embolization, a thin tubular, flexible instrument (catheter) is inserted into the main artery of the thigh (femoral artery) through a puncture made with a needle or through a tiny incision. Before the procedure, a local anesthetic is given to numb the insertion site. The catheter is threaded to the artery that supplies the fibroid. Small synthetic particles are injected. They travel to the small arteries supplying the fibroid. There,

they block blood flow, causing the fibroid to shrink. Whether the fibroid will regrow (because blocked arteries reopen or new arteries form) and whether the woman can become pregnant are unknown. The most common problems after this procedure are pain and infection.

After these procedures, fibroids may grow back, or if they could not be completely removed, they may continue to grow. In such cases, a woman may need to have a hysterectomy.

CHAPTER 247

Vaginal Infections

In the United States, vaginal infections are one of the most common reasons women see their doctor, accounting for more than 10 million visits each year. Usually, vaginal infections cause only discomfort, although the discomfort may be substantial. However, these infections occasionally are or become serious.

Vaginal infections are a type of vaginitis, or inflammation of the lining (mucosa) of the vagina. Inflammation may result from chemical or mechanical irritants, such as hygiene products, bubble bath, laundry detergents, contraceptive foams and jellies, and synthetic underwear, as well as from bacterial, yeast, and viral infections.

In women, anything that reduces the acidity (increases the pH) of the vagina increases the likelihood of infection. Acidity may be reduced by hormonal changes shortly before and during menstrual periods or during pregnancy. Frequent douching, use of spermicides, and semen can also reduce acidity.

Many bacteria normally reside in the vagina. One type, called lactobacilli, normally maintains the acidity of the vagina. By doing so, lactobacilli help keep the lining of the vagina healthy and prevent the growth of bacteria or yeasts that cause infections. Bacterial vaginosis, the most common vaginal infection, results when the number of protective lactobacilli decreases and the number of other

normally occurring bacteria (such as *Gardnerella* and *Peptostreptococcus*) increases. The reason for these changes is unknown. Bacterial vaginosis is more common among women who have a sexually transmitted disease, who have several sex partners, or who use an intrauterine device (IUD). But it is not a sexually transmitted disease. It can also occur in sexually inexperienced, lesbian, or monogamous women.

In women, yeast infections due to the fungus *Candida albicans* (candidiasis) are particularly common. *Candida albicans* normally resides on the skin or in the intestines. From these areas, the organism can spread to the vagina. Yeast infections are not transmitted sexually. They are common among pregnant women, obese women, and women who have diabetes. Yeast infections are more likely to occur during menstrual periods. Yeast infections are also more likely to develop if the immune system is suppressed by drugs (such as corticosteroids or chemotherapy drugs) or impaired by a disorder (such as AIDS). Antibiotics taken by mouth tend to kill the bacteria in the vagina that normally suppress the growth of yeast. Thus, the use of antibiotics increases the risk of developing vaginal infections. After menopause, women who take hormone replacement therapy are more likely to develop yeast infections.

Some vaginal infections are sexually transmitted.▲ Sexually transmitted diseases that can affect the vagina include chlamydial infections, genital herpes,■ gonorrhea, syphilis,

▲ see page 1176   ■ see page 1160

and trichomoniasis (a protozoan infection). Genital warts usually develop on the vulva but can develop in the vagina or on the cervix.

In children, vaginal infections are most commonly due to an object (such as a toy) inserted in the vagina and to bacteria. Yeast infections are less common. Children may develop a sexually transmitted vaginal infection as a result of sexual abuse.

Tight, nonabsorbent underclothing may irritate the genital area and trap moisture, making infection by bacteria or yeast more likely. Not keeping the genital area clean (for example, inadequately or improperly cleaning it after urinating or defecating) and fingering the genital area (which young girls may do) may make infection more likely.

Symptoms and Diagnosis

Typically, vaginal infections produce a vaginal discharge and irritation in the genital area. The appearance and amount of the discharge vary depending on the cause. Soreness and swelling are less common. Some infections can make sexual intercourse painful and make urination painful and more frequent. Rarely, the folds of skin around the vaginal and urethral openings become stuck together. However, vaginal infections sometimes produce minimal or no symptoms. Some vaginal infections, if untreated, may lead to complications that are sometimes serious.

Because a vaginal discharge, itching, and odor may have different causes, children or women who have such symptoms should see a doctor. Information about a vaginal discharge, if present, can help the doctor determine the cause. The doctor may ask about possible causes of the discharge, such as lotions or creams used to try to relieve the symptoms (including home remedies), as well as hygiene. Other questions include when the discharge began, whether it is accompanied by itching, burning, pain, or a sore in the genital area, when it occurs in relation to the menstrual period, whether the discharge comes and goes or is always present, and, if the woman has had an abnormal discharge before, how it responded to treatment. The woman may be asked about her past and current use of birth control, pain after sexual intercourse, previous vaginal infections, and the possibility of sexually transmitted diseases. The doctor also asks whether the sex partner has symptoms and whether anyone else in the household has itching in the genital area. This information

Nearby Infections: Vulvitis and Bartholinitis

The vulva is the area surrounding the opening of the vagina and containing the external female genital organs. Vulvitis is inflammation of the vulva. When both the vulva and vagina are inflamed, the disorder is called vulvovaginitis. Vulvitis may result from allergic reactions to substances that come in contact with the vulva (such as soaps, bubble bath, fabrics, and perfumes), from skin disorders (such as dermatitis), or from infections, including candidiasis and sexually transmitted diseases (such as herpes). The vulva may be infested by pubic lice (a disorder called pediculosis pubis).

Vulvitis causes itching, soreness, and redness. Rarely, the folds of skin around the vaginal and urethral openings (labia) become stuck together. Long-standing (chronic) vulvitis may result in sore, scaly, thickened, or whitish patches on the vulva. If chronic vulvitis does not respond to treatment, doctors usually perform a biopsy to look for the cause, such as cancer.

Bartholin's glands are located beside the opening of the vagina. Bartholinitis—infection of one or both glands or their ducts—may develop when bacteria from the vagina enter the glands. Rarely, bartholinitis is due to a sexually transmitted disease. The surrounding tissues (vulva) may swell. Pus accumulates in the gland, causing a painful abscess. Taking an antibiotic usually clears the infection in a few days, but the infection may recur. Analgesics may relieve the pain. An abscess or cyst needs to be drained.

If the ducts become blocked, the gland may swell but cause no pain—a disorder called Bartholin's cyst. In women younger than 50, a cyst that causes no symptoms does not require treatment. In women 50 and older, a biopsy of the cyst is recommended.

helps the doctor identify the cause of the woman's symptoms and determine whether other people require treatment.

A pelvic examination is performed. While examining the vagina, the doctor takes a sample of the discharge, if present, with a cotton-tipped swab. The sample is examined under a microscope or cultured to identify bacteria or other organisms. To determine whether the infection has spread outside the vagina, the

SOME VAGINAL INFECTIONS

INFECTION	SYMPTOMS	COMPLICATIONS	TREATMENT
Bacterial vaginosis	A thin, white, gray or yellowish cloudy discharge with a foul or fishy odor that may become stronger after sexual intercourse Itching and irritation	Pelvic inflammatory disease Infections of the membranes around the fetus Infections of the uterus after delivery of a baby or after surgery	Metronidazole (used first; taken as a vaginal gel or by mouth) Clindamycin
Chlamydial infection	Usually, no symptoms A yellow, puslike discharge A frequent need to urinate Pain during urination Abnormal vaginal bleeding	Pelvic inflammatory disease Infection and scarring of the fallopian tubes	Azithromycin Doxycycline Ofloxacin Tetracycline
Genital herpes	Painful blisters that form sores in the genital area, in the vagina, and on the cervix Itching Sometimes a fever and flu-like symptoms	If present during delivery, possibly serious infection in the newborn	Acyclovir Famciclovir Valacyclovir
Gonorrhea	A puslike discharge A frequent need to urinate Pain during urination Fever Pelvic pain	Pelvic inflammatory disease Infection of the fallopian tubes Arthritis	Ceftriaxone with azithromycin or doxycycline
Syphilis	Painless sore on the vagina or vulva Later, a fever and flu-like symptoms	Rarely, serious heart or brain disorders	Penicillin
Trichomoniasis	A usually profuse, greenish yellow, frothy, fishy-smelling discharge Itching and irritation	No known serious complications	Metronidazole (given by mouth only)
Yeast infection (candidiasis)	Thick, white, clumpy discharge (like cottage cheese) Moderate to severe itching and burning (but not always) Redness and swelling of the genital area	No serious complications	Butoconazole Clotrimazole Econazole Fluconazole Ketoconazole Miconazole Terconazole Tioconazole

doctor checks the uterus and ovaries by inserting the index and middle fingers of one gloved hand into the vagina and pressing on the outside of the lower abdomen with the other hand. If this maneuver causes substantial pain or if a fever is present, the infection may have spread.

Prevention

Keeping the genital area clean and dry can help prevent infections. Washing every day with a mild soap (such as glycerin soap) and rinsing and drying thoroughly are recommended. Wiping front to back after urinating or defecating prevents bacteria from the anus from being moved to the vagina. Children should be taught proper hygiene.

Wearing loose, absorbent clothing, such as cotton or cotton-lined underpants, allows air to circulate and helps keep the genital area dry. Douching frequently and using medicated douches are discouraged. These measures can reduce the acidity of the vagina, making infections, including pelvic inflammatory disease, more likely. Practicing sex safe and limiting the number of sex partners are important preventive measures.

Treatment

Treatment varies according to the cause.

Bacterial vaginosis is treated with an antibiotic taken by mouth or applied as a vaginal gel or cream. Bacterial vaginosis usually resolves in a few days but commonly recurs. If it recurs often, antibiotics may have to be taken for a long time. Propionic acid jelly may be used to make the vaginal secretions more acidic and thus discourage the growth of bacteria. For sexually transmitted diseases, both sex partners are treated at the same time to prevent reinfection.

Yeast infections are treated with antifungal drugs applied as a cream to the affected area, inserted into the vagina as a suppository, or taken by mouth. Several antifungal creams and suppositories are available without a prescription. A single dose of an antifungal drug taken by mouth is usually as effective as vaginal creams and suppositories. However, if infections recur often, several doses may be needed.

For trichomoniasis, a single dose of metronidazole cures up to 95% of women. However, a single dose is more likely to cause nausea and vomiting than treatment with several smaller doses. During sexual intercourse, condoms should be used until the infection resolves.

To relieve symptoms, a woman can use a premeasured vinegar-and-water douche, but only for a brief time. Occasionally, placing ice packs against the genital area, applying cool compresses, or sitting in a cool sitz bath may reduce soreness and itching. A sitz bath is taken in the sitting position with the water covering only the genital and rectal area. Flushing the genital area with lukewarm water squeezed from a water bottle may also provide relief.

Women who are at high risk of a yeast infection, such as those who have an impaired immune system, who have diabetes, or who are taking antibiotics for a long time (as for a urinary tract infection), may need to take an antifungal drug to prevent other infections from developing.

CHAPTER 248

Pelvic Inflammatory Disease

Pelvic inflammatory disease is an infection of the upper female reproductive organs.

Pelvic inflammatory disease can affect the cervix (causing mucopurulent cervicitis), the uterus (causing endometritis), the fallopian tubes (causing salpingitis), and sometimes the ovaries (causing oophoritis). Pelvic inflammatory disease is the most common preventable cause of infertility in the United States. Infertility occurs in about one of five women with pelvic inflammatory disease. About one third of women who have had pelvic inflammatory disease develop the infection again.

Pelvic inflammatory disease usually occurs in sexually active women. It rarely affects girls before their first menstrual period (menarche) or women during pregnancy or after menopause. Risk is increased for women who are younger than 24 and who do not use a barrier contraceptive (such as a condom or diaphragm), who have many sex partners, who have a sexually transmitted disease or bacterial vaginosis, or who use an intrauterine device (IUD).

Infection is usually caused by bacteria that enter the vagina, most commonly, during sexual intercourse. Usually, pelvic inflammatory disease is caused by the bacteria that cause gonorrhea (*Neisseria gonorrhoeae*) or chlamydial infection (*Chlamydia trachomatis*), which are sexually transmitted diseases.▲ Bacteria may also enter the vagina during douching. Less commonly, bacteria enter the vagina during a vaginal delivery, an abortion, or a medical procedure, such as dilation and curettage (D and C).

Pelvic inflammatory disease typically starts in the cervix and uterus. Usually, both fallopian tubes are infected, although symptoms may be worse on one side. The ovaries are not usually infected, unless the infection is severe.

Symptoms

Pelvic inflammatory disease tends to cause symptoms cyclically, toward the end of the menstrual period or for a few days afterward. For many women, the first symptoms are a low fever, mild to moderate abdominal pain (often aching), irregular vaginal bleeding, and a vaginal discharge with a bad odor. As the infection spreads, pain in the lower abdomen becomes increasingly severe and may be accompanied by nausea or vomiting. Later, the fever becomes higher, and the discharge often becomes puslike and yellow-green. However, a chlamydial infection may not produce a discharge or any other noticeable symptoms.

Sometimes infected fallopian tubes become blocked. Blocked tubes may swell because fluid is trapped. If the infection is not treated, pain in the lower abdomen may persist and irregular bleeding may occur. The infection can spread to surrounding structures, including the membrane that lines the abdominal cavity and covers the abdominal organs (causing peritonitis). Peritonitis can cause sudden, severe pain in the entire abdomen.

If infection of the fallopian tubes is due to gonorrhea or a chlamydial infection, it may spread to the tissues around the liver. Such an infection may cause pain in the upper right side of the abdomen that resembles a gallbladder disorder or stones. This complication is called the Fitz-Hugh–Curtis syndrome.

A collection of pus (abscess) forms in the fallopian tubes or ovaries of about 15% of women who have infected fallopian tubes. An abscess sometimes ruptures, and pus spills into the pelvic cavity (causing peritonitis). A rupture causes severe pain in the lower abdomen, quickly followed by nausea, vomiting, and very low blood pressure (shock). The infection may spread to the bloodstream (a condition called sepsis) and can be fatal.

Pelvic inflammatory disease often produces a puslike fluid, which can result in scarring and the formation of abnormal bands of scar tissue (adhesions) in the reproductive organs or between organs in the abdomen. Infertility may result. The longer and more severe the inflammation and the more often it recurs, the higher the risk of infertility and other complications. The risk increases each time a woman develops the infection.

Women who have had pelvic inflammatory disease are 6 to 10 times more likely to have a tubal pregnancy, in which the fetus grows in a fallopian tube rather than in the uterus. This type of pregnancy threatens the life of the woman, and the fetus cannot survive.

Prevention

Prevention of pelvic inflammatory disease is essential to the health and fertility of a woman. The best way to prevent the infection is abstaining from sex. However, if a woman has sexual intercourse with only one partner, the risk of pelvic inflammatory disease is very low, as long as neither person has a sexually transmitted disease. Refraining from douching is also helpful.

Barrier methods of birth control (such as condoms) and spermicides (such as vaginal foams) used with a barrier method can help prevent pelvic inflammatory disease.

Diagnosis and Treatment

A doctor suspects the diagnosis based mainly on the severity and location of the pain. A physical examination, including a pelvic examination, is performed. A sample is usually taken from the cervix and tested to determine whether the woman has gonorrhea or a chlamydial infection. Other symptoms and laboratory test results help confirm the diagnosis. The white blood cell count is usually high. Ultrasonography of the pelvis may be performed. If the diagnosis is still uncertain or if the woman does not respond to treatment, the doctor may insert a viewing tube (laparoscope) through a small incision near the navel to view the inside of the abdominal cavity.

As soon as possible, antibiotics are usually given. Typically, two different antibiotics that are effective against a variety of organisms are

▲ see pages 1179 and 1180

used. Most women are treated at home. However, hospitalization is usually necessary if the infection does not improve within 48 hours, if symptoms are severe, if the woman may be pregnant, or if an abscess is detected.

If abscesses persist despite treatment with antibiotics, surgery may be necessary. A ruptured abscess requires emergency surgery.

Women should refrain from sexual intercourse until antibiotic therapy is completed and a doctor confirms that the infection is completely eliminated, even if symptoms disappear. All recent sex partners should be tested for infection and treated. If pelvic inflammatory disease is diagnosed and treated promptly, a full recovery is more likely.

CHAPTER 249

Pelvic Floor Disorders

Pelvic floor (pelvic support) disorders involve a dropping down (prolapse) of the bladder, rectum, or uterus caused by weakness of or injury to the ligaments, connective tissue, and muscles of the pelvis.

Pelvic floor disorders occur only in women and become more common with age. About 1 of 11 women needs surgery for a pelvic floor disorder during her lifetime.

The pelvic floor is a network of muscles, ligaments, and tissues that act like a hammock to support the organs of the pelvis: the uterus, bladder, and rectum. If the muscles become weak or the ligaments or tissues are stretched or damaged, the pelvic organs may drop down and protrude into the wall of the vagina. If the disorder is severe, tissues may protrude all the way through the vagina and outside the body.

Pelvic floor disorders usually result from a combination of factors. Being pregnant and having a vaginal delivery may weaken or stretch some of the supporting structures in the pelvis. Pelvic floor disorders are more common among women who have had several vaginal deliveries, and the risk may increase with each delivery. The delivery itself may damage nerves, leading to muscle weakness. Delivery by cesarean section may reduce the risk of developing a pelvic floor disorder.

Obesity, chronic coughing (for example, due to a lung disorder or smoking), frequent straining during bowel movements, and heavy lifting can also contribute to pelvic floor disorders. Other causes include a hysterectomy, nerve disorders, injuries, and tumors. Some women are born with weak pelvic tissues. As women age, the supporting structures in the pelvis may weaken, making pelvic floor disorders more likely to develop.

Types and Symptoms

All pelvic floor disorders are essentially hernias, in which tissue protrudes abnormally because another tissue is weakened. The different types of pelvic floor disorders are named according to the organ affected. Often, a woman has more than one type. In all types, the most common symptom is a feeling of heaviness or pressure in the area of the vagina—a feeling that the uterus, bladder, or rectum is dropping out.

Symptoms tend to occur when the woman is upright and to disappear when she is lying down. For some women, sexual intercourse is painful. Mild cases may not cause symptoms until a woman is older.

A **rectocele** develops when the rectum drops down and protrudes into the back wall of the vagina. It results from weakening of the muscular wall of the rectum and the connective tissue around the rectum. A rectocele can make having a bowel movement difficult and may cause a sensation of constipation. Some women need to place a finger in the vagina to have a bowel movement.

An **enterocele** develops when the small intestine and the lining of the abdominal cavity (peritoneum) bulge downward between the uterus and the rectum or, if the uterus has been removed, between the bladder and the rectum. It results from weakening of the connective tissue and ligaments supporting the uterus. An enterocele often causes no symptoms. But some women have a sense of fullness or feel pressure or pain in the pelvis. Pain may also be felt in the lower back.

A **cystocele** develops when the bladder drops down and protrudes into the front wall of the vagina. It results from weakening of the connective tissue and supporting structures around the bladder. A **cystourethrocele** is similar but develops when the upper part of the urethra (bladder neck) also drops down. Either of these disorders may cause stress incontinence (passage of urine during coughing, laughing, or any other maneuver that suddenly increases pressure within the abdomen) or overflow incontinence (passage of urine when the bladder becomes too full). After urination, the bladder may not feel completely empty. Sometimes a urinary tract infection develops. Because the nerves to the bladder or urethra can be damaged, women who have these disorders may develop urge incontinence (an intense, irrepressible urge to urinate, resulting in passage of urine).

In **prolapse of the uterus** (procidentia), the uterus drops down into the vagina. It usually results from weakening of the connective tissue and ligaments supporting the uterus. The uterus may bulge only into the upper part of the vagina, into the middle part, or all the way through the opening of the vagina, causing total uterine prolapse. Prolapse of the uterus may cause pain in the lower back or over the tailbone, although many women have no symptoms. Total uterine prolapse, which is obvious, can cause pain during walking. Sores may develop on the protruding cervix and cause bleeding, a discharge, and infection. Prolapse of the uterus may cause a kink in the urethra. A kink may hide urinary incontinence if present or make urinating difficult. Women with total uterine prolapse may also have difficulty having a bowel movement.

In **prolapse of the vagina,** the upper part of the vagina drops down into the lower part, so that the vagina turns inside out. The upper part may drop part way through the vagina or all the way through, protruding outside the body and causing total vaginal prolapse. Prolapse of the vagina occurs only in women who have had a hysterectomy. Total vaginal prolapse may cause pain while sitting or walking. Sores may develop on the protruding vagina and cause bleeding and a discharge. Prolapse of the vagina may cause a compelling or frequent need to urinate. Or it may cause a kink in the urethra. A kink may hide urinary incontinence if present or make urinating difficult.

Having a bowel movement may also be difficult.

Diagnosis

Doctors can usually diagnose pelvic floor disorders by performing a pelvic examination, using a speculum (an instrument that spreads the walls of the vagina apart). A doctor may insert one finger in the vagina and one finger in the rectum to determine how severe a rectocele is.

A woman may be asked to bear down (as when having a bowel movement) or to cough while standing. She may be examined while standing. The resulting pressure in the pelvis may make a pelvic floor disorder more obvious.

Procedures to determine how well the bladder and rectum are functioning, such as urine tests, may be performed. These procedures help doctors determine whether drugs or surgery is the best treatment. If a woman has a problem with the passage of urine or urinary incontinence, doctors may use a flexible viewing tube to view the inside of the bladder (a procedure called cystoscopy) or the urethra (a procedure called urethroscopy). Also, the amount of urine that the bladder can hold without leakage and the rate of urine flow may be measured. Doctors may determine whether prolapse of the uterus may be preventing urinary incontinence.

Treatment

If prolapse is mild, performing Kegel exercises can help by strengthening the pelvic floor muscles. Kegel exercises target the muscles around the vagina, urethra, and rectum—the muscles used to stop a stream of urine. These muscles are tightly squeezed, held tight for about 10 seconds, then relaxed for about 10 seconds. The exercise is repeated 10 to 20 times in a row. Performing the exercises several times a day is recommended. Women can do Kegel exercises when sitting, standing, or lying down.

If prolapse is severe, a pessary may be used to support the pelvic organs. A pessary may be shaped like a diaphragm, cube, or doughnut. Pessaries are especially useful for women who are waiting for surgery or who cannot have surgery. A doctor fits the pessary to the woman by inserting and removing different sizes until the right one is found. A pessary can be worn for many weeks before it needs to be removed and cleaned with soap and water. Women are taught how to insert and remove

When the Bottom Falls Out: Prolapse in the Pelvis

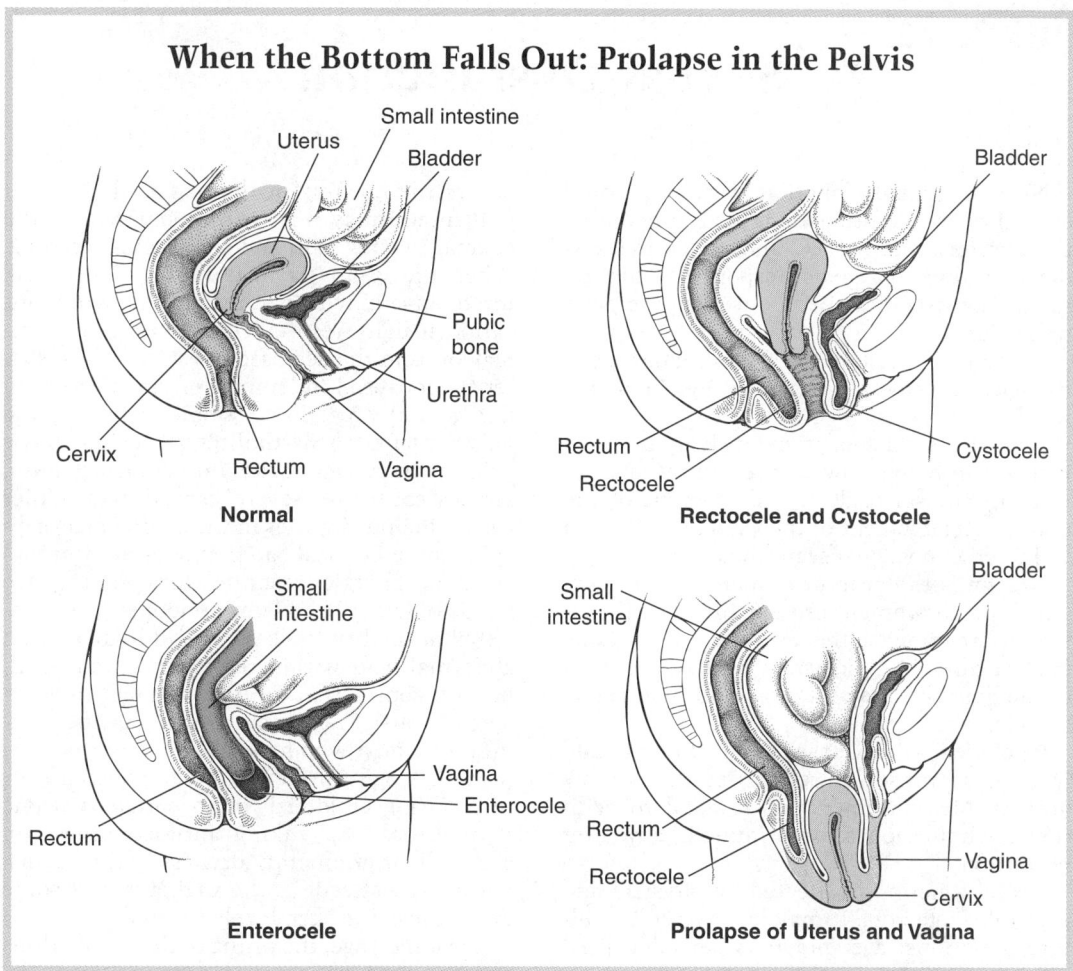

Normal

Small intestine
Uterus
Bladder
Pubic bone
Urethra
Cervix
Rectum
Vagina

Rectocele and Cystocele

Bladder
Rectum
Rectocele
Cystocele

Enterocele

Small intestine
Vagina
Enterocele
Rectum

Prolapse of Uterus and Vagina

Bladder
Small intestine
Rectum
Rectocele
Vagina
Cervix

the pessary for monthly cleaning. If they prefer, they may go to the doctor's office periodically to have the pessary cleaned. Pessaries can irritate the vaginal tissues and cause a foul-smelling discharge. Women who have this problem can use a vaginal deodorizer to mask the odor. As long as no other problems occur, these women may continue to use the pessary, removing it for cleaning each month. These women should also see their doctor every 6 to 12 months.

Estrogen vaginal suppositories or cream may be used. These preparations can help keep vaginal tissues healthy and can prevent sores from forming.

Surgery is often needed but is usually performed only after a woman has decided not to have any more children. Surgery usually involves inserting instruments into the vagina.

The weakened area is located, and the tissues around it are built up to prevent the organ from dropping through the weakened area.

For severe prolapse of the uterus or vagina, the surgery may require an incision in the abdomen. The upper part of the vagina is attached with stitches to a nearby bone in the pelvis. Often, a catheter is inserted to drain the urine for 1 to 2 days. If urinary incontinence is a problem or would occur after prolapse of the uterus is repaired, surgery to correct incontinence can usually be performed at the same time. In such cases, the catheter may be left in place longer. Heavy lifting, straining, and standing for a long time should be avoided for at least 3 months after surgery.

If prolapse of the rectum makes having a bowel movement difficult, surgery may be necessary.

CHAPTER 250

Sexual Dysfunction

Normal sexual function involves mind (thoughts and emotions) and body (including the nervous, circulatory, and endocrine systems), leading to a sexual response. Sexual response consists of desire, arousal, orgasm, and resolution.

Desire is the wish to engage in sexual activity. Desire may be triggered by thoughts, words, sights, smells, or touch.

Arousal is sexual excitement. It involves an increase in blood flow to the genital area. In women, arousal leads to enlargement of the clitoris, engorgement of the vaginal walls, and an increase in vaginal secretions.

Orgasm is the peak or climax of sexual excitement. In women, orgasm involves rhythmic contraction of the muscles surrounding the vagina. At orgasm, muscle tension throughout the body increases, and the pelvic muscles contract.

Resolution is a sense of well-being and widespread muscular relaxation that follow orgasm. Many women can respond to additional stimulation almost immediately after resolution.

Sexual function is affected by physical and psychologic factors. It may be affected by culture, emotions, age, previous sexual experiences, use of drugs, and the presence of disorders. Sexual dysfunction may involve pain during intercourse or a disturbance in sexual response, affecting desire, arousal, or orgasm. About 30 to 50% of women experience sexual dysfunction at some time during their life.

Dyspareunia

Dyspareunia is pain during sexual intercourse.

The pain of dyspareunia may be superficial, occurring in the genital area (in the vulva, including the opening of the vagina), or deep, occurring within the pelvis due to pressure on internal organs. The pain may be burning, sharp, or cramping.

Superficial pain during sexual intercourse has many causes. When women have sexual intercourse the first time, the membrane that covers the opening of the vagina (hymen), if still intact, may tear as the penis enters the vagina, causing pain and sometimes bleeding. When the vagina is inadequately lubricated, intercourse may be painful. (Inadequate lubrication usually results from insufficient foreplay or from the decrease in estrogen levels after menopause.) Inflammation or infection in the genital area (for example, affecting the vulva, vagina, or Bartholin's glands) or in the urinary tract can make intercourse painful. Herpes can cause severe genital pain. Other causes include injuries in the genital area, a diaphragm or cervical cap that does not fit properly, an allergic reaction to contraceptive foams or jellies or to latex condoms, a congenital abnormality (such as a rigid hymen or an abnormal wall within the vagina), and involuntary contraction of the vaginal muscles (vaginismus). Sexual intercourse may be painful for women who have had surgery that narrows the vagina (for example, to repair tissues torn during childbirth or to correct a pelvic floor disorder▲). Taking antihistamines can cause slight, temporary dryness of the vagina. During breastfeeding, the vagina may become dry because estrogen levels are low.

As women age, the lining of the vagina thins and becomes dry because estrogen levels decrease. This condition is called atrophic vaginitis. As a result, intercourse may be painful.

Deep pain after sexual intercourse may result from an infection of the cervix, uterus, or fallopian tubes. Other causes include endometriosis, pelvic inflammatory disease (including pelvic abscess), pelvic tumors (including ovarian cysts), and bands of scar tissue (adhesions) that have formed between organs in the pelvis after an infection or surgery. Sometimes one of these disorders results in the uterus bending backward (retroversion). The ligaments, muscles, and other tissues that hold the uterus in place may weaken, resulting in the uterus dropping down toward the vagina (prolapse).■ Such changes in position can result in pain during intercourse. Radiation therapy for cancer may cause changes in the tissues that make intercourse painful.

Psychologic factors can cause superficial or deep pain. Examples are anger or repulsion to-

---

▲ see page 1379   ■ see art on page 1381

ward a sex partner, fear of intimacy or pregnancy, a negative self-image, and a traumatic sexual experience (including rape). However, psychologic factors may be difficult to identify.

Diagnosis and Treatment

The diagnosis is based on symptoms: when and where the pain occurs and when intercourse began to be painful. To try to identify the cause, a doctor asks the woman about her medical and sexual history and performs a pelvic examination.

Women should abstain from intercourse until the problem resolves. However, sexual activity that does not involve vaginal penetration can continue.

Superficial pain can be reduced by applying an anesthetic ointment and by taking sitz baths. Liberally applying a lubricant before intercourse may help. Water-based lubricants rather than petroleum jelly or other oil-based lubricants are preferable. Oil-based products tend to dry the vagina and can damage latex contraceptive devices such as condoms and diaphragms. Spending more time in foreplay may increase vaginal lubrication. Deep pain may be reduced by using a different position for intercourse. For example, a position that gives the woman more control of penetration (such as being on top) or that involves less deep thrusting may help.

More specific treatment depends on the cause. If the cause is thinning and drying of the vagina after menopause, using a topical estrogen cream or suppository or taking estrogen by mouth (as part of hormone therapy▲) can help.

Inflammation and infection are treated with antibiotics, antifungal drugs, and other drugs as appropriate.■ If the cause is inflammation of the vulva (vulvitis), applying wet dressings of aluminum acetate solution may help. Surgery may be needed to remove cysts or abscesses, open a rigid hymen, or repair an anatomic abnormality. A poorly fitting diaphragm should be replaced with one that fits and is comfortable, or a different method of birth control should be tried.

If the cause of pain is the position of the uterus, a pessary, which resembles a diaphragm and is inserted into the vagina, can support and reposition the uterus. Using a pessary reduces the pain in some women.

Vaginismus

Vaginismus is an involuntary contraction of muscles around the opening of the vagina

that makes sexual intercourse painful or impossible.

Vaginismus may result from a woman's unconscious desire to prevent sexual intercourse. Pain experienced in the past during sexual intercourse can lead to vaginismus. Other reasons women do not want to engage in intercourse include fear of becoming pregnant, of being controlled by their partner, or of losing control. Sometimes vaginismus is caused by a physical disorder, such as a pelvic infection or scarring of the vaginal opening (due to injury, childbirth, or surgery). Irritation (due to douches, spermicides, or latex in condoms) may also cause vaginismus.

Because of the pain, some women who have vaginismus cannot tolerate sexual intercourse (that is, penetration of the vagina by the penis). However, sexual activity that does not involve penetration may be pleasurable. Some women cannot tolerate the insertion of a tampon and may need an anesthetic when a doctor performs a pelvic examination.

Diagnosis and Treatment

The diagnosis is based on the woman's description of the problem, her medical history, and the physical examination, including her reaction to a pelvic examination.

Physical disorders that may be causing or contributing to vaginismus are treated. If the cause is psychologic, counseling for the woman and her partner is usually helpful.

If vaginismus persists, the woman is taught a technique to relax the muscle spasms. The technique involves gradually widening (dilating) the vagina. The woman begins by inserting very small, lubricated plastic rods (dilators) into her vagina. The woman inserts slightly but progressively larger dilators as her level of comfort increases. Once the woman can tolerate having large dilators inserted without discomfort, she and her partner may try to have sexual intercourse again.

Kegel exercises, which strengthen the pelvic muscles, can be helpful if performed while the dilators are in place. For these exercises, the muscles around the vagina, urethra, and rectum—the muscles used to stop the flow of urine—are repeatedly squeezed hard and then relaxed 10 to 20 times. Performing the exercises several times a day is recommended. These exercises enable the woman to develop

▲ see page 1358   ■ see table on page 1376

Kegel Exercises: Squeeze and Relax

Kegel exercises help strengthen the pelvic muscles, primarily those around the vagina, urethra, and rectum. Performing them regularly can help improve sexual function and prevent or reduce the involuntary loss of urine (urinary incontinence) or stool (fecal incontinence).

To perform these exercises, a woman squeezes the muscles used to stop the flow of urine for about 10 seconds, then relaxes them for about 10 seconds. The exercise is repeated 10 to 20 times in a row at least 3 times a day. Muscle tone usually improves in 2 to 3 months. Kegel exercises can be performed anywhere, whether a woman is sitting, standing, or lying down.

Finding the right muscles to squeeze can be difficult. The muscles can be identified by inserting a finger into the vagina and squeezing or by trying to stop the flow of urine. If pressure is felt around the finger or urine flow stops, the right muscles are being squeezed.

a sense of control over the muscles that were contracting involuntarily.

Vulvodynia

Vulvodynia is chronic discomfort in the vulva—the area containing the external genital organs.

Vulvodynia typically begins suddenly, then becomes a chronic problem, lasting months to years. The cause is unknown. It may be triggered by irritation of or injury to the nerves supplying the vulva (as may occur during cryotherapy or laser therapy). Vulvodynia tends to be more common among women who have infections (especially yeast infections and sexually transmitted diseases), skin disorders, diabetes, precancerous conditions, cancer, or spasms of the muscles that support the pelvic organs. Certain substances (such as soaps, feminine hygiene sprays, menstrual pads, laundry detergents, and synthetic fibers) may cause an allergic reaction or irritate the area, increasing the likelihood of developing

vulvodynia. Women who are undergoing hormonal changes or who have a history of sexual abuse are also more likely to develop vulvodynia. Eating certain foods, such as greens, chocolate, berries, beans, and nuts, produces urine that can be irritating.

The vulva may burn or sting. It may feel raw, irritated, or painful. The pain ranges from mild to debilitating and may be constant or intermittent. It can interfere with daily activities, limiting physical and sexual activity. It may make walking and sitting uncomfortable. The vulva may appear swollen and red, or it may appear normal.

Doctors diagnose vulvodynia by ruling out other disorders that can cause similar symptoms. The goal of treatment is to relieve symptoms. Potential irritants should be avoided. Wearing cotton underwear may help reduce irritation in the area. Tight-fitting, restrictive clothing, such as pantyhose, should not be worn. Foods that may produce irritating urine should not be eaten. Physical therapy, including exercises to improve tone in the pelvic muscles, biofeedback, and relaxation exercises, often help, as do support groups.

Topical anesthetics such as viscous lidocaine may reduce the pain. Topical corticosteroids may be rubbed into the skin 2 or 3 times a day to control symptoms.

Disorders that may be contributing to vulvodynia, such as infections, are treated. Some women benefit from tricyclic antidepressants▲ or anticonvulsants.■

Decreased Libido

Decreased libido is a reduction in the sex drive.

A temporary reduction in sex drive is common, often caused by temporary conditions, such as fatigue. Sex drive that continues to be reduced can distress a woman or her partner.

Sex drive is controlled in part by sex hormones, such as estrogen and testosterone. Fluctuations in the levels of these hormones, which occur monthly and during pregnancy, can affect sex drive. In postmenopausal women, sex drive may be reduced because estrogen levels decrease. Sex drive may also be reduced in women who have had both ovaries removed.

A reduction in sex drive may result from depression, anxiety, stress, or problems in a relationship. Use of certain drugs, including anticonvulsants,★ chemotherapy drugs (such as

---

▲ see table on page 618
■ see table on page 500
★ see table on page 500

tamoxifen), beta-blockers,▲ and oral contraceptives, can also reduce the sex drive, as can drinking excessive amounts of alcohol.

The diagnosis is based on the woman's description of the problem. A doctor asks the woman about stress and other lifestyle problems and her sexual and medical history, including use of drugs. Levels of sex hormones may be measured in a blood sample.

Treatment depends on the cause. Drugs that may be contributing are discontinued if possible. If psychologic factors are involved, counseling may be recommended. If the cause is low levels of sex hormones, a low dose of testosterone combined with estrogen may be given by mouth. In addition to increasing sex drive, testosterone may also increase muscle strength, prevent loss of bone density, and improve energy.

Sexual Arousal Disorder

Sexual arousal disorder is the persistent or recurring inability to attain or to maintain adequate vaginal lubrication and other physical responses of sexual excitement before or during sexual intercourse.

Usually, when a woman is sexually stimulated, the vagina releases lubricating secretions, the labia and clitoris of the vulva swell, and the breasts enlarge slightly. In sexual arousal disorder, these responses do not occur despite sufficiently long and intense sexual stimulation.

If the disorder has been present since puberty, the woman may not know how the genital organs (particularly the clitoris) function or what arousal techniques are effective. The lack of knowledge leads to anxiety, which worsens the problem. Many women who have sexual arousal disorder associate sex with sinfulness and sexual pleasure with guilt. Fear of intimacy and a negative self-image may also contribute.

If the disorder develops after a period of adequate sexual functioning, it may be due to a problem in the current sexual relationship, such as constant fighting or arguing. Depression is a common cause, and stress may contribute.

Physical causes include inflammation of the vagina (vaginitis), inflammation of the bladder (cystitis), endometriosis, an underactive thyroid gland (hypothyroidism), diabetes mellitus, multiple sclerosis, and muscular dystrophy.

Sex Therapy: Sensate Focus Technique

The sensate focus technique may help couples that are having sexual difficulties because of psychologic rather than physical factors. The technique aims to make both partners aware of what each finds pleasurable and to reduce anxiety about performance. It is often used in the treatment of decreased libido, sexual arousal disorder, orgasmic disorder, and erectile dysfunction (impotence).

The technique has three steps. Both partners must become comfortable at each level of intimacy before proceeding to the next step.

- The first step focuses on the sensation of touching, rather than the likelihood of sexual arousal or intercourse. Each partner takes turns touching any part of the other's body, except the genitals and breasts.
- The second step allows partners to touch any part of the other's body, including the genitals and breasts. However, the focus remains the same—on the sensation of touching, not on sexual response. Intercourse is not allowed.
- The third step involves mutual touching, eventually leading to sexual intercourse as the couple becomes more comfortable with touching and being touched. The focus is on enjoyment rather than on orgasm.

Sexual arousal disorder may develop as women age. As menopause approaches, the lining of the vagina thins and becomes dry because the estrogen level decreases. As a result, the ability to become aroused declines, partly because sexual intercourse may be painful.

Taking drugs such as oral contraceptives, antihypertensives, antidepressants, or sedatives can cause sexual arousal disorder. Surgical removal of the uterus (hysterectomy) or breast (mastectomy) may damage a woman's sexual self-image, contributing to sexual arousal disorder.

Many women with sexual arousal disorder also lack sexual desire. Because the vagina does not become lubricated, sexual intercourse is usually painful or uncomfortable.

▲ see table on page 138

Diagnosis and Treatment

The diagnosis is based on the woman's description of the problem. To determine the severity of the disorder and identify the cause, a doctor asks the woman about her sexual and medical history (including use of drugs) and performs a physical examination. Tests to detect physical disorders, if thought to be the cause, may be performed.

If the cause is psychologic, counseling for the woman, usually with her partner, often helps. Individual psychotherapy or group therapy is sometimes useful. Physical disorders, if present, are treated. Postmenopausal women may benefit from treatment with estrogen or male hormones such as testosterone. Estrogen creams and suppositories reduce the thinning and drying of the lining of the vagina and thus may help with lubrication during intercourse. The use of testosterone in treating women with sexual arousal disorder is controversial.

Sensate focus exercises for couples can help relieve a couple's anxiety about intimacy and sexual intercourse. Learning about how the genital organs function can help. A woman can learn which arousal techniques are effective for her and her partner. Performing Kegel exercises can help because they strengthen the muscles involved in sexual intercourse.

Orgasmic Disorder

Orgasmic disorder is the delay in or absence of sexual climax (orgasm) despite sufficiently long and intense sexual stimulation.

The amount and type of stimulation required for orgasm varies greatly from woman to woman. Most women can reach orgasm when the clitoris is stimulated, but only about half of women regularly reach orgasm during sexual intercourse. About 1 of 10 women never reach orgasm. Orgasmic disorder occurs when problems with orgasm are persistent and frequent, interfering with sexual function and causing distress.

Usually, women who have learned how to reach orgasm do not lose that ability unless poor sexual communication, conflict in a relationship, a traumatic experience, or a physical or psychologic disorder intervenes. Physical and psychologic causes are similar to those of sexual arousal disorder. Depression is a common cause.

Orgasmic disorder may result from lovemaking that consistently ends before the woman reaches orgasm. The woman may not reach orgasm because foreplay is inadequate, because one or both partners do not understand how the genital organs function, or because ejaculation is premature. Such lovemaking produces frustration and may result in resentment and occasionally in distaste for anything sexual. Some women who become aroused may not reach orgasm because they fear "letting go," especially during intercourse. This fear may be due to guilt after a pleasurable experience, fear of abandoning oneself to pleasure that depends on the partner, or fear of losing control.

Certain drugs, particularly selective serotonin reuptake inhibitors such as fluoxetine, ▲ may inhibit orgasm.

Orgasmic disorder may be temporary, may occur after years of normal sexual function, or may be lifelong. It may occur all the time or only in certain situations. Most women who have a problem reaching orgasm also have a problem being aroused.

Diagnosis and Treatment

The diagnosis is based on the woman's description of the problem. To identify the cause, a doctor asks the woman about her sexual and medical history, including use of drugs, and performs a physical examination.

If the cause is psychologic, counseling for the woman, usually with her partner, often helps. Psychotherapy for the woman or the couple may be recommended. Physical disorders, if present, are treated.

Other useful measures include sensate focus exercises for couples, information about how the genital organs function, and Kegel exercises.

▲ see table on page 618

CHAPTER 251

Breast Disorders

Breast disorders may be noncancerous (benign) or cancerous (malignant). Most are noncancerous and not life threatening. Often, they do not require treatment. In contrast, breast cancer can mean loss of a breast or of life. Thus, for many women, breast cancer is their worst fear. However, potential problems can be detected early when women regularly examine their breasts themselves and have mammograms.

Symptoms

Common symptoms include breast pain, lumps, and a discharge from the nipple. Breast symptoms do not necessarily mean that a woman has breast cancer or another serious disorder. However, if a woman has any of the following symptoms, she should see her doctor:

• a lump that feels distinctly different from other breast tissue or that does not go away
• swelling that does not go away
• puckering or dimpling in the skin of the breast
• scaly skin around the nipple
• changes in the shape of the breast
• changes in the nipple, such as turning inward
• discharge from the nipple, especially if it is bloody

Breast Pain: Many women experience breast pain (mastalgia). Breast pain may be related to hormonal changes. For example, it may occur during or just before a menstrual period (as part of the premenstrual syndrome) or early in pregnancy. Women who take oral contraceptives or who take hormone therapy after menopause commonly have this kind of pain. The pain is due to growth of breast tissue. Such pain is usually diffuse, making the breasts tender to touch. Pain related to the menstrual period may come and go for months or years.

Other causes of breast pain include breast cysts, infections, and abscesses. In these cases, breast pain is usually felt in a particular place. Fibrocystic breast disease can also cause breast pain. Breast pain is occasionally due to breast cancer, but breast cancer does not usually cause pain. Breast pain that persists for more than 1 month should be evaluated.

Mild breast pain usually disappears eventually, even without treatment. Pain that occurs during menstrual periods can usually be relieved by taking acetaminophen or a nonsteroidal anti-inflammatory drug (NSAID).

For certain types of severe pain, danazol (a synthetic hormone related to testosterone) or tamoxifen (a drug used to treat breast cancer) may be used. These drugs inhibit the activity of estrogen and progesterone, which affect the breast. Because long-term use of these drugs causes side effects, the drugs are usually given for only a short time. Tamoxifen has fewer side effects than danazol. Tamoxifen is used mainly for postmenopausal women but may benefit younger women.

If a specific disorder is identified as the cause, the disorder is treated. For example, if a cyst is the cause, draining the fluid from the cyst usually relieves the pain.

Breast Lumps: Lumps in the breasts are relatively common and are usually not cancerous. But because they may be cancerous, they should be evaluated by a doctor without delay. Lumps may be fluid-filled sacs (cysts) or solid masses, which are usually fibroadenomas.▲

Other solid breast lumps include hardened glandular tissue (sclerosing adenosis) and scar tissue that has replaced injured fatty tissue (fat necrosis). Neither is cancerous. However, these lumps can be diagnosed only by biopsy. They require no treatment.

Nipple Discharge: One or both nipples sometimes discharge a fluid. A nipple discharge occurs normally during milk production (lactation) after childbirth or as a result of mechanical stimulation of the nipple by fondling, suckling, or irritation from clothing. During the last weeks of pregnancy, the breasts may produce a milky discharge (colostrum). A normal nipple discharge is a thin, cloudy, whitish or almost clear fluid that is not sticky. However, during pregnancy or breastfeeding, a slightly bloody discharge sometimes occurs normally.

Several disorders can cause an abnormal discharge. Abnormal discharges vary in appearance depending on the cause. A bloody dis-

▲ see page 1388

Inside the Breast

The female breast is composed of milk-producing glands (lobules) surrounded by fatty tissue and some connective tissue. Milk secreted by the glands flows through ducts to the nipple. Around the nipple is an area of pigmented skin called the areola.

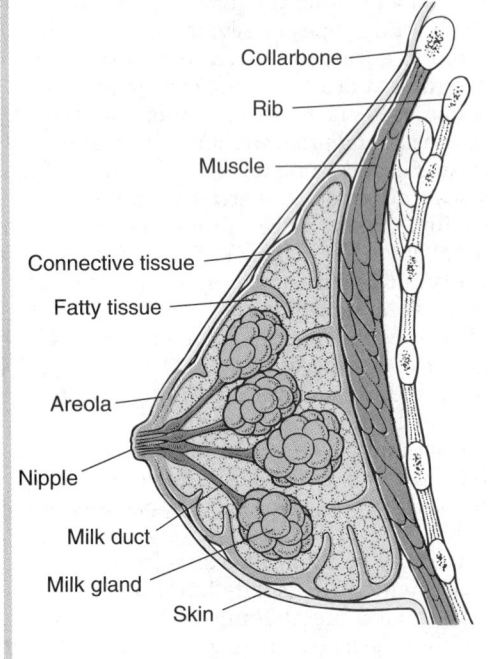

Collarbone

Rib

Muscle

Connective tissue

Fatty tissue

Areola

Nipple

Milk duct

Milk gland

Skin

charge may be caused by a noncancerous breast tumor (such as a tumor in a milk duct, called an intraductal papilloma) or, less commonly, by breast cancer. Among women who have an abnormal discharge, breast cancer is the cause in fewer than 10%. A greenish discharge is usually due to a fibroadenoma, a noncancerous solid lump. A discharge that contains pus and smells foul may result from a breast infection. A large amount of milky discharge in women who are not breastfeeding may result from galactorrhea. ▲ Tumors of the pituitary gland or brain, encephalitis (a brain infection), and head injuries can also cause a nipple discharge. Taking certain drugs, such as antidepressants and certain antihypertensives,

▲ see page 946

can cause a nipple discharge. Taking oral contraceptives may cause a watery discharge.

A discharge from one breast is likely to be caused by a problem with that breast, such as a noncancerous or cancerous breast tumor. A discharge from both breasts is more likely to be caused by a problem outside the breast, such as a pituitary tumor, or by drugs.

If a nipple discharge persists for more than one menstrual cycle or seems unusual to the woman, she should see a doctor. Postmenopausal women who have a nipple discharge should see a doctor promptly. Doctors examine the breast, looking for abnormalities. Mammography and blood tests to measure hormone levels may be performed. Computed tomography (CT) or magnetic resonance imaging (MRI) of the head may be performed. The woman is asked for a complete list of drugs she is taking. Sometimes a specific cause cannot be identified.

If a disorder is the cause, the disorder is treated. If a noncancerous tumor is causing a discharge from one breast, the duct that the discharge is coming from may be removed.

Breast Cysts

Breast cysts are fluid-filled sacs that develop in the breast.

Breast cysts are common. In some women, many cysts develop frequently, sometimes as part of fibrocystic breast disease. However, in other women, cysts never develop. The cause of breast cysts is unknown, although injury may be involved. Breast cysts can be tiny or several inches in diameter.

Cysts sometimes cause breast pain. To relieve the pain, a doctor may drain fluid from the cyst with a thin needle. The fluid is examined under a microscope to check for cancer. The color and amount are noted. If the fluid is bloody, brown, or cloudy or if the cyst does not disappear or reappears within 12 weeks after it is drained, the entire cyst is removed surgically, because cancer in the cyst wall, although rare, is possible.

Fibroadenomas

Fibroadenomas are small, solid, rubbery noncancerous lumps composed of fibrous and glandular tissue.

Fibroadenomas usually appear in young women, including teenagers. The cause is unknown.

The lumps are easy to move and have clearly defined edges that can be felt during self-examination. They may feel like small, slippery marbles. These characteristics indicate to a doctor that the lumps are less likely to be cancerous. Nonetheless, to be sure that they are not cancerous, the doctor usually removes the lumps. A local anesthetic is used. Fibroadenomas often recur. If several lumps have been removed and found to be noncancerous, a woman and her doctor may decide against removing new lumps that develop.

Fibrocystic Breast Disease

Fibrocystic breast disease is characterized by breast pain, cysts, and noncancerous lumpiness.

Most women have some general lumpiness in the breasts, usually in the upper outer part, near the armpit. In the United States, about 30% of women have this kind of lumpiness with breast pain and breast cysts—a condition called fibrocystic breast disease.

Normally, the levels of the female hormones estrogen and progesterone fluctuate during the menstrual cycle. Milk glands and ducts enlarge and breasts retain fluid when levels increase, and the breasts return to normal when levels decrease. (These fluctuations partly explain why breasts are swollen and more sensitive during a particular time of each menstrual cycle.) Fibrocystic changes may result from repeated stimulation by these hormones.

In women with fibrocystic breast disease, the lumpy areas may enlarge, causing a feeling of heaviness, discomfort, tenderness to the touch, or a burning pain. The symptoms tend to subside after menopause. Fibrocystic breast disease may increase the risk of breast cancer very slightly. Also, this condition may make breast cancer more difficult to detect.

Lumps may be removed and a biopsy may be performed. Sometimes cysts are drained, but they tend to recur. No specific treatment is available or required.

Breast Infection and Abscess

A breast infection (mastitis) is rare, except around the time of childbirth▲ or after an injury or surgery. The most common symptom is a swollen, red area that feels warm and tender. An uncommon type of breast cancer called inflammatory breast cancer■ can pro-

duce similar symptoms. A breast infection is treated with antibiotics.

A breast abscess, which is even rarer, is a collection of pus in the breast. An abscess may develop if a breast infection is not treated. An abscess is treated with antibiotics and is usually drained surgically.

Breast Cancer

Breast cancer is the second most common cancer among women after skin cancer and, of cancers, is the second most common cause of death among women after lung cancer. In 2001, breast cancer was diagnosed in about 200,000 women in the United States. About one fifth of them will die of it.

Many women fear breast cancer, because it is common. However, some of the fear about breast cancer is based on misunderstanding. For example, the statement, "One of every eight women will get breast cancer," is misleading. That figure is an estimate based on women from birth to age 95. It means that theoretically, one of eight women who live to age 95 or older will develop breast cancer. However, a 40-year-old woman has only a 1 in 1,200 chance of developing breast cancer during the next year and about a 1 in 120 chance of developing it during the next decade. But as she ages, her risk increases.

Other factors also affect the risk of developing breast cancer. Thus, for some women, the risk is much higher or lower than average. Most factors that increase risk, such as age, cannot be modified. However, regular exercise, particularly during adolescence and young adulthood, and possibly weight control may slightly reduce the risk of developing breast cancer. Regularly drinking alcoholic beverages may increase the risk.

Far more important than trying to modify risk factors is being vigilant about detecting breast cancer so that it can be diagnosed and treated early, when it is more likely to be cured. Early detection is more likely when women have mammograms and perform breast self-examinations regularly.★

Staging

Staging involves assigning a stage to a cancer when it is diagnosed. The stage is based on

▲ see page 1479   ■ see page 1391

★ see page 1392 and art on page 1395

WHAT ARE THE RISKS OF DEVELOPING OR DYING OF BREAST CANCER?

AGE (YEARS)	RISK (%)					
	IN 10 YEARS		IN 20 YEARS		IN 30 YEARS	
	DEVELOP	DIE	DEVELOP	DIE	DEVELOP	DIE
30	0.4	0.1	2.0	0.6	4.3	1.2
40	1.6	0.5	3.9	1.1	7.1	2.0
50	2.4	0.7	5.7	1.6	9.0	2.6
60	3.6	1.0	7.1	2.0	9.1	2.6
70	4.1	1.2	6.5	1.9	7.1	2.0

Based on information from Feuer EJ et al.: "The lifetime risk of developing breast cancer." *Journal of the National Cancer Institute* 85(11):892–897, 1993.

how advanced the cancer is. The stage helps doctors determine the most appropriate treatment and the prognosis. Stages of breast cancer may be generally described as in situ (not invasive), localized invasive, regional invasive, or distant (metastatic) invasive. Or, stages may be described in detail and designated by a number (0 through IV).

Carcinoma in situ means cancer in place. It is the earliest stage of breast cancer. Carcinoma in situ may be large and may even affect a substantial area of the breast, but it has not invaded the surrounding tissues or spread to other parts of the body. More than 15% of all breast cancers diagnosed in the United States are carcinoma in situ. It is usually detected during mammography.

Localized invasive cancer has invaded surrounding tissues but is confined to the breast.

Regional invasive cancer has invaded tissues near the breasts, including the chest wall and lymph nodes.

Distant (metastatic) invasive cancer has spread from the breast to other parts of the body. Cancer tends to move into the lymphatic vessels in the breast. Most lymphatic vessels in the breast drain into lymph nodes in the armpit (axillary lymph nodes). One function of lymph nodes is to filter out and destroy abnormal or foreign cells, such as cancer cells. If cancer cells get past these lymph nodes, the cancer can spread anywhere in the body. Breast cancer can also spread through the bloodstream to other parts of the body. Breast cancer tends to spread to bones and the brain but can spread to any area, including the lungs, liver, and skin. Breast cancer can appear

in these areas years or even decades after it is first diagnosed and treated. If the cancer has spread to one area, it probably has spread to other areas, even if it is not detected right away.

Types

Breast cancer is usually classified by the kind of tissue in which the cancer starts and by the extent of its spread. Breast cancer that starts in the milk ducts is called ductal carcinoma. About 90% of all breast cancers are this type. Breast cancer that starts in the milk-producing glands (lobules) is called lobular carcinoma. Breast cancer that starts in fatty or connective tissue, a rare type, is called sarcoma.

Ductal carcinoma in situ is confined to the milk ducts of the breast. It does not invade surrounding breast tissue, but it can spread along the ducts and gradually affect a substantial area of the breast. This type accounts for 20 to 30% of breast cancers.

Lobular carcinoma in situ grows within the milk-producing glands of the breast. It often occurs in several areas of both breasts. Women with lobular carcinoma in situ have a 30% chance of developing invasive breast cancer in the same or other breast during the next 24 years. This type accounts for 1 to 2% of breast cancers.

Invasive ductal carcinoma begins in the milk ducts but breaks through the wall of the ducts, invading the surrounding breast tissue. It can also spread to other parts of the body. It accounts for 65 to 80% of breast cancers.

Invasive lobular carcinoma begins in the milk-producing glands of the breast but invades surrounding breast tissue and spreads to other parts of the body. It is more likely than other types of breast cancer to occur in both breasts. It accounts for 10 to 15% of breast cancers.

Inflammatory breast cancer is fast growing and often fatal. Cancer cells block the lymphatic vessels in the skin of the breast, causing the breast to appear inflamed: swollen, red, and warm. Usually, inflammatory breast cancer spreads to the lymph nodes in the armpit. The lymph nodes can be felt as hard lumps. However, often no lump may be felt in the breast itself because this cancer is dispersed throughout the breast. Inflammatory breast cancer accounts for about 1% of breast cancers.

Paget's disease of the nipple is a type of ductal breast cancer. The first symptom is a crusty or scaly nipple sore or a discharge from the nipple. Slightly more than half of the women who have this cancer also have a lump in the breast that can be felt. Paget's disease may be in situ or invasive. Because this disease usually causes little discomfort, a woman may ignore it for a year or more before seeing a doctor. The prognosis depends on how invasive and how large the cancer is as well as whether it has spread to the lymph nodes.

Less common types of invasive ductal breast cancers include medullary carcinoma, tubular carcinoma, and mucinous (colloid) carcinoma. Mucinous carcinoma tends to develop in older women and to be slow growing. Women with these types of breast cancer have a much better prognosis than women with other types of invasive breast cancer.

Cystosarcoma phyllodes is a relatively rare type of breast cancer. It originates in breast tissue around milk ducts and milk-producing glands. It spreads to other parts of the body in fewer than 5% of women who have it.

Characteristics

All cells, including breast cancer cells, have molecules on their surfaces called receptors. A receptor has a specific structure that allows only particular substances to fit into it and thus affect the cell's activity. Whether breast cancer cells have certain receptors affects how quickly the cancer spreads and how it should be treated.

Some breast cancer cells have receptors for estrogen. The resulting cancer, described as estrogen receptor–positive, is stimulated by estrogen. This type of cancer is more common

among postmenopausal women than among younger women. Some breast cancer cells have receptors for progesterone. The resulting cancer, described as progesterone receptor–positive, is stimulated by progesterone. Estrogen receptor–positive breast cancers grow more slowly than estrogen receptor–negative breast cancers, and the prognosis is better. The same is true for progesterone receptor–positive and progesterone receptor–negative breast cancers. The prognosis is better with cancer that is both estrogen and progesterone receptor–positive than with cancer that is one or the other.

Cells have receptors called HER-2/*neu* receptors that help them grow. Breast cancer cells with too many HER-2/*neu* receptors tend to be very fast growing. In about 20 to 30% of breast cancers, the cancer cells have too many HER-2/*neu* receptors.

Symptoms

At first, a woman who has breast cancer has no symptoms. Most commonly, the first symptom is a lump, which usually feels distinctly different from the surrounding breast tissue. In more than 80% of breast cancer cases, the woman discovers the lump herself. Usually, scattered lumpy changes in the breast, especially the upper outer region, are not cancerous and indicate fibrocystic breast disease. A firm, distinctive thickening that appears in one breast but not the other may indicate cancer.

In the early stages, the lump may move freely beneath the skin when it is pushed with the fingers. In more advanced stages, the lump usually adheres to the chest wall or the skin over it. In these cases, the lump cannot be moved at all or it cannot be moved separately from the skin over it. One way to detect even slight adherence of a cancer to the chest wall or skin is to lift the arms over the head while standing in front of a mirror. A breast containing cancer may show skin puckering or another shape abnormality compared with the other breast. In advanced cancer, swollen bumps or festering sores may develop on the skin. Sometimes the skin over the lump is dimpled and leathery and looks like the skin of an orange (peau d'orange) except in color.

The lump may be painful, but pain is an unreliable sign. Pain without a lump is rarely due to breast cancer.

Lymph nodes, particularly those in the armpit on the affected side, may feel like hard

Risk Factors for Breast Cancer

Age

Increasing age is an important risk factor. About 60% of breast cancers occur in women older than 60. Risk is greatest after age 75.

Previous Breast Cancer

At highest risk are women who have had in situ or invasive breast cancer. After the diseased breast is removed, the risk of developing cancer in the remaining breast is about 0.5 to 1.0% each year.

Family History of Breast Cancer

Breast cancer in a first-degree relative (mother, sister, or daughter) increases a woman's risk by 2 to 3 times, but breast cancer in more distant relatives (grandmother, aunt, or cousin) increases the risk only slightly. Breast cancer in two or more first-degree relatives increases a woman's risk by 5 to 6 times.

Breast Cancer Gene

Recently, two separate genes for breast cancer (BRCA1 and BRCA2) have been identified in two separate small groups of women. These genes are present in fewer than 1% of women. If a woman has one of these genes, her chances of developing breast cancer are very high, possibly as high as 50 to 85% by age 80. However, if such a woman develops breast cancer, her chances of dying of breast cancer are not necessarily greater than those of any other woman with breast cancer. Women likely to have one of these genes are those who have a strong family history of breast cancer. Usually, several women in each of three generations have had breast cancer. For this reason, routine screening for these genes does not appear necessary, except in women who have such a family history. The incidence of ovarian cancer is increased in families with both breast cancer genes. The incidence of breast cancer in men is increased in families with the BRCA2 gene.

Fibrocystic Breast Disease

Having fibrocystic breast disease seems to increase risk only in women who have an increased number of cells in the milk ducts. For these women, the risk is moderate un-

---

small lumps. The lymph nodes may be stuck together or adhere to the skin or chest wall. They are usually painless but may be slightly tender.

In inflammatory breast cancer, the breast is warm, red, and swollen, as if infected (but it is not). The skin of the breast may become dimpled and leathery, like the skin of an orange, or may have ridges. The nipple may turn inward (invert). A discharge from the nipple is common. Often, no lump can be felt in the breast.

Screening

Because breast cancer rarely produces symptoms in its early stages and because early treatment is more likely to be successful, screening is important. Screening is the hunt for a disorder before any symptoms occur.

Routine self-examination enables a woman to detect lumps at an early stage. Self-examination does not reduce the death rate from breast cancer or detect as many early cancers as routine screening with mammography. With tumors detected by self-examination, the prognosis is usually better, and breast-conserving surgery can usually be performed rather than mastectomy.

A breast examination is a routine part of a physical examination. A doctor inspects the breasts for irregularities, dimpling, tightened skin, lumps, and a discharge. The doctor feels (palpates) each breast with a flat hand and checks for enlarged lymph nodes in the armpit—the area most breast cancers invade first—and also above the collarbone. Normal lymph nodes cannot be felt through the skin, so those that can be felt are considered enlarged. However, noncancerous conditions can also cause lymph nodes to enlarge. Lymph nodes that can be felt are checked to see if they adhere to the skin or chest wall and if they are matted together.

Mammography uses low-level x-rays to detect abnormal areas in the breast. It is one of the best ways to detect breast cancer early.▲ Mammography is designed to be sensitive enough to detect the possibility of cancer at an early stage. For this reason, the procedure may indicate cancer when none is present—a false-positive result. Typically, when the result is positive, more specific follow-up procedures, usually a breast biopsy, are scheduled to confirm the result. Mammography may miss up to 15% of breast cancers.

Having a mammogram every 1 to 2 years can reduce the rate of death due to breast cancer by 25 to 35% among women aged 50 and

---

▲ see art on page 1355

less abnormal tissue structure (atypical hyperplasia) is detected during a biopsy or the woman has a family history of breast cancer.

Age at Puberty, First Pregnancy, and Menopause

The earlier menstruation begins, the greater the risk of developing breast cancer. The risk is 1.2 to 1.4 times greater for women who first menstruated before age 12 than for those who first menstruated after age 14. The later menopause occurs and the later the first pregnancy, the greater the risk. Never having had a baby also doubles the risk of developing breast cancer during a woman's lifetime. These factors probably increase risk because they involve longer exposure to estrogen, which stimulates the growth of certain cancers. (Pregnancy, although it results in high estrogen levels, may reduce the risk of breast cancer.)

Prolonged Use of Oral Contraceptives or Estrogen Therapy

Most studies do not show any relationship between the use of oral contraceptives and the later development of breast cancer, except possibly for women who took them for many years. After menopause, taking estrogen therapy for 5 to 10 years may slightly increase risk. Taking hormone therapy that combines estrogen with a progestin increases the risk (although it reduces the risk of cancer of the uterus).

Obesity After Menopause

Risk is somewhat higher for obese postmenopausal women. However, there is no proof that a high-fat diet contributes to the development of breast cancer. Some studies suggest that obese women who are still menstruating are less likely to develop breast cancer.

Radiation Exposure

Radiation exposure (such as radiation therapy for cancer or significant exposure to x-rays) before age 30 increases risk.

older. As yet, no study has shown that having mammograms regularly can reduce the death rate among women younger than 50. However, evidence may be harder to obtain because breast cancer is not common among younger women. Many experts recommend that women aged 40 to 49 have mammograms every 1 to 2 years. All experts recommend yearly mammograms for women aged 50 and older.

Diagnosis

When a lump or another suspicious change is detected in the breast during a physical examination or by a screening procedure, other procedures are necessary. Mammography is performed first if it was not the way the abnormality was detected.

Ultrasonography is sometimes used to help distinguish between a fluid-filled sac (cyst) and a solid lump. This distinction is important because cysts are usually not cancerous. Cysts may be monitored (with no treatment) or drained with a small needle and syringe. Rarely, when cancer is suspected, cysts are removed. If the abnormality is a solid lump, which is more likely to be cancerous, a biopsy is performed. Often, an aspiration biopsy is performed: Some cells are removed from the lump through a needle attached to a syringe. If this procedure detects cancer, the diagnosis is confirmed. If no cancer is detected, removal of an additional piece of tissue (incisional biopsy) or of the entire lump (excisional biopsy) is necessary to be sure that the aspiration biopsy did not miss the cancer. Most women do not need to be hospitalized for these procedures. Usually, only a local anesthetic is needed.

If Paget's disease of the nipple is suspected, a biopsy of nipple tissue is performed. Sometimes this cancer can be diagnosed by examining a sample of the nipple discharge under a microscope.

A pathologist examines the biopsy samples under the microscope to determine whether cancer cells are present. Generally, a biopsy confirms cancer in one of four women in whom mammography detects an abnormality. If cancer cells are detected, the sample is analyzed to determine the characteristics of the cancer cells, such as whether the cancer cells have estrogen or progesterone receptors, how many HER-2/*neu* receptors are present, and how quickly the cancer cells are dividing. This information helps doctors estimate how rapidly the cancer may spread and which treatments are more likely to be effective.

A chest x-ray is taken and blood tests to evaluate liver function are performed to determine whether the cancer has spread. If the tu-

STAGES OF BREAST CANCER

STAGE	DESCRIPTION
0	The tumor is confined to a milk duct or milk-producing gland and has not invaded surrounding breast tissue (in situ carcinoma).
I	The tumor is less than ¾ inch (2 cm) in diameter and has not spread beyond the breast.
II	The tumor is larger than ¾ inch but smaller than 2 inches (5 cm) in diameter and/or has spread to at least one lymph node in the armpit on the same side as the tumor.
III	The tumor is larger than 2 inches in diameter and/or has spread to lymph nodes that are stuck to one another or to surrounding tissues, or the tumor, regardless of size, has spread to the skin, the chest wall, or the lymph nodes that are beneath the breast inside the chest.
IV	The tumor, regardless of size, has spread to distant organs or tissues, such as the lungs or bones, or to lymph nodes distant from the breast.

mor is large or if the lymph nodes are enlarged, x-rays of bones throughout the body (a bone scan) may be taken.

Treatment

Usually, treatment begins after the woman's condition has been thoroughly evaluated, about a week or more after the biopsy. Treatment options depend on the stage and type of breast cancer. However, treatment is complex because the different types of breast cancer differ greatly in growth rate, tendency to spread (metastasize), and response to treatment. Also, much is still unknown about breast cancer. Consequently, doctors may have different opinions about the most appropriate treatment for a particular woman.

The preferences of a woman and her doctor affect treatment decisions. A woman with breast cancer should ask for a clear explanation of what is known about the cancer and what is still unknown, as well as a complete description of treatment options. Then, a woman can consider the advantages and disadvantages of the different treatments and ac-

cept or reject the options offered. Losing some or all of a breast can be emotionally traumatic. A woman must consider how she feels about this treatment, which can deeply affect her sense of wholeness and sexuality.

Doctors may ask a woman with breast cancer to participate in research studies investigating a new treatment, which may improve her chances of survival or her quality of life. All women who participate in a research study are treated, because a new treatment is compared with other effective treatments. A woman should ask her doctor to explain the risks and possible benefits of participation, so that she can make a well-informed decision.

Treatment usually involves surgery and may include radiation therapy, chemotherapy, or hormone-blocking drugs. Often, a combination of these treatments is used.

Surgery: The cancerous tumor and varying amounts of the surrounding tissue are removed. There are two main options for removing the tumor: breast-conserving surgery and removal of the breast (mastectomy).

Breast-conserving surgery leaves as much of the breast intact as possible. There are several types:

• Lumpectomy is removal of the tumor with a small amount of surrounding normal tissue

• Wide excision or partial mastectomy is removal of the tumor and a somewhat larger amount of surrounding normal tissue

• Quadrantectomy is removal of one fourth of the breast

Removing the tumor with some normal tissue provides the best chance of preventing cancer from recurring within the breast. Breast-conserving surgery is usually combined with radiation therapy.

The major advantage of breast-conserving surgery is cosmetic: This surgery may help preserve body image. Thus, when the tumor is large in relation to the breast, this type of surgery is less likely to be useful. In such cases, removing the tumor plus some surrounding normal tissue means removing most of the breast. Breast-conserving surgery is usually more appropriate when tumors are small. In about 15% of women who undergo breast-conserving surgery, the amount of tissue removed is so small that little difference can be seen between the treated and untreated breasts. However, in most women, the treated breast shrinks somewhat and may change in contour.

How to Perform a Breast Self-Examination

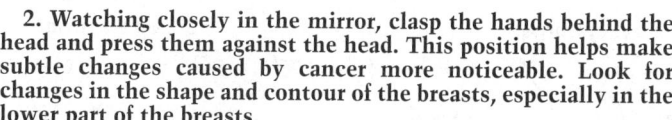

1. While standing in front of a mirror, look at the breasts. The breasts normally differ slightly in size. Look for changes in the size difference between the breasts and changes in the nipple, such as turning inward (an inverted nipple) or a discharge. Look for puckering or dimpling.

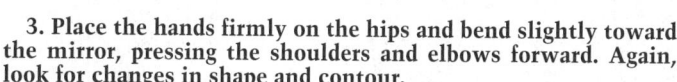

2. Watching closely in the mirror, clasp the hands behind the head and press them against the head. This position helps make subtle changes caused by cancer more noticeable. Look for changes in the shape and contour of the breasts, especially in the lower part of the breasts.

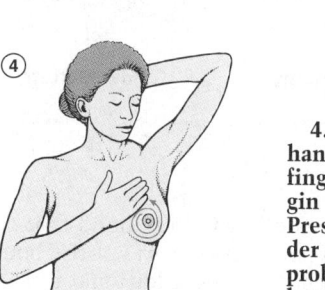

3. Place the hands firmly on the hips and bend slightly toward the mirror, pressing the shoulders and elbows forward. Again, look for changes in shape and contour.

Many women perform the next part of the examination in the shower because the hand moves easily over wet, slippery skin.

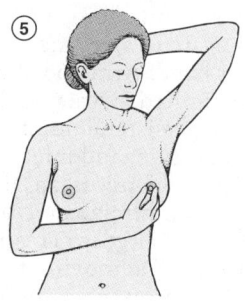

4. Raise the left arm. Using three or four fingers of the right hand, probe the left breast thoroughly with the flat part of the fingers. Moving the fingers in small circles around the breast, begin at the outer edge and gradually move in toward the nipple. Press gently but firmly, feeling for any unusual lump or mass under the skin. Be sure to check the whole breast. Also, carefully probe the armpit and the area between the breast and armpit for lumps.

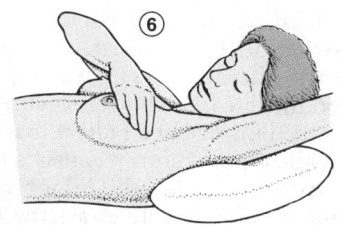

5. Squeeze the left nipple gently and look for a discharge. (See a doctor if a discharge appears at any time of the month, regardless of whether it happens during a breast self-examination.)

Repeat steps 4 and 5 for the right breast, raising the right arm and using the left hand.

6. Lie flat on the back with a pillow or folded towel under the left shoulder and with the left arm overhead. This position flattens the breast and makes it easier to examine. Examine the breast as in steps 4 and 5. Repeat for the right breast.

A woman should repeat this procedure at the same time each month. For menstruating women, 2 or 3 days after their period ends is a good time because the breasts are less likely to be tender and swollen. Postmenopausal women may choose any day of the month that is easy to remember, such as the first.

Adapted from a publication of the National Cancer Institute.

Surgery for Breast Cancer

Surgery for breast cancer consists of two main options: Breast-conserving surgery (in which only the tumor and an area of normal tissue surrounding it is removed) and mastectomy (in which all breast tissue is removed). Breast-conserving surgery includes lumpectomy (in which a small amount of surrounding normal tissue is removed), wide excision or partial mastectomy (in which a somewhat larger amount of the surrounding normal tissue is removed), and quadrantectomy (in which one fourth of the breast is removed).

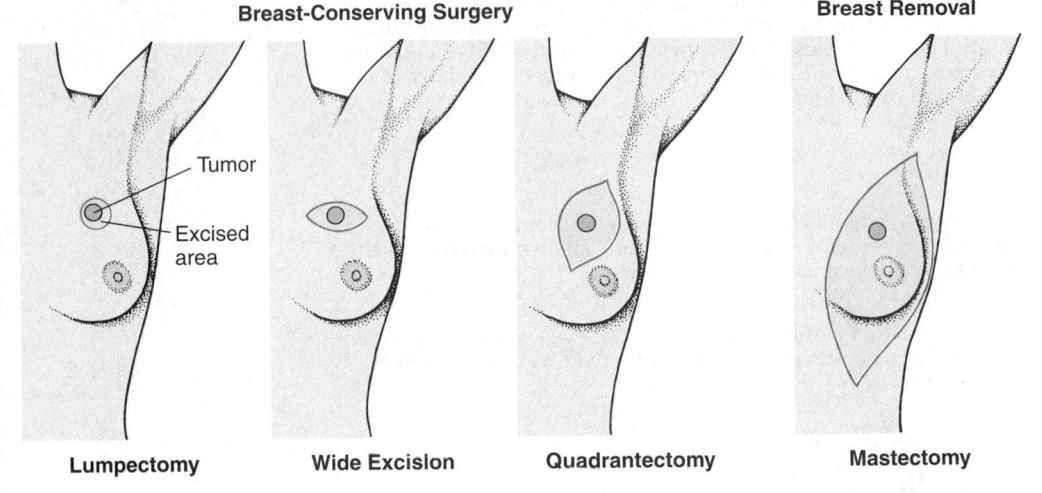

Breast-Conserving Surgery   **Breast Removal**

Tumor
Excised area

Lumpectomy   **Wide Excision**   **Quadrantectomy**   **Mastectomy**

Mastectomy is the other main surgical option. There are several types:

• Simple mastectomy consists of removing all breast tissue but leaving the muscle under the breast and enough skin to cover the wound. Reconstruction of the breast is much easier if these tissues are left. A simple mastectomy, rather than breast-conserving surgery, is usually performed when there is a substantial amount of cancer in the milk ducts.

• Modified radical mastectomy consists of removing all breast tissue and some lymph nodes in the armpit but leaving the muscle under the breast. This procedure is usually performed instead of a radical mastectomy.

• Radical mastectomy consists of removing all breast tissue plus the lymph nodes in the armpit and the muscle under the breast. This procedure is rarely performed now.

Lymph node surgery (lymph node dissection) is also performed if the cancer is or is suspected to be invasive. Nearby lymph nodes (usually about 10 to 20) are removed and examined to determine whether the cancer has spread to them. If cancer cells are detected in the lymph nodes, the likelihood that the cancer has spread to other parts of the body is increased. In such cases, additional treatment is needed. Removal of lymph nodes often causes problems, because it affects the drainage of fluids in tissues. As a result, fluids may accumulate, causing persistent swelling (lymphedema) of the arm or hand. Arm and shoulder movement may be limited. Other problems include temporary or persistent numbness, a persistent burning sensation, and infection.

A **sentinel lymph node biopsy** is an alternative approach that may minimize or avoid the problems of lymph node surgery. This procedure involves locating and removing the first lymph node (or nodes) into which the tumor drains. If this node contains cancer cells, the other lymph nodes are removed. If it does not, the other lymph nodes are not removed. Whether this procedure is as effective as standard lymph node surgery is being studied.

Breast reconstruction surgery may be performed at the same time as a mastectomy or later. A silicone or saline implant or tissue taken from other parts of the woman's body

HOW LYMPH NODE STATUS INFLUENCES SURVIVAL

Lymph Node Status	Chances of Surviving 5 Years	Chances of Surviving 10 Years	Chances of Surviving 10 Years Without Recurrence
No cancer in any node	Better than 90%	Better than 80%	Better than 70%
Cancer in one to three nodes	About 60 to 70%	About 40 to 50%	About 25 to 40%
Cancer in four or more nodes	About 40 to 50%	About 25 to 40%	About 15 to 35%

may be used. The safety of silicone implants, which sometimes leak, has been questioned. However, there is almost no evidence suggesting that silicone leakage has serious effects.

Radiation Therapy: This treatment is used to kill cancer cells at the site from which the tumor was removed and in the surrounding area, including nearby lymph nodes. Side effects include swelling in the breast, reddening and blistering of the skin in the treated area, and fatigue. These effects usually disappear within several months, up to about 12 months. Fewer than 5% of women treated with radiation therapy have rib fractures that cause minor discomfort. In about 1% of women, the lungs become mildly inflamed 6 to 18 months after radiation therapy is completed. Inflammation causes a dry cough and shortness of breath during physical activity that last for up to about 6 weeks.

To improve radiation therapy, doctors are studying several experimental procedures. In one procedure, tiny radioactive seeds are inserted through a catheter to the tumor site. Radiation therapy can be completed in only 5 days. In another procedure, a tiny coil that emits radiation is implanted in the space left by the tumor. Radiation therapy can be completed in 25 minutes.

Drugs: Chemotherapy and hormone-blocking drugs are used to suppress the growth of cancer cells throughout the body. Chemotherapy and sometimes hormone-blocking drugs are used in addition to surgery and radiation therapy if cancer cells are detected in the lymph nodes and often if they are not. These drugs are often started soon after breast surgery and are continued for several months. Some, such as tamoxifen, may be continued for up to 5 years. These drugs delay the recurrence of cancer and prolong survival in most women.

Chemotherapy is used to kill rapidly multiplying cells or slow their multiplication. Chemotherapy alone cannot cure breast cancer; it must be used with surgery or radiation therapy. Chemotherapy drugs are usually given intravenously in cycles. Sometimes they are given by mouth. Typically, a day of treatment is followed by several weeks of recovery. Using several chemotherapy drugs together is more effective than using a single drug. The choice of drugs depends partly on whether cancer cells are detected in nearby lymph nodes. Commonly used drugs include cyclophosphamide, doxorubicin, epirubicin, fluorouracil, methotrexate, and paclitaxel.▲ Side effects (such as vomiting and nausea, hair loss, and fatigue) vary depending on which drugs are used. Chemotherapy can also cause infertility and early menopause by destroying the eggs in the ovaries.

Hormone-blocking drugs interfere with the actions of estrogen or progesterone, which stimulate the growth of cancer cells that have estrogen or progesterone receptors. These drugs may be used when cancer cells have these receptors. Tamoxifen, given by mouth, is the most commonly used estrogen-blocking drug. In women who have estrogen receptor–positive cancer, use of tamoxifen increases the likelihood of survival during the first 10 years after diagnosis by about 20 to 25%. Tamoxifen, which is related to estrogen, has some of the benefits and risks of estrogen therapy taken after menopause.■ For example, it may decrease the risk of developing osteoporosis and it may increase the risk of developing cancer of the uterus (endometrial cancer). However, unlike estrogen therapy, tamoxifen may worsen the

▲ see table on page 1045   ■ see also page 1358

What Is a Sentinel Lymph Node?

A network of lymphatic vessels and lymph nodes drain fluid from the tissue in the breast. The lymph nodes are designed to trap foreign or abnormal cells (such as bacteria or cancer cells) that may be contained in this fluid. Sometimes cancer cells pass through the nodes and spread to other parts of the body by moving through the lymphatic vessels. Usually, the fluid from breast tissue drains through a single nearby lymph node first, but it may drain through more than one. Such lymph nodes are called sentinel lymph nodes.

Doctors can identify the sentinel lymph node by injecting blue dye or a radioactive substance in the fluid surrounding the breast cells. The dye can be seen or the radioactive substance detected with a Geiger counter as it reaches the first lymph node. The sentinel lymph node is then removed and examined to determine whether it contains cancer cells. If it does, other nearby lymph nodes are removed. If the sentinel lymph node does not contain cancer cells, the other lymph nodes are not removed. In about 2 to 3% of women, cancer has spread to other lymph nodes when the sentinel lymph node is clear.

Sentinel node

Lymph vessels

Tumor

Nipple

vaginal dryness or hot flashes that occur after menopause.

Biologic response modifiers are natural substances or slightly modified versions of natural substances that are part of the body's immune system. These drugs enhance the immune system's ability to fight cancer. They include interferons, interleukin-2, lymphocyte-activated killer cells, tumor necrosis factor, and monoclonal antibodies. Trastuzumab, a monoclonal antibody, is used to treat metastatic breast cancer only when the cancer cells have too many HER-2/*neu* receptors. This drug binds with HER-2/*neu* and thus prevents it from promoting the growth of cancer cells. Herceptin can cause heart problems by weakening the heart muscle. Other biologic response modifiers are sometimes tried experimentally as treatment for breast cancer,▲ but their role has not been established.

Tumor Ablation: In an experimental procedure called tumor ablation, doctors insert a multipronged probe into the tumor. Then a highly focused beam of light (laser), high-energy radio waves, or cold is used to destroy only the cancer cells.

Treatment of Noninvasive Cancer (Stage 0)

For **ductal carcinoma in situ,** treatment usually consists of a simple mastectomy or lumpectomy and sometimes radiation therapy.

For **lobular carcinoma in situ,** treatment is less clear-cut. For most women, the preferred treatment is close observation with no treatment. Observation consists of a physical examination every 6 to 12 months for 5 years and once a year thereafter plus mammography once a year. No treatment is usually needed. Although invasive breast cancer may develop (the risk is 1.3% per year or 26% for 20 years), the invasive cancers that develop are usually not fast growing and can usually be treated effectively. Furthermore, because invasive cancer is equally likely to develop in either breast, the only way to eliminate the risk of breast cancer for women with lobular carcinoma in situ is removal of both breasts (bilateral mastectomy). Some women, particularly those who are at high risk of developing invasive breast cancer, choose this option.

Alternatively, tamoxifen, a hormone-blocking drug, may be given for 5 years. It reduces

▲ see page 1046

Rebuilding a Breast

After a general surgeon removes a breast tumor and the surrounding breast tissue (mastectomy), a plastic surgeon may reconstruct the breast. A silicone or saline implant may be used. Or in a more complex operation, tissue may be taken from other parts of the woman's body, usually the abdomen. Reconstruction may be performed at the same time as the mastectomy—a choice that involves being under anesthesia for a longer time—or later—a choice that involves being under anesthesia a second time.

In many women, a reconstructed breast looks more natural than one that has been treated with radiation therapy, especially if the tumor was large. If a silicone or saline implant is used and enough skin was left to cover it, the sensation in the skin over the implant is relatively normal. However, neither type of implant feels like breast tissue to the touch. If tissue from other parts of the body is used, much of the sensation in the skin is lost since the skin is also from another part of the body. However, tissue from other parts of the body feels more like breast tissue than does a silicone or saline implant.

Silicone occasionally leaks out of its sack. As a result, an implant can become hard, cause discomfort, and appear less attractive. Also, silicone sometimes enters the bloodstream. Some women are concerned about whether the leaking silicone causes cancer in other parts of the body or rare diseases such as lupus (systemic lupus erythematosus). There is almost no evidence suggesting that silicone leakage has these serious effects, but because it might, the use of silicone implants has decreased, especially among women who have not had breast cancer.

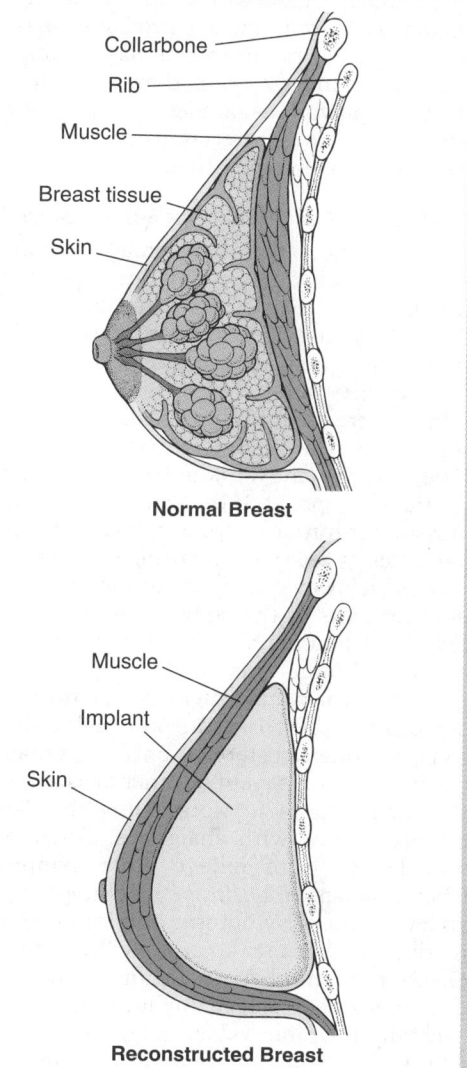

Normal Breast

Reconstructed Breast

but does not eliminate the risk of developing invasive cancer.

Treatment of Localized or Regional Invasive Cancer (Stages I through III)

For cancers that have not spread beyond nearby lymph nodes, treatment almost always includes surgery to remove as much of the tumor as possible and nearby lymph nodes or the sentinel lymph node.

A simple mastectomy is commonly used to treat invasive cancer that has spread extensively within the milk ducts (invasive ductal carcinoma), because this type of cancer often recurs when breast-conserving surgery is used. A modified radical mastectomy may also be used. A radical mastectomy, in which the underlying chest muscles and other tissues are also removed, does not improve life expectancy. Women who have had a simple or a modified radical mastectomy live as long as women who have had a radical mastectomy.

Whether radiation therapy, chemotherapy, or both are used after surgery depends on how large the tumor is and how many lymph nodes contain cancer cells. Sometimes, when the tumor is large, chemotherapy is given before surgery to reduce the size of the tumor. If chemotherapy reduces the size of the tumor, doctors can sometimes perform breast-conserving surgery rather than a mastectomy. After surgery and radiation therapy, additional chemotherapy is usually given, and women who have estrogen receptor–positive cancer are usually given tamoxifen.

Treatment of Cancer That Has Spread (Stage IV)

Breast cancer that has spread beyond the lymph nodes is rarely cured, but most women who have it live at least 2 years and a few live 10 to 20 years. Treatment extends life only slightly but may relieve symptoms and improve quality of life.

Initial treatment almost always includes surgery to remove the primary tumor, even though such removal is unlikely to cure cancer that has spread. If the cancer recurs in the breast after initial treatment, breast surgery is not usually repeated. Instead, radiation may be tried. However, surgery to remove tumors in other parts of the body (such as the brain) may be recommended, because such surgery can relieve symptoms.

Other treatments, such as chemotherapy, especially if they have uncomfortable side effects, are often postponed until a woman develops symptoms (pain or other discomfort) or the cancer starts to worsen quickly. Pain is usually treated with analgesics. Other drugs may be given to relieve other symptoms. Chemotherapy or hormone-blocking drugs are given to relieve symptoms and improve quality of life rather than to prolong life. The most effective chemotherapy regimens for breast cancer that has spread include capecitabine, cyclophosphamide, docetaxel, doxorubicin, epirubicin, gemcitabine, paclitaxel, and vinorelbine.

Hormone-blocking drugs are preferred to chemotherapy in certain situations. For example, these drugs may be preferred when the cancer is estrogen receptor–positive, when cancer has not recurred for more than 2 years after diagnosis and initial treatment, or when cancer is not immediately life threatening. Hormone-blocking drugs are especially effective for women in their 40s who are still menstruating and producing a lot of estrogen, as well as for those who are at least 5 years past menopause. However, these guidelines are not absolute. For women who are still menstruating, tamoxifen is usually the first hormone-blocking drug used because it has few side effects. For postmenopausal women who have

estrogen receptor–positive breast cancer, aromatase inhibitors (such as anastrozole, letrozole, and exemestane) may be more effective as a first treatment than tamoxifen. These drugs inhibit the enzyme aromatase (which converts some hormones to estrogen), possibly reducing estrogen production. Progestins, such as medroxyprogesterone or megestrol, may be used instead of aromatase inhibitors and tamoxifen and have almost as few side effects. Fulvestrant, a new drug, may be used when tamoxifen is no longer effective. It destroys the estrogen receptors in cancer cells. The most common side effect is stomach upset. Alternatively, for women who are still menstruating, surgery to remove the ovaries, radiation to destroy them, or drugs to inhibit their activity may be used to stop estrogen production.

The monoclonal antibody trastuzumab can be combined with paclitaxel as initial treatment for breast cancer that has spread throughout the body. Trastuzumab can be combined with hormone-blocking drugs to treat women who have estrogen receptor–positive breast cancer. Sometimes trastuzumab can be used to treat women who do not respond to chemotherapy.

In some situations, radiation therapy may be used instead of or before drugs. For example, if only one area of cancer is detected in a bone, without any other evidence of recurrences, radiation to that bone might be the only treatment used. Radiation therapy is usually the most effective treatment for cancer that has spread to bone, sometimes keeping it in check for years. It is also often the most effective treatment for cancer that has spread to the brain.

Treatment of Specific Types of Breast Cancer

For inflammatory breast cancer, treatment usually consists of both chemotherapy and radiation therapy. Mastectomy is usually performed.

For Paget's disease of the nipple, treatment usually consists of a simple mastectomy and removal of the lymph nodes. Less commonly, the nipple with some surrounding normal tissue is removed.

For cystosarcoma phyllodes, treatment usually consists of wide excision mastectomy, in which the tumor and a large amount of surrounding normal tissue are removed. If the tumor is large in relation to the breast, a simple mastectomy may be performed. After surgical removal, about 20 to 35% of cancers recur near the same site.

Follow-up Care

After treatment is completed, follow-up physical examinations, including examination of the breasts, chest, neck, and armpit, are performed every 3 months for 2 years, then every 6 months for 5 years from the date the cancer was diagnosed. Regular mammograms and breast self-examinations are also important. A woman should report any changes in her breasts to her doctor immediately. Other symptoms should also be reported. They include pain, loss of appetite or weight, changes in menstruation, bleeding from the vagina (if not associated with the menstrual period), and blurred vision. Any symptoms that seem unusual or that persist should also be reported. Diagnostic procedures, such as chest x-rays, blood tests, bone scans, and computed tomography (CT), are not needed unless a woman has symptoms suggesting recurrence of the cancer.

The effects of treatment for breast cancer cause many changes in a woman's life. Support from family members and friends can help, as can support groups. Counseling may be helpful.

End-of-Life Issues

For a woman with metastatic breast cancer, quality of life may deteriorate and the possibilities for further treatment may become limited. Staying comfortable may eventually become more important than trying to prolong life. Cancer pain can be adequately controlled with appropriate drugs.▲ So if a woman is having pain, she should ask her doctor for treatment to relieve it. Psychologic and spiritual counseling may also help.

A woman with metastatic breast cancer should prepare advance directives indicating the type of care she desires in case she is no longer able to make such decisions.■ Also, making or updating a will is important.

CHAPTER 252

Cancers of the Female Reproductive System

Cancers can occur in any part of the female reproductive system—the vulva, vagina, cervix, uterus, fallopian tubes, or ovaries. These cancers are called gynecologic cancers.

Gynecologic cancers can directly invade nearby tissues and organs or spread (metastasize) through the lymphatic vessels and lymph nodes (lymphatic system) or bloodstream to distant parts of the body.

Diagnosis

Regular pelvic examinations and Papanicolaou (Pap) tests or other similar tests★ can lead to the early detection of certain gynecologic cancers, especially cancer of the cervix and uterus. Such examinations can sometimes prevent cancer by detecting abnormalities (precancerous conditions) before they develop into cancer.

If cancer is suspected, a biopsy can usually confirm or rule out the diagnosis. If cancer is

diagnosed, one or more procedures may be performed to determine the stage of the cancer. The stage is based on how large the cancer is and how far it has spread. Some commonly used procedures include ultrasonography, computed tomography (CT), magnetic resonance imaging (MRI), chest x-rays, and bone and liver scans using radioactive substances.

Staging a cancer helps doctors choose the best treatment. Doctors often determine the stage of cancer after they remove the cancer and perform biopsies of the surrounding tissues, including lymph nodes. For cancers of the uterus and ovaries, stages range from I (the earliest) to IV (advanced). For the other gynecologic cancers, stage 0 is the earliest stage, when the cancer is confined to a surface of the

---

▲ see page 48   ■ see page 54

★ see page 1353

STAGING CANCERS OF THE FEMALE REPRODUCTIVE SYSTEM*

TYPE	STAGE 0	STAGE I	STAGE II	STAGE III	STAGE IV
Endometrial cancer	—	Only in the upper part of the uterus (not the cervix)	Spread to the cervix	Spread to nearby tissues but still within the pelvic area	A: Spread to the bladder or rectum B: Spread to distant organs
Ovarian cancer	—	Only in one or both ovaries	Spread to the uterus, fallopian tubes, and/or nearby tissues within the pelvis	Spread outside the pelvis to the lymph nodes or other organs in the abdomen (such as the surface of the liver or intestine)	Spread outside the abdomen or to the inside of the liver
Cervical cancer	Only on the surface of the cervix	Only in the cervix	Spread to nearby tissues but still within the pelvic area	Spread throughout the pelvic area, sometimes blocking the ureters	A: Spread to the bladder or rectum B: Spread to distant organs
Vulvar cancer	Only on the surface of the vulva	Only in the vulva and/or the area between the opening of the rectum and vagina (perineum); ¾ inch (2 centimeters) or smaller	In the vulva and/or perineum, but larger than ¾ inch	In the vulva and/or perineum and spread to nearby tissues and/or lymph nodes	Spread beyond nearby tissues to the bladder, to the intestine, or to more distant lymph nodes
Vaginal cancer	Only in the lining of the vagina	Only in the vagina but deeper (in the wall)	Spread to nearby tissues but still within the pelvic area	Spread throughout the pelvic area and possibly to nearby organs and lymph nodes	A: Spread to the bladder or rectum B: Spread to distant organs
Fallopian tube cancer	Only in the lining of the fallopian tubes	Only in the fallopian tubes but deeper (in the wall)	Spread to nearby tissues but still within the pelvic area	Spread throughout the pelvic area and possibly to nearby organs and lymph nodes	Spread to distant organs

*Simplified from the International Federation of Gynecology and Obstetrics staging system.

affected organ. For some cancers, further distinctions, designated by letters of the alphabet, are made within stages.

Treatment

The main treatment of gynecologic cancer is surgical removal of the tumor. Surgery may be followed by radiation therapy or chemotherapy. Radiation therapy may be external (using a large machine) or internal (using radioactive implants placed directly on the can-

cer). External radiation therapy is usually given several days a week for several weeks. Internal radiation therapy involves staying in the hospital for several days while the implants are in place.

Chemotherapy may be given by injection or by mouth. Chemotherapy is given for 5 days to 6 weeks (depending on the drugs) followed by a recovery period of several weeks without chemotherapy. The cycle may be repeated several times. A woman may have to remain at the hospital while she receives chemo-therapy.

When a gynecologic cancer is very advanced and a cure is not possible, radiation therapy or chemotherapy may still be recommended to reduce the size of the cancer or its metastases and to relieve pain and other symptoms. Women with incurable cancer should estab-lish advance directives.▲ Because end-of-life care has improved, more and more women with incurable cancer are able to die comfort-ably at home.■ Appropriate drugs can be used to relieve the anxiety and pain commonly ex-perienced by people with incurable cancer.

Cancer of the Uterus

Cancer of the uterus begins in the lining of the uterus (endometrium) and is more precisely termed endometrial cancer (carcinoma). It is the most common gynecologic cancer and the fourth most common cancer among women. This cancer usually develops after menopause, most often in women aged 50 to 60.

Risk factors for endometrial cancer include the following:

• early menarche (the start of menstrual pe-riods), menopause after age 52, or both
• menstrual problems (such as excessive bleeding, spotting between menstrual periods, or long intervals without periods)
• never having had children
• tumors that produce estrogen
• high doses of drugs that contain estrogen, such as estrogen therapy without a progestin (synthetic drugs similar to the hormone pro-gesterone), taken after menopause
• use of tamoxifen
• obesity
• high blood pressure
• diabetes
• family history of cancer of the breast, ovaries, large intestine (colon), or lining of the uterus.

Many of these conditions increase the risk of endometrial cancer because they result in a high level of estrogen but not progesterone. Estrogen promotes the growth of tissue and rapid cell division in the lining of the uterus (endometrium). Progesterone helps balance the effects of estrogen. Levels of estrogen are high during part of the menstrual cycle. Thus, having more menstrual periods during a life-time may increase the risk of endometrial can-cer. Tamoxifen, a drug used to treat breast can-cer, blocks the effects of estrogen in the breast,

but it has the same effects as estrogen in the uterus. Thus, this drug may increase the risk of endometrial cancer. Taking oral contracep-tives that contain estrogen and a progestin ap-pears to reduce the risk of endometrial cancer.

More than 80% of endometrial cancers are adenocarcinomas, which develop from gland cells. About 5% are sarcomas, which develop from connective tissue and tend to be more ag-gressive.

Symptoms and Diagnosis

Abnormal bleeding from the vagina is the most common early symptom. Abnormal bleeding includes bleeding after menopause or between menstrual periods and periods that are irregular, heavy, or longer than normal. One of three women with vaginal bleeding after menopause has endometrial cancer. Women who have vaginal bleeding after menopause should see a doctor promptly. A watery, blood-tinged discharge may also oc-cur. Postmenopausal women may have a vagi-nal discharge for several weeks or months, fol-lowed by vaginal bleeding.

If doctors suspect endometrial cancer or if Pap test results are abnormal, doctors perform an endometrial biopsy in their office. This test accurately detects endometrial cancer more than 90% of the time. If the diagnosis is still uncertain, doctors perform dilation and curet-tage (D and C),★ in which tissue is scraped from the uterine lining. At the same time, doctors may view the interior of the uterus using a thin, flexible viewing tube inserted through the vagina and cervix into the uterus in a procedure called hysteroscopy.

If endometrial cancer is diagnosed, some or all of the following procedures may be per-formed to determine whether the cancer has spread beyond the uterus: blood tests, liver function tests, a chest x-ray, and computed to-mography (CT) or magnetic resonance imag-ing (MRI). Other procedures are sometimes re-quired. Staging is based on information obtained from these procedures and during surgery to remove the cancer.

Prognosis and Treatment

If endometrial cancer is detected early, nearly 90% of women who have it survive at least 5 years, and most are cured. The progno-sis is better for women whose cancer has not

---

▲ see page 54   ■ see also page 45
★ see page 1354

Understanding Hysterectomy

A hysterectomy is the removal of the uterus. Usually, the uterus is removed through an incision in the lower abdomen. Sometimes the uterus can be removed through the vagina. Either method usually takes about 1 to 2 hours and requires a general anesthetic. Afterward, vaginal bleeding and pain may occur. The hospital stay is usually 2 to 3 days, and recovery may take up to 6 weeks. When the uterus is removed through the vagina, less bleeding occurs, recovery is faster, and there is no visible scar.

In addition to treatment of certain gynecologic cancers, a hysterectomy may be performed to treat prolapse of the uterus, endometriosis, or fibroids (if causing severe symptoms). Sometimes it is performed to treat cancer of the colon, rectum, or bladder.

There are several types of hysterectomy. The type used depends on the disorder being treated. For a subtotal hysterectomy, only the upper part of the uterus is removed, but the cervix is not. The fallopian tubes and ovaries may or may not be removed. For a total hysterectomy, the entire uterus including the cervix is removed. For a radical hysterectomy, the entire uterus plus the surrounding tissues, ligaments, and lymph nodes are removed. Both fallopian tubes and ovaries are usually also removed in women older than 45.

After a hysterectomy, menstruation stops. However, a hysterectomy does not cause menopause unless the ovaries are also removed. Removal of the ovaries has the same effects as menopause, so hormone therapy may be recommended.▲ Many women anticipate feeling depressed or losing interest in sex after a hysterectomy. However, hysterectomy rarely has these effects unless the ovaries are also removed.

▲ see page 1358

spread beyond the uterus. If the cancer grows relatively slowly, the prognosis is also better. Fewer than one third of women who have this cancer die of it.

Hysterectomy, the surgical removal of the uterus, is the mainstay of treatment for women who have endometrial cancer. If the cancer has not spread beyond the uterus, removal of the uterus plus removal of the fallopian tubes and ovaries (salpingo-oophorectomy)

almost always cures the cancer. Nearby lymph nodes are usually removed at the same time. These tissues are examined by a pathologist to determine whether the cancer has spread and, if so, how far it has spread. With this information, doctors can determine whether additional treatment (chemotherapy, radiation therapy, or a progestin) is needed after surgery.

Chemotherapy may be given after surgery, even when the cancer does not appear to have spread, in case some undetected cancer cells remain. More than half of women with cancer limited to the uterus do not need radiation therapy. However, if the cancer has spread, radiation therapy is usually needed after surgery.

A progestin is often effective. (Progestins are synthetic drugs similar to the hormone progesterone, which blocks the effects of estrogen on the uterus.) If the cancer has spread beyond the uterus, higher doses may be needed. In 15 to 30% of women who have cancer that has spread, a progestin reduces the cancer's size and controls its spread for 2 to 3 years or longer. A progestin may be continued as long as it seems to be working well. Side effects may include mood changes and weight gain due to water retention.

If the cancer has spread, is not responding to a progestin, or recurs, chemotherapy drugs (such as cisplatin, cyclophosphamide, doxorubicin, and paclitaxel) may be used instead of or sometimes with radiation therapy. These drugs are much more toxic than progestins and cause many side effects. However, they reduce the cancer's size and control its spread in more than half of women treated.

Cancer of the Ovaries

Cancer of the ovaries (ovarian carcinoma) develops most often in women aged 50 to 70. This cancer eventually develops in about 1 of 70 women. It is the second most common gynecologic cancer. However, more women die of ovarian cancer than of any other gynecologic cancer.

The risk of this cancer is higher in industrialized countries because the diet tends to be high in fat. Risk is increased for women who were unable to become pregnant, who had their first child late in life, who started menstruating early, or who reached menopause late. Risk is also increased for women who have a family history of cancer of the uterus, breast, or large intestine (colon). Less than 5% of ovarian cancer cases are related to the

BRCA1 gene, which is also related to breast cancer. Use of oral contraceptives significantly decreases risk.

There are many types of ovarian cancer. They develop from the many different types of cells in the ovaries. Cancers that start on the surface of the ovaries (epithelial carcinomas) account for more than 80%. Most other ovarian cancers are germ cell tumors (which start from the cells that produce eggs) and stromal cell tumors (which start in connective tissue). Germ cell tumors are much more common among women younger than 30. Sometimes cancers from other parts of the body spread to the ovaries.

Ovarian cancer can spread directly to the surrounding area and through the lymphatic system to other parts of the pelvis and abdomen. It can also spread through the bloodstream, eventually appearing in distant parts of the body, mainly the liver and lungs.

Symptoms and Diagnosis

Ovarian cancer causes the affected ovary to enlarge. In young women, enlargement of an ovary is likely to be caused by a noncancerous fluid-filled sac (cyst). However, after menopause, an enlarged ovary is often a sign of ovarian cancer.

Many women have no symptoms until the cancer is advanced. The first symptom may be vague discomfort in the lower abdomen, similar to indigestion. Other symptoms may include bloating, loss of appetite (because the stomach is compressed), gas pains, and backache. Ovarian cancer rarely causes vaginal bleeding.

Eventually, the abdomen may swell because the ovary enlarges or fluid accumulates in the abdomen. At this stage, pain in the pelvic area, anemia, and weight loss are common. Rarely, germ cell or stromal cell tumors produce estrogens, which can cause tissue in the uterine lining to grow excessively and breasts to enlarge. Or these tumors may produce male hormones (androgens), which can cause body hair to grow excessively, or hormones that resemble thyroid hormones, which can cause hyperthyroidism.

Diagnosing ovarian cancer in its early stages is difficult, because symptoms usually do not appear until the cancer is quite large or has spread beyond the ovaries and because many less serious disorders cause similar symptoms.

If doctors detect an enlarged ovary during a physical examination, they order ultrasonography, computed tomography (CT), or magnetic resonance imaging (MRI) to help distin-

---

What Is an Ovarian Cyst?

An ovarian cyst is a fluid-filled sac in or on an ovary. Such cysts are relatively common. Most are noncancerous and disappear on their own. Cancerous cysts are more likely to occur in women older than 40.

Most noncancerous ovarian cysts do not cause symptoms. However, some cause pressure, aching, or a feeling of heaviness in the abdomen. Pain may be felt during sexual intercourse. If a cyst ruptures or becomes twisted, severe stabbing pain is felt in the abdomen. The pain may be accompanied by nausea and fever. Some cysts produce hormones that affect menstrual periods. As a result, periods may be irregular or heavier than normal. In postmenopausal women, such cysts may cause vaginal bleeding. Women who have any of these symptoms should see a doctor.

Diagnosis begins with a pelvic examination. Ultrasonography or computed tomography (CT) may be performed to confirm the diagnosis. If the cyst appears to be noncancerous, a woman may be asked to return periodically for pelvic examinations as long as the cyst remains. If the cyst could be cancerous, the ovaries may be examined through a laparoscope, inserted through a small incision just below the navel. Blood tests can help confirm or rule out cancer.

For noncancerous cysts, no treatment is necessary. But if a cyst is larger than about 2 inches (5 centimeters) and persists or if cancer cannot be ruled out, the cyst may be removed. Sometimes the affected ovary is also removed. Cancerous cysts plus the affected ovary and fallopian tube are removed.

---

guish an ovarian cyst from a cancerous mass. If cancer seems unlikely, doctors reexamine the woman every few months. If doctors suspect cancer or test results are unclear, the ovaries are examined using a thin, flexible viewing tube (laparoscope) inserted through a small incision just below the navel. Also, tissue samples are removed using instruments threaded through the laparoscope. In addition, blood tests are usually performed to measure levels of substances that may indicate the presence of cancer (tumor markers), such as cancer antigen 125 (CA 125). Abnormal marker levels alone do not confirm the diagnosis of cancer, but when combined with other information, they can help confirm it.

If fluid has accumulated in the abdomen, it can be drawn out (aspirated) through a needle and tested to see whether cancer cells are present.

Prognosis and Treatment

If ovarian cancer is suspected or confirmed, surgery is performed to remove the mass and to determine how far the cancer has spread (its stage). The prognosis is based on the stage.▲ With treatment, 70 to 100% of women with stage I cancer and 50 to 70% of those with stage II cancer are alive 5 years after diagnosis. Only 5 to 40% of women with stage III or IV cancer are alive after 5 years.

The extent of surgery depends on the type of ovarian cancer and the stage. If the cancer has not spread beyond the ovary, removal of only the affected ovary and the adjoining fallopian tube may be sufficient. When cancer has spread beyond the ovary, both ovaries and fallopian tubes and the uterus are removed, as are nearby lymph nodes and surrounding structures that the cancer typically spreads through. If a woman has stage I cancer that affects only one ovary and she wishes to become pregnant, doctors may remove only the affected ovary and fallopian tube. For more advanced cancers that have spread to other parts of the body, removing as much of the cancer as possible improves the prognosis.

After surgery, women with stage I epithelial carcinomas usually require no further treatment. For other stage I cancers or for more advanced cancers, chemotherapy may be used to destroy any small areas of cancer that may remain. Chemotherapy consists of paclitaxel combined with cisplatin or carboplatin. Most women with advanced germ cell tumors can be cured with combination chemotherapy, usually with bleomycin, etoposide, and cisplatin. Radiation therapy is rarely used.

Advanced ovarian cancer usually recurs. So after chemotherapy, doctors typically measure levels of cancer markers. If the cancer recurs, chemotherapy (using such drugs as topotecan, hexamethylmelamine, ifosfamide, doxorubicin, or etoposide) is given.

Cancer of the Cervix

The cervix is the lower part of the uterus. It extends into the vagina. Of gynecologic cancers, cervical cancer (cervical carcinoma) is the third most common among all women and the most common among younger women. It usually affects women aged 35 to 55, but it can affect women as young as 20.

This cancer is caused by the human papillomavirus which is transmitted during sexual intercourse. This virus also causes genital warts.■ The younger a woman was the first time she had sexual intercourse and the more sex partners she has had, the higher her risk of cervical cancer.

About 85% of cervical cancers are squamous cell carcinomas, which develop in the scaly, flat, skinlike cells covering the cervix. Most other cervical cancers are adenocarcinomas, which develop from gland cells, or adenosquamous carcinomas, which develop from a combination of cell types.

Cervical cancer begins on the surface of the cervix and can penetrate deep beneath the surface. The cancer can spread directly to nearby tissues, including the vagina. Or it can enter the rich network of small blood and lymphatic vessels inside the cervix, then spread to other parts of the body.

Symptoms and Diagnosis

In the early stages, cervical cancer usually causes no symptoms. It may cause spotting or heavier bleeding between periods, bleeding after intercourse, or unusually heavy periods. In later stages, such abnormal bleeding is common. Other symptoms may include a foul-smelling discharge from the vagina, pain in the pelvic area or lower back, and swelling of the legs. The urinary tract may be blocked; without treatment, kidney failure and death can result.

Routine Papanicolaou (Pap) tests or other similar tests can detect the beginnings of cervical cancer.★ Cervical cancer begins with slow, progressive changes in normal cells on the surface of the cervix. These changes are called dysplasia. Untreated, these cells may become cancerous with time, sometimes after years. When performing a Pap test, doctors look for these changes as well as for cancer. Women with dysplasia should be checked again in 3 to 4 months.

A Pap test can accurately and inexpensively detect up to 90% of cervical cancers, even before symptoms develop. Consequently, the number of deaths due to cervical cancer has been reduced by more than 50% since Pap tests were introduced. Doctors often recommend that women have their first Pap test

---

▲ see box on page 1402   ■ see page 1183
★ see page 1353

when they become sexually active or reach the age of 18 and that a Pap test be performed annually. If test results are normal for 3 consecutive years, women may schedule Pap tests every 2 or 3 years as long as they do not change their sexual lifestyle. Any woman who has had cervical cancer or dysplasia should continue to have Pap tests at least annually. If all women had Pap tests on a regular basis, deaths from this cancer could be virtually eliminated. However, about 50% of American women are not tested regularly.

If a growth, a sore, or another abnormal area is seen on the cervix during a pelvic examination or if a Pap test detects an abnormality or cancer, a biopsy is performed. Usually, doctors use an instrument with a binocular magnifying lens (colposcope) to examine the cervix and to choose the best biopsy site. Two different types of biopsy are performed. In a punch biopsy, a tiny piece of the cervix, selected using the colposcope, is removed. In endocervical curettage, tissue that cannot be viewed is scraped from inside the cervix. These biopsies cause little pain and a small amount of bleeding. The two together usually provide enough tissue for pathologists to make a diagnosis.

If the diagnosis is not clear, doctors perform a cone biopsy to remove a larger cone-shaped piece of tissue. Usually, a thin wire loop with an electrical current running through it is used. This procedure is called the loop electrosurgical excision procedure (LEEP). Alternatively, a laser (using a highly focused beam of light) can be used. Either procedure requires only a local anesthetic and can be performed in the doctor's office. A cold (nonelectric) knife is sometimes used, but this procedure requires an operating room and an anesthetic.

If cervical cancer is diagnosed, its exact size and locations (its stage) are determined. Staging begins with a physical examination of the pelvis and various procedures (such as cystoscopy, a chest x-ray, intravenous urography, and sigmoidoscopy) to determine whether the cancer has spread to nearby tissues or to distant parts of the body. Other procedures, such as computed tomography (CT), magnetic resonance imaging (MRI), a barium enema, and bone and liver scans, may be performed.

Prognosis and Treatment

Prognosis depends on the stage of the cancer.▲ With treatment, 80 to 90% of women

with stage I cancer and 50 to 65% of those with stage II cancer are alive 5 years after diagnosis. Only 25 to 35% of women with stage III cancer and 15% or fewer of those with stage IV cancer are alive after 5 years.

Treatment also depends on the stage. If only the surface of the cervix is involved, doctors can often completely remove the cancer by removing part of the cervix using the loop electrosurgical excision procedure, a laser, or a cold knife. Or cryotherapy may be used to destroy the cancer by freezing it. These treatments preserve a woman's ability to have children. Because cancer can recur, doctors advise women to return for examinations and Pap tests every 3 months for the first year and every 6 months after that. Rarely, removal of the uterus (hysterectomy) is necessary.

If the cancer has begun to spread within the pelvic area, hysterectomy plus removal of surrounding tissues, ligaments, and lymph nodes (radical hysterectomy) is necessary. The ovaries may be removed. Normal, functioning ovaries in younger women are not removed. Alternatively, radiation therapy may be used. It usually causes few or no immediate side effects, but it may irritate the bladder or rectum. Later, as a result, the intestine may become blocked, and the bladder and rectum may be damaged. Also, the ovaries usually stop functioning. With either radical hysterectomy or radiation therapy, about 85 to 90% of women are cured.

If the cancer has spread further within the pelvis or to other organs, radiation therapy is preferred. This treatment is ineffective in about 40% of women with large or extensive cancers.

When the cancer has spread extensively or recurs, chemotherapy, usually with cisplatin and ifosfamide, is sometimes recommended. However, chemotherapy reduces the cancer's size and controls its spread in only 25 to 30% of women treated, and this effect is usually temporary.

Cancer of the Vulva

The vulva refers to the area that contains the external female reproductive organs. Cancer of the vulva (vulvar carcinoma) is the fourth most common gynecologic cancer, accounting for only 3 to 4% of these cancers. Vulvar cancer usually occurs after menopause. The average age at diagnosis is 70 years. As

▲ see box on page 1402

more women live longer, this cancer is likely to become more common.

The risk of developing vulvar cancer is increased for women who have persistent itching of the vulva, have genital warts due to human papillomavirus (HPV), or have had cancer of the vagina or cervix.

Most vulvar cancers are skin cancers that develop near or at the opening of the vagina. About 90% of vulvar cancers are squamous cell carcinomas, and 5% are melanomas. The remaining 5% include basal cell carcinomas and rare cancers such as Paget's disease and cancer of Bartholin's gland.

Vulvar cancer begins on the surface of the vulva. Most of these cancers grow slowly, remaining on the surface for years. However, some grow quickly. Untreated, vulvar cancer can eventually invade the vagina, the urethra, or the anus and spread into lymph nodes in the area.

Symptoms and Diagnosis

White, brown, or red patches on the vulva are precancerous; that is, they may indicate that cancer is likely to eventually develop. Vulvar cancer is usually seen and felt as unusual lumps or flat, red sores that do not heal. Sometimes scaly patches develop or the area becomes discolored. The surrounding tissue may contract and pucker. Usually, vulvar cancer causes little discomfort, but itching is common. Eventually, the lump or sore may bleed or produce a watery discharge (weep). These symptoms should be evaluated promptly by a doctor. About one fifth of women have no symptoms, at least at first.

Doctors diagnose vulvar cancer by performing a biopsy of the abnormal skin. The biopsy can identify whether the abnormal skin is cancerous or just infected or irritated. It also identifies the type of cancer, if present, so that doctors can develop a treatment plan. Sometimes doctors apply stains to the sores to help determine where to take a sample of tissue for a biopsy. Sometimes an instrument with a binocular magnifying lens (colposcope) is used to examine the surface of the vulva.

Prognosis and Treatment

If vulvar cancer is detected early, about 3 of 4 women have no sign of cancer 5 years after diagnosis. If the lymph nodes are involved, less than one third of women survive for 5 years.

Because most vulvar cancers can spread quickly, surgical removal of the vulva (vulvec-

tomy) is usually necessary. Depending on the extent of the cancer, all or part of the vulva is removed. Sometimes nearby lymph nodes are also removed. Treatment with radiation therapy, chemotherapy, or both may be used to shrink very large cancers so that they can be surgically removed. Sometimes the clitoris must be removed. Doctors work closely with the woman to develop a treatment plan that is best suited to her and takes into account her age, sexual lifestyle, and any other medical problems. Sexual intercourse is usually possible after vulvectomy.

For some small vulvar cancers that do not extend below the skin, treatment consists of removal with a highly focused beam of light (laser surgery), surgical removal of only the skin, or use of an ointment containing a chemotherapy drug (such as fluorouracil). Some small cancers are treated with radiation therapy alone.

Because basal cell carcinoma of the vulva does not tend to spread (metastasize) to distant sites, surgery usually involves removing only the cancer. The whole vulva is removed only if the cancer is extensive.

Cancer of the Vagina

Only about 1% of gynecologic cancers occur in the vagina. Cancer of the vagina (vaginal carcinoma) usually affects women older than 45. The average age at diagnosis is 60 to 65.

More than 95% of vaginal cancers are squamous cell carcinomas. Vaginal squamous cell carcinoma may be caused by human papillomavirus (HPV), the same virus that causes genital warts and cervical cancer. Most other vaginal cancers are adenocarcinomas. One rare type, clear cell carcinoma, occurs almost exclusively in women whose mothers took the drug diethylstilbestrol (DES), prescribed to prevent miscarriage during pregnancy. (In 1971, the drug was banned in the United States.)

Depending on the type, vaginal cancer may begin on the surface of the vaginal lining. If untreated, it continues to grow and invades surrounding tissue. Eventually, it may spread to other parts of the body.

Symptoms and Diagnosis

The most common symptom is bleeding from the vagina, which may occur during or after sexual intercourse, between menstrual periods, or after menopause. Sores may form on the lining of the vagina. They may bleed and become infected. Other symptoms include a watery discharge and pain during sexual intercourse. A few women have no symptoms. Large cancers can also affect the bladder, causing a frequent urge to urinate and pain during urination. In advanced cancer, abnormal connections (fistulas) may form between the vagina and the bladder or rectum.

Doctors may suspect vaginal cancer on the basis of symptoms, abnormal areas seen during a routine pelvic examination, or an abnormal Pap test result. Doctors may use an instrument with a binocular magnifying lens (colposcope) to examine the vagina. To confirm the diagnosis, doctors scrape cells from the vaginal wall to examine under a microscope. They also perform a biopsy on any growth, sore, or other abnormal area seen during the examination.

Prognosis and Treatment

The prognosis depends on the stage of the cancer.▲ If the cancer is limited to the vagina, about 65 to 70% of women survive at least 5 years after diagnosis. If the cancer has spread beyond the pelvis or to the bladder or rectum, only about 15 to 20% survive.

Treatment also depends on the stage. For most vaginal cancers, surgery is the treatment of choice, with or without radiation therapy. Radiation therapy may be internal (using radioactive implants placed inside the vagina) or external (directed at the pelvis from outside the body). Radiation therapy is often combined with or followed by surgical removal of the cancer. For cancer in the upper third of the vagina, a hysterectomy with removal of lymph nodes in the pelvis and the upper part of the vagina may be needed. For very advanced cancer, surgery is often not possible. In such cases, radiation therapy and chemotherapy are usually used.

Intercourse may be difficult or impossible after treatment for vaginal cancer, although sometimes a new vagina can be constructed with skin grafts or part of the intestine.

Cancer of the Fallopian Tubes

The fallopian tubes lead from the ovaries to the uterus. Less than 1% of gynecologic cancers are fallopian tube cancers. Most often, cancer that affects the fallopian tubes is cancer that has spread from the ovaries rather than started in the fallopian tubes. Fallopian tube cancer usually affects women aged 50 to

60. Occasionally, it appears to be associated with having been infertile.

More than 95% of fallopian tube cancers are adenocarcinomas, which develop from gland cells. A few are sarcomas, which develop from connective tissue. Fallopian tube cancer spreads in much the same way as ovarian cancer.

Symptoms and Diagnosis

Symptoms include vague abdominal discomfort, bloating, and pain in the pelvic area or abdomen. Some women have a watery or blood-tinged discharge from the vagina. Usually, an enlarged mass is found in the pelvis.

The diagnosis is made by viewing the fallopian tubes and surrounding tissues through a thin viewing tube (laparoscope) inserted through a small incision just below the navel or by performing surgery to remove the mass. Biopsies of the surrounding tissues are performed.

Prognosis and Treatment

The prognosis is similar to that for women who have ovarian cancer. Treatment almost always consists of removal of the uterus (hysterectomy) and removal of the ovaries and fallopian tubes (salpingo-oophorectomy), adjacent lymph nodes, and surrounding tissues. Chemotherapy (as for ovarian cancer) is usually necessary after surgery. For some cancers, radiation therapy is useful. For cancer that has spread to other parts of the body, removing as much of the cancer as possible improves the prognosis.

Hydatidiform Mole

A hydatidiform mole is growth of an abnormal fertilized egg or an overgrowth of tissue from the placenta.

Most often, a hydatidiform mole is an abnormal fertilized egg. The abnormal egg develops into a hydatidiform mole rather than a fetus (a condition called molar pregnancy). However, a hydatidiform mole can develop from cells that remain in the uterus after a miscarriage or a full-term pregnancy. Rarely, a hydatidiform mole develops when the fetus is normal.

About 80% of hydatidiform moles are not cancerous and disappear spontaneously. About 15 to 20% invade the surrounding tissue and tend to persist. Of these invasive moles, 2 to 3% become cancerous and spread throughout

▲ see box on page 1402

the body; they are then called choriocarcinomas. Choriocarcinomas can spread quickly through the lymphatic vessels or bloodstream.

The risk of hydatidiform moles is highest for women who become pregnant before age 17 or in their late 30s or later. Hydatidiform moles occur in about 1 of 2,000 pregnancies in the United States and, for unknown reasons, are nearly 10 times more common among Asian women.

Symptoms and Diagnosis

Women who have a hydatidiform mole feel as if they are pregnant. But because hydatidiform moles grow much faster than a fetus, the abdomen becomes larger much faster than it does in a normal pregnancy. Severe nausea and vomiting are common, and vaginal bleeding may occur. These symptoms indicate the need for prompt evaluation by a doctor. Hydatidiform moles can cause serious complications, including infections, bleeding, and preeclampsia or eclampsia.▲

Often, doctors can diagnose a hydatidiform mole shortly after conception. No fetal movement and no fetal heartbeat are detected. As parts of the mole decay, small amounts of tissue that resemble a bunch of grapes may pass through the vagina. After examining this tissue under a microscope, a pathologist can confirm the diagnosis.

Ultrasonography may be performed to be sure that the growth is a hydatidiform mole and not a fetus or amniotic sac (which contains the fetus and fluid around it). Blood tests to measure the level of human chorionic gonadotropin (HCG—a hormone normally produced early in pregnancy) may be performed.

If a hydatidiform mole is present, the level is usually very high because the mole produces a large amount of this hormone.

Treatment

The cure rate for a hydatidiform mole is virtually 100% if the mole has not spread. The cure rate is 60 to 80% if the hydatidiform mole has spread widely. Most women can have children afterwards and do not have a higher risk of having complications, a miscarriage, or children with birth defects. About 1% of women who have had a hydatidiform mole have another one. So for women who have had a hydatidiform mole, ultrasonography is performed early during subsequent pregnancies.

A hydatidiform mole that does not disappear spontaneously is completely removed usually by dilation and curettage (D and C) with suction.■ Only rarely is removal of the uterus (hysterectomy) necessary.

If the hydatidiform mole is detected, a chest x-ray is performed after surgery to make sure that it has not become cancerous (that is, a choriocarcinoma) and spread to the lungs. After surgery, the level of human chorionic gonadotropin in the blood is measured to determine whether the hydatidiform mole was completely removed. When removal is complete, the level returns to normal, usually within 8 weeks, and remains normal. Women who have had a mole removed are advised not to become pregnant for 1 year.

Hydatidiform moles do not require chemotherapy, but choriocarcinomas do. Usually, only one drug (methotrexate or dactinomycin) is needed. Sometimes both or another combination of chemotherapy drugs is needed.

CHAPTER 253

Violence Against Women

Violence against women is broadly defined as any act that is likely to cause physical, sexual, or psychologic harm or extreme suffering to a woman. Violence can occur in the home, workplace, or community. Two common

forms of violence against women are domestic violence and rape.

Domestic Violence

Domestic violence includes physical, sexual, and psychologic abuse between intimate partners. It occurs among people of all cul-

---

▲ see page 1452   ■ see page 1354

tures, races, occupations, income levels, and ages. In the United States, as many as 30% of marriages are considered physically aggressive.

Women are more commonly victims of domestic violence than are men. About 95% of people who seek medical attention as a result of domestic violence are women, and 30 to 40% of women's visits to the emergency department are for injuries related to domestic violence. Women are more likely to be severely assaulted or killed by a male partner than by anyone else. Each year in the United States, about 2 million women are severely beaten by their partner.

Physical abuse is the most obvious form of domestic violence. It may include hitting, slapping, kicking, punching, breaking bones, pulling hair, pushing, and twisting arms. The victim may be deprived of food or sleep. Weapons, such as a gun or knife, may be used to threaten or cause injury.

Sexual assault is also common: 33 to 50% of women who are physically assaulted by their partner are also sexually assaulted by their partner. Sexual assault involves the use of threats or force to obtain unwanted sexual contact.

Psychologic abuse may be even more common than physical abuse and may precede it. Psychologic abuse involves any nonphysical behavior that undermines or belittles the victim or that enables the perpetrator to control the victim. Psychologic abuse can include abusive language, social isolation, and financial control. Usually, the perpetrator uses language to demean, degrade, humiliate, intimidate, or threaten the victim in private or in public. The perpetrator may make the victim think she is crazy or make her feel guilty or responsible, blaming her for the abusive relationship. The perpetrator may also humiliate the victim in terms of her sexual performance, physical appearance, or both.

The perpetrator may try to partly or completely isolate the victim by controlling the victim's access to friends, relatives, and other people. Control may include forbidding direct, written, telephone, or e-mail contact with others. The perpetrator may use jealousy to justify his actions.

Often, the perpetrator withholds money to control the victim. The victim may depend on the perpetrator for most or all of her money. The perpetrator may maintain control by preventing the victim from getting a job, by keep-

Children Who Witness Domestic Violence

Each year, at least 3.3 million children are estimated to witness physical or verbal abuse in their homes. These children may develop problems such as excessive anxiety or crying, fearfulness, difficulty sleeping, depression, social withdrawal, and difficulty in school. Also, children may blame themselves for the situation. Older children may run away from home. Boys who see their father abuse their mother may be more likely to become abusive adults. Girls who see their father abuse their mother may be more likely to tolerate abuse as adults. The perpetrator may also physically hurt the children. In homes where domestic violence is present, children are much more likely to be physically mistreated.

ing information about their finances from her, and by taking money from her.

Effects

A victim of domestic violence may be physically injured. Physical injuries can include bruises, black eyes, cuts, scratches, broken bones, lost teeth, and burns. Injuries may prevent the victim from going to work regularly, causing her to lose her job. Injuries, as well as the abusive situation, may embarrass the victim, causing her to isolate herself from family and friends. The victim may also have to move often—a financial burden—to escape the perpetrator. Sometimes the perpetrator kills the victim.

As a result of domestic violence, many victims have psychologic problems. Such problems include posttraumatic stress disorder, substance abuse, anxiety, and depression. About 60% of battered women are depressed. Women who are more severely battered are more likely to develop psychologic problems. Even when physical abuse decreases, psychologic abuse often continues, reminding the woman that she can be physically abused at any time. Abused women may feel that psychologic abuse is more damaging than physical abuse. Psychologic abuse increases the risk of depression and substance abuse.

Management

In cases of domestic violence, the most important consideration is safety. During a violent incident, the victim should try to move away from areas in which she can be trapped or in which the perpetrator can obtain weapons, such as the kitchen. If she can, the victim should promptly call 911 or the police and leave the house. The victim should have any injuries treated and documented with photographs.

Developing a safety plan is important. It should include where to go for help, how to get away, and how to access money. The victim should also make and hide copies of official documents (such as children's birth certificates, social security cards, insurance cards, and bank account numbers). She should keep an overnight bag packed in case she needs to leave quickly.

Sometimes the only solution is to leave the abusive relationship permanently, because domestic violence tends to continue, especially among very aggressive men. Also, even when physical abuse decreases, psychologic abuse may persist. The decision to leave is not simple. After the perpetrator knows the victim has decided to leave, the victim's risk of serious harm may be greatest. At this time, the victim should take additional steps (such as obtaining a restraining or protection order) to protect herself and her children. Help is available through shelters for battered women, support groups, and the courts.

Rape

Rape is typically considered to be unwanted penetration of the victim's vagina, anus, or mouth. In victims younger than the age of consent, such penetration—whether wanted or not—is considered rape (statutory rape). Sexual assault is a broader term, including the use of force and threats to coerce sexual contact. The reported percentage of women who have been raped during their lifetime varies widely: from 2% to almost 30%. The reported percentage of children who are sexually abused is similarly high.▲ Reported percentages are probably lower than the actual percentages, because rape and sexual abuse are less likely to be reported to the police than are other crimes.

Men are also raped. For men as for women, injuries may occur and the psychologic effects can be devastating.

▲ see page 1644

■ see page 612

Symptoms

Physical injuries resulting from a rape may include tears in the upper part of the vagina and injuries to other parts of the body, such as bruises, black eyes, cuts, and scratches.

The psychologic effects of a rape are often more devastating than the physical. Shortly after a rape occurs, almost all women have symptoms of posttraumatic stress disorder (which can occur after any stressful event).■ Women feel fearful, anxious, and irritable. They may feel angry, depressed, or guilty (wondering whether they may have done something to provoke the rape or could have done something to avoid it). They may have intrusive, upsetting thoughts about or mental images of the assault, and they may relive the rape. Or they may stifle thoughts and feelings about the rape. They may avoid situations that remind them of the rape. Difficulty sleeping and nightmares are common. These symptoms may last for months, interfering with social activities and work. However, for most women, symptoms lessen substantially over a period of months.

In addition to her own feelings, the rape victim may have to handle negative, sometimes judgmental or derisive reactions of friends, family members, and officials. These reactions can interfere with the victim's recovery.

After a rape, there is a risk of infection with sexually transmitted diseases (such as gonorrhea, chlamydial infection, and syphilis) and hepatitis B and C. Infection with the human immunodeficiency virus (HIV) is a particular concern, even though the chances of acquiring it in a single encounter are low. Rarely, a woman becomes pregnant.

Evaluation

Having a thorough medical evaluation after a rape is important. Whenever possible, women who have been raped or sexually assaulted are taken to a sexual assault evaluation treatment center that is separate from the emergency department and that is staffed by trained, concerned support personnel.

After a rape, doctors are required by law to notify the police and to examine the victim. The examination provides evidence for prosecution of the rapist and is necessary before medical care of the victim can begin. The best evidence is obtained when the rape victim goes to the hospital as soon as possible, without showering, without changing clothes, and, if possible, without even urinating. The medical record resulting from this examination is sometimes admissible in court as evidence. However, the medical record cannot be released unless the victim gives her consent in writing or a subpoena is issued. The record may also help the victim recall details of the rape if her testimony is required later.

Immediately after a rape, a woman may be afraid of undergoing a physical examination. If possible, a female doctor examines the woman. If not, a female nurse or volunteer is present to help allay any anxiety the woman may be feeling. Before beginning the examination, the doctor should ask the woman's permission to proceed. The woman should feel no pressure to consent, although consent is generally in her best interest. The woman can ask the doctor to explain what will happen during the examination so that she knows what to expect.

The doctor asks the woman to describe the events to help guide the examination and treatment. However, talking about the rape is often frightening for the woman. She may request to give a complete description later, after her immediate needs have been met. She may first need to be treated for injuries, to clean up, and to have some time for calming down. The woman, if she wishes, is provided with bathroom facilities so that she can wash.

To help determine the likelihood of pregnancy, the doctor asks the woman when her last menstrual period was and whether she uses a contraceptive. To help interpret the analysis of any sperm samples, the doctor asks the woman if she recently had sex before the rape and, if so, when.

The doctor notes physical injuries, such as cuts and scrapes, and may examine the vagina for injuries. Photographs of injuries are taken. Because some injuries such as bruises become apparent later, a second set of photographs may be taken later. A swab is used to take samples of semen and other body fluids for evidence. Other samples, such as samples of the perpetrator's hair, blood, or skin (sometimes found under the woman's nails), are collected. Sometimes DNA testing of the samples is performed to identify the perpetrator.

If the woman consents, blood tests are performed to check for infections, including HIV infection. If the initial test results for gonorrhea, chlamydial infection, syphilis, and hepatitis are negative, the woman is tested again within 6 weeks. If results for syphilis and hepatitis are still negative, tests are repeated at 6

months. Blood tests for HIV infection may be repeated after 90 and 120 days.

Usually, a pregnancy test (to measure the level of human chorionic gonadotropin in the urine▲) is performed within a few days and again within 6 weeks. If the woman may have been pregnant before the rape, the urine test is performed during the initial examination. The test cannot detect a pregnancy that has just occurred. Thus, performed at this time, the test would detect a preexisting pregnancy, but not one that resulted from the rape.

Treatment

Most physical injuries are easily treated. Severe injuries may require surgery. For preventing infections, the woman is given antibiotics, typically one dose of ceftriaxone injected into a muscle, one dose of metronidazole given by mouth, and doxycycline given by mouth for 7 days. If test results for HIV were positive, treatment for HIV is started immediately.■

If pregnancy is a concern, emergency contraception may be used. A high dose of an oral contraceptive is given immediately, then repeated 12 hours later.★ This treatment is 99% effective if given within 72 hours of the rape. If the woman may have been pregnant before the rape, the oral contraceptive is given only if results from the pregnancy test do not detect pregnancy. If pregnancy results from the rape, abortion can be considered.

Common psychologic reactions to the rape (such as excessive anxiety or fear) are explained to the woman. As soon as feasible, a person trained in rape crisis intervention meets with her. The woman is referred to a rape crisis team if one is located in the area. This team can provide helpful medical, psychologic, and legal support. For the woman, talking about the rape and her feelings about it can help her recover. If symptoms of posttraumatic stress disorder persist, psychotherapy or antidepressants can be effective.● If necessary, the woman can be referred to a psychologist, social worker, or psychiatrist.

Family members and friends may have some of the same feelings as the victim: anxiety, anger, or guilt. They may irrationally blame the victim. Family members or close friends may benefit from meeting with a

---

▲ see page 1434   ■ see page 1173
★ see page 1423   ● see page 612

member of the rape crisis team or sexual assault evaluation unit to discuss their feelings and how they can help the victim. Usually, listening supportively to the victim and not expressing strong feelings about the rape are most helpful. Blaming or criticizing the victim may interfere with her recovery. A support network of health care workers, friends, and family members can be very helpful to the victim.

CHAPTER 254

Infertility

Infertility is the inability of a couple to achieve a pregnancy after repeated intercourse without contraception for 1 year.

Infertility affects about one of five couples in the United States. It is becoming increasingly common because people are waiting longer to marry and to have a child. Nevertheless, up to 60% of the couples who have not conceived after a year of trying do conceive eventually, with or without treatment. The goal of treatment is to reduce the time needed to conceive or to provide couples who might not otherwise conceive the opportunity to do so. Before treatment is begun, counseling that provides information about the treatment process (including its duration) and the chances of success is beneficial.

The cause of infertility may be due to problems in the man, the woman, or both. Problems with sperm, ovulation, or the fallopian tubes each account for almost one third of infertility cases. In a small percentage of cases, infertility is caused by problems with mucus in the cervix or by unidentified factors. Thus, the diagnosis of infertility problems requires a thorough assessment of both partners.

Age is a factor, primarily for women. As women age, becoming pregnant becomes more difficult and the risk of complications during pregnancy increases. Also, women, particularly after age 35, have a limited time to resolve infertility problems before menopause.

Even when no cause of infertility can be identified, the couple may still be treated. In such cases, the woman may be given drugs to stimulate several eggs to mature and be released—so-called fertility drugs.▲ Examples are clomiphene and human gonadotropins. A woman's chances of becoming pregnant are about 10 to 15% with each month of treatment. Alternatively, an artificial insemination technique that selects only the most active sperm may be tried.

While a couple is undergoing treatment for infertility, one or both partners may experience frustration, emotional stress, feelings of inadequacy, and guilt. They may alternate between hope and despair. Feeling isolated and unable to communicate, they may become angry at or resentful toward each other, family members, friends, or the doctor. The emotional stress can lead to fatigue, anxiety, sleep or eating disturbances, and an inability to concentrate. In addition, the financial burden and time commitment involved in diagnosis and treatment can cause marital strife.

These problems can be lessened if both partners are involved in and are given information about the treatment process, regardless of which one has the diagnosed problem. Knowing what the chances of success are, as well as realizing that treatment may not be successful and cannot continue indefinitely, can help a couple cope with the stress. Information about when to end treatment, when to seek a second opinion, and when to consider adoption is also helpful. Counseling and psychologic support, including support groups such as RESOLVE and the American Infertility Association, can help.

Problems With Sperm

To be fertile, a man must be able to deliver an adequate quantity of normal sperm to a woman's vagina, and sperm must be able to fertilize the egg. Conditions that interfere with this process can make a man less fertile.

▲ see page 1416

Conditions that increase the temperature of the testes (where sperm are produced) can greatly reduce the number of sperm and the vigor of sperm movement and can increase the number of abnormal sperm. Temperature may be increased by exposure to excessive heat, disorders that produce a prolonged fever, undescended testes (a rare abnormality present at birth),▲ and varicose veins in the testes (varicocele).

Certain hormonal or genetic disorders may interfere with sperm production. Hormonal disorders include hyperprolactinemia, hypothyroidism, hypogonadism, and disorders of the adrenal gland (which produces testosterone and other hormones) or pituitary gland (which controls testosterone production). Genetic disorders involve an abnormality of the sex chromosomes, as occurs in Klinefelter syndrome.

Other causes of reduced sperm production include mumps that affect the testes (mumps orchitis), injury to the testes, exposure to industrial or environmental toxins, and drugs. Drugs include androgens (such as testosterone), aspirin when taken for a long time, chlorambucil, cimetidine, colchicine, corticosteroids (such as prednisone), cotrimoxazole, cyclophosphamide, drugs used to treat malaria, estrogens taken to treat prostate cancer, marijuana, medroxyprogesterone, methotrexate, monoamine oxidase inhibitors (MAOIs—a type of antidepressant), nicotine, nitrofurantoin, opioids (narcotics), spironolactone, and sulfasalazine. Use of anabolic steroids may affect hormone levels and thus also interfere with sperm production. Excessive consumption of alcohol may reduce sperm production.

Some disorders result in the complete absence of sperm (azoospermia) in semen. They include serious disorders of the testes and blocked or missing vasa deferentia, missing seminal vesicles, and blockage of both ejaculatory ducts.

Occasionally, semen, which contains the sperm, moves in the wrong direction (into the bladder instead of down the penis). This disorder, called retrograde ejaculation,■ is more common among men who have diabetes or who have had pelvic surgery, such as prostate removal. Infertility may result.

Diagnosis

Doctors ask the man about his medical history and perform a physical examination to try to identify the cause. Doctors check for physical abnormalities, such as undescended testes, and for signs of hormonal or genetic disorders that can cause infertility. Levels of hormones (including testosterone) may be measured in the blood.

Often, a semen analysis, the main screening procedure for male infertility, is needed. For this procedure, the man is asked not to ejaculate for 2 to 3 days before the analysis. Then he is asked to ejaculate, usually by masturbation, into a clean glass jar, preferably at the laboratory site. For men who have difficulty producing a semen sample this way, special condoms that have no lubricants or chemicals toxic to sperm can be used to collect semen during intercourse. An analysis based on two or three samples, obtained at least 2 weeks apart, is more reliable than an analysis based on a single sample.

The volume of the semen sample is measured. Whether the color and consistency of semen are normal is determined. The sperm are examined under a microscope to determine whether they are abnormal in shape, size, movement, or number.

If the semen sample is abnormal, the analysis may be repeated because samples from the same man normally vary greatly. If the semen still seems to be abnormal, the doctor tries to identify the cause. However, a low sperm count may indicate only that too little time had elapsed since the last ejaculation or that only some of the semen was deposited in the collection jar. Furthermore, a low sperm count does not mean that fertility is reduced, and a normal sperm count does not guarantee fertility.

Tests of sperm function and quality can be performed. One test detects antibodies to sperm. Another determines whether sperm membranes are intact. Still others can determine the sperm's ability to bind to an egg and penetrate it. Sometimes a biopsy of the testes is performed to obtain more detailed information about sperm production and the function of the testes.

Treatment

Clomiphene, a drug used to trigger (induce) ovulation in women, may be used to try to increase sperm counts in men. However, clomiphene does not improve the sperm's ability to move or reduce the number of abnormal sperm, and it has not been proved to increase fertility.

▲ see page 1535　■ see page 1340

For men who have a low sperm count with normal sperm, artificial insemination may slightly increase their partner's chances of pregnancy. This technique uses the first portion of the ejaculated semen, which has the greatest concentration of sperm. A technique that selects only the most active sperm (washed sperm) is somewhat more successful. In vitro fertilization, often with intracytoplasmic sperm injection (the injection of a single sperm into a single egg), and gamete intrafallopian tube transfer (GIFT) are much more complex and costly procedures. They are successful in treating many types of male infertility.

For men who produce no sperm, inseminating the woman with sperm from another man (a donor) may be considered. Because of the danger of contracting sexually transmitted diseases, including infection with human immunodeficiency virus (HIV), fresh semen samples from donors are no longer used. Instead, frozen sperm samples are obtained from a certified sperm bank, which has tested the donors for sexually transmitted diseases.

Varicoceles can be treated with surgery. Sometimes fertility improves as a result.

The partner of a man who has fertility problems may be treated with human gonadotropins, to stimulate several eggs to mature and be released.▲

Problems With Ovulation

In women, a common cause of infertility is an ovulation problem—that is, the ovaries do not release an egg each month.■ Ovulation problems result when one part of the system that controls reproductive function malfunctions. This system includes the hypothalamus (an area of the brain), pituitary gland, adrenal glands, thyroid gland, and genital organs. For example, the ovaries may not produce enough progesterone, the female hormone that causes the lining of the uterus to thicken in preparation for a potential fetus. Ovulation may not occur because the hypothalamus does not secrete gonadotropin-releasing hormone, which stimulates the pituitary gland to produce the hormones that trigger ovulation (luteinizing hormone and follicle-stimulating hormone). High levels of prolactin (hyperprolactinemia), a hormone that stimulates milk production, may

result in low levels of the hormones that trigger ovulation. Prolactin levels may be high because of a pituitary gland tumor (prolactinoma), which is almost always noncancerous. Ovulation problems may be due to polycystic ovary syndrome, thyroid gland disorders, adrenal gland disorders, excessive exercise, diabetes, weight loss, obesity, or psychologic stress. Sometimes the cause is early menopause—when the supply of eggs has run out early.

Ovulation is often the problem in women who have irregular periods or no periods (amenorrhea★). It is sometimes the problem in women who have regular menstrual periods but do not have premenstrual symptoms, such as breast tenderness, lower abdominal swelling, and mood changes.

Diagnosis

To determine if or when ovulation is occurring, doctors may ask a woman to take her temperature at rest (basal body temperature) each day. Usually, the best time is immediately after awakening. A low point in basal body temperature suggests that ovulation is about to occur. An increase of more than 0.9° F (0.5° C) in temperature usually indicates that ovulation has occurred. However, basal body temperature does not reliably or precisely indicate when ovulation occurs. At best, it predicts ovulation only within 2 days. More accurate techniques include ultrasonography and ovulation predictor kits (which detect an increase in luteinizing hormone in the urine 24 to 36 hours before ovulation). These kits are used at home to test urine on several consecutive days. Also, the level of progesterone in the blood or saliva or the level of one of its by-products in the urine may be measured. A marked increase in these levels indicates that ovulation has occurred.

To determine whether ovulation is occurring normally, doctors may perform an endometrial biopsy. A small sample of tissue is removed from the lining of the uterus 10 to 12 days after ovulation is thought to have occurred. The sample is examined under a microscope. If changes that normally occur after ovulation are seen, ovulation has occurred normally. If the normal changes appear delayed, the problem may be inadequate production or inactivity of progesterone.

Treatment

A drug to trigger ovulation may be used. The particular drug is selected based on the

---

▲ see page 1417   ■ see page 1346
★ see page 1364

specific problem. If ovulation has not occurred for a long time, clomiphene with medroxyprogesterone is usually preferred. First, the woman takes medroxyprogesterone, usually by mouth, to trigger a menstrual period. Then she takes clomiphene by mouth. Usually, she ovulates 5 to 10 days after clomiphene is discontinued and has a period 14 to 16 days after ovulation. Clomiphene is not effective for all causes of ovulation problems. It is most effective when the cause is polycystic ovary syndrome.

If a woman does not have a period after treatment with clomiphene, she takes a pregnancy test. If she is not pregnant, the treatment cycle is repeated. A higher dose of clomiphene is used in each cycle until ovulation occurs or the maximum dose is reached. When the dose that triggers ovulation is determined, the woman takes that dose for at least three to four more treatment cycles. Most women who become pregnant do so by the fourth cycle in which ovulation occurs. About 75 to 80% of women treated with clomiphene ovulate, but only about 40 to 50% become pregnant. About 5% of pregnancies in women treated with clomiphene involve more than one fetus, primarily twins.

Side effects of clomiphene include hot flashes, abdominal bloating, breast tenderness, nausea, vision problems, and headaches. About 5% of women treated with clomiphene develop ovarian hyperstimulation syndrome. In this syndrome, the ovaries enlarge greatly and a large amount of fluid moves out the bloodstream into the abdomen. This syndrome may be life threatening. To try to prevent it, doctors prescribe the lowest effective dose of clomiphene, and if the ovaries enlarge, they discontinue the drug.

If a woman does not ovulate or become pregnant during treatment with clomiphene, hormonal therapy with human gonadotropins, injected into a muscle or under the skin, can be tried. Human gonadotropins stimulate the follicles of the ovaries to mature. Follicles are fluid-filled cavities, each of which contain an egg. ▲ Blood tests to measure estrogen levels and ultrasonography can detect when the follicles are mature. Then, the woman is given an injection of a different hormone, human chorionic gonadotropin, to trigger ovulation. When human gonadotropins are used appropriately, more than 95% of women treated with them ovulate, but only 50 to 75% become pregnant. About 10 to 30% of pregnancies in women

treated with human gonadotropins involve more than one fetus, primarily twins.

Human gonadotropins can have severe side effects, so doctors closely monitor the woman during treatment. About 10 to 20% of women treated with human gonadotropins develop ovarian hyperstimulation syndrome (which can also occur with clomiphene). If hyperstimulation occurs (if the ovaries enlarge markedly or if estrogen levels increase too much), doctors do not give the woman human chorionic gonadotropin to trigger ovulation. Human gonadotropins are also expensive.

If the cause of infertility is early menopause, neither clomiphene nor human gonadotropins can stimulate ovulation.

If the hypothalamus does not secrete gonadotropin-releasing hormone, a synthetic version of this hormone, called gonadorelin, may be useful. This drug, like the natural hormone, stimulates the pituitary gland to produce the hormones that trigger ovulation. The risk of ovarian hyperstimulation is low with this treatment, so close monitoring is not needed. However, this drug is not available in the United States.

When the cause of infertility is high levels of the hormone prolactin, the best drug is one that acts like dopamine, called a dopamine agonist, such as bromocriptine or cabergoline. (Dopamine is a chemical messenger that generally inhibits the production of prolactin.)

Problems With the Fallopian Tubes

The fallopian tubes may be abnormal in structure or function. If they are blocked, the egg cannot move from the ovary to the uterus. Causes of fallopian tube problems include previous infections (such as pelvic inflammatory disease), endometriosis, a ruptured appendix, and surgery in the pelvis. A mislocated (ectopic) pregnancy in the fallopian tubes can also cause damage. Structural disorders can block the fallopian tubes. These disorders include birth defects of the uterus and fallopian tubes, fibroids in the uterus, and bands of scar tissue between normally unconnected structures (adhesions) in the uterus or pelvis.

Diagnosis and Treatment

To determine whether the fallopian tubes are blocked, doctors can use hysterosalpingog-

▲ see page 1345

raphy. In this procedure, x-rays are taken after a radiopaque dye is injected through the cervix. The dye outlines the interior of the uterus and fallopian tubes. This procedure is performed shortly after a woman's menstrual period ends. This procedure can detect structural disorders that can block the fallopian tubes. However, in about 15% of cases, hysterosalpingography indicates that the fallopian tubes are blocked when they are not—called a false-positive result. After hysterosalpingography with normal results, fertility appears to be slightly improved, possibly because the procedure temporarily widens (dilates) the tubes or clears the tubes of mucus. Therefore, doctors may wait to see if a woman becomes pregnant after this procedure before additional tests of fallopian tube function are performed.

Another procedure (called sonohysterography) is sometimes used to determine whether the fallopian tubes are blocked. A salt (saline) solution is injected into the interior of the uterus through the cervix during ultrasonography so that the interior is distended and abnormalities can be seen. If the solution flows into the fallopian tubes, the tubes are not blocked. This procedure is quick and does not require an anesthetic. It is considered safer than hysterosalpingography because it does not require radiation or injection of a dye. However, it is not as accurate.

If an abnormality within the uterus is detected, doctors examine the uterus with a viewing tube called a hysteroscope, which is inserted through the cervix into the uterus. If adhesions, a polyp, or a small fibroid is detected, the hysteroscope may be used to dislodge or remove the abnormal tissue, increasing the chances that the woman will become pregnant.

If evidence suggests that the fallopian tubes are blocked or that a woman may have endometriosis, a small viewing tube called a laparoscope is inserted in the pelvic cavity through a small incision just below the navel. Usually, a general anesthetic is used. This procedure enables doctors to directly view the uterus, fallopian tubes, and ovaries. The laparoscope may also be used to dislodge or remove abnormal tissue in the pelvis.

Treatment depends on the cause. Surgery can be performed to repair a damaged fallopian tube caused by an ectopic pregnancy or an infection. However, after such surgery, the chances of a normal pregnancy are small, and those of an ectopic pregnancy are great. Con-

sequently, surgery is not often recommended. In vitro fertilization is recommended for most couples.

Problems With Mucus in the Cervix

Normally, mucus in the cervix (the lower part of the uterus that opens into the vagina) is thick and impenetrable to sperm until just before release of an egg (ovulation). Then, just before ovulation, the mucus becomes clear and elastic (because the level of the hormone estrogen increases). As a result, sperm can move through the mucus into the uterus to the fallopian tubes, where fertilization can take place. If the mucus does not change at ovulation (usually because of an infection), pregnancy is unlikely. Pregnancy is also unlikely if the mucus contains antibodies to sperm, which kill sperm before they can reach the egg.

Diagnosis and Treatment

A postcoital test, performed between 2 and 8 hours after sexual intercourse, involves evaluating cervical mucus and determining whether sperm can survive in the mucus. The test is scheduled for the midpoint of the menstrual cycle, when the estrogen level is highest and the woman is ovulating. A sample of mucus is taken with forceps or a syringe. The thickness and elasticity of the mucus and the number of sperm in the mucus are determined. Abnormal results include overly thick mucus, no sperm, and sperm clumping together because the mucus contains antibodies to the sperm. However, abnormal results do not always indicate that there is a problem with the mucus or that pregnancy cannot occur. Sperm may be absent only because they were not deposited into the vagina during intercourse, and the mucus may be overly thick only because the test was not performed at the proper time in the menstrual cycle.

Treatment may include intrauterine insemination, in which semen is placed directly in the uterus to bypass the mucus. Drugs to thin the mucus, such as guaifenesin, may be used. However, there is no proof that either treatment increases the chances of pregnancy.

Fertilization Techniques

If treatment has not resulted in pregnancy after four to six menstrual cycles, fertilization techniques, such as in vitro fertilization or gamete intrafallopian tube transfer, may be considered.

In vitro (test tube) fertilization involves stimulating the ovaries, retrieving released eggs, fertilizing the eggs, growing the resulting embryos in a laboratory, and then implanting the embryos in the woman's uterus.

Typically, a woman's ovaries are stimulated with human gonadotropins and a gonadotropin-releasing hormone agonist or antagonist (drugs that prevent ovulation from occurring until after several eggs have matured). As a result, many eggs usually mature. Guided by ultrasonography, a doctor inserts a needle through the woman's vagina into the ovary and removes several eggs from the follicles. The eggs are placed in a culture dish and fertilized with sperm selected as the most active. After about 3 to 5 days, two or three of the resulting embryos are transferred from the culture dish into the woman's uterus through the vagina. Additional embryos can be frozen in liquid nitrogen to be used later if pregnancy does not occur. Despite the transfer of several embryos, the chances of producing one full-term baby are only about 18 to 25% each time eggs are placed in the uterus.

Intracytoplasmic sperm injection may be used with in vitro fertilization to improve the chances that the woman will become pregnant, particularly when the man has a very low sperm count. In this procedure, a single sperm is injected into a single egg. With this procedure, the chances of producing a full-term baby are about the same as those with in vitro fertilization alone.

Gamete intrafallopian tube transfer (GIFT) can be performed if the fallopian tubes are functioning normally. Eggs and selected active sperm are obtained as for in vitro fertilization, but the eggs are not fertilized with the sperm in the laboratory. Instead, the eggs and sperm are transferred to the far end of the woman's fallopian tube through the abdomen (using a laparoscope) or the vagina (guided by ultrasonography), so that the egg can be fertilized in the fallopian tube. Thus, this procedure is more invasive than in vitro fertilization. For each transfer, the chances of producing a full-term baby are about the same as those with in vitro fertilization.

Variations of in vitro fertilization and GIFT include the transfer of a more mature embryo (blastocyst transfer), use of eggs from another woman (donor), and transfer of frozen embryos to a surrogate mother. These techniques raise moral and ethical issues, including questions about the disposal of stored embryos (especially in cases of death or divorce), legal parentage if a surrogate mother is involved, and selective reduction of the number of implanted embryos (similar to abortion) when more than three develop.

CHAPTER 255

Family Planning

Family planning involves using various methods to control the number and timing of pregnancies. A couple may use contraception to avoid pregnancy temporarily or sterilization to avoid pregnancy permanently. Abortion may be used to end an unwanted pregnancy when contraception has failed or not been used.

Contraception

Contraception is prevention of the fertilization of an egg by a sperm (conception) or the attachment of the fertilized egg to the lining of the uterus (implantation).

There are several methods of contraception. None is completely effective, but some methods are far more reliable than others. Each contraceptive method has advantages and disadvantages. Choice of method depends on a person's lifestyle and preferences and on the degree of reliability needed.

HORMONAL METHODS

The hormones used to prevent conception include estrogen and progestins (drugs similar to the hormone progesterone). Hormonal methods prevent pregnancy mainly by stop-

HOW EFFECTIVE IS CONTRACEPTION?

METHOD	PERCENTAGE OF WOMEN WHO BECOME PREGNANT DURING THE FIRST YEAR OF USE
Oral contraceptives:	
Combination estrogen-progestin tablets	0.1–5
Progestin-only tablets	0.5–5
Implants	0.1
Injections of medroxyprogesterone	0.3
Condom:	
Male	3–14
Female	5–21
Diaphragm with spermicide	6–20
Cervical cap with spermicide	9–40
Intrauterine device (IUD)	0.1–0.6
Natural family planning (rhythm) method	1–25
Withdrawal method	4–19

ping the ovaries from releasing eggs or by keeping the mucus in the cervix thick so that sperm cannot pass through the cervix into the uterus. Thus, hormonal methods prevent the egg from being fertilized.

Oral Contraceptives

Oral contraceptives, commonly known as the pill, contain hormones—either a combination of a progestin and estrogen or a progestin alone.

Combination tablets are typically taken once a day for 3 weeks, not taken for a week (allowing the menstrual period to occur), then started again. Inactive tablets may be included for the week when combination tablets are not taken to establish a routine of taking one tablet a day. Fewer than 0.2% of women who take combination tablets as instructed become pregnant during the first year of use. However, the chances of becoming pregnant increase if a woman skips or forgets to take a tablet, especially the first ones in a monthly cycle.

The dose of estrogen in combination tablets varies. Usually, combination tablets with a low dose of estrogen (20 to 35 micrograms) are used because they have fewer serious side effects than those with a high dose (50 micrograms). Healthy women who do not smoke can take low-dose estrogen combination contraceptives without interruption until menopause.

Progestin-only tablets are taken every day of the month. They often cause irregular bleeding. About 0.5 to 5% of women who take these tablets become pregnant. Progestin-only tablets are usually prescribed only when taking estrogen may be harmful. For example, these tablets may be prescribed for women who are breastfeeding because estrogen reduces the amount and quality of breast milk produced. Progestin-only tablets do not affect breast milk production.

Before starting oral contraceptives, a woman should have a physical examination, including measurement of blood pressure, to make sure she has no health problems that would make taking the contraceptives risky for her. If she or a close relative has had diabetes or heart disease, a blood test is usually performed to measure levels of cholesterol, other fats (lipids), and sugar (glucose). If the cholesterol or sugar level is high or other lipid levels are abnormal, doctors may still prescribe a low-dose estrogen combination contraceptive. However, they periodically perform blood tests to monitor the woman's lipid and sugar levels. Three months after starting oral contraceptives, the woman should have another examination to be sure her blood pressure has not changed. After that, she should have an examination at least once a year.

Also before starting oral contraceptives, a woman should discuss with her doctor the advantages and disadvantages of oral contraceptives for her situation.

Advantages: The main advantage is reliable, continuous contraception if oral contraceptives are taken as instructed. Also, taking oral contraceptives reduces the occurrence of menstrual cramps, premenstrual syndrome, irregular bleeding, anemia, breast cysts, ovarian cysts, mislocated (ectopic) pregnancies (almost always in the fallopian tubes), and infections of the fallopian tubes. Also, women who have taken oral contraceptives are less likely to develop rheumatoid arthritis or osteoporosis.

Taking oral contraceptives reduces the risk of developing several types of cancer, including uterine (endometrial) cancer, ovarian, colon, and rectal cancers. The risk is reduced for many years after the contraceptives are discontinued. Breast cancer is slightly more likely to be diagnosed in women while they are taking oral contraceptives but not after the contraceptives are discontinued, even in women who have a family history of breast cancer.

Oral contraceptives taken early in a pregnancy do not harm the fetus. However, they should be discontinued as soon as the woman realizes she is pregnant. Oral contraceptives do not have any long-term effects on fertility, although a woman may not release an egg (ovulate) for a few months after discontinuing the drugs.

Disadvantages: The disadvantages of oral contraceptives may include bothersome side effects. Irregular bleeding is common during the first few months of oral contraceptive use but usually stops as the body adjusts to the hormones. Also, taking oral contraceptives every day, without any breaks, for several months can reduce the number of bleeding episodes.

Some side effects are related to the estrogen in the tablet. They may include nausea, bloating, fluid retention, an increase in blood pressure, breast tenderness, and migraine headaches. Others are related mostly to the type or dose of the progestin. They may include mood disorders, weight gain, acne, and nervousness. Some women who take oral contraceptives gain 3 to 5 pounds because of fluid retention. They may gain even more because appetite also increases. Some women have headaches and difficulty sleeping. Many of these side effects are uncommon with the low-dose tablets.

In some women, oral contraceptives cause dark patches (melasma) on the face, similar to those that may occur during pregnancy.▲ Exposure to the sun darkens the patches even more. If the woman discontinues oral contraceptives, the dark patches slowly fade.

Taking oral contraceptives increases the risk of developing some disorders. The risk of developing blood clots in the veins is higher for women who take combination oral contraceptives than for those who do not. The risk is 7 times higher with tablets containing a high dose of estrogen. However, the risk is 2 to 4 times higher with tablets containing a low dose of estrogen: This risk is half of that dur-

ing pregnancy. Because surgery also increases the risk of developing blood clots, a woman must discontinue oral contraceptives a month before major elective surgery and not take them again until a month afterward. Because the risk of developing blood clots in leg veins is high during pregnancy and for a few weeks after delivery, doctors recommend that women wait 2 weeks after delivery before they take oral contraceptives. For healthy women who do not smoke, taking low-dose estrogen combination tablets does not increase the risk of having a stroke or heart attack.

Use of oral contraceptives, particularly for more than 5 years, may increase the risk of developing cervical cancer. Women who are taking oral contraceptives should have a Papanicolaou (Pap) test at least once a year. Such tests can detect precancerous changes in the cervix early—before they lead to cancer.

The likelihood of developing gallstones increases during the first few years of oral contraceptive use, then decreases.

For women in certain situations, the risk of developing certain disorders is substantially increased if they take oral contraceptives. For example, women who are older than 35 and who smoke should not use oral contraceptives because the risk of heart attack is increased. For women who have certain disorders, risks are increased if they take oral contraceptives. But if closely monitored by a health care practitioner, such women may be able to take oral contraceptives.

Some sedatives, antibiotics, and antifungals can reduce the effectiveness of oral contraceptives. Women taking oral contraceptives may become pregnant if they simultaneously take one of these drugs.

Skin Patches and Vaginal Rings

Skin patches and vaginal rings that contain estrogen and a progestin are used for 3 of 4 weeks. In the fourth week, no contraception is used to allow the menstrual period to occur.

A contraceptive skin patch is placed on the skin once a week for 3 weeks. The patch is left in place for 1 week, then removed, and a new patch is placed on a different area of the skin. During the fourth week, no patch is used. Exercise and use of saunas or hot tubs do not displace the patches.

▲ see page 1215

When Taking Oral Contraceptives Is Restricted*

A woman must not take oral contraceptives if any of the following situations apply:

- She smokes and is older than 35
- She has an active liver disorder or liver tumors
- She has very high triglyceride levels (250 mg/dL or higher)
- She has untreated high blood pressure
- She has diabetes with blocked arteries
- She has a kidney disorder
- She has had blood clots
- She has a leg immobilized (as in a cast)
- She has coronary artery disease
- She has had a stroke
- She has had cholestasis (jaundice) of pregnancy or jaundice while she was previously taking oral contraceptives
- She has breast or uterine (endometrial) cancer
- She has had a heart attack

A woman may take oral contraceptives with a doctor's supervision if any of the following situations apply:

- She is depressed
- She has premenstrual syndrome
- She frequently has migraine headaches (but no numbness in the limbs)
- She smokes cigarettes but is younger than 35
- She has had hepatitis or another liver disorder and has fully recovered
- She has high blood pressure that is controlled with treatment
- She has varicose veins
- She has a seizure disorder that is being treated with drugs
- She has fibroids in the uterus
- She has been treated for precancerous abnormalities or cancer of the cervix
- She is obese
- She has close relatives who have had blood clots

*These restrictions apply only when estrogen and a progestin are used together.

mg/dL = milligrams per deciliter of blood.

A vaginal ring is a small plastic device that is placed in the vagina and left there for 3 weeks. Then it is removed for 1 week. A woman can place and remove the vaginal ring herself. The ring comes in one size and can be placed anywhere in the vagina. Usually, the ring is not felt by the woman's partner during intercourse. A new ring is used each month.

With either method, a woman has a regular menstrual period. Spotting or bleeding between periods (breakthrough bleeding) is uncommon. Side effects and restrictions on use are similar to those of combination oral contraceptives.

Contraceptive Implants

Contraceptive implants are plastic capsules or rods containing a progestin. After numbing the skin with an anesthetic, a doctor makes a small incision or uses a needle to place the implants under the skin of the inner arm above the elbow. No stitches are necessary. The implants release the progestin slowly into the bloodstream. No implants are currently available in the United States. A single plastic implant, which is inserted through a needle and is effective for 3 years (but must be removed through an incision), will soon be available.

The most common side effects are irregular or no menstrual periods during the first year of use. After that, periods frequently become regular. Headaches and weight gain may also occur. These side effects prompt some women to have the implants removed. Because the implants do not dissolve in the body, a doctor has to remove them. Removal is more difficult than insertion because tissue under the skin thickens around the implants. Removal may result in a minor scar. As soon as the implants are removed, the ovaries return to their normal functioning, and the woman becomes fertile again.

Contraceptive Injections

Two contraceptive formulations are available as injections. Each is injected by a health care practitioner into a muscle of the arm or buttocks, and each is very effective as a contraceptive.

Medroxyprogesterone acetate, a progestin, is injected once every 3 months. Medroxyprogesterone acetate can completely disrupt the menstrual cycle. About one third of women using this contraceptive have no menstrual bleeding during the 3 months after the first injection, and another third have irregular bleeding and spotting for more than 11 days each month. After this contraceptive is used for a while, irregular bleeding occurs less often. After 2 years, about 70% of the women have no bleeding at all. When the injections are discontinued, a regular menstrual cycle resumes in about half of the women within 6 months and in about three fourths within 1 year. Fertility may not return for up to a year after injections are discontinued.

Side effects include a slight weight gain and a temporary decrease in bone density. Bones usually return to their previous density after the injections are discontinued. Medroxyprogesterone acetate does not increase the risk of developing any cancer, including breast cancer. It greatly reduces the risk of developing uterine (endometrial) cancer. Interactions with other drugs are uncommon.

The other formulation is a once-a-month injection. It contains estrogen and a much smaller amount of medroxyprogesterone acetate than the injections given every 3 months. Consequently, bleeding usually occurs regularly about 2 weeks after each injection is given, and bone density does not decrease. Because the dose of medroxyprogesterone acetate is lower, fertility returns much more rapidly after the injections are discontinued.

Emergency Contraception

Emergency contraception, the so-called morning-after pill, involves the use of hormones within 72 hours after one act of unprotected sexual intercourse or after one occasion when a contraceptive method fails (for example, if a condom breaks).

Two regimens are available. The more effective regimen consists of one dose of levonorgestrel, a progestin, followed by another dose 12 hours later. With this regimen, about 1% of women become pregnant, and fewer side effects occur than with the other regimen. Alternatively, two tablets of a combination oral contraceptive are taken within 72 hours of the unprotected intercourse. Then two more tablets are taken 12 hours later. With this regimen, only about 2% of women become pregnant, but as many as 50% have nausea and 20% vomit. Antiemetic drugs, such as hydroxyzine taken by mouth, are given to prevent nausea and vomiting.

BARRIER CONTRACEPTIVES

Barrier contraceptives physically block the sperm's access to a woman's uterus. They include the condom (male or female), diaphragm, and cervical cap.

Condoms made of latex are the only contraceptives that provide protection against sexually transmitted diseases, including those due to bacteria (such as gonorrhea and syphilis) as well as those due to viruses (such as HIV—human immunodeficiency virus—infection). However, this protection, though considerable, is not complete. Male condoms made of polyurethane also provide protection, but they are thinner and more likely to tear. Male condoms made of lambskin do not protect against viral infections such as HIV infection and thus are not recommended.

Condoms must be used correctly to be effective.▲ With some male condoms, the tip needs to be positioned so that it extends about $1/2$ inch beyond the penis to provide a space to collect semen. Other male condoms have a reservoir at the tip for this purpose. Immediately after ejaculation, the penis should be withdrawn while the condom's rim is held firmly against the base of the penis to prevent the condom from slipping off and spilling semen. The condom should then be removed carefully. If semen is spilled, sperm could enter the vagina, resulting in pregnancy. A new condom should be used after each ejaculation, and the condom should be discarded if its integrity is in doubt. A spermicide, which may be included in the condom's lubricant or inserted separately into the vagina, increases the effectiveness of condoms.

The female condom is held in the vagina by a ring. It resembles a male condom but is larger and is not as effective.

The **diaphragm,** a dome-shaped rubber cup with a flexible rim, is inserted into the vagina and positioned over the cervix. A diaphragm prevents sperm from entering the uterus.

Diaphragms come in various sizes and must be fitted by a health care practitioner, who also teaches the woman how to insert it. A diaphragm should cover the entire cervix without causing discomfort. Neither the woman nor her partner should notice its presence. A contraceptive cream or jelly should always be used with a diaphragm, in case the

▲ see box on page 1178

Blocking Access: Barrier Contraceptives

Barrier contraceptives prevent sperm from entering a woman's uterus. They include condoms, diaphragms, and cervical caps. Some condoms contain spermicides. Spermicides should be used with condoms and other barrier contraceptives that do not already contain them.

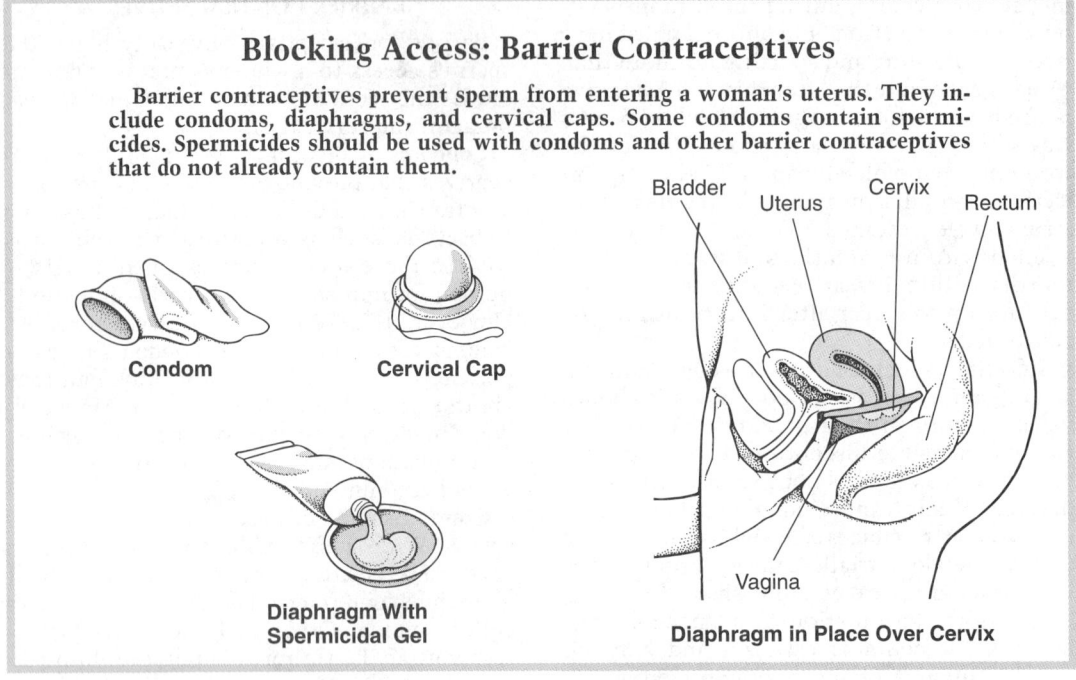

Condom

Cervical Cap

Bladder   Uterus   Cervix   Rectum

Vagina

Diaphragm With Spermicidal Gel

Diaphragm in Place Over Cervix

diaphragm is displaced during intercourse. The diaphragm is inserted before intercourse and should remain in place for at least 8 hours but no more than 24 hours afterward. If sexual intercourse is repeated while the diaphragm is in place, additional spermicide should be inserted into the vagina to continue protection. If a woman has gained or lost more than 10 pounds, has had a diaphragm for more than a year, or has had a baby or an abortion, she must be refitted for a diaphragm because the vagina's size and shape may have changed. During the first year of diaphragm use, the percentage of women who become pregnant varies from about 3% when the diaphragm is used correctly to about 14% when it is used the way most people use it.

The **cervical cap** resembles the diaphragm but is smaller and more rigid. It fits snugly over the cervix. Cervical caps must be fitted by a health care practitioner. A contraceptive cream or jelly should always be used with a cervical cap. The cap is inserted before intercourse and left in place for at least 8 hours after intercourse, up to 48 hours at a time.

SPERMICIDES

Spermicides are preparations that kill sperm on contact. They are available as vaginal foams, creams, gels, and suppositories and are placed in the vagina before sexual intercourse. These contraceptives also provide a physical barrier to sperm. No single type of preparation seems to be more effective than another. They are best used in combination with a barrier contraceptive, such as a male condom, female condom, or diaphragm.

INTRAUTERINE DEVICES

Intrauterine devices (IUDs) are small, flexible plastic devices that are inserted into the uterus. An IUD is left in place for 5 or 10 years, depending on the type, or until the woman wants the device removed. IUDs must be inserted and removed by a doctor or other health care practitioner. Insertion takes only a few minutes. Removal is also quick and usually causes minimal discomfort. IUDs kill or immobilize sperm and prevent fertilization of the egg.

Two types of IUDs are currently available in the United States. One type, which releases a progestin, is effective for 5 years. The other, which releases copper, is effective for at least 10 years. One year after removal of an IUD, 80 to 90% of women who try to conceive do so.

An IUD inserted up to 1 week after one act of unprotected sexual intercourse is nearly

100% effective as a method of emergency contraception.

The uterus is briefly contaminated with bacteria at the time of insertion, but an infection rarely results. After the first month of use, an IUD does not increase the risk of a pelvic infection.

Bleeding and pain are the main reasons that women have IUDs removed, accounting for more than half of all removals before the usual replacement time. The copper-releasing IUD increases the amount of menstrual bleeding. In contrast, the progestin-releasing IUD reduces or, after 6 months of use, completely prevents menstrual bleeding.

About 10% of IUDs are expelled during the first year after insertion, often during the first few months. A plastic string is usually attached to the IUD so that a woman can check every so often, especially after a period, to make sure that the IUD is still in place. If she cannot find the string, she should use another contraceptive method until she can see her health care practitioner to determine whether the IUD is still in place. If another IUD is inserted after one has been expelled, it usually stays in place.

Rarely, the uterus is perforated during insertion. Usually, perforation does not cause symptoms. It is discovered when a woman cannot find the plastic string and ultrasonography or x-rays show the IUD located outside the uterus. An IUD that perforates the uterus and passes into the abdominal cavity must be surgically removed to prevent it from injuring and scarring the intestine.

The risk of miscarriage is about 55% in women who become pregnant with an IUD in place. If a woman wishes to continue the pregnancy and the string of the IUD is visible, a doctor removes the IUD to reduce the risk of miscarriage. For women who conceive with an IUD in place, the likelihood of having a mislocated (ectopic) pregnancy is about 5%—5 times higher than usual. Nonetheless, the risk of an ectopic pregnancy is much lower for women using IUDs than for those not using a contraceptive method, because IUDs prevent pregnancy effectively.

TIMING METHODS

Some contraceptive methods depend on timing rather than on drugs or devices.

Natural Family Planning Methods

Natural family planning (rhythm) methods depend on abstinence from sexual intercourse during the woman's fertile time of the month.

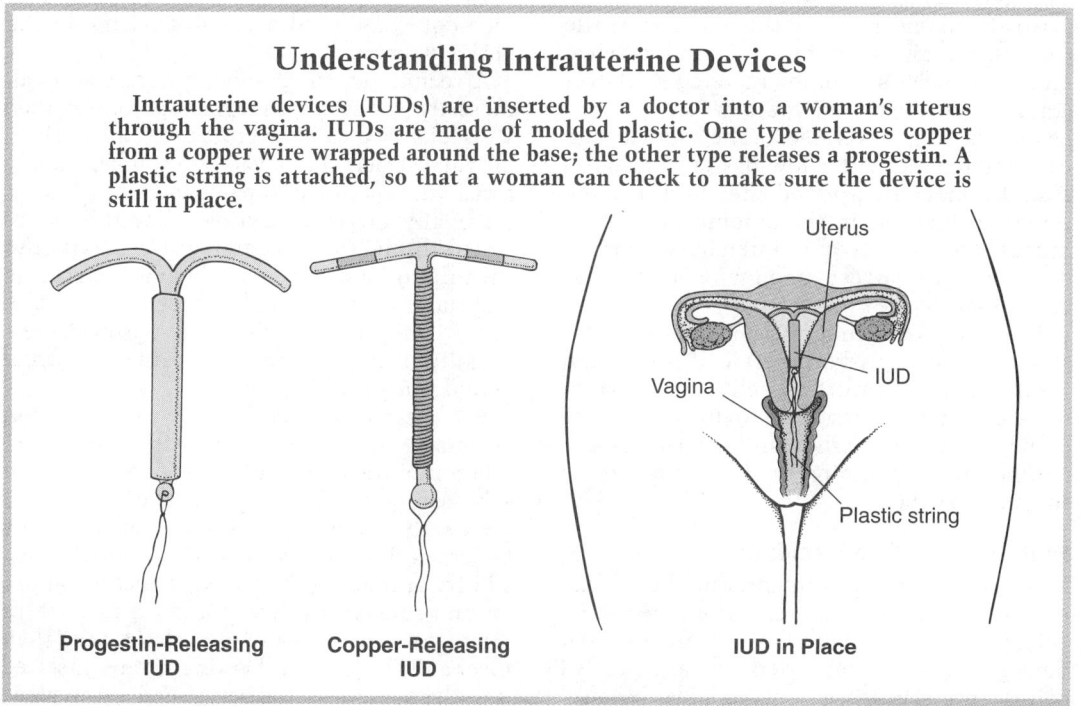

Understanding Intrauterine Devices

Intrauterine devices (IUDs) are inserted by a doctor into a woman's uterus through the vagina. IUDs are made of molded plastic. One type releases copper from a copper wire wrapped around the base; the other type releases a progestin. A plastic string is attached, so that a woman can check to make sure the device is still in place.

Uterus

Vagina

IUD

Plastic string

Progestin-Releasing IUD   **Copper-Releasing IUD**   **IUD in Place**

In most women, the ovary releases an egg about 14 days before the start of a menstrual period. Although the unfertilized egg survives only about 12 hours, sperm can survive for as long as 6 days after intercourse. Consequently, fertilization can result from intercourse that occurred up to 6 days before the release of the egg.

The calendar method is the least effective natural family planning method, even for women who have regular menstrual cycles. To calculate when to abstain from intercourse, women subtract 18 days from the shortest and 11 days from the longest of their previous 12 menstrual cycles. For example, if a woman's cycles last from 26 to 29 days, she must avoid intercourse from day 8 through day 18 of each cycle.

Other, more effective natural family planning methods include the temperature, mucus, and symptothermal methods.

For the temperature method, a woman determines the temperature of the body at rest (basal body temperature) by taking her temperature each morning before she gets out of bed. This temperature decreases before the egg is released and increases slightly after the egg is released. The couple avoids intercourse from the beginning of the woman's menstrual period until at least 48 hours after the day her basal body temperature increased.

For the mucus method, the woman's fertile period is established by observing cervical mucus, which is usually secreted in larger amounts and becomes more watery shortly before the egg is released. The woman can have intercourse with a low risk of conception after her menstrual period ends until she observes an increase in the amount of cervical mucus. She then avoids intercourse until 4 days after the largest amount of mucus has been observed.

The symptothermal method involves observing changes in both cervical mucus and basal body temperature as well as other symptoms that may be associated with the release of the egg, such as slight cramping pain. Of the natural family planning methods, this one is the most reliable.

Withdrawal Before Ejaculation

To prevent sperm from entering the vagina, a man can withdraw the penis from the vagina before ejaculation, when sperm are released during orgasm. This method, also called coitus interruptus, is not reliable because sperm may be released before orgasm. It also requires that the man have a high degree of self-control and precise timing.

Abortion

Induced abortion is the intentional ending of a pregnancy by medical means.

Worldwide, the status of abortion varies from being legally banned to being available on request. About two thirds of the women in the world have access to legal abortion. In the United States, laws regarding how late in the pregnancy elective abortion can be performed vary from state to state. In the United States, about 25% of all pregnancies are ended by elective abortion, making it one of the most common surgical procedures performed.

Abortion methods include use of surgery (surgical evacuation) and use of drugs. The method used depends in part on how long a woman has been pregnant. The length of the pregnancy may be hard to estimate if any bleeding has occurred after conception, if the woman is overweight, or if the uterus points backward rather than forward. In these situations, ultrasonography is usually performed to estimate the length of the pregnancy.

Surgical evacuation involves removing the contents of the uterus through the vagina. It is used for about 95% of abortions. Different techniques are used depending on the length of the pregnancy.

A technique called suction curettage is almost always used for pregnancies of less than 12 weeks. Typically, doctors use a small, flexible tube attached to a vacuum source, usually a machine suction pump or hand pump but occasionally a vacuum syringe. The tube is inserted through the opening of the cervix into the interior of the uterus, which is then gently and thoroughly emptied. Sometimes this procedure does not terminate the pregnancy, especially in the first week after the menstrual period is missed.

For pregnancies of 4 to 6 weeks, suction curettage can be performed with little or no dilation of the cervix, because a small suction tube can be used. For pregnancies of 7 to 12 weeks, the cervix is usually dilated because a larger suction tube is used. To reduce the possibility of injuring the cervix, a doctor can use natural substances that absorb fluids, such as dried seaweed stems (laminaria), rather than mechanical devices. Laminaria are inserted into the opening of the cervix and left in place for at least 4 to 5 hours, usually overnight. As the laminaria absorb large amounts of fluid from the body, they expand and stretch the opening of the cervix. Drugs such as prostaglandins can also be used to dilate the cervix.

For pregnancies of more than 12 weeks, a technique called dilation and evacuation is most commonly used. After the cervix is dilated, suction and forceps are used to remove the fetus and placenta. Then the uterus may be gently scraped to make sure everything has been removed. This technique results in fewer minor complications than do the drugs used to induce abortion. However, for pregnancies of more than 18 weeks, dilation and evacuation can cause serious complications, such as damage to the uterus or intestine.

Drugs used to induce abortions include mifepristone (RU-486) and prostaglandins, such as misoprostol. Mifepristone, given by mouth, blocks the action of the hormone progesterone, which prepares the lining of the uterus to support the fetus. Mifepristone is approved only for pregnancies of 7 weeks or less. Prostaglandins are hormonelike substances that stimulate the uterus to contract. They are given by mouth, placed in the vagina, or given by injection. After mifepristone is given, a prostaglandin is given. The regimen now used involves taking 1 to 3 tablets of mifepristone and, 2 days later, taking a prostaglandin (misoprostol) by mouth or vaginally. This regimen causes abortion in about 95% of cases. If abortion does not occur, surgical evacuation is performed.

Complications

In general, abortion has a higher risk of complications than contraception or sterilization, especially for young women. The risk of complications from an abortion is related to the length of the pregnancy and the abortion method used. The longer a woman has been pregnant, the greater the risk. However, complications are uncommon when an abortion is performed by a trained health care practitioner in a hospital or clinic.

The uterus is perforated by a surgical instrument in 1 of 1,000 abortions. Sometimes the intestine or another organ is also injured. Severe bleeding occurs during or immediately after the procedure in 6 of 10,000 abortions. Some techniques can tear the cervix, especially during the 2nd trimester of pregnancy.

Later, infections or blood clots in the legs may develop. Bleeding can occur if part of the

placenta is left in the uterus. Very rarely, sterility results from scarring of the uterine lining due to the procedure or a subsequent infection—a disorder called Asherman's syndrome. If the fetus has Rh-positive blood, a woman who has Rh-negative blood may produce Rh antibodies—as in any pregnancy, miscarriage, or delivery. Such antibodies may endanger subsequent pregnancies unless the woman is given injections of $Rh_0(D)$ immune globulin.▲

Sterilization

Sterilization involves making a person incapable of reproduction.

About one third of all married couples in the United States who use family planning methods choose sterilization. Sterilization should always be considered permanent. However, an operation that reconnects the appropriate tubes (reanastomosis) can be performed to restore fertility. Reanastomosis is less likely to be effective in men than in women. For couples, pregnancy rates are 45 to 60% after reanastomosis in men and 50 to 80% after reanastomosis in women.

Vasectomy is performed to sterilize men. It involves cutting and sealing the vasa deferentia (the tubes that carry sperm from the testes). A vasectomy, which is performed by a urologist in the office, takes about 20 minutes and requires only a local anesthetic. Through a small incision on each side of the scrotum, a section of each vas deferens is removed and the open ends of the tubes are sealed off. A man who has had a vasectomy should continue contraception for a while. Usually, he does not become sterile until about 15 to 20 ejaculations after the operation, because many sperm are stored in the seminal vesicles. A laboratory test can be performed to be sure that ejaculates are free of sperm.

Complications of vasectomy include bleeding (in fewer than 5% of men), an inflammatory response to sperm leakage, and spontaneous reopening (in fewer than 1%), usually shortly after the procedure. Sexual activity, with contraception, may resume as soon after the procedure as the man desires. Fewer than 1% of women become pregnant after their partner is sterilized.

▲ see page 1453

Disrupting the Tubes: Sterilization in Women

Both fallopian tubes (which carry the egg from the ovaries to the uterus) are cut, sealed, or blocked so that sperm cannot reach the egg to fertilize it.

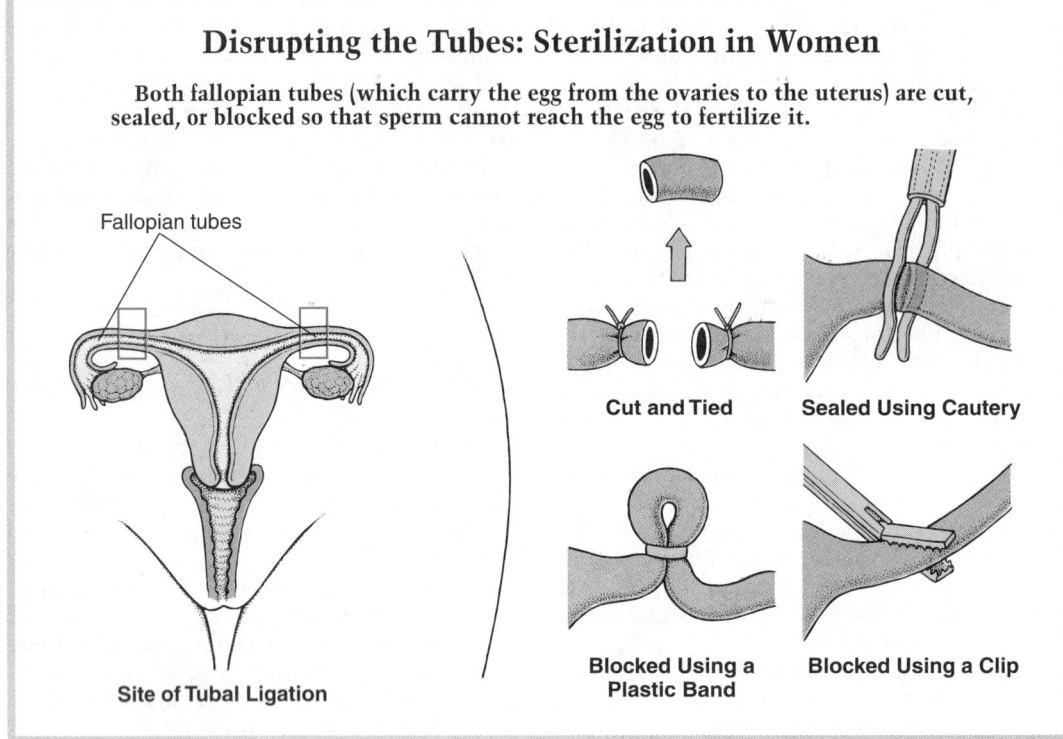

Fallopian tubes

Cut and Tied

Sealed Using Cautery

Blocked Using a Plastic Band

Blocked Using a Clip

Site of Tubal Ligation

Tubal ligation is used to sterilize women. It involves cutting and tying or blocking the fallopian tubes, which carry the egg from the ovaries to the uterus. More complicated than vasectomy, tubal ligation requires an abdominal incision and a general or regional anesthetic. Women who have just delivered a child can be sterilized immediately after childbirth or on the following day, without staying in the hospital any longer than usual. Sterilization also may be planned in advance and performed as elective surgery.

Sterilization for women is often performed by laparoscopy. Working through a thin tube inserted through a small incision in the woman's abdomen, a doctor cuts the fallopian tubes and ties off the cut ends. Or a doctor may use electrocautery (a device that produces an electrical current to cut through tissue) to seal off about 1 inch of each tube. The woman usually goes home the same day. After la-

paroscopy, up to 6% of women have minor complications, such as a skin infection at the incision site or constipation. Fewer than 1% have major complications, such as bleeding or punctures of the bladder or intestine. About 2% of women become pregnant during the first 10 years after they are sterilized. About one third of these pregnancies are mislocated (ectopic) pregnancies that develop in the fallopian tubes.

Various mechanical devices, such as plastic bands and spring-loaded clips, can be used to block the fallopian tubes instead of cutting or sealing them. Sterilization is easier to reverse when these devices are used because they cause less tissue damage. However, reversal is successful in only about three fourths of the women.

Surgical removal of the uterus (hysterectomy) results in sterility. This procedure is usually performed to treat a disorder rather than as a sterilization technique.

CHAPTER 256

Detection of Genetic Disorders

A big concern of prospective parents is whether their baby will be healthy. Some problems that occur in babies are due to genetic disorders. These disorders may result from abnormalities in one or more genes or in chromosomes.▲ Abnormalities may be hereditary or may occur spontaneously. A spontaneous abnormality may result from exposure before birth to drugs, chemicals, or other damaging substances (such as x-rays) or may occur by chance.

To determine whether the risk of having a baby with a hereditary genetic disorder is increased, a couple who is thinking of having a baby can undergo genetic screening. If a couple is considered at increased risk, procedures to test the fetus during the pregnancy (prenatal diagnostic testing) can be performed.

Genetic Screening

Genetic screening is used to determine whether a couple is at increased risk of having a baby with a hereditary genetic disorder. Genetic screening is not for everyone. Counseling is recommended when one or both partners know they have a genetic disorder or have family members who have or may have a genetic disorder. Genetic screening involves assessing the couple's family history and may involve determining whether a prospective parent who does not have symptoms of a particular disorder has a gene for that disorder (carrier screening).

Family History Assessment

To determine whether having a baby with a genetic disorder is likely, doctors ask the couple about disorders that family members have had and about the cause of death in family members. Information about three generations is usually needed. Doctors also ask about the health of all living first-degree relatives (parents, siblings, and children) and second-degree relatives (aunts, uncles, and grandparents). Information about miscarriages, stillborn babies, or babies who have died soon after birth is also helpful, as is information about intermarriages among relatives and ethnic background. If the family history is complicated, information about more distant rela-

tives may be needed. Sometimes doctors review the medical records of relatives who may have had a genetic disorder.

Carrier Screening

Carrier screening involves testing people who do not have symptoms of a particular disorder but may have one nonsex (autosomal) recessive gene for that disorder and one normal gene.■ (If a disorder results from an abnormal autosomal recessive gene, a person must have two of the abnormal genes to develop the disorder and have symptoms.) Prospective parents are screened if they have a family history of certain disorders or characteristics (such as ethnic background) that increase the risk of having certain disorders.

Screening is performed only if the following criteria are met:

- The disorder is very debilitating or lethal
- A reliable screening test is available
- One or both parents are likely to be a carrier because the disorder runs in the family or is common in their ethnic, racial, or geographic group
- The fetus can be treated, or reproductive options (such as abortion or elective sterilization) are available and acceptable to the parents.

In the United States, sickle cell anemia, the thalassemias, Tay-Sachs disease, and cystic fibrosis meet these criteria.

Screening usually consists of analyzing a blood sample. But sometimes a sample of cells from the inside of the cheek is analyzed. The person provides the sample by swishing a special fluid in the mouth, then spitting it into a specimen container. If both parents carry one abnormal autosomal recessive gene for the same disorder, their baby may be born with the disorder. In such cases, the chance of a baby receiving an abnormal recessive gene from each parent is 1 in 4 for each pregnancy.

If carrier screening indicates that both parents have an autosomal recessive gene for the same disorder, the parents may decide to have prenatal diagnostic testing. That is, the fetus may be tested for the disorder before birth. If

---

▲ see pages 9 and 1527

■ see page 11

SOME GENETIC DISORDERS THAT CAN BE DETECTED BEFORE BIRTH

DISORDER	INCIDENCE	INHERITANCE PATTERN
Cystic fibrosis	1 of 3,300 white people	Autosomal recessive
Congenital adrenal hyperplasia	1 of 10,000	Autosomal recessive
Duchenne's muscular dystrophy	1 of 3,500 male births	X-linked recessive
Hemophilia A	1 of 8,500 male births	X-linked recessive
Alpha- and beta-thalassemia	Varies widely by ethnic and racial group	Autosomal recessive
Huntington's disease	4 to 7 of 100,000	Autosomal dominant
Polycystic kidney disease (adult type)	1 of 3,000	Autosomal dominant
Sickle cell anemia	1 of 400 black people in the United States	Autosomal recessive
Tay-Sachs disease (GM_2 gangliosidosis)	1 of 3,600 Ashkenazi Jews and French Canadians; 1 of 400,000 in other groups	Autosomal recessive

the fetus has the disorder, treatment of the fetus may be possible, or termination of the pregnancy may be considered.

Prenatal Diagnostic Testing

Prenatal diagnostic testing involves testing the fetus before birth (prenatally) to determine whether it has a certain hereditary or spontaneous genetic disorder. The most common tests used to detect abnormalities in a fetus include ultrasonography, chorionic villus sampling, amniocentesis, and percutaneous umbilical blood sampling. Most of these tests are offered primarily to couples with an increased risk of having a baby with a genetic abnormality (particularly neural tube defects) or a chromosomal abnormality (particularly when the woman is aged 35 or older). In the United States, ultrasonography is often performed as part of routine prenatal care.

Neural Tube Defects: Prenatal diagnostic testing is commonly used to detect neural tube defects, which are birth defects of the brain or spinal cord.▲ Examples are spina bifida (in which the spine does not completely enclose the spinal cord) and anencephaly (in which a large part of the brain and skull is missing). In the United States, neural tube de-

fects occur in 1 of 500 to 1,000 births. Most of these defects are caused by abnormalities in several genes. A few result from abnormalities in a single gene, chromosomal abnormalities, or exposure to drugs. Prenatal diagnosis by amniocentesis and ultrasonography is recommended for couples who have at least a 1% risk of having a baby with a neural tube defect.

The risk of having a baby with a neural tube defect is increased by having a family history (including the couple's own children) of such defects. For couples who have had a baby with spina bifida or anencephaly, the risk of having another baby with one of these defects is 2 to 3%. For couples who have had two children with these defects, the risk is 5 to 10%. However, about 95% of neural tube defects occur in families without a history of the defects.

Risk also depends on where a person lives. For example, the risk is higher in the United Kingdom than in the United States. Risk may also be increased by a diet that is low in folic acid. Therefore, folic acid supplements are now routinely recommended for all women of childbearing age.

Chromosomal Abnormalities: Chromosomal abnormalities occur in about 1 of 200 live births and account for at least half of all miscarriages that occur during the 1st trimester. Most fetuses that have chromosomal abnormalities die before birth. Tests to diagnose chromosomal abnormalities before

▲ see page 1525

A WOMAN'S AGE AND HER RISK OF HAVING A BABY WITH A CHROMOSOMAL ABNORMALITY

AGE OF WOMAN	RISK OF DOWN SYNDROME	RISK OF ANY CHROMOSOMAL ABNORMALITY	AGE OF WOMAN	RISK OF DOWN SYNDROME	RISK OF ANY CHROMOSOMAL ABNORMALITY
20	1 in 1,667	1 in 526	36	1 in 294	1 in 156
22	1 in 1,429	1 in 500	38	1 in 175	1 in 102
24	1 in 1,250	1 in 476	40	1 in 106	1 in 66
26	1 in 1,176	1 in 476	42	1 in 64	1 in 42
28	1 in 1,053	1 in 435	44	1 in 38	1 in 26
30	1 in 952	1 in 384	46	1 in 23	1 in 16
32	1 in 769	1 in 323	48	1 in 14	1 in 10
34	1 in 500	1 in 238			

Data based on information in Hook EB: "Rates of chromosome abnormalities at different maternal ages." *Obstetrics and Gynecology* 58:282–285, 1981; and Hook EB, Cross PK, Schreinemachers DM: "Chromosomal abnormality rates at amniocentesis and in live-born infants." *Journal of the American Medical Association* 249(15):2034–2038, 1983.

birth are considered if a couple has an increased risk of having a baby with a chromosomal abnormality. However, diagnostic tests can have risks, although very small, particularly for the fetus. For some couples, the risks outweigh the benefits of knowing whether their baby has a chromosomal abnormality, so they choose not to be tested.

Several factors increase the risk of having a baby with a chromosomal abnormality. The risk of having a baby with Down syndrome increases with a woman's age—steeply after age 35.▲ (Down syndrome is the most common chromosomal abnormality among live-born babies.) Testing for chromosomal abnormalities in the fetus is usually offered to women who will be 35 or older when they give birth and may be offered to younger women, such as those who have already had a child with Down syndrome. The couple's anxiety, regardless of the woman's age, often justifies prenatal diagnostic testing.

Having a family history (including the couple's own children) of a chromosomal abnormality also increases the risk. If a couple has had one baby with the most common form of Down syndrome (trisomy 21) and the woman is younger than 30, the risk of having another baby with a chromosomal abnormality is increased to about 1%.

Having had a live-born or stillborn baby with a birth defect—even when no one knows whether the baby had a chromosomal abnormality—increases the risk of having a baby with a chromosomal abnormality. About 30% of babies born with a birth defect and 5% of apparently normal stillborn babies have a chromosomal abnormality.

A chromosomal abnormality in one or both parents increases the risk, even if the parent is only a carrier, is healthy, and has no physical sign of the abnormality.

Having had several miscarriages may increase the risk of having a baby with a chromosomal abnormality. If the fetus in a first miscarriage has a chromosomal abnormality, a fetus in subsequent miscarriages is also likely to have one, although not necessarily the same one. If a woman has had several miscarriages, the couple's chromosomes should be analyzed before they try to have another baby. If abnormalities are identified, the couple may choose to have prenatal diagnostic testing early in the next pregnancy.

Abnormal levels of certain substances in a pregnant woman's blood indicate that a chromosomal abnormality in the fetus is more likely. Such substances are called markers. An important marker is alpha-fetoprotein (a protein produced by the fetus). Other markers include estriol (an estrogen) and human chorionic gonadotropin (a hormone produced by the placenta). For pregnant women, measuring marker levels is part of routine prenatal care.

▲ see also box on page 1346

Interpreting Abnormal Alpha-Fetoprotein Levels

Doctors routinely offer pregnant women blood tests to screen for various birth defects. Certain substances (called markers) in the blood indicate that a chromosomal abnormality in the fetus is more likely. Results are most accurate when the blood sample is taken between 16 and 18 weeks of pregnancy. Normal levels of these substances do not guarantee a normal fetus, and abnormal levels can have different meanings.

A high level of alpha-fetoprotein in a pregnant woman's blood indicates that the risk of having a baby with a brain defect (anencephaly) or spinal cord defect (spina bifida) is increased. A high level may also indicate that more than one fetus is present, a miscarriage is likely, or the fetus has died. A low level of alpha-fetoprotein in a pregnant woman's blood suggests other chromosomal abnormalities, including Down syndrome.

If a woman has a high alpha-fetoprotein level, ultrasonography is performed to determine whether an abnormality is present. If ultrasonography cannot determine the cause, amniocentesis is usually performed to measure the alpha-fetoprotein level in the fluid that surrounds the fetus (amniotic fluid), and chromosomes may be analyzed. If the alpha-fetoprotein level in the amniotic fluid is high, the level of an enzyme called acetylcholinesterase is also measured. In most cases of anencephaly and spina bifida, the alpha-fetoprotein level is high and acetylcholinesterase is detected in the amniotic fluid. A high level of alpha-fetoprotein in the amniotic fluid, with or without acetylcholinesterase, may indicate abnormalities in other organs, such as the esophagus and stomach. A high alpha-fetoprotein level in the amniotic fluid also indicates an increased risk of complications during pregnancy, such as slowed growth or death of the fetus and early detachment of the placenta (placental abruption).

PROCEDURES

Several procedures can be used to detect genetic and chromosomal abnormalities.

Ultrasonography

Ultrasonography is commonly performed during pregnancy.▲ It has no known risks for the woman or fetus. After the third month, ultrasonography can be used to detect whether the fetus has certain obvious structural birth defects. Ultrasonography is often used to check for abnormalities in the fetus when a pregnant woman has a high or low alpha-fetoprotein level or a family history of birth defects. However, normal results do not guarantee a normal baby, because no test is completely accurate.

Ultrasonography is performed before chorionic villus sampling and amniocentesis to confirm the length of the pregnancy. Chorionic villus sampling and amniocentesis can then be performed at the appropriate time during the pregnancy. Ultrasonography can also locate the placenta and indicate whether the fetus is alive. Ultrasonography is used to monitor the fetus and to guide placement of instruments during chorionic villus sampling or amniocentesis.

Chorionic Villus Sampling

In chorionic villus sampling, a doctor removes a small sample of the chorionic villi, which are tiny projections that make up part of the placenta.■ This procedure is used to diagnose some disorders in the fetus, usually between 10 and 12 weeks of pregnancy. Chorionic villus sampling may be used instead of amniocentesis unless a sample of amniotic fluid is needed. For example, a sample is needed when the alpha-fetoprotein level in amniotic fluid must be measured.

The main advantage of chorionic villus sampling is that its results are available much earlier in the pregnancy than those of amniocentesis. Thus, if no abnormality is detected, the couple's anxiety can be relieved earlier. If an abnormality is detected earlier, simpler, safer methods can be used to terminate the pregnancy. Also, early detection of an abnormality may be necessary for appropriate treatment of the fetus before birth. For example, a pregnant woman may be given a corticosteroid to prevent male characteristics from developing in a female fetus that has congenital adrenal hyperplasia. In this hereditary disorder, the adrenal glands are enlarged and produce excessive amounts of male hormones (androgens).

Before the procedure, ultrasonography is performed to determine whether the fetus is alive, to confirm the fetus's age, to check for obvious abnormalities, and to locate the placenta.

▲ see page 1354   ■ see art on page 1437

Detecting Abnormalities Before Birth

Chorionic villus sampling and amniocentesis are used to detect abnormalities in a fetus. During both procedures, ultrasonography is used for guidance.

In chorionic villus sampling, a sample of chorionic villi (part of the placenta) is removed by one of two methods. In the transcervical method, a doctor inserts a flexible tube (catheter) through the vagina and cervix into the placenta. In the transabdominal method, a doctor inserts a needle through the abdominal wall into the placenta. In both methods, a sample of the placenta is suctioned out with a syringe and analyzed.

In amniocentesis, a doctor inserts a needle through the abdominal wall into the amniotic fluid. A sample of fluid is withdrawn for analysis.

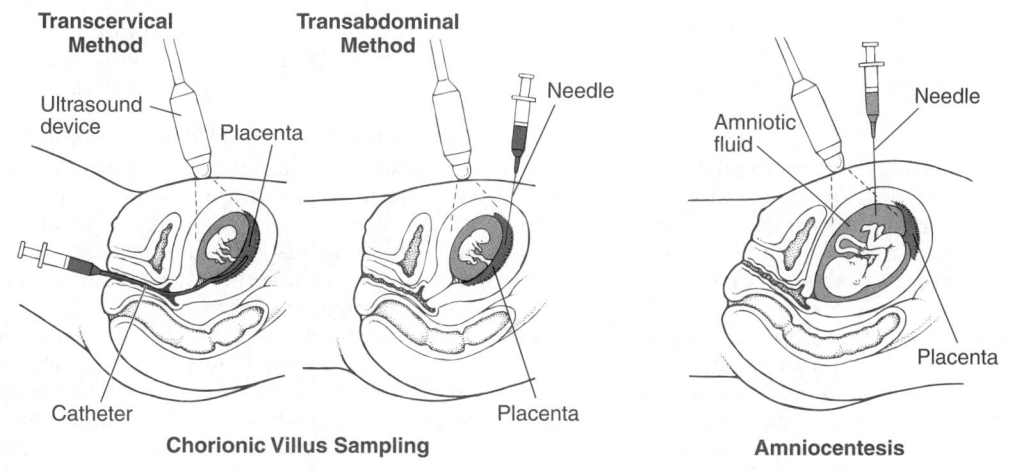

Transcervical Method

Ultrasound device
Placenta
Catheter

Transabdominal Method

Needle
Placenta

Chorionic Villus Sampling

Needle
Amniotic fluid
Placenta

Amniocentesis

A sample of the chorionic villi can be removed through the cervix (transcervically) or the abdominal wall (transabdominally). With both methods, ultrasonography is used for guidance and the tissue sample is suctioned into a catheter with a syringe and then analyzed.

To remove tissue through the cervix, a doctor inserts a thin flexible tube (catheter) through the vagina and the cervix into the placenta. The woman lies on her back with her hips and knees bent, usually supported by heel or knee stirrups, as for a pelvic examination. For most women, the procedure feels very similar to a Papanicolaou (Pap) test, but a few women find it more uncomfortable. This method cannot be used in women who have a certain abnormality of the cervix or an active genital infection, such as genital herpes, gonorrhea, or chronic inflammation of the cervix.

To remove tissue through the abdominal wall, a doctor anesthetizes an area of skin over the abdomen and inserts a needle through the abdominal wall into the placenta. Most women do not find this procedure painful. But for some women, the area over the abdomen feels slightly sore for an hour or two afterward.

After chorionic villus sampling, most women who have Rh-negative blood and who do not have antibodies to Rh factor are given an injection of $Rh_0(D)$ immune globulin to prevent them from producing antibodies to Rh factor.▲ A woman with Rh-negative blood may produce these antibodies if the fetus has Rh-positive blood that comes into contact with her blood, as it may during chorionic villus sampling. These antibodies can cause problems in the fetus. The injection is not needed if the father also has Rh-negative blood, because the fetus will have Rh-negative blood.

The risks of chorionic villus sampling are comparable to those of amniocentesis, except

▲ see page 1453

the risk of injuring the fetus's hands or feet may be slightly higher. Such injury occurs in 1 of 3,000 fetuses. Rarely, the diagnosis is unclear after chorionic villus sampling, and amniocentesis may be necessary. In general, the accuracy of the two procedures is comparable.

Amniocentesis

One of the most common procedures for detecting abnormalities before birth is amniocentesis. In this procedure, a sample of the fluid that surrounds the fetus (amniotic fluid) is removed. Amniocentesis is usually performed at 14 weeks of pregnancy or later. If the reason for performing amniocentesis is a high alpha-fetoprotein level in the woman's blood, the procedure is best performed between 15 and 17 weeks of pregnancy. Amniocentesis enables doctors to measure the alpha-fetoprotein level in the amniotic fluid. This measurement more reliably indicates whether the fetus has a brain or spinal cord defect than measurement of this level in the woman's blood.

After anesthetizing an area of skin over the abdomen, a doctor inserts a needle through the abdominal wall into the amniotic fluid. During the procedure, ultrasonography is performed so that the fetus can be monitored and the needle guided into place. Fluid is withdrawn, and the needle is removed. Results are usually available in 1 to 3 weeks. Women who have Rh-negative blood are given $Rh_0(D)$ immune globulin after the procedure to prevent them from producing antibodies to Rh factor, which can cause problems in a fetus with Rh-positive blood.▲

Amniocentesis rarely causes any problems for the woman or the fetus. Some women feel slightly sore for an hour or two afterward. About 1 to 2% of the women have spotting of blood or leakage of amniotic fluid from the vagina, but these effects do not last long and usually stop without treatment. After amniocentesis, the chance of miscarriage due to the procedure is about 1 in 200. Needle injuries to the fetus are very rare. Amniocentesis can usually be performed when a woman is pregnant with twins or even more fetuses.

Percutaneous Umbilical Blood Sampling

Percutaneous umbilical blood sampling is used when rapid chromosome analysis is needed, particularly toward the end of pregnancy when ultrasonography has detected abnormalities in the fetus. Often, results can be available within 48 hours.

The doctor first anesthetizes an area of skin over the abdomen. Guided by ultrasonography, the doctor then inserts a needle through the abdominal wall into the umbilical cord. A sample of the fetus's blood is withdrawn and analyzed, and the needle is removed. Percutaneous umbilical blood sampling is an invasive procedure and has risks for the woman and fetus.

CHAPTER 257

Normal Pregnancy

Pregnancy begins when an egg is fertilized by a sperm. For about 9 months, a pregnant woman's body provides a protective, nourishing environment in which the fertilized egg can develop into a fetus. Pregnancy ends at delivery, when a baby is born.

Detecting and Dating a Pregnancy

If a menstrual period is a week or more late in a woman who usually has regular men-

strual periods, she may be pregnant. Sometimes a woman may guess she is pregnant because she has typical symptoms. They include enlarged and tender breasts, nausea with occasional vomiting, a need to urinate frequently, unusual fatigue, and changes in appetite.

When a menstrual period is late, a woman may wish to use a home pregnancy test to determine whether she is pregnant. Home pregnancy tests detect human chorionic gonadotropin (HCG) in the urine. Human chorionic gonadotropin is a hormone produced by the placenta. Results of home pregnancy tests are

▲ see page 1453

accurate about 97% of the time. If results are negative but the woman still suspects she is pregnant, she should repeat the home pregnancy test a few days later. The first test may have been performed too early (before the next menstrual period is expected to start). If results are positive, the woman should contact her doctor, who may perform another pregnancy test to confirm the results.

Doctors test a sample of blood or urine from the woman to determine whether she is pregnant. These tests are very accurate. One of these tests, called an enzyme-linked immunosorbent assay (ELISA), can quickly and easily detect a low level of human chorionic gonadotropin in the urine. Some tests can detect the very low level that is present about $1\frac{1}{2}$ weeks after fertilization (before a menstrual period is missed). Results may be available in about half an hour. During the first 60 days of a normal pregnancy with one fetus, the level of human chorionic gonadotropin in the blood approximately doubles about every 2 days. Measurement of these levels during the pregnancy can be used to determine whether the pregnancy is progressing normally.

After pregnancy is confirmed, the doctor asks the woman when her last menstrual period was. Pregnancies are conventionally dated in weeks, starting from the first day of the last menstrual period. The doctor calculates the approximate date of delivery by counting back 3 calendar months from the first day of the last menstrual period and adding 1 year and 7 days. Only 10% or fewer of pregnant women give birth on the calculated date, but 50% give birth within 1 week and almost 90% give birth within 2 weeks (before or after the date). Delivery between 3 weeks before and 2 weeks after the calculated date is considered normal.

Ovulation usually occurs about 2 weeks after a woman's menstrual period starts, and fertilization usually occurs shortly after ovulation. Consequently, the embryo is about 2 weeks younger than the number of weeks traditionally assigned to the pregnancy. In other words, a woman who is 4 weeks pregnant is carrying a 2-week-old embryo. If a woman's periods are irregular, the actual difference may be more or less than 2 weeks. Pregnancy lasts an average of 266 days (38 weeks) from the date of fertilization (conception) or 280 days (40 weeks) from the first day of the last menstrual period if the woman has regular 28-day periods. Pregnancy is divided into three 3-month periods, based on the date of the last

menstrual period. They are called the 1st trimester (0 to 12 weeks of pregnancy), 2nd trimester (13 to 24 weeks), and 3rd trimester (25 weeks to delivery).

If a woman and her doctor cannot confidently calculate when she became pregnant based on her menstrual period, ultrasonography may be performed to measure the fetus and thus establish the date. For the most accurate measurements, ultrasonography is performed during the first 12 weeks of a pregnancy. An accurate date helps doctors determine whether the pregnancy is progressing normally.

Stages of Development

A baby goes through several stages of development, beginning as a fertilized egg. The egg develops into a blastocyst, an embryo, then a fetus.

Fertilization

During each normal menstrual cycle, one egg (ovum) is usually released from one of the ovaries, about 14 days before the next menstrual period. Release of the egg is called ovulation. The egg is swept into the funnel-shaped end of one of the fallopian tubes.

At ovulation, the mucus in the cervix becomes more fluid and more elastic, allowing sperm to enter the uterus rapidly. Within 5 minutes, sperm may move from the vagina, through the cervix into the uterus, and to the funnel-shaped end of a fallopian tube—the usual site of fertilization. The cells lining the fallopian tube facilitate fertilization.

If a sperm penetrates the egg, fertilization results. Tiny hairlike cilia lining the fallopian tube propel the fertilized egg (zygote) through the tube toward the uterus. The cells of the zygote divide repeatedly as the zygote moves down the fallopian tube. The zygote enters the uterus in 3 to 5 days. In the uterus, the cells continue to divide, becoming a hollow ball of cells called a blastocyst. If fertilization does not occur, the egg degenerates and passes through the uterus with the next menstrual period.

If more than one egg is released and fertilized, the pregnancy involves more than one fetus, usually two (twins). Such twins are fraternal. Identical twins result when one fertilized egg separates into two embryos after it has begun to divide.

Development of the Blastocyst

Between 5 and 8 days after fertilization, the blastocyst attaches to the lining of the uterus, usually near the top. This process, called implantation, is completed by day 9 or 10.

The wall of the blastocyst is one cell thick except in one area, where it is three to four cells thick. The inner cells in the thickened area develop into the embryo, and the outer cells burrow into the wall of the uterus and develop into the placenta. The placenta produces several hormones that help maintain the pregnancy. For example, the placenta produces human chorionic gonadotropin, which prevents the ovaries from releasing eggs and stimulates the ovaries to produce estrogen and progesterone continuously. The placenta also carries oxygen and nutrients from mother to fetus and waste materials from fetus to mother.

The wall of the blastocyst becomes the outer layer of membranes (chorion) surrounding the embryo. An inner layer of membranes (amnion) develops by about day 10 to 12, forming the amniotic sac. The amniotic sac fills with a clear liquid (amniotic fluid) and expands to envelop the developing embryo, which floats within it.

As the placenta develops, it extends tiny hairlike projections (villi) into the wall of the uterus. The projections branch and rebranch in a complicated treelike arrangement. This arrangement greatly increases the area of contact between the wall of the uterus and the placenta, so that more nutrients and waste materials can be exchanged. The placenta is fully formed by 18 to 20 weeks but continues to grow throughout pregnancy. At delivery, it weighs about 1 pound.

Development of the Embryo

The next stage in development is the embryo, which develops under the lining of the

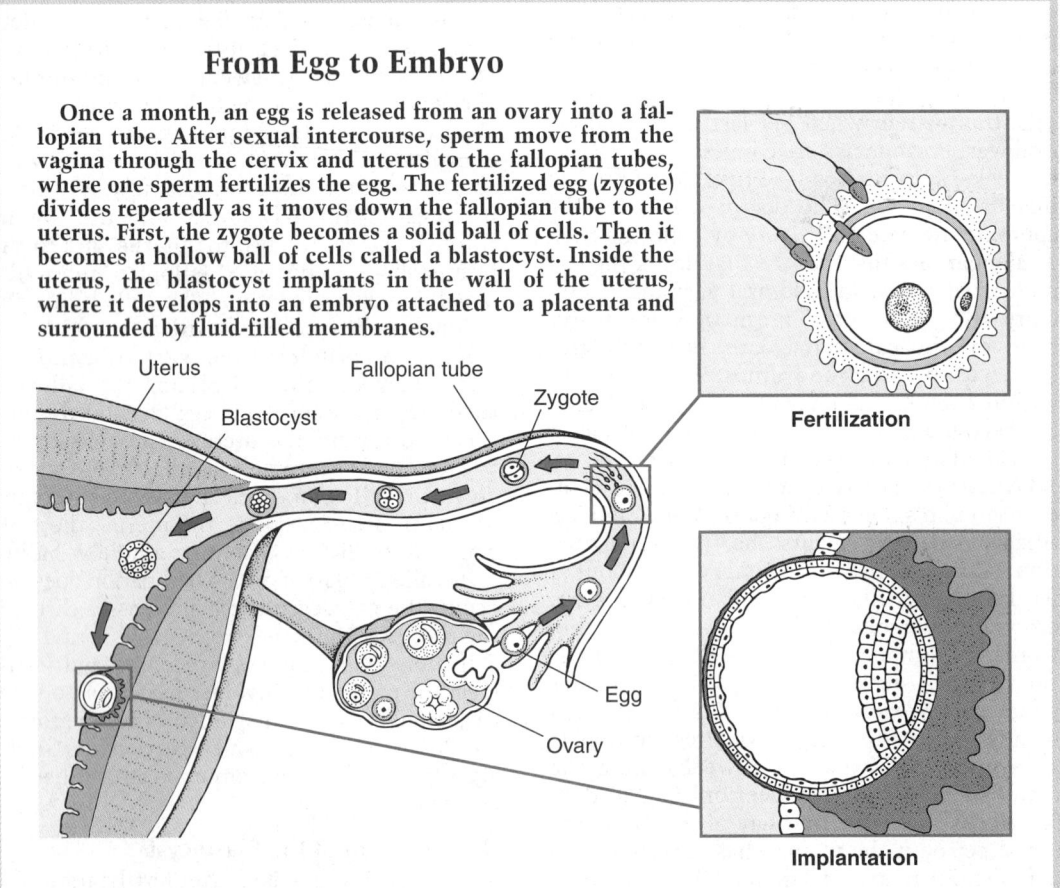

From Egg to Embryo

Once a month, an egg is released from an ovary into a fallopian tube. After sexual intercourse, sperm move from the vagina through the cervix and uterus to the fallopian tubes, where one sperm fertilizes the egg. The fertilized egg (zygote) divides repeatedly as it moves down the fallopian tube to the uterus. First, the zygote becomes a solid ball of cells. Then it becomes a hollow ball of cells called a blastocyst. Inside the uterus, the blastocyst implants in the wall of the uterus, where it develops into an embryo attached to a placenta and surrounded by fluid-filled membranes.

Uterus

Blastocyst

Fallopian tube

Zygote

Egg

Ovary

Fertilization

Implantation

Placenta and Embryo at 8 Weeks

At 8 weeks of pregnancy, the placenta and fetus have been developing for 6 weeks. The placenta forms tiny hairlike projections (villi) that extend into the wall of the uterus. Blood vessels from the embryo, which pass through the umbilical cord to the placenta, develop in the villi. A thin membrane separates the embryo's blood in the villi from the mother's blood that flows through the space surrounding the villi (intervillous space). This arrangement allows materials to be exchanged between the blood of the mother and that of the embryo.

The embryo floats in fluid (amniotic fluid), which is contained in a sac (amniotic sac). The amniotic fluid provides a space in which the embryo can grow freely. The fluid also helps protect the embryo from injury. The amniotic sac is strong and resilient.

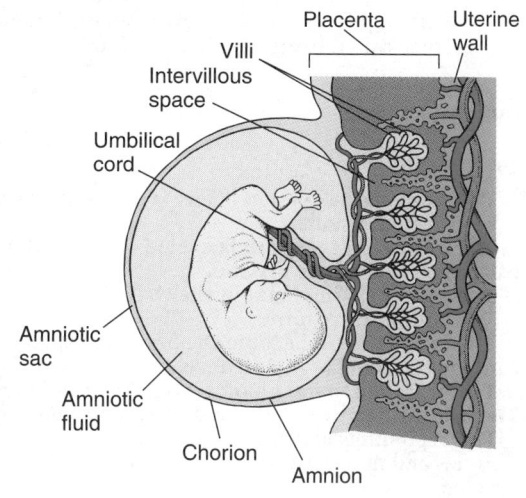

uterus on one side. This stage is characterized by the formation of most internal organs and external body structures. Organ formation begins about 3 weeks after fertilization, when the embryo is first recognizable as having a human shape. Shortly thereafter, the area that will become the brain and spinal cord (neural tube) begins to develop. The heart and major blood vessels begin to develop by about day 16 or 17. The heart begins to pump fluid through blood vessels by day 20, and the first red blood cells appear the next day. Blood vessels continue to develop in the embryo and placenta.

Almost all organs are completely formed by about 8 weeks after fertilization (which equals 10 weeks of pregnancy). The exceptions are the brain and spinal cord, which continue to mature throughout pregnancy. Most malformations occur during the period when organs are forming. During this period, the embryo is most vulnerable to the effects of drugs, radiation, and viruses. Therefore, a pregnant woman should not be given any live-virus vaccinations or take any drugs during this period unless they are considered essential to protect her health.▲

Development of the Fetus

At the end of the 8th week after fertilization (10 weeks of pregnancy), the embryo is considered a fetus. During this stage, the structures

that have already formed grow and develop. By 12 weeks of pregnancy, the fetus fills the entire uterus. By about 14 weeks, the sex can be identified. Typically, the pregnant woman can feel the fetus moving at about 16 to 20 weeks. Women who have been pregnant before typically feel movements about 2 weeks earlier than women who are pregnant for the first time. By about 23 to 24 weeks, the fetus has a chance of survival outside the uterus.

The lungs continue to mature until near the time of delivery. The brain accumulates new cells throughout pregnancy and the first year of life after birth.

Physical Changes in a Pregnant Woman

Pregnancy causes many changes in a woman's body. Most of them disappear after delivery. In some women, certain disorders, such as a skin rash or gestational diabetes,■ develop during pregnancy. Some symptoms should be immediately reported to a doctor if they occur during pregnancy. They include the following:

- persistent headaches
- persistent nausea and vomiting
- dizziness

▲ see page 1458   ■ see page 1452

Stages of Pregnancy

Although pregnancy involves a continuous process, it is divided into three 3-month periods called trimesters (weeks 0 to 12, 13 to 24, and 25 to delivery).

EVENTS	WEEKS OF PREGNANCY	

1st Trimester

The woman's last period before fertilization occurs.	0	
Fertilization occurs.	2	
The fertilized egg (zygote) develops into a hollow ball of cells called the blastocyst.		
The blastocyst implants in the wall of uterus.	3	
The amniotic sac forms.		
The area that will become the brain and spinal cord (neural tube) begins to develop.	5	
The heart and major blood vessels are developing. The beating heart can be seen during ultrasonography.	6	
The beginnings of arms and legs appear.	7	
Bones and muscles form. The face and neck develop.	9	

3 months

Most organs are formed. Brain waves can be detected.

The skeleton is formed. Fingers and toes are fully defined.

The kidneys begin to function.   10

The fetus can move and respond to touch (when prodded through the woman's abdomen).

The woman has gained some weight, and her abdomen may be slightly enlarged.

2nd Trimester

The fetus's sex can be identified.   14

The fetus can hear.

The fetus's fingers can grasp. The fetus moves more   16
vigorously, so that the mother can feel it.

The fetus's body begins to fill out as fat is deposited beneath the skin. Hair appears on the head and skin. Eyebrows and eyelashes are present.

The placenta is fully formed.

The fetus has a chance of survival outside the   23–24
uterus.

The woman begins to gain weight more rapidly.

6 months

3rd Trimester

The fetus is active, changing positions often.   25

The lungs continue to mature.

The fetus's head moves into position for delivery. On average, the fetus is about 20 inches long and weighs about 7 pounds. The woman's enlarged abdomen causes the navel to bulge.

DELIVERY   37–42

9 months

- disturbances of eyesight
- pain or cramps in the lower abdomen
- contractions
- vaginal bleeding
- leakage of amniotic fluid (described as "the water breaks")
- swelling of the hands or feet
- decreased or increased urine production
- any illness or infection

General Health: Fatigue is common, especially in the first 12 weeks and again in late pregnancy. Getting enough rest is important.

Reproductive Tract: By 12 weeks of pregnancy, the enlarging uterus may cause the woman's abdomen to protrude slightly. The uterus continues to enlarge throughout pregnancy. The enlarging uterus extends to the level of the navel by 20 weeks and to the lower edge of the rib cage by 36 weeks.

The amount of normal vaginal discharge, which is clear or whitish, commonly increases. This increase is usually normal. However, if the discharge has an unusual color or smell or is accompanied by vaginal itching and burning, a woman should see her doctor. Such symptoms may indicate a vaginal infection. Some vaginal infections, such as trichomoniasis (a protozoan infection) and candidiasis (a yeast infection), are common during pregnancy and can be easily treated.▲

Breasts: The breasts tend to enlarge because hormones (mainly estrogen) are preparing the breasts for milk production. The breasts enlarge because the glands that produce milk gradually increase in number and become able to produce milk. The breasts may feel firm and tender. Wearing a bra that fits properly and provides support may help.

During the last weeks of pregnancy, the breasts may produce a thin, yellowish or milky discharge (colostrum). Colostrum is also produced during the first few days after delivery, before breast milk is produced. This fluid, which is rich in minerals and antibodies, is the breastfed baby's first food.

Heart and Blood Flow: During pregnancy, the woman's heart must work harder because as the fetus grows, the heart must pump more blood to the uterus. By the end of pregnancy, the uterus is receiving one fifth of the woman's blood supply. During pregnancy, the amount of blood pumped by the heart (cardiac output) increases by 30 to 50%. As cardiac output increases, the heart rate at rest speeds up from a normal prepregnancy rate of about 70 beats per minute to 80 or 90 beats per

minute. During exercise, cardiac output and heart rate increase more when a woman is pregnant than when she is not. During labor, cardiac output increases by an additional 10%. After delivery, cardiac output decreases rapidly at first, then more slowly. It returns to the prepregnancy level about 6 weeks after delivery.

Certain heart murmurs and irregularities in heart rhythm may appear because the heart is working harder. Sometimes a pregnant woman may feel these irregularities. Such changes are normal during pregnancy. However, certain abnormal heart rhythms, which occur more often in pregnant women, may require treatment.

Blood pressure usually decreases during the 2nd trimester but may return to a normal prepregnancy level in the 3rd trimester.

The volume of blood increases by 50% during pregnancy. The amount of fluid in the blood increases more than the number of red blood cells (which carry oxygen). The result is mild anemia, which is normal. For reasons not clearly understood, the number of white blood cells (which fight infection) increases slightly during pregnancy and markedly during labor and the first few days after delivery.

The enlarging uterus interferes with the return of blood from the legs and the pelvic area to the heart. As a result, swelling (edema) is common, especially in the legs. Varicose veins commonly develop in the legs and in the area around the vaginal opening (vulva), sometimes causing discomfort. Clothing that is loose around the waist and legs is more comfortable and does not restrict blood flow. Wearing elastic support hose, resting frequently with the legs elevated, or lying on the left side usually reduces leg swelling and may ease the discomfort caused by varicose veins. Varicose veins may disappear after delivery.

Urinary Tract: Like the heart, the kidneys work harder throughout pregnancy. They filter the increasing volume of blood. The volume of blood filtered by the kidneys reaches a maximum between 16 and 24 weeks and remains at the maximum until immediately before delivery. Then, pressure from the enlarging uterus may slightly decrease the blood supply to the kidneys.

The activity of the kidneys normally increases when a person lies down and decreases

▲ see page 1374

when a person stands. This difference is amplified during pregnancy—one reason a pregnant woman needs to urinate frequently while trying to sleep. Late in pregnancy, lying on the side, particularly the left side, increases kidney activity more than lying on the back. Lying on the left side relieves the pressure that the enlarged uterus puts on the main vein that carries blood from the legs. As a result, blood flow improves and kidney activity increases.

The uterus presses on the bladder, reducing its size so that it fills with urine more quickly than usual. This pressure also makes a pregnant woman need to urinate more often and more urgently.

Respiratory Tract: The increased production of the hormone progesterone signals the brain to lower the level of carbon dioxide in the blood. As a result, a pregnant woman breathes faster and more deeply to exhale more carbon dioxide and keep the carbon dioxide level low. The circumference of the woman's chest enlarges slightly.

Virtually every pregnant woman becomes somewhat more out of breath when she exerts herself, especially toward the end of pregnancy. During exercise, the breathing rate increases more when a woman is pregnant than when she is not.

Because more blood is being pumped, the lining of the airways receives more blood and swells somewhat, narrowing the airways. As a result, the nose occasionally feels stuffy, and the eustachian tubes (which connect the middle ear and back of the nose) may become blocked. The tone and quality of the woman's voice may change slightly.

Digestive Tract: Nausea and vomiting, particularly in the mornings (morning sickness), are common. They may be caused by the high levels of estrogen and human chorionic gonadotropin (HCG), two hormones that help maintain the pregnancy. Nausea and vomiting may be relieved by changing the diet or patterns of eating. For example, drinking and eating small portions frequently, eating before getting hungry, and eating bland foods (such as bouillon, consommé, rice, and pasta) may help. Eating plain soda crackers and sipping a carbonated drink may relieve nausea. Keeping crackers by the bed and eating one or two before getting up may relieve morning sickness.

No drugs specifically designed to treat morning sickness are currently available. If nausea and vomiting are so intense or persistent that dehydration, weight loss, or other problems develop, a woman may need to be treated with antiemetic drugs or be hospitalized temporarily and given fluids intravenously.▲

Heartburn and belching are common, possibly because food remains in the stomach longer and because the ringlike muscle (sphincter) at the lower end of the esophagus tends to relax, allowing the stomach's contents to flow backward into the esophagus. Heartburn can be relieved by eating smaller meals, by not bending or lying flat for several hours after eating, and by taking antacids. However, the antacid sodium bicarbonate should not be used because it contains so much salt (sodium). Heartburn during the night can be relieved by not eating for several hours before going to bed and by raising the head of the bed or using pillows to raise the head and shoulders.

The stomach produces less acid during pregnancy. Consequently, stomach ulcers rarely develop during pregnancy, and those that already exist often start to heal.

As pregnancy progresses, pressure from the enlarging uterus on the rectum and the lower part of the intestine may cause constipation. Constipation may be worsened because the high level of progesterone during pregnancy slows the automatic waves of muscular contractions in the intestine, which normally move food along. Eating a high-fiber diet, drinking plenty of fluids, and exercising regularly can help prevent constipation.

Hemorrhoids, a common problem, may result from the pressure of the enlarging uterus or from constipation. Stool softeners, an anesthetic gel, or warm soaks can be used if hemorrhoids hurt.

Pica, a craving for strange foods or nonfoods (such as starch or clay), may develop. Occasionally, pregnant women, usually those who also have morning sickness, have excess saliva. This symptom may be distressing but is harmless.

Skin: Mask of pregnancy (melasma) is a blotchy, brownish pigment that may appear on the skin of the forehead and cheeks. The skin surrounding the nipples (areolae) may also darken. A dark line commonly appears down the middle of the abdomen. These changes may occur because the placenta produces a hormone that stimulates melano-

▲ see page 1451

cytes, the cells that make a dark brown skin pigment (melanin).

Pink stretch marks sometimes appear on the abdomen. This change probably results from rapid growth of the uterus and an increase in levels of adrenal hormones.

Small blood vessels may form a red spider-like pattern on the skin, usually above the waist. These formations are called spider angiomas. Thin-walled, dilated capillaries may become visible, especially in the lower legs.

Hormones: Pregnancy affects virtually all hormones in the body, mostly because of the effects of hormones produced by the placenta. For example, the placenta produces a hormone that stimulates the woman's thyroid gland to become more active and produce larger amounts of thyroid hormones. When the thyroid gland becomes more active, the heart may beat faster, causing the woman to become aware of her heartbeat (have palpitations). Perspiration may increase, mood swings may occur, and the thyroid gland may enlarge. The disorder hyperthyroidism, in which the thyroid gland is truly overactive, develops in fewer than 1% of pregnancies.

Levels of estrogen and progesterone increase early in pregnancy because human chorionic gonadotropin, the main hormone the placenta produces, stimulates the ovaries to continuously produce them. After 9 to 10 weeks of pregnancy, the placenta itself produces large amounts of estrogen and progesterone. Estrogen and progesterone help maintain the pregnancy.

During pregnancy, changes in hormone levels affect how the body handles sugar. Early in pregnancy, the sugar (glucose) level in the blood may decrease slightly. But in the last half of pregnancy, the level may increase. More insulin (which controls the sugar level in the blood) is needed and is produced by the pancreas. Consequently, diabetes, if already present, may worsen during pregnancy. Diabetes can also begin during pregnancy. This disorder is called gestational diabetes.▲

Joints and Muscles: The joints and ligaments (fibrous cords and cartilage that connect bones) in the woman's pelvis loosen and become more flexible. This change helps make room for the enlarging uterus and prepare the woman for delivery of the baby. As a result, the woman's posture changes somewhat.

Backache in varying degrees is common, because the spine curves more to balance the

Skin Rashes During Pregnancy

Two intensely itchy rashes, urticaria of pregnancy and herpes gestationis, occur only during pregnancy.

Urticaria of pregnancy is common. The cause is unknown. Red, irregularly shaped, flat or slightly raised patches appear on the abdomen. The patches sometimes have tiny fluid-filled blisters in the center. Often, the skin around them is pale. The rash spreads to the thighs, buttocks, and occasionally the arms. Hundreds of itchy patches may develop. Typically, the rash appears during the last 2 to 3 weeks of pregnancy and occasionally during the last few days. However, it may occur at any time after the 24th week. Itching is bothersome enough to keep the woman awake at night. Usually, the rash clears up promptly after delivery and does not recur during subsequent pregnancies. Doctors may have difficulty making a definite diagnosis.

Herpes gestationis is thought to be caused by abnormal antibodies that attack the body's own tissues—an autoimmune reaction. Blisters often form on the abdomen first, then spread. The blisters are small or large, irregularly shaped, and fluid-filled. The rash can appear any time after the 12th week of pregnancy or immediately after delivery. Typically, the rash worsens soon after delivery and disappears within a few weeks or months. It often reappears during subsequent pregnancies. The baby may be born with a similar rash, which usually disappears without treatment within a few weeks. This rash is diagnosed by removing a tiny piece of affected skin and testing it for abnormal antibodies.

For either rash, applying a corticosteroid cream (such as triamcinolone acetonide) directly to the skin often helps. For more widespread rashes, a corticosteroid (such as prednisone) is given by mouth.

weight of the enlarging uterus. Avoiding heavy lifting, bending the knees (not the waist) to pick things up, and maintaining good posture can help. Wearing flat shoes with good support or a lightweight maternity girdle may reduce strain on the back.

▲ see page 1452

Medical Care During Pregnancy

Ideally, a couple who is thinking of having a baby should see a doctor or other health care practitioner to discuss steps that they can take to help make the pregnancy as healthy as possible. The woman should ask the doctor about factors that could impair her health or the health of the developing fetus. Knowing about and dealing with such factors before pregnancy may help reduce the risk of problems during pregnancy.▲ These factors include the use of tobacco or alcohol and exposure to possibly harmful substances. For example, a pregnant woman should avoid exposure to secondhand smoke because it may harm the fetus. A pregnant woman should avoid contact with cats or cat feces unless the cats are strictly confined to the home and are not exposed to other cats. Such contact can transmit toxoplasmosis, an infection by a protozoan that can damage the fetus's brain. Rubella (German measles) can cause birth defects. In addition, the woman can discuss her diet and her social, emotional, and medical concerns with the doctor.

When a woman sees a doctor or other health care practitioner before she is pregnant, she can be given any needed vaccines, such as the rubella vaccine. She can also start taking prenatal multivitamins containing folic acid. If needed, genetic screening can be performed to determine whether the woman and her partner are at increased risk of having a baby with a hereditary genetic disorder.■

After pregnancy is confirmed, the woman should have a physical examination, preferably between 6 and 8 weeks of pregnancy. At this time, the length of the pregnancy can be estimated and the date of delivery can be predicted as accurately as possible.

The first physical examination during pregnancy is very thorough. Weight, height, and blood pressure are measured. The doctor performs a pelvic examination, noting the size and position of the uterus.

A sample of blood is taken and analyzed. Analysis includes a complete blood cell count, tests for infectious diseases (such as syphilis and hepatitis), and tests for evidence of immunity to rubella. Blood type, including Rh factor status (positive or negative), is determined. A test for the human immunodeficiency virus (HIV) is recommended. Other routine tests include an extensive analysis of a sample of the woman's urine and a Papanicolaou (Pap) test for cancer of the cervix. A sample from the cervix may be obtained to test for sexually transmitted diseases, such as gonorrhea and chlamydial infection.

Other tests may be performed, depending on the woman's situation. If the woman has Rh-negative blood, it is tested for antibodies to the Rh factor.★ Having Rh antibodies can cause severe problems (even death) for a fetus who has Rh-positive blood. If antibodies in a pregnant woman's blood are detected early, the doctor can take measures to protect the fetus.

Women of African descent are tested for sickle cell trait or disease if they have not been tested previously. Skin tests for tuberculosis are advisable for all women. X-rays are not routinely taken early in pregnancy, but they can be taken safely when necessary. If an x-ray is required, the fetus is shielded by placing a lead-filled garment over the woman's lower abdomen to cover the uterus.

After the first examination, a pregnant woman should see her doctor every 4 weeks until 32 weeks of pregnancy, then every 2 weeks until 36 weeks, then once a week until delivery. At each examination, the woman's weight and blood pressure are usually recorded, and the size of the uterus is noted to determine whether the fetus is growing normally. The ankles are examined for swelling.

At each visit, urine is tested for sugar. Sugar in the urine may indicate diabetes. Women who have sugar in the urine should be screened for diabetes at 24 to 28 weeks of pregnancy, as should women who have had large babies or unexplained stillbirths, who are overweight, who are older than 25, who have a close relative with diabetes, or who have polycystic ovary syndrome. At each visit, the urine is also tested for protein. Protein in the urine may indicate preeclampsia (a type of high blood pressure that develops during pregnancy).●

For women who have a high risk of conceiving a baby with a genetic disorder, prenatal diagnostic testing is performed.◆

Many doctors believe that ultrasonography, the safest imaging procedure, should be performed at least once during a pregnancy to make sure the fetus is normally formed and to verify the expected date of delivery. For the procedure, a device that produces sound waves (transducer) is placed on the woman's abdo-

▲ see page 1444   ■ see page 1429

★ see page 1453   ● see page 1452

◆ see page 1430

men. The sound waves are processed to form an image that is displayed on a monitor. Sometimes doctors use an ultrasound device that can be inserted in the vagina. Ultrasonography produces high-quality images, including live-action images that show the fetus in motion. These images provide the doctor with useful information and can reassure a pregnant woman.

Before ultrasonography of the abdomen is performed, especially early in pregnancy, a woman must drink a lot of water. A full bladder pushes the uterus out of the pelvis so that a clearer image of the fetus can be obtained. When a vaginal ultrasound device is used, the bladder does not have to be full, and a doctor can detect pregnancy even earlier.

Ultrasonography can show the fetus's beating heart at 6 weeks of pregnancy and thus can confirm that the fetus is alive. Doctors may periodically use an ultrasound device to listen to the fetus's heartbeat. Or they may use a stethoscope designed to listen to a fetus's heartbeat (fetoscope). The fetoscope can detect the heartbeat as early as 18 to 20 weeks of pregnancy.

Ultrasonography can identify the sex of the fetus at 14 weeks of pregnancy. Ultrasonography is also used to see whether a woman is carrying more than one fetus and to identify abnormalities, such as a mislocated placenta (placenta previa) or an abnormal position of the fetus. Ultrasonography is used for guidance during certain procedures, such as prenatal diagnostic testing.

Toward the end of pregnancy, ultrasonography may be used to identify premature rupture of the fluid-filled membranes containing the fetus. Ultrasonography can provide information that helps doctors decide whether to perform a cesarean section.

Experts recommend that all pregnant women be vaccinated against the influenza virus during the influenza (flu) season.

Self-Care During Pregnancy

There is much a pregnant woman can do to take care of herself during pregnancy. If she has any questions about diet, the use of drugs or nutritional supplements, physical activity, and sexual intercourse during pregnancy, she can talk with her doctor.

Diet and Weight: During pregnancy, the woman's diet should be adequate and nutritious. Most women should add about 250 calo-

ries to their daily diet to provide nourishment for the developing fetus. The diet should be well balanced, including fresh fruits, grains, and vegetables. High-fiber, sugar-free cereals are a good choice. The fetus has first choice of nutrients, but the pregnant woman must make sure that the fetus has something worthwhile to choose from. In the United States, most women get enough salt in their diet, without adding salt to their food at the table. Commercially prepared foods often contain excessive amounts of salt and should be consumed sparingly. Dieting to lose weight during pregnancy is not recommended, even for obese women, because some weight gain is essential for the fetus to develop normally. Dieting reduces the supply of nutrients to the fetus.

An average-size woman should gain about 25 to 30 pounds during pregnancy. Gaining more than 30 to 35 pounds puts fat on the woman and the fetus. Because controlling weight gain is more difficult later in pregnancy, a woman should try to avoid gaining most of the weight during the first months. On the other hand, not gaining weight is an ominous sign, especially if the total weight gain is less than 10 pounds. Growth of the fetus may be slowed or inadequate.

Sometimes a pregnant woman gains weight because she is retaining fluid. Fluid may be retained because when she stands, the enlarging uterus interferes with blood flow from the legs back to the heart. Lying on one side, preferably the left side, for 30 to 45 minutes 2 or 3 times a day may relieve this problem.

Drugs and Dietary Supplements: Generally, avoiding drugs during pregnancy is best. However, drugs must sometimes be used.▲ A pregnant woman should check with her doctor before taking any drug—including nonprescription (over-the-counter) drugs, such as aspirin, or medicinal herbs—particularly during the first 3 months.

Pregnancy doubles the amount of iron needed. Most pregnant women need an iron supplement, because the average woman does not absorb enough iron from food to meet the requirements of pregnancy, even when iron from food is combined with iron already stored in her body. If a woman has anemia or develops anemia during pregnancy, she may need to take a larger dose of iron than other

▲ see page 1458

pregnant women. Iron supplements may cause mild stomach upset and constipation.

All pregnant women should take a folic acid supplement (usually included in prenatal vitamins) daily. Ideally, the folic acid supplement is begun before pregnancy. A deficiency of folic acid increases the risk of having a baby with a birth defect of the brain or spinal cord, such as spina bifida. Women who have had a baby with spina bifida should start taking a high dose of folic acid before they become pregnant. Excessive ultraviolet (UV) light exposure, particularly in fair-skinned women, can decrease folic acid levels. Women who have taken oral contraceptives are more likely to develop a folic acid deficiency, but there is no proof that they are more likely to have a baby with spina bifida.

If the diet is adequate, other vitamin supplements may not be needed, although most doctors recommend that pregnant women take a prenatal multivitamin containing iron and folic acid daily.

Physical Activity: Many pregnant women are concerned about moderating their activities. However, most women can continue their usual activities and exercises throughout pregnancy. Mildly strenuous sports, such as swimming and brisk walking, are good choices. Vigorous activities, such as running and horseback riding, are also possible if performed cautiously. But contact sports should be avoided.

Sexual Intercourse: Sexual desire may increase or decrease during pregnancy. Sexual intercourse is safe throughout pregnancy unless a woman has vaginal bleeding, pain, leakage of amniotic fluid, or uterine contractions. In such cases, sexual intercourse should be avoided.

Preparing for Breastfeeding: Women who are planning to breastfeed do not need to do anything to prepare their nipples for breastfeeding during pregnancy.▲ Expressing fluids from the breast manually before delivery may lead to an infection of the breast (mastitis) or even early labor. The body prepares the areola and nipple for breastfeeding by secreting a lubricant to protect the surface. This lubricant should not be rubbed off. Observing and talking with women who have breastfed successfully may be instructive and encouraging.

CHAPTER 258

High-Risk Pregnancy

There is no formal or universally accepted definition of a "high-risk" pregnancy. Generally, however, a high-risk pregnancy involves at least one of the following: The woman or baby is more likely to become ill or die than usual, or complications before or after delivery are more likely to occur than usual.

Certain conditions or characteristics, called risk factors, make a pregnancy high risk. Doctors identify these factors and use a scoring system to determine the degree of risk for a particular woman. Identifying high-risk pregnancies ensures that women who most need medical care receive it.

Risk Factors Present Before Pregnancy

Some risk factors are present before women become pregnant. These risk factors include certain physical and social characteristics of women, problems that have occurred in previous pregnancies, and certain disorders women already have.

Physical Characteristics

The age, weight, and height of women affect risk during pregnancy. Girls aged 15 and younger are at increased risk of preeclampsia (a type of high blood pressure that develops during pregnancy). Young girls are also at increased risk of having underweight (small-for-gestational-age) or undernourished babies. Women aged 35 and older are at increased risk of problems such as high blood pressure, gestational diabetes (diabetes that develops during pregnancy), and complications during labor.

Women who weigh less than 100 pounds before becoming pregnant are more likely to have small, underweight babies. Obese women are more likely to have very large babies, which may be difficult to deliver. Also, obese

▲ see page 1486

women are more likely to develop gestational diabetes and preeclampsia.

Women shorter than 5 feet are more likely to have a small pelvis, which may make movement of the fetus through the pelvis and vagina (birth canal) difficult during labor. For example, the fetus's shoulder is more likely to lodge against the pubic bone. This complication is called shoulder dystocia.▲ Also, short women are more likely to have preterm labor and a baby who has not grown as much as expected.

Structural abnormalities in the reproductive organs increase the risk of a miscarriage. Examples are a double uterus or a weak (incompetent) cervix that tends to open (dilate) as the fetus grows.

Social Characteristics

Being unmarried or in a lower socioeconomic group increases the risk of problems during pregnancy. The reason these characteristics increase risk is unclear but is probably related to other characteristics that are more common among these women. For example, these women are more likely to smoke and less likely to consume a healthy diet and to obtain appropriate medical care.

Problems in a Previous Pregnancy

When women have had a problem in one pregnancy, they are more likely to have a problem, often the same one, in subsequent pregnancies. Such problems include having had a premature baby, an underweight baby, a baby that weighed more than 10 pounds, a baby with birth defects, a previous miscarriage, a late (postterm) delivery (after 42 weeks of pregnancy), Rh incompatibility that required a blood transfusion to the fetus, or a delivery that required a cesarean section. If women have had a baby who died shortly after birth, they are also more likely to have problems in subsequent pregnancies.

Women may have a condition that tends to make the same problem recur. For example, women with diabetes are more likely to have babies that weigh more than 10 pounds at birth.

Women who had a baby with a genetic disorder or birth defect are more likely to have another baby with a similar problem. Genetic testing of the baby, even if stillborn, and of both parents may be appropriate before another pregnancy is attempted.■ If these women become pregnant again, tests such as ultrason-ography, chorionic villus sampling, and amniocentesis may help determine whether the fetus has a genetic disorder or birth defect.

Having had six or more pregnancies increases the risks of very rapid labor and excessive bleeding after delivery. It also increases the risk of a mislocated placenta (placenta previa).★

Disorders Present Before Pregnancy

Before becoming pregnant, women may have a disorder that can increase the risk of problems during pregnancy. These women should talk with a doctor and try to get in the best physical condition possible before they become pregnant. After they become pregnant, they may need special care, often from an interdisciplinary team. The team may include an obstetrician (who may also be a specialist in the disorder), a specialist in the disorder, and other health care practitioners (such as nutritionists).

Heart Disease: Most women who have heart disease—including heart valve disorders (such as mitral valve prolapse) and some birth defects of the heart—can safely give birth to healthy children, without any permanent ill effects on heart function or life span. However, women who have heart failure before pregnancy are at considerable risk of problems.

Pregnancy requires the heart to work harder. Consequently, pregnancy may worsen heart disease or cause heart disease to produce symptoms for the first time. Usually, serious problems, including death of the woman or fetus, occur only when heart disease is severe before the woman becomes pregnant. About 1% of women who have severe heart disease before becoming pregnant die as a result of the pregnancy, usually because of heart failure.

The risk of problems increases throughout pregnancy as demands on the heart increase. Pregnant women with heart disease may become unusually tired and may need to limit their activities. Rarely, women with severe heart disease are advised to have an abortion early in pregnancy. Risk is also increased during labor and delivery. After delivery, women with severe heart disease may not be out of danger for at least 6 months, depending on the type of heart disease.

▲ see page 1473   ■ see page 1429

★ see page 1455

Heart disease in pregnant women may affect the fetus. The fetus may be born prematurely. Women with birth defects of the heart are more likely to have children with similar birth defects. Ultrasonography can detect some of these defects before the fetus is born. If severe heart disease in a pregnant woman suddenly worsens, the fetus may die.

During labor, women who have severe heart disease may be given an epidural anesthetic, which blocks sensation in the lower spinal cord and prevents women from pushing. Pushing during labor strains the heart, because it increases the amount of blood returning to the heart. Because pushing is not possible, the baby may have to be delivered with forceps.

For women with some types of heart disease, pregnancy is inadvisable because it so increases their risk of death. Primary pulmonary hypertension and Eisenmenger's syndrome are examples. If women who have one of these disorders become pregnant, doctors advise them to terminate the pregnancy as early as possible.

High Blood Pressure: Women who have high blood pressure (chronic hypertension) before they become pregnant are more likely to have potentially serious problems during pregnancy. These problems include preeclampsia (a type of high blood pressure that develops during pregnancy),▲ worsening of high blood pressure, a fetus that does not grow as much as expected, premature detachment of the placenta from the uterus (placental abruption), and stillbirth.

For most women with moderately high blood pressure (140/90 to 150/100 millimeters of mercury [mm Hg]), treatment with antihypertensive drugs is not recommended. Such treatment does not seem to reduce the risk of preeclampsia, premature detachment of the placenta, or a stillbirth nor to improve the growth of the fetus. However, some women are treated to prevent pregnancy from causing episodes of even higher blood pressure (which require hospitalization).

For women whose blood pressure is higher than 150/100 mm Hg, treatment with antihypertensive drugs is recommended.■ Treatment can reduce the risk of stroke and other complications due to very high blood pressure. Treatment is also recommended for women who have high blood pressure and a kidney disorder because if high blood pressure is not controlled well, the kidneys may be damaged further.

Most antihypertensive drugs used to treat high blood pressure can be used safely during pregnancy. However, angiotensin-converting enzyme (ACE) inhibitors are discontinued during pregnancy, particularly during the last two trimesters. These drugs can cause severe kidney damage in the fetus. As a result, the baby may die shortly after birth.

During pregnancy, women with high blood pressure are monitored closely to make sure blood pressure is well controlled, the kidneys are functioning normally, and the fetus is growing normally. However, premature detachment of the placenta cannot be prevented or anticipated. Often, a baby must be delivered early to prevent stillbirth or complications due to high blood pressure (such as stroke) in the woman.

Anemia: Having a hereditary anemia, such as sickle cell disease, hemoglobin S-C disease, and some thalassemias, increases the risk of problems during pregnancy. Before delivery, blood tests are routinely performed to check for hemoglobin abnormalities in women who are at increased risk of having these abnormalities because of race, ethnic background, or family history. Chorionic villus sampling or amniocentesis may be performed to detect a hemoglobin abnormality in the fetus.

Women who have sickle cell disease are particularly at risk of developing infections during pregnancy. Pneumonia, urinary tract infections, and infections of the uterus are the most common. About one third of pregnant women who have sickle cell disease develop high blood pressure during pregnancy. A sudden, severe attack of pain, called sickle cell crisis, may occur during pregnancy as at any other time. Heart failure and blockage of arteries of the lungs by blood clots (pulmonary embolism), which may be life threatening, may also occur. Bleeding during labor or after delivery may be more severe. The fetus may grow slowly or not as much as expected. The fetus may even die. The more severe sickle cell disease was before pregnancy, the higher the risk of health problems for pregnant women and the fetus and the higher the risk of death for the fetus during pregnancy. With regular blood transfusions, women are less likely to have sickle cell crises but are more likely to reject the transfused blood. This condition, called alloimmunization, can be life threatening. Also,

---

▲ see page 1452   ■ see table on page 138

transfusions to pregnant women do not reduce risks for the fetus.

Kidney Disorders: Women with a severe kidney disorder before pregnancy are more likely to have problems during pregnancy. Kidney function may rapidly worsen during pregnancy. High blood pressure, which often accompanies a kidney disorder, may also worsen, and preeclampsia (a type of high blood pressure that develops during pregnancy) may develop. The fetus may not grow as much as expected or may be stillborn. In pregnant women who have a kidney disorder, kidney function and blood pressure are monitored closely as is the growth of the fetus. Often, the baby must be delivered early.

Women who have had a kidney transplant that has been in place for 2 or more years are usually able to safely give birth to healthy babies if their kidneys are functioning normally, if they have had no episodes of rejection, and if their blood pressure is normal. Many women who have a kidney disorder and who undergo hemodialysis regularly can also give birth to healthy babies.

Seizure Disorders: For most women who take anticonvulsants to treat a seizure disorder, the frequency of seizures does not change during pregnancy. However, sometimes the dose of the anticonvulsant must be increased.

Taking anticonvulsants increases the risk of birth defects.▲ Women who take anticonvulsants should discuss the risk of birth defects with an expert in the field, preferably before they become pregnant. Some women may be able to safely discontinue anticonvulsants during pregnancy, but most women should continue to take the drugs. The risks resulting from not taking the drugs (resulting in more frequent seizures, which can harm the fetus and the woman) usually outweigh the risks resulting from taking them during pregnancy.

Sexually Transmitted Diseases: Women who have a sexually transmitted disease may have problems during pregnancy. Chlamydial infection may cause preterm labor and premature rupture of the membranes containing the fetus. It can also cause conjunctivitis in newborns, as can gonorrhea. Syphilis in pregnant women may be transmitted to the fetus through the placenta. Syphilis can cause several birth defects.

About one fourth of pregnant women who have untreated human immunodeficiency virus (HIV) infection, which causes AIDS, transmit it to their baby.■ Experts recommend that women with HIV infection take antiretroviral drugs during pregnancy. When pregnant women take these drugs, the risk of transmitting HIV to their baby is reduced to less than 2%. For some women with HIV infection, delivery by cesarean section, planned in advance, may further reduce the risk of transmitting HIV to the baby. Pregnancy does not seem to accelerate the progress of HIV infection in women.

Genital herpes can be transmitted to a baby during a vaginal delivery. A baby who is infected with herpes can develop a life-threatening brain infection called herpes encephalitis. If herpes produces sores in the genital area late in pregnancy, women are usually advised to give birth by cesarean section, so that the virus is not transmitted to the baby. If no sores are present, the risk of transmission is very low.

Diabetes: For women who have diabetes before they become pregnant, the risks of complications during pregnancy depend on how long diabetes has been present and whether complications of diabetes, such as high blood pressure and kidney damage, are present. (In some women, diabetes develops during pregnancy; this disorder is called gestational diabetes.★)

The risk of complications during pregnancy can be reduced by controlling the level of sugar (glucose) in the blood. The level should be kept as nearly normal as possible throughout pregnancy. Measures to control the blood sugar level (such as diet, exercise, and insulin) should be started before pregnancy.● Most pregnant women are asked to measure their blood sugar level several times a day at home. Controlling diabetes is particularly important late in pregnancy. Then, the blood sugar level tends to increase because the body becomes less responsive to insulin. A higher dose of insulin is usually needed.

If diabetes is poorly controlled very early in the pregnancy, the risks of early miscarriage and significant birth defects are increased. When diabetes is poorly controlled later in pregnancy, the fetus is large and the risk of stillbirth is increased. A large fetus is less likely to pass easily through the vagina and is

▲ see table on page 1460
■ see page 1573
★ see page 1452
● see page 965

more likely to be injured during vaginal delivery. Consequently, delivery by cesarean section is often necessary. The risk of preeclampsia (a type of high blood pressure that occurs during pregnancy) is also increased for women with diabetes.

The fetus's lungs tend to mature slowly. If an early delivery is being considered (for example, because the fetus is large), the doctor may remove and analyze a sample of the fluid that surrounds the fetus (amniotic fluid). This procedure, called amniocentesis, helps the doctor determine whether the fetus's lungs are mature enough for the newborn to breathe air.

Newborns of women with diabetes are at increased risk of having low sugar, low calcium, and high bilirubin levels in the blood. Hospital staff members measure the levels of these substances and observe the newborns for symptoms of these abnormalities.

For women with diabetes, the requirement for insulin drops dramatically immediately after delivery. But the requirement usually returns to what it was before pregnancy within about 1 week.

Liver and Gallbladder Disorders: Women who have chronic viral hepatitis or cirrhosis (scarring of the liver) are more likely to miscarry or to give birth prematurely. Cirrhosis can cause varicose veins to develop around the esophagus (esophageal varices). Pregnancy slightly increases the risk of massive bleeding from these veins, especially during the last 3 months of pregnancy.

Pregnant women who develop gallstones are closely monitored. If a gallstone blocks the gallbladder or causes an infection, surgery may be necessary. This surgery is usually safe for pregnant women and the fetus.

Asthma: In about half of the women who have asthma and become pregnant, the frequency or severity of asthma attacks does not change during pregnancy. About one fourth of the women improve during pregnancy, and about one fourth get worse. If pregnant women with severe asthma are treated with prednisone, the risk that the fetus will not grow as much as expected or will be born prematurely is increased.

Because asthma can change during pregnancy, doctors may ask women with asthma to use a peak flow meter to monitor their breathing more often. Pregnant women with asthma should see their doctor regularly so that treatment can be adjusted as needed. Maintaining good control of asthma is impor-

tant. Inadequate treatment can result in serious problems. Cromolyn, bronchodilators (such as albuterol), and corticosteroids (such as beclomethasone) can be taken during pregnancy. Inhalation is the preferred way for taking these drugs. When inhaled, the drugs affect mainly the lungs and affect the whole body and the fetus less. Aminophylline (taken by mouth or given intravenously) and theophylline (taken by mouth) are occasionally used during pregnancy. Corticosteroids are taken by mouth only when other treatments are ineffective. Being vaccinated against the influenza virus during the influenza (flu) season is particularly important for pregnant women with asthma.

Autoimmune Disorders: The abnormal antibodies produced in autoimmune disorders can cross the placenta and cause problems in the fetus. Pregnancy affects different autoimmune disorders in different ways.

Systemic lupus erythematosus (lupus) may appear for the first time, worsen, or become less severe during pregnancy. How a pregnancy affects the course of lupus cannot be predicted, but the most common time for flare-ups is immediately after delivery.

Women who develop lupus often have a history of repeated miscarriages, fetuses that do not grow as much as expected, and preterm delivery. If women have complications due to lupus (such as kidney damage or high blood pressure), the risk of death for the fetus or newborn is increased.

In pregnant women, lupus antibodies may cross the placenta to the fetus. As a result, the fetus may have a very slow heart rate, anemia, a low platelet count, or a low white blood cell count. However, these antibodies gradually disappear over several weeks after the baby is born, and the problems they cause resolve except for the slow heart rate.

In **Graves' disease,** antibodies stimulate the thyroid gland to produce excess thyroid hormone. These antibodies can cross the placenta and stimulate the thyroid gland in the fetus. As a result, the fetus may have a rapid heart rate and may not grow as much as expected. The fetus's thyroid gland may enlarge, forming a goiter. Very rarely, a goiter may be so large that it interferes with delivery through the vagina.

Usually, women with Graves' disease take the lowest possible effective dose of propylthiouracil, which slows the activity of the thyroid gland. Physical examinations and measurements of thyroid hormone levels are performed regularly because propylthiouracil crosses the placenta and may prevent the fetus from producing enough thyroid hormone. Often, Graves' disease becomes less severe during the 3rd trimester, so the dose of propylthiouracil can be reduced or stopped. If necessary, the thyroid gland of pregnant women may be removed during the 2nd trimester. These women must begin taking thyroid hormone 24 hours after surgery. Taking this hormone causes no problems for the fetus.

Myasthenia gravis, which causes muscle weakness, does not usually cause serious or permanent complications during pregnancy. However, very rarely during labor, women who have myasthenia gravis may need help with breathing (assisted ventilation). The antibodies that cause this disorder can cross the placenta. So about one of five babies born to women with myasthenia gravis is born with the disorder. However, the resulting muscle weakness in the baby is usually temporary, because the antibodies from the mother gradually disappear and the baby does not produce antibodies of this type.

Idiopathic thrombocytopenic purpura can cause bleeding problems in pregnant women and their babies. If not treated during pregnancy, the disorder tends to become more severe. Corticosteroids, usually prednisone given by mouth, can increase the platelet count and improve blood clotting in pregnant women with this disorder. However, prednisone increases the risk that the fetus will not grow as much as expected or will be born prematurely. High doses of gamma globulin may be given intravenously shortly before delivery. This treatment temporarily increases the platelet count and improves blood clotting. As a result, labor can proceed safely, and women can have a vaginal delivery without uncontrolled bleeding. Pregnant women are given platelet transfusions only when delivery by a cesarean section is needed or when the platelet count is so low that severe bleeding may occur. Rarely, when the platelet count remains dangerously low despite treatment, the spleen, which normally traps and destroys old blood cells and platelets, is removed. The best time for this surgery is during the 2nd trimester.

The antibodies that cause the disorder may cross the placenta to the fetus, resulting rarely in a dangerously low platelet count before and immediately after birth. The baby may then bleed during labor and delivery and may, as a result, be injured or die, especially if bleeding occurs in the brain. The antibodies disappear within several weeks, and the baby's blood then clots normally.

Rheumatoid arthritis does not affect the fetus, but delivery may be difficult for women if arthritis has damaged their hip joints or lower (lumbar) spine. The symptoms of rheumatoid arthritis may lessen during pregnancy, but they usually return to their original level after pregnancy.

Fibroids: Fibroids in the uterus,▲ which are relatively common noncancerous tumors, may increase the risk of preterm labor, abnormal presentation of the fetus, a mislocated placenta (placenta previa), and repeated miscarriages. Rarely, fibroids interfere with the movement of the fetus through the vagina during labor.

Cancer: Because cancer tends to be life threatening and because delays in treatment may reduce the likelihood of successful treatment, cancer is usually treated the same way whether women are pregnant or not. Some of the usual treatments (surgery, chemotherapy drugs, and radiation therapy) may harm the fetus. Thus, some women may consider abortion. However, treatments can sometimes be timed so that risk to the fetus is reduced.

Risk Factors That Develop During Pregnancy

During pregnancy, a problem may occur or a condition may develop to make the pregnancy high risk. For example, pregnant women may be exposed to something that can produce birth defects (teratogens), such as radiation, certain chemicals, drugs, or infections. Or a disorder may develop. Some disorders are related to (are complications of) pregnancy.

Drugs

Some drugs taken during pregnancy cause birth defects.■ Examples are alcohol, isotretinoin (used to treat severe acne), some anticonvulsants, lithium, some antibiotics (such as streptomycin, kanamycin, and tetracycline), thalidomide, warfarin, and angiotensin-converting enzyme (ACE) inhibitors (taken during the last two trimesters). Taking drugs that block the actions of folic acid (such as the

---

▲ see page 1372   ■ see page 1458

immunosuppressant methotrexate or the antibiotic trimethoprim) can also cause birth defects (a deficiency of folic acid increases the
risk of having a baby with a birth defect). Using cocaine may cause birth defects, premature detachment of the placenta (placental
abruption), and premature birth. Smoking
cigarettes increases the risk of having a baby
with a low birth weight. Early in pregnancy,
women are asked if they are using any of these
drugs. Of particular concern are alcohol, cocaine, and cigarette smoking.

Disorders That Develop During Pregnancy

During pregnancy, women may develop disorders that are not directly related to pregnancy. Some disorders increase the risk of
problems for pregnant women or the fetus.
They include disorders that cause a high fever,
infections, and disorders that require abdominal surgery. Certain disorders are more likely
to occur during pregnancy because of the
many changes pregnancy causes in a woman's
body. Examples are thromboembolic disease,
anemia, and urinary tract infections.

Fevers: A disorder that causes a temperature
greater than 103° F (39.5° C) during the 1st
trimester increases the risk of a miscarriage
and defects of the brain or spinal cord in the
baby. Fever late in pregnancy increases the
risk of preterm labor.

Infections: Some infections that occur coincidentally during a pregnancy can cause birth
defects. German measles (rubella) can cause
birth defects, particularly of the heart and inner ear. Cytomegalovirus infection can cross
the placenta and damage the fetus's liver and
brain. Other viral infections that may harm
the fetus or cause birth defects include herpes
simplex and chickenpox (varicella). Toxoplasmosis, a protozoal infection, may cause miscarriage, death of the fetus, and serious birth
defects. Listeriosis, a bacterial infection, can
also harm the fetus. Bacterial infections of the
vagina (such as bacterial vaginosis) during
pregnancy may lead to preterm labor or premature rupture of the membranes containing
the fetus. Treatment of infections with antibiotics may reduce the likelihood of these problems.

Disorders That Require Surgery: During
pregnancy, a disorder that requires emergency
surgery involving the abdomen may develop.
This type of surgery increases the risk of
preterm labor and can cause a miscarriage, especially early in pregnancy. Thus, surgery is
usually delayed as long as possible unless the
woman's long-term health may be affected.

If appendicitis develops during pregnancy,
surgery to remove the appendix (appendectomy) is performed immediately because a
ruptured appendix may be fatal. An appendectomy is not likely to harm the fetus or cause a
miscarriage. However, appendicitis may be
difficult to recognize during pregnancy. The
cramping pain of appendicitis resembles uterine contractions, which are common during
pregnancy. The appendix is pushed higher in
the abdomen as the pregnancy progresses, so
the location of pain due to appendicitis may
not be what is expected.

If an ovarian cyst persists during pregnancy,
surgery is usually postponed until after the
12th week of pregnancy. The cyst may be producing hormones that are supporting the pregnancy and often disappears without treatment. However, if a cyst or another mass is
enlarging, surgery may be necessary before the
12th week. Such a mass may be cancerous.

Obstruction of the intestine during pregnancy can be very serious. If obstruction leads
to gangrene of the intestine and peritonitis
(inflammation of the membrane that lines the
abdominal cavity), a woman may miscarry
and her life is endangered. Exploratory surgery
is usually performed promptly when pregnant
women have symptoms of intestinal obstruction, particularly if they have had abdominal
surgery or an abdominal infection.

Thromboembolic Disease: In the United
States, thromboembolic disease is the leading
cause of death in pregnant women. In thromboembolic disease, blood clots form in blood
vessels. They may travel through the bloodstream and block an artery. The risk of developing thromboembolic disease is increased for
about 6 to 8 weeks after delivery. Most complications due to blood clots result from injuries that occur during delivery. The risk is
much greater after a cesarean section than after vaginal delivery.

Blood clots usually form in the superficial
veins of the legs as thrombophlebitis or in the
deep veins as deep vein thrombosis. Symptoms include swelling, pain in the calves, and
tenderness. The severity of the symptoms
does not correlate with the severity of the disease. A clot can move from the legs to the
lungs, where it may block one or more arteries
in the lungs. This blockage, called pulmonary
embolism, can be life threatening. If a clot

blocks an artery supplying the brain, a stroke can result. Blood clots can also develop in the pelvis.

Women who have had a blood clot during a previous pregnancy may be given heparin (an anticoagulant) during subsequent pregnancies to prevent blood clots from forming. If women have symptoms suggesting a blood clot, Doppler ultrasonography may be performed to check for clots. If a blood clot is detected, heparin is started without delay. Heparin may be injected into a vein (intravenously) or under the skin (subcutaneously). Heparin does not cross the placenta and cannot harm the fetus. Treatment is continued for 6 to 8 weeks after delivery, when the risk of blood clots is high. After delivery, warfarin may be used instead of heparin. Warfarin can be taken by mouth, has a lower risk of complications than heparin, and can be taken by women who are breastfeeding.

If pulmonary embolism is suspected, a lung ventilation and perfusion scan▲ may be performed to confirm the diagnosis. This procedure involves injecting a tiny amount of a radioactive substance into a vein. The procedure is safe during pregnancy because the dose of the radioactive substance is so small. If the diagnosis of pulmonary embolism is still uncertain, pulmonary angiography is required.

Anemia: Most pregnant women develop some degree of anemia because they have an iron deficiency. The need for iron doubles during pregnancy, because iron is needed to make red blood cells in the fetus. Anemia may also develop during pregnancy because of a folic acid deficiency. Anemia can usually be prevented or treated by taking iron and folic acid supplements during pregnancy. However, if anemia becomes severe and persists, the blood's capacity to carry oxygen is decreased. As a result, the fetus may not receive enough oxygen, which is needed for normal growth and development, especially of the brain. Pregnant women who have severe anemia may become excessively tired, short of breath, and light-headed. The risk of preterm labor is increased. A normal amount of bleeding during labor and delivery can cause the anemia in these women to become dangerously severe. Women with anemia are more likely to develop infections after delivery. Also, if folic acid is deficient, the risk of having a baby with a birth defect of the brain or spinal cord, such as spina bifida, is increased.

Urinary Tract Infections: Urinary tract infections are common during pregnancy, probably because the enlarging uterus slows the flow of urine by pressing against the tubes that connect the kidneys to the bladder (ureters). When urine flow is slow, bacteria may not be flushed out of the urinary tract, increasing the risk of an infection. These infections increase the risk of preterm labor and premature rupture of the membranes containing the fetus. Sometimes an infection in the bladder or ureters spreads up the urinary tract and reaches a kidney, causing an infection there.■ Treatment consists of antibiotic therapy.

Pregnancy Complications

Pregnancy complications are problems that occur only during pregnancy. They may affect the woman, the fetus, or both and may occur at different times during the pregnancy. For example, complications such as a mislocated placenta (placenta previa) or premature detachment of the placenta from the uterus (placental abruption) can cause bleeding from the vagina during the last 3 months of pregnancy. Women who bleed at this time are at risk of losing the baby or of bleeding excessively (hemorrhaging) or dying during labor and delivery. However, most pregnancy complications can be effectively treated.

Some problems that result from hormonal changes during pregnancy cause only minor, transient symptoms in pregnant women. For example, the normal hormonal effects of pregnancy can slow the movement of bile through the bile ducts. Cholestasis of pregnancy may result. The most obvious symptom is itching all over the body (usually in the last few months of pregnancy). No rash develops. If itching is intense, cholestyramine may be given. The disorder usually resolves after delivery but tends to recur in subsequent pregnancies.

Hyperemesis Gravidarum: Hyperemesis gravidarum is extremely severe nausea and excessive vomiting during pregnancy. Hyperemesis gravidarum differs from ordinary morning sickness. If women vomit often and have nausea to such an extent that they lose weight and become dehydrated, they have hyperemesis gravidarum. If women vomit occasionally but gain weight and are not dehydrated, they do not have hyperemesis gravidarum. The cause of hyperemesis gravidarum is unknown.

Because hyperemesis gravidarum can be life threatening to pregnant women and the fetus,

---

▲ see page 287   ■ see page 1479

women who have it are hospitalized. An intravenous line is inserted into a vein to give fluids, sugar (glucose), electrolytes, and occasionally vitamins. Women who have this complication are not allowed to eat or drink anything for at least 24 hours. Sedatives, antiemetics, and other drugs are given as needed. After women are rehydrated and vomiting has subsided, they can begin eating frequent, small portions of bland foods. The size of the portions is increased if they can tolerate more food. Usually, vomiting stops within a few days. If symptoms recur, the treatment is repeated. Rarely, if weight loss continues and symptoms persist despite treatment, women are fed via a tube passed through the nose and down the throat to the small intestine for as long as necessary.

Preeclampsia: About 5% of pregnant women develop preeclampsia (toxemia of pregnancy). In this complication, an increase in blood pressure is accompanied by protein in the urine (proteinuria). Preeclampsia usually develops between the 20th week of pregnancy and the end of the first week after delivery. The cause of preeclampsia is unknown. But it is more common among women who are pregnant for the first time, who are carrying two or more fetuses, who have had preeclampsia in a previous pregnancy, who already have high blood pressure or a blood vessel disorder, or who have sickle cell disease. It is also more common among girls aged 15 and younger and among women aged 35 and older.

A variation of severe preeclampsia, called the HELLP syndrome, occurs in some women. It consists of the following:

• *h*emolysis (the breakdown of red blood cells)

• *e*levated levels of *l*iver enzymes, indicating liver damage

• *l*ow *p*latelet count, making blood less able to clot and increasing the risk of bleeding during and after labor.

In 1 of 200 women who have preeclampsia, blood pressure becomes high enough to cause seizures; this condition is called **eclampsia.** One fourth of the cases of eclampsia occur after delivery, usually in the first 2 to 4 days. If not treated promptly, eclampsia may be fatal.

Preeclampsia may lead to premature detachment of the placenta from the uterus (placental abruption). Babies of women who have preeclampsia are 4 or 5 times more likely to have problems soon after birth than babies of women who do not have this complication. Babies may be small because the placenta malfunctions or because they are born prematurely.

If mild preeclampsia develops early in the pregnancy, bed rest at home may be sufficient, but such women should see their doctor frequently. If preeclampsia worsens, women are usually hospitalized. There, they are kept in bed and monitored closely until the fetus is mature enough to be delivered safely. Antihypertensives may be needed.▲ A few hours before delivery, magnesium sulfate may be given intravenously to reduce the risk of seizures. If preeclampsia develops near the due date, labor is usually induced and the baby is delivered.

If preeclampsia is severe, the baby may be delivered by cesarean section, which is the quickest way, unless the cervix is already opened (dilated) enough for a prompt vaginal delivery. A prompt delivery reduces the risk of complications for women and the fetus. If blood pressure is high, drugs to lower blood pressure, such as hydralazine or labetalol, may be given intravenously before delivery is attempted. Treatment of the HELLP syndrome is usually the same as that of severe preeclampsia.

After delivery, women who have had preeclampsia or eclampsia are closely monitored for 2 to 4 days because they are at increased risk of seizures. As their condition gradually improves, they are encouraged to walk. They may remain in the hospital for a few days, depending on the severity of the preeclampsia and its complications. After returning home, these women may need to take drugs to lower blood pressure. Typically, they have a checkup at least every 2 weeks for the first few months after delivery. Their blood pressure may remain high for 6 to 8 weeks. If it remains high longer, the cause may be unrelated to preeclampsia.

Gestational Diabetes: About 1 to 3% of pregnant women develop diabetes during pregnancy. This disorder is called gestational diabetes. Unrecognized and untreated, gestational diabetes can increase the risk of health problems for pregnant women and the fetus and the risk of death for the fetus. Gestational diabetes is more common among obese women and among certain ethnic groups, particularly Native Americans, Pacific Islanders, and women of Mexican, Indian, and Asian descent.

▲ see table on page 1460

Most women with gestational diabetes develop it because they cannot produce enough insulin as the need for insulin increases late in the pregnancy. More insulin is needed to control the increasing level of sugar (glucose) in the blood. Some women may have had diabetes before becoming pregnant, but it was not recognized until they became pregnant.

Some doctors routinely screen all pregnant women for gestational diabetes. Other doctors screen only women who have risk factors for diabetes, such as obesity and certain ethnic backgrounds. A blood test is used to measure the blood sugar level. Women who have gestational diabetes are usually taught to measure their blood sugar levels with a home blood sugar monitoring device.

Treatment consists of eliminating high-sugar foods from the diet, eating to avoid excess weight gain during the pregnancy, and, if the blood sugar level is high, taking insulin. After delivery, gestational diabetes usually disappears. However, many women who have gestational diabetes develop type 2 diabetes as they become older.

Rh Incompatibility: Rh incompatibility occurs when a pregnant woman has Rh-negative blood and the fetus has Rh-positive blood, inherited from a father who has Rh-positive blood. In about 13% of marriages in the United States, the man has Rh-positive blood and the woman has Rh-negative blood.

The Rh factor is a molecule that occurs on the surface of red blood cells of some people. Blood is Rh-positive if red blood cells have the Rh factor and Rh-negative if they do not. Problems can occur if the fetus's Rh-positive blood enters the woman's bloodstream. The woman's immune system may recognize the fetus's red blood cells as foreign and produce antibodies, called Rh antibodies, to destroy the fetus's red blood cells. The production of these antibodies is called Rh sensitization.

During a first pregnancy, Rh sensitization is unlikely, because no significant amount of the fetus's blood is likely to enter the woman's bloodstream until delivery. So the fetus or newborn rarely has problems. However, once a woman is sensitized, problems are more likely with each subsequent pregnancy in which the fetus's blood is Rh-positive. In each pregnancy, the woman produces Rh antibodies earlier and in larger amounts.

If Rh antibodies cross the placenta to the fetus, they may destroy some of the fetus's red blood cells. If red blood cells are destroyed

faster than the fetus can produce new ones, the fetus can develop anemia. Such destruction is called hemolytic disease of the fetus (erythroblastosis fetalis) or of the newborn (erythroblastosis neonatorum).▲ In severe cases, the fetus may die.

At the first visit to a doctor during a pregnancy, women are screened to determine whether they have Rh-positive or Rh-negative blood. If they have Rh-negative blood, their blood is checked for Rh antibodies and the father's blood type is determined. If he has Rh-positive blood, Rh sensitization is a risk. In such cases, the blood of pregnant women is checked for Rh antibodies periodically during the pregnancy. The pregnancy can proceed as usual as long as no antibodies are detected.

If antibodies are detected, steps may be taken to protect the fetus, depending on how high the antibody level is. If the level becomes too high, amniocentesis may be performed. In this procedure, a needle is inserted through the skin to withdraw fluid from the amniotic sac. The level of bilirubin (a yellow pigment resulting from the normal breakdown of red blood cells) is measured in the fluid sample. If this level is too high, the fetus is given a blood transfusion. Usually, additional transfusions are given until the fetus is mature enough to be safely delivered. Then labor is induced. The baby may need additional transfusions after birth. Sometimes no transfusions are needed until after birth.

As a precaution, women who have Rh-negative blood are given an injection of Rh antibodies at 28 weeks of pregnancy and within 72 hours after delivery of a baby who has Rh-positive blood, even after a miscarriage or an abortion. The antibodies given are called $Rh_0(D)$ immune globulin. This treatment destroys any red blood cells from the baby that may have entered the bloodstream of the women. Thus, there are no red blood cells from the baby to trigger the production of antibodies by these women, and subsequent pregnancies are usually not endangered.

Fatty Liver of Pregnancy: This rare disorder occurs toward the end of pregnancy. The cause is unknown. Symptoms include nausea, vomiting, abdominal discomfort, and jaundice. The disorder may rapidly worsen, and liver failure may develop. Diagnosis is based on results of liver function tests and may be con-

▲ see box on page 1506

Problems With the Placenta

Normally, the placenta is located in the upper part of the uterus, firmly attached to the uterine wall until after delivery of the baby. In placental abruption (abruptio placentae), the placenta detaches from the uterine wall prematurely, causing the uterus to bleed and reducing the fetus's supply of oxygen and nutrients. Women who have this complication are hospitalized, and the baby may be delivered early. In placenta previa, the placenta is located over or near the cervix, in the lower part of the uterus. It may cause painless bleeding that suddenly begins late in pregnancy. The bleeding may become profuse. The baby is usually delivered by cesarean section.

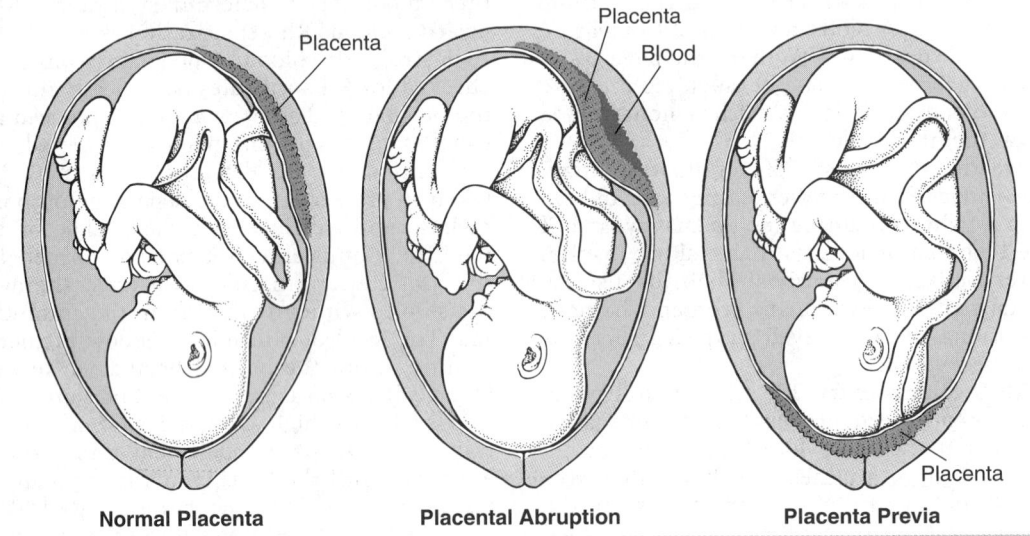

Placenta

Placenta
Blood

Placenta

Placenta

Normal Placenta   **Placental Abruption**   **Placenta Previa**

firmed by a liver biopsy. The doctor may advise immediate termination of the pregnancy. The risk of death for pregnant women and the fetus is high, but those who survive recover completely. Usually, the disorder does not recur in subsequent pregnancies.

Peripartum Cardiomyopathy: The heart's walls may be damaged late in pregnancy or after delivery, causing peripartum cardiomyopathy. The cause is unknown. Peripartum cardiomyopathy tends to occur in women who have had several pregnancies, who are older, who are carrying twins, or who have preeclampsia. In some women, heart function does not return to normal after pregnancy. They may develop peripartum cardiomyopathy in subsequent pregnancies. These women should not become pregnant again. Peripartum cardiomyopathy can result in heart failure,▲ which is treated.

▲ see page 150

Problems With Amniotic Fluid: Too much amniotic fluid (polyhydramnios) in the membranes containing the fetus (amniotic sac) stretches the uterus and puts pressure on the diaphragm of pregnant women. This complication can lead to severe breathing problems for the women or to preterm labor.

Too much fluid tends to accumulate when pregnant women have diabetes, are carrying more than one fetus (multiple pregnancy), or produce Rh antibodies to the fetus's blood. Another cause is birth defects in the fetus, especially a blocked esophagus or defects of the brain and spinal cord (such as spina bifida). About half the time, the cause is unknown.

Too little amniotic fluid (oligohydramnios) can also cause problems. If the amount of fluid is greatly reduced, the fetus's lungs may be immature and the fetus may be compressed, resulting in deformities; this combination of conditions is called Potter's syndrome.

Too little amniotic fluid tends to develop when the fetus has birth defects in the urinary tract, has not grown as much as expected, or dies. Other causes include the use of angiotensin-converting enzyme (ACE) inhibitors, such as enalapril or captopril, in the 2nd and 3rd trimesters. These drugs are given during pregnancy only when they must be used to treat severe heart failure or high blood pressure. Taking nonsteroidal anti-inflammatory drugs (NSAIDs) late in pregnancy can also reduce the amount of amniotic fluid.

Placenta Previa: Placenta previa is implantation of the placenta over or near the cervix, in the lower rather than the upper part of the uterus. The placenta may completely or partially cover the opening of the cervix. Placenta previa occurs in 1 of 200 deliveries, usually in women who have had more than one preg-

nancy or who have structural abnormalities of the uterus, such as fibroids.

Placenta previa can cause painless bleeding from the vagina that suddenly begins late in pregnancy. The blood may be bright red. Bleeding may become profuse, endangering the life of the woman and the fetus.

Ultrasonography helps doctors identify placenta previa and distinguish it from a placenta that has detached prematurely (placental abruption).

When bleeding is profuse, women may be hospitalized until delivery, especially if the placenta is located over the cervix. Women who bleed profusely may need repeated blood transfusions. When bleeding is slight and delivery is not imminent, doctors typically ad-

---

Ectopic Pregnancy: A Mislocated Pregnancy

Normally, an egg is fertilized in the fallopian tube and becomes implanted in the uterus. However, if the tube is narrowed or blocked, the egg may move slowly or become stuck. The fertilized egg may never reach the uterus, resulting in an ectopic pregnancy. Ectopic pregnancies usually develop in one of the fallopian tubes (as a tubal pregnancy) but may develop in other locations. A fetus in an ectopic pregnancy cannot survive.

One of 100 to 200 pregnancies is an ectopic pregnancy. Risk factors for an ectopic pregnancy include having had a disorder of the fallopian tubes, pelvic inflammatory disease, a previous ectopic pregnancy, exposure to diethylstilbestrol as a fetus, or a tubal ligation (a sterilization procedure) that was unsuccessful or has been surgically reversed.

Symptoms include unexpected vaginal bleeding and cramping. The fetus may grow enough to rupture the structure containing it. If the fallopian tube ruptures (typically after about 6 to 8 weeks), a woman usually feels severe pain in the lower abdomen and may faint. If the tube ruptures later (after about 12 to 16 weeks), the risk of death for the woman is increased, because the fetus and placenta are larger and more blood is lost.

If a woman is unsure she is pregnant, a pregnancy test is performed. If she is pregnant, ultrasonography is performed to determine the location of the fetus. If the uterus is empty, doctors may suspect an ectopic pregnancy. If ultrasonography shows the fetus in a location other than the uterus, the diagnosis is confirmed. Doctors may use a viewing tube called a laparoscope, inserted through a small incision just below the navel, to view the ectopic pregnancy directly.

An ectopic pregnancy must be ended as soon as possible to save the life of the woman. In most women, the fetus and placenta in an ectopic pregnancy must be removed surgically, usually with a laparoscope but sometimes through an incision in the abdomen (in a procedure called laparotomy). Rarely, the uterus is so damaged that a hysterectomy is required. Sometimes, the drug methotrexate, usually given in a single injection, can be used instead of surgery. The drug causes the ectopic pregnancy to shrink and disappear. Occasionally, surgery is needed in addition to methotrexate.

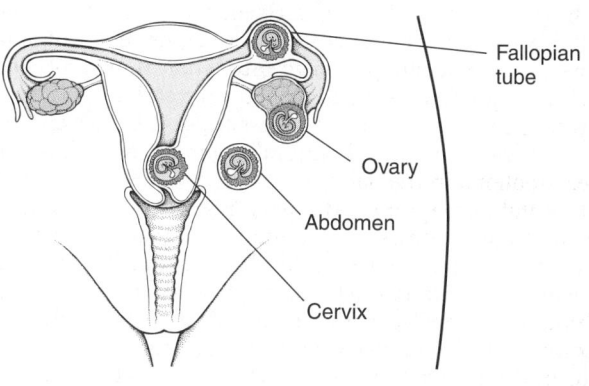

Fallopian tube

Ovary

Abdomen

Cervix

Understanding the Language of Loss

Doctors may use the term *abortion* to refer to a miscarriage (spontaneous abortion) that occurs before 24 weeks of pregnancy as well as to medical termination of pregnancy (induced abortion). After 24 weeks of pregnancy, delivery of a fetus that has died is called a stillbirth. Other terms include the following:

Therapeutic (induced) abortion: An abortion that is brought about by medical means (drugs or surgery)

Threatened abortion: Bleeding or cramping during the first 24 weeks of pregnancy, indicating that the fetus may be lost

Inevitable abortion: Pain or bleeding with opening (dilation) of the cervix, indicating that the fetus will be lost

Complete abortion: Expulsion of all of the fetus and placenta in the uterus

Incomplete abortion: Expulsion of only part of the contents of the uterus

Habitual abortion: Three or more consecutive spontaneous abortions (miscarriages)

Missed abortion: Retention of a dead fetus in the uterus for 4 weeks or longer

Septic abortion: Infection of the contents of the uterus before, during, or after an abortion

sure (including preeclampsia) and among women who use cocaine.

The uterus bleeds from the site where the placenta was attached. The blood may pass through the cervix and out the vagina as an external hemorrhage, or it may be trapped behind the placenta as a concealed hemorrhage. Symptoms depend on the degree of detachment and the amount of blood lost (which may be massive). Symptoms may include sudden continuous or crampy abdominal pain, tenderness when the abdomen is pressed, and shock. Premature detachment of the placenta can lead to widespread clotting inside the blood vessels (disseminated intravascular coagulation), kidney failure, and bleeding into the walls of the uterus, especially in pregnant women who also have preeclampsia. When the placenta detaches, the supply of oxygen and nutrients to the fetus may be reduced.

Doctors suspect premature detachment of the placenta on the basis of symptoms. Ultrasonography can confirm the diagnosis.

Women with premature detachment of the placenta are hospitalized. The usual treatment is bed rest. If symptoms lessen, women are encouraged to walk and may be discharged from the hospital. If bleeding continues or worsens (suggesting that the fetus is not getting enough oxygen) or if the pregnancy is near term, an early delivery is often best for the woman and the baby. If vaginal delivery is not possible, a cesarean section is performed.

vise bed rest in the hospital. If the bleeding stops, women are usually encouraged to walk. If bleeding does not recur, they are usually sent home, provided that they can return to the hospital easily. A cesarean section is almost always performed before labor begins. If women with placenta previa go into labor, the placenta tends to become detached very early, depriving the baby of its oxygen supply. The lack of oxygen may result in brain damage or other problems in the baby.

Placental Abruption (Abruptio Placentae): Placental abruption is the premature detachment of a normally positioned placenta from the wall of the uterus. The placenta may detach incompletely (sometimes just 10 to 20%) or completely. The cause is unknown. Detachment of the placenta occurs in 0.4 to 3.5% of all deliveries. This complication is more common among women who have high blood pres-

Miscarriage

A miscarriage (spontaneous abortion) is the loss of a fetus due to natural causes before 24 weeks of pregnancy.

Miscarriage is a common end to a high-risk pregnancy. A miscarriage occurs in about 15% of recognized pregnancies. Many more miscarriages may be unrecognized because they occur before women know they are pregnant. About 85% of miscarriages occur during the first 12 weeks of pregnancy. Most miscarriages that occur during this time are thought to occur because something was wrong with the fetus, such as a birth defect or a genetic disorder.

The remaining 15% of miscarriages occur during weeks 13 to 24. For about one third of these miscarriages, no cause is identified. The other two thirds of them result from problems in the women. A miscarriage may occur because women have structural abnormalities of the reproductive organs, such as a double uterus or an incompetent cervix, which tends to open (dilate) as the uterus enlarges. A miscarriage can also occur if women use cocaine, are injured, or have certain disorders. These disorders include an underactive thyroid gland (hypothyroidism), diabetes, infections (such as a cytomegalovirus infection or rubella), and connective tissue disorders (such as lupus). Rh incompatibility (when a pregnant woman has Rh-negative blood and the fetus has Rh-positive blood) also increases risk. Emotional disturbances in women are not linked with miscarriages.

A miscarriage is more likely for women who have had a miscarriage or preterm labor in a previous pregnancy. For women who have had three consecutive miscarriages during the 1st trimester, the chance of having another miscarriage is about 1 in 4. Before trying to become pregnant again, women who have had repeated miscarriages may want to be checked for genetic or structural abnormalities and for other disorders that increase the risk of a miscarriage. An imaging procedure (such as hysteroscopy, hysterosalpingography, or ultrasonography) may be performed to look for structural abnormalities. If the cause of a previous miscarriage is identified, treatment may correct the problem.

Symptoms

A miscarriage is usually preceded by spotting or more obvious bleeding and a discharge from the vagina. The uterus contracts, causing cramps. About 20 to 30% of pregnant women have some bleeding or cramping at least once during the first 20 weeks of pregnancy. About half of these episodes result in a miscarriage.

Early in a pregnancy, the only sign of a miscarriage may be a small amount of vaginal bleeding. Later in a pregnancy, a miscarriage may cause profuse bleeding, and the blood may contain mucus or clots. Cramps become more severe until eventually, the uterus contracts enough to expel the fetus and placenta.

Sometimes the fetus dies but no miscarriage occurs. In such cases, the uterus does not enlarge. Rarely, the dead tissues in the uterus become infected before, during, or after a miscarriage. Such an infection may be serious, causing fever, chills, and a rapid heart rate. Affected women may become delirious, and blood pressure may fall.

Diagnosis and Treatment

If a pregnant woman has bleeding and cramping during the first 20 weeks of pregnancy, a doctor examines her to determine whether a miscarriage is likely. The doctor examines the cervix to determine whether it is dilating. If it is not, the pregnancy may be able to continue. If it is dilating, a miscarriage is more likely.

Ultrasonography is usually also performed. It may be used to determine whether a miscarriage has already occurred or, if not, whether the fetus is still alive. If a miscarriage has occurred, ultrasonography can show whether the fetus and the placenta have been expelled.

If the fetus is alive and a miscarriage seems likely, bed rest is advised to help reduce bleeding and cramping. If possible, the woman should not work but should stay off her feet at home. Refraining from sexual intercourse is advised, although intercourse has not been definitely connected with miscarriages.

If a miscarriage has occurred and the fetus and the placenta have been expelled, no treatment is needed. If some of these tissues remain in the uterus, suction curettage▲ is performed to remove them.

If the fetus dies but remains in the uterus, suction curettage is usually used to remove the fetus and the placenta. If the fetus dies late in the pregnancy, a drug that can induce labor (such as oxytocin) may be given intravenously instead. Oxytocin stimulates the uterus to contract and expel the fetus. Afterward, curettage may be needed to remove pieces of the placenta.

After a miscarriage, women may feel grief, sadness, anger, guilt, or anxiety about subsequent pregnancies. Grief for a loss is a natural response and should not be suppressed or denied. Talking about their feelings with another person may help women deal with their feelings and gain perspective. Women who have had a miscarriage may wish to talk with their doctor about the likelihood of a miscarriage in subsequent pregnancies. Although having a miscarriage increases the risk of having another one, most women who have a miscarriage do not have problems in subsequent pregnancies.

▲ see page 1426

CHAPTER 259

Drug Use During Pregnancy

More than 90% of pregnant women take prescription or nonprescription (over-the-counter) drugs or use social drugs, such as tobacco and alcohol, or illicit drugs at some time during pregnancy. In general, drugs, unless absolutely necessary, should not be used during pregnancy, because many can harm the fetus. About 2 to 3% of all birth defects result from the use of drugs.

However, drugs are sometimes essential for the health of the pregnant woman and the fetus. In such cases, a woman should talk with her doctor or other health care practitioner about the risks and benefits of taking the drugs. Before taking any drug (including non-prescription drugs) or dietary supplement (including medicinal herbs), a pregnant woman should consult her health care practitioner. A health care practitioner may recommend that a woman take certain vitamins and minerals during pregnancy.

Drugs taken by a pregnant woman reach the fetus primarily by crossing the placenta, the same route taken by oxygen and nutrients, which are needed for the fetus's growth and development. Drugs that a pregnant woman takes during pregnancy can affect the fetus in several ways:

- They can act directly on the fetus, causing damage, abnormal development (leading to birth defects), or death.
- They can alter the function of the placenta, usually by constricting blood vessels and reducing the supply of oxygen and nutrients to the fetus from the mother and thus sometimes resulting in a baby that is underweight and underdeveloped.
- They can cause the muscles of the uterus to contract forcefully, indirectly injuring the fetus by reducing its blood supply or triggering preterm labor and delivery.

How a drug affects a fetus depends on the fetus's stage of development and the strength and dose of the drug. Certain drugs taken early in pregnancy (before the 20th day after fertilization) may act in an all-or-nothing fashion, killing the fetus or not affecting it at all. During this early stage, the fetus is highly resistant to birth defects. However, the fetus is particularly vulnerable to birth defects between the 3rd and the 8th week after fertilization, when its organs are developing. Drugs reaching the fetus during this stage may cause a miscarriage, an obvious birth defect, or a permanent but subtle defect that is noticed later in life. Drugs taken after organ development is complete are unlikely to cause obvious birth defects, but they may alter the growth and function of normally formed organs and tissues.

The Food and Drug Administration (FDA) classifies drugs according to the degree of risk they pose for the fetus if they are used during pregnancy. Some drugs are highly toxic and should never be used by pregnant women because they cause severe birth defects. One example is thalidomide. Several decades ago, this drug caused extreme underdevelopment of arms and legs and defects of the intestine, heart, and blood vessels in the babies of women who took the drug during pregnancy. Some drugs cause birth defects in animals, but the same effects have not been seen in people. One example is meclizine, frequently taken for motion sickness, nausea, and vomiting.

Often, a safer drug can be substituted for one that is likely to cause harm during pregnancy. For example, doctors prefer to use insulin rather than oral hypoglycemic drugs, for treatment of diabetes in pregnant women. Insulin cannot cross the placenta and controls diabetes better. Oral hypoglycemic drugs can cross the placenta, sometimes resulting in a very low blood sugar level in the newborn. For an overactive thyroid gland, propylthiouracil is usually preferred. For prevention of blood clots, the anticoagulant heparin is preferred. For anxiety disorders, meprobamate and chlordiazepoxide, which do not appear to cause birth defects or brain damage, are preferred. Several safe antibiotics, such as penicillin, are available.

Some drugs can cause effects after they are discontinued. For example, etretinate, a drug used to treat skin disorders, is stored in fat beneath the skin and is released slowly. Etretinate can cause birth defects 6 months or longer after women discontinue it. Therefore, women are advised to wait at least 1 year after

How Drugs Cross the Placenta

Some of the fetus's blood vessels are contained in tiny hairlike projections (villi) of the placenta that extend into the wall of the uterus. The mother's blood passes through the space surrounding the villi (intervillous space). Only a thin membrane (placental membrane) separates the mother's blood in the intervillous space from the fetus's blood in the villi. Drugs in the mother's blood can cross this membrane into blood vessels in the villi and pass through the umbilical cord to the fetus.

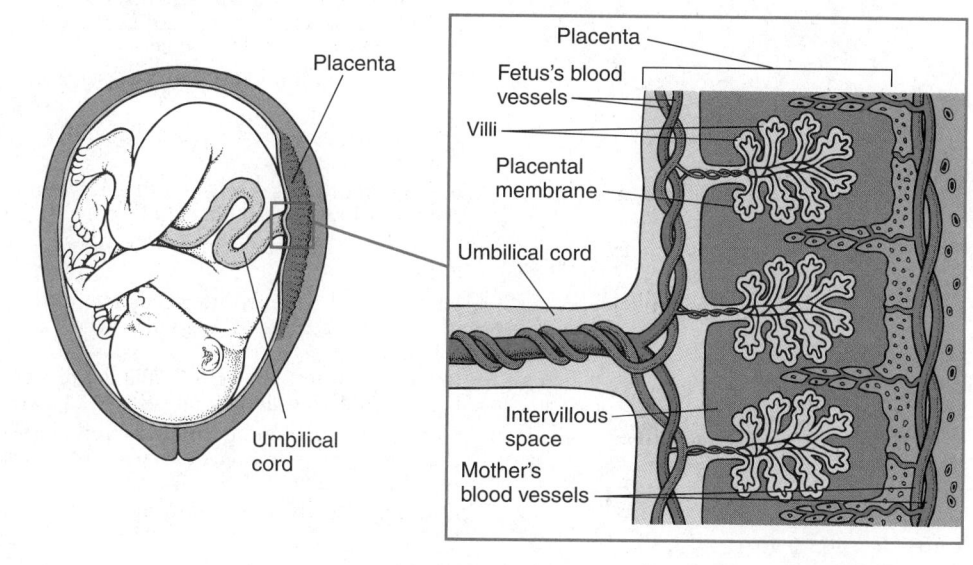

discontinuing the drug before they become pregnant.

Unless unavoidable, vaccines made with a live virus are not given to women who are or might be pregnant. Other vaccines (such as those for cholera, hepatitis A and B, plague, rabies, tetanus, diphtheria, and typhoid) are given to pregnant women only if they are at substantial risk of developing that particular infection. However, all pregnant women should be vaccinated against the influenza virus during the influenza (flu) season.

Drugs to lower high blood pressure (antihypertensives) may be needed by pregnant women who have had high blood pressure or who develop it during pregnancy (a complication called preeclampsia▲). Antihypertensives commonly used to treat preeclampsia can markedly reduce blood flow to the placenta if they lower blood pressure too rapidly in pregnant women. So pregnant women who have to take these drugs are closely monitored. Angiotensin-converting

enzyme (ACE) inhibitors and thiazide diuretics are usually not given to pregnant women because these drugs can cause serious problems in the fetus.

Digoxin, used to treat heart failure and some abnormal heart rhythms, readily crosses the placenta. But it typically has little effect on the baby before or after birth.

Most antidepressants appear to be relatively safe when used during pregnancy.

Social Drugs

Cigarette Smoking: Although cigarette smoking harms both pregnant women and the fetus, only about 20% of women who smoke quit during pregnancy. The most consistent effect of smoking on the fetus during pregnancy is a reduction in birth weight: The more a woman smokes during pregnancy, the less the baby is likely to weigh. The average birth

▲ see page 1452

SOME DRUGS THAT CAN CAUSE PROBLEMS DURING PREGNANCY*

TYPE	EXAMPLES	PROBLEM
Antianxiety drug	Diazepam	When the drug is taken late in pregnancy, depression, irritability, shaking, and exaggerated reflexes in the newborn
Antibiotics	Chloramphenicol	Gray baby syndrome In women or fetuses with glucose-6-phosphate dehydrogenase (G6PD) deficiency, the breakdown of red blood cells
	Ciprofloxacin	Possibility of joint abnormalities (seen only in animals)
	Kanamycin	Damage to the fetus's ear, resulting in deafness
	Nitrofurantoin	In women or fetuses with G6PD deficiency, the breakdown of red blood cells
	Streptomycin	Damage to the fetus's ear, resulting in deafness
	Sulfonamides	Jaundice and possibly brain damage in the newborn (much less likely with sulfasalazine) In women or fetuses with G6PD deficiency, the breakdown of red blood cells
	Tetracycline	Slowed bone growth, permanent yellowing of the teeth, and increased susceptibility to cavities in the baby Occasionally, liver failure in the pregnant woman
Anticoagulants	Heparin	When the drug is taken a long time, osteoporosis and a decrease in the number of platelets (which help blood clot) in the pregnant woman
	Warfarin	Birth defects Bleeding problems in the fetus and the pregnant woman
Anticonvulsants	Carbamazepine Phenobarbital Phenytoin	Some risk of birth defects Bleeding problems in the newborn, which can be prevented if pregnant women take vitamin K by mouth every day for a month before delivery or if the newborn is given an injection of vitamin K soon after birth Some risk of birth defects
	Trimethadione Valproate	Increased risk of miscarriage in the woman Increased risk of birth defects in the fetus, including a cleft palate and abnormalities of the heart, face, skull, hands, or abdominal organs (the risk is 70% with trimethadione and 1% with valproate)
Antihypertensives	Angiotensin-converting enzyme (ACE) inhibitors (see table on page 139)	When the drugs are taken late in pregnancy, kidney damage in the fetus, a reduction in the amount of fluid around the developing fetus (amniotic fluid), and deformities of the face, limbs, and lungs
	Thiazide diuretics	A decrease in the levels of oxygen and potassium and the number of platelets in the fetus's blood

SOME DRUGS THAT CAN CAUSE PROBLEMS (*Continued*)

TYPE	EXAMPLES	PROBLEM
Chemotherapy drugs	Busulfan Chlorambucil Cyclophosphamide Mercaptopurine Methotrexate	Birth defects such as less-than-expected growth before birth, underdevelopment of the lower jaw, cleft palate, abnormal development of the skull bones, spinal defects, ear defects, and clubfoot
Mood-stabilizing drug	Lithium	Birth defects (mainly of the heart), lethargy, reduced muscle tone, poor feeding, underactivity of the thyroid gland, and nephrogenic diabetes insipidus in the newborn
Nonsteroidal anti-inflammatory drugs (NSAIDs)	Aspirin Other salicylates	When the drugs are taken in large doses, a delay in the start of labor, premature closing of the connection between the aorta and artery to the lungs (ductus arteriosus), jaundice, and (occasionally) brain damage in the fetus and bleeding problems in the woman during and after delivery and in the newborn When the drugs are taken late in pregnancy, a reduction in the amount of fluid around the developing fetus
Oral hypoglycemic drugs	Chlorpropamide Tolbutamide	A very low level of sugar in the blood of the newborn Inadequate control of diabetes in the pregnant woman
Sex hormones	Danazol Synthetic progestins (but not the low doses used in oral contraceptives)	Masculinization of a female fetus's genitals, sometimes requiring surgery to correct
	Diethylstilbestrol (DES)	Abnormalities of the uterus, menstrual problems, and an increased risk of vaginal cancer and complications during pregnancy in daughters Abnormalities of the penis in sons
Skin treatments	Etretinate Isotretinoin	Birth defects, such as heart defects, small ears, and hydrocephalus (sometimes called water on the brain)
Thyroid drugs	Methimazole Propylthiouracil Radioactive iodine	An overactive and enlarged thyroid gland in the fetus An underactive thyroid gland in the fetus
Vaccines	Live-virus vaccines such as those for measles, mumps, German measles (rubella), polio, chickenpox, and yellow fever	With rubella vaccine, potential infection of the placenta and developing fetus; with other vaccines, potential but unknown risks

* Unless absolutely necessary, drugs should not be used during pregnancy. However, drugs are sometimes essential for the health of the pregnant woman and the fetus. In such cases, a woman should talk with her health care practitioner about the risks and benefits of taking the drugs.

Taking Drugs While Breastfeeding

When new mothers who are breastfeeding have to take a drug, they wonder whether they should stop breastfeeding. The answer depends on how much of the drug appears in the milk, whether the drug is absorbed by the baby, how the drug affects the baby, and how much milk the baby consumes. How much milk the baby consumes depends on the baby's age and the amount of other foods and liquids in the baby's diet. Some drugs, such as epinephrine, heparin, and insulin, do not appear in breast milk and are thus safe to take. Most drugs appear in breast milk but usually in tiny amounts. However, even in tiny amounts, some drugs can harm the baby. Some drugs appear in breast milk, but the baby usually absorbs so little of them that they do not affect the baby. Examples are the antibiotics gentamicin, kanamycin, streptomycin, and tetracycline.

Drugs that are considered safe include most nonprescription (over-the-counter) drugs. Exceptions are antihistamines (commonly contained in cough and cold remedies, allergy drugs, motion sickness drugs, and sleep aids) and, if taken in large amounts for a long time, aspirin and other salicylates. Acetaminophen and ibuprofen, taken in usual doses, appear to be safe.

Drugs that are applied to the skin, eyes, or nose or that are inhaled are usually safe. Most antihypertensive drugs do not cause significant problems in breastfed babies. Warfarin is considered compatible with breastfeeding a full-term, healthy baby. Caffeine and theophylline do not harm breastfed babies but may make them irritable. Even though some drugs are reportedly safe for breastfed babies, women who are breastfeeding should consult a health care practitioner before taking any drug, even a nonprescription drug, or a medicinal herb. Drug labels should be checked because they contain warnings against use during breastfeeding, if applicable.

Some drugs require a doctor's supervision during their use. Taking them safely while breastfeeding may require adjusting the dose, limiting the length of time the drug is used, or timing when the drug is taken in relation to breastfeeding. Most antianxiety drugs, antidepressants, and antipsychotic drugs require a doctor's supervision, even though they are unlikely to cause significant problems in the baby. However, these drugs stay in the body a long time. During the first few months of life, babies may have difficulty eliminating the drugs, and the drugs may affect the baby's nervous system. For example, the antianxiety drug diazepam (a benzodiazepine) causes lethargy, drowsiness, and weight loss in breastfed babies. Babies eliminate phenobarbital (an anticonvulsant and a barbiturate) slowly, so this drug may cause excessive drowsiness. Because of these effects, doctors reduce the dose of benzodiazepines and barbiturates as well as monitor their use by women who are breastfeeding.

Some drugs should not be taken while breastfeeding. They include atropine, chemotherapy drugs (such as doxorubicin and methotrexate), chloramphenicol, ergotamine, lithium, methimazole, methysergide, radioactive drugs for diagnostic procedures, thiouracil, vaccines, and illicit drugs such as cocaine, heroin, and phencyclidine (PCP). Other drugs should not be taken because they may suppress milk production. They include bromocriptine, estrogen, oral contraceptives that contain high-dose estrogen and a progestin, and levodopa.

If women who are breastfeeding must take a drug that may harm the baby, they must stop breastfeeding. But they can resume breastfeeding after they discontinue the drug. While taking the drug, women can maintain their milk supply by pumping breast milk, which is then discarded.

weight of babies born to women who smoke during pregnancy is 6 ounces less than that of babies born to women who do not smoke. The reduction in birth weight seems to be greater among the babies of older smokers.

Birth defects of the heart, brain, and face are more common among babies of smokers than among those of nonsmokers. Also, the risk of sudden infant death syndrome (SIDS) may be increased. A mislocated placenta (placenta previa), premature detachment of the placenta (placental abruption), premature rupture of the membranes, preterm labor, uterine infections, miscarriages, stillbirths, and premature births are also more likely. In addition, children of women who smoke have slight but measurable deficiencies in physical growth and in intellectual and behavioral development. These effects are thought to be caused by carbon monoxide and nicotine. Carbon monoxide may reduce the oxygen supply to the body's tissues. Nicotine stimulates the release of hormones that constrict the vessels supplying blood to the uterus and placenta, so that less oxygen and fewer nutrients reach the fetus.

Pregnant women should avoid exposure to secondhand smoke because it may similarly harm the fetus.

Alcohol: Drinking alcohol during pregnancy is the leading known cause of birth defects. Because the amount of alcohol required to cause fetal alcohol syndrome is unknown, pregnant women are advised to abstain from drinking alcohol altogether. The range of effects of drinking during pregnancy is great.

The risk of miscarriage almost doubles for women who drink alcohol in any form during pregnancy, especially if they drink heavily. Often, the birth weight of babies born to women who drink during pregnancy is substantially below normal. The average birth weight is about 4 pounds for babies exposed to significant amounts of alcohol, compared with 7 pounds for all babies. Newborns of women who drank during pregnancy may not thrive and are more likely to die soon after birth.

Fetal alcohol syndrome is one of the most serious consequences of drinking during pregnancy. It occurs in about 2 of 1,000 live births. This syndrome includes inadequate growth before or after birth, facial defects, a small head (probably caused by inadequate growth of the brain), mental retardation, and abnormal behavioral development. Less commonly, the position and function of the joints are abnormal and heart defects are present.

Babies or developing children of women who drank alcohol during pregnancy may have severe behavioral problems, such as antisocial behavior and attention deficit disorder. These problems can occur even when the baby has no obvious physical birth defects.

Caffeine: Whether consuming caffeine during pregnancy harms the fetus is unclear. Evidence seems to suggest that consuming caffeine in moderation during pregnancy poses little or no risk to the fetus. Caffeine, which is contained in coffee, tea, some sodas, chocolate, and some drugs, is a stimulant that readily crosses the placenta to the fetus. Thus, it may stimulate the fetus, increasing the heart and breathing rates. Caffeine also may decrease blood flow across the placenta and decreases the absorption of iron (possibly increasing the risk of anemia▲). Whether drinking more than seven or eight cups of coffee a day increases the risk of having a stillbirth,

premature birth, low-birth-weight baby, or miscarriage is also unclear. Some experts recommend limiting coffee consumption to two or three cups a day and drinking decaffeinated beverages when possible.

Aspartame: Aspartame, an artificial sweetener, appears to be safe during pregnancy when it is consumed in small amounts, such as in amounts used in artificially sweetened foods and beverages.

Illicit Drugs

Use of illicit drugs (particularly cocaine and opioids) during pregnancy can cause complications during pregnancy and serious problems in the developing fetus and the newborn. For pregnant women, injecting illicit drugs also increases the risk of infections that can affect or be transmitted to the fetus. These infections include hepatitis and sexually transmitted diseases (including AIDS). Also, growth of the fetus is more likely to be inadequate, and premature births are more common.

Cocaine: Cocaine readily crosses the placenta and affects the fetus. It constricts blood vessels, possibly reducing blood flow (and the oxygen supply) to the fetus. The reduced blood and oxygen supply to the fetus can slow the growth of the fetus, particularly of the bones and the intestine. Babies are more likely to be small and to have a small head. Rarely, use of cocaine results in birth defects of the brain, eyes, kidneys, and genital organs.

Use of cocaine during pregnancy can also cause complications during pregnancy. Among women who use cocaine throughout pregnancy, about 31% have a preterm delivery and 15% have premature detachment of the placenta (placental abruption). The chances of a miscarriage are also increased. About 19% have a baby who did not grow as much as normally expected before birth. If women stop using cocaine after the first 3 months of pregnancy, the risks of a preterm delivery and premature detachment of the placenta are still increased, but the fetus's growth will probably be normal.

Newborns may have withdrawal symptoms. Their behavior is also affected. Newborns interact less with other people. Babies of cocaine users may be hyperactive, tremble uncontrollably, and have difficulty learning (which may continue through age 5 years or even longer).

▲ see page 1451

Opioids: Opioids, such as heroin, methadone, and morphine, readily cross the placenta. Consequently, the fetus may become addicted to them and may have withdrawal symptoms 6 hours to 8 days after birth.▲ However, use of opioids rarely results in birth defects. Use of opioids during pregnancy increases the risk of complications during pregnancy, such as miscarriage, abnormal presentation of the baby, and preterm delivery. Babies of heroin users are more likely to be small.

Amphetamines: Use of amphetamines during pregnancy may result in birth defects, especially of the heart.

Marijuana: Whether use of marijuana during pregnancy can harm the fetus is unclear. The main ingredient of marijuana, tetrahydrocannabinol, can cross the placenta and thus may affect the fetus. If marijuana is used heavily during pregnancy, newborns may have behavioral problems.

Drugs Used During Labor and Delivery

Local anesthetics, opioids, and other analgesics usually cross the placenta and can affect the newborn. For example, they can weaken the newborn's urge to breathe. Therefore, if these drugs are needed during labor, they are given in the smallest effective doses.

CHAPTER 260

Normal Labor and Delivery

Although each labor and delivery is different, most follow a general pattern. Therefore, an expectant mother can have a general idea of what changes will occur in her body to enable her to deliver the baby and what procedures will be followed to help her. She also has several choices to make, such as whether to have the father present and where to have the baby.

An expectant mother may want the baby's father to remain with her during labor. His encouragement and emotional support may help her relax, sometimes reducing her need for drugs to relieve pain. In addition, sharing the meaningful experience of childbirth has emotional and psychologic benefits, such as creating strong family bonds. Childbirth education classes prepare both father and mother for the entire process. On the other hand, an expectant mother may prefer privacy during labor, the father may not want to be present, or another partner may be more appropriate or supportive.

In the United States, almost all babies are born in hospitals, but some women want to have their babies at home. However, because unexpected complications can occur during or shortly after labor, most experts do not advise

delivery at home. Women who prefer a homelike setting and fewer rules (for example, no limit on the number of visitors or on visiting hours) may choose birthing centers. Such centers provide an informal, personal experience of childbirth but are much safer than delivery at home. Birthing centers are part of a hospital or have an arrangement with a nearby hospital. Thus, birthing centers can provide a medical staff, emergency equipment, and full hospital facilities, if needed. If complications develop during labor, birthing centers immediately transfer the woman to the hospital.

Some hospitals have private rooms in which a woman stays from labor until discharge. These rooms are called LDRPs for labor, delivery, recovery, and postpartum (after delivery).

Regardless of the choices a woman makes, knowing what to expect helps prepare her for labor and delivery.

Labor

Labor is a series of rhythmic, progressive contractions of the uterus that gradually move the fetus through the lower part of the uterus (cervix) and birth canal (vagina) to the outside world.

Labor occurs in three main stages. The first stage (which has two phases: initial and ac-

---

▲ see also page 652

tive) is labor proper. In it, contractions cause the cervix to open gradually (dilate) and to thin and pull back (efface) until it merges with the rest of the uterus. These changes enable the fetus to pass through the vagina. The second and third stages constitute delivery of the baby and the placenta.

Labor usually starts within 2 weeks of (before or after) the estimated date of delivery. Exactly what causes labor to start is unknown. Toward the end of pregnancy (after 36 weeks), a doctor may perform a pelvic examination to try to predict when labor will start. On average, labor lasts 15 to 16 hours in a woman's first pregnancy and tends to be shorter, averaging 6 to 8 hours, in subsequent pregnancies. A woman who has had rapid deliveries in previous pregnancies should notify her doctor as soon as she thinks she is going into labor.

All pregnant women should know what the main signs of the start of labor are: contractions in the lower abdomen at regular intervals and back pain. However, other clues may precede or accompany these signs. A small discharge of blood mixed with mucus from the vagina (bloody show) is usually a clue that labor is about to start. The bloody show may appear as early as 72 hours before contractions start.

Occasionally, the fluid-filled membranes that contain the fetus (amniotic sac) rupture before labor starts, and the amniotic fluid flows out through the vagina. This event is commonly described as "the water breaks." When a woman's membranes rupture, she should contact her doctor or midwife immediately. About 80 to 90% of women whose membranes rupture before but near their due date go into labor spontaneously within 24 hours. If labor has not started after 24 hours and the baby is due, women are usually admitted to the hospital, where labor is artificially started (induced) to reduce the risk of infection. After the membranes rupture, bacteria from the vagina can enter the uterus more easily and cause an infection in the woman, the fetus, or both. Oxytocin (which causes the uterus to contract) or a similar drug, such as a prostaglandin, is used to induce labor. If the membranes rupture prematurely, doctors do not induce labor until the fetus is more mature.▲

When the contractions in the lower abdomen first start, they may be weak, irregular and far apart. They may feel like menstrual cramps. As time passes, abdominal contractions become longer, stronger, and closer to-

gether. When strong contractions occur 5 minutes apart or less and the cervix is dilated more than 1½ inches (4 centimeters), the woman is admitted to the hospital or birthing center. The strength, duration, and frequency of contractions are noted. Her weight, blood pressure, heart and breathing rates, and temperature are measured, and samples of urine and blood are taken for analysis. Her abdomen is examined to estimate how big the fetus is, whether the fetus is facing rearward or forward (position), and whether the head, face, buttocks, or shoulder is leading the way out (presentation).

The presentation and position of the fetus affect how the fetus passes through the vagina. The most common and safest combination is facing rearward (toward the woman's back), with the face and body angled toward the right or left, and head first, with the neck bent forward, chin tucked in, and arms folded across the chest.■ Head first is called a vertex or cephalic presentation. During the last week or two before delivery, most fetuses turn so that the back of the head presents first. If the presentation is buttocks first (breech) or shoulder first or the fetus is facing forward, delivery is considerably more difficult for the woman, fetus, and doctor. Cesarean delivery is recommended.

Usually, the vagina is examined to determine if the membranes have ruptured and how dilated and effaced the cervix is, but this examination may be omitted if the woman is bleeding or if the membranes have ruptured spontaneously. The color of the amniotic fluid is noted. The fluid should be clear and have no significant odor. If the membranes rupture and the amniotic fluid is green, the discoloration results from the fetus's first stool (fetal meconium).

Soon after the woman is admitted to the hospital, the doctor or another health care practitioner listens to the fetus's heartbeat directly using a fetal stethoscope (fetoscope) or uses an ultrasound device to monitor heartbeats (a procedure called electronic fetal heart monitoring).

During the first stage of labor, the heart rates of woman and fetus are monitored periodically or continuously. Monitoring the fetus's heart rate, with a fetal stethoscope or electronic fetal heart monitoring, is the easi-

---

▲ see page 1470   ■ see art on page 1472

Stages of Labor

FIRST STAGE

From the beginning of labor to the full opening (dilation) of the cervix—to about 4 inches (10 centimeters).

Initial (Latent) Phase

Contractions become progressively stronger and more rhythmic.

Discomfort is minimal.

The cervix thins and opens to about 1½ inches (4 centimeters).

This phase lasts an average of 12 hours in a first pregnancy and 5 hours in subsequent pregnancies.

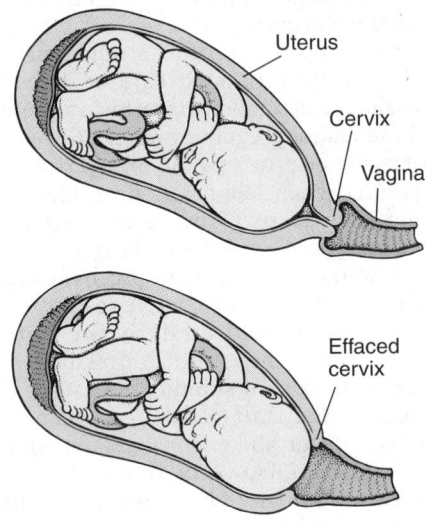

Active Phase

The cervix opens from about 1½ inches (4 centimeters) to the full 4 inches (10 centimeters).

The presenting part of the baby, usually the head, begins to descend into the woman's pelvis.

The woman begins to feel the urge to push as the baby descends.

This phase averages about 3 hours in a first pregnancy and 2 hours in subsequent pregnancies.

SECOND STAGE

From the complete opening of the cervix to delivery of the baby. This stage averages about 45 to 60 minutes in a first pregnancy and 15 to 30 minutes in subsequent pregnancies.

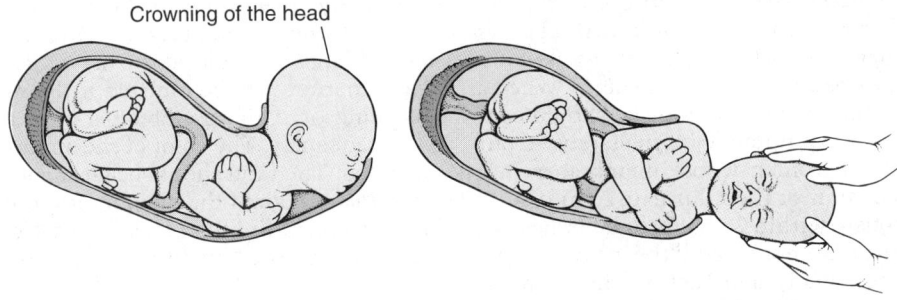

Crowning of the head

THIRD STAGE

From delivery of the baby to delivery of the placenta. This stage usually lasts only a few minutes but may last up to 30 minutes.

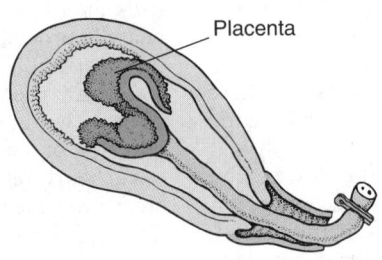

Placenta

est way to determine whether the fetus is receiving enough oxygen. An abnormal heart rate (too fast or too slow) may indicate that the fetus is in distress.▲ During the second stage of labor, the woman's heart rate and blood pressure are monitored regularly. The fetus's heart rate is monitored after every contraction or, if electronic monitoring is used, continuously.

During labor in a hospital, an intravenous line is usually inserted into the woman's arm. This line is used to give the woman fluids to prevent dehydration and, if needed, to give drugs immediately. When fluids are given intravenously, the woman does not have to eat or drink during labor, although she may choose to drink some fluids and eat some light food early in labor. An empty stomach during delivery makes the woman less likely to vomit and to inhale vomit. Inhaling vomit, although very rare, can cause respiratory distress, a potentially life-threatening disorder in which the lungs are inflamed. Usually, a woman is given an antacid by mouth to neutralize stomach acid when she is admitted to the hospital and every 3 hours after that. Antacids reduce the risk of damage to the lungs if vomit is inhaled.

Pain Relief: With the advice of her doctor or midwife, a woman usually plans an approach to pain relief long before labor starts. She may choose natural childbirth, which relies on relaxation and breathing techniques to deal with pain, or she may plan to use analgesics or a particular type of anesthetic (local, regional, or general) if needed. After labor starts, these plans may be modified, depending on how labor progresses, how the woman feels, and what the doctor or midwife recommends.

A woman's need for pain relief during labor varies considerably, depending to some extent on her level of anxiety. Attending childbirth preparation classes helps prepare the woman for labor and delivery. Such preparation and emotional support from the people attending the labor tend to lessen anxiety and often markedly reduce her need for drugs to relieve pain.

If a woman requests analgesics during labor, they are usually given to her. However, because some of these drugs can slow (depress) breathing and other functions of the newborn, the amount given is as small as possible. Most commonly, meperidine or morphine is given intravenously to relieve pain. These drugs can slow the initial phase of the first stage of labor, so they are usually given during the active phase of the first stage. In addition, because

Monitoring the Fetus

Electronic monitoring is routinely used to monitor the fetus's heart rate and the contractions of the uterus. Certain changes in the fetus's heart rate during contractions can indicate that the fetus is not receiving enough oxygen. The fetus's heart rate can be monitored externally by attaching an ultrasound device (which transmits and receives ultrasound waves) to the woman's abdomen or internally by inserting an electrode through the woman's vagina and attaching it to the fetus's scalp. The internal approach is usually used only when problems during labor appear likely or when signals detected by the external device cannot be recorded.

In a high-risk pregnancy, electronic monitoring is sometimes used as part of a nonstress test, in which the fetus's heart rate is monitored as the fetus lies still and as it moves. If the heart rate does not increase with movement, a contraction stress test may be performed. To start uterine contractions, oxytocin (a hormone that causes the uterus to contract during labor) is usually given intravenously. The fetus's heart rate is monitored during these contractions to determine whether the fetus will be able to withstand labor.

When a problem is detected, fetal scalp blood sampling may be performed. During labor, a small amount of blood is removed from the fetus's scalp to measure the acidity (pH) of the blood. This measurement helps doctors determine whether the fetus is receiving enough oxygen.

On the basis of such tests, a doctor may allow labor to continue or may perform a cesarean section immediately.

these drugs have the greatest effect during the first 30 minutes after they are given, the drugs are often not given when delivery is imminent. To counteract the sedating effects of these drugs on the newborn, a doctor can give the newborn the drug naloxone immediately after delivery.

Local anesthesia numbs the vagina and the tissues around its opening. Commonly, this area is numbed by injecting a local anesthetic through the wall of the vagina and around the pudendal nerve (which supplies sensation to the lower genital area). This procedure, called

▲ see page 1471

Natural Childbirth

Natural childbirth uses relaxation and breathing techniques to control pain during childbirth. Natural childbirth often helps reduce or eliminate the need for analgesics or anesthetics during labor and delivery.

To prepare for natural childbirth, a pregnant woman and her partner take childbirth classes, usually six to eight sessions over several weeks, to learn how to use the relaxation and breathing techniques. They also learn what happens in the various stages of labor and delivery.

The relaxation technique involves consciously tensing a part of the body and then relaxing it. This technique helps a woman relax the rest of her body while the uterus is contracting during labor and relax her whole body between contractions.

The breathing technique involves several types of breathing, which are used at different times during labor. During the first stage of labor, before the woman begins to push, the following types of breathing may help:

- Deep breathing to help the woman relax at the beginning and end of a contraction
- Fast, shallow breathing (panting) in the upper chest at the peak of a contraction
- A pattern of panting and blowing to help the woman refrain from pushing when she has an urge to push before the cervix is completely dilated

In the second stage of labor, the woman alternates between pushing and panting.

The woman and her partner should practice relaxation and breathing techniques regularly during pregnancy. During labor, the woman's partner can help her by reminding her of what she should be doing at a particular stage and by noticing when she is tense, in addition to providing emotional support. The partner may massage the woman to help her relax more.

The most well-known method of natural childbirth is probably the Lamaze method. Another method, the Leboyer method, includes birth in a darkened room and immersion of the baby into lukewarm water immediately after delivery.

a pudendal block, is used only late in labor, when the baby's head is about to emerge from the vagina. Another common but less effective procedure involves injecting a local anesthetic at the opening of the vagina. With both procedures, the woman can remain awake and push, and the fetus's functions are unaffected. These procedures are useful for deliveries that have no complications.

Regional anesthesia numbs a larger area. It may be used for women who want more complete pain relief. A lumbar epidural injection is almost always used. This procedure involves injecting an anesthetic in the lower back—into the space between the spine and the outer layer of tissue covering the spinal cord (epidural space). Alternatively, a catheter is placed in the epidural space, and opioids, such as fentanyl and sufentanil, are continuously and slowly given through the catheter. Another procedure (spinal anesthesia) involves injecting an anesthetic into the space between the middle and inner layers of tissue covering the spinal cord (subarachnoid space). A spinal injection is typically used for cesarean sections when there are no complications. Neither an epidural nor a spinal injection prevents the woman from pushing adequately. Occasionally, use of either procedure causes a fall in blood pressure. Consequently, if one of these procedures is used, the woman's blood pressure is measured frequently.

General anesthesia makes a woman temporarily unconscious. This method is rarely necessary and infrequently used because it may slow the function of the fetus's heart, lungs, and brain. Although this effect is usually temporary, it can interfere with the newborn's adjustment to life outside the uterus. General anesthesia is typically used for emergency cesarean sections because it is the quickest way to anesthetize the woman.

Delivery

Delivery is the passage of the fetus and placenta (afterbirth) from the uterus to the outside world.

For delivery in a hospital, a woman may be moved from a labor room to a birthing or delivery room, a room used only for deliveries. Usually, the father or other support people are encouraged to accompany her. If she is already in an LDRP (for labor, delivery, recovery, and postpartum), she remains there. The intravenous line remains in place.

When a woman is about to give birth, she may be placed in a semi-upright position, between lying down and sitting up. Her back can be supported by pillows or a backrest. The semi-upright position uses gravity: The downward pressure of the fetus helps the vagina and surrounding area stretch gradually, decreasing the risk of tearing. This position also puts less strain on the woman's back and pelvis. Some women prefer to deliver lying down. However, with this position, delivery may take longer.

As delivery progresses, the doctor or midwife examines the vagina to determine the position of the fetus's head. The woman is asked to bear down and push with each contraction to help move the fetus's head down through her pelvis and to widen the vaginal opening so that more and more of the head appears. When about $1\frac{1}{2}$ to 2 inches of the head appears, the doctor or midwife places a hand over the fetus's head during a contraction to control the fetus's progress. As the head crowns (when the widest part of the head passes through the vaginal opening), the head and chin are eased out of the vaginal opening to prevent the woman's tissues from tearing.

Forceps are metal instruments, similar to tongs, with rounded edges that fit around the fetus's head.▲ Forceps are used when the fetus is in distress, when the woman is having difficulty pushing, or when labor is not progressing well.

An episiotomy is no longer considered a routine procedure. It is used only when necessary for immediate delivery. For this procedure, the doctor injects a local anesthetic to numb the area and makes an incision in the area between the openings of the vagina and anus. If the muscle around the opening of the anus (rectal sphincter) is damaged during an episiotomy or is torn during delivery, it usually heals well if the doctor repairs it immediately.

After the baby's head has emerged, the body is rotated sideways so that the shoulders can emerge easily, one at a time. The rest of the baby usually slips out quickly. Mucus and fluid are suctioned out of the baby's nose, mouth, and throat. The umbilical cord is clamped and cut. The baby is then wrapped in a lightweight blanket and placed on the woman's abdomen or in a warmed bassinet.

After delivery of the baby, the doctor or midwife places a hand gently on the woman's abdomen to make sure the uterus is contracting. After delivery, the placenta usually detaches from the uterus within 3 to 10 minutes, and a gush of blood soon follows. Usually, the woman can push the placenta out on her own. If she cannot and particularly if she is bleeding excessively, the doctor or midwife applies firm downward pressure on the woman's abdomen, causing the placenta to detach from the uterus and come out. If the placenta has not been delivered within 30 minutes of delivery, the doctor or midwife may insert a hand into the uterus, separating the placenta from the uterus and removing it.

After the placenta is removed, it is examined for completeness. Fragments left in the uterus prevent the uterus from contracting. Contractions are essential to prevent further bleeding from the area where the placenta was attached to the uterus. So if fragments remain, bleeding can occur after delivery and may be substantial. Infections can also occur. If the placenta is incomplete, the doctor or midwife may remove the remaining fragments by hand. Sometimes fragments have to be surgically removed.

In many hospitals, as soon as the placenta is delivered or removed, the woman is given oxytocin (intravenously or intramuscularly), and her abdomen is periodically massaged to help the uterus contract.

The doctor stitches up any tears in the cervix, vagina, or nearby muscles and, if an episiotomy was performed, the episiotomy incision. The woman is then moved to the recovery room or remains in the LDRP. Often, a baby who does not need further medical attention stays with the mother. Typically, the woman and her baby remain together in a warm, private area for 3 to 4 hours so that bonding can begin. Many women wish to begin breastfeeding soon after delivery. Later, the baby may be taken to the hospital nursery. In many hospitals, the woman may choose to have the baby remain with her—a practice called rooming-in. All hospitals with LDRPs require it. With rooming-in, the baby is usually fed on demand, and the woman is taught how to care for the baby before they leave the hospital. If a woman needs a rest, she may have the baby taken to the nursery.

Because most complications, particularly bleeding, occur within the first 24 hours after delivery, nurses and doctors carefully observe the woman and baby during this time.

▲ see art on page 1475

CHAPTER 261

Complications of Labor and Delivery

Usually, labor and delivery occur without any problems. Serious problems are relatively rare, and most can be anticipated and treated effectively. However, problems sometimes develop suddenly and unexpectedly. Regular visits to a doctor or certified midwife during pregnancy make anticipation of problems possible and improve the chances of having a healthy baby and safe delivery.

Problems With the Timing of Labor

Labor may start too early (before the 37th week of pregnancy) or may start late (after the 41st to 42nd week of pregnancy). As a result, the health or life of the fetus may be endangered. Labor may start too early or late when the woman or fetus has a medical problem or the fetus is in an abnormal position.

No more than 10% of women deliver on their specified due date (usually estimated to be about 40 weeks of pregnancy). About 50% of women deliver within 1 week (before or after), and almost 90% deliver within 2 weeks of the due date. Determining the length of pregnancy can be difficult, because the precise date of conception often cannot be determined. Early in pregnancy, an ultrasound examination, which is safe and painless, can help determine the length of pregnancy. In mid to late pregnancy, ultrasound examinations are less reliable in determining length of pregnancy.

Premature Rupture of the Membranes: In about 10% of normal pregnancies, the fluid-filled membranes containing the fetus rupture before labor begins. Contractions usually begin within 12 to 48 hours. Rupture of the membranes is commonly described as "the water breaks." The fluid within the membranes (amniotic fluid) then flows out from the vagina. The flow varies from a trickle to a gush. As soon as the membranes have ruptured, a woman should contact her doctor or midwife.

If labor does not begin within 24 to 48 hours, the risk of infection of the uterus and fetus increases. Therefore, a doctor or certified midwife usually artificially starts (induces) labor, depending on whether or not the fetus is mature enough for delivery. The doctor may analyze the amniotic fluid to determine if the fetus's lungs are mature enough. If they are, labor is induced and the baby is delivered. If they are not, the doctor usually does not induce labor.

The woman's temperature and pulse rate are usually recorded at least twice daily. An increase in temperature or pulse rate may be an early sign of infection. If an infection develops, labor is promptly induced and the baby is delivered. Very rarely, if the amniotic fluid stops leaking and contractions stop, the woman may be able to go home. In such cases, the woman should be seen by her doctor at least once a week.

Preterm Labor: Because babies born prematurely can have significant health problems,▲ doctors try to prevent or stop labor that begins before the 34th week of pregnancy. What causes preterm labor is not well understood. However, a healthy lifestyle and regular visits to the doctor or midwife during pregnancy are helpful. Preterm labor is difficult to stop. If vaginal bleeding occurs or the membranes rupture, allowing labor to continue is often best. If vaginal bleeding does not occur and the membranes are not leaking amniotic fluid, the woman is advised to rest and to limit her activities as much as possible, preferably to sedentary ones. She is given fluids and may be given drugs that can slow labor. These measures can often delay labor for a brief time.

Drugs that can slow labor include magnesium sulfate and terbutaline. Magnesium sulfate given intravenously stops preterm labor in many women. However, if the dose is too high, it may slow the woman's heart and breathing rates. Terbutaline given by injection under the skin also can be used to stop preterm labor. However, as a side effect, it increases the heart rate in the woman, fetus, or both. Sometimes ritodrine is used instead of terbutaline.

If the cervix opens (dilates) beyond 2 inches (5 centimeters), labor usually continues until the baby is born. If doctors think that premature delivery is inevitable, a woman may be given a corticosteroid such as betamethasone. The corticosteroid helps the fetus's lungs and other organs mature more quickly and reduces the risk that after birth, the baby will have difficulty breathing (neonatal respiratory distress syndrome).

Postterm Pregnancy and Postmaturity: In most pregnancies that go a little beyond 41 to 42 weeks, no problems develop. However, problems may develop if the placenta cannot continue to maintain a healthy environment for the fetus. This condition is called postmaturity.

Typically, tests are started at 41 weeks to evaluate the fetus's movement and heart rate and the amount of amniotic fluid, which decreases markedly in postmature pregnancies. The fetus's rate of breathing and heart sounds may also be monitored. Doctors can check on the fetus's well-being with electronic fetal heart monitoring.▲ Typically, at 42 weeks, labor is induced, or the baby is delivered by cesarean section.

Labor That Progresses Too Slowly: If labor is progressing too slowly, the fetus may be too big to move through the birth canal (pelvis and vagina). Delivery by forceps, a vacuum extractor, or cesarean section may be necessary. If the birth canal is big enough for the fetus but labor is not progressing, the woman is given oxytocin intravenously to stimulate the uterus to contract more forcefully. If oxytocin is unsuccessful, a cesarean section is performed. If the baby is already in position to be delivered, forceps or a vacuum extractor may be used instead.

Problems Affecting the Fetus or Newborn

If labor does not proceed normally, the fetus or newborn may have problems.

Fetal Distress: Fetal distress is an uncommon complication of labor. It typically occurs when the fetus has not been receiving enough oxygen. The most sensitive indicator of fetal distress is an abnormal heart rate pattern in the fetus. Throughout labor, the fetus's heart rate is monitored with a fetal stethoscope—every 15 minutes during early labor and after each contraction during late labor. Or the fetus's heart rate is monitored continuously with electronic fetal heart monitoring. If a sig-

nificant abnormality in the heart rate is detected, it can usually be corrected by such measures as giving the woman oxygen, increasing the amount of fluids given intravenously to the woman, and turning the woman on her left side. If these measures are not effective, the baby is delivered as quickly as possible by forceps, a vacuum extractor, or cesarean section. If the amniotic fluid appears green after the membranes have ruptured, the fetus may be in distress (but usually is not). This discoloration is caused by the fetus's first stool (fetal meconium). Fetal distress may be associated with postmaturity (when the placenta malfunctions in a postterm pregnancy) or with complications of pregnancy or labor that affect the woman and therefore also affect the fetus.

Breathing Problems: Rarely, a baby does not start to breathe at birth, even though no problems were detected before delivery. Then the baby requires resuscitation. Personnel skilled in resuscitating babies may attend the delivery for this reason.

Abnormal Position and Presentation of the Fetus: Position refers to whether the fetus is facing rearward (toward the woman's back, or face down) or forward (face up). Presentation refers to the part of the fetus's body that leads the way out through the birth canal. The most common and safest combination is head first (called a vertex or cephalic presentation) and facing down, with the face and body angled toward the right or left and with the neck bent forward, chin tucked in, and arms folded across the chest. If the fetus is in a different position or presentation, labor may be more difficult and delivery through the vagina may not be possible.

When a fetus faces up (an abnormal position), the neck is often straightened rather than bent, and the head requires more space to pass through the birth canal. Delivery by forceps, a vacuum extractor, or cesarean section may be necessary.

There are several abnormal presentations. In face presentation, the neck arches back so that the face presents first. In brow presentation, the neck is moderately arched so that the brow presents first. Usually, fetuses do not stay in these presentations; they correct themselves.

▲ see box on page 1467

Position and Presentation of the Fetus

Toward the end of pregnancy, the fetus moves into position for delivery. Normally, the position of a fetus is facing rearward (toward the woman's back) with the face and body angled to one side and the neck flexed, and presentation is head first. An abnormal position is facing forward, and abnormal presentations include face, brow, breech, and shoulder.

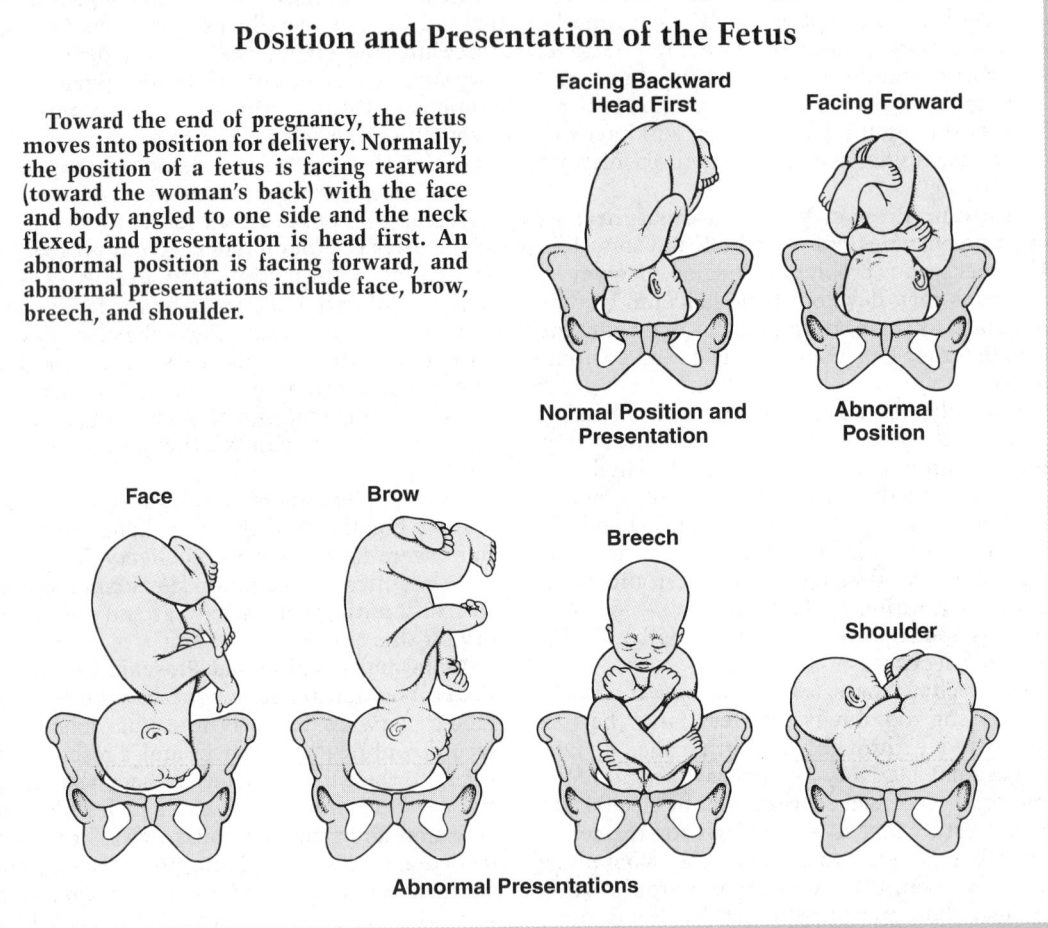

Facing Backward Head First

Facing Forward

Normal Position and Presentation

Abnormal Position

Face

Brow

Breech

Shoulder

Abnormal Presentations

Breech presentation, in which the buttocks present first, occurs in 2 to 3% of full-term deliveries. When delivered vaginally, babies that present buttocks first are more likely to be injured than those that present head first. Such injuries may occur before, during, or after birth and include death. Complications are less likely when breech presentation is detected before labor or delivery.

Sometimes the doctor can turn the fetus to present head first by pressing on the woman's abdomen before labor begins, usually at the 37th or 38th week of pregnancy. However, if labor begins and the fetus is in breech presentation, problems may occur. The passageway made by the buttocks in the birth canal may not be large enough for the head (which is wider) to pass through. In addition, when the head follows the buttocks, it cannot be molded to fit through the birth canal, as it nor-

mally is. Thus, the baby's body may be delivered and the head may be caught inside the woman. As a result, the spinal cord or other nerves may be stretched, leading to nerve damage. When the baby's navel is first seen outside the woman, the umbilical cord is compressed between the baby's head and the birth canal, so that very little oxygen can reach the baby. Brain damage due to lack of oxygen is more common among babies presenting buttocks first than among those presenting head first. In a first delivery, these problems are worse because the woman's tissues have not been stretched by previous deliveries. Because the baby could be injured or die, delivery by cesarean section is preferred when the fetus is in breech presentation.

Occasionally, a fetus lying horizontally across the birth canal presents shoulder first. A cesarean section is performed, unless the fetus is the second in a set of twins. In such a case, the fetus may be turned to be delivered through the vagina.

Multiple Births: The number of twin, triplet, and other multiple births has been increasing during the last two decades. During pregnancy, the number of fetuses can be confirmed by ultrasonography.

Carrying more than one fetus overstretches the uterus, and an overstretched uterus tends to start contracting before the pregnancy reaches full term. As a result, the babies are usually born prematurely and are small. In some cases, the overstretched uterus does not contract well after delivery, causing bleeding in the woman after delivery. Because the fetuses can be in various positions and presentations, vaginal delivery can be complicated. Also, the contraction of the uterus after delivery of the first baby may shear away the placenta of the remaining baby or babies. As a result, the baby or babies that follow the first may have more problems during delivery and later.

For these reasons, doctors may decide in advance how to deliver twins: vaginally or by cesarean section. Occasionally, the first twin is delivered vaginally, but a cesarean section is considered safer for the second twin. For triplets and other multiple births, doctors usually perform a cesarean section.

Shoulder Dystocia: Shoulder dystocia occurs when one shoulder of the fetus lodges against the woman's pubic bone, and the baby is therefore caught in the birth canal. The head comes out, but it is pulled back tightly against the vaginal opening. The baby cannot breathe because the chest is compressed by the birth canal. As a result, oxygen levels in the baby's blood decrease. This complication is more common with large fetuses, particularly when labor has been difficult or when forceps or a vacuum extractor has been used because the fetus's head has not fully descended in the pelvis.

When this complication occurs, the doctor quickly tries various techniques to free the shoulder so that the baby can be delivered vaginally. In extreme circumstances, if the techniques are unsuccessful, the baby may be pushed back into the vagina and delivered by cesarean section.

Prolapsed Umbilical Cord: The umbilical cord precedes the baby through the vagina (prolapses) in about 1 of 1,000 deliveries. When the umbilical cord prolapses, it may

constrict so that the fetus's blood supply is cut off. This complication may be obvious (overt) or not (occult).

Prolapse is overt when the membranes have ruptured and the umbilical cord protrudes into or out of the vagina before the baby emerges. Overt prolapse usually occurs when a baby emerges buttocks first (breech presentation). But it can occur when the baby emerges head first, particularly if the membranes rupture prematurely or the fetus has not descended into the woman's pelvis. If the fetus has not descended, the rush of fluid as the membranes rupture can carry the cord out ahead of the fetus. If the cord prolapses, immediate delivery, almost always by cesarean section, is necessary to prevent the blood supply to the fetus from being cut off. Until surgery begins, a nurse or doctor holds the fetus's body off the cord so that the blood supply through the prolapsed cord is not cut off.

In occult prolapse, the membranes are intact and the cord is in front of the fetus or trapped in front of the fetus's shoulder. Usually, occult prolapse can be identified by an abnormal pattern in the fetus's heart rate. Changing the woman's position or raising the fetus's head to relieve pressure on the cord usually corrects the problem. Occasionally, a cesarean section is necessary.

Nuchal Cord: The umbilical cord is wrapped around the fetus's neck in about one fourth of deliveries. Normally, the baby is not harmed. Before birth, a nuchal cord can sometimes be detected by ultrasonography, but no action is required. Doctors routinely check for it as they deliver the baby. If they feel it, they can slip the cord over the baby's head.

Problems Affecting the Woman

Preeclampsia: Preeclampsia is a complication of pregnancy. It involves high blood pressure that develops late in pregnancy or shortly after delivery. Preeclampsia may lead to premature detachment of the placenta from the uterus (placental abruption)▲ and problems in the newborn.

Amniotic Fluid Embolism: Very rarely, a volume of amniotic fluid—the fluid that surrounds the fetus in the uterus—enters the woman's bloodstream, usually during a particularly difficult labor. The fluid travels to the

▲ see page 1456

woman's lungs and may cause the arteries in the lungs to constrict. This constriction may result in a rapid heart rate, irregular heart rhythm, collapse, shock, or even cardiac arrest and death. Widespread blood clotting (disseminated intravascular coagulation) is a common complication, requiring emergency care.▲

Uterine Bleeding: After the baby is delivered, excessive bleeding (postpartum hemorrhage) from the uterus is a major concern. Ordinarily, the woman loses about 1 pint of blood after delivery. Blood is lost because some blood vessels are opened when the placenta detaches from the uterus. The contractions of the uterus help close these vessels until the vessels can heal.

Loss of more than 1 pint of blood during or after the third stage of labor (when the placenta is delivered) is considered excessive. Severe blood loss usually occurs soon after delivery but may occur even as late as 1 month afterward.

Excessive bleeding may result when the contractions of the uterus after delivery are impaired. Then, the blood vessels that were opened when the placenta detached continue to bleed. Contractions may be impaired if the uterus has been stretched too much—for example, by too much amniotic fluid in the uterus, by several fetuses, or by a very large fetus. Contractions may also be impaired when a piece of placenta remains inside the uterus after delivery, when the labor was prolonged or abnormal, when a woman has been pregnant several times, or when a muscle-relaxing anesthetic was used during labor and delivery. Excessive bleeding can result if the vagina or cervix is torn or cut during delivery or the blood level of fibrinogen (which helps blood to clot) is low. Excessive bleeding after one delivery may increase the risk of excessive bleeding after subsequent deliveries.

Before a woman goes into labor, doctors take steps to prevent or to prepare for excessive bleeding after delivery. For example, they determine whether the woman has any conditions that increase the risk of bleeding, such as too much amniotic fluid. If the woman has an unusual blood type, doctors make sure that her type of blood is available. After delivery of the placenta, the woman is monitored for at least 1 hour to make sure that the uterus has contracted and to assess vaginal bleeding.

If severe bleeding occurs, the woman's lower abdomen is massaged to help the uterus contract, and she is given oxytocin continuously through an intravenous line to help the uterus contract. If bleeding continues, prostaglandins can be injected into the uterine muscle to help the uterus contract. The woman may need a blood transfusion.

Doctors look for the cause of excessive bleeding. The uterus may be examined for retained fragments of the placenta. Dilation and curettage may be performed to remove these fragments. In this procedure, a small, sharp instrument (curet) is passed through the cervix (which is usually still open from the delivery).■ The curet is used to remove the retained fragments. This procedure requires an anesthetic. The cervix and vagina are examined for any tears.

If the uterus cannot be stimulated to contract and bleeding continues, the arteries supplying blood to the uterus may have to be closed off. The procedures used usually have no lasting ill effects, such as infertility or abnormalities in menstruation. Removal of the uterus (hysterectomy) is rarely necessary to stop the bleeding.

Inverted Uterus: Very rarely, the uterus is turned inside out, so that it protrudes through the cervix, into or through the vagina. An inverted uterus is a medical emergency that must be treated promptly. Doctors return the uterus to its normal position (reinvert it) by hand. Usually, the woman recovers fully after this procedure.

Procedures Used During Labor

Induction of labor is the artificial starting of labor. Usually, labor is induced by giving the woman oxytocin, a hormone that makes the uterus contract more frequently and more forcefully. The oxytocin given is identical to the oxytocin produced by the pituitary gland. It is given intravenously with an infusion pump, so that the amount of drug given can be controlled precisely. Sometimes prostaglandins, which help the cervix dilate, are also given to help start labor. Throughout induction and labor, the fetus's heart rate is monitored electronically. At first, a monitor is placed on the woman's abdomen. After the membranes are ruptured, an internal monitor may be inserted through the vagina and attached to the fetus's scalp. If induction is unsuccessful, the baby is delivered by cesarean section.

▲ see page 1001   ■ see page 1354

Augmentation of labor is the artificial hastening of labor that is proceeding ineffectively or too slowly. Oxytocin is used to augment labor. Labor is augmented when a woman has contractions that are not effectively moving the fetus through the birth canal.

Slowing of labor is the artificial delaying of labor that is proceeding too forcefully. Very rarely, a woman has contractions that are too strong, too close together, or both. If contractions are caused by the use of oxytocin, the drug is discontinued immediately. The woman may be repositioned and given analgesics. If the contractions occur spontaneously, a drug that can slow labor (such as terbutaline or ritodrine) may be given to stop or slow the contractions.

Forceps are metal surgical instruments, similar to tongs, with rounded edges that fit around the fetus's head. Forceps are occasionally used in a normal labor to ease delivery. Forceps may be required when the fetus is in distress or abnormally positioned, when the woman is having difficulty pushing, or when labor is prolonged. (Sometimes doctors perform a cesarean section instead.) If forceps delivery is tried and is unsuccessful, a cesarean section is performed. Rarely, using forceps bruises the baby's face or tears the woman's vagina.

A **vacuum extractor** can be used instead of forceps to help with delivery. A vacuum extractor consists of a small cup made of a rubberlike material that is connected to a vacuum. It is inserted into the vagina and uses suction to attach to the fetus's head. Rarely, a vacuum extractor bruises the baby's scalp.

Cesarean section is surgical delivery of a baby by incision through a woman's abdomen and uterus. Doctors perform this procedure when they think it is safer than vaginal delivery for the woman, the baby, or both. In the United States, about one fourth of deliveries are cesarean sections. An obstetrician, an anesthesiologist, nurses, and sometimes a pediatrician are involved in this surgical procedure. Use of anesthetics, intravenous drugs, antibiotics, and blood transfusions helps make a cesarean section safe. Having the woman walk around soon after surgery reduces the risk of pulmonary embolism, in which blood clots that form in the legs or pelvis travel to the lungs and block arteries there. Compared with a vaginal delivery, delivery by cesarean section results in more overall pain afterward, a longer hospital stay, and a longer recovery time.

For a cesarean section, an incision is made in the upper or lower part of the uterus. A lower incision is more common. The lower

Using Forceps or a Vacuum Extractor

Forceps or a vacuum extractor may be used to help with delivery. Forceps are placed around the baby's head. A vacuum extractor uses suction to adhere to the baby's head. With either device, the baby is gently pulled out as the woman pushes.

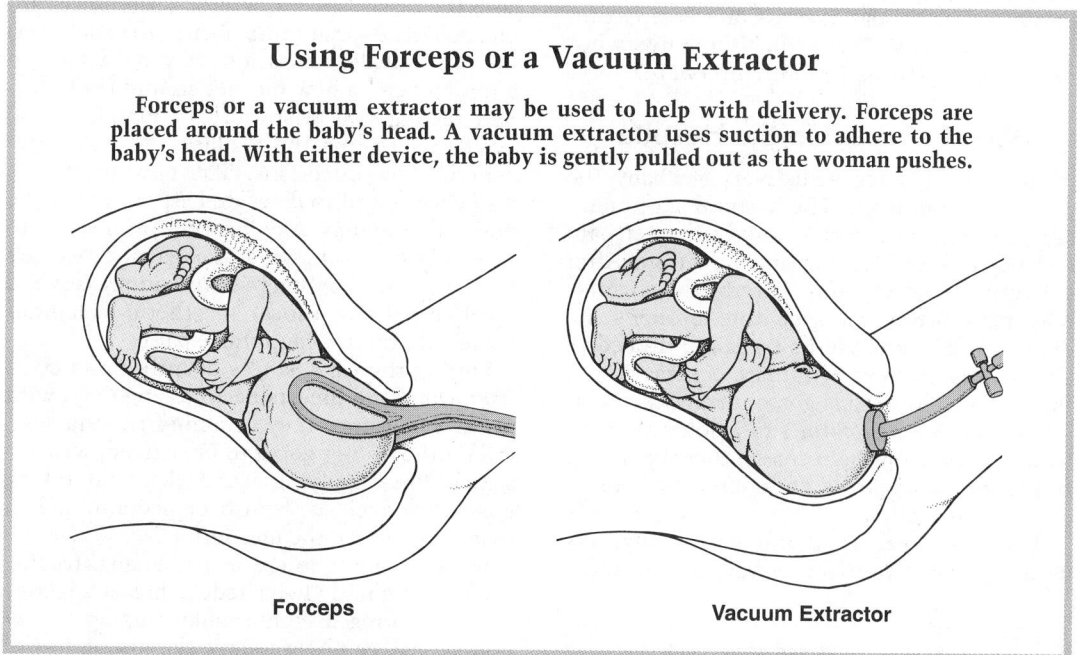

Forceps   Vacuum Extractor

part of the uterus has fewer blood vessels, so that less blood is usually lost. Also, the healed scar is stronger, so that it is less likely to open in subsequent deliveries. A lower incision may be horizontal or vertical. Usually, an upper incision is used when the placenta covering the cervix (a complication called placenta previa), when the fetus lies horizontally across the birth canal, or when the fetus is very premature.

The choice of having a vaginal delivery or a repeat cesarean section is usually offered to women who have had a lower incision. Vaginal delivery is successful in about three fourths of these women. However, such women should plan to have their baby in facilities equipped to rapidly perform a cesarean section, because there is a very small chance that the incision from the previous cesarean section will open during labor.

CHAPTER 262

Postdelivery Period

The postdelivery (postpartum) period is the 6 to 8 weeks after delivery of a baby, when the mother's body returns to its prepregnancy state.

After delivery, the mother can expect to have some symptoms, but they are usually mild and temporary. Complications are rare. Nonetheless, the doctor, hospital staff members, or health care plan usually sets up a home visit or close follow-up program. The most common complications are excessive bleeding (postpartum hemorrhage▲); bladder, kidney, or breast infections; problems with breastfeeding;■ and depression. Postpartum hemorrhage may occur soon after delivery but may occur as late as 1 month afterward.

What to Expect in the Hospital

Immediately after the delivery of a baby, the mother is monitored. The hospital staff members make every effort to minimize her pain and the risk of bleeding and infection. After delivery of the placenta (afterbirth), a nurse may periodically massage the mother's abdomen to help the uterus contract. If needed, oxytocin is given to stimulate contraction of the uterus. The drug is given intravenously as a continuous infusion for 1 to 2 hours after delivery. These steps help ensure that the uterus contracts and remains contracted to prevent excessive bleeding.

When a general anesthetic (used rarely) was used during delivery, the mother is monitored

for 2 to 3 hours after delivery, usually in a well-equipped recovery room with access to oxygen, blood that matches the mother's, and intravenous fluids.

Within the first 24 hours, the mother's pulse rate drops, her temperature may rise slightly, and the number of white blood cells temporarily increases. A bloody vaginal discharge occurs for 3 or 4 days. During the next 10 to 12 days, the discharge becomes pale brown, then yellowish white. The discharge may continue for up to about 6 weeks after delivery. Sanitary pads, changed frequently, may be used to absorb the discharge. Urine production often increases greatly, but temporarily, after delivery. Because bladder sensation may be decreased after delivery, a new mother should try to urinate regularly, at least every 4 hours. Doing so avoids overfilling the bladder and helps prevent bladder infections. The new mother is also encouraged to defecate before leaving the hospital. She may take laxatives, if needed, to avoid constipation, which can cause or worsen hemorrhoids. Applying warm compresses and a gel containing a local anesthetic to hemorrhoids, if present, can relieve pain.

During the early stages of milk production (lactation), the breasts become engorged with milk. Sometimes they become firm and sore. If a mother is not going to breastfeed, wearing a tight bra, applying ice packs, and taking analgesics such as aspirin or acetaminophen may help relieve the discomfort.

For mothers who are breastfeeding, feeding the baby regularly helps reduce breast engorgement. Wearing a comfortable nursing bra 24 hours a day can help relieve the discomfort. If

---

▲ see page 1474   ■ see page 1486

the breasts are very swollen, the mother may have to express her milk manually just before breastfeeding to enable the baby's mouth to fit around the areola (the pigmented area of skin around the nipple). If the mother is uncomfortable between feedings, she can express milk by hand in a warm shower to relieve the pressure. However, expressing milk between feedings tends to result in continued engorgement and should be done only when necessary for relief.

After the first 24 hours, recovery is rapid. The mother can have a regular diet as soon as she wants it, sometimes shortly after delivery. She should get up and walk as soon as possible. If delivery was vaginal, a new mother can start exercises to strengthen abdominal muscles, often after 1 day. Sit-ups with bent knees, done in bed, are effective. However, most new mothers are too tired to start exercising so soon after delivery.

Before the mother leaves the hospital, she is examined. If she has never had German measles (rubella) or the German measles vaccine, she is vaccinated. If she has Rh-negative blood and the baby has Rh-positive blood, she is given $Rh_0(D)$ immune globulin within 3 days of delivery. This drug destroys any of the baby's red blood cells that may have passed to the mother and may trigger the production of antibodies by the mother. Such antibodies may endanger subsequent pregnancies.▲ The new mother is examined again 6 weeks later. Also before leaving the hospital, she is given information about changes to expect in her body and the type of contraception that can be used as her body recovers from having a baby.

If mother and baby are healthy, they commonly leave the hospital within 48 hours after vaginal delivery and within 96 hours after a cesarean section.

What to Expect at Home

The uterus, still enlarged, continues to contract for some time, becoming progressively smaller during the next 2 weeks. These contractions are irregular and often painful. Contractions are intensified by breastfeeding. Breastfeeding triggers the production of the hormone oxytocin. Oxytocin stimulates the flow of milk (called the let-down reflex) and uterine contractions. Normally, after 5 to 7 days, the uterus is firm and no longer tender but is still somewhat enlarged, extending to halfway between the pubic bone and the navel. By 2 weeks after delivery, the uterus returns to its normal size. However, the new mother's abdomen does not become as flat as it was before the pregnancy for several months, even if she exercises. Stretch marks may not lighten for a year.

A new mother may take showers or baths, but she should refrain from vaginal douching for at least 2 weeks after delivery. Washing the area around the vagina with warm water 2 or 3 times a day helps reduce tenderness. Warm sitz baths can relieve pain resulting from an episiotomy or from hemorrhoids. Sitz baths are taken in a sitting position with water covering only the hips and buttocks.

Mothers who are not breastfeeding may take drugs to help them sleep or to relieve pain. For pain, they are usually given acetaminophen or a nonsteroidal anti-inflammatory drug (NSAID). Mothers who are breastfeeding are given limited amounts of such drugs because most drugs appear in breast milk.■

Mothers who are breastfeeding need to learn how to position the baby during feeding.★ If the baby is not positioned well, the mother's nipples may become sore. Sometimes the baby draws in its lower lip and sucks it, irritating the nipple. In such cases, the mother can ease the baby's lip out of its mouth with her thumb. After a feeding, she should let the milk dry naturally on the nipples rather than wipe or wash them. If she wishes, she can dry her nipples with a hair dryer set on low. In very dry climates, hypoallergenic lanolin or ointment can be applied to the nipples. Plastic bra liners should be avoided.

As long as a mother is breastfeeding, she needs extra nourishment, especially calcium. Dairy products are an excellent source of calcium. Nuts and green leafy vegetables may be substituted if the mother cannot tolerate dairy products. Or she may take calcium supplements. Vitamin supplements are not necessary if the mother's diet is well balanced, particularly if it includes sufficient amounts of vitamins B_6, B_{12}, and C.

A new mother may resume normal daily activities when she feels ready. She may resume sexual intercourse as soon as she desires it and it is comfortable. Use of contraceptives is rec-

▲ see page 1453

■ see box on page 1462

★ see art on page 1487

ommended because pregnancy is possible as soon as the mother begins to release an egg from the ovary (ovulate) again. Mothers who are not breastfeeding usually begin to ovulate again about 4 weeks after delivery, before their first period. However, ovulation can occur earlier. Mothers who are breastfeeding tend to start ovulating and menstruating somewhat later, usually 10 to 12 weeks after delivery. The interval depends on how much food other than breast milk the baby consumes. If more than four fifths of the baby's food is breast milk, ovulation is unlikely to occur. Occasionally, a mother who is breastfeeding ovulates, menstruates, and becomes pregnant as quickly as a mother who is not breastfeeding.

Full recovery after pregnancy takes about 1 to 2 years. So doctors usually advise a new mother to wait before becoming pregnant again (although she may choose not to follow that advice). At her first doctor's appointment after delivery, a new mother can discuss contraceptive options▲ with her doctor and choose one that suits her situation. A new mother who has just been vaccinated against German measles (rubella) must wait at least 1 month before becoming pregnant again to avoid endangering the fetus.

Postpartum Infections

Immediately after delivery, the woman's temperature often increases. A temperature of 101° F (38.3° C) or higher during the first 12 hours after delivery could indicate an infection but usually does not. Nonetheless, in such cases, the woman should be evaluated by her doctor or midwife. A postpartum infection is usually diagnosed after 24 hours have passed since delivery and the woman has had a temperature of 100.4° F (38° C) or higher on two occasions at least 6 hours apart. Postpartum infections are rare, because doctors try to prevent or treat conditions that can lead to infections. However, infections may be serious. Thus, if a woman has a temperature of more than 100.4° F at any time during the first week after delivery, she should call the doctor.

Postpartum infections may be directly related to delivery (occurring in the uterus or the area around the uterus) or indirectly related (occurring in the kidneys, bladder, breasts, or lungs).

INFECTIONS OF THE UTERUS

Postpartum infections usually begin in the uterus. If an infection of the membranes containing the fetus (amniotic sac) caused a fever during labor, an infection of the uterine lining (endometritis), uterine muscle (myometritis), or areas around the uterus (parametritis) may result.

Causes and Symptoms

Bacteria that normally live in the healthy vagina can cause an infection after delivery. Conditions that make a woman more likely to develop to infection include anemia, preeclampsia,■ repeated vaginal examinations, a delay of longer than 18 hours between rupture of the membranes and delivery, prolonged labor, a cesarean section, placental fragments remaining in the uterus after delivery, and excessive bleeding after delivery (postpartum hemorrhage).

Symptoms commonly include paleness, chills, headache, a general feeling of illness or discomfort, and loss of appetite. The heart rate is rapid, and the number of white blood cells is abnormally high. The uterus is swollen, tender, and soft. Typically, there is a malodorous discharge from the vagina, which varies in amount.

When the tissues around the uterus are infected, they swell, holding the swollen, tender uterus rigidly in place. The woman has severe pain and a high fever.

The abdominal lining can become inflamed, causing peritonitis. Blood clots may form in the pelvic veins, causing pelvic thrombophlebitis. A blood clot may travel to the lung and block an artery there, causing pulmonary embolism. Poisonous substances (toxins) produced by the infecting bacteria may reach high levels in the bloodstream, leading to toxic shock. In toxic shock, blood pressure falls dramatically and the heart rate is very rapid. Toxic shock may result in severe kidney damage and even death.

Diagnosis and Treatment

An infection is usually diagnosed based on results of a physical examination. Samples of urine, blood, and the vaginal discharge are cultured for bacteria.

If the uterus is infected, the woman is usually given an antibiotic intravenously until she has had no fever for 48 hours. For a few days afterward, she may be given antibiotics by mouth.

▲ see page 1419   ■ see page 1452

BLADDER AND KIDNEY INFECTIONS

A bladder infection (cystitis) sometimes develops when a catheter is placed in the bladder to relieve a buildup of urine during and after labor. Or bacteria may be present in the bladder during pregnancy but cause no symptoms until after delivery. A kidney infection (pyelonephritis) is caused by bacteria spreading from the bladder to the kidney after delivery.

Symptoms may include a fever and painful or frequent urination. Infection that has reached the kidneys may cause pain in the lower back or side, a general feeling of illness or discomfort, and constipation.

Typically, a woman is given an antibiotic. If there is no evidence that the bladder infection has spread to the kidneys, antibiotics may be given for only a few days. If a kidney infection is suspected, antibiotics are given until the woman has had no fever for 48 hours. Urine samples are cultured to identify the bacteria. After culture results are available, the antibiotic may be changed to one that is more effective against the bacteria present. Drinking plenty of fluids helps keep the kidneys functioning well and flushes bacteria out of the urinary tract. Another urine sample is cultured 6 to 8 weeks after delivery to verify that the infection is cured.

BREAST INFECTION

A breast infection (mastitis▲) can occur after delivery, usually during the first 6 weeks and almost always in women who are breastfeeding. If the skin of or around the nipples becomes cracked, bacteria from the skin can enter the milk ducts and cause an infection. An infected breast usually appears red and swollen and feels warm and tender. The woman may have a fever. A fever that develops later than 10 days after delivery is often caused by a breast infection, although it may be caused by a bladder infection.

Breast infections are treated with antibiotics. Women who have a breast infection and are breastfeeding should continue to breastfeed. Breastfeeding decreases the risk of a breast abscess (a collection of pus), which is rare. Breast abscesses are treated with antibiotics and are usually drained surgically.

Blood Clots

The risk of developing blood clots (thromboembolic disease) is increased after delivery. Typically, blood clots occur in the legs or pelvis (a disorder called thrombophlebitis). A fever that develops between 4 and 10 days after delivery may be caused by a blood clot.

Treatment consists of warm compresses (to reduce discomfort), compression bandages applied by a doctor or nurse, and bed rest with the leg elevated (by raising the foot of the bed 6 inches). Anticoagulants may be necessary.

Thyroid Disorders

In 4 to 7% of women, the thyroid gland malfunctions during the first 6 months after delivery. Thyroid hormone levels may be high or low, usually temporarily. Women who have a family history of thyroid disorders or diabetes are particularly susceptible. In women who already have a thyroid disorder, such as a goiter or Hashimoto's thyroiditis, the disorder may become worse. Treatment may be required.

Postpartum Depression

Postpartum depression is a feeling of extreme sadness and related psychologic disturbances during the first few weeks or months after delivery.

The baby blues—feeling sad or miserable within 3 days of delivery—is common after delivery. New mothers should not be overly concerned about these feelings because they usually disappear within 2 weeks. Postpartum depression is a more serious mood change. It lasts weeks or months. This form affects about 1% of women. An even more severe, very rare form, called postpartum psychosis, includes psychotic behavior.

The causes of sadness or depression after delivery are unclear. The sudden decrease in levels of hormones, particularly estrogen and progesterone, may contribute. Depression that was present before pregnancy is likely to evolve into postpartum depression. Women who have had depression before they became pregnant should tell their doctor or midwife about it during the pregnancy. The stresses of having and caring for a baby may also contribute. Such stresses include difficulties during labor and delivery, lack of sleep, and feelings of isolation and incompetence. Women who develop postpartum depression may have had depression or another psychologic disorder before pregnancy, or they may have close

▲ see also page 1389

relatives with depression. Lack of social support and marital discord increase the likelihood of developing postpartum depression.

Symptoms may include frequent crying, mood swings, and irritability as well as feelings of sadness. Less common symptoms include extreme fatigue, difficulty concentrating, sleep problems, loss of interest in sex, anxiety, appetite changes, and feelings of inadequacy or hopelessness. These symptoms interfere with the woman's daily activities. A woman with postpartum depression may show no interest in her baby.

▲ see table on page 618
■ see table on page 645
★ see box on page 1462

In postpartum psychosis, depression may be combined with suicidal or violent thoughts, hallucinations, or bizarre behavior. Sometimes postpartum psychosis includes a desire to harm the baby.

If the woman is sad, support from family members and friends is usually all that is needed. But if depression is diagnosed, professional help is also needed. Typically, a combination of counseling and antidepressants▲ is recommended. A woman who has postpartum psychosis may need to be hospitalized, preferably in a unit that allows the baby to remain with her. She may need antipsychotic drugs ■ as well as antidepressants. A woman who is breastfeeding should consult with her doctor before taking any of these drugs to determine whether she can continue to breastfeed.★

CHILDREN'S HEALTH ISSUES

263 Normal Newborns and Infants...1483

Initial Care ▪ Physical Examination ▪ First Few Days ▪ Feeding ▪ Stools and Urine ▪ Sleeping ▪ Physical Development ▪ Behavioral, Social, and Intellectual Development ▪ Promoting Optimal Development ▪ Preventive Health Care Visits ▪ Vaccinations

264 Problems in Newborns 1494

Birth Injury ▪ Prematurity ▪ Postmaturity ▪ Small for Gestational Age ▪ Large for Gestational Age ▪ Respiratory Distress Syndrome ▪ Transient Tachypnea ▪ Meconium Aspiration Syndrome ▪ Persistent Pulmonary Hypertension ▪ Pneumothorax ▪ Bronchopulmonary Dysplasia ▪ Apnea of Prematurity ▪ Retinopathy of Prematurity ▪ Necrotizing Enterocolitis ▪ Hyperbilirubinemia ▪ Anemia ▪ Polycythemia ▪ Disorders of the Thyroid Gland ▪ Neonatal Sepsis

265 Birth Defects...1511

Heart Defects ▪ Urinary Tract Defects ▪ Genital Defects ▪ Digestive Tract Defects ▪ Bone and Muscle Defects ▪ Brain and Spinal Cord Defects

266 Chromosomal and Genetic Abnormalities 1527

Down Syndrome ▪ Fragile X Syndrome ▪ Turner Syndrome ▪ Noonan Syndrome ▪ Triple X Syndrome ▪ Klinefelter Syndrome ▪ XYY Syndrome ▪ Long QT Syndrome

267 Problems in Infants and Very Young Children 1531

Fussiness, Excessive Crying, and Colic ▪ Teething ▪ Feeding Problems ▪ Bowel Problems ▪ Separation Anxiety ▪ Skin Rashes ▪ Undescended and Retractile Testes ▪ Fever ▪ Failure to Thrive ▪ Sudden Infant Death Syndrome

268 Normal Preschool and School-Aged Children 1538

Physical Development ▪ Intellectual Development ▪ Social and Emotional Development ▪ Promoting Optimal Health and Development ▪ Preventive Health Care Visits

269 Behavioral and Developmental Problems in Young Children 1543

Eating Problems ▪ Bed-Wetting ▪ Encopresis ▪ Sleep Problems ▪ Temper Tantrums ▪ Breath-Holding Spells ▪ School Avoidance ▪ Attention Deficit/Hyperactivity Disorder ▪ Learning Disorders ▪ Dyslexia

270   Normal Adolescents 1552

Physical Development ▪ Intellectual and Behavioral
Development ▪ Social Development ▪ Development of
Sexuality ▪ Preventive Health Care Visits

271   Problems in Adolescents 1555

Delayed Sexual Maturation ▪ Short Stature ▪ Obesity ▪
School Problems ▪ Behavioral Problems ▪ Drug and Substance
Use and Abuse ▪ Contraception and Adolescent Pregnancy

272   Bacterial Infections...1561

Occult Bacteremia ▪ Bacterial Meningitis ▪ Diphtheria ▪
Retropharyngeal Abscess ▪ Epiglottitis ▪ Pertussis ▪
Rheumatic Fever ▪ Urinary Tract Infection

273   Viral Infections 1568

Central Nervous System Infections ▪ Chickenpox ▪ Erythema
Infectiosum ▪ Human Immunodeficiency Virus Infection ▪
Measles ▪ Mumps ▪ Polio ▪ Respiratory Tract Infections ▪
Roseola Infantum ▪ Rubella ▪ Subacute Sclerosing
Panencephalitis

274   Respiratory Disorders 1583

Asthma ▪ Bronchiolitis ▪ Croup

275   Digestive Disorders 1586

Gastroenteritis ▪ Gastroesophageal Reflux ▪ Peptic Ulcer ▪
Intussusception ▪ Appendicitis ▪ Meckel's Diverticulum ▪
Constipation ▪ Recurring Abdominal Pain

276   Ear, Nose, and Throat Disorders 1593

Middle Ear Infections ▪ Serous Otitis Media ▪ Pharyngitis ▪
Enlarged Tonsils and Adenoids ▪ Hearing Deficits ▪ Objects in
the Ears and Nose ▪ Neck Masses ▪ Laryngeal Papillomas

277   Eye Disorders 1600

Amblyopia ▪ Strabismus

278   Bone Disorders 1603

Scoliosis ▪ Kyphosis ▪ Slipped Capital Femoral Epiphysis ▪
Legg-Calvé-Perthes Disease ▪ Osgood-Schlatter Disease ▪
Chondromalacia Patellae

279   Hereditary Connective Tissue Disorders 1607

Ehlers-Danlos Syndrome ▪ Marfan Syndrome ▪
Pseudoxanthoma Elasticum ▪ Cutis Laxa ▪
Mucopolysaccharidoses ▪ Osteogenesis Imperfecta ▪
Chondrodysplasias ▪ Osteopetroses

280   Juvenile Rheumatoid Arthritis 1612

281   **Diabetes Mellitus** **1613**

282   **Hereditary Disorders of Metabolism** **1616**
Carbohydrate Metabolism Disorders ▪ Amino Acid Metabolism
Disorders ▪ Lipid Metabolism Disorders ▪ Pyruvate Metabolism
Disorders

283   **Childhood Cancers** **1622**
Wilms' Tumor ▪ Neuroblastoma ▪ Retinoblastoma

284   **Cerebral Palsy** **1624**

285   **Mental Retardation**...**1626**

286   **Mental Health Disorders** **1630**
Autism ▪ Asperger's Disorder and Pervasive Developmental
Disorder Not Otherwise Specified ▪ Rett's Disorder ▪
Childhood Disintegrative Disorder ▪ Childhood Schizophrenia ▪
Depression ▪ Manic-Depressive Illness ▪ Suicidal Behavior ▪
Conduct Disorder ▪ Oppositional Defiant Disorder ▪
Separation Anxiety Disorder ▪ Somatoform Disorders

287   **Social Issues Affecting Children and Their Families** **1638**
Illness and Death in Infants ▪ Illness in Children ▪ Divorce ▪
Childcare ▪ Foster Care ▪ Adoption

288   **Child Neglect and Abuse** **1643**

—————————————— CHAPTER 263 ——————————————

Normal Newborns and Infants

The successful transition of a fetus, immersed in amniotic fluid and totally dependent on the placenta for nutrition and oxygen, to a squalling, air-breathing baby is a source of wonder. Healthy newborns (age birth to 1 month) and infants (age 1 month to 1 year) need good care to ensure their normal development and continued health.

Initial Care

Immediately after a baby is born, the doctor or nurse gently clears mucus and other material from the mouth, nose, and throat with a suction bulb. The newborn is then able to take a breath. Two clamps are placed on the newborn's umbilical cord, side by side, and the umbilical cord is then cut between the clamps. The newborn is dried and laid carefully on a sterile warm blanket or on the mother's abdomen.

The newborn is then weighed and measured. The doctor examines the newborn for any obvious abnormalities or signs of distress; a full physical examination comes later. The newborn's overall condition is recorded at 1 minute and at 5 minutes after birth using the Apgar score. A low Apgar score is a sign that

Cutting the Umbilical Cord

Soon after a baby is born, two clamps are placed on the umbilical cord, and the cord is cut between the clamps. The clamp on the cord's stump is removed within 24 hours after birth. The stump should be kept clean and dry. Some doctors recommend applying an alcohol solution to the stump daily. The stump falls off on its own in a week or two.

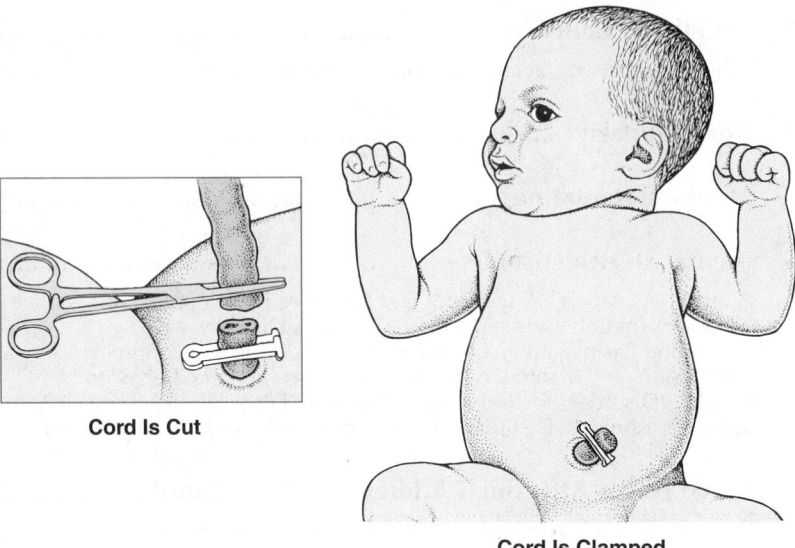

Cord Is Cut

Cord Is Clamped

the newborn is having difficulty and may need extra assistance with breathing or blood circulation. However, contrary to what people may think, babies with low Apgar scores are not more likely to develop certain problems, such as cerebral palsy or permanent disabilities.

Keeping the newborn warm is critical. As soon as possible, the newborn is wrapped in lightweight clothing (swaddled), and the head is covered to reduce the loss of body heat. A few drops of an antibiotic are placed into the eyes to prevent infection from any harmful organisms that the newborn may have had contact with during delivery.

The mother, father, and newborn usually recover together in the delivery room. If the delivery is in a birth center, the mother, father, and newborn remain together in the same room. If the mother is breastfeeding, she puts the infant to her breast within the first 30 minutes. Once transported to the nursery, the newborn is placed on his side in a small crib and kept warm. Placing the baby on his side prevents fluid or mucus from blocking the airway and impeding breathing. Because all ba-

bies are born with low levels of vitamin K, a doctor or nurse administers an injection of vitamin K to prevent bleeding (hemorrhagic disease of the newborn).

About 6 hours or more after birth, the newborn is bathed. The nurse tries not to wash off the whitish greasy material (vernix caseosa) that covers most of the newborn's skin, because this material helps protect against infection.

Physical Examination

The doctor usually gives the newborn a thorough physical examination within the first 12 hours of life. The examination begins with a series of measurements, including weight, length, and head circumference. The average weight at birth is 7 pounds, and the average length is 20 inches. Then the doctor examines the baby's skin, head and face, heart and lungs, nervous system, abdomen, and genitals.

The skin is usually reddish, although the fingers and toes may have a bluish tinge because of poor blood circulation during the first few hours. Occasionally, the skin has several hard lumps (subcutaneous fat necrosis) where pressure from bones destroyed some fatty tissue. Such lumps are most common on the head, cheek, and neck—particularly if forceps were used during delivery. The lumps may break through to the skin surface, releasing a clear yellow fluid, but they usually heal fairly quickly.

A normal head-first delivery leaves the head slightly misshapen for several days. The bones that form the skull overlap, which allows the head to become compressed for delivery. Some swelling and bruising of the scalp is typical. Sometimes bleeding from one of the bones of the skull and its outer covering causes a small bump on the head that disappears in a few weeks. When the baby is delivered buttocks first (breech delivery), the head usually does not become misshapen; however, the buttocks, genitals, or feet may become swollen and bruised instead.

Pressure during a vaginal delivery may bruise the newborn's face. In addition, compression through the birth canal may make the face initially appear asymmetrical. This asymmetry sometimes results when one of the nerves supplying the face muscles is damaged during delivery. Recovery is gradual over the next few weeks.

The doctor listens to the heart and lungs through a stethoscope to detect any abnormality. The doctor inspects the newborn's skin color and general condition for any sign of a problem. The strength of the pulse is checked.

The doctor looks for any abnormalities of the nerves and tests the baby's reflexes. A newborn's most important reflexes are the Moro, rooting, and sucking reflexes.

Many serious disorders that are not apparent at birth can nonetheless be detected by blood tests in newborns. Because of this, all states require a number of blood tests in newborns. Early diagnosis and prompt treatment can reduce or prevent disorders that may interfere with an infant's healthy development.

The doctor examines the general shape of the abdomen and also checks the size, shape, and position of internal organs, such as the kidneys, liver, and spleen. Enlarged kidneys may indicate an obstruction to the outflow of urine.

The doctor examines the flexibility and mobility of the arms, legs, and hips, and checks to see if the newborn has dislocated hips.

The doctor examines the genitals to ensure the urethra is open and in the proper location.

Three Common Reflexes of Newborns

> In the **Moro reflex,** when the newborn is startled, the arms and legs swing out and forward in a slow movement with fingers outstretched. In the **rooting reflex,** when either side of the mouth is touched, the newborn turns his head toward that side. This reflex enables the newborn to find the nipple. In the **sucking reflex,** when an object is placed in the newborn's mouth, sucking begins immediately.

In a boy, the testes should be present in the scrotum. In a girl, the labia are prominent; exposure to the mother's hormones causes them to be swollen for the first few weeks. The doctor examines the anus to make sure the opening is not sealed shut.

First Few Days

Immediately after a normal birth, the mother and father are encouraged to hold their newborn. Breastfeeding may be initiated at this time if the mother plans to breastfeed. Some experts believe that early physical contact with the newborn helps establish bonding. However, parents can bond well with their newborn even when the first hours are not spent together. Mother and baby spend a day or two in the hospital during which time new parents are taught to feed, bathe, and dress the baby and become familiar with the baby's activities and sounds. In the United States, discharge from the hospital within 24 hours is common.

The plastic cord clamp on the umbilical cord is removed within 24 hours after birth. Some doctors recommend that the stump be moistened daily with an alcohol solution to speed drying and reduce the chance of infection; an antibiotic ointment should not be used because it can prolong the drying process. The stump falls off on its own in a week or two.

Circumcision, if desired, generally is performed within the first few days of life before the newborn is discharged. The decision about having a newborn circumcised usually depends on the parents' religious beliefs or personal preferences. The main medical reason for circumcision is to remove an unusually tight foreskin that is obstructing the flow of urine. Although circumcised males also have a lower risk of cancer of the penis and urinary tract infections, these risks can be minimized with proper hygiene. Circumcision can result in infection, excessive bleeding, scarring, and very rarely in accidental amputation of the penis tip. About 2 to 20 boys per 1,000 require a minor surgical procedure later to correct various problems resulting from circumcision. An equal number of uncircumcised males require a circumcision later in life.

Circumcision should not be performed if the boy has not voided, or if the penis is abnormal in any way, because the foreskin may be needed for any plastic surgical repair that may be needed later. Circumcision must be delayed if, during the pregnancy, the mother had been taking drugs that increase the risk of bleeding, such as anticoagulants or aspirin; the doctor waits until all such drugs have been eliminated from the newborn's circulation.

Most newborns have a mild skin rash sometime during the first week after birth. The rash usually appears in areas of the body rubbed by clothing—the arms, legs, and back—and rarely on the face. It tends to disappear on its own without treatment. Applying lotions or powders, using perfumed soaps, and putting plastic pants over the diapers are likely to make the rash worse, especially in hot weather. Dryness and some skin peeling often occur after a few days, especially in the creases at the wrists and ankles.

Newborns who are otherwise normal may develop a yellow color to their skin (jaundice) after the first day. Jaundice that appears before 24 hours of age is of particular concern.

The first urine produced by a newborn is concentrated and often contains chemicals called urates, which can turn the diaper pink. If a newborn does not urinate within the first 24 hours of life, the doctor tries to find out why. Delay in starting to urinate is more common in boys.

The first bowel movement is a sticky greenish black substance (meconium). Every baby should pass meconium within the first 24 hours after birth. Failure to pass a bowel movement is usually caused by a hardened plug of meconium inside the baby's intestine, which can usually be removed by one or more gentle enemas. A birth defect may cause a more serious blockage.

After a few days in the hospital, the newborn is able to go home. Having a new baby in a household requires a great deal of adjustment for all involved. For a household that has had no children, changes in lifestyle may be dramatic. When other children are present, jealousy can be a problem. Preparing other children for the newcomer and being careful to pay attention to them and include them can ease the transition. Pets may also need some extra attention to help them adjust to the baby. In some cases, keeping pets away from the baby may be necessary.

Feeding

A normal newborn has active rooting and sucking reflexes and can start eating immediately after birth. If the baby has not been placed at the mother's breast immediately after birth, feedings are ordinarily begun within 4 hours after birth.

Most babies swallow air along with their milk. Because they cannot usually burp on their own, parents help the baby expel the air by holding him upright leaning against the parent's chest with his head against the shoulder and patting gently on his back. The combination of patting and pressure against the shoulder usually leads to an audible burp, often accompanied by spitting up of a small amount of milk. Many experts recommend exclusive breast or formula feeding for 6 months.

BREASTFEEDING

Breast milk is the ideal food for newborns. Besides providing the necessary nutrients in the most easily digestible and absorbable form, breast milk contains antibodies and white blood cells that protect the baby against infection. Breast milk favorably changes the pH of the stool and intestinal flora, thus protecting the baby against bacterial diarrhea. Because of the protective qualities of breast milk, many types of infections occur less often in babies who are breastfed rather than bottle-fed. Breastfeeding offers many advantages to the mother as well; for example, it helps her to bond and feel close to her baby in a way that bottle-feeding cannot. About 60% of mothers in the United States breastfeed their babies, and this proportion is steadily increasing. Mothers who work may breastfeed while at home and have the baby bottle-feed pumped breast milk or formula during the hours they are away. Most doctors recommend giving daily vitamin D supplements to breastfed infants after 2 months of age.

A thin yellow fluid, called colostrum, flows from the nipple before breast milk is produced. Colostrum is rich in calories, protein, and antibodies. The antibodies are absorbed directly into the body from the stomach, protecting the baby against many infections.

To begin breastfeeding, the mother settles into a comfortable, relaxed position, either seated or lying almost flat, and turns from one side to the other to offer each breast. The baby faces the mother. The mother supports her breast with her thumb and index finger on top and other fingers below and brushes her nipple against the middle of the baby's lower lip. This stimulates the baby to open his mouth—the rooting reflex—and grasp the breast. As the mother eases the nipple and areola into the baby's mouth, she makes sure the nipple is centered, which helps keep the nipple from becoming sore. Before removing the baby from the breast, the mother breaks the suction by inserting her finger into the baby's mouth and gently pressing the baby's chin down. Sore nipples result from poor positioning and are easier to prevent than to cure.

Initially, the baby tends to feed for several minutes at each breast. The resulting reflex (let-down reflex) in the mother triggers milk production. The production of milk depends on sufficient suckling time, so feeding times should be long enough for milk production to be fully established. During the first few weeks, the infant should be encouraged to nurse on both breasts with each feeding; however, some infants fall asleep while feeding at the first breast. The breast used last should be used first for the next feeding. For a first baby, full milk production is usually established in 72 to 96 hours. Less time is needed for subsequent babies. If the mother is particularly tired during the first night, one middle of the night feeding may be replaced with water. However, no more than 6 hours should elapse between feeding sessions during the first few days in order to stimulate the production of breast milk. Feeding should be on demand (the baby's, that is) rather than by the clock. Similarly, the length of each breastfeeding session should be adjusted to meet the baby's needs. Babies nurse 8 to 12 times in a 24-hour period, but this guideline varies widely.

The mother should take the baby, especially a first baby, to the doctor 3 to 5 days after delivery so that the doctor can find out how breastfeeding is going and answer any questions. A doctor may need to see the baby ear-

Positioning a Baby to Breastfeed

The mother settles into a comfortable, relaxed position. She may sit or lie almost flat, and she may hold the baby in several different positions. A mother should find the position that works best for her and her baby. She may wish to alternate among different positions.

A common position is holding the baby on the lap so that the baby is stomach to stomach with the mother. The mother supports the baby's neck and head with her left arm when the baby is feeding on the left breast. The baby is brought to the level of the breast, not the breast to the baby. Support for the mother and the baby is important. Pillows can be placed behind the mother's back or under her arm. Placing her feet on a footstool or coffee table may help keep her from leaning over the baby. Leaning over may strain her back and result in sore nipples. A pillow or folded blanket may be placed under the baby for added support.

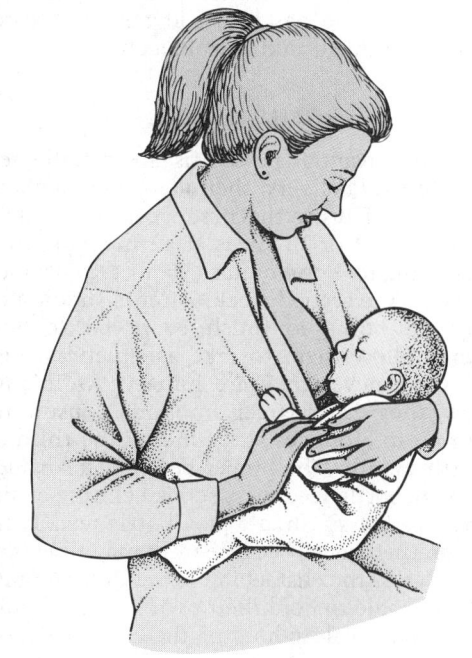

lier if the baby was discharged within 24 hours, is not feeding well, or if the parents have a particular concern. Because mothers cannot tell exactly how much milk a baby takes, doctors use frequency of feeding and weight gain to tell whether milk production is adequate. Babies that are hungry and feed every hour or two but fail to gain weight appropriately for their age and size are probably not getting enough milk.

When to stop breastfeeding (wean the infant) depends on the needs and desires of both mother and baby. Breastfeeding exclusively for at least 6 months and breastfeeding along with solid foods until age 12 months are considered most desirable. Gradual weaning over weeks or months is easier for both the baby and mother than stopping suddenly. Mothers initially replace one to three breastfeeding sessions a day with a bottle or cup of fruit juice, expressed breast milk, or formula. Some feedings, particularly those at mealtimes, should be replaced by solid food. Learning to drink from a cup is an important developmental milestone, and weaning to a cup can be completed by age 10 months. Mothers gradually replace more and more breastfeedings, although many infants continue one or two breastfeedings daily until the age of 18 to 24 months or longer. When breastfeeding continues longer, the child should also be eating solid foods and drinking from a cup.

BOTTLE-FEEDING

In the hospital, newborns are usually fed shortly after delivery, then ideally on demand thereafter. During the first week after birth, babies take 1 or 2 ounces at a time, gradually increasing to 3 or 4 ounces about 6 to 8 times a day by the second week. Parents should not urge newborns to finish every bottle but, rather, allow them to take as much as they want whenever they are hungry. As infants grow, they drink larger amounts, consuming up to 6 to 8 ounces at a time by the third or fourth month. The proper position for babies who are bottle-feeding is semi-reclining or sitting up. Babies should not bottle-feed lying flat on their backs because milk may flow into the nose or the eustachian tube. Older infants who are able to hold their own bottles should not be put to sleep holding the bottle because the continuous exposure to milk or juice can damage their teeth and lead to cavities.

Commercial baby formulas containing a proper balance of nutrients, calories, and vitamins are available in ready-to-feed, sterile bottles, cans of concentrated formula that must be diluted with water, and powder. Formulas are available both with and without an iron supplement; most doctors recommend a for-

mula that contains iron. Parents who use concentrated formula or powders must carefully follow the directions for preparation on the container. Formulas are usually made from cow's milk, although soy-based formulas—which are of benefit to infants who cannot tolerate cow's milk—are also available. There are no long-term health differences in infants fed either type of formula. Plain cow's milk, however, is not an appropriate food during the first year of life.

To minimize the infant's exposure to microorganisms, formula must be fed from a sterile container. Disposable plastic liners eliminate the need to sterilize bottles. Nipples for the bottles should be sterilized in a pot of boiling water for 5 minutes. Parents should warm formula feedings to body temperature. Filled bottles—or formula containers, if disposable liners are used—are placed in a *warm* water bath and allowed to come to body temperature. Babies may be seriously burned if formula is too hot, so parents need to shake the bottle gently to even out the temperature and then check the temperature by placing a few drops on the sensitive skin inside their wrist. Formula at body temperature should feel neither warm nor cold to the touch. Microwave ovens may dangerously overheat formula and are not recommended for warming formula or baby food.

The size of the nipple opening is important. In general, formula should drip slowly out of a bottle held upside down. Larger, older infants want larger volumes of liquid and can tolerate a larger nipple opening.

STARTING SOLID FOODS

The time to start solid food depends on the infant's needs and readiness. Generally, infants need solids when they are large enough to need a more concentrated source of calories than formula. This is recognized when an infant takes a full bottle and is satisfied, but then is hungry again in 2 or 3 hours. This typically occurs by the age of 6 months. Infants younger than this cannot easily swallow solid food, although some can swallow solids at younger ages if the food is placed on the back of the tongue. Some parents coax very young infants to eat large amounts of solid food so that they will sleep through the night. This is unlikely to work, and forcing an infant to eat early can cause aspiration pneumonia and feeding problems later. Many infants take solids after a breastfeeding or bottle-feeding, which both satisfies their need to suck and quickly relieves their hunger.

Infants develop food allergies or intolerance easier than older children or adults. If many different foods are given in a brief period, it is difficult to tell which one may have been responsible for a reaction. Because of this, parents should introduce new foods one at a time, no more than one new food a week. Once it is clear a food is tolerated, another one may be introduced.

Single-grain cereals are begun first, followed by fruits and vegetables. Meats, which are a good source of protein, should be introduced later, after about 7 months. Many infants initially reject meat.

The food should be offered on a spoon so that the infant learns the new feeding technique. By age 6 to 9 months, infants are able to grasp food and bring it to their mouths, and they should be encouraged to help feed themselves. However, babies easily choke on food in small, hard bits (such as peanuts, raw carrots, candies, and small crackers), so these foods should be avoided. Pureed home foods are less expensive than commercial baby foods and offer adequate nutrition.

Although infants enjoy sweet foods, sugar is not an essential nutrient and should be given only in small quantities, if at all. Sweetened dessert baby foods have no benefit for babies. Honey must be avoided during the first year because it may contain the spores of *Clostridium botulinum,* which are harmless to older children and adults but can cause botulism in infants.

Stools and Urine

Infants typically urinate 15 to 20 times per day. The urine varies in color from nearly clear to dark yellow. Stools vary a great deal from infant to infant in frequency, color, and consistency depending on the nature of the individual infant and the contents of his diet. The number of times infants defecate varies—from once every other day to 6 or 8 times a day. Stool consistency ranges from firm and formed to soft and runny. Stool color ranges from mustard yellow to dark brown. The stool of breastfed babies tends to be softer and of lighter color than that of formula-fed babies.

Diapers must be changed often to keep the underlying skin dry. Wet skin chafes more eas-

ily than dry skin and is more likely to develop diaper rash. Modern, super-absorbent disposable diapers contain a layer of gel that absorbs liquid and keeps it away from the skin. These diapers keep skin drier than cloth diapers after small to moderate amounts of urine, but diapers of any type should be changed when the skin is exposed to wetness. Bacteria normally present in stool can break down urea, a substance in urine, resulting in an alkaline pH that irritates the skin, so diapers should be checked frequently for stool and changed immediately. There are several environmental considerations related to diapers. Disposable diapers consume larger amounts of material than cloth and contribute a significant volume of landfill waste. Cloth diapers consume large amounts of energy and chemicals in the laundering process.

Baby powders help keep skin dry when the baby is sweating slightly, but they do not help keep the skin dry from urine or stool and are not essential. Powder made of talcum may cause lung problems if inhaled by infants, so parents should purchase baby powders that contain cornstarch instead.

Sleeping

Because the nervous system of newborns is immature, newborns sleep a great deal, but only for an hour or two at a time, independent of day or night. By 4 to 6 weeks of age, many infants are on a cycle of waking for 4 hours and sleeping for 4 hours. Only by 2 to 3 months of age are infants capable of adopting a pattern of nighttime sleeping. By 1 year of age, most infants sleep 8 to 9 hours continuously through the night.

Parents can assist infants to sleep at night by handling and stimulating the child less in the late evening and keeping the child's room dark at night, which is important in the development of normal vision. Infants should be encouraged at an early age to fall asleep on their own and not in a parent's arms. In this way, they will be able to quiet themselves when they wake in the middle of the night.

To minimize the risk of sudden infant death syndrome (SIDS), infants should sleep on their back, rather than on their stomach. This recommendation has helped reduce the incidence of SIDS in recent years. Also, infants should not sleep with soft pillows, toys, or heavy blankets, which may obstruct their breathing.

Physical Development

An infant's physical development depends on heredity, nutrition, and environment. Physical and psychologic abnormalities can also influence growth. Optimal growth requires optimal nutrition and health.

A newborn normally loses 5 to 7% of his birth weight during the first few days of life. Newborns who are breastfeeding can lose up to 7% of their birth weight. This weight is regained by the end of the first 2 weeks as the newborn starts to eat more. After this, an infant typically gains around one ounce per day during the first two months, and a pound per month after that. This generally results in a doubling of birth weight by age 5 months and a tripling by 1 year. An infant's length increases about 30% by age 5 months and more than 50% by 1 year.

An Infant's First Year: Physical Development

During the first year of life, an infant's weight and length are charted at each doctor's visit to make sure that growth is proceeding at a steady rate. Percentiles are a way of comparing infants of the same age. For an infant at the 10th percentile for weight, 10% of infants weigh less and 90% weigh more. For an infant at the 90th percentile, 90% of infants weigh less and 10% weigh more. For an infant at the 50th percentile, 50% of infants weigh less and 50% weigh more. Of more significance than the actual percentile is any significant change in percentile between doctor's visits.

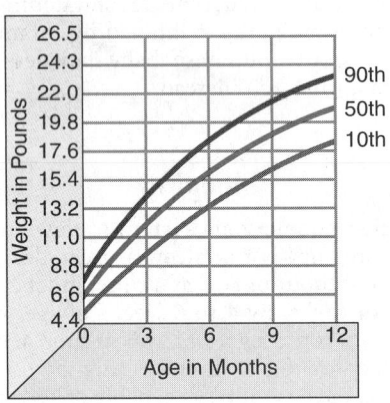

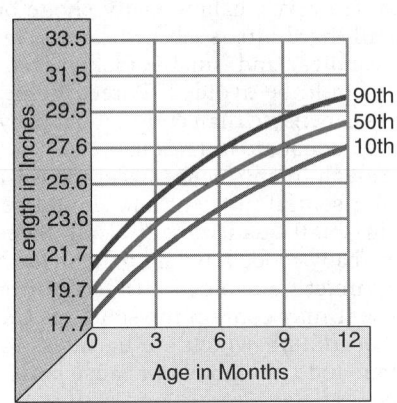

GIRLS

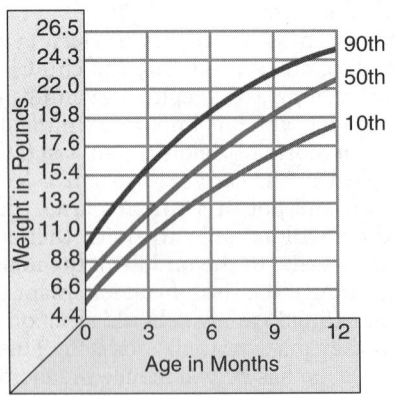

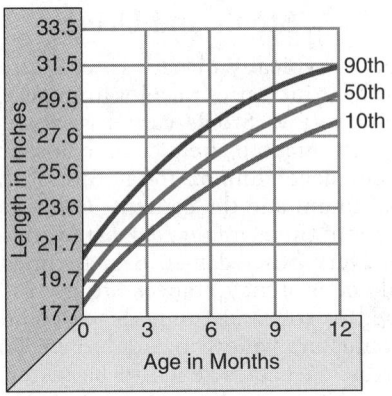

BOYS

AN INFANT'S FIRST YEAR: DEVELOPMENTAL MILESTONES

AGE	MILESTONE	AGE	MILESTONE
1 month	Brings hands toward eyes and mouth	7 months	Sits without support
	Moves head from side to side when lying on stomach		Bears some weight on legs when held upright
	Follows an object moved in an arch about 6 inches above face to the midline (straight ahead)		Transfers objects from hand to hand
			Looks for dropped object
	Responds to a noise in some way, such as startling, crying, or quieting		Responds to own name
			Responds to being told "no"
	May turn toward familiar sounds and voices		Babbles, combining vowels and consonants
	Focuses on a face		Wiggles with excitement in anticipation of playing
3 months	Raises head 45 degrees (possibly 90 degrees) when lying on stomach		Plays peekaboo
	Opens and shuts hands	9 months	Works to get a toy that is out of reach
	Pushes down when feet are placed on a flat surface		Objects if toy is taken away
	Swings at and reaches for dangling toys		Crawls or creeps on hands and knees
	Follows an object moved in an arch above face from one side to the other		Pulls self up to standing position
			Stands holding on to someone or something
	Watches faces intently		Says "mama" or "dada" indiscriminately
	Smiles at sound of mother's voice		
	Begins to make speechlike sounds	12 months	Gets into a sitting position from stomach
5 months	Holds head steady when upright		Walks by holding furniture; may walk one or two steps without support
	Rolls over one way, usually from stomach to back		
	Reaches for objects		Stands for a few moments at a time
	Recognizes people at a distance		Says "dada" and "mama" to the appropriate person
	Listens intently to human voices		
	Smiles spontaneously		Drinks from a cup
	Squeals in delight		Claps hands and waves bye-bye

Different organs grow at different rates. For example, the reproductive system has a brief growth spurt just after birth, then changes very little until just before puberty. In contrast, the brain grows almost exclusively during the early years of life. At birth, the brain is one fourth of its future adult size. By 1 year, the brain is three fourths of its adult size. The kidneys function at the adult level by the end of the first year.

Lower front teeth begin to appear at the age of 5 to 9 months. Upper front teeth begin to appear at 8 to 12 months.

Behavioral, Social, and Intellectual Development

The rate of behavioral, social, and intellectual development varies considerably from infant to infant. Some infants develop faster, although certain patterns may run in families, such as late walking or talking. Environmental factors, such as lack of sufficient stimulation, can slow development; conversely, stimulation can hasten development. Physical factors, such as deafness, can also slow development. Although a child's development is usually continuous, temporary pauses may occur in the development of a particular function, such as speech.

Crying is one means of communication. Infants cry because they are hungry, uncomfortable, distressed, and for many other reasons that may not be obvious. Infants cry most—typically 3 hours a day—at 6 weeks of age, usually decreasing to an hour a day by 3 months of age. Parents generally offer a crying baby food, change the diaper, and look for a source of pain or discomfort. If this does not work, holding or walking with the baby sometimes helps. Occasionally nothing works. Parents should not force food on a crying infant, who will readily eat if hunger is the cause of his distress.

Promoting Optimal Development

Babies obviously require appropriate food and shelter for their physical growth. If their physical needs are met regularly and consistently, infants quickly learn that their caretaker is a source of satisfaction, creating a firm bond of trust and attachment.

In addition to their physical needs, babies need affection and stimulation to develop emotionally and intellectually. Some parents provide a highly organized, structured environment for their infant using a variety of toys and gadgets. However, the particular content of the environment is less important than the existence of a pleasant, positive interaction enjoyed by both parent and baby. Parents who provide smiling faces, frequent amiable speech, physical contact, and love but who do not buy a variety of toys and gadgets are not short-changing their baby's development.

Preventive Health Care Visits

Healthy infants should be seen by their doctor often during the first year of life. Visits typically take place by 1 to 2 weeks, and at 2, 4, 6, 9, and 12 months of age. During these visits, the doctor monitors the child's growth and development by measuring the child's length, weight, and head circumference, and asking the parents questions about various developmental milestones. The doctor also examines the child for various abnormalities, including signs of hereditary disorders. Hearing and vision are tested. An infant who was born prematurely (after spending less than 37 weeks in the uterus) is regularly examined for retinopathy of prematurity, an eye disease.▲ Finally, on many visits, the doctor vaccinates the child against various illnesses.

Healthcare visits also allow the doctor to educate the parents about eating, sleeping, behavior, child safety, and good health habits. In addition, the doctor advises the parents what changes to expect in their child by the next visit.

Vaccinations

Children should be vaccinated to protect them against infectious diseases. Vaccination has eliminated smallpox and nearly eliminated other infections, such as polio and measles, that were once common childhood scourges in the United States. Despite this success, it is important for health care professionals to continue to vaccinate children. Many of the diseases prevented by vaccination are still present in the United States and remain common in other parts of the world. These diseases can spread rapidly among unvaccinated children, who will also be at particular risk when traveling to other countries.

No vaccine is 100% effective and 100% safe. A few vaccinated children fail to become immune, and a few develop side effects. Most often, the side effects are minor, such as pain at the injection site, an itchy rash, or a mild fever. Very rarely, there are more serious problems. The oral polio vaccine, which is made of a live, weakened virus, can cause polio if the weakened virus mutates, which happens once in every 2.4 million children. Although this is an extremely small chance, it led doctors in the United States to recommend completely switching to an inactivated, injectable polio vaccine. Also, the pertussis component of the older whole-cell diphtheria, tetanus, and pertussis vaccine (DTP) occasionally led to febrile seizures■ in about 1 in 10,000 children, and more rarely confusion and fainting. Although these episodes do not leave any lasting damage, they are distressing to parents. Doctors now recommend a newer version of the vaccine using *acellular* pertussis (DTaP), which has a much lower chance of these reactions. Simi-

▲ see page 1504   ■ see page 502

larly, febrile seizures have occurred in about 3 in 10,000 children following the measles, mumps, rubella (MMR) vaccine. Although the public press has reported concerns that the MMR vaccine may produce autism, scientific evidence shows that this does not happen.

To help people evaluate the risks of vaccination, the federal government requires doctors to give parents a *Vaccine Information Statement* each time a child is vaccinated. Also, a federal Vaccine Injury Compensation Program was established to compensate anyone suffering permanent consequences of vaccination.

Vaccination Schedule for Infants and Children

Vaccinations play an important role in keeping infants and children healthy. Shown are the routinely recommended ages for having an infant or child vaccinated with specific vaccines. There is a range of acceptable ages for many vaccines. A child's own doctor can provide specific recommendations, which may vary depending on the circumstances. For example, if an infant is born to a woman with the hepatitis B surface antigen in her blood, a doctor typically recommends that the infant be given the first dose of hepatitis B vaccine within 12 hours of birth. However, other infants should be given the first dose of hepatitis B vaccine at their first doctor's visit and at least by age 2 months. Often, combination vaccines are used, so that a child receives fewer injections.

●   Single dose of vaccine

▲   "Catch-up" vaccination for children not previously vaccinated (or, in the case of varicella-zoster virus, for those who have not had chickenpox by age 13)

▬   Range of acceptable ages for a single dose of vaccine

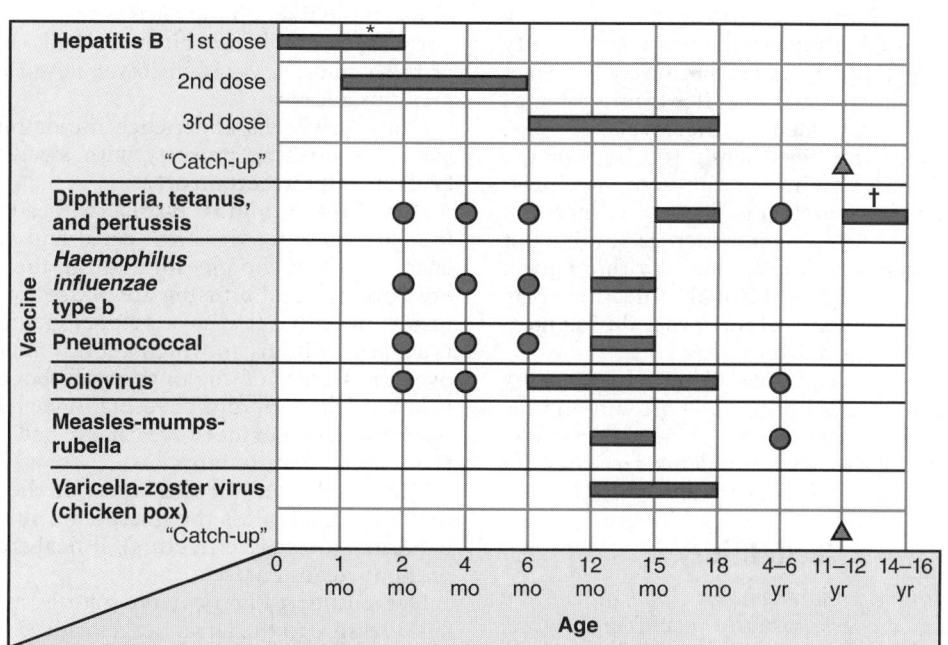

* The first dose may be given by age 2 months only if the mother does not have hepatitis B surface antigen in her blood.
† A booster dose for diphtheria and tetanus (but not pertussis) is recommended between the ages of 11 and 16 if at least 5 years have elapsed since the last dose.

This program was established because doctors and health authorities want as many children as possible to be protected from life-threatening diseases. When considering the risks of vaccination, parents must remember that their child is at much greater risk from the diseases that vaccinations prevent.

Most doctors follow the vaccination schedule recommended by the American Academy of Pediatrics, which begins during the first week after birth with the hepatitis B vaccine. The recommended ages for vaccinations should not be construed as absolute. For example, 2 months can mean 6 to 10 weeks. Although parents should try to have their children vaccinated according to the schedule, a

slight delay does not interfere with the final immunity achieved nor does it entail restarting the series of injections from the beginning. Vaccination need not be delayed, however, if the infant has a slight fever from a mild infection such as an ordinary cold. Some vaccines are recommended only under special circumstances.

More than one vaccine may be given during a visit to the doctor's office, but several vaccines are often combined into one injection, for example, pertussis, diphtheria, tetanus, and *Haemophilus influenzae* type b vaccines. A combination vaccine reduces the number of injections needed but does not reduce the safety or effectiveness of the vaccines.

CHAPTER 264

Problems in Newborns

After birth, a newborn may have a number of problems. Some problems may be due to difficulties during the birthing process; many of these problems affect the newborn's ability to breathe properly. A newborn may be bigger or smaller than usual or suffer from problems affecting blood, such as the levels of sugar (glucose) in the blood being too high or too low. Birth defects may be present.▲ A newborn may have problems due to the mother's health and health habits, such as smoking or use of alcohol or drugs (especially those given immediately before birth■). Infection may pass from mother to child, either during pregnancy or during delivery.

Doctors may be able to anticipate many problems by monitoring fetal growth and development, particularly using ultrasound. Many newborns with problems are cared for in a neonatal intensive care unit (NICU).

Birth Injury

Birth injury is damage sustained during the birthing process, usually occurring during transit through the birth canal.

A difficult delivery, with the risk of injury to the fetus, may occur if the birth canal is too

small or the fetus is too large (as sometimes occurs when the mother has diabetes). Injury is also more likely if the fetus is lying in an abnormal position before birth. Overall, the rate of birth injuries is much lower now than in previous decades.

Many newborns experience minor injuries from the birthing process, with swelling or bruising only in certain areas.

Head Injury: In most births, the head is the first part to enter the birth canal and experiences much of the pressure during the delivery. Swelling and bruising are not serious and resolve within a few days. Cephalohematoma is a bleeding injury in which a soft lump forms over the surface of one of the skull bones but below its thick fibrous covering. A cephalohematoma does not need treatment and disappears over weeks to months.

Very rarely, one of the bones of the skull may fracture. Unless the fracture forms an indentation (depressed fracture), it heals rapidly without treatment.

Nerve Injury: Rarely, nerve injuries may occur. Pressure to the facial nerves caused by forceps can result in weakness of the muscles on one side of the face. This injury is evident when the newborn cries and the face appears asymmetric. No treatment is needed, and the newborn usually recovers within a few weeks.

▲ see page 1527 ■ see also page 1458

What Is a Neonatal Intensive Care Unit?

Often referred to as the "NICU," this specialized facility brings together the medical team and technology needed to care for newborns with a variety of disorders. The largest group of newborns needing such care is those born very prematurely. Other newborns need care because of sepsis or pneumonia, respiratory disorders, and birth defects that require surgery. These newborns are cared for in incubators to keep them warm or they are placed under overhead radiant warmers, which provide warmth while allowing increased access to the newborn by the staff. Newborns are attached to monitors that can continuously measure their heart rate, breathing, blood pressure, and oxygen levels in the blood. They may have catheters placed inside the artery and vein running inside the umbilical cord to permit continuous blood pressure monitoring, to allow repeated blood sampling, and to administer intravenous fluids and drugs.

The NICU tends to be a very busy place. This is sometimes at odds with the parents' need for time and space to become acquainted with their newborn, to learn the newborn's personality, likes and dislikes, and ultimately to learn any special care that they will need to provide at home. A trend to make the NICU quieter and to design units to allow families increased privacy has helped. Visiting hours have been greatly extended so that families can spend much more time with their newborns, and often hospitals arrange for nearby sleeping facilities for the parents.

Sometimes, parents feel that they have little to offer to a newborn in a NICU. However, their presence, including stroking, speaking, and singing, is very important.

The newborn has heard his mother's voice even before birth and is accustomed to it, and he often responds better to his own parents' attempts to calm him. Skin-to-skin contact (also termed kangaroo care), in which the newborn is allowed to lie directly on the mother or father's chest, is comforting to the newborn and enhances bonding. Increasing evidence indicates that premature newborns fed breast milk are significantly protected from developing necrotizing enterocolitis and infections and that breastfeeding is otherwise beneficial.

Parents need to be kept informed of their newborn's condition and the doctor's plans, as well as the expected course and time of discharge. Regular meetings with the doctors and nurses are essential. Many NICUs have a social worker who can help to see that parents are kept informed.

In a difficult delivery of a large infant, some of the larger nerves to one or both of the newborn's arms can be stretched and injured. Weakness (paralysis) of the newborn's arm or hand results. Occasionally, the nerve going to the diaphragm (the muscle that separates the organs of the chest from those of the abdomen) is damaged, resulting in paralysis of the diaphragm on the same side. In this case, the newborn may have difficulty breathing. Injury of the nerves to the newborn's arm and diaphragm usually resolves completely within a few weeks. Extreme movements at the shoulder should be avoided to allow the nerves to heal. Very rarely, the arm and possibly the diaphragm remain weak after several months. In this case, surgery may be needed to reattach torn nerves.

Injuries to the spinal cord due to overstretching during delivery are extremely rare. These injuries can result in paralysis below where the injury occurred. Damage to the spinal cord is often permanent.

Bone Injury: Rarely, bones may be broken (fractured) during a difficult delivery. A fracture of the collarbone is most common. Fractures of bones in the newborn are splinted and almost always heal completely and rapidly.

Prematurity

A premature newborn is a newborn delivered before 37 weeks in the uterus; such a newborn has underdeveloped organs.

About 8% of newborns are born prematurely (preterm). Many of these newborns are born just a few weeks early and do not experience problems related to their prematurity. However, the more prematurely newborns are born, the more they are prone to a number of serious and even life-threatening complications. Very premature birth is the single most common cause of death in the newborn. Also, newborns born very prematurely are at high risk for chronic problems, especially delayed development and learning disorders. Such disorders occur because the internal organs have not had time to develop adequately before birth.

Common Birthmarks and Minor Skin Conditions in the Newborn

There are a number of skin conditions that are considered normal in the newborn. There may be bruises or marks from forceps on the newborn's face and scalp, or bruising of the feet following a breech delivery, all of which resolve within just a few days. Pink marks that are due to dilated capillaries under the skin may be seen on the forehead just above the nose, in the upper eyelids, or at the back of the neck (where it is called "stork-bite"). This type of birthmark fades as the infant grows but in some people remains as a faint mark that becomes brighter when the person becomes excited or upset. Some newborns have a few acne pimples, especially over the cheeks and forehead. These go away, and the only recommended action is to keep the skin clean and not to use creams or lotions.

Milia are tiny, pearly white cysts that are normally found over the nose and upper cheeks. Milia become smaller or disappear over a period of weeks. Similar white cysts are sometimes found on the gums or in the midline of the roof of the mouth (Epstein's pearls) and are also of no consequence.

Mongolian spots are bluish gray, flat areas that usually occur over the lower back or buttocks. At first glance they appear to be bruises but are not. They are usually seen in black or Asian newborns and are of no consequence.

A **"strawberry hemangioma"** is a common birthmark. It is a flat, slightly pink or red area anywhere on the skin. Over a period of weeks, it becomes darker red and also becomes raised up over the surface of the skin, appearing much as a strawberry. After several years, strawberry hemangiomas shrink and become fainter, so that by the time the child reaches school age, most are no longer visible. For this reason, surgery is not needed.

The reason for a premature birth cannot usually be determined. However, the risk of premature birth is higher in women who are poor, have little education, and have poor nutrition or health or untreated illnesses or infections during pregnancy. The risk is lower in women who had early prenatal care. For unknown reasons, black women are significantly more likely than women of other racial groups to have a premature delivery. Other women at increased risk for premature delivery are those carrying more than one fetus and those who have serious or life-threatening disorders, including severe high blood pressure or kidney disease, preeclampsia or eclampsia,▲ or infection of the uterus (chorioamnionitis).

Symptoms

Premature newborns usually weigh less than $5\frac{1}{2}$ pounds. Physical features help doctors determine the newborn's gestational age (length of time spent in the uterus after the egg is fertilized).

Underdeveloped Lungs: The lungs of the premature newborn may not have had enough time to fully develop before birth. Such newborns are likely to have respiratory distress syndrome. Respiratory distress syndrome occurs if the lungs are not mature enough to produce surfactant, a mixture of lipids (fats) and proteins that allows the air sacs of the lungs to remain open.■

Underdeveloped Brain: The part of the brain that controls regular breathing may be so immature that the newborn has inconsistent breathing, with short pauses in breathing or periods during which breathing stops for 20 seconds or longer (apnea). The parts of the brain that control the mouth and throat are immature so the newborn cannot suck and swallow normally and will have difficulty coordinating feeding with breathing.

Brain Hemorrhage: Newborns born very prematurely are at increased risk of bleeding (hemorrhage) in the brain. Bleeding typically begins in an area called the germinal matrix and may extend into spaces within the brain called the ventricles. This form of hemorrhage is most likely to occur in those born very prematurely (before 32 weeks of pregnancy) and if there were problems during labor or delivery or breathing problems (such as respiratory distress syndrome) after birth. Depending on the size of the hemorrhage, newborns may have no symptoms or may experience lethargy, seizures, or even persistent unconsciousness (coma). Newborns with small or moderate-sized hemorrhages usually develop normally. Those with very large hemorrhages are at higher risk of dying or of having learning disorders or other brain-related problems later in life.

▲ see page 1452   ■ see page 1499

Abnormal Blood Sugar: Because premature newborns have difficulty maintaining normal blood sugar (glucose) levels, they are often treated with intravenous glucose solutions or given small frequent feedings. Without regular intake of sugar, a newborn may develop low blood sugar levels (hypoglycemia). Most newborns with hypoglycemia do not develop symptoms. Others may become listless with poor muscle tone, feed poorly, or become jittery. Rarely, seizures may develop. These newborns are also prone to developing high blood sugar levels (hyperglycemia) if they receive too much sugar intravenously. Most newborns with hyperglycemia do not develop symptoms.

Underdeveloped Immune System: Newborns who are born very prematurely have low levels of antibodies, which cross the placenta from mother to the fetus during the latter part of pregnancy and offer protection from infection. Therefore, the risk of developing infections, especially infection in the blood (sepsis), is higher in premature newborns. The use of special devices for treatment, such as catheters and ventilators, further increases the newborn's risk of developing serious infections.

Underdeveloped Kidneys: Before delivery, waste products produced in the fetus are removed by the placenta and then excreted by the mother's kidneys. After delivery, the newborn's kidneys must take over these functions. Kidney function is poor in newborns who are born very prematurely but improves as the kidneys mature. A newborn with underdeveloped kidneys is likely to have difficulty regulating the amount of salt and water in the body.

Underdeveloped Digestive Tract and Liver: Initially, premature newborns may have difficulty with feedings. Not only do they have immature sucking and swallowing reflexes, but also their small stomach empties slowly. Very premature newborns may develop a serious injury to the inner surface of the intestines (necrotizing enterocolitis▲).

In premature newborns, the excretion of bilirubin may be impaired. Thus, premature newborns, even more than term newborns, tend to become jaundiced in the first few days after birth because of the build-up of bilirubin in their blood. Usually, the jaundice is mild and resolves as the newborn takes larger amounts of feedings and has more frequent bowel movements. Rarely, very high levels of bilirubin accumulate and put the newborn at

Physical Features of a Premature Newborn

- Small size
- Large head relative to rest of the body
- Little fat under the skin
- Thin, shiny, pink skin
- Veins visible beneath the skin
- Few creases on soles of feet
- Scant hair
- Soft ears, with little cartilage
- Underdeveloped breast tissue
- Boys: Small scrotum with few folds. Testicles may be undescended in very premature newborns
- Girls: Labia majora not yet covering labia minora
- Rapid breathing with brief pauses (periodic breathing), often apnea spells (pauses lasting greater than 20 seconds)
- Weak, poorly coordinated sucking and swallowing reflexes
- Reduced physical activity (a premature newborn tends not to draw up the arms and legs as does a full-term newborn)
- Sleeping for most of the time

risk for developing kernicterus, a form of brain damage caused by deposits of bilirubin in the brain.

Difficulty Regulating Body Temperature: Because premature newborns have a large skin surface area relative to their weight, they tend to lose heat rapidly, especially if they are in a cool room or if there is a draft. A lowering of body temperature results in a markedly increased rate of the body's metabolism, as the newborn attempts to maintain normal body temperature.

Prevention

The best way for premature birth to be prevented is for the expectant mother to take good care of her own health. She should eat a nutritious diet and avoid cigarettes, alcohol, and drugs. Ideally, she should receive early and regular prenatal care so that any complications of pregnancy can be recognized and treated. If it seems probable that early labor is about to start, an obstetrician may administer

▲ see page 1504

drugs (such as magnesium sulfate or ritodrine) to the mother to slow or stop contractions. Corticosteroids such as betamethasone or dexamethasone may also be given to the mother to accelerate maturation of the fetus's lungs. Corticosteroids also significantly reduce the risk of brain hemorrhage if the newborn is born prematurely.

Treatment and Prognosis

Treatment involves managing the complications, such as respiratory distress syndrome and high bilirubin levels. Very premature newborns are fed intravenously until they can tolerate tube feedings and finally feedings by mouth. A premature newborn may need to be hospitalized for days, weeks, or months. Over recent decades, the survival of premature newborns has improved dramatically. For most premature newborns, the long-term prognosis is very good, and they develop normally. However, those born extremely early (often before 28 weeks of pregnancy) are at an increased risk of death and of serious problems, including mental retardation, cerebral palsy, epilepsy, or blindness. Fortunately, only a minority of extremely premature newborns who survive have these problems. A larger percentage have normal intelligence, but many have learning disorders that eventually require special help.

Postmaturity

A postmature newborn is a newborn delivered after more than 42 weeks in the uterus.

Postmature (postterm) delivery is much less common than premature (preterm) delivery. The reason for a pregnancy to continue beyond term is usually unknown.

Reduced function of the placenta is the greatest risk to fetuses who go beyond term. Near the end of a term pregnancy, the placenta begins to shrink. As it shrinks, the placenta becomes less able to provide adequate nutrients to the fetus. To compensate, the fetus begins to use its own fat and carbohydrates to provide energy. As a result, its growth rate slows, and occasionally its weight may decrease. If the placenta shrinks sufficiently, it may not provide adequate oxygen to the fetus, particularly during labor. A lack of adequate oxygen may result in fetal distress▲ and, in extreme cases, may result in injury to the fetal

brain and other organs. Fetal distress may cause the fetus to pass stools (meconium) into the amniotic fluid. The fetus may also take deep, gasping breaths triggered by the distress and thereby inhale the meconium-containing amniotic fluid into the lungs before or during birth. As a result, the newborn may have difficulty breathing after delivery (meconium aspiration syndrome).

Symptoms

A postmature newborn has dry, peeling, loose skin and may appear emaciated, especially if the function of the placenta was severely reduced. The newborn often appears alert. The skin and nail beds may be stained green if meconium was present in the amniotic fluid. A postmature newborn is prone to developing low blood sugar levels (hypoglycemia) after delivery, especially if oxygen levels were low during labor.

Treatment

The postmature newborn who experienced low oxygen levels and fetal distress may need resuscitation at birth. If meconium has been breathed into the lungs, a ventilator may be needed. Intravenous glucose solutions or frequent breast milk or formula feedings are given to prevent hypoglycemia.

If these problems do not occur, the major goal is to provide good nutrition so that the newborn can catch up to the weight that is appropriate for him.

Small for Gestational Age

A newborn, whether delivered preterm, term, or postterm, whose weight is less than that of 90% of babies of the same gestational age at birth (below the 10th percentile) is considered small for gestational age.

There are several causes for this condition. In many cases, the newborn may be small simply because of genetic factors, such as having small parents (less commonly, a specific genetic syndrome associated with small stature may be involved). In other cases, the placenta may have functioned poorly, so that the fetus did not receive adequate nutrients and growth was impaired. This may happen if the mother has high blood pressure, preeclampsia, kidney disease, or long-standing diabetes. A viral infection, such as cytomegalovirus acquired before birth, may be responsible. Fetal growth may also have been impaired

▲ see page 1471

if the mother smoked or used alcohol or illicit drugs during the pregnancy.▲ Unless they have a genetic syndrome or viral infection, most small-for-gestational-age newborns have no symptoms. If the fetal growth was impaired because of poor placental function and inadequate nutrition, the newborn's growth may accelerate when provided with good nutrition after delivery. Some small-for-gestational-age newborns remain small as children and adults.

Large for Gestational Age

A newborn, whether delivered preterm, term, or postterm, whose weight is above that of 90% of babies of the same gestational age at birth (above the 90th percentile) is considered large for gestational age.

Some newborns are large for gestational age because of genetic factors, such as having large parents. Another cause is diabetes in the mother.

If the mother has diabetes during pregnancy, a large amount of glucose (sugar) crosses the placenta and results in high levels of glucose in the fetus's blood, with the release of increased amounts of insulin. The result is accelerated growth of the fetus, including almost all organs with the exception of the brain, which grows normally. Vaginal delivery of a very large-for-gestational-age fetus may be problematic, increasing the risk of injury. Therefore, such a fetus may have to be delivered by caesarean section.

The large-for-gestational-age newborn born to a diabetic mother typically has a florid (reddish) complexion and appears obese and sometimes lethargic. Large-for-gestational-age newborns born to mothers who do not have diabetes are large, but not reddish or lethargic. After birth, when the supply of glucose from the placenta stops, the continuing rapid production of insulin leads to low levels of glucose (hypoglycemia). Often hypoglycemia produces no symptoms. Sometimes, the newborn is listless, limp, or jittery. Despite their large size, newborns of diabetic mothers often do not feed well for the first few days. Occasionally, newborns born to diabetic mothers have an abnormally high red blood cell count. As the red blood cells are broken down, bilirubin is formed, and these newborns tend to have high bilirubin levels, resulting in jaundice.■

Large-for-gestational-age newborns born prematurely to diabetic mothers are also more likely to have immature lungs and to develop respiratory distress syndrome, even when born only a few weeks before full term. They also have a higher rate of birth defects than other newborns.

Testing the amniotic fluid in mothers with diabetes before delivery can be performed to determine lung maturity and the likelihood of the newborn developing respiratory distress syndrome after birth. If labor appears imminent, a corticosteroid may be given to increase lung maturity.

To treat hypoglycemia in the newborn, intravenous glucose or frequent feedings by mouth or by tube into the stomach are often needed. Treatment of other complications, such as respiratory distress syndrome, is needed.

Large-for-gestational-age newborns born to diabetic mothers are likely to be significantly overweight later in childhood and as adults, which puts them at risk for type 2 diabetes.★

Respiratory Distress Syndrome

Respiratory distress syndrome is a breathing disorder of premature newborns in which the air sacs (alveoli) in a newborn's lungs do not remain open because the production of surfactant is absent or insufficient.

For a newborn to be able to breathe easily, the air sacs in the lungs must be able to remain open and filled with air. Normally, the lungs produce a mixture of lipids (fats) and proteins called surfactant. Surfactant acts as a wetting agent and lines the surface of the air sacs, where it lowers the surface tension and allows the air sacs to remain open throughout the respiratory cycle. Usually, production of surfactant begins after about 34 weeks of pregnancy. The more premature the newborn, the greater the likelihood that respiratory distress syndrome will develop after birth. Respiratory distress syndrome occurs almost exclusively in premature newborns and is more common in those whose mother has diabetes.

Symptoms and Diagnosis

In an affected newborn, the lungs are stiff and the air sacs tend to collapse completely, emptying the lungs of air. In some very premature newborns, the lungs may be so stiff that the newborn is unable to begin breathing at birth. More commonly, the newborn tries to

---

▲ see page 1458   ■ see page 1497

★ see page 962

breathe, but because the lungs are so stiff, severe respiratory distress occurs. Respiratory distress is manifested by visibly labored breathing, including retractions of the chest below the rib cage, flaring of the nostrils during breathing in, and "grunting" during breathing out. Because a good portion of the lung is airless, the newborn has low blood oxygen levels, which cause a bluish discoloration to the skin (cyanosis). Over a period of hours, the respiratory distress tends to become more severe, as the small amount of surfactant in the lungs is used up and increasing numbers of air sacs collapse and also as the muscles used for breathing tire and become weak. Eventually, without treatment, the newborn may suffer damage to the brain and other organs from a lack of oxygen or may die.

Diagnosis of respiratory distress syndrome is based on the symptoms and on abnormal chest x-ray results in a premature newborn.

Prevention and Treatment

The risk of respiratory distress syndrome is greatly reduced if delivery can be safely delayed until the fetal lungs have produced sufficient surfactant. The obstetrician can perform amniocentesis, in which some amniotic fluid is withdrawn into a syringe and analyzed for the adequacy of surfactant production. If production is not adequate but premature delivery cannot be avoided, the obstetrician may give the mother injections of a corticosteroid drug (betamethasone or dexamethasone). The corticosteroid crosses the placenta into the fetus and accelerates the production of surfactant. Within 48 hours of starting the injections, the fetal lungs mature to the point that respiratory distress syndrome will not develop after delivery or, if it does, is likely to be milder.

After delivery, a newborn with mild respiratory distress syndrome may require only supplemental oxygen, which is given through an oxygen hood or through a tube placed in the nose. A newborn with severe respiratory distress syndrome may require oxygen delivered by continuous positive airway pressure (CPAP—breathing spontaneously against positive pressure oxygen or air administered through tubes placed in both nostrils). In a very sick infant, a tube may need to be passed into the windpipe (intubation), and the infant's breathing supported with mechanical ventilation.

Use of a surfactant preparation can be lifesaving and reduces complications, such as rupture of the lungs (pneumothorax). The surfactant preparation acts in the same way that natural surfactant does. Surfactant may be given immediately after birth in the delivery room to attempt to prevent respiratory distress syndrome or in the early hours after birth to a premature newborn who already has symptoms of this disorder. A newborn who is intubated can receive surfactant through the tube in the windpipe.

Surfactant treatments may be repeated several times over the first days until respiratory distress syndrome resolves.

Transient Tachypnea

Transient tachypnea of the newborn (transient rapid breathing, neonatal wet-lung syndrome) is temporary difficulty with breathing and low blood oxygen levels due to excessive fluid in the lungs after birth.

This disorder usually occurs in newborns born a few weeks before term or at term. It is more common after a caesarean section delivery. It is especially likely to occur if the mother has not been in labor before delivery (for example, a mother who has a scheduled caesarean section).

Before birth, the air sacs of the lungs are filled with fluid. Immediately after birth, the fluid must be cleared from the lungs so that the air sacs can fill with air and the newborn can establish normal breathing. Some of the fluid is squeezed out of the lungs by pressure on the chest during a vaginal delivery. More of the fluid is rapidly reabsorbed directly by the cells lining the air sacs and from which it is immediately transported into the bloodstream. If this fluid transfer does not occur rapidly, then the air sacs continue to be partially filled with fluid and the newborn has difficulty breathing.

A newborn with transient tachypnea has respiratory distress with rapid breathing, drawing in of the chest wall during breathing in and "grunting" during breathing out, and may develop a bluish discoloration of the skin (cyanosis) if the blood oxygen levels become low. A chest x-ray shows abnormal results.

Most newborns with transient tachypnea recover completely within 2 to 3 days. Treatment with oxygen is usually needed, although some newborns may need continuous positive airway pressure (CPAP—breathing spontaneously against positive pressure oxygen or air administered through tubes placed in the newborn's nostrils) or assistance with a ventilator.

Meconium Aspiration Syndrome

Meconium aspiration syndrome is respiratory distress in a newborn who has breathed (aspirated) meconium into the lungs before or around the time of birth.

Meconium is the dark green fecal material that is produced in the intestines before birth. Normally, meconium is expelled after birth when a newborn starts to feed. However, in response to stress, such as an inadequate blood oxygen level, the fetus may pass meconium into the amniotic fluid. The same stress causes the fetus to take forceful gasps, so that the meconium-containing amniotic fluid may be breathed into the lungs. After delivery, the aspirated meconium may block the airways leading to portions of the newborn's lungs, which may cause them to collapse. Alternatively, when some airways are only partially blocked, air may be able to reach the parts of the lung beyond the block but may be prevented from being breathed out. Thus, the involved lung may become over-expanded. Progressive over-expansion of a portion of the lung can eventually result in rupture and then collapse of the lung. Air may then accumulate within the chest cavity around the lung (pneumothorax). Meconium breathed into the lungs may also cause inflammation of the lungs (pneumonitis).

Meconium aspiration syndrome is often most severe in postmature newborns because the meconium is very concentrated in a smaller amount of amniotic fluid and it causes more irritation than in a term newborn.▲ Newborns with meconium aspiration syndrome are also at increased risk for developing persistent pulmonary hypertension.

An affected newborn suffers from respiratory distress, in which he breathes rapidly, draws in his lower chest wall while breathing in, and grunts during breathing out. The newborn's skin may be bluish (cyanotic) if the blood levels of oxygen are reduced.

A doctor makes the diagnosis based on the observation of thick meconium in the amniotic fluid at the time of birth, respiratory distress in the newborn, and abnormal chest x-ray results.

At delivery, if the newborn is covered with meconium, the newborn's mouth, nose, and throat are immediately suctioned to remove any meconium. If the newborn is lethargic or unresponsive, a tube may need to be passed into the windpipe to suction as much meconium as possible from the respiratory tract.

The newborn is treated with oxygen and placed on a ventilator if necessary. If the newborn needs intubation, then repeated suctioning is performed to try to remove more of the meconium. A newborn on a ventilator is observed closely for serious complications, such as pneumothorax or persistent pulmonary hypertension.

Most newborns with meconium aspiration syndrome survive. However, if the disorder is severe and especially if it leads to persistent pulmonary hypertension, it can be fatal.

Persistent Pulmonary Hypertension

Persistent pulmonary hypertension is a serious disorder in which the newborn's arteries to the lungs remain constricted after delivery, thus limiting the amount of blood flow to the lungs and therefore the amount of oxygen in the bloodstream.

Normally, the blood vessels to the lungs are tightly constricted during fetal life. The lungs do not need much blood flow before birth because the placenta eliminates carbon dioxide and transports oxygen to the fetus. Immediately after birth, the umbilical cord is cut and the newborn's lungs must take over the role of oxygenating the blood and removing carbon dioxide. To achieve this, it is necessary not only that the fluid filling the air sacs be replaced by air, but that the arteries bringing blood to the lungs widen (dilate) so that an adequate amount of blood flows through the lungs.

In response to severe respiratory distress, or as a consequence of certain drugs taken by the mother before delivery (such as large doses of aspirin), the blood vessels to the lungs may not dilate as they normally should. As a result, there is insufficient blood flow to the lungs and not enough oxygen reaches the blood.

Persistent pulmonary hypertension is more common in newborns who are term or postterm and in newborns whose mothers were regular users of aspirin or indomethacin during pregnancy. In many newborns, the respiratory distress that initiates persistent pulmonary hypertension results from other lung diseases, such as meconium aspiration syn-

▲ see page 1498

drome or pneumonia, but persistent pulmonary hypertension can also develop in newborns with no other lung disorder.

Symptoms and Diagnosis

Sometimes persistent pulmonary hypertension is present from birth; other times, it develops over the first day or two. Breathing is usually rapid, and there may be severe respiratory distress if the newborn has an underlying lung disease.▲ The most prominent feature is a bluish discoloration of the skin (cyanosis) due to low blood oxygen levels. Sometimes low blood pressure (hypotension) leads to symptoms such as weak pulses and a pale, grayish hue to the skin.

A doctor may suspect persistent pulmonary hypertension if the mother used aspirin or indomethacin during pregnancy or had a stressful delivery, or if the newborn has severe respiratory distress and measurement of oxygen levels is unexpectedly low. A chest x-ray is performed, but definitive diagnosis requires an echocardiogram.

Treatment

Treatment involves placing the newborn in an environment with 100% oxygen to breathe. Alternatively, a ventilator providing 100% oxygen may be needed. A high percentage of oxygen in the blood helps open the arteries going to the lungs. To make the blood slightly alkaline, which may also open these arteries, the newborn is often given intravenous sodium bicarbonate.

In more severe cases, a very small concentration of the gas nitric oxide may be added to the oxygen that the newborn is breathing. Inhaled nitric oxide opens the arteries in the newborn's lungs and reduces pulmonary hypertension. This treatment may be needed over several days. If all other treatments fail, extracorporeal membrane oxygenation (ECMO) can be used. In this procedure, blood from the newborn is circulated through a machine that adds oxygen and removes carbon dioxide and then returns the blood to the newborn. ECMO has been life-saving, allowing many newborns to survive until the pulmonary hypertension resolves.

Pneumothorax

Pneumothorax is a collection of air within the chest cavity surrounding a lung that develops when air leaks out of the lung.

▲ see page 1499

Pneumothorax most often occurs in a newborn with stiff lungs, such as a newborn with respiratory distress syndrome or meconium aspiration syndrome. Occasionally, it occurs as a complication from the use of continuous positive airway pressure (CPAP) or a ventilator. If the pneumothorax is under pressure, it can result in collapse of the lung and in difficulty breathing. Also, if under pressure, the pneumothorax can compress the veins bringing blood to the heart. As a result, less blood fills the chambers of the heart, the output of the heart decreases, and the newborn's blood pressure decreases.

Air that leaks from the lungs into the soft tissues in front of the heart is called pneumomediastinum. Unlike pneumothorax, this condition usually does not affect breathing.

Diagnosis and Treatment

Pneumothorax is suspected when a newborn with underlying lung disease, or a newborn on continuous positive airway pressure (CPAP) or a ventilator, develops worsening respiratory distress or a drop in blood pressure. When examining the newborn, a doctor notices a diminished sound of air entering and leaving the lung on the side of the pneumothorax. In premature newborns, a fiber-optic light may be used to light up the affected side of the newborn's chest while in a darkened room (positive transillumination); this procedure is used to look for air in the pleural cavity. A chest x-ray provides a definitive diagnosis.

No treatment is needed in newborns who do not have symptoms. A term newborn with mild symptoms may be placed in an oxygen hood. However, if the newborn's breathing is labored, and particularly if the circulation of blood is impaired, the air must be rapidly removed from the pleural cavity, which can be done using a needle and syringe. If the newborn is in significant distress, is receiving CPAP, or is on a ventilator, a doctor may need to place a chest tube to continuously suction and remove air from the chest cavity. The tube can usually be removed after several days.

A pneumomediastinum can be seen on an x-ray; no treatment is needed.

Bronchopulmonary Dysplasia

Bronchopulmonary dysplasia (chronic lung disease) is a disorder due to repetitive lung injury.

Bronchopulmonary dysplasia occurs most often in premature newborns who had severe lung disease at birth, such as respiratory distress syndrome, particularly in those who needed treatment with a ventilator for more than a few weeks after birth. The delicate tissues of the lungs can become injured when the air sacs are over-stretched by the ventilation or by high oxygen levels. As a result, the lungs become inflamed and additional fluid accumulates within the lungs. Full-term newborns who have lung disease (such as pneumonia) occasionally develop bronchopulmonary dysplasia.

Symptoms and Diagnosis

Affected newborns usually breathe rapidly and may have respiratory distress, with drawing in of the lower chest while breathing in and low levels of oxygen in the blood, causing a bluish discoloration of the skin (cyanosis). Some newborns with severe cases exhale air from the lungs slowly and develop "air trapping," in which the chest appears to be over-expanded.

Although a few newborns with very severe bronchopulmonary dysplasia die even after months of care, most newborns survive. Over several years, the lung injury heals. However, later these children are at increased risk of developing asthma and viral pneumonia, such as that caused during winter months by respiratory syncytial virus (RSV).

The diagnosis of bronchopulmonary dysplasia is made in the premature newborn who has received ventilation for a prolonged time and who has signs of respiratory distress and a prolonged need for supplemental oxygen. Measurement of low levels of oxygen in the blood and results of a chest x-ray support the diagnosis.

Prevention and Treatment

Ventilators are used only when absolutely necessary, and then as gently as possible to avoid injury to the lungs. The newborn is taken off the ventilator as early as is safe.

In a newborn with bronchopulmonary dysplasia, supplemental oxygen may be needed initially to prevent cyanosis.

Good nutrition is important to help the newborn's lungs grow and to keep the new lung tissue healthy. Thus, the damaged areas of lung become less and less important relative to the overall size of the newborn's lungs.

Because fluid tends to accumulate in the inflamed lungs, sometimes the daily intake of fluids is restricted, and diuretics may be used to increase the rate of excretion of fluid in the urine.

After discharge from the hospital, newborns with bronchopulmonary dysplasia should not be exposed to cigarette smoke or fumes from a space heater or wood-burning stove. They should be protected from exposure to people who have upper respiratory tract infections. In certain cases, doctors can give them partial immunity to RSV infection by administering doses of a specific antibody to that virus. This antibody must be injected monthly during the fall and winter.

Apnea of Prematurity

Apnea of prematurity is a pause in breathing that lasts for more than 20 seconds.

Apnea of prematurity commonly occurs in newborns who are born before 34 weeks of pregnancy, increasing in frequency and severity among the most prematurely born. In these newborns, the part of the brain that controls breathing (respiratory center) has not matured fully. As a result, the newborns may have repeated episodes of normal breathing alternating with brief pauses in breathing. In very tiny premature newborns, apnea can be caused by temporary obstruction of the pharynx due to low muscle tone or a bending forward of the neck; this is called obstructive apnea. Over time, as the respiratory center matures, episodes of apnea become less frequent, and by the time the newborn approaches term, they no longer occur.

Symptoms and Diagnosis

Premature newborns are routinely attached to a monitor that sounds an alarm if the newborn stops breathing for a prolonged time or if the heart rate slows. Depending on the length of the episodes, stoppage of breathing may decrease the oxygen levels in the blood, which results in a bluish discoloration of the skin (cyanosis). Low levels of oxygen in the blood may slow the heart rate (bradycardia).

Apnea can sometimes be a sign of a disorder, such as infection of the blood (sepsis), low blood sugar (hypoglycemia), or a low body temperature (hypothermia). Therefore, the doctor evaluates the newborn to rule out these disorders when there is a sudden or unexpected increase in frequency of episodes.

Treatment

Treatment of apnea depends on the cause. Apnea caused by obstruction of the pharynx may be decreased by keeping the newborn lying on his back or side with his head in the midline position. If episodes of apnea become frequent, and especially if the newborn has cyanosis, the newborn may be treated with a drug that stimulates the respiratory center, such as caffeine or aminophylline. If these treatments fail to prevent frequent and severe episodes of apnea, the premature newborn may need treatment with continuous positive airway pressure (CPAP) or a ventilator.

Virtually all premature newborns stop having episodes of apnea several weeks before they reach term. Although a few infants are discharged from the hospital and placed on home monitors before they have completely outgrown their episodes of apnea, this practice is not standard or generally accepted. An association between apnea in the premature newborn and the risk for sudden infant death syndrome (SIDS),▲ which usually occurs months after birth, has not been proven. Likewise, there is no proof that discharging an infant home on an apnea monitor decreases the risk of SIDS.

Retinopathy of Prematurity

Retinopathy of prematurity is a disease in which the small blood vessels in the back of the eye (retina) grow abnormally.

In newborns born very prematurely, growth of the blood vessels supplying the retina may stop for a period of time. When growth resumes, it occurs in a disorganized fashion. During disorganized rapid growth, the small blood vessels may bleed and eventually lead to scarring. In the most severe cases, this process may ultimately result in detachment of the retina from the back of the eye and loss of vision. High blood oxygen levels may also increase the risk of retinopathy of prematurity.

The newborn who is developing retinopathy of prematurity does not have symptoms, and diagnosis depends on careful examination of the back of the eyes by an eye specialist (ophthalmologist). Routinely, therefore, an ophthalmologist examines the eyes of premature newborns who weigh less than 1,500 grams at birth starting 4 or more weeks after delivery. Eye examinations are repeated every 1 to 2 weeks as needed, until growth of the blood vessels in the retina is complete. Infants who develop severe retinopathy must have eye ex-

aminations, at least yearly, for the rest of their lives. If detected early, retinal detachment can occasionally be treated to avoid complete loss of vision in the affected eye.

Prevention, Treatment, and Prognosis

In a premature newborn who needs oxygen, the oxygen use is monitored carefully to prevent excessive oxygen levels in the blood that would put the newborn at increased risk of retinopathy of prematurity. Alternatively, the oxygen levels can be indirectly monitored using a pulse oximeter, which measures the level of oxygen in the blood going through a finger or toe.

Retinopathy is usually mild and resolves spontaneously, but the eyes need to be monitored by an ophthalmologist until blood vessel growth is mature.

For very severe retinopathy of prematurity, laser treatment is applied to the outermost portions of the retina. This treatment stops the abnormal growth of blood vessels and decreases the risk of retinal detachment and loss of vision.

Necrotizing Enterocolitis

Necrotizing enterocolitis is injury to the inner surface of the intestine.

Necrotizing enterocolitis usually occurs in premature newborns. The cause is not understood. Diminished blood flow to the intestine in a sick premature newborn may result in injury to the inner layers of the intestine, allowing bacteria that normally exist within the intestine to invade the damaged intestinal wall. If the injury progresses through the entire thickness of the bowel wall and the intestinal wall perforates, intestinal contents leak into the abdominal cavity and cause peritonitis. Necrotizing enterocolitis can also lead to infection of the blood (sepsis). In the most severe cases, necrotizing enterocolitis can be fatal.

Newborns with necrotizing enterocolitis may develop swelling of the abdomen. They may vomit bile-stained intestinal fluid, and blood may be visible in the stools. These newborns soon appear very sick and lethargic and have low body temperature and repeated pauses of breathing (apnea spells). The diagnosis of necrotizing enterocolitis is confirmed by abdominal x-rays. Blood samples are taken for blood cultures to identify the bacteria responsible for the infection.

▲ see page 1538

Prevention, Treatment, and Prognosis

Feeding the premature newborn breast milk rather than formula appears to provide some protection. In tiny or sick premature newborns, the risk may also be reduced by delaying feedings for several days and then increasing the amount of feedings slowly. Feedings are stopped if necrotizing enterocolitis is suspected. A suction tube is passed into the newborn's stomach to remove pressure from swallowed air and formula, thereby decompressing the intestine. Intravenous fluids are given to maintain hydration, and antibiotics are begun after blood cultures have been obtained.

About 70% of newborns with necrotizing enterocolitis do not need surgery. If the intestine perforates, then surgery is needed. Surgery may also be needed if the condition progressively worsens despite treatment.

In the tiniest and sickest newborns, "peritoneal drains" are placed into the abdominal cavity on each side of the lower abdomen. The drains allow stool and peritoneal fluid to drain from the abdominal cavity and, along with antibiotics, may allow symptoms to improve. The condition of many newborns treated with drains stabilizes, so that an operation can be performed more safely at a later time. In some cases, the newborns recover completely without needing additional surgery.

Larger infants need surgery in which portions of the bowel are removed and the ends of the healthy bowel are brought out to the skin surface to create a temporary opening for the excretion of bodily wastes (ostomy).

Intensive medical treatment and surgery when needed have improved the prognosis for newborns with necrotizing enterocolitis. More than two thirds of such newborns survive.

Hyperbilirubinemia

Hyperbilirubinemia is an abnormally high level of bilirubin in the blood.

Aging red blood cells are removed by the spleen, and the hemoglobin from these red blood cells is broken down and recycled. The heme portion of the hemoglobin molecule is converted into a yellow pigment called bilirubin, which is carried in the blood to the liver where it is chemically modified and then excreted in the bile into the newborn's digestive tract. It is removed from the body when the newborn passes stools. Bilirubin in the stools of newborns gives them their yellow color.

In most newborns, the level of bilirubin in the blood increases in the first days after birth, causing the newborn's skin and the whites of the eyes to appear yellow (jaundice). If feedings are delayed for any reason, as occurs when newborns are sick or have a digestive tract problem, blood levels of bilirubin can become high. Also, breastfed newborns tend to have somewhat higher blood levels of bilirubin during the first week or two.

Hyperbilirubinemia may also occur when a newborn has a serious medical disorder, such as infection in the blood (sepsis). It may also be caused by hemolysis (rapid breakdown of red blood cells), as occurs with Rh incompatibility▲ or ABO incompatibility.

In the large majority of cases, elevated levels of bilirubin in the blood are not serious. However, very high bilirubin levels can produce brain damage (kernicterus). Very premature and critically ill newborns are at higher risk for developing kernicterus. In almost all cases, moderately elevated blood levels of bilirubin due to breastfeeding are not of concern. However, newborns who are slightly premature and are breastfeeding, especially if discharged early from the hospital, must be monitored closely for hyperbilirubinemia because they can develop kernicterus if the bilirubin level becomes very high.

Symptoms and Diagnosis

Newborns with hyperbilirubinemia have a yellow color to their skin and the whites of their eyes (jaundice). It may be more difficult to recognize jaundice in dark-skinned newborns. Jaundice usually first appears on the newborn's face and then, as the bilirubin level increases, progresses downward to involve the chest, abdomen, and finally the legs and feet.

Newborns with hyperbilirubinemia who are showing symptoms of kernicterus may become lethargic and feed poorly; these newborns should be examined immediately by a doctor. The later stages of kernicterus involve irritability, muscle stiffening or seizures, and a fever.

It is important that a doctor assess the degree of jaundice in all newborns during the first days of life. Some newborns have developed dangerously high levels of bilirubin after being discharged from the hospital on the first day after birth before their blood level of

---

▲ see page 1453

bilirubin had risen. Therefore, it is very important that newborns discharged early be examined at home by a visiting nurse or in the doctor's office within a few days after discharge to assess their bilirubin levels. This is especially true for newborns born a few weeks prematurely and those breastfeeding.

A doctor first examines the newborn under good lighting and then measures the level of jaundice by holding a specialized piece of equipment (bilirubinometer) against the newborn's skin or by testing a small sample of blood.

Treatment

Mild hyperbilirubinemia does not require special treatment. Offering frequent feedings accelerates the passage of stools, thus reducing the reabsorption of bilirubin from the intestinal contents and lowering the bilirubin level. Moderate hyperbilirubinemia can be treated with phototherapy, in which the newborn is placed without clothes under fluorescent bilirubin lights. The light exposure alters the composition of the bilirubin in the newborn's skin, changing it to a form that is more readily excreted by the liver and kidneys. The newborn's eyes are shielded with a blindfold. Newborns can also be treated at home by having them lie on a fiber-optic "bilirubin blanket," which exposes their skin to bright light. These newborns need to have their blood levels of bilirubin tested repeatedly until they decrease.

Rarely, it may be necessary for a mother to change from breastfeeding to formula feeding temporarily to ensure that the newborn is obtaining adequate volumes with each feeding. The mother should resume breastfeeding as soon as the bilirubin levels start to decrease. Moderate hyperbilirubinemia sometimes continues for weeks in infants who are breastfed, a normal phenomenon that poses no problems for the infant and that does not usually require withholding of breastfeeding.

If the newborn's blood level of bilirubin approaches a dangerous level, it can be lowered rapidly by performing an exchange blood

What Is Hemolytic Disease of the Newborn?

Hemolytic disease of the newborn (also called erythroblastosis fetalis) is a condition in which red blood cells are broken down or destroyed more rapidly than is normal. The newborn's red blood cells are destroyed by antibodies that were produced by the mother and crossed the placenta from the mother's circulation into the fetal circulation before delivery. A mother who is Rh-negative may have produced antibodies against Rh-positive blood cells after she was exposed to red blood cells of a previous fetus that was Rh-positive. Such exposure may occur during pregnancy or labor, but may also occur if the mother had been accidentally transfused with Rh-positive blood at any time earlier in life.

The mother's body responds to the "incompatible blood" by producing antibodies to destroy the "foreign" Rh-positive cells. These antibodies cross the placenta during a subsequent pregnancy. If the fetus she is carrying is Rh-negative, there is no consequence. However, if the fetus has Rh-positive red blood cells, the mother's antibodies attach to, and start to destroy, the fetal red blood cells, leading to anemia of varying degrees. This anemia begins in the fetus and continues after delivery.

Sometimes other blood group incompatibilities may lead to similar hemolytic diseases. For example, if the mother is blood type O and the fetus has blood type A or B, then the mother's body produces anti-A or anti-B antibodies that can cross the placenta, attach to fetal red blood cells, and lead to their breakdown (hemolysis). Rh incompatibility usually leads to more severe anemia than ABO incompatibility.

Prevention of hemolytic disease due to Rh incompatibility involves injecting the mother with a $Rh_0(D)$ immune globulin preparation at about 28 weeks of pregnancy and again immediately after delivery. Injection of this immune globulin rapidly destroys any Rh-positive fetal red blood cells that have entered the mother's circulation before they stimulate the mother's body to produce antibodies.

Severe anemia caused by hemolytic disease of the newborn is treated in the same way as any other anemia. The doctor also observes the newborn for jaundice, which is likely to occur because hemoglobin from the red blood cells that are being rapidly broken down is converted to the yellow pigment, bilirubin, giving the newborn's skin and whites of the eyes a yellow appearance. Jaundice can be treated by exposing the newborn to bright lights (phototherapy) or by having the newborn undergo an exchange blood transfusion. Very high levels of bilirubin in the blood can lead to brain damage (kernicterus).

transfusion. In this procedure, a sterile catheter is placed into the umbilical vein located in the cut surface of the umbilical cord. The newborn's bilirubin-containing blood is removed and replaced with equal volumes of fresh blood.

Anemia

Anemia is a disorder in which there are too few red blood cells in the blood.

Normally, the newborn's bone marrow does not produce new red blood cells between birth and 3 or 4 weeks of age. Anemia can occur when red blood cells are broken down too rapidly, too much blood is lost, or more than one of these processes occurs at the same time.

Any process that leads to red blood cell destruction, if sufficiently severe, results in anemia and high levels of bilirubin (hyperbilirubinemia). Hemolytic disease of the newborn may cause the newborn's red blood cells to be destroyed rapidly. The red blood cells may also be rapidly destroyed if the newborn has a hereditary abnormality of the red blood cells. An example is hereditary spherocytosis, in which the red blood cells appear small and spherical in shape when viewed under a microscope.

Infections acquired before birth, such as toxoplasmosis, rubella, cytomegalovirus, herpes simplex, or syphilis, may also rapidly destroy red blood cells, as can bacterial infections of the newborn acquired during or following birth.

Another cause of anemia is blood loss. Blood loss can occur in many ways, for example, if there is a large transfusion of the fetal blood across the placenta and into the mother's circulation (fetal-maternal transfusion) or if too much blood gets trapped in the placenta at delivery, when the umbilical cord is clamped. The placenta may separate from the uterine wall before delivery (placental abruption), leading to hemorrhage of the fetal blood. Rarely, anemia may result from a failure of the fetal bone marrow to produce red blood cells. One example of this is a genetic disorder called Fanconi's anemia. Another rare example is that due to exposure of the mother and fetus to certain drugs used during pregnancy.

Symptoms and Treatment

A newborn who has suddenly lost a large amount of blood during labor or delivery may appear pale and have a rapid heart rate and low blood pressure, along with rapid, shallow breathing. Milder anemia may result in lethargy, poor feeding, or no symptoms. When the anemia is a result of rapid breakdown of red blood cells, there is also increased production of bilirubin, and the newborn's skin and the whites of the eyes appear yellow (jaundice).

A newborn who has rapidly lost a large amount of blood, often during labor and delivery, is treated with intravenous fluids followed by a blood transfusion. Very severe anemia caused by hemolytic disease may also require a blood transfusion, but the anemia is more often treated with an exchange blood transfusion, in which part of the newborn's blood is gradually removed and replaced with equal volumes of fresh donor blood. The exchange transfusion also removes bilirubin in the circulation and thus treats the hyperbilirubinemia.

Polycythemia

Polycythemia is an abnormally high concentration of red blood cells.

A markedly increased concentration of red blood cells may result in the blood being too thick, which slows the flow of blood through small blood vessels and interferes with the delivery of oxygen to tissues. A newborn who is born postmaturely or whose mother has severe high blood pressure, smokes, or lives at a high altitude is more likely to have polycythemia. Polycythemia may also result if the newborn receives too much blood from the placenta at birth, as may occur if the newborn is held below the level of the placenta for a period of time before the umbilical cord is clamped.

The newborn with polycythemia may have a ruddy or dusky color. Most such newborns do not have other symptoms. However, the newborn may be sluggish, feed poorly, have rapid heart and respiratory rates, and, rarely, may have seizures. If the newborn has such symptoms and a blood test indicates too many red blood cells (high hematocrit), a partial exchange blood transfusion is performed, in which the newborn's blood is removed and replaced with equal volumes of albumin solution or saline, thus diluting the remaining red blood cells and correcting the polycythemia.

Disorders of the Thyroid Gland

These disorders occur if the thyroid gland produces too little thyroid hormone (hypothy-

SOME INFECTIONS OF NEWBORNS

INFECTION	MODE OF INFECTION	SYMPTOMS	TREATMENT/ PREVENTION
Herpes	Usually, the virus (herpes simplex) infects the fetus after rupture of the membranes during labor and delivery	Usually, a skin rash of small fluid-filled blisters appears; infection may be widespread, affecting many organs, such as eyes, lungs, liver, brain, and skin	Antiviral drugs are given intravenously; eye infections are treated with trifluridine drops
Hepatitis B	Usually, the virus infects the fetus after rupture of the membranes during labor and delivery	Chronic liver infection (chronic hepatitis) develops but usually does not produce symptoms until young adulthood	A newborn born to an infected mother is given both hepatitis B virus vaccine and hepatitis B immune globulin within 24 hours of birth.
Cytomega-lovirus infection	The virus is thought to cross the placenta from the mother during pregnancy or during delivery (a risk of 1%); after birth, a newborn may become infected from infected breast milk or contaminated blood from a transfusion	Most newborns do not have symptoms; about 10% have low birth weight, a small head, jaundice, small bruises, and an enlarged liver and spleen; deafness may occur	The infection cannot be cured; ganciclovir may help some symptoms; newborns should have repeated hearing evaluations during the first year
Rubella	The virus may cross the placenta during pregnancy (rare because vaccination is now routine); infection is more severe if the fetus is infected early in pregnancy	Effects on the fetus range from death before birth to birth defects or hearing loss without other symptoms; newborns may have low birth weight, brain inflammation, cataracts, damage to retina, heart defects, an enlarged liver and spleen; bruising, bluish red skin lesions, enlarged lymph nodes, and pneumonia	No specific treatment is available; to prevent infection in the mother, all women of childbearing age should be vaccinated before pregnancy; immune globulin is sometimes injected if a pregnant woman who has not been immunized comes into close contact with an infected person early in pregnancy
Toxoplas-mosis	The parasite (*Toxoplasma gondii*) may cross the placenta during pregnancy; infection is more severe if the fetus is infected early in pregnancy	The fetus may grow slowly and be born prematurely; the newborn may have a small head, brain inflammation, jaundice, an enlarged liver and spleen, and inflammation of the heart, lungs, or eyes; rashes may occur	Women should avoid handling cat litter during pregnancy; transmission from the mother to the fetus may be prevented if the mother takes spiramycin; pyrimethamine and

SOME INFECTIONS OF NEWBORNS (*Continued*)

INFECTION	MODE OF INFECTION	SYMPTOMS	TREATMENT/ PREVENTION
			sulfonamides may be taken later in pregnancy if the fetus is infected; infected newborns with symptoms are treated with pyrimethamine, sulfadiazine, and leucovorin; corticosteroids can be used for inflammation of heart, lungs, or eyes
Syphilis	The bacterium (*Treponema pallidum*) crosses the placenta during pregnancy if the mother acquires syphilis during pregnancy or if she has been inadequately treated for syphilis in the past	Stillbirth or premature birth may occur. The newborn may have no symptoms; in the first month of life, the newborn may develop large fluid-filled blisters or flat copper-colored rash on palms and soles, with raised bumps around the nose and mouth and in the diaper area; usually lymph nodes, liver, and spleen are enlarged; the newborn may not grow well and have a characteristic "old man" look, with cracks around the mouth; mucus, pus, or blood may run from the nose; rarely, meningitis occurs	Before birth, the mother is treated with penicillin. After birth, if still infected, the mother and newborn are treated with penicillin
Conjunctivitis	The bacteria (most commonly *Chlamydia* or *Neisseria gonorrhoeae*) infects the fetus after rupture of the membranes during labor or delivery	**When caused by *Chlamydia*:** Conjunctivitis usually begins 5 to 12 days after delivery but sometimes 6 weeks after, as watery discharge from eyes containing increasing amounts of pus **When caused by *Neisseria gonorrhoeae*:** Conjunctivitis begins usually 2 to 3 days after, but sometimes up to 7 days after, delivery, as discharge of pus from eyes	**When caused by *Chlamydia*:** Erythromycin is given as eye ointment and also as tablets by mouth **When caused by *Neisseria gonorrhoeae*:** An eye ointment containing polymyxin and bacitracin, erythromycin, or tetracycline is used. An antibiotic such as ceftriaxone is also given intravenously
Human papillomavirus infection	Usually newborns become infected during delivery	Symptoms are an altered cry; sometimes difficulty breathing or even significant obstruction of the airways due to warts that grow inside the windpipe; lung infection	Warts are removed surgically; recurrence can be reduced by use of interferon

roidism) or too much thyroid hormone (hyperthyroidism).

Hypothyroidism: If untreated, hypothyroidism in the newborn results in poor growth and mental delay, eventually resulting in mental retardation. The most common cause of hypothyroidism in the newborn is complete absence or underdevelopment of the thyroid gland. Initially, the newborn has no symptoms. Later, the newborn may have lethargy, poor appetite, constipation, a hoarse cry, umbilical hernia (a bulging of the abdominal contents where the umbilicus penetrates the abdominal wall), and slow growth. Eventually, the infant may develop coarse facial features and an enlarged tongue.

Early treatment can prevent mental retardation. For this reason, a blood test is performed in the hospital after birth on all newborns to measure thyroid hormone levels. Treatment is with thyroid hormone.

Hyperthyroidism: Rarely, a newborn may have hyperthyroidism, or neonatal Graves' disease. This generally occurs if the mother has Graves' disease during pregnancy or has been treated for it before pregnancy. In Graves' disease,▲ the woman's body produces antibodies that stimulate the thyroid gland to produce increased blood levels of thyroid hormone. These antibodies cross the placenta and similarly affect the fetus. The result in an affected newborn is too high a metabolic rate, with rapid heart rate and breathing, irritability, and excessive appetite with poor weight gain.

The newborn, like the mother, may have bulging eyes (exophthalmos). If the newborn has an enlarged thyroid gland (goiter), the gland may press against the windpipe and interfere with breathing. A very rapid heart rate can lead to heart failure. Graves' disease is potentially fatal if not recognized and treated.

Doctors suspect hyperthyroidism by the typical symptoms and confirm the diagnosis by measuring elevated levels of thyroid hormone and the thyroid-stimulating antibodies from the mother in the newborn's blood.

Newborns with hyperthyroidism are treated with drugs, such as propylthiouracil, that slow the production of thyroid hormone by the thyroid gland. Treatment is needed for only a few months because the antibodies that cross the placenta from the mother only last in the infant's bloodstream for this long.

Neonatal Sepsis

Sepsis is bacterial infection in the blood.

Newborns, especially premature ones, are at much higher risk of sepsis than are children and adults because of their immature immune system. Premature newborns also lack certain antibodies against specific bacteria; these antibodies usually cross the placenta from the mother late in pregnancy. Another important risk factor for sepsis is the use of intravenous lines and ventilators.

The most common type of bacteria causing sepsis in the newborn around the time of birth is Group B streptococcus. Sepsis that occurs later while the newborn is being cared for in the neonatal intensive care unit (NICU) is most likely to be caused by a type of staphylococcus (coagulase negative).

Symptoms and Diagnosis

A newborn with sepsis is usually listless, does not feed well, and often has a low body temperature. Other symptoms may include pauses in breathing (apnea), fever, pale color, and poor skin circulation, with cool extremities, abdominal swelling, and jaundice.

Because newborns have decreased immunity against infection, bacteria in the bloodstream may invade and infect various organs. One of the most serious complications of sepsis is infection of the membranes surrounding the brain (meningitis). A newborn with meningitis may have extreme lethargy, coma, seizures, or bulging of the fontanelle (the soft spot between the skull bones). A doctor can rule out or diagnose meningitis by performing a spinal tap (lumbar puncture), examining the cerebrospinal fluid, and culturing a sample of this fluid. Infection of a bone (osteomyelitis) may cause pain and swelling of an arm or leg, often suspected because the newborn does not move that extremity. Infection of a joint may cause swelling, warmth, redness, and tenderness over the joint, again with little or no movement of that joint. If joint infection is suspected, a sample of fluid from the infected site is removed by needle and cultured.

Treatment and Prognosis

While awaiting blood culture results, a doctor gives intravenous antibiotics to a newborn with suspected sepsis. Once the specific or-

▲ see page 1449

ganism has been identified, the type of antibiotic can be adjusted. In addition to antibiotic therapy, other treatments may be needed, such as use of a ventilator, intravenous fluids, and support of the blood pressure and circulation.

Sepsis is the major cause of mortality in premature newborns after the first week. Newborns who recover from sepsis should not have long-term problems, except those with meningitis, who may have mental delay, cerebral palsy, seizures, or hearing loss later in life.

CHAPTER 265

Birth Defects

Birth defects, also called congenital anomalies, are physical abnormalities that occur before a baby is born; they are usually obvious at birth or by 1 year of age.

Birth defects can involve any part of any organ in the body. Some birth defects are more common than others. Birth defects are the leading cause of death in infants in the United States. A birth defect is evident in about 7.5% of all children by age 5 years, although many of these are minor. Major birth defects are evident in about 3 to 4% of newborns. Several birth defects can occur together in the same infant.

Causes and Risks

It is not surprising that birth defects are fairly common, considering the complexities involved in the development of a single fertilized egg into the millions of specialized cells that constitute a human being. Although the cause of most birth defects is unknown, certain genetic and environmental factors increase the chance of birth defects developing. These factors include exposure to radiation, certain drugs (for example, isotretinoin, which is used to treat severe acne), alcohol, nutritional deficiencies, some infections in the mother, injuries, and hereditary disorders. Some risks are avoidable. Others occur no matter how strictly a pregnant woman adheres to healthful living practices.

Exposure to Harmful Substances (Teratogens): A teratogen is any substance that can cause or increase the chance of a birth defect. Radiation (including x-rays), certain drugs, and toxins (including alcohol) are teratogens. Most pregnant women who are exposed to teratogens have newborns without abnormalities. Whether or not a birth defect occurs depends on when, how much, and how long the pregnant woman was exposed to the teratogen. Exposure to a teratogen most commonly affects the fetal organ that is developing at the time of exposure. For example, exposure to a teratogen during the time that certain parts of the brain are developing is more likely to cause a defect in those areas than exposure before or after this critical period. Many birth defects develop before a woman knows she is pregnant.

Nutrition: Keeping a fetus healthy requires maintaining a nutritious diet. For example, insufficient folic acid (folate) in the diet increases the chance that a fetus will develop spina bifida or other abnormalities of the brain or spinal cord known as neural tube defects.▲ Maternal obesity also increases the risk of a neural tube defect.

Genetic and Chromosomal Factors: Chromosomes and genes may be abnormal. These abnormalities may be inherited from the parents, who can be affected by the condition or who can be carriers without symptoms.■ However, many birth defects are caused by seemingly random and unexplained changes (mutations) in the genes of the child. Most birth defects caused by genetic factors include more than just the obvious malformation of a single body part.

Infections: Certain infections in pregnant women can cause birth defects. Whether an infection causes a birth defect depends on the age of the fetus. The infections that most often cause birth defects are cytomegalovirus, herpesvirus, parvovirus (fifth disease), rubella (German measles), varicella (chickenpox), tox-

▲ see page 1430   ■ see page 12

OTHER BIRTH DEFECTS

Major System	Birth Defect	What Happens	Treatment
Heart	Hypoplastic left heart syndrome	Underdevelopment of the left ventricle, leading to inability to pump blood to the body	Separate operations to rebuild the left ventricle
Digestive tract	Omphalocele and gastroschisis	Hole or weakening of abdominal muscles, allowing internal abdominal organs to protrude externally	Surgery to close the abdomen
Musculo-skeletal	Congenital torti-collis	Abnormal twisting of the head and neck	Physical therapy, surgery, or injections of botulinum toxin
	Prune-belly syndrome	Missing layers of abdominal muscles, causing the abdomen to bulge; urinary system defects often develop	Surgery if a urinary system defect blocks urine flow
Neurologic	Porencephaly	Brain tissue is missing and is replaced with fluid-filled sacs	No treatment is available; ventricular shunt may decrease pressure
	Hydranencephaly	Severe porencephaly with little remaining brain tissue	No treatment is available
Genital	Vanishing testes (bilateral anorchia; testicular regression)	Both testes are absent at birth	Supplemental male hormone (testosterone) beginning before puberty
Eye	Congenital glaucoma	Glaucoma is present at birth; pressure is raised in the eyeball (usually both); the eye may enlarge, and its normal appearance may be distorted	Surgery usually performed soon after birth; eye drops used until surgery; if the glaucoma is not treated, blindness can result
	Congenital cataracts	Cataracts (cloudy areas) in the lens of the eye are present at birth; usually vision is impaired	Surgery to remove the cataract as soon as possible is the best chance of normal vision

oplasmosis (which can be transmitted in cat litter), and syphilis. A woman can have such an infection and not know it, because these infections can produce few or no symptoms in adults.

Diagnosis

During pregnancy, doctors assess whether a woman is at increased risk of having a baby with a birth defect.▲ The chance is higher for women who are older than 35 years, have had frequent miscarriages, or have had other children with chromosomal abnormalities, birth defects, or who died for unknown reasons. These women may need special tests to find out if their baby is normal.

A prenatal ultrasound can often detect specific birth defects. Sometimes blood tests can also help; for example, a high level of alpha-fetoprotein in the mother's blood may indicate a defect of the brain or spinal cord.■ Amniocentesis (removing fluid from around the fetus) or chorionic villus sampling (removing tissue from the sac around the developing baby) may be necessary to confirm a suspected diagnosis. Increasingly, birth defects are being diagnosed before the baby is born.

▲ see page 1430   ■ see box on page 1432

Heart Defects

One of 120 babies is born with a heart defect. Some are severe, but many are not. Defects may involve abnormal formation of the heart's walls or valves or of the blood vessels that enter or leave the heart.

Before birth, a fetus uses oxygen obtained from the mother's blood through the placenta. The fetus does not breathe. Also, the path by which blood circulates through the heart and lungs is different in a fetus. After birth, a newborn must obtain oxygen using his own lungs. Therefore, many changes occur in the heart and blood vessels soon after birth.

Before birth, blood that has not yet traveled to the lungs (venous blood) mixes with blood that has already traveled to the lungs (arterial blood). Such mixing occurs in the foramen ovale, a hole between the right and left atria (the upper chambers of the heart that receive blood), and the ductus arteriosus, a blood vessel connecting the pulmonary artery and the aorta. In the fetus, both venous and arterial blood contain oxygen, so mixing arterial and venous blood does not affect how much oxygen gets pumped to the body. After birth, arterial blood and venous blood do not normally mix. The foramen ovale and ductus arteriosus normally close within days to a couple of weeks after birth.

Two general processes account for most of the symptoms resulting from heart defects. One is that blood flow gets altered or re-routed (shunting). Another is that not enough blood gets pumped to the body, usually because of a blockage.

Shunting can cause oxygen-poor blood to mix with oxygen-rich blood that is pumped to the body tissues (right-to-left shunt). The more oxygen-poor blood (which is blue) that flows to the body, the more blue the body appears, particularly the skin and lips. Many heart defects are characterized by a bluish discoloration of the skin (called cyanosis); cyanosis indicates that not enough oxygen-rich blood is reaching the tissues where it is needed.

Shunting can also mix oxygen-rich blood, which is pumped under high pressures, with oxygen-poor blood being pumped through the pulmonary artery to the lungs (left-to-right shunt). This deprives the body of oxygen-rich blood and increases the pressure in the pulmonary artery. The high pressure damages the pulmonary artery and lungs. The shunt also eventually leads to an insufficient amount of blood being pumped to the body (heart failure).

In heart failure, blood also backs up, often in the lungs. Heart failure can also develop when the heart pumps too weakly (for example, when a baby is born with a weak heart muscle) or when blood is blocked from flowing to the baby's body.

Blockages may develop in the valves of the heart or in the blood vessels leading away from the heart. Blood may be impeded from flowing to the lungs because of narrowing of the pulmonary valve (pulmonary valve stenosis) or narrowing within the pulmonary artery itself (pulmonary artery stenosis). Blood may be impeded from flowing through the aorta to the body because of narrowing of the aortic valve (aortic valve stenosis) or blockage within the aorta itself (coarctation of the aorta).

Symptoms and Diagnosis

Often, heart defects produce few or no symptoms and are not detectable even during a physical examination of the child. Some mild defects produce symptoms only later in life. However, many heart defects do result in symptoms during childhood. Because oxygen-rich blood is necessary for normal growth, development, and activity, infants and children with heart defects may fail to grow or gain weight normally. They may not be able to exercise fully. In more severe cases, cyanosis may develop, and breathing or eating may be difficult. Abnormal blood flow through the heart usually produces an abnormal sound (murmur) that can be heard using a stethoscope; however, the vast majority of heart murmurs that occur during childhood are not caused by heart defects and are not indicative of any problems. Heart failure makes the heart beat rapidly and often causes fluid to collect in the lungs or liver.

Many heart defects can be diagnosed before birth using ultrasound. After birth, heart defects are suspected when symptoms develop or when particular heart murmurs are heard.

Diagnosing heart defects in children involves the same techniques used for diagnosing heart problems in adults.▲ A doctor may be able to diagnose the defect after asking the family specific questions and performing a physical examination, electrocardiography (ECG), and a chest x-ray. Ultrasound (echocardiography) is used to diagnose almost all of the

▲ see page 118

specific defects. Cardiac catheterization often can show small abnormalities that are not detected with echocardiography or can further illuminate the details of the abnormality.

Treatment

Many significant heart defects are effectively corrected using open-heart surgery. When to perform the operation depends on the specific defect, its symptoms, and severity. For example, it may be better to postpone surgery until the child is a little older. However, severe symptoms resulting from a heart defect are most effectively relieved with immediate surgery.

A narrowing can sometimes be relieved by passing a thin tube (catheter) through a blood vessel in the arm or leg into the narrowed area. A balloon attached to the catheter is inflated and widens the narrowing, usually in a valve (a procedure called balloon valvuloplasty) or blood vessel (a procedure called balloon angioplasty▲). These balloon procedures spare the child from general anesthesia and open-heart surgery. However, balloon procedures are not usually as effective as surgery.

If the aorta or pulmonary artery is severely blocked, a temporary shunt can sometimes be created to keep an adequate amount of blood flowing. A shunt can be created with a catheter balloon (for example, between the right and left atria—balloon septostomy). Or the drug prostaglandin E_1 (alprostadil) can be given to keep the ductus arteriosus open, shunting blood between the aorta and pulmonary artery. In rare cases, when no other treatment helps, a heart transplant is performed, but the lack of donor hearts limits the availability of this procedure.

Most children who have significant heart defects are at increased risk for developing life-threatening bacterial infections of the heart and its valves (endocarditis). They need to take antibiotics before certain treatments and procedures.■

PATENT DUCTUS ARTERIOSUS

In patent ductus arteriosus, the blood vessel connecting the pulmonary artery and the aorta (ductus arteriosus) fails to close as it usually does within the first 2 weeks after birth; a left-to-right shunt causes extra blood flow, and pressure in the lungs may damage the lung tissue. Premature newborns are especially susceptible to patent ductus arteriosus and lung damage.

Most often, the defect causes no symptoms. When symptoms do occur, they are usually difficulty breathing or cyanosis, which may be present at birth or not for several weeks after birth. When the infant has no symptoms, doctors most often suspect the defect when they hear a heart murmur.

Use of indomethacin, a drug that inhibits the production of chemicals called prostaglandins, closes the defect in 80% of infants. Indomethacin is most effective if given in the first 10 days after birth and is more effective in premature newborns than in full-term newborns. If the defect does not close after several doses of indomethacin, it is closed surgically.

ATRIAL AND VENTRICULAR SEPTAL DEFECTS

Atrial and ventricular septal defects are holes in the walls (septa) that separate the heart into the left and right sides. Atrial septal defects are located between the heart's upper chambers (atria), which receive blood. Ventricular septal defects are located between the lower chambers (ventricles), which pump blood. These holes typically cause left-to-right shunting of blood. Many atrial septal defects close by themselves, especially in the first year of life; many ventricular septal defects close within the first 2 years.

Infants and most older children with atrial septal defects have no symptoms. In more severe cases, children may develop heart murmurs, fatigue, and difficulty breathing. The symptoms caused by atrial septal defects increase as the person ages. For example, heart failure may develop during middle age.

Ventricular septal defects can vary from small holes, which may cause a heart murmur but no symptoms and usually close by themselves, to larger holes that cause symptoms in infants. Significant ventricular septal defects usually cause more severe symptoms than atrial septal defects, because there is more shunting of blood. Because of the way lungs develop, shunting increases during the first 6 weeks after birth. Usually the murmur becomes louder, and symptoms, typically rapid breathing, sweating, and difficulty feeding, worsen. Mild symptoms of a ventricular septal defect may be treated with diuretics (such as furosemide) or drugs that decrease resistance to the flow of blood to the body (such as capto-

▲ see art on page 208   ■ see page 184

Patent Ductus Arteriosus: Failure to Close

The ductus arteriosus is a blood vessel that connects the pulmonary artery and aorta. In the fetus, it enables blood to bypass the lungs. The fetus does not breathe air, and thus blood does not need to pass through the lungs to be oxygenated. After birth, blood needs to be oxygenated in the lungs, and normally, the ductus arteriosus closes quickly, usually within days up to 2 weeks. In patent ductus arteriosus, this connection does not close, allowing some oxygenated blood, intended for the body, to return to the lungs. As a result, the blood vessels in the lungs may be overloaded and the body may not receive enough oxygenated blood.

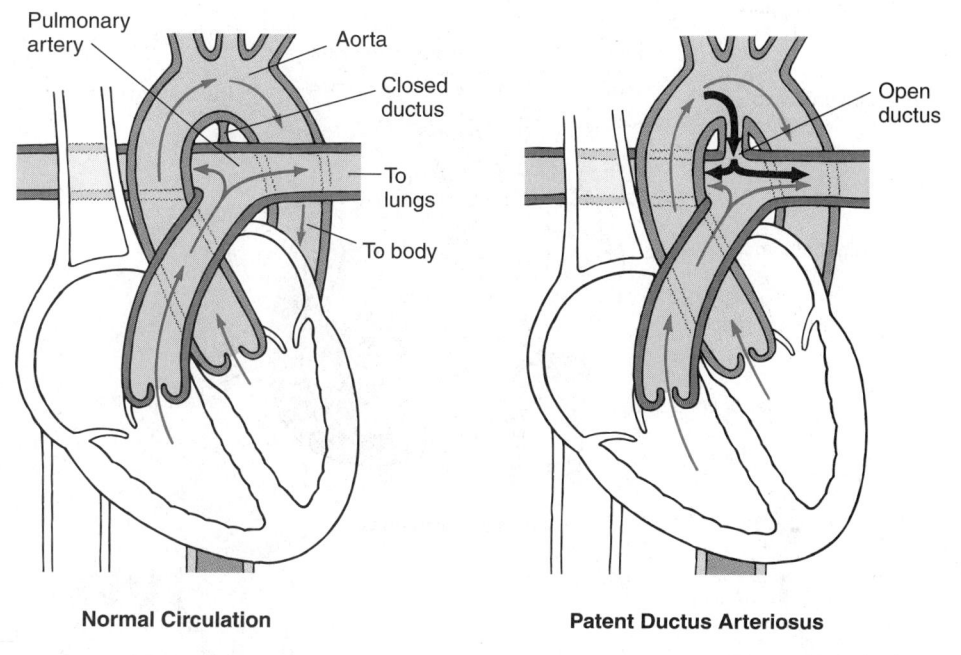

Normal Circulation   **Patent Ductus Arteriosus**

pril). If atrial and ventricular septal defects are large or cause symptoms, they are closed, usually surgically.

TETRALOGY OF FALLOT

In tetralogy of Fallot, four specific heart defects occur together. The defects are a large ventricular septal defect, displacement of the aorta that allows oxygen-poor blood to flow directly from the right ventricle to the aorta (causing a right-to-left shunt), a narrowing of the outflow passage from the right side of the heart, and a thickening of the wall of the right ventricle.

In infants with tetralogy of Fallot, the narrowed passage from the right ventricle restricts blood flow to the lungs. The restricted blood flow causes the oxygen-poor blood in the right ventricle to pass through the septal defect to the left ventricle and into the aorta (right-to-left shunt). The most important symptom is cyanosis, which can be mild or severe. Some infants have life-threatening attacks (hypercyanosis or "tet" spells), in which cyanosis suddenly worsens in response to activity, such as crying or having a bowel movement. The infant becomes very short of breath and may lose consciousness. Infants with tetralogy of Fallot usually have a heart murmur. Echocardiography confirms the diagnosis.

When an infant has a hypercyanotic spell, oxygen and morphine may provide relief. The infant may breathe more easily when the

Septal Defect: A Hole in the Heart's Wall

A septal defect is a hole in the wall (septum) that separates the heart into the left and right sides. Atrial septal defects are located between the heart's upper chambers (atria). Ventricular septal defects are located between the lower chambers (ventricles). In both types, some oxygenated blood, intended for the body, is short-circuited. It is returned to the lungs rather than pumped to the rest of the body.

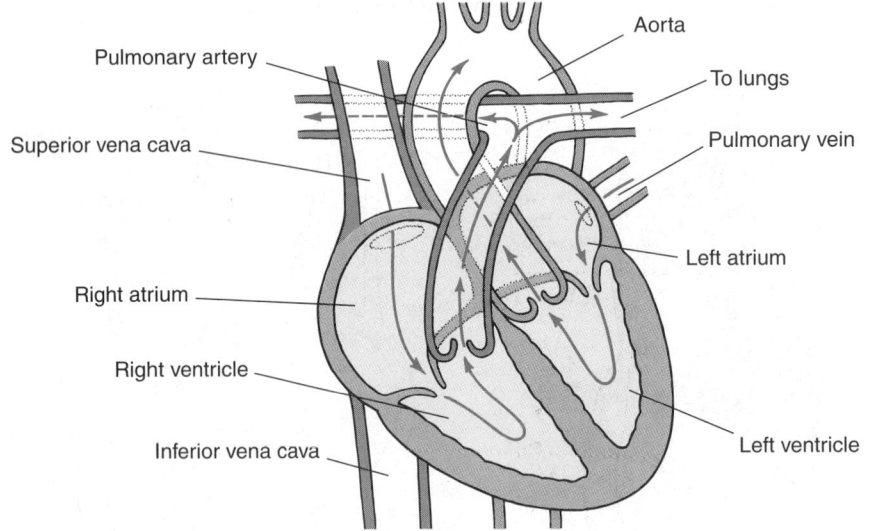

Pulmonary artery

Aorta

To lungs

Superior vena cava

Pulmonary vein

Left atrium

Right atrium

Right ventricle

Inferior vena cava

Left ventricle

Normal Circulation

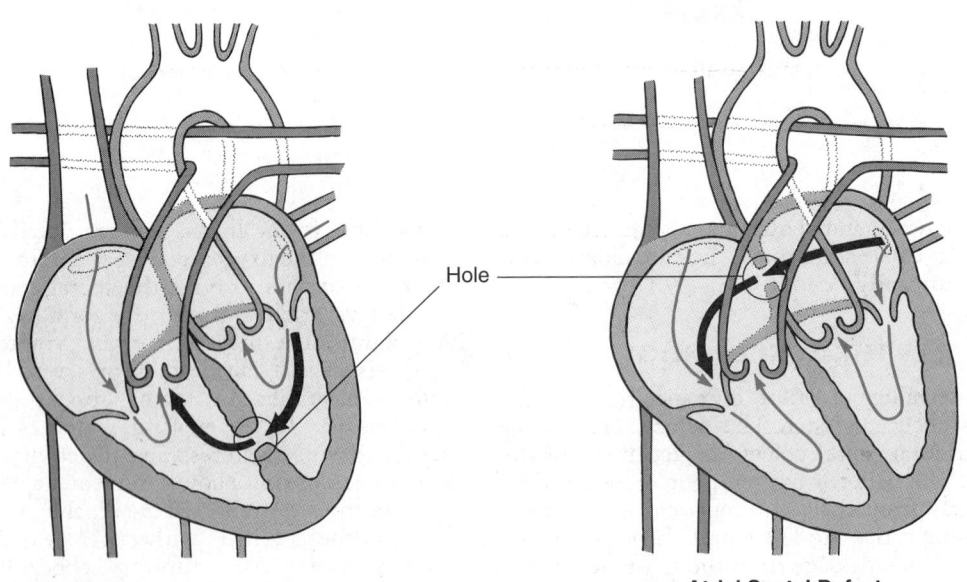

Hole

Ventricular Septal Defect

Atrial Septal Defect

knees are close to the chest (knee-chest position). Giving intravenous fluids or a drug such as phenylephrine, both of which increase resistance to the flow of blood to the body, may be helpful. A doctor may give the infant propranolol to prevent future spells.

Infants with tetralogy of Fallot eventually need surgery. Surgery can be delayed until later in infancy if the child has few symptoms. However, if the symptoms develop often or are severe, surgery should be performed soon. The ventricular septal defect is closed, the narrowed passageway from the right ventricle and the narrowed pulmonary valve are widened, and any abnormal connections between the aorta and pulmonary artery are closed.

TRANSPOSITION OF THE GREAT ARTERIES

Transposition of the great arteries is a reversal of the normal connections of the aorta and the pulmonary artery with the heart. Oxygen-poor blood returning from the body flows from the right atrium to the right ventricle as usual, but then flows to the aorta and the body, bypassing the lungs. Oxygenated blood travels back and forth between the heart and lungs (from the lungs to the pulmonary vein, then left atrium and ventricle, then the pulmonary artery) but is not transported to the body. The body cannot survive without oxygen. However, infants with this defect may survive briefly after birth because the foramen ovale (a hole between the right and left atria) and the ductus arteriosus (a blood vessel connecting the pulmonary artery with the aorta▲) are still open at birth. These openings allow oxygen-rich blood to mix with oxygen-poor blood, sometimes supplying enough oxygen to the body to keep the infant alive. Transposition of the great arteries is often accompanied by a ventricular septal defect.

Transposition of the great arteries usually results in severe cyanosis and difficulty breathing, beginning at birth. A doctor performs a physical examination, x-ray, electrocardiography, and echocardiography to confirm the diagnosis. Usually, surgery is performed within the first few days of life. Surgery consists of attaching the aorta and pulmonary artery to the appropriate ventricles and reimplanting the heart's coronary arteries in the aorta after the aorta is repositioned. Giving alprostadil or performing a balloon septostomy can shunt the blood, which can keep the infant alive until surgery can be performed.

Tetralogy of Fallot: Four Defects

Narrowed pulmonary valve

Thickened right ventricle

Ventricular septal defect

Displaced aorta

AORTIC VALVE STENOSIS

Aortic valve stenosis is a narrowing of the valve that opens to allow blood to flow from the left ventricle into the aorta and then to the body. To propel blood through the narrowed aortic valve, the left ventricle must pump under very high pressures. Sometimes, not enough blood is pumped to supply the body with oxygenated blood.

Most children with aortic valve stenosis do not develop symptoms other than a heart murmur. In some older children, the defect causes fatigue, chest pain, shortness of breath, or fainting. In adolescents, severe aortic valve stenosis may lead to sudden death, presumably because of an erratic heart rhythm caused by poor blood flow through the coronary arteries to the heart. A few infants who have aortic valve stenosis develop irritability, an unnatural lack of color to the skin (pallor), low blood pressure, sweating, rapid heartbeat, and severe shortness of breath.

▲ see page 1514

A doctor suspects aortic valve stenosis after detecting a particular murmur or if the child develops symptoms. Cardiac catheterization is often used to determine the severity of the narrowing.

For older children with severe narrowing or symptoms, the aortic valve must be replaced or widened. Usually the valve is opened surgically (using a procedure called balloon valvulotomy) or replaced with an artificial one. Children with an artificial valve must take an anticoagulant drug, such as warfarin, to prevent blood clots from forming. Infants with heart failure must have emergency treatment, usually including drugs and emergency surgery or balloon valvoplasty.

PULMONARY VALVE STENOSIS

Pulmonary valve stenosis is a narrowing of the pulmonary valve, which opens to allow blood to flow from the right ventricle to the lungs. In most children with pulmonary valve stenosis, the valve is mildly to moderately narrowed, making the right ventricle pump harder and at a higher pressure to propel blood through the valve. Severe narrowing increases pressure in the right ventricle and prevents almost any blood from reaching the lungs. When pressure in the right ventricle becomes extremely high, oxygen-poor blood is forced through abnormal paths (usually a hole in the atrial wall [atrial septal defect]) instead of the pulmonary artery, causing right-to-left shunting.

Most children with pulmonary valve stenosis have no symptoms other than a heart murmur. However, severe cyanosis or heart failure is possible. Moderate symptoms, such as difficulty breathing with exertion and fatigue, may develop as the child gets older. Occasionally, cardiac catheterization is needed to assess the severity of the narrowing.

If the valve is moderately narrowed, it may be opened with balloon valvuloplasty. If the valve is not well formed, it can be surgically reconstructed.

Severe disease that causes cyanosis in newborns is treated by giving alprostadil, which opens the ductus arteriosus, until a surgeon can create another way to open or bypass the pulmonary valve. For some of these newborns, more surgery is needed when they are older.

COARCTATION OF THE AORTA

Coarctation of the aorta is a narrowing of the aorta, usually just before the ductus arteriosus joins the aorta. Coarctation reduces blood flow to the lower half of the body; therefore, the blood pressure is lower than normal in the legs and tends to be higher than normal in the arms. Coarctation can cause heart murmurs. Without treatment, coarctation eventually strains and enlarges the heart, causing heart failure; it also causes high blood pressure. It predisposes the child to rupture of the aorta, bacterial endocarditis, and bleeding in the brain. Children with coarctation often have other heart defects, such as aortic valve stenosis or an atrial or ventricular septal defect.

For most infants, mild or moderate coarctation does not cause symptoms. Rarely, children with coarctation have headaches or nosebleeds because of high blood pressure in the arms, or leg pains during exercise because of insufficient blood and oxygen to the legs.

With a severe coarctation in infancy, blood can flow only to the lower portion of the aorta (at a point past its narrowing) through the open connection between the aorta and the pulmonary artery, the ductus arteriosus. Symptoms usually do not occur until the ductus closes, usually when the newborn is a few days to about 2 weeks old. After the closure, the blood supplied through the ductus disappears, sometimes causing sudden loss of almost the entire blood supply to the lower body. Sudden, catastrophic heart failure and low blood pressure can result.

Coarctation is usually suspected only when a doctor notices a heart murmur or differences in pulses or blood pressures between the arms and legs when performing a physical examination. X-rays, electrocardiography, and echocardiography are usually used to confirm the diagnosis.

Coarctation that does not cause severe symptoms should be surgically repaired in early childhood, usually when the child is about 3 to 5 years old. Infants with severe symptoms from coarctation require emergency treatment, including giving alprostadil to reopen the ductus arteriosus, other drugs to strengthen the heart's pumping, and emergency surgery to widen the narrowing. Some infants who undergo emergency surgery need more surgery when they are older. Sometimes, instead of surgery, doctors use balloon angioplasty to relieve coarctation.

Urinary Tract Defects

Birth defects are more common in the kidney and urinary system than in any other system of the body. Defects can develop in the kidneys, the tubes that transport urine from the kidneys to the bladder (ureters), the bladder, or the tube that expels urine from the bladder (urethra). Any birth defect that blocks or slows the flow of urine can cause urine to stagnate, which can result in infections or formation of kidney stones. Blockage also causes urine pressure to increase, which damages the kidneys and ureters over time.

Symptoms

Many urinary tract defects cause no symptoms. Some, such as kidney defects, may cause blood in the urine after minor injuries. Infections due to defects can develop anywhere in the urinary system and cause symptoms. Kidney damage results from blockage, but it usually causes symptoms only when very little kidney function remains. Then, kidney failure develops. Kidney stones may develop and cause severe, crampy pain in the side between the ribs and the hip (flank) or groin, or blood in the urine.

Diagnosis and Treatment

The techniques used to diagnose abnormalities of the urinary tract include physical examination, ultrasound, computed tomography (CT), nuclear scans, intravenous urography, and rarely, cystoscopy.▲ Defects that cause symptoms or those that lead to increased pressure on the kidneys usually need to be surgically corrected.

KIDNEY AND URETER DEFECTS

A number of defects may result in abnormal formation of the kidneys. The kidneys may be in the wrong place (ectopia), in the wrong position (malrotation), joined together (horseshoe kidney), or missing (kidney agenesis). In Potter's syndrome, which causes death, both kidneys are missing. Kidney tissue may also develop abnormally. For example, a kidney may contain many cysts (fluid-filled sacs), as in polycystic kidney disease.■ If an abnormality blocks an infant's urine flow, the affected kidney may swell so that it becomes visible and can be felt by a doctor.

Many birth defects involving the kidney do not cause symptoms and are never detected. Some defects may interfere with the function of the kidneys, leading to kidney failure, which can require dialysis or kidney transplantation.

Abnormalities of the tubes that connect the kidneys to the bladder (ureters) include formation of extra ureters, misplaced ureters, and narrowed or widened ureters. A narrowed ureter prevents urine from passing normally from the kidney to the bladder.

BLADDER AND URETHRA DEFECTS

The bladder may not close completely, so that it opens out onto the surface of the abdomen (exstrophy). The wall of the bladder may develop outpouchings (diverticula) where urine can stagnate, sometimes causing urinary tract infections. The bladder outlet (the passageway from the bladder to the urethra) may be narrowed, causing the bladder to empty incompletely. In this case, the urine stream is weak.

The urethra may be abnormal or missing altogether. In posterior urethral valves, abnormal tissue blocks (usually partially) the flow of urine from the bladder. Affected infants have a weak urinary stream and urinary tract infections; they may fail to gain weight normally or may have anemia. Less severe defects may not cause symptoms until childhood. In this case, the symptoms that develop are also milder. Surgery to open the blockage must be performed in infants.

In boys, the opening of the urethra may be in the wrong place, such as on the underside of the penis (hypospadias). In boys with hypospadias, the penis may bend downward (chordee). Both hypospadias and chordee can be repaired surgically. The urethra in the penis may lie open as a channel rather than closed as a tube (epispadias). In both boys and girls, a narrowed urethra may obstruct the flow of urine.

Genital Defects

Defects of the external genital organs (penis, testes, or clitoris) usually result from abnormal levels of sex hormones in the blood before birth. Congenital adrenal hyperplasia (a metabolic disorder) and chromosomal abnormalities commonly cause genital defects.

A child may be born with genitals that are not clearly male or female (ambiguous genitals, or intersex state). Most children with ambiguous genitals are pseudohermaphrodites—that is, they have ambiguous external genital organs but either ovaries or testes (not both).

▲ see page 823   ■ see page 854

Pseudohermaphrodites are genetically male or female.

Diagnostic evaluation of a child with ambiguous genitals includes physical examination and blood tests to analyze the chromosomes (the XY chromosome pattern is male and XX is female) and hormone levels (pituitary hormones and male sex hormones, or androgens, such as testosterone). X-rays and ultrasound of the pelvis may help identify internal sex organs. Treatment with testosterone may help enlarge the penis so that assignment to a male sex is more realistic.

Most experts believe that the child's sex must be assigned quickly. Otherwise, bonding by the parents to the child may become more difficult and the child may develop a gender identity disorder.▲ Surgery to correct the ambiguous genitals can be performed later, especially if the defect is complex. The underlying problem causing pseudohermaphroditism may also need treatment.

MALE GENITAL DEFECTS

Pseudohermaphroditism in the male is usually caused by a deficiency of male sex hormones (androgens) or a chromosomal abnormality. The penis and testes may be absent if androgen deficiency develops before the 12th week of pregnancy. If androgen deficiency develops later in pregnancy, a male fetus may have an abnormally small penis (microphallus) or testes that do not descend fully into the scrotum.■ Pseudohermaphroditism may also result from an inability to respond to androgens. After they develop, the testes produce most of the male body's androgens. Absent or underdeveloped testes causes androgen deficiency.

Androgen deficiency during childhood causes incomplete sexual development. An affected boy retains a high-pitched voice and has poor muscle development for his age. The penis, testes, and scrotum are underdeveloped. Pubic and underarm hair is sparse, and the arms and legs are abnormally long.

Androgen deficiency can be treated with testosterone. The testosterone is usually given by injection or through a skin patch. Injection and skin application cause fewer side effects than taking testosterone by mouth. Testosterone stimulates growth, sexual development, and fertility.

▲ see page 628

■ see also page 1535

FEMALE GENITAL DEFECTS

Female pseudohermaphroditism (also called virilization) is caused by exposure to high levels of male hormones. The most common cause is enlarged adrenal glands (congenital adrenal hyperplasia) that overproduce male hormones because an enzyme is missing. The male hormones cannot be converted to female hormones as occurs in normal females. Sometimes, male hormones enter the placenta from the mother's blood; for example, the mother may have been given drugs such as progesterone to prevent a miscarriage, or she may have had a hormone-producing tumor, although this is much less common.

A female pseudohermaphrodite has female internal organs but has an enlarged clitoris that resembles a small penis.

If the child is assigned to the female gender, surgery is performed to create female-appearing genitals. This surgery can include reduction of the clitoris, formation or repair of a vagina (vaginoplasty), and repair of the urethra.

Congenital adrenal hyperplasia can be life-threatening because it can cause serious abnormalities of electrolytes (sodium and potassium) in the blood. These are diagnosed with blood tests and treated with corticosteroids.

Digestive Tract Defects

A birth defect can occur anywhere along the length of the digestive tract—in the esophagus, stomach, small intestine, large intestine, rectum, or anus. In many cases, an organ is not fully developed or is abnormally positioned, which often causes narrowing or blockage (obstruction). The internal or external muscles surrounding the abdominal cavity may weaken or develop holes. The nerves to the intestines may also fail to develop (Hirschsprung disease, or congenital megacolon).

Blockages (obstructions) that develop in the intestines, rectum, or anus can cause rhythmic, crampy abdominal pain, abdominal swelling, and vomiting.

Most digestive tract defects require surgery. Generally, obstructions are surgically opened. Weakenings or holes in the muscles surrounding the abdominal cavity are sewn shut.

ESOPHAGEAL ATRESIA AND TRACHEOESOPHAGEAL FISTULA

Normally, the esophagus, a long tubelike organ, connects the mouth to the stomach. In esophageal atresia, the esophagus narrows or

Atresia and Fistula: Defects in the Esophagus

In esophageal atresia, the esophagus narrows or comes to a blind end. It does not connect with the stomach as it normally does. A tracheoesophageal fistula is an abnormal connection between the esophagus and the trachea (which leads to the lungs).

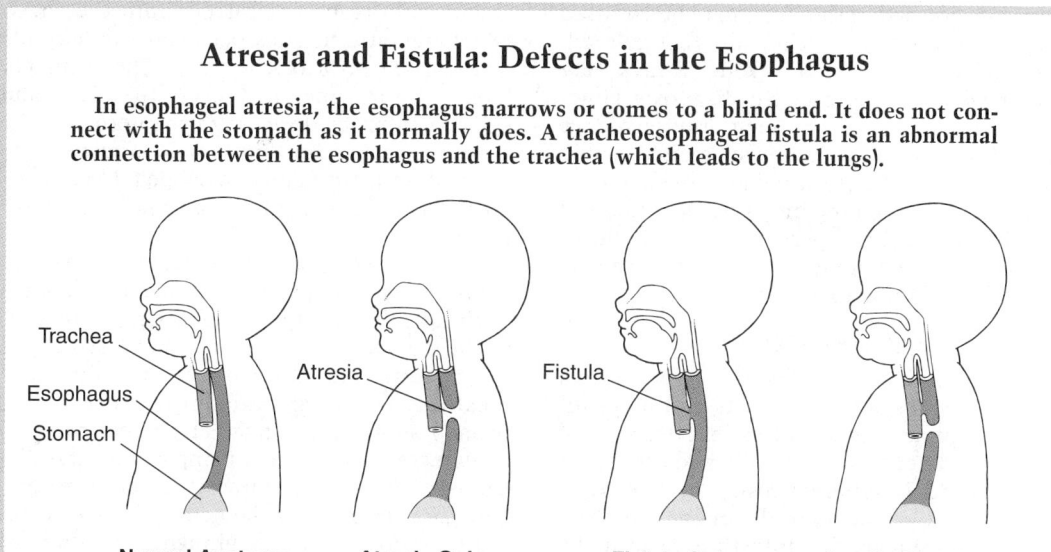

Trachea

Esophagus

Stomach

Atresia

Fistula

Normal Anatomy   **Atresia Only**   **Fistula Only**   **Atresia Plus Fistula**

comes to a blind end; food is delayed or prevented from going from the esophagus to the stomach. Most newborns with esophageal atresia also have a tracheoesophageal fistula, an abnormal connection between the esophagus (below the narrowing) and the trachea. Swallowed food and saliva travel through the fistula to the lungs, leading to coughing, choking, difficulty breathing, and possibly pneumonia. Food or fluid in the lungs may impair oxygenation of blood, leading to a bluish discoloration of the skin (cyanosis). Characteristically, a newborn with esophageal atresia coughs and drools after attempting to swallow. Many children with esophageal atresia and tracheoesophageal fistula have other abnormalities, such as heart defects.

To detect a blockage, x-rays are taken as a tube is passed down the esophagus.

The first steps in treatment are withholding oral feedings and placing a tube in the upper esophagus to continuously suction out saliva before it can reach the lungs. The infant is fed intravenously. Surgery needs to be performed soon to establish a normal connection between the esophagus and stomach and to close the connection between the esophagus and the trachea.

ANAL ATRESIA

Anal atresia is narrowing or blockage of the anus. Most infants with anal atresia develop some type of abnormal connection (fistula) between the anus and either the urethra, the area between the urethra and anus (the perineum), the vagina, or the bladder.

Infants with anal atresia fail to defecate normally after birth. Eventually, intestinal obstruction develops. However, doctors often detect the abnormality by looking at the anus when they first examine the baby after birth, before symptoms develop.

Using x-rays, a radiologist can see the path of a fistula. Anal atresia usually requires immediate surgery to open a passage for feces and to close the fistula. Sometimes, a temporary colostomy (making a hole in the abdomen and connecting it to the colon to allow stool to flow into a plastic bag on the abdominal wall) may be necessary.

INTESTINAL MALROTATION

Intestinal malrotation (abnormal rotation of the intestines) is a potentially life-threatening defect in which the intestines develop incompletely or abnormally. Malrotation can cause the intestines to later twist (volvulus), cutting off their blood supply. Infants with intestinal malrotation can suddenly develop symptoms of vomiting, diarrhea, and abdominal swelling; these symptoms can also come and go. If the blood supply to the middle of the intestine is completely cut off (mid-gut volvulus), sudden, severe pain and vomiting develop. Bile, a substance formed in the liver, may be vomited and appear yellow, green, or rust-colored. Eventually, the abdomen swells. X-rays may help the doctor determine the diagnosis. However, the volvulus can be seen only on x-rays taken after placing barium, a substance visible on the x-ray, in the rectum (barium enema).

Treatment, including intravenous fluids and usually emergency surgery, must begin within hours. If not treated rapidly, the defect can result in loss of intestinal tissue or death.

BILIARY ATRESIA

Bile, a fluid secreted by the liver, carries away the liver's waste products and helps digest fats in the small intestine. Bile ducts within the liver collect the bile and carry it to the intestine. In biliary atresia, the bile ducts are destroyed—either partially or completely—so bile cannot reach the intestine. Eventually, the bile accumulates in the liver and then escapes into the blood, causing a yellowish discoloration of the skin (jaundice). Progressive, irreversible scarring of the liver, called biliary cirrhosis, starts by the age of 2 months if the defect is not treated.

In infants with biliary atresia, the urine becomes dark, the stools become pale, and the skin becomes increasingly jaundiced. These symptoms and an enlarged, firm liver are usually first noticed about 2 weeks after birth. By the time the infant is 2 to 3 months old, he may have stunted growth, be itchy and irritable, and have large veins visible on his abdomen, as well as a large spleen.

To prevent biliary cirrhosis, the diagnosis of biliary atresia must be made before the age of 2 months. To make the diagnosis, a doctor performs a series of blood tests. Ultrasound may be helpful. If the defect is still suspected after these tests, surgery (which consists of examination of the liver and bile ducts and a liver biopsy) is performed to diagnose the defect.

Surgery is needed to create a path for bile to drain from the liver. Constructing replacement bile ducts that flow into the intestine is best, and this kind of operation is possible in 40 to 50% of infants. Most of the infants with replacement bile ducts can lead normal lives. Infants who cannot have replacement bile ducts constructed usually require liver transplantation by age 2 years.

DIAPHRAGMATIC HERNIA

A diaphragmatic hernia is a hole or weakening in the diaphragm that allows some of the abdominal organs to protrude into the chest. Diaphragmatic hernias occur on the left side of the body 90% of the time. The stomach, loops of intestine, and even the liver and spleen can protrude through the hernia. If the hernia is large, the lung on the affected side is usually incompletely developed. Many children with diaphragmatic hernias also have heart defects.

After delivery, as the newborn cries and breathes, the loops of intestine quickly fill with air. This rapidly enlarging structure pushes against the heart, compressing the other lung and causing severe difficulty breathing, often right after birth. A chest x-ray usually shows the defect. The defect can also be detected before birth using ultrasound. Diagnosis before birth allows the doctor to prepare for treatment of the defect. Surgery is required to repair the diaphragm. Measures to deliver oxygen, such as a breathing tube and ventilator, may be needed.

HIRSCHSPRUNG DISEASE

The large intestine depends on a network of nerves within its wall to synchronize rhythmic contractions and move digested material toward the anus, where the material is expelled as feces. In Hirschsprung disease (congenital megacolon), a section of the large intestine is missing the nerve network that controls the intestine's rhythmic contractions.

Children with Hirschsprung disease can have symptoms that suggest intestinal obstruction—bile-stained vomit, a swollen abdomen, and refusal to eat. If only a small section of the intestine is affected, a child may have milder symptoms and may not be diagnosed until later in childhood. These children may have ribbonlike stools and a swollen abdomen; they often fail to gain weight. In rare cases, constipation is the only symptom. Delayed passage of stool (meconium) by a newborn raises the suspicion of Hirschsprung disease.

Hirschsprung disease can also lead to life-threatening toxic enterocolitis, which produces sudden fever, a swollen abdomen, and explosive and, at times, bloody diarrhea.

A barium enema is often performed. Rectal biopsy and measurement of the pressure inside the rectum (manometry) are the only tests that can reliably be used to diagnose Hirschsprung disease.

Severe Hirschsprung disease must be treated quickly to prevent toxic enterocolitis.

Hirschsprung disease is usually treated with surgery to remove the abnormal section of intestine and to connect the normal intestine to the rectum and anus. In some cases, for example, if the child is quite ill, the surgeon connects the lower end of the normal part of the intestine to an opening made in the abdominal wall (colostomy). Stool can thus pass through the opening into a collection bag, restoring normal movement of food through the intestines. The abnormal section of intestine is left disconnected from the rest of the intestine. The normal part of the intestine can be reconnected to the rectum and anus when the child is older.

Bone and Muscle Defects

Birth defects can occur in any bone or muscle, although the bones and muscles of the skull, face, spine, hips, legs, and feet are affected most often. Bones and muscles may develop incompletely. Also, structures that normally align together may be separated or misaligned. Usually bone and muscle defects result in abnormal appearance and function of the affected part of the body. Most of these defects are repaired surgically if symptoms are troublesome. Often, the surgery is complex and involves reconstructing deformed or absent body parts.

FACIAL DEFECTS

The most common defects of the skull and face are cleft lip and cleft palate. **Cleft lip** is a separation of the upper lip, usually just below the nose. **Cleft palate** is a split in the roof of the mouth resulting in a passageway into the nose. Cleft lip and cleft palate often occur together.

Cleft lip is disfiguring and prevents the infant from closing his lips around a nipple. A cleft palate interferes with eating and speech. A dental device can temporarily seal the roof of the mouth so the infant can suckle better. Cleft lip and cleft palate can be permanently corrected with surgery. The likelihood of cleft lip and cleft palate can be reduced if a woman takes folic acid before pregnancy and through the 1st trimester of pregnancy.

Another type of facial defect is a small lower jaw (mandible). Pierre Robin and Treacher Collins syndromes, which are characterized by several defects in the head and face, are among the causes of a small lower jaw. If the lower jaw is too small, the infant may have

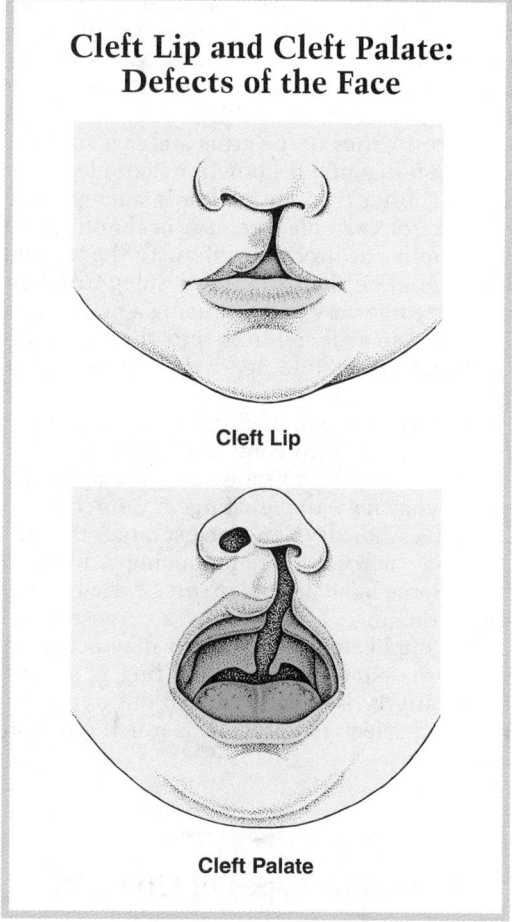

Cleft Lip and Cleft Palate: Defects of the Face

Cleft Lip

Cleft Palate

difficulty eating or breathing. Surgery may correct or diminish the problem.

LIMB AND JOINT DEFECTS

Limbs or joints can be missing, deformed, or incompletely developed at birth. A child with one limb or joint abnormality is more likely to have another related abnormality. Limbs and joints may form abnormally; for example, bones in the hand and forearm may be missing because of a genetic defect. Normal development of a limb can also become disrupted in the womb; for example, a finger can stop growing because the finger gets constricted by fibers. Another cause for limb and joint abnormalities is mechanical force; for example, pressure may cause the hip to dislocate. Chromosomal abnormalities can cause limb and joint abnormalities. Sometimes the cause is unknown. The drug thalidomide, which was taken by some pregnant women in the late 1950s and early 1960s for morning sickness, caused a variety of limb defects—usually short, poorly functioning appendages developed in place of arms and legs.

Abnormalities of the arms and legs may occur in a horizontal fashion (for example, if the arm is shorter than normal) or in a lengthwise fashion (for example, the arm is abnormal on the thumb side [from the elbow to the thumb] but normal on the little finger side). Children often become very adept at using a malformed limb, and an artificial limb (prosthesis) can often be constructed to make the limb easier to use.

Hand defects are common. Sometimes a hand does not form completely; part or all of the hand may be missing. For example, the person may have too few fingers. Sometimes a hand does not develop; for example, the fingers may not separate, producing a weblike hand. Some hand defects involve extra fingers; the little fingers or thumbs are most commonly duplicated. Overgrowth may occur, in which the hands or individual fingers are too large. Surgery is usually carried out to correct the hand defect and provide as much function as possible.

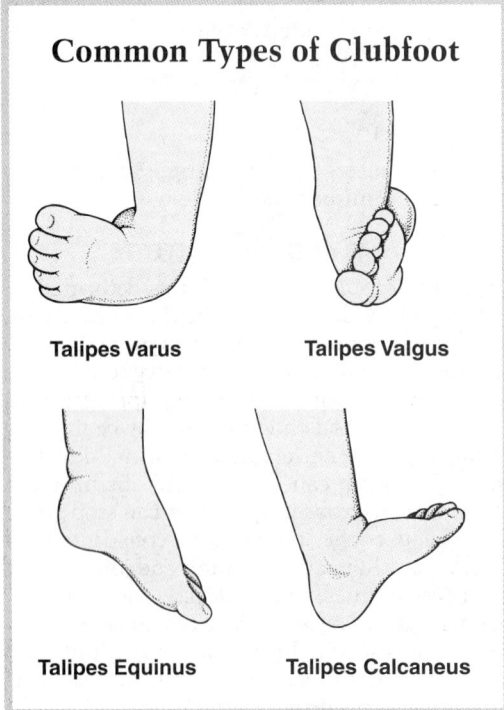

Common Types of Clubfoot

Talipes Varus

Talipes Valgus

Talipes Equinus

Talipes Calcaneus

In **congenital dislocation of the hip,** also called developmental dysplasia of the hip, the newborn's hip socket and the thighbone (femoral head), which normally form a joint, become separated, often because the hip has a socket that is not deep enough to hold the head of the femur. Dislocation of the hip is a disorder more common in girls, in newborns born in a breech (buttocks-first) position, and in newborns who have close relatives with the disorder. The right and left legs or hips often look different from each other in newborns with the defect.

The doctor can detect the defect when examining the newborn. In infants younger than 4 months, an ultrasound of the hips can confirm the diagnosis; in infants older than 4 months, an x-ray can be used. The use of triple diapers (an older treatment) is not recommended. The best treatment is use of the Pavlik harness. The Pavlik harness is a soft brace that holds the infant's knees spread outward and up toward the chest. However, if the defect persists past the age of 6 months, surgery to fix the hip in the normal position is usually needed.

Clubfoot (talipes equinovarus) is a defect in which the foot and ankle are twisted out of shape or position. The usual clubfoot is a down and inward turning of the hind foot and ankle, with twisting inward of the forefoot. Sometimes the foot only appears abnormal because it was held in an unusual position in the uterus (positional clubfoot). In contrast, true clubfoot is a structurally abnormal foot. With true clubfoot, the bones of the leg or foot or the muscles of the calf are often underdeveloped.

Positional clubfoot can be corrected by immobilizing the joints in a cast and by using physical therapy to stretch the foot and ankle. Early treatment with immobilization is beneficial for true clubfoot, but surgery, often complex, is also generally needed.

In **metatarsus adductus,** the foot appears turned inward. Mobility of the joints of the foot and ankle may be limited. Treatment depends on the severity of the deformity and immobility of the foot. Most mild cases resolve spontaneously. Corrective shoes or splints may be needed in more severe cases. Surgery is required only in exceptional instances.

In **arthrogryposis multiplex congenita,** some joints become "frozen" and consequently cannot bend. Many children with this defect have weakened muscles. It is likely that decreased movement of the muscles and joints before

Spina Bifida: A Defect of the Spine

In spina bifida, the bones of the spine (vertebrae) do not form normally. Spina bifida can vary in severity. In the least severe, most common type, one or more vertebrae do not form normally, but the spinal cord and the layers of tissues (meninges) surrounding it are not affected. The only symptom may be a tuft of hair, a dimpling, or a pigmented area on the skin over the defect. In a meningocele, a more severe type of spina bifida, the meninges protrude through the incompletely formed vertebrae, resulting in a fluid-filled bulge under the skin. The most severe type is a meningomyelocele, in which the spinal cord protrudes. The affected area appears raw and red, and the infant is likely to be severely disabled.

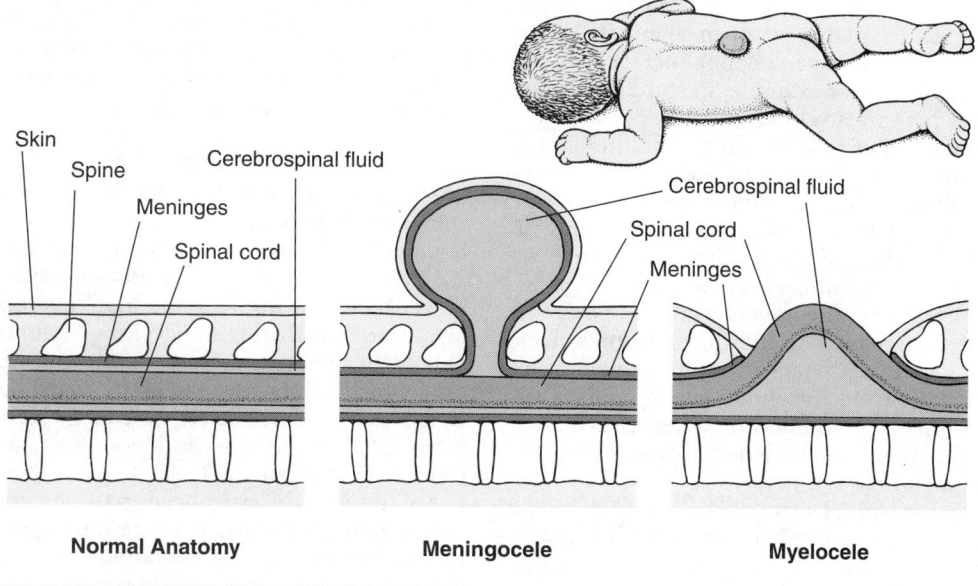

Normal Anatomy **Meningocele** **Myelocele**

birth causes the decreased movement of the joints after birth. The cause is unknown. Sometimes the nerves that would normally move the bones in the affected joints are also impaired. Infants with the defect may also have dislocated hips, knees, or elbows. Placing the limbs in a cast and performing physical therapy, in which the stiff joints are carefully manipulated, may improve joint movements. Surgically freeing the bones from attached tissue sometimes results in more normal joint movement.

Brain and Spinal Cord Defects

Of the many possible defects in the brain and spinal cord, those known as neural tube defects develop within the first weeks of pregnancy. Others, such as porencephaly and hydranencephaly, develop later in pregnancy.

Many brain and spinal cord defects result in visible abnormalities in the head or back.

Symptoms of brain or spinal cord damage may develop if the defect affects brain or spinal cord tissue. Brain damage can be fatal or result in mild or severe disability, which may include mental retardation, seizures, and paralysis. Spinal cord damage can result in paralysis, incontinence, and loss of sensation to areas of the body reached by nerves below the level of the defect.▲ Computed tomography (CT) and magnetic resonance imaging (MRI) can reveal brain and spinal cord defects by showing pictures of the internal structures of those organs.

Some defects, such as those that cause visible openings or swellings, can be repaired surgically. However, brain or spinal cord damage from the defect is usually permanent.

▲ see box on page 562

NEURAL TUBE DEFECTS

The brain and spinal cord develop as a groove that folds over to become a tube (the neural tube). Layers of tissue that come from this tube normally cover the brain and spinal cord (meninges). Sometimes the neural tube does not develop normally, which may affect the brain, spinal cord, and meninges. In the most severe form of neural tube defect, the brain tissue may fail to develop (anencephaly); this defect is fatal. Another type of defect results when the neural tube fails to close completely and remains an open channel. In its mildest form, an open channel defect may affect only bone; for example, in spina bifida occulta (which means hidden spine split in two), the bony spine fails to close, but the spinal cord and meninges are unaffected. This common abnormality usually causes no symptoms. Sometimes, a meningocele develops in which the meninges and other tissue, such as brain tissue (meningoencephalocele) or spinal cord tissue (meningomyelocele), can protrude out of the opening. Sometimes the meninges are not involved when tissue protrudes from the brain (encephalocele) or spinal cord (myelocele). Damage to brain or spinal cord tissue is much more likely when tissue protrudes than when it does not.

In occult spinal dysraphism, newborns are born with visible abnormalities on their lower backs. These include birthmarks, overly pigmented areas (hemangioma and flame nevus), tufts of hair, openings in the skin (dermal sinus), or small lumps (masses). The underlying spinal cord may be connected to the surface, which exposes it to bacteria, greatly increasing the chance for development of meningitis. The nerves of the spinal cord may become damaged as the child grows. Or, the spinal cord may have a fatty tumor (lipoma) on it, which also can lead to nerve damage. Therefore, newborns who have these abnormalities should have the underlying soft tissue and spinal cord evaluated using ultrasound or magnetic resonance imaging (MRI).

Genetic factors can make neural tube defects more likely. The defect often develops before the mother knows she is pregnant. Most symptoms from neural tube defects result from brain or spinal cord damage. A defect may be so inconsequential that it is never recognized or so severe that it is fatal. Meningo-

encephaloceles and meningomyeloceles cause severe disability. These include hydrocephalus, learning disabilities, paralysis with bone and joint abnormalities, decreased sensation of the skin, and bowel and urinary problems.

Many neural tube defects can be detected before birth. A high level of alpha-fetoprotein in the woman's blood or amniotic fluid may indicate a neural tube defect in the fetus.▲ Ultrasound performed late in pregnancy may show the defect or characteristic abnormalities. Folic acid taken just before a woman gets pregnant through the first three months of pregnancy can decrease the risk of neural tube defects by as much as 70%. Neural tube defects are usually closed surgically.

HYDROCEPHALUS

The fluid surrounding the brain (cerebrospinal fluid) is produced in spaces within the brain called ventricles. The fluid must drain to a different area, where it is absorbed into the blood. When the fluid cannot drain, hydrocephalus (water on the brain) develops. Hydrocephalus often increases the pressure in the ventricles, which compresses the brain. Many conditions, such as a birth defect, bleeding within the brain, or brain tumors can block drainage and cause hydrocephalus.

An abnormally large head may be a symptom of hydrocephalus. The infant usually fails to develop normally. Computed tomography (CT), ultrasound, or magnetic resonance imaging (MRI) of the head reveals the diagnosis as well as the degree of brain compression.

The goal of treatment is to keep pressure normal within the brain. A permanent alternate drainage path (shunt) for cerebrospinal fluid decreases the pressure and volume of the fluid inside the brain. A doctor places the shunt in the ventricles in the brain and runs it under the skin from the head to another site, usually the abdomen (ventriculoperitoneal shunt). The shunt contains a valve that allows fluid to leave the brain if the pressure becomes too high. Although a few children can eventually do without the shunt as they get older, shunts are rarely removed.

If needed, pressure within the brain can often be temporarily reduced with drugs (such as acetazolamide or furosemide) or repeated spinal taps (lumbar punctures) until a shunt is placed.

Some children with hydrocephalus develop normal intelligence. Others are mentally retarded or have learning disabilities.

▲ see page 1430

CHAPTER 266

Chromosomal and Genetic Abnormalities

Chromosomes are structures within cells that contain a person's genes. Abnormalities in chromosomes are always genetic abnormalities. Some genetic abnormalities affect the genes, but do not alter the structure of the chromosomes.▲ Thus, doctors often discuss chromosomal abnormalities separately from the broader category of genetic abnormalities. Some genetic abnormalities, such as sickle cell disease and cystic fibrosis, are very common.

A person normally has 23 pairs of chromosomes, each containing hundreds of genes. The sex chromosomes are one of these pairs of chromosomes. Normal people have 2 sex chromosomes; each is either an X or a Y chromosome. Normal females have two X chromosomes (XX), and normal males have one X and one Y chromosome (XY).

Chromosomal abnormalities can affect any chromosome, including the sex chromosomes. A chromosomal or other genetic abnormality can affect the number of chromosomes, the structure of certain chromosomes, or the composition of chromosomes (for example, genetic material from one chromosome may be attached to another). If the material found in chromosomes is balanced so that the expected amount is found in each cell, no abnormalities occur. If too much (addition) or too little (deletion) genetic material is found within each cell, abnormalities occur. These abnormalities can have profound physical effects.

The older a pregnant woman is, the greater the chance that her fetus will have a chromosomal abnormality.■ The chance of chromosomal abnormalities increases by a barely noticeable degree if the father is older. A marriage between close relatives increases the chance of developing some genetic abnormalities, but usually not chromosomal abnormalities.

Chromosomal abnormalities can cause a wide range of abnormalities or effects, usually birth defects★ or death of the embryo or fetus before birth. Genetic abnormalities can cause birth defects or diseases (for example, sickle cell disease) or have many different effects.

A person's chromosomes can be analyzed with a sample of blood. A fetus can be tested for chromosomal abnormalities before birth, for example, using amniocentesis or chorionic villus sampling.● If the fetus is found to have a chromosomal abnormality, further tests may be performed to detect specific birth defects. Although chromosomal abnormalities cannot be corrected, some of the defects can sometimes be prevented or treated.

Down Syndrome

Down syndrome (trisomy 21) is a chromosomal disorder resulting in mental retardation and physical abnormalities.

An extra chromosome, making three of a kind, is called trisomy. The most common trisomy in a newborn is trisomy 21 (three copies of chromosome 21). Trisomy 21 causes about 95% of the cases of Down syndrome. Older mothers, especially those older than 35, contribute an extra chromosome more often than do younger mothers. As a result, they more often bear children with Down syndrome.◆ However, the extra chromosome may come from the father.

Symptoms

In Down syndrome, physical and mental development is delayed. Infants with Down syndrome tend to be quiet, passive, and have somewhat limp muscles. The intelligence quotient (IQ) among children with Down syndrome varies but averages about 50, compared with normal children, whose average IQ is 100. Children with Down syndrome have better visual motor skills (such as drawing) than skills that require hearing. Thus, their language skills typically develop slowly. Early intervention with educational and other services improves the functioning of young children with Down syndrome.

Children with Down syndrome tend to have a small head, a face that is broad and flat with slanting eyes and a short nose. The tongue is

---

▲ see page 11   ■ see page 1431
★ see page 1511   ● see page 1432
◆ see also page 1430

large. The ears are small and set low in the head. The hands are short and broad, with a single crease across the palm. The fingers are short; the fifth finger, which often has two instead of three sections, curves inward. A space is visible between the first and second toes.

Children with Down syndrome often have heart defects. Many people with Down syndrome develop thyroid disease. They are prone to hearing problems because of recurring ear infections and the associated accumulation of inner ear fluid (serous otitis). They are also prone to vision problems because of problems in their corneas and lenses. Many people with Down syndrome develop symptoms of Alzheimer-like dementia in their 30s, such as memory loss, further lowering of intellect, and personality changes.

Diagnosis

The diagnosis of Down syndrome can often be made before birth.▲ An infant with Down syndrome has a physical appearance that suggests the diagnosis. A doctor confirms the diagnosis by testing the infant's chromosomes for trisomy 21 or other disorders of the 21st chromosome. After the diagnosis is made, doctors use tests, such as ultrasound and blood tests, along with examinations by specialists, to detect abnormalities associated with Down syndrome. Treating abnormalities that are detected can often prevent them from impairing health.

Prognosis

Most children with Down syndrome survive to adulthood. Life expectancy for a child with Down syndrome with mild or moderate retardation is 55 years and with profound mental retardation is 45 years. Many have progressively worsening mental functioning. Heart abnormalities are often treatable with drugs or surgery. Heart disease and leukemia account for most deaths among children with Down syndrome.

Fragile X Syndrome

Fragile X syndrome is a genetic abnormality in an X chromosome that leads to delayed development and other symptoms.

The symptoms of fragile X syndrome are caused by abnormalities in DNA on the X chromosome. Usually, affected boys inherit the condition from their mothers.

Many children with the syndrome have normal intelligence. However, the syndrome is the most commonly diagnosed genetic cause of mental retardation besides Down syndrome. The severity of symptoms, including mental retardation, is worse in boys than in girls with the disorder. Symptoms, which are often subtle, include delayed development; large, protuberant ears; a prominent chin and forehead; and, in boys, large testes (most apparent after puberty). The joints may be abnormally flexible, and heart disease (mitral valve prolapse) may occur. Features of autism may develop. Women may experience menopause in their mid 30s.

The presence of abnormal DNA on the fragile X chromosome can be detected by tests before or after birth. The greater the number of abnormal repetitions of DNA found, the more likely the child will have symptoms.

Early intervention, including speech and language therapy and occupational therapy, can help children with fragile X syndrome to maximize their abilities. Stimulants, antidepressants, and antianxiety drugs may be beneficial for some children.

Turner Syndrome

In Turner syndrome (gonadal dysgenesis), girls are born with one of the two X chromosomes partially or completely missing.

Many newborns with Turner syndrome have swelling (lymphedema) on the backs of their hands and tops of their feet. Swelling or loose folds of skin are often evident over the back of the neck. Many other abnormalities often develop, including a webbed neck (wide skin attachment between the neck and shoulders), a low hairline at the back of the neck, a broad chest with wide-spaced nipples, and poorly developed nails.

As a girl with Turner syndrome gets older, she has no menstrual periods (amenorrhea), and the breasts, vagina, and labia remain childlike rather than undergoing the changes of puberty. The ovaries usually do not contain developing eggs. A girl or woman with Turner syndrome is virtually always short; obesity is common.

Other disorders often develop. Heart defects include narrowing of part of the aorta (coarctation of the aorta■). Kidney and eye defects, di-

▲ see also page 1430   ■ see page 1518

abetes mellitus, and thyroid diseases are common. Occasionally, abnormal blood vessels in the intestine cause bleeding.

Many girls with Turner syndrome have difficulty in assessing visual and spatial relationships and have problems with planning and attention. They tend to score poorly on certain performance tests and in mathematics, even if they achieve average or above-average scores on verbal intelligence tests. Mental retardation is uncommon.

A doctor may suspect the diagnosis because of the newborn's abnormal appearance. However, suspicion often does not develop until the teenage years, when the girl fails to mature sexually. Analysis of the chromosomes confirms the diagnosis.

Treatment with a hormone normally secreted from the brain (growth hormone) can stimulate growth. Treatment with the female hormone estrogen is usually not started until after satisfactory growth has been achieved. Estrogen treatment may improve planning, attention, and assessment of visual and spatial relationships as well as stimulating sexual maturation.

Noonan Syndrome

Noonan syndrome is a genetic defect that causes a number of physical abnormalities, usually including short stature, heart defects, and an abnormal appearance.

Noonan syndrome can be inherited or can develop unpredictably in children whose parents have normal genes. Although children with the syndrome have normal chromosomal structure, they have many characteristics typical of Turner syndrome. In the past, Noonan syndrome was called "male Turner syndrome." Boys or girls can be affected. The gene responsible for Noonan syndrome has been localized to chromosome 12.

Symptoms may include webbing of the neck, low-set ears, droopy eyelids, short stature, shortened fourth (ring) fingers, a high-arched palate, and heart and blood vessel abnormalities. Intelligence may be impaired. Most affected people are short. Boys may have underdeveloped or undescended testes. In girls, the ovaries may be underactive or stop working. Puberty may be delayed, and infertility may develop.

Growth may be improved by treatment with growth hormone. After satisfactory growth, testosterone treatment may help boys whose

When Part of a Chromosome Is Missing

A number of syndromes can occur in infants who are missing part of a chromosome. These syndromes are called **chromosome deletion syndromes.**

In the rare **cri du chat syndrome** (cat's cry syndrome, 5p minus syndrome), part of chromosome 5 is missing. An infant with this syndrome is usually underweight at birth; has a small head with many abnormal features, including a round face, small jaw, wide nose, widely separated eyes, and ears set low in the head; and has a high-pitched cry that sounds like a kitten crying. Often the infant seems limp. The high-pitched cry occurs immediately after birth, lasts several weeks, and then disappears. Heart defects are common. Mental and physical development are greatly retarded. Despite these abnormalities, many children with cri du chat syndrome survive to adulthood.

In **Prader-Willi syndrome,** another chromosomal deletion syndrome, mental retardation is common. Many symptoms vary according to the child's age. Newborns with the defect feel limp, feed poorly, and gain weight slowly. Eventually these symptoms resolve. Then, between the ages of 1 and 6, appetite increases, often becoming insatiable. Obsessive-compulsive behaviors are common. Weight gain is excessive, which can lead to other health problems. Obesity can be severe enough to require gastric bypass surgery.

testes are underdeveloped. Testosterone stimulates the development of a more masculine appearance.

Triple X Syndrome

Triple X (trisomy X) syndrome is a rare disorder in which female infants are born with three X chromosomes.

Girls with triple X syndrome tend to have slightly lower intelligence and particular problems with verbal skills. Sometimes the syndrome causes infertility, although some women with triple X syndrome have given birth to physically normal children who had normal chromosomes.

Extremely rare cases of infants with four or even five X chromosomes have been identified. The more X chromosomes the girl has, the greater the chance of mental retardation and physical abnormalities.

Klinefelter Syndrome

Klinefelter syndrome is a disorder in which male infants are born with an extra X chromosome (XXY).

Klinefelter syndrome is relatively common. Most boys with Klinefelter syndrome have normal or slightly decreased intelligence. Many have speech and reading disabilities and difficulties with planning. Most have problems with language skills. Early problems with language may lead to problems with social interactions that affect behavior, and these children often get into trouble at school. Although their physical characteristics can vary greatly, most are tall with long arms but otherwise normal in appearance.

Puberty usually occurs at the normal time, but the testes remain small. At puberty, growth of facial hair is often sparse, and the breasts may enlarge somewhat (gynecomastia). Men and boys with the syndrome are usually infertile. Men with Klinefelter syndrome develop diabetes mellitus, chronic lung disease, varicose veins, hypothyroidism, and breast cancer more often than other men.

The syndrome is usually first suspected at puberty, when most of the symptoms develop. Analysis of the chromosomes confirms the diagnosis.

Boys with Klinefelter syndrome usually benefit from speech and language therapy and eventually can do well in school. Some men benefit by taking supplemental male hormones such as testosterone. The hormones improve bone density, making fractures less likely, and stimulate development of a more masculine appearance.

XYY Syndrome

The XYY syndrome is a disorder in which a male infant is born with an extra Y chromosome.

Boys with XYY syndrome tend to be tall and have difficulties with language. The IQ tends to be slightly lower than that of other family members. Learning disabilities, attention deficit disorder, and minor behavioral disorders can develop. The XYY syndrome was once thought to cause aggressive or violent criminal behavior, but this theory has been disproved.

Long QT Syndrome

Long QT syndrome is an abnormality of the heart's electrical system,▲ which may cause loss of consciousness or sudden death.

Long QT syndrome may affect as many as 1 of 7,000 people. In the United States, it may cause sudden death in 3,000 to 4,000 children and young adults each year. In children, this disorder is usually due to a genetic abnormality. A person with the disorder may have family members who died suddenly and inexplicably. In most adults, long QT syndrome is caused by use of a drug or a disorder.

People who have long QT syndrome are predisposed to developing an unusually fast heart rate, which often occurs during physical activity or emotional excitement. When the heart rate is too fast, the brain may not receive enough blood. The result is loss of consciousness. Some people with long QT syndrome are also born deaf. But about one third of people have no symptoms. Long QT syndrome can cause sudden death at a young age.

Doctors may recommend electrocardiography (ECG)■ for children or young adults who have suddenly and inexplicably lost consciousness. The procedure may be performed with the person at rest or after receiving intravenous drugs or the person may be asked to walk on a treadmill or pedal an exercise bicycle in a procedure called exercise stress testing.

Beta-blockers are effective for most children and adults. Some adults may benefit from mexiletine, an antiarrhythmic drug. For children and adults who do not respond to drugs, a pacemaker or a combination pacemaker-internal defibrillator may be tried. An internal defibrillator can shock the heart, reviving the person, whenever the heart develops a lethal rhythm abnormality. Occasionally, as an alternative, a nerve in the neck is cut in a procedure called cervicothoracic sympathectomy. Cutting this nerve can help prevent the fast heart rate that causes sudden death.

▲ see page 163

■ see box on page 122

CHAPTER 267

Problems in Infants and Very Young Children

Few children make it through their first years without minor problems. Crying, problems with feeding, and an occasional fever are common. These problems become health concerns only when they are extreme—for example, when children cry too much, when they are not growing well, or when they have high fevers that do not go away. Most childhood problems are not severe. Many children experience rashes. Very rarely, families face the tragedy of sudden infant death syndrome (SIDS).

Fussiness, Excessive Crying, and Colic

Fussiness is the inability of an infant to settle down or be soothed. Excessive crying is crying over long hours by a healthy infant whose basic needs are met. Colic is a pattern of excessive crying over weeks that is loud, piercing, constant, and that occurs at intervals, between which the infant acts normally.

Fussiness, excessive crying, and colic occur most commonly between the second week and third month of life. Their cause is usually unknown, but excessive crying is sometimes associated with excess air in the digestive tract (for example, from not burping after eating or from swallowing air while crying). Excessive crying can be due to an infection, such as an ear or urinary tract infection or meningitis. Other causes of crying are gastroesophageal reflux,▲ milk allergy, eruption of a tooth, a hair caught around a finger or toe (hair tourniquet), or a corneal abrasion.

Parents of children with excessive crying or colic should consult a doctor if there is nothing they can do to stop the child's crying or if the child has other symptoms, such as fever or poor feeding. Doctors try to diagnose and treat known causes of fussiness and crying. Infections may or may not require antibiotics. Gastroesophageal reflux can be treated by a number of strategies.■ Air in the digestive tract can be diminished by adequately burping the child. A change of formula may treat symptoms of milk allergy; however, parents should

consult with their doctor before changing the formula. Crying from teething improves with time. A hair tourniquet needs to be removed. Corneal abrasions are treated with an antibiotic ointment or drops to prevent infection.

If there is no medical reason for an infant's crying, the doctor may diagnose excessive crying or colic. There is no specific treatment. If mothers who are breastfeeding notice that certain foods lead to increased crying in their infants, they should avoid eating these foods. Many infants get some relief from being held, rocked, or patted or from the "white noise" and vibration of a fan, washing machine, or car ride. A pacifier or swaddling clothes may also be comforting. Feeding sometimes soothes the child, but parents should avoid overfeeding in an attempt to stop the crying. If left alone, some children will cry themselves to sleep.

Excessive crying and colic can be exhausting and stressful for parents. Parents should take advantage of nighttime crying interludes to lay the infant on his back in his crib to encourage self-soothing and sleep. Emotional support from friends, family, neighbors, and doctors is key to coping. Parents should ask for whatever help they need (with siblings, errands, or child care) and share their feelings and fears. Overwhelmed parents can take comfort in the fact that, despite the extreme distress the crying or colicky infant appears to be in, excessive crying and colic usually disappear by 3 to 4 months of age and cause no long-term harm.

Teething

A child's first tooth usually appears by 6 months of age, and a complete set of 20 primary or first teeth usually develops by age 3. Before a tooth appears, the child may cry, be irritable, and sleep and eat poorly. The child may drool, have red and tender gums, and constantly chew on food and objects during tooth eruption. During teething, the child may have a mildly elevated temperature (below 100° F).

▲ see page 1588   ■ see page 1588

Children with higher temperatures and those who are especially fussy should be evaluated by a doctor because these symptoms are not due to teething.

Teething infants get some relief from chewing on hard, cold objects, such as a frozen bagel or banana. Parents should prevent the infant from biting off large pieces, which can choke the child. Firm rubber teething rings and teething biscuits are also useful. Massaging the child's gums with or without ice may help. Teething gels may provide relief for a few minutes. If a child is extremely uncomfortable, acetaminophen or ibuprofen is usually effective for pain.

Feeding Problems

Feeding problems in infants and young children are usually minor but sometimes have serious consequences.

Spitting up (burping up) is the effortless return of swallowed formula or breast milk through the mouth or nose after feeding. Almost all infants spit up, because infants cannot sit upright during and after feedings. Also, the valve (sphincter) that separates the esophagus and stomach is immature and does not keep all of the stomach's contents in place. Spitting up gets worse when an infant eats too fast or swallows air. Spitting up usually stops between the ages of 7 and 12 months.

Spitting up can be reduced by feeding an infant before he gets very hungry, burping him every 4 to 5 minutes, placing him in an upright position during and after feeding, and making certain the bottle nipple lets out only a few drops with pressure or when the bottle is upside down. Spitting up that seems to cause an infant discomfort, interferes with feeding and growth, or persists into early childhood is called gastroesophageal reflux and may require medical attention.▲ If the material that is spit up is green (indicating bile), bloody, or causes any coughing or choking, medical attention is needed.

Vomiting is the uncomfortable, forced throwing up of feedings. It is never normal. Vomiting in infants is most often the result of viral gastroenteritis. It can also be caused by infections elsewhere in the body. Less commonly, vomiting occurs because of a serious medical

disorder. Infants between the ages of 2 weeks and 4 months may rarely have forceful (projectile) vomiting after feedings because of a blockage at the stomach outlet (hypertrophic pyloric stenosis). Vomiting can also be caused by life-threatening disorders, such as meningitis, intestinal blockage, and appendicitis. These disorders usually cause severe pain, lethargy, and continuous vomiting that does not get better with time.

Most vomiting caused by gastroenteritis stops on its own. Giving the child fluid and electrolytes (such as sodium and chloride) from solutions available in stores or pharmacies prevents or treats dehydration. Older children can be given popsicles or gelatin, although red versions of these foods can be confused with blood if the child vomits again. A doctor should see any child who has severe abdominal pain, is unable to drink and retain fluids, is lethargic or acting extremely ill, vomits for more than 12 hours, vomits blood or green material (bile), or is unable to urinate. These symptoms may signal dehydration or a more severe condition.

Overfeeding is the provision of more nutrition than a child needs for healthy growth. Overfeeding occurs when children are automatically fed as a response to crying, when they are given a bottle as a distraction or activity, or when they are allowed to keep a bottle with them at all times. Overfeeding also occurs when parents reward good behavior with food or expect a child to finish his food even if he is not hungry. In the short term, overfeeding causes spitting up and diarrhea. In the long term, overfed children can become obese.■

Underfeeding is the provision of less nutrition than a child needs for healthy growth. It is one of many causes of failure to thrive★ and may be related to the child or the caregiver. Underfeeding may result when a fussy or distracted infant does not sit well for feedings or has difficulty sucking or swallowing. Underfeeding can also result from improper feeding techniques and errors in formula preparation.● Poverty and poor access to nutritious food are major reasons for underfeeding. Occasionally, abusive parents and parents with mental health disorders purposely withhold food from their children.

Community social agencies (such as the Women, Infants and Children [WIC] program) can help parents purchase formula and can teach them proper techniques for formula preparation and feeding. If an infant is so far

---

▲ see page 1588   ■ see page 1557

★ see page 1537   ● see page 1488

below expected weight that he needs supervised feedings, then the doctor may admit the child to a hospital for evaluation. If the parents are abusive or neglectful, child protective services may be called.

Dehydration is caused by excess fluid loss, such as from vomiting and diarrhea, or by inadequate fluid intake, such as when an infant does not take in enough milk through breastfeeding. Children who are moderately dehydrated are less interactive or playful, cry without tears, have a dry mouth, and urinate fewer than 2 or 3 times a day. Children who are severely dehydrated become sleepy or lethargic. Sometimes dehydration causes the concentration of salt in the blood to fall or rise abnormally. Changes in salt concentration make the symptoms of dehydration worse and can worsen lethargy. In severe cases, the child can have seizures or suffer brain damage and die.

Dehydration is treated with fluids and electrolytes, such as sodium and chloride. In severe cases, intravenous fluids are needed.

Bowel Problems

The number and consistency of stools for a healthy child vary with age and diet. For example, infants who are breastfed normally have mustard-colored stools that are soft and seedy. However, repeated watery bowel movements for a time lasting longer than 12 hours are never normal.

Diarrhea is frequent, watery bowel movements. Acute diarrhea starts suddenly and improves in one to several days. Acute diarrhea is most often caused by viral gastroenteritis, which is especially likely when vomiting accompanies the diarrhea. Typically, vomiting occurs at the beginning of the illness and then tapers off, while diarrhea continues. Acute diarrhea can also be caused by a bacterial or parasitic infection; an infection elsewhere in the body, such as an ear or respiratory tract infection; and as a side effect from the use of antibiotics. Acute diarrhea is a concern mainly because it can cause dehydration. Therefore, the main treatment is administering fluids and electrolytes. Bacterial infections are treated with antibiotics. Antibiotics that cause diarrhea may be discontinued, but only after consultation with a doctor.

Chronic diarrhea lasts for weeks or months. The most common causes of chronic diarrhea in infants and young children are cystic fibrosis, celiac disease, giardiasis, sugar malabsorp-

Treating Dehydration

Minor illnesses that cause vomiting and diarrhea can lead to dehydration in children. In infants, dehydration is treated by encouraging an infant to drink fluids that contain electrolytes. Breast milk contains all the fluids and electrolytes an infant needs and is the best treatment. If an infant is not breastfeeding, oral electrolyte solutions should be given. These can be bought as powders or liquids at drug or grocery stores without a prescription. The amount of solution to give a child depends on the child's age, but generally should be about 1½ to 2½ ounces of solution in a 24-hour period for each pound the child weighs.

Children older than 1 year may try small sips of juices or clear soups, clear sodas diluted to half-strength with water, or popsicles. Plain water, juice, and colas are not good for treating dehydration at any age because the salt content of water is too low and because juice and colas have a high sugar content and ingredients that irritate the digestive tract.

Treatment of dehydration at any age is more effective if children are first given small, frequent sips of fluids about every 10 minutes. The amount of fluid can slowly be increased and given at less frequent intervals if the child can keep the fluid down without vomiting or getting severe diarrhea. Infants who digest fluids over 12 to 24 hours can then resume drinking formula from a bottle. Older children can try broths or soups and bland foods (for example, bananas, toast, rice). Infants and young children who are unable to digest any fluids, or who develop listlessness and other serious signs of dehydration, may require more intensive treatment with intravenous fluids or electrolyte solutions given through a nasogastric tube.

tion, and food allergy. In less developed countries, malnutrition is the most common cause of chronic diarrhea.

Constipation is the infrequent passing of hard, dry stools.▲ Constipation may be difficult to recognize because some infants and young children have bowel movements only once every 3 to 4 days. In general, children are constipated when they have not had a bowel movement in 5 or more days, when the stools

---

▲ see also page 1591

are hard or cause pain, or when drops of blood are seen in the diaper or stool.

Constipation in infants is usually caused by dehydration, insufficient fiber in the diet, or a change in feeding patterns. Rarely, medical disorders, such as inadequate nerve supply to the large intestine (Hirschsprung disease), low thyroid hormone levels, or calcium or potassium abnormalities cause constipation. The use of certain drugs (such as antihistamines, anticholinergic drugs, and opioids) is another rare cause.

Treatment of constipation varies with the age of the child. Infants younger than 2 months of age who consume adequate amounts of formula or breast milk can be given a teaspoon of light corn syrup in their morning and evening bottles. Apple or prune juice is good for infants between 2 and 4 months of age. Infants between 4 months and 1 year can get relief from high-fiber cereals or from strained apricots, prunes, or plums. Children older than 1 year should be given high-fiber foods, such as fruits, peas, cereals, graham crackers, beans, and spinach. Parents should not give their child a laxative, suppository, or enema without first consulting a doctor. For older children with significant constipation, doctors may use various drugs. Treatment of rare disorders includes surgery for Hirschsprung disease, thyroid hormone replacement for low thyroid hormone levels, and calcium supplements for abnormal calcium levels.

Separation Anxiety

Separation anxiety is the fear young children have that their parents will leave them.

Children with separation anxiety panic and cry when a parent leaves them, even if only to go into an adjacent room. Separation anxiety is normal for infants at about 8 months of age, is most intense between 10 and 18 months of age, and generally resolves by 2 years of age. The intensity and duration of a child's separation anxiety vary and depend partly on the child-parent relationship. For example, separation anxiety in a child with a strong and healthy attachment to a parent resolves sooner than in a child whose connection is less strong.

Separation anxiety occurs at a time when infants start to become aware that their parents are unique individuals. Because they have incomplete memory and no sense of time, these young children fear the departure of their parents may be permanent. Separation anxiety resolves as a young child develops a sense of memory and keeps an image of the parents in mind when they are gone. The child recollects that in the past the parents returned.

Parents should not limit or forego separations in response to separation anxiety; this could compromise the child's maturation and development. When parents leave the home (or leave the child at a childcare center), they should encourage the person with whom they are leaving the child to create distractions. The parent should then leave without responding at length to a child's crying. If the parents are staying at home but in a different room, they should not return immediately in response to crying, but instead call to the child from the other room. This teaches the child that parents are still present even though the child cannot see them. Separation anxiety may be worse when a child is hungry or tired, so feeding the child and letting him nap before leaving may also help.

Separation anxiety at the normal age causes no long-term harm to the child. Separation anxiety that lasts beyond age 2 may or may not be a problem depending on the extent to which it interferes with the child's development. It is normal for children to feel some fear upon leaving for preschool or kindergarten. This feeling should diminish with time. Rarely, excessive fear of separations inhibits a child from attending childcare or preschool or keeps him from playing normally with peers. This anxiety is probably abnormal (separation anxiety disorder▲). In this case, the parents should seek medical attention for the child.

Skin Rashes

Skin rashes in infants and young children are not usually serious and can have various causes.

Diaper rash (diaper dermatitis) is a bright red rash caused by irritation from prolonged skin contact with urine or stool anywhere beneath a child's diaper. Typically, the areas of the skin that touch the diaper are most affected. Diaper rash can also be caused by infection with the fungus *Candida*, typically causing a bright red rash in the creases of the skin and small red spots. Less often, diaper rash is caused by bacteria. Diaper rash does not always bother the

▲ see page 1636

child. It can be prevented or minimized by using diapers with absorbent gel, by avoiding restrictive plastic diapers or pants that trap moisture, and by frequent changing of diapers when they are soiled. Breastfed babies tend to have fewer diaper rashes because their stools contain fewer enzymes and other substances that can irritate the skin.

The main treatment for diaper rash is frequent removal or change of a child's diapers. The child's skin should be washed gently with mild soap and water. Often the rash improves with these measures alone. Use of a skin moisturizer and barrier ointment, such as zinc, petroleum jelly, or vitamin A & D cream, may help. Antifungal cream may be necessary if the doctor diagnoses a *Candida* infection. Antibiotic cream can be used if the rash is caused by bacteria.

Eczema (atopic dermatitis) is a red, scaly, dry rash that tends to appear in patches, and comes and goes. Although the cause is unknown, eczema tends to run in families and in many cases is thought to be due to an allergy. Most children outgrow eczema, but for others eczema is a life-long condition. Children with severe cases may develop infections intermittently of some particularly affected areas. Treatment includes use of skin moisturizers, gentle soaps, humidified air, corticosteroid creams, and anti-itch drugs. Efforts to control dust mites and other triggers of a child's allergies may occasionally improve the condition.

Cradle cap (seborrheic dermatitis) is a red and yellow scaling, crusty rash that occurs on an infant's head and occasionally in the skin folds. The cause is not known. Cradle cap is harmless and disappears in most children by 6 months of age. Cradle cap can be treated by regularly shampooing and massaging mineral oil into the scalp. The scales may be worked off with a fine comb. Cradle cap that does not improve with these measures may need further treatment, such as selenium shampoo or corticosteroid creams.

Tinea is a fungal infection of the skin. In children, infections of the scalp (tinea capitis) and body (tinea corporis, or "ringworm") are most common. The diagnosis and treatment of tinea are the same in children and adults.▲ Some children have an inflammatory reaction to the fungal infection that leads to a scalp mass (kerion), which may require additional treatment.

Molluscum contagiosum is a cluster of flesh-colored pearly pimples or bumps caused by a

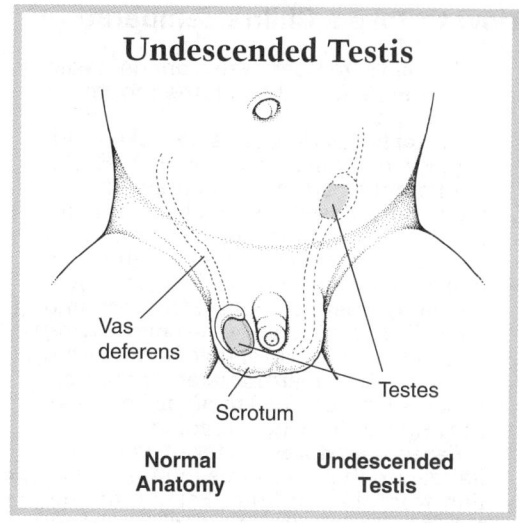

Undescended Testis

Vas deferens

Scrotum

Testes

Normal Anatomy   **Undescended Testis**

viral skin infection■ that usually disappears without treatment.

Milia are small pearly cysts on the face of newborns caused by the first secretions of the child's oil glands. Like newborn acne,★ milia require no treatment and disappear soon after birth.

Other skin rashes in young children are often caused by viral infections. Rashes caused by roseola and erythema infectiosum (fifth disease) are harmless and generally improve without treatment.● Rashes caused by measles, rubella, and chickenpox are becoming less common or rare because children are receiving vaccines.

Undescended and Retractile Testes

Undescended testes (cryptorchidism) are testes that remain in the abdomen instead of descending into the scrotum just before birth. About 3 of every 100 boys have undescended testes at birth. Most testes descend on their own within about 6 months. Boys born prematurely are much more likely to have the condition; so are boys whose family members had undescended testes. Half of the boys with the condition have an undescended testis only on the right, and one fourth are affected on both sides.

Undescended testes cause no symptoms. However, undescended testes can become

▲ see page 1225   ■ see page 1229
★ see box on page 1496   ● see page 1572

How to Take a Child's Temperature

A child's temperature can be taken from the rectum, the ear, the mouth, or the armpit.

Rectal temperatures can be taken with a glass or digital thermometer. Rectal temperatures are most accurate; that is, they come closest to the child's true internal body temperature. To take a rectal temperature, a thermometer with a coat of petroleum jelly around the bulb should be gently inserted about ½ to 1 inch into the child's rectum while the child is lying face down. The child should be kept from moving. The thermometer should be kept in place for 2 to 3 minutes before removing it and taking a reading.

Ear temperatures are taken with a digital device that measures infrared radiation from the eardrum. Ear thermometers are unreliable in infants younger than 3 months of age. To take an ear temperature, the person should form a seal around the opening of the ear with the thermometer probe and press the start button. A digital readout provides the temperature.

Oral temperatures are taken by placing a glass or digital thermometer under the child's tongue for 2 to 3 minutes. Oral temperatures provide reliable readings but are difficult to take in young children, who usually cannot keep their mouth gently closed around the thermometer to get an accurate reading.

Armpit temperatures are taken by placing a glass or digital thermometer in the child's armpit for 4 to 5 minutes. Armpit temperatures are least accurate because the armpit is cooler than the rectum, ear, or mouth.

twisted in the abdomen (testicular torsion▲), impair sperm production later in life, and increase the risk of hernia and testicular cancer. Surgery is generally performed to bring the testes down into the scrotum if the testes remain undescended at 1 year of age.

Retractile (hypermobile) testes are descended testes that easily move back and forth between the scrotum and the abdomen. Retractile testes do not lead to cancer or other complications. The testes usually stop retracting by puberty and do not require surgery or other treatment.

▲ see page 1327   ■ see also page 1090

★ see page 1561   ● see page 502

Fever

Fever is a rise in body temperature in response to infection, injury, or inflammation.■

Body temperatures vary, and temperature elevations up to 100.3° F (about 38° C) can be normal in healthy children. Therefore, minor temperature elevations that do not distress a child do not require medical attention. Temperatures of 100.4° F and higher are considered abnormal and generally deserve attention, particularly in infants younger than 3 months.

Causes and Symptoms

Fever is usually the result of common infections, such as colds and "stomach flu" (gastroenteritis). These infections are usually viral and get better without treatment. Less commonly, fever develops because of infection in the ear, lung, bladder, or kidney; these are usually bacterial infections that require antibiotics. In infants on rare occasions, fever may be the only sign of a bloodstream infection (occult bacteremia★), which can lead to meningitis and overwhelming infection (sepsis), two life-threatening conditions. These children usually appear ill. Many conditions besides infection cause fever in children, but all are rare. Unlike fevers that occur with common infections, these fevers persist for more than a few days.

Fevers can occur after routine vaccinations and are not a reason to avoid recommended vaccines. Giving the infant acetaminophen or ibuprofen at the time of vaccination and afterward minimizes the risk of getting a fever or lowers the fever itself.

Infants with fever are usually irritable and may not sleep or feed well. Older children lose their interest in play, although sometimes children with high fevers appear surprisingly well. The irritability and disinterest that fever usually causes worsen the higher the fever gets. Occasionally, a rapidly rising fever can cause seizures (febrile seizures),● and even more rarely, a fever gets so high that children become lethargic and unresponsive.

Diagnosis and Treatment

Detecting fever is not a challenge, but determining its cause can be. If the fever is low grade (100.3° F or below) and of short duration, no testing or treatment may be needed. In other cases, knowledge of the child's symptoms and a thorough examination help doctors find the cause. In general, any infant with a temperature of 100.4° F or higher should be seen by a doctor, as should older children with higher or recurring fevers.

In infants younger than 2 months of age who have a fever, doctors may order blood and urine tests and perform a spinal tap (lumbar puncture)▲ to look for occult bacteremia and meningitis. The reason for these tests is that in infants, the source of fever is difficult to determine. They are also at risk of serious infection compared with older children because of their immature immune system. Doctors may also order an x-ray if the infant's breathing is abnormal. After 2 months of age, testing may not be needed, but many doctors order blood and urine tests and perform a spinal tap if the source of the fever is not obvious and the child appears ill. For children 3 months of age and older, doctors rely more on the child's behavior and physical examination to determine which tests to order. Doctors may order blood and urine tests for children younger than 3 years old with high fevers if they cannot determine the source of fever after examining the child.

Most fevers do not require treatment except to make the child feel better. Acetaminophen and ibuprofen are used. Aspirin is not safe for lowering fever because it can interact with certain viral infections and cause a serious condition called Reye's syndrome.■ A warm (not cold) bath can sometimes make an older child feel better by reducing the fever. Rubbing the child down with alcohol or witch hazel is not recommended. The fumes can be harmful; in addition, it may come into contact with the eyes or the child might accidentally ingest it.

Additional treatment depends on the child's age and cause of the fever. Rarely, fevers persist and doctors are unable to determine their source even after extensive testing; this is called fever of unknown origin.★

Failure to Thrive

Failure to thrive is a delay in physical growth and weight gain that can lead to delays in development and maturation.

Failure to thrive is a diagnosis given to children who are consistently underweight or who do not gain weight for unclear reasons. There are many causes. Failure to thrive may be the result of environmental, emotional, physical, and medical factors that prevent a child from growing normally.

Many environmental and social factors can interact to keep the child from getting the nu-

trition he needs. Parental neglect or abuse, parental mental health disorders, and chaotic family situations in which routine, nutritious meals are insufficiently provided, may all blunt a child's growth, appetite, and intake of food. The amount of money a family has to spend on food and the nutritional value of the food they buy also affect growth. Inadequate intake of food may reflect inadequate parenting and environmental stimulation.

Sometimes failure to thrive is caused by a medical disorder in the child; sometimes the disorder is as minor as difficulty chewing or swallowing. Medical disorders, such as gastroesophageal reflux, narrowing of the esophagus, or intestinal malabsorption, may also affect a child's ability to retain, absorb, or process food. Infection, tumor, hormonal or metabolic disorders, heart disease, kidney disease, genetic disorders, and human immunodeficiency virus (HIV) infection are other physical reasons for failure to thrive.

Diagnosis

Doctors diagnose failure to thrive when a child's weight or rate of growth is well below what it should be when compared with past measurements or standard height-weight charts.● If the rate of growth is adequate, the child may be small for his or her age but still growing normally.

To determine why a child may be failing to thrive, doctors ask parents specific questions about feeding; bowel habits; social and financial stability of the family, which might affect the child's access to food; and illnesses that the child has had or that run in the family. The doctor examines the child, looking for signs of conditions that could explain the child's growth delay. The doctor makes decisions about blood and urine tests and x-rays based on this evaluation. More extensive testing is performed only if the doctor suspects an underlying disease.

Treatment and Prognosis

Treatment depends on the underlying cause. If a physical cause is found, specific treatment is given. Otherwise, treatment depends on how far below normal the child's weight is. Mild to moderate failure to thrive is treated with nutritious, high-calorie feedings given on a regular schedule. Parents may be counseled about fam-

▲ see art on page 443   ■ see box on page 1572
★ see page 1091   ● see art on page 1541

ily interactions that are damaging to the child and about financial and social resources available to them. Severe failure to thrive is treated in the hospital where social workers, nutritionists, feeding specialists, psychiatrists, and other specialists work together to determine the most likely causes of the child's failure to thrive and the best approach to feeding.

Because the first year of life is important for brain development, children who become undernourished during this time may fall permanently behind their peers, even if their physical growth improves. In about half of these children, mental development, especially verbal skills, remains below normal, and these children often have social and emotional problems in adulthood.

Sudden Infant Death Syndrome

Sudden infant death syndrome (SIDS) is the sudden, unexpected death of a seemingly healthy infant during sleep.

Although SIDS (also called crib death) is very rare, it is the most common cause of death in infants between the ages of 2 weeks and 1 year. It most often affects children between the second and fourth month of life. The syndrome occurs worldwide. SIDS is more common in premature infants, those who were small at birth, those that previously needed resuscitation, and those with upper respiratory tract infections. For unknown reasons, Black and American Indian infants are at a higher risk. It is more common among infants in families with low incomes, whose mothers are single or who used cigarettes or illicit drugs during pregnancy, and who had brothers or sisters who also died of SIDS.

The cause of SIDS is unknown. It may be due to an abnormality in the control of breathing. Some infants with SIDS show signs of having had low levels of oxygen in their blood and having had periods when they stopped breathing. Laying infants down to sleep on their stomach has been linked to SIDS.

Despite the known risk factors for SIDS, there is no certain way to prevent it. However, putting an infant to sleep on his back on a firm mattress prevents many but not all cases. The number of SIDS deaths has decreased as more parents have put their infants to sleep on their back. Parents should also remove pillows, bumper guards, and toys that could block an infant's breathing. Protecting the infant from overheating may also help but is not proven. Preventing infants from breathing second-hand cigarette smoke may help and clearly has other health benefits.

Most parents who have lost an infant to SIDS are grief-stricken and unprepared for the tragedy. They usually feel guilty. They may be further traumatized by investigations conducted by police, social workers, or others. Counseling and support from specially trained doctors and nurses and other parents who have lost an infant to SIDS are critical to helping parents cope with the tragedy. Specialists can recommend reading materials, web sites, and support groups to assist parents.

CHAPTER 268

Normal Preschool and School-Aged Children

Between the ages of 1 and 13, children's physical, intellectual, and emotional capabilities expand tremendously. Children progress from barely tottering to running, jumping, and playing organized sports. At age 1, most children can utter only a few recognizable words; by age 10, most can write book reports and use computers. Physical, intellectual, and social development, however, proceed at an individual pace.

Physical Development

Physical growth begins to slow at around age 1. At the same time, parents may notice a decrease in appetite. Some children seem to eat virtually nothing yet continue to grow and thrive. Children who are beginning to walk have an endearing physique, with the belly sticking forward and the back curved. They may also appear to be quite bow-legged. By 3

MILESTONES FROM AGES 18 MONTHS TO 6 YEARS

AGE	GROSS MOTOR SKILLS	FINE MOTOR SKILLS
18 months	Walks well	Draws vertical stroke Makes a tower of 4 cubes
2 years	Runs with coordination Climbs on furniture	Handles a spoon well Makes a tower of 7 cubes
2½ years	Jumps Walks upstairs	Scribbles in a circular pattern Opens doors
3 years	Mature gait in walking Rides tricycle	Favors using one hand over the other Copies a circle
4 years	Walks downstairs, alternating feet Hops	Copies a cross Dresses self
5 years	Skips	Copies a square Draws a person in 6 parts
6 years	Walks along a straight line from heel to toe	Writes name

years of age, muscle tone increases and the proportion of body fat decreases, so the body begins to look leaner and more muscular. Most children are physically able to control their bowels and bladder at this time.

During the preschool and school years, growth in height and weight is steady. The next major growth spurt occurs in early adolescence. During the years of steady growth, most children follow a predictable pattern. The doctor reports how the child is growing in relation to other children his age and monitors the child's weight gain compared to his height. Some children can become obese at an early age. Doubling the child's height at age 24 months fairly accurately predicts his adult height.

Intellectual Development

At the age of 2, most children understand the concept of time in broad terms. Many 2- and 3-year-olds believe that anything that happened in the past happened "yesterday," and anything that will happen in the future will happen "tomorrow." A child at this age has a vivid imagination but has difficulty distinguishing fantasy from reality. By age 4, most children have a more complicated understanding of time. They realize that the day is divided into morning, afternoon, and night. They can even appreciate the change in seasons.

From 18 months to 5 years of age, a child's vocabulary quickly expands from about 50 words to several thousand words. Children can begin to name and to actively ask about objects and events. By age 2, they begin to put two words together in short phrases, progressing to simple sentences by age 3. Pronunciation improves, with speech being half-understandable to a stranger by age 2 and fully understandable by age 4. A 4-year-old child can tell simple stories and can engage in conversation with adults or other children.

Even before 18 months of age, children can listen to and understand a story being read to them. By age 5, children are able to recite the alphabet and to recognize simple words in print. These skills are all fundamental to learning how to read simple words, phrases, and sentences. Depending on exposure to books and natural abilities, most children begin to read by age 7.

By age 7, a child's intellectual capabilities have become more complex. By this time, a child becomes increasingly able to focus on more than one aspect of an event or situation at the same time. For example, a school-aged child can appreciate that a tall, slender container can hold the same amount of water as a short, broad one. He can appreciate that medicine can taste bad but can make him feel better, or that his mother can be mad at him but can still love him. The child is increas-

Toilet Teaching

Most children can be taught to use the toilet when they are between 2 and 3 years of age. Using the toilet to defecate is usually accomplished first. By age 5, the average child can go to the toilet alone, managing all aspects of dressing, undressing, wiping, and handwashing. However, about 30% of healthy 4-year-olds and 10% of 6-year-olds have not yet achieved regular nighttime bladder control.

Recognizing signs of the child's readiness is the key to toilet teaching. Readiness is signaled when the child:

- Has dry periods lasting several hours
- Wants to be changed when wet
- Shows an interest in sitting on a potty chair or toilet
- Is able to follow simple commands

Children are usually ready to start training between the ages of 18 and 24 months. Despite physical readiness to use the toilet, some children may not be emotionally ready. To avoid a lengthy struggle over toileting, it is best to wait until the child indicates emotional readiness. When he is ready, he will ask for help in the bathroom or make his way to his potty chair on his own.

The timing method is the most commonly used method of toilet teaching. A child who seems ready is introduced to the potty chair and gradually asked to sit on it briefly while fully clothed. The child is then encouraged to practice taking his pants down, sitting on the potty chair for no more than 5 or 10 minutes, and redressing. Simple explanations are given repeatedly and are reinforced by placing wet or dirty diapers in the potty bowl. Praise or a reward is given for successful behavior. Anger or punishment for accidents or for lack of success may be counterproductive. The timing method works well for children with predictable bowel and urine schedules. Teaching children with unpredictable schedules is better delayed until they can anticipate the need to visit the bathroom on their own.

A child who resists sitting on the toilet may be allowed to get up and try again after a meal. If resistance continues for days, postponing the teaching for several weeks is the best strategy. Giving praise or a reward for sitting on the toilet and producing results is effective. Once the pattern is established, rewards can be given for every other success and then gradually withdrawn. Power struggles are unproductive and may strain the parent-child relationship.

ingly able to understand another person's perspective and so learns the essentials of taking turns in games or conversations. In addition, a school-aged child is able to follow agreed-upon rules of games. The child is also increasingly able to reason using the powers of observation and multiple points of view.

Social and Emotional Development

Emotion and behavior are based on the child's developmental stage and on his temperament. Every child has an individual temperament, or mood. Some children may be cheerful and adaptable and easily develop regular routines of sleeping, waking, eating, and other daily activities; these children tend to respond positively to new situations. Other children are not very adaptable and may have great irregularities in their routine; these children tend to respond negatively to new situations. Still other children are in between.

At about 9 months of age, infants normally become more anxious about being separated from their parents. Separations at bedtime and at childcare may be difficult and can be marked by temper tantrums; this behavior can last for many months. For many older children, a special blanket or stuffed animal serves at this time as a "transitional object" that acts as a symbol for the absent parent.

At 2 to 3 years of age, a child begins to test his limits and do what he has been forbidden to do, simply to see what will happen. The frequent "nos" that children hear from parents reflect the struggle for independence at this age. Although distressing to both the parent and child, tantrums are normal because they help children express their frustration during a time when they cannot verbalize their feelings well. Parents can help decrease the number of tantrums by not letting the child become overtired or unduly frustrated, and by predicting the child's behavior and avoiding situations that are likely to induce tantrums. Rarely, temper tantrums need to be evaluated by a doctor.▲ Some young children have particular difficulty controlling their impulses and need their parents to set stricter limits around which there can be some safety and regularity in their world.

At age 18 months to 2 years, children typically begin to establish gender identity.■ Dur-

▲ see page 1547   ■ see page 627

Height and Weight Charts for Boys and Girls

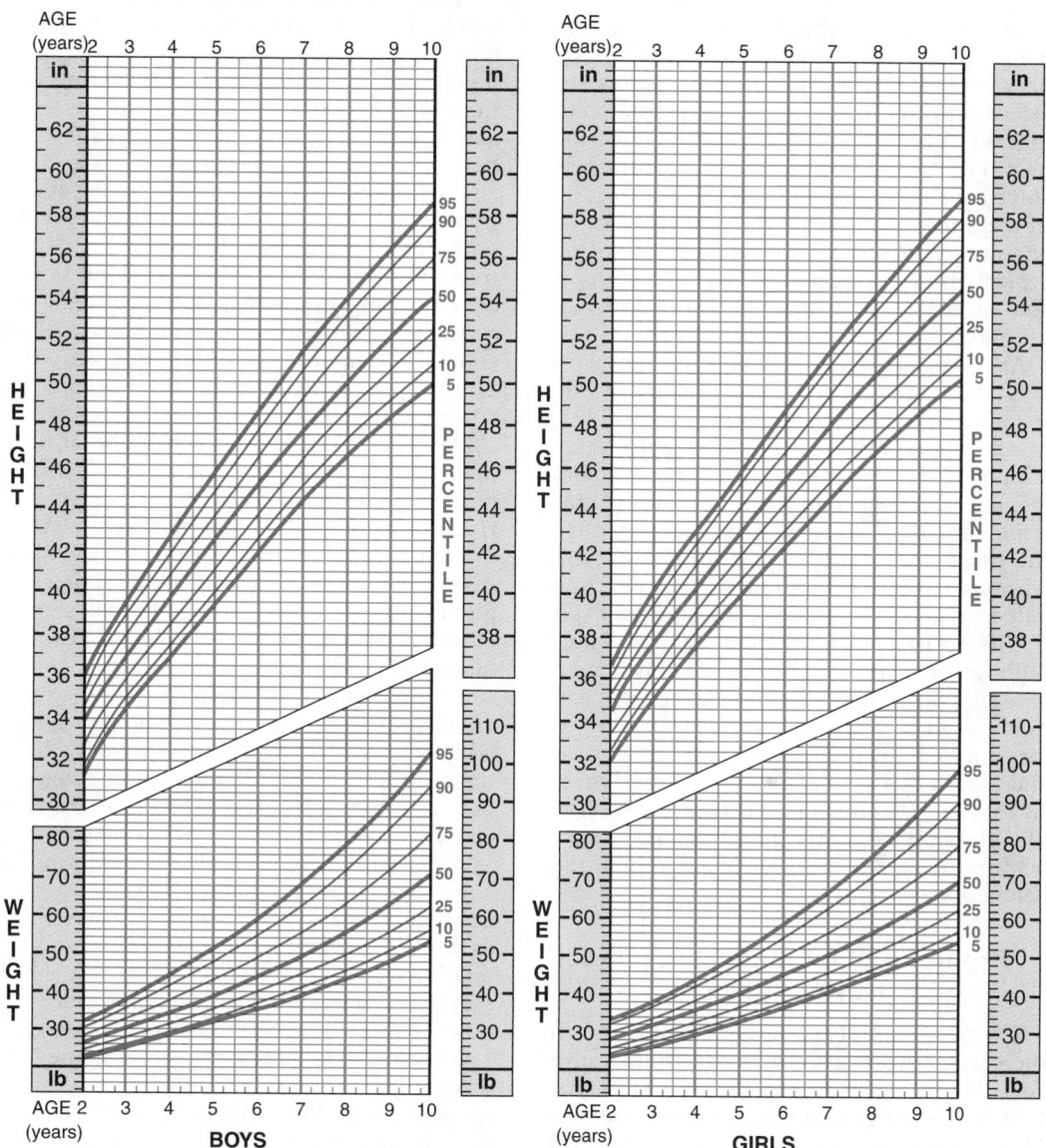

Source: The National Center for Health Statistics in collaboration with the National Center for Chronic Disease Prevention and Health Promotion (2000). http://www.cdc.gov/growthcharts

ing the preschool years, children also acquire a notion of gender role, of what boys and girls typically do. Exploration of the genitals is expected at this age and signals that children are beginning to make a connection between gender and body image.

Between 2 and 3 years of age, children begin to play more interactively with other children. Although they may still be possessive about toys, they may begin to share and even take turns in play. Asserting ownership of toys by saying, "That is mine!" helps establish the sense of self. Although children of this age strive for independence, they still need their parents nearby for security and support; for example, they may walk away from their parents when they feel curious only to later hide behind their parents when they are fearful.

At 3 to 5 years of age, many children become interested in fantasy play and imaginary friends. Fantasy play allows children to safely act out different roles and strong feelings in acceptable ways. Fantasy play also helps children grow socially; they learn to resolve conflicts with parents or other children in ways that will help them vent frustrations and maintain self-esteem. Also at this time, typical childhood fears like that of "the monster in the closet" emerge. These fears are normal.

At 7 to 12 years of age, children work through numerous issues: self-concept, the foundation for which is laid by competency in the classroom; relationships with peers, which are determined by the ability to socialize and fit in well; and family relationships, which are determined in part by the approval the child gains from his parents and siblings. Although many children seem to place a high value on the peer group, they still look primarily to parents for support and guidance. Siblings can serve as role models and as valuable supports and critics in what can and cannot be done. This period of time is very active for children, who engage in many activities and are eager to explore new activities. At this age, children are eager learners and often respond well to advice about safety, healthy lifestyles, and avoidance of high-risk behaviors.

Promoting Optimal Health and Development

There are a number of ways parents can help their children achieve the best possible health. For example, obesity can be prevented with healthy eating patterns and regular exercise. The child should consume a variety of healthy foods, including fruits and vegetables along with protein. Regular meals and small nutritious snacks encourage healthy eating in even a picky preschooler. Although the child may avoid some healthy foods, such as broccoli or beans, for a period of time, it is important to continue to offer healthy foods. In addition, parents should limit intake of fruit juices. Some children lose their appetite for food at mealtime if they drink too much fruit juice. A child who drinks from a bottle should be weaned by about 1 year of age to prevent ex-

cess juice and milk intake and to avoid tooth decay.

Promoting optimal development in a child works best if approached with flexibility, keeping the individual child's age, temperament, developmental stage, and learning style in mind. A coordinated approach involving parents, teachers, and the child usually works best. Throughout these years, children need an environment that promotes lifelong curiosity and learning. The child should be provided with books and music. A routine of daily interactive reading, with parents asking as well as answering questions, helps children pay attention, read with comprehension, and encourages their interest in learning activities. Limiting television and electronic games encourages more interactive play.

Playgroups and preschool have benefits for many young children. Children can learn important social skills, such as sharing. In addition, they may begin to recognize letters, numbers, and colors; learning these skills makes the transition to school smoother. Importantly, in a structured preschool setting, potential developmental problems can be identified and addressed early.

Parents who are in need of childcare may wonder what the best environment is and whether care by others may actually harm their child. Available information suggests that young children can do well both in their own home and in care out of the home, as long as the environment is loving and nurturing. By closely watching the child's response to a given childcare setting, parents are better able to choose the best environment. Some children thrive in a childcare environment where there are many children; others may fare better in their own home or in a smaller group.

When the child begins to receive homework assignments, parents can help by showing interest in the child's work, by being available to sort through questions but not finishing the work themselves, by providing a quiet work environment at home for the child, and by communicating with the teacher about any concerns. As the school years progress, parents need to consider their child's needs when selecting extracurricular activities. Many children thrive when offered the opportunity to participate in team sports or learn a musical instrument. These activities may also provide a venue for improving social skills. On the other hand, some children become stressed if they are "over-scheduled" and expected to participate in too many activities. Children need to be encouraged and supported in their extracurricular activities without having unrealistic expectations placed on them.

Preventive Health Care Visits

Scheduled visits to the doctor provide parents with information about their child's growth and development. Such visits also give parents an opportunity to ask questions and seek advice. The American Academy of Pediatrics recommends that after the first year of life children see their doctor for preventive health care visits at 12, 15, 18, and 24 months of age and then yearly until age 6. It is then recommended that the child come for a visit at age 8 and again at age 10. Visits can be made more often based on the advice of the doctor or the needs of the family.

A variety of measurements, screening procedures, and vaccinations are performed▲ at each visit. Height and weight are checked. Good growth is one indicator that the child is generally healthy. Head circumference is not routinely measured after the age of 18 months. Beginning at age 3, blood pressure is measured at each visit.

Preventive visits may include a check of vision and hearing. Some children may need to have their blood checked for anemia or an increased level of lead.■ The age of the child and various other factors determine which tests are performed. Some doctors also recommend that the child's urine be checked, although the value of such testing has not been established.

The doctor also asks questions to see how the child has progressed intellectually since the last visit. For example, the doctor may want to know if an 18-month-old has begun to speak or if a 7-year-old has begun to read. In the same way, doctors often ask age-appropriate questions about the child's behavior. Does the 18-month-old child have tantrums? Does the 2-year-old sleep through the night? Does the 6-year-old wet the bed at night? Parents and doctors can discuss these types of behavioral and developmental issues during the preventive health care visits and together design approaches to any behavioral or developmental problems.

Child safety is discussed during preventive visits. Specific safety concerns are based on the age of the child. For a 6-month-old, the doctor may wish to talk about childproofing the house to prevent unintentional poisonings or injury. For a 5-year-old, the discussion might be focused on the potential hazards of guns in the home and gun safety. Parents should take the opportunity to bring up topics that are most relevant to their unique family situation. As the child gets older, he can be an active participant in these discussions.

Finally, the doctor performs a complete physical examination. In addition to examining the child from head to toe, including the heart, lungs, abdomen, genitals, and head and neck, the doctor may ask the child to perform some age-appropriate tasks. To check gross motor skills (such as walking and running), the doctor may ask a 4-year-old to hop on one foot. To check fine motor skills (manipulating small objects with the hands), the child may be asked to draw a picture or copy some shapes.

CHAPTER 269

Behavioral and Developmental Problems in Young Children

Children acquire many skills as they grow. Some skills, such as controlling urine and stool, depend mainly on the level of maturity of the child's nerves and brain. Others, such as behaving appropriately at home and in school, are the result of a complicated interaction between the child's physical and intellectual (cognitive) development, health, tempera-

ment, and relationship with parents, teachers, and caregivers.

Behavioral and developmental problems can become so troublesome that they threaten normal relationships between the child and

---

▲ see art on page 1493   ■ see page 1680

Behavioral Problems due to Parenting Problems

A number of relatively minor problems of behavior may be due to parenting problems.

Child-parent interactional problems are difficulties in the relationship between a child and his parents, which may begin during the first few months of life. The relationship may be strained because of a difficult pregnancy or delivery or due to the mother suffering from depression after delivery or receiving inadequate support from the father, relatives, or friends. Contributing to the strain are a baby's unpredictable feeding and sleeping schedules. Most babies do not sleep through the night until 3 to 4 months of age. Poor relationships may slow the child's development of mental and social skills and cause failure to thrive.

A doctor or nurse can discuss the temperament of an individual baby and offer the parents information on the development of infants and helpful tips for coping. The parents may then be able to develop more realistic ex-pectations, accept their feelings of guilt and conflict as normal, and try to rebuild a healthy relationship. If the relationship is not repaired, the child may continue to have problems later.

A vicious circle pattern is a cycle of negative (naughty) behavior by the child that causes a negative (angry) response from the parent or caregiver, followed by further negative behavior by the child, leading to a further negative response from the parent. Vicious circles usually begin when a child is aggressive and resistant. The parents or caregivers respond by scolding, yelling, and spanking. Vicious circles may also result when parents react to a fearful, clinging, or manipulative child with overprotection and over-permissiveness.

The vicious circle pattern may be broken if parents learn to ignore bad behavior that does not affect the rights of others, such as temper tantrums or refusals to eat. For behavior that cannot be ignored, distraction or a time-out procedure can be tried. Parents should also praise the child for good behavior.

Discipline problems are inappropriate behaviors that develop when discipline is ineffective. Efforts to control a child's behavior through scolding or physical punishments such as spanking may work briefly if used sparingly. However, these approaches generally tend not to alter the bad behavior sufficiently and may reduce the child's sense of security and self-esteem. Moreover, spanking can get out of hand when the parent is angry. A time-out procedure can be helpful. However, punishments become ineffective when overused. Furthermore, threats that the parents will leave or send the child away can be psychologically damaging.

Praise and reward can reinforce good behavior. Because most children prefer attention for inappropriate behavior to no attention at all, the parents should create special times each day for pleasant interactions with the child.

others. Some behavioral problems, such as bed-wetting, can be mild and resolve quickly. Other behavioral problems, such as those that arise in children with attention deficit/hyperactivity disorder (ADHD), can require ongoing treatment. Most of the problems described in this chapter arise out of developmentally normal bad habits that children easily acquire. The goal of treatment is to change the bad habits by getting the child to want to change his behavior. This goal often takes persistent changes in actions by the parents, which in turn result in improved behaviors by the child.

Eating Problems

Some eating problems can be behavorial in nature.

Undereating: A decrease in appetite, caused by a slowing growth rate, is common in children around 1 year of age. However, an eating problem may develop if a parent or caregiver tries to coerce the child to eat or shows too much concern about the child's appetite or eating habits. When parents coax and threaten, children with eating problems may refuse to eat the food in their mouths. Some children may respond to parental attempts at force-feeding by vomiting.

Decreasing the tension and negative emotions surrounding mealtimes may be helpful. Emotional scenes can be avoided by putting food in front of the child and removing it in 20 to 30 minutes without comment. The child should be allowed to eat whatever he chooses from offered food at mealtimes and scheduled snacks in the morning and afternoon. Food and fluids other than water should be restricted at all other times. Young children should be offered 3 meals and 2 to 3 snacks each day. Mealtimes should be scheduled at a time when other family members are eating;

distractions, such as television, should be avoided. Sitting at a table is encouraged. Using these techniques balances the child's appetite, amount of food eaten, and nutritional needs.

Overeating: Overeating is another problem. Overeating can lead to childhood obesity.▲ Once fat cells form, they do not go away. Thus, obese children are more likely than children of normal weight to be obese as adults. Because childhood obesity can lead to adult obesity, it should be prevented or treated.■

Bed-Wetting

About 30% of children still wet the bed at age 4, 10% at age 6, 3% at age 12, and 1% at age 18. Bed-wetting is more common in boys than in girls and seems to run in families.

Bed-wetting is usually caused by slow maturation of the nerves that supply the bladder, so that the child fails to awaken appropriately when the bladder fills and needs emptying. Bed-wetting can accompany such sleep disorders as sleepwalking and night terrors.★ A physical disorder—usually a urinary tract infection—is found in only 1 to 2% of children who wet the bed. Other disorders, such as diabetes, rarely cause bed-wetting. Bed-wetting occasionally is caused by psychologic problems, either in the child or in another family member, and is occasionally part of a constellation of symptoms that suggests the possibility of sexual abuse.

Sometimes bed-wetting stops and then begins again. The relapse usually follows a psychologically stressful event or condition, but a physical cause, especially a urinary tract infection, may be responsible.

Treatment

Parents and the child need to know that bed-wetting is quite common, that it can be corrected, and that nobody should feel guilty about it. An older child who has bed-wetting can take responsibility by limiting fluids after dinner (especially caffeinated beverages), urinating before going to bed, recording wet and dry nights, and changing clothing and bedding when wet. Parents may choose to give the child age-appropriate rewards (positive reinforcement) for dry nights.

For children younger than 6, parents can avoid giving the child fluids 2 to 3 hours before bedtime and encourage the child to urinate just before going to bed. In most children of this age, time and physical maturation solve the problem.

For children older than 6 to 7 years, some form of treatment is often indicated. Bed-wetting alarms, which awaken a child when a few drops of urine are detected, are the most effective treatment available. They cure bed-wetting in about 70% of the children, and only about 10 to 15% of children start wetting the bed again after the alarms are discontinued. Alarms are relatively inexpensive and are easy to set up. In the first few weeks of use, the child awakens only after fully urinating. In the next few weeks, the child awakens after urinating a small amount and may wet the bed less often. Eventually, the need to urinate wakes the child before the bed is wet. Most parents find that the alarm can be removed after a 3-week dry period.

If bed-wetting persists in an older child after alarms and age-appropriate rewards have been tried, the doctor may prescribe imipramine. Imipramine is an antidepressant drug but is used to treat bed-wetting because it relaxes the bladder and tightens the sphincter that blocks urine flow. If imipramine is going to work, it usually does so in the first week of treatment. This rapid response is the only real advantage of the drug, particularly if the parents and child feel they need to cure the problem quickly. After 1 month without bed-wetting, the drug dose is decreased over 2 to 4 weeks, then discontinued. However, about 75% of children eventually start wetting the bed again. If this happens, a 3-month course of the drug may be tried.

An increasingly popular drug for bed-wetting is desmopressin tablets or nasal spray. This drug reduces the output of urine, which reduces bed-wetting. This drug is used for a 1- to 3-month period and then discontinued as soon as possible. It can be used intermittently, such as when the child goes to camp.

Encopresis

Encopresis is the accidental passing of bowel movements that is not caused by illness or physical abnormality.

About 17% of 3-year-olds and 1% of 4-year-olds have encopresis, most often from resistance to toilet teaching. However, chronic constipation, which stretches the bowel wall and reduces the child's awareness of a full

---

▲ see also page 1557   ■ see page 914
★ see page 1546

bowel, impairing muscle control, sometimes causes encopresis.

A doctor first tries to determine the cause. If the cause is constipation, a laxative is prescribed and other measures are instituted to ensure regular bowel movements. Once regular bowel movements are achieved, the leakage often stops. If these measures fail, diagnostic tests may be performed, such as abdominal x-rays and rarely a biopsy of the rectal wall, in which a tissue sample is taken and examined under a microscope. If a physical cause is found, it often can be treated. In the most severe cases, psychologic counseling may be needed for children whose encopresis is the result of resistance to toilet teaching or other behavioral problems.

Sleep Problems

For most children, sleep problems are intermittent or temporary and often do not need treatment.

Nightmares: Nightmares are frightening dreams that occur during rapid eye movement (REM) sleep.▲ A child having a nightmare can awaken fully and can vividly recall the details of the dream. Nightmares are not a cause for alarm, unless they occur very often. They can occur more often during times of stress, or even when the child has seen a video containing aggressive content. If nightmares occur often, parents can keep a diary to see if they can identify the cause.

Night Terrors and Sleepwalking: Night terrors, episodes of incomplete awakening with extreme anxiety shortly after falling asleep, are most common between the ages of 3 and 8. The child screams and appears frightened, with a rapid heart rate and rapid breathing. The child does not seem to be aware of the parents' presence and does not talk. He may thrash around violently and does not respond to comforting. After a few minutes, he goes fully back to sleep. Unlike with nightmares, the child is not able to recall these episodes. Night terrors are dramatic because the child screams and is inconsolable during the episode. About one third of children with night terrors also experience sleepwalking (rising from bed and walking around while apparently asleep, also called somnambulism■). About 15% of children be-

tween the ages of 5 and 12 have at least one episode of sleepwalking.

Night terrors and sleepwalking★ almost always stop on their own, although occasional episodes may occur for years; usually, no treatment is needed. If a disorder persists into adolescence or adulthood and is severe, treatment may be necessary. In children who need treatment, night terrors may sometimes respond to a sedative or certain antidepressants; however, these drugs are potent and can have side effects. Installing a lock on the outside of the bedroom door keeps a child from wandering but may frighten the child.

Resistance to Going to Bed: Children, particularly between the ages of 1 and 2, often resist going to bed. Young children often cry when left alone in their cribs, or they climb out and seek their parents. This behavior is related to separation anxiety● and, in older children, to the child's attempts to control more aspects of his environment.

Resistance to going to bed is not helped if parents stay in the room at length to provide comfort or let the child get up. To control the problem, a parent may have to sit quietly in the hallway in sight of the child and make sure the child stays in bed. The child then learns that getting out of bed is not allowed. The child also learns that the parents cannot be enticed into the room for more stories or play. Eventually, the child settles down and goes to sleep. Providing the child with an attachment object (like a teddy bear) is often helpful.

Awakening During the Night: Children often awaken during the night, but they usually fall back to sleep on their own. Repeated night awakening often follows a move, an illness, or another stressful event. Sleeping problems may be worsened when the child takes long naps late in the afternoon or is overstimulated by playing before bedtime.

Allowing the child to sleep with the parents because of the night awakening is likely only to prolong the problem. Also counterproductive are playing with or feeding the child during the night, spanking, and scolding. Returning the child to bed with simple reassurance is usually more effective. A bedtime routine that includes reading a brief story, offering a favorite doll or blanket, and using a small nightlight (in children who are older than 3) is often helpful. Parents and other caregivers should also try to keep to a routine each night, so that the child learns what is expected. If the child

---

▲ see page 474   ■ see also page 474

★ see also page 474   ● see page 1534

is physically healthy, allowing him to cry for 20 to 30 minutes often teaches him that he needs to settle himself down, which will diminish the night awakening.

Temper Tantrums

Temper tantrums are common in childhood. They usually appear toward the end of the first year, are most common between the ages of 2 and 4, and are typically infrequent after age 5. If tantrums are frequent after age 5, they may persist throughout childhood.

Causes include frustration, tiredness, or hunger. Children may also have temper tantrums to seek attention or to manipulate parents to obtain something, or to avoid doing something. Parents often place the blame on themselves (because of imagined poor parenting) when the real cause is often a combination of the child's personality, immediate circumstances, and developmentally normal behavior. An underlying psychologic, medical, or social problem may rarely be the cause and is more likely if a tantrum lasts for more than 15 minutes or if tantrums occur multiple times each day.

A child who is having a temper tantrum may shout, scream, cry, thrash about, roll on the floor, stamp with his feet, and throw things. Some of the behavior may be ragelike and potentially harmful; he may become red in the face and hit or kick.

To stop a tantrum, parents should first ask the child simply and firmly to do so. If that fails and if the behavior is sufficiently disruptive, the child may have to be removed physically from the situation. At this point, a time-out procedure can be very effective. A time-out procedure is a discipline technique used by parents to interrupt the child's disruptive behavior. A time-out is most effective in children 2 and older. After repeatedly misbehaving, the child is calmly sent or taken to a chair for a set period—1 minute for each year of age, up to a maximum of 5 minutes. If the child gets up early or does not quiet down within the set period, the timer is reset.

Breath-Holding Spells

A breath-holding spell is an episode in which the child stops breathing and loses consciousness for a short period immediately after a frightening or emotionally upsetting event.

Breath-holding spells occur in 5% of otherwise healthy children. They usually begin in the second year of life. They disappear by age 4 in 50% of children and by age 8 in about 83% of children. The 17% of children who continue to have spells as adults lose consciousness as a reaction to emotional stress. Breath-holding spells can take one of two forms.

The **cyanotic form** of breath-holding, which is most common, is initiated subconsciously by young children often as a component of a temper tantrum or in response to a scolding or other upsetting event. Episodes peak at about 2 years and are rare after 5 years. During the episode, a child holds his breath (without necessarily being aware he is doing so) until he loses consciousness. Typically, the child cries out, breathes out, then stops breathing. Shortly afterward, the child's skin begins to turn blue and he becomes unconscious. A seizure may occur. After the loss of consciousness (which generally lasts for seconds only), breathing resumes and normal skin color and consciousness return. It may be possible to interrupt the episode by placing a cold rag on the child's face when the spell begins. Despite the frightening nature of the episode, the parents must try to avoid reinforcing the initiating behavior in the cyanotic form. As the child recovers, parents should put the child safely in bed. Parents should enforce household rules; the child cannot have "free rein" of the house just because these spells follow temper tantrums. Distracting the child and avoiding situations that will likely lead to tantrums are good strategies.

The **pallid form** typically follows a painful experience, such as falling and banging the head or being suddenly startled. The brain sends out a signal (via the vagus nerve) that severely slows the heart rate, producing loss of consciousness. Thus, in this form, the loss of consciousness and stoppage of breathing (which are both temporary) result from a nerve response to being startled that leads to slowing of the heart.

The child stops breathing, rapidly loses consciousness, and becomes pale and limp. A seizure may occur. The heart typically beats very slowly during an attack. After the attack, the heart speeds up again, breathing restarts, and consciousness returns without any treatment. Because this type is rare, if the attacks occur often, further diagnostic evaluation and treatment may be needed.

School Avoidance

Avoiding school occurs in about 5% of all school-aged children and affects girls and boys

What Are Stress-Related Behaviors?

Each child handles stress differently. Certain behaviors that help children deal with stress include thumb sucking, nail biting, and, sometimes, head banging.

Thumb sucking (or sucking a pacifier) is a normal part of early childhood, and most children stop by the time they are 1 or 2 years old, but some continue into their school-age years. Occasional thumb sucking is normal at times of stress, but habitual sucking past the age of about 5 can alter the shape of the roof of the mouth, cause misalignment of teeth, and lead to teasing from other children. Occasionally, persistent thumb sucking can be the sign of an underlying emotional disorder.

All children eventually stop thumb sucking. Parents should intervene only if their child's dentist advises them to, or if they feel their child's thumb sucking is socially unhealthy. Parents need to gently encourage the child to understand why it would be good to stop. Once the child signals a willingness to stop, gentle verbal reminders are a good start. These can be followed by symbolic rewards put directly on the thumb, such as a colored bandage, fingernail polish, or a star drawn with a nontoxic colored marker. If necessary, additional measures, such as a plastic guard over the thumb, overnight elbow splinting to prevent a child from bending it, or "painting" the thumbnail with a bitter substance can be used. However, none of these measures should be used against the child's will.

Nail biting is a common problem in young children. The habit typically disappears as the child gets older, but is typically related to stress and anxiety. Children who are motivated to stop can be taught to substitute other habits (for example, twirling a pencil).

Head banging and **rhythmic rocking** are common among healthy toddlers. While alarming to parents, the children do not seem to be in distress and actually appear to derive comfort from the activity.

Children usually outgrow rocking, rolling, and head banging between 18 months and 2 years of age, but repetitive actions sometimes still occur in older children and adolescents.

Children with autism and certain other developmental problems also may bang their heads. However, these conditions have additional symptoms that make their diagnosis apparent.

Although children almost never damage themselves by these behaviors, this possibility (and the noise) can be reduced by pulling the crib away from the wall, taking off the wheels or placing carpet protectors under them, and applying a padded crib bumper to the inside of the crib.

---

equally. It is most likely to occur between ages 5 and 6 and between ages 10 and 11.

The cause is often unclear, but psychologic factors (such as anxiety and depression) and social factors (such as having no friends, feeling rejected by peers, or being bullied) may contribute. A sensitive child may be overreacting with fear to a teacher's strictness or rebukes. Younger children tend to fake illness or make other excuses to avoid school. The child may complain of a stomachache, nausea, or other symptoms that justify staying home. Some children directly refuse to go to school. Alternatively, the child may go to school without difficulty but become anxious or develop various symptoms during the school day, often going regularly to the nurse's office. This behavior is unlike that of adolescents, who may decide not to attend school (truancy, playing "hooky").▲

School avoidance tends to result in poor academic performance, family difficulties, and difficulties with the child's peers. Most children recover from school avoidance, although some develop it again after a real illness or a vacation.

Home tutoring is generally not a solution. A child with school avoidance should return to school immediately, so that he does not fall behind in his schoolwork. If school avoidance is so intense that it interferes with the child's activity and if the child does not respond to simple reassurance by parents or teachers, referral to a psychologist or psychiatrist may be warranted.

Treatment should include communication between parents and school personnel, regular attendance at school, and sometimes therapy involving the family and child with a psychologist. Therapy includes treatment of underly-

▲ see page 1558

ing causes as well as behavioral techniques to cope with the stresses at school.

Attention Deficit/Hyperactivity Disorder

Attention deficit/hyperactivity disorder (ADHD) is poor or short attention span and impulsiveness inappropriate for the child's age; some children also manifest hyperactivity.

Although there is considerable controversy about incidence, it is estimated that ADHD affects 5 to 10% of school-aged children and is diagnosed 10 times more often in boys than in girls. Many features of ADHD are often noticed before age 4 and invariably before age 7, but they may not interfere significantly with academic performance and social functioning until the middle school years. ADHD was previously just called "attention deficit disorder"; however, the common occurrence of hyperactivity in affected children—which is really a physical extension of attention deficit—led to a change in the current terminology.

ADHD can be inherited. Recent research indicates that the disorder is caused by abnormalities in neurotransmitters (substances that transmit nerve impulses within the brain). The symptoms of ADHD range from mild to severe and can become exaggerated or become a problem in certain environments, such as in the child's home or at school. The constraints of school and organized lifestyles make ADHD a problem, whereas in prior generations, the symptoms may not have interfered significantly with children's functioning because such restraints were often much fewer. Although some of the symptoms of ADHD also occur in children without ADHD, they are more frequent and severe in children with ADHD.

Symptoms

ADHD is primarily a problem with sustained attention, concentration, and task persistence (ability to finish a task). The child may also be overactive and impulsive. Many preschool children are anxious, have problems communicating and interacting, and behave poorly. They seem inattentive. They may fidget and squirm. They may be impatient and answer out of turn. During later childhood, such children may move their legs restlessly, move and fidget their hands, talk impulsively,

Signs of ADHD

All signs do not have to be present for a diagnosis of attention deficit/hyperactivity disorder (ADHD). However, signs of inattention must always be present for a diagnosis. Signs must be present in two or more situations (for example, home and school) and must interfere with social or academic functioning.

Signs of inattention:
- Often fails to pay close attention to details
- Has difficulty sustaining attention in work and play
- Does not seem to listen when spoken to directly
- Often does not follow through on instructions and fails to finish tasks
- Often has difficulty organizing tasks and activities
- Often avoids, dislikes, or is reluctant to engage in tasks that require sustained mental effort
- Often loses things
- Is easily distracted by extraneous stimuli
- Is often forgetful

Signs of hyperactivity:
- Often fidgets with hands or feet or squirms
- Often leaves seat in classroom and elsewhere
- Often runs about or climbs excessively
- Has difficulty playing or engaging in leisure activities quietly
- Is often on the go or acts as if "driven by a motor"
- Often talks excessively

Signs of impulsivity:
- Often blurts out answers before questions have been completed
- Often has difficulty awaiting his turn
- Often interrupts or intrudes on others

forget easily, and they may be disorganized. They are generally not aggressive.

About 20% of children with ADHD have learning disabilities and about 80% have academic problems. Work may be messy, with careless mistakes and an absence of considered thought. Affected children often behave as if their mind is elsewhere and they are not listening. They often do not follow through on

ADHD: Epidemic or Over-Diagnosis?

An increasing number of children are diagnosed with attention deficit/hyperactivity disorder (ADHD). However, there is a growing concern among doctors and parents that many children are misdiagnosed. A high activity level may be completely normal and be simply an exaggeration of normal childhood temperament. Alternatively, it may have a variety of causes, including emotional disorders or abnormalities of brain function, such as ADHD.

Generally, 2-year-olds are active and seldom stay still. A high activity and noise level is common up until age 4. In these age groups, such behavior is normal. Active behavior can cause conflicts between parents and child and may worry parents. It also can create problems for others who supervise such children, including teachers.

Determining whether a child's activity level is abnormally high should not simply depend on how tolerant the annoyed person is. However, some children are clearly more active than average. If the high activity level is combined with short attention span and impulsivity, it may be defined as hyperactivity and considered part of ADHD.

Scolding and punishing children whose high activity level is within normal limits usually backfires, increasing the child's activity level. Avoiding situations in which the child has to sit still for a long time or finding a teacher skilled in coping with such children may help. If simple measures do not help, a medical or psychologic evaluation may be useful to rule out an underlying disorder such as ADHD.

requests or complete schoolwork, chores, or other duties. There may be frequent shifts from one incomplete task to another.

About 40% of affected children may have issues with self-esteem, depression, anxiety, or opposition to authority by the time they reach adolescence. About 60% of young children have such problems as temper tantrums, and most older children have a low tolerance for frustration.

Diagnosis

The diagnosis is based on the number, frequency, and severity of symptoms. Symptoms must be present in at least two separate environments (typically, home and school)—occurrence of symptoms just at home or just at school and nowhere else does not qualify as ADHD. Often, diagnosis is difficult because it depends on the judgment of the observer. There is no laboratory test for ADHD. Questionnaires about various aspects of behavior can help the doctor make the diagnosis. Because learning disabilities are common, many children receive psychologic testing both to help determine if ADHD exists and to detect the presence of specific learning disabilities.

Treatment and Prognosis

To minimize the effects of ADHD, structures, routines, a school intervention plan, and modified parenting techniques are often needed. Some children who are not aggressive and who come from a stable and supportive home environment may benefit from drug treatment alone. Behavior therapy conducted by a child psychologist is sometimes combined with drug treatment. Psychostimulant drugs are the most effective drug treatment.

Methylphenidate is the psychostimulant drug most often prescribed. It is as effective as other psychostimulants (such as dextroamphetamine) and is probably safer. A number of slow-release (longer-acting) forms of methylphenidate are available in addition to the regular form and allow for one time per day dosing. Side effects of methylphenidate include sleep disturbances, such as insomnia, appetite suppression, depression or sadness, headaches, stomachaches, and high blood pressure. All of these side effects disappear if the drug is discontinued; however, most children have no side effects except perhaps a decreased appetite. However, if taken in large doses for a long time, methylphenidate can occasionally slow the child's growth; therefore, doctors monitor weight gain.

A number of other drugs can be used to treat inattentiveness and behavioral symptoms. These include clonidine, amphetamine-based drugs, antidepressants, and antianxiety drugs. Sometimes, combinations of drugs are used.

Children with ADHD generally do not outgrow their inattentiveness, although those with hyperactivity tend to become somewhat less impulsive and hyperactive with age. However, most adolescents and adults learn to adapt to their inattentiveness. Other problems that emerge or persist in adolescence and adulthood include poor academic achievement, low self-esteem, anxiety, depression, and difficulty in learning appropriate social behaviors. Importantly, the vast majority of children with ADHD become productive adults, and people who have ADHD seem to adjust better to work than to school situations. However, if the disorder is untreated in childhood, the risk of alcohol or substance abuse or suicide may increase.

Learning Disorders

Learning disorders involve an inability to acquire, retain, or broadly use specific skills or information, resulting from deficiencies in attention, memory, or reasoning and affecting academic performance.

Learning disorders are quite different from mental retardation and occur in children with normal or even high intellectual function. Learning disorders affect only certain functions, whereas in a child with mental retardation, difficulties affect cognitive functions broadly. There are three main types of learning disorders: reading disorders, disorders of written expression, and mathematics disorders. Thus, a child with a learning disorder may have significant difficulty understanding and learning math, but have no difficulty reading, writing, and performing well in other subjects. Dyslexia is the best known of the learning disorders. Learning disorders do not include learning problems that are due primarily to problems of vision, hearing, coordination, or emotional disturbance.

Although the causes of learning disorders are not fully understood, they include abnormalities in the basic processes involved in understanding or in using spoken or written language or numerical and spatial reasoning.

An estimated 3 to 15% of school children in the United States may need special educational services to compensate for learning disorders. Boys with learning disorders may outnumber girls five to one, although girls are often not recognized or diagnosed as having learning disorders.

Many children with behavioral problems perform poorly in school and are tested by educational psychologists for learning disorders. However, some children with certain types of learning disorders hide their deficits well, avoiding diagnosis, and therefore treatment, for a long time.

Symptoms

A young child may be slow to learn the names of colors or letters, to assign words to familiar objects, to count, and to progress in other early learning skills. Learning to read and write may be delayed. Other symptoms may be a short attention span and distractibility, halting speech, and a short memory span. The child may have difficulty with activities that require fine motor coordination, such as printing and copying.

A child with a learning disorder may have difficulty communicating. Some children initially become frustrated and later develop behavioral problems, such as being easily distracted, hyperactive, withdrawn, shy, or aggressive.

Diagnosis and Treatment

Children who are not reading or learning at the grade level expected for their verbal or intellectual abilities should be evaluated. Testing of hearing and eyesight should be carried out, because problems with these senses can also interfere with reading and writing skills.

A doctor examines the child for any physical disorders. The child takes a series of intelligence tests, both verbal and nonverbal, and academic tests of reading, writing, and arithmetic skills.

The most useful treatment for a learning disorder is education that is carefully tailored to the individual child. Measures such as eliminating food additives, taking large doses of vitamins, and analyzing the child's system for trace minerals are often tried but unproven. No drug treatment has much effect on academic achievement, intelligence, and general learning ability. Because some children with a learning disorder also have ADHD, certain drugs, such as methylphenidate, may improve attention and concentration, enhancing the child's ability to learn.

Dyslexia

Dyslexia is a specific reading disorder involving difficulty separating single words from groups of words and parts of words (phonemes) within each word.

Dyslexia is a particular type of learning disorder that affects an estimated 3 to 5% of children. It is identified in more boys than girls; however, it may simply go unrecognized more often in girls. Dyslexia tends to run in families.

Dyslexia occurs when the brain has difficulty making the connection between sounds and symbols (letters). This difficulty is caused by poorly understood problems with certain connections in the brain. The problems are present from birth and may cause spelling and writing errors and reduced speed and accuracy when reading aloud. People with dyslexia do not have problems understanding spoken language.

Symptoms and Diagnosis

Preschool children with dyslexia may be late in speaking, have speech articulation problems, and have difficulty remembering the names of letters, numbers, and colors. Dyslexic children often have difficulty blending sounds, rhyming words, identifying the positions of sounds in words, segmenting words into sounds, and identifying the number of sounds in words. Delays or hesitations in choosing words, making word substitutions, and naming letters and pictures are early indicators of dyslexia. Problems with short-term memory for sounds and for putting sounds in the correct order are common.

Many children with dyslexia confuse letters and words with similar ones. Reversing the letters while writing—for instance, *on* instead of *no,* and *saw* instead of *was*—or confusing letters—for instance, *b* instead of *d, w* instead of *m, n* instead of *h*—is common. However, many children without dyslexia will reverse letters in kindergarten or first grade.

Children who are not progressing in word learning skills by the middle or end of first grade should be tested for dyslexia.

Treatment

The best treatment for word recognition is direct instruction that incorporates multisensory approaches. This type of treatment consists of teaching phonics with a variety of cues, usually separately and, when possible, as part of a reading program.

Indirect instruction for word recognition is also helpful. This instruction usually consists of training to improve word pronunciation or reading comprehension. Children are taught how to process sounds by blending sounds to form words, by separating words into segments, and by identifying the positions of sounds in words.

Component-skills instruction for word recognition is also helpful. It consists of training to blend sounds to form words, to segment words into word parts, and to identify the positions of sounds in words.

Indirect treatments, other than those for word recognition, may be used but are not recommended. Indirect treatments can include using tinted lenses that allow words and letters to be read more easily, eye movement exercises, or visual perceptual training. Drugs such as piracetam have also been tried. The benefits of most indirect treatments have not been proved and may provide unrealistic expectations and delay the teaching that is needed.

CHAPTER 270

Normal Adolescents

During adolescence (usually encompassing ages 10 to 21), children become young adults. They mature socially and physically. Notably, they become sexually mature and socially independent. During this time, the adolescent develops a sense of who he or she is and learns to form intimate relationships with people who are not members of the family.

Physical Development

Normal growth during adolescence includes sexual maturation and an increase in body size. The timing and speed with which these changes occur vary and are affected by both heredity and environment. Physical maturity begins at an earlier age today than it did a century ago. For example, girls have their first menstrual period at a considerably younger age than their counterparts did 100 years ago. The reason is probably improvements in nutrition, general health, and living conditions.

During adolescence, most boys and girls reach adult height and weight, although there is considerable variation in when this occurs. The growth spurt in boys occurs between the ages of 13 and 15½ years; a gain of 4 inches can be expected in the year of maximum growth. The growth spurt in girls occurs between the ages of 11 and 13½ years; a gain of

Milestones in Sexual Development

During puberty, sexual development usually occurs in a set sequence. The tempo of change varies from person to person but occurs within a range of ages, indicated by a box in the diagram. The average age at which a change begins is indicated by a dot.

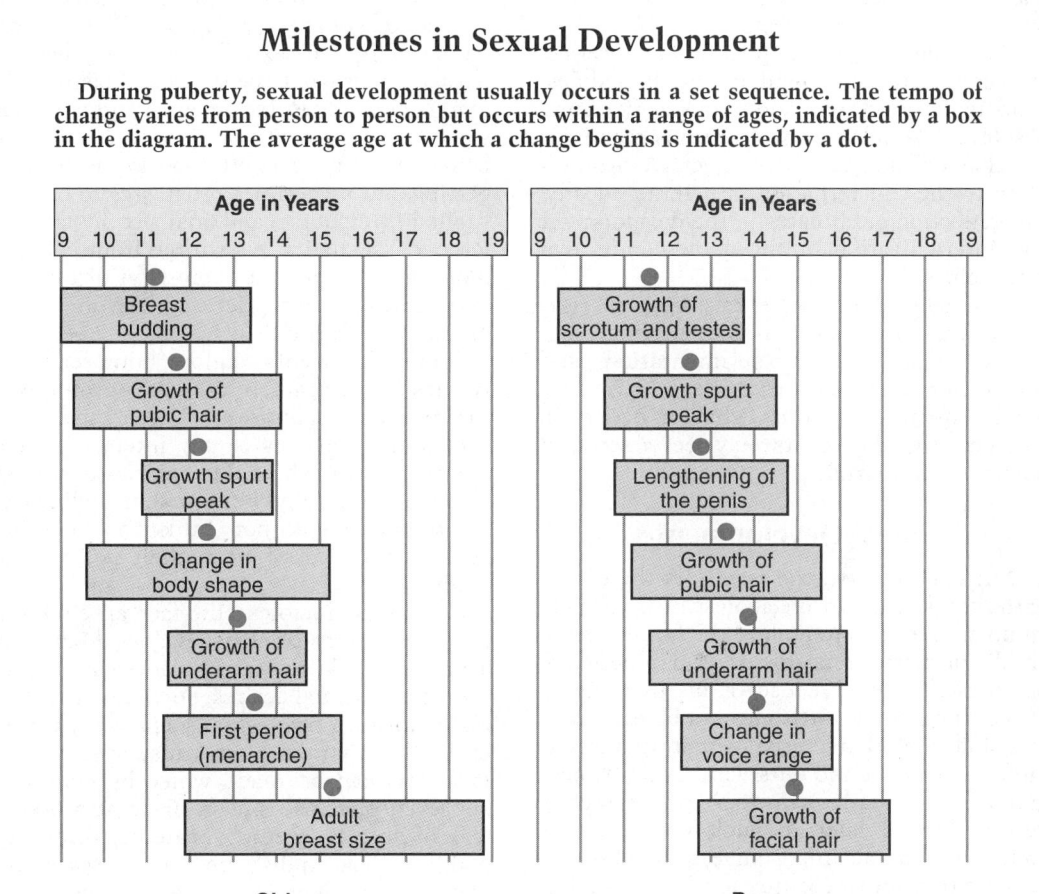

Girls

Boys

3½ inches can be expected in the year of maximum growth. In general, boys become heavier and taller than girls. By age 18, boys have about ¾ inch of growth remaining and girls have slightly less.

In boys, the first changes in sexual characteristics are enlargement of the scrotum and testes, followed by lengthening of the penis. Internally, the seminal vesicles and prostate gland enlarge. Next, pubic hair appears. Hair grows on the face and in the underarms about 2 years after it appears in the pubic area. The first ejaculation usually occurs between the ages of 12½ and 14, about 1 year after the penis begins to lengthen. Breast enlargement on one side or both is common in young adolescent boys and usually disappears within a year.

In the majority of girls, the first visible sign of sexual maturation is breast budding, closely

followed by the growth spurt. Soon afterward, pubic and underarm hair appears. The first menstrual period generally starts about 2 years after the breasts begin to enlarge. Height increases most before menstruation begins.

Intellectual and Behavioral Development

In early adolescence, a child begins to develop the capacity for abstract, logical thought. This increased sophistication leads to an enhanced awareness of self and the ability to reflect on one's own being. Because of the many noticeable physical changes of adolescence, this self-awareness often turns into self-consciousness, with an accompanying feeling of awkwardness. The adolescent also has a preoccupation with physical appearance and attractiveness and a heightened sensitivity to differences from peers.

The adolescent also applies his new reflective capabilities to moral issues. Pre-adolescents understand right and wrong as fixed and absolute. The adolescent questions standards of behavior and frequently rejects tradition—often to the consternation of parents. Ideally, this reflection culminates in the development and internalization of the adolescent's own moral code.

Many adolescents begin to engage in risk-taking behaviors, such as fast driving, substance abuse, sexual experimentation, and sometimes, theft and other illegal activities. Some experts think this behavior occurs in part because adolescents may feel a sense of power and immortality.

Social Development

During childhood, the family is the center of the child's life. During adolescence, the peer group often begins to replace the family as the child's primary social focus. Peer groups are often established because of distinctions in dress, appearance, attitudes, hobbies, interests, and other characteristics that may appear profound or trivial to outsiders. Initially, peer groups are usually same-sex but typically become mixed later in adolescence. These groups assume an importance to adolescents because they provide validation for the adolescent's tentative choices and support in stressful situations.

Those adolescents who, for various reasons, find themselves without a peer group often develop intense feelings of being different and alienated. Although these feelings often have little permanent effect, they may worsen any potential for dysfunctional or antisocial behavior. At the other extreme, the peer group assumes too much importance for some adolescents. Gang membership and behavior are more common when the home and social environments are unable to counterbalance the often dysfunctional demands of the peer group.▲

Development of Sexuality

During early adolescence, an increasing interest in sexual anatomy and pubertal changes

develops. These changes (or lack thereof) often are a source of anxiety. As adolescents mature emotionally and sexually, they may begin to engage in sexual behaviors. Masturbation among boys is nearly universal and is perhaps somewhat less common among girls. Sexual behavior with others often begins as extended petting, but sometimes progresses to oral sex, vaginal intercourse, and anal sex. By late adolescence, sexuality has shifted from being exploratory to being an expression of intimacy and sharing. Appropriate advice on safe-sex practices is essential.

Some adolescents explore homosexual activities but ultimately do not continue to be interested in same-sex relationships. Other adolescents never have any interest in opposite-sex relationships. Doctors do not understand exactly why homosexual feelings develop, but they do not think it is something adolescents "learn" from their peers or the media.

Homosexual adolescents face an emotional burden as their sexuality develops. Many teenagers are made to feel unwanted if they express homosexual desires. Such pressure (especially during a time when social acceptance is critically important) can cause severe stress. Problems can be made worse by comments and even physical threats made at school. A fear of abandonment by parents, sometimes real, may lead to dishonest or at least incomplete communication between adolescents and their parents. Threats of physical violence should be taken seriously and reported to school officials.

The emotional development of homosexual adolescents is best helped by supportive friends and family members. Family and friends should express the same interest and involvement as they would for heterosexual adolescents.

Preventive Health Care Visits

Annual health care visits allow a doctor to continue monitoring the adolescent's physical growth and sexual maturation. In most cases, the parent is not present during the examination. Examination of the skin (checking for acne), evaluation of the degree of sexual maturation, and examination of the back for scoliosis are particularly important in adolescence. Screening for sexually transmitted diseases should be performed for adolescents who are sexually active.

▲ see page 1558

Other appropriate screening tests might include a blood cholesterol level for adolescents whose families have a history of high cholesterol or heart disease and tuberculosis testing for adolescents with a history of exposure to tuberculosis. The doctor also makes sure the adolescent has had all appropriate vaccinations,▲ particularly hepatitis B, which may not have been given in childhood, and tetanus, which requires a booster.

The bulk of the doctor's visit with the adolescent encompasses discussions and questions about developmental, psychosocial, and behavioral issues. Typically, the doctor asks questions about an adolescent's home environment, academic achievement and goals, activities and hobbies, engagement in risk-taking behaviors, and emotional health. Equally important is counseling about physi-

cal and psychosocial development, healthy lifestyles, and injury prevention. Other discussions include the importance of wearing seatbelts, the dangers of drinking and driving, peer pressure, potential for becoming dependent on drugs or alcohol, readiness for parenthood, responsible sexual behavior, and avoiding violence. The doctor may provide a list of resources (for example, books, phone numbers, web sites) for the adolescent.

The doctor should also ask the parents about how they are handling the changes that come with adolescence. Specific questions about limit-setting, spending quality time with the adolescent, and discussion of expectations for behavior are typically included in the interview with the parents. Typically, the adolescent is not present for the interview with the parents.

CHAPTER 271

Problems in Adolescents

The most common problems adolescents face relate to growth and development, childhood illnesses that continue into adolescence, and experimentation with risky or illegal behavior. As adolescents try new behaviors, they become vulnerable to injury, legal consequences, and sexually transmitted diseases. Heterosexually active girls are at risk of becoming pregnant. Traumatic injuries, particularly from car and motorcycle accidents, are the leading cause of death and disability among adolescents. Interpersonal violence has become a particular problem among adolescents.

Adolescence is a time when mental health disorders, such as depression and schizophrenia,■ can become apparent, leading to a risk of suicide. Eating disorders, such as anorexia nervosa and bulimia nervosa,★ are particularly common in adolescent girls.

Delayed Sexual Maturation

Delayed sexual maturation is a delay in the onset of puberty and the development of the sexual organs.

The onset of sexual maturation (puberty) takes place when one part of the brain, the hy-

pothalamus, sends a chemical signal to another part of the brain, the pituitary gland. This signal tells the pituitary gland to begin releasing hormones called gonadotropins, which stimulate the growth of the sex organs (the testicles in boys and the ovaries in girls). The growing organs secrete sex hormones, such as testosterone (in boys) and estrogen (in girls). These hormones cause the development of sexual characteristics, including pubic and axillary hair in both sexes, facial hair and muscle mass in boys, and breast growth in girls, and of sexual desire (libido).

Some adolescents do not start their sexual development at the usual age. A delay may be perfectly normal, and in some families sexual maturation tends to occur later. In such adolescents, the growth rate before puberty is usually normal, and they otherwise appear healthy. Although the growth spurt and sexual maturation are delayed, they eventually proceed normally.

▲ see art on page 1493
■ see page 1632
★ see page 624

Various disorders, such as diabetes mellitus, inflammatory bowel disease, kidney disease, cystic fibrosis, and anemia, can delay or prevent sexual development. Development may be delayed in adolescents receiving radiation therapy or cancer chemotherapy. Adolescents, particularly girls, who become very thin because of excessive exercise or dieting often have delayed sexual maturation, including an absence of menstruation.

There are many uncommon causes of delayed sexual maturation. Chromosomal abnormalities (such as Turner syndrome in girls▲ and Klinefelter syndrome in boys■) and other genetic disorders can affect production of hormones. A tumor that damages the pituitary gland or the hypothalamus can lower the levels of gonadotropins or stop production of the hormones altogether. A mumps infection can damage the testicles and prevent puberty.

Symptoms and Diagnosis

In boys, the symptoms of delayed sexual maturation are lack of testicular enlargement by age 13½, lack of pubic hair by age 15, or a time lapse of more than 5 years from the start to the completion of genital enlargement. In girls, the symptoms are lack of breast development by age 13, more than 5 years from the beginning of breast growth to the first menstrual period, lack of pubic hair by age 14, or failure to menstruate by age 16. A short height (short stature) may indicate delayed maturation in both boys and girls.

Although adolescents are typically uncomfortable about being different from their peers, boys in particular are likely to feel psychologic stress and embarrassment from delayed puberty. Girls who remain smaller and less sexually mature than their peers are not stigmatized as quickly.

If an adolescent appears healthy and has no signs of any disorder—particularly if other family members were slow to mature—the doctor may elect to wait 6 to 12 months before conducting extensive testing. After this time, x-rays are often used to evaluate bone maturity. Adolescents whose bone maturity is delayed are probably just slow overall developers. Those with age-appropriate bone maturity are more likely to have delayed sexual maturation. They require blood tests to measure vari-

ous hormone levels, as well as tests for diabetes, anemia, and other disorders that can delay sexual development. Sometimes a chromosomal analysis may be performed. Computed tomography (CT) or magnetic resonance imaging (MRI) may be performed to ensure that there is no brain tumor.

Treatment

The treatment for delayed sexual maturation depends on its cause. Once a chronic underlying disorder has been treated, maturation usually proceeds. An adolescent who is naturally late in developing needs no treatment, although if the adolescent is severely stressed by the lack of development or development is extremely delayed, some doctors may give supplemental sex hormones to begin the process sooner. A genetic disorder cannot be cured, although replacing hormones may help sexual characteristics develop. Surgery may be needed for adolescents with tumors.

Short Stature

Short stature is height below normal for the child's age (according to standard charts for age and height).

The pituitary gland regulates the amount of growth hormone produced, which is an important factor in determining stature. If the pituitary gland produces too little growth hormone, abnormally slow growth and short stature with normal proportions (pituitary dwarfism) can result. Most short children, however, have normally functioning pituitary glands and are short because their growth spurt is late or their parents are relatively short. Chronic illnesses that affect the heart, lungs, kidneys, or intestine can also result in short stature. Abnormalities in the bone can also lead to very short stature.

Pituitary dwarfism is treated with growth hormone. Growth hormone is also used sometimes to increase height in children who have short stature but normally functioning pituitary glands, but this use is controversial. Some parents feel that short stature is a disorder, but most doctors do not approve of the use of growth hormone in these children. Regardless of the cause of short stature, pituitary hormone is effective only if given before the growth plates in the long bones become inactive. X-rays can help determine whether the growth plates are inactive.

▲ see page 1528   ■ see page 1530

When Puberty Starts Too Early

Precocious puberty and pseudoprecocious puberty are sexual maturation that begins before age 7 in a girl or before age 9 in a boy. True precocious puberty is caused by the early release of certain sex hormones (gonadotropins) from the pituitary gland. These hormones cause the ovaries or testes to develop and begin secreting other sex hormones, such as estrogen or testosterone. The estrogen or testosterone causes the development of puberty and the appearance of adult physical characteristics. This early hormone release may be caused by a tumor or other abnormality in the pituitary gland or the hypothalamus (the region of the brain that controls the pituitary gland).

In pseudoprecocious puberty, high levels of testosterone or estrogen are produced by a tumor or other abnormality in the adrenal gland or in a testis or ovary. These hormones do not cause the testes or ovaries themselves to mature but do cause a child to look more like an adult.

In both conditions, pubic and underarm hair grows, adult body odor develops, and the child's body shape changes. Acne may appear.

A boy develops facial hair, his penis lengthens, and his appearance becomes more masculine. A girl develops breasts and may start to have menstrual periods, especially if she has true precocious puberty. Height increases rapidly but stops at an early age. Therefore, the final height is shorter than would be expected. In true precocious puberty, the sex glands (ovaries or testes) also mature and enlarge, whereas in pseudoprecocious puberty, the sex glands remain immature. True precocious puberty is 2 to 5 times more common in girls.

Testotoxicosis is a rare hereditary form of pseudoprecocious puberty that affects boys; it results directly from maturation of the testes, independent of the hypothalamus or pituitary gland. Similarly, McCune-Albright syndrome is a genetic (but not hereditary) disorder that results in pseudoprecocious puberty; this disorder is more common in girls.

Doctors measure blood hormone levels and take x-rays of the hand and wrist to estimate bone maturity. They perform an ultrasound of the pelvis and adrenal glands and computed tomography (CT) or magnetic resonance imaging (MRI) of the head to check for tumors in the adrenal glands, hypothalamus, or pituitary gland. A test to measure the effect of gonadotropin-releasing hormone on pituitary hormone levels can help doctors diagnose the cause.

In true precocious puberty, taking a drug such as long-acting injections of leuprolide (synthetic gonadotropin-releasing hormone) or daily injections of deslorelin or histrelin stops the pituitary gland from producing sex hormones by desensitizing it to the effects of the body's own gonadotropin-releasing hormone. In pseudoprecocious puberty, a doctor may try to inhibit the action of the sex hormones with various drugs. The antifungal drug ketoconazole reduces the levels of testosterone circulating in the blood in boys who have testotoxicosis. A drug called testolactone reduces the levels of estrogen in adolescents who have McCune-Albright syndrome. In both of these conditions, spironolactone or cyproterone may also be useful.

When a tumor is responsible for true precocious or pseudoprecocious puberty, removing it may cure the condition.

Obesity

Obesity is the accumulation of excessive body fat.

Obesity is twice as common in adolescents as it was 30 years ago. Although most of the complications of obesity occur in adulthood,▲ obese adolescents are more likely than other adolescents to have high blood pressure and type 2 diabetes. Although fewer than one third of obese adults were obese as adolescents, most obese adolescents remain obese in adulthood.

The factors that influence obesity among adolescents are the same as those among adults. Parents often are concerned that obesity is the result of some type of endocrine disease, such as hypothyroidism, but such disorders are rarely the cause. Adolescents with weight gain caused by endocrine disorders are usually of small stature and have other signs of the underlying condition. Most obese adolescents simply eat too much and exercise too little. Because of society's stigma against obesity, many obese adolescents have a poor self-image and become increasingly sedentary and socially isolated.

Intervention for obese adolescents should be focused on developing healthy eating and ex-

▲ see page 917

ercise habits rather than on losing a specific amount of weight. Caloric intake is reduced by establishing a well-balanced diet of ordinary foods, making permanent changes in eating habits, and increasing physical activity. Summer camps for obese adolescents usually help them lose a significant amount of weight, but without continuing effort, the weight is usually regained. Counseling to help adolescents cope with their problems, including poor self-esteem, may be helpful.

Drugs that help reduce weight are generally not used during adolescence because of concerns about safety and possible abuse. One exception is for obese adolescents with a strong family history of type 2 diabetes; they are at high risk for developing diabetes. The drug metformin, which is used to treat diabetes, may help them lose weight and also lower their risk of becoming diabetic.

School Problems

School constitutes a large part of an adolescent's existence. Difficulties in almost any area of life often manifest as school problems.

School problems during the adolescent years may be the result of rebellion and a need for independence. Less commonly, they may be caused by mental health disorders, such as anxiety or depression. Substance use, abuse, and family conflict also are common contributors to school problems. Sometimes, inappropriate academic placement—particularly in adolescents with a learning disability or mild mental retardation that was not recognized early in life—causes school problems. In general, adolescents with significant school problems should undergo educational testing and a mental health evaluation. Specific problems are treated as needed, and general support and encouragement are provided.

Particular school problems include fear of going to school, truancy, dropping out, and academic underachievement. Problems that developed earlier in childhood, such as attention deficit/hyperactivity disorder (ADHD) and learning disorders,▲ may continue to cause school problems for adolescents.

Between 1% and 5% of adolescents develop fear of going to school. This fear may be generalized or related to a particular person (a

teacher or another student) or event at school (such as physical education class). The adolescent may develop physical symptoms, such as abdominal pain, or may simply refuse to go to school. School personnel and family members should identify the reason, if any, for the fear and encourage the adolescent to attend school.

Adolescents who are repeatedly truant or drop out of school have made a conscious decision to miss school. These adolescents generally have poor academic achievement and have had little success or satisfaction from school-related activities. They often have engaged in high-risk behaviors, such as having unprotected sex, taking drugs, and engaging in violence. Adolescents at risk for dropping out should be made aware of other educational options, such as vocational training and alternative programs.

Behavioral Problems

Adolescence is a time for developing independence. Typically, adolescents exercise their independence by questioning their parents' rules, which at times leads to rule breaking. Parents and doctors must distinguish occasional errors of judgment from a degree of misbehavior that requires professional intervention. The severity and frequency of infractions are guides. For example, drinking habitually, fighting often, frequent truancy and theft are much more significant than isolated episodes of the same activities. Other warning signs include deterioration of performance at school and running away from home.

Children occasionally engage in physical confrontation. However, during adolescence, the frequency and severity of violent interactions increase. Although episodes of violence at school are highly publicized, adolescents are much more likely to be involved with violence (or more often the threat of violence) at home and outside of school. Many factors, including developmental issues, gang membership, access to firearms, substance use, and poverty, contribute to an increased risk of violence for adolescents. Of particular concern are adolescents who, in an altercation, cause serious injury or use a weapon.

Because adolescents are much more independent and mobile than they were as children, they are often out of the direct physical control of adults. In these circumstances, adolescents' behavior is determined by their own moral and behavioral code. The parents guide

▲ see pages 1549 and 1551

rather than directly control the adolescents' actions. Adolescents who feel warmth and support from their parents are less likely to engage in risky behaviors. Also, parents who convey clear expectations regarding their adolescents' behavior and who demonstrate consistent limit setting and monitoring are less likely to have adolescents who engage in risky behaviors. Authoritative parenting, as opposed to harsh or permissive parenting, is most likely to promote mature behaviors.

Authoritative parents typically use a system of graduated privileges, in which the adolescent is initially given small bits of responsibility and freedom (such as caring for a pet, doing household chores, picking out clothing, or decorating his room). If the adolescent handles this responsibility appropriately over a period of time, freedom is increased. Abuses of freedom are dealt with by taking away privileges. Each increase in freedom requires close attention by parents to make sure the adolescent is where and with whom he is supposed to be, returns at the proper time, and so forth.

Some parents and their adolescents clash over almost everything. In these situations, the core issue is really control—adolescents want to feel in control of their lives and parents want adolescents to know they still make the rules. In these situations, everyone may benefit from the parents focusing their efforts on the adolescents' actions (attending school, complying with household responsibilities) rather than on expressions (dress, hairstyle, preferred entertainment).

Adolescents whose behavior is still dangerous or otherwise unacceptable despite their parents' best efforts may need professional intervention. Substance abuse is a common trigger of behavioral problems and often requires specific therapy. Behavioral problems may be the first sign of depression or other mental health disorders. Such disorders typically require treatment with drugs as well as counseling. In extreme cases, some adolescents may also need legal intervention in the form of probation.

Drug and Substance Use and Abuse

Substance use among adolescents occurs on a spectrum from experimentation to dependence.▲ The consequences range from none to life threatening, depending on the substance, the circumstances, and the frequency of use.

However, even occasional use can produce significant harm, such as overdose, motor vehicle collision, and unwanted pregnancy. Although experimentation and occasional usage are common, actual drug dependence is not.

Alcohol is the substance most often used among adolescents. About 80% of high school seniors reported trying alcohol; some engage in binge drinking, which is defined as having more than 5 drinks in a row. There are risk factors for whether an adolescent will try alcohol. Genetics may be a factor; adolescents who have a family member who is an alcoholic should be made aware of the risk. Adolescents whose friends and siblings drink excessively may think this behavior is acceptable. Society and the media often model drinking as being acceptable. Despite these influences, parents can make a difference by conveying clear expectations to their adolescent regarding drinking, setting limits consistently, and monitoring the adolescent.

The majority of adults who smoke cigarettes begin smoking during adolescence. Nearly one fifth of ninth graders report smoking regularly. If an adolescent reaches the age of 18 to 19 years without becoming a smoker, it is highly unlikely that he will become a smoker as an adult. Factors that increase the likelihood of an adolescent smoking are having parents who smoke (the single most predictive factor), peers who smoke, and poor self-esteem. Using other illegal substances is also a factor. Parents can prevent their adolescent from smoking by not smoking themselves (or quitting), by openly discussing the hazards of tobacco, and by convincing adolescents who already smoke to quit and to seek medical assistance in quitting if necessary.

Use of illegal substances in adolescents, although decreasing overall in the last few years, remains high. In the year 2000, about 54% of 12th graders had used illegal drugs at some time in their life. About 62% of 12th graders reported having been drunk; 49% reported use of marijuana; 16%, amphetamines; 13%, hallucinogens; 9%, barbiturates; 9%, cocaine; and 2%, heroin. Use of methylenedioxymethamphetamine (Ecstasy), unlike the other drugs mentioned, increased dramatically in the last few years, with 11% of 12th graders reporting use at some time.

▲ see also page 646

Up to 6% of boys in high school, including a number of non-athletes, have used anabolic steroids at least once. A particular problem with anabolic steroid use in adolescents is early closure of the growth plates at the ends of bones, resulting in permanent short stature. Other side effects are common to both adolescents and adults.▲

Adolescents as young as 12 to 14 years of age may be involved in substance use. Although there are risk factors for adolescents engaging in substance use, it is difficult to predict which adolescents will engage in the most serious forms of abuse. Parents should look for erratic behavior in their adolescent, mood swings, a change in friends, and declining school performance. If parents notice any of these behaviors, they should discuss their concerns with the adolescent and his doctor.■

The doctor can help assess whether an adolescent has a problem with substance use. Some parents simply bring the adolescent into a doctor demanding that he perform a urine drug test. There are a few points for a parent to keep in mind: The doctor cannot force the adolescent to take a drug test if he refuses. Results of a urine test may be falsely negative; factors influencing results are the metabolism of the drug and the time it was last used. Most importantly, in an atmosphere of accusation and confrontation, it will be difficult for the doctor to obtain a history from the adolescent, which is key to making the diagnosis.

If the doctor thinks the adolescent does have a problem, he can refer the adolescent to a professional with expertise in substance abuse; this person can make the diagnosis and determine the treatment needed. Treatment for adolescents is similar to that of adults★ but is typically conducted in a setting with other adolescents.

Contraception and Adolescent Pregnancy

Although adolescents may engage in sexual activity, many sexually active adolescents are not fully informed about contraception, pregnancy, and sexually transmitted diseases, including human immunodeficiency virus (HIV) infection. Impulsivity, lack of planning, and concurrent drug and alcohol use decrease the likelihood that adolescents will use birth control and barrier protection.

Any of the adult contraceptive methods may be used by adolescents.● Problems with adolescents and contraception revolve around adherence. For example, many adolescent girls who are taking oral contraceptives forget to take them regularly or stop using them for various reasons—often not substituting another form of birth control. Some girls do not feel empowered to ask their male partners to use condoms during sex. Boys generally prefer not to use condoms.

Because adolescence is a transitional stage in life, pregnancy can add significant emotional stress. Pregnant adolescents and their partners tend to drop out of school or job training, thus worsening their economic status, lowering their self-esteem, and straining personal relationships.

Pregnant adolescents, particularly the very young and those who are not receiving prenatal care, are more likely than women in their 20s to have medical problems such as anemia and toxemia. Infants of young mothers (especially mothers younger than 15 years) are more likely to be born prematurely and to have a low birth weight. However, with proper prenatal care, older adolescents have no higher risk of pregnancy problems than adults from similar backgrounds.

Having an abortion◆ does not remove the psychologic problems of an unwanted pregnancy—either for the adolescent girl or her partner. Emotional crises may occur when the pregnancy is diagnosed, when the decision to have an abortion is made, immediately after the abortion is performed, when the baby would have been born, and on the anniversaries of that date. Family counseling and education about contraceptive methods, for both the girl and her partner, can be very helpful.

Parents may have different reactions when their daughter says she is pregnant or their son says his girlfriend is pregnant. Emotions may range from apathy to disappointment and anger. It is important for parents to express their support and willingness to help the adolescent sort through his or her choices. Parents and adolescents need to communicate openly about abortion, adoption, and parenthood—all tough options for the adolescent to struggle with alone.

▲ see box on page 648

■ see also box on page 1639

★ see page 646   ● see page 1419

◆ see page 1426

CHAPTER 272

Bacterial Infections

Bacteria are microscopic, single-celled organisms▲; only some bacteria cause disease in people. The most common bacterial infections among children are skin infections (including impetigo), ear infections, and throat infections (strep throat). These disorders are treated similarly in adults and children. Other infections occur at all ages but have particular treatment considerations in children.

Certain children are at particular risk for bacterial infections. These children include infants younger than 2 months of age, children who have no spleen or who have an immune system disorder, and children who have sickle cell disease.

Sometimes doctors diagnose bacterial infections by the typical symptoms they produce. Usually, however, bacteria must be identified in samples of tissue or body fluids, such as blood, urine, pus, or cerebrospinal fluid. Sometimes bacteria from these samples can be recognized under a microscope or identified with a rapid detection test. Usually, however, they are too few or too small to see, so doctors must try to grow them in the laboratory. It typically takes 24 to 48 hours to grow (culture) the organism. Cultures can also be used to test the susceptibility of a microorganism to various antibiotics; the results can help a doctor determine which drug to use in treating an infected child. Doctors may treat certain potentially serious childhood infections with antibiotics, preemptively while culture results are pending and then change or discontinue the antibiotics when results are obtained.

Occult Bacteremia

Occult (hidden) bacteremia is the presence of bacteria in the bloodstream of a child who has a fever but who may not appear particularly sick and who has no apparent other source of infection.

Children younger than 3 years commonly develop fevers. Most of the time, they have other symptoms, such as a cough and runny nose, which allow doctors to diagnose the cause. About one third of the time, children have no other symptoms besides fever. Most of these children have viral infections that go away without treatment. However, 2 to 4% of such children have bacteria circulating in the bloodstream (bacteremia). *Streptococcus pneumoniae* is the most common type of bacteria causing occult bacteremia. Circulating bacteria are almost never present in older children or adults with fever but no other symptoms. These circulating bacteria may attack various organs and result in serious illnesses, such as pneumonia or meningitis. Although only about 10 to 15% of children with occult bacteremia develop these serious problems, doctors perform blood cultures to identify the bacteria before such problems develop. An elevated white blood cell count indicates a higher risk of bacterial infection; in this case, a doctor may choose to start antibiotics before blood culture results are available.

Because doctors cannot tell with certainty which febrile children have bacteremia, doctors may perform complete blood cell counts and blood cultures on some children younger than 3 years whose temperature is higher than 102° F and who do not have an apparent reason for their fever. Because occult bacteremia is much less common in children older than 3, these children do not require blood cultures.

For children who may have occult bacteremia, doctors reevaluate them in 24 to 48 hours, when culture results are available. Children with positive culture results are given antibiotics by mouth at home if they do not appear very ill. Children who show signs of serious illness are typically given intravenous antibiotics in the hospital. Sometimes doctors treat certain children, such as those with an elevated white blood cell count, with a single injection of an antibiotic, such as ceftriaxone, while awaiting the results of blood cultures.

A new vaccine against *Streptococcus pneumoniae*, given to infants, will greatly reduce the chance of occult bacteremia in vaccinated children. The *Haemophilus influenzae* type b vaccine, now given to nearly all children in the United States, has nearly eliminated occult bacteremia due to *Haemophilus influenzae* type b.

▲ see page 1095

Bacterial Infections Preventable With Routine Immunization*

- Diphtheria
- Infection with *Haemophilus influenzae* type b (meningitis, epiglottitis, some severe eye infections, occult bacteremia)
- Infection with *Streptococcus pneumoniae* (pneumonia, meningitis, occult bacteremia, ear infections)
- Pertussis
- Tetanus

*Note: Many viral infections can also be prevented with routine immunization.▲

Bacterial Meningitis

Bacterial meningitis is infection of the layers of tissue covering the brain and spinal cord (meninges).

Meningitis can occur at any age. Meningitis is similar in older children, adolescents, and adults■ but different in newborns and infants.

Children at particular risk for meningitis include those with sickle cell disease and those lacking a spleen. Children with congenital deformities of the face and skull may have defects in the bones that allow bacteria access to the meninges. Children who have a weakened immune system, such as those with AIDS or those who have received chemotherapy, are more susceptible to meningitis.

Causes

Meningitis in newborns is typically caused by bacteria acquired from the birth canal. The most common such bacteria are group B streptococci, *Escherichia coli*, and *Listeria monocytogenes*. Older children usually develop infection from contact with respiratory secretions from infected people. Bacteria that infect older children include *Streptococcus pneumoniae* and *Neisseria meningitidis*. *Haemophilus influenzae* type b was the most common cause of meningitis, but the widespread use of vaccination against that organism has now made it a rare cause. A new, improved vaccine against *Streptococcus pneumoniae* also should make this organism a rare cause of childhood meningitis.

▲ see box on page 1493 ■ see page 529
★ see art on page 443

Symptoms and Diagnosis

Older children and adolescents with meningitis typically have a few days of increasing fever, headache, confusion, and a stiff neck. They may have an upper respiratory tract infection that is unrelated to the meningitis. Newborns and infants rarely develop a stiff neck and are unable to communicate specific discomfort. These younger children become fussy and irritable (particularly when they are held) and stop feeding—important signs that should alert parents to a possibly serious problem. Sometimes newborns and infants have fever, vomiting, or a skin rash. One third have seizures. The nerves controlling some eye and facial movements may be damaged, causing an eye to turn inward or outward or the facial expression to become lopsided. In about 25% of newborns with meningitis, increased pressure of the fluid around the brain may make the fontanelles (the soft spots between the skull bones) bulge or feel firm. These symptoms usually develop over at least 1 to 2 days, but some infants, particularly those between birth and 3 or 4 months old, become ill very rapidly, progressing from health to near death in less than 24 hours.

Pockets of pus (abscesses) may rarely form within the brain of infants with meningitis because of certain germs. As the abscesses grow, pressure on the brain increases, resulting in vomiting, head enlargement, and bulging fontanelles.

A doctor diagnoses bacterial meningitis by examining and culturing a sample of cerebrospinal fluid obtained through a spinal tap (lumbar puncture).★ Doctors also perform blood cultures to look for bacteria in the bloodstream. Ultrasound examination or computed tomography (CT) may be used to determine if an abscess is present.

Prevention, Prognosis, and Treatment

Health care professionals can help prevent bacterial meningitis by ensuring that all children receive the *Haemophilus influenzae* type b and *Streptococcus pneumoniae* vaccines.

Even with timely, appropriate treatment, as many as 30% of newborns with bacterial meningitis die. In older infants and children, mortality varies from 3 to 5% when the cause is *Haemophilus influenzae* type b, 5 to 10% when the cause is *Neisseria meningitidis*, and 10 to 15% when the cause is *Streptococcus pneumoniae*. Nearly 25% of children with a brain abscess die.

Of the infants who survive, 10 to 20% develop serious brain and nerve damage, such as enlargement of the ventricles (hydrocephalus), deafness, cerebral palsy, and mental retardation. Up to 50% have mild residual problems, such as learning disorders, mild hearing loss, or occasional seizures.

Doctors give high doses of antibiotics intravenously as soon as they suspect meningitis. Very sick children receive antibiotics even before a spinal tap is performed. A doctor chooses an antibiotic based on the type of bacteria causing the meningitis. Children older than 6 weeks of age sometimes are given corticosteroids to help prevent permanent neurologic problems.

Diphtheria

Diphtheria is a contagious, sometimes fatal, infection of the upper respiratory tract caused by the bacterium Corynebacterium diphtheriae.

Years ago, diphtheria was one of the leading causes of death among children. Today, diphtheria is rare in developed countries, primarily because of widespread vaccination. Fewer than five cases occur in the United States each year, but diphtheria bacteria still exist in the world and can cause outbreaks if vaccination is inadequate.

The bacteria that cause diphtheria are usually spread in droplets of moisture coughed into the air. Usually the bacteria multiply on or near the surface of the mucous membranes of the mouth or throat, where they cause inflammation. Some types of *Corynebacterium diphtheriae* release a potent toxin, which can damage the heart, nerves, kidneys, and brain.

Symptoms and Diagnosis

The illness begins 1 to 4 days after exposure to the bacteria. Symptoms begin abruptly with sore throat, a general feeling of illness (malaise), and a fever up to 103° F. The child also may have a fast heart rate, nausea, vomiting, chills, and a headache. The lymph nodes in the neck may swell. The inflammation may make the throat swell, narrowing the airway and making breathing extremely difficult.

Typically, the bacteria form a tough, gray pseudomembrane—a sheet of material composed of dead white blood cells, bacteria, and other substances—near the tonsils or other parts of the throat. The pseudomembrane narrows the airway and may suddenly become detached and block the airway completely, preventing the child from being able to breathe. The toxin produced by diphtheria bacteria generally affects certain nerves, producing symptoms, such as swallowing difficulty, weakness of eye muscles, and trouble moving the arms and legs. The bacterial toxin may also damage the heart muscle (myocarditis), sometimes causing heart failure and death.

A doctor suspects diphtheria in a sick child who has a sore throat with a pseudomembrane, particularly if there is paralysis of muscles of the face or throat, and if the child was not vaccinated. The diagnosis is confirmed by culture of material from the child's throat.

Prevention and Treatment

Children are routinely immunized against diphtheria. The diphtheria vaccine is usually combined with vaccines for tetanus and pertussis (whooping cough).▲

A child with symptoms of diphtheria is typically hospitalized in an intensive care unit and given antibodies to neutralize the diphtheria toxin. Doctors also give antibiotics, such as penicillin or erythromycin, to kill the diphtheria bacteria.

Recovery from severe diphtheria is slow, and a child with the infection must avoid resuming activities too soon. Even normal physical exertion may harm an inflamed heart.

Retropharyngeal Abscess

A retropharyngeal abscess is a collection of pus in the lymph nodes at the back of the throat.

Because the lymph nodes at the back of the throat disappear after childhood, a retropharyngeal abscess almost never occurs in adults. An abscess is usually caused by a bacterial infection that has spread from the tonsils, throat, sinuses, adenoids, nose, or middle ear. Many infections are caused by a combination of bacteria. An injury to the back of the throat from a sharp object, such as a fish bone, occasionally causes a retropharyngeal abscess. Rarely, tuberculosis can also cause a retropharyngeal abscess.

Symptoms and Diagnosis

The main symptoms are pain when swallowing, a fever, and enlargement of the lymph

▲ see page 1493

nodes in the neck. The voice is muffled, and the child drools. The abscess can block the airway, causing difficulty in breathing. The child tends to lie on his back, tilt his head and neck back, and raise his chin to make breathing easier.

Complications include bleeding around the abscess, rupture of the abscess into the airway (which can block the airway), and pneumonia. The larynx may go into spasm and further interfere with breathing. Blood clots may form in the jugular veins of the neck. Infection may spread down into the chest.

After observing the symptoms, a doctor orders x-rays and computed tomography (CT) scans of the neck to confirm the diagnosis.

Treatment and Prognosis

Retropharyngeal abscesses often need to be drained, which a doctor does surgically by cutting open the abscess and allowing the pus to drain out. Penicillin plus metronidazole, clindamycin, cefoxitin, or other antibiotics is given, at first intravenously, and then by mouth. Most children do well with prompt treatment.

Epiglottitis

Epiglottitis is a severe bacterial infection of the epiglottis, which can block the windpipe, obstructing air flow.

The epiglottis is the structure that closes the entrance to the voice box and windpipe (larynx and trachea) during swallowing. Epiglottitis is most common in children 2 to 5 years old. It is uncommon in children younger than 2 but may affect people of any age, including adults.▲ In the past, most cases of childhood epiglottitis were caused by the bacterium *Haemophilus influenzae* type b. Now that most children are vaccinated against *Haemophilus influenzae* type b, the disease is quite rare and is typically caused by *Streptococcus pneumoniae*, other streptococci, and staphylococci. Children with epiglottitis often have bacteria in the bloodstream (bacteremia), which sometimes spreads the infection to the lungs, the joints, the tissues covering the brain (meninges), the sac around the heart, or the tissue beneath the skin.

Symptoms

The infection usually begins suddenly and progresses rapidly. A previously healthy child

▲ see page 1268

develops a sore throat, and often a high fever. Difficulties in swallowing and breathing are common. The child usually drools, breathes rapidly, and has a loud noise while inhaling (called stridor). The difficulty in breathing often causes the child to lean forward while stretching the neck backward to try to increase the amount of air reaching the lungs. Labored breathing may lead to a buildup of carbon dioxide and low oxygen levels in the bloodstream, causing agitation and confusion followed by sluggishness (lethargy). The swollen epiglottis makes coughing up mucus difficult. Epiglottitis can quickly become fatal because swelling of the infected tissue may block the airway and cut off breathing.

Prevention, Diagnosis, and Treatment

Prevention of epiglottitis is better than treatment. Prevention is achieved by ensuring that all children receive the *Haemophilus influenzae* type b and *Streptococcus pneumoniae* vaccines.

Epiglottitis is an emergency, and a child is hospitalized immediately when a doctor suspects it. If the child does not have all of the typical symptoms of epiglottitis and does not appear seriously ill, the doctor sometimes takes an x-ray of the neck, which can show an enlarged epiglottis. The doctor does not hold the child down or use a tongue depressor to look in the throat, because these manipulations may cause throat spasm and complete airway blockage in a child with epiglottitis.

If an enlarged epiglottis is seen on x-ray or the child appears seriously ill, doctors examine the child under anesthesia in the operating room using a laryngoscope. If the examination shows epiglottitis or triggers throat spasm, the doctor inserts a plastic tube (endotracheal tube) into the airway to keep it open. If the airway is too swollen to allow placement of an endotracheal tube, the doctor cuts an opening through the front of the neck (tracheostomy) and inserts the tube. This tube is left in place for several days until the swelling of the epiglottis goes down. The child also receives antibiotics, such as ceftriaxone or ampicillin-sulbactam. Once the child's airway is opened, the prognosis is good.

Pertussis

Pertussis (whooping cough) is a highly contagious infection caused by the bacterium Bordetella pertussis, which results in fits of coughing that usually end in a prolonged, high-pitched, deeply indrawn breath (the whoop).

Pertussis was once rampant in the United States but is now uncommon. However, pertussis remains a major problem throughout the world. Local epidemics among unimmunized people occur every 3 to 5 years. A person may develop pertussis at any age, although nearly two thirds of cases occur in children younger than 5 years. One attack of pertussis does not always give full immunity for life, but a second attack, if it occurs, is usually mild and not always recognized as pertussis. In fact, some adults with "walking pneumonia" actually have pertussis. Pertussis is most serious in children younger than 2 years.

An infected person spreads pertussis organisms into the air in droplets of moisture produced by coughing. Anyone nearby may inhale these droplets and become infected. Pertussis usually is not contagious after the third week of the infection.

Symptoms

The illness lasts about 6 weeks, progressing through three stages: mild cold-like symptoms, severe coughing fits, and gradual recovery. Cold-like symptoms include sneezing, runny nose, and a general feeling of illness (malaise). After 1 or 2 weeks, the person develops typical coughing fits. These fits typically consist of 5 to 15 or more rapid consecutive coughs followed by the whoop (a prolonged, high-pitched, deeply indrawn breath). After a fit, breathing is normal, but another coughing fit follows shortly thereafter. The cough often produces large amounts of thick mucus (usually swallowed by infants and children or seen as large bubbles from the nose). In younger children, vomiting often follows a prolonged fit of coughing. In infants, choking spells and pauses in breathing (apnea), possibly causing the skin to turn blue, can occur.

About one fourth of children develop pneumonia, resulting in difficulty breathing. Ear infections (otitis media) also frequently develop as a result of pertussis. Rarely, pertussis affects the brain of infants. Bleeding, swelling, or inflammation of the brain may cause seizures, confusion, brain damage, and mental retardation.

After several weeks, the coughing fits gradually subside, but for many weeks or even months the person has a lingering, persistent cough.

Diagnosis and Prognosis

Doctors suspect pertussis because of the typical whooping cough or other symptoms and confirm the diagnosis by culture of a sample of mucus from the back of the nose or throat. Culture results often are negative after several weeks of illness; other diagnostic tests performed on samples from the nose or throat may be helpful (polymerase chain reaction or rapid detection test).

The majority of children with pertussis recover completely, although slowly. About 1 to 2% of the children younger than 1 year die.

Prevention and Treatment

Children are routinely vaccinated against pertussis. The pertussis vaccine is usually combined with vaccines for diphtheria and tetanus.▲ The antibiotic erythromycin (or sometimes clarithromycin or azithromycin) is given as a preventive measure to children exposed to pertussis.

Severely ill infants are usually hospitalized because their breathing difficulty may become so severe that they require mechanical ventilation through a tube placed in their windpipe. Others may need extra oxygen and intravenous fluids. Older children who have mild disease are treated at home. Cough medicines are of questionable value and are not usually used.

The antibiotic erythromycin, clarithromycin, or azithromycin is usually used to eradicate the bacteria causing pertussis. Antibiotics are also used for infections that accompany the pertussis, such as pneumonia and ear infection.

Rheumatic Fever

Rheumatic fever is inflammation of the body's organ systems, especially the joints and the heart, resulting from a complication of streptococcal infection of the throat.

Although rheumatic fever follows a streptococcal infection, it is not an infection. Rather, it is an inflammatory reaction to the infection. Most people with rheumatic fever recover, but the heart is permanently damaged in a small percentage of people.

In the United States, rheumatic fever rarely develops before age 4 or after age 18 and is much less common than in developing coun-

---

▲ see page 1493

tries, probably because antibiotics are widely used to treat streptococcal infections at an early stage. However, the incidence of rheumatic fever sometimes rises and falls in a particular area for unknown reasons. Overcrowded living conditions seem to increase the risk of rheumatic fever, and heredity seems to play a part. In the United States, a child who has a streptococcal throat infection but is not treated has only a 0.4 to 1% chance of developing rheumatic fever. About half of the children who previously had rheumatic fever will develop it again with another streptococcal throat infection. Rheumatic fever follows streptococcal infections of the throat but not those of the skin (impetigo) or other areas of the body; the reasons are not known.

Symptoms

Rheumatic fever affects many parts of the body, such as the joints, heart, and skin. Symptoms of rheumatic fever vary greatly, depending on which parts of the body become inflamed. Typically, symptoms begin several weeks after the disappearance of strep throat. The most common symptoms of rheumatic fever are joint pain, fever, chest pain or palpitations caused by heart inflammation, jerky uncontrollable movements (Sydenham's chorea), a rash, and small bumps (nodules) under the skin. A child may have one symptom or several.

Joint pain and fever are the most common first symptoms. One or several joints suddenly become painful and feel tender when touched. They may also be red, hot, and swollen and may contain fluid. Ankles, knees, elbows, and wrists are commonly affected; the shoulders, hips, and small joints of the hands and feet also may be affected. As pain in one joint improves, pain in another starts (migratory pain). Joint pains may be mild or severe, and typically last 2 to 4 weeks. Long-term joint damage from rheumatic fever does not develop.

Sometimes, children with heart inflammation have no symptoms, and the past inflammation is recognized years later when heart damage is discovered. Some children feel their heart beating rapidly. Others have chest pain caused by inflammation of the sac around the heart. Heart failure may develop, causing the child to feel tired and short of breath, with

nausea, vomiting, stomachache, or a hacking cough.

Heart inflammation disappears gradually, usually within 5 months. However, it may permanently damage the heart valves, resulting in rheumatic heart disease. The likelihood of rheumatic heart disease varies with the severity of the initial heart inflammation. About 1% of people who had no heart inflammation develop rheumatic heart disease, compared to 30% with mild inflammation and 70% with severe inflammation. In rheumatic heart disease, the valve between the left atrium and ventricle (mitral valve) is most commonly damaged. The valve may become leaky (mitral valve regurgitation), abnormally narrow (mitral valve stenosis), or both.▲ Valve damage causes the characteristic heart murmurs that enable a doctor to diagnose rheumatic fever. Later in life, usually in middle age, the valve damage may cause heart failure■ and atrial fibrillation, an abnormal heart rhythm.★

A flat painless rash with a wavy edge (erythema marginatum) may appear as the other symptoms subside. It lasts for only a short time, sometimes less than a day. In children with heart inflammation, small, hard nodules may form under the skin. The nodules are usually painless and disappear without treatment.

Jerky uncontrollable movements (Sydenham's chorea) may begin gradually in children with rheumatic fever, but usually only after all other symptoms have improved. A month may go by before the movements become so intense that the child is taken to a doctor. By then, the child typically has rapid, purposeless, sporadic movements that disappear during sleep. The movements may involve any muscle except those of the eyes. Facial grimacing is common. In mild cases, the child may seem clumsy and may have slight difficulties in dressing and eating. In extreme cases, the child may have to be protected from injuring himself with his flailing arms or legs. The chorea lasts between 4 and 8 months.

Diagnosis

A doctor bases the diagnosis of rheumatic fever mainly on the characteristic combination of symptoms. Blood tests showing high levels of antibodies to streptococci may be helpful, but low levels of these antibodies are present in many children who do not have rheumatic fever. Abnormal heart rhythms

---

▲ see pages 175 and 178   ■ see page 150

★ see page 163

caused by heart inflammation can be seen on an electrocardiogram (ECG—a recording of the heart's electrical activity). An echocardiogram (an image of structures in the heart produced by ultrasound waves) may be used to diagnose abnormalities of the heart valves.

Prevention and Treatment

The best way to prevent rheumatic fever is with prompt and complete antibiotic treatment of any streptococcal throat infection. In addition, children who have had rheumatic fever should be given penicillin by mouth every day, or by monthly injections into the muscle, to help prevent another streptococcal infection. This preventive treatment should be continued until adulthood, and some doctors feel that it should be continued for life.

Treatment of rheumatic fever has three goals: curing any residual streptococcal infection; reducing inflammation, particularly in the joints and heart; and limiting physical activity that might aggravate the inflamed structures.

Doctors give children with rheumatic fever an injection of a long-acting penicillin to eliminate any remaining infection. Aspirin is given in high doses to reduce inflammation and pain, particularly if inflammation has reached the joints and heart. It is unclear whether other nonsteroidal anti-inflammatory drugs (NSAIDs) are as effective as aspirin. Analgesics, such as codeine, are sometimes used in addition to aspirin. If heart inflammation is severe, corticosteroids such as prednisone may be given to further reduce inflammation.

Bed rest may help by avoiding stress on the painful, inflamed joints. When the heart is inflamed, more rest is generally suggested.

If the heart valves become damaged, the risk of developing a valve infection (endocarditis) remains throughout life.▲ Those who have heart damage must always take an antibiotic before undergoing any surgery, including dental surgery, even in adulthood.

Urinary Tract Infection

A urinary tract infection (UTI) is a bacterial infection of the urinary bladder (cystitis) or the kidneys (pyelonephritis).

Urinary tract infections (UTIs) are common in childhood. Nearly all UTIs are caused by bacteria that enter the urethral opening and move upward to the urinary bladder and sometimes the kidneys. Among infants, boys are more likely to develop UTIs; after infancy, girls are much more likely to develop them. UTIs are more common in girls because their short urethras make passage of bacteria easier. Uncircumcised infant boys (who tend to accumulate bacteria under the foreskin) and young children with severe constipation also are more prone to UTIs.

UTIs in older school-aged children and adolescents differ little from UTIs in adults.■ Younger infants and children who have UTIs, however, more commonly have various developmental abnormalities of their urinary system that make them more susceptible to urinary infection. These abnormalities include vesicoureteral reflux (an abnormality of the tube connecting the kidney to the bladder that allows urine to pass backward from the bladder up to the kidney) and a number of conditions that produce obstruction to the flow of urine. Such abnormalities occur in as many as 50% of newborns and infants with a UTI, and in 20 to 30% of school-aged children with a UTI.

Up to 65% of infants and preschool children with a UTI—particularly those with fever—have both bladder and kidney infections. If the kidney is infected and there is severe reflux, up to 50% of children go on to have some scarring of the kidneys. If there is little or no reflux, very few children have scarring of the kidneys. Scarring is a concern because it may lead to high blood pressure and poor kidney function in adulthood.

Symptoms and Diagnosis

Newborns and infants with a UTI may have no symptoms other than a fever. Sometimes they do not eat well and have sluggishness (lethargy), vomiting, or diarrhea. Older children with bladder infections usually have pain or burning with urination, increased urinary frequency, and pain in the bladder region. Children with kidney infections typically have pain in the side or back over the affected kidney, fever, and a general feeling of illness (malaise).

A doctor diagnoses a UTI by examining the urine. Toilet-trained children may provide a urine sample by urinating into a cup after thoroughly cleaning the urethral opening. Doctors obtain urine from younger children and infants by inserting a thin, flexible, sterile tube (catheter) through the urethral opening

---

▲ see page 184   ■ see page 866

into the bladder. In infants, the doctor sometimes withdraws urine from the bladder with a needle inserted through the skin just above the pubic bone. Urine collected in plastic bags taped to the child's genital region is not helpful because it is often contaminated with bacteria and other material from the skin.

To detect white blood cells and bacteria in the urine, which occur in UTI, the laboratory examines the urine under a microscope and performs several chemical tests. The laboratory also performs a culture of the urine to grow and identify any bacteria present. The culture is the most significant of these tests.

In general, boys of all ages and girls younger than 2 to 3 years who develop even a single UTI need further tests to look for structural abnormalities of the urinary system. Such tests are also performed on older girls who have had recurring infections. The tests include ultrasound, which identifies kidney abnormalities and obstruction; and voiding cystourethrography, which further identifies abnormalities of the kidneys, ureters, and bladder and can also identify when the flow of urine is partially reversed (reflux). For voiding cystourethrography, a catheter is passed through the urethra into the bladder, a dye is instilled through the catheter, and x-rays are taken before and after urinating. Another test, radiocontrast cystourethrography, is similar to voiding cystourethrography, except that a radioactive agent is placed in the bladder and images are taken using a nuclear scanner. This procedure exposes the child's ovaries or testes to less radiation than voiding cystourethrography. However, radiocontrast cystourethrography is much more useful for following the healing of reflux rather than in its initial diagnosis, because it does not outline the structures as well. Another type of nuclear scan may be used to confirm the diagnosis of pyelonephritis and identify scarring of the kidneys.

Prevention and Treatment

Prevention of UTIs is difficult, but proper hygiene may help. Girls should be taught to wipe themselves from front to back (as opposed to back to front) after passing a bowel movement to minimize the chance of bacteria entering the urethral opening. Frequent bubble baths may irritate the skin around the urethral opening of both boys and girls at risk for UTIs. Circumcision of boys lowers their risk of UTIs during infancy by about 10 times, although it is not clear that this improvement by itself is a sufficient reason for circumcision. Regularly urinating and regular bowel movements may lessen the risk of UTIs.

Children with UTIs are given antibiotics. Children who are very ill and all newborns receive antibiotics by injection either intramuscularly or intravenously. Other children are given antibiotics by mouth. Treatment typically lasts 7 to 14 days. Children who require tests to diagnose developmental abnormalities often continue antibiotic treatment at a lower dose until tests are complete.

Some children with structural abnormalities of the urinary tract require surgery to correct the problem. Others need to take antibiotics daily to prevent infection. Certain mild abnormalities go away on their own and require no treatment.

CHAPTER 273

Viral Infections

A number of viral infections are common in children. Most childhood viral infections are not serious, and most children get better without treatment. Many viral infections are so distinctive that a doctor can diagnose them based on their symptoms. A doctor usually does not need to have a laboratory identify the specific virus involved.

Most viral infections result in fever and body aches or discomfort. Aspirin is not given to children or adolescents with these symptoms, because it increases the risk of Reye's syndrome in those who might have a viral infection; acetaminophen or ibuprofen is given instead. Viral infections range from mild (for example, a cold) to a life-threatening infection

SOME VIRAL INFECTIONS AT A GLANCE

INFECTION	PERIOD OF INCUBATION	PERIOD OF CONTAGIOUSNESS	SITE OF RASH	NATURE OF RASH
Measles (rubeola)	7 to 14 days	From 2 to 4 days before the rash appears until 2 to 5 days after	Starts around the ears and on the face and neck; in more severe cases, spreads over the trunk, arms, and legs	Irregular, flat, red areas that soon become raised; begins 3 to 5 days after the onset of symptoms; lasts 4 to 7 days
German measles (rubella)	14 to 21 days	From shortly before the onset of symptoms until the rash disappears; infected newborns are usually contagious for many months	Starts on the face and neck; spreads to the trunk, arms, and legs	Fine, pinkish, flat rash; begins 1 or 2 days after the onset of symptoms; lasts 1 to 3 days
Roseola infantum	About 5 to 15 days	Unknown	The chest and abdomen, with moderate involvement of the face, arms, and legs	Red and flat, possibly with raised areas; begins on about the 4th day, appearing as body temperature drops suddenly to normal; lasts 1 or 2 days
Erythema infectiosum (fifth disease)	4 to 14 days	From before the onset of the rash until a few days after	Starts on the cheeks; spreads to the arms, legs, and trunk	Red and flat with raised areas, often blotchy and with lacy patterns; begins shortly after the onset of symptoms; lasts 5 to 10 days; may recur for several weeks
Chickenpox (varicella)	14 to 21 days	From a few days before the onset of symptoms until all spots have crusted	Usually appears first on the trunk; later on the face, neck, arms, and legs; infrequently on the palms and soles	Small, flat, red sores that become raised and form round, fluid-filled blisters against a red background before finally crusting; appears in crops, so various stages are present simultaneously; begins shortly after the onset of symptoms; lasts a few days to 2 weeks

(for example, encephalitis). Generally, parents can discern if their child is ill with a potentially serious infection and needs immediate medical care. This is particularly true for children beyond infancy.

Central Nervous System Infections

Central nervous system infections are extremely serious infections; **meningitis** *affects the membranes surrounding the brain and spinal cord;* **encephalitis** *affects the brain itself.*

Viruses that infect the central nervous system (brain and spinal cord) include herpesviruses, arboviruses, coxsackieviruses, echoviruses, and enteroviruses. Some of these infections primarily affect the meninges (the tissues covering the brain) and result in meningitis; others primarily affect the brain and result in encephalitis; many affect both the meninges and brain and result in meningoencephalitis. Meningitis is far more common in children than is encephalitis.

Viruses affect the central nervous system in two ways. They directly infect and destroy cells during the acute illness. After recovery from the infection, the body's immune response to the infection sometimes causes secondary damage to the cells around the nerves. This secondary damage (**postinfectious encephalomyelitis**) results in the child having symptoms several weeks after recovery from the acute illness.

Children become infected through various routes. Newborns can develop herpesvirus infections through contact with infected secretions in the birth canal. Other viral infections are acquired by breathing air contaminated with virus-containing droplets exhaled by an infected person. Arbovirus infections are acquired from bites by infected insects.

The symptoms and treatment of viral meningitis and encephalitis in older children and adolescents are similar to those in adults.▲ Because the immune system is still developing in newborns and infants, different infections can occur, and the inability of infants to communicate directly makes it difficult to understand their symptoms. Usually, however, infants with central nervous system infections have some of the symptoms described below.

Symptoms

Viral central nervous system infections in newborns and infants usually begin with fever. Newborns may have no other symptoms and may initially not otherwise appear ill. Infants older than a month or so typically become irritable and fussy and refuse to eat. Vomiting is common. Because irritation of the meninges is worsened by movement, an infant with meningitis may cry more, rather than calm down, when he is picked up and rocked. Some infants develop a strange, high-pitched cry. Infants with encephalitis often have seizures or bizarre movements. An infection with herpes simplex virus, which often concentrates in only one part of the brain, may lead to seizures or weakness appearing in only one part of the body. Infants with severe en-

cephalitis may become lethargic and comatose and then die.

Postinfectious encephalomyelitis may produce many neurologic problems, depending on the part of the brain that is damaged. Children may have weakness of an arm or leg, vision or hearing loss, mental retardation, or recurring seizures. These symptoms may not be apparent until the child is old enough for the problem to appear on testing. Often the symptoms resolve with time; occasionally they are permanent.

Diagnosis

Doctors are concerned about the possibility of meningitis or encephalitis in every newborn who has a fever, as well as in an older infant who has a fever, is irritable, or is otherwise not acting normally. These infants undergo a spinal tap (lumbar puncture)■ to obtain cerebrospinal fluid (CSF) for laboratory analysis. In viral infections, the number of lymphocytes (a type of white blood cell) is increased in the cerebrospinal fluid, and no bacteria are seen. Immunologic tests that detect antibodies against viruses in samples of cerebrospinal fluid may be performed, but these tests take days to complete. Polymerase chain reaction (PCR) techniques are used to identify organisms such as herpesviruses and enteroviruses.

A test of brain waves (electroencephalogram)★ can be used to help diagnose encephalitis caused by herpesvirus. Very rarely, a biopsy of brain tissue is needed to determine whether herpesvirus is the cause.

Prognosis and Treatment

Prognosis varies greatly with the type of infection. Many types of viral meningitis and encephalitis are mild, and the child recovers quickly and completely. Other types are severe. Infection with herpes simplex virus is particularly grave. Even with treatment, 15% of newborns with herpes simplex infection of the brain die. If the herpes infection involves other parts of the body as well as the brain, mortality is as high as 50%. Nearly two thirds of the survivors have permanent neurologic disability of some kind.

Most infants require only supportive care—they need to be kept warm and given plenty of fluids. Antiviral drugs are not effective for most central nervous system infections. However, infections caused by herpes simplex virus can be treated with acyclovir given intravenously.

▲ see page 532   ■ see page 443

★ see page 445

Chickenpox

Chickenpox (varicella) is a highly contagious infection with the varicella-zoster virus that produces a characteristic itchy rash, consisting of small, raised, blistered or crusted spots.

Chickenpox is a highly contagious disease of childhood. Before the introduction of a vaccine in 1995, about 90% of children developed chickenpox by age 15. Now, the use of the vaccine has decreased the number of cases of chickenpox per year by about 70%. The disease is spread by airborne droplets of moisture containing the varicella-zoster virus. A person with chickenpox is most contagious just after symptoms start but remains contagious until the last blisters have crusted.

Although most people with chickenpox simply have sores on the skin and in the mouth, the virus sometimes infects the lungs, brain, heart, or joints. Such serious infections are more common in newborns, adults, and people with an impaired immune system.

A person who has had chickenpox develops immunity and cannot contract it again. However, the varicella-zoster virus remains dormant in the body after an initial infection with chickenpox, sometimes reactivating in later life, causing shingles.

Symptoms and Diagnosis

Symptoms begin 10 to 21 days after infection. They include mild headache, moderate fever, loss of appetite, and a general feeling of illness (malaise). Younger children often do not have these symptoms, but symptoms are often severe in adults.

About 24 to 36 hours after the first symptoms begin, a rash of small, flat, red spots appears. The spots usually begin on the trunk and face, later appearing on the arms and legs. Some children have only a few spots; others have them almost everywhere, including on the scalp and inside the mouth. Over 6 to 8 hours, each spot becomes raised; forms an itchy, round, fluid-filled blister against a red background; and finally crusts. Spots continue to develop and crust for several days. The spots may become infected by bacteria,▲ causing erysipelas, pyoderma, cellulitis, or bullous impetigo. New spots usually stop appearing by the fifth day, the majority are crusted by the sixth day, and most disappear in fewer than 20 days.

Spots in the mouth quickly rupture and form raw sores (ulcers), which often make swallowing painful. Raw sores may also occur on the eyelids and in the upper airways, rectum, and vagina. Spots in the voice box (larynx) and upper airways may occasionally cause severe difficulty in breathing. Lymph nodes at the side of the neck may become enlarged and tender. The worst part of the illness usually lasts 4 to 7 days.

Lung infection occurs in about 1 out of 400 people, especially adolescents and adults, resulting in cough and difficulty breathing. Brain infection (encephalitis) is less common and produces unsteadiness in walking, headache, dizziness, confusion, and seizures. Heart infection sometimes causes a heart murmur. Joint inflammation produces joint pain.

Reye's syndrome, a rare but very severe complication that occurs almost only in those younger than 18, may begin 3 to 8 days after the rash begins.

A doctor is usually certain of the diagnosis of chickenpox because the rash and the other symptoms are so typical. Measurement of the levels of antibodies in the blood and laboratory identification of the virus are rarely needed.

Prevention

In the United States, children are routinely vaccinated against varicella-zoster beginning at 12 months of age.■ Anyone without immunity may also be vaccinated. Susceptible people who are at high risk of complications—such as those with an impaired immune system and pregnant women—and have been exposed to someone with chickenpox may be given antibodies against the varicella virus (varicella-zoster immune globulin). Isolation of an infected person helps prevent the spread of infection to people who have not had chickenpox.

Prognosis and Treatment

Healthy children nearly always recover from chickenpox without problems; only about 2 of 100,000 children die. However, even this low rate means that before routine immunization, 100 children died annually in the United States because of complications of chickenpox. The infection is more severe in adults, of whom about 30 of 100,000 die. Chickenpox is fatal in up to 15% of people with an impaired immune system.

▲ see page 1220   ■ see page 1493

What Is Reye's Syndrome?

Reye's syndrome is a very rare but life-threatening disorder that causes inflammation and swelling of the brain and degeneration of the liver.

The cause of Reye's syndrome is unknown, although it typically occurs after infection by certain viruses, such as influenza or varicella (chickenpox), particularly in children who take aspirin. Because of this increased risk of Reye's syndrome, aspirin is not recommended for children, except for the treatment of a few specific diseases. Now that aspirin use has declined—in large part because of the possibility of triggering Reye's syndrome—fewer than a dozen children a year develop this disorder. The condition occurs mainly in children between the ages of 4 and 12 years, in late fall and winter.

Reye's syndrome begins with the symptoms of a viral infection, such as an upper respiratory tract infection, influenza, or chickenpox. After 4 or 5 days, the child suddenly develops very severe nausea and vomiting. Within a day, the child becomes confused, followed by disorientation, agitation, and sometimes seizures, coma, and death. Degeneration of the liver may lead to blood clotting problems and bleeding. The severity of illness varies greatly.

The child's prognosis depends on the amount of swelling in the brain. The overall chances that the child will die are about 20%, but range from less than 2% among children with mild disease to more than 80% among those in a deep coma.

Children who survive the acute phase of the illness usually recover fully. Those with more severe symptoms may later show some evidence of brain damage, such as mental retardation, a seizure disorder, abnormal muscle movement, or damage to specific nerves. Reye's syndrome rarely affects a child twice.

There is no specific treatment for Reye's syndrome. Children are placed in intensive care. Vitamin K or fresh frozen plasma is given to help prevent bleeding. Drugs such as mannitol, corticosteroids, or barbiturates may be used to help reduce the pressure within the brain.

Mild cases of chickenpox require only the treatment of symptoms. Wet compresses on the skin help soothe itching, which may be intense, and prevent scratching, which may spread the infection and cause scars. Because of the risk of bacterial infection, the skin is bathed often with soap and water, the hands are kept clean, the nails are clipped to minimize scratching, and clothing is kept clean and dry. Drugs that relieve itching, such as antihistamines, are sometimes given by mouth. If a bacterial infection develops, antibiotics may be needed.

Doctors may use antiviral drugs, such as acyclovir, valacyclovir, and famciclovir, for adolescents and adults as well as for groups at high risk of complications—premature infants and children with immune system disorders. The drugs must be given within 24 hours of onset of disease to be effective. These antiviral drugs are not given to pregnant women.

Erythema Infectiosum

Erythema infectiosum (fifth disease) is a contagious viral infection that causes a blotchy or raised red rash with mild illness.

Erythema infectiosum is caused by human parvovirus B19 and occurs most often during the spring months, often in geographically limited outbreaks among children and adolescents. Infection is spread mainly by breathing in small droplets that have been breathed out by an infected person. The infection can also be transmitted from mother to fetus during pregnancy; it rarely causes stillbirth or severe anemia and excess fluid and swelling (edema) in the fetus (hydrops).

Symptoms begin about 4 to 14 days after infection. Symptoms can vary, and some children have none. However, a child with erythema infectiosum typically has a low fever, feels mildly ill, and develops red cheeks that often look like they have been slapped. Within a day or two, a rash appears, especially on the arms, legs, and trunk but not usually on the palms or soles. The rash can be itchy and consists of raised, blotchy red areas and lacy patterns, particularly on areas of the arms not covered by clothing, because the rash may be worsened by exposure to sunlight.

The illness generally lasts 5 to 10 days. Over the next several weeks, the rash may temporarily reappear in response to sunlight, exercise, heat, fever, or emotional stress. In adolescents, mild joint pain and swelling may remain or come and go for weeks to months.

Erythema infectiosum can also present in a different way, particularly in children with sickle cell disease, or immunodeficiency diseases, such as acquired immunodeficiency syndrome (AIDS). The virus can affect the bone marrow and produce severe anemia.

A doctor makes the diagnosis based on the characteristic appearance of the rash. Blood tests can help identify the virus, although these are rarely performed. Treatment is aimed at relieving the fever and pain.

Human Immunodeficiency Virus Infection

Human immunodeficiency virus (HIV) infection is a viral infection that progressively destroys the white blood cells and causes acquired immunodeficiency syndrome (AIDS).

Only about 2% of the people infected with HIV in the United States are children or adolescents. Worldwide, HIV is a much more common problem in children.

The two human immunodeficiency viruses—HIV-1 and HIV-2—progressively destroy certain types of white blood cells called lymphocytes, which are an important part of the body's immune defenses. When these lymphocytes are destroyed, the body becomes susceptible to attack by many other infectious organisms. Many of the symptoms and complications of HIV infection, including death, are the result of these other infections and not of the HIV infection itself. HIV infection may lead to various troublesome infections with organisms that do not ordinarily infect healthy people. These are termed opportunistic infections; these infections may result from viruses, parasites, and—in children, unlike in adults—bacteria.

Acquired immunodeficiency syndrome (AIDS) is the most severe form of HIV infection. A child with HIV infection is considered to have AIDS when at least one complicating illness develops or there is a significant decline in the body's ability to defend itself from infection.

Transmission of Infection

In young children, HIV infection is nearly always acquired from the mother. Less than 7% of children now living with AIDS acquired the infection from other sources, including blood transfusion (from blood products used to treat hemophilia) or sexual abuse. Because of improved safety measures in blood and blood products, very few current infections result from these mechanisms.

As many as 7,000 HIV-infected women give birth each year in the United States. Without

preventive measures, one fourth to one third of them would transmit the infection to their baby. The risk is highest in mothers who acquire the infection during pregnancy, who have more virus in their bodies, or who are severely ill. Transmission often takes place during labor and delivery.

The virus also can be transmitted in breast milk; 10 to 15% of babies not infected at birth acquire HIV infection if they breastfeed from an HIV-infected mother. Most often, transmission occurs in the first few weeks or months of life, although transmission may occur later. Transmission is more likely in mothers who acquire the infection while breastfeeding or who have infection of the breast (mastitis).

In adolescents, transmission is the same as in adults: through sexual intercourse—both heterosexual and homosexual—and through sharing of infected needles while injecting drugs.

The virus is *not* transmitted through food, water, household articles, or social contact in a home, workplace, or school. In very rare cases, HIV has been transmitted by contact with infected blood on the skin. In almost all such cases, the skin surface was broken by scrapes or open sores. Although saliva may contain the virus, transmission of infection by kissing or biting has never been confirmed.

Symptoms

Children born with HIV infection rarely have symptoms for the first few months. If the children remain untreated, only about 20% develop problems during the first or second year of life; for the remaining 80% of children, problems may not appear until age 3 or later even without treatment. With the use of effective anti-HIV drugs, children with HIV infection do not necessarily develop any signs or symptoms of HIV infection. The symptoms of HIV infection acquired during adolescence are similar to those in adults.▲

The first signs of HIV infection in children are usually slowed growth and a delay of maturation, recurring diarrhea, lung infections, or a fungal infection of the mouth (thrush). Sometimes children have repeated episodes of bacterial infections, such as otitis media, sinusitis, or pneumonia.

A variety of symptoms and complications can appear as the child's immune system dete-

▲ see page 1170

riorates. About one third of HIV-infected children develop lung inflammation (lymphocytic interstitial pneumonitis), with cough and difficulty breathing.

Children born with HIV infection commonly have at least one episode of *Pneumocystis* pneumonia in the first 15 months of life if they are not receiving anti-HIV drugs. More than half of untreated children infected with HIV develop the pneumonia at some time. *Pneumocystis* pneumonia is a major cause of death among children and adults with AIDS.

In a significant number of HIV-infected children, progressive brain damage prevents or delays developmental milestones, such as walking and talking. These children also may have impaired intelligence and a head that is small in relation to their body size. Up to 20% of untreated infected children progressively lose social and language skills and muscle control. They may become partially paralyzed or unsteady on their feet, or their muscles may become somewhat rigid.

Anemia (a low red blood cell count) is common in HIV-infected children; because of anemia, they become weak and tire easily. About 20% of untreated children develop heart problems, such as rapid or irregular heartbeat, or heart failure.

Less commonly, untreated children develop inflammation of the liver (hepatitis) or kidneys (nephritis). Cancers are uncommon in children with AIDS, but non-Hodgkin's lymphoma and lymphoma of the brain may occur somewhat more often than in uninfected children. Kaposi's sarcoma, an AIDS-related cancer that affects the skin and internal organs, is extremely rare in children.

Diagnosis

The diagnosis of HIV infection among children begins with the identification of HIV infection in pregnant women through routine prenatal screening. Newborns of mothers with HIV infection or of mothers who are at risk for HIV infection because of lifestyle should be tested. Such infants should be tested at frequent intervals—typically in the first 2 days of life, at 2 weeks of age, between 1 and 2 months, and between 3 and 6 months. Such frequent testing identifies most HIV-infected infants by 6 months of age.

In infants, the standard adult blood tests for HIV antibodies are not helpful, because an infant's blood almost always contains HIV antibodies if the mother is HIV-infected (even if the infant is not). To definitively diagnose HIV infection in children younger than 18 months of age, special blood tests that identify the virus in the blood are used. The standard blood tests are used to diagnose HIV infection in children older than 18 months and in adolescents.

Prevention

The most effective means of preventing infection in newborns is for HIV-infected women to avoid pregnancy. If an infected woman does become pregnant, anti-HIV drugs are fairly effective at minimizing transmission. Women not already taking drugs are given zidovudine (AZT) by mouth during the 2nd and 3rd trimesters (last 6 months) of pregnancy; zidovudine is also given intravenously during labor and delivery. Zidovudine is then given daily to the newborn for 6 weeks. This treatment reduces the rate of transmission from about 33% to about 8%. The rate may be as low as 1 to 2% in women receiving combination therapy with three anti-HIV drugs. Also, delivery by cesarean section reduces the baby's risk of acquiring HIV infection.

In countries where good infant formulas and clean water are readily available, HIV-infected mothers should bottle-feed their babies. In countries where the risks of malnutrition or infectious diarrhea from unclean water are high, the benefits of breastfeeding outweigh the risk of HIV transmission.

Because a child's HIV status may not be known, all schools and day care centers should adopt special procedures for handling accidents, such as nosebleeds, and for cleaning and disinfecting surfaces contaminated with blood. During cleanup, personnel are advised to avoid having their skin come in contact with blood. Latex gloves should be routinely available, and hands should be washed after the gloves are removed. Contaminated surfaces should be cleaned and disinfected with a freshly prepared bleach solution containing 1 part of household bleach to 10 to 100 parts of water.

Prevention for adolescents is the same as for adults.▲ All adolescents should be taught how HIV is transmitted and how it can be avoided, including abstaining from sex or using safe-sex practices.

▲ see page 1173

Treatment and Prognosis

Children are treated with most of the same anti-HIV drugs as adults,▲ typically a combination of two or more reverse-transcriptase inhibitors and a protease inhibitor. However, not all of the drugs used for adults are available to small children, in part because some are not available in liquid form. It may be difficult for parents and children to follow complicated drug regimens, which can limit the effectiveness of therapy. In general, children develop the same types of side effects as adults but usually at a much lower rate; however, the side effects of drugs may also limit the treatment. A doctor monitors the effectiveness of treatment by regularly measuring the amount of virus present in the blood and the child's CD4+ count.■ Increased numbers of virus in the blood may be a sign of the development of resistance of HIV to the drugs or a lack of taking the drugs. In either case, the doctor may need to change the drugs.

To prevent *Pneumocystis* pneumonia, trimethoprim-sulfamethoxazole is given to infants older than 1 month who were born to HIV-infected women and children with a significantly impaired immune system. Children with serious allergic reactions to this drug may be given dapsone or atovaquone. Children with a significantly impaired immune system also are given azithromycin or clarithromycin to prevent *Mycobacterium avium complex* infection. Children with recurring bacterial infections may be given intravenous immune globulin once a month.

Nearly all HIV-infected children should receive the routine childhood vaccinations, except usually the measles-mumps-rubella and varicella vaccines. Both of these vaccines contain live virus and can cause a severe or fatal illness in the most immunologically compromised children with HIV, but they are recommended for children with HIV infection whose immune system is not severely compromised. However, the effectiveness of any vaccination will be less in children with HIV infection.

For children who need foster care, childcare, or schooling, a doctor can help assess the child's risk of exposure to infectious diseases. In general, transmission of infections, such as chickenpox, to the HIV-infected child (or to any child with an impaired immune system) is more of a danger than is transmission of HIV from that child to others. A young child with HIV infection who has open skin sores or who engages in potentially dangerous behavior, such as biting, should not attend childcare.

HIV-infected children should participate in as many routine childhood activities as their physical condition allows. Interaction with other children enhances social development and self-esteem. Because of the stigma associated with the illness and the fact that transmission of the infection to other children is extremely unlikely, there is no need for anyone other than the parents, the doctor, and perhaps the school nurse to be aware of the child's HIV status.

As a child's condition worsens, treatment is best given in the least restrictive environment possible. If home health care and social services are available, the child can spend more time at home rather than in a hospital.

With current drug therapy, 75% of children born today with HIV infection are alive at 5 years, and 50% are alive at 8 years. The average age at death is still about 10 years for HIV-infected children, but more and more children are surviving well into adolescence and early adulthood.

Measles

Measles (rubeola, 9-day measles) is a highly contagious viral infection that produces various symptoms and a characteristic rash.

Children become infected with measles by breathing in small airborne droplets of moisture coughed out by an infected person or by touching items contaminated by such droplets. Measles is contagious from 2 to 4 days before the rash appears until the rash disappears.

Before vaccination became widely available, measles epidemics occurred every 2 or 3 years, particularly in preschool-aged and school-aged children, with small localized outbreaks during intervening years. Although measles is still common in other countries, only about 100 people a year in the United States develop measles. A woman who has had measles or has been vaccinated passes immunity (in the form of antibodies) to her child; this immunity lasts most of the first year of life. Thereafter, however, susceptibility to measles is high unless vaccination is given. A person who has had measles develops immunity and cannot contract it again.

▲ see page 1173 and table on page 1175
■ see page 1170

Enteroviral Infections: Common in Childhood

The enteroviruses include numerous strains of coxsackievirus, echovirus, and others. These viruses are responsible for illness in 10 to 30 million people each year in the United States, primarily in the summer and fall. Infections are highly contagious and typically affect many people in a community, sometimes reaching epidemic proportions. Enteroviral infections are most common in children, particularly those living in conditions of poor hygiene.

The infection begins when material contaminated with the virus is swallowed; the virus then reproduces in the digestive tract. The body's immune defenses stop many infections at this stage; the result is few or no symptoms. Sometimes, the virus survives and spreads into the bloodstream, resulting in fever, headache, sore throat, and vomiting. People often refer to such illnesses as the "summer flu," although they are not influenza. Some strains of enterovirus also produce a generalized, non-itchy rash on the skin or sores inside the mouth. This type of illness is by far the most common enteroviral infection. Rarely, an enterovirus will progress from this stage to attack a particular organ. The virus can attack many different organs, and the symptoms and severity of disease depend on the specific organ infected. Several diseases are caused by enteroviruses:

- **Hand-foot-and-mouth disease** affects the skin and mucous membranes; painful sores appear inside the mouth and on the hands and feet.

- **Herpangina** also affects the skin and mucous membranes, producing painful sores on the tongue and the back of the throat.

- **Aseptic meningitis** affects the central nervous system, causing severe headache, stiff neck, and sensitivity to light.

- **Encephalitis** causes confusion, weakness, seizures, and coma.

- **Paralytic illness** leads to weakness of various muscles.

- **Myocarditis** affects the heart, causing weakness and shortness of breath with exertion.

- **Epidemic pleurodynia** affects the muscles, leading to intermittent painful spasms of muscles in the wall of the lower chest (adults), or upper abdomen (children).

- **Acute hemorrhagic conjunctivitis** affects the eyes, causing painful, red, runny eyes; bleeding under the conjunctiva; and swollen eyelids.

Enteroviral infections usually resolve completely, but infections of the heart or central nervous system are occasionally fatal. There is no cure. Treatment is directed at relieving symptoms.

Symptoms and Diagnosis

The symptoms of measles begin about 7 to 14 days after infection. The infected child first develops a fever, runny nose, sore throat, hacking cough, and red eyes. Sometimes, the eyes are sensitive to bright light. Tiny white spots (Koplik's spots) appear inside the mouth 2 to 4 days later.

A mildly itchy rash appears 3 to 5 days after the start of symptoms. The rash begins in front of and below the ears and on the side of the neck as irregular, flat, red areas that soon become raised. The rash spreads within 1 to 2 days to the trunk, arms, and legs, as it begins to fade on the face.

At the peak of the illness, the child feels very sick, the rash is extensive, and the temperature may exceed 104° F. In 3 to 5 days, the temperature falls, the child begins to feel better, and any remaining rash quickly fades. The diagnosis is based on the typical symptoms and characteristic rash. No special tests are performed.

Brain infection (encephalitis) occurs in about 1 of 1,000 children with measles. If encephalitis occurs, it often starts with a high fever, seizures, and coma, usually 2 days to 3 weeks after the rash appears. The illness may be brief, with recovery in about 1 week, or it may be prolonged, resulting in brain damage or death.

Secondary bacterial infections, such as pneumonia (especially in infants) or a middle ear infection (otitis media), occur fairly often, and children with measles are especially susceptible to infection with streptococci bacteria. Rarely, blood platelet levels become so low that the child bruises and bleeds.

Prognosis, Prevention, and Treatment

In healthy, well-nourished children, measles is rarely serious. However, secondary bacterial infections, particularly pneumonia, can occasionally be fatal. In rare cases, subacute sclerosing panencephalitis—a serious complication of measles—occurs months to years later, resulting in brain damage.▲

Measles vaccine, one of the routine immunizations of childhood, is given between 12 and 15 months of age.■ Children (and adults) who are exposed to measles and do not have immunity may be protected by vaccination within 2 days of the exposure. Pregnant women and infants younger than 1 year should not receive the vaccine and are given measles immune globulin for protection.

There is no specific treatment for measles. Some doctors in the United States give vitamin A to children aged 6 months to 2 years hospitalized with measles, because vitamin A has reduced the number of deaths from measles in countries where vitamin A deficiency is common. A child with measles is kept warm and comfortable. Acetaminophen or ibuprofen may be given to reduce fever. If a secondary bacterial infection develops, an antibiotic is given.

Mumps

Mumps is a contagious viral infection that causes painful enlargement of the salivary glands; the infection may also affect the testes, brain, and pancreas, especially in adults.

Children become infected with mumps by breathing in small airborne droplets of moisture coughed out by an infected person or by having direct contact with objects contaminated by infected saliva. Mumps is less contagious than measles or chickenpox. In heavily populated areas, it occurs year-round but is most frequent in late winter and early spring. Epidemics may occur when people without immunity are crowded together. Although the infection may occur at any age, most cases occur in children 5 to 15 years old. The infection is unusual in children younger than 2 years. One infection with the mumps virus usually provides lifelong immunity.

Symptoms and Diagnosis

Symptoms begin 14 to 24 days after infection. Most children develop chills, headache, poor appetite, a general feeling of illness (malaise), and a low to moderate fever. These symptoms are followed in 12 to 24 hours by swelling of the salivary glands, which is most prominent on the second day. Some children simply have swelling of the salivary glands without the other symptoms; this results in pain when chewing or swallowing, particularly when swallowing acidic liquids, such as citrus fruit juices. The glands are tender when touched. At this stage, the temperature usually rises to 103 or 104° F.

About 20% of men who become infected after puberty develop inflammation of one or both testes (orchitis). Inflammation of the testes produces severe pain. On healing, the affected testis may be smaller. If both testes are damaged, sterility may result.

Mumps leads to viral inflammation of the brain or its covering (meningoencephalitis) in 10% of people. Meningoencephalitis causes headache, stiff neck, drowsiness, coma, or seizures. Most people recover completely, but some have permanent nerve or brain damage, such as nerve deafness or paralysis of the facial muscles, usually affecting only one side of the body.

Inflammation of the pancreas (pancreatitis) may occur toward the end of the first week of infection. This disorder causes abdominal pain, nausea, and vomiting, which varies from mild to severe. These symptoms disappear in about a week, and the person recovers completely.

Doctors diagnose mumps based on the typical symptoms, particularly when they occur during an outbreak of mumps. Laboratory tests can identify the mumps virus and its antibodies, but such tests are rarely needed to make the diagnosis.

Prognosis, Prevention, and Treatment

Almost all children with mumps recover fully without problems, but in rare cases symptoms may worsen again after about 2 weeks.

Vaccination against mumps is routine in childhood, beginning at 12 to 15 months of age,★ and fewer than 1,000 cases occur each year. Once the infection has started, it just has to run its course. To minimize discomfort, children should avoid foods that require much chewing or are acidic. Analgesics, such as acetaminophen and ibuprofen, may be used for headache and discomfort.

Boys or men with inflammation of the testes need bed rest. The scrotum may be supported

---

▲ see page 1582   ■ see page 1493
★ see page 1493

with an athletic supporter or by an adhesive tape bridge connected between the thighs. Ice packs may be applied to relieve pain.

If pancreatitis causes severe nausea and vomiting, intravenous fluids may be given, and intake by mouth should be avoided for a few days. Children with meningoencephalitis may need intravenous fluids and acetaminophen or ibuprofen for a fever or headache. If seizures develop, anticonvulsant drugs may be needed.

Polio

Polio (poliomyelitis) is a highly contagious, sometimes fatal, viral infection that affects nerves and can produce permanent muscle weakness, paralysis, and other symptoms.

Polio is caused by poliovirus, an enterovirus, which is spread by swallowing material contaminated by the virus. The infection spreads from the intestine to the parts of the brain and spinal cord that control the muscles. In the early 20th century, polio was widespread throughout the United States. Today, because of extensive vaccination, polio outbreaks have largely disappeared, and most doctors have never seen a new polio infection. The last case of wild poliovirus infection in the United States occurred in 1979. The Western Hemisphere was certified polio-free in 1994. A global polio eradication program is under way. Unimmunized people of all ages are susceptible to polio. In the past, polio outbreaks occurred mainly in children and adolescents, because many older people had already been exposed to the virus and developed immunity.

Symptoms and Diagnosis

Fewer than 1 of 100 infected people develop any symptoms. Of those with symptoms, 80 to 90% simply have fever, mild headache, sore throat, and a general feeling of illness (malaise). This mild illness resolves completely in 24 to 72 hours. The remaining 10 to 20% of people have more serious symptoms (major polio). Major polio is more likely in older children and adults. The symptoms, which usually appear 7 to 14 days after infection, include fever, severe headache, a stiff neck and back, and deep muscle pain. Sometimes areas of skin develop odd sensations, such as pins and needles or unusual sensitiv-

ity to pain. Depending on which parts of the brain and spinal cord are affected, the disease may progress no further, or weakness or paralysis may develop in certain muscles. The person may have difficulty in swallowing and may choke on saliva, food, or fluids. Sometimes fluids go up into the nose, and the voice may develop a nasal quality. Sometimes the part of the brain responsible for breathing is affected, causing weakness or paralysis of the chest muscles. Some people are completely unable to breathe.

A doctor can diagnose polio from its symptoms. Diagnosis is confirmed by identifying poliovirus in a stool sample and by detecting high levels of antibodies to the virus in the blood.

Prevention

Polio vaccine is included among the routine childhood immunizations.▲ Two types of vaccine are available worldwide: an inactivated poliovirus vaccine (Salk vaccine) given by injection and a live poliovirus vaccine (Sabin vaccine) taken by mouth. The live oral vaccine provides better immunity but can mutate and cause polio in about 1 in every 2.4 million children. Although this is very uncommon, because live polio was eradicated in the United States, doctors recommend only the injected vaccine for children in this country. The oral vaccine is used for rapid treatment of unprotected people in local outbreaks in other parts of the world.

A first vaccination of people older than 18 is not routinely recommended because the risk of acquiring polio as an adult is extremely low in the United States. Adults who have never been immunized and who are traveling to an area where polio is still a health risk should be vaccinated. Local and state health departments have information about which areas have polio.

Prognosis and Treatment

About 50% of people with major polio recover without paralysis. Another 25% have mild permanent disability, and 25% have permanent severe paralysis. Some children, even those who apparently recovered completely, develop a return or worsening of muscle weakness 15 or more years after an attack of polio. This condition (postpolio syndrome) often results in severe disability.■

Polio cannot be cured, and available antiviral drugs do not affect the course of the dis-

▲ see page 1493   ■ see page 576

ease. A ventilator may be needed if the muscles used in breathing are weakened. Often, the need for a ventilator is temporary.

Respiratory Tract Infections

Respiratory tract infections affect the nose, throat, and airways and may be caused by any of several different viruses.

Children develop on average six viral respiratory tract infections each year. Viral respiratory tract infections include the common cold and influenza.▲ Doctors often refer to these as upper respiratory infections (URIs), because they produce symptoms mainly in the nose and throat. In small children, viruses also commonly cause infections of the lower respiratory tract—the windpipe, airways, and lungs. These infections include croup, bronchiolitis, and pneumonia. Children sometimes have infections involving both the upper and lower respiratory tracts.

In children, rhinoviruses, influenza viruses (during annual winter epidemics), parainfluenza viruses, respiratory syncytial virus (RSV), and certain strains of adenovirus are the main causes of viral respiratory infections.

Most often, viral respiratory tract infections spread when a child's hands come into contact with nasal secretions from an infected person. These secretions contain viruses. When the child touches his mouth, nose, or eyes, the viruses gain entry and produce a new infection. Less often, infections spread when a child breathes air containing droplets that were coughed or sneezed out by an infected person. For various reasons, nasal or respiratory secretions from children with viral respiratory tract infections contain more viruses than those from infected adults. This increased output of viruses, along with typically lesser attention to hygiene, makes children more likely to spread their infection to others. The possibility of transmission is further enhanced when many children are gathered together, such as in childcare centers and schools. Contrary to what people may think, other factors, such as becoming chilled, wet, or tired, do not cause colds or increase a child's susceptibility to infection.

Symptoms and Complications

When viruses invade cells of the respiratory tract, they trigger inflammation and production of mucus. This situation leads to nasal congestion, a runny nose, scratchy throat, and

cough, which may last up to 14 days. Fever, with a temperature as high as 101 to 102° F, is common. The child's temperature may even rise to 104° F. Other typical symptoms in children include decreased appetite, lethargy, and a general feeling of illness (malaise). Headaches and body aches develop, particularly with influenza. Infants and young children are usually not able to communicate their specific symptoms and just appear cranky and uncomfortable.

Because newborns and young infants prefer to breathe through their nose, even moderate nasal congestion can create difficulty breathing. Nasal congestion leads to feeding problems as well, because infants cannot breathe while suckling from the breast or bottle. Because infants are unable to spit out mucus that they cough up, they often gag and choke.

The small airways of young children can be significantly narrowed by inflammation and mucus, making breathing difficult. These children breathe rapidly and may develop a high-pitched noise heard on breathing out (wheezing) or a similar noise heard on breathing in (stridor). Severe airway narrowing may cause children to gasp for breath and turn blue (cyanosis). Such airway problems are most common with infection caused by parainfluenza viruses and RSV; affected children need to be seen urgently by a doctor.

Some children with a viral respiratory tract infection also develop an infection of the middle ear (otitis media) or the lung tissue (pneumonia). Otitis media and pneumonia may be caused by the virus itself or by a bacterial infection that develops because the inflammation caused by the virus makes tissue more susceptible to invasion by other germs. In children with asthma, respiratory tract infections often lead to an asthma attack.

Diagnosis

Doctors and parents recognize respiratory tract infections by their typical symptoms. Generally, otherwise healthy children with mild upper respiratory tract symptoms do not need to see a doctor unless they have trouble breathing, are not drinking, or have a fever for more than a day or two. X-rays of the neck and chest may be taken in children who have difficulty breathing, stridor, wheezing, or audible lung congestion. Blood tests and tests of respiratory secretions are rarely helpful.

▲ see pages 1155 and 1159

Prevention and Treatment

The best preventive measure is practicing good hygiene. A sick child and the people in the household should wash their hands frequently. In general, the more intimate physical contact (such as hugging, snuggling, or bed sharing) that takes place with an ill child, the greater the risk of spreading the infection to other family members. Parents must balance this risk with the need to comfort an ill child. Children should stay home from school or childcare until the fever is gone and they feel well enough to attend.

Influenza is the only viral respiratory infection preventable by vaccination. Children with heart or lung disease (including asthma), diabetes, kidney failure, or sickle cell disease should receive the vaccine. Additionally, children whose immune system is compromised (including children with HIV infection and those undergoing chemotherapy) should receive the vaccine.

Antibiotics are not necessary to treat viral respiratory tract infections. Children with respiratory tract infections need additional rest and increased fluids. Acetaminophen or nonsteroidal anti-inflammatory drugs (NSAIDs), such as ibuprofen, can be given for fever and aches. School-aged children may take a nonprescription decongestant for bothersome nasal congestion, although the drug often does not help. Infants and younger children are particularly sensitive to the side effects of decongestants and may experience agitation, confusion, hallucinations, lethargy, and rapid heart rate. In infants and young children, congestion may be relieved somewhat by using a cool-mist vaporizer to humidify the air and by suctioning the mucus from the nose with a rubber suction bulb.

Doctors may give certain children at high risk of developing a severe RSV infection monthly injections of palivizumab, which contains antibodies against RSV. Children who receive palivizumab are less likely to need hospitalization, but doctors are not sure whether this treatment prevents death or serious complications.

Children who have difficulty breathing are taken to a hospital. Depending on their condition, doctors may treat them with oxygen and drugs, such as albuterol or epinephrine, to open the airways (bronchodilators). Ribavirin is sometimes given to children with severe RSV pneumonia; however, the benefit of this drug is not clear.

Roseola Infantum

Roseola infantum is a contagious viral infection of infants or very young children that causes a high fever followed by a rash.

Roseola infantum occurs most often in the spring and fall, sometimes in local outbreaks. The usual cause is herpesvirus 6, one of the many herpesviruses. Most children who develop roseola infantum are between 6 months and 3 years old.

Symptoms begin about 5 to 15 days after infection. A fever of 103 to 105° F begins abruptly and lasts for 3 to 5 days. In 5 to 15% of children, seizures occur as a result of high fever, particularly as the fever begins and rises quickly. Despite the high fever, the child is usually alert and active. A few children have a mild runny nose, sore throat, or an upset stomach. The lymph nodes at the back of the head, the sides of the neck, and behind the ears may be enlarged. The fever usually disappears on the fourth day.

About 30% of children develop a rash within a few hours to at most a day after the temperature falls. The rash is red and flat, but it may have raised areas, mostly on the chest and abdomen and less extensively on the face, arms, and legs. The rash is not itchy and may last from a few hours to 2 days.

A doctor makes the diagnosis based on the symptoms. Antibody tests and a culture of the virus are rarely needed.

Fever is treated with acetaminophen or ibuprofen. The seizures and rash do not require any specific treatment. But since they are frightening, most parents bring their child to the doctor for evaluation.

Rubella

Rubella (German measles, 3-day measles) is a contagious viral infection that produces mild symptoms, such as joint pain and a rash.

Rubella is a typically mild childhood infection that may, however, have devastating consequences for infants infected prior to birth. A woman infected during the first 16 weeks (particularly the first 8 to 10 weeks) of pregnancy often passes the infection to the fetus. This fetal infection causes miscarriage, stillbirth, or severe birth defects.▲

▲ see page 1511

What Is Kawasaki Syndrome?

Kawasaki syndrome produces inflammation in the walls of blood vessels throughout the body. The cause is unknown, but evidence suggests a virus or other infectious organism. Inflammation of blood vessels in the heart causes the most serious problems.

Most children with Kawasaki syndrome range from 2 months to 5 years old, although adolescents can be affected. Roughly twice as many boys as girls are affected. The illness is more common in children of Asian descent. Several thousand cases of Kawasaki syndrome are estimated to occur in the United States every year.

The illness begins with fever—usually above 102° F —which rises and falls over 1 to 3 weeks. Within a day, a red, patchy rash usually appears over the trunk and around the diaper area. Within several days, the rash appears on mucous membranes, such as the lining of the mouth or vagina. The child has a red throat; reddened, dry, cracked lips; and a strawberry-red tongue. The eyes become red but without any discharge. Also, the palms and soles turn red or purplish red, and the

hands and feet often swell. The skin on the fingers and toes begins to peel 10 to 20 days after the illness starts. The lymph nodes in the neck are often swollen and slightly tender.

About 50% of children develop problems involving the heart, such as a rapid or irregular heart beat, usually beginning 2 to 4 weeks after the onset of illness. Half of the children with heart problems develop the most serious heart problem, coronary artery aneurysm (a bulge in the wall of the coronary artery). These aneurysms can rupture or provoke a blood clot, leading to a heart attack and sudden death. Other problems include inflammation of the tissues lining the brain (meningitis), joints, and gallbladder. These symptoms eventually resolve without causing permanent damage. Doctors perform ultrasound of the heart to detect coronary artery aneurysms.

Children recover completely if their coronary arteries are not affected within the first 8 weeks of illness. For those with coronary artery problems, survival varies with the severity of disease, but overall between 0.05% and 0.1% of children

with Kawasaki syndrome die, even with treatment. Of these, most die in the first few months, but death can occur decades afterward. About half of the aneurysms resolve within 1 to 2 years. The remaining half are permanent. Even the ones that resolve may lead to an increased risk of heart problems in adulthood.

Treatment given within 10 days of symptoms significantly reduces the risk of coronary artery damage and speeds the resolution of fever, rash, and discomfort. For 1 to 4 days, high doses of immunoglobulin are given intravenously, and high doses of aspirin are given by mouth. Once the fever is gone, a lower dose of aspirin is usually continued for several weeks to months. If the child contracts influenza or chickenpox, dipyridamole is sometimes used temporarily instead of aspirin to lessen the risk of Reye's syndrome.

Children with large coronary aneurysms may be treated with anticoagulant drugs. Some children may even require coronary artery angioplasty, stent placement, or coronary artery bypass grafting.

Rubella was once common during the springtime, with major epidemics every 6 to 9 years infecting millions of people. The disease is now rare in the United States because of widespread vaccination. Nonetheless, some young adult women have never had rubella or rubella vaccination and are thus at risk of having children with serious birth defects if they become infected during early pregnancy.

Rubella is spread mainly by breathing in small virus-containing droplets of moisture that have been coughed into the air by an infected person. Close contact with an infected person can also spread the infection. The infection is contagious from 1 week before the

rash appears until 1 week after the rash disappears. An infant infected before birth can spread the infection for many months after birth.

Symptoms and Diagnosis

Symptoms begin about 14 to 21 days after infection. Some children feel mildly ill for a few days, with a runny nose, cough, and painless, rose-colored spots on the roof of the mouth. These spots later merge with each other into a red blush extending over the back of the throat. In most children, particularly older ones, the first sign of illness is the development of swollen lymph nodes in the neck and back of the head. A characteristic rash develops about a day later and lasts about 3 days. The rash begins on the face and neck and quickly spreads to the trunk, arms, and legs. As the rash appears, a mild reddening of the skin (flush) occurs, particularly on the face.

Up to one third of older girls and women develop arthritis or joint pain with rubella. In rare instances, a middle ear infection (otitis media) develops. Brain infection (encephalitis) is a very rare but occasionally fatal complication.

The diagnosis is based on the typical symptoms. A definite diagnosis, necessary during pregnancy, can be made by measuring levels of antibodies to rubella virus in the blood.

Prevention and Treatment

Rubella vaccine, one of the routine immunizations of childhood, is given beginning at 12 months of age.▲ A person who has had rubella develops immunity and cannot contract it again.

Most children with rubella recover fully without treatment. A middle ear infection■ can be treated with antibiotics. No treatment is available for encephalitis, which must just run its course with supportive care.

Subacute Sclerosing Panencephalitis

Subacute sclerosing panencephalitis, a progressive and usually fatal disorder, is a rare complication of measles that appears months or years later and produces mental deterioration, muscle jerks, and seizures.

Subacute sclerosing panencephalitis results from a long-term brain infection with the measles virus. The virus sometimes enters the brain during a measles infection. It may cause immediate symptoms of brain infection (encephalitis), or it may remain in the brain for a long time without causing problems.

Subacute sclerosing panencephalitis occurs because the measles virus reactivates; in the United States for reasons that are not known, the disorder occurs in about 1 or 2 people per 1 million who previously had measles. In very rare cases, a person who never had measles but received live measles vaccine may develop subacute sclerosing panencephalitis.

The number of people with subacute sclerosing panencephalitis is declining in the United States and Western Europe. Males are affected more often than females.

Symptoms and Diagnosis

The disorder usually begins in children or young adults, generally before age 20. The first symptoms may be poor performance in schoolwork, forgetfulness, temper outbursts, distractibility, sleeplessness, and hallucinations. Sudden muscular jerks of the arms, head, or body may occur. Eventually, seizures may occur, together with abnormal uncontrollable muscle movements. Intellect and speech continue to deteriorate. Later, the muscles become increasingly rigid, and swallowing may become difficult. The swallowing difficulty sometimes causes the person to choke on his saliva, resulting in pneumonia. The person may become blind. In the final phases, the body temperature may rise, and the blood pressure and pulse become abnormal.

A doctor makes the diagnosis based on the symptoms. The diagnosis may be confirmed by a blood test that reveals high levels of antibody to the measles virus, by an abnormal electroencephalogram (EEG), or by magnetic resonance imaging (MRI) or computed tomography (CT) scans that show brain abnormalities.

Prognosis and Treatment

The disease is nearly always fatal within 1 to 3 years. Although the cause of death is usually pneumonia, the pneumonia results from the extreme weakness and abnormal muscle control caused by this disease.

Nothing can be done to halt progression of the disease. Anticonvulsant drugs may be taken to control or reduce seizures.

▲ see page 1493

■ see page 1593

CHAPTER 274

Respiratory Disorders

Respiratory disorders commonly affect children. The most serious and common are asthma, bronchiolitis, and croup.

Asthma

Asthma is a recurring condition in which certain stimuli trigger the airways to temporarily narrow, resulting in difficulty breathing. ▲

Although asthma can develop at any age, it most commonly begins in children, particularly in the first 5 years of life. Some children continue to have asthma into the adult years; in others, it resolves. More children than ever have asthma. Doctors are not sure why this is so, although there are theories. More than 6% of children in the United States have been diagnosed with asthma, a 75% increase in recent decades. The rate soars to 40% among some populations of urban children.

Most children with asthma are able to participate in normal childhood activities, except during flare-ups. A smaller number of children have moderate or severe asthma and need to take daily preventive drugs to enable them to engage in sports and normal play.

For unknown reasons, children with asthma respond to certain stimuli (triggers) in ways that children without asthma do not. There are many potential triggers, and most children respond to only a few. Triggers include indoor irritants, such as strong odors and irritating fumes (perfume, tobacco smoke); outdoor pollution; cold air; exercise; emotional distress; viral respiratory infections; and various substances to which the child is allergic, such as animal dander, dust or house dust mites, molds, and outdoor pollen. In some children, specific triggers for flare-ups cannot be identified.

These triggers all result in a similar response; certain cells in the airways release chemical substances. These substances cause the airways to become inflamed and swollen and stimulate the muscle cells in the walls of the airways to contract. Repeated stimulation by these chemical substances increases mucus production in the airways, causes shedding of the cells lining the airways, and enlarges the muscle cells in the walls of the airways. Each of these responses contributes to a sudden narrowing of the airways (asthma attack). In most children, the airways return to normal between asthma attacks.

Risk Factors

Doctors do not completely understand why some children develop asthma, but a number of risk factors are recognized. A child with one asthmatic parent has a 25% risk of developing asthma; if both parents have asthma, the risk increases to 50%. Children whose mothers smoked during pregnancy are more likely to develop asthma. In the United States, children in urban environments are more likely to develop asthma, particularly if they are from lower socioeconomic groups. Although asthma affects a higher percentage of black children than white, the role that genetic aspects of race play in the increasing rate of asthma is controversial because black children are also more likely to live in urban areas. Children who are exposed to high concentrations of allergens, such as dust mites or cockroach feces, at an early age are more likely to develop asthma. Children who have bronchiolitis ■ at an early age often wheeze with subsequent viral infections. The wheezing may at first be interpreted as asthma, but these children are no more likely than others to have asthma during adolescence.

Symptoms and Diagnosis

As the airways narrow in an asthma attack, the child develops difficulty breathing, typically accompanied by wheezing. Wheezing is a high-pitched noise heard when the child breathes out. Not all asthma attacks produce wheezing, however. Mild asthma, particularly in very young children, may result only in a cough; some older children with mild asthma tend to cough only when exercising or when exposed to cold air. Also, children with extremely severe asthma may not wheeze because there is too little air flowing to make a noise. In a severe attack, breathing becomes visibly difficult, wheezing usually becomes louder, the child breathes faster and with greater effort, and the ribs stand out when the child breathes in (inspiration). With very se-

---

▲ see also page 274   ■ see page 1585

vere attacks, the child gasps for breath and sits upright, leaning forward. The skin is sweaty and pale or blue-tinged.

Children with frequent severe attacks sometimes have a slowing of their growth, but their growth usually catches up to that of other children by adulthood.

A doctor suspects asthma in children who have repeated episodes of wheezing, particularly when family members are known to have asthma or allergies. Children with frequent wheezing episodes may be tested for other disorders, such as cystic fibrosis or gastroesophageal reflux. Older children sometimes undergo pulmonary function tests,▲ although in most children, pulmonary function is normal between flare-ups.

Prognosis, Prevention, and Treatment

One half or more of children with asthma outgrow the condition. Those with more severe disease are more likely to have asthma as adults.

Asthma flare-ups can often be prevented by avoiding whatever triggers a particular child's attacks. Parents of children with allergies usually are advised to remove feather pillows, carpets, drapes, upholstered furniture, stuffed toys, and other potential sources of dust and allergens from the child's room. Secondhand tobacco smoke often worsens symptoms in children with asthma. If a particular allergen cannot be avoided, a doctor may try to desensitize the child using allergy shots, although the benefits of allergy shots for asthma are not well known. Because exercise is so important for a child's development, doctors usually recommend that a child not avoid exercise, but rather use an asthma drug immediately before exercising if needed.

Older children or adolescents known to have asthma often use a peak flow meter—a small device that records how fast a person can blow out air—to measure the degree of airway obstruction. This measurement can be used as an objective assessment of the child's condition.

Treatment of an acute attack consists of opening the airways (bronchodilation) and stopping inflammation. A variety of inhaled drugs open the airways (bronchodilators■). Typical examples are albuterol and ipra-

tropium. Older children and adolescents usually can take these drugs using a metered-dose inhaler. Children younger than 8 years or so often find it easier to use an inhaler with a spacer or holding chamber attached.★ Infants and very young children sometimes can use an inhaler and spacer if an infant-sized mask is attached. Those who cannot use inhalers may receive inhaled drugs at home through a mask connected to a nebulizer, a small device that creates a mist of drug using compressed air. Inhalers and nebulizers are equally effective at delivering the drug. Albuterol also can be taken by mouth, although this route is less effective than inhalation and is usually used only in infants who do not have a nebulizer. Children with moderately severe attacks also may be given corticosteroids by mouth.

Children with very severe attacks are treated in the hospital with bronchodilators given in a nebulizer at least every 20 minutes initially. Sometimes doctors use injections of epinephrine, a bronchodilator, in children with very severe attacks if they are not able to breathe enough of the nebulized mist. Doctors usually give corticosteroids intravenously to children having a severe attack.

Children who have mild, infrequent attacks usually take drugs only during an attack. Children with more frequent or severe attacks also need to take drugs even when they are not having attacks. Different drugs are used depending on the frequency and severity of the child's attacks. Children with infrequent attacks that are not very severe usually use inhaled drugs, such as cromolyn or nedocromil, or a low dose of an inhaled corticosteroid every day to help prevent attacks. These drugs block the release of the chemical substances that inflame the airways, and they reduce inflammation. Long-acting theophylline preparations are a less expensive alternative for prevention in some children. Children with more frequent or more severe attacks also receive one or more other drugs, including long-acting bronchodilators such as salmeterol, leukotriene modifiers such as zafirlukast or montelukast, and inhaled corticosteroids. If these drugs do not prevent severe attacks, children may need to take corticosteroids by mouth. Children who experience attacks mainly during exercise usually inhale a dose of bronchodilator just before exercising.

Because asthma is a long-term condition with a variety of treatments, doctors work with parents and children to make sure they understand the condition as well as possible. Parents and children should learn how to determine the severity of an attack, when to use drugs and a peak flow meter, when to call the doctor, and when to go to the hospital.

Parents and doctors should inform school nurses, childcare providers, and others of the child's condition and drugs being used. Some children may be permitted to use inhalers in school as needed, and others must be supervised by the school nurse.

Bronchiolitis

Bronchiolitis is a contagious viral infection of the airways of infants and young children that causes difficulty in breathing, especially breathing out.

Bronchiolitis is most often caused by the respiratory syncytial virus, although other viruses, such as the parainfluenza and adenoviruses, are sometimes involved. Infection with these viruses causes inflammation of the airways. The inflammation causes the airways to narrow, obstructing the flow of air into and out of the lungs.

Bronchiolitis typically affects children younger than 18 months of age and is most common in infants younger than 6 months. During the first year of life, bronchiolitis affects about 11 of every 100 children, although during some epidemics a much higher proportion of infants is affected. Winter and early spring are the peak seasons for bronchiolitis. The disease may be more common in infants whose mothers smoke cigarettes, particularly those who smoked during pregnancy, and it appears to be less common among breastfed infants. Parents and older siblings can be infected with the same virus, but for them the virus usually causes only a mild cold.

Symptoms and Diagnosis

Bronchiolitis starts with symptoms of a cold—runny nose, sneezing, mild fever, and some coughing. After several days, the child develops difficulty breathing, with a worsened cough. Usually the child has a high-pitched sound on breathing out (wheezing). In most infants, the symptoms are mild; even though the infant may breathe somewhat rapidly and be very congested, he is alert, happy, and eating well. Other infants are more severely affected, breathing rapidly, shallowly, and with difficulty. Sometimes the child turns blue from a lack of oxygen. The rapid breathing creates a

difficulty in drinking, which may result in dehydration.

A doctor bases the diagnosis on the symptoms and the physical examination. Sometimes the doctor swabs mucus from deep inside the nose to try to identify the virus in the laboratory.

Prognosis and Treatment

Most children recover at home in 3 to 5 days. During the illness, frequent small feedings of clear fluids may be given. Increasing difficulty in breathing, bluish skin discoloration, fatigue, and dehydration indicate that the child should be hospitalized. Children with congenital heart or lung disease or an impaired immune system may be hospitalized sooner and are far more likely to become quite ill from bronchiolitis. With proper care, the chance of dying of bronchiolitis is low, even for children who need to be hospitalized.

In the hospital, oxygen levels are monitored with a sensor on a finger, toe, or an earlobe, and oxygen is given by an oxygen tent or face mask. A ventilator may be needed to assist breathing. Intravenous fluids are given if the child cannot drink adequately. Inhaled drugs that open the airways (bronchodilators) may be tried, although their effectiveness in bronchiolitis is questionable. The antiviral drug ribavirin may be given by nebulizer to infants who are premature or who have other conditions that put them at high risk for severe breathing problems, such as congenital heart or lung disease, cystic fibrosis, or AIDS. Antibiotics are not helpful.

Croup

Croup (laryngotracheobronchitis) is a contagious viral infection of the upper airways that causes cough and sometimes difficulty breathing, especially breathing in.

Croup is a viral infection that causes swelling of the lining of the airways, particularly the area just below the voice box (larynx). Parainfluenza virus is the most common cause, but croup can be caused by other viruses, such as the respiratory syncytial virus or an influenza virus. Although croup is most common in the fall and winter, it occurs throughout the year. Croup primarily affects children 6 months to 3 years of age, although it occasionally affects those younger or older. Croup caused by an influenza virus may be particularly severe and is more likely to occur in children between the ages of 3 and 7. The disease is usually spread by breathing in airborne droplets containing viruses or by having contact with objects contaminated by these droplets.

Symptoms and Diagnosis

Croup usually starts with symptoms of a cold—runny nose, sneezing, mild fever, and some coughing. Then the child develops a frequent, unusual-sounding cough, which is described as "brassy" or barking. Sometimes swelling of the airway causes difficulty breathing, which is most noticeable on breathing in (inspiration). In severe croup, there may be a loud squeaking noise (stridor) heard with each inspiration. All symptoms are typically much worse at night and may awaken the child from sleep. The child's condition often improves in the morning and worsens again the next night. A doctor distinguishes croup by its characteristic symptoms, especially the sound of the cough.

Treatment

A child who is mildly ill with croup may be cared for at home and usually recovers in 3 to 4 days. The child should be made comfortable, given plenty of fluids, and allowed to rest because fatigue and crying can worsen the condi-

tion. Home humidifying devices (for example, cool-mist vaporizers or humidifiers) may reduce drying of the upper airways and ease breathing. The humidity can be raised quickly by running a hot shower to steam up the bathroom. Carrying the child outside to breathe cold night air may also open the airways significantly—something parents often discover when the child's breathing returns to normal by the time they arrive at the hospital.

Children who do not respond to these measures need to be taken to the hospital. Children with increasing or continuing difficulty in breathing, rapid heart rate, fatigue, or bluish skin discoloration need to be hospitalized. In the hospital, oxygen is given when levels of oxygen in the blood are low. Doctors usually treat the child with epinephrine given in a nebulizer and corticosteroids given by mouth or injection. These drugs help shrink swollen tissue in the airways. Children who improve with these treatments may be sent home, although children with more severe cases should remain in the hospital. Antibiotics are used only in the rare situation when a child with croup also develops a bacterial infection. Rarely, a ventilator is needed. Fortunately, the vast majority of children with croup recover completely.

CHAPTER 275

Digestive Disorders

Children can develop a variety of digestive disorders. All digestive disorders involve varying degrees of pain, vomiting, or changes in appetite and bowel function. The challenge for parents is to provide information that will help their doctors distinguish serious from nonserious disorders and, in some cases, to help their children adjust to chronic disorders that need medical attention over time.

Gastroenteritis

Gastroenteritis is inflammation of the digestive tract that results in vomiting and diar-

rhea, sometimes accompanied by fever or abdominal cramps.

Gastroenteritis, sometimes called "stomach flu," is common in children.▲ Severe gastroenteritis results in dehydration and an imbalance of blood chemicals (electrolytes) because of a loss of body fluids in the vomit and diarrhea. Although gastroenteritis is rarely serious when proper medical care is available, in developing countries it can be extremely serious; millions of children die each year from diarrhea caused by gastroenteritis.

Causes

A wide variety of viruses, bacteria, and parasites cause gastroenteritis. However, viruses (such as rotavirus) are a far more common

▲ see also page 719

cause than are bacteria (such as *Escherichia coli, Vibrio cholerae, Salmonella,* or *Shigella*) or parasites (such as *Giardia*).

Children usually contract viral gastroenteritis from other children who have had or who have been exposed to it, such as those in childcare centers, schools, and other crowded settings. Viral gastroenteritis is generally spread from hand to mouth but can also be spread by sneezing and spitting. It spreads particularly easily because of the way children play—putting hands and fingers in and near their mouths and then touching toys and each other.

Children can contract bacterial gastroenteritis from eating mayonnaise, dairy products, meat, and other foods that have not been refrigerated. Improper preparation of food, especially undercooking, can lead to gastroenteritis. Gastroenteritis contracted in this way is sometimes called "food poisoning."▲ Children can also contract bacterial or parasitic gastroenteritis from swallowing contaminated water, such as from wells, streams, and swimming pools, and while traveling in developing countries.

Occasionally, gastroenteritis results when children eat things they are not supposed to, such as plants and vitamin pills. Rarely, gastroenteritis results because of an allergic condition (eosinophilic gastroenteritis) or from contact with animals at petting zoos.

Symptoms and Diagnosis

Symptoms are usually a combination of vomiting, diarrhea, abdominal cramps, fever, and poor appetite. Usually, vomiting predominates early in the illness, and diarrhea becomes more prominent later, but some children have both at the same time. The stools may be bloody if certain bacteria are a cause. These symptoms eventually improve in children who drink enough fluids. Children who are slightly dehydrated are thirsty, but seriously dehydrated children become listless, irritable, or lethargic, and may stop drinking. Infants are much more likely than older children to develop these serious side effects.

A doctor bases the diagnosis of gastroenteritis on the child's symptoms and on the parents' responses to questions about what the child has been exposed to. Diagnostic tests are not usually needed because most forms of gastroenteritis get better by themselves over a short time. Doctors who suspect a bacterial or parasitic infection may order additional tests, including stool and blood tests, and ones that measure white blood cells. Dehydrated children require blood tests to help doctors guide treatment.

Prevention and Treatment

The best way to prevent gastroenteritis is to encourage children to wash their hands and to teach them to avoid improperly prepared or stored foods. A vaccine to prevent rotavirus infection is available in developing countries, but its use was discontinued in the United States because of side effects.

Once a child has gastroenteritis, parents should encourage the child to take frequent sips of water and to try to take small amounts of juices and soups, which contain both fluids and electrolytes. If gastroenteritis persists longer than 12 to 24 hours, or the child cannot hold down juice, electrolytes usually should be replaced. Electrolyte replacement is done at home using nonprescription electrolyte solutions available as powders and liquids in pharmacies and some grocery stores.

For a vomiting child, the parents wait about 10 minutes and give the child a few sips of a liquid. If the liquid is not vomited, the sips are repeated every 10 or 15 minutes, increasing the amount given to an ounce or two after an hour or so. These larger amounts can be given less often, about every hour. Liquids are absorbed very quickly, so if the child vomits more than 10 minutes after drinking, most of the fluid was absorbed and fluids should be continued. The amount of liquid to give a child depends on the child's age, but generally should be about $1\frac{1}{2}$ to $2\frac{1}{2}$ ounces of solution for each pound the child weighs in a 24-hour period. If the child's vomiting or diarrhea improves while drinking electrolyte solutions, parents may try resuming a diet of juice, soups, and soft foods like bananas and applesauce the next day.

Children with diarrhea but little vomiting are fed their normal diet, with extra liquid given to make up for the fluid lost in the diarrhea.

Danger signs include inability to keep down even sips of liquid or signs of dehydration (such as lethargy, dry mouth, lack of tears, and no output of urine for 6 hours or more). Such children should see the doctor immediately. Children without such signs should see the

▲ see page 724

doctor if symptoms last more than 1 or 2 days. If the dehydration is severe the doctor may give the child intravenous fluids.

Antidiarrheal drugs such as loperamide are not usually recommended for children; there is reason to think these may slow the resolution of infection by preventing the body from flushing the virus, bacteria, or parasites out with the stools. Antibiotics are of no value when a viral infection is the cause of gastroenteritis. Doctors give antibiotics only for certain bacteria that are known to respond to these drugs. Antiparasitic drugs may be given for a parasitic infection.

Gastroesophageal Reflux

Gastroesophageal reflux is the backward movement of food and acid from the stomach into the esophagus and sometimes into the mouth.▲

Nearly all infants have episodes of gastroesophageal reflux; "burping up" that babies do after feeding is considered normal. Gastroesophageal reflux becomes a concern when it interferes with feeding and nutrition, causes poor weight gain, damages the esophagus, leads to breathing difficulties, or continues beyond infancy into childhood.

Causes

Healthy infants have reflux for many reasons. The circular band of muscle that normally keeps stomach contents from entering the esophagus (lower esophageal sphincter) is not fully developed in infants, allowing stomach contents to move backward into the esophagus. Being held flat during a feeding (instead of more upright) or lying down after a feeding promotes reflux. Overfeeding predisposes to reflux, as does exposure to cigarette smoke or caffeine in breast milk, both of which relax the lower esophageal sphincter and can cause the child to become irritable and eat poorly. Less commonly, children may have an anatomic abnormality, such as narrowing of the esophagus or abnormal position of the intestines (malrotation), which makes reflux even more likely. Immaturity of the nerves that control stomach emptying can also lead to gastroesophageal reflux. Milk allergy is a rare cause.

Symptoms

The most obvious symptoms of gastroesophageal reflux in infants are vomiting and excessive spitting up. Less obviously, the infant may be irritable, may not eat well, or may have "spells" of twisting and posturing that may be confused with seizures.

Reflux usually improves gradually until the age of 1 or 2 years, when the child starts eating solid foods and is able to eat on his own in an upright position. However, reflux occasionally leads to complications. Some infants lose weight. Some develop a low red blood cell count (anemia) because of bleeding from the esophagus, and some inhale (aspirate) stomach acid and food into their lungs. Aspiration of stomach contents can cause pneumonia, asthma, periods when breathing stops (apnea), a slow heart rate, and, extremely rarely, infant death.

Older children are usually able to describe chest pain or heartburn when they have gastroesophageal reflux. Chronic cough, hoarseness, hiccups, ear pain, and high-pitched breathing (stridor) may also be subtle signs of reflux in older children. In some children, reflux may be a cause of chronic ear infection (serous otitis media■).

Diagnosis and Treatment

Diagnosis of gastroesophageal reflux can be difficult when the symptoms are not obvious. Some doctors recommend simple measures to see if an infant's symptoms improve before ordering more extensive tests. For example, a doctor may recommend thicker, smaller, and more frequent feedings with more frequent burpings. Eliminating a child's exposure to cigarette smoke and caffeine also helps. Laying the child to sleep on the stomach or on an angle with the head elevated also reduces reflux. This is one of the few exceptions to the general recommendation that infants be put to sleep on their back and should be done only when a doctor specifically recommends it. Occasionally, doctors recommend a change of formula to determine if cow's milk or a formula ingredient is contributing to the infant's problem.

Some doctors recommend that infants whose symptoms do not improve with these measures and most older children try drug treatment for a short time before undergoing diagnostic testing. Drugs for reflux are generally safe and effective. Antacids neutralize stomach acid, and histamine-2 blockers and

---

▲ see also page 717   ■ see page 1594

proton pump inhibitors suppress acid production by the stomach and improve reflux symptoms, at least temporarily. Promotility drugs, such as metoclopramide, stimulate the stomach to move its contents forward rather than backward and may tighten the lower esophageal sphincter.

Various tests can be used to diagnose reflux. X-rays taken after swallowing barium help doctors determine if the anatomy of the esophagus and stomach is normal. In addition, a diary can be kept to record the child's symptoms. Information from this diary, combined with monitoring of the level of acid in the esophagus through a small flexible tube that has been passed through the nose, helps doctors determine if reflux episodes are the cause of the symptoms. A form of radionuclide imaging called a gastric emptying study can reveal to what degree stomach contents move forward appropriately or reflux backward. Examination of the esophagus using a flexible viewing tube (endoscopy) allows doctors to see if the esophagus is inflamed or bleeding. Examination of the voice box (larynx) and airways through a flexible viewing tube (bronchoscopy▲) gives information that helps doctors decide if reflux is a likely cause of lung or breathing problems.

Peptic Ulcer

A peptic ulcer is erosion of the lining of the stomach or duodenum due to excess stomach acid, breakdown of the stomach's protective lining, or both.

Peptic ulcers are much less common in children than in adults. As with adults, use of nonsteroidal anti-inflammatory drugs (NSAIDs) and infection with *Helicobacter pylori* bacteria can lead to the formation of peptic ulcers.■ Children whose parents have peptic ulcers are more likely to have ulcers, as are those whose parents smoke. Adolescents who drink alcohol or smoke are also more likely to develop ulcers. Children of any age can develop ulcers when they are extremely sick, such as after severe burns, injuries, and illnesses.

Infants with ulcers may be fussy and irritable around feedings. Ulcers in older children usually cause abdominal pain. At any age, peptic ulcers can perforate, bleed, or lead to obstruction. The diagnosis and treatment of peptic ulcers and their complications are the same in children as in adults.

Intussusception

Intussusception is the telescoping of one portion of the intestine into another, causing obstruction of the bowel and blockage of its blood flow.

Intussusception is an uncommon cause of abdominal pain that typically affects children between the ages of 6 months and 2 years. It can occasionally affect older children. In most cases, the cause is unknown. Rarely, thickening of the intestinal wall due to a diverticulum, polyp, or tumor may lead to intussusception.

Symptoms

Intussusception usually causes sudden pain in a child who is otherwise healthy. The pain initially comes and goes, and the child may pull his legs up to his trunk during pain spasms. The child may return to normal activities between episodes, but the pain eventually becomes constant. Some children simply become irritable or listless and apathetic between episodes of pain. After a time, the child may vomit, pass stools with blood and mucus ("currant jelly" stools), or develop a fever. If unrecognized and untreated, intussusception can cause death of bowel tissue, which spreads bacteria from the gut into the bloodstream.

Diagnosis and Treatment

A doctor may suspect intussusception based on the child's symptoms and a physical examination. X-rays may be useful, but results are normal about one third of the time. Ultrasound is better, but a barium enema can both diagnose and treat intussusception. With a barium enema, the doctor instills barium and air into the child's rectum and then takes x-rays. The pressure of the barium and air pushes the collapsed portion of the intestine back into place. Sometimes just air without barium is used. When this procedure is successful, the child can be sent home from the hospital after a short time. Parents are advised to watch for symptoms because intussusception can recur in the next 1 to 2 days.

Surgery is needed if the barium enema is not successful in correcting the intussusception, if the child is too ill to tolerate a barium enema, if the child has recurrences of the condition, or if complications occur. In the case of a re-

▲ see page 256   ■ see page 713

currence, surgery is performed not only to correct the condition but also to look for a polyp, tumor, or other abnormality that could explain why the intussusception recurred.

Appendicitis

Appendicitis is inflammation and infection of the appendix.

The appendix is a small finger-length portion of intestine that does not appear to have any essential bodily function.▲ Appendicitis is a medical emergency that requires surgery. Appendicitis is rare in children younger than 1 year but becomes more common as children grow older and is most common in adolescents.

Appendicitis seems to develop when the appendix becomes blocked either as a result of infection in the digestive tract or elsewhere in the body or, less commonly, as a result of obstruction with hard feces. In either case, the appendix becomes infected. If an infected appendix is unrecognized or untreated, the appendix can rupture, creating a pocket of infection outside the intestine (abscess) or spilling contents of the intestines into the abdomen (peritonitis).

Symptoms and Diagnosis

Appendicitis almost always causes pain. The pain may start in the middle of the abdomen, near the navel, and gradually move to the lower right area of the abdomen. However, children younger than 2 years are often not able to complain of pain and are therefore more likely to be irritable or listless. They may lose consciousness partly or completely if a delay in diagnosis has led to rupture of the appendix with peritonitis. Older children sometimes develop diffuse abdominal pain rather than pain in the specific area of the appendix.

The diagnosis of appendicitis in children can be challenging for many reasons. The child can have gastroenteritis, Meckel's diverticulum, intussusception, or Crohn's disease, all of which may cause symptoms similar to those of appendicitis. The child may not have a fever or elevated white blood cell count, which are signs of infection. And the child may ask for food rather than avoid it in the way adults with appendicitis typically do.

Doctors who suspect appendicitis usually give intravenous fluids and antibiotics while waiting for results of blood tests. They may order ultrasound or computed tomography (CT) scans to see inside the abdomen. Repeated physical examinations help a doctor determine whether the condition is improving or getting worse and make a decision about treatment.

Treatment

The best treatment for appendicitis is surgical removal of the inflamed appendix (appendectomy). Appendectomy is fairly simple and safe, requiring a hospital stay of 2 to 3 days. If the appendix has ruptured, the doctor removes it and may wash out the abdomen with fluid, give antibiotics for several days, and watch for complications, such as infection and bowel blockage. About 10 to 20% of the time, surgeons discover a normal appendix while performing an appendectomy. This is not considered a medical error because the consequences of delaying surgery when appendicitis is suspected are serious. When the appendix is found to be normal, the surgeon looks within the abdomen for another cause of the pain. The doctor may remove the normal appendix so that the child will never develop appendicitis.

Meckel's Diverticulum

Meckel's diverticulum is a saclike outpouching of the wall of the small intestine present in some children at birth.

About 3% of infants are born with Meckel's diverticulum. People can live their whole lives without ever knowing they have Meckel's diverticulum, but occasionally the abnormality can cause problems.

Symptoms and Diagnosis

Most children with Meckel's diverticulum have no symptoms, and many adults learn they have the condition only after surgeons discover it while performing surgery for another reason. The most common symptom in children younger than 2 years is painless rectal bleeding, which comes from ulcers in the small intestine caused by acid secreted by the diverticulum. Because of the bleeding, stools may appear bright red or brick- or currant jelly–colored because of a mixture of blood and mucus. Or they may appear black because of the breakdown of blood. Only rarely is the bleeding so severe that the child needs emergency attention.

Sometimes, the diverticulum can become inflamed or infected, a condition called diver-

▲ see art on page 695

ticulitis. Diverticulitis caused by a Meckel's diverticulum causes severe pain, abdominal tenderness, and sometimes vomiting and can easily be confused with appendicitis.

It is often difficult for doctors to diagnose Meckel's diverticulum. Blood tests, x-rays, computed tomography (CT), and barium enemas are not usually helpful. The best test is an imaging study called a Meckel radionuclide scan, in which a substance is given intravenously and is taken up by the diverticulum and detected by a camera.

Treatment

No treatment is needed for a diverticulum that does not cause symptoms. A bleeding diverticulum or one that causes symptoms must be surgically removed. If a Meckel's diverticulum is found in a child during an operation being performed for another reason, it is generally removed to prevent future complications.

Constipation

Constipation is the difficult and infrequent passing of hard, dry stools.

Parents often worry about how often their children have bowel movements. However, constipation generally does not have any serious consequences and should be a concern only when passing stools becomes painful and leads to withholding of stools, or when constipation causes other symptoms.

Causes and Symptoms

Constipation is extremely common in children. The most common cause is insufficient amounts of fruits, vegetables, and whole grains (fiber) in the child's diet.

Children who are constipated often report intermittent abdominal discomfort. After a time, parents may notice soiling of the child's underwear because liquid stool from the intestine involuntarily leaks around hard stool in the rectum. Small amounts of blood may appear from small erosions (fissures) caused by the passage of hard stools. Occasionally, constipation can lead to difficulty with urination.

Treatment

Minor cases of constipation can be treated by increasing the child's dietary fiber, either with whole grains and fruits or with a supplement such as psyllium. Good hydration is important. Sometimes, reducing the intake of milk helps constipation. Children become distracted and typically do not sit long enough on

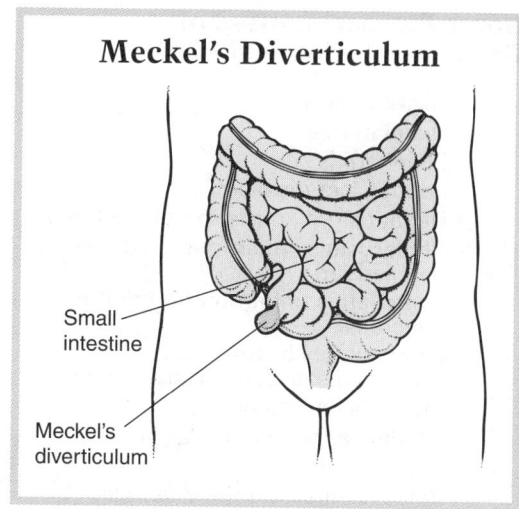

Meckel's Diverticulum

Small intestine

Meckel's diverticulum

the toilet to pass constipated stools. They need to be guided to sit an adequate time on the toilet at regular intervals—at least twice a day—so they can establish a routine that gives them the opportunity to defecate fully. Parents can use enemas and stool softeners, such as mineral oil or milk of magnesia, to facilitate this process if necessary.

Children accustomed to withholding their stools may need several months of stool softeners to get them reconditioned to soft, comfortable stools.

Recurring Abdominal Pain

Recurring abdominal pain is abdominal pain that occurs 3 or more times over a period of at least 3 months.

About 1 in 10 school-aged children has recurring abdominal pain. It is most common in children between the ages of 8 and 10 and is rare in those younger than 4. Recurring abdominal pain is slightly more common among girls than boys and is fairly common among girls in early adolescence.

Causes

In most children, recurring abdominal pain is caused by anxiety and other psychologic distress that is a result of stress at school, with friends, between parents, or within a family. A significant number of children with the condition are depressed. About 1 in 10 have an identifiable physical cause, usually from a digestive or genitourinary tract disorder. The absence of a physical cause in most children is sometimes frustrating for parents.

Some Physical Causes of Recurring Abdominal Pain

Intestinal disorders
- Hiatal hernia
- Esophagitis
- Peptic ulcer disease
- Hepatitis (inflammation of the liver)
- Cholecystitis (inflammation of the gallbladder)
- Pancreatitis (inflammation of the pancreas)
- Inflammatory bowel disease (Crohn's disease, ulcerative colitis)
- Meckel's diverticulum
- Chronic appendicitis
- Intussusception
- Parasitic infection (for example, giardiasis)
- Tuberculosis of the intestine
- Celiac sprue
- Constipation
- Lactase deficiency

Genitourinary disorders
- Structural anomalies
- Urinary tract infection
- Normal monthly ovulation (in girls)
- Menstrual cramps (in girls)
- Pelvic inflammatory disease (in girls)
- Ovarian cysts (in girls)
- Endometriosis (in girls)

General illnesses
- Heavy metal poisoning (lead)
- Henoch-Schönlein purpura
- Sickle cell disease
- Food allergy
- Porphyria
- Familial Mediterranean fever
- Hereditary angioedema
- Abdominal migraine

When recurring abdominal pain has no physical cause, concerned responses from parents and teachers can make the pain better or worse to the extent that it favorably alters stressful situations to which the child is responding. For example, pain that distracts family members from arguing, garners attention for the child, or takes the child away from school or other stressful settings may be an effective way for a child to relieve anxieties he could otherwise not control. Importantly, most children do not intentionally use their symptoms to communicate distress to their parents or teachers. Rather, it is a symptom of true and significant emotional discomfort.

The most serious cause of recurring abdominal pain is sexual abuse. However, routine stresses at school or home are far more common causes of recurring abdominal pain than is sexual abuse.

Symptoms

Recurring abdominal pain caused by a physical condition generally recurs at predictable times or in the same location. It may be brought on by certain activities or foods and may worsen over days to months. Often, although not always, the pain may awaken the child from sleep. The child may also have other symptoms, such as loss of appetite, weight loss, changes in the form and color of bowel movements, constipation or diarrhea, vomiting of food or blood, swelling of the abdomen, recurring or persistent fever, jaundice, blood in the stools, or discomfort with urination.

Recurring abdominal pain without a clear physical cause is generally less likely to recur at predictable times and in the same location. It is often described in vague terms and occasionally disappears for weeks or months. It seldom disturbs a child during sleep but may wake him up early. The child can often be distracted from the pain by activities he enjoys; this is less likely to be the case when there are physical causes of the pain.

Diagnosis

The doctor asks the parent and child a series of questions about the character of the pain and about any symptoms that occur with it. The doctor also performs a physical examination, including a rectal examination, looking for clues for a physical cause. The interview and examination give the doctor the information to decide what additional tests, if any, the child should undergo. Often, the doctor may strongly suspect a psychologic cause just from the child's answers to questions and from observing the child and parents in the interview.

Some possible tests for recurring abdominal pain range from urine and blood tests, which can detect infection, to more invasive procedures, such as colonoscopy, which can detect inflammation and other abnormalities within the large intestine. However, invasive tests are rarely needed. Given the frequency with which depression or anxiety accompanies symptoms of recurring abdominal pain, many doctors consider psychologic assessment to be the most important test.

Treatment

Physical causes of recurring abdominal pain are treated for the specific disorder responsible. When a physical cause for the child's symptoms cannot be found, a doctor may suspect a psychologic cause. Treatment then depends on good communication and a trusting relationship with the doctor as well as periodic monitoring of the child's symptoms.

The child should be supported in efforts to return to a full range of activities, including school. Teachers have a large role to play in limiting the child's withdrawal from activities with peers and in helping the child resolve conflicts related to school. A child who needs to leave class because of pain should be allowed to visit the school nurse for only a limited time. With the parents' permission, the nurse can give the child a mild pain reliever, such as ibuprofen or acetaminophen, if neces-

sary. Typically, a child will request time in the nurse's office 1 or more times a day during the first week or two of treatment. Over time, the behavior becomes less frequent. Generally, when the parents stop treating the child as different or ill, pain with a psychologic cause initially worsens but then improves.

A child whose abdominal pain has no physical cause may be helped by seeing the doctor at regular intervals—weekly, monthly, or every other month—depending on the child's needs. In some cases, the doctor may prescribe antidepressants or antianxiety drugs. This treatment may result in a reduction or disappearance of the child's symptoms, but it is not always successful. Some children may develop new physical symptoms or emotional difficulties, or they may express unresolved emotional difficulties with new symptoms, such as a headache. If the pain persists despite all efforts, especially if the child is severely depressed or if there are significant psychologic problems at home, the child may need to see a mental health professional.

CHAPTER 276

Ear, Nose, and Throat Disorders

Ear, nose, and throat disorders are extremely common in children. Ear infections occur almost as often as the common cold. They can occur behind the eardrum (in the middle ear, otitis media) or in front of the eardrum (in the outer ear, otitis externa▲). Throat infections are not usually serious, but they make children uncomfortable and can lead to missed school days and multiple doctor visits. Other disorders, such as hearing deficits and neck masses, affect fewer children but are potentially serious. In general, any abnormality of a child's ear, nose, or throat that does not improve within several days should be evaluated by a doctor.

Middle Ear Infections

Middle ear infections are extremely common between the ages of 3 months and 3 years and often accompany the common cold. Young children are susceptible to middle ear infections for several reasons. The eustachian

tube, which balances pressure within the ear, connects the middle ear with the nasal passages.■ In older children and adults, the tube is more vertical, wider, and fairly rigid, and secretions that pass into it from the nasal passages drain easily. But in younger children, the eustachian tube is more horizontal, narrower, and less rigid. The tube is more likely to become obstructed by secretions and to collapse, trapping those secretions in or close to the middle ear and impairing middle ear ventilation. Any viruses or bacteria in the secretions then multiply, causing infection. Viruses and bacteria can move back up the short eustachian tube of infants, causing middle ear infections.

Besides differences in anatomy of the ear, infants at about the age of 6 months become more susceptible to infection because they lose protection from their mother's antibod-

---

▲ see page 1253   ■ see art on page 1257

ies, which they received through the placenta before birth. Breastfeeding appears to partially protect children from ear infections because the mother's antibodies are contained in breast milk. Children also become more sociable around this time and may develop viral infections by touching other children and objects and putting their fingers in their mouth and nose; these infections may in turn lead to middle ear infections. Exposure to cigarette smoke further increases the risk for middle ear infections, as does the use of a pacifier, both of which may impair the function of the eustachian tube and affect middle ear ventilation. Attendance at childcare centers increases the risk of exposure to the common cold and hence to otitis media.

Middle ear infections can resolve relatively quickly (acute), or they can recur or persist over a long time (chronic).

ACUTE MIDDLE EAR INFECTION

Acute middle ear infection (also called acute otitis media▲) is most often caused by the same viruses that cause the common cold. Acute infection may also be caused by bacteria found in the mouth and nose, such as *Streptococcus pneumoniae, Haemophilus influenzae,* and *Moraxella catarrhalis.* An infection initially caused by a virus sometimes leads to a bacterial infection.

Infants with acute middle ear infections have fever, crying or irritability that sometimes cannot be explained, and disturbances in sleep. They may also have a runny nose, cough, vomiting, and diarrhea. Infants and children who cannot fully communicate may pull at their ears. Older children are usually able to tell parents that their ear hurts or that they cannot hear well.

Commonly, fluid may accumulate behind the eardrum and persist after the acute infection has resolved (serous otitis media). Rarely, acute middle ear infection leads to more serious complications. Rupture of the eardrum can cause drainage of blood or fluid from the ear. Infection of the bone surrounding the ear (mastoiditis) can cause pain; infection of the inner ear (labyrinthitis) can cause dizziness and deafness; and infection of the tissues surrounding the brain (meningitis) or brain abscesses (collections of pus) can cause sei-

---

▲ see also page 1257

■ see also page 1258

zures and other neurologic problems. Recurring infections can promote growth of skinlike tissue through the eardrum (cholesteatoma). Cholesteatoma can damage the bones of the middle ear and cause hearing loss.

Doctors diagnose acute middle ear infections by looking for bulging and redness of the eardrum with an otoscope. They may need to clean wax from the ear first so they can see more clearly. Doctors may use a rubber bulb and tube attached to the otoscope to squeeze air into the ear to see if the eardrum moves. If the eardrum does not move or moves only slightly, then infection may be present.

Acetaminophen or ibuprofen is effective for fever and pain. Doctors used to give antibiotics to all children with acute middle ear infections. However, they now realize that many acute middle ear infections improve without antibiotics. Thus, many doctors use antibiotics (such as amoxicillin with or without clavulanate, or trimethoprim with sulfamethoxazole) only when the child does not improve after a brief period of time or if there are signs that the infection is not getting better.

CHRONIC MIDDLE EAR INFECTION

Chronic middle ear infection occurs as a result of repeated acute infection or when recurring infections damage the eardrum or lead to formation of a cholesteatoma, which in turn promotes more infection. Chronic ear infections are more likely among children who are exposed to cigarette smoke, use pacifiers, and attend group day care centers. For children with chronic ear infections, doctors may recommend daily antibiotics for several months. If infection persists or recurs despite the use of antibiotics, or if chronic infections have led to eardrum damage or formation of cholesteatoma, doctors may recommend ventilating (tympanostomy) tubes, eardrum repair, or surgical removal of the cholesteatoma.

Serous Otitis Media

Serous otitis media is fluid accumulation behind the eardrum.■

Serous otitis media often occurs after acute otitis media. The fluid that has accumulated behind the eardrum during the acute infection remains after the infection resolves. Serous otitis media may also occur without preceding infection, and may be due to gastroesophageal reflux disease or a blockage of the eustachian tube by infection or enlarged adenoids. Serous

Ventilating Tubes: Treating Recurring Ear Infections

Ventilating (tympanostomy) tubes are tiny, hollow plastic or metal tubes that are placed in the eardrum through a small slit. These tubes equalize the pressure between the environment and the middle ear. Doctors recommend ventilating tubes for children who have had recurring ear infections (acute otitis media) or chronic fluid collections in their middle ears (serous otitis media).

Placement of ventilating tubes is a common surgical procedure, performed in a hospital or doctor's office. After the procedure, children usually go home within a few hours. The tubes usually fall out on their own after a few months, although some types stay in for a year or more. Children with ventilating tubes may wash their hair and go swimming, but some doctors recommend that the children not submerge their head completely in water without using earplugs. Drainage of fluid from the ears indicates an infection and the doctor should be notified.

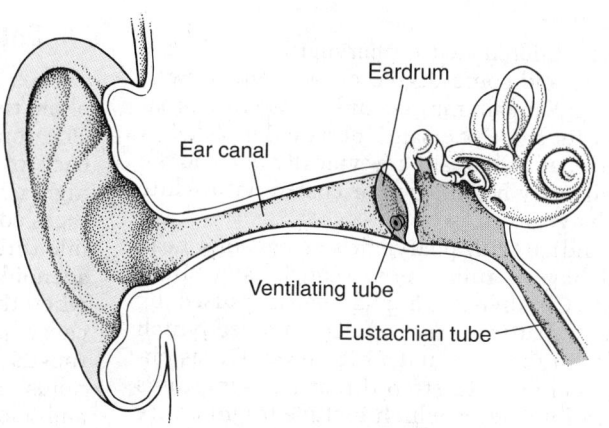

otitis media is extremely common in children between the ages of 3 months and 3 years.

Although serous otitis media is painless, the fluid can impair hearing, understanding of speech, language development, learning, and behavior.

Doctors diagnose serous otitis media by looking for changes in the color and appearance of the eardrum and by squeezing air into the ear to see if the eardrum moves. If the eardrum does not move but there is no redness or bulging and the child has few symptoms, then serous otitis media is likely.

Serous otitis media often does not improve when treated with antibiotics or other drugs, such as decongestants, antihistamines, or nasal sprays. The condition often resolves by itself after weeks or months.

If the condition persists without improvement after 3 months, surgery may help. In the United States, doctors perform myringotomy, in which they make a tiny slit in the eardrum, remove the fluid, and insert a small ventilating (tympanostomy) tube in the slit to provide drainage from the middle to the outer ear. Some doctors may perform a myringotomy to remove fluid but not to insert ventilating tubes; this procedure is called tympanocentesis.

Pharyngitis

Pharyngitis is infection of the throat (pharynx) and sometimes the tonsils.

Most pharyngitis is caused by the same viruses that cause the common cold. Like the common cold, viral pharyngitis gets better by itself and is a problem only because it makes children miserable and causes them to miss school. Streptococcus bacteria are a less common but more serious cause of pharyngitis ("strep throat"); strep throat is unusual in children younger than 2 years. Pharyngitis is also rarely caused by unusual infections, such as infectious mononucleosis or—in countries with low vaccination rates—diphtheria.

The tonsils (patches of lymphoid tissue at the back of the throat) also can become infected in children with pharyngitis. A doctor may use the term tonsillitis when the tonsils are particularly enlarged. Occasionally, the tonsils remain infected, inflamed, or enlarged (chronic tonsillitis) after an episode of pharyngitis.

Bacterial pharyngitis can cause persistent inflammation, infection, and enlargement of the tonsils (chronic tonsillitis); pus within folds of the tonsils (cryptic tonsillitis); and abscesses in the tissues to the side of the pharynx (lateral pharyngeal abscesses), behind the pharynx (retropharyngeal abscesses), or around the tonsils (peritonsillar abscesses▲). Some rare complications of streptococcal pharyngitis include rheumatic fever,■ glomerulonephritis, or life-threatening infection of the tissues (necrotizing fasciitis) and bloodstream (toxic shock syndrome).

Symptoms

All children with pharyngitis have sore throats and some degree of pain when swallowing. Ear pain may occur because the throat and ears share the same nerves. The back of the throat and tonsils are typically red, and the tonsils may be enlarged or coated with white discharge.

Children with pharyngitis as part of a head cold have a runny nose, cough, and slight fever. Children with pharyngitis caused by strep throat may have tender, enlarged lymph nodes in the neck and a high fever. Occasionally, a child with strep throat has symptoms of scarlet fever,★ which include bright white or red changes of the tongue ("strawberry tongue") and a distinctive red skin rash (scarlatiniform rash).

Children with chronic tonsillitis may have a sore throat or discomfort or pain with swallowing.

Diagnosis and Treatment

Doctors suspect pharyngitis when they see redness and white discharge or pus in the back of the throat and when the lymph nodes in the neck are enlarged.

If doctors suspect strep throat, they may take a swab from the back of the throat and send it for two tests: rapid antigen testing and a bacterial culture. Rapid antigen testing can detect strep throat within minutes. If the result of a rapid test is positive, the bacterial culture is not needed. However, if the result of the rapid test is negative, most doctors perform a culture, which takes about 1 to 2 days for results.

Strep throat is usually treated with penicillin, either in a single injection or over 10 days by mouth. If the child is allergic to penicillin, the doctor may give erythromycin or another antibiotic. Treatment of strep throat and viral pharyngitis includes giving ibupro-

fen or acetaminophen for pain and fever and encouraging the child to drink fluids. Providing soup is a good way to keep the child well hydrated and nourished when swallowing is painful and before the appetite has returned. Gargling with salt water or using an anesthetic throat spray may also help to temporarily relieve pain.

Enlarged Tonsils and Adenoids

Tonsils and adenoids are collections of lymphoid tissue that help the body fight infection. The tonsils are located on both sides of the back of the throat. The adenoids are located higher and further back, where the nasal passages connect with the throat, and are not visible through the mouth. However, tonsils and adenoids can become enlarged—for example, when they become infected with bacteria that cause pharyngitis. When this happens, the tonsils become more prominent and the adenoids may block the nose. Usually, the tonsils and adenoids return to normal size once the infection is over. Sometimes they remain enlarged, particularly in children who have had frequent or chronic infections. Although extremely rare, cancer sometimes causes enlarged tonsils or adenoids in children.

Symptoms

Most enlarged tonsils and adenoids cause no symptoms; some degree of tonsillar enlargement is even considered normal in preschool and adolescent children. However, children with enlarged tonsils or adenoids can experience sore throat and discomfort or pain with swallowing. Enlarged adenoids can give the voice a "pinched nose" quality and lead to changes in the shape of the child's palate and the position of the teeth.

Enlarged tonsils and adenoids are considered a problem when they cause more serious effects. They can cause chronic ear infections and hearing loss due to obstruction of the eustachian tube and fluid accumulation in the middle ear. They can also cause recurring sinus infections and nosebleeds. Some children have obstructive sleep apnea,● with snoring and brief periods without breathing; this can cause low oxygen levels in the blood, frequent waking, and daytime sleepiness. Rarely, obstructive sleep apnea caused by enlarged tonsils and adenoids can lead to serious complications, such as high blood pressure in the lungs (pulmonary hypertension) and changes in the

▲ see page 1267   ■ see page 1565
★ see page 1113   ● see page 472

heart that result from pulmonary hypertension (cor pulmonale▲).

Children with enlarged tonsils can also lose or fail to gain weight, either because of pain and difficulty eating or because of the constant physical effort it takes for them to breathe.

Diagnosis and Treatment

Doctors do not rely on the size of the tonsils alone to make the diagnosis. Very large tonsils may be normal, and chronically infected tonsils may be normal-sized. Instead, doctors look for redness of the tonsils, enlargement of lymph nodes at the jaw and in the neck, and the effect of the tonsils on breathing. The diagnosis of obstructive sleep apnea is suspected when parents report frequent periods without breathing. Doctors may also recommend a polysomnogram, in which oxygen in the blood is measured and the child is observed while sleeping.

Doctors may give antibiotics if they think a bacterial infection may be the cause of the enlarged tonsils. If antibiotics are not effective or if doctors think antibiotics will not be useful, they may recommend the surgical removal of the tonsils and adenoids (tonsillectomy and adenoidectomy).

Tonsillectomy and adenoidectomy used to be very common operations performed on children in the United States, but they are much less common now that doctors are more aware of which children will benefit from the operation. Children who benefit from surgery include those with obstructive sleep apnea and those whose talking and breathing are extremely uncomfortable. Doctors may also recommend surgery if they think cancer might be a cause of the enlargement, or if the child has had multiple throat or ear infections (defined by some as seven or more infections in 1 year, five or more infections a year over 2 years, or three or more a year over 3 years). A doctor may recommend adenoidectomy alone for ear infections, recurring nasal congestion, or sinus infections.

Tonsillectomy and adenoidectomy have not been shown to decrease the frequency or severity of colds, cough, and other symptoms. These procedures should be performed at least 3 weeks after any infection has cleared.

Tonsillectomy and adenoidectomy are usually performed on an outpatient basis. The surgical complication rate is low, but postoperative pain and difficulty swallowing may

last up to a week. Bleeding is a less common complication but may occur anytime from the first day of surgery to the tenth day after surgery.

Hearing Deficits

About 3 in every 1,000 children are born with severe hearing deficits. One in ten may be born with deficits that are less severe, and many more who have normal hearing at birth develop hearing deficits before adulthood. Failure to recognize and treat a deficit can seriously impair a child's ability to speak and understand language. The impairment can lead to failure in school, teasing by peers, social isolation, and emotional difficulties.

Causes

Genetic defects are the most common cause of hearing deficits in newborns. Ear infections, including serous otitis media, are the most common cause of hearing deficits in older children, along with accumulation of earwax. Other causes in older children are head trauma,

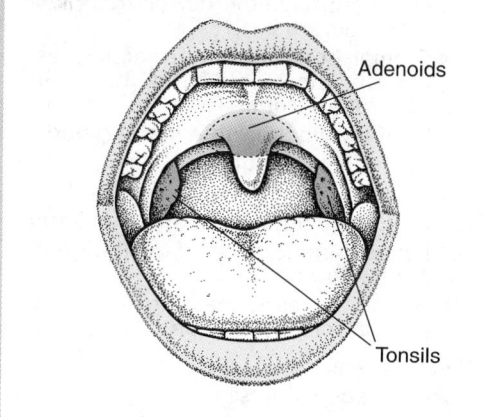

Locating the Tonsils and Adenoids

The tonsils are two areas of lymphoid tissue located on either side of the throat. The adenoids, also lymphoid tissue, are located higher and further back, behind the palate, where the nasal passages connect with the throat. The adenoids are not visible through the mouth.

Adenoids

Tonsils

▲ see box on page 323

Risk Factors for Hearing Deficits in Children

Newborns

- Low birth weight (especially less than 3.3 pounds)
- Low Apgar score (lower than 5 at 1 minute or lower than 7 at 5 minutes)
- Low blood oxygen or seizures resulting from a difficult delivery
- Infection with rubella, syphilis, herpes, cytomegalovirus, or toxoplasmosis before birth
- Cranial or facial abnormalities, especially those involving the outer ear and ear canal
- High level of bilirubin in the blood
- Bacterial meningitis
- Bloodstream infection (sepsis)
- Prolonged time spent on a ventilator
- Drugs (aminoglycoside antibiotics, some diuretics)
- History of early hearing loss in a parent or close relative

Older children

All the above, plus:

- Head trauma with skull fracture or loss of consciousness
- Chronic otitis media with cholesteatoma
- Some neurologic disorders, such as neurofibromatosis and neurodegenerative disorders
- Exposure to noise
- Perforation of the eardrum from infection or trauma

loud noise (including loud music), use of aminoglycoside antibiotics (such as gentamicin) or thiazide diuretics, certain viral infections (for example, mumps), tumors or traumas that damage the auditory nerve, trauma from pencils or other foreign objects that get stuck deep in the ear, and rarely, autoimmune disease.

Symptoms

Parents may suspect a severe hearing deficit if the child does not respond to sounds or if the child has difficulty talking or delayed speech. Less severe hearing deficits can be more subtle and lead to symptoms that are misinterpreted by parents and doctors. Children who ignore their parents or other people who are talking to them some, but not all of

the time, may be doing so because of modest hearing deficits. Children who talk and hear well at home but not in school may have a mild or moderate hearing deficit that is a problem only in the midst of the background noise of a classroom. In general, children who are developing well in one setting but who have significant social, behavioral, language, or learning difficulties in a different setting should be screened for hearing deficits.

Screening and Diagnosis

Because hearing plays such an important role in a child's development, many doctors recommend that all newborns be tested for hearing deficits by the age of 3 months. This testing is required by law in many states.

Screening is usually done in two parts. First, the child is tested for echoes produced by healthy ears in response to soft clicks made by a handheld device (evoked otoacoustic emissions testing). If this test raises questions about a child's hearing, a second test measures electrical signals from the brain in response to sounds (the auditory brain stem response test [ABR]). The ABR is painless and usually performed while the child is sleeping; it can be performed on children of any age. If results of the ABR are abnormal, the test is repeated in 1 month. If hearing loss is still detected, the child may be fitted with hearing aids and may benefit from placement in an educational setting responsive to children with hearing deficits.

Several different tools are used to diagnose hearing deficits in older children. One involves asking a series of questions to detect delays in a child's normal development or to assess a parent's concern about language and speech development. The child's ears may also be examined for abnormalities. Children between the ages of 6 months and 2 years may be tested for their response to various sounds. Additionally, the response of the eardrum to a range of sound frequencies (tympanometry) may indicate if there is fluid in the middle ear. After the age of 2 years, children can usually demonstrate that they hear and understand speech by following simple commands, and they can be tested for responses to sounds using earphones.

Treatment

Some causes of hearing loss can be treated so that a child can regain hearing. For example, ear infections can be treated with antibiotics or surgery, earwax can be manually removed or dissolved with ear drops, and cholesteatomas can be surgically removed.

Most often, however, the cause of a child's hearing loss cannot be reversed, and treatment involves use of a hearing aid to compensate for the deficit as much as possible.

Hearing aids are available for children as young as 2 months. Children with a mild or moderate hearing deficit that occurs only in the classroom may also respond well to radio systems that transmit a teacher's voice directly to a set of speakers, hearing aids, or earphones. Cochlear implants (devices placed in the inner ear to stimulate the auditory nerve with an electrical current in response to sounds) are used for children with severe hearing deficits.▲

A sense of pride has grown in recent years among people in deaf communities concerning their rich culture and alternative forms of communication. Many people oppose the aggressive treatment of hearing deficits on the grounds that it denies children the opportunities available in those communities. Families who wish to consider this approach should discuss it with their doctor.

Objects in the Ears and Nose

Cotton, pieces of pencils, paper, pebbles, and beans are just a few of the many objects children put in their ears and nose. Insects sometimes crawl into ears and cause significant pain.

Objects in the ear can be removed by flushing with sterile water or saline, using suction, or with forceps or other tools. A doctor may remove an insect by putting a topical anesthetic or mineral oil in the ear, which kills the insect, stops pain, and makes removal easier. Younger, more frightened children may need sedation or general anesthesia for these procedures.

Sharp objects, such as pencils, can perforate the child's eardrum. Perforations require evaluation by an ear specialist, but most heal by themselves over time without loss of hearing.

Objects stuck up the nose are of greater concern because they can obstruct the child's airway, cause infection, and be difficult to remove. Children are often scared to admit they put an object in their nose; many parents become aware of the problem only after the child develops persistent bleeding, a runny nose, a

foul-smelling discharge, or difficulty breathing on one side of the nose only.

Doctors use a topical anesthetic and attempt to remove the object using suction or forceps. If these measures do not work, the doctor may need to sedate the child or give general anesthesia to remove the object.

Neck Masses

Neck masses are swellings that change the shape of the neck.

Neck masses are extremely common in children. The most common cause of a neck mass is one or more enlarged lymph nodes.■ A lymph node may enlarge if it is infected (lymphadenitis) or if there is an infection nearby, such as the throat. Some neck masses are the result of a cyst (a fluid-filled sac) present from birth that is noticed only after it becomes inflamed or infected. Other causes include swelling due to trauma to the neck, inflammation of the salivary glands, or noncancerous (benign) tumors. Rarely, lymphoma and thyroid tumors or other cancerous (malignant) tumors are causes.

Most neck masses cause no symptoms and are of greater concern to parents than to the children who have them. However, infected lymph nodes or cysts are tender and painful.

Because many neck masses are caused by viral infections and disappear without treatment, tests are usually not needed unless a mass persists for several weeks. However, doctors may take a swab from the back of the throat to test for a bacterial infection, or they may perform blood tests to look for such conditions as infectious mononucleosis, leukemia, hyperthyroidism, or bleeding problems. Doctors may also perform x-rays and computed tomography (CT) to determine if the mass is a tumor or a cyst and to determine more precisely how big it is and where it extends. A skin test may determine if tuberculosis is a likely cause, and a biopsy gives the doctor information about whether a cancerous tumor is present.

Treatment of a neck mass depends on the cause. Antibiotics are useful for lymphadenitis and other bacterial infections. Masses caused by viral infections and swelling from trauma gradually disappear with time. Tumors and cysts generally require surgery.

▲ see also page 1252

■ see also box on page 1273

Laryngeal Papillomas

Laryngeal papillomas are rare noncancerous (benign) tumors of the voice box (larynx).

Laryngeal papillomas are caused by human papillomavirus. Although they can occur at any age, papillomas mostly affect children between the ages of 1 and 4 years. Papillomas are suspected when parents notice hoarseness, a weak cry, or other changes in the child's voice. Papillomas recur often and occasionally spread into the windpipe and lungs, obstructing the airway. Rarely, they become cancerous.

Laryngeal papillomas are detected using a laryngoscope to view the voice box. Doctors perform a biopsy in which they take a sample of the papilloma to confirm the diagnosis. Surgery is the usual treatment. Drug treatment is available for papillomas that rapidly recur or spread beyond the larynx. Many children require numerous procedures through childhood to remove the tumors as they reappear. At puberty, some papillomas may disappear on their own.

CHAPTER 277

Eye Disorders

Congenital glaucoma and congenital cataracts▲ are rare disorders that can affect a newborn. Although disorders that most often blur vision, such as nearsightedness, farsightedness, and astigmatism (refractive errors), do develop in children, they more often require treatment among adults. Certain disorders, including misalignment between the two eyes (strabismus), occur more often among children. Refractive errors and strabismus can cause a loss of vision (amblyopia).

Amblyopia

Amblyopia is loss of vision that occurs because the brain ignores the image from the eye.

In amblyopia, vision loss is usually caused by the abnormal functioning of the brain, not of the eye. It develops only during childhood. Amblyopia is the most common cause of vision loss in children.

People have depth perception because the two images—one from each eye—are recorded from slightly different angles. The brain combines, or fuses, the separate images into one, three-dimensional picture. The brain develops the ability to fuse images only during childhood. When the input to the brain from one eye is of poor quality, such as a relatively blurred image or a double image, the brain suppresses the images, actually ignoring the input from that eye. The person is unaware of the image from one eye even though the eye itself is normal.

Causes

One of the most common causes of amblyopia is misalignment between the two eyes (strabismus). With strabismus, the eyes do not point to the same object, so the brain sees two very different images. These images are too different to be fused. In adults, seeing two different images results in double vision (diplopia). However, in children, if the ability to fuse images has not yet developed, the brain learns to ignore the image from the misaligned eye.

Similarly, poor vision in one eye (due to severe nearsightedness, farsightedness, or even congenital cataract) can impair a child's ability to fuse images. If the images the brain receives from the eyes are vastly different from each other, the brain learns to ignore the image that is more blurred.

Symptoms and Diagnosis

Children with amblyopia may be too young to describe symptoms. Or, a child may not realize that there is a problem, such as not being able to see out of one eye. Because only one image is perceived, the child lacks depth perception, although the child may not realize it.

▲ see table on page 1512

In addition to performing a routine eye examination, doctors examine children at the earliest possible age for strabismus and refractive errors, which can cause amblyopia.

Prognosis and Treatment

Sometimes amblyopia is mild and temporary. Amblyopia is more likely to be permanent when it begins at an early age or persists for a long time. Amblyopia from any cause that has not been treated by the age of 10 usually cannot be fully reversed.

The sooner treatment is begun, the more likely amblyopia can be prevented or corrected. Treatment entails forcing the brain to use the visual images from the problem eye. Sometimes this is accomplished by correcting the vision in the problem eye with eyeglasses. The most effective way is to "handicap" the normal, stronger eye by putting a patch over it or giving eye drops that blur vision, such as atropine.

Strabismus

Strabismus (squint, cross-eyes, wandering eye) is a misalignment or wandering of one eye so that its line of vision is not pointed at the same object as the other eye.

The causes of strabismus are varied and include an imbalance in the pull of muscles that control the position of the eyes or poor vision in one eye.

There are several different types of strabismus, each developing in different ways. Some types of strabismus are characterized by inward turning of the eye (esotropia) and some by outward turning (exotropia). Others are characterized by upward turning (hypertropia) or downward turning (hypotropia).

Parents sometimes notice strabismus because the child's eyes appear to be positioned abnormally. Strabismus may cause double vision (diplopia) in the older child or amblyopia in the younger child.

The child should be examined periodically to detect strabismus, beginning at the age of a few months. To examine an infant, a doctor shines a light into the eyes to see if the light reflects back from the same location on each pupil. Older children can be examined more thoroughly; they may be asked to stare at objects, sometimes with one eye covered. The more thorough examination may reveal mild strabismus that would otherwise be impossible to detect. Children with strabis-

Refractive Errors in Children

Refractive errors, such as nearsightedness, farsightedness, and astigmatism, are conditions that result in blurring of vision because the eye cannot focus images precisely on the retina. If only one eye is affected, loss of vision (amblyopia) may develop.

The symptoms of refractive errors are the same in children as adults,▲ although young children are often not able to make their vision problems known. Sometimes a teacher or school nurse may be the first to notice a child is having a problem seeing correctly.

All children need to be checked for refractive errors. Diagnosis is generally similar in children and adults. Children as young as 3 or 4 years can read charts with pictures, figures, or letters used to test vision. Vision is tested in each eye separately to detect loss of vision that affects only one eye. The eye not being tested is covered with a patch or other object.

Refractive errors are generally treated with eyeglasses in children and adults. However, contact lenses are not used often in children. Many children are not able to care for and clean their contact lenses; inadequate cleaning or sterilization of contact lenses can lead to eye infections. In addition, some children tend to lose contact lenses.

mus need frequent examinations by an eye doctor.

If strabismus is mild, treatment may not be needed. However, if strabismus is severe or worsening, treatment is usually required. Treatment depends on the particular characteristics of the strabismus.

Phoria is a tendency for misalignment of the eyes. The tendency is so minor that, for most of the day, the eye muscle and brain can completely correct any misalignment and maintain fusion. Phoria usually does not cause symptoms, but if sufficiently severe, it can lead to strabismus and double vision. Eye doctors can perform tests to diagnose phoria. Usually, no treatment is needed for phorias without symptoms.

Infantile Esotropia: Infantile esotropia is inward turning of the eyes that develops before 6 months of age; it often runs in families and

▲ see page 1286

Strabismus: A Misaligned Eye

There are several types of strabismus. In the most common types, an eye turns inward (esotropia or cross-eye) or outward (exotropia or walleye). In this illustration, the child's right eye is affected.

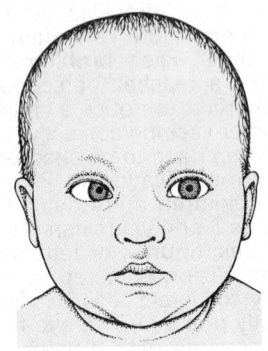

Esotropia

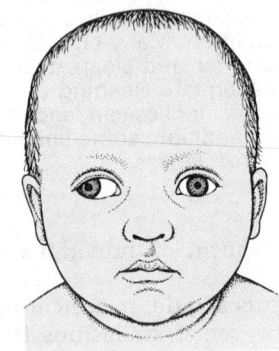

Exotropia

tends to be severe. The eyes often begin to turn in by 3 months of age. The inward turning tends to be constant and is easily noticeable.

Surgery, which is accomplished by changing the pull of the eye muscles, is usually needed to realign the eyes. Repeated operations may be necessary. Rarely, even the best possible treatment may not fully correct strabismus. Occasionally, amblyopia can develop by the age of 2, even with treatment.

Accommodative Esotropia: Accommodative esotropia is inward turning of the eyes that develops between the ages of 6 months and 7 years, most often in 2- to 3-year-olds and is related to optical focusing (accommodation) of the eyes.

The misalignment is the result of how the eyes move when focusing on nearby or distant objects. Children with accommodative esotropia are often farsighted. Although everyone's eyes turn inward when focusing on very close objects, eyes that are farsighted also turn inward when looking at distant objects. In mild cases, the eyes may turn too far inward only when looking at nearby objects. In more severe cases, the eyes turn too far inward all the time. With treatment, accommodative esotropia can usually be corrected. The first treatment tried is usually eyeglasses, which can help the child focus on objects, reducing the tendency for the eyes to turn inward when viewing those objects. Many children outgrow farsightedness and eventually do not need eyeglasses.

Occasionally, drugs (such as echothiophate eye drops) are used to help the eyes to focus on nearby objects. If eyeglasses and eye drops fail to properly align the eyes, surgery may help. Permanent amblyopia develops less often in children with accommodative esotropia than in children with infantile esotropia.

Paralytic Strabismus: In paralytic strabismus, one or more of the eye muscles that move the eye in a different direction become paralyzed. As a result, the muscles no longer work in balance. The eye muscle paralysis is usually caused by a disorder affecting the nerves to the eye muscles. For example, brain injuries or tumors can increase pressure within the skull, compressing nerves to the eye muscles.

In children with paralytic strabismus, movement of the affected eye is impaired only when the eye tries to move in a specific direction, not in all directions. Amblyopia or double vision may develop. The double vision is made worse by looking in directions normally controlled by the paralyzed eye muscles.

Paralytic strabismus may be treated with eyeglasses that contain prism lenses, which bend the light so that both eyes receive nearly the same image. It may heal by itself over time. Alternatively, surgery may be needed. If paralytic strabismus results from another condition affecting the nerves, such as a brain tumor, the other condition also needs to be treated.

Intermittent Exotropia: Exotropia is outward turning of the eyes. The eyes turn out only sometimes (intermittently), usually when the child is looking at distant objects. Intermittent exotropia is detectable after the age of 6 months.

Intermittent exotropia that does not cause troublesome symptoms, such as double vision, may not need treatment. Amblyopia rarely develops. If symptoms are occasionally troublesome, eyeglasses may help. Rarely, a doctor may recommend exercises for the eye muscles. If symptoms worsen despite the use of eyeglasses, surgery may be effective.

CHAPTER 278

Bone Disorders

Although most bone disorders affecting children are similar to those affecting adults, there are some differences. Children's bones are continually growing and extensively reshaping themselves (remodeling). Growth proceeds from a vulnerable part of the bone called the growth plate. In remodeling, old bone tissue is gradually replaced by new bone tissue.▲ Children's bones can remodel more extensively than adults' can. Also, in children, bones heal more rapidly, and scarring and stiffening develop less often. Most childhood bone disorders are minor and do not cause permanent problems.

Causes

Bone disorders in children can develop from any of the causes that affect adults, such as injuries and infections. Causes that affect mainly children include gradually developing misalignment of bones. In children, the bones in the legs can be very curved, which usually results from the way the legs were positioned in the uterus before birth.

Poor blood supply can also damage the growth plate, as can separation from the rest of the bone or even minor misalignment. Damage to the growth plate suppresses the growth of bones, distorts the joint, and can cause long-standing joint damage (arthritis).

Certain rare hereditary disorders of connective tissue affect the bones, such as Marfan syndrome, mucopolysaccharidoses, osteogenesis imperfecta, chondrodysplasias, and osteopetroses.■

Symptoms and Diagnosis

Children usually experience the same symptoms as adults. Pain is common and may develop slowly, over weeks or longer. Infants and very young children may be unable to communicate their pain. Bone disorders sometimes cause painless deformities. Some deformities may affect a child's ability to walk or use the limbs. Diagnosis of bone disorders is similar in children and adults.

Treatment

Treatment of most bone disorders, such as fractures and infections, is usually similar in children and adults.

If the growth plate becomes damaged, surgery may help. Accurately realigning separated or misaligned ends of the growth plate surgically may restore normal bone growth. By decreasing the irritation caused by misalignment, surgery may prevent the development of arthritis in the joint.

If a bone disorder causes a physical deformity, the child may become anxious or depressed. Some treatments for bone disorders may also be psychologically difficult to accept. For example, adolescents may be reluctant to wear a back brace for treatment of scoliosis, because doing so makes them appear different from peers. Professional counseling may relieve anxiety or depression. Counseling may also help a child go through with difficult treatments.

Scoliosis

Scoliosis is abnormal curvature of the spine.

Scoliosis is very common, especially among girls. Scoliosis may result from a birth defect or develop later in life, most often in adolescence. Usually, the cause cannot be found.

▲ see page 335   ■ see page 1607

Scoliosis: A Curved Spine

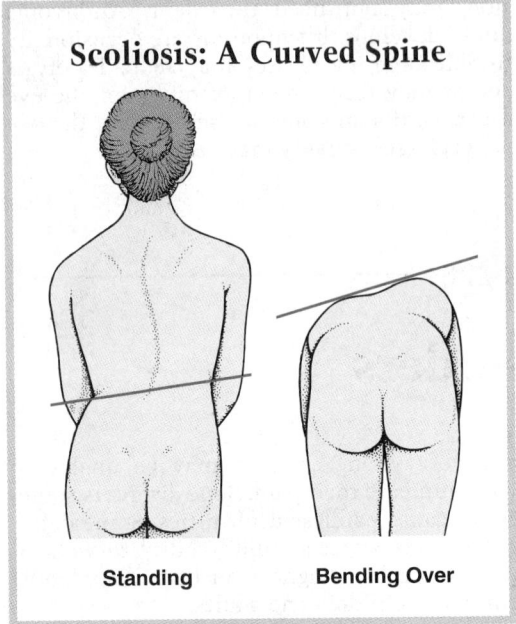

Standing   **Bending Over**

The spine usually bulges toward the right when the curvature is in the upper back and to the left when it is in the lower back. The result is that the right shoulder is usually higher than the left. One hip may be higher than the other. Scoliosis often develops in children with kyphosis (kyphoscoliosis).

Symptoms and Diagnosis

Mild scoliosis usually produces no symptoms. Sometimes the back becomes sore or stiff after the child sits or stands for a long period of time. Mild or more severe pain may eventually follow.

Mild scoliosis may be discovered during a routine physical examination. A parent, teacher, or doctor may suspect scoliosis when one of the child's shoulders seems higher than the other or when the child's clothes do not hang straight.

In about half of affected children, scoliosis is likely to worsen. The more severe the curve, the greater the likelihood of it worsening. Likewise, the more symptoms that develop, the greater the likelihood that scoliosis will worsen.

Because scoliosis tends to worsen when the child reaches puberty, the earlier it develops, the longer it has to worsen. Thus, a small curve in a 10-year-old is of much greater concern than that same curve in a 16-year-old.

Worsening scoliosis may eventually cause permanent problems, such as noticeable deformities or chronic pain. Severe scoliosis may even affect internal organs, for example, deforming and damaging the lungs. Sometimes, scoliosis can worsen even if symptoms have not developed.

To diagnose the condition, a doctor asks the child to bend forward and views the spine from behind, because the abnormal spinal curve can be seen more easily in this position. X-rays show the precise angles of curvature. If doctors think scoliosis may worsen, they may examine the child several times a year. Special devices may be used to more precisely measure the curve of the spine.

Prognosis and Treatment

In the vast majority of children who have scoliosis, the curvature will not progress more but rather remain small. However, it needs to be followed by a doctor regularly. Scoliosis that causes symptoms, is worsening, or is severe may need to be treated. The earlier treatment is begun, the better the chance of preventing a severe deformity.

A brace or object fashioned to hold the spine (orthosis) may be worn to keep the spine straight. In the most severe cases, the vertebrae need to be bonded together surgically; a metal rod may be inserted during surgery to keep the spine straight until the vertebrae have bonded permanently.

Kyphosis

In kyphosis (Scheuermann disease), changes in the cartilages of the vertebrae (osteochondritis) cause a humpback.

Some amount of kyphosis is common and begins in adolescence, affecting boys more often than girls. The cause is unknown. The vertebrae curve forward on each other, usually in the upper back. As a result, the back develops a hump. Scoliosis also often develops in children with kyphosis (kyphoscoliosis).

Kyphosis often produces no symptoms. Sometimes, mild, persistent back pain develops. Kyphosis may be noticed only because it alters the body's appearance. The shoulders may appear rounded. The upper spine may appear more curved than normal, or a hump may be visible. Mild kyphosis that does not produce symptoms is sometimes detected only during a routine physical examination. A doctor confirms the diagnosis by taking x-rays of

Kyphosis: A Humpback

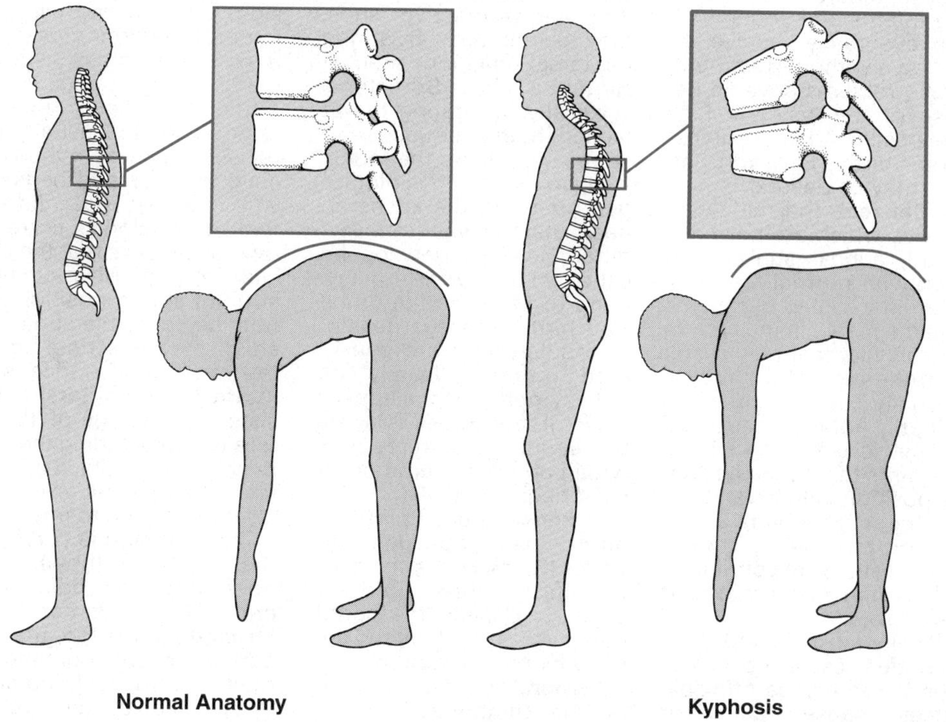

Normal Anatomy

Kyphosis

the spine, which show the curve and the deformity of the vertebrae.

Treatment most often consists of wearing a spinal brace or sleeping on a rigid bed. In mild kyphosis, the spine may straighten slightly with treatment, although symptoms may not improve. It is unclear whether treating mild kyphosis prevents the curve from worsening. When kyphosis is more severe, treatment may improve symptoms and prevent the curve from worsening. Rarely, despite treatment, kyphosis worsens to such an extent that surgery is needed to straighten the spine.

Slipped Capital Femoral Epiphysis

Slipped capital femoral epiphysis is a separation within the thighbone (femur) at its growth plate in the hip joint.

Slipped capital femoral epiphysis usually develops in overweight adolescents, most commonly boys. The cause is not known. However, the disorder may result from a

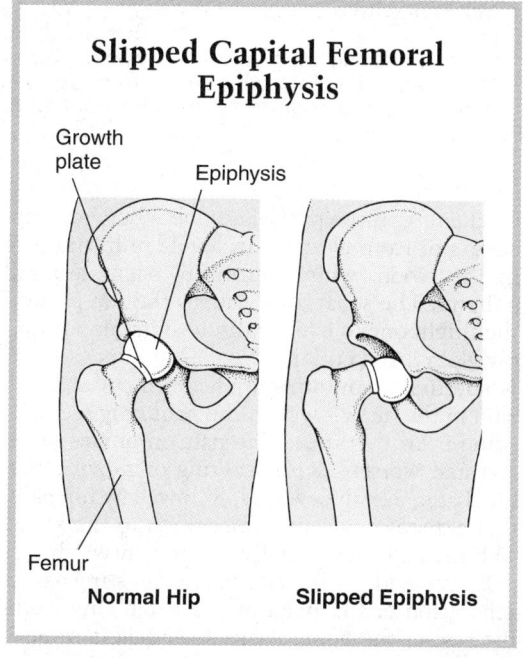

Slipped Capital Femoral Epiphysis

Growth plate

Epiphysis

Femur

Normal Hip

Slipped Epiphysis

Common Foot, Knee, and Leg Disorders in Infants and Young Children

Many knee and foot problems that parents notice in their infants and young children eventually resolve on their own without treatment. Some problems develop because of the way the legs were positioned in the uterus before birth. Rarely, treatment may be needed.

In **flat feet,** the middle of the feet, which are normally arched, appear sunken. An infant with normal feet may appear flat-footed because a fat pad appears in the arch of the foot. Flat feet may result when the arch of the foot is unusually flexible **(flexible flatfeet).** Another cause of flat feet is stiffening of the foot joints that fixes the foot in a position with a flattened arch **(tarsal coalition).** Tarsal coalition may be a birth defect or result from conditions such as injuries or prolonged swelling.

Usually fat pads and flexible flatfeet cause no symptoms. Sometimes flexible flatfeet cause pain or cramps in the feet. Tarsal coalition may cause pain or cramping. Feet with tarsal coalition are stiff, which can interfere with walking or running.

Fat pads do not require treatment. Flexible flatfeet usually do not require treat-ment. However, if an older child has pains or cramps in the feet, corrective shoes may be needed. Treatment for tarsal coalition often includes a cast. Sometimes surgically separating the attached internal structures restores mobility to the foot.

In **bowlegs** (physiological genu varum), the knees appear rotated away from each other. Bowlegs develop because of the way the legs bend to fit in the uterus before birth. Bowlegs develop in toddlers and are considered normal. Usually the only symptom is the appearance of the knees. Usually the condition corrects itself within about a year after the child begins to walk.

In **knock knees** (genu valgum), the knees point inward. Knock knees most often affect children aged 3 to 5 years. Usually the condition corrects itself by the age of 10 without treatment.

Femoral torsion is curving of the thighbone (femur). With internal femoral torsion, the thighs curve inward. The knees, and usually the toes, point toward each other. With external femoral torsion, the thighs curve outward. The knees and toes point away from each other. Internal femoral torsion de-velops much more often than external femoral torsion. Children with internal femoral torsion sometimes have abnormally flexible joints and ligaments.

Internal and external femoral torsion usually correct themselves when the child is older and begins to walk. Sometimes, internal femoral torsion is corrected by making sure that the child sits straight. Maintaining a straight sitting position may not be possible until the child reaches school age. In the rare circumstance when internal femoral torsion persists past the age of 10, surgically straightening the bone may be necessary. It can take years for internal or external femoral torsion to improve.

Tibial torsion is curving of the shinbone (tibia). Tibial torsion develops before birth and is very common. In internal tibial torsion, the tibia curves inward, pointing the toes toward each other. In external tibial torsion, the shinbone curves outward, pointing the toes away from each other. Tibial torsion is often noticed during the second year of life when the child begins to walk. The shinbone appears curved but gradually straightens after the child begins walking.

thickening in the part of a bone where growth occurs or from changes in levels of hormones in the blood, which normally occur around puberty. The separation causes the top part of the thighbone to eventually lose its blood supply, decay, and collapse.

The first symptom may be stiffness or mild pain in the hip. However, the pain may seem to come from the knee. The pain improves with rest and worsens with walking or moving the hip. Later, a limp develops, followed by hip pain that extends down the inner thigh to the knee. The affected leg is usually twisted outward.

X-rays of the affected hip show a slippage or separation of the head of the thighbone from the rest of the bone. Early diagnosis is impor-tant because treatment becomes more difficult and gives less satisfactory results later.

Surgery is usually needed to align the separated ends of the thighbone and to fasten them together with metal pins. The hip is immobilized in a cast for several weeks to 2 months.

Legg-Calvé-Perthes Disease

Legg-Calvé-Perthes disease is destruction of the growth plate of the thighbone.

Legg-Calvé-Perthes disease develops most commonly in boys between the ages of 5 and 10. It is caused by a poor blood supply to the upper growth plate of the thighbone. The reason for the poor blood supply is not known.

Legg-Calvé-Perthes disease can cause severe hip damage without causing severe symptoms at first. The severe damage may, however, lead to permanent arthritis of the hip. The first symptom is often hip or thigh pain. Pain begins gradually and progresses slowly. The pain tends to worsen when moving the hip or walking. A limp can develop, sometimes before the child experiences much pain. Eventually, joint movement becomes restricted, and the thigh muscles may become wasted (atrophied) from lack of use. X-rays may show changes around the growth plate, such as a fracture or destruction of the bone.

Treatment includes prolonged immobilization of the hip. Sometimes the partial immobilization provided by bed rest is sufficient. Sometimes nearly total immobilization for 12 to 18 months is necessary, requiring traction, slings, plaster casts, or splints. Such treatments keep the legs rotated outward. Physical therapy is also given to keep the muscles from contracting and wasting away. If a child is older than 6 and has moderate or severe bone destruction, surgery may be helpful. Regardless of how it is treated, Legg-Calvé-Perthes disease usually takes at least 2 years to heal.

Osgood-Schlatter Disease

Osgood-Schlatter disease is inflammation of the bone and cartilage at the top of the shinbone (tibia).

Osgood-Schlatter disease develops between the ages of 10 and 15, usually in boys. The cause is thought to be repetitive, excessive pulling by the tendon of the kneecap (patellar tendon) on its point of attachment at the top of the shinbone (tibia). This point of attachment is called the tibial tubercle.

The major symptom is pain at the tibial tubercle. The pain worsens with activity and is relieved with rest. Swelling and tenderness eventually develop at the site. X-rays of the knee may show enlargement or fragmentation of the tibial tubercle.

Avoiding sports and excessive exercise helps reduce pain. Avoiding deep knee bending is particularly helpful. Use of nonsteroidal anti-inflammatory drugs (NSAIDs) may help the pain. Several weeks or months may be required for healing. Occasionally, the entire leg, from the ankle to the upper thigh, must be immobilized in a plaster cast for several weeks.

Chondromalacia Patellae

Chondromalacia patellae is damage to the cartilage under the kneecap (patella).

Chondromalacia patellae typically develops in adolescents. Joggers are especially susceptible. The cause is probably a minor, repetitive injury resulting from misalignment of the kneecap. The misalignment causes the cartilage on the underside of the kneecap to grate against other bones when the knee bends.

Dull, aching pain is felt all around and behind the knee. Climbing, especially going up or down stairs, and running usually worsen the pain. Prolonged sitting may also worsen the pain. A doctor makes the diagnosis based on the symptoms and physical examination and may recommend exercises to strengthen the quadriceps muscles, which straighten, or extend, the knee joint. Increasing knee flexibility with stretching exercises helps. Activities that worsen the pain should be avoided. Analgesic or non-steroidal anti-inflammatory drugs (NSAIDs), such as ibuprofen or naproxen, can help relieve symptoms.

CHAPTER 279

Hereditary Connective Tissue Disorders

Muscles, bones, cartilage, ligaments, and tendons are built mostly of connective tissue. Connective tissue is also found in other parts of the body, such as the skin and internal organs. Connective tissue is strong and thus able to support weight and tension.▲

Certain hereditary disorders cause connective tissue throughout the body to form abnormally. In general, the hereditary connective tissue disorders develop in childhood but last throughout life. Muscular dystrophies are a group of hereditary muscle disorders that lead to muscle weakness.■

▲ see page 334   ■ see page 412

Most hereditary connective tissue disorders are diagnosed by their symptoms and findings on a physical examination. Analysis of genes, usually from a blood test, may help doctors diagnose some hereditary disorders. Biopsy (removal of a tissue sample for examination under a microscope) can also help; the tissue is usually removed using local anesthesia. X-rays can reveal bone abnormalities.

Ehlers-Danlos Syndrome

Ehlers-Danlos syndrome is a rare disorder of connective tissue that results in unusually flexible joints, very elastic skin, and fragile tissues.

Ehlers-Danlos syndrome is caused by an abnormality in one of the genes that controls the production of connective tissue. There are several variations (with widely varying severity), each affecting a different gene and producing slightly different changes. The result is abnormally fragile connective tissue, which causes problems in joints and bones and may weaken internal organs.

Children with Ehlers-Danlos syndrome usually have very flexible joints. Some develop small, hard, round lumps under the skin; a humpback with an abnormal curve of the spine (kyphoscoliosis); or flat feet. The skin can be stretched several inches but returns to its normal position when released.

Ehlers-Danlos syndrome may alter the body's response to injuries. Minor injuries may result in wide gaping wounds. Although these wounds usually do not bleed excessively, they leave wide scars. Sprains and dislocations develop easily.

In a small number of children with Ehlers-Danlos syndrome, the blood clots poorly. Bleeding from minor wounds may be difficult to stop.

The intestines can bulge through the abdominal wall (hernias), and abnormal outpouchings (diverticula) can develop in the intestine. Rarely, a fragile intestine bleeds or ruptures (perforates).

If a pregnant woman has Ehlers-Danlos syndrome, delivery may be premature. If the fetus has Ehlers-Danlos syndrome, its surrounding membranes may rupture early (premature rupture of membranes). A mother or baby who has Ehlers-Danlos syndrome can bleed excessively around the time of delivery.

A doctor makes the diagnosis based on the symptoms and results of a physical examina-

tion. The doctor can confirm the diagnosis of some types of Ehlers-Danlos syndrome by taking a sample of skin to examine under a microscope.

Treatment and Prognosis

There is no way to cure Ehlers-Danlos syndrome or correct the abnormalities in the connective tissue. Injuries can be treated, but it may be difficult for a doctor to stitch cuts because stitches tend to tear out of the fragile tissue. Usually, using an adhesive tape or medical skin glue closes cuts more easily and leaves less scarring.

Special precautions should be taken to prevent injuries. For example, protective clothing and padding may be worn in children with severe forms; surgery requires special techniques that minimize injury and ensure that a large supply of blood is available for transfusion.

Despite the many and varied complications people with Ehlers-Danlos syndrome may have, their life span is usually normal. However, in a few people with one specific type of Ehlers-Danlos syndrome, complications (usually bleeding) are fatal.

Marfan Syndrome

Marfan syndrome is a rare disorder of connective tissue, resulting in abnormalities of the eyes, bones, heart, and blood vessels.

In Marfan syndrome, which is caused by a dominant gene, some fibers and other parts of connective tissue undergo changes that ultimately weaken the tissue. The weakening affects bones and joints as well as internal structures, such as the heart, blood vessels, eyes, and intestines. Weakened tissues stretch, distort, and can even tear. For example, the aorta may weaken, bulge, or tear. Connective tissues that join structures may weaken or break, separating formerly attached structures. For example, the eye's lens or retina may separate from its normal attachments.

Symptoms can range from mild to severe. Many people with Marfan syndrome never notice symptoms. In some people, symptoms may not become apparent until adulthood. People with Marfan syndrome are taller than expected for their age and family. Their arm span (the distance between fingertips when the arms are outstretched) is greater than their height. Their fingers are long and thin. Often, the breastbone (sternum) is deformed and pushed either outward or inward. The joints may be very flexible. Flat feet and a humpback with an abnormal curve of the spine (kyphoscoliosis) are common; so are hernias. Usually, the person has little fat under the skin. The roof of the mouth is often high.

The most dangerous complications develop in the heart and lungs. Weakness may develop in the connective tissue of the wall of the body's main artery, the aorta. The weakened wall may result in blood seeping between the layers of the aorta's wall (aortic dissection) or a bulge (aneurysm), which can rupture.▲ Pregnancy increases the risk of dissection. Delivery by caesarean section is often recommended to minimize the risk.

If the aorta gradually widens, the aortic valve, which leads from the heart into the aorta, may begin to leak (aortic regurgitation). The mitral valve, which is located between the left atrium and ventricle, may leak or become prolapsed (bulge backward into the left atrium■). These heart valve abnormalities can impair the heart's ability to pump blood. Abnormal heart valves can also develop serious infections (infective endocarditis). Air-filled sacs (cysts) may develop in the lungs. The cysts may rupture, bringing air into the space that surrounds the lungs (pneumothorax★).

The lens of one or both eyes may be displaced in Marfan syndrome. The light-sensitive area at the back of the eye (retina) may detach from the rest of the eye. Displacement of the lens and detachment of the retina may cause permanent loss of vision.

Doctors may suspect the diagnosis if an unusually tall, thin person has any of the characteristic symptoms, or if Marfan syndrome has been recognized in other family members.

It is most important for doctors to monitor for complications that can cause serious symptoms. Echocardiography is used to evaluate the heart and aorta and is usually repeated yearly. The eyes are usually examined yearly. Echocardiography and eye examinations are also performed whenever symptoms develop.

Treatment and Prognosis

There is no cure for Marfan syndrome nor any way to correct the abnormalities in the connective tissue. Treatment is aimed at fixing abnormalities before dangerous complications develop. Some doctors prescribe drugs, such as beta-blockers, that make blood flow more gently through the aorta. However, whether these drugs help is controversial. If the aorta has widened or developed an aneurysm, the affected section can be repaired or replaced surgically. A displaced lens or retina can usually be reattached surgically.

Years ago, most people with Marfan syndrome died in their 40s. Now, most people with Marfan syndrome live until their 60s. Prevention of aortic dissection and rupture probably explains why the life span has been lengthened.

Pseudoxanthoma Elasticum

Pseudoxanthoma elasticum is a disorder of connective tissue that causes abnormalities in the skin, eyes, and blood vessels.

Pseudoxanthoma elasticum stiffens the fibers that enable tissue to stretch and then spring back into place (elastic fibers). Elastic fibers are in the skin and various other tissues throughout the body, including blood vessels. The blood vessels may stiffen, losing their normal ability to expand and allow more blood to flow as needed; stiffness also prevents the blood vessels from contracting.

The skin of the neck, underarms, groin, and around the navel eventually becomes thick, grooved, inflexible, and loose. Yellowish, pebbly bumps give the skin an appearance similar to an orange or a plucked chicken. The change in appearance may be mild and overlooked during early childhood but becomes more noticeable as the child ages.

Stiff blood vessels lead to high blood pressure. Nosebleeds and bleeding in the brain, uterus, and intestine may occur. Too little blood flow may result in chest pain (angina) and leg pain while walking (intermittent claudication). Bleeding may continue for prolonged periods. Damage to the back of the eye (retina) can cause severe loss of vision or blindness.

Treatment and Prognosis

There is no cure for pseudoxanthoma elasticum nor any way to correct the abnormalities in the connective tissue. Treatment is aimed at preventing complications. People should avoid drugs that may cause stomach or intestinal bleeding, such as aspirin, other nonsteroidal anti-inflammatory drugs (NSAIDs), and anticoagulants. People with pseudoxan-

▲ see art on page 230

■ see page 178

★ see page 316

thoma elasticum should avoid contact sports because of the risk of injury to the eye. Complications often limit life span.

Cutis Laxa

Cutis laxa is a rare disorder of connective tissue that causes the skin to stretch easily and hang in loose folds.

In cutis laxa, the elastic fibers contained in the connective tissue become loose. Sometimes only the skin is affected, but connective tissues throughout the body can be affected. Cutis laxa is usually hereditary. In some kinds of cutis laxa, the abnormal genes cause problems unrelated to connective tissues—for example, mental retardation.

Cutis laxa can be mild, affecting only a person's appearance, or severe, affecting the internal organs. The skin may be very loose at birth, or it may become loose later. The loose skin is often most noticeable on the face, resulting in a prematurely aged appearance. The lungs, heart, intestines, or arteries may be affected with a variety of severe impairments.

Although symptoms often become noticeable shortly after birth, they may begin suddenly in children and adolescents, sometimes with a fever and rash. In some people, symptoms develop gradually in adulthood.

A doctor can usually diagnose cutis laxa by examining the skin. Sometimes, a skin biopsy is necessary.

Treatment and Prognosis

Plastic surgery can often improve the appearance of the skin, although the improvement may be only temporary. Severe impairments of the heart, lungs, arteries, or intestines can be fatal.

Mucopolysaccharidoses

The mucopolysaccharidoses are a group of hereditary disorders affecting the connective tissue that result in a characteristic facial appearance and abnormalities of the bones, eyes, liver, and spleen, sometimes accompanied by mental retardation.

Mucopolysaccharides are essential parts of connective tissue. In the mucopolysaccharidoses, the body lacks enzymes needed to break down and store mucopolysaccharides. As a re-

sult, excess mucopolysaccharides enter the blood and are deposited in abnormal locations throughout the body.

During infancy and childhood, short stature, hairiness, and abnormal development become noticeable. The face may appear coarse. Some types of mucopolysaccharidoses cause mental retardation to develop over several years. In some types, vision or hearing may become impaired. The arteries or heart valves can be affected. Finger joints are often stiff.

A doctor usually bases the diagnosis on the symptoms and findings on a physical examination. The presence of a mucopolysaccharidosis in other family members also suggests the diagnosis. Urine tests may help but are sometimes inaccurate. X-rays may show characteristic bone abnormalities. Mucopolysaccharidoses can be diagnosed before birth using amniocentesis or chorionic villus sampling.▲

Treatment and Prognosis

In one type of mucopolysaccharidosis, attempts at replacing the abnormal enzyme have had limited, temporary success. Bone marrow transplantation may help some people. However, death or disability often results, and this treatment remains controversial.

The prognosis depends on the type of mucopolysaccharidosis. A normal life span is possible. Some types, usually those that affect the heart, cause premature death.

Osteogenesis Imperfecta

Osteogenesis imperfecta is a group of disorders of bone formation that make the bones abnormally fragile.

Osteogenesis imperfecta is the best known of a group of disorders that disturb bone growth; these disorders are called osteodysplasias. In osteogenesis imperfecta, synthesis of collagen, one of the normal components of bone, is impaired. The bones become weak and fracture easily. There are several types of osteogenesis imperfecta.

Osteogenesis imperfecta can range from mild to severe. Most people with osteogenesis imperfecta have fragile bones and hearing loss. Infants with severe osteogenesis imperfecta are usually born with many broken bones; the skull may be so soft that the brain is not protected from pressure applied to the head during childbirth. With moderate osteogenesis imperfecta, bones often break after very minor injuries, usually when the child begins to

▲ see art on page 1433

walk. Children with mild osteogenesis imperfecta may sustain few broken bones during childhood and even fewer after puberty, when bones strengthen. Sometimes heart or lung diseases develop in children with osteogenesis imperfecta.

X-rays may show abnormal bone structure that suggests osteogenesis imperfecta. A bone biopsy is used to confirm the diagnosis. A test called audiometry is performed often throughout childhood to monitor hearing.

Treatment

Bisphosphonate drugs (such as pamidronate, alendronate, etidronate, and risedronate) may strengthen bones. Treatment of broken bones is similar for children with osteogenesis imperfecta as for children without the disorder. However, broken bones can become deformed or fail to grow. As a result, body growth can become permanently stunted in children with many broken bones, and deformities are common. Bones may require stabilization with metal rods (intramedullary rods). Taking measures to avoid even minor injuries can help prevent fractures.

Chondrodysplasias

The chondrodysplasias are a group of rare disorders of cartilage that cause the skeleton to develop abnormally.

In chondrodysplasias, the growth plate, which contains cartilage, does not make new bone cells. Thus, growth of bone is impaired.

Each type of chondrodysplasia produces different symptoms. Chondrodysplasias usually cause short stature (dwarfism). Some cause more shortening of the limbs than the trunk (short-limbed dwarfism); others cause more shortening of the trunk than the limbs. Some children and adults have short limbs, bowlegs, a bulky forehead, an unusually shaped nose (saddle nose), and an arched back. Sometimes, joints do not develop the capacities for their full range of motion.

A doctor usually makes the diagnosis based on the symptoms, physical examination, and x-rays of the bones. Sometimes the abnormal genes responsible for chondrodysplasias can be detected, usually by a blood test. Analyzing the genes is most helpful for predicting the disease before birth. Diagnosis of severe types before birth is also possible using other methods; in some cases, the fetus can be directly viewed with a flexible scope (fetoscopy), or an

ultrasound is performed. Surgery may be needed to replace joints that have severely restricted movement with artificial ones.

Osteopetroses

The osteopetroses are a group of rare disorders that increase the density of bones.

In osteopetroses (sometimes called marble bone diseases), the body fails to recycle old bone cells. The result is increased density of the bones. The increased density makes bones weaker than normal. The dense bone tissue also crowds out the bone marrow.

The osteopetroses range from mild to severe and can even be life threatening. Symptoms may begin in infancy (early onset) or later in life (delayed onset).

Although the osteopetroses are different disorders, many of the same symptoms develop in most of them. Bone growth is usually impaired. Bones thicken and break easily. Formation of blood cells may be impaired because of a lack of bone marrow, leading to anemia, infection, or bleeding. Bone overgrowth in the skull can compress nerves, causing facial paralysis or loss of vision or hearing, and can distort the face and teeth.

Doctors usually establish the diagnosis based on the symptoms and the appearance of very dense bone on x-rays. When the person has no symptoms, osteopetrosis is sometimes detected only by chance, after a doctor sees very dense bones on x-rays taken for an unrelated purpose.

Treatment and Prognosis

There is no cure. Corticosteroids, such as prednisone, decrease formation of new bone cells and may increase the rate of removal of old bone cells, strengthening bones. Bone marrow transplantation appears to have cured some infants with early-onset disease. However, the long-term prognosis after transplantation is unknown.

Fractures, anemia, bleeding, and infection require treatment. If nerves leaving the skull are compressed, surgery may be required to release the nerve. Orthodontic treatment may be needed.

Early-onset osteopetrosis that is not treated with bone marrow transplantation usually causes death during infancy or early childhood. Death usually results from anemia, infection, or bleeding. Late-onset osteopetrosis is often very mild.

CHAPTER 280

Juvenile Rheumatoid Arthritis

Juvenile rheumatoid arthritis is persistent or recurring inflammation of the joints similar to rheumatoid arthritis▲ but beginning before age 16.

Juvenile rheumatoid arthritis is an uncommon disease characterized by inflammation of joints or connective tissue. The cause is unknown. Although juvenile rheumatoid arthritis is not considered a hereditary disorder, hereditary factors may increase a child's chance of developing it.

Symptoms and Complications

There are several types of juvenile rheumatoid arthritis, each with different characteristics. The type of juvenile rheumatoid arthritis is determined by which symptoms develop during the first months of the disease and how many joints are affected.

In pauciarticular juvenile rheumatoid arthritis, four or fewer joints, usually those of the leg, are affected. The knee is usually the first joint affected. The hip and shoulder are usually spared. Occasionally, a single toe, a finger, a wrist, or the jaw becomes stiff and swollen. The back may also be involved. The joint pain and swelling may persist or come and go.

In polyarthritis, five or more (sometimes as many as 20 to 40) joints are affected. The inflammation usually affects the same joint on both sides of the body—for example, both knees or both hips. The jaw, neck joints, and wrists may be affected. Symptoms may develop slowly; fever and enlargement of the spleen or lymph glands can occur. Inflammation may develop in the tendons and connective tissues around joints (tenosynovitis), causing pain, swelling, and warmth.

In systemic disease (Still's disease), any number of joints can be involved. Inflammation also occurs at sites other than the joints. The liver, spleen, and lymph nodes may enlarge, and sometimes inflammation develops in the membrane surrounding the heart (pericarditis). Rarely, the kidneys become inflamed. A high fever and rash may appear before joint pain and swelling. The fever comes and goes, usually for at least 2 weeks. Temperature is usually highest in the afternoon or evening (often 103° F or higher), then returns rapidly to normal. A child with fever may feel tired and less energetic. A rash made up of flat, pink or salmon-colored patches—mainly on the trunk and the upper part of the legs or arms—appears for hours (often in the evening). The rash can reappear days later on a different part of the body.

With any type of juvenile rheumatoid arthritis, the joints may be stiff when the child awakens. Joints often become swollen and warm. Later, joints may become painful, but the pain may be milder than expected from the amount of swelling. Pain may become worse when the joint is moved. A child may be reluctant to walk. Joint pain tends to persist for weeks or months.

Any type of juvenile rheumatoid arthritis can interfere with physical growth. Joint deformities often develop. When juvenile rheumatoid arthritis interferes with growth of the jaw, a small chin (micrognathia) can result. Long-standing (chronic) joint inflammation can eventually cause deformities or permanent damage of the affected joint.

Inflammation of the iris in the eye (iridocyclitis) can develop with any kind of juvenile rheumatoid arthritis, but most often iridocyclitis develops with pauciarticular juvenile rheumatoid arthritis or polyarthritis. Iridocyclitis may cause eye redness, eye pain, or loss of vision, but it can develop without any symptoms. If untreated, iridocyclitis can lead to permanent eye damage.

Diagnosis

A doctor diagnoses juvenile rheumatoid arthritis based on the child's symptoms and the results of a physical examination. There is no single, definitive laboratory test for juvenile rheumatoid arthritis. Blood is tested for rheumatoid factor and antinuclear antibodies, which are present in some people with rheumatoid arthritis and related diseases (for example, autoimmune diseases, such as lupus, polymyositis, or scleroderma). However, many children with juvenile rheumatoid arthritis do not have rheumatoid factor or antinuclear an-

▲ see page 370

tibodies in their blood. Also, children with many other conditions can have rheumatoid factor or antinuclear antibodies in their blood. X-rays eventually may show characteristic changes in the bones or joints. The child must be examined regularly by an ophthalmologist for iridocyclitis regardless of whether symptoms are present.

Treatment and Prognosis

The types of juvenile rheumatoid arthritis are treated similarly, and the drugs used to reduce pain and inflammation are the same as for rheumatoid arthritis.▲ However, children with juvenile rheumatoid arthritis often also need treatment for iridocyclitis. Iridocyclitis is treated with corticosteroid eye drops or ointments, which suppress inflammation. Eye drops that widen (dilate) the pupil can decrease eye pain from iridocyclitis. Both types of drugs can prevent glaucoma and blindness. For unusually severe iridocyclitis, eye surgery may be needed.

As in rheumatoid arthritis in adults, non-drug therapies are also used in children; for example, splinting and flexibility exercises, to prevent permanent stiffening of joints.

Symptoms of juvenile rheumatoid arthritis completely disappear in a high proportion of affected children. Up to half of the children with pauciarticular juvenile rheumatoid arthritis and about one quarter or more of children with polyarthritis or systemic disease have a complete remission.

CHAPTER 281

Diabetes Mellitus

Diabetes mellitus is a disorder in which blood sugar (glucose) levels are abnormally high because the body does not produce enough insulin.

The symptoms, diagnosis, and treatment of diabetes are similar in children and adults.■ However, treatment of diabetes in children may be more complex and must be tailored to the child's physical and emotional maturity level.

Insulin is a hormone released by the pancreas that controls the amount of sugar in the blood. A child with diabetes has high blood sugar levels either because the pancreas produces little or no insulin (type 1 diabetes, formerly called juvenile-onset diabetes) or because the body is insensitive to the amount of insulin that is produced (type 2 diabetes). In either case, the amount of insulin available is insufficient for the body's needs.

Type 1 diabetes occurs throughout childhood, even in infancy, with a usual age of onset between 6 and 13 years. Type 2 diabetes occurs mainly in adolescents.

Up until the 1990s, more than 95% of children who developed diabetes had type 1, usually as a result of an attack by the immune system on the cells in the pancreas that make insulin (islet cells). Recently, the number of children, especially adolescents, with type 2 diabetes has been steadily increasing. Today, 10 to 40% of children newly diagnosed with diabetes have type 2. The increase in childhood type 2 diabetes has been particularly prominent among Native Americans, blacks, and Hispanics. Obesity and a family history of type 2 diabetes are major factors in the development of type 2 diabetes (but not type 1).

Symptoms

High blood sugar levels are responsible for a variety of immediate symptoms and long-term complications.

Symptoms develop quickly in type 1 diabetes, usually over 2 to 3 weeks or less, and tend to be quite obvious. High blood sugar levels cause the child to urinate excessively. This fluid loss causes an increase in thirst and the consumption of fluids. Some children become dehydrated, resulting in weakness, lethargy, and a rapid pulse. Vision may become blurred.

Diabetic ketoacidosis occurs at the beginning of the disease in about one third of children with type 1 diabetes. Without insulin, cells cannot use the sugar that is in the blood. Cells switch to a back-up mechanism to obtain en-

---

▲ see page 371   ■ see page 962

ergy and break down fat, producing compounds called ketones as byproducts. Ketones make the blood too acidic (ketoacidosis), causing nausea, vomiting, fatigue, and abdominal pain. The ketones make the child's breath smell like nail polish remover. Breathing becomes deep and rapid as the body attempts to correct the blood's acidity.▲ The increase of ketones in the blood leads to diabetic ketoacidosis. Diabetic ketoacidosis can progress to coma and death, sometimes within a few hours. Children with ketoacidosis often have other chemical imbalances in the blood, such as an abnormal level of potassium and high levels of lipids (fats).

Symptoms in children with type 2 diabetes are milder than those in type 1 and develop more slowly—over weeks or even a few months. Parents may notice an increase in the child's thirst and urination or only vague symptoms, such as fatigue. Typically, children with type 2 diabetes do not develop ketoacidosis or severe dehydration.

Diagnosis

Doctors suspect diabetes when children have typical symptoms or when a urine test done during a routine physical examination reveals sugar. The diagnosis is confirmed by measurement of the blood sugar level. Preferably, the blood test is done after fasting overnight. A child is considered to have diabetes if the fasting blood sugar level is 126 milligrams per deciliter (mg/dL) or higher. Rarely, doctors order a blood test that detects antibodies to islet cells to help distinguish type 1 diabetes from type 2; however, this information is rarely useful.

Because prompt measures (such as dietary changes, an increase in physical activity, and weight loss) may help prevent or delay the onset of type 2 diabetes, children at risk should be screened with a blood test. Nothing can be done to prevent type 1 diabetes.

Treatment

The main goal of treatment is to keep blood sugar levels as close to the normal range as can be done safely. To control blood sugar, children with diabetes take drugs (such as insulin or drugs given by mouth) and change their lifestyle. Changes include adjustments in diet, regular exercise, and, for overweight children, weight loss.

When type 1 diabetes is first diagnosed, children are usually hospitalized. Children with diabetic ketoacidosis are treated in an intensive care unit. Children with type 1 diabetes always require insulin because nothing else is effective. They typically receive two or more daily injections of insulin, although a few may receive insulin continuously delivered under the skin by a pump. Insulin treatment is usually begun in the hospital so that blood sugar levels can be tested often and doctors can change insulin dosage in response. Rarely, treatment is started at home.

Children with type 2 diabetes do not usually need to receive treatment in the hospital. They do require treatment with diabetic drugs taken by mouth. The drugs used for adults with type 2 diabetes■ are safe for children, although some of the side effects—particularly diarrhea—cause more problems in children. Some children with type 2 diabetes need insulin. A few children who lose weight, improve their diet, and exercise regularly may be able to stop taking the drugs.

Nutritional management and education are particularly important for all children with diabetes. Because carbohydrates in food are turned into glucose by the body, variations in carbohydrate intake cause variations in blood sugar levels. Thus, children with diabetes need to eat meals on a regular schedule; long periods between eating should be avoided because blood sugar may fall too low. Large amounts of sugar, such as soda, candy, and pastries, are discouraged because blood sugar may rise too high. Parents and older children are taught how to gauge the carbohydrate content of food and adjust what children eat as needed to maintain a consistent daily intake of carbohydrates. Children of all ages find it difficult to consistently follow a properly balanced meal plan (consumed at regular intervals) and avoid the temptations of sugary snacks. Infants and preschool-aged children present a particular challenge to parents because of the concern arising from the dangers of frequent and severe low blood sugar (hypoglycemia).

Emotional issues affect children with diabetes and their families. The realization that they have a lifelong condition may cause some children to become sad, angry, and sometimes even deny that they have an illness. A doctor needs to address these emotions to secure the child's cooperation in complying with the required regimen of meal plan, physical activity, blood glucose testing, and drugs. Failure to re-

▲ see page 930   ■ see table on page 968

solve these issues can lead to difficulties with glucose control.

Summer camps for children with diabetes allow these children to share their experiences with one another while learning how to become personally more responsible for their condition.

If treating the diabetes is difficult, the doctor may enlist the aid of a team of other professionals, possibly including a pediatric endocrinologist, dietitian, diabetes educator, social worker, or psychologist. Family support groups may also help. The doctor may provide parents with information to bring to school so that school personnel understand their roles.

Monitoring Treatment: Children and parents are taught to monitor the blood sugar level at least 4 times a day using a blood sample obtained by pricking a fingertip or the forearm with a small implement called a lancet. Once experience is gained, parents and many children can adjust the insulin dose as needed to achieve the best control. In general, by 10 years of age, children start to become interested in testing their blood sugar levels and injecting insulin themselves. Parents should encourage this independence but make sure the child is being responsible. Doctors teach most children how to adjust their insulin dosage in accordance with the patterns of their home blood glucose records.

Children with diabetes typically see their doctor 4 times a year. The doctor evaluates their growth and development, reviews blood sugar records that the family member keeps, provides guidance and counseling about nutrition, and measures glycosylated hemoglobin (hemoglobin A_{1c})—a substance in the blood that reflects blood glucose levels over the long term. The doctor screens for long-term complications▲ once a year by measuring protein in the urine, assessing function of the thyroid gland, and performing neurologic and eye examinations.

Some children with diabetes do very well and control their diabetes without undue effort or conflict. In others, diabetes becomes a constant source of stress within the family, and control of the condition deteriorates. Adolescents in particular often find it difficult to follow the proper treatment routine given the demands on their schedule and the limitations on their freedom that arise from diabetes. An adolescent benefits if the doctor considers the adolescent's desired schedule and activities and takes a flexible approach to problem solving—working with the adolescent rather than imposing solutions.

Which Children Are at Risk for Type 2 Diabetes?

Children and adolescents meeting these criteria should be tested with a fasting blood sugar test every 2 years beginning at about age 10:

- Being overweight (weighing more than 85% of children of similar age, sex, and height **or** weighing more than 120% of the ideal weight for height)

Plus any two of the following factors:

- Having a close relative with type 2 diabetes
- Being Native American, black, Hispanic, Asian/Pacific Islander
- Having high blood pressure, high blood levels of lipids (fats), or polycystic ovary syndrome

Complications of Treatment and Illness: No treatment completely maintains blood sugar at normal levels. The goal of treatment is to avoid blood sugar levels that are too high and too low. The complications of diabetes include heart disease, kidney failure, blindness, peripheral vascular disease, and other serious disorders. Although these events take years to develop, the better the control of diabetes, the less likely that complications will ever occur.

Low blood sugar (hypoglycemia■) occurs when too much insulin or diabetic drugs are taken or when the child does not eat regularly. Hypoglycemia produces weakness, confusion, and even coma. In adults, adolescents, and older children, episodes of hypoglycemia rarely cause long-term problems. However, frequent episodes of hypoglycemia in children younger than 5 may permanently impair intellectual development. Young children also may not be aware of the warning symptoms of hypoglycemia. To minimize the possibility of hypoglycemia, doctors and parents monitor young children with diabetes particularly closely and also use a slightly higher target range for their blood sugar level.

Children and adolescents with type 1 diabetes who miss insulin injections may develop diabetic ketoacidosis within days. The long-term insufficient or inadequate use of insulin can lead to a syndrome of stunted growth, delayed puberty, and an enlarged liver (Mauriac syndrome).

▲ see page 964   ■ see also page 970

CHAPTER 282

Hereditary Disorders of Metabolism

Most of the foods and drinks people ingest are complex materials that the body must break down into simpler substances. This process may involve several steps. The simpler substances are then used as building blocks, which are assembled into the materials the body needs to sustain life. The process of creating these materials may also require several steps. The major building blocks are carbohydrates, amino acids, and fats (lipids). This complicated process of breaking down and converting the substances ingested is called metabolism.

Metabolism is carried out by chemical substances called enzymes, which are made by the body. If a genetic abnormality affects the function of an enzyme or causes it to be deficient or missing altogether, various disorders can occur. The disorders usually result from an inability to break down some substance that should be broken down—so that some intermediate substance that is toxic builds up—or from an inability to produce some essential substance. Metabolic disorders are classified by the particular building block that is affected.

Some hereditary disorders of metabolism (such as phenylketonuria and the lipidoses) can be diagnosed in the fetus using amniocentesis or chorionic villus sampling.▲ Usually, the diagnosis of a hereditary disorder of metabolism is made using a blood test or an examination of a tissue sample to determine whether a specific enzyme is deficient or missing.

Carbohydrate Metabolism Disorders

Carbohydrates are sugars. Some sugars are simple, and others are more complex. Sucrose (table sugar) is made of two simpler sugars called glucose and fructose. Lactose (milk sugar) is made of glucose and galactose. Both sucrose and lactose must be broken down into their component sugars by enzymes before the body can absorb and make use of them. The carbohydrates in bread, pasta, rice, and other carbohydrate-containing foods are long chains of simple sugar molecules. These longer molecules must also be broken down by the body. If an enzyme needed to process a certain sugar is missing, the sugar can accumulate in the body, causing problems.

GLYCOGEN STORAGE DISEASES

Glycogen is made of many glucose molecules linked together. The sugar glucose is the body's main source of energy for the muscles (including the heart) and brain. Any glucose that is not immediately used for energy is held in reserve in the liver, muscles, and kidneys in the form of glycogen and released when needed by the body.

There are many different glycogen storage diseases (also called glycogenoses), each identified by a roman numeral. These diseases are caused by a hereditary lack of one of the enzymes that is essential to the process of forming glucose into glycogen and breaking down glycogen into glucose. About 1 in 20,000 infants has some form of glycogen storage disease.

Some of these diseases cause few symptoms; others are fatal. The specific symptoms, age at which symptoms start, and their severity vary considerably among these diseases. For types II, V, and VII, the main symptom is usually weakness. For types I, III, and VI, symptoms are low levels of sugar in the blood and protrusion of the abdomen (because excess or abnormal glycogen may enlarge the liver). Low levels of sugar in the blood cause weakness, sweating, confusion, and sometimes seizures and coma. Other consequences for children may include stunted growth, frequent infections, or sores in the mouth and intestines. Glycogen storage diseases tend to cause uric acid, a waste product, to accumulate in the joints (which can cause gout) and in the kidneys (which can cause kidney stones). In type I glycogen storage disease, kidney failure is common in the second decade of life or later.

The specific diagnosis is made when a chemical examination of a sample of tissue, usually muscle or liver, determines that a specific enzyme is missing.

▲ see page 1432

TYPES AND CHARACTERISTICS OF GLYCOGEN STORAGE DISEASES

NAME	AFFECTED ORGANS	SYMPTOMS
Type O	Liver, muscle	Enlarged liver with accumulation of fat inside the liver cells (fatty liver); episodes of low blood sugar levels (hypoglycemia) when fasting
von Gierke's disease (Type IA)	Liver, kidney	Enlarged liver and kidney; slowed growth; very low blood sugar levels; abnormally high levels of acid, fats, and uric acid in blood
Type IB	Liver, white blood cells	Same as in von Gierke's disease but may be less severe; low white blood cell count; recurring mouth and intestinal infections or Crohn's disease
Pompe's disease (Type II)	All organs	Enlarged liver and heart, muscle weakness
Forbes' disease (Type III)	Liver, muscle, heart, white blood cells	Enlarged liver or cirrhosis; low blood sugar levels; muscle damage and heart damage in some people
Andersen's disease (Type IV)	Liver, muscle, most tissues	Cirrhosis in juvenile type; muscle damage and heart failure in adult (late-onset) type
McArdle's disease (Type V)	Muscle	Muscle cramps or weakness during physical activity
Hers' disease (Type VI)	Liver	Enlarged liver; episodes of low blood sugar when fasting; often no symptoms
Tarui's disease (Type VII)	Skeletal muscle, red blood cells	Muscle cramps during physical activity; red blood cell destruction (hemolysis)

Treatment depends on the type of glycogen storage disease. For many people, eating many small carbohydrate-rich meals every day helps prevent blood sugar levels from dropping. For people who have glycogen storage diseases that produce low blood sugar, glucose levels are maintained by giving uncooked cornstarch every 4 to 6 hours around the clock. Sometimes carbohydrate solutions are given through a stomach tube all night to prevent low blood sugar levels from occurring at night.

GALACTOSEMIA

Galactosemia (a high blood level of galactose) is caused by lack of one of the enzymes necessary for metabolizing galactose, a sugar present in lactose (milk sugar). A metabolite builds up that is toxic to the liver and kidneys and also damages the lens of the eye, causing cataracts.

A newborn with galactosemia seems normal at first but within a few days or weeks loses his appetite, vomits, becomes jaundiced, has diarrhea, and stops growing normally.

White blood cell function is affected, and serious infections can develop. If treatment is delayed, affected children remain short and become mentally retarded or may die.

Galactosemia is detectable with a blood test. This test is performed as a routine screening test on newborns in nearly all states in the United States and particularly in those with a family member known to have the disorder.

Galactosemia is treated by completely eliminating milk and milk products—the source of galactose—from an affected child's diet. Galactose is also present in some fruits, vegetables, and sea products, such as seaweed. Doctors are not sure whether the small amounts in these foods cause problems in the long term. People who have the disorder must restrict galactose intake throughout life.

If galactosemia is recognized at birth and adequately treated, the liver and kidney problems do not develop, and initial mental development is normal. However, even with proper treatment, children with galactosemia often have a lower intelligence quotient (IQ) than their siblings, and they often have speech problems. Girls often have ovaries that do not function, and only a few are able to conceive naturally. Boys, however, have normal testicular function.

HEREDITARY FRUCTOSE INTOLERANCE

In this disorder, the body is missing an enzyme that allows it to use fructose, a sugar present in table sugar (sucrose) and many fruits. As a result, a by-product of fructose accumulates in the body, blocking the formation of glycogen and its conversion to glucose for use as energy. Ingesting more than tiny amounts of fructose or sucrose causes low blood sugar levels (hypoglycemia), with sweating, confusion, and sometimes seizures and coma. Children who continue to eat foods containing fructose develop kidney and liver damage, resulting in jaundice, vomiting, mental deterioration, seizures, and death. Chronic symptoms include poor eating, failure to thrive, digestive symptoms, liver failure, and kidney damage.

The diagnosis is made when a chemical examination of a sample of liver tissue determines that the enzyme is missing. Treatment involves excluding fructose (generally found in sweet fruits), sucrose, and sorbitol (a sugar substitute) from the diet. Acute attacks respond to glucose given intravenously; milder attacks of hypoglycemia are treated with glucose tablets, which should be carried by anyone who has hereditary fructose intolerance.

Amino Acid Metabolism Disorders

Amino acids are the building blocks of proteins and have many functions in the body. Hereditary disorders of amino acid processing can be the result of defects either in the breakdown of amino acids or in the body's ability to get the amino acids into cells. Because these disorders produce symptoms early in life, newborns are routinely screened for several common ones. In the United States, newborns are commonly screened for phenylketonuria, maple syrup urine disease, homocystinuria, tyrosinemia, and a number of other inherited disorders, although screening varies from state to state.

PHENYLKETONURIA

Phenylketonuria (PKU) is a disorder that causes a buildup of the amino acid phenylala-

nine, which is an essential amino acid that cannot be synthesized in the body but is present in food. Excess phenylalanine is normally converted to tyrosine, another amino acid, and eliminated from the body. Without the enzyme that converts it to tyrosine, phenylalanine builds up in the blood and is toxic to the brain, causing mental retardation.

PKU occurs in most ethnic groups. If PKU runs in the family and DNA is available from an affected family member, amniocentesis or chorionic villus sampling with DNA analysis can be performed to determine whether a fetus has the disorder.

Most affected newborns are detected during routine screening tests. Newborns with PKU rarely have symptoms right away, although sometimes an infant is sleepy or eats poorly. If not treated, affected infants progressively develop mental retardation over the first few years of life, which eventually becomes severe. Other symptoms include seizures, nausea and vomiting, an eczema-like rash, lighter skin and hair than their family members, aggressive or self-injurious behavior, hyperactivity, and sometimes psychiatric symptoms. Untreated children often give off a "mousy" body and urine odor as a result of a by-product of phenylalanine (phenylacetic acid) in their urine and sweat.

To prevent mental retardation, phenylalanine intake must be restricted (but not eliminated altogether as people need some phenylalanine to live) beginning in the first few weeks of life. Because all natural sources of protein contain too much phenylalanine for children with PKU, affected children cannot have meat, milk, or other common foods that contain protein. Instead, they must eat a variety of phenylalanine-free processed foods, which are specially manufactured. Low-protein natural foods, such as fruits, vegetables, and restricted amounts of certain grain cereals, can be eaten.

A restricted diet, if started early and maintained well, allows for normal development. However, if very strict control of the diet is not maintained, affected children may begin to have difficulties in school. Dietary restrictions started after 2 to 3 years of age may control extreme hyperactivity and seizures and raise the child's eventual IQ but do not reverse mental retardation. Recent evidence suggests that functioning of some mentally retarded adults with PKU (born before newborn screening tests were available) may improve when they follow the PKU diet.

A phenylalanine-restricted diet should continue for life or intelligence may decrease and neurologic and psychiatric problems may ensue.

MAPLE SYRUP URINE DISEASE

Children with maple syrup urine disease are unable to metabolize certain amino acids. By-products of these amino acids build up, causing neurologic changes, including seizures and mental retardation. These by-products also cause body fluids, such as urine and sweat, to smell like maple syrup. This disease is most common among Mennonite families.

There are many forms of maple syrup urine disease; symptoms vary in severity. In the most severe form, infants develop neurologic abnormalities, including seizures and coma, during the first week of life and can die within days to weeks. In the milder forms, children initially appear normal but develop vomiting, staggering, confusion, coma, and the odor of maple syrup particularly during physical stress, such as infection or surgery.

In some states, newborns are routinely screened for this disease with a blood test.

Infants with severe disease are treated with dialysis.▲ Some children with mild disease benefit from injections of the vitamin B_1 (thiamin). After the disease has been brought under control, children must always consume a special artificial diet that is low in the particular amino acids that are affected by the missing enzyme.

HOMOCYSTINURIA

Children with homocystinuria are unable to metabolize the amino acid homocysteine, which, along with certain toxic by-products, builds up to cause a variety of symptoms. Symptoms may be mild or severe, depending on the particular enzyme defect.

Infants with this disorder are normal at birth. The first symptoms, including dislocation of the lens of the eye, causing severely decreased vision, usually begin after 3 years of age. Most children have skeletal abnormalities, including osteoporosis; the child is usually tall and thin with a curved spine, elongated limbs, and long, spiderlike fingers. Psychiatric and behavioral disorders and mental retardation are common. Homocystinuria makes the blood more likely to spontaneously clot, resulting in strokes, high blood pressure, and many other serious problems.

In a few states, children are screened for homocystinuria at birth with a blood test. The diagnosis is confirmed by a test measuring enzyme function in liver or skin cells.

Some children with homocystinuria improve when given vitamin B_6 (pyridoxine) or vitamin B_{12} (cobalamin).

TYROSINEMIA

Children with tyrosinemia are unable to completely metabolize the amino acid tyrosine. By-products of this amino acid build up, causing a variety of symptoms. In some states, the disorder is detected on the newborn screening tests.

There are two main types of tyrosinemia: I and II. Type I tyrosinemia is most common in children of French-Canadian or Scandinavian descent. Children with this disorder typically become ill sometime within the first year of life with dysfunction of the liver, kidneys, and nerves, resulting in irritability, rickets, or even liver failure and death. Restriction of tyrosine in the diet is of little help. An experimental drug, which blocks production of toxic metabolites, may help children with type I tyrosinemia. Often, children with type I tyrosinemia require a liver transplant.

Type II tyrosinemia is less common. Affected children sometimes have mental retardation and frequently develop sores on the skin and eyes. Unlike type I tyrosinemia, restriction of tyrosine in the diet can prevent problems from developing.

Lipid Metabolism Disorders

Fats (lipids) are an important source of energy for the body. The body's store of fat is constantly broken down and reassembled to balance the body's energy needs with the food available. Groups of specific enzymes help the body break down and process fats. Certain abnormalities in these enzymes can lead to the buildup of specific fatty substances that normally would have been broken down by the enzymes. Over time, accumulations of these substances can be harmful to many organs of the body. Disorders caused by the accumulation of lipids are called lipidoses. Other enzyme abnormalities result in the body being unable to properly convert fats into energy. These abnormalities are called fatty acid oxidation disorders.

▲ see page 833

GAUCHER'S DISEASE

In Gaucher's disease, glucocerebrosides, which are a product of fat metabolism, accumulate in tissues. Gaucher's disease is the most common lipidosis. The disease is most common in Ashkenazi (Eastern European) Jews. Gaucher's disease leads to an enlarged liver and spleen and a brownish pigmentation of the skin. Accumulations of glucocerebrosides in the eyes cause yellow spots called pingueculae to appear. Accumulations in the bone marrow can cause pain and destroy bone.

Most people who have Gaucher's disease develop type 1, the chronic form, which results in an enlarged liver and spleen and bone abnormalities. Most are adults, but children also may have type 1. Type 2, the infantile form, develops in infancy; infants with the disease have an enlarged spleen and severe nervous system abnormalities and usually die within a year. Type 3, the juvenile form, can begin at any time during childhood. Children with the disease have an enlarged liver and spleen, bone abnormalities, and slowly progressive nervous system abnormalities. Children who survive to adolescence may live for many years.

Many people with Gaucher's disease can be treated with enzyme replacement therapy, in which enzymes are given intravenously, usually every 2 weeks. Enzyme replacement therapy is most effective for people who do not have nervous system complications.

TAY-SACHS DISEASE

In Tay-Sachs disease, gangliosides, which are products of fat metabolism, accumulate in tissues. The disease is most common in families of Eastern European Jewish origin. At a very early age, children with this disease become progressively retarded and appear to have floppy muscle tone. Spasticity develops and is followed by paralysis, dementia, and blindness. These children usually die by age 3 or 4. Tay-Sachs disease can be identified in the fetus by chorionic villus sampling or amniocentesis. The disease cannot be treated or cured.

NIEMANN-PICK DISEASE

In Niemann-Pick disease, the deficiency of a specific enzyme results in the accumulation of sphingomyelin (a product of fat metabolism) or cholesterol. Niemann-Pick disease has several

forms, depending on the severity of the enzyme deficiency and thus accumulation of sphingomyelin or cholesterol. The most severe forms tend to occur in Jewish people. The milder forms occur in all ethnic groups.

In the most severe form (type A), children fail to grow properly and have multiple neurologic problems. These children usually die by age 3. Children with type B disease develop fatty growths in the skin, areas of dark pigmentation, and an enlarged liver, spleen, and lymph nodes; they may be mentally retarded. Children with type C disease develop symptoms in childhood, with seizures and neurologic deterioration.

Some forms of Niemann-Pick disease can be diagnosed in the fetus by chorionic villus sampling or amniocentesis. After birth, the diagnosis can be made by a liver biopsy (removal of a tissue specimen for examination under a microscope). None of the types of Niemann-Pick disease can be cured, and children tend to die of infection or progressive dysfunction of the central nervous system.

FABRY'S DISEASE

In Fabry's disease, glycolipid, which is a product of fat metabolism, accumulates in tissues. Because the defective gene for this rare disorder is carried on the X chromosome, the full-blown disease occurs only in males.▲ The accumulation of glycolipid causes noncancerous skin growths (angiokeratomas) to form over the lower part of the trunk. The corneas become cloudy, resulting in poor vision. A burning pain may develop in the arms and legs, and the person may have episodes of fever. People with Fabry's disease eventually develop kidney failure and heart disease, although most often they live into adulthood. Kidney failure may lead to high blood pressure, which may result in stroke.

Fabry's disease can be diagnosed in the fetus by chorionic villus sampling or amniocentesis. The disease cannot be cured or even treated directly, but researchers are investigating a treatment in which the deficient enzyme is replaced by transfusion. Treatment consists of taking analgesics to help relieve pain and fever. People with kidney failure may need a kidney transplant.

FATTY ACID OXIDATION DISORDERS

Several enzymes help break fats down so that they may be turned into energy. An inher-

▲ see page 11

ited defect or deficiency of one of these enzymes leaves the body short of energy and allows breakdown products, such as acyl-CoA, to accumulate. The enzyme most commonly deficient is medium chain acyl-CoA dehydrogenase (MCAD). MCAD deficiency is one of the most common inherited disorders of metabolism, particularly in people of Northern European descent.

Symptoms usually develop between birth and age 3. Children are most likely to develop symptoms if they go without food for a period of time (which depletes other sources of energy) or have an increased need for calories because of exercise or illness. The level of sugar in the blood drops significantly, causing confusion or coma. The child becomes weak and may have vomiting or seizures. Over the long term, children have delayed mental and physical development, an enlarged liver, heart muscle weakness, and an irregular heartbeat. Sudden death may occur.

Some states screen newborns for MCAD deficiency with a blood test. Immediate treatment is with intravenous glucose. For long-term treatment, the child must eat often, never skipping meals, and consume a diet high in carbohydrates and low in fats. Supplements of the amino acid carnitine may be helpful. The long-term outcome is generally good.

Pyruvate Metabolism Disorders

Pyruvate is a substance formed in the processing of carbohydrates and proteins that serves as an energy source for cells. Problems with pyruvate metabolism can limit a cell's ability to produce energy and allow a buildup of lactic acid, a waste product. Many enzymes are involved in pyruvate metabolism. A hereditary deficiency in any one of these enzymes results in one of a variety of disorders, depending on which enzyme is missing. Symptoms may develop any time between early infancy and late adulthood. Exercise and infections can worsen symptoms, leading to severe lactic acidosis. These disorders are diagnosed by measuring enzyme activity in cells from the liver or skin.

Pyruvate dehydrogenase complex deficiency is a lack of a group of enzymes needed to process pyruvate. This deficiency results in a variety of symptoms, ranging from mild to severe. Some newborns with this deficiency have brain malformations. Other children appear normal at birth but develop symptoms, in-

Other Rare Hereditary Disorders of Lipid Metabolism

Wolman's disease is a disorder that results when specific types of cholesterol and glycerides accumulate in tissues. This disease causes enlargement of the spleen and liver. Calcium deposits in the adrenal glands cause them to harden, and fatty diarrhea (steatorrhea) also occurs. Infants with Wolman's disease usually die by 6 months of age.

Cerebrotendinous xanthomatosis occurs when cholestanol, a product of cholesterol metabolism, accumulates in tissues. This disease eventually leads to uncoordinated movements, dementia, cataracts, and fatty growths (xanthomas) on tendons. The disabling symptoms often appear after age 30. If started early, the drug chenodiol helps prevent progression of the disease, but it cannot undo any damage already done.

In **sitosterolemia,** fats from fruits and vegetables accumulate in blood and tissues. The buildup of fats leads to atherosclerosis, abnormal red blood cells, and fatty deposits on tendons (xanthomas). Treatment consists of reducing the intake of foods that are rich in plant fats, such as vegetable oils, and taking cholestyramine resin.

In **Refsum's disease,** phytanic acid, which is a product of fat metabolism, accumulates in tissues. A buildup of phytanic acid leads to nerve and retinal damage, spastic movements, and changes in the bone and skin. Treatment involves avoiding eating green fruits and vegetables that contain chlorophyll. Plasmapheresis, in which phytanic acid is removed from the blood, may be helpful.

cluding weak muscles, seizures, poor coordination, and a severe balance problem, later in infancy or childhood. Mental retardation is common. This disorder cannot be cured, but some children are helped by a diet that is high in fat and low in carbohydrates.

Absence of pyruvate carboxylase, an enzyme, is a very rare condition that interferes with or blocks the production of glucose from pyruvate in the body. Lactic acid and ketones build up in the blood. Often this disease is fatal. Children who survive have seizures and severe mental retardation, although there are recent reports of children with milder symptoms. There is no cure, but some children are helped by eating frequent carbohydrate-rich meals and restricting dietary protein.

CHAPTER 283

Childhood Cancers

Cancer is a rare disease among children, occurring in only 1 of 5,000 children every year. Although the most common childhood cancers are leukemia, lymphoma, and brain tumors, these cancers also occur in adults, and the diagnosis and treatment are similar in adults and children. Several of the more common cancers that occur mainly in children are Wilms' tumor, neuroblastoma, and retinoblastoma.

In contrast to many adult cancers, cancers in children tend to be much more curable. About 75% of children with cancer survive at least 5 years. Nonetheless, cancer kills over 2,000 children each year.

As in adults, doctors use a combination of treatments, including surgery, chemotherapy, and radiation therapy. However, because children are still growing, these treatments may have side effects that do not occur in adults. For example, in a child, an arm or leg that received radiation may not grow to full size. Children who receive radiation to the brain may not have normal intellectual development.

Children who survive cancer have more years than adults to develop long-term consequences of chemotherapy and radiation therapy, such as infertility, poor growth, damage to the heart, and even development of second cancers (which occurs in 3 to 12% of children who survive cancer). Because of these significant possible consequences and the complexity of treatment, children with cancer are best treated in centers with expertise in childhood cancers.

The impact of being diagnosed with cancer and the intensity of the treatment are overwhelming to the child and family. It is difficult for the health care team and the family to maintain a sense of normalcy for the child, especially considering the child's frequent hospitalizations and office visits for treatment of the cancer and its complications. Overwhelming stress is typical, as parents struggle to continue to work, be attentive to siblings, and still attend to the many needs of the child with cancer.▲ The situation is even more difficult when the child is being treated at a specialty center far from home. The treatment team should include pediatric cancer specialists, other needed specialists, and the primary care doctor. Other essential personnel are a so-

cial worker (who can provide emotional support and help with financial aspects of care), a teacher (who can work with the child, the school, and the health care team to ensure that the child's education continues), and a psychologist (who can help the child, siblings, and parents throughout treatment). Many centers also include a parent advocate—a parent who had a child with cancer who can offer guidance to family members.

Wilms' Tumor

Wilms' tumor (nephroblastoma) is a specific kind of cancer of the kidneys.

Wilms' tumor usually develops in children younger than 5 years of age, although it occasionally occurs in older children and rarely in adults. Very rarely, it develops before birth and appears in the newborn. In about 4% of cases, Wilms' tumor occurs simultaneously in both kidneys.

The cause of Wilms' tumor is not known, although a genetic abnormality may be involved in some cases. Children with certain birth defects, such as absence of the irises or excessive growth of one side of the body, both of which may be caused by a genetic abnormality, have an increased risk of developing Wilms' tumor. However, most children with Wilms' tumor have no such recognizable abnormalities.

Symptoms and Diagnosis

Symptoms include a large abdomen (for example, a rapid change to a larger diaper size), abdominal pain, fever, poor appetite, nausea, and vomiting. Blood appears in the urine in 15 to 20% of cases. Because the kidneys are involved in controlling blood pressure, Wilms' tumor may cause high blood pressure. This cancer can spread to other parts of the body, especially the lungs. Involvement of the lungs can lead to a cough and shortness of breath.

The first sign of Wilms' tumor, a painless mass in their child's abdomen, is most often noticed by the parents. A doctor is usually able to feel a lump (mass) in the child's abdomen. If the doctor suspects Wilms' tumor, ultrasound, computed tomography (CT), or magnetic resonance imaging (MRI) is performed to determine the nature and size of the lump.

▲ see also page 1638

Prognosis and Treatment

Younger children, children with smaller tumors, and children whose tumor has not spread tend to fare better. In general, Wilms' tumor is very curable; about 70 to 95% of children with Wilms' tumor survive, depending on how widespread the disease is. Even older children and children with widespread tumors have a very good prognosis. However, one particular type of Wilms' tumor (present in less than 5% of cases) is more resistant to treatment. Children with this type of tumor, which is recognized by its microscopic appearance, have a poorer prognosis.

Doctors treat Wilms' tumor by removing the kidney that contains the tumor. During the operation, the other kidney is examined to determine whether it also has a tumor. After surgery, doctors give the child chemotherapy drugs—most commonly actinomycin D, vincristine, and doxorubicin. Children with larger or widespread tumors also receive radiation therapy. Sometimes the tumor cannot be removed initially; in that case, the child is first treated with chemotherapy and radiation, and the tumor is removed when it is smaller.

Neuroblastoma

Neuroblastoma is a common childhood cancer that grows in parts of the nervous system.

A neuroblastoma develops in a certain kind of nerve tissue located in many places of the body. It usually originates in nerves in the abdomen or chest, most commonly in the adrenal glands (located above each kidney). Very rarely, a neuroblastoma originates in the brain.

Neuroblastoma is the most common cancer in infants and one of the most common tumors in children of any age. About 80% of all neuroblastomas occur in children younger than 5 years. Although its cause is not known, this cancer sometimes runs in families.

Symptoms and Diagnosis

The symptoms depend on where the neuroblastoma originated and whether it has spread. For cancers originating in the abdomen, the first symptoms include a large abdomen, a sensation of fullness, and abdominal pain. Cancers in the chest may cause cough or difficulty breathing. In over half of the children, the cancer has spread beyond the original location by the time the child sees a doctor. Symptoms in these children relate to spread of the cancer. For example, cancer that has invaded the bones causes pain. Cancer that has reached the

bone marrow may reduce the number of various types of blood cells. A reduced number of red blood cells (anemia) causes a weak and tired feeling; a reduced number of platelets causes bruising; and a reduced number of white blood cells lowers the resistance to infection. The cancer can spread to the skin, where it produces lumps, or to the spinal cord, where it may cause weakness of the arms or legs. About 90% of neuroblastomas produce hormones, such as epinephrine, which can increase heart rate and cause anxiety.

Early diagnosis of a neuroblastoma is not easy. If the cancer grows large enough, the doctor may be able to feel a lump (mass) in the abdomen. A doctor who suspects a neuroblastoma may suggest an ultrasound examination, computed tomography (CT), or magnetic resonance imaging (MRI) of the chest and abdomen. A urine sample can be tested for excessive production of epinephrine-like hormones. To see if the cancer has spread, the doctor may obtain a bone scan, take x-rays of bones, or examine tissue samples from the liver, lung, skin, bone marrow, or bone.

Prognosis and Treatment

Children younger than 1 year and children with small cancers have a very good prognosis. If the cancer has not spread, it usually can be removed by surgery. Nearly all children receive chemotherapy drugs such as vincristine, cyclophosphamide, doxorubicin, etoposide, and cisplatin. Also, radiation therapy may be used. In children older than 1 year, the cure rate is low for cancer that has spread.

Retinoblastoma

Retinoblastoma is a cancer of the retina, the light-sensing area at the back of the eye.

Retinoblastomas represent about 2% of childhood cancers and almost always occur before age 4. They occur in both eyes at the same time in 20 to 30% of children. This cancer is the result of damage to specific, known genes that control eye development. Sometimes a damaged gene is inherited from a parent or becomes damaged very early during embryonic development. Children with this type of damage may pass the defective gene on to their offspring, who may also develop retinoblastoma. Other times, genes are damaged later in embryonic development only in the embryo's eye cells. This damage cannot be passed on to offspring. Retinoblastoma is hereditary in all of the children with cancer in both eyes and in 15 to 20% of children with cancer in one eye.

Retinoblastoma usually spreads to the brain along the optic nerve (the nerve that leads from the eye to the brain). However, it also may spread to other organs, such as the bone marrow.

Symptoms and Diagnosis

Symptoms of a retinoblastoma can include a white pupil or strabismus (cross-eyes). Retinoblastomas of sufficient size also may affect vision but tend to produce few other symptoms.

If a doctor suspects a retinoblastoma, the child is given general anesthesia and both eyes are examined by looking at the retina through the lens and iris; general anesthesia is necessary because small children are not able to cooperate during the careful, time-consuming examination required to diagnose retinoblastoma. The cancer can also be identified by computed tomography (CT) or magnetic resonance imaging (MRI). Both tests help determine whether the cancer has spread to the brain. Doctors also look for cancer cells in a sample of cerebrospinal fluid (taken by spinal tap [lumbar puncture]); finding cancer cells is further evidence that the cancer has spread to the brain. Because the cancer can spread to the bone marrow, a sample of bone marrow is obtained for examination.

Prognosis and Treatment

Without treatment, most children with retinoblastoma die within 2 years. However, with treatment, children with retinoblastoma are cured more than 90% of the time. When only one eye is affected and that eye has little or no vision, doctors usually remove the entire eyeball along with part of the optic nerve. When there is significant vision in the affected eye, or the cancer affects both eyes, doctors sometimes give chemotherapy and try to avoid surgery in an attempt to spare the eyeballs. Chemotherapy drugs include etoposide, carboplatin, vincristine, and cyclophosphamide. The chemotherapy may completely eliminate the cancer and often shrinks it enough that the remainder may be removed with lasers, freezing (cryogenic) probes, or patches containing radioactive material. If these treatments do not eliminate the cancer, doctors may remove the eyeball or give radiation therapy. Sometimes, both eyeballs must be removed. Chemotherapy is also used when the cancer has spread beyond the eye or if the cancer returns after initial treatment.

Radiation therapy to the eye has significant consequences, such as cataracts, decreased vision, chronic dry eye, and wasting of the tissue around the eye. The bones of the face may fail to grow normally, resulting in a deformed appearance.

After treatment, doctors re-examine the eyes every 2 to 4 months to determine whether the cancer has returned. Children with the hereditary type of retinoblastoma have a particularly high risk of having the cancer recur. Furthermore, within 50 years from the time of diagnosis, as many as 50% of those with a hereditary retinoblastoma develop a second cancer, such as soft tissue sarcomas, melanomas, and osteosarcomas. Doctors recommend that immediate family members of any child with a retinoblastoma have regular eye examinations. Other young children in the family need to be examined for a retinoblastoma, and adults need to be examined for a retinocytoma, a noncancerous tumor caused by the same gene. Family members who have no evidence of cancer can have their DNA analyzed to see if they carry the retinoblastoma gene.

CHAPTER 284

Cerebral Palsy

Cerebral palsy is poor muscle control, spasticity, paralysis, and other neurologic problems resulting from brain injury before, during, or shortly after birth.

Cerebral palsy affects 2 to 4 of every 1,000 infants, but it is 10 times more common in premature infants. It is particularly common in infants of very low birth weight.

Cerebral palsy is not a disease; it is a constellation of symptoms that result from damage to the parts of the brain that control muscle movements (motor areas). Sometimes children with cerebral palsy have damage to other parts of the brain as well. The brain damage that results in cerebral palsy may occur during pregnancy, during birth, after birth, or in early childhood. Once the brain damage has occurred, it does not get worse even though the child's symptoms may change with growth and maturation. Brain damage occurring after age 5 is not considered cerebral palsy.

Causes

Many different types of injury to the brain can cause cerebral palsy, and most often a specific cause cannot be identified. Birth injuries and poor oxygen supply to the brain before, during, and immediately after birth cause 10 to 15% of cases. Prenatal infections, such as rubella, toxoplasmosis, or cytomegalovirus infection, sometimes result in cerebral palsy. Premature infants are particularly vulnerable, possibly in part because the blood vessels of the brain are poorly developed and bleed easily. High levels of bilirubin in the blood can lead to a form of brain damage called kernicterus. During the first years of life, severe illness, such as inflammation of the tissues covering the brain (meningitis), sepsis, trauma, and severe dehydration, can cause brain injury and result in cerebral palsy.

Symptoms

The symptoms of cerebral palsy can range from barely noticeable clumsiness to severe spasticity that contorts the child's arms and legs, requiring mobility aids, such as braces, crutches, and wheelchairs.

There are four main types of cerebral palsy: spastic, choreoathetoid, ataxic, and mixed. In all forms of cerebral palsy, speech may be hard to understand because the child has difficulty controlling the muscles involved in speech. Because non-motor parts of the brain also may be affected, many children with cerebral palsy have other disabilities, such as mental retardation, behavioral problems, difficulty seeing or hearing properly, and seizure disorders.

In the spastic type, which occurs in about 70% of children with cerebral palsy, the muscles are stiff and weak. The stiffness may affect both arms and both legs (quadriplegia), mainly the legs (diplegia), or only the arm and leg on one side (hemiplegia). The affected arms and legs are poorly developed, stiff, and weak. Children with spastic quadriplegia are the most severely affected. They commonly have mental retardation (sometimes severe)

along with seizures and trouble swallowing. Trouble with swallowing makes these children prone to choking on secretions from the mouth and stomach (aspiration). Aspiration injures the lungs, causing difficulty breathing. Repeated aspiration can permanently damage the lungs. Children with spastic diplegia usually have normal mental development and rarely have seizures. About one fourth of children with spastic hemiplegia have below-normal intelligence, and one third have seizures.

In the choreoathetoid type, which occurs in about 20% of children with cerebral palsy, the muscles spontaneously move slowly and without normal control. Movements of the arms, legs, and body may be writhing, abrupt, and jerky. Strong emotion makes the movements worse; sleep makes them disappear. These children usually have normal intelligence and rarely have seizures.

In the ataxic type, which occurs in about 10% of children with cerebral palsy, coordination is poor and movements are shaky. These children also have muscle weakness and trembling. Children with this disorder have difficulty making rapid or fine movements and walk unsteadily, with their legs widely spaced.

In the mixed type, two of the above types, most often spastic and choreoathetoid, are combined. This type occurs in many children with cerebral palsy.

Diagnosis

Cerebral palsy is difficult to diagnose during early infancy. As the baby matures, poor development, weakness, spasticity, or lack of coordination becomes noticeable. Although laboratory tests cannot identify cerebral palsy, a doctor may perform blood tests, electrical studies of muscle (electromyography), a muscle biopsy, and computed tomography (CT) or magnetic resonance imaging (MRI) of the brain to clarify the nature of the brain damage and to look for other disorders. The doctor might recommend additional testing if the child's symptoms appear to be evolving in a way not typical of cerebral palsy. The specific type of cerebral palsy often cannot be distinguished before the child is 18 months old.

Prognosis and Treatment

The prognosis usually depends on the type of cerebral palsy and on its severity. More than 90% of children with cerebral palsy survive into adulthood. Only the most severely affected—those incapable of any self-care—have a substantially shortened life expectancy.

Cerebral palsy cannot be cured; its problems are lifelong. However, much can be done to improve a child's mobility and independence. Physical therapy, occupational therapy, and braces may improve muscle control and walking, particularly when rehabilitation is started as early as possible. Surgery may be performed to cut or lengthen tendons of the stiff muscles that limit motion. Sometimes cutting certain nerve roots coming from the spinal cord improves the spasticity. Speech therapy may make speech much clearer and help with swallowing problems. Seizures can be treated with anticonvulsant drugs. Drugs taken by mouth, such as dantrolene and baclofen, are sometimes used to help spasticity, but their benefits are limited by side effects. New treatments deliver drugs directly to the nerves and muscles that are affected. Botulinum toxin can be injected into spastic muscles.

Children with cerebral palsy grow normally and attend regular schools if they do not have severe intellectual and physical disabilities. Other children require extensive physical therapy, need special education, and are severely limited in activities of daily living, requiring some type of lifelong care and assistance. However, even severely affected children can benefit from education and training.

Information and counseling are available to parents to help them understand their child's condition and potential and to assist with problems as they arise. Loving parental care combined with assistance from public and private agencies, such as community health agencies and vocational rehabilitation organizations, can help a child reach his highest potential.

CHAPTER 285

Mental Retardation

Mental retardation is significantly subaverage intellectual functioning present from birth or early infancy, causing limitations in the ability to conduct normal activities of daily living.

Mental retardation is not a specific medical disorder like pneumonia or strep throat, and it is not a mental health disorder. A person with mental retardation has significantly below average intellectual functioning that limits his ability to cope with two or more activities of normal daily living (adaptive skills). These activities include the ability to communicate; live at home; take care of oneself, including making decisions; participate in leisure, social, school, and work activities; and be aware of personal health and safety.

People with mental retardation have varying degrees of impairment. While recognizing each person's individuality, doctors find it helpful to classify a person's level of functioning. Intellectual functioning levels can be based on the results of intelligence quotient (IQ) tests or on the level of support a person requires. Support is categorized as intermittent, limited, extensive, or pervasive. Intermittent means occasional support; limited means support such as a day program in a sheltered workshop; extensive means daily, ongoing support; pervasive means a high level of support for all activities of daily living, possibly including full-time nursing care.

Based only on IQ test scores, about 3% of the total population are considered to have mental retardation. However, if classification is based on the need for support, only about 1% of people have significant retardation.

Causes

A wide variety of medical and environmental conditions can cause mental retardation. Some are genetic; some are present before or at the time of conception; others occur during pregnancy, during birth, or after birth. The common factor is that something interferes with the growth and development of the brain. However, doctors can identify a specific cause in only about one third of people with mild mental retardation and in two thirds of people with moderate to profound mental retardation.

Symptoms

Some children with mental retardation have abnormalities apparent at birth or shortly thereafter. These abnormalities may be physi-

LEVELS OF MENTAL RETARDATION

LEVEL	INTELLIGENCE QUOTIENT (IQ) RANGE	ABILITY AT PRESCHOOL AGE (BIRTH TO 5 YEARS)	ABILITY AT SCHOOL AGE (6 TO 20 YEARS)	ABILITY AT ADULT AGE (21 YEARS AND OLDER)
Mild	52–68	Can develop social and communication skills; motor coordination is slightly impaired; often not diagnosed until later age	Can learn up to about the 6th-grade level by late teens; can be expected to learn appropriate social skills	Can usually achieve enough social and vocational skills for self-support, but may need guidance and assistance during times of unusual social or economic stress
Moderate	36–51	Can talk or learn to communicate; social awareness is poor; motor coordination is fair; can profit from training in self-help	Can learn some social and occupational skills; can progress to elementary school level in schoolwork; may learn to travel alone in familiar places	May achieve self-support by performing unskilled or semiskilled work under sheltered conditions; needs supervision and guidance when under mild social or economic stress
Severe	20–35	Can say a few words; able to learn some self-help skills; has limited speech skills; motor coordination is poor	Can talk or learn to communicate; can learn simple health habits; benefits from habit training	May contribute partially to self-care under complete supervision; can develop some useful self-protection skills in controlled environment
Profound	19 or below	Extremely retarded, little motor coordination; may need nursing care	Some motor coordination; limited communication skills	May achieve very limited self-care; usually needs nursing care

cal as well as neurologic and may include unusual facial features, a head that is too large or too small, deformities of the hands or feet, and various other abnormalities. Sometimes such children have an outwardly normal appearance but have other signs of serious illness, such as seizures, lethargy, vomiting, abnormal urine odor, and failure to feed and grow normally. During their first year, many children with more severe mental retardation have delayed development of motor skills, being slow to roll, sit, and stand.

However, most children with mental retardation do not develop symptoms that are noticeable until the preschool period. Symptoms become apparent at a younger age in those more severely affected. Usually, the first problem parents notice is a delay in language development. Children with mental retardation are slower to use words, put words together, and speak in complete sentences. Their social development is sometimes slow, because of

cognitive impairment and language deficiencies. Children with mental retardation may be slow to learn to dress and feed themselves. Some parents may not consider the possibility of retardation until the child is in school or preschool and is unable to keep up with age-appropriate expectations.

Children with mental retardation are somewhat more likely than other children to have behavioral problems, such as explosive outbursts, temper tantrums, and physically aggressive behavior. These behaviors are often related to specific frustrating situations compounded by an impaired ability to communicate and control impulses. Older children may be gullible and easily taken advantage of or led into minor misbehavior.

About 10 to 40% of people with mental retardation also have a mental health disorder (dual diagnosis). In particular, depression is common, especially in children who are aware that they are different from their peers or who

Some Causes of Mental Retardation

Before or At Conception
- Inherited disorders (such as phenylketonuria, hypothyroidism, fragile X syndrome)
- Chromosome abnormalities (for example, Down syndrome)

During Pregnancy
- Severe maternal malnutrition
- Infections with HIV, cytomegalovirus, herpes simplex; toxoplasmosis, rubella
- Toxins (alcohol, lead, methylmercury)
- Drugs (phenytoin, valproate, isotretinoin, cancer chemotherapy)
- Abnormal brain development (spina bifida, myelomeningocele)

During Birth
- Insufficient oxygen (hypoxia)
- Extreme prematurity

After Birth
- Brain infections (meningitis, encephalitis)
- Severe head injury
- Malnutrition of the child
- Severe emotional neglect or abuse
- Toxins (lead, mercury)
- Brain tumors and their treatments

are maligned and mistreated because of their disability.

Diagnosis

Many children are evaluated by teams of professionals, including a pediatric neurologist or developmental pediatrician, a psychologist, speech pathologist, occupational or physical therapist, special educator, social worker, or nurse.

Doctors evaluate a child suspected of having mental retardation by testing intellectual functioning and looking for a cause. Even though mental retardation is usually irreversible, identifying a disorder that caused the retardation may allow doctors to predict the child's future course, plan any interventions that can increase the child's level of function-

ing, and counsel parents on the risk of having another child with that disorder.

Newborns with physical abnormalities or other symptoms suggestive of a condition associated with mental retardation often need laboratory tests to help detect metabolic and genetic disorders. Imaging tests, such as computed tomography (CT) or magnetic resonance imaging (MRI), may be performed to look for structural problems within the brain.

Some children who are delayed in learning language and mastering social skills have conditions other than mental retardation. Because hearing problems interfere with language and social development, a hearing evaluation is typically performed. Emotional problems and learning disorders also can be mistaken for mental retardation. Children who have been severely deprived of normal love and attention▲ for long periods of time may appear retarded. A child with delays in sitting or walking (gross motor skills) or in manipulating objects (fine motor skills) may have a neurologic disorder not associated with mental retardation.

Because mild developmental problems are not always noticed by parents, doctors routinely perform developmental screening tests during well-child visits. Doctors use simple tests, such as the Denver Developmental Screening Test, to quickly evaluate the child's cognitive, verbal, and motor skills. Questions can be asked of the parents to help the doctor determine the child's level of functioning. Children who perform significantly below their age level on these screening tests are referred for formal testing.

Formal testing has three components: interviews with parents, observations of the child, and norm-referenced tests. Some tests, such as the Wechsler Intelligence Scale for Children-III (WISC-III), measure intellectual ability. Other tests, such as the Vineland Adaptive Behavior Scales, assess areas such as communication, daily living skills, social abilities, and motor skills. Generally, these formal tests accurately compare a child's intellectual and social abilities with those of others his age. However, children of different cultural backgrounds, non-English speaking families, and very low socioeconomic status are more likely to perform poorly on these tests. Because of this, a diagnosis of mental retardation requires that the doctor integrate the test data with information obtained from parents and direct observations of the child. A diagnosis of men-

▲ see page 1645

tal retardation is appropriate only when both intellectual and adaptive skills are significantly below average.

Prevention and Prognosis

Prevention mainly applies to genetic and infectious disorders and to accidental injuries. Doctors may recommend genetic testing for people with a family member or other child with a known inherited disorder, particularly ones related to mental retardation, such as phenylketonuria, Tay-Sachs disease, or fragile X syndrome. Identification of a gene for an inherited disorder allows genetic counselors to help parents evaluate the risk of having an affected child. Women who plan to get pregnant should receive necessary vaccinations, particularly against rubella. Women who are at risk for infectious disorders that may be harmful to a fetus, such as rubella and HIV, should be tested for these before getting pregnant.

Proper prenatal care lowers the risk of having a child with mental retardation. Folic acid, a vitamin supplement, taken before conception and early in pregnancy can help prevent certain kinds of brain abnormalities. Advances in the practices of labor and delivery and in the care of premature infants have helped to reduce the rate of mental retardation related to prematurity.

Certain tests, such as ultrasound, amniocentesis, chorionic villus sampling, and various blood tests, can be performed during pregnancy to identify conditions that often result in mental retardation. Amniocentesis or chorionic villus sampling is often used for women at high risk of having a baby with Down syndrome. A few conditions, such as hydrocephalus and severe Rh incompatibility,▲ may be treated during pregnancy. Most conditions, however, cannot be treated, and early recognition can serve only to prepare the parents and allow them to consider the option of abortion.

Because mental retardation sometimes coexists with serious physical problems, the life expectancy of children with mental retardation may be shortened, depending on the specific condition. In general, the more severe the retardation and the more physical problems the child has, the shorter the life expectancy. However, a child with mild mental retardation has a relatively normal life expectancy.

Treatment

The child with mental retardation is best cared for by a multidisciplinary team consisting of the primary care doctor, social workers, speech and physical therapists, psychologists, educators, and others. Together with the family, these people develop a comprehensive, individualized program for the child, which is begun as soon as the diagnosis of mental retardation is suspected. The parents and siblings of the child also need emotional support, and the whole family should be an integral part of the program.

The full array of a child's strengths and weaknesses must be considered in determining what kind of support is needed. Factors such as physical disabilities, personality problems, mental illness, and interpersonal skills all help determine how much support is needed.

All children with mental retardation benefit from education. The Federal Individuals with Disabilities Education Act requires public schools to provide free and appropriate education to children and adolescents with mental retardation or other developmental disorders. Education must be provided in the least restrictive, most inclusive setting possible— where the children have every opportunity to interact with non-disabled peers as well as equal access to community resources.

A child with mental retardation usually does best living at home. However, some families cannot provide care at home, especially for children with severe, complex disabilities. This decision is difficult and requires extensive discussion between the family and their entire support team. Having a child with severe disabilities at home can be disruptive and requires dedicated care that many parents may not be able to provide. The family may need psychologic support. A social worker can organize services to assist the family. Help can be provided by day care centers, housekeepers, child caregivers, and respite care facilities. Most adults with mental retardation live in community-based residences that provide services appropriate to the person's needs, with work and recreational opportunities.

▲ see page 1453

CHAPTER 286

Mental Health Disorders

Several important mental health disorders, such as depression, often develop in childhood. Some disorders, such as autism, develop only in childhood.

With a few exceptions, the symptoms of mental health disorders tend to be similar to feelings that every child experiences, such as sadness, anger, suspicion, excitement, withdrawal, and loneliness. The difference between a disorder and a normal feeling is the extent to which the feeling becomes so powerful as to overwhelm and interfere with the activities of normal life and cause the child to suffer. Because of this, doctors must use a significant degree of judgment to determine when particular thoughts and emotions stop being a normal component of childhood experience and become a disorder.

In children, some disorders affect both mental health and the child's overall development. These are called the pervasive developmental disorders, which include autism, Asperger's disorder, pervasive developmental disorder not otherwise specified (PDD-NOS), Rett's disorder, and childhood disintegrative disorder. The pervasive developmental disorders comprise a group of related conditions that all involve some combination of impaired social relationships, stereotyped or ritualistic behavior, abnormal language development and use, and in some cases, intellectual impairment.

Autism

Autism is a disorder in which a young child cannot develop normal social relationships, uses language abnormally or not at all, behaves in compulsive and ritualistic ways, and may fail to develop normal intelligence.

Autism, the most common of the pervasive developmental disorders,▲ occurs in 5 of 10,000 children. Symptoms of autism may appear in the first 2 years of life and always before age 3. The disorder is 2 to 4 times more common in boys than in girls. Autism is different from mental retardation, although many children with autism have both.

The specific cause of autism is not fully understood, although it is clearly a biologically determined disorder. Several chromosomal abnormalities, such as fragile X syndrome, contribute to the development of autism. Prenatal infections, for example, viral infections such as rubella or cytomegalovirus, may also play a role. It is clear, however, that autism is *not* caused by poor parenting, adverse childhood conditions, or vaccination.

Symptoms

Autistic children develop symptoms in at least 3 of the following areas: social relationships, language, behavior, and sometimes intelligence. Symptoms range from mild to severe and often keep children from functioning independently in school or society. In addition, about 20 to 40% of autistic children, particularly those with an intelligence quotient (IQ) less than 50, develop seizures before reaching adolescence.

Social Relationships: An autistic infant does not cuddle and avoids eye contact. Although some autistic infants become upset when separated from their parents, they may not turn to parents for security as do other children. Older autistic children often prefer to play by themselves and do not form close personal relationships, particularly outside of the family. When interacting with other children, they do not use eye contact and facial expressions to establish social contact, and they are not able to interpret the moods and expressions of others.

Language: About 50% of autistic children never learn to speak. Those who learn do so much later than normal and use words in an unusual way. They often repeat words spoken to them (echolalia) or reverse the normal use of pronouns, particularly using *you* instead of *I* or *me* when referring to themselves. These children rarely have an interactive dialogue with others. Autistic children often speak with an unusual rhythm and pitch.

Behavior: Autistic children are very resistant to changes, such as new food, toys, furniture arrangement, and clothing. They often become excessively attached to particular inanimate objects. They often repeat certain

---

▲ see also page 1631

acts, such as rocking, hand flapping, or spinning objects in a repetitive manner. Some may injure themselves through repetitive behaviors such as head banging or biting themselves.

Intelligence: About 70% of children with autism have some degree of mental retardation (an IQ less than 70). Their performance is uneven; they usually do better on tests of motor and spatial skills than on verbal tests. Some autistic children have idiosyncratic or "splinter" skills, such as the ability to perform complex mental arithmetic or advanced musical skills. Unfortunately, such children are often not able to use these skills in a productive or socially interactive way.

Diagnosis

The diagnosis is made by close observation of the child in a playroom setting and careful questioning of parents and teachers. Standardized tests, such as the Childhood Autism Rating Scale, may help the evaluation. In addition to giving standardized tests, a doctor should perform certain tests to look for underlying treatable or inherited medical disorders (such as hereditary disorders of metabolism▲ and fragile X syndrome■).

Prognosis and Treatment

The symptoms of autism generally persist throughout life. The prognosis is strongly influenced by how much usable language the child has acquired by age 7. Autistic children with below-normal intelligence—for example, those who score below 50 on standard IQ tests—are likely to need full-time institutional care as adults.

Autistic children may benefit from certain intensive behavioral modification techniques. Children whose IQs are normal may be helped by psychotherapy aimed at correcting social difficulties. Special education is crucial and often includes speech, occupational, physical, and behavioral therapy within a program equipped to manage children with autism.

Drug therapy cannot change the underlying disorder. However, the selective serotonin reuptake inhibitors (SSRIs), such as fluoxetine, paroxetine, and fluvoxamine, are often effective in reducing ritualistic behaviors of autistic children. Antipsychotic drugs, such as risperidone, may be used to reduce self-injurious behavior, although the risk of side effects (such as movement disorders) must be considered.

Although some parents try special diets, gastrointestinal therapies, or immunologic therapies, currently there is no good evidence that any of these therapies helps children with autism.

Asperger's Disorder and Pervasive Developmental Disorder Not Otherwise Specified

These pervasive developmental disorders are closely related to autism but are less severe.

Children with Asperger's disorder have impaired social interactions similar to those of children with autism, as well as stereotyped or repetitive behaviors and mannerisms and nonfunctional rituals. However, language skills are normal and sometimes superior to those of an average child, and IQ is normal.

Children who have significantly impaired social interactions or stereotyped behaviors without all of the features of autism or Asperger's disorder are considered to have pervasive developmental disorder not otherwise specified (abbreviated as PDD-NOS). Children with Asperger's disorder or PDD-NOS tend to function at a higher level than children with autism and may be able to function independently. Children with Asperger's disorder often respond well to psychotherapy.

Rett's Disorder

Rett's disorder is a rare genetic disorder occurring in girls that causes impaired social interactions, loss of language skills, and repetitive hand movements.

A girl with Rett's disorder appears to develop normally until some time between the age of 5 months and 4 years. When the disorder begins, the growth of her head slows and her language and social skills deteriorate. Typically, she displays repetitive hand motions resembling washing or wringing. Purposeful hand movements are lost, walking is impaired, and trunk movements are clumsy. Mental retardation develops and is usually severe.

Slight spontaneous improvements in social interaction may occur in late childhood and early adolescence, but the language and behavior problems progress. Most girls with Rett's

▲ see page 1616   ■ see page 1528

disorder need full-time care and specialized educational programs. There is no cure.

Childhood Disintegrative Disorder

In childhood disintegrative disorder, an apparently normal child begins to act younger (regress) after age 3.

In most children, physical and mental development occur in spurts. It is common for children to take a step backward; for example, a toilet-trained child occasionally wets himself. Childhood disintegrative disorder, however, is a rare serious disorder in which a child older than age 3 stops developing normally and regresses to a much lower level of functioning, typically following a serious illness, such as an infection of the brain and nervous system.

The typical child with childhood disintegrative disorder develops normally until age 3 or 4, learning speech, becoming toilet trained, and displaying appropriate social behavior. Then, after a period of a few weeks or months during which time the child is irritable and moody, the child undergoes obvious regression. He may lose previously acquired language, motor, or social skills, and he may no longer have control over his bladder or bowels. In addition, the child develops difficulties in social interaction and begins performing repetitive behaviors similar to those that occur in children with autism. Quite often the child gradually deteriorates to a severely retarded level. A doctor makes the diagnosis based on the symptoms and searches for an underlying disorder.

Childhood disintegrative disorder cannot be specifically treated or cured, and most children, particularly those who are severely retarded, need lifelong care.

Childhood Schizophrenia

Childhood schizophrenia is a chronic disorder involving abnormal thought and social behavior.

Schizophrenia is quite rare in childhood; it typically develops in late adolescence and early adulthood.▲ When schizophrenia does develop in childhood, it usually begins between the age of 7 and the start of adolescence.

Schizophrenia probably occurs because of chemical abnormalities in the brain. Doctors do not know what causes these abnormalities, although it is clear that there is an inherited vulnerability and that it is not caused by poor parenting or adverse childhood conditions.

Symptoms and Diagnosis

A child with schizophrenia typically becomes withdrawn, loses interest in activities, and develops distorted thinking and perception. These symptoms may continue for some time before progressing. As with adults, children with schizophrenia are likely to develop hallucinations, delusions, and paranoia, often fearing that others are planning to harm them or are controlling their thoughts. Children with schizophrenia typically have blunted emotions—neither their voice nor facial expressions change in response to emotional situations. Events that would normally make people laugh or cry may produce no response. In adolescents, use of illicit drugs may mimic symptoms of schizophrenia.

There is no specific diagnostic test for schizophrenia. A doctor bases the diagnosis on a thorough assessment of the symptoms over time, psychologic tests, and lack of evidence of an underlying medical condition, such as drug abuse, a brain tumor, and other disorders.

Treatment

Childhood schizophrenia cannot be cured, although hallucinations and delusions may be controlled with antipsychotic drugs, such as haloperidol, olanzapine, quetiapine, and risperidone.■ Children are particularly susceptible to the side effects of antipsychotic drugs, such as tremors, slowed movements, and movement disorders. Psychologic and educational support for the child and counseling for family members are essential to help everyone cope with the illness and its consequences.

Children with schizophrenia may need to be hospitalized at times when the symptoms worsen, so that drug doses can be adjusted and their safety can be assured.

Depression

Depression is a feeling of intense sadness; it may follow a recent loss or other sad event but is out of proportion to that event and persists beyond an appropriate length of time.★

▲ see page 640   ■ see table on page 645
★ see also page 614

Sadness and unhappiness are common human emotions, particularly in response to troubling situations. For children, such situations may include the death of a parent, divorce, a friend moving away, difficulty in adjusting to school, and difficulty making friends. Sometimes, however, feelings of sadness are out of proportion to the event or persist far longer than might be expected. In this case, particularly when the negative feelings cause difficulties in day-to-day functioning, the child may have depression. Like adults, some children become depressed even without unhappy life events. This is more common if there is a family history of mood disorders.

Depression occurs in 1 to 2% of children and as many as 8% of adolescents. Doctors do not know exactly what causes depression, but chemical abnormalities in the brain are probably involved. Some tendency to depression is inherited. A combination of factors, both life experience and genetic vulnerability, appear to contribute. Sometimes, a medical disorder, such as an underactive thyroid, is the cause.

Symptoms and Diagnosis

The symptoms of depression in children relate to feelings of overwhelming sadness, worthlessness, and guilt. The child loses interest in activities that normally give him pleasure, such as playing sports, watching television, playing video games, or playing with friends. Appetite may be increased or decreased, often leading to significant weight changes. Sleep is usually disturbed, with either insomnia or excessive sleeping. Depressed children often are not energetic or physically active. However, particularly in younger children, depression is sometimes masked by seemingly contradictory symptoms, such as overactivity and aggressive, antisocial behavior. Symptoms typically interfere with the child's ability to think and concentrate, and schoolwork usually suffers. Suicidal thoughts, fantasies, and attempts are common. The doctor must always assess the risk of suicide in depressed children.

To diagnose depression, a doctor relies on several sources of information, including an interview with the child or adolescent and information from parents and teachers. Sometimes, structured questionnaires▲ help distinguish depression from a normal reaction to an unfortunate situation. A doctor tries to find out whether family or social stresses may

Symptoms of Depression in Children

- Sad mood
- Apathy
- Withdrawal from friends and social situations
- Reduced capacity for pleasure
- Feeling rejected and unloved
- Sleep disturbance, nightmares
- Self-blame
- Poor appetite, weight loss
- Thoughts of suicide
- Giving away valued possessions
- New physical complaints
- Falling grades

have precipitated the depression and also determines whether a physical disorder, such as an underactive thyroid, is the cause.

Treatment

As with adults, there is a wide range of severity of depression, and the intensity of treatment depends on the severity of the symptoms.

Antidepressant drugs correct chemical imbalances in the brain. Serotonin reuptake inhibitors (SSRIs), such as fluoxetine, sertraline, and paroxetine,■ are the drugs most commonly prescribed to depressed children and adolescents. The tricyclic antidepressants, such as imipramine, are much less effective in children than adults and have more side effects, and so are rarely used in children.

Treatment of depression requires more than drug therapy. Individual psychotherapy, group therapy, and family therapy may all be beneficial. Suicidal children must be hospitalized, usually briefly until they are no longer at risk to themselves.

Manic-Depressive Illness

Manic-depressive illness is a disorder in which periods of intense elation and excitation alternate with periods of depression and despair.

Children normally have fairly rapid mood swings, going from happy and active to glum and withdrawn. These swings rarely indicate

▲ see page 616   ▲ see table on page 618

mental illness of any kind. Manic-depressive illness (also called bipolar disorder) is far more severe than these normal mood changes and is rare in children, but more common than previously thought. More typically, it begins in adolescence or early adulthood.▲

The cause is unknown, but a tendency to the disorder can be inherited. Rarely, drugs with stimulant effects, such as amphetamines, which are sometimes used for attention deficit/hyperactivity disorder (ADHD),■ produce symptoms in children similar to manic-depressive illness.

Symptoms

Many children with manic-depressive illness exhibit a mixture of mania—a state of elation, excitation, racing thoughts, irritability, and grandiosity (in which the child feels he has some great talent or has made an important discovery)—and depression. The mania and depression occur simultaneously or in rapid alteration. During manic episodes, sleep is disturbed, the child may become aggressive, and school performance often deteriorates. Children with manic-depressive illness appear normal between episodes, in contrast to children with hyperactivity, who have a constant state of increased activity. Because ADHD can produce some similar symptoms, differentiating between the two conditions is important.

Treatment

Manic-depressive illness is treated with mood-stabilizing drugs, such as lithium, carbamazepine, and valproate. Individual and family psychotherapy help children and their families cope with the consequences of the disorder.

Suicidal Behavior

Suicidal behavior, an action intended to harm oneself, encompasses both suicide attempts and completed suicide.

Suicide is rare in children before puberty and is mainly a problem of adolescence, particularly between the ages of 15 and 19, and of adulthood.★ However, child suicide does occur and must not be overlooked in preadolescents. After accidents, suicide is the leading cause of death in adolescents, resulting in 2,000 deaths per year in the United States. It is also likely that a number of the deaths attributed to accidents, such as from motor vehicles and firearms, are actually suicides.

Many more young people attempt suicide than actually succeed. A survey performed by the Centers for Disease Control and Prevention found that 28% of high school students had suicidal thoughts and 8.3% had attempted suicide.

Among adolescents in the United States, boys outnumber girls in completed suicide by more than four to one. Girls, however, are 2 to 3 times more likely to attempt suicide than boys.

Risk Factors

Multiple factors typically interact before suicidal thoughts become suicidal behavior. Very often, there is an underlying mental health problem and a triggering stressful event. Examples of stressful events include the death of a loved one, loss of a boyfriend or girlfriend, a move from familiar surroundings (school, neighborhood, friends), humiliation by family or friends, failure at school, and trouble with the law. Stressful events such as these are fairly common among children, however, and rarely lead to suicidal behavior if there are no other underlying problems. The two most common underlying problems are depression and alcohol or drug abuse. Adolescents with depression have feelings of hopelessness and helplessness that limit their ability to consider alternative solutions to immediate problems. The use of alcohol or drugs lowers inhibitions against dangerous actions and interferes with anticipation of consequences. Finally, poor impulse control is a common factor in suicidal behavior. Adolescents attempting suicide are commonly angry with family members or friends, are unable to tolerate the anger, and turn the anger against themselves.

Sometimes suicidal behavior results when a child imitates the actions of others. For instance, a well-publicized suicide, such as that of a celebrity, is often followed by other suicides or suicide attempts. Suicides may cluster in families with a genetic vulnerability to mood disorders.

Prevention, Diagnosis, and Treatment

Parents, doctors, teachers, and friends may be in a position to identify children who might attempt suicide, particularly those who have

▲ see page 620   ■ see page 1549

★ see page 622

had any recent change in behavior. Children and adolescents often confide only in their peers, who must be encouraged not to keep a secret that could result in the tragic death of the suicidal child. Children who express overt thoughts of suicide such as "I wish I'd never been born" or "I'd like to go to sleep and never wake up" are at risk, but so are children with more subtle signs, such as social withdrawal, falling grades, or parting with favorite possessions. Health care professionals have two key roles: evaluating a suicidal child's safety and need for hospitalization, and treating underlying conditions, such as depression or substance abuse.

Directly asking an at-risk child about suicidal thoughts and plans reduces, rather than increases, the risk that the child will attempt suicide because identifying suicidal thinking can lead to interventions. Crisis hot lines, offering 24-hour assistance,▲ are available in many communities, and provide ready access to a sympathetic person who can give immediate counseling and assistance in obtaining further care. Although it is difficult to prove that these services actually reduce the number of deaths from suicide, they are helpful in directing children and families to appropriate resources.

Children who attempt suicide need urgent evaluation in a hospital emergency department. Any type of suicide attempt must be taken seriously, because one third of those who completed suicide had a previous suicidal attempt—sometimes apparently trivial, such as making a few shallow scratches to the wrist or swallowing a few pills. When parents or caretakers belittle or minimize an unsuccessful suicide attempt, children may see this as a challenge, and the risk of subsequent suicide increases.

Once the immediate threat to life has been removed, the doctor decides whether the child should be hospitalized. The decision depends on the degree of risk in remaining at home and the family's capacity to provide support and physical safety for the child. The seriousness of a suicide attempt can be gauged by a number of factors, including whether the attempt was carefully planned rather than spontaneous, whether steps were taken to prevent discovery, the type of method used, and whether any injury was actually inflicted. It is critical to distinguish intent from actual consequences; for example, an adolescent who ingests harmless pills he or she believes to be

Risk Factors for Child and Adolescent Suicide

- Preoccupation with morbid themes
- Poor hygiene and self-care (if an abrupt change)
- Access to firearms and prescription drugs
- Alcohol or drug abuse
- Family history of suicide
- Dramatic changes in mood, peer contact, grades
- Depressed mood, appetite or sleep disturbance
- Previous attempt at suicide

lethal should be considered at extreme risk. If hospitalization is not needed, families of children going home must ensure that firearms are removed from the home altogether and that drugs and sharp objects are removed or securely locked.

Conduct Disorder

A conduct disorder is characterized by a repetitive pattern of behavior in which the basic rights of others are violated.

Although some children are better behaved than others, children who repeatedly and persistently violate rules and the rights of others in ways inappropriate for their age have a conduct disorder. The problem usually begins in late childhood or early adolescence and is more common among boys than girls. Evaluation of conduct must take the child's social environment into account. Misconduct developed by children as an adaptation to life in war-torn areas, settings of civil unrest, or other highly stressed environments is not a conduct disorder.

In general, children with a conduct disorder are selfish, do not relate well to others, and lack an appropriate sense of guilt. They tend to misperceive the behavior of others as threatening and react aggressively. They may engage in bullying, threatening, and frequent fights and may be cruel to animals. Other children with conduct disorder damage property, especially by setting fires. They may be deceit-

▲ see box on page 623

Effects of Stress on Children

A stressful change in a child's life, such as a geographic move, divorce of the parents, or the death of a family member or pet, can trigger an **adjustment disorder**. Adjustment disorder is an acute but time-limited response to environmental stress. The child may have symptoms of anxiety (for example, nervousness, worries, and fears), symptoms of depression (for example, tearfulness or feelings of hopelessness), or behavioral problems. The symptoms and problems abate as the stress diminishes.

Posttraumatic stress disorder is a much more extreme response and may occur after a natural disaster (such as a hurricane, tornado, or earthquake), an accident, death, or a senseless act of violence,▲ including child abuse. The child usually fails in his attempts to avoid remembering the event, suffers a persistent state of anxiety, and may reexperience the traumatic event while awake (flashback) or asleep (nightmares). Crisis intervention is usually necessary, in the form of an extended period of individual, group, or family therapy. Treatment with anxiety-reducing drugs may be needed.

ful or engage in theft. Seriously violating rules is common and includes running away from home and frequent truancy from school. Girls with conduct disorder are less likely than boys to be physically aggressive; they typically run away, lie, abuse substances, and sometimes engage in prostitution.

About half of the children with conduct disorder stop such behaviors by adulthood. The younger the child is when the conduct disorder began, the more likely the behavior is to continue. Adults in whom such behaviors persist often encounter legal trouble, chronically violate the rights of others, and are often diagnosed with antisocial personality disorder.■

Treatment

Treatment is very difficult because children with conduct disorder rarely perceive anything wrong with their behavior. Often the most successful treatment is to separate the

child from a troubled environment and to provide a strictly structured setting, in either a mental health or a juvenile justice setting.

Oppositional Defiant Disorder

Oppositional defiant disorder is a recurring pattern of negative, defiant, and disobedient behavior.

Children with oppositional defiant disorder are stubborn, difficult, and disobedient without being physically aggressive or actually violating the rights of others. Many preschool and early adolescent children occasionally display oppositional behaviors, but oppositional defiant disorder is diagnosed only if behaviors persist for 6 months or more and are serious enough to interfere with social or academic functioning. Most often, children develop this disorder by age 8.

Typical behaviors of children with oppositional defiant disorder include arguing with adults; losing their temper; actively defying rules and instructions; blaming others for their own mistakes; and being angry, resentful, and easily annoyed. These children do know the difference between right and wrong and feel guilty if they do anything that is seriously wrong.

Oppositional defiant disorder is best treated through behavior management techniques, which include a consistent approach to discipline and appropriate reinforcement of desired behavior. Parents and teachers can be instructed in these techniques by the child's counselor or therapist.

Separation Anxiety Disorder

Separation anxiety disorder is characterized by excessive anxiety about being away from home or separated from people to whom the child is attached.

Some degree of separation anxiety is normal and occurs in almost all children, especially in very young children.★ In contrast, separation anxiety disorder is excessive anxiety that goes beyond that expected for the child's developmental level. Separation anxiety is considered a disorder if it lasts at least a month and causes significant distress or impairment in functioning. The duration of the disorder reflects its severity.

Some life stress, such as the death of a relative, friend, or pet or a geographic move or change in schools, may trigger the disorder.

▲ see also page 612   ■ see page 632
★ see page 1534

Genetic vulnerability to anxiety also typically plays a key role.

Symptoms

Children with this disorder experience great distress when separated from home or from people to whom they are attached. They often need to know the whereabouts of these people and are preoccupied with fears that something terrible will happen either to them or to their loved ones. Traveling by themselves makes them uncomfortable, and they may refuse to attend school or camp or to visit or sleep at friends' homes. Some children are unable to stay alone in a room, clinging to a parent or "shadowing" the parent around the house.

Difficulty at bedtime is common. Children with separation anxiety disorder may insist that someone stay in the room until they fall asleep. Nightmares may disclose the children's fears, such as destruction of the family through fire or another catastrophe.

Treatment

Because a child who has this disorder often avoids school, an immediate goal of treatment is enabling the child to return to school. Doctors, parents, and school personnel must work as a team to ensure the child's prompt return to school. Individual and family psychotherapy and anxiety-reducing drugs may play an important role.

Somatoform Disorders

Somatoform disorders are a group of disorders in which an underlying psychologic problem causes distressing or disabling physical symptoms.

A child with a somatoform disorder may have a number of symptoms, including pain, difficulty breathing, and weakness, without evidence of a physical cause. Often, a child develops psychologically based physical symptoms when another family member is seriously ill. These physical symptoms are thought to develop unconsciously in response to a psychologic stress or problem.▲ It is clear that the symptoms are not consciously fabricated, and the child is actually experiencing the symptoms he describes.

Somatoform disorders are further classified as conversion disorder, somatization disorder,

body dysmorphic disorder, and hypochondriasis.■ In **conversion disorder,** the child may seem to have a paralyzed arm or leg, become deaf or blind, or have shaking activity resembling seizures. These symptoms begin suddenly, usually in relation to a precipitating event, and may or may not resolve abruptly. A **somatization disorder** is similar to conversion disorder, but the child develops numerous symptoms that are more vague, such as headaches, abdominal pain,★ and nausea. These symptoms may come and go for long periods of time. In **body dysmorphic disorder,** the child becomes preoccupied with an imagined defect in appearance, such as the size of his nose or ears, or develops a markedly excessive concern with a minor abnormality, such as a wart. In **hypochondriasis,** the child has no specific, ongoing symptoms but is obsessed with bodily functions, such as heartbeat, digestion, and sweating, and is convinced that he has a serious disease when nothing is actually wrong.

Somatoform disorders are equally common among young boys and young girls, but they are more common among adolescent girls than adolescent boys.

Diagnosis

Before establishing the diagnosis of a somatoform disorder, the doctor makes sure that the child does not have a physical illness that could account for the symptoms. However, extensive laboratory tests are generally avoided because they may further convince the child that a physical problem exists and unnecessary diagnostic tests may themselves traumatize the child. If no physical illness can be found, the doctor then talks to the child and family members to try to identify underlying psychologic problems or troubled family relationships.

Treatment

A child may balk at the idea of visiting a psychotherapist because to the child his symptoms are purely physical. However, an approach combining individual and family psychotherapy and physical rehabilitation has been shown to be effective in many cases.

▲ see box on page 604   ■ see also page 603
★ see also page 1591

CHAPTER 287

Social Issues Affecting Children and Their Families

In order to thrive, a child must experience the consistent and ongoing care of a loving, nurturing caregiver, whether it be a parent or someone else. The security and support that such an adult can provide give a child the self-confidence and resiliency to cope effectively with stress.

In order to mature emotionally and socially, children must interact with people outside the home. These interactions typically occur with close relatives; friends; neighbors; and people at childcare sites, schools, churches, and sports teams or other activities. By coping with the minor stresses and conflicts of these interactions, children gradually acquire the skills to handle more significant ones.

However, certain major events, such as illness and divorce, may challenge a child's abilities to cope. These events may also interfere with the child's emotional and social development. For example, a chronic illness may prevent a child from participating in activities and also impair performance in school.

Events affecting the child may also have adverse consequences for people close to the child. Everyone who cares for a sick child is under stress. The consequences of such stress vary with the nature and severity of the illness and with the family's emotional and other resources and supports.

Illness and Death in Infants

The medical needs of ill or premature newborns and infants often require that these children be separated from their parents temporarily. Although doctors may allow parents to hold their infant some of the time, medical care often sharply limits the opportunity for parents to interact with their infant. In addition, parents are usually emotionally distressed by their infant's condition. The separation and parental distress can interfere with bonding,▲ particularly in severely ill infants who are hospitalized for a long time. Parents need to see, hold, and interact with their infant as soon as it is practical. Even with severely ill infants, parents often can help to feed, bathe, and change their infant. Breast-feeding may be possible, even if the infant must be fed through a tube at first.

If an infant has a birth defect, parents may experience guilt, sadness, anger, or even horror. Many feel even more guilt because they have such feelings. Seeing and touching the child can help the parents look beyond the birth defect and see the infant as a whole person; this helps the bonding process begin. Information about the condition, possible treatments, and the infant's prognosis can help the parents adjust psychologically and plan for the best medical care.

Death of an infant is always traumatic for parents. However, if a newborn dies before being seen or touched by the parents, the parents may feel as though they never had a baby. Although painful, holding or seeing the dead baby can help parents begin to grieve and begin the process of closure. Emptiness, lost hopes and dreams, and fear may overwhelm parents, who may become depressed. Parents tend to feel guilty, blaming themselves even when they are not responsible for the death. The grief and guilt that follow may strain the relationship between parents.

Many families whose infants are severely ill or who have died can benefit from counseling from psychologic or religious personnel. Parent and family support groups also may help.

Illness in Children

Severe illness, even if temporary, can provoke a great deal of anxiety for children. Chronic illness or disability usually causes even more emotional distress.

Coping with illness may require coping with pain, undergoing tests, taking drugs, and changing diet and lifestyle. Chronic illness often interferes with a child's education because of frequent absences from school. The illness as well as side effects from treatments may impair the child's ability to learn. Parents and teachers may have lower academic expectations of ill children; however, it is important for them to maintain the challenges and encouragement children need to achieve their best.

▲ see page 1485

Talking With Children About Difficult Topics

Many life events, including illness or death of someone close, divorce, and bullying, are scary or unpleasant for children. Even events that do not directly affect the child, such as natural disasters, war, or terrorism, may cause anxiety. Fears about all of these, rational or irrational, can preoccupy a child.

Children often have difficulty talking about unpleasant topics. However, open discussion can help the child deal with difficult or embarrassing topics and dispel irrational fears. A child needs to know that anxiety is normal and will get better.

Parents should discuss difficult topics during a quiet time, in a private place, and when the child is interested. Parents should remain calm, present factual information, and give the child undivided attention. Acknowledging what was said with phrases such as, "I understand," or with a quiet nod encourages the child to confide; so does reflecting back what was said. For example, if a child mentions anger about a divorce, one could say, "So, the divorce makes you angry," or "Tell me more about that." Asking how the child feels can also encourage him to discuss sensitive emotions or fears—for example, fear of abandonment by the noncustodial parent during a divorce or guilt for causing the divorce.

By disclosing their own feelings, parents encourage children to acknowledge their fears and concerns. For example, about a divorce, a parent might say, "I am sad about the divorce, too. But, I also know it is the right thing for mommy and daddy to do. Even though we cannot live together anymore, we will both always love you and take care of you." By doing this, parents are able to discuss their own feelings, offer reassurance, and explain that divorce is the right choice for them. Sometimes children, particularly younger ones, need to hear the same message repeatedly.

Sometimes a parent must raise a difficult topic with a child, such as telling the child about a serious illness in a relative or friend. If tragedy affects someone else, children may feel more confident, and less helpless, if they can contribute—for example, by picking flowers; writing or drawing a card; wrapping a present; or collecting food, clothing, money, or toys. When a child appears withdrawn or sad, refuses to engage in usual activities, or becomes aggressive, the parent should seek professional help.

A parent may also have to address a difficult aspect of the child's own behavior. For example, a parent who suspects the child or adolescent of using drugs or alcohol should address the issue directly with the child. A parent might say "I am worried that you are using drugs. I feel this way because . . ." The parent should then calmly list the behaviors that concern him, limiting the list to three or four behaviors. If the child denies there is a problem, the parent should restate the concerns calmly and explain to the child that there is a plan of action in place (such as an appointment with a pediatrician or counselor).

Throughout any discussion, the parent should reassure the child that he is loved and will be supported.

Illness and hospitalization deprive children of opportunities to play with other children. Other children may even reject or taunt an ill child because of physical differences and limitations. A child can become self-conscious if illness changes his body, particularly when the change occurs during childhood or adolescence rather than being present from birth. Parents and family members may overprotect the child, discouraging independence.

Chronic illness places enormous psychologic and physical burdens on parents. Sometimes the parents become closer by working together to overcome these burdens. However, often the burdens can strain the relationship. Parents may feel guilty about the illness, particularly if it is genetic, resulted from complications during pregnancy, or was caused by an accident (such as a motor vehicle collision), or a behavior of a parent (such as smoking). In addition, medical care can be expensive and can cause the parents to miss work. Sometimes, one parent assumes the burden of the care, which can lead to feelings of resentment in the caregiving parent or feelings of isolation in the other. Parents may feel angry with health care providers, themselves, each other, or the child. The emotional distress involved in providing care can also make it difficult to form a deep attachment to a disabled or seriously ill child.

Parents who spend a lot of time with an ill child often have less time to devote to other children in the family. Siblings may resent the extra attention the ill child receives and then feel guilty for feeling that way. The ill child may feel guilty about hurting or burdening the family. Parents may be too lenient with the ill

The Changing Structures of Families

> Most people picture a traditional family as a married man and woman and their biological children. However, a family may consist of a gay couple, single parent, or even a group of unrelated adults who live and rear children together.
>
> During the last several decades, increasing numbers of families have deviated from the traditional model. Divorces force many children into single parent families or blended families created by remarriage. About one third of children are born to single mothers; about 10% of children are born to single teenage mothers. Many children are reared by grandparents or other relatives. About one million children live with adoptive parents.
>
> Even traditional families have changed. Often both parents work outside the home, requiring many children to receive regular care outside of the family setting. Because of school and career commitments, many couples postpone having children until their 30s and even 40s. Changing cultural expectations have resulted in fathers spending increasing amounts of time rearing children.
>
> Conflicts develop in every family, but healthy families are strong enough to resolve conflicts or thrive despite them. Whatever their makeup, healthy families provide children with a sense of belonging and meet children's physical, emotional, developmental, and spiritual needs. Members of healthy families express emotion and support for each other in ways consistent within their own culture and family traditions.

child, or they may enforce discipline inconsistently, particularly if the symptoms come and go.

Hospitalization is a frightening event for children even under the best circumstances, and it should be avoided whenever possible. If hospitalization is needed, it should be as brief as possible, preferably in a part of the hospital used exclusively for children. In many hospitals, parents are able to stay with their children, even during painful or fear-provoking procedures. Despite their parents' presence, children often become clingy or dependent (regress) while in the hospital.

Although a child's illness is always stressful for the entire family, there are several steps a parent can take to help lessen the impact. Parents should learn as much as possible about their child's illness from reliable sources, such as the child's doctors and reliable medical resources. Information obtained from some Internet sources is not always accurate, and parents should check with their doctors about the information they read. A support group or another family that has already faced similar issues can provide information and emotional support; doctors can often refer parents to such people.

Services needed by the child may involve care by medical specialists, nurses, home health personnel, mental health personnel, and personnel from a variety of other services. A case manager may be needed to help coordinate medical care for children with complex chronic illnesses. The child's doctor, nurse, social worker, or other professional can serve as the case manager. The case manager can also ensure that the child receives training in social skills and that the family and child receive appropriate counseling, education, and psychologic and social support, such as respite care.

Divorce

Separation and divorce interrupt the stability and predictability that children need. Other than the death of an immediate family member, divorce is the most stressful event that can affect a family. Because the world as they know it has ended, children may feel a great loss as well as anxiety, anger, and sadness. Children may fear being abandoned or losing their parents' love. For many reasons, parenting skills often worsen around the time of the divorce. Parents are usually preoccupied and may be angry and hostile toward each other. Regardless of whether they contributed to the divorce, children may feel guilty about causing it. If parents ignore children or visit sporadically and unpredictably, children feel rejected.

Once parents decide to separate and divorce, family members move through several stages of adjustment. In the acute stage (the period when parents decide to separate, including the time preceding the divorce), turmoil is often maximal. This stage may last up to 2 years. During the transitional stage (the weeks around the actual divorce), the child has more control over change and adjusts to the new relationship between the parents, visitation, and the new relationship with the noncustodial parent. After the divorce (the post-divorce stage), stability usually returns.

During the divorce, schoolwork may seem unimportant to children and adolescents, and school performance often worsens. Children may have fantasies that parents will reconcile. Children aged 2 to 5 years may have difficulty sleeping, temper tantrums, and separation anxiety. Toileting skills may deteriorate. Children aged 5 to 12 years can experience sadness, grief, intense anger, and irrational fears (phobias). Adolescents often feel insecure, lonely, and sad. Some engage in risk-taking behaviors such as drug and alcohol use, sex, theft, and violence. Others may develop eating disorders, become defiant, skip school, or join peers who are engaging in risk-taking behaviors.

Children need to be able to express their feelings to an adult who listens attentively. Counseling can provide children with a caring adult who, unlike their parents, will not be upset by their feelings.

Children adjust best when parents cooperate with each other and focus on the child's needs. Parents must remember that a divorce only severs their relationship as husband and wife, not their relationship as parents of their children. Whenever possible, parents should live close to each other, try not to anger each other, maintain the other's involvement in the child's life, and consider the child's wishes regarding visitation. Older children and adolescents should be given increasing say in living arrangements. Parents should never suggest that their children take sides and should try not to express negative feelings about the other parent to their children. Parents should discuss issues openly, honestly, and calmly with their children; remain affectionate with them; continue to discipline consistently; and maintain normal expectations regarding chores and schoolwork. Most children regain a sense of security and support within about a year after divorce if the parents adjust and work to meet the child's needs.

For a child, remarriage of either parent can restore a sense of stability and permanency but can also create new conflict. Some children feel disloyal to one parent by accepting the other parent's new spouse.

Childcare

About 80% of children receive childcare outside the home before they start school. Many children aged 5 to 12 also receive care outside the home before or after school. Sources of care include relatives, neighbors, licensed and unli-censed private homes, and childcare centers. Care can also be provided in the home by a relative or nanny. Childcare centers can be licensed, accredited, or both. Accreditation usually requires that the center meet higher standards than those required for licensing.

Care outside of the home varies in quality; while some is excellent, some is poor. Care outside of the home can also have benefits. Children whose parents—particularly single parents—are not able to spend much time interacting with them can benefit from the social and academic stimulation of quality childcare.

Early exposure to music, books, art, and language stimulates a child's intellectual and creative development. Group play stimulates social development. Outdoor and occasional vigorous play help dissipate pent-up physical energy and stimulate muscle development. Opportunities to initiate their own activities help children develop independence. Nutritious meals or snacks should be available every few hours. Television and videos contribute little to the child's development and are best avoided. If they are used, the content should be age-appropriate and supervised by an adult.

Foster Care

Foster care is care provided for children whose families are temporarily unable to care for them. The local government determines the process of arranging foster care. Foster care is surprisingly common in the United States; around 750,000 children are in the foster care system each year.

The foster parent assumes day-to-day care for the child. However, the birth parents usually remain the child's legal guardians. This means that the birth parents still make legal decisions for the child. For example, if the child needs an operation, only the birth parents can provide consent.

Most children in foster care are from poor families. About 70% of the children in foster care are put there by child protective services because the child has been abused or neglected. Most of the remaining 30% are adolescents placed in care by the juvenile justice system. Very few children are placed voluntarily by their parents. Most children in foster care live with foster families, although many adolescents live in group homes or residential treatment facilities.

Removal from their family is enormously painful to children. In foster care, children

What Is Bullying?

Bullying is repeated physical or psychologic attacks that are performed to dominate or humiliate. Although it typically involves only two people, bullying can involve groups. Bullying hurts and demeans the victim. In addition, the bully often unknowingly repels his friends and peers, hurting himself.

Although they sometimes tell family members or friends, victims are often too embarrassed and frightened to disclose bullying to an adult. Occasionally, a teacher informs a parent. Victims may refuse to go to school, appear sad or withdrawn, or become moody.

Victims need reassurance that bullying is always unacceptable. Parents can demonstrate ways a victim can respond to the bully—for example, telling an adult, walking away, changing their routines to avoid the bully, or engaging in counseling. Although it is usually not advisable (for safety reasons) to directly confront the bully, teaching the child to ignore and actually not be bothered by the bully will reduce the bully's satisfaction and eventually lessen the bullying. Praising the victim's courage for reporting bullying can begin to rebuild the child's self-esteem.

If bullying occurs at school, parents should inform school officials. The victim's parents should also inform the bully's parents but should avoid confrontation, which could be counterproductive by making the bully's parents defensive. Victims may fear that telling the bully's parents will worsen bullying, but it often stops bullying, particularly if the discussion is positive and not accusatory, but instead focuses on the harmful behavior.

The bully's parents should make it clear to their child that bullying is not acceptable. These parents should insist that the bully apologize and make amends to the victim. Doing so can help the bully learn right from wrong, can make the bully more sensitive to the victim, and can make others see the bully more sympathetically. Adults should watch the child closely to ensure that bullying stops. Counseling can sometimes help the child who is doing the bullying, who often is expressing his or her unmet needs or who is modeling the aggressive behavior of a parent or older sibling.

may have frequent visits with their families or only limited, supervised visits. Children in foster care leave behind their neighborhoods, communities, schools, and most of their belongings. Many children and adolescents in foster care feel anxious, uncertain, and helpless to control their lives. Many feel angry, rejected, and pained by the separation, or they develop a profound sense of loss. Some feel guilty, believing that they caused the disruption of their birth family. Peers often tease children about being in foster care, reinforcing perceptions that they are somehow different or unworthy. Children in foster care have more chronic illnesses and behavioral, emotional, and developmental problems than do other children. Yet, most children in foster care adjust well as long as the foster family nurtures the child's emotional needs. Most children in foster care benefit from counseling.

About half of the children eventually return to their birth families. About 20% of children in foster care are eventually adopted, most often by their foster family. Other children return to a relative or become too old for foster care. A small number of children are later transferred to another foster care agency.

Adoption

Adoption is the legal process of adding a person to an existing family. Adoption, unlike foster care, is meant to be permanent. The goal of adoption is to provide lifelong security to a child and the family.

Children who are orphaned are obvious candidates for adoption. In the United States, children can be adopted if the parents give up the child voluntarily, or if the child is freed involuntarily through the court process known as termination of parental rights. International adoption (adoption of children from other countries, for example, from foreign orphanages) is also often possible.

Depending on the type, adoption can sometimes cost tens of thousands of dollars. Having experienced legal representation, often from a lawyer, helps the adoptive parents regardless of the type of adoption.

Sometimes, adoptive parents connect with birth parents. The parties may already be related in some way. For example, a stepparent can adopt a spouse's birth child, or grandparents can adopt their grandchildren. In other cases, parents may connect through word of mouth or newspaper advertisements.

In some cases, birth parents may appreciate the chance to visit the child. Also, knowing the birth parents may make adoptive parents less likely to worry that the birth parents will try to reclaim the child. In addition, sometimes there are benefits for the child. All such issues are often best discussed with an expert (such as a mental health and a legal professional) before making decisions.

Most adopted children, including those previously in foster care or foreign orphanages, adjust well and develop few problems. However, as children age, they may develop feelings of rejection because they were given up by their birth family. During adolescence and young adulthood, in particular, an adopted person may be very curious about his birth parents, even if he does not ask about them. Some adopted people seek information about, or seek out, their birth parents, and some birth parents seek out their birth children.

Withholding the fact that children were adopted can hurt them later. Children adjust best if told by about age 7. If asked, adoptive parents should tell the child about the birth parents in a comforting manner. For example, if the child was abused or neglected, parents can say the child was removed because the birth parent had problems or was ill and could not provide proper care. Children need reassurance that they are loved and always will be loved. If children have contact with their birth families, it helps for parents to tell the child that two sets of parents love them.

If birth parents request anonymity, there is controversy about whether children should be able to find information about them. Some states provide a web site for birth parents and children to post their identity. If both do so, then they will be placed in touch with each other. Contact cannot be initiated unless both parties agree.

CHAPTER 288

Child Neglect and Abuse

Children can be mistreated by having essential things withheld from them (neglect) or by having harmful things done to them (abuse). Neglect involves not meeting children's basic needs: physical, medical, educational, and emotional. Emotional neglect is a part of emotional abuse. Abuse can be physical, sexual, or emotional. The different forms of abuse sometimes occur together. Child neglect and abuse often occur together and with other forms of family violence, such as spousal abuse. In addition to immediate harm, neglect and abuse cause long-lasting problems, including mental health problems and substance abuse. Also, adults who were physically or sexually abused as children are more likely to abuse their own children.

In the United States, more than 800,000 children are neglected or abused every year, and about 1,100 of them die. Neglect is about 3 times more common than physical abuse.

Neglect and abuse result from a complex combination of individual, family, and social factors. Being a single parent, being poor, having problems with drug or alcohol abuse, or having a mental health problem (such as a per-

sonality disorder or low self-esteem) can make a parent more likely to neglect or abuse a child. Neglect is 12 times more common among children living in poverty.

Doctors and nurses are required by law to promptly report cases of suspected child neglect or abuse to a local Child Protective Services agency. Depending on the circumstances, the local law enforcement agency may also be notified. Prompt reporting is also required from all people whose job places children younger than 18 in their care. Such people include teachers, childcare workers, and police and legal services personnel. Anyone else who knows of or suspects neglect or abuse is encouraged to report it but is not required to do so.

All reported cases of child abuse are investigated by representatives of the local Child Protective Services agency, who determine the facts and make recommendations. Agency representatives may recommend social services (for the child and family members), temporary hospitalization, temporary foster care, or permanent termination of parental rights. Doctors and social workers help the representatives from the Child Protective Services agency decide what to do based on the immediate medical needs of the child, the seriousness of the harm, and the likelihood of further neglect or abuse.

Types

There are a number of different types of child neglect and abuse.

Physical Neglect: Not meeting a child's essential needs for food, clothing, and shelter is the most basic form of neglect. But there are many other forms. Parents may not obtain preventive dental or medical care for the child, such as vaccinations and routine physical examinations. Parents may delay obtaining medical care when the child is ill, putting the child at risk of more severe illness and even death. Parents may not make sure the child attends school or is privately schooled. Parents may leave a child in the care of a person who is known to be abusive, or may leave a young child unattended.

Physical Abuse: Physically mistreating or harming a child, including inflicting excessive physical punishment, is physical abuse. Children of any age may be physically abused, but infants and toddlers are particularly vulnerable. Physical abuse is the most common cause of serious head injury in infants. In toddlers, physical abuse is more likely to result in abdominal injuries, which may be fatal. Physical abuse (including homicide) is among the 10 leading causes of death in children. Generally, a child's risk of physical abuse decreases during the early school years and increases during adolescence.

Most perpetrators of physical abuse are males known by the children. Children who are born in poverty to a young, single parent are at highest risk. Family stress contributes to physical abuse. Stress may result from unemployment, frequent moves to another home, social isolation from friends or family members, or ongoing family violence. Children who are difficult (irritable, demanding, hyperactive, or handicapped) may be more likely to be physically abused. Physical abuse is often triggered by a crisis in the midst of other stresses. A crisis may be a loss of a job, a death in the family, a discipline problem, or even a toileting accident.

Sexual Abuse: Any action with a child that is for the sexual gratification of an adult or a significantly older child is considered sexual abuse. It includes penetrating the child's vagina, anus, or mouth, touching the child with sexual intention but without penetration, exposing the genitals or showing pornography to a child, and using a child in the production of pornography. Sexual abuse does not include sexual play. In sexual play, children who are less than 4 years apart in age view or touch each other's genital area without force or coercion.

By the age of 18, about 12 to 25% of girls and 8 to 10% of boys have been sexually abused. Most perpetrators of sexual abuse are people known by the children, commonly a stepfather, an uncle, or the mother's boyfriend. Female perpetrators are less common.

Certain situations increase the risk of sexual abuse. For example, children who have several caregivers or a caregiver with several sex partners are at increased risk. Being socially isolated, having low self-esteem, having family members who are also sexually abused, or being associated with a gang also increases risk.

Emotional Abuse: Using words or acts to psychologically mistreat a child is emotional abuse. Emotional abuse makes children feel that they are worthless, flawed, unloved, unwanted, in danger, or valuable only when they meet another person's needs.

Emotional abuse includes spurning, exploiting, terrorizing, isolating, and neglecting. Spurning means belittling the child's abilities and accomplishments. Exploiting means encouraging deviant or criminal behavior, such as committing crimes or abusing alcohol or drugs. Terrorizing means bullying, threatening, or frightening the child. Isolating means not allowing the child to interact with other adults or children. Emotionally neglecting a child means ignoring and not interacting with the child; the child is not given love and attention. Emotional abuse tends to occur over a long period of time.

Münchausen by Proxy: In this unusual type of child abuse, a caregiver, usually the mother, exaggerates, fakes, or causes an illness in the child.▲

Symptoms

The symptoms of neglect and abuse vary depending partly on the nature and duration of the neglect or abuse, on the child, and on the particular circumstances. In addition to obvious physical injuries, symptoms include emotional and mental health problems. Such prob-

---

▲ see box on page 602

lems may develop immediately or later and may persist.

Physical Neglect: Physically neglected children may appear undernourished, tired, or dirty or may lack appropriate clothing. They may frequently be absent from school. In extreme cases, children may be found living alone or with siblings, without adult supervision. Physical and emotional development may be slow. Some neglected children die of starvation or exposure.

Physical Abuse: Bruises, burns, welts, or scrapes are common. These marks often have the shape of the object used to inflict them, such as a belt or lamp cord. Cigarette or scald burns may be visible on the arms or legs. Severe injuries to the mouth, eyes, brain, or other internal organs may be present but not visible. Children may have signs of old injuries, such as broken bones, that have healed. Sometimes injuries result in disfigurement.

Toddlers who have been intentionally dunked into a hot bathtub have scald burns. These burns may be located on the buttocks and may be shaped like a doughnut. The splash of hot water may cause small burns on other parts of the body.

Infants who are shaken may have shaken baby (shaken impact) syndrome. This syndrome is caused by violent shaking, often followed by throwing the infant. Infants who are shaken may have no visible signs of injury and may appear to be sleeping deeply. This sleepiness is due to brain damage and swelling, which may result from bleeding between the brain and skull (subdural hemorrhage). Infants may also have bleeding in the retina (retinal hemorrhage) at the back of the eye. Ribs and other bones may be broken.

Children who have been abused for a long time are often fearful and irritable. They often sleep poorly. They may be depressed and anxious. They are more likely to act in violent, criminal, or suicidal ways.

Sexual Abuse: Changes in behavior are common. Such changes may occur abruptly and be extreme. Children may become aggressive or withdrawn or develop phobias or sleep disorders. Children who are sexually abused may behave in sexual ways inappropriate for their age. Children who are sexually abused by a parent or other family member may have conflicted feelings. They may feel emotionally close to the offender, yet betrayed.

Sexual abuse may also result in physical injuries. Children may have bruises, tears, or bleeding in areas around the genitals, rectum, or mouth. Injuries in the genital and rectal areas may make walking and sitting difficult. Girls may have a vaginal discharge. A sexually transmitted disease, such as gonorrhea, chlamydial infection, or sometimes human immunodeficiency virus (HIV) infection, may be present.

Emotional Abuse: In general, children who are emotionally abused tend to be insecure and anxious about their attachments to other people because they have not had their needs met consistently or predictably. Infants who are emotionally neglected may seem unemotional or uninterested in their surroundings. Their behavior may be mistaken for mental retardation or a physical disorder. Children who are emotionally neglected may lack social skills or be slow to develop speech and language skills. Children who are spurned may have low self-esteem. Children who are exploited may commit crimes or abuse alcohol or drugs. Children who are terrorized may appear fearful and withdrawn. They may be distrustful, unassertive, and extremely anxious to please adults. Children who are isolated may be awkward in social situations and have difficulty forming normal relationships. Older children may not attend school regularly or may not perform well when they do attend.

Diagnosis

Neglect and abuse are often difficult to recognize unless children appear severely undernourished or are obviously injured or unless neglect or abuse is witnessed by other people. Neglect and abuse may not be recognized for years. There are many reasons for this difficulty. Abused children may feel that abuse is a normal part of life and may not mention it. Physically and sexually abused children are often reluctant to volunteer information about their abuse because of shame, threats of retaliation, or even a feeling that they deserved the abuse. Physically abused children often describe what happened to them if asked directly, but sexually abused children may be sworn to secrecy or so traumatized that they do not.

When doctors suspect neglect or any type of abuse, they look for signs of other types of abuse. They also fully evaluate the physical, environmental, emotional, and social needs of the child.

Physical Neglect: A neglected child is usually identified by health care practitioners or social workers during evaluation of an unrelated issue, such as an injury, an illness, or a behavioral problem. Doctors may notice that a child is not developing physically or emotionally at a normal rate or has missed many vaccinations or appointments. Teachers may identify a neglected child because of frequent unexplained absences from school. If neglect is suspected, doctors often check for anemia, infections, and lead poisoning, which are common among neglected children.

Physical Abuse: Physical abuse may be suspected when an infant who is not yet walking has bruises or serious injuries. Abuse may be suspected when a toddler or older child has certain types of bruises, such as bruises on the back of the legs, buttocks, and torso. When children are learning to walk, bruises often result, but such bruises typically occur on prominent bony areas on the front of the body, such as the knees, shins, forehead, chin, and elbows.

Abuse may also be suspected when parents appear to know little about their child's health or to be unconcerned about an obvious injury. Parents who abuse their child may be reluctant to describe to the doctor or friends how an injury occurred. The description may not fit the age and nature of the injury or may change each time the story is told.

If doctors suspect physical abuse, they obtain accurate drawings and photographs of the injuries. Sometimes x-rays are taken to look for signs of previous injuries. If a child is younger than 2 years, x-rays of all bones are often taken to check for fractures.

Sexual Abuse: Often, sexual abuse is diagnosed on the basis of the child's or a witness's account of the incident. However, because many children are reluctant to talk about sexual abuse, it may be suspected only because the child's behavior becomes abnormal. If a child has been sexually abused within 72 hours, doctors examine the child to collect legal evidence of sexual contact, such as swabs of body fluids and hair samples from the genital area. Photographs of any visible injuries are taken. In some communities, health care practitioners who are specially trained to evaluate sexual abuse of children perform this examination.

Emotional Abuse: Emotional abuse is usually identified during evaluation of another problem, such as poor performance in school or a behavioral problem. Children who are emotionally abused are checked for signs of physical and sexual abuse.

Treatment

A team of doctors, other health care practitioners, and social workers try to deal with the causes and effects of neglect and abuse. The team helps family members understand the child's needs and helps them access local resources. For example, a child whose parents cannot afford health care may qualify for medical assistance from the state. Other community and government programs can provide assistance with food and shelter. Parents with substance abuse or mental health problems may be directed to appropriate treatment programs. Parenting programs are available in some areas.

All physical injuries and disorders are treated. Some children are hospitalized for treatment of injuries, severe undernutrition, or other disorders. Some severe injuries require surgery. Infants with shaken baby syndrome usually need to be admitted to a pediatric intensive care unit. Sometimes healthy children are hospitalized to protect them from further abuse until appropriate home care can be ensured.

Some children who have been sexually abused are given drugs to prevent sexually transmitted diseases, sometimes including HIV infection. Children who appear to be very upset need immediate counseling and support. Sexually abused children, even those who appear unaffected initially, are referred to a mental health care practitioner, because long-lasting problems are common. Long-term psychologic counseling is often needed. Doctors refer other children for counseling if behavioral or emotional problems develop.

The goal of treatment is to return children to a safe, healthy family environment. Depending on the nature of the abuse and the abuser, children may go home with their family or may be removed from their home and placed with relatives or in foster care. This placement is often temporary, for example, until the parents can obtain housing or employment or until regular home visits by a social worker are established. In severe cases of neglect or abuse, the parents' rights may be permanently terminated. In such cases, the child remains in foster care until the child is adopted or becomes an adult.▲

▲ see pages 1641 and 1642

ACCIDENTS AND INJURIES

289 Burns 1648

290 Heat Disorders 1652
Heat Cramps ▪ Heat Exhaustion ▪ Heatstroke

291 Cold Injuries 1654
Hypothermia ▪ Nonfreezing Tissue Injuries ▪ Frostbite

292 Radiation Injury 1657

293 Electrical and Lightning Injuries 1661

294 Near Drowning 1665

295 Diving and Compressed Air Injuries 1666
Barotrauma ▪ Decompression Sickness

296 Altitude Illness 1672

297 Poisoning 1674
Acetaminophen Poisoning ▪ Aspirin Poisoning ▪ Carbon
Monoxide Poisoning ▪ Poisoning With Caustic Substances ▪
Hydrocarbon Poisoning ▪ Insecticide Poisoning ▪ Iron
Poisoning ▪ Lead Poisoning

298 Bites and Stings 1681
Animal Bites ▪ Human Bites ▪ Poisonous Snake Bites ▪
Poisonous Lizard Bites ▪ Spider Bites ▪ Bee, Wasp, Hornet, and
Ant Stings ▪ Insect Bites ▪ Tick and Mite Bites ▪ Centipede
and Millipede Bites ▪ Scorpion Stings ▪ Marine Animal Stings
and Bites

299 First Aid 1687
Priorities During Emergency First Aid ▪ Cardiac Arrest ▪
Choking ▪ Internal Bleeding ▪ Wounds ▪ Soft Tissue
Injuries ▪ Severed or Constricted Limbs or Digits

CHAPTER 289

Burns

Burns are injuries to tissue that result from heat, electricity, radiation, or chemicals.

Burns are usually caused by heat (thermal burns), such as fire, steam, tar, or hot liquids. Burns caused by chemicals are similar to thermal burns, whereas burns caused by radiation,▲ sunlight,■ and electricity★ tend to differ significantly.

Thermal and chemical burns usually occur because heat or chemicals contact part of the body's surface, most often the skin. Thus, the skin usually sustains most of the damage. However, severe surface burns may penetrate to deeper body structures, such as fat, muscle, or bone.

When tissues are burned, fluid leaks into them from the blood vessels, causing swelling and pain. In addition, damaged skin and other body surfaces are easily infected because they can no longer act as a barrier against invading organisms.

More than 2 million people in the United States require treatment for burns each year, and between 3,000 and 4,000 die of severe burns. Older people and young children are particularly vulnerable.

Classification

Doctors classify burns according to strict, widely accepted definitions. These definitions may not correspond to a person's understanding of those terms. For example, a doctor may classify a burn as serious even though the person regards it as minor. The definitions classify the burn's depth and the extent of tissue damage.

The depth of injury from a burn is described as first, second, or third degree. First-degree burns are the most shallow (superficial). They affect only the top layer of skin (epidermis). Second-degree burns extend into the middle layer of skin (dermis). Third-degree burns involve all three layers of skin (epidermis, dermis, and fat layer), usually destroying the sweat glands, hair follicles, and nerve endings as well.

Burns are classified as minor, moderate, or severe. The severity determines how they are predicted to heal and whether complications are likely. Doctors determine the severity of the burn by estimating the percentage of the body surface that has been burned. Special charts are used to show what percentage of the body surface various body parts comprise. For example, in an adult, the arm constitutes about 9% of the body. Separate charts are used for children, because their body proportions are different. All first-degree burns as well as second-degree burns that involve less than about 15% of the body surface usually are classified as minor, although they may seem severe to the person. A third-degree burn may

When Chemicals Burn the Skin

Chemical burns are caused by caustic substances that contact the skin. Caustic substances are sometimes found in household products, including those containing lye (in drain cleaners and paint removers), phenols (in deodorizers, sanitizers, and disinfectants), sodium hypochlorite (in disinfectants and bleaches), and sulfuric acid (in toilet bowl cleaners). Many chemicals used in industry and during armed conflicts can cause burns. Wet cement left on the skin can cause severe burns as well.

The first step in stopping chemical burns is to remove contaminated clothing and brush away any dry particles. Next, the area is rinsed with large amounts of water. Because chemicals can continue to inflict damage long after first contacting the skin, rinsing should continue for at least 30 minutes. In rare cases involving certain industrial chemicals (for example, metal sodium), water should not be used because it can actually worsen the burn. In addition, some chemicals have specific treatments that can further reduce skin damage. Further treatment of chemical burns is the same as that for thermal burns.

If more information is needed concerning treatment of a burn caused by a specific chemical, the local Poison Control Center can be contacted.

▲ see page 1657   ■ see page 1230

★ see page 1661

be classified as minor if it involves less than 5% of the body surface, unless it involves the face, hands, feet, or genitals. Burns involving these areas or involving deeper layers of skin over larger areas of the body are classified as moderate or, more often, as severe.

Symptoms and Diagnosis

First-degree burns are red, moist, swollen, and painful. The burned area whitens (blanches) when lightly touched but does not develop blisters. Second-degree burns are red, swollen, and painful, and they develop blisters that may ooze a clear fluid. The burned area may blanch when touched. Third-degree burns usually are not painful because the nerves have been destroyed. The skin becomes leathery and may be white, black, or bright red. The burned area does not blanch when touched, and hairs can easily be pulled from their roots without pain. No blisters develop. The appearance and symptoms of deep burns can worsen during the first hours or even days after the burn.

Complications

Most minor burns are superficial and do not cause complications. However, deep second-degree and third-degree burns swell and take more time to heal. In addition, deeper burns can cause scar tissue to form. This scar tissue shrinks (contracts) as it heals. If the scarring occurs at a joint, the resulting contracture may restrict movement.

Severe burns can cause serious complications due to extensive fluid loss and tissue damage. Complications from severe burns may take hours to develop. The longer the complication is present, the more severe are the problems it tends to cause. Young children and older adults tend to be more seriously affected by complications than other age groups.

Dehydration eventually develops in people with widespread burns, because fluid seeps from the blood to the burned tissues. Shock develops if dehydration is severe.▲ Destruction of muscle tissue (rhabdomyolysis) occurs in deep third-degree burns. The muscle tissue releases myoglobin, one of the muscle's proteins, into the blood. If present in high concentrations, myoglobin harms the kidneys. Rhabdomyolysis can be diagnosed from tests of the blood and urine.

Thick, crusty surfaces (eschars) are produced by deep third-degree burns. Eschars can

Smoke Inhalation

Many people who have been burned in fires have also inhaled smoke. Sometimes people inhale smoke without sustaining skin burns. Smoke inhalation often causes no serious, lasting effects. However, if the smoke is unusually hot or dense or if inhalation is prolonged, serious problems can develop. The hot smoke can burn the windpipe (trachea), resulting in swelling. As the swelling narrows the trachea, airflow into the lungs is obstructed. Inhalation of chemicals released in the smoke, such as hydrogen chloride, phosgene, sulfur dioxide, and ammonia, can swell and damage the lungs and trachea. Eventually, the small airways leading to the lungs narrow, further obstructing airflow. Smoke can also contain chemicals that poison the body's cells, such as carbon monoxide■ and cyanide.

Damage to the trachea or the lungs can cause shortness of breath, which can take up to 24 hours to develop. Obstruction of airflow due to swelling of the airways can produce wheezing and worsen shortness of breath. The person may have soot in the mouth or nose, singed nasal hairs, or burns around the mouth. Lung damage may cause chest pain, coughing, and wheezing. If the oxygen supply is depleted due to smoke, the person may pass out. High levels of carbon monoxide in the blood may cause confusion or disorientation or may even be fatal.

To assess the extent of a tracheal burn, a doctor may pass a flexible viewing tube (bronchoscope) into the trachea. A doctor may assess lung damage with a chest x-ray or with a test that determines the level of oxygen in the blood.

A person who has inhaled smoke is given oxygen through a face mask. If a tracheal burn is suspected, a breathing tube is inserted through the person's nose or mouth in case the trachea later swells and obstructs airflow. If the person begins to wheeze, drugs that open small airways, such as albuterol, may be given, usually as a mist that is combined with oxygen and inhaled through a face mask. If lung damage causes shortness of breath that persists despite use of a face mask and albuterol, a ventilator may be necessary. Relieving the stress of breathing conserves the person's energy and usually allows faster recovery and healing.

▲ see page 148   ■ see page 1677

Small, Shallow Burns

Most people who sustain small burns attempt to treat them at home rather than visit the doctor. Indeed, simple first-aid measures may be all that is necessary to treat small, shallow burns that are clean. In general, a clean burn is one that affects only clean skin and that does not contain any dirt particles or food. Running cold water over the burn can relieve pain. Covering the burn with an over-the-counter antibiotic ointment and a nonstick, sterile bandage can prevent infection.

Generally, a doctor's examination and treatment are recommended if a tetanus vaccination is needed. Likewise, a doctor should examine a burn if it has any of the following characteristics:

- Is larger than about the size of the person's palm
- Contains blisters
- Darkens or breaks the skin
- Involves the face, hand, foot, genitals, or skinfolds
- Is not completely clean
- Causes pain that is not relieved by acetaminophen
- Causes pain that does not improve within one day after the burn was sustained

become too tight, cutting off blood supply to healthy tissues or impairing breathing.

Treatment

Before burns are treated, the burning agent must be stopped from inflicting further damage. For example, fires are extinguished. Clothing—especially any that is smoldering (such as melted synthetic shirts), covered with hot tar, or soaked with chemicals—is immediately removed.

Hospitalization is sometimes necessary for optimal care of burn injuries. For example, elevating a severely burned arm or leg above the level of the heart to prevent swelling is more easily accommodated in a hospital. In addition, burns that prevent a person from performing essential daily functions, such as walking or eating, make hospitalization necessary. Severe burns, deep second- and third-

degree burns, burns occurring in the very young or the very old, and burns involving the hands, feet, face, or genitals are usually best treated at burn centers. Burn centers are hospitals that are specially equipped and staffed to care for burn victims.

Superficial Minor Burns: Superficial minor burns are immersed immediately in cool water if possible. The burn is carefully cleaned to prevent infection. If dirt is deeply embedded, a doctor can give analgesics or numb the area by injecting a local anesthetic and then scrub the burn with a brush.

Often, the only treatment required is application of an antibiotic cream, such as silver sulfadiazine. The cream prevents infection and forms a seal to prevent further bacteria from entering the wound. A sterile bandage is then applied to protect the burned area from dirt and further injury. A tetanus vaccination is given if needed.▲

Care at home includes keeping the burn clean to prevent infection. In addition, many people are given analgesics, often opioid analgesics, for at least a few days. The burn can be covered with a nonstick bandage or with sterile gauze. The gauze can be removed without sticking by first being soaked in water.

Deep Minor Burns: As with more superficial burns, deep minor burns are treated with antibiotic cream. However, any dead skin and broken blisters must be removed before the antibiotic cream is applied. In addition, keeping a deeply burned arm or leg elevated above the heart for the first few days reduces swelling and pain. The burn may require frequent re-examination at a hospital or doctor's office, possibly as often as daily for the first few days.

A skin graft may be needed. Most skin grafts replace the burned skin. Other skin grafts help by temporarily covering and protecting the skin as it heals on its own. In a skin grafting procedure, a piece of healthy skin is taken from an unburned area of the person's body (autograft), from another living or dead person (allograft), or from another species (xenograft)—usually pigs because their skin is most similar to human skin. The skin graft is surgically sewn over the burned area after removing any dead tissue and ensuring that the wound is clean. Autografts are permanent. Allografts and xenografts, however, are rejected after 10 to 14 days by the person's immune system. Artificial skin has been developed recently and can also be used to replace the

▲ see page 1093

burned skin. Burned skin can be replaced anytime within several days of the burn.

Physical and occupational therapy usually are needed to prevent immobility caused by scarring around the joints. Stretching exercises are started within the first few days after the burn. Splints are applied to ensure that joints that are likely to be immobile rest in positions that are least likely to lead to contractures. The splints are left in place except when the joints are moved. If a skin graft has been used, however, therapy is not started for the first 5 to 10 days after the grafts are attached so that the healing graft is not disturbed. Bulky dressings that put pressure on the burn can prevent large scars from developing.

Severe Burns: Severe, life-threatening burns require immediate care. Dehydration is treated with large amounts of fluids given intravenously. A person who has gone into shock as a result of dehydration is also given oxygen through a face mask.

Destruction of muscle tissue is also treated with large amounts of fluids given intravenously. The fluids dilute the myoglobin in the blood, preventing extensive damage to the kidneys. Sometimes a chemical, sodium bicarbonate, is given intravenously to help dissolve myoglobin and thus also prevent further damage to the kidneys.

Eschars that cut off blood supply to an extremity or that impair breathing are cut open in a surgical procedure called escharotomy. Escharotomy usually causes some bleeding, but because the burn causing the eschar has destroyed the nerve endings in the skin, there is little pain.

Keeping the burned area clean is important, because the damaged skin is easily infected. Cleaning may be accomplished by gently running water over the burns periodically. Wounds are cleaned and bandages changed 1 to 3 times per day.

A proper diet that includes adequate amounts of calories, protein, and nutrients is important for healing. People who cannot consume enough calories may drink nutritional supplements or receive them by way of a tube inserted through the nose into the stomach (a nasogastric tube), or nutrition may be given intravenously. Additional vitamins and minerals are usually given.

Because severe burns take a long time to heal, sometimes years, and can cause disfig-

Estimating the Extent of a Burn

To determine the severity of a burn, doctors estimate what percentage of the body's surface has been burned. For adults, doctors use the rule of nines. This method divides almost all of the body into sections of 9% or of 2 times 9% (18%). For children, doctors use charts that adjust these percentages according to the child's age (Lund-Browder charts). Adjustment is needed because different areas of the body grow at different rates.

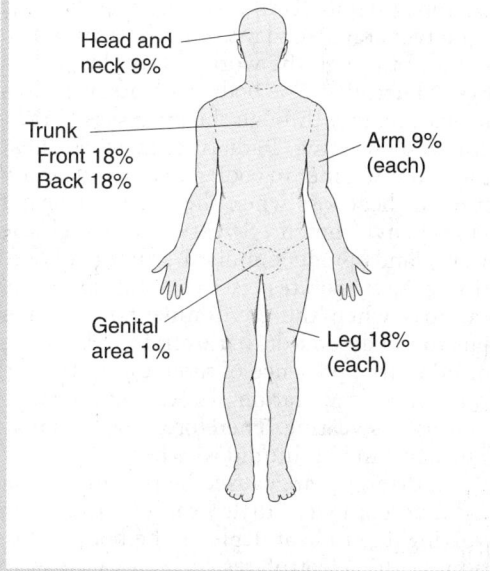

Head and neck 9%

Trunk
Front 18%
Back 18%

Arm 9% (each)

Genital area 1%

Leg 18% (each)

urement, the person can become depressed. Depression often can be relieved with drugs or psychotherapy or both.

Prognosis

First- and second-degree burns heal in days to weeks without scarring. Deep second-degree and small (less than 1 inch) third-degree burns take weeks to heal and usually cause scarring. Larger third-degree burns require skin grafting. Burns that involve more than 90% of the body surface, or more than 60% in an older person, usually are fatal.

CHAPTER 290

Heat Disorders

Humans, who are warm-blooded animals, maintain their body temperature within a narrow range (within 1 or 2 degrees of 98.6° F) despite large fluctuations in external temperatures. This internal temperature range must be maintained for the body to function normally. Body temperature that gets too high or too low can result in serious injury to organs or death.

The body regulates its temperature by balancing heat production and heat loss. One way the body produces heat is through chemical reactions (metabolism) resulting mostly from the conversion of food into energy. Heat is also produced through the work of muscles during physical activity. The body cools itself by losing heat, mainly through the processes of radiation and sweating. Radiation, in which heat flows from warmer to cooler areas, is the main source of heat loss when the body is warmer than its environment. Sweating, in which the sweat glands produce moisture that cools the skin as it evaporates, is the main source of heat loss when the environment is warmer than the body and during exercise. However, humidity (the presence of moisture in the air) slows water evaporation, decreasing the effectiveness of sweating. Therefore, heat loss may be difficult in hot, humid weather.

Heat disorders are caused by too much heat production or by too little heat loss. Excessive sweating due to heat depletes the body of fluids and salts (electrolytes), which can lead to low blood pressure and painful muscle contractions. Which heat disorder develops depends on the severity of body fluid and salt depletion. Heat cramps result from mild or moderate depletion; heat exhaustion, from moderate or severe depletion; and heatstroke, the most serious of the heat disorders, often from severe depletion.

Ineffective heat loss most commonly occurs in hot, humid conditions. Several factors contribute greatly to ineffective heat loss. Wearing heavy, tight, waterproof clothing that does not breathe (that is, that does not allow air and moisture to pass through easily) prevents sweat from evaporating from the skin surface, thus impairing cooling. Sweating can be impaired by certain drugs, most often antipsychotic drugs and drugs with anticholinergic effects▲; by some diseases that affect the skin, such as cystic fibrosis, scleroderma, psoriasis, and eczema; and by severe sunburns. Obesity impairs sweating as well because it requires the heart to work harder, thereby depleting the reserve needed to increase pumping for sweating. Also, a thick layer of fat slows heat loss from internal organs, which may sustain damage from prolonged heat exposure. Alcohol interferes with sensible responses that could prevent heat disorders. For example, an inebriated person may not move to a cool environment, remove heavy clothing, or turn on an air conditioner.

Excessive heat production is most often caused by fever, increased thyroid activity, extreme exertion, and certain stimulant drugs, such as cocaine and amphetamines. Strenuous muscular activity occurs by choice or results from medical conditions such as seizures, agitation, or alcohol or drug withdrawal.

The chance of developing heat disorders increases when exposure to heat occurs suddenly, such as when a child is left in a closed car on a hot summer day. When a person is exposed to longer periods of heat and humidity, the body gradually adjusts and is better able to maintain normal body temperature. This process is called acclimatization. Acclimatization occurs no more rapidly in young or physically active people than in older or physically inactive people.

Prevention

Using common sense is the best way to prevent heat disorders. For example, strenuous exertion in a very hot environment should be avoided. During hot, humid weather, it is best to wear light, loose-fitting clothing made of cloth that breathes (that is, that allows air and moisture to pass through easily), such as cotton. Fluids and salts lost through sweating can be replaced by consuming lightly salted foods and beverages, such as salted tomato juice or cool bouillon. Many commercially available drinks contain extra salt. To replace adequate

▲ see box on page 79

amounts of fluids, drinking must continue even after thirst is quenched. When exertion in a hot environment cannot be avoided, drinking plenty of fluids and frequently cooling the skin by misting or wetting it with cool water can help keep body temperature near normal.

People engaged in outdoor activities who drink large quantities of water may dilute the sodium in the blood. Consuming salt, even in salty "junk" food, along with the water can alleviate this problem.

Enclosed, poorly ventilated spaces, such as a car, can heat up rapidly. In hot weather, the interior of a closed car can heat from 80 to 120° F in 15 minutes. Children and pets should never be left in such an environment, even for a few minutes.

Heat Cramps

Heat cramps are severe muscle spasms resulting from a combination of prolonged exercise, heavy sweating, and excessive water replacement in extreme heat.

During sweating, salts (electrolytes) and fluids are lost, but drinking large quantities of water dilutes the salts, causing cramps. Heavy sweating is most likely to occur on warm days, especially during strenuous exertion. Heat cramps are common among manual laborers, such as engine-room personnel, steelworkers, roofers, and miners. Heat cramps may also develop in athletes, especially mountain climbers or skiers, whose many layers of clothing may keep them from noticing their heavy sweating. Cramps are common in tennis players and runners who do not take time to replace salts lost in sweat.

Heat cramps are rhythmic contractions in muscles of the hands, calves, feet, thighs, or arms. The contractions cause muscles to become hard, tense, and painful.

Mild heat cramps can be treated by drinking beverages that contain salt or eating salty food. Severe heat cramps are treated with fluids and salts given intravenously.

Heat Exhaustion

Heat exhaustion is excessive loss of salts (electrolytes) and fluids due to heat, leading to decreased blood volume that causes many symptoms, sometimes including fainting or collapse.

Heat exhaustion is more severe than heat cramps. Fluids and salts are more depleted, and symptoms are more severe.

Symptoms and Diagnosis

Dizziness, light-headedness, weakness, fatigue, headache, blurred vision, muscle aches, or nausea and vomiting may develop. A person may feel faint or even lose consciousness when standing. Drenching sweats are common. Mild confusion may develop. The heart rate and breathing rate may become rapid; blood pressure may become low. Body temperature can be normal or high but not higher than 104° F.

Heat exhaustion usually can be diagnosed on the basis of the symptoms and occurrence after exposure to heat.

Treatment

Treatment involves replacing fluids (rehydration) and salts and removing the person from the hot environment. If symptoms are mild, sipping cool, slightly salty beverages every few minutes may be all that is needed. Removing or loosening clothing and applying wet cloths or ice packs to the skin also aid cooling.

If symptoms include loss of consciousness, confusion, rapid breathing or heartbeat, or low blood pressure, then fluids are given intravenously. After rehydration, a person usually recovers rapidly and fully. If left untreated, heat exhaustion can lead to heatstroke.

Heatstroke

Heatstroke is a life-threatening condition that results in very high body temperature and dysfunction of many organ systems.

Heatstroke is the most severe form of heat-induced illness. Two features distinguish heatstroke from other heat disorders: body temperature usually is higher than 104° F, and symptoms of brain damage develop. Heatstroke may occur when a person is exerting himself in extreme heat or is in a closed, hot environment. For example, heatstroke can develop during prolonged periods of hot weather when people stay in rooms that are not air-conditioned. Older people and young children are most vulnerable to heatstroke.

Heatstroke occurs because the body cannot lose heat rapidly enough in extreme heat. Because the body cannot cool itself, body temperature continues to rise rapidly to dangerously high levels. Certain skin disorders and certain drugs increase the risk.

Heatstroke can temporarily or permanently damage vital organs, such as the heart, lungs, kidneys, liver, and brain. The higher the temperature, especially when higher than 106° F, the more rapidly problems develop. Death may occur.

Symptoms and Diagnosis

Heatstroke typically develops in older, sedentary people living in poorly ventilated rooms during a heat wave. Heatstroke may develop slowly over hours to days or quickly, especially in people exerting themselves in hot, humid environments. Dizziness, lightheadedness, weakness, fatigue, headache, blurred vision, muscle aches, nausea, and vomiting (which are also symptoms of heat exhaustion) are common warning symptoms.

During heatstroke, the skin becomes hot, flushed, and dry. Sweating may not occur despite the heat. A person may become confused and disoriented and may have seizures or lapse into a coma. The heart rate and breathing rate increase. The pulse rate is usually rapid. The blood pressure may be high or low. Body temperature usually exceeds 104° F and may be so high that it exceeds the markings on a typical thermometer.

Treatment

The body must be cooled immediately. While awaiting transportation to the hospital, a person should be wrapped in cold, wet bedding or clothing; immersed in a lake, stream, or cool bathtub; or cooled with ice. At the hospital, body cooling is usually accomplished by removing the clothes and covering the exposed skin with water or ice. To speed evaporation and body cooling, a fan may be used to blow air on the body. Body temperature is measured frequently, often constantly. Cooled fluids may be given intravenously. To avoid overcooling, cooling is stopped when the body temperature is reduced to about 102° F.

Seizures or coma may also need treatment. Heatstroke is best treated in an intensive care unit of a hospital. After recovery, body temperature may fluctuate abnormally for weeks. The brain may not fully recover, leaving a person with personality changes, clumsiness, or poor coordination.

CHAPTER 291

Cold Injuries

The skin and the tissues under it are kept at a constant temperature (about 98.6° F) by the circulating blood. The blood gets its heat mainly from the energy given off by cells when they burn (metabolize) food—a process that requires a steady supply of food and oxygen. A normal body temperature is necessary for proper functioning of all the cells and tissues in the body. In a person with low body temperature, most organs, especially the heart and brain, become sluggish and eventually stop working.

Body temperature falls when the skin is exposed to colder surroundings. In response to this, the body uses several protective mechanisms to generate additional heat. For example, the muscles produce additional heat through shivering. Also, the small blood vessels in the skin narrow (constrict), so that more blood is diverted to vital organs, such as the heart and brain. However, as less warm blood reaches the skin, body parts such as the fingers, toes, ears, and nose cool more rapidly. If body temperature falls much below about 88° F, these protective mechanisms stop working and the body cannot rewarm itself. If body temperature falls below 83° F, death is likely.

Cold injuries usually do not occur, even in extremely cold weather, if the skin, fingers, toes, ears, and nose are well protected or are exposed only briefly. The risk of cold injuries increases when the flow of blood is impeded, when food intake is inadequate, or when insufficient oxygen is available, as occurs at high altitudes.

Keeping warm in a cold environment requires several layers of clothing—preferably wool or synthetics such as polypropylene, because these materials insulate even when wet. Because the body loses a large amount of heat from the head, a warm hat is essential. Eating enough food and drinking enough fluids (particularly warm fluids) also help. Food provides fuel to be burned, and warm fluids directly provide heat and prevent dehydration. Alcoholic beverages should be avoided, because alcohol widens (dilates) blood vessels in the skin, which makes the body temporarily feel warm but actually causes greater heat loss.

Cold injuries include hypothermia, frostnip, chilblains, immersion foot, and frostbite. Other problems related to the cold include Raynaud's disease and Raynaud's phenomenon▲ and allergic reactions to the cold.■

Hypothermia

Hypothermia is a dangerously low body temperature.

Hypothermia results when the body loses more heat than can be replaced by increasing metabolism (through exercise) or by increasing warming from external sources, such as a fire or the sun. Wind increases heat loss, as does sitting or lying on a cold surface or being immersed in water. Sudden immersion in very cold water may cause fatal hypothermia in 5 to 15 minutes; however, a few people, mostly infants, have survived for as long as 1 hour completely submerged in ice water. The shock shuts off all systems, essentially protecting the body. Hypothermia may also occur after prolonged exposure in only moderately cool water.

People at greatest risk are those who are lying immobile in a cold environment—such as those who have had a stroke or who are unconscious from intoxication or injury. Because they are not moving, these people generate less heat and also are unable to leave the cold environment. Such people are at risk of becoming hypothermic even when the surrounding temperature may be only as cold as 55 or 60° F. The very young and the very old are at particular risk. People in these age groups often do not compensate for cold as well as young adults and are dependent on others to

anticipate their needs and keep them warm. Very old people quite often become hypothermic from sitting immobile in a cold room for hours. Infants lose body heat rapidly and are particularly susceptible to hypothermia.

Symptoms

The symptoms of hypothermia usually develop so gradually that neither the person himself nor others realize what is happening. Initial symptoms include intense shivering and teeth chattering. As body temperature falls further, shivering stops and movements become slow and clumsy, reaction time is longer, thinking is blurred, and judgment is impaired. The person may fall, wander off, or simply lie down to rest. If body temperature continues to fall, shivering stops, which is an ominous sign. At that point, the person becomes more sluggish and slips into a coma. The heart and breathing rates become slower and weaker. Eventually the heart stops.

The lower the body temperature, the higher the risk of death. Death may occur at body temperatures below 88° F but is most likely to occur below 83° F.

Diagnosis and Treatment

Doctors diagnose hypothermia by measuring body temperature, typically with a rectal thermometer. Conventional thermometers do not record below 94° F, thus special thermometers are needed to measure temperatures in severe hypothermia.

In the early stages, changing into warm dry clothing or drinking hot beverages can bring about recovery. If the person is found unconscious, further heat loss is prevented by wrapping the person in a warm dry blanket and, if possible, moving him to a warm place while arrangements are made for immediate transportation to a hospital. Often, no pulse can be felt and no heartbeat can be heard, although the heart may be beating weakly. The person must be handled gently, because a sudden jolt may cause an irregular heart rhythm (arrhythmia) that could be fatal. For this reason, if the person appears to be breathing, even very shallowly, cardiopulmonary resuscitation (CPR) is not recommended outside of a hospital. Because it is so difficult for untrained people to detect very faint respirations and heartbeats,

▲ see page 224   ■ see page 1070

some doctors do not recommend CPR for any hypothermic person outside a hospital.

In the hospital, doctors warm the person with warmed oxygen and heated fluids given intravenously or passed into the abdominal or chest cavity through plastic tubes inserted into those areas. In addition, the blood may be warmed through the process of hemodialysis (in which the blood is pumped out of the body, through a filter with a heating attachment, and back into the body) or with a heart-lung machine (which pumps blood out of the body, heats the blood, adds oxygen, and then returns the blood to the body).

Because some people with hypothermia who have arrived at the hospital with no signs of life have recovered, doctors usually continue resuscitation efforts until the person is warmed but still shows no signs of life.

Nonfreezing Tissue Injuries

In nonfreezing tissue injuries, parts of the skin are chilled but not frozen.

Nonfreezing tissue injuries include frostnip, immersion foot, and chilblains.

Frostnip is a cold injury in which the chilled areas of skin become numb, swollen, and red. The only treatment needed is warming the area for a few minutes. During warming, the area may hurt or itch intensely. No permanent damage results, although sometimes the area is particularly sensitive to cold for months or years afterward.

Immersion foot (trench foot) is a cold injury that develops when a foot is kept in wet, cold socks and boots for several days. The foot is pale, clammy, and cold. After warming, the foot becomes red and painful to the touch. Sometimes blisters develop, which may become infected. Treatment consists primarily of gently warming, drying, and cleaning the foot; elevating it; and keeping it dry and warm. Some doctors give antibiotics to prevent infection. A tetanus booster is given if the person's tetanus vaccination is not current. Rarely, this type of injury occurs in the hands. Immersion foot can often be prevented by changing socks and drying the feet at least daily.

Chilblains (pernio) is an uncommon reaction that may occur with repeated exposure to cold. Symptoms include itching, pain, and, in rare cases, discolored areas or blisters on the affected area (usually the leg). The condition is uncomfortable and recurrent but not serious. Preventing exposure to cold is the best treatment. The drug nifedipine, taken by mouth, sometimes relieves symptoms.

Frostbite

Frostbite is a cold injury in which an area of the body is frozen.

The damage caused by frostbite results from a combination of factors. Freezing kills some cells: others survive. Because cold causes blood vessels to narrow, tissue that is near the frozen area but not itself frozen may be damaged as a result of the decreased blood flow. Sometimes cold also causes clots to form in small blood vessels in this tissue. These clots may limit blood flow so much that the tissue dies. When blood flow returns to the affected area, the damaged tissues release a number of chemical substances that promote inflammation; inflammation worsens the damage caused by the cold. In addition, toxic substances are released into the bloodstream as frozen tissue is warmed. These toxins may cause irregular heart rhythms (arrhythmias). Therefore, doctors monitor heart function and blood levels of these toxins.

Exposure to below-freezing temperatures puts any part of the body at risk of frostbite. The risk of frostbite damage depends on how cold it is and how long the part was exposed. People at greatest risk of developing frostbite are those who have poor circulation because of diabetes or arteriosclerosis, blood vessel spasm (which may be caused by smoking, some neurologic disorders, or certain drugs), or constriction of blood flow by gloves or boots that are too tight. Exposed hands and feet and an exposed face are most vulnerable. Contact with wetness or metal accelerates freezing and is particularly dangerous.

Symptoms

Symptoms vary with the depth and amount of tissue frozen. Shallow frostbite results in a numb white patch of skin that peels after warming. Slightly deeper frostbite causes blisters and swelling of the affected area. Deeper freezing causes the extremity to feel numb, cold, and hard. The area is pale and cold. Blisters often appear. Blisters filled with clear fluid indicate milder damage than do blisters filled with bloodstained fluid.

The extremity may become gray and soft (wet gangrene). If wet gangrene develops, in many cases the extremity must be amputated. More frequently, the area becomes black and leathery (dry gangrene).

Diagnosis and Treatment

Frostbite is diagnosed by its typical appearance and occurrence after significant exposure to cold.

A person who has frostbite should be covered with a warm blanket and given a hot beverage, because people with frostbite may also have hypothermia. The frostbitten area should be warmed as quickly as possible by immersing it in warm water that is no hotter than can be comfortably tolerated by the caregiver (100 to 104° F). Rubbing the area (particularly with snow) leads to further tissue damage. Because the area has no sensation, it should not be warmed in front of a fire or with a heating pad or electric blanket. The frostbitten area becomes extremely painful on warming; thus an injection of an opioid analgesic may be necessary. Blisters should not be broken. If blisters break, they should be covered with antibiotic ointment.

It is more damaging to thaw and refreeze tissue than to allow it to remain frozen. Thus, if a person with frostbite must be reexposed to freezing conditions, particularly if he must walk on frostbitten feet, the tissue should not be thawed. Thawed feet are more vulnerable to damage from walking. If the person must walk on thawed feet to reach help, every effort should be made to protect the damaged tissue from rubbing, constriction, or further damage.

Once the tissue is warmed, the frostbitten area should be gently washed, dried, wrapped in sterile bandages, and kept meticulously clean and dry to prevent infection. Anti-inflammatory drugs, such as ibuprofen by mouth, or aloe vera gel applied topically helps relieve the inflammation. Infection requires use of antibiotics, although some doctors give antibiotics to all people with deep frostbite. Some doctors also use drugs given intravenously, such as low-molecular-weight dextrans, heparin, or phenoxybenzamine, to improve circulation to the affected area, although these forms of treatment are beneficial only in the first few days after injury.

Most people slowly improve over several months, although amputation is sometimes necessary to remove the dead tissue. Because frostbite may appear to affect a larger area and to be more severe than it will weeks or months later, the decision to amputate is usually postponed for several months until the area has had time to heal.

CHAPTER 292

Radiation Injury

Radiation injury is damage to tissues caused by exposure to radiation.

In general, radiation refers to high-energy electromagnetic waves (x-rays, gamma rays) or particles (alpha particles, beta particles, neutrons). Radiation is emitted by radioactive substances (radioisotopes), such as uranium, radon, and plutonium. Radiation is also produced by man-made sources, such as x-ray and radiation therapy machines.

Radiation dose is measured in several different units, but all relate to the amount of energy deposited. The units include the roentgen (R), the gray (Gy), and the sievert (Sv). The sievert and gray are similar, except the sievert takes into account the biologic effects of different types of radiation.

The two main types of radiation exposure are irradiation and contamination. Many radiation accidents expose a person to both.

Irradiation is exposure to radiation waves that pass directly through the body from outside the body. Irradiation can make a person sick immediately (acute radiation illness). Additionally, irradiation, particularly in high doses, can damage a person's genetic material (DNA), causing chronic (delayed) disorders, such as cancer and birth defects. However, irradiation does not make the person or his tissues radioactive.

Contamination is contact with and retention of radioactive material, typically in the form of a dust or liquid. The radioactive material may stay on the skin, where it can fall or be rubbed off, contaminating other people and objects. The material also may be absorbed by the body through the lungs, digestive tract, or breaks in the skin. The absorbed material is transported to various sites in the body, such as the bone marrow, where it continues to release radiation. This internalized radiation does not cause acute radiation illness but may produce chronic disorders such as cancer.

Causes

People are constantly exposed to low levels of natural radiation (background radiation). Radiation comes from outer space (cosmic radiation), although much of it is blocked by the earth's atmosphere. Exposure to cosmic radiation is greater for people living at high altitudes. Radioactive elements, particularly radon gas, also are present in many rocks and minerals. These elements end up in a variety of substances, including food and construction materials. Radon exposure is a greater risk in basements because of their proximity to the ground. In addition, people are exposed to radiation from man-made sources, including the environmental radiation that results from nuclear weapons testing and radiation from various medical tests and treatments. The average person receives a total of about 3 to 4 mSv (1 mSv = 1/1000 Sv) per year from natural radiation and man-made sources. People who work with radioactive materials and with x-ray sources are at risk of exposure to higher levels of radiation. People who are receiving radiation treatments for cancer may receive very high levels of radiation.

Rarely, radiation has been released from nuclear power plants, including the Three Mile Island plant in Pennsylvania in 1979 and the Chernobyl plant in the Ukraine in 1986. The Three Mile Island accident did not result in major radiation exposure; in fact, anyone living within 1 mile of the plant received only about 0.08 mSv additional radiation. However, people living near the Chernobyl plant were exposed to about 430 mSv of radiation. More than 30 people died, many more were injured, and radiation from that accident reached other parts of Europe, Asia, and the United States. In total, radiation exposure from reactors in the first 40 years of nuclear energy use, excluding Chernobyl, has resulted in 35 serious exposures with 10 deaths, but none were associated with power plants.

Nuclear weapons release massive amounts of radiation. These weapons have not been used against people since 1945. However, a number of nations now possess nuclear weapons, and several terrorist groups have also tried to obtain them, raising the possibility that these weapons could once again be used.

The damaging effects of radiation depend on several factors, including the amount (dose) and duration of exposure. A single, rapid dose of radiation to the entire body can be fatal, but the same total dose given over a period of weeks or months may have much less effect. For a given dose, genetic damage is more likely with rapid exposure. The effects of radiation also depend on how much of the body is exposed. For example, more than 6 Gy generally causes death when the radiation is distributed over the entire body; however, when concentrated in a small area, as in radiation therapy for cancer, 3 or 4 times this amount can be given without serious harm.

The distribution of radiation is also important, because certain parts of the body are more sensitive to radiation. Organs and tissues in which cells are multiplying quickly, such as the intestines and bone marrow, are harmed more easily by radiation than those in which cells multiply more slowly, such as muscles and tendons. The genetic material of sperm and egg cells can be damaged by radiation. During radiation therapy for cancer, therefore, every attempt is made to shield the more vulnerable parts of the body from radiation so that high doses can be delivered primarily to the cancer.

Symptoms

Radiation exposure produces two types of injury: acute (immediate) and chronic (delayed). Radiation therapy for cancer mainly produces symptoms in the part of the body that receives radiation. For example, in radiation therapy for rectal cancer, abdominal cramping and diarrhea are common because of the effects of radiation on the small intestine.

Acute Radiation Illness: Acute radiation illness generally occurs in people whose entire body has been exposed to radiation. Acute radiation illness progresses through several stages, beginning with early symptoms (prodrome) and followed by a symptom-free period (latent stage). Various syndromes (patterns of symptoms) follow, depending on the amount of radiation the person received. The greater the amount of radiation, the more severe the symptoms and the quicker the progression from the early symptoms to the actual syndrome. The symptoms and time course are consistent from person to person for a given amount of radiation exposure. Doctors can predict a person's radiation exposure from the timing and nature of the symptoms. Doctors divide acute radiation syndromes into three groups based on the main organ system affected, although there is overlap among these groups.

The **hematopoietic syndrome** is caused by the effects of radiation on the bone marrow, spleen, and lymph nodes—the primary sites of blood cell production (hematopoiesis). Loss of appetite (anorexia), lethargy, nausea, and vomiting begin 2 to 12 hours after exposure to 2 Gy or more of radiation. These symptoms resolve within 24 to 36 hours after exposure, and the person feels well for a week or more. During this symptom-free period, the blood-producing cells in the bone marrow, spleen, and lymph nodes begin to waste away and are not replaced, leading to a severe shortage of white blood cells, followed by a shortage of platelets and then red blood cells. The shortage of white blood cells can lead to severe infections. The shortage of platelets may cause uncontrolled bleeding. The shortage of red blood cells (anemia) causes fatigue, weakness, paleness, and difficulty breathing with physical exertion. After 4 to 5 weeks, if the person survives, blood cells begin to be produced once more, but the person feels weak and tired for months.

The **gastrointestinal syndrome** is due to the effects of radiation on the cells lining the digestive tract. Severe nausea, vomiting, and diarrhea begin 2 to 12 hours after exposure to 4 Gy or more of radiation. The symptoms may lead to severe dehydration, but they resolve after 2 days. During the next 4 or 5 days, the person feels well, but the cells lining the digestive tract, which normally act as a protective barrier, die and are shed. After this time, severe diarrhea—often bloody—returns, once more resulting in dehydration. Bacteria from the digestive tract invade the body, producing severe infections. People who have received this much radiation also develop the hematopoietic syndrome, which results in bleeding and infection and increases their risk of death.

The **cerebrovascular (brain) syndrome** occurs when the total dose of radiation exceeds 20 to 30 Gy. A person rapidly develops confusion, nausea, vomiting, bloody diarrhea, and shock. Within hours, blood pressure falls, accompanied by seizures and coma. The cerebrovascular syndrome is always fatal.

ANNUAL RADIATION EXPOSURE IN THE UNITED STATES

SOURCE	AVERAGE DOSE (MILLISIEVERTS)
Naturally occurring sources	
Radon gas	2.00
Other terrestrial sources	0.28
Radiation from outer space	0.27
Natural internal radioactive elements	0.39
Subtotal	2.94
Man-made sources	
Diagnostic x-rays (for average person)	0.39
Nuclear medicine	0.14
Consumer products	0.10
Fallout from weapons testing	less than 0.01
Nuclear industry	less than 0.01
Subtotal	0.63
Total annual exposure	**3.6**
Other sources of exposure	
Airline travel	0.005 mSv/ hour of flight
Dental x-rays	0.09
Chest x-ray	0.10
Barium enema	8.75

Chronic Effects of Radiation: Chronic effects of radiation result from damage to the genetic material in dividing cells. These alterations may cause abnormalities of cell growth, such as cancer. In severely irradiated animals, damage to reproductive cells has been shown to lead to defective offspring (birth defects). However, no deformities resulting from irradiation have been observed in the offspring of survivors of the nuclear blasts in Japan. It may be that radiation exposure below a certain (unknown) level does not alter genetic material enough to cause birth defects.

Radiation Therapy for Cancer: Radiation therapy for cancer can be either internal or external. In internal therapy, small pellets of radioactive material are implanted directly into the cancer. In external therapy, a beam of radiation is transmitted through the person's body into the cancer.

External radiation therapy for cancer produces a number of symptoms, depending on the amount of radiation and the area of the body treated. Nausea, vomiting, and loss of appetite may occur during or shortly after irradiation of the brain or abdomen. Large amounts of radiation to a limited area of the body often damage the skin over that area. Skin changes include hair loss, redness, peeling, sores, and, eventually, thinning of the skin and dilated blood vessels just beneath the skin's surface (spider veins). These changes increase the likelihood of skin cancer years later. Radiation to the mouth and jaw can cause permanent dry mouth, resulting in an increased number of dental caries and damage to the jawbone. Pus-filled pockets of infection (abscesses) may then develop. Radiation to the lungs can cause lung inflammation (radiation pneumonitis), and large amounts may cause severe scarring (fibrosis) of lung tissue, which can be fatal. The heart and its protective sac (pericardium) can become inflamed after extensive radiation to the breastbone and chest. High accumulated doses of radiation to the spinal cord can cause catastrophic damage, leading to paralysis. Extensive radiation to the abdomen (for lymph node, testicular, or ovarian cancer) can lead to chronic ulcers, scarring, and narrowing or perforation of the intestines.

Prolonged or repeated exposure to low doses of radiation from radioactive implants or because of job-related duties (as occurs with some health care professionals) may cause cessation of menstrual periods (amenorrhea) in women, decreased fertility or sterility, and decreased sex drive (libido).

Occasionally, severe injuries develop long after the completion of radiation therapy. Kidney function may decline 6 months to a year after a person has received extremely large amounts of radiation, resulting in anemia and high blood pressure. High accumulated doses of radiation to muscles may cause a painful condition that includes muscle wasting (atrophy) and calcium deposits in the irradiated muscle. Very rarely, these changes result in a cancerous (malignant) muscle tumor. Radiation-induced cancers typically occur 10 or more years after exposure.

Diagnosis

Exposure to radiation is usually obvious from the history.

Irradiation injury is suspected when a person becomes ill after receiving radiation therapy or being exposed to radiation in an accident. No specific tests are available to diagnose the condition, although certain tests may be used to detect infection, low blood count, or organ malfunction. To determine the severity of radiation exposure, doctors measure the number of lymphocytes (a type of white blood cell) in the blood. The lower the lymphocyte count 48 hours after exposure, the worse the radiation exposure.

Radioactive contamination, unlike irradiation, can be determined by surveying a person's body with a Geiger counter, a device that detects radiation. Swabs from the nose, throat, and any wounds also are checked for radioactivity.

Prognosis and Treatment

The outcome depends on the dose, dose rate (how quickly the exposure has occurred), and distribution over the body as well as on the person's underlying state of health. In general, most people who have received more than 6 Gy of radiation at once die. Because doctors are unlikely to know the measured amount of radiation a person has received, they usually judge outcome by the person's symptoms. The cerebrovascular syndrome is fatal within hours to a few days. The gastrointestinal syndrome generally is fatal within 3 to 10 days, although some people survive for a few weeks. Many people who receive proper medical care survive the hematopoietic syndrome, depending on their total amount of radiation; those who do not survive typically die after 8 to 50 days.

Irradiation has no emergency treatment, but doctors closely monitor the person for the development of the various syndromes and treat the symptoms as they arise.

Contamination requires immediate removal of the radioactive material to prevent it from being taken up by the body. Skin contaminated by radioactive materials should be scrubbed immediately with large amounts of soap and water or with a solution designed for this purpose, when available. Small puncture wounds should be cleaned vigorously to remove all radioactive particles, even though scrubbing may cause pain. Contaminated hair is clipped off, not shaved—shaving may abrade the skin and allow contamination to enter the body. Scrubbing continues until the Geiger counter shows that the radioactivity is gone. If a person has recently swallowed radioactive material, vomiting is induced. Some radioactive materials have specific antidotes that can prevent absorption of swallowed material. Most such antidotes are given only to people exposed to significant radioactive contamination, such as from a major reactor accident or nuclear explosion. Potassium iodide prevents the thyroid gland from absorbing radioactive iodine and lowers the risk of thyroid cancer. Other drugs, such as pentetic acid (DTPA), ethylenediaminetetraacetic acid (EDTA), and penicillamine, can be given intravenously to remove certain radioactive elements after they have been absorbed.

When contamination is not suspected, nausea and vomiting can be reduced by taking drugs to prevent vomiting (antiemetics); such drugs are routinely given to people undergoing radiation therapy. Dehydration is treated with fluids given intravenously.

People with the gastrointestinal or hematopoietic syndrome are kept isolated so that they do not contact infectious microorganisms. Blood transfusions and injections of growth factors (such as erythropoietin and colony-stimulating factor) that stimulate blood cell production are given to decrease bleeding and increase blood counts. If the bone marrow is severely damaged, these growth factors are ineffective, and sometimes a bone marrow transplantation is performed, although the success rate is low.

People with the gastrointestinal syndrome require antiemetics, fluids given intravenously, and sedatives. Some people may be able to eat a bland diet. Antibiotics, such as neomycin, are given by mouth to kill bacteria in the intestine that may invade the body. Antibiotics as well as antifungal and antiviral drugs also are given intravenously when necessary.

Treatment for the cerebrovascular syndrome is geared toward providing comfort by relieving pain, anxiety, and breathing difficulties. Drugs are given to control seizures.

People with chronic effects of radiation or disorders caused by radiation therapy receive treatment directed at their symptoms. Sores or ulcers can be removed or repaired surgically and can be helped to heal with the use of high-pressure (hyperbaric) oxygen therapy. Radiation-induced leukemia is treated with chemotherapy. Blood cells can be replaced through transfusions. No treatment can reverse sterility, but low levels of sex hormones as a result of abnormal ovarian and testicular functioning can be treated with replacement hormones. Investigators are currently exploring ways to prevent or reduce radiation-induced normal tissue injury using cytokines, growth factors, and various other therapies. Amifostine has been shown to decrease the severity of dry mouth (xerostomia) in people with head and neck cancer treated with radiation therapy.

CHAPTER 293

Electrical and Lightning Injuries

Injuries can result from spontaneous atmospheric electricity (lightning injuries) or generated electricity, such as household or industrial electrical currents (electrical injuries). Electrical current passing through the body generates heat, which burns and destroys tissues. Burns can affect internal tissues as well as the skin. An electrical shock can short-circuit the body's own electrical systems, causing nerves to stop transmitting impulses or to transmit impulses erratically. Abnormal impulse transmission can affect the muscles, causing them to contract violently; the heart, causing it to stop beating (cardiac arrest); or the brain, causing seizures, loss of consciousness, or other abnormalities.

Electrical Injuries

An electrical injury occurs when a current passes through the body, interfering with the function of an internal organ or sometimes burning tissue.

Electrical injury may result from contact with faulty electrical appliances or machinery or inadvertent contact with household wiring or electrical power lines. Electrical injury can also occur from lightning.▲ The severity of the injury ranges from minor to fatal and is determined by the intensity of the current, the

▲ see page 1663

type of current, the pathway of the current through the body, the duration of exposure to the current, and electrical resistance to the current.

The intensity of the current is measured in volts. Ordinary household current in the United States is 110 to 220 volts. Anything over 500 volts is considered high voltage. High voltage can jump (arc) through the air anywhere from an inch up to several feet, depending on the voltage. Thus a person may be injured simply by coming too close to a high-voltage line. High voltage causes more severe injuries than low voltage and is more likely to cause internal damage. Kidney damage may result when high voltage burns large amounts of muscle, which releases a chemical into the blood (rhabdomyolysis).▲

Electrical current is categorized as direct current (DC) or alternating current (AC). Direct current, such as current generated by batteries, flows in the same direction constantly. Alternating current, such as current available through household wall sockets, changes direction periodically. Alternating current, which is used in most households in the United States, is more dangerous than direct current. Direct current tends to cause a single muscle contraction often strong enough to force the person away from the current's source. Alternating current causes a continuing muscle contraction, often preventing people from releasing their grip on the current's source. As a result, exposure may be prolonged. Even a small amount of alternating current—barely enough to be felt as a mild shock—may cause a person's grip to freeze. Slightly more alternating current can cause the chest muscles to contract, making breathing impossible. Still more current can cause deadly heart rhythms.

The path that the current takes through the body determines which tissues are affected. The most common entry point for electricity is the hand; the second most common is the head. The most common exit point is the foot. A current that travels from arm to arm or from arm to leg may go through the heart and is much more dangerous than a current that travels between a leg and the ground. A current that travels through the head may affect the brain.

Tissues differ in susceptibility to electrical damage. For example, nerves, blood vessels, and muscle tend to be more easily damaged than bone and tendon. A current passing through a leg or an arm is likely to cause more internal damage than the same current passing across the trunk.

Resistance is the ability to impede the flow of electricity. Most of the body's resistance is concentrated in the skin. The thicker the skin, the greater its resistance. A thick, callused palm or sole, for example, is much more resistant to electrical current than an area of thin skin, such as an inner arm. The skin's resistance decreases when broken (for example, punctured or scraped) or when wet. If skin resistance is high, more of the damage is local, causing only skin burns. If skin resistance is low, more of the damage affects the internal organs. Thus, the damage is mostly internal if a person who is wet comes in contact with electrical current, for example, when a hair dryer falls into a bathtub or a person steps in a puddle that is in contact with a downed electrical line.

Symptoms

Often, the main symptom of an electrical injury is a skin burn,■ although not all electrical injuries cause external damage. High-voltage injuries may cause massive internal burns. If muscle damage is extensive, a limb may swell so much that its arteries become compressed (compartment syndrome★), cutting off blood supply to the limb. If a current travels close to the eyes, it may lead to cataracts. Cataracts can develop within days of the injury or years later.

Toddlers who bite or suck on extension cords can burn their mouth and lips. These burns may cause facial deformities and growth problems of the teeth, jaw, and face. An added danger is that severe bleeding from an artery in the lip may occur when the scab falls off, usually 7 to 10 days after the injury.

A minor shock may cause muscle pain and may trigger mild muscle contractions or startle a person, causing a fall. Severe shocks can cause abnormal heart rhythms, ranging from inconsequential to immediately fatal. The heart's pumping may also become impaired. Severe shocks can also trigger powerful muscle contractions sufficient to throw a person to the ground or to cause joint dislocations, bone fractures, and other blunt injuries. The nerves and brain can be injured in various ways, causing seizures, brain hemorrhages,

---

▲ see page 1649   ■ see page 1648

★ see page 349

poor short-term memory, personality changes, irritability, or difficulty sleeping. Damage to the nerves in the body or spinal cord may cause weakness, paralysis, numbness, tingling, uncontrollable loss of urine (incontinence), and chronic pain.

Prevention

Education about and respect for electricity are essential. Making sure that all electrical devices are properly designed, installed, and maintained helps prevent electrical injuries at home and work. Electrical wiring should be installed and serviced by properly trained people.

Any electrical device that touches or may be touched by the body should be properly grounded. Three-pronged outlets are safest. Cutting off the lower (ground) prong of a power cord with 3 prongs (so that it will fit older two-pronged plugs) is dangerous and increases the chances of electrical injury. Circuit breakers that interrupt (trip) circuits when current as low as 5 milliamperes leaks are advisable in areas that get wet, such as kitchens, bathrooms, and outdoors.

To avoid injury from current that jumps (arcing injury), ladders should not be used near high-voltage power lines.

Treatment

First the person must be separated from the current's source. The safest way to do so is to shut off the current—for example, by throwing a circuit breaker or switch or by disconnecting the device from an electrical outlet. *No one should touch the person until the current has been shut off, particularly if high-voltage lines could be involved.* High-voltage and low-voltage lines are difficult to distinguish, especially outdoors. Shutting off current to high-voltage lines is done by the local power company. Many well-meaning rescuers have been injured by electricity when trying to free a person.

Once the person can be safely touched, the rescuer should check to see if the person is breathing and has a pulse. If the person is not breathing and has no pulse, cardiopulmonary resuscitation (CPR) should be started immediately.▲ Emergency medical assistance should be called for anything more than a minor injury. At the hospital, a doctor checks the person for fractures, dislocations, and spinal cord or other injuries. People with rhabdomyolysis receive large amounts of fluids containing

sodium bicarbonate, which is given intravenously. A tetanus shot is given if needed.

Because the extent of an electrical burn may be deceptive, medical assistance should be sought if any doubt exists regarding severity.

Skin burns are treated with burn cream (such as silver sulfadiazine, bacitracin, or sterile aloe vera) and sterile dressings. A person with only minor skin burns can be treated at home. If the injury is more severe, the person is admitted to the hospital, ideally a burn center. An electrocardiogram (ECG) is performed to monitor the heartbeat and to look for heart damage. If the results of the ECG are abnormal or if the person has lost consciousness, has symptoms of a heart problem (for example, chest pain, shortness of breath, awareness of heartbeats [palpitations]), or has other severe injuries, he is kept in the hospital for 12 to 24 hours. Toddlers who bite or suck on extension cords should be referred to an orthodontist, an oral surgeon, or a surgeon who specializes in burns for follow-up care.

Lightning Injuries

A lightning injury occurs after brief exposure to the very intense current of the strike.

Lightning delivers a massive, very hot electrical pulse over a fraction of a millisecond. The brief duration of the exposure frequently limits the damage to the outer layer of skin. In addition, lightning is much less likely to cause internal burns than generated electricity. However, it can kill a person by instantaneously short-circuiting the heart or brain. Lightning is the second most frequent cause of storm-related deaths in the United States.

Lightning tends to strike tall objects, including trees, gazebos, towers, shelters, flagpoles, bleachers, and fences. A person may be the tallest object in an open field. Metal objects and water easily transmit electricity. Electricity from lightning can travel from outdoor power or telephone lines to electrical equipment or telephone lines inside a house.

Lightning can injure a person in several ways. Lightning can strike a person directly. In addition, electricity can reach a person who is touching or near an object that has been struck. Current can also reach a person through the ground. The shock can also throw a person, producing blunt injuries.

▲ see page 1689

Symptoms

After a person has been struck by lightning, the heart may stop beating or may beat erratically, and breathing often stops. The heart may beat again on its own, but if breathing has not restarted, the body is deprived of oxygen. The lack of oxygen and, possibly, nervous system damage can cause the heart to stop beating again.

Brain injury usually causes loss of consciousness. If brain damage is severe, coma may develop. Typically, the person awakens but does not remember what happened before the injury. The person may be confused, think slowly, and have difficulty concentrating and remembering recent events. Personality changes may occur.

The eardrums are often perforated. Many eye injuries can develop, including cataracts. Often both legs become temporarily paralyzed, blue, and numb (keraunoparalysis). The skin may sustain minor burns that have a feathering, branching pattern, consist of clusters of tiny pinpoint spots like a cigarette burn, or consist of streaks where sweat has been turned into steam.

Prevention

During the thunderstorm season, listening to weather reports, which is particularly important for organizers of outdoor events, can help in deciding whether to cancel outdoor activities and in planning for any emergencies than may develop.

High winds, rain, and clouds may mean that a thunderstorm is imminent. If thunder from a distant storm becomes louder or if the interval between lightning and thunder becomes less than 30 seconds, shelter should be sought. Shelter in small open structures, such as a gazebo, is not safe. Shelter is safer inside large, enclosed buildings or enclosed metal vehicles—such as cars, vans, or trucks—with the vehicle's windows closed. It is not safe to resume outdoor activities until 30 minutes after the last sound of thunder is heard or lightning is seen.

To prevent lightning injury when outdoors, a person should avoid high ground, metal objects, water, and open spaces, such as a field. If escape from the open is not possible, a person should squat to make himself as low as possible but should not lie on the ground. Staying at least 15 feet away from other people is also advised, as is seeking shelter in the middle of a grove of trees (but not under a solitary tree).

To prevent lightning injuries when indoors, a person should avoid contact with water, talking on the telephone, working on a computer, or using headsets attached by a cable to a sound system. Being away from windows and doors increases safety, as does turning off and unplugging electrical equipment before the thunderstorm arrives.

Treatment and Prognosis

Lightning injuries are often unwitnessed and may be suspected when a person is found unconscious outside during a thunderstorm.

A person struck by lightning does not retain electricity, so there is no danger in providing first aid. People without a heartbeat and who are not breathing need cardiopulmonary resuscitation (CPR) immediately.▲ Simply providing artificial respiration to a person struck by lightning may provide enough oxygen to keep the heart beating. Many people struck by lightning are in good general health and are more likely to recover if given timely CPR. In the hospital, an electrocardiogram (ECG) is performed to determine whether the heart is beating normally. Burns and other injuries are treated as needed. If resuscitation efforts are not successful within the first 40 minutes, they are unlikely to be.

About 10% of people with lightning injuries die. Almost all deaths result from cardiac arrest and cessation of breathing. Most people whose heartbeat and breathing resume survive. If memory of recent events is impaired or thinking is slow, the person may have permanent brain injury. Keraunoparalysis usually resolves within several hours.

▲ see page 1689

CHAPTER 294

Near Drowning

Near drowning is severe oxygen deprivation (suffocation) caused by submersion in water but not resulting in death; when death occurs, the event is called drowning.

When a person is submerged under water, water enters the lungs. The vocal cords may go into severe spasm, temporarily preventing water from reaching the lungs. When filled with water, the lungs cannot efficiently transfer oxygen to the blood. The decrease in the level of oxygen in the blood that results may lead to brain damage and death. Water in the lungs, particularly water that is contaminated by bacteria, algae, sand, dirt, chemicals, or a person's vomit, can cause lung injury.

Children younger than 4 years are at greatest risk of near drowning because their energy and curiosity can easily lead them to fall into water, including bathtubs and large buckets, from which they cannot escape. In teenagers and adults, near drowning is common in those who are intoxicated, who have taken sedatives, who have had a seizure, or who are physically impaired because of a medical condition. Spinal injuries and paralysis caused by diving accidents, which are likely to occur when diving into shallow water, increase the chances of near drowning. People who intentionally hold their breath under water for extended periods may pass out and be unable to surface, thus increasing the risk of near drowning as well.

Submersion in cold water has both good and bad effects. Cooling of the muscles makes swimming difficult, and dangerously low body temperature (hypothermia) can impair judgment. Cold, however, protects tissues from the ill effects of oxygen deprivation. In addition, cold water may stimulate the mammalian diving reflex, which may prolong survival in cold water. The diving reflex slows the heartbeat and redirects the flow of blood from the hands, feet, and intestine to the heart and brain, thus helping to preserve these vital organs. The diving reflex is more pronounced in children than in adults; thus children have a greater chance of surviving prolonged submersion in cold water than adults.

Symptoms and Diagnosis

People who are drowning and struggling to breathe are usually unable to call for help. Children who are unable to swim may become submerged in less than 1 minute compared with adults, who may struggle longer.

People who are rescued may have symptoms ranging from anxiety to near death. They may be alert, drowsy, or comatose. Some may not be breathing. People who are breathing may gasp for breath or vomit, cough, or wheeze. The skin may appear blue (cyanosis), indicating insufficient oxygen in the blood. In some cases, respiratory problems may not become evident for several hours after near drowning.

A doctor diagnoses near drowning based on the events and the person's symptoms. Measurement of the level of oxygen in the blood and chest x-rays help reveal the extent of lung damage.

Prevention

Swimming pools should be adequately fenced, because they are one of the most common sites of near-drowning accidents. In addition, all doors and gates leading to the pool area should be locked. Children in or near any body of water, including pools and bathtubs, need constant supervision, regardless of whether flotation devices are used. Because a child can drown in only a few inches of water, even water-filled containers, such as buckets or ice chests, can be hazardous.

A person should not engage in swimming or boating when under the influence of alcohol or sedatives. Swimming should be curtailed if a person feels or looks very cold. People who have seizures that are well controlled need not avoid swimming but should be careful near water, whether boating, showering, or bathing.

To decrease the risk of drowning, a person should not swim alone and should swim only in areas patrolled by lifeguards. Ocean swimmers should learn to escape rip currents (strong currents that pull away from the shore) by swimming parallel to the beach rather than by swimming toward the beach. Wearing life jackets when in boats is encouraged for everyone and is required for nonswimmers and for small children, who should also wear a life jacket when playing near bodies of water. Spinal injuries can be prevented by not diving into shallow water.

Treatment

Immediate on-site resuscitation is the key to increasing the chance of survival without brain damage. Attempts should be made to revive the person even when the time under water is prolonged. Artificial respiration and CPR should be provided as necessary.▲ The neck should be moved as little as possible if there is a chance of spinal injury. Anyone who nearly drowns must be transported to a hospital, by ambulance if possible.

In the hospital, most people need supplemental oxygen, in some cases given with the help of a ventilator. A ventilator can deliver oxygen using high pressures to reinflate collapsed sections of the lungs. If wheezing develops, bronchodilator drugs can help. In some cases, treatment with oxygen in a high-pressure (hyperbaric) chamber may be tried.

If the water was cold, the person may have a dangerously low body temperature (hypothermia) and may need warming.■ Spinal injury requires special treatment.★

If a person who was submerged has only mild symptoms, discharge home may be possible, but only after several hours of observation in the emergency department. If symptoms persist for a few hours, or if the level of oxygen in the blood is low, the person needs to be admitted to the hospital.

Prognosis

The factors that most influence the chances of survival without permanent brain and lung damage are the duration of submersion, the water temperature (cold water accidents can have a better outcome), the person's age (children are more likely to have a better outcome), and how soon resuscitation begins. People who have consumed alcoholic beverages before submersion are especially likely to die or develop brain or lung damage. Survival is possible after submersion for as long as 40 minutes. Almost all people who are alert and conscious upon their arrival at the hospital recover fully. Many people who need CPR can also recover fully.

CHAPTER 295

Diving and Compressed Air Injuries

People who engage in deep-sea or scuba diving are at risk of a number of injuries. Diving in cold water can rapidly lead to hypothermia (dangerously low body temperature), which causes clumsiness and poor judgment. Cold water can also trigger fatal heartbeat irregularities in people with coronary heart disease. Other potential diving hazards include drowning; bites and stings from various marine life; sunburn and heat disorders; cuts and bruises; and motion sickness. Drugs (both legal and illegal) and alcohol may have unanticipated, dangerous effects at depth.

Most diving-related disorders, however, are associated with changes in pressure. These disorders also can affect people who work in underwater tunnels or caissons (watertight enclosures used for construction work). Such structures contain air under high pressure to keep out water.

High pressure under water is caused by the weight of the water above, just as barometric (atmospheric) pressure on land is caused by the weight of the air above. In diving, underwater pressure is often expressed in units of depth (feet or meters) or atmospheres absolute. Pressure in atmospheres absolute includes the weight of the water, which at about 33 feet is 1 atmosphere (14.7 pounds per square inch), plus the atmospheric pressure at

---

▲ see page 1689   ■ see page 1655

★ see page 561

the surface, which is 1 atmosphere. So a diver at a depth of 33 feet is exposed to a total pressure of 2 atmospheres absolute, or twice the atmospheric pressure at the surface. With each additional 33 feet of depth, the pressure increases by 1 atmosphere.

Diving disorders can be divided into two categories: Those that result from expansion or compression of gas-filled spaces in the body (barotrauma) and those that result from dissolved nitrogen in the blood and tissues (decompression sickness).

Barotrauma

Barotrauma is tissue injury caused by a change in pressure, which compresses or expands gas contained in various body structures.

Increased pressure outside the body is transmitted equally throughout the blood and body tissues, which do not compress because they are composed mainly of liquid. Thus, a person's leg, for example, does not feel squeezed as water pressure increases. However, gases (such as the air inside the lungs, sinuses, or middle ear or inside a face mask or goggles) compress or expand as outside pressure increases or decreases. This compression and expansion can cause pain and damage to tissue.

NONPULMONARY BAROTRAUMA

Nonpulmonary barotrauma is injury to gasfilled parts of the body other than the lungs caused by increasing pressure that occurs during descent.

At 2 atmospheres absolute pressure (a depth of about 33 feet), air in gas-filled structures of the body is compressed to one half its original volume. If the pressure inside these structures is not equalized with surrounding water pressure, the pressure difference can strain and damage the surrounding tissue.

Symptoms

Divers often use the term "squeeze" for injuries caused by differences in pressure. If a diver does not properly equalize pressure in the face mask, the relatively lower pressure inside the mask causes it to act like a suction cup applied to the eyes. The difference in pressure inside and outside the mask causes blood vessels near the surface of the eyes to dilate, leak fluid, and finally burst and bleed. Al-

though the eyes appear red and bloodshot, vision is not affected.

If pressure in the middle ear becomes lower than the water pressure, the resulting stress causes a painful inward bulge of the eardrum.▲ When the pressure becomes high enough, the eardrum ruptures, resulting in a rush of cold water into the middle ear, causing vertigo (severe dizziness with a spinning sensation), disorientation, nausea, and sometimes vomiting. These symptoms may place the diver at risk of drowning. The vertigo diminishes as the water in the ear reaches body temperature. A ruptured eardrum impairs hearing and may lead to a middle ear infection, causing pain and producing discharge from the ear. The inner ear can be injured as well, causing a sudden loss of hearing, buzzing in the ear (tinnitus), and vertigo.

Pressure differences have similar effects on the sinuses (air-filled pockets in the bones around the nose), causing facial pain or headaches, and on the air-filled pockets in or under a tooth or filling, causing toothache.

People who dive while holding their breath may feel a sensation of their chest being squeezed when descending. This sensation is not experienced by those who breathe compressed air while diving.

Prevention and Treatment

Pressure in the lungs and airways is automatically equalized with outside pressure when a supply of pressurized air is available at depth, as from a diving helmet or air tank. This pressurized air also equalizes pressure in the sinuses, as long as the openings to the sinuses are not narrowed by inflammation due to allergies or an upper respiratory tract infection. Pressure in a face mask is equalized by blowing out air from the nose into the mask. Divers equalize pressure differences in the middle ear by yawning or swallowing, which opens the tube connecting the middle ear and the back of the throat (eustachian tube).

Wearing earplugs or a tight-fitting wet suit hood creates a closed space between the earplug and the eardrum in which pressure cannot be equalized. The pressure inside goggles cannot be equalized either. Therefore, neither earplugs nor goggles should be worn during diving.

▲ see art on page 1257

When nasal congestion prevents pressure in the ears and sinuses from being equalized, decongestants (such as pseudoephedrine taken by mouth before diving) may temporarily unclog blocked nasal passages, eustachian tubes, or sinuses.

A ruptured eardrum usually heals by itself, although a middle ear infection requires antibiotics given by mouth or as eardrops. A rupture between the middle and inner ear may require prompt surgical repair to prevent permanent damage.

PULMONARY BAROTRAUMA

Pulmonary barotrauma is injury caused by the expansion of air held in the lungs due to decreasing pressure during ascent.

Because air under high pressure is compressed, each breath taken at depth contains many more molecules than a breath taken at the surface. At 33 feet (2 atmospheres absolute), for example, each breath contains twice as many molecules as a breath taken at the surface (and therefore depletes an air tank twice as rapidly). As pressure decreases, air expands—its volume increases. So if a diver fills his lungs with compressed air at 33 feet and ascends without freely exhaling, the volume of air doubles, causing the lungs to overinflate.

Overinflation of the lungs can rupture small air sacs, allowing air to leak out. Air bubbles can enter the blood (air embolism▲) and travel to any organ in the body and block small blood vessels, most commonly those of the brain and heart. At best, air embolism places the diver at risk of drowning. At worst, the diver may die within minutes. Air embolism is a leading cause of death among divers.

Air that leaks out of the lungs can be trapped in the space between the lungs and the chest wall, causing the lung to collapse (pneumothorax■). Alternatively, air may be forced out of the lungs into the tissues surrounding the heart (pneumomediastinum) and under the skin of the neck and upper chest (subcutaneous emphysema).

The most common cause of pulmonary barotrauma is breath-holding during an ascent from a scuba dive, typically resulting from running out of air at depth. In panic, a diver may forget to exhale freely as air in the lungs expands during the ascent. Air embolism can occur in as little as 4 feet of water if a person breathing pressurized air holds his breath while ascending.

Symptoms

Symptoms of air embolism usually appear within 1 to 2 minutes of reaching the surface. Air embolism to the brain often resembles a stroke, resulting in headache, confusion, agitation, and partial paralysis. Some people have sudden loss of consciousness or seizures. Severe air embolism can block blood flow through the heart and the large arteries, leading to shock★ and death.

Pneumothorax and pneumomediastinum cause chest pain and shortness of breath. Some people cough up blood or develop bloody froth at the mouth. Air in the tissues of the neck can impair the vocal cords, causing the voice to sound different. Subcutaneous emphysema produces a crackling sensation when the affected area of skin is touched.

Prevention and Treatment

To prevent pulmonary barotrauma, divers using an air supply, such as a scuba tank, must not hold their breath during ascent. Any air inhaled at depth—even the depth of a swimming pool—must be exhaled freely during ascent.

A diver who loses consciousness during ascent or very shortly afterward is assumed to have air embolism and must be treated promptly. A person who has air embolism is given oxygen immediately and must be returned at once to a high-pressure environment, so that the air bubbles are compressed and forced to dissolve in the blood. A number of medical centers have high-pressure (recompression or hyperbaric) chambers for this purpose. Flying, even at a low altitude, reduces atmospheric pressure and allows bubbles to expand further, but it can be justified if it saves substantial time in getting the person to a suitable chamber. If possible, the person should fly in a plane pressurized to sea level, or the plane should not fly above 1,000 feet.

A small pneumothorax does not require treatment, but a large pneumothorax causes severe breathing problems and requires insertion of a plastic tube into the chest to remove the air. Treatment of pneumomediastinum and subcutaneous emphysema usually is bed rest and oxygen given through a face mask.

▲ see page 286

■ see page 316

★ see page 148

Decompression Sickness

Decompression sickness (decompression illness, caisson disease, the bends) is a disorder in which nitrogen dissolved in the blood and tissues by high pressure forms bubbles as pressure decreases.

Air is composed mainly of nitrogen and oxygen. Because air under high pressure is compressed, each breath taken at depth contains many more molecules than a breath taken at the surface. Because oxygen is used continuously by the body, the extra oxygen molecules breathed under high pressure usually do not accumulate. However, the extra nitrogen molecules do accumulate in the blood and tissues. As outside pressure decreases during ascent from a dive or when leaving a caisson, the accumulated nitrogen that cannot be exhaled immediately forms bubbles in the blood and tissues. These bubbles may expand and injure tissue, or they may block blood vessels in many organs—either directly or by triggering small blood clots. This blood vessel blockage causes pain and a variety of other symptoms. Nitrogen bubbles also cause inflammation, producing swelling and pain in muscles, joints, and tendons.

The risk of developing decompression sickness increases with increasing pressure (that is, the depth of the dive) and with the length of time spent in a pressurized environment. Other risk factors include rapid ascent, fatigue, exertion, dehydration, cold water, obesity, and older age. Because excess nitrogen remains dissolved in the body tissues for at least 12 hours after each dive, repeated dives within 1 day are more likely to cause decompression sickness than a single dive. Flying immediately after diving (such as at the end of a vacation)

Breathing Air Under High Pressure

Air is a mixture of gases, mainly nitrogen and oxygen with very small amounts of other gases. Each gas has a partial pressure, based on its concentration in the air and on the atmospheric pressure. Both oxygen and nitrogen can have harmful effects at high partial pressures.

Oxygen toxicity occurs in most people when the partial pressure of oxygen reaches 1.6 atmospheres, equivalent to slightly over 200 feet depth when breathing air. Symptoms include tingling, focal seizures (facial or lip twitching), vertigo, nausea and vomiting, and constricted vision. About 10% of people have seizures or fainting, which typically results in drowning.

Nitrogen narcosis (rapture of the deep) is caused by high partial pressures of nitrogen and resembles alcohol intoxication. People become euphoric and disoriented and show very poor judgment. They may fail to surface on time or even swim deeper, thinking they are going to the surface. This effect becomes noticeable at 100 feet in most divers breathing compressed air and is usually incapacitating at 300 feet (about 10 atmospheres absolute).

To minimize these effects, divers who must dive to great depths typically breathe a special mixture of gases rather than regular air. Low concentrations of oxygen are used, diluted with helium or hydrogen rather than nitrogen, because helium and hydrogen do not produce narcosis.

A buildup of carbon dioxide in the bloodstream is the body's signal to breathe. Divers, such as snorkelers, who hold their breath rather than use a breathing apparatus, often breathe vigorously (hyperventilate) before a dive, breathing out a large amount of carbon dioxide but adding little oxygen to the blood. This maneuver allows them to hold their breath and swim under water longer because their carbon dioxide levels are low. However, this maneuver is also hazardous because a diver can run out of oxygen and lose consciousness before the carbon dioxide reaches a level high enough to signal the need to return to the surface and breathe. This sequence of events is probably responsible for many unexplained drownings among spearfishing competitors and others who hold their breath while diving.

Some scuba divers have carbon dioxide buildup because they do not increase their breathing adequately during exertion. Others retain carbon dioxide because the compressed air at depth is denser and requires greater effort to move it through a diver's airways and breathing apparatus. High carbon dioxide levels can lead to blackouts, increase the likelihood of seizures from oxygen toxicity, and worsen the severity of nitrogen narcosis. Divers who frequently have headaches after diving or who pride themselves on using air at a low rate may be retaining carbon dioxide.

High Risk Factors for Diving

Prospective divers should be evaluated for fitness and for the following physical and mental conditions that can increase the risk of mishaps and injury during diving by a doctor who is familiar with diving:

- Alcohol or drug abuse
- Chronic or short-term congestion of the nose and sinuses
- Diabetes, type 1
- Drugs that can cause drowsiness
- Epilepsy
- Fainting spells
- Impulsive behavior; prone to accidents
- Irregular heart rhythms
- Lung problems such as asthma, lung cysts, emphysema, a history of pneumothorax
- Obesity*
- Older age*
- Open foramen ovale (a congenital heart defect)
- Physical disabilities
- Poor cardiovascular fitness
- Pregnancy
- Ruptured eardrum

Professional divers may undergo additional medical tests, such as those for heart and lung function, exercise stress, hearing, and vision, as well as bone x-rays. In addition, adequate diver training is absolutely necessary.

*Higher risk of decompression sickness.

exposes a person to an even lower atmospheric pressure, making decompression sickness slightly more likely.

Nitrogen bubbles may form in small blood vessels or in the tissues themselves. Tissues with a high fat content, such as those in the central nervous system, are particularly likely to be affected, because nitrogen dissolves very readily in fats.

Decompression sickness may affect a variety of organs and can range from mild to severe.

Symptoms

Symptoms of decompression sickness develop more slowly than do those of pulmonary barotrauma. Only half of the people with decompression sickness have symptoms within 1 hour of surfacing, but 90% have symptoms by 6 hours. Symptoms commonly begin gradually and take some time to reach their maximum effect.

The less severe type (or musculoskeletal form) of decompression sickness (type I), often called **the bends,** typically produces pain. The pain usually occurs in the joints of the arms or legs. Sometimes the location is hard to pinpoint. The pain may be mild or intermittent at first but may steadily grow stronger and become severe. The pain may be sharp or may be described as "deep" or "like something boring into bone." Less common symptoms include itching, skin mottling, and extreme fatigue. These symptoms do not threaten life but may precede more dangerous problems.

The more severe type of decompression sickness (type II) most commonly results in neurologic symptoms, which range from mild numbness to paralysis and death. The spinal cord is especially vulnerable. When the spinal cord is affected, numbness, tingling, and weakness in the arms, legs, or both may result. Mild weakness or tingling may progress over hours to irreversible paralysis. Inability to urinate may also occur. Abdominal and back pain also are common. Symptoms of brain involvement, which are similar to those of air embolism, are headache, confusion, trouble speaking, and double vision. Loss of consciousness is rare.

The nerves of the inner ear may be affected, causing severe vertigo (the "staggers"). Gas bubbles that travel through the veins to the lungs produce cough, chest pain, and progressively worsening difficulty breathing (the "chokes"). Severe cases may result in circulatory collapse and death.

Late effects of decompression sickness include the destruction of bone tissue (dysbaric osteonecrosis, avascular bone necrosis), especially in the shoulder and hip, which produces persistent pain and severe disability. These injuries are not found among recreational divers but, rather, among people who work in a compressed-air environment and divers who work in underwater habitats. These workers are exposed to high pressure for prolonged periods and may have an undetected case of the bends. Bone and joint injuries may gradually progress over months or years to severe, disabling arthritis. By the time severe joint damage has occurred, the only treatment may be joint replacement.

Permanent neurologic problems, such as partial paralysis, usually result from delayed or inadequate treatment of spinal cord symptoms. However, sometimes the damage is too severe to correct, even with appropriate treatment. Repeated treatments with oxygen in a high-pressure chamber seem to help some people recover from spinal cord damage.

Diagnosis and Treatment

Doctors recognize decompression sickness by the nature of the symptoms and their onset in relation to diving. Tests such as computed tomography (CT) or magnetic resonance imaging (MRI) sometimes show brain or spinal cord abnormalities but are not reliable. However, recompression therapy is begun before the results of a CT or MRI scan are available, except in cases in which the diagnosis is uncertain or the diver's condition is stable.

Divers reporting only itching, skin mottling, and fatigue usually do not need to undergo recompression, but they should be kept under observation, because more serious problems may follow. Breathing 100% oxygen from a close-fitting face mask may provide relief.

Any other symptoms of decompression sickness indicate the need for treatment in a high-pressure (recompression or hyperbaric oxygen) chamber, because recompression restores normal blood flow and oxygen to affected tissues. After recompression, pressure is reduced gradually, with designated pauses, allowing time for excess gases to leave the body harmlessly. Because symptoms may reappear or worsen over the first 24 hours, even people with only mild or transient pain or neurologic symptoms are treated.

Recompression therapy is beneficial for up to 48 hours after diving and should be given even if reaching the nearest chamber requires significant travel. While awaiting and during transport, oxygen is administered with a close-fitting face mask, and fluids are given by mouth or intravenously. Long delays in treatment increase the risk of permanent injury.

Prevention

A diver can usually prevent decompression sickness by restricting the total amount of gas his body absorbs. The amount can be restricted by limiting the depth and duration of dives to a range that does not need decompression stops during ascent (called no-stop limits by divers) or by ascending with decompression stops as specified in authoritative guidelines, such as the decompression table in the *United States Navy Diving Manual*. The table provides a schedule for ascent that usually allows excess nitrogen to escape without causing harm. Many divers now wear a portable dive computer that continually tracks the diver's depth and time at depth. The computer calculates the decompression schedule for a safe return to the surface and indicates when decompression stops are needed.

In addition to following a table or computer guidelines for ascent, many divers make a safety stop of a few minutes at about 15 feet below the surface.

Following these procedures, however, does not eliminate the risk of decompression sickness. About 50% of cases of decompression sickness develop after no-stop dives, and the incidence of decompression sickness has not declined despite the widespread use of dive computers. The inability to eliminate decompression sickness may be because the published tables and computer programs do not completely account for the variation in risk factors among different divers or because some people fail to obey the recommendations of the tables or computer.

Other precautions also are necessary. After several days of diving, a period of 12 to 24 hours at the surface is commonly recommended before flying or going to a higher altitude. People who have completely recovered from mild decompression sickness should refrain from diving for at least 2 weeks. People who have developed decompression sickness despite following dive table or computer recommendations should return to diving only after a thorough medical evaluation for underlying risk factors, such as a heart defect. The Divers Alert Network (919-684-8111) provides 24-hour consultation for diving-related problems.

Altitude Illness

Altitude illness occurs because of a lack of oxygen at high altitudes.

As altitude increases, the atmospheric pressure decreases, thinning the air so that less oxygen is available. For example, compared with the air at sea level, the air in Denver (about 5,300 feet above sea level) contains 20% less available oxygen; the air in Aspen, Colorado (about 8,000 feet above sea level), about 25% less oxygen; and the air near the top of Mount Everest (more than 29,000 feet above sea level), about 66% less oxygen.

Altitude illness occurs when an oxygen deficiency at high altitudes causes fluid in the blood to leak from the smallest blood vessels (capillaries) into the surrounding tissues, resulting in swelling (edema). The forms of altitude illness differ mainly in their degree of severity and where in the body the fluid accumulates. Mild fluid accumulation in the brain causes acute mountain sickness, whereas more severe fluid accumulation in the brain causes high-altitude cerebral edema. Fluid accumulation in the lungs causes high-altitude pulmonary edema. Fluid accumulation in the hands, feet, and face causes high-altitude edema.

Altitude illness is common in people visiting high altitudes. The severity of the illness depends on how high and how quickly a person ascends. For example, most people who, within a day or two, ascend to above 6,000 feet develop high-altitude edema. Acute mountain sickness develops in 10% of people who ascend too rapidly above 8,000 feet, in 25% of people above 9,000 feet, and in almost 50% of people above 14,000 feet. High-altitude pulmonary edema and high-altitude cerebral edema rarely develop at altitudes below 10,000 feet.

People who normally live at sea level or at very low altitudes are more likely to be affected by altitude illness, as are those who engage in strenuous exertion soon after ascent. People with certain lung diseases (such as chronic obstructive pulmonary disease), heart and blood vessel disorders (such as angina, heart failure, or peripheral vascular disease), or blood disorders (such as sickle cell anemia or hemoglobin S-C disease) may have particular difficulties at high altitudes. Asthma, however, does not seem to be worse at high altitudes. Spending less than a few weeks at altitudes below 10,000 feet does not appear to be dangerous for a pregnant woman or the fetus. Physical fitness has no effect on a person's risk of developing altitude illness. Fewer older people than young people develop altitude illness. People who have had high-altitude pulmonary edema and high-altitude cerebral edema previously are particularly likely to develop those conditions again after ascent.

The body eventually adjusts (acclimatizes) to higher altitudes by increasing respiration and heart activity and by producing more red blood cells to carry oxygen to the tissues. Most people can adjust to altitudes of up to 10,000 feet in a few days. Adjusting to much higher altitudes takes many days or weeks, but some people can eventually carry out normal activities at altitudes above 17,500 feet.

Symptoms and Diagnosis

Acute mountain sickness is a mild form of altitude illness. Symptoms usually develop within 4 to 12 hours of ascent and include headache, light-headedness, and, particularly with exercise, shortness of breath. Loss of appetite and nausea and vomiting may follow, along with fatigue, weakness, and irritability. Some people describe the symptoms as similar to those of a hangover. People who stay overnight at a high altitude may have trouble sleeping. Symptoms usually last 24 to 36 hours. However, acute mountain sickness may progress to more severe forms of altitude illness.

High-altitude edema causes swelling of the hands, the feet, and, on awakening, the face. The swelling causes little discomfort and usually subsides in a few days.

High-altitude pulmonary edema may progress from a mild illness to a life-threatening one within a few hours. Symptoms often develop during the second night after ascent, are worse at night, and can become progressively more severe. Mild symptoms usually include a dry cough and shortness of breath after only mild exertion. Moderate symptoms include shortness of breath at rest; confusion; pink or bloody sputum; low-grade fever; and a bluish

Other Illnesses that Develop at High Altitudes

Some illnesses develop at high altitudes for reasons unrelated to the fluid accumulation that causes altitude illness.

High-altitude retinal hemorrhages (small areas of bleeding in the retina at the back of the eye) may develop after ascent to altitudes of 8,000 feet or higher. Retinal hemorrhages rarely produce symptoms. However, if a hemorrhage occurs in the part of the eye that is responsible for central vision (the macula), the person may notice a small blind spot. High-altitude retinal hemorrhages resolve after 1 or 2 weeks without treatment. If hemorrhage involves the macula, the person should descend.

Snow blindness, which is a sunburn of the eye, often develops at high altitudes. Ultraviolet (UV) light becomes about 5% stronger every 1,000 feet above sea level. Reflection from the snow makes the light even more intense. Even on cloudy days, strong UV light burns the eye. Symptoms of snow blindness develop 6 to 12 hours after a burn is sustained. The eye becomes painful, red, swollen, and sensitive to light and feels gritty. Analgesics, cool compresses, and eye patches usually help. Anesthetic drops should not be used; instead, a drop of mineral oil may relieve pain. Symptoms disappear within about 24 hours. To prevent snow blindness, strong sunglasses with side shields should be worn.

High-altitude pharyngitis and bronchitis often develop at altitudes higher than 10,000 feet. The dry, cold air irritates the throat and lungs, causing a sore throat and a hacking cough. The cough can become severe enough to fracture ribs. Drinking a lot of fluids and increasing salivation by sucking hard candies can relieve symptoms. Masks made of silk or similar materials may also help by trapping moist, hot exhaled air within the mouth and nose. Antibiotics rarely help.

Chronic mountain sickness (Monge's disease) is an uncommon illness that develops in some people who live at altitudes higher than 12,000 feet for many months or years. In these people, the body overcompensates for the lack of oxygen by overproducing red blood cells (secondary polycythemia▲). The extra red blood cells make the blood so thick that it cannot pass easily through small blood vessels. Symptoms include headache, muddled thinking, difficulty sleeping, drowsiness, aches and pains, and shortness of breath. Blood clots may form in the legs and lungs, and the heart may become unable to pump enough blood. Periodic removal of a pint of blood (phlebotomy) provides temporary relief, but the only effective treatment is descent to sea level. Complete recovery can take months.

---

tinge to the skin, lips, and nails (cyanosis). Severe symptoms include gasping for breath and making gurgling sounds while breathing.

High-altitude cerebral edema is present in a mild form in other types of altitude illness but may become severe. It causes headache, confusion, walking that is unsteady and uncoordinated (ataxia), and coma. These symptoms may progress rapidly from mild to life-threatening within a few hours.

A doctor diagnoses altitude illness based mainly on the symptoms. In high-altitude pulmonary edema, fluid can sometimes be heard in the lungs through a stethoscope. An x-ray of the chest and measurement of the amount of oxygen in the blood can help confirm the diagnosis.

Treatment

People with acute mountain sickness must stop their ascent and rest. They should not ascend to higher altitudes until symptoms disappear. Most people with acute mountain sickness improve within a day or two. Acetazolamide or corticosteroids, such as dexamethasone, may help relieve symptoms. Acetaminophen or nonsteroidal anti-inflammatory drugs (NSAIDs)■ help relieve headache.

If symptoms are more severe, supplemental oxygen should be provided through a face mask. If supplemental oxygen is unavailable, however, or if symptoms persist or worsen despite treatment, the person should descend to a lower altitude, preferably at least 2,500 feet lower.

If high-altitude edema is troublesome, diuretics, such as hydrochlorothiazide, can be helpful. However, the swelling resolves after descent, regardless of treatment.

People with high-altitude pulmonary edema should receive oxygen and, if there is no rapid improvement, descend as soon as possible. However, unnecessary exertion should be

---

▲ see box on page 1024   ■ see page 452

avoided, because it increases the body's need for oxygen, thus worsening symptoms of high-altitude pulmonary edema. Therefore, the person should be carried to a lower altitude, if possible, and kept warm. The drug nifedipine may temporarily help by decreasing blood pressure in the arteries to the lungs.

If high-altitude cerebral edema develops, the person should descend as far down and as soon as possible. Supplemental oxygen and dexamethasone should be given.

When prompt descent to a lower altitude is not possible, a hyperbaric bag can be used. This device, which consists of a lightweight, portable fabric bag or tent and a manually operated pump, simulates an increase in atmospheric pressure. The person is placed in the bag, which is then tightly sealed. The bag's internal pressure is then increased with the pump. The person remains in the bag for 2 or 3 hours. The hyperbaric bag is as beneficial as supplemental oxygen, which often is not available when mountain climbing.

Prevention

The best way to prevent altitude illness is to ascend slowly, taking 2 days to reach 8,000 feet and another day for each 1,000 to 2,000 additional feet. The altitude at which a person sleeps is more important than the maximum height reached during the day. The pace of as-

cent should be slowed if symptoms of altitude illness develop.

Acetazolamide taken at the start of the ascent can prevent altitude illness. If taken after the illness has begun, acetazolamide may help lessen symptoms. Acetazolamide should be continued for a few days after ascent. Some doctors believe that dexamethasone can also prevent altitude illness and lessen its symptoms. Ginkgo, a medicinal herb, has proved to be moderately effective in preventing altitude illness. If a person has had previous episodes of high-altitude pulmonary edema, nifedipine, given at the start of ascent, may prevent a recurrence.

Avoiding strenuous exertion for a day or two after arrival may prevent altitude illness, as may eating frequent, small high-carbohydrate meals instead of fewer large meals, and drinking at least 4 quarts of noncaffeinated fluids per day. Alcohol and sedatives, which can cause symptoms similar to acute mountain sickness, should be avoided.

Athletes residing at sea level can take certain steps to prepare for competitions held at high altitudes. For brief, high-intensity competitions such as sprints or jumps, for example, performance is best if the person arrives less than 1 day before the event. For endurance competitions, performance is best if for several weeks beforehand the person trains at low altitudes but sleeps at high altitudes.

CHAPTER 297

Poisoning

Poisoning is the harmful effect that occurs when a toxic substance is swallowed, is inhaled, or comes in contact with the skin, eyes, or mucous membranes, such as those of the mouth or nose.

Poisoning is the most common cause of nonfatal accidents in the home. More than 2 million people suffer some type of poisoning each year in the United States. Drugs—prescription, nonprescription, and illegal—are the most common source of serious poisonings

and poisoning-related deaths. Other common poisons include gases, household products, agricultural products, plants, industrial chemicals, vitamins, and foods (particularly certain species of mushrooms and fish▲). However, almost any substance ingested in sufficiently large quantities can be toxic.

Young children are particularly vulnerable to accidental poisoning in the home, as are older people, often from confusion about their drugs. Also vulnerable to accidental poisoning are hospitalized people (from drug errors) and industrial workers (from exposure to toxic chemicals). Poisoning may also be a deliberate

---

▲ see page 725

attempt to commit murder or suicide. Most adults attempting suicide by poisoning take more than one drug and also consume alcohol.

The damage caused by poisoning depends on the poison, the amount taken, and the age and underlying health of the person who takes it. Some poisons are not very potent and cause problems only with prolonged exposure or repeated ingestion of large amounts. Other poisons are so potent that just a drop on the skin can cause severe damage.

Some poisons produce symptoms within seconds, whereas others produce symptoms only after hours or even days. Some poisons produce few obvious symptoms until they have damaged vital organs—such as the kidneys or liver—sometimes permanently.

First Aid and Prevention

Anyone exposed to a toxic gas should be removed from the source quickly, preferably out into fresh air.

In chemical spills, all contaminated clothing should be removed immediately. The skin should be thoroughly washed with soap and water. If the eyes have been exposed, they should be thoroughly flushed with water. Rescuers must be careful to avoid contaminating themselves.

If the person appears very sick, emergency medical assistance (911 in most areas of the United States) should be called. Bystanders should perform cardiopulmonary resuscitation (CPR) if needed.▲ If the person does not appear very sick, family members or coworkers can contact the nearest poison center for advice. In the United States, the local poison center can be reached at 800-222-1222. If the caller knows the identity of the poison and the amount ingested, treatment can often be managed at home.

Containers of the poisons or the drugs taken should be saved and given to the doctor. If the poisoning could be serious, the person must be treated as soon as possible. The poison center may recommend giving activated charcoal■ at home and, occasionally, may recommend giving syrup of ipecac to induce vomiting, particularly if the person must travel far to reach the hospital. To prevent accidental poisoning, drugs should be kept in their original child-resistant containers. Expired drugs should be flushed down the toilet. In addition, drugs and poisonous substances should be kept out of sight and beyond a child's reach, preferably in a locked cabinet.

Nontoxic Household Products*

Adhesives	Magic markers
Antacids	Matches
Bath oil	Mineral oil
Bleach (less than 5% sodium hypochlorite)	Modeling clay
	Newspaper
Body conditioners	Perfumes
Bubble bath soaps (detergents)	Petroleum jelly
	Sachets (essential oils, powders)
Chalk (calcium carbonate)	Shaving creams and lotions
Colognes	Soap and soap products
Cosmetics	
Deodorants	Suntan preparations
Deodorizers, spray and refrigerant	
	Sweetening agents (saccharin, aspartame)
Fabric softeners	
Hand lotions and creams	Toothpaste with or without fluoride
3% hydrogen peroxide, medicinal	
	Water colors
Incense	Wax or paraffin
Indelible markers	Zinc oxide
Ink (black, blue)	Zirconium oxide
"Lead" pencils (which are really made of graphite)	

*Almost any substance can be toxic if ingested in sufficient amounts.

All labels should be read before taking or giving any drugs.

Diagnosis and Treatment

Identifying the poison is crucial to successful treatment. Labels on bottles and other information from the person, family members, or coworkers best enables the doctor or the poison center to identify poisons. Urine and blood tests may help in identification as well. Sometimes, blood tests can reveal how serious the poisoning is.

Many people who have been poisoned must be hospitalized. The principles for the treatment of all poisoning are the same: prevent additional absorption; increase elimination of the poison; give specific antidotes (substances

---

▲ see page 1689   ■ see page 1676

that eliminate, inactivate, or counteract the effects of the poison), if available; and prevent reexposure. With prompt medical care, most people recover fully. The usual goal of hospital treatment is to keep the person alive until the poison disappears or is inactivated. Eventually, most poisons are inactivated by the liver or are passed into the urine.

Stomach emptying may be attempted if an unusually dangerous poison is involved or if the person appears very sick. In this procedure, a tube is inserted through the mouth or nose into the stomach. Water is poured into the stomach through the tube and is then drained out (gastric lavage). This procedure is repeated several times.

For many swallowed poisons, hospital emergency departments usually give activated charcoal. Activated charcoal binds to the poison that is still in the digestive tract, preventing its absorption into the blood. Charcoal is usually taken by mouth but may have to be given through a tube that is inserted through the nose into the stomach. Sometimes doctors give charcoal every several hours to help cleanse the body of the poison.

If a poisoning remains life threatening despite the use of charcoal and antidotes, more complicated treatments may be needed. The most common involve filtering poisons directly from the bloodstream—hemodialysis (which uses an artificial kidney [dialyzer] to filter the poisons▲) or charcoal hemoperfusion (which uses charcoal to help eliminate the poisons). For either of these methods, small tubes (catheters) are inserted into blood vessels, one to drain blood from an artery and another to return blood to a vein. The blood is passed through special filters that remove the toxic substance before being returned to the body.

Poisoning often requires additional treatment. For example, a person who becomes very drowsy or comatose may need a breathing tube inserted into the windpipe. The tube is then attached to a ventilator, which mechanically supports the person's breathing. The tube prevents vomit from entering the lungs, and the ventilator ensures adequate breathing. Treatment also may be needed to control seizures, abnormal heart rhythms, low blood pressure, high blood pressure, fever, or vomiting.

If the kidneys stop working, hemodialysis is necessary. If liver damage is extensive, treat-ment for liver failure may be necessary. If the liver or kidneys sustain permanent, severe damage, organ transplantation may be needed.

People who attempt suicide by poisoning need mental health evaluation and appropriate treatment.

Acetaminophen Poisoning

More than 100 products contain acetaminophen, a common over-the-counter pain reliever.■ If several similar products are consumed at a time, a person may inadvertently take too much acetaminophen. Many preparations intended for use in children are available in liquid, tablet, and capsule form, and a parent may try several preparations simultaneously or within several hours, not realizing they all contain acetaminophen.

Acetaminophen usually is a very safe drug, but it is not harmless. To cause poisoning, several times the recommended dose of acetaminophen must be taken. For example, a person who weighs 150 pounds generally needs to take at least 20 325-mg tablets before toxic effects due to a single overdose are possible. Death is extremely unlikely unless the person takes more than 40 325-mg tablets. In toxic doses, acetaminophen can damage the liver. Liver failure can follow.

Symptoms and Diagnosis

Most overdoses produce no immediate symptoms. The level of acetaminophen in the blood, measured 2 to 4 hours after ingestion, predicts the severity of the liver damage accurately. If the overdose is very large, symptoms develop in four stages. In stage 1 (after several hours), the person may vomit but does not seem ill. Many people have no symptoms until stage 2 (after 24 hours), when nausea, vomiting, and abdominal pain may develop. At this stage, blood tests show that the liver is functioning abnormally. In stage 3 (after 2 to 5 days), vomiting becomes worse. Tests show that the liver is functioning poorly, and jaundice and bleeding develop. In stage 4 (after 5 days), the person either recovers quickly or experiences liver failure, which may prove fatal.

Treatment

If acetaminophen was taken within the previous several hours, activated charcoal is usually given.

If the level of acetaminophen in the blood is high, acetylcysteine is generally given by

▲ see page 834   ■ see page 95

mouth or intravenously to reduce the toxicity of the acetaminophen. Acetylcysteine is given repeatedly, for one to several days. Treatment for liver failure may also be necessary.

Aspirin Poisoning

Ingestion of aspirin and similar drugs (salicylates) can lead to rapid poisoning due to an overdose. The dose necessary to produce rapid poisoning, however, is quite large. A person weighing about 150 pounds would have to consume more than 30 325-mg tablets to develop even mild poisoning. An aspirin overdose, therefore, is seldom accidental.

Gradual aspirin poisoning can develop unintentionally by taking aspirin repeatedly at much lower doses. Children with fever who are given only slightly higher than the prescribed dose of aspirin for several days may develop poisoning. Adults, many of them elderly, can develop poisoning gradually after several weeks of use. The dosage of aspirin recommended to people with coronary artery disease to reduce the risk of heart attack (1 baby aspirin, $\frac{1}{2}$ of an adult aspirin, or 1 full adult aspirin daily) is too small to cause gradual poisoning.

The most toxic form of salicylate is oil of wintergreen (methyl salicylate). Methyl salicylate is a component of products such as liniments and solutions used in hot vaporizers. A young child can die from swallowing less than 1 teaspoonful of pure methyl salicylate. Far less toxic are over-the-counter products containing bismuth subsalicylate (used to treat infections of the digestive tract), which can cause poisoning after several doses.

Symptoms

The first symptoms of rapid aspirin poisoning are usually nausea and vomiting followed by rapid breathing, ringing in the ears, sweating, and sometimes fever. Later, if poisoning is severe, the person can develop light-headedness, drowsiness, confusion, seizures, and difficulty breathing.

The symptoms of gradual aspirin poisoning develop over days or weeks. Drowsiness, confusion, and hallucinations are the most common symptoms. Light-headedness, rapid breathing, and shortness of breath can develop.

Diagnosis and Treatment

A blood sample is taken to measure the precise level of aspirin in the blood. Measurement of the blood pH and the level of carbon dioxide or bicarbonate in the blood also can help determine the severity of poisoning. Tests are usually repeated during treatment to reveal whether the person is recovering.

Activated charcoal reduces aspirin absorption. For moderate or severe poisoning, fluids containing sodium bicarbonate are given intravenously; unless there is kidney damage, potassium is added to the fluid. This mixture moves aspirin from the bloodstream into the urine. If the person's condition is worsening despite other treatments, hemodialysis can remove aspirin from the blood. Vitamin K may be given to treat bleeding problems.

Carbon Monoxide Poisoning

Carbon monoxide is a colorless, odorless gas that, when inhaled, prevents the blood from carrying oxygen and prevents the tissues from using oxygen effectively. Small amounts are not usually harmful, but poisoning occurs if levels of carbon monoxide in the blood become too high. Carbon monoxide disappears from the blood after several hours.

Smoke from fires commonly contains carbon monoxide, particularly when combustion of fuels is incomplete. If improperly vented, automobiles, furnaces, hot water heaters, gas heaters, kerosene heaters, and stoves (including wood stoves and stoves with charcoal briquettes) can cause carbon monoxide poisoning. Inhaling tobacco smoke produces carbon monoxide in the blood, but usually not enough to result in symptoms of poisoning.

Symptoms and Diagnosis

Mild carbon monoxide poisoning causes headache, nausea, vomiting, drowsiness, and poor coordination. Most people who develop mild carbon monoxide poisoning recover quickly when moved into fresh air. Moderate or severe carbon monoxide poisoning causes confusion, unconsciousness, chest pain, shortness of breath, and coma. Thus, most victims are not able to move themselves and must be rescued. Severe poisoning is often fatal. Rarely, weeks after apparent recovery from severe carbon monoxide poisoning, symptoms such as memory loss, poor coordination, and uncontrollable loss of urine (which are referred to as delayed neuropsychiatric symptoms) develop.

Carbon monoxide is dangerous because a person may not recognize drowsiness as a symptom of poisoning. Consequently, someone with mild poisoning can go to sleep and continue to breathe the carbon monoxide until severe poisoning or death occurs. Some people with long-standing, mild carbon monoxide poisoning caused by furnaces or heaters may mistake their symptoms for other conditions, such as the flu or other viral infections.

Carbon monoxide poisoning is diagnosed by measuring the level of carbon monoxide in the blood.

Treatment and Prevention

For mild poisoning, fresh air may be all that is needed. To treat more severe poisoning, high concentrations of oxygen are given, usually through a face mask. Oxygen hastens the disappearance of carbon monoxide from the blood and relieves symptoms. The value of high-pressure oxygen treatment (in a hyperbaric chamber) remains uncertain.

To prevent poisoning, sources of indoor combustion, such as gas space heaters and wood stoves, require properly installed ventilation. If such ventilation is impractical, an open window can limit carbon monoxide accumulation by allowing it to escape from the building. Exhaust pipes attached to furnaces and other heating appliances need periodic inspections for cracks and leaks. Chemical detectors are available for the home that can sense carbon monoxide in the air and sound alarms when it is present. Constant monitoring with such detectors can identify carbon monoxide before poisoning develops. Like smoke detectors, carbon monoxide detectors are recommended for all homes.

Poisoning With Caustic Substances

Caustic substances (strong acids and alkalies), when swallowed, can burn the tongue, mouth, esophagus, and stomach. These burns may cause perforation (piercing) of the esophagus or stomach. Food and saliva leaking from a perforation cause severe, sometimes deadly infection within the chest (mediastinitis or empyema) or abdomen (peritonitis). Burns that do not perforate can result in scarring of the esophagus and stomach.

Industrial products are usually the most damaging because they are highly concentrated. However, some common household products, including drain and toilet bowl cleaners and some dishwasher detergents, contain damaging caustic substances, such as sodium hydroxide and sulfuric acid.

Caustic substances are available as solids and liquids. The burning sensation of a solid particle sticking to a moist surface (such as the lips) may prevent a person from consuming much of the product. Because liquids do not stick, it is easier to consume more of the product, and the entire esophagus can be damaged.

Symptoms

Pain in the mouth and throat develops rapidly, usually within minutes, and can be severe, particularly with swallowing. Coughing, drooling, an inability to swallow, and shortness of breath may occur. In severe cases involving strong caustic substances, a person may develop very low blood pressure (shock), difficulty breathing, or chest pain, possibly leading to death.

Perforation of the esophagus or stomach may occur during the first week after ingestion, often after vomiting or severe coughing. The esophagus may perforate into the area between the lungs (the mediastinum) or into the area surrounding the lungs (the pleural cavity). Either circumstance causes chest pain, fever, rapid heart rate, very low blood pressure, and the development of an abscess (a collection of pus) that requires surgery. Peritonitis results in severe abdominal pain.

Scarring of the esophagus results in narrowing (stricture), which causes difficulty in swallowing. Strictures usually develop weeks after the burn, sometimes in burns that initially caused only mild symptoms.

Diagnosis and Treatment

The mouth is examined for chemical burns. Because the esophagus and stomach may be burned without the mouth being burned, the doctor may insert an endoscope (a flexible viewing tube) down the esophagus to look for burns, particularly if the person drools or has difficulty swallowing. Directly inspecting the area allows the doctor to determine the severity of the injury and possibly to predict the risk of subsequent narrowing and the possible need for surgical repair of the esophagus.

The extent of damage determines treatment. People with severe burns sometimes need immediate surgery to remove severely damaged tissue. Corticosteroids and antibiotics are used to try to prevent strictures and infections, but whether these drugs are helpful is not clear.

Because caustic substances can cause as much damage returning up the esophagus as they did when swallowed, a person who has swallowed a caustic substance should not be made to vomit.

If burns are mild, the person may be encouraged to begin drinking fluids fairly soon during recovery. Otherwise, fluids are given intravenously until drinking is possible. If strictures develop, a bypass tube (stent) may be placed in the narrowed portion of the esophagus to prevent esophageal closure and to allow for future widening (dilation). Repeated widening may be needed for months or years. For severe strictures, surgery to rebuild the esophagus may also be necessary.

Hydrocarbon Poisoning

Petroleum products, cleaning products, and glues contain hydrocarbons (substances composed largely of hydrogen and carbon). Many children younger than age 5 are poisoned by swallowing petroleum products, such as gasoline, kerosene, and paint thinners, but most recover. At greater risk are teenagers who intentionally breathe the fumes of these products to become intoxicated, a type of drug abuse called huffing, sniffing, glue sniffing, or volatile substance use.▲

Swallowed hydrocarbons can enter and irritate the lungs, a serious condition in itself (chemical pneumonitis), and can lead to severe pneumonia. Lung involvement is a particular problem with thin, easy-flowing hydrocarbons such as mineral seal oil, which is used in furniture polish. Serious poisoning also can affect the brain, heart, bone marrow, and kidneys.

Symptoms

A person usually coughs and chokes after swallowing hydrocarbons. A burning sensation can develop in the stomach, and the person may vomit. If the lungs are affected, the person continues to cough intensely; breathing becomes rapid, and the skin may become bluish (cyanosis) because of low levels of oxygen in the blood.

Hydrocarbon ingestion also produces neurologic symptoms, including drowsiness, poor coordination, stupor or coma, and seizures. Inhalation of hydrocarbons may induce fatal irregular heartbeats or cardiac arrest, especially after exertion or stress.

Diagnosis and Treatment

Hydrocarbon poisoning is diagnosed based on a description of the events and the characteristic odor of petroleum on the person's breath. Pneumonia and chemical pneumonitis are diagnosed with a chest x-ray and by measuring the level of oxygen in the blood.■

To treat poisoning, contaminated clothing should be removed, and the skin should be washed. If the person has stopped coughing and choking, particularly if the ingestion was small and accidental, treatment at home is possible. This should be discussed with someone at a poison center. People with breathing problems are hospitalized. If pneumonia or chemical pneumonitis develops, hospital treatment can include oxygen, and, if severe, a ventilator. Antibiotics help if pneumonia develops. Recovery from pneumonia typically takes about a week.

Insecticide Poisoning

The properties that make insecticides deadly to insects can sometimes make them poisonous to humans. Most serious insecticide poisonings result from the organophosphate and carbamate types of insecticides, particularly when used in suicide attempts. These compounds are derived from nerve gases. Pyrethrins and pyrethroids, which are commonly used insecticides derived from flowers, usually are not poisonous to humans.

Many insecticides can cause poisoning after being swallowed, inhaled, or absorbed through the skin. Some insecticides are odorless, thus the person is unaware of being exposed to them. Organophosphate and carbamate insecticides make certain nerves "fire" erratically, causing many organs to become overactive and eventually to stop functioning. Pyrethrins can occasionally cause allergic reactions. Pyrethroids rarely cause any problems.

Symptoms

Organophosphates and carbamates cause eye tearing, blurred vision, salivation, sweating, coughing, vomiting, and frequent bowel movements and urination. Breathing may become difficult, and muscles twitch and become weak. Rarely, shortness of breath or muscle weakness is fatal. Symptoms last hours to days after exposure to carbamates but

▲ see page 659   ■ see page 255

can last for weeks after exposure to organophosphates.

Pyrethrins can cause sneezing, eye tearing, coughing, and occasional difficulty breathing. Serious symptoms rarely develop.

Diagnosis and Treatment

The diagnosis of insecticide poisoning is based on the symptoms and on a description of the preceding events. Blood tests can confirm organophosphate or carbamate poisoning.

If an insecticide might have contacted the skin, clothing is removed and the skin is washed. Anyone with symptoms of organophosphate poisoning should see a doctor. Atropine, given intravenously, can relieve most of the symptoms. Pralidoxime, given intravenously, can speed up recovery of nerve function, eliminating the cause of the symptoms. Symptoms of carbamate poisoning are also relieved by atropine but usually not by pralidoxime. Symptoms of pyrethrin poisoning resolve without treatment.

Iron Poisoning

Pills containing iron are commonly used to treat certain kinds of anemia. Iron also is included in many multiple vitamin supplements. People—especially toddlers—who overdose on these pills may develop iron poisoning. Because many households contain multiple vitamin supplements for adults that contain iron, iron overdose is common. However, overdose of iron-containing vitamins, particularly children's chewable vitamins, usually does not involve enough iron to cause serious poisoning. Overdose of pure iron supplements, however, may cause serious iron poisoning.

Serious iron poisoning is uncommon. It first irritates the stomach and digestive tract. Within hours, iron poisons the cells, interfering with their internal chemical reactions. Within days, the liver can be damaged. Weeks after recovery, the stomach, digestive tract, and liver can develop scars due to the previous irritation.

Symptoms

Serious iron poisoning usually causes symptoms within 6 hours of the overdose. The symptoms of iron poisoning typically occur in

four stages. In stage 1 (within 6 hours after the overdose), symptoms include vomiting, diarrhea, abdominal pain, drowsiness, unconsciousness, and seizures. The stomach may bleed. If poisoning is very serious, rapid breathing, a rapid heart rate, and low blood pressure may develop. In stage 2 (8 to 24 hours after the overdose), the person's condition can appear to improve. In stage 3 (6 to 48 hours after the overdose), very low blood pressure (shock), bleeding, jaundice, liver failure, seizures, confusion, and coma can develop. Sugar levels in the blood can decrease. In stage 4 (2 to 6 weeks after the overdose), the stomach or intestines can become blocked by constricting scars. Scarring in either organ can cause crampy abdominal pain and vomiting. Severe scarring of the liver (cirrhosis▲) can develop later.

Diagnosis and Treatment

The diagnosis of iron poisoning is based on the person's history, symptoms, and the amount of iron in the blood. If many pills have been swallowed, they can sometimes be seen on x-rays of the stomach or intestines.

People with symptoms or high levels of iron in the blood need hospitalization. To remove any iron remaining in the stomach, gastric lavage may be necessary. However, a large amount of iron can remain in the stomach even after gastric lavage or vomiting. A special saltwater solution may be given by mouth or through a stomach tube to wash the contents of the stomach and intestines (whole bowel irrigation), although its effectiveness is unclear. Injections of deferoxamine, which binds iron in the blood, are given.

Lead Poisoning

Although it is far less common since paint containing lead pigment was banned in 1977 and lead was eliminated from most gasoline, lead poisoning (plumbism) is still a major public health problem in U.S. cities on the East Coast. Workers in industries that handle lead are at risk of lead poisoning, as are children who live in older houses that contain peeling lead paint or lead pipes. Young children may eat enough paint chips to develop symptoms of lead poisoning. Lead affects many parts of the body, including the brain, nerves, kidneys, liver, blood, digestive tract, and sex organs. Children are particularly susceptible because lead produces the most damage in nervous systems that are still developing.

▲ see page 797

If the level of lead in the blood is high for days, symptoms of sudden brain damage (encephalopathy) usually develop. Lower blood levels that are sustained for longer periods of time sometimes produce long-term intellectual deficits.

Symptoms and Diagnosis

Many people with mild lead poisoning have no symptoms. Symptoms that do occur usually develop over several weeks or longer. Sometimes symptoms flare up periodically.

Typical symptoms of lead poisoning include personality changes, headaches, loss of sensation, weakness, a metallic taste in the mouth, uncoordinated walking, poor appetite, vomiting, constipation, crampy abdominal pain, bone or joint pains, and anemia.▲ Kidney damage often develops without symptoms.

Young children may become cranky and play less frequently over the course of several weeks. Encephalopathy can then begin suddenly and worsen over the next several days, resulting in persistent, forceful vomiting; confusion; sleepiness; and, finally, seizures and coma.

Adults often develop loss of sex drive, infertility, and, in men, erectile dysfunction (impotence). Encephalopathy rarely develops in adults.

Some symptoms may diminish if exposure to lead is stopped, only to worsen again if exposure is resumed.

Lead poisoning is diagnosed with a blood test. Adults whose jobs involve handling lead need frequent blood tests. Children living in communities with many older houses, where peeling lead-based paint is common, should also undergo blood tests for lead. In children, bone and abdominal x-rays often show evidence of lead poisoning.

Treatment and Prognosis

Treatment consists of stopping exposure to lead and removing accumulated lead from the body. Doctors remove lead from the body by giving drugs that bind with the lead (chelation therapy), allowing it to pass into the urine. All drugs that remove lead work slowly and can cause serious side effects.

People with mild lead poisoning are given succimer by mouth. People with more serious lead poisoning are treated in the hospital with injections of chelating drugs, such as dimercaprol, succimer, penicillamine, and edetate calcium disodium. Because chelating drugs also can remove beneficial minerals, such as zinc, copper, and iron, from the body, the person often is given supplements of these minerals.

Even after treatment, many children with encephalopathy develop some degree of permanent brain damage. Kidney damage is also sometimes permanent.

Prevention

Commercially available kits can be used to test household paint, ceramics, and water supplies for lead content. Dusting affected windowsills weekly with a damp cloth removes some dust that could contain lead from paint. Chipped leaded paint should be repaired. Larger renovation projects to remove leaded paint can release large quantities of lead into the house and should be done professionally. Commercially available faucet filters can remove most lead from drinking water.

CHAPTER 298

Bites and Stings

Many creatures, including humans, bite when frightened or provoked. Bites may cause injuries ranging from superficial scratches to extensive wounds and often become infected with bacteria from the mouth of the biting creature.

Certain animals can inject venom (poison) through mouthparts or a stinger. These venoms range in toxicity from mild to life threat-

---

▲ see page 987

ening. Even mildly toxic venoms may cause serious allergic reactions.

Animal Bites

Although any animal may bite, dogs and, to a lesser extent, cats account for most bites in the United States. Owing to their popularity as household pets, dogs account for the majority of bites as a result of protecting their owners and territory. About 10 to 20 people, mostly children, die from dog bites each year. Cats do not defend territory and bite mainly when humans restrain them for various reasons or attempt to intervene in a cat fight. Domestic animals, such as horses, cows, and pigs, bite infrequently, but their size and strength are such that serious wounds may result. Wild animal bites are rare.

Dog bites typically have a ragged, torn appearance. Cat bites involve deep puncture wounds that frequently become infected. Infected bites are painful, swollen, and red. Rabies▲ may be transmitted from animals (most commonly bats) infected with that organism. Rabies is rare among pets in the United States because of vaccination.

Treatment

After receiving routine first-aid treatment,■ victims of animal bites should see a doctor immediately. If possible, the offending animal should be penned up by its owner. If the animal is loose, the person who has been bitten should not try to capture it. The police should be notified so that the proper authorities can observe the animal for signs of rabies.

A doctor cleans an animal bite with sterile salt water (saline) or soap and water. Sometimes tissue is trimmed from the edge of the bite wound, particularly if the tissue is crushed or ragged. Facial bite wounds are surgically closed (sutured). However, minor wounds, puncture wounds, and bite wounds to the hands are not closed. Antibiotics are given by mouth to prevent infection. Infected bites sometimes require antibiotics given intravenously.

Human Bites

Because human teeth are not particularly sharp, most human bites cause a bruise and only a shallow tear (laceration), if any. Excep-

tions are on fleshy appendages, such as the ears, nose, and penis, which may be severed. The clenched-fist injury, or "fight bite," which occurs on the knuckles of a person who punches another person in the mouth, is likely to become infected.★ This cut frequently lacerates the finger tendon that passes over the knuckle. Sometimes the biting person transmits diseases, such as hepatitis, to the victim. HIV transmission, however, is extremely unlikely.

Symptoms and Diagnosis

Bites are painful and usually produce a mark on the skin with the pattern of the teeth. Fight bites leave only a small, straight cut over a knuckle. A lacerated finger tendon results in difficulty moving the finger in one direction. Infected bites become very painful, red, and swollen.

Treatment

Human bites, like animal bites, are cleaned with sterile salt water (saline) or soap and water. Severed parts can be reattached,● and tears, except those involving the hand, are surgically closed. All people with human bites that have broken the skin are given antibiotics by mouth to prevent infection. Infected bites are treated with antibiotics and often must be opened surgically to examine and clean the wound. If the biting person is known or suspected to have a disease that may be spread by biting, preventive treatment may be necessary.

Poisonous Snake Bites

About 25 species of venomous (poisonous) snakes are native to the United States. The venomous snakes include pit vipers (rattlesnakes, copperheads, and cottonmouths) and coral snakes. Of the roughly 45,000 snakebites in the United States each year, fewer than 8,000 are by venomous snakes, and about six people die. In about 25% of all pit viper bites, venom is not injected. Most deaths occur in children, older people, and people who are untreated or treated inappropriately. Rattlesnakes account for about 70% of poisonous snakebites in the United States and for almost all of the deaths. Copperheads and, to a lesser extent, cottonmouths account for most other poisonous snakebites. Coral snake bites and those from imported snakes are rare.

The venom of rattlesnakes and other pit vipers damages tissue around the bite. Rat-

---

▲ see page 535   ■ see page 1691

★ see page 402   ● see box on page 1083

tlesnake venom may produce changes in blood cells, prevents blood from clotting, and damages blood vessels, causing them to leak. These changes can lead to internal bleeding and to heart, respiratory, and kidney failure. The venom of coral snakes affects nervous system activity but causes little damage to tissue around the bite. Most bites occur on the hand or foot.

Symptoms

The symptoms of snake venom poisoning vary widely, depending on the size and species of snake, the amount and toxicity of the venom injected, the bite's location, and the victim's age and underlying medical problems. Usually, bites by most pit vipers rapidly cause pain. Redness and swelling usually follow within 20 to 30 minutes and can progress to affect the entire leg or arm within several hours. The person bitten by a rattlesnake may experience tingling and numbness in the fingers or toes or around the mouth and a metallic or rubbery taste in the mouth. Other symptoms include fever, chills, general weakness, faintness, sweating, and nausea and vomiting. Breathing difficulties can develop, particularly after Mojave rattlesnake bites. The person may have a headache, blurred vision, drooping eyelids, and a dry mouth.

Moderate or severe pit viper poisoning commonly causes bruising of the skin 3 to 6 hours after the bite. The skin around the bite appears tight and discolored; blisters, often filled with blood, may form in the bite area. Without treatment, tissue around the bite may be destroyed. The bitten person's gums may bleed, and blood may appear in the person's vomit, stools, and urine.

Coral snake bites usually cause little or no immediate pain and swelling. More severe symptoms may take several hours to develop. The area around the bite may tingle, and nearby muscles may become weak. Muscle incoordination and severe general weakness may follow. Other symptoms include visual disturbances and increased saliva production, with speech and swallowing difficulties. Breathing problems, which may be extreme, may follow.

Diagnosis

Emergency medical personnel must try to determine whether the snake was poisonous, what species it was, and whether venom was injected. The bite marks sometimes suggest whether the snake was poisonous. The fangs of a poisonous snake usually produce one or two large punctures, whereas the teeth of nonpoisonous snakes usually leave multiple small rows of scratches. Without a detailed description of the snake, the doctor may have difficulty determining the particular species that caused the bite. Envenomation is recognized by the development of characteristic symptoms. People who are bitten are generally kept in the hospital for 8 to 12 hours to see if any symptoms develop. Doctors perform various tests to assess the effects of the venom.

Treatment and Prognosis

Anyone bitten by a poisonous snake should be moved beyond the snake's striking distance, kept as calm and still as possible, and taken to the nearest medical facility immediately. The bitten limb should be loosely immobilized and kept positioned below heart level. Rings, watches, and tight clothing should be removed from the area of the bite. Alcohol and caffeine should be avoided. Tourniquets, ice packs, and cutting the, bite open are not recommended and are dangerous.

If no venom was injected, treatment is the same as for any puncture wound.▲ If venom was injected and symptoms indicate a serious bite, venom antidote (antivenom) is the most important part of treatment and is more effective the sooner it is given. Antivenom neutralizes venom's toxic effects. It is given intravenously and is available for all native poisonous snakes. Pit viper antivenom made from horse serum frequently causes serum sickness (an immune system reaction against foreign protein); newer antivenom made of purified antibody fragments from sheep is much safer.

A person with low blood pressure is given fluids intravenously. If problems with blood clotting develop, the person is given fresh frozen plasma, concentrated clotting factors (cryoprecipitate), or platelet transfusions.

Prognosis depends on the person's age and overall health and on the location and venom content of the bite. Almost everyone bitten by a poisonous snake survives if treated early with appropriate amounts of antivenom.

Poisonous Lizard Bites

The only two lizards known to be poisonous are the beaded lizard of Mexico and the Gila

▲ see page 1691

What Is Serum Sickness?

Serum sickness is a reaction by the immune system against large amounts of foreign protein that have entered the bloodstream. A common source of such foreign protein is horse serum, an ingredient found in many venom antidotes (antivenoms) that are used to treat poisonous snake and spider bites and scorpion stings. Symptoms of serum sickness include fever, rash, and joint pains. Rarely, kidney damage and death can occur. Doctors treat serum sickness with antihistamines, such as diphenhydramine, and corticosteroids. Antivenoms that do not contain horse serum are unlikely to result in serum sickness.

monster, found in Arizona; Sonora, Mexico; and adjacent areas. The venom of these lizards is somewhat similar in content and effect to that of some pit vipers, although symptoms tend to be much less severe, and bites are almost never fatal. Unlike most snakes, the Gila monster clamps on firmly when it bites and chews the venom into its victim rather than injecting it through fangs. The lizard may be difficult to dislodge.

Common symptoms include pain, swelling, and discoloration in the area around the bite as well as swollen lymph nodes. Weakness, sweating, thirst, headache, and ringing in the ears (tinnitus) may develop. In severe cases, blood pressure may fall.

Various suggestions for removing Gila monsters include forcing the jaws open with pliers, applying a flame under the lizard's chin, and immersing the lizard and body extremity under water. Once the lizard has been detached, tooth fragments often remain in the skin and must be removed. Treatment of low blood pressure or blood clotting problems is similar to that of pit viper bites. A specific antivenom is not available.

Spider Bites

Almost all spiders are poisonous. Fortunately, the fangs of most species are too short or too fragile to penetrate human skin. Although at least 60 species in the United States have been implicated in biting people, serious injury occurs mainly from only two types of spiders: the black widow and the brown recluse (fiddleback, or violin) spiders. Although tarantulas are considered dangerous, their bites do not seriously harm people. Spider bites cause fewer than three deaths a year in the United States, usually in children.

Symptoms

The bite of a **black widow spider** usually causes a sharp pain, somewhat like a pinprick, followed by a dull, sometimes numbing, pain in the area around the bite. Cramping pain and muscle stiffness, which may be severe, develop in the abdomen or the shoulders, back, and chest. Other symptoms may include nausea, vomiting, sweating, restlessness, anxiety, headache, drooping and swelling of the eyelids, skin rash and itching, severe breathing problems, increased saliva production, and weakness.

The bite of a **brown recluse spider** may cause little or no immediate pain, but some pain develops in the area around the bite within about an hour. Pain may be severe and may affect the entire injured area, which may become red and bruised and may itch. The rest of the body may itch as well. A blister forms, surrounded by a bruised area or by a more distinct red area that resembles a bull's-eye. Then the blister enlarges, fills with blood, and ruptures, forming an open sore (ulcer) that may leave a large craterlike scar. Nausea and vomiting, aches, fatigue, chills, sweats, blood disorders, and kidney failure may develop, but the bite is rarely fatal.

Diagnosis and Treatment

There is no way to identify a particular spider on the basis of its bite mark. Therefore, a specific diagnosis can be made only if the spider can be observed. Black widow spiders are recognized by a red or orange hourglass-shaped marking on the abdomen. Brown recluse spiders have a violin-shaped marking on their back.

The only first-aid measure of any value for a spider bite is placing an ice cube on the bite to reduce pain. For a black widow spider bite, muscle pain and spasms can be relieved with muscle relaxants and opioid analgesics. Hot baths may relieve mild pain. Antivenom is given for severe poisoning. Hospitalization is usually required for people younger than 16 and older than 60 and for those with high blood pressure or heart disease. For a brown recluse spider bite, antivenom is not yet commercially available. Skin sores are cleaned daily with a povidone-iodine solution and are soaked 3 times a day in sterile salt water (saline); dead tissue is trimmed away as needed.

Bee, Wasp, Hornet, and Ant Stings

Stings by bees, wasps, and hornets are common throughout the United States. Some ants also sting. The average person can safely tolerate 10 stings for each pound of body weight. This means that the average adult could withstand more than 1,000 stings, whereas 500 stings could kill a child. However, one sting can cause death from an anaphylactic reaction (a life-threatening allergic reaction in which blood pressure falls and the airway closes▲) in a person who is allergic to such stings. In the United States, 3 or 4 times more people die from bee stings than from snakebites. A more aggressive type of honeybee, called the Africanized killer bee, has reached some southern states as these bees travel north from South America. By attacking their victim in swarms, these bees cause a more severe reaction than do other bees.

In the South, particularly in the Gulf region, fire ants sting up to 40% of the people who live in infested areas each year, causing at least 30 deaths.

Symptoms

Bee stings produce immediate pain and a red, swollen area about $1/2$ inch across. In some people, the area swells to a diameter of 2 inches or more over the next 2 or 3 days. This swelling is sometimes mistaken for infection, which is rare after bee stings.

The fire ant sting usually produces immediate pain and a red, swollen area, which disappears within 45 minutes. A blister then forms, rupturing in 2 to 3 days, and the area often becomes infected. In some cases, a red, swollen, itchy patch develops instead of a blister. Isolated nerves may become inflamed, and seizures may occur.

Treatment

A bee may leave its stinger in the skin. The stinger should be removed as quickly as possible without concern for the method of removal. An ice cube placed over the sting reduces the pain. A cream containing a combination of an antihistamine, an analgesic, and a corticosteroid is often useful. People who are allergic to stings should always carry a preloaded syringe of epinephrine, which blocks anaphylactic or allergic reactions.

People who have had a severe allergic reaction to a bee sting sometimes undergo desensitization (allergen immunotherapy),■ which may help prevent future allergic reactions.

Insect Bites

Among the more common biting and sometimes bloodsucking insects in the United States are sand flies, horseflies, deerflies, mosquitoes, fleas, lice, bedbugs, kissing bugs, and certain water bugs. The bites of these insects may be irritating because of the components of their saliva. Most bites result in nothing more than a small, red, itchy bump. Sometimes, a person develops a large sore (ulcer), with swelling and pain. The most severe reactions occur in people who are allergic to the bites or who develop an infection after being bitten.

The bite should be cleaned, and an ointment containing a combination of an antihistamine, an analgesic, and a corticosteroid may be applied to relieve itching, pain, and inflammation. People with multiple bites can take an antihistamine by mouth. People who are allergic to the bite should seek medical attention immediately or use an emergency allergy kit containing a preloaded syringe of epinephrine.

Tick and Mite Bites

Ticks carry many diseases (for example, deer ticks may carry the bacteria that cause Lyme disease★; other types of ticks may carry the bacteria that cause rickettsial or ehrlichial infections.● The bites of pajaroello ticks, which are found in Mexico and the southwestern United States, produce pus-filled blisters that break, leaving open sores that develop scabs.

Mite infestations are common and are responsible for chiggers (an intensely itchy rash caused by mite larvae under the skin), scabies,◆ and a number of other diseases. The effects on the tissues around the bite vary in severity.

Treatment

Ticks should be removed as soon as possible. Removal is best accomplished by grasping the tick with curved tweezers as close to the

---

▲ see page 1072   ■ see page 1064
★ see page 1105   ● see page 1132
◆ see page 1218

Tick Paralysis

> In North America, some tick species secrete a toxin that causes tick paralysis. A person with tick paralysis feels restless, weak, and irritable. After a few days, a progressive paralysis develops, moving up from the legs. The muscles that control breathing also may become paralyzed.
>
> Tick paralysis is cured rapidly by finding and removing the tick. If breathing is impaired, oxygen therapy or a mechanical ventilator may be needed to assist with breathing.

skin as possible and pulling it directly out. The tick's head, which may not come out with the body, should be removed, because it can cause prolonged inflammation. Most of the folk methods of removing a tick, such as applying alcohol, fingernail polish, or a hot match, are ineffective and may cause the tick to expel infected saliva into the bite site.

Mite infestations are treated by applying a cream containing permethrin or a solution of lindane. After treatment with permethrin or lindane, a cream containing a corticosteroid is sometimes used for a few days to reduce the itching until all the mites are gone.

Centipede and Millipede Bites

Some of the larger centipedes can inflict a painful bite, causing swelling and redness. Symptoms rarely persist for more than 48 hours. Millipedes do not bite but may secrete a toxin that is irritating, particularly when accidentally rubbed into the eye.

An ice cube placed on a centipede bite usually relieves the pain. Toxic secretions of millipedes should be washed from the skin with large amounts of soap and water. If a skin reaction develops, a corticosteroid cream should be applied. Eye injuries should be flushed with water (irrigated) immediately.

Scorpion Stings

The stings of North American scorpions are rarely serious and usually result in pain, minimal swelling, tenderness, and warmth at the sting site. However, the bark scorpion (*Centruroides exilicauda* or *sculpturatus*), which is found in Arizona and New Mexico and on the California side of the Colorado River, has a much more toxic sting. The sting is painful, sometimes causing numbness or tingling in the area around the sting. Serious symptoms are more common in children and include abnormal head, eye, and neck movements; increased saliva production; sweating; and restlessness. Some people develop severe involuntary twitching and jerking of muscles. Breathing difficulties may occur.

The stings of most North American scorpions require no special treatment. Placing an ice cube on the wound reduces pain, as does an ointment containing a combination of an antihistamine, an analgesic, and a corticosteroid. *Centruroides* stings that result in serious symptoms may require the use of sedatives, such as midazolam, given intravenously. *Centruroides* antivenom rapidly relieves symptoms, but it may cause a serious allergic reaction or serum sickness. The antivenom is available only in Arizona.

Marine Animal Stings and Bites

Stingrays contain venom in spines located on the back of their tail. Injuries usually occur when a person steps on a stingray while wading in shallow ocean surf. The stingray thrusts its tail spine into the victim's foot or leg, releasing venom. Fragments of the spine's covering may remain in the wound, increasing the risk of infection.

The wound from the spine is usually jagged and bleeds freely. Pain is immediate and severe, gradually diminishing over 6 to 48 hours. Fainting spells, weakness, nausea, and anxiety are common. Vomiting, diarrhea, sweating, generalized cramps, and breathing difficulties are less common.

Because stingray venom is inactivated by heat, pain can be relieved by immersing the injured limb in water as hot as the person can tolerate for 30 to 90 minutes. A doctor cleans the wound thoroughly and removes any fragments of the spine or its covering to prevent infection. The wound may require surgical closure. Infected stingray wounds require antibiotics, and the doctor may reopen the wound to look for any retained fragments of the spines.

A few **mollusks,** which include snails, octopuses, and bivalves (such as clams, oysters, and scallops), are venomous. The California cone (*Conus californicus*) is the only dangerous mollusk in North American waters. Its sting may cause pain, swelling, and numbness in the area of the sting and may be followed by difficulty speaking, blurred vision, paralysis of muscles, respiratory failure, and cardiac arrest. The bites of North American octopuses are rarely serious. However, the bite of the blue-ringed octopus—found in Australian waters—although painless, produces weakness and paralysis that may be fatal.

First-aid measures seem to provide little benefit for injuries from *Conus* stings and blue-ringed octopus bites. However, these injuries may require intensive medical support because of possible respiratory paralysis.

Sea urchins are covered with long, sharp, venom-coated spines. Touching or stepping on these spines typically produces a painful puncture wound. The spines commonly break off in the skin and cause chronic pain and inflammation if not removed. Joint and muscle pain and skin rashes may develop.

Sea urchin spines should be removed immediately. Because vinegar dissolves most sea urchin spines, several vinegar soaks or compresses may be all that is needed to remove spines that have not penetrated deeply. Surgical removal may be required for imbedded spines. Because sea urchin venom is inactivated by heat, soaking the injured body part in hot water often relieves the pain.

Many **coelenterates,** which include corals, sea anemones, jellyfish, and the Portuguese man-of-war, have highly developed stinging units (nematocysts) on their tentacles; a single tentacle may contain thousands. The severity of the sting depends on the type of animal.

The sting of most species results in a painful, itchy rash. The rash may develop into blisters that fill with pus and then rupture. Other symptoms include weakness, nausea, headache, muscle pain and spasms, runny eyes and nose, excessive sweating, and chest pain that worsens with breathing. Stings from the Portuguese man-of-war, including those that occur in North American waters, have caused death.

Most coelenterate stings require no more than cleaning. The following general treatment is suggested:

1. Pour ocean (not fresh) water over the injured area.
2. Soak the injured area in a solution of vinegar for 30 to 60 seconds. (This inactivates the nematocysts of box jellyfish.)
3. Remove the tentacles with a tweezer or a gloved hand.
4. Pour flour or baking soda over the wound and carefully scrape the powder off with a sharp knife.
5. Soak the area in vinegar again.
6. Apply an ointment containing a combination of an antihistamine, an analgesic, and a corticosteroid.

People with more serious reactions may require oxygen therapy or other assistance in breathing. Painful muscle spasms and severe pain are treated with drugs given intravenously. Antivenom is available for the stings of certain Australian species, but it is ineffective for stings of North American species.

CHAPTER 299

First Aid

The goal of first aid is to save life, to prevent an injury or illness from worsening, or to help speed recovery. First aid for cardiac arrest, choking, bleeding, minor wounds, and minor soft tissue injuries are discussed in this chapter. Other chapters discuss first aid for near drowning, heat stroke, low body temperature (hypothermia), serious allergic reactions (anaphylaxis), spinal cord injuries, low blood sugar (hypoglycemia), poisoning, seizures, stings, bite wounds, chemical burns of the eyes, fractures, frostbite, nosebleeds, sprains, and loose teeth.

Priorities During Emergency First Aid

The first priority is to assess a person's airway, breathing, and circulation (the ABCs). A problem in any of these areas is always fatal if

Basic First-Aid Supplies

The medicine chest or first-aid kit should always be kept well stocked. The following basic supplies should be included:

- Adhesive tape
- Antiseptic cream (such as bacitracin)
- Aspirin or acetaminophen
- Bandages or surgical tape
- Cotton-tipped swabs
- First-aid manual
- Sharp scissors
- Soap
- Sterile adhesive or gauze bandages in several sizes
- Thermometer
- Thin, translucent gloves
- Tissues
- Tweezers

not corrected. The airway (A)—the passage through which air travels to the lungs—can become blocked. Various illnesses and injuries can cause breathing (B) to cease. Cardiac arrest—cessation of the heartbeat—stops blood from circulating (C) through the body.

The next priority is usually to get professional medical assistance by calling for emergency medical care (except in cases of choking and some instances of cardiac arrest, in which treatment should be started before calling for help). Most people in the United States access care by calling 911. The caller should rapidly give the dispatcher a full description of the person's condition and how the injury or illness developed. The caller should not hang up until told to do so. If several lay people (rescuers) are present, one should call for help while another begins assessment and first aid.

After calling for medical assistance, the ABCs are corrected before any other treatment is started. Cardiopulmonary resuscitation (CPR)▲ is provided, if necessary.

If many people are injured, the most seriously injured person should be treated first. Determining who is in most urgent need of treatment may be difficult; someone screaming in pain may be less seriously injured than someone who cannot breathe or whose heart has stopped and, therefore, is quiet. Assess-

ment should take less than 1 minute per injured person. In each case, the rescuer should consider whether the situation is life threatening, urgent but not life threatening, or not urgent. Cardiac arrest and massive bleeding are life threatening; a broken bone can wait for treatment, no matter how painful.

If the injured person is unable to convey information about his medical condition, information should be obtained in other ways. For example, if an unconscious person is found near an empty bottle of pills, the bottle should be given to the emergency medical personnel. A description of how a person became injured and other information from bystanders, family members, or rescuers can be essential to the person's treatment. After these steps have been taken, reassurance and simple measures, such as supplying a blanket and keeping the person calm and warm, can provide comfort.

Serious diseases, such as HIV and hepatitis B, can be transmitted through blood. Rescuers should avoid contact with the blood from wounds, especially the blood of strangers whose medical history is unknown. Latex examination gloves afford the best protection. If gloves are not available, plastic can be used. For example, the rescuer can place his hands inside a plastic food storage bag or anything waterproof. If contaminated with blood, the hands—including the area under the fingernails—should be washed vigorously with soap and water or a mild solution of bleach (about 1 tablespoon of bleach per quart of water) as soon as possible. Contact with saliva and urine is much less likely to result in disease transmission than is contact with blood.

Cardiac Arrest

Cardiac arrest is what happens when a person dies; the heart does not beat and breathing ceases, which starves the body of oxygen. Sometimes a person can be revived during the first several minutes after suffering cardiac arrest. However, the more time that passes, the less likely it is that the person can be revived and, if revived, the more likely it is that he will have brain damage.

A person in cardiac arrest lies motionless without breathing and does not respond to questions or to stimulation, such as shaking. A rescuer who encounters someone who fits this description first determines whether the person is conscious by loudly asking, "Are you OK?" If there is no response, the rescuer turns

▲ see page 1689

Automated External Defibrillator:
Jump-Starting the Heart

An automated external defibrillator (AED) is a device that can detect and correct a specific type of abnormal heart rhythm called ventricular fibrillation. Ventricular fibrillation causes cardiac arrest. If cardiac arrest occurs, an AED, if available, should be used immediately. An AED is used before calling for help and before attempting cardiopulmonary resuscitation (CPR) because an AED is more likely to save lives. If the AED detects ventricular fibrillation, it provides an electrical shock (defibrillation) that can restore normal heart rhythm and start the heart beating again. If a person remains in cardiac arrest after an AED is used, help should be called and CPR should be performed.

AEDs are easy to use. The American Red Cross provides half-day training sessions on the use of AEDs. Different AEDs have somewhat different instructions for use. The instructions that are written on the AED being used should be carefully followed. AEDs are available in many public gathering places, such as stadiums and concert halls. People who are told by their doctor that they are likely to develop ventricular fibrillation may want to purchase an AED for home use by family members.

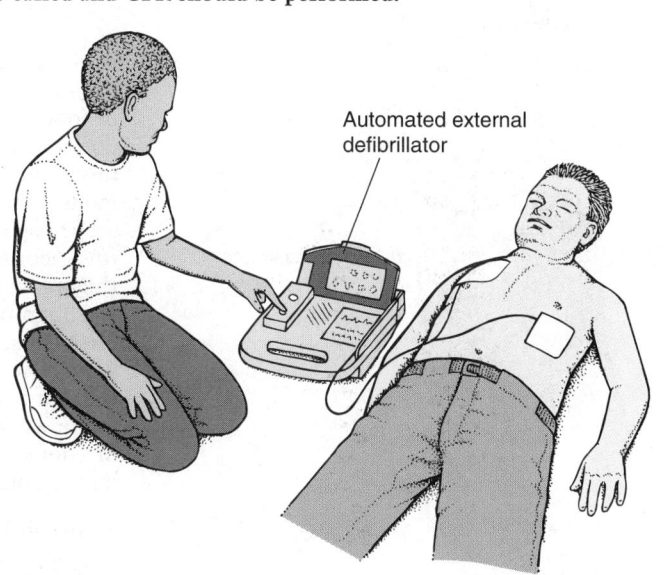

Automated external defibrillator

the person on his back and uses the "look, listen, and feel" approach to determine whether breathing has stopped: looking to see whether the chest moves up and down, listening for sounds of breathing, and feeling for air movement over the person's mouth. If the person is not breathing, the rescuer checks for airway blockage by looking into the mouth and throat for any visible objects.

First-Aid Treatment

First aid for cardiac arrest should proceed as quickly as possible. If an automated external defibrillator (a device that can start the heart beating again) is available, it should be used immediately. The next step is to call for professional medical assistance. Next, if the person has not resumed breathing, cardiopulmonary resuscitation (CPR) should be started. CPR combines artificial respiration, which supplies oxygen to the lungs, with chest compressions, which circulate oxygen to the brain and other vital organs by forcing blood out of the heart.

Skill in CPR is best obtained through a training course. The American Heart Association, American Red Cross, and many local fire departments and hospitals offer CPR training courses. Because procedures may change over time, it is important to stay up to date on training and to repeat courses as recommended.

To begin CPR, the rescuer lays the person on his back, rolling the head, body, and limbs at the same time. The rescuer then removes any object visibly blocking the airway. Next, the rescuer tilts the person's head back slightly and lifts the chin, which sometimes opens a blocked airway. If breathing does not resume, the rescuer covers the person's mouth with his own and begins artificial respiration (mouth-to-mouth resuscitation, rescue breathing) by slowly exhaling air into the person's

Performing the Heimlich Maneuver

The rescuer encircles the person's abdomen. With one hand, the rescuer forms a fist and clasps the other hand around the fist. The rescuer places the hands halfway between the breastbone and navel and thrusts the hands inward and upward.

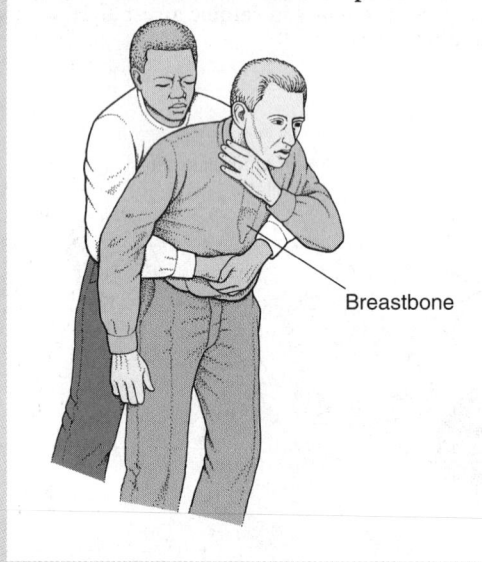

Breastbone

performed by one person (who alternately performs artificial respiration and chest compressions) or by two people (one to perform artificial respiration and one to perform chest compressions). Breaths are given about 15 to 20 times per minute (once every 3 or 4 seconds), and chest compressions are performed about 80 to 100 times per minute. The rescuer continues CPR until medical assistance arrives, he is too tired to continue, or the person recovers.

Choking

Maneuvers to relieve choking are frequently life saving. Adults most often choke on a piece of food, such as a large piece of meat. Infants do not have well-developed swallowing reflexes and may choke if given small, rounded foods such as peanuts or hard candies. Children, especially toddlers, also may choke on toys, coins, and other inedible objects that they place in their mouth.

Coughing may be the first symptom and is often so severe that the person cannot ask for help. The person may grasp both hands near the throat. Breathing and speaking can become weak or stop. There can be high-pitched or snoring sounds. The person can turn blue, have a seizure, or faint.

First-Aid Treatment

Treatment for a person who is choking takes precedence over calling for emergency medical care.

A strong cough often expels the object from the airway. A person with a strong cough should be allowed to continue coughing. A person who can speak normally usually still has a strong cough. If a person who is choking cannot cough, the Heimlich maneuver should be performed. The Heimlich maneuver produces increased pressure in the abdomen and chest, which expels the object.

If the person is conscious, the rescuer approaches from behind, then circles his hands around the person's abdomen. The rescuer forms a fist, with the thumb pointing inward, and places it between the breastbone and navel, toward the person. The other hand is then placed firmly over the fisted hand. The hands are then thrust inward and upward forcefully, 5 times in succession. Less force should be used if the person is a child. Series of thrusts should be repeated until the object is expelled. If the person loses consciousness, the rescuer should stop the thrusts.

lungs. To prevent air from escaping from the person's nose, the rescuer pinches the nose shut as he is exhaling into the mouth.

Artificial respiration is very similar in children and adults. However, with an infant, the rescuer places his mouth over the infant's mouth and nose. To prevent damaging the infant's smaller lungs, the rescuer exhales with less force than with adults.

Failure of the chest to rise after artificial respiration indicates that the person's airway is blocked. If the chest rises, the rescuer gives two deep, slow breaths.

Next, chest compressions are performed. The rescuer kneels to one side and, with arms held straight, leans over the person and places both hands, one on top of the other, on the lower part of the breastbone. The rescuer compresses the chest to a depth of $1\frac{1}{2}$ to 2 inches in an adult, less deeply in a child. For an infant, the rescuer uses two fingers to compress the infant's breastbone just below the nipples to a depth of $\frac{1}{2}$ to 1 inch. CPR can be

If the person loses consciousness, steps are taken to open the airway and provide artificial respiration.▲ Failure of the chest to rise indicates that the airway is still blocked. The rescuer checks the airway for, and removes, visible objects. If none are found, the rescuer inserts his finger into the person's mouth to find and remove any hidden objects present. Artificial respiration is then resumed.

For an infant, the Heimlich maneuver is not performed. Instead, the infant is turned face down, the chest resting on the rescuer's hand, with the head lower than the body. The rescuer then strikes the infant between the shoulder blades 5 times using the heel of the hand (back blows). The strikes should be firm but not hard enough to cause injury. The rescuer then checks the mouth, removing any visible objects. If the airway remains blocked, the rescuer turns the infant face up with the head down, thrusts his second and third fingers inward and upward on the breastbone 5 times (chest thrusts), then checks the mouth again.

Internal Bleeding

Heavy internal bleeding may occur in the abdominal cavity, chest cavity, digestive tract, or tissues surrounding broken bones.

Initially, internal bleeding itself causes no symptoms, although an injured organ that is bleeding is often painful. However, the person may be distracted from this pain by other injuries or may be unable to express pain because of confusion, drowsiness, or unconsciousness. Eventually, internal bleeding usually becomes apparent. For example, blood in the digestive tract may be vomited or passed from the rectum. Extensive blood loss causes low blood pressure, making the person feel weak and dizzy. The person may faint when standing or even sitting and, if blood pressure is very low, lose consciousness.

First-Aid Treatment

A lay person cannot stop internal bleeding. If extensive bleeding causes light-headedness or symptoms of shock,■ the person should be laid down and the legs elevated. Professional help should be summoned as quickly as possible.

Wounds

Cuts or tears in tissue (lacerations), scrapes (abrasions), and puncture wounds can be

Clearing a Blocked Airway in an Infant

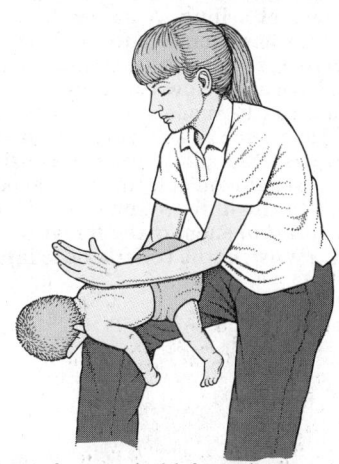

The infant is held face down with the chest resting on the rescuer's hand. Then, the rescuer strikes the infant's back between the shoulder blades.

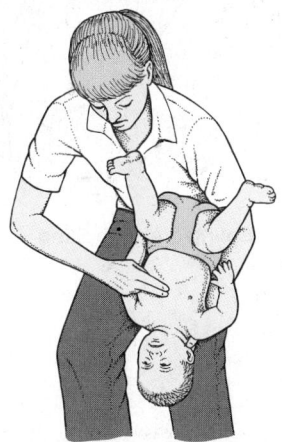

The infant is turned face up with the head lower than the body. Then, the rescuer places the second and third fingers on the infant's breastbone and thrusts inward and upward.

caused by bites★ or other injuries. Wounds that are not caused by bites usually heal rapidly without any problems. However, some

▲ see page 1689   ■ see page 148
★ see page 1681

Commonly Used Splints

A splint can be anything that prevents movement of a limb. A splint is used to prevent further damage and limit pain. To be effective, a splint must immobilize the joints above and below the injury.

Splints can be made from readily available objects, such as a magazine or stack of newspapers. But splints usually consist of a rigid, straight object, such as a board, strapped to the limb. A sling may be used with a splint to support the forearm when an arm, a wrist, or the collarbone is injured.

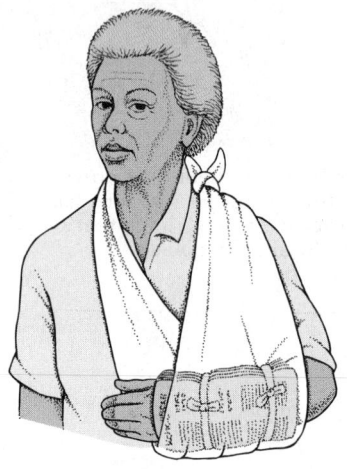

Splinted Arm in Sling

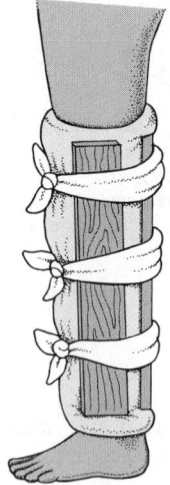

Splinted Leg

wounds can cause extensive blood loss. Others can become complicated by infection or injury to deeper structures, such as nerves, tendons, or blood vessels. A piece of foreign material can also remain hidden inside a puncture wound.

Shallow cuts to most areas of the skin rarely bleed much and often stop bleeding on their own. Cuts to the hand and scalp as well as cuts to arteries and larger veins often bleed vigorously.

Infection can develop when a wound is contaminated with dirt and bacteria. Although any wound can become infected, infection is particularly likely in deep scrapes, which grind dirt into the skin, and in puncture wounds, which introduce contamination deep under the skin. Also, wounds that contain foreign material (such as splinters, glass, or clothing fragments) almost always become infected. The longer a wound remains contaminated, the more likely it is that infection will develop.

Wounds can be painful at first, but usually the pain lessens after the first day. If a cut affects a nerve or tendon, the person may be unable to move the body part fully. Some nerve injuries cause numbness. If a foreign object remains inside a puncture wound, usually the part of the wound near the object is painful when touched.

Pain that worsens a day or more after the injury is often the first sign of infection. Later, an infected wound becomes red and swollen and may ooze pus. A fever may develop.

First-Aid Treatment

The first step in treating a cut is to stop the bleeding. Visible bleeding can almost always be stopped by firmly compressing the bleeding area with a finger or hand for at least 5 minutes. Whenever possible, the bleeding part is elevated above the level of the heart—for example, by raising a limb. Because tourniquets shut off all blood flow to a body part and deprive it of oxygen, they are rarely used.

To prevent infection, dirt and particles are removed and the wound is washed. Large, visible particles are picked off. Smaller dirt and particles that cannot be seen are removed by washing with mild soap and tap water. Dirt and particles that remain after washing often can be removed with a more highly pressured stream of warm tap water. Harsher agents, such as alcohol, iodine, and peroxide, are not recommended. These solutions can damage tissue, impairing the capacity to heal. Scrubbing is required to clean deep scrapes. After cleaning, antibiotic ointment and a bandage are applied. If a wound is very small, it can be kept closed with certain commercially available tapes. Stitches may be needed for deep or large cuts.

Professional medical assistance is needed under the following circumstances:

• If a cut is longer than about ⅓ inch, is on the face, appears deep, or has edges that separate

• If bleeding does not stop within several minutes or after pressure is applied

• If there are symptoms of a nerve or tendon injury

• If a scrape is deep or has dirt and particles that are difficult to remove

• If there is a puncture wound, particularly if a foreign object in the wound is likely

• If the person has not had a tetanus vaccination within the past 5 years.

All wounds, whether treated at home or by medical professionals, should be observed for symptoms of infection during the first several days after treatment. If any symptoms of infection develop, professional medical assistance should be sought within several hours. Most small wounds heal within a few days.

Soft Tissue Injuries

Soft tissue injuries include bumps and bruises (contusions) and small tears of muscles (minor strains) or of ligaments and tendons near joints (minor sprains).

Contusions, mild strains, and mild sprains produce mild to moderate pain and swelling. The swelling can become discolored, turning purple after a day and becoming yellow or brown days later. The person usually can continue using the body part. People with more severe symptoms, such as pain, deformity, or an inability to walk or use an injured part may have a mild strain or sprain. However, they may also have a complete separation of bones that were attached within a joint (dislocation), partial separation of bones that were attached within a joint (subluxation), fracture,▲ or other severe injury. People with severe symptoms usually need professional medical care to determine the nature of the injury.

First-Aid Treatment

Contusions, mild strains, and mild sprains can be treated at home with *rest*, *ice*, *compression*, and *elevation* (RICE),■ which speeds recovery and decreases pain and swelling. If a fracture, severe strain, severe sprain, subluxation (partial dislocation), or dislocation is a possibility, a splint should be applied until professional help is available.

Severed or Constricted Limbs or Digits

Body parts such as fingers and toes can become severed. Also, tissue may die because blood flow has been cut off by rings or other constricting devices. Rings cut off blood flow when parts of the body near the ring swell, often as the result of an injury or simply because of constriction by the ring.

Severed body parts, if properly preserved, can sometimes be reattached in the hospital. To prolong tissue life, the severed part should be put in a sealed, dry plastic bag, and the bag should be put in a container with ice. Dry ice should not be used.

A ring or other object that encircles any body part, such as a finger or arm, must be removed before the limb swells. Sustained, gentle traction can be used to remove rings. Soap and water may reduce friction, easing removal. Otherwise, prompt medical care is needed.

▲ see also box on page 350   ■ see page 421

SPECIAL SUBJECTS

300 Medical Decision Making 1695

Sources of Information ▪ Decisions About Medical Tests ▪
Decisions About Treatment ▪ Participating in Medical Decision
Making ▪ Realities of Decision Making

301 Surgery..1698

302 Complementary and Alternative Medicine 1704

Effectiveness and Safety ▪ Alternative Medical Systems ▪ Mind-
Body Techniques ▪ Biologically Based Therapies ▪ Body-Based
Therapies ▪ Energy Therapies

303 Travel and Health 1708

Preparations Before Travel ▪ Problems That Occur in Transit ▪
Specific Medical Conditions and Travel ▪ Problems After Arrival ▪
Problems After Arriving Home

304 Amyloidosis 1715

305 Familial Mediterranean Fever 1716

306 Diseases of Unknown Cause 1717

Chronic Fatigue Syndrome ▪ Gulf War Syndrome ▪ Multiple
Chemical Sensitivity Syndrome ▪ Sick Building Syndrome

CHAPTER 300

Medical Decision Making

Making decisions about medical care is most effective when a doctor and a patient work together. The best and most appropriate decisions are reached when the doctor's experience and knowledge of medicine are combined with the person's knowledge, wishes, and values. However, there are many challenges that can interfere.

Sources of Information

Most doctors rely heavily on their experience: what they have learned from diagnosing and treating people with similar problems. However, doctors also read medical books and journals, consult with colleagues, and refer to other resources such as health sites on the Internet for more information on specific problems and to keep up with new information generated by medical research. They may also review recommendations (practice guidelines) published by groups of experts.

People who need health information rely most heavily on their doctors. But many people also turn to an ever-growing number of resources in print and on the Internet.

As new research findings are published, a doctor evaluates studies and considers how their findings might be applied. Different types of studies provide different types of information.

A cross-sectional study compares groups of people at the same point in time. Such a study compares test results of people who do and do not have a given disease and is often used to evaluate how well tests help diagnose diseases. A case-control study compares the histories of people who are similar except for the condition that is being studied. Such a study is often used to understand the cause or causes of a disease. In a cohort study, people are studied for a similar period of time, which varies from hours to decades, depending on what is being studied. A cohort study might be used to determine the effect of a disease on people over time (prognosis).

A clinical trial is considered the most rigorous type of study. In a controlled clinical trial, one group of people gets a particular treatment or test while the other groups (control groups) get different treatments or tests or no treatment or test at all. People may be assigned to the groups at random in a randomized controlled clinical trial. Conditions in a clinical trial are restricted, so only people with similar characteristics participate.

Sometimes studies are done to compare the relative costs of different approaches to diagnosis and treatment. These are called cost-effectiveness and cost-benefit studies. They may help a doctor consider the effects of decisions from society's perspective, but they may be less helpful when the doctor is considering decisions for a particular person.

Because of differences in the way studies are planned and carried out, even studies that are intended to evaluate the same thing may produce conflicting results. One method to try to resolve these conflicts is to prepare a summary of the findings of all studies that pertain to the topic and rigorously compare and evaluate them. This type of study is called a systematic review. Another method that tries to resolve conflicting results of studies is called

meta-analysis; a meta-analysis combines the studies' results mathematically and then compares them.

Decisions About Medical Tests

Tests are performed to screen for disease, diagnose disease, classify and measure the severity of disease, and monitor the course of a disease, especially its response to treatment.

Screening uses tests to try to detect a disease when there is no evidence that a person has the disease. For example, measuring cholesterol levels helps determine the risk of cardiovascular disease in people who have no symptoms of cardiovascular disease. To be useful, tests used for screening must be accurate, be relatively inexpensive, pose little risk, and cause little or no discomfort.

Diagnosis, on the other hand, uses tests to confirm or rule out a disease when there is suspicion that a person has the disease. For example, a doctor who suspects serious heart disease might recommend cardiac catheterization. This test would not be a good screening test because it is expensive, can produce side effects, and is uncomfortable. However, these drawbacks are outweighed by the need for this test when the presence or absence of disease must be confirmed.

Tests are used to classify and measure the severity of a disease that has already been diagnosed. Results may lead to more specific and effective choices for treatment. For example, after a diagnosis of breast cancer is confirmed, additional tests are performed to determine if and where the cancer has spread.

Tests are also used to monitor the course of a disease over time, often to determine the response to treatment. For example, blood tests are performed periodically in people with insufficient production of thyroid hormone (hypothyroidism) to determine whether they are receiving a dose of replacement thyroid hormone that best meets their needs. A decision is made about how often such testing is needed for a person.

When deciding whether to recommend testing for a disease, especially for diagnosis, the doctor estimates how likely it is that a person has the disease. In coming up with an estimate for a specific person (the pre-test probability of disease), the doctor may consider information about the disease in the area where he practices, including how common the disease is (prevalence) and how many new cases of the disease occur during a specific period of time (incidence). The doctor also considers whether the person has particular characteristics (risk factors) that make him more or less likely to be affected. With this information, the doctor can then select the best test to confirm the presence of the disease.

When deciding whether to perform a test, a doctor must determine what its results may mean. Unfortunately, tests are not perfect. They may sometimes produce normal results for people who have the disease being tested for; that is, they produce false-negative results. They may sometimes produce abnormal results for people who do not have the disease being tested for; that is, they produce false-positive results. Therefore, important characteristics of a test are its sensitivity (the likelihood that it will produce abnormal results for people with the disease being tested for) and its specificity (the likelihood that it will produce normal results for people without that disease). A doctor can mathematically combine the pre-test probability of disease with the results of the test and with information about the test's sensitivity and specificity to come up with a more accurate estimate of the likelihood that the person has the disease (post-test probability).

Another characteristic of a test is its reliability. A highly reliable test gives the same result when a person undergoes the test more than once, unless the disease being tested for has actually improved or worsened. Results from a less reliable test may change randomly.

Before performing a test, a doctor weighs the potential harm of the test against the potential benefit of the information the test may provide. He must also consider how the results will be used. It may not be useful to perform a test if the results will not change the treatment that is recommended. For example, if a test is being considered to determine if a particular treatment would be an option for a person, but the person has already decided he does not want that treatment, then the test need not be performed.

Decisions About Treatment

Doctors weigh the potential harm of a treatment against its potential benefit before recommending a course of action. Sometimes the benefit of treatment is improvement of symptoms, for example, reduction of pain. Benefit may also be improvement in function, for ex-

ample, being able to walk farther. At times, benefit is cure of a disease. At other times, a treatment reduces the future likelihood of undesirable events, such as complications of a disease. Then, the benefit is a decrease in the risk of the event that people want to avoid.

Risk is the likelihood that a harmful outcome will occur. For example, a doctor may consider recommending a drug to reduce the risk of a stroke. A controlled clinical trial might show that of 1,000 people given this particular drug, 20 have a stroke despite taking the drug. The study might also show that of 1,000 people who are not given the drug, 40 have a stroke. The results of the study could be expressed as showing that the drug cut the risk of stroke in half, because 20 is half of 40 (relative decrease in risk). However, the results could also be expressed as showing that only 20 people of 1,000 had their risk of a stroke eliminated, because the difference between 40 and 20 is 20 (absolute decrease in risk). Cutting the risk of stroke in half sounds impressive, but the doctor has to consider whether a treatment that benefits only 20 of every 1,000 people who take it is the right choice for the person being treated. In determining whether it is the right choice to use the drug, both the doctor and the person being treated may consider a variety of information, such as how likely the drug is to cause serious side effects.

Research studies provide information about how much a treatment reduces the risk of a harmful outcome on average. But average effects do not always tell the doctor how an individual person will respond to a treatment.

Participating in Medical Decision Making

To participate fully in the medical decision making process, a person needs to work closely with his doctor. A person may wish to obtain additional information about a recommended test or treatment before making a decision. Information can be obtained from pamphlets, brochures, and other materials the doctor provides; publications such as books, newsletters, and magazines designed to explain medical information to consumers; and from the Internet. The person should read the information carefully, keeping in mind the potential sources of bias in the information. For example, anecdotal information may indicate a treatment is helpful, but it may not be helpful for everyone. These resources may generate additional questions for the person to discuss with his doctor.▲ The person may also want to consult with another doctor, particularly one who has additional expertise (second opinion).

The person should also be very clear in expressing his choices to the doctor, especially if he has a condition, such as a terminal illness, that may make it impossible for him to express his wishes at some point later on.■

Realities of Decision Making

Whenever a decision must be made about diagnosis or treatment, two tasks must be accomplished. The first is to choose from a variety of information resources to help determine the best course of action. The second is to apply what is learned from those information resources to the individual person's situation.

There are several challenges. One challenge is time. Many decisions must be made quickly. Doctors and patients may not have enough time to gather and evaluate all the information available. The doctor must also help patients weigh the quality of information from several sources. For example, the doctor may feel that his personal experience merits more trust than results from a clinical trial.

The doctor must judge the potential effects of any diagnostic recommendations. He must help the person weigh the consequences of overlooking a serious condition even if the diagnosis is unlikely.

The same type of reasoning is used in deciding about treatments. If a person has a mild condition that will eventually get better on its own, a doctor will probably not recommend a treatment that may cause serious side effects. Conversely, if the person's condition is grave, such side effects may be worth the risk.

The doctor and the person may not share the same perceptions of risk. A person who hears about a possible side effect of a drug may be very concerned because the side effect is serious, regardless of how often the side effect occurs. The doctor may not be as concerned if the possibility of that side effect is remote. Or the doctor may not understand that what might seem to be a relatively minor side effect for most people may cause great problems for a particular person. For example, if a person drives for a living, it may be difficult for him to regularly take a drug that causes drowsiness.

Often, however, the balance between the risk of the disease and its treatment is not so clear-cut. A doctor may judge the risks and benefits of a treatment differently than the person being treated does. Understanding risks can also help a person weigh options. A doctor may outline several approaches and ask the person to decide among them. By evaluating the relative and absolute risks of the various choices and then factoring in his own values, a person can make more informed choices about medical care.

CHAPTER 301

Surgery

Surgery is the term traditionally used for treatments that involve cutting or stitching tissue. However, advances in surgical techniques have made the definition more complicated: Sometimes lasers, rather than scalpels, are used to cut tissue, and wounds may be closed without stitches. In modern medical care, distinguishing between a surgical and

medical procedure is not always easy; however, making that distinction is not important as long as the doctor performing the procedure is well trained and experienced.

Surgery is a broad area of care and involves many different techniques. In some surgical procedures, tissue is removed. In others, blockages are opened. In still others, arteries and veins are attached in new places to provide additional blood flow to areas that do not receive enough. Grafts, sometimes made of artificial

---

▲ see page 21   ■ see page 54

materials, may be implanted to replace skin, and metal rods may be inserted into bone to replace broken parts.

Surgery is sometimes used to aid in the diagnosis of a problem. A biopsy, in which a piece of tissue is removed for examination under a microscope, is the most common type of diagnostic surgery. In some emergencies, in which there is no time for diagnostic tests, surgery is used for both diagnosis and treatment. For example, surgery may be needed to quickly identify and repair organs that are bleeding from a gunshot wound.

Three categories of surgery are often described—emergency, urgent, and elective. Emergency surgery, such as stopping rapid internal bleeding, is performed as soon as possible; minutes can make a difference. Urgent surgery, such as removal of an inflamed appendix, is best performed within hours. Elective surgery, such as replacement of a knee joint, can be delayed for some period of time, until everything has been done to optimize a person's chances of doing well during and after the surgical procedure.

Anesthesia: Because surgery is generally painful, it is almost always proceeded by the administration of some type of anesthesia. Anesthesia blocks the perception of pain. Anesthesia may be local, regional, or general.

Local and regional anesthesia consist of injections of drugs, such as lidocaine or bupivacaine, that numb only specific parts of the body. In local anesthesia, the drug is injected under the skin of the site to be cut, numbing only that site. In regional anesthesia, which numbs a larger area of the body, the drug is injected into one or more nerves and numbs an area of the body supplied by those nerves. For example, injecting a drug into certain nerves can numb fingers, toes, or large parts of limbs. One type of regional anesthesia involves injecting a drug into a vein (intravenous regional anesthesia). A device such as a woven elastic bandage or blood pressure cuff compresses the area where the limb joins the body, trapping the drug within the veins of that limb. Intravenous regional anesthesia can numb an entire limb.

During local and regional anesthesia, the person remains awake. However, doctors sometimes give antianxiety drugs intravenously to calm and relax the person. Local and regional anesthesia are generally considered safer than general anesthesia because they usually do not affect the vital organs, such as the heart, lungs, brain, liver, and kidneys. Rarely, numbness,

Cosmetic Surgery

Cosmetic surgery involves a wide variety of operations, including removing facial and neck wrinkles (rhytidectomy); removing fat and wrinkles from the abdomen (abdominoplasty); enlarging or reducing breasts (mammoplasty); restoring scalp hair (hair replacement surgery); altering the appearance of facial features, such as the jaw (mandibuloplasty), eyelids (blepharoplasty), and nose (rhinoplasty); removing body fat (liposuction); and eliminating varicose veins (sclerotherapy).

Popular and tempting as cosmetic surgery may be, it is also expensive. In addition, cosmetic surgery poses risks, including serious health risks as well as the possibility that appearance may be less pleasing to the person than it was originally. Because obtaining the best results requires close adherence to instructions after the operation, cosmetic surgery is recommended only for highly motivated people. A person should choose a doctor who has met a medical specialty's standards for practice (board certification) and who has extensive experience with the procedure.

tingling, or pain can persist in the numbed area for days or even weeks.

Spinal and epidural anesthesia are specific types of regional anesthesia in which a drug is injected around the spinal cord in the lower back. Depending on the site of the injection and position of the body, a large area (such as from the waist to the toes) can be numbed. Spinal and epidural anesthesia are useful for operations of the lower body, such as hernia repairs and prostate, rectal, bladder, leg, and some gynecologic operations. Spinal and epidural anesthesia can also be useful for childbirth. Headaches occasionally develop in the days after spinal anesthesia but usually can be treated effectively.

In general anesthesia, a drug that circulates throughout the bloodstream is administered, rendering the person unconscious. The drug can be given intravenously or inhaled. Because a general anesthetic slows breathing, the anesthesiologist may insert a breathing tube in the windpipe. For short operations, however, such a tube may not be necessary; instead, the anesthesiologist can support breathing using a hand-held breathing mask. For longer opera-

Surgery Through a Keyhole

Technical advances now make it possible to perform surgery with smaller incisions and less tissue disruption than occurs with traditional surgery. Surgeons can insert tiny lights, video cameras, and surgical instruments through keyhole-sized incisions. The surgeons can then perform procedures using the images transmitted to video monitors as guides for manipulating the surgical instruments. This kind of surgery is called laparoscopic surgery when performed in the abdomen, arthroscopic surgery when performed in joints, and thoracoscopic surgery when performed in the chest.

Because it causes less tissue damage than traditional surgery, keyhole surgery has several advantages, including a briefer hospital stay (in most cases), less pain after the operation, earlier return to work, and a tendency toward smaller scars. However, the disadvantages of keyhole surgery often are underestimated, both by surgeons and by people undergoing the surgery. Because surgeons are using a video monitor, they are seeing only a two-dimensional view of the site on which they are operating. Also, the surgical instruments used have long handles and are controlled from outside of the person's body, so the surgeon may find that using them feels less natural than using traditional surgical instruments. For these reasons, keyhole surgery often takes longer than traditional surgery. More importantly, especially when a procedure is new, errors are more likely to occur than with traditional approaches because of the complexity of keyhole surgery. Finally, although keyhole surgery may cause less pain than traditional surgery, pain still occurs, often more than anticipated.

Because keyhole surgery is technically difficult, a person should choose a highly experienced surgeon. The person should establish that surgery is necessary and should ask the surgeon how pain will be treated.

Major and Minor Surgery: A distinction is sometimes made between major and minor surgery, although many surgical procedures have characteristics of both.

Major surgery usually involves the use of general anesthesia. Major surgery often involves opening one of the major body cavities—the abdomen (laparotomy), the chest (thoracotomy), or the skull (craniotomy)—and can stress vital organs. The surgery is usually performed in an operating room by a team of doctors. A stay of at least one night in the hospital is usually needed after major surgery.

Minor surgery can involve the use of local, regional, or general anesthesia. Major body cavities are not opened. Minor surgery may be performed in an emergency department, an ambulatory surgical center, or a doctor's office. Vital organs usually are not stressed, and surgery can be performed by a single doctor, who may or may not be a surgeon. Usually, the person can return home on the same day that minor surgery is performed.

Second Opinion: The choice to undergo surgery is not always clear, and there may be several options for the kind of surgical procedure. Thus, a person may seek the opinion of more than one doctor. Some medical insurance plans require a second opinion for elective surgery.

Some experts advise establishing up front that the doctor giving the second opinion will not perform the operation, so that there is no conflict of interest. Others advise obtaining a second opinion from a doctor who is not a surgeon, to eliminate any bias toward surgery when nonsurgical treatment is an option. However, some experts recommend that another surgeon give the second opinion, believing that a surgeon knows more about the advantages and disadvantages of surgery than would a nonsurgeon.

Preparing for the Day of Surgery

Various preparations are made in the days and weeks before surgery. It is often recommended that physical conditioning and nutrition be improved as much as possible, because good general health helps a person recover from the stress of surgery.

Eliminating or minimizing tobacco and alcohol use before undergoing surgery that involves general anesthesia can increase safety. Recent tobacco use makes abnormal heart rhythms more likely to develop during general anesthesia and impairs lung function. Exces-

tions, the breathing tube and a ventilator breathe for the person. General anesthetics affect vital organs, so the anesthesiologist closely monitors the heart rate, heart rhythm, breathing, body temperature, and blood pressure until the drugs wear off. Fortunately, serious side effects are very rare.

sive alcohol consumption can damage the liver, causing heavy bleeding during surgery and unpredictably increasing or decreasing the effect of the drugs used for general anesthesia. Alcohol consumption should be decreased gradually, however, because a sudden decrease before undergoing general anesthesia can cause harmful effects, such as fever and abnormalities of blood pressure or heart rhythm.

The doctor performs a physical examination and takes a medical history, which includes the person's recent symptoms, past medical conditions, use of tobacco and alcohol, and allergies. The person is also asked to list all drugs currently being taken. Nonprescription as well as prescription drugs must be disclosed, or serious health problems could result. For example, the use of aspirin, which a person may consider too trivial to mention, can increase bleeding during surgery.

Tests performed before surgery (preoperative testing) may include blood and urine tests, an electrocardiogram, x-rays, and pulmonary function tests. These tests determine how well the vital organs are functioning. If organs are functioning poorly, the stress of surgery or anesthesia can cause problems. Preoperative tests may also reveal an inapparent temporary illness, such as an infection, which would require the postponement of surgery.

A person may wish to store his own blood in case a blood transfusion is needed during surgery. Use of one's own blood (autologous blood transfusion▲) eliminates the risk of infections and most transfusion reactions. A pint of blood can be withdrawn from the person—several times, if necessary—and preserved until surgery. The body replaces the missing blood during the weeks after the blood donation.

The anesthesiologist may meet the person before the day of surgery to review test results and identify any medical conditions that might affect the choice of anesthetic. The safest and most effective types of anesthesia may be discussed as well.

A durable power of attorney for health care and a living will■ should be prepared before surgery in case the person becomes unable to communicate or incapacitated after surgery.

Sometime before the surgery, the surgeon obtains the person's permission to perform the operation, a process called informed consent. The surgeon discusses risks and benefits of the operation and answers questions. The person reads and signs a form documenting consent.

In cases of emergency surgery in which the person is unable to provide informed consent, doctors try to contact the family. Rarely, emergency surgery must proceed before the family is contacted.

Because some of the drugs given during surgery may cause vomiting, the person should generally not eat or drink anything for at least 8 hours beforehand. Specific guidelines should be given and vary depending on the kind of surgery. The person should ask the doctor which of his regularly prescribed drugs should be taken before surgery. People undergoing surgery involving the intestines are given laxatives for a day or two before the operation.

Because the device that monitors the level of oxygen in the blood is attached to a finger, nail polish and artificial nails should be removed before going to the hospital. Then, this device can perform more accurately. Also, valuables should be left at home.

The Day of Surgery

Before most operations, a person removes all clothing, jewelry, hearing aids, false teeth, and contact lenses or eyeglasses and puts on a hospital gown. The person is taken to a specially designated room (the holding area) or to the operating room itself for final preparations before surgery. The skin that will be cut (operative site) is scrubbed with an antiseptic, which removes bacteria, helping to prevent infection. A health care practitioner may shave the operative site. A plastic tube (catheter) is inserted in one of the veins of the hand or arm, through which fluids and drugs are given. A drug may be given intravenously for sedation.

If the final preparations are done in the holding area, the person is then taken to the operating room. At this point, the person may still be awake, although groggy, or may already be asleep. The person is moved to the operating table, over which are specially designed surgical lights. Doctors, nurses, and other personnel who will be near or touching the operative site thoroughly scrub their hands with antiseptic soap, which minimizes the number of bacteria and viruses in the operating room. For surgery, they also wear scrub suits, caps, masks, shoe covers, sterile gowns, and sterile gloves.

▲ see page 985

■ see page 55

In the Operating Room

The operating room provides a sterile environment in which the operating team can perform surgery.

The operating team consists of the chief surgeon, who directs the surgery; one or more assistant surgeons, who help the chief surgeon; the anesthesiologist, who controls the supply of anesthetic and monitors the person closely; the scrub nurse, who passes instruments to the surgeon; and the circulating nurse, who provides extra equipment to the operating team.

The operating room typically contains a monitor that displays vital signs, an instrument table, and an operating lamp. Anesthetic gases are piped into the anesthetic machine. A catheter attached to a suction machine removes excess blood and other fluids, which can prevent surgeons from seeing the tissues clearly. Intravenous fluids, started before the person enters the operating room, are continued.

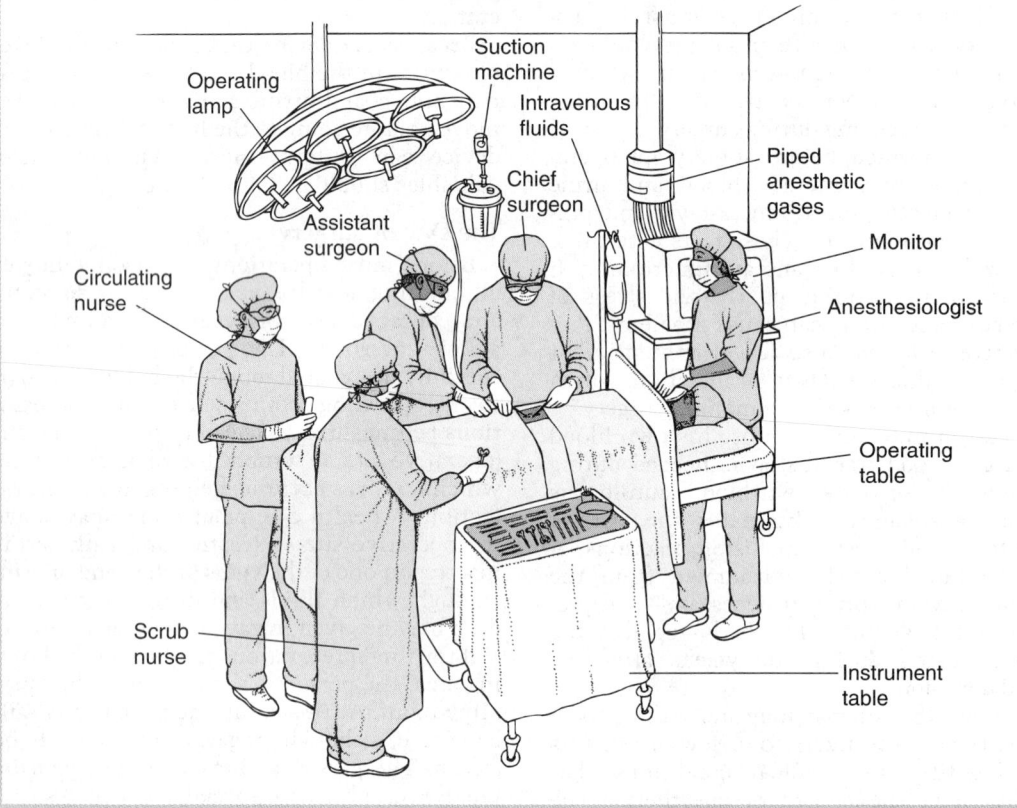

Anesthesia—local, regional, or general—is given.

After Surgery

After the operation is completed and anesthesia begins to wear off, the person is taken to a recovery room to be closely watched for about 1 or 2 hours. Most people feel groggy when awakening, particularly after major sur-

gery. Some people are nauseated for a short while. Some may feel cold.

Depending on the nature of the surgery and the type of anesthesia, a person may go home directly from the recovery room or be admitted to the hospital, sometimes in an intensive care unit (ICU). A person being sent home must be thinking clearly, breathing normally, able to drink fluids, able to urinate, able to walk, and be free of severe pain. The operative site should be free of bleeding and unexpected swelling.

A person who is admitted to the hospital may awaken to find many tubes and devices in and on him. For example, there may be a breathing tube in the throat, adhesive pads on the chest to monitor the heartbeat, a tube in the bladder, a device attached to a finger to measure the level of oxygen in the blood, a dressing on the operative site, a tube in the nose or mouth, and one or more tubes in the veins.

Pain is expected after most operations and can almost always be relieved. Drugs that relieve pain (analgesics) can be given intravenously, by mouth, by injection into the muscle, or applied to the skin as a patch. If epidural anesthesia was administered, the anesthesiologist may leave a plastic tube in the person's back through which opioid analgesics, such as morphine, can be injected. A person staying in the hospital may be given a device with which he can control the amount of analgesia he receives (patient-controlled analgesia). If pain persists, additional treatment can be requested.▲ Repeated use of opioid analgesics often causes constipation. To prevent constipation, a stimulant laxative or stool softener may be given.

Complications such as fever, blood clots, and infection can develop during the days after surgery. Common causes of fever include collapse of small parts of the lungs (atelectasis), urinary tract infections, and infections at the operative site. Atelectasis often can be prevented by periodically breathing forcefully in and out of a hand-held device (incentive spirometry).

Lying immobile during and after surgery sometimes causes clots to develop in the legs (deep vein thrombosis). The clots can dislodge from the legs and travel through the bloodstream to the lungs, where they can block blood from circulating through the lungs (pulmonary embolism). As a result, the oxygen supply to the rest of the body may be decreased, and sometimes blood pressure may fall. For certain operations after which blood clots are particularly likely, and for those people who are likely to have to lie still without much movement, doctors give preventive anticoagulants, such as low-molecular-weight heparin, or put elastic stockings on the person's legs to improve blood circulation.

If surgery makes eating impossible for more than several days, an alternative source of nutrition can speed recovery and prevent problems. People who had surgery of the digestive tract may be given nutrients through one of the body's large veins (parenteral nutrition). People whose digestive tracts are functioning but who are otherwise unable to eat may be given nutrients through a tube placed into the stomach. Such a tube may be passed through the nose, mouth, or abdominal wall.

To decrease the risk of infection, the surgical incision is dressed after surgery. The dressing includes a sterile bandage and usually includes an antibiotic ointment. The bandage absorbs fluids that ooze from the incision. Because prolonged exposure to these fluids can infect the incision, the dressing is changed often, usually daily.

Occasionally, the edges of the operative site that were stitched together begin to separate (dehiscence). The operative site can also become infected. An infected site can become increasingly painful 1 or more days after surgery and become red and warm or drain pus or fluid. Fever can develop. If symptoms of dehiscence or infection develop, the doctor should be seen as soon as possible.

Before being discharged home, a person should schedule a follow-up visit with the doctor, should know what drugs to take, and should know what activities to avoid or limit. Examples of activities that may need to be avoided temporarily include climbing stairs, driving a car, lifting heavy objects, and having sexual intercourse. A person should know what symptoms necessitate contacting the doctor before the scheduled follow-up visit.

During recovery from surgery, the person gradually resumes normal activity. Some people need rehabilitation, which involves special exercises and activities, to improve strength and flexibility.■ For example, rehabilitation after hip replacement surgery can involve learning ways to walk, stretch, and exercise.

▲ see page 450

■ see page 36

CHAPTER 302

Complementary and Alternative Medicine

Complementary and alternative medicine includes a variety of healing approaches and therapies taken from around the world. Many aspects of complementary and alternative medicine are rooted in ancient systems of healing, such as those of China, India, Tibet, and Africa. Complementary and alternative medicine includes treatments and health care practices that generally are not taught in most medical schools, used in hospitals, or reimbursed by insurance companies.

Complementary and alternative medicine practices may be used alone (alternative medicine) or in conjunction with conventional medicine (complementary medicine). For simplicity, however, the term alternative medicine is used in the remainder of this chapter.

Although the distinction between conventional and alternative medicine is not always easy to determine, a basic philosophical difference exists. Conventional medicine generally defines health as the absence of disease. The main causes of disease are usually considered to be isolated factors, such as pathogens (bacteria or viruses) or biochemical imbalances, and treatment often involves drugs or surgery. In contrast, alternative medicine practices often define health as a balance of body systems—physical, emotional, and spiritual—involving the whole person, that is, a holistic approach. Disharmony between these systems is thought to cause illness. Treatment involves strengthening the body's own defenses and restoring these balances. Alternative medicine also emphasizes preventing health problems before they arise.

An increasing number of people in Western countries are exploring alternative medicine as part of their medical care. In 1997, Americans made more than 629 million visits to alternative medicine practitioners, a 47% increase since 1990. This number substantially exceeds the 386 million visits made to all primary care doctors in the same year. The conditions for which people are most likely to seek alternative medicine treatments include chronic lower back pain, stress, migraine headaches, and arthritis. Some people also seek alternative medicine treatment when conventional treatment offers little hope, especially at the end of life.

Effectiveness and Safety

In 1992, the Office of Alternative Medicine within the National Institutes of Health (NIH) was formed to research the effectiveness and safety of alternative therapies. This office became the National Center for Complementary and Alternative Medicine in 1999.

The effectiveness of alternative medicine treatments is an important consideration. Some therapies have been shown to be effective for specific conditions, although these therapies are applied more broadly. Many forms of alternative medicine have not undergone thorough evaluation. However, a lack of proof does not mean that a therapy is ineffective, but rather, that its effectiveness has not been established. If an alternative therapy has been proved ineffective, its use cannot be further advocated scientifically. The greatest risk occurs when a person is treated by an alternative medicine approach in place of a proven conventional medicine approach, although data suggest this is rarely the case.

Safety is another important consideration. Some alternative medicine therapies can pose potential harm. Because herbal medicines are not regulated by the Food and Drug Administration (FDA), their manufacturers do not have to prove their safety.▲ Also, harm can be done by alternative therapies that involve manipulation of the body or other nonchemical interventions. In most cases of alternative medicine, harm has not been established or excluded, but in some cases potential harm has been demonstrated.

Types of Alternative Medicine

Alternative medicine can be classified into five major domains of practice: alternative medical systems, mind-body techniques, biologically based therapies, body-based therapies, and energy therapies. Some approaches

---

▲ see also page 106

are understandable within the concepts of modern science. Others are nearly incomprehensible within that paradigm.

Alternative Medical Systems

A number of alternative medical systems exist, including traditional Chinese medicine, Ayurveda, and unconventional Western practices of natural healing.

Traditional Chinese Medicine: Originating in China thousands of years ago, this system is based on the theory that illness results from the improper flow of the life force (qi) through the body. Qi is restored by balancing the opposing forces of yin and yang, which manifest in the body as heat and cold, external and internal, and deficiency and excess. Various practices are used to preserve and restore health, including herbal remedies, massage, meditation, and acupuncture.

Acupuncture is one of the most widely accepted alternative medicine techniques in the Western world. Licensed practitioners do not necessarily have a medical degree, although some medical doctors, often pain specialists, are trained and licensed to perform acupuncture. Acupuncture involves stimulating specific points on the body, usually by inserting very fine needles into the skin and underlying tissues. Sometimes, additional stimulation is added with a very low voltage electrical current or by warming the needle. Stimulating these specific points is believed to unblock the flow of qi along energy pathways (meridians) and thus restore balance between yin and yang. The procedure is not painful but may cause a tingling sensation. (A variation of acupuncture, called acupressure, uses localized massage instead of needles.)

Research has shown that acupuncture releases various chemical messengers in the brain (neurotransmitters), including serotonin, that serve as natural painkillers. Besides its potential effectiveness as a pain reliever, acupuncture may help relieve the nausea and vomiting that commonly occur after surgery. However, acupuncture has been ineffective in helping people to stop smoking or lose weight.

Side effects of acupuncture are uncommon if the procedure is performed correctly. Infection is one of the greatest risks but is extremely rare. Most practitioners use disposable needles; reusable ones must be sterilized properly. Worsening of symptoms (usually temporary) and fainting are the most common side effects reported by people who have undergone acupuncture.

Ayurveda: Ayurveda is the traditional medical system of India, originating more than 4,000 years ago. It is based on the theory that illness results from the imbalance of the body's life force, or prana. The balancing of this life force is determined by the equilibrium of the three bodily qualities, called doshas: vata, pitta, and kapha. Most people have a dominant dosha; the specific balance is unique to each person. Ayurveda uses herbs, massage, yoga, and internal cleansing to restore balance within the body and with nature.

Homeopathy: Homeopathy, which was developed in Germany in the late 1700s, is based on the principle that "like cures like" (thus the name homeo [Greek for "like"] and patho [Greek for "disease"]). In other words, a substance that in large doses causes illness is believed to cure the same illness if given in minute doses.

The remedies used in homeopathy are derived from naturally occurring substances, such as plant extracts and minerals. These substances are used to stimulate the body's innate capacity to heal. The more dilute the homeopathic medicine, the stronger it is considered to be.

Traditional scientists can find no scientific explanation for how the diluted remedies used in homeopathy might cure illness. There are few risks associated with homeopathy. However, side effects, such as allergic and toxic reactions, can occur.

Naturopathy: Naturopathy, which draws its practices from many cultures, began as a formal health care system in the United States in the early 1900s. Founded on the notion of the healing power of nature, naturopathy emphasizes prevention and treatment of disease through a healthy lifestyle, treatment of the whole person, and use of the body's natural healing abilities. This system also focuses on finding the cause of the disease rather than merely treating symptoms.

Naturopathy uses a combination of therapies, including nutrition, herbal medicine, homeopathy, physical medicine, exercise therapy, counseling, stress management, acupuncture, natural childbirth, and hydrotherapy.

Mind-Body Techniques

Mind-body techniques are based on the theory that mental and emotional factors can influence physical health. Behavioral, psychologic, social, and spiritual methods are used to preserve health and prevent or cure disease.

Because of the abundance of scientific evidence backing the benefits of mind-body techniques, many of the approaches are now considered mainstream. Methods such as relaxation, cognitive-behavioral therapy, meditation, imagery, biofeedback, and hypnosis, for example, are used in the treatment of coronary artery disease, headaches, difficulty sleeping (insomnia), and loss of urinary control (incontinence). These methods are also used as an aid in childbirth, in coping with the disease-related and treatment-related symptoms of cancer, and in preparing patients before surgery. Mind-body techniques are also used in the treatment of high blood pressure, asthma, arthritis, pain, and ringing in the ears (tinnitus), although with less success.

There are few known risks associated with the use of mind-body techniques.

Meditation: Meditation focuses on stilling the mind and allowing for greater self-awareness. It usually involves sitting or resting quietly, often with the eyes closed. Sometimes, it involves the repetitive sounding of a phrase (a mantra) meant to help the person focus. Most meditation practices were developed within a religious or spiritual context and held as their ultimate goal some type of spiritual growth, personal transformation, or transcendental experience. As a health care intervention, however, meditation may be effective regardless of the person's cultural or religious background. Meditation has been shown to offer numerous health benefits, including relieving stress and pain.

Relaxation Techniques: Relaxation techniques are practices specifically designed to relieve tension and strain. The specific technique may be aimed at lowering blood pressure, easing muscle tension, slowing metabolic processes, or altering brain wave activity.

Guided Imagery: Guided imagery involves the use of mental images to promote relaxation and wellness or to facilitate healing of a particular ailment, such as cancer or psychologic trauma. The images can involve any of the senses and may be self-directed or guided by a practitioner, sometimes in a group setting. For example, a person with cancer might be told to imagine an army of white blood cells fighting against the cancer cells.

Hypnotherapy: In hypnotherapy, a person is put into an advanced state of relaxation in which he is relatively unaware, but not entirely unconscious, of his surroundings. A

hypnotized person becomes absorbed in the images presented by the hypnotherapist and tends not to be consciously aware of the experiences he is undergoing. Hypnosis can be used to treat some conditions, such as certain pain syndromes and conversion disorders, in which apparent physical illness is actually due to psychologic stress and conflict. It has been used with some success to help people stop smoking and lose weight. Some people are able to learn to hypnotize themselves.

Biofeedback: Biofeedback involves the use of electronic devices to measure and report information about a person's biologic functions, such as heart rate, blood pressure, and muscle tension. The person can then understand why these functions change and can learn how to regulate them. Biofeedback typically is used to treat pain,▲ stress, difficulty sleeping (insomnia), headache, and muscle injuries.

Biologically Based Therapies

Biologically based therapies involve the use of chemicals, although typically these chemicals are derived from natural sources.

Herbal Medicine: Herbal medicine, the oldest known form of health care, uses plants to treat disease and promote health. Either a single herb or a mixture of different herbs can be used. In the case of Chinese herbal medicine, mixtures can also contain minerals and animal parts. Unlike conventional drugs, in which the active substance is extracted from the herb, herbal medicine usually makes use of the herb in its whole form. Herbal medicines are available as extracts (solutions obtained by steeping or soaking a substance, usually in water), tinctures (usually alcohol-based preparations, with the alcohol acting as a natural preservative), infusions (the most common method of internal herbal preparation, usually referred to as a tea), decoctions (similar to an infusion), pills, and powders and even in a moistened cloth applied to the skin. In the United States, the government has very little oversight of herbal products and places few regulations on the industry.■

Orthomolecular Medicine: Orthomolecular medicine focuses on the use of proper nutrition to maintain and restore health. It uses combinations of vitamins, minerals, and amino acids normally found in the body to treat specific conditions. Sometimes referred to as megavitamin therapy, orthomolecular therapy emphasizes supplementing the diet with large quantities of vitamins. Some of the more common

---

▲ see also page 455   ■ see page 106

orthomolecular treatments make use of shark cartilage to treat cancer, chelation therapy (removal of toxic materials from the bloodstream) to treat cardiovascular disease, and glucosamine or chondroitin (substances occurring naturally in the body) to treat osteoarthritis (for which there is good evidence of its effectiveness).

Body-Based Therapies

Body-based therapies include techniques that treat various conditions through bodily manipulation.

Chiropractic: In chiropractic, the relationship between the structure of the spine and the function of the nervous system is seen as key to maintaining or restoring health. The main method for achieving this balance is spinal manipulation.

Studies have shown chiropractic to be effective in treating low back pain. In addition, spinal manipulation may be useful in treating a variety of headaches. In general, however, the effect of manipulation on conditions not directly related to the musculoskeletal system has not been established. Serious complications resulting from spinal manipulation are rare but include low back pain from damage to nerve roots at the end of the spine (cauda equina syndrome▲) and blockage of blood supply to the brain from damage to arteries supplying the brain (cerebrovascular artery dissection). Other side effects include local discomfort, headache, and fatigue, which usually disappear within 24 hours.

Massage Therapy: Massage therapy is the manipulation of body tissues to promote wellness and reduce pain and stress. It involves a variety of techniques, from stroking and kneading (as used in Swedish massage) to applying pressure to specific points (as used in Shiatsu, acupressure, and neuromuscular massage). These techniques are claimed to help the musculoskeletal, nervous, and circulatory systems of the body.

Massage has been shown to be helpful in relieving pain, such as that caused by back injuries, muscle soreness, fibromyalgia, and anxiety in people with cancer. Massage has also been effective in treating low-birth-weight infants, preventing injury to the mother's genitals during childbirth, relieving chronic constipation, and controlling asthma. Massage may lower stress and anxiety.

Massage therapy should not be used in people who have infectious or contagious skin diseases, open wounds, burns, high fever, tumors, or a low platelet count.

Rolfing: Rolfing, also called structural integration, is based on the theory that good health depends on proper body alignment. It is a form of deep tissue massage that is typically performed over a series of sessions. Proper alignment of bone and muscle is achieved by manipulating and stretching fascia (fibrous tissue that surrounds certain body organs, such as muscles).

Reflexology: In reflexology, manual pressure is applied to specific areas of the foot that are believed to correspond to different organs or systems of the body. Stimulation of these areas is believed to eliminate the blockage of energy responsible for pain or disease in the corresponding body part.

Postural Reeducation: Postural reeducation uses movement and touch to help people relearn healthy posture. The therapies involved seek to release habitual, harmful ways of holding the body by focusing on awareness through movement.

Energy Therapies

Energy therapies focus on the energy fields thought to exist in and around the body (biofields). They also encompass the use of external energy sources (electromagnetic fields) to influence health and healing. All energy therapies are based on a core belief in the existence of a universal life force or subtle energy that resides in and around the body.

Practitioners of energy therapies typically place their hands on or near the body and use their energy to affect the energy field of the person.

Bioelectromagnetic-based Therapies: Bioelectromagnetic-based therapies use pulsed fields, magnetic fields, or alternating- or direct-current fields. Magnets, in particular, have become a popular treatment for various musculoskeletal conditions. Magnets have been marketed in clothing, jewelry, and mattresses to relieve pain, although there has been very little scientific investigation of their effectiveness.

Reiki: Reiki is a technique of Japanese origin in which the practitioner channels energy through his hands and into the person's body to promote healing.

Therapeutic Touch: Often referred to as "laying on of hands" even though actual touch is not needed, this therapy uses the therapist's healing energy to identify and repair imbalances in a person's biofield.

▲ see box on page 565

CHAPTER 303

Travel and Health

Health concerns are no longer a significant barrier to travel. However, all travel carries some risks. Therefore, smart travelers plan appropriately, address health concerns in transit and while away from home, and seek proper medical attention when symptoms or questions arise after returning home.

Preparations Before Travel

Preparation is crucial to ensuring that health concerns do not interfere with travel. Even people who are healthy need to plan appropriately to safeguard their health. Proper preparations are inexpensive relative to the costs of getting sick while away from home.

Travel Kits

Travel kits containing first-aid supplies; pain relievers, such as acetaminophen or non-steroidal anti-inflammatory drugs; decongestants; antacids; and antidiarrheal drugs, such as loperamide, are useful for minor injuries and illnesses. More significant problems can often be prevented with common-sense precautions. Detailed medical information, including written information about vaccinations and medications, may be the most valuable thing a person can have in a medical emergency.

Health and Travel Insurance

Health insurance is important for domestic and international travel. Some plans, however, limit coverage for emergency health care away from home; thus, the traveler should know the limitations of his policy.

Coverage is more often a problem for international travel. Some domestic insurance plans limit coverage for vaccinations and preventive drugs for international travel, even though some vaccinations are required for entry into certain countries. Likewise, Medicare does not cover the cost of any treatment given outside the United States. In addition, most domestic health insurance plans are not recognized in foreign countries. Instead, a cash deposit or payment in full may be required in some international hospitals before care is provided.

To avoid high costs or inability to obtain care, travelers should determine in advance what international coverage, if any, their health plan offers, how to seek prior authorization for international care, and how to make a claim after an emergency. Travel health insurance, including insurance for emergency evacuation, is available through many travel services and credit card companies. Elements of care for which travelers might want to purchase insurance include emergency care, transportation for care within foreign countries, transportation for care to the United States, medical equipment and personnel during transport, dental care, prenatal or postnatal care, lost or stolen prescription drugs, and medical translators.

Travelers can turn to other helpful resources as well. Directories listing English-speaking doctors in foreign countries are available from several organizations and Internet (Web) sites.▲ United States consulates may help travelers identify and secure emergency medical services.

Vaccinations

Vaccinations are important for travel to most developing countries and are required by some countries for entry. Common infections for which vaccines are available include hepatitis A and B, polio, and yellow fever. Some vaccines take up to 6 months to achieve their maximum effect, so early planning is necessary. An International Certificate of Vaccination is the best place to document the names and dates of all vaccinations. The certificate is easy to carry and can be obtained from many travel clinics or from the Superintendent of Documents at the U.S. Government Printing Office.■

Traveling With a Medical Condition

Traveling with a medical condition requires special preparation. People with a medical condition should visit their doctor before departure to ensure that their condition is stable and to determine if any changes in drugs are needed. A letter summarizing the person's medical history, including drug names and doses and dates of treatment, is invaluable in an emergency away from home. A medical

---

▲ see page 1768   ■ see page 1768

VACCINES FOR INTERNATIONAL TRAVEL [*, †, ‡]

INFECTION	REGIONS WHERE VACCINE IS RECOMMENDED	COMMENTS
Hepatitis A	Central and South America, Africa, Middle East and Asia, Eastern Europe	Requires 4 weeks for full immunity; should be given with hepatitis immune globulin if departure is less than 4 weeks away. Safe for pregnant women.
Hepatitis B	Alaska, Yukon and Northern Territories; Western Arctic Circle Islands; Southern and Western Pacific Islands; Amazon River Basin; Sub-Saharan Africa; China; Central and Southeast Asia	Recommended primarily for travelers anticipating sexual contact with residents or contact with their blood or blood products. Safe for pregnant women.
Japanese B encephalitis	Central and Southeast Asia, Far East; Torres Strait in Australia	Recommended only for people spending 1 or more months in rural areas of Asian countries during transmission seasons. Not recommended for pregnant women.
Meningococcus	Northern Sub-Saharan Africa	Travelers are at low risk even when traveling in epidemic areas, but vaccine adds protection. Required for entry to Saudi Arabia during Hajj. Safe for pregnant women.
Rabies	All countries, including United States	Recommended for travelers at risk of animal bites, including rural campers, veterinarians, field workers, and people living in remote areas. Does not eliminate need for additional vaccinations after animal bite for added protection.
Typhoid fever	Central and South America, Africa, Middle East and Asia, Eastern Europe	Offers good but imperfect protection. Protection is improved with close attention to food, water, and hygiene. Revaccination necessary after 5 years. Available as pill and injection. Pill containing weakened virus is not safe for pregnant women.
Yellow fever	South America, Africa	The disease is rare, but many countries require vaccination for entry. Not safe for pregnant women.

*See also Chapter 189.

†In addition to the listed vaccinations, travelers should be up to date on vaccinations for measles, mumps, rubella, tetanus, diphtheria, polio, pneumococcal disease, influenza, and varicella. Influenza vaccine is recommended for all adults who are traveling to the tropics, who are traveling to the Southern hemisphere between April and September, and who are traveling in large groups.

‡All recommendations are subject to change. For the latest recommendations, consult the Centers for Disease Control and Prevention.

identification tag or bracelet serves a similar function. Travelers should also carry proof of medical insurance.

Necessary drugs should remain in their original bottles so that the precise names of the drugs and the instructions for taking them can be reviewed in an emergency. The generic name of a drug is more useful than its brand name, because brand names differ among countries.

Travelers should also pack an extra supply of drugs in carry-on bags in case checked bags get lost, stolen, or delayed in transit or if the return trip is delayed. Because opioids, syringes, and large amounts of any drug are likely to raise the suspicions of security or customs officers, travelers should have a doctor's note explaining the medical need for the supplies. In addition, syringes should be packed together with the drugs that are dispensed in them. Travelers should also check with airports, airlines, or embassies to determine what additional documentation is helpful in making travel with these supplies go smoothly.

Problems That Occur in Transit

Several conditions are common even among healthy people while in transit.

Motion Sickness

Motion sickness during air, sea, rail, bus, or car travel occurs when the brain receives conflicting signals about movement.▲ Motion sickness is often triggered by turbulence and vibration and made worse by warmth, anxiety, hunger, or overeating. The main symptoms are stomach upset, nausea, vomiting, sweating, and dizziness.

Motion sickness can be minimized before and during travel by moderating intake of food, fluids, and alcohol. Fixing the eyes on a stationary object or on the horizon can help, as can lying down and keeping the eyes closed. Other measures include choosing a seat where motion is felt least (for example, in the center of an airplane, over the wing), refraining from reading, and sitting by an open window or an air vent if possible. A cabin in the middle of a ship close to water level may reduce motion sickness in some people. A scopolamine patch (which requires a prescription) or antihistamines are often useful, especially if taken before travel. These drugs often cause drowsiness, light-headedness, and dry mouth and can result in confusion, falls, and other problems in older people.

Blood Clots

Blood clots can occur when people sit for long periods during air, rail, bus, or car travel. Blood clots generally affect older people; people who are overweight, smoke, have varicose veins, or are taking estrogen; pregnant women; people who have recently undergone surgery or who have had blood clots previously; and people who have been inactive or immobile. Blood clots form in leg or pelvic veins (deep vein thrombosis■) and occasionally dislodge and travel to the lungs (pulmonary emboli★). Some blood clots in the legs do not cause symptoms,

whereas others cause cramping, swelling, and color changes of the calves and feet. Pulmonary emboli are much more serious than leg blood clots; people may first develop a sensation of not feeling well, followed by shortness of breath, chest pain, or fainting. Pulmonary emboli are sometimes fatal.

Blood clots can be prevented by changing position, straightening and moving the legs frequently while seated, and getting up to walk and stretch every 1 to 2 hours. Prolonged leg crossing may decrease leg circulation and should be avoided. Drinking fluids; avoiding smoking, caffeine, and alcohol; and refraining from wearing stockings, pantyhose, or pants that have constrictive bands at the top of the calves or thighs also help. Elastic support stockings improve circulation in the legs and may help as well.

Ear and Sinus Pressure

Ear and sinus pressure while flying is the result of changes in air pressure (cabin pressure). Normally, as an airplane takes off, cabin pressure decreases, and small pockets of air trapped in the sinuses and middle ear expand, leading to ear pressure, ear "popping," and mild sinus pressure or discomfort. As an airplane descends, cabin pressure increases, and similar symptoms occur. These mild sensations usually disappear as air pressure in the sinuses and ears equalizes with cabin pressure.

Swallowing frequently or yawning during takeoff and descent helps equalize pressure. These actions are normally sufficient to relieve minor ear and sinus discomfort. With allergies, sinus problems, and head colds, however, the passages that connect the ears and sinuses to the nose and mouth become inflamed and obstructed by mucus, which prevents air pressure from equalizing normally. People with these problems may experience significant discomfort and benefit from taking decongestants before flying or by blowing hard against a closed mouth and pinched nostrils to equalize air pressure. People with severe nasal and sinus congestion, whatever the cause, should consider postponing air travel.

Children are particularly susceptible to the pain of unequal air pressure. They should chew gum, suck hard candy, or be given something to drink during takeoff and descent to encourage swallowing. Babies can be breastfed or given a bottle or pacifier. In general, infants may fly safely after the age of 7 days.

▲ see also page 465   ■ see page 232
★ see page 285

Sleep Disturbance

Sleep disturbance (jet lag) is common with air travel across more than three time zones. Sleep disturbance does not occur with sea, rail, or car travel because travelers have time to adjust to time zone changes. The most obvious symptom is fatigue on arrival; other symptoms include irritability, difficulty sleeping (insomnia), headache, and difficulty concentrating. Jet lag can be minimized by adjusting sleep and wake times 1 or 2 days before departure to coincide with those of the destination time zone. In flight, a person should drink plenty of fluids and avoid smoking, caffeine, and excessive alcohol. Some people also benefit from supplements of melatonin, a sleep-inducing hormone normally produced by the body during periods of darkness. Melatonin induces sleep without a "hangover" effect when taken about 1 hour before regularly scheduled bedtime. Melatonin is more effective when traveling east, because the duration of daylight during travel is less, and nightfall arrives earlier. Other short-acting sedatives may also be helpful but may cause side effects, such as daytime drowsiness, amnesia, and nighttime insomnia. Long-acting sedatives, such as diazepam, can also cause confusion and falls in older people and should be avoided. On arrival, travelers should minimize napping, maximize exposure to sunlight, and remain physically active until evening.

Dehydration

Dehydration while flying is common because of the low humidity in airplanes. Dehydration tends to affect older people and people with certain medical conditions, such as diabetes and disorders requiring treatment with diuretic drugs. The main symptoms are light-headedness, drowsiness, confusion, and, occasionally, fainting. Dehydration can also cause dry skin. Dehydration can be prevented by drinking fluids and by avoiding alcohol and caffeine. Dry skin can be treated with moisturizers.

Spread of Infection

Spread of infection on airplanes and cruise ships often receives media attention but is relatively uncommon. Concern is greatest for influenza, viral diarrhea, and bacterial meningitis. Travelers can minimize their risk of influenza by making sure they have received the most current influenza vaccine. They can minimize their risk of diarrhea by washing their hands frequently. There is no reliable way to prevent bacterial meningitis. Some

cruise ships offer antibiotics to passengers who have been in close contact with passengers who have these infections.

Minor Injuries

Minor injuries are common. Unaccustomed lifting of heavy luggage is a common cause of shoulder injuries. Luggage falling out of overhead storage bins can cause other significant injuries. During ship travel, injuries can be prevented by wearing shoes that provide good traction on wet surfaces; using handrails and removing sunglasses before entering ship stairwells; and remaining alert in unfamiliar surroundings. A flashlight at night is useful for preventing falls as well.

Anxiety

Anxiety affects many people who travel. Fear of flying, fear of confined spaces, and worries about medical conditions worsening during flight are common sources of anxiety. Anxiety can cause insomnia, making jet lag worse. Companionship with a seasoned traveler or caretaker may help relieve anxiety. Cognitive therapy and desensitization programs may also help. Sedatives or antianxiety drugs may be necessary as well.▲

Specific Medical Conditions and Travel

People with specific medical conditions encounter special problems in transit.

Heart Disease

People with angina pectoris, heart failure, or rhythm disturbances that cause symptoms at rest or with minimal exertion should not travel. People who have had a heart attack within the past 14 days or a heart attack causing shock or heart failure within the past 8 weeks are also advised not to travel.

All travelers with heart disease should carry a copy of a recent electrocardiogram. People with pacemakers, implantable defibrillators, or coronary stents should carry a card or doctor's letter documenting the presence, kind, location, and electronic characteristics of the implanted device. An implanted metal device may trigger an alarm as the person passes through electronic security. Electronic security devices do not generally affect implant-

▲ see table on page 607

able defibrillators, but travelers are advised to avoid standing in walk-through metal detectors for more than 15 seconds. Hand-held metal detectors are also safe for people with defibrillators, but prolonged contact, such as holding the detector over the defibrillator for more than 5 seconds, should be avoided.

Most major airlines can provide low-sodium, low-fat meals on flights with regular meal service if given 24-hours' notice. Many cruise lines can also provide these meals if notified in advance.

Lung Disease

Travelers with lung cysts, severe emphysema, a large collection of fluid around the lungs (pleural effusion), recent chest surgery, or recent lung collapse can develop complications from airplane pressure changes and should not fly without approval from their doctor.

Other travelers with lung disease may need supplemental oxygen while aboard an airplane. A doctor determines a person's need for in-flight oxygen by measuring the level of oxygen in the blood. Airlines will provide in-flight oxygen if given a doctor's prescription and 48-hours' notice; travelers are not allowed to carry oxygen in any form aboard an airplane. Travelers who need oxygen during airport layovers must make their own arrangements, although most oxygen vendors will assist their regular customers without charge. Other respiratory equipment, such as continuous positive airway pressure devices, can be accommodated on an airplane provided the equipment does not exceed the size allowed for carry-on luggage. However, travelers who need this equipment should allow extra time for security checks.

Travel at high altitudes may present special problems because there is less oxygen available than at sea level. In general, people with mild or moderate lung problems do not experience any difficulty at altitudes below 5,000 feet, but the greater the altitude, the greater the chance of problems. People with lung disease traveling in or through such areas should take the same precautions that they would if they were flying.

Bus, train, car, and ship travel is safe for people with lung disease but requires planning to ensure a supply of oxygen. Commercial services can coordinate oxygen deliveries for travelers anywhere in the world.

People with asthma, emphysema, or bronchitis may find that their symptoms worsen in cities where air pollution is significant. They

may need additional treatments from their inhalers or additional drugs, such as corticosteroids, to control symptoms adequately.

Diabetes

Blood sugar levels are best managed in transit by frequent testing, with adjustments of food intake and drug doses as needed. Travelers with diabetes should pack sugar (glucose) supplements in their carry-on bags or carry juice, crackers, and fruit for when blood sugar levels are low. If travel plans incur time changes of more than a few hours, people with diabetes, especially those people taking insulin, should consult with a doctor on how best to schedule their drugs. Insulin can be stored without refrigeration for many days but should be kept out of extreme heat.

Most major airlines provide special meals for people with diabetes if given 24-hours' notice. Measures to prevent dehydration while in flight are important.

Blood sugar levels should be monitored frequently on arrival, because activities and diet often differ from those at home. Diabetic travelers should adhere to established diets despite temptations to try new foods and to eat more frequently or off schedule. They should wear comfortable socks and shoes, check their feet daily, and avoid walking barefoot so as to prevent minor injuries that might become infected or be slow to heal.

Pregnancy

Pregnancy generally is not affected by travel. However, pregnant women close to their due date (over 34 weeks) and those at risk of miscarriage, premature delivery, or placental abruption should avoid flying and traveling long distances. Most airlines have policies regarding travel for pregnant women, and these policies should be checked before tickets are purchased. Pregnant women traveling long distances should take precautions to reduce the risk of blood clots (such as getting up often when traveling by airplane and stopping to take short walks when traveling by car) and dehydration. Seat belts should be fastened low across the thighs, not over the abdomen, to prevent injury to the fetus.

Vaccines that contain a virus that has been weakened but not killed—such as yellow fever, Japanese B encephalitis, inactivated polio vaccine, and measles-mumps-rubella—are not safe for pregnant women. But all vaccines are safe for women who are breastfeeding.

Pregnant women should avoid prolonged use of water purification tablets that contain iodine, because iodine can affect development of the fetal thyroid gland.

Pregnant women who cannot postpone travel to regions of the world where malaria is common must weigh the risks of taking protective drugs whose effects on pregnancy are not well known against those of traveling without adequate protection. Malarial infection is more likely to be serious and life threatening in pregnant women than in women who are not pregnant, even with preventive drugs.

Pregnant women are also at risk of contracting hepatitis E infection, a viral liver infection rare in the United States but common in Asia, the Middle East, North Africa, and Mexico.▲ Miscarriage, liver failure, or death may result. There is no treatment, so postponing travel to regions where hepatitis E is common should be considered. Those who cannot postpone travel should be vigilant about handwashing.

Other Conditions

Travel and transit also affect other medical conditions.

Some travelers with sickle cell disease, for example, are at risk of experiencing pain (sickle cell crisis) when exposed to the low humidity and oxygen of airplane cabins. This risk can be minimized with proper hydration and oxygen.

People with a colostomy should wear a large bag or bring extra supplies, because fecal output may increase with expansion of intestinal gas during flight. Because gas expands in flight, water should be substituted for air in devices secured by air-filled cuffs or balloons, such as feeding tubes and urinary catheters.

People who wear contact lenses may want to wear eyeglasses en route or wet their lenses frequently to compensate for low humidity in the airplane. In general, bringing an extra set of eyeglasses or lenses, or a prescription in case replacements are necessary, is a good idea. Extra batteries for hearing aids may also be useful.

Travelers with serious mental health disorders, such as poorly controlled schizophrenia, may pose a risk to themselves or others and should be accompanied by a responsible attendant.

Most airlines provide disabled travelers with wheelchairs and stretchers on commercial flights. Some airlines accommodate travelers who need special equipment, such as intravenous lines or ventilators, as long as trained personnel accompany them and arrangements have been made in advance.

General advice about traveling with various medical conditions can be obtained from the medical departments of major airlines, from the Federal Aviation Administration, from on-line travel information sources,■ or from local travel clinics.

Problems After Arrival

Problems after arrival are especially important in international settings. Though many people are most concerned about infection when considering a trip overseas, heart disease is the most common cause of death among international travelers. Heart disease is the most common cause of death among nontravelers as well, suggesting that proper attention to health before leaving home is the best way to prevent illness while away.

Injuries

Injuries are the second most common cause of death overseas, most often due to motor vehicle or water accidents. Commonsense measures can be taken to prevent many such injuries. For example, people uncomfortable with unfamiliar traffic patterns (such as driving on the left side of the road in England versus the right side in the United States) can take public transportation or hire drivers familiar with local roads and traffic laws. Travelers should avoid overcrowded taxis, ferries, or other transports and avoid nighttime driving and swimming in poorly lit areas. Travelers should wear seat belts even as passengers. Also, alcohol should never be consumed before driving or swimming, even where laws do not formally prohibit such actions or where laws that do exist are not enforced.

Many cities are unsafe after dark, and some are unsafe even during the day. A traveler should avoid walking alone on ill-lit or deserted streets in such cities, especially in countries where the traveler is obviously a stranger.

Traveler's Diarrhea

Traveler's diarrhea★ is one of many infectious diseases that affect international travelers. Traveler's diarrhea may be prevented by drinking and brushing the teeth with bottled,

---

▲ see table on page 805   ■ see page 1768

★ see page 725

filtered, boiled, or chlorinated water; avoiding ice in drinks; eating freshly prepared foods heated to steaming temperatures; eating only those fruits and vegetables that can be peeled or shelled; avoiding food from street vendors; washing the hands frequently; and avoiding all foods likely to have been exposed to flies.

In most cases, traveler's diarrhea subsides by itself and requires only the steady intake of fluids to prevent dehydration. Other measures, though not always necessary, may be helpful. Bismuth subsalicylate taken 4 times a day may both prevent and treat traveler's diarrhea, though it should not be used by children and by people taking aspirin. Traveler's diarrhea can also be treated with the antidiarrheal drug loperamide (which is available without a prescription), the antibiotic ciprofloxacin or ofloxacin (which requires a prescription), or both. Children with traveler's diarrhea are given the antibiotic trimethoprim-sulfamethoxazole.

Powdered rehydration mixes are available for travel. If these are unavailable, rehydration solutions can be made with small amounts of salt, baking soda, and sugar or honey mixed in water.

Malaria

Malaria▲ is common in Africa, Southeast Asia, and some parts of South America. The best treatment is prevention. Malaria is prevented by wearing long-sleeved shirts and long trousers (especially at dawn and dusk, when mosquitoes are most active), sleeping under a mosquito net, and wearing clothing impregnated with permethrin. Insect repellants that contain diethyl-methylbenzamide (DEET) are also important and can help prevent other mosquito-borne diseases such as dengue and yellow fever. Even with these measures, antimalarial drugs (such as mefloquine, chloroquine, or atovaquone/proguanil) are necessary before, during, and after travel.

▲ see page 1140   ■ see page 1142

★ see pages 1218 and 1219

● see box on page 1178

Schistosomiasis

Schistosomiasis is a common and potentially serious infection caused by a parasite that lives in still water in Africa, Southeast Asia, China, and eastern South America. Schistosomiasis can be prevented by wearing footwear and socks when walking through water and by avoiding freshwater activities in areas in which schistosomiasis is common.■

Lice and Scabies

Lice and scabies are common in crowded or underdeveloped accommodations and can be treated with permethrin, malathion, or lindane lotions.★ However, these lotions should not be used preventively.

Sexually Transmitted Diseases

Sexually transmitted diseases, including HIV, gonorrhea, syphilis, trichomoniasis, and sometimes hepatitis B, are more common in developing countries. All can be prevented through abstinence or with proper, consistent use of a condom.● Because HIV and hepatitis B are also transmitted through blood and needles, an international traveler should never accept a blood transfusion without assurance that the blood has been tested for infection. Also, injections should be accepted only through one-time-only disposable needles.

Problems After Arriving Home

Symptoms or problems that developed during travel and that have not subsided by the time a person has returned home warrant medical attention. Some symptoms may develop weeks or months after a person has returned; fever after international travel is especially common. Although the connection between travel and new symptoms often is not apparent, information about recent travel can be the key element in making a diagnosis.

People with medical conditions should refill prescription drugs immediately if the drugs were lost or used up while away from home.

CHAPTER 304

Amyloidosis

Amyloidosis is a rare disease in which a protein called amyloid accumulates in various tissues and organs, impairing normal function.

Amyloidosis causes few or no symptoms in some people, while producing severe symptoms and fatal complications in other people. The severity of the disease depends on which organs are affected by amyloid deposits. Amyloidosis is twice as common in men as in women and is more common among older people.

Many forms of amyloidosis exist, and the disease can be classified into four groups: primary amyloidosis, secondary amyloidosis, hereditary amyloidosis, and amyloidosis associated with normal aging.

Primary amyloidosis (light chain amyloidosis) occurs with abnormalities of plasma cells, and some people with primary amyloidosis also have multiple myeloma (cancer of the plasma cells▲). Typical sites of amyloid buildup in primary amyloidosis are the heart, lungs, skin, tongue, thyroid gland, intestines, liver, kidneys, and blood vessels.

Secondary amyloidosis may develop in response to various diseases that cause persistent infection or inflammation, such as tuberculosis, rheumatoid arthritis, and familial Mediterranean fever. Typical sites of amyloid buildup in secondary amyloidosis are the spleen, liver, kidneys, adrenal glands, and lymph nodes.

Hereditary amyloidosis has been noted in some families, particularly those from Portugal, Sweden, and Japan. The amyloid-producing defect occurs because of mutations in specific proteins in the blood. Typical sites for amyloid buildup in hereditary amyloidosis are the nerves, heart, blood vessels, and kidneys.

Amyloidosis associated with normal aging usually affects the heart. What causes amyloid to build up in the heart, other than age, usually is not known. Amyloid also accumulates in the brain of people with Alzheimer's disease and is thought to play a role in causing Alzheimer's.

Symptoms and Diagnosis

The accumulation of large amounts of amyloid can disturb the normal functioning of

EFFECTS OF AMYLOID BUILDUP

Organ Affected	Possible Consequences
Brain	Alzheimer's disease
Heart	Heart failure, abnormal heart rhythms (arrhythmias), enlarged heart
Kidneys	Kidney failure; fluid accumulation in the tissues, causing swelling (edema)
Nervous system	Numbness, tingling, weakness
Digestive system	Intestinal obstruction, poor nutrient absorption, enlarged tongue
Blood and blood vessels	Easy bruising
Lungs	Difficulty breathing
Skin	Skin papules, bruises, enlarged lymph nodes
Thyroid gland	Enlarged thyroid gland
Liver	Enlarged liver
Musculoskeletal system	Carpal tunnel syndrome
Lymph nodes	Enlarged lymph nodes

many organs. Many people have few symptoms, whereas others develop severe, life-threatening disease. Common symptoms are fatigue and weight loss. Other symptoms of amyloidosis depend on where the amyloid builds up.

Amyloidosis is sometimes difficult for doctors to recognize because it produces so many different problems. However, a doctor may suspect amyloidosis when several organs fail; when fluid accumulates in the tissues, causing swelling (edema); or when unexplained bleeding occurs, especially in the skin. The hereditary form is suspected when an inherited peripheral nerve disorder is discovered in a family.

The diagnosis is generally made by testing a small amount of abdominal fat obtained through a needle inserted near the navel. Al-

▲ see page 1007

ternatively, the doctor can perform a biopsy by taking a sample of tissue from the skin, rectum, gums, kidney, or liver and examining it under a microscope with the use of special stains.

Prognosis and Treatment

There is no cure for amyloidosis. However, in secondary amyloidosis, treating the underlying disease usually slows or reverses the amyloidosis. Primary amyloidosis with or without multiple myeloma has a bleak prognosis; most people who have both diseases die within 1 to 2 years. People with amyloidosis who develop heart failure have a poor prognosis as well.

Treatment to decrease or control symptoms and complications of amyloidosis has been only modestly successful for most people. Chemotherapy (prednisone and melphalan, sometimes combined with colchicine) and stem cell transplantation offer relief to some people. Colchicine alone may help relieve amyloidosis that is triggered by familial Mediterranean fever. Accumulations of amyloid in a specific area of the body can sometimes be removed surgically.

Organ transplants (for example, of a kidney or the heart) have extended the lives of a small number of people with organ failure due to amyloidosis. The disease usually continues to progress, however, and eventually the transplanted organ accumulates amyloid. The exception is liver transplantation,▲ which usually stops the progression of amyloidosis in the hereditary form of the disease.

CHAPTER 305

Familial Mediterranean Fever

Familial Mediterranean fever (familial paroxysmal peritonitis) is an inherited disorder characterized by episodes of high fever together with abdominal pain or, less commonly, chest pain, joint pain, or a rash.

Familial Mediterranean fever occurs most commonly among people of Mediterranean origin (for example, Sephardic Jews, Arabs, Armenians, and Turks). However, in the United States, about 50% of people with familial Mediterranean fever have no known family history of the disorder.

Familial Mediterranean fever is an inherited disorder caused by an abnormal recessive gene.■ The abnormal gene results in the production of a defective form of pyrin, a protein that regulates inflammation. Some people with familial Mediterranean fever who do not receive proper treatment develop amyloidosis, in which an unusually shaped protein called amyloid is deposited in many organs and tissues, impairing their function.★

Symptoms and Diagnosis

Symptoms usually begin between the ages of 5 and 15. The person experiences irregularly occurring attacks of abdominal pain accompanied by fever as high as 104° F. The painful attacks usually last 24 to 72 hours but occasionally may last as long as a week. Attacks may occur as often as twice a week or as seldom as once a year. The severity and frequency of the attacks tend to decrease with age and during pregnancy. Sometimes the attacks stop completely for a number of years, only to resume later.

Recurring abdominal pain occurs in 95% of people with familial Mediterranean fever. The pain is caused by inflammation of the lining of the abdominal cavity (peritonitis). The pain usually starts in one part of the abdomen and then spreads throughout the entire abdomen. The severity of the pain may vary with each attack. Chest pain occurs in fewer than 50% of people with familial Mediterranean fever in the United States. Chest pain is caused by inflammation of the membranes surrounding the lungs (pleuritis) or, in extremely rare cases, by inflammation of the sac surrounding the heart (pericarditis). Inflammation of the large joints (arthritis), such as the knees, occurs in about

---

▲ see page 1077   ■ see art on page 12
★ see page 1715

10% of people with familial Mediterranean fever in the United States; the percentage is higher in other parts of the world, such as North Africa. Also comparatively rare in the United States is a painful red rash that usually appears near the ankles. People in whom amyloidosis affects the kidneys may experience fluid retention, weakness, and loss of appetite.

A doctor usually makes a diagnosis based on the typical symptoms. However, the abdominal pain of familial Mediterranean fever is virtually indistinguishable from that of other abdominal emergencies, particularly a ruptured appendix. Thus, some people with this condition undergo urgent surgery before the correct diagnosis is made. No routine laboratory test is by itself diagnostic, but such tests can be useful in excluding other conditions. Blood tests to determine a hereditary component can aid in making the diagnosis.

Prognosis, Prevention, and Treatment

Despite the severity of symptoms during attacks, people rapidly recover and remain free of illness until their next attack. However, if the disorder is not treated, some people develop kidney damage and eventually kidney failure because of amyloid deposited in the kidneys.

The daily use of colchicine, taken by mouth, eliminates or markedly reduces the number of attacks of pain in about 85% of people and virtually eliminates the risk of kidney failure due to amyloidosis. For people with infrequent attacks, colchicine can be withheld until symptoms first occur but then must be taken promptly.

Although mild analgesics, such as nonsteroidal anti-inflammatory drugs (NSAIDs),▲ may relieve pain sufficiently, opioids, such as meperidine, are usually needed.

CHAPTER 306

Diseases of Unknown Cause

Many people suffer greatly from disorders for which no specific cause has been identified. Some doctors believe these disorders are due to psychologic factors. Others believe that the disorders are caused by physical agents, such as viruses and toxic chemicals, or by abnormalities of the immune system. Although a cause has not been proved for any of these disorders, many people undergo considerable testing and try unproved treatments in time-consuming and costly attempts to diagnose and relieve their symptoms.

Chronic Fatigue Syndrome

Chronic fatigue syndrome refers to long-standing severe and disabling fatigue without a proven physical or psychologic cause.

Chronic fatigue syndrome may occur in up to 40 of 10,000 people in the United States; it affects people primarily between the ages of 20 and 50 and is about 1½ times more common in women than in men.

Cause

Despite considerable research, the cause of chronic fatigue syndrome remains unknown. Controversy exists as to whether there is a single cause or many causes and whether the cause is physical or psychologic.

Earlier studies have suggested infection with the Epstein-Barr virus, rubella, herpesvirus, or human immunodeficiency virus (HIV) as a possible cause of chronic fatigue syndrome. However, current research indicates that viral infections probably do not cause this syndrome, although in some cases they may hasten the onset of symptoms.

Some evidence suggests abnormalities of the immune system as a possible cause. Other suggested causes include allergies (about 65% of people with chronic fatigue syndrome report previous allergies), hormonal abnormalities, low blood pressure, decreased blood flow

---

▲ see page 452

Diagnosis of Chronic Fatigue Syndrome

According to the Centers for Disease Control and Prevention, a diagnosis of chronic fatigue syndrome requires the following:

1. Medically unexplained persistent or recurring fatigue of at least 6 months' duration that is new or had a definite beginning, is not due to exercise, is not substantially relieved by rest, and substantially interferes with work-related, educational, social, or personal activities.

2. At least four of the following symptoms:

- Poor memory for recent events or reduced concentration severe enough to interfere with work-related, educational, social, or personal activities
- Sore throat
- Tender lymph nodes in the neck or armpits
- Muscle pain
- Pain in more than one joint without joint swelling or tenderness
- Headaches that differ from previous headaches in terms of type, pattern, or severity
- Unrefreshing sleep
- Persistent feeling of illness for at least 24 hours after exercise

These symptoms must have been present persistently or recurrently during, but not before, the period of fatigue.

to the brain, and lack of certain nutrients in the diet.

Chronic fatigue syndrome seems to run in families, which may support an infectious agent as a cause. Alternatively, members of the same family may respond similarly to physical and psychosocial stress.

Some researchers have suggested that prolonged bedrest during convalescence from an illness may play a role in causing this disorder.

Symptoms and Diagnosis

The most important symptom is fatigue, usually lasting at least 6 months, that is severe enough to interfere with daily activities. Severe fatigue is present even on awakening and persists throughout the day. The fatigue often worsens with physical exertion or psychologic stress. However, evidence of muscle weakness or of joint or nerve abnormalities is

rare. Symptoms often begin after a coldlike illness that involves swollen lymph nodes that are tender or painful; extreme fatigue begins with a fever, runny nose, and chest congestion (accumulation of fluid within the air sacs).

Other symptoms that may occur are difficulty in concentrating and sleeping, sore throat, headache, joint pains, muscle pains, and abdominal pain.

No laboratory tests are available to confirm a diagnosis of chronic fatigue syndrome. Doctors therefore must rule out other diseases that may cause similar symptoms, such as thyroid disease, psychosis, and alcoholism. The diagnosis of chronic fatigue syndrome is made only if no other cause, including side effects of drugs, is found to explain the fatigue.

Treatment

In most cases, symptoms of chronic fatigue syndrome lessen over time.

Regular aerobic exercise, such as walking, swimming, cycling, or jogging, under close medical supervision may reduce fatigue and improve physical function. Psychotherapy, including individual and group behavioral therapy, may be helpful as well.

Drug therapy has had mixed results. Antidepressants and corticosteroids have been useful in some cases, although their safety and effectiveness in the treatment of chronic fatigue syndrome have not been established. A number of other treatments, including use of interferons and antiviral drugs, have been mostly disappointing. Dietary supplements, such as evening primrose oil, fish oil supplements, and high-dose vitamins, are commonly used, but their benefits remain unproved. Intramuscular injections of magnesium sulfate have been shown to improve mood and energy levels in a few cases. Intravenous injections of immunoglobulin have benefitted some people, but the side effects of this drug can be very harmful.

Excessive periods of prolonged rest may worsen symptoms of chronic fatigue syndrome.

Gulf War Syndrome

Gulf War syndrome consists of a group of symptoms experienced by more than 100,000 American, British, and Canadian veterans of the Persian Gulf War (1992).

Gulf War syndrome is poorly understood. Within a few months of returning from the Persian Gulf, veterans from different military units in the United States, Britain, and Canada began reporting a variety of symptoms, including headache, fatigue, difficulty sleeping, joint pain, chest pain, skin rashes, and diarrhea. In most cases, however, the symptoms reported by the person, such as headache and nausea, could not be objectively confirmed by a doctor. Even when symptoms could be confirmed, such as a skin rash, no specific cause could be attributed to them.

The cause of Gulf War syndrome is unknown. Gulf War veterans may have been exposed to a number of potentially toxic substances, including chemical weapons, biological warfare, depleted uranium weapons, insecticides, and smoke from burning oil wells. Veterans may also have been exposed to irritant petroleum products, decontamination solutions, and a variety of airborne substances that may have produced allergies. Vaccination with the anthrax vaccine,▲ which was given to U.S. military personnel involved in the Gulf War as protection against biological warfare, has also been proposed as a cause, although this vaccine has not caused symptoms in other recipients. The use of pyridostigmine tablets to help prevent the lethal effects of chemical weapons has been suggested as a possible cause as well. However, none of these agents has been convincingly linked to Gulf War syndrome.

Symptoms

Symptoms predominantly involve the nervous system. These include problems with memory, reasoning, concentration, and attention; difficulty falling asleep; depression; fatigue; and headache. Other symptoms may include disorientation, dizziness, erectile dysfunction (impotence), muscle pains, muscle fatigue, weakness, pins-and-needles sensations, diarrhea, skin rashes, cough, and chest pain.

Diagnosis, Treatment, and Prognosis

Diagnosis and treatment have not been established; therefore, doctors focus on relieving the symptoms.

Veterans who have Gulf War syndrome do not have a higher hospitalization or death rate than anyone else of the same age.

Multiple Chemical Sensitivity Syndrome

Multiple chemical sensitivity syndrome is a disorder that appears to be triggered by low-

Reported Triggers for Multiple Chemical Sensitivity Syndrome

- Alcohol and drugs
- Caffeine and food additives
- Carpet and furniture odors
- Fuel odors and engine exhaust
- Painting materials
- Perfume and other scented products
- Pesticides and herbicides

level exposure to multiple chemical substances commonly found in the environment.

Multiple chemical sensitivity syndrome is more common among women than men. In addition, 40% of people with chronic fatigue syndrome and 16% of people with fibromyalgia have multiple chemical sensitivity syndrome as well.

Some doctors consider this disorder to be psychologic in cause, probably a type of anxiety disorder similar to agoraphobia (fear of going out in public) or a panic attack.■ Others believe the disorder may be a type of allergic reaction.★ Indeed, various changes in the immune system may occur, supporting the idea of an allergic reaction. However, there is no consistent pattern of such changes among people who have this syndrome, and the cause remains unknown.

Symptoms and Diagnosis

Some people start having symptoms after a single exposure to high levels of various toxic substances. Sufferers blame their symptoms on exposure to these substances, but evidence is usually lacking.

Symptoms include a rapid heart rate, chest pain, sweating, shortness of breath, fatigue, flushing, dizziness, nausea, choking, trembling, numbness, coughing, hoarseness, and difficulty concentrating.

A doctor makes the diagnosis of multiple chemical sensitivity based on the symptoms. The diagnosis is supported if the symptoms recur after repeated exposure to the chemical substance; recur after exposure to levels much lower than those that have been tolerated previously or that are commonly tolerated by others; subside when the person leaves the of-

▲ see page 1098   ■ see page 608
★ see page 1063

fending environment; and develop in response to a wide variety of unrelated chemical substances.

A blood test may be performed to measure red and white blood cell counts and antibody levels but is of no proven value.

Treatment

Treatment usually involves trying to avoid the toxic substances thought to cause the symptoms. However, avoidance may be difficult, because many of these substances are widespread. Psychotherapy is sometimes helpful.

Sick Building Syndrome

Sick building syndrome refers to a group of symptoms that affects several workers in a particular building and is not caused by an identifiable specific illness. It may be caused by exposure to various harmful agents that exist in small concentrations within such buildings.

Sick building syndrome generally affects people employed in office or other buildings that house many workers in close proximity. Most frequently, it occurs in newer office buildings, which are designed to be energy-efficient, have windows that do not open, and usually have heating and cooling ducts that originate from a common source.

Elevated levels of carbon dioxide, which occur most commonly in such buildings, are a frequent cause of sick building syndrome. Chemicals present in renovation materials, cleaning solutions, and office machinery may also be causes. Molds and bacteria that grow in older poorly maintained buildings as a result of water leakage can also cause sick building syndrome. Trucks and other vehicles idling near the air intakes may also result in excessive exposure to carbon monoxide and diesel fumes. Poor lighting, excessive noise, and uncomfortable temperatures within the work environment may worsen symptoms in affected office workers.

Affected people become anxious, breathe rapidly (hyperventilate), and may experience muscle spasms and severe shortness of breath. They may also experience headaches, fatigue, sore throat, cough, dry eyes, skin rash, and itching. Some people report smelling strange odors.

Treatment and Prognosis

Symptoms subside when the person leaves the offending environment. The suspected building should be evaluated and improvements made as needed. Adequate ventilation should be provided.

There are no known permanent complications of sick building syndrome.

APPENDIXES

I   Weights and Measures 1721

II   Common Medical Tests 1724

III   Drug Names: Generic and Trade 1732

IV   Resources for Help and Information 1756

APPENDIX I

Weights and Measures

In medicine, precise measurements are necessary—for example, when various substances are measured in laboratory tests to evaluate health or make a diagnosis. Different units of measure may be used depending on the substance. Usually, the metric system, based on multiples of 10, is used to measure mass, volume, and length. Grams measure mass, the amount of matter in an object. Mass is similar to weight, but weight is affected by gravity. Liters measure volume, the amount of space an object occupies. Meters measure length.

Prefixes, indicating which multiple of 10 is meant, can be attached to the basic unit, such as meter (m), liter (L), or gram (g). Using prefixes helps make a number more readable. Commonly used prefixes include kilo (k), deci (d), centi (c), milli (m), and micro (μ).

Other units measure different properties of a substance. For example, a mole (mol) is the number of particles (molecules or ions) in a substance. Regardless of the substance, 1 mole always equals the same number of particles. However, the number of grams in 1 mole varies greatly from substance to substance. One mole equals the molecular (atomic) weight of a substance in grams. For example, the molecular weight of calcium is 40, and 1 mole of calcium equals 40 grams. Osmoles (Osm) and milliosmoles (mOsm) refer to the number of particles in a specific amount of liquid. Equivalents (Eq) and milliequivalents (mEq) measure a substance's ability to combine with another substance. A milliequivalent is roughly equivalent to a milliosmole.

Formulas are used to convert a measurement from one unit to another. The same amount can be expressed in terms of different units. For example, the concentration of calcium in the blood is normally about 10 milligrams in a deciliter (mg/dL), 2.5 millimoles in a liter (mmol/L), or 5 milliequivalents in a liter (mEq/L).

PREFIXES IN THE METRIC SYSTEM

Prefix	Multiple of 10	Comparison	
kilo (k)	1000	1 kilometer (km) = 1000 meters (m)	1 meter = 0.001 kilometer
deci (d)	0.1	1 deciliter (dL) = 0.1 liter (L)	1 liter = 10 deciliters
centi (c)	0.01	1 centimeter (cm) = 0.01 meter	1 meter = 100 centimeters
milli (m)	0.001	1 milliliter (mL) = 0.001 liter	1 liter = 1000 milliliters
micro (μ)	0.000001	1 microliter (μL) = 0.000001 liter	1 liter = 1 million microliters
pico (p)	0.000000000001	1 picoliter (pL) = 0.000000000001 liter	1 liter = 1 trillion picoliters

EQUIVALENTS FOR WEIGHT, VOLUME, AND LENGTH

Nonmetric to Metric	Metric to Nonmetric

Weight
  1 pound (lb) = 16 ounces (oz) = 0.454 kilogram (kg)   1 kilogram = 2.2 pounds
  1 ounce = 28.35 grams (g)   1 gram = 0.035 ounce

Volume
  1 gallon (gal) = 4 quarts (qt) = 3.785 liters (L)   1 liter = 1.057 quarts
  1 quart = 2 pints (pt) = 0.946 liter
  1 pint = 16 fluid ounces (fl oz) = 0.473 liter
  1 cup = 8 fluid ounces = 16 tablespoons (tbsp)
  1 fluid ounce = 29.573 milliliters (mL)
  1 tablespoon = ½ fluid ounce = 3 teaspoons (tsp)

Length
  1 mile (mi) = 1,760 yards (yd) = 1.609 kilometers (km)   1 kilometer = 0.62 mile
  1 yard = 3 feet (ft) = 0.914 meter (m)   1 meter = 39.37 inches (in)
  1 foot = 12 inches = 30.48 centimeters (cm)   1 centimeter = 0.39 inch
  1 inch = 2.54 centimeters   1 millimeter (mm) = 0.039 inch

EQUIVALENTS FOR HEIGHT AND WEIGHT

HEIGHT		WEIGHT	
ft-in	**cm**	**lb**	**kg**
4′ 10″	147.3	100	45.4
4′ 11″	149.9	110	49.9
5′ 0″	152.4	120	54.5
5′ 1″	154.9	130	59.0
5′ 2″	157.5	140	63.6
5′ 3″	160.0	150	68.1
5′ 4″	162.6	160	72.6
5′ 5″	165.1	170	77.2
5′ 6″	167.6	180	81.7
5′ 7″	170.2	190	86.3
5′ 8″	172.7	200	90.8
5′ 9″	175.3	210	95.3
5′ 10″	177.8	220	99.9
5′ 11″	180.3	230	104.4
6′ 0″	182.9	240	109.0
6′ 1″	185.4	250	113.5
6′ 2″	188.0	260	118.0
6′ 3″	190.5	270	122.6
6′ 4″	193.0	280	127.1

EQUIVALENTS FOR TEMPERATURE

To convert Fahrenheit to centigrade: Subtract 32, then multiply by $5/9$ or 0.555.

To convert centigrade to Fahrenheit: Multiply by $9/5$ or 1.8, then add 32.

	DEGREES	
	Centigrade (C)	**Fahrenheit (F)**
Freezing	0	32.0
Body temperature range	36.0	96.8
	36.5	97.7
	37.0	98.6
	37.5	99.5
	38.0	100.4
	38.5	101.3
	39.0	102.2
	39.5	103.1
	40.0	104.0
	40.5	104.9
	41.0	105.8
	41.5	106.7
	42.0	107.6
Boiling	100.0	212.0

Common Medical Tests

A large number of tests are widely available. Many tests are specialized for a particular disease or group of related diseases. Generally, specialized tests are described with the appropriate diseases in this book. However, other tests are used commonly for a wide range of diseases.

Tests are performed for a variety of reasons, including screening, diagnosing a disease, evaluating the severity of a disease so that treatment can be planned, and monitoring the response to treatment. Sometimes, a test may be used for more than one purpose. A blood test may reveal that a person has too few red blood cells (anemia), and then the same test may be repeated after treatment to check that the number of red blood cells has returned to normal. In some instances, a condition can be treated at the same time a screening or diagnostic test is performed. For example, when colonoscopy, a test in which a flexible viewing tube is used to examine the inside of the large intestine, reveals growths (polyps), they can be removed before colonoscopy is completed.

Types of Tests

Medical tests generally fall into one of six categories: analysis of body fluids, imaging tests, endoscopy, measurement of body functions, biopsy, and analysis of genetic material in cells. In many instances, the lines that separate the categories become blurred. For example, endoscopy of the stomach enables the examiner to view the inside of the stomach as well as obtain tissue samples for examination in a laboratory.

Analysis of body fluids most often consists of tests of the blood, urine, and fluid that surrounds the spinal cord and brain (cerebrospinal fluid). Less often, fluids such as sweat and saliva and fluid from the digestive tract (for example, gastric juices) are analyzed. Sometimes, the fluids analyzed are present only if a disease is present, such as when fluid collects in the abdomen (ascites) or in the space between the two membranes covering the lungs (pleural effusion).

Imaging consists of tests that provide a picture of the inside of the body, either in its entirety or only of certain parts. Ordinary x-rays are the most common imaging tests, but others include ultrasound, radioisotope (nuclear) scans, computed tomography (CT) scans, magnetic resonance imaging (MRI) scans, and positron emission tomography (PET) scans.

Endoscopy is the use of a viewing tube to directly observe the inside of body organs or spaces (cavities). Most often, the endoscope is flexible, although a few types are rigid. The tip of the endoscope is usually equipped with a light and a camera, so images can be seen on a television monitor while the examiner is observing through the endoscope. Tools are often passed through a channel in the endoscope. One type of tool is used to cut and remove tissue samples.

Endoscopy usually consists of passing the viewing tube through an existing body opening. For example, esophagogastroduodenoscopy (EGD) is accomplished by passing a viewing tube through the mouth. Colonoscopy involves passing a viewing tube through the anus. However, sometimes an opening in the body must be created. This can be done by making a small cut (incision) through the skin and through layers of tissue beneath the skin, so that the endoscope can be passed into a body cavity. For example, in arthroscopy, an endoscope is passed through an incision to view a joint, such as the knee or shoulder.

Measurement of body functions often involves recording and analyzing the activity of various body organs. For example, electrical activity of the heart is measured with electrocardiography (ECG), and electrical activity of the brain is measured with electroencephalography (EEG).

Biopsy involves removing tissue samples and examining them, usually with a microscope. The examination often focuses on finding abnormal cells that might provide evidence of inflammation or of a disease, such as cancer. Tissues that are commonly examined include skin, breast, lung, liver, kidney, and bone.

Analysis of genetic material usually involves testing cells from skin, blood, or bone marrow. Genetic testing consists of an examination for abnormalities of chromosomes, genes, or both. Examination of genes includes analysis of DNA. Fetuses may undergo genetic testing to determine whether they have a genetic disorder. Children and young adults often undergo genetic testing to determine whether they themselves have a disease or are at risk of a disease. Adults sometimes undergo genetic testing to help determine the likelihood that their relatives, such as children or grandchildren, will develop certain diseases.

Risks and Results

Every test has some risk. The risk may be only the need for further testing if the result is abnormal, or it may be the possibility of injury during the test. Doctors weigh the risk of a test against the usefulness of the information it will provide.

Normal test result values are expressed as a range, which is based on the average values in a healthy population; 95% of healthy people have values within this range, but average values are slightly different for women and men and also may vary by age. These values also vary somewhat among laboratories.

BLOOD TESTS*

Test	Reference Range/Threshold (conventional units†)
Acidity (pH)	7.35–7.45
Alcohol (ethanol)	0 mg/dL (more than 0.1 mg/dL usually indicates intoxication)
Ammonia	15–50 units/L
Amylase	53–123 units/L
Antinuclear antibodies (ANA; other antibodies can also be identified)	0 (negative result)
Ascorbic acid	0.4–1.5 mg/dL
Bicarbonate (carbon dioxide content)	18–23 mEq/L
Bilirubin	*Direct:* up to 0.4 mg/dL *Total:* up to 1.0 mg/dL
Blood volume	8.5–9.1% of body weight
Calcium	8.5–10.5 mg/dL (slightly higher in children)
Carbon dioxide pressure (expressed as a comparison with how high the level of mercury [Hg] rises in a tube due to air pressure at sea level)	35–45 mm Hg
Carboxyhemoglobin (carbon monoxide in hemoglobin)	Less than 5% of total hemoglobin
CD4 cell count	500–1500 cells/μL
Ceruloplasmin	15–60 mg/dL
Chloride	98–106 mEq/L
Complete blood cell count (CBC)	*See individual tests:* Hemoglobin, hematocrit, mean corpuscular hemoglobin, mean corpuscular hemoglobin concentration, mean corpuscular volume, platelet count, white blood cell count

Table continues on the following page.

BLOOD TESTS* *(Continued)*

TEST	REFERENCE RANGE/THRESHOLD (CONVENTIONAL UNITS†)
Copper	70–150 µg/dL
Creatine kinase (CK or CPK)	*Male:* 38–174 units/L *Female:* 96–140 units/L
Creatine kinase isoenzymes	5% MB or less
Creatinine	0.6–1.2 mg/dL
Electrolytes	*See individual tests:* Electrolytes routinely tested include calcium, chloride, magnesium, potassium, and sodium
Erythrocyte sedimentation rate (ESR)	*Male:* 1–13 mm/hr *Female:* 1–20 mm/hr
Glucose	*Fasting:* 70–110 mg/dL
Hematocrit	*Male:* 45–52% *Female:* 37–48%
Hemoglobin	*Male:* 13–18 gm/dL *Female:* 12–16 gm/dL
Iron	60–160 µg/dL (higher in males)
Iron-binding capacity	250–460 µg/dL
Lactate (lactic acid)	*Venous:* 4.5–19.8 mg/dL *Arterial:* 4.5–14.4 mg/dL
Lactic dehydrogenase	50–150 units/L
Lead	20 µg/dL or less (much lower in children)
Lipase	10–150 units/L
Lipids: Cholesterol	Less than 225 mg/dL (for age 40–49 yr; increases with age)
High-density lipoprotein (HDL)	30–70 mg/dL
Low-density lipoprotein (LDL)	60 mg/dL
Triglycerides	40–200 mg/dL (higher in males)
Liver function tests	Include bilirubin (total), phosphatase (alkaline), protein (total and albumin), transaminases (alanine and aspartate), prothrombin
Magnesium	1.5–2.0 mg/dL
Mean corpuscular hemoglobin (MCH)	27–32 pg/cell
Mean corpuscular hemoglobin concentration (MCHC)	32–36% hemoglobin/cell
Mean corpuscular volume (MCV)	76–100 cu µm
Osmolality	280–296 mOsm/kg plasma
Oxygen pressure (expressed as a comparison with how high the level of mercury [Hg] rises in a tube due to air pressure at sea level)	83–100 mm Hg

BLOOD TESTS* *(Continued)*

TEST	REFERENCE RANGE/THRESHOLD (CONVENTIONAL UNITS†)
Oxygen saturation (arterial)	96–100%
Partial thromboplastin time (PTT)	30–45 seconds
Phosphatase (alkaline)	50–160 units/L (higher in infants and adolescents, lower in females)
Phosphorus	3.0–4.5 mg/dL
Platelet count	150,000–350,000/mL
Potassium	3.5–5.0 mEq/L
Prostate-specific antigen (PSA)	0–4 ng/mL (increases with age)
Protein:	
Total	6.0–8.4 gm/dL
Albumin	3.5–5.0 gm/dL
Globulin	2.3–3.5 gm/dL
Prothrombin time (PT)	10–13 seconds
Red blood cell (RBC) count	4.2–5.9 million/mL
Sodium	135–145 mEq/L
Thyroid-stimulating hormone (TSH)	0.5–5.0 m units/L
Transaminase:	
Alanine (ALT)	1–21 units/L
Aspartate (AST)	7–27 units/L
Troponin:	
I	Less than 1.6 ng/mL
T	Less than 0.1 ng/mL
Urea nitrogen (BUN)	7–18 mg/dL
Uric acid	3.0–7.0 mg/dL
Vitamin A (other vitamins can also be measured)	30–65 µg/dL
White blood cell (WBC) count	4,300–10,800 /mL

*Blood can be tested for many other substances as well.
†Units are explained in Appendix I. Conventional units can be converted to international units by using a conversion factor. International units (IU), a different system, is sometimes used by laboratories.

DIAGNOSTIC PROCEDURES

PROCEDURE	BODY AREA OR SAMPLE TESTED	DESCRIPTION	MORE INFORMATION (PAGE NUMBER)
Amniocentesis	Fluid from the sac surrounding the fetus	Analysis of fluid to detect an abnormality in the fetus	1433 (box), 1434
Arteriography (angiography)	Any artery in the body; commonly in the brain, heart, kidneys, aorta, or legs	X-ray study in which radiopaque dye is used to detect and outline or highlight a blockage or defect of an artery	128, 130, 256, 445, 789, 828
Audiometry	Ears	Assessment of the ability to hear and distinguish sounds at specific pitches and volumes	1249
Auscultation	Heart	Listening with a stethoscope for abnormal heart sounds	121
Barium x-ray studies	Esophagus, stomach, intestine, rectum	X-ray study to detect ulcers, tumors, or other abnormalities	703
Biopsy	Any tissue in the body	Removal and examination of tissue sample under a microscope for cancer or another abnormality	256, 257, 343, 790, 828, 1041, 1354
Blood pressure measurement	Usually an arm	Test for high or low blood pressure	135 (box)
Blood tests	Usually a blood sample from an arm	Measurement of substances in the blood to evaluate organ function and to help diagnose and monitor various disorders	342, 789 (box), 980, 981 (box)
Bone marrow aspiration	Hipbone or breastbone	Examination of marrow under a microscope for abnormalities of blood cells	981, 982 (box)
Bronchoscopy	Airways of the lungs	Direct examination for a tumor or other abnormality	256
Cardiac catheterization	Heart	Study of heart function and structure	128
Chorionic villus sampling	Placenta	Examination of a sample under a microscope for an abnormality in the fetus	1432, 1433 (box)
Chromosomal analysis	Blood	Examination under a microscope to detect a genetic disease or to determine a fetus's sex	1430
Colonoscopy	Large intestine	Direct examination for a tumor or other abnormality	703
Colposcopy	Cervix	Direct examination of the cervix with a magnifying lens	1353
Computed tomography (CT)	Any part of the body	Computer-enhanced x-ray study to detect structural abnormalities	125, 255, 342, 443, 705, 789, 827
Cone biopsy	Cervix	Removal and examination of a cone-shaped piece of tissue	1407

DIAGNOSTIC PROCEDURES (*Continued*)

PROCEDURE	BODY AREA OR SAMPLE TESTED	DESCRIPTION	MORE INFORMATION (PAGE NUMBER)
Culture	Sample from any area of the body (usually a fluid such as blood or urine)	Examination of microorganisms grown from a sample to identify infection with bacteria or fungi	366, 826
Dilation and curettage (D and C)	Cervix and uterus	Examination of a sample under a microscope for an abnormality of the uterine lining	1354 (box)
Dual X-ray absorptiometry (DEXA)	Skeleton, focusing on specific regions, usually hip, spine, and wrist	Study of thickness of bones using a type of x-ray	342
Echocardiography	Heart	Study of heart structure and function using sound waves	125
Electrocardiography (ECG)	Heart	Study of the heart's electrical activity	122
Electroencephalography (EEG)	Brain	Study of brain's electrical function	445
Electromyography	Muscles	Recording of a muscle's electrical activity	342, 446
Electrophysiologic testing	Heart	Test to evaluate rhythm or electrical conduction abnormalities	124
Endoscopic retrograde cholangiopancreatography (ERCP)	Biliary tract	X-ray study of the biliary tract after injection of a radiopaque dye using a flexible viewing tube to reach the biliary tract	789, 790 (box)
Endoscopy	Digestive tract	Direct examination of internal structures using a flexible viewing tube	703, 704 (box)
Enzyme-linked immunosorbent assay (ELISA)	Usually blood	The sample is mixed with a sample of allergens or microorganisms to test for the presence of specific antibodies	1172
Fluoroscopy	Digestive tract, heart, lungs	A continuous x-ray study that allows a doctor to see the inside of an organ as it functions	125, 704
Hysteroscopy	Uterus	Direct examination of the inside of the uterus with a flexible viewing tube	1354
Intravenous urography	Kidneys, urinary tract	X-ray study of the kidneys and urinary tract after intravenous injection of a radiopaque dye	827
Joint aspiration	Joints between bones, especially shoulder, elbow, fingers, hips, knees, ankles, toes	Examination of fluid from the space within joints for blood cells, crystals formed from minerals, and microorganisms	342

Table continues on the following page.

DIAGNOSTIC PROCEDURES *(Continued)*

PROCEDURE	BODY AREA OR SAMPLE TESTED	DESCRIPTION	MORE INFORMATION (PAGE NUMBER)
Laparoscopy	Abdomen	Direct examination for diagnosis and treatment of abnormalities in the abdomen	703, 1355
Magnetic resonance imaging (MRI)	Any part of the body	Magnetic imaging test for any structural abnormality	126, 255, 342, 443, 705, 789, 827
Mammography	Breasts	X-ray study for breast cancer	1355 (box)
Mediastinoscopy	Chest	Direct examination of the area of the chest between the lungs	258
Myelography	Spinal column	Simple or computer-enhanced x-ray of the spinal column after injection of a radiopaque dye	445
Nerve conduction study	Nerves	Test to determine how fast an impulse travels	342, 446
Occult blood test	Large intestine	Test to detect blood in the stool	705
Ophthalmoscopy	Eyes	Direct examination to detect abnormalities inside the eye	1283, 1284 (box)
Papanicolaou (Pap) test	Cervix	Examination under a microscope of cells scraped from the cervix to detect cancer	1353
Paracentesis	Abdomen	Insertion of a needle into the abdominal cavity to remove fluid for examination	705
Percutaneous transhepatic cholangiography	Liver, biliary tract	X-ray study of the liver and biliary tract after injection of a radiopaque dye into the liver	789
Positron emission tomography (PET)	Brain and heart	Radioactive imaging to detect abnormality of function	127, 444
Pulmonary function tests	Lungs	Tests to measure the lungs' capacity to hold air, to move air in and out of the body, and to exchange oxygen and carbon dioxide	254
Radionuclide imaging	Many organs	Radioactive imaging to detect abnormalities of blood flow, structure, or function	127, 255, 342, 789, 828
Reflex tests	Tendons	Tests to detect abnormalities of nerve function	440
Retrograde urography	Bladder, ureters	X-ray study of the bladder and ureters after infusion of a radiopaque dye	827

DIAGNOSTIC PROCEDURES *(Continued)*

PROCEDURE	BODY AREA OR SAMPLE TESTED	DESCRIPTION	MORE INFORMATION (PAGE NUMBER)
Sigmoidoscopy	Rectum and last portion of the large intestine	Direct examination to detect tumors or other abnormalities	703
Skin allergy tests	Usually an arm or the back	Tests for allergies	1063, 1188
Spinal tap (lumbar puncture)	Spinal canal	Test for abnormalities of spinal fluid	442, 443 (box)
Spirometry	Lungs	Test of lung function that involves blowing into a measuring device	254 (box)
Stress test (exercise tolerance)	Heart	Test of heart function with exertion	123
Thoracentesis	The space that surrounds the lungs (pleural space)	Removal of fluid from the chest with a needle to detect abnormalities	256
Thoracoscopy	Lungs	Examination of the pleura and the pleural space through a viewing tube	258
Tympanometry	Ears	Measurement of the impedance (resistance to pressure) of the middle ear, which helps in determining the cause of hearing loss	1249
Ultrasonography (ultrasound scanning)	Any part of the body	Ultrasound imaging to detect structural or functional abnormalities	125, 255, 445, 704, 788, 826, 1354, 1432
Urinalysis	Kidneys and urinary tract	Chemical analysis of urine sample to detect protein, sugar, ketones, and blood cells	825
Venography	Veins	X-ray study to detect blockage of a vein	848

Drug Names: Generic and Trade

Most prescription drugs placed on the market are given trade names (also called proprietary, brand, or specialty names) to distinguish them as being produced and marketed exclusively by a particular manufacturer. In the United States, these names are usually registered as trademarks with the Patent Office; this gives the registrant certain legal rights with respect to the use of the name. A trade name may be registered for a product containing a single active ingredient, with or without additives, or for one containing two or more active ingredients.

A drug marketed by several companies may have several trade names. A drug manufactured in one country and marketed in many countries may have different trade names in each country.

Throughout this book, generic (nonproprietary) names have been used whenever possible. However, because trade names are used commonly and may be more readily recognized, the generic drugs mentioned in this book are listed below in alphabetic order along with many of their trade names. A second table follows, listing the trade names in alphabetic order along with their generic name.

With few exceptions, the trade names in these tables are limited to those marketed in the United States. These tables are by no means all-inclusive, and no effort has been made to list every trade name in current use for each drug. The inclusion of a drug in these tables does not indicate approval of a drug's use, nor does it imply that a drug is effective or safe. Many drugs are marketed almost exclusively under their generic name. Including a trade name of such a drug in these tables does not indicate an endorsement or preference for the trade name version over the generic version.

Whether it is best to use a trade or a generic version of a drug may be a complex decision. It is best to discuss such matters with a doctor or pharmacist.

Rx   SOME TRADE NAMES OF GENERIC DRUGS*

GENERIC NAME	TRADE NAME	GENERIC NAME	TRADE NAME
Abacavir	ZIAGEN	Amprenavir	AGENERASE
Abciximab	REOPRO	Anagrelide	AGRYLIN
Acarbose	PRECOSE	Anastrozole	ARIMIDEX
Acebutolol	SECTRAL	Anisindione	MIRADON
Acetaminophen	TYLENOL	Anistreplase	EMINASE
Acetazolamide	DIAMOX	Anthralin	ANTHRA-DERM
Acetohexamide	DYMELOR	Apraclonidine	IOPIDINE
Acetylcysteine	MUCOMYST	Argatroban	ARGATROBAN
Acetylsalicylic acid	See Aspirin	Asparaginase	ELSPAR
		Aspirin	ECOTRIN, ASPERGUM
ACTH	See Corticotropin	Atenolol	TENORMIN
Acyclovir	ZOVIRAX	Atorvastatin	LIPITOR
Adapalene	DIFFERIN	Atovaquone	MEPRON
Adenosine	ADENOCARD	Atovaquone-Proguanil	MALARONE
Albendazole	ALBENZA		
Albuterol	PROVENTIL, VENTOLIN	Atracurium	TRACRIUM
Alclometasone	ACLOVATE	Auranofin	RIDAURA
Alemtuzumab	CAMPATH	Azatadine	OPTIMINE
Alendronate	FOSAMAX	Azathioprine	IMURAN
Allopurinol	LOPURIN, ZYLOPRIM	Azelaic acid	AZELEZ, FINEVIN
Almotriptan	AXERT	Azelastine	OPTIVAR
Alprazolam	XANAX	Azithromycin	ZITHROMAX
Alprostadil	CAVERJECT, PROSTIN VR	Aztreonam	AZACTAM
		Bacitracin	AK-TRACIN
Aluminum hydroxide	AMPHOGEL, ALU-CAP	Baclofen	LIORESAL
		Balsalazide	COLAZAL
Amantadine	SYMMETREL	Basiliximab	SIMULECT
Amcinonide	CYCLOCORT	Beclomethasone	BECONASE, VANCENASE
Amikacin	AMIKIN		
Amiloride	MIDAMOR	Benazepril	LOTENSIN
Aminocaproic acid	AMICAR	Benzathine penicillin	BICILLIN
Aminophylline	PHYLLOCONTIN	Benzonatate	TESSALON
Amiodarone	CORDARONE	Benzoyl peroxide	BENZAC, DESQUAM
Amitriptyline	ELAVIL, ENDEP	Benzphetamine	DIDREX
Amlodipine	NORVASC	Benztropine	COGENTIN
Amorolfine†	LOCERYL	Bepridil	VASCOR
Amoxapine	ASENDIN	Betamethasone	CELESTONE, UTICORT, VALISONE
Amoxicillin	AMOXIL, POLYMOX, TRIMOX		
		Betaxolol	BETOPTIC, KERLONE
Amphetamine	ADDERAL	Bethanechol	URECHOLINE
Amphotericin B	FUNGIZONE	Bleomycin	BLENOXANE
Ampicillin	OMNIPEN, POLYCILLIN, PRINCIPEN	Bicalutamide	CASODEX

℞ SOME TRADE NAMES OF GENERIC DRUGS*

GENERIC NAME	TRADE NAME	GENERIC NAME	TRADE NAME
Bimatoprost	LUMIGAN	Caspofungin	CANEIDAS
Bisacodyl	DULCOLAX	Castor oil	NEOLOID, EMULSOIL
Bismuth subgallate	DEVROM	Cefaclor	CECLOR
Bismuth subsalicylate	PEPTO-BISMOL	Cefadroxil	DURICEF
		Cefamandole	MANDOL
Bisoprolol	ZEBETA	Cefazolin	ANCEF, KEFZOL, ZOLICEF
Bitolterol	TORNALATE		
Botulinum toxin	BOTOX	Cefdinir	OMNICEF
Bretylium	BRETYLOL	Cefditoren	SPECTRACEF
Brimonidine	ALPHAGAN	Cefepime	MAXIPIME
Brinzolamide	AZOPT	Cefixime	SUPRAX
Bromocriptine	PARLODEL	Cefoperazone	CEFOBID
Brompheniramine	DIMETANE	Cefotaxime	CLAFORAN
Budesonide	RHINOCORT	Cefotetan	CEFOTAN
Bumetanide	BUMEX	Cefoxitin	MEFOXIN
Buprenorphine	BUPRENEX	Cefpodoxime	VANTIN
Bupropion	WELLBUTRIN	Cefprozil	CEFZIL
Buspirone	BUSPAR	Ceftazidime	FORTAZ, TAZICEF, TAZIDIME
Busulfan	MYLERAN		
Butenafine	MENTAX	Ceftibuten	CEDAX
Butoconazole	FEMSTAT	Ceftizoxime	CEFIZOX
Butorphanol	STADOL	Ceftriaxone	ROCEPHIN
Cabergoline	DOSTINEX	Cefuroxime	CEFTIN, ZINACEF
Calcitonin	MIACALCIN, CALCIMAR	Celecoxib	CELEBREX
		Cephalexin	KEFLEX
Calcitriol	ROCALTROL	Cephradine	VELOSEF
Calcium carbonate	TUMS, CALTRATE, OSCAL	Cetirizine	ZYRTEC
		Chlorambucil	LEUKERAN
Candesartan	ATACAND	Chloramphenicol	CHLOROMYCETIN
Capsaicin	ZOSTRIX, CAPSIN, CAPZASIN	Chlordiazepoxide	LIBRIUM
		Chlorhexidine	HIBICLENS
Captopril	CAPOTEN	Chlormezanone	TRANCOPAL
Carbachol	MIOSTAT, CARBASTAT	Chloroquine	ARALEN
Carbamazepine	TEGRETOL	Chlorothiazide	DIURIL
Carbenicillin	GEOCILLIN	Chlorotrianisene	TACE
Carbidopa	LODOSYN	Chlorpheniramine	CHLOR-TRIMETON, TELDRIN
Carbimazole	NEO-MERCAZOLE		
Carboplatin	PARAPLATIN	Chlorpromazine	THORAZINE
Carisoprodol	SOMA	Chlorpropamide	DIABINESE
Carteolol	CARTROL, OCUPRESS	Chlorthalidone	HYGROTON
Carvedilol	COREG	Chlorzoxazone	PARAFLEX, PARAFON FORTE

℞   SOME TRADE NAMES OF GENERIC DRUGS*

GENERIC NAME	TRADE NAME	GENERIC NAME	TRADE NAME
Cholestyramine	QUESTRAN	Cyclobenzaprine	FLEXERIL
Choline magnesium trisalicylate	TRILISATE	Cyclopentolate	CYCLOGYL
Ciclopirox	LOPROX	Cyclophosphamide	CYTOXAN
Cidofovir	VISTIDE	Cycloserine	SEROMYCIN
Cilostazol	PIETAL	Cyclosporine	SANDIMMUNE, NEORAL
Cimetidine	TAGAMET	Cyproheptadine	PERIACTIN
Ciprofloxacin	CILOXAN, CIPRO	Cytarabine	CYTOSAR-U
Cisplatin	PLATINOL	Dacarbazine	DTIC
Citalopram	CELEXA	Daclizumab	ZENAPAX
Clarithromycin	BIAXIN	Dactinomycin	COSMEGEN
Clemastine	TAVIST	Dalfopristin	See Quinapristin
Clidinium	QUARZAN	Danazol	DANOCRINE
Clindamycin	CLEOCIN	Dantrolene	DANTRIUM
Clocortolone	CLODERM	Darbepoietin alpha	ARANESP
Clofazimine	LAMPRENE	Daunorubicin	CERUBIDINE
Clofibrate	ATROMID-S	Deferoxamine	DESFERAL
Clomiphene	CLOMID, SEROPHENE	Delavirdine	RESCRIPTOR
Clomipramine	ANAFRANIL	Demecarium	HUMORSOL
Clonazepam	KLONOPIN	Demeclocycline	DECLOMYCIN
Clonidine	CATAPRES	Desipramine	NORPRAMIN, PERTOFRANE
Clopidogrel	PLAVIX		
Clorazepate	TRANXENE	Desmopressin	DDAVP, STIMATE
Clotrimazole	LOTRIMIN, MYCELEX	Deslorelin	SOMAGARD
Cloxacillin	TEGOPEN	Desonide	TRIDESILON, DESOWEN
Clozapine	CLOZARIL		
Coal tar	FOTOTAR, ZETAR	Desoximetasone	TOPICORT
Colesevelam	WELCHOL	Dexamethasone	DECADRON, HEXADROL
Colestipol	COLESTID		
Colistin	COLY-MYCIN	Dexbrompheniramine	DRIXORAL
Corticotropin (ACTH)	ACTHAR	Dexchlorpheniramine	POLARAMINE
Cortisol	CORTEF, HYDROCORTONE	Dextrans	PROMIT, MACRODEX, GENTRAN
Cosyntropin	CORTROSYN	Dextroamphetamine	DEXADRINE
Co-trimoxazole	See Trimethoprim-sulfamethoxazole	Dextromethorphan	BENYLIN DM, DELSYM
Cromolyn	CROLOM, INTAL, NASALCROM	Diazepam	VALIUM, DIASTAT
Cyclandelate	CYCLOSPASMOL	Diazoxide	HYPERSTAT, PROGLYCEM
Cyclizine	MARAZINE		

℞ SOME TRADE NAMES OF GENERIC DRUGS*

GENERIC NAME	TRADE NAME	GENERIC NAME	TRADE NAME
Diclofenac	CATAFLAM, VOLTAREN	Doxylamine	NYQUIL
Dicloxacillin	DYCILL, DYNAPEN, PATHOCIL	Dronabinol	MARINOL
Dicyclomine	BENTYL	Drotrecogin alfa (activated)	XIGRIS
Didanosine (ddl)	VIDEX	Dyclonine	DYCLONE
Diethylcarbama-zine	HETRAZAN	Dyphylline	DILOR, LUFYLLIN
		Echothiophate	PHOSPHOLINE
Diethylpropion	TENUATE, TEPANIL	Econazole	SPECTAZOLE
Diethylstilbestrol	STILPHOSTROL	Edetate calcium disodium	CALCIUM DISODIUM VERSENATE
Diethyltoluamide (DEET)	OFF	Edrophonium	TENSILON
Diflorasone	MAXIFLOR	Efavirenz	SUSTIVA
Diflunisal	DOLOBID	Eflornithine	VANIQA
Digitoxin†	DIGITALINE	Emedastine	EMADINE
Digoxin	LANOXIN	Enalapril	VASOTEC
Dihydroergota-mine	D.H.E. 45, MIGRANAL	Enoxacin	PENETREX
		Enoxaparin	LOVENOX
Diltiazem	CARDIZEM, DILACOR	Entacapone	COMTAN
Dimenhydrinate	DRAMAMINE	Epinephrine	ADRENALIN
Dimercaprol	BAL	Epirubicin	ELLENCE
Dimethyl sulfoxide	RIMSO-50	Eprosartan	TEVETEN
		Eptifibatide	INTEGRILLIN
Diphenhydramine	BENADRYL, NYTOL, SOMINEX	Ergocalciferol	DRISDOL
Diphenoxylate with atropine	LOMOTIL, MOTOFEN	Ergotamine	ERGOMAR
		Ertapenem	INVANZ
Dipivefrin	PROPINE, AK Pro	Erythromycin	E-MYCIN, ERYTHROCIN, ILOSONE
Dipyridamole	PERSANTINE		
Dirithromycin	DYNABAC	Erythropoietin	EPOGEN, PROCRIT
Disopyramide	NORPACE	Escitalopram	CIPRALEX
Disulfiram	ANTABUSE	Estrogens	PREMARIN
Divalproex	DEPAKOTE	Etanercept	ENBREL
Dobutamine	DOBUTREX	Ethacrynic acid	EDECRIN
Docetaxel	TAXOTERE	Ethambutol	MYAMBUTOL
Docosanol	ABREVA	Ethosuximide	ZARONTIN
Docusate	COLACE	Ethylenediamine-tetraacetic acid (EDTA)	ENDRATE, VERSENATE
Donepezil	ARICEPT		
Dopamine	INTROPIN	Etidronate	DIDRONEL
Dorzolamide	TRUSOPT	Etodolac	LODINE
Doxazosin	CARDURA	Etretinate	TEGISON
Doxepin	SINEQUAN, ZONALON	Famciclovir	FAMVIR
Doxorubicin	ADRIAMYCIN	Famotidine	PEPCID
Doxycycline	VIBRAMYCIN		

Rx   SOME TRADE NAMES OF GENERIC DRUGS*

GENERIC NAME	TRADE NAME
Felbamate	FELBATOL
Felodipine	PLENDIL
Fenoprofen	NALFON
Fentanyl	SUBLIMAZE
Ferrous sulfate	FEOSOL
Fexofenadine	ALLEGRA
Finasteride	PROSCAR
5-fluorouracil	EFUDEX
Flecainide	TAMBOCOR
Fluconazole	DIFLUCAN
Flucytosine	ANCOBON
Fludarabine	FLUDARA
Fludrocortisone	FLORINEF
Flunisolide	NASALIDE
Fluocinolone	SYNALAR
Fluocinonide	LIDEX
Fluorouracil	ADRUCIL
Fluorouracil (topical)	EFUDEX
Fluoxetine	PROZAC
Fluoxymesterone	HALOTESTIN
Fluphenazine	PERMITIL, PROLIXIN
Flurandrenolide	CORDRAN
Flurazepam	DALMANE
Flurbiprofen	ANSAID, OCUFEN
Flutamide	EULEXIN
Fluticasone	CUTIVATE, FLONASE, FLOVENT
Fluvastatin	LESCOL
Fluvoxamine	LUVOX
Fomivirsen	VITRAVENE
Foscarnet	FOSCAVIR
Fosfomycin	MONUROL
Fosinopril	MONOPRIL
Fosphenytoin	CEREBYX
Fulvestrant	FASLODEX
Furazolidone	FUROXONE
Furosemide	LASIX
Gabapentin	NEURONTIN
Galantamine	REMINYL
Gallium nitrate	GANITE
Ganciclovir	CYTOVENE

GENERIC NAME	TRADE NAME
Gatifloxacin	TEQUIN
Gemcitabine	GEMZAR
Gemfibrozil	LOPID
Gemtuzumab-zogamicin	MYLOTARG
Gentamicin	GARAMYCIN
Glatiramer	COPAXONE
Glimepiride	AMARYL
Glipizide	GLUCOTROL
Glyburide	DIABETA, MICRONASE
Gold	MYOCHRYSINE
Goserelin	ZOLADEX
Granisetron	KYTRIL
Griseofulvin	FULVICIN
Guaifenesin	ROBITUSSIN
Guanabenz	WYTENSIN
Guanadrel	HYLOREL
Guanfacine	TENEX
Guanethidine	ISMELIN
Halcinonide	HALOG
Halobetasol	ULTRAVATE
Haloperidol	HALDOL
Haloprogin	HALOTEX
Hexachlorophene	PHISOHEX
Hexobarbital	SOMBULEX
Histrelin	SUPPRELIN
Hydralazine	APRESOLINE
Hydrochlorothiazide	ESIDRIX, HydroDIURIL, ORETIC
Hydrochlorothiazide-triamterene	DYAZIDE, MAXZIDE
Hydrocortisone	See Cortisol
Hydroflumethiazide	DIUCARDIN
Hydromorphone	DILAUDID
Hydroxychloroquine	PLAQUENIL
Hydroxyurea	HYDREA
Hydroxyzine	ATARAX, VISTARIL
Hyoscyamine	LEVSIN, ANASPAZ, LEVBID
Ibuprofen	ADVIL, MOTRIN, NUPRIN

Rx SOME TRADE NAMES OF GENERIC DRUGS*

GENERIC NAME	TRADE NAME	GENERIC NAME	TRADE NAME
Ibutilide	CORVENT	Ketorolac	TORADOL
Idarubicin	IDAMYCIN	Labetalol	NORMODYNE, TRANDATE
Imatinib	GLEEVEC	Lactulose	CEPHULAC, CHRONULAC
Imipenem-cilastatin	PRIMAXIN		
Imipramine	TOFRANIL	Lamivudine (3TC)	EPIVIR
Imiquimod	ALDARA	Lamotrigine	LAMICTAL
Indapamide	LOZOL	Lansoprazole	PREVACID
Indinavir	CRIXIVAN	Latanoprost	XALATAN
Indomethacin	INDOCIN	Lecithin	PhosChol, PERTROPIN
Infliximab	REMICADE	Leflunomide	ARAVA
Insulin	HUMULIN, NOVOLIN	Lepirudin	REFLUDAN
Interferon-alfacon-1	INFERGEN	Leucovorin	WELLCOVORIN
		Leuprolide	LUPRON
Interferon-alpha-2a	ROFERON-A	Levarterenol	See Norepinephrine
		Levetiracetam	KEPPRA
Interferon-alpha-2b	INTRON A	Levobetaxolol	BETAXON
		Levobunolol	BETAGAN
Interferon-alpha-2b and ribavirin	REBETRON	Levodopa	DOPAR, LARODOPA
		Levodopa-carbidopa	SINEMET
Interferon-alpha-N3	ALFERON N	Levofloxacin	QUIXIN, LEVAQUIN
Interferon-beta-1A	REBIF, AVONEX	Levonorgestrel	NORPLANT
Interferon-beta-1B	BETASERON	Levorphanol	LEVO-DROMORAN
Interferon-gamma-1B	ACTIMMUNE	Lidocaine	XYLOCAINE
		Lindane	KWELL
Ipratropium	ATROVENT	Linezolid	ZYVOX
Irbesartan	AVAPRO	Lisinopril	PRINIVIL, ZESTRIL
Irinotecan	CAMPTOSAR	Lithium	LITHANE, LITHONATE
Isoniazid	INH, NYDRAZID	Lomefloxacin	MAXAQUIN
Isoproterenol	ISUPREL	Loperamide	IMODIUM
Isosorbide	ISORDIL, SORBITRATE	Lopinavir-Ritonavir	KALETRA
Isosorbide dinitrate	ISORDIL, SORBITATE	Loracarbef	LORABID
Isosorbide nitrate	ISMO, IMDUR, ISOTRATE ER	Loratadine	CLARITIN
		Lorazepam	ATIVAN
Isotretinoin	ACCUTANE	Losartan	COZAAR
Isradipine	DYNACIRC	Lovastatin	MEVACOR
Itraconazole	SPORANOX	Loxapine	LOXITANE
Kanamycin	KANTREX	Lysine	L-LYSINE, ENISYL
Kaolin	KAOPECTATE	Mafenide	SULFAMYLON
Ketoconazole	NIZORAL	Magnesium hydroxide	MILK OF MAGNESIA
Ketoprofen	ORUDIS, ORUVAIL		

℞   SOME TRADE NAMES OF GENERIC DRUGS*

GENERIC NAME	TRADE NAME	GENERIC NAME	TRADE NAME
Maprotiline	LUDIOMIL	Metoclopramide	REGLAN
Mazindol	MAZANOR, SANOREX	Metolazone	MYKROX, ZAROXOLYN
Mebendazole	VERMOX	Metronidazole	FLAGYL
Meclizine	ANTIVERT, BONINE	Metoprolol	LOPRESSOR, TOPROL-XL
Meclofenamate	MECLOMEN	Mexiletine	MEXITIL
Medroxyproges-terone	PROVERA	Miconazole	MICATIN, MONISTAT
Mefenamic acid	PONSTEL	Midazolam	VERSED
Mefloquine	LARIAM	Midodrine	PROAMATINE
Megestrol	MEGACE	Mifepristone	MIFEPREX
Meloxicam	MOBIC	Miglitol	BLYSERT
Melphalan	ALKERAN	Milrinone	PRIMACOR
Meperidine	DEMEROL	Minocycline	MINOCIN
Meprobamate	EQUANIL, MILTOWN	Minoxidil	LONITEN, ROGAINE
Mercaptopurine	PURINETHOL	Mirtazapine	REMERON
Meropenem	MERREM	Misoprostol	CYTOTEC
Mesalamine	ASACOL, ROWASA, CANASA	Mitomycin	MUTAMYCIN
Mesoridazine	SERENTIL	Mitoxantrone	NOVANTRONE
Metaproterenol	ALUPENT, METAPREL	Modafinil	PROVIGIL
Metaxalone	SKELAXIN	Moexipril	UNIVASC
Metformin	GLUCOPHAGE	Molindone	MOBAN
Methadone	DOLOPHINE	Mometasone	NASONEX, ELOCON
Methamphetamine	DESOXYN	Montelukast	SINGULAIR
Methazolamide	NEPTAZANE, GLAUC	Moricizine	ETHMOZINE
Methenamine	HIPREX, MANDELAMINE	Morphine	MS CONTIN, ORAMORPH
Methicillin	STAPHCILLIN	Moxifloxacin	AVELOX
Methimazole	TAPAZOLE	Mupirocin	BACTROBAN
Methocarbamol	ROBAXIN	Muromonab-CD3	ORTHOCLONE OKT3
Methotrexate	RHEUMATREX	Mycophenolate mofetil	CELLCEPT
Methoxsalen	OXSORALEN	Nabumetone	RELAFEN
Methylcellulose	CITRUCEL	Nadolol	CORGARD
Methyldopa	ALDOMET	Nafcillin	UNIPEN
Methylphenidate	RITALIN, CONCERTA, METHYLIN	Naftifine	NAFTIN
Methylpredniso-lone	MEDROL	Naloxone	NARCAN
		Naltrexone	REVIA
		Naphazoline	VASOCON, NAPHCON
		Naproxen	ALEVE, ANAPROX
Methyltestosterone	ORETON	Naratriptan	AMERGE
Methysergide	SANSERT	Nateglinide	STARLIX
Metipranolol	OPTIPRANOLOL	Nedocromil	TILADE

R̃ₓ **SOME TRADE NAMES OF GENERIC DRUGS***

GENERIC NAME	TRADE NAME	GENERIC NAME	TRADE NAME
Nefazodone	SERZONE	Oxytetracycline	TERRAMYCIN
Nelfinavir	VIRACEPT	Oxytocin	PITOCIN, SYNTOCINON
Netilmicin	NETROMYCIN		
Nevirapine	VIRAMUNE	Paclitaxel	TAXOL
Nicardipine	CARDENE	Palivizumab	SYNAGIS
Niclosamide	NICLOCIDE	Pamidronate	AREDIA
Nicotine	NICORETTE, NICOTROL	Pancuronium	PAVULON
		Pantoprazole	PROTONIX
Nifedipine	ADALAT, PROCARDIA	Papaverine	PAVABID
Nilutamide	NILANDRON	Paromomycin	HUMATIN
Nimodipine	NIMOTOP	Paroxetine	PAXIL
Nisoldipine	SULAR	Peginterferon alpha-2b	PEG-INTRON
Nitrazepam†	MOGADON		
Nitrofurantoin	FURADANTIN, MACRODANTIN	Pemirolast	ALAMAST
		Pemoline	CYLERT
Nitroglycerin	NITRO-BID, NITROL	Penbutolol	LEVATOL
Nitroprusside	NIPRIDE	Penciclovir	DENAVIR
Nizatidine	AXID	Penicillamine	CUPRIMINE
Norepinephrine	LEVOPHED	Penicillin V	PEN-VEEK, VEETIDS
Norfloxacin	NOROXIN	Pentamidine	NEBUPENT, PENTAM 300
Nortriptyline	AVENTYL		
Nystatin	MYCOSTATIN, NILSTAT	Pentazocine	TALWIN
Octreotide	SANDOSTATIN	Pentobarbital	NEMBUTAL
Ofloxacin	FLOXIN, OCUFLOX	Pentosan poly-sulfate	ELMIRON
Olanzapine	ZYPREXA		
Olopatadine	PATANOL	Pentostatin	NIPENT
Olsalazine	DIPENTUM	Pentoxifylline	TRENTAL
Omeprazole	PRILOSEC	Pergolide	PERMAX
Orlistat	XENICAL	Perindopril	ACEON
Oseltamivir	TAMIFLU	Permethrin	NIX, RID
Oxacillin	PROSTAPHLIN	Perphenazine	TRILAFON
Oxaprozin	DAYPRO	Phenazopyridine	PYRIDIUM, URISTAT
Oxazepam	SERAX	Phendimetrazine	BONTRIL, PRELU-2
Oxcarbazepine	TRILEPTAL	Phenelzine	NARDIL
Oxiconazole	OXISTAT	Phenindamine	NOLAHIST
Oxybutynin	DITROPAN	Pheniramine	TUSSIREX
Oxycodone	OXYCONTIN	Phenobarbital	LUMINAL
Oxymetazoline	AFRIN	Phenoxybenza-mine	DIBENZYLINE
Oxymetholone	ANADROL	Phentermine	IONAMIN
Oxymorphone	NUMORPHAN	Phentolamine	REGITINE

℞ SOME TRADE NAMES OF GENERIC DRUGS*

GENERIC NAME	TRADE NAME	GENERIC NAME	TRADE NAME
Phenylephrine	NEO-SYNEPHRINE	Pyrantel pamoate	ANTIMINTH
Phenytoin	DILANTIN	Pyridostigmine	MESTINON
Physostigmine	ANTILIRIUM	Pyrimethamine	DARAPRIM
Pilocarpine	ISOPTOCARPINE, PILOCAR	Quetiapine	SEROQUEL
Pimozide	ORAP	Quinacrine	ATABRINE
Pindolol	VISKEN	Quinapril	ACCUPRIL
Pioglitazone	ACTOS	Quinidine	CARDIOQUIN, QUINAGLUTE
Piperacillin	PIPRACIL	Quinupristin- dalfopristin	SYNERCID
Piracetam	NOOTROPIL	Rabeprazole	ACIPHEX
Piroxicam	FELDENE	Ramipril	ALTACE
Pleconaril	PICOVIR	Ranitidine	ZANTAC
Plicamycin	MITHRACIN	Repaglinide	PRANDIN
Podophyllin toxin	PODOFIN	Reteplase	RETAVASE
Polycarbophil	FIBERCON, EQUALACTIN, MITROLAN	Ribavirin	VIRAZOLE
		Rifabutin	MYCOBUTIN
Potassium iodide	SSKI, PIMA	Rifampin	RIFADIN, RIMACTANE
Pralidoxime	PROTOPAM	Rimantadine	FLUMADINE
Pramipexole	MIRAPEX	Risperidone	RISPERDAL
Pravastatin	PRAVACHOL	Ritodrine	YUTOPAR
Praziquantel	BILTRICIDE	Ritonavir	NORVIR
Prazosin	MINIPRESS	Rituximab	RITUXAN
Prednisolone	DELTA-CORTEF, HYDELTRASOL	Rizatriptan	MAXALT
Prednisolone tebutate	PREDNISOL TBA	Rivastigmine	EXELON
		Rofecoxib	VIOXX
Prednisone	DELTASONE, METICORTEN	Ropinirole	REQUIP
		Rosiglitazone	AVANDIA
Primidone	MYSOLINE	Salmeterol	SEREVENT
Probenecid	BENEMID	Salmeterol- fluticasone	ADVAIR
Procainamide	PROCAN SR, PRONESTYL	Salsalate	DISALCID, SALFLEX
Procarbazine	MATULANE	Saquinavir	INVIRASE, FORTOVASE
Prochlorperazine	COMPAZINE	Scopolamine	ISOPTO HYOSCINE
Promethazine	PHENERGAN	Secobarbital	SECONAL
Propafenone	RYTHMOL	Selegiline	ELDEPRYL
Propantheline	PRO-BANTHINE	Selenium sulfide	SELSUN
Propoxyphene	DARVON, DOLENE	Senna sennosides	SENOKOT
Propranolol	INDERAL	Sertraline	ZOLOFT
Protriptyline	VIVACTIL	Sibutramine	MERIDIA
Pseudoephedrine	AFRINOL, SUDAFED	Sildenafil	VIAGRA
Psyllium	METAMUCIL, KONSYL	Silver sulfadiazine	SILVADENE

℞ SOME TRADE NAMES OF GENERIC DRUGS*

GENERIC NAME	TRADE NAME	GENERIC NAME	TRADE NAME
Simethicone	MYLICON, PHAZYME	Tetracycline	ACHROMYCIN V, TETRACYN, SUMYCIN
Simvastatin	ZOCOR	Thalidomide	THALOMID
Sirolimus	RAPAMUNE	Theophylline	BRONKODYL, THEOLAIR
Sotalol	BETAPACE	Thiabendazole	MINTEZOL
Spectinomycin	TROBICIN	Thiopental	PENTOTHAL
Spiramycin	ROVAMYCINE	Thioridazine	MELLARIL
Spironolactone	ALDACTONE	Thiothixene	NAVANE
Stanozolol	WINSTROL	Thyrotropin	THYTROPAR
Stavudine (d4T)	ZERIT	Tiagabine	GABITRIL
Streptokinase	STREPTASE	Ticarcillin	TICAR
Streptozocin	ZANOSAR	Ticlopidine	TICLID
Succimer	CHEMET	Timolol	BLOCADREN, TIMOPTIC
Sucralfate	CARAFATE	Tioconazole	MONOSTAT, VAGISTAT
Sulbactam-ampicillin	UNASYN	Tiopronin	THIOLA
Sulconazole	EXELDERM	Tirofiban	AGGRASTAT
Sulfacetamide	BLEPH-10, SULAMYD	Tizanidine	ZANAFLEX
Sulfadoxine-pyrimethamine	FANSIDAR	Tobramycin	NEBCIN, TOBREX
Sulfamethoxazole	GANTANOL	Tocainide	TONOCARD
Sulfasalazine	AZULFIDINE	Tolazamide	TOLINASE
Sulfinpyrazone	ANTURANE	Tolbutamide	ORINASE
Sulfisoxazole	GANTRISIN	Tolcapone	TASMAR
Sulindac	CLINORIL	Tolmetin	TOLECTIN
Sumatriptan	IMITREX	Tolnaftate	TINACTIN
Tacrine	CONEX	Tolterodine	DETROL
Tacrolimus	PROGRAF	Topiramate	TOPAMAX
Tamoxifen	NOLVADEX	Torsemide	DEMADEX
Tamsulosin	FLOMAX	Trandolapril	MAVIX
Tazarotene	TAZORAC	Tranylcypromine	PARNATE
Telmisartan	MICARDIS	Trastuzumab	HERCEPTIN
Temazepam	RESTORIL	Travoprost	TRAVATAN
Tenofovir	VIREAD	Trazodone	DESYREL
Terazosin	HYTRIN	Tretinoin	RETIN-A, AVITA, RENOVA
Terbinafine	LAMISIL AT	Triamcinolone	ARISTOCORT, KENACORT, KENALOG
Terbutaline	BRETHINE, BRICANYL	Triamcinolone hexacetonide	ARISTROSPAN
Terconazole	TERAZOL	Triamterene	DYRENIUM
Terfenadine	SELDANE	Triazolam	HALCION
Testolactone	TESLAC	Trichlormethiazide	NAQUA, METAHYDRIN
Testosterone	DELATESTRYL, DEPO-TESTOSTERONE		
Tetracaine	CEPACOL, VIRACTIN		

℞ SOME TRADE NAMES OF GENERIC DRUGS*

GENERIC NAME	TRADE NAME	GENERIC NAME	TRADE NAME
Trichloroacetic acid	TRI-CHLOR	Valproate	DEPARENE
Trifluoperazine	STELAZINE	Valsartan	DIOVAN
Triflupromazine	VESPRIN	Vancomycin	VANCOCIN
Trifluridine	VIROPTIC	Vasopressin	PITRESSIN
Trihexyphenidyl	ARTANE	Venlafaxine	EFFEXOR
Trimeprazine	TEMARIL	Verapamil	CALAN, ISOPTIN
Trimethadione	TRIDIONE	Vidarabine	VIRA-A
Trimethobenza-mide	TIGAN	Vigabatrin	SABRIL
Trimethoprim	PROLOPRIM, TRIMPEX	Vinblastine	VELBAN
Trimethoprim-polymyxin	POLYTRIM	Vincristine	ONCOVIN
		Vinorelbine	NAVELBINE
Trimethoprim-sulfamethoxazole	BACTRIM, SEPTRA	Voriconazole	VFEND
		Warfarin	COUMADIN
Trimipramine	SURMONTIL	Xylometazoline	OTRIUIN
Tripelennamine	PBZ-SR	Yohimbine	YOCON
Triprolidine	ACTIFED	Zafirlukast	ACCOLATE
Troleandomycin	TAO	Zalcitabine (ddC)	HIVID
Tropicamide	MYDRIACIL	Zanamivir	RELENZA
Trovafloxacin	TROVAN	Zidovudine (AZT)	RETROVIR
2-chlorodeoxy-adenosine	CLADRIBINE	Zileuton	ZYFLO
Undecylenate	DESENEX	Ziprasidone	GEODON
Unoprostone	RESCULA	Zoledronic acid	ZOMETA
Ursodiol	ACTIGALL	Zolmitriptan	ZOMIG
Valacyclovir	VALTREX	Zolpidem	AMBIEN
Valdecoxib	BEXTRA	Zonisamide	ZONEGRAN
Valganciclovir	VALCYTE		

*Some drugs mentioned in this book are manufactured only as generics and therefore have no trade name and are not included in this table.

†Not available in the United States.

℞ GENERIC NAMES FOR SOME TRADE NAME DRUGS*

TRADE NAME	GENERIC NAME	TRADE NAME	GENERIC NAME
ABREVA	Docosanol	AMARYL	Glimepiride
ACCOLATE	Zafirlukast	AMBIEN	Zolpidem
ACCUPRIL	Quinapril	AMERGE	Naratriptan
ACCUTANE	Isotretinoin	AMICAR	Aminocaproic acid
ACEON	Perindopril	AMIKIN	Amikacin
ACHROMYCIN V	Tetracycline	AMOXIL	Amoxicillin
ACIPHEX	Rabeprazole	AMPHOGEL	Aluminum hydroxide
ACLOVATE	Alclometasone	ANADROL	Oxymetholone
ACTHAR	Corticotropin (ACTH)	ANAFRANIL	Clomipramine
ACTIFED	Triprolidine	ANAPROX	Naproxen
ACTIGALL	Ursodiol	ANASPAZ	Hyoscyamine
ACTIMMUNE	Interferon-gamma-1B	ANCEF	Cefazolin
ACTOS	Pioglitazone	ANCOBON	Flucytosine
ADALAT	Nifedipine	ANSAID	Flurbiprofen
ADDERAL	Amphetamine	ANTABUSE	Disulfiram
ADENOCARD	Adenosine	ANTHRA-DERM	Anthralin
ADRENALIN	Epinephrine	ANTILIRIUM	Physostigmine
ADRIAMYCIN	Doxorubicin	ANTIMINTH	Pyrantel pamoate
ADRUCIL	Fluorouracil	ANTIVERT	Meclizine
ADVAIR	Salmeterol-fluticasone	ANTURANE	Sulfinpyrazone
ADVIL	Ibuprofen	APRESOLINE	Hydralazine
AFRIN	Oxymetazoline	ARALEN	Chloroquine
AFRINOL	Pseudoephedrine	ARANESP	Darbepoietin alpha
AGENERASE	Amprenavir	ARAVA	Leflunomide
AGGRASTAT	Tirofiban	AREDIA	Pamidronate
AGRYLIN	Anagrelide	ARGATROBAN	Argatroban
AK Pro	Dipivefrin	ARICEPT	Donepezil
AK-TRACIN	Bacitracin	ARIMIDEX	Anastrozole
ALAMAST	Pemirolast	ARISTOCORT	Triamcinolone
ALBENZA	Albendazole	ARISTROSPAN	Triamcinolone hexacetonide
ALDACTONE	Spironolactone		
ALDARA	Imiquimod	ARTANE	Trihexyphenidyl
ALDOMET	Methyldopa	ASACOL	Mesalamine
ALEVE	Naproxen	ASENDIN	Amoxapine
ALFERON N	Interferon-alpha-N3	ASPERGUM	Aspirin
ALKERAN	Melphalan	ATABRINE	Quinacrine
ALLEGRA	Fexofenadine	ATACAND	Candesartan
ALPHAGAN	Brimonidine	ATARAX	Hydroxyzine
ALTACE	Ramipril	ATIVAN	Lorazepam
ALU-CAP	Aluminum hydroxide	ATROMID-S	Clofibrate
ALUPENT	Metaproterenol	ATROVENT	Ipratropium

℞ GENERIC NAMES FOR SOME TRADE NAME DRUGS*

TRADE NAME	GENERIC NAME	TRADE NAME	GENERIC NAME
AVANDIA	Rosiglitazone	BRONKODYL	Theophylline
AVAPRO	Irbesartan	BUMEX	Bumetanide
AVELOX	Moxifloxacin	BUPRENEX	Buprenorphine
AVENTYL	Nortriptyline	BUSPAR	Buspirone
AVITA	Tretinoin	CALAN	Verapamil
AVONEX	Interferon-beta-1A	CALCIMAR	Calcitonin
AXERT	Almotriptan	CALCIUM DISODIUM VERSENATE	Edetate calcium disodium
AXID	Nizatidine		
AZACTAM	Aztreonam	CALTRATE	Calcium carbonate
AZELEZ	Azelaic acid	CAMPATH	Alemtuzumab
AZOPT	Brinzolamide	CAMPTOSAR	Irinotecan
AZULFIDINE	Sulfasalazine	CANASA	Mesalamine
BACTRIM	Trimethoprim-sulfamethoxazole	CANEIDAS	Caspofungin
		CAPOTEN	Captopril
BACTROBAN	Mupirocin	CAPSIN	Capsaicin
BAL	Dimercaprol	CAPZASIN	Capsaicin
BECONASE	Beclomethasone	CARAFATE	Sucralfate
BENADRYL	Diphenhydramine	CARBASTAT	Carbachol
BENEMID	Probenecid	CARDENE	Nicardipine
BENTYL	Dicyclomine	CARDIOQUIN	Quinidine
BENYLIN DM	Dextromethorphan	CARDIZEM	Diltiazem
BENZAC	Benzoyl peroxide	CARDURA	Doxazosin
BETAGAN	Levobunolol	CARTROL	Carteolol
BETAPACE	Sotalol	CASODEX	Bicalutamide
BETASERON	Interferon-beta-1B	CATAFLAM	Diclofenac
BETAXON	Levobetaxolol	CATAPRES	Clonidine
BETOPTIC	Betaxolol	CAVERJECT	Alprostadil
BEXTRA	Valdecoxib	CECLOR	Cefaclor
BIAXIN	Clarithromycin	CEDAX	Ceftibuten
BICILLIN	Benzathine penicillin	CEFIZOX	Ceftizoxime
BILTRICIDE	Praziquantel	CEFOBID	Cefoperazone
BLENOXANE	Bleomycin	CEFOTAN	Cefotetan
BLEPH-10	Sulfacetamide	CEFTIN	Cefuroxime
BLOCADREN	Timolol	CEFZIL	Cefprozil
BLYSERT	Miglitol	CELEBREX	Celecoxib
BONINE	Meclizine	CELESTONE	Betamethasone
BONTRIL	Phendimetrazine	CELEXA	Citalopram
BOTOX	Botulinum toxin	CELLCEPT	Mycophenolate mofetil
BRETHINE	Terbutaline	CEPACOL	Tetracaine
BRETYLOL	Bretylium	CEPHULAC	Lactulose
BRICANYL	Terbutaline		

R_x GENERIC NAMES FOR SOME TRADE NAME DRUGS*

TRADE NAME	GENERIC NAME	TRADE NAME	GENERIC NAME
CEREBYX	Fosphenytoin	CROLOM	Cromolyn
CERUBIDINE	Daunorubicin	CUPRIMINE	Penicillamine
CHEMET	Succimer	CUTIVATE	Fluticasone
CHLOROMYCE-TIN	Chloramphenicol	CYCLOCORT	Amcinonide
		CYCLOGYL	Cyclopentolate
CHLOR-TRIMETON	Chlorpheniramine	CYCLOSPASMOL	Cyclandelate
		CYLERT	Pemoline
CHRONULAC	Lactulose	CYTOSAR-U	Cytarabine
CILOXAN	Ciprofloxacin	CYTOTEC	Misoprostol
CIPRALEX	Escitalopram	CYTOVENE	Ganciclovir
CIPRO	Ciprofloxacin	CYTOXAN	Cyclophosphamide
CITRUCEL	Methylcellulose	D.H.E. 45	Dihydroergotamine
CLADRIBINE	2-chlorodeoxyadenosine	DALMANE	Flurazepam
CLAFORAN	Cefotaxime	DANOCRINE	Danazol
CLARITIN	Loratadine	DANTRIUM	Dantrolene
CLEOCIN	Clindamycin	DARAPRIM	Pyrimethamine
CLINORIL	Sulindac	DARVON	Propoxyphene
CLODERM	Clocortolone	DAYPRO	Oxaprozin
CLOMID	Clomiphene	DDAVP	Desmopressin
CLOZARIL	Clozapine	DECADRON	Dexamethasone
COGENTIN	Benztropine	DECLOMYCIN	Demeclocycline
COLACE	Docusate	DELATESTRYL	Testosterone
COLAZAL	Balsalazide	DELSYM	Dextromethorpan
COLESTID	Colestipol	DELTA-CORTEF	Prednisolone
COLY-MYCIN	Colistin	DELTASONE	Prednisone
COMPAZINE	Prochlorperazine	DEMADEX	Torsemide
COMTAN	Entacapone	DEMEROL	Meperidine
CONCERTA	Methylphenidate	DENAVIR	Penciclovir
CONEX	Tacrine	DEPAKOTE	Divalproex
COPAXONE	Glatiramer	DEPARENE	Valproate
CORDARONE	Amiodarone	DEPOTESTOS-TERONE	Testosterone
CORDRAN	Flurandrenolide		
COREG	Carvedilol	DESENEX	Undecylenate
CORGARD	Nadolol	DESFERAL	Deferoxamine
CORTEF	Cortisol	DESOWEN	Desonide
CORTROSYN	Cosyntropin	DESOXYN	Methamphetamine
CORVENT	Ibutilide	DESQUAM	Benzoyl peroxide
COSMEGEN	Dactinomycin	DESYREL	Trazodone
COUMADIN	Warfarin	DETROL	Tolterodine
COZAAR	Losartan	DEVROM	Bismuth subgallate
CRIXIVAN	Indinavir	DEXADRINE	Dextroamphetamine

℞   GENERIC NAMES FOR SOME TRADE NAME DRUGS*

TRADE NAME	GENERIC NAME	TRADE NAME	GENERIC NAME
DIABETA	Glyburide	DYRENIUM	Triamterene
DIABINESE	Chlorpropamide	ECOTRIN	Aspirin
DIAMOX	Acetazolamide	EDECRIN	Ethacrynic acid
DIASTAT	Diazepam	EFFEXOR	Venlafaxine
DIBENZYLINE	Phenoxybenzamine	EFUDEX	5-fluorouracil
DIDREX	Benzphetamine	EFUDEX	Fluorouracil (topical)
DIDRONEL	Etidronate	ELAVIL	Amitriptyline
DIFFERIN	Adapalene	ELDEPRYL	Selegiline
DIFLUCAN	Fluconazole	ELLENCE	Epirubicin
DIGITALINE†	Digitoxin	ELMIRON	Pentosan polysulfate
DILACOR	Diltiazem	ELOCON	Mometasone
DILANTIN	Phenytoin	ELSPAR	Asparaginase
DILAUDID	Hydromorphone	EMADINE	Emedastine
DILOR	Dyphylline	EMINASE	Anistreplase
DIMETANE	Brompheniramine	EMULSOIL	Castor oil
DIOVAN	Valsartan	E-MYCIN	Erythromycin
DIPENTUM	Olsalazine	ENBREL	Etanercept
DISALCID	Salsalate	ENDEP	Amitriptyline
DITROPAN	Oxybutynin	ENDRATE	Ethylenediaminetetra-acetic acid (EDTA)
DIUCARDIN	Hydroflumethiazide		
DIURIL	Chlorothiazide	ENISYL	Lysine
DOBUTREX	Dobutamine	EPIVIR	Lamivudine (3TC)
DOLENE	Propoxyphene	EPOGEN	Erythropoietin
DOLOBID	Diflunisal	EQUALACTIN	Polycarbophil
DOLOPHINE	Methadone	EQUANIL	Meprobamate
DOPAR	Levodopa	ERGOMAR	Ergotamine
DOSTINEX	Cabergoline	ERYTHROCIN	Erythromycin
DRAMAMINE	Dimenhydrinate	ESIDRIX	Hydrochlorothiazide
DRISDOL	Ergocalciferol	ETHMOZINE	Moricizine
DRIXORAL	Dexbrompheniramine	EULEXIN	Flutamide
DTIC	Dacarbazine	EXELDERM	Sulconazole
DULCOLAX	Bisacodyl	EXELON	Rivastigmine
DURICEF	Cefadroxil	FAMVIR	Famciclovir
DYAZIDE	Hydrochlorothiazide-triamterene	FANSIDAR	Sulfadoxine-pyrimethamine
DYCILL	Dicloxacillin	FASLODEX	Fulvestrant
DYCLONE	Dyclonine	FELBATOL	Felbamate
DYMELOR	Acetohexamide	FELDENE	Piroxicam
DYNABAC	Dirithromycin	FEMSTAT	Butoconazole
DYNACIRC	Isradipine	FEOSOL	Ferrous sulfate
DYNAPEN	Dicloxacillin	FIBERCON	Polycarbophil

℞ GENERIC NAMES FOR SOME TRADE NAME DRUGS*

TRADE NAME	GENERIC NAME	TRADE NAME	GENERIC NAME
FINEVIN	Azelaic acid	HIPREX	Methenamine
FLAGYL	Metronidazole	HIVID	Zalcitabine (ddC)
FLEXERIL	Cyclobenzaprine	HUMATIN	Paromomycin
FLOMAX	Tamsulosin	HUMORSOL	Demecarium
FLONASE	Fluticasone	HUMULIN	Insulin
FLORINEF	Fludrocortisone	HYDELTRASOL	Prednisolone
FLOVENT	Fluticasone	HYDREA	Hydroxyurea
FLOXIN	Ofloxacin	HYDROCOR-TONE	Cortisol
FLUDARA	Fludarabine		
FLUMADINE	Rimantadine	HYDRODIURIL	Hydrochlorothiazide
FORTAZ	Ceftazidime	HYGROTON	Chlorthalidone
FORTOVASE	Saquinavir	HYLOREL	Guanadrel
FOSAMAX	Alendronate	HYPERSTAT	Diazoxide
FOSCAVIR	Foscarnet	HYTRIN	Terazosin
FOTOTAR	Coal tar	IDAMYCIN	Idarubicin
FULVICIN	Griseofulvin	ILOSONE	Erythromycin
FUNGIZONE	Amphotericin B	IMDUR	Isosorbide nitrate
FURADANTIN	Nitrofurantoin	IMITREX	Sumatriptan
FUROXONE	Furazolidone	IMODIUM	Loperamide
GABITRIL	Tiagabine	IMURAN	Azathioprine
GANITE	Gallium nitrate	INDERAL	Propranolol
GANTANOL	Sulfamethoxazole	INDOCIN	Indomethacin
GANTRISIN	Sulfisoxazole	INFERGEN	Interferon alfacon-1
GARAMYCIN	Gentamicin	INH	Isoniazid
GEMZAR	Gemcitabine	INTAL	Cromolyn
GENTRANS	Dextrans	INTEGRILLIN	Eptifibatide
GEOCILLIN	Carbenicillin	INTRON A	Interferon-alpha-2b
GEODON	Ziprasidone	INTROPIN	Dopamine
GLAUC	Methazolamide	INVANZ	Ertapenem
GLEEVEC	Imatinib	INVIRASE	Saquinavir
GLUCOPHAGE	Metformin	IONAMIN	Phentermine
GLUCOTROL	Glipizide	IOPIDINE	Apraclonidine
HALCION	Triazolam	ISMELIN	Guanethidine
HALDOL	Haloperidol	ISMO	Isosorbide nitrate
HALOG	Halcinonide	ISOPTIN	Verapamil
HALOTESTIN	Fluoxymesterone	ISOPTO HYOSCINE	Scopolamine
HALOTEX	Haloprogin		
HERCEPTIN	Trastuzumab	ISOPTOCARPINE	Pilocarpine
HETRAZAN	Diethylcarbamazine	ISORDIL	Isosorbide dinitrate
HEXADROL	Dexamethasone	ISORDIL	Isosorbide
HIBICLENS	Chlorhexidine		

R̶ GENERIC NAMES FOR SOME TRADE NAME DRUGS*

TRADE NAME	GENERIC NAME	TRADE NAME	GENERIC NAME
ISOTRATE ER	Isosorbide nitrate	LOMOTIL	Diphenoxylate with atropine
ISUPREL	Isoproterenol		
KALETRA	Lopinavir-RITONAVIR	LONITEN	Minoxidil
KANTREX	Kanamycin	LOPID	Gemfibrozil
KAOPECTATE	Kaolin	LOPRESSOR	Metoprolol
KEFLEX	Cephalexin	LOPROX	Ciclopirox
KEFZOL	Cefazolin	LOPURIN	Allopurinol
KENACORT	Triamcinolone	LORABID	Loracarbef
KENALOG	Triamcinolone	LOTENSIN	Benazepril
KEPPRA	Levetiracetam	LOTRIMIN	Clotrimazole
KERLONE	Betaxolol	LOVENOX	Enoxaparin
KLONOPIN	Clonazepam	LOXITANE	Loxapine
KONSYL	Psyllium	LOZOL	Indapamide
KWELL	Lindane	LUDIOMIL	Maprotiline
KYTRIL	Granisetron	LUFYLLIN	Dyphylline
LAMICTAL	Lamotrigine	LUMIGAN	Bimatoprost
LAMISIL AT	Terbinafine	LUMINAL	Phenobarbital
LAMPRENE	Clofazimine	LUPRON	Leuprolide
LANOXIN	Digoxin	LUVOX	Fluvoxamine
LARADOPA	Levodopa	MACRODANTIN	Nitrofurantoin
LARIAM	Mefloquine	MACRODEX	Dextrans
LASIX	Furosemide	MALARONE	Atovaquone-Proguanil
LESCOL	Fluvastatin	MANDELAMINE	Methenamine
LEUKERAN	Chlorambucil	MANDOL	Cefamandole
LEVAQUIN	Levofloxacin	MARAZINE	Cyclizine
LEVATOL	Penbutolol	MARINOL	Dronabinol
LEVBID	Hyoscyamine	MATULANE	Procarbazine
LEVO-DROMORAN	Levorphanol	MAVIX	Trandolapril
		MAXALT	Rizatriptan
LEVOPHED	Norepinephrine	MAXAQUIN	Lomefloxacin
LEVSIN	Hyoscyamine	MAXIDE	Hydrochlorothiazide-triamterene
LIBRIUM	Chlordiazepoxide		
LIDEX	Fluocinonide	MAXIFLOR	Diflorasone
LIORESAL	Baclofen	MAXIPIME	Cefepime
LIPITOR	Atorvastatin	MAZANOR	Mazindol
LITHANE	Lithium	MECLOMEN	Meclofenamate
LITHONATE	Lithium	MEDROL	Methylprednisolone
L-LYSINE	Lysine	MEFOXIN	Cefoxitin
LOCERYL†	Amorolfine	MEGACE	Megestrol
LODINE	Etodolac	MELLARIL	Thioridazine
LODOSYN	Carbidopa	MENTAX	Butenafine

℞ GENERIC NAMES FOR SOME TRADE NAME DRUGS*

TRADE NAME	GENERIC NAME	TRADE NAME	GENERIC NAME
MEPRON	Atovaquone	MUCOMYST	Acetylcysteine
MERIDIA	Sibutramine	MUTAMYCIN	Mitomycin
MERREM	Meropenem	MYAMBUTOL	Ethambutol
MESTINON	Pyridostigmine	MYCELEX	Clotrimazole
METAHYDRIN	Trichlormethiazide	MYCOBUTIN	Rifabutin
METAMUCIL	Psyllium	MYCOSTATIN	Nystatin
METAPREL	Metaproterenol	MYDRIACIL	Tropicamide
METHYLIN	Methylphenidate	MYKROX	Metolazone
METICORTEN	Prednisone	MYLERAN	Busulfan
MEVACOR	Lovastatin	MYLICON	Simethicone
MEXITIL	Mexiletine	MYLOTARG	Gemtuzumab-zogamicin
MIACALCIN	Calcitonin	MYOCHRYSINE	Gold
MICARDIS	Telmisartan	MYSOLINE	Primidone
MICATIN	Miconazole	NAFTIN	Naftifine
MICRONASE	Glyburide	NALFON	Fenoprofen
MIDAMOR	Amiloride	NAPHCON	Naphazoline
MIFEPREX	Mifepristone	NAQUA	Trichlormethiazide
MIGRANAL	Dihydroergotamine	NARCAN	Naloxone
MILK OF MAGNESIA	Magnesium hydroxide	NARDIL	Phenelzine
		NASALCROM	Cromolyn
MILTOWN	Meprobamate	NASALIDE	Flunisolide
MINIPRESS	Prazosin	NASONEX	Mometasone
MINOCIN	Minocycline	NAVANE	Thiothixene
MINTEZOL	Thiabendazole	NAVELBINE	Vinorelbine
MIOSTAT	Carbachol	NEBCIN	Tobramycin
MIRADON	Anisindione	NEBUPENT	Pentamidine
MIRAPEX	Pramipexole	NEMBUTAL	Pentobarbital
MITHRACIN	Plicamycin	NEOLOID	Castor oil
MITROLAN	Polycarbophil	NEO-MERCAZOLE	Carbimazole
MOBAN	Molindone	NEORAL	Cyclosporine
MOBIC	Meloxicam	NEO-SYNEPHRINE	Phenylephrine
MOGADON†	Nitrazepam		
MONOPRIL	Fosinopril	NEPTAZANE	Methazolamide
MONISTAT	Miconazole	NETROMYCIN	Netilmicin
MONOSTAT	Tioconazole	NEURONTIN	Gabapentin
MONUROL	Fosfomycin	NICLOCIDE	Niclosamide
MOTOFEN	Diphenoxylate with atropine	NICORETTE	Nicotine
		NICOTROL	Nicotine
MOTRIN	Ibuprofen	NILANDRON	Nilutamide
MS CONTIN	Morphine	NILSTAT	Nystatin

℞   GENERIC NAMES FOR SOME TRADE NAME DRUGS*

TRADE NAME	GENERIC NAME	TRADE NAME	GENERIC NAME
NIMOTOP	Nimodipine	ORUDIS	Ketoprofen
NIPENT	Pentostatin	ORUVAIL	Ketoprofen
NIPRIDE	Nitroprusside	OSCAL	Calcium carbonate
NITRO-BID	Nitroglycerin	OTRIUIN	Xylometazoline
NITROL	Nitroglycerin	OXISTAT	Oxiconazole
NIX, RID	Permethrin	OXSORALEN	Methoxsalen
NIZORAL	Ketoconazole	OXYCONTIN	Oxycodone
NOLAHIST	Phenindamine	PARAFLEX	Chlorzoxazone
NOLVADEX	Tamoxifen	PARAFON FORTE	Chlorzoxasone
NOOTROPIL	Piracetam	PARAPLATIN	Carboplatin
NORMODYNE	Labetalol	PARLODEL	Bromocriptine
NOROXIN	Norfloxacin	PARNATE	Tranylcypromine
NORPACE	Disopyramide	PATANOL	Olopatadine
NORPLANT	Levonorgestrel	PATHOCIL	Dicloxacillin
NORPRAMIN	Desipramine	PAVABID	Papaverine
NORVASC	Amlodipine	PAVULON	Pancuronium
NORVIR	Ritonavir	PAXIL	Paroxetine
NOVANTRONE	Mitoxantrone	PBZ-SR	Tripelennamine
NOVOLIN	Insulin	PEG-INTRON	Peginterferon alpha-2b
NUMORPHAN	Oxymorphone	PENETREX	Enoxacin
NUPRIN	Ibuprofen	PENTAM 300	Pentamidine
NYDRAZID	Isoniazid	PENTOTHAL	Thiopental
NYQUIL	Doxylamine	PEN-VEEK	Penicillin V
NYTOL	Diphenhydramine	PEPCID	Famotidine
OCUFEN	Flurbiprofen	PEPTO-BISMOL	Bismuth subsalicylate
OCUFLOX	Ofloxacin	PERIACTIN	Cyproheptadine
OCUPRESS	Carteolol	PERMAX	Pergolide
OFF	Diethyltoluamide (DEET)	PERMITIL	Fluphenazine
OMNICEF	Cefdinir	PERSANTINE	Dipyridamole
OMNIPEN	Ampicillin	PERTROPHANE	Desipramine
ONCOVIN	Vincristine	PERTROPIN	Lecithin
OPTIMINE	Azatadine	PHAZYME	Simethicone
OPTIPRANOLOL	Metipranolol	PHENERGAN	Promethazine
OPTIVAR	Azelastine	PHISOHEX	Hexachlorophene
ORAMORPH	Morphine	PhosChol	Lecithin
ORAP	Pimozide	PHOSPHOLINE	Echothiophate
ORETIC	Hydrochlorothiazide	PHYLLOCONTIN	Aminophylline
ORETON	Methyltestosterone	PICOVIR	Pleconaril
ORINASE	Tolbutamide	PIETAL	Cilostazol
ORTHOCLONE OKT3	Muromonab-CD3	PILOCAR	Pilocarpine
		PIMA	Potassium iodide

℞ GENERIC NAMES FOR SOME TRADE NAME DRUGS*

TRADE NAME	GENERIC NAME	TRADE NAME	GENERIC NAME
PIPRACIL	Piperacillin	PROTONIX	Pantoprazole
PITOCIN	Oxytocin	PROTOPAM	Pralidoxime
PITRESSIN	Vasopressin	PROVENTIL	Albuterol
PLAQUENIL	Hydroxychloroquine	PROVERA	Medroxyprogesterone
PLATINOL	Cisplatin	PROVIGIL	Modafinil
PLAVIX	Clopidogrel	PROZAC	Fluoxetine
PLENDIL	Felodipine	PURINETHOL	Mercaptopurine
PODOFIN	Podophyllin toxin	PYRIDIUM	Phenazopyridine
POLARAMINE	Dexchlorpheniramine	QUARZAN	Clidinium
POLYCILLIN	Ampicillin	QUESTRAN	Cholestyramine
POLYMOX	Amoxicillin	QUINAGLUTE	Quinidine
POLYTRIM	Trimethoprim-polymyxin	QUIXIN	Levofloxacin
		RAPAMUNE	Sirolimus
PONSTEL	Mefenamic acid	REBETRON	Interferon-alpha-2b and Ribavirin
PRANDIN	Repaglinide		
PRAVACHOL	Pravastatin	REBIF	Interferon-beta-1A
PRECOSE	Acarbose	REFLUDAN	Lepirudin
PREDNISOL TBA	Prednisolone tebutate	REGITINE	Phentolamine
PRELU-2	Phendimetrazine	REGLAN	Metoclopramide
PREMARIN	Estrogens	RELAFEN	Nabumetone
PREVACID	Lansoprazole	RELENZA	Zanamivir
PRILOSEC	Omeprazole	REMERON	Mirtazapine
PRIMACOR	Milrinone	REMICADE	Infliximab
PRIMAXIN	Imipenem-cilastatin	REMINYL	Galantamine
PRINCIPEN	Ampicillin	RENOVA	Tretinoin
PRINIVIL	Lisinopril	REOPRO	Abciximab
PROAMATINE	Midodrine	REQUIP	Ropinirole
PRO-BANTHINE	Propantheline	RESCRIPTOR	Delavirdine
PROCAN SR	Procainamide	RESCULA	Unoprostone
PROCARDIA	Nifedipine	RESTORIL	Temazepam
PROCRIT	Erythropoietin	RETAVASE	Reteplase
PROGLYCEM	Diazoxide	RETIN-A	Tretinoin
PROGRAF	Tacrolimus	RETROVIR	Zidovudine (AZT)
PROLIXIN	Fluphenazine	REVIA	Naltrexone
PROLOPRIM	Trimethoprim	RHEUMATREX	Methotrexate
PROMIT	Dextrans	RHINOCORT	Budesonide
PRONESTYL	Procainamide	RIDAURA	Auranofin
PROPINE	Dipivefrin	RIFADIN	Rifampin
PROSCAR	Finasteride	RIMACTANE	Rifampin
PROSTAPHLIN	Oxacillin	RIMSO-50	Dimethyl sulfoxide
PROSTIN VR	Alprostadil	RISPERDAL	Risperidone

℞ GENERIC NAMES FOR SOME TRADE NAME DRUGS*

TRADE NAME	GENERIC NAME	TRADE NAME	GENERIC NAME
RITALIN	Methylphenidate	SORBITATE	Isosorbide dinitrate
RITUXAN	Rituximab	SORBITRATE	Isosorbide
ROBAXIN	Methocarbamol	SPECTAZOLE	Econazole
ROBITUSSIN	Guaifenesin	SPECTRACEF	Cefditoren
ROCALTROL	Calcitriol	SPORANOX	Itraconazole
ROCEPHIN	Ceftriaxone	SSKI	Potassium iodide
ROFERON-A	Interferon-alpha-2a	STADOL	Butorphanol
ROGAINE	Minoxidil	STAPHCILLIN	Methicillin
ROVAMYCINE	Spiramycin	STARLIX	Nateglinide
ROWASA	Mesalamine	STELAZINE	Trifluoperazine
RYTHMOL	Propafenone	STILPHOSTROL	Diethylstilbestrol
SABRIL	Vigabatrin	STIMATE	Desmopressin
SALFLEX	Salsalate	STREPTASE	Streptokinase
SANDIMMUNE	Cyclosporine	SUBLIMAZE	Fentanyl
SANDOSTATIN	Octreotide	SUDAFED	Pseudoephedrine
SANOREX	Mazindol	SULAMYD	Sulfacetamide
SANSERT	Methysergide	SULAR	Nisoldipine
SECONAL	Secobarbital	SULFAMYLON	Mafenide
SECTRAL	Acebutolol	SUMYCIN	Tetracycline
SELDANE	Terfenadine	SUPPRELIN	Histrelin
SELSUN	Selenium sulfide	SUPRAX	Cefixime
SENOKOT	Senna sennosides	SURMONTIL	Trimipramine
SEPTRA	Trimethoprim-sulfamethoxazole	SUSTIVA	Efavirenz
		SYMMETREL	Amantadine
SERAX	Oxazepam	SYNAGIS	Palivizumab
SERENTIL	Mesoridazine	SYNALAR	Fluocinolone
SEREVENT	Salmeterol	SYNERCID	Quinupristin-dalfopristin
SEROMYCIN	Cycloserine	SYNTOCINON	Oxytocin
SEROPHENE	Clomiphene	TACE	Chlorotrianisene
SEROQUEL	Quetiapine	TAGAMET	Cimetidine
SERZONE	Nefazodone	TALWIN	Pentazocine
SILVADENE	Silver sulfadiazine	TAMBOCOR	Flecainide
SIMULECT	Basiliximab	TAMIFLU	Oseltamivir
SINEMET	Levodopa-carbidopa	TAO	Troleandomycin
SINEQUAN	Doxepin	TAPAZOLE	Methimazole
SINGULAIR	Montelukast	TASMAR	Tolcapone
SKELAXIN	Metaxalone	TAVIST	Clemastine
SOMA	Carisoprodol	TAXOL	Paclitaxel
SOMAGARD	Deslorelin	TAXOTERE	Docetaxel
SOMBULEX	Hexobarbital	TAZICEF	Ceftazidime
SOMINEX	Diphenhydramine	TAZIDIME	Ceftazidime

℞ GENERIC NAMES FOR SOME TRADE NAME DRUGS*

TRADE NAME	GENERIC NAME	TRADE NAME	GENERIC NAME
TAZORAC	Tazarotene	TRANDATE	Labetalol
TEGISON	Etretinate	TRANXENE	Clorazepate
TEGOPEN	Cloxacillin	TRAVATAN	Travoprost
TEGRETOL	Carbamazepine	TRENTAL	Pentoxifylline
TELDRIN	Chlorpheniramine	TRI-CHLOR	Trichloroacetic acid
TEMARIL	Trimeprazine	TRIDESILON	Desonide
TENEX	Guanfacine	TRIDIONE	Trimethadione
TENORMIN	Atenolol	TRILAFON	Perphenazine
TENSILON	Edrophonium	TRILEPTAL	Oxcarbazepine
TENUATE	Diethylpropion	TRILISATE	Choline magnesium trisalicylate
TEPANIL	Diethylpropion	TRIMOX	Amoxicillin
TEQUIN	Gatifloxacin	TRIMPEX	Trimethoprim
TERAZOL	Terconazole	TROBICIN	Spectinomycin
TERRAMYCIN	Oxytetracycline	TROVAN	Trovafloxacin
TESLAC	Testolactone	TRUSOPT	Dorzolamide
TESSALON	Benzonatate	TUMS	Calcium carbonate
TETRACYN	Tetracycline	TUSSIREX	Pheniramine
TEVETEN	Eprosartan	TYLENOL	Acetaminophen
THALOMID	Thalidomide	ULTRAVATE	Halobetasol
THEOLAIR	Theophylline	UNASYN	Sulbactam-ampicillin
THIOLA	Tiopronin	UNIPEN	Nafcillin
THORAZINE	Chlorpromazine	UNIVASC	Moexipril
THYTROPAR	Thyrotropin	URECHOLINE	Bethanechol
TICAR	Ticarcillin	URISTAT	Phenazopyridine
TICLID	Ticlopidine	UTICORT	Betamethasone
TIGAN	Trimethobenzamide	VAGISTAT	Tioconazole
TILADE	Nedocromil	VALCYTE	Valganciclovir
TIMOPTIC	Timolol	VALISONE	Betamethasone
TINACTIN	Tolnaftate	VALIUM	Diazepam
TOBREX	Tobramycin	VALTREX	Valacyclovir
TOFRANIL	Imipramine	VANCENASE	Beclomethasone
TOLECTIN	Tolmetin	VANCOCIN	Vancomycin
TOLINASE	Tolazamide	VANIQA	Eflornithine
TONOCARD	Tocainide	VANTIN	Cefpodoxime
TOPAMAX	Topiramate	VASCOR	Bepridil
TOPICORT	Desoximetasone	VASOCON	Naphazoline
TOPROL-XL	Metoprolol	VASOTEC	Enalapril
TORADOL	Ketorolac	VEETIDS	Penicillin V
TORNALATE	Bitolterol	VELBAN	Vinblastine
TRACRIUM	Atracurium	VELOSEF	Cephradine
TRANCOPAL	Chlormezanone		

℞   GENERIC NAMES FOR SOME TRADE NAME DRUGS*

TRADE NAME	GENERIC NAME	TRADE NAME	GENERIC NAME
VENTOLIN	Albuterol	XYLOCAINE	Lidocaine
VERMOX	Mebendazole	YOCON	Yohimbine
VERSED	Midazolam	YUTOPAR	Ritodrine
VERSENATE	Ethylenediaminetetra-acetic acid (EDTA)	ZANAFLEX	Tizanidine
		ZANOSAR	Streptozocin
VESPRIN	Triflupromazine	ZANTAC	Ranitidine
VFEND	Voriconazole	ZAROXOLYN	Metolazone
VIAGRA	Sildenafil	ZARONTIN	Ethosuximide
VIBRAMYCIN	Doxycycline	ZEBETA	Bisoprolol
VIDEX	Didanosine (ddl)	ZENAPAX	Daclizumab
VIOXX	Rofecoxib	ZERIT	Stavudine (d4T)
VIRA-A	Vidarabine	ZESTRIL	Lisinopril
VIRACEPT	Nelfinavir	ZETAR	Coal tar
VIRACTIN	Tetracaine	ZIAGEN	Abacavir
VIRAMUNE	Nevirapine	ZINACEF	Cefuroxine
VIRAZOLE	Ribavirin	ZITHROMAX	Azithromycin
VIREAD	Tenofovir	ZOCOR	Simvastatin
VIROPTIC	Trifluridine	ZOLADEX	Goserelin
VISKEN	Pindolol	ZOLICEF	Cefazolin
VISTARIL	Hydroxine	ZOLOFT	Sertraline
VISTIDE	Cidofovir	ZOMETA	Zoledronic acid
VITRAVENE	Fomivirsen	ZOMIG	Zolmitriptan
VIVACTIL	Protriptyline	ZONALON	Doxepin
VOLTAREN	Diclofenac	ZONEGRAN	Zonisamide
WELCHOL	Colesevelam	ZOSTRIX	Capsaicin
WELLBUTRIN	Bupropion	ZOVIRAX	Acyclovir
WELLCOVORIN	Leucovorin	ZYFLO	Zileuton
WINSTROL	Stanozolol	ZYLOPRIM	Allopurinol
WYTENSIN	Guanabenz	ZYPREXA	Olanzapine
XALATAN	Latanoprost	ZYRTEC	Cetirizine
XANAX	Alprazolam	ZYVOX	Linezolid
XENICAL	Orlistat		
XIGRIS	Drotrecogin alfa (activated)		

*Some drugs mentioned in this book are manufactured only as generics and therefore have no trade name and are not included in this table.

†Not available in the United States.

Resources for Help and Information

The following list is selective and restricted largely to national organizations in the United States, many of which have local chapters. Sites chosen are generally not-for-profit and usually offer information or support rather than advocacy. Telephone numbers and web sites are included as appropriate; however, such information changes frequently. Additional information is available through health care professionals, local libraries, telephone listings, and the Internet.

AGING

Administration on Aging
Washington, DC
800-438-4380 (information on Alzheimer's disease)
800-677-1116
800-877-8339 (TTY)
202-619-7501
www.aoa.gov

American Association of Retired People
Washington, DC
800-424-3410
202-434-2277
www.aarp.org

Benefits Check Up
The National Council on the Aging
www.benefitscheckup.org

Health and Age
Novartis Foundation for Gerontology
www.healthandage.com

Infoaging.org (AFAR)
New York, NY
212-703-9977
www.infoaging.org

National Association of Area Agencies on Aging
Washington, DC
202-296-8130
www.n4a.org

National Council on the Aging
Washington, DC
202-479-1200
202-479-6674 (TDD)
www.ncoa.org

National Institute on Aging
Bethesda, MD
800-222-2225
800-222-4225 (TTY)
301-496-1752
www.nia.nih.gov

Older Women's League
Washington, DC
800-825-3695
202-783-6686
www.owl-nation.org

Senior Options
Online Guide to Senior Services
www.senioroptions.com

AIDS

AIDS Action
Washington, DC
202-530-8030
www.aidsaction.org

The American Foundation for AIDS Research
New York, NY
800-342-2437
212-806-1600
www.amfar.org

CDC National AIDS/HIV Hotline
800-342-2437
www.ashastd.org/nah

Gay Men's Health Crisis
New York, NY
800-243-7692
212-807-6655
212-645-7470 (TTY)
www.gmhc.org

National Association for People With AIDS
Washington, DC
202-898-0414
www.napwa.org

Project Inform
San Francisco, CA
800-822-7422
415-558-9051
415-558-8669
www.projinf.org

Universal Fellowship of Metropolitan Community Churches AIDS Ministry
Los Angeles, CA
213-464-5100
www.thebody.com/ufmcc/ufmcc.html

Women Alive
Los Angeles, CA
800-554-4876
323-965-1564
www.women-alive.org

ALCOHOLISM

(see also Drug Abuse)

Al-Anon Family Group Headquarters
Virginia Beach, VA
800-356-9996
757-563-1600
www.al-anon.alateen.org

Alcoholics Anonymous
New York, NY
212-870-3400
www.alcoholics-anonymous.org

National Clearinghouse for Alcohol & Drug Information
Rockville, MD
800-729-6686
800-487-4889 (TDD)
www.health.org

National Council on Alcoholism & Drug Dependence
New York, NY
800-622-2255
212-269-7797
www.ncadd.org

LifeRing Recovery
Oakland, CA
510-763-0779
www.lifering.org

ALLERGY & ASTHMA

Allergy and Asthma Network/Mothers of Asthmatics, Inc.
Fairfax, VA
800-878-4403
703-573-7794
www.aanma.org

American Academy of Allergy, Asthma, and Immunology
Milwaukee, WI
414-272-6071
www.aaaai.org

Asthma & Allergy Foundation of America
Washington, DC
800-717-8462
202-466-7643
www.aafa.org

ALZHEIMER'S DISEASE & OTHER DEMENTIAS

Alzheimer's Association
Chicago, IL
800-272-3900
312-335-8700
www.alz.org

Alzheimer's Disease Education & Referral Center
Silver Spring, MD
800-438-4380
www.alzheimer.org

The Alzheimer's Society
London, UK
www.alzheimers.org.uk

The Alzheimer's Society CJD Support Group
London, UK
www.alzheimers.org.uk/cjd

AMPUTATION

(see also Disabilities & Rehabilitation)

The American Amputee Foundation, Inc.
Little Rock, AR
501-666-2523

National Amputation Foundation
Malverne, NY
516-887-3600
www.nationalamputation.org

AMYLOIDOSIS

Amyloidosis Network International, Inc.
Houston, TX
888-269-5643
www.amyloidosis.org

AMYOTROPHIC LATERAL SCLEROSIS

The ALS Association
Calabasas Hills, CA
800-782-4747 (patients only);
818-880-9007
www.alsa.org

ANKYLOSING SPONDYLITIS

Spondylitis Association of America
Sherman Oaks, CA
800-777-8189
818-981-1616
www.spondylitis.org

ARTHRITIS

American Juvenile Arthritis Organization
Atlanta, GA
800-283-7800
404-965-7514

Arthritis Foundation
Atlanta, GA
800-283-7800;
www.arthritis.org

ASTHMA

(see Allergy & Asthma)

ATTENTION DEFICIT DISORDER

Attention Deficit Disorder Association
Highland Park, IL
847-432-2332
www.add.org

Children and Adults With Attention Deficit Disorders
Landover, MD
800-233-4050
www.chadd.org

Learning Disabilities Association of America
Pittsburgh, PA
412-341-1515
www.ldanatl.org

AUTISM

Autism Research Institute
San Diego, CA
619-563-6840
www.autism.tv

Autism Society of America
Bethesda, MD
800-328-8476
301-657-0881
www.autism-society.org

National Autism Hotline/Autism Services Center
Huntington, WV
304-525-8014

BALDING

National Alopecia Areata Foundation
San Rafael, CA
415-472-3780
www.alopeciaareata.com

BEREAVEMENT

(see Death & Bereavement)

BIRTH DEFECTS

(see also Cleft Palate; Spina Bifida)

Federation for Children With Special Needs
Boston, MA
800-331-0688
617-236-7210
www.fcsn.org

March of Dimes Birth Defects Foundation
White Plains, NY
888-663-4637
914-428-7100
www.modimes.org

National Foundation for Jewish Genetic Diseases, Inc.
New York, NY
212-371-1030
www.nfjgd.org

BLINDNESS & VISION PROBLEMS

American Association of the Deaf-Blind
Silver Spring, MD
800-735-2258
301-495-4403
301-495-4402 (TTY)
www.aadb.org

Association for Macular Diseases
New York, NY
212-605-3719
www.macula.org

American Council of the Blind
Washington, DC
800-424-8666
202-467-5081
www.acb.org

American Foundation for the Blind
New York, NY
800-232-5463
212-502-7600
www.afb.org

Association for the Education & Rehabilitation of the Blind & Visually Impaired
Alexandria, VA
703-823-9690
www.aerbvi.org

Fight for Sight
New York, NY
212-679-6060
www.fightforsight.com

The Foundation Fighting Blindness
Owing Mills, MD
888-394-3937
800-683-5551 (TDD);
410-568-0150
www.blindness.org

Glaucoma Research Foundation
San Francisco, CA
800-826-6693
415-986-3162
www.glaucoma.org

Helen Keller Services for the Blind
Sands Point, NY
800-255-0411
516-944-8637 (TTY)
www.helenkeller.org/national

National Association for Visually Handicapped
New York, NY
212-255-2804
www.navh.org

Prevent Blindness America
Schaumburg, IL
800-331-2020
847-843-2020
www.preventblindness.org

BLOOD DISORDERS

Leukemia Society of America
White Plains, NY
800-955-4572
914-949-5213
www.leukemia.org

National Hemophilia Foundation
New York, NY
212-219-8180
www.hemophilia.org

Sickle Cell Disease Association of America, Inc.
Culver City, CA
800-421-8453
www.sicklecelldisease.org

Thalassemia Action Group
Flushing, NY
800-522-7222
718-321-2873
www.thalsite.com/tag

BRAIN DISORDERS

(see also Cancer & Other Tumors;
Alzheimer's Disease & Other Dementias;
Epilepsy)

Brain Injury Association of America
Alexandria, VA
800-444-6443 (Family Helpline)
703-236-6000
www.biausa.org

National Institute of Neurological Disorders & Stroke
Bethesda, MD
800-352-9424
www.ninds.nih.gov

CANCER & OTHER TUMORS

American Cancer Society
Atlanta, GA
800-227-2345
404-320-3333
www.cancer.org

Cancer Care, Inc.
New York, NY
800-813-4673
212-712-8080
212-302-2400
www.cancercare.org

National Cancer Institute
Bethesda, MD
800-422-6237
301-496-5583
www.cancer.gov

National Coalition for Cancer Survivorship
Silver Spring, MD
301-650-9127
www.canceradvocacy.org

Patient Advocates for Advanced Cancer Treatments, Inc.
Grand Rapids, MI
616-453-1477
www.paactusa.org

BRAIN

Acoustic Neuroma Association
Cumming, GA
770-205-8211
www.anausa.org

American Brain Tumor Association
Des Plains, IL
800-886-2282
847-827-9910
www.abta.org

Brain Tumor Society
Watertown, MA
800-770-8287
617-924-9997
www.tbts.org

The Children's Brain Tumor Foundation
New York, NY
866-228-4673 (toll free)
212-448-9494
www.cbtf.org

National Brain Tumor Foundation
Oakland, CA
800-934-2873
www.braintumor.org

Pituitary Network Association
Thousand Oaks, CA
805-499-9973
www.pituitary.com

BREAST

National Alliance of Breast Cancer Organizations
New York, NY
888-806-2226
www.nabco.org

The Susan G. Komen Breast Cancer Foundation
Dallas, TX
800-462-9273
972-855-1600
www.komen.org

Y-ME: National Breast Cancer Organization
Chicago, IL
800-221-2141
312-986-8338
www.y-me.org

PROSTATE

US-TOO International
Downers Grove, IL
800-808-7866
630-795-1002
www.ustoo.com

SKIN

The Skin Cancer Foundation
New York, NY
800-754-6490
www.skincancer.org

CARDIOVASCULAR DISORDERS

American Heart Association
Dallas, TX
800-242-8721
214-373-6300
www.americanheart.org

Heart and Stroke Foundation of Canada
Toronto, Ontario, Canada
416-489-7111
www.heartandstroke.ca

National Heart, Lung, and Blood Institute
Bethesda, MD
301-251-1222
www.nhlbi.nih.gov

National Stroke Association
Englewood, CO
800-787-6537
303-649-9299
www.stroke.org

Sister Kenny Institute
Minneapolis, MN
612-863-4457
www.sisterkennyinstitute.com

Vascular Disease Foundation
Lakewood, CO
866-723-4636 (toll free)
303-949-8337
www.vdf.org

CEREBRAL PALSY

United Cerebral Palsy Associations, Inc.
Washington, DC
800-872-5827
202-776-0406
202-973-7197 (TTY)
www.ucpa.org

CHILD ABUSE & NEGLECT

American Humane Association, Children's Division
Englewood, CO
800-227-4645
303-792-9900
www.amerhumane.org

Kempe Children's Center
Denver, CO
303-864-5252
www.kempecenter.org

CHILDBIRTH/PREGNANCY

(see also Family Planning; Infertility)

America's Crisis Pregnancy Helpline
Dallas, TX
800-672-2296
www.thehelpline.org

Maternity Center Association
New York, NY
212-777-5000
www.maternitywise.org

CLEFT PALATE

Cleft Palate Foundation
Chapel Hill, NC
800-242-5338
www.cleftline.org

Wide Smiles
Stockton, CA
209-942-2812
www.widesmiles.org

CYSTIC FIBROSIS

Cystic Fibrosis Foundation
Bethesda, MD
800-344-4823
301-951-4422
www.cff.org

DEAFNESS & HEARING DISORDERS

Alexander Graham Bell Association for the Deaf and Hard of Hearing
Washington, DC
800-432-7543
202-337-5220
202-337-5221 (TTY)
www.agbell.org

American Association of the Deaf-Blind
Silver Spring, MD
800-735-2258
301-495-4403
301-495-4402 (TTY)
www.aadb.org

American Society for Deaf Children
Gettysburg, PA
800-942-2732 (Parent Hotline)
717-334-7922
www.deafchildren.org

American Tinnitus Association
Portland, OR
800-634-8978
503-248-9985
www.ata.org

Deafness Research Foundation
Washington, DC
800-829-5934
202-289-5850
www.drf.org

The Ear Foundation
Nashville, TN
800-545-4327
615-284-7807
www.earfoundation.org

Helen Keller National Center
Sands Point, NY
800-255-0411
516-944-8637 (TTY)
www.helenkeller.org/national

National Association of the Deaf
Silver Spring, MD
301-587-1788
301-587-1789 (TTY)
www.nad.org

DEATH & BEREAVEMENT

Aiding Mothers and Fathers Experiencing Neonatal Death (AMEND)
St. Louis, MO
314-487-7582
www.amendgroup.com

The Compassionate Friends
Oak Brook, IL
877-969-0010
630-990-0010
www.compassionatefriends.org

The Hemlock Society USA
Denver, CO
800-247-7421
www.hemlock.org

Hospice Education Institute
Machiasport, ME
800-331-1620
207-255-8800
www.hospiceworld.org

National Hospice Foundation
Alexandria, VA
703-516-4928
www.hospiceinfo.org

Partnership for Caring
Washington, DC
800-989-9455
202-296-8071
www.partnershipforcaring.org

DEMENTIA
(see Alzheimer's Disease & Other Dementias)

DEPRESSION
(see also Psychiatric Disease)

Depression and Related Affective Disorders Association (DRADA)
Baltimore, MD
410-955-4647
www.drada.org

National Depressive and Manic-Depressive Association
Chicago, IL
800-826-3632
312-642-0049
www.ndmda.org

Recovery, Inc.
Chicago, IL
312-337-5661
www.recovery-inc.com

DIABETES

American Diabetes Association
Alexandria, VA
800-342-2383
www.diabetes.org

The Juvenile Diabetes Foundation International
New York, NY
800-533-2873
212-785-9500
www.jdrf.org

National Institute of Diabetes & Digestive & Kidney Diseases
Bethesda, MD
301-654-3327
301-435-0714
www.niddk.nih.gov

DIGESTIVE DISORDERS

Crohn's & Colitis Foundation of America
New York, NY
800-343-3637
www.ccfa.org

Digestive Disease National Coalition
Washington, DC
202-544-7497
www.ddnc.org

International Foundation for Functional Gastrointestinal Disorders
Milwaukee, WI
889-964-2001
414-964-1799
www.iffgd.org

Intestinal Disease Foundation
Pittsburgh, PA
877-587-9606
412-261-5888
www.intestinalfoundation.org

National Digestive Diseases Information Clearinghouse
Bethesda, MD
800-891-5389
301-654-3810
www.niddk.nih.gov

United Ostomy Association
Irvine, CA
800-826-0826
949-660-8624
www.uoa.org

DISABILITIES & REHABILITATION

(see also Amputation; Mental Retardation)

Disabled American Veterans
Cold Springs, KY
877-726-2838
859-441-7300
www.dav.org

Easter Seals
Chicago, IL
800-221-6827
312-726-6200
312-726-4258 (TTY)
www.easter-seals.org

National Organization on Disability
Washington, DC
202-293-5960
www.nod.org

National Rehabilitation Information Center
Lanham, MD
800-346-2742
www.naric.com

National Rehabilitation Association
Alexandria, VA
888-258-4295
703-836-0850
www.nationalrehab.org

Paralyzed Veterans of America
Washington, DC
800-424-8200
202-872-1300
www.pva.org

DOWN SYNDROME

Association for Children With Down Syndrome
Plainview, NY
516-933-4700
www.acds.org

National Down Syndrome Congress
Atlanta, GA
800-232-6372
770-604-9500
www.ndsccenter.org

National Down Syndrome Society
New York, NY
800-221-4602
www.ndss.org

DRUG ABUSE

(see also Alcoholism)

Cocaine Anonymous World Service
Los Angeles, CA
800-347-8998
310-559-5833
www.ca.org

Hazelden
Center City, MN
800-257-7810
651-213-4000
www.hazelden.org

Narcotics Anonymous
Van Nuys, CA
818-997-3822
www.na.org

EAR

(see Deafness & Hearing Disorders)

EATING DISORDERS

National Association of Anorexia Nervosa and Associated Disorders
Highland Park, IL
847-831-3438
www.anad.org

Overeaters Anonymous
Rio Rancho, NM
505-891-2664
www.overeatersanonymous.org

ENDOCRINE DISORDERS

(see also Diabetes)

National Adrenal Diseases Foundation
Great Neck, NY
516-487-4992
www.medhelp.org/nadf

Thyroid Foundation of America
Boston, MA
800-832-8321
617-726-8500
www.tsh.org

EPILEPSY

Epilepsy Foundation of America
Landover, MD
800-332-1000
www.efa.org

ERECTILE DYSFUNCTION (IMPOTENCE)

Impotents Anonymous
Maryville, TN
615-983-6064

EYE

(see Blindness & Vision Problems)

FAMILY PLANNING

(see also Childbirth/Pregnancy; Infertility)

Planned Parenthood Federation of America
New York, NY
212-541-7800
www.plannedparenthood.org

GAUCHER'S DISEASE

National Gaucher Foundation
Rockville, MD
800-925-8885
800-428-2437
www.gaucherdisease.org

GENERAL

American Academy of Family Physicians
Leawood, KS
www.familydoctor.org

American Academy of Neurology
1080 Montreal Avenue
Saint Paul, MN
800-879-1960
www.aan.com

American Academy of Pediatrics
Elm Grove Village, IL
847-434-4000
www.aap.org

American Medical Association
Chicago, IL
312-464-5000
www.ama-assn.org

Centers for Disease Control and Prevention
Atlanta, GA
800-311-3435
404-639-3311
www.cdc.gov

The Merck Manuals
Merck & Co., Inc.
West Point, PA
www.merckmanuals.com

National Institutes of Health
Bethesda, MD
301-496-4000
www.nih.gov

US Department of Health and Human Services
Washington, DC
877-696-6775
202-619-0257
www.os.dhhs.gov

US Food and Drug Administration
Office of Consumer Affairs Inquiry Information Line
Rockville, MD
888-463-6332
www.fda.gov

Electronic Orange Book
Approved Drug Products With Therapeutic Equivalence Evaluations
www.fda.gov/cder/ob/default

GENETIC DISEASES
(see also Birth Defects)

Alliance of Genetic Support Groups
Washington, DC
202-966-5557
www.geneticalliance.org

HEADACHE

**American Council
  for Headache Education**
Mt. Royal, NJ
800-255-2243
856-423-0258
www.achenet.org

National Headache Foundation
Chicago, IL
888-643-5552
773-388-6399
www.headaches.org

HEAD INJURY
(see Brain Disorders)

HEARING
(see Deafness & Hearing Disorders)

HEART DISORDERS
(see Cardiovascular Disorders)

HEMOCHROMATOSIS

American Hemochromatosis Society
Lake Mary, FL
407-829-4488
www.americanhs.org

Hemochromatosis Foundation, Inc.
Albany, NY
518-489-0972
www.hemochromatosis.org

Iron Overload Diseases Association
North Palm Beach, FL
561-840-8512
www.ironoverload.org

HOME CARE

National Association for Home Care
Washington, DC
202-547-7424
www.nahc.org

HOSPICES
(see Death & Bereavement)

IMPOTENCE
(see Erectile Dysfunction)

INCONTINENCE

National Association for Continence
Spartanburg, SC
800-252-3337
864-579-7900
www.nafc.org

The Simon Foundation for Continence
Wilmette, IL
800-237-4666

INFERTILITY
(see also Childbirth/Pregnancy; Family
Planning)

American Society for Reproductive Medicine
Birmingham, AL
202-978-5000
www.asrm.org

Ferre Institute, Inc.
Binghamton, NY
607-724-4308
www.ferre.org

Resolve: The National Infertility Association
Somerville, MA
888-623-0744
www.resolve.org

IRON OVERLOAD
(see Hemochromatosis)

KIDNEY DISORDERS

American Association of Kidney Patients
Tampa, FL
800-749-2257
www.aakp.org

American Kidney Fund
Rockville, MD
800-638-8299
www.akfinc.org

National Kidney Foundation
New York, NY
800-622-9010
212-889-2210
www.kidney.org

**National Kidney and Urologic Diseases
Information Clearinghouse**
Bethesda, MD
800-891-5390
301-654-4415
www.niddk.nih.gov

LEARNING DISABILITIES
(see also Attention Deficit Disorder)

American Association on Mental Retardation
Washington, DC
800-424-3688
202-387-1968
www.aamr.org

Learning Disabilities Association
Pittsburgh, PA
412-341-1515
www.ldanatl.org

National Center for Learning Disabilities
New York, NY
888-575-7373
212-545-7510
www.ncld.org

LEPROSY

American Leprosy Foundation
Rockville, MD
301-984-1336
www.charity.org/alf.html

LIVER DISORDERS

American Liver Foundation
New York, NY
800-465-4837
212-668-1000
www.liverfoundation.org

LUNG DISORDERS
(see Respiratory Disorders)

LUPUS

Lupus Foundation of America
Rockville, MD
800-558-0121
301-670-9292
www.lupus.org

MEDIC ALERT

MedicAlert Foundation
Turlock, CA
888-633-4298
209-668-3333
www.medicalert.org

MENTAL HEALTH
(see Depression and Psychiatric Disease)

MENTAL RETARDATION
(see also Learning Disabilities)

**The ARC of the United States (formerly
Association for Retarded Citizens of the
United States)**
Silver Spring, MD
301-565-3842
www.thearc.org

FRAXA Research Foundation
Newburyport, MA
978-462-1866
www.fraxa.org

The Joseph P. Kennedy, Jr. Foundation
Washington, DC
202-393-1250
www.jpkf.org

**National Association of Developmental
Disabilities Councils**
Washington, DC
202-347-1234
www.naddc.org

Voice of the Retarded
Rolling Meadows, IL
847-253-6020
www.vor.net

MOVEMENT DISORDERS
(see also Parkinson's Disease)

We Move
204 West 84th Street
New York, NY 10024
www.wemove.org

MULTIPLE SCLEROSIS

National Multiple Sclerosis Society
New York, NY
800-344-4867
212-986-3240
www.nmss.org

MUSCULAR DYSTROPHY

Muscular Dystrophy Association-USA
Tucson, AZ
800-572-1717
www.mdausa.org

MYASTHENIA GRAVIS

Myasthenia Gravis Foundation of America
Minneapolis, MN
800-541-5454
952-545-9438
www.myasthenia.org

NUTRITION

American Dietetic Association
Chicago, IL
800-877-1600
312-899-0040
www.eatright.org

OSTEOPOROSIS

National Osteoporosis Foundation
Washington, DC
202-223-2226
www.nof.org

PAGET'S DISEASE

The Paget Foundation
New York, NY
800-237-2438
212-509-5335
www.paget.org

PAIN RELIEF

American Chronic Pain Association
Baltimore, MD
888-615-7246
www.painfoundation.org

PARKINSON'S DISEASE

American Parkinson Disease Association
Staten Island, NY
800-223-2732
718-981-8001
www.apdaparkinson.com

National Parkinson Foundation
Miami, FL
800-327-4545
800-433-7022 (in FL)
www.parkinson.org

Parkinson's Action Network
Alexandria, VA
800-850-4726
703-518-8877
www.parkinsonsaction.org

Parkinson's Disease Foundation
New York, NY
800-457-6676
212-923-4700
www.pdf.org

PRADER-WILLI SYNDROME

Prader-Willi Syndrome Association (USA)
Sarasota, FL
800-926-4797
941-312-0400
www.pwsausa.org

PREGNANCY

(see Childbirth/Pregnancy)

PROSTATE DISORDERS

(see also Cancer & Other Tumors)

The Prostatitis Foundation
Smithshire, IL
888-891-4200
www.prostatitis.org

PSORIASIS

National Psoriasis Foundation
Portland, OR
800-723-9166
503-244-7404
www.psoriasis.org

PSYCHIATRIC DISEASE

(see also Depression)

National Alliance for the Mentally Ill
Arlington, VA
800-950-6264
703-524-7600
www.nami.org

National Institute of Mental Health
Bethesda, MD
301-443-4513
www.nimh.nih.gov

National Mental Health Association
Alexandria, VA
800-969-6642
800-443-5959 (TTY)
703-684-7722
www.nmha.org

Metanoia
800-784-2433
www.metanoia.org/suicide

Survivors of Suicide
www.thewebpager.com/sos

RARE DISORDERS

National Organization for Rare Disorders
Danbury, CT
800-999-6673
203-744-0100
www.rarediseases.org

RESPIRATORY (LUNG) DISORDERS

American Lung Association
New York, NY
800-586-4872
212-315-8700
www.lungusa.org

Asthma & Allergy Foundation of America
Washington, DC
800-727-8462
202-466-7643
www.aafa.org

REYE'S SYNDROME

National Reye's Syndrome Foundation
Bryan, OH
800-233-7393
419-636-2679
www.reyessyndrome.org

SJÖGREN'S SYNDROME

National Sjögren's Syndrome Association
Bethesda, MD
800-475-6473
www.sjogrens.org

SLEEP DISORDERS

American Sleep Apnea Association
Washington, DC
202-293-3650
www.sleepapnea.org

American Sleep Disorders Association
Rochester, MN
708-492-0930
www.asda.org

SPINA BIFIDA

Spina Bifida Association of America
Washington, DC
800-621-3141
202-944-3285
www.sbaa.org

SPINAL CORD INJURY

National Spinal Cord Injury Association
Bethesda, MD
800-962-9629
301-588-6959
www.spinalcord.org

STUTTERING & OTHER SPEECH DISORDERS

National Council on Stuttering & Foundation for Fluency
Dekalb, IL
815-756-6986

National Stuttering Association
Anaheim Hills, CA
800-364-1677
www.nsastutter.org

Stuttering Foundation of America
Memphis, TN
800-992-9392
901-452-7343
www.stuttersfa.org

SUDDEN INFANT DEATH SYNDROME

SIDS Network
Ledyard, CT
www.sids-network.org

Sudden Infant Death Syndrome Alliance
Baltimore, MD
800-221-7437
410-653-8226
www.sidsalliance.org

TAY-SACHS DISEASE

National Tay-Sachs & Allied Diseases Association
Brighton, MA
800-906-8723
www.ntsad.org

TRANSPLANTATION

United Network for Organ Sharing
Richmond, VA
888-894-6361
www.unos.org

TRAVEL HEALTH

CDC National Center for Infectious Diseases
Travelers' Health
888-394-8747
www.cdc.gov/travel

Federal Aviation Administration
Information for the Air Traveler With a
   Disability
www.faa.gov

**International Association for Medical
   Assistance to Travelers**
Lewiston, NY
716-754-4883
www.iamat.org

International SOS
Trevose, PA
800-523-8930
215-244-1500
www.internationalsos.org

International Society of Travel Medicine
www.istm.org

Travel Health Online
www.tripprep.com

US Government Printing Office
International Certificate of Vaccination as
   Approved by the World Health Organization
www.access.gpo.gov

US State Department
Help for Americans Abroad
www.travel.state.gov/acs

World Health Organization
International Travel and Health
www.who.int/ith

WOMEN'S HEALTH

(see also Aging)

**American College of Obstetricians and
   Gynecologists**
Washington, DC
202-638-5577
202-863-2518
www.acog.org

National Women's Health Network
Washington, DC
202-347-1140
www.womenshealthnetwork.org

INDEX

Note: Page numbers in *italics* refer to illustrations, tables, or sidebars.

A

Abacavir, *1175*
Abdomen, 694–698, *695*
  abscess of, 778–779
  examination of
    in aortic aneurysm, 227
    in ascites, 795
    in digestive system disorders, 702
    in gynecologic disorders, 1352
    in heart disease, 121
    in high blood pressure, 136
    in newborn, 1485
    in superior mesenteric artery disease,
      218
  fat accumulation in, 918
  fluid in (ascites), 794–795
    peritonitis and, 782
    removal of (paracentesis), 705, 783, 795
  pain in, 700–701, 702
    in appendicitis, 781–782, 1590
    in constipation, 751
    in Crohn's disease, 739
    in familial Mediterranean fever, 1716
    in infants, 1532
    in intestinal obstruction, 780
    in intussusception, 1589
    in ischemic colitis, 783
    in pancreatic cancer, 774
    in pancreatitis, 730, 732
    in peptic ulcers, 714, *715*
    in porphyria, 935
    recurring, in children, 1591–1593, *1592*
    in ruptured spleen, 1029
    in splenic enlargement, 1028
  radiation injury to, 1660
  stretch marks on, during pregnancy, 1441
Abdominal aorta, aneurysm of, 226–228,
  227
Abdominal cavity, 694
Abducens nerve, 589, *590*
Abetalipoproteinemia, 927
ABO incompatibility, *1506*
Abortion, 1426–1427, *1456*
  for adolescent, 1560
  spontaneous (*see* Miscarriage)
Abrasions, 22, 1691–1693
Abruptio placentae, 1451, *1454*, 1456, 1507
Abscess
  abdominal, 778–779, 1097
  anus and rectum, 761
  Bartholin's gland, *1375*

Abscess (*continued*)
  brain, 539–540
    coma with, *492*
    with ear infection, 1594
    headache with, *459*
    in meningitis, 1562
  breast, 1112, 1389
  in chancroid, 1182
  chest, 1097
  face, 1097
  fallopian tube, 1378
  hand, 402–403
  jaw, 1097
  lacrimal sac, 1293
  liver, 1136
  lung, 265, 272–273, 1112
  pharyngeal, 1596
  pilonidal, 763
  retroperitoneal, 779
  skin, 1112, 1220, 1224
    in acne, *1205*, 1206
  sweat gland, 1224
  throat (retropharyngeal), 1563–1564, 1596
  tonsillar, 1267–1268, 1596
  tooth, 680
  urethral, 868
Absence (petit mal) seizures, 497, *498*
Abuse
  child, *639*, 1179, 1643–1646
    foster care for, 1641–1642
    information resources on, 1760
  domestic, 1410–1412, *1411*
  drug (*see* Drugs, abuse of)
  psychologic, 1411
  sexual, 1411, 1412–1413, 1592, 1644, 1645,
    1646
Acalculous cholecystitis, 815, 816
Acarbose, *968*
Accessory nerve, *591*
Accidents (*see* Injury [injuries])
Acclimatization, 1652
Accommodative esotropia, 1602
ACE (*see* Angiotensin-converting enzyme)
Acetaminophen, 95, 97, 454
  in common cold, *1158*
  hepatitis with, 803
  poisoning with, 1676–1677
  in respiratory tract infection, 1580
Acetazolamide
  in altitude illness, 1674
  in glaucoma, *1308*
Acetohexamide, *968*

Acetylcholine receptors, *71–72*, 578
Acetylcholinesterases, in amniotic fluid, *1432*
Acetylsalicylic acid (*see* Aspirin)
N-Acetyltransferase, 74
Achalasia, 709
Achilles tendon
  bursitis of, 408–409, *408*
  tendinitis of, 424–425
Acid
  burns from, 1648–1651, 1678–1679
  stomach, 696
    in gastrinoma, 775
    gastritis from, 711–713
    peptic ulcers from, 713–717, *715, 718*
    reflux of, 706, 717–719, 1588–1589
    in Zollinger-Ellison syndrome, *717*, 775
Acid-base balance, 930–933, *932*
Acidity
  blood, 930–932, *930, 932*
    reference range for, *1725*
  urine, 826
Acidosis
  in diabetes mellitus, 963, 966
  in Fanconi's syndrome, 852
  in kidney failure, 831
  metabolic, 931–932, *932*
  renal tubular, 849–850, *850*
  respiratory, 931–932
Acitretin, 1203
Acne, 1204–1208, *1205, 1207*
  in newborn, *1496*
Acoustic nerve, *590*
Acoustic neuroma, 1260–1261
Acoustic reflex, 1244
Acquired immunodeficiency syndrome (*see* HIV infection)
Acrocyanosis, 225
Acrodermatitis enteropathica, 914
Acromegaly, 945–946
ACTH (*see* Corticotropin)
Acting out, *634*
Actinic keratoses, *1231*
Actinomycosis, 1097–1098
Activated charcoal, 1676
Activated protein C resistance, 1000
Acupressure, 1705
Acupuncture, 38, 455, 1705
Acute disseminated encephalomyelitis, 560
Acute intermittent porphyria, 934–936
  hormone replacement therapy and, 1359
Acute respiratory distress syndrome, 326–328, *327*
Acute transverse myelitis, 567
Acyclovir, *1156*, 1162
Adam (methylenedioxymethamphetamine), 656
Adam's apple, 244
Adapalene, *1207*
Addiction, drug, 647 (*see also* Drugs, abuse of)

Addison's disease, 942, 956–958
  high potassium levels in, 911
  low sodium levels in, 912–913
  oral color changes with, *663*
Adenocarcinoma (*see also* Cancer)
  esophagus, 764–766
  large intestine, 770–773
  pancreas, 773–774
  small intestine, 768
  stomach, 766–768
Adenoidectomy, 1250, 1597
Adenoids, *1246, 1597*
  enlargement of, 1596–1597
Adenoma
  adrenal, 958, 959, 960
  brain, *520*
  liver, 810
  parathyroid, *904*
  pituitary, *521, 522, 523*, 941, 943–944
    acromegaly with, 945–946
    Cushing's syndrome with, 958
    galactorrhea with, 946–947
  salivary gland, 671
  thyroid, 950
Adenomyosis, *1365*
Adenosine, *167*
Adenosine deaminase deficiency, 1061–1062
Adenosis, vaginal, 1366
Adenovirus infection
  in children, 1579–1580, 1585
  eye (keratoconjunctivitis), *1297*
  immunization for, *1094*
ADHD (attention deficit/hyperactivity disorder), 1549–1551, *1549, 1550*
  information resources on, *1758*
Adherence (compliance), with drug treatment, 63, 76, 81, 86–88, *87*
Adjustment disorder, *1636*
Adolescents, 1552–1555 (*see also* Puberty)
  development of, 1552–1554, *1553*
  preventive health care for, 1554–1555
  problems in, 1555–1560, *1557*
  sexual behavior in, 1554
  suicidal behavior in, 1634–1635, *1635*
Adoption, 1642–1643
Adrenal crisis, 957
Adrenal glands, *938, 939, 956, 957*
  adenoma of, 958, 959, 960
  congenital hyperplasia of, *1430*, 1520
  corticosteroid suppression of, *958*
  overactive
    aldosterone overproduction, 960, *961*
    androgen overproduction (virilization), 959–960
    catecholamine overproduction (pheochromocytoma), 960–961, 973
    corticosteroid overproduction, 958–959
    (*see also* Cushing's syndrome)

Adrenal glands *(continued)*
  removal of, 959, *959*
  transplantation of, 1083
  tumors of
    in Cushing's syndrome, 958, 959
    in hyperaldosteronism, 960
    in multiple endocrine neoplasia, 973
    pheochromocytoma, 960–961
  underactive, *942, 943,* 956–958 *(see also*
    Addison's disease)
Adrenaline *(see* Epinephrine)
Adrenergic blockers
  in high blood pressure, *138,* 139
  urinary incontinence with, *859*
Adrenocorticotropin (ACTH) *(see*
  Corticotropin)
Adrenoleukodystrophy, 560
Adrenomyeloneuropathy, 560
Adult respiratory distress syndrome, 326–328,
  327
Advance directive, 22, 48, 51, *53,* 54–56
Adynamic ileus, 781
Aerobes, 1096
Aerobic exercise, 33, 35–36
  in high blood pressure, 137
  in pain prevention, 572
Aerophagia, 701, 758, 1486, 1531
Affect, in schizophrenia, 641
Affective disorders, 613 *(see also* Depression;
  Mania)
Aflatoxins, 811
AFP (alpha-fetoprotein)
  in birth defects, 1431, *1432,* 1512, 1526
  as tumor marker, *1039*
Afterbirth *(see* Placenta)
Agammaglobulinemia, X-linked (Bruton's),
  1059
Ageusia, 596
Aging, 16–21, *18–19*
  acceleration of, 21
  blood pressure changes with, 117–118
  bodily changes with, 17–19, *18–19,* 79
  bone marrow changes with, 979
  breast changes with, 1348
  cancer and, 1033
  dental changes with, 663
  digestive system changes with, 698, 751
  vs. disease, 17
  drugs and, 79–81, *80–81,* 84–85
  ear changes with, 1246–1247
  eye changes with, 1278, 1310–1311
  female reproductive system changes with,
    1348
  heart changes with, 117–118
  illness and, 19–21
  immune system changes with, 1056
  information resources on, 1756
  liver changes with, 788
  lung changes with, 248

Aging *(continued)*
  male reproductive system changes with,
    1324
  nose changes with, 1246–1247
  skin changes with, 1187–1188
  successful (healthy), 16–17
  throat changes with, 1246–1247
  urinary tract changes with, 822–823, 857
  water imbalance with, 930
Agnogenic myeloid metaplasia, 1025
Agnosia, 478–479
Agonists, drugs as, 70–72, *71–72*
Agoraphobia, 609–610
AIDS *(see* HIV infection)
Air
  in blood, 825
  in chest (pneumothorax), 316–317, *316*
    in asthma, 276
    in COPD, 282–283
    diving-related, 1668
    in meconium aspiration syndrome, 1501
    in newborn, 1502
  compressed, injuries with, 1666–1671,
    1669, 1670
  embolism of, 286, 289, 1668
  swallowing of, 701, 758, 1486, 1531
  in urine, 869
Air conditioner lung, 309, *309*
Air travel, 1708–1714
  air pressure changes with, 1244, 1256–1257,
    1257, 1710
  blood clot prevention during, 287–288, 1710
  information resources on, 1768
  motion sickness with, 465, 1710
Airways *(see also specific parts, eg,* Nose;
    Throat [pharynx])
  biology of, 244–248, *245, 246, 247*
  defense mechanisms of, 247–248,
    1087–1088
  disorders of, 243–331 *(see also* Lungs *and*
    terms starting with* Bronch-)
  in emergency first aid, 1687–1688
  hyperreactivity of, in bronchitis, 263
  obstruction of
    in asthma, 274–281, *275*
    chronic, 281–285
    respiratory failure in, *325*
    wheezing with, 251–252
Alanine transaminase, *1727*
Albinism, 1214
Albumin, 978
  blood levels of, 889, *1727*
Albuterol
  in asthma, 70, *278,* 279–280, 1584
  in COPD, 283
Alcohol
  blood, *1725*
  cleansing with, 1190
Alcoholics Anonymous, *651*

Alcohol use and abuse, 647, 649–652, *650*
  by adolescents, 1559, 1636
  consciousness alterations with, *492*
  coronary artery disease and, 200
  in essential tremor, 546
  folic acid deficiency with, 899
  head injury and, 518
  heat disorders with, 1652
  in high blood pressure, 137
  information resources on, 1757
  liver disease in, 797–799, *799*
  niacin deficiency with, 897
  obesity and, 915
  optic neuropathy with, 1316
  oral cancer and, 672
  over-the-counter drug precautions and, *102*
  pancreatitis and, 729–733
  during pregnancy, 1463
  preoperative decrease in, 1700–1701
  suicide and, 623
  urinary incontinence with, *859*
  vitamin B_1 deficiency with, 896
  Wernicke-Korsakoff syndrome with,
    479–480, 650, 896
  withdrawal from, 649, 651–652, *651*
Aldosterone, 912, *939*, 956
  deficiency of, 956
    high potassium levels with, 911
  excess of, 960, *961*
    low potassium levels with, 910
Alendronate
  food interactions with, 77
  in osteogenesis imperfecta, 1610
  in osteoporosis, 345, 346, *1360*
  in Paget's disease of bone, 347–348
Alkali, burns from, 1648–1651, 1678–1679
Alkaline phosphatase, *1727*
Alkalinity, blood, 930–931, *930*, 932–933, *932*
Alkalosis
  metabolic, 932–933, *932*
  respiratory, 932–933
Alkylating agents, *1045*
ALL (acute lymphocytic/lymphoblastic
  leukemia), *20*, 1011–1012
Allergens, 1063
  anaphylactic reactions to, 1065, 1068,
    1072–1073
  in asthma, 274–275, 276, 277
  in contact dermatitis, 1193–1194, *1193*
  immunotherapy against, 1064, 1066–1067
  skin testing for, 1063–1064, 1068
Allergic purpura, 996–997
Allergy and allergic reactions, 1063–1073
  anaphylactic (*see* Anaphylactic reactions)
  to antibiotics, 1125
  aspergillosis, 311–312
  to aspirin, 453–454
  asthma (*see* Asthma)
  bee sting, 1685

Allergy and allergic reactions *(continued)*
  to blood transfusion, 986
  conjunctivitis, 1066, 1067, 1298–1299
  dermatitis, 1193–1194, *1193*
  diagnosis of, 1063–1064
  to drugs, 85, 843–844, 1064,
    1198–1199
  eosinophilic pneumonia, 310–311
  exercise-induced, 1070–1071
  eyelid swelling with, 1293–1294
  to food, 1068–1069
    in infant, 1489
  to gases and chemicals, 300
  to grass pollen, 1065–1067
  to house dust, 1067–1068
  in IgA deficiency, 1060
  immunoglobulin E in, 1063
  information resources on, 1757
  to insulin, 968
  lip swelling with, 664, 1071
  in lungs, 308–312
  mastocytosis, 1069–1070
  to milk, in infant, 1531
  multiple chemical sensitivity syndrome,
    1719–1720, *1719*
  nasal polyps in, 1067, 1068
  nephrotic syndrome, 840, *840*
  occupational, *297*, 299–300
  over-the-counter drugs for, 98–99
  photosensitivity, 1232–1233 (*see also*
    Photosensitivity)
  physical, 1070
  pneumonitis, 308–310, *309*
  to pollen, 1065–1067, 1298–1299
  prevention of, 1064, 1067–1068
  to radiopaque dyes, *827*, *1069*
  rhinitis, 1065–1067, 1264
  seasonal, 1065–1067
  sinusitis, 1266–1267, *1266*
  skin testing in, 276, 1063–1064, 1188,
    1731
  symptoms of, 1063
  treatment of, 1064–1065, *1065*
  tubulointerstitial nephritis (kidney disease),
    843–844
  year-round, 1067–1068
Alloimmunization, in sickle cell disease,
  1446–1447
Allopurinol, *393*, 394
All-*trans*-retinoic acid, 1014
Alopecia (baldness), 1212–1214
Alpha-agonists
  in glaucoma, *1308*
  in high blood pressure, *138*, 139
  urinary incontinence with, *859*
Alpha$_1$-antitrypsin
  deficiency of, 282, 285, 801
  in intestinal lymphangiectasia, 738
Alpha-beta blockers, *138*, 139

Alpha-blockers
    in benign prostatic hyperplasia, 1330
    in high blood pressure, *138, 139*
Alpha-fetoprotein (AFP)
    in birth defects, 1431, *1432,* 1512, 1526
    as tumor marker, *1039*
Alpha heavy chain disease, 1010
Alpha-thalassemia, 994
Alport's syndrome, 856
Alprostadil
    in coarctation of aorta, 1518
    in congenital artery blockage, 1514
    in erectile dysfunction, 1338
    in pulmonary valve stenosis, 1518
ALS (amyotrophic lateral sclerosis),
        575–577
    information resources on, 1757
Alternative medicine, 1704–1707
    for cancer, 1046
    for postmenopausal symptoms, 1361
Altitude illness, 1672–1674
Aluminum acetate (Burow's solution), 1194
Aluminum antacids, 99, 716, 718
Aluminum chloride, 1211
Alveolar cell carcinoma, 328
Alveoli, 245, *245,* 246
    bleeding from, *307*
    inflammation of (alveolitis), 308–310,
        309
    macrophages of, 248
    proteinosis of, 306, 308
Alzheimer's disease, *20,* 487–488 (*see also*
        Dementia)
    information resources on, 1757
Amanita phalloides (mushroom) poisoning,
        725, 726
Amantadine, *1156*
    in influenza, 1160
    in Parkinson's disease, *549,* 550
Amblyopia, 1600–1601
    nutritional, 1316
    toxic, 1316
Ambulation exercise, 39
    after hip fracture, 43
Amebiasis, 1135–1136
Ameboma, 1136
Amenorrhea, *1362,* 1364–1365
    with galactorrhea, 946
American Sign Language, 1253
Amifostine, 1661
Amikacin, *1122*
Amino acids
    in cystinuria, 851–852
    essential, 882
    in Fanconi's syndrome, 852
    in Hartnup disease, 853
    metabolism of, disorders of, 1618–1619
Aminoglycosides, *1122*
    hearing loss with, 1248

Aminosalicylates, *741*
Amitriptyline, in elderly persons, *80*
AML (acute myelocytic leukemia),
        1012–1014, *1013*
Ammonia
    inhalation of, 300–301
    reference range for, *1725*
Amnesia, 479–480 (*see also* Memory)
    dissociative, 636–637
Amniocentesis, *1433,* 1434, *1728*
    in birth defect diagnosis, 1512, 1629
    in fetal lung evaluation, 1448, 1499, 1500
    in Rh incompatibility, 1453
Amnion, 1436, *1437*
Amniotic fluid, *1437*
    acetylcholinesterase in, *1432*
    alpha-fetoprotein in, *1432*
    color of, 1465
    embolism of, 286, 289, 1473–1474
    meconium in, 1498
    problems with, 1454–1455
    tests on (*see also* Amniocentesis)
        in immunodeficiency disorders, 1059
Amniotic sac, *1437*
    rupture of, 1465
        premature, 1470
Amoxicillin, *1123*
    in peptic ulcer, 718
Amphetamines, 656
    during pregnancy, 1464
Amphotericin B, *1152*
Ampicillin, *1123*
Amprenavir, *1175*
Amputation
    after frostbite, 1657
    information resources on, 1757
    of leg, 222, 964
    rehabilitation after, 43–44
Amsler grid, 1283
Amygdala, 434
Amylase, 697
    in acute pancreatitis, 731
    reference range for, *1725*
Amyl nitrite, *659*
Amyloidosis, 162, 1714–1716, *1714*
    heart failure in, 152–153
    information resources on, 1757
Amyotrophic lateral sclerosis (ALS),
        575–577
    information resources on, 1757
Anabolic steroids, *647* (*see also* Androgens)
    adolescent use of, 1560
    coronary artery disease and, 200
Anaerobes, 1096–1097, *1097*
Anaerobic exercise, 33, 36
Anaerobic infections (*see specific infections*)
Anagrelide
    in polycythemia vera, 1025
    in thrombocythemia, 1026–1027

Analgesics, 450–455
  in common cold, *1158*
  in elderly persons, *80*
  in labor and delivery, 1464, 1467
  in migraine headache, *460*
  nonopioid, 452–454, *453, 454*
  opioid, 450–452, *451*
  over-the-counter, 94–95, *97*
  patient-controlled, 452, 1703
  postoperative, 1703
Anaphylactic reactions, 1063, 1072–1073
  vs. anaphylactoid reactions, *1069*
  exercise-induced, 1070–1071
  in food allergy, 1068
  in selective IgA deficiency, 1060
  treatment of, 1065, 1073
Anaphylactoid reactions, *1069*
  in mastocytosis, 1069
Anastomosis, ileo-anal, 744
Anatomy, 2–7, *3*
  adenoids, *1597*
  adrenal glands, 956, *957*
  anus, *695, 698, 759*
  aorta, *227*
  appendix, *695, 698*
  bile ducts, 786–788, *787*
  biliary tract, *695, 697*
  bladder, *821, 822*
  bones, 334–335, *336, 337*
  brain, 433–435, *435*
  breast, *1388*
  bursas, 335
  digestive system, 694–698, *695*
  disease and, 8
  duodenum, *696*
  ear, 1244–1245, *1245*
  endocrine system, 937–940, *938, 939*
  esophagus, *695, 696*
  eye, 1276–1277, *1276, 1277*
  gallbladder, *695, 697,* 786–788, *787*
  heart, 114–117, *115, 116*
    electrical pathway and, 163–164
  ileum, *696*
  jejunum, *696*
  joints, 336–339, *338*
  kidney, 820, *821, 845*
  large intestine, *695,* 697–698
  ligaments, 335–336
  liver, *695, 697,* 786, *787*
  lung, 244–245, *245*
  lymphatic system, *1053*
  mouth, 661–662, *662*
  muscles, 335, *336, 337*
  nerve roots, *436*
  nervous system, 433–438, *435, 436, 437*
  nose and sinuses, 1245–1246, *1246, 1265*
  optic nerve, 1315, *1316*
  pancreas, *695,* 696–697, 729, *730, 787*
  pituitary gland, 940, *941*

Anatomy *(continued)*
  pleura, 312, *313*
  rectum, *695,* 698, 759
  reproductive system
    female, 1343–1345, *1344, 1345*
    male, 1321–1323, *1322*
  retina, 1309–1310, *1310*
  salivary glands, 666, *667*
  skin, 1186–1187, *1187*
  small intestine, *695, 696*
  spinal cord, 435–437, *436*
  spleen, 1027, *1027*
  stomach, *695, 696*
  tear system, *1293*
  temporomandibular joint, 685–686, *686*
  tendons, 335
  throat, 694, *695, 696,* 1246, *1246*
  thyroid gland, 948–949, *948*
  tonsils, *1597*
  tooth, 662–663
  ureter, *821,* 822
  urethra, *821,* 822
  urinary tract, 820–823, *821*
Ancylostoma duodenale infection
    (hookworm), 1138–1140, *1139*
Ancylostomiasis, 1138–1140, *1139*
Andersen's disease, *1617*
Androgens
  coronary artery disease and, 200
  deficiency of, in children, 1520
  excess of, 959–960
  in female, 1343
  in hair growth, 1212
Anemia(s), 978, 980, 987–994
  angina in, 203
  aplastic, *991,* 1002
  autoimmune, 991–992, *1074*
  with cancer treatment, 1047
  causes of, 987, *988, 989*
  in chronic disease, 987, *988,* 991
  in decreased red blood cell production, 987,
      988, 989–990
  drug-related, 83
  in excessive bleeding, 987–989, *988*
  in fetus, 1453
  in folic acid deficiency, 899, 990–991
  in gastritis, 712
  in gastroesophageal reflux, 1588
  heart failure with, 152
  in hemoglobin abnormalities, 992–994
  hemolytic, 987, *988, 989*
    autoimmune, 991–992, *1074*
  in HIV infection, 1574
  in Hodgkin's disease, *1017*
  in hookworm infection, 1139
  in increased red blood cell destruction, *988,*
      989, 991–992
  in increased red blood cell production, 987
  iron deficiency, 708, 907–908, 989–990

Anemia(s) *(continued)*
  in kidney failure, 833
  in leukemia, 1015
  in macroglobulinemia, 1009
  in multiple myeloma, 1008
  in myelofibrosis, 1025
  in newborn, *1506,* 1507
  in non-Hodgkin's lymphoma, 1020, *1021*
  oral discoloration with, *663, 665*
  in paroxysmal nocturnal hemoglobinuria, *989*
  pernicious, 898, *1074*
  during pregnancy, 1439, 1443–1444, 1446–1447, 1451
  radiation injury and, 1659
  shortness of breath in, 251
  in sickle cell disease, 992–994, *993*
  spleen enlargement and, *989*
  in stomach cancer, 767
  in thalassemia, 994
  in vitamin B$_{12}$ deficiency, 898, 990–991
Anencephaly, 1430, *1432,* 1526
Anesthesia, 66, 1699–1700
  muscle sensitivity to, 75
Anesthetics
  for canker sores, 668
  in labor and delivery, 1464, 1467–1468
  topical, 455
Aneurysm
  aortic, 20, 119, 226–229, *227*
    in Marfan syndrome, 1608
    in syphilis, 1177
  cerebral artery, 229
    coma with, *492*
    in polycystic kidney disease, 855
    rupture of, 511, 512
  coronary artery, in Kawasaki syndrome, *1581*
  dissecting, 229–231, *230*
  femoral artery, 229
  of heart, *212*
  hepatic artery, 807
  popliteal artery, 229
Angel dust (phencyclidine), 658
Angina, 118, 202–210, *206–207, 208, 210*
  Ludwig's, 670
  sexual activity and, *1337*
  travel and, 1711–1712
Angina decubitus, 203
Angioedema, 1063, 1070, 1071–1072
  hereditary, 664, *1072*
Angiography (arteriography), 128, *1728*
  cerebral (brain), 445, 508, 512
  computed tomography, 125, 287
  coronary (heart), 129, 204
  digital substraction, 130
  hepatic (liver), 789
  intestinal, 768
  magnetic resonance, 127, 444

Angiography (arteriography) *(continued)*
  peripheral artery, 130, 219
  pulmonary (lung), 256, 287
  renal (kidney), 828
  retinal (eye), 1285, 1312
  selective, 130
Angioma, 1235–1236, *1235*
  spider, 1236
    during pregnancy, 1441
Angioplasty, 128
  of carotid artery, 507
  of coronary arteries, 149, 208–209, *208*
    in infants, 1514
  of peripheral arteries, 220
  of renal artery, 846
Angiosarcoma, 812
Angiotensin, 937–938, *939*
Angiotensin-converting enzyme (ACE), in sarcoidosis, 305
Angiotensin-converting enzyme (ACE) inhibitors
  after heart attack, 215
  in coronary artery disease, 205
  fetal effects of, 1446
  in heart failure, *156,* 157
  in high blood pressure, 139, *139*
  in nephrotic syndrome, 841
  oligohydramnios with, 1455
  during pregnancy, 1459, *1460*
  urinary incontinence with, *859*
Angiotensin II, 132, *133*
Angiotensin II blockers
  in heart failure, *156,* 157
  in high blood pressure, 139, *139*
Angular cheilitis, 664
Anhedonia, 641
Animal bites, 1682
Ankle
  fracture of, 354
  sprain of, 405–407, *406*
  swelling of (edema) of, 153, 912 (*see also* Swelling)
Ankylosing spondylitis, 377, 569
  information resources on, 1757
Ankylosis, of temporomandibular joint, 687
Anomia, 477
Anorchia, *1512,* 1520
Anorexia, 701
Anorexia nervosa, 624–626, 1365
Anoscopy, 703, *704,* 759
Anosmia, 596
Antacids, 99
  in elderly persons, 101
  in flatulence, 758–759
  in gastritis, 713
  in gastroesophageal reflux, 719, 1588
  in peptic ulcer, 716, *718*
Antagonists, drugs as, 70–72, *71–72*

Anterior chamber, of eye, *1276*, 1277
  bleeding into, 1290
  paracentesis of, 1312
Anthrax, *1089*, 1098
  immunization for, *1094*, 1098
Antiallergy drugs (*see also* Antihistamines)
  over-the-counter, 98–99
Antianxiety drugs, 600, 607, *607*
  abuse of, 653–654, *654*
  during breastfeeding, *1462*
  in elderly persons, *81*
  during pregnancy, *1460*
  in recurring abdominal pain, 1593
  withdrawal from, 654
Antiarrhythmic drugs, 161, 165, *166–167*
Antiasthmatic drugs, 276–281, *278*, *279*
  generic substitutions for, *90*
  during pregnancy, 1448
Antibiotics, 1120–1125, *1122–1124* (*see also*
    specific antibiotics and diseases)
  in acne, 1206, *1207*
  administration of, 1121, 1124
  bacterial resistance to, 78, 1112, 1121
  in bladder infection, 870, *870*
  in cellulitis, 1221
  colitis with, *720*, 745–746, 1125
  combinations of, 1121
  in Crohn's disease, 740–741
  in ear infection, 1594
  in endocarditis, 186–187
  in gastroenteritis, 723
  in immunodeficiency disorders, 1059
  intravenous administration of, 1121, 1124
  in kidney infection, 872
  in peptic ulcer, *718*
  during pregnancy, *1460*
  preventive use of, 1091, 1121
    before surgery, 186, *187*
  selection of, 1120–1121, *1122–1124*
  side effects of, 1124–1125
  in splenic disorders, 1063
Antibodies, 1050, *1052*, 1055–1056, *1055*,
    1088, 1090 (*see also* Immunoglobulin[s])
  ABO, *1506*
  antinuclear, 379, 1612–1613, *1725*
  autoimmune (*see* Autoimmune disorders)
  to clotting factors, 1000
  deficiency of
    in common variable immunodeficiency,
      1060
    in infant, 1060
    in premature infant, 1497
    in severe combined immunodeficiency,
      1060–1062
    in X-linked agammaglobulinemia, 1059
  in infants, 1056
  in kidney disease, 837
  in Lyme disease, 1106
  mitochondrial, 800

Antibodies (*continued*)
  monoclonal, 1006
    in cancer treatment, 1044–1046, *1045*
    in non-Hodgkin's lymphoma, 1022
    in transplantation, *1079*
  in nephritis, 837
  in organ transplantation, 1076
  in pemphigus, 1216
  Rh, 1427, 1433, 1442, 1453, 1477, *1506*
  in rheumatoid arthritis, 371
  ribonucleoprotein, 384–385
  to self (*see* Autoimmune disorders)
  SS-B, 382
  transfusion of, 985
  to tumors, 1034
Anticancer drugs (*see* Chemotherapy)
Anticholinergic drugs
  in asthma, *278*, 280
  in collagenous colitis, 745
  in COPD, 283
  in Crohn's disease, 740
  in elderly persons, 79, *79*
  in lymphocytic colitis, 745
  in Parkinson's disease, 549, 550
  in ulcerative colitis, 743
  urinary incontinence with, *859*
Anticlotting drugs (*see* Anticoagulants)
Anticoagulants, 996
  after surgery, 288
  in atrial fibrillation and atrial flutter, 170
  in coronary artery disease, *206*
  in deep vein thrombosis prevention, 234
  dental procedures and, 692
  food interactions with, 77
  gastrointestinal bleeding and, 777
  in heart failure, 157, *157*
  during pregnancy, *1460*
  in pulmonary embolism, 288
  in pulmonary embolism prevention, 234
  in renal artery thrombosis, 846
  in renal vein thrombosis, 849
  in stroke, 509
  in thrombophilia, 1001
Anticonvulsants, 499, *500–501*
  folic acid deficiency with, 899
  generic substitutions for, *90*
  in head injury, 515
  in manic-depressive illness, 621
  for pain, 455
  during pregnancy, 1447, *1460*
Antidepressants, 600, 617–619, *618*
  after menopause, 1359, *1360*
  in anorexia nervosa, 626
  in anxiety disorders, 607
  during breastfeeding, *1462*
  in bulimia nervosa, 627
  in children, 1633
  drug interactions with, 103
  in elderly persons, *80*

Antidepressants *(continued)*
  food interactions with, 77
  generic substitutions for, *90*
  in manic-depressive illness, 621
  for obsessive-compulsive disorder, 612
  for pain, 455
  in panic attacks and panic disorder, 609
  in posttraumatic stress disorder, 613
  during pregnancy, 1459
  in premenstrual syndrome, 1363
  in recurring abdominal pain, 1593
  in sleep disorders, *471*
  in social phobia, 610
  urinary incontinence with, *859*
Antidiabetic drugs, 968–969, *968*
  in children, 1614
  in elderly persons, *80*
  generic substitutions for, *90*
  in pancreatitis, 733
  during pregnancy, *1461*
Antidiarrheal drugs, 756, *756*
  in children, 1588
  in collagenous colitis, 745
  in Crohn's disease, 740
  in lymphocytic colitis, 745
  in ulcerative colitis, 743
Antidiuretic hormone (vasopressin), 822, *913,*
    939, 940, 941, 956
  in blood volume regulation, 912
  in diabetes insipidus, 851, 944–945
  inappropriate secretion of, 912, *913,* 929
  in water balance, *928*
Antidotes
  for monoamine oxidase inhibitors, 618
  for radioactive materials, 1660
Antiemetic drugs, in elderly persons, *80*
Antifungal drugs, 1148–1149, *1152*
  topical, 1226, *1226*
Antigens, 1049, *1052*
  B lymphocyte interaction with, 1054–1055
  T lymphocyte recognition of, *1051*
  tumor, 1034
Antiglobulin test (Coombs test), 992
Antihistamines, 98, 1064, *1065*
  in allergic conjunctivitis, 1067
  in allergic rhinitis, 1066, 1264
  in common cold, 1158, *1158,* 1264
  in cough remedies, 250
  in elderly persons, *80,* 101
  in food allergy, 1069
  in itching, 1190, 1192
  in motion sickness, 99
  over-the-counter, 96–97, 98–99
  precautions with, 96–97
  side effects of, 96
  as sleep aid, 100
Antihyperglycemic drugs, oral, 968–969, *968*
Antihypertensive drugs, *138–139,* 139–140
  in elderly persons, *80*

Antihypertensive drugs *(continued)*
  generic substitutions for, *90*
  postprandial hypotension and, 147
  during pregnancy, 1446, 1459, *1460*
Anti-infective agents, 1191 *(see also*
    Antibiotics)
Anti-inflammatory drugs
  in collagenous colitis, 745
  in Crohn's disease, 740, *741*
  in lymphocytic colitis, 745
  nonsteroidal *(see* Nonsteroidal anti-
    inflammatory drugs)
  over-the-counter, 94–95, 97
  in proctitis, 762
  steroidal *(see* Corticosteroids)
  topical, 1190–1191
  in ulcerative colitis, 743
Antilymphocyte globulin, *1078*
Antimetabolites, *1045*
Antimitotics, *1045*
Antioxidant, 882–883
  selenium as, 911
  vitamin C as, 900
  vitamin E as, 895
Antiphospholipid (anticardiolipin) syndrome,
    1000
Antiplatelet drugs
  in coronary artery disease, *206,* 207–208
  in peripheral artery disease, 222
  in stroke prevention, 505
Antipsychotic drugs, 600, *643*
  in autism, 1631
  during breastfeeding, *1462*
  in childhood schizophrenia, 1632
  in dementia, 486
  in elderly persons, *80,* 486
  generic substitutions for, *90*
  in manic-depressive illness, 621
  in schizophrenia, 643–644, *643, 645*
  side effects of, 643, *644*
  swallowing problems with, 708
  in Tourette's syndrome, 552
  urinary incontinence with, *859*
Antipyretic drugs, 1091
  in common cold, *1158*
Antiseizure drugs *(see* Anticonvulsants)
Antisense technology, 16
Antishock trousers, 149
Antisocial personality, 632
Antispasmodic drugs, *81*
  in irritable bowel syndrome, 757
Antithrombin deficiency, 1000
Antithymocyte globulin, *1078*
Antitussive drugs, 249
Antivenom
  for coelenterate sting, 1687
  serum sickness with, *1684*
  for snake bite, 1683
  for spider bite, 1684

Antiviral drugs, 1155, *1156*
in chickenpox, 1572
in hepatitis, 805
in herpes simplex virus infection, 1162, 1302
in herpes zoster ophthalmicus, 1302
in immunodeficiency disorders, 1059
in influenza, 1160
in Parkinson's disease, *549, 550*
Ant stings, 1685
Anuria, 829
Anus, *695, 698, 1344*
abscess of, 761
atresia of, 1521
biology of, 698, 759
bleeding from, 776–778, *777*
cancer of, 773
examination of, 702
exercises for, 757–758
fissure of, 760
in Crohn's disease, 739
fistula of, 761, *762*
foreign objects in, 764
hemorrhoids of, 759–760, *761*
itching around, 760, 763–764, 1198
muscles of, problems with, 751, 762
in newborn, 1485
rectal prolapse in, 763
Anvil (incus), 1244, *1245*
Anxiety, 605–613, *607*
alkalosis with, 932–933
drugs for (*see* Antianxiety drugs)
in dying person, 50
dyspepsia and, 700
hyperventilation syndrome and, 251
irritable bowel syndrome and, 756
medical disorders and, 608
in panic attacks and panic disorder, 608–609, *609*
performance and, *606*
in personality disorders, 633
in phobic disorders, 609–611, *611*
in posttraumatic stress disorder, 612–613
separation, in children, 1534, 1540, 1636–1637
social, 610–611
during travel, 1711
Anxiolytics (*see* Antianxiety drugs)
Aorta
aneurysm of, *20,* 119, 226–229, *227*
in Marfan syndrome, 1608
in syphilis, 1177
angiography of, 130
atherosclerosis of, and atheroembolic kidney disease, 846–847
coarctation of, 1518
congenital blockage of, 1514
dissection of, 119, 229–231, *230*
in Marfan syndrome, 1608

Aorta (*continued*)
obstruction of, 217–218, 222
in tetralogy of Fallot, 1515, *1517*
transposition of, 1517
Aortic valve, 114, *115*
bicuspid, 180, 181
regurgitation, 180–181
in Marfan syndrome, 1608
stenosis, 181–182
in children, 1517–1518
sexual activity and, *1337*
in syphilis, 1177
Aortography, 130
Apgar score, 1483–1484
Aphasia, 477–478, *477*
rehabilitation for, 44
Aplastic anemia, *991,* 1002
Apnea
in newborn, 1496
in premature infant, 1503–1504
sleep, 255, 472–474, 917, 1596–1597
Apolipoprotein E (apo E), 487
Appendicitis, 781–782
in children, 1590
during pregnancy, 1450
Appendix, *695, 698*
immune function of, 1050–1051, *1053*
inflammation of (*see* Appendicitis)
Appetite
in dying person, 49
loss of, 701
in young children, 1544–1545
Applanation tonometry, 1285
Apprehension (*see* Anxiety)
Apraclonidine, *1308*
Apraxia, 478
rehabilitation for, 44–45
Aqueous humor, 1277, 1306, *1307*
Arachnoid mater, 435, *435, 436*
Arbovirus infection, 537–538, 1167
Arcus senilis, 1278
Arenavirus infection, 538, 1165–1167
Argon plasma coagulator
in colorectal cancer, 773
in proctitis, 762
Argyll Robertson pupils, 1281
Aripiprazole, *645*
Arm
amputation of, rehabilitation after, 43–44
artery to, blockage of, 217
birth defects of, 1523–1524
fracture of, 358
injury to, in newborn, 1495
lymphedema in, 240
pain in (thoracic outlet syndrome), 582–583
reattachment of, *1083*
severed or constricted, 1693
splint for, *1692*

Aromatase inhibitors, 1400
Arrhythmias, 163–175, *164, 166–167, 168*
　atrial fibrillation and atrial flutter,
　　169–170
　atrial premature beats, 168–169
　bundle branch block, 175
　in electrical injury, 1662
　electrophysiologic testing in, 124
　in frostbite, 1656
　in heart attack, 211
　heart block, 174–175
　heart failure with, 152
　paroxysmal supraventricular tachycardia,
　　170–171
　in potassium abnormalities, 911
　sexual activity and, *1337*
　travel and, 1711–1712
　ventricular fibrillation, 173–174
　ventricular premature beats, 172
　ventricular tachycardia, 172–173
　in Wolff-Parkinson-White syndrome,
　　171–172
Arsenic, angiosarcoma and, 812
Arterial blood gas analysis, 255
Arteriography *(see Angiography)*
Arterioles, 117
　in blood pressure control, 141
　dilatation of (erythromelalgia), 225
　in Raynaud's disease and Raynaud's
　　phenomenon, 224–225
　in syndrome X, 202
Arteriolosclerosis, *195*
Arteriosclerosis, 195, *195 (see also*
　　Atherosclerosis)
　high blood pressure and, 133–134
　high phosphate levels and, 910
Arteriovenous fistula, 238–239
　in hemodialysis, 834, *836*
Arteriovenous malformation
　in brain, 511
　in digestive system, 776
　in eye, 1319
　in spine, 565–566
Arteritis
　Takayasu's, *387*
　temporal (giant cell), *387, 388, 389,* 1316
　　headache with, *459*
Artery (arteries), 117
　cerebral, *503*
　　aneurysm of, 511, 512
　　bleeding of *(see Stroke, hemorrhagic)*
　　blood clots in *(see Stroke, ischemic)*
　coronary *(see Coronary arteries)*
　great, transposition of, 1517
　hardening of, 194–198, *195, 196 (see also*
　　Atherosclerosis)
　hepatic (liver), 786, 787, 806, *807*
　　aneurysm of, 807
　　occlusive disease of, 806–807

Artery (arteries) *(continued)*
　oxygen saturation of, *1727*
　peripheral
　　angiography of, 130
　　computed tomography angiography of,
　　　125
　　functional disease of, 224–225
　　magnetic resonance angiography of,
　　　127
　　occlusive disease of, 216–223, *219, 221,*
　　　222
　　Raynaud's disease and Raynaud's
　　　phenomenon of, 224–225
　　spasm of, 225
　in polyarteritis nodosa, 387–388, *387*
　renal (kidney), 820, *821, 845*
　　obstruction of, 844–846, *846*
　in Takayasu's arteritis, *387*
　in temporal (giant cell) arteritis, *387, 388,*
　　389
Arthritis
　degenerative *(see Osteoarthritis)*
　in gout, 392
　infectious (septic), 365–366, 687, 688, 689
　information resources on, 1758
　in Lyme disease, 1106, 1107
　psoriatic, 375–376, 1202
　reactive (Reiter's syndrome), 376–377
　rheumatoid, 370–375, *372, 374*
　　juvenile, 1612–1613
　in rubella, 1582
　septic, 365–366, 687, 688, 689
　in Sjögren's syndrome, 382
　of temporomandibular joint, 686, 688, 689
Arthritis-dermatitis syndrome, 1179
Arthrography, 342
Arthrogryposis multiplex congenita,
　　1524–1525
Arthroplasty (joint replacement), 352–353
　in avascular necrosis, 363
　hip, 355–356, *357, 370*
　infection and, 365
　knee, *369, 370*
Arthroscopy, 343, *1700, 1724*
Artificial insemination, 1416
Artificial tears, 1301
Asbestosis, 296, *297*
Ascariasis, 1136–1137
Ascites, 794–795
　peritonitis and, 782
　in portal hypertension, 794
　removal of (paracentesis), 705, 783, 795
Ascorbic acid *(see Vitamin C)*
Aseptic meningitis, *535, 1576*
Aseptic necrosis, 362–363, *363*
　of lunate bone (Kienböck's disease), 400
Asherman's syndrome, 1365, 1427
Asociality, 641
Aspartame, during pregnancy, 1463

Aspartate transaminase, *1727*
Asperger's disorder, 1631
Aspergilloma, 1149
Aspergillosis, 271, 311–312, 1149
Aspiration
   age-associated, 1247
   in cerebral palsy, 1625
   in gastroesophageal reflux, 1588
   meconium, 1498, 1501
   pneumonia with, 271–272, 890
   pneumonitis with, *307*
Aspiration (needle)
   bone marrow, 981–982, *982*, *1728* (*see also*
      Bone marrow, examination of)
   breast, 1393
   joint, 342–343, *1729*
   of pleural fluid, 256
Aspirin, 94–95, 453–454
   anaphylactoid reactions to, *1069*
   in common cold, 1158, *1158*
   dental procedures and, 692
   drug interactions with, 103
   gastrointestinal side effects of, 64, 453, 711,
      714, 777
   for heart attack, *206*, 214
   in heart attack prevention, *206*, 207–208
   in Kawasaki syndrome, *1581*
   in peripheral arterial disease, 222
   poisoning with, 1677
   during pregnancy, *1461*, 1501
   Reye's syndrome and, 95, 1537, 1568, *1572*
      information resources on, 1767
   in rheumatic fever, 1567
   in rheumatoid arthritis, 372–373, *372*
   side effects of, 453–454
   in stroke prevention, 505
   in systemic lupus erythematosus, 380
   tinnitus and, 1261
Assisted suicide, 624
Asterixis (flapping tremor), 545–546, 796
Asthenia, 341
Asthma, 274–281, *275, 277, 278, 279, 280*
   allergic, 274–275, *277*, 1593, 1584
   aspirin and, 453–454
   cardiac, 154
   in children, 1583–1585
   exercise-induced, 276, 1070–1071
   information resources on, 1757
   occupational, *297*, 299–300
   over-the-counter drug precautions in, *102*
   during pregnancy, 1448
   wheezing in, 251–252
Astigmatic keratotomy, 1289
Astigmatism, 1279, *1282*
   in children, *1601*
Astrocytoma, *520, 522, 527*
Ataxia, 556
   in cerebral palsy, 1625

Ataxia-telangiectasia, 556, 1061
Atelectasis, 292–294
   postoperative, 1703
Atenolol (*see* Beta-blockers)
Atheroma, 195, *196*
Atherosclerosis, 194–198, *195, 196*
   cholesterol in, 921–922
   of coronary arteries, 199–215 (*see also*
      Coronary arteries, disease of)
   in diabetes mellitus, *963, 964*
   estrogen and, 1358
   in familial hypercholesterolemia, 926
   homocysteine level and, *899*
   kidney failure and, 832
   of peripheral arteries, 216–223, *219, 221,
      222*
   progestin and, 1359
   of renal arteries, 844–846
   stroke and, 504
Athetosis, 552–553
Athlete's foot (tinea pedis), 1225
Athletic heart syndrome, 32
Atkins Diet, 887
Atonic seizures, 497
Atopic dermatitis, 1194–1196
   in food allergy, 1068
   in infants and young children, 1535
Atorvastatin, *925*
Atovaquone-proguanil, 1141
Atresia
   anal, 1521
   bile duct, 1522
   esophageal, 1520–1521, *1521*
Atrial fibrillation, 169–170
   in mitral regurgitation, 177
   in mitral stenosis, 180
   in Wolff-Parkinson-White syndrome, 171
Atrial flutter, 169–170
Atrial premature beats, 168–169
Atrial septal defect, 1514–1515, *1516*
Atrium (atria), 114, 115–116, *115*
Atrophic gastritis, 711, 712, 713
Atrophic rhinitis, 1264–1265
Atrophy
   muscular, 341, 575–577
      peroneal (Charcot-Marie-Tooth disease),
         587
      spinal, 587–588
   skin, *1189*
   tongue, 594
   urethral, *20*
   vaginal, *20*, 1348, 1357, 1382
Attention deficit/hyperactivity disorder
   (ADHD), 1549–1551, *1549, 1550*
   information resources on, 1758
Atypical moles (dysplastic nevi), 1234
Audiometry, 1249, *1728*
Auditory brain stem response, 1250, 1598

Auditory nerve, *1245*
  tumors of, 1260–1261
Augmentation cystoplasty, *860*
Aura
  of migraine headache, 459
  of seizure disorders, 495
Auricle (outer ear), 1244, *1245*
  disorders of, 1253–1255
Auscultation, *1728*
Autism, 1630–1631
  information resources on, 1758
Autoantibodies (*see* Autoimmune disorders)
Autoimmune disorders, 378–386, 1073–1075,
    1074 (see also specific disorders)
  acute transverse myelitis, 567
  allergic (Henoch-Schönlein) purpura,
    996–997
  alopecia areata, 1213
  aplastic anemia, *991*
  brachial neuritis, 582
  bullous pemphigoid, 1217
  causes of, 1074
  dermatitis herpetiformis, 1217–1218
  dermatomyositis, 383–384
  Eaton-Lambert syndrome, 581, *1037*
  eosinophilic fasciitis, 385–386
  Goodpasture's syndrome, 312
  Guillain-Barré syndrome, 584–586
  hearing loss in, 1248
  hemolytic anemia, 991–992, *1074*
  hepatitis, 803, 806
  mixed connective tissue disease, 384–385
  multiple sclerosis, 557–560, *558*
  myasthenia gravis, 577–579, *1074*
  pemphigus, 1216–1217
  peripheral ulcerative keratitis, 1302
  polyglandular deficiency syndrome,
    943
  polymyositis, 383–384
  in pregnancy, 1448–1449
  relapsing polychondritis, 385
  rheumatoid arthritis, 370–375
  scleroderma, 380–382
  Sjögren's syndrome, 382–383
  streptococcal infection, 1113
  systemic lupus erythematosus, 378–380,
    379, 1074
  tests for, 1074
Automated external defibrillator, 167, 1689,
    1689
Autonomic nervous system, 5, 437
  in blood pressure control, 132
  in Shy-Drager syndrome, 550–551
  testing of, 441
Autopsy, 52
Avascular necrosis
  of bone, 362–363, *363*
  of lunate bone (Kienböck's disease), 400

Avoidant personality, 633
Axon, *437*
Ayurveda, 1705
Azatadine, *1065*
Azathioprine
  in autoimmune hepatitis, 806
  in Crohn's disease, 740, *741*
  in rheumatoid arthritis, *372*, 374–375
  in transplantation, *1078*
  in ulcerative colitis, 744
Azelaic acid, *1207*
Azelastine, 1066
Azithromycin, *1123*
Azoospermia, 1415, 1416
Azotemia, 824
Aztreonam, *1123*

B

Babesiosis, 1137
Babinski's sign, 441
Baby blues, 1479–1480
Bacille Calmette-Guérin (BCG)
  in bladder cancer, 878
  in tuberculosis prevention, 1130
Bacilli, *1096*
Bacitracin, *1123*
Back pain, 568–574, *571*
  in ankylosing spondylitis, 377
  in disk disease, 569, *570, 571*, 574
  in esophageal disorders, 706
  in kidney disorders, 823
  during pregnancy, 1441
  prevention of, 572, *573*
  in spinal cord circulation interruption,
    567
  in splenic enlargement, 1028
  with swallowing, 701
  in transverse myelitis, 567
  in vertebral fracture, 344–345
  with weight lifting, 569
Bacteremia, 1118–1119
  in *Campylobacter* infection, 1099
  in children, 1561
  in epiglottitis, 1564
  in gonorrhea, 1179
  staphylococcal, 1112
Bacteria, *1087*, 1095–1097 (*see also* Bacterial
    infections)
  aerobic, 1096
  anaerobic, 1096–1097, *1097*
  antibiotic resistance of, 78, 1112,
    1121
  gram-negative, 1095–1096
  gram-positive, 1096
  intestinal, 698
  shapes of, 1095, *1096*

Bacterial infections, *1087,* 1095–1118,
*1102–1103 (see also specific infections
and organisms)*
   bacillary, *1096,* 1098, 1099–1100, 1104,
     1110, 1117–1118
   coccal, *1096,* 1108–1109, 1111–1112
   in infants and children, 1561–1568
   lung (*see* Pneumonia)
   meninges, 529–531, 1562–1563
   skin, 1220–1224
   spirochetal, *1096,* 1099, 1104–1105,
     1176–1179
Bad breath (halitosis), *684*
Bagassosis, *309*
Baker's cyst, 419
Baking soda (sodium bicarbonate)
   as antacid, 99
   in renal tubular acidosis, 850
Balance
   disorders of, 461–467, 1259–1260
   testing of, 462
   vestibular system and, 1244, *1245*
Balanitis, 376, 1324
Balanoposthitis, 1324
Baldness, 1212–1214
   information resources on, 1758
Balloon catheterization
   in coronary angioplasty, 208–209, *208*
     in infants, 1514
   in renal artery angioplasty, 846
   in valvuloplasty, 180, 182
     in infants, 1514
Balloon septostomy, 1514
Balsalazide
   in Crohn's disease, 740, *741*
   in ulcerative colitis, 743
Bandage
   after surgery, 1703
   Barton's, 691, *691*
   hydrocolloid, 1190
Barbiturates
   abuse of, 653–654
     in adolescents, 1559–1560
   in elderly persons, *81*
   side effects of, 63
   in sleep disorders, *471*
   warfarin interaction with, 76
Barium studies, 703–704, *1728*
   in achalasia, 709
   in Crohn's disease, 740
   in diverticulitis, 748
   in esophageal cancer, 766
   in esophageal spasm, 708
   in gastroesophageal reflux, 718, 1589
   in intestinal malrotation, 1522
   in intussusception, 1589
   in peptic ulcers, 715
Baroreceptors, 142
Barotrauma, 1256–1257, *1257,* 1667–1668

Barr body, 11
Barrett's esophagus, 717, 719
   cancer and, 765
Barrier(s)
   body surface, 5, 7
   natural, against infection, 7, 1050,
     1087–1088
Barrier contraceptives, 1423–1424,
   1424
Bartholinitis, *1375*
Bartholin's cyst, *1375*
Bartholin's glands, 1343
Bartonella infection, *1102*
Barton's bandage, 691, *691*
Bartter's syndrome, 853–854, 910
Basal cell carcinoma, 1238, *1239*
   ear, 1255
   eyelid, 1295
   vulva, 1408
Basal ganglia, 434
   disorders of, 546–556, *549*
Basiliximab, *1079*
Basophils, 978, *1052,* 1054
   disorders of, 1006
Battle's sign, 516
BCG (bacille Calmette-Guérin)
   in bladder cancer, 878
   in tuberculosis prevention, 1130
Beard
   ingrown hairs of, 1214, 1224
   ringworm of, 1226
Becker muscular dystrophy, 412–413
Bedbug bites, 1685
Bedsores (*see* Pressure sores)
Bed-wetting (enuresis), 824, 1545
Beef tapeworm, 1143–1144, *1143*
Bee stings, 1685
Behavior
   in adolescents, 1553–1554
     problems in, 1558–1559
   in autism, 1630–1631
   bullying, *1642*
   in children, 1540–1542, 1543
     mental retardation and, 1627, 1628
     problems in, 1543–1544, *1544, 1548,*
     1549, 1550
   in conduct disorder, 1635–1636
   development of (*see under* Development)
   in oppositional defiant disorder, 1636
Behavior therapy, 601 (*see also* Cognitive-
     behavior therapy)
   in attention deficit/hyperactivity disorder,
     1550
   in erectile dysfunction, 1339
   in personality disorders, 635
   in premature ejaculation, *1339,* 1340
Behçet's syndrome, 390–391
   mouth sores in, 670
Bejel, 1099

Belching, 701, 758
  during pregnancy, 1440
Belladonna alkaloids, 81
Bell's palsy, 591–593
Bence Jones protein, 1007
Bends (decompression sickness), 1669–1671,
    1669, 1670
Benign intracranial hypertension, 523
  papilledema and, 1315
Benign paroxysmal positional vertigo,
    465–467, 466
Benign prostatic hyperplasia (BPH), 20,
    1329–1331
Benzodiazepines
  abuse of, 653–654
  in anxiety, 607, 607
  in elderly persons, 81
  food interactions with, 77
  in mania, 620
  in panic attacks and panic disorder,
    609
  in sleep disorders, 471
Benzonatate, 249, 1158
Benzoyl peroxide, 1207
Benzphetamine, 919
Benztropine, 549, 550
Bereavement, 613
  information resources on, 1761
Beriberi, 896
Beryllium disease (berylliosis), 297,
    298–299
Beta-agonists
  in asthma, 277, 278, 279–280, 279
  in COPD, 283
Beta-blockers, 70, 72
  in acute intermittent porphyria, 935
  after heart attack, 215
  in arrhythmias, 166
  in coronary artery disease, 205, 206
  in glaucoma, 1308
  in heart failure, 156, 157
  in high blood pressure, 138, 139
  in hyperthyroidism, 951, 952
  in hypertrophic cardiomyopathy, 162
  in long QT syndrome, 1530
  in Parkinson's disease, 549
  in pheochromocytoma, 961
Beta-carotene, 891
  in porphyria, 936
Beta-human chorionic gonadotropin (b-HCG),
  as tumor marker, 1039
Beta-interferon, 559
Betamethasone, 1471
Beta$_2$-microglobulin, 1039
  in multiple myeloma, 1008
Beta-thalassemia, 994
Beverly Hills Diet, 887
Bezoars, 727–729, 751
Bicalutamide, 1045, 1334

Bicarbonate (blood), 1725
  deficiency of, acidosis in, 931–932
  excess of, alkalosis in, 932–933
Bicycle riding, 35
Biguanides, 968–969, 968
Bile, 697, 786–788
  age-associated changes in, 788
  drug excretion in, 69
  obstructed flow of (cholestasis), 792–793
    in hepatitis, 802
Bile acids and salts, 786–788
  drug binding of, cholesterol reduction with,
    925
  in gallstone treatment, 815
Bile ducts (biliary tract), 695, 697
  atresia of, 1522
  biology of, 786–788, 787
  cancer of, 800, 801, 811–812, 817
  cirrhosis of, 799–800
    in children, 1522
  inflammation of, 799–800
    in ulcerative colitis, 743
  ischemia of, 807
  obstruction of, 791, 792, 807
    by cancer, 817
    in pancreatic cancer, 774
    by stone, 813–814, 816
  primary sclerosing cholangitis of, 800–801
  replacement of, 1522
  stones in (choledocholithiasis), 813–815
  tests for, 788–791, 790
Bilharziasis (schistosomiasis), 1142–1143
Biliary tract (see Bile ducts)
Bilirubin, 697, 791
  in jaundice (see Jaundice)
  in newborns, 1505–1507, 1506
  reference range for, 1725
  in Rh incompatibility, 1453
Bilirubin blanket, 1506
Bimatoprost, 1308
Binge eating disorder, 627
Bingeing, in bulimia nervosa, 626
Bioelectric impedance analysis, 881
Bioelectromagnetic-based therapies, 1707
Biofeedback, 1706
  in anal sphincter training, 758
  in temporomandibular joint disorders,
    689
Biological warfare, 1089
Biologic response modifiers, 1045, 1046
  in breast cancer, 1398
Biopsy, 343, 1699, 1724, 1728
  bone, 359
  bone marrow, 981–982, 982
  brain, 524, 540
  breast, 1393
  in cancer staging, 1041
  cervix, 1354, 1407
  digestive tract, 703

Biopsy *(continued)*
  endometrium, 1354, 1403, 1416
  heart, 192
  in Hodgkin's disease, 1018
  intestine, 734
  kidney, 828, 832, 839, 847
  liver, 790–791, 805, 809, 811, 812
  lung, 256, 257, 258, 302, 303
  lymph node, in breast cancer, 1396, *1398*
  pancreas, 774
  pericardium, 191
  pleura, 256, 298, 315
  prostate gland, 1331–1332
  scalp, 1213
  skin, 1188
  spinal cord, 526
  temporal artery, *389*
  thyroid gland, 955
  vagina, 1354
  vulva, 1354, 1408
Biotin, *893*
Bipolar disorder (manic-depressive illness),
    620–621
  in children, 1633–1634
Bird fancier's lung, *309*
Birth *(see* Labor and delivery)
Birth canal *(see* Vagina)
Birth control *(see* Contraception and
    contraceptives)
Birth defects, 1511–1526, *1512 (see also*
    Genetics, disorders of)
  anencephaly, 1430, *1432,* 1526
  anticonvulsants and, 1447
  bladder, 1567
  brain, *1512,* 1525–1526
  causes of, 1511–1512
  chromosomal *(see* Chromosome[s],
      abnormalities of)
  digestive system, *1512,* 1520–1521, *1521*
  drugs and, 1449–1450, *1460–1461*
  etretinate and, 1458–1459
  eye, *1512*
  fetal alcohol syndrome, 1463
  genital, *1512,* 1519–1520
  heart, *1512,* 1513–1518, *1515, 1516, 1517*
  infections and, 1450
  information resources on, 1758
  intersex, 1519–1520
  maternal diabetes and, 1447–1448
  maternal infection and, 1511–1512
  maternal rubella and, 1450
  maternal smoking and, 1462–1463
  musculoskeletal system, *1512,* 1523–1524,
      1523, 1524
  neural tube, 1430, *1432, 1525,* 1526
  nutrition and, 1511
  parental response to, 1638
  prenatal testing for, 1512
  spina bifida, 1430, *1432, 1525,* 1526

Birth defects *(continued)*
  spinal, 1525–1526, *1525*
  syphilis and, 1447
  teratogens and, 1511
  testing for, 1445
  thalidomide and, 1458, 1523–1524
  urinary tract, 1518–1519, 1567
  Wilms' tumor and, 1622
Birthing center, 1464
Birthmarks, 1235, *1496*
Bisacodyl, 752–753, *753*
Bisexuality, 628
Bismuth subsalicylate
  in diarrhea, *756*
  in peptic ulcer, *718*
  poisoning with, 1677
Bisphosphonates
  in multiple myeloma, 1008
  in osteogenesis imperfecta, 1610
  in osteoporosis, 345, 346, 1359, *1360*
  in Paget's disease of bone, 347–348
Bites and stings, 1681–1687
  anaphylactic reactions to, 1072–1073
  animal, 1682
  ant, 1685
  bee, 1685
  centipede, 1686
  disease transmission in
    arbovirus infection, 537–538, 1167
    babesiosis, 1137
    dengue fever, 1167
    ehrlichioses, 1134–1135
    Lyme disease, 1105–1107, *1107*
    malaria, 1140–1142
    rabies, 535–537, *536*
    rat-bite fever, *1103*
    relapsing fever, *1103*
    rickettsial infections, 1132–1134, *1133*
    tularemia, 1116–1117
    yellow fever, 1167
  hornet, 1685
  human, 402, 1682
  insect, 1685
  lizard, 1683–1684
  marine animal, 1686–1687
  millipede, 1686
  mite, 1685–1686
  scorpion, 1686
  snake, 1682–1683
  spider, 1684–1685
  tick, 1685–1686, *1686*
  wasp, 1685
Bitot's spots, 891
Black cohash, 1361
Black eye, 1290
Blackheads, 1205, *1205*
Black lung, 296, *297*
Blackwater fever, 1140
Black widow spider bite, 1684–1685

Bladder, *1345*
  age-associated changes in, *18*, 823, 857
  biology of, *821, 822*
  birth defects of, 1519, 1567
  cancer of, 877–878
  cystoscopy of, 828
  diverticula of, 1519
  fistula of
    in cystitis, 868, 869
    in diverticulitis, 748–749, *749*
  imaging of, 826–828, *827*
  incontinence of (*see* Incontinence, urinary)
  infection of, 868–871, *870*
    after childbirth, 1479
    in children, 1567–1568
  in infection prevention, 1088
  inflammation of, 869, *869*
  injury to, 874
  neurogenic, 858, *860*
  overactive, 858, *860*
  pain in, 823
  pressure in, 861
  prolapse of, 1348, 1379–1381
  removal of, 878
  schistosomiasis of, 867
  stones in, 864–866
  tumors of, 877–878
  underactive, *860*
  x-ray of, *827*
Blast crisis, 1015, 1016
Blastocyst, 1435–1436, *1436*
  transfer of, 1419
Blastomycosis
  North American, 1149–1150
  pneumonia and, 271
  South American, 1153
Bleaching
  of skin, 1215
  of teeth, *677*
Bleeding, 117 (*see also* Blood)
  after labor and delivery, 1474
  after liver biopsy, 791
  after oral surgery, 692
  in allergic purpura, 996–997
  alveolar, *307*
  in anemia, 987–989, *988*
  anus, 776–778, *777*
  aspirin and, 453
  blood pressure response to, 142–143
  brain, 510–512, *511*, 517–519
    coma with, *492*
    in premature infant, 1496
  in cancer, 1035–1036
  in colorectal cancer, 770
  conjunctiva, 1280–1281
  from cut, 1692
  digestive system, 699–700, 705, 776–778, 777
  disorders of (*see* Clotting, disorders of)

Bleeding *(continued)*
  in disseminated intravascular coagulation, 1001
  in diverticulosis, 747
  drugs and, 777
  in Ehlers-Danlos syndrome, 1608
  epidural, *511*, 518
  from esophageal varices, 794, 808, 809
  in esophagitis, 717
  esophagus, 776–778, *777*
  in eye, 1290, *1673*
  with fracture, 348–349
  in hemolytic-uremic syndrome, 998
  in hemophilia, 999–1000
  of hemorrhoids, 760
  in hereditary hemorrhagic telangiectasia (Rendu-Osler-Weber disease), 996
  internal, 1691
  iron deficiency with, 907–908
  large intestine, 776–778, *777*
  in Mallory-Weiss syndrome, 710
  menstrual, 1345, 1346–1348, *1347*
    disorders of, 1361–1366, *1362, 1363, 1365, 1366*
  in nephrotic syndrome, 840–841
  in newborn, 1449, 1485, 1494
  nose, 1263
  in peptic ulcers, *715*
  in polycythemia vera, 1023
  postmenopausal, *1362*
  during pregnancy, 1451, 1455, 1456, 1457
  in pseudoxanthoma elasticum, 1609
  rectum, 776–778, *777*
    in Meckel's diverticulum, 1590
  retina, at high altitudes, *1673*
  shock in, 148
  small intestine, 776–778, *777*
  stomach, 776–778, *777*
    drug-related, *83*
  in stress gastritis, 712, 713
  subarachnoid, 511–512, *511*
  subdural, *511*, 518
  in thrombocytopenia, 997–999
  in ulcerative colitis, 742
  uterine (*see also* Menstrual cycle)
    dysfunctional, 1367
  vaginal, 1350, 1366–1367, 1403, 1408–1409
  in vitamin C deficiency, 900
  in vitamin K deficiency, 895
  in Von Willebrand's disease, 999
  in Wiskott-Aldrich syndrome, 1062
Bleeding time, 981
Blepharitis (eyelid inflammation), 1294
Blepharospasm, 554
Blindness, 1279, *1280* (*see also* Vision, loss of)
  cataract and, 1303–1305, *1304*
  color, 1280, *1281*, 1283
  information resources on, 1758–1759
  in Leber's hereditary optic neuropathy, 560

Blindness *(continued)*
  night, 891, 1280
  rehabilitation for, 45
  in retinitis pigmentosa, 1312
  snow, *1673*
  trachoma and, 1297–1298
  in vitamin A deficiency, 891
Blind spot, 1283
Blisters, *1189*, 1216–1218
  in bullous pemphigoid, 1217
  in cellulitis, 1221
  in contact dermatitis, 1194
  in dermatitis herpetiformis, 1217–1218
  in erythema multiforme, 1200
  in frostbite, 1656
  genital
    in chancroid, 1181–1182
    in lymphogranuloma venereum, 1181
  in herpes simplex virus infection, 668–669,
      1161
  in impetigo, 1222
  in necrotizing skin infection, 1222
  in nummular dermatitis, 1196
  in pemphigus, 1216–1217
  in pompholyx, 1198
  in porphyria cutanea tarda, 934
  in shingles, 1163
  in Stevens-Johnson syndrome, 1199–1200
  in toxic epidermal necrolysis, 1199–1200
  in tularemia, 1116
Bloating, 701, 758
Blood, 6 *(see also* Bleeding)
  acidity of, 930–932, *930, 932*
    reference range for, *1725*
  age-associated changes in, *19*
  alcohol level in, *1725*
  alkalinity of, 930–931, *930,* 932–933, *932*
  anemia and *(see* Anemia[s])
  bacteria in *(see also* Bacteremia; Sepsis)
  biology of, 978–979
  cancer of *(see* Leukemia; Lymphoma)
  cells of *(see also* Red blood cells; White
      blood cells)
  components of, 978–979
  coughing up of, 252–253, *307*
  dialysis of *(see* Dialysis)
  disorders of, 987–1029 *(see also specific
      disorders, eg,* Anemia[s]; Bleeding;
      Leukemia)
    diagnosis of, 980–982
    information resources on, 1759
    symptoms of, 979–890
  glucose levels of *(see* Sugar[s], blood)
  hyperviscosity of, in macroglobulinemia,
      1009
  liver processing of, 697
  occult, *29,* 705, 770, *1038, 1041, 1730*
  in phlegm, 252–253, *307*

Blood *(continued)*
  in pleural space (hemothorax), 314, 316
  purification of (hemapheresis), *986*
  radiation effects on, 1659
  red cell deficiency of *(see* Anemia[s])
  Rh factor in, 1427, 1433, 1442, 1453, 1477
  in sputum, 252–253, *307*
  stem cells from, 1081–1083 *(see also* Stem
      cells)
  in stool, 699, 705, 754, *1038,* 1041
  testing of, 980–981, *981, 983, 984,*
      1725–1727, 1728
    from fetus, 1434, *1467*
    in pregnancy, 1435
  transfusion of *(see* Blood transfusion)
  typing of, 981, *984*
  umbilical cord, sampling from, 1434
  in urine (hematuria), 825, 826, 875–876, 877
  volume of, 912, 981, *1725*
    overhydration and, 929
    during pregnancy, 1439
  in vomit, 699, 702, 705
Blood-brain barrier, 433–434
Blood clots *(see also* Embolism)
  after childbirth, 1479
  after heart attack, *212*
  after surgery, 1703
  in aneurysm, 226
  in atherosclerosis, 195
  in Budd-Chiari syndrome, 808–809
  of deep veins, 232–236, *235*
  in disseminated intravascular coagulation,
      1001
  formation of
    drug effects on, *996*
    in hemostasis, 995–996, *995*
  in frostbite, 1656
  in heart attack, 211, 214
  in mountain sickness, *1673*
  in nephrotic syndrome (kidney disease), 840
  oral contraceptives and, 1421
  in peripheral arterial disease, 216
  portal vein, 809
  in pregnancy, 1450–1451
  prevention of, 287–288 *(see also*
      Anticoagulants)
  pulmonary artery *(see* Pulmonary
      embolism)
  renal artery, 844–846
  renal vein, 848–849
  risks for, *287*
  in skin infection, 1221
  of superficial veins (thrombophlebitis), 232,
      236
  in thrombophilia, 1000–1001
  travel and, 1710
Blood flow *(see* Circulation)
Blood flukes, 540

Blood gas analysis, 255
Bloodletting (phlebotomy)
  in hemochromatosis, *909*
  in polycythemia vera, 1024
  in porphyria cutanea tarda, 934
Blood pressure
  age-associated changes in, 117–118, 131, *132*
  classification of, *137*
  control of, 131–132, *133*, 141–143, 822
  high (*see* High blood pressure)
  low (*see* Low blood pressure)
  measurement of, 124, 131, 134–136, *135*,
    1728
  in peripheral arterial disease, 218
  during pregnancy, 1439
  in preventive care, *29*
  stress effects on, 134
  24–hour monitoring of, 136
  variations in, *132*
Blood test (*see* Blood, testing of)
Blood thinners (*see* Anticoagulants)
Blood transfusion, 982–986
  adverse reactions to, 986
  autologous, 985, 1701
  directed donation for, 985
  donation process for, 983–984, *983, 984, 986*
  graft-versus-host reaction in, 986
  in hemophilia, 1000
  HIV transmission with, 1169
  in hyperbilirubinemia, 1506–1507
  in kidney failure, 833
  leukocyte reduction in, 986
  in newborn anemia, 1507
  precautions for, 985
  in Rh incompatibility, 1453
  types of, 984–985
Blood urea nitrogen (BUN), 826, *1727*
Blood vessels, 117 (*see also* Artery [arteries];
    Vein[s])
  age-associated changes in, 117–118
  aneurysm of, 119, 226–229, *227*, 492, 511,
    512 (*see also* Aneurysm)
  atherosclerosis of (*see* Atherosclerosis)
  cerebral, 433, *503*
  collateral, 794
    in portal vein thrombosis, 809
  disorders of, 118–130 (*see also specific*
    disorders, eg, High blood pressure)
  dissection of, 119, 229–231, *230*
  eye, 1277, 1310, *1310*, 1312
  fistula of, 238–239
  inflammation of (vasculitis), 371, 386–391,
    387, 389
  kidney, 820–822, 844–849, *845*
  liver, 786, 787, 806–810, *807*
  phlebitis of, 232, 236
  in pseudoxanthoma elasticum, 1609
  skin, 1187, *1187*, 1235–1236

Blood vessels (*continued*)
  spinal, blockage of, 567–568
  thrombosis of, 232–236 (*see also* Blood
    clots)
  varicose (*see* Varicose veins)
Bloody show, 1465
B lymphocytes, 978, 1050, 1054–1055
  in ataxia-telangiectasia, 1061
  high levels of (leukocytosis), 1004–1005
  leukemia of, 1014–1015
  low levels of (lymphocytopenia), 1004
  in phagocytosis, *1056*
  in X-linked agammaglobulinemia, 1059
Body (*see* Human body)
Body dysmorphic disorder, 604–605
  in children, 1637
Body mass index, *881*, 914–915, *916–917*
Boils, 1112, 1224
  of ear, 1253–1255
  of nose, 1263–1264
Bonding (dental), *677*
Bonding, with newborn, 1485, *1495*, 1520
Bone(s)
  age-associated changes in, 338
  avascular necrosis of, 362–363, *363*, 400
    in decompression sickness, 1670
  biology of, 334–335, *336, 337*
  density of
    evaluation of, 342, 345
    increase in, 1611
    in osteoporosis, 343–346, *344, 345*, 1357
  disorders of, 343–365
    in children, 1603–1607, *1604, 1605, 1606*
    diagnosis of, 341–343
    in kidney failure, 832
  of ear, 1244, *1245*
  examination of, 341
  exercise effects on, 31
  fluoride accumulation in, 906
  fracture of (*see* Fracture)
  fragility of, in osteogenesis imperfecta,
    1610–1611
  grafts of, 353
    in avascular necrosis, 363
  healing of, *349*, 353
  infection of (osteomyelitis), 364–365
  kidney effects on, 822
  metastatic tumors of, 361
  in nail-patella syndrome, 856
  in osteoporosis, 20, 343–346, *344, 345*, 1357
  Paget's disease of, 346–348
  pain in, 339
    in children, 1603
    in sickle cell disease, 993
  remodeling of, 335, 343, *349*, 1603
  transplantation of, 1083
  tumors of, 359–361
  in vitamin D–resistant rickets, 852–853

Bone marrow, 335, 1050, *1053*
 age-associated changes in, 979
 aspiration of, *1728*
 biopsy of (*see* Bone marrow, examination of)
 blood cell formation in, 979
 cancer of (*see* Leukemia)
 examination of, 981–982, *982, 1728*
  in iron deficiency, 907–908
  in macroglobulinemia, 1010
  in multiple myeloma, 1008
  in neutropenia, 1003
 failure of, *991*
  in fetus, 1507
 fibrosis of, *1023*, 1025–1026
 radiation effects on, 1659
 transplantation of, 1081–1083
  in myelofibrosis, 1026
  in osteopetroses, 1611
  radiation therapy before, 1077
  in sickle cell disease, 994
Borborygmi (intestinal sounds), 700, 702, 780
Borderline personality, 633
Borrelia infection
 Lyme disease, 1105–1107, *1107*
 relapsing fever, *1103*
Bosentan, 324
Bottle-feeding, 1488
Botulin
 in achalasia, 709
 in dystonia, 555
 in facial spasms, 593
 in spasmodic torticollis, 555–556
 in Tourette's syndrome, 552
Botulism, 579–581, 1489
Bouchard's nodules, 368, 397
Boutonnière deformity, *396*, 397
Bowel (*see* Large intestine; Small intestine)
Bowel movements, 698
 in colorectal cancer, 770
 disorders of, 750–759, *753, 755, 756* (*see also* Constipation; Diarrhea)
  in infants and young children, 1533–1534, 1545–1546
 hygiene for, 1568
 incontinence of, 757–758
  in dying person, 49
 in infant, 1489
 in newborn, 1486
 toilet teaching for, *1540*
Bowel sounds (borborygmi), 700, 702, 780
Bowen's disease, 1239, 1325
Bowlegs, *1606*
Bowman's capsule, 820, *821*
BPH (benign prostatic hyperplasia), *20*, 1329–1331
Braces (orthodontic therapy), 662, 681
Brachial neuritis, 582
Brachial plexus, 581–582, *581*
Brachytherapy, 1334

Bradyarrhythmias, 164
Bradycardia, 163, 174
 in apnea of prematurity, 1503
Bradycardia-tachycardia syndrome, 174
Brain
 abscess of, 539–540
  with ear infection, 1594
  headache with, *459*
  in meningitis, 1562
 age-associated changes in, *18*, 438
 in Alzheimer's disease, 487–488
 anencephaly of, 1430, *1432*
 aneurysm of, 511, 512
 biology of, 433–435, *435*
 biopsy of, 524, 540
 birth defects of, 1430, *1432, 1512,* 1525–1526
 bleeding in/around, 510–512, *511,* 517–519
 bruise of, 517
 cancer of, 519–526, *520–521, 522, 525, 528*
  headache with, *458, 521*
 circulation of, 433, 438, *503*
  testing of, 441–442
 cysts of, 540
 damage to (*see* Brain, injury to)
 death of, 494
 in dementia, 484–490 (*see also* Dementia)
 demyelination of, 557–560
 development of, 1491
 diagnostic tests for, 442–446, *443*
 digestive system and, 694
 dysfunction of, 475–480, *476, 477*
  in cancer, 1036–1037, *1036*
  coma with, *492*
  in dehydration, 928–929
  in hyperbilirubinemia, 1505
  in hypercalcemia, 905
  in hypernatremia, 914
  in hypocalcemia, 903
  in hypoglycemia, 971
  in hyponatremia, 913
  in overhydration, 929
  in vitamin B_1 deficiency, 896
 electrical injury to, 1662–1663
 hemorrhage in, 510–512, *511, 515,* 517–519
  in premature infant, 1496
 herniation of, 510, 513, *515,* 523
 imaging of, 443–445
 infection of, 529–540, *533*
  childhood disintegrative disorder and, 1632
  fungal, 1153
  seizures with, *496*
 inflammation of (*see* Encephalitis; Encephalopathy)
 injury to, 513–519, *514, 515*
  in cerebral palsy, 1624–1626
  in children, 514, *516*
  in HIV infection, 1574
  information resources on, 1759

Brain *(continued)*
  injury to *(continued)*
    from radiation, 528
    rehabilitation after, 41
    seizures with, *496*
  laceration of, 517
  lightning effects on, 1664
  malaria effects on, 1140
  in movement, *576*
  in newborn, 1496
  prion diseases of, 541–543, *542*
  radiation effects on, 1659
  retinoblastoma spread to, 1624
  in seizures *(see* Seizures)
  in stroke *(see* Stroke)
  swelling (edema) of
    in head injury, 513, *515*
    at high altitudes, 1673
    in Reye's syndrome, *1572*
    seizures with, *496*
    in stroke, 508
  syphilis effects on, 1177
  in taste sensation, *595*
  trauma to *(see* Brain, injury to)
  tumors of, 519–526, *520–521, 522, 525,* 528
    headache with, *458, 521*
  water on *(see* Hydrocephalus)
Brain death, 494
Brain stem, 434, *435*
  nerve degeneration in, 587–588
  syrinx of, 566
Brain waves *(see* Electroencephalography)
Bran, 752, *753*
Breakbone fever, 1167
Breastfeeding, 1477–1478, 1486–1488, *1487*
  colostrum in, 1439
  discomfort with, 1476–1477
  drug use and, 85, 101–102, *1462*
  high bilirubin levels and, 1505, 1506
  HIV transmission with, 1573
  of newborn, 1484, 1485
  preparation for, 1444
Breast milk, 1486
  abnormal production of (galactorrhea),
    946–947
  absence of, 942
  production of, 1476–1477
Breasts
  abscess of, 1112, 1389
  after childbirth, 1476–1477
  age-associated changes in, 1348
  anatomy of, *1388*
  biopsy of, 1393
  cancer of, 1389–1401, *1394*
    hormone replacement therapy and,
      1358–1359
    in male, *1323*
    metastatic, 1390, *1394,* 1400, 1401
    nipple discharge in, 1387–1388
    oral contraceptives and, 1421

Breasts *(continued)*
  cancer of *(continued)*
    receptors in, 1391
    risk factors for, 1389, *1390, 1392–1393*
    screening for, *29, 1038,* 1040, *1392–1393,*
      1395
    staging of, *1040,* 1041, 1389–1390, *1394*
    treatment of, 1046, 1394–1401,
      1396–1397, *1396, 1397, 1399*
  cystosarcoma phyllodes of, 1391,
    1400–1401
  cysts of, 1388
  development of, 1346
  discharge from, 1387–1388
    during pregnancy, 1439
  disorders of, 1387–1401
  engorgement of, 1476–1477
  enlargement of (gynecomastia), *1323*
    in squamous cell carcinoma, *1037*
  examination of, *29, 1038,* 1352, 1392, *1395*
  fibroadenoma of, 1388–1389
  fibrocystic disease of, 1389
  infection of, 1389
    after childbirth, 1479
  lump(s) in, 1387, 1388–1389, 1391
  mammography of, *29, 1038,* 1040,
    1355–1356, *1355,* 1392–1393, *1730*
  milk production in, 1476–1477
  Paget's disease of, 1241, 1391, 1393, 1400
  pain in, 1351, 1387
  physician examination of, 1392
  during pregnancy, 1439
  reconstruction of, 1396–1397, *1399*
  self-examination of, *1038,* 1041, 1392, *1395*
Breath *(see also* Breathing)
  bad (halitosis), *684*
  holding of
    by children, 1547
    by scuba diver, 1668
  shortness of, 250–251
    in asbestosis, 297
    in asthma, 275–276
    in cancer, 1037
    in COPD, 282, 283
    in coronary artery disease, 119, 211
    in dilated cardiomyopathy, 160
    in heart failure, 119, 153–154
    in Hodgkin's disease, *1017*
    in hypertrophic cardiomyopathy, 161
    in mitral stenosis, 179
    in non-Hodgkin's lymphoma, *1021*
    in obesity, 917
    in pulmonary embolism, 286
    in pulmonary hypertension, 323–324
    pulmonary rehabilitation for, 259–262
    in scoliosis, 250
    in silicosis, 295
    smoke inhalation and, *1649*
    stridor with, 252
    in tuberculosis, 1127

Breathing (*see also* Breath)
  cessation of (apnea)
    in newborn, 1496
    in premature infant, 1503–1504
    in sleep, 472–474, 917
  in chest examination, 254
  control of, 246–247, *247*
  in dying person, 48–49
  emergency-related evaluation of, 1689
  in epiglottitis, 1268, 1564
  exercises for, 261–262
  for natural childbirth, *1468*
  in newborn, 1471, 1495, 1496
    problems with, 1499–1500
  periodic (Cheyne-Stokes), 154, 473, 491
  in pneumonia prevention, 266
  during pregnancy, 1440
  pursed-lip, 261–262
  in respiratory tract infection, 1579
  shortness of (*see* Breath, shortness of)
  stopping of, by children, 1547
  stridor during, 252
    in croup, 1586
    in epiglottitis, 1564
    in respiratory tract infection, 1579
  in stroke, 504
  wheezing during, 251–252, 1583–1584
Breech (buttocks-first) presentation, 1465,
    1472, *1472*, 1485
Bridges, dental, 679, *679*
Brief psychotic disorder, *642*
Bright light therapy, in insomnia, 469
Brimonidine, *1308*
Brinzolamide, *1308*
Broca's aphasia, *477*, 478
Bromhidrosis, 1210–1211
Bromocriptine
  in acromegaly, 946
  in ovulation problems, 1417
  in Parkinson's disease, *549*
  in prolactinoma, 944, 947
Brompheniramine, *1065, 1158*
Bronchi, 244–245, *245*
  in asthma (*see* Asthma)
  dilatation of (*see* Bronchiectasis)
  infection of (*see* Bronchitis)
  lung cancer origin in, 328
  obstruction of, atelectasis with, 292–294
Bronchial artery, embolization of, 252
Bronchiectasis, 289–292, *290, 291*
Bronchioles, 245, *245*
Bronchiolitis, 1579–1580, 1583, 1585–1586
  idiopathic, 303
  with interstitial lung disease, *307*
Bronchitis
  acute, 262–264, *263*
  chronic, 281–285
  at high altitudes, *1673*

Bronchoalveolar lavage, 257
Bronchodilators, 250
  in asthma, 277, *278*, 279–280, *279*
    in children, 1584
  in bronchiolitis, 1585
  in bronchitis, 264
Bronchogenic carcinoma, 328–331, *329*
Bronchopulmonary aspergillosis, 271, 311–312
Bronchopulmonary dysplasia, 1502–1503
Bronchoscopy, 256–257, *257, 1728*
  in gastroesophageal reflux, 1589
  in lung abscess, 273
  in pulmonary alveolar proteinosis, 308
Brown recluse spider bite, 1684–1685
Brown-Séquard syndrome, 528
Brucellosis, *1102*
Bruises
  in allergic purpura, 996–997
  bladder, 874
  brain, 517
  in child abuse, 1645
  first aid for, 1693
  kidney, *873*
  in leukemia, 1011
  in newborn, 1485, *1496*
  in thrombocytopenia, 998
  urethral, 875
Bruits, 121
  liver, 810, 811
Bruton's agammaglobulinemia, 1059
Bruxism (teeth grinding), 674, 686
Bubble boy syndrome, 1061–1062
Bubonic plague, 1107–1108
Budd-Chiari syndrome, 808–809
Budesonide, 740, *741*
Buerger's disease, 223–224
Bugs (*see* Insects)
Bulbar palsy, 575–577
Bulimia nervosa, 626–627
Bulking agents, 752, *753*
Bullae (*see* Blisters)
Bullous keratopathy, 1302
Bullous pemphigoid, 670, *1074*, 1217
Bullying, *1642*
BUN (blood urea nitrogen), 826, *1727*
Bundle branch block, 175
Bunion, 410–411, *411*
Buprenorphine, 653
Bupropion, 655
Burkitt's lymphoma, *1020*
Burning mouth syndrome, *665*
Burns, 1648–1651, *1648, 1650, 1651*
  chemical, 1648, *1648*, 1678–1679
  in child abuse, 1645
  electrical, 1661–1664
  eye, 1292
  infection and, 1092
  tracheal, *1649*

Burow's solution (aluminum acetate), 1194
Burping, in infants, 1486, 1532
Bursas, 335
Bursitis, 417–418
   Achilles tendon, 408–409, *408*
   metatarsal, 404
Buspirone
   in anxiety, 607, *607*
   in premenstrual syndrome, 1363
Butter, vs. margarine, *201*, 923
Bypass surgery
   in coronary artery disease, 209–210, *210*
   in peripheral artery disease, 220, *221*
Byssinosis, *297*, 300

C

CA 15–3 (carbohydrate antigen 15–3), *1039*
CA 19–9 (carbohydrate antigen 19–9), *1039*
CA-125 (carbohydrate antigen 125), *1039*
Cabergoline, 944, 947
   in ovulation problems, 1417
Cachexia, 889
Café au lait spots, 527
Caffeine
   in apnea of prematurity, 1504
   headache and, 457
   during pregnancy, 1463
Caisson disease, 1669–1671, *1669, 1670*
Calcitonin
   in calcium regulation, 901
   in medullary thyroid cancer, 955
   in osteoporosis, 346
   in Paget's disease of bone, 348
Calcitriol, 822 (*see also* Vitamin D)
Calcium, 901–905, *902*
   dietary
      during breastfeeding, 1477
      deficiency of, *735*
      in celiac disease, 736
   high blood levels of (hypercalcemia),
      904–905, *904* (*see also* Hypercalcemia)
      in vitamin D excess, 894
   in hyperkalemia, 911
   kidney regulation of, 822
   in kidney stones, 864–866
   low blood levels of (hypocalcemia), 901, 903–904
      in DiGeorge anomaly, 1061
   in osteoporosis, 346
   in osteoporosis prevention, 345
   reference range for, *1725*
Calcium carbonate
   in antacids, 99
   in kidney failure, 831
   in peptic ulcer, 716, *718*

Calcium channel blockers, 60
   in arrhythmias, *166*
   in cardiomyopathy, 162
   in coronary artery disease, 205, *206–207*
   food interactions with, 77
   gingivitis and, 682
   in high blood pressure, 139, *139*
   urinary incontinence with, *859*
Calcium gluconate, 909
Calcium polycarbophil, *753*
Calcium pyrophosphate dihydrate crystal
   deposition disease (pseudogout), 394–395
Calculi (*see* Stones)
Calculus (tartar), 674
Calendar method, in family planning, 1426
California cone sting, 1686–1687
California encephalitis, 537
Calix, 820, *821*
Calluses, 410
Caloric testing, 464
Calories, 883, *883*
   deficiency of, 887–890, *888, 889*
   exercise and, *34*
   requirements for, 883
Calorimetry, *883*
Calymmatobacterium granulomatis
   infection, 1182
Campylobacter infection, *720*, 1099–1100, 1183–1184
Cancer, 1031–1034, *1034*
   age and, 1033
   alternative medicine for, 1046
   anus, 773
   bile duct, 800, 801, 811–812, 817
   bladder, 877–878
   bleeding in, 1035–1036
   blood cell (*see* Leukemia)
   bone, 359–361
   bone marrow (*see* Leukemia)
   brain, 519–526, *520–521, 522, 525, 528*
      headache with, *458, 521*
   breast, 1389–1401 (*see also* Breasts, cancer
      of)
   carcinoid, 974–975
   cardiac, 194
   cervix, 1350, *1402*, 1406–1407, 1421 (*see
      also* Cervix, cancer of)
   chemical causes of (carcinogens),
      1031–1032, 1033, *1033*
   chemotherapy for, 1043–1044, *1045* (*see
      also* Chemotherapy)
   childhood, 1622–1624
   chronic meningitis with, 532
   colorectal, 770–773, *771*
      ulcerative colitis and, 742–743
   complications of, *1036, 1037*
   depression in, 1036
   development of, 1031–1032, *1033*

Cancer *(continued)*
  diagnosis of, 1037–1041, *1038, 1039, 1040*
  digestive system, 764–776, *765, 767, 769,*
      771, 774, 778
    carcinoid, 974–975
  drug resistance in, 78
  ear, 1255
  embolism with, 286
  endometrium, 1350, *1402,* 1403–1404, *1404*
    hormone replacement therapy and, 1358
  environmental factors in, 1033–1034
  esophagus, 764–766, *765*
  eye, 1314
  eyelid, 1295
  fallopian tube, *1402,* 1409
  family history and, 1032–1033
  fatigue in, 1036
  gastrin production and, *717*
  genes in, 14
  genetic factors and, 1032–1033
  geographic variation in, 1033
  hypercalcemia and, 904
  immune system and, 1034
  immunotherapy for, 1044–1046
  information resources on, 1759–1760
  jaw, 672–673
  kidney, 875–876
  in kidney transplant recipient, 1077
  larynx, 1271–1272, *1272*
  lip, 673
  liver, 798, 811–813
  lung, 328–331, *329* (*see also* Lungs, cancer of)
  lymphatic system (*see* Lymphoma)
  lymph nodes in, 1036, *1273*
  lymphocytic leukocytosis in, 1004
  markers of, *1039,* 1041
  metastatic (*see* Metastasis)
  in monoclonal gammopathy, 1006–1007
  mouth, 671–674
  in multiple endocrine neoplasia (*see*
      Multiple endocrine neoplasia)
  neck lump in, *1273*
  nervous system, 519–528, *520–521, 522,*
      525, 527
    in children, 1623
  neurologic symptoms of, 1036–1037
  nose, 1273
  oral color changes with, *663*
  orbit, 1319
  ovary, *1402,* 1404–1405
  pain in, 1035
  pancreas, 773–774, *774*
  paranasal sinus, 1272
  paraneoplastic syndromes in, 330, 904,
      1035, *1037*
  penis, 1325
  peritoneum, 296–297, 298
  pineal gland, *521, 522*
  pituitary gland, *521, 522,* 523, 1279

Cancer *(continued)*
  plasma cell, 1007–1009, *1009*
  pleura, 296–297, 298, 315–316
  plexus disorders with, 581–582
  during pregnancy, 1449
  prevention of, *27,* 1042, *1043*
  prostate, *20,* 1331–1332, *1333* (*see also*
      Prostate gland, cancer of)
  radiation exposure and, 125
  radiation therapy for, 1043, 1046,
      1659–1660 (*see also* Radiation therapy)
  renal pelvis, 876–877
  respiratory symptoms of, 1037
  retina, 1314
    in children, 1623–1624
  risk factors for, 1032–1034, *1034*
  salivary gland, 667, 672–673
  screening for, 1037–1041, *1038* (*see also*
      Screening tests, for cancer)
  skin, 1230, *1231,* 1238–1241, *1239, 1240,*
      1325 (*see also* Skin, cancer of)
  small intestine, 768, *769*
  spinal cord, 526, *527*
  spread of, 1032
  staging of, *1040,* 1041
  stomach, 766–768, *767*
    ulcers and, 714
  surgery for, 1042–1043, 1046
  symptoms of, 1035–1037
  terminology for, *1032*
  testis, 1326
  tests for, 1037–1041, *1038, 1039*
  throat, 1273
  thymus gland, 578, *579*
  thyroid gland, 949, 954–955
    radiation accident and, 906
  tongue, 665, 672
  tonsils, 1273
  treatment of, 1042–1047, *1044, 1045* (*see*
      also Chemotherapy; Immunotherapy;
      Radiation therapy)
    side effects of, 1046–1047
  types of, 1032
  ureter, 876–877
  urethra, 878
  urinary tract, 875–878
  uterus, 1350, 1358, *1402,* 1403–1404, *1404*
      (*see also* Uterus, cancer of)
  vagina, 1350, *1402,* 1408–1409
  viral infection and, *1155*
  vocal cord, *1269*
  vulva, *1402,* 1407–1408
  warning signs of, 1035, *1035, 1240*
  weight loss in, 1036
Candidiasis, 1150–1151
  in diaper rash, 1534–1535
  genital, 1227, 1350, 1374, *1376,* 1377
  in HIV infection, *1172*
  mucocutaneous, chronic, 1060–1061

Candidiasis *(continued)*
  oral (thrush), 666, 682, 1057, 1227
  skin, 1226–1227
  urinary tract, 867
Cane, *42*
Canker sores, 668, 1161
Cannabis (marijuana), 655–656
  adolescent use of, 1559–1560
  in HIV infection, 1174
Capacity, 53–54
Capillaries, 117
  alveolar, 245, *246*
  of blood-brain barrier, 433–434
  enlargement of (spider veins), 236–237, 238,
    1236
    in ataxia-telangiectasia, 1061
  malformation of (port-wine stain), 1236
  in newborn, *1496*
  of skin, *1187*
Caplan's syndrome, 296
Capsaicin cream, 455
Carbachol, *1308*
Carbamate poisoning, 1679–1680
Carbamazepine
  in central diabetes insipidus, 945
  in manic-depressive illness, 621
  during pregnancy, *1460*
  in seizure disorders, *500*
Carbapenems, *1122*
Carbecephem, *1122*
Carbenicillin, *1123*
Carbidopa, 548
Carbimazole, *951*, 952
Carbohydrate antigen 15–3 (CA 15-3), *1039*
Carbohydrate antigen 19–9 (CA 19-9), *1039*
Carbohydrate antigen 125 (CA-125), *1039*
Carbohydrates, 881
  diet-related restriction of, 886
  hypoglycemic reaction to, 971
  metabolism of (see also Diabetes mellitus;
    Hyperglycemia; Hypoglycemia)
  hereditary disorders of, 1616–1618
Carbon dioxide
  in acid-base regulation, 930
  blood transport of, 978
  in diver, *1669*
  in lungs, 245–246, *246*
  measurement of, in blood, 255, *1725*
  pressure, *1725*
  in sick building syndrome, 1720
Carbonic anhydrase inhibitors, *1308*
Carbon monoxide
  diffusing capacity test for, 255
  in hemoglobin, *1725*
  poisoning with, *492*, 1677–1678
Carboplatin, *1045*
Carboxyhemoglobin, *1725*
Carbuncles (skin abscesses), 1112, *1205*, 1206,
  1220, 1224

Carcinoembryonic antigen (CEA), 771, *1039*
Carcinogens, 1031–1032, 1033, *1033*
Carcinoid tumor and carcinoid syndrome,
    974–975
  in lung cancer, *1037*
  of small intestine, *769*
Carcinoma, 1032 (see also Cancer)
  alveolar cell, 328
  basal cell, 1238, *1239*, 1255
  bronchogenic, 328–331, *329*
  fibrolamellar, 811
  hepatocellular (hepatoma), 798, 811
  renal cell, 875–876
  squamous cell (see Squamous cell
    carcinoma)
  transitional cell, of renal pelvis, 876–877
Cardiac arrest, 173, 1688–1690, *1689*
  coma with, *492, 494*
Cardiac asthma, 154
Cardiac catheterization, 128–129
  in angioplasty, 208–209, *208*
  in congenital heart defects, 1514
  in dilated cardiomyopathy, 160
  in pericarditis, 191
Cardiac tamponade, *189*
  in cancer, *1036*
Cardialgia (see Indigestion)
Cardiomyopathy, 144, 158–163, *159*
  peripartum, 1454
  in selenium deficiency, 912
  sexual activity and, *1337*
Cardiopulmonary resuscitation (CPR), 56,
    1689–1690
  in electrical injury, 1663
  in hypothermia, 1655–1656
  in lightning injury, 1664
  in near drowning, 1666
  order against, 48, 57
Cardiospasm, 709
Cardiovascular system, 4, 6 (see also Blood
    vessels; Heart)
Cardioversion, 124, 167
Caries, 675–679, *676, 678, 679,* 906
Carotenoids, 891
Carotid arteries
  aneurysm of, 229
  in ischemic stroke, 507
  in transient ischemic attack, 506–507
Carotid sinus stimulation, 145
Carpal tunnel syndrome, 398–399, *399*
Carrier screening, 1429–1430
Carrots, excess ingestion of, 792
Car sickness (see Motion sickness)
Cartilage, 337
  in chondrodysplasias, 1611
  in osteoarthritis, *20*
  in relapsing polychondritis, 385
  transplantation of, 1083
Cascara, 752–753, *753*

Case-control study, 1696
Caspofungin, *1152*
Cast, 351–352, *352*
  pressure sores with, 353
Castor oil, 752–753, *753*
Cataplexy, 471
Cataract, *20*, 1303–1305, *1304*
  congenital, *1512*
  in electrical injury, 1662
  in galactosemia, 1617
Catatonia, in schizophrenia, 641, 642
Cat bite, 1682
Catecholamines, 960–961
Catheter(ization)
  for antibiotic administration, 1121, 1124
  cardiac, 128–129, *1728*
    in angioplasty, 208–209, *208*
    in congenital heart defects, 1514
    in dilated cardiomyopathy, 160
    in pericarditis, 191
  central venous, 130
  in hemodialysis, 834
  infection of, 1111
  in liver biopsy, 791
  in peritoneal dialysis, 834
  in poisoning, 1676
  pulmonary artery, 129–130, 252
  for tube feeding, 890
  urinary
    in bladder injury, 874
    in hydronephrosis, 863
    in overflow incontinence, *860*, 862
    for sample collection, 861, 1567–1568
CAT scan (*see* Computed tomography)
Cat-scratch disease, *1102*
Cat's cry syndrome, *1529*
Cauda equina, *436*
Cauda equina syndrome, *565*
Cauliflower ear, 1255
Causalgia, 449
Caustic burns, 1648–1651, *1648*, 1678–1679
Cavernous hemangioma, 1235
Cavernous sinus thrombosis, *1318*
Cavities, 675–679, *676*, *678*, *679*
  fluoride and, 906
CBC (complete blood count), 980–981, *981*,
    1725
  in acute lymphocytic leukemia, 1011
C-(cesarean) section, 1475–1476
CD4 lymphocytes, *1725*
  in HIV infection, 1169–1170, 1172, 1174
CEA (carcinoembryonic antigen), 771, *1039*
Cecum, 697–698
Cefaclor, *1122*
Cefadroxil, *1122*
Cefamandole, *1122*
Cefazolin, *1122*
Cefdinir, *1122*
Cefditoren, *1122*

Cefepime, *1122*
Cefixime, *1122*
Cefmetazole, *1122*
Cefonicid, *1122*
Cefoperazone, *1122*
Cefotazime, *1122*
Cefotetan, *1122*
Cefoxitin, *1122*
Cefpodoxime, *1122*
Cefprozil, *1122*
Ceftazidime, *1122*
Ceftibuten, *1122*
Ceftizoxime, *1122*
Ceftriaxone, *1122*
Cefurozime, *1122*
Celiac disease, 736–737
  in dermatitis herpetiformis, 1217–1218
Cell(s), 2, *4*, *1052*
  blood (*see also* Blood, cells of; Red blood
      cells; White blood cells)
  Langerhans', 1186
  membrane of, 2
  receptors of, 2, 70–72, *70*, *71–72*, *73*
  Reed-Sternberg, 1018
  stem (*see* Stem cells)
  types of, 2, *4*
Cellophane maculopathy, 1311
Cellulase, for foreign objects, 729
Cellulitis, 1220–1221
  necrotizing, 1221–1222
  oral, 680
  orbital, 1318
  staphylococcal, 1112
  streptococcal, 1113
  tonsillar, 1267–1268
Cementum, 663
Centigrade temperature scale, 1722
Centipede bites, 1686
Central nervous system (*see also* Brain;
    Spinal cord)
  age-associated changes in, 438
  biology of, 433–435, *435*, *436*
  diagnostic tests for, 442–446, *443*
  viral infection of, 532–539
    in children, 1569–1570
Central sleep apnea, 472, 474
Central venous pressure, 130
Cephalexin, *1122*
Cephalic (head-first) presentation, 1465, *1472*,
    1485
Cephalohematoma, 1494
Cephalosporins, *1122*
Cephapirin, *1122*
Cephradine, *1122*
Cerebellar degeneration, subacute, 1037
Cerebellum, 435, *435*
  disorders of, coordination problems and,
      556
  herniation of, 513, *515*

Cerebral (see Brain)
Cerebral arteries, 503
  aneurysm of, 229, 511, 512
    in polycystic kidney disease, 855
  bleeding of (see Stroke, hemorrhagic)
  blood clots in (see Stroke, ischemic)
Cerebral hemispheres, 434, 476 (see also
  Brain)
Cerebral palsy, 1624–1626
  information resources on, 1760
Cerebrospinal fluid (CSF)
  accumulation of (hydrocephalus), 523,
    524–525, 525
    congenital, 1526
  biology of, 435
  sample collection of, 442, 443 (see also
    Spinal tap)
Cerebrotendinous xanthomatosis, 1621
Cerebrovascular accident (see Stroke)
Cerebrovascular syndrome, 1659, 1661
Cerebrum, 435
  biology of, 434
  dysfunction of, 476–477, 476
Ceruloplasmin, 906, 1725
Cerumen (earwax), 1253, 1254
Ceruminoma, 1255
Cervical cap, 1420, 1424, 1424
Cervical dystonia, 555–556
Cervical plexus, 581–582, 581
Cervical spondylosis, 564–565
Cervicitis, 1377
Cervicothoracic sympathectomy, in long QT
  syndrome, 1530
Cervix, 1344–1345, 1345
  biopsy of, 1354, 1407
  cancer of, 1406–1407, 1421
    screening for, 26, 29, 1038, 1040, 1353,
      1353, 1406–1407
    staging of, 1040, 1402
  chlamydial infection of, 1180–1181
  colposcopy of, 1353–1354
  conization of, 1728
  curettage of, 1354
  dilation of, 1465, 1466
  examination of, 1353, 1353
  gonococcal infection of, 1179–1180
  in labor, 1465, 1466
  loop electrical excision procedure on, 1354
  mucus of, 1418, 1426
Cesarean section, 1475–1476
Cetirizine, 1065
Chagas' disease (Trypanosoma cruzi
  infection), 1146
Chalazion, 1295
Chamomile, 104, 107
Chancre, 670, 1176–1177
Chancroid, 1181–1182
Charcoal, in poisoning, 1676
Charcot-Marie-Tooth disease, 587

Charcot's joints, 585
Charleyhorse, 339
Chédiak-Higashi syndrome, 1058
Cheese washer's lung, 309
Cheilitis, 664
Chelation therapy, 1681
Chemical(s)
  burns from, 1648–1651, 1648, 1650, 1651
    of esophagus, 1678–1679
    of eye, 1292
  in cancer risk, 1031–1032, 1033, 1033
  dermatitis from, 1193, 1193
  inhalation of
    hypersensitivity pneumonitis from, 297,
      308–310, 309
    occupational lung disease from, 300–301
  photosensitivity reactions from, 1232, 1232
  poisoning from, in food, 722, 725–726
  sensitivity to, 1719–1720, 1719
  in sick building syndrome, 1720
  vaginal discharge from, 1350
  vaginal itching from, 1349
Chemical pneumonitis, 272
Chemical worker's lung, 309
Chemotaxis, 1052, 1053
Chemotherapy, 1043–1044, 1045
  for acute lymphocytic leukemia, 1012
  for acute myelocytic leukemia, 1014
  for amyloidosis, 1716
  for brain tumor, 524, 525
  for breast cancer, 1397, 1400
  for carcinoid tumors, 975
  for cervical cancer, 1407
  for chronic lymphocytic leukemia, 1015
  for chronic myelocytic leukemia, 1016
  combination, 1046
  for endometrial cancer, 1404
  for gynecologic cancer, 1402–1403
  hair loss with, 1213
  for Hodgkin's disease, 1019
  for liver cancer, 811, 812–813
  for lung cancer, 331
  for macroglobulinemia, 1010
  for multiple myeloma, 1008
  for neuroblastoma, 1623
  for non-Hodgkin's lymphoma, 1022
  for ovarian cancer, 1405
  for pheochromocytoma, 961
  during pregnancy, 1461
  for retinoblastoma, 1624
  side effects of, 1047
  for Wilms' tumor, 1623
Cherry hemangioma, 1235
Chest
  abscess of, 1097
  air in (pneumothorax), 316–317, 316
    in asthma, 276
    in barotrauma, 1668
    in COPD, 282–283

Chest *(continued)*
air in (pneumothorax) *(continued)*
in meconium aspiration syndrome, 1501
in newborn, 1502
compression of, in CPR, 1690
examination of, 121, 254
imaging of, 255–256
in aspergillosis, 311
in black lung, 296
in eosinophilic pneumonia, 310
in heart disease, 125
in idiopathic pulmonary fibrosis, 302
in lung cancer, 330, *1038*
in pericarditis, 191
in pneumonia, 265
in pneumonitis, 303
in pulmonary embolism, 287
in silicosis prevention, 295
in tuberculosis, 1128
pain in
in angina, 203
in aortic stenosis, 181
in coronary artery disease, 202–210,
206–207, 208, 210
in esophageal disorders, 706, 708
in familial Mediterranean fever,
1716–1717
in heart attack, 211
in pleurisy, 313
in respiratory disorders, 251
in sickle cell disease, 993
with swallowing, 701
physical therapy for, 261–262
Chest cavity, 245
Chest tube, 315, 317
Chest wall
pain in, 251, 313 *(see also* Chest, pain in)
in respiratory failure, *325*
Cheyne-Stokes respiration, 154, 473, 491
Chickenpox, 1162, *1569,* 1571–1572
immunization for, *265, 1094, 1095, 1493*
pneumonia, 269
Chiggers, 1685
Chilblains, 1656
Childbirth *(see* Labor and delivery)
Childcare, 1542, 1641
HIV-related precautions for, 1574, 1575
Childhood disintegrative disorder, 1632
Children *(see also* Infant[s])
abuse of, *639,* 1179, 1643–1646
information resources on, 1760
adverse drug reactions in, 84
air travel by, 1710
bacterial infections in, 1561–1568
behavioral problems in, 1543–1544, *1544,
1548, 1549, 1550*
bone disorders in, 1603–1607, *1604, 1605,
1606*
cancer in, 1622–1624

Children *(continued)*
connective tissue disorders in, 1607–1611
development of *(see* Development, child)
diabetes mellitus in, 1613–1615, *1615*
digestive system disorders in, 1586–1593,
1591, 1592
dissociative identity disorder in, 638–639,
639
domestic violence and, *1411*
drug dosage for, 101
drug safety and, 86
ear, nose, and throat disorders in,
1593–1600, *1595, 1597, 1598*
eye disorders in, 1600–1603, *1601, 1602*
foster care for, 1641–1642
head injury in, 514, *516*
immunization for, 1492–1494, *1493*
mental health disorders in, 1630–1637,
1633, 1635, 1636
mental retardation in, 1626–1629, *1627, 1628*
metabolic disorders in, 1616–1621, *1617,
1621*
Münchausen syndrome and, *602*
neglect of, 1643–1646
over-the-counter drugs for, 100–101
respiratory disorders in, 1583–1586
rheumatoid arthritis in, 1612–1613
seizures in, 502
social issues affecting, 1638–1643, *1639,
1642*
suicidal behavior in, 1634–1635, *1635*
tooth eruption in, 662
toxoplasmosis in, 1145
treatment compliance in, 86
tumors in, 1622–1624
very young, problems in, 1531–1543, *1533,
1535, 1536*
viral infection in, 1568–1582, *1569, 1572,
1576, 1581*
Wolff-Parkinson-White syndrome in, 172
Chinese alternative medicine, 1705
Chinese restaurant syndrome (MSG
sensitivity), *726*
Chiropractic, 1707
Chlamydial infection
cervix (cervicitis), 1180–1181, *1181*
eye (conjunctivitis), 1296
in newborn, *1509*
gonorrhea with, 1180
lymphogranuloma venereum, 1181
parrot fever, *268*
pneumonia, 269
during pregnancy, 1447
trachoma, 1297–1298
urethritis in, 868
vaginitis, *1376*
Chloral hydrate
abuse of, 653–654
in sleep disorders, *471*

Chlorambucil
in cancer, *1045*
during pregnancy, *1461*
Chloramphenicol, *1124*
in infants, 84
during pregnancy, *1460*
Chlordiazepoxide, in elderly persons, *81*
Chlorhexidine, 678
Chloride, *902, 1725*
Chlorine, inhalation of, 300–301
Chloroma, 1013
Chloroquine
in malaria, 1141
in porphyria, 934
Chlorpheniramine, *1065*
in common cold, *1158*
in elderly persons, *80*
Chlorpromazine, in elderly persons, *80*
Chlorpropamide
in diabetes insipidus, 945
in diabetes mellitus, 968
in elderly persons, *80*
during pregnancy, *1461*
Chlorzoxazone, in elderly persons, *81*
Choking, 1690–1691, *1690, 1691*
with infant feeding, 1489
Cholangiocarcinoma, 800, 801, 811–812
Cholangiography
operative, 789, *790*
percutaneous transhepatic, 789, *790*, 801
Cholangitis
bacterial, 800, 801, 814
primary sclerosing, 800–801
Cholecalciferol (vitamin D$_3$), 894
Cholecystectomy (gallbladder removal),
814–815, 816
Cholecystitis, 815–817
Cholecystokinin, *939*
Choledocholithiasis (bile duct stones),
813–815, 816
Cholelithiasis (*see* Gallstones)
Cholera, *720, 721*, 1100–1101
immunization for, *1094*
Cholescintigraphy, 789, 816
Cholestasis (bile flow obstruction), 792–793
in hepatitis, 802
during pregnancy, 1451
Cholesteatoma, 1258–1259, 1594
Cholesterol, 920, *921, 1726*
in atherosclerosis, 197, 920, 921–922
in cerebrotendinous xanthomatosis, *1621*
coronary artery disease and, 200
desirable blood levels of, *922*
estrogen and, 1358
exercise effects on, 31
in gallstone formation, 813
HDL, 197, 202, 920, *921, 922*
high blood levels of, 920, 921–926, *924, 925*
hereditary, 926

Cholesterol *(continued)*
LDL, 197, 202, 920, *921, 922*
estrogen and, 1358
progestin and, 1359
liver production of, 697, 786
low blood levels of, 926–927
lowering of, 922–923, *923, 924, 925*
in coronary artery disease prevention,
202
oral contraceptive use and, 1420
in preventive care, *29*
progestin and, 1359
reference range for, *1726*
VLDL, 920, *921*
in Wolman's disease, *1621*
Cholestyramine, 793, *925*
Cholinergic agents, *1308*
Chondroblastoma, 360
Chondrodysplasias, 1611
Chondroitin sulfate, 422
Chondroma, 360
Chondromalacia patellae, 1607
Chondromyxoid fibroma, 360
Chondrosarcoma, 360, 361
Chordee, 1519
Chordoma, *520*
Chorea, 552–553
Huntington's, 552, 553–554, *553*
Sydenham's, 552, 1566
Chorea gravidarum, 552–553
Choreoathetosis, 552, 1625
Choriocarcinoma, 1409–1410
Choriomeningitis, 538
Chorion, 1436, *1437*
Chorionic villus sampling, 1432–1434, *1433*,
1512, 1629, *1728*
Chorioretinitis, 1305–1306
Choroid, 1305, *1306*, 1310
melanoma of, 1314
metastases to, 1314
Choroiditis, 1305–1306
Chromium picolinate, 107
Chromosome(s), *4, 9, 10*, 1527
abnormalities of, 1511, 1527–1530,
1529
parental age and, *1346*, 1527
prenatal testing for, 1430–1431, *1431*,
1527
analysis of, *1728*
deletions of, *1529*
in leukemia, 1010
mitochondrial, 14
Philadelphia, 1016
sex, *9, 11*, 1527, 1528–1530 (*see also* X
chromosome; Y chromosome)
Chronic deep vein insufficiency, 233
Chronic fatigue syndrome, 1717–1718,
1718
Chronic granulomatous disease, 1062

Chronic obstructive pulmonary disease (COPD), 281–285
  prevention of, 27
  pulmonary hypertension in, 323
  pulmonary rehabilitation in, 259–262, 284–285
Chylomicrons, 920, *921*
  deficiency of (abetalipoproteinemia), 927
  excess of, 925–926
Chylothorax, 314, 316
Chyluria, 867–868
Ciclopirox, 1226
Cidofovir, *1156*
Cigarette smoking (*see* Smoking)
Ciguatera poisoning, 725–726
Cilia
  of airways, 248, 1088
  of fallopian tubes, 1345
  of hair cells, 1244–1245
  of nose and sinuses, 1245
  of smell receptors, 1246
  of throat cells, 1246
Ciliary body, 1305, 1306, *1306, 1307*
Cilostazol, 221
Cimetidine
  drug interactions of, 76
  in elderly persons, 81
  in peptic ulcer, 716, *718*
Cineangiography, 129
Cine-computed tomography, 125
Cineradiography, 708, 710
C1 inhibitor deficiency, *1072*
Ciprofloxacin, *1123*
  drug interactions of, 76
  during pregnancy, *1460*
Circle of Willis, *503*
Circulation
  blood, 115–116, *115*
    in fetus, 1513
  cerebral, 433, 438, *503*
    testing of, 441–442
  coronary, 116–117, *116*
    during pregnancy, 1439
  spinal, 567–568
Circumcision, 1485–1486, 1568
Cirrhosis, 797–799, *799*
  in children, 1522
  liver cancer and, 811
  during pregnancy, 1448
  primary biliary, 799–800
Cisplatin, *1045*
CK-MB enzyme, 213
Clap (*see* Gonorrhea)
Clarithromycin, *1123*
Claudication, 217, 221
Clavicle, fracture of, 358
Clean-catch urine sample, 826, *826*
Cleansing agents, 1189–1190
Clear cell carcinoma, 1408

Cleft lip and palate, 1523, *1523*
  information resources on, 1760
Clemastine, *1065, 1158*
Clidinium-chlordiazepoxide, in elderly persons, 81
Climacteric (*see* Menopause)
Clindamycin, *1124, 1207*
Clinical trial, 1696
Clitocybe (mushroom) poisoning, 725
Clitoris, 1343, *1344*
CLL (chronic lymphocytic leukemia), 1014–1015
Clofibrate, 945
Clomiphene
  in low sperm count, 1415
  in ovulation problems, 1417
  in polycystic ovary syndrome, 1368
Clonazepam, *500*
Clonidine
  for hot flashes, 1359, *1360*
  in opioid withdrawal, 653
  in Tourette's syndrome, 552
Cloning, 15
Clonorchiasis (liver fluke infection), *1146*
Clopidogrel
  for heart attack, *206*
  in peripheral arterial disease, 222
  in stroke prevention, 505
Clostridial infection, *746, 1097*
  antibiotic-associated colitis, *720,* 745–746
  botulism, 579–581
  food poisoning, *721,* 724–725
  gas gangrene, 1101
  tetanus, 1114–1115
    immunization for, 1093, *1094,* 1115, *1115*
Clotting, 995–996, *995* (*see also* Anticoagulants; Blood clots)
  in allergic purpura, 996–997
  bleeding time test of, 981
  disorders of, 980, 996–1001, *997*
  in disseminated intravascular coagulation, 1001
  drug effects on, *996* (*see also* Anticoagulants)
  in hemolytic-uremic syndrome, 998
  in hemophilia, 999–1000
  in hereditary hemorrhagic telangiectasia (Rendu-Osler-Weber disease), 996
  in homocystinuria, 1619
  in thrombocytopenia, 997–999, *997*
  in thrombophilia, 1000–1001
  in Von Willebrand's disease, 999
Clotting factors
  deficiency of, 980, 999–1000
  testing of, 981
  transfusion of, 984–985, 1000
Cloxacillin, *1123*

Clozapine
  monitoring of, 63
  in schizophrenia, 644, *645*
Clubbing, of fingers, 253, *253*
Clubfoot, 1524, *1524*
Cluster headache, *458*, 461
CML (chronic myelocytic leukemia),
    1015–1016
Coal workers' pneumoconiosis, 296, *297*
Coarctation of aorta, 1518
Cobalamin (vitamin B$_{12}$), *893*, 898–899, *899*
  deficiency of, 898–899, 990–991
  in homocystinuria, 1619
  supplementation with, 990
Cocaine, 656–657
  adolescent use of, 1559–1560
  during pregnancy, 1450, 1463
Coccal infection, *1096*, 1108–1109,
    1111–1112 *(see also specific infections)*
Coccidioidomycosis, 1151
  pneumonia and, 270–271
Cochlea, 1244–1245, *1245*
Cochlear implant, 1252, *1252*, 1599
Codeine, *451*
  in cough remedies, 98, 249, *1158*
  in diarrhea, *756*
Coelenterate sting, 1687
Coenurosis, 540
Coffee worker's lung, *309*
Cognitive-behavior therapy, 601
  in anxiety, 607
  in bulimia, 626–627
Cognitive impairment
  after stroke, 41
  in Alzheimer's disease, 487–488
  in delirium, 481–482
  in dementia, 485
  in schizophrenia, 641
Cohort study, 1696
Coke *(see Cocaine)*
Colchicine
  in amyloidosis, 1716
  in familial Mediterranean fever, 1717
  in gout, 393, *393*
  in pseudogout, 395
Cold, common, 1155, 1157–1159, 1264
  in children, 1579–1580
  remedies for, 22, 95–98, 1157–1159, *1158*
Cold antibody hemolytic anemia, 992
Cold environment
  allergy to, 1070
  injury from, 1654–1657
  keeping warm in, 1655
Cold sores, 668–669, 1161
Cold therapy (cryotherapy), 37
  after dental treatment, 691–692
  in ankle sprain, 406
  in cervical cancer, 1407
  in heat stroke, 1654

Cold therapy *(continued)*
  in sports injuries, 421–422
  in wart removal, 1229
Colesevelam, *925*
Colestipol, *925*
Colic
  biliary (gallbladder pain), 788, 814, 816
  in infants, 1531
  renal, 823, 863, 865
Colistin, *1123*
Colitis *(see also Crohn's disease)*
  antibiotic-associated, *720*, 745–746, 1125
  collagenous, 744–745
  diversion, 745
  hemorrhagic, 723–724
  ischemic, 783
  lymphocytic, 744–745
  toxic, 742, 744
  ulcerative, 742–744
Collagenous colitis, 744–745
Colles' fracture, 345, 358
Colon *(see Large intestine)*
Colonic enema, 753–754
Colonic inertia, 751
Colonoscopy, 703, *704*, 1724, *1728*
  in cancer screening, *1038*
  in Crohn's disease, 740
  in diverticulitis, 748–750
  in intestinal polyps, 769
  in small intestine cancer, 768
  in ulcerative colitis, 742–743
Color blindness, 14, 1280, *1281*
  testing for, 1283
Colorectal cancer, 770–773, *771*
  ulcerative colitis and, 742–743
Colostomy, *772*
  in colorectal cancer, 772
  diversion colitis after, 745
  in diverticulitis, 750
  in fecal incontinence, 758
  in Hirschsprung disease, 1523
  travel with, 1713
Colostrum, 1439, 1487
Colposcopy, 1353–1354, *1728*
Coma, 490–494, *492–493*
  diabetic, 964, 966
  hepatic, 649–650, 795–796
  myxedema, 953
Common bile duct, *695*, 787
Common cold *(see Cold, common)*
Common hepatic duct, *695, 697, 787*
Common variable immunodeficiency, 1060
Communicable diseases *(see Infection)*
Communication
  with dying person, *46*
  with health care professionals, 21–24, 47,
      54, 87
    in medical decision-making, 1695–1698
  parent-child, *1639, 1642*

Compartment syndrome, 349, 353
  in electrical injury, 1662
Competency, 53–54, *53*
Complementary medicine, 1704–1707
Complement system, 1050, *1052*, 1054
Complete blood count (CBC), 980–981, *981*,
  1725
Complex partial (psychomotor) seizures,
  496–497
Complex regional pain syndrome, 449
Compliance (adherence), with drug
  treatment, *63*, *76*, 81, 86–88, *87*
Compressed air injuries, 1666–1671, *1669*,
  1670
Compression bandages
  in deep vein thrombosis, 234–235
  in leg ulcers, 235
Compulsions, 611–612
Computed tomography (CT), 8, *1728*
  in acromegaly, 946
  in cancer staging, 1041
  in Crohn's disease, 740
  in digestive system disorders, 705
  of eye, 1286
  of fracture, 350
  in heart disease, 125
  in Hodgkin's disease, 1018
  in idiopathic pulmonary fibrosis, 302
  in kidney and urinary tract disorders,
    827
  of liver, 789
  in lung cancer, 330, *1038*
  in lung disorders, 255
  in musculoskeletal disorders, 342
  in neurologic disorders, 443
  in pancreatitis, 731, 733
Computed tomography angiography (CTA),
  125, 287
Computer keyboard, hand position at, *399*
Conception (*see* Fertilization)
Conchae, nasal, 1245, *1246*
Concussion, 513, 517
Condom, 1176, *1178*, *1420*, 1423, *1424*
Conduct disorder, 1635–1636
Conduction aphasia, *477*
Condylomata acuminata, 1183, 1325
Condylomata lata, 1177, 1325
Cones, 1276
Confidentiality, 54
Confusion, *481*
  in delirium, 481
  drug-related, *83*
  in dying person, 50
Congenital adrenal hyperplasia, *1430*, 1520
Congenital disorders (*see* Birth defects;
    Chromosome[s], abnormalities of;
    Genetics, disorders of)
Congestive heart failure (*see* Heart failure)
Conization, *1728*

Conjunctiva, 1276, *1276*, 1277, 1296
  bleeding in, 1280–1281
  dark spots on, 1281
  disorders of, 1296–1299
  inflammation of (*see* Conjunctivitis)
  noncancerous growths on, 1299
  sarcoidosis of, 305
Conjunctivitis, 1296–1297, *1297*
  allergic, 1066, 1067, 1298–1299
  gonococcal, 1179
  granular, 1297–1298
  hemorrhagic, *1576*
  inclusion, 1296
  in newborn, *1509*
  in Reiter's syndrome, 376
Connective tissue, 2, 334
  disorders of
    autoimmune, 378–386, *379*
    in diabetes mellitus, *963*
    hereditary, 1607–1611
    mixed, 384–385
    pulmonary hypertension with, 324
    vasculitic, 386–391, *387*, *389*
Conn's syndrome, 960
Consciousness, 491 (*see also* Coma;
    Confusion)
  in breath-holding spells, 1547
  in concussion, 517
  in delirium, 480–484
  in head injury, 513
  in heat exhaustion, 1653
  in heatstroke, 1654
  in lightning injury, 1664
  in low blood pressure, 143–146
  in nitrogen narcosis, *1669*
  in respiratory failure, 325
  in seizures, 145, 495
Consent, 54, 1701
Constipation, 699, 750–754, *753*
  in dying person, 49
  in dyschezia, 751, 752
  in infants and children, 1533–1534, 1591
  in infants and young children,
    1545–1546
  in irritable bowel syndrome, 756–757
  during pregnancy, 1440
  psychogenic, 751
Constriction devices, in erectile dysfunction,
  1338–1339
Consumption (*see* Tuberculosis)
Contact dermatitis, 1193–1194, *1193*, *1195*
Contact lenses, 1287–1288
  travel with, 1713
Contagious diseases (*see* Infection)
Continuous ambulatory electrocardiography,
  123–124, *124*
  in angina evaluation, 204
  in arrhythmias, 165
  in fainting, 145

Continuous positive airway pressure
(CPAP)
in apnea of prematurity, 1504
in atelectasis, 294
in obstructive sleep apnea, 473
in respiratory distress syndrome, 1500
in transient tachypnea of newborn, 1500
during travel, 1712
Contraception and contraceptives,
1419–1426, *1420*
for adolescents, 1560
after childbirth, 1477–1478
barrier, *1420,* 1423–1424, *1424*
condoms, *1420,* 1423, *1424*
effectiveness of, *1420*
emergency, 1423
hormonal methods for, 1419–1423, *1420,*
1422
implants in, *1420,* 1422
injectable, *1420,* 1422–1423
intrauterine devices in, *1420,* 1424–1425,
1425
oral, 1420–1421, *1420 (see also* Oral
contraceptives)
rhythm methods in, *1420,* 1425–1426
skin patches in, 1421–1422
sterilization in, 1427–1428, *1428*
vaginal rings in, 1421–1422
withdrawal method in, *1420*
Contractions
after childbirth, 1474, 1477
in labor (*see* Labor and delivery)
Contracture
after amputation, 43
Dupuytren's, 397–398
Contrast agents, problems with, *827, 1069*
Contusion
bladder, 874
brain, 517
eye, 1290
first aid for, 1693
kidney, *873*
urethra, 875
Conversion disorder, 603, 1637
Conversion symptoms, *604*
Convulsions (*see* Seizures)
Coombs test, 992
Coordination
disorders of, 556
testing of, 441
COPD (chronic obstructive pulmonary
disease), 281–285
prevention of, *27*
pulmonary hypertension in, 323
pulmonary rehabilitation in, 284–285
rehabilitation for, 259–262
Coping mechanisms, *634*
Copper, *902,* 905–906, *905*
deficiency of, 905–906

Copper (*continued*)
excess of, 906
liver accumulation of (Wilson's disease),
905
hepatitis and, 803
reference range for, *1726*
Copperhead snake bite, 1682–1683
Copper IUD, 1424–1425, *1425*
Coprolalia, 552
Coral snake bite, 1682–1683
Coral sting, 1687
Cord (*see* Umbilical cord)
Corkscrew esophagus, 708–709
Cork worker's lung, *309*
Cornea, 1276, *1276*
abrasion of, in infant, 1531
age-associated changes in, 1278
disorders of, 1299–1302
drying of, 1301
herpes simplex virus infection of, 1161,
1301–1302
pain in, 1281
shape changes in, 1302
swelling of, 1302
thickness of, 1286
transplantation of, *1082,* 1083
ulcers of, 1288, 1300, 1302
Corns, 410
Cornstarch, 1190, 1489
Coronary arteries, 116–117, *116*
aneurysm of, in Kawasaki syndrome,
1581
angiography of, 129, 204
angioplasty of, 128, 149, 208–209, *208*
bypass surgery of, 209–210, *210*
catheterization of, 128–129
disease of, 118, 199–215, *210*
after menopause, 1357
angina in, 202–210, *206–207, 208*
in cardiomyopathy, 159
in dilated cardiomyopathy, 161
in familial hypercholesterolemia, 926
heart failure with, 152
prevention of, 200–202
risk factors for, 199–200
radionuclide imaging of, 127
spasm of, 203
Coronary artery bypass graft (CABG) surgery,
149
Coronary stent, travel and, 1711–1712
Coronary thrombosis (*see* Heart attack)
Corpora cavernosa, 1321
Cor pulmonale, 322, *323*
Corpus luteum, *1347,* 1348
Corpus spongiosum, 1321
Corti, organ of, 1244–1245
Cortical necrosis, 847
Corticobasal ganglionic degeneration,
547

Corticosteroids, *374*, 1190–1191 (*see also*
   Immunosuppressive drugs
   [immunomodulators])
   in Addison's disease, 957
   adrenal gland suppression by, *958*
   in allergic conjunctivitis, 1067
   in allergic rhinitis, 1066
   in allergy, 1065
   in aspergillosis, 312
   in asthma, 277, *278*, 281, 1584
   in autoimmune disorders, 806, 992, 1075
   in Behçet's syndrome, 391
   in Bell's palsy, 592
   in bronchitis, 264
   in canker sores, 668
   control of, 956
   in COPD, 284
   in Crohn's disease, 740, *741*
   in croup, 1586
   in Cushing's disease, 958–959
   in cystic fibrosis, 321
   deficiency of, 956–958 (*see also* Addison's
      disease)
   depression with, 615
   in dermatomyositis, 384
   in eosinophilic fasciitis, 386
   in eosinophilic gastritis, 713
   in eosinophilic pneumonia, 311
   in fetal lung immaturity, 1498, 1500
   in fungal infection, 1226
   generic substitutions for, *90*
   in gout, 393, *393*
   in idiopathic pulmonary fibrosis, 302
   in itching, 1192
   in lichen planus, 1204
   in meningitis, 531
   in mixed connective tissue disease, 385
   in multiple myeloma, 1008
   in multiple sclerosis, 559
   in muscular dystrophy, 413
   in nasal polyps, 1265
   in nephrotic syndrome, 843
   in osteopetroses, 1611
   overproduction of (Cushing's syndrome),
      958–959
   over-the-counter, 98–99
   in pancreatitis, 733
   in pemphigus, 1217
   in polyarteritis nodosa, 388
   in polymyalgia rheumatica, 389
   in polymyositis, 384
   in preterm labor, 1471
   in rapidly progressive glomerulonephritis,
      839
   in rheumatoid arthritis, *372*, 373
   in sarcoidosis, 306
   in seborrheic dermatitis, 1196
   in spinal cord injury, 563
   in sports injuries, 422

Corticosteroids *(continued)*
   in Stevens-Johnson syndrome, 1200
   in systemic lupus erythematosus, 380
   in temporal (giant cell) arteritis, 388
   in tendinitis, 418
   in thyroiditis, 954
   topical, 1190–1191
   in toxic epidermal necrolysis, 1200
   in transplantation, *1078*
   in ulcerative colitis, 743–744
   in Wegener's granulomatosis, 390
Corticotropin (ACTH), *939*, 940, *941*, 956
   in Addison's disease, 957
   deficiency of, 942
   measurement of, 943
   overproduction of, 958
Corticotropin-releasing hormone, 956
Cortisol, *939* (*see also* Corticosteroids)
Cortisone (*see* Corticosteroids)
Corynebacterium minutissimum infection,
      1222–1223
Coryza (*see* Cold, common)
Cosmetic dentistry, *677*
Cosmetics, dermatitis from, 1193–1194,
      1193
Cosmetic surgery, *1699*
Cost-benefit study, *1696*
Cottonmouth snake bite, 1682–1683
Cough, 249–250
   in asthma, 1583
   blood in, 252–253, *307*
   in bronchiectasis, 290
   in COPD, 282
   in croup, 1586
   in cystic fibrosis, 319
   fainting with, 144
   in Hodgkin's disease, *1017*
   remedies for, 98, 249–250, *1158*, 1159
   in tuberculosis, 1127
   whooping (pertussis), 1564–1565
      immunization for, 1093, *1094*, 1492,
         1493, 1562
Counseling
   for children of divorce, 1641
   genetic, 1429–1430
   in immunodeficiency disorders, 1059
   in macular degeneration, 1311
   in muscular dystrophy, 413
   in neurofibromatosis, 528
   in pulmonary medicine, 260
   in sickle cell disease, 994
Coup contrecoup injury, 517
Coxibs (*see* Cyclooxygenase-2 [COX-2]
      inhibitors)
Coxiella burnetii infection (Q fever),
      1133
COX-2 inhibitors (*see* Cyclooxygenase-2
      [COX-2] inhibitors)
Coxsackie B virus infection, 160

CPR (cardiopulmonary resuscitation), *56,* 1689–1690
  do-not-resuscitate order against, 48
  in electrical injury, 1663
  in hypothermia, 1655–1656
  in lightning injury, 1664
  in near drowning, 1666
  order against, 57
Crabs (pubic lice), 1219, *1219*
Crack cocaine, 656–657
Cradle cap (seborrheic dermatitis), 1196, 1535
Cramps
  in Buerger's disease, 223
  heat, 1653
  intestinal, 699, 755
  muscle, 415
Cranberry, 107–108
Cranial nerves, 437–438
  disorders of, 588–594, *592, 593*
  sarcoidosis of, 305
  testing of, 439, *590–591*
Craniopharyngioma, *520*
Craniotomy, *525*
Cravings, food, 1440
C-reactive protein
  in multiple myeloma, 1008
  in osteomyelitis, 365
Creams, 1189
  estrogen, 1359
  in itching, 1192
Creatine, as nutraceutical, 108
Creatine kinase, 342
  reference range for, *1726*
Creatinine, *1726*
Creatinine clearance test, 826, 829
Creeping eruption, 1220
CREST syndrome, 381
Creutzfeldt-Jakob disease, 490, 541–543, *542*
Crib death, 1489, 1504, 1538
Cri du chat syndrome, *1529*
Crohn's disease, 738–742, *741*
Cromolyn, 1064–1065
  in allergic conjunctivitis, 1067
  in allergic rhinitis, 1066
  in asthma, 278, 280–281, 1584
Cross-dressing, 629
Cross-eyes (strabismus), 1601–1603, *1602*
Cross-sectional study, 1696
Crotalaria leaves, 808
Croup, 1579–1580, 1585–1586
Crowns, dental, *679*
Crust (scab), *1189*
Crying, in infants, 1492, 1531, 1570
Cryofibrinogen, 1070
Cryoglobulinemia, 1009, *1009*
Cryoglobulins, 1070
Cryomyolysis, 1373
Cryopexy, 1311–1312

Cryotherapy, 37
  after dental treatment, 691–692
  in ankle sprain, 406
  in cervical cancer, 1407
  in heat stroke, 1654
  in sports injuries, 421–422
  in wart removal, 1229
Cryptococcosis, 1151–1152
  with HIV infection, *1172*
  pneumonia and, 271
Cryptogenic organizing pneumonitis, 303
Cryptorchidism, 1327, 1535–1536, *1535*
Cryptosporidium infection, *721, 722,* 1137–1138
  with HIV infection, *1172*
Crystal (methamphetamine), 656
Crystal deposition
  in gout, 391–394, *392, 393*
  in pseudogout, 394–395
CSF (*see* Cerebrospinal fluid)
CT (*see* Computed tomography)
Cubital tunnel syndrome, 399–400
Culture, *1088, 1729*
  in bacteremia, 1561
  in sepsis, 1119
  in strep throat, 1596
  urine, 826, 1568
Curettage
  for abortion, 1426–1427
  endocervical, 1354
Curvature, spinal, 1603–1604, *1604*
  in Scheuermann disease, 1604–1605, *1605*
Cushing's syndrome, 958–959
  in lung cancer, *1037*
  obesity in, 916
  potassium deficiency with, 910
Cutaneous larva migrans, 1220
Cuticle, infection of (paronychia), 402
Cutis laxa, 1610
Cuts, 22, 1691–1693 (*see also* Laceration)
Cyanosis, 253
  in apnea of prematurity, 1503
  in breath-holding spells, 1547
  in carcinoid tumors, 974
  in congenital heart defects, 1513
  of hands and feet, 225
  in heart disease, 120
  in meconium aspiration syndrome, 1501
  in persistent pulmonary hypertension, 1502
  in pulmonary valve stenosis, 1518
  in respiratory disorders, 253
  in respiratory tract infection, 1579
  in shock, 148
  in tetralogy of Fallot, 1515
  in tracheoesophageal fistula, 1521
  in transient tachypnea of newborn, 1500
  in transposition of great arteries, 1517

Cyclobenzaprine, in elderly persons, *81*
Cyclooxygenase-2 (COX-2) inhibitors (coxibs),
    454
  in gout, 393, *393*
  in osteoarthritis, 369
  in rheumatoid arthritis, *372,* 373
Cyclophosphamide
  in cancer, *1045*
  during pregnancy, *1461*
  in rheumatoid arthritis, *372,* 374–375
  in transplantation, *1078*
Cyclosporine
  in Behçet's syndrome, 391
  in Crohn's disease, *741*
  food interactions with, 77
  gingivitis and, 682
  in psoriasis, 1202
  in rheumatoid arthritis, *372*
  in transplantation, *1079*
  in ulcerative colitis, 744
Cyclothymic disorder, 620
Cyproheptadine, *1065*
  in elderly persons, *80*
  in physical allergy, 1070
Cyproterone, 1368
Cyst(s)
  Baker's, 419
  Bartholin's, *1375*
  brain, 540
  breast, 1388
  dermoid, *520*
  epidermal, 1237
  ganglion, 395
  kidney, 854–855, *855*
  neck, 1599
  oral, 671
  ovarian, 959, 960, 1367–1368, *1405*
    during pregnancy, 1450
  popliteal, 419
  pulmonary, in Marfan syndrome, 1608
  sebaceous, 1255
Cystadenocarcinoma, *774*
Cystectomy, 878
Cystic duct, 697, *787*
  blockage of, 814
Cysticercosis, 540, 1143–1144
Cystic fibrosis, 250, 317–322, *318, 1430*
  information resources on, 1760
Cystic medial necrosis, 228
Cystine
  in kidney stones, 864–866
  in urine (cystinuria), 851–852
Cystitis, 868–871, *869, 870*
  after childbirth, 1479
  in children, 1567–1568
Cystocele, 1380, *1381*
Cystography, 827
Cystoplasty, *860*
Cystosarcoma phyllodes, 1391, 1400–1401

Cystoscopy, 828
  in urethral stricture, 1325
Cystourethrocele, 1380
Cystourethrography
  in urinary tract infection, 1568
  voiding, 870
Cytapheresis, *986*
Cytarabine, *1045*
Cytokines, 1050, *1052,* 1054, 1119
Cytomegalovirus infection, 1164–1165
  with HIV infection, *1172*
  in newborn, *1508*
  during pregnancy, 1450
Cytopenia, 1047
Cytoplasm, 2, *4*
Cytotoxic drugs (*see* Chemotherapy)

D

Daclizumab, *1079*
Dacryoadenitis, 1318
Dacryocystitis, 1293
Dacryostenosis, 1293
Dairy products, intolerance to, 698, 735–736,
    754
Danazol
  in breast pain, 1387
  in endometriosis, 1370, *1371*
  in fibroids, 1373
  during pregnancy, *1461*
D and C (dilation and curettage), 1354, *1354,*
    1729
  after childbirth, 1474
  in dysfunctional uterine bleeding, 1367
D and E (dilation and evacuation), 1427
Dandruff, 1196
Dapsone, 1131
  in dermatitis herpetiformis, 1218
Darbepoietin
  abuse of, *647*
  in kidney failure, 833
  in multiple myeloma, 1008
Dawn phenomenon, 969
Daycare, 1542, 1641
  HIV-related precautions for, 1574, 1575
Daytop Village, 653
D-dimer test, 287
Deafness (*see* Hearing, loss of)
Death and dying, 45–52 (*see also* Legal
    issues)
  advance directive for, 51, *53,* 54–56
  anxiety and, 50
  in breast cancer, 1401
  breathing during, 48–49
  confusion and, 50
  in COPD, 285
  depression and, 50
  digestive system disorders during, 49

Death and dying *(continued)*
  disability and, 50
  fatigue and, 50
  of fetus, 1457
  financial concerns and, 50–51, 57
  health care choices and, 47–48
  in heart failure, 158
  incontinence and, 49
  of infant, 1638
    SIDS and, 1489, 1504, 1538
      information resources on, 1767
  information resources on, 1761
  legal issues and, 51
  in leukemia, 1011
  in lung cancer, 331
  in multiple myeloma, 1008
  obesity and, 918
  pain in, 48
  preparation for, 51
  pressure sores and, 49–50
  signs of, 52
  suicide and, 51
  time course of, 46–47
  treatment options and, 47–48
  unconsciousness and, 50
Death certificate, 52
Death rattle, 52
Death With Dignity Act (1998), 51
Decay, tooth (cavities), 675–679, *676, 678,*
    679
Decision making
  medical, 1695–1698
  surrogate, 56–57, 487
Decompression sickness, 1669–1671, *1669,*
    1670
Decongestants, 97–98, 250, *1158*
  in allergic rhinitis, 1066
  for children, 1580
  before diving, 1668
  urinary incontinence with, *859*
Decubitus ulcers *(see* Pressure sores)
Deep-sea diving injuries, 1666–1671, *1669,*
    1670
Deep vein thrombosis, 232–236, *235*
  after surgery, 1703
  in pregnancy, 1450–1451
  in thrombophilia, 1000
Deer fly bites, 1685
Deer fly fever (tularemia), 1116–1117,
    1116
DEET (diethyltoluamide), *1107,* 1134
Defecation *(see* Bowel movements)
Defense mechanisms, *634*
  against disease, 1050 *(see also* Immune
      system)
  against infection, 1087–1092
  of lungs, 247–248
Deferoxamine, 908, 1680
Defibrillation, 167

Defibrillator
  external, 1689, *1689*
  implantable
    in long QT syndrome, 1530
    travel and, 1711–1712
Deformities *(see* Birth defects)
Dehydration, 928–929
  in Addison's disease, 956
  during air travel, 1711
  body response to, 5
  in burn injury, 1649, 1651
  in cholera, 1100–1101
  constipation and, 751
  in cystic fibrosis, 319
  in diabetes insipidus, 851, 944
  in diarrhea, 755, 756
  in elderly persons, 930
  fainting with, 144
  in gastroenteritis, 722, 723, 1587–1588
  in heat exhaustion, 1653
  in infants and children, 1532, 1533, *1533,*
      1587–1588
  during labor and delivery, 1467
  orthostatic hypotension with, 146
  in premature infant, 930
  in radiation illness, 1659
  in shigellosis, 1111
Dehydroepiandrosterone (DHEA), *939,*
    1361
  in Addison's disease, 956
  as nutraceutical, 108
Dejection *(see* Depression)
Delavirdine, *1175*
Delirium, 480–484, *481*
  vs. dementia, *483*
  in mania, 619
  vs. psychosis, 482, *482*
Delirium tremens (DTs), 649
Delivery *(see* Labor and delivery)
Delta-aminolevulinic acid, 935
Delusions, 644–646
  in depression, 616
  in schizophrenia, 641
Demecarium, *1308*
Demeclocycline, *1123*
Dementia, 20, 481, 484–490, *487, 488*
  Alzheimer's, 487–488
  vs. delirium, *483*
  depression and, 484
  information resources on, 1757
  Lewy body, 489
  sleep disorders with, 475
  vascular, 489–490
Dementia pugilistica, 490
Demyelination, 557–560, *558*
Dendrite, *437*
Dendritic cells, *1052,* 1055
Dengue fever, 1167
Denial, *604*

Dental caries (cavities), 675–679, *676, 678, 679*
Dental hygiene (*see* Oral hygiene)
Dental problems (*see* Tooth [teeth])
Dentin, 663
Dentist
  examination by, 677
  language of, *675*
  tooth repair techniques of, *677, 678–679, 678, 679*
Deoxyribonucleic acid (DNA), 8–9, *10*
  cell transfer of (gene therapy), 15–16
  laboratory copying of, 15
  mitochondrial, 14
Dependence, drug, 450, 646–647 (*see also* Drugs, abuse of)
Dependent personality, 633
Depersonalization, 638, 639–640
Depilatory, 1212, 1214
Depression, 614–619, *614, 618*
  in adolescents, 1636
  alcohol and, 650
  in anorexia, 626
  in burn injury, 1651
  in cancer, 1036
  in children, 1632–1633, *1633*
  constipation in, 751
  drugs for (*see* Antidepressants)
  in dying person, 50
  in elderly persons, 19
  information resources on, 1761
  mental retardation and, 1627–1628
  physical disorders and, 615, *615*
  postpartum (after childbirth), 1479–1480
  pseudodementia of, 484
  suicide and, 616, 623
  transient, 615
Depth perception, 1279
DeQuervain's syndrome, 419
Derealization, 638
Dermabrasion, 1208
Dermatitis, 1193–1198
  of anus, 763–764
  atopic, 1194–1196
  chronic, 1193, 1198
  contact, 1193–1194, *1193, 1195*
  diaper, 1534–1535
  exfoliative, 1196–1197
  in food allergy, 1068
  hot-tub, 1223–1224
  in infants and young children, 1535
  nummular, 1196
  perioral, 1198
  poison ivy, *1195*
  scratch, 1198
  seborrheic, 1196, 1294
  stasis, 1197–1198
Dermatitis herpetiformis, 1217–1218
  in celiac disease, 736, 1217
Dermatofibroma, 1234–1235

Dermatomes, *563*
Dermatomyositis, 383–384
  in cancer, *1037*
Dermatophytid eruption, 1225
Dermatophytoses (fungal skin infection), 1225–1228
Dermis, 1187, *1187* (*see also* Skin)
Dermoid cyst, *520*
DES (diethylstilbestrol), 1408, *1461*
Desensitization (immunotherapy), 1064, 1066–1067
Desert rheumatism, 1151
Deslorelin, *1557*
Desmopressin
  in bed-wetting, 1545
  in central diabetes insipidus, 945
  in nephrogenic diabetes insipidus, 851
Desquamative gingivitis, 682–683
Desquamative interstitial pneumonia, 302–303
Detergents, 1189–1190
Detoxification
  in alcohol abuse, 651–652
  in antianxiety drug dependence, 654
  in cocaine abuse, 657
  in opioid dependence, 653
Development
  adolescent
    behavioral, 1553–1554
      problems in, 1558–1559
    intellectual, 1553–1554
    physical, 1552–1553, *1553*
    social, 1554
  child
    behavioral, 1540–1542, 1543
      mental retardation and, 1627, 1628
    intellectual, 1539–1540, 1543
    normal, 1538–1543, *1539*
    pervasive disorders of, 1630–1632
    physical, 1538–1539, *1540, 1541*
    problems in, 1543–1544, *1544, 1548, 1549*
  infant
    behavioral, 1491–1492, *1491*
    intellectual, 1491–1492, *1491*
    physical, 1490–1491, *1490*
Deviated septum, 1262
Dexamethasone (*see also* Corticosteroids)
  in canker sores, 668
  in transplantation, *1078*
Dexamethasone suppression test, 959, 960
DEXA (dual-energy x-ray absorptiometry) scan, 342, 345, 881, *1729*
Dexchlorpheniramine, *1065*
  in elderly persons, *80*
Dextromethorphan, 98, 249, *1158*
Diabetes insipidus
  central, 944–945
  high sodium levels in, 913
  nephrogenic, 851, 945
  urine output in, 824

Diabetes mellitus, 962–969
   atherosclerosis in, 197, 964
   in children, 1613–1615, *1615*
   cholesterol levels in, 921
   complications of, *963, 964,* 1615
   coronary artery disease in, 200
   eye problems (retinopathy) in, *963, 964,*
      1313–1314
   foot care in, 222, *222,* 964, *965*
   gestational, 1441, 1452–1453
   infection in, 964, *965*
   information resources on, 1761–1762
   insulin-dependent (type I), 962, *1074*
      in children, 1613
   ketoacidosis in, *963,* 966
      in children, 1613–1614, 1615
   kidney problems in, 840, 964
   low blood sugar (hypoglycemia) in, 966,
      970–972, 1615
   nerve problems (neuropathy) in, 584, *963,*
      964
   non–insulin-dependent (type II), *20,* 962
      in children, 1613, *1615*
   oral contraceptive use and, 1420
   over-the-counter drug precautions in, *102*
   pancreatitis and, 733
   during pregnancy, 1441, 1447–1448,
      1452–1453
      fetal effects of, 1499
      screening for, 1453
   prevention of, *27*
   tests for, 964–965
   travel and, 1712
   treatment of, 965–969
      in children, 1614–1615
      insulin for, 966–968, *967,* 1614
      oral drugs for, 968–969, *968,* 1614
      pancreas transplantation in, 1080–1081
   urine output in, 824
Diagnostic and Statistical Manual of Mental
   Disorders (DSM), 599
Diagnostic tests, 1724–1725, *1728–1731*
Dialysis
   hemodialysis, 831, 833–837, *834, 836*
   in hypercalcemia, 905
   in maple syrup urine disease, 1619
   peritoneal, 833–837, *835, 836*
      peritonitis and, 782
   in poisoning, 1676
   reasons for, *833*
Diapering, 1489
Diaper rash, 1534–1535
Diaphragm (contraceptive), *1420,* 1423–1424,
   1424
   bladder infection with, 868
Diaphragm (respiratory muscle), 247, *247*
   age-associated changes in, 248
   hernia of, 727, *728,* 1522
   paralysis of, in newborn, 1495
   spasms of (hiccups), *545*

Diarrhea, *699,* 754–756, *755*
   in amebiasis, 1136
   antibiotic-associated, 745–746
   in carcinoid tumors, 974
   in cholera, 1100–1101
   in *Clostridium difficile* infection, 746
   in *Clostridium perfringens* food poisoning,
      724–725
   in collagenous colitis, 744–745
   in Crohn's disease, 739
   in cryptosporidiosis, 1137–1138
   dehydration in, 755, 756, 928–929
   drug-induced, *723*
   drugs for, 756, *756*
   in *Escherichia coli* infection, 723–724
   exudative, 754
   in food poisoning, 724–726
   in gastroenteritis, 719–726, *720–721,*
      1587
   in giardiasis, 1138
   in infants and young children, 1533
   in irritable bowel syndrome, 756–757
   in lactose intolerance, 735–736
   in lymphocytic colitis, 744–745
   osmotic, 754
   in radiation illness, 1659
   in salmonellosis, *1089,* 1110
   secretory, 754
   in shigellosis, 1110–1111
   in staphylococcal food poisoning, 724
   traveler's, 725, 1713–1714
   in ulcerative colitis, 742–744
Diazepam, *607*
   during breastfeeding, *1462*
   in elderly persons, *81*
   during pregnancy, *1460*
DIC (disseminated intravascular coagulation),
   1001
   in labor and delivery, 1474
   in placental abruption, 1456
Dicloxacillin, *1123*
Dicyclomine, in elderly persons, *81*
Didanosine (ddI), *1175*
Diet, 884–887 (*see also* Food; Nutrition)
   bland, *723*
   during breastfeeding, 1477
   in burn injury, 1651
   cancer risk and, 1033
   in celiac disease, 736–737
   coronary artery disease and, 200
   in Crohn's disease, 741
   in cystic fibrosis, 321
   in diabetes mellitus, 965–966, 1614
   in dialysis, 835
   in diverticulosis, 747
   elimination, 1068–1069
   fad, 886–887
   food-combining and food-cycling, 887
   food guide pyramid for, 884, *885*
   in fructose intolerance, 1618

Diet *(continued)*
  in galactosemia, 1617
  in gastroenteritis, 723
  gluten-free, 736–737
  in Hartnup disease, 853
  high-fiber, 886
    in constipation, 752
    in coronary artery disease, 201
  high protein–low carbohydrate,
      885–886
  information resources on, 1766
  in irritable bowel syndrome, 757
  in kidney failure, 831, 832–833
  liquid, 886
  in liver encephalopathy, 796
  in liver failure, 796
  low-carbohydrate, 886
  low-cholesterol, 922–923, *923, 924*
  low-fat, 886, 922–923, *923, 924*
    in coronary artery disease, 200, *201*
  low-fiber, 751
  in MCAD deficiency, 1621
  in nephrotic syndrome, 841
  obesity and, 915
  in osteoporosis prevention, 345
  in pancreatitis, 733
  in Parkinson's disease, 548
  in peptic ulcer, 716
  in phenylketonuria, 1618–1619
  in porphyria, 935
  during pregnancy, 1443
  in rheumatoid arthritis, 371
  stomach cancer and, 767
  tooth decay and, 677–678
  in ulcerative colitis, 743
  in urinary tract stones, 866
  vegetarian, 898
  weight loss, 884–887, 918
Dietary Supplement Health Education Act
    (1994), 106
Dietary supplements, 103–112
  drug interactions with, 76, 78, *104–106,*
      107
Diethylpropion, 919
Diethylstilbestrol (DES), 1408, *1461*
Diethyltoluamide (DEET), *1007,* 1134
Diffusing capacity of lung, 255
Diffusion, in gas exchange, 246
DiGeorge anomaly, 1061, 1083
Digestive system, 4–5, *6*
  age-associated changes in, 698
  air in, 1486, 1531
  anthrax infection of, 1098
  biology of, 694–698, *695*
  birth defects of, *1512,* 1520–1521, *1521*
  bleeding in, 699–700, 705, 776–778, *777*
  blockage of, 700, 707–708, 751, 770,
      779–781, *780*
  Campylobacter infection of, 1099–1100

Digestive system *(continued)*
  cancer of, 764–776, *765, 767, 769, 771, 774*
    bleeding in, 778
    carcinoid, 974–975
    staging of, *1040*
  disorders of, 699–783 (*see also specific*
      structures, eg, Esophagus; Stomach)
    in children, 1586–1593, *1591, 1592*
    in diabetes mellitus, *963,* 971
    in dying person, 49
    emergency, 776–783
    information resources on, 1762
    in multiple endocrine neoplasia, 973
    in non-Hodgkin's lymphoma, *1021*
    in premature infant, 1497
    symptoms of, 699–702
    tests for, 703–706, *704*
  diverticular disease of, 747–750, *748, 749,*
      751–752
  examination of, 702–706, *704*
  foreign objects in, 727–729, 751
  hormones of, 938, *939*
  indigestion and (*see* Indigestion)
  infection of (*see* Gastroenteritis)
  in infection prevention, 1088
  inflammatory disorders of, 738–745, *741*
  malabsorption in, 734–738, *735*
  in niacin deficiency, 897
  radiation effects on, 1659
  sexually transmitted diseases of, 1183–1184
  tumors of, 764–776
    carcinoid, 974–975
Digital substraction angiography, 130
Digits (*see* Finger[s]; Toe[s])
Digoxin
  in arrhythmias, *167*
  in elderly persons, *81*
  food interactions with, 77
  generic substitutions for, *90, 92*
  in heart failure, 156, *157*
  in mitral stenosis, 180
  in pregnancy, 1459
Dihydrotestosterone, 1212
Dilated (congestive) cardiomyopathy,
    158–161, *159*
Dilation and curettage (D and C), 1354, *1354,*
    1729
  after childbirth, 1474
  in dysfunctional uterine bleeding, 1367
Dilation and evacuation (D and E), 1427
Dimenhydrinate, *471*
Dimercaprol, 1681
2,5-Dimethoxy-4-methylamphetamine,
    657–658
Dimethyl sulfoxide, *869*
Diphenhydramine, *1065*
  in common cold, *1158*
  in elderly persons, *80*
  in sleep disorders, *471*

Diphenoxylate, *756*
Diphtheria, 1563
  immunization for, 1093, *1094*, 1492, *1493,*
    1562
Diphyllobothriasis (fish tapeworm infection),
  1143–1144
Dipivefrin, *1308*
Diplopia (double vision), 1279
  in Graves' disease, 950, 952
Dipyridamole
  in Kawasaki syndrome, *1581*
  in stroke prevention, 505
Directive to doctor (living will), *53, 55*
Dirithromycin, *1123*
Disability, information resources on, 1762
Discharge
  nipple, 1387–1388
  vaginal, 1349–1350, 1375
    after childbirth, 1476
    during pregnancy, 1439
Discipline problems
  in adolescents, 1559
  in children, *1544*
  time-out procedure for, 1547
Disclosure, 54
Discoid lupus erythematosus, 378
Discrimination testing, of hearing, 1249
Disinfecting agents, 1191
Diskectomy, 574
Disks, intervertebral, *436*
  degeneration of, 564–565
  herniated (ruptured, "slipped"), 569, *570,*
    571, 574
Disopyramide, in elderly persons, *81*
Dissection, aortic, 119, 229–231, *230*
  in Marfan syndrome, 1608
Disseminated intravascular coagulation
  (DIC), 1001
  in labor and delivery, 1474
  in placental abruption, 1456
Dissociative identity disorder, 638–639,
  639
Disulfiram, 651–652
Diuretics
  abuse of, *647*
  dehydration with, 144, 928–929
  in diabetes insipidus, 851, 945
  in heart failure, 155–157, *156*
  in high blood pressure, *138,* 139
  in mitral stenosis, 180
  orthostatic hypotension with, 146
  potassium deficiency with, 910
  during pregnancy, 1459, *1460*
  urinary incontinence with, *859*
  in urinary tract stones, 866
Divalproex
  in manic-depressive illness, 621
  in seizure disorders, *500*
Diversion colitis, 745

Diverticula (*see also* Diverticulitis;
    Diverticulosis)
  bladder, 1519
  in Ehlers-Danlos syndrome, 1608
  esophageal, 709–710
  Meckel's, 1590–1591, *1591*
Diverticulitis, 748–750, *749*
  in Meckel's diverticulum, 1590–1591
  surgery for, *749,* 750
Diverticulosis, 747–748, *748, 749*
Diving
  air embolism with, 286, 289
  barotrauma with, 1256–1257, *1257*
  decompression sickness (bends) with,
    1669–1671, *1669, 1670*
  injuries with, 1666–1671, *1669, 1670*
  risk factors for, *1670*
Diving reflex, 1665
Divorce, 1640–1641, *1640*
Dix-Hallpike maneuver, 464
Dizziness, 461–467 (*see also* Vertigo)
  tilt table for, 39
DNA, 8–9, *10*
  cell transfer of (gene therapy), 15–16
  laboratory copying of, 15
  mitochondrial, 14
Doctor (*see* Physician)
Docusate, 752, *753*
Dog bite, 1682
DOM (2,5-dimethoxy-4-
    methylamphetamine), 657–658
Domestic violence, 1410–1412
  effects on children, *1411*
Donation
  of blood, 983–984, *983, 985, 986*
  of organs, 1075–1076
Dong quai, 1361
Do-not-resuscitate order, 48, *56, 57*
Dopamine
  in chorea, 552
  in Parkinson's disease, 546–550
  in pheochromocytoma, 960–961
Doppler ultrasonography
  in deep vein thrombosis, 233
  in heart disease, 126
  in neurologic disorders, 445
  in peripheral arterial disease, 218–219
Dornase alfa, 250
  in cystic fibrosis, 321
Dorzolamide, *1308*
Double vision, 1279
Douching, 1377
Dowager's hump, 345
Down syndrome, 1527–1528
  accelerated aging in, 21
  information resources on, 1762
  prenatal testing for, 1431
  risk for, *1431*
Doxazosin, 1330

Doxepin, in elderly persons, *80*
Doxorubicin, *1045*
Doxycycline, *1123*
  in acne, 1206, *1207*
  in malaria, 1141
Drainage
  of lung (postural), 261
  of skin abscess, 1224
Dressing
  after surgery, 1703
  occlusive, 1191
  for pressure sores, 1209
Dressler's syndrome, 188, 213, 215
Dronabinol
  in HIV infection, 1174
  in undernutrition, 890
Drotrecogin alfa, 1119
Drowning, near, 1665–1666
Drugs, 60–112 *(see also specific drugs)*
  for abortion, 1427
  absorption of, 67–68
  abuse of, 60, 646–659, *647*
    by adolescents, 1559–1560, 1636
    alcohol *(see* Alcohol use and abuse)
    amphetamines, 656, 1464
    antianxiety drugs, 653–654, *654*
    cocaine, 656–657, 1463
    definition of, 646
    endocarditis and, 184
    gamma hydroxybutyrate, 658–659
    hallucinogens, 657–658
    HIV infection transmission and,
      1168–1169
    information resources on, 1762
    ketamine, 658
    marijuana, 655–656, 1464
    opioids, 652–653, 1464
    phencyclidine, 658
    during pregnancy, 1463–1464
    prescription drugs, 653–654, *654*
    sedatives, 653–654, *654*
    sleep aids, 653–654, *654*
    solvent inhalants, 658, 659, *659*
  action of, 72–73
  addiction to, 647 *(see also* Drugs,
    abuse of)
  administration of, 64–67
  adverse reactions to, 62, 82–86, *83,*
    1198–1200, 1232, *1232*
    in elderly persons, 79
  aging and, 79–81, *80–81*
  allergic reactions to, 85, 843–844, 1064,
    1069, 1072–1073
  anesthetic, 1699–1700
  antidiuretic hormone secretion with, *913*
  anxiety reaction with, 606, 608
  benefits vs. risks of, 84
  bioequivalence of, 91–92
  during breastfeeding, *1462*

Drugs *(continued)*
  classification of, 60
  clotting effects of, *996*
  compliance issues in, *63,* 76, 81, 86–88, *87*
  consciousness alterations with, 491, *492*
  constipation with, 751
  contact dermatitis with, *1193*
  delirium with, 481
  dependence on, 450, 646–647 *(see also*
    Drugs, abuse of)
  depressive reaction with, 615, *615*
  dermatitis with, 1197
  design and development of, 60–61, 91
  diarrhea with, 745–746
  dietary supplement interactions with, 76,
    78, *104–106,* 107
  digestive tract bleeding with, 777
  disease interactions with, 78
  distribution of, 68, 70–72
  dry mouth and, 666
  for dying persons, 48
  dynamics of, 69–73
  effectiveness of, 63
  efficacy of, 73
  in elderly persons, 79–81, *80–81,* 84–85,
    101, 788
  elimination of, 69
  fetal effects of, 1458–1464, *1459, 1460–1461*
  folic acid deficiency with, 899
  food interactions with, 77, 78
  formulations of, 67–68
  galactorrhea with, 946
  gastroenteritis with, *723*
  generic, 60, 88–92, *89, 90–91*
  gingivitis with, 682
  hair loss with, 1213
  hearing loss with, 1248
  heat disorders with, 1652
  hepatitis with, 803
  homocysteinemia with, 198
  immunosuppressive *(see* Immunosuppressive
    drugs [immunomodulators])
  for indigestion, 99
  for inflammation, 97
  injection of, 64–66, *65*
  interactions between, 75–76, *76,* 102–103
  kinetics of, 64
  during labor and delivery, 1464
  manic reaction with, *620*
  metabolism of, 68–69
  multiple, 84
  names of, 60, 88–89, *89*
  nephrotic syndrome with, 840, *840*
  optimal benefit from, *63*
  oral color changes with, *663*
  orthostatic hypotension with, 146
  overdose toxicity of, 85–86
  over-the-counter, 22, 92, 93–103, *94, 96, 97,*
    98, 100, 102

Drugs *(continued)*
  patent for, 89
  pericarditis from, 188
  photosensitivity reactions with, 1232, *1232*
  placebos, 61, *61*
  potassium levels and, 910–911
  potency of, 73
  during pregnancy, 85, 1443, 1449–1450,
    1458–1464, *1459, 1460–1461*
  rash with, 1198–1199
  response to, 73–78, *74*
  risk-benefit analysis of, 1697, 1698
  safety of, 63
  seizures with, *496*
  side effects of *(see* Drugs, adverse reactions
    to)
  site selectivity of, 70–72, *70, 71–72, 73*
  for sleep problems, 100
  sperm problems with, 1415
  Steven-Johnson syndrome with, 1199–1200
  storage of, 67–68
  testing of, *62*
  tolerance to, 78
  topical, 66, 1188–1191
  toxic epidermal necrolysis with, 1199–1200
  trade names of, 60, *1733–1755*
  for travel, 1709–1710
  undernutrition and, 888
  urinary incontinence with, *859*
  weight gain and, 916
Dry eye, 1282, 1300–1301
  in Sjögren's syndrome, 382–383
Drying agents, 1190
Dry mouth, 666
  in dying person, 49
  radiation therapy and, 1660
  in Sjögren's syndrome, 382–383
Dry skin, 1191–1192, *1192*
Dry socket, 692
DSM *(Diagnostic and Statistical Manual of
  Mental Disorders)*, 599
DTs (delirium tremens), 649
Dual-energy x-ray absorptiometry (DEXA),
  342, 345, *881, 1729*
Duchenne's muscular dystrophy, 412–413,
  1430
Duck-bill deformity, 396–397
Ductus arteriosus, 1513
  coarctation of aorta and, 1518
  patent, 1514, *1515*
Duodenum, 696
  blockage of, 779
  gastrinoma of, 775–776
  ulcers of, 713–717, *715, 718*
    in children, 1589
Dupuytren's contracture, 397–398
Durable power of attorney for health care, *53,*
  55–56, 1701
Dura mater, 435, *435, 436*

Dusts
  asbestos, 296, *297*
  in asthma, 274–275, *277*
  beryllium, *297,* 298–299
  coal, 296, *297*
  fiber, *297, 299,* 300
  house, 1067–1068
  organic, 308–310
  silica (quartz), 295–296, *297*
Dwarfism, 942, 1556, 1611
Dwarf tapeworm, *1146*
Dyclonine, 668
Dyes
  food, 1068
  radiopaque (contrast), *827*
    anaphylactoid reactions to, *1069*
Dying *(see* Death and dying)
Dysarthria, 478, 556
  rehabilitation for, 44
Dysbetalipoproteinemia, 926
Dyschezia, 751, 752
Dyschromatopsia *(see* Color blindness)
Dysentery *(see also* Diarrhea)
  bacillary (shigellosis), 1110–1111
Dysesthesia, oral (burning mouth syndrome),
  665
Dysfunctional uterine bleeding, 1367
Dysgeusia, 596
Dysgraphia, 478
Dyshidrosis, 1198
Dyslexia, 1551–1552
Dysmenorrhea, *1362,* 1364
Dysmetria, 556
Dysosmia, 596
Dyspareunia, 1382–1383
Dyspepsia, 700, 712
Dysphagia *(see* Swallowing, difficulty in)
Dysphagia lusoria, 707
Dysphonia, 554
Dysplastic nevi (atypical moles), 1234, 1240
Dyspnea *(see* Breath, shortness of)
Dysthymia, 616
Dystocia, shoulder, 1473
Dystonia, 554–556
Dystrophin, 412–413

E

E. coli infection *(see Escherichia coli*
  infection)
Earache, *1258*
Eardrum, 1244, *1245*
  examination of, 1594, 1595, 1598
  infection of, 1257
  perforation of, 1256, 1258–1259, 1599
  pressure damage to, 1256–1257, *1257,* 1667
  rupture of, 1594, 1667
  ventilating tubes for, *1595*

Ears (*see also* Hearing)
   acoustic neuroma of, 1260–1261
   age-associated changes in, 17, *18*,
      1246–1247
   aspergillosis of, 1149
   biology of, 1244–1245, *1245*
   blockage of, 1253, *1254*
      in nasopharyngeal cancer, 1273
   cancer of, 1255
   disorders of, 1247–1253, *1254, 1257, 1258,
      1261* (*see also specific disorders, eg,*
      Hearing, loss of)
      in vertigo, 463, 465–467
   foreign objects in, 1253, 1599
   infection of, 1248, 1253–1255, 1257–1259,
      1258
      in children, 1593–1594, *1595*
      pseudomonal, 1109
   injury to, 1255
      from pressure, 1256–1257, *1257*
   insect in, 1253
   irrigation of, 1253, *1254*
   pain in (earache), *1258*
   popping of, 1244
   pressure in
      in air travel, 1244, 1256–1257, 1710
      injuries from, 1256–1257, *1257*, 1667
   ringing in (tinnitus), 1259, 1261
   swimmer's, 1109, 1110, 1253–1255
   temperature taking from, *1536*
   tumors of, 1255
   wax in, 1253, *1254*
Earwax, 1253, *1254*
Eastern equine encephalitis, 537
Eating disorders, 624–627
   information resources on, 1763
   menstrual problems and, 1365
   in young children, 1544–1545
Eaton-Lambert syndrome, 581, *1037*
Ebola virus infection, 1165
ECG (*see* Electrocardiography)
Echinacea, *104*, 108, 1157
Echinococcosis (hydatid disease), 540, *1146*
Echocardiography, 125–126, 154, *1729*
   in aortic stenosis, 182
   in coronary artery disease, 204
   in endocarditis, 186
   in fainting, 145
   in heart attack, 213
   in heart defects, 1513–1514
   in heart tumors, 192
   in mitral regurgitation, 177
   in pericarditis, 191
   in pulmonary hypertension, 324
   in rheumatic fever, 1567
Echoencephalography, 444
Echolalia, 552, 1630
Echothiophate, *1308*
   in esotropia, 1602

Eclampsia, 1452
ECMO (extracorporeal membrane
      oxygenation), in persistent pulmonary
      hypertension, 1502
Ecstasy (methylenedioxymethamphetamine),
      656
   adolescent use of, 1559–1560
Ectopic corticotropin syndrome, 958
Ectopic pregnancy, *1455*
Ectropion (turned-out eyelid), 1278, 1295, *1295*
Eczema (*see* Dermatitis)
Eczema herpeticum, 1161, 1195
Edema (*see* Swelling)
Edetate calcium disodium, 1681
EEG (*see* Electroencephalography)
Efavirenz, *1175*
Effusion
   around the heart (pericardial), 190–191
   around the lungs (pleural), 251, 314–316,
      315
      aspiration of, 256
      in cancer, 329, *1036*
      in non-Hodgkin's lymphoma, *1021*
      in tuberculosis, 1127
Eflornithine cream, 1212, 1350
Eggs (human), 1345, *1346*
   donor, 1419
   fertilization of (*see* Fertilization)
   release of (*see* Ovulation)
Egyptian ophthalmia, 1297–1298
Ehlers-Danlos syndrome, 1608
Ehrlichioses, 1134–1135
Eighth nerve tumor, 1260–1261
Eisenmenger's syndrome, 1446
Ejaculation, 1323–1324, 1336
   premature, *1339*, 1340
   retrograde, 1340, 1415
   withdrawal before, *1420*, 1426
EKG (*see* Electrocardiography)
Elastic stockings
   in deep vein thrombosis, 234, 235
   in varicose veins, 237
Elation, 613–614
   in mania, 619–620
Elbow
   drug abuser's (myositis ossificans), 652
   fracture of, 358
   nerve damage at, 399–400
   tennis, 427–429, *427, 428*
Elderly persons (*see also* Aging)
   antacids for, 101
   antihistamines for, *80*, 101
   blood pressure changes in, 117–118, 131, *132*
   compliance in, 87
   dehydration in, 928–929, 930
   depression in, 616–617
   diseases in, 19–21, *20*
   drug use in, 79–81, *80–81*, 84–85, 788
   heart changes in, 117–118

Elderly persons *(continued)*
  heatstroke in, 1653–1654
  high sodium levels in, 913–914
  liver encephalopathy in, 796
  over-the-counter drugs for, 101
  undernutrition in, 887, 888
  vitamin D deficiency in, 894
Electrical injuries, 1661–1663
Electrical shock, for cardioversion, 124, 167
Electrical stimulation, of muscles, 37–38
Electrocardiography (ECG, EKG), 122–123,
    122, 1724, *1729*
  in arrhythmias, 165
  continuous ambulatory, 123–124, *124*
    in angina evaluation, 204
  in electrical injury, 1663
  in fainting, 145
  in heart attack, 213
  in heart failure, 154
  in long QT syndrome, 1530
  in pericarditis, 188
  in rheumatic fever, 1566–1567
  in stroke, 509
Electrocochleography, 1250
Electroconvulsive therapy, 600, 619
Electroencephalography, 445–446, 1724, *1729*
  in brain death, 494
  in encephalitis, 1570
  in liver encephalopathy, 796
  in seizures, 498, *498*
Electrolarynx, *1272*
Electrolysis, 1212, 1350
Electrolytes, 900–914, *902–903 (see also
    specific substances)*
  abnormal levels of, 901
    in anorexia, 625
    in Bartter's syndrome, 853–854
    in dehydration, 929
    in delirium, 481
    in diarrhea, 722, 755, 1587
    in Fanconi's syndrome, 852
    in heat cramps, 1653
    in heat exhaustion, 1653
    in Liddle's syndrome, 854
    water balance and, 928
  functions of, 901
  reference range for, *1726*
Electromyography, 342, 446, *1729*
Electronic fetal heart monitoring, 1465, 1467,
    1467, 1471
Electronystagmography, 464
Electrophoresis
  in multiple myeloma, 1007
  in sickle cell disease, 993
Electrophysiologic testing, 124, 165, *1729*
Electroretinography, 1285
Electroversion, 167
Elephantiasis, 240, 868
Elimination diet, 1068–1069

ELISA test, *1729*
  for HIV infection, 1172
  for pregnancy, 1435
Elliptocytosis, hereditary, *989*
Embolism
  air, 286, 289, 1668
  amniotic fluid, 286, 289, 1473–1474
  from aneurysm, 226
  brain (cerebral), 154
  from cardiac tumors, 192, 193
  in cardiomyopathy, 160
  from deep veins, 232–233
  in endocarditis, 185
  fat, 195, 286, 289, 507
  in heart attack, 211
  lung *(see* Pulmonary embolism)
  of renal arteries, 846–847
  tumor, 286
Embolization, uterine artery, 1374
Embryo
  development of, 1436–1437, *1436, 1437*
  transfer of, 1419
Emergency, 22 *(see also* Cardiopulmonary
    resuscitation [CPR]; Injury [injuries];
    Poisoning)
  first aid for, 1687–1693, *1688*
Emergency contraception, 1423
Emesis *(see* Vomiting)
EMG *(see* Electromyography)
Emollients, 1190
Emotion(s)
  in childhood schizophrenia, 1632
  in children, 1540–1542
  disease and, 7–8
  disorders of *(see* Mental health disorders)
Emphysema, 281–285
  in alpha$_1$-antitrypsin deficiency, 801
  over-the-counter drug precautions in, *102*
Empty sella syndrome, 947–948
Empyema, 314, 315
  subdural, 540
Enamel, tooth, 662–663, 675
Encephalitis, 532–538
  arbovirus, 537–538
  California, 537
  in children, 1569–1570
    enteroviral, *1576*
    herpes, 1570
    measles, 1576, 1582
    varicella-zoster virus, 1571
  equine, 537
  herpes, 534, 535, 1162
  immunization for, *1709*
  Japanese, *1094*
  parainfectious (postinfectious), 533
  rabies, 535–537, *536*
  rubella, 1582
  in toxoplasmosis, 1145
  West Nile, 537

Encephalocele, 1526
Encephalomyelitis, 560, 1570
Encephalopathy
  in chronic kidney failure, 831
  hypertensive, 134, 141
  lead, 1681
  liver (hepatic), 795–796
    coma with, *492*
  radiation therapy and, 528
  spongiform (prion disease), 541–543, *542*
  traumatic, 490
  Wernicke's, 479–480, 650, 896
Encopresis, 1545–1546
Endarterectomy, 506–507
Endocarditis, 184–187, *186*
  antibiotic prevention of, *187*
  gonococcal, 1179
  heart valve disease and, 178
  Löffler's, 1005
  noninfective, *185*
  Pseudomonas, 1110
  in rheumatic fever, 1566
  staphylococcal, 1112
  streptococcal, 1113
Endocervical curettage, 1354
Endocrine system, 5, 6, 937–940 (*see also*
    Gland[s]; Hormone[s])
Endolymphatic shunt procedure, 1260
Endometrioma, 1368
Endometriosis, 1369–1372, *1370, 1371*
Endometritis, 1377
Endometrium, 1345, *1345*
  biopsy of, 1354, 1403, 1416
  cancer of, 1350, 1358, 1403–1404, *1404*
    staging of, *1402*
  dilation and curettage of, 1354, *1354*
  menstrual cycle of, 1346–1348, *1347*
  uterine ingrowth of (adenomyosis), *1365*
Endophthalmitis, 1314
Endorphins, 32, 940, *941*
Endoscopic retrograde
    cholangiopancreatography (ERCP), 789,
    790, 1729
  in bile duct cancer, 817
  in gallstones, 815
  in pancreatitis, 732, 733
  in primary sclerosing cholangitis, 801
Endoscopy, 703, *704,* 1724, *1729*
  in esophageal cancer, 765
  in gastroesophageal reflux, 718, 1589
  in intestinal obstruction, 781
  in peptic ulcers, 714–715
  in small intestine cancer, 768
  in stomach cancer, 767
  ultrasound with, 705
  of urinary tract, 828
Enemas, 753–754
Energy (*see also* Calories)
  in food, 883
  requirements for, 883

Energy therapies, 1707
Enkephalins, *941*
Enoxacin, *1123*
Entacapone, *549*
Entamoeba histolytica infection, *720,*
    1135–1136
Enteral feeding, 889–890
Enteric fever, *1094,* 1117–1118
Enteritis (*see also* Gastroenteritis)
  regional (Crohn's disease), 738–742, *741*
Enterobacteriaceae infection, 1101, 1103
Enterobacter infection, 1103
Enterobiasis (pinworm infection), 1142
Enterocele, 1379–1380, *1381*
Enterocolitis
  necrotizing, 1504–1505
  toxic, 1522
Enterohepatic circulation, 697
Enteropathy, gluten (celiac disease),
    736–737
Enteroviral infections, *1576*
  polio, 1578–1579
Entropion (turned-in eyelid), 1295, *1295*
Enuresis (bed-wetting), 824, 1545
Envenomation, 1682–1683
Environmental factors
  in cancer, 1033–1034
  in child development, 1542–1543
  in dementia, 486, *487*
  in infant development, 1492
  in risk assessment, 25, *26*
Enzymes, 1616
  digestive, 697, 731, 733, 734
    tests for, 735
  drug effects on, 72
  in drug metabolism, 68, 74
  in heart attack, 213
  liver, *789*
  in porphyrias, 933–936
Eosinophil(s), 978, *1052,* 1053–1054
  in asthma, 274
  in chronic granulomatous disease, 1062
  disorders of, 1005
  in infection, 1088
Eosinophilic fasciitis, 385–386
Eosinophilic gastritis, 711, 713
Eosinophilic granuloma, 304
Eosinophilic pneumonia, 310–311
Ependymoma, *520, 527*
Epicondylitis, 427–429, *427, 428*
Epidemic pleurodynia, *1576*
Epidemic typhus, *1133*
Epidermal cyst, 1237
Epidermis, 1186, *1187*
Epidermoid tumor, *520*
Epidermophyton infection (ringworm),
    1225–1226
Epididymis, 1322, *1322*
Epididymitis, 1328
Epididymo-orchitis, 1328

Epidural block, in labor and delivery, 1468
Epidural hemorrhage, *511, 518*
Epiglottis, 244, *245*, 696, 1246, *1246*
Epiglottitis, 1268
　in children, 1564
Epilepsia partialis continua, 497
Epilepsy, 495–502, *500–501*
　information resources on, 1763
　posttraumatic, 513–514
　reflex, 495
Epinephrine (adrenaline), 5, *939*
　in anaphylactic (allergic) reactions, 1065,
　　1073
　in asthma, 1584
　in blood pressure control, 132
　in croup, 1586
　in food allergy, 1069
　in glaucoma, *1308*
　in heart failure, 153
　in hypoglycemia, 971
　in pheochromocytoma, 960–961
　receptors for, *71*
Epiphora, 1293
Epiretinal membrane, 1311
Episcleritis, 1299
Episiotomy, 1469
Epispadias, 1519
Epistaxis, 1263
Epley maneuver, *466*, 467
Epstein-Barr virus infection, 1163–1164
　in Burkitt's lymphoma, *1020*
　cancer and, *1155*
　in head and neck cancer, 1273
　in Hodgkin's disease, 1017
Epstein's pearls, *1496*
Equine encephalitis, 537
Erb's muscular dystrophy, 413
ERCP (*see* Endoscopic retrograde
　cholangiopancreatography)
Erectile dysfunction, 1336–1339
　in acromegaly, 945
　in galactorrhea, 946
　information resources on, 1763
Erection, 1323, 1336
　distorted (Peyronie's disease), 1326
　failure of (*see* Erectile dysfunction)
　persistent (priapism), 1325–1326
Ergocalciferol (vitamin D$_2$), 894
Ergotamine, *460*, 461
Erosive gastritis, 711, 712, 713
Ertapenem, *1122*
Erysipelas, 1221
Erysipelothricosis, *1102*
Erythema infectiosum, 1535, *1569,*
　1572–1573
Erythema marginatum, 1566
Erythema migrans, 1106
Erythema multiforme, 1200
Erythema nodosum, *387*, 1200–1201
Erythrasma, 1222–1223

Erythroblastosis fetalis, 1453, *1506*, 1507
Erythroblastosis neonatorum, 1453
Erythrocyte (*see* Red blood cells)
Erythrocyte sedimentation rate, 342, 1074,
　1726
Erythroderma, 1196–1197
Erythrodermic psoriasis, 1202
Erythromelalgia, 225
Erythromycin, *1123*
　in acne, 1206, *1207*
　drug interactions of, 76
　topical, *1207*
Erythroplakia, 671
Erythroplasia of Queyrat, 1325
Erythropoietic protoporphyria, 936
Erythropoietin, 822, *939*, 979
　abuse of, *647*
　in kidney failure, 829, 833
　in multiple myeloma, 1008
　in polycythemia vera, 1024
Eschar, 1649–1650
Escharotomy, 1651
Escherichia coli infection, *720*
　intestine, 721, 723–724, 1101, 1103
　kidneys, 871–872
　meninges, 529
Esomeprazole, *718*
Esophageal incoordination, 708
Esophageal speech, *1272*
Esophagitis, 710, 717
　in HIV infection, *1172*
Esophagogastroduodenoscopy, 1724
Esophagoscopy, 703, *704*
　in achalasia, 709
Esophagus, *695, 696, 706–707, 707, 1246*
　achalasia of, 709
　acid reflux into, 706, 707, 717–719,
　　1588–1589
　age-associated changes in, 698, 706
　Barrett's, 717, 719
　　cancer and, 765
　bleeding from, 776–778, *777*, 794, 809
　blockage of, 700, 707–708
　cancer of, 764–766, *765*
　chemical burns of, 1678–1679
　compression of, 707
　corrosive injury of, 710, 1678–1679
　development abnormalities (atresia) of,
　　1520–1521, *1521*
　dilation of, 709
　disorders of, 706–710
　　pain with, 701
　diverticula of, 709–710
　endoscopy of, 765
　fistula of, 1520–1521, *1521*
　foreign objects in, 727–729
　globus sensation in, 700
　inflammation of (*see* Esophagitis)
　injury to, 710, 1678–1679
　manometry of, 706, 708–709, 718–719

Esophagus *(continued)*
  narrowing of (stricture), 717, 719
    in poisoning, 1678, 1679
  perforation of, 710, 1678
  pouches of, 709–710
  rings in, 707
  rupture of, 709, 710
  in scleroderma, 381
  spasm of, 708–709
  stuck food sensation (globus) in, 700
  swallowing difficulty in, 700, 706, 708–710
  tumors of, 329, 764–766, 765
  ulcers of, 717
  varicose veins of, 707, 776, 778, 794
    in Budd-Chiari syndrome, 808, 809
    in cirrhosis, 798
    in portal vein thrombosis, 809
    during pregnancy, 1448
    in veno-occlusive disease, 808
  webs in, 707–708
Esotropia, 1601–1602, 1602
ESR (erythrocyte sedimentation rate), 342,
    1074, 1726
Essential tremor, 544–545, 546
Estrogens, 939, 940, 1343
  breast cancer and, 1358–1359
  clot formation and, 996
  cream formulation of, 1359
  in dysfunctional uterine bleeding, 1367
  food interactions with, 77
  generic substitutions for, 90
  menopause and, 1356–1357
  in menstrual cycle, 1346, 1347
  migraine headache and, 457
  in oral contraceptives, 1420
  in porphyria, 934
  during pregnancy, 1441
  in prolactinoma, 947
  receptors for, 1391
  replacement therapy with, 1358–1359, 1360
    in osteoporosis prevention, 345
    in Turner syndrome, 1529
  skin patch formulation of, 1421–1422
  tablet formulation of, 1359
  vaginal ring formulation of, 1421–1422
Etanercept, 372, 375, 1075 (*see also*
    Immunosuppressive drugs
    [immunomodulators])
Ethambutol, 1124, 1129
Ethical issues, 53–57 (*see also* Legal issues)
  in death and dying, 51
Ethmoid sinus, 1245–1246, 1265
Ethosuximide, 500
Etidronate, 347–348, 1610 (*see also*
    Bisphosphonates)
Etretinate, 1458–1459, 1461
Eumelanin, 1212
Eustachian tube, 1244, 1245
  blockage of, 1256–1257, 1257
  in children, 1593

Euthyroid sick syndrome, 949
Evening primrose, 1361
Evoked otoacoustic emissions testing,
    1598
Evoked responses, 446, 559
Ewing's sarcoma, 361
Examination (*see* Physical examination)
Excoriation, 1189
Exercise, 31–36
  aerobic, 33, 35
  after hip fracture, 43
  after menopause, 1358
  allergy to, 1070–1071
  ambulation, 39
  anaerobic, 33, 36
  in ankylosing spondylitis, 377
  asthma with, 276, 1070–1071
  in back pain prevention, 573
  benefits of, 31–32
  breathing, 261–262
  calories burned during, 34
  conditioning, 39
  cooling down for, 34, 421
  coordination, 39
  in COPD, 259–260
  in coronary artery disease prevention,
    197–198, 202
  with dieting, 884, 918–919
  in elderly persons, 32
  fainting with, 143–144
  in fracture, 353
  heartbeats (heart rate) in, 33
  in heart failure, 155
  heat disorder and, 1652–1653
  in high blood pressure, 137
  injury prevention during, 34
  Kegel, 1384
    in pelvic floor disorders, 1380
    in urinary incontinence, 861, 1358
    in vaginismus, 1383–1384
  in multiple sclerosis, 560
  muscle-strengthening, 39, 421 (*see also*
    Strength exercise)
  in osteoarthritis, 368
  in osteoporosis prevention, 345
  in pain prevention, 572
  in peripheral arterial disease, 221
  during pregnancy, 1444
  in pulmonary rehabilitation, 259–260
  range-of-motion, 38–39, 38
  shortness of breath in, 250
  spray and stretch, in temporomandibular
    joint disorders, 689
  stretching for, 34, 421
  warming up for, 34, 421
Exercise stress testing, 123, 127, 204,
    1731
Exertional (effort) syncope, 143–144
Exfoliative dermatitis, 1196–1197
Exhibitionism, 630

Exophthalmos (bulging eyes), 1281, 1319
  in Graves' disease, 950, 952
  in newborn, 1510
Exotropia, 1601–1603, *1602*
Expectant mother (*see* Pregnancy)
Expectorants, 250, *1158*
Exposure therapy, *609*
  for agoraphobia, 610
  for obsessive-compulsive disorder, 612
  for panic attacks and panic disorder, 609
  for phobias, 611
  for social phobia, 610
Exstrophy, of bladder, 1519
External auditory meatus, 1244, *1245*
Extracorporeal membrane oxygenation
    (ECMO), 1502
Extracorporeal shock wave lithotripsy, *865*, 866
Exudative diarrhea, 754
Eye(s) (*see also* Vision)
  age-associated changes in, 17, *18*, 1278
  appearance of, changes in, 1280–1281
  barotrauma to, 1667
  in Behçet's syndrome, 390
  in Bell's palsy, 592
  biology of, 1276–1278, *1276, 1277*
  birth defects of, *1512*
  bleeding in, 1290
  bulging (exophthalmos), 950, 952, 1281, 1319
    in newborn, 1510
  burns to, 1292
  cancer of, 1314, 1623–1624
  in coma, 493
  crossed (strabismus), 1601–1603, *1602*
  disorders of, *1280, 1281, 1282,* 1286–1319
    in children, 1600–1603, *1601, 1602*
    diagnosis of, 1282–1286, *1284, 1285*
    in multiple sclerosis, 558
    symptoms of, 1278–1280
  droopy (Horner's syndrome), *592*
  drug administration to, 66
  dry, 1282, 1300–1301
    in Sjögren's syndrome, 382–383
  foreign objects in, 1291–1292
  in Gaucher's disease, 1620
  glaucoma of, 20, 1279, 1281, 1306–1309,
      1307, 1308 (*see also* Glaucoma)
  Horner's syndrome of, 592
  infection of, 1313 (*see also* Conjunctivitis)
    from contact lenses, 1288
    in gonorrhea, 1179, 1296–1297
    herpes simplex virus, 1161, 1301–1302
  injury to, 1290–1292
  in juvenile rheumatoid arthritis, 1612, 1613
  in Marfan syndrome, 1608
  misalignment of (phoria), 1601
  movement disorders of, 588–589
  muscle weakness of, 588
  in myasthenia gravis, 578
  of newborn, 1484, *1509*
  in newborn meningitis, 1562

Eye(s) (*continued*)
  pink-, *1297* (*see also* Conjunctivitis)
  in premature infant, 1504
  pressure elevation (glaucoma) in, *20,* 1279,
      1281, 1306–1309, *1307, 1308*
  in progressive supranuclear palsy, 550
  protective features of, 1277–1278, *1277*
  refractive disorders of, 1286–1290,
      1287
    in children, *1601*
  sarcoidosis of, 305
  Sjögren's syndrome and, 382–383, 666
  socket of (orbit), 1276, *1277*
    disorders of, 1317–1319
  spasms of, in neuroblastoma, *1037*
  strabismus of, 1601–1603, *1602*
  sunburn of (snow blindness), *1673*
  tumors of, 1314
  ulcers of, 1288, 1300, 1302
    contact lenses and, 1288
    Pseudomonas and, 1109, 1110
  in vitamin A deficiency, 891
Eye chart, 1283
Eye drops, *1295*
  in allergic conjunctivitis, 1067
  in glaucoma, 1309
  in infectious conjunctivitis, 1297
  in injury, 1291
Eyeglasses, 1287–1288
  in amblyopia, 1601
  in esotropia, 1602
  in strabismus, 1602
Eyelashes, 1277, *1277*
  infection of, 1281
Eyelids, 1277, *1277,* 1292
  age-associated changes in, 1278
  burns to, 1292
  cancer of, 1295
  disorders of, 1293–1294
  droopy, 1281
  in Graves' disease, 950
  inflammation of, 1294
  spasm of (blepharospasm), 554
  swelling of, 1281, 1293–1294
  tumors of, 1295

F

Fabry's disease, 1620
Face (*see also* Ears; Eye(s); Mouth; Nose)
  birth defects of, 1523, *1523*
  brown pigmentation of (melasma),
      1215–1216, 1421, 1440–1441
  moon, 958
  of newborn, 1485, 1494–1495
  pain in, *593*
    in Bell's palsy, 591–593
    in trigeminal neuralgia, 589, 591
  spasm of, 593

Facial muscles
  in Bell's palsy, 591–593
  in Parkinson's disease, 547
Facial nerve
  in ear disorders, *1261*
  palsy of (Bell's palsy), 591–593
  testing of, *590*
Facioscapulohumeral (Landouzy-Dejerine)
    muscular dystrophy, 413
Factor IX deficiency, 999–1000
Factor VIII deficiency, 999–1000
Factor V Leiden, 1000
Fad diets, 886–887
Fahrenheit temperature scale, 1722
Failure to thrive, 1537–1538
Fainting, 120, 143–146
  in aortic stenosis, 181–182
  in arrhythmias, 165
  in cardiomyopathy, 161
  in esophageal injury, 710
  parade ground, 120
  tilt table testing in, 124, 145
Falciparum malaria, 1140, 1141
Fallopian tubes, 1344, 1345, *1345*
  cancer of, *1402*, 1409
  infection of, 1378
  in infertility, 1417–1418
  inflammation of, 1180, 1377
  ligation of, 1427, *1428*
  pelvic inflammatory disease and, 1378
  pregnancy in, *1455*
Fallot, tetralogy of, 1515, 1517, *1517*
Falls, prevention of, *358*
Famciclovir, *1156*, 1162
Familial hypercholesterolemia, 197
Familial hypophosphatemic rickets, 13
Familial insomnia, fatal, 543
Familial Mediterranean fever, 1716–1717
Familial polyposis, 768, 769
Family planning, 1419–1428, *1420, 1422,*
    1424 (*see also* Contraception and
    contraceptives; Oral contraceptives)
  information resources on, 1763
Family relationships, 1542, 1638–1643
  adoption and, 1642–1643
  in autism, 1630
  changing structures of, *1640*
  childhood illness and, 1622, 1638–1640
  divorce and, 1640–1641, *1640*
  foster care and, 1641–1642
  infant illness and death and, 1638
  parent-child discussions and, *1639,*
    1642
  problems in, *1544*
Family therapy, 598
Famotidine, 716, *718*
  in elderly persons, *81*
Fanconi's syndrome, 852, 910
Fantasizing, *634*

Fantasy play, 1542
Farmer's lung, 309, *309*
Farsightedness (hyperopia), 1279, 1286,
  1287
  in children, *1601*
Farting (flatus), 701, 758
Fasciitis
  eosinophilic, 385–386
  necrotizing, 1113, 1221–1222
  plantar, 407–408
Fasciola hepatica infection, *1146*
Fasciotomy, 353
Fasting, hypoglycemia with, 970
Fat
  cholesterol (*see* Cholesterol)
  dietary, 882
    in coronary artery disease, 200, *201*
    restriction of, 886, 922–923, *923, 924*
  embolism of, 195, 286, 289, 507
  high blood levels of, 921–926, *922*
    in nephrotic syndrome, 841
  in liver (fatty liver), 797, *798, 799,*
    1453–1454
  metabolism of, disorders of, 1619–1621,
    1621
  in stool (steatorrhea), 734, 793, 927
  types of, 882, *923*
Fat (body)
  age-associated changes in, 17
  in Cushing's syndrome, 958
  estimation of, *881,* 916–917
  gain of, 883, 914–920 (*see also* Obesity)
  hormones of, *939*
  loss of
    with dieting, 884–887
    with undernutrition, 889
  under skin, 1187, *1187*
Fatal familial insomnia, 543
Fatal illness (*see* Death and dying; Terminal
    illness)
Fatigue
  in cancer, 1036
  chronic, 1717–1718, *1718*
  in dying person, 50
  in heart disease, 119
  in kidney disorders, 823–824, 831
Fat pads, of foot, *1606*
Fatty acids
  essential, 882
  oxidation of, disorders of, 1620–1621
Fatty liver, 797, *798, 799*
  of pregnancy, 1453–1454
Fear (*see also* Anxiety)
  exaggerated (phobia), 609–611, *611*
  of marketplace (agoraphobia), 609–610
  of school, 1558
Febrile seizures, 495, 502
  immunization and, 1492–1494
Feces (*see* Stool)

Feeding (*see also* Diet; Nutrition)
  enteral, 889–890
  of infants, 1486–1489, *1487* (*see also*
      Breastfeeding)
    problems in, 1532–1533
  intravenous, 890
  in necrotizing enterocolitis, 1505
  of premature infant, 1497, 1498
  tube, 889–890
    for cancer patient, 1047
    for dying person, 49
  in undernutrition, 889–890
Felbamate, *500*
Felon (fingertip infection), 402
Felty's syndrome, 371
Female-pattern baldness, 1212–1213
Femoral artery, aneurysm of, 229
Femur (thighbone)
  fracture of, 355
  in Legg-Calvé-Perthes disease, 1606–1607
  separation of (slipped capital femoral
      epiphysis), 1605–1606, *1605*
  torsion of, *1606*
Fenfluramine (fen-phen), 919
Fenofibrate, *925*
Fentanyl, *451*
Ferritin, 907, 990
Ferrochelatase deficiency, 936
Ferrous sulfate, in elderly persons, *81*
Fertility problems, 1414–1419
Fertilization, 1435, *1436*
  most likely time for, 1345
  in vitro, 1416, 1419
Fetal alcohol syndrome, 1463
Fetal tissue implant, 550, 1083
Fetishism, 629
Fetoscopy, 1465, 1467, 1471
Fetus
  alcohol effect on, 1463
  amniocentesis from, *1433*, 1434 (*see also*
      Amniocentesis)
  anemia in, 1507
  anticonvulsant effects on, 1447
  blood loss in, 1507
  blood sampling from, 1434, *1467*
  caffeine effects on, 1463
  chorionic villus sampling from, 1432–1434,
      1433, 1512, 1629, *1728*
  circulation of, 1513
  death of, 1457
  development of, *1436*, 1437
  distress of, 1471, 1498
  drug effects on, 1206, 1449–1450,
      1458–1464, *1459*, *1460–1461*
  Graves' disease effects on, 1448
  heartbeats of, 1443, 1465, 1467, *1467*, 1471
  hemolytic disease of, 1453
  infections in, *1508–1509*
  lungs of, 1448, 1454, 1498

Fetus (*continued*)
  lupus antibodies of, 1448
  maternal diabetes and, 1447–1448
  maternal heart disease effects on, 1446
  monitoring of, *1467*
  multiple, 1473
  nutrition for, 1511
  prenatal testing of, 1430–1434, *1430*, *1431*,
      1432, *1433*
  presentations of, 1465, 1471–1473, *1472*
  toxoplasmosis in, 1144–1145
  ultrasound examination of, 1355, 1432,
      1433, 1435, 1442–1443
  umbilical cord injury of, 1473
Fever, 1090–1091, *1090*
  after childbirth, 1478
  after immunization, 1536
  after surgery (postoperative), 1703
  in childhood respiratory tract infection,
      1579
  in cholecystitis, 816
  coma with, *493*
  in infants and children, 1536–1537, *1536*,
      1561
  in juvenile rheumatoid arthritis, 1612
  in kidney disorders, 823
  in malaria, 1140
  Mediterranean, familial, 1716–1717
  in pancreatitis, 730
  Pel-Ebstein, 1017
  during pregnancy, 1450
  seizures with, *496*, 502
  of unknown origin, 1091
Fever blisters (herpes simplex virus infection),
      668–669
Feverfew, *104*, 108–109
Fexofenadine, *1065*
Fiber, dietary, 201, 883, 923
  in constipation, 751, 752, 1591
  in irritable bowel syndrome, 757
  in ulcerative colitis, 743
  in weight loss diet, 886
Fibric acid derivatives, *925*
Fibrin, 995, *995*
Fibrinogen, 995
Fibrinolytic therapy (*see* Thrombolytic
      therapy)
Fibroadenoma, breast, 1388–1389
Fibroblasts, 1025
Fibrocystic breast disease, 1389
Fibrodysplasia, *846*
Fibroids, 1372–1374
  in pregnancy, 1449
Fibrolamellar carcinoma, 811
Fibroma
  chondromyxoid, 360
  heart, 191–193
  small intestine, 768
  uterine, 1372–1374

Fibromatosis, palmar, 397–398
Fibromyalgia, 415–417, *416*
Fibromyoma, 1372–1374
Fibrosarcoma, 361
Fibrosis
 bone marrow, *1023*, 1025–1026
 cystic, 317–322, *318*
 idiopathic pulmonary, 301–302
 lung, 296, 301–302, 323
 premacular (macular pucker), 1311
Fibrous histiocytoma, 361
Fiddleback spider bite, 1684–1685
Fifth disease, 1535, *1569, 1572–1573*
Fight-or-flight response, 5, 437
Filariasis
 lymphedema in, 240
 urinary tract, 867–868
Filiform warts, 1229
Fillings, tooth, 678–679
Filovirus infection, 1165
Filter, in pulmonary embolism prevention,
 234, *235*, 289
Filtration surgery, for glaucoma, 1309
Finasteride, 1213, 1330
Finger(s) (*see also* Hand)
 birth defects of, 1523, 1524
 blue discoloration (acrocyanosis) of, 225
 clubbing of, 253, *253*
 deformities of, 395–398, *396*
 dislocations of, *401*
 fracture of, 359
 infections of, 402–403
 injuries to, 359, *401*, 402, 1693
 mallet, 359, 396, *396*
 Raynaud's disease and Raynaud's
  phenomenon of, 224–225
 reattachment of, *1083*
 in scleroderma, 380
 severed or constricted, 1693
 trigger, *398*
Finkelstein test, 419
Fire ant stings, 1685
First aid, 1687–1693, *1688, 1689*
 for cardiac arrest, 1689–1690, *1689*
 for choking, 1690–1691, *1690, 1691*
 for internal bleeding, 1691
 for soft tissue injuries, *1692*, 1693
 for wounds, 1691–1693
Fish oils, 882
Fish poisoning, 725–726
Fish tapeworm, 1143–1144
Fissure, anal, 760
 in Crohn's disease, 739
Fistula
 anus-rectum (anorectal), 761, 762, 1521
 artery-vein (arteriovenous), 238–239
  in hemodialysis, 834, *836*
 bladder-intestine (vesicoenteric), 869
 in Crohn's disease, 739

Fistula *(continued)*
 in diverticulitis, 748, *749*
 trachea-esophagus (tracheoesophageal),
  1520–1521, *1521*
 urinary tract, 825
Fistulotomy, 762
Fitness, 31–36 (*see also* Exercise)
Fits (*see* Seizures)
Fitz-Hugh-Curtis syndrome, 1378
Flapping tremor, 545–546
Flashbacks, LSD-induced, 657
Flashing (flickering) lights, 1280
Flat feet, *1606*
Flatulence, 701, 758
Flat warts, 1229
Flatworm infection (schistosomiasis),
 1142–1143
Flea bites, 1685
 rickettsial infections from, 1132–1134, *1133*
Flesh-eating disease, 1221–1222
Floaters, 1278, 1280, 1305
Flock worker's lung, *297*, 299
Flow rate (lung), 254, *254*
Flow volume (lung), 254
Flu
 respiratory (*see* Influenza)
 stomach (*see* Gastroenteritis)
Fluconazole, *1152*
Flucytosine, *1152*
Fludarabine, *1045*
Fludrocortisone, 147, 958
Fluid retention (*see* Swelling [edema])
Fluid therapy
 in burn injury, 1651
 in cholera, 1100–1101
 in cystinuria, 852
 in dehydration, 929
 in excessive sweating, 1652–1653
 in gastroenteritis, 723, 1532, *1533*, 1587
 in heat cramps, 1653
 in heat exhaustion, 1653
 in hemorrhagic colitis, 724
 in hypernatremia, 914
 in infants and children, 1532, *1533*
 in kidney failure, 830–831
 in labor and delivery, 1467
 in shigellosis, 1111
Flukes, 540, 1142–1143, *1146*
Fluoride, *902, 906*
 in cavity prevention, 678, 906
 in osteoporosis, 346
Fluoroscopy, *1729*
 in digestive disorders, 704
 in heart disease, 125
Fluorosis, 906
Fluorouracil, *1231*
Flurazepam, in elderly persons, *81*
Flutamide, 1334
Fluvastatin, *925*

Flying (*see* Air travel)
Focal segmental glomerulosclerosis, *842*
Folded lung syndrome, 293, 294
Folic acid (folate), *893, 899, 899*
  deficiency of, *735,* 899
    anemia with, 990–991
    birth defects and, 1430, 1511
  excess of, 899
  during pregnancy, 1444, 1526, 1629
Follicle-stimulating hormone, *939, 940, 941,*
    1343
  deficiency of, 942
  measurement of, 943
  in menstrual cycle, 1346, *1347*
Folliculitis, 1112, 1223–1224
  hot-tub, 1109
Fomivirsen, *1156,* 1165
Fontanelles, in newborn meningitis, 1562
Food (*see also* Diet; Nutrition)
  additives to, 1068
  allergy to, 1068–1069, 1072–1073
    in infant, 1489
  aspiration of, 890
  calories in, 883
  composition of, 880
  contamination of, 724–726, 1110, 1587
  cravings for, 1440
  diarrhea with, 754, *755*
  drug interactions with, 77, 78
  gas-producing, 758
  gastroenteritis from, 724–726, 1110, 1587
  glycemic index of, 885–886
  hypoglycemic reaction to, 971
  infection from, 540, 1117–1118, 1137–1138,
    1143–1148, *1143*
  intolerance to, 1068
    in infant, 1489
  in irritable bowel syndrome, 756
  malabsorption of, 734–738, *735*
  poisoning from (*see* Food poisoning)
  prion contamination of, 542, *542*
  propulsion of, problems with, 708–710
  pyramid of, 884, *885*
  serotonin in, 974
  solid, for infant, 1488–1489
  spitting up of (regurgitation), 700
    in children, 1486, 1532, 1588–1589
  swallowing of (*see* Swallowing)
Food, Drug, and Cosmetic Act (1938), 93
Food and Drug Administration, 60, 62, 91, 93
Food guide pyramid, 884, *885*
Food poisoning, *720–721*
  chemical, 725–726
  Clostridium botulinum (botulism),
    579–581, 1489
  Clostridium perfringens, 721, 724–725
  fish, 725–726
  mushroom, 725, 726
  plant, 725

Food poisoning (*continued*)
  seafood, 725–726
  staphylococcal, *721,* 724
Foot (*see also* Toe[s]; Toenails)
  asleep, *583*
  athlete's, 1225
  ball of, pain in, 403–404
  birth defects of, 1524–1525, *1524*
  blue discoloration (acrocyanosis) of, 225
  calluses of, 410
  care for, 222, *222,* 964, *965*
  in diabetes mellitus, 964, *965*
  disorders of, 403–411, *405, 406, 408, 411*
  erythromelalgia of, 225
  fat pads of, *1606*
  flat, *1606*
  fracture of, 353–354, *354,* 422–423, *422*
  immersion, 1656
  pain in, 403–405
  pronation of, 420
  swelling (edema) of, 153, 912 (*see also*
    Swelling)
  trench, 1656
  ulcer of, 222
  warts on, 1228–1229
Foramen ovale, 1513
Forbes' disease, *1617*
Forceps delivery, 1469, 1475, *1475*
Foreign objects
  in anus and rectum, 764
  in digestive tract, 727–729, 751
  in ear, 1253, 1599
  in eye, 1291–1292
  in nose, 1599
  in vagina, 1350
Foreign travel (*see* Air travel; Travel)
Foreskin
  inflammation of (balanoposthitis), 1324
  removal of (circumcision), 1485–1486, 1568
  tightness of (phimosis), 1324–1325
Forgetfulness (*see* Amnesia; Dementia;
    Memory)
Formulas, for bottle-feeding, 1488
Foscarnet, *1156*
Fosfomycin, *1124*
Fosphenytoin, *500*
Foster care, 1641–1642
Fracture, 348–359, *349, 350, 352*
  ankle, 354
  arm, 358
  boxer's, 359
  ear canal, 1255
  elbow, 358
  eye socket, 1317–1318
  foot, 353–354, *354,* 422–423, *422*
  hand, 359, *401*
  hip, 349–350, 355–356, *356, 357*
    rehabilitation after, 43
  jaw, 691, *691*

Fracture *(continued)*
 leg, 354–355
 mandible, 691, *691*
 maxilla, 691, *691*
 in newborn, 1494, 1495
 nose, 1262
 in osteogenesis imperfecta, 1610–1611
 in osteoporosis, 344–345, 346, 569
 pelvis, 356–357
 penis, 1326
 prevention of, *358*
 shoulder, 358
 skull, 515–517
  in newborn, 1494
 temporal bone, 1260
 tooth, 690
 vertebrae, 344–345, 346, 357–358, 571–572
 wrist, 345, 349, 358, *401*
Fragile X syndrome, 1528, *1628*, 1629
Frambesia, 1099
Francisella tularensis infection (tularemia),
  1116–1117, *1116*
Freckles, 1214
 around lip, 664
Free radicals, 882–883
Freezing therapy *(see* Cryotherapy)
French disease *(see* Syphilis)
Frenzel glasses, 464
Frequency, of urination, 824
Friction massage, in temporomandibular joint
  disorders, *689*
Friedreich's ataxia, 556
Fright *(see* Anxiety; Fear)
Frigidity (sexual arousal disorder), 1385–1386
Frontal lobe, 434, *435*
 injury to, 476–477, *476*
Frontal sinus, 1245–1246, *1246*, *1265*
Frostbite, 1656–1657
Frostnip, 1656
Fructose intolerance, 1618
Fugue, 637–638
Fulvestrant, 1400
Fungal balls, *1266*
Fungal infection, *1087*, 1148–1154 *(see also*
  specific infections, eg, Aspergillosis)
 bone, 364, 365
 brain, 532
 drugs for, 1148–1149, *1152*
 gums, 682
 nails (onychomycosis), 409–410
 pneumonia, 270–271
 risk factors for, *1149*
 sinuses, *1266*
 skin, 1225–1228, *1226*, 1535
 stomach, 711
 urinary tract, 867
Furuncles (boils), 1112, 1224
 of ear, 1253–1255
 of nose, 1263–1264
Fussiness, 1531

G

Gabapentin, *500*
Gait *(see* Walking)
Galactorrhea, 946–947
 in acromegaly, 945
Galactosemia, 1617–1618
Galantamine, 489
Gallbladder, *695*, 697
 age-associated changes in, 698
 biology of, 786–788, *787*, 813
 in cystic fibrosis, 319
 disorders of, 813–817
 inflammation of (cholecystitis), 815–817
 removal of (cholecystectomy), 814–815, 816
 stones in *(see* Gallstones)
 tests for, 788–791
Gallium scan
 in Hodgkin's disease, 1018
 in sarcoidosis, 305
Gallop rhythm, 121
Gallstones, 788, 813–815, *814*
 hormone replacement therapy and, 1359
 indigestion and, 700
 oral contraceptives and, 1421
 pancreatitis and, 729–733
 during pregnancy, 1448
 x-rays of, 790
Gamekeeper's thumb, *401*
Gamete intrafallopian tube transfer (GIFT),
  1416, 1419
Gamma globulin, 1004
Gamma heavy chain disease, 1010
Gamma hydroxybutyrate, 658–659
Gamma knife surgery, *525*
Gammopathy, monoclonal, *20*
Ganciclovir, *1156*
 in cytomegalovirus infection, 1165
Ganglia (ganglion cyst), 395
Ganglioside accumulation (Tay-Sachs
  disease), *1430*, 1620
Gangrene
 in frostbite, 1656–1657
 gas, 1101
 in intestinal strangulation, 780
Gardner's syndrome, 671, 768–769
Garlic, *104*, 109
Gas(es)
 in digestive system, 701, 758, 781
 exchange of, in lungs, 245–246, *246*
 laughing, 659
 in necrotizing skin infection, 1222
 pressure changes in, diving injuries and,
  1666–1671, *1669*, *1670*
 toxic, 300–301
 in urine, 825
Gas gangrene, 1101
Gasoline poisoning, 1679
Gastrectomy, 711, 712
Gastric bypass surgery, 919–920, *919*

Gastric emptying study, 1589
Gastrinoma, 754, 775–776
Gastritis, 711–713, *712*
Gastroenteritis, 719–726, *720–721, 723*
  Campylobacter, 1099
  in children, 1586–1588
  Enterobacteriaceae, 1101, 1103
  in infants, 1532
  Salmonella, 1110
Gastroesophageal reflux, 706, 717–719
  in infants and children, 1532, 1588–1589
Gastrointestinal syndrome, in acute radiation
    illness, 1659, 1661
Gastrointestinal system *(see specific
    digestive system organs)*
Gastroplasty, 919–920
Gastroschisis, *1512*
Gastroscopy, 703, *704*
Gatifloxacin, *1123*
Gaucher's disease, 1620
  information resources on, 1763
Gels, 1189
Gemfibrozil, *925*
Gemtuzumab ozogamicin, 1046
  in cancer, *1045*
  in leukemia, 1014
Gender identity, 628–629, 1540–1541
  disorders of, 1520
Gene(s), 9, 11, *11*, 12, *12*
  abnormalities of, 11–14, *11, 12, 13*
    gene therapy for, 15–16
  cancer, 14
  expression of, 11–14
  mitochondrial, 14
  radioactive labeling of, 15
  tumor suppressor, 14
  X-linked, 11, 12–14, *13*
Generalized exfoliative dermatitis, 1196–1197
Generic drugs, 60, 88–92, *89, 90–91*
  names of, *1732–1755*
Gene therapy, 15–16
  in cystic fibrosis, 321
  in severe combined immunodeficiency,
    1062
  in sickle cell disease, 994
Genetics, 8–16
  of Alport's syndrome, 856
  of Alzheimer's disease, 487
  of Bartter's syndrome, 853–854
  of cancer, 1032–1033
  cloning experiments in, *15*
  of diabetes insipidus, 851
  disorders of, 11–14, *11, 12, 13*, 1527–1530
    information resources on, 1764
    prenatal testing for, 1430–1434, *1430,
      1431, 1432, 1433*
    screening for, 1429–1430
  drug response and, 74–75
  of Hartnup disease, 853
  of Huntington's disease, *553*

Genetics *(continued)*
  of hypophosphatemic rickets (vitamin
    D–resistant rickets), 853
  longevity and, 17
  of multiple sclerosis, 557
  of muscular dystrophy, 412
  of obesity, 915
  of polycystic kidney disease, 854
  of retinoblastoma, 1623–1624
  of Wilms' tumor, 1622
Genetic testing, 1725
  in cystic fibrosis, 320
  in Huntington's disease, *553*
  in immunodeficiency disorders, 1059
  in mental retardation, 1629
  in sickle cell disease, 994
Genital herpes, 1160–1162, *1376*
  pregnancy and, 1447
Genitals *(see also specific parts, eg,* Penis)
  ambiguous, 1519–1520
  birth defects of, 1519–1520
  development of, 1553, *1553*, 1556
Genital warts, 1183, 1229, 1325, *1376*
Genitourinary tract *(see* Reproductive
    system; Urinary tract)
Genotype, 9
Gentamicin, *1122*
  in Meniere's disease, 1260
Genu valgum, *1606*
Genu varum, *1606*
Geographic tongue, 665
GERD *(see* Gastroesophageal reflux)
Geriatrics, 19–21, *20 (see also* Elderly
    persons)
German measles *(see* Rubella)
Germ cell tumor, *520*
Germline gene therapy, 16
Germs *(see* Microorganisms)
Gerstmann-Sträussler-Scheinker disease,
    543
Gestational diabetes, 1441, 1452–1453
GHB (gamma hydroxybutyrate), 658–659
Ghrelin, *939*
Giant cell (temporal) arteritis, 387, 388, *389*,
    1316
  headache with, *459*
Giant cell tumor, 360
Giant diverticulum, *748*
Giardia lamblia infection (giardiasis), 721,
    722, 1138
  sexually transmitted, 1183–1184
GIFT (gamete intrafallopian tube transfer),
    1416, 1419
Gigantism, 945–946
Gila monster bite, 1683–1684
Gilbert's syndrome, 791
Gilchrist's disease, 1149–1150
Ginger, *104*, 109
Gingivitis, 681–685, *683*
Gingivostomatitis, herpetic, 682, 1161

Ginkgo, *104,* 109
　in altitude illness, 1674
Ginseng, *104–105,* 109–110, 1361
Glands *(see also specific glands and*
　　hormones)
　biology of, 937–940, *938, 939*
　disorders of, 940–969
　hormones of, 938–940, *939*
Glare, 1280
Glatiramer acetate
　in multiple sclerosis, 559
　in transplantation, *1079*
Glaucoma, *20,* 1306–1309, *1307, 1308*
　congenital, *1512*
　headache with, *458*
　over-the-counter drug precautions in, *102*
　pain in, 1281, 1307
　vision loss in, 1279
Gleason score, 1332
Glimepiride, *968*
Glioblastoma multiforme, *520*
Glioma, *520*
Glipizide, *968*
Globulins, *1078, 1727*
Globus sensation (globus hystericus), 700
Glomerulonephritis, 837, 838–843, *840, 842*
　acute (acute nephritic syndrome),
　　838–839
　membranoproliferative, *842*
　membranous, *842*
　mesangial proliferative, *842*
　postinfectious (acute nephritic syndrome),
　　838–839
　rapidly progressive, 838–839
Glomerulosclerosis, *842*
Glomerulus, 820, *821, 845*
　age-associated changes in, 822–823
　inflammation of (see Glomerulonephritis)
Glossitis, 665
Glossopharyngeal nerve, *590,* 593–594
Glucagon, 697, *939*
　in hypoglycemia, 966, 972
Glucagon-like peptide, *939*
Glucagonoma, 776
Glucocerebrosides, accumulation of
　　(Gaucher's disease), 1620
Glucosamine, 422
Glucose, 1616
　in blood, *1726* (see also Sugar[s], blood)
　in coma, 493
　in high potassium levels (hyperkalemia),
　　911
　in low blood sugar levels (hypoglycemia),
　　966, 971–972
　in porphyria, 935
　in urine (glucosuria), 825, 850–851
Glucose-6–phosphate dehydrogenase
　　deficiency, 75, 989
Glucose tolerance test, 946, 965
Glucosidase inhibitors, 968–969, *968*

Glues, poisoning from, 1679
Gluten enteropathy (celiac disease), 736–737
　in dermatitis herpetiformis, 1217–1218
Glutethimide, 653–654
Glyburide, *968*
Glycemic index, 885–886
Glycogen, 881
　storage diseases of (glycogenoses),
　　1616–1617, *1617*
Glycolated hemoglobin, 965, 969, 1615
Glycolipid, accumulation of (Fabry's disease),
　　1620
Glycoprotein IIb/IIIa inhibitors, *206*
Goiter, 906, 907
　in fetus, 1448
　toxic diffuse (Graves' disease), 949–951, *952*
　　in newborn, 1510
　　in pregnancy, 1448–1449
　toxic multinodular (Plummer's disease), 950
Gold compounds, *372, 373*
Goldenseal, *105,* 110
Goldmann perimeter, 1283
Golfer's dystonia (yips), 554
Gonadorelin, 1417
Gonadotropin-releasing hormone, 1343
Gonadotropin-releasing hormone agonists
　in endometriosis, 1370, *1371*
　in premenstrual dysphoric disorder, 1363
　in uterine fibroids, 1373
Gonadotropins, *939, 940, 941*
　deficiency of, 942
　measurement of, 943
　in ovulation problems, 1417
Gonads (see Ovary [ovaries]; Testis [testes])
Gonioscopy, 1308
Gonorrhea, 1179–1180, *1376*
　in eye, 1296–1297
　in traveler, 1714
　urethritis in, 868
Goodpasture's syndrome, 312
Goserelin, 1334
Gout, 391–394, *392, 393*
　generic drug substitutions in, *90*
Grafts
　for aneurysm repair, 228, 229
　bone, 353, 363
　bone marrow (see Bone marrow,
　　transplantation of)
　skin, 1083, 1210, 1650
Graft-versus-host reaction, 986, 1082
Grain worker's lung, 300
Gram-negative infection, 270, 1095–1096
Gram-positive infection, 1096
Grand mal (tonic-clonic) seizures, 497, *498*
Granuloma
　eosinophilic, 304
　formation of, *1056*
　pyogenic, 1236
　sarcoid, 304–306
　in yaws, 1099

Granuloma annulare, 1201
Granuloma inguinale, 1182
Granulomatosis, 303–304
  Wegener's, 389–390, 829, 1318
Granulomatous ileitis (Crohn's disease),
  738–742, *741*
Grapefruit diet, 886–887
Graves' disease, 949–951, *952, 1074,* 1319
  in pregnancy, 1448–1449, 1510
Gray baby syndrome, 84
Great arteries, transposition of, 1517
Grief, 51, 613
  information resources on, 1761
Grinding, of teeth, 674
Griseofulvin, 1226
Ground itch (hookworm infection), 1139
Growth, 1538–1539
  in adolescent, 1552–1553, *1553*
  asthma and, 1584
  charts for, *1541*
  delays in, in infants and young children,
    1537–1538
  in diabetes mellitus, 1615
  in girls, 1346
  heart defects and, 1513
  in infant, 1490–1491, *1490*
  in juvenile rheumatoid arthritis, 1612
Growth hormone, *939, 940, 941*
  abuse of, *647*
  deficiency of, 942
  excess of, 945–946
  measurement of, 943, 946
  in Noonan syndrome, 1529
  pituitary regulation of, 1556
  replacement of, 944
  in short stature, 1556
  in Turner syndrome, 1529
  in undernutrition, 890
Growth plate, 335, 1603
  in chondrodysplasias, 1611
  femoral
    in Legg-Calvé-Perthes disease,
      1606–1607
    in slipped capital femoral epiphysis,
      1605–1606, *1605*
  injury to, 1603
Guaiac test, 705
Guaifenesin, 98, 250, *1158*
Guided imagery, 1706
Guillain-Barré syndrome, 584–586
Gulf War syndrome, 1718–1719
Gummas, 1177
Gums, *662*
  color changes of, *663,* 673
  infection of, 670
  inflammation of (gingivitis), 681–685
  lump on, 670–671
  recession of, 685
  tooth impaction in, 680
Gut *(see specific digestive system organs)*

Gynecology, 1349–1356 (*see also specific
  topics, eg,* Pregnancy)
  evaluation for, 1351–1356, *1353, 1354,*
    1401–1402
  information resources on, 1768
Gynecomastia (male breast enlargement),
  1323
  in cancer, *1037*

H

Haemophilus ducreyi infection (chancroid),
  1181–1182
Haemophilus infection, 1104
  in epiglottitis, 1268
  immunization for, *265,* 1093, *1094, 1493,*
    1561, *1562*
  pneumonia, 267
Hair, *1187,* 1211–1212
  bezoars of, 727–729
  excess, 1212, 1350
    in polycystic ovary syndrome, 1368
  growth of, 1212
  ingrown, 1214, 1224
  lice in, 1219, *1219*
  loss of (balding), 1212–1214
    information resources on, 1758
  pulling of, 1213
  removal of, 1212
  transplantation of, 1213
Hair cells, in ear, 1244–1245
Hair follicles, *1187,* 1211
  infection of, 1223–1224
  keratosis pilaris of, 1204
  staphylococcal infection of, 1112
Hairy cell leukemia, 1014, 1015
"Hairy" tongue, 664
Halitosis, *684*
Hallucinations
  alcoholic, 649
  in delirium, 481–482
  in depression, 616
  in narcolepsy, 471–472
  in schizophrenia, 641
  smell-related (olfactory), 596
Hallucinogens, 657–658
  adolescent use of, 1559–1560
Hallux (big toe)
  arthritis of, 404
  displacement of, 410–411, *411*
  fracture of, 354, *354*
  gout in, 391
Hallux rigidus, 404
Hallux valgus, 410–411, *411*
Haloperidol
  in elderly persons, *80*
  in mania, 620
  in Tourette's syndrome, 552
Halos, 1280

Hamate bone, fracture of, *401*
Hammer (malleus), 1244, *1245*
Hammer toe, 411, *411*
Hamstring injury, 426
Hand (*see also* Finger[s]; Wrist)
  abscess of, 402–403
  arthritis of, 397
  birth defects of, 1523, 1524
  bite injury to, 402
  blue discoloration (acrocyanosis) of,
      225
  carpal tunnel syndrome of, 398–399, *399*
  computer keyboard position for, *399*
  deformities of, 395–398, *396*
  Dupuytren's contracture of, 397–398
  erythromelalgia of, 225
  fracture of, 359
  ganglia of, 395
  infections of, 402–403
  injuries to, *401*, 402
  Kienböck's disease of, 400
  laying on of, 1707
  Raynaud's disease and Raynaud's
      phenomenon of, 224–225, 380, 383,
      384
  reattachment of, *1083*
  reflex sympathetic dystrophy of (shoulder-
      hand syndrome), 400
  severed or constricted, 1693
Hand-foot-and-mouth disease, *1576*
Hand-Schüller-Christian disease, 303–304
Hand washing, 1091
Hansen's disease (leprosy), 1130–1132
Hantavirus infection, 1167
Hardening, of arteries (*see* Atherosclerosis)
Hartnup disease, 853, 897
Hashimoto's thyroiditis, 950, 952, 953–954,
    1074
Hay fever, 1065–1067
HCG (*see* Human chorionic gonadotropin)
β-HCG (beta–human chorionic gonadotropin),
    1039
HDL cholesterol, 197, 202, 920, *921*, 922,
    1726
  progestin and, 1359
Head (*see also* Brain)
  banging of, *1548*
  injury to, 513–519, *514, 515*
    in children, 514, *516*
    coma with, 494
    consciousness alterations with, 491, *492*
    dementia with, 490
    in newborn, 1494
  in Paget's disease, 347
Headaches, 456–461, *458–459*
  after spinal tap, 442
  in brain hemorrhage, 512
  in brain tumor, *458*, 521
  cluster, *458*, 461
  information resources on, 1764

Headaches (*continued*)
  migraine, 457–461, *458, 460*
  tension-type, 457, *458*
Health care professionals
  communication with, 21–24, 47, 54, 87
  decision making by, 1695–1698
  disclosure by, 54
  mental health, *599*, 600
  needlestick injury in, 1169, 1173
  prevention and, 30
Health insurance, 24
  drug policies of, 92
  for dying person, 47
Hearing
  age-associated changes in, 17, *18*, 1247
  loss of, 1247–1253
    after eardrum perforation, 1256
    age-related (presbycusis), 1247
    aids for, 1250–1252, *1251*
    in Alport's syndrome, 856
    in autoimmune disorders, 1248
    in children, 1597–1599, *1598*
    conductive, 1247, *1248*
    drug-related, 1248
    in ear infection, 1248
    information resources on, 1761
    noise-related, 1245, 1248, 1250
    in osteogenesis imperfecta, 1610
    in otosclerosis, 1247–1248, 1250
    prevention of, 1250
    rehabilitation for, 45, 1253
    sensorineural, 1247, *1248*
    tests for, 1249–1250, *1249*
    treatment of, 1250, *1251, 1252*
  temporary threshold shift in, 1248
  testing of, *29*, 1249–1250, *1249*
Hearing aids, 1250–1252, *1251*
  for children, 1599
Heart (*see also entries at* Cardiac *and*
    Cardio-)
  abnormal rhythms of, 163–175, *164,
      166–167, 168* (*see also* Arrhythmias;
      Heartbeats)
  age-associated changes in, *18*, 117–118
  anatomy of, 114–117, *115, 116*
  aneurysm of, *212*
  angina of, 202–210, *206–207, 208, 210*
    travel and, 1711–1712
  arteries of (*see* Coronary arteries)
  of athlete, 32
  auscultation of, 121, *1728*
  biopsy of, 192
  birth defects of, *1512*, 1513–1518, *1515,
      1516, 1517*
  blood flow in, 115–116, *115*
    during pregnancy, 1439
  bypass surgery of, 209–210, *210*
  cancer of, 194
  catheterization of, 128–129, *1728*
    in angioplasty, 208–209, *208*

Heart *(continued)*
  catheterization of *(continued)*
    in cardiomyopathy, 160
    in pericarditis, 191
  coronary artery disease of, 199–215,
    206–207, 208, 210
  disease of
    diagnosis of, 120–130, *122, 124,* 145
    in DiGeorge anomaly, 1061
    fainting in, 143
    information resources on, 1760
    in Kawasaki syndrome, *1581*
    low blood pressure with, 143
    oral contraceptive use and, 1420
    over-the-counter drug precautions in, *102*
    pericardial, 188–191, *189*
    in pregnancy, 1445–1446, 1454
    prevention of, 27
    rehabilitation for, 40–41
    sexual activity and, *1337*
    shock in, 148
    symptoms of, 118–120
    during travel, 1711–1712
  electrical pathway of, 163–164, *164*
  enlargement of, 125, 134
    in acromegaly, 945
  failure of *(see* Heart failure)
  inflammation (infection) of *(see*
    Endocarditis; Pericarditis)
  lightning effects on, 1664
  murmurs of *(see* Murmurs)
  muscle of (myocardium), 335
    blood supply of (coronary arteries),
      116–117, *116*
      inadequate, 118
    dysfunction of, 158–163, *159*
    inflammation of, 152, 159–160
      in rheumatic fever, 1566
    rupture of, *212*
  radiation injury to, 1660
  rupture of, *212*
  sarcoidosis of, 305
  scar tissue of, *212*
  sounds of, 114–115
    fourth, 136
    in high blood pressure, 136
  transplantation of, 1079–1080
    in heart defects, 1514
    in heart failure, 157–158
  tumors of, 191–194, *193,* 329
  valves of, 114, *115*
    in cardiomyopathy, 160, 161
    disease of, 119, 175–183, *176*
      in children, 1517–1518
      in heart failure, 152, 153
    infection of (endocarditis), 184–187, *186,*
      187, 1110, 1112, 1113
    in Marfan syndrome, 1608
    replacement of, 177–178, *179,* 181, 182
    valvuloplasty of, 128, 180, 182

Heart attack, 210–215
  cholesterol level and, 922
  complications of, 211–213, *212*
  estrogen and, 1358
  in hypercholesterolemia, 926
  mitral regurgitation with, 177
  oral contraceptives and, 1421
  pericarditis after, 188
  radionuclide imaging after, 127
  rehabilitation after, 40–41
  shock with, 149
  ventricular fibrillation after, 173
  ventricular premature beats after, 172
Heartbeats (heart rate), 117, 163
  in apnea of prematurity, 1503
  in atrial fibrillation and flutter, 169–170
  awareness of (palpitations), 119–120
    in arrhythmias, 164, 165
    in mitral regurgitation, 177
  control of, 163
  electrocardiogram of, 122–123, *122 (see also*
    Electrocardiography)
  in exercise, 33
  fetal, 1443, 1465, 1467, *1467,* 1471
  in heart block, 174–175
  in heart disease, 119–120, 121
  in long QT syndrome, 1530
  in pacemaker dysfunction, 174
  in paroxysmal supraventricular tachycardia,
    170–171
  during pregnancy, 1439, 1441
  premature
    atrial, 168–169
    ventricular, 172
  in sick sinus syndrome, 174
  in ventricular fibrillation, 173–174
  in ventricular tachycardia, 172–173
  in Wolff-Parkinson-White syndrome,
    171–172
Heart block, 174–175
Heartburn
  in gastroesophageal reflux, 717
  during pregnancy, 1440
  remedies for, 99
  in scleroderma, 381
Heart failure, 150–158, *151*
  acute, 158
  after heart attack, *212*
  in aortic regurgitation, 181
  in cardiomyopathy, 161, 162
  diastolic, 150, *151,* 152–153
  drugs for, *156–157*
  gallop rhythm in, 121
  in heart defects, 1513
  in kidney failure, 831
  liver damage in, 810
  in mixed connective tissue disease, 384
  in Paget's disease of bone, 347
  pregnancy and, 1445–1446
  in rheumatic fever, 1566

Heart failure *(continued)*
  in septic shock, 1120
  sexual activity and, *1337*
  systolic, 150, *151*, 152
  thrombophilia in, 1000
  travel and, 1711–1712
  in vitamin B₁ deficiency, 896
Heart rate (*see* Heartbeats)
Heat
  allergy to, 1070
  disorders from, 1652–1654
  injury from (*see* Burns)
Heat cramps, 1653
Heat exhaustion, 1653
Heatstroke, 1653–1654
Heat therapy, 37
Heavy chain disease, 1010
Heberden's nodes, 368, 397
Heel
  bursitis in, 408–409, *408*
  pain in, 407–408
  spurs of, 404–405, *405*, 408
Height
  in adolescent, 1552–1553
  children's charts for, *1541*
  metric equivalents for, 1723
  pregnancy and, 1445
  in preventive care, *29*
  short, 942, 1556, 1611
Height-weight chart, *880*
Heimlich maneuver, 1690, *1690*
Helicobacter pylori
  chamomile effect on, 107
  in gastritis, 711, *712*
  indigestion and, 700
  in peptic ulcer, 712, 714, 715
HELLP syndrome, 1452
Helper T cells, *1052*, 1055
Hemangioblastoma, 519, *520*
Hemangioma, 810, 1235–1236, *1235*, *1496*
Hemapheresis, *986*
Hematemesis, 699, 705
Hematochezia, 699, 705
Hematocrit, *1726*
  measurement of, *981*
  in polycythemia vera, 1024
Hematoma
  brain (intracranial), *459*, 517–519
  dissecting, 229–231, *230*
  ear, 1255
  spinal, 565–566
Hematopoietic syndrome, 1659, 1661
Hematuria, 825, 826, 875–876, 877
  asymptomatic proteinuria with, 843
Heme, 907, 933
Hemianopia, *1317*
Hemiballismus, 553
Hemifacial spasm, 593

Hemochromatosis, 908, *909*
  information resources on, 1764
Hemodialysis, 831, 833–837, *833, 834, 836*
  in hypercalcemia, 905
  in maple syrup urine disease, 1619
  in poisoning, 1676
Hemoglobin, 907, 978, *1726*
  abnormalities of, 992–994
  carbon monoxide in, *1725*
  deficiency of (*see* Anemia[s])
  measurement of, *981*
  in polycythemia, 1024
  in urine, 825
Hemoglobin A₁C, 965, 969, 1615
Hemoglobin C disease, 994
Hemoglobin E disease, 994
Hemoglobin S-C disease, 994
Hemoglobinuria, paroxysmal nocturnal, 989
Hemolytic anemia, 987, *988, 989*
  autoimmune, 991–992, *1074*
Hemolytic disease of newborn, *1506*, 1507
Hemolytic reaction, with blood transfusion, 986
Hemolytic-uremic syndrome, 723–724, 998
Hemoperfusion, charcoal, in poisoning, 1676
Hemophilia, 999–1000
  prenatal testing for, *1430*
  transfusion-related HIV infection in, 1169
Hemophilus infection (*see Haemophilus* infection)
Hemoptysis, 252–253
Hemorrhage, 7 (*see also* Bleeding)
  cerebral (*see* Stroke)
Hemorrhagic colitis, 723–724
Hemorrhagic conjunctivitis, *1576*
Hemorrhagic disease of the newborn, 895
Hemorrhagic fevers, 1165–1167
Hemorrhagic telangiectasia, hereditary (Rendu-Osler-Weber disease), 996
Hemorrhoids, 759–760, *761*
  during pregnancy, 1440
Hemostasis, 995–996, *995* (*see also* Clotting)
  drug effects on, *996*
Hemothorax, 314, 316
Henoch-Schönlein purpura, *387*, 996–997
Hen worker's lung, *309*
Heparin, *996*
  after surgery, 288
  in hemodialysis, 834
  during pregnancy, 1451, *1460*
  in pulmonary embolism, 288
  in stroke, 509
Hepatic arteries, 786, 787, 806, *807*
  aneurysm of, 807
  occlusive disease of, 218, 223, 806–807
Hepatic coma, 649–650

Hepatic ducts, *695, 697, 787*
Hepatic encephalopathy (coma), 795–796
Hepatic veins, 786, 787, 806, *807*
  in Budd-Chiari syndrome, 808–809
  in heart failure, 810
  occlusive disease of, 807–808
Hepatitis, 802–806, *804–805*
  acute, 802–803
  alcoholic, *799*
  autoimmune, 803, 806
  cancer and, *1155*
  chronic, 803–806
  immunization for, 29–30, 1093, *1094, 1493,*
    1709
  ischemic, 806–807
  liver cancer and, 811
  in newborn, *1508*
  during pregnancy, 1448, 1713
  prevention of, *27,* 1688
  sexually transmitted, 1183–1184
  transfusion-acquired, *983*
  in traveler, 1714
Hepatoblastoma, 812
Hepatocellular adenoma, 810
Hepatocellular carcinoma (hepatoma), 798,
  811
Hepatomegaly, 793
Hepatorenal syndrome, 796
Herbal medicine, 1706
Herbs, medicinal, 103–112, *104–106*
  for cancer, 1046
Hereditary angioedema, 664, *1072*
Hereditary diseases *(see* Gene[s]; Genetics;
  and specific diseases)
Hereditary hemorrhagic telangiectasia
  (Rendu-Osler-Weber disease), 810, 996
Hereditary (familial) spastic paraparesis,
  566–567
HER-2/*neu,* 1391, 1398
Hernia and herniation
  brain, 510, 513, *515,* 523
  diaphragm, 1522
  in Ehlers-Danlos syndrome, 1608
  hiatus, 727, *728*
  inguinal, 1328, *1328*
  intervertebral disk, 569, *570,* 571, 574
  intestinal, 780, *780*
Heroin, 652–653
  adolescent use of, 1559–1560
  during pregnancy, 1464
Herpangina, *1576*
Herpes gestationis, *1441*
Herpes simplex virus infection, 1160–1162
  in atopic dermatitis (eczema herpeticum),
    1195
  brain (encephalitis), 534, 535, 1570
  cornea (keratitis), 1301–1302
  erythema multiforme with, 1200
  fingertip (herpetic whitlow), 402

Herpes simplex virus infection *(continued)*
  genital, 1160–1162, *1376*
  mouth, 668–669, 682
  in newborn, *1508*
  during pregnancy, 1447
Herpesviruses, 1155
Herpesvirus 6 infection, 1580
Herpesvirus 8 infection, cancer and, *1155,*
  1240–1241
Herpes zoster (shingles), *20,* 251, 1162–1163,
  1163
  cornea, 1302
  mouth, 670
  pain after, 449, *1163*
Herpetic gingivostomatitis, 1161
Herpetic whitlow, 402
Hers' disease, *1617*
5-HIAA (5-hydroxyindoleacetic acid),
  974–975
Hiatus hernia, 727, *728*
Hiccups, *545*
Hidradenitis suppurativa, 1224
High blood pressure, 131–141 (*see also*
  Hypertension)
  arteriosclerosis and, 133–134, 197
  causes of, 132–134, *134*
  in cirrhosis, 798
  classification of, *137*
  diagnosis of, 134–136, *135*
  drug therapy in, *138–139,* 139–140
  essential (primary), 132
  eye damage and, 136, 1312
  headache with, *458*
  heart failure and, 152
  in kidney cancer, 876
  in kidney failure, 831, 833
  in Liddle's syndrome, 854
  in lungs, 322–324, *323*
  in malignant nephrosclerosis, 847–848
  measurement of, 124
  in nail-patella syndrome, 856
  in nephritic syndrome, 838
  over-the-counter drug precautions in, *102*
  in pheochromocytoma, 134, 136, 960–961
  in polycystic kidney disease, 854–855
  in portal vein, 793–794, 808, 809
  in pregnancy, 1446, 1452, 1459, 1473
  in pseudoxanthoma elasticum, 1609
  in renal artery stenosis, *846*
  retinopathy in, 136, 1312
  secondary, 132
  sexual activity and, *1337*
  systolic, isolated, 118, 131
  treatment of, 136–141, *138–139*
Hip
  avascular necrosis of, 362
  congenital dislocation (developmental
    dysplasia) of, 1524
  degeneration of, 362

Hip *(continued)*
  fracture of, 349–350, 355–356, *356, 357*
    rehabilitation after, 43
  in Legg-Calvé-Perthes disease, 1606–1607
  in newborn, 1485
  pain in
    in Calvé-Perthes disease, 1607
    in slipped capital femoral epiphysis, 1606
  replacement of, 355–356, *357,* 363, 370
Hippocampus, 434
Hirschsprung disease, 1522–1523
Hirsutism (excess hair), 1212, 1350
  in polycystic ovary syndrome, 1368
Histamine (*see also* Antihistamines)
  fish, poisoning from, 726
  receptors for, 72
Histamine-2 blockers
  in elderly persons, *81*
  in gastritis, 713
  in gastroesophageal reflux, 1588–1589
  in indigestion, 99, 1588–1589
  in peptic ulcer, 716, 718
Histiocytoma, 361
Histiocytosis, 303–304
Histocompatibility, *1052*
Histoplasmosis, 1152–1153
  pneumonia and, 270
Histrionic (hysterical) personality, 631–632
Hives, 1063, 1071–1072, *1189*
  in solar urticaria, 1232
HIV infection (human immunodeficiency
    virus infection, AIDS), 533, 1168–1175,
    1169, 1171
  CD4+ lymphocyte count in, 1170
  dementia with, 490
  erythema infectiosum in, 1572–1573
  heart inflammation in, 188
  in infants and children, 1573–1575
  infections in, 1092, 1127, 1145, *1172,* 1174
  information resources on, 1756–1757
  Kaposi's sarcoma in, *663, 672,* 1240–1241
  low white blood cell count and, 1004
  meningitis in, 532, *534*
  opioid abuse and, 652
  Pneumocystis carinii pneumonia in, 271,
    1574, 1575
  during pregnancy, 1447, 1574
  prevention of, 1173, *1173*
  prognosis for, 1174–1175
  toxoplasmosis in, 1145
  transfusion-acquired, *983*
  transmission of, 1168–1169, *1170,* 1573,
    1688
  treatment of, 1173–1174, *1175*
  tuberculosis in, 1127
HLA (human leukocyte antigen), 1050, *1052*
  in organ transplantation, 1076
HLA-B27, 377
HMG-CoA reductase inhibitors, *925*
  food interactions with, 77

Hoarseness
  in laryngitis, 1268
  in vocal cord disorders, 1269
Hodgkin's disease, 1017–1018, *1017, 1019*
  paraneoplastic syndromes in, *1037*
Holter monitoring, 123–124, *124*
  in angina evaluation, 204
  in arrhythmias, 165
  in fainting, 145
Home care, *47*
  antibiotic administration in, 1121, 1124
  information resources on, 1764
  oxygen therapy in, 260–261
Homeopathy, 1705
Homeostasis, 5
Home pregnancy test, 1434–1435
Homework, 1542
Homocysteinemia
  atherosclerosis and, 198, *899*
  thrombophilia and, 1000, 1001
Homocystinuria, 1619
Homosexuality, 627–628
  in adolescents, 1554
Honey, 1489
Hook of hamate bone, *401*
Hookworm infection, 1138–1140, *1139*
  of skin (creeping eruption), 1220
Hordeolum, 1294–1295
Hormone(s), 5, 938–940, *939*
  in anorexia, 625
  disorders of, 940–969 *(see also specific
    hormones)*
  generic substitutions for, *90*
  marijuana effects on, 655
Hormone, sex (*see* Estrogens; Testosterone)
Hormone replacement therapy, 1358–1359,
    1360
Horner's syndrome, 228, 329, 592
  in esophageal cancer, 765
Hornet stings, 1685
Horsefly bites, 1685
Horse serum, *1684*
Hospice care, *47*
Hospitalization
  for burns, 1650
  for children, 1640
  delirium and, 480–481
Host defenses (*see* Immune system)
Hot flashes, 1356–1357, *1360*
  prevention of, 1358
Hot-tub folliculitis, 1109, 1223–1224
House dust, allergy to, 1067–1068
Household products
  burns with, 1678–1679
  nontoxic, *1675*
HTLV (human T-cell lymphotropic virus)
    infection
  leukemia and, 1011
  lymphoma and, 1020
  myelopathy and, 539, 560

Human body, 2–8
  aging of, 16–21, *18–19*, 79
  anatomy of, 2–7, *3, 8* (*see also* Anatomy)
  barriers of, 5, 7
  cells of, 2, *4* (*see also* Cell[s])
  composition of, 880, *881*
  mind interactions with, 7–8
  organ systems of, 3–5, *3, 6*
  tissues of, 2–3
Human chorionic gonadotropin, 1348
  in hydatidiform mole, 1410
  in ovulation problems, 1417
  in pregnancy detection, 1434–1435
β–Human chorionic gonadotropin (β-HCG), *1039*
Human Genome Project, 14
Human leukocyte antigen (HLA), 1050, *1052*
  in organ transplantation, 1076
Human papillomavirus infection
  cancer and, *1155*, 1406
  genital warts and, 1183
  of newborn, *1509*
  skin warts and, 1228–1229
Human parvovirus infection, 1572–1573
Human T-cell lymphotropic virus (HTLV)
    infection
  leukemia and, 1011
  lymphoma and, 1020
  myelopathy and, 539, 560
Humerus, fracture of, 358
Humidifier, 249
  in croup, 1586
Humpback (kyphosis), 1604–1605, *1605*
Hunger (*see* Appetite)
Huntington's disease, 12, 552, 553–554, *553, 1430*
Hutchinson-Gilford syndrome, 21
Hyaluronate injection, 369–370
Hydatid disease (echinococcosis), 540, *1146*
Hydatidiform mole, 1409–1410
Hydranencephaly, *1512*
Hydrocarbon poisoning, 1679
Hydrocele, 1328–1329
Hydrocephalus, 524–525, *525*
  brain tumor and, 523
  congenital, 1526
  normal-pressure, 490
Hydrochloric acid, in stomach, 696
Hydrocolloid dressings, 1190, 1209
Hydrocortisone
  in fungal infection, 1226
  in itching, 1192
  over-the-counter, 98–99
  in proctitis, 762
  in skin disorders, 1191
Hydrofluoric acid, 300–301
Hydrogen peroxide, in trench mouth, 685
Hydrogen sulfide, 300–301
Hydromorphone, *451*
Hydronephrosis, 829, 862–864, *863*

Hydrophobia (rabies), 535–537, *536*
Hydrops (*see* Swelling [edema])
Hydroquinone cream, 1215
Hydrostatic (underwater) weighing, *881*
Hydroxyapatite, 335
Hydroxychloroquine
  in porphyria, 934
  in rheumatoid arthritis, 372, 373
5-Hydroxyindoleacetic acid (5-HIAA), 974–975
Hydroxymethylbilane synthase deficiency
    (acute intermittent porphyria), 934–936
5-Hydroxytryptamine (5-HT, triptans), 460–461, *460*
Hydroxyurea
  in polycythemia, 1024–1025
  in sickle cell disease, 993–994
  in thrombocythemia, 1026–1027
Hydroxyzine, *1065*
  in elderly persons, *80*
  in physical allergy, 1070
Hymen, 1344, *1344*
Hymenolepis nana infection, *1146*
Hyoscyamine, in elderly persons, *81*
Hypacusis, 1250
Hyperactivity, in children, 1549–1551, *1549, 1550*
  information resources on, 1758
Hyperaldosteronism, 960, *961*
Hyperbaric oxygen therapy, 1668
  in altitude illness, 1674
  in decompression sickness, 1671
Hyperbilirubinemia, 1505–1507 (*see also* Jaundice)
Hypercalcemia, 904–905, *904*
  in cancer, *1037*
  constipation in, 751
  in multiple myeloma, 1007
  in Paget's disease of bone, 347, 348
  in sarcoidosis, 305
  in vitamin D excess, 894
Hypercalciuria, 866
Hypercholesterolemia (*see* Cholesterol, high blood levels of)
Hyperchylomicronemia, 925–926
Hyperemesis gravidarum, 1451–1452
Hypereosinophilic syndrome, 1005
Hyperglycemia (*see also* Diabetes mellitus)
  coma with, *493*
  in premature infant, 1497
Hyperhidrosis, 1210–1211
Hyperhomocysteinemia, 1000, 1001
  atherosclerosis and, 198
Hyperimmunoglobulinemia E syndrome, 1062
Hyperinsulinemia, 916
Hyperkalemia, 911
  in kidney failure, 832, 833
  periodic paralysis with, 414

Hyperlipoproteinemia (hyperlipidemia), 921–926, *922, 924, 925*
  hereditary, 925–926
Hypermagnesemia, 909
Hypernatremia, 913–914
  coma with, *493*
Hyperopia (farsightedness), 1279, 1286, *1287*
  in children, *1601*
Hyperosmia, 596
Hyperparathyroidism, 904–905, *904, 972, 973*
Hyperphosphatemia, 910
  in kidney failure, 833
Hyperproteinemia, idiopathic (intestinal lymphangiectasia), 737–738
Hypersensitivity (*see* Allergy and allergic reactions)
Hypersensitivity pneumonitis, *297,* 308–310, *309*
Hypersensitivity vasculitis, *387*
Hypersomnia, 470
Hypersplenism, 1028
Hypertension, 131–141 (*see also* High blood pressure)
  intracranial, *523,* 1315
  malignant, 131, 134, 141
    kidney failure in, 847–848
  portal, 793–794, 809
  pulmonary, 152, 179, 322–324, *323*
    in newborn, 1501–1502
    pregnancy and, 1446
  renovascular, 223
  secondary, 139
  white coat, 134
Hyperthermia, malignant, 75
Hyperthyroidism, 907, 949–952, *951, 952*
  after childbirth, 1479
  apathetic, 950
  arrhythmias in, 164
  in cancer, *1037*
  in elderly persons, 19
  heart failure with, 152
  masked, 950
  in newborn, 1510
  over-the-counter drug precautions in, *102*
  during pregnancy, 1441
  in thyroiditis, 954
Hypertriglyceridemia (*see* Triglycerides, high blood levels of)
Hypertrophic osteoarthropathy, *1037*
Hypertrophic pyloric stenosis, 1532
Hyperuricemia, 391–394, *392, 393*
Hyperventilation
  alkalosis with, 932–933
  in diver, *1669*
Hyperventilation syncope, 144
Hyperventilation syndrome, 251
Hyperviscosity syndrome, 1009
Hyphema, 1290

Hypnosis, 601, 1706
  in conversion disorder, 603
  in dissociative amnesia, 636–637
  in dissociative identity disorder, 639
  for pain, 455
Hypoalphalipoproteinemia, 927
Hypobetalipoproteinemia, 927
Hypocalcemia, 901, 903–904
  in DiGeorge anomaly, 1061
Hypochondriasis, 603–604, *634*
  in children, 1637
Hypogammaglobulinemia, in infants, 1060
Hypogeusia, 596
Hypoglossal nerve, *591, 594*
Hypoglycemia, 966, 970–972
  in children, 1615
  coma with, *493*
  in large-for-gestational-age infant, 1499
  in pancreatitis, 733
  in postmature newborn, 1498
  in premature infant, 1497
Hypokalemia, 910–911 (*see also* Potassium, low blood levels of)
Hypolipoproteinemia, 926–927
Hypomagnesemia, 908–909
  low calcium levels and, 901
Hypomania, 619–620, *620*
Hypomenorrhea, *1362*
Hyponatremia, 912–913
  coma with, *493*
  in gastroenteritis, 722
  in lung cancer, *1037*
Hypopharynx, 1246, *1246*
Hypophosphatemia, 909–910
  rickets and, 852–853
Hypopituitarism, 942–944, *942*
Hypoplastic left heart syndrome, *1512*
Hyposmia, 596
Hypospadias, 1519
Hypotension, 141–147 (*see also* Low blood pressure)
  orthostatic, 39
    in anemia, 988
    in dehydration, 929
    idiopathic (Shy-Drager syndrome), 550–551
Hypothalamic-pituitary axis, 938, 940
Hypothalamus, 434, *938*
  in body temperature regulation, 1090
  in female reproductive function, 1343
  in hormone control, 938, 940, 956
Hypothermia, 1655–1656
  coma with, *493*
Hypothyroidism, 942, 943, 952–953
  after childbirth, 1479
  after thyroid removal, 952
  arrhythmias in, 164
  cholesterol levels in, 921
  constipation in, 751
  in elderly persons, 19, *20*

Hypothyroidism (continued)
  heart failure with, 152
  in newborn, 1510
  in thyroiditis, 954
Hysterectomy, 1356, 1373, 1404
  in cervical cancer, 1407
  in endometrial cancer, 1404
  in fallopian tube cancer, 1409
  in vaginal cancer, 1409
Hysteria (see Conversion disorder)
Hysterical fainting, 145
Hysterosalpingography, 1355, 1417–1418
Hysteroscopy, 1354, 1418, 1729

I

Ibuprofen, 95, 97, 454
ICD-10–CM (International Classification of
  Disease, 10th Revision, Clinical
  Modification), 599
Ichthyosis, 1192
ICU (intensive care unit) psychosis, 480
Identity disorder, 638–639, 639
Idiopathic bronchiolitis obliterans, 303
Idiopathic hypereosinophilic syndrome, 1005
Idiopathic hyperproteinemia (intestinal
  lymphangiectasia), 737–738
Idiopathic pulmonary fibrosis, 301–302
Idiopathic thrombocytopenic purpura, 997,
  998
  pregnancy and, 1449
Id reaction, 1225
IgA (immunoglobulin A), 1056
  selective deficiency of, 1060
IgD (immunoglobulin D), 1056
IgE (immunoglobulin E), 1056
  in allergic reactions, 1063
  high levels of, 1062
IgG (immunoglobulin G), 1056
IgM (immunoglobulin M), 1055–1056
Ileitis, 738–742, 741
Ileo-anal anastomosis, 744
Ileocolitis (Crohn's disease), 738–742, 741
Ileostomy, 744
  in antibiotic-associated colitis, 746
  diversion colitis after, 745
Ileum, 696
Ileus, 781
  gallstone, 814
  meconium, 319
Iliac arteries, 217–218, 222
Iloprost, 324
Imagery, guided, 1706
Imatinib, 767, 1016, 1045
Imipenem/cilastatin, 1122
Imipramine, 1545
Imiquimod, 1229
Immersion foot, 1656

Immobilization
  in fracture treatment, 351–352, 353
  high calcium levels with, 904–905
Immune globulin
  in ataxia-telangiectasia, 1061
  in immunodeficiency disorders, 1059, 1060
  in pemphigus, 1217
  Rh$_O$(D), 1433, 1453, 1477
  in transient hypogammaglobulinemia of
    infancy, 1060
  varicella-zoster, 1571
  in X-linked agammaglobulinemia, 1059
Immune system, 1049–1056, 1051, 1052,
  1055, 1056
  age-associated changes in, 18, 1056
  in allergy (see Allergy and allergic
    reactions)
  cancer and, 1034
  disorders of, 1050, 1057–1075 (see also
    Allergy and allergic reactions;
    Autoimmune disorders;
    Immunodeficiency)
  lymphoid organs of, 1050–1051, 1053
  in premature infant, 1497
  response of, 1049–1051, 1051, 1052, 1053,
    1089–1090
  suppression of (see Immunodeficiency;
    Immunosuppressive drugs
    [immunomodulators])
    for transplantation, 1076–1077,
    1078–1079
Immunity (see also Immune system)
  nonspecific (innate), 1050, 1051–1054
  specific (adaptive), 1050, 1054–1056
Immunization, 1092–1095, 1094, 1562
  adenovirus, 1094
  in adults, 29–30
  anthrax, 1094, 1098
  in bronchiectasis prevention, 291
  chickenpox, 265, 1493
  cholera, 1094
  in cystic fibrosis, 320–321
  diphtheria, 1093, 1094, 1492, 1493, 1562
  fever after, 1536
  Haemophilus influenzae type b, 265, 1093,
    1094, 1493, 1561, 1562
  hepatitis, 802, 804–805, 1093, 1094, 1493,
    1709
  in HIV-infected children, 1575
  in immunodeficiency disorders, 1059
  in infants and children, 1492–1494, 1495,
    1536
  influenza, 265, 269, 1094, 1094, 1159–1160,
    1160, 1580
    for pregnant women, 1443, 1448
  Japanese encephalitis, 1094, 1709
  measles, 1093, 1094, 1493, 1493, 1577
  meningococcal meningitis, 1094, 1709
  mumps, 1093, 1094, 1493, 1493, 1577

Immunization *(continued)*
  Neisseria meningitidis, 531
  in non-Hodgkin's lymphoma, 1022
  in older adults, 30
  pertussis (whooping cough), 1093, *1094,*
      1492, *1493*
  plague, *1094*
  pneumococcal infection, *265, 266,* 1094,
      1094, 1109, *1493,* 1561, *1562*
  polio, 1094, *1094,* 1492, *1493,* 1578
  during pregnancy, 1459, *1461*
  rabies, 536, *536, 1094, 1709*
  rotavirus, *1094,* 1587
  rubella, 1093, *1094,* 1442, 1477, 1493, *1493,*
      1582
  side effects of, 1492–1494
  smallpox, *1094,* 1095, *1166*
  spleen removal and, 1029
  tetanus, 1093, *1094,* 1115, *1115, 1493,* 1562
  for travelers, 1095, 1708, *1709*
  tuberculosis, *1094*
  typhoid, *1094,* 1117, *1709*
  varicella-zoster virus, *1094,* 1095, *1493*
  yellow fever, *1094, 1709*
Immunodeficiency, 1057–1063 *(see also* HIV
      infection; Immunosuppressive drugs)
  acquired, 1057 *(see also* HIV infection)
  ataxia-telangiectasia, 1061
  causes of, 1057, *1058*
  chronic granulomatous disease, 1062
  common variable, 1060
  congenital, 1057, *1058*
  cytomegalovirus infection in, 1164–1165
  diagnosis of, 1058–1059
  DiGeorge anomaly, 1061, 1083
  herpes simplex virus infection in, 1161
  hyperimmunoglobulinemia E syndrome,
      1062
  mucocutaneous candidiasis, 1060–1061
  Pneumocystis carinii pneumonia in, 271
  pneumonia and, 264
  prevention of, 1059
  selective antibody deficiency, 1060
  severe combined, 1061–1062
  in splenic disorders, 1062–1063
  symptoms of, 1057–1058
  toxoplasmosis in, 1145
  transient hypogammaglobulinemia of
      infancy, 1060
  treatment of, 1059
  Wiskott-Aldrich syndrome, 1062
  X-linked (Bruton's) agammaglobulinemia,
      1059
Immunoelectrophoresis, 1007
Immunoglobulin(s), *1052,* 1055–1056, *1055*
      (see also Antibodies)
  transfusion of, 985
Immunoglobulin A (IgA), 1056
  selective deficiency of, 1060

Immunoglobulin D (IgD), 1056
Immunoglobulin E (IgE), 1056
  in allergic reactions, 1063
  high levels of, 1062
Immunoglobulin G (IgG), 1056
Immunoglobulin M (IgM), 1055–1056
Immunosuppressive drugs
      (immunomodulators)
  in autoimmune disorders, 1075
  in Crohn's disease, 740, *741*
  in dermatomyositis, 384
  immunodeficiency disorder with, 1057
  in polymyositis, 384
  in rheumatoid arthritis, *372,* 374–375
  in systemic lupus erythematosus, 380
  in transplantation, 1076–1077, *1078–1079*
  in ulcerative colitis, 744
  in Wegener's granulomatosis, 390
Immunotherapy
  in allergy, 1064, 1066–1067
  in cancer, 1044–1046
Impaction
  stool, 699, 752, 757
  tooth, 680, 683
Impetigo, 1112, 1222–1223
Implant(s)
  cochlear (ear), 1252, *1252,* 1599
  contraceptive, *1420,* 1422
  defibrillator, 146, 167
  dental, *679*
  for heart, 146, 167
  hip, 355–356, *357*
  joint, 352–353
  knee, *369*
  pacemaker, 146, 165, 167, *168,* 175
  penile, 1339
Implantation, in pregnancy, 1435–1436, *1436*
Impotence *(see* Erectile dysfunction)
Incapacity, 53–54, *53*
Incentive spirometry, 261
Inclusion conjunctivitis, 1296
Incompetency, 53, *53*
Incontinence
  fecal, 757–758
    in dying person, 49
  urinary, *20,* 824, 857–862
    after menopause, 1357
    causes of, 857–858, *859, 860*
    in dying person, 49
    information resources on, 1764
Incus (anvil), 1244, *1245*
Indigestion, 699 *(see also* Heartburn; Nausea;
      Vomiting)
  remedies for, 99
Indinavir, *1175*
Indomethacin
  in elderly persons, *80*
  in patent ductus arteriosus, 1514
  during pregnancy, 1501

Infant(s) (*see also* Children)
  adverse drug reactions in, 84
  antibodies in, 1056
  bacterial infections in, 1561–1568
  botulism in, 579, 580, 1489
  breathing (respiratory) disorders in,
    1583–1586
  choking in, 1691, *1691*
  death of, 1638
    SIDS and, 1489, 1504, 1538
    information resources on, 1767
  development of
    behavioral, 1491–1492, *1491*
    intellectual, 1491–1492, *1491*
    physical, 1490–1491, *1490*
  feeding of, 1486–1489, *1487*
    problems in, 1532–1533
  immunization for, 1492–1494, *1493*
  large-for-gestational-age, 1499
  meningitis in, 1562–1563
  myasthenia in, 578
  normal, 1483–1494
  premature, 1470–1471 (*see also* Premature
    infant)
  preventive health care for, 1492
  problems in, 1531–1543, *1533, 1535,*
    1536
  small-for-gestational-age, 1498–1499
  transient hypogammaglobulinemia in,
    1060
  undernutrition in, 887–888
  viral infection in, 1568–1582, *1569, 1572,*
    1576, 1581
  vitamin deficiencies in, 894, 895
Infantile esotropia, 1601–1602
Infantile spasms (salaam seizures), 502
Infarction
  brain (*see* Stroke)
  kidney, 844–846
  lung, 285, 286
  myocardial (*see* Heart attack)
Infection
  abdominal, 778–779, 782–783
  after childbirth, 1478–1479
  after rape, 1412, 1413
  anus and rectum, 761
  in atherosclerosis, 195
  bacterial, 1095–1118, *1102–1103* (*see also*
    Bacterial infections)
    in children, 1561–1568
  Bartholin's gland, *1375*
  in biological warfare, *1089*
  biology of, 1086–1092, *1087, 1088, 1090*
  bladder (cystitis), 868–871
    after childbirth, 1479
    in children, 1567–1568
  bloodstream, 1118–1119
    in children, 1561
    in newborn, *1508–1509,* 1510–1511

Infection (*continued*)
  bone (osteomyelitis), 364–365
  with bone marrow transplantation, 1082
  brain, 529–540, *533, 536*
    childhood disintegrative disorder and,
      1632
    coma with, *492*
    seizures with, *496*
  breast, 1389
    after childbirth, 1479
  bronchus (bronchitis), 262–264, *263*
  during cancer treatment, 1047
  conjunctiva (*see* Conjunctivitis)
  coronary artery disease and, 200
  cuticle (paronychia), 402
  in cystic fibrosis, 321
  defenses against, 1050, 1087–1092 (*see also*
    Immune system)
  development of, 1086–1087, *1091*
  in diabetes mellitus, *963, 964, 965*
  diverticula, 748–750
  ear, 1248, 1253–1255, 1257–1259, *1258*
    in children, 1593–1594, *1595*
  ehrlichial, 1134–1135
  epiglottis, 1268
  eye, 1299–1300, 1301–1302, 1313 (*see also*
    Conjunctivitis)
  eyelash, 1281
  eyelid, 1294
  fever in, 1090–1091, *1090,* 1536
  finger, 402–403
  fungal, 1148–1154 (*see* Fungal infection)
  gastroenteritis, 719–726, *720–721*
    in children, 1586–1588
    in infants, 1532
  gums, 682
  hand, 402–403
  heart (endocarditis), 184–187, *186, 187*
  in Hodgkin's disease, *1017*
  immunization against (*see* Immunization)
  in immunodeficiency disorders, 1057–1058,
    1059
  joint, 365–366
    temporomandibular, 687, 688, 689
  kidney (pyelonephritis), 871–872
    after childbirth, 1479
    in children, 1567–1568
  liver (hepatitis), 802–806, *804–805*
  lung (*see* Pneumonia)
  lymph node, 240–241
  mastoid, 1259
  from medical devices, *1091,* 1092
  meninges (*see* Meningitis)
  mouth, 670, 680
  in multiple myeloma, 1008
  in neutropenia, 1002–1003
  in newborns, *1508–1509*
  in non-Hodgkin's lymphoma, *1021*
  nose, 1263–1264

Infection *(continued)*
  opportunistic
    in HIV infection, *1172*, 1174
    in immunosuppressed person, 1092
  orbit, 1318
  pancreas, 731
  parasitic, 1135–1148 *(see also* Parasitic
    infection)
  peritoneum *(see* Peritonitis)
  during pregnancy, 1447, 1450, 1451, 1463,
    1511–1512
  in premature infant, 1497
  in pressure sores, 1209, 1210
  prevention of, 1091
  prostate gland, 868–869, 1335
  reactive arthritis (Reiter's syndrome) with,
    376–377
  rectum, 762
  respiratory, 1155–1160 *(see also*
    Pneumonia)
  rickettsial, 1132–1134
  in sickle cell disease, 993
  sinus, 1266–1267, *1266*
  skin *(see* Skin, infection of)
  spinal cord, 529–540, *533*
  in spleen disorders, 1029, 1062–1063
  stomach, 711, *712*
  tear (lacrimal) sac, 1293
  throat, 1113, 1268, 1595, 1596
  toenail (onychia), 410
  tonsil, 1267–1268, 1595
  tooth, 680
  transfusion-acquired, *983*
  travel and, 1711
  tube feeding and, 890
  ureter (ureteritis), 871
  urethra (urethritis), 868
  urinary tract, 866–872, *867* *(see also*
    Urinary tract, infection of)
  uterus, after childbirth, 1478
  vagina, 1349, 1353, 1374–1377, *1376*
  viral, 1154–1167 *(see also* Viral infection)
    in children, 1568–1582
  vulva, *1375*
  wound, 1692–1693
Infectious mononucleosis, 1155,
  1163–1164
Infertility, 1414–1419
  information resources on, 1764
Infiltrative lung diseases, 301–308, *302,
  307*
Inflammation, 1088–1089
  alveoli (alveolitis), allergic, 308–310, *309*
  appendix (appendicitis), 781–782
    in children, 1590
    during pregnancy, 1450
  in atherosclerosis, 195
  bile duct, 799–800
    in ulcerative colitis, 743

Inflammation *(continued)*
  bladder, 869, *869*
  blood vessels (vasculitis), 223, 232, 236,
    371, 386–391, *387, 389*
  brain *(see* Encephalitis; Encephalopathy)
  bronchus (bronchitis), 262–264, *263*
  bursa, 417–418
  cancer and, 1034
  cervix, 1179–1180
  choroid (choroiditis), 1305–1306
  conjunctiva *(see* Conjunctivitis)
  diverticula (diverticulitis), 748–750, *749,*
    751–752
  epididymis (epididymitis), 1328
  esophagus (esophagitis), 717
    erosive, 710
  eye, 1299, 1305–1306, 1318 *(see also*
    Conjunctivitis)
  eyelid (blepharitis), 1294
  fallopian tube, 1180, 1377
  gallbladder (cholecystitis), 815–817
  gums (gingivitis), 681–685
  heart
    endocarditis, 184–187, *185, 186, 187*
    myocarditis, 152, 159–160
    pericarditis, 118–119, 153, 188–191, *189,*
      211, 213
  iris (iritis), 1305–1306
  joint, 339, 370–377 *(see also* Arthritis)
  kidney (nephritis), 837–844
  large intestine, 738–745, *741* *(see also*
    Colitis)
  larynx (laryngitis), 1268–1269
  in leprosy, 1131
  lip (cheilitis), 664
  liver *(see* Hepatitis)
  lymphatic vessels (lymphangitis), 241
  lymph nodes (lymphadenitis), 240–241
  muscle (myositis), 339
  nose (rhinitis), 1264–1265
  optic nerve (optic neuritis), 1315–1316
  orbit, 1318–1319
  pancreas (pancreatitis), 729–733
    in mumps, 1577
  penis (balanoposthitis), 1324–1325
  pericardium *(see* Pericarditis)
  peritoneum (peritonitis), 782–783
  plantar fascia, 407–408
  pleura (pleurisy), 251, 313–314, *314*
  prostate gland (prostatitis), 1335
  pulp (pulpitis), 679–680
  rectum (proctitis), 762
    ulcerative, 742, 743, 744
  sclera (scleritis), 1299, 1318
  sesamoid, 411
  sinus (sinusitis), 1245–1246, 1266–1267
  skin, 1193–1198, *1193, 1195* *(see also*
    Dermatitis)
    drugs for, 1190–1191

Inflammation *(continued)*
  small and medium-sized arteries (Buerger's
    disease), 223–224
  spinal cord (transverse myelitis), 567
  spine (ankylosing spondylitis), 569
  stomach (gastritis), 711–713, *712*
  superficial veins (thrombophlebitis), 232,
    236
  sweat gland, 1224
  tear gland (dacryoadenitis), 1318
  tendon (tendinitis), 418, 424–425, 429, *429*
  tendon sheath (tenosynovitis), 406, 418
  testis (orchitis), 1328, 1577
  thumb tendon (De Quervain's syndrome),
    419
  thyroid gland (thyroiditis), 950, 952,
    953–954
  tibia, 1607
  toenail (onychia), 410
  tongue (glossitis), 665
  tooth, 679–680
  treatment of, 37–38, 94–95, 97
  urethra *(see* Urethritis)
  uvea (uveitis), 1305–1306
  vagina (vaginitis), 1349–1350, 1374–1377,
    1376
  veins, 223
  vertebrae (ankylosing spondylitis), 377
Inflammatory bowel disease, 738–745, *741*
Inflammatory breast cancer, 1391, 1392,
  1400
Inflammatory demyelinating polyneuropathy
  (Guillain-Barré syndrome), 584–586
Inflammatory orbital pseudotumor, 1318
Infliximab *(see also* Immunosuppressive
  drugs)
  in autoimmune disorders, 1075
  in Crohn's disease, 740, *741*
  in rheumatoid arthritis, *372,* 375
  in transplantation, *1079*
Influenza, 1159–1160
  in children, 1579–1580
  immunization for, 29, 30, *265,* 269, 1094,
    1094, 1159–1160, *1160*
    in children, 1580
    in pregnant women, 1443, 1448
  vs. lymphocytic choriomeningitis, 538
  pneumonia and, 269
  prevention of, 27
Informed consent, 54, 1701
Ingrown hair, 1214, 1224
Ingrown toenail, 409
Inguinal hernia, 1328, *1328*
Inhalants, *658, 659, 659*
Inhalation
  drug administration by, 66
  dust, 294–301, *297*
  gas or chemical, *297,* 300–301, 308–310,
    309

Inhaler
  in allergy, 1064–1065
  in asthma, 279–280, *279,* 1584
  in COPD, 283
Inheritance *(see* Gene[s]; Genetics)
Injections
  of contraceptive, *1420,* 1422–1423
  of drugs, 64–66, *65*
  of insulin, 966–968, *967*
Injection sclerotherapy
  for esophageal varices, 778
  for hemorrhoids, 760
  for varicose veins, 238
Injury (injuries)
  acute stress gastritis and, 712
  altitude illness, 1672–1674
  arm, in newborn, 1495
  arteriovenous fistula with, 238–239
  atelectasis after, 293
  birth, 1494–1495
    in cerebral palsy, 1624–1626
  bite *(see* Bites and stings)
  bladder, 874
  body part reattachment after, *1083*
  bone *(see* Fracture)
  brain *(see* Brain, injury to)
  burn, 1648–1651, *1648, 1649, 1650, 1651,*
    1661–1664
    in child abuse, 1645
    to esophagus, 1678–1679
    to eye, 1292
  in child abuse, 1643–1646
  cold, 1654–1657
  compressed air, 1666–1671, *1669, 1670*
  diving, 1666–1671, *1669, 1670*
  domestic violence, 1410–1412
  ear, 1255, 1256–1257, *1257*
  in Ehlers-Danlos syndrome, 1608
  esophagus, 710
  exercise-related, prevention of, 34
  eye, 1290–1292
  first aid for, 1687–1693, *1688, 1689*
  hand, *401, 402*
  head *(see* Head, injury to)
  heat, 1652–1654
  high potassium levels with, 911
  intestine, in newborn, 1504–1505
  kidney, 872–873, *873*
  lightning, 1663–1664
  lung, in newborn, 1502–1503
  mouth, 669–670
  muscle, 349, 353
  near drowning, 1665–1666
  needlestick, 1169, 1173
  nerve, 583–585, *585*
    in newborn, 1494–1495
  nose, 1262
  penis, 1326
  poisoning *(see* Poisoning)

Injury *(continued)*
  prevention of, *27*, 421
  radiation, 1657–1661
  rape, 1412–1413
  salivary gland, 667
  scrotum, 1326
  soft tissue, first aid for, *1692, 1693*
  spinal cord, 561–563, *562–563*
    incontinence after, *860*
    information resources on, 1767
    in newborn, 1495
    rehabilitation after, 41–43
  sports, 419–429
  stings *(see* Bites and stings)
  stress gastritis and, 711
  stress reaction after, 612–613
  testes, 1326
  tongue, 664–666
  tooth, 690
  during travel, 1711, 1713
  ureter, 874
  urethra, 874–875
  urinary tract, 872–875, *873*
Inner ear, 1244–1245, *1245*
  disorders of, 1255–1261, *1261*
Inocybe (mushroom) poisoning, 725
Inotropic drugs, *157*
Insanity *(see* Mental health disorders)
Insecticide poisoning, 1679–1680
Insects *(see also specific insects)*
  bites by, 1685
  in ear, 1253, 1599
Insemination
  artificial, 1416
  intrauterine, 1418
Insomnia, 468–470
  drugs for, 100
    in elderly persons, *81*
  fatal familial, 543
Insulin, 697, *939, 962*
  in diabetes mellitus, 966–968, *967*, 1614
  high blood levels of (hyperinsulinemia),
    obesity and, 916
  in high potassium levels (hyperkalemia),
    911
  insufficiency of *(see* Diabetes mellitus)
  low blood sugar (hypoglycemia) with,
    970
  meal frequency and, 884
  in pancreatitis, 733
  in polycystic ovary syndrome, 1368
  during pregnancy, 1441
  receptor binding of, 2
  resistance to, *922*, 967–968
  sensitivity to, 968
  during travel, 1712
Insulin-like growth factor I (IGF-I), 943,
  946
Insulinoma, 775, 971, *972*

Insurance plans, 24
  drug policies of, 92
  for dying person, 47
  for travel, 1708
Intellectual development
  adolescent, 1553–1554
  child, 1539–1540, 1543
    galactosemia and, 1617–1618
    low blood sugar levels (hypoglycemia)
      and, 1615
  infant, 1491–1492, *1491*
Intelligence quotient (IQ)
  in autism, 1631
  in Down syndrome, 1527
  evaluation of, 1628–1629
  in mental retardation, 1626, *1627*
Intention (cerebellar) tremor, 545, 546
Intercourse *(see* Sexual function)
Interferon-alpha, 1046, *1156*
  in cancer, *1045*
  in decreased platelets (thrombocythemia),
    1026–1027
  in hepatitis, 805
  in polycythemia, 1025
Interferon-gamma, 1062
Interleukin, *1052*
  in kidney cancer, 876
Intermittent claudication, 217, 221
Intermittent exotropia, 1602–1603
Intermittent porphyria, 934–936
  hormone replacement therapy and, 1359
International Classification of Disease,
  10th Revision, Clinical Modification
  (ICD-10–CM), 599
International travel *(see* Air travel; Travel)
Internet, for research, 24
Internuclear ophthalmoplegia, 558, 588
Interpersonal therapy, 601
Intersex states, 1519–1520
Interstitial cystitis, 869, *869*
Interstitial lung disease, 301–308, *302, 307*
  bronchiolitis-associated, *307*
  drug-induced disease of, *307*
Interstitial pneumonia
  desquamative, 302–303
  lymphoid, 303
Interstitial pneumonitis, in HIV infection,
  1574
Intervertebral disks, *436*
  degenerative disease of, 368
  herniation of, 569, *570, 571,* 574
Intestinal lipodystrophy (Whipple's disease),
  737
Intestinal lymphangiectasia, 737–738
Intestine, *695 (see also* Large intestine; Small
    intestine)
  age-associated changes in, *18*
  death (necrosis) of, in premature infant,
    1504–1505

Intestine *(continued)*
  inguinal hernia of, 1328, *1328*
  ischemia of, 218, *219*, 223
  malrotation of, 1521–1522
  obstruction of
    in dying person, 49
    during pregnancy, 1450
Intoxication *(see* Alcohol use and abuse;
    Poisoning; Toxins)
Intracerebral hemorrhage, 510–511, *511*, 519
Intracranial hemorrhage, 510–512, *511, 515*,
    517–519
Intracranial hypertension, *523*
Intramuscular route, of drug administration,
    65, *65*
Intraocular lens, implantation of, 1289,
    1304
Intraocular pressure, *20*
  increased (glaucoma), 1306–1309, *1308* (see
    also Glaucoma)
  measurement of, 1307
Intrathecal route, of drug administration,
    65–66
Intrauterine device (IUD), *1420*, 1424–1425,
    1425
Intrauterine insemination, 1418
Intravenous route
  for drug administration, 65, *65*, 1121, 1124
  for nutrient administration, 890
Intravenous urography, 827, 863, 865, *1729*
Intrinsic factor, 712
Introitus, 1343, *1344*
Intubation *(see* Tube)
Intussusception, 780, *780*
  in children, 1589–1590
In vitro fertilization, 1416, 1419
Iodine, *902*, 906–907
  deficiency of, 906, 953
  excess of, 906–907
  in hyperthyroidism, *951, 952*
  during pregnancy, *1461*
  in thyroid hormone formation, 948
Iontophoresis, 1211
Ipecac syrup, abuse of, *647*
Ipratropium
  in asthma, 70, *278*, 280, 1584
  in COPD, 283
IQ (intelligence quotient)
  in autism, 1631
  in Down syndrome, 1527
  evaluation of, 1628–1629
  in mental retardation, 1626, *1627*
Iridocyclitis
  in juvenile rheumatoid arthritis, 1612,
    1613
  relapsing, 390
Irinotecan, *1045*
Iris, 1276, *1276*, 1305, *1306*
  dark spots on, 1281

Iritis, 1305–1306
  headache with, *458*
Iron, *902*, 907–908
  deficiency of, 735, 907–908
    anemia with, 708, 989–990
  excess of, 908, *909*
  poisoning with, 1680
  reference range for, *1726*
  supplementation with, 908, 990
    in elderly persons, *81*
    during pregnancy, 1443–1444
Iron-binding capacity, *1726*
Irradiation therapy *(see* Radiation therapy)
Irregularity *(see* Constipation)
Irritable bowel syndrome, 756–757
Isaac's syndrome, *577*
Ischemia
  bone (avascular necrosis), 362–363, *363*, 400
  brain, 507–510, *508* (see *also* Stroke)
  heart, 118, 202–210, *206–207, 208, 210*
  intestine, 218, *219*, 223
  liver, 806–807
  in peripheral arterial disease, 216
Ischemic colitis, 783
Ishihara plates, 1283
Islet cells, transplantation of, 1080–1081
Isomaltase deficiency, 735
Isoniazid, *1124*
  hepatitis with, 803
  in tuberculosis, 1129, 1130
Isosorbide, 205, *207*
Isotretinoin, 891
  in acne, 1206, *1207*
  during pregnancy, *1461*
Itching, 1191–1193
  anus, 760, 763–764
  in chickenpox, 1572
  in cholestasis, 793
  in contact dermatitis, 1194
  dermatitis from, 1198
  eyes, 1282
  in food allergy, 1068
  in hay fever, 1066
  in hives, 1071
  in hookworm infection, 1139
  in impetigo, 1222–1223
  in kidney disorders, 823–824
  in lice infestation, 1219
  in lichen planus, 1204
  in pancreatic cancer, 773
  in perennial allergies, 1067
  in pityriasis rosea, 1203
  during pregnancy, *1441*, 1451
  in ringworm, 1225
  in scabies, 1218–1219
  in schistosomiasis, 1143
  treatment of, 1190
  vaginal, 1349
Itraconazole, *1152*, 1226

IUD (intrauterine device), *1420*, 1424–1425, *1425*
Ivermectin, 1218

J

Jacksonian seizures, 496
Jail fever (*see* Typhus)
Jakob-Creutzfeldt disease, 490, 541–543, *542*
Jamaican vomiting sickness, 725
Japanese encephalitis, *1094*, *1709*
Jarisch-Herxheimer reaction, 1178–1179
Jaundice, 791–792
    in biliary atresia, 1522
    in cholestasis, 793
    in cirrhosis, 798
    in hepatitis, 802
    in Hodgkin's disease, *1017*
    in newborn, 1486, 1505–1507, *1506*
    in pancreatic cancer, 773
    in premature infant, 1497
    ultrasound in, 788–789
Jaw
    abscess of, 1097
    cancer of, 672–673
    congenital smallness of, 1523
    dislocation of, 691
    fracture of, 691, *691*
    hypermobility of, 687, 688, 689–690
    infection of, 1097
    in malocclusion, 680–681
    motion device for, 689
    physical therapy for, 688, *689*
    temporomandibular joint disorders of,
        685–690, *686*
    torus of, 671
JC virus infection, 538–539
Jejunum, 696
Jellyfish sting, 1687
Jet lag, 468, 469, 1711
Job-Buckley syndrome, 1062
Jock itch, 1225
Joint(s), 336–339
    age-associated changes in, 338
    in ankylosing spondylitis, 377
    arthroscopy of, 343
    aspiration of, 342–343, *1729*
    birth defects of, 1523–1524
    Charcot's, *585*
    degenerative disease of (osteoarthritis),
        367–370, *368*, *369*, 404
    disorders of, 365–366 (*see also* Arthritis)
    in Ehlers-Danlos syndrome, 1608
    exercise effects on, 31
    in gout, 392
    infection of, 365–366 (*see also* Septic
        arthritis)
    inflammation of, 339 (*see also* Arthritis)

Joint(s) (*continued*)
    noises in, 341
    pain in, 339
        in rheumatic fever, 1566
        in rubella, 1582
        in pseudogout, 394–395
    range of motion of, 341–342
    in Reiter's syndrome, 376–377
    replacement of, 352–353, 355–356, *357*
        in avascular necrosis, 363
        infection and, 365
        in osteoarthritis, *369*, 370
    sampling of, 342–343, *1729*
    in scleroderma, 381
    stiffness of, 341
    in systemic lupus erythematosus, 378
    temporomandibular, 685–690, *686*
    x-ray of, 342
Joint tenancy, 57
Juvenile rheumatoid arthritis, 1612–1613

K

Kallmann's syndrome, 942
Kanamycin, *1122*
    during pregnancy, *1460*
Kangaroo care, *1495*
Kaolin, *756*
Kaposi's sarcoma, 1240–1241
    in HIV infection, 1172
    in mouth, *663*, 672
Kava, 607
Kawasaki syndrome, 664, 665, *1581*
Kearns-Sayre syndrome, 413
Kegel exercises, 861, *1384*
    in pelvic floor disorders, 1380
    in urinary incontinence, 861, 1358
    in vaginismus, 1383–1384
Keloids, 1237, 1255
Keratectomy, 1289
Keratitis
    herpes simplex, 1161, 1301–1302
    peripheral ulcerative, 1302
    superficial punctate, 1299–1300
    xerotic, 1301
Keratoacanthoma, 671, 1237
Keratoconjunctivitis
    epidemic, *1297*
    herpes simplex, 1301–1302
Keratoconjunctivitis sicca (dry eye),
        1300–1301
Keratoconus, 1302
Keratoderma blennorrhagicum, 376
Keratomalacia, 1301
Keratopathy, bullous, 1302
Keratoses
    actinic, *1231*
    seborrheic, 1237

Keratosis pilaris, 1204
Keratotomy, 1289
Keraunoparalysis, 1664
Kerion, 1225
Kernicterus, 1505
Kerosene poisoning, 1679
Keshan disease, 911–912
Ketamine, 658
Ketoacidosis, 963, 966
  in children, 1613–1614, 1615
Ketoconazole, *1152*
  in precocious puberty, *1557*
Ketones
  in blood, 964
  in urine, 826
Ketoprofen, 95, 97, 454
Ketosis, with low-carbohydrate diet, 886
Keyhole surgery, *1700*
Kidney failure, 828–837
  acute, 829–831, *830*
  in atheroembolic kidney disease, 846–847
  cholesterol levels in, 921
  chronic, 831–833
  coma with, *492*
  in cortical necrosis, 847
  in Fabry's disease, 1620
  in Goodpasture's syndrome, 312
  in malaria, 867
  in malignant hypertension, 847–848
  in multiple myeloma, 1007
  in nephrotic syndrome, 840
  in septic shock, 1120
  shortness of breath with, 251
Kidneys, *939*
  absence of, 1519
  in acid-base regulation, 930–931
  age-associated changes in, *18*, 822–823
  in asymptomatic proteinuria and hematuria
    syndrome, 843
  atheroembolic disease of, 846–847
  biology of, 820–823, *821*
  biopsy of, 828, 832, 839, 847
  birth defects of, 1519, 1567
  in blood pressure control, 132, 822
  blood vessels of, 820–822, *845*
    blockage of, 218, 222–223, 844–846, *846*
    disorders of, 844–849
  cancer of, 875–876
    in children, 1622–1623
  cysts in, 854–855, *855*
  in diabetes insipidus, 851
  dialysis of (*see* Dialysis)
  disorder/dysfunction of, 828–856, 875–876
    (*see also* Kidney failure)
    in diabetes mellitus, *963*, 964
    heart failure with, 152
    in high blood pressure, 136
    information resources on, 1764–1765
    in low blood pressure, 143

Kidneys *(continued)*
  disorder/dysfunction of *(continued)*
    in multiple myeloma, 1007
    over-the-counter drug precautions in,
      102
    during pregnancy, 1447
    in premature infant, 1497
    symptoms of, 823–825
    tests for, 825–828, *827*
    in vitamin D excess, 894
  distention of, 862–864, *863*
  drug elimination by, 69
  drug-related damage to, *83*
  failure of (*see* Kidney failure)
  functions of, 820–822, 849
  in heart failure, 153
  infection of (pyelonephritis), 871–872
    after childbirth, 1479
    in children, 1567–1568
  inflammation of (nephritis), 837–844
  injury to, 872–873, *873*
  necrosis of, 847
  in nephritic syndrome, 838–839
  in nephrotic syndrome, 839–843, *840*, *842*
  polycystic, 854–855, *855*, *1430*, 1519
  during pregnancy, 1439–1440
  radiation effects on, 1660
  radiopaque dye toxicity to, *827*
  in renal tubular acidosis, 849–850, *850*
  stones in, 823, 851–852, 864–866, *865*
    birth defects and, 1519
    in gout, 392, 394
  transplantation of, 1077
    pregnancy and, 1447
  tubules of, 820, *821*
    disorders of, 849–854, *850*
  in tubulointerstitial nephritis, 843–844
  urine backup in (hydronephrosis), 829,
    862–864, *863*
Kienböck's disease, 400
Killer (cytotoxic) T cells, *1052*, 1055,
  1089–1090
Kissing bug bites, 1685
Klebsiella infection, 1103
  meninges, 529
Klinefelter syndrome, 1530, 1556
Knee, 337–338, *338*
  avascular necrosis of, 362
  Baker's (popliteal) cyst of, 419
  knock, 420, *1606*
  in Lyme disease, 1106
  in Osgood-Schlatter disease, 1607
  replacement of, *369*, 370
  runner's (patellofemoral stress syndrome),
    425–426, *425*, *426*
Kneecap (patella), *338*
  chondromalacia of, 1607
  in nail-patella syndrome, 856
Knee jerk reflex, *442*, 561

Knock knees, 420, *1606*
Koplik's spots, *663*, 1576
Korsakoff's syndrome, 479–480, 650, 896
Kuru, 543
Kwashiorkor, 888
Kyphoplasty, 346
Kyphosis, 357, 1604–1605, *1605*

L

Labia majora, 1343, *1344*
  in newborn, 1485
Labia minora, 1343, *1344*
Labor and delivery, 1464–1469
  amniotic fluid embolism in, 1473–1474
  birthing centers for, 1464
  cerebral palsy after, 1624–1626
  cesarean section for, 1475–1476
  complications of, 1470–1476, *1472, 1475*
  disseminated intravascular coagulation in,
    1456, 1474
  drug use during, 1464
  fetal problems during, *1467*, 1471–1473,
    1472, 1507
  forceps for, 1469, 1475, *1475*
  induction of, 1470, 1474
  infection after, 1478–1479
  inverted uterus with, 1474
  maternal heart disease and, 1446
  monitoring after, 1476–1477
  of multiple births, 1473
  natural, *1468*
  newborn injury during, 1494–1495
  pain relief during, 1467–1468
  position for, 1469
  postdelivery period and, 1476–1480
  postterm, 1498
  in preeclampsia, 1473
  presentations for, 1465, 1471–1473, *1472*,
    1485
  preterm, 1470–1471, 1495–1496, *1497*
  shoulder dystocia in, 1473
  slow progression of, 1471
  stages of, 1464–1465, *1466*
  timing problems in, 1470–1471
  of twins, 1473
  umbilical cord prolapse in, 1473
  uterine bleeding after, 1474
  vacuum extractor for, 1475, *1475*
Labyrinth (inner ear), 1244–1245, *1245*
  disorders of, 1255–1261, *1261*
Labyrinthectomy, 1260
Labyrinthitis, 463
  in children, 1594
Laceration
  bladder, 874
  cerebral, 517
  ear, 1255

Laceration *(continued)*
  esophagus, 710
  eye, 1290–1291
  first aid for, 1691–1693
  kidney, 872–873, *873*
  liver, 791
Lacrimal nerve, 1277
Lacrimal system, *1293* (*see also* Tears and
    tear system)
Lactase deficiency, 698, 735–736, 754
Lactate (lactic acid), *1726*
Lactate dehydrogenase, *1039*
Lactation (*see also* Breastfeeding)
  abnormal (galactorrhea), 946–947
Lactic acid (lactate), *1726*
Lactic hydrogenase, *1726*
Lactobacilli, of vagina, 1374
Lactose, 1616
Lactose intolerance, 698, 735–736, 754
Lactulose
  in constipation, *753*
  in liver encephalopathy, 796
L-alpha-acetylmethadol (LAAM), 653
Lamaze method, *1468*
Laminaria, 1426–1427
Laminectomy, 574
Lamivudine (3TC), *1175*
Lamotrigine
  in manic-depressive illness, 621
  in seizure disorders, *500*
Landouzy-Dejerine (facioscapulohumeral)
    muscular dystrophy, 413
Langerhans' cell, 1186
Langerhans' cell granulomatosis, 303–304
Language
  in autism, 1630
  in brain injury, 477–478, *477*
  development of, 1539
  in dyslexia, 1551–1552
  in hearing loss in children, 1598
  in Klinefelter syndrome, 1530
  in mental retardation, 1627
  in Rett's disorder, 1631–1632
Lansoprazole, *718*
Laparoscopy, 703, 1355, 1418, *1700, 1730*
Laparotomy, in cancer staging, 1041
Large-for-gestational-age infant, 1499
Large intestine, *695*, 697–698
  age-associated changes in, *18*, 698, 751
  amebiasis of, 1135–1136
  bleeding in, 776–778, *777*
  blockage (obstruction) of, 751, 770,
    779–781, *780*
    in children, 1589–1590
  cancer of, 770–773, *771*
    screening for, *1038*
    ulcerative colitis and, 742–743
  Crohn's disease of, 738–742, *741*
  diverticulitis of, 748–750, *749*, 751–752

Large intestine *(continued)*
  diverticulosis of, 747–748, *748*
  endoscopy of, 703, *704*
  Escherichia coli infection of, 723–724
  examination of (sigmoidoscopy), *29*
  fistula of, 748–749, *749*
  hemorrhagic colitis of, 723–724
  Hirschsprung disease of, 1522–1523
  inertia of, 751
  inflammatory disease of, 738–745, *741* (*see also* Colitis)
  ischemia of, 218, *219*, 223, 783
  polyps of, 768–769
  rapid stool transit in, 754
  slowed stool transit in, 750–751
  spastic (irritable bowel syndrome), 756–757
  strangulation of, 780, *780*
  surgical removal of, 744
  tumors of, 768–769
  ulcerative colitis of, 742–744
Larva migrans
  cutaneous, 1220
  visceral (toxocariasis), 1144
Laryngitis, 1268–1269
Laryngoceles, 1270
Laryngotracheobronchitis, 1579–1580, 1585–1586
Larynx (voice box), 244, *245*, 1246, *1246*
  cancer of, 1271–1272, *1272*
  outpouchings of (laryngoceles), 1270
  papilloma of, 1600
Laser epithelial keratomileusis (LASEK), 1290
Laser in situ keratomileusis (LASIK), 1289
Laser therapy
  for arteriovenous fistula, 239
  for birthmarks, *1235*
  for diabetic retinopathy, 1313–1314
  for endometriosis, 1371
  for glaucoma, 1309
  for hair removal, 1212
  for macular degeneration, 1311
  for retinal detachment, 1311–1312
  for retinopathy of prematurity, 1504
  for varicose veins, 238
  for vision (refractive) disorders, 1288–1290
  for wart removal, 1229
Laser thermal keratoplasty (LTK), 1289–1290
LASIK (laser in situ keratomileusis), 1289
Lassa fever, 1165–1167
Latanoprost, *1308*
Lateral epicondylitis (backhand tennis elbow), 427–428, *427, 428*
Laughing gas, *659*
Lavage, bronchoalveolar, 257
Laws (*see* Legal issues)
Laxatives, 752, *753*
  abuse of, *647*
Lazy bowel syndrome, 752–753

LDL cholesterol, 197, 202, 920, *921, 922, 1726*
  after menopause, 1357
  estrogen and, 1358
  progestin and, 1359
Lead
  poisoning with, 1680
  reference range for, *1726*
Learning disorders, 1551
  in ADHD, 1549–1550
  information resources on, 1765
Leber's hereditary optic neuropathy, 14, 560
Leboyer method, *1468*
Leflunomide, 372, 375
Leg
  amputation of, 222, 964
    rehabilitation after, 43–44
  arterial disease of, 216–223, *221, 222*
  birth defects of, 1523–1524
  bowing of, *1606*
  chilblains of, 1656
  claudication in, 217, 221
  deep vein thrombosis in, 232–236, *235*
  fracture of, 354–355
  lymphatic vessel deficiency in, 240
  lymphedema in, 240
  pain in
    in Buerger's disease, 223
    when walking, 217, 221
  popliteus tendinitis of, 424
  reattachment of, *1083*
  sciatica of, *571*
  severed or constricted, 1693
  shin splints in, 423–424, *423, 424*
  splint for, *1692*
  stasis dermatitis of, 1197–1198
  swelling (edema) in, 153, 240
  thrombophlebitis of, 232, 236
  torsion of, *1606*
  ulcers of, 217, 235–236
  varicose veins of, 236–238, *237*
  veins of, 231–232, *232*
Legal issues, 53–57
  advance directive, 22, 48, 51, *53*, 54–56
  capacity, 53–54
  in child abuse and neglect, 1643–1644
  competency, 53–54, *53*
  confidentiality, 54
  in death and dying, 51
  disclosure, 54
  do-not-resuscitate order, 48, 57
  durable power of attorney for health care, *53*, 55–56
  informed consent, 54
  joint tenancy, 57
  living will, *53*, 55
  power of attorney, 57
  property management, 57
  revocable (living) trust, 57
  surrogate decision making, 56–57

Legg-Calvé-Perthes disease, 1606–1607
Legionnaires' disease, 267–268
Leiomyoma
  esophagus, 764
  small intestine, 768
  uterus, 1372–1374
Leiomyosarcoma
  esophagus, 765
  small intestine, 769
  stomach, 767
Length
  of infant, 1490, *1490*
  metric equivalents for, 1722
  of newborn, 1484
Lens(es), 1276, *1276*
  age-associated changes in, 1278
  cloudiness of (cataract), *20*, 1303–1305,
      1304
    congenital, *1512*
    in electrical injury, 1662
    in galactosemia, 1617
  dislocation of, in homocystinuria, 1619
  intraocular, implantation of, 1289, 1304
Leprosy, 1130–1132
  information resources on, 1765
Leptin, 915, *939*
Leptospirosis, 1104–1105
Leriche's syndrome, 217–218
Let-down reflex, 1477, 1487
Letterer-Siwe disease, 303–304
Leukemia, 1010–1016, 1032
  acute lymphocytic (lymphoblastic), *20*,
      1011–1012
  acute myelocytic (myeloid, myelogenous,
      myeloblastic, myelomonocytic),
      1012–1014, *1013*
  acute promyelocytic, 1013, 1014
  adult T-cell, 1011
  chronic lymphocytic (lymphoblastic),
      1014–1015
  chronic myelocytic (myeloid, myelogenous,
      granulocytic), 1015–1016
  gingivitis in, 683
  hairy cell, 1014, 1015
  T-cell, 1014
Leukocyte (*see* White blood cells)
Leukocyte adhesion defects, *1058*
Leukocyte esterase, 826
Leukocyte glucose-6-phosphate
    dehydrogenase deficiency, *1058*
Leukocytosis, 979, 1002
  lymphocytic, 1004–1005
  neutrophilic, 1003
Leukoedema, *663*
Leukoencephalopathy, progressive multifocal,
    538–539
Leukopenia, 979, 980, 1002
  with cancer treatment, 1047
Leukoplakia, 671

Leukotriene modifiers, *278*, 280, 1584
Leuprolide
  in precocious puberty, *1557*
  in prostate cancer, 1334
Levetiracetam, *500*
Levobetaxalol, *1308*
Levobunolol, *1308*
Levodopa, 548, *549*
Levofloxacin, *1123*
Levorphanol, *451*
Lewy body dementia, 489
Leyden-Möbius muscular dystrophy, 413
Lhermitte's sign, 558–559
Libido (sex drive)
  female, 1382, 1384–1385
  male, 1336, 1339–1340
    in erectile dysfunction, 1337
Lice, 1219, *1219*, 1685
  rickettsial infections from, 1132–1134,
      1133
  in traveler, 1714
Lichenification, *1189*
Lichen planus, 670, 1203–1204
Lichen sclerosus, 1349
Lichen simplex chronicus (localized scratch
    dermatitis), 1198
Licorice, *105*, 110, *961*
Liddle's syndrome, 854, 910
Lidocaine
  for canker sores, 668
  in chronic pancreatitis, 733
  topical, 455, 668
Life expectancy, 17
Life span, 17
Lifestyle
  aging and, 19, 20
  longevity and, 17
  in risk assessment, 25, 26, *26*
Life-sustaining treatment, 47–48, *56*
Lifting technique, 572
Ligament(s), 335–336
  ankle, 405–407, *406*
  scapholunate, *401*
Light
  depression (seasonal affective disorder) and,
      614
  sensitivity to (photophobia), 1281–1282
  sun (*see* Sunlight; Ultraviolet light)
Lightheadedness, 461–462
  in heart disease, 120
Lightning injury, 1663–1664
Light therapy
  for manic-depressive illness, 621
  for seasonal affective disorder, *614*
Limb-girdle muscular dystrophy, 413
Limbic system, 434
Limbs (*see also* Arm; Leg)
  birth defects of, 1523–1524
  severed or constricted, 1693

Lindane, 1219
Linea alba, of gum, *663*
Linezolid, *1124*
Lip, 661
  cancer of, 673
  cleft, 1523, *1523*
  color changes in, 664
  inflammation of (cheilitis), 674
  keratoacanthoma of, 671
  sores on, 664
  sunlight damage to, 664
  swelling of, 664
Lipase, 697, 731, *1726*
Lipid (*see* Fat; Lipoproteins)
Lipid-lowering drugs, 923–925, *925*
  after menopause, 1359, *1360*
Lipidoses, 1619–1620, *1621*
Lipodystrophy, intestinal (Whipple's disease),
  737
Lipoma, 1234
  small intestine, 768
  spinal cord, 1526
Lipoproteins, 920, *921*
  after menopause, 1357
  in atherosclerosis, 197, 920, 921–922
  coronary artery disease and, 200
  desirable blood levels of, *922*
  HDL, 197, 202, 920, *921*, *922*, *1726*
    estrogen and, 1358
    progestin and, 1359
  high blood levels of, 920, 921–926, *924*, *925*
  inhibitors of, *925*
  LDL, 197, 202, 920, *921*, 922, *1726*
    estrogen and, 1358
    progestin and, 1359
  lowering of, 922–923, *923*, *924*, *925*
    in coronary artery disease prevention,
      202
  oral contraceptive use and, 1420
  VLDL, 920, *921*
Liposuction, *1699*
  in gynecomastia, *1323*
Lip reading, 1252–1253
Liquid diet, 886
Liquor (*see* Alcohol use and abuse)
Listeria monocytogenes infection (listeriosis),
  1105
  meninges, 529
  during pregnancy, 1450
Lithium
  in mania, 620
  in manic-depressive illness, 621
  during pregnancy, *1461*
Lithotripsy, *865*, 866
Liver, *695*, 697
  abscess of, 779, 1136
  adenoma of, 810
  age-associated changes in, *18*, 698, 788
  alcohol effects on, 649–650

Liver *(continued)*
  in alpha$_1$-antitrypsin deficiency, 801
  angiosarcoma of, 812
  in ascites, 794–795
  biology of, 786, 787, *807*
  biopsy of, 790–791, 805, 809, 811, 812
  blood supply of, 786, 806, *807*
    disorders of, 218, 223, 806–810
  cancer of, 798, 811–813
  cholangiocarcinoma of, 811–812
  in cholestasis, 792–793
  cirrhosis of, 797–799, *799*
    during pregnancy, 1448
  colorectal cancer spread to, 772
  copper accumulation in (Wilson's disease),
    905
  disease of *(see also specific diseases)*
    cholesterol levels in, 921
    clinical manifestations of, 791–796, *792*
    hormone replacement therapy and, 1359
    information resources on, 1765
    during pregnancy, 1448
    prevention of, *27*
    in Reye's syndrome, *1572*
    tests for, 788–791, *789*
    in ulcerative colitis, 743
  drug metabolism by, 68, 69, 74, 75, 76, 788
  drug-related damage to, 83, 1676
  in encephalopathy, 795–796
  enlargement of, 793
    in heart disease, 121
    in myelofibrosis, 1025
    in polycythemia, 1023
  failure of, 796
    bad breath and, *684*
    in Budd-Chiari syndrome, 808–809
    coma with, *492*
  fatty, 797, *798*, *799*
    of pregnancy, 1453–1454
  function tests of, *1726*
  gonococcal infection of, 1179
  hemangioma of, 810
  hepatoblastoma of, 812
  hepatoma of, 798, 811
  in hereditary hemorrhagic telangiectasia,
    810
  immune function of, 1050–1051, *1053*
  infection of, 779, 1136 (*see also* Hepatitis)
  inflammation of (*see* Hepatitis)
  in jaundice, 791–792
  metastasis to, 812–813
  palpation of, 793
  in polycystic kidney disease, 854
  in portal hypertension, 793–794
  of premature infant, 1497
  primary biliary cirrhosis of, 799–800
  primary sclerosing cholangitis of, 800–801
  sarcoidosis of, 305
  tests for, 788–791, *789*, *1726*

Liver *(continued)*
  transplantation of, 1077–1079
    in alpha₁-antitrypsin deficiency, 801
    in cirrhosis, 799
    in hepatitis, 806
    in portal vein thrombosis, 809
    in primary sclerosing cholangitis, 801
  tumors of, 810–813
Liver fluke infection, *1146*
Living trust (revocable trust), 57
Living will, *53, 55*
Lizard bites, 1683–1684
Localized scratch dermatitis, 1198
Locked-in state, 494
Lockjaw *(see Tetanus)*
Löffler's endocarditis, 1005
Löffler's syndrome, 310
Lomefloxacin, *1123*
Longevity, 17
Long QT syndrome, 1530
Loop electrical excision procedure, 1354, 1407
Loop of Henle, 820, *821*
Loperamide, *756*
Lopinavir, *1175*
Loracarbef, *1122*
Loratadine, *1065*
Lorazepam, *500*
Lorenzo's oil, 560
Lotions, 1189
Loudness, measurement of, *1249*
Lou Gehrig's disease (amyotrophic lateral sclerosis), 575–577
  information resources on, 1757
Lovastatin, 72, *925*
Low back pain *(see Back pain)*
Low blood pressure, 141–147
  after eating, 144, 147
  in anemia, 988
  causes of, *142,* 143
  in dehydration, 929
  fainting with, 143–146
  in persistent pulmonary hypertension, 1502
  during pregnancy, 1439
  in shock, 148–149
  upon standing, 144, 146–147
Low blood sugar *(see Hypoglycemia)*
Low-molecular-weight heparin, 288
LSD (lysergic acid diethylamide), 657–658
LTK (laser thermal keratoplasty), 1289–1290
Ludwig's angina, 670
Lumbago *(see Back, pain in)*
Lumbar plexus, 581–582, *581*
Lumbar puncture *(see Spinal tap)*
Lumbar strain, 569
Lump *(see also Tumor[s])*
  in breast, 1387, 1388–1389, 1391
  in neck, *1273*
    in children, 1599

Lump *(continued)*
  in newborn skin, 1485
  in throat, 700
  in vulva, 1408
Lumpectomy, 1394, *1396*
Lumpy jaw, 1097
Lunacy *(see Mental health disorders)*
Lunate bone, avascular necrosis of (Kienböck's disease), 400
Lungs *(see also Breathing)*
  abscess of, 265, 272–273, 1112
  age-associated changes in, *18,* 248
  air conditioner, 309, *309*
  anthrax infection of, 1098
  asbestosis of, 296, *297*
  aspergillosis of, 1149
  atelectasis of, 292–294
  barotrauma to, 1668
  beryllium disease of, *297,* 298–299
  biology of, 244–248, *245, 246, 247*
  biopsy of, 256, 257, 258, 302, 303
  bird fancier's, *309*
  black, 296, *297*
  blood flow in, 115–116, *115*
  byssinosis of, *297,* 300
  cancer of, 328–331, *329*
    abscess with, 272
    asbestosis and, 297
    coughing up blood in, 252
    paraneoplastic syndromes in, *1037*
    positron emission tomography in, 256
    screening for, 330, *1038*
    staging of, *1040*
    toxic gas exposure and, 300
  cheese washer's, *309*
  chemical exposure and, 300–301, *309*
  in chickenpox, 1571
  cigarettes and *(see Smoking)*
  coffee worker's, *309*
  congestion of *(see Pneumonia; Pulmonary edema)*
  cork worker's, *309*
  cystic fibrosis of, 317–322, *318*
  cysts of, in Marfan syndrome, 1608
  defense mechanisms of, 247–248
  diffusing capacity of, 255
  disorders of, 243–331 *(see also specific disorders, eg, Pneumonia)*
    allergic, 308–312, *309*
    coma with, *492*
    diagnosis of, 253–258, *254, 257*
    infiltrative, 301–308, *302, 307*
    information resources on, 1767
    in newborn, 1499–1500
    occupational, 294–301, *297*
    in opioid abuse, 652
    rehabilitation for, 259–262, 284–285
    symptoms of, 248–253
    travel and, 1712

Lungs *(continued)*
  drug-induced disease of, *307*
  dysplasia of, in newborn, 1502–1503
  embolism of (*see* Pulmonary embolism)
  failure of, 325–326, *325*
  farmer's, 309, *309*
  fetal, 1448, 1454, 1498
  fibrosis of, 323
    in black lung, 296
    cystic, 317–322, *318*
    idiopathic, 301–302
  flock worker's, *297*, 299
  flow rate of, 254, *254*
  fluid accumulation in, in heart failure,
    153–154, 158
  fluke infection of, *1146*
  function testing of, 254–255, *254*
  gas exchange in, 245–246, *246*
  grain worker's, 300
  hantavirus infection of, 1167
  histoplasmosis of, 1152–1153
  imaging of, 255–256
  infection of (*see* Bronchitis, acute;
    Pneumonia *and specific infections*)
  inflammation of (*see* Pneumonitis)
  irritation of (*see* Pneumonitis)
  of large-for-gestational-age infant, 1499
  malt worker's, *309*
  maple bark stripper's, *309*
  miller's, *309*
  mushroom worker's, *309*
  occupational diseases of, 294–301, *297*
  pain in, 251
  pleural effusion and, 251, 314–316, *315*
  pleurisy and, 119, 251, 313–314, *314*
  postural drainage of, 261
  in premature infant, 1496, 1499–1500
  radiation injury to, 1660
  reduction surgery for, 292
  respiratory distress syndrome of, 326–328,
    327
  scan of, 255–256, 287
  shortness of breath and, 250
  silicosis of, 295–296, *297*
  silo filler's disease of, *297*, 300
  smoke-related injury to, *1649*
  suctioning of, 258, 261
  surgery on
    in bronchiectasis, 292
    in COPD, 285
    in cystic fibrosis, 321
    in lung cancer, 330–331
  thoracoscopy for, 258
  thoracotomy for, 258
  transplantation of, 292, 321, 324, 1080
  tuberculosis of, 1125–1130
  woodworker's, *309*
Lung volume, 254, *254*
Lupus anticoagulant, 1000

Lupus erythematosus
  discoid, 378
  information resources on, 1765
  systemic, 378–380, *379*, *1074*
    in pregnancy, 1448
Luteinizing hormone, *939*, 940, *941*, 1343,
    1368
  deficiency of, 942
  measurement of, 943
  in menstrual cycle, 1346, 1347, *1347*
Lye burns, *1648*
Lyme disease, 1105–1107, *1107*
Lymph, 239
  accumulation of (lymphedema), 240
  urinary, 867–868
Lymphadenitis, 240–241, 1599
Lymphangiectasia, intestinal, 737–738
Lymphangioma, 1236
Lymphangitis, 241
Lymphatic system, 1050–1051, *1053* (*see also*
    Lymph nodes)
  cancer of (*see* Lymphoma)
  disorders of, 239–241
  injury to, 314, 316
  vessels of, 239, *1053*
    inflammation of (lymphangitis), 241
Lymphedema, 240
  of scrotum, 1329
  in Turner syndrome, 1528
Lymph nodes, 239, *1053*
  abscess of, 1563–1564
  in breast cancer, 1391–1392, 1396, *1397*
  in cancer, 1036, *1273*
  in Hodgkin's disease, 1017, 1018
  inflammation of (lymphadenitis), 240–241
  of neck, *1273*, 1599
  in non-Hodgkin's lymphoma, 1020
  radiation effects on, 1659
  sentinel, 1396, *1398*
  in tuberculosis, 1127
Lymphoblasts, 1004
Lymphocytes, 978, 1050, *1051*, *1052*,
    1054–1055 (*see also* B lymphocytes;
    T lymphocytes)
  formation of, 979
  high levels of (leukocytosis), 1004–1005
  low levels of (lymphocytopenia), 1004,
    1004
Lymphocytic choriomeningitis, 538
Lymphocytic colitis, 744–745
Lymphocytic interstitial pneumonitis,
    1574
Lymphocytic (lymphoblastic) leukemia
  acute (ALL), 1011–1012
  chronic (CLL), 1014–1015
Lymphocytic leukocytosis, 1004–1005
Lymphocytopenia, 1004, *1004*
Lymphogranuloma venereum, 1181
Lymphoid interstitial pneumonia, 303

Lymphoma, 1016–1022, 1032
  Burkitt's, *1020*
  Hodgkin's, 1017–1018, *1017, 1019*
    paraneoplastic syndromes in, *1037*
  in kidney transplant recipient, 1077
  non-Hodgkin's, 1019–1022, *1020, 1021*
    bone, 361
    celiac disease and, 737
    esophagus, *765*
    small intestine, *769*
    stomach, 767
  in Sjögren's syndrome, 382
  staging of, *1040*
Lysergic acid diethylamide (LSD), 657–658

M

Maceration, of skin, 1190
Macroglobulinemia, 1009–1010, *1009*
Macrolides, *1123*
  in transplantation, *1078*
Macrominerals, 900 *(see also specific minerals)*
Macronutrients, 880–882
Macrophages, *1052*
  alveolar, 248
  in chronic granulomatous disease, 1062
  in immune response, 1051–1052
Macula, 1276, *1276, 1310*
  degeneration of, 1279, 1310–1311
Macular pucker, 1311
Macules, *1189*
  melanotic, 664
Maculopathy
  age-related, 1310–1311
  cellophane, 1311
Mad cow disease, *542*
Madness (*see* Mental health disorders)
Mafenide, *1123*
Magic mushroom, 657–658
Magnesium, *902,* 908–909
  in antacids, 99
  deficiency of, *735*
  high blood levels of (hypermagnesemia), 909
  low blood levels of (hypomagnesemia), 908–909
    low calcium levels and, 901
  reference range for, *1726*
Magnesium citrate, *753*
Magnesium hydroxide
  in constipation, *753*
  in peptic ulcer, 716, *718*
Magnesium sulfate, 1452, 1470
Magnetic resonance angiography (MRA), 127
Magnetic resonance cholangiopancreato-graphy (MRCP), 789

Magnetic resonance imaging (MRI), 8, *1730*
  in acromegaly, 946
  of biliary tract, 789
  of brain, 508, 539
  in cancer staging, 1041
  of digestive system, 705
  of eye, 1286
  of fracture, 350
  of heart, 126–127, 191
  of kidney and urinary tract, 827
  of lung, 255
  in multiple sclerosis, 559
  of musculoskeletal system, 342
  in neurologic disorders, 443–444
  in stroke, 508
  in vertigo, 464
Major histocompatibility complex (MHC), 1050, *1052*
  in organ transplantation, 1076
Malabsorption, 734–738, *735*
  in vitamin B_{12} deficiency, 898
Malaria, 1140–1142, 1714
  kidney damage and, 867
  during pregnancy, 1713
Malassezia furfur infection, 1227–1228
Malathion, 1219
Mal de mer (sea sickness) (*see* Motion sickness)
Male-pattern baldness, 1212–1213
Malformations (*see* Birth defects)
Malignancy (*see* Cancer)
Malignant fibrous histiocytoma, 361
Malignant hypertension, 131, 134, 141
  kidney failure in, 847–848
Malignant hyperthermia, 75
Malignant melanoma (*see* Melanoma)
Malignant nephrosclerosis, 847–848
Malingering, 637
Mallet finger, 359, 396, *396*
Malleus (hammer), 1244, *1245*
Mallory-Weiss syndrome, 710
Malnutrition, 887–890, *888, 889*
  in immunodeficiency disorders, 1057
  in infants and young children, 1537–1538
  in nephrotic syndrome, 840
  optic neuropathy and, 1316
  pressure sores and, 1208
Malocclusion, 680–681
Maltase deficiency, 735
Malt worker's lung, *309*
Mammary glands (*see* Breasts)
Mammography, *29, 1038,* 1040, 1355–1356, *1355,* 1392–1393, *1730*
Managed care, 24
  drug policies of, 92
  for dying person, 47
Mandible (*see also* Jaw)
  congenital smallness of, 1523
  dislocation of, 691
  fracture of, 691, *691*

Mania, 619–620, *620*
Manic-depressive illness, 620–621
  in children, 1633–1634
Mannitol, 515
Manometry, 706
  in esophageal spasm, 708–709
  in gastroesophageal reflux, 718–719
MAOIs (*see* Monoamine oxidase inhibitors)
Maple bark stripper's lung, *309*
Maple syrup urine disease, 1619
Marasmus, 887–888
Marble bone disease, 1611
Marburg virus infection, 1165
Marchiafava-Bignami disease, 650
Marfan syndrome, 1608–1609
  aortic aneurysm in, 228
Margarine, *201, 923*
Marijuana
  adolescent use of, 1559–1560
  dependence on, 655–656
  in HIV infection, 1174
  during pregnancy, 1464
Marine animal bites and stings, 1686–1687
Markers, tumor, 1034, *1039*, 1041
Marketplace, fear of (agoraphobia), 609–610
Marsh fever (*see* Malaria)
Masculinization, 1368
Mask of pregnancy, 1215–1216, 1421,
    1440–1441
Masochism, 630
Massage, 38, 1707
  in temporomandibular joint disorders, *689*
MAST (military [medical] antishock trousers),
    149
Mastalgia, 1387
Mast cells, *1052*, 1069
  in allergic reactions, 1063
  in asthma, 274
Mastectomy, 1396, *1396*
  breast reconstruction after, 1396–1397,
    1399
Master gland (*see* Pituitary gland)
Mastitis, 1112, 1389, 1479
Mastocytoma, 1069
Mastocytosis, 1069–1070
Mastoiditis, 1259, 1594
Masturbation, 627, 1554
Mathematics, learning disorders in, 1551
Maturation (*see* Puberty)
Mauriac syndrome, 1615
Maxilla (*see* Jaw)
Maxillary sinus, 1245–1246, *1265*
Mazindol, 919
MCAD (medium chain acyl-CoA
    dehydrogenase) deficiency, 1621
McArdle's disease, *1617*
McCune-Albright syndrome, *1557*
MDMA (methylenedioxymethamphetamine),
    656

Mean corpuscular hemoglobin (MCH), *1726*
Mean corpuscular hemoglobin concentration
    (MCHC), *1726*
Mean corpuscular volume (MCV), *981, 1726*
Measles (rubeola), *1569*, 1575–1577
  immunization for, 1093, *1094*, 1493, *1493*,
    1577
  in HIV-infected children, 1575
  Koplik's spots of, *663*
  subacute sclerosing panencephalitis with,
    1582
Measles, German (*see* Rubella)
Measurements, tables for, 1721–1725
Mechanical ventilation, 285, 326, 327 (*see
    also* Ventilation, mechanical)
Meckel's diverticulum, 1590–1591, *1591*
Meconium, 1465, 1486
  aspiration of, 1498, 1501
  ileus with, in cystic fibrosis, 319
Medial epicondylitis (forehand tennis elbow),
    427, 428–429, *428*
Median nerve compression (carpal tunnel
    syndrome), 398–399, *399*
Mediastinoscopy, 258, *1730*
Mediastinum, 245
Medical decision making, 1695–1698
MedicAlert Foundation, 1765
Medical information, 1695–1696, 1697–1698
Medical records, 23–24
Medications (*see* Drugs)
Meditation, 1706
Mediterranean fever, familial, 1716–1717
Medium chain acyl-CoA dehydrogenase
    (MCAD) deficiency, 1621
Medroxyprogesterone
  in contraception, *1420*, 1422–1423
  in ovulation problems, 1417
  in undernutrition, 890
Medullary cystic disease, 855
Medullary sponge kidney, 855–856
Medulloblastoma, *521*
Mefloquine, 1141
Megacolon
  congenital, 1522–1523
  toxic, 742, 744
Megaesophagus, 709
Megestrol, 1174
Meglitinides, 968–969, *968*
Melanin, 1186, 1211–1212, 1214, 1230
  absence of (albinism), 1214
Melanocytes, 1186, *1187*, 1214
  loss of (vitiligo), 1215
Melanocyte-stimulating hormone, 940, *941*
Melanoma, 1239–1240
  choroid, 1314
  dysplastic nevi and, 1234
  mole changes and, 1234
  in mouth, 672
  warning signs of, *1240*

Melanosis, smoker's, *663*
Melanosis coli, 752–753
Melasma, 1215–1216, 1421, 1440–1441
Melatonin
   in insomnia, 469–470
   in jet lag, 1711
   as nutraceutical, 110–111
Melena, 699, 705, 754
Melphalan, *1045*
Membrane(s)
   amniotic, rupture of, 1465
      premature, 1470
   cell, 2
   epiretinal, 1311
   mucous (*see also* Mucous membranes)
      barrier function of, 1087
      drug-related blistering of, 1199–1200
Membranoproliferative glomerulonephritis,
   842
Membranous glomerulonephritis, *842*
Memory
   age-associated changes in, 484
   alcohol and, 479–480, 650
   in dementia, 485
   in Korsakoff's syndrome, 479–480, 650
   loss of, 479–480
      in dissociative amnesia, 636–637
      in dissociative fugue, 637–638
      in dissociative identity disorder, 638
      in temporal lobe injury, 477
Memory aids, for drug compliance, 88
Menaquinone, 895
Menarche, 1346
Ménétrier's disease, 711, 712
Meniere's disease, 463, 1259–1260
Meninges, 435, *435, 436*
Meningioma, *521, 522, 527*
Meningitis
   arenavirus, 538
   aseptic, *535*
   bacterial, 529–531
   in children, 1569–1570
      aseptic, *1576*
      bacterial, 1562–1563
   chronic, 532, *533, 534*
   Cryptococcus neoformans, 1151–1152
      with HIV infection, *1172*
   with ear infection, 1594
   headache with, 456, *459*
   meningococcal, immunization for, *1094,
      1709*
   in newborn, 1510
   noninfectious, *534*
   in syphilis, 1177
   tuberculous, 1128
   viral, 532–535
Meningocele, 1526
Meningoencephalitis, mumps, 1577, 1578

Meningoencephalocele, 1526
Meningomyelocele, 1526
Meniscoid body, 406
Menometrorrhagia, *1362*
Menopause, 1348, 1356–1361, *1360*
   artificial, 1356
   bleeding after, *1362*
   gingivitis after, 682–683
   hormone replacement therapy for,
      1358–1359, *1360*
   osteoporosis after, 343–346, *344, 345*
   premature, 1356, 1361
   vaginal bleeding after, 1366, 1403
   weight gain after, 916
Menorrhagia, *1362*
Menstrual cycle, 1345, 1346–1348, *1347*
   in acromegaly, 945
   discharge during, 1349
   disorders of, 1361–1366, *1362, 1363, 1365,
      1366*
   first (menarche), 1346
   galactorrhea and, 946
   during perimenopause, 1356
Mental health disorders, 597–659
   anxiety disorders, 605–613
   Asperger's disorder, 1631
   autism, 1630–1631
   bipolar disorder, 1633–1634
   childhood disintegrative disorder, 1632
   in children, 1630–1637, *1633, 1635, 1636*
   classification of, 599
   deinstitutionalization and, 598
   depression, 614–619, *614, 618* (*see also*
      Depression)
   digestive system disorders and, 702–703
   dissociative disorders, 636–640
   eating disorders, 624–627
   health care professionals for, *599, 600*
   information resources on, 1766–1767
   mania, 619–620, *620*, 1633–1634
   manic-depressive disorder (bipolar disorder),
      620–621, 1633–1634
   with marijuana use, 655
   mental retardation and, 1627–1628
   overview of, 598–601
   personality disorders, 631–635, *632, 634*
   pervasive developmental disorder not
      otherwise specified, 1631
   Rett's disorder, 1631–1632
   schizophrenia, 640–644, *643, 645*, 1632
   sexual disorders, 627–630
   social aspects of, 598–599
   somatoform disorders, 601–605, *604*,
      1637
   suicidal behavior, 622–624, *622, 623*,
      1634–1635, *1635*
   travel and, 1713
   treatment of, 599–601

Mental retardation, 1626–1629, *1627, 1628*
   in Down syndrome, 1527–1528
   in fragile X syndrome, 1528
   information resources on, 1765
   in phenylketonuria, 1618
Mental status examination, 439, *441*
Meperidine, *451*
   in elderly persons, *80*
Meprobamate
   abuse of, 653–654
   in elderly persons, *81*
   in sleep disorders, *471*
Mercaptopurine, *1045*
   in Crohn's disease, 740, *741*
   during pregnancy, *1461*
   in ulcerative colitis, 744
Meropenem, *1122*
Mesalamine
   in Crohn's disease, 740, *741*
   in proctitis, 762
   in ulcerative colitis, 743
Mesangial proliferative glomerulonephritis,
   842
Mescaline, 657–658
Mesenteric artery, blockage of, 218, *219,*
   223
Mesothelioma, 296–297, 298
Meta-analysis, 1696
Metabisulfite, 1068
Metabolic acidosis, 931–932, *932*
Metabolic alkalosis, 932–933, *932*
Metabolic syndrome, *922*
Metabolism, 1616
   age-associated changes in, *18*
   disorders of
      carbohydrate (*see* Diabetes mellitus)
      in children, 1616–1621, *1617, 1621*
      seizures with, *496*
   drug, 68–69
Metacarpal bones, fracture of, 359
Metal, dermatitis from, *1193,* 1194
Metal fume fever, 914
Metaplasia, gastric, 712
Metastasis, 1032 (*see also* Cancer)
   to bile ducts, 817
   from bladder cancer, 878
   to bone, 361
   to brain, 519, 521, 525
   from breast cancer, 1390, 1398, 1400,
      1401
   to choroid, 1314
   from colorectal cancer, 772
   from esophageal cancer, 765
   to esophagus, *765*
   to heart, 192, 194
   hypercalcemia and, 904
   from kidney cancer, 876
   to liver, 812–813

Metastasis *(continued)*
   to lung, 328, 331
   from lung cancer, 329–330
   from melanoma, 1240
   from oral cancer, 673
   from ovarian cancer, 1405
   from prostate cancer, 1331
   from retinoblastoma, 1624
   to spinal cord, 526
   from stomach cancer, 767
Metatarsal bones
   fracture of, 354, *354*
   stress fracture of, 422–423, *422*
Metatarsalgia, 404
Metatarsus adductus, 1524
Metaxalone, in elderly persons, *81*
Metered-dose inhaler
   in asthma, 279–280, *279,* 1584
   in COPD, 283
Metformin, *968*
Methadone, *451*
   in opioid withdrawal, 653
   during pregnancy, 1464
Methamphetamine (speed, crystal), 656
Methazolamide, *1308*
Methimazole, *951,* 952
   during pregnancy, *1461*
Methocarbamol, *81*
Methotrexate, *1045*
   in Crohn's disease, 740, *741*
   folic acid deficiency with, 899
   during pregnancy, *1461*
   in psoriasis, 1202
   in rheumatoid arthritis, *372,* 375
   in transplantation, *1078*
Methoxsalen, 376
Methylcellulose, *753*
Methyldopa
   in elderly persons, *80*
   hepatitis with, 803
Methylenedioxymethamphetamine, 656
   adolescent use of, 1559–1560
Methylphenidate, 1550
Methylprednisolone
   in multiple sclerosis, 559
   in spinal cord injury, 563
Methyl salicylate poisoning, 1677
Methylxanthines
   in asthma, *278,* 280
   in COPD, 284
Methysergide, *460*
Metipranolol, *1308*
Metoprolol, *951*
Metric measurement, 1721–1725
Metronidazole, *1124, 1182,* 1377
   in amebiasis, 1136
   in Crohn's disease, 740–741
   in peptic ulcer, *718*

Metrorrhagia, *1362*
Mexiletine
  in long QT syndrome, 1530
  for pain, 455
Mezlocillin, *1123*
MHC (major histocompatibility complex),
    1050, *1052*
  in organ transplantation, 1076
Microbes (*see* Microorganisms)
β$_2$-Microglobulin, *1039*
  in multiple myeloma, 1008
Micronutrients, 880, 882–883, 890–914,
    892–893, 902–903 (see also specific
    vitamins and minerals)
Microorganisms, 1086, *1087 (see also*
    Bacteria; Infection; Viral infection)
  body invasion by, 1086–1087
  identification of, *1088*
Microphallus, 1520
Microsporum infection (ringworm),
    1225–1226
Micturition (*see* Urination)
Micturition syncope, 144
Midazolam, *501*
Middle ear, 1244, *1245*
  disorders of, 1255–1261, *1258, 1261*
Middle lobe syndrome, 293, 294
Midodrine, 147
Mifepristone, 1427
Miglitol, *968*
Migraine headache, 457–461, *458, 460*
  vision loss in, 1279
Migratory phlebitis, 223, 236
Milia, *1496,* 1535
Miliaria, 1210, *1211*
Military (medical) antishock trousers,
    149
Milk
  allergy to, in infant, 1531
  breast (*see* Breast feeding; Breast milk)
  in galactosemia, 1617
  in hypophosphatemia, 910
  intolerance to, 698, 735–736, 754
  for weight loss diet, 886
Milk-alkali syndrome, 904
Milk thistle, *105,* 111
Miller-Fisher syndrome, 586
Miller's lung, *309*
Millipede bites, 1686
Mind-body
  interactions of, 7–8
  therapeutic techniques for, 1705–1706
Minerals, 882–883, 900–914, *902–903*
    (*see also specific minerals, eg,* Iron;
    Zinc)
Minimal change disease, *842*
Minocycline, *1123*
  in acne, 1206, *1207*
  teeth discoloration with, *663*
Minoxidil, 1213

Miscarriage, 1456–1457
  alcohol use and, 1463
  chromosomal abnormalities and, 1431
  IUD use and, 1425
  pelvic abnormalities and, 1445
Misconduct, 1635–1636
Misoprostol
  in abortion, 1427
  in peptic ulcer, 716, *718*
Mites, 1218–1219
  bites by, 1685–1686
  rickettsial infections from, 1132–1134, *1133*
Mitochondrial antibodies, 800
Mitochondrial myopathy, 413
Mitochondrion (mitochondria), 2, *4*
  genes of, 14
Mitotic inhibitors, *1078*
Mitoxantrone, 559
Mitral valve, 114, *115*
  in cardiomyopathy, 161
  in Marfan syndrome, 1608
  prolapse of, 119, 178
  regurgitation at, 175–178, *176*
    in children, 1566
  stenosis of, *176,* 178–180
    in children, 1566
Mittleschmerz, 1347
Mixed connective tissue disease, 384–385
Mixed sleep apnea, 472
Mohs' technique, 673, 1238, *1239*
Moisturizers, 1190, 1192
Molar pregnancy, 1409–1410
Mole(s)
  hydatidiform, 1409–1410
  skin, 1233–1234, 1240
Molecule, *1052*
Molluscum contagiosum, 1229, 1325
  in children, 1535
Mollusk sting, 1686–1687
Mönckeberg's arteriosclerosis, *195*
Monge's disease, *1673*
Mongolian spots, *1496*
Mongolism (*see* Down syndrome)
Moniliasis (*see* Candidiasis)
Monoamine oxidase inhibitors, 617–618, *618*
  drug interactions with, 103
  food interactions with, 77
  in Parkinson's disease, 548, *549*
Monoclonal antibodies, 1006
  in cancer, 1044–1046, *1045*
  in non-Hodgkin's lymphoma, 1022
  in transplantation, *1079*
Monoclonal gammopathies (plasma cell
    disorders), 20, 1006–1010, *1009*
Monocytes, 978
  in chronic granulomatous disease, 1062
  disorders of, 1005
  in immune response, 1051–1052
  in infection, 1088
Mononeuritis multiplex, 584

Mononeuropathy, 583, *583*
Mononucleosis, 1163–1164
Monosodium glutamate (MSG) sensitivity, *726*, 1068
Mons pubis, 1343
Montelukast, *278*, *280*, 1584
Mood disorders, 613–614 (*see also* Depression; Mania)
Mood stabilizers, 600
    during pregnancy, *1461*
Morning-after pill, 1423
Morning sickness, 1440
Moro reflex, *1485*
Morphine, *451*, 452
    in coronary artery disease, *207*
    in heart attack, 214
    during pregnancy, 1464
Morton's neuroma, 403–404
Mosquito bites, 1685
    dengue fever from, 1167
    encephalitis from, 537–538
    malaria from, 1140–1142
    protection against, 1141
    yellow fever from, 1167
Motion, range of, 341
Motion sickness, 465, 1710
    drugs for, 99–100, *100*
    vertigo and, 463
Motor nerves, 438
    hereditary neuropathies of, 586–587
    muscle stimulation disorders and, 575–577
    testing of, 439
Mountain sickness, 1672–1674, *1673*
Mouth (*see also* Lip; Tooth [teeth]; Tongue)
    abscess of, 680
    age-associated changes in, *18*, 663
    bacterial infection of, 670, 680
    biology of, 661–663, *662*
    bleeding from, after oral surgery, 692
    burning, *665*
    cancer of, 671–674
    candidiasis of, 666, 682, 1150–1151, 1227
    chemical burns of, 1678–1679
    color changes in, *663*, 671, 673
    dermatitis around, 1198
    drugs by, 64
    dry, 49, 666
        radiation therapy and, 1660
        in Sjögren's syndrome, 382–383
    growths in, 670–674
    herpes simplex virus infection of, 668–669, 1160–1162
    lichen planus of, 1204
    precancerous lesions of, 671
    radiation injury to, 1660
    rose-colored spots in, 1581
    sores of, 667–670, 1041
        during cancer treatment, 1047

Mouth (*continued*)
    sores of (*continued*)
        in herpes simplex virus infection, 668–669, 1161
        in pemphigus, 1216
        temperature taking from, *1536*
        trench, 685
    Mouth rinses
        for canker sores, 668
        for cavity prevention, 678
        for cold sores, 669
    Movement
        brain-muscle communication in, *576*
        disorders of, 544–545, *545*, *549*, *553*
        information resources on, 1765
    Moxifloxacin, *1123*
    M-protein, 1006
    MRI (*see* Magnetic resonance imaging)
    MS (multiple sclerosis), 557–560, *558*
    MSG (monosodium glutamate) sensitivity, *726*, 1068
    Mucocele, 1293
    Mucolytics, 250
    Mucopolysaccharidoses, 1610
    Mucormycosis, 1153
        pneumonia and, 271
    Mucous membranes
        barrier function of, 1087
        drug-related blistering of, 1199–1200
        of larynx, 1270
        of nose, 1245
        of sinuses, 1245
        of throat, 1246, 1270
        of vagina, 1344
    Mucus
        cervical, 1344–1345, 1418, 1426
        in infection prevention, 1087–1088
        in stomach, 696
        vaginal, in newborns, 1349
    Mu heavy chain disease, 1010
    Multi-infarct dementia, 489–490
    Multiple births, 1473
    Multiple chemical sensitivity syndrome, 1719–1720, *1719*
    Multiple endocrine neoplasia, 972–974
        gastrinoma in, 775
        hyperparathyroidism and, *904*
        pheochromocytoma in, 961
        thyroid cancer in, 955
    Multiple myeloma, 360, 1007–1009
        high calcium levels and, 904
    Multiple organ system failure, 327
    Multiple personality disorder, 638–639, *639*
    Multiple sclerosis, 557–560, *558*
        information resources on, 1765
    Mumps, 1577–1578
        in adult male, 1329, 1415, 1577
        immunization for, 1093, *1094*, 1493, *1493*, 1577
        in HIV-infected children, 1575

Münchausen syndrome, *602, 970,* 1644
Murine typhus, *1133*
Murmurs, 121
  in athlete, 32
  in heart defects, 1513, 1514
  machinery, 239
  in mitral regurgitation, 177
  in mitral stenosis, 180
  during pregnancy, 1439
Muromonab, in transplantation, *1079*
Muscarine poisoning, 725
Muscle(s) (*see also* Musculoskeletal system)
  age-associated changes in, 338
  anal, 751, 752
  anesthetic effects on, 75
  atrophy of, 341
  biology of, 335, *336, 337*
  brain communication with, *576*
  breathing (respiratory), 254–255
  burn-related injury to, 1649, 1651
  in cerebral palsy, 1624–1626
  clostridial infection of, 1101
  cramps of, 415
  disorders of, 339–341, *340,* 412–419
  electrical stimulation of, 37–38
  examination of, 341
  exercise for, 31, 39
  eye, 1277
    in neuroblastoma, *1037*
    weakness and paralysis of, 588–589
  facial, weakness and paralysis of, 591–593
  in fibromyalgia, 415–417, *416*
  in Gerstmann-Sträussler-Scheinker disease, 543
  hypertrophy of, 341
  inflammation of (myositis), 339
  jaw, 686, 687, 688
  low calcium level effects on, 903–904
  in movement disorders, 544–545, *545, 549, 553*
  in nerve stimulation dysfunction, 575–577
  in neuromuscular junction disorders, 577–581
  pain in, 339
  in Parkinson's disease, 546–550, *549*
  passive resistance of, 341–342
  in polymyalgia rheumatica, 388–389
  in polymyositis, 383–384
  radiation effects on, 1660
  sarcopenia of, 338
  skeletal, 335
  smooth, 335
  spasm of (*see* Spasm)
  in sports injury, 420, 423–424, *423, 424, 426, 427*
  swelling of (compartment syndrome), 349, 353
  throat, 708
  weakness of (*see* Weakness, muscle)

Muscle relaxants
  in elderly persons, *81*
  in low back pain, 574
Muscular atrophy
  generalized, 341
  peroneal (Charcot-Marie-Tooth disease), 587
  progressive, 575–577
  spinal, 587–588
Muscular dystrophy, 412–413, *1430*
  information resources on, 1766
Musculoskeletal system, 5, 6, 334–338, *336, 337* (*see also* Bone[s]; Joint[s]; Ligament[s]; Muscle[s]; Sports, injuries in; *and specific disorders*)
  birth defects of, *1512,* 1523–1524, *1523, 1524*
  disorders of, 343–365
    diagnosis of, 341–343
    symptoms of, 339–341, *340*
Mushroom poisoning, 725, 726
Mushroom worker's lung, *309*
Mutation, 11
Myasthenia gravis, 577–579, *1074*
  information resources on, 1766
  pregnancy and, 1449
Mycobacterium avium complex (MAC) infection, *1126, 1172*
Mycobacterium bovis infection, 1126
Mycobacterium fortuitum infection, *1126*
Mycobacterium leprae infection (leprosy), 1130–1132
Mycobacterium tuberculosis infection (*see* Tuberculosis)
Mycophenolate mofetil, *1079*
Mycoplasma pneumoniae infection, 268–269
Mycosis fungoides, 1014, *1020*
Myectomy, 162
Myelin sheath, *437,* 556–557, *557*
  disorders of, 557–560, *558*
Myelitis, transverse, 567
Myeloblasts, 1003
Myelocele, 1526
Myelocytic (myeloid, myelogenous, myeloblastic, myelomonocytic) leukemia
  acute (AML), 1012–1014, *1013*
  chronic (CML), 1015–1016
Myelodysplastic syndromes, *1013*
Myelofibrosis, *1023,* 1025–1026
Myelography, 445, *1730*
Myeloma, multiple, 360, 1007–1009
  high calcium levels and, 904
Myelopathy
  in human T-cell lymphotropic virus infection, 539
  radiation, 528
Myeloperoxidase deficiency, *1058*
Myeloproliferative disorders, 1023–1027, *1023*
Myocardial infarction (*see* Heart attack)

Myocarditis, 159–160
  in enteroviral infection, *1576*
  heart failure with, 152
  in rheumatic fever, 1566
Myocardium, 335
  blood supply of (coronary arteries),
    116–117, *116*
    inadequate, 118, 199 (*see also* Heart
      attack)
  dysfunction of, 158–163, *159*
  inflammation of (*see* Myocarditis)
  rupture of, *212*
  weakness (aneurysm) of, *212*
Myoclonic seizures, 497
Myoclonus, 544
  in neuroblastoma, *1037*
Myofascial pain syndrome, 416, 686, 687,
  688
Myofibroma, 1372–1374
Myokymia, *577*
Myolysis, 1373
Myoma, 1372–1374
Myomectomy, 1373
Myonecrosis, 1101
Myopathy (*see also* Muscle[s])
  mitochondrial, 413
  myotonic, 413–414
Myopia (nearsightedness), 1279, 1286, *1287*
  in children, *1601*
Myositis, 339
Myositis ossificans, 652
Myotomy, 709
Myotonia congenita (Thomsen's disease),
  413–414
Myotonic dystrophy (Steinert's disease), 414
Myotonic myopathy, 413–414
Myringitis, 1257
Myringotomy, 1258, 1595
Myxedema, 952
  coma in, 953
Myxoma, 191, 193–194, *193*
Myxomatous degeneration, of mitral valve,
  177

N

Nafcillin, *1123*
Nail-patella syndrome, 856
Nails
  biting of, *1548*
  candidiasis of, 1227
  infection of (onychomycosis), 409–410,
    1225, 1226
  inflammation of (onychia), 410
  ingrown, 409
  spoon, 907
  thickening of (onychauxis and
    onychogryphosis), 410

Naltrexone, 652, 653
Naphazoline, *1158*
Naproxen, 95, 97, 454
Narcissistic personality, 632
Narcoanalysis, 603
Narcolepsy, 470–472
Narcosis, nitrogen, *1669*
Narcotics (*see* Opioids)
Nasal (*see also* Nose)
Nasal septum, 1245
  deviation of, 1262
  perforation of, 1262–1263
Nasal sprays, 97–98, 1264
Nasoenteric tube, 706
Nasogastric tube, 705–706, 890
Nasolacrimal duct, *1293*
  blockage of, 1293
Nasopharynx, 1246, *1246*
  cancer of, 1273
Nateglinide, *968*
Natural childbirth, *1468*
Natural killer cells, 978, *1052*, 1054
  low levels of, 1004
Naturopathy, 1705
Nausea, 701–702
  in cancer patient, 1047
  in dying person, 49
  in food poisoning, *720–721*
  in gastritis, 712
  in kidney disorders, 823–824
  in motion sickness, 465, 1710
  during pregnancy, 1440, 1451–1452
  in radiation illness, 1659
Near drowning, 1665–1666
Nearsightedness (myopia), 1279, 1286, *1287*
  in children, *1601*
Nebulizer
  in allergy, 1064–1065
  in asthma, 280, 1584
  in COPD, 283–284
Necator americanus infection (hookworm),
  1138–1140, *1139*
Neck
  lump in, *1273*
    in children, 1599
    in thyroid cancer, 955
  spasms of, 555–556
  spinal cord compression at, 564–565
  stiff, in meningitis, 530
  umbilical cord around, 1473
Necrolysis, toxic epidermal, 1199–1200
Necrolytic migratory erythema, 776
Necrosis
  avascular, 362–363, *363*
    in decompression sickness, 1670
    of lunate bone (Kienböck's disease), 400
  fat, in newborn, 1485
  of kidneys, 847
  skin, 1221–1222

Necrotizing cellulitis, 1221–1222
Necrotizing enterocolitis, 1504–1505
Necrotizing fasciitis, 1113, 1221–1222
Necrotizing pancreatitis, 731
Necrotizing sialometaplasia, 670
Nedocromil, *278, 280–281, 1584*
Needle biopsy (*see* Biopsy)
Needlestick injury, 1169, 1173
Neglect, child, 1643–1646
    information resources on, 1760
Neisseria infection, *1102*
    conjunctivitis, 1296–1297
        of newborn, *1509*
    gonorrhea, 1179–1180, *1376*
    meninges, 529–531
    in traveler, 1714
    urethra, 868
Nelfinavir, *1175*
Nelson's syndrome, *959*
Neobladder, orthotopic, 878
Neomycin, *1122*
    in liver encephalopathy, 796
Neonatal intensive care unit, *1495*
Neonatal wet-lung syndrome, 1500
Neonate (*see* Infant[s])
Nephritic syndrome, 838–839
Nephritis, 837–844, *840, 842* (*see also*
        Glomerulonephritis)
    hereditary (Alport's syndrome), 856
Nephroblastoma, 1622–1623
Nephrogenic diabetes insipidus, 851, 945
Nephrolithiasis, 864–866
Nephrons, 820, *821, 845*
    age-associated changes in, 822–823
    inflammation of (*see* Glomerulonephritis;
        Nephritis)
Nephrosclerosis, malignant, 847–848
Nephrotic syndrome, 824, 839–843, *840,
    842*
    congenital and infantile, *842*
Nephroureterectomy, 877
Nerve(s) (*see also* Brain; Nervous system)
    in acromegaly, 945
    alcohol injection into, 591
    biology of, 437–438, *437*
    conduction study of, 446
    cranial, 437–438
        disorders of, 588–594, *592, 593*
        testing of, 439, *590–591*
    disorders of, 575–588 (*see also* Neuropathy)
    electrical injury to, 1662–1663
    inflammation of (*see* Neuritis)
    injury to, in newborn, 1494–1495
    in leprosy, 1130–1132
    motor, 438
        hereditary neuropathy of, 586–587
        testing of, 439
    in multiple sclerosis, 557–560, *558*
    in muscle stimulation disorders, 575–577

Nerve(s) (*continued*)
    myelin sheath of, 556–557, *557*
        disorders of, 557–560, *558*
    at neuromuscular junction, 577
    in neuropathy (*see* Neuropathy)
    pain and (*see* Neuralgia)
    palsy of (*see* Palsy)
    peripheral, 437–438, *576*
        disorders of, 575–588, *577, 583, 585*
    plexuses of, 438, 581, *581*
    radiation injury to, 528
    sensory, 438
        hereditary neuropathy of, 586–587
        testing of, 439–440
    in skin, 1187, *1187*
    spinal, *436*, 437–438, 561 (*see also* Spinal
        cord)
    tests of, 342, 439–440, 446, *590–591, 1730*
Nerve block, 455
    in labor and delivery, 1467–1468
Nerve cell (neuron), 433, 434, 437, *437*
    age-associated changes in, 438
Nerve conduction study, 342, 446, *1730*
Nerve roots, *436*, 438, 561
    compression of, 563–564, 570, 571–572, 574
    dermatomes of, *563*
Nervousness (*see* Anxiety)
Nervous system, 6, 433–438, *435, 436, 437*
    (*see also* Nerve[s])
    age-associated changes in, 438
    assessment of, 439–446, *440, 441, 442, 443*
    autonomic, 5, 437 (*see also* Autonomic
        nervous system)
        in blood pressure control, 132
        testing of, 441
    central (*see* Brain; Central nervous system;
        Spinal cord)
    peripheral, 437–438 (*see also* Peripheral
        nerves)
    radiation injury to, 528
    somatic, 437
    tumors of, 519–528, *520–521, 522, 525, 527*
        in children, 1623
Netilmicin, *1122*
Neuralgia
    in ankle sprain, 406
    glossopharyngeal, 593–594
    postherpetic, 449, *1163*
    trigeminal, 589, 591, *593*
Neural tube defects, *1525,* 1526
    folic acid deficiency and, 1511
    prenatal testing for, 1430, *1432*
Neurinoma, acoustic, 1260–1261
Neuritis
    brachial, 582
    optic, 1315–1316
        in multiple sclerosis, 558
Neuroblastoma, 1623
    paraneoplastic syndromes in, *1037*

Neurodermatitis (localized scratch dermatitis), 1198
Neuroendovascular surgery, 512
Neurofibroma, small intestine, 768
Neurofibromatosis, 527–528
  pheochromocytoma in, 961
Neurogenic bladder, 858, *860*
Neuroleptic malignant syndrome, 643, *644*
Neurologic examination, 439–446, *440, 441, 442*
Neuroma
  acoustic, 1260–1261
  Morton's, 403–404
  in multiple endocrine neoplasia, 973
Neuromuscular junction, 577
  disorders of, 577–581
Neuron (nerve cell), 433, 434, 437, *437*
  age-associated changes in, 438
Neuronitis, vestibular, 1260
Neuropathic pain, 449
Neuropathy
  in cancer, *1037*
  in diabetes, 584, *963, 964*
  hereditary, 586–587
  inflammatory demyelinating (Guillain-Barré syndrome), 584–586
  in Lyme disease, 1106
  multiple-nerve (polyneuropathy), 584–586
  optic, 1316–1317
    Leber's hereditary, 560
  single-nerve (mononeuropathy), 583, *583*
  in vitamin B$_{12}$ deficiency, 898
Neurosyphilis, 1177
Neurotoxins, 579, 726
Neurotransmitters, 433
Neutropenia, 1002–1003
  with cancer treatment, 1047
Neutrophil(s), 978, *1052*, 1053
  in chronic granulomatous disease, 1062
  high levels of (leukocytosis), 1003
  in hyperimmunoglobulinemia E syndrome, 1062
  in infection, 1088
  low levels of (neutropenia), 1002–1003
    with cancer treatment, 1047
Neutrophilic leukocytosis, 1003
Nevi (moles), 1233–1234, 1240
Nevi flammeus, 1236
Nevirapine, *1175*
Newborn (*see also* Infant[s])
  birth defects in, 1511–1526, *1512, 1515, 1516, 1517, 1521, 1523, 1524, 1525*
  birth injury to, 1494–1495
  bleeding in, 1449, 1485, 1494
  cocaine withdrawal in, 1463
  cytomegalovirus infection in, 1164–1165
  development of, 1490, *1490, 1491*
  feeding of, 1486–1489, *1487*
    in necrotizing enterocolitis, 1505

Newborn (*continued*)
  hemolytic disease of, 1453, *1506*, 1507
  hemorrhagic disease of, 895
  herpes simplex virus infection in, 1162
  HIV infection in, 1447
  infections in, *1508–1509*
  initial care of, 1483–1484, *1484*
  jaundice in, 1505–1507, *1506*
  meningitis in, 1562–1563
  normal, 1483–1494, *1485*
  physical examination of, 1484–1485, *1485*
  problems in, 1494–1511, *1495, 1496, 1497*
  resuscitation of, 1471
  toxoplasmosis in, 1145
  vaginal discharge in, 1349
Niacin (nicotinic acid), 893, 897
  deficiency of, *735*, 897
    gingivitis with, 682
    red tongue with, 665
  excess of, 897
  in hyperlipoproteinemia, *925*
Niacinamide deficiency, 853
Nickel, dermatitis from, *1193*, 1194
Nicotinamide (*see* Niacin [nicotinic acid])
Nicotine (*see* Smoking)
NICU (neonatal intensive care unit), *1495*
Niemann-Pick disease, 1620
Nifedipine, gingivitis and, 682
Night blindness, 891, 1280
Nightmares, 474, 1546
Night terrors, 474, 1546
Nilutamide, 1334
Nipple
  in breastfeeding, 1477
  discharge from, 1387–1388
  Paget's disease of, 1241, 1391, 1393, 1400
Nitrates
  in coronary artery disease, 205, *207*
  in urine, 826
Nitrazepam, in elderly persons, *81*
Nitric oxide, 1502
Nitrofurantoin, *1124*
  hepatitis with, 803
  during pregnancy, *1460*
Nitrogen, in decompression sickness, 1669–1671
Nitrogen dioxide, inhalation of, 300–301
Nitrogen narcosis, *1669*
Nitroglycerin, 205, *207*, 214
Nitrous oxide, *659*
Nits, 1219
Nizatidine
  in elderly persons, *81*
  in peptic ulcer, 716, *718*
Nocardiosis, *1102*
Nociceptive pain, 449
No code (do-not-resuscitate order), 48, *56, 57*

Nocturia, 824
in benign prostatic hyperplasia, 1330
in kidney failure, 831
Nocturnal dyspnea, 119
Nocturnal ischemia, 202
Nodules
in ankle ligament, 406
Bouchard's, 368, 397
in rheumatoid arthritis, 371
skin, *1189*
in acne, *1205, 1206*
in dermatofibroma, 1234–1235
in erythema nodosum, 1200–1201
in granuloma annulare, 1201
thyroid, 949, 950, 955
vocal cord, 1269, *1269*
Noise
in ear (tinnitus), 1261
hearing loss from, 1245, 1248, 1250
in joints, 341
measurement of, *1249*
Non-Hodgkin's lymphoma, 1019–1022, *1020, 1021* (*see also* Lymphoma, non-Hodgkin's)
Nonketotic hyperglycemic-hyperosmolar coma, 966
Non-nucleoside reverse transcriptase inhibitors, 1173–1174, *1175*
Nonprescription drugs (*see* Over-the-counter [nonprescription] drugs)
Non-REM (rapid eye movement) sleep, 467, *468*
Nonsteroidal anti-inflammatory drugs (NSAIDs), 452–454, *453, 454*
allergic reactions to, *1069*
in ankylosing spondylitis, 377
in common cold, *1158*
in dysmenorrhea, 1364
in endometriosis, 1370
gastrointestinal side effects of, 64, 452, 711, 714, 777
in gout, 393, *393*
oligohydramnios with, 1455
in osteoarthritis, 369
over-the-counter, 94–95, 97
during pregnancy, *1461*
in pregnancy, 101–102
in respiratory tract infection, 1580
in rheumatoid arthritis, 372–373, *372*
side effects of, 452–453
in systemic lupus erythematosus, 380
in uterine fibroids, 1373
Nontropical sprue (celiac disease), 736–737
Noonan syndrome, 1529
Norepinephrine, *939*
in blood pressure control, 132
in heart failure, 153
in pheochromocytoma, 960–961
receptors for, *71*
Norfloxacin, *1123*

Normal-pressure hydrocephalus, 490
North American blastomycosis, 1149–1150
Nose
age-associated changes in, 1246–1247
anatomy of, 1245–1246, *1246*
broken, 1262
cancer of, 1273
decongestant spray for, 97–98, *1158*
deviated septum in, 1262
disorders of, 1262–1267, *1264*
drug administration by, 66
foreign object in, 1599
mucormycosis of, 1153
packing of, 1263
polyps of, *1264*, 1265
in allergic rhinitis, 1067, 1068
in rosacea, 1203
runny, 1264–1265
in allergic rhinitis, 1066
saddle, 1611
tumors of, 1273
vestibulitis of, 1263–1264
Nosebleeds, 1263
NSAIDs (*see* Nonsteroidal anti-inflammatory drugs)
Nuchal cord, 1473
Nuclear power plants, 1658
Nuclear scan (*see* Radionuclide imaging)
Nuclear weapons, 1658
Nucleoside reverse transcriptase inhibitors, 1173–1174, *1175*
Nucleus, 2, *4*
Numbness, in leprosy, 1131
Nummular dermatitis, 1196
Nursing (*see* Breastfeeding)
Nursing home, 47
Nutraceuticals, 103–112, *104–106*, 1046
Nutrients, 880–883
deficiencies of, *735*
malabsorption of, 734–738
requirements for, 883–884, *885*
Nutrition, 880–887, *880, 881* (*see also* Diet; Food)
in anorexia, 625–626
in burns, 1651
for children, 1542
counseling on
in lung disease, 260
in obesity, 918
in cystic fibrosis, 321
in diabetes mellitus, 1614
disorders of, 887–890, *888, 889* (*see also* Malnutrition)
for dying person, 49
enteral, 889–890
for fetus, 1511
food guide pyramid for, 884, *885*
for infant, 1486–1489, *1487*, 1532–1533 (*see also* Breastfeeding)

Nutrition *(continued)*
  information resources on, 1766
  minerals in, 882–883, 900–914, *902–903*
    (*see also specific minerals, eg,* Iron;
    Zinc)
  obesity and (*see* Obesity)
  in orthomolecular medicine, 1706–1707
  parenteral, 890, 1703
  salt in (*see* Salt [sodium chloride])
  vitamins in, 882–883, 890–900, *892–893*
    (*see also specific vitamins*)
Nystagmus, 1260
  in vertigo, 463, 464
Nystatin, 682

O

Obesity, 914–920, *916–917, 919*
  in adolescents, 1557–1558
  apnea and, 472
  atherosclerosis and, 197
  in children, 915–916, 1545
  diabetes mellitus and, 962
  dieting in, 918
  heart failure and, 155
  heat disorders with, 1652
  hypertension and, 134, 137
  in polycystic ovary syndrome, 1368
  pregnancy and, 1444–1445
  prevention of, 1542
Obesity-hypoventilation syndrome
    (pickwickian syndrome), 473
Ob gene, 915
Obsessive-compulsive disorder, 611–612
Obsessive-compulsive personality, 633
Obstetrics (*see* Labor and delivery; Pregnancy)
Obstipation (*see* Constipation)
Obstructive sleep apnea, 472, 473
  with enlarged tonsils and adenoids,
    1596–1597
Occipital lobe, 434, *435*
  injury to, *476, 477*
Occlusive dressing, 1191
Occult bacteremia, 1561
Occult blood, *29,* 705, 770, *1038,* 1041,
    1730
Occupational lung disorders, 294–301, *297*
  allergic, *297,* 299–300
  chemical, 300–301
  psittacosis, *268*
Occupational therapy, 39–40
  in burn injury, 1651
Octopus bite, 1687
Octreotide
  in acromegaly, 946
  in glucagonoma, 776
Oculomotor nerve, 589, *590*
Odontoma, 671

Odors
  in bad breath (halitosis), *684*
  in excessive sweating, 1210–1211
  in maple syrup urine disease, 1619
  perception of, *595, 662*
    disorders of, 594–596
  in phenylketonuria, 1618
  of urine, 825
Ofloxacin, *1123*
Oil of wintergreen poisoning, 1677
Ointments, 1189, 1190
Olfaction, *595, 662*
  age-associated changes in, *18*
  disorders of, 594–596
Olfactory bulb, *1246*
Olfactory nerve, *590, 1246*
Oligodendroglioma, *520, 522*
Oligohydramnios, 1454–1455
Oligomenorrhea, *1362*
Oliguria, 829
Olopatadine, 1067
Olsalazine
  in Crohn's disease, 740, *741*
  in ulcerative colitis, 743
Omeprazole, 73, *718*
Omphalocele, *1512*
Oncogenes, 14
One-and-a-half syndrome, 588
Onychauxis, 410
Onychia, 410
Onychogryphosis, 410
Onychomycosis, 409–410, 1225, 1226
Oocytes, 1345, *1346*
Oophoritis, 1377
Operation (*see* Surgery)
Ophthalmic artery, 1277
Ophthalmoplegia, internuclear, 588
Ophthalmoscopy, 1283–1284, *1284, 1730*
  in heart disease, 121
  in high blood pressure, 136, 1313
  in premature infant, 1504
  in retinal vessel blockage, 1312
  before spinal tap, 442
Opioids, 450–452, *451*
  abuse of, 652–653
    during pregnancy, 1464
  in coronary artery disease, *207*
  in cough remedies, 98, 249
  dependence on, 450
  for dying persons, 48
  in heart failure, *157*
  side effects of, 450
  urinary incontinence with, *859*
  withdrawal from, 653
Opium, tincture of (paregoric), in diarrhea,
    756
Oppositional defiant disorder, 1636
Opsoclonus, *1037*
Optic chiasm, 1315, *1316*

Optic nerve, 1276, *1276*, 1277, 1309–1310, *1310*, 1315, *1316*
  disorders of, 1315, *1317*
    in glaucoma, 1306–1309, *1308*
  inflammation of, 1315–1316
  in malignant hypertension, 848
  swelling of, 1315
  testing of, 442, *590*
Optic nerve sheath, *523*
Optic neuritis, 1315–1316
  in multiple sclerosis, 558
Optic neuropathy, 1316–1317
  Leber's hereditary, 560
Oral antihyperglycemic drugs, 968–969, *968*, 1614
  in pancreatitis, 733
  during pregnancy, *1461*
Oral cavity (*see* Mouth)
Oral contraceptives, 1420–1421, *1420*
  after rape, 1413
  in dysfunctional uterine bleeding, 1367
  in dysmenorrhea, 1364
  for emergency contraception, 1423
  in endometriosis, 1370, *1371*
  food interactions with, 77
  gingivitis and, 682
  liver tumors and, 810
  melasma (brown skin patches) with, 1215–1216
  in polycystic ovary syndrome, 1368
  in premenstrual syndrome, 1363
  in prolactinoma, 947
  restrictions on, *1422*
  rifampin interaction with, 72
  side effects of, 1421
  in uterine fibroids, 1373
Oral hygiene, *29*, 677
  after oral cancer treatment, 674
Oral hypoglycemic drugs (*see* Oral antihyperglycemic drugs)
Orbit (eye socket), 1276, *1277*
  disorders of, 1317–1319
Orchiectomy, 1327, 1334
Orchitis, 1328, 1415, 1577
Organ donation, 48
Organisms, microscopic (*see* Microorganisms)
Organ of Corti, 1244–1245
Organophosphate poisoning, 1679–1680
Organ systems, 3–5, *3, 6*
Organ transplantation (*see* Transplantation)
Orgasm
  female, 1357, 1382
    delay in or absence of, 1386
  male, 1323–1324, 1336 (*see also* Ejaculation; Erectile dysfunction)
Orlistat, 919
Oropharynx, 1246, *1246*
Orthodontic therapy (braces), 662, 681
Orthomolecular medicine, 1706–1707

Orthopnea, 251
Orthostatic hypotension, 144, 146–147
  in anemia, 988
  in dehydration, 929
  idiopathic (Shy-Drager syndrome), 550–551
  tilt table for, 39
Orthotics, shoe, 421
Orthotopic neobladder, 878
Oseltamivir, *1156*
  in influenza, 1160
Osgood-Schlatter disease, 1607
Osmolality, *1726*
  urine, 826
Osmotic agents, in constipation, 752, *753*
Osmotic diarrhea, 754
Ossicles (ear bones), 1244, *1245*
Osteoarthritis, *20*, 367–370, *368, 369*
  of big toe, 404
  erosive (inflammatory), of hand, 397
  low back pain with, 569
  in obesity, 917
  of temporomandibular joint, 686, 688, 689
Osteoarthropathy, hypertrophic, *1037*
Osteochondritis dissecans, 362–363, *363*
  of lunate bone (Kienböck's disease), 400
Osteochondroma, 359–360
Osteodystrophy, renal, 832
Osteogenesis imperfecta, 1610–1611
Osteoma, *521*
  of ear, 1255
  osteoid, 360
Osteomalacia, 894
Osteomyelitis, 364–365
  staphylococcal, 1112
Osteonecrosis, 362–363, *363*
  after diving, 1670
  of lunate bone (Kienböck's disease), 400
Osteopetroses, 1611
Osteoporosis, *20*, 343–346, *344, 345*
  information resources on, 1766
  low back pain with, 569
  in macroglobulinemia, 1009
  menopause and, 1357, *1360*
  in multiple myeloma, 1007
Osteosarcoma, 360–361, *521*
Osteotomy, 363
Otitis externa (swimmer's ear), 1109, 1110, 1253–1255
Otitis media
  acute, 1257–1258, *1258*, 1594
  chronic, 1258–1259, 1594, *1595*
  hearing loss from, 1248
  in measles, 1576
  in respiratory tract infection, 1579
  in rubella, 1582
  serous, 1258, 1594–1595
Otoacoustic emissions test, 1250

Otosclerosis, 1247–1248, 1250
Otoscope, 1594
Oval window, 1244, *1245*
Ovarian hyperstimulation syndrome, 1417
Ovary (ovaries), *938, 939*, 1344, 1345, *1345*
  cancer of, 1404–1405
    screening for, *1038*
    staging of, *1040, 1402*
  cysts of, *1405*
    during pregnancy, 1450
    virilization with, *959, 960*
  enlargement of, *1405*
  failure of (menopause), 1356–1361, *1360*
    bleeding after, *1362*
    premature, 1361
  palpation of, 1353
  polycystic, 1367–1368
    obesity and, 916
  radiation effects on, 1659, 1660
Overdose, of drugs, 85–86, 103
Overeating, by young child, 1545
Overfeeding, of children, 1532
Overflow incontinence, 858, *860*, 861–862
Overhydration, 929–930
Over-the-counter (nonprescription) drugs, 93–103, *94, 98*
  for allergy, 98–99, 1064, *1065*
  during breastfeeding, *1462*
  in children, 100–101
  for colds, 22, 95–98, 1157–1159, *1158*
  in elderly persons, 101
  generic, 92
  for inflammation, 94–95
  interactions of, 102–103
  labels of, *94, 96*
  for motion sickness, 99–100, *100*
  overdoses of, 103
  for pain, 94–95, *97*
  precautions with, 100–103
  in pregnancy, 101–102
  vs. prescription drugs, 60
  safety of, 93, *95*
  for sleep problems, 100, *471*
Overweight (*see* Obesity)
Ovulation, 1347, *1347*
  after childbirth, 1478
  cervical mucus in, 1344–1345
  monitoring of, 1425–1426
  problems with, 1416–1417
Oxacillin, *1123*
Oxalate, urinary, 866
Oxcarbazepine, *501*
Oximetry, 253, 255
  in premature infant, 1504
Oxybutynin
  in elderly persons, *81*
  in urge incontinence, 861

Oxycodone, *451*
Oxygen
  in blood, *1727*
    deficiency of (*see also* Ischemia)
      in anemia, 988
      in brain (*see* Stroke)
      at high altitudes, 1672–1674
      in polycythemia, *1024*
      seizures with, *496*
      in sickle cell disease, 992
    measurement of, 255, *1727*
    pressure of, *1726*
    transport of, 978
  in lungs, 245–246, *246*
  toxicity of, *1669*
Oxygen therapy, 260–261
  in acute respiratory distress syndrome, 327
  in altitude illness, 1673
  in bronchiolitis, 1585
  in carbon monoxide poisoning, 1678
  in COPD, 284
  in decompression sickness, 1671
  in diving injury, 1668
  in meconium aspiration syndrome, 1501
  in near drowning, 1666
  in pulmonary hypertension, 324, 1502
  in respiratory distress syndrome, 1500
  in respiratory failure, 325–326
  retinopathy of prematurity and, 1504
  in secondary polycythemia, *1024*
  in smoke inhalation, *1649*
  in transient tachypnea of newborn, 1500
  during travel, 1712
Oxymetazoline, *1158*
Oxymorphone, *451*
Oxytetracycline, *1123*
Oxytocin, *939, 940, 941*
  after childbirth, 1469
  for labor, 1465, 1474–1475

P

Pacemaker
  artificial, 146, 165, 167, *168*, 175
    travel and, 1711–1712
  escape, 174
  natural, 117, 163
    dysfunction of, 174
Pachymetry, 1286, 1302
Paclitaxel, *1045*
Paget's disease
  of bone, 346–348
    hypercalcemia and, 904
  information resources on, 1766
  of nipple, 1391, 1393, 1400
  of penis, 1325
  of skin, 1241

Pain, 447–455, *448, 451, 453, 454*
  abdominal, 700–701, 702 (*see also*
    Abdomen, pain in)
  in ankylosing spondylitis, 377
  in aortic aneurysm, 119
  in aortic dissection, 119, 230
  in appendicitis, 1590
  arm, in thoracic outlet syndrome, 582–583
  in atherosclerosis, 198
  back (*see* Back pain)
  in bladder infection, 823
  bone, 339, 359
    in children, 1603
    with fracture, 348
  breakthrough, 448
  breast, 1351, 1387
  in cancer, 1035
  with canker sores, 668
  chest (*see* Chest, pain in)
  in chondromalacia patellae, 1607
  with cold sores, 669
  in dying person, 48
  ear, *1258*
  in erythromelalgia, 225
  evaluation of, 447–448
  eye, 1281
  face
    in Bell's palsy, 591–593
    in trigeminal neuralgia, 589, 591, *593*
  in fibromyalgia, 416
  foot, 403–405
  gallbladder, 788, 814, 816
  in headache, 456–461, *458–459, 460*
  in heart attack, 211
  in heart disease, 118–119
  heel, 404–405, *405,* 407–408
  hip
    in Calvé-Perthes disease, 1607
    in fracture, 355
    in slipped capital femoral epiphysis, 1606
  information resources on, 1766
  joint, 339
    in rheumatic fever, 1566
    in rubella, 1582
  in kidney disorders, 823, 863, 865
  during labor and delivery, 1467–1468
  leg
    in Buerger's disease, 223
    when walking, 217, 221
  in mitral valve prolapse, 119
  muscle, 339
  nerve (*see* Neuralgia)
  neuropathic, 449
  nociceptive, 449
  at ovulation (mittleschmerz), 1347
  pelvic, 1350–1351, *1351*
    in endometriosis, 1368
    during menstrual period, 1364
    in pelvic congestion syndrome, *1366*

Pain (*continued*)
  in pericarditis, 118–119
  phantom limb, 44, 449
  pleuritic, 251, 313
  postoperative, 1703
  psychogenic, 449–450
  referred, 447, *448,* 569–570, 572
  sciatic, *571*
  during sexual intercourse, 1382–1383
  in shingles, 449
  shoulder, in thoracic outlet syndrome,
    582–583
  in thoracic aortic aneurysm, 228–229
  throat, in glossopharyngeal neuralgia,
    593–594
  toe, 404
  tooth, 674, 676, 680, 690
  treatment of, 37–38, 450–455
    nondrug, 455
    nonopioid, 452–454, *453, 454*
    opioid, 450–452, *451*
    over-the-counter drugs for, 94–95, *97*
  during urination, 868, 869
  vulvar, 1384
Pain relievers (*see* Analgesics)
Paint thinner, poisoning from, 1679
Palate, 661, *662*
  cleft, 1523, *1523*
    information resources on, 1760
  necrotizing sialometaplasia of, 670
  torus of, 671
Palivizumab, 1580
Palliative care, *56*
Pallidotomy, 550
Palpitations, 119–120, 164, 165 (*see also*
  Arrhythmias)
  in mitral regurgitation, 177
Palsy
  abducens nerve, 589
  Bell's (facial nerve), 591–593
  bulbar, 575–577
  cerebral, 1624–1626
    information resources on, 1760
  oculomotor nerve, 589
  peroneal nerve, 583
  pseudobulbar, 575–577
  radial nerve, 583
  supranuclear, 550
  trochlear, 589
  ulnar nerve, 583
Pamidronate
  in multiple myeloma, 1008
  in osteogenesis imperfecta, 1610
  in osteoporosis, 346
  in Paget's disease of bone, 347–348
Pancoast syndrome, 329
Pancreas, *695,* 696–697, *729, 730,* 787, *938,*
  939
  abscess of, 779

Pancreas *(continued)*
   age-associated changes in, 698
   cancer of, 773–774, *774*
      in multiple endocrine neoplasia, 972–973
   function tests of, 735
   gastrinoma of, 775–776
   glucagonoma of, 776
   infection of, 731
   inflammation of *(see* Pancreatitis)
   insulinoma of, 775, 971, 972
   pseudocyst of, 731, 733
   transplantation of, 969, 1080–1081
   tumors of, 775–776, 971, 972
Pancreatic duct, *695, 697, 787*
   obstruction of, 814, 816
   in pancreatitis, 732, 733
   tumor of, *774*
Pancreatitis, 729–733
   acute, 729–733, *731*
   chronic, 732–733
   with endoscopic retrograde
      cholangiopancreatography, 789
   in hyperlipoproteinemia, 921, 926
   in mumps, 1577
   necrotizing, 731
Panencephalitis, subacute sclerosing, 1577,
   1582
Panic attacks and panic disorder, 608–609,
   609
Pantoprazole, 718
Pantothenic acid, *893*
Papilledema, *523*, 1315
Papillitis, headache with, *458*
Papilloma, laryngeal, 1600
Pap test, 26, *29*, 1040, 1353, *1353*, 1406–1407,
   1421, *1730*
   recommendations for, *1038*
Papule, *1189*
Paracentesis, 705, 783, 795, *1730*
   anterior chamber, 1312
Paracetamol *(see* Acetaminophen)
Paracoccidioidomycosis, 1153
Parade ground syncope (fainting), 120
Parainfectious (postinfectious) encephalitis,
   533
Parainfectious (acute disseminated)
   encephalomyelitis, 560
Parainfluenza virus infection, 1579–1580,
   1585
Paralysis
   in botulism, 579
   in decompression sickness, 1670
   of diaphragm, in newborn, 1495
   facial, 591–593
   in lightning injury, 1664
   in locked-in state, 494
   periodic, 414
   in polio, 1578
   in rabies, 536

Paralysis *(continued)*
   sleep, 471
   in spinal cord injury, 561
   in stroke, 504
   tick, *1686*
   Todd's, 495
   vocal cord, *1269*, 1270
Paralytic ileus, 781
Paralytic illness, *1576*
Paralytic strabismus, 1602
Paranasal sinuses, *1265*
   anatomy of, 1245–1246, *1246*
   cancer of, 1272
   disorders of, *1264*, 1266–1267, *1266* (*see*
      also Sinusitis)
   pressure trauma to, 1710
Paraneoplastic syndromes, 330, 904, 1035,
   1037
Paranoia
   in personality disorder, 631
   in schizophrenia, 642
Paraparesis, spastic
   hereditary, 566–567
   tropical, 539
Paraphilias, 629–630
Paraphimosis, 1325
Paraplegia (*see* Spinal cord, injury to)
Parasitic infection, *1087*, 1135–1148, *1139,
   1143, 1146–1147* (*see also specific
   infections*)
   brain, 540
   cancer and, 1034
   skin, 1218–1219, *1219*
   urinary tract, 867–868
Parasomnias, 474
Parathyroid glands, *938, 939*
   absence of, 1061
   in polyglandular deficiency syndrome, *943*
   tumors of, 972
Parathyroid hormone, 901, *939*
   excess of, 904–905, *904*, 972, 973
   low levels of, 901
   in osteoporosis, 346
Paregoric, *756*
Parenteral nutrition, 890, 1703
Paresthesia, *583*
Parietal lobe, 434, *435*
   injury to, *476, 477*
Parkinsonism, 546–547
Parkinson's disease, *20*, 546–550, *549*
   constipation in, 751
   dementia in, 490
   information resources on, 1766
Paronychia, 402, 1227
Parotid glands, 662, 666, *667*
   in mumps (*see* Mumps)
Paroxysmal nocturnal dyspnea, 154, 251
Paroxysmal nocturnal hemoglobinuria, *989*
Paroxysmal peritonitis, familial, 1716–1717

Paroxysmal positional vertigo, benign, 465–467, *466*
Paroxysmal supraventricular tachycardia, 170–171
  in Wolff-Parkinson-White syndrome, 171
Parrot fever, *268*
Partial seizures, 495–496
Partial thromboplastin time (PPT), 981, *1727*
Parvovirus B19 infection (erythema infectiosum, fifth disease), 1535, *1569*, 1572–1573
Patch
  contraceptive, 1421–1422
  drug administration by, 66–67
  eye, in amblyopia, 1601
Patch test, 1188, 1194
Patella (kneecap), *338*
  chondromalacia of, 1607
  in nail-patella syndrome, 856
Patellofemoral stress syndrome (runner's knee), 425–426, *425, 426*
Patent, for drugs, 89
Patent ductus arteriosus, 1514, *1515*
Pavlik harness, 1524
PCP (phencyclidine), 658
PCR (polymerase chain reaction), 15
PDD-NOS (pervasive developmental disorder not otherwise specified), 1631
Peak flow meter, 254, 276, 1584
Pectin, *756*
Pediatric patients (*see* Children; Infant[s])
Pediculosis (lice), 1219, *1219*
Pedophilia, 629–630
Peeing (*see* Urination)
Peeling (skin)
  in staphylococcal scalded skin syndrome, 1223
  in toxic epidermal necrolysis, 1199
Peer relationships, 1542, 1554
Pel-Ebstein fever, 1017
Pellagra, 897
  gingivitis in, 682
  red tongue in, 665
Pelvic congestion syndrome, *1366*
Pelvic examination, 1352–1353, *1353*
  for cancer screening, *1038*
  in vaginal infection, 1375–1376
Pelvic floor disorders, 1379–1381, *1381*
Pelvic inflammatory disease, 1377–1379
  peritonitis and, 782
Pelvis
  abscess in, 779
  fracture of, 356–357
  pain in, 1350–1351, *1351*
    in endometriosis, 1368
    during menstrual period, 1364
    in pelvic congestion syndrome, *1366*
    varicose veins in (pelvic congestion syndrome), *1366*

Pemphigoid, bullous, 670, *1074*, 1217
Pemphigus, 670, *1074*, 1216–1217
Penciclovir, *1156*, 1162
Penetrance, genetic, 14
Penicillamine
  in lead poisoning, 1681
  in rheumatoid arthritis, *372, 373*
  in scleroderma, 381
Penicillin, 63, *1123*
  in pneumococcal infection, 1109
  in strep throat, 1596
  in syphilis, 1178
Penis, 1321, *1322*
  absence of, 1520
  cancer of, 1325
  candidiasis of, 1227
  circumcision of, 1485–1486, 1568
  erection of, 1323, 1336
    distorted (Peyronie's disease), 1326
    failure of (erectile dysfunction, impotence), 1336–1339
      in acromegaly, 945
      in galactorrhea, 946
      information resources on, 1763
    persistent (priapism), 1325–1326
  fibrous thickening of (Peyronie's disease), 1326
  growths on, 1325
  infections of (*see* Sexually transmitted diseases)
  inflammation of, 1324–1325
  injury to, 1326
  prosthetic, 1339
  small, 1520
  urethra opening misplacement in, 1519
Pentamidine, 971
Pentazocine, *451*
  in elderly persons, *80*
Pentosan polysulfate, *869*
Pentoxifylline, 221
P-450 enzymes, 68, 75, 76
Pepsin, 696
Peptic ulcers, 698, *712*, 713–717, *718*
  in children, 1589
  complications of, *715*
  drug-related, *83*
  gastrinoma and, 775
  stomach cancer and, 767
Percutaneous balloon pericardiotomy, *189*, 190
Percutaneous transhepatic cholangiography, 789, *790*, 801, *1730*
Percutaneous transluminal coronary angioplasty (PTCA), 149, 208–209, *208*
Percutaneous transluminal renal angioplasty, 846
Perforation
  of eardrum, 1256, 1258–1259, 1599
  of nasal septum, 1262–1263
  of uterus, 1425, 1427

Performance, anxiety and, *606*, 610–611
Perfusion, in gas exchange, 246
Perfusion scan, lung, 255–256, 287
  in pregnancy, 1451
Pergolide
  in Parkinson's disease, *549*
  in prolactinoma, 947
Periapical abscess, 680
Pericardial rub, 188
Pericardiocentesis, *189*
Pericardiotomy, *189, 190*
Pericarditis, 118–119, 153, 188–191, *189*
  after heart attack, 213
  in kidney failure, 831–832
  in tuberculosis, 1128, 1129
Pericardium, 187–188
  defects of, 187–188
  inflammation of (*see* Pericarditis)
  radiation injury to, 1660
Perichondritis, 1254–1255
Pericoronitis, 683
Perimenopause, 1356
Perineum, 1343, *1344*
Period (menstrual), 1345, 1346–1348, *1347*,
    1349
  disorders of, 1361–1366, *1362, 1363, 1365,
    1366*
  first (menarche), 1346
  during perimenopause, 1356
Periodic paralysis, 414
Periodontal diseases, 663, 681–685, *683*
Periodontitis, 683–685, *683*
Periosteum, 335
Peripheral arteries (*see* Artery [arteries],
    peripheral)
Peripheral nerves, 437–438, *576*
  age-associated changes in, 438
  disorders of, 575–588, *577, 583, 585*
Peripheral ulcerative keratitis, 1302
Peristalsis, esophageal, *707*
  disorders of, 708–710
Peritoneal dialysis, 833–837, *833, 835, 836*
  peritonitis and, 782
Peritoneal drains, 1505
Peritoneum, 694
Peritonitis, 782–783
  in ascites, 795
  paroxysmal, familial, 1716–1717
  in pelvic inflammatory disease, 1378
Perlèche, 1227
Permethrin, 1218, 1219
Pernicious anemia, 898, *1074*
Pernio, 1656
Peroneal muscular atrophy (Charcot-Marie-
    Tooth disease), 587
Peroneal nerve palsy, 583
Peroneal tenosynovitis, 406
Persistent pulmonary hypertension,
    1501–1502

Personality disorders, 631–635, *632, 634*
  multiple personalities, 638–639, *639*
Pertussis (whooping cough), 1564–1565
  immunization for, 1093, *1094*, 1492, *1493,
    1562*
Pervasive developmental disorder not
    otherwise specified (PDD-NOS), 1631
Pessary, 1380–1381
Pessimism, health and, 7–8
Pestis minor, 1108
PET (*see* Positron emission tomography)
Petit mal (absence) seizures, 497, *498*
Petroleum jelly
  in atopic dermatitis, 1196
  cleansing with, 1190
Petroleum products, poisoning from, 1679
Peutz-Jeghers syndrome, 664, 769
Peyer's patches, 1051, *1053*
Peyote (mescaline), 657–658
Peyronie's disease, 1326
pH, *930*
  blood, 930–933, *1725*
  esophageal, 706, 719
  vaginal, 1374
Phagocytes, *1052, 1053, 1056*
  in lung, 248
Phagocytosis, *1052*, 1053, *1056*
Phalloidine poisoning, 725, 726
Phallus (*see* Penis)
Phantom limb, 44
  pain in, 449
Pharmacist, communication with, 88
Pharmacodynamics, 69–73
Pharmacokinetics, 64
Pharmacological stress testing, 123, 127
Pharyngitis (*see also* Sore throat)
  in children, 1595–1596
  at high altitudes, *1673*
Pharynx (*see* Throat)
Phencyclidine, 658
Phendimetrazine, 919
Phenobarbital
  during breastfeeding, *1462*
  in elderly persons, *81*
  folic acid deficiency with, 899
  during pregnancy, *1460*
  in seizure disorders, *501*
  warfarin interaction with, 76
Phenol burns, *1648*
Phenotype, 9
Phenoxybenzamine, 961
Phentermine, 919
Phentolamine, 1338
Phenylephrine, 250, *1158*
Phenylketonuria (PKU), 1618–1619
Phenytoin
  folic acid deficiency with, 899
  gingivitis and, 682
  during pregnancy, *1460*

Phenytoin *(continued)*
  in seizure disorders, *501*
  selective IgA deficiency with, 1060
Pheochromocytoma, 960–961
  in cardiomyopathy, 162
  high blood pressure in, 134, 136
  in multiple endocrine neoplasia, 973
Pheomelanin, 1212
Pheromones, 1343
Philadelphia chromosome, 1016
Phimosis, 1324–1325
Phlebitis, 223, 236
Phlebotomy (bloodletting)
  in hemochromatosis, *909*
  in polycythemia, 1024
  in porphyria, 934
Phlegm (sputum), 249
  blood in, 252–253
  in bronchitis, 262, 263
  in COPD, 282
  for lung cancer screening, *1038*
  in tuberculosis, 1128
Phobias, 609–611, *611*
  school, 1558
Phoenix House, 653
Phoria, 1601
Phoropter, 1283
Phosgene, 300–301
Phosphatase (alkaline), *1727*
Phosphorus and phosphate, *903,* 909–910
  high blood levels of (hyperphosphatemia),
    910
    in kidney failure, 833
  kidney regulation of, 822
  low blood levels of (hypophosphatemia),
    909–910
    rickets and, 852–853
  radioactive, 1025
  reference range for, *1727*
Photoallergic contact dermatitis, 1194
Photodynamic therapy
  in angioma, *1235*
  in esophageal cancer, 766
  in macular degeneration, 1311
Photophobia, 1281–1282
Photoreceptors, 1276
  electroretinography of, 1285
Photorefractive keratectomy, 1289
Photosensitivity, 1232–1233
  drug-related, 1199, 1232, *1232*
  in pellagra, 897
  in porphyrias, 933, 936
Phototherapy, *1202*
  for atopic dermatitis, 1196
  for granuloma annulare, 1201
  for hyperbilirubinemia, 1506
  for lichen planus, 1204
  for manic-depressive illness, 621
  for psoriasis, 1202

Phototherapy *(continued)*
  for seasonal affective disorder, *614*
  for vitiligo, 1215
Phototoxic contact dermatitis, 1194
Phycomycosis, 1153
Phylloquinone, 895
Physical activity
  atherosclerosis and, 197–198
  cholesterol lowering with, 923
  in heart disease, 119
  obesity and, 915
Physical allergy, 1070
Physical examination
  in child's preventive care, 1543
  in digestive system disorders, 702
  in gynecologic disorders, 1352–1353
  in heart and blood vessel disorders,
    120–121
  in kidney disorders, 825
  in musculoskeletal disorders, 341–342
  in neurologic disorders, 439–442, *440, 441,*
    442
  of newborn, 1484–1485, *1485*
  during pregnancy, 1442
Physical punishment (for children), *1544*
Physical therapy, 38–39, *38* (*see also*
    Rehabilitation)
  in burn injury, 1651
  chest, 261–262
  in osteoarthritis, 369
  in sports injuries, 422
  in temporomandibular joint disorders, 688,
    689
Physician
  communication with, 21–24, 47, 54, 87
  decision making by, 1695–1698
  for dying person, 47
  general organizations for, 1763–1764
  medical record release by, 23–24
  prevention and, 30
  primary care, 22
  visit to, 22–23
Physostigmine, *1308*
Phytanic acid, accumulation of (Refsum's
    disease), *1621*
Pia mater, 435, *435, 436*
Pica, 907, 1440
Pick's disease, 490
Pickwickian syndrome (obesity-
    hypoventilation syndrome), 473
PID (pelvic inflammatory disease), 1377–1379
Pierre Robin syndrome, 1523
Pigeon breeder's lung, *309*
Pigment, of skin, 1214–1216
Pill
  the (*see* Oral contraceptives)
  in esophagus, 710
Pilocarpine, *1308*
  in esotropia, 1602

Pilonidal disease, 763
Pimples
  in acne, 1204–1208, *1205*
  in newborn, *1496*
  in rosacea, 1203
  in seborrheic dermatitis, 1196
Pinealoma, *521, 522*
Pinguecula, 1299
  in Gaucher's disease, 1620
Pinkeye, *1297* (*see also* Conjunctivitis)
Pinna (external ear), 1244, *1245*
  disorders of, 1253–1255, *1254*
Pins-and-needles, *583*
Pinta, 1099
Pinworm infection, 1142
Pioglitazone, *968*
Piperacillin, *1123*
Pitcher's shoulder, 429, *429*
Pituitary gland, *938, 939*, 940–948, *941*
  adenoma of, 941, 943–944
    acromegaly with, 945–946
  dysfunction of, 941
    in diabetes insipidus, 944
    in hyperthyroidism, 950
  in empty sella syndrome, 947–948
  enlargement of, 941–942
  in growth, 1556
  in hormone control, 938, 940
  imaging of, 941, 943
  in puberty, 1324
  sarcoidosis of, 305
  tumors of, *521, 522*, 523, 941, 943–944
    acromegaly with, 945–946
    Cushing's syndrome with, 958
    galactorrhea with, 946–947
    in multiple endocrine neoplasia, 973
    in Nelson's syndrome, *959*
    vision loss with, 1279
  underactive (hypopituitarism), 942–944,
    942
Pit viper bite, 1682–1683
Pityriasis rosea, 1203
Pityriasis versicolor, 1227–1228
PKU (phenylketonuria), 1618–1619
Placebos, 61, *61*
Placenta, *1437, 1454*
  delivery of, *1466*, 1469
  detachment of (placental abruption), 1451,
    1454, 1456, 1507
  drug transport across, *1459*
  mislocation of (placenta previa), 1451,
    1454, 1455–1456
  of postmature fetus, 1498
Placenta previa, 1451, *1454*, 1455–1456
Plague, 1107–1108
  immunization for, *1094*
Plane travel (*see* Air travel)
Plantar fasciitis, 407–408
Plantar warts, 1228–1229

Plants
  dermatitis from, *1193, 1195*
  poisoning from, 725
Plaque (dental), 674
  in gingivitis, 681–682
  in periodontitis, 683–684, *683*
Plaque (skin), *1189*
Plasma, 978
  exchange of (plasmapheresis), *986* (*see also*
    Plasmapheresis)
  low levels of, in relative polycythemia, *1024*
  transfusion of, 985
Plasma cell, 1054–1055
  disorders of, *20*, 1006–1010, *1009*
Plasma cell gastritis, 711
Plasmapheresis, *986*
  in autoimmune disorders, 1075
  in autoimmune hemolytic anemia, 992
  in Goodpasture's syndrome, 312
  in macroglobulinemia, 1010
  in multiple sclerosis, 560
  in thrombocythemia, 1027
  in thrombotic thrombocytopenic purpura,
    998–999
Plasmodium infections (malaria), 1140–1142,
  1714
  kidney damage and, 867
  during pregnancy, 1713
Platelet(s), 979
  aspirin and, 452–453
  bleeding time test of, 981
  in clot formation, 995, *995*
  count of, 980–981, *981*, *1727*
  donation of, 985
  formation of, 979
  high levels of (thrombocythemia), 979,
    1023, 1026–1027, *1026*
  low levels of (thrombocytopenia), 979, 980,
    997–999, *997*
    with cancer treatment, 1047
    in Wiskott-Aldrich syndrome, 1062
  mean volume of, *981*
  in polycythemia, 1023
  radiation effects on, 1659
  splenic entrapment of (hypersplenism),
    1028
  transfusion of, 984, 985
    for pregnant women, 1449
Plateletpheresis, 985
Platinum derivatives, in cancer, *1045*
Play, 1541–1542
Pleura, 245
  anatomy of, 312, *313*
  biopsy of, 256, 298, 315
  disorders of, 312–317
  inflammation of (pleurisy), 119, 251,
    313–314, *314*
  mesothelioma of, 296–297, 298
  pain in, 251

Pleural effusion, 251, 314–316, *315*
  aspiration of, 256
  in cancer, 329, *1036*
  in non-Hodgkin's lymphoma, *1021*
  in tuberculosis, 1127
Pleural rub, 313
Pleurisy, 119, 251, 313–314, *314*
Pleurodesis, 315–316
Pleurodynia, epidemic, *1576*
Plexus, 438, 581, *581*
  disorders of, 581–582
Plummer's disease, 950
Plummer-Vinson syndrome, 707–708
5p minus syndrome, *1529*
PMS (premenstrual syndrome), 1362–1364,
    1362, 1363
Pneumatic sleeve, 240
Pneumatic stockings, 234, 240
Pneumaturia, 869
Pneumococcal (*Streptococcus pneumoniae*)
    infection, 1108–1109
  immunization for, *265*, 1094, *1094*, 1109,
    1493, 1561, *1562*
  meninges, 529–531, 1109
  occult bacteremia, 1561
  pneumonia, 267
Pneumoconiosis, 294–301, *297*
  benign, *297*, 300
  coal workers', 296, *297*
  organic dust, 308–310, *309*
Pneumocystis carinii pneumonia, 271, *1172*
  in children, 1574, 1575
Pneumomediastinum
  in barotrauma, 1668
  in newborn, 1502
Pneumonia, 264–272, *265, 266, 268*
  abscess with, 265, 272–273
  Aspergillus, 311
  aspiration, 271–272, 890
  Chlamydia pneumoniae, 269
  Chlamydia psittaci, 268
  eosinophilic, 310–311
  fungal, 270–271
  gram-negative, 270
  Haemophilus influenzae, 267
  in influenza, 1159
  interstitial
    desquamative, 302–303
    lymphoid, 303
  in Legionnaires' disease, 267–268
  in measles, 1576
  mycoplasmal, 268–269
  pneumococcal, 29, 30, 267, 1108–1109
  Pneumocystis carinii, 271, *1172*, 1575
    in children, 1574
  prevention of, 27
  in respiratory tract infection, 1579
  staphylococcal, 269–270, 1112
  in subacute sclerosing panencephalitis,
    1582

Pneumonia (*continued*)
  in tularemia, 1116
  in typhoid fever, 1117
  viral, 267, 269, *269*, 1159
    in children, 1579–1580
Pneumonitis
  aspiration, *307*
  chemical, 272, 1679
  in HIV infection, 1574
  hypersensitivity, *297*, 308–310, *309*
  in meconium aspiration syndrome, 1501
  organizing, cryptogenic, 303
Pneumothorax, 316–317, *316*
  in asthma, 276
  in barotrauma, 1668
  in COPD, 282–283
  in meconium aspiration syndrome, 1501
  in newborn, 1502
Podagra, 391
Poisoning, 1674–1681, *1675*
  acetaminophen, 1676–1677
  aspirin, 1677
  carbon monoxide, 1677–1678
  caustic substances, 1678–1679
  fish, 725–726, 1100–1101
  food (*see* Food poisoning)
  hydrocarbon, 1679
  insecticide, 1679–1680
  iron, 1680
  lead, 1680
  lizard-bite, 1683–1684
  mushroom, 725, 726
  plant, 725
  seafood, 725–726, 1100–1101
  shellfish, *720, 721*, 726, 1100–1101
  snake-bite, 1682–1683
  spider-bite, 1684–1685
  toadstool, 725
Poison ivy, *1195*
Polio, 1578–1579
  immunization for, 1094, *1094*, 1492, *1493,*
    1578
  muscle weakness after, 576
Pollen, 1065–1067
Polyarteritis nodosa, 387–388, *387*
Polychondritis, relapsing, 385
Polycystic kidney disease, 854–855, *855,*
    1430, 1519
Polycystic ovary syndrome, 1367–1368
  obesity in, 916
Polycythemia, 322, 978
  in chronic mountain sickness, *1673*
  in newborn, 1507
  primary (polycythemia vera), 1023–1025,
    1023
  relative, *1024*
  secondary, *1024*
Polydipsia
  in diabctes insipidus, 944
  in diabetes mellitus, 963

Polyglandular deficiency syndromes, *943*
Polyhydramnios, 1454
Polymenorrhea, *1362*
Polymerase chain reaction (PCR), 15
Polymorphous light eruption, 1232
Polymyalgia rheumatica, 388–389
Polymyositis, 383–384
  in cancer, *1037*
Polymyxin B, *1123*
Polyneuropathy, 584–586
  in cancer, *1037*
  diabetic, 964
Polyp(s)
  familial, 768, 769
  large intestine, 768–769
  nasal, 1067, 1068, *1264*, 1265
  stomach, 766, 767
  vocal cord, 1269, *1269*
Polypeptide antibiotics, *1123*
Polysomnography, 255, 468, *469*, 1597
Polyuria
  in diabetes insipidus, 944–945
  in diabetes mellitus, 963
Polyvinyl chloride, 812
Pompe's disease, *1617*
Pompholyx, 1198
Popliteal artery, aneurysm of, 229
Popliteal cyst, 419
Popliteus tendinitis, 424
Porcelain veneers, *677*
Porencephaly, *1512*
Pork tapeworm, 540, 1143–1144
Porphobilinogen, 935
Porphobilinogen deaminase deficiency (acute
    intermittent porphyria), 934–936
Porphyria cutanea tarda, 933–934
Porphyrias, 933–936, *934*
  hormone replacement therapy and, 1359
Porphyrins, 933
Portal-systemic encephalopathy, 795–796
Portal-systemic shunt, 794
Portal vein, 786, 787, 806, *807*
  high blood pressure in, 793–794, 808, 809
  thrombosis of, 809
Portuguese man-of-war sting, 1687
Port-wine stain, 1236
Positron emission tomography (PET), *1730*
  in cancer staging, 1041
  in heart disease, 127–128
  in Hodgkin's disease, 1018
  in lung disorders, 256
  in neurologic disorders, 444
Postcoital test, 1418
Postconcussion syndrome, 513, 517
Postdrome, of migraine headache, 459
Posterior chamber, of eye, *1276*, 1277
Posterior tibial nerve, compression of (tarsal
    tunnel syndrome), 407
Posterior urethral valves, 1519
Postherpetic neuralgia, 449, *1163*

Posthitis, 1324
Postinfectious (parainfectious) encephalitis,
    533
Postinfectious (acute disseminated)
    encephalomyelitis, 560
Postmature infant, 1498
Postmaturity, of pregnancy, 1471
Post–myocardial infarction syndrome, 188,
    213, 215
Postpartum depression, 1479–1480
Postpartum period, 1476–1480
Postpolio syndrome, 576, 1578
Postprandial hypotension, 144, 147
Post-streptococcal glomerulonephritis,
    838–839
Postterm pregnancy, 1471
Posttraumatic stress, 612–613, *1636*
Postural drainage, 261
Postural (orthostatic) hypotension, 144,
    146–147
Posture, 572, 1707
Potassium, *903*, 910–911
  high blood levels of (hyperkalemia), 911
    in kidney failure, 832, 833
    periodic paralysis with, 414
  low blood levels of (hypokalemia), 910–911
    in Bartter's syndrome, 853–854, 910
    in Cushing's syndrome, 910
    in gastroenteritis, 722
    in hyperaldosteronism, 960
    in Liddle's syndrome, 854, 910
    periodic paralysis with, 414
  reference range for, *1727*
  supplementation with, 911
    generic substitutions for, *91*
Potassium channel blockers, *166*
Potassium citrate
  in cystinuria, 852
  in urinary tract stones, 866
Potassium iodide, 1660
Potency, of drugs, 73
Potter's syndrome, 1454, 1519
Pouches, esophageal, 709–710
Powders, 1189, 1190
Power of attorney, for health care, *53*, 55–56,
    57, 1701
Poxvirus infection (molluscum contagiosum),
    1229
Prader-Willi syndrome, *1529*
  information resources on, 1766
Pralidoxime, 1680
Pramipexole, *549*
Pravastatin, *925*
Precocious puberty, 812, 1366, *1557*
Prednisolone (*see* Corticosteroids;
    Prednisone)
Prednisone (*see also* Corticosteroids)
  adrenal gland suppression by, *958*
  in allergic bronchopulmonary aspergillosis,
    312

Prednisone *(continued)*
  in autoimmune disorders, 1075
  in autoimmune hemolytic anemia, 992
  in Behçet's syndrome, 391
  in Bell's palsy, 592
  in canker sores, 668
  in Crohn's disease, 740, *741*
  in dermatomyositis, 384
  in eosinophilic pneumonia, 311
  in gout, 393, *393*
  in idiopathic pulmonary fibrosis, 302
  in meningitis, 531
  in multiple sclerosis, 559
  in muscular dystrophy, 413
  in osteopetroses, 1611
  in polyarteritis nodosa, 388
  in polymyalgia rheumatica, 389
  in polymyositis, 384
  in rheumatoid arthritis, *372, 373*
  in systemic lupus erythematosus, 380
  in temporal (giant cell) arteritis, 388
  in transplantation, *1078*
  in ulcerative colitis, 743–744
Preeclampsia, 1452, 1459, 1473
Pregnancy, 1434–1444, *1436, 1437, 1438,*
    1441 (see also Embryo; Fetus)
  ABO incompatibility in, *1506*
  in adolescents, 1560
  after premature menopause, 1361
  age considerations in, 1444
    Down syndrome and, 1431, *1431*
  alcohol use during, 650, 1463
  amniocentesis during, *1433*, 1434
  anemia in, 1439, 1443–1444, 1446–1447,
    1451
  anticonvulsant use during, 499, 1447
  appendicitis during, 1450
  aspartame use during, 1463
  aspirin use during, 1501
  asthma during, 1448
  autoimmune disorders in, 1448–1449
  bleeding during, 1451, 1455, 1456, 1457
  caffeine consumption during, 1463
  cancer during, 1449
  cardiomyopathy with, 1454
  cholestasis during, 1451
  chorea in, 552–553
  chorionic villus sampling during,
    1432–1434, *1433*
  cocaine use during, 657, 1450, 1463
  complications of, 1451–1456
  cortical necrosis during, 847
  cystitis during, 870
  cytomegalovirus infection during, 1165
  dating of, 1435
  detection of, 1434–1435
  diabetes mellitus during, 1441, 1447–1448,
    1452–1453, 1499
  Down syndrome and, 1431, *1431*

Pregnancy *(continued)*
  drug addiction during, 647
  drug use in, 85, 101–102, 1449–1450,
    1458–1464, *1459, 1460–1461*
    alcohol, 650, 1463
    cocaine, 657, 1450, 1463
    marijuana, 655
    opioid, 652–653, 1464
  eclampsia in, 1452
  ectopic, *1455*
  Ehlers-Danlos syndrome and, 1608
  fatty liver of, 1453–1454
  fertilization in (*see* Fertilization)
  fever during, 1450
  fibroids during, 1372
  folic acid and, 899, 1526, 1629
  gallstones during, 1448
  genetic screening before, 1429–1430
  gingivitis during, 682
  Graves' disease in, 1448–1449, 1510
  heart disease in, 1445–1446
  HELLP syndrome in, 1452
  hepatitis during, 1448, 1713
  herpes gestationis in, *1441*
  herpes simplex virus infection during,
    1162, 1447
  high blood pressure during, 1446, 1459,
    1473
  high-risk, 1444–1457
  HIV infection during, 1169, 1447, 1574
  hydronephrosis during, 863
  idiopathic thrombocytopenic purpura in,
    1449
  immunization during, 1459, *1461*
  indomethacin use during, 1501
  infection during, 871, 1105, 1447, 1450,
    1451, 1463, 1511–1512
  information resources on, 1760, 1764
  iodine deficiency during, 906
  iron supplementation during, 908,
    1443–1444
  IUD use and, 1425
  kidney disorders in, 1447
  kidney infection during, 871
  listeriosis during, 1105
  liver disease during, 1448
  loss of (*see* Abortion; Miscarriage)
  malaria during, 1713
  Marfan syndrome and, 1608
  marijuana use during, 655
  mask of (melasma), 1215–1216, 1440–1441
  medical care during, 1442–1443
  miscarriage of (*see* Miscarriage)
  molar, 1409–1410
  myasthenia gravis in, 1449
  nausea and vomiting during, 1451–1452
  nipple discharge during, 1387
  number of, 1445
  oligohydramnios in, 1454–1455

Pregnancy *(continued)*
opioid use during, 652–653, 1464
physical changes during, 1437–1441, *1438, 1441*
placental problems in, 1451, *1454,* 1455–1456
polyhydramnios in, 1454
portal vein thrombosis during, 809
postterm, 1471
preeclampsia in, 1452, 1459, 1473
prenatal testing for, 1430–1434, *1430, 1431, 1432, 1433*
prevention of *(see* Contraception and contraceptives; Oral contraceptives)
previous pregnancies and, 1445
problems achieving (infertility), 1414–1419
rape and, 1413
rheumatoid arthritis during, 1449
Rh incompatibility in, 1427, 1433, 1442, 1453, 1477, *1506*
risk factors in, 1444–1457
rubella during, 1580
seizures during, 1447
self-care during, 1443–1444
sexually transmitted disease during, 1447
sickle cell disease and, 1446–1447
smoking during, 1450, 1459, 1462–1463
stages of, *1438*
surgery during, 1450
systemic lupus erythematosus and, 380, 1448
termination of *(see* Abortion; Miscarriage)
thyroiditis after, 954
toxemia of (preeclampsia), 1452, 1459, 1473
toxoplasmosis during, 1144–1145
travel during, 1712–1713
tubal, 1378
ultrasonography during, 1355, 1432, *1433,* 1435, 1442–1443
umbilical cord blood sampling during, 1434
uterine fibroids in, 1449
vaccination during, 1459, *1461*
vitamin A during, 891
vitamin D deficiency during, 894
weight gain in, 916
Premacular fibrosis, 1311
Premature ejaculation, *1339,* 1340
Premature infant, 1470–1471, 1495–1496, *1497 (see also* Labor and delivery, preterm)
apnea in, 1503–1504
dehydration in, 930
eye problems (retinopathy) in, 1492, 1504
infection in, *1508–1509,* 1510–1511
intestinal problems (necrotizing enterocolitis) in, 1504–1505
lung development problems (bronchopulmonary dysplasia) in, 1502–1503

Premature infant *(continued)*
respiratory distress syndrome in, 1499–1500
sepsis in, 1510–1511
vitamin E deficiency in, 895
Premature labor *(see* Labor and delivery, preterm)
Premature menopause, 1361
Premenstrual dysphoric disorder, 1362, 1363
Premenstrual syndrome (PMS), 1362–1364, *1362, 1363*
Prenatal testing, 1430–1434, *1430, 1431, 1432, 1433,* 1512, 1527, 1629
Presbycusis, 17, 1247
Presbyesophagus, 706
Presbyopia, 17, 1279, 1286
Preschool, 1542, 1641
Prescription drugs, 60 *(see also* Drugs)
abuse of, 653–654, *654*
Preservatives, for food, 1068
Pressure
bladder, 861
blood *(see* Blood pressure; High blood pressure; Low blood pressure)
carbon dioxide, *1725*
in diving, 1666–1671, *1669, 1670*
ear, 1244, 1256–1257, *1257,* 1710
eye (intraocular), 20
anterior chamber paracentesis for, 1312
increased (glaucoma), 1279, 1281, 1306–1309, *1308*
measurement of, 1307
oxygen, *1726*
Pressure sores, *20,* 1208–1210, *1209*
casts and, 353
in dying person, 49–50
prevention of, 1209
Preterm labor and delivery *(see* Labor and delivery, preterm; Premature infant)
Prevention, 25–31, *26, 27, 29*
in adolescents, 1554–1555
in adults, 28–30, *29*
barriers to, 30–31
cancer, 1042, *1043*
in children and teenagers, 28, 1543, 1554–1555
components of, 26–30, *27*
doctor visits for, 22
exercise for, 31–36 *(see also* Exercise)
in infants, 1492
of obesity, 1542
in older adults, 30
of premature birth, 1497–1498
primary, 28
risk assessment in, 25, *26*
secondary, 28
tertiary, 28
value of, 25–26
Priapism, 1325–1326

Prickly heat, 1210, *1211*
Primaquine, 1141
Primary biliary cirrhosis, 799–800
Primary care doctor, 22
Primary lateral sclerosis, 575–577
Primary sclerosing cholangitis, 800–801
Prion diseases, 541–543, *542*
Prisms
  in amblyopia, 1601
  in strabismus, 1602
Pritikin diet, 887
PRK (photorefractive keratectomy), 1289
Probenecid, *393*, 394
Procidentia, 763, 1380, *1381*
Proctitis, 762
  ulcerative, 742, 743, 744
Prodrome, of migraine headache, 459
Progeroid syndromes, 21
Progesterone, *939*, 1343
  in menstrual cycle, 1346, *1347*, 1348
  during pregnancy, 1441
  in premenstrual syndrome, 1362
  receptors for, 1391
Progestin
  in breast cancer, 1400
  in endometrial (uterine) cancer, 1404
  in endometriosis, 1370, *1371*
  implant formulation of, 1422
  injectable, 1422–1423
  in IUD, 1424–1425, *1425*
  in oral contraceptives, 1420
  in polycystic ovary syndrome, 1368
  during pregnancy, *1461*
  replacement therapy with, 1358–1359, *1360*
  skin patch formulation of, 1421–1422
  in uterine fibroids, 1373
  vaginal ring formulation of, 1421–1422
Prognathism, 945
Progressive bulbar palsy, 575–577
Progressive massive fibrosis, in black lung, 296
Progressive multifocal leukoencephalopathy, 538–539, *1172*
Progressive muscular atrophy, 575–577
Progressive pseudobulbar palsy, 575–577
Progressive supranuclear palsy, 550
Projection, as defense mechanism, *634*
Prolactin, *939*, 940, *941*, 1343
  deficiency of, 942
  galactorrhea and, 946–947
Prolactinoma, 946–947
Prolapse
  bladder, 1348, 1379–1381, *1381*
  mitral valve, 119, 178
  rectal, 763, 1348, 1379–1381, *1381*
  small intestine, 1379–1380, *1381*
  umbilical cord, 1473
  urethra, 1380
  uterus, 1348, 1379–1381, *1381*
  vagina, 1348, 1380, *1381*

Promethazine, *1065*
  in elderly persons, *80*
Promyelocytic leukemia, 1013
Propantheline, in elderly persons, *81*
Propionibacterium acnes, 1205
Propionic acid, 1377
Propoxyphene, *451*
  in elderly persons, *80*
Propranolol (*see* Beta-blockers)
Propylthiouracil, *951*
  in hyperthyroidism, 952, 1510
  during pregnancy, *1461*
Prostacyclin, 324
Prostaglandin analogues
  in abortion, 1427
  in congenital artery blockage, 1514
  in glaucoma, *1308*
  in labor and delivery, 1474
Prostate gland, *1322*, 1323
  benign hyperplasia of, *20*, 825, 1329–1331
    over-the-counter drug precautions in, *102*
    urination problems with, 824
  cancer of, *20*, 1331–1332, *1333*
    screening for, 29, *1038*, 1040–1041, 1331
    staging of, *1040*
  enlargement of (*see* Prostate gland, benign hyperplasia of)
  examination of, 825
  infection of, 868–869, 1335
  inflammation of (prostatitis), 1335
  information resources on, 1766
  removal of (prostatectomy), 1333
  swelling of, 1335
  testosterone replacement effects on, *1322*
  transurethral resection of (TURP), 1330
Prostate-specific antigen (PSA), 29, *1038*, *1039*, 1040–1041, 1330, 1331, 1334
  reference range for, *1727*
Prostatitis, 1335
  information resources on, 1766
Protease inhibitors, 1173–1174, *1175*
Protein(s)
  Bence Jones, 1007
  dietary, 881
    deficiency of, *735*, 887–890, *888*, *889*
    in phenylketonuria, 1618–1619
    in weight loss diet, 885–886
  plasma, 978
  reference range for, *1727*
  urinary (proteinuria), 825
    hematuria with, 843
    in nephrotic syndrome, 839–840
    during pregnancy, 1442
Protein C deficiency, 1000
Proteinosis, alveolar, 306, 308
Protein S deficiency, 1000
Proteus infection, 1103
Prothrombin time (PT), 981, *1727*

Proton pump inhibitors
  in gastritis, 713
  in gastroesophageal reflux, 719, 1589
  in peptic ulcer, 716, *718*
Protoporphyria, 936
Prune-belly syndrome, *1512*
Pruritus (*see* Itching)
Pruritus ani, 760, 763–764, 1198
Pruritus vulvae, 1198
PSA (prostate-specific antigen), 29, *1038*,
    1039, 1040–1041, 1330, 1331, 1334
  reference range for, *1727*
Pseudobulbar palsy, progressive, 575–577
Pseudocholinesterase, 75
Pseudocyst, pancreatic, 731, 733
Pseudodementia, 484, 616–617
Pseudoephedrine, *1158*
Pseudofolliculitis barbae, 1214, 1224
Pseudogout, 394–395
Pseudohermaphroditism, 1519–1520
Pseudohypertension, 136
Pseudohypoparathyroidism, 901
Pseudomembrane, in diphtheria, 1563
Pseudomonas infection, 1109–1110
  of skin, 1223–1224
Pseudoprecocious puberty, *1557*
Pseudotumor, orbital, 1318
Pseudotumor cerebri, *523*, 1315
Pseudoxanthoma elasticum, 1609–1610
Psilocybin, 657–658
Psittacosis, *268*
Psoralens, *1202*
  in granuloma annulare, 1201
  in lichen planus, 1204
  in psoriasis, 1202
  in psoriatic arthritis, 376
  in vitiligo, 1215
Psoriasis, 1201–1203
  arthritis with, 375–376, 1202
  information resources on, 1766
Psychiatric disorders (*see* Mental health
    disorders)
Psychoanalysis, 600–601, 635
Psychogenic halitosis, *684*
Psychogenic hypacusis, 1250
Psychogenic incontinence, 859
Psychogenic pain, 449–450
Psychologic abuse, 1411
Psychologic issues (*see also* Family
    relationships; Mental health disorders)
  after childbirth, 1479–1480
  for caregiver, *488*
  in childhood cancer, 1622
  in chronic childhood illness, 1638–1640
  in constipation, 751
  in diabetes mellitus, 1614–1615
  in dialysis, 836–837
  digestive system and, 694, 702–703
  in dyspareunia, 1382–1383
  in elderly persons, 21

Psychologic issues (*continued*)
  in erectile dysfunction, 1339
  in globus sensation, 700
  in infertility, 1414
  in irritable bowel syndrome, 756, 757
  in lung disease, 260
  in obesity, 916, 918
  in rape, 1412, 1413
  in recurring abdominal pain, 1591–1593
  in vomiting, 702
Psychomotor (complex partial) seizures,
    496–497
Psychopathic personality, 632
Psychosis (*see also* Mental health disorders)
  after childbirth, 1479, 1480
  amphetamine-induced, 656
  brief, *642*
  vs. delirium, 482, *482*
  ICU (intensive care unit), 480
  Korsakoff's amnesic, 650
  LSD-induced, 657
  in schizophrenia, 640–644, *643*, *645*
  toxic, 655, 656, 657
Psychosomatic disorders, 601–605, *604*
Psychostimulants, *618*, 619
  in attention deficit/hyperactivity disorder,
    1550
Psychotherapy, 600–601
  in depression, 619
  in dissociative identity disorder, 639
  in erectile dysfunction, 1339
  in manic-depressive illness, 621
  in panic attacks and panic disorder, 609
  in personality disorders, 635
  in posttraumatic stress disorder,
    612–613
  in schizophrenia, 644
Psychotic behavior (*see* Psychosis; Mental
    health disorders)
Psyllium, 752, *753*
  in irritable bowel syndrome, 757
Pterygium, 1299
Ptomaine poisoning (*see* Food poisoning)
Ptosis, 1281
Puberty
  delayed, 1364–1365, 1555–1556
  in female, 1345–1346, 1553, *1553*
  in male, 1324, 1553, *1553*
  precocious, 812, 1366, *1557*
Pubic bone, *1345*
Pubic lice, 1219, *1219*
Pudendal block, 1467–1468
Puffer fish poisoning, 726
Pulmonary alveolar proteinosis, 306, 308
Pulmonary artery
  angiography of, 256
  catheterization of, 129–130, 252
  in heart disease, 125
  stenosis of, in children, 1513, 1514
  transposition of, 1517

Pulmonary edema, 250–251
in heart failure, 153–154, 158 (see also
Heart failure)
at high altitudes, 1672–1673
Pulmonary embolism, 285–289, *287*
after fracture, 349–350, 353
after surgery, 1703
in deep vein thrombosis, 232–233, 234
heart failure with, 152
in pregnancy, 1450–1451
prevention of, 234
Pulmonary fibrosis, idiopathic, 301–302
Pulmonary function testing, 254–255, *254,
276, 1730*
Pulmonary hypertension, 322–324, *323*
heart failure with, 152
mitral stenosis and, 179
persistent, 1501–1502
pregnancy and, 1446
Pulmonary infiltrates with eosinophilia
syndrome, 310–311
Pulmonary rehabilitation, 259–262
in chronic lung disease, 284–285
Pulmonary valve, 114, *115*
stenosis of, 183
in children, 1518
Pulpitis, 679–680
Pulse
in aortic regurgitation, 181
in heart disease, 120–121
in pacemaker dysfunction, 174
in peripheral arterial disease, 218
Puncture wound, 1691–1693
Punishment, for children, *1544*
Pupils, 1276, *1276*
age-associated changes in, 1278
in coma, 493
size changes in, 1281
Purging, in bulimia nervosa, 626
Purine nucleosides, *167*
Purpura
allergic (Henoch-Schönlein),
387, 996–997
thrombocytopenic
idiopathic, 997, *998*
pregnancy and, 1449
thrombotic, 997, *998*
Pursed-lip breathing, 261–262
Pus (see also Abscess)
around brain (subdural empyema), 540
around lung (pleural empyema), 314, *315*
in skin (abscess), 1224
Pustule, *1189*
PUVA therapy, *1202*
in granuloma annulare, 1201
in lichen planus, 1204
in psoriasis, 1202
in psoriatic arthritis, 376
in vitiligo, 1215

Pyelonephritis, 871–872
after childbirth, 1479
in children, 1567–1568
Pyloric stenosis, hypertrophic, 1532
Pyoderma gangrenosum, 744
Pyogenic granuloma, 1236
Pyorrhea (periodontitis), 683–685, *683*
Pyrazinamide, *1124*
in tuberculosis, 1129, 1130
Pyridostigmine, 578
Pyridoxine (vitamin B_6), *893,* 897–898, *899*
deficiency of, 897
excess of, 897–898
in homocystinuria, 1619
Pyrogens, 1090
Pyruvate, metabolism of, 1621
Pyruvate carboxylase deficiency, 1621
Pyruvate dehydrogenase complex deficiency,
1621

Q

Q fever, *1133*
Quadrantectomy, 1394, *1396*
Quadriplegia (see Spinal cord, injury to)
Quaking (see Tremor)
Queasiness (see Nausea; Vomiting)
Quinine
adverse effects of, 652
hypoglycemia with, 971
in malaria, 1141
Quinolones, *1123*
Quinupristin/dalfopristin, *1124*

R

Rabbit fever, 1116–1117, *1116*
Rabeprazole, *718*
Rabies, 535–537, *536*
immunization for, *1094, 1709*
Raccoon's eyes, 516
Radial keratotomy, 1289
Radial nerve
compression of (radial tunnel syndrome),
400
palsy of, 583
Radial tunnel syndrome, 400
Radiation (see also Radiation therapy)
annual exposure to, 1658, *1659*
in cancer development, 1032, 1033
injury from, 1657–1661
Radiation accident, 1657–1661
thyroid cancer and, 906
Radiation therapy, 1043, 1046, 1659–1660
for acromegaly, 946
for brain tumor, 524, *525,* 528
for breast cancer, 1397, 1400

Radiation therapy *(continued)*
  for cervical cancer, 1407
  dry mouth and, 666
  for eye cancer, 1624
  gastritis and, 711, 712
  for gynecologic cancer, 1402
  for Hodgkin's disease, 1018–1019
  hyperparathyroidism and, *904*
  for leukemia, 1016
  for lung cancer, 331
  for lymphoma, 1018–1019
  for multiple myeloma, 1008
  nervous system damage from, 528
  for neuroblastoma, 1623
  in oral cancer, 673–674
  for pituitary tumor, 943–944
  proctitis and, 762
  for prolactinoma, 947
  for prostate cancer, 1333–1334
  for retinoblastoma, 1624
  side effects of, 240, 528, 666, 711, 712, 762,
    1047
  swelling after, 240
  for throat (laryngeal) cancer, 1271–1272
  in transplantation, 1077
  for vaginal cancer, 1409
  for Wilms' tumor, 1623
Radioactive iodine
  in hyperthyroidism, *951,* 952–953
  during pregnancy, *1461*
Radioallergosorbent test (RAST), 1064
Radiocontrast cystourethrography, 1568
Radiofrequency ablation, 168
  in atrial fibrillation and atrial flutter, 170
  in ventricular tachycardia, 173
  in Wolff-Parkinson-White syndrome, 172
Radiology *(see also* Computed tomography;
    Magnetic resonance imaging;
    Radionuclide imaging; Ultrasonography)
  in heart disease, 125
  in lung disorders, 255, 265
  in musculoskeletal disorders, 342
Radionuclide imaging, *1730*
  of bile ducts, 789
  in bone infection (osteomyelitis), 365
  in carcinoid tumors, 975
  in coronary artery disease, 204
  in esophageal spasm, 708
  of fractures, 351
  in heart attack, 213
  in heart disease, 127, 204, 213
  in Hodgkin's disease, 1018
  in kidney and urinary tract disorders, 828
  of liver, 789
  in lung disorders, 255–256
  in musculoskeletal disorders, 342
Radiopaque dyes, *827, 1069*
Radiosurgery, for brain tumor, *525*
Radon, 1033, 1658

Raloxifene, 1359, *1360*
  in osteoporosis prevention, 345
Ram's horn nail, 410
Range of motion, 341
  exercise for, 38–39, *38*
Ranitidine, 716, *718*
  in elderly persons, *81*
Rape, 1412–1413
  statutory, 630
Rapid antigen testing, in strep throat, 1596
Rapid eye movement (REM) sleep, 467, *468*
Rapidly progressive glomerulonephritis,
    838–839
Rapid plasma reagin (RPR) test, 1178
Rare disorders, information resources on,
    1767
Rash, 1191
  in allergic reactions, 1063
  around mouth, 1198
  in chickenpox, 1571
  in coelenterate sting, 1687
  in dermatitis, 1194, 1195, 1196
  in dermatomyositis, 383
  diaper, 1534–1535
  drug-related, 1198–1199
  in enteroviral infection, *1576*
  in erythema infectiosum, 1535, 1572
  in erythema multiforme, 1200
  in food allergy, 1068
  on glans penis (balanitis circinata), 376
  in glucagonoma, 776
  in Hartnup disease, 853
  in hot-tub folliculitis, 1109, 1223–1224
  in infants and young children,
    1534–1535
  in juvenile rheumatoid arthritis, 1612
  in Kawasaki syndrome, *1581*
  in kidney failure, 829
  in leprosy, 1131
  in lichen planus, 1203–1204
  in Lyme disease, 1106
  in measles, 1576
  in meningitis, 530
  in mite infestations, 1685
  in newborn, 1486
  on palms and soles (keratoderma
    blennorrhagicum), 376
  in pellagra, 897
  during pregnancy, *1441*
  in prickly heat, 1210
  in rheumatic fever, 1566
  in Rocky Mountain spotted fever, 1134
  in roseola, 1535, 1580
  in rubella, 1582
  in scarlet fever, 1113, 1596
  in Stevens-Johnson syndrome, 1199–1200
  in syphilis, 1177
  in systemic lupus erythematosus, 378
  in toxic epidermal necrolysis, 1199–1200

RAST (radioallergosorbent test), 1064
Rat-bite fever, *1103*
Rattlesnake bite, 1682–1683
Raynaud's disease (and phenomenon),
   224–225, 324
   in mixed connective tissue disease, 384
   in polymyositis, 383
   in scleroderma, 380
Reactive arthritis (Reiter's syndrome),
   376–377
Reading, 1539, 1542, 1551
Receptor(s)
   of airways, 274
   cell, 2, *1052*
      for drugs, 70–72, *70, 71–72, 73*
      for hormones, 938, 1391
   pain, 447
   for smell, 1246
Recommended dietary allowance (RDA)
   for minerals, *902–903*
   for vitamins, *892–893*
Recompression therapy, 1668, 1671
Rectocele, 1379, *1381*
Rectovaginal examination, 1353
Rectum, *695, 698, 1345* (*see also* Anus)
   abscess of, 761
   age-associated changes in, 698
   biology of, 759
   bleeding in, 776–778, *777*
      in Meckel's diverticulum, 1590
   cancer of, 770–773
      screening for, *1038*
   drug administration by, 66
   examination of, 702, 705, 825, *1038*
      in benign prostatic hyperplasia, 1330
      in prostate cancer, 1331
   fistula of, 761, 762
   foreign objects in, 764
   hemorrhoids of, 759–760, *761*
   inflammation of (*see* Proctitis)
   polyps of, 768–769
   prolapse of, 763, 1348, 1379–1381, *1381*
   temperature taking from, *1536*
Red blood cells
   babesiosis of, 1137
   biology of, 978
   deficiency of (*see* Anemia[s])
   examination of, 980, *981*
   excess of (polycythemia), 978, 1023–1025,
      1023, 1024
      in newborn, 1507
   formation of, 979
   hemoglobin in (*see* Hemoglobin)
   in kidney cancer, 876
   malaria effects on, 1140–1142
   radiation effects on, 1659
   reference range for, *1727*
   shape of, *993*
   sickle-shaped, 992–994, *993*
   transfusion of, 984

Red color
   in mouth, 671
   of tongue, 665
Red eye, 1280–1281
Red-green color blindness, 14
Reed-Sternberg cell, 1018
Referred pain, 447, *448*, 569–570, 572
Reflex epilepsy, 495
Reflexes, *442, 1730*
   acoustic, 1244
   diving, 1665
   knee jerk, *442*, 561
   let-down, 1477, 1487
   in newborn, 1485, *1485*
   rooting, *1485*, 1487
   in spinal cord injury, 561
   testing of, 440–441, *442*
Reflexology, 1707
Reflex sympathetic dystrophy, 449
   ankle, 407
   shoulder-hand, 400
Reflux
   acid, 706, 717–719
      in infants and children, 1532, 1588–1589
   urine (vesicoureteral), 1567
Refractive disorders, 1279, 1286–1290, *1287*
   in children, *1601*
   diagnosis of, 1282–1283
Refsum's disease, *1621*
Regional enteritis (Crohn's disease), 738–742,
   741
Regurgitation
   aortic valve, 180–181
      in Marfan syndrome, 1608
   of food, 700, 1486, 1532, 1588–1589 (*see
      also* Nausea; Vomiting)
   mitral valve, 175–178, *176*, 1566
   of stomach acid, 706, 717–719
   tricuspid valve, 182–183
Rehabilitation, 36–45, *38, 42* (*see also*
   Physical therapy)
   after amputation, 43–44
   after brain injury, 41
   after fracture, 353
   after heart attack, 215
   after hip fracture, 43
   after spinal cord injury, 41–43
   after stroke, 41, 44–45, 505
   in alcohol abuse, 651–652
   for blindness, 45
   in chronic lung disease, 259–262, 284–285
   cognitive, 41
   for drug dependence, 653, 654
   for hearing loss, 45, 1253
   for heart disease, 40–41
   information resources on, 1762
   in schizophrenia, 644
   for speech disorders, 44–45
Rehydration solutions, 1100–1101
Reiki, 1707

Reiter's syndrome, 376–377
Relapsing fever, *1103*
Relapsing iridocyclitis, 390
Relapsing polychondritis, 385
Relaxation techniques, 1706
Reliability, of test, 1697
REM (rapid eye movement) sleep, 467, *468*
Renal arteries, 820, *821, 845*
    blockage (occlusive disease) of, 218,
        222–223, 844–846, *846*
Renal cell carcinoma, 875–876
Renal failure (*see* Kidney failure)
Renal pelvis, transitional cell carcinoma of,
    876–877
Renal tubular acidosis, 849–850, *850*
Renal veins, 820, *821, 845*
    blockage (thrombosis) of, 848–849
    metastasis of, 876
Rendu-Osler-Weber disease (hereditary
    hemorrhagic telangiectasia), 810, 996
Renin, 132, *133*, 822, 937–938, *939*
Renin-angiotensin-aldosterone system, 132,
    133, 822, 956, 960
Renovascular hypertension, 223
Repaglinide, *968*
Reproductive system
    birth defects of, 1519–1520
    development of, 1491
    failure of (infertility), 1414–1419
    female, 6, 1343–1348, *1344, 1345, 1347*
        age-associated changes in, *19*, 1348
        cancer of, 1401–1410, *1402*
        evaluation of, 1351–1356
        information resources on, 1768
    male, 6, 1321–1324, *1322*
        age-associated changes in, *18*, 1324
        birth defects of, *1512*
    maturation of (*see* Puberty)
    radiation effects on, 1659, 1660
Reserpine, in elderly persons, *80*
Resident flora, 1086
Resistance
    to disease (*see* Immune system;
        Immunization)
    drug, 78
Resistance training, 36
Resistin, *939*
Respiration (*see also* Breath; Breathing)
    artificial (*see* Resuscitation,
        cardiopulmonary [CPR])
    Cheyne-Stokes, 154, 473, 491
Respirator (*see* Ventilation, mechanical)
Respiratory acidosis, 931–932
Respiratory alkalosis, 932–933
Respiratory center, in premature infant, 1503
Respiratory distress syndrome, 326–328, *327*
    in large-for-gestational-age infant, 1499
    in premature infant, 1496, 1499–1500
Respiratory failure, 325–326, *325*
    in septic shock, 1120
Respiratory infections, 1155–1160 (*see also*
    Bronchitis; Pneumonia)
    in children, 1579–1580
Respiratory syncytial virus (RSV) infection,
    1579–1580, 1585
    in newborn, 1503
Respiratory system, 6, 244–245 (*see also*
    Airways; Lungs)
Respiratory therapy, 261–262
    in cystic fibrosis, 321
Respite care, *47*
Resting tremor, 545, 546
Restless legs syndrome, 474
Restraints, for delirious person, 483–484
Resuscitation
    cardiopulmonary (CPR), 56, 1689–1690
        in electrical injury, 1663
        in hypothermia, 1655–1656
        in lightning injury, 1664
        in near drowning, 1666
        order against, 48, 57
    of newborn, 1471
Retardation, mental (*see* Mental retardation)
Retching (*see* Nausea; Vomiting)
Reticulocyte count, 981
Reticulum cell sarcoma, 361
Retina, 1276, *1276,* 1309–1310, *1310* (*see also*
    Eye[s])
    age-associated changes in, 1278
    bleeding in, at high altitudes, *1673*
    cancer of, 1314, 1623–1624
    cytomegalovirus infection in, 1165
    degeneration of, 1312 (*see also* Retinopathy)
    detachment of, 1280, 1290, 1305, 1311–1312
        in Marfan syndrome, 1608
    diabetes and, 963, 964, 1313–1314
    disorders of, 1310–1314 (*see also*
        Retinopathy)
    electroretinography of, 1285
    examination of, 1283–1284, *1284*
        in heart disease, 121
        in high blood pressure, 136, 1313
        in premature infant, 1504
        in retinal vessel blockage, 1312
    high blood pressure and, 136, 1313
    macular degeneration of, 1310–1311
    membrane over, 1311
Retinal artery, 1277, 1310, *1310*
    blockage of, 1312
Retinal vein, *1310*
    blockage of, 1312
Retinitis pigmentosa, 1312
Retinoblastoma, 1623–1624
Retinocytoma, 1624
Retinoic acid, 1014
Retinol (vitamin A), 891, *892*
    deficiency of, 891
        corneal disorders with, 1300, 1301
    excess of, 891
    reference range for, *1727*

Retinopathy (*see also* Retina)
in diabetes, *963*, 964, 1313–1314
in high blood pressure, 136, 1312
of prematurity, 1492, 1504
Retractile testes, 1536
Retrograde ejaculation, 1340
Retrograde urethrography, 870
Retrograde urography, 827–828, 865, *1730*
Retroperitoneal abscess, 779
Retropharyngeal abscess, 1563–1564, 1596
Retrovirus, *1169*
Rett's disorder, 1631–1632
Reverse-transcriptase inhibitors, 1575
Revocable trust (living trust), 57
Reye's syndrome, 84, 95, 1537, 1568, 1571, *1572*
information resources on, 1767
Rhabdomyolysis, 1649, 1651
Rhabdomyoma, 191–193
Rheumatic fever, 1565–1566
aortic regurgitation in, 180
aortic stenosis in, 181
heart infection (endocarditis) in, 184
mitral regurgitation in, 177
mitral stenosis in, 177
tricuspid stenosis in, 183
Rheumatism (*see* Arthritis; Rheumatoid arthritis)
Rheumatoid arthritis, 370–375, *372*, *374*
juvenile, 1612–1613
peripheral ulcerative keratitis and, 1302
in pregnancy, 1449
of temporomandibular joint, 687, 689
Rheumatoid factor, 371, 1612–1613
Rh incompatibility, 1427, 1433, 1442, 1453, 1477, *1506*
Rhinitis, 1264–1265
allergic, 1065–1067
Rhinophyma, 1203
Rhinovirus infection (*see* Cold, common)
$Rh_O(D)$ immune globulin, 1433, 1453, 1477
Rhythmic rocking, *1548*
Rhythm method, for family planning, *1420*, 1425–1426
Rhythms, of heart (*see* Arrhythmias)
Ribavirin, *1156*
in bronchiolitis, 1585
in hepatitis, 805
in respiratory syncytial virus infection, 1580
Riboflavin (vitamin B_2), *892*, 896
deficiency of, *735*, 896
Ribonucleic acid (RNA), 9
Ribs, 245
Rice diet, 887
RICE treatment
in ankle sprain, 406
in sports injuries, 421–422
Richard Simmons diet, 887

Rickets, 894
familial, 13
hypophosphatemic (vitamin D–resistant), 852–853
Rickettsial infections, 1132–1134, *1133*
Rickettsialpox, *1133*
Rifampin, *1124*
in leprosy, 1131
oral contraceptive interaction with, 72
in tuberculosis, 1129, 1130
Rigidity, muscular, 546–550, *549*
Rimantadine, *1156*, 1160
Ringing, in ear (tinnitus), 1259, 1261
Rings, esophageal, 707
Ringworm, 1225–1226, *1226*, 1535
Rinne tuning fork test, 1249–1250
Risedronate
in osteogenesis imperfecta, 1610
in osteoporosis, 345, 346, *1360*
in Paget's disease of bone, 347–348
Risk-taking behavior, by adolescents, 1554, 1558
Ritonavir, *1175*
Rituals, 611–612
Rituximab
in cancer, *1045*, 1046
in non-Hodgkin's lymphoma, 1022
Rivastigmine, 489
RNA, 9
Rocking, by children, *1548*
Rocky Mountain spotted fever, 1133–1134
Rods (of eye), 1276
Roentgenotherapy (*see* Radiation therapy)
Rolfing, 1707
Romberg test, 441
Rooming-in, 1469
Root canal treatment, 678, 679
Rooting reflex, *1485*, 1487
Ropinirole, *549*
Rosacea, 1203
Rosary bead esophagus, 708–709
Roseola, 1535, *1569*, 1580
Rosiglitazone, *968*
Rotator cuff tendinitis, 429, *429*
Rotavirus infection, *1094*, 1587
Rounded atelectasis, 293, 294
Roundworms, 1136–1137, 1142, 1145, *1146*, 1147
allergic reaction to, 711
Rowing, 36
RPR (rapid plasma reagin) test, 1178
RU 486, 1427
Rubber band ligation
in esophageal varices, 778
in hemorrhoids, 760, *761*
Rubella (German measles), *1569*, 1580–1582
immunization for, 1093, *1094*, 1442, 1477, 1493, *1493*, 1582
in HIV-infected children, 1575

Rubella *(continued)*
  in newborn, *1508*
  during pregnancy, 1450, 1580
Rubeola (measles), *1569*, 1575–1577
  immunization for, 1093, *1094*, 1493, *1493*,
    1577
    in HIV-infected children, 1575
  Koplik's spots of, *663*
  subacute sclerosing panencephalitis with,
    1582
Rule of nines, *1651*
Rumination, 700
Runner's knee, 425–426, *425*, *426*
Running
  Achilles tendinitis with, 424–425
  foot fracture with, 422–423, *422*
  knee problems with, 425–426, *425*, *426*
  popliteus tendinitis with, 424
  pronation and, 420
  shin splints with, 423–424, *423*, *424*
  shoes for, 421
Runs (*see* Diarrhea)
Rupture
  of amniotic sac, 1465, 1470
  of Baker's (popliteal) cyst, 419
  of cerebral aneurysm, 511, 512
  of eardrum, 1594, 1667
  of esophagus, 709, 710
  of heart muscle, *212*
  of scapholunate ligament, *401*
  of spleen, 1029

S

Sacral plexus, 581–582, *581*
Saddle nose, 1611
Sadism, 630
Sadness (*see* Depression)
Safety
  of alternative medicine therapies, 1704
  of child's environment, 1543
  of dietary supplements, 106
  of drugs, 63, 93, *95*
St. John's wort, *105–106*, 111–112, 619,
    1361
St. Vitus' dance (Sydenham's disease), 552
  in rheumatic fever, 1566
St. Louis encephalitis, 537
Salaam seizures (infantile spasms), 502
Salicylates (*see* Aspirin)
Salicylic acid, 1196
Saliva, 662, 663
Salivary glands, 662, 666, *667* (*see also*
    Parotid glands)
  malfunction of, 666
  swelling of, 666–667
  tumors of, 667, 671, 672–673

Salmeterol
  in asthma, *278*, 279–280, 1584
  in COPD, 283
Salmonella infection
  gastroenteritis, *720*, *1089*, 1110
  sexually transmitted, 1183–1184
  typhoid fever, 1117–1118
Salpingitis, 1377
Salt (sodium chloride)
  in cystic fibrosis, 319, 320
  in dehydration, 929
  in excessive sweating, 1652–1653
  in heart failure, 155
  in high blood pressure, 137
  in kidney failure, 832
  in orthostatic hypotension, 147
Sand fly bites, 1685
San Joaquin fever, 1151
Saphenous vein, removal of, 237–238
Saquinavir, *1175*
Sarcoidosis, 304–306
Sarcoma, *521*, *527*, 1032
  of bone (osteogenic), 360–361
  Ewing's, 361
  Kaposi's, 1240–1241
    in HIV infection, 1172
    in mouth, *663*, 672
  reticulum cell, 361
Sarcopenia, 338
Sarcoptes scabiei infestation, 1218–1219
Saturday night palsy, 583
Saw palmetto, *105*, 111
Scab, *1189*
Scabies, 1218–1219
  in traveler, 1714
Scalded skin syndrome, 1112, 1223
Scaling, of skin, *1189*
  in athlete's foot, 1225
  in dermatitis, 1196–1197
  in dry skin (ichthyosis), *1192*
  in pityriasis rosea, 1203
  in psoriasis, 1202
Scalp
  hair loss from, 1212–1214
  lice of, 1219
  ringworm of, 1225
  seborrheic dermatitis of, 1196
Scaphoid bone, fracture of, *401*
Scapholunate ligament, rupture of, *401*
Scarlet fever, 665, 1113, 1596
Scarring, *1189* (*see also* Fibrosis; Sclerosis)
  in acne, 1206, 1208
  in burn injury, 1649
  in deep vein thrombosis, 233
  hair loss with, 1213
  of heart muscle, *212*
  keloids, 1237
  of lymphatic vessels, 240
  in scleroderma, 381

Schatzki's ring, 707
Scheuermann disease, 1604–1605, *1605*
Schilling test, 898–899
Schirmer test, 382, 1301
Schistosomiasis, 1142–1143
 brain, 540
 in traveler, 1714
 urinary tract, 867
Schizoaffective disorder, *642*
Schizoid personality, 631
Schizophrenia, 640–644, *643, 645*
 childhood, 1632
Schizophreniform disorder, *642*
Schizotypal personality, 631, *642*
School, 1542
 abdominal pain during, 1593
 adolescents' problems with, 1558
 avoidance of, 1547–1548
 chronic childhood illness and, 1638
 fear of, 1558
 HIV-related precautions for, 1574, 1575
 learning disorders and, 1551
 for mentally retarded children, 1629
 in separation anxiety disorder, 1637
Schwannoma, *527*
 ear (vestibular), 1260–1261
Sciatica, *571*
Sclera, 1276, *1276*, 1296
 age-associated changes in, 1278
 disorders of, 1299
Scleritis, 1281, 1299, 1318
Sclerodactyly, 380
Scleroderma, 380–382
Sclerosis (*see also* Scarring)
 amyotrophic lateral, 575–577
 limited cutaneous (CREST syndrome),
  381
 multiple, 557–560, *558*
 primary lateral, 575–577
 systemic (scleroderma), 380–382
Sclerotherapy
 for esophageal varices, 778
 for hemorrhoids, 760
 for varicose veins, 238
Scoliosis, 1603–1604, *1604*
 shortness of breath with, 250
Scorpion stings, 1686
Scrapes, 1691–1693
Scrapie, 540, *542*
Scratch dermatitis, 1198
Scratching (*see* Itching)
Screening tests, 26
 for adolescents, 1554–1555
 for cancer, 1037–1041, *1038*
  breast, 29, *1038*, 1040, 1392–1393,
   1395
  cervical, 26, *29, 1038*, 1040, 1353, *1353*,
   1406–1407
  colon, *1038*

Screening tests (*continued*)
  liver, 811
  lung, 330, *1038*
  ovarian, *1038*
  prostate, 29, *1038*, 1040–1041, 1331
  rectal, *1038*
  skin, *1038*
  testicular, *1038*
  uterus (endometrium), *1038*
 decisions about, 1696–1697
 for diabetes during pregnancy, 1453
 for genetic disorders, 1429–1430
 for glaucoma, 1307–1308
 for hearing, 1598
 for mental and behavioral development,
  1628–1629
 for Rh antibodies, 1453
Scrotum, 1321–1322, *1322* (*see also* Testis
 [testes])
 injury to, 1326
 swelling of, 1329
 varicocele of, 1329
Scrub typhus, *1133*
Scuba diving, 1666–1671, *1669, 1670*
Scurvy, 900
Sea anemone sting, 1687
Seafood poisoning, 725–726, 1100–1101
Sealants, in cavity prevention, 678
Sea sickness (*see* Motion sickness)
Seasonal affective disorder, *614*
Seasonal allergies, 1065–1067, 1298–1299
Sea urchin injury, 1687
Sebaceous cyst, 1255
Sebaceous glands, 1187, *1187*, 1205
 disorders of, 1204–1208, *1205*
Seborrheic dermatitis, 1196, 1294
 in infants and young children, 1535
Seborrheic keratoses, 1237
Sebum, 1205
Secobarbital, in elderly persons, *81*
Second opinion, for surgery, 1700
Secretin test, *717*
Secretory diarrhea, 754
Sedatives
 abuse of, 653–654, *654*
 in elderly persons, *81*
 urinary incontinence with, *859*
Seeing (*see* Eye[s]; Vision)
Seizures, 495–502, *500–501*
 after head trauma, 513–514
 brain activity during, *498*
 causes of, 495, *496*
 coma with, *492*
 electroencephalography (EEG) in, 445–446,
  498
 vs. fainting, 145
 with fever (febrile), 502, 1492–1494
 immunization and, 1492–1494
 information resources on, 1763

Seizures *(continued)*
  pregnancy and, 1447
  in roseola infantum, 1580
  salaam (infantile spasms), 502
  in shigellosis, 1111
Selective antibody deficiency, 1060
Selective estrogen receptor modulators, 1359, *1360*
Selective serotonin reuptake inhibitors, 617, *618*
  in autism, 1631
  in bulimia, 627
  in children, 1633
Selegiline, 548, *549*
Selenium, *903*, 911–912
  deficiency of, 911–912
  excess of, 912
Selenium sulfide, 1228
Self-concept, 1542
Self-tanning lotion, *1231*
Sella turcica, 940
  enlargement of (empty sella syndrome), 947–948
Semen, 1323
  analysis of, 1415
  ejaculation of *(see* Ejaculation)
Semicircular canals, 1245, *1245*
  in benign paroxysmal positional vertigo, 465–467, *466*
Seminal vesicles, *1322*, 1323
Senecio leaves, 808
Senescence, 16 *(see also* Aging)
Senile chorea, 552
Senna, 752–753, *753*
Sensate focus exercises, *1385*, 1386
  in erectile dysfunction, 1339
Sensation
  dizziness, 120, 461–467
  fainting, 120
  hearing *(see* Hearing)
  lightheadedness, 120
  pain *(see* Pain)
  sight *(see* Vision)
  smell *(see* Smell)
  taste *(see* Taste)
  throat sticking, 700
  touch, testing of, 440
  whirling *(see* Vertigo)
Sensitivity
  to allergens *(see* Allergy and allergic reactions)
  of test, 1697
Sensory nerves, 438
  hereditary neuropathies of, 586–587
  testing of, 439–440
Sentinel lymph node, in breast cancer, 1396, *1398*
Separation anxiety, 1534, 1540, 1636–1637

Sepsis, 1118–1119
  heart infection (endocarditis) and, 184
  in newborn, *1508–1509*, 1510–1511
Septic arthritis, 365–366
  of temporomandibular joint, 687, 688, 689
Septic shock, 149, 1119–1120
Septostomy, 1514
Septum
  cardiac, hole in, 1514–1515, *1516*
  nasal, 1245
    deviated, 1262
    perforation of, 1262–1263
Sequoiosis, *309*
Serratia infection, 1103
Serum sickness, 1683, *1684*
Sesamoid bones, fracture of, 354, *354*
Sesamoiditis, 411
Severe combined immunodeficiency, 1061–1062
Sex chromosomes, 9, 11, 1527 *(see also* X chromosome; Y chromosome)
  abnormalities of, 1528–1530
Sex drive (libido)
  female, 1382, 1384–1385
  male, 1336, 1339–1340
    in erectile dysfunction, 1337
Sex hormones *(see* Estrogens; Testosterone)
Sex organs *(see* Reproductive system)
Sex reassignment surgery, 629
Sexual abuse, 1179, 1411, 1412–1413
  of children, 1592, 1644, 1645, 1646
  recurring abdominal pain and, 1592
Sexual activity *(see also* Sexuality)
  bisexual, 628
  with different partners, 628
  heart disease and, *1337*
  HIV transmission with, 1168–1169, *1170*
  homosexual, 627–628
  in paraphilias, 629–630
  during pregnancy, 1444
Sexual arousal disorder, 1385–1386
Sexual development, 1553, *1553*
  delay of, 1555–1556
  early, *1557*
Sexuality *(see also* Sexual activity)
  in adolescents, 1554
  development of, 1553, *1553*
  disorders of, 627–630
  female, 1382
    disorders of, 1382–1386
  male, 1323–1324, 1336
    disorders of, 1335–1340, *1336*
    heart disease and, *1337*
Sexually transmitted diseases, 868, 1176–1184, *1177*, 1374–1375 *(see also* HIV infection)
  pregnancy and, 1447
  prevention of, 27, 1176, *1178*

Sexually transmitted diseases *(continued)*
    proctitis and, 762
    reactive arthritis (Reiter's syndrome) with, 376–377
    in traveler, 1714
Sézary syndrome, 1014, *1020*
Shaken baby syndrome, 1645
Shampoos
    in lice infestation, 1219
    in seborrheic dermatitis, 1196
    for skin cleansing, 1190
    in tinea versicolor, 1228
Sheehan's syndrome, 942
Sheep liver fluke infection, *1146*
Shellfish poisoning, *720, 721, 726*
Shigella infection (shigellosis), *720,*
    1110–1111, 1183–1184
Shingles (herpes zoster), *20, 251,* 1162–1163,
    1163, 1302
    pain after, 449
Shin splints, 423–424, *423, 424*
Shock, 143, 148–149
    septic, 1119–1120
    in toxic shock syndrome, 1115–1116
Shock (electrical), for cardioversion, 124,
    167
Shock (electroconvulsive) therapy, 600,
    619
Short bowel syndrome, 734
Shortness of breath *(see* Breath, shortness of)
Short stature, 942, 1556, 1611
Shoulder
    avascular necrosis of, 362
    bursitis of, 418
    degeneration of, 362
    fracture of, 358
    range of motion of, *38*
    strengthening exercise for, *429*
    tendinitis of, 429, *429*
    in thoracic outlet syndrome, 582–583
Shoulder dystocia, 1473
Shoulder-hand syndrome, 400
Shoulder impingement syndrome, 429,
    429
Shoulder presentation, for delivery,
    1472–1473, *1472*
Shrub poisoning, 725
Shunt
    in congenital artery blockage, 1514
    in hydrocephalus, 514–515, *515,* 1526
    in portal hypertension, 794
    in portal vein thrombosis, 809
Shy-Drager syndrome, 550–551
SIADH (syndrome of inappropriate secretion
    of antidiuretic hormone), 912, *913,* 929
Sialometaplasia, necrotizing, 670
Sibutramine, 919
Sicca complex (syndrome), 382
Sick building syndrome, 1720

Sickle cell disease, 992–1094, *993, 1430*
    erythema infectiosum in, 1572–1573
    liver damage in, 810
    pregnancy and, 1446–1447
    travel and, 1713
Sick sinus syndrome, 174
Sideropenic dysphagia, 707–708
SIDS (sudden infant death syndrome), 1489,
    1538
    apnea of prematurity and, 1504
    information resources on, 1767
Sight *(see* Eye[s]; Vision)
Sigmoidoscopy, *29,* 703, *704,* 759, *1038, 1731*
    in colorectal cancer, 770
    in diarrhea, 755
    in intestinal polyps, 769
    in ulcerative colitis, 743
Sign language, 1253
Sildenafil, *1337,* 1338
Silent ischemia, 118, 202
Silicosis, 295–296, *297*
Silo filler's disease, *297,* 300
Silver sulfadiazine cream, 1650
Simethicone, 758–759
Simvastatin, *925*
Single photon emission computed
    tomography (SPECT), 127, 444–445
Sinoatrial node, 163
Sinus arrest, 174
Sinus bradycardia, 174
Sinuses, 1245–1246, *1246, 1265*
    cancer of, 1272
    disorders of, *1264,* 1266–1267, *1266*
    infection of *(see* Sinusitis)
    irrigation of, 1068
    pressure injury to, 1667, 1710
Sinusitis, 1245–1246, 1266–1267, *1266*
    chronic, 1067, 1068, 1266
    headache with, *458*
    toothache with, 690
Sinus (sinoatrial) node, 117, 174
Sinus tarsi syndrome, 407
Sinus tract, pilonidal, 763
Sirolimus, *1078*
Sitosterolemia, *1621*
Sitz bath, 760, 1377
Sjögren's syndrome, 382–383, 666
    information resources on, 1767
Skeleton, 334–335, *336, 337 (see also* Bone[s])
Skiing, cross-country, 36
Skin, 6 *(see also* Hair; Nails)
    abscess of, 1112, *1205,* 1206, 1220, 1224
    in acromegaly, 945
    age-associated changes in, *18,* 1187–1188
    artificial, 1650–1651
    atrophic, *1189*
    barrier function of, 1050, 1087
    biology of, 1186–1187, *1187*
    biopsy of, 1188

Skin *(continued)*
  bleeding in, 998
  blisters of *(see* Blisters)
  burns of *(see* Burns)
  café au lait spots of, 527
  cancer of, 1230, *1231,* 1238–1241, *1239,*
      1240
    of ear, 1255
    of penis, 1325
    screening for, *1038*
    of vulva, 1408
  candidiasis of, 1150–1151
  color of, 1214
    in Addison's disease, 957
    at birth, 1484–1485
    in carcinoid tumors, 974
    disorders of, 1214–1216
    in erythromelalgia, 225
    in heart disease, 120
    in jaundice, 791–792
    in newborn, 1486, *1496*
    in shock, 148
    in tinea versicolor, 1227–1228
  cyanosis of *(see* Cyanosis)
  decontamination of, in radiation exposure,
      1660
  dermatitis of *(see* Dermatitis)
  dermatomes of, *563*
  in dermatomyositis, 383
  in diabetes mellitus, *963,* 964
  disorders of, 1188–1241, *1189 (see also*
      specific disorders)
    diagnosis of, 1188
    terminology for, *1189*
    topical drugs for, 1188–1191
  dry, 1191–1192, *1192*
  elastic
    in cutis laxa, 1610
    in Ehlers-Danlos syndrome, 1608
  in eosinophilic fasciitis, 385–386
  frostbite injury to, 1656–1657
  grafts of, 1083, 1210, 1650
  in Graves' disease, 950
  infection of
    anthrax, 1098
    bacterial, 1111–1112, 1220–1224
    fungal, 1150–1151, 1153–1154,
        1225–1228, *1226,* 1535
    parasitic, 1218–1219, *1219*
    prevention of, 1220
    risk for, 1220
    spirochetal, 1099
    viral, 1160–1162, 1228–1229
  inflammation of, 1193–1198, *1193, 1195*
      (see also Dermatitis)
  itching of *(see* Itching)
  jaundice of, 791–792 *(see also* Jaundice)
  in leprosy, 1130–1132
  limited sclerosis of (CREST syndrome), 381

Skin *(continued)*
  maceration of, 1190
  in neurofibromatosis, 527–528
  of newborn, 1484, 1486, *1496*
  noncancerous growths of, 1233–1237
  in non-Hodgkin's lymphoma, *1021*
  pigmentation of, 1214
    disorders of, 1214–1216
  postmenopausal changes in, 1357
  in postterm fetus, 1498
  during pregnancy, 1440–1441, *1441*
  purple-black spots of, in *Pseudomonas*
      infection, 1110
  radiation effects on, 1660
  resistance of, to electricity, 1662
  in sarcoidosis, 304–305
  in scleroderma, 380–381
  sclerosis of, 380–381
  stiffness of, in pseudoxanthoma elasticum,
      1609–1610
  sunlight effects on *(see* Sunlight)
  in systemic lupus erythematosus,
      378–379
  tags of, 1234
  tanning of, *1231*
  tumors of, 1230, *1231,* 1238–1241, *1239,*
      1240
  ulcers of, *20, 1189 (see also* Pressure sores)
    of leg and foot, 217, 222, *222,* 235
  warts of, 1228–1229
  yeast infection of, 1150–1151
  yellow color of *(see* Jaundice)
Skinfold thickness, 881
Skin testing
  in allergy, 1063–1064, 1068, 1188, *1731*
  in asthma, 276
  in immunodeficiency disorders, 1058–1059
  in tuberculosis, 1128, *1128*
Skull
  fracture of, 515–517
    in newborn, 1494
  in newborn meningitis, 1562
  in Paget's disease, 347
  tumors of, *521*
SLE *(see* Systemic lupus erythematosus)
Sleep
  apnea in, 255, 472–474, 917
    with enlarged tonsils and adenoids,
        1596–1597
  in children, 1546–1547
  contact lens use during, 1288
  in depression, 616, 617
  disorders of, 467–475, *469, 470, 471*
    drugs for *(see* Sleep aids)
    information resources on, 1767
    travel-related, 1711
  excessive, 470–472
  improvement of, *470*
  in infant, 1489

Sleep *(continued)*
  paralysis during, 471
  requirements for, 467
  stages of, 467, *468*
Sleep aids, 469, *471*
  abuse of, 653–654, *654*
  in elderly persons, *81*
  over-the-counter, 100
Sleep apnea, 255, 472–474, 917, 1596–1597
Sleeping sickness (*Trypanosoma brucei* infection), *1147*
Sleepwalking, 474, 1546
Sling, 351
Slipped capital femoral epiphysis, 1605–1606, *1605*
Slit lamp examination, 1284, *1285*
Small-for-gestational-age infant, 1498–1499
Small intestine, *695*, 696
  age-associated changes in, 698
  biopsy of, 734
  bleeding in, 776–778, *777*
  cancer of, 768, *769*
  Crohn's disease of, 738–742, *741*
  gallstone in, 814
  lymphangiectasia of, 737–738
  malabsorption in (*see* Malabsorption)
  Meckel's diverticulum of, 1590–1591, *1591*
  obstruction of, 779–781, *780*
  prolapse of, 1379–1380, *1381*
  transplantation of, 1083
  Tropheryma whippelii infection of (Whipple's disease), 737
  tumors of, 768, *769*
Smallpox (variola), *1166*
  immunization for, *1094*, 1095
Smell, 585, 662, 1246
  age-associated changes in, *18*, 1247
  disorders of, 584–586
  in Parkinson's disease, 547
Smoke inhalation, *1649*
Smoking
  by adolescents, 1559
  atherosclerosis and, 196–197
  bronchiolitis and, 1585
  Buerger's disease and, 223
  cancer risk and, 1033
  cessation of, 197, 200, 654–655
    in COPD, 283
    preoperative, 1700–1701
    weight gain with, 916
  COPD and, 282
  coronary artery disease and, 200
  Crohn's disease and, 739
  dependence on, 644–645
  desquamative interstitial pneumonia and, 302–303
  drug effectiveness and, 76
  lung cancer and, 328

Smoking *(continued)*
  lung disease and, 282, 302–303, 328, 1585
  oral cancer and, 672
  oral melanosis with, *663*
  peptic ulcers and, 714
  during pregnancy, 1450, 1459, 1462–1463
  ulcerative colitis and, 742
Snake bites, 1682–1683
Snellen chart, 1283
Snow blindness, *1673*
Soap, 1189–1190
Soap-suds enema, 753
Social diseases (*see* Sexually transmitted diseases)
Social factors, in risk assessment, 25, *26*
Social phobia, 610–611
Social relationships (*see also* Family relationships)
  in autism, 1630
  in Rett's disorder, 1631–1632
Sociopathic personality, 632
Socket, dry, after tooth extraction, 692
Sodium, *903*, 912–914 (*see also* Salt)
  high blood levels of (hypernatremia), 913–914
    coma with, *493*
  low blood levels of (hyponatremia), 912–913
    coma with, *493*
    in gastroenteritis, 723
    in lung cancer, *1037*
  reference range for, *1727*
Sodium bicarbonate, 697
  in antacids, 99
  in aspirin poisoning, 1677
  in burn injury, 1651
  in cystinuria, 852
  in gout, 394
  in peptic ulcer, 716, *718*
  in renal tubular acidosis, 850
Sodium channel blockers, *166*
Sodium hypochlorite burns, *1648*
Sodium phosphate, *753*
Sodium polystyrene sulfonate, 831
Sodium urate crystal deposition, 391–394, *392*, *393*
Solar keratoses, *1231*
Solar urticaria, 1232
Solutions, 1189
Solvent
  cleansing with, 1190
  inhalation of, *658*, 659, *659*
Somatic gene therapy, 15–16
Somatic nervous system, 437
Somatization disorder, 602–603
  in children, 1637
Somatoform disorders, 601–605, *604*
  in children, 1637

Somatostatin, 697
Somnambulism, 474
Sonography (*see* Ultrasonography)
Sonohysterography, 1355, 1418
Sorbitol, *753*
Sores
  canker, 668
  cold, 668–669, 1161
  genital
    in chancroid, 1181–1182
    in syphilis, 1176–1177
  lip, 664
  mouth, 667–670, 1041
    in pemphigus, 1216
  pressure (*see* Pressure sores)
  tongue, 665
  in tularemia, 1116, *1116*
Sore throat
  in children, 1595–1596
  in diphtheria, 1563
  gonococcal, 1179
  strep, 1113, 1595–1596
    nephritic syndrome after, 838–839
    rheumatic fever after, 1565–1566
Sounds, heart (*see* Heart, sounds in;
    Murmurs, heart)
South American blastomycosis, 1153
South American hemorrhagic fever,
    1165–1167
Southern blot test, 15
Spanking, *1544*
Spasm(s)
  anus, 760
  artery, 225
  in cerebral palsy, 1625
  coronary artery, 203
  diaphragm (hiccups), *545*
  esophagus, 708–709
  eyelid (blepharospasm), 554
  face, 593
  in heat cramps, 1653
  in Huntington's disease, 553
  infantile, 502
  intestine
    in diverticulosis, 747
    in irritable bowel syndrome, 756–757
  muscle (tetany), 904
    in DiGeorge anomaly, 1061
  neck, in torticollis, 555–556
  in neuroblastoma, *1037*
  in rabies, 536
  ureteral, 871
  vagina (vaginismus), 1383–1384
  in vitamin D deficiency, 894
  vocal cord (spasmodic dysphonia), 554
Spasmodic dysphonia, 554
Spasmodic torticollis, 555–556
Spastic colon (irritable bowel syndrome),
    756–757

Spastic paraparesis
  hereditary, 566–567
  tropical, 539, 560
Special K (ketamine), 658
Specific gravity, of urine, 826
Specificity, of test, 1697
SPECT (*see* Single photon emission computed
    tomography)
Spectinomycin, *1124*
Speech
  in autism, 1630
  in brain injury, 477–478, *477*
  disorders of
    information resources on, 1767
    rehabilitation for, 44–45
  in dysarthria, 556
  in schizophrenia, 641
  in spasmodic dysphonia, 554
  in stroke, 44–45, 504
  in Tourette's syndrome, 552
  without vocal cords, *1272*
Speech reading, 1252–1253
Speech threshold audiometry, 1249
Speed (methamphetamine), 656
Spells (*see* Seizures)
Sperm, 1321
  donor, 1416
  infertility-related problems with,
    1414–1415
  intracytoplasmic injection of, 1419
  sac of (spermatocele), 1329
Spermatocele, 1329
Spermicides, 1424
Sphenoid sinus, 1245–1246, *1246*
Spherocytosis, hereditary, *989*
Sphincter(s)
  anal, 698, 759
    exercises for, 757–758
    spasm of, 760
  esophageal, 696, 706, *707*
    in achalasia, 709
    incoordination of, 708
    in infant, 1588
Sphincter of Oddi, *695*, 786, 787
  abnormal function of, 816–817
Sphincterotomy, in gallstones, 815
Sphingomyelin accumulation (Niemann-Pick
    disease), 1620
Sphygmomanometer, *135*
Spider angioma, 1236
  during pregnancy, 1441
Spider bites, 1684–1685
Spider veins, 236–237, 238
  in ataxia-telangiectasia, 1061
  radiation therapy and, 1660
Spina bifida, *1432*, 1511, *1525*, 1526
  information resources on, 1767
  prenatal testing for, 1430
Spinal anesthesia, in labor and delivery, 1468

Spinal column (*see* Spine; Vertebrae)
Spinal cord
  age-associated changes in, 438
  biology of, 435–437, *436*, 561
  biopsy of, 526
  birth defects of, 1430, 1525–1526, *1525*
  blood accumulation around (hematoma),
    565–566
  blood flow to, interruption of, 567–568
  compression of, 563–564, *565*
    in cancer, *1036*
    in cervical spondylosis, 564–565
    in disk disease, 569, *570*, 571, 574
    in hematoma, 565–566
  damage to (*see* Spinal cord, injury to)
  degeneration of, 568
  demyelination of, 557–560, *558*
  infection of, 529–540, *533*
    human T-cell lymphotropic virus type I,
      539, 560
    rabies, 535–537, *536*
  inflammation of (transverse myelitis), 567
  injury to, 561–563, *562–563*
    in decompression sickness, 1670
    incontinence after, *860*
    information resources on, 1767
    in newborn, 1495
    radiation-related, 1660
    rehabilitation after, 41–43
  lipoma of, 1526
  nerve degeneration in, 587–588
  nerve roots of, *436*, 438
  spina bifida of, *1432*
  syrinx of, 566
  tumors of, 526, *527*
  viral infection of, 1569–1570
  in vitamin B_{12} deficiency, 568
  x-ray of, 445
Spinal fluid (*see* Cerebrospinal fluid)
Spinal hematoma, 565–566
Spinal muscular atrophy, 587–588
Spinal nerves, 437–438, 561
  compression of, 571–572
  degeneration of, 587–588
Spinal stenosis, 569, 571, 574
Spinal tap (lumbar puncture), 442, *443*,
  1731
  in bacterial meningitis, 530–531, 1562
  in brain tumor, 524
  complications of, 510
  in encephalitis, 1570
  in infants and young children, 1537, 1570
  in multiple sclerosis, 559
  in neurosyphilis, 1178
  in newborn, 1510
  in papilledema, 1315
  in retinoblastoma, 1624
  in stroke, 509
  in tuberculous meningitis, 1128

Spine, 569 (*see also* Spinal cord)
  arthritis of, 368
  biology of, *436*
  curvature of, 1603–1604, *1604*
    in Scheuermann disease, 1604–1605,
      1605
  fracture of, 344–345, 346, 357–358
  inflammation of (ankylosing spondylitis),
    377, 569
  osteoarthritis of, 569
  osteoporosis of, 344–345, 569
  stenosis of, 569, 571, 574
Spirituality, 51
Spirochetes, *1096*
  infection with, 1099, 1104–1105,
    1176–1179 (*see also* Syphilis)
Spirometry, 254–255, *254*, *1731*
  in asthma, 276
  in COPD, 283
  incentive, 261
Spironolactone, 960
  in polycystic ovary syndrome, 1368
Spitting up (regurgitation), 700, 1486, 1532,
  1588–1589
Spleen, 1027, *1027*, *1053*
  abscess of, 779
  absence of, 1062–1063
  disorders of, 1027–1029
  enlargement of, 1028–1029, *1028*
    anemia with, 989
    in Epstein-Barr virus infection, 1164
    in myelofibrosis, 1025
    in polycythemia, 1023
    in portal hypertension, 794
    in rheumatoid arthritis, 371
    in sickle cell disease, 993
  radiation effects on, 1659
  removal of, 1027, 1029
    in autoimmune hemolytic anemia, 992
    in idiopathic thrombocytopenic purpura,
      998
  rupture of, 1029
Splenectomy (*see* Spleen, removal of)
Splenic arteries, 218, 223
Splenomegaly (*see* Spleen, enlargement of)
Splint, 351, *1692*
  in burn injury, 1651
  in temporomandibular joint disorders, 688
Splitting, as defense mechanism, *634*
Spondylitis, ankylosing, 377, 569
Spondylosis, cervical, 564–565
Spongiform encephalopathies (prion diseases),
  541–543, *542*
Spontaneous pneumothorax, 316–317
Sporotrichosis, 1153–1154
Sports injuries, 419–429
  Achilles tendinitis, 424–425
  foot fracture, 422–423, *422*
  hamstring injury, 426, *427*

Sports injuries *(continued)*
  popliteus tendinitis, 424
  rotator cuff tendinitis, 429, *429*
  runner's knee (patellofemoral stress
      syndrome), 425–426, *425, 426*
  shin splints, 423–424, *423, 424*
  tennis elbow, 427–429, *427, 428*
Spotted fever, 1133–1134
Sprain, *1692*
  ankle, 405–407, *406*
  first aid for, 1693
  washerwoman's (De Quervain's syndrome),
      419
Spray and stretch exercise, in
    temporomandibular joint disorders, *689*
Spring-summer hypomania, *614*
Sprue
  nontropical (celiac disease), 736–737
  tropical, 737
Spur, heel, 404–405, *405*, 408
Sputum (*see* Phlegm)
Squamous cell carcinoma, 1238–1239
  anus, 773
  cervix, 1406
  ear, 1255
  esophagus, 764–766
  eyelid, 1295
  mouth, 672
  paraneoplastic syndromes in, *1037*
  penis, 1325
  vagina, 1408–1409
  vulva, 1408
Squeamishness (*see* Nausea; Vomiting)
Squint (strabismus), 1601–1603, *1602*
Staghorn stone, 865
Staging, of cancer, *1040,* 1041
  breast, 1389–1390, *1394*
  gynecologic, 1401–1402, *1402*
  prostate, 1332
Stapedius muscle, 1244
Stapes (stirrup), 1244, *1245*
Staphylococcal infection, 1111–1112
  antibiotic resistance in, 1112
  bone, 364
  food poisoning, *721,* 724
  impetigo, 1222–1223
  pneumonia, 269–270
  skin, 1220–1221, 1223–1224
  stye, 1294–1295
Staphylococcal scalded skin syndrome, 1223
Starvation, 883, 888, *889*
Stasis dermatitis, 1197–1198
Statins, *925*
Status asthmaticus, *280*
Status epilepticus, 497, 499
Statutory rape, 630, 1412–1413
Stavudine (d4T), *1175*
STD (*see* Sexually transmitted diseases)
Steam inhalation, 249

Steatorrhea, 734
  in abetalipoproteinemia, 927
  in cholestasis, 793
Steinert's disease (myotonic dystrophy), 414
Stein-Leventhal syndrome, 1367–1368
Stem cells, 979, *1081*
  in neutropenia, 1003
  transfusion of, 985
  transplantation of, 1081–1083
    in chronic granulomatous disease,
        1062
    in Hodgkin's disease, 1019
    in immunodeficiency disorders, 1059
    in leukemia, 1012, 1016
    in myelofibrosis, 1026
    in sickle cell disease, 994
    in Wiskott-Aldrich syndrome, 1062
Stenosis
  aortic valve, 181–182, 1517–1518
  mitral valve, *176,* 178–180, 1566
  pulmonary valve, 183, 1518
  pyloric, hypertrophic, 1532
  renal artery, *846*
  spinal, 569, 571, 574
  tricuspid valve, 183
Stents
  for abdominal aneurysm, 228
  for coronary artery disease, 209, 1711–1712
  for ureter, 864
Stereotactic surgery, for brain tumor, *525*
Sterilization, for family planning, 1427–1428,
    1428
Steroids
  anabolic, *647*
    adolescent use of, 1560
    coronary artery disease and, 200
  cortico- (*see* Corticosteroids)
Stethoscope, 121, *135*
Steven-Johnson syndrome, 1199–1200
Stiffness, 341
  in osteoarthritis, 367
  in polymyalgia rheumatica, 388–389
Stiff-person syndrome, *577*
Still's disease, 1612
Stingray injury, 1686
Stings (*see* Bites and stings)
Stirrup (stapes), 1244, *1245*
Stockings (*see also* Support hose)
  elastic, 234, 235, 237
  pneumatic, 234, 240
Stomach, *695, 696*
  acid in (*see* Acid, stomach)
  age-associated changes in, 698
  bezoars of, 727–729
  bleeding from, 776–778, *777*
    drug-related, *83*
  blockage of, *715,* 1532
  bypass surgery on, in obesity, 919–920,
    919

Stomach *(continued)*
  cancer of, 766–768, *767*
    ulcers and, 714
  chemical burns of, 1678–1679
  emptying of, in poisoning, 1676
  foreign objects in, 727–729
  hernia of, 727, *728*
  infection of, 711, *712*, 719–726, *720–721*
    in children, 1586–1588
  inflammation of (gastritis), 711–713, *712*
  metaplasia of, 712
  polyps of, 766, 767
  removal of, 775–776
  stapling of, 919–920, *919*
  tumors of, 766–768, *767*
  ulcers of, 712, 713–717, *715*, *718*
    in children, 1589
  upset *(see* Indigestion)
Stomach flu *(see* Gastroenteritis)
Stomatodynia (burning mouth syndrome),
  665
Stomatopyrosis (burning mouth syndrome),
  665
Stones
  bile duct (choledocholithiasis), 813–815,
    816
  bladder, 864–866
  gallbladder *(see* Gallstones)
  kidney, 823, 851–852, 864–866, *865*
    birth defects and, 1519
    in gout, 392, 394
  salivary gland, 666–667, *667*
  urinary tract, 823, 851–852, 864–866, *865*
Stool
  blood in, *29*, 699, 705, 754, 770, *1038*, 1041,
    1589
  in constipation *(see* Constipation)
  in diarrhea *(see* Diarrhea)
  in diverticulosis, 747
  examination of, 755
  fat in (steatorrhea), 734
    in abetalipoproteinemia, 927
    in cholestasis, 793
  impaction of, 699, 752 *(see also*
    Constipation)
  in infant, 1489
  in malabsorption, 734
  passing of *(see* Bowel movements)
  softeners for, 752, *753*
Stop-and-start technique, in premature
  ejaculation, *1339*
Stork-bite, *1496*
STP (2,5-dimethoxy-4-methylamphetamine),
  657–658
Strabismus, 1601–1603, *1602*
  in amblyopia, 1600
Strain, *1692*
  first aid for, 1693
  lumbar, 569

Strangulation, intestinal, 780, *780*
Stratum corneum, 1186, *1187*
Strawberry hemangioma, 1235, *1496*
Strawberry tongue, 665, 1596
Strength exercise, 39, 421
  in back pain prevention, 572, *573*
  in fracture, 353
  hamstring, *427*
  inner thigh, *425*
  shoulder, *429*
  wrist muscles, *428*
Strep throat, 1113, 1595, 1596
  nephritic syndrome after, 838–839
  rapid test for, 1596
  rheumatic fever after, 1565–1566
Streptobacillus moniliformis (rat-bite fever),
  1103
Streptococcal infection, 1112–1113
  nephritic syndrome after, 838–839
  pneumococcal infection *(see* Pneumococcal
    infection)
  rheumatic fever after, 1565–1566
  skin (cellulitis), 1220–1221
  skin (impetigo), 1222–1223
  strep throat, 1113, 1595, 1596
Streptococcus pneumoniae infection *(see*
  Pneumococcal infection)
Streptomycin, *1122*
  during pregnancy, *1460*
  in tuberculosis, 1129
Stress
  acute, 613
  in Addison's disease, 957
  amenorrhea and, 1365
  angina and, 203
  anxiety and, 606
  blood pressure effects of, 134
  children's responses to, *1548*, *1636*
    overscheduling and, 1542–1543
  disease and, 7
  family, in childhood illness, 1622,
    1638–1640
  gastritis and, 711, 712, 713
  hair loss with, 1213
  irritable bowel syndrome and, 756
  obesity and, 916
  peptic ulcers and, 713
  posttraumatic, 612–613, *1636*
  prevention of, *27*
  psychosomatic disorders and, *604*
  suicidal behavior and, 1636
Stress fracture, foot, 422–423, *422*
Stress incontinence, 858, 861
  after menopause, 1357
Stress testing, 123, 127, 204, *1731*
Stretching exercise, 34, 421
  after burn injury, 1651
  in back pain prevention, 572, *573*
Stretch marks, during pregnancy, 1441

Stridor, 252
 in croup, 1586
 in epiglottitis, 1564
 in respiratory tract infection, 1579
Stroke, *20*, 502–512, *505*
 atrial fibrillation and, 170
 brain impairment after, 41
 cholesterol level and, 922
 coma with, *492*
 dementia with, 489–490
 estrogen and, 1358
 fainting with, 144
 hemorrhagic, 510–512
 ischemic, 507–510, *508*
 prevention of, *27*, 505
 recognition of, *508*
 rehabilitation after, 41, 44–45, 505
 speech disorders after, 44–45, 504
 vision loss in, 1279
Strongyloides (threadworm) infection, *1146*
Structural integration (rolfing), 1707
Strümpel-Lorrain disease, 566–567
Struvite stones, 864, 866
Stupor, 482, 490–494, *492–493*
Stuttering, information resources on, 1767
Stye, 1294–1295
Subacute cerebellar degeneration, *1037*
Subacute combined degeneration of spinal
  cord, 568
Subacute sclerosing panencephalitis, 1577,
  1582
Subacute spongiform encephalopathy
  (Creutzfeldt-Jakob disease), 541–543
Subarachnoid hemorrhage, 511–512, *511*
 headache with, *459*
Subarachnoid space, 435, *435*
Subcision, in scar treatment, 1208
Subcutaneous fat necrosis, in newborn,
  1485
Subcutaneous route, of drug administration,
  64–65, *65*
Subdural bleeding (hematoma, hemorrhage),
  459, *511*, 518
Subdural empyema, 540
Suberosis, *309*
Sublingual glands, 662, 666, *667*
Sublingual route, of drug administration,
  66
Submandibular glands, 662, 666, *667*
Substance abuse (*see* Alcohol use and abuse;
  Drugs, abuse of)
Subxiphoid pericardiotomy, *189*, 190
Succimer, 1681
Succinylcholine, 75
Sucking reflex, *1485*
Sucralfate, 716, *718*
Sucrase deficiency, 735
Suction curettage, 1426–1427
Suctioning, of respiratory tract, 258, 261

Sudden infant death syndrome (SIDS), 1489,
  1538
 apnea of prematurity and, 1504
 information resources on, 1767
Sudeck's atrophy, 407
Suffocation, in near drowning, 1665–1666
Sugar(s), 881 (*see also* Glucose)
 blood, 962, 963, 964
  in children, 1614
  in glycogen storage disease, 1616–1617
  high levels of (*see* Diabetes mellitus;
    Hyperglycemia)
  in large-for-gestational-age infant,
    1499
  levels of, *1726*
  low levels of, 966, 970–972 (*see also*
    Hypoglycemia)
  measurement of, 964–965, 969, 971
  monitoring of, 969, 1615
  oral contraceptives and, 1420
  in postmature newborn, 1498
  during pregnancy, 1441
  in premature infant, 1497
  reference range for, *1726*
  during travel, 1712
 diarrhea with, *755*
 for infants, 1489
 intolerance to, 698, 735–736
 metabolism of (*see also* Diabetes mellitus)
  hereditary disorders of, 1616–1618
 tooth decay and, 677–678
 urine, 969
  during pregnancy, 1442
Sugar disease (*see* Diabetes mellitus)
Suicide, 51, 622–624, *622*, *623*
 assisted, 624
 centers for prevention of, *623*, 1635
 in children and adolescents, 1634–1635,
   1635
 in depression, 616, 623
Suitcase elbow, 428–429
Sulfacetamide, *1123*
Sulfamethizole, *1123*
Sulfasalazine, *1123*
 in Crohn's disease, 740, *741*
 folic acid deficiency with, 899
 in rheumatoid arthritis, *372*, 373
 in ulcerative colitis, 743
Sulfinpyrazone, *393*, 394
Sulfisoxazole, *1123*
Sulfonamides, *1123*
 during pregnancy, *1460*
Sulfonylureas, 968–969, *968*
 hypoglycemia with, 970
Sulfur dioxide, 300–301
Sulfuric acid burns, *1648*
Sunblock, 1231
Sunburn, 1230–1232
 of eyes (snow blindness), *1673*

Sunlight, 1230
  allergy to, 1070, 1232–1233
  cancer and, 1230, 1238
  damage from, *1231*
  epidermal cyst growth and, 1237
  lip damage from, 664
  mole development and, 1234
  sensitivity to, 1230, 1232–1233, 1281–1282
    in albinism, 1215
    in contact dermatitis, 1194
    drug-related, 1199, 1232, *1232*
    in pellagra, 897
    in porphyria, 933, 936
  skin damage from, 1188, 1230–1232, *1231*
Sunscreens, 1231
Suntan, *1231*
Superficial punctate keratitis, 1299–1300
Superior mesenteric artery, 218, *219*, 223
Superior vena cava syndrome
  in cancer, *1036*
  in Hodgkin's disease, *1017*
  in lung cancer, 329
Super K (ketamine), 658
Supernumerary teeth, 662
Support groups
  for illness information, 24
  for mental health disorders, 598–599
Support hose
  in deep vein thrombosis, 234, 235
  in stasis dermatitis, 1197
  in varicose veins, 237
Suppositories, for drug administration, 66
Suppressor T cells, *1052*, 1055
Supranuclear palsy, progressive, 550
Supraventricular tachycardia, paroxysmal, 170–171
  in Wolff-Parkinson-White syndrome, 171
Surfactant deficiency, 293, 294, 1499–1500
Surgery, 1698–1703, *1699*, *1700*, *1702*
  antibiotics before, 186, *187*
  anticoagulants before, 234
  atelectasis after, 293
  for cancer, 1042–1043, 1046
  clot prevention after, 288
  endocarditis and, 184
  in hemophilia patient, 1000
  Mohs', 1238, *1239*
  opioid analgesics after, 452
  second opinion for, 1700
Surrogate decision making, 56–57, 487
Surrogate mother, 1419
Swallowing, 694, 696, *707*
  of air (aerophagia), 701, 758, 1486, 1531
  difficulty in (dysphagia), 700, 706, 708–710
    in cerebral palsy, 1625
    in dying person, 49

Swallowing *(continued)*
  difficulty in *(continued)*
    in muscle stimulation dysfunction, 576
    in Parkinson's disease, 547
    in subacute sclerosing panencephalitis, 1582
  in scleroderma, 381
Swan-neck deformity, 396–397, *396*
Sweat glands, 1187, *1187*, *1211*
  inflammation of, 1224
Sweating, 927, 1652
  dehydration with, 928–929
  disorders of, 1210–1211, *1211*
  excessive, 1210–1211, 1652
    heat cramps with, 1653
    in heat exhaustion, 1653
  fluid replacement for, 1652–1653
  impairment of, 1652
    in heatstroke, 1653–1654
  during perimenopause, 1357
  in tuberculosis, 1127
Sweat test, 320
Swelling (edema), 120, 912
  of abdomen (*see* Ascites)
  after dental treatment, 691–692
  in allergic reactions, 1063
  ankle, 153, 912
  brain
    in head injury, 513, *515*
    at high altitudes, 1673
    in Reye's syndrome, *1572*
    seizures with, *496*
    in stroke, 508
  cornea, 1302
  in deep vein thrombosis, 233, 234–235
  eyelid, 1281, 1293–1294
  foot, 153, 912
  in heart failure, 153, 155, 158
  at high altitudes, 1672–1674
  in Hodgkin's disease, *1017*
  in kidney disorders, 824, 838, 840
  in kidney failure, 829
  lip, 664
  in lymphatic system obstruction, 240
  muscle (compartment syndrome), 349, 353
  in non-Hodgkin's lymphoma, *1021*
  optic nerve, 1315
  in pericarditis, 190
  during pregnancy, 1439, 1443
  prostate gland, 1335
  pulmonary (*see* Pulmonary edema)
  in pulmonary hypertension, 324
  salivary gland, 666–667
  testes, 1329
Swimmer's ear, 1109, 1110, 1253–1255
  prevention of, 1254
Swimmer's itch, 1143

Swimmer's shoulder, 429, *429*
Swimming, 35
  contact lens use during, 1288
  near drowning and, 1665–1666
Sydenham's disease (St. Vitus' dance), 552
  in rheumatic fever, 1566
Sympathectomy
  in long QT syndrome, 1530
  in Raynaud's disease and Raynaud's
    phenomenon, 225
Sympathetic ophthalmia, 1291
Synapse, 433, *437*
Syncope (*see* Fainting)
Syndrome of inappropriate secretion of
  antidiuretic hormone (SIADH), 912, *913*,
  929
Syndrome X, 202
Synovial fluid, 337, *338*
Synovial tissue, 337, *338*
Syphilis, 1176–1179, *1376*
  aortic valve regurgitation in, 180
  Argyll Robertson pupils in, 1281
  chancre in, 670
  endemic (bejel), 1099
  in newborn, *1509*
  penile growths in, 1325
  during pregnancy, 1447
  tongue cancer and, 672
  transfusion-acquired, *983*
  in traveler, 1714
Syringes, for travel, 1709–1710
Syringobulbia, 566
Syringomyelia, 566
Syrinx, 566
Systemic lupus erythematosus, 378–380, *379*,
  1074
  information resources on, 1765
  kidney disease in, 840
  in pregnancy, 1448
Systemic sclerosis (scleroderma), 380–382
Systolic hypertension, isolated, 118, 131

T

T$_3$ (triiodothyronine) (*see* Thyroid hormones)
T$_4$ (thyroxine) (*see* Thyroid hormones)
Tabes dorsalis, 1177
Tablet, 67
Tachyarrhythmias, 164
Tachycardia, 163
  supraventricular (atrial), paroxysmal,
    170–171
  ventricular, 172–173
Tachypnea (*see also* Breathing)
  in newborn, 1500
Tacrine, 489
Tacrolimus, *1078*

Taenia saginata (beef tapeworm) infection,
  1143–1144, *1143*
Taenia solium (pork tapeworm) infection,
  1143–1144
Tags (skin), 1234
Takayasu's arteritis, *387*
Talcum powder, 1190
Talipes equinovarus (clubfoot), 1524, *1524*
Tamoxifen, 1359
  in breast cancer, 1397–1398, 1400
  in breast pain, 1387
  in cancer, *1045*
  endometrial (uterine) cancer and, 1403
Tamponade, *189*
  in cancer, *1036*
Tampons, in toxic shock syndrome,
  1115–1116
Tamsulosin, 1330
Tangent screen, 1283
Tanning, *1231*
Tantrums, 1540, 1547
Tapeworms, 540, 1143–1144, *1143, 1146*
Tap water iontophoresis, 1211
Tarsal coalition, *1606*
Tarsal tunnel syndrome, 407
Tartar, 674
Tartrazine, 1068
Tarui's disease, *1617*
Taste, *595*, 662, 1246
  age-associated changes in, *18*, 663
  disorders of, 594–596
Tay-Sachs disease, *1430*, 1620
  information resources on, 1767
Tazarpteme, *1207*
TB (*see* Tuberculosis)
T-cell leukemia, 1014
Tears and tear system, 1277–1278, *1277*,
  1293
  age-associated changes in, 1278
  disorders of, 1292–1293, 1300–1301
  infection of, 1293
  inflammation of, 1318
  in Sjögren's syndrome, 382
Technetium scanning
  of fractures, 351
  in musculoskeletal disorders, 342
  in osteomyelitis, 365
Teething, 1531–1532
Telangiectasia, *1189*
  hereditary hemorrhagic (Rendu-Osler-
    Weber disease), 810, 996
Telangiectasia-ataxia, 1061
Telephone, for hearing aid user, 1252
Telephone calls, to physician, 22
Telomeres, 9
Temperature (body)
  in children, 1536–1537, *1536*
  high (*see* Fever)

Temperature *(continued)*
  low (hypothermia), 1655–1656
    coma with, *493*
  maintenance of, 1652, 1654
  measurement scales for, 1722
  in ovulation determination, 1348, 1416,
    1426
  of premature infant, 1497
  regulation of, 1090
  of testes, 1415
Temper tantrums, 1540, 1547
Temporal (giant cell) arteritis, *387*, 388, *389*
  headache with, *459*
Temporal artery, biopsy of, *389*
Temporal bone, fracture of, 1260
Temporal lobe, 434, *435*
  injury to, 476, 477
Temporomandibular joint, 685–686, *686*
  disorders of, 685–690, *689*
  internal derangement of, 686, 687,
    688–689
  in myofascial pain syndrome, 416, 686, 687,
    688
Tender points, in fibromyalgia, 416, *416*
Tendinitis, 418
  Achilles, 424–425
  popliteus, 424
  rotator cuff, 429, *429*
Tendons, 335
  abscess of, in hand, 402–403
  inflammation of (*see* Tendinitis)
Tendon sheath
  infection of, in hand, 403
  inflammation of (tenosynovitis), 406,
    418
Tenesmus, 824
Tennis elbow, 427–429, *427*, *428*
Tennis shoulder, 429, *429*
Tenofovir, *1175*
Tenosynovitis, 418
  peroneal, 406
TENS (transcutaneous electrical nerve
    stimulation), 37–38, 455, 574
  in temporomandibular joint disorders,
    689
Tension pneumothorax, 316–317, *316*
Tension-type headache, 457, *458*
Tensor tympani muscle, 1244
Teratogens, 1511
Terazosin, 1330
Terbinafine, 1226
Terbutaline, 1470
Terminal illness (*see also* Death and dying)
  advance directive for, 48, 51, *53*, 54–56
  suicide and, 51
  symptoms during, 48–50
Terpin hydrate, 250
Terrorism, biological, *1089*

Test(s), 1724–1731
  airway function, 254–255, *254*
  allergy, 1063–1064, 1068, 1188
  autonomic nervous system, 441
  balance, 462
  biliary tract, 788–791, *790*
  blood, 980–981, *1725–1727*, *1728*
    complete blood count, 980–981, *981*, *1725*
    on donated blood, 981, 983, 984
  of blood circulation, 441–442
  blood sugar, 964–965
  brain function, 442–446, *443*
  caloric, 464
  cancer, 1037–1041, *1038*, *1039*, *1040*
  coordination, 441
  cranial nerve, *590–591*
  decisions about, 1696–1697
  diagnostic, 1724–1725, *1728–1731*
  digestive tract, 703–706, *704*
  ear, 464, 1249–1250
  eye, 1282–1286
  eye pressure, 1307
  gallbladder, 788–791
  genetic (*see* Genetic testing)
  hearing, 1249–1250
  joints, 341–342
  liver, 788–791, *789*
  lung function, 254–255, *254*
  mental status, 439, *441*
  muscle function, 341
  nerve function, 342, 439–442, *441*, *442*
  in newborns, 1485
  occult blood, 705, 770
  pancreas, 735
  Pap, 1353, *1353*, 1406–1407, 1421, *1730*
  for pituitary hormones, 941, 943
  pregnancy, 1434–1435
  prenatal, 1430–1434, *1430*, *1431*, *1432*,
    1433, 1512, 1527, 1629
  preoperative, 1701
  pulmonary function, 254–255, *254*
  reflex, 440–441, *442*
  Romberg, 441
  screening (*see* Screening tests)
  secretin, *717*
  sensation, 440
  skin (allergy), 276
  stress, 123, 127, 204
  syphilis, *1178*
  thyroid function, 949, 955
  types of, 1724–1725
  urinary tract, 825–828, *827*, 861
Testis (testes), 938, *939*, 1322, *1322* (*see also*
    Scrotum)
  absence of (anorchia), *1512*, 1520
  cancer of, 1326
    screening for, *1038*
    staging of, *1040*

Testis *(continued)*
  hydrocele of, 1328–1329
  inflammation of (orchitis), 1328, 1577
  injury to, 1326
  in newborn, 1485
  radiation effects on, 1659, 1660
  regression of, *1512*
  removal of (orchiectomy), 1327, 1334
  retractile, 1536
  self-examination of, *1038*, 1041
  swelling of, 1329
  temperature effects on, 1415
  torsion of, 1327–1328, *1327*
  tumors of, 1326
  undescended (cryptorchidism), 1327,
    1535–1536, *1535*
  varicocele of, 1329
Testolactone, *1557*
Testosterone, *939, 940*
  coronary artery disease and, 200
  excess of, in virilization, 959–960
  in hair growth, 1212
  low levels of, in erectile dysfunction,
    1337
  marijuana effects on, 655
  postmenopausal use of, 1359, *1360,*
    1361
  at puberty, 1324
  replacement therapy with, *1322*
    in erectile dysfunction, 1338
    in Klinefelter syndrome, 1530
    in pseudohermaphroditism, 1520
Testotoxicosis, *1557*
Test tube (in vitro) fertilization, 1416,
  1419
Tetanus (lockjaw), 1114–1115
  immunization for, 1093, *1094,* 1115, *1115,*
    1493, 1562
Tetany (muscle spasm), 904
  in DiGeorge anomaly, 1061
Tetracycline, *1123*
  in acne, 1206, *1207*
  for canker sores, 668
  in children, 84
  dental effects of, 675
  food interactions with, 77
  during pregnancy, *1460*
Tetralogy of Fallot, 1515, 1517, *1517*
Tetraodon poisoning, 726
Thalamus, 434
  in tremor, 546
Thalassemias, *1430*
  pregnancy and, 1446
Thalidomide, 1458, 1523–1524
Theophylline
  in asthma, *278, 280,* 1584
  in COPD, 284
  drug interactions of, 76

Thiabendazole, 1220
Thiamin (vitamin B$_1$), *892,* 895–896
  deficiency of, *735,* 896
    in maple syrup urine disease, 1619
    in Wernicke's encephalopathy, 480
Thiazide diuretics (*see also* Diuretics)
  in diabetes insipidus, 851
  in high blood pressure, *138, 139*
  during pregnancy, 1459, *1460*
  in urinary tract stones, 866
Thiazolidinediones, 968–969, *968*
Thiersch procedure, 763
Thighbone (femur), fracture of, 355
Thigh muscles
  injury to, 426
  strengthening of, *425, 427*
Thioridazine, in elderly persons, *80*
Thiothixene, in elderly persons, *80*
Thirst, *928, 928*
  in diabetes insipidus, 851, 944
  in diabetes mellitus, 963
Thomsen's disease (myotonia congenita),
    413–414
Thoracentesis, 256, 314–315, *1731*
Thoracic aorta, aneurysm of, *227,*
    228–229
Thoracic outlet syndrome, 216, 582–583
Thoracoscopy, 258, *1700, 1731*
Thoracotomy, 258
Thought disorder, in schizophrenia, 641
Threadworm (strongyloides) infection,
    1146
Three-day measles (*see* Rubella)
Throat (pharynx), 244, *245,* 694, *695, 696*
  age-associated changes in, 1246–1247
  anatomy of, 1246, *1246*
  cancer of, 1273
  in diphtheria, 1563
  disorders of, 1267–1270
  lump in (globus sensation), 700
  pain in
    in glossopharyngeal neuralgia, 593–594
    in strep throat, 1113, 1595, 1596
  propulsion disorders of, 708
  retropharyngeal abscess of, 1563–1564
  sore (*see* Sore throat)
  strep, 1113, 1595, 1596
    nephritic syndrome after, 838–839
    rheumatic fever after, 1565–1566
Thrombin, 995
Thromboangiitis obliterans (Buerger's
    disease), 223–224
Thrombocytes (*see* Platelet[s])
Thrombocythemia, 979, *1023,* 1026–1027,
    1026
Thrombocytopenia, 979, 980, 997–999, *997*
  with cancer treatment, 1047
  in Wiskott-Aldrich syndrome, 1062

Thrombocytopenic purpura
  idiopathic, 997, 998
    pregnancy and, 1449
  thrombotic, 997, 998
Thrombolytic therapy, *996*
  in deep vein thrombosis, 234
  in heart disease, *207, 214*
  in kidney disease, 846
  in pulmonary embolism, 288
  in stroke, 509
Thrombophilia, 1000–1001
Thrombophlebitis, 232, 236
  after childbirth, 1479
  in pregnancy, 1450–1451
Thromboplastin time (PPT), 981
Thrombosis (*see* Blood clots)
  cavernous sinus, *1318*
  coronary (*see* Heart attack)
  deep vein (*see* Deep vein thrombosis)
Thrombotic thrombocytopenic purpura, 997,
  998
Throwing up (*see* Nausea; Vomiting)
Thrush, 666, 682, 1057, 1150, 1227
Thumb
  birth defects of, 1524
  dislocation of, *401*
  duck-bill deformity of, 396–397
  gamekeeper's, *401*
  sucking of, *1548*
  tendon inflammation of (De Quervain's
    syndrome), 419
Thymoma, 578, 579
Thymus gland, 1050, *1053*
  absence of (DiGeorge anomaly), 1061,
    1083
  in myasthenia gravis, 578
  transplantation of, 1059, 1083
  tumor of, 578, 579
Thyroidectomy, 952
Thyroid gland, *938, 939, 948–955, 948*
  absence of, 1510
  adenoma of, 950
  biopsy of, 955
  cancer of, 949, 954–955
    in multiple endocrine neoplasia, 973, 974
    radiation accident and, 906
  enlargement of (goiter), 906, 907, 949–951,
    952
    in fetus, 1448
    in newborn, 1510
  in euthyroid sick syndrome, *949*
  hormones of (*see* Thyroid hormones)
  inflammation of (thyroiditis), 950, 952,
    953–954, *1074*
  overactive (hyperthyroidism), 907, 949–952,
    951, 952 (*see also* Hyperthyroidism)
  in polyglandular deficiency syndromes, *943*
  during pregnancy, 1441
  removal of, 952

Thyroid gland (*continued*)
  scan of, 949, 955
  tumors of, 954–955
    in multiple endocrine neoplasia, 973, 974
  underactive (hypothyroidism), 942, 943,
    952–953 (*see also* Hypothyroidism)
Thyroid hormones, *939, 948–949* (*see also*
    Thyroid-stimulating hormone)
  deficiency of (hypothyroidism), 942,
    952–953 (*see also* Hypothyroidism)
  in euthyroid sick syndrome, *949*
  excess of (hyperthyroidism), 907, 949–952,
    951, 952 (*see also* Hyperthyroidism)
    sudden, extreme (thyroid storm), *952*
  formation of, 948
  generic substitutions for, *90*
  replacement of, 953
Thyroiditis, 950, 952, 953–954, *1074*
Thyroid-stimulating hormone, *939, 940, 941,*
    948–949
  deficiency of, 942, 943
  measurement of, 949, 950, 953, 955
  reference range for, *1727*
Thyroid storm, *952*
Thyrotropin-releasing hormone, 948
Thyroxine (T$_4$) (*see* Thyroid hormones)
Thyroxine-binding globulin, 949
TIA (transient ischemic attack), 503, 507
  vertigo with, 463
Tiagabine, *501*
Tibia
  fracture of, 354–355
  Osgood-Schlatter disease of, 1607
  torsion of, *1606*
Tibial nerve compression (tarsal tunnel
    syndrome), 407
Ticarcillin, *1123*
Tic douloureux (trigeminal neuralgia), 589,
    591
Tick fever, 1133–1134
Ticks
  babesiosis from, 1137
  bites by, 1685–1686, *1686*
  ehrlichioses from, 1134–1135
  Lyme disease from, 1105–1107
  paralysis and, *1686*
  protection against, *1107*, 1134
  relapsing fever from, *1103*
  removal of, *1107*
  rickettsial infections from, 1132–1134
  Rocky Mountain spotted fever from,
    1133–1134
  tularemia from, 1116–1117
Tick typhus, 1133–1134
Ticlopidine, 505
Tics, 551
Tilt table testing, 39, 124, 145
Tiludronate, 347–348
Time-out procedure, 1547

Timing method, of toilet teaching, *1540*
Timolol, *1308*
Tinea infections (ringworm), 1225–1226, *1226*
  in children, 1535
Tinea versicolor, 1227–1228
Tinnitus, 1261
  in Meniere's disease, 1259
TIPS (transjugular intrahepatic portal-
    systemic shunting), 794
Tissue matching, 1076
Tissue plasminogen activator (tPA), 509
Tissues, body, 2–3
  drug distribution to, 68, 70–72, *70*, *71–72*
  matching of, 1076
T lymphocytes, 978, 1050, *1052*, 1055 (*see
    also* White blood cells)
  antigen recognition by, *1051*
  in ataxia-telangiectasia, 1061
  in chronic mucocutaneous candidiasis,
      1060–1061
  in DiGeorge anomaly, 1061
  high levels of (leukocytosis), 1004–1005
  in HIV infection, 1169–1170
  killer, *1052*, 1055, 1089–1090
  leukemia of, 1014–1015
  low levels of (lymphocytopenia), 1004
  in severe combined immunodeficiency,
      1060–1062
  in Wiskott-Aldrich syndrome, 1062
TMJ (*see* Temporomandibular joint)
Toadstool poisoning, 725
Tobacco (*see* Smoking)
Tobramycin, *1122*
Todd's paralysis, 495
Toe(s)
  big (hallux)
    displacement of, 410–411, *411*
    fracture of, 354, *354*
    osteoarthritis of, 404
  blue discoloration (acrocyanosis) of, 225
  corns of, 410
  fracture of, 354, *354*
  gout in, 391–394, *392*, *393*
  hammer, 411, *411*
  Morton's neuroma of, 403–404
  pain in, 404
  Raynaud's disease and Raynaud's
      phenomenon of, 224–225
  severed or constricted, 1693
Toenails
  infection of (onychomycosis), 409–410
  inflammation of (onychia), 410
  ingrown, 409
  thickening of (onychauxis and
      onychogryphosis), 410
Toilet teaching, *1540*
Tolazamide, *968*
Tolbutamide, *968*
  during pregnancy, 1461

Tolcapone, *549*
Tolerance, to drug, 78
Tolterodine, 861
Tongue, 661–662, *662*
  atrophy of, 594
  cancer of, 672
  chemical burns of, 1678–1679
  color changes of, 664–665, 673
  disorders of, 664–666
  drug administration under, 66
  geographic, 665
  "hairy," 664
  inflammation of (glossitis), 665
  strawberry, 665, 1596
  taste receptors of, *595*
  temperature taking under, *1536*
  tumors of, 665
  white-strawberry, 1113
Tonic-clonic (grand mal) seizures, 497, *498*
Tonometry, 1284–1285, 1307
Tonsillectomy, 1597
Tonsillitis, 1595–1597
Tonsils, 1050–1051, *1053*, 1246, *1246*, *1597*
  cancer of, 1273
  enlargement of, 1596–1597
  infection of, 1267–1268, 1595
  tumors of, 1273
Tooth (teeth), 662–663, *662*, *675*
  abscess of, 680
  ache in (*see* Toothache)
  after dental treatment, 691–692
  age-associated changes in, 663
  brushing of, 677
  cavities in, 675–679, *676*, *678*, *679*
    fluoride deficiency and, 906
  clenching of, 674
  cosmetic treatments for, 677
  discoloration of, 675
  disorders of, 674–681
  emergency problems of, 690–692
  eruption of, 662, 1491, 1531–1532
  examination of, *29*, 677
  extraction of, 679, 680, 692
  fluorosis of, 906
  fracture of, 690
  grinding of, 674, 686
  impaction of, 680, 683
  infection of, 670, 675
  inflammation of (pulpitis), 679–680
  injury to, 690
  in jaw fracture, 691
  knocked-out, 690
  loosened, 690
  loss of
    in periodontitis, 683–685, *683*
    prevention of, *27*
  malocclusion of, 680–681
  misshapen, 675
  pain in (*see* Toothache)

Tooth *(continued)*
  in periodontal diseases, 681–685
  in periodontitis, *683*
  reimplantation of, 690
  root canal treatment in, *678, 679*
  sensitivity of, 676, 680, 685
  tetracycline effect on, 84, 675
  wisdom, 662, 680
Toothache, 674, 676, 690
  in pulpitis, 680
Tophi, 392, 394
Topical drugs, 66, 1188–1191
Topiramate, *501*
Topoisomerase inhibitors, *1045*
Torsion
  femoral, *1606*
  testicular, 1327–1328, *1327*
  tibial, *1606*
Torsion dystonia, 554
Torticollis, 555–556, *1512*
Torus, 671
Total parenteral nutrition, 890
Touch
  sense of, testing of, 440
  therapeutic, 1707
Tourette's syndrome, 551–552
Toxemia of pregnancy (preeclampsia), 1452,
    1459, 1473
Toxic alopecia, 1213
Toxic amblyopia, 1316
Toxic colitis, 742, 744
Toxic diffuse goiter (Graves' disease),
    949–951, 952
  in pregnancy, 1448–1449
Toxic enterocolitis, 1522
Toxic epidermal necrolysis, 1112, 1199–1200
Toxicity, drug, 85–86
Toxic megacolon, 742, 744
Toxic multinodular goiter (Plummer's
    disease), 950
Toxic shock syndrome, 1115–1116
  after childbirth, 1478
Toxins
  bacterial, 1087
  in cholera, 1100
  Clostridium difficile, 746
  in diphtheria, 1563
  foodborne
    in botulism, 579–581
    chemical, 722, 725–726
    in cholera, 1100
    in gastroenteritis, 721
  in frostbite, 1656
  liver processing of, 786
  in optic neuropathy, 1316
  radiopaque dye, *827*
  in scarlet fever, 1113
  secretory diarrhea and, 754
  in tetanus, 1114–1115
  in toxic shock syndrome, 1115–1116

Toxocariasis, 1144
Toxoplasmosis, 1144–1145
  with HIV infection, *1172*
  in newborn, *1508–1509*
  during pregnancy, 1450
tPA (tissue plasminogen activator), 509
Trabeculectomy, 1309
Trace minerals, 882, 900
Trachea (windpipe), 244, *245*, 1246,
    1246
  burns of, *1649*
  fistula of, 1520–1521, *1521*
Tracheoesophageal puncture, *1272*
Tracheostomy
  in epiglottitis, 1564
  in vocal cord paralysis, 1270
Trachoma, 1297–1298
Traction, 38, 352
Traction diverticulum, 710
Trade names, of drugs, 60, 88–89, *89*,
    1733–1743
  generic names for, *1744–1755*
Train sickness (*see* Motion sickness)
Transaminases, *1727*
Transcutaneous electrical nerve stimulation
    (TENS), 37–38, 455, 574
  in temporomandibular joint disorders,
    689
Transdermal route (drug administration),
    66–67
Transesophageal echocardiography, 186
Transesophageal ultrasonography, 126
Transferrin, 907, 990
Transfer training, 39
Transfusion, blood (*see* Blood transfusion)
Transient depression, 615
Transient flora, 1086
Transient global amnesia, 479
Transient hypogammaglobulinemia of
    infancy, 1060
Transient ischemic attack (TIA), 503, 507
  vertigo with, 463
Transient tachypnea, 1500
Transillumination, 1502
Transitional cell carcinoma, of renal pelvis,
    876–877
Transjugular intrahepatic portal-systemic
    shunting (TIPS), 794
Transplantation, 1075–1083
  adrenal gland, 1083
  in amyloidosis, 1716
  body part, *1083*
  bone, 1083
  bone marrow, 1081–1083
    in myelofibrosis, 1026
    in osteopetroses, 1611
    radiation therapy before, 1077
    in sickle cell disease, 994
  cartilage, 1083
  cornea, *1082*, 1083

Transplantation *(continued)*
  donors for, 48, 1075–1076
  fetal tissue, 550, 1083
  gene therapy in, 16
  hair, 1213
  heart, 157–158, 1079–1080
    in congenital heart defects, 1514
  heart-lung, 1080
  immune system suppression in,
      1076–1077, *1078–1079*
  immunosuppressive drugs for,
      1076–1077
  information resources on, 1767
  islet cell, 1080–1081
  kidney, 1077
    pregnancy and, 1447
  liver, 1077–1079 *(see also* Liver,
      transplantation of)
  lung, 292, 321, 324, 1080
  pancreas, 969, 1080–1081
  rejection of, 1076–1077, *1078–1079*
  skin, 1083
  small intestine, 1083
  stem cell, 1081–1083 *(see also* Stem cells,
      transplantation of)
  thymus, 1083
    in immunodeficiency disorders, 1059
  tissue matching and, 1076
Transposition of great arteries, 1517
Transsexualism, 628–629
Transurethral resection of prostate (TURP),
    1330
Transvenous liver biopsy, 791
Transverse myelitis, 567
Transvestic fetishism, 629
Trastuzumab, *1045*, 1046
  in breast cancer, 1400
  in metastatic breast cancer, 1398
Trauma *(see* Injury [injuries])
Travel, 1708–1714
  air *(see* Air travel)
  immunization for, 1095, 1708, *1709*
  information resources on, 1768
Traveler's diarrhea, 725, 1713–1714
Travel insurance, 1708
Travoprost, *1308*
Treacher Collins syndrome, 1523
Tremor, 544–546
  in alcohol abuse, 650
  in orthostatic hypotension, 550–551
  in Parkinson's disease, 547
Trench foot, 1656
Trench mouth, 685, 1150
Treponema infection, 1099, 1176–1179 *(see
    also* Syphilis)
Tretinoin
  in acne, 1206, *1207*
  in cancer, *1045*
Triamcinolone hexacetonide, *393*
Trichinosis, 1145, 1147

Trichomoniasis, 1182, 1350, *1376*, 1377
  in traveler, 1714
  urinary tract, 867–868
Trichophyton infection (ringworm),
    1225–1226
Trichotillomania, 1213
Trichuriasis, 1147–1148
Tricuspid valve, 114, *115*
  regurgitation at, 182–183
  stenosis of, 183
Tricyclic antidepressants, 617, *618*
  in children, 1633
Trifluridine, *1156*
Trigeminal nerve, testing of, *590*
Trigeminal neuralgia, 589, 591, *593*
Trigger finger, 398
Triglycerides, 920, *1726*
  desirable blood levels of, *922*
  high blood levels of, 920, 921–926, *922,
      924, 925*
Trihexyphenidyl, *549*, 550
Triiodothyronine (T$_3$) *(see* Thyroid
    hormones)
Trimethadione, during pregnancy, *1460*
Trimethobenzamide, in elderly persons,
    80
Trimethoprim-sulfamethoxazole, *1123*
  folic acid deficiency with, 899
  in *Pneumocystis carinii* pneumonia,
      1575
Tripelennamine, in elderly persons, *80*
Triplets, 1473
Triple X syndrome, 11, 1529–1530
Triprolidine, *1065*
Triptans (5-hydroxytryptamine [5-HT]),
    460–461, *460*
Trisodium citrate, 394
Trisomy 21 *(see* Down syndrome)
Trochlear nerve, 589, *590*
Troleandomycin, *1123*
Tropheryma whippelii infection (Whipple's
    disease), 737
Tropical eosinophilia, 310
Tropical spastic paraparesis, 539, 560
Tropical sprue, 737
Troponin, *1727*
Trots *(see* Diarrhea)
Trousseau's syndrome, 236
Trovafloxacin, *1123*
Truancy, 1558
Trust, revocable (living), 57
Trypanosoma brucei infection (sleeping
    sickness), 1147
Trypanosoma cruzi infection (Chagas'
    disease), *1146*
Trypsin, 697
  in cystic fibrosis, 320
Tryptophan deficiency, of Hartnup disease,
    853
Tubal ligation, 1427, *1428*

Tube (*see also* Catheter[ization])
　chest, 315, 317
　endotracheal, 1268, 1564
　feeding, 889–890
　　for cancer patient, 1047
　　for dying person, 49
　nasoenteric, 706
　nasogastric, 705–706
　ventilating (tympanostomy), *1595*
Tuberculin skin test, 1128, *1128*
Tuberculosis, 1125–1130
　diseases resembling, *1126*
　extrapulmonary, *1127*, 1128
　in HIV infection, 1127, *1172*
　immunization for, *1094*
　miliary, *1129*
　pericarditis in, 188, 190, 1128, 1129
　prevention of, 1129–1130
　in silicosis, 295
　testing for, *1128*
　treatment of, 1129
Tubes, fallopian (*see* Fallopian tubes)
Tubules, kidney, 820, *821*
　disorders of, 849–854, *850*
Tubulointerstitial nephritis, 837–838,
　843–844
Tularemia, 1116–1117, *1116*
Tumor(s) (*see also* Cancer)
　adrenal gland, 958, 959
　　in hyperaldosteronism, 960
　　in multiple endocrine neoplasia, 973
　　pheochromocytoma, 960–961
　antibodies to, 1034
　antigens of, 1034
　anus, 773
　auditory nerve, 1260–1261
　bile duct, 800, 801, 811–812, 817
　bladder, 877–878
　bone, 359–361
　brain, 519–526, *520–521, 522, 525,* 528
　　coma with, *492*
　　headache with, *458, 521*
　breast, 1387, 1388, 1389, 1391 (*see also*
　　Breasts, cancer of)
　carcinoid, 974–975
　childhood, 1622–1624
　chronic meningitis with, 532
　definition of, 1031
　digestive system, 764–776, 778
　　carcinoid, 974–975
　ear, 1255
　embolism of, 286
　esophagus, 764–766, *765*
　eye, 1314
　eyelid, 1295
　gastrin production and, *717*
　heart, 191–194, *193*
　high calcium levels and, 904
　information resources on, 1759–1760

Tumor(s) *(continued)*
　jaw, 672–673
　kidney, 875–876
　　in children, 1622–1623
　large intestine, 768–769
　　ulcerative colitis and, 742–743
　larynx, 1271–1272, *1272*
　lip, 673
　liver, 798, 810–813
　lung, 328–331, *329* (*see also* Lungs, cancer
　　of)
　markers of, 1034, *1039,* 1041
　metastatic (*see* Metastasis)
　mouth, 670–674
　in multiple endocrine neoplasia, 972–974
　　(*see also* Multiple endocrine neoplasia)
　nasopharynx, 1273
　nervous system, 519–528, *520–521, 522,*
　　525, 527
　　in children, 1623
　nose, 1273
　oral color changes with, *663*
　orbit, 1319
　pancreas, 773–774, *774*
　　hypoglycemia with, 971, 972
　　in multiple endocrine neoplasia, 972–973
　parathyroid gland, 972
　peritoneum, 296–297, 298
　pineal gland, *521, 522*
　pituitary gland, *521, 522,* 523, 941,
　　943–944, 1279 (*see also* Pituitary gland,
　　tumors of)
　plasma cell, 1007–1009, *1009*
　pleura, 296–297, 298, 315–316
　plexus disorders with, 581–582
　renal pelvis, 876–877
　retina, 1314, 1623–1624
　salivary gland, 667, 671, 672–673
　sinus, 1272
　skin, 1230, *1231,* 1238–1241, *1239, 1240,*
　　1325
　small intestine, 768, *769*
　spinal cord, 526, *527*
　stomach, 766–768, *767*
　　ulcers and, 714
　testis, 1326
　thymus gland, 578, 579
　thyroid gland, 949, 954–955
　　in multiple endocrine neoplasia, 973,
　　　974
　　radiation accident and, 906
　tongue, 665, 672
　tonsils, 1273
　ureter, 876–877
　urethra, 878
　urinary tract, 875–878
　uterus, 1372–1374
　viral infection and, *1155*
　vocal cord, *1269*

Tumor ablation procedure, in breast cancer, 1398
Tumor suppressor genes, 14
Tuning fork test, 1249–1250
Turista (traveler's diarrhea), 725
Turner syndrome, 11, 1528–1529, 1556
TURP (transurethral resection of prostate), 1330
Twins, 1435, 1473
Tympanic cavity, *1245*
Tympanic membrane, 1244 (*see also* Eardrum)
Tympanocentesis, 1595
Tympanometry, 1249, 1598, *1731*
Tympanostomy, 1250, *1595*
Typhoid fever, 1117–1118
    immunization for, *1094, 1709*
Typhus
    epidemic, *1133*
    murine, *1133*
    scrub, *1133*
    tick, 1133–1134
Tyrosinemia, 1619

U

Ulcer(s)
    cornea, 1288, 1300, 1302
    decubitus (*see* Pressure sores)
    duodenal, 698, 712, 713–717 (*see also* Peptic ulcers)
    esophageal, 717
    eye
        contact lenses and, 1288
        Pseudomonas and, 1109, 1110
    foot, 222, *222*
    gastric, 698, 712, 713–717 (*see also* Peptic ulcers)
    genital, in syphilis, 1176–1177
    leg, 217, 235–236
    mouth, 668, 669–670
        during cancer treatment, 1047
    nasal, 1262–1263
    peptic, 698, *712*, 713–717 (*see also* Peptic ulcers)
    skin, *1189* (*see also* Pressure sores; Skin, ulcers of)
    stomach, 698, 712, 713–717 (*see also* Peptic ulcers)
    vocal cord, 1269–1270, *1269*
    in Zollinger-Ellison syndrome, *717*
Ulcerative colitis, 742–744
Ulcerative proctitis, 742, 743, 744
Ulnar nerve
    compression of (cubital tunnel syndrome), 399–400
    palsy of, 583

Ultrasonography, *1731*
    of abdomen, 227, 704–705
    of arteries, 218–219
    of bile ducts, 788–789
    of breast, 1393
    in cancer staging, 1041
    Doppler (*see* Doppler ultrasonography)
    of eye, 1285–1286
    of fallopian tubes, 1418
    of fetus, 1435
    of gallbladder, 788–789, 814
    of heart (*see* Echocardiography)
    in hydatidiform mole, 1410
    in kidney and urinary tract disorders, 826–827
    of liver, 788–789
    in lung disorders, 255
    in miscarriage, 1457
    in placental problems, 1455
    during pregnancy, 1432, *1433*, 1442–1443
    of thyroid gland, 949
    in urinary tract infection, 1568
    of uterus, 1354
Ultraviolet light, 1230 (*see also* Sunlight)
    psoralens with, *1202*
        in granuloma annulare, 1201
        in lichen planus, 1204
        in psoriasis, 1202
        in psoriatic arthritis, 376
        in vitiligo, 1215
Umbilical cord, *1437*
    around fetus's neck, 1473
    blood sampling from, 1434
    cutting and clamping of, 1483, *1484*
    prolapse of, 1473
    stump of, 1485
Umbrella filter, 234, *235*, 289
Unconsciousness (*see also* Coma)
    in dying person, 50
Undereating, by young child, 1544–1545
Underfeeding, 1532–1533
Undernutrition, 887–890, *888, 889* (*see also* Nutrition)
    in immunodeficiency disorders, 1057
Underwater (hydrostatic) weighing, *881*
Units of measure, 1721–1725
Unna's boot, 1197
Unoprostone, *1308*
Unstable angina, 203, 205
Urate crystal deposition, 391–394, *392, 393*
Ureaplasma urealyticum infection, 1180, *1181*
Ureter, *821, 822*
    birth defects of, 1519
    cancer of, 876–877
    infection of (ureteritis), 871
    injury to, 874
    stents for, 864
    stones in, 823, 864–866, *865*

Urethra, *821, 822,* 1088
  age-associated changes in, 823
  atrophy of, *20*
  birth defects of, 1519
  blockage of, 824
  cancer of, 878
  female, 1343, *1344, 1345*
    prolapse of, 1380
  infection of (*see* Urethritis)
  injury to, 874–875
  male, *1321, 1322,* 1323
    birth defects of, 1519
    stricture of, 1325
  in newborn, 1485
Urethritis, 868
  atrophic, *20*
  gonococcal, 1179–1180
  nongonococcal, 1180–1181, *1181*
  in Reiter's syndrome, 376
  in trichomoniasis, 1182
Urethrography, retrograde, 870
Urethrotomy, 1325
Urge incontinence, 858, 861, 869, 1357
Uric acid
  in glycogen storage disease, 1616
  in gout, 391–394, *392, 393*
  in kidney stones, 864–866
  reference range for, *1727*
Urinalysis (*see* Urine, testing of)
Urinary incontinence (*see* Incontinence,
    urinary)
Urinary tract, 6 (*see also* Bladder; Kidneys;
    Ureter; Urethra)
  age-associated changes in, 822–823, 857
  biology of, 820–823, *821*
  birth defects of, 1518–1519, 1567
  blockage of, 824, 862–866
    in benign prostatic hyperplasia, 1329,
      1330
    in urethral stricture, 1325
  cancer of, 875–878
  disorders of, 823–878
    symptoms of, 823–825
    tests for, 825–828, *827*
  infection of, 866–872, *867*
    after childbirth, 1479
    in children, 1567–1568
    during pregnancy, 1451
    prevention of, 1568
    stones and, 865
  injury to, 872–875, *873*
  stones in, 823, 851–852, 864–866, *865*
Urination, 927 (*see also* Urine)
  after childbirth, 1476
  after menopause, 1357
  in benign prostatic hyperplasia, 1329, 1330
  by children, problems with, 1545
  control of, 857
  in diabetes insipidus, 851, 944
  in diabetes mellitus, 963

Urination (*continued*)
  fainting with (micturition syncope), 144
  frequency of, 824
  hesitating with, 824
  incontinence of (*see* Incontinence,
      urinary)
  by infant, 1489
  in kidney failure, 829
  mechanisms of, 822, 857
  by newborn, 1486
  at night, 824, 831
  pain during, 868, 869
  during pregnancy, 1439–1440
  in prostatitis, 1335
  straining during, 824
  toilet teaching for, *1540*
  in urethral stricture, 1325
  urgency of, 824, 858, 869, 1357
Urine (*see also* Urination)
  acidity of, 826
  air in, 869
  backup of (hydronephrosis), 829, 862–864,
    863
  blood in (hematuria), 825, 826, 875–876,
    877
  calcium in, 866
  cloudy, 825
  color of, 825
  concentration of, 826
  culture of, 826, 1568
  cystine in, 851–852
  cytology of, 828
  in diabetes insipidus, 944–945
  diversion of, 878
  in Fanconi's syndrome, 852
  formation of, 820–822
  gas in, 825
  glucose in (*see* Urine, sugar in)
  incontinence of (*see* Incontinence, urinary)
  of infant, 1489
  ketones in, 826
  in kidney failure, 829, 832
  lymph in, 867–868
  of newborn, 1486
  nitrates in, 826
  odor of, 825
  output of, 824
  oxalate in, 866
  protein in (proteinuria)
    hematuria with, 843
    in nephrotic syndrome, 839–840
    during pregnancy, 1442
  residual, 857, 860–861
  retention of, in benign prostatic
      hyperplasia, 1329, 1330
  sample collection of, 826, *826*
    from children, 1567–1568
  sediment in, 826
  sugar in, 825, 850–851, 963, 969
    during pregnancy, 1442

Urine *(continued)*
   testing of, 825–826, *826, 1731*
      in high blood pressure, 136
      in kidney disease, 841, 843
      for marijuana use, 655–656
      during pregnancy, 1442
   uncontrolled loss of (*see* Incontinence,
      urinary)
Urodynamic testing, 861
Urography
   intravenous, 827, 863, 865, *1729*
   retrograde, 827–828, 865, *1730*
Urolithiasis, 392, 394, 864–866
Ursodeoxycholic acid, 815
Urticaria, 1071–1072
   during pregnancy, *1441*
   solar, 1232
Urticaria pigmentosa, 1069
Usher's syndrome, 1312
Uterine artery, embolization of, 1374
Uterus, 1344, 1345, *1345*
   adenomyosis of, *1365*
   blastocyst implantation in, 1435–1436,
      1436
   bleeding from, 1367
      after labor and delivery, 1474
   cancer of, 1350, 1358, 1403–1404, *1404*
      screening for, *1038*
      staging of, *1040, 1402*
   contractions of
      after childbirth, 1474, 1477
      in labor (*see* Labor and delivery)
   fibroids of, 1372–1374
      in pregnancy, 1449
   hysterosalpinography of, 1355
   hysteroscopy of, 1354, 1418
   infection of, after childbirth, 1478
   inverted, 1474
   laparoscopy of, 1355
   palpation of, 1353
   perforation of, 1425, 1427
   prolapse of, 1348, 1379–1381
   removal of, 1356, *1404* (*see also*
      Hysterectomy)
   size of, during pregnancy, 1439
   tumors of, 1372–1374
   ultrasonography of, 1354
Uvea, 1305, *1306*
Uveitis, 1305–1306
   pain in, 1281
   in sarcoidosis, 305
Uvula, *662, 663,* 1246

V

Vaccination (*see* Immunization)
Vaccine Injury Compensation Program,
   1493–1494
Vacuum devices, in erectile dysfunction, 1339

Vacuum extractor, for delivery, 1475, *1475*
Vagina, 1344, *1344, 1345*
   adenosis of, 1366
   atrophy of, *20,* 1348, 1357, 1382
   biopsy of, 1354
   bleeding from, 1366–1367, 1403, 1408–1409
      abnormal, 1350
      in children, 1366
   cancer of, 1350, *1402,* 1408–1409
   candidiasis of, 1150–1151, 1227, 1350,
      1374, *1376,* 1377
   dilation of, 1383
   discharge from, 1349–1350, 1375
      after childbirth, 1476
      during pregnancy, 1439
   drug administration in, 66
   examination of, 1352–1353
   foreign object in, 1350
   inflammation/infection of (*see* Vaginitis)
   itching around, 1198, 1349
   pH of, 1374
   prolapse of, 1348, 1380, *1381*
   rectal prolapse into, 763
   spasms of (vaginismus), 1383–1384
   trichomoniasis of, 1182, 1350, *1376,* 1377
   yeast infection of, 1150–1151, 1227, 1350,
      1374, *1376,* 1377
Vaginal ring, 1421–1422
Vaginismus, 1383–1384
Vaginitis, 1374–1377, *1376*
   atrophic, *20*
   in children, 1375
   culture for, 1353
   discharge in, 1349–1350
   in trichomoniasis, 1182
Vaginosis, 1350, 1374, *1376,* 1377
   during pregnancy, 1450
Vagus nerve
   stimulation of
      fainting with, 144, 145
      in paroxysmal supraventricular
         tachycardia, 171
      in seizure disorders, 502
   testing of, *591*
Valacyclovir, *1156,* 1162
Valerian, *106,* 112, 607
Valganciclovir, *1156*
Valley fever, 1151
Valproate
   during pregnancy, *1460*
   in seizure disorders, *501*
Valves
   heart (*see* Heart, valves of)
   urethral, 1519
   in veins, 231, *232*
Valvuloplasty, 128
   in aortic stenosis, 182
   in heart defects, 1514
   in mitral stenosis, 180
Valvulotomy, 1518

Vancomycin, *1124*
Vanishing testes, *1512*
Vaporizer, 249, 1580
  in croup, 1586
Variant angina, 203
Variant Creutzfeldt-Jakob disease, 542,
  542
Varicella-zoster virus infection, 1162–1163,
  1163
  in children, *1569*, 1571–1572
  corneal, 1302
  immunization for, *1094*, 1095, *1493*
  in HIV-infected children, 1575
Varices (*see* Varicose veins)
Varicocele, 1329
Varicose veins, 236–238, *237*
  esophageal, 707, 776, 778, 794
    in Budd-Chiari syndrome, 808, 809
    in cirrhosis, 798
    in portal vein thrombosis, 809
    during pregnancy, 1448
    in veno-occlusive disease, 808
  pelvic, *1366*
  during pregnancy, 1439
  scrotal, 1329
Variola (smallpox), *1166*
  immunization for, *1094*, 1095
Vascular dementia, 489–490
Vasculitis, 371, 386–391, *387*, *389*
Vas deferens, *1322*
Vasectomy, 1427
Vasodilators
  in heart failure, *156*, 157
  in high blood pressure, 139, *139*
  orthostatic hypotension with, 146
  in pulmonary hypertension, 324
Vasomotor rhinitis, 1265
Vasopressin (*see* Antidiuretic hormone)
Vasovagal (vasomotor) syncope, 144, 145
Vastus medialis muscles, strengthening of,
  425
VDLR (*see* Venereal Disease Research
  Laboratory [VDLR] test)
Vegetarian diet, 898
Vegetative state, 494
Vein(s), 117
  blockage of (*see* Deep vein thrombosis)
  in blood pressure control, 141
  disorders of, 231–239, *235*, *237*
  filters in, 234, *235*, 289
  in heart disease, 121
  inflammation of, 223
  liver (hepatic), 786, 787, 806, *807*
    in Budd-Chiari syndrome, 808–809
    in heart failure, 810
    occlusive disease of, 807–808
  renal, *820*, *821*, *845*
    metastasis of, 876
    thrombosis of, 848–849

Vein(s) (*continued*)
  spider, 236–237, 238
    in ataxia-telangiectasia, 1061
    radiation therapy and, 1660
  stripping of, 237–238
  valves in, 231, *232*
  varicose, 236–238, *237* (*see* Varicose veins)
Vena cava
  lung cancer spread to, 329
  metastasis of, 876
Venereal disease, 1176–1184, *1177* (*see also*
  HIV infection)
  prevention of, 1176, *1178*
Venereal Disease Research Laboratory (VDRL)
  test, 1178
Venography, *1731*
Venomous snake bites, 1682–1683
Veno-occlusive disease, of liver, 807–808
Ventilating (tympanostomy) tubes, *1595*
Ventilation, mechanical, 285, 326, 327 (*see*
  also Breath; Breathing)
  in apnea of prematurity, 1504
  in bronchiolitis, 1585
  bronchopulmonary dysplasia with,
    1502–1503
  in meconium aspiration syndrome, 1501
  in persistent pulmonary hypertension,
    1502
  in poisoning, 1676
Ventilation scan, 255–256, 287
  in pregnancy, 1451
Ventricles, 114, 115–116, *115*
  aneurysm of, *212*
  in tetralogy of Fallot, 1515, *1517*
  thickening of, 153, 161–162
Ventricular fibrillation, 173–174
Ventricular premature beats, 172
Ventricular septal defect, 1514–1515, *1516*
  in tetralogy of Fallot, 1515, *1517*
Ventricular tachycardia, 172–173
Ventriculography, 129
Venules, 117
Verbal apraxia, 478
  rehabilitation for, 44–45
Vernal conjunctivitis, 1298
Vernix caseosa, 1484
Verrucae (*see* Warts)
Vertebrae, 435–437, *436*, 569 (*see also* Spine)
  degenerative disease of, 368, 569
  fracture of, 344–345, 346, 357–358, 571–572
  infection of, 364, 365
  inflammation of (ankylosing spondylitis),
    377, 569
  osteoporosis and, 344–345, 569
  in Paget's disease, 347
Vertebrobasilar insufficiency, 463
Vertebroplasty, 346
Vertex presentation, for delivery, 1465, *1472*,
  1485

Vertigo, 462–464
  after diving, 1667
  benign positional, 465–467, *466*
  in decompression sickness, 1670
  in Meniere's disease, 1259–1260
  in vestibular neuronitis, 1260
Vesicles, *1189*
Vesicoenteric fistula, 869
Vesicoureteral reflux, 1567
Vestibular nerve
  surgery on, 1260
  tumors of, 1260–1261
Vestibular neuronitis, 1260
Vestibular schwannoma, 1260–1261
Vestibular system, 1244, *1245*
Vestibulitis, nasal, 1263–1264
Vibrio infection, *720*, 721, 1100–1101
  immunization for, *1094*
Vicious circle, in behavioral problems, *1544*
Vidarabine, *1156*
Vigabatrin, *501*
Vincent's infection, 685
Vincristine, *1045*
Vinorelbine, *1045*
Violence
  among adolescents, 1558
  against self (suicide), 616, 622–624, *622*,
    623
  toward children, 1643–1646
  against women, 1410–1414, *1411*
Violin spider bite, 1684–1685
Vipoma, 754
Viral infection, *1087*, 1154–1167, *1156 (see
    also specific viral infections)*
  AIDS *(see* HIV infection)
  arbovirus, 537–538
  arenavirus, 538
  brain, 532–538, 1585–1586
  bronchial, 262–264, *263*, 1579–1580,
    1585–1586
  cancer and, 1034, *1155*
  central nervous system, 532–539,
    1569–1570
  common cold *(see* Cold, common)
  conjunctivitis, 1296–1297, *1297*
  encephalitis, 532–538, *536*
  eye, 1296–1297, *1297*
  gastritis, 711
  gastroenteritis, *721*, 722, 1586–1588
  gums, 682
  heart, 159–160
  hepatitis, 802–806, *804–805*
  herpes *(see* Herpes simplex virus infection)
  HIV *(see* HIV infection)
  in infants and children, 1568–1582, *1569*,
    1572, 1576, 1581
  inner ear (labyrinthitis), 463
  JC virus, 538–539
  keratitis, 1301–1302

Viral infection *(continued)*
  laryngitis, 1268–1269
  lung, 262–264, *263*, 267, 269, *269*,
    1579–1580, 1585–1586
  meningitis, 532–535
  myocardial, 159–160
  nephrotic syndrome with, 840
  in newborn, *1508–1509*
  pneumonia, 267, 269, *269*
  during pregnancy, 1450
  rabies, 535–537, *536*
  rectal, 762
  sexually transmitted, 1168–1175, 1183 *(see
    Sexually transmitted diseases)*
  skin, 1228–1229
  stomach, 711, *721*, 722, 1586–1588
  subacute painful thyroiditis, 954
  urinary tract, 867
Viral load, in HIV infection, 1170, 1172
Virchow's triad, 233
Virilization, 959–960
  in congenital adrenal hyperplasia, 1520
  in polycystic ovary syndrome, 1368
Virulence, of infection, 1087
Viscera *(see* Digestive system *and specific
    organs)*
Visceral larva migrans, 1144
Vision *(see also* Blindness; Eye[s])
  acuity of, 1283, 1286
  age-associated changes in, 17, *18*, 1278
  astigmatic, 1279, *1282*
  in benign intracranial hypertension, *523*
  distortion of, 1280–1281
  double (diplopia), 1279
    in Graves' disease, 950, 952
  in Leber's hereditary optic neuropathy, 560
  loss of, 1279, *1280*
    in acromegaly, 945
    in cataract, 1303–1305, *1304*
    in children, 1600–1601
    in diabetes mellitus, *963*, 964, 1313
    in endophthalmitis, 1313
    in glaucoma, 1307
    information resources on, 1758–1759
    in macular degeneration, 1310–1311
    in optic nerve disorders, 1315, 1316,
      1317
    in papilledema, 1315
    in pituitary gland enlargement, 941–942,
      946
    in prolactinoma, 946
    in retinal artery blockage, 1312
    in retinal detachment, 1311
    in retinal vein blockage, 1312
    in retinitis pigmentosa, 1312
    trachoma and, 1297–1298
    in vitamin A deficiency, 891
  in multiple sclerosis, 558
  refractive disorders and, 1279, 1282–1283

Visual field testing, 1283, 1307–1308
Vitamin(s), 882–883, 890–900, *892–893*
  deficiency of *(see specific vitamins)*
  supplements of *(see specific vitamins)*
Vitamin A (retinol), 891, *892*
  acute promyelocytic leukemia and,
    1014
  deficiency of, *735,* 891
    corneal disorders with, 1300, 1301
  excess of, 891
  leukemia and, 1013
  reference range for, *1727*
Vitamin B$_1$ (thiamin), *892,* 895–896
  deficiency of, *735,* 896
  in maple syrup urine disease, 1619
  in Wernicke's encephalopathy, 480
Vitamin B$_2$ (riboflavin), *892,* 896
  deficiency of, *735,* 896
Vitamin B$_3$ (niacin), deficiency of, *735*
  gingivitis with, 682
  red tongue with, 665
Vitamin B$_6$ (pyridoxine), *893,* 897–898, *899*
  deficiency of, 897
  excess of, 897–898
  in homocystinuria, 1619
Vitamin B$_{12}$ (cobalamin), *893,* 898–899,
    899
  deficiency of, *735,* 898–899
    anemia with, 990–991
    in celiac disease, 736
    in gastritis, 712
    spinal cord degeneration with, 568
  in homocystinuria, 1619
  supplementation with, 990
Vitamin C (ascorbic acid), *893,* 900
  in common cold, 1157
  deficiency of, *735,* 900
    gingivitis with, 682
  drug interactions of, 76
  reference range for, *1725*
Vitamin D, *892,* 894
  deficiency of, *735,* 894
  excess of, 894
  kidney metabolism of, 822
  for newborn, 1486
  in osteoporosis, 346
  in osteoporosis prevention, 345
  overdose of, 904
  in Paget's disease of bone, 348
Vitamin E, *892,* 895
  deficiency of, 895
  excess of, 895
Vitamin K, *892,* 895
  deficiency of, *735,* 895
  for newborn, 1484
Vitiligo, 1215
Vitrectomy, 1313
Vitreous humor, 1277
VLDL cholesterol, 920, *921*

Vocal cords, 1246
  cancer of, *1269*
  contact ulcers of, 1269–1270, *1269*
  examination of, *1269*
  in Hodgkin's disease, *1017*
  nodules of, 1269, *1269*
  paralysis of, *1269,* 1270
  polyps of, 1269, *1269*
  spasm of, 554
  speech without, *1272*
Vocal tics, in Tourette's syndrome, 552
Voice (*see also* Larynx)
  changes in, 1268, 1269, 1270
  vocal cord problems and, 1269–1270, *1269*
Voice box (*see* Larynx)
Voiding (*see* Urination)
Voiding cystourethrography, 870, 1568
Volume, metric equivalents for, 1722
Volvulus, 780, *780*
  in children, 1521–1522
Vomiting, 702
  blood with, 699, 702, 705
  in bulimia, 626
  in cancer patient, 1047
  dehydration with, 928–929
  in dying person, 49
  in gastritis, 712
  in gastroenteritis, 1587
  in infants, 1532
  in kidney disorders, 823–824
  during labor and delivery, 1467
  during pregnancy, 1440, 1451–1452
  in radiation illness, 1659
Von Gierke's disease, *1617*
Von Hippel-Lindau disease, 961
Von Recklinghausen's disease, 527–528
  pheochromocytoma in, 961
Von Willebrand factor, 995
Von Willebrand's disease, 999
Voriconazole, *1152*
Voyeurism, 630
Vulva, *1344*
  biopsy of, 1354, 1408
  cancer of, *1402,* 1407–1408
  infection of, *1375*
  pain in, 1384
  removal of (vulvectomy), 1408
Vulvitis, *1375*
Vulvodynia, 1384

W

Waldenström's macroglobulinemia,
    1009–1010, *1009*
Walking, 35 (*see also* Running)
  for amputee, 44
  assistive devices for, *42*
  in ataxia-telangiectasia, 1061

Walking *(continued)*
  cane for, *42*
  in children, 1538–1539, *1539*
  cholesterol lowering with, 923
  exercise improvement of, 39
    after hip fracture, 43
  with frostbite, 1657
  obesity effects on, 917
  pain with, 217, 221
  in Parkinson's disease, 547
  pronation and, 420
  in pulmonary rehabilitation, 260
  test of (gait), 441
Wandering eye (strabismus), 1601–1603, *1602*
Warfarin, *996*
  after surgery, 288
  barbiturate interaction with, 76
  monitoring of, 63
  during pregnancy, *1460*
  in pulmonary embolism, 288
Warm antibody hemolytic anemia, 991–992
Warming therapy
  in frostbite, 1657
  in hypothermia, 1656
  in stingray injury, 1686
Warts, 1228–1229
  genital, 1183, 1325
  oral, 671
  plantar, 1228–1229
  seborrheic, 1237
Washerwoman's sprain, 419
Wasp stings, 1685
Water (amniotic fluid), breaking of, 1465
  premature, 1470
Water (body)
  balance of, 927–930, *928*
  on brain (*see* Hydrocephalus)
  deficiency of (*see* Dehydration)
  excess of, 929–930
  excretion of, 927
  retention of (*see* Swelling [edema])
Water (dietary)
  daily requirement for, 927
  fluoridation of, 678, 906
  in gastroenteritis, 723
  in hemorrhagic colitis, 724
Water (environmental)
  amebiasis from, 1135–1136
  ascariasis from, 1136–1137
  cholera from, 1100–1101
  contamination of, 721, 722, 1587
  cryptosporidiosis from, 1137–1138
  diving injuries in, 1666–1671, *1669, 1670*
  drowning in, 1665–1666
  filters for, 1138
  giardiasis from, 1138
  schistosomiasis from, 1142–1143
Water aerobics, 35–36
Water bug bites, 1685

Water deprivation test, 944–945
Waterhouse-Friderichsen syndrome, 530
WBCs (*see* White blood cells)
Weakness, muscle, 339–341, *340*
  in acute intermittent porphyria, 935
  age-related (sarcopenia), 338
  in amyotrophic lateral sclerosis, 575
  in Bell's palsy, 591–593
  in botulism, 579–581
  in brachial plexus disorders, 582
  in Brown-Séquard syndrome, 528
  in Charcot-Marie-Tooth disease, 587
  in Guillain-Barré syndrome, 584–586
  in kidney failure, 831
  in muscular dystrophy, 412–413
  in myasthenia gravis, 577–579
  in myotonic dystrophy, 414
  in periodic paralysis, 414
  in polymyositis, 383
  in progressive supranuclear palsy, 550
  in respiratory failure, *325*
  in spinal muscular atrophy, 587–588
  testing of, 341
  in vitamin B_{12} deficiency, 898
Weaning, of infant, 1488
Webs, esophageal, 707–708
Wegener's granulomatosis, 389–390, 829, 1318
Weight
  of adolescent, 1552–1553, 1557–1558
  body composition and, *881*
  children's charts for, *1541*
  gain of, 883, 914–920 (*see also* Obesity)
    in infant, 1490, *1490*, 1537–1538
    during pregnancy, 1443
  vs. height, *880*
  loss of, 883, 918–920
    in anorexia, 624–626
    in cancer, 1036
    in coronary artery disease prevention, 202
    diets for, 884–887, 918
    drugs for, 919
    in high blood pressure, 137
    in HIV infection, 1172
    in polycystic ovary syndrome, 1368
    surgery for, 919–920, *919*
    in undernutrition, 889
  metric equivalents for, 1722, 1723
  of newborn, 1484, 1490
  of premature infant, 1496
  pre-pregnancy, 1444
  in preventive care, *29*
Weight lifter's back, 569
Weight lifter's syncope, 144
Weight lifting, 36
Weights and measures, 1721–1725
Weil's syndrome, 1104
Well-child visits, 1492, 1543, 1554–1555

Werdnig-Hoffmann disease, 587–588
Werner's syndrome, 21
Wernicke-Korsakoff syndrome, 479–480, 650, 896
Wernicke's aphasia, *477, 478*
Wernicke's encephalopathy, 479–480, 650, 896
Western equine encephalitis, 537
West Nile encephalitis, 537
Wet-lung syndrome, 1500
Wheals, 1071–1072, *1189*
  in allergy skin test, 1064
Wheezing, 251–252
  in asthma, 275, 1583–1584
  in bronchiolitis, 1583
  in respiratory tract infection, 1579
Whipple's disease, 737
Whipworm infection, 1147–1148
Whirling sensation (*see* Vertigo)
White blood cells, *1052*
  biology of, 978–979, 1001–1002
  cancer of (*see* Leukemia)
  count of, 980, *981*, 1002, 1091, *1727*
  disorders of, 1001–1006, *1004*
  drug-related decrease in, *83*
  formation of, 979, 1002
  high levels of (leukocytosis), 979, 1002
  in infection, 1050, 1088
  low levels of (leukopenia), 979, 980, 1002
    with cancer treatment, 1047
  in nonspecific (innate) immunity, 1051–1054
  during pregnancy, 1439
  radiation effects on, 1659
  transfusion of, 985
White coat hypertension, 134
White color
  in mouth, *663, 671*
  of tongue, 665
White plague (*see* Tuberculosis)
White sponge nevus, *663*
Whooping cough (pertussis), 1564–1565
  immunization for, 1093, *1094*, 1492, *1493, 1562*
Wide excision surgery, in breast cancer, 1394, *1396*
Will, living, 53, 55
Wilms' tumor, 1622–1623
Wilson's disease, *905*
  hepatitis in, 803
Windpipe (*see* Trachea)
Wintergreen oil poisoning, 1677
Wisdom teeth, 662
  impaction of, 680
Wiskott-Aldrich syndrome, 1062
Withdrawal (*see* Drugs, abuse of)
Withdrawal method, for family planning, *1420*, 1426

Wohlfart-Kugelberg-Welander disease, 587–588
Wolff-Parkinson-White syndrome, 171–172
Wolman's disease, *1621*
Womb (*see* Uterus)
Wood's light examination, 1188, 1215
Woodworker's lung, *309*
Woolsorter's disease, 1098
Word recognition, in dyslexia, 1551–1552
Workplace diseases (*see* Occupational disorders)
Worm infection, 1136–1137, 1138–1140, *1139*, 1142–1144, *1143*, 1145, *1146*, 1147
Worry (*see* Anxiety)
Wound
  botulism in, 579
  first aid for, 1691–1693
  surgical, 1703
Wrinkles, 17
Wrist (*see also* Hand)
  carpal tunnel syndrome of, 398–399, *399*
  fracture of, 345, 349, 358
  ganglia of, 395
  Kienböck's disease of, 400
  strengthening exercise for, *428*
Writing, learning disorders in, 1551
Wry neck, 555–556

X

Xanthelasma, 1295
Xanthomas, 921, 925, 926
Xanthomatosis, *1621*
X chromosome, 9, 11, 1527
  in fragile X syndrome, 1528
  genes on, 11, 12–14, *13*
  inactivation of, 11
  in Klinefelter syndrome, 1530
  in triple X syndrome, 1529–1330
  in Turner syndrome, 1528–1529
Xerophthalmia, 891, 1301
Xerosis (dry skin), 1191–1192, *1192*
Xerostomia (*see* Dry mouth)
X-linked agammaglobulinemia, 1059
X-linked lymphoproliferative syndrome, *1058*
X-rays, 8
  in bone infection (osteomyelitis), 365
  chest, 255 (*see also* Chest, imaging of)
  in digestive disorders, 703–704
  dye-related allergic reactions with, *1069*
  in epiglottitis, 1564
  of fracture, 350
  of gallstones, 790
  in intestinal malrotation, 1522
  in kidney and urinary tract disorders, 826

X-rays *(continued)*
  in musculoskeletal disorders, 342
  in oral cancer, 673
  in osteoarthritis, 368
  in slipped capital femoral epiphysis, 1606
  spinal, 445
  therapeutic *(see* Radiation therapy)
  of uterus, 1355
Xylometazoline, *1158*
XYY syndrome, 1530

Y

Yaws, 1099
Y chromosome, 9, 11, 1527
  in XYY syndrome, 1530
Yeast infection *(see* Candidiasis)
Yellow color (jaundice), 791–792 *(see also*
    Jaundice)
Yellow dye, 1068
Yellow fever, 1167
  immunization for, *1094, 1709*
Yersinia pestis infection (plague),
    1107–1108

Yips (golfer's dystonia), 554
Yohimbine, 1338

Z

Zafirlukast, *278,* 280, 1584
Zalcitabine (ddC), *1175*
Zanamivir, *1156,* 1160
Zenker's diverticulum, 710
Zidovudine (AZT), *1175*
  during pregnancy, 1574
Zileuton, *278,* 280
Zinc, *903,* 914
  in common cold, 1157, *1158*
  deficiency of, 914
  excess of, 914
  in stasis dermatitis, 1197
Zoledronic acid, 1008
Zollinger-Ellison syndrome, *717,* 775
Zonisamide, *501*
Zoster (shingles), *20,* 251, 1162–1163, *1163,*
    1302
  pain after, 449
Zygote, 1435, *1436*

The Merck Manual of Medical Information—Second Home Edition is set in 9 point Trump Medieval, with heads set in Optima Bold. The original draft was produced using Microsoft Word and transmitted on disks to Nesbitt Graphics, Inc. in Fort Washington, Pennsylvania, where it was electronically assembled into pages using Quark. The original pen and ink illustrations were scanned and digitized at Nesbitt Graphics, using Adobe Illustrator. The 8-page color insert was printed by the web offset printing process on 50-pound paper at Quebecor World Eusey Press in Leominster, Massachusetts. The book was printed by the web offset printing process on 27-pound paper at Quebecor World in Taunton, Massachusetts.